ABPI Data Sheet Compendium

1986–87

Datapharm Publications Limited
12 Whitehall, London SW1A 2DY

Responsibility for Data Sheets

The data sheets in this Compendium are prepared independently by each participating company and each proof is checked and the text confirmed as correct by the participant concerned. Neither Datapharm Publications Limited nor the Association of the British Pharmaceutical Industry (ABPI) give any guarantee whatsoever as to the accuracy of the information contained in the data sheets and accept no liability whatsoever in respect of any loss, damage or expense arising from any such information or for any error or omission in the data sheets and in particular (but without prejudice to the generality of the foregoing) shall not be liable for any consequential damages or expenses or any loss of profit or any liability to third parties incurred by anyone relying on the information contained in the data sheets appearing in this Compendium.

ISBN 0 907102 00 X
ISSN 0306–9133

It is anticipated that the next edition of
the ABPI Data Sheet Compendium will be published in January 1988

Published by Datapharm Publications Limited

Compiled by Gillian Walker
Produced by David Massam

Printed and bound in Great Britain
by William Clowes Limited, Beccles and London

The Compendium

For the convenience of users of the Compendium, physiological values for certain body fluids, tables of weights for men and women and an obstetric table can be found in the tinted section at the back of the volume.

Indexes

An alphabetical index of products, an index of non-proprietary names and a directory of participating companies (together with their telephone numbers) are provided in the tinted section at the back of the Compendium.

A list is also provided of products which are the subject of data sheets in this edition of the Compendium but which were not included in the 1985–86 edition.

Data sheets

Data sheets are supplied to practitioners in order to comply with the requirements of the Medicines Act 1968.

They are prepared by the individual companies concerned and, in consequence, vary somewhat in style. All follow, however, the requirements which are laid down by 'The Medicines (Data Sheet) Regulations 1972'.

Participation in the Compendium is open to all companies manufacturing medicinal products intended for use under medical supervision.

Further information

The regulations which relate to data sheets restrict the scope of the material which may be given under the heading 'Further information' and require insertion of the word 'Nil' in any data sheet where there is no entry under that heading. Manufacturers are, of course, none the less always willing to provide additional information on their products upon request.

Enquiries should be directed to the companies concerned.

Legal category

The following abbreviations are used under the heading 'Legal category' in entries in the Compendium.

GSL	A preparation which is included in the General Sale List.
P	A pharmacy sale medicine which can be sold only from a retail pharmacy.
POM	A prescription only medicine.
CD	A preparation controlled by the Misuse of Drugs Act 1971 and Regulations. The CD is followed by (Sch 1), (Sch 2), (Sch 3), (Sch 4) or (Sch 5) depending on the schedule to the Misuse of Drugs Regulations 1985 in which the preparation is included.

Doctors are reminded that certain of the particulars must be in their own handwriting on prescriptions for preparations coming within Schedule 2 and Schedule 3 (except phenobarbitone) to the Misuse of Drugs Regulations 1985.

Date of preparation

The data sheets included in this Compendium were prepared or reviewed during the first quarter of 1986 and the compendium itself was published in October 1986.

Revised data sheets

Individual participating companies may issue loose leaf data sheets which supersede those included in this Compendium.

It is advisable to retain any such revised data sheets which are received and to indicate that fact on the corresponding data sheets in the Compendium.

Trade marks

An asterisk by the name of a product indicates that the name is a trade mark. The company symbols which appear in certain participants' sections are also trade marks.

Code of Practice for the Pharmaceutical Industry

Revised Sixth Edition (January 1986)

For many years members of The Association of the British Pharmaceutical Industry have voluntarily agreed to observe the principles set out in a *Code of Practice for the Pharmaceutical Industry*; a Code which regulates the standards of conduct to be followed in the marketing of medicines intended for use under medical supervision.

The Code was first published in 1958 and has been regularly revised to take account of changes in marketing practices. A revised sixth edition was introduced in 1986, publication following consultation with the British Medical Association and the Department of Health and Social Security. The Code embodies the basic principles and procedures which the pharmaceutical industry believes to be essential for the conduct of its marketing activities and for the maintenance of standards which are in the interests alike of the public, the medical and allied professions and the industry.

On occasion, the criticism has been made that members of the medical profession were not aware of the provisions of the Code and, consequently, that the Code had been less effective than might otherwise have been the case. To ensure that these provisions become better known, the revised sixth edition of the Code has been reproduced in its entirety below.

Those who feel that the promotion of a medical speciality product has fallen below the standards which are required by the Code may write, if they so wish, to the Secretary, Code of Practice Committee, The Association of the British Pharmaceutical Industry, 12 Whitehall, London SW1A 2DY, and ask that the matter be investigated.

INTRODUCTION

a This Code of Practice for the Pharmaceutical Industry has been drawn up after consultation with the British Medical Association and the Department of Health and Social Security.

b The Code owes its origin to the determination of the Association of the British Pharmaceutical Industry to secure the acceptance and adoption of high standards of conduct in the marketing of medical products designed for use under medical supervision.

c Medical products usually owe their existence to research carried out by their manufacturers or to the development by them of results of academic research. Before a medical product is placed on the market the manufacturer will have accumulated considerable toxicological, pharmacological and clinical evidence and will have met all the statutory requirements for the testing, manufacture and marketing of that product. Comprehensive legislation has been introduced to safeguard the public by ensuring that all products meet standards of quality, efficacy and safety which are acceptable in the state of present knowledge and experience.

d It is necessary, however, for the manufacturer, operating as he does in a keenly competitive industry and serving professions for which freedom of choice is essential, to draw attention to the existence and nature of a particular product; for example, by appropriate promotional measures and the dissemination of further knowledge and experience gained in widespread use.

e While it is possible to legislate satisfactorily for the testing, manufacture and control of medical products, the Association believes that appropriate standards of marketing conduct cannot be defined by the same means. For this reason, members of the Association have concurred in the promulgation of the Code of Practice and submitted to its restraints.

f The Code emphasises the importance in the public interest of providing the medical and allied professions with accurate, fair and objective information on medical products so that rational prescribing decisions can be made. Moreover, the Code accepts the principle that such information should be presented in a form and by ways and means which conform not only to legal requirements but also to ethical standards and canons of good taste.

The industry recognises its obligations to provide information about medical products to the pharmaceutical profession and the principles set out in this Code, therefore, apply equally to communications addressed to that profession. However, there may be instances where compliance with every provision of the Code would be inappropriate; for example, in connection with promotional material the purpose of which is to convey information of a commercial nature to pharmacists or pharmaceutical distributors.

g The Code, therefore, represents an act of self-discipline. Acceptance and observance of its provisions are a condition of membership of the Association of the British Pharmaceutical Industry. Member companies also acknowledge that the Code itself is to be applied in the spirit, as well as in the letter.

Pharmaceutical companies outside the Association are invited to accept and observe the Code because it is considered that high ethical standards should be followed throughout the whole industry if it is to maintain the confidence of all the interests which it serves.

h The Code is administered by a Committee established by the Board of Management of the Association. The Committee, with an independent legally qualified Chairman from outside the industry, consists of two independent members who are medically qualified persons not engaged in the industry, and twelve members who are drawn from the senior management of member companies, including at least four medical directors or medically qualified persons of equivalent status.

The Chairman has general authority to obtain expert assistance in any field, and has an original and a casting vote.

i The Committee meets regularly to deal with complaints, to secure compliance with the Code, and to make such recommendations as it deems fit for the amendment of the provisions of the Code.

j An outstanding feature has been the success of voluntary compliance with the provisions of the Code and acceptance of the rulings of the Committee. It has not been found necessary to apply sanctions to secure compliance because members of the Association are anxious to ensure that their marketing activities conform to the highest standard.

k It is important, therefore, that the Code should accurately reflect that standard and for this reason it is kept under constant review by the Board of Management and amended from time to time where necessary to clarify it and bring it up to date. Notes for the guidance of member companies are issued periodically to keep them informed of the rulings and recommendations of the Committee and of any alterations to the Code.

l This edition of the Code supersedes all previous issues and is the sixth edition since the Code was established in 1958. It embodies the basic principles and provisions which the pharmaceutical industry believes are essential for the conduct of its marketing activities and for the maintenance of standards which are in the interests alike of the public, the medical and allied professions and the industry.

PROVISIONS OF THE CODE

The supplementary text, which appears in italics, is intended to give guidance as to the interpretation of the Code.

1 Definition of certain terms

1.1 The term 'promotion' means those informational and marketing activities, undertaken by a pharmaceutical company or with its authority, the purpose of which is to induce the prescribing, supply or administration of its medical products.

It includes the activities of representatives and all other aspects of sales promotion in whatever form, such as journal and direct mail advertising; participation in exhibitions; the use of audio-cassettes, films, records, tapes and video recordings; the use of viewdata systems and data storage devices such as memory discs accessed and reproduced on television apparatus, visual display units and the like; the provision of samples, gifts and hospitality.

The term 'promotion' does not extend to:

(i) Replies made in response to enquiries from particular doctors or to replies in response to a specific communication, whether of enquiry or comment, including letters published in a medical journal.

(ii) Announcements of pack changes, adverse reaction warnings or recall of products provided they contain no product claims.

(iii) 'Trade advertisements' as defined in the Medicines (Advertising of Medicinal Products) Regulations 1975, i.e. catalogues, price lists or other documents issued with a view to wholesale dealing but not containing any reference to product usage other than a therapeutic classification.

By 'wholesale dealing' is meant the sale of a product to a person who, during the course of his business or professional practice, buys it for the purpose of selling it or administering it or causing it to be administered to one or more human beings.

1.2 The term 'medical product' means any unbranded or branded pharmaceutical product intended for use in humans which is promoted to the medical profession rather than directly to the lay public.

1.3 The term 'medical profession', 'practice of medicine', 'practitioner' and 'doctor' should be interpreted to extend to the dental profession and be construed accordingly.

1.4 The term 'medical representative' means a representative whose duties comprise or include calling upon members of the medical profession.

2 Methods of promotion

Methods of promotion must never be such as to bring discredit upon, or reduce confidence in, the pharmaceutical industry.

The issue of rubber stamps to doctors for use as aids to prescription writing is one of the methods of promotion barred by this clause.

3 Grant of product licence

A medical product must not be promoted prior to the grant of the product licence authorising its sale or supply.

This prohibition does not apply to any product which is exempt from the need to be the subject of a product licence.

4 Nature and availability of information

4.1 Upon reasonable request, the company concerned shall promptly provide members of the medical profession with accurate and relevant information about the medical products which the company markets.

4.2 Information about medical products should accurately reflect current knowledge or responsible opinion.

4.3 Information about medical products must be accurate, balanced and must not mislead either directly or by implication.

Claims for superior potency per unit weight are meaningless and best avoided unless they can be linked with some practical advantage, e.g. reduction in side-effects or cost of effective dosage.

4.4 Information must be capable of substantiation, such substantiation being provided without delay at the request of members of the medical profession.

5 Claims and comparisons

5.1 Claims for a medical product must be based on an up-to-date evaluation of all the evidence and must reflect this evidence accurately and clearly.

5.2 Exaggerated or all-embracing claims must not be made and superlatives must not be used. Claims should not imply that a medical product, or an active ingredient, has some special merit, quality or property unless this can be substantiated.

5.3 Any statement about side-effects should be specific and based on data submitted with the licence application or notified to the licensing authority, or on published data to which references are given. It should not be stated that a product has no side-effects, toxic hazards or risks of addiction. The word 'safe' must not be used without qualification.

5.4 The word 'new' should not be used to describe any product or presentation which has been generally available, or any therapeutic indication which has been generally promoted, for more than twelve months in the United Kingdom.

5.5 Comparisons of products must be factual, fair, and capable of substantiation. In presenting a comparison, care must be taken to ensure that it does not mislead by distortion, by undue emphasis, or in any other way.

'Hanging' comparatives, which merely claim that a product is 'better' or 'stronger', etc, must not be used.

5.6 Brand names of products of other companies must not be used unless the prior consent of the proprietors has been obtained.

6 Disparaging references

6.1 The products or services of other companies should not be disparaged either directly or by implication.

Substantiated comparative claims inviting fair comparisons with a group of products or with other products in the same field are permissible, provided that such claims are not presented in a way which is likely to mislead, whether by distortion, undue emphasis or otherwise.

6.2 The clinical and scientific opinions of members of the medical and allied professions should not be disparaged either directly or by implication.

7 Printed promotional material

7.1 The Medicines Act 1968 requires a pharmaceutical company to provide a practitioner with a data sheet before promoting a product directly to him. The content of such data sheets is determined by Regulations made under the Medicines Act.

Data Sheets for many prescription products are published in the ABPI Data Sheet Compendium which is issued at regular intervals. Copies of the Compendium are supplied to members of the medical and pharmaceutical professions.

7.2 All other printed material (including journal advertising) which is issued for promotional purposes by the product licence holder or with his authority must include certain information specified in this Code.

The requirements of Clause 7.3 or 7.4, as appropriate, must be complied with in any advertising directed towards the medical profession even if it is of a general nature, e.g. prestige advertisements listing a company's products.

An advertisement which would not otherwise conform with the Code should not be regarded as doing so by reason only of the fact that the content of the data sheet is reproduced as part of the advertisement or because a data sheet is sent with the advertisement.

7.3(i) Except for 'abbreviated advertisements', as defined in Clause 7.4, the following information must be given clearly and concisely on printed promotional material:

a The number of the relevant product licence and the name and address of the holder of the licence, or the business name and address of the part of his business responsible for the sale of the product.

b A quantitative list of the active ingredients, using approved names where such exist, or other non-proprietary names; alternatively, the non-proprietary name of the product if it is the subject of an accepted monograph.

Attention is drawn to the fact that the Medicines (Advertising to Medical and Dental Practitioners) Regulations 1978 (SI 1978 No. 1020) impose additional requirements which relate to the position and type size of this information.

c At least one authorised indication for use consistent with the data sheet.

d A succinct statement of the information in the data sheet relating to the dosage and method of use relevant to the indications quoted in the advertisement and, where not otherwise obvious, the route of administration.

e A succinct statement of the side-effects, precautions and contra-indications relevant to the indications in the advertisement, giving, in an abbreviated form, the substance of the relevant information in the data sheet.

f Any warning issued by the Medicines Commission, a committee appointed under Section 4 of the Medicines Act 1968 or the licensing authority, which is required to be included in advertisements.

g The cost of a product, except in the case of advertisements in journals which have an appreciable proportion of their circulation outside the United Kingdom.

The cost of a product is the cost (excluding value added tax) of either a specified package of the product, or a specified quantity or recommended daily dose, calculated by reference to any specified package of the product.

Attention is drawn to the fact that the Medicines (Advertising to Medical and Dental Practitioners) Regulations 1978 (SI 1978 No. 1020) impose a specific requirement to that proportion of the circulation of a journal which has to be outside the United Kingdom in order to qualify for the exception to this requirement.

7.3(ii) The information required by Clause 7.3 (i) (d), (e) and (f) must be printed in such type and in such a position that its relationship to the claims and indications is readily appreciated by the reader.

7.4(i) The requirements of Clause 7.3 do not apply in the case of an 'abbreviated advertisement'. An 'abbreviated advertisement' is one, the text of which contains in relation to the product no more than:

a The brand name of the product.

b The approved names of the active ingredients, where such names exist, or other non-proprietary names; alternatively, the non-proprietary name of the product if it is the subject of an accepted monograph.

Attention is drawn to the fact that the Medicines (Advertising to Medical and Dental Practitioners) Regulations 1978 (SI 1978 No. 1020), impose additional requirements which relate to the position and type of this information.

c The name and address of the product licence holder, or the business name and address of the part of his business responsible for the sale of the product.

d One indication for use, or more than one indication provided that these are related, consistent with the data sheet.

e A concise statement, consistent with the data sheet, giving the reason why the product is recommended for such indication or indications.

f A form of words which indicates clearly that further information is available on request to the licence holder or is to be found in the data sheet relating to the product.

7.4(ii) An 'abbreviated advertisement' must always contain the information required by Clause 7.4(i) (a), (b), (c) and (f). The information required by Clause 7.4(i) (d) and (e) is optional. An 'abbreviated advertisement' must not include any illustration which is likely to convey any information about the product or imply claims which are additional to those provided in accordance with Clause 7.4(i) (a) to (e) inclusive.

7.4(iii) An 'abbreviated advertisement' directed towards a doctor is permissible only when it constitutes an advertisement appearing in a publication sent or delivered wholly or mainly to doctors. A loose insert included in such a publication cannot be an 'abbreviated advertisement'.

Attention is drawn to the fact that the Medicines (Advertising to Medical and Dental Practitioners) Regulations 1978 (SI 1978 No. 1020) impose additional requirements which relate to the maximum permitted size of an 'abbreviated advertisement'.

7.4(iv) An 'abbreviated advertisement' is not permissible where the Medicines Commission, a committee appointed under Section 4 of the Medicines Act 1968 or the licensing authority, have required a warning to be included in any advertisement relating to the medical product, and the licensing authority have issued a direction that 'abbreviated advertisements' should not be issued.

7.5 Promotional material, such as mailings and journal advertisements, must not be designed to disguise its real nature.

Doctors rightly resent receiving promotional material in the guise of personal communications, as when advertisements are enclosed in a plain envelope or are addressed in real or facsimile handwriting on letters or postcards.

Envelopes should not be used for the dispatch of promotional material if they bear words implying that the contents are non-promotional, e.g. that the contents provide information relating to safety.

It is advisable to use first class mail only for important communications of a non-promotional nature such as notifications of warnings or cautions or the withdrawal or recall of a product.

Advertisements in journals should not be designed so as to resemble editorial matter.

7.6 Promotional material should conform, both in text and illustration, to canons of good taste and should recognise the professional standing of the recipients.

Representations of the nude female form (even in silhouette) or partly clothed figures should not be used in promotional material in such a way as to arouse a visual or emotional response in order to attract attention to the text.

Displays of part of the naked body which are necessary to illustrate pictorially the message of the text are permissible provided that they conform to the dictates of decency and good taste.

7.7 Doctors' names or photographs must not be used in a prominent manner in promotional material or in any other way that is contrary to the ethical code of the medical profession.

7.8 Promotional material should not imitate the devices, copy, slogans or general layout adopted by other companies in a way that is likely to mislead or confuse.

7.9 Where appropriate, for example, in technical and other informative material, the date of printing or the last review should be stated.

7.10 Extremes of format, size or cost of printed material should be avoided.

Large size mailings which cannot be put through letter boxes are a source of irritation to doctors and should be avoided as far as possible.

7.11 Postcards, other exposed mailings, envelopes or wrappers should not carry matter which might be regarded as advertising to the lay public or which could be considered unsuitable for public view.

Postcards and other exposed mailings should not contain copy or illustrations which ought not to be read or seen by lay persons.

7.12 'Telemessages' and 'Telex' must not be used for promotional purposes.

7.13 In a multi-page press advertisement only one page need include the information required by Clause 7.3 of the Code, provided that each of the other pages (except the page on which, or facing which, the information is printed) includes a reference, on an outer edge, in at least 8 point type, indicating on which page that information appears. No initial recto or final verso must be false or misleading if read in isolation.

A loose insert included in a journal is not regarded as a 'multi-page press advertisement' for the purpose of this clause.

By 'multi-page press advertisement' is meant an advertisement in a journal in which the pages follow on from one another without interruption. It does not include, for example, promotional material which appears on a series of successive right-hand pages. Where the pages of an advertisement do not follow on without interruption each individual page, or uninterrupted group of pages, is to be regarded as a separate advertisement.

7.14 In a multi-page advertisement other than a press advertisement, the information required by Clause 7.3 of the Code must appear on one or more continuous pages and, where such an advertisement consists of more than four pages, the advertisement must include a clear indication as to where this information may be found.

8 References to official bodies

Promotional material should not include any reference to the Medicines Commission, a committee appointed under Section 4 of the Medicines Act 1968 or the licensing authority, unless this is specifically required by the licensing authority.

9 References to the National Health Service

9.1 Where reference is made to the prescribing of a product under the National Health Service, the phrase 'freely prescribable' or similar phrases suggesting a lack of restriction or restraint must not be used.

This clause was inserted in the first edition of the Code in deference to the wishes of the then Ministry of Health. 'Freely' in this context means 'without restriction or restraint'.

Although NHS doctors are free to prescribe whatever medicines they consider necessary for the treatment of a patient, they are nevertheless required to exercise due economy.

9.2 Reproductions of official documents, such as prescription form FP 10, should not be used for promotional purposes unless the agreement of the appropriate Government department has been received.

The term 'reproduction' includes any depiction which simulates or might be taken to simulate the document in question.

10 Artwork, graphs, illustrations, etc.

10.1 Illustrations must not mislead as to the nature of the claims or comparisons being made, nor as to the purposes for which the product is used; nor should illustrations detract from warnings or contra-indications.

10.2 Artwork and graphs must conform to the letter and the spirit of the Code. Graphs and tables should be presented in such a way as to give a clear, fair, balanced view of the matters with which they deal, and should only be included if they are strictly relevant to the claims or comparisons being made.

10.3 Graphs and tables must not be used in any way which might mislead; for example, by their incompleteness or by the use of suppressed zeros or unusual scales.

11 Reprints, abstracts and quotations

This clause is included to accord with the views of the Ethical Committee of the British Medical Association; its object is to avoid the risk of contravention of the BMA Code of Ethics.

11.1 Reprints of articles by members of the medical profession must not be included in mailings but may be supplied to individual doctors on request. It is permissible to include in promotional material reasonably brief abstracts of, or quotations from, articles by members of the medical profession and to include in such material reference to doctors' names in a bibliography of published works. In no case, however, should doctors' names be used in a prominent manner in promotional material.

Quotations from public broadcasts, e.g. radio and television, may not be used in promotional material. It is permissible to use quotations from private occasions, e.g. medical conferences or symposia, with the written permission of the speaker.

11.2 Quotations from medical literature, or from personal communications received from doctors, must accurately reflect the meaning of the author and the significance of the study.

11.3 The utmost care must be taken to avoid ascribing claims or views to medical authors when such claims or views no longer represent, or may not represent, the current views of the author concerned.

12 Distribution of printed promotional material

12.1 Promotional material should only be sent or distributed to those categories of persons whose need for, or interest in, the particular information can reasonably be assumed.

12.2 Any information designed to encourage the use of medical products in clinics, industrial concerns, clubs or schools must be addressed to the medical adviser or medical officer or to medical auxiliary staff.

12.3 Restraint should be exercised on the frequency of distribution and on the volume of promotional material distributed.

The style of mailings is relevant to their acceptability to doctors and criticism of their frequency is most likely to arise where their informational content is limited or where they appear to be elaborate and expensive. A higher frequency rate will be accepted for mailings on 'new' products than for others.

12.4 Mailing lists must be kept up to date. Requests from doctors to be removed from promotional mailing lists must be complied with promptly and no name may be restored except at the doctor's request or with his permission.

13 Audio-visual material

13.1 Audio-visual material must comply with all relevant requirements of the Code, with the exception of Clause 7.3.

13.2 When audio-visual material is used to promote a product, copies of the relevant data sheet, or a document with the same content, must be made available to all persons present or to whom the material is sent or delivered.

The expression 'audio-visual material' is to be interpreted as including material which consists either of sound only or of projected moving or still pictures only. It includes sound recordings, cinematograph films, tape-slide presentations, video-recordings and sound or television broadcasting. It does not include information reproduced on television apparatus, visual display units and the like which comes within the scope of Clause 14.

13.3 Audio-visual promotional material is subject to the certification requirements of Clause 15.

14 Material reproduced on television apparatus, visual display units and the like

14 (i) Promotional material which is made available to hospitals, doctors, pharmacists etc., by systems which enable the material to be accessed and reproduced on to television apparatus, visual display units and the like, must comply with all relevant requirements of the Code, with the exception of Clauses 7.3 and 7.14.

Such material includes viewdata systems, memory discs and the like, but not video-tapes, which come within the scope of Clause 13.

14 (ii) The obligatory information required by Clause 7.3(i)(a)–(f) must be available through the system conveying the promotional material and instructions for accessing that information must be displayed with the promotional material

14 (iii) Promotional material made available in this way is subject to the certification requirements of Clause 15.

Copies of promotional information made available in this way must be made in permanent form and retained for not less than three years.

15 Certification of printed promotional material

15.1 No promotional material shall be issued unless the final text and layout have been certified by two persons on behalf of the company in the manner provided by this Clause. One of the two persons shall be a doctor. The other shall be a pharmacist or some other appropriately qualified person or a senior official of the company. The doctor, pharmacist or other qualified person must be a senior employee of the company or an appropriately qualified person whose services are retained for that purpose.

15.2 The names of those nominated, together with their qualifications, shall be notified in advance to the licensing authority. The names and qualifications of designated alternative signatories must also be given. Changes in the names of nominees must be promptly notified.

15.3 The certificate shall certify that the signatories have examined the material in its final form and that in their belief it is in accordance with the requirements of the relevant advertising regulations and this Code of Practice, is consistent with the product licence and the data sheet, and is a fair and truthful presentation of the facts about the product.

15.4 Companies shall preserve all certificates, together with the material in the form certified, for not less than three years and produce them upon request from the licensing authority or the Association at the instance of the Code of Practice Committee.

15.5 The foregoing procedure shall apply, with the necessary variations, to audio-visual material prepared by or on behalf of companies in accordance with Clause 13, to promotional material provided by or with the authority of companies for reproduction on television apparatus, visual display units and the like in accordance with Clause 14 and to briefing material for representatives prepared in accordance with Clause 17.12.

16 Suspension of advertisements

In the event of the Code of Practice Committee requiring a company either:

(i) to suspend the use of an advertisement pending its decision on a complaint by the licensing authority relevant to the safe or proper use of the product, in accordance with paragraph 8 of the 'Constitution and Procedure for the Code of Practice Committee', or,

(ii) to discontinue a practice or suspend the use of an advertisement until a review has been completed, in accordance with paragraph 13 of the 'Constitution and Procedure for the Code of Practice Committee',

the company shall at once make every possible endeavour to comply.

17 Medical representatives

17.1 Medical representatives must be adequately trained and possess sufficient medical and technical knowledge to present information on the company's products in an accurate and responsible manner.

17.2 Medical representatives should at all times maintain a high standard of ethical conduct in the discharge of their duties.

17.3 The requirements of the Code which aim at accuracy, fairness, balance, and good taste apply to oral representations as well as printed material.

17.4 Unfair or misleading comparisons or comparisons implying a therapeutic advantage which is not in fact justified must be avoided by medical representatives.

17.5 Claims made for products by medical representatives must be limited to the indications permitted by the product licence.

17.6 Medical representatives must not employ any inducement or subterfuge to gain an interview. No payment of a fee should be made for the grant of an interview.

The practice of gaining or extending an interview on the pretext of carrying out a survey is to be avoided. This does not preclude the use of medical representatives to obtain bona fide survey information, but it is essential that the survey should be devised and conducted so as to leave no doubt in the doctor's mind that the survey will produce medically useful information.

17.7 Medical representatives must ensure that the frequency, timing and duration of calls on doctors, or on hospitals, together with the manner in which they are made, do not cause inconvenience. The wishes of an individual doctor, or the arrangements in force at any particular establishment, must be observed by medical representatives.

The number of calls made on a medical practitioner and the intervals between successive visits are relevant to the determination of frequency.

Companies should arrange that intervals between visits do not cause inconvenience to practitioners and the number of calls made by a medical representative each year should not normally exceed, on average, three visits to each doctor.

Averages are to be calculated separately for general practitioners and other members of the medical profession to whom visits are made.

The calculation should exclude:

(i) Attendance by a medical representative at a scientific meeting or an audio-visual presentation given to a group of doctors.

(ii) A visit which is requested by a doctor or a call which is made in order to respond to a specific enquiry.

(iii) A visit to follow up a report of an adverse reaction.

A medical representative should not stay in a surgery in which another medical representative is already waiting, except with the doctor's or receptionist's approval.

Medical representatives must always endeavour to treat the doctor's time with the utmost respect and give him no cause to believe that his time might have been wasted. If, for any unavoidable reasons, an appointment with a doctor cannot be kept, the longest possible notice must be given.

Calls on hospital medical staff should generally be limited to matters likely to be of specific interest to them. The majority are specialists and medical representatives should ensure that their specialised interests are borne in mind. It is preferable for most hospital staff to be seen only after making a prior appointment, at which time subjects for discussion should be identified.

17.8 Medical representatives must take adequate precautions to ensure the security of medical products in their possession.

17.9 Medical representatives must not use the telephone to promote products to the medical profession unless prior arrangement has been made with individual doctors.

17.10 Medical representatives should be paid on the basis of a fixed basic salary, and any addition proportional to sales of prescription medicines should not constitute an undue proportion of their remuneration.

17.11 When discussion about a product is initiated by a medical representative, he should place before the doctor for reference either a data sheet in respect of that product or another document with the same content. If, however, the doctor asks a question about a different product, then the medical representative will not be required to produce such data in respect of that other product.

17.12 Companies must prepare detailed briefing material for medical representatives on the technical aspects of any product which the medical representative is to promote. A copy of such material must be made available to the licensing authority on request. Briefing material must comply with the relevant requirements of the Code and, in particular, is subject to the certification requirements of Clause 15.

17.13 Medical representatives should not make a claim for a product based on the regulatory treatment of that product, or of competing products, or based on any warnings issued in relation to other products, unless in accordance with a specific requirement. However, a medical representative may refer to such matters in answer to a specific question.

17.14 A company may only employ as medical representatives persons who have passed the examination established by the Association except that:

17.14(i) Persons with an acceptable professional qualification, e.g. in pharmacy, medicine or nursing, who were employed as medical representatives at any time before 1 October 1984 are exempt from this requirement.

17.14(ii) Persons who were employed as medical representatives on 1 October 1979 are exempt from this requirement.

17.14(iii) Trainee medical representatives may be employed for a period of up to two years from the date of commencing training as a medical representative.

18 Samples

18.1 Samples intended for treatment should be provided to a doctor only in response to a signed request.

A company may make available to a doctor a pre-printed request form or card; such a form or card may bear no more than the doctor's name, the company's name and address and an identifying reference, together with guidance as to the further information which the doctor himself must add. This limitation as to the provision of information on a pre-printed request form or card does not apply, however, in the case of a product controlled under the Misuse of Drugs Act 1971.

If such a pre-printed form or card is presented by a representative, then the doctor himself must complete the form by inserting the requisite information.

Wherever practicable, an individual sample should not represent more than four days' treatment for a single patient.

18.2 A signed request is not required when samples are provided to assist doctors in the recognition or identification of a product, or to demonstrate the use of a particular apparatus or equipment. Only the minimum quantity necessary for this purpose should be supplied.

18.3 No samples should be mailed to doctors except in response to a request. Samples which are sent by post must be packed so as to be reasonably secure against the package being opened by young children.

18.4 Where samples of products restricted by law to supply on prescription are distributed by a representative, the sample must be handed direct to the doctor or given to a person authorised to receive the sample on his behalf. A similar practice must be adopted for products which it would be unsafe to use except under medical supervision.

18.5 Samples of products restricted by law to supply on prescription, which are made available to representatives for distribution, should be strictly limited in quantity and an adequate system of accountability should be established.

18.6 Distribution of samples in hospitals should comply with individual hospital regulations, if any.

19 Gifts and inducements

19.1 Subject to Clause 19.2 no gift or financial inducement shall be offered or given to members of the medical profession for purposes of sales promotion.

Schemes designed to test the extent to which mailings are opened and read and which involve a reward, e.g. a reward for the return of a voucher included in the mailing, are unacceptable if the gift is one which would not come within Clause 19.2.

19.2 Gifts in the form of articles designed as promotional aids, whether related to a particular product or of general utility, may be distributed to members of the medical and allied professions provided the gift is inexpensive and relevant to the practice of medicine or pharmacy.

Amongst other items, nail brushes, book matches and pens have been held to be reasonable gifts. Gifts of table mats have been held to be in contravention of the Code as being irrelevant to the practice of medicine or pharmacy.

19.3 The requirements of Clause 7.3 or Clause 7.4 do not apply if a promotional aid of the type mentioned in Clause 19.2 bears no more than one or more of the following particulars:

(i) The name of the product.

(ii) The name of the product licence holder or the name of that part of his business responsible for the sale of the product.

(iii) The address of the product licence holder or the address of the part of his business responsible for the sale of the product.

(iv) An indication that the product name is a trade mark.

If a promotional aid consists of a note pad in which the individual pages bear advertising material, there is no need for the individual pages to comply with Clause 7 provided that the information required by the clause is given elsewhere in the pad; for example, on the cover.

20 Hospitality

Entertainment or other hospitality offered to members of the medical and allied professions for purposes of sales promotion should always be secondary to the main purpose of the meeting. It should not extend beyond members of the professions. The level of hospitality should be appropriate and not out of proportion to the occasion; its cost should not exceed that level which the recipients might normally adopt when paying for themselves.

Medical and group meetings are desirable and are to be encouraged. Both the British Medical Association and the Association share the opinion that such meetings should only take place if the advertising content is supported by a clear educational content. If hospitality is offered at meetings attendance should be restricted to members of the medical and allied professions.

It follows, therefore, that invitations to such medical and group meetings should not be extended to wives or husbands unless they themselves are practising members of the medical or allied professions.

When organising a meeting at which hospitality will be offered, a factor to be taken into account is the impression which will be created in the minds of the recipients or those who hear about it. Hospitality which becomes little more than pure entertainment has limited value in terms of the provision of information and promotion; such hospitality can only be regarded, therefore, as irrelevant and wasteful.

21 Marketing research

Marketing research is the collection and analysis of information and must be unbiased and non-promotional. The use to which the statistics or information is put may be promotional. The two phases should be kept distinct.

21.1 Methods used for marketing research must never be such as to bring discredit upon, or to reduce confidence in, the pharmaceutical industry. The following provisions apply whether the research is carried out directly by the company concerned or by an organisation acting on the company's behalf.

21.2 The following information must be made available to the informant at first approach:

(i) The nature of the survey.

(ii) The name and address of the organisation carrying out the work.

(iii) The identity of the interviewer.

(iv) The nature and length of the interview.

The requirement in Clause 21.2(ii) does not mean that the organisation is also obliged to reveal the identity of its client. This must depend upon the contract between the client and the organisation.

21.3 Questions intended to solicit disparaging references to competing products or companies must be avoided.

21.4 Any written or oral statement given or made to an informant in order to obtain co-operation must be both factually correct and honoured.

21.5 Any incentives offered to the informants should be kept to a minimum and be commensurate with the work involved.

21.6 Marketing research must not in any circumstances be used as a disguised form of sales promotion and the research *per se* must not have as a direct objective the influencing of the opinions of the informant.

21.7 The identity of an informant must be treated as being confidential, unless he has specifically agreed otherwise.

In the absence of this agreement it follows that the information provided (as distinct from the overall results of the research) must not be used as the basis upon which a subsequent approach is made to that informant for the purpose of sales promotion.

21.8 Precautions should be taken to ensure that no embarrassment results for informants following on from an interview, or from any subsequent communication concerning the research project.

22 Relations with the general public and lay communication media

22.1 Requests from individual members of the public for information or advice on personal medical matters must always be refused and the enquirer recommended to consult his or her own doctor.

22.2 Medicines which cannot legally be sold or supplied to the public otherwise than in accordance with a prescription, or which are legally limited to promotion for sale or supply only on prescription, must not be advertised to the general public.

Posters or notices issued for display in doctor's surgeries, pharmacies or anywhere to which the public have access must not include any message likely to arouse a demand for any particular product.

22.3 Statements must never be designed or made for the purpose of encouraging members of the public to ask their doctor to prescribe a product.

22.4 Information about medical products or matters related thereto, including scientific discoveries or advances in treatment, should not in general be made available to the general public either directly or through any lay medium.

The intention is to ensure that arrangements made for a press conference, or the extent of a press release, are such as to confine the disclosure of information about medical products or matters relating thereto to persons who are capable of evaluating the information responsibly and not concerned to exaggerate or even sensationalise its significance.

22.5 The importance of such information and the existence of legitimate public interest in acquiring it may exceptionally justify holding a press conference or the issue of a press release.

Invitations to attend such a conference, or the distribution of such a press release, should be confined to persons who are either medically qualified or established as the representatives of the medical, pharmaceutical or scientific press, or as the medical correspondents of a responsible medium.

In the circumstances set out above as to the significance of the information, and in response to an unsolicited enquiry from a person of the standing described, information may also be released in an informal manner.

22.6 A further exception may arise when there exists a genuine mutual interest of a financial or commercial nature justifying the disclosure of information about medical products or related matters privately or to a restricted public. Examples are the interests of shareholders, financial advisers, employees and creditors.

When releasing information, it is essential to bear in mind the provisions of Clause 5.3 and, in particular, the extreme caution required in any reference to side-effects; it should also be emphasised that the treatment of a particular individual is solely a matter for decision by his medical practitioner.

22.7 On all occasions the information whether written, or communicated by other means, must be presented in a balanced way so as to avoid the risk of raising unfounded hopes of successful treatment or stimulating the demand for prescription of the particular product.

22.8 An announcement of the introduction of a new medical product must not be made by press conference or formal press release until the appropriate steps have been taken to inform the medical profession of its availability.

23 Operative date

This Revised Sixth Edition of the Code shall take effect on 1 January 1986.

The reporting of adverse reactions

Suspected adverse reactions to any therapeutic agents should be reported. These agents include drugs, vaccines, blood products, X-ray contrast media, dental or surgical materials, intra-uterine contraceptive devices, absorbable sutures, contact lens fluids.

Newer drugs marked ▼

Doctors are asked to report any adverse or unexpected event, however minor, which could conceivably be attributed to the drug. Reports should be made despite uncertainty in the doctor's mind about a causal relationship, irrespective of whether the reaction is well recognised, and even if other drugs have been given concurrently.

Established drugs

Doctors are asked to report any suspected adverse drug reaction which was potentially dangerous, incapacitating or lethal. These should be reported even though the toxic effect is well recognised. Examples include anaphylaxis, blood dyscrasias, endocrine disturbances, effects on fertility, haemorrhage from any site, renal impairment, jaundice, ophthalmic disorders, severe CNS effects, severe skin reactions, reactions in pregnant women, and any drug interactions. For established drugs doctors are asked not to report well known, relatively minor side effects such as dry mouth with tricyclic antidepressants, constipation with opiates, or nausea with digoxin.

Special problems

(i) Delayed drug effects Doctors are reminded that some reactions (e.g., the development of cancers, chloroquine retinopathy and retroperitoneal fibrosis) may become manifest months or years after drug exposure. Please report any suspicion of such an association.

(ii) Drugs in the elderly Doctors are asked to be particularly alert to the possibility of adverse reactions when drugs are given to the elderly.

(iii) Congenital abnormalities When an infant is born with a congenital abnormality or there is a malformed aborted fetus, doctors are asked to consider the possibility that this might be an adverse reaction to a drug and to report all drugs (including self-medication) taken by the mother during pregnancy.

(iv) Adverse reactions to vaccines Doctors are asked to report all suspected reactions to both new and established vaccines. The balance between risks and benefits from vaccines is liable to change and needs to be kept under continuous review.

Special postage-paid forms ('yellow cards') are provided for reports. Supplies of these can be obtained from the Committee on Safety of Medicines at Market Towers, 1 Nine Elms Lane, London SW8 5NQ, telephone 01-720 2188.

The above statement and the symbols marking certain products have been included in the Compendium at the request of the Medicines Division of the Department of Health and Social Security.

The individual companies concerned would find it helpful to be informed by practitioners of any adverse reactions to their products which are reported.

Abbott Laboratories Limited
Queenborough
Kent ME11 5EL

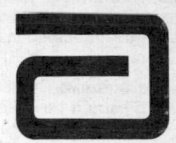

CORDILOX*

Presentation
Cordilox tablets 40 mg: Yellow, biconvex, film-coated Verapamil Hydrochloride Tablets BP imprinted with 'Cordilox' and '40' on one face and 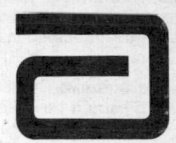 on the other containing 40 mg Verapamil Hydrochloride BP per tablet.

Cordilox tablets 80 mg: Yellow, biconvex, film-coated Verapamil Hydrochloride Tablets BP imprinted with 'Cordilox' and '80' on one face and 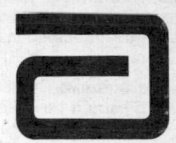 on the other containing 80 mg Verapamil Hydrochloride BP per tablet.

Cordilox tablets 120: Yellow, biconvex, film-coated Verapamil Hydrochloride Tablets BP imprinted with 'Cordilox' and '120' on one face and 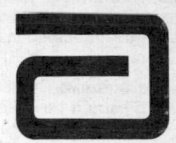 on the other containing 120 mg Verapamil Hydrochloride BP per tablet.

Cordilox 160: Yellow, biconvex, film-coated Verapamil Hydrochloride Tablets BP imprinted with 'Cordilox' and '160' on one face and 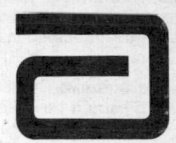 on the other containing 160 mg Verapamil Hydrochloride BP per tablet.

Cordilox IV: Colourless glass 2 ml ampoules with break-line containing 5 mg Verapamil Hydrochloride BP per ampoule.

Uses
Cordilox tablets:
(1) The treatment of mild to moderate hypertension and renal hypertension, used alone or in conjunction with other antihypertensive therapy.
(2) The treatment and prophylaxis of angina pectoris, and variant angina.
(3) The treatment and prophylaxis of supraventricular tachycardia (paroxysmal tachycardia, premature supraventricular contractions, atrial fibrillation and flutter) and paroxysmal supraventricular tachycardia of the reciprocating type associated with the Wolff-Parkinson-White syndrome.

Cordilox IV: The treatment of supraventricular arrhythmias.

Mode of Action: Cordilox is a calcium channel blocker which inhibits the inward movement of calcium in smooth muscle cells of the systemic and coronary arteries and in the cells of cardiac muscle and the intracardiac conduction system.

Cordilox lowers peripheral vascular resistance with little or no reflex tachycardia. Its efficacy in reducing both raised systolic and diastolic blood pressure is thought to be primarily due to this mode of action.

The decrease in systemic and coronary vascular resistance and the sparing effect on intracellular oxygen consumption appear to explain the anti-anginal properties of the product.

Because of its effect on the movement of calcium in the intracardiac conduction system, it reduces automaticity, decreases conduction velocity and increases the refractory period.

Dosage and administration
Hypertension (oral administration)
Adults: The usual dosage is 160 mg twice a day. However, a minority of patients may be successfully controlled on 120 mg b.d. while others may require up to 480 mg daily given in divided doses. A further reduction in blood pressure may be obtained by combining Cordilox with other antihypertensive agents, e.g. thiazide diuretics. For concomitant administration of beta-blockers, see 'Precautions'.
Children: Up to 10 mg/kg/day orally in divided doses according to the severity of disease.

Angina (oral administration)
Adults: The usual dosage is 120 mg three times a day. 80 mg t.d.s. can be completely satisfactory in some patients with angina of effort. Less than 120 mg t.d.s. is not likely to be effective in angina at rest and variant angina.
Children: No data available.

Supraventricular arrhythmias
Non-acute (oral administration)
Adults: 40–120 mg t.d.s. according to the severity of the condition.
Children: Up to 2 years: ½ 40 mg tablet 2–3 times a day. 2 years and above: 1–3 40 mg tablets 2–3 times a day according to age.

Acute (IV injection)
Adults: For the treatment of tachyarrhythmias, 5–10 mg (1–2 ampoules) should be injected intravenously over a period of 30 seconds with continuous observation of the patient and, preferably, with simultaneous ECG monitoring.

In cases of paroxysmal tachyarrhythmias a further 5 mg may, if necessary, be injected 5–10 minutes after the first injection with the same precautions being observed.

Higher doses are not usually necessary.
Children: Newborn: 0.75–1 mg (0.3–0.4 ml)
Infants: 0.75–2 mg (0.3–0.8 ml)
1–5 years: 2–3 mg (0.8–1.2 ml)
6–15 years: 2.5–5 mg (1.0–2.0 ml).
In many cases smaller doses than those mentioned above are sufficient. The injection should be stopped at the onset of the desired effect.

For concomitant administration with beta-blockers see 'Precautions'.

Elderly: No special dosage recommendations except in those patients with impaired liver function or cardiac conduction disturbances (see 'Precautions').

Contra-indications, warnings, etc
Contra-indications: Hypotension, marked bradycardia

(less than 50 beats/minute), second and third degree atrioventricular block, sick sinus syndrome, uncompensated heart failure. Combination with beta-blockers is contra-indicated in patients with poor ventricular function.

Precautions: Cordilox may affect impulse conduction and should be used with caution in patients with first degree atrioventricular block. The effects of Cordilox and beta-blockers or other drugs with a cardio-depressive action may be additive both with respect to conduction and contraction, therefore care must be exercised when these are administered concurrently or closely together. This is especially true when either drug is administered intravenously.

Patients with atrial fibrillation/flutter and an accessory pathway with anterograde conduction (e.g. W-P-W syndrome), when receiving Cordilox IV, may rarely develop increased conduction across the anomalous pathway and ventricular tachycardia may be precipitated.

Cordilox may have an additive effect with other antihypertensive drugs. Thus, in many cases, with Cordilox, a reduction in the dose of the other antihypertensive drug may be possible.

Cordilox may affect left ventricular contractility as a result of its mode of action. This effect is small and normally not important but cardiac failure may be precipitated or aggravated if it exists. In cases of poor ventricular function therefore, Cordilox should only be given after appropriate therapy for cardiac failure such as digitalis, etc.

Verapamil hydrochloride has been shown to increase the serum concentration of digoxin and caution should be exercised with regard to digitalis toxicity.

Caution should be observed in the acute phase of myocardial infarction.

In patients with impaired liver function, particular attention should be paid to the dosage because of reduced drug metabolism.

Use in pregnancy: Although animal studies have not shown any teratogenic effect, Cordilox should not be given during pregnancy (especially in the first trimester) unless, in the clinician's judgement, it is essential for the welfare of the patient.

Side-effects:
Oral administration: Cordilox is generally well tolerated. Constipation is not uncommon, flushing is observed occasionally, headaches rarely. Nausea and vomiting have seldom been reported and allergic reactions even more rarely. On very rare occasions a reversible impairment of liver function characterised by an increase in transaminases and/or alkaline phosphatase, may occur during verapamil treatment and is most probably a hypersensitivity reaction.

Parenteral administration: Cordilox is well tolerated and does not exert a bronchoconstrictor effect.

Due to its mode of action, undesired effects on atrioventricular conduction and blood pressure are possible. This applies particularly to patients with atrioventricular block and/or considerably impaired myocardial function. On rare occasions the intravenous administration of Cordilox may lead to an undesired blocking of conduction and, in extreme cases, to asystole. The asystole is usually of short duration and normally sinus rhythm returns spontaneously after a few seconds. However, if on rare occasions asystole persists, treatment should be carried out as described below.

Intravenous administration of Cordilox may lead to a slight transient fall in blood pressure due to a reduction in peripheral resistance. Rarely this may result in severe hypotension.

Treatment of acute cardiovascular side-effects: If acute complications occur after intravenous injection of Cordilox (asystole, atrioventricular block or ventricular fibrillation) the usual emergency measures should be applied, e.g. cardiac massage, mechanical ventilation, the intravenous injection of adrenaline, and the intravenous injection of 10–20 ml of calcium gluconate 10% solution. Hypotension following intravenous injection of Cordilox may, if necessary, be controlled without difficulty by the use of vasoconstrictor substances.

Overdosage
Oral administration: Usual emergency measures for acute cardiovascular side-effects should be followed as above. In the case of second and third degree AV block, atropine, isoprenaline or a temporary pace-maker may be necessary. If myocardial insufficiency occurs, dopamine, dobutamine, cardiac glycosides or calcium gluconate (10–20 ml of a 10% solution) may be required. Appropriate positioning of the patient and vasoconstrictor drugs may be indicated in the case of hypotension.

Parenteral administration: See 'Treatment of acute cardiovascular side-effects'.

Pharmaceutical precautions Nil.

Legal category POM.

Package quantities

Cordilox 40 mg:	Containers of 100 tablets
Cordilox 80 mg:	Containers of 100 tablets
Cordilox 120:	Containers of 100 and 500 tablets
Cordilox 160:	Blister packs of 56 tablets
Cordilox IV:	Containers of 5 × 2 ml ampoules.

Further information
Metabolisable carbohydrate:

Cordilox 40 mg:	3.2 mg/tablet
Cordilox 80 mg:	6.4 mg/tablet
Cordilox 120:	9.6 mg/tablet
Cordilox 160:	12.8 mg/tablet
Cordilox IV:	Nil.
Cordilox IV:	Sodium content: 0.30 mmol/ampoule (0.15 mmol/ml).

Product licence numbers

Cordilox 40 mg:	0037/0098
Cordilox 80 mg:	0037/0085
Cordilox 120:	0037/0084
Cordilox 160:	0037/0131
Cordilox IV:	0037/5903

DOPAMINE HYDROCHLORIDE IN 5% DEXTROSE INJECTION

Presentation Dopamine hydrochloride in 5% dextrose solution is a sterile, nonpyrogenic solution for administration by intravenous infusion. It is presented in 250 ml flexible containers of 200 mg (800 mcg/ml), 400 mg (1600 mcg/ml) and 800 mg (3200 mcg/ml) Dopamine Hydrochloride USP in 5% dextrose injection.

It is intended for use as a single-dose injection.

Uses Dopamine administered intravenously is a positive myocardial inotropic agent, which also may increase mesenteric and renal blood flow plus urinary output.

Dopamine hydrochloride in 5% dextrose is indicated in patients with poor perfusion, low cardiac output, impending renal failure and for the correction of haemo-dynamic imbalances present in shock due to myocardial infarction, trauma, endotoxic septicaemia, open heart surgery, renal failure and chronic cardiac decompensation as in refractory congestive failure.

Dosage and administration Where appropriate, the circulating blood volume must be restored with a suitable plasma expander or whole blood, prior to administration of dopamine hydrochloride.

Begin infusion of dopamine hydrochloride solution at doses of 2.5 mcg/kg/min in patients who are likely to respond to modest increments of heart force and renal perfusion.

In more seriously ill patients, begin infusion of dopamine hydrochloride at doses of 5 mcg/kg/min and increase gradually using 5 to 10 mcg/kg/min increments up to a rate of 20 to 50 mcg/kg/min as needed. If doses in excess of 50 mcg/kg/min are required, it is advisable to check urine output frequently. Should urinary flow begin to decrease in the absence of hypotension, reduction of dopamine dosage should be considered. It has been found that more than 50% of patients have been satisfactorily maintained on doses less than 20 mcg/kg/min.

In patients who do not respond to these doses, additional increments of dopamine may be given in an effort to achieve adequate blood pressure, urine flow and perfusion generally.

Treatment of all patients requires constant evaluation of therapy in terms of blood volume, augmentation of cardiac contractility, and distribution of peripheral perfusion and urinary output.

Dosage of dopamine should be adjusted according to the patient's response, with particular attention to diminution of established urine flow rate, increasing tachycardia or development of new dysrhythmias as indications for decreasing or temporarily suspending the dosage.

Contra-indications, warnings, etc
Contra-indications: Dopamine hydrochloride should not be used in patients with phaeochromocytoma. Dextrose solutions without electrolytes should not be administered simultaneously with blood through the same infusion set because of the possibility that pseudoagglutination of red cells may occur.

Warnings: Dopamine should not be administered in the presence of uncorrected tachyarrhythmias or ventricular fibrillation.

Patients who have been treated with monoamine oxidase (MAO) inhibitors prior to administration of dopamine should receive substantially reduced dosage of the latter. The starting dose in such patients should be reduced to at least one-tenth (1/10) of the usual dose.

Excess administration of potassium-free solutions may result in significant hypokalaemia.

The intravenous administration of these solutions can cause fluid and/or solute overloading resulting in dilution of serum electrolyte concentrations, overhydration, congested states or pulmonary oedema.

Precautions: Hypovolaemia should be corrected where necessary prior to treatment with dopamine.

If a disproportionate rise in diastolic pressure (i.e. a marked decrease in pulse pressure) is observed, the infusion rate should be decreased and the patients observed carefully for further evidence of predominant vasoconstriction activity, unless such an effect is desired.

Patients with a history of peripheral vascular disease should be closely monitored for any changes in colour or temperature of the skin of the extremities. If a change of skin colour or temperature occurs and is thought to be the result of compromised circulation to the extremities, the benefits of continued dopamine infusion should be weighed against the risk of possible necrosis. These changes may be reversed by decreasing the rate or discontinuing the infusion.

Dopamine hydrochloride in 5% dextrose injection should be infused into a large vein whenever possible to prevent the possibility of infiltration of perivascular tissue adjacent to the infusion site. Extravasation may cause necrosis and sloughing of the surrounding tissue. Ischaemia can be reversed by infiltration of the affected area with 10–15 ml of saline containing 5 to 10 mg phentolamine mesylate. A syringe with a fine hypodermic needle should be used to liberally infiltrate the ischaemic area as soon as extravasation is noted.

Dopamine should be used with extreme caution in patients inhaling cyclopropane or halogenated hydro-carbon anaesthetics due to the arterial arrhythmogenic potential.

Dextrose solutions should be used with caution in patients with known subclinical or overt diabetes mellitus.

Adverse reactions: The most frequently reported adverse reactions to dopamine have been ectopic beats, tachycardia, nausea, vomiting, anginal pain, palpitations, dyspnoea, headache, hypotension and vasoconstriction.

Very rarely reported reactions include aberrant conduction, bradycardia, piloerection, widened QRS complex, azotaemia and elevated blood pressure.

Usage in pregnancy: Animal studies have shown no evidence of teratogenic effects with dopamine. The drug may be used in pregnant women when, in the judgment of the physician, the expected benefits outweigh the potential risk to the foetus.

Usage in children: Safety and effectiveness in children have not been established.

Overdosage: Accidental overdosage as evidenced by excessive blood pressure elevation can be controlled by dose reduction or discontinuing the administration for a short period until the patient's condition stabilises.

If these measures fail, an infusion of phentolamine mesylate should be considered.

Pharmaceutical precautions Do not add sodium bicarbonate or other alkaline substances, since dopamine is inactivated in alkaline solution.

Do not administer unless solution is clear and seal is intact. Discard unused portion.

Additive medications should not be delivered via this solution.

Recommended storage: Room temperature (25°C). Store away from heat. Protect from freezing.

Legal category POM.

Package quantities 250 ml flexible containers containing: Dopamine hydrochloride 200 mg in 5% dextrose injection.

Dopamine hydrochloride 400 mg in 5% dextrose injection.

Dopamine hydrochloride 800 mg in 5% dextrose injection.

Further information Nil.

Product licence numbers 200 mg 0037/0145
400 mg 0037/0146   800 mg 0037/0147

ENDURON*

Presentation Each square, pink tablet engraved with a bisect line on one face and the ⊃ logo on the other, contains 5 mg methyclothiazide, an oral diuretic.

Uses Enduron is indicated as a primary measure in the treatment of mild to moderate hypertension and as an adjunct to other drugs in the treatment of resistant hypertension. It is also indicated in the same clinical situations in which thiazides are of value. It is used in the treatment and control of oedema associated with congestive heart failure, the nephrotic syndrome, hepatic cirrhosis, pre-menstrual tension and the administration of steroids. The use of Enduron permits a reduction in the dosage of more potent antihypertensive agents with a consequent reduction in side-effects.

Dosage and administration The usual adult oral dose is 2.5–5 mg daily. This may be increased to 10 mg once daily, if necessary, but doses larger than 10 mg have little additional therapeutic effect. Enduron is not recommended for use in children.

Elderly: No special dosage recommendations except in those patients with renal or hepatic disease (see 'Contra-indications'). Borderline renal or hepatic insufficiency may be unpredictably aggravated by thiazides. See also warnings.

Contra-indications, warnings, etc

Contra-indications: Known sensitivity to thiazide derivatives. It should not be administered in the presence of severe renal or hepatic disease, Addison's disease, hypercalcaemia and concurrent lithium therapy.

Warnings:
1. Diabetes may be precipitated or aggravated.
2. Gout may be precipitated or aggravated.
3. Renal function should be monitored.
4. Patients on corticosteroids, or with impending hepatic coma, cirrhotic oedema or ascites may require potassium supplements, and should be carefully evaluated clinically.
5. Pancreatitis may be precipitated.
6. Particular caution is needed in the case of elderly patients because of their likely susceptibility to electrolyte imbalance.
7. Pregnancy warning:
 (i) Diuretics are best avoided for the management of oedema in pregnancy or hypertension in pregnancy as their use may be associated with hypovolaemia, increased blood viscosity and reduced placental perfusion.
 (ii) There is inadequate evidence of safety in human pregnancy and some workers have described foetal bone marrow depression and thrombocytopaenia. Foetal and neonatal jaundice have also been reported.
8. Lactation warning: As diuretics pass into breast milk they should be avoided in mothers who wish to breast feed.

Precautions and side-effects: Although the incidence of side-effects with Enduron is extremely low, it is a benzothiadiazine derivative, and the physician should be alert for the side-effects inherent in this type of medication. If potassium depletion occurs, potassium or a potassium sparing drug should be given. Myocardial sensitivity to digitalis is increased in the presence of reduced potassium and signs of digitalis intoxication may be produced by formerly tolerated doses of digitalis. Hypokalaemia can cause an increase in arrhythmias.

Hypochloraemic alkalosis is a possibility with any potent benzothiadiazine, but remote with Enduron because it produces approximately equivalent sodium and chloride excretion. Elevation of the blood urea nitrogen, serum uric acid, blood sugar have occurred with the use of thiazide drugs. In common with other thiazides impotence may occur. Blood dyscrasias including thrombocytopenia with purpura, agranulocytosis and aplastic anaemia have also been reported but are rare.

Overdosage: Symptoms: Electrolyte imbalance; dehydration; hypotension; signs of potassium deficiency including confusion; dizziness; muscular weakness and gastro-intestinal disturbances may occur.

Treatment: Employ general supportive measures. Blood pressure and fluid/electrolyte balance should be monitored. Replacement of fluids and electrolytes may be indicated. For recent ingestion gastric lavage or emesis should be considered.

Pharmaceutical precautions Nil.

Legal category POM.

Package quantities Enduron is supplied in containers of 100 tablets.

Further information Metabolisable carbohydrate content: Approx. 0.18 g per tablet.

Product licence number 0037/5028.

ERYTHROCIN* 250
ERYTHROCIN* 500

Presentation Erythrocin 250 and Erythrocin 500 are white, film-coated tablets containing respectively 250 mg and 500 mg of erythromycin as Erythromycin Stearate BP. They are Erythromycin Stearate Tablets BP.

Uses For the prophylaxis and treatment of infections caused by erythromycin-sensitive organisms.

Clinical indications:
1. Upper respiratory tract infections.
2. Lower respiratory tract infections.
3. Skin and soft tissue infections.
4. Bone infections.
5. Sexually transmitted diseases.
6. Oral/dental infections.
7. Eye infections.
8. Gastro-intestinal infections.
9. Prophylaxis.

Microbiological indications: Erythromycin has been shown to be active in vitro against the following organisms: Staphylococci, Streptococci, *Haemophilus influenzae*, L-forms, *Mycoplasma pneumoniae*, *Legionella pneumophila*, *Branhamella catarrhalis*, *Bordetella pertussis*, *Corynebacterium diphtheriae* (as an adjunct to antitoxin), Neisseria, *Treponema pallidum*, *Chlamydia trachomatis*, Clostridia, *Ureaplasma urealytica*, Campylobacter.

Dosage and administration

Adults and children over 8 years: For mild to moderate infections 1–2 g daily in divided doses. For severe infections this may be increased to 4 g daily in divided doses. Tablets should be taken before or with meals.

Elderly: No special dosage recommendations.

Children under 8 years: Erythroped suspension is recommended.

Period of dosing with regard to indication

Upper respiratory tract infections	5–10 days.
Lower respiratory tract infections	7–14 days or until signs and symptoms indicate a cure. Legionnaires' disease may require prolonged treatment. Initially administration of erythromycin lactobionate by the intravenous route is recommended.
Skin and soft tissue infections	5–10 days. Acne may require prolonged treatment.
Sexually transmitted diseases	
NGU and syphilis	10–21 days. Some conditions may require prolonged treatment.
Oral/dental infections (see below for dental procedures)	At least 5 days.
Eye infections	
Chlamydial inclusion conjunctivitis	3 weeks.
Gastro-intestinal infections	
Campylobacter	Minimum 5 days.
Prophylaxis of bacterial endocarditis with oral surgery	Erythromycin stearate 1.5 g one hour before procedure, then 500 mg six hours later.

Contra-indications, warnings, etc
Contra-indications: Known sensitivity to erythromycin.

Precautions: Erythromycin is excreted principally by the liver, so caution should be exercised in administering the antibiotic to patients with impaired hepatic function or concomitantly receiving potentially hepatotoxic agents.

The administration of erythromycin has been infrequently associated with the occurrence of reversible cholestatic jaundice.

The use of erythromycin in patients who are receiving digoxin, warfarin, carbamazepine and high doses of theophylline may result in the potentiation of their effects due to reduction in the rates of excretion.

Use in pregnancy: There is no evidence of hazard from erythromycin in human pregnancy. It has been in wide use for many years without apparent ill consequence. Animal studies have shown no hazard.

Side-effects: Occasional side-effects such as nausea, abdominal discomfort, vomiting and diarrhoea may be experienced. Reversible hearing loss associated with doses of erythromycin usually greater than 4 g per day has been reported. Allergic reactions are rare and mild, although anaphylaxis has occurred extremely rarely. There are no reports implicating erythromycin products with abnormal tooth development and only rare reports of damage to the blood, kidneys, liver or central nervous system.

Overdosage: Symptoms: Hearing loss, severe nausea, vomiting and diarrhoea.

Treatment: Gastric lavage, general supportive measures.

Pharmaceutical precautions Keep bottle tightly closed. Protect from light. Store below 25°C.

Legal category POM.

Package quantities Erythrocin 250: Containers of 100, 500 and 1000 tablets.

Erythrocin 500: Containers of 100 and 500 tablets and blister packs of 10 and 15 tablets.

Further information Erythrocin 250 and 500 contain no dyes. They contain respectively 0.07 g and 0.15 g Maize Starch BP.

Product licence number
Erythrocin 250   0037/5079
Erythrocin 500   0037/5044

ERYTHROCIN* IV LACTOBIONATE

Presentation A sterile, white, lyophilised presentation of 1.0 g of erythromycin as erythromycin lactobionate in a vial.

When reconstituted with 20 ml Water for Injections BP provides 22 ml of solution. Deliberate overage ensures that each 20 ml of this solution contains 1.0 g of erythromycin as erythromycin lactobionate with 180 mg benzyl alcohol as preservative.

The solution must be further diluted prior to intravenous administration (see dosage and administration).

Erythrocin IV Lactobionate is not suitable for intramuscular use.

Uses
Clinical indications: Erythromycin is highly effective in the treatment of a great variety of clinical infections. It is indicated in severe and immunocompromised cases of infections caused by sensitive organisms where high blood levels are required at the earliest opportunity or when the oral route is compromised.

1. Upper respiratory tract infections.
2. Lower respiratory tract infections.
3. Skin and soft tissue infections.
4. Bone infections.
5. Sexually transmitted diseases.
6. Gastro-intestinal and biliary infections.
7. Prophylaxis: Peri-operative secondary infection prophylaxis, severe trauma and burns secondary infection prophylaxis, endocarditis prophylaxis (dental procedures).
8. Endocarditis.
9. Septicaemia.
10. Oral/dental infections.
11. Eye infections.

Microbiological indications: Erythromycin has been shown to be active in vitro against the following organisms: Staphylococci, Streptococci, *Haemophilus influenzae*, L-forms, *Mycoplasma pneumoniae*, *Legionella pneumophila*, *Branhamella catarrhalis*, *Bordetella pertussis*, Corynebacterium diphtheriae (as an adjunct to antitoxin), Neisseria, *Treponema pallidum*, *Chlamydia trachomatis*, Clostridia, *Ureaplasma urealytica*, Campylobacter.

Dosage and administration
Recommended dosage
Adults, children and neonates: Severe and immunocompromised infections, 50 mg/kg/day, preferably by continuous infusion (equivalent to 4 g per day for adults).

Mild to moderate infections (oral route compromised) 25 mg/kg/day.

Elderly: No special dosage recommendations.

Recommended administration: Continuous intravenous

infusion with an erythromycin concentration of 1 mg/ml (0.1% solution) is recommended.

If required, solution strengths up to 5 mg/ml (0.5% solution) may be used, but should not be exceeded. Higher concentrations may result in pain along the vein

Bolus injection is not recommended

However, if it is decided to administer the daily dose as 4 doses once every 6 hours, then the erythromycin concentration should not exceed 5 mg/ml and the time of each infusion should be between 20 and 60 minutes.

Preparation of solution for intravenous administration

Step 1: Inject 20 ml of Water for Injections BP into the vial and shake to dissolve contents. Do not use saline or other diluents. This will give 22 ml of solution.

20 ml of this solution will contain 1.0 g erythromycin (50 mg erythromycin/ml).

Use within 24 hours of preparation. Keep in a refrigerator between 2°C and 8°C.

This solution must be further diluted before administration, see Step 2.

Step 2: Solutions for administration are prepared with Sodium Chloride Intravenous Infusion BP 0.9% w/v (see also below).

Dose required	Volume from Step 1	Volume of sterile 0.9% saline	Total volume	Erythromycin concentration
1.0 g	20 ml	1000 ml	1020 ml	1.0 mg/ml
500 mg	10 ml	500 ml	510 ml	
1.0 g	20 ml	500 ml	520 ml	1.9 mg/ml
500 mg	10 ml	250 ml	260 ml	
1.0 g	20 ml	200 ml	220 ml	4.6 mg/ml
500 mg	10 ml	100 ml	110 ml	

If, for clinical reasons, 0.9% saline is not suitable, then neutralised Glucose Intravenous Infusion BP 5% w/v may be used. Neutralised glucose solution is prepared by the addition of 5 ml of sterile 8.4% w/v sodium bicarbonate solution to each litre of Glucose Intravenous Injection BP 5% w/v.

It is necessary to buffer the glucose solution in this way because the stability of Erythrocin IV Lactobionate is adversely affected below pH 5.5.

To ensure potency, all solutions for administration should be used within 8 hours of preparation.

Contra-indications, warnings, etc

Contra-indications: Known sensitivity to erythromycin.

Precautions: Erythromycin is excreted principally by the liver, so caution should be exercised in administering the antibiotic to patients with impaired hepatic function or concomitantly receiving potentially hepatotoxic agents.

The administration of erythromycin has been infrequently associated with the occurrence of reversible cholestatic jaundice.

The use of erythromycin in patients who are receiving digoxin, warfarin, carbamazepine and high doses of theophylline may result in the potentiation of their effects due to reduction in the rates of excretion.

Use in pregnancy: There is no evidence of hazard from erythromycin in human pregnancy. It has been in wide use for many years without apparent ill consequence. Animal studies have shown no hazard.

Side-effects: Occasional side-effects such as nausea, abdominal discomfort, vomiting and diarrhoea may be experienced. Reversible hearing loss associated with doses of erythromycin usually greater than 4 g per day has been reported. Allergic reactions are rare and mild, although anaphylaxis has occurred extremely rarely. There are no reports implicating erythromycin products with abnormal tooth development and only rare reports of damage to the blood, kidneys, liver or central nervous system.

Overdosage: Symptoms: Hearing loss, severe nausea, vomiting and diarrhoea.

Treatment: General supportive measures.

Pharmaceutical precautions The powder is stable at room temperature.

Legal category POM.

Package quantities 1 g vials of Erythrocin IV Lactobionate.

Further information Contains no sodium. Compatibility with other IV additives has not been established.

Product licence number 0037/0092.

ERYTHROMID*
ERYTHROMID DS*

Presentation Erythromid and Erythromid DS are orange-coloured, enteric-coated, film-coated tablets containing respectively 250 mg and 500 mg of Erythromycin BP. They are Erythromycin Tablets BP.

Uses For the prophylaxis and treatment of infections caused by erythromycin-sensitive organisms.

Clinical indications:
1. Upper respiratory tract infections.
2. Lower respiratory tract infections.
3. Skin and soft tissue infections.
4. Bone infections.
5. Sexually transmitted diseases.
6. Oral/dental infections.
7. Eye infections.
8. Gastro-intestinal infections.
9. Prophylaxis.

Microbiological indications: Erythromycin has been shown to be active in vitro against the following organisms: Staphylococci, Streptococci, *Haemophilus influenzae*, L-forms, *Mycoplasma pneumoniae, Legionella pneumophila, Branhamella catarrhalis, Bordetella pertussis, Corynebacterium diphtheriae* (as an adjunct to antitoxin), Neisseria, *Treponema pallidum, Chlamydia trachomatis*, Clostridia, *Ureaplasma urealytica*, Campylobacter.

Dosage and administration

Adults and children over 8 years: For mild to moderate infections 1–2 g daily in divided doses. For severe infections this may be increased to 4 g daily in divided doses. Tablets should be taken before or with meals.

Elderly: No special dosage recommendations.

Children under 8 years: Erythroped suspension is recommended.

Period of dosing with regard to indication

Upper respiratory tract infections	5–10 days.
Lower respiratory tract infections	7–14 days or until signs and symptoms indicate a cure. Legionnaires' disease may require prolonged treatment. Initially administration of erythromycin lactobionate by the intravenous route is recommended.
Skin and soft tissue infections	5–10 days. Acne may require prolonged treatment.
Sexually transmitted diseases	
NGU and syphilis	10–21 days. Some conditions may require prolonged treatment.
Oral/dental infections (see below for dental procedures)	At least 5 days.
Eye infections	
Chlamydial inclusion conjunctivitis	3 weeks.
Gastro-intestinal infections	
Campylobacter	Minimum 5 days.
Prophylaxis of bacterial endocarditis with oral surgery	Erythromycin stearate 1.5 g one hour before procedure, then 500 mg six hours later.

Contra-indications, warnings, etc

Contra-indications: Known sensitivity to erythromycin.

Precautions: Erythromycin is excreted principally by the liver, so caution should be exercised in administering the antibiotic to patients with impaired hepatic function or concomitantly receiving potentially hepatotoxic agents.

The administration of erythromycin has been infrequently associated with the occurrence of reversible cholestatic jaundice.

The use of erythromycin in patients who are receiving digoxin, warfarin, carbamazepine and high doses of theophylline may result in the potentiation of their effects due to reduction in the rates of excretion.

Use in pregnancy: There is no evidence of hazard from erythromycin in human pregnancy. It has been in wide use for many years without apparent ill consequence. Animal studies have shown no hazard.

Side-effects: Occasional side-effects such as nausea, abdominal discomfort, vomiting and diarrhoea may be experienced. Reversible hearing loss associated with doses of erythromycin usually greater than 4 g per day has been reported. Allergic reactions are rare and mild, although anaphylaxis has occurred extremely rarely. There are no reports implicating erythromycin products with abnormal tooth development and only rare reports of damage to the blood, kidneys, liver or central nervous system.

Overdosage: Symptoms: Hearing loss, severe nausea, vomiting and diarrhoea.

Treatment: Gastric lavage, general supportive measures.

Pharmaceutical precautions Keep bottle tightly closed. Protect from light. Store below 25°C.

Legal category POM.

Package quantities Erythromid: Containers of 25, 50, 100, 500 and 1000 tablets.

Erythromid DS: Containers of 25, 50, 100 and 500 tablets.

Further information Erythromid and Erythromid DS each contain two azo dyes (not tartrazine), E110 and E124. No metabolisable carbohydrate is present.

Product licence numbers

Erythromid	0037/5019
Erythromid DS	0037/0121

ERYTHROPED* A
ERYTHROPED* PI
ERYTHROPED*
ERYTHROPED* FORTE

Presentation

Erythroped A: Oval, yellow film coated tablet. Each tablet contains 500 mg erythromycin as erythromycin ethylsuccinate.

Suspensions: Erythromycin in the form of granules which, when reconstituted, make a banana flavour suspension. It is available in three strengths:

1. Erythroped PI which contains 125 mg erythromycin per 5 ml.
2. Erythroped, containing 250 mg erythromycin per 5 ml.
3. Erythroped Forte, containing 500 mg erythromycin per 5 ml.

In addition single dose sachet presentations are available for each of the three strengths.

Uses For the prophylaxis and treatment of infections caused by erythromycin sensitive organisms.

Clinical indications:

1. Upper respiratory tract infections.
2. Lower respiratory tract infections.
3. Skin and soft tissue infections.
4. Bone infections.
5. Sexually transmitted diseases.
6. Oral/dental infections.
7. Eye infections.
8. Gastro-intestinal infections.
9. Prophylaxis.

Microbiological indications: Erythromycin has been shown to be active in vitro against the following organisms: Staphylococci, Streptococci, *Haemophilus influenzae*, L-forms, *Mycoplasma pneumoniae*, *Legionella pneumophila*, *Branhamella catarrhalis*, *Bordetella pertussis*, *Corynebacterium diphtheriae* (as an adjunct to antitoxin), Neisseria, *Treponema pallidum*, *Chlamydia trachomatis*, Clostridia, *Ureaplasma urealytica*, Campylobacter.

Dosage and administration

Adults and children over 8 years: For mild to moderate infections 2 g daily in divided doses. Up to 4 g daily in severe infections.

Elderly: No special dosage recommendations.

Children: Aged 2–8 years: For mild to moderate infections 1 g daily in divided doses.

Infants and babies up to 2 years: For mild to moderate infections 500 mg daily in divided doses.

For severe infections doses may be doubled.

Period of dosing with regard to indication

Upper respiratory tract infections	5–10 days.
Lower respiratory tract infections	7–14 days or until signs and symptoms indicate a cure. Legionnaires' disease may require prolonged treatment. Initially administration of erythromycin lactobionate by the intravenous route is recommended.
Skin and soft tissue infections	5–10 days. Acne may require prolonged treatment.
Sexually transmitted diseases	
NGU and syphilis	10–21 days. Some conditions may require prolonged treatment.
Oral/dental infections (see below for dental procedures)	At least 5 days.
Eye infections	
Chlamydial inclusion conjunctivitis	3 weeks.
Gastro-intestinal infections	
Campylobacter	Minimum 5 days.
Prophylaxis of bacterial endocarditis with oral surgery	Erythromycin stearate 1.5 g one hour before procedure, then 500 mg six hours later.

Contra-indications, warnings, etc

Contra-indications: Known sensitivity to erythromycin.

Precautions: Erythromycin is excreted principally by the liver, so caution should be exercised in administering the antibiotic to patients with impaired hepatic function or concomitantly receiving potentially hepatotoxic agents.

The administration of erythromycin has been infrequently associated with the occurrence of reversible cholestatic jaundice.

The use of erythromycin in patients who are receiving digoxin, warfarin, carbamazepine and high doses of theophylline may result in the potentiation of their effects due to reduction in the rates of excretion.

Use in pregnancy: There is no evidence of hazard from erythromycin in human pregnancy. It has been in wide use for many years without apparent ill consequence. Animal studies have shown no hazard.

Side-effects: Occasional side-effects such as nausea, abdominal discomfort, vomiting and diarrhoea may be experienced. Reversible hearing loss associated with doses of erythromycin usually greater than 4 g per day has been reported. Allergic reactions are rare and mild, although anaphylaxis has occurred extremely rarely. There are no reports implicating erythromycin products with abnormal tooth development and only rare reports of damage to the blood, kidneys, liver or central nervous system.

Overdosage: Symptoms: Hearing loss, severe nausea, vomiting and diarrhoea.

Treatment: Gastric lavage, general supportive measures.

Pharmaceutical precautions Erythroped suspensions should be stored in a cool place and the container kept tightly closed. The suspensions should be used within 14 days of dispensing. Shake well before using.

Legal category POM.

Package quantities Erythroped A: Bottles of 50, 100 and 500 tablets.

Erythroped suspensions: 100 ml bottles and single dose sachets.

Further information Contains dye E104 (non-azo).
Sugar content:

Erythroped PI	3.4 g/5 ml,	0.7 g per sachet
Erythroped	3.2 g/5 ml,	1.5 g per sachet
Erythroped Forte	2.9 g/5 ml,	2.9 g per sachet

Product licence numbers

Erythroped PI	125 mg/5 ml	0037/0149
	125 mg/sachet	0037/0156
Erythroped	250 mg/5 ml	0037/0150
	250 mg/sachet	0037/0157
Erythroped Forte	500 mg/5 ml	0037/0151
	500 mg/sachet	0037/0158
Erythroped A		0037/0137

ERYTHROPED* SUGAR FREE

Presentation Sachets containing 250 mg erythromycin as erythromycin ethylsuccinate in disaccharide- and dye-free granules. When dispersed in a little water, immediately before taking, the entire contents of one sachet provide a unit dose in the form of a fine cherry flavour suspension.

Uses For the prophylaxis and treatment of infections caused by erythromycin sensitive organisms.

Clinical indications:
1. Upper respiratory tract infections.
2. Lower respiratory tract infections.
3. Skin and soft tissue infections.
4. Bone infections.
5. Sexually transmitted diseases.
6. Oral/dental infections.
7. Eye infections.
8. Gastro-intestinal infections.
9. Prophylaxis.

Microbiological indications: Erythromycin has been shown to be active in vitro against the following organisms: Staphylococci, Streptococci, *Haemophilus influenzae*, L-forms, *Mycoplasma pneumoniae*, *Legionella pneumophila*, *Branhamella catarrhalis*, *Bordetella pertussis*, *Corynebacterium diphtheriae* (as an adjunct to antitoxin), Neisseria, *Treponema pallidum*, *Chlamydia trachomatis*, Clostridia, *Ureaplasma urealytica*, Campylobacter.

Dosage and administration
Adults and children over 8 years: For mild to moderate infections 2 g daily in divided doses. Up to 4 g daily in severe infections.

Elderly: No special dosage recommendations.

Children: Aged 2–8 years: For mild to moderate infections 1 g daily in divided doses.

Infants and babies up to 2 years: For mild to moderate infections 500 mg daily in divided doses.

For severe infections doses may be doubled.

Period of dosing with regard to indication

Upper respiratory tract infections	5–10 days.
Lower respiratory tract infections	7–14 days or until signs and symptoms indicate a cure. Legionnaires' disease may require prolonged treatment. Initially administration of erythromycin lactobionate by the intravenous route is recommended.
Skin and soft tissue infections	5–10 days. Acne may require prolonged treatment.
Sexually transmitted diseases	
NGU and syphilis	10–21 days. Some conditions may require prolonged treatment.
Oral/dental infections (see below for dental procedures)	At least 5 days.
Eye infections	
Chlamydial inclusion conjunctivitis	3 weeks.
Gastro-intestinal infections	
Campylobacter	Minimum 5 days.
Prophylaxis of bacterial endocarditis with oral surgery	Erythromycin stearate 1.5 g one hour before procedure, then 500 mg six hours later.

Contra-indications, warnings, etc

Contra-indications: Known sensitivity to erythromycin.

Precautions: Erythromycin is excreted principally by the liver, so caution should be exercised in administering the antibiotic to patients with impaired hepatic function or concomitantly receiving potentially hepatotoxic agents.

The administration of erythromycin has been infrequently associated with the occurrence of reversible cholestatic jaundice.

The use of erythromycin in patients who are receiving digoxin, warfarin, carbamazepine and high doses of theophylline may result in the potentiation of their effects due to reduction in the rates of excretion.

Use in pregnancy: There is no evidence of hazard from erythromycin in human pregnancy. It has been in wide use for many years without apparent ill consequence. Animal studies have shown no hazard.

Side-effects: Occasional side-effects such as nausea, abdominal discomfort, vomiting and diarrhoea may be experienced. Reversible hearing loss associated with doses of erythromycin usually greater than 4 g per day has been reported. Allergic reactions are rare and mild, although anaphylaxis has occurred extremely rarely. There are no reports implicating erythromycin products with abnormal tooth development and only rare reports of damage to the blood, kidneys, liver or central nervous system.

Overdosage: Symptoms: Hearing loss, severe nausea, vomiting and diarrhoea.

Treatment: Gastric lavage, general supportive measures.

Pharmaceutical precautions Store below 30°C.

Legal category POM.

Package quantities Cartons of 20 sachets.

Further information Nil.

Product licence number 0037/0135.

ĒTHRANE* ▼

Presentation Ēthrane (enflurane) is an inhalation anaesthetic with a pleasant ethereal odour. No additives or stabilisers are present.

Uses Ēthrane may be used for induction and maintenance of general anaesthesia. Adequate data are not available yet to establish its full place in obstetric anaesthesia other than in caesarean section. High concentrations of Ēthrane may produce marked uterine relaxation.

Ēthrane may be used for outpatient and dental anaesthesia in view of the rapidity of action and recovery, with stability of the cardiovascular system. Ēthrane can be used in children.

Actions: Induction and recovery are rapid. It does not stimulate excessive salivation, tracheobronchial secretions or cause bronchial constriction. Pharyngeal and laryngeal reflexes are diminished quickly. The level of anaesthesia changes rapidly with Ēthrane. Tachypnoea does not usually occur. Spontaneous respiration becomes depressed as the depth of anaesthesia increases.

Ēthrane provokes a 'sigh' response reminiscent of that seen with diethyl ether.

During induction there is a decrease in blood pressure followed by a return to near normal levels, which may or may not be associated with surgical stimulation.

Blood pressure tends to fall in direct relation to the depth of anaesthesia but cardiac rate and rhythm remain stable. Ēthrane appears to 'sensitise' the myocardium to adrenaline in man to a lesser extent than halothane. Available data indicate that subcutaneous injections of adrenaline may be safely administered to humans in concentrations of 1:100,000 or less at a dose of 10 ml in any given 10 minute period and not more than 30 ml/hour. All the usual precautions in the use of vasoconstrictor substances must be observed.

Good muscular relaxation is obtained with Ēthrane, but should greater relaxation be necessary minimal doses of an intravenous muscle relaxant may be used with measures to ensure adequate ventilation.

All commonly used intravenous muscle relaxants are compatible with Ēthrane.

Note: Ēthrane potentiates the effect of the non-depolarising muscle relaxants which should therefore be used in reduced dosage. Neostigmine does not reverse the direct effect of Ēthrane.

Ēthrane produces little post-operative analgesia.

Metabolism of Ēthrane in the human body proceeds at a low rate; inorganic fluoride is formed but serum levels in healthy individuals have not been shown to rise to significant levels.

Dosage and administration Vaporisers calibrated specifically for Ēthrane should be used so that the concentration being delivered is known.

The inspired concentration required to achieve clinical anaesthesia depends upon the age of the patient and to a minimal extent on body temperature. The MAC value is higher in children and decreases with advancing age, falling from an average in oxygen of 2.4% in the newborn and 2.5% at puberty, to 1.9% in young adults, and 1.7% at middle age. As with other agents, lesser concentrations of Ēthrane are normally required to maintain surgical anaesthesia in elderly patients. MAC values increase with increasing body temperature.

Premedication: Drugs used for premedication should be selected for each individual patient. The use of anticholinergic drugs is a matter of choice.

Induction: To avoid excitement a short acting barbiturate or other intravenous induction agent should be administered, followed by inhalation of the Ēthrane mixture. Ēthrane and oxygen alone or oxygen-nitrous oxide mixtures may be used.

It is recommended that Ēthrane induction be initiated at a concentration of 0.4% and gradually increased by 0.5% increments after every few breaths until surgical anaesthesia is achieved.

The maximum inspired concentration during induction should be no more than 4.5%. High inspired concentrations should be lowered as rapidly as possible to maintenance levels to prevent overdosage, and the blood pressure carefully observed.

Maintenance: In conjunction with nitrous oxide, surgical levels of anaesthesia may be maintained with a 0.5%–3% concentration of Ēthrane. A 3% concentration should not be exceeded for maintenance during spontaneous respiration. With controlled respiration techniques, during prolonged operations, single or supplementary doses of muscle relaxants may be used if required, bearing in mind the possibility of some slight potentiation. Ventilation to maintain the carbon dioxide tension in arterial blood in the the 4.7–6.0 kPa (35–45 mmHg) range is preferred to hyper- or hypoventilation, in order to minimise the possibility of CNS excitation.

Blood pressure levels during maintenance depend on Ēthrane concentration in the absence of other complicating factors. Excessive decreases (unless related to hypovolaemia) may be due to depth of anaesthesia and in such instances should be corrected by reducing the inspired Ēthrane concentration.

Elderly: As with other agents, lesser concentrations of Ēthrane are normally required to maintain surgical anaesthesia in elderly patients.

Contra-indications, warnings, etc

Contra-indications: Known sensitivity to Ēthrane.

Precautions: Ēthrane should be used with caution in patients who, by virtue of medical or drug history, may be considered more susceptible to cerebral stimulation produced by this drug. Increasing depth of anaesthesia with Ēthrane may produce changes in the electroencephalogram characterised by high voltage, fast frequency waves progressing through spike-dome complexes alternating with periods of electrical silence to frank seizure activity patterns. The latter may or may not be associated with motor movement. Motor activity, when encountered, generally consists of twitching or 'jerks' of various muscle groups; it is self-limiting and can be terminated by lowering the anaesthetic concentration. This electroencephalographic pattern associated with deep anaesthesia may be exacerbated by hyperventilation producing low arterial carbon dioxide tension. The pattern serves as a warning that depth of anaesthesia is excessive. Cerebral blood flow and metabolism studies in normal volunteers during seizure patterns show no evidence of cerebral hypoxia, and recovery appears to be uncomplicated.

Since levels of anaesthesia may be altered easily and rapidly, only vaporisers which deliver a predictable output with reasonable accuracy should be used. Hypotension and respiratory exchange can serve as a guide to anaesthetic depth. With deep levels of anaesthesia, more marked hypotension and respiratory depression are encountered.

The action of non-depolarising relaxants is augmented by Ēthrane, so less than the usual amounts of those drugs should be used.

Overdosage or unduly rapid absorption of adrenaline administered topically or by subcutaneous or submucosal injection during Ēthrane anaesthesia may give rise to cardiac arrhythmias (see 'Actions' section). Care must be taken to avoid intravenous injection.

Bromsulphthalein (BSP) retention is mildly raised post-operatively in some cases. There is some elevation of blood glucose and white blood cell count intra-operatively.

Use in pregnancy: Reproduction studies have been performed in rats and rabbits. Following single and multiple maternal administrations, no evidence of teratogenicity due to Ēthrane was found in the developing foetuses in these species. The relevance of these studies to the human is not known. Since there is no adequate experience in pregnant women who have received the drug, safety in pregnancy has not been established.

Adverse reactions:

1. Motor activity exemplified by movement of various muscle groups and seizures may be encountered with deep levels of Ēthrane anaesthesia, particularly with hyperventilation.

2. Hypotension, respiratory depression and arrhythmias have been reported.

3. Elevation of the white blood cell count has been observed. It has not been determined whether this is related to Ēthrane or to surgical stress.

4. A mild increase in serum glucose concentration has been observed in some normal and diabetic patients, as with other anaesthetic agents. There seems to be no contra-indication to the use of the agent in these patients for whom rapid recovery is advantageous.

5. Hepatic enzyme changes occur less frequently and to a lesser degree after multiple Ēthrane anaesthetics when compared with multiple exposures to halothane. While jaundice and significant hepatic enzyme increases occasionally occur after halothane anaesthesia, this is extremely rare after the administration of Ēthrane in the absence of complicating factors such as blood transfusion or concomitant administration of hepatotoxic drugs.

6. Increased serum inorganic fluoride levels have been found during and immediately after Ēthrane anaesthesia due to biodegradation of the agent. These levels normally remain well below the postulated threshold for nephrotoxicity and, after reaching a peak within eight hours of the end of the anaesthetic, rapidly return to preoperative values.

Although there is no evidence that Ēthrane anaesthesia adversely affects the normal or diseased kidney it may be prudent to avoid its use in cases of chronic renal failure.

Side-effects: Nausea, vomiting, hiccups or shivering may occur occasionally.

Pharmaceutical precautions Store away from heat. Keep well closed.

Legal category P.

Package quantities Ēthrane is supplied in bottles of 250 ml.

Further information Nil.

Product licence number 0037/0053.

FERROGRAD*

Presentation Each red Filmtab* (film-coated tablet Abbott) contains Dried Ferrous Sulphate BP 325 mg (equivalent to 105 mg elemental iron) in a sustained release form (Gradumet*).

Uses For the prevention and treatment of iron-deficiency anaemia.

The Gradumet device allows sustained release of the active ingredient over a number of hours, which increases iron utilisation and reduces gastro-intestinal intolerance.

The device consists of an inert plastic matrix, honey-combed by thousands of narrow passages which contain the active drug together with a water-soluble channelling agent. As the tablet passes down the gastro-intestinal tract the iron is leached out. The spent matrix is finally excreted in the stools.

Dosage and administration *Recommended adult oral dosage:* 1 tablet daily before food. As gastro-intestinal intolerance is not a problem with Ferrograd it should be given on an empty stomach, when iron is most effectively absorbed.

Children: Not recommended for children under 12 years of age.

Elderly: The sustained release tablet and its inert plastic matrix may cause a safety hazard in some elderly or other patients suffering from delayed intestinal transit.

Contra-indications, warnings, etc *Contra-indications:* Intestinal diverticula or any intestinal obstruction.

Precautions: As with all iron preparations Ferrograd should be given with care in patients with haemochromatosis, haemolytic anaemia or haemoglobinopathies. Interaction (chelation) with tetracyclines. Ferrograd tablets should be kept out of children's reach. The sustained release tablet and its inert plastic matrix may cause a safety hazard in some elderly or other patients suffering from delayed intestinal transit. There may also be further delay in release of the iron.

Side-effects: Those associated with conventional oral iron preparations, such as nausea, vomiting, diarrhoea and/or constipation, are less likely to occur because of the sustained release pattern of the formulation.

Overdosage: Initial symptoms of iron overdosage include nausea, vomiting, abdominal pain, diarrhoea, haematemesis and rectal bleeding. However, following a massive overdosage of Ferrograd, these initial symptoms may be absent due to its sustained release characteristics. Therefore if overdosage is suspected treatment should not be delayed by the absence of symptoms. A latent phase followed by a relapse 24–48 hours after ingestion manifest by hypotension, coma and hepatocellular necrosis may occur.

Treatment: The ingested Gradumet matrix cannot be readily aspirated through a stomach tube and there is no known chemical which will dissolve the Gradumet without harming the gastric mucosa. Accordingly, when overdosage is discovered early, the following procedure is recommended.

1. Administer an emetic by stomach tube.
2. Withdraw the stomach tube and wait for the patient to vomit.
3. Keep the patient under constant surveillance to detect possible aspiration of vomitus; maintain suction apparatus and standby emergency oxygen in case of need.
4. Examine the vomitus for returned Gradumet tablets.

5. Administer a saline purgative. By the time toxic signs have appeared, Gradumet tablets are in most cases past the pylorus so that emesis is of no value. Gastric lavage may be considered to remove the drug already released in the stomach. A saline purgative then should be given to speed the Gradumet tablets along the alimentary canal so as to minimise or prevent further absorption of the medication.

6. The use of an iron chelating agent such as oral desferrioxamine should be considered. In severe cases parenteral desferrioxamine may be necessary.

Pharmaceutical precautions Nil.

Legal category P.

Package quantities Ferrograd is supplied in 5 carton packs, each carton containing 30 (3 × 10) tablets.

Further information *Metabolisable carbohydrate content:* Approx. 0.02 g per tablet.

Product licence number 0037/5000.

FERROGRAD* C

Presentation Each two-layered, red Filmtab* (film-coated tablet Abbott) contains Dried Ferrous Sulphate BP 325 mg (equivalent to 105 mg elemental iron) in a sustained release form (Gradumet*) and 500 mg vitamin C, as sodium ascorbate.

Uses For the prevention and treatment of iron-deficiency anaemia and for the simultaneous treatment of vitamin C deficiency.

Ferrograd C combines the advantages of ferrous sulphate in the Gradumet matrix with a large dose of sodium ascorbate further to enhance absorption and is indicated in iron-deficiency anaemia, especially when poor absorption is a problem, and to promote haemopoiesis in patients where an underlying Vitamin C deficiency limits optimal haemoglobin formation. In patients whose haemoglobin has returned to normal, Ferrograd C may be of particular value in replenishing the depleted stores of iron.

The Gradumet device allows sustained release of ferrous sulphate over a number of hours, which increases iron utilisation and reduces gastro-intestinal intolerance. The Gradumet consists of an inert plastic matrix honey-combed by thousands of narrow passages which contain the active drug together with a water-soluble channelling agent. As the tablet passes down the gastro-intestinal tract the iron is leached out. The spent matrix is finally excreted in the stools.

Dosage and administration *Recommended adult oral dosage:* 1 tablet a day before food.

Children: not recommended for children under 12 years of age.

Elderly: The sustained release tablet and its inert plastic matrix may cause a safety hazard in some elderly or other patients suffering from delayed intestinal transit.

Contra-indications, warnings, etc *Contra-indications:* Intestinal diverticula or any intestinal obstruction.

Warning: The administration of therapeutic doses of sodium ascorbate may interfere with the Clinistix test for glycosuria giving a false negative result.

Precautions: As with all iron preparations Ferrograd C should be given with care in patients with haemochromatosis, haemolytic anaemias or haemoglobinopathies. There is an interaction (chelation) with tetracyclines. Ferrograd C tablets should be kept out of children's reach.

The sustained release tablet and its inert plastic matrix may cause a safety hazard in some elderly or other patients suffering from delayed intestinal transit. There may also be further delay in release of the iron.

Side-effects: Those associated with conventional oral iron preparations, such as nausea, vomiting, diarrhoea and/or constipation, are less likely to occur because of the sustained release pattern of the formulation.

Overdosage: Initial symptoms of iron overdosage include nausea, vomiting, abdominal pain, diarrhoea, haematemesis and rectal bleeding. However, following a massive overdosage of Ferrograd C, these initial symptoms may be absent due to its sustained release characteristics. Therefore if overdosage is suspected treatment should not be delayed by the absence of symptoms. A latent phase followed by a relapse 24–48 hours after ingestion manifest by hypotension, coma and hepatocellular necrosis may occur.

Vitamin C overdosage may cause acidosis and haemolytic anaemia in predisposed individuals (glucose 6 – phosphate dehydrogenase deficiency). Renal failure may occur in massive Vitamin C overdosage.

Treatment: The ingested Gradumet matrix cannot be readily aspirated through a stomach tube and there is no known chemical which will dissolve the Gradumet without harming the gastric mucosa. Accordingly, when overdosage is discovered early, the following procedure is recommended:

1. Administer an emetic by stomach tube.
2. Withdraw the stomach tube and wait for the patient to vomit.
3. Keep the patient under constant surveillance to detect possible aspiration of vomitus; maintain suction apparatus and standby emergency oxygen in case of need.
4. Examine the vomitus for returned Gradumet tablets.
5. Administer a saline purgative. By the time toxic signs have appeared, Gradumet tablets are in most cases past the pylorus so that emesis is of no value. Gastric lavage may be considered to remove the drug already released in the stomach. A saline purgative should then be given to speed the Gradumet tablets along the alimentary canal so as to minimise or prevent further absorption of the medication.
6. The use of an iron chelating agent such as oral desferrioxamine should be considered. In severe cases parenteral desferrioxamine may be necessary.

Pharmaceutical precautions Nil.

Legal category P.

Package quantities Ferrograd C is supplied in 5 carton packs, each carton containing 30 (3 × 10) tablets.

Further information *Metabolisable carbohydrate contents:* Approx. 0.01 g per tablet.

Product licence number 0037/5001.

FERROGRAD* FOLIC

Presentation A two-layered (red and yellow), round, bi-convex Filmtab* (film-coated tablet Abbott). Each tablet contains Dried Ferrous Sulphate BP 325 mg (equivalent to 105 mg elemental iron) in a sustained release form (red half – Gradumet*) and 350 mcg Folic Acid BP (yellow half).

Uses Ferrograd Folic* is indicated:
1. For the prevention and treatment of iron-deficiency anaemia of pregnancy.
2. For the prophylaxis of megaloblastic anaemia of pregnancy.

Folic acid requirements in pregnancy can be met with supplements of between 300 and 400 mcg daily. Without such supplements folate deficiency may develop leading to megaloblastic anaemia with attendant obstetric risks. Doses over 400 mcg may mask undiagnosed primary B_{12} deficiency.

In the extremely unlikely event of this condition occurring in a pregnant woman, the safe prophylactic dose is considered to be 350 mcg.

The Gradumet device allows sustained release of ferrous sulphate over a number of hours, which increases iron utilisation and reduces gastro-intestinal intolerance. The device consists of an inert plastic matrix, honeycombed by thousands of narrow passages which contain the active drug together with a water-soluble channelling agent. As the tablet passes down the gastro-intestinal tract the iron is leached out. The spent matrix is finally excreted in the stools.

Dosage and administration *Recommended adult oral dosage:* 1 tablet daily before food throughout pregnancy and during the first month of the puerperium.

Children: Not recommended for children under 12 years of age.

Elderly: The sustained release tablet and its inert plastic matrix may cause a safety hazard in some elderly or other patients suffering from delayed intestinal transit.

Contra-indications, warnings, etc
Contra-indications: Megaloblastic anaemia due to primary vitamin B_{12} deficiency. Intestinal diverticula or any intestinal obstruction.

Precautions: As with all iron preparations, Ferrograd Folic should be given with care in patients with haemochromatosis, haemolytic anaemias or haemoglobinopathies. There is an interaction (chelation) with tetracyclines. Ferrograd Folic tablets should be kept out of children's reach. The sustained release tablet and its inert plastic matrix may cause a safety hazard in some elderly or other patients suffering from delayed intestinal transit. There may also be further delay in release of the iron.

Side-effects: Those associated with conventional oral iron preparations such as nausea, vomiting, diarrhoea and/or constipation, are less likely to occur, because of the sustained release pattern of the formulation.

Overdosage: Initial symptoms of iron overdosage include nausea, vomiting, abdominal pain, diarrhoea, haematemesis and rectal bleeding. However, following a massive overdosage of Ferrograd Folic, these initial symptoms may be absent due to its sustained release characteristics. Therefore if overdosage is suspected treatment should not be delayed by the absence of symptoms. A latent phase followed by a relapse 24–48 hours after ingestion manifest by hypotension, coma and hepatocellular necrosis may occur.

Treatment: The ingested Gradumet matrix cannot be readily aspirated through a stomach tube and there is no known chemical which will dissolve the Gradumet without harming the gastric mucosa. Accordingly, when overdosage is discovered early, the following procedure is recommended:

1. Administer an emetic by stomach tube.
2. Withdraw the stomach tube and wait for the patient to vomit.
3. Keep the patient under constant surveillance to detect possible aspiration of vomitus; maintain suction apparatus and standby emergency oxygen in case of need.
4. Examine the vomitus for returned Gradumet tablets.
5. Administer a saline purgative. By the time toxic signs have appeared, Gradumet tablets are in most cases past the pylorus so that emesis is of no value. Gastric lavage may be considered to remove the drug already released in the stomach. A saline purgative then should be given to speed the Gradumet tablets along the alimentary canal so as to minimise or prevent further absorption of the medication.
6. The use of an iron chelating agent such as oral desferrioxamine should be considered. In severe cases, parenteral desferrioxamine may be necessary.

Pharmaceutical precautions Store below 20°C.

Legal category POM.

Package quantities Ferrograd Folic is supplied in 5 carton packs, each carton containing 30 (3 × 10) tablets.

Further information *Metabolisable carbohydrate content:* Approx. 0.3 g per tablet.

Product licence number 0037/5002.

FORANE* ▼

Presentation Forane (isoflurane) is an inhalation anaesthetic with a mildly pungent ethereal odour. No additive or stabiliser is present.

Uses Inhalation anaesthesia.

Actions: Induction and particularly recovery are rapid. Although slight pungency may limit the rate of induction, excessive salivation and tracheobronchial secretions are not stimulated. Pharyngeal and laryngeal reflexes are diminished quickly. Levels of anaesthesia change rapidly with Forane. Heart rhythm remains stable. Spontaneous respiration becomes depressed as depth of anaesthesia increases and should be closely monitored.

During induction there is a decrease in blood pressure which returns towards normal with surgical stimulation.

Blood pressure tends to fall during maintenance in direct relation to depth of anaesthesia, but cardiac rhythm remains stable. With controlled respiration and normal $PaCO_2$, cardiac output tends to be maintained despite increasing depth of anaesthesia, primarily through a rise in heart rate. With spontaneous respiration, the resulting hypercapnia may increase heart rate and cardiac output above awake levels.

Cerebral blood flow remains unchanged during light Forane anaesthesia but tends to rise at deeper levels. Increases in cerebrospinal fluid pressure may be prevented or reversed by hyperventilating the patient before or during anaesthesia.

Electroencephalographic changes and convulsions are extremely rare with Forane.

Forane appears to sensitise the myocardium to adrenaline to an even lesser extent than enflurane. Limited data suggest that subcutaneous infiltration of up to 50 ml

of 1:200,000 solution adrenaline does not induce ventricular arrhythmias in patients anaesthetised with Forane.

Muscular relaxation may be adequate for some intra-abdominal operations at normal levels of anaesthesia, but should greater relaxation be required small doses of intravenous muscle relaxants may be used. All commonly used muscle relaxants are markedly potentiated by Forane, the effect being most profound with non-depolarising agents. Neostigmine reverses the effects of non-depolarising muscle relaxants but has no effect on the relaxant properties of Forane itself. All commonly used muscle relaxants are compatible with Forane.

Forane may be used for the induction and maintenance of general anaesthesia. Adequate data are not available to establish its place in pregnancy, obstetrics or in children under two years of age.

Relatively little metabolism of Forane occurs in the human body. In the post-operative period only 0.17% of the isoflurane taken up can be recovered as urinary metabolites. Peak serum inorganic fluoride values usually average less than 5 micromol/litre and occur about four hours after anaesthesia, returning to normal levels within 24 hours. No signs of renal injury have been reported after Forane administration.

Dosage and administration Vaporisers specially calibrated for Forane should be used so that the concentration of anaesthetic delivered can be accurately controlled.

MAC values for Forane diminish with age, falling from an average in oxygen of 1.28% in the mid-twenties to 1.15% in the mid-forties, to 1.05% in the mid-sixties age group.

Premedication: Drugs used for premedication should be selected for the individual patient, bearing in mind the respiratory depressant effect of Forane. The use of anticholinergic drugs is a matter of choice.

Induction: A short-acting barbiturate or other intravenous induction agent is usually administered followed by inhalation of the Forane mixture. Alternatively, Forane with oxygen or with an oxygen/nitrous oxide mixture may be used.

It is recommended that induction with Forane be initiated at a concentration of 0.5%. Concentrations of 1.5 to 3.0% usually produce surgical anaesthesia in 7 to 10 minutes.

Maintenance: Surgical levels of anaesthesia may be maintained with 1.0–2.5% Forane in oxygen/nitrous oxide mixtures. An additionally 0.5–1.0% Forane may be required when given with oxygen alone.

Arterial pressure levels during maintenance tend to be inversely related to alveolar Forane concentrations in the absence of other complicating factors. Excessive falls in blood pressure may be due to depth of anaesthesia and, in these circumstances, should be corrected by reducing the inspired Forane concentration.

Elderly: As with other agents, lesser concentrations of Forane are normally required to maintain surgical anaesthesia in elderly patients. See above for MAC values.

Contra-indications, warnings, etc
Contra-indications: Known sensitivity to Forane, or history of malignant hyperpyrexia following its administration should be considered contra-indications.

Precautions: Since levels of anaesthesia may be altered quickly and easily with Forane, only vaporisers which deliver a predictable output with reasonable accuracy, or techniques during which inspired or expired concentrations can be monitored, should be used. The degree of hypotension and respiratory depression may provide some indication of anaesthetic depth.

Clinical experience with Forane to date has not shown evidence of liver toxicity, even after prolonged administration. However, experience with repeated exposure to Forane is limited and it is not yet possible to determine the effects of this on liver function.

As with other halogenated agents, Forane must be used with caution in patients with increased intracranial pressure. In such cases hyperventilation may be necessary.

The action of non-depolarising relaxants is markedly potentiated with Forane.

Use in pregnancy: Reproduction studies have been carried out on animals after repeated exposure to anaesthetic concentrations of Forane. Studies with the rat demonstrated no effect on fertility, pregnancy or delivery or on the viability of the offspring. No evidence of teratogenicity was revealed. Comparable experiments in rabbits produced similar negative results. The relevance of these studies to the human is not known. Safety in pregnancy has not been established. Blood losses comparable with those found following anaesthesia with other inhalation agents have been observed with Forane in patients undergoing induced abortion. Adequate data have not been developed to establish the safety of Forane in obstetric anaesthesia.

Adverse reactions
1. Arrhythmias have been occasionally reported.
2. Elevation of the white blood cell count has been observed, even in the absence of surgical stress.
3. Minimally raised levels of serum inorganic fluoride occur during and after Forane anaesthesia, due to biodegradation of the agent. It is unlikely that the low levels of serum inorganic fluoride observed (mean 4.4 micromol/l in one study) could cause renal toxicity, as these are well below the proposed threshold levels for kidney toxicity.

Side-effects: As with other halogenated anaesthetics, hypotension and respiratory depression have been observed. Close monitoring of blood pressure and respiration is recommended. Supportive measures may be necessary to correct hypotension and respiratory depression resulting from excessively deep levels of anaesthesia. Undesirable effects during recovery (shivering, nausea and vomiting) are minor in nature and comparable in incidence with those found with other anaesthetics.

Pharmaceutical precautions Store away from heat. Keep container well closed.

Legal category P.

Package quantities Forane is supplied in bottles of 100 ml.

Further information Nil.

Product licence number 0037/0115.

HARMOGEN*

Presentation Peach-coloured, flat, elongated, scored tablets marked LV. Each tablet contains 1.5 mg Estropipate USP (piperazine oestrone sulphate), equivalent to 0.93 mg oestrone.

Uses Oestrogen replacement therapy for the relief of oestrogen deficiency symptoms during or after the menopause and following oophorectomy, e.g. vasomotor symptoms, senile atrophic vaginitis, vulvitis and urethral syndrome, postmenopausal osteoporosis, depression, irritability and sleep disturbances.

Dosage and administration
Adults: 1.5–4.5 mg daily, taken as a single or divided oral dose. It may be necessary to divide the dose if gastro-intestinal irritation becomes a problem.

Clinical studies indicate that two Harmogen tablets daily is a satisfactory starting dose. For maintenance, the lowest effective dose should be used for a period of 3–4 weeks followed by a rest period of 5–7 days. Unless the patient has undergone hysterectomy Harmogen should be given clinically and accompanied by the administration of a progestogen. Withdrawal bleeding may occur towards the end of the rest period.

Elderly: As for adults.

Children: Not recommended.

Contra-indications, warnings, etc
Contra-indications: Oestrogen dependent carcinomas; history of thromboembolic disease; disorders of carbohydrate or lipid metabolism; undiagnosed bleeding from the genital tract; pregnancy; hepatic and renal disease; porphyria; history of herpes gestationis.

Precautions: The occurrence of abnormal, irregular bleeding at the commencement of, or during, therapy should be thoroughly investigated. Possible causes include incorrect dosage, fibroids or carcinoma.

Oestrogens may cause fluid retention, therefore caution should be exercised in patients with epilepsy, hypertension, migraine or cardiac disease.

Use with caution in patients with the combined factors of obesity, hypertension and smoking.

Prolonged exposure to unopposed oestrogens may increase the risk of the development of endometrial carcinoma.

Adverse effects of oestrogen therapy on blood pressure and gall bladder function have been reported.

In the unlikely event of the use of Harmogen in breast-feeding women, it should be remembered that oestrogens are excreted in the breast milk and inhibit milk flow.

Side-effects: The incidence of side-effects with Harmogen is low. Nausea is the most frequently reported side-effect; less common side-effects include fluid retention, breast swelling and tenderness, anorexia, vomiting, headaches, changes in liver function and breakthrough bleeding. Rare reactions include allergies, jaundice and changes in glucose metabolism and in libido. Oestrogens may precipitate porphyria cutanea tarda.

Overdosage: Overdosage is unlikely to cause serious problems. However, gastric lavage or emesis may be used when considered appropriate.

Pharmaceutical precautions Nil.

Legal category POM.

Package quantities Harmogen is supplied in containers of 100 tablets.

Further information Metabolisable carbohydrate content: Approx. 0.2 g per tablet.

The amount of piperazine in Harmogen is not sufficient

to exert a pharmacological action, but its addition ensures solubility, stability and uniform potency.

Product licence number 0037/5064.

IROFOL* C

Presentation Each two-layered, red Filmtab* (film-coated tablet Abbott) contains Dried Ferrous Sulphate BP 325 mg (equivalent to 105 mg elemental iron) in a sustained release form (the Gradumet*), 500 mg vitamin C (as sodium ascorbate) and 350 mcg Folic Acid BP.

Uses
1. For the prevention and treatment of iron-deficiency anaemia during pregnancy.
2. For the prophylaxis of megaloblastic anaemia during pregnancy.
3. For the simultaneous treatment of vitamin C deficiency.

Irofol C combines the advantages of ferrous sulphate in the slow release form with a large dose of sodium ascorbate further to enhance iron absorption, and to produce haemopoiesis in patients where an underlying vitamin C deficiency limits optimal haemoglobin formation.

During pregnancy folic acid requirements can be met with between 300–400 mcg daily. Without such supplementation folate deficiency may develop leading to undiagnosed primary B_{12} deficiency, in the extremely unlikely event of this condition occurring in a pregnant woman, so the safe prophylactic dose is considered to be 350 mcg.

The Gradumet device allows sustained release of ferrous sulphate over a number of hours which increases iron utilisation and reduces gastro-intestinal intolerance. The device consists of an inert plastic matrix, honeycombed by thousands of narrow passages which contain the active drug together with a water soluble chanelling agent. As the tablet passes down the gastro-intestinal tract the iron is leached out. The spent matrix is finally excreted in the stools.

Dosage and administration

Recommended adult oral dosage: 1 tablet a day before food throughout pregnancy.

Children: Not recommended for children under 12 years of age.

Elderly: The sustained release tablet and its inert plastic matrix may cause a safety hazard in some elderly or other patients suffering from delayed intestinal transit.

Contra-indications, warnings, etc

Contra-indications: Megaloblastic anaemia due to vitamin B_{12} deficiency. Intestinal diverticula or any intestinal obstruction.

Warning: Administration of therapeutic doses of sodium ascorbate may interfere with the Clinistix* test for glucosuria giving a false negative result.

Precautions: As with all iron preparations Irofol C should be given with care in patients with haemochromatosis, haemolytic anaemia or haemoglobinopathies. There is an interaction (chelation) with tetracyclines. Irofol C should be kept out of children's reach. The sustained release tablet and its inert plastic matrix may cause a safety hazard in some elderly or other patients suffering from delayed intestinal transit. There may also be further delay in release of the iron.

Side-effects: Those associated with conventional oral iron preparations, such as nausea, vomiting, diarrhoea and/or constipation, are less likely to occur because of the sustained release pattern of the formulation.

Overdosage: Initial symptoms of iron overdosage include nausea, vomiting, abdominal pain, diarrhoea, haematemesis and rectal bleeding. However, following a massive overdosage of Irofol C, these initial symptoms may be absent due to its sustained release characteristics. Therefore if overdosage is suspected treatment should not be delayed by the absence of symptoms. A latent phase followed by a relapse 24–48 hours after ingestion manifest by hypotension, coma and hepatocellular necrosis may occur.

Vitamin C overdosage may cause acidosis and haemolytic anaemia in predisposed individuals (glucose 6-phosphate dehydrogenase deficiency). Renal failure may occur in massive vitamin C overdosage.

Treatment: The ingested Gradumet matrix cannot be readily aspirated through a stomach tube and there is no known chemical which will dissolve the Gradumet without harming the gastric mucosa. Accordingly, when overdosage is discovered early, the following procedure is recommended:
1. Administer an emetic by stomach tube.
2. Withdraw the stomach tube and wait for the patient to vomit.
3. Keep the patient under constant surveillance to detect possible aspiration of vomitus; maintain suction apparatus and standby emergency oxygen in case of need.
4. Examine the vomitus for returned Gradumet tablets.
5. Administer a saline purgative. By the time toxic signs have appeared, Gradumet tablets are in most cases past the pylorus so that emesis is of no value. Gastric lavage may be considered to remove the drug already released in the stomach. A saline purgative should then be given to speed the Gradumet tablets along the alimentary canal so as to minimise or prevent further absorption of the medication.
6. The use of an iron chelating agent such as oral desferrioxamine should be considered. In severe cases parenteral desferrioxamine may be necessary.

Pharmaceutical precautions Nil.

Legal category POM.

Package quantities Irofol C is supplied in 5 carton packs, each carton containing 30 (3 × 10) tablets.

Further information Metabolisable carbohydrate content: Approx. 0.01 g per tablet.

Product licence number 0037/5003.

NORMETIC*

Presentation Flat, pale peach, bisected tablets with bevelled edges, 8.5 mm diameter and marked Normetic, containing Amiloride Hydrochloride BP equivalent to 5 mg anhydrous amiloride hydrochloride and 50 mg Hydrochlorothiazide BP.

Uses Antihypertensive and diuretic with potassium conserving properties. Indicated in the care of patients with hypertension, congestive heart failure, or hepatic cirrhosis with ascites, or where potassium depletion may occur. The amiloride hydrochloride in Normetic reduces the possibility of excessive potassium loss during prolonged and vigorous diuresis. Normetic is recommended in those conditions where potassium balance is particularly important, for example in patients with congestive heart failure receiving digitalis.

In hepatic cirrhosis and ascites, Normetic is likely to provide satisfactory diuresis with diminished potassium loss, thus lessening the risk of metabolic alkalosis.

Dosage and administration The rate of weight loss and the level of serum electrolytes should determine the dosage. The ideal target for weight loss after initiation of diuresis being in the range of 0.5–1.0 kg per day.

Hypertension: Usually 1 or 2 tablets once a day or in divided doses, which may be increased up to a maximum of 4 tablets per day.

Normetic may be used alone or in conjunction with other antihypertensive drugs. Since Normetic enhances the action of such agents, the antihypertensive dosage regimen may have to be altered to obviate any hypotensive reaction.

Hepatic cirrhosis with ascites: Starting with 1 tablet per day, dosage may be increased if required until there is effective diuresis provided the dose does not exceed 4 tablets per day. Ideally, a gradual weight loss is preferred in cirrhotic patients to minimise the occurrence of untoward reactions associated with diuretic therapy (your attention is drawn to the precautions section). Maintenance doses are sometimes less than the dosage necessary to initiate diuresis; consequently, the patient's weight should be stabilised before attempting to reduce dosage.

Congestive heart failure: The starting dose is 1 or 2 tablets per day, which may be altered if necessary to a maximum of 4 tablets per day. Serum potassium levels and diuretic response will establish the optimal dosage. On the establishment of initial diuresis, maintenance therapy is possible with a dosage reduction, or by the use of intermittent therapy.

Paediatric dosage: Normetic is not recommended for use in children since the safety of amiloride hydrochloride in this age group has not been established.

Use in the elderly: The dosage should be carefully adjusted according to renal function and clinical response. Where patients require reduced dosage, tablets may be halved by breaking along the bisect line.

Dosage in pregnancy: See 'Contra-indications, warnings, etc'.

Contra-indications, warnings, etc
Contra-indications: Hyperkalaemia (serum potassium over 5.5 mmol/litre); hypercalcaemia (serum calcium [total] over 2.6 mmol/litre; other potassium-conserving diuretics and potassium supplements; acute renal failure; severe progressive renal disease; diabetic nephropathy; hepatic failure; Addisons disease; anuria; patients with blood urea over 10 mmol/litre or serum creatinine over 130 micromol/litre in whom serum electrolyte and blood urea levels cannot be monitored with satisfaction and frequency; a known sensitivity to amiloride hydrochloride or hydrochlorothiazide.

The risk of lithium toxicity with patients combined on lithium and diuretics is very high and lithium should not be administered concurrently with Normetic.

In renal impairment, use of a potassium conserving agent may result in rapid development of hyperkalaemia.

Precautions: Diabetes Mellitus: Hyperkalaemia has been widely reported in diabetic patients on amiloride hydrochloride, mainly associated with chronic renal disease or pre-renal azotaemia. Renal function status should be established before prescribing Normetic to known or suspected diabetics. The taking of Normetic should be stopped prior to giving a glucose-tolerance test. Restabilising the insulin requirements of diabetic patients may be necessary. Latent diabetes mellitus may become manifest during thiazide therapy.

Metabolic or respiratory acidosis: severely ill patients likely to experience respiratory or metabolic acidosis on induction of potassium-conserving therapy, should be treated with caution. Categories such as decompensated diabetics or cardiopulmonary cases should be assessed for shifts in acid-base balance which may alter the balance of extracellular-intracellular potassium, and the development of acidosis may be associated with a marked rise in serum potassium.

Blood urea increases and electrolyte imbalance: Very infrequently, amiloride hydrochloride and hydrochlorothiazide, as combined in Normetic, fail to overcome any chloride deficit. Normal salt intake will, in the main, prevent any problem in this area.

Hyperkalaemia (serum potassium level over 5.5 mmol/litre): It has been noted that hyperkalaemia may be present in patients receiving amiloride hydrochloride either alone or in combination with other diuretics, especially in such categories as diabetics; the aged; congestive heart failure cases with known renal involvement; patients suffering from hepatic cirrhosis, or those subjected to vigorous diuretic therapy or the seriously ill. Careful observation of such categories of patients for manifestation of hyperkalaemia, using clinical, laboratory and ECG evidence should be undertaken as hyperkalaemia is not always accompanied by an abnormal ECG. In any development of hyperkalaemia, Normetic therapy should be stopped forthwith and, should it be desirable, reduction of serum potassium levels to normal values should be actively instituted. Reversible increases in blood urea have been reported in association with vigorous diuresis, notably in cases of hepatic cirrhosis with ascites and metabolic alkalosis or resistant oedema. In these cases, serum electrolyte and blood urea levels should be carefully monitored. Caution is advised in the use of Normetic with patients suffering renal impairment (see 'Contra-indications'). Care should be observed to avoid cumulative or toxic effects due to a reduced excretion of its components. Azotaemia may be precipitated or increased by hydrochlorothiazide. Normetic should be discontinued if increased azotaemia and oliguria occur during treatment.

Effects in cirrhotic patients: Patients with hepatic cirrhosis and ascites are more likely to experience adverse reactions during oral diuretic therapy owing to the fact that these patients are intolerant of acute shifts in electrolyte balance and because they may be subject to pre-existing hypokalaemia due to associated aldosteronism. Hepatic encephalopathy is characterised by coma, confusion and tremors has been reported with patients receiving amiloride hydrochloride and subjects receiving Normetic with no liver complications should be assessed for these conditions. A tenuous relationship between amiloride hydrochloride and a deepening of jaundice in cirrhotic patients has been postulated.

Additional precautions: Thiazides may produce sensitivity reactions in patients with or without a record of allergy or bronchial asthma. The action of other antihypertensive agents is potentiated by hydrochlorothiazide and a reduced dosage may be necessary at the introduction of Normetic. Reports indicate that there exists a possibility that thiazides may activate or exacerbate systemic lupus erythematosus.

Hydrochlorothiazide may reduce arterial responsiveness to noradrenaline, but not to such a degree as to prevent the effectiveness of noradrenaline in therapeutic usage. Thiazides may enhance the responsiveness to tubocurarine. In post-sympathectomy patients, the antihypertensive action of thiazides may be enhanced. Should orthostatic hypotension occur, it may be potentiated by narcotics, barbiturates and alcohol.

In some patients receiving thiazides, gout may be precipitated or hyperuricaemia may occur.

Acute pancreatitis associated with the use of hydrochlorothiazide has been reported.

Prolonged thiazide therapy has provoked isolated reports of pathological changes in the parathyroid glands accompanied by hypophosphataemia and hypercalcaemia. Serum BPI levels may be reduced by thiazide administration although not characterised by thyroid disturbance. The common complications of hyperparathyroidism have not been recorded. To establish parathyroid function, first discontinue thiazide administration.

As with any recently introduced preparations, patients should be monitored for possible signs of blood dyscrasias, liver dysfunction and idiosyncratic reactions.

Pregnancy and lactation warning: Owing to the limited clinical experience, the use of Normetic is not recommended during pregnancy and, as thiazides are found in breast milk, the patient should be instructed to stop nursing if contamination of the drug is thought to be essential. In general, as thiazides do cross the placental barrier and can be found in cord blood, the overall benefits of Normetic should be assessed against any potential harm to the foetus where pregnancy is present or suspected. Such problems noted have been thrombocytopaenia, foetal bone marrow depression, neonatal or foetal jaundice with the possibility of other side-effects associated with adult treatment. Diuretics are best avoided for the management of oedema of pregnancy or hypertension in pregnancy as their use may be associated with hypovolaemia, increased blood viscosity and reduced placental perfusion.

Side-effects: Related to diuresis: Orthostatic hypotension, muscle cramps, susceptibility to fatigue, weakness, dizziness, vertigo, salivary gland inflammation, transient blurred vision, paraesthesia, thirst, dry mouth.

Gastro-intestinal: Constipation and diarrhoea, pain, cramps, gastric irritation, abdominal fullness, vomiting, nausea, anorexia.

Additional side-effects: Side-effects associated with thiazide therapy are hyperuricaemia, glycosuria, hyperglycaemia, yellow vision, jaundice (intrahepatic cholestatic jaundice), restlessness, headache. Fever, necrotising angiitis (vasculitis, cutaneous vasculitis), photosensitivity, urticaria, rash, purpura, haemolytic anaemia, aplastic anaemia, agranulocytosis, leucopenia, thrombocytopenia, impotence, respiratory distress including pneumonitis and anaphylactic reactions have also been reported.

There have been a few reports of gastro-intestinal bleeding in subjects with a background of gastrointestinal disease receiving amiloride hydrochloride alone; a causal relationship to amiloride, however, has not been established. Rare reversible abnormalities, possibly relating to Amiloride Hydrochloride, have been noted in liver function tests.

In the case of moderate or severe side-effects, the dosage of Normetic should be reduced or withdrawn altogether.

Treatment of overdosage: There is no specific antidote.

Dehydration, electrolyte imbalance and hepatic coma are treated by the established procedures. If ingestion is recent, gastric lavage should be performed or emesis induced. Treatment is symptomatic and supportive. If hyperkalaemia occurs, prompt measures should be taken to lower the serum potassium levels. For respiratory impairment, oxygen or artificial respiration should be administered.

Pharmaceutical precautions Keep container tightly closed; store in a cool place, protected from light.

Legal category POM.

Package quantities Containers of 8, 50, 100 and 500 tablets.

Further information Oral potassium supplements must not be given with Normetic.

Onset of diuretic action begins within two to four hours after administration of Normetic, and reaches a peak at about the fourth hour; there is detectable activity for about 24 hours.

Product licence number 0037/0148.

PLEGISOL*

Presentation Plegisol is a sterile, pyrogen-free solution of electrolytes in water enclosed in a 1 litre flexible container. The solution contains 1.2 mmol calcium, 160 mmol chloride, 16 mmol magnesium, 16 mmol potassium and 110 mmol sodium per litre.

It is intended for single use only.

Uses Plegisol, when suitably buffered with Sodium Bicarbonate Injection BP 8.4% (10 ml per litre of Plegisol) is used in combination with total body hypothermia to induce cardiac arrest and protect the myocardium from ischaemic damage while the aorta is cross clamped during cardiopulmonary bypass.

Dosage and administration 10 ml of 8.4% Sodium Bicarbonate Injection BP must be added to each litre of Plegisol immediately before use. The buffered solution should not be kept longer than 24 hours.

Following institution of cardiopulmonary bypass at perfusate temperatures of 28°–30°C and after cross-clamping of the aorta, the buffered Plegisol (cooled to 4°C) should be rapidly infused into the aortic root at a rate of 300 ml/sq.m. body surface area/min for 1 to 2 minutes. Should myocardial activity persist, a further 300 ml/sq.m/min may be infused for one minute. Further infusions of smaller volumes of the solution may be repeated at intervals of 15–30 minutes or less. If myocardial temperature rises above 15°–20°C or returning cardiac activity is observed, supplementary doses of Plegisol can be administered. Additives may be incompatible. When introducing additives, mix thoroughly and use the solution promptly.

The volumes suggested may be varied according to duration and type of procedure.

Elderly: No special dosage recommendations.

Contra-indications, warnings, etc
Contra-indications: Plegisol must not be administered without the addition of sodium bicarbonate.

Warnings: If large volumes are infused and allowed to enter the heart/lung bypass machine and hence the general circulation, plasma magnesium and potassium levels may rise. Venting of the solution and removal by suction from the right heart is therefore recommended, if large volumes of Plegisol are used, or in the absence of satisfactory diuresis.

Precautions: Before use, check for minute leaks by squeezing the container. If leaks are found, the solution should be discarded. Do not use unless the solution is clear and colourless. Discard the unused portion.

Myocardial temperature should be monitored to confirm adequate hypothermia throughout surgery. Continuous ECG monitoring is desirable to detect changes in myocardial activity during the procedure.

Complications: Spontaneous recovery of normal cardiac activity may be delayed or absent. In those with ventricular fibrillation/tachycardia direct current defibrillation will be required. Transient heart block can also occur and may necessitate the use of a pacemaker. Myocardial function may be impaired following cardiopulmonary bypass and the administration of inotropic and vasoactive drugs, or even intra-aortic balloon counter pulsation, may be required.

Usage in pregnancy: Animal reproduction studies have not been conducted with Plegisol. It is not known whether the solution affects either the growing foetus or reproductive capacity.

Safety in pregnancy has not been established.

Overdosage: Excessive infusion of the solution may result in dilatation of the coronary vasculature, and possibly cardiac oedema, thereby impairing myocardial performance. Treatment is as outlined above.

Pharmaceutical precautions Protect from freezing and extreme heat. Do not store above 40°. Do not remove the overwrap until immediately before use.

Legal category POM.

Package quantities Plegisol is supplied in 1000 ml flexible containers (without sodium bicarbonate solution).

Further information The flexible container is made from PVC. Small quantities of moisture may permeate from the container inside the overwrap, but not in amounts sufficient to significantly alter the composition of the solution.

The osmolarity of the buffered solution is approximately 280 mOsm/litre.

Product licence number 0037/0144.

THEOGRAD*

Presentation Each white Filmtab* (film-coated tablet Abbott) contains 350 mg Theophylline BP in a sustained release form (Gradumet*).

Uses For the prevention or relief of bronchospasm. The Gradumet consists of a plastic matrix, honeycombed by thousands of narrow passages which contain the active drug together with a water soluble channelling agent. As the tablet passes down the gastro-intestinal tract, the theophylline is leached out; this action is quite independent of intestinal variables such as pH and enzyme effect, viscosity, ion concentration, surface tension and motility. The spent matrix is finally excreted in the stools.

Quite apart from providing a more uniform and prolonged clinical effect, the controlled release of theophylline reduces gastric irritation, often a problem with conventional preparations, to a minimum.

Dosage and administration Usual adult dosage: 1 tablet every 12 hours. In patients with acute symptoms 2 tablets initially, followed by 1 tablet at 12-hourly intervals.

Patients may require to have the dose titrated to produce the desired therapeutic effect, which is usually obtained with a serum concentration of 10–20 mcg/ml.

Children: Not recommended.

Elderly: Theophylline should be administered with caution to elderly patients and to those with cardiac and liver disease. A reduction in dosage may be necessary. The sustained release tablet and its inert plastic matrix may cause a safety hazard in some elderly or other patients suffering from delayed intestinal transit.

Contra-indications, warnings, etc
Contra-indications: Intestinal diverticula or any intestinal obstruction.

Precautions: As with all adrenergic stimulants, Theograd should be used with caution in patients with cardiac arrhythmias.

The sustained release tablet and its inert plastic matrix may cause a safety hazard in some elderly or other patients suffering from delayed intestinal transit. There may also be further delay in release of the active ingredient.

Recent studies reveal that the use of erythromycin in patients who are receiving high doses of theophylline may be associated with an increase of serum theophylline levels and potential theophylline toxicity.

In case of theophylline toxicity and/or elevated serum theophylline levels, the dose of theophylline should be reduced while the patient is receiving erythromycin therapy.

Pregnancy and lactation: The safety of theophylline in human pregnancy has not been established. Theophylline crosses the placental barrier and is excreted in breast milk.

Side-effects: As with all theophylline preparations, some patients may experience gastro-intestinal side-effects. However, the incidence has been reduced to a minimum by the sustained release formulation.

Overdosage: Symptoms: The delayed release of the theophylline gives extra time in which gastric lavage and general treatment may be instituted. Treatment should not be delayed, therefore, even if immediate symptoms are absent. Symptoms may include nausea, vomiting, gastro-intestinal irritation, tachycardia, hypotension.

Treatment: The ingested Gradumet cannot be readily aspirated through a stomach tube and there is no known chemical which will dissolve the Gradumet without harming the gastric mucosa. Accordingly, when overdosage is discovered early, the following procedure is recommended:

1. Administer an emetic by stomach tube.
2. Withdraw the stomach tube and wait for the patient to vomit.
3. Keep the patient under constant surveillance to detect possible aspiration of vomitus; maintain suction apparatus and standby emergency oxygen in case of need.
4. Examine vomitus for returned Gradumet tablets.
5. Administer a saline purgative.

By the time toxic signs have appeared, Gradumet tablets are in most cases past the pylorus so that emesis is of no value. Gastric lavage may be considered to remove the drug already released in the stomach. A saline purgative then should be given to speed the Gradumet tablets along the alimentary canal so as to minimise or prevent further absorption of the medication.

General supportive measures should be employed.

Pharmaceutical precautions Nil.

Legal category P.

Package quantities Theograd is supplied in 5 carton packs, each carton containing 30 (3 × 10) tablets.

Further information *Metabolisable carbohydrate content:* Approx. 0.02 g per tablet.

Product licence number 0C37/5059.

UREAPHIL*

Presentation Ureaphil is supplied as 40 g of anhydrous, lyophilised, non-pyrogenic, sterile urea powder in a 150 ml container.

Uses

1. To reduce cerebral oedema and raised intracranial pressure resulting from trauma, surgery or disease.

2. To counteract oliguria following burns, surgery or other trauma.

3. To promote an abundant flow of urine following prostatectomy and so reduce the need for frequent irrigation of the bladder.

4. To induce therapeutic abortion in the mid-trimester of pregnancy.

Note: Although urea acts as an osmotic diuretic, it is not considered the drug of choice for the management of oedema in cardiac failure.

Dosage and administration

Administration: Ureaphil is administered by slow intravenous infusion. The rate of injection should not exceed 4 ml per minute. Extreme care is essential to prevent accidental extravasation of the solution at the site of injection, since this may cause local reactions ranging from mild irritation to tissue necrosis. Ureaphil may be reconstituted by the addition of 5 or 10% glucose solution.

It is administered in hypertonic concentrations of 30% (w/v) or 4% (w/v) depending upon clinical indications. To prepare a 30% solution 105 ml of diluent are added to the contents of one 40 g bottle producing 135 ml of solution. To prepare a 4% solution, the contents of one 40 g container should be dissolved in situ by aseptically transferring approximately 100 ml of the diluent from a 1 litre IV solution bag, shaking to dissolve and then reinjecting the urea solution back into the IV bag – final volume 1030 ml. Since the dissolution is an endothermic reaction, the diluent should be warmed slightly or the solution allowed to reach room temperature, before use. Urea will decompose if the diluent is warmed above 40°C.

Dosage: The amount to be administered is generally estimated on the basis of 1 g of urea per kg of body weight. The dosage must also take into account the clinical condition of the patient, especially the state of hydration, electrolyte balance and integrity of renal function. The total daily dose should not exceed 120 g of urea.

1. *Increased intracranial or cerebrospinal fluid pressure:* For the reduction of cerebral oedema, and increased intracranial or cerebrospinal fluid pressure, a 30% solution is usually employed. The adult dose ranges from 1.0 to 1.5 g (3.3 to 5.0 ml) per kg of body weight.

In children the dosage is from 0.5 to 1.5 g/kg of body weight. In young children up to 2 years of age as little as 0.1 g/kg can be effective.

2. *Oliguria:* To combat antidiuresis following surgery, burns or other trauma a 4% solution has produced satisfactory results. In the adult, the dose ranges from 1.0 to 1.5 g/kg body weight. This is approximately equivalent to a volume of 1,500–3,000 ml.

In children up to 5 years of age, the usual dose of the 4% solution is 1 g/kg/day, administered by slow intravenous drip. Larger doses may be required in older children.

3. *Prostatectomy:* Following prostatectomy, urea is employed as a 4% solution. Depending upon clinical circumstances, 3 litres of solution may be administered daily for three days following surgery. This is equivalent to a daily dose of 120 g of urea.

Dosage in the elderly: No special dosage recommendation but see under 'Contra-indications' and 'Precautions'.

4. *Therapeutic abortion:* Methods: A sterile, suprapubic, drainage catheter is passed into the amniotic cavity, the liquor drained off and the volume measured.

(1) Ureaphil alone: 200 ml of a 40% w/v solution (80 g Ureaphil in 140 ml of 5% glucose solution) is given through the cannula into the amniotic cavity.
Note: Some clinicians have increased the amount of 5% glucose solution to 210 ml (final volume 270 ml).
The time required to induce therapeutic abortion can be reduced by the addition of either oxytocin or prostaglandin E_2 given by methods described below:

(2) Combined intra-amniotic Ureaphil: 200 ml of a 40% w/v solution (80 g Ureaphil in 140 ml of 5% glucose solution) and a simultaneous intravenous infusion of oxytocin (100–200 units in 500 ml Compound Sodium Lactate Injection BP – Hartmann's solution).

(3) Intra-amniotic Ureaphil: 140 ml of a 57% w/v solution (80 g Ureaphil dissolved in 80 ml Hartmann's solution). When the administration of the Ureaphil solution is complete either 2.5 mg, 5 mg or 10 mg of prostaglandin E_2 in alcohol is injected. This method is particularly successful in inducing mid-trimester abortion within 24 hours.

Contra-indications, warnings, etc

Contra-indications: Urea should not be used in patients with severely impaired renal function, active intracranial bleeding or marked dehydration. Frank liver failure is also a contra-indication for use. Ureaphil should not be infused in the veins of the lower limbs of elderly patients, since phlebitis and thrombosis of superficial veins may occur.

Precautions: Urea may cause depletion of electrolytes, which can result in hyponatraemia and hypokalaemia. Early signs of such depletion may indicate the need for supplementation before serum levels are reduced. An indwelling urethral catheter should be used in comatose patients receiving Ureaphil, to ensure bladder emptying. The rapid intravenous administration of a hypertonic solution of urea may be associated with haemolysis as well as a direct effect on the cerebral vasomotor centres, and as a result there may be increased capillary bleeding. These effects usually can be avoided by not exceeding an infusion rate of 4 ml per minute. Solutions of urea should not be administered through the same set by which blood is being infused. Although arterial oozing has been reported as a nuisance when intracranial surgery is performed on patients after they have been treated with urea, it has not been a significant problem.

However, Ureaphil should not be used in the presence of active intracranial bleeding unless such use is preliminary to prompt surgical intervention to control haemorrhage. It should be borne in mind that the reduction in brain oedema induced by urea may result in reactivation of intracranial bleeding.

In the presence of kidney disease, urea should be administered with caution. Mild elevation of non-protein nitrogen does not preclude its acute or chronic use, but frequent laboratory studies should be made to determine if kidney function is adequate to eliminate the infused urea, as well as that produced endogenously.

Patients exhibiting a temporary reduction in urine volume are generally able to maintain a satisfactory elimination of urea. However, if diuresis does not follow the injection of urea in such patients within 6–12 hours, the drug should be withdrawn pending further evaluation of renal function. As with other infused solutions, Ureaphil may temporarily maintain circulatory volume and blood pressure in spite of considerable blood loss. Consequently, when excessive blood loss occurs within a short period of time, blood replacement should be adequate and simultaneous with the infusion of urea.

Hypothermia when used with urea infusion may increase the risk of venous thrombosis and haemoglobinuria.

Usage in pregnancy and lactation: It has not been established whether or not sterile urea can cause foetal harm when given to pregnant women or can affect reproductive capacity. Ureaphil should be given in pregnancy only if clearly needed. Urea may be excreted in human milk following Ureaphil administration, hence caution should be exercised when used in nursing mothers.

Side-effects: Headaches (reported to be similar to those which occur in some patients following lumbar puncture), nausea, vomiting, occasional syncope and disorientation have been known to follow intravenous administration of urea. Less often reported is a transient agitated confusional state. No serious reactions have been noted when solutions have been infused slowly provided renal function is not seriously impaired and there is no evidence of active intracranial bleeding. Chemical phlebitis and thrombosis near the site of injection have been reported infrequently.

Overdosage: In the event of overdosage as reflected by unusually elevated blood urea nitrogen levels, discontinue administration of the drug, evaluate the patient and institute corrective measures as indicated. See 'Precautions' and 'Dosage'.

Pharmaceutical precautions Ureaphil should be used immediately after reconstitution. It should not be stored for any length of time, even in a refrigerator.

Legal category POM.

Package quantities Ureaphil is supplied in 150 ml Abbott single-use containers containing 40 g.

Further information Small quantities of sodium hydroxide may have been added to some batches for adjustment of pH.

Product licence number 0037/5072.

*Trade Mark

Alcon Laboratories (U.K.) Limited
Imperial Way
Watford
Hertfordshire, WD2 4YR

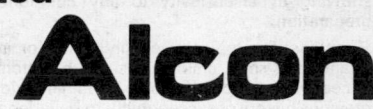

BALANCED SALT SOLUTION ALCON BSS*

Presentation A sterile physiological balanced salt solution which is isotonic to the tissues of the eye. It is a lint free solution containing essential ions for normal cell metabolism. Each ml contains Sodium Chloride 0.64%, Potassium Chloride 0.075%, Calcium Chloride 0.048%, Magnesium Chloride Hexahydrate 0.030%, Sodium Acetate 0.39%, Sodium Citrate 0.17% and Water for Injection.

Uses As a physiologic irrigating solution.

Dosage and administration Sufficient to produce the required irrigation. The adaptor plug is designed to accept an ophthalmic irrigating needle. Intra-ocular tissue may be irrigated by attaching the needle to the Steri-Unit Drop-Tainer Bottle as follows:
1. Aseptically remove the Drop-Tainer by peeling off the paper backing.
2. Snap on surgical irrigator needle. Push well to ensure it is firmly in place.
3. Test patency of the assembly.
Squeeze out several drops before inserting into the anterior chamber. The needle should be removed from the chamber prior to releasing pressure to prevent suction.

Contra-indications, warnings, etc
Contra-indication: There are no specific contra-indications for this product.

Warning: If the blister or paper backing is damaged or broken sterility of the enclosed bottle cannot be assured. Open under aseptic conditions only.

Pharmaceutical precautions This solution contains no preservative and should not be re-used.
Store in a cool place.

Legal category P.

Package quantities 15 ml Steri-Unit Drop-Tainer dispenser.

Further information The enclosed Steri-Unit Drop-Tainers are sterile and may be safely handled by the surgeon.

Product licence number 0649/0007.

ISOPTO* ALKALINE

Presentation Isopto Alkaline is a sterile clear, colourless solution containing hydroxypropyl methylcellulose (Hypromellose) 1.0%, preserved with benzalkonium chloride 0.01%.

Uses Isopto Alkaline is an emollient solution used as a physiologic ophthalmic vehicle or suspending agent, and as a tear replacement in tear deficiency, Keratoconjunctivitis sicca and for ocular lubrication.

Dosage and administration It is suitable for use both by adults and children. The dose depends upon the desired amount of lubrication, the usual dosage being one or two drops to be instilled into the eyes three times daily, or as needed.

Contra-indications, warnings, etc If an irritation persists or increases use of the drops should be discontinued. In order to help preserve sterility the dropper should not be allowed to touch the eyelashes or any other surface. This product contains benzalkonium chloride and should not be used when soft contact lenses are being worn.

Pharmaceutical precautions The eyedrops should be stored in a cool place. Discard one month after opening.

Legal category P.

Package quantities 10 ml containers.

Further information Isopto Alkaline eye-drops are contained in an unbreakable semi-rigid plastic dropper bottle with a screw-on cap.

Product licence number 0649/5900.

ISOPTO* ATROPINE 1.0%

Presentation Isopto Atropine is a clear, colourless, sterile solution containing atropine sulphate 1.0% and hydroxypropyl methylcellulose (hypromellose) 0.5% and preserved with benzalkonium chloride 0.01%.

Uses Atropine is a powerful mydriatic and cycloplegic. It is used in refraction, especially in children, and in uveitis.

Dosage and administration *Adults:* For refraction, administer one or two drops topically to the eye(s) one hour before refracting. For uveitis, administer one or two drops topically to the eye(s) up to four times daily.

Children: For refraction, administer one drop to each eye twice daily for one to three days prior to examination. For uveitis, administer one drop to each eye up to three times daily.

Prescribing in the elderly: In the elderly and others where increased intra-ocular pressure may be encountered, mydriatics and cycloplegics should be used cautiously. To avoid inducing angle closure glaucoma, an estimation of the depth of the angle of the anterior chamber should be made.

Contra-indications, warnings, etc
Contra-indications: Contra-indicated in persons with

primary glaucoma or a tendency toward glaucoma, e.g. narrow anterior chamber angle, and in those persons showing hypersensitivity to any component of this preparation.

Warnings: For topical use only – not for injection. In infants and small children, use with extreme caution. Excessive use in children or in certain individuals with a previous history of susceptibility to belladonna alkaloids may produce systemic symptoms of atropine poisoning. This product contains benzalkonium chloride and should not be used when soft contact lenses are being worn.

Precautions: To avoid excessive systemic absorption, the lacrimal sac should be compressed by digital pressure for one minute after instillation.

Patient warning: Patients should be advised not to drive or engage in other hazardous activities while pupils are dilated. Patients may experience sensitivity to light and should protect eyes in bright illumination during dilation. Parents should be warned not to get this preparation in their child's mouth and to wash their own hands and the child's hands following administration.

Adverse reactions: Prolonged use may produce local irritation characterized by follicular conjunctivitis, vascular congestion, oedema, exudate and an exczematoid dermatitis. Severe reactions are manifested by hypotension with progressive respiratory depression. Coma and death have been reported in the very young.

Overdosage: Systemic atropine toxicity is manifested by flushing and dryness of the skin (a rash may be present in children), blurred vision, a rapid and irregular pulse, fever, abdominal distention in infants, mental aberration (hallucinosis) and loss of neuromuscular co-ordination. Physostigmine should be administered parenterally (for dosage refer to Goodman & Gilman or other pharmacology reference). In infants and small children, the body surface must be kept moist.

Pregnancy warning: There is insufficient evidence as to drug safety in human pregnancy. This product should therefore only be used during pregnancy if considered essential by the physician.

Pharmaceutical precautions Isopto Atropine should be stored in a cool place away from direct sunlight. Keep the container tightly closed. The contents should be discarded one month after opening.

Legal category POM.

Package quantities 5 ml containers.

Further information Isopto Atropine eye drops are contained in an unbreakable semi-rigid, plastic dropper bottle with screw-on cap.

Product licence number 0649/5901.

ISOPTO* CARBACHOL 3%

Presentation Isopto Carbachol is a clear colourless sterile solution, containing 3% Carbachol and 1% hydroxypropyl methylcellulose (hypromellose), and preserved with benzalkonium chloride 0.005%.

Uses To reduce intraocular pressure. May be used to control intraocular pressure where control by pilocarpine has been lost or in cases of pilocarpine sensitivity.

Dosage and administration Instil two drops topically into the eye(s) up to four times daily. For adult use only.

Contra-indications, warnings, etc
Contra-indications: Miotics are contra-indicated where constriction is undesirable such as in acute iritis. Contra-indicated in those persons showing hypersensitivity to any component of this preparation.

Warnings: For topical use only. Not for injection. Carbachol should be used with caution in the presence of corneal abrasion to avoid excessive penetration which can produce systemic toxicity, and in patients with acute cardiac failure, bronchial asthma, active peptic ulcer, hyperthyroidism, gastrointestinal spasm, urinary tract obstruction and Parkinson's disease. As with all miotics, retinal detachment has been reported when used in certain susceptible individuals. The causal relationship has not been established. This product contains benzalkonium chloride and should not be used when soft contact lenses are being worn.

Precautions: Avoid overdosage. The miosis usually causes difficulty in dark adaptation. Patients should be advised to exercise caution in night driving and other hazardous occupations in poor light.

Adverse reactions: This preparation is capable of producing systemic symptoms of a cholinesterase inhibitor even when the epithelium is intact. Transient ciliary and conjunctival injection, headache and ciliary spasm with resultant temporary decrease of visual acuity may occur. Salivation, syncope, cardiac arrhythmia, gastrointestinal cramping, vomiting, asthma and diarrhoea may occur.

Overdosage: Atropine should be administered parenterally (for dosage refer to Goodman & Gilman or other pharmacology reference).

Pregnancy warning: There is insufficient evidence as to drug safety in human pregnancy. This product should therefore only be used during pregnancy if considered essential by the physician.

Pharmaceutical precautions Isopto Carbachol eye drops should be stored in a cool place away from direct sunlight. Keep the container tightly closed. Contents should be discarded one month after opening.

Legal category POM.

Package quantities 10 ml containers.

Further information Isopto Carbachol eye drops are contained in an unbreakable semi-rigid plastic dropper bottle with screw-on cap.

Product licence number 0649/5902.

ISOPTO* CARPINE
0.5%, 1.0%, 2.0%, 3.0%, 4.0%

Presentation Isopto Carpine is a clear, colourless, sterile solution available in five strengths; containing 0.5, 1, 2, 3 or 4% pilocarpine hydrochloride and 0.5% hydroxypropyl methylcellulose (hypromellose), and preserved with benzalkonium chloride 0.01%.

Uses Isopto Carpine is a miotic and its main use is in the treatment of glaucoma.

Dosage and administration Two drops topically in the eye(s) up to three or four times daily. Under selected conditions, more frequent instillations may be indicated. Individuals with heavily pigmented irides may require larger doses.

Contra-indications, warnings, etc
Contra-indications: Miotics are contra-indicated where

constriction is undesirable such as in acute iritis; in those persons showing hypersensitivity to any of their components; and in pupiliary block glaucoma.

Warnings: For topical use only. Not for injection. This product contains benzalkonium chloride and should not be used when soft contact lenses are worn.

Precautions: The miosis usually causes difficulty in dark adaptation. Patients should be advised to exercise caution in night driving and other hazardous occupations in poor illumination.

Adverse reactions: Ciliary spasms, conjunctival vascular congestion, temporal or supraorbital headache, and induced myopia may occur. This is especially true in younger individuals who have recently started administration. Reduced visual acuity in poor illumination is frequently experienced by older individuals with lens opacity. As with all miotics, rare cases of retinal detachment have been reported when used in certain susceptible individuals. Lens opacity may occur with prolonged use of pilocarpine.

Overdosage: Systemic reactions following topical administration are extremely rare.

Pregnancy warning: There is insufficient evidence as to the drug safety in human pregnancy. This product should therefore only be used during pregnancy if considered essential by the physician.

Pharmaceutical precautions Isopto Carpine should be stored in a cool place away from direct sunlight. Keep the container tightly closed. The contents should be discarded one month after opening.

Legal category POM.

Package quantities 10 ml containers.

Further information Isopto Carpine eye drops are contained in an unbreakable semi-rigid, plastic dropper bottle with screw-on cap.

Product licence numbers
0.5% 0649/5903
1.0% 0649/5904
2.0% 0649/5905
3.0% 0649/5906
4.0% 0649/5907

ISOPTO* CETAMIDE 15%

Presentation Isopto Cetamide is a clear, colourless sterile solution, containing sulphacetamide sodium 15% and 0.5% hydroxypropyl methylcellulose (hypromellose), and preserved with methylparaben 0.05% and propylparaben 0.01%.

Uses As an anti-infective.

Dosage and administration Two drops to be instilled into the eye every 4 hours or as prescribed. In acute infections the dose should be increased to two drops every 2 hours. Isopto Cetamide is suitable for use by both adults and children.

Contra-indications, warnings, etc

Contra-indications: Contra-indicated in those persons who have shown hypersensitivity to sulphonamide preparations or any component of this product.

Warnings: As with all sulphonamide preparations, severe sensitivity reactions, e.g. Stevens-Johnson syndrome, fever, skin rash, gastrointestinal disturbance and bone marrow depression have been identified in individuals with no prior history of sulphonamide hyersensitivity.

Precautions: Non-susceptible organisms, including fungi, may proliferate with the use of this preparation. Sulponamides are inactivated by the aminobenzoic acid present in purulent exudates.

Pregnancy warning: There is insufficient evidence as to the drug safety in human pregnancy. This product should therefore only be used during pregnancy if considered essential by the physician.

Pharmaceutical precautions Isopto Cetamide eye drops should be stored in a cool place away from direct sunlight. Keep the container tightly closed. Contents should be discarded one month after opening.

Legal category POM.

Package quantities 10 ml.

Further information Isopto Cetamide eye drops are contained in an unbreakable semi-rigid container.

Product licence number 0649/5909.

ISOPTO* EPINAL
0.5% and 1.0%

Presentation Isopto Epinal is a clear, colourless to light yellow, sterile, aqueous solution containing 0.5% or 1% adrenaline (as the borate complex), hydroxypropyl methylcellulose (hypromellose) 0.5%, and preserved with benzalkonium chloride 0.01%.

Uses Isopto Epinal is indicated for the control of simple open angle glaucoma. It may be used with miotics. Carbonic Acid Anhydrase inhibitors may be used with this drug in selected cases.

Dosage and administration The dosage must be adjusted to tonometric readings before and during therapy. The usual dosage is one drop in the eye(s) once or twice daily. When used to complement miotic therapy this drug should be instilled 5 to 10 minutes after the miotic drug.

Contra-indications, warnings, etc Do not use in narrow angle glaucoma. Do not use until the diagnosis of glaucoma has been verified. For ophthalmic use only. Not for injection.

Treatment of severe reaction: A severe reaction to adrenaline is rapid in onset and of short duration. In such an event give individuals I.V. injection of quick acting α-adrenergic blocking agent such as 5 to 10 mg pentolamine mesylate, followed by a β-blocking agent such as 2.5 to 5 mg propranolol.

Adverse Reactions: Isopto Epinal drops should be used with caution in patients with hypertensive cardiovascular disease. Prolonged use may produce extra-cellular pigmentation. On rare occasions systemic side-effects have been observed such as headaches, palpitation, pallor, tachycardia, trembling and perspiration. Stinging may occur after instillation with rebound redness. This product contains benzalkonium chloride and should not be used when soft contact lenses are worn.

Pregnancy warning: There is insufficient evidence as to the drug safety in human pregnancy. This product should therefore only be used during pregnancy if considered essential by the physician.

Pharmaceutical precautions Contents should be

discarded one month after opening. After dispensing, the patient is advised to observe the following precautions:

1. Store the bottle in an up-right position with the dropper tightly sealed.

2. Protect from excessive heat and light. Keep in a cool, dark place.

3. Prevent the dropper tip from touching the eye-lid or other surfaces since this may contaminate the solution. Do not rinse the dropper in tap water.

4. If the clear solution changes colour, obtain a fresh supply from the pharmacist.

Legal category P.

Package quantities 7.5 ml amber glass bottles with dropper.

Further information Nil.

Product licence numbers
1% 0649/0001
0.5% 0649/0002

ISOPTO* FRIN 0.12%

Presentation Isopto Frin is a clear, colourless sterile solution, containing Phenylephrine Hydrochloride 0.12% and hydroxypropyl methylcellulose (hypromellose) 0.5%, and preserved with benzethonium chloride 0.01%.

Uses As an emollient lubricant with vasoconstrictive effect.

Dosage and administration One or two drops three times a day or as necessary.

Isopto Frin is suitable for use by both adults and children.

Contra-indications, warnings, etc If the irritation persists or increases its use should be discontinued. Slight dilation of the pupil may occur in some patients. For this reason it should be used with care where narrow angle glaucoma may be present, since its use may precipitate angle closure, or in those with a shallow anterior chamber. This product contains benzethonium chloride and should not be used when soft contact lenses are being worn.

Pregnancy Warning: This product should only be used during pregnancy if considered essential by the physician.

Precautions: Care should be exercised in its use in small children, pressure should be put on the inner canthus of the eye for a few minutes after instillation to decrease systemic absorption via the naso lacrimal duct.

Use with caution on an inflamed eye, as hyperaemia greatly increases the rate of systemic absorption through the conjunctiva.

Pharmaceutical precautions Isopto Frin eye drops should be stored in a cool place away from direct sunlight. Keep the container tightly closed. Contents should be discarded one month after opening.

Legal category P.

Package quantities 10 ml containers.

Further information Isopto Frin eye drops are contained in an unbreakable semi-rigid plastic dropper bottle with screw-on cap.

Product licence number 0649/5911.

ISOPTO* PLAIN

Presentation Isopto Plain is a sterile, clear, colourless solution containing hydroxypropyl methylcellulose (Hypromellose) 0.5%, and preserved with benzalkonium chloride 0.01%.

Uses Isopto Plain is a soothing emollient solution used in cases of tear deficiency as a lubricant, and as an artificial tear.

Dosage and administration It is suitable for use both by adults and children. The dose is one or two drops topically instilled into the eyes three times daily as needed, or as prescribed by the doctor.

Contra-indications, warnings, etc If an irritation persists or increases, use of the drops should be discontinued. In order to help preserve sterility the dropper should not be allowed to touch the eyelids or any other surface. This product contains benzalkonium chloride, and should not be used when soft contact lenses are being worn.

Pharmaceutical precautions The eye-drops should be stored in a cool place (8° to 25°C). Keep the container tightly closed. Keep out of reach of children. Discard contents one month after opening.

Legal category P.

Package quantities 10 ml containers.

Further information Isopto Plain eye-drops are contained in an unbreakable semi-rigid plastic dropper bottle with a screw-on cap.

Product licence number 0649/5920.

MAXIDEX*

Presentation Dexamethasone 0.1% in a vehicle containing 0.5% hydroxypropyl methylcellulose (hypromellose). A sterile, isotonic, ophthalmic suspension, preserved with benzalkonium chloride 0.01%.

Uses Steroid responsive inflammatory conditions of the palpebral and bulbar conjunctiva, cornea and anterior segment of the globe. These include allergic conjunctivitis, acne rosacea, superficial punctate keratitis, herpes zoster keratitis, iritis, cyclitis, selected infective conjunctivitides, corneal injury from chemical, radiation, or thermal burns, or penetration of foreign bodies when the inherent hazard of steroid use is accepted to obtain an advisable diminution in oedema and inflammation. May be used to suppress graft reaction after keratoplasty.

Dosage and administration One or two drops topically in the conjunctival sac(s). In severe disease, drops may be used hourly, being tapered to discontinuation as the inflammation subsides. In mild disease, drops may be used up to four to six times daily.

Contra-indications, warnings, etc
Contra-indications: Contra-indicated in epithelial herpes simplex (dendritic keratitis), vaccinia, varicella, and most other viral diseases of the cornea and conjunctiva; tuberculosis of the eye; and in those persons who have shown hypersensitivity to any component of this preparation.

Warnings: Use in the treatment of herpes simplex requires great caution. This drug is not effective in the treatment of Sjorgen's keratoconjunctivitis. Prolonged use may result in glaucoma, damage to the optic nerve, defects in visual acuity and visual field; cataract formation; or may aid in the establishment of secondary ocular infection from pathogens due to suppression of host response. In acute purulent infections of the eye, infection appears to be enhanced with the presence of steroids. In those diseases causing thinning of the cornea or sclera, perforation has been known to occur with the use of topical steroids. It is advisable that the intraocular pressure be checked frequently. This product contains benzalkonium chloride and should not be used when soft contact lenses are being worn.

Precautions: As fungal infections of the cornea are particularly prone to develop coincidentally with long-term local steroid application, fungus invasion must be suspected in any persistent corneal ulceration where a steroid has been used or is in use.

Adverse reactions: Glaucoma with optic nerve damage, visual acuity and field defects; cataract formation; secondary ocular infection following suppression of host response; and perforation of the globe may occur.

Pregnancy Warning: Although topical steroids have not been reported to have an adverse effect on pregnancy, the safety of their use in pregnancy has not been absolutely established, therefore it is advisable not to use this product for long term treatment of pregnant patients.

Pharmaceutical precautions Maxidex should be stored in a cool place away from direct sunlight. Keep the container tightly closed. The contents should be discarded one month after opening. Shake well before using.

Legal category POM.

Package quantities 5 ml and 10 ml containers.

Further information Maxidex eye drops are contained in an unbreakable semi-rigid, plastic dropper bottle with a screw-on cap, containing 5 ml or 10 ml of the preparation. Maxidex is a highly penetrating form of dexamethasone, a 0.1% microfine suspension especially formulated to provide maximum corneal absorption.

Product licence number 0649/5914.

MAXITROL* EYE DROPS
MAXITROL* EYE-OINTMENT

Presentation *Drops:* Dexamethasone BP 0.1% Poly-myxin B Sulphate USP 6,000 units/ml and Neomycin Sulphate equivalent to Neomycin 3.5 mg/ml in a vehicle containing 0.5% hydroxypropyl methycellulose (hypromellose). A sterile, isotonic, ophthalmic suspension, preserved with benzalkonium chloride 0.004%.

Ointment: Dexamethasone BP 0.1% Polymyxin B Sulphate USP 6,000 units/g and Neomycin Sulphate equivalent to Neomycin 3.5 mg/g in an ointment base, preserved with methylparaben 0.05% and propylparaben 0.01%.

Uses For steroid responsive inflammatory ocular conditions for which a corticosteroid is indicated and where bacterial infection or ocular infection exists.

Ocular steroids are indicated in inflammatory conditions of the palpebral and bulbar conjunctiva, cornea and anterior segment of the globe where the inherent risk of steroid use is accepted to obtain a diminution in oedema and inflammation. They are also indicated in chronic anterior uveitis and corneal injury from chemical, radiation or thermal burns, or penetration of foreign bodies.

The use of a combination drug with an anti-infective component is indicated where the risk of infection is high or where there is an expectation that potentially dangerous numbers of bacteria will be present in the eye.

The particular anti-infective drugs in this product are active against the following common bacterial eye pathogens: *Staphylococcus aureus, Escherichia coli, Haemophilus influenzae,* Klebsiella/Enterobacter species, Neisseria species and Pseudomonas aeruginosa.

This product does not provide adequate coverage against: *Serratia marcescens* and Streptococci including *Streptococcus pneumoniae.*

Dosage and administration *Maxitrol Suspension:* One or two drops topically in the conjunctival sac(s). In severe disease, drops may be used hourly, being tapered to discontinuation as the inflammation subsides. In mild disease, drops may be used up to four to six times daily.

Maxitrol Ointment: Apply a small amount into the conjunctival sac(s) up to three or four times daily or, may be used adjunctively with drops at bedtime.

Not more than 20 ml or 8 g should be prescribed initially and the prescription should not be refilled without further evaluation as outlined in 'Precautions' below.

Contra-indications, warnings, etc
Contra-indications: Epithelial herpes simplex keratitis (dendritic keratitis); vaccinia; varicella, and most other diseases of the cornea and conjunctiva. Mycobacterial infection of the eye. Fungal diseases of ocular structures. Hypersensitivity to a component of the medication. (Hypersensitivity to the antibiotic component occurs at a higher rate than for other components.) The use of these combinations is always contra-indicated after uncomplicated removal of a corneal foreign body.

Warnings: Not for injection. Prolonged use may result in glaucoma with damage to the optic nerve, defects in visual acuity and fields of vision, and posterior subcapsular cataract formation. Prolonged use may suppress the host response and thus increase the hazard of secondary ocular infections in those diseases causing thinning of the cornea or sclera, perforations have been known to occur with the use of topical steroids. In acute purulent conditions of the eye, steroids may mask infection or enhance existing infection. If these products are used for 10 days or longer, intraocular pressure should be routinely monitored even though it may be difficult in children and uncooperative patients.

Products containing neomycin sulphate may cause cutaneous sensitization. Employment of steroid medication in the treatment of herpes simplex requires great caution. Maxitrol drops contain benzalkonium chloride and should not be used when soft contact lenses are being worn.

Precautions: The initial prescription and renewal of the medication order beyond 20 ml or 8 g should be made by a physician only after examination of the patient with the aid of magnification, such as slit lamp biomicroscopy and where appropriate, fluorescein staining. The possibility of persistent fungal infections of the cornea should be considered after prolonged steroid dosing.

Adverse reactions: Adverse reactions have occurred with steroid/anti-infective combination drugs which can be attributed to the steroid component, the anti-infective component, or the combination.

Reactions occurring most often from the presence of the anti-infective ingredient are allergic sensitizations. The reactions due to the steroid component are: elevation of intraocular pressure (IOP) with possible development of glaucoma and infrequent optic nerve damage; posterior subcapsular cataract formation and delayed wound healing.

Secondary infection: The development of secondary infection has occurred after use of combinations containing steroids and antimicrobials. Fungal infections of the cornea are particularly prone to develop coincidentally with long-term applications of steroid. The possibility of fungal invasion must be considered in any persistent corneal ulceration where steroid treatment has been used.

Secondary bacterial ocular infection following supression of host responses also occurs.

Pregnancy Warning: Although topical steroids have not been reported to have an adverse effect on pregnancy, the safety of their use in pregnancy has not been absolutely established, therefore it is advisable not to use this product for long term treatment of pregnant patients.

Pharmaceutical precautions Maxitrol eye-drops and eye-ointment should be stored in a cool place away from direct sunlight. Keep the container tightly closed. Contents should be discarded one month after opening. Drops should be well shaken before use.

Legal category POM.

Package quantities *Drops:* 5 ml container
Ointment: 3.5 g

Further information *Drops:* Maxitrol eye-drops are contained in an unbreakable semi-rigid, plastic dropper bottle with screw-on cap.

Ointment: Maxitrol eye-ointment is contained in a tube with a screw-on cap.

Product licence numbers
Maxitrol Eye-Drops 0649/5915
Maxitrol Eye-Ointment 0649/5916

MYDRIACYL 0.5% w/v and 1.0% w/v

Presentation Mydriacyl is a sterile clear, colourless solution containing Tropicamide 0.5% w/v or 1.0% w/v, packed in 5 ml Droptainers, and preserved with benzalkonium chloride 0.01%.

Uses As a mydriatic and cycloplegic.

Dosage and administration For refraction, 1 or 2 drops of 1.0% solution instilled into the eye(s), repeated in 5 minutes. If patient is not seen within 20 to 30 minutes, an additional drop may be instilled to prolong mydriatic effect. For examination of fundus, 1 or 2 drops of 0.5% solution 15 or 20 minutes prior to examination. Individuals with heavily pigmented irides may require larger doses.

Prescribing in the elderly: In the elderly and others where increased intra-ocular pressure may be encountered, mydriatics and cycloplegics should be used cautiously. To avoid inducing angle closure glaucoma, an estimation of the depth of the angle of the anterior chamber should be made.

Contra-indications, warnings, etc
Contra-indications: Contra-indicated in narrow-angle glaucoma and in persons showing hypersensitivity to any component of this preparation.

Warnings: For topical use only – not for injection. This preparation may cause CNS disturbances which may be dangerous in infants and children. Possibility of occurrence of psychotic reaction and behavioural disturbance due to hypersensitivity to anticholinergic drugs should be borne in mind. This product contains benzalkonium chloride and should not be used when soft contact lenses are being worn.

Precautions: The lacrimal sac shoud be compressed by digital pressure for 1 minute after instillation to avoid excessive systemic absorption.

Patient warning: Patient should be advised not to drive or engage in other hazardous activities while pupils are dilated. Patient may experience sensitivity to light and should protect eyes in bright illumination during dilation. Parents should be warned not to get this preparation in their child's mouth and to wash their own hands and the child's hands following administration.

Adverse reactions: Increased intraocular pressure. Psychotic reactions, behavioural disturbances, and cardiorespiratory collapse in children with this class of drug have been reported. Transient stinging, dryness of the mouth, blurred vision, photophobia with or without corneal staining, tachycardia, headache, parasympathetic stimulation, or allergic reaction may occur.

Pregnancy Warning: There is no evidence as to the drug safety in human pregnancy, nor is there evidence from animal work that it is free from hazard. This product should only be used during pregnancy if considered essential by the physician.

Treatment of Severe Reaction: A severe reaction to tropicamide is rapid in onset and of short duration. In such an event give immediate I.V. injection of quick acting α-adrenergic blocking agent such as 5 to 10 mg pentolamine mesylate, followed by a β-blocking agent such as 2.5 mg of propranolol.

Pharmaceutical precautions Mydriacyl eye drops should be stored in a cool place, away from direct sunlight, but do not refrigerate. Keep the container tightly closed. Discard one month after opening.

Legal category POM.

Package quantities 5 ml containers.

Further information Mydriacyl eye drops are contained in a semi-rigid plastic dropper bottle with a screw-on cap.

Product licence numbers 0649/5917
0649/5918

ALCON OPULETS* ATROPINE 1%

Presentation Single-dose, clear, colourless, sterile eye drops containing 1% w/v atropine sulphate.

Uses Atropine is a powerful mydriatic and cycloplegic. It is used in refraction, especially in children, and in uveitis.

Dosage and administration *Adults:* For refraction, administer one or two drops topically to the eye(s) one hour before refracting. For uveitis, administer one or two drops topically to the eye(s) up to four times daily.

Children: For refraction, administer one drop to each eye twice daily for one to three days prior to examination. For uveitis, administer one drop to each eye up to three times daily.

Prescribing in the elderly: In the elderly and others where increased intra-ocular pressure may be encountered, mydriatics and cycloplegics should be used cautiously. To avoid inducing angle closure glaucoma, an estimation of the depth of the angle of the anterior chamber should be made.

Contra-indications, warnings, etc
Contra-indications: Contra-indicated in persons with primary glaucoma or a tendency toward glaucoma, e.g. narrow anterior chamber angle, and in those persons showing hypersensitivity to any component of this preparation.

Warnings: For topical use only – not for injection. In infants and small children, use with extreme caution. Excessive use in children or in certain individuals with a previous history or susceptibility to belladonna alkaloids may produce systemic symptoms of atropine poisoning.

Precautions: To avoid excessive systemic absorption, the lacrimal sac should be compressed by digital pressure for one minute after instillation.

Patient warning: Patients should be advised not to drive or engage in other hazardous activities while pupils are dilated. Patients may experience sensitivity to light and should protect eyes in bright illumination during dilation. Parents should be warned not to get this preparation in their child's mouth and to wash their own hands and the child's hands following administration.

Adverse reactions: Prolonged use may produce local irritation characterized by follicular conjunctivitis, vascular congestion, oedema, exudate and an exczematoid dermatitis. Severe reactions are manifested by hypotension with progressive respiratory depression. Coma and death have been reported in the very young.

Overdosage: Systemic atropine toxicity is manifested by flushing and dryness of the skin (a rash may be present in children), blurred vision, a rapid and irregular pulse, fever, abdominal distention in infants, mental aberration (hallucinosis) and loss of neuromuscular co-ordination. Physostigmine should be administered parenterally (for dosage refer to Goodman & Gilman or other pharmacology reference). In infants and small children, the body surface must be kept moist.

Pregnancy warning: There is insufficient evidence as to the drug safety in human pregnancy. This product should therefore only be used during pregnancy if considered essential by the physician.

Pharmaceutical precautions Alcon Opulets should be stored in a cool place and protected from strong light.

Legal category POM.

Package quantities Alcon Opulets are available in packs of 20 units each containing 0.5 ml.

Further information Nil.

Product licence number 0649/0061.

ALCON OPULETS* BENOXINATE

Presentation Single dose, clear, colourless sterile eye drops containing 0.4% w/v Oxybuprocaine hydrochloride (Benoxinate).

Uses Local anaesthetic.

Dosage and administration One drop.
  Benoxinate is less irritant than amethocaine in similar concentrations.

Tonometry: One drop is sufficient to anaesthetise the surface of the eye to allow tonometry after 60 seconds.

Fitting Contact Lenses: A further drop after 90 seconds provides adequate anaesthesia for the fitting of contact lenses.

Removal of Foreign Body and/or Incision of Meibomian Cyst: Three drops at 90 second intervals provides sufficient anaesthesia after five minutes for a foreign body to be removed from the corneal epithelium or incision of a Meibomian cyst through the conjunctival surface. Corneal sensitivity is normal again after about one hour.

Children: Dosage is at the discretion of the physician.

Contra-indications, warnings, etc The anaesthetised eye should be protected from dust and bacterial contamination. Prolonged application of anaesthetic eye drops may damage the cornea.

Pregnancy warning: There is insufficient evidence as to the drug safety in human pregnancy. This product should therefore only be used during pregnancy if considered essential by the physician.

Pharmaceutical precautions Alcon Opulets should be stored in a cool place and protected from strong light.
  Solutions of Benoxinate and fluorescein sodium should not be mixed as a precipitate may be formed.

Legal category POM.

Package quantities Alcon Opulets are available in packs of 20 units each containing 0.5 ml.

Further information Benoxinate produces very little conjunctival irritation or hyperaemia and has no effect on the pupil.
  The sensitivity of the cornea returns to normal about one hour after administration of Benoxinate drops.

Product licence number 0649/0056.

ALCON OPULETS* CHLORAMPHENICOL 0.5%

Presentation Single dose, clear, colourless, sterile eye drops containing 0.5% w/v Chloramphenicol BP.

Uses Chloramphenicol is a broad spectrum bacteriostatic antibiotic effective against a wide range of Gram negative and Gram positive organisms.

Dosage and administration *Adult:* One or more drops as required.
Children: One drop as required.

Contra-indications, warnings, etc Treatment should be discontinued on the appearance of toxic symptoms or allergic skin rashes. Such a general allergy should be treated with antihistamines by mouth.
  Aplastic anaemia, in some cases fatal, has been reported following the topical use of chloramphenicol, but this is very rare.

Pregnancy warning: This product should not be used during pregnancy unless considered essential by the physician.

Pharmaceutical precautions Alcon Opulets containing Chloramphenicol should be stored below 15°C and away from strong light.

Legal category POM.

Package quantities Alcon Opulets are available in packs of 20 units each containing 0.5 ml.

Further information Nil.

Product licence number 0649/0047.

ALCON OPULETS* CYCLOPENTOLATE 1%

Presentation Single-dose, clear, colourless, sterile eye drops containing 1% w/v Cyclopentolate hydrochloride.

Uses As a mydriatic and cycloplegic.

Dosage and administration One or two drops as required. Maximum effect is achieved 30–60 minutes after instillation. This preparation should not be used in very young infants as they are particularly prone to CNS and cardiopulmonary side-effects from systemic absorption of cyclopentolate.

Prescribing in the elderly: In the elderly and others where increased intra-ocular pressure may be encountered, mydriatics and cycloplegics should be used cautiously. To avoid inducing angle closing glaucoma, an estimation of the depth of the angle of the anterior chamber should be made.

Contra-indications, warnings, etc
Contra-indications: Should not be used when narrow angle glaucoma or anatomical narrow angles are present, or where there is hypersensitivity to any component of this preparation.

Warnings: For topical use only – not for injection. This preparation may cause CNS disturbances. This is especially true in younger age groups, but may occur at any age.

Precautions: The lacrimal sac should be compressed by digital pressure for one minute after instillation to avoid excessive systemic absorption.

Information for patients: Patients should be advised not to drive or engage in other hazardous activities while pupils are dilated. Patients may experience sensitivity to light and should protect eyes in bright illumination during dilation. Parents should be warned not to get this preparation in their child's mouth and to wash their own hands and the child's hands following administration.

Adverse reactions: Increased intraocular pressure. Use of cyclopentolate has been associated with psychotic reactions and behavioural disturbances, usually in children, especially with a 2% concentration. These disturbances include ataxia, incoherent speech, restlessness, hallucinations, hyperactivity, seizures, disorientation as to time and place and failure to recognise people. This drug produces reactions similar to those of other anticholinergic drugs, but the central nervous system manifestations as noted above are more common. Other toxic manifestations of anticholinergic drugs are tachycardia, hyperpyrexia, vasodilation, urinary retention, diminished gastrointestinal motility and decreased secretion in salivary and sweat glands, pharynx, bronchii and nasal passages. Severe manifestations of toxicity include coma, medullary paralysis and death.

Overdosage: In case of severe manifestations of toxicity the antidote of choice is physostigmine salicylate. Paediatric dose: Slowly inject intravenously 0.5 mg. If toxic symptoms persist and no cholinergic symptoms are produced repeat at five minute intervals to a maximum dose of 2.0 mg. Adolescent and adult: Slowly inject 2.0 mg intravenously. A second dose of 1–2 mg may be given after 20 minutes if no reversal of toxic manifestations has occurred. Physostigmine salicylate can be administered subcutaneously.[1,2]

References:
1. Rumack B. H.: Anticholinergic Poisoning: Treatment with Physostigmine. Pediatrics 52(6) 449–551, 1973.
2. Duvoisin R. C. and Katz R.: Reversal of Central Anticholinergic Syndromes in Man by Physostigmine. J. Am. Med. Assn. 206 (9) 1963–65, 1968.

Pregnancy warning: There is no evidence as to the drug safety in human pregnancy, nor is there evidence from animal work that it is free from hazard. This product should only be used during pregnancy if considered essential by the physician.

Pharmaceutical precautions Alcon Opulets should be stored in a cool place and protected from strong light.

Legal category POM.

Package quantities Alcon Opulets are available in packs of 20 units each containing 0.5 ml.

Further information Recovery of accommodation occurs within 24 hours, but may be achieved more rapidly if 1 or 2 drops of a 2% w/v solution of pilocarpine hydrochloride are instilled.

Product licence number 0649/0058.

ALCON OPULETS* FLUORESCEIN SODIUM 1%

Presentation Single dose, clear orange/red sterile solution of 1% w/v Fluorescein sodium BP.

Uses As a diagnostic stain. Fluorescein does not stain the normal cornea.
Corneal and conjunctival abrasions or ulcers are stained a bright green and foreign bodies are surrounded by a green ring.

Dosage and administration Sufficient solution should be applied to stain the damaged areas. Excess solution may be washed away with sterile saline solution.

Contra-indications, warnings, etc Special care should be taken to avoid bacterial contamination.

Pharmaceutical precautions Alcon Opulets should be stored in a cool place and not exposed to strong light.

Legal category P.

Package quantities Alcon Opulets are available in packs of 20 units each containing 0.5 ml.

Further information The use of single dose contained preparations of fluorescein sodium are to be preferred according to Martindale (Extra Pharmacopoeia).

Product licence number 0649/0048.

ALCON OPULETS* PILOCARPINE

Presentation Single-dose, clear, colourless, sterile eye drops. Three strengths are available containing Pilocarpine hydrochloride 1%, 2% and 4% w/v in a buffered aqueous solution.

Uses Pilocarpine is a parasympathomimetic agent which decreases intraocular pressure in glaucoma and detachment of the retina. Pilocarpine is also used as the miotic of choice for counteracting the weaker mydriatics.

Dosage and administration To produce miosis one drop of a 1% solution is usually sufficient. In the treatment of glaucoma, instillation 4–6 times daily is usually necessary to obtain control.

Contra-indications, warnings, etc
Contra-indications: Miotics are contra-indicated where constriction is undesirable such as in acute iritis; in those persons showing hypersensitivity to any of their components; and in pupillary block glaucoma.

Warnings: For topical use only. Not for injection.

Precautions: The miosis usually causes difficulty in dark adaptation. Patients should be advised to exercise caution in night driving and other hazardous occupations in poor illumination.

Adverse reactions: Ciliary spasms, conjunctival vascular congestion, temporal or supraorbital headache, and induced myopia may occur. This is especially true in younger individuals who have recently started administration. Reduced visual acuity in poor illumination is frequently experienced by older individuals with lens opacity. As with all miotics, rare cases of retinal detachment have been reported when used in certain susceptible individuals. Lens opacity may occur with prolonged use of pilocarpine.

Overdosage: Systemic reactions following topical administration are extremely rare.

Pregnancy warning: There is insufficient evidence as to the drug safety in human pregnancy. This product should therefore only be used during pregnancy if considered essential by the physician.

Pharmaceutical precautions Alcon Opulets should be stored in a cool place away from strong light.

Legal category POM.

Package quantities Alcon Opulets are available in packs of 20 units each containing 0.5 ml.

Further information Nil.

Product licence numbers 1% 0649/0052
2% 0649/0053
4% 0649/0054

ALCON OPULETS* SODIUM CHLORIDE

Presentation Single dose, clear, colourless, sterile eye drops containing 0.9% w/v sodium chloride BP.

Uses Irrigating agent for the eye.

Dosage and administration Use sufficient solution to adequately irrigate the eye.

Contra-indications, warnings, etc None.

Pharmaceutical precautions Alcon Opulets should be stored in a cool place and should not be exposed to strong light.

Legal category P.

Package quantities Alcon Opulets are available in packs of 20 units each containing 0.5 ml.

Further information Nil.

Product licence number 0649/0055.

TEARS Naturale*

Presentation Tears Naturale is a clear, colourless sterile solution, presented in a 15 ml Drop-Tainer Dispenser, and contains the Duasorb water soluble polymeric system Dextran 70 0.1% and Hydroxypropyl Methylcellulose (Hypromellose) 0.3%, and preserved with benzalkonium chloride 0.01% and disodium edetate 0.05%.

Uses A soothing solution for use as an artificial tear and lubricant in the relief of dry eye syndromes associated with deficient tear secretion or deficient mucous.

Dosage and administration Instill 1 or 2 drops into the eye(s), as frequently as to relieve eye irritation symptoms.

Contra-indications, warnings, etc
Contra-indications: This product contains benzalkonium chloride, and should not be used when soft contact lenses are being worn.

Precautions: If irritation persists, discontinue use.

Pharmaceutical precautions To avoid contaminating the solution, do not let the dropper tip touch any surface. Keep the container tightly closed. Discard the contents 1 month after opening.

Legal category P.

Package quantities 15 ml.

Further information Tears Naturale eye-drops are contained in an unbreakable semi-rigid plastic dropper bottle with a screw-on cap.

Product licence number 0649/0031.

TOBRALEX* ▼

Presentation A sterile, clear, colourless to very pale yellow ophthalmic solution containing tobramycin 0.3% w/v, preserved with 0.01% benzalkonium chloride.

Uses Tobralex (tobramycin) Sterile Ophthalmic Solution is a bactericidal topical antibiotic indicated in the treatment of external bacterial conditions of the eye and its appendages. The spectrum of activity covers a wide range of Gram-positive organisms and many Gram-negative organisms.
A significant bacterial population resistant to tobramycin has not yet been reported. However, there is the possibility that bacterial resistance may develop following prolonged use.

Dosage and administration Adults and children: In mild to moderate cases, instil one or two drops into the affected eye every four hours. For severe infections, instil two drops into the eye hourly until there is an improvement and then reduce treatment, prior to discontinuation.

Contra-indications, warnings, etc
Contra-indications: Persons with known sensitivity to tobramycin or gentamicin.

Warnings: Sensitivity may occur in some patients. If so, discontinue use. Transient irritation may occur with some susceptible patients.
Tobralex ophthalmic solution is not for injection.

Precautions: As with other antibiotics, prolonged use may result in the overgrowth of non-susceptible organisms, including fungi. If super-infection occurs, appropriate therapy should be initiated.

Use in pregnancy: Reproduction studies in animals at doses up to thirty-three times the normal human systemic dose have revealed no evidence of impaired fertility or harm to the foetus due to tobramycin. There are, however, no adequate and well-controlled studies in pregnant women. Because animal studies are not always predictive of human response, this drug should be used during pregnancy only if clearly needed.

Nursing mothers: Because of the potential for adverse reactions in nursing infants from Tobralex, a decision should be made whether to discontinue nursing the infant or discontinue the drug, taking into account the importance of the drug to the mother.

Adverse reactions: The most frequent adverse reactions to Tobralex Ophthalmic Solution are localized ocular toxicity and hypersensitivity, including lid itching and swelling, and conjunctival erythema. These reactions occur in less than 3% of patients treated with Tobralex. Similar reactions may occur with the topical use of other aminoglycoside antibiotics. Other adverse reactions have not been reported from Tobralex therapy, however, if topical ocular tobramycin is administered concomitantly with systemic aminoglycoside antibiotics, care should be taken to monitor the total serum concentration.

Overdosage: Clinically apparent signs and symptoms of an overdose of Tobralex Ophthalmic Solution (punctate keratitis, erythema, increased lacrimation, oedema and lid itching) may be similar to adverse reaction effects seen in some patients.

Pharmaceutical precautions Store at 8°C to 25°C. Do not freeze. Keep the container tightly closed. Discard contents one month after opening.
Sterile until opened.

Legal category POM.

Package quantities 5 ml.

Further information Tobralex eye drops are contained in an unbreakable semi-rigid plastic dropper bottle with screw-on cap.

Product licence number 0649/0044.

ZINCFRIN*

Presentation Zincfrin is a clear, colourless sterile solution containing Zinc Sulphate 0.25% w/v and Phenylephrine Hydrochloride 0.12% w/v, preserved with benzalkonium chloride 0.01% w/v.

Uses For the treatment of mild, non-specific conjunctivitis, ocular irritation and allergies.

Dosage and administration 1 or 2 drops in the eyes 3 times daily for adults, and children or as directed by physician.
Zincfrin is suitable for use in both adults and children.

Contra-indications, warnings, etc If irritation persists or increases the use of Zincfrin should be discontinued. It causes slight dilatation of the pupil and should be used with care in cases of narrow angle glaucoma, since its use may precipitate angle closure, or in those with a shallow anterior chamber.
This product contains benzalkonium chloride and should not be used when soft contact lenses are being worn.

Pregnancy Warning: This product should only be used during pregnancy if considered essential by the physician.

Precautions: Care should be exercised in its use in small children, pressure should be put on the inner canthus of the eye for a few minutes after instillation to decrease systemic absorption via the naso-lacrimal duct.
Use with caution on an inflamed eye, as hyperaemia greatly increases the rate of systemic absorption through the conjunctiva.

Pharmaceutical precautions Zincfrin eye drops should be stored in a cool place away from direct sunlight. Keep the container tightly closed. Discard contents one month after opening.

Legal category P.

Package quantities 10 ml containers.

Further information Zincfrin eye drops are contained in an unbreakable semi-rigid plastic dropper bottle with screw-on cap.

Product licence number 0649/5921.

ALCODERM* CREAM/LOTION

Presentation *Cream:* A white, thick smooth cream.

Lotion: A creamy white, smooth, viscous lotion.
Alcoderm contains liquid paraffin, purified water, cetylalcohol, stearyl alcohol, sodium lauryl sulphate, carbomer, polysorbate 60, triethanolamine, methylparaben, propylparaben.

Uses Dry, chafed or irritated skin – Alcoderm is indicated in any condition where the moisture content of the horny layer has decreased below the normal level and the skin is no longer soft and pliable.

Also recommended:
(a) in acute inflammatory conditions where the skin is intact, such as sunburn and windburn.
(b) as a smoothing, hydrating agent in certain inflammatory skin conditions where there is dryness and scaling, such as ichthyosis, atopic eczema, winter itch etc.
(c) as a vehicle for other active constituents.

Additional information: Alcoderm is a specially formulated emulsion with a double acting moisturizing effect. The lotion is suitable for large areas of skin, the cream for smaller drier areas. Alcoderm has a double moisturizing action which can be provided only by oil-in-water emulsions. It hydrates rapidly the surface layers of the skin, and at the same time the oil droplets form a thin, protective layer on the skin. This film gives Alcoderm its special characteristics; it is highly hydrostatic and protects the skin against excessive evaporation of the water. Only 0.6% of the film-forming surface active agents in Alcoderm are water-soluble. No other oil-in-water emulsion contains such a small quantity of water soluble ingredients.

Administration Apply topically to the skin as required or as directed by a doctor.

Contra-indications, warnings, etc Avoid contact with the eyes.

Legal category P.

Package quantities
Cream: 60 g
Lotion: 120 ml

Further information Nil.

Product licence numbers
0649/0004 Cream
0649/0005 Lotion

DEBROXIDE*

Presentation Debroxide is a topical aqueous gel containing Benzoyl peroxide 5%/10%, dioctyl sodium sulfosuccinate, edetate disodium, poloxamer 182, carbomer 940, propylene glycol, silicon dioxide, purified water, citric acid and/or sodium hydroxide to adjust pH.

Uses Debroxide is recommended for adjunctive topical treatment of acne vulgaris. Benzoyl peroxide is an established and effective keratolytic agent with antibacterial properties. It has been shown to be effective in reducing the local population of Propionibacterium acnes leading to a reduction in the production of irritant fatty acids in the sebaceous glands.

Administration After washing with a mild cleanser and water, apply once or twice daily to the affected area. The degree of drying and peeling can be adjusted by modification of the dosage schedule.

Contra-indications, warnings, etc
Contra-indication: Persons having known sensitivity to benzoyl peroxide.
Precaution: Avoid contact with the eyes, eyelids and other mucous surfaces.
Warning: May bleach hair and coloured fabrics.
Overdosage: The skin may become excessively red and sore during the first few days of treatment. Apply less often until this phase has passed.

Pharmaceutical precautions Store at room temperature.

Legal category P.

Package quantities Debroxide 5–60 g plastic tubes. Debroxide 10 – 60 g plastic tubes.

Further information Nil.

Product licence numbers
Debroxide 5   0649/0051
Debroxide 10   0649/0062

IONAX* SCRUB

Presentation A pale yellow semi-translucent abradant gel with a fresh odour of lemon. The active ingredients are polyethylene granules, benzalkonium chloride, macrogol (4) lauryl ether, macrogol (23) lauryl ether, alcohol and foaming agents in an aqueous gel base.

Uses An abradant cleanser for the control and hygiene of acne. Use Ionax Scrub to cleanse skin prior to acne or oily skin treatment.

Administration Apply to wet face. Massage on the skin for one or two minutes, then rinse thoroughly.
Use once or twice daily, or as directed by your physician.

Contra-indications, warnings, etc *Caution:* Avoid contact with the eyes.
Upon accidental contact, flush with water and avoid rubbing.

If the skin gets too dry or too reddened discontinue use temporarily.

Pharmaceutical precautions There are no special pharmaceutical precautions.

Legal category P.

Package quantities 60 g packs in plastic collapsible tubes with plastic screw caps.

Further information Nil.

Product licence number 0649/0006.

IONIL T* SHAMPOO

Presentation A clear brown liquid shampoo with a slight odour of coal tar. It contains Salicylic acid, Benazalkonium chloride, coal tar solution 5% with polyoxyethylene ethers in an hydro-alcoholic shampoo base.

Uses For seborrhoeic dermatitis of the scalp.

Administration Massage Ionil T Shampoo into wet hair.
Do not expect much initial lather as the shampoo is formulated for low foaming.
Rinse, and then apply Ionil T shampoo again and massage into a lather. Allow to remain in the hair for about five minutes before rinsing.
This shampoo may be used daily or as directed by the physician.
For best results do not use soap, detergent or other shampoo on the hair immediately before or after using Ionil T.

Contra-indications, warnings, etc *Caution:* Avoid contact with the eyes.
Upon accidental contact, flush with clear water.

Pharmaceutical precautions Store away from internal preparations and foods.

Legal category P.

Package quantities 120 ml and 240 ml in cylindrical plastic containers with plastic screw caps.

Further information Nil.

Product licence number 0649/0003.

NUTRAPLUS* Cream

Presentation A smooth white, unperfumed cream. It contains 10% Urea, purified water, blend of light mineral oil, glyceryl monostearate, propylene glycol, methylparaben, propylparaben.

Uses An emollient, moisturising and protective cream for the treatment of dry or damaged skin. The presence of 10% urea in the product assists in providing a 'moisturising' effect lasting 5-6 hours, as shown by experiments measuring 'trans-epidermal water loss', in addition to providing the recognised actions of urea for dermatological purposes.

Dosage and administration Apply evenly to dry skin areas 2 to 3 times daily, or as necessary.

Contra-indications, warnings, etc If irritation occurs to any ingredient, discontinue use temporarily. Avoid contact with eyes.

Pharmaceutical precautions Store in a cool place. Replace cap after use.

Legal category P.

Package quantities 60 g.

Further information Nil.

Product licence number 0649/0041.

PSORIGEL*

Presentation A clear thin brown gel with a slight characteristic odour of tar. It contains Solution of Coal Tar 7.5%, 33% alcohol, carbomer 946, propylene glycol, ethanol, laureth 4, diisopropanolamine, and purified water. The hydroalcoholic gel base which is emollient, provides a moist film with the minimum of tar odour and staining potential.

Uses For the relief and treatment of inflammatory manifestations of tar responsive dermatoses. Among these are eczema, psoriasis, inflammation, erythema, scaling, pruritus and induration that accompanies various forms of dermatitis.

It also helps to relieve the itching that accompanies psoriasis, and eczema, and helps control the flaking and scaling as well.

Dosage and administration Rub into the affected areas once or twice daily. The gel may be applied more frequently if necessary.

Rub in well, allow to dry and remove any excess by patting with a paper tissue.

Contra-indications, warnings, etc *Caution:* Avoid contact with eyes. Upon accidental contact, flush with water.

After using, avoid exposure to direct sunlight, unless its action is specifically required.

Do not use on highly inflamed or broken skin.

The product contains alcohol.

If undue irritation develops, reduce the frequency of use, or suspend use until irritation subsides.

The staining potential of the product is minimal, but if it does occur, standard laundry procedure will remove most stains.

Pharmaceutical precautions There are no special pharmaceutical precautions.

Legal category P.

Package quantities 90 g in plastic collapsible tubes.

Further information Nil.

Product licence number 0649/0039.

*Trade Mark

Allen & Hanburys Limited
Horsenden House
Oldfield Lane North
Greenford, Middlesex UB6 0HB

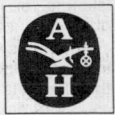

AMINOGRAN* FOOD SUPPLEMENT

Presentation Aminogran Food Supplement provides a mixture of L-amino acids, including all the essential amino acids except phenylalanine. It is intended for use with Aminogran Mineral Mixture (see separate Data Sheet for Aminogran Mineral Mixture).

Content per 100 g = 1,675 kJ (400 calories)

	g	mmol
L-Alanine	2.44	27.4
L-Arginine (as glutamate)	4.20	24.1
L-Aspartic acid	6.10	45.8
L-Cystine	1.45	6.0
L-Glutamic acid (total)	12.19	82.9
Glycine	6.10	81.3
L-Histidine (as monohydrochloride)	3.40	21.9
L-Isoleucine	8.53	65.0
L-Leucine	9.95	75.9
L-Lysine (as glutamate)	6.61	45.2
L-Methionine	2.96	19.8
L-Proline	4.26	37.0
L-Serine	8.39	79.8
L-Threonine	5.71	47.9
L-Tryptophan	1.45	7.1
L-Tyrosine	6.42	35.4
L-Valine	7.01	59.8

Aminogran Food Supplement is packed as 500 g in a white polythene bag in a cylindrical plastic container with cardboard carton. The mixture is a white powder. A white measuring scoop is provided which contains 5 g when levelled with a knife edge.

Uses Aminogran Food Supplement is indicated in conjunction with Aminogran Mineral Mixture for the dietary management of phenylketonuria in infants and children, and in phenylketonuric women during pregnancy. It may be used for bottle feeding phenylketonuric infants, but if available, a preparation based on a low-phenylalanine protein hydrolysate is more practicable. Prior to weaning bottle feeds can more easily be prepared from a preparation based on a low-phenylalanine protein hydrolysate, together with carbohydrates and fats to supply energy requirements. Once weaning is started a gradual change to Aminogran should be made, as it proves more acceptable than the protein hydrolysate and reduces feeding problems.

Dosage and administration The aim of treatment with Aminogran preparations is to provide an adequate diet in which there is a reduced intake of phenylalanine so that the blood levels of this amino acid are maintained at 0.2–0.5 mmol/litre (3–8 mg/100 ml).

In sucklings this is best obtained with a preparation based on a low-phenylalanine protein hydrolysate as there are practical difficulties associated with the administration of Aminogran in bottle form due to its low energy value and high osmolarity. However, once spoon-feeding is started Aminogran has the advantages of smaller bulk and superior palatability. Aminogran Food Supplement and Aminogran Mineral Mixture can be used, in appropriately reduced dosage, in conjunction with low-phenylalanine protein hydrolysate during weaning. As the quantity of Aminogran is increased so the low-phenylalanine protein hydrolysate is decreased and eventually omitted once adequate energy is being taken from solids. Thereafter Aminogran preparations are given mixed as a paste or drink as described for older children. Gradually the Aminogran paste can be spoon-fed and given at feed times with the other foods necessary for the phenylalanine and the energy content of the diet.

For older children Aminogran Food Supplement, in the required calculated quantity for the day, together with the daily dose of Aminogran Mineral Mixture, is mixed into a drink or paste with water and/or an appropriate volume of natural vegetable oil or a 50% vegetable oil emulsion (Prosparol*; Duncan, Flockhart & Co. Ltd), sugar and/or natural or synthetic protein-free flavouring, such as milk-shake syrup or concentrate. Sugar or milk-shake flavouring must be added if the oil or emulsion is used, to counteract the ketogenic effect of the fat content. The mixture is divided into three equal portions with one portion being given within 20 minutes of each of the three main meals, which should contain a proportion of the daily phenylalanine allowance. A separate drink should be given if the Aminogran mixture is administered as a paste because of the high solute content of the mixture. Administration with a meal is important as some phenylalanine is necessary to ensure that the amino-acid mixture (dietary nitrogen) is utilised for growth.

From school age the Aminogran mixture may be more practically given as two doses daily with two meals.

The daily requirements of energy, Aminogran Food Supplement and phenylalanine are shown in the table on following page.

The daily dose of Aminogran Food Supplement is calculated on the actual body weight in kilograms. The required quantity can be easily measured with the scoop provided, which, when levelled off with a knife edge, contains 5 g. Aminogran Food Supplement should be prescribed to the nearest half-scoop measurement. Aminogran Food Supplement is phenylalanine free so that it is essential it is not used as the sole source of protein nitrogen but that the diet should contain sources of phenylalanine from natural foods together with low-protein foods and energy foods such as sugar, protein-free starches, fat or oil. Special low-protein foods such as breads and biscuits are also available. As phenylalanine is an essential amino acid it is of particular importance that the growing child is not exposed to phenylalanine deficiency which can easily arise from an increased requirement in association with accelerated growth rate, inadequate absorption of phenylalanine due to vomiting, refusal of diet or inadequate replacement of phenylalanine, or inaccurate measurement of concentrated phenylalanine sources.

Infections or any other situation causing catabolism increases blood phenylalanine levels. It is recommended that the dietary phenylalanine be continued along with a source of easily digested calories such as sugary drinks if the infection continues for more than two or three days, though the Aminogran Food Supplement can be temporarily omitted.

Because of the preponderance of synthetic foods in the diet adequate vitamin supplementation is essential. Rashes, failure to thrive, and even death can result from a deficiency of phenylalanine or vitamins such as choline chloride, calcium pantothenate, inositol, biotin, α-tocopherol, vitamin B_{12} and folic acid. A complete vitamin supplement is provided by 3 Ketovite* Tablets (Paines & Byrne Ltd) plus 5 ml of Ketovite Liquid each day. For young children Ketovite Tablets should be crushed, suspended in the Ketovite Liquid and given once daily as a medicine.

The aim of dietary management in children with Aminogran is to maintain the blood phenylalanine concentration between 0.2 and 0.5 mmols/litre (3 and 8 mg/100 ml). For this the blood phenylalanine levels should be monitored at regular intervals and the phenylalanine (natural protein) allowance adjusted as necessary.

Women with phenylketonuria in pregnancy: The children of mothers with untreated phenylketonuria have a very high incidence of congenital abnormalities, including mental retardation, intrauterine and postnatal retardation of growth, microcephaly, skeletal, cardiac and ocular manifestations. Patients treated from early life are now reaching reproductive age and it is suggested that all their pregnancies should be planned and dietary restriction together with Aminogran Food Supplement and Mineral Mixture should commence before stopping the contraceptive method and prior to conception. Even then it is impossible to guarantee that the child will be normal at birth.

Although the exact threshold levels of maternal blood phenylalanine that can prove injurious to the fetus are not known it is recommended that blood phenylalanine levels of 0.2–0.5 mmols/litre (3–8 mg/100 ml) be maintained throughout pregnancy of women with phenylketonuria. Ideally, the blood phenylalanine level should be maintained within the recommended range prior to the onset of pregnancy but when this has not been planned the diet with Aminogran preparations should be instituted as soon as pregnancy is suspected. It should be then continued until the onset of labour. More frequent monitoring of the blood phenylalanine level during pregnancy is mandatory because of the increasing demand for phenylalanine by the growing fetus. This is of particular importance during the third trimester of pregnancy.

Initially a protein plus amino acid intake of 1 g/kg body weight using Aminogran Food Supplement is the suggested dose provided that the total intake of protein is not less than 50 g per day. Phenylalanine from natural foods should be given as indicated by previous tolerance. Initially 15 mg/kg is suggested, adjusted according to tolerance and increasing with fetal growth. The total diet should provide the energy requirement to maintain satisfactory weight gain and any weight loss should be avoided as it causes blood phenylalanine levels to rise.

Contra-indications, warnings, etc

Contra-indications: Aminogran Food Supplement is prepared solely for the dietary management of phenylketonuria and is unsuitable for the dietary management of any other disorder or to form part of the nutrition of normal persons.

Precautions: Aminogran Food Supplement when mixed with Aminogran Mineral Mixture presents a high osmolar load that requires an adequate fluid intake, especially in infants and young children.

Care should be taken to ensure all patients taking the Aminogran diet consume the full calculated diet which must contain adequate energy foods. If the diet is insufficient in energy the blood phenylalanine concentration will show an increase due to catabolism of body protein. The existence of an infection will also cause a rise in blood phenylalanine but under these circumstances appetite should be the guide to nutritional intake. The priority will be for high-energy protein-free drinks and the phenylalanine allowance, in foods such as milk, is only a secondary consideration. Only if milk is acceptable should the mixture of Aminogran Food

Guide to daily requirements in dietary management of classical phenylketonuria

Age (years)	Energy per kg actual body weight kilo Joules (Calories)	Aminogran Food Supplement per kg actual body weight (g)	Initial dose of phenylalanine* per kg actual body weight from other foods (mg)
0–1	420–630 (100–150)	3	50 to 60 and if necessary up to 110
1–2	380–420 (90–100)	2–3	30–40
2–4	330–420 (80–100)	2	25–40
4–6	330–420 (80–100)	2	25
6–8	290–380 (70–90)	2	15–25
8–14	230–310 (55–75)	see footnote 1	As tolerance
Over 14	190 (45)	see footnote 2	As tolerance

* This suggested initial starting dose must subsequently be adjusted according to the results of initially very frequent and then regular tests of blood phenylalanine levels.

1. Approximately 1 to 1.5 g or as appropriate according to natural protein intake to give 1.5 to 2.0 g protein plus amino acids per kg per day.

2. Approximately 1 g or as appropriate according to natural protein intake to give 1.5 g protein plus amino acids per kg per day.

Supplement and Aminogran Mineral Mixture be administered. A temporary period without Aminogran, as in any child not eating during an infection, does no harm and blood level control of phenylalanine returns when the infection is over.

Side-effects: No side-effects arise from administration of Aminogran Food Supplement so long as there is correct dietary management to avoid too high or too low a blood level of phenylalanine. The high osmolarity may give rise to vomiting and/or diarrhoea but can be overcome by additional fluid. Parental or patient anxiety over the dietary regime and/or diagnosis may cause similar effects so careful frequent supervision and monitoring of the diet is essential.

Overdosage: The high osmolarity may give rise to vomiting and/or diarrhoea. Treatment is administration of fluids by the oral or, if necessary, parenteral routes.

Pharmaceutical precautions Store in a cool dry place and ensure that the container lid is always replaced securely.

Legal category P.

Package quantities Aminogran Food Supplement is supplied in containers of 500 g.

Further information A booklet describing the use of Aminogran preparations is available on request. It is advisable that this be consulted before Aminogran Food Supplement is prescribed.

Product licence number 0045/0114.

AMINOGRAN* MINERAL MIXTURE

Presentation Aminogran Mineral Mixture contains all the necessary minerals for balanced nutrition in the correct proportions for human needs and is intended for use with Aminogran Food Supplement (see separate Data Sheet for Aminogran Food Supplement).

Content per 100 g and per 8 g dose

		per 100 g		per 8 g dose	
Potassium	8.3 g	0.21 mol	0.66 g	17 mmol
Calcium	8.1 g	0.20 mol	0.65 g	16 mmol
Phosphorus	6.0 g	0.19 mol	0.48 g	15 mmol
Sodium	4.0 g	0.17 mol	0.32 g	14 mmol
Magnesium	0.97 g	40 mmol	77 mg	3.2 mmol
Iron	63 mg	1 mmol	5 mg	90 micromol
Zinc	48 mg	0.7 mmol	4 mg	59 micromol
Copper	13 mg	0.2 mmol	1 mg	16 micromol
Manganese	4 mg	81 micromol	0.4 mg	6 micromol
Iodine				
Aluminium				
Cobalt	} Trace quantities			
Molybdenum				

Aminogran Mineral Mixture is packed as 250 g in a yellow polythene bag in a cylindrical plastic container with cardboard carton. The mixture is a mottled white powder. A yellow measuring scoop is provided which contains 2.7 g when levelled with a knife edge. Three scoopfuls provide the usual daily dose of 8 g.

Uses Aminogran Mineral Mixture is indicated in conjunction with Aminogran Food Supplement for the dietary management of phenylketonuria. Aminogran Mineral Mixture is also indicated as an adjuvant in the treatment of the following conditions:

1. Other disorders of amino-acid metabolism such as maple syrup urine disease and homocystinuria.
2. Urea cycle defects. These include carbamyl phosphate synthetase deficiency, ornithine carbamyl transferase deficiency, argininosuccinate synthetase deficiency (citrullinaemia), argininosuccinase deficiency (argininosuccinicaciduria), arginase deficiency (hyperargininaemia), hyperlysinaemia and other urea cycle defects as they are recognised.
3. Organicacidurias. These include hypervalinaemia, isovalericacidaemia, beta-methylcrotonylglycinuria, alpha-methylacetoaceticaciduria and propionicacidaemia.
4. In conjunction with artificial diets used in the treatment of food intolerance with malabsorption.
5. In any diet in infants and children where there is severe restriction of natural food, such as in some ketogenic diets for the treatment of epilepsy.

Dosage and administration Used for the dietary management of phenylketonuria, with Aminogran Food Supplement, it is recommended that the total daily intake of Aminogran Mineral Mixture is 8 g per day, provided that the patient's body weight is not less than 5.5 kg. For infants under 5.5 kg body weight the dosage is calculated on the basis of 1.5 g/kg/day. Solutions with a high osmolarity may cause vomiting, abdominal pain and diarrhoea in young infants so that it is advised that each gram of Aminogran Mineral Mixture should be diluted for infants with at least 100 ml of fluid. The usual method of administration is to prepare a drink or paste of Aminogran Food Supplement, in the required daily quantity (see separate Data Sheet for this product), together with three level, unpacked scoopfuls (8 g) of Aminogran Mineral Mixture. The drink or paste may be prepared with water and/or a vegetable oil or emulsion (Prosparol; Duncan, Flockhart & Co. Ltd) sugar and/or protein-free flavouring such as fruit, milk-shake, syrup or concentrate. If the oil is included then sugar should be added. The drink or paste is divided into three equal portions and one portion taken with each of the three main meals of the day like a dose of medicine and washed down with water or fruit juice. For older children the preparation may be divided into two portions with each portion taken with a convenient main meal. Some food containing natural protein must be consumed at the time of administration to supply the phenylalanine necessary for utilisation of the amino acids for growth.

Aminogran Mineral Mixture may be similarly used in the other conditions for which it is indicated.

Contra-indications, warnings, etc

Contra-indications: Aminogran Mineral Mixture is unsuitable for use where trace element supplementation only is required. If used for infants of less than 5.5 kg body weight the total daily dose should not exceed 1.5 g per kg body weight.

Precautions: When used in infants under the age of six months each 1 g of Aminogran Mineral Mixture must be diluted with at least 100 ml of fluid. For older children a drink to follow is satisfactory.

Pregnancy: See separate Data Sheet for Aminogran Food Supplement.

Side-effects: Mineral solutions with high osmolarity may cause vomiting, abdominal pain and diarrhoea. This may be avoided by dilution as advised under 'Precautions'.

Overdosage: If Aminogran Mineral Mixture is inadvertently given to infants in excess of the recommended dose of 1.5 g/kg/day or inadequately diluted to at least

1 g per 100 ml, symptoms of hyperosmolarity may occur and the serum electrolytes should be checked. Treatment is administration of fluids by the oral or, if necessary, parenteral routes.

Pharmaceutical precautions Store below 25°C in a dry place and ensure that the container lid is always replaced securely.

Legal category P.

Package quantities Aminogran Mineral Mixture is supplied in containers of 250 g.

Further information It is essential that the Data Sheet for Aminogran Food Supplement is consulted for a full understanding of the use of Aminogran preparations in the dietary management of phenylketonuria. A booklet describing the use of Aminogran preparations in phenylketonuria is available on request and it is advisable that it should be read before the products are prescribed.

Product licence number 0045/0115.

BECLOFORTE* INHALER

Presentation Becloforte Inhaler is a metered-dose aerosol which delivers 250 micrograms Beclomethasone Dipropionate BP per actuation into the mouthpiece of a specially designed actuator.

Uses Beclomethasone Dipropionate BP given by inhalation has a potent glucocorticoid anti-inflammatory action within the lungs without the side effects observed when steroids are administered systemically.

Becloforte Inhaler is indicated for those asthmatic patients who have been shown to require high doses (greater than 800 micrograms to 1,000 micrograms daily) of Becotide* Inhaler (Beclomethasone Dipropionate BP 50 micrograms per actuation) to control their symptoms. It may also be indicated for those patients whose asthma is no longer controlled by maximum maintenance doses of bronchodilators and Becotide Inhaler.

Some patients with severe asthma require oral corticosteroid therapy in addition to Becotide Inhaler for the adequate control of their symptoms. Many of these patients may, on transfer to Becloforte Inhaler, be able to reduce significantly or eliminate their requirement for additional oral corticosteroids.

Dosage and administration
Adults: Two inhalations (500 micrograms) twice daily, or one inhalation (250 micrograms) four times daily, is the recommended maintenance dosage. If necessary, dosage may be increased to two inhalations (500 micrograms) three or four times daily, according to response.

Children: Becloforte Inhaler is not indicated for use in children.

Contra-indications, warnings, etc
Contra-indications: Hypersensitivity to Becloforte Inhaler is a contra-indication; and special care is necessary in patients with active or quiescent pulmonary tuberculosis.

Pregnancy: Unnecessary administration of drugs during the first trimester of pregnancy is undesirable.

Precautions: The patients' inhaler technique should be checked to make sure that aerosol actuation is synchronised with inspiration of breath for optimum dispersal of drug within the lungs.

Patients should also be made aware of the prophylactic nature of therapy with Becloforte Inhaler and that it should be taken regularly even when they are asymptomatic.

Patients being treated with Becotide Inhaler may be transferred directly to treatment with Becloforte Inhaler.

In the majority of patients no significant adrenal suppression occurs until doses of 1,500 micrograms per day are exceeded. Some patients receiving 2,000 micrograms of Becloforte per day may show a degree of adrenocortical suppression although short term adrenal reserve remains intact. In such patients the risks of developing adrenal suppression should be balanced against the therapeutic advantages and precautions should be taken to provide systemic steroid cover in situations of prolonged stress.

Patients being treated with oral corticosteroids should be in a stable state before having Becloforte Inhaler added to their current therapy. Gradual withdrawal of the systemic steroid may be attempted after a week or two. Patients who have been treated with systemic steroids for long periods of time or at a high dose may have adrenocortical suppression. With these patients adrenocortical function should be monitored regularly and their dose of systemic steroid reduced cautiously.

Patients recently transferred from oral steroids to Becloforte Inhaler together with those still receiving oral steroids, should be warned that they may need to increase the dosage of oral steroids in times of stress, e.g., surgery, chest infections or worsening asthmatic attacks, but that this can be reduced again after the stress has been resolved. A small supply of oral steroids can be given to them for emergency use.

Treatment with Becloforte Inhaler should not be stopped abruptly.

Side-effects: No serious side-effects have been reported with the recommended doses of Becloforte Inhaler. Candidiasis of the mouth and throat occurs in some patients but the incidence is no greater than that with Becotide Inhaler. Patients with high blood levels of Candida precipitins, indicating a previous infection, are more likely to develop this complication. Such patients may find it helpful to rinse their mouth with water after using the Inhaler. Symptomatic candidiasis can be treated with topical anti-fungal therapy whilst still continuing with the Becloforte Inhaler.

Overdosage: If Becloforte Inhaler is used excessively over a long period, this could lead to adrenal suppression. In such cases, the patient should be transferred to oral corticosteroid therapy and when the condition has stabilised, be returned to the inhaled therapy at the recommended dose. To guard against the unexpected event of adrenal suppression regular tests of adrenal function are advised.

Pharmaceutical precautions Becloforte Inhaler should be stored at a temperature below 30°C. Direct sunlight and heat should be avoided. The canister should not be punctured, broken or burnt even when apparently empty.

Legal category POM.

Package quantities Each canister of Becloforte Inhaler provides 200 inhalations.

Further information Nil.

Product licence number 0045/0125.

BECONASE* AQUEOUS NASAL SPRAY

Presentation Beconase Aqueous Nasal Spray is a presentation of an aqueous suspension of microfine Beclomethasone Dipropionate BP delivered by a metering, atomising pump. Each 100 mg spray delivered by the nasal applicator contains 50 micrograms Beclomethasone Dipropionate BP.

Uses Beconase Aqueous Nasal Spray is indicated for the prophylaxis and treatment of perennial and seasonal allergic rhinitis including hay fever, and vasomotor rhinitis. Beclomethasone Dipropionate BP has a potent anti-inflammatory effect within the respiratory tract at doses which are not systemically active.

Dosage and administration Beconase Aqueous Nasal Spray is for administration by the intranasal route only.

Adults and children: The recommended dosage is two sprays into each nostril twice daily. For some patients, a dosage regimen of a single spray into each nostril three or four times daily may be preferred. Total daily administration should not normally exceed eight sprays.

For full therapeutic benefit regular usage is essential. The co-operation of the patient should be sought to comply with the regular dosage schedule and it should be explained that maximum relief may not be obtained within the first few doses.

For children under six years old, there are insufficient clinical data to recommend use.

Contra-indications, warnings, etc

Contra-indications: Beconase Aqueous Nasal Spray is contra-indicated in patients with a history of hypersensitivity to any of its components.

Precautions: Infections of the nasal passages and paranasal sinuses should be appropriately treated but do not constitute a specific contra-indication to treatment with Beconase Aqueous Nasal Spray.

Care must be taken while transferring patients from systemic steroid treatment to Beconase Aqueous Nasal Spray if there is any reason to suppose that their adrenal function is impaired.

Although Beconase Aqueous Nasal Spray will control seasonal allergic rhinitis in most cases, an abnormally heavy challenge of summer allergens may in certain instances necessitate appropriate additional therapy particularly to control eye symptoms.

Pregnancy: Unnecessary administration of drugs during the first trimester of pregnancy is undesirable.

Side-effects: No major side-effects attributable to Beconase Aqueous Nasal Spray have been reported.

Overdosage: The only harmful effect that follows inhalation of large amounts of the drug over a short time period is suppression of hypothalamic-pituitary-adrenal (HPA) function. No special emergency action need be taken. Treatment with Beconase Aqueous Nasal Spray should be continued at the recommended dose. HPA function recovers in a day or two.

Pharmaceutical precautions Beconase Aqueous Nasal Spray should be protected from light and stored below 25°C. Do not refrigerate.

Legal category POM.

Package quantities Beconase Aqueous Nasal Spray is supplied in an amber glass bottle fitted with a metering, atomising pump and nasal applicator. Each bottle contains 22 grams of suspension and provides approximately 200 metered sprays in recommended use.

Further information Beconase Aqueous Nasal Spray is an alternative intranasal presentation of Beclomethasone Dipropionate BP to Beconase Nasal Spray and is available for those who may prefer an aqueous product.

Product licence number 0045/0127.

BECONASE* NASAL SPRAY

Presentation Beconase Nasal Spray is a metered-dose aerosol which delivers 50 micrograms Beclomethasone Dipropionate BP per actuation into a specially designed nasal applicator.

Uses Beconase is indicated for the prophylaxis and treatment of perennial and seasonal allergic rhinitis, including hay fever, and vasomotor rhinitis. Beclomethasone Dipropionate BP has a potent anti-inflammatory effect within the respiratory tract at doses which are not systemically active.

Dosage and administration Beconase is for administration by the intranasal route only. The recommended dosage is two applications into each nostril twice daily (400 micrograms/day).

For some patients, a dosage regimen of a single application into each nostril three or four times daily may be preferred. Total daily administration should not normally exceed 8 puffs.

For full therapeutic benefit regular usage is essential. The co-operation of the patient should be sought to comply with the regular dosage schedule and it should be explained that maximum relief may not be obtained within the first few applications. For children under six years old, there are insufficient clinical data to recommend use.

Contra-indications, warnings, etc

Contra-indications: Beconase Nasal Spray is contra-indicated in patients with a history of hypersensitivity to any of its components.

Precautions: Infections of the nasal passages and paranasal sinuses should be appropriately treated but do not constitute a specific contra-indication to treatment with Beconase.

Care must be taken while transferring patients from systemic steroid treatment to Beconase if there is any reason to suppose that their adrenal function is impaired.

Although Beconase Nasal Spray will control seasonal allergic rhinitis in most cases, an abnormally heavy challenge of summer allergens may in certain instances necessitate appropriate additional therapy particularly to control eye symptoms.

Pregnancy: Unnecessary administration of drugs during the first trimester of pregnancy is undesirable.

Side-effects: No major side-effects attributable to Beconase have been reported, but occasionally sneezing attacks have followed immediately after the use of the aerosol.

Overdosage: The only harmful effect that follows inhalation of large amounts of the drug over a short time period is suppression of hypothalamic-pituitary-adrenal (HPA) function. No special emergency action need be taken. Treatment with Beconase Nasal Spray should be continued at the recommended dose. HPA function recovers in a day or two.

Pharmaceutical precautions Beconase should be stored at a temperature below 30°C but protected from frost. Exposure to direct sunlight or heat should be avoided. The canister should not be punctured, broken or burnt even if it is apparently empty.

Legal category POM.

Package quantities Beconase Nasal Spray is a metered-dose aerosol with a specially designed nasal applicator. Each canister provides 200 sprays.

Further information When Beconase is administered as two applications into each nostril the first puff should be directed at the upper and the second at the lower part of the nasal cavity.

Product licence number 0045/0093.

BECOTIDE* INHALER

Presentation Becotide Inhaler is a metered-dose aerosol which delivers 50 micrograms Beclomethasone Dipropionate BP per actuation into the mouthpiece of a specially designed actuator.

Uses Beclomethasone Dipropionate BP given by inhalation has a potent glucocorticoid anti-inflammatory action within the lungs but does not cause adverse systemic glucocorticoid effects at therapeutic doses. Becotide Inhaler therefore is indicated for a wide range of patients with bronchial asthma.

These patients include: those whose asthma is becoming worse and the relief provided by bronchodilators is less effective; those who are inadequately controlled by sodium cromoglycate in addition to bronchodilators; those with severe asthma who are dependent on systemic corticosteroids, or adrenocorticotrophic hormone (ACTH) or its synthetic equivalent.

Becotide Inhaler is particularly important for managing severe asthma in children because good control can be achieved without retardation of growth.

Dosage and administration *Adults:* 2 inhalations (100 micrograms) three or four times a day is the usual maintenance dose. Alternatively, the total daily dose may be administered as two divided doses. In severe cases dosage may be started at 600–800 micrograms per day and subsequently reduced when the patient begins to respond.

Children: 1 or 2 inhalations (50–100 micrograms) should be given two, three or four times daily, according to the response.

Contra-indications, warnings, etc
Contra-indications: Hypersensitivity to Becotide Inhaler is a contra-indication; and special care is necessary in patients with active or quiescent pulmonary tuberculosis.

Precautions: Patients should be instructed on the proper use of the inhaler to ensure that the drug reaches the target areas within the lungs. They should also be made aware that Becotide Inhaler has to be used regularly for optimum benefit.

The maximum daily intake of Becotide Inhaler should not exceed 20 inhalations (1 mg); significant reduction of plasma cortisol levels has been reported in patients who received twice this amount.

Pregnancy: Unnecessary administration of drugs during the first trimester of pregnancy is undesirable.

Patients inadequately controlled by bronchodilator therapy: The use of Becotide Inhaler in patients who have never taken steroids or taken only occasional courses of steroids is straightforward. An improvement in respiratory function is obvious within a week. The few patients who do not respond during this period usually have excessive mucus in their bronchi so that the drug is unable to penetrate to its site of action. In such cases a short course of systemic steroid in relatively high dosage should be given to control secretion of mucus and other inflammatory changes in the lungs. Continuation of treatment with Becotide Inhaler usually maintains the improvement achieved, the oral steroid being gradually withdrawn. Exacerbation of asthma caused by infection is usually controlled by appropriate antibiotic treatment, by increasing the dose of Becotide Inhaler and if necessary by giving a systemic steroid.

Steroid-dependent patients: The transfer of steroid-dependent patients to Becotide Inhaler and their subsequent management needs special care mainly because recovery from impaired adrenocortical function, caused by prolonged systemic steroid therapy, is slow. The patient should be in a reasonably stable state before being given Becotide Inhaler in addition to his usual maintenance dose of systemic steroid. After about a week, gradual withdrawal of the systemic steroid is started by reducing the daily dose by 1 mg prednisolone, or its equivalent of other corticosteroid, at not less than weekly intervals. Patients treated with systemic steroids for long periods of time or who have received high doses may have adrenocortical suppression. With these patients adrenocortical function should be monitored regularly and their dose of systemic steroid reduced cautiously. Some patients feel unwell during the withdrawal phase despite maintenance or even improvement of respiratory function. They should be encouraged to persevere with the inhaler and withdrawal of systemic steroid continued, unless there are objective signs of adrenal insufficiency. Most patients can be successfully transferred to Becotide Inhaler with maintenance of good respiratory function, but special care is necessary for the first months after the transfer until the pituitary-adrenal system has sufficiently recovered to enable the patient to cope with emergencies such as trauma, surgery or infections. Transferred patients whose adrenocortical function is impaired should carry a warning card indicating that they need supplementary systemic steroid during periods of stress. They should also be given a supply of oral steroid to use in emergency, for example when the asthma worsens as a result of a chest infection. The dose of Becotide Inhaler should be increased at this time and then reduced to the maintenance level after the systemic steroid has been discontinued.

Replacement of systemic steroid treatment with Becotide Inhaler sometimes unmasks allergies such as allergic rhinitis or eczema previously controlled by the systemic drug. These allergies should be symptomatically treated with antihistamine and/or topical preparations.

Side-effects: No major side-effects attributable to the use of recommended doses of Becotide Inhaler have been reported. Candidiasis of the mouth and throat (thrush) occurs in some patients, the incidence of which is increased with doses greater than 400 micrograms beclomethasone dipropionate per day. Patients with high blood levels of Candida precipitins, indicating a previous infection, are more likely to develop this complication.

Such patients may find it helpful to rinse their mouth with water after using the Inhaler. Symptomatic candidiasis can be treated with topical anti-fungal therapy whilst still continuing with the Becotide Inhaler.

Overdosage: The acute toxicity of beclomethasone dipropionate is low. The only harmful effect that follows inhalation of large amounts of the drug over a short time period is suppression of hypothalamic-pituitary-adrenal (HPA) function. No special emergency action need be taken. Treatment with Becotide Inhaler should be continued at the recommended dose to control the asthma; HPA function recovers in a day or two.

Reduction of plasma cortisol levels has been reported in patients who received twice the recommended maximum dose of Becotide Inhaler. In the unlikely event of grossly excessive intake of beclomethasone dipropionate for weeks or months on end a degree of adrenocortical atrophy could occur in addition to suppression of HPA function. The patient should be treated as steroid-dependent and transferred to a suitable maintenance dose of a systemic steroid such as prednisolone. Once the patient's condition is stabilised he should be transferred to Becotide Inhaler by the method recommended in this Data Sheet.

Pharmaceutical precautions Becotide Inhaler should be stored at a temperature below 30°C. Direct sunlight and heat should be avoided.

The canister should not be punctured, broken or burnt even if it is apparently empty.

Legal category POM.

Package quantities Becotide Inhaler is a metered-dose aerosol with a specially designed actuator. Each canister provides 200 inhalations.

Further information Nil.

Product licence number 0045/0089.

BECOTIDE* ROTACAPS*

Presentation Becotide Rotacaps, an alternative inhalation form of Beclomethasone Dipropionate to Becotide Inhaler, are especially valuable for treating patients who are unable to use pressurised inhalers effectively or who might use them incorrectly.

Becotide Rotacaps contain a mixture of microfine beclomethasone dipropionate and larger particle lactose in buff or chocolate-brown/colourless hard gelatine cartridges. Each Rotacap contains 100 micrograms (buff) or 200 micrograms (chocolate-brown) of beclomethasone dipropionate and is marked Becotide 100 or Becotide 200. The contents of a Rotacap are inhaled using a specially developed device called a Rotahaler*, which separates the cartridge into halves that rotate and release the drug when the patient inhales. This breath actuation is very sensitive and so the drug is fully available even at the lowest inspiratory flow rates. The Rotahaler is therefore a more reliable drug delivery system for many patients but a rather larger unit dose relative to Becotide Inhaler is necessary for the same therapeutic effect.

Uses Beclomethasone Dipropionate BP given by inhalation has a potent glucocorticoid anti-inflammatory action within the lungs but does not cause adverse systemic glucocorticoid effects at therapeutic doses. Becotide Rotacaps therefore are indicated for a wide range of patients with bronchial asthma. These patients include: those whose asthma is becoming worse and the relief provided by bronchodilators is less effective; those who are inadequately controlled by sodium cromoglycate in addition to bronchodilators; those with severe asthma who are dependent on systemic corticosteroids, or adrenocorticotrophic hormone (ACTH) or its synthetic equivalent.

Becotide Rotacaps are particularly important for managing severe asthma in children because good control can be achieved without retardation of growth.

Dosage and administration Becotide Rotacaps are for inhalation use only, using a Becotide Rotahaler. For optimum results Becotide Rotacaps should be used regularly.

Adults: One 200 microgram Rotacap three or four times a day is the usual maintenance dose. Alternatively, the total daily dose may be administered as two divided doses.

Children: One 100 microgram Rotacap two, three or four times a day, according to the response.

Contra-indications, warnings, etc
Contra-indications: Hypersensitivity to Becotide Rotacaps is a contra-indication; and special care is necessary in patients with active or quiescent pulmonary tuberculosis.

Precautions: Patients should be instructed in the proper use of the Rotahaler to ensure that the drug reaches the target areas within the lungs. They should also be made aware that Becotide Rotacaps have to be used regularly for optimum benefit.

The maximum daily intake of beclomethasone dipropionate should not exceed 1 mg; significant reduction of plasma cortisol levels has been reported in patients who received twice this amount.

Pregnancy: Unnecessary administration of drugs during the first trimester of pregnancy is undesirable.

Patients inadequately controlled by bronchodilator therapy: The use of Becotide Rotacaps in patients who have never taken steroids or taken only occasional courses of steroids is straightforward. An improvement in respiratory function is obvious within a week. The few patients who do not respond during this period usually have excessive mucus in their bronchi so that the drug is unable to penetrate to its site of action. In such cases a short course of systemic steroid in relatively high dosage should be given to control secretion of mucus and other inflammatory changes in the lungs. Continuation of treatment with Becotide Rotacaps usually maintains the improvement achieved, the oral steroid being gradually withdrawn. Exacerbation of asthma caused by infection is usually controlled by appropriate antibiotic treatment, by increasing the dose of Becotide Rotacaps and if necessary by giving systemic steroid.

Steroid-dependent patients: The transfer of steroid-dependent patients to Becotide Rotacaps and their subsequent management needs special care mainly because recovery from impaired adrenocortical function, caused by prolonged systemic steroid therapy, is slow. The patient should be in a reasonably stable state before being given Becotide Rotacaps in addition to his usual maintenance dose of systemic steroid. After about a week, gradual withdrawal of the systemic steroid is started by reducing the daily dose by 1 mg prednisolone, or its equivalent of other corticosteroid, at not less than weekly intervals. Patients treated with systemic steroids for long periods of time or who have received high doses may have adrenocortical suppression. With these patients adrenocortical function should be monitored regularly and their dose of systemic steroid reduced cautiously. Some patients feel unwell during the withdrawal phase despite maintenance or even improvement of respiratory function. They should be encouraged to persevere with the Rotacaps and withdrawal of systemic steroid continued unless there are objective signs of adrenal insufficiency. Most patients can be successfully transferred to Becotide Rotacaps with maintenance of good respiratory function, but special care is necessary for the first months after the transfer until the pituitary-adrenal system has sufficiently recovered to enable the patient to cope with emergencies such as trauma, surgery or infections. Transferred patients whose adrenocortical function is impaired should carry a warning card indicating that they need supplementary systemic steroid during periods of stress. They should also be given a supply of oral steroid to use in emergency, for example when the asthma worsens as a result of a chest infection. The dose of Becotide Rotacaps should be increased at this time and then reduced to the maintenance level after the systemic steroid has been discontinued.

Replacement of systemic steroid treatment with Becotide Rotacaps sometimes unmasks allergies such as allergic rhinitis or eczema previously controlled by the systemic drug. These allergies should be symptomatically treated with antihistamine and/or topical preparations.

Side-effects: No major side-effects attributable to the use of recommended doses of Becotide Rotacaps have been reported. Candidiasis of the mouth and throat (thrush) occurs in some patients; patients with high blood levels of Candida precipitins, indicating a previous infection, are more likely to develop this complication. Such patients may find it helpful to rinse their mouth with water after using the Rotahaler. Symptomatic candidiasis can be treated with topical anti-fungal therapy whilst still continuing with the Becotide Rotacaps.

Overdosage: The acute toxicity of beclomethasone dipropionate is low. The only harmful effect that follows inhalation of large amounts of the drug over a short time period is suppression of hypothalamic-pituitary-adrenal (HPA) function. No special emergency action need be taken. Treatment with Becotide Rotacaps should be continued at the recommended dose to control the asthma; HPA function recovers in a day or two.

Reduction of plasma cortisol levels has been reported in patients who received twice the recommended maximum dose of beclomethasone dipropionate. In the unlikely event of grossly excessive intake of beclomethasone dipropionate for weeks or months on end a degree of adrenocortical atrophy could occur in addition to suppression of HPA function. The patient should be treated as steroid-dependent and transferred to a suitable maintenance dose of a systemic steroid such as prednisolone. Once the patient's condition is stabilised he should be transferred to Becotide Rotacaps by the method recommended in this Data Sheet.

Pharmaceutical precautions To keep the Rotacaps in good condition it is important that they are stored in a dry place where they will not be exposed to extremes of temperature. A convenient supply may be carried in the special container for the Rotahaler. The Rotacaps should only be inserted in the Rotahaler immediately prior to use. Failure to observe this instruction may affect the operation of the Rotahaler.

Legal category POM.

Package quantities Becotide Rotacaps 100 micrograms and 200 micrograms are supplied in containers of 100.

Further information Nil.

Product licence numbers
Becotide Rotacaps 100 micrograms   0045/0119
Becotide Rotacaps 200 micrograms   0045/0120

BECOTIDE* SUSPENSION FOR NEBULISATION

Presentation Becotide Suspension for Nebulisation is an aqueous suspension of Beclomethasone Dipropionate BP adjusted with a buffer to about pH 4.5. The concentration of beclomethasone dipropionate is 50 micrograms per ml of suspension.

Uses Becotide Suspension for Nebulisation is indicated for the management of infants and children whose asthma is inadequately controlled by bronchodilators and/or sodium cromoglycate, thus necessitating additional treatment with steroids, and who are unable to use a pressurised inhaler (e.g., Becotide Inhaler) effectively or unable to inhale the drug in powder form (e.g., Becotide Rotacaps).

Becotide Suspension for Nebulisation is not a substitute for injectable or oral corticosteroids in emergency situations.

Dosage and administration Becotide Suspension for Nebulisation should be administered as an aerosol produced by a nebuliser with an adequate flow rate and using a suitable mouthpiece to enable delivery of the drug.

The exact dose delivered to the patient varies slightly depending on the equipment used (e.g., driving source, nebuliser chamber).

For optimum results Becotide Suspension for Nebulisation should be used according to a regular daily schedule.

Infants: (Up to one year) 1 ml (50 micrograms) administered two, three or four times daily is the usual maintenance dose.

Children: (One to 12 years) 2 ml (100 micrograms) administered two, three or four times daily is the usual maintenance dose.

Becotide Suspension for Nebulisation should be used with a respirator or nebuliser only under the close supervision of a physician. Patients receiving treatment with Becotide Suspension for Nebulisation must be warned that if their clinical condition deteriorates they should not increase the dose or the frequency of administration but should seek medical advice.

To aid administration of small volumes of the suspension it may be diluted immediately before use with up to an equal volume of normal saline.

Adults: Because of the large volumes which would be necessary, Becotide Suspension for Nebulisation is not suitable for administering high doses of beclomethasone dipropionate.

Contra-indications, warnings, etc
Contra-indications: Hypersensitivity to Becotide Suspension for Nebulisation is a contra-indication; and special care is necessary in patients with active or quiescent pulmonary tuberculosis.

Precautions: Becotide Suspension for Nebulisation is not a substitute for injectable or oral corticosteroids if these are indicated, and it should not be injected or administered orally. It is advisable to administer the suspension via a mouthpiece to avoid the possibility of atrophic changes of facial skin which may occur with prolonged use with a face-mask. Patients and/or parents should be made aware that Becotide Suspension for Nebulisation has to be used regularly for optimum benefit.

The daily intake of Becotide Suspension for Nebulisation should not exceed 20 ml (1,000 micrograms).

Pregnancy: Unnecessary administration of drugs during the first trimester of pregnancy is undesirable.

Patients inadequately controlled by bronchodilator therapy: The use of Becotide Suspension for Nebulisation in patients who have never taken steroids or taken only occasional courses of steroids is straightforward. The few patients who do not respond to Becotide Suspension for Nebulisation usually have excessive mucus in their bronchi so that the drug is unable to penetrate to its site of action. In such cases a short course of systemic steroid in relatively high dosage should be given to control secretion of mucus and other inflammatory changes in the lungs. Continuation of treatment with Becotide Suspension for Nebulisation usually maintains the improvement achieved, the oral steroid being gradually withdrawn. Exacerbation of asthma caused by infection is usually controlled by appropriate antibiotic treatment, by increasing the dose of Becotide Suspension for Nebulisation and, if necessary, by giving a systemic steroid.

Steroid-dependent patients: The transfer to Becotide Suspension for Nebulisation of steroid-dependent patients unable to use an aerosol or Rotahaler and their subsequent management needs special care mainly because recovery from impaired adrenocortical function, caused by prolonged systemic steroid therapy, is slow. Initially, patients should be given Becotide Suspension for Nebulisation in addition to their usual maintenance dose of systemic steroid. After about a week, gradual withdrawal of the systemic steroid is started by reducing the daily dose by 1 mg of prednisolone, or its equivalent, at not less than weekly intervals. Patients treated with systemic steroids for long periods of time or who have received high doses may have adrenocortical suppression. With these patients adrenocortical function should be monitored regularly and the dose of systemic steroid reduced cautiously. Some patients feel unwell during the withdrawal phase despite maintenance or even improvement of respiratory function. Unless there are objective signs of adrenal insufficiency they should be encouraged to persevere with Becotide Suspension for Nebulisation and withdrawal of systemic steroids should be continued. Most patients can be successfully transferred to Becotide Suspension for Nebulisation with maintenance of good respiratory function, but special care is necessary for the first months after the transfer until the hypothalamic-pituitary-adrenal system has sufficiently recovered to enable the patient to cope with emergencies such as trauma, surgery or infections. Transferred patients whose adrenocortical function is impaired should carry a warning card indicating that they need supplementary systemic steroid during periods of stress. They should also be given a supply of oral steroid to use in emergency, for example when the asthma worsens as a result of a chest infection. The dose of Becotide Suspension for Nebulisation should be in-creased by the physician at this time and then reduced to the maintenance level after the systemic steroid has been discontinued.

Replacement of systemic steroid treatment with Becotide Suspension for Nebulisation may unmask allergies such as allergic rhinitis or eczema previously controlled by the systemic drug. These allergies should be symptomatically treated with antihistamines and/or topical preparations.

Side-effects: No major side effects attributable to the use of recommended doses of Becotide Suspension for Nebulisation have been reported. Candidiasis of the mouth and throat (thrush) is known to occur in some patients treated with beclomethasone dipropionate. Patients with high blood levels of Candida precipitins, indicating a previous infection, are the most likely to develop this complication. The condition usually responds to topical anti-fungal therapy without discontinuing treatment with Becotide Suspension for Nebulisation.

Overdosage: If Becotide Suspension for Nebulisation is used excessively over a long period this could lead to adrenal suppression. In such a case, the patient should be transferred to oral corticosteroid therapy and when the condition has stabilised, be returned to the inhaled therapy at the recommended dose. Oral steroids should then be withdrawn slowly, as for steroid dependent patients.

Pharmaceutical precautions Becotide Suspension for Nebulisation should be stored in a cool place and protected from light.

The suspension may be diluted immediately before use with up to an equal volume of normal saline.

The suspension should not be mixed with other agents.

Once the bottle has been opened the contents should be discarded after one month. Any unused suspension in the chamber of the nebuliser should be discarded.

Legal category POM.

Package quantities Becotide Suspension for Nebulisation is supplied in screw-capped amber glass bottles of 10 ml.

Further information Nil.

Product licence number 0045/0126

EUDEMINE* TABLETS 50 mg
EUDEMINE* INJECTION

Presentation Eudemine Tablets 50 mg are white, sugar-coated tablets each containing Diazoxide BP 50 mg. Identification code AH/8D.

Eudemine Injection. Ampoules of 20 ml containing Diazoxide BP 300 mg in an aqueous, colourless solution with sodium hydroxide at pH 11.6.

Uses Diazoxide is a benzothiadiazine analogue which has two main therapeutic actions. Clinically it is used in the treatment of intractable hypoglycaemia, and for the treatment of severe hypertension associated with renal disease and for patients resistant to conventional hypotensive agents. Diazoxide also causes salt and water retention.

Hypoglycaemia: Eudemine administered orally is indicated for the treatment of intractable hypoglycaemia with severe symptoms from a variety of causes including: idiopathic hypoglycaemia in infancy, leucine-sensitive or unclassified; functional islet-cell tumours both malignant and benign if inoperable, extra-pancreatic neoplasms producing hypoglycaemia; glycogen storage disease; hypoglycaemia of unknown origin.

Hypertensive emergencies: Eudemine Injection is used particularly for the emergency treatment of acute hypertensive crises, especially those occurring in association with acute hypertensive encephalopathy, congestive heart failure, acute glomerular nephritis, eclampsia or pre-eclampsia.

Severe hypertension: It is also indicated for the control of severe hypertension associated with renal disease.

In hypertensive patients requiring such diagnostic procedures as renal biopsy, arteriography or cardiac catheterisation, Eudemine Injection may be given to facilitate the procedure and reduce the danger of haemorrhage due to hypertension. Eudemine Injection is also indicated in patients who have failed to respond to other hypotensive agents.

Eudemine Tablets may be used to treat patients with severe hypertension associated with renal disease or where the conventional hypotensive agents have failed. It is also possible that Eudemine Tablets may be used as maintenance therapy in patients who have had their hypertension controlled initially with Eudemine Injection.

Dosage and administration *Hypoglycaemia:* In hypoglycaemia the dosage schedule of Eudemine Tablets is determined according to the clinical needs and the response of the individual patient. For both adults and children a starting oral dose of 5 mg/kg body weight divided into 2 or 3 equal doses per 24 hours will establish the patient's response and thereafter the dose can be increased until the symptoms and blood glucose level respond satisfactorily. Regular determinations of the blood glucose in the initial days of treatment are essential. In children with leucine-sensitive hypoglycaemia, a dosage range of 15–20 mg/kg/day is suggested.

In adults with benign or malignant islet-cell tumours producing large quantities of insulin, high dosages of up to 1,000 mg per day have been used.

Hypertensive emergencies and severe hypertension: In the treatment of hypertension, Eudemine Injection is administered by the intravenous route only and it should never be given intramuscularly or subcutaneously.

Adults: A full dose of 300 mg in 20 ml will be required by most patients. However, an adequate fall in blood pressure in some patients may be obtained with as little as 150 mg. Patients must be recumbent during the injection which must be rapid and not exceed 30 seconds.

Children: On the rare occasions that Eudemine Injection is indicated for hypertension in children the dosage should be based on a level of 5 mg per kg body weight by injection.

A response occurs within five minutes and usually persists for at least four hours. One injection is usually effective, but further injections may be required, particularly in hypertensive crises or in accelerating disease refractory to other hypotensive agents. Up to four ampoules of 300 mg may be given in 24 hours. An initial dose of 600 mg is recommended only in life-threatening situations. Once the blood pressure is controlled by Eudemine Injection, treatment with anti-hypertensive agents designed for maintenance therapy can be initiated. It appears that if hypertensive patients treated with Eudemine Injection are allowed an unrestricted sodium

intake then the subsequent response to oral hypotensive agents will be improved.

When Eudemine Tablets are used in the treatment of hypertension the dosage ranges from 400 mg to 1,000 mg daily, given in 2 or 3 divided doses. Apart from obtaining control over hypertension, dosage adjustment may also be occasioned by the development of side-effects.

Contra-indications, warnings, etc
Contra-indications: In the treatment of hypoglycaemia, Eudemine is contra-indicated in all cases which are amenable to surgery or other specific therapy.

There are no absolute contra-indications to Eudemine for the relief of hypertension but it should be used with discretion. Agents which can be given by infusion, such as hydralazine or labetalol, should have been shown to be ineffective before a bolus injection of diazoxide is given.

Precautions: Each of the two main therapeutic actions of Eudemine tend to be unwanted effects when the product is used for the alternative main indication. Thus in the treatment of hypoglycaemia it is necessary that the blood pressure be monitored regularly, whilst in the treatment of hypertension long-term therapy with Eudemine necessitates regular monitoring of the blood glucose levels.

In either indication, retention of sodium and water is likely to necessitate therapy with an oral diuretic such as frusemide or ethacrynic acid. The dosage of either of the diuretics mentioned may be up to 1 g daily. It must be appreciated that if diuretics are employed then both the hypotensive and the hyperglycaemic activities of diazoxide will be potentiated and it is likely that the dosage of diazoxide will require adjustment downwards. In patients with severe renal failure it is desirable to maintain, with diuretic therapy, urinary volumes in excess of 1 litre daily. Hypokalaemia should be avoided by adequate potassium replacement.

In the long-term treatment of hypertension with oral diazoxide it is advisable to employ four-hourly diabetic urine testing in the initial stages. Explosive forms of hyperglycaemia will occur early, if at all, so that with maintenance therapy diabetic urine testing will only be required twice daily. Control of hyperglycaemia is usually effected with tolbutamide, of which the dosage should be regulated by the results of regular monitoring of the blood sugar.

Whenever Eudemine is given over a prolonged period regular haematological examinations are indicated to exclude changes in white blood cell and platelet counts. Also in children, there should be regular assessment of growth, bone and psychological maturation.

With Eudemine Injection the high alkalinity of the solution necessitates that great care is taken to ensure that the injection is given directly into a vein without leakage into surrounding tissues.

The very rapid, almost complete protein binding of diazoxide requires cautious dosage to be used in patients whose plasma proteins may be lower than normal.

Pregnancy: Eudemine Tablets are only to be used in pregnant women when the indicated condition is deemed to put the mother's life at risk. Prolonged oral therapy of Eudemine during pregnancy has been reported to cause alopecia in the newborn.

Side-effects: In the treatment of hypertension the hyperglycaemia induced by diazoxide is generally inevitable. Each injection of diazoxide usually means a transient rise in blood sugar of about 10%. Fortunately the hyperglycaemia in hypertensive patients can be readily controlled with tolbutamide, or exceptionally with insulin. A hypotensive effect in normotensive patients is of minor importance and rarely requires any specific therapy. An oral diuretic may be indicated to control sodium and water retention.

With Eudemine Injection reflex tachycardia is not uncommon in the first few minutes after injection and is more frequent in digitalised patients. Orthostatic hypotension is unlikely but it may occur in those recently treated with adrenergic blocking agents. When it is used during labour for the treatment of toxaemia, the smooth muscle relaxant effect can cause delay in the second stage. This should be counteracted with oxytocic agents.

With oral therapy nausea is common in the first two or three weeks and may require relief with an anti-nauseant. Prolonged therapy has given rise to reports of hypertrichosis lanuginosa, anorexia and hyperuricaemia. In the treatment of hypertension with oral Eudemine a recent report has confirmed the extrapyramidal side-effects which have been reported with oral diazoxide in the treatment of hypoglycaemia. In oral hypotensive therapy, it was found that extra-pyramidal effects, such as Parkinsonian tremor, cogwheel rigidity and oculogyric crises, could be easily suppressed by intravenous injection of an anti-Parkinsonian drug such as procyclidine and that they could be prevented by maintenance therapy with such a drug given orally.

Other adverse effects of Eudemine which have been reported are hyperosmolar non-ketotic coma, cardiomegaly, leucopenia and thrombocytopenia.

Drugs potentiated by diazoxide therapy include: oral diuretics, antihypertensive agents and anticoagulants.

Overdosage: Excessive dosage of Eudemine can result in hyperglycaemia which will respond to insulin; or to hypotension which will necessitate maintenance of blood volume with intravenous fluids.

Pharmaceutical precautions No special storage conditions are needed for Eudemine Tablets.

It is particularly important that Eudemine Injection is protected from light.

Eudemine Injection should never be mixed with other drugs and it should not be diluted.

Legal category POM.

Package quantities Eudemine Tablets 50 mg are packed in containers of 100.

Eudemine Injection is in ampoules individually boxed in packs of five.

Further information Nil.

Product licence numbers
Eudemine Tablets 50 mg   0045/5081
Eudemine Injection   0045/0084

FENTAZIN* TABLETS
FENTAZIN* INJECTION

Presentation
Fentazin Tablets 2 mg each contain Perphenazine BP 2 mg. Identification code is AH/1C.

Fentazin Tablets 4 mg each contain Perphenazine BP 4 mg. Identification code is AH/2C.

Fentazin Tablets 8 mg each contain Perphenazine BP 8 mg. Identification code is AH/4C.

All are white, sugar-coated tablets.

Fentazin Injection contains 5 mg Perphenazine BP in each ampoule of 1 ml. It is colourless.

Uses Fentazin is a potent tranquilliser and anti-emetic of the phenothiazine group. It is indicated in the following: as an adjunct to the short-term management of anxiety, severe psychomotor agitation, excitement, violent or dangerously impulsive behaviour; schizophrenia, treatment of symptoms and prevention of relapse, other psychoses, especially paranoid, mania and hypomania; nausea and vomiting. Because of the hazard of severe extrapyramidal reactions, Fentazin is not indicated for the treatment of agitation and restlessness in the elderly.

Fentazin Injection is indicated in cases where rapid control of symptoms is essential or when oral administration is impracticable.

Fentazin Injection can also be used as premedication and for the control of post-operative vomiting.

It may be of value in the control of intractable hiccough.

Dosage and administration
Adults: Fentazin Tablets are administered orally in a usual dosage of 4 mg perphenazine three times daily. As there may be great variability of individual response and dosage requirement, the dose may have to be adjusted upwards or downwards according to patient response. The total daily dose should not exceed 24 mg.

Treatment should be started and dosage increased under close supervision. Treatment should be reviewed at intervals so as to avoid indiscriminate or unduly prolonged use.

Fentazin Injection is administered intramuscularly. The usual initial dose is 5 to 10 mg, which may be followed by further 5 mg doses at six-hourly intervals. Patients should be transferred to oral administration as soon as clinically appropriate. Care is necessary at this time because comparative potency of different formulations or routes of administration is not absolutely predictable.

Elderly: One quarter or one half the recommended starting dose for adults may be sufficient for therapeutic response in the elderly.

Children: Fentazin should not be given to children under the age of fourteen years.

Contra-indications, warnings, etc
Contra-indications: Fentazin should not be administered to patients with leucopenia or in association with drugs liable to cause bone-marrow depression or to patients in comatose states.

Precautions: The possibility of suicide in depressed patients remains during treatment and until significant remission occurs. Fentazin should be used with caution in patients with liver disease; cardiac arrhythmias; congestive cardiac failure; coronary artery disease; severe respiratory disease; renal failure; epilepsy, conditions predisposing to epilepsy (e.g., alcohol withdrawal or brain damage); Parkinson's disease; patients who have shown hypersensitivity to other phenothiazines; personal or family history of narrow-angle glaucoma; hypothyroidism; myasthenia gravis; phaeochromocytoma; prostatic hypertrophy. Since temperature regulation may be impaired, care should be taken in extremely hot weather, and in cold weather, especially in the elderly and frail because of risk of hypothermia.

Pregnancy: The safety of perphenazine in pregnancy has not yet been established.

Drug interactions: Fentazin can increase the central nervous system depression produced by other CNS-depressant drugs including alcohol, hypnotics, sedatives or strong analgesics. It may antagonise the action of adrenaline and other sympathomimetic agents and reverses the blood pressure-lowering effects of adrenergic-blocking agents such as guanethidine and clonidine. It may impair the metabolism of tricyclic antidepressants, the anti-parkinson effects of levodopa and the effects of anti-convulsants.

Undesirable anticholinergic effects can be enhanced by anti-parkinson or other anticholinergic drugs. Phenothiazines may enhance the cardiac-depressant effects of quinidine, the effect of diazoxide and of neuromuscular blocking agents and the absorption of corticosteroids and digoxin.

Fentazin may affect the control of the diabetes and the action of anticoagulants. The possibility of interactions with lithium should be born in mind.

Fentazin should not be taken with tea or coffee as absorption may be impaired by the formation of insoluble precipitates. Antacids can also impair its absorption.

Side-effects: Not all the following side effects have been reported with this specific drug; however, pharmacological similarities with other phenothiazine derivatives require that each be considered. Many of these side effects may be prevented by a reduction in dosage.

Drowsiness, sedation, dry mouth and nasal stuffiness may occur, particularly with high dosage and at the start of treatment. Dose-related postural hypotension may occur, particularly in the elderly and after intramuscular injections. Other dose-related anticholinergic-type side effects including blurring of vision, tachycardia, constipation and urinary hesitancy or retention. Adynamic ileus rarely occurs with phenothiazine therapy, but is of particular concern in psychiatric patients who may fail to seek treatment of the condition.

Perphenazine may impair alertness, especially at the start of treatment. These effects may be potentiated by alcohol. Patients should be warned of the risks of sedation and advised not to drive or operate machinery during treatment, until their susceptibility is known.

Extrapyramidal reactions may occur even at low dosage. Acute dystonias may occur early in treatment. Parkinsonian rigidity, tremor, akathisia tend to appear less rapidly. Oculogyric crises have been reported. Anti-parkinson agents should not be prescribed routinely, because of the possible risks of aggravating anticholinergic side effects of perphenazine, of precipitating toxic-confusional states or of impairing its therapeutic efficacy. They should only be given as required.

Tardive dyskinesia is a syndrome of irregularly repetitive involuntary movements which may occur during administration or after withdrawal of perphenazine and other neuroleptic drugs. It is characterised by abnormal writhing movements or protrusions of the tongue with lip-smacking, puckering or chewing movements and facial grimaces. Choreoathetoid movements of the extremities or repetitive movements of the neck or trunk may accompany the orofacial dyskinesia or can occur alone. The syndrome is common among patients treated with moderate to high doses of antipsychotic drugs for prolonged periods of time and may prove irreversible, particularly in patients over the age of 50. It is unlikely to occur in the short term when low or moderate doses are used as recommended, but since its occurrence may be related to duration of treatment as well as daily dose, perphenazine should be given in the minimal effective dose for the minimum possible time, unless it is established that long-term administration for the treatment of schizophrenia is required. The potential seriousness and unpredictability of tardive dyskinesia and the fact that it has occasionally been reported to occur when neuroleptic antipsychotic drugs have been prescribed for relatively short periods in low dosage means that the prescribing of such agents requires especially careful assessment of risks versus benefit. Tardive dyskinesia can be precipitated or aggravated by anti-parkinson drugs. Short-lived dyskinesias may occur after abrupt drug withdrawal.

In schizophrenia, the response to antipsychotic drug treatment may be delayed. If drugs are withdrawn, recurrence of symptoms may not become apparent for several weeks or months. Perphenazine may also cause abnormalities of cerebrospinal fluid proteins.

Perphenazine, even in low dosage in susceptible (especially non-psychotic) individuals, may cause unpleasant subjective feelings of being mentally dulled or slowed down, nausea, dizziness, headache or paradoxical effects of excitement, agitation or insomnia. Confusional states or epileptic fits can occur. The elderly are more susceptible to the sedative and hypotensive effects.

The effects of phenothiazines on the heart are dose-related. ECG changes with prolongation of the QT interval and T-wave changes have been reported commonly in patients treated with moderate to high dosage; they are reversible on reducing the dose. In a very small number of cases, they have been reported to precede serious arrhythmias, including ventricular tachycardia and fibrillation, which have also occurred after overdosage.

Hormonal effects of antipsychotic neuroleptic drugs include hyperprolactinaemia, which may cause galactorrhoea, gynaecomastia and oligo or amenorrhoea. Sexual function, including erection and ejaculation is sometimes impaired by perphenazine. Weight gain may occur. Oedema has been reported with phenothiazine medication. Perphenazine administration may also result in false-positive pregnancy tests.

Agranulocytosis has been reported very rarely, most commonly in the first three months of treatment, but occasionally later. Blood counts should be performed if the patient develops signs of a persistent infection. Transient leucopenia can also occur. The occurrence of antinuclear antibodies has been reported with phenothiazines. Systemic lupus erythematosus has very rarely occurred.

Raised serum cholesterol and rarely hyperglycaemia have been reported in association with phenothiazines.

Perphenazine rarely causes increased susceptibility to sunburn and patients should be warned to avoid excessive exposure. Skin rashes have occurred rarely. Fine deposits in the cornea and lens and pigmented retinopathy have been reported after long-term therapy.

Perphenazine may impair body temperature-regulation and cases of severe hypothermia or hyperpyrexia have been reported, usually in association with moderate or high dosage of phenothiazines. The elderly or hypothyroid patient may be particularly susceptible to hypothermia. The hazard of hyperthermia may be increased by especially hot or humid weather or by drugs, such as anti-parkinson agents, which impair sweating.

Perphenazine can very rarely cause obstructive jaundice associated with stasis in biliary canaliculi. It has been thought to be a hypersensitivity reaction. Transient abnormalities of liver function tests may occur in the absence of jaundice.

Withdrawal: Acute withdrawal symptoms including

nausea, vomiting and insomnia, have very rarely been described after abrupt cessation of high doses of phenothiazines. Gradual withdrawal is advisable.

Overdosage: With oral preparations of Fentazin, gastric lavage is recommended. Emetics are likely to be of little value because of the potent anti-emetic activity of the drug. Hypotension is not usually a problem, especially if the patient is passing urine satisfactorily. Severe hypotension may require fluid infusion therapy. If a vasopressor is needed, norepinephrine may be used. Central nervous system depression is best treated conservatively; analeptics should not be used. Rewarming measures should not be employed unless the body temperature falls below 30°C. Convulsions may be controlled with standard methods, but the use of barbiturates should be avoided. Cardiac monitoring for at least 48 hours is recommended.

Pharmaceutical precautions
Storage: Fentazin Injection should be protected from light.

Dilution: Fentazin Injection should not be mixed with other agents as this may affect the stability of the solution.

Legal category POM.

Package quantities
Fentazin Tablets 2 mg, 4 mg and 8 mg are issued in cartons each containing 100 tablets in 10 foil strips of 10 (5 × 2) tablets.

Fentazin Injection is available in boxes of 5 and 100 ampoules of 1 ml each containing 5 mg.

Further information
Perphenazine is a phenothiazine with piperazine side chain. Its pharmacological profile of activity includes moderate sedative and hypotensive properties and a fairly pronounced tendency to cause extrapyramidal reactions.

Product licence numbers
Fentazin Tablets 2 mg	0045/5082R
Fentazin Tablets 4 mg	0045/5083R
Fentazin Tablets 8 mg	0045/5084R
Fentazin Injection	0045/5055R

ISOGEL*
Presentation Isogel is a preparation of Ispaghula Husk BP, which consists of the epidermis and collapsed adjacent layers removed from the dried ripe seeds of *Plantago ovata* Forssk.

Isogel is supplied as small, reddish-pink granules in containers of 200 g.

Uses Isogel is not absorbed from the gastrointestinal tract, but it adsorbs water to form a mucilaginous mass. This results in a purely mechanical stimulus to mass peristalsis without any purgative effect. It is for this reason that Isogel is not only an effective remedy for constipation but is also of value in the treatment of diarrhoea, the irritable bowel syndrome and the management of patients with a colostomy. Isogel is indicated in habitual constipation, including cases due to spastic colon, dietary insufficiencies and in patients with haemorrhoids or diabetes. It can be used to normalise the bowel movement in patients with mucous or ulcerative colitis.

Isogel is a help to patients with colostomy as the formation of a well-formed, easily passed stool assists in the maintenance of cleanliness and the establishment of control.

Dosage and administration The required quantity of Isogel should be stirred briskly into half a glass of water and swallowed at once. An aerated water is frequently preferred and may be easier to swallow.

Adults: 2 teaspoonfuls once or twice daily, preferably at mealtimes.

Children: 1 teaspoonful once or twice daily, preferably at mealtimes.

The above dosage is only a general guide and it should be adjusted to suit the needs of each individual patient.

In diarrhoea the dose, usually 1 teaspoonful, is taken three times daily until symptoms abate.

Contra-indications, warnings, etc
Contra-indications: Nil.

Precautions: A few cases of inhalation of the mucilaginous mass which forms on allowing an Isogel/water mixture to stand have been reported. In consequence, it is important that Isogel should be swallowed immediately after mixing, and elderly or debilitated patients should be supervised whilst taking it.

Pregnancy: Unnecessary administration of drugs during the first trimester of pregnancy is undesirable.

Side-effects: Nil.

Overdosage: As Isogel is not absorbed and it has no purgative action the problem of overdosage does not arise.

Pharmaceutical precautions No special storage precautions are necessary.

Legal category GSL.

Package quantities Isogel is supplied in containers of 200 g.

Further information Nil.

Product licence number 0045/5028.

PIRITON* TABLETS
PIRITON* SPANDETS*
PIRITON* SYRUP
PIRITON* INJECTION

Presentation Piriton is a potent antihistamine (Chlorpheniramine Maleate BP) presented as tablets, sustained-action tablets, syrup and injection.

Piriton Tablets: Round, biconvex, cream tablets each containing Chlorpheniramine Maleate BP 4 mg. Identification engraved Piriton AH.

Piriton Spandets: Cream and white, round, layered tablets each containing Chlorpheniramine Maleate BP 12 mg. After swallowing, 4 mg Chlorpheniramine Maleate BP is released immediately from the cream layer and then a further 8 mg chlorpheniramine maleate is gradually released from the special porous matrix comprising the white layer. Identification engraved Piriton AH Spandet.

Piriton Syrup: Each 10 ml of Piriton Syrup contains Chlorpheniramine Maleate BP 4 mg. It is colourless.

Piriton Injection: Each 1 ml of Piriton Injection contains Chlorpheniramine Maleate BP 10 mg. It is colourless.

Uses The oral preparations of Piriton are indicated for symptomatic control of all allergic conditions responsive to antihistamines, including hay fever, vasomotor rhinitis, urticaria, angioneurotic oedema, food allergy, drug and serum reactions, pruritus ani et vulvae, insect bites.

Piriton Injection is indicated for acute urticaria, control of allergic reactions to insect bites and stings, angioneurotic oedema, drug and serum reactions, desensitisation reactions, hay fever, vasomotor rhinitis, severe pruritus of non-specific origin.

Dosage and administration *Piriton Tablets:*

Adults: 1 tablet three or four times a day.

Children: (aged 6–12 years): $\frac{1}{2}$–1 tablet three or four times a day.

Piriton Spandets: Adults: 1 Spandet every 8–12 hours.

Children (over 12 years of age): 1 Spandet daily.

Piriton Spandets must be swallowed whole and not chewed.

Piriton Syrup: Adults: Two 5 ml spoonfuls three or four times a day.

Children (up to 1 year): $\frac{1}{2}$ spoonful (2.5 ml) twice daily.

Children (1–5 years): $\frac{1}{2}$–1 spoonful (2.5–5 ml) three times daily.

When Piriton Syrup is dispensed to meet prescriptions involving doses of 2.5 ml it should be diluted with an equal quantity of unpreserved Syrup BP. The resultant mixture should be used within 14 days.

Piriton Injection: The injection may be subcutaneous, intramuscular or intravenous. The latter is recommended when a rapid effect is desired as in anaphylactic reactions. For the intravenous route Piriton should be diluted in the syringe with 5–10 ml of blood and then injected slowly over a period of one minute. Any drowsiness, giddiness or hypotension which may follow is usually transitory.

The usual dose of Piriton Injection for adults is 10–20 mg, but not more than 40 mg should be given per 24 hours.

In the event of a blood transfusion reaction a dose of 10–20 mg of Piriton should be given by the subcutaneous route. This can be repeated to a total of 40 mg per 24 hours or oral forms of Piriton may be given until the symptoms subside. Though Piriton may be helpful in the prevention of delayed reactions to penicillin and other drugs it cannot be relied on to prevent anaphylactic reactions in patients known to be allergic to a particular drug. Piriton Injection 10 mg should be injected separately by the intramuscular route immediately prior to injection of any other drug.

In the event of an anaphylactic reaction Piriton Injection 10–20 mg may be given by slow intravenous injection in addition to the emergency therapy of adrenaline, corticoids, oxygen and supportive therapy.

Contra-indications, warnings, etc
Contra-indications: There are no known definite contra-indications to therapy with Piriton.

Precautions: All antihistamines, given in effective dosage, may cause dizziness or drowsiness. In consequence, until the effect of the treatment is known, patients treated with Piriton should be warned not to take charge of vehicles or machinery. The sedative action of alcohol may be potentiated by antihistamines so that drowsiness can occur in patients not otherwise subject to it if alcohol is taken.

Pregnancy: Unnecessary administration of drugs during the first trimester of pregnancy is undesirable.

Side-effects: Drowsiness and dizziness may occur. Some patients have reported a stinging or burning sensation at the site of injection. Rapid intravenous injection may cause transitory hypotension or CNS stimulation.

Overdosage: The estimated lethal dose of Piriton is 25–50 mg per kg body weight. Treatment should include gastric lavage if massive overdosage has been by the oral route. In the event of convulsions sedate with intramuscular paraldehyde. Severe respiratory depression may necessitate mechanical ventilation. Severe hypotension may require fluid replacement.

Pharmaceutical precautions *Storage:* There are no special storage conditions needed for Piriton Tablets. Piriton Spandets require a cool dry place and Piriton Syrup a cool dark place. Piriton Injection should be protected from light.

Dilution: If it is necessary to dilute Piriton Syrup then the suitable diluent is unpreserved Syrup BP. The resulting mixture will keep for 14 days at room temperature.

Legal category Tablets P.
Spandets P.
Syrup P.
Injection POM.

Package quantities Piriton Tablets are supplied in containers of 50 and 500.
Piriton Spandets are supplied in containers of 100.
Piriton Syrup is supplied in bottles of 150 ml.
Piriton Injection is supplied in boxes of 5 and 100 ampoules.

Further information No Piriton preparation contains tartrazine.

Product licence numbers
Piriton Tablets   0045/5077
Piriton Spandets   0045/5078
Piriton Syrup   0045/5019
Piriton Injection   0045/5056

PROPADERM* CREAM
PROPADERM* OINTMENT
PROPADERM*-FORTE CREAM

Presentation Propaderm Cream, Ointment and Propaderm-Forte Cream are topical preparations of Beclomethasone Dipropionate BP. Beclomethasone Dipropionate BP is a potent anti-inflammatory steroid when applied topically to the skin.

Propaderm Cream: Beclomethasone Dipropionate BP 0.025% in a cream base.

Propaderm Ointment: Beclomethasone Dipropionate BP 0.025% in an ointment base.

Propaderm-Forte Cream: Beclomethasone Dipropionate BP 0.5% in a cream base.

Propaderm Cream and Propaderm-Forte Cream are all white in colour; Propaderm Ointment is yellowish.

Uses Propaderm Cream and Ointment are indicated for the local treatment of the various forms of eczema and dermatitis; the various forms of psoriasis; neurodermatoses including lichen simplex; intertrigo; discoid lupus erythematosus.

Propaderm Cream is preferred for weeping conditions or where the skin is usually moist or hairy.

Propaderm Ointment is suitable for dry, lichenified or scaly conditions or for use under occlusive dressings.

Propaderm-Forte Cream is used for resistant dermatoses, including pustular psoriasis of palms and soles, discoid lupus erythematosus, pemphigus erythematosus, mycosis fungoides, and some unusual conditions such as pretibial myxoedema, necrobiosis lipoidica, granuloma annulare.

Dosage and administration Propaderm preparations should be applied thinly over the whole of the affected area and gently rubbed in. Initial application is made twice daily, but when improvement is seen the intervals between applications may be extended and treatment eventually stopped. If the condition recurs, treatment should be re-instituted. Subsequent re-appearance of the condition is likely to be avoided by application of Propaderm every third or fourth day. Propaderm-Forte Cream may have to be applied three times daily in the initial stages until improvement is observed. The beneficial effect may be enhanced by preliminary use of hot soaks, or by intermittent applications of occlusive dressings.

Contra-indications, warnings, etc
Contra-indications: Propaderm should not be applied to the eyes. Infections of the skin should receive specific therapy, and the steroid withdrawn if the response is delayed. Propaderm is contra-indicated in the presence of tuberculosis of the skin, chickenpox, vaccinia, herpes virus infections and, also, for the treatment of varicose ulcers or any other stasis ulcers.

Precautions: When Propaderm, and in particular Propaderm-Forte Cream, is used under occlusive dressings over extensive areas there is the possibility of systemic absorption which could lead to side-effects and adrenal suppression. For this reason it is inadvisable to use more than 2 g of Propaderm-Forte Cream under occlusive dressings per application.

In infants there is the possibility of adrenal suppression with long-term application of Propaderm even without occlusion.

Pregnancy: Topical administration of steroids to pregnant animals can cause abnormalities of fetal development. The relevance of this finding to human beings has not been established; however, topical steroids should not be used extensively in pregnancy, i.e. in large amounts or for prolonged periods.

Side-effects: A single case of skin atrophy has been reported in a patient who had continuous therapy with Propaderm Ointment for 700 days. In the event of adverse effects occurring the preparation should be withdrawn.

Overdosage: Should systemic corticosteroid effects arise from excessive application of Propaderm preparations topical treatment should be discontinued. If adrenal function is impaired the patient will need to be protected from any harmful effects of stress with oral corticosteroid preparations until normal adrenal function is established.

Pharmaceutical precautions *Storage:* All Propaderm preparations should be stored at a temperature below 25°C and protected from light.

Dilution: Propaderm Cream may be diluted, if necessary, with Cetomacrogol Cream Formula A BPC. For Propaderm Ointment dilution can be effected with White Soft Paraffin BP.

Legal category POM.

Package quantities Propaderm Cream is available in tubes of 15 g and 50 g; Propaderm Ointment in tubes of 15 g and 50 g; and Propaderm-Forte Cream in tubes of 5 g.

Further information No Propaderm preparation contains lanolin or parabens.

Product licence numbers
Propaderm Cream   0045/5000
Propaderm Ointment   0045/5005
Propaderm-Forte Cream 0045/5001

PROPADERM*-A OINTMENT

Presentation Propaderm-A Ointment contains Beclomethasone Dipropionate BP 0.025% and Chlortetracycline Hydrochloride BP 3.0%. It is pale yellow in colour.

Beclomethasone Dipropionate BP is a potent anti-inflammatory steroid when applied topically to the skin. Chlortetracycline Hydrochloride BP is a broad-spectrum antibiotic unlikely to cause skin sensitisation reactions.

Uses Propaderm-A Ointment is indicated for skin conditions which respond to therapy with an anti-inflammatory steroid where infection is present or is likely to occur, e.g. infective eczema of various types, seborrhoeic dermatitis and infective intertrigo. The combination of an anti-inflammatory steroid with an antibacterial is frequently preferred when occlusive dressings are used in conjunction with topical steroid therapy.

Occlusive dressings of an impermeable material such as polythene film can enhance the effect of Propaderm-A Ointment in certain resistant conditions such as fissured and lichenified eczema and neurodermatoses, hypertrophic lichen planus, chronic discoid lupus erythematosus, and psoriasis on the elbows and knees.

Dosage and administration Propaderm-A Ointment should be applied thinly over the whole of the affected area and gently rubbed in. Initially application should be twice daily, but when improvement is seen the intervals between applications may be extended and treatment eventually stopped. If the condition recurs, treatment should be re-instituted. Subsequent re-appearance of the condition can usually be avoided by application of Propaderm-A Ointment every third or fourth day.

Contra-indications, warnings, etc
Contra-indications: Propaderm-A Ointment should not be applied to the eyes. Infections of the skin failing to respond necessitate withdrawal of Propaderm-A and use of specific therapy. Propaderm-A Ointment is contra-indicated in the presence of tuberculosis of the skin, chickenpox, vaccinia, herpes virus infections, fungal infections and, also, for the treatment of varicose ulcers or any other stasis ulcers.

Precautions: When Propaderm-A Ointment is used under occlusive dressings over extensive areas there is the possibility that this could lead to side-effects and adrenal suppression. In infants long-term continuous topical steroid therapy could cause adrenal suppression even without occlusion.

Propaderm-A Ointment may stain hair, skin or fabric, and the application should be covered with a dressing to protect clothing.

Pregnancy: Topical administration of steroids to pregnant animals can cause fetal abnormalities. The relevance of this finding to human beings has not been established; however, topical steroids should not be used extensively in pregnancy, i.e. in large amounts or for prolonged periods.

Side-effects: Chlortetracycline very occasionally causes sensitisation. A single case of skin atrophy has been reported in a patient who had continuous therapy with Propaderm Ointment for 700 days. If adverse effects occur the preparation should be withdrawn.

Overdosage: Should systemic corticosteroid effects arise from excessive application of Propaderm preparations topical treatment should be discontinued. If adrenal function is impaired the patient will need to be protected from any harmful effects of stress with oral corticosteroid preparations until normal adrenal function is established.

Pharmaceutical precautions Store at a temperature not exceeding 25°C and protect from light.

Propaderm-A Ointment may be diluted, if necessary, with White Soft Paraffin BP.

Legal category POM.

Package quantities Propaderm-A Ointment is available in tubes of 15 g and 50 g.

Further information No lanolin or parabens included in the formula of Propaderm-A Ointment.

Product licence number 0045/5006.

PROPADERM*-C CREAM
PROPADERM*-C OINTMENT

Presentation Propaderm-C Cream and Ointment are topical preparations of Beclomethasone Dipropionate BP and Clioquinol BP.

Propaderm-C Cream contains Beclomethasone Dipropionate BP 0.025% and Clioquinol BP 3.0%. Propaderm-C Ointment contains Beclomethasone Dipropionate BP 0.025% and Clioquinol BP 3.0%. Both Propaderm-C Cream and Ointment are pale yellow in colour.

Beclomethasone Dipropionate BP is a potent anti-inflammatory steroid when applied topically to the skin. Clioquinol BP has a wide range of antibacterial and antifungal activity.

Uses Propaderm -C Cream and Ointment are indicated for skin conditions which respond to topical steroid therapy where infection is present or is likely to occur, particularly where the infection is fungal.

Propaderm-C Cream is preferred for weeping conditions or where the skin is usually moist or hairy. Propaderm-C Ointment is suitable for dry, lichenified or scaly conditions or for use under occlusive dressings.

Dosage and administration Propaderm-C should be applied thinly over the whole of the affected area and gently rubbed in. Initial application is made twice daily, but when improvement is seen the intervals between the applications may be extended and treatment eventually stopped.

If the condition recurs, treatment should be reinstituted. Subsequent re-appearance of the condition can usually be avoided by application of Propaderm-C every third or fourth day.

Contra-indications, warnings, etc
Contra-indications: Propaderm-C should not be applied to the eyes. Infections of the skin failing to respond necessitate withdrawal of Propaderm-C and use of specific therapy. Propaderm is contra-indicated in the presence of tuberculosis of the skin, chickenpox,

vaccinia, herpes virus infections and, also, for the treatment of varicose ulcers or any other stasis ulcers.

Precautions: When Propaderm-C is used under occlusive dressings over extensive areas there is the possibility of systemic absorption which could lead to side-effects and adrenal suppression.

In infants there is the possibility of adrenal suppression with long-term application of Propaderm-C even without occlusion.

Propaderm-C Cream and Ointment may stain hair, skin or fabric, and the application should be covered with a dressing to protect clothing.

Pregnancy: Topical administration of steroids to pregnant animals can cause fetal abnormalities. The relevance of this finding to human beings has not been established; however, topical steroids should not be used extensively in pregnancy, i.e. in large amounts or for prolonged periods.

Side-effects: Sensitisation reactions to clioquinol have been reported. Where there is unexplained relapse with continued treatment this possibility may be responsible.

A single case of skin atrophy has been reported in a patient who had continuous therapy with Propaderm Ointment for 700 days. If adverse effects occur the preparation should be withdrawn.

Overdosage: Should systemic corticosteroid effects arise from excessive application of Propaderm preparations topical treatment should be discontinued. If adrenal function is impaired the patient will need to be protected from any harmful effects of stress with oral corticosteroid preparations until normal adrenal function is established.

Pharmaceutical precautions Store at a temperature below 25°C and protect from light.

Propaderm-C Cream may be diluted, if necessary, with Cetomacrogol Cream Formula A BPC and Propaderm-C Ointment with White Soft Paraffin BP.

Legal category POM.

Package quantities Propaderm-C Cream and Ointment are available in tubes of 15 g.

Further information Propaderm-C Cream and Ointment do not contain lanolin or parabens.

Product licence numbers
Propaderm-C Cream   0045/5002
Propaderm-C Ointment 0045/5007

STERISPON*

Presentation Sterispon is Absorbable Gelatin Sponge BP and an effective haemostatic. It is not friable and may be cut into any desired shape or size or moulded with the fingers. Sterispon is prepared sterile and specially packed ready for use in the operating theatre. It is white in colour.

Uses For control of capillary oozing and venous bleeding in most forms of surgery (for exceptions, see Contra-indications). Sterispon may be used as a material for the obliteration of surgical 'dead spaces'.

Dosage and administration The sponge should be removed from the packings with sterile forceps and, if necessary, cut into pieces of the desired size and shape. It may be used in the dry state or moistened with normal saline. If the latter state is required, place the sponge in normal saline and remove the air by gentle squeezing before use. Sterispon is applied to the site of bleeding with sufficient pressure to enable adherence of the sponge and control of bleeding. Since Sterispon is completely absorbed by normal phagocytosis it is usually left *in situ* and the wound closed.

Contra-indications, warnings, etc

Contra-indications: Sterispon is contra-indicated for use in stapedectomy or other aural surgery where it could come into contact with fluid from the internal ear. In ophthalmic surgery it is inadvisable to use Sterispon in operations where the aqueous or vitreous humours are exposed.

Precautions: It is not advisable to apply Sterispon in the usual manner in the presence of infection, but it may be used to control haemorrhage if treated as a removable pack.

Side-effects: None.

Overdosage: Not applicable.

Pharmaceutical precautions Sterispon cannot be resterilised once the container has been opened without alteration to the properties of the sponge.

Storage: Store at a temperature not exceeding 25°C.

Legal category P.

Package quantities Sterispon is supplied sterile in the following sizes:

Size No. 1	Strips, $6 \times 2 \times 0.7$ cm, in glass tubes each containing one piece.
Size No. 2	Strips, $20 \times 10 \times 0.1$ cm, in glass tubes each containing one piece.
Size No. 3	Thin wafers, $2 \times 2 \times 0.1$ cm, in glass tubes each containing six pieces.
Size No. 4	Strips, $10 \times 10 \times 0.5$ cm, in envelopes containing one piece in packs of six envelopes.
Size No. 5	For dental use. Pieces, $2 \times 2 \times 1$ cm, in glass tubes each containing six pieces.

Further information Nil.

Product licence number 0045/5063.

TRIPTAFEN*
TRIPTAFEN*-M

Presentation Triptafen are sugar-coated pink tablets, coded AH/1D, each containing Amitriptyline Hydrochloride BP 25 mg and Perphenazine BP 2 mg.

Triptafen-M are sugar-coated, light salmon pink tablets, coded AH/2D, each containing Amitriptyline Hydrochloride BP 10 mg and Perphenazine BP 2 mg.

Uses Amitriptyline hydrochloride is a tricyclic compound with antidepressive activity. Perphenazine is a piperazine derivative of phenothiazine which has potent tranquillising activity.

Triptafen and Triptafen-M are indicated for the treatment of mild to moderate depression associated with anxiety.

Dosage and administration Triptafen preparations are administered orally.

Adults: Triptafen: 1 tablet three times daily with a further tablet at night if necessary.

Triptafen-M: 1 tablet three times daily with a further tablet at night if necessary.

Failure to respond within four weeks is an indication to review treatment. In all cases treatment should not continue beyond three months without reassessment.

Children: Triptafen preparations are not suitable for administration to children under fourteen years of age.

Contra-indications, warnings, etc

Contra-indications: Glaucoma; urinary retention; congestive heart failure; coronary artery disease; epilepsy; severely impaired liver function; concurrent administration of other antidepressive drugs, particularly monoamine oxidase inhibitors (MAOIs). No Triptafen preparation should be given to patients with leucopenia or in association with drugs liable to cause bone-marrow depression.

Precautions: Triptafen or Triptafen-M should not be given in conjunction with MAOIs and, because of the persistent action of the latter, an interval of at least fourteen days should be allowed to elapse between withdrawal of an MAOI and the introduction of a Triptafen preparation.

Persistent oral dyskinesia has been reported occasionally, particularly in elderly female patients, after long-term treatment with potent phenothiazine drugs including perphenazine. Consequently, Triptafen preparations should be prescribed with regular patient reassessments.

Pregnancy: Unless there are compelling reasons, these preparations should not be used during pregnancy, especially during the first and last trimesters. There is inadequate evidence of safety of these preparations in human pregnancy, although they have been in wide use for many years without apparent ill-effect. There is evidence of harmful effects in pregnancy in animals when given in exceptionally high doses.

Side-effects: Amitriptyline may give rise to dryness of the mouth, drowsiness and occasionally tachycardia and blurred vision. Perphenazine may cause mild drowsiness and a slight fall in blood pressure and in addition tremor and extrapyramidal side effects have been reported. Idiosyncratic side-effects, such as pruritus, nausea, diarrhoea and indigestion may occur.

Overdosage: Gastric lavage should be performed as soon as possible. If convulsions occur or threaten they should be controlled with standard methods, but barbiturates should be avoided. In severe cases haemodialysis may be performed if practicable. It is recommended that patients who have taken an overdose of Triptafen should be observed for at least 48 hours even if symptoms are not severe.

Pharmaceutical precautions
Storage: No special storage conditions are necessary for either of the Triptafen preparations.

Legal category POM.

Package quantities Triptafen Tablets and Triptafen-M Tablets are issued in cartons containing 100 tablets in foil strips of 10.

Further information Nil.

Product licence numbers
Triptafen Tablets	0045/0128
Triptafen-M Tablets	0045/0129

VENTIDE* INHALER ▼

Presentation Ventide Inhaler is a metered-dose aerosol which delivers 100 micrograms Salbutamol BP and 50 micrograms Beclomethasone Dipropionate BP per actuation, into the mouthpiece of a specially designed actuator.

Uses This association of Salbutamol BP with Beclomethasone Dipropionate BP is specially provided for those patients who require regular doses of both drugs for treatment of their obstructive airways disease. Ventide Inhaler is not intended for use as a first-line treatment but is for use once the need for inhaled corticosteroid therapy has been established.

Dosage and administration *Adults:* 2 inhalations (200 micrograms salbutamol and 100 micrograms beclomethasone dipropionate) three or four times a day.

Children: 1 or 2 inhalations (100 micrograms to 200 micrograms salbutamol and 50 micrograms to 100 micrograms beclomethasone dipropionate) two, three or four times a day.

Contra-indications, warnings, etc
Contra-indications: Although intravenous salbutamol and occasionally salbutamol tablets are used in the management of uncomplicated premature labour, Ventide should not be used for threatened abortion during the first and second trimesters of pregnancy.

Ventide Inhaler is contra-indicated in patients with a history of hypersensitivity to any of its components.

Precautions: Patients should be instructed in the proper use of the inhaler to ensure that the drugs reach the target areas within the lungs.

Patients should be made aware that Ventide Inhaler should be used regularly for optimum benefit. However, patients should be regularly reassessed so that their continuing need for corticosteroid therapy can also be reviewed.

Ventide Inhaler is not for use in acute attacks but for routine long-term management so some patients will require a separate Ventolin* Inhaler for relief of acute bronchospasm. However, should the effect of the additional Ventolin Inhaler or the relief provided by the Ventide Inhaler last for less than four hours, patients should be advised that this may indicate that their asthma is worsening and to seek medical advice in case treatment with inhaled corticosteroids needs to be increased or treatment with systemic corticosteroids needs to be started or increased.

The maximum daily intake of inhaled beclomethasone dipropionate should not exceed 1 mg. Significant reduction of plasma cortisol levels has been reported in some patients who received twice this amount.

For those patients who are steroid-dependent it is advisable to commence therapy with beclomethasone dipropionate as the separate aerosol, Becotide Inhaler. Instructions regarding the introduction of Becotide Inhaler as full or part replacement for systemic steroids are given in the Data Sheet for Becotide Inhaler.

Patients who have been weaned in the previous few months from long-term systemic corticosteroids need special consideration until the hypothalamic-pituitary-adrenal system has recovered sufficiently to enable the patient to cope with emergencies such as trauma, surgery or infections. Such patients should carry a warning indicating that they need supplementary systemic steroid during periods of stress, until their adrenocortical function has become normal. These patients should also be given a supply of oral steroid to use in emergency when their airways obstruction worsens.

Special care is necessary in patients with active or quiescent pulmonary tuberculosis.

Ventide Inhaler should be administered cautiously to patients suffering from thyrotoxicosis.

Pregnancy: Unnecessary administration of drugs during the first trimester of pregnancy is undesirable.

Side-effects: No major side effects have been reported in patients taking salbutamol and beclomethasone dipropionate by inhalation from the metered-dose device. Candidiasis of the mouth and throat (thrush) occurs in some patients inhaling beclomethasone dipropionate. Patients with high blood levels of Candida precipitins, indicating a previous infection, are more likely to develop this complication. The incidence of candidiasis is increased with doses greater than 400 micrograms beclomethasone dipropionate per day. The condition usually responds to topical antifungal therapy without discontinuing treatment with Ventide Inhaler.

Overdosage: The preferred antidote for overdosage with Ventide Inhaler is a cardio-selective, beta-blocking agent, to counteract the salbutamol component, but beta-blocking drugs should be used with caution in patients with a history of bronchospasm. The acute toxicity of beclomethasone dipropionate is low. The only harmful effect that follows inhalation of large amounts of the drug over a short time period is suppression of hypothalamic-pituitary-adrenal (HPA) function. No special emergency action need be taken. Treatment with Ventide Inhaler should be continued at the recommended dose to control the asthma; HPA function recovers in a day or two.

Reduction of plasma cortisol levels has been reported in patients who received twice the recommended maximum dose of beclomethasone dipropionate. In the unlikely event of grossly excessive intake of beclomethasone dipropionate for weeks or months a degree of adrenocortical atrophy could occur in addition to suppression of HPA function. The patient should be treated as steroid-dependent and transferred to a suitable maintenance dose of a systemic steroid such as prednisolone. Once the patient's condition is stabilised the reintroduction of inhaled corticosteroids should be considered.

Pharmaceutical precautions *Storage:* Ventide Inhaler should be stored in a cool place, protected from direct sunlight and heat.

The canister should not be punctured, broken or burnt even if it is apparently empty.

Legal category POM.

Package quantities Ventide Inhaler is a metered-dose aerosol with a specially designed actuator. Each canister provides 200 inhalations.

Further information Products containing salbutamol do not cause difficulty in micturition because, unlike sympathomimetic drugs such as ephedrine, salbutamol does not stimulate alpha-adrenoreceptors. Salbutamol products are not contra-indicated in patients under treatment with monoamine oxidase inhibitors (MAOIs).

Product licence number 0045/0122.

VENTOLIN* INHALER

Presentation Metered-dose aerosol delivering 100 micrograms Salbutamol BP per actuation, with a specially designed actuator.

Uses Salbutamol BP is a beta-adrenergic stimulant

which has a highly selective action on the receptors in bronchial muscle and, in therapeutic dosage, little or no action on the cardiac receptors.

Salbutamol is also highly active in preventing antigen-induced release of histamine and slow-reacting substance of anaphylaxis, SRS(A), from mast cells in human lung sensitised with IgE antibody. Such Type I hypersensitivity reactions are generally considered to be the primary triggers of the allergic asthma syndrome.

Ventolin Inhaler is, therefore, indicated both for the treatment and prophylaxis of bronchial asthma, and also for the treatment of other conditions, such as bronchitis and emphysema, with associated reversible airways obstruction. Because Ventolin Inhaler is long-acting it is ideally suited for routine maintenance therapy in chronic asthma and chronic bronchitis. The inhaler drug-delivery system, using salbutamol in microgram dosage, avoids the skeletal muscle tremor sometimes associated with oral therapy.

Ventolin Inhaler acts rapidly and may be used when necessary to relieve attacks of acute dyspnoea. Doses may be taken prophylactically before exertion or to prevent exercise-induced asthma.

Because of its selective action on the bronchi and its lack of effects on the cardiovascular system, Ventolin Inhaler is suitable for treating bronchospasm in patients with coexisting heart disease or hypertension, including those taking beta-blocking drugs which often impair respiratory function.

Dosage and administration *Adults:* For the relief of acute bronchospasm and for managing intermittent episodes of asthma, one or two inhalations may be administered as a single dose. The recommended dose for chronic maintenance or prophylactic therapy is two inhalations three or four times a day.

To prevent exercise-induced bronchospasm, two inhalations should be taken before exertion.

Children: One inhalation is the recommended dose for the relief of acute bronchospasm, in the management of episodic asthma or before exercise.

One inhalation should be administered three or four times a day for routine maintenance or prophylactic therapy. These doses may be increased to two inhalations, if necessary.

For optimum results, in most patients, Ventolin Inhaler should be used regularly.

The bronchodilator effect of each administration of inhaled Ventolin lasts for at least four hours, except in patients whose asthma is becoming worse. Such patients should be warned not to increase their usage of inhaler but should seek medical advice in case treatment with an inhaled and/or systemic glucocorticosteroid is indicated.

Contra-indications, warnings, etc
Contra-indications: Although intravenous salbutamol and occasionally salbutamol tablets are used in the management of uncomplicated premature labour, Ventolin presentations should not be used for threatened abortion during the first or second trimesters of pregnancy.

Ventolin Inhaler is contra-indicated in patients with a history of hypersensitivity to any of its components.

Precautions: In the event of a previously effective dose of Ventolin Inhaler failing to give relief for at least three hours, the patient should be advised to seek medical advice in order that any necessary additional steps may

be taken. Ventolin should be administered cautiously to patients suffering from thyrotoxicosis.

Pregnancy: Unnecessary administration of drugs during the first trimester of pregnancy is undesirable.

Side-effects: No important side-effects have been reported following Ventolin Inhaler therapy.

Overdosage: The preferred antidote for overdosage with Ventolin Inhaler is a cardioselective beta-blocking agent, but beta-blocking drugs should be used with caution in patients with a history of bronchospasm.

Pharmaceutical precautions Ventolin Inhaler should be stored in a cool place, protected from frost and direct sunlight. The canister should not be broken, punctured or burnt, even when apparently empty.

Legal category POM.

Package quantities Ventolin Inhaler is a metered-dose aerosol with a specially designed actuator. Each canister provides 200 inhalations.

Further information Ventolin does not cause difficulty in micturition because, unlike sympathomimetic drugs such as ephedrine, it does not stimulate alpha-adrenoceptors. Ventolin is not contra-indicated in patients under treatment with monoamine oxidase inhibitors (MAOIs).

Product licence number 0045/5022R.

VENTOLIN* NEBULES* 2.5 mg ▼

Presentation Ventolin Nebules 2.5 mg are a plastic ampoule presentation containing an aqueous, colourless solution of Salbutamol BP as the sulphate. The concentration, which is expressed in terms of Salbutamol BP is 0.1% (1 mg Salbutamol BP as the sulphate in 1 ml). Each Nebule contains 2.5 ml of solution equivalent to 2.5 mg salbutamol. The solution is adjusted with acid to pH 4.0.

Uses Ventolin Nebules 2.5 mg are indicated for use in the routine management of chronic bronchospasm unresponsive to conventional therapy and in the treatment of acute severe asthma.

Dosage and administration
Adults and children: A suitable starting dose of salbutamol by wet aerosol is 2.5 mg (one Nebule) but this may be increased to 5 mg.

Treatment may be repeated up to four times daily by means of a nebuliser. Delivery of the aerosol may be by face mask or 'T' piece.

Ventolin Nebules 2.5 mg are intended to be used undiluted. However, if prolonged delivery time is desirable (more than 10 minutes) dilution with normal saline for injection may be required.

Contra-indications, warnings, etc
Contra-indications: Although intravenous salbutamol and occasionally salbutamol tablets are used in the management of uncomplicated premature labour, Ventolin presentations should not be used for threatened abortion during the first or second trimesters of pregnancy.

Ventolin Nebules are contra-indicated in patients with a history of hypersensitivity to any of their components.

Precautions: Ventolin Nebules 2.5 mg should be used with care in patients known to have received large doses of other sympathomimetic drugs. They should be administered cautiously to patients suffering from thyrotoxicosis.

Ventolin Nebules 2.5 mg are to be used with a nebuliser, only under the direction of a physician. The solution should not be injected or administered orally.

Patients receiving treatment at home with Ventolin Nebules 2.5 mg must be warned that if either the usual relief is diminished or the usual duration of action reduced, they should not increase the dose or its frequency of administration, but should seek medical advice.

Pregnancy: Unnecessary administration of drugs during the first trimester of pregnancy is undesirable.

Side-effects: A small increase in heart rate may occur in patients who inhale large doses of Ventolin. This is not usually accompanied by any changes in the electrocardiogram.

Other side-effects which occur with very high doses of Ventolin by inhalation are peripheral vasodilatation and fine tremor of skeletal muscle.

Overdosage: The preferred antidote to overdosage with Ventolin Nebules 2.5 mg is a cardioselective beta-blocking agent, but beta-blocking drugs should be used with caution in patients with a history of bronchospasm.

Pharmaceutical precautions
Storage: Ventolin Nebules 2.5 mg should be stored at a temperature below 25°C and protected from light.

Dilution: Ventolin Nebules 2.5 mg may be diluted with Sodium Chloride Injection BP (normal saline). Solutions in nebulisers should be replaced daily.

Legal category POM.

Package quantities Each box contains 20 Nebules in strips of 5.

Further information Ventolin does not cause difficulty in micturition because, unlike sympathomimetic drugs such as ephedrine, it does not stimulate alpha-adrenoceptors. Ventolin is not contra-indicated in patients under treatment with monoamine oxidase inhibitors (MAOIs).

Ventolin Nebules 2.5 mg are suitable for treating bronchospasm in patients with co-existing heart disease or hypertension.

Product licence number 0045/0123.

VENTOLIN* PARENTERAL PREPARATIONS
VENTOLIN* INJECTION 500 microgram (0.5 mg) in 1 ml (500 microgram/ml)
VENTOLIN* INJECTION 250 microgram (0.25 mg) in 5 ml (50 microgram/ml)
VENTOLIN* SOLUTION FOR INTRAVENOUS INFUSION 5 mg in 5 ml (1 mg/ml)

Presentation Ventolin Injection 500 microgram (0.5 mg) in 1 ml (500 microgram/ml) is presented as ampoules of 1 ml each containing 500 microgram Salbutamol BP as Salbutamol Sulphate BP, in a sterile isotonic solution adjusted to pH 3.5 with sulphuric acid.

Ventolin Injection 250 microgram (0.25 mg) in 5 ml (50 microgram/ml) is presented as ampoules of 5 ml each containing 250 microgram Salbutamol BP as Salbutamol Sulphate BP, in a sterile isotonic solution adjusted to pH 3.5 with sulphuric acid.

Ventolin Solution for Intravenous Infusion 5 mg in 5 ml (1 mg/ml) is presented as ampoules of 5 ml each containing 5 mg Salbutamol BP as Salbutamol Sulphate BP, in a sterile isotonic solution adjusted to pH 3.5 with sulphuric acid.

The ampoules are of clear, neutral glass and the solution is colourless or faintly straw coloured.

Uses Salbutamol BP is a beta-adrenergic stimulant that has a selective action on the $beta_2$-adrenoceptors in the bronchi and uterus and much less action on the $beta_1$-adrenoceptors in the heart.

Ventolin parenteral preparations are indicated for two distinct clinical situations:

1. For the relief of severe bronchospasm associated with asthma or bronchitis and for the treatment of status asthmaticus.

2. For the management of uncomplicated premature labour in the last trimester of pregnancy.

Dosage and administration 1. *In severe bronchospasm and status asthmaticus*

Subcutaneous route: Adults: 500 micrograms (8 micrograms/kg body weight) and repeated every four hours as required.

Intramuscular route: Adults: 500 micrograms (8 micrograms/kg body weight) and repeated every four hours as required.

Intravenous route: Adults: 250 micrograms (4 micrograms/kg body weight) injected slowly. If necessary the dose may be repeated. Ventolin Injection 250 microgram in 5 ml (50 microgram/ml) is a suitably dilute preparation for slow intravenous injection, but if Ventolin Injection 500 microgram in 1 ml (500 microgram/ml) is used the injection may be facilitated by dilution with Water for Injections BP.

Infusion: In status asthmaticus, infusion rates of 3–20 micrograms per minute are generally adequate, but in patients with respiratory failure, higher dosage has been used with success. A starting dose of 5 micrograms per minute is recommended with appropriate adjustment in dosage according to patient response.

A suitable solution for infusion may be prepared by diluting 5 ml of Ventolin Solution for Intravenous Infusion in 500 ml of an infusion solution such as Sodium Chloride and Dextrose Injection BP to provide a salbutamol dose of 10 micrograms/ml of solution.

Children: At present there is insufficient evidence to recommend a dosage regimen for routine use in children.

2. *In the management of premature labour*
For this indication Ventolin Solution for Intravenous Infusion is recommended using a solution prepared as in 1. above.

Infusion rates of 10–45 micrograms per minute are generally adequate to control uterine contractions but greater or lesser infusion rates may be required according to the strength and frequency of contractions. A starting rate of 10 micrograms per minute is recommended, increasing the rate at 10-minute intervals until there is evidence of patient response shown by diminution in strength, frequency or duration of contractions. Thereafter the infusion rate may be increased slowly until contractions cease. The maternal pulse rate should be monitored and the infusion rate adjusted to avoid excessive maternal heart rates (above 140 beats per minute). Once uterine contractions have ceased the infusion rate should be maintained at the same level for one hour and then reduced by 50% decrements at six-hourly intervals. Treatment may be continued orally with Ventolin Tablets 4 mg given three or four times daily.

As an alternative procedure or to counteract inadvertent overdosage with oxytocic drugs Ventolin Injection may be administered as a single injection by the intravenous or intramuscular routes. The usual recommended dose is 100–250 micrograms of salbutamol. The dose may be repeated according to the response of the patient.

Note. The contents of the ampoules of Ventolin Solution for Intravenous Infusion must not be injected undiluted.

Ventolin parenteral preparations should not be administered in the same syringe or infusion as any other medication.

Contra-indications, warnings, etc

Contra-indications: Although intravenous salbutamol and occasionally salbutamol tablets are used in the management of uncomplicated premature labour, their use in premature labour associated with toxaemia of pregnancy or antepartum haemorrhage from whatever cause is contra-indicated. Ventolin presentations should not be used for threatened abortion during the first or second trimesters of pregnancy.

Ventolin Parenteral preparations are contra-indicated in patients with a history of hypersensitivity to any of their components.

Precautions: The use of Ventolin parenteral preparations in the treatment of severe bronchospasm or status asthmaticus does not obviate the requirement for glucocorticoid steroid therapy as appropriate. When practicable, administration of oxygen concurrently with parenteral Ventolin is recommended, particularly when it is given by intravenous infusion to hypoxic patients. In common with other beta-adrenoceptor agonists, Ventolin can induce reversible metabolic changes. These are most pronounced during infusions of the drug when an increase in blood glucose is likely. The diabetic patient may be unable to compensate for this and the development of ketoacidosis has been reported. Concurrent administration of corticosteroids can exaggerate this effect. Therefore diabetic patients and those concurrently receiving corticosteroids should be monitored frequently during intravenous infusion of Ventolin so that remedial steps (e.g. an increase in insulin dosage) can be taken to counter any metabolic change occurring. For these patients it may be preferable to dilute Ventolin Solution for Intravenous Infusion in Sodium Chloride Injection BP rather than Sodium Chloride and Dextrose Injection BP.

Ventolin should be administered cautiously to patients suffering from thyrotoxicosis. In patients being treated to inhibit uterine contractions in premature labour by intravenous infusion of salbutamol, increases in maternal heart rate of the order of 20 to 50 beats per minute usually accompany the infusion. The maternal pulse rate should be monitored and not normally allowed to exceed a steady rate of 140 beats per minute. Maternal blood pressure may fall slightly during the infusion; the effect being greater on diastolic than on systolic pressure. Falls in diastolic pressure are usually within the range of 10–20 mmHg. The effect of infusion on fetal heart rate is less marked, but increases of up to 20 beats per minute may occur. In the treatment of premature labour, before Ventolin parenteral preparations are given to any patient with known heart disease, an adequate assessment of the patient's cardiovascular status should be made by a physician experienced in cardiology. Unnecessary administration of drugs during the first trimester of pregnancy is undesirable.

Side-effects: Intramuscular use of the undiluted injection may produce slight pain or stinging. Enhancement of physiological tremor may occur with Ventolin. This effect is caused by a direct action on skeletal muscle and is common to all beta-adrenergic stimulants.

Ventolin parenteral preparations may dilate some peripheral arterioles leading to a small reduction in arterial pressure and a compensatory increase in cardiac rate. Increases in heart rate are more likely to occur in patients with normal heart rates and these increases are dose-dependent. In patients with pre-existing sinus tachycardia, especially those in status asthmaticus, the heart rate tends to fall as the condition of the patient improves.

In the management of premature labour, intravenous infusion of Ventolin has occasionally been associated with nausea, vomiting and headaches.

Overdosage: The preferred antidote for overdosage with Ventolin is a cardioselective beta-blocking agent. Beta-blocking drugs should be used with caution in patients with a history of bronchospasm.

Pharmaceutical precautions Ventolin parenteral preparations may be diluted with Water for Injections BP, Sodium Chloride Injection BP, Sodium Chloride and Dextrose Injection BP or Dextrose Injection BP. These are the only recommended diluents.

Ventolin parenteral preparations should not be administered in the same syringe or infusion as any other medication.

The contents of the ampoule of Ventolin Solution for Intravenous Infusion must not be injected in the undiluted form; the concentration should be reduced by at least 50% before administration.

Storage: Ventolin parenteral preparations should be protected from light and stored at a temperature below 30°C.

Legal category POM.

Package quantities Ventolin Injection 500 microgram (0.5 mg) in 1 ml (500 microgram/ml) is available in boxes of 5 ampoules.

Ventolin Injection 250 microgram (0.25 mg) in 5 ml (50 microgram/ml) is available in boxes of 10 ampoules.

Ventolin Solution for Intravenous Infusion 5 mg in 5 ml (1 mg/ml) is available in boxes of 10 ampoules.

Further information Ventolin does not cause difficulty in micturition because, unlike sympathomimetic drugs such as ephedrine, it does not stimulate alpha-adrenoceptors. Ventolin is not contra-indicated in patients under treatment with monoamine oxidase inhibitors (MAOIs).

Product licence numbers
Ventolin Injection 500 microgram (0.5 mg) in 1 ml
(500 microgram/ml)   0045/0102
Ventolin Injection 250 microgram (0.25 mg) in 5 ml (50 microgram/ml)   0045/0108
Ventolin Solution for Intravenous Infusion 5 mg in 5 ml
(1 mg/ml)   0045/0103

VENTOLIN* RESPIRATOR SOLUTION

Presentation Ventolin Respirator Solution is an aqueous, colourless solution of Salbutamol Sulphate BP adjusted with acid to pH 3.5. The concentration, which is expressed in terms of Salbutamol BP, is 0.5% or 5 mg per ml of solution.

Uses Ventolin Respirator Solution is indicated for the treatment of severe acute asthma (status asthmaticus) and other forms of bronchospasm.

Dosage and administration *1. By intermittent administration. Adults:* Ventolin Respirator Solution 0.5–1.0 ml (2.5–5.0 mg of salbutamol) should be diluted to a final volume of 2.0 to 4.0 ml with normal saline for injection. The resulting solution is inhaled from a suitably driven nebuliser until aerosol generation ceases. Using a correctly matched nebuliser and driving source this should take about ten minutes.

Ventolin Respirator Solution may be used undiluted for intermittent administration. For this, 2.0 ml of Ventolin Respirator Solution (10.0 mg salbutamol) is placed in the nebuliser and the patient allowed to inhale the nebulised solution until bronchodilatation is achieved. This usually takes 3–5 minutes.

Some adult patients may require higher doses of salbutamol, up to 10 mg, in which case nebulisation of the undiluted solution may continue until aerosol generation ceases.

Children: The same mode of administration for intermittent administration is also applicable to children. The usual dosage for children under the age of twelve years is 0.5 ml (2.5 mg salbutamol) diluted to 2.0 to 4.0 ml with normal saline for injection. Some children may however require higher doses of salbutamol up to 5.0 mg.

Intermittent treatment may be repeated four times daily.

2. By continuous administration: Ventolin Respirator Solution is diluted with normal saline for injection to contain 50–100 micrograms of salbutamol per ml, (1–2 ml solution made up to 100 ml with diluent). The diluted solution is administered as an aerosol by a suitably driven nebuliser. The usual rate of administration is 1–2 mg per hour.

Delivery of the aerosol may be by facemask, 'T' piece or via an endotracheal tube. Intermittent positive pressure ventilation may be used but is rarely necessary. When there is a risk of anoxia through hypoventilation, oxygen should be added to the inspired air.

Contra-indications, warnings, etc
Contra-indications: Although intravenous salbutamol and occasionally salbutamol tablets are used in the management of uncomplicated premature labour, Ventolin presentations should not be used for threatened abortion during the first or second trimesters of pregnancy.

Ventolin Respirator Solution is contra-indicated in patients with a history of hypersensitivity to any of its components.

Precautions: Ventolin Respirator Solution should be used with care in patients known to have received large doses of other sympathomimetic drugs.

It should be administered cautiously to patients suffering from thyrotoxicosis.

Ventolin Respirator Solution is to be used with a respirator or nebuliser only, under the direction of a physician. It is not to be injected or administered orally.

Patients receiving treatment at home with Ventolin Respirator Solution must be warned that if either the usual relief is diminished or the usual duration of action reduced, they should not increase the dose or its frequency of administration, but should seek medical advice.

Pregnancy: Unnecessary administration of drugs during the first trimester of pregnancy is undesirable.

Side-effects: A small increase in heart rate may occur in patients who inhale large doses of Ventolin. This is not usually accompanied by any changes in the electrocardiogram. Other side-effects which may occur with very high doses of Ventolin by inhalation are peripheral vasodilatation and fine tremor of skeletal muscle.

Overdosage: During continuous administration of Ventolin Respirator Solution any signs of overdosage can usually be counteracted by withdrawal of the drug.

The preferred antidote for overdosage with Ventolin Respirator Solution is a cardioselective beta-blocking agent, but beta-blocking drugs should be used with caution in patients with a history of bronchospasm.

Pharmaceutical precautions *Storage:* Ventolin Respirator Solution should be stored at a temperature below 25°C and protected from light. Once the bottle has been opened the contents should be discarded after one month.

Dilution: Ventolin Respirator Solution may be diluted with Sodium Chloride Injection BP (normal saline).

Solutions in nebulisers should be replaced daily.

Legal category POM.

Package quantities Ventolin Respirator Solution is supplied in screw-capped bottles of 20 ml.

Further information Ventolin does not cause difficulties in micturition because, unlike sympathomimetic drugs such as ephedrine, it does not stimulate alpha-adrenoceptors. Ventolin is not contra-indicated in patients under treatment with monoamine oxidase inhibitors (MAOIs).

Ventolin Respirator Solution is suitable for treating bronchospasm in patients with coexisting heart disease or hypertension.

Product licence number 0045/5023R.

VENTOLIN* ROTACAPS*

Presentation Ventolin Rotacaps, an alternative inhalation form of salbutamol to Ventolin Inhaler, are especially valuable for treating patients who are unable to use pressurised inhalers effectively or who might use them unwisely.

Ventolin Rotacaps contain a mixture of microfine salbutamol sulphate and larger particle lactose in blue/colourless hard gelatine cartridges. Each Rotacap contains 200 micrograms (light blue) or 400 micrograms (dark blue) of salbutamol (as sulphate) and is marked Ventolin 200 or Ventolin 400. The contents of a Rotacap are inhaled using a specially developed device called a Rotahaler*, which separates the cartridge into halves that rotate and release the drug when the patient inhales. This breath actuation is very sensitive and so the drug is fully available even at the lowest inspiratory flow rates. The Rotahaler is, therefore, a more reliable drug delivery system for many patients, but a rather larger unit dose relative to Ventolin Inhaler is necessary for the same therapeutic effect.

Uses Salbutamol BP is a beta-adrenergic stimulant which has a highly selective action on bronchial beta-adrenoceptors and little or no effect on cardiac beta-receptors at therapeutic doses.

Salbutamol is also highly active in preventing antigen-induced release of histamine and slow-reacting substance of anaphylaxis, SRS(A), from mast cells in human lung sensitised with IgE antibody. Such Type I hypersensitivity reactions are generally considered to be the primary triggers of the allergic asthma syndrome.

Ventolin Rotacaps are therefore indicated both for the treatment and prevention of bronchial asthma, and also for the treatment of other conditions, such as bronchitis and emphysema, with associated reversible airway obstruction. Inhaled salbutamol has a long duration of action and Ventolin Rotacaps are ideally suited for routine maintenance therapy and prophylaxis in chronic asthma, both to relieve persistent bronchospasm and to suppress the allergic response within the lungs. Their regular use is also indicated for controlling persistent bronchospasm in chronic bronchitis.

Ventolin Rotacaps act rapidly and may be used when necessary to relieve attacks of acute dyspnoea. Rotacaps may also be used before exertion to prevent exercise-induced asthma or before exposure to a known unavoidable allergen challenge.

The effective dose of salbutamol from Rotacaps is only one tenth of the usual oral dose and so the skeletal muscle tremor sometimes associated with oral therapy does not occur.

The selective action of salbutamol on the bronchi and its lack of effects on the cardiovascular system make Ventolin Rotacaps particularly suitable for treating patients with coexisting heart disease or hypertension, including those taking beta-blocking drugs which often impair respiratory function.

Dosage and administration Ventolin Rotacaps are for inhalation use only, using a Ventolin Rotahaler.

Adults: For the relief of acute bronchospasm and for managing intermittent episodes of asthma, 200 micrograms or 400 micrograms may be administered as a single dose.

The recommended dose for chronic maintenance or prophylactic therapy is 400 micrograms three or four times a day.

To prevent exercise-induced bronchospasm, 400 micrograms should be taken before exertion.

Children: 200 micrograms is the recommended dose for the relief of acute bronchospasm, in the management of episodic asthma or before exercise.

200 micrograms should be administered three or four times a day for routine maintenance or prophylactic therapy.

For optimum results, in most patients Ventolin Rotacaps should be used regularly.

The bronchodilator effect of each administration of inhaled Ventolin lasts for at least four hours, except in patients whose asthma is becoming worse. Such patients should be warned not to increase their usage of Rotacaps but should seek medical advice in case treatment with an inhaled and/or systemic glucocorticosteroid is indicated.

Contra-indications, warnings, etc
Contra-indications: Although intravenous salbutamol and occasionally salbutamol tablets are used in the management of uncomplicated premature labour, Ventolin presentations should not be used for threatened abortion during the first or second trimesters of pregnancy.

Ventolin Rotacaps are contra-indicated in patients with a history of hypersensitivity to any of their components.

Precautions: In the event of a previously effective dose of inhaled Ventolin failing to give relief lasting at least three hours, the patient should be advised to seek medical advice in order that any necessary additional steps may be taken. Ventolin should be administered cautiously to patients suffering from thyrotoxicosis.

Pregnancy: Unnecessary administration of drugs during the first trimester of pregnancy is undesirable.

Side-effects: No important side effects have been reported following treatment with Ventolin Rotacaps.

Overdosage: The preferred antidote for overdosage with salbutamol is a cardioselective beta-blocking agent, but beta-blocking drugs should be used with caution in patients with a history of bronchospasm.

Pharmaceutical precautions To keep the Rotacaps in good condition it is important that they are stored in a dry place where they will not be exposed to extremes of temperature. A convenient supply may be carried in the special container for the Rotahaler. The Rotacaps should only be inserted in the Rotahaler immediately prior to use. Failure to observe this instruction may affect the operation of the Rotahaler.

Legal category POM.

Package quantities Ventolin Rotacaps 200 micrograms and 400 micrograms are supplied in containers of 100.

Further information Ventolin does not cause difficulty in micturition because, unlike sympathomimetic drugs such as ephedrine, it does not stimulate alpha-adrenoceptors. Ventolin is not contra-indicated in patients under treatment with monoamine oxidase inhibitors (MAOIs).

Product licence numbers
Ventolin Rotacaps 200 micrograms   0045/0116
Ventolin Rotacaps 400 micrograms   0045/0117

VENTOLIN* TABLETS 2 mg and 4 mg
VENTOLIN* SYRUP
VENTOLIN* SPANDETS*

Presentation *Ventolin Tablets 2 mg:* Pink tablets each containing Salbutamol BP 2 mg as sulphate. Engraved VENTOLIN AH around the perimeter of one side and the number 2 in the centre.

Ventolin Tablets 4 mg: Pink tablets each containing Salbutamol BP 4 mg as sulphate. Engraved VENTOLIN AH around the perimeter of one side and the number 4 in the centre.

Ventolin Syrup: Salbutamol BP 2 mg as sulphate in each 5 ml of a fruit-flavoured, sugar-free syrup, which is devoid of artificial colouring agents.

Ventolin Spandets: Salbutamol BP 8 mg as sulphate in a specially designed, two-layered pink and white tablet. Salbutamol is released immediately from the pink layer and gradually from the porous matrix in the white layer. Engraved VENTOLIN SPANDET around the perimeter of one side and AH in the centre.

Uses Salbutamol BP is a beta-adrenergic stimulant which has a highly selective action on the receptors in bronchial muscle and, in therapeutic dosage, little or no action on the cardiac receptors.

Ventolin Tablets 2 mg and 4 mg, Syrup and Spandets

are indicated for the relief of bronchospasm in bronchial asthma of all types, chronic bronchitis and emphysema.

Ventolin Syrup is suitable oral therapy for children or for those adults who prefer liquid medicines.

Ventolin Spandets are sustained-action tablets, particularly suitable when nocturnal bronchospasm is a problem.

Because of their selective action on the bronchi and their lack of effects on the cardiovascular system, Ventolin oral preparations are suitable for treating bronchospasm in patients with coexisting heart disease or hypertension.

The selective action of salbutamol on the β_2-adrenoceptors has led to the use of parenteral Ventolin, usually as a continuous intravenous infusion, for the management of premature labour during the third trimester of pregnancy. Once the uterine contractions have ceased and the infusion of Ventolin has been gradually withdrawn, maintenance therapy can be effected with Ventolin Tablets.

Dosage and administration *Ventolin Tablets 2 mg and 4 mg and Syrup: Adults:* The usual effective dose is 4 mg (one tablet 4 mg or 10 ml of syrup) three or four times per day. If adequate bronchodilation is not obtained each single dose may be gradually increased to as much as 8 mg.

However, it has been established that some patients obtain adequate relief with 2 mg three or four times daily. In elderly patients or in those known to be unusually sensitive to beta-adrenergic stimulant drugs, it is advisable to initiate treatment with 2 mg three or four times per day.

Children: The following doses should be administered three or four times daily:

2–6 years: 1–2 mg as 2.5–5 ml of syrup or $\frac{1}{2}$–1 tablet 2 mg.

6–12 years: 2 mg as 5 ml of syrup or 1 tablet 2 mg.

Over 12 years: 2–4 mg as 1 tablet 2 mg or 1 tablet 4 mg.

The drug is well tolerated by children so that, if necessary, these doses may be cautiously increased.

In the management of premature labour, after uterine contractions have been controlled by intravenous infusion of Ventolin and the infusion has been withdrawn, maintenance therapy can be continued with oral Ventolin. The usual dosage is 4 mg three or four times daily.

Ventolin Spandets: Adults: 1 Spandet night and morning. In severe cases the dose may be increased to 4 Spandets per 24 hours.

Children over 12 years: 1 Spandet every 12 hours.

Ventolin Spandets must be swallowed whole and not chewed.

Contra-indications, warnings, etc

Contra-indications: Although intravenous salbutamol and occasionally salbutamol tablets are used in the management of uncomplicated premature labour, Ventolin presentations should not be used for threatened abortion during the first or second trimesters of pregnancy.

Ventolin oral preparations and beta-blocking drugs, such as propranolol, should not usually be prescribed together.

Ventolin oral preparations are contra-indicated in patients with a history of hypersensitivity to any of their components.

Precautions: Ventolin should be administered cautiously to patients suffering from thyrotoxicosis. Unnecessary administration of drugs during the first trimester of pregnancy is undesirable.

Side-effects: The only side-effect of significance with oral Ventolin is a fine tremor of skeletal muscle which occurs in some patients, usually the hands are most obviously affected. This effect is dose related and is common to all beta-adrenergic stimulants. A few patients feel tense; this is also due to the effects on skeletal muscle and not to direct CNS stimulation. With doses of Ventolin higher than those recommended or in patients who are unusually sensitive to beta-adrenergic stimulants, peripheral vasodilatation and a compensatory small increase in heart rate may occur. Occasionally headaches have been reported.

Overdosage: The preferred antidote for overdosage with Ventolin is a cardioselective beta-blocking agent, but beta-blocking drugs should be used with caution in patients with a history of bronchospasm.

Pharmaceutical precautions *Storage:* Ventolin Tablets 2 mg and 4 mg, Ventolin Spandets and Ventolin Syrup should be stored at a temperature not exceeding 30°C.

Ventolin Syrup should be protected from light.

Dilution: Ventolin Syrup does not contain sugars. It may be diluted with Purified Water BP. The resulting mixture should be protected from light and used within 28 days. A 50% v/v dilution of Ventolin Syrup has been shown to be adequately preserved against microbial contamination. However, to avoid the possibility of introducing excessive microbial contamination, the Purified Water used for dilution should be recently prepared or alternatively it should be boiled and cooled immediately before use. Dilution of Ventolin Syrup with Syrup BP or Sorbitol solution is not recommended as this may result in precipitation of the cellulose thickening agent. Admixture of Ventolin Syrup with other liquid preparations is not recommended.

Legal category POM.

Package quantities Ventolin Tablets 2 mg are supplied in containers of 100 and 500.

Ventolin Tablets 4 mg are supplied in containers of 100 and 500.

Ventolin Syrup is supplied in bottles of 150 ml and 2 litres.

Ventolin Spandets are supplied in containers of 50.

Further information The Syrup preparation does not contain sugars, so it is unlikely to predispose to dental caries with long-term use.

Ventolin does not cause difficulty in micturition because, unlike sympathomimetic drugs such as ephedrine, it does not stimulate alpha-adrenoceptors.

Ventolin is not contra-indicated in patients under treatment with monoamine oxidase inhibitors (MAOIs).

Product licence numbers
Ventolin Tablets 2 mg   0045/5079R
Ventolin Tablets 4 mg   0045/0088
Ventolin Syrup   0045/5024R
Ventolin Spandets   0045/0083

*Trade Mark

Allergan Ltd
Turnpike Road
Cressex Industrial Estate
High Wycombe
Buckinghamshire HP12 3NR

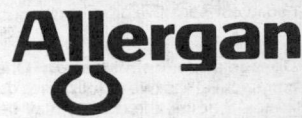

EPIFRIN* 1%

Presentation Clear, colourless to very slightly straw coloured, sterile, aqueous ophthalmic solution containing 1.0% Adrenaline, present as the hydrochloride, and 0.004% benzalkonium chloride as preservative.

Uses Chronic simple glaucoma. In many cases control of intraocular pressure can be obtained when miotics have failed, and is most useful in combination with miotics to obtain better control.

Dosage and administration The usual dosage is one drop in affected eye(s) once daily. However the dosage should be adjusted to meet the needs of the individual patient.

Contra-indications, warnings, etc Should not be used in closed-angle glaucoma, since the dilation of the pupil may precipitate an acute attack. Undesirable side reactions may include eye pain or ache, brow ache, headache, conjunctival hyperemia and allergic lid reactions. Adrenachrome deposits in the conjunctiva and cornea after prolonged adrenaline therapy have been reported. Adrenaline has been reported to produce macular oedema in some aphakic patients and should be used with caution in these patients.

Pharmaceutical precautions Protect from excessive light. If the solution discolours or a precipitate forms it should be discarded.

Legal category POM.

Package quantities Epifrin 1% is available in a 10 ml plastic dropper bottle.

Further information Nil.

Product licence number 0426/0018R.

FML*

Presentation White microfine sterile ophthalmic suspension containing 0.1% fluorometholone and 0.004% benzalkonium chloride as preservative.

Uses Topical ophthalmic suspension for steroid responsive inflammation of the palpebral and bulbar conjunctiva, cornea and anterior segment of the globe.

Dosage and administration 1 to 2 drops instilled into the conjunctival sac two to four times daily. During the initial 24 to 48 hours the dosage may be safely increased to 2 drops every hour. Care should be taken not to discontinue therapy prematurely.

Contra-indications, warnings, etc
Contra-indications: Acute superficial herpes simplex keratitis. Fungal diseases of ocular structures. Vaccinia, varicella and most other viral diseases of the cornea and conjunctiva. Tuberculosis of the eye. Hypersensitivity to the constituents of this medication.

Warnings: Steroid medication in the treatment of herpes simplex keratitis (involving the stroma) requires great caution: frequent slit-lamp microscopy is mandatory. Prolonged use may result in glaucoma, damage to the optic nerve, defects in visual acuity and fields of vision, posterior subcapsular cataract formation, or may aid in the establishment of secondary ocular infections from fungi or viruses liberated from ocular tissue.

In those diseases causing thinning of the cornea or sclera, perforation has been known to occur with use of topical steroids.

Safety and effectiveness have not been demonstrated in children of the age group two years or below.

This preparation contains benzalkonium chloride and should be used with caution in association with hydrophilic contact lenses.

Use in pregnancy: Safety of the use of topical steroids during pregnancy has not been established.

Precautions: As fungal infections of the cornea are particularly prone to develop coincidentally with long-term local steroid applications, fungus invasion must be suspected in any persistent corneal ulceration where a steroid has been used or is in use.

Intraocular pressure should be checked frequently.

Adverse reactions: Glaucoma with optic nerve damage, visual acuity or field defects, posterior subcapsular cataract formation, secondary ocular infection from pathogens liberated from ocular tissues, perforation of the globe.

Local side-effects of steroid therapy, i.e. skin atrophy, striae and telangiectasia, are especially likely to affect facial skin.

Pharmaceutical precautions Protect from freezing.

Legal category POM.

Package quantities Supplied in plastic dropper bottles of 5 ml and 10 ml.

Further information Nil.

Product licence number 0426/0028.

FML-NEO*

Presentation Sterile, white, microfine ophthalmic suspension containing fluorometholone NF 0.1% and neomycin sulphate, BP 0.5% (equivalent to 0.35% neomycin base).

Uses FML-Neo is indicated for the management of steroid responsive inflammation of the palpebral or bulbar conjunctiva, cornea and anterior segment of the globe, when threatened or complicated by infection with neomycin-sensitive organisms.

Dosage and administration One to two drops in the conjunctival sac two to four times daily. During the initial 24 to 48 hours, the dosage may be safely increased to one drop every hour. Care should be taken not to discontinue treatment prematurely. Shake well before using.

Contra-indications, warnings, etc Acute untreated purulent ocular infections. Acute superficial herpes simplex (dendritic keratitis), vaccinia, varicella and most other viral diseases of the conjunctiva and cornea. Ocular tuberculosis, fungal diseases of the eye and hypersensitivity to any of the components of the drug.

Warnings: In diseases due to micro-organisms resistant to neomycin, infection may be masked, enhanced or activated by the steroid. Prolonged use may result in overgrowth of nonsusceptible organisms.

Articles in current medical literature indicate an increase in the prevalence of persons sensitive to neomycin. The possibility of such a reaction should be borne in mind.

If sensitivity or other untoward reactions occur, discontinue the medication.

As fungal infections of the cornea have been reported coincidentally with long-term steroid applications, fungal invasion may be suspected in any persistent corneal ulceration where a steroid has been used, or is in use, over a prolonged period of time.

In those diseases causing thinning of the cornea, perforation has been known to have occurred with the use of topical steroids.

Acute purulent untreated infections of the eye may be masked, enhanced or activated by the presence of steroid medication. Secondary ocular infection may occur from pathogens liberated from ocular tissues.

Use of steroid medication in the presence of stromal herpes simplex requires great caution; frequent slit lamp microscopy is required.

Reports in the literature indicate that posterior subcapsular lenticular opacities have occurred after heavy or protracted use of topical ophthalmic corticosteroids.

Eye drops containing corticosteroids should not be used for more than one week except under strict ophthalmic supervision with regular determination of intraocular pressure.

This preparation contains benzalkonium chloride and should be used with caution in association with hydrophilic contact lenses.

Precautions: Patients with histories of herpes simplex keratitis should be treated with caution. Use of topical steroids may increase intraocular pressure.

Safety of intensive or protracted use of topical steroids during pregnancy has not been substantiated.

Local side effects of steroid therapy, i.e. skin atrophy, striae and telangiectasia, are especially likely to affect facial skin.

Pharmaceutical precautions Shake well before using. Do not freeze.

Legal category POM.

Package quantities Available in 5 ml plastic dropper bottles.

Further information Nil.

Product licence number 0426/0043.

KERECID* OPHTHALMIC OINTMENT
KERECID* OPHTHALMIC SOLUTION

Presentation An off-white, translucent ophthalmic ointment containing 0.5% w/w idoxuridine.

A clear, colourless and odourless aqueous ophthalmic solution containing 0.1% w/v idoxuridine, 0.004% benzalkonium chloride as a preservative with Liquifilm* (polyvinyl alcohol) 1.4%.

Uses Kerecid is an antiviral agent active against herpes simplex virus and certain other DNA viruses. It is indicated in herpes simplex keratitis, particularly in acute dendritic ulcers; infections with stromal involvement may respond less favourably.

Dosage and administration Adults and children.

Kerecid ophthalmic ointment: Apply approximately every 4 hours, five times a day, with the last dose at bedtime. The ointment should be placed inside the conjunctival sac of the infected eye.

Kerecid ophthalmic solution: For optimal results, the infected tissues should be kept 'saturated' with Kerecid ophthalmic solution. One of the following schedules is recommended:

1. Instil one drop in the infected eye(s) every hour during the day. At night, the dosage may be reduced to one drop every other hour.

2. Instil one drop every minute for 5 minutes. This schedule should be repeated every 4 hours – night and day.

To minimise recurrences, continue treatment for five to seven days after healing appears to be complete, that is, after complete loss of corneal staining with fluorescein. Treatment should not usually be continued for more than 21 days.

Observe patients frequently during treatment. Improvement in dendritic keratitis and other superficial infections is generally seen within a week, but may occasionally occur much earlier. Some strains of herpes simplex virus appear resistant to the action of idoxuridine. If superficial infections show no sign of improvement after seven to eight days, alternative treatment is indicated. A faint dendritic pattern in the deeper epithelial layers that neither stains nor produces symptoms may persist for two to four weeks. This does not indicate failure of treatment or a need for continued therapy.

Antibiotics may be used to control secondary infections; and atropine preparations may be given if needed. Do not, however, mix Kerecid ophthalmic solution with these adjuvant medications.

Contra-indications, warnings, etc

Contra-indications: Hypersensitivity to the active ingredient or other components of this medication. Do not administer boric acid during treatment as it may cause irritation in the presence of Kerecid.

Precautions: Caution is required with concomitant use of topical corticosteroids which may encourage the spread of viral infection. They should not be used in the presence of active corneal ulceration, but may be considered when the stromal disease seriously affects vision, or when oedema or uveitis is present. Kerecid should be continued for several days after corticosteroid treatment has been completed.

In common with other antiviral agents, idoxuridine is potentially mutagenic.

Use in pregnancy: One isolated study has indicated that idoxuridine may have embryotoxic effects in rabbits, but these effects were not confirmed in extensive repeat studies. Other work has shown very high parenteral doses to be embryotoxic in mice and rats. Kerecid* has been available since 1963 and no other experimental or clinical evidence of any associated hazard to the foetus has emerged. While local application to the eye is unlikely to produce significant levels within the body, Kerecid should not be administered in pregnancy unless essential, especially during the first trimester; or in women with childbearing potential.

Adverse reactions: Transient irritation and pain on administration may occur; itching, inflammation, oedema and, rarely, allergic reactions and occlusions of the lachrymal puncta, have been reported.

Overdosage: Excessive use may damage the corneal epithelium. Toxic effects are unlikely to follow ingestion.

Pharmaceutical precautions Store ophthalmic ointment at a temperature not exceeding 30°C. Store ophthalmic solution at controlled room temperature (15–30°C) and protect from light. The contents are sterile until the pack is opened; discard any unused contents one month after opening.

Legal category POM.

Package quantities Ophthalmic ointment in tubes of 4 g. Ophthalmic solution in polythene bottles with integral dropper, each containing 15 ml.

Further information Nil.

Product licence numbers
Kerecid ophthalmic ointment   0426/0055
Kerecid ophthalmic solution   0426/0019

LACRI-LUBE*

Presentation Sterile, bland, non-medicated ophthalmic ointment, for topical administration to humans, containing white petrolatum mineral oil, non-ionic lanolin derivatives with chlorobutanol 0.5% as a preservative.

Uses Useful as adjunctive therapy to lubricate and protect the eye in conditions characterized by exposive keratitis, decreased corneal sensitivity, recurrent corneal erosions, keratitis sicca.

Dosage and administration For topical administration. Pull lower lid down to form pocket. Apply small amount as needed.

Contra-indications, warnings, etc No known contra-indications.

Pharmaceutical precautions Store away from heat. To avoid contamination during use, do not touch tip to any surface.

Legal category P.

Package quantities Available in 3.5 g ophthalmic ointment tubes.

Further information Nil.

Product licence number 0426/0041.

LIQUIFILM* TEARS

Presentation Clear, colourless to slightly straw coloured, sterile, aqueous ophthalmic solution, containing 1.4% polyvinyl alcohol and 0.5% chlorobutanol as preservative.

Uses For dry eyes, especially where natural mucus is absent, or deficient, also as an ocular lubricant.

Dosage and administration 1 drop in the eye as needed, or as directed.

Contra-indications, warnings, etc Not for use with soft contact lenses. If irritation increases or persists, discontinue use.

Pharmaceutical precautions Nil.

Legal category P.

Package quantities Liquifilm Tears is available in plastic dropper bottles containing 15 ml.

Further information Nil.

Product licence number 0426/0009.

PROPINE* ▼

Presentation Sterile ophthalmic solution containing dipivefrin hydrochloride (0.1%).

Uses For the control of intraocular pressure in chronic open angle glaucoma or ocular hypertensive patients with anterior chamber open angles.

Dosage and administration The usual dosage is one drop in the affected eye(s) every 12 hours.

Contra-indications, warnings, etc
Use in pregnancy: The safety of the intensive or protracted use of dipivefrin during pregnancy has not been substantiated.
Contra-indications: Patients suffering from closed angle glaucoma.
Precautions: Dipivefrin should be used with caution in patients with narrow angles since dilation of the pupil may trigger an attack of angle closure glaucoma. Macular oedema is a rare occurrence with adrenaline use in aphakic patients. Prompt reversal generally follows discontinuance of the drug. Macular oedema with dipivefrin does present as a possibility in the aphakic patient.
Adverse reactions: Rebound vasodilation and allergic blepharoconjunctivitis are rarely observed following treatment with dipivefrin. Dipivefrin has been used successfully in patients who have demonstrated such intolerance to adrenaline. Adrenochrome deposits have been rarely observed following the use of dipivefrin. Very slight transitory stinging may occur upon instillation in some patients.

This product contains benzalkonium chloride and should not be used in conjunction with soft contact lenses.

Pharmaceutical precautions Store at a temperature of 4–23°C; however, it can be stored for up to 30°C for a short period of time (a few days).

Legal category POM.

Package quantities Supplied in plastic dropper bottles containing 10 ml.

Further information Nil.

Product licence number 0426/0040.

*Trade Mark

American Hospital Supply (UK) Limited
Wallingford Road
Compton, Nr Newbury
Berkshire RG16 0QW

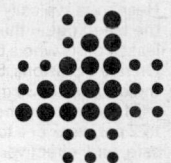

HESPAN* ▼

Presentation Hespan is a 6% colloidal solution for plasma volume expansion.

Composition:
Each 100 ml contains:

Hestastarch	6.0 g
Sodium Chloride BP	0.9 g
Water for Injections BP	qs

pH adjusted with Sodium Hydroxide. Concentration of Electrolytes (mEq/litre): Sodium 154, Chloride 154. pH: Approx. 5.5.
Calculated Osmolarity: Approx. 310 mOsm/litre

Weight average molecular weight	450,000
Number average molecular weight	70,000
Degree of substitution	0.7

Description: Hetastarch is an artificial colloid derived from a waxy starch composed almost entirely of amylopectin. Hydroxyethyl ether groups are introduced into the glucose units of the starch and the resultant material is hydrolyzed to yield a product with a molecular weight suitable for use as a plasma expander. Clinical Hetastarch is characterized by its molecular weight and its degree of substitution. The weight average molecular weight is approximately 450,000 with 90% of the polymer units falling within the range of 10,000 to 1,000,000. The degrees of substitution is 0.7 which means Hetastarch has 7 hydroxyethyl groups for every 10 glucose units. The polymerized glucose units in Hetastarch are joined primarily by 1–4 linkages with hydroxyethyl groups being attached primarily at the No. 2 position. The polymer closely resembles glycogen.

The Hetastarch dosage form is a clear, pale yellow to amber solution. Exposure to prolonged adverse storage conditions (temperatures above 25°C or below freezing) may result in a change to turbid deep brown or the formation of a crystalline precipitate. Do not use the solution if these conditions are evident.

Uses *Actions:* The colloidal properties of 6% Hetastarch approximate those of human albumin. Intravenous infusion of Hetastarch results in expansion of plasma volume slightly in excess of the volume infused, which decreases from this maximum over the succeeding 24 to 36 hours. This expansion of plasma volume may improve the haemodynamic status for 24 hours and longer.

Hetastarch molecules below 50,000 molecular weight are rapidly eliminated by renal excretion with approximately 40% of a given total dose appearing in the urine in 24 hours. This is a variable process but generally results in an intravascular Hetastarch concentration of less than 1% of the total dose injected by two weeks. The hydroxyethyl group is not cleaved by the body, but remains intact and attached to glucose units when excreted.

The addition of Hetastarch to whole blood increases the erythrocyte sedimentation rate. Therefore, Hetastarch is used to improve the efficiency of granulocyte collection by centrifugal means.

Indications:
(1) As a plasma volume expander in cases of hypovolaemia due to:
   (a) Haemorrhage
   (b) Acute trauma
   (c) Burns
   (d) Sepsis
   (e) Water and electrolyte loss in acute gastrointestinal disturbances
   (f) Surgery
(2) Leucapheresis
(3) Extracorporeal circulation

Contra-indications, warnings, etc There are no absolute contraindications to the use of Hespan but Hespan should be used with caution in patients with established renal failure since Hespan is excreted primarily in the urine. In common with all plasma volume expanders, Hespan can produce dilutional effects on fibrinogen and prothrombin activity. In large volumes Hespan may alter the coagulation mechanism and produce a transient prolongation of the clotting time. Hespan should be used with caution in patients with severe bleeding disorders.

Hespan should be used with caution in patients vulnerable to vascular overloading (congestive cardiac failure, renal disease, etc.). Caution should be observed before administering Hespan to patients with a history of liver disease in view of slightly raised indirect bilirubin levels observed on very rare occasions in volunteers.

Hespan is non-antigenic, nor is its administration associated with raised plasma histamine levels. Mild allergic or sensitivity reactions have been occasionally reported consisting of peri-orbital oedema, urticaria or wheezing. If such reactions occur, they are readily controlled by discontinuation of the drug and, if necessary, administration of an antihistaminic agent.

Dosage and administration
Plasma volume expansion: Hespan should be administered by intravenous infusion only, in an initial volume approximately equal to half the estimated blood loss.

In adults the amount usually administered is 500 ml to 1,000 ml. Total dosage does not usually exceed 1,500 ml per day or 20 ml per kg of bodyweight for a typical 70 kg patient, but in common with other colloids, the limiting dose will depend on circulating volume and haematocrit.

In acute haemorrhagic shock, an initial administration rate approximately 20 ml/kg/hr may be recommended; in burns or septic shock, it is usually administered at slower rates. However, both the rate of infusion and the total dosage will be dependent upon the condition of the patient.

Leucapheresis: In leucapheresis procedures 250–700 ml Hespan is typically added to the Y junction just above the bleed out in the ratio of 1 part citrated Hespan to at least 8 parts whole blood; ratios of 1:20 have been used. On rare occasions, 500 ml Hespan has been infused into the donors 15–30 minutes before collection.

Multiple leucapheresis procedures using Hespan of up to 2 per week or a total of 7–10 have been reported to be safe and effective. The safety of more frequent or a greater number of procedures has not yet been established.

Pharmaceutical precautions The safety and compatability of additives have not been established.

Handling and Storage: Follow instructions for use of Steriflex bags: (instruction leaflet enclosed with package insert/data sheet).

Do not freeze. Do not store above 25°C.

Legal category POM.

Package quantities Hespan is supplied in 500 ml Steriflex bags.

Further information Intravenous infusion of Hydroxyethyl starch results in expansion of plasma volume slightly in excess of the volume infused which decreases from this maximum over the succeeding 24–36 hours.

Isovolaemic substitution with Hespan up to 20% does not interfere with cross-matching determinations. Higher dilutions may lead to rouleaux formation which can easily be distinguished from agglutination by the addition of isotonic saline solution.

Usage in pregnancy: Reproduction studies have been done in mice with no evidence of fetal damage. Relevance to humans is not known since Hetastarch has not been given to pregnant women. Therefore, it should not be used in pregnant women, particularly during early pregnancy, unless in the judgement of the physician the potential benefits outweigh the potential hazards.

Usage in Children: No data available pertaining to use in children.

Hespan is also known as Volex or Plasmasteril.

Product licence number 2737/0042.

INTROPIN*

Presentation Intropin 800 mg/5 ml ampoules; each ml contains 160 mg dopamine hydrochloride and 1% sodium bisulphite. Intropin 200 mg/5 ml ampoules and prefilled syringes; each ml contains 40 mg dopamine hydrochloride and 1% sodium bisulphite. The solutions are clear and practically colourless.

Uses *Actions:* Intropin exerts its beneficial haemodynamic effects by its action on different receptors; at 1–5 mcg/kg/min Intropin dilates the renal and mesenteric vascular beds by its unique action on 'dopaminergic' receptors, causing increases in glomerular filtration rate, renal blood flow, sodium excretion, and urine output.

At 5–20 mcg/kg/min Intropin exerts a direct inotropic effect on the myocardium causing dose related increases in cardiac output with minimal effect on heart rate. Blood pressure usually rises and further increases in the urine output are seen.

At 20 mcg/kg/min and above there are further increases in cardiac output and Intropin raises blood pressure by its alpha adrenergic action on peripheral blood vessels, however, even at these doses, renal blood flow is higher than prior to therapy.

Preparation: Transfer 800 mg Intropin by aseptic technique to 500 ml of one of the following sterile intravenous solutions:

1. Sodium Chloride Injection
2. 5% Dextrose Injection
3. 5% Dextrose and 0.9% Sodium Chloride Injection
4. 5% Dextrose in 0.45% Sodium Chloride Solution
5. 5% Dextrose in Lactated Ringer Solution
6. Sodium Lactate (1/6 Molar) Injection
7. Lactated Ringer's Injection.

This gives a concentration of 1,600 micrograms/ml of Intropin.

Intropin is stable for a minimum of 24 hours after dilution in the above solutions, however dilution should be made just before administration.

Do NOT add Intropin to 5% sodium bicarbonate or other alkaline solution since the drug is inactivated.

Administration: Intropin, after dilution, is administered intravenously through an intravenous catheter or needle in as large a vein as possible. An I.V. drip chamber or infusion pump is essential for controlling the infusion rate in drops/minute. The infusion rate should be titrated to the optimum patient response and constantly evaluated in terms of patient's changing condition.

Indications: Intropin is indicated for the correction of poor perfusion, low cardiac output, impending renal failure and shock associated with: Myocardial infarction, Trauma, Endotoxic septicaemia, Open heart surgery, Heart failure.

Dosage and administration *Warning:* This is a potent drug. It must be diluted before administration.

Dosage: Where appropriate, restoration of blood volume with a suitable plasma expander should be started or completed before Intropin therapy. Begin infusion of Intropin therapy at 2 mcg/kg/min in patients who are likely to respond to modest increments in heart force and renal perfusion. In more seriously ill patients begin infusion of Intropin at 5 mcg/kg/min, and in both cases the infusion rate should be titrated upwards in 5–10 mcg/kg/min increments until the optimum dose for the patient is achieved as judged by increases in blood pressure, urine flow, and perfusion generally. Doses of 50 mcg/kg/min and above have been successfully used, although urine output should be checked frequently, and should it fall, dosage reduction of Intropin should be considered.

Contra-indications, warnings, etc

Contra-indications: Intropin should not be used in patients with phaeochromocytoma.

Warnings: Intropin should not be used in the presence of uncorrected tachyarrhythmias or ventricular fibrillation.

Patients who have been treated with monoamine oxidase (MAO) inhibitors prior to Intropin should be given reduced doses; the starting dose should be one tenth ($\frac{1}{10}$) of the usual dose.

Usage in Pregnancy: Animal studies have shown no evidence of teratogenic effects with Intropin. The drug may be used in pregnant women when the expected benefits outweigh the potential risk to the foetus.

Usage in children: The safety and efficacy of Intropin use in children has not been established.

Precautions: Hypovolaemia should be corrected where necessary prior to Intropin infusion. Vasoconstriction can occur due to the alpha adrenergic actions of Intropin, especially in patients with a history of occlusive vascular disease. If desired, this condition can be rapidly reversed by dose reduction or discontinuing the infusion, since Intropin has a half-life of less than 2 minutes in the body.

Extravasation of Intropin at the infusion site can cause local vasoconstriction, hence the desirability of infusing into a large vein. The resulting ischaemia can be reversed by infiltration of the affected area with 10–15 ml of saline containing 5 to 10 mg phentolamine mesylate. A syringe with a fine hypodermic needle should be used to liberally infiltrate the ischaemic area as soon as extravasation is noted.

Adverse reactions: Adverse reactions to Intropin are entirely related to its pharmacological action; immune mediated reactions are not seen since dopamine is a normal body product. The most frequently reported reactions to Intropin have been ectopic beats, tachycardia, anginal pain, palpitations, dyspnoea, nausea, vomiting, hypotension and vasoconstriction. Very rarely reported reactions include aberrant conduction, bradycardia, piloerection, widened QRS complex, azotaemia and hypertension. Vomiting is rare with Intropin, but should it occur, electrolyte replacement should be given.

Overdosage: Accidental overdosage as evidenced by excessive blood pressure elevation can be controlled by dose reduction or discontinuing the Intropin infusion for a short period, since the duration of action of Intropin is short.

Should these measures fail, an infusion of phentolamine mesylate should be considered.

Pharmaceutical precautions Do not add Intropin to 5% sodium bicarbonate or other alkaline solution since the drug is inactivated. Protect from light, do not use if discoloured. Avoid contact with solutions of alkalis.

Legal category POM.

Package quantities Ampoules containing 200 mg dopamine hydrochloride, 20 ampoules per outer carton. Ampoules containing 800 mg dopamine hydrochloride 20 ampoules per outer carton. Pre-filled syringes containing 200 mg dopamine hydrochloride, 5 syringes per outer carton.

Further information Nil.

Product licence numbers
Intropin 200 mg   2737/0040
Intropin 800 mg   2737/0043

TRIDIL*

Presentation Tridil 50 mg is supplied as a sterile, non-pyrogenic, practically colourless solution containing 5 mg/ml nitroglycerin in 30% alcohol and 30% propylene glycol and water for injection. Each 10 ml ampoule contains 50 mg nitroglycerin for intravenous infusion.

Tridil 5 mg is supplied as a sterile, non-pyrogenic solution containing 0.5 mg/ml nitroglycerin stabilized by alcohol BP 10% v/v, lactose and monobasic sodium phosphate. Each 10 ml glass ampoule contains 5 mg nitroglycerin for intravenous use.

Actions: Nitroglycerin causes relaxation of vascular smooth muscle. In a dose related manner nitroglycerin produces dilatation of both the arterial and venous vascular beds, however, the venous effects predominate. Dilatation of the post capillary vessels including large veins results in peripheral pooling and a reduction in venous return. Therapeutic doses of Tridil given intravenously produce a reduction in left ventricular end diastolic volume, left ventricular end diastolic pressure and myocardial wall tension. Myocardial oxygen consumption, as measured by the rate pressure product and tension time index is decreased.

Pulmonary vascular resistance, systemic vascular resistance and arterial pressure are all reduced by Tridil administration. Although the predominant clinical benefits result from the peripheral venodilating effects and the resultant reduction in myocardial oxygen demand, some effect on oxygen supply may occur by direct coronary vasodilatation. A re-distribution of blood from normal to ischaemic areas of the myocardium has been demonstrated.

Uses *Surgery:* Tridil may be used for the prompt control of hypertension encountered during cardiac surgery.

Tridil may be used to reduce blood pressure and maintain controlled hypotension during surgical procedures.

Tridil may be used to control myocardial ischaemia during and after cardiovascular surgery.

Unresponsive Congestive Cardiac Failure Secondary to Acute Myocardial Infarction: Tridil may be used to reduce elevated left ventricular filling pressure in patients with unresponsive congestive cardiac failure secondary to acute myocardial infarction.

Unstable Angina: Tridil infusion can reduce myocardial oxygen demand in proportion to the reduction in pre-load and after-load. Tridil may be indicated for the control of anginal episodes in patients with unstable angina who are refractory to treatment with standard therapy.

Patients with recurrent myocardial ischaemia not responsive to beta-blockers or sublingual nitrates may benefit from the intravenous Tridil infusion prior to surgery or angiography.

Frequent monitoring of blood pressure and pulse rate are recommended during the infusion.

Dosage and administration Tridil is a concentrated pharmacological drug which should be diluted in 5% Dextrose in Water or 0.9% Sodium Chloride prior to its infusion.

It is recommended that the drug is diluted to give a final concentration of 400 mcg/ml or less according to the dosage requirements of the patient. Most patients respond to doses between 10–200 mcg/min, although doses up to 400 mcg/min may be required during some surgical procedures.

Compatibility: (See also Pharmaceutical Precautions) Tridil is compatible with glass infusion bottles. Tridil has also been shown to be compatible with certain rigid infusion packs made of polyethylene; these include the Boots polyfusor and the bottlepack distributed by Dylade, Cheshire U.K. (bottlepak; flatpak) or Antigen Ltd., Roscrea, S. Ireland (Braun). Tridil can be administered as an infusion using one of these recommended infusion bottles/packs.

Tridil is not compatible with infusion bags made from PVC and loss of activity in excess of 40% may occur if contact between nitroglycerin and polyvinylchloride is prolonged. It is therefore recommended that contact with PVC bags is avoided. Some loss of activity can also occur through the infusion sets but the clinical response should be used to determine the rate of infusion and thus the dosage of the drug required by the patient.

An alternative method of administration is via a syringe pump. Tridil can be infused slowly via a syringe pump using a glass syringe or rigid plastic syringe (Gillette Sabre syringe, Brunswick Disposable, B.D. plastipak syringes). A high pressure polyethylene tubing known to be compatible with nitroglycerin is the Lectrocath tubing, Vygon, Gloucester.

The chosen method of administration should ensure that the drug is given at a constant Infusion rate.

Dosage: The recommended dosage range is 10–200 mcg/min. Doses in excess of these have been used and up to 400 mcg/min may be required during some surgical procedures.

Clinical assessment and frequent monitoring of blood pressure are essential to maintain the appropriate infusion rate. Where available, measurement of pulmonary capillary wedge pressure and cardiac output can be used to titrate dosage to response.

Surgery: For the control of hypertensive episodes the recommended starting dose is 25 mcg/min increasing in steps of 25 mcg/min at 5 minute intervals until the desired drop in B.P. is achieved. Although most patients respond to doses between 10–200 mcg/min, doses up to 400 mcg/min have been required during some surgical procedures. In the treatment of perioperative myocardial ischaemia, the recommended starting dose is 15–20 mcg/min increasing in steps of 10–15 mcg/min until the desired effect is achieved.

Unresponsive Congestive Cardiac Failure Secondary to Acute Myocardial Infarction: The recommended starting dose is 20–25 mcg/min which can be decreased to 10 mcg/min or increased in steps of 20–25 mcg/min at 15–30 minute intervals until the desired effect is achieved.

Unstable angina: The recommended starting dose is 10 mcg/min increasing in steps of 5–10 mcg/min at approximately 30 minute intervals.

Children: The safety and efficacy of Tridil has not been established in children.

Contra-indications, warnings, etc Tridil should not be given to patients with known hypersensitivity to nitrates.

Tridil should not be used in patients with marked anaemia, severe cerebral haemorrhage, uncorrected hypovolaemia or severe hypotension.

Tridil should be used with caution in patients suffering from hypothyroidism, malnutrition, severe liver or renal disease or hypothermia.

Safety for intracoronary injection has not been shown.

As with all vasodilators, Tridil should be used with caution in patients predisposed to closed angle glaucoma.

As the safety of Tridil during pregnancy and lactation has not been established, it should not be used unless considered essential by the physician.

Adverse reactions to nitrates may include hypotension, tachycardia, nausea, retching, diaphoresis, apprehension, headache, restlessness, muscle twitching, retrosternal discomfort, palpitations, dizziness, and abdominal pain. Paradoxical bradycardia has occasionally been observed.

Mild overdosage usually resulting in hypotension and tachycardia can be reversed by elevating the legs or decreasing or terminating the infusion. If severe, intravenous administration of methoxamine or phenylephrine is recommended.

Pharmaceutical precautions Opened ampoules should be used immediately and any unused diluted drug should be discarded.

Tridil solution is stable for at least 24 hours at room temperature in glass or recommended plastic containers (see compatibility). Considerable losses of nitroglycerin will occur if Tridil is in contact with polyvinylchloride (PVC) plastic infusion bags and therefore contact with PVC should be avoided. Tridil should therefore be administered in the recommended infusion bottles/packs or via a syringe pump.

Protect from strong light. Do not use if discoloured.

Legal category POM.

Package quantities Tridil 50 mg is available as either a Tridilkit (incorporating one 10 ml ampoule and a compatible infusion set—Tridilset) or in a box containing four 10 ml ampoules.

Tridil 5 mg is available in a box containing twenty 10 ml ampoules.

Further information Experience so far has shown that when given by slow infusion, the onset of action occurs within approximately 3–5 minutes.

Nitroglycerin is also known as glyceryl trinitrate, trinitroglycerin and trinitrin.

Product licence numbers
Tridil 5 mg   2737/0041
Tridil 50 mg   2737/0046

*Trade Mark

Anaquest Ltd
Dorcan Complex
Faraday Road
Swindon
Wiltshire SN3 5JB

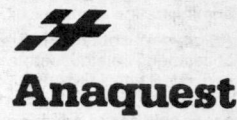

Anaquest

ÆRRANE* ▼

Presentation Ærrane (isoflurane) is a nonflammable general inhalation anaesthetic agent. Ærrane (isoflurane), which is a clear liquid, is packaged in 100 ml amber-coloured bottles.

Uses Ærrane (isoflurane) may be used for induction and maintenance of general anaesthesia. Adequate data have not been developed to establish its application in obstetrical anaesthesia.

Dosage and administration Induction and recovery from Ærrane (isoflurane) anaesthesia are rapid. Isoflurane has a mild pungency, which limits the rate of induction, although excessive salivation or tracheobronchial secretions do not appear to be stimulated. Pharyngeal and laryngeal reflexes are readily obtunded. The level of anaesthesia may be changed rapidly with isoflurane.

Premedication: Premedication should be selected according to the need of the individual patient, taking into account that secretions are weakly stimulated by Ærrane (isoflurane) and the heart rate tends to be increased. The use of anticholinergic drugs is a matter of choice.

Inspired concentration: The concentration of isoflurane being delivered from a vaporizer during anaesthesia should be known. This may be accomplished by using:
(a) vaporizers calibrated specifically for isoflurane;
(b) vaporizers from which delivered flows can be calculated, such as vaporizers delivering a saturated vapour which is then diluted. The delivered concentration from such a vaporizer may be calculated using the formula

$$\% \text{ isoflurane} = \frac{100 \, Pv \, Fv}{Ft \, (Pa - Pv)}$$

where: Pa = Pressure of atmosphere
Pv = Vapour pressure of isoflurane
Fv = Flow of gas through vaporizer (ml)
Ft = Total gas flow (ml)

Isoflurane contains no stabiliser. Nothing in the agent alters calibration or operation of these vaporizers.

Induction: Because of its mild pungency, induction with isoflurane in oxygen or in combination with oxygen-nitrous oxide mixtures may produce coughing, breath holding, or laryngospasm. These difficulties may be avoided by the use of a hypnotic dose of an ultra-short-acting barbiturate. Inspired concentrations of 1.5 to 3% isoflurane usually produce surgical anaesthesia in 7 to 10 minutes.

Maintenance: Surgical levels of anaesthesia may be sustained with a 1.0–2.5% concentration when nitrous oxide is used concomitantly. An additional 0.5% to 1.0% may be required when isoflurane is given using oxygen alone. If added relaxation is required, supplemental doses of muscle relaxants may be used.

The level of blood pressure during maintenance is an inverse function of isoflurane concentration in the absence of other complicating problems. Excessive decreases may be due to depth of anaesthesia and in such instances may be corrected by lightening anaesthesia.

Ærrane (isoflurane) does not sensitise the myocardium to exogenously administered adrenaline in the dog. Limited data indicate that subcutaneous injection of 0.25 ml of adrenaline (50 ml of 1.200,000 solution) does not produce an increase in ventricular arrhythmias in patients anaesthetized with isoflurane. At surgical levels of anaesthesia Ærrane (isoflurane) does not produce any change in EEG convulsive activity.

Ærrane (isoflurane) undergoes minimal biotransformation in man. In the post-anaesthesia period, only 0.17% of the isoflurane taken up can be recovered as urinary metabolites.

Contra-indications, warnings, etc
Contra-indications: Known sensitivity to Ærrane (isoflurane) or to other halogenated agents. Known or suspected genetic susceptibility to malignant hyperthermia.

Warnings: Since levels of anaesthesia may be altered easily and rapidly, only vaporizers producing predictable concentrations should be used. Hypotension and respiratory depression increase as anaesthesia is deepened.

Increased blood loss comparable to that seen with halothane has been observed in patients undergoing abortions.

Ærrane (isoflurane) markedly increases cerebral blood flow at deeper levels of anaesthesia. There may be a transient rise in cerebral spinal fluid pressure which is fully reversible with hyperventilation.

Precautions
General: Ærrane (isoflurane) is a profound respiratory depressant. Respiration must be monitored closely and supported when necessary. As anaesthetic dose is increased, tidal volume decreases and respiratory rate is unchanged. This depression is partially reversed by surgical stimulation, even at deeper levels of anaesthesia. Blood pressure decreases with induction of anaesthesia but returns towards normal during surgical stimulation. Progressive increases in depth of anaesthesia produce corresponding decreases in blood pressure. Nitrous oxide diminishes the inspiratory concentration of isoflurane required to reach a desired level of anaesthesia and may reduce the arterial hypotension seen with isoflurane alone. Heart rhythm remains stable.

Drug interactions: Isoflurane potentiates the muscle relaxant effect of all muscle relaxants, most notably non-depolarizing muscle relaxants, and MAC (minimum alveolar concentration) is reduced by concomitant administration of nitrous oxide.

Pregnancy: Isoflurane has been shown to have a possible anaesthetic-related foetotoxic effect in mice when given in doses 6 times the human dose. There are no adequate and well-controlled studies in pregnant women. Isoflurane should be used during pregnancy only if the potential benefit justifies the potential risk to the foetus.

Nursing mothers: It is not known whether this drug is excreted in human milk. Because many drugs are excreted in human milk, caution should be exercised when isoflurane is administered to a nursing woman.

Laboratory tests: Transient increases in BSP retention, blood glucose and serum creatinine with decrease in BUN, serum cholesterol and alkaline phosphatase have been observed.

In susceptible individuals, isoflurane anaesthesia may trigger a skeletal muscle hypermetabolic state leading to high oxygen demand and the clinical syndrome known as malignant hyperthermia. The syndrome includes non-specific features such as muscle rigidity, tachycardia, tachypnoea, cyanosis, arrhythmias, and unstable blood pressure. (It should also be noted that many of these non-specific signs may appear with light anaesthesia, acute hypoxia, etc.)

Side effects: Adverse reactions encountered in the administration of Ærrane (isoflurane) are in general dose dependent extensions of pharmacophysiologic effects and include respiratory depression, hypotension and arrhythmias.

Shivering, nausea, vomiting, and ileus have been observed in the postoperative period.

As with all other general anaesthetics, transient elevations in white blood count have been observed even in the absence of surgical stress.

Overdosage: In the event of overdosage, or what may appear to be overdosage, the following action should be taken:

Stop drug administration; establish a clear airway and initiate assisted or controlled ventilation with pure oxygen.

Pharmaceutical precautions *Storage:* Store at room temperature. Isoflurane contains no additives and has been demonstrated to be stable at room temperature for periods in excess of five years.

Legal category POM.

Package quantities 100 ml bottles of Ærrane (isoflurane) are supplied in boxes of 6 bottles.

Further information Nil.

Product licence number 5247/0002

ALYRANE* ▼

Presentation Alyrane (enflurane) is a nonflammable inhalation anaesthetic agent. Alyrane (enflurane), which is a clear liquid, is packed in 250 ml bottles.

Uses Alyrane (enflurane) may be used for induction and maintenance of general anaesthesia. Enflurane may be used to provide analgesia for vaginal delivery. Low concentrations of enflurane (see 'Dosage and Adminis-

tration') may also be used to supplement other general anaesthetic agents during delivery by Caesarean section.

Dosage and administration Induction and recovery from anaesthesia with enflurane are rapid. Enflurane has a mild sweet odour. Enflurane may provide a mild stimulus to salivation or tracheobronchial secretions. Pharyngeal and laryngeal reflexes are readily obtunded. The level of anaesthesia can be changed rapidly by changing the inspired enflurane concentration. Enflurane reduces ventilation as depth of anaesthesia increases. High $PaCO_2$ levels can be obtained at deeper levels of anaesthesia if ventilation is not supported.

The concentration of Alyrane (enflurane) being delivered from a vaporizer during anaesthesia should be known. This may be accomplished by using:
(a) vaporizers calibrated specifically for enflurane;
(b) vaporizers from which delivered flows can easily and readily be calculated.

Preanaesthetic medication: Preanaesthetic medication should be selected according to the need of the individual patient, taking into account that secretions are weakly stimulated by enflurane and that enflurane does not alter heart rate. The use of anticholinergic drugs is a matter of choice.

Surgical anaesthesia: Induction may be achieved using enflurane alone with oxygen or in combination with oxygen-nitrous oxide mixtures. Under these conditions some excitement may be encountered. If excitement is to be avoided, a hypnotic dose of an ultra-short-acting barbiturate should be used to induce unconsciousness, followed by the enflurane mixture. In general, inspired concentrations of 2–4.5 per cent enflurane produce surgical anaesthesia in 7–10 minutes.

Surgical levels of anaesthesia may be maintained with 0.5–3 per cent enflurane. Maintenance concentrations should not exceed 3 per cent. If added relaxation is required, supplemental doses of muscle relaxants may be used. Ventilation to maintain the tension of carbon dioxide in arterial blood in the 35–45 mm Hg range is preferred. Hyperventilation should be avoided in order to minimize possible CNS excitation.

The level of blood pressure during maintenance is an inverse function of enflurane concentration in the absence of other complicating problems. Excessive decreases (unless related to hypovolaemia) may be due to depth of anaesthesia and in such instances should be corrected by lightening the level of anaesthesia.

Analgesia: Enflurane 0.25 to 1 per cent provides analgesia for vaginal delivery equal to that produced by 30 to 60 per cent nitrous oxide. These concentrations normally do not produce amnesia.

Caesarean section: Enflurane should ordinarily be administered in the concentration range of 0.5 to 1 per cent to supplement other general anaesthetics.

Contra-indications, warnings, etc
Contra-indications: Known sensitivity to Alyrane (enflurane) or other halogenated anaesthetics.

Known or suspected genetic susceptibility to malignant hyperthermia.

Warnings: Increasing depth of anaesthesia with Alyrane (enflurane) may produce a change in the electroencephalogram characterized by high voltage, fast frequency, progressing through spike-dome complexes alternating with periods of electrical silence to frank seizure activity. The latter may or may not be associated with motor movement. Motor activity, when encountered, generally consists of twitching or 'jerks' of various muscle groups; it is self limiting and can be terminated by lowering the anaesthetic concentration. This electroencephalographic pattern associated with deep anaesthesia is exacerbated by low arterial carbon dioxide tension. A reduction in ventilation and anaesthetic concentrations usually suffices to eliminate seizure activity. Cerebral blood flow and metabolism studies in normal volunteers immediately following seizure activity show no evidence of cerebral hypoxia. Mental function testing does not reveal any impairment of performance following prolonged enflurane anaesthesia associated with or not associated with seizure activity.

Since levels of anaesthesia may be altered easily and rapidly, only calibrated vaporizers which measure output with reasonable accuracy should be used. Hypotension and respiratory exchange can serve as a guide to depth of anaesthesia. Deep levels of anaesthesia may produce marked hypotension and respiratory depression.

Precautions: The action of non-depolarizing relaxants is augmented by Alyrane (enflurane). Less than the usual amounts of these drugs should be used. If the usual amounts of non-depolarizing relaxants are given, the time for recovery from neuromuscular blockade will be longer in the presence of enflurane than when halothane or nitrous oxide with a balanced technique is used.

Bromsulfalein (BSP) retention is mildly elevated postoperatively in some cases. This may relate to the effect of surgery since prolonged anaesthesia (5 to 7 hours) in human volunteers does not result in BSP elevation. There is some elevation of glucose and white blood count intraoperatively. Glucose elevation should be considered in diabetic patients. Enflurane should be used with caution in patients who by virtue of medical or drug history could be considered more susceptible to cortical stimulation produced by this drug.

In susceptible individuals, enflurane anaesthesia may trigger a skeletal muscle hypermetabolic state leading to high oxygen demand and the clinical syndrome known as malignant hyperthermia. The syndrome includes non-specific features such as muscle rigidity, tachycardia, tachypnoea, cyanosis, arrhythmias, and unstable blood pressure (It should also be noted that many of these non-specific signs may appear with light anaesthesia, acute hypoxia, etc.). The syndrome of malignant hyperthermia secondary to enflurane appears to be rare.

Swiss ICR mice were given enflurane to determine whether such exposure might induce neoplasia. Enflurane was given at $\frac{1}{2}$, $\frac{1}{8}$, and $\frac{1}{32}$ MAC for four in utero exposures and for 24 exposures to the pups during the first nine weeks of life. The mice were killed at 15 months of age. The incidence of tumours in these mice was the same as in untreated control mice who were given the same background gases, but not the anaesthetic.

Exposure of mice to 20 hours of 1.2 per cent enflurane causes a small (about 0.5%) but statistically significant increase in sperm abnormalities. In contrast to these results, in vitro approaches to the study of mutagenesis (Ames test, sister chromatid exchange test, and the 8-azaguanidine system) have not shown a mutagenic effect of enflurane.

Pregnancy: Reproduction studies have been performed in rats and rabbits at doses up to four times the human dose and have revealed no evidence of impaired fertility or harm to the foetus due to enflurane. There are, however, no adequate and well-controlled studies in pregnant women. Because animal reproduction studies are not always predictive of human response, this drug should be used during pregnancy only if clearly needed.

Side effects:
1. Malignant hyperthermia.
2. Motor activity exemplified by movements of various muscle groups and/or seizures may be encountered with deep levels of Alyrane (enflurane) anaesthesia, or light levels with hypocapnia.
3. Hypotension and respiratory depression have been reported.
4. Arrhythmias, shivering, nausea, and vomiting have been reported.
5. Elevation of the white blood count has been observed.

Overdosage: In the event of overdosage, the following action should be taken: Stop drug administration; establish a clear airway and initiate assisted or controlled ventilation with pure oxygen.

Pharmaceutical precautions *Storage:* Store at room temperature. Enflurane contains no additives and has been demonstrated to be stable at room temperature for periods in excess of five years.

Legal category POM.

Package quantities 250 ml bottles of Alyrane (enflurane) are supplied in boxes of 6 bottles.

Further information Nil.

Product licence number 5247/0001.

*Trade Mark

Approved Prescription Services Limited
Whitcliffe House
Whitcliffe Road, Cleckheaton
West Yorkshire BD19 3BZ

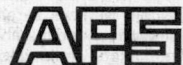

APSIFEN*
APSIFEN*-F

Presentation Apsifen is available in two presentations:
Apsifen: Plain round biconvex pink sugar-coated tablets.
Apsifen-F: Round biconvex pink film-coated tablets
marked 'APS' on one side and plain on the other side.

Both presentations contain the same active ingredient,
Ibuprofen BP, and both are available in two strengths,
200 mg and 400 mg. They comply with the monograph
for Ibuprofen Tablets BP.

Apsifen-F is also available in a 600 mg strength; this
tablet is pink, capsule-shaped, plain, biconvex and film-
coated.

Uses Ibuprofen is a non-steroidal anti-inflammatory
agent with analgesic and anti-pyretic activity. Its principal effects are to relieve pain and stiffness and to reduce
swelling.

Apsifen and Apsifen-F may therefore be used in the
management of:
(a) Rheumatoid Arthritis including Still's disease;
(b) Osteoarthrosis and seronegative (non rheumatoid)
arthropothies;
(c) Ankylosing Spondylitis.

Like other similar agents, ibuprofen has also been used
in non-articular rheumatic conditions and in soft-tissue
injuries, and for the relief of mild to moderate pain such
as dysmenorrhoea, dental and post-operative pain.

Dosage and administration (Oral)
Adults: Initially 1200 mg per day in divided doses. In
severe conditions up to 1800 mg per day may be given
until the acute phase of the condition has been brought
under control. Some patients may be maintained on
doses in the range 600–1200 mg per day. Under no
circumstances should the dose of ibuprofen exceed
2400 mg in any 24 hours.

Children: 20 mg/kg of body weight given daily in divided
doses. The tablets are not suitable for children weighing
less than 20 kg and no more than two 200 mg tablets
should be given in 24 hours to those weighing less than
30 kg.

The Elderly: A separate dosage schedule is not recommended because ibuprofen is well tolerated and overdosage is not usually dangerous, but see precaution (d)
below.

Contra-indications, warnings, etc
Contra-indications: Ibuprofen should not be used in
patients with:

(a) active peptic ulceration;
(b) a history of severe peptic ulceration.

Precautions: Special care must be taken when using
ibuprofen in the following situations:

(a) In patients with asthma;
(b) In allergic patients or in patients who have developed bronchospasm with other non-steroidal anti-
inflammatory agents;
(c) Pregnancy: As with other agents the use of ibuprofen during pregnancy should be avoided if possible;
(d) In elderly patients, in whom increased tissue levels
may result from the normal processes of ageing with
an attendant increase in the risk of adverse reactions
(which are more likely to be masked by concurrent
therapy or disease in the elderly).

Adverse Reactions: As with other non-steroidal anti-
inflammatory agents, the most common unwanted
effects with ibuprofen include dyspepsia, gastro-intestinal intolerance and bleeding. Other unwanted effects
include a variety of skin rashes and, less commonly,
thrombocytopaenia. A few cases of toxic amblyopia
which recovered on withdrawal of treatment have been
reported. Signs of intolerance or unwanted effects are
indications for stopping treatment.

Overdosage: There is no specific antidote to ibuprofen.
Management usually includes gastric lavage associated
with special care of plasma electrolytes and any other
appropriate symptomatic relief.

Pharmaceutical precautions Apsifen and Apsifen-F
Tablets should be stored at room temperature in a dry
place and protected from light.

Legal category POM.

Package quantities
Apsifen and Apsifen-F 200 mg: polypropylene tubes of
100 and 500 tablets.

Apsifen and Apsifen-F 400 mg: polypropylene tubes of
100 and 250 tablets.

Apsifen-F 600 mg: polypropylene tubes of 100 tablets.

Further information Nil.

Product licence numbers
Apsifen Tablets 200 mg   0289/0029
Apsifen Tablets 400 mg   0289/0037
Apsifen-F Tablets 200 mg 0289/0062
Apsifen-F Tablets 400 mg 0289/0063
Apsifen-F Tablets 600 mg 0289/0069

APSIN* VK

Presentation Apsin VK is available in two presentations, tablets and granules for syrup.

Apsin VK Tablets are white, round, biconvex, film-
coated, scored on one side and marked 'APS' on the
other side. The tablets are also marked with the strength
(250) and code number (2102) on the scored side. They
contain the equivalent of 250 mg penicillin V (as the

potassium salt) per tablet and comply with the monograph for Phenoxymethylpenicillin Tablets BP.

Apsin VK Syrups are prepared by adding water to the granules to produce an orange coloured and flavoured clear syrup. Each 5 ml syrup contains the equivalent of 125 mg or 250 mg penicillin V (as the potassium salt). The products comply with the specification for Penicillin V Elixir BPC.

Uses Phenoxymethylpenicillin is a bactericidal agent active against penicillin-sensitive Gram-positive bacteria.

Apsin VK may therefore be used in the management of infections due to penicillin-sensitive organisms, in particular streptococci and staphylococci.

As with other similar agents phenoxymethylpenicillin has occasionally been used prophylactically, when appropriate before and after surgery or dental treatment in patients at risk from bacterial endocarditis owing to congenital or acquired cardiac valvular disease – eg. rheumatic heart disease.

Dosage and administration (Oral).
Adults: 250 mg every 4 hours, or for prophylaxis 125 mg every 12 hours.
Children: aged 6 to 12 years, 250 mg every six hours; aged 1 to 5 years, 125 mg every six hours.
Infants: under 12 months old should receive 62.5 mg every six hours.
The Elderly: Phenoxymethylpenicillin is erratically absorbed from the gastro-intestinal tract, and this phenomenon is likely to be exaggerated in the elderly, so the efficacy of treatment may be less predictable in these patients. A separate dosage schedule is not recommended.

It is recommended that doses are taken 30 minutes before food.

In patients with beta-haemolytic streptococcal infection, it is usual to continue treatment at the full dosage for 10 days in order to minimise the occurrence of secondary complications such as acute nephritis and rheumatic fever.

Contra-indications, warnings, etc
Contra-indications: Phenoxymethylpenicillin should not be used in patients with:
(a) chronic or deep-seated infections such as subacute bacterial endocarditis, meningitis or syphilis.
(b) hypersensitivity to penicillins.
Precautions: Special care must be taken when using phenoxymethylpenicillin in patients with a history of allergy, as they are more likely to develop hypersensitivity reactions. For this reason, penicillin should not be used for trivial infections.
Adverse Reactions: Occasionally patients suffer from transient diarrhoea. Hypersensitivity reactions such as urticaria are less common and usually milder than those associated with penicillins given by injection. However, as with all penicillins, anaphylaxis can occur in susceptible hypersensitive individuals and is an acute emergency. Normally, sensitivity reactions may be controlled with antihistamines or, if these fail, with systemic corticosteroids or pressor amines such as adrenaline.
Overdosage: There are no serious sequelae reported, and management should be symptomatic.

Pharmaceutical precautions
Storage: Apsin VK Tablets and granules for Syrup should

be stored below 20°C in a dry place, not in a refrigerator. The tablets should be dispensed in airtight containers.

Apsin VK Syrups, when reconstituted, should be used within seven days. They will retain potency for this period if stored below 15°C.
Dilution: Apsin VK Syrups can be diluted with Syrup BP if required. Such dilutions must be freshly prepared.

Legal category POM.

Package quantities
Apsin VK Tablets: polypropylene tubes of 1000.

Apsin VK Syrups: granules to produce 100 ml of Syrup when reconstituted with 60 ml water for 250 mg/5 ml Syrup or 65 ml water for 125 mg/5 ml Syrup.

Further information Nil.

Product licence numbers
Apsin VK Tablets 250 mg	0289/5130
Apsin VK Syrup 125 mg/5 ml	0289/5278
Apsin VK Syrup 250 mg/5 ml	0289/5279

APSOLOL*

Presentation Apsolol is presented as pink, round, biconvex, film-coated tablets scored on one side and marked 'APS' on the other side. The tablets are also marked with the strength and code number on the scored side. They contain Propranolol Hydrochloride BP and comply with the monograph for Propranolol Tablets BP. Four strengths are available:

Apsolol 10 mg (of Propranolol Hydrochloride BP) marked '10/0212'
Apsolol 40 mg (of Propranolol Hydrochloride BP) marked '40/0213'
Apsolol 80 mg (of Propranolol Hydrochloride BP) marked '80/0214'
Apsolol 160 mg (of Propranolol Hydrochloride BP) marked '160/0215'

Uses Propranolol is a beta adrenergic receptor blocking agent. Its principal effects are on the cardiovascular system.

Apsolol may therefore be used in the management of:

(a) Angina Pectoris;
(b) Hypertension;
(c) Some forms of Cardiac Dysrhythmias;
(d) Anxiety and Anxiety-induced Tachycardia;
(e) Hypertrophic Obstructive Cardiomyopathy;
(f) Essential Tremor.

Beta adrenergic blocking agents, including propranolol, are also used in the prophylaxis of migraine and as an adjunct to the management of Thyrotoxicosis and Cardiac Dysrhythmias associated with anaesthesia.

Dosage and administration (Oral)
Adults: Angina Pectoris, Anxiety, Migraine and Essential Tremor: Initially 40 mg two to three times per day increased at weekly intervals to suit the patient's requirements. The usual dose for angina is in the range 120–240 mg per day and for anxiety, migraine and essential tremor in the range 80–160 mg per day.
Adults: Hypertension: The usual initial dose is 80 mg twice daily and may be increased at weekly intervals as necessary. Most patients will be managed with a dose in the range 160–320 mg per day. It is usual to add a suitable diuretic to the management of most hypertensives who require the higher doses of a beta-blocker.

Adults: Dysrhythmias, Anxiety-induced Tachycardia, Hypertrophic Obstructive Cardiomyopathy and Thyrotoxicosis: Initially 10–40 mg three to four times per day. This dose may be increased to achieve the desired effect.

Children: Occasionally beta-blockers have been given to children for the management of dysrhythmias. There is no accepted dosage scheme, but a useful guide is 0.25–0.50 mg/kg body weight three to four times per day.

The Elderly: Older patients tend to be more susceptible to the effects of beta blockade, so reduced dosages should be used initially. The presence of minor complaints such as cold extremities should be considered as a reason for using alternative treatment regimes if available. Patients already stabilised on beta blockade may require reduced dosage with increasing age.

Contra-indications, warnings, etc

Contra-indications: Propranolol should not be used:

(a) In patients with 2nd or 3rd degree heart-block.
(b) In patients with a history of bronchospasm (Asthma).
(c) In patients with marked bradycardia (less than 55 b/minute).
(d) In patients with cardiogenic shock or uncontrolled heart failure.
(e) In patients receiving VERAPAMIL or other calcium antagonists. Several days should be allowed for complete elimination of one agent before administering the other.

Precautions: Special care must be taken when using beta-blockers such as propranolol in the following situations:

(a) *Cardiac Failure:* If there is evidence of cardiac failure this must be controlled before initiating and during treatment with propranolol.
(b) *Pulse Rate:* If the pulse rate falls below 50 b/min, treatment should be withdrawn temporarily and resumed at a lower dose.
(c) *Metabolic Disorders:* In patients with metabolic disorders including alcoholism and diabetic acidosis, great care should be taken in the administration of propranolol. Treatment with beta-blockers is liable to mask symptoms and deepen the underlying abnormality in hypoglycaemia and other disorders of carbohydrate metabolism. In patients with labile or insulin-dependent diabetes in whom it is proposed to initiate beta-blocker treatment, it may prove necessary to adjust the dosage of the antidiabetic therapy.
(d) *High Doses:* When high doses of a beta-blocker such as propranolol are used, excessive reduction in blood pressure or pulse rate may occur, particularly when used in conjunction with other hypotensive agents such as neurone blocking agents, vasodilators, reserpine or diuretics.
(e) *Pregnancy:* Many beta-blockers such as propranolol have been known to cause bradycardia in the foetus, and this may persist after birth. As with all treatment during pregnancy, labour and lactation, extra care should be taken, and as far as possible treatment should be avoided during these periods, to protect the foetus or the suckling new-born child.
(f) *Other Anti-arrhythmic Agents:* Care should be exercised during co-administration or sequential administration, because serious interactions have been reported between some beta-blocking agents

and other anti-arrhythmics/cardiac depressants besides verapamil.

(g) *Anaesthesia:* Should treatment with propranolol be continued over the period of anaesthesia, then atropine (1–2 mg intravenously) should be included in the pre-medication and special care taken to avoid anaesthetics with negative inotropic activity or that encourage vagal dominance, such as ether, cyclopropane, halothane and trichloroethylene. Otherwise withdrawal should be gradual and completed 24 hours before anaesthesia.

(h) *Renal Failure:* An increased interval between doses may be required to avoid accumulation of propranolol.

(i) *Elderly Patients:* See the entry under *Dosage and administration.*

Adverse Reactions: Like other beta-blockers, propranolol is well tolerated in normal use. In general untoward effects are minor and include dizziness, headache, insomnia, drowsiness, excitability, gastrointestinal disturbances and rarely bradycardia. Like other beta-blockers, propranolol may precipitate bronchospasm, heart failure, or be associated with cold extremities, and occasionally paraesthesia of the hands, skin rashes and/or dry eyes. The occurrence of these latter symptoms is a reason for discontinuing treatment. (See next paragraph about stopping teatment).

Cessation of Treatment: Withdrawal should be gradual, as several beta-blockers, including propranolol, have been associated with a significant increase in symptoms of angina or increase in blood pressure following abrupt withdrawal. If clonidine is co-prescribed, then clonidine should not be withdrawn until several days after Apsolol withdrawal has been completed. (Please refer to prescribing information on clonidine for further information).

Overdosage: Excessive bradycardia and hypotension may be treated with atropine 1–2 mg intravenously and, if necessary, this may be followed by a beta-receptor stimulant such as isoprenaline hydrochloride 25 micrograms intravenously. Where cardiogenic shock has supervened, glucagon 5–10 mg intravenously has been reported to be useful. Bronchospasm may be countered by appropriate beta$_2$ receptor stimulants such as salbutamol, either by inhalation or 4 micrograms/kg body weight by slow intravenous injection.

Pharmaceutical precautions Apsolol Tablets should be stored at room temperature in a dry place and protected from light.

Legal category POM.

Package quantities
Apsolol 10, 40 and 80 mg: polypropylene tubes of 500 tablets
Apsolol 160 mg: polypropylene tubes of 100 tablets

Further information Hypertension is a condition which can benefit from the use of both a beta-blocking agent as contained in Apsolol and a thiazide diuretic such as bendrofluazide. This is because their separate pharmacological actions are complementary in hypertension and may allow adequate treatment with smaller doses of each than would be required if either were to be used alone.

The time-to-peak plasma level in fasted healthy young human volunteers following a single dose of Apsolol is approximately 2 hours, and the excretion half-life of propranolol in plasma is about $2\frac{1}{2}$ hours. However, as with most other beta-blocking agents the onset of biological activity is delayed and the duration is prolonged relative to the plasma concentration. The decay half-life of the biological effect following a single-dose in normal volunteers has been reported to be 11 hours for propranolol, the measure of 'effect' being the reduction in exercise-induced double product (maximum heart rate × systolic blood pressure).†

Product licence numbers

Apsolol Tablets	10 mg	0289/0034
Apsolol Tablets	40 mg	0289/0035
Apsolol Tablets	80 mg	0289/0036
Apsolol Tablets	160 mg	0289/0044

†Vukovich R. A. et al. *Br. J. Clin. Pharmacol.* 1979; 7 Supp 2: 167S–172S.

APSOLOX*

Presentation Apsolox is presented as round, biconvex, film-coated tablets marked 'APS' on one side, while the strength and code number are marked on the other side. The tablets contain Oxprenolol Hydrochloride BP and comply with the monograph for Oxprenolol Tablets BP. Four strengths are available:

Apsolox 20 mg (of Oxprenolol Hydrochloride BP) marked '20/0220' and coloured white.

Apsolox 40 mg (of Oxprenolol Hydrochloride BP) marked '40/0221' and coloured white.

Apsolox 80 mg (of Oxprenolol Hydrochloride BP) marked '80/0222' and coloured yellow.

Apsolox 160 mg (of Oxprenolol Hydrochloride BP) marked '160/0223' and coloured orange.

Uses Oxprenolol is a beta adrenergic receptor blocking agent. As with propranolol its principal effects are on the cardiovascular system. However, oxprenolol is dissimilar in having partial agonist activity (sometimes termed intrinsic sympathomimetic activity).

Apsolox may therefore be used in the management of:

(a) Angina Pectoris
(b) Hypertension
(c) Some forms of Cardiac Dysrhythmias
(d) Anxiety-induced Tachycardia
(e) Hypertrophic Obstructive Cardiomyopathy

Beta adrenergic blocking agents, including oxprenolol, are also used as an adjunct to the management of Thyrotoxicosis and Cardiac Dysrhythmias associated with anaesthesia.

Dosage and administration (Oral)

Adults: Angina Pectoris: The usual dose range is 120–480 mg per day in divided doses to suit the patient's requirements.

Adults: Hypertension: The usual initial dose is 80 mg twice daily and may be increased at weekly intervals as necessary. Most patients will be managed with a dose in the range 160–320 mg per day. It is usual to add a suitable diuretic to the management of most hypertensives who require the higher doses of a beta-blocker.

Adults: Dysrhythmias, Anxiety-induced Tachycardia, Hypertrophic Obstructive Cardiomyopathy and Thyrotoxicosis: Initially 20–40 mg three times per day. This dose may be increased up to 480 mg per day (in divided doses) to achieve the desired effect.

Children: Occasionally beta-blockers have been given to children for the management of dysrhythmias. There is no accepted dosage scheme, but it has been found useful to start with a dose based on 1 mg/kg body weight per day.

The Elderly: Older patients tend to be more susceptible to the effects of beta blockade, so reduced dosages should be used initially. The presence of minor complaints such as cold extremities should be considered as a reason for using alternative treatment regimes if available. Patients already stabilised on beta blockade may require reduced dosage with increasing age.

Contra-indications, warnings, etc

Contra-indications: Oxprenolol should not be used:

(a) In patients with 2nd or 3rd degree heart-block.
(b) In patients with a history of bronchospasm (Asthma).
(c) In patients with marked bradycardia (less than 55 b/minute).
(d) In patients with cardiogenic shock or uncontrolled heart failure.
(e) In patients receiving verapamil or other calcium antagonists. Several days should be allowed for complete elimination of one agent before administering the other.

Precautions: Special care must be taken when using beta-blockers such as oxprenolol in the following situations:

(a) *Cardiac Failure:* If there is evidence of cardiac failure this must be controlled before initiating and during treatment with oxprenolol.

(b) *Pulse Rate:* If the pulse rate falls below 50 b/min, treatment should be withdrawn temporarily and resumed at a lower dose.

(c) *Metabolic Disorders:* In patients with metabolic disorders including alcholism and diabetic acidosis, great care should be taken in the administration of oxprenolol. Treatment with beta-blockers is liable to mask symptoms and deepen the underlying abnormality in hypoglycaemia and other disorders of carbohydrate metabolism. In patients with labile or insulin-dependent diabetes in whom it is proposed to initiate beta-blocker treatment, it may prove necessary to adjust the dosage of the antidiabetic therapy.

(d) *High Doses:* When high doses of a beta-blocker such as oxprenolol are used, excessive reduction in blood pressure or pulse rate may occur, particularly when used in conjunction with other hypotensive agents such as neurone blocking agents, vasodilators, reserpine or diuretics.

(e) *Pregnancy:* Many beta-blockers such as oxprenolol have been known to cause bradycardia in the foetus, and this may persist after birth. As with all treatment during pregnancy, labour and lactation, extra care should be taken, and as far as possible treatment should be avoided during these periods, to protect the foetus or the suckling new-born child.

(f) *Other Anti-arrhythmic Agents:* Care should be exercised during co-administration or sequential administration, because serious interactions have been reported between some beta-blocking agents and other antiarrhythmics/cardiac depressants besides verapamil.

(g) *Anaesthesia:* Should treatment with oxprenolol be continued over the period of anaesthesia, then atropine (1–2 mg intravenously) should be included in the pre-medication and special care taken to avoid anaesthetics with negative inotropic activity or that encourage vagal dominance, such as ether, cyclopropane, halothane and trichloroethylene. Similarly, some muscle relaxants – for example suxamethonium – may also increase bradycardia. Otherwise withdrawal should be gradual and completed 24 hours before anaesthesia.

(h) *Renal Failure:* An increased interval between doses may be required to avoid accumulation of oxprenolol.

(i) *Elderly Patients:* See the entry under *Dosage and administration.*

Adverse Reactions: Like other beta-blockers, oxprenolol is well tolerated in normal use. In general untoward effects are minor and include dizziness, headache, insomnia, drowsiness, excitability, gastrointestinal disturbances and rarely bradycardia. Like other beta-blockers, oxprenolol may precipitate bronchospasm, heart failure, or be associated with cold extremities, skin rashes and/or dry eyes. The occurrence of any of these latter symptoms is a reason for discontinuing treatment. (See next paragraph about stopping treatment).

Cessation of Treatment: Withdrawal should be gradual, as several beta-blockers, including oxprenolol, have been associated with a significant increase in symptoms of angina or increase in blood pressure following abrupt withdrawal. If clonidine is co-prescribed, then clonidine should not be withdrawn until several days after Apsolox withdrawal has been completed. (Please refer to prescribing information on clonidine for further information).

Overdosage: Excessive bradycardia and hypotension may be treated with atropine 1–2 mg intravenously and, if necessary, this may be followed by a beta receptor stimulant such as isoprenaline hydrochloride 25 micrograms intravenously. Where cardiogenic shock has supervened, glucagon 5–10 mg intravenously has been reported to be useful. Bronchospasm may be countered by appropriate beta$_2$ receptor stimulants such as salbutamol, either by inhalation or 4 micrograms/kg body weight by slow intravenous injection.

Pharmaceutical precautions Apsolox Tablets should be stored at room temperature in a dry place. The 80 mg and 160 mg strengths should be protected from light.

Legal category POM.

Package quantities
Apsolox 20 and 160 mg: polypropylene tubes of 100 tablets.
Apsolox 40 and 80 mg: polypropylene tubes of 100 and 500 tablets.

Further information Hypertension is a condition which can benefit from the use of both a beta-blocking agent as contained in Apsolox and a thiazide diuretic such as bendrofluazide. This is because their separate pharmacological actions are complementary in hypertension and may allow adequate treatment with smaller doses of each than would be required if either were to be used alone.

The time-to-peak plasma level in fasted healthy young human volunteers following a single dose of Apsolox is approximately 1½–2 hours, and the excretion half-life of oxprenolol in plasma is about 1½ hours. However, as with most other beta-blocking agents the onset of biological activity is delayed and the duration is prolonged relative to the plasma concentration. The decay half-life of the biological effect following a single-dose in normal

volunteers has been reported to be 13 hours for oxprenolol, the measure of 'effect' being the reduction in exercise-induced double product (maximum heart rate × systolic blood pressure).†

Product licence numbers

Apsolox Tablets	20 mg	0289/0050
Apsolox Tablets	40 mg	0289/0051
Apsolox Tablets	80 mg	0289/0052
Apsolox Tablets	160 mg	0289/0053

† Vukovich R. A. et al. *Br. J. Clin. Pharmacol.* 1979; 7 Supp 2: 167S–172S.

ASMAVEN*

Presentation
Asmaven Tablets are pink, round, flat-faced with bevelled edges, marked 'APS' on one side, while the strength and code number are marked on the other side. The tablets contain Salbutamol BP as the sulphate and comply with the monograph for Salbutamol Tablets BP. Two strengths are available:
Asmaven 2 mg (of Salbutamol BP) marked '2/1507'.
Asmaven 4 mg (of Salbutamol BP) marked '4/1508'.

Asmaven Inhaler (not available in the UK at the time of writing) is a metered-dose metal aerosol canister mounted in a specially-designed blue plastic actuator with white plastic cap. It delivers 100 micrograms of Salbutamol BP to the patient per actuation and contains sufficient for at least 200 metered inhalations. The whole is enclosed in a carton with an instruction leaflet for the patient. Asmaven Inhaler complies with the monograph for Salbutamol Aerosol Inhalation BPC.

Uses *Tablets and Inhaler:* Salbutamol is a beta-adrenergic stimulant which has a selective action on the beta-adrenergic receptors in bronchial muscle and, in therapeutic dosage, little or no action on the cardiac beta-adrenergic receptors. In view of the selective action on the bronchi, salbutamol preparations are suitable for treating bronchospasm in patients with co-existing heart disease or hypertension.

Salbutamol is also active, when used locally in human lung sensitised with IgE antibody, in preventing antigen-induced release of histamine and slow reacting substance of anaphylaxis, SRS(A), from mast cells. Such Type I hypersensitivity reactions are generally considered to be the primary triggers of the allergic asthma syndrome.

The inhaler delivers a much smaller dose than the tablets. The small dose is effective because it is delivered locally to the tissues responsible for bronhco-constriction, but it minimises the unwanted systemic effects such as the skeletal muscle tremor sometimes associated with the higher systemic doses arising from tablet usage. The increased therapeutic ratio when salbutamol is used locally makes the inhaler suitable for use in those patients also receiving beta-blocking agents. The inhaler also has the advantage of a rapid local onset of action and a relatively prolonged duration of effect.

Asmaven preparations (tablets or inhaler) may therefore be used in the management of:
(a) Bronchial Asthma
(b) Other conditions with associated reversible airways obstruction such as Bronchitis and Emphysema ⎫ including patients with co-existing heart disease or hypertension.

The Asmaven Inhaler is particularly suitable for:

(a) Relieving attacks of Acute Dyspnoea

(b) Routine maintenance therapy in Chronic Asthma

(c) Routine maintenance therapy in Chronic Bronchitis

(d) Prophylaxis before exertion to prevent exercise-induced Asthma

including patients also receiving beta-blocking agents.

Tablets in Premature Labour: Asmaven Tablets may be used following the administration of salbutamol as a continuous intravenous infusion for the management of premature labour during the third trimester of pregnancy. Once the uterine contractions have ceased and the infusion has been withdrawn, maintenance therapy may be continued with Asmaven Tablets.

Dosage and administration (Oral)
Asmaven Tablets.

Adults: The usual effective dose is 4 mg three or four times per day. If adequate bronchodilation is not obtained, each single dose may be gradually increased to as much as 8 mg. However, it has been established that some patients obtain adequate relief with 2 mg three or four times daily.

Children: The following doses should be administered three or four times daily:
2–6 years: ½ to 1 of the 2 mg tablets.
6–12 years: 1 of the 2 mg tablets.
Over 12 years: 1–2 of the 2 mg tablets or 1 of the 4 mg tablets.

Salbutamol is well tolerated by children so that, if necessary, these doses may be cautiously increased.

The Elderly: In elderly patients or in those known to be unusually sensitive to beta-adrenergic stimulants, it is advisable to initiate treatment with 2 mg three or four times per day.

Premature Labour: In the management of premature labour, after uterine contractions have been controlled by intravenous salbutamol and the infusion has been withdrawn, maintenance therapy may be continued with Asmaven Tablets. The usual dosage is 4 mg three or four times daily.

Asmaven Inhaler
Adults: Acute Bronchospasm and intermittent episodes of Asthma: One or two inhalations as a single dose.

Adults: Chronic Maintenance or Prophylactic Therapy: Two inhalations three or four times a day.

Adults: Prevention of Exercise-induced Bronchospasm: Two inhalations before exertion.

Children: Acute Bronchospasm, Episodic Asthma, or before exercise: One inhalation.

Children: Routine Maintenance or Prophylactic Therapy: One inhalation three or four times a day.

These doses may be increased to two inhalations if necessary.

Duration of effect: The bronchodilator effect of each administration of inhaled salbutamol lasts at least four hours except in patients whose asthma is worsening. Such patients should be warned not to increase their usage of inhaler but to seek medical advice in case treatment with a glucocorticoid is indicated.

Contra-indications, warnings, etc
Contra-indications
Pregnancy: Although intravenous salbutamol and salbutamol tablets are used in the management of premature labour, these preparations should not be used for threatened abortion during the first or second trimester of pregnancy.

Beta-blocking Agents: Salbutamol tablets should not usually be prescribed for patients under treatment with beta-blocking agents, but note that the inhaler may be prescribed for such patients.

Precautions: Thyrotoxicosis: Care should be taken when administering salbutamol preparations to patients suffering from thyrotoxicosis.

Pregnancy: As with other agents the use of salbutamol during pregnancy should be avoided if possible (except for the management of premature labour).

Duration of Inhaler Action: Patients using salbutamol inhaler should be warned to seek medical advice if a previously effective dose fails to continue relief for at least three hours; treatment with a glucocorticoid may then be indicated.

Adverse Reactions: The only side-effect of significance with salbutamol tablets is a fine tremor of skeletal muscle which occurs in some patients; usually the hands are most obviously affected. This effect is dose related and is common to all beta-adrenergic stimulants. A few patients feel tense; this is also due to the effects on skeletal muscle and not to direct CNS stimulation. With doses of salbutamol higher than those recommended or in patients who are unusually sensitive to beta-adrenergic stimulants peripheral vasodilation and a compensatory small increase in heart rate may occur. Occasionally headaches have been reported.

No important adverse reactions have been reported following therapy with salbutamol inhaler. This is presumably due to the small size of the effective dose and the correspondingly increased therapeutic ratio.

Overdosage: The preferred antidote for overdosage with salbutamol is a cardioselective beta-blocking agent, but such agents should be used with caution in patients with a history of bronchospasm.

Pharmaceutical precautions
Asmaven Tablets should be stored at a temperature not exceeding 30°C.

Asmaven Inhaler should be stored in a cool place, protected from frost, direct heat and sunlight. The canister should not be broken, punctured or burnt even when apparently empty.

Legal category POM.

Package quantities
Asmaven Tablets 2 mg and 4 mg: Polypropylene tubes of 500 tablets.

Asmaven Inhaler: One aerosol canister mounted in a plastic actuator and enclosed in a carton with an instruction leaflet. The inhaler is not available in the U.K at the time of writing.

Further information Unlike sympathomimetic agents such as ephedrine, salbutamol does not stimulate alpha-adrenoceptors and, therefore, does not cause difficulty in micturition. Therefore salbutamol is not contra-indicated in patients under treatment with monoamine oxidase inhibitors (MAOIs).

Product licence numbers

Asmaven Tablets 2 mg	0289/0066
Asmaven Tablets 4 mg	0289/0067
Asmaven Inhaler	0289/0068

LIBANIL*

Presentation Libanil is presented as white biconvex tablets marked 'APS' on one side and with the strength and code number on the other side. They contain Glibenclamide BP and comply with the monograph for Glibenclamide Tablets BP. Two strengths are available:
2.5 mg – round tablets coded 3103;
  5 mg – elongated tablets coded 3104 with a break-line.

Uses Glibenclamide is an oral hypoglycaemic agent. Libanil may therefore be used in the management of non-insulin-dependent diabetes mellitus in patients who have responded poorly to dietary measures alone.

Dosage and administration (Oral)
Adults: Previously untreated Diabetes Mellitus: Treatment should be started with 5 mg daily, taken during or immediately following breakfast or the first main meal of the day. It is wise to start at a lower dose of 2.5 mg daily if the patient is elderly or debilitated – see 'Contra-indications, warnings, etc.' If control of diabetic symptoms remains inadequate, the daily dose may be increased not more frequently than weekly in steps of 2.5 mg (usual) or 5 mg (maximum) daily to a maximum dose not exceeding 15 mg daily. This is normally given as a single dose during or immediately after breakfast or the first main meal of the day. However, care should be taken to apportion the diet with the daily activity schedule and the final dosage schedule for each individual patient.

Adults: Changing from other oral sulphonyl-urea hypoglycaemic agents: These changes may be made without any formal break in treatment. Where the patient is already well controlled, Libanil treatment should commence with one 5 mg dose daily, adjusted weekly in increments not exceeding 5 mg to a maximum of 15 mg daily – see above. Where control has not been adequate on previous therapy, Libanil treatment may be started on the approximately equivalent dose provided this does not exceed 10 mg daily. It may then be raised at weekly intervals to a maximum dose of 15 mg daily.

  5 mg of Glibenclamide BP is approximately equivalent to:

Tolbutamide	1 g
Glymidine	1 g
Acetohexamide	500 mg
Tolazamide	250 mg
Chlorpropamide	250 mg
Glibonuride	25 mg
Glipizide	5 mg

Adults: Changing from biguanides such as metformin: Libanil treatment should be started at a dose of 2.5 mg daily and the biguanide then withdrawn. To achieve control the dose of Libanil should be adjusted at weekly intervals in increments of 2.5 mg daily but not exceeding the maximum dose of 15 mg daily.

Adults: Combination Therapy with biguanides: Where control of diabetic symptoms has not been achieved with a single oral hypoglycaemic agent such as glibenclamide at the maximum dosage of 15 mg daily, control may often be achieved by adding a biguanide derivative to the regime.

Adults: Changing from an insulin regime: A few patients with very low daily insulin requirements may remain controlled if transferred to glibenclamide and should be treated as new patients. Tablets should always be taken with or immediately after the first main meal of the day, and the insulin dose should be reduced further with each increased dose level of glibenclamide.

Children: Juvenile-onset diabetes mellitus is normally insulin-dependent, and consequently glibenclamide is not suitable for use in children.

Contra-indications, warnings, etc
Contra-indications: Glibenclamide should not be used:
  (a) in patients suffering from or with a history of diabetic keto-acidosis.
  (b) in patients with serious impairment of function in the kidneys, liver or adrenal glands.
  (c) in patients undergoing surgery.
  (d) in pregnant patients, for whom insulin treatment is normally preferred.

Warning: The hypoglycaemic effect of glibenclamide may be ENHANCED (occasionally dramatically) by:
  (a) coumarin anticoagulants.
  (b) monoamine oxidase inhibitors.
  (c) beta-adrenergic blocking agents.
  (d) sulphonamides.
  (e) phenylbutazone.
  (f) chloramphenicol
  (g) cyclophosphamide
  (h) salicylates e.g., aspirin.

Conversely the hypoglycaemic effect of glibenclamide may be DIMINISHED by:
  (a) sympathomimetic agents e.g., adrenalin.
  (b) steroids including oral contraceptives.
  (c) thiazide diuretics.

Precautions: Special care must be taken when using glibenclamide in the following situations:
  (a) *Elderly or Debilitated Patients:* These patients are more likely to suffer from hypoglycaemia – see treatment of overdosage.
  (b) *Pregnancy and Lactation:* There is no adequate information on the use of glibenclamide in human pregnancy. It is normal practice to manage diabetes in pregnant patients with insulin, although there appear to be no specific reasons to stop a pre-existing regime which includes glibenclamide. There is no evidence of teratogenicity in animal experiments. However, as with other sulphonylurea hypoglycaemic agents, it is wise to assume that glibenclamide is present in human breast milk. Consequently, its use is best avoided where the patient expresses a desire to breast-feed.

Adverse Reactions: Like other oral hypoglycaemic agents, glibenclamide is well tolerated in normal use. Untoward effects are usually mild and rarely require treatment to be discontinued. Among these mild effects are gastro-intestinal symptoms (anorexia, diarrhoea and nausea) and allergic-type skin reactions. Leucopaenia and thrombocytopaenia have been reported, and are reversible on stopping treatment. Transient changes in liver enzymes and function tests have been reported during glibenclamide treatment, although a definite relationship to treatment has yet to be established. As with all other oral hypoglycaemic agents, an over-response to treatment may occur, especially in relation to unexpected heavy exercise. These hypoglycaemic attacks are not usually prolonged and should be managed as for overdosage.

Overdosage: Conscious Patients with early signs of hypoglycaemia – faintness, nausea, cold-sweats and/or palpitation – may be treated with glucose water or 3–4 lumps of sugar (sucrose) with water. This treatment may be repeated as necessary and, if symptoms continue to recur at intervals, may be supplemented with half a pint of milk after successful management of the current recurrence of symptoms.

Overdosage: Comatose Patients should receive glucose administered as a continuous intravenous infusion, because a bolus injection may lead to a more severe and prolonged rebound hypoglycaemia. An alternative approach is to administer 1 mg of glucagon as a subcutaneous or intramuscular injection. The objective of both treatments is to achieve rapid recovery of consciousness, when further 'feeding' should be instituted, as above.

Pharmaceutical precautions Libanil Tablets should be stored below 25°C.

Legal category POM.

Package quantities
Libanil 2.5 mg: polypropylene tubes of 100 tablets.
Libanil 5 mg: polypropylene tubes of 100 and 500 tablets.

Further information Nil.

Product licence numbers
Libanil Tablets 2.5 mg   0289/0047
Libanil Tablets   5 mg   0289/0048

STILBOESTROL TABLETS BP

Presentation APS Stilboestrol Tablets are available in two presentations:

Plain, round, biconvex, white tablets
Plain, round, biconvex, pink, sugar-coated tablets.

Both presentations contain the same active ingredient, Stilboestrol BP, and both are available in two strengths, 1 mg and 5 mg. They comply with the monograph for Stilboestrol Tablets BP.

Uses Stilboestrol is a synthetic non-steroidal oestrogen hormone. It has been in use for many years. However, it has carcinogenic potential, so its use is now only justified in the management of malignant disease.

It may be used to suppress androgenic hormonal activity in the management of androgen-dependent carcinomas such as carcinoma of the prostate in males and some post-menopausal carcinomas such as breast cancer in females.

APS Stilboestrol Tablets may therefore be used in:
(a)   Carcinoma of the Prostate;
(b)   Post-menopausal Carcinoma of the Breast.

Dosage and administration (Oral)
Adults: Management of prostatic carcinoma 1–3 mg daily.
Adults: Management of post-menopausal breast carcinoma 10–20 mg daily.
Children: Not suitable.
The Elderly: As the conditions for which stilboestrol is indicated primarily occur in the elderly, the recommended dosage remains unchanged.

Contra-indications, warnings, etc
Contra-indications: Stilboestrol is contra-indicated in:

(a)   pregnancy – it is not suitable for pre-menopausal women;
(b)   children;
(c)   any oestrogen-dependent neoplasms especially of the genital tract;
(d)   pre-menopausal carcinoma of the breast;

or where there is:

(e)   undiagnosed vaginal bleeding;
(f)   a history of herpes gestationis;
(g)   porphyria;
(h)   severe hypertension;
(i)   active liver disease;
(j)   a history of thrombo-embolism or conditions predisposing to it such as sickle cell anaemia, untreated polycythaemia and pulmonary hypertension.

Precautions: Care should be taken when administering stilboestrol preparations to patients with:

(a)   cardiac failure;
(b)   hypertension;
(c)   diabetes;
(d)   epilepsy;
(e)   migraine;
(f)   depression;
(g)   contact lenses.

Pregnancy: Stilboestrol is NOT indicated for pre-menopausal women.

Children: Stilboestrol is NOT suitable for children.

Adverse Reactions: As high doses of stilboestrol in early pregnancy have caused vaginal carcinoma in female offspring 16–20 years later, it should not be used in pre-menopausal women.

As with other oestrogens the following hormonal disturbances may occur – fluid retention, headache, nausea and vomiting, weight gain, hypertension, breast discomfort, chloasma and cholestatic jaundice. Venous thrombosis and possibly cerebral and coronary thrombosis are also risks.

In men there will be some feminization – e.g. gynaecomastia and testicular atrophy, and impotence.

Other effects may be withdrawal bleeding in women and an increased incidence of cholelithiasis. In the event of prolonged usage there is an increased risk of endometrial carcinoma.

Overdosage: There is no specific antidote to stilboestrol. The commonest symptoms of overdosage are nausea and vomiting. Management may include gastric lavage associated with special care of plasma electrolytes and any other appropriate symptomatic relief. Should the overdose (abuse) be in female children, an oestrogen-withdrawal bleed may be induced.

Pharmaceutical precautions APS Stilboestrol Tablets should be stored in a dry place below 25°C and protected from light.

Legal category POM.

Package quantities
APS Stilboestrol Tablets uncoated 1 mg: polypropylene tubes of 500 tablets.
APS Stilboestrol Tablets uncoated 5 mg: polypropylene tubes of 250 tablets.
APS Stilboestrol Tablets sugar-coated 1 mg: polypropylene tubes of 100 and 500 tablets.

APS Stilboestrol Tablets sugar-coated 5 mg: polypropylene tubes of 100 and 500 tablets.

Further information Stilboestrol should not be used in children or young adults because it has carcinogenic potential.

In prostatic carcinoma and post-menopausal breast carcinoma, stilboestrol causes temporary disease regression in approximately 80% and 30% of patients respectively.

Product licence numbers

APS Stilboestrol Tablets uncoated 1 mg	0289/5188
APS Stilboestrol Tablets uncoated 5 mg	0289/5189
APS Stilboestrol Tablets sugar-coated 1 mg	0289/5247
APS Stilboestrol Tablets sugar-coated 5 mg	0289/5248

'Trade Mark

Armour Pharmaceutical Company Limited
St. Leonards House
St. Leonards Road
Eastbourne
East Sussex BN21 3YG

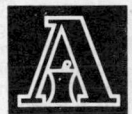

AAA* MOUTH AND THROAT SPRAY

Presentation The can contains 7.5 g with a valve providing 60 metered doses.
Each metered dose contains:

Benzocaine PhEur   1.5 mg
Cetalkonium Chloride   0.0413 mg.
in an inert flavoured propellant.

Uses Treatment of sore throats caused by cold, post-nasal drip and other irritants, and minor infections of the mouth and throat.

Dosage and administration Shake can before use.
Adults: 2 shots every two to three hours if required (not more than 16 shots in 24 hours or as directed by the physician).
Children aged 6–12: 1 shot every two to three hours if required (not more than 8 shots in 24 hours or as directed by the physician).

Contra-indications, warnings, etc
Side-effects: Hypersensitivity reactions to benzocaine have been reported.
Precautions: Avoid spraying into eyes.
Contents under pressure – do not puncture.
Keep away from heat and flames – do not throw finished container into fire.
Contra-indications: Known hypersensitivity to Benzocaine.

Pharmaceutical precautions Store in a cool place. Shelf-life 3 years. Shake can before use.

Legal category P.

Package quantities Single can containing 7.5 g with a valve providing 60 × 100 mg metered doses (shots).

Further information Published clinical studies have demonstrated antibacterial activity by the reduction in the population of pathogenic organisms of the buccal mucosa. Together with the spray's local anaesthetic activity, this has been found of value in the treatment of pain and infection following tonsillectomy.

Product licence number 0231/5026.

ACTHAR* GEL

Presentation Corticotrophin Gelatin Injection BP in vials containing 20, 40 and 80 i.u./ml for subcutaneous or intramuscular use only.

Uses Rheumatic and Collagen diseases. Asthma. Diseases of the GI tract (e.g. ulcerative colitis). Nephrotic syndrome. Diseases of the CNS (e.g. Bell's Palsy, Retrobulbar Neuritis and Multiple Sclerosis). Adrenal function tests. Chronic skin and allergic conditions responsive to corticosteroids (e.g. psoriasis and certain eczemas and refractory hay fever unresponsive to conventional treatment).

Dosage and administration General information on dosage for therapeutic use. The aim of treatment with Acthar Gel is to obtain a satisfactory therapeutic effect with minimal dosage, the clinical response being the sole measure of adequate dosage. Therapeutic effects may appear within hours, although with some chronic diseases improvement may not show for several days.

Because patients' adrenal glands vary in their sensitivity to ACTH and because disease conditions vary in their response to corticosteroids, no specific uniform dose can be equally effective for all individuals. Some conditions, e.g. acute exacerbations of asthma and multiple sclerosis may require high doses initially to obtain a remission. Once the disease is under control the total daily dosage should be decreased as rapidly as possible. Dosage reduction should be consistent with maintaining clinical improvement. Some conditions, e.g. rheumatoid arthritis, nephrotic syndrome and chronic asthma may need long-term maintenance therapy. Again, the aim is to obtain satisfactory therapeutic effect with minimal dosage. If the treatment regimen is started on a daily basis once the smallest daily maintenance dose has been established (e.g. 20 i.u.), attempts should be made to lengthen the dosage intervals. If at any step of dosage reduction symptoms reappear, a return to the previous effective schedule is necessary before a further attempt at dosage reduction is made. On occasions Acthar Gel can be completely withdrawn as the patient experiences a remission.

Instead of starting with daily injections, it may be more convenient to commence with an initial higher fixed unit dosage (say 40 i.u. per injection) twice or thrice weekly.

Suggested practical regimens for specific conditions are given below. These are guidelines only, the dosage should be titrated to the patient's response.

Conditions needing maintenance therapy
Rheumatoid arthritis: Initially a dose of 40 i.u. should be given daily. Review the dosage at intervals of three days and adjust according to the clinical response. The dosage should be increased or decreased bearing in mind that the ideal dosage is the minimum necessary to relieve symptoms.

Chronic asthma: Initially a dose of 40–80 i.u. should be given daily for a period of five days. Reduce by steps of 10 i.u. until symptoms are satisfactorily controlled. On remission of symptoms, treatment may be withdrawn completely. In some patients, however, continued therapy may be necessary.

Still's disease: 40 i.u. Acthar Gel daily for three days reducing to 20 i.u. on alternate days. Suppression of symptomatology without the appearance of 'cushingoid signs' is the aim of therapy. The administration of ACTH to children should be confined to early morning (approximately 10 a.m.) to reduce the incidence of 'growth interference'.

Conditions requiring short – medium term therapy
Acute exacerbation of asthma: 200 i.u. Acthar Gel repeated at a 72-hour interval gives remission in the majority of cases. Upon remission the dosage should be reduced to maintenance levels (see chronic asthma).

Very high levels of corticosteroids may be needed rapidly in cases of status asthmaticus, and the delay in achieving this by corticotrophin treatment may render this form of therapy inappropriate, at least initially.

Hay fever: Acthar Gel should be reserved for patients with refractory hay fever unresponsive to conventional treatment, e.g. antihistamines and topical medication, who may benefit from treatment with Acthar Gel. The dosage and duration of treatment will depend upon the severity of the condition. In adults, dosages of up to 40–80 i.u. once or twice weekly during the pollen season can be given. In children under the age of seven, the use of ACTH treatment for hay fever is not recommended unless absolutely necessary. In children over the age of seven, the dosage should not exceed 40–80 i.u. Acthar Gel given in the early morning once or twice weekly during the pollen season. The child should be carefully monitored during the course of therapy for side-effects including diminution of growth velocity and hypothalamic pituitary suppression.

Bell's palsy: Treatment should commence as soon as possible after the onset of paralysis.

Acthar Gel 80 i.u. daily for five days, reducing to 60 i.u. on day 6, 40 i.u. on day 7, 20 i.u. on day 8 and 10 i.u. on days 9 and 10.

Alternatively a simplified regimen of 40 i.u. daily for 10 days, or until signs of improvement occur, can be employed.

Retrobulbar neuritis: Acthar Gel 40 i.u. daily for a period of 30 days.

Ulcerative colitis and Crohn's disease: For the treatment of acute exacerbations of Crohn's disease and ulcerative colitis, a short course of treatment is generally used. The starting dose should be 80–120 units daily and should be rapidly reduced consistent with maintaining clinical remission. Maintenance therapy with other agents may then be necessary.

Multiple sclerosis: For the treatment of exacerbations of multiple sclerosis a diminishing dosage regimen is generally used. The initial dosage should be between 80–120 i.u. daily for the first week. Subsequently daily dosages should be reduced on a weekly basis over three-six weeks to 10–20 i.u. and then stopped.

Nephrotic syndrome: For the treatment of nephrotic syndrome, a short course of treatment is generally used. Administer Acthar Gel 60–80 i.u. daily for 10–12 days and then stop treatment abruptly to allow spontaneous diuresis. If diuresis is inadequate repeat treatment after 5 days.

Adrenal function tests: Withdraw 5–8 ml venous blood into a heparinised tube, then inject intramuscularly 40 i.u. Acthar Gel. After approximately 4 hours withdraw a further 5–8 ml into a heparinised tube, centrifuge the blood specimen and measure plasma hydroxycorticosteroids.

Contra-indications, warnings, etc
Precautions and contra-indications: The contra-indications to ACTH are those of corticosteroids but are rarely absolute. Only after careful consideration should ACTH be given to patients suffering from: active tuberculosis, peptic ulcer, acute psychosis, hypertension, diabetes mellitus, congestive heart failure, Cushing's syndrome, osteoporosis or in pregnancy.

As with corticosteroids, ACTH may increase susceptibility to infections.

Side-effects: Side-effects such as hyperglycaemia, psychological disturbances, hypertension, sodium retention, potassium loss, peptic ulcer formation and osteoporosis may occur. The occurrence of these side effects may be a sign of overdosage and may be reversed either by reducing the dosage or withdrawing therapy. Some side-effects, such as peptic ulceration and osteoporosis are thought to be less common with ACTH than with corticosteroid therapy.

Warnings: Hypersensitivity reactions may occur.

Pharmaceutical precautions *Acthar Gel:* Should be stored between 2–8°C and protected from light. Shelf-life 18 months.

Legal category POM.

Package quantities For intramuscular and subcutaneous use.
5 ml vial 20 i.u. per ml
2 ml vial 40 i.u. per ml
5 ml vial 40 i.u. per ml
5 ml vial 80 i.u. per ml

Further information
To replace corticosteroids with Acthar Gel:
1. To establish adrenal responsiveness: Administer 80–120 i.u. daily together with current steroid dosage until therapeutic or biochemical response or overdosage effects occur.

Clinical: Increased weight, sense of well-being and increased appetite, flushing of the face, and major reduction of disease symptoms.

Biochemical: Raised plasma cortisol levels or raised urinary excretion of 17-hydroxycorticosteroids.

2. As soon as adrenal response is established, reduce steroids by 25% of the original dose each day, maintaining the above dosage pattern of Acthar Gel.

3. When steroids are safely withdrawn, reduce Acthar Gel dosage to maintenance level.

To replace tetracosactrin depot with Acthar Gel: Substitute 40 units of Acthar Gel for each 0.5 mg of the tetracosactrin depot preparation. There should be no necessity to increase the frequency of injections.

Unduly large or small injection volumes are obviated by the comprehensive range of Acthar Gel strengths which are available.

Product licence numbers
20 iu/ml   0231/5000
40 iu/ml   0231/5051
80 iu/ml   0231/5052

ALBUMINAR*-5

Presentation Albuminar-5 is a sterile aqueous solution of Normal Serum Albumin (Human) 5% obtained from large pools of adult human venous plasma. Each 100 ml of Albuminar-5 contains 5 g of human serum albumin which is osmotically equivalent to normal human plasma.

The product conforms to the monograph for Normal Serum Albumin (Human) USP.

Indications Albuminar-5 is indicated in: The emergency treatment of shock and in other conditions where the restoration of blood volume is urgent.

Serious burns to prevent haemoconcentration and to combat fluid and sodium losses.

Clinical situations associated with low plasma protein (Hypoproteinaemia) with or without oedema, provided that sodium restriction is not imperative.

Therapeutic Plasma Exchange as a replacement fluid for phoresed plasma.

Dosage and administration (a) *Administration*: Albuminar-5 is for intravenous infusion.

Albuminar-5 may be given intravenously without further dilution; 5% solution is approximately isotonic and isosmotic with citrated plasma.

When albumin solution is administered to patients with normal blood volume, particular attention should be given to the rate of infusion so that the plasma volume is not expanded too rapidly.

(b) *Standard dose: Urgent restoration of blood volume:* In the emergency treatment of shock, the amount of albumin and duration of therapy must be based on the responsiveness of the patient as indicated by blood pressure, central venous pressure, degree of pulmonary congestion and haematocrit. The initial dose may be followed by additional albumin within 15–30 minutes if the response is deemed inadequate. If there has been considerable loss of blood, transfusion with whole blood is indicated, or if there is continued loss of protein, blood or plasma it may also be desirable to give whole blood and/or other blood fractions.

Burns: Albuminar-5 may be used to prevent marked haemoconcentration and to maintain appropriate electrolyte balance. An optimal regimen involving the use of albumin, crystalloids and water has not been established. Suggested therapy in the treatment of burns includes administration of large volumes of crystalloid solution during the first 24 hours to maintain an adequate plasma volume, even when albumin is infused. Continuation of therapy beyond 24 hours usually requires more albumin and less crystalloid solution. Duration of treatment varies depending on the extent of protein loss through renal excretion, denuded areas of skin and decreased albumin synthesis. Attempts to raise the albumin level above 40 g/litre may only result in an increased rate of catabolism.

Conditions associated with hypoproteinaemia: In these conditions, 1,000 to 1,500 ml of Albuminar-5 may be required to reduce oedema and to bring serum protein values to normal. Since such patients usually have approximately normal blood volume, doses of more than 500 ml of Albuminar-5 should not be given faster than 500 ml in 30–45 minutes to avoid circulatory embarrassment. If slower administration is desired, e.g. in patients with hypertension or cardiac insufficiency, 1,000 ml of Albuminar-5 may be administered by continuous drip at a rate of 100 ml of this solution per hour. Unless the pathological condition responsible for the hypoproteinaemia can be corrected, albumin in any form can afford only symptomatic or supportive relief. The 5% solution should not be administered in situations where sodium restriction is imperative.

Therapeutic plasma exchange: In plasma exchange procedures the volume of plasma removed may be replaced with an equivalent volume of Albuminar-5.

(c) *Children:* The amount of albumin given and the duration of therapy must be determined by the child's condition, response and other parameters, as stated under '*Standard Dose*'. However, when treating children, their body weight should also be taken into account.

Use in pregnancy: There is some experience of albumin being used in the treatment of pre-eclampsia and eclampsia. However, there is very little experience of the use of albumin in the early stages of pregnancy. There is no evidence either in human pregnancy or in animal work that administration of albumin is free from hazard.

Pharmacology: Action: Albuminar-5 is active osmotically and is therefore important in regulating the volume of circulating blood. When the circulating blood volume has been depleted, the haemodilution following albumin administration persists for many hours. In individuals with normal blood volumes, it usually lasts only a few hours.

Contra-indications, warnings, etc *Contra-indications:* Albuminar-5 may be contra-indicated in patients with severe anaemia or cardiac failure.

Precautions: If dehydration is present additional fluids must accompany or follow the administration of Albuminar-5.

The rise in blood pressure which may follow rapid administration of albumin necessitates careful observation of the injured patient to detect bleeding points, which failed to bleed at the lower blood pressure; otherwise new haemorrhage and shock may occur.

Albuminar-5 should be administered with caution to patients with low cardiac reserve or with no albumin deficiency, because a rapid increase in plasma volume may cause circulatory embarrassment or pulmonary oedema. In cases of hypertension or cardiac insufficiency, a slower rate of administration is desirable, at a rate of 5 g of albumin (100 ml) per hour. A careful watch must be kept for the possible development of pulmonary oedema. Should pulmonary oedema occur, the infusion must be stopped immediately.

Warnings and adverse effects: Do not use if the solution is turbid or contains a deposit. Since the solution contains no preservative, it should be used within 3 hours after entering the vial.

The incidence of adverse reactions to Normal Serum Albumin (Human) 5% is low, although nausea, vomiting, increased salivation and febrile reactions may occasionally occur.

Toxicity and treatment of overdosage: Administration of large quantities of albumin should be supplemented with red cell concentrates or replaced by whole blood to combat the relative anaemia which would follow such use. If circulatory embarrassment or pulmonary oedema should develop, the infusion must be stopped immediately and specific treatment given.

Pharmaceutical precautions
(a) *Presentation and Composition:* Albuminar-5 is a sterile, clear, brownish, slightly viscous aqueous solution of human serum albumin. It is stabilised with 0.004 M sodium acetyltryptophanate and 0.004 M sodium caprylate and the pH of the solution is adjusted with sodium bicarbonate or acetic acid. The solution contains approximately 130–160 mmol/l of sodium and not more than

1 mmol/l of potassium. The solution contains no preservative.

(b) *Storage:* Albuminar-5 should be stored at a temperature between 2° and 25°C. Freezing will not harm the solution, but might damage the container and allow contamination of the contents.

Protect solution from light.

When stored as directed Albuminar-5 has a shelf-life of 3 years.

Legal category POM.

Package quantities
Albuminar-5 is supplied as a 5% solution in:
    250 ml glass vials containing 12.5 grams of albumin
    500 ml glass vials containing 25.0 grams of albumin
1,000 ml glass vials containing 50.0 grams of albumin.

Further information Albuminar-5 is prepared from blood that was non-reactive for hepatitis B surface antigen (HBsAg) when tested with licensed reagents. The likelihood of the presence of viable hepatitis viruses has been further minimised by pasteurising the product at 60°C for 10 hours. Such treatment has been shown to be effective in this respect even when prepared from plasma known to be infective and albumin so prepared, unlike whole blood or plasma, is considered free of the danger of homologous serum hepatitis. Albuminar-5 may be given in conjunction with other parenteral fluids, such as whole blood, plasma, saline, dextrose, or sodium lactate. It is convenient to use, since no cross-matching is required and the absence of cellular elements removes the danger of sensitisation with repeated infusions.

Albuminar-5 contains none of the recognised components of the clotting mechanism of normal blood or plasma. It does not interfere with the normal clotting of blood.

Product licence number 0231/0056.

ALBUMINAR-20

Presentation Albuminar-20 is a sterile aqueous solution of Normal Serum Albumin (Human) 20% obtained from large pools of adult human venous plasma. Each 100 ml of Albuminar-20 contains 20 g of human serum albumin which is osmotically equivalent to 400 ml of normal human plasma.

The product conforms to the monograph for Human Albumin BP.

Indications Albuminar-20 is indicated in: The emergency treatment of shock and in other conditions where the restoration of blood volume is urgent.

Serious burns to prevent haemoconcentration and to combat fluid and sodium losses.

Clinical situations associated with low plasma protein (hypoproteinaemia) with or without oedema.

As an adjunct to exchange transfusion for the treatment of hyperbilirubinaemia in haemolytic disease of the newborn.

In priming heart lung machines for cardiopulmonary by-pass surgery.

Dosage and administration
(a) *Administration:* Albuminar-20 is for intravenous infusion.

Albuminar-20 may be given intravenously without dilution or it may be diluted with normal saline or 5% dextrose before administration. 250 ml per litre gives a solution which is approximately isotonic and isosmotic with citrated plasma.

When undiluted albumin solution is administered to patients with normal blood volume, particular attention should be given to the rate of infusion so that the plasma volume is not expanded too rapidly.

(b) *Standard dose: Urgent restoration of blood volume:* In these conditions effectiveness of Albuminar-20 depends on its ability to draw tissue fluid into the blood stream, when such fluid is available. Therefore, if dehydration is present, other fluids must be administered by any available route, either with albumin or following it. In the emergency treatment of shock, the amount of albumin and duration of therapy must be based on the responsiveness of the patient as indicated by blood pressure, central venous pressure, degree of pulmonary congestion and haematocrit. The initial dose may be followed by additional albumin within 15–30 minutes if the response is deemed inadequate. If there has been considerable loss of blood, transfusion with whole blood is indicated, or if there is continued loss of protein, blood or plasma it may also be desirable to give whole blood and/or other blood fractions.

Burns: Albuminar-20 may be used in conjunction with normal saline or dextrose to prevent marked haemoconcentration and to maintain appropriate electrolyte balance. An optimal regimen involving the use of albumin, crystalloids and water has not been established. Suggested therapy in the treatment of burns includes administration of large volumes of crystalloid solution during the first 24 hours to maintain an adequate plasma volume, even when albumin is infused. Continuation of therapy beyond 24 hours usually requires more albumin and less crystalloid solution. Duration of treatment varies depending on the extent of protein loss through renal excretion, denuded areas of skin and decreased albumin synthesis. Attempts to raise the albumin level above 40 g/litre may only result in an increased rate of catabolism.

Conditions associated with hypoproteinaemia: In these conditions, 200 to 300 ml of Albuminar-20 may be required to reduce oedema and to bring serum protein values to normal. Since such patients usually have approximately normal blood volume, doses of more than 100 ml of Albuminar-20 should not be given faster than 100 ml in 30–45 minutes to avoid circulatory embarrassment. If slower administration is desired, e.g. in patients with hypertension or cardiac insufficiency, 250 ml of Albuminar-20 may be mixed with 250 ml of 10% dextrose solution and administered by continuous drip at a rate of 100 ml of this dextrose solution per hour. Unless the pathological condition responsible for the hypoproteinaemia can be corrected, albumin in any form can afford only symptomatic or supportive relief.

Hyperbilirubinaemia in haemolytic disease of the newborn: In neonates, with serum bilirubin levels above 20 mg per 100 ml severe cerebral damage can develop due to kernicterus. In hypoalbuminaemia the reserve binding capacity for bilirubin is decreased and consequently bilirubin toxicity increases and with it the risk of cerebral damage. The risk of cerebral damage can be reduced by correction of the bilirubin binding capacity with Albuminar-20.

If immediate protection of the patient is required an intravenous injection of 1.0–1.5 g/kg albumin (5–7 ml Albuminar-20/kg bodyweight) can be given. Following this injection the exchange transfusion procedure should be instituted within 6 hours.

If albumin is intended for increasing the removal of bilirubin during exchange transfusion, it is suggested that 1.5–2.5 g albumin (7–12 ml Albuminar-20) is added to each 100 ml donor blood during exchange transfusion.

In Priming Heart Lung Machines for Cardiopulmonary By-Pass Surgery: Pre-operative dilution of the blood by use of a pump prime consisting of only albumin and crystalloid has been shown to be well tolerated during clinical studies. An albumin concentration of 5 g per cent has been widely used. A commonly employed programme is an albumin and crystalloid pump prime adjusted so as to achieve a haematocrit reading of 20 per cent and a plasma albumin level of 2.5 g/100 ml in the patient.

(c) *Children*: The amount of albumin given and the duration of therapy must be determined by the child's condition, response and other parameters, as stated under '*Standard Dose*'. However, when treating children, their body weight should also be taken into account.

Use in pregnancy: There is some experience of albumin being used in the treatment of pre-eclampsia and eclampsia. However, there is very little experience of the use of albumin in the early stages of pregnancy. There is no evidence either in human pregnancy or in animal work that administration of albumin is free from hazard.

Pharmacology: Action: Albuminar-20 is active oncotically and is therefore important in regulating the volume of circulating blood. When injected intravenously, 50 ml of Albuminar-20 draws approximately 3 volumes of additional fluid into the circulation within 15 minutes, except in the presence of marked dehydration. This extra fluid reduces haematocrit and blood viscosity. The degree of volume expansion is dependent on the initial blood volume. When circulating blood volume has been depleted, the haemodilution following albumin administration persists for many hours. In individuals with normal blood volume, it usually lasts only a few hours.

Contra-indications, warnings, etc

Contra-indications: Albuminar-20 may be contra-indicated in patients with severe anaemia or cardiac failure.

Precautions: If dehydration is present additional fluids must accompany or follow the administration of Albuminar-20.

The rise in blood pressure which may follow rapid administration of albumin necessitates careful observation of the injured patient to detect bleeding points, which failed to bleed at the lower blood pressure; otherwise new haemorrhage and shock may occur.

Albuminar-20 should be administered with caution to patients with low cardiac reserve or with no albumin deficiency, because a rapid increase in plasma volume may cause circulatory embarrassment or pulmonary oedema. In cases of hypertension or cardiac insufficiency, a slower rate of administration is desirable: 250 ml of Albuminar-20 may be mixed with 250 ml of 10% dextrose solution and administered at a rate of 10 g of albumin (100 ml) per hour. A careful watch must be kept for the possible development of pulmonary oedema. Should pulmonary oedema occur, the infusion must be stopped immediately.

Warnings and adverse effects: Do not use if the solution is turbid or contains a deposit. Since the solution contains no preservative, it should be used within 3 hours after entering the vial.

The incidence of adverse reactions to Normal Serum Albumin (Human) 20% is low, although nausea, vomit-ing, increased salivation and febrile reactions may occasionally occur.

Toxicity and treatment of overdosage: Administration of large quantities of albumin should be supplemented with red cell concentrates or replaced by whole blood to combat the relative anaemia which would follow such use.

If circulatory embarrassment or pulmonary oedema should develop, the infusion must be stopped immediately and specific treatment given.

Pharmaceutical precautions

(a) *Presentation and composition:* Albuminar-20 is a sterile, clear, brownish, slightly viscous aqueous solution of human serum albumin. It is stabilised with 0.016 M sodium acetyltryptophanate and 0.016 M sodium caprylate and the pH of the solution is adjusted with sodium bicarbonate or acetic acid. The solution contains not more than 130 mmol/l of sodium and not more than 1 mmol/l of potassium. The solution contains no preservative.

(b) *Storage:* Albuminar-20 should be stored at a temperature between 2° and 25°C. Freezing will not harm the solution, but might damage the container and allow contamination of the contents. Protect solution from light.

When stored as directed, Albuminar-20 has a shelf-life of 3 years.

Legal category POM.

Package quantities
Albuminar-20 is supplied as a 20% solution in:
50 ml vials containing 10.0 grams of albumin;
100 ml vials containing 20.0 grams of albumin.

Further information
Albuminar-20 is prepared from blood that was non-reactive for hepatitis B surface antigen (HBsAg) when tested with licensed reagents. The likelihood of the presence of viable hepatitis viruses has been further minimised by pasteurising the product at 60°C for 10 hours. Such treatment has been shown to be effective in this respect even when prepared from plasma known to be infective and albumin so prepared, unlike whole blood or plasma, is considered free of the danger of homologous serum hepatitis.

Albuminar-20 may be given in conjunction with other parenteral fluids, such as whole blood, plasma, saline, dextrose, or sodium lactate. It is convenient to use, since no cross-matching is required and the absence of cellular elements removes the danger of sensitisation with repeated infusions.

Albuminar-20 contains none of the recognised components of the clotting mechanism of normal blood or plasma. It does not interfere with the normal clotting of blood.

Product licence number 0231/0057

ALBUMINAR-25

Presentation Albuminar-25 is a sterile aqueous solution of Normal Serum Albumin (Human) 25% obtained from large pools of adult human venous plasma. Each 100 ml of Albuminar-25 contains 25 g of human serum albumin which is osmotically equivalent to 500 ml of normal human plasma.

The product conforms to the monograph for Normal Serum Albumin (Human) USP.

Indications Albuminar-25 is indicated in: The emergency treatment of shock and in other conditions where the restoration of blood volume is urgent.

Serious burns to prevent haemoconcentration and to combat fluid and sodium losses.

Clinical situations associated with low plasma protein (hypoproteinaemia) with or without oedema.

As an adjunct to exchange transfusion for the treatment of hyperbilirubinaemia in haemolytic disease of the newborn.

In priming heart-lung machines for cardiopulmonary by-pass surgery.

Dosage and administration

(a) *Administration:* Albuminar-25 is for intravenous infusion.

Albuminar-25 may be given intravenously without dilution or it may be diluted with normal saline or 5% dextrose before administration; 200 ml per litre gives a solution which is approximately isotonic and isosmotic with citrated plasma.

When undiluted albumin solution is administered to patients with normal blood volume, particular attention should be given to the rate of infusion so that it is slow enough to prevent too rapid expansion of plasma volume.

(b) *Standard dose: Urgent restoration of blood volume:* In these conditions effectiveness of Albuminar-25 depends on its ability to draw tissue fluid into the blood stream, when such fluid is available. Therefore, if dehydration is present, other fluids must be administered by any available route, either with albumin or following it. In the emergency treatment of shock, the amount of albumin and duration of therapy must be based on the responsiveness of the patient as indicated by blood pressure, central venous pressure, degree of pulmonary congestion and haematocrit. The initial dose may be followed by additional albumin within 15–30 minutes if the response is deemed inadequate. If there has been considerable loss of blood, transfusion with whole blood is indicated, or if there is continued loss of protein, blood or plasma it may also be desirable to give whole blood and/or other blood fractions.

Burns: Albuminar-25 may be used in conjunction with normal saline or dextrose to prevent marked haemoconcentration and to maintain appropriate electrolyte balance. An optimal regimen involving the use of albumin, crystalloids and water has not been established. Suggested therapy in the treatment of burns includes administration of large volumes of crystalloid solution during the first 24 hours to maintain an adequate plasma volume, even when albumin is infused. Continuation of therapy beyond 24 hours usually requires more albumin and less crystalloid solution. Duration of treatment varies depending on the extent of protein loss through renal excretion, denuded areas of skin and decreased albumin synthesis. Attempts to raise the albumin level above 40 g/litre may only result in an increased rate of catabolism.

Conditions associated with hypoproteinaemia: In these conditions, 200 to 300 ml of Albuminar-25 may be required to reduce oedema and to bring serum protein values to normal. Since such patients usually have approximately normal blood volume, doses of more than 100 ml of Albuminar-25 should not be given faster than 100 ml in 30–45 minutes to avoid circulatory embarrassment. If slower administration is desired, e.g. in patients with hypertension or cardiac insufficiency, 200 ml of Albuminar-25 may be mixed with 300 ml of 10% dextrose

solution and administered by continuous drip at a rate of 100 ml of this dextrose solution per hour. Unless the pathological condition responsible for the hypoproteinaemia can be corrected, albumin in any form can afford only symptomatic or supportive relief.

Hyperbilirubinaemia in haemolytic disease of the newborn: In neonates with serum bilirubin levels above 20 mg per 100 ml severe cerebral damage can develop due to kernicterus. In hypoalbuminaemia the reserve binding capacity for bilirubin is decreased and consequently bilirubin toxicity increases and with it the risk of cerebral damage. The risk of cerebral damage can be reduced by correction of the bilirubin binding capacity with Albuminar-25.

If immediate protection of the patient is required an intravenous injection of 1.0–1.5 g/kg albumin (4–6 ml Albuminar-25/kg bodyweight) can be given. Following this injection the exchange transfusion procedure should be instituted within 6 hours.

If albumin is intended for increasing the removal of bilirubin during exchange transfusion, it is suggested that 1.5–2.5 g albumin (6–10 ml Albuminar-25) is added to each 100 ml donor blood during exchange transfusion.

In Priming Heart Lung Machines for Cardiopulmonary By-Pass Surgery: Pre-operative dilution of the blood by use of a pump prime consisting of only albumin and crystalloid has been shown to be well tolerated during clinical studies. An albumin concentration of 5 g per cent has been widely used. A commonly employed programme is an albumin and crystalloid pump prime adjusted so as to achieve a haematocrit reading of 20 per cent and a plasma albumin level of 2.5 g/100 ml in the patient.

(c) *Children:* The amount of albumin given and the duration of therapy must be determined by the child's condition, response and other parameters, as stated under 'Standard Dose'. However, when treating children, their body weight should also be taken into account.

Use in pregnancy: There is some experience of albumin being used in the treatment of pre-eclampsia and eclampsia. However, there is very little experience of the use of albumin in the early stages of pregnancy. There is no evidence either in human pregnancy or in animal work that administration of albumin is free from hazard.

Pharmacology: Action: Albuminar-25 is active oncotically and is therefore important in regulating the volume of circulating blood. When injected intravenously, 50 ml of Albuminar-25 draws approximately 175 ml of additional fluid into the circulation within 15 minutes, except in the presence of marked dehydration. This extra fluid reduces haematocrit and blood viscosity. The degree of volume expansion is dependent on the initial blood volume. When circulating blood volume has been depleted, the haemodilution following albumin administration persists for many hours. In individuals with normal blood volume, it usually lasts only a few hours.

Contra-indications, warnings, etc

Contra-indications: Albuminar-25 may be contra-indicated in patients with severe anaemia or cardiac failure.

Precautions: If dehydration is present additional fluids must accompany or follow the administration of Albuminar-25.

The rise in blood pressure which may follow rapid administration of albumin necessitates careful observation of the injured patient to detect bleeding points, which failed to bleed at the lower blood pressure; otherwise new haemorrhage and shock may occur.

Albuminar-25 should be administered with caution to patients with low cardiac reserve or with no albumin deficiency, because a rapid increase in plasma volume may cause circulatory embarrassment or pulmonary oedema. In cases of hypertension or cardiac insufficiency, a slower rate of administration is desirable: 200 ml of Albuminar-25 may be mixed with 300 ml of 10% dextrose solution and administered at a rate of 10 g of albumin (100 ml) per hour. A careful watch must be kept for the possible development of pulmonary oedema. Should pulmonary oedema occur, the infusion must be stopped immediately.

Warnings and adverse effects: Do not use if the solution is turbid or contains a deposit. Since the solution contains no preservative, it should be used within 3 hours after entering the vial.

The incidence of untoward reactions to Normal Serum Albumin (Human) 20% is low, although nausea, vomiting, increased salivation and febrile reactions may occasionally occur.

Toxicity and treatment of overdosage: Administration of large quantities of albumin should be supplemented with red cell concentrates or replaced by whole blood to combat the relative anaemia which would follow such use.

If circulatory embarrassment or pulmonary oedema should develop, the infusion must be stopped immediately and specific treatment given.

Pharmaceutical precautions
(a) *Presentation and composition:* Albuminar-25 is a sterile, clear, brownish, slightly viscous aqueous solution of human serum albumin. It is stabilised with 0.02 M sodium acetyltryptophanate and 0.02 M sodium caprylate and the pH of the solution is adjusted with sodium bicarbonate or acetic acid. The solution contains approximately 130–160 mmol/l of sodium and not more than 1 mmol/l of potassium. The solution contains no preservative.

(b) *Storage:* Albuminar-25 should be stored at a temperature between 2° and 25°C. Freezing will not harm the solution, but might damage the container and allow contamination of the contents. Protect solution from light.

When stored as directed, Albuminar-25 has a shelf-life of 3 years.

Legal category POM.

Package quantities Albuminar-25 is supplied as a 25% solution in:
  20 ml vials containing 5.0 grams of albumin.
  50 ml vials containing 12.5 grams of albumin;
100 ml vials containing 25.0 grams of albumin.

Further information Albuminar-25 is prepared from blood that was non-reactive for hepatitis B surface antigen (HBsAg) when tested with licensed reagents. The likelihood of the presence of viable hepatitis viruses has been further minimised by pasteurising the product at 60°C for 10 hours. Such treatment has been shown to be effective in this respect even when prepared from plasma known to be infective and albumin so prepared, unlike whole blood or plasma, is considered free of the danger of homologous serum hepatitis.

Albuminar-25 may be given in conjunction with other parenteral fluids, such as whole blood, plasma, saline, dextrose, or sodium lactate. It is convenient to use, since no cross-matching is required and the absence of cellular elements removes the danger of sensitisation with repeated infusions.

Albuminar-25 contains none of the recognised components of the clotting mechanism of normal blood or plasma. It does not interfere with the normal clotting of blood.

Product licence number 0231/0045

ARVIN*

Presentation A sterile clear colourless aqueous solution of ancrod for intravenous and subcutaneous injection. Each ml contains 70 international units put up in isotonic saline. pH is 6.8, phosphate content approximately 0.0025M and chlorbutol approximately 0.005%.

The international unit is defined as the specific biological activity contained in 0.307 mg of the international standard for ancrod.

Uses *Controlled defibrination for:*
1. The prevention of deep vein thrombosis following surgical repair of fractured neck of femur and hip replacement.
2. The treatment of deep vein thrombosis, central retinal and branch vein thrombosis, priapism, pulmonary hypertension of embolic origin, embolism after insertion of prosthetic cardiac valves, rethrombosis after thrombolytic therapy and rethrombosis after vascular surgery.
3. Peripheral arterial insufficiency.

Dosage and administration
Subcutaneous dosage:
1. Prophylaxis of deep vein thrombosis in:
(a) Patients undergoing surgical repair for fractured neck of femur – 4 × 1 ml ampoules as a single s.c. injection immediately after surgery then 1 ampoule daily for the next 4 days.
(b) Hip replacement – 4 × 1 ml ampoules as a single s.c. injection immediately after surgery then 1 ampoule daily for the next 8 days.

With these prophylactic regimes, Arvin normally produces predictable defibrination. Occasionally however, the clinical situation may warrant the measurement of fibrinogen levels.

2. Peripheral arterial insufficiency – 1 unit/kg body weight as a single injection into the anterior abdominal wall or thigh each day for four days to lower the plasma fibrinogen to 50 mg% or more; then 4 units/kg as a single injection every three or four days to maintain the fibrinogen at this level. This subcutaneous regimen may be used for up to one month in patients with chronic peripheral arterial insufficiency. Fibrinogen levels should be monitored prior to administration of the next dose.

Intravenous dosage:
Treatment of established thrombo-embolic conditions:

Induction dose: 2–3 units/kg body weight in 50–500 ml Sodium Chloride Injection BP by slow intravenous drip over a period of four to twelve hours. Administration of this dose should not take place over a period of less than 4 hours.

Maintenance doses: 2 units/kg body weight in 10–50 ml Sodium Chloride Injection BP by intravenous injections at twelve-hour intervals, given slowly, taking about five minutes over each injection. Fibrinogen levels should be monitored daily by standard laboratory procedures to facilitate accurate control of dosage.

Contra-indications, warnings, etc

Contra-indications: Severe infections and diffuse intra-vascular coagulation.

Pregnancy.

Gastro-intestinal ulcers liable to bleed such as peptic ulcer, ulcerative colitis.

Ulcerogenic drugs.

Haematological defects which interfere with haemostasis such as platelet count of < 100,000/cu mm.

Patients in receipt of plasma expanders such as dextrans or antifibrinolytic agents such as EACA should not be treated with Arvin.

Precautions: Pretreatment investigations such as blood film, platelet count and fibrinogen should be made before treatment.

The intravenous induction dose of Arvin must not be given in less than 4 hours as if given rapidly the fibrin degradation products may produce a rise in blood viscosity.

Warnings: Haemorrhage may occur and can be rapidly reversed by the specific antidote although this is rarely necessary as fibrinogen levels return to haemostatic values within a few hours of cessation of therapy.

Defibrination may complicate malignant hypertension; acute pericarditis, sub-acute bacterial endocarditis, retinopathy (grade 3 or worse), diabetic retinopathy, resting diastolic pressure > 120 mm Hg and may cause bleeding in uraemia > 100 mg%, renal colic with calculus, cerebrovascular accidents, history of neurosurgery.

Migraine – a few patients with a history of migraine have experienced headaches after Arvin injections.

ESR – during treatment with Arvin, the erythrocyte sedimentation rate falls to about 1 mm/hour and cannot be used as an index of pathological activity.

Platelets – although Arvin has no specific effect on platelets the fibrin degradation products produce reduced platelet aggregation.

Treatment of overdosage or excessive bleeding: A specific antidote has been prepared of which 1 ml neutralises 70 units of Arvin *in vivo*.

The following procedure is recommended for the use of the antidote.

1. 1 in 1,000 adrenaline should be available on the giving tray.
2. Give 0.2 ml antidote subcutaneously and observe for an erythematous reaction for half hour.
3. If satisfactory, give 0.8 ml antidote intramuscularly and observe for a nodular reaction for a further half hour.
4. If satisfactory, give 1 ml intravenously.
5. Give 5 g human fibrinogen intravenously (available from the Regional Blood Transfusion Centre). If this is not available give 1 litre fresh plasma or whole blood.

The whole procedure takes about one hour and will restore the plasma fibrinogen to normal in this time.

In emergencies the intramuscular dose may be ignored but the subcutaneous test dose should not be omitted. In the case of a reaction after the subcutaneous dose, more antidote should not be administered but substituted by fresh plasma or whole blood unless the bleeding is life threatening. *When immediate neutralisation of the Arvin effect is essential, the highly purified nature of the antidote allows intravenous injection without the usual trial doses, with a normal supportive corticosteroid/antihistamine regime ready if anaphylactic shock develops. Fibrinogen should also be administered.*

Pharmaceutical precautions Store under refrigeration between 4°C and 8°C. Do not freeze.

Legal category POM.

Package quantities Ampoules 1 ml containing 70 international units ancrod per ml. Pack of 4.

Further information *Clinical effects:* The properties of Arvin provide *controlled therapeutic defibrination* to prevent the formation and extension of thrombi and the dissemination of emboli. Despite marked hypocoagulability, spontaneous haemorrhage is rarely observed, although serosanguineous oozing or frank haemorrhage may be seen in incompletely healed surgical wounds. Consistent clinical features include the absence of thromboembolic events during treatment, normal menstruation, absence of fibrinogen rebound and a very low incidence of rethrombosis after treatment is stopped. The plasma fibrinogen returns to haemostatic levels within 12 hours and to normal levels usually around the 10th post-treatment day, but in a few patients this may be delayed for a further 10 days. Apart from apparently avoiding rebound hypercoagulation, this slow return of fibrinogen allows a smooth change over to oral anticoagulants when necessary. While Arvin does not lyse established thrombi, rapid resolution of secondary oedema has been noted frequently and is believed to result from improved flow in the micro-circulation.

Arvin antidote: Ampoules of Arvin antidote are available free of charge for *clinical use* in hospitals. Laboratories may order the antidote for in vitro use.

Product licence numbers
Arvin   0152/0099
Antidote   0152/0128

CALCITARE*

Presentation *For intramuscular or subcutaneous use only.* Each vial contains 160 international units Calcitonin (Pork) BP.

Uses *Paget's disease of bone*

Hypercalcaemia: The calcium lowering effect of calcitonin is usually rapid. Treatment should be regarded as an adjunct to more specific long-term measures. The fall in serum calcium is more pronounced in hypercalcaemic patients with a raised bone turnover, e.g. Paget's disease and thyrotoxicosis. Treatment may also be beneficial in patients with hypercalcaemia due to immobilisation in Paget's disease, malignancy, vitamin D intoxication and hyperparathyroidism. Calcitonin is of particular value when such patients have concurrent renal or cardiac failure.

Dosage and administration Calcitare can be given subcutaneously or intramuscularly.

1. *Paget's disease of bone:* Clinical and biochemical improvement has been observed with dosage regimens ranging from 80 international units three times a week to 160 international units daily in single or divided doses.

Daily injections of 80 international units or 160 international units are recommended for three to six months in patients with bone pain or nerve compression syndromes.

Clinical improvement is usually seen within three months but may occasionally be delayed for as long as a year. When clinical improvement occurs, an attempt to reduce the dose and/or frequency of injection may be made, consistent with maintaining a remission. Alternatively, treatment can be stopped and restarted at a later date when necessary.

Biochemical improvement is shown by a reduction in serum alkaline phosphatase and urinary hydroxyproline excretion, the fall in urinary hydroxyproline often occurring in a matter of days. The fall in serum alkaline phosphatase occurs in a matter of weeks. Serum alkaline phosphatase and urinary hydroxyproline levels return slowly towards pre-treatment values (at different rates) on withdrawal of calcitonin therapy. Long-term treatment with calcitonin may be needed in those asymptomatic patients with rapidly advancing and potentially disabling disease.

Radiological and histological improvement has also been observed with long-term treatment and this reconstructive action of calcitonin on bone has been shown to be dose-dependent.

When changing from synthetic salmon calcitonin (Calsynar) to porcine calcitonin (Calcitare), 80 international units of Calcitare may be conveniently substituted for 50 international units of Calsynar and 160 international units for 100 international units respectively.

2. *Hypercalcaemia:* The optimum dosage pattern must essentially be gauged by the magnitude of the hypocalcaemic response obtained in a particular patient. In general the greatest response will be observed in cases of rapid bone turnover. Four international units per kg per day of Calcitare may produce a fall in serum calcium. However, larger doses of calcitonin may be necessary, but are inconvenient to administer as Calcitare, in which case treatment with Calsynar is advised.

Contra-indications, warnings and side-effects

Calcitonin may cause nausea, vomiting, facial flushing and tingling of the hands. An unpleasant taste and inflammatory reactions at the injection site have been reported. The nausea and flushing are usually transient and rarely necessitate withdrawal of treatment. If necessary, the injections can be administered at night with an antiemetic.

In any patient with a history of allergy, a scratch (or intradermal) test should be conducted prior to administration of Calcitare using a 1:100 dilution in Sodium Chloride Injection BP. To detect gelatin sensitivity a similar test should be carried out using gelatin diluent in the same dilution.

Some patients will develop porcine calcitonin binding antibodies after several months of treatment. The antibodies are generally of low titre and are more likely to occur in patients on the higher doses. The development of these antibodies is not usually related to loss of clinical efficacy. It is possible that this may be analogous to treated diabetic patients in whom insulin binding antibodies frequently develop, but who rarely manifest clinical resistance to insulin. The presence of these antibodies appears to bear no relationship to allergic reactions which are very rare. Secondary hyperparathyroidism is not thought to occur following calcitonin therapy.

Reproductive studies performed with salmon calcitonin showed a decrease in foetal birth weight in rabbits when given in doses of 14–56 times the dose recommended for human use. Since calcitonin does not cross the placental barrier this finding may be due to metabolic effects of calcitonin on the pregnant animal. There are no studies in pregnant women. Salmon calcitonin, and by inference porcine calcitonin, should be used only when clearly needed in women who are or who may become pregnant.

Calcitonin has been shown to inhibit lactation in animals and should not be administered to nursing mothers.

Following injections of calcitonin serum calcium levels may be transiently lowered to below normal values. This effect is noted most frequently on therapy where bone turnover is abnormally high, but diminishes as osteoclastic activity is reduced with Calcitare. Whilst this phenomenon does not usually give rise to complications, care should be exercised in patients who are receiving concurrent cardiac glycosides as dosage adjustments of these drugs may be necessary in view of the fact that their effect may be modified by changes in cellular electrolyte concentrations. Trace amounts of T_3/T_4 are present in Calcitare. Experience over a number of years has not revealed any significant metabolic effects due to T_3 and T_4, when Calcitare has been given at the maximum recommended dose for Paget's disease of 160 international units daily. At higher doses (e.g. 8 i.u./kg) used in the treatment of hypercalcaemia, the amounts of T_3/T_4 normally detected in the product are most unlikely to have any adverse effect, except in highly susceptible patients such as those with significant ischaemic heart disease.

Pharmaceutical precautions Calcitare is presented as a sterile, lyophilised powder providing 160 international units porcine calcitonin per vial. Calcitare should normally be used immediately after aseptic reconstitution. The reconstituted product will, however, maintain its potency for up to 24 hours at room temperature or 7 days in a refrigerator (2–8°C).

The lyophilised powder when stored at less than 25°C will retain its potency for three years.

Legal category POM.

Package quantities *For intramuscular or subcutaneous use:* Boxes of 5 vials Calcitare 160 international units per vial sterile, lyophilised, with 5 vials gelatin diluent, sterile.

Boxes of 10 vials Calcitare 160 international units per vial sterile, lyophilised, with 10 vials gelatin diluent, sterile.

Further information The calcium lowering ability of the calcitonins is measured in international units. The international unit is based on a rat bioassay in which one fortieth of the weight of salmon calcitonin, as compared with weights of porcine and human calcitonin, produces the same fall in serum calcium. The weights of pure calcitonin equivalent to 100 international units in this assay are: human calcitonin, 1 mg. porcine calcitonin, 1 mg, and salmon calcitonin, 0.025 mg.

Product licence number 0231/0011.

CALSYNAR* (Salcatonin Injection BP)

Presentation *Multidose vials:* Each multidose vial contains 400 international units of synthetic salmon calcitonin in 2 ml of saline acetate diluent (i.e. 200 international units of approximately 0.05 mg synthetic salmon calcitonin per ml). For subcutaneous or intramuscular use only.

Ampoules: Each clear glass ampoule contains 100 international units of synthetic salmon calcitonin in 1 ml saline acetate diluent. For subcutaneous or intramuscular use only.

Uses *Postmenopausal Osteoporosis:* Studies based on total body calcium determinations have indicated that

Calsynar may be effective in the prevention of progressive loss of bone mass in the treatment of postmenopausal osteoporosis.

Paget's disease of bone.
Hypercalcaemia: The calcium lowering effect of calcitonin is usually rapid. Treatment should be regarded as an adjunct to more specific long-term measures. The fall in serum calcium is more pronounced in hypercalcaemic patients with a raised bone turnover, e.g. Paget's disease and thyrotoxicosis. Treatment may also be beneficial in patients with hypercalcaemia due to immobilisation in Paget's disease, malignancy, vitamin D intoxication and hyperparathyroidism.

Calcitonin is of particular value when such patients have concurrent renal or cardiac failure.

Pain associated with metastatic bone cancer: Calsynar has been reported to be beneficial in some patients in the relief of moderately severe or severe bone pain associated with metastases in advanced malignant disease.

Dosage and administration (a) *Postmenopausal osteoporosis:* The recommended dose of Calsynar is 100 i.u. per day given subcutaneously or intramuscularly. Patients should also receive supplementary calcium (equivalent to 600 mg elemental calcium daily) and vitamin D (400 units daily). An adequate diet is also essential. (See also 'Further Information').
(b) *Paget's disease of bone:* Clinical and biochemical improvement has been observed with dosage regimens ranging from 50 international units three times a week to 100 international units daily in single or divided doses given subcutaneously or intramuscularly.

Daily injections of 50 international units or 100 international units are recommended for three to six months in patients with bone pain or nerve compression syndromes.

Clinical improvement is usually seen within three months but may occasionally be delayed for as long as a year. When clinical improvement occurs, an attempt to reduce the dose and/or frequency of the injections may be made, consistent with maintaining a remission. Alternatively, treatment can be stopped and restarted at a later date when necessary.

Biochemical improvement is shown by a reduction in serum alkaline phosphatase and urinary hydroxyproline excretion, the fall in urinary hydroxyproline often occurring in a matter of days, the fall in serum alkaline phosphatase occurring in a matter of weeks. Serum alkaline phosphatase and urinary hydroxyproline levels return slowly towards pre-treatment values (at different rates) on withdrawal of calcitonin therapy. Long-term treatment with calcitonin may be needed in those asymptomatic patients with rapidly advancing and potentially disabling disease.

Radiological and histological improvement has also been observed with long-term treatment and this reconstructive action of calcitonin on bone has been shown to be dose-dependent.

When changing from porcine calcitonin (Calcitare) to synthetic salmon calcitonin (Calsynar) 50 international units of Calsynar may be conveniently substituted for 80 international units of Calcitare and 100 international units for 160 international units of Calcitare.

(c) *Hypercalcaemia:* Calsynar should be given by subcutaneous or intramuscular injection. Treatment should be adjusted to the patient's clinical and biochemical response.

Severe hypercalcaemia may require high doses of Calsynar and initially 400 international units may be given six or eight-hourly. Lower doses may be satisfactory in some patients and dosage may be adjusted according to the patient's clinical and biochemical response. There is no additional benefit to be gained from doses in excess of 8 international units per kg six-hourly.

(d) *Pain associated with metastatic bone cancer:* Administer Calsynar subcutaneously or intramuscularly at a dose of 200 iu six-hourly or 400 iu twelve-hourly for 48 hours. Concomitant analgesic medication may be reduced as appropriate. The treatment course may be repeated at the discretion of the physician.

Many patients with advanced malignant disease already suffer from anorexia and nausea. In these cases, prior administration of anti-emetic therapy may reduce the incidence of nausea and vomiting sometimes associated with calcitonin therapy.

Contra-indications, warnings, etc Calcitonin may cause nausea, vomiting, facial flushing, tingling of the hands, and an unpleasant taste. Inflammatory reactions at the injection site have been reported. The nausea and flushing are usually transient and rarely necessitate withdrawal of treatment. If necessary, the injections can be administered at night with an antiemetic.

In any patient with a history of allergy, a scratch (or intradermal) test should be conducted prior to administration of Calsynar using a 1:100 dilution in Sodium Chloride Injection BP.

Some patients will develop salmon calcitonin binding antibodies after several months of treatment. The antibodies are generally of low titre and are more likely to occur in patients on the higher doses. The development of these antibodies is not usually related to loss of clinical efficacy. It is possible that this may be analogous to treated diabetic patients in whom insulin binding antibodies frequently develop, but who rarely manifest clinical resistance to insulin. The presence of antibodies appears to bear no relationship to allergic reactions which are very rare.

Secondary hyperparathyroidism is not thought to occur following calcitonin therapy.

Salmon calcitonin has been shown to cause decrease in foetal birth weight in rabbits when given in doses of 14–56 times the dose recommended for human use. Since calcitonin does not cross the placental barrier this finding may be due to metabolic effects of calcitonin on the pregnant animal. Studies have not been carried out in pregnant women. Whenever possible, treatment should be avoided in women of child-bearing potential. Calcitonin has been shown to inhibit lactation in animals and should not be administered to nursing mothers.

Following injections of calcitonin serum calcium levels may be transiently lowered to below normal values. This effect is noted most frequently on initiation of therapy where bone turnover is abnormally high, but diminishes as osteoclastic activity is reduced with Calsynar. Whilst this phenomenon does not usually give rise to complications, care should be exercised in patients who are receiving concurrent cardiac glycosides as dosage adjustments of these drugs may be necessary in view of the fact that their effect may be modified by changes in cellular electrolyte concentrations.

Pharmaceutical precautions Calsynar multidose vials, when stored between 2–8°C will retain their potency for 3 years. Do not freeze.

Calsynar ampoules 100 iu when stored between 2–8°C will retain their potency for 2 years. Do not freeze.

Legal category POM.

Package quantities Box of 1 and cartons of 4 multidose vials of Calsynar 400 international units per vial in 2 ml saline acetate diluent.

Cartons of 5 ampoules, each ampoule containing 100 international units in 1 ml saline acetate diluent.

Further information
Postmenopausal osteoporosis: There is evidence from published literature on postmenopausal osteoporosis that cyclical therapy with Calsynar may be useful in some patients.

Units and potency: The calcium lowering ability of the calcitonins is measured in international units. The international unit is based on a rat bioassay in which one fortieth of the weight of salmon calcitonin, as compared with weights of porcine and human calcitonin, produces the same fall in serum calcium. The weights of pure calcitonin equivalent to 100 international units in this assay are approximately: human calcitonin 1 mg; porcine calcitonin 1 mg; and salmon calcitonin, 0.025 mg.

Product licence numbers
Multidose vials: 0231/0027.
Ampoules: 0231/0055.

CHYMOCYCLAR*

Presentation Each pink, gelatin capsule contains:
50,000 Armour units of proteolytic activity supplied by a purified enzyme concentrate containing trypsin and chymotrypsin.
250 mg Tetracycline Hydrochloride BP.

Uses Infections due to tetracycline-sensitive organisms.

Dosage and administration
For administration to adults only: One or two capsules to be taken four times a day, half an hour before meals. The capsules should be swallowed whole since damage to the enteric coated core results in loss of proteolytic activity.

Absorption of tetracycline is impaired by the concomitant administration of food or drugs of high calcium content.

Contra-indications, warnings, etc
Precautions: In the presence of renal or hepatic impairment accumulation of tetracycline may occur and special attention to dosage is necessary. If possible, serum antibiotic levels should be controlled in such patients. Special care should be exercised with the use of tetracycline during pregnancy.

Side-effects: Tetracycline is known to produce gastrointestinal disturbances and may facilitate monilial infection in some cases. Although no specific reports relating to Chymocyclar have been received, tetracycline has been recorded as causing haemolytic anaemia, eosinophilia, thrombocytopenia, hepatotoxicity, allergic skin reactions and photosensitivity.

Tetracycline has also been reported to reduce the efficacy of oral steroid contraceptives.

Contra-indications: Patients with known sensitivities to enzymes and tetracycline. During the period of tooth development, last trimester of pregnancy and early childhood, it is possible that tetracycline may cause yellowish brown discolouration of the teeth and enamel hyperplasia in prolonged high dosage.

Pharmaceutical precautions Chymocyclar should be stored in a cool dry place, protected from light – Shelf-life 3 years.

Legal category POM.

Package quantities Securitainers of 30, 100 and 500 capsules.

Further information In conditions where inflammatory oedema is associated with infections, the administration of the proteolytic enzymes may be directly advantageous, and the beneficial clinical results obtained with combination therapy of this nature have been reported in the literature.

Product licence number 0231/5001.

CHYMORAL*
CHYMORAL* FORTE

Presentation Enteric-coated tablets containing a purified proteolytic enzyme concentrate providing trypsin and chymotrypsin activity.
Chymoral – 50,000 Armour units.
Chymoral Forte – 100,000 Armour units.

Uses Resolution of acute, inflammatory oedema associated with: Accidental and surgical trauma. Episiotomies. Intervertebral disc herniation (sciatica). Thrombophlebitis. Vasectomies. Reduction in viscosity of mucus and sputum associated with bronchitis, rhinitis and sinusitis.

Dosage and administration *Chymoral:* 2 tablets four times a day. Children 1 tablet four times a day.

Chymoral Forte: 1 tablet four times a day. Not for administration to children.

The tablets must be taken half an hour before meals and swallowed whole without crushing, since damage to the enteric coating rapidly causes loss of potency.

Contra-indications, warnings, etc
Precautions: Patients with known sensitivity to enzymes.

After many years of widespread clinical use, there is no reason to believe that Chymoral is, or may be, teratogenic in humans. However, it is a sound medical principle to exercise precaution in prescribing any medication during the first three months of pregnancy.

Side-effects: Occasional slight gastric disturbance.

Pharmaceutical precautions The tablets should be stored in a cool dry place – shelf-life is three years for both Chymoral and Chymoral Forte.

Legal category P.

Package quantities *Chymoral:* Securitainers of 50 and 500 tablets.

Chymoral Forte: Securitainers of 30, 200 and 500 tablets.

Further information Nil.

Product licence numbers

Chymoral	0231/5021
Chymoral Forte	0231/5020

DIORALYTE*
DIORALYTE* CHERRY
DIORALYTE* PINEAPPLE

Presentation Compound Sodium Chloride and Glucose Powder BP in foil-laminate sachets each containing:

Sodium Chloride BP	0.20 g
Potassium Chloride BP	0.30 g
Sodium Bicarbonate BP	0.30 g
Glucose BP	8.00 g

Uses Oral correction of fluid and electrolyte loss in infants, children and adults.

Treatment of watery diarrhoea of varying aetiologies, including gastroenteritis, in all age groups.

Dosage and administration *Reconstitution:* The contents of each sachet should be dissolved in 200 ml (approximately 7 fluid ounces) of drinking water. Use fresh drinking water for adults and children. For infants, and where drinking water is unavailable, the water should be freshly boiled and cooled. The solution should be made up immediately before use. If refrigerated, the solution may be stored for up to 24 hours, otherwise any solution remaining an hour after reconstitution should be discarded. The solution must not be boiled.

The actual volume of reconstituted Dioralyte which should be taken should be decided by the clinician, taking into consideration the weight of the patient and the stage and severity of the condition. A basic principle of treatment of diarrhoea is to replace lost fluid and then to maintain sufficient fluid intake to replace fluid loss from stools.

Daily intake may be based on a volume of 150 ml/kg body weight for infants and 20–40 ml/kg body weight for adults and children. A reasonable approximation is:

Infants – One to one and a half times the usual feed volume.

Children – One sachet after every loose motion.

Adults – One or two sachets after every loose motion.

More may be required initially to ensure early and full volume repletion.

Day	Volume of Dioralyte solution (ml)	Volume of artificial milk feed (ml)	Total volume in 24 hours (ml)
1	150 × wt*	0	150 × wt
2	120 × wt	30 × wt	150 × wt
3	90 × wt	60 × wt	150 × wt
4	60 × wt	90 × wt	150 × wt
5	30 × wt	120 × wt	150 × wt
6	0	150 × wt	150 × wt

* Weight in kilograms.

In the initial stages of treatment of diarrhoea all foods, including cow's or artificial milk, should be stopped. However, breast milk need not be witheld. In breast fed infants it is suggested that the infant is given the same volume of Dioralyte as the normal feed and then put to the breast until satisfied. Expression of residual milk from the breasts may be necessary during this period. After 24–48 hours, when symptoms have subsided, the normal diet should be resumed but this should be gradual to avoid exacerbation of the condition. A suggested regimen for the treatment of severe infantile diarrhoea based on body weight in kilograms is given in previous column.

Where vomiting is present with the diarrhoea it is advisable that small amounts of Dioralyte be taken frequently. However, it is important that the whole of the required volume of Dioralyte is taken. Where the kidneys are functioning normally, it is difficult to overhydrate by mouth and where there is doubt about the exact dosage, more rather than less should be taken.

Contra-indications, warnings, etc There are no known contra-indications to Dioralyte. However, there may be a number of conditions where treatment with Dioralyte will be inappropriate eg intestinal obstruction requiring surgical intervention.

Precautions: For oral administration only.

Dioralyte should not be reconstituted in diluents other than water.

Each sachet should always be dissolved in 200 ml of water. A weaker solution than recommended will not contain the optimal glucose and electrolyte concentration and a stronger solution than recommended may give rise to electrolyte imbalance.

If the diarrhoea does not improve promptly, the patient should be reassessed.

Warning: Cow's milk and artificial milk feeds in infants should be stopped for 24 hours and gradually reintroduced when the diarrhoea has lessened. However, breast feeding should be continued.

Pharmaceutical precautions The sachet should be stored in a cool, dry place. Shelf-life 3 years.

Legal category P.

Package quantities Packs of 20 sachets.

Further information The composition of Dioralyte is based on the observation that a correctly balanced, isotonic solution of glucose and sodium stimulates intestinal water absorption.

A litre of made up solution (5 sachets, 5 × 200 ml quantities) contains: 35 mmol Sodium (Na^+); 20 mmol Potassium (K^+); 37 mmol Chloride (Cl^-); 18 mmol Bicarbonate (HCO_3); 200 mmol Dextrose.

The total osmolarity is 310 mmol per litre.

Each sachet of Dioralyte contains 8 g of glucose which is equivalent to 30.5 kcal.

Product licence numbers

Dioralyte	0231/0043.
Dioralyte Cherry	0231/0067
Dioralyte Pineapple	0231/0068

FACTORATE* HEAT TREATED ▼

Presentation Dried Human Antihaemophilic Fraction Factorate Heat Treated is a stable lyophilised concentrate of Factor VIII (AHF, AHG) prepared from pooled human plasma.

Each vial contains the labelled amount of antihaemophilic activity in International Units (one International Unit is the activity equivalent to the average Factor VIII content of 1 ml aliquots of 167 samples of fresh normal plasma, as determined in an international collaborative study). Each vial also contains sufficient sodium chloride to make the reconstituted solution approximately isotonic when sterile Water for Injections BP is added as directed.

This product has been heated at 60°C for 30 hours. This step has been introduced in order to reduce the risk of transmission of infectious agents.

All units of source plasma are tested for antibodies to human T cell lymphotropic virus type III (HTLV III) and found to be negative.

Uses For use in therapy of classic haemophilia (Haemophilia A).

Dosage and administration Factorate Heat Treated is for intravenous administration only. As a general rule one unit of Factor VIII activity per kg will increase by 2% the circulating Factor VIII level, and although dosage must be adjusted according to the needs of the patient (weight, severity of haemorrhage, presence of inhibitors) the following general dosages are suggested.

1. Overt bleeding: Initially 20 units per kg of body weight followed by 10 units per kg every eight hours for the first 24 hours and the same dose every 12 hours for the next 3 or 4 days. For massive wounds, give until bleeding stops and maintain with 20 units per kg 8-hourly to achieve a minimum Factor VIII level of 40%.

2. Muscle haemorrhages: (a) Minor haemorrhages in extremities or non-vital areas: 10 units per kg once a day for 2 or 3 days.

(b) Massive haemorrhages in non-vital areas: 10 units per kg by infusion at 12 hour intervals for 2 days and then once a day for 2 more days.

(c) Haemorrhages near vital organs (neck, throat, subperitoneal): 20 units per kg, initially; then 10 units per kg every 8 hours. After 2 days the dose may be reduced by one-half.

3. Joint haemorrhages: 10 units per kg every 8 hours for a day; then twice daily for 1 or 2 days. If aspiration is carried out, 10 units per kg just prior to aspiration with additional infusions of 10 units per kg 8 hours later and again on the following day.

4. Surgery: Dosages of 30 to 40 units per kg body weight prior to surgery are recommended. After surgery 20 units per kg every 8 hours should be administered. Close laboratory control to maintain the blood level of Factor VIII above 40% of normal for at least 10 days post-operatively is suggested.

5. Dental extractions: For simple extractions a pre-operative dose of 20–25 units per kg sufficient to raise the Factor VIII level to 50% should be given, followed by intravenous administration of tranexamic acid. For multiple extractions further doses of Factor VIII may be advisable 24 or 36 hours after the operation.

Recommended reconstitution: Reconstitute Factorate Heat Treated using the appropriate quantity of Water for Injections BP as shown below using standard aseptic precautions.

Nominal amount of antihaemophilic activity (International Units)	Quantity of Water for Injections BP (ml)
250	20(10†)
500	40 (20†)
1000	60 (30†)

† In some circumstances, where a small volume is required, it may be preferable to reconstitute Factorate Heat Treated with a lower volume of Water for Injections BP, however the content of sodium and citrate ions will not comply with the BP. These volumes are given in brackets in the table above.

Warm both diluent and Factorate Heat Treated vials to between 20°C and 25°C. Direct diluent down the side of the vial and gently rotate the vial until contents are dissolved. DO NOT SHAKE VIAL. Vigorous shaking will cause frothing and prolong the reconstitution time. Complete solution usually takes less than 5 minutes. The solution is now ready for administration. If a gel forms on reconstitution, the preparation should not be used.

Administration: Standard aseptic techniques should be used at all times.

Intravenous injections: Plastic disposable syringes are recommended with Factor VIII solution. The ground glass surfaces of all-glass syringes tend to stick with solutions of this type.

1. Attach a filter needle to a sterile disposable syringe. Insert filter needle into stopper of Factor VIII vial; inject air and withdraw the reconstituted solution from the vial.

2. Discard the filter needle and attach a suitable intravenous needle.

3. Administer solution by slow intravenous injection (20 ml in about five minutes).

Intravenous infusion: The infusion equipment used should comply with that described in sections 3 or 4 of British Standard 2463:1962, Transfusion Equipment for Medical Use.

1. Prepare solution of Factorate Heat Treated as recommended under '*Reconstitution*'.

2. Attach suitable infusion set.

3. If more than one vial is to be administered to the same patient the infusion set may be transferred to a second vial.

4. When infusion of Factorate Heat Treated is complete, the infusion set may be flushed with sterile isotonic saline to avoid loss of any of the reconstituted solution.

5. After use, discard infusion set, needles and vials together with any unused solution.

Contra-indications, warnings, etc

Warning: Factor VIII is prepared from human plasma, each donation of which has been found negative for hepatitis B surface antigen (HBsAg) by the radio-immunoassay (RIA) method. In addition, each batch, after reconstitution as recommended, has been tested and found negative by the RIA method. However, since no completely reliable laboratory test is yet available to detect all potentially infectious plasma donations, the risk of transmitting viral hepatitis is still present.

Side-effects: Products of this type are known to cause mild chills, nausea or stinging at the infusion site.

Contra-indications: There are no known contra-indications to antihaemophilic fraction.

Precautions: Factor VIII contains low levels of group A and B isohaemagglutinins. When large volumes are given to patients of blood groups A, B or AB, the possibility of intravascular haemolysis should be considered. Such patients should be monitored by means of a haematocrit and direct Coombs test for signs of progressive anaemia.

Pharmaceutical precautions Factorate Heat Treated is to be stored at refrigerator temperature (2°C–6°C). When stored as directed, it will maintain its labelled potency for the dating period indicated on the label but within this period may be stored at room temperature (not exceeding 30°C or 86°F) for up to six months.

Legal category POM.

Package quantities Factorate Heat Treated is supplied in single dose vials (potency is stated on each vial label).

Further information Haemophilia A, a hereditary disorder of blood coagulation occurring almost exclusively in males results in profuse bleeding in joints, muscles or internal organs as a result of minor trauma. The disease appears to be due to a deficiency of a specific plasma protein, antihaemophilic factor, Factor VIII: Factorate Heat Treated provides temporary replacement of the missing clotting factor.

Affected Individuals frequently require therapy following minor trauma. Surgery, when required in such individuals must be preceded by temporary correction of the clotting abnormality with fresh plasma transfusions, cryoprecipitate or by injections of Factor VIII concentrates. Obvious advantages of the use of concentrates of Factor VIII are the avoidance of hyper-proteinaemia, overloading the circulatory system and possible kidney dysfunction resulting from large volume transfusions.

Several different concentrations of Factor VIII have been used successfully. These range from Fraction 1 of Cohn to highly purified potent preparations. Dried Human Antihaemophilic Fraction – Factorate Heat Treated is in an intermediate category, being purified cryoglobulin complying with the standards of the BP.

Product licence number 0231/0038.

HIGH POTENCY FACTORATE* HEAT TREATED ▼

Presentation Dried Human Antihaemophilic Fraction High Potency Factorate Heat Treated is a stable lyophilised concentrate of Factor VIII (AHF, AHG) prepared from pooled human plasma. It conforms to the monograph for Dried Human Antihaemophilic Factor BP.

Each vial contains the labelled amount of antihaemophilic activity in International Units (one International Unit is the activity equivalent to the average Factor VIII content of 1 ml aliquots of 167 samples of fresh normal plasma, as determined in an international collaborative study). Each vial also contains sufficient sodium chloride to make the reconstituted solution approximately isotonic when Water for Injections BP is added as directed.

This product has been heated at 60°C for 30 hours. This step has been introduced in order to reduce the risk of transmission of infectious agents.

All units of source plasma are tested for antibodies to human T cell lymphotropic virus type III (HTLV III) and found to be negative.

Uses For use in therapy of classic haemophilia (Haemophilia A).

Dosage and administration High Potency Factorate Heat Treated is for intravenous administration only. As a general rule one unit of Factor VIII activity per kg will increase by 2% the circulating Factor VIII level, and although dosage must be adjusted according to the needs of the patient (weight, severity of haemorrhage, presence of inhibitors) the following general dosages are suggested.

1. Overt bleeding: Initially 20 units per kg of body weight followed by 10 units per kg every eight hours for the first 24 hours and the same dose every 12 hours for the next 3 or 4 days. For massive wounds, give until bleeding stops and maintain with 20 units per kg 8-hourly to achieve a minimum Factor VIII level of 40%.

2. Muscle haemorrhages: (a) Minor haemorrhages in extremities or non-vital areas: 10 units per kg once a day for 2 or 3 days.

(b) Massive haemorrhages in non-vital areas: 10 units per kg by infusion at 12 hour intervals for 2 days and then once a day for 2 more days.

(c) Haemorrhages near vital organs (neck, throat, subperitoneal), 20 units per kg, initially; then 10 units per kg every 8 hours. After 2 days the dose may be reduced by one-half.

3. Joint haemorrhages: 10 units per kg every 8 hours for a day; then twice daily for 1 or 2 days. If aspiration is carried out, 10 units per kg just prior to aspiration with additional infusions of 10 units per kg 8 hours later and again on the following day.

4. Surgery: Dosages of 30 to 40 units per kg body weight prior to surgery are recommended. After surgery 20 units per kg every 8 hours should be administered. Close laboratory control to maintain the blood level of Factor VIII above 40% of normal for at least 10 days post-operatively is suggested.

5. Dental extractions: For simple extractions a preoperative dose of 20–25 units per kg sufficient to raise the Factor VIII level to 50% should be given, followed by intravenous administration of tranexamic acid. For multiple extractions further doses of Factor VIII may be advisable 24 or 36 hours after the operation.

Recommended reconstitution: Reconstitute High Potency Factorate Heat Treated using the appropriate quantity of Water for Injections BP as shown below, using standard aseptic precautions.

Nominal amount of antihaemophilic activity (International Units)	Quantity of Water for Injections BP (ml)
250	10
500	20
1000	30
2000	60

Warm both diluent and High Potency Factorate Heat Treated vials to between 20°C and 25°C. Direct diluent down the side of the vial and gently rotate the vial until contents are dissolved. DO NOT SHAKE VIAL. Vigorous shaking will cause frothing and prolong the reconstitution time. Complete solution usually takes approximately 10 minutes. The solution is now ready for administration. If a gel forms on reconstitution, the preparation should not be used. The solution should be used within 3 hours of reconstitution.

Administration: Standard aseptic techniques should be used at all times.

Intravenous injections: Plastic disposable syringes are recommended with Factor VIII solution. The ground glass surfaces of all-glass syringes tend to stick with solutions of this type.

1. Attach a filter needle to a sterile disposable syringe. Insert filter needle into stopper of Factor VIII vial; inject air and withdraw the reconstituted solution from the vial.

2. Discard the filter needle and attach a suitable intravenous needle.

3. Administer solution by slow intravenous injection, at a rate comfortable to the patient, and not exceeding 2 ml per minute.

Intravenous infusion: The infusion equipment used should comply with that described in sections 3 or 4 of British Standard 2463:1962, Transfusion Equipment for Medical Use.

1. Prepare solution of High Potency Factorate Heat Treated as recommended under 'Reconstitution'.

2. Attach suitable infusion set.

3. If more than one vial is to be administered to the same patient the infusion set may be transferred to a second vial.

4. When infusion of High Potency Factorate Heat Treated is complete, the infusion set may be flushed with sterile isotonic saline to avoid loss of any of the reconstituted solution.

5. After use, discard infusion set, needles and vials together with any unused solution.

Contra-indications, warnings, etc

Warning: Factor VIII is prepared from human plasma, each donation of which has been found negative for hepatitis B surface antigen (HBsAg) by the radio-immunoassay (RIA) method. In addition, each batch, after reconstitution as recommended, has been tested and found negative by the RIA method. However, since no completely reliable laboratory test is yet available to detect all potentially infectious plasma donations, the risk of transmitting viral hepatitis is still present.

Side-effects: Products of this type are known to cause mild chills, nausea or stinging at the infusion site.

Contra-indications: There are no known contra-indications to antihaemophilic fraction.

Precautions: Factor VIII contains low levels of group A and B isohaemagglutinins. When large volumes are given to patients of blood groups A, B or AB, the possibility of intravascular haemolysis should be considered. Such patients should be monitored by means of a haematocrit and direct Coombs test for signs of progressive anaemia.

Pharmaceutical precautions High Potency Factorate Heat Treated is to be stored at refrigerator temperature (2°C–6°C). When stored as directed, it will maintain its labelled potency for the period indicated on the label but within this period it may be stored at room temperature (not exceeding 30°C or 86°F) for up to six months.

Legal category POM.

Package quantities High Potency Factorate is supplied in single dose vials (potency is stated on each vial label).

Further information Haemophilia A, a hereditary disorder of blood coagulation occurring almost exclusively in males, results in profuse bleeding in joints, muscles or internal organs as a result of minor trauma. The disease appears to be due to a deficiency of a specific plasma protein, antihaemophilic factor, Factor VIII; High Potency Factorate Heat Treated provides temporary replacement of the missing clotting factor.

Affected individuals frequently require therapy following minor trauma. Surgery, when required in such individuals, must be preceded by temporary correction of the clotting abnormality with fresh plasma transfusions, cryoprecipitate or by injections of Factor VIII concentrates. Advantages of the use of concentrates of Factor VIII are the avoidance of hyperproteinaemia, overloading the circulatory system and possible kidney dysfunction resulting from large volume transfusions.

Several different concentrations of Factor VIII have been used successfully. These range from Fraction 1 of Cohn to highly purified potent preparations. Dried Human Antihaemophilic Fraction – High Potency Factorate Heat Treated is a purified preparation with lower levels of fibrinogen and other non-AHF protein per international unit than 'Intermediate Purity' AHF preparations.

Product licence number 0231/0044.

KALSPARE* ▼

Presentation Orange film coated tablet marked 'A' on one side and with a breakline on the reverse. Each tablet contains 50 mg Chlorthalidone BP and 50 mg Triamterene BP. Presented in calendar packs.

Uses Kalspare is a long acting potassium sparing diuretic and antihypertensive of particular value in conditions where potassium conservation is an important consideration.

Management of mild to moderate hypertension, oedema associated with congestive cardiac failure, nephrosis, corticosteroid or oestrogen therapy and ascites associated with hepatic cirrhosis.

Dosage and administration

Hypertension: Usually one tablet daily taken after breakfast. If necessary the dose may be increased to two tablets taken once daily.

Oedema: The usual dose is one tablet daily taken after breakfast. If oedema persists after seven to ten days the dose may be increased to two tablets daily.

Dosage in children has not been established and Kalspare is recommended for the treatment of adults only.

Contra-indications, warnings, etc

Contra-indications: Hypersensitivity to the individual components or to other sulphonamide-derived drugs.

Progressive renal failure (see also Precautions).

Concomitant lithium therapy.

Kalspare should not be used in the presence of hyperkalaemia (plasma potassium above 5.0 mmol/litre) or in patients receiving other potassium-sparing agents, such as spironolactone or amiloride.

Warnings: Caution should be exercised in patients with severe kidney disease, impaired liver function or progressive liver disease.

As with thiazide diuretics and chlorthalidone, treatment with Kalspare may result in hyperuricaemia or the precipitation of acute gout in certain patients.

Potassium supplements should not be given with Kalspare except in the presence of hypokalaemia.

Chlorthalidone has, in common with other sulphonamide diuretics, occasionally aggravated or precipitated Diabetes mellitus. This effect is usually reversible on cessation of therapy.

Chlorthalidone and related drugs may decrease serum protein bound iodine levels without signs of thyroid disturbance.

Triamterene may cause a decreasing alkali reserve, with the possibility of metabolic acidosis.

Precautions: Although no clinically significant hyperkalaemia has occurred in studies with Kalspare, all potassium conserving diuretic combinations can cause an abnormal elevation of plasma potassium. It is recommended that measurements of potassium are made at the time of dosage adjustments and at appropriate intervals during therapy, particularly in elderly or diabetic patients with confirmed or suspected renal insufficiency.

Signs or symptoms of hyperkalaemia include paraesthesia, muscular weakness, fatigue, flaccid paralysis of the extremities, bradycardia, shock and ECG abnormalities. If hyperkalaemia occurs in patients taking Kalspare, the drug should be withdrawn, a diuretic substituted and potassium intake restricted. If the plasma potassium level exceeds 6.5 mmol per litre, active measures should be taken to reduce it. Such measures include the intravenous administration of sodium bicarbonate solution or oral or parenteral glucose with a rapid-acting insulin preparation.

If progressive renal impairment becomes evident, Kalspare therapy should be withdrawn and alternative therapy instituted if necessary.

Use in pregnancy and lactation: Thiazide diuretics have been shown to cross the placenta and also to appear in breast milk. In rare instances, thrombocytopenia, pancreatitis or hypokalaemia have been reported in newborn infants of mothers treated with thiazide diuretics. The use of Kalspare in pregnant women or nursing mothers should therefore be avoided unless essential.

Side effects: Side-effects are similar to those that have been associated with thiazide therapy and include nausea, dry mouth, constipation, leg cramp, headaches, dizziness and fatigue.

Rare cases of megaloblastic anaemia have been reported in association with triamterene.

Drug interactions: Kalspare may add to or potentiate the action of other antihypertensive drugs.

Any tendency to orthostatic hypotension on Kalspare treatment may be aggravated by concomitant alcohol, barbiturates or narcotics.

Chlorthalidone and related drugs may increase the responsiveness to tubocurarine.

Overdose: The stomach contents should be emptied immediately. Treatment should be symptomatic and supportive with correction of electrolyte imbalance and fluid depletion. No specific antidote exists for Kalspare.

Pharmaceutical precautions Store in a cool dry place. Protect from light.

Legal category POM.

Package quantities Calendar packs of 2 × 14 tablets.

Further information The potassium conserving action of Kalspare has been shown to reduce the need for additional potassium in the maintenance of normal plasma levels. It is therefore particularly valuable where dietary potassium intake is low, and for patients on digitalis. Kalspare is highly effective baseline therapy for hypertension and may be used with other antihypertensive drugs such as beta-blockers. Its prolonged duration of action ensures smooth 24 hour antihypertensive control from once daily administration.

Product licence number 0231/0064.

*Trade Mark

Astra Pharmaceuticals Limited
Home Park Estate
Kings Langley
Herts WD4 8DH

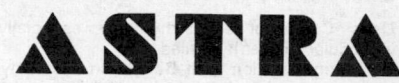

BETALOC*

Presentation White tablets containing either 50 mg metoprolol tartrate coded A/BB or 100 mg metoprolol tartrate coded A/ME.

Uses In the management of hypertension and angina pectoris. Cardiac arrhythmias, especially supraventricular tachyarrhythmias. Adjunct to the treatment of thyrotoxicosis.

Early intervention with Betaloc in acute myocardial infarction reduces infarct size and the incidence of ventricular fibrillation. Pain relief may also decrease the need for opiate analgesics.

Betaloc has been shown to reduce mortality when administered to patients with acute myocardial infarction.

Prophylaxis of migraine.

Dosage and administration The dose must always be adjusted to the individual requirements of the patient. The following are guide lines:

Hypertension: Total daily dose 100–400 mg to be given as a single or twice daily dose.

The starting dose is 100 mg per day. This may be increased by 100 mg per day at weekly intervals.

If full control is not achieved using a single daily dose, a b.d. regimen should be initiated. Combination therapy with a diuretic or other hypotensive agent may also be considered.

Angina: Usually 50–100 mg twice or three times daily.

Cardiac arrhythmias: 50 mg b.i.d. or t.i.d. should usually control the condition. If necessary the dose can be increased up to 300 mg per day in divided doses.

Following the treatment of an acute arrhythmia with Betaloc injection, continuation therapy with Betaloc tablets should be initiated 4–6 hours later. The initial oral dose should not exceed 50 mg t.i.d.

Thyrotoxicosis: 50 mg four times a day.

Myocardial infarction: Early intervention. To achieve optimal benefits from intravenous Betaloc, suitable patients should present within 12 hours of the onset of chest pain. Therapy should commence with 5 mg i.v. every 2 minutes to a maximum of 15 mg total as determined by blood pressure and heart rate. Orally, therapy should commence 15 minutes after the injection with 50 mg every 6 hours for 48 hours. Patients who fail to tolerate the full intravenous dose should be given half the suggested oral dose.

The usual maintenance dose is 200 mg daily.

Migraine prophylaxis: 100–200 mg daily given in divided doses.

Elderly: In healthy elderly volunteers there was no significant difference in the volume of distribution, elimination half life, total body clearance or bioavailability of metoprolol. Because metoprolol undergoes biotrans-formation in the liver, severe hepatic failure may mean that the lower dosage recommendations will be more appropriate.

Contra-indications, warnings, etc

Contra-indications: A V block. Digitalis refractory heart failure.

Warnings: In labile and insulin-dependent diabetes it may be necessary to adjust the hypoglycaemic therapy.

Betaloc therapy must be reported to the anaesthetist prior to general anaesthetic.

Digitalisation and/or diuretics should be considered for patients with a previous history of heart failure, or patients known to have a poor cardiac reserve.

Betaloc has proved safe in a large number of asthmatic patients; although it is a selective beta-blocker it is prudent to exercise care in the treatment of patients with chronic obstructive pulmonary disease.

Until further clinical experience is available, it is recommended that treatment with Betaloc be avoided during pregnancy.

There have been reports of skin rashes and/or dry eyes associated with the use of beta-adrenoceptor blocking drugs. The reported incidence is small and in most cases the symptoms have cleared when treatment was withdrawn. Discontinuation of the drug should be considered if any such reaction is not otherwise explicable. Cessation of therapy with a beta-blocker should be gradual.

Side-effects: These are mild and have been infrequently reported. The commonest appear to be lassitude, GI disturbances, and disturbance of sleep pattern. In many cases these effects have been transient, or have disappeared after a reduction in dosage.

Pharmaceutical precautions Protect from light, heat and moisture.

Legal category POM.

Package quantities Blister packs of 100 and Securitainers of 500.

Further information *Treatment of overdosage:* Marked bradycardia may be treated by intravenous atropine sulphate (0.25–2.0 mg) and in severe cases by slow intravenous infusion of about 5 mcg per minute of isoprenaline.

Metoprolol undergoes biotransformation in the liver and thereafter is mainly excreted as inactive metabolites by the kidney.

Product licence numbers
Tablets 50 mg   0017/0073
Tablets 100 mg   0017/0074

BETALOC* I.V. INJECTION ▼

Presentation *Ampoules:* Each ampoule of 5 ml contains 5 mg metoprolol tartrate.

Uses Control of tachyarrhythmias, especially supraventricular tachyarrhythmias.

Early intervention with Betaloc in acute myocardial infarction reduces infarct size and the incidence of ventricular fibrillation. Pain relief may also decrease the need for opiate analgesics.

Dosage and administration Initially up to 5 mg injected i.v. at a rate of 1–2 mg per minute. The injection can be repeated at 5 minute intervals until a satisfactory response has been obtained.

A total dose of 10–15 mg generally proves sufficient. Because of the risk of a pronounced drop of blood pressure, the i.v. administration of Betaloc to patients with a systolic blood pressure below 100 mm Hg should only be given with special care.

During anaesthesia: 2–4 mg injected slowly i.v. at induction is usually sufficient to prevent the development of arrhythmias during anaesthesia. The same dosage can also be used to control arrhythmias developing during anaesthesia. Further injections of 2 mg may be given as required to a maximum overall dose of 10 mg.

Myocardial infarction: Early intervention. To achieve optimal benefits from intravenous Betaloc, suitable patients should present within 12 hours of the onset of chest pain. Therapy should commence with 5 mg i.v. every 2 minutes to a maximum of 15 mg total as determined by blood pressure and heart rate. Orally, therapy should commence 15 minutes after the injection with 50 mg every 6 hours for 48 hours. Patients who fail to tolerate the full intravenous dose should be given half the suggested oral dose.

Elderly: In healthy elderly volunteers there was no significant difference in the volume of distribution, elimination half life or total body clearance of metoprolol. Because metoprolol undergoes biotransformation in the liver, severe hepatic failure may mean that the lower dosage recommendations will be more appropriate.

Contra-indications, warnings, etc
Contra-indications: AV Block. Digitalis refractory heart failure. Severe bradycardia. Cardiogenic shock.

Warnings: In labile and insulin dependent diabetes, it may be necessary to adjust the hypoglycaemic therapy.

Betaloc therapy must be reported to the anaesthetist prior to general anaesthetic.

Digitalisation and/or diuretics should be considered for patients with a previous history of heart failure, or patients known to have a poor cardiac reserve.

Betaloc has proved safe in a large number of asthmatic patients; although it is a selective beta-blocker it is prudent to exercise care in the treatment of patients with chronic obstructive pulmonary disease. In patients suffering from asthma, additional therapy with a β_2-stimulant (e.g. terbutaline) may be advisable.

There have been reports of skin rashes and/or dry eyes associated with the use of beta-adrenoceptor blocking drugs. The reported incidence is small and in most cases the symptoms have cleared when treatment was withdrawn. Discontinuation of the drug should be considered if any such reaction is not otherwise explicable. Cessation of therapy with a beta-blocker should be gradual.

Betaloc therapy should be avoided during pregnancy. If there are overwhelming clinical reasons for its use during the second or third trimesters, particular attention should be paid to its β-blocking effects (especially bradycardia) in the mother, foetus and neonate.

In a patient under beta-blockade, the anaesthetic selected should be one exhibiting as little negative inotropic activity as possible (e.g. halothane/nitrous oxide).

Side-effects: As in the case of other beta-blockers, a marked fall in blood pressure may sometimes occur following intravenous injection of Betaloc.

Pharmaceutical precautions Protect from light.

Legal category POM.

Package quantities 4×5 ml ampoules.

Further information *Treatment of overdosage:* Marked bradycardia may be treated by intravenous atropine sulphate (0.25 to 2.0 mg) and in severe cases by slow intravenous infusion of about 5 mcg/minute of isoprenaline.

Betaloc is a cardioselective β_1-receptor blocker exhibiting no intrinsic sympathomimetic activity. Betaloc injection is suitable for the treatment of cardiac arrhythmias, especially supraventricular tachyarrhythmias. Its use often re-establishes normal sinus rhythm in patients with paroxysmal atrial tachycardia or reduces the ventricular rate. Also where atrial fibrillation or flutter exists it can not only reduce ventricular rate but may also restore sinus rhythm. It also reduces the number of ventricular extrasystoles.

Product licence number 0017/0072.

BETALOC*-SA

Presentation White tablets (coded A MD) containing 200 mg metoprolol tartrate as Durules* (sustained release tablets).

Uses In the management of angina pectoris and hypertension.

Prophylaxis of migraine.

Dosage and administration *Angina pectoris and hypertension:* Oral, once daily in the morning. In rare cases two tablets may be indicated.

Prophylaxis of migraine: One tablet daily in the morning.

Administration of Betaloc-SA results in a controlled release of active substance which means that the peak plasma levels are reduced. Compared to Betaloc tablets the absorption phase is prolonged and the duration of effect is extended. The substance is completely absorbed and the maximal beta-blocking effect is reached after about four hours.

These factors may lead to a more convenient dosage and an improved degree of beta$_1$ – selectivity.

The effect on the pulse and blood pressure remain pronounced 24 hours after administration.

Betaloc-SA tablets should be swallowed whole and not broken or chewed.

Metoprolol undergoes bio-transformation in the liver and thereafter is mainly excreted as inactive metabolites by the kidney.

Elderly: In healthy elderly volunteers there was no significant difference in the volume of distribution, elimination half life, total body clearance or bioavailability of metoprolol. Because metoprolol undergoes biotransformation in the liver, severe hepatic failure may mean that the lower dosage recommendations will be more appropriate.

Contra-indications, warnings, etc
Contra-indications: AV block. Digitalis refractory heart failure.

Warnings: In labile and insulin-dependent diabetes, it may be necessary to adjust the hypoglycaemic therapy.

Betaloc therapy must be reported to the anaesthetist prior to general anaesthetic.

Digitalisation and/or diuretics should be considered for patients with a previous history of heart failure or patients known to have a poor cardiac reserve.

Betaloc has proved safe in a large number of asthmatic patients; although it is a selective beta-blocker it is prudent to exercise care in the treatment of patients with chronic obstructive pulmonary disease. Use of a beta$_2$-bronchodilator may be advisable in some asthmatics.

There have been reports of skin rashes and/or dry eyes associated with the use of beta-adrenoceptor blocking drugs. The reported incidence is small and in most cases the symptoms have cleared when treatment was withdrawn. Discontinuation of the drug should be considered if any such reaction is not otherwise explicable. Cessation of therapy with a beta-blocker should be gradual.

Until further clinical experience is available, it is recommended that treatment with Betaloc-SA be avoided during pregnancy.

Side-effects: These are mild and have been infrequently reported. The commonest appear to be lassitude, GI disturbances and disturbances of sleep pattern. In many cases these effects have been transient, or have disappeared after a reduction in dosage.

Pharmaceutical precautions Store in a cool dry place.

Legal category POM.

Package quantities Calendar pack of 28 tablets. Securitainers of 300 tablets.

Further information *Treatment of overdosage:* Marked bradycardia may be treated by intravenous atropine sulphate (0.25–2.0 mg) and in severe cases by slow intravenous infusion of about 5 mcg per minute of isoprenaline.

Product licence number 0017/0093.

BRICANYL* INHALER
BRICANYL* SPACER INHALER

Presentation *Bricanyl Inhaler:* Metered dose aerosol delivering 0.25 mg terbutaline sulphate per actuation.

Bricanyl Spacer Inhaler: Metered dose aerosol with extended mouthpiece delivering 0.25 mg terbutaline sulphate per actuation.

Bricanyl Refill Canister: Canister containing 400 doses of terbutaline sulphate 0.25 mg. For use with the Nebuhaler or as a refill for Bricanyl Spacer Inhaler.

Nebuhaler: 750 ml plastic cone with a one-way valve. For use in conjunction with Bricanyl refill canister.

Uses A selective beta$_2$-adrenergic stimulant recommended for prophylactic treatment and relief of an acute attack of allergic, intrinsic and exercise induced asthma, chronic bronchitis, emphysema and other bronchopulmonary disorders on which bronchospasm is a complicating factor.

Dosage and administration *Bricanyl Inhaler: Adults and children:* Prophylaxis and relief of acute attack. One or two inhalations as required, with a short interval between each inhalation. Not more than 8 inhalations should be necessary in any 24 hours.

See package insert for simple operating instructions.

Bricanyl Spacer Inhaler: Bricanyl Spacer Inhaler is particularly recommended to enable patients with difficulty coordinating conventional aerosols to derive greater therapeutic benefit.

Adults and children: Prophylaxis and relief of acute attack. One or two inhalations as required, with a short interval between each inhalation. Not more than 8 inhalations should be necessary in any 24 hours.

See package insert for simple operating instructions.

Nebuhaler: The Nebuhaler is recommended to enable patients with difficulty coordinating conventional aerosols to derive greater therapeutic benefit.

Adults and children: Prophylaxis and relief of acute attack. One or two inhalations as required, with a short interval between each inhalation. Not more than 8 inhalations should be necessary in any 24 hours.

Bricanyl via the Nebuhaler may also be used in conditions such as severe bronchospasm and severe acute asthma which are normally managed by administration of nebulised bronchodilators.

Adults: The dose must always be adjusted to patient response and severity of the bronchospasm. Patients must be instructed to actuate the aerosol and breathe in slowly and deeply through the mouthpiece. Ideally two inspirations per actuation are required to empty the Nebuhaler. For hospital use in acute asthma, the initial dose should be 2 mg (8 actuations); this may be repeated up to a total dose of 8 mg in one hour. Thereafter a dose of up to 4 mg may be given four times daily. A similar dosage range can be used for domiciliary use, but patients should be warned that if either the usual relief or duration of action is diminished, they should seek medical advice immediately.

See package insert for simple operating instructions.

Elderly: Dosage as for adults. Because of the difficulty experienced by many elderly patients, in coordinating inhalation with actuation, Bricanyl Spacer inhaler or use via the Nebuhaler will provide a more certain delivery of drug.

Contra-indications, warnings, etc No contra-indications are known. Care should be taken with patients suffering from myocardial insufficiency or thyrotoxicosis. Although no teratogenic effects have been observed in animal experiments, caution is recommended during the first trimester of pregnancy.

Side-effects: The frequency of side-effects is low, and those which have been recorded, e.g. tremor and palpitations, are all characteristic of sympathomimetic amines. Whenever these have occurred the majority have resolved spontaneously within the first week of treatment.

Pharmaceutical precautions None.

Legal category POM.

Package quantities *Bricanyl Inhaler:* Aerosol containing 400 metered doses.

Bricanyl Spacer Inhaler: Aerosol containing 400 metered doses complete with extended mouthpiece.

Bricanyl Refill Canister: Canister containing 400 doses:

Nebuhaler: 750 ml plastic cone with a one-way valve.

Further information Bricanyl is also available as Respirator Solution, Tablets, Syrup, Injection, Expectorant and Compound Tablets.

Product licence number 0017/0061

BRICANYL* TABLETS
BRICANYL* SYRUP

Presentation *Bricanyl Tablets:* Off-white scored tablet containing terbutaline sulphate 5 mg.

Bricanyl Syrup: Clear aqueous solution containing 0.3 mg terbutaline sulphate per ml.

Uses A bronchodilator recommended for relief of allergic and intrinsic asthma, chronic bronchitis, emphysema and other broncho-pulmonary disorders in which bronchospasm is a complicating factor. Bricanyl Expectorant is recommended in these conditions where secretion is a complicating factor.

Dosage and administration
Bricanyl Tablets: Adults: 1 tablet twice a day; or three times a day at eight-hourly intervals.

Children: 7–15 years: ½ tablet twice a day; or three times a day at eight-hourly intervals.

Bricanyl Syrup: Adults: 2–3 × 5 ml spoonfuls three times a day at eight-hourly intervals.

Children: 7–15 years: 1–2 × 5 ml spoonfuls three times a day at eight-hourly intervals.

3–7 years: ½–1 × 5 ml spoonful three times a day at eight-hourly intervals.

Elderly: Dosage as for adults.

Contra-indications, warnings, etc No contra-indications are known. Care should be taken with patients suffering from myocardial insufficiency or thyrotoxicosis. Although no teratogenic effects have been observed in animal experiments, caution is recommended during the first trimester of pregnancy.

Side-effects: The frequency of side-effects is low, and those which have been recorded, e.g. tremor and palpitations, are all characteristic of sympathomimetic amines. Whenever these have occurred, the majority have been spontaneously reversible within the first week of treatment.

Pharmaceutical precautions No special storage conditions are necessary for any of the Bricanyl preparations. The recommended diluent for Bricanyl Syrup is water.

Legal category POM.

Package quantities *Bricanyl Tablets:* Bottles of 100 and 500 tablets.

Bricanyl Syrup: Bottles of 300 ml and 1 litre.

Further information When Bricanyl is prescribed orally a suitable regime for providing eight-hourly administration is: on rising, in the mid-afternoon, on retiring.

Product licence numbers
Bricanyl Tablets	0017/0047
Bricanyl Syrup	0017/0058

BRICANYL* INJECTION
Presentation Clear aqueous solution for injection containing 0.5 mg terbutaline sulphate per ml.

Uses
1. *For bronchodilatation.* A selective β_2 adrenergic stimulant recommended for the relief of allergic and intrinsic asthma, chronic bronchitis, emphysema and other broncho-pulmonary disorders in which bronchospasm is a complicating factor.

2. *For the management of uncomplicated premature labour.*

Dosage and administration
1. *For bronchodilatation.* When a rapid therapeutic response is required, Bricanyl can be administered by any of the three standard parenteral routes: subcutaneous, intramuscular, or i.v. bolus. The preferred routes will usually be subcutaneous or intramuscular. When given as an i.v. bolus the injection must be made slowly noting patient response.

Adults: ½–1 ampoule (0.25–0.5 mg) up to four times a day.

Children: 2–15 years. 0.01 mg/kg body weight to a maximum of 0.3 mg total.

Age	Average weight		mg terbutaline	ml volume
	kg	(lb)		
<3	10	(22)	0.1	0.2
3	15	(33)	0.15	0.3
6	20	(44)	0.2	0.4
8	25	(55)	0.25	0.5
10+	30+	(66+)	0.3	0.6

By infusion: 3 to 5 ampoules (1.5–2.5 mg) in 500 ml dextrose, saline or dextrose/saline solution given by continuous intravenous infusion at a rate of 10–20 drops (0.5–1 ml) per minute for 8 to 10 hours. Corresponding reduction in dosage should be made for children.

Elderly: Dosages as for adults.

2. *For management of premature labour.* The dose must be individually titrated with reference to suppression of contractions, increase in pulse rate and changes in blood pressure, which are limiting factors.

These parameters should be carefully monitored during treatment. A maternal heart rate of more than 135 beats/min should be avoided. 10 mcg/min i.v. should be infused during the first hour. This can be increased by 5 mcg/min at 10 min intervals until the contractions stop. The highest dose should be 25 mcg/min. During the next seven hours, the dose should be decreased in 30 minute periods by 5 mcg/min to the lowest maintenance dose that produces continued suppression of the contractions. After this initial treatment, subcutaneous injections (0.25 mg) should be given four times a day for three days. During this period, oral treatment should be started (5 mg three times a day). The oral treatment should be continued until the end of the 36th week of pregnancy. Suggestion for dilution: 5 mg (10 ampoules) in 1,000 ml of dextrose solution (40 drops contain approximately 10 mcg).

Contra-indications, warnings, etc
1. *For bronchodilatation.* No contra-indications are known. Care should be taken with patients suffering from myocardial insufficiency or thyrotoxicosis. Although no teratogenic effects have been observed in animal experiments, caution is recommended during the first trimester of pregnancy.

Side-effects: When used as a bronchodilator the frequency of side-effects is low, and those which have been recorded, e.g. tremor and palpitations, are all characteristic of sympathomimetic amines. Whenever these have occurred, the majority have resolved spontaneously within the first week of treatment.

Precautions: When used for bronchodilatation care should be taken when aminophylline or related compounds are given to patients receiving Bricanyl by injection.

2. *For management of premature labour.* The following are contra-indications: ante-partum haemorrhage due to any cause, toxaemia of pregnancy, cord compression. Any condition of the mother or foetus in which prolongation of pregnancy is hazardous.

In premature labour in a patient with known or suspected cardiac disease a physician experienced in cardiology should assess the suitability of treatment before i.v. infusion with Bricanyl.

Warnings: In treatment of premature labour, hyperglycaemia and ketoacidosis have been found in pregnant women with diabetes after treatment with β_2-stimulants. It may therefore be necessary to adjust the insulin dose when β_2-stimulants are used in the treatment.

During infusion treatment in pregnant women with β_2-stimulants in combination with corticosteroids a rare complication with a pathological picture resembling pulmonary oedema, has been reported.

Increased tendency to uterine bleeding has been reported in connection with Caesarian section. However, this can be effectively stopped by propranolol 1–2 mg injected intravenously.

Pharmaceutical precautions No special storage conditions are necessary. The recommended diluent is water for injection, or sterile saline or dextrose.

Legal category POM.

Package quantities Packs of 5 × 1 ml ampoules.

Further information Nil.

Product licence number 0017/0048.

BRICANYL* COMPOUND TABLETS
BRICANYL* EXPECTORANT

Presentation *Compound Tablets:* Plain white tablets each containing:

Terbutaline sulphate	2.5 mg
Guaiphenesin	100 mg

Expectorant: Clear aqueous solution containing:

Terbutaline sulphate	0.3 mg/ml
Guaiphenesin	13.3 mg/ml

Uses Bronchodilator and expectorant recommended for relief of bronchial asthma, bronchitis, emphysema and other broncho-pulmonary disorders where bronchospasm and secretion are complicating factors.

Dosage and administration *Compound Tablets:* Two tablets three times daily at eight-hourly intervals. Not recommended for children.

Expectorant: Adults: 2–3 × 5 ml spoonfuls three times daily at eight-hourly intervals. Not recommended for children.

Elderly: Dosage as for adults.

Contra-indications, warnings, etc No contra-indications are known. Care should be taken with patients suffering from myocardial insufficiency or thyrotoxicosis. Although no teratogenic effects have been observed in animal experiments, caution is recommended during the first trimester of pregnancy.

Side-effects: The frequency of side-effects is low. Those which have been recorded, e.g. tremor and palpitations, are all characteristic of sympathomimetic amines. Whenever these have occurred, the majority have been spontaneously reversible within the first week of treatment.

Pharmaceutical precautions No special storage conditions required. Recommended diluent for Expectorant is water.

Legal category POM.

Package quantities *Compound Tablets:* Bottles of 100.

Expectorant: Bottles of 300 ml and 1 litre.

Further information Bricanyl is also available as ampoules, plain tablets, syrup, pressurised aerosol and respirator solution.

Product licence numbers
Compound Tablets	0017/0067
Expectorant	0017/0068

BRICANYL* RESPIRATOR SOLUTION

Presentation A clear aqueous solution for nebulisation.

Single dose unit ampoules containing 5 mg terbutaline sulphate in 2 ml. Multidose bottles containing 10 mg/ml.

Uses For the relief of severe bronchospasm.

Dosage and administration *Adults:* The usual dose of terbutaline by wet aerosol is 2–5 mg or in severe cases up to 10 mg. Administration of terbutaline solution can be via a nebuliser or an IPPV machine.

The terbutaline solution must be diluted with sterile physiological saline to ensure delivery of the correct dose. Such dilution will depend on two factors: the period of time over which the dose of terbutaline is to be delivered; the design of the equipment used to deliver the solution – its capacity, dead-space, etc.

For example, administration over a short period of time in a machine capable of completely utilising small volumes of liquid (e.g. Bird Respirator) may indicate little if any dilution (e.g. 3–5 ml). At the other extreme, use of a nebuliser such as Ventimask, Wright's or De Vilbiss would require a dilution suited to the equipment and administration time. For such chronic administration terbutaline should be given at a rate of 1–2 mg per hour in a solution of 100 mcg/ml (1 : 100 dilution).

Children: Acute usage: The doses in the table below are based on the adult dosage for severe bronchospasm of 10 mg terbutaline.

Age	Average weight		mg terbutaline	ml undiluted solution
	kg	lb		
<3	10	22	2.0	0.2
3	15	33	3.0	0.3
6	20	44	4.0	0.4
8	25	55	5.0	0.5
10+	30+	66+	6.0	0.6

Chronic usage: Pro rata to adult chronic administration.

Elderly: Dosage as for adults.

Contra-indications, warnings, etc No contra-indications are known. Care should be taken with patients suffering from myocardial insufficiency or thyrotoxicosis. Although no teratogenic effects have been observed in animal experiments, caution is recommended during the first trimester of pregnancy.

Side-effects: The frequency of side-effects is low and those which have been recorded, e.g. tremor and palpitations, are all characteristic of sympathomimetic amines. Whenever these have occurred, the majority have been spontaneously reversible within the first week of treatment.

Pharmaceutical precautions Bricanyl Respirator Solution should be stored in a cool place away from light.

Whilst the usual diluent will be sterile physiological saline, water for injection can also be used.

Solution in nebulisers should be replaced daily.

Legal category POM.

Package quantities Single dose unit ampoules. Packs of 50 × 2 ml ampoules. Multidose bottles: 10 ml bottles.

Further information Nil.

Product licence numbers
Single dose ampoules   0017/0114
Multidose bottles   0017/0078

BRICANYL* SA

Presentation White tablet with engraving $\frac{A}{BD}$ containing 7.5 mg terbutaline sulphate in a sustained-release formulation.

Uses For relief of bronchospasm in bronchial asthma and in chronic bronchitis, emphysema and other pulmonary disorders in which bronchospasm is a complicating factor.

Dosage and administration *Adults:* 1 tablet morning and evening. The tablet may not be divided or chewed, but must be swallowed whole together with liquid.

Elderly: Dosage as for adults.

Contra-indications, warnings, etc Care should be taken with patients suffering from myocardial insufficiency, thyrotoxicosis and diabetes. Bricanyl is contraindicated when there is known hypersensitivity to sympathomimetic amines.

Although no teratogenic effects have been observed in animal experiments, caution is recommended during the first trimester of pregnancy. It is not known if terbutaline sulphate passes over to maternal milk.

Side-effects: The frequency of side effects is low and those which have been recorded, e.g. tremor and palpitations are all characteristic of sympathomimetic amines. Whenever these have occurred the majority have been spontaneously reversible within the first week of treatment.

As with other β-stimulants cramps may occur in hands and feet at high dosage.

Pharmaceutical precautions No special storage conditions are necessary.

Legal category POM.

Package quantities Glass bottles containing 60 tablets.

Further information The inactive components in Bricanyl SA form a matrix which is insoluble in the digestive juices. The empty matrix may sometimes pass through the digestive system unchanged and be excreted.

Product licence number 0017/0110.

CITANEST*

Presentation A sterile clear aqueous solution of prilocaine hydrochloride 0.5%, 1.0%. Each ml contains prilocaine hydrochloride 5 mg; 10 mg.

Uses Citanest is a local anaesthetic solution for use in infiltration anaesthesia, intravenous regional anaesthesia and nerve blocks.

Dosage and administration The dose is adjusted according to the response of the patient and the site of administration. The lowest concentration and smallest dose producing the required effect should be given. The maximum dose for healthy adults should not exceed 400 mg.

Children and elderly or debilitated patients require smaller doses, commensurate with age and physical status.

Contra-indications, warnings, etc Known hypersensitivity to anaesthetics of the amide type. Citanest should be avoided in patients with anaemia or congenital or acquired methaemoglobinaemia.

Precautions In common with other local anaesthetics, Citanest should be used cautiously in patients with epilepsy, impaired cardiac conduction, impaired respiratory function, and in patients with liver or kidney damage, if the dose or site of administration is likely to result in high blood levels.

Facilities for resuscitation should be available when local anaesthetics are administered.

The effect of local anaesthetics may be reduced if an injection is made into an inflamed or infected area.

Use in pregnancy: Although there is no evidence from animal studies of harm to the foetus, as with all drugs, Citanest should not be given during early pregnancy unless the benefits are considered to outweigh the risks.

Adverse reactions: In common with other local anaesthetics, adverse reactions to Citanest are rare and are usually the result of excessively high blood concentrations due to inadvertent intravascular injection, excessive dosage, rapid absorption or occasionally to hypersensitivity, idiosyncracy or diminished tolerance on the part of the patient. In such circumstances systemic effects occur involving the central nervous system and/or the cardiovascular system.

CNS reactions are excitatory and/or depressant, and may be characterised by nervousness, dizziness, blurred vision and tremors, followed by drowsiness, convulsions, unconsciousness and possibly respiratory arrest. The excitatory reactions may be very brief or may not occur at all, in which case the first manifestations of toxicity may be drowsiness, merging into unconsciousness and respiratory arrest. Cardiovascular reactions are depressant, and may be characterised by hypotension, myocardial depression, bradycardia and possibly cardiac arrest.

Allergic reactions are extremely rare. They may be characterised by cutaneous lesions, urticaria, oedema or anaphylactoid reactions. Detection of sensitivity by skin testing is of doubtful value.

Hypotension may occur as a physiological response to central nerve blocks.

Clinically significant levels of methaemoglobin may occur with cyanosis when doses of prilocaine exceed 600 mg. Methaemoglobinaemia may be treated by the intravenous administration of a 1% solution of methylene blue in a dose of 1 mg/kg.

Pharmaceutical precautions Store at room temperature.

Legal category POM.

Package quantities
Single dose vial: 0.5%: Packs of 5 × 50 ml.
Multidose vials: 0.5%, 1.0%: Packs of 5 × 20 ml and packs of 5 × 50 ml.

Further information Citanest 0.5% SDV (single dose vial) is preservative free and should therefore be used on one occasion only.

Citanest multidose vials contain methylhydroxybenzoate 1 mg/ml.

Product licence numbers
0.5% (multi-dose vial)	0017/5047
1.0% (multi-dose vial)	0017/5048
0.5% (single-dose vial)	0017/0208

CITANEST* 3% WITH OCTAPRESSIN*

Presentation Sterile clear aqueous solution for dental anaesthesia; prilocaine hydrochloride 30 mg/ml, felypressin 0.03 i.u. per ml.

Uses Local anaesthetic solution with vasoconstrictor for dental infiltration anaesthesia where there is no necessity for profound ischaemia in the area injected. For all dental nerve-block techniques.

Dosage and administration 1–2 ml should be sufficient for the majority of procedures. The addition of Octapressin decreases the rate of absorption of the injected solution. For this reason the recommended maximum dosage for Citanest with Octapressin is higher than that recommended for a plain solution, but total dosage of Citanest should not exceed 600 mg in a healthy adult of body weight 70 kg. The total dose should not exceed 20 ml. In aged and debilitated patients the dose must be reduced. In children the maximum dose is considerably less and should be calculated in relation to body weight.

Contra-indications, warnings, etc In known cases of ischaemic heart disease not more than four cartridges should be used at one sitting.

Known sensitivity to local anaesthetics of the amide type.

Adverse reactions: The type of toxic reaction is unpredictable and depends on dosage, route of administration and state of the patient. The reactions are primarily of two types, and typified by stimulation and depression of the cerebral cortex and medulla respectively. Slow onset – stimulation leading to nervousness, dizziness, blurred vision, nausea, tremors, convulsions and respiratory arrest. Rapid onset – depression leading to respiratory arrest, cardiovascular collapse and cardiac arrest. Symptoms occur rapidly and with little warning.

Precautions: Adequate resuscitation equipment must be available whenever local or general anaesthesia is administered. Though clinical tolerance is remarkably good, overdosage or accidental intravenous injection may give rise to toxic reactions. Care should be observed in patients suffering from epilepsy.

Pharmaceutical precautions Store at room temperature.

Legal category POM.

Package quantities Glass cartridges of 2.2 ml standard, and 2.2 ml self-aspirating, in boxes of 100.

Further information Citanest 3% with Octapressin solutions contain methylhydroxybenzoate 1 mg/ml.

Product licence number 0017/5003.

CITANEST* 4%

Presentation Sterile clear aqueous solution. Each millilitre contains prilocaine hydrochloride 40 mg.

Uses Local anaesthetic solution without vasoconstrictor for dental infiltration anaesthesia where there is no necessity for profound ischaemia in the area injected. For all dental nerve-block techniques. For all dental injections where a vasoconstrictor is contra-indicated.

Dosage and administration 1–2 ml. In a healthy adult of a normal body weight (70 kg) the maximum dose should not exceed 400 mg. In aged and debilitated patients the dose must be reduced, and in children the maximum dose should be calculated in relation to body weight, i.e. 3 mg per lb or 6 mg per kg.

Contra-indications, warnings, etc Known hypersensitivity to anaesthetics of the amide type.

Side-effects: Systemic effects due to the use of Citanest in dental practice are practically unknown due to the small dosages employed.

Adverse reactions: The type of toxic reaction is unpredictable, and depends on dosage, route of administration and state of patient. Reactions are primarily of two types typified by stimulation and depression of the cerebral cortex and medulla respectively. Slow onset – stimulation leading to nervousness, dizziness, blurred vision, nausea, tremors, convulsions and respiratory arrest. Rapid onset – depression leading to respiratory arrest, cardiovascular collapse and cardiac arrest. Symptoms occur rapidly and with little warning.

Precautions: Though clinical tolerance is remarkably good, overdosage or accidental intravenous injection may give rise to toxic reactions. These are best avoided by aspiration before making an injection, in order to avoid accidental intravascular injection. Care should be observed in patients suffering from epilepsy.

Pharmaceutical precautions Store at room temperature.

Legal category POM.

Package quantities Glass cartridges of 2.2 ml standard cartridges in boxes of 100.

Further information Nil.

Product licence number 0017/5050.

CO-BETALOC*

Presentation White scored tablets (coded A/MH) containing 100 mg metoprolol tartrate and 12.5 mg hydrochlorothiazide.

Uses In the management of mild or moderate hypertension. The combination product may be suitable for use when satisfactory control of arterial blood pressure cannot be obtained with either a diuretic or a beta-adrenoreceptor blocking drug used alone.

Dosage and administration The dose will depend on patient response. Usually 1–3 tablets per day as a single or in divided dose.

Elderly: In healthy elderly volunteers there was no significant difference in the volume of distribution, elimination half life, total body clearance or bioavailability of metoprolol. Because metoprolol undergoes biotransformation in the liver, severe hepatic failure may mean that the lower dosage recommendations will be more appropriate.

Contra-indications, warnings, etc
Contra-indications: AV block.
　Digitalis refractory heart failure.
　Severe kidney and liver failure.
　Manifest gout.
　Anti-diuretic effect has been reported following concomitant treatment with diuretics and lithium. As with all products which contain diuretics, Co-Betaloc is contra-indicated during lithium therapy.

Warnings: In labile and insulin dependent diabetes, it may be necessary to adjust the hypoglycaemic therapy.
　Co-Betaloc therapy must be reported to the anaesthetist prior to general anaesthetic.
　Digitalisation should be considered for patients with a previous history of heart failure, or patients known to have a poor cardiac reserve.
　Metoprolol has proved safe in a large number of asthmatic patients; although it is a selective beta-blocker it is prudent to exercise care in the treatment of patients with chronic obstructive pulmonary disease.
　There have been reports of skin rashes and/or dry eyes associated with the use of beta-adrenoceptor blocking drugs. The reported incidence is small and in most cases the symptoms have cleared when treatment was withdrawn. Discontinuation of the drug should be considered if any such reaction is not otherwise explicable. Cessation of therapy with a beta-blocker should be gradual.
　Until further evidence is available Co-Betaloc therapy should be avoided in pregnancy.

Side-effects: Are mild and infrequent. The most common are gastro-intestinal disturbance, lassitude and disturbances of sleep pattern. In many cases these effects are transient or have disappeared with a reduction in dosage. The familiar side-effects of thiazide diuretics may be expected.

Pharmaceutical precautions Store in a cool dry place.

Legal category POM.

Package quantities Calendar packs of 28 tablets. Securitainers of 300 tablets.

Further information The use of a colootivo beta blocker in this combination may counteract the tendency to hyperglycaemia which the diuretic may provoke.

Treatment of overdosage: Marked bradycardia may be treated by intravenous atropine sulphate (0.25–2.0 mg) and in severe cases by slow intravenous infusion of about 5 mcg per minute of isoprenaline.

Product licence number 0017/0092.

CO-BETALOC* SA ▼

Presentation Yellow, biconvex, film coated tablets engraved $\dfrac{A}{MC}$

　Each tablet contains metoprolol tartrate 200 mg embedded in a white tablet layer, from which release takes place slowly, and hydrochlorothiazide 25 mg, in a yellow layer, which is rapidly released.

Uses In the management of mild or moderate hypertension. Co-Betaloc SA may be suitable for use when satisfactory control of arterial blood pressure cannot be obtained with either a diuretic or a beta-adrenoreceptor blocking drug used alone.

Dosage and administration The dose will depend on patient response. Usually 1 tablet daily.

Elderly: In healthy elderly volunteers there was no significant difference in the volume of distribution, elimination half life, total body clearance or bioavailability of metoprolol. Because metoprolol undergoes biotransformation in the liver, severe hepatic failure may mean that the lower dosage recommendations will be more appropriate.

Contra-indications, warnings, etc
Contra-indications: AV block. Digitalis refractory heart failure. Severe kidney and liver failure. Manifest gout.
　Anti-diuretic effect has been reported following concomitant treatment with diuretics and lithium. As with all products which contain diuretics, Co-Betaloc SA is contra-indicated during lithium therapy.

Warnings: In labile and insulin dependent diabetes, it may be necessary to adjust the hypoglycaemic therapy.
　Co-Betaloc SA therapy must be reported to the anaesthetist prior to general anaesthetic.
　Digitalisation should be considered for patients with a previous history of heart failure, or patients known to have a poor cardiac reserve.
　Metoprolol has proved safe in a large number of asthmatic patients; although it is a selective beta-blocker it is prudent to exercise care in the treatment of patients with chronic obstructive pulmonary disease.
　There have been reports of skin rashes and/or dry eyes associated with the use of beta-adrenoceptor blocking drugs. The reported incidence is small and in most cases the symptoms have cleared when treatment was withdrawn. Discontinuation of the drug should be considered if any such reaction is not otherwise explicable. Cessation of therapy with a beta-blocker should be gradual.

Until further evidence is available Co-Betaloc SA therapy should be avoided in pregnancy.

Side-effects: Are mild and infrequent. The most common are gastro-intestinal disturbance, lassitude and disturbances of sleep pattern. In many cases these effects are transient or have disappeared with a reduction in dosage. The familiar side-effects of thiazide diuretics may be expected.

Pharmaceutical precautions Store in a cool dry place.

Legal category POM.

Package quantities Calendar packs of 28 tablets.

Further information The use of a selective beta-blocker in this combination may counteract the tendency to hyperglycaemia which the diuretic may provoke.

Treatment of overdosage: Marked bradycardia may be treated by intravenous atropine sulphate (0.25–2.0 mg) and in severe cases by slow intravenous infusion of about 5 mcg per minute of isoprenaline.

Product licence number 0017/0202.

DIRYTHMIN SA* ▼

Presentation White, film-coated sustained release tablets (Durules), engraved $_D A_R$ on one side containing 150 mg disopyramide base as the phosphate.

Uses Dirythmin-SA is a Class I antiarrhythmic drug, indicated for treatment of a wide range of supraventricular and ventricular arrhythmias including:

Atrial or ventricular ectopic beats.
Paroxysmal atrial or ventricular tachycardia.
Arrhythmias associated with myocardial infarction.
Wolff-Parkinson-White syndrome.
Maintenance of sinus rhythm following electro-conversion.

Dirythmin-SA can be used in both digitilised and non-digitalised patients.

Dosage and administration The dosage should be adjusted dependant on the patient response and tolerance. The normal adult dosage is 2 tablets 12 hourly (600 mg daily). Dosage should not normally exceed 900 mg daily.

In patients with moderate renal insufficiency (creatinine clearance > 40 ml/min) or hepatic insufficiency, dosage should be limited to 1 Dirythmin-SA tablet b.d. In patients with creatinine clearance < 40 ml/min standard capsules are advised.

Dirythmin-SA tablets should be swallowed whole.

Patients treated with conventional disopyramide capsules q.i.d. can be transferred to the equivalent dosage of Dirythmin-SA e.g. 150 mg disopyramide q.i.d. is equivalent to 2 × 150 mg Dirythmin-SA tablets b.d.

Elderly: The renal function of the patient must be considered in relation to the dose as above.

Contra-indications, warnings, etc
Contra-indications: AV block II and III in absence of pacemaker. Known hypersensitivity. Cardiogenic shock.

Warnings: Disopyramide should not be administered to patients with cardiomyopathy, or uncompensated cardiac failure.

Treatment with disopyramide should be discontinued if any of the following develop: Hypotension, 2nd or 3rd degree heart block, significant QRS prolongation (> 25%) or QT prolongation.

Disopyramide has been associated with hypoglycaemia usually in patients with impaired liver function. Caution should be observed in patients with prostatic hypertrophy, glaucoma, myasthenia gravis or digitalis intoxication.

Disopyramide dosage should be reduced if 1st degree heart block develops and may require discontinuation if the block persists.

Patients should be digitalised prior to administration of disopyramide for the treatment of atrial flutter or fibrillation or blocked SVT.

Use of disopyramide with other Class I antiarrhythmics and/or beta-blockers is not recommended.

Disopyramide may be ineffective in the presence of marked hypokalaemia.

The safety and efficacy of disopyramide in children has not been established. The safety of disopyramide in pregnancy has not been established.

Side-effects: Side-effects reported are usually associated with the anticholinergic properties of disopyramide and include dry mouth, blurred vision and urinary retention.

Treatment of overdosage: Disopyramide should be discontinued and supportive or symptomatic treatment instigated.

Pharmaceutical precautions Store in a cool, dry place.

Legal category POM.

Package quantities Amber glass bottles of 100 tablets.

Further information Nil.

Product licence number 0017/0100.

HEMINEVRIN* 0.8% INFUSION

Presentation Colourless aqueous solution containing chlormethiazole edisylate 8 mg/ml BP.

Uses Heminevrin is a hypnotic and anticonvulsant used for the treatment of: Pre-eclamptic toxaemia, status epilepticus, acute alcohol withdrawal symptoms where oral administration is not practicable. As a sedative during regional anaesthesia.

Dosage and administration *Pre-eclamptic toxaemia:* An intravenous infusion is set up with 30–50 ml Heminevrin 0.8%. The solution is to run quickly at 60 drops per minute (4 ml/min) until the patient feels drowsy. The exact amount given depends on the patient's response. The drip rate is then maintained at 15 drops/minute (= 1 ml/min) or decreased to 10 drops per minute if the patient is very drowsy. As the patient responds very quickly to the change of dosage, the drop rate can be increased if the patient is restless, and reduced again once the patient is well sedated. The optimum level is sleep from which rapid awakening occurs on verbal command. The patient should be closely and constantly observed. The level of consciousness should lighten rapidly on interrupting the drip flow. It is important to continue to check the level of consciousness by decreasing or interrupting the drip flow during prolonged therapy.

Status epilepticus: Adults: 40–100 ml of Heminevrin 0.8% infusion administered over a period of 5–10 minutes will usually stop convulsions. Thereafter an intravenous infusion of Heminevrin 0.8% may be required depending on the patient's response.

Elderly: The half life of chlormethiazole may be longer in some elderly patients and less drug will be needed to achieve the required level of sedation. The response to dosage reductions may be slower in these cases.

Children: An initial infusion rate of 0.01 ml/kg/min (0.08 mg/kg/min). If seizures continue the dose is increased every 2 to 4 hours until seizures are abolished or drowsiness occurs. When seizures have ceased for 2 days the rate of infusion may be gradually reduced every 4 to 6 hours. If seizures recur the dose should be increased to the previous level at which they were controlled.

Acute alcohol withdrawal symptoms: Either of the above regimes can be utilised depending on the patient's condition but if the rapid infusion method is used it will be necessary to continue with either an infusion of Heminevrin 0.8% or oral therapy with Heminevrin capsules due to the short half life (three to four hours) of chlormethiazole. Oral therapy should be resumed as soon as possible.

Sedative during regional anaesthesia: The patient must be premedicated with atropine or similar antisialogogue to prevent nasal congestion and upper airway mucus secretion that otherwise occurs with chlormethiazole. As judged by unresponsiveness to sound and loss of eyelash reflex, unconsciousness should be induced by intravenous infusion of a fast running (approx 25 ml/min) drip for 1–2 minutes. Thereafter, maintenance must be judged on the patient's reaction but the dose required is of the order of 1–4 ml/min.

If being used to cover a regional block, e.g. spinal or epidural, the block must be fully effective before surgery begins.

Chlormethiazole has no analgesic properties and the patient will respond to painful stimuli by moving.

Contra-indications, warnings, etc

Contra-indications: Known sensitivity to chlormethiazole. Acute pulmonary insufficiency.

Pregnancy: Do not use in pregnancy, especially during the first trimester, unless there are compelling reasons. There is no evidence of safety in human pregnancy nor is there evidence from animal studies that it is entirely free from hazard.

Lactation: Chlormethiazole is excreted into breast milk. The effects of even small quantities of sedative/hypnotic and anti-convulsant drugs on the infant brain is not established. Nursing mother should be advised to stop breast feeding.

Precautions: Heminevrin should be used cautiously in patients with chronic pulmonary unsufficiency. Heminevrin may potentiate or be potentiated by centrally acting depressant drugs, including alcohol. Fatal cardio respiratory collapse has been reported when chlormethiazole was combined with other CNS depressant drugs. When used concomitantly dosage should be appropriately reduced. The patient should be kept under close and constant observation by a nurse during the period of continuous drip infusion. With too high a rate of infusion the sleep induced with Heminevrin can pass unnoticed into deep unconsciousness with the consequent risk of mechanical airway obstruction. With overdosage there is always the possibility of causing centrally induced respiratory depression and circulatory collapse. In view of the possible risk of slight respiratory depression during routine Heminevrin therapy, caution should be observed when administering the solution to patients with a history of obstructive pulmonary disease. Because of the possible danger of mechanical airway obstruction occurring in deep sleep during Heminevrin therapy, the patient should be maintained where necessary by the use of an oral airway tube. In addition, an aspirator should always be close at hand.

Warnings and adverse effects: The most common side-effect appears to be a tingling sensation in the nose and sneezing occurring immediately after the start of the intravenous infusion. Conjunctival irritation has also been noted in some cases, and occasionally these symptoms may be severe and may be associated with severe headache. Intravenous administration of Heminevrin solution may be followed by a slight but temporary decrease in blood pressure, which is less pronounced the slower the infusion is given. Rapid infusion may cause apnoea and hypotension. Thrombophlebitis may occur at the site of injection with intravenous infusion. Neither heparin nor cortisone has been shown to be helpful in preventing such reactions.

In rare cases anaphylactic reactions have occurred.

Bronchial secretions may be increased with high dosage.

There has been a report of thrombophlebitis, fever and headache in young children during prolonged Heminevrin infusion. This may have been due to interaction with plastic giving sets. For administration in small children a motor driven glass syringe should be used in preference to a drip set. A teflon intravenous cannula should be used whcih can be connected to the syringe by a polythene extension tube.

If a drip set is used in older patients, it should be changed at least every 24 hours. A teflon intravenous cannula should be used.

As Heminevrin is sorbed by PVC giving sets, there may be some loss in concentration before the drug reaches the patient. Dosage must therefore be adjusted to the patient's response and not given on a fixed milligram basis.

Status epilepticus: High fever and severe headache have been reported in children. Paradoxical worsening may occur in the Lennox-Gastaut Syndrome.

In eclampsia: The newborn infants of mothers treated with chlormethiazole may suffer from hypotonia, hypoventilation and apnoea.

In regional anaesthesia: If the regional block does not fully relieve the pain of operation it is better to convert to a non-volatile inhalation anaesthetic rather than try to increase the dosage of chlormethiazole.

The only cardiovascular effect of note is a tachycardia which seems to be largely dose dependent.

At the end of operation, stopping the chlormethiazole allows the patient to awaken usually in 1–5 minutes.

Legal category POM.

Pharmaceutical Precautions Store between 5°C–8°C.

Package quantities Bottles of 500 ml.

Further information Nil.

Product licence number 0017/5007R.

HEMINEVRIN* CAPSULES
HEMINEVRIN* SYRUP

Presentation *Capsules:* Greyish-brown gelatine capsules containing chlormethiazole (base) 192 mg in Miglyol.

Syrup: Clear, colourless, aqueous solution containing chlormethiazole edisylate 50 mg/ml.

Uses Neuropharmacological studies in animals show that Heminevrin possesses sedative/hypnotic and anticonvulsant properties. Whilst the mode of action is uncertain, the anticonvulsant effect may involve direct or indirect actions on GABA-systems in the CNS. The sedative/hypnotic properties involve actions on both catecholaminergic and gabaergic systems.

Indications: Heminevrin is indicated in the management of restlessness and agitation in the elderly, in the short term treatment of severe insomnia in the elderly and in the control of symptoms arising from acute withdrawal from alcohol where close hospital supervision is also provided.

Heminevrin is not recommended for use in children.

Dosage and administration *Severe insomnia in the elderly:* 1–2 capsules or 5–10 ml of the syrup before going to bed. The lower dose should be tried first. The doses are not strictly equivalent: one capsule contains 192 mg chlormethiazole base; 5 ml of syrup contains the equivalent of 157 mg base.

Management of restlessness and agitation in the elderly: One capsule or 5 ml syrup three times daily.

Alcohol withdrawal states: Heminevrin is *not* a treatment for 'alcoholism'. Alcohol withdrawal should be treated in hospital or, in exceptional circumstances, on an outpatient basis by specialist units when the daily dosage of Heminevrin must be monitored closely by community health staff. The dosage should be adjusted to patient response. A suggested regimen is:

Initial dose: 2 to 4 capsules, if necessary repeated after some hours.

Day 1, first 24 hours: 9 to 12 capsules, divided into 3 or 4 doses.

Day 2: 6 to 8 capsules, divided into 3 or 4 doses.

Day 3: 4 to 6 capsules, divided into 3 or 4 doses.

Days 4 to 6: A gradual reduction in dosage until final dose.

Administration for more than nine (9) days is not recommended. 5 ml of Heminevrin syrup can be substituted for each capsule administered, if desired.

Contra-indications, warnings, etc
Contra-indications: Known sensitivity to chlormethiazole. Acute pulmonary insufficiency.

Pregnancy: Do not use in pregnancy especially during the first and last trimesters, unless there are compelling reasons. There is no evidence of safety in human pregnancy, nor is there evidence from animal studies that it is entirely free from hazard.

Lactation: Chlormethiazole is excreted into the breast milk. The effect of even small quantities of sedative/hypnotic and anticonvulsant drugs on the infant brain is not established. Nursing mothers should be advised to stop breast feeding.

Precautions: Chronic pulmonary insufficiency. Chronic renal or hepatic disease. Heminevrin may potentiate or be potentiated by centrally acting depressant drugs including alcohol. Whilst the concurrent use of other central nervous system drugs should be avoided, if they are used, dosages should be appropriately reduced. Particular caution should be exercised when either chlormethiazole or another CNS depressant is given parenterally. Hypoxia, resulting from, for example, cardiac and/or respiratory insufficiency, may result in manifestations of symptoms of agitation and restlessness leading to a confusional state. Recognition and specific treatment of the cause is essential in such patients.

Side effects: The most common side-effect is nasal congestion and irritation, which may occur 15 to 20 minutes after drug ingestion. Conjunctival irritation has also been noted in some cases and, occasionally, these symptoms may be severe and may be associated with severe headache. Gastrointestinal disturbances have been reported.

In rare cases anaphylactic reactions have occurred.

Hangover effects in the elderly are uncommon but may occur.

Excessive sedation may occur, especially with higher doses or when given to the elderly for daytime sedation. Paradoxical excitement or confusion may occur rarely. Large doses of chlormethiazole depress respiration. Performance at skilled tasks and alertness may be impaired. Where relevant, patients should be warned of this hazard and advised not to drive or operate machinery during treatment.

When Heminevrin has been given at higher than recommended doses for other than recommended indications over prolonged periods of time, physical dependence, tolerance and withdrawal reactions have been reported.

Great caution is required in prescribing Heminevrin for patients with a history of chronic alcoholism, drug abuse or marked personality disorder.

Heminevrin should not be prescribed for alcoholics who continue to drink alcohol.

Overdose: The main symptoms to be expected with overdose of Heminevrin are: coma, respiratory depression, hypotension and hypothermia.

Hypothermia is thought to be due to a direct central effect as well as a result of lying unconscious for several hours. In addition, patients have increased secretion in the upper airways, which in one series was associated with a high incidence of pneumonia. The effects of overdosage are not usually severe in patients with no evidence of alcoholic liver disease, but they may be exacerbated when chlormethiazole is taken in combination with alcohol and/or CNS depressant drugs, particularly those that are metabolised by the liver. There is no specific antidote to chlormethiazole. Treatment of overdosage should therefore be carried out on a symptomatic basis, applying similar principles to those used in the treatment of barbiturate overdosage.

Further information Heminevrin has a short half life and therefore a low incidence of daytime sedation when prescribed as an hypnotic.

In the elderly, the safety and efficacy of Heminevrin has been established in controlled studies of up to three months duration. However, as with all psychotropic drugs, treatment should be kept to a minimum, reviewed regularly and discontinued as soon as possible.

Pharmaceutical precautions Heminevrin Syrup should be stored in a cool place.

Legal category POM.

Package quantities
Capsules: Bottles of 60.

Syrup: Bottles of 300 ml.

Product licence numbers
Capsules 0017/5009R
Syrup 0017/0063R

HEWLETTS* ANTISEPTIC CREAM

Presentation White scented cream: zinc oxide 8%, boric acid 2.5%, lanolin 4%.

Uses Topical ointment for nursing hygiene and care of skin.

Dosage and administration Applied as required.

Contra-indications, warnings, etc Not to be administered to large areas of broken skin.

Pharmaceutical precautions Store at room temperature.

Legal category P.

Package quantities 35 g tubes.

Further information Nil.

Product licence number 0017/5010.

JECTOFER*

Presentation Dark brown liquid for intramuscular injection; Iron Sorbitol Citric Acid Complex BP (50 mg elemental iron per ml).

Uses For the treatment of iron-deficiency anaemia and the rapid replenishment of iron stores.

Dosage and administration The recommended single dose of Jectofer is 1.5 mg per kg body weight by intramuscular injection to a maximum of 100 mg per injection. A series of daily injections of this single dose should be given to restore haemoglobin levels to normal and replenish iron stores based on the following table.

Hb gm/100 ml	5.0	6.0	7.0	8.0	9.0	10.0	11.0
Hb%	33	40	46	53	60	66	73
No. of injections	24	22	20	17	14	12	10

In patients who have a low tolerance threshold to intramuscular iron the injections should be given on alternate days. Not recommended in children under 3 kg (7 lb) body weight.

Elderly: Dosage as for adults.

Contra-indications, warnings, etc Serious liver or kidney damage. Ineffective in aplastic or hypoplastic anaemias and acute leukaemia.

Side-effects: A few cases have been reported of serious reactions of a cardiovascular type with cardiac arrhythmia.

Precautions: The importance of using the correct recommended dose in relation to body weight is emphasised, especially in patients who are already markedly underweight. Oral iron should be discontinued 24 hours before Jectofer is administered.

Pharmaceutical precautions Store at room temperature, do not refrigerate.

Legal category POM.

Package quantities 10×2 ml and 100×2 ml ampoules for intramuscular use.

Further information Nil.

Product licence number 0017/5011.

KINIDIN DURULES*

Presentation Film-coated white oval tablets, each containing 250 mg quinidine bisulphate (equivalent to 200 mg Quinidine Sulphate BP) in a sustained action form.

Uses Maintenance of sinus rhythm following cardioversion of atrial fibrillation.
Suppression of supraventricular and ventricular tachyarrhythmias.

Dosage and administration An initial test dose of one tablet should be given to detect hypersensitivity. Dosage is adjusted according to individual patient requirements.
The usual dose is 2 to 5 tablets morning and evening.
Tablets should be swallowed whole with water.

Contra-indications, warnings, etc Kinidin Durules are contra-indicated in patients with known hypersensitivity to quinidine, a history of quinidine induced thrombocytopenia or complete heart block.
Quinidine should be used with extreme caution in patients with incomplete atrio-ventricular block uncompensated cardiac failure, digitalis toxicity, myocardial damage, or myasthenia gravis.

Precautions: Hypokalaemia should be corrected prior to treatment with Kinidin.

Drug Interactions: In digitalised patients quinidine may increase the concentration of digitalis in plasma by up to 100%.
Quinidine may enhace the effects of antihypertensive agents and vasodilators, oral anticoagulants, and non depolarising skeletal muscle relaxants.
Drugs with enzyme-inducing effects may enhance the metabolism of quinidine, and thus reduce its effect.

Adverse reactions: Quinidine may cause gastro-intestinal irritation with nausea, vomiting and diarrhoea.
Signs of cinchonism with tinnitus, blurred vision, headache and dizziness may occur but are usually associated with overdosage.
Hypersensitivity reactions are rare. Symptoms include urticaria, fever, and thrombocytopenia. Granulomatous hepatitis with raised liver enzymes, reversible on stopping therapy has also been reported.
Heart block and serious disturbances of rhythm such as extrasystoles, venticular tachycardia and ventricular fibrillation can occur.
Occasional cases of photosensitivity have been reported.

Pharmaceutical precautions Store in a cool dry place.

Legal category POM.

Package quantities Securitainers of 100 and 250.

Further information The therapeutic plasma concentration is 2 to 4 µg per ml (6 to 12 µ mol per litre) when determined using method of Cramer and Isaksson, Scand. *J. Clin. Lab. Invest,* 1963, **15**, 553.

Product licence number 0017/5015R.

MARCAIN*
MARCAIN* WITH ADRENALINE

Presentation Clear, colourless, aqueous, sterile solution. 0.25%, 0.5%, with and without adrenaline and 0.75% without adrenaline.

0.25% Marcain – 10 ml ampoule containing bupivacaine hydrochloride 2.64 mg/ml.

0.25% Marcain with adrenaline – 10 ml ampoule containing bupivacaine hydrochloride 2.64 mg/ml with adrenaline 1 in 200,000.

0.5% Marcain – 10 ml ampoule containing bupivacaine hydrochloride 5.28 mg/ml.

0.5% Marcain with adrenaline – 10 ml ampoule containing bupivacaine hydrochloride 5.28 mg/ml with adrenaline 1 in 200,000.

0.75% Marcain – 10 ml ampoule containing bupivacaine hydrochloride 7.92 mg/ml.

Uses For the production of local anaesthesia by percutaneous infiltration, peripheral nerve block(s) and central neural block (caudal or epidural), that is, for specialist use in situations where prolonged anaesthesia is required. Because sensory nerve block is more marked than motor block, Marcain is especially useful in the relief of pain e.g. during labour.

Marcain 0.75% solution produces a more prolonged motor block than 0.25% or 0.5% solutions and is, therefore, recommended for epidural anaesthesia for surgical purposes. Epidural anaesthesia is usually maintained for 3 to 4 hours.

Dosage and administration The dosage varies and depends upon the area to be anaesthetised, the vascularity of the tissues, the number of neuronal segments to be blocked, individual tolerance and the technique of anaesthesia used. The lowest dosage needed to provide effective anaesthesia with Marcain solutions should be administered. For most indications, the duration of anaesthesia with Marcain solutions is such that a single dose is sufficient.

In each case, maximum dosage limit must be determined by evaluating the size and physical status of the patient and considering the usual rate of systemic absorption from a particular injection site. Experience to date indicates a single dose up to 150 mg bupivacaine hydrochloride. Doses up to 50 mg 2-hourly may subsequently be used. The doses in the following table are recommended as a guide for use in the average adult. For young, elderly or debilitated patients, these doses should be reduced.

Caudal block in children
Age 1 to 10 years
Up to lower thoracic (T10)
0.25% (2.5 mg/ml)   0.75 to 1 ml/kg
Mid-thoracic
0.25% (2.5 mg/ml)   1.00 to 1.25 ml/kg
If total amount greater than 20 ml reduce concentration to 0.2%.

Contra-indications, warnings, etc
Contra-indications: Marcain solutions are contra-indicated in patients with a known hypersensitivity to local anaesthetic agents of the amide type or to other components of the injectable formulation.

Solutions of Marcain with adrenaline should not be used in digital block because of the adrenaline content; plain solutions must be used for this purpose.

Solutions of Marcain are contra-indicated for i.v. regional anaesthesia.

Type of block	% Conc	Each dose		Motor block†
		ml	mg	
Local infiltration	0.25	up to 60	up to 150	—
Lumbar epidural Surgical operations	0.50	10 to 20	50 to 100	Moderate to complete
	0.75	10 to 20	75 to 150	Complete
Analgesia in labour	0.50	6 to 12	30 to 60	Moderate to complete
	0.25	6 to 12	15 to 30	Minimal
Caudal epidural Surgical operations	0.50	15 to 30	75 to 150	Moderate to complete
Analgesia in labour	0.50	10 to 20	50 to 100	Moderate to complete
	0.25	15 to 30	25 to 50	Moderate
Peripheral	0.50	up to 30	up to 150	Moderate to complete
	0.25	5 to max	32.5 to max	Slight to moderate
Sympathetic	0.25	20 to 50	50 to 125	—

† With continuous (intermittent) techniques, repeat doses may increase the degree of motor block.

0.75% solution is contra-indicated for epidural use in obstetrics.

Precautions: Adequate resuscitation equipment should be available whenever local or general anaesthesia is administered. Overdosage or accidental intravenous injection may give rise to toxic reactions.

The lowest dose that produces effective anaesthesia should be used. Injection of repeated doses of Marcain may cause significant increases in blood levels with each repeated dose due to slow accumulation of the drug. Tolerance varies with the status of the patient. Debilitated, elderly or acutely ill patients should be given reduced doses commensurate with their physical status. Marcain should be used with caution in patients with severe shock or heart block.

Marcain solutions should be used with caution in persons with known drug sensitivities. Patients allergic to ester-type local anaesthetic drugs (procaine, tetracaine, benzocaine, etc.) have not shown cross sensitivity to agents of the amide type such as Marcain. Since Marcain is metabolised in the liver, it should be used cautiously in patients with liver disease or with reduced liver blood flow (e.g. in severe shock).

Solutions containing adrenaline should be used with extreme caution for patients whose medical history and physical evaluation suggest the existence of hypertension, arteriosclerotic heart disease, cerebral vascular insufficiency, heart block, thyrotoxicosis or diabetes, etc. and those patients receiving drugs known to produce blood pressure alterations i.e. MAO inhibitors, tricyclic antidepressants, phenothiazines, etc., as severe and sustained hypotension or hypertension may occur.

Serious cardiac arrhythmias may occur if preparations containing a vasoconstrictor drug are employed in patients during or following the administration of chloroform, halothane, cyclopropane, trichlorethylene or other related agents.

Overdosage: Toxicity caused by Marcain solutions is similar in character to that observed with other local anaesthetic agents. It is caused by high plasma concentrations as a result of excessive dosage, rapid absorption or, most commonly, inadvertent intravascular injection. Such reactions involve the central nervous system and the cardiovascular system. CNS reactions are characterised by numbness of the tongue, lightheadedness, dizziness, blurred vision and tremors, followed by drowsiness, convulsions, unconsciousness and possibly respiratory arrest.

Cardiovascular reactions are depressant and are characterised by hypotension and myocardial depression. They may be the result of hypoxia due to convulsions and apnoea as well as a direct effect.

Treatment of overdosage: Treatment of a patient with toxic manifestations consists of arresting convulsions and assuring adequate ventilation with oxygen, if necessary by assisted or controlled ventilation (respiration). If convulsions occur they must be treated rapidly by intravenous injection of thiopentone 100 to 200 mg. Alternatively, diazepam 5 to 10 mg may be used.

Once convulsions have been controlled and adequate ventilation of the lungs ensured, no other treatment is generally required. If hypotension is present, however, a vasopressor, preferably one with inotropic activity, e.g. ephedrine 15 to 30 mg, should be given intravenously.

Pharmaceutical precautions No special requirements.

Legal category POM.

Package quantities
0.25% Marcain 10 × 10 ml sterile wrapped ampoules.
0.25% Marcain with adrenaline 10 × 10 ml sterile wrapped ampoules.
0.5% Marcain 10 × 10 ml sterile wrapped ampoules.
0.5% Marcain with adrenaline 10 × 10 ml sterile wrapped ampoules.
0.75% Marcain 10 × 10 ml sterile wrapped ampoules.

Product licence numbers
0.25% plain	0017/0116
0.25% with adrenaline	0017/0118
0.5% plain	0017/0117
0.5% with adrenaline	0017/0119
0.75%	0017/0133

MARCAIN* HEAVY ▼

Presentation Clear, colourless solution containing bupivacaine hydrochloride 5 mg per ml and glucose 80 mg per ml. The specific gravity of the solution is 1.026 at 20°C.

Uses Spinal anaesthesia for surgery (urological and lower limb surgery lasting 2–3 hours, abdominal surgery lasting 45–60 minutes). Bupivacaine is a long acting local anaesthetic agent of the amide type. Marcain Heavy has rapid onset of action and long duration. The duration of analgesia in the T_{10}–T_{12} segments is 2–3 hours.

Marcain Heavy produces a moderate muscular relaxation of the lower extremities lasting 2–2.5 hours. The motor blockade of the abdominal muscles makes the solution suitable for performance of abdominal surgery lasting 45–60 minutes. The duration of motor blockade does not exceed the duration of analgesia. The cardiovascular effects of Marcain Heavy are similar or less than those seen with other spinal agents. Bupivacaine 5 mg/ ml with glucose 80 mg/ml is exceptionally well tolerated by all tissues with which it comes in contact.

Dosage and administration The dose should be regarded as a guide for use in the average adult.

Spinal anaesthesia for surgery: 2–4 ml (10–20 mg bupivacaine hydrochloride).

The spread of anaesthesia obtained with Marcain Heavy depends on several factors, the most important being the volume of solution introduced and the position of the patient.

When injected in the L_3–L_4 interspace with the patient in the sitting position, 3 ml of Marcain Heavy spreads to the T_7–T_{10} segments.

If the patient is in the lateral position the blockade spreads to T_4. The effects of injections of Marcain Heavy exceeding 4 ml have not yet been studied and such volumes can therefore not be recommended.

Contra-indications, warnings, etc Bupivacaine is contra-indicated in patients with a known hypersensitivity to local anaesthetics of the amide type.

Side-effects: The safety of Marcain Heavy is comparable to that of other available local anaesthetics used for spinal anaesthesia. Side-effects of Marcain Heavy are extremely rare but may occur in connection with extensive (total) spinal blockade. The first manifestations of CNS-toxicity is drowsiness merging into unconsciousness and respiratory arrest. Cardiovascular reactions are depressant and may be characterised by hypotension, myocardial depression, bradycardia and possibly cardiac arrest.

Systemic side-effects are rarely associated with spinal anaesthesia but might occur after accidental intravascular injection. Systemic side-effects are characterised by numbness of the tongue, lightheadedness, dizziness and tremor followed by convulsions.

Treatment of side-effects: Treatment of extensive spinal blockade consists of assuring and maintaining a patent airway and supporting ventilation using oxygen, if necessary by assisted or controlled ventilation.

Should circulatory depression occur, a vasopressor (preferably one with inotropic activity such as ephedrine 15–30 mg) should be given intravenously.

In case of inadvertent intravascular injection resulting in convulsions, intravenous injection of thiopentone 100–200 mg or diazepam 5–10 mg should be given intravenously as soon as possible.

Pharmaceutical precautions The solution must not be stored in contact with metals, e.g. needles or metal parts of syringes, as dissolved metal ions may cause swelling at the site of the injection.

The solution should be used immediately after opening of the ampoule. Any remaining solution should be discarded.

Legal category POM.

Package quantities Sterile wrapped ampoules 4 ml.

Product licence number 0017/0139.

PROCAINAMIDE DURULES*

Presentation Slightly yellow, circular, convex tablets containing 500 mg procainamide hydrochloride.

Uses Supraventricular tachyarrhythmias (atrial premature beats, paroxysmal atrial tachycardia, atrial flutter,

atrial fibrillation, AV junctional tachycardia and premature beats).

Ventricular arrhythmias (ectopic beats, premature
beats, and tachycardia).

Digitalis induced arrhythmias.

Dystrophia myotonia; myotonia congenita (Thom-
sen).

Dosage and administration Ideally the dosage
should be adjusted to maintain a serum concentration
between 4–8 mcg per ml, usually 2–3 tablets three times
a day (3–4.5 g daily).

Guidelines: Anti-arrhythmic prophylaxis after acute
myocardial infarction, initially 3–4 Durules followed by
2–3 Durules thrice daily as maintenance. During transition from lignocaine therapy, treatment with Procainamide Durules should be initiated two hours prior to
discontinuation of infusion of lignocaine. It may occasionally be necessary to divide the daily dose into 4
doses per day.

The Durules should be swallowed whole, not broken
or chewed.

Elderly: Lower doses will be required if renal insufficiency
or heart failure are present.

Contra-indications, warnings, etc
Contra-indications: Procainamide hypersensitivity.
Second or third degree AV-block and bifascicular block
with AV-block type I if the patient does not have a
pacemaker. Bronchial asthma, myasthenia gravis and
SLE are relative contra-indications.

Precautions: In patients with renal insufficiency or heart
failure, accumulation of procainamide may occur;
caution should therefore be observed and the dose
adjusted if necessary. Accumulation leads to an impairment of hepatic and/or renal function.

Side-effects: Procainamide is generally well tolerated,
but anorexia, nausea and vomiting and diarrhoea may
occur. Occasional cases of flushing, skin rash, pruritus,
depression, vertigo, psychosis with hallucinations, shivering, fever, joint and muscle pain, 'bitter taste' and
muscle weakness have been reported. A possible lupus
erythematosus-like syndrome may occur during treatment. Serological tests for ANF should therefore be made
before commencement of treatment and regularly thereafter. The blood should also be examined for LE-type
cells at the same time. If the ANF titre rises or LE cells
appear, then cessation of treatment should be considered. Usually these increases are noted before overt
clinical symptoms are detectable. The syndrome is
usually completely reversible. Serious side-effects in the
form of leucopenia and agranulocytosis may occur
during long-term treatment.

Pharmaceutical precautions Procainamide Durules
may be stored at room temperature.

Legal category POM.

Package quantities 500 mg tablets in bottles of 100.

Further information Procainamide Durules are a
sustained release formulation which enable therapeutic
blood levels of procainamide to be conveniently attained
and maintained.

Product licence number 0017/0071.

PULMICORT* ▼

Presentation Pulmicort Inhaler is a metered dose
aerosol delivering 200 mcg budesonide per actuation via
a standard or Spacer adapter. Pulmicort Paediatric Inhaler
is a metered dose aerosol delivering 50 mcg budesonide
per actuation via a Spacer adapter.

Uses Pulmicort Inhaler and Pulmicort Paediatric Inhaler
contain the potent, non-halogenated corticosteroid
budesonide. Clinical studies have shown inhaled budesonide to possess a local anti-inflammatory action in the
lungs without giving rise to systemic corticosteroid
effects. Investigations with Pulmicort have documented
good therapeutic results in bronchial asthma, whilst
being well tolerated during prolonged treatment.

Pulmicort is, therefore, recommended in patients with
bronchial asthma who have not previously been well
controlled on bronchodilators and/or anti allergic agents.

The specially designed Spacer adaptor permits the
aerosol propellants to evaporate and the particle velocity
to decrease, resulting in reduced drug deposition in the
oral cavity. In addition the Spacer adaptor diminishes the
need for co-ordination between aerosol actuation and
inhalation, making this inhaler suitable for patients who
have difficulty using conventional inhalers.

Dosage and administration *Adults:* 200 mcg twice
daily, in the morning and in the evening. During periods
of severe asthma the daily dosage can be increased to
up to 1200 mcg.

In patients well controlled the daily dose may be
reduced below 400 mcg, but should not go below
200 mcg.

Children: 50 to 200 mcg to be given twice daily i.e.
maximum dosage 400 mcg per day.

Elderly: Dosage as for adults.

Contra-indications, warnings, etc No specific contra-indications are known, but special care is needed in
patients with lung tuberculosis, fungal and viral infections in the airways.

Precautions *Pregnancy and breast feeding:* In pregnant animals, administration of budesonide causes
abnormalities of foetal development. The relevance of
this finding to man has not been established. Administration during pregnancy should be avoided unless there
are compelling reasons. As yet there is no information
regarding the passage of budesonide into breast milk.

Patients not dependent on steroids: Treatment with the
recommended doses of Pulmicort usually gives a therapeutic benefit within 7 days. However, certain patients
may have an excessive collection of mucous secretion in
the bronchi, which reduces penetration of the active
substance into the airways. In these cases a short course
of oral corticosteroids (usually 1 to 2 weeks) should be
given in addition to the aerosol. After the course of the
oral drug the inhaler alone should be sufficient therapy.
Exacerbations of asthma caused by bacterial infections
are usually controlled by appropriate antibiotic treatment
and possibly increasing the Pulmicort dosage or if
necessary, by giving systemic steroids.

Steroid dependent patients: Transferral of patients
dependent upon oral steroids to treatment with Pulmicort
demands special care mainly due to the slow restitution
of the disturbed hypothalamic-pituitary function caused
by extended treatment with oral corticosteroids. When
the Pulmicort treatment is initiated the patient should be
in a relatively stable phase. Pulmicort is then given in

combination with the previously used oral steroid dose for about 10 days.

After this period of time the reduction of the oral corticoid dose can be started with a dose reduction corresponding to about 1 mg prednisolone per day every week. The oral dose is thus reduced to the lowest level which in combination with Pulmicort gives a stable respiratory capacity.

In many cases it may eventually be possible to withdraw completely the oral steroid with Pulmicort treatment, but other cases may have to be maintained on a low oral steroid dosage.

Some patients may experience uneasiness during the withdrawal period due to a decreased steroid effect. The physician may have to explain the reason for the Pulmicort treatment in order to encourage the patient to continue. The length of time needed for the body to regain its natural production of corticosteroid in sufficient amounts is often extensive. Thus during physically stressing situations such as severe infections, trauma and surgical operations it will be necessary to give the patient an additional oral steroid dose. Acute exacerbations, accompanied by increased mucous viscosity and mucous plugging, require complementary treatment with a short course of oral corticosteroids.

During transferal from oral therapy to Pulmicort a generally lower systemic steroid action will be experienced which may result in the appearance of allergic or arthritic symptoms such as rhinitis, eczema and muscle and joint pain. Specific treatment should be initiated for these conditions.

Side effects: Occasional cases of mild irritation in the throat and hoarseness have been reported. Due to drug deposition in the oral cavity candidiasis of the mouth and throat occurs in some patients. However, the incidence should be less with the Spacer adaptor as this reduces oral deposition. In most cases this condition responds to topical anti-fungal therapy without discontinuing treatment with Pulmicort.

Pharmaceutical precautions To be stored at room temperature.

Legal category POM.

Package quantities Pulmicort Inhaler (200 mcg/puff). Aerosol canister containing 100 metered doses complete with standard and Spacer adapters.

Pulmicort Paediatric Inhaler (50 mcg/puff). Aerosol canister containing 200 metered doses complete with Spacer delivery system.

Pulmicort (200 mcg/puff) and Pulmicort Paediatric (50 mcg/puff) refill canisters are available.

Further information Pulmicort and Pulmicort Paediatric may also be administered via the Nebuhaler.

Product licence numbers
Pulmicort Inhaler (200 mcg/puff)   0017/0128
Pulmicort Paediatric Inhaler (50 mcg/puff) 0017/0113

RHINOCORT* ▼

Presentation Rhinocort is a metered-dose aerosol for nasal application delivering 50 mcg budesonide per actuation.

Uses Seasonal and perennial, allergic rhinitis and vasomotor rhinitis.

Dosage and administration Two applications into each nostril morning and evening. (Total dose 400 mcg). When good effect has been achieved the dosage may be reduced to one application into each nostril morning and evening.

Contra-indications, warnings, etc No specific contra-indications are known, but special care is needed in fungal and viral infections in the airways, and in patients with lung tuberculosis.

Precautions: Pregnancy and breast feeding: In pregnant animals, administration of budesonide causes abnormalities of foetal developments. The relevance of this to man has not been established. Administration during pregnancy should be avoided unless there are compelling reasons. As yet there is no information regarding the passage of budesonide into breast milk.

The patient should be informed that the full effect of Rhinocort is not achieved until after a few days. Concomitant treatment with an antihistamine may sometimes be necessary to counteract potential eye symptoms caused by the allergy. In continuous long-term treatment with Rhinocort the nasal mucosa should be inspected regularly, at least once a year. Until greater experience has been achieved continuous long-term treatment of children is not recommended.

Side-effects: Occasionally, sneezing attacks may follow immediately after the use of the aerosol. Slight haemorrhagic secretions may occur.

Pharmaceutical precautions *Storage:* To be stored at room temperature.

Legal category POM.

Package quantities Rhinocort is an aerosol vial containing 7 g suspension corresponding to 200 doses.

Further information In pharmacological investigations and investigations in human beings budesonide (a non-halogenated corticosteroid) has shown a favourable relationship between anti-inflammatory effects and systemic effects due to the fact that budesonide is inactivated very rapidly in the liver after systemic absorption. With the recommended dosage of Rhinocort, an effective corticosteroid treatment of the nasal mucous membrane is attained with very little risk of systemic side-effects. The duration of action of Rhinocort is such that application morning and evening is sufficient.

Product licence number 0017/0204.

TONOCARD* ▼

Presentation Yellow, biconvex, film coated tablets containing tocainide hydrochloride, either 400 mg (coded A/TT) or 600 mg (coded A/TC).

Injection vials of 15 ml, each 1 ml of clear aqueous sterile solution for injection contains 50 mg tocainide hydrochloride.

Infusion bottles of 75 ml, each 1 ml of clear aqueous sterile solution for injection contains 10 mg tocainide hydrochloride.

Uses For the treatment of patients with life-threatening symptomatic ventricular tachyarrhythmias associated with severely compromised left ventricular function who do not respond to other therapy or for whom other therapy is contra-indicated.

Dosage and administration *Acute Treatment:* 500–750 mg by infusion or by slow intravenous injection given over 15–30 minutes, followed immediately by 600–800 mg orally.

Maintenance treatment: 8 hours after acute treatment, commence maintenance therapy with 1200 mg daily, divided into two or three oral doses.

Chronic ventricular arrhythmias: 1200 mg daily, divided into two or three oral doses.

The oral daily dosage of Tonocard may be increased to 1800–2400 mg in divided doses, if necessary.

Not to be administered to children.

Elderly: Dosage reduction may be necessary if renal disease is present.

Contra-indications, warnings, etc *Contra-indications:* Known hypersensitivity to amide drugs. Second or third degree AV block, in the absence of a pacemaker.

Precautions: Tonocard therapy should only be instituted when facilities are available for regular monitoring of blood counts.

Agranulocytosis, aplastic anaemia and thrombocytopenia have been reported in patients receiving Tonocard; the incidence of neutropenia may be as high as 1 in 300. Fatalities have occurred. Patients should be instructed to promptly report the development of bruising or bleeding and any signs of infection such as fever, sore throat or chills. Since most of these events have been noted during the first 12 weeks of therapy, it is recommended that blood counts be performed weekly during this period, and montly thereafter. If any of these haematological disorders are identified, specialist advice should be sought with a view to discontinuing Tonocard therapy and substituting other appropriate treatment.

Like other drugs, Tonocard should be used with caution in patients with severe hepatic or renal disease and in the elderly because of the potential risk of accumulation. Caution is also advised in patients with uncompensated heart failure and in patients receiving other antiarrhythmic agents.

Reproduction studies in animals have shown maternal and foetal toxicity. The safety of Tonocard in human pregnancy has not been tested and the potential benefit should be weighed against possible hazard.

Side-effects: Side effects during Tonocard treatment are generally mild and transient. Reported side effects are mainly neurological or gastro-intestinal. CNS symptoms are usually dose-related and may include tremor, dizziness, lightheadedness, paraesthesia, visual hallucinations and convulsions. Gastro-intestinal symptoms include nausea and vomiting. Rash and fever have been reported. Bradycardia and hypotension may occur after i.v. injection. Positive ANF titres, clinical manifestation of LE syndrome and fibrosing alveolitis have been reported during Tonocard therapy. Agranulocytosis, aplastic anaemia and thrombocytopenia have occurred.

Pharmaceutical precautions Recommended diluents for i.v. injection (50 mg/ml) are sodium chloride injection or 5% dextrose injection.

Legal category POM.

Package quantities *Tablets:* 400 mg, bottle of 100 tablets; 600 mg, bottle of 100 tablets.

Injection: Packs of 5 × 15 ml injection vials 50 mg/ml.

Infusion: Packs of 5 × 75 ml injection infusion 10 mg/ml.

Further information Tonocard is a primary amine analogue of lignocaine, with a high oral bioavailability.

Its electrophysiological properties are similar to lignocaine and, as such, Tonocard has been shown to be effective in the treatment of ventricular arrhythmias. In therapeutic plasma concentration, no clinically significant adverse haemodynamic changes have been reported, even in patients with acute myocardial infarction or those pre-treated with beta-blockers.

Product licence numbers

400 mg tablets	0017/0106
600 mg tablets	0017/0107
50 mg/ml I.V. Injection	0017/0108
10 mg/ml I.V. Infusion	0017/0135

XYLOCAINE*

Presentation A sterile clear aqueous solution of Lignocaine Hydrochloride BP. Each ml contains:

0.5% solution:	Lignocaine hydrochloride anhydrous 5 mg
1.0% solution:	Lignocaine hydrochloride anhydrous 10 mg
1.5% solution:	Lignocaine hydrochloride anhydrous 15 mg
2% solution:	Lignocaine hydrochloride anhydrous 20 mg

Uses Xylocaine is a local anaesthetic solution for use in infiltration anaesthesia, intravenous regional anaesthesia and nerve blocks.

Dosage and administration The dosage is adjusted according to the response of the patient and site of administration. The lowest concentration and smallest dose producing the required effect should be given. The maximum dose for healthy adults should not exceed 200 mg.

Children and elderly or debilitated patients require smaller doses, commensurate with age and physical status.

Contra-indications, warnings, etc Known hypersensitivity to anaesthetics of the amide type.

Precautions: In common with other local anaesthetics, Xylocaine should be used cautiously in patients with epilepsy, impaired cardiac conduction, bradycardia, impaired respiratory function, and in patients with impaired hepatic function, if the dose or site of administration is likely to result in high blood levels.

Facilities for resuscitation should be available when local anaesthetics are administered.

The effect of local anaesthetics may be reduced if an injection is made into an inflamed or infected area.

Use in pregnancy: Although there is no evidence from animal studies of harm to the foetus, as with all drugs, Xylocaine should not be given during early pregnancy unless the benefits are considered to outweigh the risks.

Adverse reactions: In common with other local anaesthetics, adverse reactions to Xylocaine are rare and are usually the result of excessively high blood concentrations due to inadvertent intravascular injection, excessive dosage, rapid absorption or occasionally to hypersensitivity, idiosyncracy or diminished tolerance on the part of the patient. In such circumstances systemic effects occur involving the central nervous system and/or the cardiovascular system.

CNS reactions are excitatory and/or depressant, and may be characterized by nervousness, dizziness, blurred vision and tremors, followed by drowsiness, convulsions, unconsciousness and possibly respiratory arrest. The excitatory reactions may be very brief or may not occur at all, in which case the first manifestations of toxicity may be drowsiness, merging into unconsciousness and respiratory arrest. Cardiovascular reactions are depressant, and may be characterized by hypotension, myocardial depression, bradycardia and possibly cardiac arrest.

Allergic reactions are extremely rare. They may be characterized by cutaneous lesions, urticaria, oedema or anaphylactoid reactions. Detection of sensitivity by skin testing is of doubtful value.

Hypotension may occur as a physiological response to central nerve blocks.

Pharmaceutical precautions Store at room temperature.

Legal category POM.

Package quantities
Vials:
0.5% solution – 20 ml, 50 ml. Packs of 5 vials.
1.0% solution – 20 ml, 50 ml. Packs of 5 vials.
2.0% solution – 20 ml, 50 ml. Packs of 5 vials.

Ampoules:
0.5% solution – 10 ml × 50.
1.0% solution – 2 ml × 100, 10 ml × 20.
1.5% solution – 25 ml.
2.0% solution – 5 ml × 50.

Further information Nil.

Product licence numbers
Vials
0.5% 0017/5031R
1.0% 0017/5032R
2.0% 0017/5034R

Ampoules
0.5% 0017/0218R
1.0% 0017/0219R
1.5% 0017/5033R
2.0% 0017/0220R

XYLOCAINE* WITH ADRENALINE 1 : 200,000

Presentation A sterile clear aqueous solution of Lignocaine Hydrochloride NP. Each ml contains:

0.5% solution: Lignocaine hydrochloride anhydrous 5 mg Adrenaline BP 0.005 mg
1.0% solution: Lignocaine hydrochloride anhydrous 10 mg Adrenaline BP 0.005 mg
2% solution: Lignocaine hydrochloride anhydrous 20 mg Adrenaline BP 0.005 mg

Uses Xylocaine with Adrenaline is a local anaesthetic solution for use in infiltration anaesthesia and nerve blocks.

Dosage and administration The dosage is adjusted according to the response of the patient and the site of administration. The lowest concentration and smallest dose producing the required effect should be given. The maximum single dose of Xylocaine when given with adrenaline is 500 mg.

Children and elderly or debilitated patients require smaller doses, commensurate with age and physical status.

Contra-indications, warnings, etc Known hypersensitivity to anaesthetics of the amide type.

The use of a vasoconstrictor is contra-indicated for anaesthesia of fingers, toes, tip of nose, ears and penis.

Xylocaine with adrenaline should not be given intravenously.

Precautions: In common with other local anaesthetics, Xylocaine with adrenaline should be used cautiously in patients with epilepsy, impaired cardiac conduction, impaired respiratory function, and in patients with impaired hepatic function, if the dose or site of administration is likely to result in high blood levels.

Facilities for resuscitation should be available when local anaesthetics are administered.

The effect of local anaesthetics may be reduced if an injection is made into an inflamed or infected area.

Solutions containing adrenaline should be used with caution in patients with hypertension, cardiac disease, cerebrovascular insufficiency, thyrotoxicosis, in patients taking tricyclic antidepressants, MAOI's, or receiving potent general anaesthetic agents.

Solutions containing adrenaline should be used where possible so as to prolong anaesthesia and reduce systemic absorption. This is particularly important in highly vascular areas.

Adverse reactions: In common with other local anaesthetics, adverse reactions to Xylocaine with adrenaline are rare and are usually the result of excessively high blood concentrations due to inadvertent intravascular injection, excessive dosage, rapid absorption or occasionally to hypersensitivity, idiosyncracy or diminished tolerance on the part of the patient. In such circumstances systemic effects occur involving the central nervous system and/or the cardiovascular system.

CNS reactions are excitatory and/or depressant, and may be characterized by nervousness, dizziness, blurred vision and tremors, followed by drowsiness, convulsions, unconsciousness and possibly respiratory arrest. The excitatory reactions may be very brief or may not occur at all, in which case the first manifestations of toxicity may be drowsiness, merging into unconsciousness and respiratory arrest.

Cardiovascular reactions are depressant, and may be characterized by hypotension, myocardial depression, bradycardia and possibly cardiac arrest.

Allergic reactins are extremely rare. They may be characterized by cutaneous lesions, urticaria, oedema or anaphylactoid reactions. Detection of sensitivity by skin testing is of doubtful value.

Hypotension may occur as a physiological response to central nerve blocks.

Pharmaceutical precautions Store at room temperature.

Legal category POM.

Package quantities
0.5% with adrenaline 50 ml. Packs of 5 vials
1.0% with adrenaline 20 ml, 50 ml. Packs of 5 vials
2.0% with adrenaline 20 ml, 50 ml. Packs of 5 vials

1.0% with adrenaline 10 ml. Pack of 20 ampoules.

Further information Multidose vial preparations of Xylocaine with adrenaline 1 : 200,000 contain methylhydroxybenzoate 1 mg/ml.

Product licence numbers
Vials
0.5% 0017/5028R
1.0% 0017/5029R
2.0% 0017/5030R

Ampoule
1%   0017/0214R.

XYLOCAINE* 2% WITH ADRENALINE 1 : 80,000

Presentation Sterile clear aqueous solution: lignocaine hydrochloride 20 mg/ml, Adrenaline BP 1 : 80,000.

Uses Local anaesthetic solution with vasoconstrictor for dental infiltration anaesthesia where a vasoconstrictor is indicated. For all dental nerve-block techniques.

Dosage and administration Infiltration – 1 ml. Nerve block – 1.5–2 ml. Extensive surgery – 3–5 ml. Adult maximum dose 500 mg.
In children the maximum dose is considerably less and should be calculated in relation to the body weight.

Contra-indications, warnings, etc Patients with thyrotoxicosis and cardiac disease, particularly with arrhythmia or hypertension. Known hypersensitivity to local anaesthetics of the amide type.

Adverse reactions: The type of toxic reaction is unpredictable and depends on dosage, route of administration and state of patient. The reactions are primarily of two types, typified by stimulation and depression of the cerebral cortex and medulla respectively. Slow onset – stimulation leading to nervousness, dizziness, blurred vision, nausea, tremor, convulsions and respiratory arrest. Rapid onset – depression leading primarily to respiratory arrest, cardiovascular collapse and cardiac arrest. Symptoms occur rapidly and with little warning.

Precautions: Adequate resuscitation equipment must be available whenever local or general anaesthesia is administered. Though clinical tolerance is remarkably good, overdosage or accidental intravenous injection may give rise to toxic reactions. These are best avoided by aspiration before making an injection in order to avoid accidental intravascular injection.
Care should be observed in patients taking tricyclic anti-depressants.

Pharmaceutical precautions Store in a cool place.

Legal category POM.

Package quantities Glass cartridges of 2.2 ml standard, and 2.2 ml self-aspirating, in boxes of 100.

Further information Dental cartridges of Xylocaine 2% with adrenaline 1 : 80,000 do not contain an antimicrobial agent.

Product licence number 0017/5027.

XYLOCAINE* ANTISEPTIC GEL

Presentation Clear sterile viscous gel. Each millilitre contains Lignocaine Hydrochloride BP 21.4 mg (equivalent to 20 mg lignocaine hydrochloride anhydrous), Chlorhexidine Gluconate Solution BPC 0.0025 ml in a water-miscible base.

Uses Anaesthetic gel for anaesthesia of the urethra and topical application on mucous membrane wherever an anaesthetic/antiseptic effect is required.

Dosage and administration *Men:* 10 ml injected initially, followed by 3–5 ml.

Women: 3–5 ml injected into the urethra.

Contra-indications, warnings, etc Known hypersensitivity to anaesthetics of the amide type.

Pharmaceutical precautions Store in a cool place.

Legal category P.

Package quantities 15 ml tubes.

Further information Nil.

Product licence number 0017/5035.

XYLOCAINE* GEL

Presentation Sterile clear gel. Each millilitre contains Lignocaine Hydrochloride BP 21.4 mg (equivalent to 20 mg lignocaine hydrochloride anhydrous).

Uses Gel for anaesthesia of the urethra.

Dosage and administration *Men:* 10 ml injected initially, followed by 3–5 ml.

Women: 3–5 ml injected into the urethra.

Contra-indications, warnings, etc Known hypersensitivity to anaesthetics of the amide type.

Pharmaceutical precautions Store in a cool place.

Legal category P.

Package quantities Packs of 10 × 20 g tubes and packs of 20 × 20 g Accordion syringes.

Further information Xylocaine Gel is also available in the Xylocaine Accordion, a 'bellows type' syringe in a sterile blister pack. Use of the Accordion eliminates the necessity for attaching a separate nozzle prior to urethral catheterisation. The gel in the Accordion syringe contains no antimicrobial preservative. Xylocaine Accordion Gel is available in packs of 20 × 20 g.

Product licence number 0017/5037.

XYLOCAINE* OINTMENT 5%

Presentation White cream. Each gramme contains lignocaine base 50 mg in a water-miscible vehicle.

Uses Local anaesthetic for topical use in dentistry for surface anaesthesia of the gums, and for the relief of soreness of the nipples in nursing mothers, pain relief in pruritus ani and vulvae, haemorrhoids, herpes zoster and labialis. As a lubricant for proctoscope and cystoscope.

Dosage and administration In dentistry, apply to dry gum and rub gently. For soreness of nipples, apply on a small piece of lint or gauze (to be washed off immediately before next feeding). For other indications, apply when required.

Contra-indications, warnings, etc Known hypersensitivity to anaesthetics of the amide type.

Pharmaceutical precautions Xylocaine ointment is not intended for use with aseptic techniques, nor is it bactericidal.

Legal category P.

Package quantities 15 g tubes.

Further information Nil.

Product licence number 0017/5038.

XYLOCAINE* SPRAY

Presentation Clear spray solution. Each gram contains 100 mg lignocaine base, 0.1 mg cetyl pyridinium chloride.

Uses Anaesthetic solution for surface analgesia of mucous membrane in ENT surgery, obstetrics and dental surgery.

Dosage and administration The spray is supplied in metered spray bottles. Each metered dose contains 10 mg of lignocaine base. The number of sprays needed depends upon the extent of the area to be anaesthetised. Maximum adult dosage based on body weight of 70 kg is 200 mg, equal to 20 spray doses. Maximum dosage in children is proportionately lower according to body weight.

Contra-indications, warnings, etc Known hypersensitivity to anaesthetics of the amide type.

Side-effects: Does not produce side-effects when used at the recommended dosage.

Adverse reactions: The type of toxic reaction is unpredictable and depends on dosage and state of the patient. The reactions are primarily of two types, typified by stimulation and depression of the cerebral cortex and medulla respectively.

Precautions: The spray should not come in contact with the eyes. Accidental application should be counteracted by immediate instillation of pure liquid paraffin followed by a boric acid (2–3%) wash.

Pharmaceutical precautions Store in a cool place. Keep away from excessive heat and direct sunlight. Empty container must not be thrown on to a fire or other source of heat.

Legal category P.

Package quantities Supplied in spray bottles of 80 g (approx. 800 spray doses) with a metering valve complete with adjustable spray nozzle which can be steam sterilised at 115°C or 121°C.

Further information Nil.

Product licence number 0017/5039.

XYLOCAINE* 4% TOPICAL

Presentation Clear aqueous solution. Each millilitre contains 40 mg lignocaine hydrochloride anhydrous.

Uses Anaesthesia of mucous membrane in bronchoscopy and bronchography; biopsy in the mouth and throat; puncture of the maxillary sinus or polypectomy; tonsillectomy; resection of nasal turbinates; in dentistry.

Dosage and administration *Bronchoscopy and bronchography:* With a suitable spray 2–3 ml Xylocaine 4% may be applied to the mouth, pharynx, larynx and trachea.

Biopsy: 3–4 ml may be sprayed on the area or the solution may be applied for a few minutes with a swab. Adrenaline may be added to this solution in order to produce vasoconstriction (add 1–2 drops, 0.05 ml, 1 : 1,000, solution to 5 ml Xylocaine 4% solution).

Puncture of maxillary sinus or polypectomy: A swab soaked in the solution may be applied for two to three minutes. The addition of adrenaline is advised in these procedures, made up on the lines indicated above.

The maximum adult dose (70 kg body weight) should not exceed 5 ml (200 mg). For the debilitated, the aged and children the dosage should be reduced. In children the maximum dose is calculated as 1.4 mg per lb, or 3 mg/kg.

Contra-indications, warnings, etc Known hypersensitivity to anaesthetics of the amide type.

Precautions: Adrenaline added to the solution as described above decomposes fairly rapidly. A freshly prepared solution should be made up and used within a few hours or discarded.

Pharmaceutical precautions Store at room temperature.

Legal category P.

Package quantities Bottles of 25 ml.

Further information Nil.

Product licence number 0017/5040.

XYLOCAINE* VISCOUS

Presentation Viscous clear liquid. Each millilitre contains Lignocaine Hydrochloride BP 21.4 mg (equivalent to 20 mg lignocaine hydrochloride anhydrous).

Uses Topical anaesthetic solution for:
1. Mucous membrane lesions of mouth and throat following tonsillectomy, and post-tonsillectomy sore throat.
2. Introduction of instruments and catheters into the stomach.
3. Oesophagoscopy, oesophagitis, pharyngitis and stomatitis.
4. Severe hiccough.

Dosage and administration
1. One teaspoonful (5 ml) swished around the mouth and swallowed slowly. (Not more than six times in 24 hours.)
2. One tablespoonful (15 ml).
3. One dessertspoonful (10 ml) swished around the mouth and swallowed slowly. (Not more than three times in 24 hours.)
4. One dessertspoonful (10 ml) swallowed quickly in one gulp. (Not more than three times in 24 hours.)

The maximum dose for adults of normal body weight is 15 ml. This should be reduced for debilitated and aged patients.

Contra-indications, warnings, etc Known hypersensitivity to anaesthetics of the amide type. There are no known side-effects or adverse reactions.

Precautions: No food or drink should be taken for three hours after administration. Not more than 30 ml to be administered in 24 hours. Minimal interval between doses – four hours.

Pharmaceutical precautions None.

Legal category P.

Package quantities Bottles of 150 ml.

Further information Nil.

Product licence number 0017/5041.

XYLOCARD*

Presentation *Xylocard 100 mg Intravenous bolus injection:* Clear aqueous sterile solution in pre-loaded 5 ml syringe: lignocaine hydrochloride anhydrous 20 mg/ml.

Xylocard 1 g and 2 g for addition to intravenous infusion: Sterile aqueous solution in pre-loaded 5 ml or 10 ml syringe: lignocaine hydrochloride anhydrous 200 mg/ml.

Uses Prevention of ventricular tachyarrhythmias in patients with suspected or proven acute myocardial infarction. Treatment of ventricular tachyarrhythmias associated with acute myocardial infarction. Ventricular extrasystoles and ventricular tachycardia. As anti-arrhythmic cover in cases of ventricular fibrillation being DC converted.

Dosage and administration
Adults:
Xylocard 100 mg I.V. bolus injection: 1 mg/kg body weight. Normal doses 50–100 mg (2.5–5 ml) as initial treatment to be injected slowly over a period of two minutes. When necessary injection can be repeated once or twice at 5–10 minute intervals. Effect can be observed within two minutes.

Xylocard 1 g and 2 g for addition to I.V. Infusion: A concentration of 0.2% lignocaine infusion may be recommended for most cases. This is achieved by adding 1 × Xylocard 1 g syringe (or half × Xylocard 2 g syringe) to 500 ml infusion solution. Normal dose 2–4 mg/min. Based on a concentration of 0.2% this is equivalent to an infusion rate of 1–2 ml/min.

Children: The safety and efficacy of lignocaine in children has not been established.

Elderly: In patients with cardiac failure, total plasma clearance will be reduced and lower dosages may be required.

Contra-indications, warnings, etc Lignocaine is contra-indicated in patients with a known history of hypersensitivity.
  Atrioventricular block is an absolute or relative contra-indication, according to severity.
  Other serious conduction disturbances, and cardiac decompensation not dependent on treatable tachy-arrhythmias, are also contra-indications.

Precautions: In bradycardia complicated by ventricular tachyarrhythmias, Xylocard may need to be combined with atropine or atropine-like drugs or pacemaker therapy.
  Patients with severe liver damage should be given lower doses and the effect carefully monitored. Manifest renal insufficiency calls for special care in infusion therapy.

Side-effects: Dizziness, paraesthesia or drowsiness often occur when intravenous injections of Xylocard are given too rapidly. These mild side-effects are transient and do not require special therapeutic measures.
  Central nervous side-effects: Drowsiness, persistent dizziness, paresthesiae, tinnitus, disorientation, blurred vision, tremor, convulsions, loss of consciousness and respiratory depression. Cardiovascular side-effects: Hy potension and bradycardia, which may lead to cardiac arreest.
  With the recommended dosage, central nervous and cardiovascular side-effects are rare.

Pharmaceutical precautions Store in a cool place.
  The contents of the Xylocard 1 g and 2 g syringes are for dilution in infusion fluid only. Under no circumstances are they to be administered undiluted.

Legal category POM.

Package quantities *Xylocard 100 mg 5 ml (20 mg/ml):* Pre-loaded syringe for immediate use. Box of 5.
Xylocard 1 g (5 ml) and Xylocard 2 g (10 ml) both 200 mg/ml: Pre-loaded syringe for addition to infusion bottles and bags. Box of 10.

Further information All Xylocard syringes are free of bacteriostat and preservatives.

Product licence numbers
Xylocard 100 mg I.V. bolus   0017/5018
Xylocard 1 g for I.V. infusion   0017/0064R
Xylocard 2 g for I.V. infusion   0017/0064R

XYLODASE*

Presentation White cream. Each gram contains lignocaine (base) 50 mg, Hyaluronidase BP 50 units (0.015%) in water-miscible base.

Uses Surface anaesthesia in dental procedures: surface analgesia before any injection, opening of abscesses, preparation of sensitive cervical cavities, deep scaling, extraction of deciduous teeth not embedded deeply in the bone, wiring of teeth.

Dosage and administration ½–1 g or as required.

Contra-indications, warnings, etc Known hypersensitivity to anaesthetics of the amide type.

Pharmaceutical precautions To be stored at room temperature.

Legal category P.

Package quantities Boxes of 12 × 15 g tubes.

Further information Nil.

Product licence number 0017/5042.

XYLOPROCT* OINTMENT

Presentation White water-miscible cream. Each gram contains: Xylocaine (lignocaine) 50 mg, Hydrocortisone Acetate BP 2.75 mg, Zinc Oxide BP 180 mg, aluminium acetate 35 mg.

Uses External and prolapsed haemorrhoids and other painful perianal conditions.
  Pruritus ani – pruritus vulva.

Dosage and administration To be applied several times a day according to the severity of the condition.

Contra-indications, warnings, etc There are no known contra-indications or side-effects.

Pharmaceutical precautions Store in a cool place.

Legal category POM.

Package quantities *Tubes:* 30 g ointment complete with special applicator.

Further information Nil.

Product licence number 0017/5023R.

XYLOPROCT* SUPPOSITORIES

Presentation White cone-shaped suppositories. Each suppository contains: Xylocaine (lignocaine) 60 mg, hydrocortisone Acetate BP 5 mg, Zinc Oxide BP 400 mg, Aluminium acetate 50 mg.

Uses For the treatment of internal haemorrhoids and other disorders of the anal canal such as proctitis, fissure in ano, anal fissure and anal fistula.

Dosage and administration Removing protective foil, use 1 suppository at night before retiring and repeat the treatment after each bowel action.

Contra-indications, warnings, etc There are no known contra-indications or side-effects.

Pharmaceutical precautions Store in a cool place.

Legal category POM.

Package quantities Packs containing 10 separate foil-protected suppositories.

Further information Nil.

Product licence number 0017/5024R.

*Trade Mark

Ayerst Laboratories Limited
South Way
Andover
Hampshire SP 10 5LT

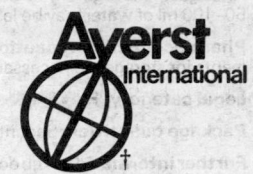

Ayerst International

ANTEPSIN* TABLETS ▼

Presentation Antepsin Tablets 1 gram are white, oblong, biconvex, uncoated tablets scored and engraved 1239 on one side and Ayerst on the other. Each tablet contains 1 gram sucralfate, a basic aluminium salt of sucrose octa sulphate.

Uses For the treatment of duodenal ulcer, gastric ulcer and chronic gastritis.

Dosage and administration For oral administration: *Adults:* Usual dose 1 gram 4 times a day to be taken 1 hour before meals and at bedtime. Maximum daily dose 8 grams. For ease of administration Antepsin tablets may be dispersed in 10–15 ml of water.

Four to six weeks' treatment is usually needed for ulcer healing but up to twelve weeks may be necessary in resistant cases.

Antacids may be used as required for relief of pain, but should not be taken half an hour before or after Antepsin.

Elderly: There are no special dosage requirements for elderly patients but as with all medicines the lowest effective dose should be used.

Safety and effectiveness in children have not been established.

Contra-indications, warnings, etc
Contra-indications: There are no known contra-indications.

Precautions: 1. The product should only be used with caution in patients with renal dysfunction.

2. *Use in pregnancy:* Although animal studies show no evidence of foetal malformations, safety in pregnant women has not been established and Antepsin should be used during pregnancy only if clearly needed.

3. It is not known whether this drug is excreted in human milk. Caution should be exercised when sucralfate is administered to a nursing woman.

Drug interactions: Concomitant administration of Antepsin may reduce the bioavailability of certain drugs as has been observed in animal studies with tetracycline, phenytoin and cimetidine, and in human studies with digoxin. Administration of Antepsin with any of these drugs should be separated by two hours.

Since Antepsin may hinder warfarin absorption, caution should be exercised when these two drugs are used together.

Side-effects: A low incidence of mild side-effects, e.g. constipation, has been reported.

Overdosage: There is no experience in humans with overdosage. Acute oral toxicity studies in animals, however, using doses up to 12 g/kg body weight, could not find a lethal dose. Risks associated with overdosage, should, therefore, be minimal.

Pharmaceutical precautions No special requirements for storage are necessary.

Legal category POM.

Package quantities Antepsin 1 gram: Securitainers of 100.

Further information Antepsin is not significantly absorbed. It forms a chemical complex which selectively binds to the ulcer site, establishing a protective barrier against the actions of pepsin, bile and gastric acid.

Product licence number 0607/0045.

BC 500* WITH IRON

Presentation BC 500 with Iron tablets contain high potency B complex and C vitamins with ferrous fumarate. Each tablet contains:

Ferrous Fumarate	200 mg
Thiamine Mononitrate	25 mg
Riboflavine	12.5 mg
Nicotinamide	100 mg
Pyridoxine Hydrochloride	10 mg
Calcium Pantothenate	20 mg
Ascorbic Acid as Sodium Ascorbate	500 mg

BC 500 with Iron is a red film-coated round biconvex tablet printed Ayerst 1143.

Uses BC 500 with Iron tablets are recommended for the treatment of iron deficiency when therapeutic doses of water soluble vitamins are also required.

Dosage and administration *Adults:* One tablet daily or as recommended by the physician.

Elderly: There are no special dosage requirements for elderly patients but as with all medicines the lowest effective dose should be used.

Children: Not recommended.

Contra-indications, warnings, etc *Precautions:* Iron chelates with tetracyclines and may impair absorption of both agents. Pyridoxine may antagonise laevodopa when given for Parkinson's Disease.

Use in pregnancy: The product has not been studied in human pregnancy. The use of BC 500 with iron requires that the anticipated benefit be weighed against possible hazard.

Side-effects: As with all iron preparations, nausea, gastro-intestinal irritation and constipation may rarely occur.

Overdose: In the event of overdose emesis and/or gastric lavage is indicated. Immediate injection of 2 g desferrioxamine mesylate in water for injection is required.

After gastric lavage 5 g of desferrioxamine mesylate in 50–100 ml of water may be left in the stomach.

Pharmaceutical precautions No special requirements for storage are necessary.

Legal category P.

Package quantities Securitainers of 100 tablets.

Further information The dose of Vitamin C is sufficient both to treat deficiency of this vitamin and to enhance the absorption of iron.

Product licence number 0607/0028.

CALTHOR* TABLETS
CALTHOR* SUSPENSION

Presentation Calthor Tablets are white, round, flat and scored one side, containing 250 mg or 500 mg ciclacillin. The 250 mg tablets are 10mm in diameter. The 500 mg tablets are 13mm in diameter.

Calthor Suspension 125 is presented as a granular off-white powder. When reconstituted, it contains 125 mg ciclacillin per 5 ml and is a pink homogeneous suspension with a characteristic fruity smell. Calthor Suspension 250 is presented as a granular off-white powder. When reconstituted, it contains 250 mg ciclacillin per 5 ml and is an off-white, homogeneous suspension with a characteristic fruity smell.

Uses Calthor is an orally active broad spectrum penicillin. Calthor is indicated for the oral treatment of a wide range of bacterial infections caused by commonly occurring pathogens.

Calthor is active against the following organisms *in vitro*: Group A beta-haemolytic streptococci, *Strep. faecalis* (enterococci), alpha-haemolytic streptococci, *Strep. pneumoniae*, non-penicillinase-producing staphylococci, *Haemophilus influenzae*, *Escherichia coli*, *Proteus mirabilis*, *Neisseria gonorrhoeae*. All strains of pseudomonas and most strains of klebsiella and enterobacter are resistant: some strains of *E. coli* and *H. influenzae* may be resistant. Calthor should not be used in any infections caused by *E. coli* and *P. mirabilis* other than urinary tract infections. Efficacy against salmonella infections has not been established.

Calthor is indicated for the treatment of the following infections, due to susceptible organisms:

Respiratory Tract infections, *e.g.*: Tonsillitis, pharyngitis, bronchitis, pneumonia,
Otitis Media,
Skin and Skin Structure (Integumentary) infections,
Urinary Tract infections.

Dosage and administration *Preparation of the suspension:* 125 mg/5 ml – add 57 ml of water to the powder for reconstitution and shake well.

250 mg/5 ml – add 74 ml of water to the powder for reconstitution and shake well.

Adults and elderly: Respiratory Tract Infections: Tonsillitis and Pharyngitis 250 mg qid in equally spaced doses.

Bronchitis and Pneumonia: Mild or moderate infections – 250 mg qid in equally spaced doses; chronic infections – 500 mg qid in equally spaced doses.

Otitis Media: 250 mg to 500 mg qid in equally spaced doses depending on severity.

Skin and Skin Structure Infections: 250 mg to 500 mg qid in equally spaced doses depending on severity.

Urinary Tract Infections: 500 mg qid in equally spaced doses.

Children: 2 months to 10 years – half adult dose. Over 10 years – adult dose.

All recommended dosages are a guide only. In severe infections dosages may be increased.

In infections caused by Group A beta-haemolytic streptococci a minimum of 10 days of treatment is recommended to guard against the risk of rheumatic fever or glomerulonephritis.

In the treatment of chronic urinary tract infection frequent bacteriological and clinical appraisal is necessary during therapy and may be required for several months afterwards. Persistent infection may require treatment for several weeks.

Calthor should not be used in children under 2 months of age.

Patients with renal failure: Each patient should be individually considered. Based on a dosage of 500 mg qid the following adjustment in dosage interval is recommended:

Patients with a creatinine clearance of 50 ml/min need no dosage interval adjustment.

Patients with a creatinine clearance of 30–50 ml/min should receive a full dose every 12 hours.

Patients with a creatinine clearance of between 15–30 ml/min should receive full doses every 18 hours.

Patients with a creatinine clearance of between 10–15 ml/min should receive full doses every 24 hours.

In patients with a creatinine clearance of < 10 ml/min or serum creatinine values > 10 mg/100 ml (850 µmol/l) serum ciclacillin levels are recommended to determine the subsequent dosage and frequency.

Contra-indications, warnings, etc

Contra-indications: Calthor should not be given to patients with a history of hypersensitivity to penicillin.

Precautions: Animal experiments show no teratogenic effect but, as with all medicines, Calthor should not be administered during pregnancy unless considered essential. Because many drugs are excreted in human milk, caution should be exercised when Calthor is administered to a nursing mother.

Prolonged use of an anti-infective may result in overgrowth of non-sensitive organisms.

Side-effects: Calthor is generally very well tolerated and side-effects are rare. Diarrhoea, nausea, vomiting and skin reactions have occasionally been observed.

Penicillins may cause an acute anaphylactic reaction which can be fatal. This reaction appears to occur more frequently in patients with bronchial asthma or other allergic disorders.

Overdosage: Since Calthor is a penicillin problems of overdosage are unlikely to be encountered.

Pharmaceutical precautions Store in a cool place.

After reconstitution the suspension should be stored in a refrigerator and the unused portion discarded after 14 days. The suspension may be diluted with Syrup BP.

Legal category POM.

Package quantities
Tablets: Cartons of 120 tablets in blister packs of twelve.
Suspension: Bottles containing powder to give 120 ml reconstituted suspension.

Further information Nil.

Product licence numbers

Calthor tablets 250 mg	0607/0036
Calthor tablets 500 mg	0607/0037
Calthor suspension 125 mg/5 ml	0607/0040
Calthor suspension 250 mg/5 ml	0607/0038

EVADYNE* TABLETS

Presentation *Evadyne Tablets 25 mg* are orange film-coated round bi-convex tablets, containing butriptyline 25 mg as the hydrochloride.

Evadyne Tablets 50 mg are pink film-coated round bi-convex tablets containing butriptyline 50 mg as the hydrochloride.

Uses Evadyne is indicated for the relief of symptoms of depressive illness.

Dosage and administration *Adults:* Initially 25 mg 3 times daily increasing daily or alternate days to a maximum of 150 mg per day.

Maintenance dose – when a satisfactory response is achieved the dose may be gradually reduced to 25 mg 3 times a day.

Elderly: 10–25 mg 3 times a day initially. The initial dose should be increased with caution under close supervision. Half the normal maintenance dose may be sufficient to produce a satisfactory clinical response.

Children: Not recommended.

If it is necessary to continue treatment beyond 3 months a full physical examination including ECG should be made.

Contra-indications, warnings, etc

Contra-indications: Recent myocardial infarction, any degree of heart block or other cardiac arrhythmias, mania, severe liver disease, during breast feeding. Safety in pregnancy has not been established although animal reproductive studies show no foetal malformations; do not use during pregnancy, especially during the first and last trimesters, unless there are compelling reasons.

Precautions: The elderly are particularly liable to experience adverse reactions, especially agitation, confusion and postural hypotension (see Dosage). Avoid if possible in patients with narrow angle glaucoma, symptoms suggestive of prostatic hypertrophy and a history of epilepsy. Patients posing a high suicidal risk require close initial supervision. Tricyclic antidepressants potentiate the central nervous depressant action of alcohol. Anaesthetics given during tri/tetracyclic antidepressant therapy may increase the risk of arrhythmias and hypotension. If surgery is necessary, the anaesthetist should be informed that a patient is being so treated.

Drug interactions: Butriptyline should not be given concurrently with, or within 2 weeks of cessation of, therapy with monoamine oxidase inhibitors.

Preliminary work with Evadyne suggests that butriptyline, unlike other tricyclic antidepressants, does not inhibit the tyramine pressor response. If confirmed, this would mean that interactions with directly acting sympathomimetic adrenergic neurone-blocking anti-hypertensive drugs such as guanethidine and bethanidine are less likely with this drug than with other tricyclic antidepressants. Meanwhile, however, it is advisable to review all hypertensive therapy from time to time during treatment.

Butriptyline should not be given with sympathomimetic agents such as adrenaline, ephedrine, isoprenaline, noradrenaline, phenylephrine and phenylpropanolamine.

Barbiturates may decrease and methyl phenidate may increase respectively the antidepressant action of butriptyline.

Warnings and side-effects: Studies have shown that butriptyline relieves anxiety within 1 or 2 weeks but improvement may not always occur during the first 2–4 weeks treatment; patients should be closely monitored during this period.

Butriptyline may initially impair alertness. Patients should be warned of the possible hazard when driving or operating machinery.

Cardiac arrhythmias and severe hypotension are likely to occur with dosage exceeding the recommended range or in deliberate overdosage. They may also occur in patients with pre-existing heart disease taking normal dosage.

The following adverse effects although not necessarily all reported with butriptyline have occurred with other tricyclic antidepressants:

Atropine-like side effects including dry mouth, disturbance of accommodation, tachycardia, constipation and hesitancy of micturition are common early in treatment, but usually lessen.

Other common adverse effects include drowsiness, sweating, postural hypotension, tremor and skin rashes. Interference with sexual functions may occur.

Psychotic manifestations, including mania and paranoid delusions, may be exacerbated during treatment with tricyclic antidepressants.

Withdrawal symptoms may occur on abrupt cessation of therapy, and include insomnia, irritability and excessive perspiration.

Adverse effects such as withdrawal symptoms, respiratory depression and agitation have been reported in neonates whose mothers had taken anti-depressants during the last trimester of pregnancy.

Serious adverse effects are rare; the following have been reported:

Depression of the bone marrow including agranulocytosis, cholestatic jaundice, hypomania, convulsions and peripheral neuropathy.

Overdosage: There is no specific antidote for overdosage with tricyclic compounds. Induced emesis and gastric lavage are recommended.

If the patient is stuporous but responds to stimuli, only close watching may be required for a few days; if comatose, supportive measures will be required. Maintain an open airway and adequate fluid intake; regulate body temperature. Anticonvulsants may be given to control convulsions. Central nervous system depression may be treated with nonconvulsant doses of CNS stimulants.

Digitalis should be considered if cardiovascular abnormalities occur. Standard measures such as oxygen and I.V. fluids may be used to manage circulatory shock.

Pharmaceutical precautions No special pharmaceutical precautions are necessary.

Legal category POM.

Package quantities
Evadyne Tablets 25 mg are packed in Securitainers of 100.

Evadyne Tablets 50 mg are packed in Securitainers of 100.

Further information Nil.

Product licence numbers
Evadyne Tablets 25 mg   0607/0019R
Evadyne Tablets 50 mg   0607/0020R

HRF AYERST*

Presentation HRF Ayerst contains leutinising hormone/follicle stimulating hormone releasing hormone

(LH/FSH-RH; gonadorelin) in a freeze-dried form. HRF Ayerst is available in 2 strengths, 100 mcg and 500 mcg with 100 mg lactose. An ampoule of sterile diluent is supplied which contains 2% benzyl alcohol and water for injection.

Uses HRF Ayerst as a single injection is indicated for evaluating the functional capacity and response of the gonadotropes of the anterior pituitary. The LH response is used in testing patients with suspected gonadotropin

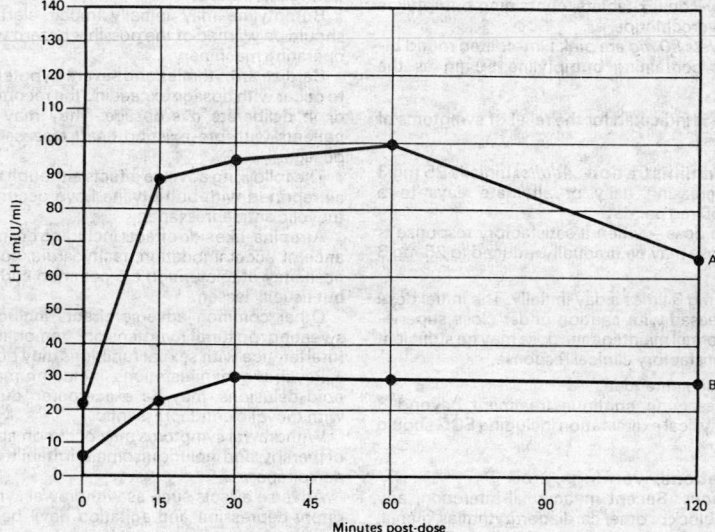

Figure 1. Normal male LH response after HRF Ayerst 100 mcg subcutaneous administration 10th and 90th percentiles.

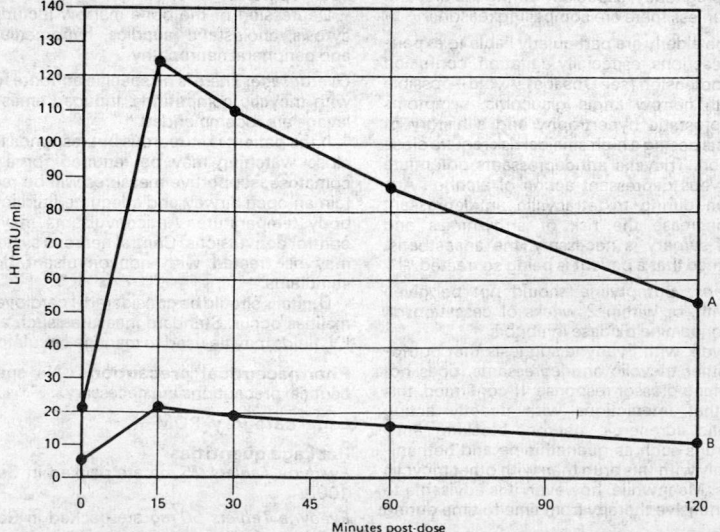

Figure 2. Normal male LH response after HRF Ayerst 100 mcg intravenous administration 10th and 90th percentiles.

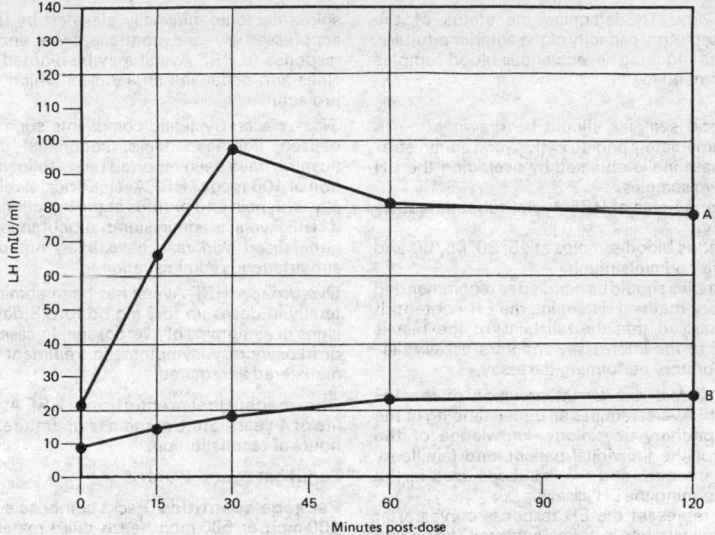

Figure 3. Normal female LH response after HRF Ayerst 100 mcg subcutaneous administration 10th and 90th percentiles.

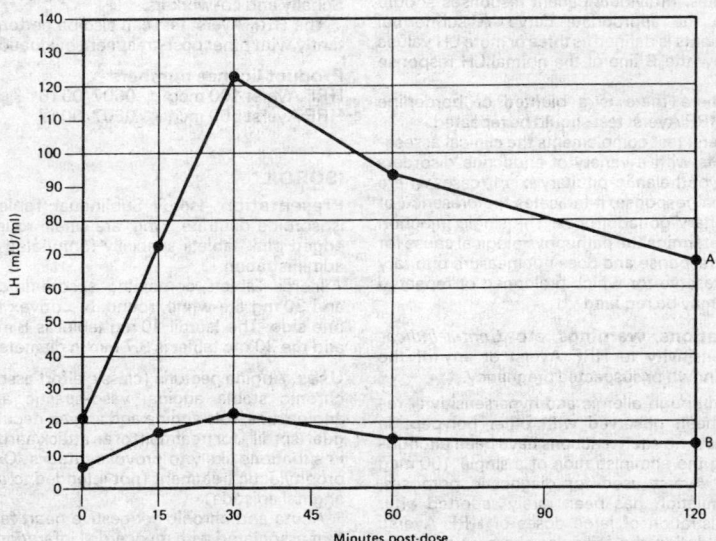

Figure 4. Normal female LH response after HRF Ayerst 100 mcg intravenous administration 10th and 90th percentiles.

deficiency, whether due to hypothalamus alone or in combination with anterior pituitary failure. HRF Ayerst is also indicated for evaluating residual gonadotropic function of the pituitary following removal of a pituitary tumour or surgery and/or irradiation.

Dosage and administration *Adults:* 100 mcg dose, subcutaneously or intravenously. In females for whom

the phase of the menstrual cycle can be established, the test should be performed in early follicular phase (days 1–7).

Refined determination of pituitary function: To determine the threshold of pituitary response, an initial dose of 25 mcg is recommended. This may be increased in steps until the pituitary threshold is determined. Doses as high as 500 mcg have been used for this purpose.

Test methodology: To determine the status of the gonadotropin secretory capacity of the anterior pituitary, a test procedure requiring seven venous blood samples for LH is recommended.

Procedure

1. Venous blood samples should be drawn at − 15 minutes and immediately prior to HRF Ayerst administration. The LH baseline is obtained by averaging the LH values of the two samples.

2. Administer a bolus of HRF Ayerst subcutaneously or intravenously.

3. Draw venous blood samples at 15, 30, 45, 60 and 120 minutes after administration.

4. Blood samples should be handled as recommended by the laboratory that will determine the LH content. It must be emphasised that the reliability of the test is directly related to the inter-assay and intra-assay reliability of the laboratory performing the assay.

Interpretation of test results: Intepretation of the LH response to HRF Ayerst requires an understanding of the hypothalamic-pituitary physiology, knowledge of the clinical status of the individual patient, and familiarity with the normal ranges and the standards used in the laboratory performing the LH assays.

Figures 1–4 represent the LH response curves after HRF Ayerst administration in normal subjects. The normal LH response curves were established between the 10th percentile (B line) and 90th percentile (A line) of all LH responses in normal subjects analysed from the results of clinical studies. Individual patient responses should be plotted on the appropriate curve. A subnormal response in patients is defined as three or more LH values which fall below the B line of the normal LH response curve.

In cases where there is a blunted or borderline response, the HRF Ayerst test should be repeated.

The HRF Ayerst test complements the clinical assessment of patients with a variety of endocrine disorders involving the hypothalamic-pituitary axis. In cases where there is a normal response, it indicates the presence of functional pituitary gonadotropes. The single injection test does not determine the pathophysiological cause for the subnormal response and does not measure pituitary gonadotropic reserve for which prolonged or repeated administration may be required.

Contra-indications, warnings, etc *Contra-indications:* Hypersensitivity to HRF Ayerst or any of the components. Known or suspected pregnancy.

Precautions: Although allergic and hypersensitivity reactions have been observed with other polypeptide hormones, to date no such reactions have been encountered following the administration of a single 100 mcg dose of HRF Ayerst used for diagnostic purposes. Antibody formulation has been rarely reported after chronic administration of large doses of HRF Ayerst. Administration during the follicular phase of a normal cycle may result in premature ovulation and appropriate measures are advised to prevent an unwanted pregnancy in these circumstances. Repetitive, high doses of HRF Ayerst may cause luteolysis and inhibition of spermatogenesis.

Drug interactions: The HRF Ayerst test should be conducted in the absence of other drugs which directly affect the pituitary secretion of the gonadotropins. These would include a variety of preparations which contain androgens, oestrogens, progestins, or glucocorticoids. The gonadotropin levels may be transiently elevated by spironolactone, minimally elevated by laevodopa, and suppressed by oral contraceptives and digoxin. The response to HRF Ayerst may be blunted by phenothiazines and dopamine antagonists which cause a rise in prolactin.

Side-effects: Systemic complaints such as headaches, nausea, lightheadedness, abdominal discomfort and flushing have been reported rarely following administration of 100 mcg of HRF Ayerst. Local swelling, occasionally with pain and pruritus at the injection site may occur if HRF Ayerst is administered subcutaneously. Local and generalised skin rash have been noted after chronic subcutaneous administration.

Overdosage: HRF Ayerst has been administered parenterally in doses up to 3 mg bd for 28 days without any signs or symptoms of overdosage. In case of overdosage or idiosyncrasy, symptomatic treatment should be administered as required.

Pharmaceutical precautions HRF Ayerst has a shelf life of 4 years. Store at room temperature. Use within 24 hours of reconstitution.

Legal category POM.

Package quantities Packs comprise a vial containing 100 mcg or 500 mcg freeze-dried material and a 2 ml ampoule of sterile diluent.

Further information HRF Ayerst is a synthetic decapeptide, identical to the LH/FSH-RH identified by Schally and co-workers.

The HRF Ayerst test can also be performed concomitantly with other post-treatment evaluations.

Product licence numbers
HRF Ayerst 100 mcg   0607/0016
HRF Ayerst 500 mcg   0607/0017

ISORDIL*

Presentation Isordil Sublingual Tablets, containing isosorbide dinitrate 5 mg, are small, round, flat, bevel-edged pink tablets specially formulated for sublingual administration.

Isordil Tablets, containing isosorbide dinitrate 10 mg and 30 mg are white, round, bi-convex tablets, scored one side. The Isordil 10 mg tablet is 8 mm in diameter and the 30 mg tablet is 9.7 mm in diameter.

Uses Angina pectoris (classic effort associated angina, chronic stable angina, vaso-spastic angina, variant angina, unstable angina and angina decubitus): Sublingual Isordil – for treatment of an attack and for prophylaxis in situations likely to provoke attacks: Oral Isordil – for prophylactic treatment (not intended to abort the acute anginal episode).

Acute and chronic congestive heart failure including that associated with myocardial infarction as adjunctive therapy.

Dosage and administration
Angina Pectoris: Acute attack or prophylactically in situations likely to provoke attacks: One or two 5 mg Isordil tablets sublingually every 2 hours or as required.

Prophylaxis: 40 to 120 g daily in divided doses or as required. In selected cases daily doses of up to 240 mg Isordil have been administered without undue adverse effects.

In order to obtain maximal therapeutic effect it is important that the dosages of sublingual and oral forms of Isordil be individualised in accordance with patients' needs, response and tolerance.

Congestive heart failure: Acute and chronic, including after myocardial infarction: Sublingual Isordil 5 to 15 mg every 2–3 hours or as needed. The oral form of Isordil may be administered in doses of 10 to 60 mg four times daily or as needed.

The therapeutic uses of Isordil in selected cases of acute and chronic congestive heart failure should be considered as an adjunct to the more conventional modes of therapy such as cardiac glycosides, diuretics and other vasodilators. In refractory cases Isordil may be used alone or concomitantly with other vasodilators. Haemodynamic monitoring of the patient under treatment is desirable and optimal dose regimens should be determined for individual cases depending on these results. Isordil therapy should begin with the lowest effective dose, based on assessment of the severity of heart failure and then adjusted as necessary. In both acute and chronic failure Isordil should be administered initially in the sublingual form to stabilise the patients' symptoms and determine the magnitude of haemodynamic response and then in the oral form for maintenance therapy.

Elderly: There are no special dosage requirements for elderly patients but as with all medicines the lowest effective dose should be used.

Children: Not recommended.

Contra-indications, warnings, etc

Contra-indications: Hypersensitivity to this drug.

Precautions:

1. Tolerance to this drug and cross tolerance to other nitrates and nitrites, may occur; withdrawal restores the original sensitivity.
2. In congestive heart failure, as a rule, pulmonary capillary pressure should not be allowed to fall below 15 mmHg or systolic blood pressure below physiological range in normal or hypertensive patients. In patients with hypotension in the range of 90–100 mmHg of systolic pressure there should be no fall at all. As with other vasodilators in sensitive patients Isordil may cause paradoxical side-effects which may increase ischaemia and may even lead to extension of myocardial damage and advanced congestive heart failure.

Use in pregnancy: The product has not been studied in human pregnancy. The use of Isordil requires that the anticipated benefit be weighed against possible hazard.

Side effects: Side effects due to Isordil are common to all nitrates used for the treatment of angina pectoris.

1. Cutaneous vasodilation with flushing.
2. Headache is common and in some patients may be severe and persistent. Analgesics have been useful in some cases.
3. Transient episodes of dizziness and weakness and other signs of cerebral ischaemia associated with postural hypotension may occur.
4. This drug can act as a physiological antagonist to noradrenaline, acetylcholine, histamine and many other agents.
5. An occasional individual exhibits a marked sensitivity to the hypotensive effects of nitrate and severe responses (nausea, vomiting, weakness, restlessness, pallor, perspiration and collapse) can occur even with the usual therapeutic dose. Alcohol may enhance this effect.

6. Drug rash and/or exfoliative dermatitis may occasionally occur.

Treatment of overdosage: The main manifestation is hypotension. In such event the drug should be withheld and the patient carefully monitored. Passive exercise and elevation of legs of the recumbent patient will promote venous return. In life threatening situations administration of vasopressors should be considered. The LD_{50} of isosorbide dinitrate in rodents is of the order of 1000 mg/kg.

Pharmaceutical precautions *Storage:* Unlike glyceryl trinitrate, Isordil Tablets are stable and no special storage conditions are necessary.

Legal category P.

Package quantities Isordil Sublingual Tablets 5 mg in Securitainers of 100.
Isordil Tablets 10 mg in Securitainers of 100.
Isordil Tablets 30 mg in Securitainers of 100.

Further information Isordil has a very high solubility compared with other nitrates and therefore acts sublingually to abort the acute attack of angina pectoris quickly. In addition, Isordil can be administered orally to give a prolonged effect. Because Isordil is physically and chemically stable it is reliable in use.

Product licence numbers
Isordil Tablets 5 mg   0607/0006
Isordil Tablets 10 mg   0607/0007
Isordil Tablets 30 mg   0607/0027

ISORDIL* TEMBIDS* CAPSULES

Presentation Isordil Tembids capsules containing isosorbide dinitrate 40 mg in a sustained release formulation are gelatin capsules with a colourless, transparent body containing white irregular pellets and opaque blue cap for oral administration.

Uses Prophylaxis of angina pectoris (classic effort associated angina, chronic stable angina, vasospastic angina, variant angina, unstable angina, nocturnal angina and angina decubitus).

Dosage and administration *Adults:* For oral administration – One capsule 2 or 3 times a day. In selected cases daily doses of up to 240 mg oral isosorbide dinitrate have been administered. Capsules should be swallowed without chewing.

Elderly: There are no special dosage requirements for elderly patients but as with all medicines the lowest effective dose should be used.

Children: Not recommended.

Contra-indications, warnings, etc

Contra-indications: Hypersensitivity to this drug.

Precaution: Tolerance to this drug, and cross-tolerance to other nitrates and nitrites may occur; withdrawal restores the original sensitivity.

Use in pregnancy: The product has not been studied in human pregnancy. The use of Isordil Tembids requires that the anticipated benefit be weighed against possible hazard.

Side effects: Side effects due to Isordil are common to all nitrates used for the treatment of angina pectoris.

1. Cutaneous vasodilation with flushing.
2. Headache is common and in some patients may be

severe and persistent. Analgesics have been useful in some cases.

3. Transient episodes of dizziness and weakness and other signs of cerebral ischaemia associated with postural hypotension may occur.

4. This drug can act as a physiological antagonist to noradrenaline, acetylcholine, histamine and many other agents.

5. An occasional individual exhibits a marked sensitivity to the hypotensive effects of nitrate and severe responses (nausea, vomiting, weakness, restlessness, pallor, perspiration and collapse) can occur even with the usual therapeutic dose. Alcohol may enhance this effect.

6. Drug rash and/or exfoliative dermatitis may occasionally occur.

Treatment of overdosage: The main manifestation is hypotension. In such event the drug should be withheld and the patient carefully monitored. Passive exercise and elevation of legs of the recumbent patient will promote venous return. In life threatening situations administration of vasopressors should be considered. The LD_{50} of isosorbide dinitrate in rodents is of the order of 1000 mg/kg.

Pharmaceutical precautions *Storage:* Unlike glyceryl trinitrate, Isordil Tembids are stable and no special storage conditions are necessary.

Legal category P.

Package quantities Securitainers of 100.

Further information Isosorbide dinitrate is released from the slow release formulation over a 6 hour period to provide up to 12 hours of sustained effect.

Product licence number 0607/0041.

LODINE* ▼

Presentation Lodine capsules containing etodolac 200 mg are hard gelatin capsules with an opaque dark grey body and light grey cap, printed with two red bands and 'Lodine 200'.

Uses Lodine (etodolac) is indicated for acute or long-term use in rheumatoid arthritis.

Dosage and administration The usual effective oral dosage of Lodine is 200 mg twice daily. However, some patients may require 600 mg daily. Patients may also respond to 400 mg or 600 mg administered as a single daily dose.

The safety of doses in excess of 600 mg per day has not been established. No occurrence of tolerance or tachyphylaxis has been reported.

Elderly: No change in initial dosage required in the elderly (*see 'Precautions'*).

Children: A paediatric dosage has not been established.

Contra-indications, warnings, etc
Contra-indications: Lodine should not be used in patients who have previously shown hypersensitivity to it. Lodine should not be used in patients with active peptic ulceration or a history of peptic ulcer disease. Due to possible cross-reactivity, Lodine should not be administered to patients who experience asthma, rhinitis or urticaria during therapy with aspirin or other non-steroidal anti-inflammatory drugs.

Pregnancy: Drugs which inhibit prostaglandin biosyn-thesis may cause dystocia and delayed parturition as evidenced by studies in pregnant animals. Safety in human pregnancy has not been established and Lodine should not be used during pregnancy. Safety of Lodine use during lactation has not been established.

Precautions: Although non-steroidal anti-inflammatory drugs do not have the same direct effect on platelets as does aspirin, all drugs which inhibit the biosynthesis of prostaglandins may interfere, to some extent, with platelet function. Patients receiving Lodine who may be adversely affected by such actions should be carefully observed.

There has been no evidence of significant changes in renal or hepatic function with the use of Lodine in man. However, impairment of renal or hepatic functions due to other causes may alter drug metabolism; patients receiving long-term therapy, especially the elderly, should be observed for potential side-effects and their drug doses adjusted as needed, or the drug discontinued.

Drug interactions: Since Lodine is extensively protein-bound, it may be necessary to modify the dosage of other highly protein-bound drugs, *e.g.* anticoagulants when these are administered concurrently.

Bilirubin tests can give a false positive result due to the presence of phenolic metabolites of Lodine in the urine.

Side-effects: Lodine is well tolerated. Most side-effects are mild and transient and have only occasionally resulted in the discontinuation of therapy. Reported side-effects include nausea, epigastric pain, diarrhoea, indigestion, heartburn, flatulence, abdominal pain, constipation, headaches, dizziness, drowsiness, tinnitus, rash and fatigue.

Overdosage: There have been no reported cases of Lodine overdosage. In the absence of experience with acute overdosage, it is reasonable to assume that the standard practices of gastric evacuation, activated charcoal administration, and general supporting therapy would apply.

Pharmaceutical precautions Store at room temperature (approximately 25°C).

Legal category POM.

Package quantities Securitainers of 60 capsules.

Further information Nil.

Product licence number 0607/0074.

MICOLETTE* MICRO-ENEMA

Presentation A disposable polyethylene tube with a 2" pliable nozzle which contains 5 ml of a clear, virtually colourless, viscous liquid, comprising 45 mg sodium lauryl sulphoacetate, 450 mg sodium citrate and 625 mg glycerol, together with potassium sorbate, citric acid, sorbitol and water.

Uses Micolette combines the action of sodium citrate, a 'peptizing' agent which liberates water present in the faeces; sorbitol which enhances this action; sodium lauryl sulphoacetate, a wetting agent, and glycerol which promotes peristalsis and evacuation of the lower bowel.

Micolette is indicated whenever an enema is necessary for chronic and acute constipation in the rectum and sigmoid colon. Also indicated for use in constipation in geriatrics, paediatrics and obstetrics.

Dosage and administration

Adults and Children Aged 3 years and Over: Lubricate the nozzle with one drop of the contents, insert full length of nozzle into the rectum and squeeze tube until total contents have been administered. Two tubes may be necessary in severe cases.

Elderly: There are no special dosage requirements for elderly patients but as with all medicines the lowest effective dose should be used.

Contra-indications, warnings, etc

Contra-indications: Inflammatory or ulcerative bowel disease. Acute gastro-intestinal conditions.

Precautions: Very occasionally, a slight cramp may occur. Prolonged use may lead to irritation of the anal canal and may interfere with the absorption of some vitamins. Excessive use of Micolette Micro-enema may cause diarrhoea and fluid loss. In such cases Micolette should be discontinued and appropriate therapy instituted.

Pharmaceutical precautions Store in a cool place.

Legal category P.

Package quantities Packs of 12.

Further information Nil.

Product licence number 0607/0042.

PHOSPHOLINE IODIDE*

Presentation Packs to provide 4 strengths of solution. Each pack contains:

1. Ecothiopate Iodide BP 1.5 mg, 3.0 mg, 6.25 mg, 12.5 mg in a sterile, freeze-dried form mixed with 40 mg potassium acetate in a vial sufficient for: 5 ml of 0.03%, or 5 ml of 0.06%, or 5 ml of 0.125%, or 5 ml of 0.25%.

2. 5 ml sterile aqueous diluent containing chlorbutanol 0.55%, mannitol 1.2%, boric acid 0.06%, exsiccated sodium phosphate 0.026%.

3. A sterile dropper.

Uses Chronic open-angle glaucoma. Chronic angle-closure glaucoma after iridectomy. Certain non-uveitic secondary types of glaucoma. Accommodative esotropia.

Dosage and administration *Early simple glaucoma:* Phospholine Iodide 0.03% instilled twice daily; before retiring, and in the morning.

Advanced simple glaucoma and glaucoma secondary to cataract surgery: These cases may respond satisfactorily to Phospholine Iodide 0.03% twice a day as above, but one of the higher strengths, 0.06%, 0.125% or 0.25%, may be needed. In this case, a brief trial with the 0.03% eyedrops will be advantageous in that the higher strengths will then be more easily tolerated. A single dose before retiring has been used, but twice daily is normal. More frequent dosage is undesirable. When a patient has been transferred from other therapy a brief trial with 0.03% may be useful.

Accommodative esotropia:

In diagnosis: One drop 0.125% once daily in both eyes on retiring, for two or three weeks. A favourable response may be noted within a few hours if the esotropia is accommodative.

In treatment: After initial period of treatment for diagnostic purposes, 0.125% every other day or 0.06% daily.

Dosage can be lowered as treatment progresses. Maximum recommended dose 0.125% once daily.

Concomitant therapy: Phospholine Iodide may be used concomitantly with adrenaline, a carbonic anhydrase inhibitor, or both.

Elderly: There are no special dosage requirements for elderly patients but as with all medicines the lowest effective dose should be used.

Children: Accommodative esotropia occurs more frequently in children and the dosage recommendations are as above.

Digital compression of the nasolacrimal ducts for a minute or two following instillation minimises drainage into the nasal chamber and hence reduces the incidence of any systemic side-effects.

Contra-indications, warnings, etc

Contra-indications: Most cases of angle-closure glaucoma. Active uveal inflammation. Hypersensitivity. Bronchial asthma.

Precautions: Gonioscopy is recommended prior to initiation of therapy. Use pilocarpine eyedrops for 2 months before high strength Phospholine Iodide in adults.

Temporarily discontinue Phospholine Iodide eyedrops if (otherwise inexplicable) persistent diarrhoea, urinary incontinence, profuse sweating, muscle weakness, cardiac irregularities, should occur.

Anticholinesterase drugs should be used with extreme caution in patients with marked vagotonia, peptic ulcer, pronounced bradycardia, hypotension, recent infarction, epilepsy, Parkinsonism, etc.

Use prior to ophthalmic surgery may increase the risk of hyphaema.

To reduce systemic effects, digital compression of the naso-lacrimal ducts for a minute following instillation is necessary.

Succinylcholine should not be used prior to general anaesthetic because of the risk of potentiation.

Use in patients with myaesthenia gravis receiving a systemic anti-cholinesterase may have additive adverse effects.

Use should be avoided in patients with a history of retinal detachment or uveitis.

The use of anticholinesterase drugs in pregnancy has not been established, nor has the absence of adverse effects on the foetus or on the respiration of the neonate.

Patients receiving Phospholine Iodide who are exposed to carbamate or organophosphate type insecticides and pesticides should be warned of the possible additive systemic effects through absorption of the pesticide through the respiratory tract or skin. Wearing masks, frequent washing and clothing changes may be advisable.

Adverse reactions: 1. Brow-ache, stinging, conjunctival reddening, and blurring due to accommodative spasm may occur when therapy is started but will disappear after 5–10 days of continuing treatment. Very few patients will be unable to tolerate the drug if reassurance is provided by the physician.

2. Lens opacities during Phospholine Iodide therapy have been reported in adults, but the cause has not been established. Lens opacities have not been reported in adults following pilocarpine therapy or when using low-strength Phospholine Iodide. Lens opacities have not been reported in children.

3. Iris cysts occur only occasionally in adults but fairly frequently in children. They usually do not interfere with

continuation of treatment and will regress on reduction of dosage, or frequency of instillation.

4. Paradoxical increase in intra-ocular pressure may follow anticholinesterase instillation. This may be alleviated by prescribing a sympathomimetic, e.g. phenylephrine.

5. Prolonged use may cause conjunctiva thickening or obstruction of the nasolacrimal canals.

6. Although the relationship, if any, of retinal detachment to the administration of Phospholine Iodide has not been established, retinal detachment has been reported in a few cases during the use of Phospholine Iodide in adult patients without a previous history of this disorder.

Overdosage: Antidotes are atropine 2 mg parenterally: pralidoxime salts 25 mg/kg intravenously: artificial respiration should be given if necessary.

Pharmaceutical precautions Phospholine Iodide has a shelf-life of 18 months in the dry form. After reconstitution the drops are stable for one month at room temperature or until the expiry date if kept in a refrigerator.

Legal category POM.

Package quantities Package for 5 ml of 0.03%. Package for 5 ml of 0.06%. Package for 5 ml of 0.125%. Package for 5 ml of 0.25%.

Further information Phospholine Iodide is a potent, long-acting miotic. It offers a great advantage over short-acting miotics in that it continues to provide a protection against rising intra-ocular pressure during the night-time hours, which may otherwise lead to permanent retinal damage and narrowing of vision. The effects of Phospholine Iodide are constant and stable, and the incidence of side-effects low once the dosage has been established.

Product licence numbers
0.03% Eye Drops   0607/5003
0.06% Eye Drops   0607/5004
0.125% Eye Drops   0607/5005
0.25% Eye Drops   0607/5006

PREMARIN* TABLETS

Presentation Premarin Tablets contain natural conjugated oestrogens.
  Premarin Tablets 0.625 mg are maroon, oval, sugar-coated tablets printed 'Ayerst'.
  Premarin Tablets 1.25 mg are yellow, oval, sugar-coated tablets printed 'Ayerst'.
  Premarin Tablets 2.5 mg are purple, oval, sugar-coated tablets printed 'Ayerst 865'.

Uses Menopausal and post-menopausal oestrogen replacement therapy for vasomotor symptoms (sweating, flushes) and allied disorders such as post-menopausal osteoporosis, atrophic vaginitis, Kraurosis vulvae, atrophic urethritis. Palliation of selected cases of breast cancer in women more than five years post menopausal. Inoperable prostatic carcinoma for palliation only.

Dosage and administration *Menopausal and post-menopausal oestrogen deficiency:* Premarin 0.625–1.25 mg daily is the usual starting dose. Cyclic administration is recommended (three weeks' on followed by one week off). For maintenance the lowest effective dose should be used. If the patient has not menstruated within the last two months or more, cyclic administration is started arbitrarily. If the patient is menstruating, cyclic administration is started on day five of bleeding.

In women with an intact uterus and in particular in women with obesity, diabetes, low parity or a familial history of endometrial carcinoma, for whom hormone replacement therapy is required, the addition of a progestogen is advisable. Long term oestrogen therapy in women should normally be accompanied by the administration of a progestogen.

Before therapy commences it is recommended that the patient is fully informed of all the relative risks and benefits, and the question of continued need of treatment should be reviewed periodically. She should have a complete physical and gynaecological examination, including customary biochemical tests and special emphasis on blood pressure, breasts, abdomen and pelvic organs, including endometrial assessment, whenever possible. Regular follow-up examinations, including endometrial assessments, where possible, are recommended every 6–12 months. Any breakthrough bleeding is an indication for endometrial evaluation.

Atrophic vaginitis, kraurosis vulvae and atrophic urethritis: Cyclically 0.625–1.25 mg daily depending on the response of the individual patient.

Post-menopausal osteoporosis: Cyclically 0.625–1.25 mg daily.

Breast cancer: In selected cases of mammary cancer oestrogens may be used for palliation in women who are at least five years post-menopausal. The suggested dose of Premarin is up to 10 mg three times a day for a period of at least three months.

Prostatic carcinoma: 1.25–2.5 mg three times daily, as palliative therapy. The effectiveness of therapy can be judged by phosphatase determinations as well as by symptomatic improvement of the patient.

Elderly: There are no special dosage requirements for elderly patients but as with all medicines the lowest effective dose should be used.

Children: Not recommended.

Contra-indications, warnings, etc
Contra-indications:
  1. Known or suspected pregnancy.
  2. Known or suspected cancer of the breast except in appropriately selected patients being treated for metastatic disease.
  3. Known or suspected oestrogen-dependent neoplasia.
  4. Undiagnosed abnormal genital bleeding.
  5. A history of, or active, thrombophlebitis, thrombosis or thromboembolic disorders (including coronary thrombosis, cerebrovascular accident etc), especially when associated with previous oestrogen use (except when used in treatment of breast or prostatic malignancy).
  6. Acute or chronic liver disease or history of liver disease where the liver function tests have failed to return to normal. Roto syndrome or Dubin-Johnson syndrome.
  7. Severe cardiac or renal disease.

Precautions:
In the male: Continuous therapy over prolonged periods of time may produce gynaecomastia, loss of libido and testicular atrophy.

In the female: There is an increased risk of endometrial carcinoma associated with oestrogen administered long-term (for more than one year); the greatest risk appears to be associated with use over five years or more. However, the addition of a progestogen to an oestrogen regimen lowers the incidence of endometrial hyperplasia and carcinoma.

Animal data appear to indicate that there is a need for caution in prescribing oestrogens for women with a strong family history of breast cancer or who have breast nodules, fibrocystic disease or abnormal mammograms.

Women who in the past received large doses of diethystilboestrol (DES) during pregnancy may be at increased risk for development of breast cancer. It is recommended that post-menopausal oestrogen replacement be used in these patients only for severe menopausal symptoms uncontrolled by other means and exposure to oestrogens be as short as possible. For women exposed to DES in utero, it is also recommended that oestrogen use be kept to a minimum.

It has been reported that there is an increase in the risk of surgically confirmed gallbladder disease in women receiving postmenopausal oestrogens.

When oestrogens are administered to patients with hypertension, supervision is necessary and blood pressure should be monitored at regular intervals. The increased risk of hypertension with oestrogen use is minimal in menopausal women. As with oral contraceptives, blood pressure returns to normal on discontinuing the drug.

Oestrogens may cause fluid retention therefore patients with epilepsy, migraine, asthma, renal or cardiac dysfunction should be carefully observed.

Diseases that are known to be subject to deterioration during pregnancy (e.g. multiple sclerosis, epilepsy, porphyria, tetancy and otosclerosis) should be carefully observed during treatment.

In a diabetic patient insulin requirement may be altered.

Consideration should be given to discontinue treatment at least four weeks prior to surgery if this entails a risk of thrombosis, or during periods of prolonged immobilisation.

If jaundice or thrombosis develops in any patient receiving oestrogen, the medication should be discontinued while the cause is investigated.

Oestrogen should be used with caution in patients with cerebral vascular or coronary artery disease.

Women of child-bearing potential should be advised to adhere to nonhormonal contraceptive methods.

Endometriosis.

In patients with diabetes, obesity, low parity or a familial history of endometrial carcinoma, for whom HRT is required, Premarin plus a progestogen should be considered in preference to unopposed oestrogen.

Since oestrogens influence the metabolism of calcium and phosphorus, they should be used with caution in patients with metabolic bone diseases that are associated with hypercalcemia or in patients with renal insufficiency.

As larger doses of oestrogen may increase thyroid binding globulin leading to increased circulating total thyroid hormone, care should be taken in providing oestrogens for patients with thyrotoxicosis.

Changed oestrogen levels may theoretically affect certain endocrine and liver function tests.

There is the possibility that oestrogen and progestogen oral contraceptives may be associated with thromboembolic disease, benign hepatic adenoma, glucose intolerance and mental depression, and that they may also occur following administration of natural oestrogens, particularly at high doses. This is questionable in the postmenopausal woman on oestrogen replacement therapy at the currently recommended low dosages. Similarly oral contraceptive use has been associated with an increased risk for non-fatal myocardial infarction in otherwise healthy women between the ages of 39 and 45 who smoke.

Because of the effects of oestrogens on epiphyseal closure they should be used judiciously in young patients in whom bone growth is not complete.

Side-effects: The following additional side-effects have been reported with oestrogen/progestogen therapy, including oral contraceptives but not necessarily with Premarin.

1. Genitourinary system – breakthrough bleeding, spotting, change in menstrual flow, dysmenorrhoea, premenstrual-like syndrome, amenorrhoea during and after treatment, increase in size of uterine fibromyomata, vaginal candidiasis, change in cervical erosion and in degree of cervical secretion, cystitis-like syndrome.

2. Breasts – tenderness, enlargement, secretion.

3. Gastrointestinal – nausea, vomiting, abdominal cramps, bloating, cholestatic jaundice.

4. Skin – chloasma or melasma which may persist when drug is discontinued, erythema multiforme, erythema nodosum, haemorrhagic eruption, loss of scalp hair, hirsuitism.

5. Eyes – steepening of corneal curvature, intolerance to contact lenses.

6. CNS – headaches, migraine, dizziness, mental depression, chorea.

7. Miscellaneous – increase or decrease in weight, reduced carbohydrate tolerance, aggravation of porphyria, oedema, changes in libido.

Acute overdosage: Numerous reports of ingestion of large doses of oestrogen-containing oral contraceptives by young children indicate that acute serious ill effects do not occur. Overdosages of oestrogen may cause nausea, and withdrawal bleeding may occur in females.

Pharmaceutical precautions No special requirements for storage are necessary.

Legal category POM.

Package quantities
Premarin 0.625 mg: Blister packs of 21 and Securitainers of 100.

Premarin 1.25 mg: Blister packs of 21 and Securitainers of 100.

Premarin 2.5 mg: Securitainers of 100.

Further information Premarin is a mixture of natural oestrogens. Amelioration of the individual's mental outlook, especially in the menopause, is generally associated with clinical improvement and is described by the patient as a gratifying sense of 'well being'.

Product licence numbers
Premarin Tablets 2.5 mg   0607/0002
Premarin Tablets 1.25 mg   0607/5001
Premarin Tablets 0.625 mg 0607/5000

PREMARIN* VAGINAL CREAM

Presentation Premarin Vaginal Cream contains 0.625 mg per gram of conjugated oestrogens in a non-liquefying base.

Uses Atrophic vaginitis and postmenopausal atrophic urethritis. Kraurosis vulvae.

Dosage and administration 1 to 2 g daily intravaginally or topically depending on the severity of the condition. A total daily dosage of 4 g should not be exceeded. Cyclic administration is recommended (three weeks on followed by one week off). For maintenance the lowest effective dose should be used. If the patient has not menstruated within the last two months or more, cyclic administration is started arbitrarily. If the patient is menstruating, cyclic administration is started on day five of bleeding. In postmenopausal surgery, therapy is suggested 10 days before and 10 days following intervention.

Before therapy commences it is recommended that the patient is fully informed of all the relative risks and benefits, and the question of continued need of treatment should be reviewed periodically. She should have a complete physical and gynaecological examination, including customary biochemical tests and special emphasis on blood pressure, breasts, abdomen and pelvic organs, including endometrial assessment, whenever possible. Regular follow-up examinations, including endometrial assessments, where possible, are recommended every 6–12 months. Any break-through bleeding is an indication for endometrial evaluation.

Elderly: There are no special dosage requirements for elderly patients, but as with all medicines, the lowest effective dose should be used.

Children: Not recommended.

Contra-indications, warnings, etc
Contra-indications:
1. Known or suspected pregnancy.
2. Known or suspected cancer of the breast except in appropriately selected patients being treated for metastatic disease.
3. Known or suspected oestrogen-dependent neoplasia.
4. Undiagnosed abnormal genital bleeding.
5. A history of, or active, thrombophlebitis, thrombosis or thromboembolic disorders (including coronary thrombosis, cerebrovascular accident etc), especially when associated with previous oestrogen use (except when used in treatment of breast malignancy).
6. Acute or chronic liver disease or history of liver disease where the liver function tests have failed to return to normal. Rotor syndrome or Dubin-Johnson syndrome.
7. Severe cardiac or renal disease.

Precautions: Due to systemic oestrogen absorption following the application of Premarin Vaginal Cream, prolonged administration might result in effects similar to those associated with prolonged use of Premarin Tablets. Therefore, the following should be considered:
There is an increased risk of endometrial carcinoma associated with oestrogen administered long-term (for more than one year); the greatest risk appears to be associated with use over five years or more. However, the addition of a progestogen to an oestrogen regimen lowers the incidence of endometrial hyperplasia and carcinoma.
Animal data appear to indicate that there is a need for caution in prescribing oestrogens for women with a strong family history of breast cancer or who have breast nodules, fibrocystic disease or abnormal mammograms.
Women in the past received large doses of diethystilboestrol (DES) during pregnancy may be at increased risk for development of breast cancer. It is recommended that post-menopausal oestrogen replacement be used in these patients only for severe menopausal symptoms uncontrolled by other means and exposure to oestrogens

be as short as possible. For women exposed to DES in utero, it is also recommended that oestrogen use be kept to a minimum.
It has been reported that there is an increase in the risk of surgically confirmed gallbladder disease in women receiving postmenopausal oestrogens.
When oestrogens are administered to patients with hypertension, supervision is necessary and blood pressure should be monitored at regular intervals. The increased risk of hypertension with oestrogen use is minimal in menopausal women. As with oral contraceptives, blood pressure returns to normal on discontinuing the drug.
Oestrogens may cause fluid retention therefore patients with epilepsy, migraine, asthma, renal or cardiac dysfunction should be carefully observed.
Diseases that are known to be subject to deterioration during pregnancy (e.g. multiple slcerosis, epilepsy, porphyria, tetancy and otosclerosis) should be carefully observed during treatment.
In a diabetic patient insulin requirement may be altered.
Consideration should be given to discontinue treatment at least four weeks prior to surgery if this entails a risk of thrombosis, or during periods of prolonged immobilisation.
If jaundice or thrombosis develops in any patient receiving oestrogen, the medication should be discontinued while the cause is investigated.
Oestrogen should be used with caution in patients with cerebral vascular or coronary artery disease.
Women of child-bearing potential should be advised to adhere to nonhormonal contraceptive methods.
Endometriosis.
Since oestrogens influence the metabolism of calcium and phosphorus, they should be used with caution in patients with metabolic bone diseases that are associated with hypercalcemia or in patients with renal insufficiency.
As larger doses of oestrogen may increase thyroid binding globulin leading to increased circulating total thyroid hormone, care should be taken in providing oestrogens for patients with thyrotoxicosis.
Changed oestrogen levels may theoretically affect certain endocrine and liver function tests.
There is the possibility that oestrogen and progestogen oral contraceptives may be associated with thromboembolic disease, benign hepatic adenoma, glucose intolerance and mental depression, and that they may also occur following administration of natural oestrogens, particularly at high doses. This is questionable in the postmenopausal woman on oestrogen replacement therapy at the currently recommended low dosages. Similarly oral contraceptive use has been associated with an increased risk for non-fatal myocardial infarction in otherwise healthy women between the ages of 39 and 45 who smoke.
Because of the effects of oestrogens on epiphyseal closure they should be used judiciously in young patients in whom bone growth is not complete.

Side-effects: The following additional side-effects have been reported with oestrogen therapy including oral contraceptives, but not necessarily with Premarin/ Premarin Vaginal Cream.
1. Genitourinary system – breakthrough bleeding, spotting, change in menstrual flow, dysmenorrhoea, premenstrual-like syndrome, amenorrhoea during and after treatment, increase in size of uterine fibromyomata,

vaginal candidiasis, change in cervical erosion and in degree of cervical secretion, cystitis-like syndrome.

2. Breasts – tenderness, enlargement, secretion.

3. Gastrointestinal – nausea, vomiting, abdominal cramps, bloating, cholestatic jaundice.

4. Skin – chloasma or melasma which may persist when drug is discontinued, erythema multiforme, erythema nodosum, haemorrhagic eruption, loss of scalp hair, hirsutism.

5. Eyes – steepening of corneal curvature, intolerance to contact lenses.

6. CNS – headaches, migraine, dizziness, mental depression, chorea.

7. Miscellaneous – Increase or decrease in weight, reduced carbohydrate tolerance, aggravation of porphyria, oedema, changes in libido.

Acute overdosage: Numerous reports of ingestion of large doses of oestrogen-containing oral contraceptives by young children indicate that acute serious ill effects do not occur. Overdosage of oestrogen may cause nausea, and withdrawal bleeding may occur in females.

Pharmaceutical precautions No special requirements for storage are necessary.

Legal category POM.

Package quantities Each pack contains 42.5 g of the non-liquefying cream with one calibrated applicator.

Further information Due to the low bulk of each application there is little likelihood of leakage.

Product licence number 0607/0005.

PREMPAK*

Presentation Prempak 0.625 consists of 21 maroon tablets containing natural conjugated oestrogens (Premarin*) 0.625 mg plus 7 white tablets containing norgestrel 0.5 mg.

Prempak 1.25 consists of 21 yellow tablets containing natural conjugated oestrogens (Premarin) 1.25 mg plus 7 white tablets containing norgestrel 0.5 mg.

Uses Menopausal and postmenopausal oestrogen replacement therapy for vasomotor symptoms (sweating, flushes) and allied disorders such as postmenopausal osteoporosis, atrophic vaginitis, Kraurosis vulvae, atrophic urethritis.

Dosage and administration
Menopausal and postmenopausal oestrogen deficiency: Premarin 0.625 mg or 1.25 mg daily, cyclically. One norgestrel tablet should be taken daily from day 15 to day 21 of Premarin therapy. This should be followed by 7 tablet free days. Therapy may be initiated with either dose depending upon severity of symptoms: for maintenance, the lowest effective dose is recommended. If the patient has not menstruated within the last two months or more, cyclic administration is commenced arbitrarily. If the patient is menstruating, cyclic administration is started on day 5 of bleeding.

In women with an intact uterus and in particular in women with obesity, diabetes, low parity or a familial history of endometrial carcinoma, for whom hormone replacement therapy is required, Prempak should be considered in preference to unopposed oestrogen therapy. Prempak provides both oestrogens and a progestogen to avoid endometrial hyperstimulation. This also provides a form of cycle regulation in women who are still menstruating but irregularly.

Before therapy commences it is recommended that the patient is fully informed of all the relative risks and benefits, and the question of continued need of treatment should be reviewed periodically. She should have a complete physical and gynaecological examination, including customary biochemical tests and special emphasis on blood pressure, breasts, abdomen and pelvic organs, including endometrial assessment, where necessary. Regular follow-up examinations, are recommended every 6–12 months. Any breakthrough bleeding is an indication for endometrial evaluation.

Elderly: There are no special dosage requirements for elderly patients, but as with all medicines, the lowest effective dose should be used.

Children: Not recommended.

Contra-indications, warnings, etc
Contra-indications:

1. Known or suspected pregnancy.

2. Known or suspected cancer of the breast except in appropriately selected patients being treated for metastatic disease.

3. Known or suspected oestrogen-dependent neoplasia.

4. Undiagnosed abnormal, genital bleeding.

5. A history of, or active, thrombophlebitis, thrombosis or thromboembolic disorders (including coronary thrombosis, cerebrovascular accident etc), especially when associated with previous oestrogen use (except when used in treatment of breast or prostatic malignancy).

6. Acute or chronic liver disease or history of liver disease where the liver function tests have failed to return to normal. Rotor syndrome or Dubin-Johnson syndrome.

7. Severe cardiac or renal disease.

Precautions: Animal data appear to indicate that there is a need for caution in prescribing oestrogens for women with a strong family history of breast cancer or who have breast nodules, fibrocystic disease or abnormal mammograms.

Women who in the past received large doses of diethystilboestrol (DES) during pregnancy may be at increased risk for development of breast cancer. It is recommended that post-menopausal oestrogen replacement be used in these patients only for severe menopausal symptoms uncontrolled by other means and exposure to oestrogens be as short as possible. For women exposed to DES in utero, it is also recommended that oestrogen use be kept to a minimum.

It has been reported that there is an increase in the risk of surgically confirmed gallbladder disease in women receiving postmenopausal oestrogens.

When oestrogens are administered to patients with hypertension, supervision is necessary and blood pressure should be monitored at regular intervals. The increased risk of hypertension with oestrogen use is minimal in menopausal women. As with oral contraceptives, blood pressure returns to normal on discontinuing the drug.

Oestrogens may cause fluid retention therefore patients with epilepsy, migraine, asthma, renal or cardiac dysfunction should be carefully observed.

Diseases that are known to be subject to deterioration during pregnancy (e.g. multiple sclerosis, epilepsy, porphyria, tetany and otosclerosis) should be carefully observed during treatment.

In a diabetic patient insulin requirement may be altered.

Consideration should be given to discontinue treatment at least four weeks prior to surgery if this entails a risk of thrombosis, or during periods of prolonged immobilisation.

If jaundice or thrombosis develops in any patient receiving oestrogen, the medication should be discontinued while the cause is investigated.

Oestrogen should be used with caution in patients with cerebral vascular or coronary artery disease.

Prempak is not an oral contraceptive, neither will it restore fertility. Women of child-bearing potential should be advised to adhere to nonhormonal contraceptive methods.

Endometriosis.

Since oestrogens influence the metabolism of calcium and phosphorus, they should be used with caution in patients with metabolic bone diseases that are associated with hypercalcemia or in patients with renal insufficiency.

As larger doses of oestrogen may increase thyroid binding globulin leading to increased circulating total thyroid hormone, care should be taken in providing oestrogens for patients with thyrotoxicosis.

Changed oestrogen levels may theoretically affect certain endocrine and liver function tests.

There is the possibility that oestrogen and progestogen oral contraceptives may be associated with thromboembolic disease, benign hepatic adenoma, glucose intolerance and mental depression, and that they may also occur following administration of natural oestrogens, particularly at high doses. This is questionable in the postmenopausal woman on oestrogen replacement therapy at the currently recommended low dosages. Similarly oral contraceptive use has been associated with an increased risk for non-fatal myocardial infarction in otherwise healthy women between the ages of 39 and 45 who smoke.

Side-effects: The following additional side-effects have been reported with oestrogen/progestogen therapy, including oral contraceptives but not necessarily with Prempak.

1. Genitourinary system – breakthrough bleeding, spotting, change in menstrual flow, dysmenorrhoea, premenstrual-like syndrome, amenorrhoea during and after treatment, increase in size of uterine fibromyomata, vaginal candidiasis, change in cervical erosion and in degree of cervical secretion, cystitis-like syndrome.

2. Breasts – tenderness, enlargement, secretion.

3. Gastrointestinal – nausea, vomiting, abdominal cramps, bloating, cholestatic jaundice.

4. Skin – chloasma or melasma which may persist when drug is discontinued, erythema multiforme, erythema nodosum, haemorrhagic eruption, loss of scalp hair, hirsutism.

5. Eyes – steepening of corneal curvature, intolerance to contact lenses.

6. CNS – headaches, migraine, dizziness, mental depression, chorea.

7. Miscellaneous – increase or decrease in weight, reduced carbohydrate tolerance, aggravation of porphyria, oedema, changes in libido.

Acute overdosage: Numerous reports of ingestion of large doses of oestrogen-containing oral contraceptives by young children indicate that acute serious ill effects do not occur. Overdosage of oestrogen may cause nausea, and withdrawal bleeding may occur in females.

Pharmaceutical precautions No special requirements for storage are necessary.

Legal category POM.

Package quantities Blister strip of 21 Premarin tablets 0.625 mg or 1.25 mg plus 7 norgestrel tablets 0.5 mg.

Further information Prempak provides oestrogen/progestogen therapy for the menopausal syndrome and associated disorders. The blister strip contains 21 tablets of Premarin. From day 15 to day 21 inclusive each bubble contains in addition one norgestrel 0.5 mg tablet. The two tablets should be taken together for these seven days. The specially designed pack avoids the use of tablets containing more than one active compound.

Product licence numbers
Prempak 0.625   0607/0029
Prempak 1.25   0607/0030

PREMPAK*-C

Presentation Prempak-C 0.625 consists of 28 maroon tablets containing natural conjugated oestrogens (Premarin) 0.625 mg plus 12 light brown tablets containing norgestrel 0.15 mg.

Prempak-C 1.25 consists of 28 yellow tablets containing natural conjugated oestrogens (Premarin) 1.25 mg plus 12 light brown tablets containing norgestrel 0.15 mg.

Uses Menopausal and postmenopausal oestrogen replacement therapy for vasomotor symptoms (sweating, flushes) and allied disorders such as postmenopausal osteoporosis, atrophic vaginitis. Kraurosis vulvae, atrophic urethritis.

Dosage and administration
Menopausal and postmenopausal oestrogen deficiency: Premarin 0.625 mg or 1.25 mg daily. One norgestrel tablet should be taken daily from day 17 to day 28 of Premarin therapy. Oestrogen administration is continued without a break in therapy. Therapy may be initiated with either dose depending upon severity of symptoms: for maintenance, the lowest effective dose is recommended. Therapy may be commenced arbitrarily although, if the patient is menstruating regularly, commencement on first day of bleeding may be preferred. In women with an intact uterus, and in particular in women with obesity, diabetes, low parity or a familial history of endometrial carcinoma, for whom hormone replacement therapy is required, Prempak-C should be considered in preference to unopposed oestrogen therapy. Prempak-C provides both oestrogens and a progestogen to avoid endometrial hyperstimulation. This also provides a form of cycle regulation in women who are still menstruating but irregularly.

Before therapy commences it is recommended that the patient is fully informed of all the relative risks and benefits, and the question of continued need of treatment should be reviewed periodically. She should have a complete physical and gynaecological examination, including customary biochemical tests and special emphasis on blood pressure, breasts, abdomen and pelvic organs, including endometrial assessment, where necessary. Regular follow-up examinations are recommended every 6-12 months. ...y breakthrough bleeding is an indication for endometrial evaluation.

Elderly: There are no special dosage requirements for elderly patients, but as with all medicines, the lowest effective dose should be used.

Children: Not recommended.

Contra-indications, warnings, etc

Contra-indications:

1. Known or suspected pregnancy.

2. Known or suspected cancer of the breast except in appropriately selected patients being treated for metastatic disease.

3. Known or suspected oestrogen-dependent neoplasia.

4. Undiagnosed abnormal genital bleeding.

5. A history of, or active, thrombophlebitis, thrombosis or thromboembolic disorders (including coronary thrombosis, cerebrovascular accident, etc.), especially when associated with previous oestrogen use (except when used in treatment of breast or prostatic malignancy).

6. Acute or chronic liver disease or history of liver disease where the liver function tests have failed to return to normal. Rotor syndrome or Dubin-Johnson syndrome.

7. Severe cardiac or renal disease.

Precautions: Animal data appear to indicate that there is a need for caution in prescribing oestrogens for women with a strong family history of breast cancer or who have breast nodules, fibrocystic disease or abnormal mammograms.

Women who in the past received large doses of diethystilboestrol (DES) during pregnancy may be at increased risk for development of breast cancer. It is recommended that post-menopausal oestrogen replacement be used in these patients only for severe menopausal symptoms uncontrolled by other means and exposure to oestrogens be as short as possible. For women exposed to DES *in utero*, it is also recommended that oestrogen be kept to a minimum.

It has been reported that there is an increase in the risk of surgically confirmed gallbladder disease in women receiving postmenopausal oestrogens.

When oestrogens are administered to patients with hypertension, supervision is necessary and blood pressure should be monitored at regular intervals. The increased risk of hypertension with oestrogen use is minimal in menopausal women. As with oral contraceptives, blood pressure returns to normal on discontinuing the drug.

Oestrogens may cause fluid retention, therefore patients with epilepsy, migraine, asthma, renal or cardiac dysfunction should be carefully observed.

Diseases that are known to be subject to deterioration during pregnancy (e.g. multiple sclerosis, epilepsy, porphyria, tetany and otosclerosis) should be carefully observed during treatment.

In a diabetic patient insulin requirement may be altered.

Consideration should be given to discontinue treatment at least four weeks prior to surgery if this entails a risk of thrombosis, or during periods of prolonged immobilisation.

If jaundice or thrombosis develops in any patients receiving oestrogen, the medication should be discontinued while the cause is investigated.

Oestrogen should be used with caution in patients with cerebral vascular or coronary artery disease.

Prempak-C is not an oral contraceptive, neither will it restore fertility. Women of child-bearing potential should be advised to adhere to non-hormonal contraceptive methods.

Endometriosis.

Since oestrogens influence the metabolism of calcium and phosphorus, they should be used with caution in patients with metabolic bone diseases that are associated with hypercalcaemia or in patients with renal insufficiency.

As larger doses of oestrogen may increase thyroid binding globulin leading to increased circulating total thyroid hormone, care should be taken in providing oestrogens for patients with thyrotoxicosis.

Changed oestrogen levels may theoretically affect certain endocrine and liver function tests.

There is the possibility that oestrogen and progestogen oral contraceptives may be associated with thromboembolic disease, benign hepatic adenoma, glucose intolerance and mental depression, and that they may also occur following administration of natural oestrogens, particularly at high doses. This is questionable in the postmenopausal woman on oestrogen replacement therapy at the currently recommended low dosages. Similarly oral contraceptive use has been associated with an increased risk for non-fatal myocardial infarction in otherwise healthy women between the ages of 39 and 45 who smoke.

Side-effects: The following additional side-effects have been reported with oestrogen/progestogen therapy, including oral contraceptives but not necessarily with Prempak-C.

1. Genitourinary system – breakthrough bleeding, spotting, change in menstrual flow, dysmenorrhoea, premenstrual-like syndrome, amenorrhoea during and after treatment, increase in size of uterine fibromyomata, vaginal canadiasis, change in cervical erosion and in degree of cervical secretion, cystitis-like syndrome.

2. Breasts – Tenderness, enlargement, secretion.

3. Gastrointestinal – nausea, vomiting, abdominal cramps, bloating, cholestatic jaundice.

4. Skin – chloasma or melasma which may persist when drug is discontinued, erythema multiforme, erythema nodosum, haemorrhagic eruption, loss of scalp hair, hirsutism.

5. Eyes – steepening of corneal curvature, intolerance to contact lenses.

6. CNS – headaches, migraine, dizziness, mental depression, chorea.

7. Miscellaneous – increase or decrease in weight, reduced carbohydrate tolerance, aggravation of porphyria, oedema, changes in libido.

Acute overdosage: Numerous reports of ingestion of large doses of oestrogen-containing oral contraceptives by young children indicate that acute serious ill effects do not occur. Overdosage of oestrogen may cause nausea, and withdrawal bleeding may occur in females.

Pharmaceutical precautions No special requirements for storage are necessary.

Legal category POM.

Package quantities Blister strip of 28 Premarin tablets 0.625 mg or 1.25 mg plus 12 norgestrel tablets 0.15 mg. There is also a triple pack of each strength containing 3 strips as above.

Further information Prempak-C provides oestrogen/ progestogen therapy for the menopausal syndrome and associated disorders. The blister strip contains 28 tablets of Premarin. From day 17 to day 28 inclusive each bubble contains in addition one norgestrel 0.15 mg tablet. The two tablets should be taken together for these twelve days. The specially designed pack avoids the use of tablets containing more than one active compound.

Product licence numbers
Prempak-C 0.625   0607/0053
Prempak-C 1.25   0607/0054

Trade Mark

Bayer UK Limited
Pharmaceutical Division
Bayer House
Strawberry Hill
Newbury, Berkshire, RG13 1JA

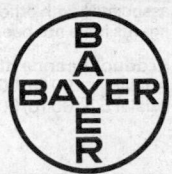

ADALAT*
ADALAT 5

Presentation *Adalat/Adalat 5:* Orange, soft gelatin capsules containing a yellow, viscous liquid. Adalat Capsules are over-printed with 'ADALAT' and contain 10 mg nifedipine. Adalat 5 Capsules are over-printed with 'ADALAT 5' and contain 5 mg nifedipine.

Uses
Mode of action: As a specific and potent calcium antagonist, Adalat's main action is to relax arterial smooth muscle both in the coronary and peripheral circulation.

In angina pectoris, Adalat capsules relax peripheral arteries so reducing the load of the left ventricle. Additionally Adalat dilates submaximally both clear and atherosclerotic coronary arteries, thus protecting the heart against coronary artery spasm and improving perfusion to the ischaemic myocardium.

Adalat capsules reduce the frequency of painful attacks and the ischaemic ECG changes irrespective of the relative contribution from coronary artery spasm or atherosclerosis.

Adalat causes a reduction in blood pressure such that the percentage lowering of blood pressure is directly related to its initial height. In normotensive individuals Adalat has little or no effect on blood pressure.

Indications: For the treatment and prophylaxis of angina pectoris, and the treatment of Raynaud's phenomenon and all grades of hypertension.

Dosage and administration For oral administration, the capsules should be taken with a little fluid during or after meals. The recommended dose is one 10 mg capsule three times daily. If necessary, up to two capsules three times daily may be taken.

If an immediate effect is required, the capsule should be bitten open and the liquid contents allowed to remain in the mouth.

Adalat 5 capsules permit titration of initial dosage in the elderly and those patients on concomitant medication. The recommended dose is one Adalat 5 capsule three times daily.

For the treatment of Raynaud's phenomenon the recommended dose is one 10 mg capsule three times a day with subsequent titration of dose according to response, to a maximum of two 10 mg capsules three times a day.

Treatment may be continued indefinitely.

Contra-indications, warnings, etc
Contra-indications: Must not be given to women capable of child-bearing.

Warnings and precautions: Adalat is not a beta-blocker and therefore gives no protection against the dangers of abrupt beta-blocker withdrawal; any such withdrawal should be by gradual reduction of the dose of beta-blocker, preferably over 8–10 days.

Adalat may be used in combination with beta-blocking drugs and other antihypertensive agents, but the possibility of an additive effect resulting in postural hypotension should be borne in mind. Adalat will not prevent possible rebound effects after cessation of antihypertensive therapy.

Adalat should be used with caution in patients whose cardiac reserve is poor.

Ischaemic pain has been reported in a small proportion of patients within 30 minutes of the introduction of Adalat therapy. Patients experiencing this effect should discontinue Adalat.

Rare cases of hypersensitivity-type jaundice have been reported.

The use of Adalat in diabetic patients may require adjustment of their control.

The antihypertensive effect of Adalat can be potentiated by simultaneous administration with cimetidine. When used in combination with nifedipine, serum quinidine levels have been shown to be suppressed regardless of dosage of quinidine.

Side-effects: Adalat is well tolerated. Minor side-effects, usually associated with vasodilatation are mainly headache, flushing and lethargy. Gravitational oedema associated with increased capillary filtration capacity has been reported. These effects are transient and invariably disappear with continued treatment.

Overdosage: Standard measures such as atropine and noradrenaline may be used for resultant bradycardia and hypotension. Intravenous calcium gluconate may be of benefit combined with metaraminol.

Pharmaceutical precautions The capsules should be protected from strong light and stored in the manufacturer's original container.

Legal category POM.

Package quantities Adalat and Adalat 5 capsules are available in foil strips of 10 in packs of 100. Hospital packs containing 500 Adalat 10 mg capsules are available.

Further information Adalat has no therapeutic antiarrhythmic effect. Since Adalat does not cause a rise in intraocular pressure, it can be used in patients with glaucoma.

In long-term treatment, none of these formulations have been shown to cause serious adverse reactions.

Metabolic disturbance, failure of ejaculation, increased incidence of Raynaud's phenomenon and bronchospasm associated with other anti-anginal and anti-hypertensive agents have not been observed.

Product licence numbers
Adalat   0010/0021
Adalat 5   0010/0079

ADALAT* RETARD

Presentation Pink-grey lacquered tablets each containing 20 mg nifedipine, on one side marked 1U, and the reverse side with the Bayer Cross.

Uses
Mode of action: Nifedipine is a specific and potent calcium antagonist. In hypertension Adalat Retard's main action is to cause peripheral vasodilatation and thus reduce peripheral resistance.

Adalat Retard twice daily provides 24 hour control of raised blood pressure. Adalat Retard causes reduction in blood pressure such that the percentage lowering of blood pressure is directly related to its initial height. In normotensive individuals Adalat Retard has little or no effect on blood pressure.

Indications: For the treatment of all grades of hypertension and the prophylaxis of angina pectoris.

Dosage and administration The recommended dose of Adalat Retard is one 20 mg tablet twice daily swallowed after food with a little fluid. If necessary the dose may be increased to 40 mg twice daily.

Treatment may be continued indefinitely.

Contra-indications, warnings, etc
Contra-indications: Must not be given to women capable of child-bearing.

Warnings and precautions: Adalat Retard is not a beta-blocker and therefore gives no protection against the dangers of abrupt beta-blocker withdrawal; any such withdrawal should be by gradual reduction of the dose of beta-blocker, preferably over 8–10 days.

Adalat Retard may be used in combination with beta-blocking drugs and other antihypertensive agents, but the possibility of an additive effect resulting in postural hypotension should be borne in mind. Adalat Retard will not prevent possible rebound effects after cessation of antihypertensive therapy.

Adalat Retard should be used with caution in patients whose cardiac reserve is poor.

Ischaemic pain has been reported in a small proportion of patients within 30 minutes of the introduction of Adalat Retard therapy. Patients experiencing this effect should discontinue Adalat Retard.

Rare cases of hypersensitivity-type jaundice have been reported.

The use of Adalat Retard in diabetic patients may require adjustment of their control.

The antihypertensive effect of Adalat Retard can be potentiated by simultaneous administration with cimetidine. When used in combination with nifedipine, serum quinidine levels have been shown to be suppressed regardless of dosage of quinidine.

Side-effects: Adalat Retard is well tolerated. Minor side effects, usually associated with vasodilatation are mainly headache, flushing, and lethargy. Gravitational oedema associated with increased capillary filtration capacity has been reported. These effects are transient and invariably disappear with continued treatment.

Overdosage: Standard measures such as atropine and noradrenaline may be used for resultant bradycardia and hypotension. Intravenous calcium gluconate may be of benefit combined with metaraminol.

Pharmaceutical precautions The tablets should be protected from strong light and stored in the manufacturer's original container.

Legal category POM.

Package quantities Adalat Retard tablets are available in foil strips of 10 in packs of 100.

Further information Adalat Retard has no therapeutic antiarrhythmic effect. Since Adalat Retard does not cause a rise in intraocular pressure, it can be used in patients with glaucoma.

In long-term treatment, Adalat Retard has not been shown to cause serious adverse reactions. Metabolic disturbance, failure of ejaculation, increased incidence of Raynaud's phenomenon and bronchospasm associated with other anti-anginal and anti-hypertensive agents have not been observed.

Product licence number 0010/0078

ALRHEUMAT*

Presentation Opaque 'off-white' hard gelatin capsules each containing 50 mg ketoprofen.

Uses Alrheumat is recommended for the management of the rheumatic diseases: rheumatoid arthritis, osteoarthrosis, ankylosing spondylitis, sero-negative (non-rheumatoid) arthropathies, non-articular rheumatism and soft tissue rheumatism.

Dosage and administration Alrheumat capsules are administered orally and should be taken with food. Dosage is usually 1 capsule (50 mg) three times daily. This dosage may be increased to 1 capsule four times daily or decreased to 1 capsule twice daily depending on the weight and clinical condition of the patient and the severity of the disease. Paediatric usage has not been established.

Contra-indications, warnings, etc
Contra-indications: Ketoprofen should not be given to patients known to be sensitive to aspirin or to other non-steroidal anti-inflammatory agents which are prostaglandin inhibitors. In such patients, and in those with a history of bronchial asthma or allergic disease, severe broncho-spasm may be precipitated.

Ketoprofen should not be given to patients with active peptic ulceration.

Side-effects: Occasional gastro-intestinal disturbances occur and in some such cases a reduction in dosage has been helpful. In common with most other anti-inflammatory agents, there have been very rare reports of gastro-intestinal haemorrhage. Skin rashes have been rare.

Precautions: Patients with a history of peptic ulcer or chronic dyspepsia should be carefully monitored. Care should also be taken in patients with a history of impaired hepatic function. Alrheumat, in common with other propionic acid derivatives, exhibits moderate plasma protein binding. Patients receiving anticoagulants, hydantoins and protein-bound sulphonamides must therefore be closely monitored. The required dose of these drugs may well be beneficially reduced if taken concurrently with Alrheumat.

No embryotoxic or teratogenic effects have been reported, but, on principle, caution should be exercised when prescribing any new medication during pregnancy and lactation.

Pharmaceutical precautions Nil.

Legal category POM.

Package quantities Alrheumat capsules are available in blister strips of 10 packed in boxes of 100 and 500 capsules.

Further information Nil.

Product licence number
Capsules 0010/0025R

BAYCARON*

Presentation A white scored tablet 7 mm × 2 mm, one side scored L/1, the reverse side with the Bayer cross, containing 25 mg mefruside.

Uses Baycaron is a diuretic agent and is intended for the treatment of hypertension and oedema.

Dosage and administration Baycaron is best taken with a little fluid after meals.
Hypertension: 25 mg to 50 mg initially for 10 to 14 days, then maintenance dose of 25 mg each morning. Alternate day dosage may also be used.
Oedema: 25 mg to 50 mg every morning increasing if necessary to 75 mg to 100 mg to obtain the desired response. For long-term therapy intermittent dosage is preferable e.g. 25 mg to 50 mg every second or third day.
Daily doses in excess of 100 mg do not usually increase diuresis further.
Paediatric dosage has not yet been established.

Contra-indications, warnings, etc
Contra-indications: Severe renal failure, hepatic coma, Addisons disease, severe hypercalcaemia.
Side-effects: Baycaron is very well tolerated. Occasionally, with daily doses of up to 100 mg, dyspepsia and nausea are encountered initially, but usually subside on continued treatment. There are no reports of postural hypotension nor of any impairment of micturition or bowel habit. Due to its profile of diuretic action Baycaron does not precipitate acute retention of urine in for example, cases of prostatic hypertrophy. Impotence is rarely associated with mefruside.
Overdosage; There is no special antidote and general supportive measures should be offered together with monitoring of blood pressure, fluid and electrolyte balance, correcting when necessary.
Warnings and Precautions: It is often necessary to give extra potassium during treatment with diuretics and potassium supplements may be necessary during long-term treatment with Baycaron, especially in patients with impaired liver function or in those also receiving cardiac glycosides. Although there is no short-term alteration of carbohydrate metabolism in normal subjects on a 50 mg daily dose, the glucose tolerance curve may be prolonged in some diabetics. After Baycaron administration serum uric acid may be raised, and therefore it should be used with caution in potential cases of gout.

Baycaron is not suitable for the treatment of acute conditions of fluid excess such as pulmonary and cerebral oedema and glaucoma. Baycaron has not been shown to produce teratogenic effects, either after administration to animals, or when used to treat toxaemia of pregnancy. However, the benefits should be carefully weighed against possible risks in the first trimester of pregnancy.

Diuretics are best avoided for the management of oedema of pregnancy or hypertension in pregnancy as their use may be associated with hypovolaemia, increased blood viscosity and reduced placental perfusion.

There is inadequate evidence of safety in human pregnancy and some workers have described foetal bone marrow depression and thrombocytopaenia. Foetal and neonatal jaundice have also been described.

Patients with known sulphonamide sensitivity may show allergic reactions to Baycaron.

Particular care is necessary in the elderly because of their susceptibility to electrolyte imbalance.

Mefruside should not be administered concurrently with lithium carbonate. Care should be exercised when prescribed with non steroidal anti-inflammatory drugs. It is always advisable to monitor renal function. Thiazide and thiazide-like diuretics have been implicated in blood dyscrasias and pancreatitis.
Lactation warning: As diuretics pass into breast milk they should be avoided in mothers who wish to breast feed.

Pharmaceutical precautions There are no special precautions or requirements regarding the storage of Baycaron.

Legal category POM.

Package quantities Bottles of 150 tablets.

Further information
Hypertension: Baycaron, with its powerful natriuretic effect is particularly suited to the treatment of hypertension, especially in the long term. Baycaron may be administered alone or in combination with other antihypertensive agents.

Oedema: By virtue of its prolonged and smooth natriuretic action, Baycaron is eminently suitable for the long-term treatment of oedematous conditions; for example oedema of cardiac, hepatic, or renal origin, and premenstrual tension. Its profile of action leads to minimum patient inconvenience. Diuresis begins two to four hours following oral administration and is maximal between six and twelve hours after administration.

Product licence number 0010/5903R.

BAYOLIN*

Presentation A white cream. Each 100 g cream contains heparinoid 'Bayer' 5,000 HDBu., glycol salicylate 10 g, benzyl nicotinate 2.5 g.

Uses Bayolin is a rubefacient used to treat all forms of muscular rheumatism, muscular stiffness due to exertion, lumbago, lumbar and cervical syndrome, local therapy of pains in muscles and joints due to rheumatic polyarthritis, arthroses and spondylosis deformans.

Dosage and administration Topical application two or three times daily, the cream being massaged gently into the affected area until absorbed.

Contra-indications, warnings, etc *Side-effects:* Occasionally a skin reaction to the nicotinic acid component of Bayolin may be seen.

Precautions: Bayolin is very well tolerated, but like any other rubefacient it can be very painful if it is allowed to get into the eyes, or come into contact with mucous membranes. It is advisable for the hands to be washed after application.

Pharmaceutical precautions There are no special requirements for storage or other precautions to be taken.

Legal category P.

Package quantities Bayolin Cream is available in 35 g tubes.

Further information Nil.

Product licence number 0010/5907.

BAYPEN*

Presentation Vials containing 0.5 g, 1 g, 2 g mezlocillin as mezlocillin sodium monohydrate. Infusion vials containing 5 g mezlocillin as mezlocillin sodium monohydrate. Baypen infusion sets containing 3 × 5 g mezlocillin, 3 × 50 ml Water for Injections and 3 transfer needles.

Uses Mezlocillin is a broad spectrum antibiotic indicated for the treatment of infections caused by sensitive organisms and prophylaxis of post-operative sepsis following abdominal surgery, including biliary, and vaginal hysterectomy.

The following Gram-positive and Gram-negative pathogens are sensitive to mezlocillin: *Escherichia coli*, species of the *Klebsiella-Enterobacter-Serratia* group, *Proteus* spp. (indole-positive and indole-negative), *Providencia* spp., *Citrobacter* spp., *Pseudomonas aeruginosa*, *Salmonella* spp. and *Shigella* spp., enterococci, staphylococci (penicillin sensitive), *Corynebacteria* and *Clostridium* spp. as well as *Bacteroidaceae*, in particular *Bacteroides fragilis*. *Haemophilus influenzae*, gonococci, meningococci, pneumococci and streptococci are particularly sensitive.

Mezlocillin is, therefore, indicated for the treatment of the following systemic and/or local infections in which the above-named organisms have been detected or are suspected: Septicaemia, infections of the urogenital tract (including gonorrhoea), respiratory and biliary tracts, meningitis, bone and soft tissue infections, peritonitis, infected wounds and burns, proven or suspected infections in patients with impaired or suppressed immunological status.

Mezlocillin is usually effective alone, but when appropriate may be used in combination with aminoglycoside antibiotics, and third generation cephalosporins or with beta-lactamase stable isoxazolyl penicillins since there is evidence of synergy in vitro.

An aminoglycoside should not be mixed in the same syringe or intravenous fluid container as mezlocillin.

Dosage and administration Mezlocillin is normally given by the intravenous route but may be given intramuscularly if required.

Intravenous administration: Mezlocillin is prepared for injection by shaking the powder with a suitable volume of Water for Injections for 30–60 seconds until completely dissolved to make a 10% solution, i.e. 0.5 g in

5 ml, 1 g in 10 ml, 2 g in 20 ml and 5 g in 50 ml. A 10% aqueous solution is isotonic.

It is recommended that the 5 g strength is given by infusion over 15–20 minutes; all other strengths by bolus injection over two to four minutes depending on the volume.

Intramuscular administration: Mezlocillin may be administered by the IM route if required as an alternative to the IV route (e.g. patients with poor veins). A single dose should not exceed 2 g, each 1 g of powder requiring 3.5 ml of water for injection to achieve complete solution.

Adults:

1. *Patients with normal renal function:* Life-threatening infections and infections due to unidentified organisms or Pseudomonas strains should be treated with 5 g, IV, six to eight hourly, by infusion over 15–20 minutes.

Non life-threatening infections due to sensitive organisms, and biliary and urinary tract infections, should be treated with 2 g, IV, six to eight hourly, as a bolus injection over two to four minutes.

If required, an intramuscular injection of 0.5–2 g may be given by deep injection into the buttocks in these cases.

For the treatment of acute gonorrhoea the dose is a single IM injection of 1 g.

Prophylactic dosage: In prolonged surgery and some colorectal procedures it may be beneficial to use 5.0 g IV pre-operatively as a single dose; or 2.0 g IV to be given pre-operatively followed by two injections of 2.0 g post-operatively at eight hourly intervals.

2. *Patients with renal insufficiency:* These patients should receive the appropriate doses outlined above but at intervals of only 12 hours. Monitoring of the serum levels is recommended to ensure that adequate and constant levels are maintained.

Children: In the dosage schedule below the individual dose for premature babies and neonates is based on 75 mg/kg twice daily as a prolonged IV infusion and for infants and older children 3 × 75 mg/kg as bolus injection or short infusion (IV).

Children over six years old, over 20 kg body weight: 1.5 g eight-hourly.

Children two to six years old, 13–20 kg body weight: 1–1.5 g eight-hourly.

Children one to two years old, 10–13 kg body weight: 0.75–1 g eight-hourly.

Infants over three months, 5–10 kg body weight: 0.4–0.75 g eight-hourly.

Infants up to three months, 3–5 kg body weight: 0.2–0.4 g eight-hourly.

Infants and premature babies, below 3 kg body weight: 75 mg/kg body weight 12 hourly corresponding to 0.2 g 12 hourly.

Duration of treatment: The duration of treatment depends upon the severity of the case and also the clinical response and bacteriological findings. In principle, treatment should be carried out for at least three days after disappearance of clinical symptoms. Duration of treatment is usually 7–10 days.

Contra-indications, warnings, etc
Contra-indications: Penicillin hypersensitivity.

As with all new drugs mezlocillin should not be used during the first three months of pregnancy.

Side effects: As for other penicillins.

Pharmaceutical precautions Mezlocillin should not be stored in temperatures exceeding 25°C.

Mezlocillin should be freshly prepared prior to administration, any unused solution being discarded.

Mezlocillin should be administered separately unless compatibility is proven.

Mezlocillin is compatible with dextrose 5% and 10%, laevulose 5%, Ringer's Solution and physiological saline during the period of administration.

Legal category POM.

Package quantities Vials containing 0.5 g, 1 g, 2 g in boxes of 5 vials.
Vials of 5 g: single vials.
Infusion Packs of 3 × 5 g with diluent and transfer needles.

Further information
Sodium content:

Each 5.0 g vial contains	9.27 mEq sodium (213.1 mg)
Each 2.0 g vial contains	3.71 mEq sodium (85.2 mg)
Each 1.0 g vial contains	1.85 mEq sodium (42.6 mg)
Each 0.5 g vial contains	0.93 mEq sodium (21.3 mg)
Displacement value	0.74 ml/g

Product licence number
Baypen 0010/0070
Water for injections BP 0010/0095

CANESTEN*

Presentation

1. *Cream:* A white cream containing 1.0% clotrimazole.

2. *Atomiser Spray:* A clear solution containing 1.0% clotrimazole in 30% isopropanol. The spray is produced by an atomiser and contains no propellent.

3. *Solution:* A clear solution containing 1.0% clotrimazole in polyethylene glycol 400.

4. *Powder:* A white powder containing 1.0% clotrimazole.

5. *Vaginal Tablets:* White convex tablets, measuring 25mm × 6.5mm × 10mm, 100 mg tablet marked 'BAYER' on one side and 'AD' on the other.
200 mg tablet marked 'BAYER' on one side and 'F9' on the other.

500 mg tablet (Canesten 1) marked 'Bayer' on one side and 'MU' on the other.

6. *Vaginal Cream:* A white cream containing 2.0% clotrimazole.

7. *Duopak:* A combination pack comprising 6 Canesten vaginal tablets (each containing 100 mg clotrimazole) plus a 20 g tube of Canesten cream (containing 1.0% clotrimazole).

Indications Clotrimazole is a broad spectrum antifungal. It also exhibits activity against Trichomonas, Staphylococci, Streptococci and Bacteroides. It has no effect on Lactobacilli:

1. *Cream:* All fungal skin infections due to dermatophytes (e.g. Trichophyton species), yeasts (e.g. Candida species), moulds and other fungi. These include ringworm (tinea) infections, athlete's foot, paronychia, pityriasis versicolor, erythrasma, intertrigo, fungal nappy rash, candida vulvitis and candida balanitis.

2. *Atomiser Spray:* As Canesten cream, recommended for infections covering large and/or hairy areas.

3. *Solution:* The solution is particularly suitable for use on hairy skin and in fungal infections of the outer ear (otitis externa).

4. *Powder:* As an adjunct to treatment with cream or atomiser spray and as a prophylactic against re-infection, particularly in infections such as athlete's foot. The powder should be applied to the lesions simultaneously and dusted inside articles of clothing in contact with infected areas.

5. *Vaginal Tablets:* Candida vaginitis and mixed vaginal infections where Trichomonas is present or suspected. Canesten is not recommended as sole treatment for pure trichomoniasis, except in cases where systemic therapy is contra-indicated.

6. *Vaginal Cream:* As for (5) above.

7. *Duopak:* Vaginal tablets for candida vaginitis; cream for associated vulvitis and to treat the sexual partner to prevent re-infection.

Dosage and administration

1. *Cream:* Canesten cream should be thinly and evenly applied to the affected area two to three times daily, and rubbed in gently.

Treatment should be continued for at least one month, or for at least two weeks after the disappearance of all signs of infection (to prevent relapse).

If the feet are infected, they should be thoroughly washed and dried, especially between the toes, before applying the cream.

2. *Atomiser Spray:* As per Canesten cream.

3. *Solution:* As per Canesten cream.

4. *Powder:* Sprinkle on to the affected areas two to three times daily after using the cream or atomiser spray. The powder may also be dusted inside articles of clothing and footwear which are in contact with the infected area.

5. *Vaginal Tablets 100 mg:* Two vaginal tablets should be inserted daily, preferably at night, for three consecutive days. Alternatively, 1 vaginal tablet daily for six days may be given.

Vaginal Tablets 200 mg: One vaginal tablet should be inserted daily, preferably at night for three consecutive days.

Vaginal tablet 500 mg: (Canesten 1). The single tablet should be inserted at night.

Using the applicator provided, each vaginal tablet should be inserted as deeply as is comfortable into the vagina. This is best achieved when lying back with the legs bent up.

6. *Vaginal Cream:* insert one filled applicator (5 g) intravaginally twice daily for three consecutive days or once daily for six consecutive days preferably at night.

7. *Duopak:* 100 mg vaginal tablets as in 5, above. The cream should be applied night and morning to the vulva and surrounding area and/or to the sexual partner's penis to prevent re-infection.

Contra-indications, warnings, etc
Contra-indications: None known.

Side-effects: Rarely patients may experience local mild burning or irritation immediately after applying cream or atomiser spray or after inserting the vaginal tablet. Very rarely, the patient may find this irritation intolerable and stop treatment.

Precautions: Canesten atomiser spray should not be used near a naked flame, should not be allowed to come into contact with the eyes, ears or mucous membranes and should not be inhaled.

Pharmaceutical precautions *Storage.*

Cream – none.
Atomiser Spray – none.
Solution – none.
Powder – none.
Vaginal Tablets – none.
Vaginal Cream – none.
Duopak – none.

Legal category

Cream   P.
Atomiser Spray   P.
Solution P.
Powder   P.
Vaginal Tablets   POM.
Vaginal Cream   POM.
Duopak   POM.

Package quantities

1. *Cream:* Each tube contains 20 g or 50 g.
2. *Atomiser Spray:* Each bottle contains 40 ml.
3. *Solution:* Each dropper bottle contains 20 ml.
4. *Powder:* Each pack contains 30 g.
5. *Vaginal Tablets:* 6 × 100 mg vaginal tablets packed in a blister strip. 3 × 200 mg vaginal tablets packed in a blister strip. 1 × 500 mg vaginal tablet packed in foil.
An applicator and patient instructions are included.
6. *Vaginal Cream:* Each tube contains 35 g and is supplied with 6 disposable applicators and a patient instruction leaflet.
7. *Duopak:* Each box contains 6 × 100 mg vaginal tablets packed in a blister strip plus a 20 g tube of cream. An applicator for the vaginal tablets and patient instructions are included.

Further information Nil.

Product licence numbers

Cream   0010/0016
Atomiser Spray   0010/0060
Solution   0010/0082
Powder   0010/0067
Vaginal Tablets 100 mg   0010/0015
Vaginal Tablets 200 mg   0010/0072
Vaginal Tablet 500 mg   0010/0083
Vaginal Cream   0010/0077
Duopak   0010/0016 & 0010/0015

CANESTEN*-HC

Presentation A white cream containing 1.0% clotrimazole and 1.0% hydrocortisone.

Uses The treatment of skin infections due to dermatophytes, yeasts, moulds and other fungi, where co-existing symptoms of inflammation e.g. itching, require rapid relief.

Dosage and administration Canesten-HC should be thinly and evenly applied to the affected area twice daily and rubbed in gently.

Contra-indications, warnings, etc

Contra-indications: Hypersensitivity to any of the ingredients.

Side-effects: Rarely patients may experience local mild irritation or burning immediately after applying cream.

Precautions: Long term continuous therapy to extensive areas of the skin and application under occlusive dressing should be avoided, particularly in infants and children. Topical administration of corticosteroids to pregnant animals can cause abnormalities of foetal development. The relevance of this to humans has not been established, but topical steroids should not be used extensively in pregnancy, i.e. in large amounts or for prolonged periods.

Pharmaceutical precautions Store in a cool place.

Legal category POM.

Package quantities 30 g.

Further information Nil.

Product licence number 0010/0120.

DTIC-DOME*

Presentation *Active ingredients:* 5-(3,3-dimethyl-1-triazeno) imidazole-4-carboxamide prepared as the citrate salt (dacarbazine).
100 mg and 200 mg vials of sterile dacarbazine.
DTIC-Dome is a colourless to ivory-coloured solid to be reconstituted with Water for Injections BP.

Uses *Actions:* Although the exact mechanism of action of dacarbazine is unknown, three hypotheses have been offered:
1. Inhibition of DNA synthesis by acting as a purine analogue.
2. Action as an alkylating agent.
3. Interaction with SH groups.

The volume of distribution of DTIC-Dome exceeds body water content, suggesting localisation in some body tissues. DTIC is only slightly (approximately 5%) protein bound. Its plasma half life after I.V. administration is approximately 35 minutes. After 6 hours in animal study, approximately 46% of radiolabelled dose was recovered from the urine. Of this 46% almost half was unchanged DTIC and a like quantity was amino-imidazole carboxamide, a metabolite. DTIC is subject to renal tubular secretion rather than glomerular filtration.

Indications: Metastatic Malignant Melanoma.
Sarcoma.
Hodgkin's Disease.
In addition, DTIC-Dome has been shown when used in combination with other cytotoxic agents, to be of value in treatment of other malignant diseases including:
Carcinoma of colon, ovary, breast, lung.
Testicular teratoma.
Solid tumours in children.

Dosage and administration *Standard dose:* The following dosage schedules are recommended:
1. 2.0–4.5 mg/kg/day for 10 days, which may be repeated at 4 week intervals.
2. 250 mg/m²/day for 5 days, which may be repeated at 3 week intervals.
3. A further alternative is to administer the total schedule dose on the first day.

Other schedules may be used at the discretion of the prescribing physician.

Children: The dosage for children is calculated on a mg/kg or mg/m² basis as per the standard dosage.

Administration: DTIC-Dome 100 mg and 200 mg vials are reconstituted with 9.9 ml and 19.7 ml, respectively, of Water for Injections BP. The resulting solution contains an equivalent of 10 mg/ml of dacarbazine. After the solution has been prepared, the calculated dose is drawn into a syringe and injected intravenously. Injection may be completed in one or two minutes.

If desired, the reconstituted solution may be further diluted with 125–250 ml of Dextrose Injection BP 5% or Sodium Chloride Injection BP 0.9% and administered by intravenous infusion over a period of 15 to 30 minutes.

Contra-indications, warnings, etc DTIC-Dome is contra-indicated in patients who have demonstrated a hypersensitivity to it in the past.

This product should not normally be administered to patients who are pregnant or to mothers who are breast feeding.

Studies have demonstrated this agent to have a carcinogenic and teratogenic effect when used on animals.

DTIC-Dome should be administered preferably to patients who are hospitalised and who can be observed carefully and frequently during and after therapy, with particular reference to the haemopoietic system.

Care must be taken to avoid extravasation of the drug subcutaneously during intravenous administration as this may result in tissue damage and severe pain.

Users should avoid contact of DTIC-Dome with the skin and eyes when reconstituting or administering.

It is recommended that DTIC-Dome be administered under the supervision of a physician experienced in the use of cancer chemotherapeutic agents. Since facilities for necessary laboratory studies must be available, hospitalisation is recommended.

Haemopoietic depression is the most common toxic side effect of DTIC-Dome and involves primarily the leucocytes and platelets, although mild anaemia may sometimes occur. Leucopaenia and thrombocytopaenia may be severe enough to cause death. The possible bone marrow depression requires careful monitoring of white blood cell, red blood cell and platelet levels. Haemopoietic toxicity may warrant temporary suspension or cessation of DTIC-Dome therapy.

Symptoms of anorexia, nausea and vomiting are the most frequently noticed side-effects. Over 90% of patients are affected with the first few doses. The vomiting lasts for 1–12 hours and may be completely but unpredictably palliated by phenobarbital and/or prochlorperazine. Rarely, DTIC-Dome causes diarrhoea. Some helpful suggestions include restricting the patient's oral intake of fluids and food for 4–6 hours prior to treatment. The rapid toleration of these symptoms suggests a central nervous system mechanism, and usually these symptoms subside after the first 1 or 2 days.

Infrequently, some patients have experienced an influenza-like syndrome of fever to 39°C, myalgias and malaise. This syndrome occurs usually after large single doses and approximately 7 days after treatment with DTIC-Dome and lasts 7–21 days, and may recur with successive treatments.

Alopecia has been noted as has facial flushing and facial paraesthesia.

Hepatic toxicity accompanied by hepatic vein thrombosis and hepatocellular necrosis resulting in death, has been reported. The incidence of such reactions has been low; approximately 0.01% of patients treated. This toxicity has been observed mostly when DTIC-Dome has been administered concomitantly with other antineoplastic drugs; however, it has also been reported in some patients treated with DTIC-Dome alone.

Anaphylaxis can occur very rarely following administration of DTIC-Dome.

Erythematous and urticarial rashes have been observed infrequently after administration of DTIC-Dome.

Rarely photosensitivity reactions may occur.

Pharmaceutical precautions Store in a refrigerator between 2° and 8°C.

DTIC-Dome, like all triazenes is sensitive to unnecessary exposure to light and the reconstituted solution should be protected from light.

After reconstitution in the vial the solution may be stored, suitably protected from light, at 4°C for 72 hours or at normal room termperature for up to 8 hours.

If the reconstituted solution is further diluted in 5% Dextrose Injection BP or Sodium Chloride Injection BP 0.9% the resulting solution may be stored at 4°C for up to 24 hours.

Legal category POM.

Package quantities Vials containing 100 mg and 200 mg DTIC-Dome as sterile dacarbazine.

Further information When reconstituted each ml of solution for injection contains:
dacarbazine 10 mg, citric acid 10 mg and mannitol 5.0 mg (100 ml vial) or 3.75 mg (200 ml vial) pH 3.0–4.0.

Product licence numbers
100 mg   0010/0127
200 mg   0010/0128

FABAHISTIN*

Presentation *Tablets:* orange-coloured sugar-coated tablets measuring approximately 8.5 mm × 5.5 mm, each tablet containing 50 mg mebhydrolin base.

Suspension: An orange-coloured suspension in a 100 ml glass bottle, each 5 ml suspension containing 50 mg mebhydrolin as mebhydrolin napadisylate.

Uses Fabahistin is an antihistamine recommended for the treatment of hay fever, urticaria, rhinitis and all other allergic disorders.

Dosage and administration Oral administration as follows:

Adults: 1 or 2 × 50 mg tablets three times a day.

Children: Over 10 years: 1 or 2 × 50 mg tablets three times a day.

Under 10 years: 1–4 × 5 ml spoonfuls of suspension daily, according to age, in divided doses after meals.

Contra-indications, warnings, etc
Contra-indications: None known.

Side-effects: Very rarely cases of granulocytopenia or agranulocytosis associated with the use of mebhydrolin have been reported.

Overdosage: No symptoms have been reported in a patient receiving 140 × 50 mg tablets.

Precautions: The substance may cause drowsiness. If affected, do not drive or operate machinery. Avoid alcoholic drinks.

No embryotoxic or teratogenic effects have been

reported, but, on principle, caution should be exercised when prescribing any new medication during pregnancy and lactation.

Pharmaceutical precautions There are no special requirements for storage.

The suspension should not be diluted with water, but a suitable suspending agent should be used such as tragacanth. Suspensions to be stored for long periods should be diluted with a suspending agent containing methyl hydroxybenzoate BP 0.07 g, sodium carboxymethyl cellulose 0.5 g in 100 ml Purified Water BP.

Legal category POM.

Package quantities Strip packs of 20 tablets. Bottles of 250 tablets. Bottles of 100 ml suspension.

Further information Nil.

Product licence numbers
Tablets   0010/5913
Suspension   0010/5915

LASONIL*

Presentation *Ointment:* A yellow-tinged transparent soft ointment contained in aluminium tubes. Each 100 g ointment contains heparinoid 'Bayer' 5,000 HDBu., hyaluronidase 15,000 i.u.

Uses Lasonil is a preparation containing heparinoid and hyaluronidase, which counteracts inflammation, promotes resorption of local oedema and extravasated blood, and locally delays blood clotting.

Ointment: Traumatic conditions: bruises, sprains, soft tissue injuries.

Varicose conditions: thrombophlebitis, superficial thrombosis, varicose ulcers.

Haemorrhoids.

Dosage and administration *Ointment: Traumatic conditions:* Unless otherwise directed, apply thickly and gently massage into the affected area two to three times daily.

Varicose conditions: In varicose ulcers Lasonil should be applied around the ulcer and gently massaged into the skin.

In thrombophlebitis and superficial thrombosis Lasonil should be massaged gently into the affected area three to five times daily.

Haemorrhoids: Apply night and morning, and after defaecation, to the anal region and inject a small quantity into the anal canal through the applicator.

There is no special dosage for children.

Contra-indications, warnings, etc *Contra-indications:* None.

Side-effects: None.

Precautions: Lasonil should not be applied to open or infected wounds.

Pharmaceutical precautions There are no special precautions or requirements regarding the storage, etc. of Lasonil.

Legal category P.

Package quantities *Ointment:* Aluminium tubes containing 14 g and 40 g Lasonil.

Further information Nil.

Product licence number 0010/5914.

MIGRAVESS*

Presentation Round, flat, white tablets, 22 mm diameter engraved with a breakline and a letter 'M' in each half of the tablet.

Each dry tablet contains:

Metoclopramide Monohydrochloride	5 mg
Aspirin BP	325 mg
Sodium Bicarbonate PhEur	1180 mg
Citric Acid PhEur	850 mg

Uses Analgesic/anti-emetic for the rapid symptomatic relief of headache and nausea associated with migraine.

Dosage and administration *Adults:* 2 tablets dissolved in water to be taken at the first symptoms of a migraine attack. If the attack persists the dose may be repeated up to a maximum of 3 doses (6 tablets) per day.

Children/young adults (10–15 years): Half the adult dose.

Migravess must be dissolved completely in half a glass of water before taking.

Contra-indications, warnings, etc True hypersensitivity to salicylates.

Migravess should not be administered concomitantly with atropine, any anticholinergic drugs or concurrent with the administration of phenothiazines or butyrophenones. If vomiting persists the patient should be reassessed to exclude the possibility of an underlying disorder e.g. cerebral irritation.

Side-effects: Various extra-pyramidal reactions to metoclopramide have been reported, particularly in the young and the elderly. The incidence may be increased if daily doses in excess of those recommended are administered. The rarely occurring reactions include: spasm of facial, extra ocular or cervical muscles. There may be a generalised increase in muscle tone. Any side-effects normally disappear within 24 hours of withdrawal of the drug.

Should treatment be required an anti-Parkinson drug of the anticholinergic type may be used to counteract these reactions.

In common with most anti-emetic drugs, metoclopramide may cause drowsiness but this is less common than with antihistamines.

Although studies in several mammalian species have demonstrated no teratogenic effects with metoclopramide, the use of Migravess is not recommended during the first trimester of pregnancy.

Each tablet contains 14 m Eq Na$^+$.

Overdosage: Treat with gastric lavage and supportive therapy. Atropine 2 mg i.m. should be given for dystonic reactions in adults.

Pharmaceutical precautions Store at room temperature in a dry place and do not remove tablets from the foil until required.

Legal category POM.

Package quantities Migravess is available in cartons of 30 tablets (15 strips of 2 tablets). The tablets are packed in moisture proof aluminium foil laminate.

Further information Migravess presents aspirin and metoclopramide in effervescent form intended to hasten gastric emptying and therefore absorption, with freedom from the side-effects often associated with ergotamine containing preparations.

Product licence number 0010/0109.

MIGRAVESS* FORTE

Presentation Round, flat, white tablets, 22 mm diameter engraved with a breakline and a letter 'f' in each half of the tablet.

Each dry tablet contains:

Metoclopramide monohydrochloride	5 mg
Aspirin BP	450 mg
Sodium Bicarbonate PhEur	1230 mg
Citric Acid PhEur	850 mg

Uses Analgesic/anti-emetic for the rapid symptomatic relief of headache and nausea associated with severe migraine.

Dosage and administration *Adults:* 2 tablets dissolved in water to be taken at the first symptoms of a migraine attack. If the attack persists the dose may be repeated up to a maximum of 3 doses (6 tablets) per day.

Children/young adults (10–15 years): Half the adult dose.

Migravess Forte must be dissolved completely in half a glass of water before taking.

Contra-indications, warnings, etc True hypersensitivity to salicylates.

Migravess Forte should not be administered concomitantly with atropine, any anticholinergic drugs or concurrent with the administration of phenothiazines or butyrophenones.

If vomiting persists the patient should be reassessed to exclude the possibility of an underlying disorder, e.g. cerebral irritation.

Side-effects: Various extra-pyramidal reactions to metoclopramide have been reported, particularly in the young and the elderly. The incidence may be increased if daily doses in excess of those recommended are administered. The rarely occurring reactions include: spasm of facila, extra ocular or cervical muscles. There may be an generalised increase in muscle tone. Any side-effects normally disappear within 24 hours of withdrawal of the drug.

Should treatment be required an anti-Parkinson drug of the anticholinergic type may be used to counteract these reactions.

In common with most anti-emetic drugs, metoclopramide may cause drowsiness but this is less common than with antihistamines.

Although studies in several mammalian species have demonstrated no teratogenic effects with metoclopramide, the use of Migravess is not recommended during the first trimester of pregnancy.

Each tablet contains 14.6 m Eq Na+.

Overdosage: Treat with gastric lavage and supportive therapy. Atropine 2 mg i.m. should be given for dystonic reactions in adults.

Pharmaceutical precautions Store at room temperature in a dry place and do not remove tablets from the foil until required.

Legal category POM.

Package quantities Migravess Forte is available in cartons of 30 tablets (15 strips of 2 tablets). The tablets are packed in moisture proof aluminium foil laminate.

Further information Migravess Forte presents aspirin and metoclopramide in effervescent form intended to hasten gastric emptying and therefore absorption, with freedom from the side-effects often associated with ergotamine containing preparations.

Product licence number 0010/0108.

NYSTAFORM*-HC OINTMENT
NYSTAFORM*-HC CREAM

Presentation *Nystaform-HC ointment: Active ingredients:* Nystatin BP 100,000 units/g; Chlorhexidine acetate BP 1.0% w/w; Hydrocortisone PhEur 1.0% w/w.

Form and appearance: Nystaform-HC ointment is a yellow ointment containing the active ingredients in a water-repellent base.

Nystaform HC cream: Active ingredients: Nystatin BP 100,000 units/g; Chlorhexidine hydrochloride BP 1.0% w/w; Hydrocortisone PhEur 0.5% w/w.

Form and appearance: Nystaform-HC cream is a light yellow cream containing the active ingredients in a water miscible base.

Uses *Actions:* Nystatin is a fungistatic and fungicidal antibiotic primarily effective against Candida albicans. Chlorhexidine has activity against a wide range of bacteria. Hydrocortisone exercises a vasoconstrictive effect, thus reducing inflammation and oedema and also has an antipruritic effect.

Indications: Nystaform-HC preparations are indicated in infected dermatoses where fungal (particularly monilial) and/or bacterial infection is present. The choice of cream or ointment presentations will depend upon the severity, physical characteristics and site of the condition, and upon the physician's preference.

Dosage and administration For topical application only. Apply liberally to infected areas 2–3 times daily. Continue application for one week after lesions have healed. This dosage is recommended for both children and adults.

Contra-indications, warnings, etc

Contra-indications: Tuberculous lesions of the skin. Known sensitivity to any of the ingredients.

Precautions: For external use only. Keep out of eyes. In infants, long term continuous topical steroid therapy should be avoided. Adrenal suppression can occur even without occlusions. As with other topical corticosteroids, systemic absorption may occur when extensive areas are treated, particularly under occlusion.

Topical administration of corticosteroids to pregnant animals can cause abnormalities of foetal development. The relevance of this finding to humans has not been established. However, topical steroids should not be used extensively in the first trimester of pregnancy, i.e. in large amounts or for prolonged periods. However, the unproven theoretical teratogenic hazard must be placed in perspective against the need to maintain the health of the patient.

Overdosage: Not applicable.

Main side-effects/adverse reactions: None reported.

Pharmaceutical precautions *Storage:* Store in a cool place.

Legal category POM.

Package quantities Nystaform-HC cream 15 g and 30 g tubes. Nystaform-HC ointment 30 g tubes.

Further information If sensitivity occurs, or if new infection appears, discontinue use and institute appropriate therapy.

The micronisation and microdispersion of the hydrocortisone in Nystaform-HC preparations ensure that the dispersal of this active ingredient over the affected area is as uniform as possible.

The water miscible base of Nystaform-HC cream is particularly easy to apply to inflamed and tender skin. It is pleasant to use and does not leave the skin feeling greasy. The water repellent base of Nystaform-HC ointment spreads easily and helps to protect against urine when used in the nappy rash area.

Product licence numbers
Nystaform-HC ointment   0010/0124
Nystaform-HC cream   0010/0123

NYSTAFORM* OINTMENT
NYSTAFORM CREAM

Presentation *Nystaform ointment: Active ingredients:* Nystatin BP 100,000 units/g; Chlorhexidine acetate BP 1.0% w/w.

Form and appearance: Nystaform ointment is a yellow ointment containing the active ingredients in a water-repellent base.

Nystaform cream: Active ingredients: Nystatin BP 100,000 units/g Chlorhexidine hydrochloride BP 1.0% w/w.

Form and appearance: Nystaform cream is a light yellow cream containing the active ingredients in a water miscible base.

Uses *Actions:* Nystatin is a fungistatic and fungicidal antibiotic primarily effective against Candida albicans. Chlorhexidine has activity against a wide range of bacteria.

Indications: For the treatment of infected skin conditions where fungal (particularly monilial) and/or bacterial infections are present.

Dosage and administration For topical application only. Apply liberally to infected area 2–3 times daily. Continue application for one week after lesions have healed.

This dosage is recommended for both children and adults.

The patient should be advised that if the condition is not better within seven days, to return to the surgery for a further consultation. In any event the duration of this treatment should not normally exceed fourteen days.

Contra-indications, warnings, etc
Contra-indications: Known sensitivity to any of the ingredients.

Precautions: For external use only. Keep out of eyes.

Overdosage: Not applicable.

Main side-effects/adverse reactions: None reported.

Pharmaceutical precautions *Storage:* Store in a cool place.

Legal category POM.

Package quantities 30 g tubes.

Further information If sensitivity occurs, or if new infection appears, discontinue use and institute appropriate therapy.

The water miscible base of Nystaform cream is particularly easy to apply to inflamed and tender skin. It is pleasant to use and does not leave the skin feeling greasy. The water repellent base of Nystaform ointment spreads easily and helps to protect against urine when used in the nappy rash area.

Product licence numbers
Nystaform ointment   0010/0122
Nystaform cream   0010/0121

SECUROPEN*

Presentation Vials containing 0.5 g, 1.0 g, 2.0 g azlocillin as azlocillin monosodium. Infusion vials containing 5.0 g as azlocillin monosodium.

Securopen infusion set containing 3×5 g azlocillin, 3×50 ml Water for Injections and 3 transfer needles.

Uses Azlocillin is a broad spectrum antibiotic with especially significant anti-pseudomonal activity. In addition to *Pseudomonas* strains the spectrum of activity of azlocillin includes the following Gram-negative and Gram-positive pathogens: *Escherichia coli, Klebsiella-Enterobacter-Serratia* group, *Proteus* (indole-positive and indole-negative), *Providencia, Citrobacter, Salmonella* and *Shigella*, enterococci, staphylococci (pencillin sensitive), *Haemophilus influenzae*, gonococci, meningococci, pneumococci, streptococci and *Corynebacterium* spp. The spectrum also includes the anaerobic organisms *Clostridia* and *Bacteroides species*, including *Bacteroides fragilis*.

Azlocillin is specifically indicated for the treatment of infections due to *Pseudomonas* strains especially those of the respiratory and urinary tracts and for septicaemia. Also for infections in other areas due to this organism.

Azlocillin may be administered concomitantly with an aminoglycoside or with beta-lactamase stable isoxazolyl-penicillins, since there is evidence of synergy with these groups.

Dosage and administration *Adult Dosage: Patients with normal renal function:* Life-threatening infections 5.0 g every 8 hours. In non life-threatening and urinary tract infections 2.0 g every 8 hours.

Patients with severely impaired renal function: i.e. with a serum creatinine above 2 mg% or with creatinine clearance less than 30 ml/minute, the unit dose should be as above but at 12 hourly intervals.

Patients on haemodialysis: Azlocillin is dialysable. On non-dialysing days, patients receive the recommended unit dose of azlocillin twice daily. Before each dialysis an additional unit dose should be given to compensate for the amount of azlocillin removed by dialysis.

Children's Dosage:

Children 1–14 years	: 3×75 mg/kg bodyweight/day
Infants > 7 days–1 year	: 3×100 mg/kg bodyweight/day
Neonates < 7 days	: 2×100 mg/kg bodyweight/day

Premature babies   : 2 × 50 mg/kg bodyweight/ day

From this the following dosages can be derived:

Children 6–14 years
(20–40 kg bodyweight)   1.5–3.0 g 3 × daily
Children 2–6 years
(13–20 kg bodyweight)   1.0–1.5 g 3 × daily
Children 1–2 years
(10–13 kg bodyweight)   0.75–1.0 g 3 × daily
Infants 7 days–1 year
(about 3–10 kg body-
weight)   0.3–1.0 g 3 × daily
Neonates 7 days
(about 3 kg bodyweight)   0.3 g 2 × daily
Premature babies up to
2.5 kg bodyweight   2.5 kg bodyweight: 125 mg
                         2 × daily
                         2.0 kg bodyweight: 100 mg
                         2 × daily
                         1.5 kg bodyweight: 75 mg
                         2 × daily.

Duration of Treatment: The duration of treatment depends upon the severity of the case and also the clinical and bacteriological course of the disease. In principle, treatment should be maintained for at least 3 days after fever or clinical symptoms have disappeared. This on average requires 7–10 days therapy.

Administration: Azlocillin is administered intravenously as a 10% solution in Water for Injections. For doses of 2.0 g or less it is administered as a bolus injection and for higher doses as an infusion over 20–30 minutes. Aminoglycosides, when given concomitantly, should not be mixed in the same syringe or infusion fluid as azlocillin.

Combination Therapy: In patients already receiving intravenous infusion therapy with other drugs, azlocillin should be infused during the intervening periods or as a parallel infusion. In order to achieve higher initial concentrations in the serum and tissues, part of the dose – up to half – may be injected slowly through the tubing of the existing infusion. Azlocillin solution is compatible with glucose solution (5% and 10%), laevulose solution (5%), Ringer's solution and physiological saline. Supplementary drugs should be injected through the drip tubing and not introduced into the bag or bottle. Injectable tetracycline derivatives, for example, have proved to be incompatible. Before administering special, rarely used solutions or drugs the compatability of the individual components must be ascertained; precipitation, cloudiness or discolouration indicates possible incompatibility.

Stability in other infusions: Azlocillin is stable in the common infusion fluids provided the solution has been freshly prepared. If azlocillin must be prepared before administration it may be kept as the 10% solution at room temperature for 6 hours without loss of efficacy.

Contra-indications, warnings, etc

Contra-indications: A history of allergy to other penicillins and cephalosporins. Securopen is inactivated by β-lactamases (penicillinases). As with all new drugs Securopen should not be used during the first 3 months of pregnancy.

Side-effects: Uncommon and typical for other injectable penicillins.

Toxicity and treatment of overdose: There have been no reports of toxic effects or overdosage.

Pharmaceutical precautions *Storage:* The shelf life is 4 years when stored below 25°C and expiry date is printed on the packaging. Azlocillin should not be stored in temperatures exceeding 25°C.

Dilution: Azlocillin should be freshly prepared immediately before administration by shaking the powder with a suitable volume of Water for Injections until completely dissolved to make a 10% solution – that is, 0.5 g in 5 ml, 1.0 g in 10 ml, 2.0 g in 20 ml and 5.0 g in 50 ml. Any unused solution should be discarded. Azlocillin is stable in 5% and 10% dextrose solution, laevulose 5%, Ringer's solution and physiological saline.

Legal category POM.

Package quantities 0.5 g, 1.0 g, 2.0 g vials packed in boxes of 5.
5.0 g vial packed singly.
Infusion pack of 3 × 5 g with diluent and transfer needles.

Further information
Sodium content:

Each 5.0 g vial contains	10.84 mEq sodium (249.1 mg)
Each 2.0 g vial contains	4.33 mEq sodium (99.6 mg)
Each 1.0 g vial contains	2.17 mEq sodium (49.8 mg)
Each 0.5 g vial contains	1.08 mEq sodium (24.9 mg)
Displacement value	0.74 ml/g

Product licence number
Securopen   0010/0075
Water for injections BP   0010/0095

TRASYLOL*

Presentation A colourless ampoule containing a solution of aprotinin for injection, each 5 ml ampoule containing 100,000 kallikrein inactivator units (KIU) and each 10 ml ampoule containing 200,000 KIU.

Uses Trasylol is a broad-spectrum protease inhibitor. Its indications are as follows:
    Traumatic, haemorrhagic, pancreatogenic, endotoxic shock and fat-embolism syndrome.
    Acute pancreatitis.
    Prophylaxis in upper abdominal surgery.
    Hyperfibrinolytic haemorrhage.

Dosage and administration *Traumatic, haemorrhagic, pancreatogenic, endotoxic shock and fat-embolism syndrome:* An initial 500,000 KIU should be administered immediately by slow i.v. injection (at a rate not exceeding 5 ml/min.) followed by 200,000 KIU four-hourly by i.v. infusion. It may be necessary to continue this dosage for three days or longer, depending on the clinical picture.

Acute pancreatitis: As above.

Prophylaxis in upper abdominal surgery: 200,000 KIU should be administered by slow i.v. injection immediately before commencing the operation. During the day of the operation, as well as during the first and second post-operative days, 200,000 KIU should be administered four-hourly by slow i.v. injection or continuous i.v. infusion.

Hyperfibrinolytic haemorrhage: Up to 500,000 KIU should be administered by slow i.v. injection within the first 30 minutes: subsequently 200,000 KIU four-hourly

should be given by continuous i.v. infusion until haemostasis has definitely been achieved. In disseminated
intravascular coagulation with secondary hyperfibrino-
lysis (consumption coagulopathy) higher dosages up to
1,000,000 KIU or more may be required. In fibrinogen
deficiency substitution may be necessary.

The dose for children should be calculated in proportion to the adult dose on the basis of body weight.

Contra-indications, warnings, etc

Contra-indications: There are no contra-indications.

Side-effects: Trasylol is very well tolerated, even in high
dosage. Local or general reactions are very rare (less
than 0.1%). However, being a polypeptide, care should
be exercised in treating patients intermittently or those
who have previously received Trasylol, since an anaphylactic reaction can occur.

Trasylol is incompatible with most corticosteroids and
nutrient solutions containing amino-acids or fat emulsions.

Overdosage: There is no special antidote or other action
to be taken.

Pharmaceutical precautions Trasylol is very stable
when stored in sealed ampoules at room temperature.
Opened ampoules, however, quickly lose activity if
bacterial contamination is not prevented.

Legal category POM.

Package quantities Trasylol is supplied in strengths
of 100,000 KIU per 5 ml ampoule and 200,000 KIU per
10 ml ampoule in boxes of 5 and 25 ampoules.

Further information Nil.

Product licence number 0010/5900.

YOMESAN*

Presentation Yellowish tablets measuring 13 mm ×
4 mm, each tablet containing 500 mg niclosamide BP.
One side marked FE, the reverse side with the Bayer
cross. The tablets are flavoured with vanilla.

Uses An anthelmintic for treatment of tapeworm
infections:

Taenia saginata	(beef tapeworm)
Taenia solium	(pork tapeworm)
Diphyllobothrium latum	(fish tapeworm)
Hymenolepis nana	(dwarf tapeworm)

It has no effect in cysticercosis and echinococcosis due
to cestode larvae (cysticerci) lodging in extra intestinal
tissues.

Dosage and administration *Taenia saginata, Taenia
solium, Diphyllobothrium latum.*

Adults and children over 6 years:	4 tablets
Children 2 to 6 years:	2 tablets
Children under 2 years:	1 tablet

In *Taenia solium* the tablets should be taken as a single
dose after a light breakfast but in the case of *Taenia
saginata* and *Diphyllobothrium latum* the dose may be
divided, half being taken after breakfast and the remainder one hour later.

An aperient should be administered two hours later

and in the case of *Taenia solium* a drastic purge should
be given.

If reinfection occurs repeat treatment.

Infection due to *Hymenolepis nana* should be treated
for 7 days:

First day:

Adults and children over 6 years:	4 tablets
Children from 2 to 6 years:	2 tablets
Children under 2 years:	1 tablet

The subsequent 6 days:

Adults and children over 6 years:	2 tablets
Children from 2 to 6 years:	1 tablet
Children under 2 years:	½ tablet

It is important that the tablets are chewed thoroughly
before washing down with water. In the case of small
children the tablets should be ground up before administration.

Contra-indications, warnings, etc

Contra-indications: there are no known contra-indications.

Side-effects: limited to occasional gastrointestinal upsets, light headedness and pruritus.

Overdosage: Yomesan is not absorbed and no cases of
overdosage have occurred.

Use in Pregnancy: In common with most drugs it is wise
to avoid treatment in the first trimester of pregnancy.
Healthy children have been born to women treated with
Yomesan in the first trimester of pregnancy.

Experimental studies in rats showed no embryotoxic
or teratogenic effects.

Warning: In infections with *Taenia solium* there is always
a danger of cysticercosis. A drastic purge is therefore
recommended after treatment to eject the lower segment
of the tapeworm containing mature eggs.

The hands should be thoroughly scrubbed after
defaecation not only on the treatment day but for several
days afterwards to avoid reinfection.

The consumption of alcohol during treatment must be
avoided.

Pharmaceutical precautions The tablets are light
sensitive and should only be stored in the original foil.

Legal category P.

Package quantities Packs of 4 tablets of 0.5 g.

Further information Unless the tapeworm is expelled
by a drastic purgative, residual parts of it may be
eliminated with the stools during the next two or three
days. Thereafter, neither tapeworm segments nor ova
should be present in the stools. In re-infection with
Taenia saginata and *Taenia solium* new tapeworm
segments or ova should only appear after three months.

In infections with *Hymenolepis nana* the follow-up
period is only 14 days as surviving scolices regenerate
very rapidly to sexually mature tapeworms and accordingly, after approx. 10 days, ova are eliminated with the
stools.

Product licence number 0010/5910.

*Trade Mark

Beecham Research Laboratories
Great West Road
Brentford
Middlesex TW8 9BD

BEECHAM RESEARCH

AMPICLOX* INJECTION

Presentation *Ampiclox Injection:* Vials containing 250 mg ampicillin as Ampicillin Sodium BP with 250 mg cloxacillin as Cloxacillin Sodium BP.

Uses Ampiclox is indicated for the immediate treatment of severe infections before the infecting organism is identified, and for mixed staphylococcal and Gram-negative infections.

Typical indications include: Bronchopneumonia, post-influenzal pneumonia and other severe respiratory infections. Post-operative chest and wound infections. Septic abortion and infections during the puerperium. Septicaemia. Infections in patients receiving immunosuppressive drugs. Prophylaxis in major surgery.

Dosage and administration *Adult dosage (including elderly patients): Intramuscular/Intravenous:* 1–2 vials four to six hourly.

Children's dosage: Up to 2 years: ¼ adult dose.†
2–10 years: ½ adult dose.

Administration: Intramuscular: Dissolve vial contents in 1.5 ml Water for Injections BP.

Intravenous: Dissolve vial contents in 10 ml Water for Injections BP and administer slowly (three to four minutes). Ampiclox may also be added to infusion fluids or injected, suitably diluted, into the drip tube over a period of three to four minutes.

Dosage may be further increased where necessary.

Contra-indications, warnings, etc
Contra-indications: Penicillin hypersensitivity; ocular administration.

Side-effects: As with other penicillins. An erythematous rash may occasionally occur, as with ampicillin. The incidence of this rash is particularly high in patients with infectious mononucleosis. If a rash is reported it is advisable to discontinue treatment.

Pharmaceutical precautions Ampiclox should be stored in a cool, dry place. Solutions for injection should be used immediately.

Ampiclox may be added to most intravenous fluids but should not be mixed with blood products or other proteinaceous fluids (e.g. protein hydrolysates). In intravenous solutions containing glucose or other carbohydrates, Ampiclox should be infused within two hours.

† Ampiclox Neonatal (regd) is recommended for the treatment of infections in neonates and premature babies.

Legal category POM.

Package quantities *Ampiclox Injection:* Boxes of 10.

Further information Nil.

Product licence number 0038/5003.

AMPICLOX* NEONATAL INJECTION
AMPICLOX* NEONATAL SUSPENSION

Presentation *Ampiclox Neonatal Injection:* Vials containing 50 mg ampicillin as Ampicillin Sodium BP with 25 mg cloxacillin as Cloxacillin Sodium BP.

Ampiclox Neonatal Suspension: Bottles containing powder for the preparation of 10 ml suspension. When reconstituted each 0.6 ml dose contains 60 mg ampicillin as Ampicillin Trihydrate BP with 30 mg cloxacillin as Cloxacillin Sodium BP. A pipette to measure the 0.6 ml dose is provided.

Uses Ampiclox Neonatal is indicated for the prophylaxis or treatment of infections in premature babies or neonates, particularly:

Suspected or confirmed infections.

Babies born of mothers with infected liquor or whose membranes ruptured more than 48 hours before delivery.

Babies requiring certain surgical procedures carrying risk of infection such as exchange transfusions.

Babies born with respiratory distress necessitating endotracheal procedures, when subsequent infection is a possible hazard.

Babies following difficult delivery, when inhalation of much liquor, mucus or meconium has occurred.

Dosage and administration *Dosage: Oral:* 0.6 ml suspension (90 mg) every four hours.
Intramuscular/Intravenous: 1 vial (75 mg) three times a day.

Administration: Ampiclox Neonatal Injection:

Intramuscular: Dissolve vial contents in 0.5 ml Water for Injections BP.
Intravenous: Dissolve vial contents in 2 ml Water for Injections BP and administer slowly (three to four minutes). Ampiclox Neonatal may also be added to infusion fluids or injected, suitably diluted, into the drip tube over a period of three to four minutes.

Contra-indications, warnings, etc
Contra-indications: Penicillin-hypersensitivity; ocular administration.

Caution should be observed when administering Ampiclox Neonatal to babies whose mothers are hypersensitive to penicillin.

Side-effects: As with other penicillins. An erythematous rash may occasionally occur, as with ampicillin. The incidence of this rash is particularly high in patients with infectious mononucleosis. If a rash is reported it is advisable to discontinue treatment.

Pharmaceutical precautions Ampiclox Neonatal should be stored in a cool, dry place.

Solutions for injection should be used immediately. Ampiclox Neonatal may be added to most intravenous fluids but should not be mixed with blood products or other proteinaceous fluids (e.g. protein hydrolysates). In intravenous solutions containing glucose or other carbohydrates, Ampiclox Neonatal should be infused within two hours.

Once dispensed, Ampiclox Neonatal Suspension remains stable for five days if kept in a cool place.

Legal category POM.

Package quantities *Ampiclox Neonatal Injection:* Boxes of 10.
Ampiclox Neonatal Suspension: 10 ml bottles.

Further information Ampiclox Neonatal Suspension is sugar-free to minimise the risk of diarrhoea in the newborn.

If tube feeding is necessary the suspension can easily be passed down a Ryle's tube.

Product licence numbers
Ampiclox Neonatal Injection   0038/5001
Ampiclox Neonatal Suspension   0038/5009

ANXON* CAPSULES

Presentation Anxon Capsules: Dark pink/light pink capsules, in two sizes containing 15 mg or 30 mg ketazolam overprinted with product name 'Anxon' and the strength.

Uses *Action:* Anxon is a benzodiazepine and shares the general characteristics of this group of products.

Indications: Anxon is indicated for the treatment of anxiety, tension, irritability and similar stress related symptoms. Anxon also possesses muscle-relaxant properties and may be used in the management of spasticity associated with conditions such as spinal cord trauma, cerebrovascular accident and multiple sclerosis.

Dosage and administration *Usual Adult Dosage:* For most patients it is recommended that treatment should commence with a single dose of 30 mg, taken before retiring.

The effective dosage is usually in the range 15–60 mg per day, taken either as a single dose before retiring or in divided doses. When treating elderly or debilitated patients (e.g. those with cerebral disorders or cardiorespiratory insufficiency), a reduced dosage should be used initially until tolerance and efficacy have been assessed.

Patients undergoing therapy with centrally active products should be periodically reviewed.

Children: Insufficient data are available to recommend the administration of Anxon to children.

Contra-indications, warnings, etc
Precautions: The usual precautions when prescribing products of the benzodiazepine group should be observed.

Anxon may potentiate other centrally acting drugs such as alcohol, tranquillisers, anti-depressants, hypnotics, analgesics and anaesthetics.

Patients should be warned to exercise care when driving or operating heavy machinery, since drowsiness and modification of their reactions may occur depending on dosage and individual sensitivity.

Usage cannot be recommended during pregnancy, labour or lactation.

Side-effects: Anxon is well tolerated; in comparative studies the overall incidence of side-effects was no greater than that observed with placebo.

As with other benzodiazepines daytime drowsiness has been reported.

Overdosage: Symptoms of overdosage may include drowsiness and ataxia, with coma in severe cases. The toxicity of the benzodiazepine group of drugs is very low, however, and symptomatic treatment only is required. Gastric lavage may be useful if performed soon after ingestion.

Pharmaceutical precautions Anxon capsules should be stored in well closed containers in a cool place.

Legal category CD (Sch 4) POM.

Package quantities
Anxon Capsules: 15 mg – packs of 100.
                            30 mg – packs of 100.

Further information Anxon is particularly appropriate for those patients for whom a simple once daily dosage and a low incidence of side-effects are important considerations.

Product licence numbers
Anxon Capsules 15 mg   0038/0252
Anxon Capsules 30 mg   0038/0253

AUGMENTIN* TABLETS ▼
AUGMENTIN* DISPERSIBLE TABLETS ▼
AUGMENTIN* JUNIOR SUSPENSION ▼
AUGMENTIN* PAEDIATRIC SUSPENSION ▼
AUGMENTIN INTRAVENOUS ▼

Presentation
Augmentin tablets: White oval film-coated tablets engraved 'Augmentin' on one side. Each tablet provides 125 mg clavulanic acid with 250 mg amoxycillin. (375 mg Augmentin.)

Augmentin Dispersible tablets: White round tablets engraved 'Augmentin'. Each tablet provides 125 mg clavulanic acid with 250 mg amoxycillin. (375 mg Augmentin.)

Augmentin Junior suspension: Bottles of powder for the preparation of 100 ml suspension. When reconstituted each 5 ml provides 62 mg clavulanic acid with 125 mg amoxycillin. (187 mg Augmentin.)

Augmentin Paediatric suspension: Bottles of powder for the preparation of 100 ml suspension. When reconstituted each 5 ml provides 62 mg clavulanic acid with 125 mg amoxycillin. (156 mg Augmentin.)

Augmentin Intravenous: Vials of sterile powder providing 100 mg clavulanic acid with 500 mg amoxycillin (600 mg Augmentin) or 200 mg clavulanic acid with 1 g amoxycillin (1.2 g Augmentin). For reconstitution as an intravenous injection or infusion.

In all the above presentations the clavulanic acid is present as potassium clavulanate.

The amoxycillin is present as amoxycillin trihydrate in Augmentin oral presentations and as amoxycillin sodium in Augmentin intravenous presentations.

Uses Augmentin is an antibiotic agent with a notably broad spectrum of activity against the commonly occurring bacterial pathogens in general practice and hospital. The β-lactamase inhibitory action of clavulanate extends the spectrum of amoxycillin to embrace a wider range of organisms, including many resistant to other β-lactam antibiotics.

Augmentin is indicated for short-term treatment of bacterial infections at the following sites:

Upper Respiratory Tract Infections (including ENT) e.g. tonsillitis, sinusitis, otitis media.

Lower Respiratory Tract Infections e.g. acute and chronic bronchitis, lobar and bronchopneumonia.

Genito-urinary Tract Infections e.g. cystitis, urethritis, pyelonephritis, female genital infections.

Skin and Soft Tissue Infections.

Bone and joint infections e.g. osteomyelitis.

Other infections e.g. septic abortion, puerperal sepsis, intra-abdominal sepsis, septicaemia, peritonitis, post-surgical infections.

Augmentin is indicated for prophylaxis against infection which may be associated with major surgical procedures such as gastro-intestinal, pelvic, head and neck, cardiac, renal, joint replacement and biliary tract.

Augmentin is bactericidal to a wide range of organisms including:

Gram-positive
Aerobes:
Streptococcus faecalis
Streptococcus pneumoniae
Streptococcus pyogenes
Streptococcus viridans
Staphylococcus aureus
Corynebacterium species
Bacillus anthracis
Listeria monocytogenes

Anaerobes:
Clostridium species
Peptococcus species
Peptostreptococcus

Gram-negative
Aerobes:
Haemophilus influenzae
Escherichia coli
Proteus mirabilis

Proteus vulgaris
Klebsiella species
Salmonella species
Shigella species
Bordetella pertussis
Brucella species
Neisseria gonorrhoeae
Neisseria meningitidis
Vibrio cholerae
Pasteurella multocida

Anaerobes:
Bacteroides spp. including B. fragilis.

Dosage and administration
Usual dosages for the treatment of infection

	Oral	Intravenous injection
Adults and children over 12 years	1 Augmentin tablet or Dispersible tablet three times a day. In severe infections this may be increased to two tablets three times a day. Therapy can be started parenterally and continued with an oral preparation.	Usually 1.2 g 8-hourly. In more serious infections, increase frequency to 6-hourly intervals.
Children 6–12 years	5 ml Augmentin Junior Suspension three times a day. In severe infections this may be increased to 10 ml three times a day.	Usually 30 mg/kg† Augmentin 8-hourly. In more serious infections, increase frequency to 6-hourly intervals.
Children 2–6 years	5 ml Augmentin Paediatric Suspension three times a day. In severe infections this may be increased to 10 ml three times a day.	
Children 9 months–2 years	5 ml half-strength Augmentin Paediatric Suspension three times a day.	
Children 3–9 months	2.5 ml half-strength Augmentin Paediatric Suspension three times a day.	
Children 0–3 months	No suitable presentation is currently available for this age group.	30 mg/kg† Augmentin every 12 hours in premature infants and in full term infants during the perinatal period, increasing to 8 hours thereafter.

†Each 30 mg Augmentin provides 5 mg clavulanic acid with 25 mg amoxycillin.

Dosage for surgical prophylaxis: Surgical prophylaxis with Augmentin should aim to protect the patient for the period of risk of infection. Accordingly, procedures lasting for less than 1 hour are covered in adults by 1.2 g Augmentin IV given at induction of anaesthesia. Longer operations require subsequent doses of 1.2 g Augmentin

IV (up to 4 doses in 24 hours), and this regime can be continued for several days if the procedure has significantly increased the risk of infection. Clear clinical signs of infection at operation will require a normal course of intravenous or oral Augmentin therapy post-operatively.

Dosage in renal impairment

Adults	Mild impairment (Creatinine clearance >30 ml/min)	Moderate impairment (Creatinine clearance 10–30 ml/min)	Severe impairment (Creatinine clearance <10 ml/min)
Oral therapy	No change in dosage.	1–2 tablets 12 hourly.	Not more than 1 tablet 12 hourly.
Injectable therapy	No change in dosage.	1.2 g IV stat. followed by 600 mg IV 12 hourly	1.2 g IV stat. followed by 600 mg IV 24 hourly. Dialysis decreases serum concentrations of Augmentin and an additional 600 mg IV dose may need to be given during dialysis and at the end of dialysis.

Children: Similar reductions in dosage should be made for children.

Each 1.2 g vial of Augmentin contains 1.0 mmol of potassium and 2.8 mmol of sodium (approx).

Each 375 mg tablet of Augmentin contains 0.63 mmol of potassium.

Administration

Oral: Tablets, dispersible tablets or suspensions. The absorption of Augmentin is unaffected by food. Dispersible tablets should be stirred into a little water before taking.

Intravenous: Augmentin Intravenous may be administered either by intravenous injection or by intermittent infusion. It is not suitable for intramuscular administration.

600 mg vial: To reconstitute dissolve in 10 ml Water for Injections B.P. (Final volume 10.5 ml.)

1.2 g vial: To reconstitute dissolve in 20 ml Water for Injections B.P. (Final volume 20.9 ml.)

Augmentin Intravenous should be given by slow intravenous injection over a period of 3–4 minutes and used within 20 minutes of reconstitution. It may be injected directly into a vein or via a drip tube.

Alternatively, Augmentin Intravenous may be infused in Water for Injections BP or Sodium Chloride Intravenous Injection BP (0.9% w/v). Add without delay 600 mg reconstituted solution to 50 ml infusion fluid or 1.2 g reconstituted solution to 100 ml infusion fluid (e.g. using a minibag or in-line burette). Infuse over 30–40 minutes and complete within 4 hours of reconstitution. For other appropriate infusion fluids: see package enclosure leaflet.

Any residual antibiotic solutions should be discarded.

Augmentin Intravenous is less stable in infusions containing glucose, dextran or bicarbonate. Reconstituted solution should, therefore, not be added to such infusions but may be injected into the drip tubing over a period of 3–4 minutes.

Augmentin Intravenous should not be mixed with blood products, other proteinaceous fluids such as protein hydrolysates or with intravenous lipid emulsions.

Treatment should not be extended beyond 14 days without review.

Contra-indications, warnings, etc

Contra-indication: Penicillin hypersensitivity.

Use in pregnancy: Animal studies with orally and parenterally administered Augmentin have shown no teratogenic effects. The product has been used orally in human pregnancy in a limited number of cases, with no untoward effect; however, use of Augmentin tablets in pregnancy is not recommended unless considered essential by the physician.

There is no experience with Augmentin IV in human pregnancy; therefore its use in pregnancy cannot be recommended.

Precautions: Changes in liver function tests have been observed in some patients receiving Augmentin IV. The clinical significance of these changes is uncertain but Augmentin should be used with care in patients with evidence of severe hepatic dysfunction.

In patients with moderate or severe renal impairment Augmentin dosage should be adjusted as recommended in the 'Dosage' section.

Side-effects: Side-effects, as with amoxycillin, are uncommon and mainly of a mild and transitory nature.

Diarrhoea, indigestion, nausea, vomiting and candidiasis have been reported. Nausea, although uncommon, is more often associated with higher oral dosages. If gastro-intestinal side-effects occur with oral therapy they may be reduced by taking Augmentin at the start of meals. Phlebitis at the site of injection has also been reported.

Urticarial and erythematous rashes sometimes occur but their incidence has been particularly low in clinical trials. Erythematous rashes have been associated with glandular fever in patients receiving amoxycillin. Treatment should be discontinued if either type of rash appears.

Pharmaceutical precautions Augmentin preparations should be stored in a dry place.

Bottles of Augmentin tablets should be kept tightly closed and the tablets dispensed in moisture-proof containers.

Once dispensed, Augmentin Junior and Paediatric suspensions remain stable for 7 days if kept in a refrigerator (but not frozen).

For administration to children up to 2 years, Augmentin Paediatric suspension should be diluted to half-strength, using water.

For Augmentin Intravenous, particulars of stability in solution and compatibilities are given under 'Administration' and in the package enclosure leaflet.

Legal category POM

Package quantities *Augmentin tablets:* Bottles of 30, 100 and 500.

Augmentin Dispersible tablets: Foil wrapped in cartons of 30 and 90.

Augmentin Junior suspension: Bottles of 100 ml.

Augmentin Paediatric suspension: Bottles of 100 ml.

Augmentin Intravenous: 600 mg Pack of 10. 1.2 g Pack of 5.

Further information Augmentin is a novel concept in antibiotic therapy.

Resistance to many antibiotics is caused by bacterial enzymes which destroy the antibiotic before it can act on the pathogen. The clavulanate in Augmentin anticipates this defence mechanism by blocking the β-lactamase enzymes, thus rendering the organisms sensitive to amoxycillin's rapid bactericidal effect at concentrations readily attainable in the body. Clavulanate by itself has little antibacterial activity; however, in association with amoxycillin as Augmentin it produces a novel antibiotic agent of broad spectrum with wide application in hospital and general practice.

The pharmacokinetics of the two components of Augmentin are closely matched. Peak serum levels of both occur about 1 hour after oral administration. Both clavulanate and amoxycillin have low levels of serum binding; about 70% remains free in the serum.

Doubling the dosage of Augmentin approximately doubles the serum levels achieved.

All Augmentin presentations are sugar-free formulations.

Product licence numbers

Augmentin Tablets	0038/0270
Augmentin Dispersible Tablets	0038/0272
Augmentin Junior suspension	0038/0274
Augmentin Paediatric suspension	0038/0298
Augmentin Intravenous 600 mg	0038/0320
Augmentin Intravenous 1.2 g	0038/0320

BACTROBAN* OINTMENT ▼

Presentation *Bactroban Ointment:* A sterile presentation of mupirocin 2% w/w in a white, translucent, water-soluble, polyethylene glycol base.

Uses
Action: Bactroban is a topical antibacterial agent, active against those organisms responsible for the majority of skin infections, e.g. *Staphylococcus aureus*, including methicillin-resistant strains, other staphylococci, streptococci. It is also active against Gram-negative organisms such as *Escherichia coli* and *Haemophilus influenzae*.

Indications: Acute primary bacterial skin infections, e.g. impetigo and folliculitis.

Dosage and administration
Adults and children: Bactroban Ointment should be applied to the affected area up to three times a day, for up to 10 days. The area may be covered with a dressing or occluded if desired.

There is no long-term experience of Bactroban in humans.

Contra-indications, warnings, etc
Contra-indications: Hypersensitivity to Bactroban or other ointments containing polyethylene glycols.

This Bactroban ointment formulation is not suitable for ophthalmic or intra-nasal use.

Use in pregnancy: Studies in experimental animals have shown mupirocin to be without teratogenic effects. However, there is inadequate evidence of safety to recommend the use of Bactroban during pregnancy.

Precautions: When Bactroban Ointment is used on the face, care should be taken to avoid the eyes.

Polyethylene glycol can be absorbed from open wounds and damaged skin and is excreted by the kidneys. In common with other polyethylene glycol based ointments, Bactroban Ointment should be used with caution if there is evidence of moderate or severe renal impairment.

Adverse reactions and side-effects: During clinical studies some minor adverse effects, localised to the area of application, were seen such as burning, stinging and itching.

Pharmaceutical precautions Bactroban Ointment may be stored at room temperature (below 25°C).

The ointment is supplied sterile; any remaining at the end of treatment should be discarded.

Legal category POM.

Package quantities Bactroban Ointment is available in a 15 g tube in a sealed carton.

Further information Bactroban is a novel antibiotic, both in chemical structure and mode of action; available only for topical application.

The active ingredient of Bactroban was previously described as pseudomonic acid in the published literature.

Bactroban Ointment is water soluble and does not stain the skin or clothing; it is easily removed by washing.

Product licence number 0038/0319.

BROXIL* CAPSULES
BROXIL* SYRUP

Presentation *Broxil Capsules* (Phenethicillin Capsules BP): Black and ivory capsules overprinted 'Broxil', containing 250 mg phenethicillin as Phenethicillin Potassium BP.

Broxil Syrup (Phenethicillin Elixir BP): Bottles containing powder for the preparation of 100 ml syrup.

When reconstituted each 5 ml contains 125 mg phenethicillin as Phenethicillin Potassium BP.

Uses Broxil is indicated for the oral treatment of infections caused by sensitive organisms. Typical indications include:

Ear, nose and throat infections: Tonsillitis, pharyngitis, sinusitis, laryngitis, otitis media, 'Strep' throat, dental abscess.

Respiratory tract infections: Acute bronchitis and lobar pneumonia.

Skin and soft tissue infections.

Dosage and administration *Adults (including elderly patients):* 250 mg orally four times a day.

Children 2 to 10: ½ adult dose.

Children under 2: ¼ adult dose.

Broxil should be given half to one hour before meals. Dosage may be doubled where necessary.

Contra-indications, warnings, etc
Contra-indication: Penicillin hypersensitivity.

Side-effects: As with other penicillins.

Pharmaceutical precautions Broxil should be stored in a cool, dry place.

Once dispensed, Broxil Syrup remains stable for seven days if kept in a cool place. If a dilution of the reconstituted syrup is required, Syrup BP should be used.

Legal category POM.

Package quantities *Broxil Capsules:* Containers of 100.

Broxil Syrup: 100 ml bottles.

Further information Nil.

Product licence numbers
Broxil Capsules   0038/5023
Broxil Syrup   0038/0094

CELBENIN* INJECTION

Presentation *Celbenin Injection* (Methicillin Injection BP 1973): Vials containing 1 g Methicillin Sodium BP 1973.

Uses Celbenin is indicated for the treatment of infections suspected or confirmed to be caused by β-lactamase-producing staphylococci.

Typical indications include: Respiratory tract infections. Skin and soft tissue infections. Osteomyelitis and septic arthritis. Staphylococcal urinary tract infections. Enteritis. Endocarditis. Meningitis. Septicaemia.

Dosage and administration *Usual adult dosage (including elderly patients):*

Intramuscular: 1 g four to six hourly.
Intravenous: 1 g four to six hourly.

All recommended dosages are a guide only. In severe infections systemic dosages may be increased.
Intra-articular: 500 mg to 1 g once daily.
Intrapleural: 500 mg to 1 g once daily.
Subconjunctival: Up to 500 mg once daily.
By nebuliser: 500 mg four times a day.

Usual children's dosage: 2–10 years: ½ adult dose.
Under 2 years: ¼ adult dose.

Administration: Intramuscular: Add 1.5 ml Water for Injections BP to 1 g vial contents.

Intravenous: Dissolve 1 g in 20 ml Water for Injections BP and give by slow injection (three to four minutes). Celbenin may also be added to infusion fluids or injected, suitably diluted, into the drip tube over a period of three to four minutes. Infusion bottles containing Celbenin should be changed every five hours.

Celbenin may be administered by other routes in conjunction with systemic therapy.

Intra-articular: Dissolve 1 g in 5 ml Water for Injections BP or 0.5% lignocaine hydrochloride solution.

Intrapleural: Dissolve 1 g in 10 ml Water for Injections BP.

Subconjunctival: Dissolve up to 500 mg in 0.5–0.75 ml of sterile water.

Nebuliser Solution: Dissolve 500 mg in 5 ml sterile water and administer by a suitable nebuliser.

Contra-indications, warnings, etc
Contra-indications: Penicillin hypersensitivity.

Side-effects: As with other penicillins.

Pharmaceutical precautions Celbenin should be kept in a cool, dry place.

Solutions should be used within 30 minutes of preparation.

Celbenin may be added to most intravenous fluids but should not be mixed with blood products or other proteinaceous fluids (e.g. protein hydrolysates).

Legal category POM.

Package quantities Celbenin vials are supplied in boxes of 10.

Further information Nil.

Product licence number 0038/5024.

FLOXAPEN* CAPSULES
FLOXAPEN* SYRUPS
FLOXAPEN* INJECTION

Presentation *Floxapen Capsules* (Flucloxacillin Capsules BP): Black and caramel capsules overprinted Floxapen, containing 250 mg or 500 mg flucloxacillin as Flucloxacillin Sodium BP.

Floxapen Vials for Injection (Flucloxacillin Injection BP): Each vial contains 250 mg, 500 mg or 1 g flucloxacillin as Flucloxacillin Sodium BP.

Floxapen Syrups (Flucloxacillin Mixture): Bottles containing powder for the preparation of 100 ml suspension. When reconstituted each 5 ml contains 125 mg or 250 mg flucloxacillin, as flucloxacillin magnesium.

Unidose sachets of powder for the preparation of a single dose of suspension. Each sachet contains 125 mg flucloxacillin as flucloxacillin magnesium.

Uses Floxapen is indicated for the treatment of infections due to Gram-positive organisms, including infections caused by β-lactamase-producing staphylococci. Typical indications include:

Skin and soft tissue infections: Boils. Abscesses. Carbuncles. Infected skin conditions, e.g. ulcer, eczema, and acne. Furunculosis. Cellulitis. Infected wounds. Infected burns. Protection for skin grafts. Otitis media and externa. Impetigo.

Respiratory tract infections: Pneumonia. Lung abscess. Empyema. Sinusitis. Pharyngitis. Tonsillitis. Quinsy.

Other infections caused by Floxapen-sensitive organisms: Osteomyelitis. Enteritis. Endocarditis. Urinary tract infection. Meningitis. Septicaemia.

Floxapen is also indicated for use as a prophylactic agent during major surgical procedures where appropriate; for example, cardiothoracic and orthopaedic surgery.

Dosage and administration
Usual adult dosage (including elderly patients)
Oral – 250 mg four times a day.
Intramuscular – 250 mg four times a day.
Intravenous – 250 mg – 1 g four times a day.

The above systemic dosages may be doubled where necessary; oral doses should be administered ½–1 hour before meals.
Osteomyelitis, endocarditis – Up to 8 g daily, in divided doses six to eight hourly.
Surgical prophylaxis – 1 to 2 g IV at induction of anaesthesia followed by 500 mg six hourly IV, IM, or orally for up to 72 hours.

Floxapen may be administered by other routes in conjunction with systemic therapy.
Intrapleural – 250 mg once daily.
By nebuliser – 125–250 mg four times a day.
Intra-articular – 250–500 mg once daily.
Intrathecal – Consult the Company's Medical Department.

Usual children's dosage
2–10 years: ½ adult dose.
Under 2 years: ¼ adult dose.

Abnormal renal function: In common with other penicillins, Floxapen usage in patients with renal impairment does not usually require dosage reduction. However, in the presence of severe renal failure (creatinine clearance

< 10 ml/min) a reduction in dose or an extension of dose interval should be considered.

Floxapen is not significantly removed by dialysis and hence no supplementary dosages need to be administered either during, or at the end of the dialysis period.

Administration

Intramuscular: Add 1.5 ml Water for Injections BP to 250 mg vial contents or 2 ml Water for Injections BP to 500 mg vial contents.

Intravenous: Dissolve 250–500 mg in 5–10 ml Water for Injections BP or 1 g in 15–20 ml Water for Injections BP. Administer by slow intravenous injection (three to four minutes). Floxapen may also be added to infusion fluids or injected, suitably diluted, into the drip tube over a period of three to four minutes.

Intrapleural: Dissolve 250 mg in 5–10 ml Water for Injections BP.

Intra-articular: Dissolve 250–500 mg in up to 5 ml Water for Injections BP or 0.5% lignocaine hydrochloride solution.

Intrathecal: An intrathecal preparation and further information may be obtained from the Company's Medical Department.

Nebuliser solution: Dissolve 125–250 mg of the vial contents in 3 ml sterile water.

Contra-indications, warnings, etc

Contra-indications: Penicillin hypersensitivity; ocular administration.

Side-effects: As with other penicillins.

Pharmaceutical precautions Floxapen Capsules and Floxapen Vials for Injection should be stored in a cool, dry place. Floxapen Syrups (bottles and sachets) should be stored in a dry place.

Once dispensed, Floxapen Syrups (bottles) remain stable for fourteen days when kept in a cool place. If a dilution of the reconstituted syrup is required, Syrup BP should be used.

Solutions for IM and direct IV injection should normally be administered within 30 minutes of preparation. However, aqueous solutions of Floxapen retain their activity for up to 24 hours at room temperature (25°C) and for up to 72 hours in a refrigerator (5°C). Reconstitution of the injection should be carried out under appropriate aseptic conditions if these extended storage periods are required.

Floxapen may be added to most intravenous fluids but should not be mixed with blood products or other proteinaceous fluids (e.g. protein hydrolysates).

If Floxapen is prescribed concurrently with an aminoglycoside, the two antibiotics should not be mixed in the syringe, intravenous fluid container or administration set; precipitation may occur.

For further information see package enclosure leaflet.

Legal category POM.

Package quantities
Capsules 250 mg: containers of 20, 100 and 500.
Capsules 500 mg: containers of 100.
Vials 250 mg or 500 mg: boxes of 10.
Vials 1 g: boxes of 5.
Syrup 125 mg/5 ml: 100 ml bottles.
Syrup Forte 250 mg/5 ml: 100 ml bottles.
Syrup 125 mg Unidose Sachets: boxes of 20 (hospital only).

Further information Floxapen syrups are now formulated using the magnesium salt of flucloxacillin, in preference to the sodium salt, in order to provide two palatable strengths of suspension.

Following oral administration Floxapen gives blood levels comparable to those achieved by intramuscular injection.

Product licence numbers
Floxapen Capsules 250 mg	0038/5055
Floxapen Capsules 500 mg	0038/5056
Floxapen Vials for Injection 250 mg	0038/5051
Floxapen Vials for Injection 500 mg	0038/5052
Floxapen Vials for Injection 1 g	0038/5053
Floxapen Syrup 125 mg/5 ml	0038/0309
Floxapen Syrup Forte 250 mg/5 ml	0038/0310
Floxapen Syrup 125 mg Unidose Sachet	0038/0311

MAGNAPEN* CAPSULES
MAGNAPEN* SYRUP
MAGNAPEN* INJECTION

Presentation *Magnapen Capsules:* Black and turquoise capsules overprinted 'Magnapen', containing 250 mg ampicillin as Ampicillin Trihydrate BP with 250 mg flucloxacillin as Flucloxacillin Sodium BP.

Magnapen Syrup: Bottles containing powder for the preparation of 100 ml suspension. When reconstituted each 5 ml contains 125 mg ampicillin as Ampicillin Trihydrate BP with 125 mg flucloxacillin as flucloxacillin magnesium.

Magnapen Vials for Injection: 500 mg Vial: containing 250 mg ampicillin as Ampicillin Sodium BP with 250 mg flucloxacillin as Flucloxacillin Sodium BP.

1 g Vial: containing 500 mg ampicillin as Ampicillin Sodium BP with 500 mg flucloxacillin as Flucloxacillin Sodium BP.

Uses Magnapen is indicated for the treatment of severe infections where the causative organism is unknown, and for mixed infections involving β-lactamase-producing staphylococci. Typical indications include:

In general practice: Chest infections, ENT infections, skin and soft tissue infections, and infections in patients whose underlying pathology places them at special risk.

In hospital (prior to laboratory results being available): Severe respiratory tract infections. Post-operative chest and wound infections. Septic abortion; puerperal fever. Septicaemia. Prophylaxis in major surgery. Infections in patients receiving immuno-suppressive therapy.

The spectrum of activity of Magnapen also makes it suitable for the treatment of many mixed infections, particularly those where β-lactamase-producing staphylococci are suspected or confirmed.

Dosage and administration
Usual adult dosage (including elderly patients):
Oral: 1 capsule or 10 ml syrup four times a day.
Intramuscular/Intravenous: 500 mg four times a day.

Usual children's dosage:
Oral: Under 10 years: 5 ml syrup four times a day.†
Intramuscular/Intravenous: Under 2 years: ¼ adult dose.†
2–10 years: ½ adult dose.

The above dosages for adults and children may be doubled where necessary.

† Ampiclox Neonatal is recommended for the treatment of infections in neonates and premature babies.

Oral doses should be administered $\frac{1}{2}$–1 hour before meals.

Administration: Intramuscular: 500 mg Vial: add 1.5 ml Water for Injections BP to vial contents. 1 g Vial: add 2 ml Water for Injections BP to vial contents.

Intravenous: Dissolve 500 mg in 10 ml Water for Injections BP, or 1 g in 20 ml Water for Injections BP. Administer by slow intravenous injection (3–4 minutes). Magnapen Injection may be added to infusion fluids or injected, suitably diluted into the drip tube over a period of 3–4 minutes.

Contra-indications, warnings, etc

Contra-indications: Penicillin hypersensitivity; ocular administration.

Side-effects: As with other penicillins. An erythematous rash may occasionally occur, as with ampicillin. The incidence of this rash is particularly high in patients with infectious mononucleosis. If a rash is reported it is advisable to discontinue treatment.

Pharmaceutical precautions Magnapen Capsules and Magnapen Vials for Injection should be stored in a cool, dry place. Magnapen Syrup should be stored in a dry place.

Once dispensed, Magnapen Syrup remains stable for 14 days when kept in a cool place. If a dilution of the reconstituted suspension is required, Syrup BP should be used.

Magnapen solutions for injection should be used immediately. Magnapen may be added to most intravenous fluids but should not be mixed with blood products or other proteinaceous fluids (e.g. protein hydrolysates). In intravenous solutions containing glucose or other carbohydrates, Magnapen should be infused within two hours.

Legal category POM.

Package quantities *Magnapen Capsules:* Containers of 20 and 100.
Magnapen Syrup: 100 ml bottles.
Magnapen Injections: Boxes of 10 vials.

Further information Infections encountered in medical practice can be of mixed bacteriology, often including β-lactamase-producing strains. Magnapen provides a broad spectrum of activity, which should be considered when dealing with such infections.

Magnapen Syrup is now formulated using the magnesium salt of flucloxacillin in preference to the sodium salt, in order to provide a more palatable suspension with extended stability.

Product licence numbers

Magnapen Capsules	0038/0090
Magnapen Syrup	0038/0324
Magnapen Vials 500 mg	0038/0089
Magnapen Vials 1 g	0038/0089

MAXOLON* TABLETS
MAXOLON* SYRUP
MAXOLON* PAEDIATRIC LIQUID
MAXOLON* INJECTION

Presentation *Maxolon Tablets:* (Metoclopramide Tablets BP): Small, white, scored tablets, engraved 'Maxolon'. Each tablet contains Metoclopramide Hydrochloride BP equivalent to 10 mg of the anhydrous substance.

Maxolon Syrup: Clear yellow, lemon/lime flavoured solution. Each 5 ml dose contains Metoclopramide Hydrochloride BP equivalent to 5 mg of the anhydrous substance.

Maxolon Paediatric Liquid: Clear, yellow, lemon/lime flavoured solution, in a bottle with a 1 ml pipette. Each 1 ml contains Metoclopramide Hydrochloride BP equivalent to 1 mg of the anhydrous substance.

Maxolon Ampoules (Metoclopramide Injection BP): Clear, colourless solution. Each 2 ml ampoule contains Metoclopramide Hydrochloride BP equivalent to 10 mg of the anhydrous substance.

Uses *Digestive disorders:* Maxolon restores normal co-ordination and tone to the upper digestive tract and relieves symptoms of gastro-duodenal dysfunction including:

Dyspepsia. Flatulence. Heartburn. Regurgitation of bile. Sickness. Pain. – associated with such conditions as:

Peptic ulcer. Reflux oesophagitis. Gastritis. Duodenitis. Hiatus hernia. Cholelithiasis and post-cholecystectomy dyspepsia.

Nausea and vomiting: Maxolon is indicated for the treatment of nausea and vomiting associated with:

Gastro-intestinal disorders. Cyclical vomiting. Intolerance to essential drugs including digitalis, antibacterial and cytotoxic drugs. Congestive heart failure. Deep X-ray or cobalt therapy. Post-anaesthetic vomiting.

Migraine: Maxolon relieves symptoms of nausea and vomiting, and overcomes gastric stasis associated with attacks of migraine. This improvement in gastric emptying assists the absorption of concurrently administered oral anti-migraine therapy (e.g. paracetamol) which may otherwise be impaired in such patients.

Post-operative conditions: Post-operative gastric hypotonia. Post-vagotomy syndrome. Maxolon promotes normal gastric emptying and restores motility in vagotomised patients, and where post-operative symptoms suggest gastro-duodenal dysfunction.

Diagnostic procedures: Radiology. Duodenal intubation. Maxolon speeds up the passage of a barium meal by decreasing gastric emptying time, co-ordinating peristalsis and dilating the duodenal bulb. Maxolon also facilitates duodenal intubation procedures.

Dosage and administration Total daily dosage of Maxolon, especially for children and young adults, should not normally exceed 0.5 mg/kg bodyweight.

Medical indications:

Oral:

Adults (including elderly patients)	10 mg three times daily
Young adults 15–20 years	5–10 mg three times daily, commencing at the lower dosage.
Children	Maxolon should only be used after careful examination to avoid masking an underlying disorder, e.g. cerebral irritation. The following dosage recommendations should be strictly adhered to if side-effects of the dystonic type are to be avoided.

5–14 years	2½–5 mg three times daily.	
3–5 years	2 mg two to three times daily.	
1–3 years	1 mg two to three times daily.	
Under 1 year	1 mg twice daily.	

Treatment of children should commence at the lower dosage.

Tablets should not be used in children under the age of 15. A liquid presentation should be used in the younger age groups: more accurate dosage is facilitated by the use of the paediatric liquid.

IM or IV:

Maxolon may be administered at the dosages stated above, either intramuscularly or by slow intravenous injection (1–2 min).

Diagnostic indications:
A single dose of Maxolon may be given 5–10 minutes before the examination.

Adults	(over 15 years)	10–20 mg
Children	5–14 years	2½–5 mg
	3–5 years	2 mg
	Under 3 years	1 mg

Abnormal renal or liver function: In patients with clinically significant degrees of renal or hepatic impairment, therapy should be initiated at half the usual dose. Subsequent dosage will depend on individual clinical response.

Contra-indications, warnings, etc

Use in pregnancy: Animal tests in several mammalian species and clinical experience have not indicated a teratogenic effect. Nevertheless, Maxolon should only be used when there are compelling reasons and is not advised during the first trimester.

Precautions: If vomiting persists the patient should be re-assessed to exclude the possibility of an underlying disorder, e.g. cerebral irritation.

Various extrapyramidal reactions to Maxolon, usually of the dystonic type, have been reported. The incidence of these reactions in children and young adults may be increased if daily dosages higher than 0.5 mg/kg body weight are administered. Reactions include: spasm of the facial muscles, trismus, rhythmic protrusion of the tongue, a bulbar type of speech, spasm of extra-ocular muscles including oculogyric crises, unnatural positioning of the head and shoulders and opisthotonos. There may be a generalised increase in muscle tone. The majority of reactions occur within 36 hours of starting treatment and the effects usually disappear within 24 hours of withdrawal of the drug. Should treatment of a dystonic reaction be required, an anticholinergic anti-Parkinsonian drug or a benzodiazepine may be used. Since extrapyramidal symptoms may occur with both Maxolon and phenothiazines, care should be exercised in the event of both drugs being prescribed concurrently.

Tardive dyskinesia has been reported during prolonged treatment in a small number of mainly elderly patients. Patients on prolonged treatment should be regularly reviewed.

Metoclopramide may induce an acute hypertensive response in patients with phaeochromocytoma.

Raised serum prolactin levels have been observed during metoclopramide therapy; this effect is similar to that noted with many other compounds.

The action of Maxolon on the gastro-intestinal tract is antagonised by anticholinergics.

Following operations such as pyloroplasty or gut anastomosis Maxolon therapy should be withheld for three or four days as vigorous muscular contractions may not help healing.

Pharmaceutical precautions Maxolon Syrup must be protected from light and should be dispensed into amber glass containers. It may be diluted with Purified Water BP but should not be stored diluted for long periods.

Once dispensed Maxolon Paediatric Liquid should be used within 14 days.

If ampoules are removed from their carton, they should be stored away from light. If inadvertent exposure occurs, ampoules showing discoloration must be discarded.

Compatibility: If the standard formulation of Maxolon is used for the treatment of nausea and vomiting associated with cytotoxic drugs, the cytotoxic agent should be administered as a separate infusion (see Further Information).

Legal category POM.

Package quantities *Tablets:* Containers of 100 and 500.
Syrup: Bottles of 200 ml and 1 litre.
Paediatric Liquid: 15 ml bottles with 1 ml pipette.
Ampoules: Boxes of 10.

Further information The action of Maxolon is closely associated with parasympathetic nervous control of the upper gastro-intestinal tract, where it has the effect of encouraging normal peristaltic action. This provides for a fundamental approach to the treatment of those conditions where disturbed gastro-intestinal motility is a common underlying factor.

The absorption of any concurrently administered oral medication may be modified by the effect of Maxolon on gastric motility.

Maxolon Syrup and Maxolon Paediatric Liquid are sugar-free formulations.

A separate parenteral formulation is available as Maxolon 'High Dose' (100 mg/20 ml) for the IV treatment of nausea and vomiting associated with cytotoxic drugs; it is specially formulated to be compatible in solution with cisplatin. This is the subject of a separate Data Sheet available from the Company.

Product licence numbers

Maxolon Tablets	0038/5041
Maxolon Syrup	0038/5040
Maxolon Paediatric Liquid	0038/0095
Maxolon Ampoules	0038/0098

MAXOLON* 'HIGH DOSE' ▼

Presentation *Maxolon 'High Dose' Ampoules:* Clear, colourless solution. Each 20 ml ampoule contains Metoclopramide Hydrochloride BP equivalent to 100 mg of the anhydrous substance.

Uses Maxolon 'High Dose' is indicated for the treatment of nausea and vomiting associated with intolerance to cytotoxic drugs.

Dosage and administration Maxolon 'High Dose' may be given in doses of up to 2 mg/kg body weight by IV infusion suitably diluted. The initial dose should be given prior to commencement of cytotoxic chemotherapy. Dosage may be repeated two-hourly up to a maximum of 10 mg/kg body weight in any 24 hour period. It is recommended that each dose be added to at least 50 ml of an appropriate diluent (see below), and infused over at least 15 minutes.

Abnormal renal or liver function: In patients with clinically significant degrees of renal or hepatic impairment, therapy should be initiated at half the usual dose. Subsequent dosage will depend on individual clinical response.

Note: The high dose ampoule presentation is not suitable for multidose use.

Compatibility with cytotoxic agents: Maxolon 'High Dose' is compatible with a number of cytotoxic drugs. However it should not be mixed in solution with therapeutic agents other than those stated.

Maxolon 'High Dose' is compatible with cisplatin, cyclophosphamide and doxorubicin hydrochloride and is stable over the concentration ranges listed below for 24 hours at room temperature when protected from light.

40–200 ml cisplatin (1 mg/ml) per 100 mg/20 ml Maxolon 'High Dose' in 1 litre of sodium chloride 0.9%.

Up to 40 mg doxorubicin hydrochloride (powder) per 100 mg/20 ml of Maxolon 'High Dose'.

Up to 4 g cyclophosphamide (1g/50 ml) per 100 mg/20 ml of Maxolon 'High Dose'.

Compatibility with morphine/diamorphine: Maxolon 'High Dose' is compatible with morphine hydrochloride and diamorphine hydrochloride and is stable over the concentration ranges listed below for 48 hours at room temperature under normal fluorescent lighting.

Up to 100 mg of morphine hydrochloride per 100 mg/20 ml of Maxolon 'High Dose'.

Up to 50 mg of diamorphine hydrochloride per 100 mg/20 ml of Maxolon 'High Dose'.

Maxolon 'High Dose' 100 mg/20 ml also remains stable for 48 hours at room temperature with 100 mg of morphine hydrochloride, or 50 mg diamorphine hydrochloride, when diluted 1 in 10 with sodium chloride 0.9%.

Stability in intravenous fluids: Ideally, intravenous solutions should be prepared at the time of infusion. However, Maxolon 'High Dose' has been shown to be stable for at least 48 hours at room temperature in the following solutions when administered in a PVC infusion bag (e.g. Viaflex* Travenol):

Sodium Chloride Intravenous Infusion BP (0.9% w/v)
Glucose Intravenous Infusion BP (5% w/v)
Sodium Chloride and Glucose Intravenous Infusion BP (sodium chloride 0.18% w/v; glucose 4% w/v)
Compound Sodium Lactate Intravenous Infusion BP (Ringer-Lactate Solution; Hartmann's Solution).

Contra-indications, warnings, etc

Use in pregnancy: Animal tests in several mammalian species and clinical experience have not indicated a teratogenic effect. Nevertheless, Maxolon should only be used when there are compelling reasons and is not advised during the first trimester.

Precautions: When given at high dose in association with cancer chemotherapy, Maxolon has been found to be well tolerated with few adverse effects, the most common being mild sedation.

Various extrapyramidal reactions to Maxolon, usually of the dystonic type, have been reported. Studies of Maxolon given in doses up to 10 mg/kg body weight/day by IV infusion report an incidence of extrapyramidal

reactions of less than 10%. The incidence of such reactions may be increased in the younger patient.

Reactions to Maxolon have included: Spasm of the facial muscles, trismus, rhythmic protrusion of the tongue, a bulbar type of speech, spasm of extra-ocular muscles including oculogyric crises, unnatural positioning of the head and shoulders and opisthotonos. There may be a generalised increase in muscle tone. The majority of reactions occur within 36 hours of starting treatment and the effects usually disappear within 24 hours of withdrawal of the drug. Should treatment of a dystonic reaction be required an anticholinergic anti-Parkinsonian drug, or a benzodiazepine may be used. Since extrapyramidal symptoms may occur with both Maxolon and phenothiazines, care should be exercised in the event of both drugs being prescribed concurrently.

Metoclopramide may induce an acute hypertensive response in patients with phaeochromocytoma.

Raised serum prolactin levels have been observed during metoclopramide therapy: this effect is similar to that noted with many other compounds.

The action of Maxolon on the gastro-intestinal tract is antagonised by anticholinergics.

Following operations such as pyloroplasty or gut anastomosis Maxolon therapy should be withheld for three or four days as vigorous muscular contractions may not help healing.

Pharmaceutical precautions If ampoules are removed from their carton they should be stored away from light. If inadvertent exposure occurs, ampoules showing discoloration must be discarded.

Legal category POM.

Package quantities 'High Dose' Ampoules: Boxes of 10.

Further information Maxolon 'High Dose' is specifically for use in the management of cytotoxic intolerance. It is specially formulated to ensure compatibility in solution with cisplatin. The 20 ml ampoule provides ease of administration.

Maxolon exerts a three-fold anti-emetic action: By inhibiting central dopamine receptors Maxolon raises the threshold of the chemoreceptor trigger zone, and reduces the reaction of the adjacent vomiting centre to centrally-acting emetics. Maxolon decreases the sensitivity of the visceral afferent nerves to the vomiting centre, reducing the effect of locally-acting emetics and irritant substances. In the upper gastro-intestinal tract Maxolon promotes normal gastric emptying and it may thus abolish gastric stasis which is part of the vomiting reflex.

The absorption of any concurrently administered oral medication may be modified by the effect of Maxolon on gastric motility.

Maxolon 'High Dose' is not intended for use in the wider range of indications for which Maxolon at standard dose is indicated. The separate Maxolon Data Sheet should be consulted for such uses.

Product licence number Maxolon 'High Dose' Ampoules for Injection: 0038/0300.

ORBENIN* CAPSULES
ORBENIN* SYRUP
ORBENIN* INJECTION

Presentation *Orbenin Capsules* (Cloxacillin Capsules BP): Orange and black capsules overprinted 'Orbenin', containing 250 mg or 500 mg cloxacillin as Cloxacillin Sodium BP.

Orbenin Syrup (Cloxacillin Elixir BP): Bottles containing powder for the preparation of 100 ml syrup.

When reconstituted each 5 ml contains 125 mg cloxacillin as Cloxacillin Sodium BP.

Orbenin Vials for Injection (Cloxacillin Injection BP): Each vial contains 250 mg, 500 mg or 1 g cloxacillin as Cloxacillin Sodium BP.

Uses Orbenin is indicated for the treatment of infections caused by Gram-positive organisms, including infections caused by β-lactamase-producing staphylococci.

Typical indications include:

Skin and soft tissue infections: Boils. Abscesses. Carbuncles. Furunculosis. Cellulitis. Infected wounds. Infected burns. Protection for skin grafts. Otitis media and externa.

Infected skin conditions, e.g. ulcer, eczema and acne.

Respiratory tract infections: Pneumonia. Lung abscess. Empyema. Sinusitis. Pharyngitis. Tonsillitis. Quinsy.

Other infections caused by Orbenin-sensitive organisms: Osteomyelitis. Enteritis. Endocarditis. Urinary tract infection. Meningitis. Septicaemia.

Dosage and administration *Usual adult dosage (including elderly patients):*
Oral: 500 mg four times a day.
Intramuscular: 250 mg four to six hourly.
Intravenous: 500 mg four to six hourly.

Systemic dosages may be doubled where necessary: oral dosages should be administered $\frac{1}{2}$–1 hour before meals.
Intrapleural: 500 mg once daily.
Intrathecal: Consult the Company's Medical Department.
Intra-articular: 500 mg once daily.
By nebuliser: 125–250 mg four times a day.

Usual children's dosage:
2–10 years: $\frac{1}{2}$ adult dose.
Under 2 years: $\frac{1}{4}$ adult dose.

Administration: Intramuscular: Add 1.5 ml Water for Injections BP to 250 mg vial contents or 2 ml Water for Injections BP to 500 mg vial contents.
Intravenous: Dissolve 500 mg in 10 ml or 1 g in 15–20 ml Water for Injections BP. Administer by slow intravenous injection (three to four minutes). Orbenin may also be added to infusion fluids or injected, suitably diluted, into the drip tube over a period of three to four minutes.

Orbenin may be administered by other routes in conjunction with systemic therapy.
Intrapleural: Dissolve 500 mg in 5–10 ml Water for Injections BP.
Intra-articular: Dissolve 500 mg in up to 5 ml Water for Injections BP or 0.5% lignocaine hydrochloride solution.

Nebuliser Solution: Dissolve 125–250 mg of the vial contents in 3 ml sterile water and administer by a suitable nebuliser.

Contra-indications, warnings, etc
Contra-indications: Penicillin hypersensitivity; ocular administration.

Side-effects: As with other penicillins.

Pharmaceutical precautions Orbenin should be stored in a cool, dry place.

Once dispensed, Orbenin Syrup remains stable for seven days if kept in a cool place. If a dilution of the reconstituted syrup is required, Syrup BP should be used.

Solutions for IM and direct IV injection should normally be administered within 30 minutes of preparation. However, aqueous solutions of Orbenin retain their activity for up to 24 hours at room temperature (25°C) and for up to 72 hours in a refrigerator (5°C). Reconstitution of the injection should be carried out under appropriate aseptic conditions if these extended storage periods are required.

Orbenin may be added to most intravenous fluids but should not be mixed with blood products or other proteinaceous fluids (e.g. protein hydrolysates).

If Orbenin is prescribed concurrently with an aminoglycoside, the two antibiotics should not be mixed in the syringe, intravenous fluid container or administration set; precipitation may occur.

For further information see package enclosure leaflet.

Legal category POM.

Package quantities *Capsules 250 mg or 500 mg:* Containers of 100.
Vials 250 mg or 500 mg: Boxes of 10.
Vials 1 g: Box of 100.
Syrup: 100 ml bottles.

Further information Nil.

Product licence numbers

Orbenin Capsules 250 mg	0038/5028
Orbenin Capsules 500 mg	0038/5029
Orbenin Vials for Injection 250 mg	0038/5025
Orbenin Vials for Injection 500 mg	0038/5026
Orbenin Vials for Injection 1 g	0038/5027
Orbenin Syrup	0038/0128

PARAMAX*

Presentation *Paramax Tablets:* White, round scored tablets, engraved 'Paramax' on one side.
Paramax Sachets: Sachets containing effervescent powder.

Each tablet or sachet contains 500 mg Paracetamol BP with Metoclopramide Hydrochloride BP equivalent to 5 mg of the anhydrous substance.

Uses *Indications:* Paramax is indicated for the symptomatic treatment of migraine.

Action: Paracetamol relieves pain. More rapid absorption is promoted by the action of metoclopramide which also relieves gastric stasis and overcomes nausea and vomiting.

Dosage and administration For oral administration only.

Paramax should be taken at the first warning of an attack. If symptoms persist, further doses may be taken at four-hourly intervals. Total dosage in any 24-hour period should not exceed the quantity stated.

Usual Recommended Dosage (Tablets or Sachets)

	Initial dose at first warning of attack	Maximum dosage in any 24-hour period
Adults (including elderly patients)	2	6
Young Adults (15–20 years)	1 or 2	5
Adolescents (12–14 years)	1	3

Children: A presentation of Paramax suitable for the treatment of children under 12 years of age is not available.

Note: Total daily dosage of metoclopramide should not exceed 0.5 mg/kg body weight.

Paramax Sachets: Empty a sachet into about $\frac{1}{4}$ of a glass of water and stir before taking.

Contra-indications, warnings, etc
Use in pregnancy: There is no evidence that metoclopramide or paracetamol by themselves have teratogenic effects. Nevertheless, Paramax should only be used when there are compelling reasons and is not advised during the first trimester.

Precautions: If vomiting persists the patient should be re-assessed to exclude the possibility of an underlying disorder, e.g. cerebral irritation.

Various extra-pyramidal reactions to metoclopramide, usually of the dystonic type, have been reported. The incidence of these reactions may be increased if the metoclopramide dosage exceeds 0.5 mg/kg body weight/day. Reactions include: spasm of the facial muscles, trismus, rhythmic protrusion of the tongue, a bulbar type of speech, spasm of extra-ocular muscles, including oculogyric crises, unnatural positioning of the head and shoulders and opisthotonos. There may be a generalised increase in muscle tone. The majority of reactions occur within 36 hours of starting treatment and the effects usually disappear within 24 hours of withdrawal of the drug. Should treatment of a dystonic reaction be required, a benzodiazepine or an anticholinergic anti-Parkinson drug may be used.

Care should be exercised in the event of Paramax being prescribed concurrently with a phenothiazine since extra-pyramidal symptoms may occur with both products. The action of metoclopramide on the gastro-intestinal tract is antagonised by anticholinergics.

Metoclopramide may induce an acute hypertensive response in patients with phaeochromocytoma.

Raised serum prolactin levels have been observed during metoclopramide therapy; this effect is similar to that noted with many other compounds.

As with other paracetamol-containing products, an overdose of Paramax can be toxic to the liver. Overdosage should be treated by gastric lavage with appropriate supportive measures. Intravenous N-acetylcysteine or oral methionine if administered within 10 hours of paracetamol overdosage appears to exert a protective effect on the liver.

Pharmaceutical precautions Protect tablets from light. Store sachets in a dry place.

Legal category POM.

Package quantities *Paramax tablets:* Pack of 108. Each pack contains 6 blister strips of 18 tablets. *Paramax sachets:* Carton of 30.

Further information An acute attack of migraine is frequently characterised by impaired absorption of analgesics even when abdominal symptoms are absent. The beneficial effect of Paramax on delayed gastric emptying, nausea and vomiting contrasts with the gastric stasis which may occur following administration of phenothiazine or antihistamine antiemetics.

Product licence numbers
Paramax Tablets   0038/0256
Paramax Sachets   0038/0257

PAYNOCIL*
Presentation *Appearance:* Flat, circular, white, scored tablet engraved on one side with the product name 'PAYNOCIL'.

Active ingredients: Each tablet contains:

Aspirin (acetylsalicylic acid)	600 mg
Glycine (aminoacetic acid)	300 mg

Uses *Principal action:* Aspirin is an analgesic, and antipyretic.

The glycine content allows the tablet to disperse instantly on the tongue and be rapidly distributed into the stomach in fine glycine-coated particles; the risk of gastric irritation is therefore minimised.

Uses: Pain and Febrile conditions in which aspirin is indicated.

Rheumatoid Arthritis and other rheumatic conditions in which high and sustained dosage with plain aspirin tablets may increase the risk of intolerance.

Dosage and administration Paynocil should be taken orally. It can be taken without water as the lemon flavoured glycine coating of the particles masks the unpleasant taste of aspirin.

Adult dosage (including elderly patients): As Paynocil contains 600 mg aspirin per tablet it is twice the strength of Aspirin Tablets BP and in equivalent dosage is twice as rapidly absorbed.

Analgesic/antipyretic: 1 tablet, every four to six hours if required.

In Rheumatoid Arthritis: for the treatment of early and recurrent rheumatoid arthritis, it is recommended that 2–3 tablets should be taken three times a day for two to three weeks. When the patient responds, the dosage should be reduced to 1–2 tablets three times a day as a maintenance dose.

Do not exceed the stated dose.

Contra-indications, warnings, etc
Contra-indications: Paynocil should not be given when aspirin is contra-indicated: e.g. hypersensitivity, peptic ulceration, haemophilia.

Use in pregnancy: As aspirin is a prostaglandin-synthetase inhibitor and may affect blood clotting, therapy should ideally be withheld at term and during labour.

Precautions: Aspirin may enhance the effects of anticoagulants, inhibit the action of uricosurics and precipitate attacks of asthma in susceptible individuals.

Side-effects: Aspirin may induce gastro-intestinal haemorrhage (occasionally severe). Gastric irritation, however, is minimised with Paynocil as the aspirin particles are coated with glycine.

Overdosage: Irrespective of the reported time interval since ingestion, gastric aspiration and lavage should be performed. Blood must be taken for plasma salicylate estimation. Forced alkaline diuresis may be needed.

Pharmaceutical precautions Store in a cool, dry place.

Legal category P.

Package quantities 30 tablets in foil strips of 6.

Further information Paynocil is rapidly absorbed and well tolerated. It is easy to take because of the glycine formulation and palatable lemon flavour.

Product licence number 0038/5081.

PENBRITIN* CAPSULES
PENBRITIN* SYRUP
PENBRITIN* SYRUP FORTE
PENBRITIN* PAEDIATRIC SUSPENSION
PENBRITIN* PAEDIATRIC TABLETS
PENBRITIN* INJECTION

Presentation *Penbritin Capsules* (Ampicillin Capsules BP): black and red capsules overprinted 'Penbritin', containing 250 mg or 500 mg ampicillin as Ampicillin Trihydrate BP.

Penbritin Syrup (Ampicillin Mixture BP): Bottles containing powder for the preparation of 100 ml cream-coloured suspension. When reconstituted each 5 ml contains 125 mg ampicillin as Ampicillin Trihydrate BP.

Penbritin Syrup Forte (Strong Ampicillin Mixture BP): Bottles containing powder for the preparation of 100 ml cream-coloured suspension. When reconstituted each 5 ml contains 250 mg ampicillin as Ampicillin Trihydrate BP.

Penbritin Paediatric Suspension: Bottles containing powder for the preparation of 25 ml pink-coloured suspension. When reconstituted each 1.25 ml contains 125 mg ampicillin as Ampicillin Trihydrate BP. A pipette to measure the 1.25 ml dose is provided.

Penbritin Paediatric Tablets (Ampicillin Tablets BP): Flavoured, off-white, scored tablets engraved 'Penbritin'. Each tablet contains 125 mg ampicillin as Ampicillin Trihydrate BP.

Penbritin Vials for Injection (Ampicillin Sodium BP for Injection): Each vial contains 250 mg or 500 mg ampicillin as Ampicillin Sodium BP.

Uses Penbritin is a broad-spectrum penicillin, indicated for the treatment of a wide range of bacterial infections caused by ampicillin-sensitive organisms.

Typical indications include: Ear, nose and throat infections. Bronchitis. Pneumonia. Urinary tract infections. Gonorrhoea. Gynaecological infections. Septicaemia. Peritonitis. Endocarditis. Meningitis. Enteric fever. Gastro-intestinal infections.

Extraperitoneal application of Penbritin to wounds can be used to prevent infection following abdominal surgery.

Dosage and administration *Usual adult dosage* (including elderly patients) – oral, except where stated:

Ear, nose and throat infections: 250 mg four times a day.
Bronchitis: Routine therapy: 250 mg four times a day.
       High-dosage therapy: 1 g four times a day.
Pneumonia: 500 mg four times a day.
Urinary tract infections: 500 mg three times a day.
Gonorrhoea: 2 g orally with 1 g probenecid as a single dose. Repeated doses are recommended for the treatment of females.
Gastro-intestinal infections: 500–750 mg three to four times daily.
Enteric: Acute: 1–2 g four times a day for two weeks.
    Carriers: 1–2 g four times a day for four to twelve weeks.

Septicaemia, endocarditis, osteomyelitis: 500 mg four to six times a day IM or IV for one to six weeks.
Peritonitis, intra-abdominal sepsis: 500 mg four times a day IM or IV.
Meningitis: Adult dosage: 2 g six-hourly IV.
Children's dosage: 150 mg/kg daily IV in divided doses. (Intrathecal therapy may be given concurrently – see below.)
Usual children's dosage (under 10 years): $\frac{1}{2}$ adult routine dosage.

All recommended dosages are a guide only. In severe infections the above dosages may be increased, or Penbritin given by injection. Oral doses of Penbritin should be taken half to one hour before meals.

Administration: Oral: Capsules, Syrups, Paediatric Suspension or Paediatric Tablets.
Intramuscular: Add 1.5 ml Water for Injections BP to 250 mg or 500 mg vial contents.
Intravenous: Dissolve 250 mg in 5 ml or 500 mg in 10 ml Water for Injections BP. Administer by slow injection (three to four minutes). Penbritin may also be added to infusion fluids or injected, suitably diluted, into the drip tube over a period of three to four minutes.

Penbritin may also be administered by other routes in conjunction with systemic therapy.
Intraperitoneal: 500 mg daily in up to 10 ml Water for Injections BP.
Intrapleural: 500 mg daily in 5–10 ml Water for Injections BP.
Intra-articular: 500 mg daily, in up to 5 ml Water for Injections BP or sterile 0.5% procaine hydrochloride solution.
Intrathecal: An intrathecal preparation and further information may be obtained from the Company's Medical Department.
Local use in abdominal surgery: 1 g sterile powder sprinkled into the wound extraperitoneally or into muscle layers to prevent wound infection post-operatively.

Contra-indications, warnings, etc
Contra-indications: Penicillin hypersensitivity.

Side-effects: Side-effects, as with other penicillins, are rare and usually of a mild, transitory nature. Two types of rashes have been observed: an urticarial rash which is usually indicative of true penicillin hypersensitivity and an erythematous rash which is generally specific to ampicillin. The incidence of this erythematous rash is particularly high in patients with infectious mononucleosis. If a rash is reported it is advisable to discontinue treatment.

Pharmaceutical precautions Penbritin should be stored in a cool dry place.

Once dispensed, Penbritin Syrups and Paediatric Suspension remain stable for seven days if kept in a cool place. If a dilution of the reconstituted syrup is required, Syrup BP should be used.

Penbritin solutions for injection should be used immediately.

Penbritin may be added to most intravenous fluids but should not be mixed with blood products or other proteinaceous fluids (e.g. protein hydrolysates). In intravenous solutions containing glucose or other carbohydrates, Penbritin should be infused within one hour of preparation.

Legal category POM.

Package quantities *Penbritin Capsules 250 mg:* Containers of 100 and 500.

Penbritin Capsules 500 mg: Containers of 100.
Penbritin Vials for Injection 250 mg, 500 mg: Boxes of 10.
Penbritin Syrup and Syrup Forte: 100 ml bottles.
Penbritin Paediatric Suspension: Bottles of 25 ml.
Penbritin Paediatric Tablets: Containers of 100.

Further information Nil.

Product licence numbers

Penbritin Capsules 250 mg	0038/5074
Penbritin Capsules 500 mg	0038/5075
Penbritin Vials for Injection 250 mg	0038/5060
Penbritin Vials for Injection 500 mg	0038/5061
Penbritin Syrup	0038/5067
Penbritin Syrup Forte	0038/5068
Penbritin Paediatric Suspension	0038/5066
Penbritin Paediatric Tablets	0038/5072

PYOPEN* INJECTION

Presentation *Pyopen 1 g Vial:* Vials containing 1 g carbenicillin as Carbenicillin Sodium BP.

Pyopen 5 g Vial: Vials containing 5 g carbenicillin as Carbenicillin Sodium BP.

Uses Pyopen is indicated primarily for the treatment of infections caused by sensitive Pseudomonas and Proteus species.

At recommended dosages, Pyopen is also effective against a wide range of other Gram-negative and Gram-positive bacteria, including: Escherichia coli, Haemophilus influenzae, Bacteroides fragilis and other anaerobes, Clostridium spp., Staphylococcus aureus (penicillin sensitive), Streptococcus spp.

Typical indications include: General Systemic Infections, Respiratory Tract Infections, Septicaemia, Urinary Tract Infections, Post-surgical Infections, Intra-abdominal sepsis, Endocarditis, Meningitis, Infected Burns, Infected Wounds.

In life-threatening infections, consideration should be given to the synergistic effects of Pyopen and a parenteral aminoglycoside; they should be given separately, at recommended dosages.

Dosage and administration *Dosage:* See table below.
Preparation
1 gram vial: Intramuscular: Add 2 ml Water for Injections BP to the contents of the vial and shake vigorously.
Intravenous: Add 5 ml Water for Injections BP to the contents of the vial and shake vigorously. Dilute to 20 ml.

5 gram vial (50 ml): Intravenous injection: Add at least 20 ml Water for Injections BP to the contents of the 5 g vial and shake vigorously.

Intravenous infusion: Add 20 ml Water for Injections BP to the contents of the 5 g vial, shake vigorously and add to a suitable volume of infusion fluid (approximately 100–150 ml).

Water for Injections BP is the preferred diluent for intravenous infusion of Pyopen. Alternatively, the antibiotic may be infused in a sterile solution of glucose of 5% or lower concentration. (The use of 0.9% sodium chloride solution as diluent will add to the sodium load of Pyopen and is, therefore, not usually recommended). The use of the appropriate diluents, when Pyopen is given intravenously, will reduce the possibility of phlebitis.

Heat is generated when Pyopen is dissolved; some warming of the contents of the vial may consequently be experienced.

N.B. Pyopen vials are not suitable for multi-dose use.

Administration: Intramuscular: Pyopen should be given every six hours.

Intravenous: Pyopen should be given every four to six hours by slow injection (three to four minutes) or by rapid infusion over 30–40 minutes (i.e. at a rate of approximately 50 drips per minute). Infusion over longer periods may result in sub-therapeutic serum concentrations.

Higher and more prolonged serum concentrations may be achieved with concurrent oral administration of probenecid (1 g three times a day in adults); however,

Dosage of Pyopen

Infection	Organism	
	Pseudomonas	Proteus spp.
Adult (incl. elderly patients) Respiratory tract infections Chronic urinary tract infections Infected wounds and burns	5 g IV four to six-hourly	2 g IM six-hourly
Systemic infections Septicaemia, endocarditis, meningitis	5 g IV four-hourly	5 g IV six-hourly
Acute uncomplicated urinary tract infections	2 g IM six-hourly	1–2 g IM six-hourly
Paediatric (daily dosage per kg body weight: to be administered in divided doses 4–8 hourly)		
Respiratory tract infections Chronic urinary tract infections Infected wounds and burns	250–400 mg per kg per day IV	100 mg per kg per day IM
Systemic infections Septicaemia, endocarditis, meningitis	400 mg per kg per day IV	250 mg per kg per day IV
Acute uncomplicated urinary tract infections	100 mg per kg per day IM	50–100 mg per kg per day IM

caution should be exercised in the administration of probenecid to patients with impaired renal function.

Pyopen may be administered by other routes in conjunction with systemic therapy.

Intra-articular: Add 2–4 ml Water for Injections BP or 0.5% lignocaine hydrochloride solution to the contents of a 1 g vial. 500 mg to 1 g once daily is a suitable dosage.

Intrapleural: Add 5 ml Water for Injections BP to the contents of a 1 g vial. Dilute to 10 ml. This dosage is normally given once daily.

Nebuliser Solution: Dissolve 250–500 mg Pyopen powder in 3–5 ml of water and administer four times daily by a suitable nebuliser.

Subconjunctival: A 25% solution (125 mg in Lignocaine and Adrenaline Injection BP) is recommended.

Local irrigation: A 0.2% solution of Pyopen should be used.

Contra-indications, warnings, etc

Contra-indication: Penicillin hypersensitivity.

Side-effects: Side-effects are uncommon and typical of other injectable penicillins. If pain at the intramuscular injection site is troublesome, the vial contents may be dissolved in 0.5% lignocaine hydrochloride solution. In rare cases, spontaneous skin and mucous membrane haemorrhages due to interference with normal clotting mechanisms have been reported.

Precautions: Except in cases of renal impairment, recommended dosages should never be reduced. Administration at less than full dosage may permit the multiplication of resistant strains, especially of Pseudomonas. Where renal function is impaired, Pyopen dosage may be reduced. However, monitoring is advisable in these cases to ensure that adequate serum antibiotic concentrations are achieved. In treating patients on sodium restriction it should be noted that each 1 g vial of Pyopen contains 5.4 mmol sodium (approx. 124 mg), and each 5 g vial contains 27.1 mmol sodium.

When Pyopen is used with an aminoglycoside the usual dosage should be adopted; concurrent therapy is not an opportunity to secure dosage reduction unless indicated for other reasons – for instance renal failure.

If Pyopen is prescribed with a parenteral aminoglycoside, the compounds should be administered separately.

Pharmaceutical precautions *Stability and storage:*
Pyopen is unstable to heat and is very hygroscopic. The vials of dry powder should be stored in a refrigerator at 5°C.

Solutions for IM and direct IV injection should normally be administered within 30 minutes of preparation. However, aqueous solutions of Pyopen retain their activity for up to 24 hours at room temperature (25°C) and for up to 72 hours in a refrigerator (5°C). Reconstitution of the injection should be carried out under appropriate aseptic conditions if these extended storage periods are required.

Compatibility: Pyopen is compatible with intravenous solutions in general use except: proteinaceous fluids (e.g. protein hydrolysates), blood and plasma, intravenous lipids.

Legal category POM.

Package quantities
Pyopen 1 g Vials: Cartons of 10.
Pyopen 5 g Vials: Cartons of 6 (50 ml vials).

Further information Pyopen continues to be effective in patients with lowered host defences.

Product licence numbers
Pyopen 1 g Vials	0038/5035
Pyopen 5 g Vials	0038/5037

TALPEN*

Presentation *Talpen Tablets:* Red film coated tablets, engraved Talpen on one side. Each tablet contains 250 mg of the ampicillin ester, talampicillin hydrochloride.

Talpen Syrup: Bottles containing powder for the preparation of 100 ml suspension. When reconstituted each 5 ml contains talampicillin napsylate (167 mg) equivalent to 125 mg talampicillin hydrochloride.

Uses Following oral administration, Talpen is particularly well absorbed and rapidly hydrolysed to give high blood levels of ampicillin. Talpen is indicated for the oral treatment of a wide range of bacterial infections caused by ampicillin-sensitive organisms, for example:

Gram-positive: Penicillin sensitive *Staph. aureus, Strep. pyogenes, Strep. faecalis, Strep. viridans, Strep. pneumoniae, Clostridium species, Bacillus anthracis, Corynebacterium diphtheriae.*

Gram-negative: Neisseria gonorrhoeae, Neisseria meningitidis, Escherichia coli, Haemophilus influenzae, Bordetella pertussis, Salmonella typhi, Salmonella paratyphi, Salmonellae (other), *Shigella* species, *Brucella* species, *Proteus mirabilis.*

Typical indications include: Acute and chronic bronchitis; Pneumonia; Ear, nose and throat infections; Gynaecological infections; Urinary tract infections; Skin and soft tissue infections; Gonorrhoea.

Dosage and administration *Usual adult oral dosage (including elderly patients):* †One Talpen tablet or 10 ml Talpen Syrup, three times a day.

Gonorrhoea: 1.5–2 g talampicillin hydrochloride as a single dose, is recommended.

Usual children's oral dosage: (2–10 years) †5 ml Talpen Syrup, three times a day. (Under two years) the equivalent of 3–7 mg talampicillin hydrochloride per kilogram body weight, three times a day.

Total ampicillin availability following oral administration of Talpen is unaffected by food.

† Dosage may be doubled in severe infections.

Contra-indications, warnings, etc
Contra-indication: Penicillin hypersensitivity.

Precaution: Talpen is not recommended for patients with severe renal or hepatic impairment.

Side-effects: As with other penicillins. These are rare and usually of a mild and transitory nature. An erythematous rash may occasionally occur. The incidence of this rash is particularly high in patients with infectious mononucleosis. Controlled clinical trials have shown that the incidence of diarrhoea as a side-effect is significantly lower following the administration of Talpen than following oral ampicillin.

Pharmaceutical precautions Talpen should be stored in tightly closed containers and kept in a cool dry place. Once dispensed, Talpen Syrup remains stable for seven days if kept in a cool place. If a dilution of the reconstituted syrup is required, Syrup BP should be used.

Legal category POM.

Package quantities
Talpen Tablets: Bottles of 100 and 500.
Talpen Syrup: Bottles of 100 ml.

Further information Following oral administration of 250 mg Talpen, ampicillin peak serum concentrations are twice those obtained from 250 mg ampicillin capsules and are usually achieved in half the time This excellent absorption is further reflected in urinary recovery studies.

Each 250 mg of talampicillin hydrochloride is chemically equivalent to 169 mg of ampicillin.

Product licence numbers
Talpen Tablets   0038/0209
Talpen Syrup   0038/0243

TICAR*

Presentation *Ticar 1 g vial:* Vials containing 1 g ticarcillin as ticarcillin sodium.

Ticar 3 g vial: Vials containing 3 g ticarcillin as ticarcillin sodium.

Ticar 5 g vial: Vials containing 5 g ticarcillin as ticarcillin sodium.

Ticar infusion: Infusion bottles containing 5 g ticarcillin as ticarcillin sodium.

Uses Ticar is an injectable broad-spectrum penicillin indicated for the treatment of a wide range of bacterial infections. Sensitive organisms include:

Streptococcus species
Staphylococcus aureus (penicillin sensitive)
Clostridium species
Bacteroides species and other anaerobes
Pseudomonas species
Proteus species
E. coli
Haemophilus influenzae

Typical indications include:

General Systemic Infections
Respiratory Tract Infections
Septicaemia
Urinary Tract Infections
Peritonitis, intra-abdominal sepsis
Endocarditis
Infected burns
Infected wounds
Post-surgical infections

Ticar acts synergistically with aminoglycosides against Pseudomonas and other organisms. When Ticar is prescribed concurrently with an aminoglycoside the two products should be administered separately, at recommended dosages.

Dosage and administration *Dosage: Adults (including elderly patients):* The usual recommended daily dosage is 15–20 g administered in divided doses, usually at 4–8 hourly intervals.

For the treatment of acute uncomplicated urinary tract infections the usual recommended daily dosage is 3–4 g in divided doses, usually at 4–8 hourly intervals.

Children: The usual recommended dosage for children is 200–300 mg/kg/day in divided doses, usually at 4–8 hourly intervals.

For acute uncomplicated urinary tract infections the recommended dosage is 50–100 mg/kg/day in divided doses, usually at 4–8 hourly intervals.

Abnormal Renal Function: If renal function is impaired as indicated by urea or creatinine levels monitoring of antibiotic serum levels is advised and a reduction in dosage may need to be considered. In renal failure an appropriate adult dose would be 2 g every 8–12 hours. In such cases the serum half life may be as long as 13 hours compared with 70 minutes in normal subjects. (Corresponding reductions in dosage should be considered for children.)

Haemodialysis removes Ticar from the blood stream therefore a supplementary 2 g dose is recommended midway through the dialysis period.

Peritoneal dialysis removes Ticar at a slower rate than haemodialysis therefore a dosage of 2 g 8 hourly is recommended.

Preparation: 1 gram vial: Intramuscular – Add 2 ml Water for Injections BP and shake vigorously.

Intravenous – Add 5 ml Water for Injections BP and shake vigorously. Dilute to 20 ml.

3 gram vial: Intravenous injection: Add 20 ml Water for Injections BP and shake vigorously.

Intravenous infusion: Add 20 ml Water for Injections BP shake vigorously and add to a suitable volume of infusion fluid (approximately 100 ml).

5 gram vial: Intravenous injection: Add 20 ml Water for Injections BP and shake vigorously.

Intravenous infusion: Add 20 ml Water for Injections BP shake vigorously and add to a suitable volume of infusion fluid (approximately 100–150 ml).

Water for Injections BP is the preferred diluent for intravenous infusion of Ticar. Alternatively, the antibiotic may be infused in a sterile glucose solution of 5% or lower concentration. (The use of 0.9% sodium chloride solution as diluent will add to the sodium load of ticarcillin and is, therefore, not usually recommended). The use of these appropriate diluents, when Ticar is given intravenously, will reduce the possibility of phlebitis.

Infusion pack: See detailed instructions on Transfer Needle leaflet and Package Enclosure leaflet.

Reconstituted solutions of Ticar are normally a pale straw colour.

Heat is generated when Ticar dissolves. Ticar vials may therefore become warm during preparation of solutions for injection.

Ticar vials are not suitable for multi-dose use.

Administration: When administered intravenously Ticar should be given by slow injection (three to four minutes) or by infusion over e.g. 30–40 minutes (i.e. at a rate of approximately 50 drops per minute). Infusion over long periods may result in subtherapeutic concentrations.

Higher and more prolonged serum concentrations may be achieved with concurrent oral administration of probenecid (1 g three times a day in adults); however, caution should be exercised in the administration of probenecid to patients with impaired renal function.

Other routes of administration: Insufficient clinical information is available to assess fully the value of Ticar by the following routes of administration. In life-threatening infections, however, the following dosage guidelines may be helpful. In all cases systemic Ticar therapy, at full dosage, should also be administered.

Nebuliser solution: Dissolve 500 mg Ticar powder in 3–5 ml water (or smaller volume if required). Administer this dosage three to four times daily by a suitable nebuliser.

Intra-articular: Add 2–4 ml Water for Injections BP or 0.5% lignocaine hydrochloride solution to the contents of a 1 g vial. 500 mg to 1 g is a suitable dosage.

Intrapleural: Add 5 ml Water for Injections BP to the contents of a 1 g vial. Dilute to 10–20 ml. This dosage is normally given once daily.

Local irrigation: A 0.2% solution of Ticar may be used.

Intrathecal: Further information may be obtained from the Company's Medical Department.

Contra-indications, warnings, etc
Contra-indication: Penicillin hypersensitivity.

Side-effects: Side-effects are uncommon and typical of other injectable penicillins. If pain at the intramuscular injection site is troublesome the vial contents may be dissolved in 0.5% lignocaine hydrochloride solution. In rare cases spontaneous skin and mucous membrane haemorrhages due to interference with normal clotting mechanisms have been reported.

Precautions: Use of Ticar at less than recommended dosages may permit multiplication of resistant strains of bacteria especially of Pseudomonas. For patients with abnormal renal function see 'Dosage and Administration'. In treating patients on sodium restriction it should be noted that each 1 g vial of Ticar contains 5.3 mmol of sodium (approx.) each 3 g vial contains 16.0 mmol of sodium (approx.) and each 5 g vial contains 26.7 mmol of sodium (approx.)

Pharmaceutical precautions *Stability and storage:* Vials of Ticar powder may be stored at room temperature (25°C or below).

Solutions for IM and direct IV injection should normally be administered within 30 minutes of preparation. However, aqueous solutions of Ticar retain their activity for up to 24 hours at room temperature (25°C) and for up to 72 hours in a refrigerator (5°C). Reconstitution of the injection should be carried out under appropriate aseptic conditions if these extended storage periods are required.

Compatibility: Ticar is compatible with intravenous solutions in general use except:

Proteinaceous fluids (e.g. protein hydrolysates)
Blood and plasma
Intravenous lipids

Details of the stability of Ticar in various fluids are given in the Package Enclosure Leaflet.

If Ticar is prescribed concurrently with an aminoglycoside the antibiotics should not be mixed in the syringe or intravenous fluid container because loss of activity of the aminoglycoside can occur under these conditions.

Legal category POM.

Package quantities *Ticar 1 g vials:* Cartons of 10. *Ticar 3 g vials:* Cartons of 6. *Ticar 5 g vials:* Cartons of 4. *Ticar infusion:* 5 g infusion bottle with diluent and transfer needle, in packs of 4.

Further information Ticar has proved to be particularly valuable in the treatment of patients with lowered host defences.

Synergy has been observed between Ticar and aminoglycosides, such as gentamicin, tobramycin and amikacin, against Pseudomonas and other organisms.

When Ticar is used with an aminoglycoside the usual recommended dosages of both products should be used. Concurrent therapy is not an opportunity to secure dosage reduction unless indicated for other reasons – for example renal failure. (See manufacturers' literature for details of aminoglycoside prescribing information.)

As with other penicillins, Ticar is eliminated by glomerular filtration and tubular secretion. It is not highly bound to serum protein (approximately 45%) and is excreted unchanged in high concentrations in the urine.

Ticar can be detected in tissues and interstitial fluid following parenteral administration. Penetration into the cerebrospinal fluid, bile and pleural fluid has been demonstrated.

Product licence numbers

1 g vial	0038/0084
3 g vial	0038/0084
5 g vial	0038/0084
5 g infusion	0038/0084
Water for Injections BP	0038/0118

UTICILLIN* TABLETS

Presentation Oval, white tablets, engraved 'Uticillin'. Each tablet contains 500 mg carfecillin sodium.

Uses Uticillin is indicated for the treatment of acute and chronic infections of the upper and lower urinary tract when these are caused by sensitive organisms, including *Escherichia coli,* Proteus spp. and *Strep. faecalis.* Uticillin is of particular value in the treatment of urinary tract infections involving Pseudomonas.

Typical indications include: Cystitis. Pyelonephritis. Asymptomatic bacteriuria.

Dosage and administration *Adults (including elderly patients):* Simple urinary tract infections – 1 tablet (500 mg) three times a day.

Complicated and recurrent urinary tract infections – 2 tablets (1 g) three times a day.

Children: 2–10 years: ½ adult dose.

Children's dosage should be in the range 30–60 mg/kg daily in 3 divided doses.

Abnormal renal function: see 'Precaution'.

Contra-indications, warnings, etc
Contra-indication: Penicillin hypersensitivity.

Side-effects: As with other penicillins.

Precaution: In mild and moderate degrees of renal impairment, the normal dosage recommendations should be followed. In patients with severe renal failure (creatinine clearance of 10 ml/min or less) carfecillin is not recommended; in such patients the levels of carbenicillin in the urine may be insufficient for therapeutic efficacy.

Pharmaceutical precautions Uticillin should be stored in a cool, dry place.

Legal category POM.

Package quantities Bottles of 30.

Further information *Pharmacology:* Following oral administration, Uticillin is rapidly absorbed in the body and hydrolysed to carbenicillin, producing high concentrations in the urine.

Product licence number 0038/0155.

*Trade Mark

Bencard
Great West Road
Brentford
Middlesex TW8 9BD

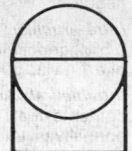

ALAVAC-P*

Presentation Alavac-P vaccine contains alum-precipitated extracts from aqueous pyridine solutions of twelve varieties of common grass pollens: (Bent, Brome, Cocksfoot, Crested Dogstail, False Oat, Fescue, Meadow Foxtail, Meadow Grass, Rye Grass, Timothy, Vernal and Yorkshire Fog).

The vaccine consists of a set of three multidose vials in graded concentrations as follows:

Vial Number	Concentration
1. (Green Label)	250 Noon units per ml.
2. (Buff Label)	2,500 Noon units per ml.
3. (Red Label)	25,000 Noon units per ml.

The aluminium hydroxide content is not more than 3 mg/ml and the preparation is preserved with Phenol BP 0.5% w/v.

Uses Indicated for the treatment of classical hayfever and pollen asthma, to give long-term protection whenever grass pollens are considered to be the sole or predominant cause.

Alavac-P is formulated from the pollens of twelve common grasses which are responsible for the majority of classical hayfever and pollen asthma cases and provides a convenient and effective preventive treatment.

Dosage and administration Please note that the section on 'Contra-Indications, Warnings, Etc.' must be studied before Alavac-P is administered.

Adrenaline Injection BP (Adrenaline 1 in 1,000) should always be kept at hand when giving any desensitising vaccine.

The administration procedures shown in the leaflet included with each course of Alavac-P should be carefully followed.

Alavac-P may be given to adults (including elderly patients) and children aged 5 years and over in accordance with the provisions given below.

Injections should be given at intervals of 7–14 days.

The vial should be shaken thoroughly immediately before withdrawing a dose.

Sterile syringes should always be used for the withdrawal of doses. Since each vial is used more than once, aseptic precautions must be sufficient to avoid the risk of microbial contamination.

Injections should be given slowly by the subcutaneous route. Do not inject into a blood vessel or intramuscularly. Do not rub the site of injection.

Treatment should be given pre-seasonally. The course should normally be started by mid-March (in the UK) to ensure completion before the onset of the grass pollen season. For continued clinical improvement it is recommended that a course should be given in each of three successive years.

Dosage schemes:

Adults
The dosage scheme should be selected according to the patient's previous history of asthma and severity of allergic symptoms as outlined below. When in doubt, treatment should be commenced at the lowest dosage.

Patient Classification		
Very sensitive	Moderately sensitive	Mildly sensitive
Severe symptoms of allergy (e.g. eczema) or any history of asthma	Moderate symptoms of allergy with no history of asthma	Mild symptoms of allergy with no history of asthma

Children
Children aged 5–14 years: treat according to the children's dosage scheme shown below. However, in the presence of a history of asthma or severe symptoms, consultant advice should be sought.

Children under five: consultant advice should be sought.

Recommended dosage schemes
Not to be used during the grass pollen season.

Commence with the No. 1 (Green label) vial then proceed to the No. 2 (Buff label) vial and the No. 3 (Red label) vial as indicated in the scheme below.

If a reaction occurs during treatment, dosage should be reduced: see 'Adjustment of Dosage'.

Adults:

Vial number	Very sensitive adult patients	Moderately sensitive adult patients	Mildly sensitive adult patients
	dosage (ml)	dosage (ml)	dosage (ml)
1. Green label	0.1 0.2 0.4 0.8	0.2 0.5	 0.5
2. Buff label	0.15 0.3 0.6	0.1 0.2 0.4 0.8	0.1 0.3 0.7
3. Red label	0.1 0.2	0.15 0.25 0.4	0.15 0.3 0.5 1.0

Children:

Vial Number	Dosage for children aged 5–14 years (ml)	Children under five
1. Green label	0.1 0.2 0.4 0.8	
2. Buff label	0.15 0.3 0.6	Children under five: consultant advice should be sought
3. Red label	0.1 0.2	

Extended treatment: when time is available before the onset of the pollen season and there is sufficient vaccine, it may be beneficial to repeat the top treatment dose at fortnightly intervals, the final dose being given two weeks before the pollen season is expected to start.

Contra-indications, warnings, etc

Contra-indications: Patients should not be given an allergy vaccine if:

(a) They have had a severe asthma attack not responding to an inhaled bronchodilator;

(b) they have suffered from a febrile condition or an acute attack of asthma in the 24 hours preceding the intended dose.

Use in pregnancy: It is advisable to avoid use during pregnancy.

Precautions: Children under five: consultant advice should be sought.

Patients should be warned not to eat a heavy meal immediately before an injection is due to be given.

In very sensitive patients, it is advantageous to give an antihistamine tablet about one hour before each injection.

Injections should be given slowly by the subcutaneous route. Do not inject into a blood vessel or intramuscularly. Do not rub the site of injection.

Adrenaline Injection BP (Adrenaline 1 in 1,000) should always be kept at hand when giving any desensitising vaccine.

All patients should be instructed to remain under observation in the surgery for at least 20 minutes after each injection and advised to contact the doctor immediately in the unlikely event of a delayed reaction.

The patient should not take any strenuous physical exercise for several hours following the injection.

Note: A patient must not be transferred from Alavac-P to an aqueous vaccine unless a complete course of the aqueous vaccine is to be given, commencing with the lowest strength (No. 1) vial.

Reactions: (see also 'Adjustment of Dosage'):
Local reactions, such as slight swelling or irritation, can sometimes occur and may require symptomatic treatment if they persist.

Mild systemic reactions such as rhinitis or urticaria may be treated with antihistamines orally, or by injection if necessary. In mild bronchospasm, a sympathomimetic bronchodilator such as salbutamol and possibly an anti-inflammatory steroid should be given. If required, 0.5 ml Adrenaline Injection BP (1 in 1,000) may be given subcutaneously.

Severe systemic reactions may occasionally arise in the form of typical allergic symptoms; anaphylaxis is rare.

Treatment of anaphylaxis:
Anaphylactic shock: characterised by bronchospasm, laryngeal oedema, urticaria and shock. Immediate attention should be given as follows:

1. The patient should be laid down and treated immediately.

2. 0.5 ml† Adrenaline Injection BP (Adrenaline 1 in 1,000) should be given intramuscularly close to the vaccine injection site. This should be repeated to a total of 2 ml† over 15 minutes if necessary. In extreme cases, 0.5 ml† Adrenaline (1 in 10,000) can be given by slow intravenous injection.

3. If bronchospasm persists, 10–20 ml† of Aminophylline Injection BP (250 mg per 10 ml) should be given by slow intravenous injection at a rate of 2 ml† per minute.

4. In addition, 200–400 mg† of Hydrocortisone Injection BP should be given intravenously. This is to combat persistent bronchospasm which can occur 6–8 hours after the initial collapse.

5. Full supportive measures should be available and employed if necessary and patients should be closely monitored for at least 24 hours after recovery.

Adjustment of Dosage (in the event of the occurrence of a reaction):

Reaction to the first injection:

Moderately sensitive or mildly sensitive adult dosage scheme: The patient should be transferred to the very sensitive adult dosage scheme.

Very sensitive adult dosage scheme and children: return the complete course to Bencard. An appropriate course of Alavac-S containing grass pollens together with a Special Dilution Vial (No. 0 – Black label, 1/10th dilution of the No. 1 vial) will be supplied free of charge. Treatment should recommence from the Special Dilution Vial according to the dosage scheme issued with it; the normal dosage scheme should then be continued, but no attempt should be made to exceed the maximum tolerated dose.

Reaction to subsequent injections:

Local
Mild reaction: Reduce the dose by one step.
Severe reaction: Reduce the dose by two steps.

Systemic
Mild reaction: Reduce the dose by two steps.

Severe reaction: Treatment should be discontinued.

Except in cases where a severe systemic reaction has occurred, the course may be continued with caution up to the top dose quoted, or to the highest dose tolerated without significant reaction.

Pharmaceutical precautions Alavac-P must be stored in a refrigerator (2–8°C). It must not be frozen. Vaccine left over from an Alavac-P course must not be used the following year.

Legal category POM.

Package quantities Each course of treatment consists of a set of three multidose vials of vaccine in graded concentrations. Ready assembled disposable syringes with attached needles and an instruction leaflet are included with each set.

Further information Alavac-P is formulated from the pollens of twelve common grasses responsible for classical hayfever and pollen asthma and offers a

† All dosages should be reduced as required for children.

fundamental alternative to symptomatic treatment. Ala-vac-P may be prescribed from case history and clinical symptoms alone, providing these reveal marked season-ality corresponding with the grass pollen season. Risk of reaction is reduced because of the slow release of active material into the system.

Alavac-P may be prescribed on NHS form FP10 and is available for immediate supply from stock.

The Bencard Medical Department will be pleased to advise on any aspect of treatment.

Product licence number 0038/5085.

ALAVAC-S*

Presentation Each course of Alavac-S is a desensitis-ing vaccine, specially prepared for an individual patient, from extracts of specific allergens, in accordance with the information obtained from the patient during case history investigations and subsequent skin tests. The vaccine comprises alum-adsorbed extracts of specific allergens precipitated from aqueous pyridine solutions. Each course is presented as three multidose vials of allergen concentrate in graded concentrations. The No. 1 and No. 2 vials are 1/100th and 1/10th dilutions respectively of the No. 3 vial.

Special Dilution Vials (No. 0, Black label, 1/10th dilution of the No. 1 vial) are available on request to initiate treatment of highly sensitive patients.

The No. 3 vial is also available in a larger size for physicians practising maintenance therapy with courses which do not contain pollen allergens (see Dosage and Administration).

For the best clinical results with Alavac-S, no more than 4 allergens should normally be included (with a maximum of 6) in any one course.

If the patient is sensitive to more than 6 allergens, those which can be avoided without undue inconveni-ence, or are of little clinical significance, should be omitted and the patient given advice on avoidance; otherwise two separate vaccines will be prepared.

The aluminium hydroxide content is not more than 3 mg/ml and the preparation is preserved with Phenol BP 0.5% w/v.

The adsorbed allergen extracts available for inclusion in Alavac-S are:

Dusts: Hay dust, House dust, Straw dust, Mixed threshings (barley, maize, oats and wheat).

Epithelials: Mixed feathers, Cat fur, Rabbit fur, Cow hair, Dog hair, Horse hair, Human hair, Sheep wool.

Fabrics: Cotton flock, Kapok.

House Dust Mite: Dermatophagoides pteronyssinus.

Fungi: Alternaria alternata, Aspergillus fumigatus, Asper-gillus niger. Candida albicans. Cladosporium herbarum, Fusarium spp., Merulius lacrymans, Neurospora sito-phila, Penicillium notatum, Rhizopus nigricans, Sporo-bolomyces roseus. Trichophytons (T. mentagrophytes and T. rubrum).

Pollens: Available individually:
Elder (*Sambucus nigra*), Hazel (*Corylus spp.*), Maize (*Zea mays*), Nettle (*Urtica dioica*), Plantain (*Plantago lanceolata*), Poplar (*Populus spp.*), Rye, Cultivated (*Secale cereale*), Silver Birch (*Betula spp.*).

Available as standard groups.
Group B2-Grass pollens containing:
Bent, Brome, Cocksfoot, Crested Dogstail, False Oat,

Meadow Fescue, Meadow Foxtail, Meadow Grass, Rye Grass, Timothy, Vernal, Yorkshire Fog.

Group B3-Tree pollens containing:
Alder, Ash, Beech, Birch, Elm, Hazel, Oak, Plane, Poplar, Willow.

Group B5-Weed and Shrub pollens containing:
Heather, Nettle, Plantain, Fat Hen, Mugwort, Orache.

The allergens used in the preparation of Alavac-S correspond with those available as Bencard Skin Testing Solutions. Alavac vaccines themselves are unsuitable for skin testing.

Uses To provide fundamental treatment for a wide variety of common allergic conditions such as asthma, perennial rhinitis, hay fever and some skin conditions.

Dosage and administration Please note that the section on 'Contra-Indications, Warnings, Etc.' must be studied before Alavac-S is administered.

Adrenaline Injection BP (Adrenaline 1 in 1,000) should always be kept at hand when giving any desensitising vaccine.

The administration procedures shown in the leaflet included with each course of Alavac-S should be carefully followed.

Alavac-S may be given to adults (including elderly patients) and children aged 5 years and over in accordance with the guidelines given below.

Children under five: consultant advice should be sought.

Injections should be given at intervals of 7–14 days unless otherwise stated.

The vial should be shaken thoroughly immediately before withdrawing a dose.

Sterile syringes should always be used for the with-drawal of doses. Since each vial is used more than once, aseptic precautions must be sufficient to avoid the risk of microbial contamination.

Injections should be given slowly by the subcutaneous route. Do not inject into a blood vessel or intramuscularly. Do not rub the site of injection.

Adults
The dosage scheme should be selected according to the patient's previous history of asthma and severity of allergic symptoms as outlined below. When in doubt, treatment should be commenced at the lowest dosage.

Patient Classification		
Very sensitive	Moderately sensitive	Mildly sensitive
Severe symptoms of allergy (e.g. eczema) or any history of asthma	Moderate symptoms of allergy with no history of asthma	Mild symptoms of allergy with no history of asthma

Children
Children aged 5–14 years: treat according to the children's dosage scheme shown below. However, in the presence of a history of asthma or severe symptoms, consultant advice should be sought.

Children under five: consultant advice should be sought.

Alavac-S: Dosage recommendations for vaccines which contain pollen allergens:
Treatment should be given pre-seasonally. The course

should be timed to end before the usual date of onset of the patient's seasonal symptoms (e.g. in the UK, by mid-May for grass pollen sensitivity and by the end of March for tree pollen sensitivity). For continued clinical improvement it is recommended that a course should be given in each of three successive years.

Recommended dosage schemes for vaccines which contain pollen allergens
Not to be used during the pollen season.

Commence with the No. 1 (Green label) vial then proceed to the No. 2 (Buff label) vial and the No. 3 (Red label) vial as indicated in the schemes below.

If a reaction occurs during treatment, dosage should be reduced: see 'Adjustment of Dosage'.

Adults:

Vial Number	Very sensitive adult patients	Moderately sensitive adult patients	Mildly sensitive adult patients
	dosage (ml)	dosage (ml)	dosage (ml)
1. Green label	0.1 0.2 0.4 0.8	0.2 0.5	0.5
2. Buff label	0.15 0.3 0.6	0.1 0.2 0.4 0.8	0.1 0.3 0.7
3. Red label	0.1 0.2	0.15 0.25 0.4	0.15 0.3 0.5 1.0

Children:

Vial Number	Dosage for children aged 5–14 years (ml)	Children under five
1. Green label	0.1 0.2 0.4 0.8	
2. Buff label	0.15 0.3 0.6	Children under five: consultant advice should be sought.
3. Red label	0.1 0.2	

Surplus vaccine must not be used the following season.

Extended treatment: when time is available before the onset of the pollen season and there is sufficient vaccine, it may be beneficial to repeat the top treatment dose at fortnightly intervals, the final dose being given two weeks before the pollen season is expected to start.

Alavac-S: Recommended dosage schemes for vaccines which do not contain pollen allergens (Initial course)
Courses may be given at any time of year.

Commence with the No. 1 (Green label) vial then proceed to the No. 2 (Buff label) vial and the No. 3 (Red label) vial as indicated in the schemes below.

If a reaction occurs during treatment, dosage should be reduced: see 'Adjustment of Dosage'.

Adults:

Vial Number	Very sensitive adult patients	Moderately sensitive adult patients	Mildly sensitive adult patients
	dosage (ml)	dosage (ml)	dosage (ml)
1. Green label	0.25 0.5 1.0	0.5 1.0	
2. Buff label	0.2 0.4 0.8	0.2 0.4 0.8	0.1 0.2 0.4 0.8
3. Red label	0.15 0.25	0.15 0.3 0.6	0.15 0.3 0.6

Maintenance treatment following the initial course is recommended.

Children:

Vial Number	Dosage for children aged 5–14 years (ml)	Children under five
1. Green label	0.25 0.5 1.0	
2. Buff label	0.2 0.4 0.8	Children under five: consultant advice should be sought.
3. Red label	0.15 0.25	

Maintenance treatment following the initial course is recommended.

Maintenance therapy: (for use only with vaccines which do not contain pollens)

Maintenance therapy, which consists of a series of boosting injections, is recommended particularly for patients with perennial symptoms provided that the initial treatment course has been well tolerated.

Maintenance therapy should commence between 1 and 2 weeks after completion of the initial course, and should follow the dosage scheme below. Treatment may be continued at the discretion of the physician, with review at appropriate intervals.

N.B. Maintenance therapy is not suitable for use with pollen-containing vaccines.

Recommended maintenance dosage schemes for vaccines which do NOT contain pollen allergens.
Injections should be given from vial No. 3.

If a reaction occurs during treatment, dosage should be reduced: see 'Adjustment of Dosage'.

Adults: Maintenance Dosage Scheme (Using No. 3 vial supplied with Initial Course).

| Injection Number | Interval since previous injection | Dosage (ml) from No. 3 vial (use maximum tolerated dose if lower) | | Duration |
		very sensitive adults	moderately or mildly sensitive adults	
First	1–2 weeks after completion of Initial Course	0.25	0.6	
2nd	1–2 weeks	0.25	0.6	Maintenance therapy may be continued at the discretion of the physician, with review at appropriate intervals.
3rd	2 weeks	0.25	0.6	
4th	2 weeks	0.25	0.6	
5th and subsequent	4 weeks	0.25	0.6	

Children: (aged 5–14 years)* Maintenance Dosage Scheme (Using No. 3 vial supplied with Initial Course).

Injection Number	Interval since previous injection	Dosage (ml) from No. 3 vial (use maximum tolerated dose if lower)	Duration
First	1–2 weeks after completion of Initial Course	0.25	
2nd	1–2 weeks	0.25	Maintenance therapy may be continued at the discretion of the physician, with review at appropriate intervals.
3rd	2 weeks	0.25	
4th	2 weeks	0.25	
5th and subsequent	4 weeks	0.25	

* Children under five: consultant advice should be sought.

N.B. Care should be taken when administering the first injection from a new No. 3 vial, as in a very few cases a local or general reaction may occur.

If a period of five to eight weeks has elapsed since the last injection, from the previous No. 3 vial, the first two doses from the new No. 3 vial should be modified according to the following recommendations:

– for very sensitive adults and for children
the first dose should be 0.05 ml and the second dose 0.15 ml
– for moderately or mildly sensitive adults
the first dose should be 0.15 ml and the second dose 0.3 ml
given at an interval of 7–14 days.

Maintenance treatment should then be continued as shown in the above tables.

If more than eight weeks have elapsed since the previous injection, it is advisable not to attempt maintenance therapy but to re-start with a complete Initial course, commencing with the lowest strength (No. 1 Green label) vial.

This regimen is unsuitable for use with pollen-containing vaccines.

Contra-indications, warnings, etc
Contra-indications: Patients should not be given an allergy vaccine if:

(a) They have had a severe asthma attack not responding to an inhaled bronchodilator;
(b) they have suffered from a febrile condition or an acute attack of asthma in the 24 hours preceding the intended dose.

Use in pregnancy: It is advisable to avoid use during pregnancy.

Precautions: Children under five: consultant advice should be sought.

Patients should be warned not to eat a heavy meal immediately before an injection is due to be given.

In very sensitive patients it is advantageous to give an antihistamine tablet about one hour before each injection.

Injections should be given slowly by the subcutaneous route. Do not inject into a blood vessel or intramuscularly. Do not rub the site of injection.

Adrenaline Injection BP (Adrenaline 1 in 1,000) should always be kept at hand when giving any desensitising vaccine.

All patients should be instructed to remain under observation in the surgery for at least 20 minutes after each injection and advised to contact the doctor immediately in the unlikely event of a delayed reaction. The patient should not take any strenuous physical exercise for several hours following the injection.

Note: A patient must not be transferred from Alavac-S

to an aqueous vaccine unless a complete course of the aqueous vaccine is to be given, commencing with the lowest strength (No. 1 Green label) vial.

Reactions (see also 'Adjustment of Dosage'):
Local reactions, such as slight swelling or irritation, can sometimes occur and may require symptomatic treatment if they persist.

Mild systemic reactions such as rhinitis or urticaria may be treated with antihistamines orally, or by injection if necessary. In mild bronchospasm, a sympathomimetic bronchodilator such as salbutamol and possibly an anti-inflammatory steroid should be given. If required, 0.5 ml Adrenaline Injection BP (Adrenaline 1 in 1,000) may be given subcutaneously.

Severe systemic reactions may occasionally arise in the form of typical allergic symptoms; anaphylaxis is rare.

Treatment of anaphylaxis:
Anaphylactic shock: characterised by bronchospasm, laryngeal oedema, urticaria and shock. Immediate attention should be given as follows:
1. The patient should be laid down and treated immediately.
2. 0.5 ml† Adrenaline Injection BP (Adrenaline 1 in 1,000) should be given intramuscularly close to the vaccine injection site. This should be repeated to a total of 2 ml† over 15 minutes if necessary. In extreme cases, 0.5 ml† Adrenaline (1 in 10,000) can be given by slow intravenous injection.
3. If bronchospasm persists, 10–20 ml† of Aminophylline Injection BP (250 mg per 10 ml) should be given by slow intravenous injection at a rate of 2 ml† per minute.
4. In addition, 200–400 mg† of Hydrocortisone Injection BP should be given intravenously. This is to combat persistent bronchospasm which can occur 6–8 hours after the initial collapse.
5. Full supportive measures should be available and employed if necessary and patients should be closely monitored for at least 24 hours after recovery.

Adjustment of Dosage (in the event of the occurrence of a reaction):
Reaction to the first injection
Moderately sensitive or mildly sensitive adult dosage scheme: The patient should be transferred to the very sensitive adult dosage scheme.

Very sensitive adult dosage scheme and children: return the complete course to Bencard. A Special Dilution Vial (No. 0 – Black label, 1/10th dilution of the No. 1 vial) will be prepared free of charge and returned with a new complete course.

Treatment should recommence from the dilute vial according to the dosage scheme issued with it; the normal dosage scheme should then be continued, but no attempt should be made to exceed the maximum tolerated dose.
Reaction to subsequent injections:
Local
Mild reaction: Reduce the dose by one step.
Severe reaction: Reduce the dose by two steps.

Systemic
Mild reaction: Reduce the dose by two steps.
Severe reaction: Treatment should be discontinued.

Except in cases where a severe systemic reaction has occurred, the course may be continued with caution up to the top dose quoted, or to the highest dose tolerated without significant reaction.

† All dosages should be reduced as required for children.

Pharmaceutical precautions Alavac-S must be stored in a refrigerator (2–8°C). It must not be frozen.
Surplus vaccine from courses of Alavac-S containing pollen allergens must not be used the following year.
Vaccine left over from the No. 3 vial of courses which do not contain pollen allergens may be used for maintenance therapy (see Maintenance therapy for vaccines which do not contain pollen allergens).

Legal category POM.

Package quantities Each course of treatment consists of a set of three multidose vials of vaccine in graded concentrations. Ready-assembled disposable syringes with attached needles and an instruction leaflet are included with each set. The No. 3 vial is also available in a larger size for maintenance therapy with Alavac-S vaccines which do not contain pollen allergens (see Dosage and Administration).
Normal delivery time for a complete course or a single vial is about two weeks to allow for individual formulation and sterility testing.

Further information Ordering procedure: FP10 forms (or other prescriptions) should be taken to a chemist who will arrange the supply of the vaccine. The prescription should be accompanied by the following information:
When available, a Skin Test Reaction Chart or a list of the allergens to be included in the vaccine with a note of the patient's sensitivity to each one, or, the reference number of a previous course.
Patient's name
Patient's date of birth and/or age
The Bencard Medical Department will be pleased to advise on any aspect of treatment.

Product licence number 0038/5086.

AMOXIL* CAPSULES
AMOXIL* DISPERSIBLE TABLETS
AMOXIL* SYRUP 125 mg
AMOXIL* SYRUP SF 125 mg
AMOXIL* SYRUP 250 mg
AMOXIL* SACHETS 3 g
AMOXIL* PAEDIATRIC SUSPENSION
AMOXIL* INJECTION

Presentation *Amoxil Capsules:* (Amoxycillin Capsules BP) Maroon and gold capsules overprinted 'Amoxil 250', each providing 250 mg amoxycillin.
Maroon and gold capsules overprinted 'Amoxil 500', each providing 500 mg amoxycillin.

Amoxil Dispersible Tablets: Flat, white circular tablets, engraved 'Amoxil 500', each providing 500 mg amoxycillin.

Amoxil Syrups and Amoxil Syrup SF: (Amoxycillin Mixture BP). Citrus flavoured syrup, providing 125 mg or 250 mg amoxycillin per 5 ml. The SF presentation is sucrose free, providing 125 mg amoxycillin per 5 ml in a sorbitol base.
Presented as powder in bottles for preparing 100 ml.

Amoxil 3 g Sachet: Each sachet provides 3 g amoxycillin for reconstitution in approximately one third of a glass of water.

Amoxil Paediatric Suspension. Citrus flavoured suspension, providing 125 mg amoxycillin per 1.25 ml (measured by the pipette supplied).
Presented as powder in bottles for preparing 20 ml.

Amoxil Vials for Injection: Each vial provides 250 mg,

500 mg or 1 g amoxycillin. Presented as powder for reconstitution.

The amoxycillin content per dose unit is present as the trihydrate in Amoxil oral preparations and as the sodium salt in Amoxil injections.

Uses *Treatment of Infection:* Amoxil is a broad spectrum antibiotic indicated for the treatment of commonly-occurring bacterial infections such as:

Upper Respiratory Tract Infections
Otitis media
Acute and Chronic Bronchitis
Lobar and Bronchopneumonia
Cystitis, Urethritis, Pyelonephritis
Bacteriuria in pregnancy
Gynaecological infections including puerperal sepsis
    and septic abortion
Gonorrhoea
Peritonitis
Intra abdominal sepsis
Septicaemia
Bacterial endocarditis
Typhoid and Paratyphoid fever
Skin and Soft Tissue Infections
Osteomyelitis

In children with urinary tract infection the need for investigation should be considered.

Prophylaxis of endocarditis: Amoxil may be used for the prevention of bacteraemia, associated with procedures such as dental extraction, in patients at risk of developing bacterial endocarditis.

The wide range of organisms sensitive to the bactericidal action of Amoxil include:

Gram-positive	*Gram-negative*
Streptococcus faecalis	Haemophilus influenzae
Streptococcus pneumoniae	Escherichia coli
Streptococcus pyogenes	Proteus mirabilis
Streptococcus viridans	Salmonella species
Staphylococcus aureus	Shigella species
(penicillin-sensitive)	Bordetella pertussis
Clostridium species	Brucella species
Corynebacterium species	Neisseria gonorrhoeae
Bacillus anthracis	Neisseria meningitidis
Listeria monocytogenes	Vibrio cholerae
	Pasteurella septica

Dosage and administration *Treatment of Infection:*

Adult dosage (including elderly patients):
Oral:

Standard adult dosage: 250 mg three times daily, increasing to 500 mg three times daily for more severe infections.

High dosage therapy (maximum recommended oral dosage 6 g daily in divided doses): A dosage of 3 g twice daily is recommended in appropriate cases for the treatment of severe or recurrent purulent infection of the respiratory tract.

Short course therapy: Simple acute urinary tract infection: two 3 g doses with 10–12 hours between the doses. Gonorrhoea: single 3 g dose.

Injectable:
500 mg IM eight hourly (or more frequently if necessary) in moderate infections.

1 g IV six hourly in severe infections.

Children's dosage (up to 10 years of age): Oral: 125 mg three times daily, increasing to 250 mg three times daily for more severe infections.

Injectable: 50–100 mg/kg body weight a day, in divided doses.

Parenteral therapy is indicated if the oral route is considered impracticable or unsuitable, and particularly for the urgent treatment of severe infection.

In renal impairment the excretion of the antibiotic will be delayed and depending on the degree of impairment it may be necessary to reduce the total daily dosage.

Prophylaxis of endocarditis: see table on next page.

Administration: Oral: Using capsules, dispersible tablets, syrups or 3 g sachets. The use of Amoxil Paediatric Suspension is recommended for children under six months of age.

Intravenous: Dissolve 250 mg in 5.0 ml Water for Injections BP.
Dissolve 500 mg in 10 ml Water for Injections BP.
Dissolve 1 g in 20 ml Water for Injections BP.
Amoxil injection, suitably diluted, may be injected directly into a vein or drip tube, taking 3–4 minutes – or added to infusion fluids, as recommended in the package enclosure leaflet, and infused over a period of $\frac{1}{2}$–1 hour.

Intramuscular: 250 mg: Add 1.5 ml Water for Injections BP† and shake vigorously.

500 mg: Add 2.5 ml Water for Injections BP† and shake vigorously.

1 g: Add 2.5 ml of 1% sterile lignocaine hydrochloride solution and shake vigorously.

†If pain is experienced on intramuscular injection, a sterile 1% solution of lignocaine hydrochloride or 0.5% solution of procaine hydrochloride may be used in place of Water for Injections.

A transient pink colouration or slight opalescence may appear during reconstitution. Reconstituted solutions are normally a pale straw colour.

Contra-indications, warnings, etc Amoxil is a penicillin and should not be given to penicillin-hypersensitive patients.

Side-effects: Side-effects, as with other penicillins, are usually of a mild and transitory nature; they may include diarrhoea, indigestion, or occasionally rash, either urticarial or erythematous. An urticarial rash suggests penicillin hypersensitivity and the erythematous type rash may arise if Amoxil is administered to patients with glandular fever. In either case treatment should be discontinued. Since Amoxil is a penicillin, problems of overdosage are unlikely to be encountered.

Pharmaceutical precautions Prior to use, oral presentations of Amoxil should be stored in a dry place. Amoxil injections should be stored in a cool, dry place. Once dispensed, Amoxil syrups and paediatric suspension should be used within the periods stated on the labels. Any remaining syrup or suspension should be discarded.

When prepared for intramuscular or direct intravenous injection, Amoxil should be administered immediately after reconstitution. The stability of Amoxil in various infusion fluids is given in the package enclosure leaflet. Amoxil should not be mixed with blood products, other proteinaceous fluids such as protein hydrolysates, or with intravenous lipid emulsions.

Legal category POM.

Package quantities *Amoxil Capsules:* 250 mg packs of 100 and 500. 500 mg packs of 100.
Amoxil Dispersible Tablets: 500 mg packs of 30.
Amoxil Syrups: 125 mg and 250 mg per 5 ml: 100 ml bottles.

Prophylaxis of Endocarditis:

Condition	Adults' Dosage (including elderly)	Children's Dosage	Notes
Dental Procedures: Prophylaxis for patients undergoing extraction, scaling or surgery involving gingival tissues, and who have not received a penicillin in the previous month. (N.B. Patients with prosthetic heart valves should be referred to hospital – see below.) Patient not having general anaesthetic.	3 g Amoxil orally, 1 hour before procedure. A second dose may be given 6 hours later, if considered necessary.	Under 10: Half adult dose. Under 5: Quarter adult dose	*Note 1.* Prophylaxis with alternative antibiotics should be considered if the patient has received a penicillin within the previous month. *Note 2.* To minimise pain on injection, Amoxil should be dissolved in sterile 1% lignocaine solution (see 'Administration').
Patient having general anaesthetic: oral antibiotics considered to be appropriate.	Initially 3 g Amoxil orally 4 hours prior to anaesthesia, followed by 3 g orally (or 1 g IM if oral dose not tolerated) 6 hours after the initial dose.	The use of Amoxil 500 mg Dispersible Tablets is recommended.	
Patient having general anaesthetic: oral antibiotics not appropriate.	1 g Amoxil IM immediately before induction; with 500 mg orally, 6 hours later.	Under 10: Half adult dose.	See Note 2. *Note 3.* Amoxil and gentamicin should not be mixed in the same syringe. *Note 4.* Please consult the appropriate data sheet for full prescribing information on gentamicin.
Dental Procedures: Patients for whom referral to hospital is recommended: (a) patients to be given a general anaesthetic who have been given a penicillin in the previous month. (b) patients to be given a general anaesthetic who have a prosthetic heart valve. (c) patients who have had one or more attacks of endocarditis.	Initially: 1 g Amoxil IM with 120 mg gentamicin IM, immediately prior to anaesthesia (if given) or 15 minutes prior to dental procedure. Followed by (6 hours later): 500 mg Amoxil orally.	Under 10: The doses of Amoxil should be half the adult dose; the dose of gentamicin should be 2 mg/kg.	
Genito-urinary Surgery or Instrumentation: Prophylaxis for patients who have no urinary tract infection and who are to have genito-urinary surgery or instrumentation under general anaesthesia. *Obstetric and Gynaecological Procedures* *Gastro-intestinal Procedures* } Routine prophylaxis is recommended only for patients with prosthetic heart valves.	Initially: 1 g Amoxil IM with 120 mg gentamicin IM, immediately before induction. Followed by (6 hours later): 500 mg Amoxil orally or IM according to clinical condition.	Under 10: The doses of Amoxil should be half the adult dose; the dose of gentamicin should be 2 mg/kg.	See Notes 2, 3 and 4 above.
Surgery or Instrumentation of the Upper Respiratory Tract Patients other than those with prosthetic heart valves.	1 g Amoxil IM immediately before induction; 500 mg Amoxil IM 6 hours later.	Under 10: Half adult dose.	See Note 2 above. *Note 5.* The second dose of Amoxil may be administered orally as Amoxil Syrup.
Patients with prosthetic heart valves.	Initially: 1 g Amoxil IM with 120 mg gentamicin IM, immediately before induction; followed by (6 hours later) 500 mg Amoxil IM.	Under 10: The doses of Amoxil should be half the adult dose; the gentamicin dose should be 2 mg/kg.	See Notes 2, 3, 4 and 5 above.

Amoxil Syrup SF: 125 mg per 5 ml: 100 ml bottles.
Amoxil 3 g Sachet: Packs of 2 and 10.
Amoxil Paediatric Suspension: 125 mg per 1.25 ml:
20 ml bottles with pipette.
Amoxil Vials for Injection: 250 mg, 500 mg and 1 g:
packs of 10, 10 and 5 respectively.

Further information Amoxil is well absorbed by the
oral and parenteral routes. Oral administration, usually at
convenient t.d.s. dosage, produces high serum levels
independent of the time at which food is taken. Amoxil
gives good penetration into bronchial secretions and
high urinary concentrations of unchanged antibiotic. It
is rapidly bactericidal and possesses the safety profile of
a penicillin.

Sucrose content: Amoxil Syrup (125 mg) 3.1 g per 5 ml;
Amoxil Syrup (250 mg) 2.9 g per 5 ml; Amoxil Paediatric
Suspension (125 mg) 0.6 g per 1.25 ml; Amoxil Sachet
(3 g) 19 g.
The following presentations of Amoxil are sucrose-
free: Amoxil Capsules, Amoxil Dispersible Tablets and
Amoxil Syrup SF.

Product licence numbers

Amoxil Capsules 250 mg	0038/0103
Amoxil Capsules 500 mg	0038/0105
Amoxil Dispersible Tablets 500 mg	0038/0277
Amoxil Syrup 125 mg per 5 ml	0038/0108
Amoxil Syrup 250 mg per 5 ml	0038/0109
Amoxil Syrup SF 125 mg per 5 ml	0038/0326
Amoxil 3 g Sachet	0038/0238
Amoxil Paediatric Suspension	
125 mg per 1.25 ml	0038/0107
Amoxil Vials for Injection 250 mg	0038/0221
Amoxil Vials for Injection 500 mg	0038/0222
Amoxil Vials for Injection 1 g	0038/0225

ASERBINE* CREAM
ASERBINE* SOLUTION

Presentation *Aserbine Cream:* White cream in a tube.
Aserbine Solution: Clear colourless liquid in a polythene
bottle.
Aserbine is prepared from:

	Aserbine cream %	Aserbine solution %
Propylene glycol	1.7	40.0
Malic acid	0.36	2.25
Benzoic acid	0.024	0.15
Salicylic acid	0.006	0.0375

Uses *Principal action:* Aserbine is a desloughing and
cleansing agent which does not affect living tissue and
has antibacterial properties to guard against wound
infection.
Indications:
1. Whenever the presence of slough delays healing:
   Chronic skin ulcers:
      Venous (varicose) ulcers and other benign chronic
      ulcers; trophic ulcers including pressure sores.
   Burns.
   Traumatic injuries:
      Crushed limb injuries; multiple lesions.
   Surgical procedures where slough may be a problem:
      Preparation for skin grafting; mastectomies; am-
      putations; post-surgical incisions.

2. Cleansing:
   Wounds and abrasions where coagulum, debris, dirt
   and grit, etc. are a problem.

Administration Aserbine is suitable for both adults
and children and should be applied topically.
For desloughing: Aserbine Cream should be applied
liberally to the wound surface and before each new
application the wound should be washed with Aserbine
Solution so that the loose slough and cream from the
previous application are removed.
Dressing the wound twice daily has been found to
produce the best results; however, more frequent
dressings may be made if necessary.
Aserbine Solution may also be applied as a wet
dressing which should be kept constantly moist.
For cleansing: Both Aserbine Cream and Solution have
proved of value as cleansing agents in casualty work for
the removal of coagulum, debris, dirt, grit, etc. from
wounds and abrasions.

Contra-indications, warnings, etc
Contra-indications: None.

Warning: For external use only.

Precautions: Care should be taken to avoid contact with
the eyes because of Aserbine's low pH.
As Aserbine Cream contains 0.015% hexachlorophane
it should not be used except on medical advice for
children under two years of age.

Overdosage: Not applicable.

Side-effects: Mild pyrexia, partially due to the absorption
of protein products of slough breakdown from the
wound, has been reported in severely burned patients.
Irritation of the hypersensitive skin surrounding the
wound may occur in a few patients. In these cases,
Aserbine should be kept away from the growing
epithelium at the periphery of the wound.
Occasionally a mild urticarial rash has been seen a
small distance around the treated area. The discomfort
was slight and readily controlled by antihistamines.

Pharmaceutical precautions Prolonged contact of
Aserbine Solution with metallic surfaces is inadvisable.

Legal category GSL.

Package quantities *Aserbine Cream:* 100 g tube.
Aserbine Solution: 500 ml bottle.

Further information The acid pH of Aserbine Cream
and Solution is such that, when applied to a wound, it
causes maximum differential swelling between the living
protein of healthy tissues and the dead protein of slough,
leading to the separation of the dead tissue (desloughing). The wound surface is cleared from the presence of
slough and debris without affecting the living tissue so
that uninterrupted normal healing can proceed. Aserbine
also has antibacterial properties which guard against
wound infection.
Dressings with Aserbine Cream are non-adherent,
odourless and do not stain the skin, clothing, etc.

Product licence numbers
Aserbine Cream	0038/5089
Aserbine Solution	0038/5090

BENCARD* SKIN TESTING SOLUTIONS

Presentation Bencard Skin Testing Solutions for the
diagnosis of allergy are available for over 200 allergens.

Prick testing is the generally recommended method. The full range of extracts is available for inclusion in SDV (specific desensitising vaccines).

The more common allergens (marked † in the list of allergens below) are also available for inclusion in Alavac-S vaccines.

Prick tests: Aqueous allergen extracts containing 50% glycerin, 6% sodium chloride (with the exception of mould extracts, which contain < 1% sodium chloride) and 0.5% phenol as a preservative. Supplied in polythene-capped vials containing approximately 2 ml of solution, sufficient for about 100 individual tests.

Intradermal tests: When these are requested they will be supplied as aqueous allergen extracts in dilute phosphate buffer with 0.5% phenol as a preservative. Supplied in vials containing approximately 2 ml of sterile solution, sufficient for about 30 individual tests.

Form and appearance: The colours of individual skin testing solutions vary depending on the characteristics of the raw material involved, e.g. pollens tend to be yellowish whilst dusts and moulds, in particular, are shades of brown.

Availability: Bencard Skin Testing Solutions are available either individually from the list specified below or as Kits (Series I and Series II) containing selections of the most important allergens.

STANDARD GROUPS OF ALLERGENS

(all allergens contained in these groups are also available individually)

† *B2 Grass pollens:* Bent; Brome; Cocksfoot; Dogstail (Crested); False oat (Oat grass); Fescue (Meadow); Foxtail (Meadow); Meadow grass; Rye grass; Timothy; Vernal (Sweet); Yorkshire fog.

† *B3 Tree pollens:* Alder; Ash; Beech; †Birch, Silver; Elm; †Hazel; Oak; Plane; †Poplar; Willow.

† *B5 Weed and shrub pollens:* Heather; †Nettle; †Plantain; Fat Hen; Mugwort; Orache.

INDIVIDUAL ALLERGENS

Dusts: Flax Dust and Fibre; †Hay; †House; †Straw; †Threshings (bran), Mixed (Barley, Maize, Oats, Wheat); Threshings (bran), Wheat.

Epithelials (feathers, fur, hair and danders): Feathers: Budgerigar; Canary; Chicken; Goose; †Mixed; Pigeon.

Fur: †Cat; Mixed (fine); (Beaver, Fox, Mink, Musquash, Squirrel); †Rabbit.

Hair: Camel; †Cow; †Dog; Goat; Guinea Pig; Hamster; †Horse; †Human; Mouse; Rat.

Pig bristle.

†Sheep wool.

Fabrics: Acrilan; †Cotton flock; Hessian (Jute); †Kapok; Linen; Nylon; Rayon; Silk; Terylene; White wool.

Flowers and foliage (mixed): Chrysanthemum (*C. morifolium*); Geranium (*Pelargonium* spp.); Grass cuttings; Primula (*Primula* spp.).

Woods (sawdust): Beech (*Fagus sylvatica*); Birch (*Betula* spp.); Cedar of Lebanon (*Cedrus libani*); Cedar, Western Red (*Thuya plicata*); Deal; (*Pinus sylvestris*); Douglas Fir (*Pseudotsuga menziesii/douglasii*); Hemlock (*Tsuga heterophylla*); Iroko (*Chlorophora* spp); Makore (*Mimusops beckelii*); Mahogany (*Khaya ivorensis*); Oak (*Quercus* spp.); Obeche (*Triplochiton scleroxylon*); Pine, Parana (*Araucaria brasiliana*); Ramin (*Gonystylus* spp.); Teak (*Tectona grandis*).

(FOODS)

Cereals (Grain, Flour, Bread): Flour, Mixed (Plain, Self-raising and Wholewheat); Plain; Rye; Wholewheat.

Grain: Barley; Maize; Oat, Rice; Rye; Wheat.

Dairy products: Cheese, Mixed (Cheddar and Dutch); Egg Whole; Milk (Cow).

Drinks: Coffee; Tea.

Fish: Cod; Herring; Plaice; Sardine.

Shellfish: Crab; Lobster; Mussel; Oyster; Shrimp.

Fruits: Apple; Banana; Grapes (Mixed black and white); Lemon; Orange; Strawberry; Tomato.

Meats: Beef-veal; Mutton-lamb; Pork-bacon.

Nuts: Mixed (Almond, Brazil, Chestnut, Hazel and Walnut).

Vegetables: Beans, Mixed (Broad, Haricot and Runner); Cabbage; Carrot; Mushroom; Onion; Pea; Potato (New); Spinach.

Unclassified: Chocolate; Mustard; Yeast (Mixed); Yeast (Bakers).

(MICRO-ORGANISMS)

House dust mite: Dermatophagoides farinae (culinae); †Dermatophagoides pteronyssinus.

Bacteria: Bramhamella/Neisseria catarrhalis; Corynebacterium hofmannii; Escherichia coli (B. coli); Haemophilus influenzae; Klebsiella pneumoniae; (Friedlander's bacillus); Pseudomonas aeruginosa; (B. pyocyaneus); Staphylococcus albus; Staphylococcus aureus; Streptococcus Lancefield Group C; Streptococcus Lancefield Group G; Streptococcus pneumoniae Type 1; Streptococcus viridans.

Fungi (moulds and yeasts): †Alternaria alternata; Aspergillus amstelodami; †Aspergillus fumigatus; †Aspergillus niger; Aspergillus terreus; Botrytis cinerea; †Candida albicans; Chaetomium globosum; †Cladosporium herbarum; Epicoccum purpurascens; †Fusarium spp.; †Merulius lacrymans (Dry rot); Mucor mucedo; Mucor racemosus; Mucor spinosus; †Neurospora sitophila; Paecilomyces marquandii (Spicaria violacea); †Penicillium notatum; Phoma betae; Pullularia pullulans; †Rhizopus nigricans; †Sporobolomyces roseus; †Trichophytons (T. mentagrophytes and T. rubrum); Trichophyton mentagrophytes (interdigitale); Trichophyton rubrum; Trichophyton verrucosum; Ustilago.

Insects: Bee (*Apis mellifera*)* – weak or strong; Flour beetle (*Tribolium confusum*); Mosquito (*Culex* spp.); Wasp (*Vespula* spp.)* – weak or strong.

* Bee/Wasp: Testing should begin (as directed in the package enclosure leaflet) using the weak solution. Only if the reaction obtained is negative or very weakly positive should the patient be tested with the strong solution.

(POLLENS)

Flower pollens: Aster (*Callistephus chinensis*); Bluebell (*Hyacinthoides non-scripta/Endymion non-scriptus*); Chrysanthemum (*C. morifolium koreanum*); Daffodil (*Narcissus* spp.); Dahlia (*Dahlia* spp.); Goldenrod (Solidago canadensis); Lupin (*Lupinus polyphyllus*); Marguerite, (*Chrysanthemum leucanthemum*); Michaelmas Daisy (*Aster novi-belgii*); Tulip (*Tulipa* spp.); Wallflower (*Cheiranthus cheiri*).

Grass pollens: Bent (*Agrostis capillaris/tenuis*); Bermuda (*Cynodon dactylon*); Brome (*Bromus* spp.); Cocksfoot (*Dactylis glomerata*); Couch (*Elymus/Agropyron repens*); Dogstail, Crested (*Cynosurus cristatus*);

False Oat (*Arrhenatherum elatius*); Fescue, Meadow (*Festuca pratensis*); Foxtail, Meadow (*Alopecurus pratensis*); †Maize (*Zea mays*); Meadow Grass (*Poa pratensis/trivialis*); Oat, Cultivated (*Avena sativa*); Oat, Wild (*Avena fatua*); †Rye, Cultivated (*Secale cereale*); Rye-grass (*Lolium perenne/multiflorum*); Timothy (*Phleum pratense*); Vernal, Sweet (*Anthoxanthum odoratum*); Wheat, Cultivated (*Triticum* spp.); Yorkshire Fog (*Holcus lanatus*).

Shrub and tree pollens: Acacia, False (*Robinia pseudoacacia*); Alder (*Alnus* spp.); Ash (*Fraxinus* spp.); Beech (*Fagus* spp.); †Birch, Silver (*Betula* spp.); †Elder (*Sambucus nigra*); Elm (*Ulmus* spp.); Hawthorn (*Crataegus* spp.); †Hazel (*Corylus* spp.); Heather (*Calluna vulgaris*); Horse-chestnut (*Aesculus* spp.); Laburnum (*L. anagyroides*); Lilac (*Syringa vulgaris*); Lime (*Tilia europea/cordata*); Mezquit (*Prosopis* spp.); Mock Orange (*Philadelphus* spp.); Oak, Common (*Quercus* spp.); Pine, Austrian (*Pinus nigra*); Pine Scots (*Pinus sylvestris*); Plane (*Platanus* spp.); †Poplar (*Populus* spp.); Privet (*Ligustrum* spp.); Rose (*Rosa* spp.); Sycamore (*Acer* spp.); Willow (*Salix* spp.).

Weed and miscellaneous pollens: Buttercup (*Ranunculus* spp.); Clover (*Trifolium* spp.); Dandelion (*Taraxacum* spp.); Fat Hen (*Chenopodium* spp.); Mugwort (*Artemisia vulgaris*); †Nettle (*Urtica dioica*); Orache (*Atriplex* spp.); †Plantain (*Plantago lanceolata*); Ragweed, Common or Short (*Ambrosia elatior*); Ragwort (*Senecio jacobaea*); Sorrel (*Rumex acetosa*); Willowherb, Rosebay (*Chamerion/Chamaenerion angustifolium*); Wormwood (*Artemisia absinthium*).

MISCELLANEOUS ITEMS:

1. Prick Test Diluent Control Solution contains 50% glycerol, 6% sodium chloride and 0.5% phenol (as a preservative). It has no allergen content.
2. Intradermal Test Diluent Control Solution contains 0.5% sodium chloride, 0.5% phenol (as a preservative), 0.14% sodium phosphate and 0.04% potassium dihydrogen phosphate. It has no allergen content.
3. Histamine dihydrochloride solution is available for assessment of histamine reactivity, as a prick test (1 mg/ml) or as an intradermal test (0.1 mg/ml). It can be of value when a patient with a case history indicating allergy gives negative skin reactions to all the allergens tested. A positive reaction to the histamine solution helps to rule out the possibility that the patient's skin reactivity may have been suppressed by concomitant antihistamine drug treatment.

SERIES I AND SERIES II KITS

The most important allergens are supplied as Series I, and the next important as Series II kits. Both kits are supplied complete with control solution, prick test instruments, Bencard Case History Charts and Skin Test Reaction Charts.

　The contents are listed below:

Series I (20 prick test solutions): †House dust mite (*D. pteronyssinus*); †House dust; †Feathers; †Horse hair and dander; †Cat fur; †Dog hair; †Sheep wool; †Human hair and dandruff; †Rabbit fur; †Cotton flock; †B2 Grass pollens; †B3 Tree pollens; †B5 Weed and shrub pollens; †Hay dust; †Straw dust; †*Cladosporium herbarum*; †*Alternaria alternata*; †Plantain pollen; †Nettle pollen; †Birch pollen.

Series II (19 prick test solutions): †Cow dander; †Kapok; †*Aspergillus niger*; †*Neurospora sitophila*; †*Rhizopus*

nigricans; †*Penicillium notatum*; †*Fusarium* spp.; †*Sporobolomyces roseus*; †Dry rot; †*Aspergillus fumigatus*; †Mixed threshings; Staph. aureus; †Hazel pollen; Whole egg; Wheat grain; Milk; Chocolate; Cod; Lobster.

Allergens marked † in the above lists are available for inclusion in both Alavac-S and SDV vaccines.

All other allergens listed are available for inclusion in SDV only.

Bencard tries to ensure that all allergens are immediately available from stock; however, in view of the large range, this may not always be possible.

The Bencard list of allergens is continually being reviewed to reflect current practice and demand.

Uses Bencard Skin Testing Solutions are used to confirm the significance of the most likely causative allergens indicated by case history and to establish their relative importance in allergic conditions.

Dosage and administration Prick testing solutions must not be used for intradermal testing.

Recommended technique for skin testing:

1. *General information:* Adrenaline Injection BP (Adrenaline 1 in 1000) and other supportive measures must always be kept at hand when skin testing with any allergens.

Antihistamines and other drugs which are likely to suppress the immediate Type 1 reaction should be discontinued 48 hours prior to testing. (In the case of long-acting antihistamines earlier discontinuation is required. Please consult the appropriate manufacturer.)

The flexor aspect of the forearm is a convenient site for testing. Clean the skin with soap and water if necessary – do not sterilize with organic solvents or strong antiseptics.

A ball point pen may be used to mark the skin (with suitable symbols) adjacent to planned test sites to identify the allergen and control solutions used.

Since each vial is used more than once, aseptic precautions must be sufficient to avoid the risk of microbial contamination.

2. *Prick testing:* Using the applicator attached to the vial cap, place one drop of the control solution on the skin.

In the same way, place one drop of each prick test solution required at about 3 cm intervals along the arm.

Hold the prick test instrument supplied almost parallel to the skin with its tip in the drop of control solution. Push until the tip just enters the superficial skin layer taking care not to draw blood. Raise the tip slightly and then withdraw the instrument.

Repeat the procedure with each test solution, either rinsing the prick test instrument in carbol saline and wiping it between each test, or using a fresh prick test instrument.

Carefully wipe any excess test solution away using a fresh piece of sterile cotton wool for each test.

3. *Intradermal testing:* Clean the rubber cap of the testing solution vial with sterile saline or 0.5% phenol solution. Do not use spirit or other strong antiseptics.

Using a tuberculin syringe with a short bevel needle, inject 0.01 to 0.02 ml of control solution intradermally. It is important to inject into the skin and not beneath it. This will raise a small bleb.

In the same way, inject 0.01 to 0.02 ml of each intradermal test required at about 3 cm intervals along the arm.

Use either a fresh syringe or clean the syringe and needle after each test by three times drawing into it and ejecting sterile saline or 0.5% phenol solution. The three washes are best drawn from three separate beakers (which should be used in the same order after each test) and each wash discarded into a fourth beaker.

4. *Interpretation of Skin Test Reactions:* Examine reactions approximately fifteen minutes after testing. (Reactions to histamine should be examined after approximately ten minutes.) Assess the strength of each reaction by the degree of erythema and the area of the weal formed. Weal size may be measured with a Bencard Skin Test Reaction Gauge. Record the strength of each reaction relative to the control on a Bencard Skin Test Reaction Chart as follows:

Prick testing

−	No weal. Erythema absent or less than 1 mm diameter.
+	Weal absent or very slight. Erythema present, not more than 3 mm diameter.
+ +	Weal not more than 3 mm diameter, with associated erythema.
+ + +	Weal between 3 mm and 5 mm diameter, with erythema.
+ + + +	Any larger reaction, possibly with pseudopodia.

Intradermal testing

−	No increase in the size of bleb since injection. No erythema.
+	An increase in the size of bleb to a weal not more than 5 mm diameter, with associated erythema.
+ +	Weal between 5 mm and 8 mm diameter, with associated erythema.
+ + +	Weal between 8 mm and 12 mm diameter, with erythema.
+ + + +	Any larger reaction, possibly with pseudopodia.

Although some patients will give a reaction to the control solution, they will usually give significantly larger reactions to the allergens to which they are clinically sensitive. In recording the reactions to these allergens, an allowance should be made for the size of the control reaction.

Contra-indications, warnings, etc
Prick testing solutions must not be used for intradermal testing.

Precautions: Although the likelihood of a systemic reaction is very low, Adrenaline Injection BP (Adrenaline 1 in 1000) and other supportive measures must always be kept at hand.

Treatment of anaphylaxis: Anaphylactic shock: characterised by bronchospasm, laryngeal oedema, urticaria and shock. Immediate attention should be given as follows:

1. The patient should be laid down and treated immediately.
2. 0.5 mlt Adrenaline Injection BP (Adrenaline 1 in 1,000) should be given intramuscularly close to the vaccine injection site. This should be repeated to a total of 2 mlt over 15 minutes if necessary. In extreme cases, 0.5 mlt Adrenaline (1 in 10,000) can be given by slow intravenous injection.

3. If bronchospasm persists, 10–20 mlt of Aminophylline Injection BP (250 mg per 10 ml) should be given by slow intravenous injection at a rate of 2 mlt per minute.
4. In addition, 200–400 mgt of Hydrocortisone Injection BP should be given intravenously. This is to combat persistent bronchospasm which can occur 6–8 hours after the initial collapse.
5. Full supportive measures should be available and employed if necessary and patients should be closely monitored for at least 24 hours after recovery.

Pharmaceutical precautions Bencard skin testing solutions should be stored between 2 and 8°C. Do not freeze.

Legal category POM.

Package quantities Prick and Intradermal Testing Solutions are prepared in 2ml multidose vials available individually or in Series I and II Skin Testing Kits.

Further information Nil.

Product licence number 0038/5000.

† All dosages should be reduced as required for children.

JUVEL* TABLETS
JUVEL* SYRUP

Presentation *Juvel Tablets:* Sugar-coated tablets overprinted in black with the product name 'JUVEL'.

Juvel Syrup: Lemon-flavoured liquid.

Active ingredients

	Tablet	5 ml syrup
Vitamin A	5,000 units	4,000 units
Vitamin D_2	500 units	400 units
Vitamin B_1 (Thiamine Hydrochloride)	2.5 mg	2 mg
Vitamin B_2 (Riboflavine)	2.5 mg	2 mg
Vitamin B_6 (Pyridoxine Hydrochloride)	2.5 mg	2 mg
Nicotinamide	50 mg	40 mg
Vitamin C (Ascorbic Acid)	50 mg	40 mg

Uses *Principal action:* Juvel is a balanced multivitamin dietary supplement.

Indications: As a course of multivitamin therapy, in the elderly on restricted diets; in patients on imposed dietary regimes; when impaired absorption is suspected; or when nutritional demand is greater than normal, during periods of rapid growth in childhood or adolescence and during pregnancy and lactation.

Dosage and administration For oral administration only.

Adults (including elderly patients): 1 tablet or one 5 ml spoonful of syrup daily.
Children: over 2 years: One 5 ml spoonful of syrup daily.
Children under 2 years: 2.5 ml of syrup daily.

Contra-indications, warnings, etc
Contra-indications: None at the recommended dosage.

Precautions: Juvel may be used in patients being treated for Parkinson's disease with a levodopa preparation which includes a dopa-decarboxylase inhibitor (e.g. carbidopa, benserazide) but should not be used with levodopa alone as pyridoxine may act as an antagonist.

Side-effects: None reported.

Overdosage: Prolonged ingestion of massive doses of vitamins A and D can lead to hypervitaminosis states. Symptoms include dry rough skin, painful joint swellings, anorexia and vomiting; these disappear when treatment is discontinued.

Pharmaceutical precautions Store in a cool place.

The syrup should be protected from strong light and be well shaken before dispensing into amber glass containers.

Syrup BP is a suitable diluent.

Legal category Tablets P.
Syrup GSL.

Package quantities *Tablets:* 100.
Syrup: 200 ml.

Further information Vitamin A is required for normal epithelial growth; vitamins of the B complex for normal intracellular carbohydrate metabolism, particularly in the brain; vitamin C for the maintenance of collagen, tissue repair and blood formation; and vitamin D for metabolism of calcium and phosphorus.

Product licence numbers
Tablets   0038/5112
Syrup   0038/5111

MIGEN*

Presentation Migen contains tyrosine-adsorbed glycerinated extract of house dust mite (*Dermatophagoides pteronyssinus*).

Initial course: Six unit-dose syringes prefilled with 0.5 ml of vaccine in graded concentrations as follows:

Syringe no.	Dose: Noon Units
1	4
2	10
3	25
4	60
5	150
6	400

Maintenance course: Six unit-dose syringes prefilled with 0.5 ml of vaccine at the top dose concentration of 400 Noon units.

The tyrosine content is 4.0% w/v; with Phenol BP as a preservative.

The D. pteronyssinus extract is adsorbed on to tyrosine, a naturally occurring amino acid, to ensure slow release of the active material, giving a prolonged and efficient desensitising effect.

Uses Indicated for the treatment of asthma and perennial rhinitis for patients in whom house dust mite is implicated as the principal allergen.

Dosage and administration Please note that the section on 'Contra-indications, warnings, etc.' must be studied before Migen is administered.

Adrenaline Injection BP (Adrenaline 1 in 1,000) should always be kept at hand when giving any desensitising vaccine.

The administration procedures shown in the leaflet included with each course of Migen should be carefully followed.

Migen may be given to adults (including elderly patients) and children of six years and over.

Migen must be removed from the refrigerator 2–3 hours before use.

The syringe should be shaken thoroughly immediately prior to giving the injection.

Injections should be given slowly by the subcutaneous route.

Do not inject into a blood vessel, or intramuscularly. Do not rub the site of injection.

Initial course: Injections should be given at intervals of 7–14 days.

If there is a break in treatment (i.e., more than 14 days between injections), it is recommended that treatment should be recommenced with a new Initial course.

Maintenance therapy: Maintenance therapy is recommended to maintain clinical improvement. The first maintenance injection should be given one month after the final injection of the initial course. Subsequent maintenance injections should be given monthly, with review at appropriate intervals, at the discretion of the physician.

If there is a break in treatment (i.e., more than 5 weeks between injections), it is recommended that treatment should be recommenced with a new Initial course.

Contra-indications, warnings, etc

Contra-indications: Patients should not be given an allergy vaccine if:

(a) They have had a severe asthma attack not responding to an inhaled bronchodilator;

(b) they have suffered from a febrile condition or an acute attack of asthma in the 24 hours preceding the intended dose.

Use in pregnancy: It is advisable to avoid use during pregnancy.

Precautions: Patients should be warned not to eat a heavy meal immediately before an injection is due to be given.

In very sensitive patients, it is advantageous to give an antihistamine tablet about one hour before each injection.

Injections should be given slowly by the subcutaneous route. Do not inject into a blood vessel or intramuscularly. Do not rub the site of injection.

Adrenaline Injection BP (Adrenaline 1 in 1,000) should always be kept at hand when giving any desensitising vaccine.

All patients should be instructed to remain under observation in the surgery for at least 20 minutes after each injection and advised to contact the doctor immediately in the unlikely event of a delayed reaction.

The patient should not take any strenuous physical exercise for several hours following the injection.

Reactions: Local reactions, such as slight swelling or irritation, can sometimes occur and may require symptomatic treatment if they persist.

Mild systemic reactions such as rhinitis or urticaria may be treated with antihistamines orally, or by injection if necessary. In mild bronchospasm, a sympathomimetic bronchodilator such as salbutamol and possibly an anti-inflammatory steroid should be given. If required, 0.5 ml Adrenaline Injection BP (Adrenaline 1 in 1,000) may be given subcutaneously.

Severe systemic reactions may occasionally arise in the form of typical allergic symptoms; anaphylaxis is rare.

Treatment of anaphylaxis: Anaphylactic shock: characterised by bronchospasm, laryngeal oedema, urticaria and shock. Immediate attention should be given as follows:

1. The patient should be laid down and treated immediately.

2. 0.5 mlt Adrenaline Injection BP (Adrenaline 1 in 1,000) should be given intramuscularly close to the vaccine injection site. This should be repeated to a total of 2 mlt over 15 minutes if necessary. In extreme cases, 0.5 mlt Adrenaline (1 in 10,000) can be given by slow intravenous injection.

3. If bronchospasm persists, 10–20 mlt of Aminophylline Injection BP (250 mg per 10 ml) should be given by slow intravenous injection at a rate of 2 mlt per minute.

4. In addition, 200–400 mgt of Hydrocortisone Injection BP should be given intravenously. This is to combat persistent bronchospasm which can occur 6–8 hours after the initial collapse.

5. Full supportive measures should be available and employed if necessary and patients should be closely monitored for at least 24 hours after recovery.

† All dosages should be reduced as required for children.

Note: A severe local reaction, or severe systemic reaction such as urticaria or asthma, indicates that the standard vaccine is unsuitable for the treatment of the particular patient, who should be referred to a consultant for advice or transferred to a suitably dilute specific desensitising vaccine (Alavac-S or SDV) containing house dust mite obtainable from Bencard.

(For full prescribing information please refer to the relevant data sheets).

Legal category POM.

Pharmaceutical precautions Migen must be stored in a refrigerator (5°C). It must not be frozen and must be removed 2–3 hours before use.

Package quantities Initial and Maintenance courses each consist of a set of 6 unit-dose syringes prefilled with vaccine, and with needles attached. An instruction leaflet is included with each set.

Further information Migen is a standard vaccine prepared from extract of Dermatophagoides pteronyssinus, the predominant species of house dust mite occurring in British homes. The house dust mite is the most commonly implicated allergen in allergic asthma and perennial rhinitis.

Desensitisation with Migen offers a fundamental approach to the management of the mite allergic patient. It should be prescribed when the mite has been implicated as the principal allergen by case history, and preferably confirmed by skin-testing. An appropriate testing solution is available from Bencard.

Patients who benefit from an Initial course of treatment are likely to maintain their clinical improvement with Maintenance therapy.

Migen may be prescribed on NHS form FP10. Both Initial and Maintenance courses are available for immediate supply from stock.

The Bencard Medical Department will advise on any aspect of treatment.

Product licence number 0038/0112.

NACTON*
NACTON FORTE*

Presentation Nacton (2 mg): White-coloured, scored tablets engraved 'NACTON 2'.

Nacton Forte (4 mg): Orange-coloured, scored tablets engraved 'NACTON 4'.

Active ingredients: Nacton: Each tablet contains 2 mg of Poldine Methylsulphate BP.

Nacton Forte: Each tablet contains 4 mg of Poldine Methylsulphate BP.

Uses Principal action: Poldine methylsulphate is a proven anticholinergic compound which at therapeutic doses acts mainly on the parietal or oxyntic cells of the stomach, causing gastric acid production to be reduced by over 50%.

Indications: Peptic ulcer; recurrent dyspepsia associated with hyperacidity; whenever acidity causes pain.

Nacton has also proved helpful in the treatment of nocturnal enuresis.

Dosage and administration Adults:

Standard dosage: 1 tablet of Nacton Forte (4 mg) four times a day (the last at bedtime). This will give effective and continuous pain relief without side-effects in the majority of patients.

If necessary (e.g. in elderly patients), optimum dosage may be determined by adjusting to individual requirements. For example, initially 1 tablet of Nacton (2 mg) four times a day (the last at bedtime) followed by review after four days.

Tailored dosage: If dose titration is required, initially 1 tablet of Nacton (2 mg) four times a day (the last at bedtime), increasing by half a Nacton tablet (1 mg) per dose after every four days. Continue until the first signs of overdosage appear and then reduce each dose by half a Nacton tablet (1 mg). This level should be the optimum therapeutic dose.

If treatment is suspended for more than a week and later resumed, the therapeutic dose should again be built up gradually. If the previous therapeutic dose was greater than 4 mg taken four times a day, the patient may resume treatment, building up from a starting dose of 4 mg four times a day.

Children: Nacton may be used for the treatment of nocturnal enuresis in children; 1 tablet (2 mg) at bedtime is a suitable dose.

Contra-indications, warnings, etc
Contra-indications and precautions: For patients in whom tachycardia, difficulty in micturition or increase in ocular tension might give rise to particular anxiety, Nacton and Nacton Forte should only be used under close supervision.

Use in pregnancy: There is no evidence that Nacton or Nacton Forte have teratogenic effects. However, treatment is not advised during the first trimester of pregnancy.

Side-effects. There are no side-effects at therapeutic doses.

Overdosage: Mild overdosage: Signs of mild overdosage are, in order of frequency, dry mouth, blurred vision, hesitancy of micturition or tachycardia. They will usually disappear if one or two doses are omitted before resuming treatment at a lower dosage level.

Gross overdosage: Gastric aspiration and lavage should be performed immediately. A short-acting barbiturate such as thiopentone sodium may be given cautiously for the stage of excitement.

Pharmaceutical precautions Store in a dry place.

Legal category POM.

Package quantities Nacton (2 mg): 50 and 250 tablets.
Nacton Forte (4 mg): 100 tablets.

Further information Nacton and Nacton Forte provide an environment for ulcer healing by halving gastric acid production. Reduction of gastric acid secretion can be maintained over several years without development of tolerance to the dosage used. Pain is controlled even at night as each dose of Nacton or Nacton Forte is effective for 8–9 hours. Nacton and Nacton Forte permit patients a liberal diet and a return to normal working life.

Product licence number
Nacton   0038/5077
Nacton Forte   0038/5078

NORMAX*

Presentation *Normax Capsules* (Co-danthrusate Capsules), containing 50 mg danthron and 60 mg docusate sodium. Dark brown capsules, overprinted with the product name 'Normax'.

Uses *Principal action:* Danthron is a mild peristaltic stimulant acting on the lower bowel to encourage normal bowel movement without causing irritation. Docusate sodium is a softening agent which prevents excessive colonic dehydration and hardening of stools.

Indications: For the short-term management of acute or chronic constipation. Constipation in geriatric practice, especially in immobilised patients. Conditions in which defaecation must be free of strain, such as cardiac failure, coronary thrombosis, episiotomy and haemorrhoids. Preparation for surgical or radiographic procedures requiring an empty colon – for example barium enema studies; also of great value in clearing the bowel of barium following diagnostic radiology. Following haemorrhoidectomy.

Dosage and administration For oral administration only.

Adults (including elderly patients): 1–3 capsules taken at bedtime.

Children: (6–12 years): 1 capsule at bedtime.

Contra-indications, warnings, etc
Contra-indications: In common with all laxatives, Normax is contra-indicated in cases of non-specific abdominal pain, and when intestinal obstruction is suspected.

Use in pregnancy: Although animal studies have not shown hazard, Normax cannot be recommended during early pregnancy.

Precautions: Prolonged use is not recommended. Danthron may appear in the milk during lactation in sufficient quantities to affect the nursing infant.

Side-effect: The griping often found with other types of laxative is not an appreciable problem with Normax. Occasionally, an orange tint in the urine may be observed, due to the danthron component.

Overdosage: The patient should be encouraged to drink fluids. An anticholinergic preparation may be used to ease excessive intestinal motility if necessary.

Pharmaceutical precautions Store in a cool dry place.

Legal category P.

Package quantities Normax is available in packs of 30 and 250.

Further information The gently effective twofold action of Normax is particularly helpful in restoring normal bowel function in the elderly and infirm. A predictable overnight action follows bedtime dosage, enabling the patient to produce soft, formed stools on rising.

Product licence number 0038/0092

NORVAL*

Presentation *Norval tablets:* Orange film coated tablets engraved 'Norval' on one side and '30' on the other. Each tablet contains 30 mg Mianserin Hydrochloride BP.

Also available, orange film coated tablets containing 10 mg and 20 mg Mianserin Hydrochloride BP. Each tablet is engraved 'Norval' on one side and '10' or '20' respectively on the reverse.

Uses Symptoms of depressive illness.

Dosage and administration *For oral administration:* The tablets should be swallowed whole without chewing.

Adults: Treatment should normally be initiated, for the first few days, at 30–40 mg a day as a single bedtime dose, or in divided doses. The effective maintenance dosage will normally lie between 30 mg and 90 mg a day as indicated in the table, though higher levels may be required in some patients.

Degree of depression	Usual daily dosage
Mild to moderate	30–60 mg nocte or in divided doses.
Moderate to severe	60–90 mg nocte or in divided doses. If higher levels are required these should be given in divided doses.

Divided daily dosages up to 200 mg are well tolerated. It is often advantageous to maintain antidepressant treatment for several months after initial clinical improvement has occurred.

Elderly: Not more than 30 mg a day initially. This starting dose should be increased with caution under close supervision. A lower maintenance dosage than is usual may be sufficient to produce a satisfactory clinical response.

Children: Not recommended.

Contra-indications, warnings, etc
Contra-indications: Use is contra-indicated in mania, severe liver disease and during breast feeding. (Breast feeding should be discontinued if antidepressant therapy is considered essential.)

Use in pregnancy: Do not use during pregnancy unless there are compelling reasons. There is no evidence of safety in human pregnancy. Animal studies have not shown hazard.

Precautions: Care should always be taken in patients with recent myocardial infarction or heart block. However, serious cardiotoxic effects appear to be rare at therapeutic dosage, even in patients with pre-existing cardiac disease, recent myocardial infarction or cardiac insufficiency.

The elderly are less liable to experience adverse reactions such as agitation, confusion and postural hypotension with Norval, than with tricyclics or bridged tricyclics, but all antidepressant therapy should be used with caution in this group of patients.

Patients posing a high suicide risk always require close initial supervision.

Avoid, if possible, in patients with epilepsy.

When treating patients with diabetes, hepatic or renal insufficiency, normal precautions should be exercised and the dosages of any concurrent therapy kept under review.

Patients with narrow angle glaucoma or symptoms suggestive of prostatic hypertrophy, should also be monitored even though anticholinergic side-effects are not anticipated with Norval therapy.

There are indications that Norval, like other anti-depressants, may precipitate hypomania in susceptible subjects with bipolar affective illness.

Norval may potentiate the central nervous depressant action of alcohol.

If surgery is necessary during Norval therapy, the anaesthetist should be informed of the treatment being given.

Drug interactions: Norval should not be given concurrently with, or within two weeks of cessation of therapy with, monoamine oxidase inhibitors.

Clinical experience has shown that Norval does not interact with the antihypertensives bethanidine, clonidine, hydralazine, guanethidine and propranolol. Nevertheless, the monitoring of blood pressure is recommended for those patients receiving concurrent antihypertensive therapy.

Phenytoin plasma levels should be monitored in patients treated concurrently with Norval.

Concurrent anticoagulant therapy of the coumarin-type (e.g. warfarin) is also permissible, but close additional monitoring should be undertaken.

Interactions have not been reported between Norval and sympathomimetic agents and are unlikely.

Warnings and adverse effects: As improvement may not occur during the first 2–4 weeks of treatment, patients should be closely monitored during this period. It may be advisable to maintain treatment for several months after initial clinical improvement has occurred.

The most commonly occurring side-effect is drowsiness, particularly during the first few days of therapy. Patients should be warned of the possible hazard in driving or operating machinery. Any drowsiness may be potentiated by alcohol.

Serious adverse effects are uncommon. A small number of cases of bone marrow depression, usually presenting as an agranulocytosis or granulocytopenia, and generally reversible on stopping treatment, have been reported. If a patient develops symptoms of infection, e.g. fever, sore throat, stomatitis or other inflammatory conditions, during treatment with Norval, treatment should be stopped and a full blood count obtained. This adverse reaction has been observed in all age groups but appears to be more common in the elderly.

Jaundice, usually mild, hypomania and convulsions have also been reported at therapeutic dosage and under such circumstances treatment should be withdrawn.

Additional adverse effects that may occur include breast disorders (gynaecomastia, nipple tenderness and non-puerperal lactation), altered liver enzyme levels, dizziness, postural hypotension, polyarthropathy, skin rash, sweating and tremor.

Psychotic manifestations including mania and paranoid delusions may be exacerbated during antidepressant therapy.

The following adverse effects although not reported with Norval can occur with tricyclics and bridged tricyclics: interference with sexual function; withdrawal symptoms in adults; withdrawal symptoms (e.g. neuromuscular irritability) in neonates whose mothers received tricyclic or bridged tricyclic antidepressants during pregnancy.

Overdosage: There is no specific antidote. Treatment is by gastric lavage with appropriate supportive therapy. Symptoms of overdosage are normally confined to prolonged sedation. Cardiac arrhythmias, severe hypotension, convulsions and respiratory depression are unlikely to occur.

Pharmaceutical precautions Protect tablets from light.

Legal category POM.

Package quantities Norval 30 mg tablets are supplied in foil packs of 30. Each pack contains three blister strips of 10 tablets. Also available in containers of 100 and 500 tablets. Norval 10 mg tablets are available in foil packs of 90 (three blister strips of 30) and in containers of 100 and 500 tablets. The 20 mg tablet is available in containers of 100 and 500.

Further information Norval is an antidepressant with a distinctive tetracyclic structure which confers important benefits over the tricyclic compounds. Norval has also been shown to possess anxiolytic properties comparable with diazepam.

Antidepressant activity is at least equal to that of amitriptyline and imipramine, but Norval may be preferred for its absence of troublesome anticholinergic side-effects; this may be of special importance when treating depressed patients who may be at concurrent risk from conditions such as glaucoma, urinary retention and prostatic hypertrophy. There is also substantial evidence that anticholinergic effects such as dry mouth can be a psychosomatic feature of depressive illness; such symptoms have been shown to be alleviated with Norval therapy. Clinical experience has confirmed that Norval is significantly less toxic than either amitriptyline or imipramine and that cardiac problems are unlikely. Norval appears to be particularly effective in improving 'pessimistic thought' and 'suicidal ideation'. Moreover, its relatively high safety margin is of considerable importance in view of the high number of suicides attributed to tricyclic overdosage.

Product licence numbers
Norval 10 mg: 0038/0230R
Norval 20 mg: 0038/0247R
Norval 30 mg: 0038/0248R

NULACIN*

Presentation Off-white coloured tablets embossed with the product name 'NULACIN'. Each tablet contains:

Whole milk combined with dextrins and maltose.

Magnesium trisilicate	230 mg
Heavy magnesium oxide	130 mg
Calcium carbonate	130 mg
Heavy magnesium carbonate	30 mg
Peppermint oil q.s.	

Calorific content per tablet: 11 calories.

Uses *Principal action:* The balanced combination of antacids and milk protein in Nulacin causes rapid and continuous neutralisation of excess gastric acid so that the gastric acidity is maintained at pH 3–4.

The milk fat in Nulacin helps to inhibit the formation of excess gastric juice.

Indications: Dyspepsia. Reflux oesophagitis. Hiatus hernia. Peptic ulcer. Whenever gastric hyperacidity causes pain.

Dosage and administration (including elderly patients) One or more tablets as required.

For continuous therapeutic effect the tablet should be allowed to disperse slowly in the mouth, placed between cheek and gum. For quicker relief the tablet should be chewed and swallowed.

Contra-indications, warnings, etc
Contra-indication: As Nulacin contains gluten, it is contra-indicated in coeliac disease.

Warnings and precautions: Nil.

Side-effects: No significant side-effects have been encountered with Nulacin.

Overdosage: Overdosage has not been reported. However, as with all antacids, there is a theoretical danger of alkalosis.

Pharmaceutical precautions Store in a cool dry place. Replace container cap after use.

Legal category GSL.

Package quantities 25 tablets.

Further information Nulacin contains effective doses of antacids to give rapid relief from gastric pain. Nulacin disperses slowly in the mouth to give continuous relief which is independent of the rate of stomach emptying. Nulacin is presented in convenient tablets which have a very acceptable malt and mint flavour.

Product licence number 0038/5079.

OROVITE* TABLETS
OROVITE* SYRUP

Presentation *Orovite Tablets:* Maroon, sugar-coated tablets overprinted in white with the product name 'OROVITE'.

Orovite Syrup: Orange-flavoured solution.

Active ingredients

	Tablet (mg)	5 ml syrup (mg)
Thiamine Hydrochloride (vitamin B$_1$)	50	20
Riboflavine (vitamin B$_2$)	5	2
Pyridoxine Hydrochloride (vitamin B$_6$)	5	2
Nicotinamide	200	80
Ascorbic Acid (vitamin C)	100	40

Uses *Principal action;* Orovite contains high concentrations of the water-soluble vitamins B and C to correct disturbed carbohydrate metabolism.

Indications: Deficiency of the B complex and C vitamins, in particular when encountered: (a) in association with alcoholism, as maintenance therapy; (b) as debility after febrile illnesses such as influenza, measles; acute bron-

chitis, tonsillitis, enteritis, viral pneumonia; (c) in confusional states in old age or following illness; (d) as debility following operation.

Orovite is also useful as oral maintenance therapy following a course of Parentrovite. (See Parentrovite data sheet.)

Dosage and administration For oral administration only.

Adults (including elderly patients): One tablet or two 5 ml spoonfuls syrup three times a day.

Children: One 5 ml spoonful syrup three times a day.

If parenteral therapy is required, treatment should be commenced with Parentrovite.

Contra-indications, warnings, etc
Contra indications: Nil.

Precautions: Orovite may be used in patients being treated for Parkinson's disease with a levodopa preparation which includes a dopa-decarboxylase inhibitor (e.g. carbidopa, benserazide) but should not be used with levodopa alone as pyridoxine may act as an antagonist.

Side-effects: Flushing of the face has been reported occasionally.

Overdosage: Nil.

Pharmaceutical precautions Store in a cool place. The syrup should be protected from strong light and be well shaken before dispensing into amber glass containers. If a dilution is required, Syrup BP should be used.

Legal category GSL.

Package quantities *Tablets:* 25, 100, 500.
Syrup: 200 ml.

Further information Vitamins of the B complex play an integral part as co-enzymes in the intracellular metabolism of carbohydrates. The efficient functioning of this metabolism is essential for normal health. Similarly, ascorbic acid plays an important part in the biochemical reactions of cells and tissues and is normally present in the highest concentrations in those parts of the brain which are the most active metabolically.

Lack of water soluble vitamins results in impairment of normal intracellular metabolism. The high concentrations of the water soluble vitamins contained in Orovite rapidly replenish depleted cellular stores and speed the return of normal intracellular metabolism.

Product licence numbers
Tablets 0038/5092
Syrup 0038/5091

OROVITE '7'*

Presentation Orange coloured granules in unit dose sachets.

Active ingredients: Each sachet provides:

Vitamin A (Palmitate)	2,500 units
Vitamin D$_2$	100 units
Vitamin B$_1$ (Thiamine Mononitrate)	1.4 mg
Vitamin B$_2$ (as Riboflavine Sodium Phosphate)	1.7 mg
Vitamin B$_6$ (Pyridoxine Hydrochloride)	2.0 mg
Nicotinamide	18 mg
Vitamin C	60 mg

Uses Orovite '7' provides a course of balanced multivitamin therapy for the management of potential vitamin deficiencies.

Dosage and administration For oral administration only.

Adults (including elderly patients) and children over 5 years of age: The contents of one sachet per day, dissolved in approximately one third of a glass of water.

Contra-indications, warnings, etc

Contra-indications: None at the recommended dosage.

Precautions: Orovite '7' may be used in patients being treated for Parkinson's disease with a levodopa preparation which includes a dopa-decarboxylase inhibitor (e.g. carbidopa, benserazide) but should not be used with levodopa alone as pyridoxine may act as an antagonist.

Side-effects: None reported.

Overdosage: Prolonged ingestion of massive doses of vitamins A and D can lead to hypervitaminosis states. Symptoms include dry rough skin, painful joint swellings, anorexia and vomiting; these disappear when treatment is discontinued.

Pharmaceutical precautions Store in a cool dry place.

Legal category GSL.

Package quantities 10 and 30 sachets.

Further information Orovite '7' provides adequate intake of essential vitamins for patients whose daily nutritional requirements may not otherwise be met, such as the elderly on restricted diets, patients on imposed dietary regimes, or in cases where impaired absorption is suspected.

Orovite '7' has a convenient and palatable once-daily sachet presentation which improves patient compliance and is especially suitable for patients who may have difficulty in swallowing tablets or measuring doses from bottles.

Product licence number 0079/0164.

PARENTROVITE* IVHP
PARENTROVITE* IMHP
PARENTROVITE* IMM

Presentation Paired amber glass ampoules for injectable administration; available in three different presentations. Intravenous High Potency (IVHP), Intramuscular High Potency (IMHP) and Intramuscular Maintenance (IMM).

Active ingredients: See table on next page.

Uses *Principal action:* Parentrovite IVHP, IMHP and IMM contain very high concentrations of the water-soluble vitamins B and C to correct disturbed carbohydrate metabolism.

Indications: Deficiency of the B complex and C vitamins, in particular that encountered: (a) in association with alcoholism; (b) in peripheral neuritis, associated with malabsorption syndromes, alcoholism or diabetic neuropathy; (c) after acute febrile illness, e.g. influenza, pneumonia; (d) in confusional states following severe illness or operation, especially in the elderly; (e) in states of acute malnutrition.

Dosage and administration

Indication	Dosage (incl. elderly)
(a) In association with alcoholism – acute alcoholic psychosis – delirium tremens – coma or delirium – post-operative confusional states.	2 to 4 pairs Intravenous High Potency ampoules, repeated 4 to 8 hourly for up to 2 days as indicated clinically, followed by 1 pair Intravenous High Potency or Intramuscular High Potency ampoules daily for 5 to 7 days.
(b) Peripheral neuritis associated with malabsorption states, alcoholism or diabetic neuropathy.	1 pair Intravenous High Potency or Intramuscular High Potency ampoules, once or twice daily for 3 to 7 days.
(c) After acute febrile illness	1 to 2 pairs Intramuscular Maintenance ampoules daily.
(d) In confusional states following severe illness especially in the elderly.	"
(e) In states of acute malnutrition.	"
Maintenance therapy for longer term treatment of the above conditions.	1 to 2 pairs Intramuscular Maintenance ampoules daily, until full health is restored, or until continuation therapy by oral route is possible (e.g. with Orovite tablets).

Children: Parenteral therapy is rarely necessary as children usually respond well to oral administration of the vitamin B complex in high dosage: e.g. with Orovite syrup. (See Orovite data sheet.) However, when parenteral administration of vitamins is required, the following dosage guidelines are recommended;

6–10 years: $\frac{1}{3}$ adult dose,

10–14 years: $\frac{1}{3}$ to $\frac{1}{2}$ adult dose.

14 years and over: adult dose.

These dosages may have to be modified in individual cases.

Administration: For parenteral administration only.

The contents of each pair of ampoules (i.e. No. 1 and No. 2) should be mixed together in a single syringe immediately prior to administration.

The intravenous and intramuscular presentations are not interchangeable. As a result of its high volume and lack of local anaesthetic, the intravenous presentation may cause unnecessary pain if administered intramuscularly. The presence of the anaesthetic in the intramuscular presentation makes it unsuitable for intravenous administration.

When given by infusion with other drugs, Parentrovite should be injected into the drip-tubing immediately after mixing.

	Intravenous		Intramuscular			
	High potency (IVHP)		High potency (IMHP)		Maintenance (IMM)	
Active ingredients of Parentrovite	No. 1 (mg)	No. 2 (mg)	No. 1 (mg)	No. 2 (mg)	No. 1 (mg)	No. 2 (mg)
Thiamine Hydrochloride (vitamin B₁)	250		250		100	
Riboflavine (vitamin B₂)	4		4		4	
Pyridoxine Hydrochloride (vitamin B₆)	50		50		50	
Nicotinamide		160		160		160
Ascorbic Acid (vitamin C)		500		500		500
Anhydrous glucose		1,000				
Benzyl Alcohol*			140		80	
				†		†
Volume per ampoule	5 ml	5 ml	5 ml	2 ml	2 ml	2 ml

* To give 2% in the mixed ampoules
† Contains 0.2% Chlorocresol

Intravenous Parentrovite – Contents of each pair of ampoules to be mixed in the syringe before injecting slowly into a vein. Dilution with normal saline may be made for drip infusion.

Intramuscular Parentrovite – Contents of each pair of ampoules to be mixed in the syringe before injecting slowly into the lateral muscles of the thigh or into the gluteal region.

Contra-indications, warnings, etc
Contra-indications: Sensitivity to any of the vitamins present.

Warnings and Precautions: Parentrovite may be used in patients being treated for Parkinson's disease with a levodopa preparation which includes a dopadecarboxylase inhibitor (e.g. carbidopa, benserazide) but should not be used with levodopa alone as pyridoxine may act as an antagonist. On very rare occasions repeated injections of preparations containing high concentrations of thiamine may give rise to anaphylactic shock. Should this occur, appropriate measures, such as the injection of adrenaline and soluble glucocorticoids (e.g. hydrocortisone) or antihistamine preparations must be taken immediately.

Side-effects: Flushing of the face has been reported occasionally.

Overdosage: Effects of overdosage are rare. It has been reported, however, that following administration of very large doses (for example over 10 pairs IVHP daily for three or more days) a state of excitement can result which is characterised by rapid mental activity. This subsides within 24 hours of stopping treatment, and there is often amnesia for the episode.

Pharmaceutical precautions Store in a cool place.

Legal category POM.

Package quantities
IV High Potency: 3 pairs, 12 pairs.
IM High Potency: 3 pairs, 12 pairs.
IM Maintenance: 3 pairs, 12 pairs.

Further Information Vitamins of the B complex play an integral part as co-enzymes in the intracellular metabolism of carbohydrates. The efficient functioning of this metabolism is essential for normal health. Similarly,

ascorbic acid plays an important part in the biochemical reactions of cells and tissues and is normally present in the highest concentrations in those parts of the brain which are the most active metabolically.

Lack of the water soluble vitamins results in impairment of normal intracellular metabolism. In some cases, such as an alcoholic who develops Wernicke's encephalopathy, lack of immediate treatment can result in permanent brain damage or even death.

The very high concentrations of the water-soluble vitamins contained in Parentrovite, rapidly replenish depleted cellular stores and speed the return of normal metabolism.

Product licence numbers
IV High Potency: 0038/5095
IM High Potency: 0038/5097
IM Maintenance: 0038/5099

POLLINEX*

Presentation Pollinex contains glutaraldehyde-modified extracts of pollen from twelve varieties of common grasses (Bent, Brome, Cocksfoot, Crested Dogstail, False Oat, Fescue, Meadow Foxtail, Meadow-grass, Rye-grass, Timothy, Vernal and Yorkshire Fog) adsorbed on to tyrosine.

Each course of treatment is presented in three unit-dose syringes each prefilled with 0.5 ml of vaccine in graded concentrations as follows:

Syringe no.	Dose: Noon Units
1	300
2	800
3	2,000

The tyrosine content is 4.0% w/v, with Phenol BP as a preservative. The grass pollen extract is modified by glutaraldehyde and adsorbed onto tyrosine, a naturally occurring amino acid, to ensure slow release of the active material, giving a prolonged and efficient desensitising effect.

Uses Indicated for the treatment of classical hayfever and pollen asthma, to give long-term protection whenever grass pollens are considered to be the sole or predominant cause.

Pollinex is formulated from the pollens of twelve common grasses which are responsible for the majority of classical hayfever and pollen asthma cases, and provides a convenient and effective preventive treatment.

Dosage and administration Please note that the section on 'Contra-indications, warnings, etc.' must be studied before Pollinex is administered.

Adrenaline Injection BP (Adrenaline 1 in 1,000) should always be kept at hand when giving any desensitising vaccine.

The administration procedures shown in the leaflet included with each course of Pollinex should be carefully followed.

The course should normally be started by mid-April (in the U.K.) in order to ensure completion before the onset of the grass pollen season. Do not use during the grass pollen season.

Pollinex may be given to adults (including elderly patients) and children of six years and over. Injections should be given at intervals of 7–14 days. Pollinex must be removed from the refrigerator 2–3 hours before use. The syringe should be shaken thoroughly immediately prior to giving the injection. Injections should be given slowly by the subcutaneous route. Do not inject into a blood vessel or intramuscularly. Do not rub the site of injection.

The three graduated doses of Pollinex constitute a complete course for one year. The administration of an initial course of treatment should produce a significant improvement during the ensuing pollen season. For continued clinical improvement, it is recommended that a course should be given in each of three successive years.

Contra-indications, warnings, etc
Contra-indications: Patients should not be given an allergy vaccine if:

(a) They have had a severe asthma attack not responding to an inhaled bronchodilator;

(b) they have suffered from a febrile condition or an acute attack of asthma in the 24 hours preceding the intended dose.

Use in pregnancy: It is advisable to avoid use during pregnancy.

Precautions: Patients should be warned not to eat a heavy meal immediately before an injection is due to be given.

In very sensitive patients, it is advantageous to give an antihistamine tablet about one hour before each injection.

Injections should be given slowly by the subcutaneous route. Do not inject into a blood vessel or intramuscularly. Do not rub the site of injection.

Adrenaline Injection BP (Adrenaline 1 in 1,000) should always be kept at hand when giving any desensitising vaccine.

All patients should be instructed to remain under observation in the surgery for at least 20 minutes after each injection and advised to contact the doctor immediately in the unlikely event of a delayed reaction.

The patient should not take any strenuous physical exercise for several hours following the injection.

Reactions:
Local reactions, such as slight swelling or irritation, can sometimes occur and may require symptomatic treatment if they persist.

Mild systemic reactions such as rhinitis or urticaria may be treated with antihistamines orally, or by injection if necessary. In mild bronchospasm, a sympathomimetic bronchodilator such as salbutamol and possibly an anti-inflammatory steroid should be given. If required, 0.5 ml Adrenaline Injection BP (Adrenaline 1 in 1,000) may be given subcutaneously.

Severe systemic reactions may occasionally arise in the form of typical allergic symptoms; anaphylaxis is rare.

Treatment of anaphylaxis:
Anaphylactic shock: characterised by bronchospasm, laryngeal oedema, urticaria and shock. Immediate attention should be given as follows:

1. The patient should be laid down and treated immediately.
2. 0.5 ml† Adrenaline Injection BP (Adrenaline 1 in 1,000) should be given intramuscularly close to the vaccine injection site. This should be repeated to a total of 2 ml† over 15 minutes if necessary. In extreme cases, 0.5 ml† Adrenaline (1 in 10,000) can be given by slow intravenous injection.
3. If bronchospasm persists, 10–20 ml† of Aminophylline Injection BP (250 mg per 10 ml) should be given by slow intravenous injection at a rate of 2 ml† per minute.
4. In addition, 200–400 mg† of Hydrocortisone Injection BP should be given intravenously. This is to combat persistent bronchospasm which can occur 6–8 hours after the initial collapse.
5. Full supportive measures should be available and employed if necessary and patients should be closely monitored for at least 24 hours after recovery.

† All dosages should be reduced as required for children.

Note: A severe local reaction, or severe systemic reaction such as urticaria or asthma, indicates that the standard vaccine is unsuitable for the treatment of the particular patient, who should be referred to a consultant for advice or transferred to a suitably dilute specific desensitising vaccine (Alavac-S or SDV) obtainable from Bencard. (For full prescribing information please refer to the relevant data sheets.)

Pharmaceutical precautions Pollinex must be stored in a refrigerator (5°C). It must not be frozen and must be removed 2–3 hours before use.

Legal category POM.

Package quantities Each course of treatment consists of a set of 3 unit-dose syringes prefilled with vaccine, and with needles attached. An instruction leaflet is included with each set.

Further information Pollinex is a short-course 3-injection vaccine which offers a practical and more permanent alternative to temporary palliatives.

Pollinex may be prescribed on the basis of case history and clinical symptoms alone, providing these reveal marked seasonality corresponding with the grass pollen season. Pollinex is prescribable on NHS form FP10 and is available for immediate supply from stock.

The Bencard Medical Department will be pleased to advise on any aspect of treatment.

Product licence number 0038/0111.

PREGNAVITE FORTE* F

Presentation Lilac, sugar coated tablets, overprinted (FPF) in white.

Active ingredients

	Each tablet contains	Hence daily dose (1 tab. three times a day) provides
Dried ferrous sulphate	84 mg (equiv. to 25.2 mg Fe)	252 mg (equiv. to 75.6 mg Fe)
Calcium phosphate	160 mg	480 mg
Vitamin A	1,333 units	4,000 units
Vitamin D$_2$	133 units	400 units
Thiamine hydrochloride (vitamin B$_1$)	0.5 mg	1.5 mg
Riboflavine (vitamin B$_2$)	0.5 mg	1.5 mg
Pyridoxine hydrochloride (vitamin B$_6$)	0.33 mg	1.0 mg
Nicotinamide	5.0 mg	15 mg
Folic acid	0.12 mg	0.36 mg
Ascorbic acid (vitamin C)	13.3 mg	40 mg

Uses Prevention of iron and folic acid deficiency anaemia and provision of mineral and vitamin support in pregnancy.

Dosage and administration For oral administration only.

Adults: 1 tablet three times daily, during or after meals.

Children: Pregnavite Forte F is not suitable for children.

Contra-indications, warnings, etc

Contra-indication: Pernicious anaemia.

Side-effects: These are rare but are occasionally encountered as mild gastro-intestinal upsets.

Precautions: Pregnavite Forte F may be used in patients being treated for Parkinson's disease with a levodopa preparation which includes a dopa-decarboxylase inhibitor (e.g. carbidopa, benserazide) but should not be used with levodopa alone as pyridoxine may act as an antagonist.

Overdosage: In the event of overdosage, the patient should be referred to hospital, where desferrioxamine may be administered, if required, to reduce plasma iron levels. For full details please refer to the desferrioxamine data sheet.

Prolonged ingestion of massive doses of vitamins A and D can lead to hypervitaminosis states. Symptoms include dry, rough skin, painful joint swellings, anorexia and vomiting, but these disappear when treatment is discontinued.

Pharmaceutical precautions Store in a cool dry place.

Legal category POM.

Package quantities *Tablets:* 60.

Further information Nil.

Product licence number 0038/5106.

PRODEXIN* TABLETS

Presentation *Appearance:* White tablet embossed with the product name PRODEXIN.

Active ingredients: Each tablet contains:

Aluminium glycinate	900 mg
Magnesium carbonate	100 mg

Uses *Principal action:* Prodexin is a fast acting buffer antacid which disperses slowly in the mouth to release a steady trickle of antacid providing the sustained action of intragastric drip techniques in a simple and convenient way.

In the stomach, aluminium glycinate hydrolyses readily to form glycine and fully active aluminium hydroxide gel; this combination is capable of maintaining the gastric pH within the desired 3–5 range.

Aluminium glycinate has a high buffering capacity, about six times greater than that of dried aluminium hydroxide gel. The glycine acts at high acid levels whereas the aluminium hydroxide is fully effective at lower acidities. These properties are not diminished by pepsin.

As aluminium compounds sometimes cause constipation, magnesium carbonate is incorporated in Prodexin to counteract this tendency.

Indications: Peptic ulcer, hyperacidity and dyspepsia; nausea and heartburn of pregnancy, hiatus hernia, reflux oesophagitis and oesophageal ulcer.

Dosage and administration (including elderly patients) *For hyperacidity, dyspepsia, pregnancy nausea and heartburn.* One or two tablets as necessary.

To prevent hyperacidity: One tablet every hour.

For peptic ulcer: One or more tablets an hour as required.

For continuous therapeutic effect 1 tablet at a time should be allowed to disperse in the sulcus between the lower jaw and the cheek.

For extra rapid relief tablets may be chewed and swallowed.

Contra-indications, warnings, etc

Contra-indications: Nil.

Warnings and precautions: Nil.

Side-effects: No significant side-effects have been encountered with Prodexin.

Overdosage: Overdosage has not been reported.

Pharmaceutical precautions Nil.

Legal category GSL.

Package quantities 30 tablets.

Further information Prodexin is a fast-acting buffer antacid which gives relief within minutes of placing a tablet on the tongue.

Prodexin tablets are conveniently small and have a pleasant peppermint taste.

Product licence number 0038/5082.

SDV
(Specific Desensitising Vaccine)

Presentation SDV is an aqueous desensitising vaccine consisting of an individually formulated set of multidose vials of allergen extracts in graded concentrations. The No. 1 and No. 2 vials are 1/64th and 1/8th dilutions respectively of the No. 3 vial.

SDV courses are available in various strengths (full, half, quarter, eighth) to meet each particular patient's requirements. If required, special reduced strength courses can also be provided. (See 'Dosage and Administration'). When a vaccine is ordered for any patient with severe symptoms of allergy or any history of asthma a Special Dilution Vial (No. 0, Black label, $\frac{1}{8}$th dilution of the No. 1 vial) will be provided automatically (except in cases where a special reduced strength course is supplied) and should be used to initiate therapy. Special Dilution Vials are also available on request for other patients.

The allergen extracts are incorporated in a base of physiological saline with Phenol BP 0.5% w/v as preservative.

Each course of SDV is specially prepared for an individual patient in accordance with the information on causative allergens revealed by case history and skin testing and recorded on Skin Test Reaction Charts or with orders.

For the best clinical results with SDV, no more than 6 allergens should normally be included (with a maximum of 8) in any one course.

If the patient is sensitive to more than eight allergens, those which can be avoided without undue inconvenience should be omitted, and the patient given advice on avoidance; otherwise two separate vaccines will be prepared.

Over 200 standard allergen extracts, including House Dust Mite, are available for inclusion and are listed in the Bencard Skin Testing Solutions Data Sheet.

Uses To provide fundamental treatment for a wide variety of common allergic conditions such as asthma, perennial rhinitis, hayfever and some skin conditions.

Dosage and administration Please note that the section on 'Contra-Indications, Warnings, Etc.' must be studied before SDV is administered.

Adrenaline Injection BP (Adrenaline 1 in 1,000) should always be kept at hand when giving any desensitising vaccine.

The administration procedures shown in the leaflet included with each course of SDV should be carefully followed.

In the dosage schemes which follow, all injections should be given at intervals of 3–7 days, unless otherwise stated.

These schemes should be followed for all SDV patients (including elderly patients), irrespective of the course strength selected.

The vial should be shaken thoroughly immediately prior to withdrawing a dose.

Sterile syringes should always be used for the withdrawal of doses. Since each vial is used more than once, aseptic precautions must be sufficient to avoid the risk of microbial contamination.

Injections should be given slowly by the subcutaneous route. Do not inject into a blood vessel or intramuscularly. Do not rub the site of injection.

If a reaction occurs, the dosage should be adjusted accordingly (see Contra-indications, warnings etc).

SDV: Selection of course strength.
The strength of course should be selected according to the patient's previous history of asthma and severity of allergic symptoms as outlined below. When in doubt, the lowest strength course should be selected, or consultant advice sought.

Adults (aged 15 years or over):

Clinical condition	Course strength
Severe symptoms of allergy (e.g. eczema) or any history of asthma	Quarter
Moderate symptoms of allergy with no history of asthma	Half
Mild symptoms of allergy with no history of asthma	Full

Children:
Alavac-S (specific vaccine-alum adsorbed allergens) is normally preferred to SDV for the treatment of children. Please refer to the product data sheet for prescribing information. SDV may be considered when a vaccine containing allergens which are not included in the Alavac-S range is required. In such cases the following dosage schemes are recommended.

8–14 years:

Clinical condition	Age	Course strength
Severe symptoms of allergy (e.g. eczema) or any history of asthma	8–14	Consultant advice should be sought. If treatment is required a course of one-eighth strength or lower (special reduced strength) can be provided
Moderate symptoms of allergy with no history of asthma	8–11	Eighth
	12–14	Quarter
Mild symptoms of allergy with no history of asthma	8–11	Quarter
	12–14	Half

Under 8 years:
The use of SDV for children under the age of 8 years is not recommended by Bencard. If, however, after taking consultant advice, treatment is considered necessary, a specially reduced strength treatment course can be provided, with a dosage schedule appropriate to the individual patient's requirements.

SDV: Dosage recommendations for vaccines which contain pollen allergens.
Treatment should be given pre-seasonally. The course should be timed to end before the usual date of onset of the patient's seasonal symptoms (e.g. in the UK, by mid-May for grass pollen sensitivity, and by the end of March for tree pollen sensitivity. For continued clinical improvement it is recommended that a course should be given in each of three successive years.

Recommended dosage scheme for vaccines which contain pollen allergens.
Not to be used during the pollen season.

Commence with the No. 1 (Green label) vial then proceed to the No. 2 (Buff label) vial and the No. 3 (Red label) vial as indicated in the scheme shown.

If a reaction occurs during treatment, dosage should be reduced: see 'Adjustment of Dosage'.

Vial Number*	Injection Number	Dosage
1. Green label	1	0.1 ml
	2	0.2 ml
	3	0.3 ml
	4	0.5 ml
	5	0.7 ml
	6	1.0 ml
2. Buff label	7	0.1 ml
	8	0.2 ml
	9	0.3 ml
	10	0.5 ml
	11	0.7 ml
	12	1.0 ml
3. Red label	13	0.1 ml
	14	0.2 ml
	15	0.3 ml
	16	0.5 ml
	17	0.7 ml
	18	1.0 ml

*When a Special Dilution Vial (No. 0, Black label) is supplied to initiate treatment, dosage instructions relating to its use are provided in an accompanying leaflet.

Surplus vaccine must not be used the following season.

Extended treatment: when time is available before the onset of the pollen season and there is sufficient vaccine, it may be beneficial to repeat the top treatment dose at fortnightly intervals, the final dose being given two weeks before the pollen season is expected to start.

SDV: Dosage recommendations for vaccines which do not contain pollen allergens (Initial course).
Courses may be given at any time of the year.

Commence with the No. 1 (Green label) vial then proceed to the No. 2 (Buff label) vial and the No. 3 (Red label) vial as indicated in the scheme shown.

If a reaction occurs during treatment, dosage should be reduced: see 'Adjustment of Dosage'.

Vial Number*	Injection Number	Dosage
1. Green label	1	0.1 ml
	2	0.2 ml
	3	0.3 ml
	4	0.5 ml
	5	0.7 ml
	6	1.0 ml
2. Buff label	7	0.1 ml
	8	0.2 ml
	9	0.3 ml
	10	0.5 ml
	11	0.7 ml
	12	1.0 ml
3. Red label	13	0.1 ml
	14	0.2 ml
	15	0.3 ml
	16	0.5 ml
	17	0.7 ml
	18	1.0 ml

*When a Special Dilution Vial (No. 0, Black label) is supplied to initiate treatment, dosage instructions relating to its use are provided in an accompanying leaflet.

Maintenance treatment following the initial course is recommended.

Maintenance Therapy (for use only with vaccines which do not contain pollens)
Maintenance therapy, which consists of a series of boosting injections, is recommended particularly for patients with perennial symptoms provided that the initial treatment course has been well tolerated.

Maintenance therapy should commence between 1 and 2 weeks after completion of the initial course and should follow the dosage scheme below. Treatment may be continued at the discretion of the physician, with review at appropriate intervals.

Maintenance Dosage Schemes. (See tables on next page.)
N.B. Care must be taken when administering the first injection from a new No. 3 vial as in a small number of cases, a local or general reaction may occur. If a reaction occurs during treatment, dosage should be reduced: see 'Adjustment of Dosage'.

Contra-indications, warnings, etc
Contra-indications: Patients should not be given an allergy vaccine if:
(a) They have had a severe asthma attack not responding to an inhaled bronchodilator;
(b) they have suffered from a febrile condition or an acute attack of asthma in the 24 hours preceding the intended dose.
Use in pregnancy: It is advisable to avoid use during pregnancy.
Precautions: Patients should be warned not to eat a heavy meal immediately before an injection is due to be given.

In very sensitive patients it is advantageous to give an antihistamine tablet about one hour before each injection.

Injections should be given slowly by the subcutaneous route. Do not inject into a blood vessel or intramuscularly. Do not rub the site of injection.

Adrenaline Injection BP (Adrenaline 1 in 1,000) should always be kept at hand when giving any desensitising vaccine.

All patients should be instructed to remain under observation in the surgery for at least 20 minutes after each injection and advised to contact the doctor immediately in the unlikely event of a delayed reaction.

The patient should not take any strenuous physical exercise for several hours following the injection.
Reactions: (see also 'Adjustment of Dosage'):
Local reactions, such as slight swelling or irritation, can sometimes occur and may require symptomatic treatment if they persist.

Mild systemic reactions such as rhinitis or urticaria may be treated with antihistamines orally, or by injection if necessary. In mild bronchospasm, a sympathomimetic bronchodilator such as salbutamol and possibly an anti-inflammatory steroid should be given. If required, 0.5 ml Adrenaline Injection BP (Adrenaline 1 in 1,000) may be given subcutaneously.

Severe systemic reactions may occasionally arise in the form of typical allergic symptoms; anaphylaxis is rare.
Treatment of anaphylaxis:
Anaphylactic shock: characterised by bronchospasm, laryngeal oedema, urticaria and shock. Immediate attention should be given as follows:
1. The patient should be laid down and treated immediately.

A. Commencement of Maintenance Therapy: (using No. 3 vial supplied with Initial Course).

Injection Number	Interval Since Previous Injection*	Dosage (ml) (From No. 3 Vial)	Duration
First Injection	1–2 weeks after completion of Initial Course	1.0 ml (or maximum tolerated dose if lower)	Continue until contents of No. 3 vial are exhausted.
Subsequent Injections	1 week	1.0 ml (or maximum tolerated dose if lower)	Then introduce new No. 3 vial as described below.

B. Continuation of Maintenance Therapy: Dosage scheme to be followed when introducing a new No. 3 vial.

Injection Number	Interval Since Previous Injection*	Dosage (ml) (From No. 3 Vial)	Duration
First	1 week	0.1 ml	Maintenance therapy may be continued at the discretion of the physician, with review at appropriate intervals.
2nd	1 week	0.2 ml	
3rd	1 week	0.4 ml	
4th	1 week	0.8 ml	
5th	1 week	1.0 ml	
6th	2 weeks	1.0 ml	
7th and subsequent	4 weeks	1.0 ml	

(This scheme may also be suitable for resumption of maintenance therapy following an interruption of treatment – see note below*).

* Special precautions are required if more than 4 weeks elapse:

(a) before initiating maintenance therapy following completion of the initial course;
(b) between maintenance injections.

In such cases, dosage must be modified as follows:

If a period of 4–8 weeks has elapsed treatment may be resumed with caution, using the dosage scheme specified above for the introduction of a new No. 3 vial.

If more than 8 weeks have elapsed since the previous injection, it is advisable not to attempt maintenance therapy but to re-start with a complete Initial course, commencing with the lowest strength (No. 1, green label) vial.

This regimen is unsuitable for use with pollen-containing vaccines.

2. 0.5 ml† Adrenaline Injection BP (Adrenaline 1 in 1,000) should be given intramuscularly close to the vaccine injection site. This should be repeated to a total of 2 ml† over 15 minutes if necessary. In extreme cases, 0.5 ml† Adrenaline (1 in 10,000) can be given by slow intravenous injection.

3. If bronchospasm persists, 10–20 ml† of Aminophylline Injection BP (250 mg per 10 ml) should be given by slow intravenous injection at a rate of 2 ml† per minute.

4. In addition, 200–400 mg† of Hydrocortisone Injection BP should be given intravenously. This is to combat persistent bronchospasm which can occur 6–8 hours after the initial collapse.

5. Full supportive measures should be available and employed if necessary and patients should be closely monitored for at least 24 hours after recovery.

Adjustment of Dosage (in the event of the occurrence of a reaction):

Reaction to the first injection:

If the patient has a significant reaction to the first dose from the No. 1 vial, the complete course should be returned direct to Bencard. A Special Dilution vial (No. 0-Black label; 1/8th dilution of the No. 1 vial) will be prepared free of charge and returned with a complete new course.

Treatment should recommence from the dilute vial according to the dosage scheme issued with it, but no attempts should be made to exceed the maximum tolerated dose.

† All dosages should be reduced as required for children.

Reactions to subsequent injections:

Local
Mild reaction: Reduce the dose by one step.
Severe reaction: Reduce the dose by two steps.

Systemic
Mild reaction: Reduce the dose by two steps.
Severe reaction: Treatment should be discontinued.

Except in cases where a severe systemic reaction has occurred, the course may be continued with caution up to the top dose quoted, or to the highest dose tolerated without significant reaction.

Pharmaceutical precautions SDV must be stored in a refrigerator (2–8°C). It must not be frozen. Vaccine left over from SDV courses containing pollen allergens must not be used the following year.

Vaccine left over from the No. 3 vial of courses which do not contain pollen allergens may be used for maintenance therapy (see Maintenance therapy for vaccines which do not contain pollen allergens).

Legal category POM.

Package quantities Each course of treatment consists of a set of three multidose vials of vaccine in graded concentrations. An instruction leaflet is supplied with each set.

The No. 3 vial is also available for physicians practising maintenance therapy with SDV courses which do not contain pollen allergens (see Dosage and Administration).

Normal delivery time for a complete course or a single vial is about two weeks to allow for individual formulation and sterility testing.

Further information Ordering Procedure: FP 10 forms (or other prescriptions) should be taken to a chemist who will arrange the supply of the vaccine.

The prescription should be accompanied by the following information:

When available a Skin Test Reaction Chart or a list of the allergens to be included in the vaccine with a note of the patient's sensitivity to each one, or the reference number of a previous course.

Patient's name

Patient's date of birth and/or age

The Bencard Medical Department will be pleased to advise on any aspect of treatment.

Product licence number 0038/5000.

VITAVEL*

Presentation

Appearance: Amber glass bottles containing powder for the preparation of 150 ml opaque yellow liquid.

Active ingredients: One 5 ml spoonful provides:

Vitamin A (Palmitate)	500 units
Vitamin D$_2$	200 units
Vitamin B$_1$ (Thiamine Mononitrate)	0.3 mg
Vitamin B$_2$ (Riboflavine)	0.4 mg
Nicotinamide	4.5 mg
Vitamin C	10 mg

in a citrus flavoured sorbitol/mannitol (sucrose-free) base.

Uses Vitavel is formulated to provide a course of balanced multivitamin therapy especially suitable for children and infants.

Dosage and administration For oral administration.

Infants: (under two years) Under 3 months: 2.5 ml daily (diluted to 5 ml with water)
Over 3 months: 5 ml daily

Children: (over two years): 10 ml daily.

Adults (including elderly patients): 20 ml daily.

Contra-indications, warnings, etc

Contra-indications: Nil.

Side-effects: None reported.

Overdosage: Prolonged ingestion of massive doses of vitamins A and D can lead to hypervitaminosis states. Symptoms include dry, rough skin, painful joint swellings, anorexia and vomiting; these disappear when treatment is discontinued.

Pharmaceutical precautions Store in a dry place. Vitavel is prepared for use by adding water (approximately 140 ml) to the level marked on the bottle.

Once prepared, Vitavel should be used within 30 days. Any remaining liquid should then be discarded.

If dilution of Vitavel liquid is required (for administration to infants under 3 months) water should be used; once Vitavel is diluted in this way, it should be stored in a refrigerator and used within 15 days.

Legal category P.

Package quantities 150 ml bottle.

Further information Vitavel is specifically formulated to provide an adequate intake of essential vitamins for children and infants in accordance with current medical practice and it thus supersedes the older product "Vitavel syrup".

Vitavel has a convenient and palatable once daily dosage.

In order to give a product of low cariogenic potential, Vitavel has been reformulated as a sucrose-free preparation.

Product licence number 0038/0306.

*Trade Mark

Bengué & Company Limited
St Ives Road
Maidenhead
Berkshire SL6 1RD

BENGUÉ'S BALSAM*

Presentation Creamy yellow, soft, greasy ointment: odour of menthol and methyl salicylate. Menthol 20%, methyl salicylate 20% in a lanolin base.

Uses Topically for the symptomatic relief of muscular pain and stiffness (including rheumatic pains, backache, lumbago, sciatica, fibrositis, muscular aches, sprains and strains, painful bruising) and chilblains where the skin is unbroken.

As a decongestant by application to the chest or by inhalation from hot water in head colds, coughs and laryngo-bronchitis.

Dosage and administration *Adults:* For topical use apply with gentle massage to the affected area up to 4 times daily. For use as a decongestant squeeze about 1 inch into a bowl of hot water and inhale the vapours, or massage Bengué's Balsam into the chest before retiring.

Children: Use as directed above. Not to be used in children under 4 years of age for skin application. Not to be used as an inhalant in children under 6 years of age.

Contra-indications, warnings, etc
Contra-indications: None known.

Precautions and warnings: For external use on unbroken skin only. Do not use near the eyes. Use as an inhalant in laryngo-bronchitis should be for symptomatic treatment only, as an adjunct to standard therapy. Bengué's Balsam should be used with caution as an inhalant in patients with asthma or chronic obstructive bronchitis since, as with any inhalant, it may exacerbate bronchospasm. Bengué's Balsam should be used sparingly if aspirin or other salicylates are used concurrently.

Side-effects: Skin sensitivity reactions have been reported rarely. Isolated cases of palindromic rheumatism have occurred.

Use in pregnancy: As with all medicines use with caution in pregnant women.

Pharmaceutical precautions Store in a cool place. Incompatible with aqueous liquids or emulsions.

Legal category GSL.

Package quantities Tubes of 25 g.

Further information Nil.

Product licence number 0102/5005.

BENGUÉ'S BALSAM SG*

Presentation White, non-greasy cream: odour of menthol and methyl salicylate. Menthol 10%, methyl salicylate 15% in a vanishing cream base.

Uses Topically for the symptomatic relief of muscular pain and stiffness (including rheumatic pains, backache, lumbago, sciatica, fibrositis, muscular aches, sprains and strains, painful bruising) and chilblains where the skin is unbroken.

As a decongestant by application to the chest or by inhalation from hot water in head colds, coughs and laryngo-bronchitis.

Dosage and administration *Adults:* For topical use apply with gentle massage to the affected area up to 4 times daily. For use as a decongestant squeeze about 1 inch into a bowl of hot water and inhale the vapours, or massage Bengué's Balsam S.G. into the chest before retiring.

Children: Over 4 years, use as directed above. Not to be used in children under 4 years of age.

Contra-indications, warnings, etc
Contra-indications: None known.

Precautions and warnings: For external use on unbroken skin only. Do not use near the eyes. Use as an inhalant in laryngo-bronchitis should be for symptomatic treatment only, as an adjunct to standard therapy. Bengué's Balsam S.G. should be used with caution as an inhalant in patients with asthma or chronic obstructive bronchitis since, as with any inhalant, it may exacerbate bronchospasm. Bengué's Balsam S.G. should be used sparingly if aspirin or other salicylates are used concurrently.

Side-effects: Skin sensitivity reactions have been reported rarely. Isolated cases of palindromic rheumatism have occurred.

Use in pregnancy: As with all medicines use with caution in pregnant women.

Pharmaceutical precautions Store in a cool place.

Legal category GSL.

Package quantities Tubes of 25 g.

Further information Nil.

Product licence number 0102/5006.

CORTENEMA*

Presentation Off-white, slightly viscous, aqueous suspension. Each 60 ml unit contains Hydrocortisone BP 100 mg.

Uses An adjunct in the treatment of idiopathic non-specific ulcerative colitis. It is most useful in cases involving the rectum and sigmoid colon where it exerts its maximum topical effect. It may also be effective in some cases involving the descending colon. Rectal steroid therapy brings about prompt symptomatic and proctological remissions in a significant proportion of patients, but it does not alter the recurrent and progressive nature of ulcerative colitis. Therefore, this form of treatment is not recommended for prophylaxis during periods of remission.

Dosage and administration *Adults (including the elderly):* The usual dose is one Cortenema retention enema daily for two to three weeks, and every second day thereafter, administered intra-rectally in the evening before retiring. Every effort should be made to retain the medication for at least one hour, preferably all night. This may be facilitated by prior sedation. If clinical or proctological improvement fails to occur within two or three weeks, this form of treatment should be discontinued.

Instruct the patient to lie on his left side during the instillation. The bottle must be shaken vigorously to ensure homogeneity. Expose the lubricated tip by removal of the protective sheath, grasping the bottle at the neck where it is most rigid. Carefully insert the lubricated tip into the rectum in the direction of the sacrum. Slowly express the contents by compression of the container. After instillation, the patient should remain on his left side for at least thirty minutes to allow distribution of the hydrocortisone.

Children: Not recommended.

Contra-indications, warnings, etc
Contra-indications: Rectal steroids are not suitable in cases where local complications, including obstruction, infection, abscesses or extensive fistulae and sinus tracts, are present. Patients with severe ulcerative disease are unsuitable because of the risks of perforation of the bowel wall. It should not be used in patients with toxic megacolon, or in those with known hypersensitivity to parabens.

Side-effects and precautions: Local pain or burning, and rectal bleeding have been reported rarely. Hydrocortisone administered rectally may be absorbed to a sufficient degree to have systemic activity. Thus, it should be borne in mind that high doses of Cortenema may cause insomnia, ecchymosis, moon face, aggravation of peptic ulcer, masking of infections etc. Disturbances of electrolyte balance and raising of blood sugar levels are less likely, but nevertheless possible.

Use in pregnancy: Topical administration of corticosteroids in pregnant animals can cause abnormalities of foetal development. The relevance of this finding to human beings has not been established; however, steroids should not be used extensively in pregnancy, i.e. in large amounts for prolonged periods.

Pharmaceutical precautions Store in a cool place. Protect the enemas from light.

Legal category POM.

Package quantities Cartons of 7 × 60 ml single-dose units.

Further information The flexible, disposable plastic container with lubricated applicator nozzle is designed for ease of self-administration for out-patient as well as in-patient use. To obtain optimum distribution of the enema it is important that patients should follow the illustrated directions enclosed in each pack.

Product licence number 0102/5010.

NESTOSYL* OINTMENT

Presentation Buff-coloured, greasy ointment; odourless. Benzocaine 2%, butyl aminobenzoate 2%, resorcin 2%, zinc oxide 10%, hexachlorophane 0.1%.

Uses Topically for the relief of local pain and irritation in lacerated skin conditions; also in haemorrhoids and anal pruritus.

Dosage and administration Apply and cover if necessary with a light dressing.

Contra-indications, warnings, etc Idiosyncrasy to aminobenzoates. Not to be used for babies.

Pharmaceutical precautions Store in a cool place. Replace cap after use. Incompatible with aqueous liquids and emulsions.

Legal category P.

Package quantities Tubes of 30 g supplied with rectal nozzles.

Further information Nil.

Product licence number 0102/5015.

OPOBYL*

Presentation Spherical pills approx. 7.5 mm diameter, coated deep blue with name of product printed in black. Desiccated liver 50 mg, sodium tauroglycocholate 50 mg, aqueous extract of boldo 10 mg, podophyllin 2 mg, alcoholic extract of euonymus 2 mg, aloes 20 mg per pill.

Uses Biliary stasis. Habitual constipation caused by intestinal sluggishness.

Dosage and administration *Adults (including the elderly):* One or two pills before or after meals.

Children: Not recommended.

Contra-indications, warnings, etc
Contra-indications: Abdominal pain of unknown origin. Inflammatory conditions of the colon. Use in pregnancy and breast-feeding: Opobyl should not be used during pregnancy or by nursing mothers.

Precautions and warnings: In case of diarrhoea or abdominal pain, the product should be discontinued. Opobyl should not be used for extended periods of time. Prolonged use can result in chronic irritation of the colon, or disturbances in blood electrolytes, particularly hypokalaemia.

Pharmaceutical precautions Nil.

Legal category POM.

Package quantities Tubes of 50 pills.

Further information Nil.

Product licence number 0102/5017.

*Trade Mark

Berk Pharmaceuticals Limited
St. Leonards House
St. Leonards Road
Eastbourne East Sussex BN21 3YG

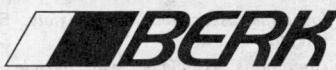

ASILONE*

Presentation *Tablets:* White, square tablets marked 'ASILONE'. Each tablet contains activated dimethicone 270 mg and the equivalent of Dried Aluminium Hydroxide BP 500 mg.

Orange Tablets: Orange, square tablets marked 'ASILONE'. Each orange flavoured tablet contains activated dimethicone 270 mg and the equivalent of Dried Aluminium Hydroxide BP 500 mg.

Suspension: White suspension containing in each 5 ml activated dimethicone 135 mg and the equivalent of Dried Aluminium Hydroxide BP 420 mg and Light Magnesium Oxide BP 70 mg.

Gel: Thick white suspension containing in each 5 ml, activated dimethicone 135 mg and the equivalent of Dried Aluminium Hydroxide BP 420 mg and Light Magnesium Oxide BP 70 mg.

Asilone for Infants: White, blackcurrant-flavoured suspension containing in each 5 ml, activated dimethicone 27 mg and the equivalent of Dried Aluminium Hydroxide BP 84 mg and Light Magnesium Oxide BP 14 mg.

Uses Mucosal protective, antiflatulent and antacid; dyspepsia, flatulence and abdominal distension; heartburn in pregnancy; heartburn in hiatus hernia; drug-induced gastritis, dietary induced gastritis; symptomatic relief in peptic ulceration.

Asilone for Infants: The treatment of wind pains, 'gripes' and regurgitation in infants over one month of age.

Dosage and administration *Tablets and orange tablets:* 1–2 tablets chewed or sucked before meals and at bedtime. For heartburn they should be sucked slowly.

Suspension & gel: One or two 5 ml spoonfuls before meals and at bedtime.

Asilone for infants: Infants 1–3 months: 2.5 ml 3 to 4 times daily before or during a feed.

3 months and over: one 5 ml spoonful three to four times daily before or during a feed.

In windy colic it may be necessary to continue dosage for 24 hours before relief is achieved. Asilone for Infants may be given at the recommended dosage for several weeks, if that is necessary, but should not be continued for more than 48 hours without medical advice, as symptoms may not be due to intestinal gas. It should not be used in infants under one month of age.

Contra-indications, warnings, etc There are no known contra-indications to Asilone, but it is probably wise to avoid taking preparations containing antacids in the first trimester of pregnancy.

Very rarely, minor disturbances of bowel function have been reported.

Asilone Tablets and Asilone Orange Tablets each contain 1 g sucrose per tablet and are therefore less suitable for diabetic patients than the Suspension and Gel which contain no sugars.

Pharmaceutical precautions *Tablets:* No special precautions.

Gel, Suspension, Infants: Do not freeze. Diluent for Asilone for Infants, Asilone Suspension and Gel: Purified Water BP.

Legal category

Tablets:	GSL.
Suspension:	GSL.
Gel:	P.
Asilone for infants:	P.
Orange tablets:	P.

Package quantities
Tablets: Packs of 12, 30 and 100.

Suspension: Bottles of 100 ml, 300 ml and 500 ml.

Gel: Bottles of 500 ml.

Asilone for Infants: Bottles of 100 ml.

Orange Tablets: Packs of 100.

Further information The sodium content of the adult Asilone range is low. Asilone is, therefore, particularly suited to the management of gastro-oesophageal conditions where there is co-existing hypertension, congestive heart failure, hepatic failure and/or renal failure.

Asilone suspension: typical sodium content 0.032 to 0.097 mmol per 10 ml.

Asilone gel: typical sodium content 0.040 to 0.090 mmol per 10 ml.

Product licence numbers

Tablets	0152/5025
Suspension	0152/5026
Gel	0152/0082
Asilone for Infants	0152/0087
Orange Tablets	0152/0139

ATENSINE*

Presentation White Diazepam Tablets BP 2 mg, marked 'BERK 2', with single break line.

Yellow Diazepam Tablets BP 5 mg, marked 'BERK 5', with single break line.

Blue Diazepam Tablets BP 10 mg, marked 'BERK 10', with single break line.

Uses Acute and chronic anxiety, tension states and muscle spasm.

Dosage and administration *Acute and chronic*

anxiety states: Mild anxiety in ambulant patients 2 mg t.i.d.

Severe anxiety states, 15–30 mg daily in divided doses.

Children: 1–5 mg daily in divided doses.

Insomnia associated with anxiety: 5–30 mg before retiring.

Conditions associated with muscle spasm: Spastic children with minimal brain damage: 2–40 mg daily in divided doses.

Cerebral palsy of adults, particularly associated with athetoid movements: 2–60 mg daily in divided doses.

Upper motor neuronic spasticity: 5–60 mg daily in divided doses.

Muscle spasm of varied aetiology, fibrositis, cervical spondylosis: 2–15 mg daily in divided doses.

Premedication for dental operations: One 5 mg tablet the night before the appointment, 5 mg on waking and 5 mg two hours before the appointment.

Atensine should be given to elderly and debilitated patients in doses half those recommended for ordinary adults.

Contra-indications, warnings, etc

Contra-indications: Known sensitivity to benzodiazepines.

Acute pulmonary insufficiency.

Acute narrow angle glaucoma.

Use in pregnancy: Not to be taken during pregnancy, especially in the first trimester, unless there are compelling reasons.

Precautions: Chronic pulmonary insufficiency.

In chronic renal or hepatic disease.

In labour. High single doses or repeated low doses have been reported to produce hypotonia, poor sucking and hypothermia in the neonate and irregularities in the foetal heart.

Avoid if possible in lactation.

The concurrent use of other CNS depressant drugs should be avoided.

Warnings and adverse effects: Common adverse effects include drowsiness, sedation, unsteadiness and ataxia.

Performance and alertness may be impaired during the first week of administration. Patients should be warned of the possible hazard when driving or operating machinery. These effects may be potentiated by alcohol.

The elderly and the debilitated are particularly liable to experience these symptoms, together with confusion, especially if organic brain symptoms are present.

Rebound insomnia has been reported following abrupt cessation of treatment.

Abnormal psychological reaction to benzodiazepines have been reported. Rare behavioural adverse effects include paradoxical aggressive outbursts, excitement, confusion, and the uncovering of depression and suicidal tendencies.

Other rare adverse effects including hypotension, gastro-intestinal and visual disturbances, skin rashes, urinary retention, headache, vertigo, changes in libido, blood dyscrasias and jaundice have also been reported.

As with any benzodiazepine, excessive or prolonged use of Atensine may result in the development of psychological dependence with withdrawal symptoms on discontinuation.

Treatment of overdosage: Ataxia is usually the most serious symptom. Gastric lavage may be carried out, followed by observation. Very occasionally a respirator may be required but Atensine generally causes few problems in overdosage. In children behavioural changes are likely.

Pharmaceutical precautions Store in a cool dry place protected from light.

Legal category CD (Sch 4) POM.

Package quantities *Tablets 2 mg:* Containers of 50, 250, 1,000 and 5,000.

Tablets 5 mg: Containers of 50, 100, 250, 1,000 and 5,000.

Tablets 10 mg: Containers of 500.

Further information Nil.

Product licence numbers
Tablets 2 mg   0152/0058
Tablets 5 mg   0152/0059
Tablets 10 mg   0152/0158

AZATHIOPRINE TABLETS BP

Presentation Each tablet contains 50 mg Azathioprine BP. The tablets are yellow and marked BERK 1D2 on one side with a breakline on the reverse.

Uses Azathioprine facilitates the survival and function of organ transplants.

Azathioprine has a significant therapeutic effect in a proportion of patients suffering from chronic active hepatitis, severe rheumatoid arthritis, systemic lupus erythematosus (SLE), idiopathic thrombocytopenic purpura, acquired haemolytic anaemia, severe cases of specified dermatological diseases (pemphigus vulgaris, dermatomyositis, polyarteritis nodosa, pyoderma gangrenosa) when these conditions are: (a) refractory to corticosteroids, or (b) when corticosteroids are contra-indicated, or (c) controlled by corticosteroids in dosages which are producing severe side-effects. In patients with such side-effects, the aim of azathioprine medication is to reduce the required maintenance dose of steroids.

In pemphigus and rheumatoid arthritis azathioprine has been shown to have significant therapeutic activity when used without corticosteroids.

The risks associated with azathioprine therapy should be considered against the severity of the patient's condition and the expected clinical effect.

The use of azathioprine in other indications must be regarded as experimental.

Dosage and administration

Adults: Transplantation: A loading dose of up to 5 mg/kg is usually given. The dosage during the first three months after transplantation is usually 1–4 mg/kg body weight per day (median 2.4 mg/kg body weight per day). 1–2.5 mg/kg body weight per day may be given intravenously as a maintenance dose, but only if oral therapy is impracticable. Cessation of azathioprine therapy, even after a period of years, carries a high risk of rejection within a few weeks.

Other conditions: For the treatment of the conditions listed under 'Uses', except for chronic active hepatitis, the dosage is usually between 2 and 2.5 mg/kg body weight per day. For the treatment of chronic active hepatitis the dosage is usually between 1 and 1.5 mg/kg body weight per day.

The dosage of azathioprine and the duration of treatment may vary according to the condition, its severity and the clinical response obtained. A therapeutic response may not be evident for a few days or even weeks after initiation of therapy. If no discernible improvement occurs in the patient's condition within three months, consideration should be given to the withdrawal of the drug. Treatment is otherwise undertaken on long-term basis unless the patient exhibits evidence of intolerance to the drug.

Children: As for adults.

Contra-indications, warnings, etc
Contra-indications: Azathioprine hypersensitivity will generally be a contra-indication to continued use.

Precautions: There are potential hazards in the use of this preparation. Therefore, it should not be prescribed unless the patient can be adequately monitored for toxic effects throughout the duration of the therapy.

During the first eight weeks of therapy with azathioprine complete blood counts, including platelet counts, must be performed at least weekly (and more frequently when higher dosages are used or in the presence of disturbed renal or hepatic function), and with decreasing frequency thereafter.

Azathioprine may be given long-term unless the patient cannot tolerate the preparation. Withdrawal of an effective dose in certain instances, e.g. SLE with nephritis, may result in a serious relapse of the condition. In other instances, such as rheumatoid arthritis and certain haematological conditions, treatment may be withdrawn after a suitable interval without any ill-effect. Withdrawal should always be a gradual process performed under close supervision.

In the presence of severe renal or hepatic impairment careful monitoring is initially required, since the dosage of azathioprine may have to be reduced.

Severe secondary infections, often with uncommon organisms, are a hazard of immunosuppressive therapy. These are seen more frequently in transplant recipients than in patients being treated for other indications.

Azathioprine is potentially mutagenic and has been shown to cause chromosome damage in man. The clinical significance of these findings is unclear since the damage is apparently reversible on withdrawal.

Azathioprine has no detectable inhibitory effect on either male or female fertility. The depression of fertility accompanying chronic uraemia is generally reversed after transplantation and its accompanying azathioprine treatment.

An increased number of malignant tumours especially lymphoreticular and epithelial has been observed in transplant recipients. The skin tumours that have occurred in transplant patients have been primarily on sun-exposed skin. Patients should be cautioned against undue sun exposure, and the skin should be examined at regular intervals. There is, however, as yet no conclusive evidence of an increased incidence to tumours in other treated subjects. In such patients the risk may be indistinguishable from that accompanying some of the diseases under treatment.

The few cases reported show a different pattern from that seen in transplantation: tumour occurrence is much less common, has an increased latency, is seen mainly after prolonged continuous therapy, is less exclusively lymphoreticular and tends to occur in those patients also treated with alkylating agents. Use with caution in hyperplenism.

Concomitant allopurinol therapy: When azathioprine and allopurinol are given concomitantly only one quarter of the usual dosage of azathioprine should be given since allopurinol has an inhibitory effect on its metabolism.

Concomitant use of cytotoxics: Azathioprine should be used with caution in patients receiving, or who have recently received, other bone marrow suppressive agents.

Concomitant use of muscle relaxants: There is clinical evidence that azathioprine antagonises the effect of non-depolarising muscle relaxants such as curare, d-tubocurarine and pancuronium. Experimental data confirm that azathioprine reverses the neuromuscular blockage caused by d-tubocurarine, and show that azathioprine potentiates the neuromuscular blockage caused by succinylcholine.

Side-effects, adverse effects: The principal side-effect of azathioprine is a dose-related, generally reversible, depression of bone marrow function expressed as leucopenia, thrombocytopenia and rarely anaemia.

An additional form of haematological toxicity in patients receiving azathioprine is megaloblastic erythropoiesis and macrocytosis.

Haematological toxicity is most frequently noted at the outset of therapy but reports of the late occurrence of leucopenia and anaemia confirm the wisdom of continuing haematological surveillance of patients even on stable long-term treatment.

The report incidence of gastro-intestinal intolerance to oral administration of azathioprine is variable. It is manifested largely as nausea and anorexia with occasional vomiting. In some instances it seems to be a dose-related phenomenon and after a brief interruption administration may often be successfully reinstituted, at a lower dose. Doses should, when possible, be taken with food. Other more serious gastro-intestinal complications of therapy have been recorded. Pancreatitis is seen most commonly in transplant recipients and has also been reported in patients with granulomatous bowel disease treated with azathioprine.

Gastro-duodenal ulcer, intestinal haemorrhage and intestinal necrosis and perforation are complications seen only after transplantation and it appears likely that they are due to concomitant steroid therapy.

Azathioprine may occasionally cause cholestatic, dose-related reversible hepatotoxicity. In such cases withdrawal is advisable. A variety of possibly allergic manifestations has been reported. Drug fever, skin rash, myalgia and arthralgia are well documented though uncommon complications. There are also single case reports of possible azathioprine-related effects including acute renal insufficiency, haemolytic anaemia, acute restrictive lung disease and unexplained meningitis reactions.

Use in pregnancy and lactation: The potential teratogenicity of azathioprine should be borne in mind. Although it has been shown to be teratogenic in laboratory animals clinical evidence suggests that the risk is not appreciable in man. There is no doubt that azathioprine and its metabolites cross the placenta. A temporary impairment of immune function has been noted following exposure 'in utero' to azathioprine combined with prednisone. The long-term consequences of these properties of azathioprine are unknown, but many children exposed 'in utero' have now completed the first decade of life without reported problems.

It has not been possible to detect azathioprine or its metabolites in the breast milk of treated patients.

Toxicity and treatment of overdosage: The most likely side-effect of overdosage is bone marrow depression, which may not reach its maximum until 9–14 days later.

A single large dose of azathioprine is less likely to have a toxic effect than a chronic minor overdosage on prescription. Although the effects of overdosage may be delayed it is not uncommon for improvement to commence after day 12 provided that the patient has not had high doses during the intervening period. If overdosage occurs the blood picture and hepatic function in particular should be monitored. Azathioprine is known to be dialysable and dialysis may be used in severe cases.

Pharmaceutical precautions Store below 25°C. Protect from light. Keep dry.

Legal category POM.

Package quantities Securitainers of 100 tablets.

Further information Nil.

Product licence number 0152/0210.

BERKATENS* TABLETS

Presentation Yellow biconvex film-coated tablets containing Verapamil Hydrochloride BP 40 mg (engraved BERK 1T1), 80 mg (engraved BERK 2T1), 120 mg (engraved BERK 3T1) and 160 mg (engraved BERK 4T1).

Uses Berkatens is indicated for the treatment and prophylaxis of angina pectoris. It may be used in the treatment and prophylaxis of supraventricular tachycardia, atrial fibrillation and atrial flutter. It may also be used in the management of mild to moderate hypertension and renal hypertension.

Dosage and administration
Angina
Adults: The usual dosage is 120 mg three times daily. 80 mg three times daily may be satisfactory in some patients with angina of effort.

Supraventricular Tachycardias
Adults: 40–120 mg three times daily according to the severity of the condition. *Children:* 2 years and above: 1–3 40 mg tablets 2–3 times daily.

Hypertension
Adults: The usual dosage is 80–160 mg three times daily. *Children:* Up to 10 mg/kg/day, in divided doses according to the severity of condition.

Contra-indications, warnings, etc
Contra-indications: Hypotension associated with cardiogenic shock, marked bradycardia, uncompensated heart failure, second or third degree atrioventricular block and sick sinus syndrome.
Precautions: Caution should be observed in the acute phase of myocardial infarction.
Care must be taken when verapamil and beta blockers are administered concurrently or closely together as their effects may be additive both with respect to conduction and contraction.
Verapamil may affect impulse conduction and should be used with caution in patients with first degree atrioventricular block.
Verapamil may affect left ventricular contractility as a result of its mode of action. Although this effect is small and normally not important, cardiac failure may be precipitated or aggravated if it exists. Thus in patients with poor ventricular function verapamil should only be

given after appropriate therapy for cardiac failure such as digitalis, etc.
Verapamil has been shown to increase the serum concentration of digoxin and caution should be exercised with regard to digitalis toxicity.
In patients with impaired liver function, particular attention should be paid to the dosage because of reduced drug metabolism.
Though there is no published evidence that verapamil has any teratogenic effect, it should not be given during the first trimester of pregnancy, unless, in the clinician's judgement, it is essential for the welfare of the patient.
Side-effects: Berkatens is generally well-tolerated. Constipation may occur, flushing is observed occasionally, headaches rarely. Nausea, vomiting and allergic reactions have seldom been reported.
Treatment of overdosage: Usual emergency measures for acute cardiovascular side-effects should be applied, e.g.: in the case of second and third degree AV block: atropine, isoprenaline and, if required, pace-maker therapy; in the case of signs of myocardial insufficiency: dopamine, dobutamine, cardiac glycosides or calcium gluconate (10–20 mg of a 10% solution); in the case of hypotension: appropriate positioning of patient, dopamine, dobutamine, noradrenaline.

Pharmaceutical precautions Nil.

Legal category POM.

Package quantities
40 mg tablets: Securitainers of 100.
80 mg tablets: Securitainers of 100.
120 mg tablets: Securitainers of 100.
160 mg tablets: Securitainers of 100.

Further information Nil.

Product licence numbers
40 mg tablets   0152/0198
80 mg tablets   0152/0199
120 mg tablets   0152/0200
160 mg tablets   0152/0217

BERKMYCEN*

Presentation Yellow film-coated Oxytetracycline Tablets BP 250 mg engraved BERK 1C5 on one side.

Uses Antibiotic.
Infections caused by oxytetracycline-sensitive organisms. These include acute and chronic bronchitis, pneumonia, urinary tract infections, brucellosis, pertussis, rickettsial fevers and psittacosis.

Dosage and administration *Adults:* 250 mg every six hours. In severe infections dosage may be increased to 250 mg every three hours after an initial loading dose of 1 g.

Contra-indications, warnings, etc 'Berkmycen' should only be given to patients with renal dysfunction or failure if its use is considered essential.
Milk, or antacids containing aluminium, magnesium or calcium, interfere with the absorption of oxytetracycline. If gastric irritation occurs the tablets should be taken with food. As with all tetracyclines, 'Berkmycen' should be used with caution in patients with hepatic or renal dysfunction.
Berkmycen should not be used in late pregnancy or given to children during the period of tooth development,

unless it is essential to use a tetracycline because of resistance to other antibiotics.

Like all tetracyclines, 'Berkmycen' may produce gastro-intestinal irritations, giving rise to nausea, abdominal discomfort and diarrhoea. Intestinal overgrowth of resistant organisms (Candida albicans in particular) may occur. Drug fever and allergic skin rashes may occur rarely.

Treatment of overdosage: Serious symptoms are unlikely. Gastric lavage might be beneficial in the first hours after ingestion followed by conservative management. Milk will reduce absorption.

Pharmaceutical precautions Store in a cool place.

Legal category POM.

Package quantities Containers of 1000 and 5000.

Further information 'Berkmycen' oxytetracycline is an antimicrobial agent active against most pathogenic bacteria, both Gram-positive and Gram-negative, except for the majority of strains of *Proteus vulgaris* and *Pseudomonas aeruginosa.* Salmonella species and *Mycobacterium tuberculosis* show resistance, as do the yeasts and fungi, but 'Berkmycen' is effective against Actinomyces, *Entamoeba histolytica, Trichomonas vaginalis,* treponemata and some rickettsias and viruses.

Product licence number 0152/0094.

BERKOLOL*

Presentation
1. Pink, film-coated, Propranolol Tablets BP 10 mg embossed BERK 1Z1, with breakline on reverse.
2. Pink, film-coated, Propranolol Tablets BP 40 mg embossed BERK 2Z1, with breakline on reverse.
3. Pink, film-coated, Propranolol Tablets BP 80 mg embossed BERK 3Z1, with breakline on reverse.
4. Pink, film-coated, Propranolol Tablets BP 160 mg embossed BERK 4Z1, quadrisected with double breakline on reverse.

Uses Berkolol is a competitive blocker of adrenergic β-receptor sites. It is used in the treatment of hypertension, angina pectoris, cardiac dysrhythmias, tachycardia, anxiety, essential tremor and for the long term prevention of sudden cardiac death in patients who have shown evidence of dysrhythmias during the acute phase of myocardial infarction. It may also be used as a prophylactic in migraine, and as adjunctive therapy in thyrotoxicosis.

Dosage and administration Dosage requires individual adjustment. A heart rate of 55/min or less is an indication that dosage should be increased no further.

Adults: Hypertension: Initially, 80 mg twice daily, increased where necessary at weekly intervals. The usual maintenance dosage is 160–320 mg daily. Lower doses may be effective when a diuretic or other antihypertensive drug is given concurrently.

Angina pectoris: Initially, 40 mg twice or thrice daily increased by the same amount at weekly intervals until control is achieved, or the maximum daily dose of 480 mg is reached.

Prophylaxis against recurrence of myocardial infarction: For long term prevention of sudden cardiac death in patients who have survived the acute phase of myocardial infarction, clinical study has shown that treatment should

be commenced four to six days after the infarction at a dose of 40 mg four times daily which should then be maintained. As the overriding principle is to maintain adequate β-blockade the dose may need to be varied for some patients.

Anxiety, migraine, essential tremor: 40 mg twice or thrice daily, increased at weekly intervals if needed to a daily total of 160 mg.

Dysrhythmias, anxiety tachycardia, hypertrophic obstructive cardiomyopathy, thyrotoxicosis: 10–40 mg three or four times daily.

Children: Dysrhythmias, thyrotoxicosis: The minimum effective dosage, based on 0.25–0.5 mg/kg body weight, three or four times daily.

Migraine: Children under the age of 12 may be given 20 mg two or three times daily. Older children may be given adult dosage.

Contra-indications, warnings, etc
Contra-indications: Second or third degree heart block; History of bronchospasm; Prolonged fasting; Metabolic acidosis.

Precautions: Although there is no evidence that propranolol is teratogenic, Berkolol should not be used in pregnancy unless it is considered essential.

Berkolol should be used with great caution in patients with heart failure, unless that is due to thyrotoxicosis alone. Concomitant therapy with digitalis and diuretics is usually desirable in heart failure.

Particular care should be taken in the elderly where hepatic clearance may be reduced thus requiring an appropriate reduction in dosage.

Berkolol should be withdrawn 24 hours before elective surgery, as it may interfere with response to stress. If this cannot be done, 1–2 mg atropine should be given intravenously before anaesthesia commences and anaesthetics such as ether, chloroform, cyclopropane and trichloroethylene, which may cause myocardial depression, should not be used.

Warnings and adverse reactions: Treatment with beta-blocking agents must not be stopped suddenly. If it is necessary to withdraw Berkolol, this should be done gradually, or another beta-blocker should be substituted.

Bradycardia and hypotension are usually a sign of overdosage, but may rarely be due to intolerance of the drug. In the latter case Berkolol should be withdrawn and, if necessary, the patient should be treated as for overdosage. Heart block and congestive heart failure have been reported due to propranolol.

Dry eyes and skin rash have been reported during treatment with β-adrenergic blocking agents. If these symptoms are not attributable to some other cause, Berkolol should be withdrawn.

Berkolol may cause or precipitate Raynaud's phenomenon, intermittent claudication or peripheral arterial insufficiency. Bronchospasm may occur, particularly in patients with a history of asthma or hay fever.

There have been rare reports of blood dyscrasias during treatment with propranolol.

Minor side-effects include cold extremities, nausea, vomiting, diarrhoea, fatigue or insomnia. These are usually transient and are less common if the drug is introduced gradually.

Treatment of overdosage: The clinical features can include bradycardia, severe hypotension, bronchospasm, hypoglycaemia, delirium and unconsciousness. Initially isoprenaline should be infused, and if marked bradycardia is present atropine should be given intravenously (0.6–3 mg; 50 mcg/kg in children): if the response is limited, glucagon therapy must be instituted (50–150 mcg/kg intravenously over one minute followed by 1–5 mg/hour infused). Bronchospasm may be treated by nebulized salbutamol or intravenous aminophylline or salbutamol.

Pharmaceutical precautions Protect from light.

Legal category POM.

Package quantities
Tablets 10 mg: containers of 100 and 500
Tablets 40 mg: containers of 100 and 1,000
Tablets 80 mg: containers of 100 and 500
Tablets 160 mg: containers of 100

Further information Nil.

Product licence numbers
Tablets 10 mg   0152/0150
Tablets 40 mg   0152/0151
Tablets 80 mg   0152/0152
Tablets 160 mg   0152/0153.

BERKOZIDE*

Presentation Plain white Bendrofluazide Tablets BP 2.5 mg and 5 mg. The 2.5 mg tablets are marked 1G5 on one side. The 5 mg tablets are marked 2G5 on one side with a breakline on the reverse.

Uses Diuretic. Oedema, cardiac failure, inhibition of lactation, hypertension.

Dosage and administration In cardiac failure, 5–10 mg daily or on alternate days, a usual maintenance dosage being 5–10 mg on three days per week. For pre-menstrual oedema, 'Berkozide' may be given 5 mg daily for three to four days before menstruation. For inhibition of lactation 5 mg in the morning and 5 mg at noon for five days is usually adequate. In hypertension the dosage should be 2.5–5 mg daily. Bendrofluazide potentiates other antihypertensive agents, the dosage of which should be reduced and then adjusted as necessary.
    Berkozide is not recommended for children.

Contra-indications, warnings, etc 'Berkozide' is contra-indicated in severe renal insufficiency and hypercalcaemia and should be used with caution in patients with renal or hepatic disorders. It may precipitate hepatic coma in advanced cirrhosis.
    Thiazide diuretics may induce water and electrolyte disturbances particularly in the elderly or when dosage is high or prolonged. Plasma electrolytes should be checked at regular intervals during therapy.
    Potassium supplements should be given (preferably on non-diuretic days) when the dosage of 'Berkozide' is high or when diet is inadequate. It may be necessary to reduce the dosage of digitalis if this is given concurrently.
    Toxic effects such as nausea, allergy, skin rashes or blood dyscrasias are rare. Hypokalaemia may develop with long use of 'Berkozide', but this risk is reduced by administration on alternate days. Like other thiazides, bendrofluazide may provoke hyperglycaemia and glycosuria in diabetic patients and may precipitate latent diabetes mellitus. It may also precipitate acute attacks of gout. Breast feeding should be avoided since thiazide diuretics are secreted in mother's milk.
Treatment of overdosage: Replace fluids with saline while monitoring plasma sodium and potassium. Potassium replacement may be required.

Pharmaceutical precautions No special precautions.

Legal category POM.

Package quantities Tablets 2.5 mg: Containers of 100 and 1,000.
Tablets 5 mg: Containers of 100 and 1,000.

Further information Bendrofluazide is an oral diuretic of the thiazide group which inhibits proximal tubular resorption of sodium chloride.

Product licence numbers
Tablets 2.5 mg   0152/5081
Tablets 5 mg   0152/5084

CAPLENAL*

Presentation
100 mg tablets: white biconvex tablets containing 100 mg of Allopurinol BP, engraved BERK 1K1 on one side with a break-line on the reverse.
300 mg tablets: white biconvex tablets containing 300 mg of Allopurinol BP, engraved BERK 2K1 on one side with a break-line on the reverse.

Uses Gout: Primary hyperuricaemia.
Secondary hyperuricaemia: Prophylaxis of uric acid and calcium oxalate stones.

Dosage and administration Adults: The initial dose is 100–200 mg. The maintenance dose is 200–600 mg/daily. Maximum single dose 300 mg. It has rarely been found necessary to exceed 900 mg per day. The dose should be adjusted by monitoring serum uric acid and/or urinary uric acid levels at appropriate intervals until the desired effect is attained, which may take one to three weeks.
Children: 10–20 mg/kg body weight/day. Use in children is mainly indicated in malignant conditions, especially leukaemia and certain enzyme disorders, for example Lesch-Nyhan syndrome.
Initiation of therapy: In the early stages of treatment with allopurinol, as with the uricosuric agents, an acute attack of gouty arthritis may be precipitated. Therefore it is advisable to give a prophylactic dose of a suitable anti-inflammatory agent or colchicine (0.5 mg three times a day) for at least one month.
Use with uricosurics: As allopurinol does not interfere with the action of uricosuric agents, they may be given concurrently. When changing from uricosuric therapy to allopurinol 1–3 weeks overlap of treatments is recommended to ensure a continuous hypouricaemic effect.
Use in neoplasia: When giving allopurinol to prevent uric acid nephropathy in neoplastic conditions, it is advisable to start treatment with allopurinol before cytotoxic therapy.
Dose recommendations in impaired renal function: Since allopurinol and its metabolites are excreted via the kidney, impairment of renal function may lead to retention of the drug and its metabolites with consequent prolongation of action. Thus, the amount and frequency of the dosage may require reduction as indicated by monitoring serum uric acid levels. The following schedule is provided for guidance in adults.
    If creatinine clearance exceeds 20 ml/minute – give standard dose.
    If creatinine clearance is between 10 and 20 ml/minute – give 100–200 mg/day.

If creatinine clearance is between 2 and 10 ml/minute – give 100 mg/day or at longer intervals.

Dose recommendations in renal dialysis: Allopurinol and its metabolites are removed by renal dialysis. If frequent dialysis is required an alternative schedule of 300–400 mg allopurinol after each dialysis with none in the interim should be considered.

Contra-indications, warnings, etc

Contra-indications: Acute gout. Known intolerance of allopurinol.

Precautions: Treatment should not be started during or immediately after an acute attack of gout. When 6-mercaptopurine or azathioprine is given concurrently with allopurinol, only one quarter of the usual dose of those drugs should be given because inhibition of xanthine oxidase will prolong their activity. There is no unequivocal evidence that allopurinol potentiates the activity of other cytotoxic drugs. If allopurinol is given concomitantly with chlorpropamide when renal function is poor, there may be an increased risk of prolonged hypoglycaemia activity.

The dosage of allopurinol should be reduced in patients with renal or hepatic diseases.

There is no evidence that allopurinol taken orally causes foetal abnormalities. However, as with all drugs, due caution should be exercised in pregnancy.

Particular care should be taken in the elderly where renal function may be reduced thus leading to a retention of the drug and its metabolites with the consequent prolongation of action.

Warnings and adverse effects: Adverse reactions in association with allopurinol are usually rare and mostly of a minor nature. The incidence is higher in the presence of renal and/or hepatic disorders. The possible potentiation of anticoagulant action should be borne in mind when a patient on anticoagulants is given allopurinol.

Skin reactions are the most common reactions and may occur at any time during treatment. They may be pruritic, maculopapular, sometimes scaly or purpuric and rarely exfoliative. Allopurinol should be withdrawn immediately should such reactions occur. After recovery from mild reactions allopurinol may, if desired, be reintroduced at a low dose (e.g. 50 mg/day) which may be gradually increased. If the rash recurs, allopurinol should be permanently withdrawn.

Exfoliative skin reactions associated with other signs of hypersensitivity including fever, lymphadenopathy, arthralgia and eosinophilia occur rarely. If they do occur, it may be at any time during treatment. Allopurinol should then be withdrawn immediately and permanently. Corticosteroids may be beneficial in overcoming such reactions. Patients manifesting generalised hypersensitivity reactions usually have pre-existing renal and/or hepatic disorders.

Nausea and vomiting have been reported. This reaction is not a significant problem and can be avoided by taking allopurinol after meals.

There have been occasional reports of transient reduction in the numbers of circulating formed elements in the blood, usually in association with pre-existing renal and/or hepatic disorders. The clinical significance has yet to be demonstrated.

Exacerbation of acute gouty attacks may occur in the early stages of hypouricaemic therapy. In those conditions where the body's miscible urate pool is greatly increased (e.g. malignant diseases and its treatment: Lesch-Nyhan syndrome), the rise in xanthine concentra-

tion resulting from the action of allopurinol may lead to tissue deposition of xanthine. Adequate hydration will reduce the risk of xanthine deposition in the kidney and fluid intake should ensure adequate urinary output. Xanthine crystals have been seen in muscle tissue of patients receiving allopurinol but this appears to have no clinical significance.

The following complaints have been reported occasionally, but do not appear to have a clear cause and effect relationship with allopurinol: fever, general malaise, headache, vertigo, somnolence, taste perversion, hepatic necrosis, granulomatous hepatitis, abnormal liver function tests, hyperlipaemia, visual disorder, cataracts, macular changes, neuropathy, impotence, diabetes mellitus, furunculosis, alopecia, hypertension, haematuria, oedema.

Treatment of overdosage: No reports of overdosage or acute intoxication with Caplenal are available.

Pharmaceutical precautions No special precautions.

Legal category POM.

Package quantities
100 mg tablets: containers of 100 and 500 tablets
300 mg tablets: containers of 100 tablets

Further information Nil.

Product licence numbers
Tablets 100 mg   0152/0154
Tablets 300 mg   0152/0176

CEPLAC

Presentation Rose coloured tablets engraved CEPLAC on one face and plain on the reverse face. Each tablet contains 6 mg erythrocine.

Uses As an aid to the efficient teaching of oral hygiene.

Dosage and administration *Adults and children:* The patient should be given a Ceplac Tablet in the surgery. This will at once demonstrate the shortcomings of his current oral hygiene techniques and make it easier to gain his co-operation.

When he has been shown the correct method of brushing his teeth, he should be sent home with a supply of Ceplac Tablets and instructions on how to use them. Ceplac will play a central role in helping him to acquire the habit of regular and correct tooth brushing.

Initially, at least once a day, the patient should crush one Ceplac Tablet between his teeth before cleaning them, and distribute saliva to all tooth and gum surfaces with the aid of the tongue for at least half a minute. He should then spit out into a bowl of running water, and rinse his mouth once or twice with water.

He should then brush his teeth in the way he has been shown until all red stain has been removed.

Once a sound brushing technique has been established the patient can use Ceplac once or twice a week after brushing, as a check on continuing proficiency.

In the same way, patients should be given Ceplac on each successive visit to the surgery, to assess their progress.

Contra-indications, warnings, etc There are no known contra-indications or adverse reactions.

Treatment of overdosage: Gastric lavage.

Pharmaceutical precautions No special precautions.

Legal category GSL.

Package quantities Packs of 14 and 1,000 tablets.

Further information Ceplac stains bacterial plaque and food debris a brilliant red. The stain is non-persistent and is easily removed from lips or clothing with soap and water.

Product licence number 0152/5032.

CREMALGIN*

Presentation Pink balm containing methyl nicotinate 1.0% w/w, capsicin 0.1% w/w, glycol salicylate 10.0% w/w.

Uses Rubefacient balm. For the symptomatic relief of rheumatism, sciatica, lumbago, fibrositis and muscular stiffness.

Dosage and administration Two or three times daily or as required. Place a sufficient quantity on the skin over the affected area and massage gently and smooth the cream through the skin. To be applied to the unbroken skin only.

Contra-indications, warnings, etc Cremalgin is contra-indicated in those patients with salicylate hypersensitivity. Erythematous reactions may occur in sensitive patients.

Pharmaceutical precautions No special precautions.

Legal category GSL.

Package quantities Tubes of 30 g.

Further information Nil.

Product licence number 0152/5019.

DOMICAL*

Presentation Round film-coated bi-convex Amitriptyline Tablets BP marked 'D': 10 mg tablets are blue, 25 mg are orange and 50 mg are red-brown.

Uses Amitriptyline is an antidepressant of the tricyclic group.

It is indicated by symptoms of a depressive illness especially when sedation is required.

Dosage and administration *Adults:* Initially 75 mg/day in divided doses or as a single dose at night, increasing to 200 mg/day according to clinical response. Maintenance dose is 50–100 mg at night.

Elderly or adolescent patients: 10–50 mg daily initially (see 'Precautions').

Children: Domical is not recommended for children under 12 years of age.

Contra-indications, warnings, etc

Contra indications: History of myocardial infarction, arrhythmias, particularly heart block of any degree, congestive cardiac failure, coronary artery insufficiency.

Receipt of monoamine oxidase inhibitors within the last two weeks.

Mania. Severe liver disease. Hypersensitivity to any tricyclic antidepressant. Breast feeding.

Precautions: Safety in pregnancy and lactation has not been established. Do not use during pregnancy nor in nursing mothers unless there are compelling reasons.

The elderly or debilitated are particularly liable to experience toxic effects, especially agitation, confusion and postural hypotension. The initial dose should be increased with great caution under close supervision. Half the normal maintenance dose may be sufficient to produce a satisfactory clinical response.

All patients with severe depression should be closely supervised, particularly during the early stages of therapy when partial response may increase the risk of suicide.

Domical should be used with great caution in patients with a history of narrow angle glaucoma, urinary retention, epilepsy or recent convulsions, hepatic insufficiency, hyperthyroidism, cardiovascular disorders or blood dyscrasias, or symptoms suggestive of prostatic hypertrophy.

Tricyclic antidepressants potentiate the central nervous depressant action of alcohol.

Anaesthetics given during tri/tetracyclic antidepressant therapy may increase the risk of arrhythmias and hypotension. If surgery is necessary, the anaesthetist should be informed that a patient is being so treated.

Drug interactions: In patients who have been treated previously with monoamine oxidase inhibitors, at least two weeks should elapse before treatment with Domical is started, with great caution, commencing with low dosage and slow increments.

Amitriptyline may decrease the antihypertensive effect of guanethidine, debrisoquine, bethanidine and possibly clonidine. It is advisable to review all antihypertensive therapy during treatment with tricyclic antidepressants.

Amitriptyline should not be given with sympathomimetic agents such as ephedrine, isoprenaline, noradrenaline, phenylephrine and phenylpropanolamine, or with ethchlorvynol.

The antidepressant action of Domical may be decreased by barbiturates and increased by methylphenidate.

The dose of thyroid hormone medication may need to be reduced if amitriptyline is given concurrently.

Warnings and adverse reactions: As improvement may not occur during the first month of therapy, patients should be closely monitored during this period.

Cardiac arrhythmias and severe hypotension are likely to occur with high dosage or in deliberate overdosage. They may also occur in patients with pre-existing heart disease taking normal dosage.

Confusion may occur at high doses or in elderly patients, requiring reduction of dosage.

Drowsiness is not uncommon in the early stages of treatment, and patients should be warned not to drive or operate machinery until it has been established that their alertness is not impaired.

The following adverse effects, although not necessarily all reported with amitriptyline, have occurred with tricyclic antidepressants:

Atropine-like side-effects including dry mouth, disturbances of accommodation, tachycardia, constipation and hesitancy of micturition are common early in treatment, but usually lessen.

Other common adverse effects include nausea, sweating, postural hypotension, dizziness, tremor and rashes. Interference with sexual function may occur.

Serious adverse effects are rare. These include bone marrow depression, agranulocytosis, cholestatic jaundice, hypomania, convulsions and peripheral neuropathy.

Withdrawal symptoms which may occur on abrupt cessation of therapy include insomnia, irritability and excessive perspiration. There have also been reports of withdrawal symptoms in neonates whose mothers received tricyclic antidepressants during the third trimester of pregnancy.

Psychotic manifestations, including mania and paranoid delusions may be exacerbated during treatment with tricyclic antidepressants.

Treatment of overdosage: The major symptoms are likely to be coma and respiratory depression. Primary therapy must be aimed at correction of hypoxia, acidosis and electrolyte imbalance. Gastric lavage should be performed and the ECG monitored. If convulsions occur they may be treated with diazepam. Serious dysrhythmias are rare and DC conversion may be preferable to anticholinesterase agents, which can exacerbate convulsions.

Pharmaceutical precautions No special precautions.

Legal category POM.

Package quantities *Tablets 10 mg:* Containers of 500.
Tablets 25 mg: Containers of 500.
Tablets 50 mg: Containers of 100.

Further information Nil.

Product licence numbers
Tablets 10 mg   0152/0065
Tablets 25 mg   0152/0066
Tablets 50 mg   0152/0114

DOPAMET*

Presentation Yellow film-coated Methyldopa Tablets BP. 125 mg (marked 'BERK 1C3'). 250 mg (marked 'BERK 2C3'). 500 mg (marked 'BERK 3C3').

Uses Hypertension.

Dosage and administration *Initiating therapy: Adults:* 250 mg twice a day for two days, increased at intervals of not less than two days by an additional 250–500 mg daily until satisfactory control is achieved. This normally follows within 12–24 hours of reaching the effective dose for the individual patient, which is generally in the range of 500–2,000 mg daily. It is seldom necessary to exceed 3,000 mg daily and, because methyldopa is largely excreted by the kidneys, patients with impaired renal function may respond to comparatively low doses.

The requirement of 'Dopamet' may be reduced by giving a thiazide diuretic concurrently: downward adjustments of dosage should likewise be made at intervals of not less than 48 hours.

In the few cases where tolerance develops, effective control can frequently be restored by increasing the dosage of 'Dopamet' or by adding a diuretic to the regimen.

When patients are on other hypotensive agents and it is desired to change them over to 'Dopamet', drug interactions must be carefully watched for.

Reserpine and other Rauwolfia alkaloids, hydrallazine and mebutamate when used alone or in any combination should be discontinued before treatment with 'Dopamet' is started.

Ganglion blocking agents and adrenergic blocking agents used alone or in combination should be withdrawn cautiously and progressively. During the first week of transfer the dosage of blocking agent should be reduced by a half and 'Dopamet' added at a dosage of 250 mg twice a day. The blocking agent is then reduced still further and the dosage of 'Dopamet' adjusted upwards by 250–500 mg stages at two- to seven-day intervals to maintain optimal control of the blood pressure.

Monoamine oxidase inhibitors should be discontinued before treatment with 'Dopamet' commences. It should then be used cautiously in case of delayed excretion of the monoamine oxidase inhibitors.

Contra-indications, warnings, etc Dopamet should not be given in cases of active liver disease, such as acute hepatitis and active cirrhosis, and in patients known to be sensitive to methyldopa. Dopamet is not recommended where phaeochromocytoma is suspected, since methyldopa fluoresces at the same wavelengths as catecholamines in urine samples; spuriously high concentrations of urinary catecholamines may be reported and this will interfere in the diagnosis of phaeochromocytoma. Dopamet should not be used with reserpine, other Rauwolfia alkaloids, hydrallazine, mebutamate and monoamine oxidase inhibitors. When methyldopa is used with other antihypertensive agents, potentiation of antihypertensive action may occur. The progress of patients should be carefully followed to detect side reactions or manifestations of drug idiosyncrasy. Patients may require reduced doses of anaesthetics when on methyldopa. If hypotension does occur during anaesthesia, it can usually be controlled by vasopressors. Since experience of methyldopa in pregnancy is still limited, Dopamet is not currently recommended for pregnant women or for nursing mothers, but in serious cases the benefits of the drug might be weighed against any potential risk.

Sedation is the most frequent side-effect and may occur even at the starting dose level. It usually wears off after an effective maintenance dosage has been established. Depression may occur and corrective treatment with tricyclic antidepressants may antagonise the therapeutic effect of Dopamet. Other minor side-effects are headache and a feeling of weakness but again these wear off with time. Symptoms of cerebrovascular insufficiency associated with effective lowering of blood pressure may also occur, including dizziness, lightheadedness and faintness. If such symptoms occur, dosage should be reduced. Symptoms due to postural hypotension are fewer and less severe with Dopamet than with other hypotensive agents and exercise hypotension rarely occurs. If such symptoms do occur, the dose of Dopamet should be reduced. Occasionally bradycardia, nasal stuffiness, mild dryness of the mouth and gastro-intestinal symptoms – including distension, constipation, flatus and diarrhoea – may occur. These are generally relieved by reducing the dosage. Vomiting has been reported in very few patients and sore or black tongue has been observed rarely. Weight gain and oedema occur infrequently and are usually relieved by administering a thiazide diuretic. If oedema becomes progressive or other signs of heart failure appear after the addition of a thiazide diuretic, Dopamet should be discontinued. On rare occasions breast enlargement, lactation, impotence, skin rash, mild arthralgia, myalgia, parasthesias, Parkinsonism, psychic disturbances – including nightmares and reversible mild psychosis – have been reported. A rise in blood urea has been found in some cases. Rarely, urine from patients receiving Dopamet may darken on exposure to air simply because of the chemical breakdown of methyldopa or its metabolites. Cases of acquired haemolytic anaemia have occurred in association with methyldopa. Should clinical symptoms suggest the possibility of anaemia, appropriate tests should be undertaken. If haemolysis is found to be present Dopamet should be discontinued. In addition some patients on continued therapy with methyldopa develop a positive direct Coombs test, but this rarely develops in the first six months of therapy and if it has not developed within 12 months it is not likely to do so. Prior knowledge of a positive Coombs reaction will aid in evaluation of cross-matching for transfusion. If a patient with a positive Coombs reaction shows an incompatible minor cross-match, an indirect Coombs test should be performed. If this is negative, transfusion with blood otherwise compatible in the major cross-match may be carried out. If positive, the advisability of transfusion should be determined by a haematologist.

A reversible thrombocytopenia has occurred on rare occasions and reversible reduction of the white blood cell count has been seen with a primary effect on the granulocytes. The granulocyte count, however, returns promptly to normal when the drug is discontinued. Rare cases of clinical agranulocytosis have been reported. On rare occasions fever occurs, usually within the first three weeks of administering methyldopa, in some cases accompanied by eosinophilia or abnormalities in one or more liver function measurements. Jaundice with or without fever may also occur, usually within the first two to three months of therapy. In some patients the findings are consistent with cholestasis. Rare cases of fatal hepatic necrosis have been reported. It is advisable to take a total and differential white blood cell count and to perform liver function tests at intervals during the first 6–12 weeks of treatment, or if the patient develops an unexplained fever. Should fever, abnormality in the liver function of jaundice occur, therapy should be withdrawn. Dialysis may remove methyldopa. Hypertension may, therefore, recur after this procedure.

Rarely involuntary choreoathetotic movements have been observed during therapy with methyldopa in patients with severe bilateral cerebrovascular disease. Should these movements occur, therapy should be discontinued.

When a thiazide diuretic is added to the dosage regimen, an excessive drop in blood pressure may occur so that the dosage of Dopamet may be reduced by half when a thiazide is used additionally. Careful observation of changes in blood pressure must be made. If Dopamet is added to the regimen of a patient taking a thiazide diuretic then the initial dosage should be limited to 375 mg per day for the first two days and the dosage increased gradually at intervals of not less than two days until adequate control of the blood pressure is obtained.

Treatment of overdosage: Gastric lavage may be helpful if carried out within a reasonable time after ingestion and can be assisted by dialysis if the overdosage has been substantial. Other treatment should be symptomatic, with general support provided to maintain cardiac output, blood volume, electrolyte balance and urinary output.

Pharmaceutical precautions Store in a cool dry place and protect from light.

Legal category POM.

Package quantities *Tablets 125 mg:* Containers of 250.

Tablets 250 mg: Containers of 250, 1,000 and 2,500.

Tablets 500 mg: Containers of 250 and 500.

Further information 'Dopamet' is an effective hypotensive agent which possesses significant advantages over the ganglion blocking and postganglion blocking agents, controlling high blood pressure throughout the day and night after a basic regimen particular to the patient has been established. It usually reduces supine as well as standing blood pressure and produces little or no postural or exertional hypotension. Normal or elevated plasma renin activity may decrease in the course of methyldopa therapy.

Product licence numbers
Tablets 125 mg 0152/0093
Tablets 250 mg 0152/5021
Tablets 500 mg 0152/0080

DRYPTAL* TABLETS 40 mg

Presentation White Frusemide Tablets BP 40 mg marked 'BERK 2B2', single break line.

Uses Diuretic. Oedema of cardiac, hepatic or renal origin. Pulmonary oedema. Toxaemia of pregnancy. Mild or moderate hypertension.

Dosage and administration The usual initial dosage is 1 tablet daily, thereafter adjusted to the minimum effective dose which may range from $\frac{1}{2}$ tablet (20 mg) on alternate days to 3 tablets (120 mg) daily.

Children: From 1 to 3 mg/kg body weight.

Contra-indications, warnings, etc Dryptal is contra-indicated in the presence of electrolyte deficiency, hepatic cirrhosis or digitalis intoxication and should be used with great caution in advanced renal failure. Patients with prostatic hypertrophy or impairment of micturition have an increased risk of developing acute retention. Cephaloridine nephrotoxicity may be increased by concomitant administration of potent diuretics such as frusemide.

During prolonged use and at high dosage a close check should be kept upon plasma electrolytes.

Dryptal may potentiate the action of cardiac glycosides and of hypotensive agents, the dosage of which may need to be reduced. Dryptal may also precipitate diabetes, or necessitate increased dosage of insulin.

Serum uric acid levels tend to rise during treatment with Dryptal and an acute attack of gout may occasionally be precipitated.

Elderly patients may be particularly susceptible to disturbances of water and electrolyte balance and micturition disorders during therapy with frusemide and particular caution should be exercised.

Other reported side-effects include nausea, gastric upset and malaise. The incidence of allergic reactions such as skin rashes is very low but when these occur treatment should be withdrawn. Bone marrow depression has been reported as a rare complication and necessitates withdrawal of treatment.

Only when it is essential should Dryptal be given in the first trimester of pregnancy or to nursing mothers.

Treatment of overdosage: Correct dehydration and electrolyte depletion. Reversible deafness may occur.

Pharmaceutical precautions Store in a cool dry place protected from light.

Legal category POM.

Package quantities Containers of 50, 250 and 1,000.

Further information Nil.

Product licence number 0152/0083.

DRYPTAL* TABLETS 500 mg

Presentation Yellow, flat, bevel-edged Frusemide Tablets BP 500 mg engraved Berk 3B2 on one side and with a double breakline on the other.

Uses Diuretic for the management of oliguria due to acute or chronic renal insufficiency with a GFR below 20 ml/minute.

Dosage and administration In patients with chronic renal insufficiency an initial daily dose of 250 mg ($\frac{1}{2}$ tablet) is employed. If a satisfactory diuresis is not produced then the dose may be increased in steps of 250 mg at four to six hourly intervals up to a maximum dose of 2,000 mg (4 tablets) as a single dose.

In cases of acute renal failure which have been initially controlled using Dryptal injection oral therapy may be substituted for parenteral therapy regarding one 500 mg tablet as approximately equal to 250 mg of injection. Appropriate dosage adjustments may then be made according to the observed clinical response.

Contra-indications, warnings, etc During treatment with high-dosage forms of Dryptal, fluid balance should be carefully controlled. In the case of patients with shock, steps should be taken to normalise blood pressure and circulating blood volume before commencing therapy. Regular checks of plasma electrolytes, particularly sodium, potassium, chloride and bicarbonate should be carried out, and electrolyte replacement therapy instituted if necessary.

Contra-indications: Dryptal tablets 500 mg are contra-indicated in renal failure as a result of poisoning by nephrotoxic or hepatotoxic agents and in renal failure associated with hepatic coma.

Warnings: The dosage of concurrently administered cardiac glycosides or antihypertensive agents may require adjustment.

Cephaloridine nephrotoxicity may be increased by concomitant administration of potent diuretics such as frusemide.

Latent diabetes may become manifest or the insulin requirements of diabetic patients may increase.

Precautions: The safety of high dosage frusemide in pregnancy has not been established and Dryptal tablets 500 mg should be used with caution, weighing potential benefit to the patient against possible hazard to the foetus.

Elderly patients may be particularly susceptible to disturbances of water and electrolyte balance and micturition disorders during therapy with frusemide and particular caution should be exercised.

Treatment of overdosage: Correct dehydration and electrolyte depletion. Reversible deafness may occur.

Side-effects: Dryptal tablets 500 mg are generally well tolerated. Side-effects of a minor nature such as nausea, malaise or gastric upset may occur but are not usually severe enough to cause withdrawal of treatment. The incidence of allergic reactions such as skin rashes is very low but when these occur treatment should be withdrawn. In common with other sulphonamide-based diuretics hyperuricaemia may occur and, in rare cases, clinical gout may be precipitated. Bone marrow depression has been reported as a rare complication and necessitates withdrawal of treatment.

Pharmaceutical precautions Store in a cool dry place protected from light.

Legal category POM.

Package quantities Containers of 100.

Further information Nil.

Product licence number 0152/0145.

DRYPTAL* INJECTION 20 mg/2 ml

Presentation Dryptal Injection 20 mg contains 20 mg Frusemide BP in 2 ml.

Uses Dryptal is a diuretic recommended for use in all indications when a prompt and effective diuresis is required. Indications include cardiac odema, renal oedema, peripheral oedema due to mechanical obstruction or changes in the walls of the veins, ascites, toxaemia of pregnancy, hypertension and miscellaneous conditions such as acute barbiturate poisoning, after prostatectomy and in cases where other diuretics have failed to produce the desired effect.

Dosage and administration Dryptal has an exceptionally wide therapeutic range the effect being proportional to the dosage. Dryptal is best given as a single dose either daily, on alternate days, or on three successive days of the week.

Parenteral administration: Intravenous injections of Dryptal **must** be given slowly. In cases of emergency or when oral therapy is precluded an initial dose of 20–40 mg (1–2 ampoules) i.m. or i.v. is recommended. Further adjustment may then be necessary according to the observed clinical response.

Parenteral doses for children range from 0.5–1.5 mg/kg body weight.

Contra-indications, warnings, etc

Contra-indications: Dryptal is contra-indicated in electrolyte deficiency and precomatose states associated with liver cirrhosis.

Warnings: Patients with prostatic hypertrophy or impairment of micturition have an increased risk of developing acute retention.

The dosage of concurrently administered cardiac glycosides or antihypertensive agents may require adjustment.

Cephaloridine nephrotoxicity may be increased by concomitant administration of potent diuretics such as frusemide.

Latent diabetes may become manifest or the insulin requirements of diabetic patients may increase.

Infusion rates in excess of 4 mg/min are associated with an increased risk of ototoxicity, usually reversible hearing loss.

Precautions: Caution should be observed in patients liable to electrolyte deficiency.

Elderly patients may be particularly susceptible to disturbances of water and electrolyte balance and micturition disorders during therapy with frusemide and particular caution should be exercised.

The use of Dryptal during the first trimester of pregnancy should be subject to the normal precautions which apply to any drug at this time. As Dryptal may inhibit lactation it should be used with caution in nursing mothers.

Treatment of overdosage: Correct dehydration and electrolyte depletion. Reversible deafness may occur.

Side-effects: Dryptal is generally well tolerated. Side-effects of a minor nature such as nausea, malaise or gastric upset may occur but are not usually severe enough to cause withdrawal of treatment.

The incidence of allergic reactions such as skin rashes is very low but when these occur treatment should be withdrawn.

In common with other sulphonamide-based diuretics hyperuricaemia may occur and, in rare cases, clinical gout may be precipitated.

Bone marrow depression has been reported as a rare complication and necessitates withdrawal of treatment.

Pharmaceutical precautions Dryptal should be stored in a cool dry place protected from light in the original containers.

Injections of Dryptal should not be mixed with any other preparation. Opened ampoules should be used immediately and any remainder discarded.

Legal category POM.

Package quantities Dryptal ampoules are available in packs of 10 × 2 ml.

Further information Dryptal produces a prompt and effective diuresis which lasts for approximately two hours following parenteral administration. Therefore the time of administration can be adjusted to suit the patient's requirements.

Product licence number 0152/0149.

DRYPTAL* INJECTION 50 mg/5 ml

Presentation Dryptal injection 50 mg contains 50 mg Frusemide BP in 5 ml.

Uses Dryptal is a diuretic recommended for use when a prompt and effective diuresis is required. The intravenous formulation is appropriate for use in emergencies. Indications include cardiac oedema, pulmonary oedema, hepatic oedema, renal oedema and cases in which other therapy has failed to produce the desired response.

Dosage and administration Dryptal injection **must** always be given slowly. The diuretic effect of Dryptal is proportional to the dosage. Up to 50 mg may be given initially; if larger doses are required, they should be given by slow infusion and titrated according to the response. In such cases the use of Dryptal 250 mg ampoules should be considered.

Contra-indications, warnings, etc Intravenous injections of Dryptal, **must** always be given slowly.

Contra-indications: Dryptal is contra-indicated in electrolyte deficiency and pre-comatose states associated with liver cirrhosis.

Warnings: Patients with prostatic hypertrophy or impairment of micturition have an increased risk of developing acute retention.

The dosage of concurrently administered cardiac glycosides or antihypertensive agents may require adjustment.

Cephaloridine nephrotoxicity may be increased by concomitant administration of potent diuretics such as frusemide.

Latent diabetes may become manifest or the insulin requirements of diabetic patients may increase.

Infusion rates in excess of 4 mg/min are associated with an increased risk of ototoxicity, usually reversible hearing loss.

Precautions: Caution should be observed in patients liable to electrolyte deficiency.

Elderly patients may be particularly susceptible to disturbances of water and electrolyte balance and micturition disorders during therapy with frusemide and particular caution should be exercised.

The use of Dryptal during the first trimester of pregnancy should be subject to the normal precautions which apply to any drug at this time.

As Dryptal may inhibit lactation it should be used with caution in nursing mothers.

Treatment of overdosage: Correct dehydration and electrolyte depletion. Reversible deafness may occur.

Side-effects: Dryptal is generally well tolerated. Side-effects of a minor nature such as nausea, malaise or gastric upset may occur but are not usually severe enough to cause withdrawal of treatment.

The incidence of allergic reactions such as skin rashes is very low but when these occur treatment should be withdrawn.

In common with other sulphonamide-based diuretics hyperuricaemia may occur and in rare cases, clinical gout may be precipitated.

Bone marrow depression has been reported as a rare complication and necessitates withdrawal of treatment.

Pharmaceutical precautions Dryptal 50 mg should be stored in a cool dry place protected from light in the original containers. Injections of Dryptal should not be mixed with any other preparations. Opened ampoules should be used immediately and any remainder discarded.

Legal category POM.

Package quantities Dryptal ampoules 50 mg are available in packs of 10 × 5 ml.

Further information Nil.

Product licence number 0152/0149.

DRYPTAL* INJECTION 250 mg/25 ml

Presentation Dryptal 250 mg ampoules contain 250 mg Frusemide BP in 25 ml.

Uses Dryptal 250 mg is a diuretic preparation for the management of oliguria due to acute or chronic renal insufficiency with a GFR below 20 ml/minute.

Dosage and administration Dryptal 250 mg should be administered by intravenous injection at a rate not exceeding 4 mg/min.

The recommended initial dose is one 25 ml ampoule (250 mg) diluted in approximately 225 ml Sodium Chloride Injection BP or Ringer's Solution for Injection administered over one hour. This gives an approximate drip rate of 80 drops/minute, ensuring that the infusion is at the level of 4 mg/minute.

If a satisfactory increase in urine output, such as 40–50 ml/hour, is not attained within the next hour a second infusion of two 25 ml ampoules (500 mg) in an appropriate infusion fluid should be given, the total volume of the infusion being governed by the patient's state of hydration. If a satisfactory output is still not achieved within one hour of the end of the second infusion, a third infusion consisting of four 25 ml ampoules (1,000 mg) can be given. The rate of infusion should not exceed 4 mg/min.

If the third infusion using the maximum intravenous

dose of 1,000 mg over four hours is not effective, then dialysis will probably be required.

In oliguric or anuric patients with significant fluid overload, it may not be practicable to administer high-dose Dryptal injection by the method suggested above. Under these circumstances, the use of a constant-rate infusion pump (e.g. Sage pump) with micrometer screw-gauge adjustment may be considered for direct admin-istration of the injection into the vein. The rate of administration should not exceed 4 mg/min.

If the Dryptal infusion produces a satisfactory response of 40–50 ml/hour, then the effective dose (up to 1,000 mg) can be repeated every 24 hours. Alternatively, maintenance therapy can be continued with oral Dryptal 500 mg tablets when one 500 mg tablet may be regarded as being approximately equal to one 250 mg ampoule. Appropriate dosage adjustments may then be made according to the observed clinical response.

Contra-indications, warnings, etc During treat-ment with high-dosage forms of Dryptal, fluid balance should be carefully controlled. In the particular case of patients with shock, steps should be taken to correct the blood pressure and circulating blood volume before commencing therapy. Regular checks of plasma electo-lytes, particularly sodium, potassium, chloride and bicar-bonate, should be carried out, and electrolyte replacement therapy instituted accordingly.

Intravenous injections of Dryptal **must** be given slowly.

Infusion rates in excess of 4 mg/min are associated with an increased risk of ototoxicity, usually reversible hearing loss.

Contra-indications: Dryptal injection 250 mg is contra-indicated in renal failure as a result of poisoning by nephrotoxic or hepatotoxic agents and in renal failure associated with hepatic coma.

Warnings: The dosage of concurrently administered cardiac glycosides or antihypertensive agents may require adjustment.

Cephaloridine nephrotoxicity may be increased by concomitant administration of potent diuretics such as frusemide.

Latent diabetes may become manifest or the insulin requirements of diabetic patients may increase.

Precautions: The safety of high dosage frusemide in pregnancy has not been established and Dryptal injection 250 mg should be used with caution depending on the severity of the condition. As Dryptal may inhibit lactation it should be used with caution in nursing mothers.

Elderly patients may be particularly susceptible to disturbances of water and electrolyte balance and micturition disorders during therapy with frusemide and particular caution should be exercised.

Treatment of overdosage: Correct dehydration and electrolyte depletion. Reversible deafness may occur.

Side-effects: Dryptal injection 250 mg is generally well tolerated. Side-effects of a minor nature such as nausea, malaise or gastric upset may occur but are not usually severe enough to cause withdrawal of treatment.

The incidence of allergic reactions such as skin rashes is very low but when these occur treatment should be withdrawn.

In common with other sulphonamide-based diuretics hyperuricaemia may occur and, in rare cases, clinical gout may be precipitated.

Bone marrow depression has been reported as a rare complication and necessitates withdrawal of treatment.

Pharmaceutical precautions Dryptal ampoules 250 mg should be stored in a cool place protected from light. Frusemide may precipitate in solutions of low pH and therefore dextrose solutions are not suitable infusion fluids for Dryptal injection 250 mg. The injection solution should not be mixed with other drugs in the infusion bottle.

Opened ampoules should be used immediately and any remainder of either the ampoule content or the prepared infusion solution should be discarded.

Legal category POM.

Package quantities Dryptal ampoules 250 mg are available in packs of 10 × 25 ml.

Further information Diuresis should commence within a few minutes and last for approximately two hours. A diuretic effect is seen during the infusion and its duration is related to the infusion time.

Product licence number 0152/0149.

ERYCEN*

Presentation Plain orange film enteric coated ery-thromycin. Tablets BP 250 mg and 500 mg (Erythromy-cin base).

Uses Infections caused by erythromycin-sensitive or-ganisms especially Gram-positive pyogenic cocci and some Gram-negative bacteria, notably Haemophilus and Neisseria groups.

Dosage and administration *Adults:* Usual oral dose 250 mg every four to six hours. This may be increased to 4 g or more per day in unusually severe infections.

Contra-indications, warnings, etc Known sensi-tivity to erythromycin. Do not use in conjunction with other anti-infectives, except when specifically war-ranted.

Precautions: Caution should be exercised in administer-ing erythromycin to patients with impaired hepatic function, since the antibiotic is excreted principally by the liver.

Side-effects are rare and usually mild. Nausea, vomiting, diarrhoea and pruritus have occurred. Allergic reactions are rare and mild, although anaphylaxis has occurred. Treatment should not usually be continued for longer than ten days. The rare possibility of superinfection caused by overgrowth of non-susceptible bacteria or fungi should be borne in mind during prolonged or repeated therapy, especially when other antibacterial agents are simultaneously employed.

Treatment of overdosage: It is unlikely that serious symptoms will occur; observation and conservative management are indicated.

Pharmaceutical precautions Store below 30°C and protect from light. Keep container tightly closed.

Package quantities Tablets 250 mg: Containers of 100 and 500.
Tablets 500 mg: Containers of 100 and 500.

Legal category POM.

Further information Erythromycin is bacteristatic and bactericidal, depending on the concentration. Its anti-microbial spectrum is similar to that of penicillin G but it shows increased activity against some Gram-negative bacteria.

Product licence numbers
Tablets 250 mg   0152/0132
Tablets 500 mg   0152/0203

FRUMIL ▼

Presentation Orange tablets with a breakline, marked Frumil each containing 40 mg Frusemide BP and 5 mg Amiloride Hydrochloride BP.

Uses Frumil is indicated where a prompt diuresis is required. It is of particular value in conditions where potassium conservation is important: congestive cardiac failure, nephrosis, corticosteroid therapy, oestrogen therapy. Ascites associated with cirrhosis.

Dosage and administration The adult dose is one to two tablets, to be taken in the morning.

Contra-indications, warnings, etc

Contra-indications: Hyperkalaemia (serum potassium >5.3 mmol/litre), Addison's disease, acute renal failure, anuria, severe progressive renal disease, electrolyte imbalance, precomatose states associated with cirrhosis, concomitant potassium supplements, known sensitivity to frusemide or amiloride.

Frumil is contra-indicated in children as safety in this age group has not been established.

Warnings: Hyperkalaemia has been observed in patients receiving amiloride hydrochloride.

Frusemide may cause latent diabetes to become manifest. It may be necessary to increase the dose of hypoglycaemic agents in diabetic patients.

Patients with prostatic hypertrophy or impairment of micturition have an increased risk of developing acute urinary retention during diuretic therapy.

Serum uric acid levels may rise during treatment with Frumil and acute attacks of gout may be precipitated.

Cephaloridine nephrotoxicity may be increased by concomitant administration of potent diuretics such as Frumil.

Precautions: Patients who are being treated with this preparation require regular supervision, with monitoring of fluid and electrolyte states to avoid excessive loss of fluid.

Frumil should be used with particular caution in elderly patients or those with potential obstruction of the urinary tract or disorders rendering electrolyte balance precarious.

Hyponatraemia, hypochloraemia and raised blood urea nitrogen may occur during vigorous diuresis, especially in seriously ill patients or the elderly. Careful monitoring of serum electrolytes and urea should therefore be undertaken in these patients.

The dosage of concurrently administered cardiac glycosides or antihypertensive agents may require adjustment.

Frumil should be discontinued before a glucose tolerance test.

Pregnancy and lactation: The safety of Frumil use during pregnancy and lactation has not been established.

Side effects: Malaise, gastric upset, nausea, vomiting, diarrhoea, and constipation may occur.

If skin rashes or pruritus occur, treatment should be withdrawn.

Rare complications may include minor psychiatric disturbances, disturbances in liver function tests and ototoxicity.

Bone marrow depression occasionally complicates treatment, necessitating withdrawal of the product. The haematopoietic state should be regularly monitored during treatment.

Treatment of overdosage: Treatment of overdosage should be aimed at reversing dehydration and correcting electrolyte imbalance, particularly hyperkalaemia. Emesis should be induced or gastric lavage performed. Treatment is symptomatic and supportive. If hyperkalaemia is seen, appropriate measures to reduce serum potassium must be instituted.

Pharmaceutical precautions Store in a cool, dry place, protect from light.

Legal category POM.

Package quantities Cartons of 28 tablets consisting of 2 calendar foils of 14 tablets.

Cartons of 56 tablets consisting of 4 calendar foils of 14 tablets.

Further information Frumil is particularly suitable for patients at risk from hypokalaemia and causes significantly less potassium excretion than frusemide during the 12 hours after administration. The daily loss of potassium with Frumil is equivalent to normal potassium excretion.

Product licence number 0152/0183.

GLIBENCLAMIDE TABLETS BP

Presentation White tablets containing 5 mg of Glibenclamide BP, marked BERK 2L7 on one face with a breakline on the reverse.

Uses Glibenclamide is a sulphonyl urea with oral hypoglycaemic action indicated for the treatment of maturity onset diabetes which cannot be adequately controlled using dietary measures alone.

Dosage and administration

1. New diabetic patients: Initial dosage should be 5 mg daily or 2.5 mg daily in debilitated or elderly patients. If proper control is not achieved at this dosage it should be increased at weekly intervals by 2.5 mg or 5.0 mg at the discretion of the physician. It is rarely necessary to exceed a daily dosage of 15 mg, and an increase of dosage above this level is unlikely to produce any further response.

The total daily dose selected should normally be given immediately at breakfast or the first main meal of the day, but due consideration should be given to the patient's dietary habits and daily activity when apportioning dosage.

2. Transfer from other oral anti-diabetic agents: It is normally possible to transfer to glibenclamide from other similar oral antidiabetic agents without any break in therapy.

Glibenclamide treatment should commence at a dose of 5 mg daily, then, if necessary, be adjusted in increments of 2.5 or 5 mg.

The following approximate equivalence data may be useful when affecting a transfer: 5 mg of glibenclamide is approximately equivalent to 1 g of tolbutamide, 250 mg chloropropamide or tolazamide, 500 mg acetohexamide, 25 mg glibornuride, or 5 mg glipizide.

3. Change-over from biguanides: Glibenclamide treatment should be started with 2.5 mg daily and the biguanide withdrawn. Dosage should then be adjusted by increments of 2.5 mg until control is achieved.

Combination with biguanides: If it is not possible to achieve control with 15 mg of glibenclamide daily and appropriate dietary measures, control can often be established by a combination of glibenclamide with a biguanide derivative.

4. Change-over from insulin: While it is appreciated that most patients who are on insulin therapy will continue to need it, there may be a few patients, particularly those on low daily doses, who will remain stabilised if transferred to glibenclamide.

No dosage recommendations can be made for the administration of glibenclamide to children.

Contra-indications, warnings, etc

Contra-indications: Glibenclamide should not be used for the treatment of juvenile or unstable diabetes, in those patients who have or have had diabetic ketoacidosis or diabetic coma or pre-coma, who have insulin dependent diabetes mellitus or serious impairment of renal, hepatic, thyroid or adrenocortical function.

Glibenclamide is also contra-indicated in conditions of unusual stress such as surgery or during pregnancy when insulin is preferable. After delivery glibenclamide therapy can be commenced or re-started.

Precautions: The hypoglycaemic action of glibenclamide may be enhanced by sulphonamides, salicylates, phenylbutazone, coumarin derivatives, betablocking agents, monoamine oxidase inhibitors, cyclophosphamide, chloramphenicol and tuberculo-statics. Hypoglycaemic activity may be diminished by adrenalin, corticosteroids, oral contraceptives, thiazide diuretics, frusemide and ethacrynic acid.

Lactation: It has not yet been established whether glibenclamide is transferred to human milk. Since other sulphonylureas have been identified in milk there is no evidence to suggest that glibenclamide differs from other members of the group in this respect.

Infection and trauma: The dose of glibenclamide may need to be increased in patients suffering from infections or trauma. Where these are severe, control of hypoglycaemia may be lost. In such cases glibenclamide should be withdrawn and diabetic control maintained with insulin. Once the patient has recovered from the infection or trauma, glibenclamide should be re-introduced.

Side-effects: Glibenclamide is well tolerated and serious side effects sufficient to necessitate withdrawal are uncommon.

Mild gastrointestinal and allergic skin reactions have been reported.

Rare incidents of reversible leucopenia and thrombocytopenia have also been reported.

Transient changes in liver enzymes and function tests have been observed during glibenclamide treatment. It has not been confirmed whether these changes are directly related to the product.

As with other oral anti-diabetic agents, hypoglycaemia can occur with glibenclamide. Debilitated or aged patients may be more liable to suffer this reaction. Hypoglycaemia is not usually prolonged and responds to appropriate therapeutic measures.

Overdosage and treatment: If a hypoglycaemic reaction should occur and the patient is conscious, it may be treated by the administration of glucose or three to four lumps of sugar with water. If necessary, this may be repeated after 15 minutes.

If the patient is comatose, sucrose or glucose may be given by stomach tube or glucose as an intravenous infusion. Bolus injections of glucose are not recommended because of the possibility of rebound hypoglycaemia.

Glucagon may be administered at a dose of 1 mg subcutaneously or intramuscularly to produce consciousness.

Pharmaceutical precautions Protect from light.

Legal category POM.

Package quantities Glibenclamide 5 mg Tablets: Securitainers of 100, 250, 500 and 1,000.

Further information When administered orally, glibenclamide is mainly absorbed and excreted in the urine as three major metabolites. These metabolites have little or no hypoglycaemic activity.

Product licence number 0152/0209.

IBUPROFEN TABLETS BP

Presentation Sugar-coated tablets containing either 200 mg or 400 mg of Ibuprofen BP. The tablets are light-magenta in colour.

Uses Ibuprofen is indicated for its analgesic and anti-inflammatory effect in the treatment of rheumatoid arthritis (including juvenile rheumatoid arthritis or Still's disease), ankylosing spondylitis, osteoarthritis and other non-rheumatoid (seronegative) arthropathies.

In the treatment of non-articular rheumatic conditions, Ibuprofen is indicated in periarticular conditions such as frozen shoulder (capsulitis), bursitis, tendinitis, tenosynovitis and low-back pain. Ibuprofen can also be used in soft-tissue injuries such as sprains and strains.

Ibuprofen is also indicated for its analgesic effect in the relief of mild to moderate pain such as dysmenorrhoea, dental and post-operative pain. In addition Ibuprofen is indicated for the relief of migraine.

Dosage and administration

Adult: The recommended initial dosage of ibuprofen is 1200 mg daily in divided doses. Some patients can be maintained on 600 to 1200 mg daily. In severe or acute conditions it can be advantageous to increase the dosage until the acute phase is brought under control, provided that the total daily dosage does not exceed 2400 mg in divided doses.

Children: The dosage of ibuprofen 20 mg per kg of bodyweight daily except in children weighing less than 30 kg the total dose given in 24 hours should not exceed 500 mg.

Contra-indications, warnings, etc Ibuprofen should not be given to patients with severe or active peptic ulceration. Whilst no teratogenic effects have been demonstrated in animal experiments, the use of ibuprofen during pregnancy should, if possible be avoided. Ibuprofen should be prescribed with caution for those with asthma and especially for patients who have developed bronchospasm with other nonsteroidal agents.

Adverse effects reported include dyspepsia, gastrointestinal intolerance and bleeding, and skin rashes of various types. Less frequently, thrombocytopenia has occurred. Toxic amblyopia has occurred very rarely but, in those cases reported, recovery occurred on cessation of treatment.

Treatment of overdosage: Gastric lavage and, if necessary, correction of blood electrolytes. There is no specific antidote to ibuprofen.

Pharmaceutical precautions No special precautions.

Legal category POM.

Package quantities
400 mg tablets: Pack of 100, 250, 500 and 1,000.
200 mg tablets: Pack of 100, 250, 500 and 1,000.

Further information Taken on an empty stomach, peak serum levels of Ibuprofen occur 45 minutes after ingestion whereas, taken after a meal the peak is delayed up to 90 minutes. Since most people can take Ibuprofen on an empty stomach without gastric discomfort the initial dose of the day will be more rapidly effective if taken before food. This is particularly valuable in providing relief of the morning stiffness associated with arthritis.

Product licence numbers
Ibuprofen Tablets 200 mg 0152/0206
Ibuprofen Tablets 400 mg 0152/0207

IMBRILON*

Presentation Opaque yellow Indomethacin Capsules BP 25 mg (marked 'BERK 1J3 25') and 50 mg (marked 'BERK 2J3 50').
Cream-coloured Indomethacin Suppositories BP 100 mg. The base is polyethylene glycol.

Uses Non steroidal analgesic and anti-inflammatory agent. Indicated in active rheumatoid arthritis, osteoarthritis, ankylosing spondylitis and acute gout. Also may be indicated in severe acute periarticular disorders such as bursitis, tendinitis, synovitis, tenosynovitis and capsulitis.

Dosage and administration Indomethacin Capsules should always be given with food, milk or an antacid to lessen the chance of gastro-intestinal disturbance.
Imbrilon Suppositories should be given singly, one night and morning.
Adults: 50–100 mg daily.
Children: Paediatric dosage not established.

Contra-indications, warnings, etc
Contra-indications: It is not known if indomethacin is safe to use in children or in pregnancy or during lactation and it should not be given to such patients.
Active peptic ulcer, a history of recurrent gastro-intestinal lesions, sensitivity to indomethacin or to aspirin are also contra-indications.

Precautions and drug interactions: Indomethacin should be used with caution in patients with hepatic or renal dysfunction. Hepatitis and jaundice have been reported rarely. Patients should be warned not to drive or operate machinery, if they become dizzy.
In common with other anti-inflammatory analgesic antipyretic agents, indomethacin may mask the signs and symptoms of infectious disease and this should be borne in mind in order to avoid delay in starting treatment for infection.
Indomethacin should be used with caution in patients with an existing, albeit controlled, infection.

Particular care should be taken with older patients who are more susceptible to side-effects from indomethacin.

Treatment of overdosage: Gastric lavage should be given if indomethacin is considered still to be part of the stomach contents.
Otherwise supportive therapy is required and a watch should be kept for gastro-intestinal bleeding for several days.

Warnings and adverse effects: It must be expected that about 20% of patients will complain of side-effects, but starting treatment at a low dosage and increasing it gradually until symptomatic relief is obtained will minimise their incidence.
The most common side-effects are headache, dizziness and dyspepsia. If headache persists, even after dosage reduction, indomethacin should be withdrawn.
Other CNS side-effects which may occur include mental confusion, depression, convulsions, coma, depersonalisation and tinnitus. These are often transient and disappear with time or on reduction of dosage.
Indomethacin may aggravate psychiatric disorders, epilepsy and Parkinsonism.
Gastro-intestinal disorders which occur most frequently are nausea, anorexia, vomiting, epigastric distress, abdominal pain and diarrhoea. Giving indomethacin with food, milk or antacids lowers the incidence of these side-effects. Ulceration of the oesophagus, stomach or duodenum may also occur, accompanied by haemorrhage and perforation (a few fatalities have been reported). Gastro-intestinal bleeding without obvious ulceration may also occur. If this happens indomethacin treatment should be discontinued.
Blood dyscrasias, particularly thrombocytopenia, have been reported.
Blurred vision and orbital and peri-orbital pain are seen infrequently. Corneal deposits and retinal disturbances have been reported in some patients with rheumatoid arthritis on prolonged therapy with indomethacin, and ophthalmic examinations are desirable in patients given prolonged treatment.
Oedema and increased blood pressure also sometimes occur, as does haematuria.
Hypersensitivity reactions include pruritus, urticaria, angiitis, erythema nodosum. Skin rash and hair loss may also occur.
Acute respiratory distress including sudden dyspnoea and asthma, have been reported on rare occasions. Bronchospasm may be precipitated in patients suffering from, or with a previous history of bronchial asthma or allergic disease.

Pharmaceutical precautions Store in a cool place and protect from light.

Legal category POM.

Package quantities *Capsules 25 mg:* Containers of 500.

Capsules 50 mg: Containers of 100.

Suppositories 100 mg: Containers of 30.

Further information Nil.

Product licence numbers

Capsules 25 mg   0152/0072
Capsules 50 mg   0152/0074
Suppositories 100 mg   0152/0127.

LADROPEN*

Presentation Opaque orange/brown capsules containing 250 mg and 500 mg flucloxacillin as Flucloxacillin Sodium BP and overprinted 'BERK 1A8' and 'BERK 2A8' in white respectively.

Uses Treatment of infections caused by Gram-positive organisms including those caused by penicillin-resistant staphylococci.

Dosage and administration Adults: Oral: 250 mg four times daily. Capsules should be taken one hour before meals. This dosage may be doubled where necessary.

Contra-indications, warnings, etc
Contra-indications: Hypersensitivity to penicillin.

Warnings: Some patients may experience gastro-intestinal symptoms but these effects usually resolve rapidly when treatment is stopped. Urticarial or erythematous rashes occasionally occur. Treatment should be discontinued if either type of rash is observed.

Precautions: Patients with a known history of allergy are more likely to develop a hypersensitivity reaction.

Pharmaceutical precautions Flucloxacillin capsules should be stored in a cool, dry place.

Legal category POM.

Package quantities Capsules 250 mg: packs of 100 and 500 capsules.
Capsules 500 mg: packs of 100 capsules.

Further information Nil.

Product licence numbers
Capsules 250 mg   0152/0184.
Capsules 500 mg   0152/0185

LORAZEPAM TABLETS BP

Presentation White, dragee shaped tablets containing 1 mg Lorazepam BP, engraved BL1 with a breakline on the reverse. Peach-orange dragee shaped tablets containing 2.5 mg Lorazepam BP, engraved BL2.5 with a breakline on the reverse.

Uses Lorazepam is indicated for the following: mild, moderate and severe anxiety states, phobic or obsessional states, moderate to severe tension states, anxiety in psychosomatic, organic or psychotic illness, insomnia associated with anxiety, premedication before operative dentistry and as a sedative for the anxious dental patient, premedication before general surgery.

Dosage and administration
Dosage: Adults: Mild anxiety – 1–4 mg daily in divided doses.
    Moderate/severe anxiety – up to 8 mg daily in divided doses.
    Severe anxiety, phobic or obsessional/compulsive state – up to 10 mg daily.
    Insomnia – 1–4 mg before retiring.
    Premedication – 2–3 mg the night before operation, 2–4 mg one to two hours before operation.

Elderly: The elderly may respond to lower doses and half the normal adult dose or less may be sufficient.

Children: Not recommended for children.

Dentistry: 1–2.5 mg, 1½–2 hours before dental treatment. For operative dentistry dosage as for premedication.

Contra-indications, warnings, etc
Contra-indications: Lorazepam should not be given to patients with a previous history of sensitivity to benzodiazepines.

Precautions and warnings:
1. Concomitant administration with central nervous system depressants, including alcohol, general anaesthetics, narcotic analgesics, monoamine oxidase inhibitors and antidepressants will result in an accentuation of their effects.
2. Prolonged or excessive use of benzodiazepines may occasionally result in the development of some psychological dependence with withdrawal symptoms on sudden discontinuation. This is more likely in patients with a history of alcoholism, drug abuse or in patients with marked personality disorders.
Treatment in all patients should be withdrawn gradually. Careful monitoring of all patients is essential.
3. As with other drugs acting on the central nervous system, patients should be cautioned against driving or operating machinery until it is established that they do not become dizzy or drowsy while taking lorazepam.
4. Lorazepam tablets should not be administered during pregnancy or lactation unless in the judgement of the physician such administration is clinically justifiable. Special care should be taken in the first three months of pregnancy.
5. This product should be used with caution in patients with impairment of renal or hepatic function.
6. Elderly patients or those suffering from cerebral vascular changes such as arteriosclerosis are likely to respond to smaller doses.
7. Lorazepam should be used with caution during labour. Respiratory depression, poor sucking and hypothermia in the neonate have occasionally been reported especially in patients who are at high risk.
8. Lorazepam does not depress respiration in most patients but the drug should be used with caution in patients with acute or chronic pulmonary insufficiency.
9. The use of benzodiazepines may release suicidal tendencies in depressed patients. Other rarely reported behavioural effects of the benzodiazepines include paradoxical aggressive outbursts, excitement and confusion.

Overdosage: As with other benzodiazepines, overdosage should not present a threat to life. General supportive measures should be used. Treatment is symptomatic and gastric lavage may be of use if performed shortly after ingestion. If the patient is conscious, an emetic such as ipecacuanha may be given. The patient is likely to sleep and a clear airway should be maintained. The usefulness of dialysis has not been determined.

Side-effects: Lorazepam is well tolerated and imbalance or ataxia is an indication of excessive dosage. Daytime drowsiness may be seen initially and is to be anticipated in the effective treatment of anxiety. It will normally diminish rapidly and may be minimised in the early days of treatment by giving the larger proportion of the day's dose before retiring.
Occasional confusion, hangover, headache on walking, dizziness, blurred vision and nausea have also been reported.

Pharmaceutical precautions Store in a cool, dry place.

Legal category CD (Sch 4) POM.

Package quantities Securitainers containing 100, 250, 500 and 1000 tablets.

Further information Lorazepam is a short acting benzodiazepine. It is rapidly absorbed from the gastro-intestinal tract and is metabolised by a simple one-step process to a pharmacologically inactive glucuronide. The elimination half-life of lorazepam is about 12 hours so that steady state plasma levels are quickly reached and there is minimal risk of excessive accumulation, giving a wide margin of safety.

Product licence numbers
Tablets 1 mg 0152/0224
Tablets 2.5 mg 0152/0225

MUCODYNE*

Presentation *Mucodyne Capsules:* Opaque yellow capsules marked 'MUCODYNE 375', each containing carbocisteine 375 mg.

Mucodyne Syrup: Clear amber syrup containing carbocisteine 250 mg in each 5 ml.

Mucodyne Syrup Forte: Opaque orange syrup containing carbocisteine 750 mg in each 5 ml.

Mucodyne Paediatric Syrup: Clear red syrup containing carbocisteine 125 mg in each 5 ml.

Uses Mucolytic agent for the adjunctive therapy of respiratory tract disorders, characterised by excessive or viscous mucus, including Glue Ear in children.

Mucodyne reduces the viscosity of bronchial secretions and facilitates expectoration. There is also evidence that during treatment with Mucodyne, the physical and chemical characteristics of the mucin components of sputum return to a more normal pattern, with reduction of fucose and sulphate content and an increase in the proportions of sialomucins.

Dosage and administration *Adults:* (Syrup, Syrup Forte and Capsules.) Dosage is based upon an initial daily dosage of 2250 mg carbocisteine in divided doses reducing to 1500 mg daily in divided doses when a satisfactory response has been obtained, e.g. for normal syrup 15 ml tds reducing to 10 ml tds.

Children: The normal daily dose is 20 mg/kg body weight in divided doses. The following dosage is recommended for the Mucodyne Paediatric syrup: 2 to 5 years: 2.5–5 ml four times a day; 5 to 12 years: 10 ml three times a day. Dosage in younger children and infants has not been established.

Contra-indications, warnings, etc Although tests in mammalian species have revealed no teratogenic effects, Mucodyne is not recommended during the first trimester of pregnancy.

There have been rare reports of skin rashes or gastro-intestinal bleeding occurring during treatment with Mucodyne.

Treatment of overdosage: Gastric lavage may be beneficial, followed by observation. Gastro-intestinal disturbance is the most likely symptom of Mucodyne overdosage.

Pharmaceutical precautions The syrups should be stored in a cool place. Mixture with linctus of pholcodeine

causes precipitation of carbocisteine from solution. Dilution of Mucodyne Syrup may be effected with unpreserved Syrup BP but diluted preparations should not be kept for more than 14 days.

Legal category POM.

Package quantities *Mucodyne Capsules:* Containers of 30 and 100.
Mucodyne Syrup: Bottles of 300 ml with dosage cap.
Mucodyne Forte Syrup: Bottles of 200 ml with dosage cap.
Mucodyne Paediatric Syrup: Bottles of 300 ml with dosage cap.

Further information Nil.

Product licence numbers
Capsules	0152/0098
Syrup	0152/0042
Forte Syrup	0152/0124
Paediatric Syrup	0152/0166

NITRADOS*

Presentation White, round, flat, bevel-edged Nitrazepam Tablets BP, marked BERK 1N4, with single break line on reverse, each containing 5 mg Nitrazepam BP.

Uses Hypnotic of the benzodiazepine group, indicated for the relief of insomnia due to anxiety or stress. It may also be used as adjunctive therapy in the treatment of sleep disturbances due to organic causes.

At therapeutic doses nitrazepam induces sleep lasting some six to eight hours, from which the sleeper may be readily aroused if necessary. There is less confusion upon awakening than is observed with the barbiturates, especially in the elderly.

Dosage and administration *Adults:* Usually 5 mg before retiring. This may be increased to 10 mg when necessary or to 20 mg in hospitalised patients.

Smaller doses, 2.5–5 mg are more suitable for elderly patients.

Children: Nitrados is not recommended for the routine treatment of children but 2.5 mg may be given when necessary to children aged one to six years and 5 mg to children aged seven years or older.

Contra-indications, warnings, etc Nitrados should only be used with great caution in patients with impairment of renal or hepatic function, or who are elderly or debilitated. Particular consideration should be given to respiratory function.

Concomitant administration with CNS depressants (including alcohol), general anaesthetics, narcotic analgesics, monoamine oxidase inhibitors and anti-depressants may result in an accentuation of their effects.

Patients should be warned of the possibility of drowsiness occurring, particularly in the first few days of therapy and advised to moderate their use of alcohol. They should also be warned not to drive or operate machinery if Nitrados affects their alertness.

Although animal experiments have revealed no teratogenic effects, nitrazepam is not recommended during the first trimester of pregnancy.

Side-effects are few at the recommended dosage, although fatigue, drowsiness or light-headedness are occasionally noted and confusion may occur in the elderly.

Excessive or prolonged use of nitrazepam may result

in the development of psychological dependence with withdrawal symptoms on discontinuance.

Treatment of overdosage: Drowsiness and ataxia will be the predominant initial symptoms and the patient may be unconscious for up to 36 hours. Gastric lavage may be useful but Nitrados causes few serious problems in overdosage. In children behavioural changes are likely.

Pharmaceutical precautions Store in a cool place. Protect from light.

Legal category CD (Sch 4) POM.

Package quantities Containers of 50 and 500 tablets.

Further information Nil.

Product licence number 0152/0130.

OXPRENOLOL TABLETS BP

Presentation White tablets each containing 20 mg oxprenolol hydrochloride, marked 1G1 BK.

White tablets each containing 40 mg oxprenolol hydrochloride, marked 2G1 BK.

Yellow tablets each containing 80 mg oxprenolol hydrochloride, marked 3G1 BERK.

Orange tablets each containing 160 mg oxprenolol hydrochloride, marked 4G1 BERK.

Uses *Mode of action:* Oxprenolol is a beta-adrenergic receptor blocking drug. Its principal effects are seen on the heart where the rate is slowed (negative chronotropic effect) with consequent reduction in heart work and myocardial oxygen consumption.

Oxprenolol provides effective prophylactic control of angina throughout the day in the majority of patients. The frequency and severity of anginal attacks are reduced, whether precipitated by exercise or emotional stress and exercise tolerance is improved. ST segment depression seen on exercise is also reduced.

Oxprenolol has partial agonist activity (PAA) also known as intrinsic sympathomimetic activity (ISA). This property means that some degree of stimulation of beta receptors is maintained. Under conditions of rest this tends to balance the negative chronotropic and negative inotropic effects. Oxprenolol blocks the effects of excessive catecholamine stimulation resulting from stress.

The mechanism of the antihypertensive effect of Oxprenolol is not clearly understood. Whilst haemodynamic effects on cardiac output and peripheral resistance appear to be factors, effects on plasma renin and/or the central nervous system may be of significance.

Indications: For the treatment of angina pectoris, all grades of hypertension and sympathetically induced cardiac arrhythmias. For the control of anxiety and anxiety tachycardia. Subsidiary indications include functional heart disorders, hypertrophic obstructive cardiomyopathy, as an adjunct to the treatment of thyrotoxicosis and dysrhythmias associated with anaesthesia.

Dosage and administration

Adults: Angina pectoris: Most patients respond to 40–160 mg three times daily. Individual patients may require more, but only rarely are doses above 480 mg daily required.

Oxprenolol is compatible with glyceryl trinitrate when the patient has become established on oxprenolol.

As with other beta-blocking drugs, sudden withdrawal

of treatment with oxprenolol may induce severe and continuous angina. Patients should, therefore, be advised to avoid interruption of established therapy and if withdrawal becomes necessary it should be done gradually.

Hypertension: Initially 80 mg twice daily. If necessary this daily dose can be increased at convenient intervals (eg weekly or fortnightly) until satisfactory blood pressure control is achieved. When used as monotherapy, doses of 480 mg/day should not be exceeded, since experience has shown that hardly any increase in the response can be achieved by this means. The addition of a diuretic will often give a quicker and more satisfactory response. Usually patients respond to a dose of 80–320 mg oxprenolol in combination with a diuretic and most of the antihypertensive effect is achieved within 2–3 days. The addition of a vasodilator will often enable control to be achieved in the minority of patients who might otherwise fail to respond.

Cardiac arrhythmias: Initial dose 20–40 mg three times daily. This may be increased if necessary to achieve the desired effect.

Anxiety states: The majority of patients will respond to a total daily dose of 160 mg. Although no evidence of habituation of tolerance has been observed with oxprenolol its effectiveness in the long term treatment of anxiety has not been established. In the treatment of transient situational anxiety a single dose of 40–80 mg of oxprenolol may be prescribed. Oxprenolol can be administered concurrently with benzodiazepines. When withdrawal of pre-existing anxiolytic therapy is indicated, this should take place gradually.

Hyperthyroidism: 40–120 mg daily in 2 or 3 divided doses.

Pre-operatively: Patients with thyrotoxicosis and phaeochromocytoma may be managed on 60 mg daily in three divided doses. Atropine must always be used pre-operatively.

In patients undergoing elective surgery, it may be considered desirable to employ a beta-blocker as premedication, by shielding the heart against the effects of stress, the beta-blocker may serve to guard against excessive sympathetic stimulation, which is liable to provoke such cardiac disturbances as arrhythmia or acute coronary insufficiency. In a patient under beta-blockade, the anaesthetic selected should be one exhibiting as little negative inotropic activity as possible, eg halothane, nitrous oxide. If, on the other hand, inhibition of sympathetic tone during the operation is regarded as undesirable, the beta-blocker can be withdrawn gradually prior to surgery.

Children: Occasionally oxprenolol has been given to children and infants to control arrhythmias. No dosage scheme has been worked out but oral oxprenolol has been given empirically on a body-weight basis of approximately 1 mg/kg.

Contra-indications, warnings, etc

Side-effects: Oxprenolol is well tolerated. However dizziness, drowsiness, headache, insomnia, excitement and gastro-intestinal disturbance may occur particularly at the start of treatment. Isolated cases of excessive bradycardia and thrombocytopenia have been reported.

As with other beta-blockers, bronchospasm and heart failure may occasionally be recipitated in susceptible patients (see 'Precautions') and exertional tiredness and feelings of coldness in the extremities have been reported on rare occasions. However, the incidence of these side-effects is low, possibly due to the partial protection afforded by the sympathomimetic effect of oxprenolol.

Oxprenolol possesses antihypertensive effects, but these are unlikely to be noted in normotensive subjects.

There have been reports of skin rashes and/or dry eyes associated with the use of beta-adrenergic blocking drugs. The reported incidence is small, and in most cases the symptoms have cleared when the treatment was withdrawn. Discontinuance of the drug should be considered if any such reaction is not otherwise explicable. Cessation of therapy with a beta-adrenergic blocker should be gradual.

Contra-indications: Oxprenolol is contra-indicated in patients with atrioventricular block, marked bradycardia, uncontrolled heart failure and cardiogenic shock.

Precautions: If there is evidence of cardiac failure, this must be controlled by digitalis and/or diuretics before and during oxprenolol therapy. Should the pulse rate fall much below 50 per minute, then treatment should be withdrawn and re-started at a lower dose. Caution should be observed when treating asthmatics, chronic bronchitics or other individuals where bronchospasm may be provoked. Oxprenolol should be given cautiously to patients with metabolic acidosis or anaesthesia with ether or chloroform (see Dosage and Administration). Treatment with a beta-blocker is liable to mask symptoms of hypoglycaemia and also to affect carbohydrate metabolism. In patients with labile or insulin dependent diabetes in particular, it may therefore be necessary to readjust the dosage of anti-diabetic medication. Like other beta-blockers, oxprenolol should not be given in combination with calcium antagonists of the verapamil type, because their concomitant use may result in bradycardia, hypotension or even cardiac arrest.

Beta-blockers may cause bradycardia in the foetus which can also persist after birth. During pregnancy and in the course of labour and during lactation beta-blockers should only be employed after the needs of the mother have been weighed against the possible risks to the foetus.

Treatment of overdosage: Overdosage with oxprenolol may lead to excessive bradycardia, hypotension, coma and convulsions. It should also be noted that severe toxicity may develop rapidly and that there may be severe hypotension and bradycardia despite a normal ECG. For sinus bradycardia and hypotension 0.5–2.0 mg of atropine should be administered slowly by intravenous infusion.

If this does not raise the heart rate sufficiently isoprenaline may be necessary. The dose of isoprenaline needs to be sufficient to reverse the blockade and should be assessed by the clinical response. A reasonable starting dose would be 25 mcg of isoprenaline hydrochloride.

In severe cardiogenic shock the treatment of choice appears to be glucagon. The initial dose should be 5–10 mg intravenously, further boluses or an infusion can be used according to the patient's condition. Transvenous pacing has been used, sometimes with success. If bronchospasm develops bronchodilators should be used. Patients should be monitored for several days as the beta-blocking effects of oxprenolol exceed its plasma half-life.

Pharmaceutical precautions The tablets should be protected from moisture.

Legal category POM.

Package quantities
20 mg tablets: Containers of 100, 250, 500 and 1,000
40 mg tablets: Containers of 100, 250, 500 and 1,000
80 mg tablets: Containers of 100, 250, 500 and 1,000
160 mg tablets: Containers of 100, 250, 500 and 1,000

Further information In hypertension, oxprenolol blocks only the beta-receptors and does not share the problems usually associated with other antihypertensive therapy, eg postural effects, failure of ejaculation, diarrhoea. Mental and physical lethargy is not a problem with oxprenolol, many patients reporting an increased sense of well-being.

Oxprenolol protects the cardiovascular system from excess adrenergic discharge and the resulting elevation of catecholamine levels, which are a known risk factor in coronary heart disease and which, in the long term, may contribute to the secondary effects of hypertension.

Oxprenolol prevents emotional tachycardia during environmental stress. In anxiety, oxprenolol does not produce sedation or cause dependence. The best response is seen in patients who have not previously received benzodiazepines.

Product licence numbers
Oxprenolol 20 mg   0152/0211
Oxprenolol 40 mg   0152/0212
Oxprenolol 80 mg   0152/0213
Oxprenolol 160 mg   0152/0214

PACITRON*

Presentation Film-coated oblong orange-yellow tablets marked 'PCT 500', each containing L-tryptophan 500 mg.

Uses L-tryptophan is a metabolic precursor of 5-hydroxytryptamine (serotonin) which acts as a neurotransmitter in the central nervous system. L-tryptophan is indicated for the short-term relief of mild to moderate depressive illness. It is recommended that therapy be reviewed at 3-monthly intervals. L-tryptophan may enhance the action of amitriptyline and other antidepressant drugs.

Dosage and administration
Adults: The usual adult dosage is 3 g daily in divided doses. Some patients may require up to 6 g daily. L-tryptophan may also be given to patients responding inadequately to monoamine oxidase inhibitors (MAOI) but when the two are given together the side-effects of both may be increased. Pacitron should therefore be introduced more slowly, beginning at 500 mg daily for the first week, 1 g daily for the second. Normal dosage may be given from the third week onwards, but Pacitron should be discontinued at once if headache or blurring of vision occurs.

Children: L-tryptophan is not recommended in children.

Contra-indications, warnings, etc
Contra-indications: The use of Pacitron should not replace standard management in patients with severe depression and/or a risk of suicide. There is no absolute contra-indication to the use of Pacitron.

Precautions: Concurrent use of MAOI may potentiate the adverse reactions of both drugs.

In patients taking Pacitron together with or after phenothiazines or benzodiazepines, there have been rare reports of sexual disinhibition and of reversible Parkinsonian-like rigidity and dyskinesias. Since these other drugs may reduce plasma binding of tryptophan it is recommended that initial dosage of Pacitron should not exceed one tablet three times daily if the patient is taking or has just finished treatment with a major tranquilliser.

Pacitron should be used with caution in patients with overt nutritional deficiency.

Pacitron is not advised, except for relatively short periods in patients with active bladder disease or known bladder lesions.

Warnings, Side-effects etc.: L-tryptophan may produce drowsiness. Patients should be warned of the possible hazard when driving or operating machinery.

Other reported side-effects include nausea, headache and light-headedness.

There is at present no information on safety and efficacy after long-term administration of Pacitron.

Abnormal tryptophan metabolism may occur in patients who are pyridoxine deficient, such deficiency may occur in women taking oral contraceptives or in elderly or undernourished patients who have an inadequate vitamin intake. Pyridoxine supplements may be advisable in patients suspected of deficiency.

Use in Pregnancy: Evidence from animal studies is insufficient to establish safety in pregnancy. Use in pregnant and nursing mothers is not advised.

Treatment of overdosage: No serious consequences are known to result from overdosage. Gastric lavage might be helpful followed by observation and general supportive measures.

Pharmaceutical precautions No special precautions.

Legal category POM.

Package quantities Containers of 100 tablets.

Further information As with other antidepressant drugs the full therapeutic effect may not be seen for two or three weeks and patients should be told this.

Product licence number 0152/0117.

PONOXYLAN*

Presentation White gel containing 10% w/w polynoxylin.

Uses Topical broad spectrum antibacterial and healing agent.

Ponoxylan Gel is indicated in all infective skin conditions including furunculosis and pustular acne. It is of great value in burns wounds and cutaneous infected conditions including staphylococcal nasal infections. It reduces inflammation in intertrigo and many eczematoid eruptions.

It is of considerable value in dermatology as an alternative to broad spectrum antibiotic therapy with or without corticosteroids.

Dosage and administration Ponoxylan Gel should be gently applied to the affected areas.

Contra-indications, warnings, etc There are no known contra-indications. There are no special precautions to be taken with Ponoxylan Gel.

Ponoxylan is virtually insoluble and is therefore not absorbed into the blood stream. Systemic toxicity is thus nil. There have been no reports of sensitivity to polynoxylin. A very occasional patient may experience stinging or pain following application.

Pharmaceutical precautions No known incompatibilities.

Legal category P.

Package quantities Tubes of 25 g.

Further information Nil.

Product licence number 0152/5042.

PRAMIDEX*

Presentation White Tolbutamide Tablets BP 500 mg marked 'BERK 5E5', single break line.

Uses As an oral hypoglycaemic agent in the treatment of mild and moderately severe uncomplicated diabetes mellitus, particularly of the maturity-onset type, where control cannot be achieved by diet alone.

The hypoglycaemic effect of tolbutamide only occurs when the β cells of the islet tissue in the pancreas are intact and when they retain some functional capacity. It is therefore presumed that tolbutamide stimulates the pancreas to a greater insulin output. It has no effect on glucose tolerance.

It follows that Pramidex has no place in the treatment of the severe diabetic, but finds its chief use in the treatment of maturity-onset diabetes, responding inadequately to dietary treatment alone. In some of these patients it can replace low doses of insulin or reduce the requirement for high doses.

Dosage and administration Pramidex should be given with or just before meals for optimum control of blood sugar.

Initial: 4–8 tablets.
2nd day: 3–6 tablets.
3rd day: 2–4 tablets.

Maintenance: 1–3 tablets daily, the exact dose being that sufficient to correct glycosuria and hyperglycaemia without producing hypoglycaemia. The full effect of therapy may take up to a week to develop.

Where a patient is already taking insulin, the change to tolbutamide may be effected directly where the dose of insulin is 15 units or less per day. Where insulin is being given in greater amounts, the number of units should be decreased over several days and a watch should be kept for glycosuria.

Contra-indications, warnings, etc Diabetes complicated by fever, trauma or gangrene and diabetic ketosis. Impaired renal, hepatic or thyroid function. Pramidex is contra-indicated during pregnancy. Sulphafurazole is thought to potentiate the action of tolbutamide and the concurrent administration of these two drugs is contra-indicated.

Gastric irritation may occur and may be reduced by giving in divided doses. Skin sensitisation, weakness, paraesthesias, tinnitus, headache, intolerance to alcohol and jaundice have all been observed. Reversible blood dyscrasias have also occurred. A very small proportion of patients are thought to have difficulty in metabolising tolbutamide and in consequence develop hypoglycaemia even on low dose.

If fever or a sore throat occurs, a white cell count should be performed and should be repeated after five days as blood abnormalities may develop slowly.

Severe hypoglycaemia has occurred with the concomitant administration of coumarins.

The possibility of thrombocytopenia should be borne in mind and a platelet count performed if indicated.

Cases which respond initially to tolbutamide may relapse at a later date and this should be considered as a possibility should glycosuria or hyperglycaemia appear.

Pramidex should not be used as a substitute for dietary treatment in obese diabetics.

Elderly patients are especially sensitive to sulphonyl-urea-induced hypoglycaemia. This may be insidious in onset and quite prolonged.

Treatment of overdosage: Gastric lavage. Hypoglycaemia may be counteracted with dextrose and, if necessary, glucagon.

Pharmaceutical precautions No special precautions.

Legal category POM.

Package quantities Containers of 500 tablets.

Further information Nil.

Product licence number 0152/0061.

PRIMPERAN*

Presentation *Tablets:* White tablet marked 'PRIMPERAN' with single break line on reverse. Each tablet contains 10 mg Metoclopramide Hydrochloride BP.

Syrup: Each 5 ml of lime-coloured syrup contains 5 mg Metoclopramide Hydrochloride BP.

Ampoules: Colourless solution for injection containing 10 mg Metoclopramide Hydrochloride BP in 2 ml.

Uses *For the relief of upper gastro-intestinal symptoms:* including heartburn, nausea, vomiting in flatulent dyspepsia, gastritis and duodenitis associated with gastrointestinal disorders including peptic ulcers, and sequelae of gastrectomy.

As an anti-emetic agent: for the treatment of nausea and vomiting accompanying the following conditions:

– intolerance to essential drugs such as digitalis, antibiotics and antibacterial agents, tuberculostatic agents, cystostatic and cytotoxic drugs.
  – malignant disease.
  – uraemic conditions.
  – post-anaesthetic vomiting.
  – post-operative gastric hypotonia.
  – post vagotomy syndrome.
  – migraine
and during deep X-ray and cobalt treatment.

In diagnosis: radiological investigation to facilitate duodenal intubation procedures; to facilitate barium meal examination.

For barium meal procedures:
(a) Where barium-meal studies are held up by spasm of the duodenal cap making examination for the presence of the ulcer difficult;
(b) To facilitate examination of the hypotonic stomach with delayed emptying, gastric stasis and pyloric channel syndrome.

Dosage and administration The daily dose level of Primperan is based upon 0.5 mg/kg body weight, in divided doses, which in normal circumstances should not be exceeded.

General therapeutic dosage:

Oral: (tablets and syrup).

Adults: 10 mg three times daily.

Young adults (15–20 years): 5–10 mg three times daily commencing at the lower dosage.

Children: Primperan should only be used following careful examination to avoid masking an underlying disorder, e.g. cerebral irritation. The stated dosage recommendations should be strictly adhered to if side effects are to be avoided.

The syrup presentation facilitates accurate dosage and tablets should not be used in children under the age of 15 years. Recommended dosages for this group are:

    5–14 years: 2½–5 mg three times daily
    3–5 years: 2 mg two to three times daily
    1–3 years: 1 mg two to three times daily
    Under 1 year: 1 mg twice daily.

Treatment of children should commence at the lower dosage.

Intramuscular or intravenous administration: The dosages stated above are applicable to parenteral administration of Primperan.

Diagnostic dosage: (barium meal examination and small bowel intubation)

Primperan may be given 5–10 minutes before examination as a single dose as under:

    Adults (15 years and over): 10–20 mg
    Children 5–14 years: 2½–5 mg
    3–5 years: 2 mg
    Under 3 years: 1 mg

Contra-indications, warnings, etc

Contra-indications: There are no absolute contra-indications to the use of Primperan.

Warnings: The recommended dosage should not be exceeded, particularly in children, young adults and other patients of low body weight, who may be more liable to dystonic reactions.

If vomiting persists the patient should be reassessed to exclude the possibility of an underlying disorder, e.g. cerebral irritation.

Since atropine effecively blocks the action of 'Primperan', the concomitant administration of this and other anticholinergic drugs should be avoided.

Precautions: As both Primperan and phenothiazines may cause benign transient dystonia, care should be exercised in the event of both drugs being prescribed concurrently.

Reduced renal clearance of metoclopramide may be observed in elderly patients with impaired kidney function; dosage may therefore need adjustment.

Pregnancy: Primperan is not recommended during pregnancy, although animal tests in several mammalian species have revealed no teratogenic effect.

Side-effects: A low incidence of side-effects has been associated with the use of Primperan with absence of serious toxicity and excellent tolerance by oral and parenteral routes. Although rare, drowsiness and dystonic reactions have been reported. These are reversible, usually disappearing within 24 hours of stopping treatment.

Symptoms which can occur include spasm of facial, extra-ocular or cervical muscles which may be constant or rhythmic. There may also be a generalised increase in muscle tone. Anti-Parkinsonian drugs of the anticholinergic type may be used to counteract these reactions.

Treatment of overdosage: Gastric lavage and intensive supportive therapy should be initiated. Dystonic symptoms are likely and may be treated in severe cases with atropine, benztropine or other anticholinergic agents. Generalised convulsions may appear in infants.

Pharmaceutical precautions No known incompatibilities.

Diluent for Syrup: Syrup BP.

Protect from light. Store in a cool place.

Legal category POM.

Package quantities *Tablets:* Containers of 100 and 500.

Syrup: Bottles of 100 ml.

Ampoules: Boxes of 10 × 2 ml.

Further information Primperan has the unique action of normalising the hypomotile stomach and small intestine and also possesses powerful antiemetic effects.

Product licence numbers
Tablets 0152/5001
Syrup 0152/5002
Ampoules 0152/5003

SPIROLONE*

Presentation White sugar coated tablets containing 100 mg Spironolactone BP (marked 100). White sugar coated tablets containing 50 mg Spironolactone BP (marked 50). White sugar coated tablets containing 25 mg Spironolactone BP (marked 25).

Uses Congestive heart failure, essential hypertension, hepatic cirrhosis, malignant ascites, idiopathic oedema and nephrotic syndrome.

Since the pharmacological action of Spironolactone is to provide diuresis by competitive inhibition of aldosterone it may also be used for the diagnosis and treatment of primary hyperaldosteronism.

Dosage and administration Spironolactone tablets should always be administered with fluid.

Adults: Congestive heart failure: Usual dose 100 mg/day. In difficult or severe cases the dosage may be gradually increased up to 400 mg/day. When oedema is controlled, the usual maintenance level is 75–200 mg/day.

Hepatic cirrhosis with ascites and oedema: If urinary Na^+/K^+ ratio is greater than 1.0, 100 mg/day. If the ratio is less than 1.0, 200–400 mg/day. Maintenance dosage should be individually determined.

Malignant ascites: Initial dose usually 100–200 mg/day. In severe cases the dosage may be gradually increased up to 400 mg/day. When oedema is controlled, maintenance dosage should be individually determined.

Nephrotic syndrome: Usual dose – 100–200 mg/day. Spironolactone has not been shown to be anti-inflammatory, nor to affect the basic pathological process. Its use is only advised if glucocorticoids by themselves are insufficiently effective.

Idiopathic oedema including premenstrual oedema: Usual dose – 100 mg/day.

Diagnosis and treatment of primary aldosteronism: Spironolactone may be employed as initial diagnostic measure to provide presumptive evidence of primary hyperaldosteronism while patients are on normal diets.

Long tests: Spironolactone is administered at a daily dosage of 400 mg for three to four weeks. Correction of hypokalaemia and of hypertension provides presumptive evidence for the diagnosis of primary hyperaldosteronism.

Short test: Spironolactone is administered at a daily dosage of 400 mg for four days. If serum potassium increases during Spironolactone administration but drops when Spironolactone is discontinued, a presumptive diagnosis of primary hyperaldosteronism should be considered.

After the diagnosis of hyperaldosteronism has been established by more definitive testing procedures, Spironolactone may be administered in doses of 100 mg to 400 mg daily in preparation for surgery. For patients who are considered unsuitable for surgery, Spironolactone may be employed for long-term maintenance therapy at the lowest effective dosage determined for the individual patient.

Essential hypertension: Usual dose – 50–100 mg/day, which for difficult or severe cases may be gradually increased at two weekly intervals up to 200 mg/day.

Treatment should be continued for two weeks or longer since an adequate response may not occur before this time. Dosage should subsequently be adjusted according to the response of the patient.

Children: Initially 1.5 to 3.0 mg per kg bodyweight in divided doses, and then the dose should be adjusted in accordance with the patient's response and tolerance of the drug. If the child experiences problems in swallowing the smallest tablet, the tablets may be crushed and taken dispersed in food or drink.

Contra-indications, warnings, etc Spironolactone Tablets BP are contra-indicated in patients with renal failure, acute renal insufficiency, in hyperkalaemia and in those patients who are hypersensitive to Spironolactone.

Spironolactone tablets should not be administered with potassium supplements except initially when there is proven hypokalaemia. If potassium supplements are considered essential, serum electrolytes should be monitored. Occasional checks on serum electrolytes are recommended even when the drug is administered without potassium supplementation. Spironolactone tablets should also not be administered with other potassium sparing diuretics.

As Spironolactone or its metabolites may cross the placental barrier, and one of the metabolites appears in breast milk, the use of Spironolactone tablets in women who are pregnant, who may become pregnant or who are breast feeding is not recommended.

Spironolactone tablets may potentiate the effect of other diuretics, their initial dosage should be reduced to half of that normally administered and then adjusted in accordance with the patient's response. Patients with hepatic dysfunction should be carefully monitored as hepatic coma may be precipitated by Spironolactone in occasional susceptible subjects.

Spironolactone has an increased half-life in elderly patients and caution should therefore be exercised during medication.

Carcinogenicity: Spironolactone has been shown to produce tumours in rats when administered at high doses over a long period of time. The significance of these findings with respect to clinical use is not certain. However, the long-term use of Spironolactone in young patients requires careful consideration of the benefits and the potential hazard involved.

Adverse effects: These are infrequent and usually mild.

Gynaecomastia may develop on rare occasions but is normally reversible once dosing is discontinued. Alterations in voice pitch may also occur on rare occasions which may not be reversible.

Other adverse reactions reported include gastrointestinal effects, drowsiness and mental confusion (especially in conjunction with alcohol), headache, skin rashes, menstrual irregularities, impotence, breast enlargement and nipple sensitivity.

Overdosage: Toxic effects following acute overdosage may be drowsiness, mental confusion, dizziness, nausea, vomiting or diarrhoea.

Chronic overdosage produces symptoms mainly as a result of hyperkalaemia including cardiac irregularities, lassitude and muscular weakness, flaccid paralysis or muscle spasm.

No specific antidote has been discovered and overdosage should be treated by ceasing therapy and general supportive measures instituted.

Hyperkalaemia should be treated with potassium excreting diuretics, and reduction of potassium intake. The use of ion-exchange resins orally or intravenous glucose with regular insulin may also be effective.

Hyperkalaemia, similar to chronic overdosage, may also be seen in patients with impaired renal function or excessive potassium intake. Treatment of the hyperkalaemia of this cause should be as for chronic overdosage.

Pharmaceutical precautions Spironolactone tablets should be stored in a cool, dry place. Protect from light.

Legal category POM.

Package quantities Containers of 100 tablets.

Further information Nil.

Product licence numbers
25 mg tablets	0152/0194
50 mg tablets	0152/0195
100 mg tablets	0152/0196

TEMAZEPAM

Presentation Green, soft gelatin capsules containing temazepam 10 mg or 20 mg in solution. The 10 mg capsules are marked 10 and the 20 mg capsules 20 in white.

Uses Temazepam is indicated for the short term treatment of insomnia.

It is also indicated for pre-medication before minor surgical and investigatory procedures, particularly for out-patients.

Dosage and administration
Insomnia: Adults: 10 to 30 mg orally half an hour before retiring. This dose will prove satisfactory for most patients but may be increased to 40 or 60 mg for those patients who do not respond to the lower dose.

Elderly patients: Half the normal adult dose may be adequate to produce a therapeutic response in the elderly, or those suffering from cerebral vascular changes. (See also 'Warnings' and 'Side-effects').

Children: Not recommended.

Pre-medication: 20–40 mg from half or one hour before the surgical or investigatory procedures are undertaken.

Contra-indications, warnings, etc
Contra-indications: Known sensitivity to benzodiazepines. Acute pulmonary insufficiency.

Warnings:
1. When used for the treatment of insomnia daytime drowsiness is unlikely to occur; however, patients should be cautioned against driving or operating machinery until it is clearly established that hangover effects are not a problem while taking temazepam.

Such effects are more liable to occur on higher doses of temazepam and in patients new to hypnotic therapy or the elderly.

2. Patients should be advised not to consume alcohol whilst taking temazepam. The effects of other CNS depressants such as general anaesthetics, antidepressant drugs and monoamine oxidase inhibitors will be accentuated.

3. Prolonged or excessive use of benzodiazepines may lead to dependence, particularly when high dosages are used or when given over long periods.

The likelihood of psychological dependence is greater in patients with a history of alcoholism, drug abuse or those with personality disorders. Regular monitoring of such patients is essential.

4. Withdrawal symptoms such as sweating, depression, nervousness, irritability, diarrhoea and rebound insomnia have been reported following sudden discontinuation, particularly of prolonged or excessive treatment. In such cases treatment should be withdrawn gradually.

Use in pregnancy: Temazepam capsules should not be administered during pregnancy, especially during the first and last trimesters, unless in the opinion of the physician there are compelling reasons.

Side-effects: Temazepam has a short half-life and its effects are generally restricted to within a few hours after ingestion. Drowsiness, dizziness and blurring of vision rarely occur. Such effects are more common in the elderly and are potentiated by alcohol.

Other rare adverse effects including hypotension, gastro-intestinal upsets, transient skin rashes, urinary retention, headache, changes in libido, blood dyscrasias and jaundice have been reported.

Precautions: Temazepam capsules should be given with caution to patients with chronic pulmonary insufficiency or renal or hepatic dysfunction. They should also be avoided, if possible, during lactation.

Overdosage: Overdosage is rarely life threatening. Treatment should be generally supportive and symptomatic. In spite of the drug's rapid absorption and short half-life, gastric lavage may be useful if performed soon after ingestion.

Pharmaceutical precautions Store in a cool, dry place. Dispense, if necessary, into well closed glass or plastic containers.

Legal category CD (Sch 4) POM.

Package quantities
10 mg – containers of 250 and 500 capsules
20 mg – containers of 250 and 100 capsules.

Further information Temazepam is a benzodiazepine compound with a short half-life of approximately 8 hours and is rapidly absorbed from the liquid filled gelatin capsule formulation. It is mainly metabolised to a pharmacologically inactive glucuronide.

These factors provide prompt induction of sleep with a low incidence of hangover effects.

The lack of accumulation and the short action of this

benzodiazepine offers advantages in the treatment of those patients where daytime alertness is desirable.

Product licence numbers
Capsules 10 mg 0152/0215
Capsules 20 mg 0152/0216

TETRACHEL*

Presentation *Tablets:* Orange film-coated Tetracycline Tablets BP 250 mg engraved BERK 3C7.

Capsules: Orange Tetracycline Capsules BP 250 mg.

Uses Infections caused by organisms sensitive to tetracycline. These include pneumonia, acute and chronic bronchitis, whooping cough, psittacosis, urinary tract infections, amoebic dysentery, brucellosis and rickettsial fevers.

Dosage and administration *Adults:* 1 tablet or capsule every six hours.

Contra-indications, warnings, etc Tetrachel is contra-indicated in patients with advanced renal insufficiency and in those hypersensitive to tetracyclines.

Administration of Tetrachel with milk, antacids, calcium or iron preparations may affect absorption.

Tetracyclines should only be administered with great caution to patients with hepatic insufficiency. Careful monitoring of dosage by serum levels is necessary.

Prolonged use of an anti-infective agent may result in the development of superinfection due to micro-organisms resistant to the anti-infective.

Tetracyclines are absorbed to some extent by developing bones and teeth and may produce staining and enamel hypoplasia. For this reason, during the second half of pregnancy, during breast feeding and in children up to the age of eight years, tetracycline should only be administered if considered essential by the physician, and for as short a treatment period as feasible. Repeated courses should be avoided. The effect appears to be related to total dosage given and not only to duration of treatment.

Tetracyclines should only be administered with great caution to patients with renal insufficiency and dosage may need to be reduced.

Tetracyclines may prolong the action of coumarin anticoagulants, and may themselves delay coagulation.

Tetracyclines should only be used with great caution in conjunction with other potentially hepatotoxic drugs.

Cross-resistance between tetracyclines may develop in micro-organisms, and cross-sensitisation in patients.

Tetrachel should not be used in conjunction with penicillins.

Side-effects may include nausea, vomiting or diarrhoea, and glossitis, stomatitis, vaginitis or pruritus ani due to candidal overgrowth. Resistant staphylococci may occasionally give rise to enterocolitis. Skin rashes and allergic reaction are rare.

Treatment of overdosage: Serious symptoms are unlikely. Gastric lavage might be beneficial in the first hours after ingestion followed by conservative management. Milk will reduce absorption.

Pharmaceutical precautions Store in a cool place.

Legal category POM.

Package quantities *Tablets:* Packs of 100 and 1,000. *Capsules:* Containers of 100 and 500.

Further information Nil.

Product licence numbers
Tablets 0152/0095
Capsules 0152/5005

TRIMOPAN*

Presentation

Trimopan 200 mg tablet: White, circular, biconvex tablets, marked 'Berk 3H7' on one side with a single breakline on the reverse. Each tablet contains 200 mg Trimethoprim BP.

Trimopan 100 mg tablets: White, circular, biconvex tablets marked 'Berk 2H7' on one side with a single break-line on the reverse. Each tablet contains 100 mg Trimethoprim BP.

Trimopan suspension: White suspension containing 50 mg Trimethoprim BP in each 5 ml.

Uses Trimopan has potent antimicrobial activity due to its selective inhibition of bacterial dihydrofolate reductase. It is effective *in-vitro* against most Gram-positive and Gram-negative aerobic organisms, including *Haemophilus influenzae. Streptococcus pneumoniae, Klebsiella pneumoniae, Staphylococcus aureus, E. coli, Enterobacter, Proteus* and *Streptococcus faecalis.*

Exceptions include anaerobic bacteria. *Mycobacterium tuberculosis, Neisseria gonorrhoeae, Pseudomonas aeruginosa* and *Treponema pallidum.*

Indications: Treatment of susceptible infections caused by trimethoprim-sensitive organisms including urinary tract and respiratory tract infections.

Prophylaxis of recurrent urinary tract infections.

Dosage and administration

Adults and children over 12 years of age: Treatment of urinary tract infections and all other susceptible infections: 200 mg twice daily.

Long-term prophylaxis of recurrent urinary tract infections: 100 mg at night.

Children 4 months to 12 years of age: Treatment of urinary tract infections and all other susceptible infections is based on a dosage of 6 mg/kg body weight daily subdivided into two equal doses. Suggested regimens are:

4 months–2 years	25 mg twice daily
2–6 years	50 mg twice daily
6–12 years	100 mg twice daily

Long-term prophylaxis of recurrent urinary tract infections is based on 2.5 mg/kg body weight daily given as a single dose at night. Suggested regimens are:

4 months–2 years	25 mg at night
2–8 years	50 mg at night
8–12 years	100 mg at night

Contra-indications, warnings, etc *Contra-indications:* Severe hepatic insufficiency. Severe renal insufficiency, unless blood trimethoprim concentrations can be monitored regularly.

Megaloblastic anaemia and other blood dyscrasias.

Trimethoprim should not be administered to pregnant women, premature infants or children under 4 months of age.

Precautions: In patients with marked impairment of renal function, care should be taken to avoid accumulation and resulting adverse haematological effects. Regular haematological tests should be undertaken in patients receiving long-term treatment and those predisposed to folate deficiency. Particular care should be exercised in the haematological monitoring of children on long-term therapy. The usual caution in prescribing any drug for women of childbearing age should be exercised with trimethoprim. Trimethoprim is excreted in breast milk but is not contra-indicated for short term use in lactating mothers.

Side-effects: Nausea, vomiting, gastrointestinal disturbance, headache, skin rashes and pruritus have been reported but are rare.

Isolated cases of megaloblastic anaemia during prolonged therapy with trimethoprim in doses higher than those recommended have been reported but these are reversible with discontinuation of therapy and administration of calcium folinate.

Treatment of overdosage: Symptomatic treatment, gastric lavage and forced diuresis can be used. Depression of haematopoiesis by trimethoprim can be counteracted by intramuscular administration of calcium folinate.

Pharmaceutical precautions The suspension should be discarded after completion of course of treatment. Protect from light.

Legal category POM.

Package quantities
200 mg tablets:	Containers of 100 tablets Cartons of 70 tablets consisting of 5 calendar foils of 14 tablets each
100 mg tablets:	Containers of 100 tablets.
10 mg/ml suspension:	Bottles of 100 ml.

Further information Nil.

Product licence numbers
200 mg tablets	0152/0162
100 mg tablets	0152/0156
10 mg/ml suspension	0152/0160.

UBRETID*

Presentation *Tablets:* White tablets marked 'UBRETID' with single break line on reverse. Each tablet contains 5 mg distigmine bromide.

Ampoules: Clear ampoules each containing 0.5 mg distigmine bromide in 1 ml.

Uses Anticholinesterase. Post-operative urinary retention. Post operative ileus and intestinal atony. To assist emptying of the neurogenic bladder. As an adjuvant in the treatment of myasthenia gravis.

'Ubretid' distigmine bromide is an anticholinesterase with a much longer duration of action than neostigmine or pyridostigmine. In man, maximum inhibition of plasma cholinesterase occurs nine hours after a single intramuscular dose of 0.5 mg 'Ubretid', and persists for approximately 24 hours returning to normal after 48 hours.

Dosage and administration *In prevention of urinary retention, ileus or intestinal atony following surgery:* 1 'Ubretid' Ampoule by intramuscular injection given 12 hours after surgery is usually adequate prophylaxis and this may be repeated at 24-hourly intervals until normal function is restored. Caution should be exercised in the timing of this initial dose, where doubt exists as to the integrity of any bowel anastamosis. When injections are not convenient, 1 'Ubretid' Tablet may be given daily half-an-hour before breakfast.

In neurogenic bladder: 1 'Ubretid' Tablet daily or on alternate days, half-an-hour before breakfast, on an empty stomach. Intramuscular injections may be given in place of tablets for the first few days of therapy.

In myasthenia gravis — tablets only should be used: Adults: Dosage to be individualised for each patient, dependent upon the severity of the condition, the degree and duration of response and the side-effects encountered. The tablets should always be taken on an empty stomach half an hour before breakfast. Dosage should commence at 1 tablet daily and may be adjusted at intervals of three to four days to a total not exceeding 4 tablets daily.

Children: Up to 2 tablets daily, according to age.

Contra-indications, warnings, etc 'Ubretid' is contra-indicated in cases of severe post-operative shock, serious circulatory insufficiency and serious spastic and mechanical ileus.

'Ubretid' should not be administered to pregnant women.

'Ubretid' should be used with caution in conditions where the potentiation of acetylcholine effects is undesirable, e.g. vagotonia, bronchial asthma, cardiac disease, peptic ulcer, epilepsy and Parkinsonism.

In myasthenia gravis, where short-acting cholinergic drugs are taken concurrently, their dosage should be reduced to the minimum required to control symptoms.

The patient should be supervised in the early stages of dosage regulation to guard against the possibility of myasthenic crisis or cholinergic crisis.

Overdosage with 'Ubretid' would be expected to give rise to the signs of anticholinesterase poisoning. Atropine (up to 2 mg i.m.) should be given at once and repeated at intervals indicated by the clinical progress until signs of mild atropinisation appear (dry mouth, mydriasis). The patient is best kept fully atropinised for 24 hours.

Muscarinic side-effects of 'Ubretid' are usually few and mild, and can be controlled with atropine, giving 2 mg intramuscularly and maintaining atropinisation for at least 24 hours.

Treatment of overdosage: Oral absorption is poor unless Ubretid is taken on a completely empty stomach. Observation may be sufficient. Generalised parasympathomimetic symptoms should be antagonised by atropine.

Pharmaceutical precautions No special precautions.

Diluent for ampoules: Water for Injection BP.

Legal category POM.

Package quantities *Tablets:* Containers of 30 and 100 tablets.

Ampoules: Boxes of 10.

Further information Nil.

Product licence numbers
Tablets	0152/5034
Ampoules	0152/5035.

VIDOPEN*

Presentation Red and pink Ampicillin Capsules BP 250 mg marked VIDOPEN 250 and 500 mg marked VIDOPEN 500.

Pink powder for Syrup 125 mg/5 ml (Ampicillin Mixture BPC), or Syrup Forte 250 mg/5 ml (strong Ampicillin Mixture BPC), wild cherry flavoured and containing ampicillin trihydrate equivalent to the stated quantities of ampicillin.

Uses Ampicillin is a broad-spectrum antibiotic active against Shigella, *Escherichia coli, Proteus mirabilis, Haemophilus influenzae, Bordetella pertussis* and other Gram-negative bacteria. *Actinomyces muris ratti* and other Actinomycetes, as well as penicillin – sensitive Gram-positive pathogens. Vidopen is therefore indicated in a wide range of infections, particularly those of the respiratory, urinary and digestive tracts where there may be multiple pathogens.

Vidopen is not effective against organisms resistant to penicillin, since it is inactivated by penicillinase.

Dosage and administration Vidopen should be taken half an hour before meals.

Adults: ENT infections: 250 mg four times daily.
Bronchitis: 250 mg four times daily, or up to 1 g four times daily in acute exacerbations.
Pneumonia: 500 mg four times daily.
Urinary tract infections: 500 mg three times daily.
Gastro-intestinal infections: 500–750 mg three or four times daily.

Children: Over 20 kg bodyweight: Adult dosage.
Under 20 kg bodyweight:
Moderately severe infections: 100 mg/kg/day in divided doses every six or eight hours.
Severe infections: 200 mg/kg/day in divided doses every six hours.

Contra-indications, warnings, etc Known sensitivity to penicillin or the cephalosporins is a contra-indication. Patients should be questioned on this before Vidopen is prescribed.

Safety in pregnancy has not been established.

A rash may occur, particularly in patients with infectious mononucleosis. If it does, Vidopen should be discontinued.

Gastro-intestinal symptoms may occur but usually resolve rapidly when treatment is stopped. If they persist they may indicate overgrowth of resistant organisms, requiring specific treatment.

Ampicillin is inactivated by penicillinase and should therefore not be used to treat infections which have survived treatment with penicillin.

Treatment of overdosage: Serious symptoms are unlikely. Observation.

Pharmaceutical precautions Store in a cool dry place.

The suspension, when made up, should be stored in a cool place and used within seven days. It may be diluted with Syrup BP.

Legal category POM.

Package quantities *Capsules 250 mg:* Containers of 250 and 1,000.

Capsules 500 mg: Containers of 100 and 500.

Syrup: Bottles of 100 ml.

Syrup Forte: Bottles of 100 ml.

Further information Nil.

Product licence numbers
Capsules 250 mg   0152/0118
Capsules 500 mg   0152/0119
Syrup 125 mg/5 ml   0152/0120
Syrup Forte 250 mg/5 ml 0152/0121.

*Trade Mark

Bioglan Laboratories Limited
Bridge Road
Letchworth, Herts SG6 4ET

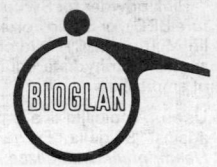

BENZAGEL* 5
BENZAGEL* 10

Presentation Benzagel 5 is a white gel containing 5% w/w micronised benzoyl peroxide.

Benzagel 10 is a white gel containing 10% w/w micronised benzoyl peroxide.

Uses Benzagel is indicated as an aid in the treatment of acne, providing drying, desquamative and antiseptic activity.

Dosage and administration *Adults and children:* Commence treatment with Benzagel 5. Wash the affected areas with soap and water, dry and apply Benzagel once or twice daily.

The therapeutic response to benzoyl peroxide differs in individual patients and, in order to provide a satisfactory drying and desquamative action, it may be necessary to increase the strength to Benzagel 10.

Contra-indications, warnings, etc
Contra-indications: Patients with a known sensitivity to benzoyl peroxide.

Warnings: For external use only. To avoid irritation, take care to keep the product away from the mouth, eyes and other mucous membranes.

Precautions: The product should be applied with caution to sensitive areas, such as the neck and shoulders. Avoid contact with clothing and fabric.

Side-effects: In normal use a mild burning sensation will probably be felt on first application, and a moderate reddening and peeling of the skin will occur within a few days. During the first few weeks of treatment, a sudden increase in peeling will occur in most patients. This is not harmful and will subside within a day or two if the treatment is temporarily discontinued.

Pharmaceutical precautions Store in a cool place.

Legal category P.

Package quantities Benzagel 5 and Benzagel 10 are supplied in plastic tubes, each containing 40 g.

Further information The formulation of Benzagel contains micronised benzoyl peroxide which ensures a uniform dispersion of the active ingredient throughout the gel. Skin penetration is provided by the gel base, which dries to an invisible film.

Product licence numbers
Benzagel 5   3384/0005
Benzagel 10   3384/0006

VITA-E* GELUCAPS
VITA-E* GELS
VITA-E* SUCCINATE TABLETS
Presentation
Vita-E Gelucaps: Yellow oval coated tablets, 14.5 mm diameter, each containing d-α-tocopheryl acetate equivalent to 75 i.u. (55 mg) of vitamin E.

Vita-E 75: Yellow oval soft gelatin capsules 11 mm diameter, each containing d-α-tocopheryl acetate equivalent to 75 i.u. (55 mg) of vitamin E.

Vita-E 200: Yellow oblong soft gelatin capsules, 16.5 mm diameter, marked 'BLE 200', each containing d-α-tocopheryl acetate equivalent to 200 i.u. (147 mg) of vitamin E.

Vita-E 400: Red oblong soft gelatin capsules, 19 mm diameter, marked 'BLE 400', each containing d-α-tocopheryl acetate equivalent to 400 i.u. (294 mg) of vitamin E.

Vita-E Succinate 50: Yellow circular scored tablets. Engraved 'BIOGLAN' on one side and '50 i.u.E.' on other, each containing d-α-tocopheryl acid succinate equivalent to 50 i.u. (41 mg) of vitamin E.

Vita-E Succinate 200: Yellow circular scored tablets. Engraved 'BIOGLAN' on one side and '200 i.u.E.' on other, each containing d-α-tocopheryl acid succinate equivalent to 200 i.u. (165 mg) of vitamin E.

Uses *Indications:* Intermittent claudication as an adjunct to specific surgery or where surgical intervention has proved inadequate or is inappropriate.

Dosage and administration
Vita-E Gelucaps: Oral – chewed and eaten during meals.
Vita-E Gels: Oral – swallowed intact and taken with meals.
Vita-E Succinate tablets: Oral – taken with meals.

Adults: 400–1600 i.u. (294 mg–1176 mg) daily.

Elderly: As for adults.

Pregnancy: Although there is no evidence of teratogenicity, use in pregnancy should be avoided unless considered essential.

The doses recommended are larger than nutritional studies would demand, but smaller dosage is generally insufficient for successful therapy. The maintenance dose equals the therapeutic dose.

Vitamin E is not recommended for self-medication since, as a therapeutic agent and when used with other medications, d-α-tocopherol may enhance/lessen the effect of those medications. A physician should be consulted.

Contra-indications, warnings, etc Fish-liver oils should not be given at the same time, as they appear to have a detrimental effect on the vitamin. If iron is indicated, separate the doses by about nine hours.

Pharmaceutical precautions Store in a cool dry place.

Legal category GSL.

Package quantities Vita-E Gelucaps are available in containers of 100.

Vita-E Gels 75, 200 and 400 are available in containers of 100 and 500.

Vita-E Succinate tablets 50 and 200 are available in containers of 100 and 500.

Product licence numbers

Vita-E Gelucaps	0041/5000
Vita-E 75	0041/5006
Vita-E 200	0041/5012
Vita-E 400	0041/5013
Vita-E Succinate 50	0041/5004
Vita-E Succinate 200	0041/5005

*Trade Mark

Boehringer Ingelheim Limited
Ellesfield Avenue
Bracknell
Berkshire RG12 4YS

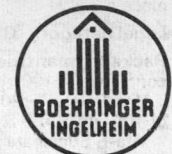

ALUPENT*

Presentation *Alupent Tablets:* White/off white compressed tablets, scored and impressed with the letters 'At' on one side and with the Company symbol on the reverse. Each tablet contains orciprenaline sulphate 20 mg.

Alupent Syrup: Clear, colourless syrup with vanilla-like flavour. Each 5 ml contains orciprenaline sulphate 10 mg.

Alupent Metered Aerosol: 15 ml vial (300 metered doses) available as complete unit with mouthpiece or as refill vial only. Each metered dose contains orciprenaline sulphate 0.75 mg (0.67 mg available to the patient).

Alupent Ampoules: Ampoules for injection. Each ampoule contains orciprenaline sulphate 0.5 mg in 1 ml.

Uses *Action:* Alupent is a sympathomimetic amine with bronchodilator properties.

Indications: Alupent is indicated for the relief of bronchospasm, as in asthma, bronchitis and emphysema.

Alupent tablets and syrup are suggested for maintenance therapy.

Alupent metered aerosol is indicated for the relief of acute attacks. Alupent ampoules are for maintenance therapy in patients unable to take other dosage forms. On occasions the ampoules have been used for treatment of acute attacks.

Dosage and administration *Orally*

	Tablets 20 mg	Syrup 10 mg in 5 ml
Adults	1 four times daily	2 × 5 ml four times daily
Children 3–12 years	½ four times daily to 1 three times daily	1 × 5 ml four times daily to 2 × 5 ml three times daily
Children 1–3 years	Syrup recommended	½ × 5 ml four times daily to 1 × 5 ml four times daily
Children 0–1 year	Syrup recommended	½ × 5 ml three times daily to 1 × 5 ml three times daily

By inhalation
Metered Aerosol 0.75 mg per puff (0.67 mg available to the patient):

Adults: 1 or 2 puffs. Not to be repeated within 30 minutes. No more than 12 puffs in 24 hours.

Children 6–12 years: 1 or 2 puffs. Not to be repeated within 30 minutes. No more than 4 doses in 24 hours.

Children under 6 years: 1 puff. Not to be repeated within 30 minutes. No more than 4 puffs in 24 hours.

By intra-muscular injection:

	Adults	Children 6–12 years	Children under 6 years
Ampoules 0.5 mg in 1 ml	1 ampoule repeated after 30 minutes if necessary	1 ampoule	½ ampoule

Diluents: Alupent Syrup may be diluted with either Syrup BP or Sorbitol Solution BP.

No specific information on the use of this product in the elderly is available. Clinical trials have included patients over 65 years and no adverse reactions specific to this age group have been reported.

Contra-indications, warnings, etc
Contra-indications: Thyrotoxicosis.

Precautions: Caution should be observed should it be necessary to administer Alupent to patients with myocardial insufficiency, angina, cardiac dysrhythmias, hypertension or hypertrophic subvalvular aortic stenosis. In view of the possible interaction between sympathomimetic amines and monoamine oxidase inhibitors, care should be exercised if it is proposed to administer an MAO inhibitor concurrently with Alupent. Caution should be observed with the use of Alupent if a patient is already receiving other sympathomimetic agents as cardiovascular effects may be additive.

Patients must be instructed in the correct use of a metered aerosol, and warned not to exceed the prescribed dose. Patients should also be warned to seek medical advice if a reduced response becomes apparent.

Although Alupent has been in wide general use for many years, there is no definite evidence of ill-consequence during human pregnancy. Only in doses much higher than the equivalent maximum therapeutic dose in man were effects on foetal development seen in animals. Alupent treatment may result in the prolongation of pregnancy and inhibition of labour. Medicines should not be used in pregnancy, especially the first trimester, unless the expected benefit is thought to outweigh any possible risk to the foetus.

Beta-adrenergic blocking agents may antagonise Alupent and reduce its bronchodilator effect if administered concurrently.

Side-effects: Transitory sympathomimetic side-effects, such as tremor, palpitation, tachycardia and headache, have occasionally been reported, as have nausea and abdominal discomfort.

Overdosage: No fatal doses have been reported but the following single doses should be considered toxic – 1.5 mg by IV injection, 3.0 mg by IM or SC injection, 0.15 mg/min by IV infusion, 200 mg orally.

Overdosage may be manifest by tachycardia, palpitation, increase in systolic blood pressure, decrease in diastolic blood pressure, tremor and anxiety. It is suggested that the patient should be treated symptomatically, but care should be taken if beta-adrenergic blocking drugs are used in patients liable to bronchospasm.

Pharmaceutical precautions Alupent preparations should be protected from heat, light and air. Aerosol vials should not be incinerated or opened even when apparently empty.

Legal category POM.

Package quantities *Tablets:* Packs of 50, 250 and 1,000
Syrup: Packs of 250 ml and 2 litres.
Metered Aerosol: 15 ml vial (300 metered doses) complete with mouthpiece. 15 ml refill vial.
Ampoules: Packs of 6.

Further information Nil.

Product licence numbers

Alupent Tablets	0015/0046
Alupent Syrup	0015/0001
Alupent Metered Aerosol	0015/5002
Alupent Ampoules	0015/5000

ATROVENT*

Presentation *Metered dose inhaler:* 10 ml vial (200 metered doses) available as complete unit with mouthpiece. Each metered dose contains ipratropium bromide 0.02 mg of which 0.018 mg is available to the patient.

Uses *Action:* Atrovent is an anticholinergic bronchodilator.

Indications: Atrovent metered dose inhaler is indicated in the treatment of chronic reversible airways obstruction, particularly in chronic bronchitis.

Dosage and administration *Adults:* Usually 1 or 2 puffs three or four times daily, although some patients may need up to 4 puffs at a time to obtain maximum benefit during early treatment.
Children: 6–12 years: usually 1 or 2 puffs three times daily. Under 6 years: usually 1 puff three times daily.
In order to ensure that the inhaler is used correctly, administration should be supervised by an adult.
No specific information on the use of this product in the elderly is available. Clinical trials have included patients over 65 years and no adverse reactions specific to this age group have been reported.

Contra-indications, warnings, etc
Contra-indications: Known hypersensitivity to atropine.
Precautions: The patient should be warned to seek medical advice should a reduced response become apparent.
Patients must be instructed in the correct use of a metered dose inhaler and warned against the accidental release of the contents into the eye. Generally, caution is advocated in the use of anticholinergic agents in patients with glaucoma or prostatic hypertrophy. However, specific studies with Atrovent in patients with glaucoma showed that inhaling cumulative doses of 0.16 mg had no effect on the eye.
Atrovent has been in general use for several years and there is no definite evidence of ill-consequence during pregnancy; animal studies have shown no hazard. Nevertheless, medicines should not be used in pregnancy, especially during the first trimester, unless the expected benefit is thought to outweigh any possible risk to the foetus.
Side-effects: Anticholinergic side-effects are unlikely to occur at therapeutic doses although dry mouth has occasionally been reported. Urinary retention and constipation have only rarely been reported with Atrovent.

There is no evidence that in the therapeutic dose range Atrovent has any adverse effect on bronchial secretion.
Overdosage: Inhaled doses of 5 mg produce an increase in heart rate and palpitation. Single doses of ipratropium bromide 30 mg by mouth caused anticholinergic side-effects but these were not severe and did not require specific reversal.

Pharmaceutical precautions Protect from heat including the sun. The vials should not be punctured or incinerated even when apparently empty.

Legal category POM.

Package quantities 10 ml vial (200 metered doses) complete with mouthpiece.

Further information There is evidence that the concurrent administration of Atrovent and sympathomimetic drugs produces a greater relief of bronchospasm than either drug given alone.
Atrovent has been shown to produce effective bronchodilatation in patients receiving beta-adrenergic blocking agents.
Patients should be informed when starting treatment that the onset of action of Atrovent is slower than that of inhaled sympathomimetic bronchodilators.
Atrovent is also available as Atrovent Forte (0.04 mg per puff) and as a nebuliser solution (0.25 mg/ml).

Product licence number Atrovent metered dose inhaler 0015/0043

ATROVENT* FORTE
METERED DOSE INHALER

Presentation Metered dose inhaler 10 ml (200 metered doses) available as complete unit with mouthpiece. Each metered dose contains ipratropium bromide 0.04 mg of which 0.036 mg is available to the patient.

Uses *Action:* Atrovent is an anticholinergic bronchodilator.

Indications: Atrovent is indicated in the treatment of chronic reversible airways obstruction, particularly in chronic bronchitis.

Dosage and administration
Adults: Usually 1 puff three or four times daily, although some patients may need 2 puffs at a time to obtain maximum benefit during early treatment.
Children: 6–12 years – usually 1 puff three times daily.
In order to ensure that the inhaler is used correctly, administration should be supervised by an adult.
No specific information on the use of this product in the elderly is available. Clinical trials with Atrovent MDI have included patients over 65 years and no adverse reactions specific to this age group have been reported.

Contra-indications, warnings, etc
Contra-indications: Known hypersensitivity to atropine.
Precautions: The patient should be warned to seek medical advice should a reduced response become apparent.
Patients must be instructed in the correct use of a metered dose inhaler and warned against accidental release of the contents into the eye. Generally, caution is advocated in the use of anticholinergic agents in patients with glaucoma or prostatic hypertrophy. However, specific studies with Atrovent in patients with glaucoma

showed that inhaling cumulative doses of 0.16 mg had no effect on the eye.

Atrovent has been in general use for several years and there is no definite evidence of ill-consequence during pregnancy; animal studies have shown no hazard. Nevertheless, medicines should not be used in pregnancy, especially during the first trimester, unless the expected benefit is thought to outweigh any possible risk to the foetus.

Side-effects: Anticholinergic side-effects are unlikely to occur at therapeutic doses, although dry mouth has occasionally been reported. Urinary retention and constipation have only rarely been reported with Atrovent. There is no evidence that in the therapeutic dose range Atrovent has any adverse effect on bronchial secretion.

Overdosage: Inhaled doses of 5 mg produce an increase in heart rate and palpitation. Single doses of ipratropium bromide 30 mg by mouth caused anticholinergic side-effects but these were not severe and did not require specific reversal.

Pharmaceutical precautions Protect from heat including the sun. The vials should not be punctured or incinerated even when apparently empty.

Legal category POM

Package quantities 10 ml vial (200 metered doses) complete with mouthpiece.

Further information There is evidence that the concurrent administration of Atrovent and sympathomimetic drugs produces a greater relief of bronchospasm than either drug given alone.

Atrovent has been shown to produce effective bronchodilatation in patients receiving beta-adrenergic blocking agents.

Patients should be informed when starting treatment that the onset of action of Atrovent is slower than that of inhaled sympathomimetic bronchodilators.

Atrovent is also available as a metered dose inhaler providing 0.02 mg per metered dose and as a nebuliser solution (0.25 mg/ml).

Product licence number 0015/0107.

ATROVENT NEBULISER SOLUTION

Presentation An isotonic solution of ipratropium bromide 0.025% (0.25 mg/ml) for administration by inhalation.

Uses

Action: Ipratropium bromide is an anticholinergic bronchodilator.

Indications: Atrovent Nebuliser Solution is indicated in the treatment of reversible airways obstruction.

Dosage and administration Atrovent Nebuliser Solution may be administered from an intermittent positive pressure ventilator or from suitable nebulisers.

The recommended dose is:

Adults: 0.4–2.0 ml solution (0.1–0.5 mg) up to 4 times daily.

Children: (3–14 years) 0.4–2.0 ml solution (0.1–0.5 mg) up to 3 times daily.

The dose of nebuliser solution may need to be diluted in order to obtain a final volume suitable for the particular nebuliser being used; if dilution is necessary use only sterile sodium chloride 0.9% solution.

The Atrovent nebuliser solution can be measured by means of the integral dropper – 20 drops are approximately equivalent to 1 ml. The dropper can easily be removed if it is not required.

There is no specific information on the use of isotonic Atrovent Nebuliser Solution in the elderly. Clinical trials with the previously available hypotonic formulation included patients over 65 years and no adverse reactions specific to this age group were reported.

Contra-indications, warnings, etc

Contra-indications: Known hypersensitivity to atropine.

Precautions: Administration of Atrovent nebuliser solution has been associated with occasional reports of paradoxical bronchospasm during early treatment. Use of the nebuliser solution should always be initiated in hospital and be subject to close medical supervision during the first week of treatment.

The patient should be advised to seek medical advice should a reduced response become apparent.

Patients must be instructed in the correct administration of Atrovent nebuliser solution and warned not to allow the solution or mist to enter the eyes. Generally, caution is advocated in the use of anticholinergic agents in patients with glaucoma or prostatic hypertrophy. However, specific studies with Atrovent metered dose inhaler in patients with glaucoma showed that inhaling cumulative doses of 0.16 mg had no effect on the eye.

Atrovent has been in general use for several years and there is no definite evidence of ill-consequence during pregnancy; animal studies have shown no hazard. Nevertheless, medicines should not be used in pregnancy, especially during the first trimester, unless the expected benefit is thought to outweigh any possible risk to the foetus.

Side-effects: Anticholinergic side-effects are unlikely at therapeutic doses, but some patients may complain of a dry mouth. Urinary retention and constipation have only rarely been reported with Atrovent.

There is no evidence that in the therapeutic dose range Atrovent has any adverse effect on bronchial secretion.

Overdosage: Inhaled doses of 5 mg produce an increase in heart rate and palpitation but single doses of 2 mg have been given to adults and 1 mg to children without causing side-effects. Single doses of ipratropium bromide 30 mg by mouth cause anticholinergic side-effects but these are not severe and do not require specific reversal.

Pharmaceutical precautions Store at room temperature. Protect from heat and light. Once the bottle has been opened, the contents should not be kept for longer than 1 month. Following dilution, Atrovent Nebuliser Solution should be used within 24 hours.

Legal category POM

Package quantities 20 ml in amber glass bottle complete with integral dropper.

Further information There is evidence that the concurrent administration of Atrovent and sympathomimetic drugs produces a greater relief of bronchospasm than either drug given alone.

Atrovent has been shown to produce effective bronchodilatation in patients receiving β-blocking agents. Atrovent is also available as a metered dose inhaler.

Product licence number 0015/0078

BEROTEC*

Presentation Pressurised metered inhaler: 10 ml vial (200 metered doses) available as complete unit with mouthpiece. Each metered dose contains fenoterol hydrobromide 0.2 mg (0.18 mg available to the patient).

Uses *Action:* Berotec is a highly potent, rapidly acting, selective beta$_2$ – adrenergic stimulant with a duration of action of 6–8 hours. The degree of selectivity coupled with administration by inhalation allows maximal bronchodilator effect with minimal side-effects.

Indications: For the treatment of reversible airways obstruction as in bronchial asthma, bronchitis and emphysema.

Dosage and administration By inhalation.

As Berotec has a longer duration of action than other bronchodilators a dosage of 1 or 2 puffs three times daily is usually sufficient to control bronchospasm in adults. If necessary this may be increased up to 2 puffs every four hours. Children (6–12 years) will normally require 1 puff three times daily but this may be increased up to 1 puff every four hours if necessary. It is recommended that administration of Berotec to children should be supervised by a responsible adult.

No specific information on the use of this product in the elderly is available. Clinical trials have included patients over 65 years and no adverse reactions specific to this age group have been reported.

Contra-indications, warnings, etc

Contra-indications: There are no absolute contra-indications to the use of Berotec.

Precautions: Caution should be observed should it be necessary to administer Berotec to patients with thyrotoxicosis, myocardial insufficiency, angina, cardiac dysrhythmias, hypertension or hypertrophic subvalvular aortic stenosis.

In view of the possible interaction between sympathomimetic amines and monoamine oxidase inhibitors or tricyclic anti-depressants, care should be exercised if it is proposed to administer these compounds concurrently with Berotec.

Berotec should be used with caution in patients already receiving other sympathomimetic agents as cardiovascular effects may be additive.

Patients must be instructed in the correct use of a metered inhaler and warned not to exceed the prescribed dose. If relief is not obtained after correct use of the inhaler, the dose should not be exceeded and the patient should contact the doctor for advice.

Although Berotec has been in wide general use for several years, there is no definite evidence of ill consequence during human pregnancy. Animal studies have shown no hazard.

Berotec treatment may result in the prolongation of pregnancy and inhibition of labour.

Medicines should not be used in pregnancy, especially in the first trimester, unless the expected benefit is thought to outweigh any possible risk to the foetus.

Beta-adrenergic blocking agents may antagonise Berotec and reduce its bronchodilator effect if administered concurrently.

A temporary dose-related decrease in serum potassium levels has been observed in some patients.

Side-effects: Transient sympathomimetic side-effects, such as palpitation, tachycardia, headache and tremor may occur, as with other beta-adrenergic agonists, but are uncommon with administration by inhaler.

Overdosage: Accidental overdosage may give rise to tachycardia, palpitation and tremor. It is suggested that the patient should be treated symptomatically.

Should the administration of a beta-adrenergic blocking agent be considered necessary to counteract the effects of overdosage, its use in a patient liable to bronchospasm should be carefully monitored.

Pharmaceutical precautions Protect from heat, including the sun.

The inhaler vial should not be incinerated or opened even when apparently empty.

Legal category POM.

Package quantities 10 ml vial (200 metered doses) complete with mouthpiece.

Further information There is evidence to suggest that Berotec may reduce the allergic response of tissues. Animal studies have shown that Berotec also produces an increase in the frequency of movement of the respiratory epithelial cilia and in the rate of mucus transport.

Long-term use has shown Berotec to be free from significant adverse effects, particularly with respect to the blood gases and general biochemistry. Tolerance is not a feature of long-term use.

Product licence number 0015/0034.

BEROTEC* NEBULISER SOLUTION

Presentation An aqueous solution of fenoterol hydrobromide 0.5% (5 mg/ml) for administration by inhalation.

Uses *Action:* Berotec is a highly potent, rapidly acting, selective beta$_2$-adrenoceptor stimulant with a long duration of action. The degree of selectivity coupled with administration by inhalation allows maximal bronchodilator effect with minimal side-effects.

Indications: For the treatment of reversible airways obstruction as in bronchial asthma, bronchitis and emphysema.

Dosage and administration Berotec nebuliser solution may be administered from an intermittent positive pressure ventilator or from suitable nebulisers.

The recommended dose per inhalation ranges from 0.5–2.5 mg and this can be achieved by nebulising 0.1 to 0.5 ml solution. These volumes may be measured using the integral dropper (20 drops are approximately equivalent to 1 ml) and diluted with sterile sodium chloride 0.9% solution for ease of administration. Dilution should be carried out just before inhalation.

Adults: 0.5 mg–2.5 mg up to four times daily. Single doses of 5.0 mg have been safely used.

Children: (6–14 years) up to 1.0 mg up to three times daily.

The final volume depends on the type of nebuliser to be used and the administration time acceptable. 2 ml is a suitable final volume for most nebulisers such as the Bird micro-nebuliser, Bennett twin-jet, Acorn/OEM and Turrett No. 51. However, if a total volume of 2 ml is not suitable for the particular nebuliser to be used, the dilution should be adjusted to give the volume recommended by the manufacturer of the nebuliser.

No specific information on the use of this product in the elderly is available. Clinical trials have included patients over 65 years and no adverse reactions specific to this age group have been reported.

Contra-indications, warnings, etc

Contra-indications: There are no absolute contra-indications to the use of Berotec.

Precautions: Caution should be observed should it be necessary to administer Berotec to patients with thyrotoxicosis, myocardial insufficiency, angina, cardiac dysrhythmias, hypertension or hypertrophic subvalvular aortic stenosis.

In view of the possible interaction between sympathomimetic amines and monoamine oxidase inhibitors or tricyclic anti-depressants, care should be exercised if it is proposed to administer these compounds concurrently with Berotec.

Berotec should be used with caution in patients already receiving other sympathomimetic agents as cardiovascular effects may be additive.

If relief is not obtained after correct use of the nebuliser solution the dose should not be exceeded and the patient should contact the doctor for advice.

Although Berotec has been in wide general use for several years, there is no definite evidence of ill-consequence during human pregnancy; animal studies have shown no hazard.

Berotec treatment may result in the prolongation of pregnancy and inhibition of labour.

Medicines should not be used in pregnancy, especially during the first trimester, unless the expected benefit is thought to outweigh any possible risk to the foetus.

Beta-adrenergic blocking agents may antagonise Berotec and reduce its bronchodilator effect if administered concurrently.

A temporary dose-related decrease in serum potassium levels has been observed in some patients.

Side-effects: As with other beta-adrenergic agonists transient sympathomimetic side-effects such as tremor, palpitation, tachycardia and headache may occur, but are uncommon with administration by inhalation.

Overdosage: Accidental overdosage may give rise to tachycardia, palpitation and tremor. It is suggested that the patient should be treated symptomatically.

Should the administration of a beta-adrenergic blocking agent be considered necessary to counteract the effects of overdose, its use in a patient liable to bronchospasm should be carefully monitored.

Pharmaceutical precautions Protect from light and heat.

Legal category POM.

Package quantities 20 ml amber glass bottle with integral dropper.

Further information There is evidence to suggest that Berotec may reduce the allergic response of tissues. Animal studies have shown that Berotec also produces an increase in the frequency of movement of the respiratory epithelial cilia and in the rate of mucus transport.

Long-term use has shown Berotec to be free from significant adverse effects, particularly with respect to the blood gases and general biochemistry.

Product licence number 0015/0082.

BUSCOPAN*

Presentation *Buscopan Tablets:* White, sugar-coated tablets, marked 'Buscopan' on one side. Each tablet contains hyoscine-N-butylbromide 10 mg.

Buscopan Ampoules: Ampoules for intramuscular or intravenous injection, each containing hyoscine-N-butylbromide 20 mg in 1 ml.

Uses *Action:* Buscopan is an antispasmodic agent, which relaxes smooth muscle of the organs of the abdominal and pelvic cavities. It is believed to act predominantly on the intramural parasympathetic ganglia of these organs.

Indications: Buscopan tablets are indicated in spasm of the gastro-intestinal or genito-urinary tracts and in spasmodic dysmenorrhoea.

Buscopan ampoules are indicated in acute spasm, as in renal or biliary colic; in radiology for differential diagnosis of obstruction and to reduce spasm and pain in pyelography, and in other diagnostic procedures where spasm may be a problem, e.g. gastro-duodenal endoscopy.

Dosage and administration *Adults: Orally:* 2 tablets four times daily. In spasmodic dysmenorrhoea, treatment should commence two days before the expected onset of the period and continue for three days after menstruation has begun.

By injection: 1 ampoule intramuscularly or intravenously repeated after half-an-hour if necessary. When used in endoscopy this dose may need to be repeated more frequently.

Children 6–12 years: Orally: 1 tablet three times daily.

Diluent: Buscopan injection solution may be diluted with dextrose or with sodium chloride 0.9% injection solutions. It is also miscible and compatible with most of the commonly used aqueous radiological contrast media such as sodium diatrizoate.

No specific information on the use of this product in the elderly is available. Clinical trials have included patients over 65 years and no adverse reactions specific to this age group have been reported.

Contra-indications, warnings, etc

Contra-indications: Because of a possible mydriatic effect, Buscopan should not be administered to patients with glaucoma.

Precautions: Although Buscopan has been in wide general use for many years, there is no definite evidence of ill-consequence during human pregnancy; animal studies have shown no hazard. Nevertheless, medicines should not be used in pregnancy, especially the first trimester, unless the expected benefit is thought to outweigh any possible risk to the foetus.

Side-effects: Dryness of the mouth, temporary loss of accommodation and tachycardia have very occasionally been reported.

Overdosage: Oral doses of up to 1090 mg produced only tiredness. Other features which may be encountered are dry mouth, loss of accommodation, tachycardia, orthostatic hypotension and Cheyne-Stokes respiration.

Gastric lavage should be employed where appropriate. Parasympathetic agents, e.g. pilocarpine or neostigmine, should be used as necessary.

Pharmaceutical precautions Buscopan tablets and ampoules should be protected from light and heat.

Legal category POM.

Package quantities *Tablets:* Packs of 100 and 500. *Ampoules:* Packs of 10.

Further information Nil.

Product licence numbers
Buscopan Tablets   0015/0047
Buscopan Ampoules 0015/5005

CATAPRES*

Presentation *Catapres Tablets 0.10 mg:* White compressed tablets impressed with the motif $\frac{c}{\circ}$ on one side and with the Company symbol on the reverse. Each tablet contains clonidine hydrochloride 0.10 mg.

Catapres Tablets 0.30 mg: White, compressed tablets impressed with the motif $\frac{03C}{03C}$ and with the Company symbol on the reverse. Each tablet contains clonidine hydrochloride 0.30 mg.

Catapres PL Perlongets: red/yellow gelatin capsules imprinted with the notation Catapres PL, 11P and the Company symbol. Each Perlonget contains 5 minitablets constituting 0.25 mg clonidine hydrochloride in sustained release form.

Catapres Ampoules: Ampoules for injection. Each ampoule contains clonidine hydrochloride 0.15 mg in 1 ml.

Uses *Action:* Catapres is an antihypertensive agent with both central and peripheral sites of action. With long-term treatment Catapres reduces the responsiveness of peripheral vessels to vasoconstrictor and vasodilator substances and to sympathetic nerve stimulation. Early in treatment, however, blood pressure reduction is associated with a central reduction of sympathetic outflow and increased vagal tone.

Clinically there may be reduced venous return and slight bradycardia resulting in reduced cardiac output. Although initially peripheral resistance may be unchanged it tends to be reduced as treatment continues. There is no interference with myocardial contractility. Studies have shown that cardiovascular reflexes, as shown by the lack of postural hypotension and exercise hypotension, are preserved.

Indications: Catapres is indicated for the treatment of all grades of essential and secondary hypertension, hypertension during pregnancy and hypertensive crises.

Catapres PL is indicated for all degrees of hypertension excluding hypertensive crises.

Dosage and administration *Catapres Tablets:* Oral treatment should commence with 0.05–0.10 mg three times daily.

This dose should be increased gradually every second or third day until control is achieved. Most patients will be controlled on divided daily doses of 0.30–1.2 mg. However, some patients may require higher doses, e.g. 1.8 mg or more.

Catapres PL Perlongets: most patients will be satisfactorily controlled on one Perlonget daily (usually given in the evening). This dosage can be increased if necessary up to 2 or 3 Perlongets daily (one in the morning and one or two at night).

Catapres may be added to an existing antihypertensive regimen where blood pressure control has not been satisfactorily achieved. If side-effects with existing therapy are troublesome the concomitant use of Catapres may allow a lower dose of the established regimen to be employed. Patients changing treatment should have their existing therapy reduced gradually whilst Catapres is added to their regimen.

Catapres Ampoules: In hypertensive crises 1 or 2 Catapres ampoules should be given by slow intravenous injection.

An effect is usually seen within 10 minutes and reaches a maximum about 30 minutes to 1 hour after administration. The duration of effect depends upon the severity of the condition and is commonly of the order of 3–7 hours. Up to 5 ampoules may be given in 24 hours to achieve and maintain the desired blood pressure.

Patients undergoing anaesthesia should continue their Catapres treatment before, during and after anaesthesia, using oral or intravenous administration according to individual circumstances.

Diluent: Catapres injection solution is compatible with 0.9% sodium chloride solution and with 5% dextrose solution.

No specific information on the use of this product in the elderly is available. Clinical trials have included patients over 65 years and no adverse reactions specific to this age group have been reported.

Contra-indications, warnings, etc
Contra-indications: There are no known absolute contra-indications to the use of Catapres.

Precautions: This product may cause drowsiness. Patients who are affected should not drive or operate machinery. Sedation due to the drug may be increased by the concomitant use of other central nervous system depressants.

Sudden withdrawal of Catapres, particularly in those patients receiving high doses, may result in rebound hypertension. Termination of long-term therapy with Catapres for any reason should therefore be performed gradually. With Catapres PL this may be achieved by progressively increasing the interval between doses. If a hypertensive episode should nevertheless occur, reintroduction of oral or intravenous Catapres should reverse any such effect. If the use of Catapres is not practical then an alpha-adrenergic blocking drug, such as phentolamine, should be used.

If Catapres is being given concurrently with a β-blocker, Catapres should not be discontinued until several days after the withdrawal of the β-blocker.

Patients with a known history of depression should be carefully supervised while under long-term treatment with Catapres as there have been occasional reports of further depressive episodes during oral treatment in such patients.

Caution should be exercised in patients with Raynaud's disease or other occlusive peripheral vascular disease. As with all drugs used in hypertension, Catapres should be used with caution in patients with cerebrovascular, coronary or renal insufficiency.

Concomitant use of diuretics or other antihypertensive agents will usually result in an increased antihypertensive effect.

Concomitant administration of tricyclic antidepressants may reduce the antihypertensive effect of Catapres.

Alpha-adrenergic blocking drugs antagonise the acute effects of Catapres.

Although clonidine has been in wide general use for many years, there is no definite evidence of hazard during human pregnancy. In animal studies involving doses higher than the equivalent maximum therapeutic dose in man, effects on foetal development were seen only in one species. Foetal malformations did not occur. Medicines should not be used in pregnancy, especially the first trimester, unless the expected benefit is thought to outweigh any possible risk to the foetus.

Catapres should only be given to breast-feeding women if considered essential by the physician. There is as yet insufficient experience to enable Catapres to be recommended for children.

Intravenous injection of Catapres should be given slowly to avoid a possible transient pressor effect. This is particularly important in patients already under treatment with other antihypertensive agents such as guanethidine or reserpine.

Side-effects: Initially, sedation or dry mouth are encountered in a few patients. These effects usually subside as treatment continues. Other drug-related side-effects which have been mentioned in the literature include dizziness, headache, nocturnal unrest, nausea, euphoria, rash, constipation, impotence (rarely) and agitation on withdrawal of long-term therapy.

There are occasional reports of fluid retention during initial stages of oral treatment. This is usually transitory and can be corrected by the addition of a diuretic.

Facial pallor has been noted following injection.

A single case of toxic hepatitis has been reported, but the authors commented that the role of Catapres in hepatotoxicity in this patient remains questionable.

Acute administration in animals or in man has occasionally induced a transient elevation of blood sugar. This is believed to be due to the initial pharmacological effect of alpha-adrenergic stimulation. Investigators agree that this has no clinical significance. The inclusion of diabetic patients in many Catapres investigations has confirmed its suitability as an antihypertensive agent for such patients.

Overdosage: Accidental overdosage may cause hypotension, bradycardia, sedation and coma. Transient hypertension may be seen if the total dose is over 10 mg.

Gastric lavage should be performed where appropriate. In most cases all that is required are general supportive measures. Forced diuresis has been employed. Where bradycardia is severe atropine will increase the heart rate. If hypotension is giving rise to concern the administration of an alpha-adrenergic blocking drug such as phentolamine may help.

Pharmaceutical precautions Catapres tablets and ampoules should be protected from light and heat.

Legal category POM.

Package quantities *Tablets 0.10 mg:* Packs of 50 and 250.

Tablets 0.30 mg: Pack of 100.

Perlongets 0.25 mg: Calendar pack of 56.

Ampoules 0.15 mg in 1 ml: Pack of 5.

Further information No adverse reaction has been reported with the concurrent administration of digoxin, aminophylline, anticonvulsants or antiarrhythmic preparations. Monitoring of haematological and hepatic status in large numbers of patients has revealed no drug-related adverse effects. Renal blood flow and glomerular filtration rates are maintained and there is no deterioration in renal function. There is evidence that plasma renin levels are reduced. Catapres does not affect the estimation of VMA levels.

Clonidine hydrochloride is also available as Dixarit 0.025 mg tablets for the prophylactic management of migraine, recurrent vascular headache and menopausal flushing.

Product licence numbers

Catapres Tablets 0.10 mg	0015/5009
Catapres Tablets 0.30 mg	0015/5041
Catapres PL Perlongets 0.25 mg	0015/0072
Catapres Ampoules 0.15 mg in 1 ml	0015/5008

CELEVAC*

Presentation Methylcellulose 450 BP as pink granules containing 64% and pink tablets containing 500 mg.

Uses *Action:* Methylcellulose is a hydrophilic colloid which absorbs water to swell to a soft gel of uniform consistency.

Indications:

1. In the control of colostomy, ileostomy and diarrhoea.

2. In the management of diverticular disease.

3. In the management of simple constipation.

4. As an aid to appetite control and as an aid in the management of obesity.

5. To prevent diarrhoea in patients receiving liquid and tube-fed diets.

Dosage and administration

1. *Colostomy and ileostomy control and for diarrhoea:* 1–2 level 5 ml spoonfuls of granules (or 3–6 tablets) twice daily with the minimum of liquid. Liquids should be avoided for 30 minutes before and after each dose. Dosage should be adjusted to give stools the required consistency.

2. *Diverticular disease:* 3–6 tablets or 1–2 level 5 ml spoonfuls of granules twice daily, adjusted according to the degree of constipation, diarrhoea or spastic pain.

3. *Simple constipation:* 1–2 level 5 ml spoonfuls of granules (or 3–6 tablets) twice daily, to be taken with at least 300 ml of liquid. The dose may be reduced as normal bowel function is restored.

4. *Appetite control and obesity:* 3 tablets, with at least 300 ml of warm liquid, half an hour before each meal, and between meals when hunger pangs are severe.

5. *Liquid diet and intragastric tube feeding:* 1 level 5 ml spoonful of granules, dispersed in hot water, added to each litre of diet mix.

No specific information on the use of this product in the elderly is available. Clinical trials have included patients over 65 years and no adverse reactions specific to this age group have been reported.

Contra-indications, warnings, etc Celevac should not be used in cases where the physician believes there is a pathological cause for the diarrhoea which would render the condition unsuitable for symptomatic medical treatment, e.g. infective bowel disease and imminent or threatened bowel obstruction. Bowel obstruction is a rare complication of treatment with any bulk-forming hydrophilic colloid.

Although Celevac has been in wide general use for many years there is no evidence of ill-consequence during human pregnancy.

Medicines should not be used in pregnancy, especially the first trimester, unless the expected benefit is thought to outweigh any possible risk to the foetus.

Overdosage: Methylcellulose is not absorbed. The features to be expected would be abdominal distension which may be followed by intestinal obstruction.

Gastric lavage should be employed where appropriate. The patient should be observed and fluids given. If obstruction develops, appropriate measures such as rectal washout must be taken.

Pharmaceutical precautions Protect from heat and moisture.

Legal category GSL.

Package quantities Granules packs of 500 g. Tablets packs of 250.

Further information Methylcellulose is a hydrophilic colloid which bonds loosely with H_2O and with H_2S, thus acting as a bulking agent and a deodorising agent. In diverticular disease its use has been associated with a fall in intracolonic pressures as well as relief of symptoms.

Product licence numbers
Celevac Granules   1416/5000
Celevac Tablets   1416/5003

DEXA-RHINASPRAY*

Presentation Dexa-Rhinaspray metered nasal spray, complete with nasal applicator. Each 9 g vial contains about 125 metered doses. One metered dose contains: tramazoline hydrochloride 0.12 mg, dexamethasone-21 isonicotinate 0.02 mg, neomycin sulphate 0.10 mg.

Uses
Action: Tramazoline hydrochloride is a sympathomimetic substance with local vasoconstrictor activity. It has a quick-acting, long-lasting decongestant effect on the nasal mucosa.

Dexamethasone-21 isonicotinate is a corticosteroid with marked anti-inflammatory and anti-allergic properties. Neomycin sulphate is locally active against a wide range of both Gram-positive and Gram-negative bacteria.
Indication: Treatment of allergic rhinitis.

Dosage and administration
Adults: 1 metered dose can be applied into each nostril up to six times in 24 hours, although 2 or 3 applications a day are usually sufficient.

Children: 5–12 years – 1 metered dose into each nostril up to twice daily.

Children: under 5 years – not recommended.

No specific information on the use of this product in the elderly is available. Clinical trials have included patients over 65 years and no adverse reactions specific to this age group have been reported.

Contra-indications, warnings, etc
Contra-indications: Its use is contra-indicated in patients hypersensitive to neomycin or tramazoline and in infants.

Precautions: Prolonged use may result in the development of superinfection due to organisms resistant to neomycin. Care should be used to avoid contact with the eyes as conjunctival irritation may occur.

Although Dexa-Rhinaspray has been in general use for many years, there is no evidence of ill-consequence during human pregnancy; animal studies have shown no hazard. Nevertheless, medicines should not be used in pregnancy, especially the first trimester, unless the expected benefit is thought to outweigh the risk to the foetus.

Side-effects: A slight burning sensation in the nose, with sneezing, has been reported when using tramazoline hydrochloride alone.

Overdosage: There have been no reports of overdosage with Dexa-Rhinaspray, but absorption of tramazoline may produce pallor, sweating, tachycardia and anxiety. These should be treated symptomatically.

Pharmaceutical precautions Protect from extremes of temperature. The vials should not be punctured or incinerated even when apparently empty.

Legal category POM.

Package quantities 9 g vial (125 doses) complete with nasal applicator.

Further information Neomycin sulphate is rarely used systemically. Local use therefore does not prejudice the patient's response to later systemic antibiotic treatment.

Product licence number 0015/5010

DIXARIT*

Presentation Blue, bi-convex, sugar-coated tablets, One side plain, the obverse marked with DIXARIT. Each tablet contains clonidine hydrochloride 0.025 mg.

Uses *Action:* Treatment with Dixarit diminishes the responsiveness of peripheral vessels to constrictor and dilator stimuli, thereby preventing the vascular changes associated with migraine. The same direct action on peripheral vessels moderates the vascular changes associated with menopausal flushing.
Indications:
1. The prophylactic management of migraine or recurrent vascular headache.
2. The management of vasomotor conditions commonly associated with the menopause and characterised by flushing.

Dosage and administration *Adults:* Initially 2 tablets twice daily. If after two weeks there has been no remission, increase to 3 tablets twice daily.

Children: Not generally recommended for administration to children under 12 years.

The duration of treatment depends upon the severity of the condition.

No specific information on the use of this product in the elderly is available. Clinical trials have included patients over 65 years and no adverse reactions specific to this age group have been reported.

Contra-indications, warnings, etc
Contra-indications: There are no known absolute contra-indications to the use of Dixarit.

Precautions: Dixarit may be unsuitable for patients who have co-existing or a previous history of depressive illness, since further depressive episodes have occasionally been reported in such patients.

Although clonidine has been in wide general use for many years there is no definite hazard during human pregnancy.

In animal studies involving doses higher than the equivalent maximum therapeutic dose in man, effects on foetal development were only seen in one species. Foetal malformations did not occur.

Medicines should not be used in pregnancy, especially

the first trimester unless the expected benefit is thought to outweigh any possible risk to the foetus.

Using higher doses than those recommended above, clonidine is an effective antihypertensive agent. Caution should therefore be observed where antihypertensive agents are being used as potentiation of hypotensive effect may occur. Provided the recommended Dixarit dosage regimen is followed, no difficulty with hypotension should arise during the routine management of patients with either migraine or menopausal flushing.

Clonidine is available for the management of hypertension as Catapres Tablets (0.10 mg and 0.30 mg), Perlongets (0.25 mg) and Ampoules (0.15 mg in 1 ml). Where Catapres is already being used Dixarit therapy is obviously illogical.

Side-effects: Initially there may be sedation or dry mouth in some patients. Dizziness, nausea and nocturnal unrest have been reported, and occasionally rashes have been attributed to Dixarit.

In the management of hypertension a single case of toxic hepatitis has been reported with clonidine. However, the role of clonidine in hepatotoxicity in this patient remains questionable. Monitoring of haematological, renal and hepatic status in large numbers of patients has revealed no drug-related adverse effects.

Overdosage: Accidental overdosage may cause hypotension, bradycardia, sedation and coma. Transient hypertension may be seen if the total dose is over 10 mg.

Gastric lavage should be performed where appropriate. In most cases all that is required are general supportive measures. Forced diuresis has been employed. Where bradycardia is severe atropine will increase the heart rate. If hypotension is giving rise to concern the administration of an alpha-adrenergic blocking drug such as phentolamine may help.

Pharmaceutical precautions Protect from heat, moisture and light.

Legal category POM.

Package quantities Packs of 100.

Further information There is no information which suggests that Dixarit will interact with any other preparation used routinely in the management of either migraine or menopausal flushing.

Product licence number 0015/5014.

DULCODOS*

Presentation White, sugar-enteric-coated tablets printed on one side with the Company symbol. Each tablet contains bisacodyl (Dulcolax*) 5 mg and docusate sodium 100 mg.

Uses *Action:* Dulcodos combines the contact laxative effect of Dulcolax with the faecal softening action of docusate sodium. Dulcodos tablets disintegrate in the small intestine, the two constituents being released simultaneously. In the colon, docusate sodium, by lowering surface tension, allows water to penetrate the faecal mass more readily, preventing normal faeces from becoming inspissated. At the same time Dulcolax, on contact with the mucosa of the large bowel, initiates a general peristaltic movement which results in the evacuation of soft, well-formed stools. Neither substance depends for its effect on systemic absorption. Dulcodos tablets, when taken after food, act in 10–12 hours.

Indications: Chronic constipation, or other conditions in which painful defaecation is a problem. Replacement of the enema, prior to surgery, labour or radiological investigation, in conjunction with Dulcolax suppositories.

Dosage and administration Dulcodos tablets are suitable for routine use in adults, and children over 10 years.

In constipation, 2 tablets at night.

For complete bowel clearance, 2 tablets at night, followed by one Dulcolax suppository next morning.

In radiology, 2 tablets on each of the two nights prior to the investigation, followed by 1 Dulcolax suppository (if necessary) 1 hour before the investigation.

No specific information on the use of this product in the elderly is available. Clinical trials have included patients over 65 years and no adverse reactions specific to this age group have been reported.

Contra-indications, warnings, etc

Contra-indications: Only those conditions where any laxative is contra-indicated.

Precautions: Because Dulcodos tablets are enteric-coated for disintegration in the intestine, they should not be crushed or chewed. For the same reason antacids should not be given within 1 hour of administering Dulcodos tablets.

Although Dulcodos has been in general use for many years, there is no evidence of ill-consequence during human pregnancy; animal studies have shown no hazard. Medicines should not be used in pregnancy, especially the first trimester, unless the expected benefit is thought to outweigh any possible risk to the foetus.

Side-effects: The mode of action of Dulcolax, and the addition of the faecal softener, docusate sodium, mean that side-effects, such as abdominal discomfort, should only rarely be encountered.

Overdosage: Colicky lower abdominal pain with possible signs of dehydration may be expected particularly in the elderly and the very young.

Gastric lavage should be performed where appropriate. Adequate hydration must be maintained and the serum potassium should be measured. Antispasmodics may be of some value. Particular care about fluid balance should be taken in the elderly and young.

Pharmaceutical precautions Dulcodos tablets should be protected from heat and light.

Legal category P.

Package quantities Blister packs of 20 and 100.

Further information Nil.

Product licence number 0015/5013.

DULCOLAX*

Presentation *Dulcolax Tablets:* Yellow sugar-enteric-coated tablets marked 'Dulcolax' on one side. Each tablet contains bisacodyl 5 mg.

Dulcolax Suppositories: White, opaque, foil-wrapped suppositories, each containing bisacodyl 10 mg.

Dulcolax Children's Suppositories: White, opaque, foil-wrapped suppositories for children, each containing bisacodyl 5 mg.

Dulcolax Rectal Solution: Buffered polyethylene glycol solution containing bisacodyl 2.74 mg/ml.

Uses *Action:* Dulcolax is a synthetic laxative which acts on contact with the mucosa of the large bowel. It is reliable and predictable in its action, producing in most cases a soft, formed stool without straining.

Dulcolax tablets taken after food act in 10–12 hours. A Dulcolax suppository will produce a motion within 20 minutes to 1 hour of insertion.

Indications: Constipation, either chronic or of recent onset, whenever a stimulant laxative is required.

Bowel clearance before surgery, labour or radiological investigation. Replacement of the evacuant enema in all its indications.

The rectal solution is indicated specifically in radiological procedures, either as a preparatory measure when given as a miniature enema to reduce flatus and faecal shadow interference, or mixed with the barium enema.

Dosage and administration Dulcolax is suitable for routine use in adults of all ages, and in children.

1. *In constipation*
(a) *Adults and children over 10 years:* 2 tablets at night, or one 10 mg suppository in the morning. (Occasionally a higher tablet dosage is required: up to 3 or 4 may be given.)
(b) *Children under 10 years:* 1 tablet at night or one 5 mg suppository in the morning.

2. *For replacement of the enema*
(a) *Adults and children over 10 years:* 2 tablets at night followed by one 10 mg suppository in the morning.
(b) *Children under 10 years:* 1 tablet at night followed by one 5 mg suppository in the morning.

3. *In preparation for radiological investigation*
(a) *Adults and children over 10 years:* 2 tablets on each of the 2 nights before the investigation and one 10 mg suppository (if necessary) 1 hour before investigation. Where needed 2–3 ml of the rectal solution may be administered, as a miniature enema.
(b) *Children under 10 years:* 1 tablet on each of the 2 nights before the investigation and one 5 mg suppository (if necessary) 1 hour before the investigation. Where needed 1–2 ml of the rectal solution may be administered, as a miniature enema.

N.B. Dulcolax rectal solution may be administered together with a barium enema, at a dose of 2–5 ml in 1–3 litres of enema solution.

No specific information on the use of this product in the elderly is available. Clinical trials have included patients over 65 years and no adverse reactions specific to this age group have been reported.

Contra-indications, warnings, etc
Contra-indications: Only those conditions where any laxative is contra-indicated.

Precautions: Because Dulcolax tablets are enteric-coated for disintegration in the intestine, they should not be crushed or chewed. For the same reason, antacids should not be given within 1 hour of administering Dulcolax tablets.

Dulcolax solution is for rectal administration only.

Although Dulcolax has been in general use for many years, there is no evidence of ill-consequence during human pregnancy; animal studies have shown no hazard. Nevertheless, medicines should not be used in pregnancy, especially the first trimester, unless the expected benefit is thought to outweigh any possible risk to the foetus.

Side-effects: As with any effective laxative, griping has

occasionally been reported after administration of Dulcolax tablets. If this occurs, it can be minimised by dosage adjustment.

Overdosage: Colicky lower abdominal pain with possible signs of dehydration may be expected particularly in the elderly and the very young.

Gastric lavage should be performed where appropriate. Adequate hydration must be maintained and the serum potassium should be measured. Antispasmodics may be of some value. Particular care about fluid balance should be taken in the elderly and young.

Pharmaceutical precautions All dosage forms should be protected from heat and light.

Legal category P.

Package quantities *Tablets:* Packs of 40, 200 and 1,000.

Suppositories 10 mg: Packs of 6, 50 and 200.

Children's Suppositories 5 mg: Packs of 6.

Rectal Solution: 250 ml bottles.

Further information Nil.

Product licence numbers
Dulcolax Tablets	0015/0048
Dulcolax Suppositories 10 mg	0015/0049
Dulcolax Children's Suppositories 5 mg	0015/0050
Dulcolax Rectal Solution	0015/5011

DUOVENT* ▼

Presentation Pressurised metered dose inhaler: 10 ml vial (200 metered doses) available as complete unit with mouthpiece. Each metered dose contains fenoterol hydrobromide 0.10 mg (0.090 mg available to the patient) and ipratropium bromide 0.04 mg (0.036 mg available to the patient).

Uses *Action:* Fenoterol hydrobromide is a highly potent, rapidly acting selective beta$_2$-adrenoceptor stimulant. The degree of selectivity coupled with administration by inhalation allows maximal bronchodilator effect with minimal side-effects.

Ipratropium bromide is an anticholinergic drug with bronchodilator properties.

There is evidence that the concurrent administration of ipratropium bromide and a sympathomimetic drug produces a greater relief of bronchospasm than either drug given alone.

Indications: For the treatment of reversible airways obstruction as in bronchial asthma, bronchitis and emphysema.

Dosage and administration *Adults:* 1 or 2 puffs three or four times daily.

Children over 6 years: 1 puff three times daily. It is recommended that administration of Duovent to children be supervised by an adult.

No specific information on the use of this product in the elderly is available. Clinical trials have included patients over 65 years and no adverse reactions specific to this age group have been reported.

Contra-indications, warnings, etc
Contra-indications: Known sensitivity to atropine.

Precautions: Caution should be observed should it be necessary to administer Duovent to patients with thyrotoxicosis, myocardial insufficiency, angina, cardiac dysrhythmias, hypertension or hypertrophic subvalvular aortic stenosis. In view of the possible interaction between sympathomimetic amines and monoamine oxidase inhibitors or tricyclic anti-depressants, care should be exercised if it is proposed to administer these compounds concurrently with Duovent. Duovent should be used with caution in patients already receiving other sympathomimetic agents as cardiovascular effects may be additive.

Generally, caution is advocated in the use of anticholinergic agents in patients with glaucoma and prostatic hypertrophy. However, specific studies with ipratropium bromide in patients with glaucoma showed that inhaling cumulative doses of 0.16 mg had no effect on the eye. Urinary retention and constipation have only rarely been reported.

Patients must be instructed in the correct use of a metered dose inhaler and warned against the accidental release of the contents into the eye. If relief is not obtained after correct use of the inhaler, the dose should not be exceeded and the patient should contact the doctor for advice.

Although both fenoterol hydrobromide and ipratropium bromide have been in general use for several years, there is no definite evidence of ill-consequence during human pregnancy; animal studies have shown no hazard. Beta-adrenergic agents have been shown to prolong pregnancy and inhibit labour although the amount in the prescribed dose of Duovent is probably insufficient to do so.

Medicines should not be used in pregnancy, especially the first trimester, unless the expected benefit is thought to outweigh any possible risk to the foetus.

Beta-adrenergic blocking agents may antagonise fenoterol hydrobromide and reduce its bronchodilator effect if administered concurrently.

A transient dose related decrease in serum potassium levels has been observed in some patients treated with fenoterol.

Side-effects: Transient sympathomimetic side-effects, such as palpitation, tachycardia, headache and tremor may occur, as with other beta-adrenergic agonists, but are uncommon with administration by inhaler.

Anticholinergic side-effects are unlikely to occur at therapeutic doses but some patients may complain of a dry mouth. There is no evidence that in the therapeutic dose range Duovent has any adverse effect on bronchial secretion.

Overdosage: Accidental overdosage may give rise to tachycardia, palpitation and tremor. It is suggested that the patient should be treated symptomatically. Should the administration of a beta-adrenergic blocking agent be considered necessary to counteract the effects of over-dosage, its use in a patient liable to bronchospasm should be carefully monitored.

Very high doses (30 mg) of ipratropium bromide by mouth have been reported to cause anticholinergic side-effects but these were not severe and did not require specific reversal.

Pharmaceutical precautions Protect from heat, including the sun. The canister should not be incinerated or opened even when apparently empty.

Legal category POM.

Package quantities 10 ml vial (200 metered doses) complete with mouthpiece.

Further information There is evidence to suggest that fenoterol may reduce the allergic response of tissues. Animal studies have shown that fenoterol also produces an increase in the frequency of movement of the respiratory epithelial cilia and in the rate of mucus transport.

Long-term use has shown fenoterol and ipratropium to be free from significant adverse effects.

Product licence number 0015/0091.

HERPID*

Presentation A clear, colourless solution containing Idoxuridine BP 5% in dimethyl sulphoxide, of spectroscopic quality.

Uses *Action:* The antiviral agent idoxuridine arrests replication of DNA viruses, e.g. varicella/zoster; herpesvirus hominis; vaccinia. The idoxuridine is dissolved in dimethyl sulphoxide which penetrates the skin and carries the antiviral agent to the deeper levels of the epidermis where the virus is replicating.

Indications: Cutaneous herpes simplex and herpes zoster (shingles).

Dosage and administration Herpid should be painted on the lesions and their erythematous bases 4 times daily for four days. Treatment should start as soon as the condition has been diagnosed, ideally within two to three days after the rash appears. Good results are less likely if treatment is not started within seven days.

No specific information on the use of this product in the elderly is available. Clinical trials have included patients over 65 years and no adverse reactions specific to this age group have been reported.

Contra-indications, warnings, etc
Contra-indications: Animal studies have shown idoxuridine to be teratogenic. Consequently, Herpid should not be prescribed for women who are pregnant or at risk of becoming pregnant. In a small number of cases of women who used Herpid inadvertently in early pregnancy and who were followed to term, the infant was normal in each case.

Known hypersensitivity to either idoxuridine or dimethyl sulphoxide.

Dermographia.

Side-effects: Patients often experience stinging when applying Herpid and a distinctive taste during a course of treatment; both effects are transient.

Skin reactions have occasionally been reported.

Over-usage of the solution may lead to maceration of the skin.

Warning: Herpid in the eye causes stinging: treat by washing out with water.

Overdosage: There is no clinical experience of overdosage. Standard supportive measures should be adopted.

Pharmaceutical precautions Herpid should be stored in its box at room temperature. Do not refrigerate as the contents of the bottle may solidify. If crystals do form, allow to redissolve before use.

Legal category POM.

Package quantities 5 ml bottle, with brush. 50 ml hospital dispensing pack.

Further information Herpid can damage some synthetic materials (e.g. artificial silk and Terylene) and printed cotton fabrics. Contact between Herpid and these materials should therefore be avoided.

The use of Herpid in children with malignant disease might be justified but, although not a contra-indication, its use in children under the age of 12 years is not recommended.

Product licence number 1416/0001.

ORGANIDIN*

Presentation Light yellow elixir containing iodinated glycerol 60 mg and alcohol (96%) 1.25 ml per 5 ml.

Uses *Action:* Mucosecretory stimulating agent.

Indications: For the treatment of diseases of the respiratory tract in which thick, tenacious mucus, or lack of mucous secretion, is an undesirable feature, e.g. bronchitis, asthma, laryngitis.

Dosage and administration *Adults and children over 12 years:* One 5 ml spoonful four times daily.

Children: Up to half the adult dosage.

Diluent: Organidin may be diluted with a 1:1 mixture of glycerol and water.

No specific information on the use of this product in the elderly is available. Clinical trials have included patients over 65 years and no adverse reactions specific to this age group have been reported.

Contra-indications, warnings, etc In view of the association of neonatal goitre and/or hypothyroidism with maternal ingestion of iodides, Organidin therapy is not advocated during pregnancy, particularly during the last two trimesters. Long-term administration of iodides to children is also best avoided because of this goitrogenic hazard. Caution is recommended in cases of known hypersensitivity to iodides. Most patients, however, will tolerate Organidin, and any adverse reactions which may occur are likely to be less severe than those resulting from inorganic iodide therapy.

Overdosage: Symptoms may be those of alcoholic intoxication or excessive salivation. Elimination of the drug may be hastened by increasing the water and sodium chloride intake or by forced diuresis with mannitol.

Pharmaceutical precautions Store in a cool place, protect from light.

Legal category P.

Package quantities Bottles of 250 ml.

Further information Nil.

Product licence number 1416/5034.

PAVACOL-D*

Presentation Dark brown, sugar-free, tartrazine-free cough mixture. Each 5 ml contains Papaverine Hydrochloride BP 1 mg and Pholcodine BP 5 mg, together with balsam of tolu, oil of clove, tincture of ginger, oil of aniseed, tincture of capsicum, oil of peppermint, alcohol and chloroform.

Uses *Action:* Pholcodine exerts an inhibitory action on the cough centre, and has been found to be as effective as heroin as a cough suppressant. It is not a drug of addiction, and does not cause constipation.

Papaverine is a myotropic spasmolytic. It relaxes the bronchi by direct action on the smooth muscle of their walls.

Indications: For the symptomatic treatment of cough due to upper respiratory tract infection, influenza, bronchitis, pulmonary tuberculosis, carcinoma of the bronchus, etc, particularly in diabetic patients who require strict control of carbohydrate intake. It is also suitable for patients who are on a weight-reducing diet.

Dosage and administration *Adults:* One or two 5 ml spoonfuls as required.

The above dosage is adequate for most patients, but higher doses can safely be prescribed if necessary.

Children: from 6 to 12 years: One 5 ml spoonful four or five times daily.

From 3 to 5 years: One 5 ml spoonful three times daily.

From 1 to 2 years: Half a 5 ml spoonful three or four times daily.

Pavacol-D may be diluted with Sorbitol Solution BPC.

No specific information on the use of this product in the elderly is available. Clinical trials have included patients over 65 years and no adverse reactions specific to this age group have been reported.

Contra-indications, warnings, etc Hypersensitivity to papaverine has been recorded. Nausea and drowsiness occur occasionally after pholcodine.

Although Pavacol-D has been in general use for many years, there is no evidence of ill-consequence during human pregnancy.

Medicines should not be used in pregnancy, especially the first trimester, unless the expected benefit is thought to outweigh any possible risk to the foetus.

Overdosage: Overdosage may be manifest by drowsiness or nausea and should be treated by emesis or gastric lavage followed by oral hydration.

Pharmaceutical precautions Store in a cool place and protect from light.

Legal category P.

Package quantities Bottles of 150 ml and 1 litre.

Further information A sugar-free, tartrazine-free mixture suitable for both diabetic and non-diabetic patients.

Product licence number 1416/5039.

PERSANTIN*

Presentation Persantin tablets 25 mg: orange sugar-coated tablets, marked 'Persantin 25' on one side, containing dipyridamole 25 mg.

Persantin tablets 100 mg: white sugar-coated tablets, marked 'Persantin 100' on one side, containing dipyridamole 100 mg.

Uses
Action: Dipyridamole has an antithrombotic action based on its ability to modify various aspects of platelet function, such as platelet aggregation, adhesion and survival, which have been shown to be factors associated with the initiation of thrombus formation.

Dipyridamole modifies platelet function by enhancing prostacyclin effect through a strong inhibition of phosphodiesterase and mild stimulation of adenyl cyclase formation. It has also been shown to inhibit the formation of thromboxane A_2 which is known to cause platelet adhesion and aggregation.

Indications:
 (i) An adjunct to oral anticoagulation for prophylaxis of thromboembolism associated with prosthetic heart valves.
 (ii) In co-administration with aspirin for:
   (a) prophylaxis of deep venous thrombosis as an alternative to subcutaneous heparin, other than in hip surgery;
   (b) prophylaxis of recurrent deep venous thrombosis resistant to oral anticoagulation;
   (c) prophylaxis of occlusion following prosthetic arterial grafts and coronary artery bypass grafts.

Dosage and administration

Adults: 300–600 mg daily in three or four doses

Children: The normal total oral daily dose is 5 mg/kg in divided doses.

Persantin should usually be taken before meals.

Contra-indications, warnings, etc

Contra-indications: There are no absolute contra-indications to the administration of Persantin.

Precautions: Persantin is a potent vasodilator and should therefore be used with caution in patients with rapidly worsening angina, subvalvular aortic stenosis or haemodynamic instability associated with a recently sustained myocardial infarction.

There is inadequate evidence of safety in human pregnancy but Persantin has been used for many years without apparent ill-consequence. Medicines should not be used in pregnancy, especially the first trimester, unless the expected benefit is thought to outweigh any possible risk to the foetus.

The concurrent administration of antacids may reduce the efficacy of Persantin.

It is possible that Persantin may enhance the effects of oral anticoagulants.

Persantin should be used with caution in patients with coagulation disorders.

Side-effects: If these occur it is usually during the early part of treatment and they are often dose-related. The vasodilating properties of Persantin may occasionally produce a vascular headache which normally disappears with dosage reduction. Dizziness, faintness, dyspepsia, mild diarrhoea and rash have also been reported occasionally.

Overdosage: Overdosage may lead to headache, gastrointestinal symptoms and hypotension. Coronary vasodilatation may cause chest pain in patients with ischaemic heart disease.

General supportive measures should be employed. Coronary vasodilatation may be reversed by administering aminophylline by slow IV injection.

Pharmaceutical precautions   Protect from heat, light and moisture.

Legal category   POM.

Package quantities   Packs of 100 and 1000 tablets.

Further information   There is evidence that the effects of aspirin and dipyridamole on platelet behaviour are synergistic.

Product licence number
Persantin tablets 25 mg   0015/0052
Persantin tablets 100 mg   0015/5016

TRANXENE⁺

Presentation   Tranxene Capsules 15 mg: Pink/grey hard gelatin capsules imprinted with the notation 15 mg and the Company symbol. Each capsule contains dipotassium clorazepate 15 mg.

Tranxene Capsules 7.5 mg: Maroon/grey hard gelatin capsules imprinted with the product name, 7.5 mg and the Company symbol. Each capsule contains dipotassium clorazepate 7.5 mg.

Uses

Action: Tranxene is a tranquilliser exhibiting many characteristics of the benzodiazepine group of preparations. Particular features which distinguish Tranxene from other members of this group are the rapid appearance in the blood of the anxiolytic compound nordiazepam, the maintenance of satisfactory therapeutic effect in most patients with once daily administration, and little sedation.

Indications: Relief of all forms of anxiety, tension and agitation in acute and chronic anxiety states. Tranxene is compatible with all antidepressants in the treatment of anxiety accompanied by depression.

Dosage and administration   Adults only, not generally recommended for children under 16 years. Tranxene 15 mg: one capsule daily, usually administered at night. Tranxene 7.5 mg: one capsule up to three times daily.

Half the normal dose may be sufficient for a therapeutic response in the elderly.

Contra-indications, warnings, etc

Contra-indications: Known hypersensitivity to benzodiazepines; acute pulmonary insufficiency.

Precautions: As sole treatment, Tranxene is not recommended for acute primary depressive states or major psychoses. The action of Tranxene may potentiate other preparations with central nervous system depressant effects such as barbiturates, narcotics, phenothiazines and alcohol.

Although sedation has not proved to be a problem with Tranxene, in accordance with general principles patients should be advised that their ability to drive or to operate dangerous machinery may be impaired.

There is no evidence as to drug safety in human pregnancy nor is there evidence from animal work that it is free from hazard. Do not use during pregnancy, especially during the first and last trimesters, unless there are compelling reasons.

Tranxene and its metabolites are excreted in human milk in minimal quantities and therefore use during lactation should be avoided if possible. In labour, high single doses or low repeated doses of benzodiazepines have been reported to produce irregularities of the foetal heart and hypotonia, and poor suckling and hypothermia in the neonate. Caution should be exercised in patients suffering from chronic pulmonary insufficiency, or chronic renal or hepatic disease.

Side-effects: Side-effects, which have been reported only rarely, include dizziness, gastro-intestinal upset, nervousness, blurred vision, dry mouth, headache, skin rashes and jaundice. Drowsiness has occasionally been reported but does not constitute a major problem.

Hypotension, urinary retention, changes in libido and blood dyscrasias have also been reported for benzodiazepines in general.

Abnormal psychological reactions to benzodiazepines have been reported. Rare behavioural adverse effects include paradoxical aggressive outbursts, and mental confusion together with excitement and the uncovering of depression with suicidal tendencies.

Excessive or prolonged use may occasionally result in the development of some psychological dependence with withdrawal symptoms on sudden discontinuation of the benzodiazepine, particularly in patients with a history of drug abuse or alcoholism or in patients with marked personality disorders. In such patients treatment should be monitored closely and routine prescriptions avoided, with gradual drug withdrawal when appropriate. The symptoms of benzodiazepine withdrawal have included depression, nervousness, rebound insomnia, irritability, sweating and diarrhoea. Normal usage seldom results in the development of dependence.

Overdosage: An overdose of 900 mg has been reported, causing drowsiness, ataxia, respiratory depression and coma. If vomiting has not occurred spontaneously, it should be induced. Gastric lavage is recommended. General supportive therapy is indicated and specific measures to counteract central nervous system depressant effects may be necessary. Prolonged administration of doses as high as 120 mg daily has not given rise to organ toxicity. Abrupt withdrawal of excessive doses of benzodiazepines has been reported as occasionally producing confusion, toxic psychosis, convulsion or a condition resembling delerium tremens.

Pharmaceutical precautions Tranxene capsules should be protected from heat, light and moisture.

Legal category POM.

Package quantities Packs of 100 and 20 in aluminium foil strips.

Further information In common with other benzodiazepines, Tranxene has a central muscle-relaxant effect, and synergism with peripherally acting muscle relaxants is a theoretical possibility.

Product licence numbers
Tranxene capsules 15 mg   0015/0057.
Tranxene capsules 7.5 mg   0015/0045,

VILLESCON* LIQUID

Presentation Red, raspberry-flavoured liquid. Each 5 ml contains:

Prolintane hydrochloride	2.5 mg
Thiamine hydrochloride	1.67 mg
Riboflavine-5-phosphate sodium	1.36 mg
Pyridoxine hydrochloride	0.5 mg
Nicotinamide	5.0 mg

Uses *Action:* The principal ingredient of Villescon, prolintane hydrochloride, is a sympathomimetic amine with two main actions. It stimulates appetite and has a mild central action which produces an increased feeling of well-being in debilitated patients.

Indications: Villescon is indicated as a tonic after illness, surgery or labour, for apathy and anorexia in elderly patients, for institutional neuroses and for anorexia and lassitude following radiotherapy.

Dosage and administration *Adults:* 2 × 5 ml twice daily.

Children 5–12 years: ½ × 5 ml twice daily to 2 × 5 ml twice daily.

The normal course of treatment is 1–2 weeks.

It is recommended that the second daily dose be taken before four o'clock in the afternoon.

Diluent: Villescon Liquid may be diluted with purified water.

No specific information on the use of this product in the elderly is available. Clinical trials have included patients over 65 years and no adverse reactions specific to this age group have been reported.

Contra-indications, warnings, etc
Contra-indications: Thyrotoxicosis, epilepsy.

Precautions: Although no interaction between Villescon and MAO inhibitors has ever been demonstrated, the theoretical possibility of such an interaction should be borne in mind if these preparations are co-prescribed. It should be noted that even in very small quantities pyridoxine hydrochloride (vitamin B6) inhibits the activity of levodopa.

There exists a proportion of patients whose ill-defined symptoms reflect a basic inadequacy of personality. Such patients are liable to misuse any drug with central activity, and it is advised that in these cases the recurrent prescription of Villescon should be avoided.

Although Villescon liquid has been in wide general use for many years, there is no definite evidence of ill-consequence during human pregnancy; animal studies have shown no hazard. Nevertheless, medicines should not be used in pregnancy, especially the first trimester, unless the expected benefit is thought to outweigh any possible risk to the foetus.

Side-effects: Tachycardia, nausea and colicky abdominal pains have been reported. Sleeplessness may be caused if Villescon is taken late in the day.

Overdosage: Accidental overdosage has been reported only rarely and may give rise to restlessness, insomnia, tachycardia and increase of blood pressure. An overdose of 300 mg prolintane has been reported in a young female who made a full recovery. Treatment should include gastric lavage and general supportive measures. Sedation may be required to treat restlessness and insomnia.

Pharmaceutical precautions Villescon preparations should be protected from heat, light and moisture.

Legal category POM.

Package quantities Bottles of 250 ml and 1 litre.

Further information Nil.

Product licence number 0015/0054.

VILLESCON* TABLETS

Presentation Orange, sugar-coated tablets, with the Company symbol on one side. Each tablet contains:

Prolintane hydrochloride	10.0 mg
Thiamine mononitrate	5.0 mg
Riboflavine	3.0 mg
Pyridoxine hydrochloride	1.5 mg
Nicotinamide	15.0 mg
Ascorbic acid	50.0 mg

Uses *Action:* The principal ingredient of Villescon, prolintane hydrochloride, is a sympathomimetic amine with two main actions. It stimulates appetite and has a mild central action which produces an increased feeling of well-being in debilitated patients.

Indications: Villescon is indicated as a tonic after illness, surgery or labour, for apathy and anorexia in elderly patients, for institutional neuroses and for anorexia and lassitude following radiotherapy.

Dosage and administration *Adults:* 1 tablet twice daily.

Children over 8 years: 1 tablet after breakfast.

The normal course of treatment is 1–2 weeks. It is recommended that the second daily dose be taken before four o'clock in the afternoon.

No specific information on the use of this product in the elderly is available. Clinical trials have included patients over 65 years and no adverse reactions specific to this age group have been reported.

Contra-indications, warnings, etc
Contra-indications: Thyrotoxicosis, epilepsy.

Precautions: Although no interaction between Villescon and MAO inhibitors has ever been demonstrated, the theoretical possibility of such an interaction should be borne in mind if these preparations are co-prescribed. It should be noted that even in very small quantities pyridoxine hydrochloride (vitamin B_6) inhibits the activity of levodopa.

There exists a proportion of patients whose ill-defined symptoms reflect a basic inadequacy of personality. Such patients are liable to misuse any drug with central activity, and it is advised that in these cases the recurrent prescription of Villescon should be avoided.

Although Villescon tablets have been in wide general use for many years there is no definite evidence of ill-consequence during human pregnancy; animal studies have shown no hazard. Medicines should not be used in pregnancy, especially the first trimester, unless the expected benefit is thought to outweigh any possible risk to the foetus.

Side-effects: Tachycardia, nausea and colicky abdominal pains have been reported. Sleeplessness may be caused if Villescon is taken late in the day.

Overdosage: Accidental overdosage has been reported only rarely and may give rise to restlessness, insomnia, tachycardia and increase of blood pressure. An overdose of 300 mg prolintane has been reported in a young female who made a full recovery. Treatment should include gastric lavage and general supportive measures. Sedation may be required to treat restlessness and insomnia.

Pharmaceutical precautions Villescon preparations should be protected from heat, light and moisture.

Legal category POM.

Package quantities Packs of 20 and 100.

Further information Nil.

Product licence number 0015/0055.

*Trade Mark

Boehringer Ingelheim Hospital Division
A Division of Boehringer Ingelheim Limited
Ellesfield Avenue
Bracknell
Berkshire RG12 4YS

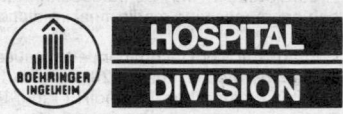

ENDOXANA*

Presentation White, compression-coated tablets containing Cyclophosphamide BP 10 mg or 50 mg; marked WBP E1 on one side and either 10 or 50 on the reverse. White powder for injection in vials containing Cyclophosphamide BP 107 mg, 214 mg, 535 mg or 1,069 mg (equivalent to 100 mg, 200 mg, 500 mg or 1,000 mg anhydrous cyclophosphamide respectively) and sodium chloride sufficient to render isotonic when diluted with Water for Injections using the volume recommended for each strength.

Uses *Action:* Cyclophosphamide is inert until activated by microsomal enzymes. This occurs mainly in the liver, producing potent alkylating cytotoxic metabolites.

Indications: Endoxana is a cytotoxic drug for the treatment of malignant disease.

As a single agent it has successfully produced an objective remission in a wide range of malignant conditions. Endoxana is also frequently used in combination with other cytotoxic drugs.

Dosage and administration Endoxana should only be used by clinicians experienced in the use of cancer chemotherapy.

Dosage: The dose, route of administration and frequency of administration should be determined by the tumour type, tumour stage, the general condition of the patient and whether other chemotherapy or radiotherapy is to be administered concurrently.

A guide to the dosage regimens used for most indications is given below:

Conventional dose: 100–300 mg daily as a single i.v. or oral dose, or 500 mg–1 g as a single i.v. dose weekly.

High dose: 20–40 mg/kg as a single i.v. dose or short infusion, given at 10–20 day intervals.

Administration: Endoxana is inert until activated by enzymes in the liver. However, as with all cytotoxics, it is suggested that reconstitution should be performed by trained personnel, in a designated area. Those handling the preparation should wear protective gloves. Care should be taken to avoid splashing material into the eyes. The material should not be handled by women who are pregnant. Adequate care and precautions should be taken in the disposal of items (syringes, needles etc.) used to reconstitute cytotoxic drugs. The dry contents of a vial should be dissolved in sterile water (5 ml per 100 mg Endoxana) and used within eight hours. The pH of an aqueous solution is between 4.5 and 5.5. Endoxana is usually given directly into the vein over one or two minutes or directly into the tubing of a fast running i.v. infusion with the patient supine. Care should be taken

that extravasation does not take place, however, should it occur, no specific measures need be taken. Endoxana injection may also be given intraperitoneally or intrapleurally, but these routes offer no therapeutic advantages over the i.v. route. For further information contact Boehringer Ingelheim Hospital Division. Endoxana has been given intra-arterially and by local perfusion. These routes should only be used by clinicians experienced in these procedures.

A minimum urine output of 100 ml/hr should be maintained during therapy with conventional doses. If the larger doses are used an output of at least this level should be maintained for 24 hours following administration, if necessary by a forced diuresis. Alkalinisation of the urine is not recommended. Endoxana should be given early in the day and the bladder voided frequently. The patient should be well hydrated and maintained in fluid balance. Mesna (Uromitexan) can be used concurrently to reduce urotoxic effects (see Uromitexan data sheet). Anti-emetics given before and during therapy may reduce nausea and vomiting.

If the leucocyte count is below 4,000/mm^3 or the platelet count is below 100,000/mm^3, treatment with Endoxana should be temporarily withheld until the blood count returns to normal levels.

An elixir may be prepared by dissolving the contents of the dry powder vials in Aromatic Elixir USP shortly before oral administration.

No specific information on the use of this product in the elderly is available. Clinical trials have included patients over 65 years and no adverse reactions specific to this age group have been reported.

Contra-indications, warnings, etc
Contra-indications: Endoxana should only be administered where there are facilities for regular monitoring of clinical, biochemical and haematological parameters before during and after administration and under the direction of a specialist oncology service.

Endoxana is contra-indicated in patients with known hypersensitivity, with acute infections, with bone marrow aplasia, with acute urinary tract infection or with acute urothelial toxicity from cytotoxic chemotherapy or radiation therapy.

Endoxana should not be used in the management of non-malignant disease, except for immuno-suppression in life-threatening situations.

Contraception in both sexes is advised during Endoxana therapy. Patients should receive counselling with respect to subsequent pregnancies. Endoxana should not be used in pregnancy, especially the first trimester, unless the expected benefit is thought to outweigh the substantial risk to the foetus. Mothers should not breast-feed while being treated with Endoxana.

Precautions: Care should be exercised in patients who are elderly, debilitated, have diabetes mellitus or evidence of myelosuppression or who have recently received or are receiving concurrent treatment with radiotherapy or cytotoxic agents.

Cardiotoxicity may be induced in patients who have had or are receiving mediastinal irradiation or doxorubicin.

Endoxana is not recommended in patients with plasma creatinine greater than 120 µmol/l (1.5mg/100 ml), bilirubin greater than 17 µmol/l (1 mg/100 ml), or with transaminases or alkaline phosphatase more than 2–3 times the normal value.

Increased myelosuppression may be seen following concurrent administration of other marrow depressant drugs.

Endoxana potentiates the hypoglycaemic effects of the sulphonylurea compounds. An alteration in carbohydrate metabolism may be seen in patients on Endoxana; hyperglycaemia has been reported.

Side-effects: Nausea and vomiting. This may be reduced by the prior administration of an anti-emetic agent.

Alopecia occurs to some degree in about 20% of patients receiving over 100 mg daily and is inevitable following high doses. Epilation commences usually after the first three weeks of treatment but regrowth is evident after three months in most patients even though they remain on treatment.

The reticulo-endothelial system is depressed, granulopoiesis and lymphopoiesis being more affected than thrombopoiesis and erythropoiesis but this depression is reversible. When a single dose is given, the fall in the peripheral white cell count reaches its nadir within 5 to 10 days. Recovery is seen at 10–14 days following administration, with full recovery in most cases by 21–28 days. The fall in the peripheral count and the time taken to recover may increase with increasing doses of Endoxana. If the peripheral white cell count is very low, an increased risk of infection should be considered but since recovery is usually spontaneous, steroids are not recommended.

Haematuria may occur during or after therapy with Endoxana.

An adequate output of urine (2–3 L/day) should be maintained. Adequate hydration with frequent emptying of the bladder is recommended. The administration of a diuretic may sometimes be necessary to achieve this, particularly when higher doses of Endoxana are used. Mesna (Uromitexan) may be considered to reduce the urotoxicity and if used, frequent emptying of the bladder should be avoided. Endoxana should be withheld from patients with cystitis from whatever cause, until it has been treated.

Amenorrhoea and azoospermia often occur but can be reversible. Endoxana may have an effect on pre-pubertal gonads and appropriate counselling should be given.

Cardiotoxicity has been observed with high doses of Endoxana. Endoxana should be discontinued and appropriate treatment given.

Other side-effects such as pigmentation, macrocytosis, water retention, and induction of hyperglycaemia or hypoglycaemia have been reported. Following large doses ECG changes and elevation of LDH, SGOT and CPK have been reported in some patients. Pneumonitis and pulmonary fibrosis have also occasionally been associated with Endoxana therapy. Side-effects have occasionally occurred after cessation of treatment.

Endoxana has been shown to be mutagenic, terato-genic and carcinogenic in certain laboratory tests, and, as with other cytotoxic agents, there have been reports of possible drug-induced neoplasia.

Overdosage: The most serious consequences of over-dosage are myelosuppression and haemorrhagic cystitis. The former usually recovers spontaneously, but until it does, administration of a broad spectrum antibiotic may be advisable. Transfusion of whole-blood, platelets or white cells are rarely necessary.

If the overdose is recognised within the first 24 hours and possibly up to 48 hours, i.v. mesna may be beneficial in ameliorating damage to the urinary system. Normal supportive measures such as analgesics and maintenance of fluid balance should be instituted. If despite these measures the cystitis does not resolve, more intensive treatment may be necessary and a urological opinion should be sought. No further courses should be given until the patient has fully recovered.

Pharmaceutical precautions Store below 25°C; protect from light. The solution for parenteral use should be used within eight hours of preparation.

Legal category POM.

Package quantities
10 mg tablets in containers of 100.
50 mg tablets in containers of 100.
100 mg dry vials in boxes of 10.
200 mg dry vials in boxes of 10.
500 mg dry vials, singles.
1,000 mg dry vials, singles.

Further information The dosage regimen for Uromitexan varies according to the dose of Endoxana administered. In general, Uromitexan is given as 60% w/w of the dose of i.v. Endoxana in three equal doses of 20% at 0, 4 and 8 hours. With the higher doses of Endoxana, the dose and frequency of administration may need to be increased. Full prescribing information is available on the Uromitexan data sheet or on request from Boehringer Ingelheim Hospital Division.

Product licence numbers

Tablets of 10 mg	1416/5011
Tablets of 50 mg	1416/5012
Vials of 100 mg	1416/5013
Vials of 200 mg	1416/5014
Vials of 500 mg	1416/5015
Vials of 1,000 mg	1416/5016.

HONVAN*

Presentation White tablets marked $\frac{WBP}{H}$ on one side containing tetrasodium fosfestrol 100 mg and 5 ml ampoules containing tetrasodium fosfestrol 276 mg.

Uses *Action:* Honvan is a water-soluble synthetic oestrogen which is inert until activated by dephosphorylation at sites of high phosphatase (particularly acid phosphatase) activity, releasing high local concentrations of oestrogen which have been demonstrated to exert a cytotoxic effect in animals. The localisation of activity reduces systemic effects, in particular adrenal hypertrophy, often associated with conventional hormonal treatment. Honvan administered in lower oral doses is comparable with conventional hormonal therapy.

Indications: Honvan is a cytotoxic drug for the treatment of all stages of prostatic carcinoma. Honvan may be used as an adjuvant to surgery, in inoperable cases and for the reduction of pain due to metastases. Patients who are resistant to conventional hormone therapy have responded to Honvan. Where acute retention has occurred the use of Honvan may reduce the need for transurethral resection.

Dosage and administration Honvan is inert until activated by dephosphorylation. However, as with all cytotoxics, it is suggested that reconstitution should be performed by trained personnel in a designated area. Those handling the preparation should wear protective gloves. Care should be taken to avoid splashing materials into the eyes. The material should not be handled by women who are pregnant. Adequate care and precautions should be taken in the disposal of items (syringes, needles, etc.) used to reconstitute cytotoxic drugs.

Initial therapy: Acute retention of urine and Relapse: 2–4 ampoules Honvan intravenously as a single injection daily for at least five days or until a response has been obtained (seven to ten days). The patient should preferably be lying down and the injection given slowly, directly into the vein. Slow infusions are not recommended as high local cytotoxic levels may not be achieved.

Maintenance: 1 ampoule intravenously one to four times weekly.

Oral maintenance therapy is usually 1–6 tablets daily in divided doses. The initial dose should be up to 2 tablets three times daily for the first week, reducing over the next two weeks to the lowest dose that will control the disease which is usually from 1 to 3 tablets daily in divided doses.

No specific information on the use of this product in the elderly is available. Clinical trials have included patients over 65 years and no adverse reactions specific to this age group have been reported.

Contra-indications, warnings, etc There are no absolute contra-indications to the use of Honvan. Honvan should only be administered under the direction of a specialist oncology service having facilities for the regular monitoring of clinical, biochemical and haematological effects during and after administration.

Caution is advised when using Honvan in patients with poor cardiac reserve or fluid retention, and in these cases concomitant diuretic therapy may be indicated. In rare cases hypersensitivity to Honvan has been noted.

Honvan should not be administered to pregnant women as oestrogens have been shown to produce a teratogenic effect in the female foetus.

Side-effects: A burning in the perineum and pain in bony metastases may occur during or immediately after intravenous injection. Perineal discomfort may be reduced by prior administration of a sedative.

Nausea and vomiting may occur, but will be less severe than with hormone therapy; oedema and lung congestion have been reported, but there is no evidence of an increased incidence of cardiovascular disease. After prolonged high dosage, feminising side-effects which may occur, due to leak of oestrogen from sites of dephosphorylation, will be less marked than those occurring during conventional hormonal therapy.

Honvan is non-irritant to the veins and should an injection accidentally enter the paravenous tissue no specific action is necessary.

Overdosage: In the event of overdosage, monitoring for fluid retention should be undertaken and in patients with

cardiac disease, the administration of diuretics and digitalis should be considered.

Pharmaceutical precautions Store in a cool place. Incompatible with aqueous solutions of pH less than 7 and solutions containing calcium or magnesium ions.

Legal category POM.

Package quantities Ampoules in boxes of 10 × 5 ml. Tablets in containers of 100.

Further information Response to treatment with Honvan may be objectively assessed by the degree of reduction in plasma acid phosphatase concentrations and by the reduction in size of: the primary prostatic tumour, cutaneous, subcutaneous or lymph node metastases, bone lesions or visceral metastases. Subjective assessment may be made by the reduction in pain, improvement in urinary function and improvement in patient well-being.

Product licence numbers
Honvan Tablets   1416/5023
Honvan Ampoules   1416/5022

MEXITIL*

Presentation *Mexitil Capsules 200 mg:* Red/red hard gelatin capsules imprinted with the notation 200 mg and the Company symbol. Each capsule contains mexiletine hydrochloride 200 mg.

Mexitil Capsules 50 mg: Red/purple hard gelatin capsules imprinted with the notation 50 mg and the Company symbol. Each capsule contains mexiletine hydrochloride 50 mg.

Mexitil Ampoules: Ampoules for intravenous injection. Each ampoule contains mexiletine hydrochloride 250 mg in 10 ml.

Uses *Action:* Mexitil is an anti-arrhythmic agent which depresses the maximum rate of depolarisation with little or no modification of resting potentials or the duration of action potentials.

Indications: For the treatment of existing or anticipated ventricular arrhythmias and ectopic beats such as those found after myocardial infarction and in ischaemic heart disease. Also for ventricular arrhythmias induced by digitalis or other drugs and for idiopathic and other ventricular arrhythmic states. It has been given in conjunction with, or after, other anti-arrhythmic preparations and also other drugs acting on the cardiovascular system.

Dosage and administration

1. *Intravenous Mexitil:*

(a) *Loading dose:* IV injection of 4–10 ml (100–250 mg) Mexitil given at a suggested rate of 1 ml per minute (25 mg per minute).
Then
add 500 mg (2 ampoules) Mexitil to 500 ml of a suitable infusion solution (see 'Pharmaceutical Precautions'). Administer the first 250 ml by IV infusion over 1 hour (4 ml per minute).
Then
administer the second 250 ml by IV infusion over 2 hours (2 ml per minute).

(b) *Maintenance dose:* Add 250 mg (1 ampoule) Mexitil to 500 ml of a suitable infusion solution (see 'Pharmaceutical Precautions'). Administer by IV infusion at a suggested rate of 1 ml per minute (0.5 mg per minute), according to patient response. Continue for as long as required or until oral maintenance therapy is commenced.

2. *Oral Mexitil*

(a) *Loading dose:* Give 400 mg Mexitil.

(b) *Maintenance dose:* Give 200–250 mg Mexitil three to four times daily commencing 2 hours after the loading dose. The usual daily dose is between 600–800 mg in divided doses.

Note: In acute myocardial infarction and particularly when opiates have been given, absorption may be delayed and therefore a larger loading dose e.g. 600 mg may be preferable.

3. *Alternative loading dose regimes*

(a) *Combination IV Mexitil and Oral Mexitil loading dose:* IV injection of 8 ml (200 mg) Mexitil given at a suggested rate of 1 ml per minute. On completion of injection or infusion give 400 mg Mexitil orally.
    Maintenance dose.
    As in 2b.

(b) *Combination IV Lignocaine and Oral Mexitil loading dose:* Give IV lignocaine according to manufacturer's instructions.
    On completion of injection give 400 mg Mexitil orally.
    Maintenance dose.
    As in 2b.

4. *Change over from IV to Oral Mexitil maintenance:* On discontinuing the IV infusion commence the maintenance dose. Give 200–250 mg Mexitil orally three or four times a day.

Notes:

1. The loading dose regime is designed to compensate for the rapid phase of tissue distribution which occurs especially with IV loading.

2. Side-effects are more likely to be encountered during the initial tissue loading phase in which case the rate of infusion should be reduced.

3. If the optimum therapeutic effect is not achieved the rate of infusion or oral dosage may be increased, side-effects permitting.

4. Gastric emptying time may be delayed in patients with myocardial infarction and/or to whom opiates have been given and thus it may be necessary to titrate the dose against therapeutic effects and side-effects.

5. The 50 mg capsule is available in order that a more precise dose titration may be undertaken should this be required. Smaller increments will also reduce the incidence of side-effects.

No specific information on the use of this product in the elderly is available. Clinical trials have included patients over 65 years and no adverse reactions specific to this age group have been reported.

Contra-indications, warnings, etc

Contra-indications: In view of the conditions in which ventricular arrhythmias may be encountered there are no specific exclusions or contra-indications. However, if the drug is used in the following situations, the patient should be carefully monitored; sinus node dysfunction, conduction defect, bradycardia, hypotension or cardiac, renal or hepatic failure. There may be potentiation of tremor in patients with Parkinsonism.

Precautions: Because of the conditions in which Mexitil is used, patients will usually be under observation with particular regard to ECG and blood pressure. Routine laboratory monitoring is also advisable although disturbance of renal and hepatic function or appearance of anti-nuclear factor have not been a feature even of long-term treatment.

The duration of treatment required in any patient is of necessity variable, and although no precise guide can be given, withdrawal of treatment may be attempted after a suitable period free of arrhythmia. Gradual withdrawal, i.e. over 1–2 weeks, is preferable as arrhythmias which have been satisfactorily controlled may recur.

Although Mexitil has been in general use for several years, there is no definite evidence of ill-consequence during human pregnancy; animal studies have shown no hazard. Nevertheless, medicines should not be used in pregnancy, especially the first trimester, unless the expected benefit is thought to outweigh any possible risk to the foetus.

Side-effects: Side-effects are mainly related to blood concentration and may therefore be seen during the initial phases of both IV and oral treatment when fluctuation may occur before the blood and tissue concentrations reach equilibrium. Reducing the rate of injection or infusion or delaying the next oral dose allows the blood concentration to fall and usually reduces side-effects. Generally side-effects are of three types:

Gastro-intestinal – nausea, vomiting, indigestion, unpleasant taste, hiccoughs.

Central nervous system – light-headedness, drowsiness, confusion, dizziness, diplopia, blurred vision, nystagmus, dysarthria, ataxia, tremor, paraesthesiae, convulsion, psychiatric disorders.

Cardiovascular – hypotension, sinus bradycardia, atrial fibrillation, palpitation.

Rash and jaundice have also been reported.

Side-effects can usually be reversed by reducing dosage. When hypotension has occurred this has tended to be in patients with severe illness who have already been given a variety of anti-arrhythmic or other preparations and, if associated with bradycardia, may be reversed by the use of atropine. Animal studies using toxic doses have shown that benzodiazepines (diazepam) reduce the CNS effects.

Overdosage: The minimum fatal dose is unknown but 4.40 g proved fatal in a healthy young adult.

The clinical features include nausea, vomiting, drowsiness, confusion, ataxia and convulsions. Blurred vision and paraesthesiae have also been reported. Hypotension, sinus bradycardia, atrial fibrillation and cardiac arrest are more specific effects.

Gastric lavage should be performed where appropriate and the patient should be transferred to an intensive/coronary care unit for possible cardiopulmonary support. Arrhythmias should be treated as appropriate and diazepam may be useful to control convulsions.

Pharmaceutical precautions Mexitil solution for injection is known to be compatible with the following infusion solutions: sodium chloride 0.9%; sodium chloride 0.9% with potassium chloride 0.3% or 0.6%; dextrose 5%; sodium bicarbonate 1.4%; sodium lactate (M/6).

Legal category POM.

Package quantities

    Capsules 200 mg: pack of 100.
    Capsules 50 mg: pack of 100.

Ampoules 250 mg in 10 ml: pack of 5.

Further information Mexitil has been used successfully within a few hours of myocardial infarction. Concomitant IV therapy with other local anaesthetic type anti-arrhythmic agents such as lignocaine or procainamide is not recommended, although no problems have been encountered using oral mexiletine in conjunction with these drugs. Mexitil may be used concurrently with digoxin and beta-adrenergic blocking drugs.

Mexitil is also available as Mexitil PL Perlongets, each containing 360 mg mexiletine hydrochloride in sustained release form.

Product licence numbers

Mexitil Capsules 200 mg	0015/0064
Mexitil Capsules 50 mg	0015/0062
Mexitil Ampoules 250 mg in 10 ml	0015/0065

MEXITIL* PL PERLONGETS*

Presentation Mexitil PL Perlongets: Turquoise/scarlet hard gelatin capsules. Each Perlonget contains 5 mini-tablets constituting 360 mg mexiletine hydrochloride in sustained release form.

Uses
Action: Mexitil is an anti-arrhythmic agent which depresses the maximum rate of depolarisation with little or no modification of resting potentials or the duration of action potentials.

Indications: For the treatment of existing or anticipated ventricular arrhythmias and ectopic beats such as those found after myocardial infarction and in ischaemic heart disease. Also for ventricular arrhythmias induced by digitalis or other drugs and for idiopathic and other ventricular arrhythmic states. It has been given in conjunction with, or after, other anti-arrhythmic preparations and also other drugs acting on the cardiovascular system.

Dosage and administration One Mexitil PL capsule twice daily (twelve hourly) will maintain therapeutic blood levels of mexiletine. If this regimen is used initially in new patients, therapeutic blood levels of mexiletine will be achieved after about 36 hours. If a more rapid effect is required, one of the following loading doses may be used:

(a) Two Mexitil PL capsules. This will give therapeutic blood levels of mexiletine within 6 hours.

(b) One Mexitil PL capsule together with 250 mg Mexitil as conventional capsules. This will give therapeutic blood levels of mexiletine within 2½ hours.

(c) Intravenous loading dose. See Mexitil capsules and injection data sheet for details. This will give therapeutic blood levels of mexiletine within 5 minutes.

No specific information on the use of this product in the elderly is available. Clinical trials have included patients over 65 years and no adverse reactions specific to this age group have been reported.

Contra-indications, warnings, etc
Contra-indications: In view of the conditions in which ventricular arrhythmias may be encountered there are no specific exclusions or contra-indications. However, if the drug is used in the following situations, the patient should be carefully monitored: sinus node dysfunction; conduction defect; bradycardia; or cardiac, renal or hepatic failure. There may be potentiation of tremor in patients with Parkinsonism.

Precautions: Because of the conditions in which Mexitil is used, patients will usually be under observation with particular regard to ECG and blood pressure.

Routine laboratory monitoring is also advisable although disturbance of renal and hepatic function or appearance of anti-nuclear factor have not been a feature even of long-term treatment.

The duration of treatment required in any patient is of necessity variable, and although no precise guide can be given, withdrawal of treatment may be attempted after a suitable period free of arrhythmia.

Gradual withdrawal, i.e. over one to two weeks, is preferable as arrhythmias which have been satisfactorily controlled may recur.

Although Mexitil has been in general use for several years, there is no definite evidence of ill-consequence during human pregnancy; animal studies have shown no hazard. Nevertheless, medicines should not be used in pregnancy, especially the first trimester, unless the expected benefit is thought to outweigh the risk to the foetus.

Side-effects: Side-effects of Mexitil are mainly related to blood concentration and may therefore be seen during the initial phases of treatment when fluctuation may occur before the blood and tissue concentrations reach equilibrium. Delaying the next oral dose allows the blood concentration to fall and usually reduces side-effects. Generally, side-effects are of three types:

gastro-intestinal – nausea, vomiting, indigestion, unpleasant taste, hiccoughs.

central nervous system – light-headedness, drowsiness, confusion, dizziness, diplopia, blurred vision, nystagmus, dysarthria, ataxia, tremor, paraesthesiae, convulsion, psychiatric disorders.

cardiovascular – hypotension, sinus bradycardia, atrial fibrillation, palpitation

Rash and jaundice have also been reported.

Side-effects can usually be reversed by reducing dosage. When hypotension has occured this has tended to be in patients with severe illness who have already been given a variety of anti-arrhythmic or other preparations and, if associated with bradycardia, may be reversed by the use of atropine. Animal studies using toxic doses have shown that benzodiazepines (diazepam) reduce the CNS effects.

Overdosage: The minimum fatal dose is unknown but 4.40 g (as conventional Mexitil capsules) proved fatal in a healthy adult.

The clinical features include: nausea, vomiting, drowsines, confusion, ataxia and convulsion. Blurred vision and paraesthesiae have also been reported. Hypotension, sinus bradycardia, atrial fibrillation and cardiac arrest are more specific effects.

Gastric lavage should be performed where appropriate and the patients should be transferred to an intensive/coronary care unit for possible cardio-pulmonary support. Arrhythmias should be treated as appropriate and diazepam may be useful to control convulsions.

Legal category POM.

Package quantities 60 capsules in blister strips of 10.

Further information Mexitil has been used successfully within a few hours of myocardial infarction. No problems have been encountered using oral mexiletine in conjunction with other local anaesthetic type anti-arrhythmic agents such as lignocaine or procainamide, but their concurrent IV use is not recommended. Mexitil may be used concurrently with digoxin and β-adreno-ceptor blocking drugs.

Mexitil is also available as capsules containing 50 mg or 200 mg mexiletine hydrochloride, and as ampoules for intravenous administration containing 250 mg mexiletine hydrochloride in 10 ml

Product licence number Mexitil PL Perlongets 0015/0084

MITOXANA*

Presentation White powder for injection in vials containing ifosfamide 500 mg, 1 g or 2 g for dissolving in Water for Injections using the volume recommended for each strength.

Uses *Action:* Mitoxana is an alkylating agent which is inert until activated by microsomal enzymes. This occurs mainly in the liver, producing antitumour metabolites.

Indications: Clinical experience so far has shown Mitoxana to be effective in tumours of lung, ovary, cervix, breast and testis and in soft tissue sarcoma. Responses have also been reported in osteosarcoma, malignant lymphomas, carcinoma of the pancreas, and in head and neck tumours.

Mitoxana has been used as a single agent and in combination with radiotherapy, surgery and other cyto-toxic agents.

Dosage and administration Mitoxana should be used only by clinicians experienced in the use of cytotoxic drugs. Mitoxana is inert until activated by enzymes in the liver. However, as with all cytotoxics, it is suggested that reconstitution should be performed by trained personnel, in a designated area. Those handling the preparation should wear protective gloves. Care should be taken to avoid splashing material into the eyes. The material should not be handled by women who are pregnant. Adequate care and precautions should be taken in the disposal of items (syringes, needles, etc.) used to reconstitute cytotoxic drugs.

Dosage: Mitoxana should not be used without the concurrent administration of mesna (Uromitexan). The dosage of mesna is discussed under Further information.

The dose of Mitoxana varies considerably depending on the clinical indication and the regimen employed. The usual total dose for each course is either 8–10 g/m², which is equally fractionated as single daily doses over five days, or 5–6 g/m² (maximum 10 g) given as a twenty-four hour infusion. Courses are normally repeated at intervals of 2–4 weeks for intermittent therapy or 3–4 weeks for 24-hour infusions depending on the haematological and biochemical status of the patient. The white cell count should not be less than 4000/mm³ or the platelet count less than 100,000/mm³ before the start of each course. There should be no signs or symptoms of urothelial toxicity or renal or hepatic impairment.

The usual number of courses given is four but up to seven (six by 24-hour infusion) courses have been given. Re-treatment has been given following relapse.

Experience in children is limited and involves the five day regimen only.

Administration: The dry contents of a vial should be dissolved in Water for Injections as follows:

500 mg vial:	add 6.5 ml of Water for Injections.	
1 g	vial:	add 12.5 ml of Water for Injections.
2 g	vial:	add 25 ml of Water for Injections.

The resultant solution of 8% ifosfamide should not be injected directly into the vein. The solution may be:

1. diluted to less than a 4% solution and injected directly into the vein, with the patient supine, or
2. infused in 5% dextrose-saline or normal saline over 30–120 mins or
3. injected directly into a fast-running infusion or
4. made up in 3 litres of dextrose-saline or normal saline and infused over 24 hours. Each litre should be given over eight hours, and should be freshly made up immediately before infusion.

Should the drug accidentally be given extravenously, local tissue damage is unlikely and no specific measures need to be taken. Repeated intravenous injections of large doses of Mitoxana have resulted in local irritation.

Mesna (Uromitexan) should be used to prevent urothelial toxicity. Patients should be maintained in fluid balance, replacement fluids being given as necessary to achieve this. The fluid intake of patients on the intermittent regimen should not be less than 2L in 24 hours. As Mitoxana may exert an antidiuretic effect, a diuretic may be necessary to ensure an adequate urinary output.

Urine should be sent for laboratory analysis before, and at the end of, each course of treatment, and the patient should be monitored for output and evidence of proteinuria and haematuria at regular intervals (4-hourly if possible) throughout the treatment period. The patient should be instructed to report any signs or symptoms of cystitis.

Antiemetics administered before and during treatment may reduce nausea and vomiting. Oral hygiene is important.

No specific information on the use of this product in the elderly is available. Clinical trials have included patients over 65 years and no adverse reactions specific to this age group have been reported.

Contra-indications, warnings, etc

Contra-indications: Mitoxana is contra-indicated in patients with known hypersensitivity, bone marrow aplasia, myelosuppression, infections including urinary tract infections or acute urothelial toxicity, renal impairment (serum creatinine above 120 μmol/l i.e. 1.5 mg/100 ml), or hepatic impairment (bilirubin above 17 μmol/l i.e. 1 mg/100 ml, with alkaline phosphatase or transaminases more than 2–3 times normal).

Contraception in both sexes is advised during Mitoxana therapy. Patients should receive counselling with respect to subsequent pregnancies. Mitoxana should not be given in pregnancy, especially the first trimester, unless the expected benefit is thought to outweigh the substantial risk to the foetus. Mothers should not breast-feed whilst being treated with Mitoxana.

Precautions: Mitoxana has been shown to be mutagenic, teratogenic and carcinogenic in laboratory tests and there is a risk of drug-induced neoplasia following long-term treatment. Amenorrhoea and azoospermia can occur. Patients should be warned of a potential risk to future progeny.

Mitoxana is a potent immunosuppressive drug and the increased risk to a patient should be borne in mind.

Care should be exercised in patients who are elderly, debilitated, have diabetes mellitus or evidence of myelosuppression or who have recently received radiotherapy or cytotoxic drugs. Caution is necessary in patients who have undergone nephrectomy.

Side-effects: Urothelial toxicity is the usual dose-limiting factor. This can be largely prevented by the concurrent administration of mesna.

Urotoxicity can affect the efferent urinary tract as well as the bladder. The usual symptoms are frequency, dysuria, or haematuria, but oliguria, raised uric acid and creatinine, glycosuria and changes in serum proteins and electrolytes have also been reported.

Nausea and vomiting. Anti-emetic administration before and during treatment may reduce this.

Large doses of Mitoxana give rise to a predictable marrow toxicity. The white cell count reaches its nadir 5–10 days after commencing treatment, recovery commencing after 10–14 days and usually returning to normal within 2–3 weeks. About 30% of patients would be expected to have a fall in haemoglobin of greater than 2 g/100 ml and a white cell count less than 2000/mm^3 but only 5% would be expected to have a platelet count less than 100,000/mm^3. There have been only occasional reports of coagulation disorders.

Central nervous system side effects may occur. Confusion and lethargy have been most commonly reported but tonic-clonic spasms, motor unrest, emotional lability and disorientation have also been noted. These resolve spontaneously 1–2 days after cessation of the therapy.

A much rarer event involving EEG changes, fever, tachycardia, confusion, echolalia, disorientation, some aggression and depression of consciousness has been reported. Occasionally this has been fatal. If such effects occur, the drug should be stopped and supportive therapy given.

Alopecia occurs frequently but is usually reversible.

Reversible changes in liver function have been reported and jaundice has occurred in one patient. Other side-effects reported are stomatitis, diarrhoea, pulmonary fibrosis, allergy, dermatitis, and venous irritation.

Overdosage: The most serious consequences of overdosage are haemorrhagic cystitis and myelosuppression. The latter usually recovers spontaneously but until it does, administration of a broad spectrum antibiotic may be advisable. Transfusions of whole blood should be given as necessary.

If the overdose is recognised within the first 24 hours and possibly up to 48 hours, i.v. mesna may be beneficial in ameliorating damage to the urinary system.

Normal supportive measures such as analgesics and maintenance of fluid balance should be instituted. If despite these measures the cystitis does not resolve, more intensive treatment may be necessary and a urological opinion should be sought. No further courses should be given until the patient has fully recovered.

Pharmaceutical precautions Store below 25˚C; protect from light.

Legal category POM.

Package quantities 500 mg, 1 g and 2 g dry vials, singles.

Further information Mitoxana is not recommended for use in non-malignant conditions. The dosage of mesna (Uromitexan) varies according to its route of administration and the dose and route of administration of Mitoxana. The Uromitexan data sheet shoud be consulted for full prescribing information before comm-

encing treatment. Further information is available from Boehringer Ingelheim Hospital Division.

Product licence numbers
Vials of 500 mg   1416/0015
Vials of 1 g   1416/0016
Vials of 2 g   1416/0017

MYDRILATE*

Presentation Isotonic, sterile, aqueous solutions of Cyclopentolate Hydrochloride BP 0.5% and 1.0% w/v buffered to pH5 and containing 0.01% w/v benzalkonium chloride.

Uses *Action:* A cycloplegic and mydriatic agent: it produces paralysis of the iris sphincter and ciliary muscle by local anticholinergic action.

Indications: The primary indication is refraction, but Mydrilate may be used whenever mydriasis is required for diagnosis or treatment, e.g. in corneal ulceration, keratitis, iritis, iridocyclitis, choroiditis, especially where atropine or homatropine cannot be used.

Dosage and administration *Refraction: Adults (16 and over):* 1 drop of 0.5% solution. Repeat in 15–20 minutes only if no apparent effect is produced.

Children (6 to 16 years): 1 drop of 1% solution. Repeat in five minutes. Refraction can be carried out 40–50 minutes after instillation.

Under 6 years: 1 or 2 drops of 1% solution 40–50 minutes before refraction. It may sometimes by necessary to instil 1 drop in the evening before examination.

Mydriasis: 1 drop of 0.5% or 1% solution as required.

Treatment: 1–2 drops of 0.5% or 1% solution as required.

Cycloplegia following administration is quick in onset and short-lived. Maximal cycloplegia is achieved within 15–45 minutes of instillation, and lasts on average about 20 minutes. Recovery normally takes place in about four hours, but very occasionally some effect persists for up to 24 hours.

Mydriasis is produced very rapidly and an average pupil diameter of 7 mm is usually reached 15–30 minutes after instillation of 1 drop of 0.5% solution. Complete recovery from the mydriatic effect generally occurs spontaneously in not more than 20 hours.

No specific information on the use of this product in the elderly is available. Clinical trials have included patients over 65 years and no adverse reactions specific to this age group have been reported.

Contra-indications, warnings, etc Where intraocular pressure is high, caution should be observed, but the effect on tension is less and does not last as long as that produced by conventional cycloplegic mydriatic drugs.

Caution should be observed when drugs of this group are administered to patients with prostatic enlargement, coronary insufficiency or cardiac failure. They are contra-indicated in patients with paralytic ileus. Systemic side-effects have rarely been reported, but have included ataxia and other atropine-like effects. Physostigmine Eye Drops BNF or any miotic agent will reverse the effect of Mydrilate.

Although Mydrilate has been in wide general use for many years, there is no evidence of ill-consequence during human pregnancy.

Medicines should not be used in pregnancy especially the first trimester, unless the expected benefit is thought to outweigh any possible risk to the foetus.

Overdosage: Symptoms of overdose include dry mouth,

tachycardia, dilated pupils, ataxia, nightmares and other atropine-like effects. Treat with gastric lavage where appropriate. Neostigmine by injection may be necessary.

Pharmaceutical precautions Store in a cool place. The BPC recommends that when eye drops are dispensed for domiciliary use a caution should be given to the user to avoid contamination during use and not to use the eye drops later than one month after first opening the container. When eye drops are used in hospital wards, a separate container should be provided for each patient, and, when both eyes are being treated, a separate container for each eye. They should be discarded not later than one week after first opening the container. In out-patient and casualty departments, opened containers should be discarded at the end of each day, but each patient who has undergone out-patient surgery should be treated with a separate supply of the drops. In operating theatres, a previously unopened container should be used for each patient.

Legal category POM.

Package quantities 5 ml dropper bottles of 0.5% and 1.0% solutions.

Further information Mydrilate is non-irritant and sensitivity reactions are uncommon. The onset of cycloplegia is at least as fast as that obtained by any other preparation for the purpose. In the normal eye it has little or no effect on intra-ocular tension.

Product licence numbers
Mydrilate 0.5%   1416/5030
Mydrilate 1.0%   1416/5031

UROMITEXAN* ▼

Presentation Clear, glass ampoules containing a clear, colourless, aqueous solution of mesna (sodium 2-mercapto-ethanesulphonate) 400 mg in 4 ml and 1000 mg in 10 ml.

Uses *Action:* Mesna is a sulphydryl-containing compound which is excreted in the urine. Co-administration with oxazaphosphorine alkylating agents such as ifosfamide (Mitoxana) and cyclophosphamide (Endoxana) significantly reduces the troublesome urotoxic effects of these by reacting with the causal metabolites, including acrolein, in the urinary system. No reduction in the antitumour activity of these oxazaphosphorine compounds has been detected.

Indications: For the prophylaxis of urothelial toxicity in patients treated with ifosamide and cyclophosphamide.

Dosage and administration Sufficient mesna must be given to protect the patient adequately from the urotoxic effects of the oxazaphosphorine. When calculating the dose of mesna the quantity should be rounded up to the nearest whole ampoule.

Urinary output should be maintained and the urine monitored for haematuria and proteinuria throughout the treatment period.

Where ifosfamide or cyclophosphamide is used as an i.v. bolus: Mesna is given by intravenous injection over 15–30 minutes as 20% of the simultaneously administered oxazaphosphorine on a weight for weight basis (w/w). The same dose of mesna is repeated after 4 and 8 hours. The total dose of mesna is 60% (w/w) of the oxazaphosphorine dose. This is repeated on each occasion that the cytotoxic agents are used.

If necessary the dose of mesna can be increased to 40% of the oxazaphosphorine dose given four times at three hourly intervals (0, 3, 6 and 9 hours). (Total dose = 160% (w/w) of the oxazaphosphorine dose). This larger dose is recommended in children, in patients whose urothelium may be damaged from previous treatment with oxazaphosphorine or pelvic irradiation, or in patients who are not adequately protected by the standard dose of mesna.

Where ifosfamide is used as a 24-hour infusion: Mesna can be used as a concurrent infusion. An initial 20% (w/w) of the total ifosfamide dose is given as an i.v. bolus, then an infusion of 100% (w/w) of the ifosfamide over 24 hours, followed by a further 12-hour infusion of 60% (w/w) of the ifosfamide dose. (Total mesna dose = 180% of the ifosfamide dose).

The final 12-hour infusion of mesna may be replaced by boluses at 28, 32 and 36 hours, each of 20% (w/w) of the ifosfamide dose, or by oral mesna (see below). Mesna can be mixed in the same infusion bag as the ifosfamide.

Oral use of mesna: Mesna has been shown to be effective when taken orally with intermittent oxazaphosphorine therapy or following the 24-hour infusion of ifosfamide and mesna. The first dose of 40% (w/w) of the oxazaphosphorine is given with the oxazaphosphorine or as the infusion is stopped, and repeated after 4 and 8 hours. Mesna should be taken immediately the ampoule is opened, in a soft drink (e.g. orange juice).

No specific information on the use of this product in the elderly is available. Clinical trials have included patients over 65 years and no adverse reactions specific to this age group have been reported.

Contra-indications, warnings, etc
Contra-indications: There are no absolute contra-indications to the use of mesna.

Precautions: As mesna counteracts only the urotoxic side-effects of cyclophosphamide and ifosfamide, other side-effects of cytotoxic therapy e.g. myelosuppression, nausea, vomiting, alopecia, may still be expected. No other interaction between mesna and these alkylating agents has been demonstrated.

Side-effects: Because patients receive potent cytotoxic agents concurrently, the side-effect profile of mesna is difficult to define. However, in healthy volunteers the following side-effects occurred at single doses of 60–70 mg/kg per day, nausea, vomiting, colic diarrhoea, fatigue, headache, limb pains, depression, irritability, lack of energy and rash.

Overdosage: There is no clinical experience of overdosage. Standard supportive measures should be adopted.

Pharmaceutical precautions Protect from light, store below 30°C. Mesna is stable for up to 24-hours in a solution of sodium chloride 0.9% and of ifosfamide in sodium chloride 0.9%.

Legal category POM.

Package quantities 4 ml ampoules in boxes of 15. 10 ml ampoules in boxes of 15.

Further information There is evidence that the long term urothelial toxicity of the oxazaphosphorines can be almost totally prevented by the concurrent administration of mesna in the appropriate dosage.

A false positive test for urinary ketones (e.g. Rothera's test, N-Multistix reagent strip) may arise in patients treated with mesna. The colour is red-violet rather than violet and it will fade immediately on the addition of glacial acetic acid.

Product licence number
4 ml and 10 ml ampoules 0015/0083

WARFARIN WBP

Presentation Compressed tablets containing Warfarin Sodium BP, impressed with the letters $\frac{WBP}{W}$ one side and coloured according to strength; 1 mg–brown; 3 mg–blue, 5 mg–pink.

Uses *Action:* Oral anticoagulant.

Indications: For prophylaxis against venous thrombosis and pulmonary embolism, and for use in the treatment of these conditions to prevent their extension. For the prophylaxis of systemic embolisation in patients with rheumatic heart disease and atrial fibrillation.

Dosage and administration Effective blood levels are rapidly reached by administering an *initial loading dose* usually of the order of 0.45–0.50 mg/kg for adults.

Maintenance dosage is started when the peak effect of the initial dosage is passed, usually after 48 hours. Its size depends on the prothrombin time or other appropriate coagulation tests. The single daily maintenance requirement is usually between 5 mg and 12 mg, but can vary between 2 mg and 30 mg.

The maintenance dose is omitted if the prothrombin time is excessively prolonged. Once the maintenance dose is stabilised in the therapeutic range it is rarely necessary to alter it.

Use in elderly patients: The elderly are generally more sensitive to the effects of warfarin and often require a smaller dose on a weight for weight basis than younger patients.

Contra-indications, warnings, etc
Contra-indications: Animal studies have shown warfarin to be teratogenic and there have been reports of foetal death associated with its administration during human pregnancy. Warfarin should not be prescribed for pregnant women.

Warfarin should not be given to patients within three days of surgery.

The use in patients known to be hypersensitive to warfarin is contra-indicated.

Warnings: When warfarin therapy is first introduced, patients should be told what to do if bleeding occurs.

Warfarin should be given with caution to patients with impaired liver or kidney function or in severe hypertension.

Warfarin should be given with caution to patients where there is a risk of serious haemorrhage such as haemorrhagic blood dyscrasias, haemophilia, ulcerative disorders, threatened abortion, subacute bacterial endocarditis, in the presence of extensive surgical wounds and after recent surgery to the eye and central nervous system.

Prothrombin times should be determined at least twice weekly for the first two weeks and subsequently at longer intervals (every two to three weeks).

Overdose: Overdosage may be manifest by haematuria or spontaneous bruising. This should be treated with vitamin K_1 (5–10 mg) intravenously. Significant correction occurs within four hours. Haemorrhage or severe overdose should be treated with an infusion of fresh frozen plasma (or whole blood if the former is not available). Intravenous vitamin K_1 (5–10 mg) may be used to supplement specific therapy with factor concentrations or before minor procedures such as dental extractions. The administration of vitamin K_1 may make the patient resistant to anticoagulation for some days. For this reason, fresh frozen plasma should be administered to those patients with prosthetic heart valves.

Many factors *potentiate* the effect of warfarin:
1. Warfarin in the circulation is firmly bound to plasma protein and will have an increased effect if displaced by other drugs such as diuretics, oral anti-diabetic agents, anti-inflammatory agents and amiodarone.
2. Certain drugs, for example D-thyroxine, potentiate the effects of warfarin by increasing its affinity for the hepatic receptor site.
3. Alcohol may inhibit liver enzymes, leading to a reduced dosage requirement of warfarin.
4. Other drugs which may potentiate the effect of warfarin include anabolic steroids, cimetidine, aspirin, clofibrate, sulphinpyrazone, chloral hydrate, some aminoglycoside antibiotics, chloramphenicol, disulfiram and paracetamol.
5. Renal damage may reduce the rate of excretion of warfarin and thus decrease the dose requirement.
6. Acute illness, weight loss and a decreased intake of vitamin K will exaggerate the response.

Other factors may *decrease* the effect of warfarin:
1. Warfarin is metabolised in the liver by microsomal enzymes. These enzymes are induced by drugs such as barbiturates and phenytoin leading to rapid metabolism of warfarin and necessitating an increased dose.
2. Oestrogens and oral contraceptives increase the concentration of vitamin K-dependent factors. Increased doses of warfarin may therefore be required.
3. Cholestyramine may absorb warfarin and thus reduce its effect.
4. Weight gain, gastro-intestinal upset and increased intake of vitamin K will necessitate an increase in maintenance dosage of warfarin.
5. Carbamazepine, glutethimide, phenazone, griseofulvin and rifampicin also diminish the effect of warfarin.

Pharmaceutical precautions Protect from heat, light and moisture.

Legal category POM.

Package quantities 1 mg, 3 mg and 5 mg tablets in containers of 100 and 500.

Further information Nil.

Product licence numbers
Tablets 1 mg   1416/5060
Tablets 3 mg   1416/5061
Tablets 5 mg   1416/5062

*Trade Mark

The Boots Company PLC
1 Thane Road West
Nottingham NG2 3AA

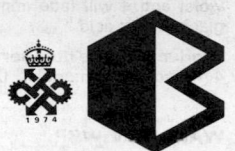

ABICOL*

Presentation Abicol is presented as pink, scored tablets, each containing Reserpine BP 0.15 mg and Bendrofluazide BP 2.5 mg.

Uses Abicol is indicated for all grades of hypertension, either alone or in conjunction with other hypotensive agents.

Dosage and administration For most cases of hypertension, half to one tablet morning and evening. If necessary, dosage may be increased up to two tablets morning and evening. When Abicol is added to an existing regimen of antihypertensive drugs, the dosage of the latter should be reduced initially.

Because of the reserpine content, Abicol is not recommended for use in the elderly.

Contra-indications, warnings, etc

Electrolyte imbalance: All the thiazide diuretics can produce some degree of electrolyte imbalance, especially in patients with renal or hepatic impairment, or when dosage is high or prolonged. Serum electrolyte levels should be checked for abnormalities, particularly hypokalaemia, this being corrected by the addition of a potassium supplement to the regimen.

Digitalis intoxication: Sensitivity to digitalis may be increased by the kaliuretic effect of concurrent bendrofluazide and patients should be observed for signs of digitalis intoxication. Should these appear, the dosage of digitalis should be reduced temporarily and a potassium supplement given to restore stability.

Uric acid retention: Thiazide diuretics may raise serum uric acid levels with consequent exacerbation of gout in susceptible subjects.

Diabetes: Thiazide derivatives sometimes lower carbohydrate tolerance and it may be necessary to adjust the insulin dosage of the diabetic patient. Care is also necessary when bendrofluazide is administered to those with a known pre-disposition to diabetes.

Pregnancy: Thiazides cross the placental barrier and it is, therefore, reasonable to assume that side-effects occurring in the adult may also develop in the foetus.

Other side-effects which may be encountered are those associated with reserpine, i.e. lethargy, vertigo, tremor, gastro-intestinal upset and nasal congestion.

Treatment of overdosage: Symptomatic and supportive; there is no specific antidote.

Pharmaceutical precautions Recommended storage conditions: 5°C to 20°C.

Legal category POM.

Package quantities Containers of 100 and 500 tablets.

Further information Bendrofluazide is an oral diuretic and antihypertensive agent which augments the antihypertensive activity of reserpine, thus allowing a smaller dose of the latter to be used. In this way, the side-effects associated with the normal therapeutic dose of reserpine are less likely to occur or are reduced in severity.

Product licence number 0014/5126.

APRINOX*

Presentation Aprinox is Bendrofluazide BP, an oral diuretic of the benzothiadiazine group. Aprinox is available as white tablets in two strengths, 2.5 mg and 5 mg.

Uses Aprinox is indicated in all cases where the reduction of fluid retention by diuresis is required – oedema of cardiac, renal or hepatic origin; premenstrual, iatrogenic and all other types of oedema.

Aprinox will produce a moderate but usefully prolonged fall of blood pressure in hypertensive patients and often gives adequate control when used alone; if necessary, Aprinox can be administered concurrently with other specific hypotensive agents, allowing a reduction in the dosage of the latter.

Aprinox will effectively inhibit lactation without the hormonal effects attendant upon stilboestrol or other oestrogens.

Dosage and administration *Diuretic:* Initially 5-10 mg once daily or on alternate days. Maintenance: 5-10 mg once or twice weekly. The dose should be taken early in the morning so as to complete diuresis by bedtime.

Hypotensive: 2.5–5 mg once daily. When Aprinox is used concurrently with other specific hypotensive agents the dose of the latter should be halved.

A suggested dosage for inhibition of lactation is 5 mg in the morning and 5 mg at midday for about five days.

Dosage in children should be at the discretion of the attending physician.

The dosage of thiazide diuretics may need to be reduced in the elderly, particularly when renal function is impaired.

Contra-indications, warnings, etc *Electrolyte imbalance:* All the thiazide diuretics can produce a degree of electrolyte imbalance, especially in patients with renal or hepatic impairment, or when dosage is high or prolonged. Serum electrolyte levels should be checked for abnormalities, particularly hypokalaemia, and the latter corrected by the addition of a potassium supplement to the regimen.

Note: Apinox does not contain a potassium supplement.

Digitalis intoxication: Sensitivity to digitalis may be increased by the kaliuretic effect of concurrent bendrofluazide. Patients should be observed for signs of digitalis intoxication; if these appear, the dosage of digitalis should be temporarily reduced and a potassium supplement given to restore stability.

Uric acid retention: The thiazide diuretics may raise serum uric acid levels with consequent exacerbation of gout in susceptible subjects.

Diabetes: Thiazide derivatives sometimes lower carbohydrate tolerance and the insulin dosage of the diabetic patient may require adjustment. Care is necessary when bendrofluazide is administered to those with a known predisposition to diabetes.

Pregnancy: Thiazides cross the placental barrier; therefore it is reasonable to assume that side-effects occurring in the adult may also appear in the neonate.

Pharmaceutical precautions Recommended storage conditions: 5–20°C.

Legal category POM.

Package quantities Bottles of 100 and 500 tablets.

Further information A single dose of Aprinox will induce a diuresis extending over 12–18 hours – a period which can be contained within the patient's normal working day, leaving the night undisturbed. Simple dosage schedules, a low incidence of side-effects and economy in prescribing have established Aprinox as one of the most useful general-purpose diuretics.

Product licence numbers
Aprinox 2.5 mg   0014/5117
Aprinox 5 mg   0014/5118

BRUFEN*

Presentation Brufen is available as sugar-coated tablets containing either 200 mg or 400 mg of Ibuprofen BP. It is also available as Brufen 600, film-coated tablets each containing 600 mg of Ibuprofen BP.

The tablets are light-magenta in colour. The 200 mg tablets bear the overprint 'Brufen' in black; the 400 mg tablets are overprinted 'Brufen 400' and the 600 mg tablets 'Brufen 600' also in black.

For children, and for adults who have a difficulty in swallowing tablets, Brufen is presented as Brufen Syrup, an orange flavoured liquid containing 100 mg of Ibuprofen BP in each 5 ml.

Uses Brufen is indicated for its analgesic and anti-inflammatory effect in the treatment of rheumatoid arthritis (including juvenile rheumatoid arthritis or Still's disease), ankylosing spondylitis, osteoarthritis and other non-rheumatoid (seronegative) arthropathies.

In the treatment of non-articular rheumatic conditions, Brufen is indicated in periarticular conditions such as frozen shoulder (capsulitis), bursitis, tendinitis, tenosynovitis and low-back pain; Brufen can also be used in soft-tissue injuries such as sprains and strains.

Brufen is indicated for its analgesic effect in the relief of mild to moderate pain such as dysmenorrhoea, dental and post-operative pain and in the relief of migraine.

Dosage and administration

Adult: The recommended initial dosage of Brufen is 1200 mg daily in divided doses. Some patients can be maintained on 600 to 1200 mg daily. In severe or acute conditions it can be advantageous to increase the dosage until the acute phase is brought under control, provided that the total daily dosage does not exceed 2400 mg in divided doses.

Children: The daily dosage of Brufen is 20 mg per kg of body-weight in divided doses. In juvenile rheumatoid arthritis up to 40 mg per kg of body-weight daily in divided doses may be taken. In children weighing less than 30 kg the total dose given in 24 hours should not exceed 500 mg.

Elderly: No special dosage modifications are required for elderly patients, unless renal or hepatic function is impaired, in which case dosage should be assessed individually.

Contra-indications, warnings, etc Brufen should not be given to patients with severe or active peptic ulceration. Bronchospasm may be precipitated in patients suffering from, or with a previous history of, bronchial asthma. Brufen should not be given to patients in whom aspirin and other non-steroidal anti-inflammatory drugs induce the symptoms of asthma, rhinitis or urticaria.

Adverse effects reported include: Dyspepsia, gastrointestinal intolerance and bleeding, and skin rashes of various types. Less frequently, thrombocytopenia has occurred.

Use in pregnancy and lactation: Whilst no teratogenic effects have been demonstrated in animal experiments, the use of Brufen during pregnancy should, if possible, be avoided. In the limited studies so far available, Brufen appears in the breast milk in very low concentration and is unlikely to affect the breast-fed infant adversely.

Drug interactions: In therapeutic doses, no evidence of interaction with other commonly used drugs has so far been observed. However, as with other non-steroidal anti-inflammatory agents, caution should be exercised in patients receiving β-blockers and thiazide diuretics.

Interference with laboratory tests: There is no evidence so far that ibuprofen interferes with laboratory tests.

Treatment of overdosage: Gastric lavage and, if necessary, correction of serum electrolytes. There is no specific antidote to Brufen.

Pharmaceutical precautions Brufen 600 (600 mg tablets) and Brufen Syrup should be stored below 25°C.

Legal category POM.

Package quantities
Brufen 600 (600 mg tablets): pack of 100
Brufen 400 (400 mg tablets): pack of 100, pack of 250
Brufen Tablets (200 mg): pack of 100, pack of 500
Brufen Syrup: Bottle of 200 ml.

Further information Taken on an empty stomach, peak serum levels of Brufen occur 45 minutes after ingestion whereas, taken after a meal, the peak is delayed up to 90 minutes. Since most people can take Brufen on an empty stomach without gastric discomfort, the initial dose of the day will be more rapidly effective if taken before food. This is particularly valuable in providing relief of the morning stiffness associated with arthritis.

Product licence numbers
Brufen 600 Tablets   0014/0264
Brufen 400 Tablets   0014/0158

Brufen Tablets 200 mg   0014/5132
Brufen Syrup   0014/0217

CHLORPROPAMIDE – BOOTS

Presentation Chlorpropamide – Boots is available as white, scored tablets each containing either 100 mg (7 mm diameter) or 250 mg (9.5 mm diameter) of Chlorpropamide BP.

Uses Chlorpropamide is indicated for the treatment of mild or moderately severe uncomplicated diabetes mellitus of the stable, non-ketotic, maturity-onset or adult type. It should not be used to replace dietetic therapy in the obese diabetic patient.

Dosage and administration Generally, chlorpropamide should be given as a single dose each morning before breakfast. The initial dose is 250–500 mg daily and this should be reduced to a maintenance level as soon as possible. In elderly patients, a smaller dose is advisable.

In establishing the optimal dosage for a particular patient, it should be borne in mind that it may take four to seven days for the hypoglycaemic response to become maximal. It may take several weeks to achieve adequate control.

Note: The daily dosage of chlorpropamide should not exceed 500 mg.

Contra-indications, warnings, etc Chlorpropamide is contra-indicated in juvenile diabetes mellitus and in unstable or severely 'brittle' type diabetes; in maturity-onset type diabetes when complicated by ketosis, fever, trauma, gangrene, or by serious impairment of renal, hepatic or thyroid function. It is also contra-indicated in pregnancy.

Caution: Chlorpropamide may cause hypoglycaemic reactions, which should be treated similarly to those occurring during insulin therapy. The hypoglycaemic effects of chlorpropamide are enhanced by dicoumarol, monoamine oxidase inhibitors, beta-blockers and salicylates; conversely, the action may be diminished by adrenalin, corticosteroids, oral contraceptives and thiazide diuretics. Alcohol should be avoided since it may cause a disulfiram-like reaction.

Side-effects: These include skin sensitisation, gastrointestinal disturbance, paraesthesias, tinnitus and headache. A rare reaction to chlorpropamide is impairment of liver function. Isolated cases of bone-marrow aplasia, including aplastic anaemia and agranulocytosis have been reported.

Treatment of overdosage: Hypoglycaemia should be treated by infusion of dextrose; treatment may have to be prolonged.

Pharmaceutical precautions None.

Legal category POM.

Package quantities *100 mg Tablets:* Bottle of 500. *250 mg Tablets:* Bottle of 500.

Product licence numbers
100 mg Tablets   0014/0175
250 mg Tablets   0014/0176

CORTISTAB*

Presentation Cortistab is available as tablets and as an injection. The tablets are Cortisone Tablets BP, containing Cortisone Acetate BP, 5 mg and 25 mg; the injection is Cortisone Injection BP containing Cortisone Acetate Injection BP 25 mg per ml.

Uses Cortisone Acetate has both glucocorticoid and mineralocorticoid properties and is used mainly for replacement therapy in chronic adrenocortical insufficiency. It can be used for other conditions requiring corticosteroid therapy.

Dosage and administration As with other corticosteroids, the dosage of Cortistab should be adjusted according to the severity, prognosis and anticipated duration of the disease, and the response of the individual patient.

In replacement therapy, the normal daily requirement is 12.5–50 mg of cortisone acetate by mouth in divided doses increased during infectious trauma or stress. In other conditions, a suggested regimen is 100 to 300 mg daily by intramuscular injection or 25 to 75 mg four times daily by mouth. When the desired degree of response has been achieved, reduce the dosage *gradually* to the lowest dose which maintains remission, usually from 25 mg to 100 mg daily. In chronic conditions, it is often better to maintain a sub-optimal response with small doses than to give high doses and produce signs of hormonal excess. After prolonged corticosteroid treatment, the function of the patient's own adrenal cortices is often suppressed. To allow normal adrenal function to be restored, Cortistab dosage should be reduced gradually, e.g. by 5 to 12.5 mg every few days. Cortisone acetate is ineffective when injected into joint capsules.

Elderly: Steroids should be used cautiously in the elderly, since adverse effects are enhanced by old age.

Contra-indications, warnings, etc The contra-indications to Cortistab therapy are those common to all forms of corticosteroid therapy. These include severe infections (unless there is adequate chemotherapy), peptic ulcer, osteoporosis, a history of recent psychotic illness and chronic renal insufficiency.

Caution is necessary in patients with diabetes mellitus, congestive heart failure or hypertension. During treatment, the patient should be observed for psychotic reactions, muscular weakness, electrocardiographic changes, hypertension and untoward hormonal effects.

Side-effects: Corticosteroids exert hormonal and metabolic effects and prolonged treatment may be attended by such side-effects as moonface, hirsutism, psychosis and gastro-intestinal disturbance.

Treatment of overdosage: Treatment is symptomatic but is unlikely to be required.

Pharmaceutical precautions Cortistab Tablets should be protected from light. Cortistab injection should be kept at a temperature not exceeding 25°C, it should not be allowed to freeze. Protect from light.

Legal category POM.

Package quantities Cortistab Tablets 5 mg: Bottle of 100. Cortistab Tablets 25 mg: Bottle of 100. Cortistab Injection: Ampoule of 10 ml.

Further information Nil.

Product licence numbers
Cortistab Tablets, 5 mg: 0014/5044.
Cortistab Tablets, 25 mg: 0014/5045.
Cortistab Injection: 0014/5408.

DELTASTAB* INJECTION

Presentation Deltastab Injection is a sterile suspension of 25 mg per ml of Prednisolone Acetate BP 1963.

Uses Deltastab Injection is intended primarily for the local treatment by intra-articular or peri-articular injection of arthritic conditions such as rheumatoid arthritis and osteoarthrosis when few joints are involved, and in traumatic arthritis, except when associated with fractures into the joint. In addition to articular use, Deltastab Injection injected into inflamed tendon sheaths and bursae will provide symptomatic treatment.

Deltastab Injection is suitable for parenteral administration by the intramuscular route in conditions requiring systemic corticosteroids.

Dosage and administration For articular use, 5 to 25 mg depending upon the size of the joint; the injections may be repeated when relapse occurs. Not more than three joints should be treated in any one day.

For parenteral use by intramuscular injection, the dosage of Deltastab Injection will depend upon the clinical circumstances and the judgement of the physician.

Suggested dosage: 25 to 100 mg once or twice weekly.

Elderly: Steroids should be used cautiously in the elderly, since adverse effects are enhanced by old age.

Contra-indications, warnings, etc Intra-articular and peri-articular injections of Deltastab Injection are contra-indicated when the joint or surrounding tissues are infected. The presence of infection also precludes injection into tendon sheaths and bursae. Deltastab Injection must not be injected directly into tendons, nor should it be injected into the spinal joints or any other than true diarthrodial joints.

Precautions: It should be borne in mind that joints and tissues injected with corticosteroids have an increased susceptibility to infection and full aseptic precautions should be observed when making local injections of Deltastab.

Side-effects: With intra-articular and other local injections, the principal side-effect encountered is a temporary local exacerbation with increased pain and swelling. Normally, this subsides after a few hours. Particularly after high or prolonged local administration corticosteroids can be absorbed in amounts sufficient to produce systemic effects.

Note: When being given by intramuscular injection, the precautions, side-effects, contra-indications and withdrawal symptoms associated with the systemic use of corticosteroids become relevant to Deltastab Injection.

Treatment of overdosage: Treatment is symptomatic, but is unlikely to be required.

Pharmaceutical precautions Store between 15°C to 20°C. Protect from light. Shake well before use.

Legal category POM.

Package quantities Vial of 5 ml.

Further information Nil.

Product licence number 0014/5137.

DIALAFLEX* SOLUTIONS 61, 62, 63

Presentation Dialaflex Solutions 61, 62 and 63 are sterile solutions specially formulated for peritoneal dialysis and are available in transparent, collapsible plastic containers of 1 litre.

The formulae of the solutions are as follows:

	Dialaflex 61 g/litre	Dialaflex 62 g/litre	Dialaflex 63 g/litre
Dextrose BP	13.6	63.6	13.6
Sodium Lactate	5.0	5.0	5.0
Sodium Chloride BP	5.6	5.6	5.0
Calcium Chloride BP	0.26	0.26	0.26
Magnesium Chloride for Dialysis BP	0.15	0.15	0.15
Sodium Metabisulphite (antioxidant)	0.05	0.12	0.05

The following table gives the solutions in terms of mEq/litre and mmol/litre:

	mEq/litre	g/litre	mmol/litre
Diaflex 61			
Sodium	140.92		140
Calcium	3.6		1.8
Magnesium	1.5		0.75
Total Chloride	100.8		100
Lactate	44.6		45
Dextrose		13.6	75
Total			364.37
Dialaflex 62			
Sodium	140.92		140
Calcium	3.6		1.8
Magnesium	1.5		0.75
Total Chloride	100.8		100
Lactate	44.6		45
Dextrose		63.6	353
Total			642.91
Dialaflex 63			
Sodium	130.52		130
Calcium	3.6		1.8
Magnesium	1.5		0.75
Total Chloride	90.5		90
Lactate	44.6		45
Dextrose		13.6	75
Total			343.67

Dialaflex Solutions are colourless.

Indications Dialaflex Solutions are indicated only for use in peritoneal dialysis. This is employed as an alternative to haemodialysis in: Acute renal failure, chronic renal failure, prolonged post-operative anuria, intractable oedema, chronic congestive heart failure, poisoning due to ingestion of dialysable poisons.

Dialaflex 61 Solution is slightly hypertonic to avoid the dangers of increased hydration by absorption of water from the peritoneal cavity. It is indicated for routine dialyses which are not intended to remove excessive fluid from the body. Dialaflex 62 Solution is markedly hypertonic and is indicated when rapid removal of oedematous fluid is indicated. Dialaflex 63 Solution has a lower sodium content than Dialaflex 61. It is indicated for use in maintenance dialysis where removal of sodium is often desirable.

Dosage and administration Administration of Diala-flex Solutions necessitates the use of a special giving set to allow delivery of the solutions to and from the peritoneal cavity. This is done through a peritoneal catheter which is generally advised to be inserted in the mid-line between the umbillicus and the symphysis pubis at the junction of the middle and lower thirds.

Adults: For each dialysis 2 litres of Dialaflex Solution, ready warmed to body temperature, should be allowed to flow into the peritoneal cavity. After 20 minutes the solution is syphoned out and the procedure is repeated as often as is warranted by the situation and the condition of the patient.

Children: Each dialysis is usually performed with a volume of 1 litre of Dialaflex Solution.

Elderly: Caution should be exercised in elderly patients due to their inability to tolerate acute changes in fluid and electrolyte balance.

Contra-indications, warnings, etc
Contra-indications: Peritoneal dialysis should not be employed if there has been recent injury to abdominal organs or in the presence of severe peritonitis.

Precautions: If full aseptic precautions are observed the danger of infection during peritoneal dialysis is slight. However, additional precautions against this possibility may be achieved by addition of antibiotics to the dialysis solution or by parenteral antibiotic administration.

Introduction of the trocar to enable the insertion of the catheter may carry the rare possibility of intestinal perforation.

Protein loss has been reported following prolonged period of peritoneal dialysis.

In patients with normal or depleted plasma potassium levels oral potassium supplements should be given or four millimoles potassium added to each litre of Dialaflex Solution.

Side-effects: Selection of the most suitable Dialaflex Solution and proper supervision of the peritoneal dialysis should ensure no untoward effects occur.

Overdosage: As peritoneal dialysis is invariably performed under supervision the question of overdosage is unlikely to arise.

Pharmaceutical precautions *Storage:* Dialaflex Solutions should be stored at 2°C–25°C. The shelf-life is two years.

Legal category POM.

Package quantities Plastic containers of 1 litre of Dialaflex Solutions are available in packs of 10.

Further information The volume of fluid recovered after dialysis should usually exceed the volume administered. The latter can be calculated by weighing the bags before and after dialysis. The weight per ml of solution is 1.009 g for Dialaflex 61 and Dialaflex 63, and 1.028 g for Dialaflex 62. Any deficiency in fluid balance may be corrected by either the oral or intravenous routes.

Product licence numbers
61 0014/0198
62 0014/0199
63 0014/0200

DIMERCAPROL INJECTION

Presentation Dimercaprol Injection BP (B.A.L. Injection) is a sterile solution of dimercaprol in arachis oil containing 10% V/V benzyl benzoate. It is presented in 2 ml ampoules, and each ml of the injection contains 50 mg of Dimercaprol BP.

Uses Dimercaprol Injection is indicated in the treatment of acute poisoning by certain heavy metals – arsenic, mercury, gold, bismuth, antimony and possibly thallium. Although dimercaprol has not been successful in the treatment of lead poisoning when used alone, there is evidence that, used in conjunction with sodium calcium edetate, it can be used successfully in the treatment of lead poisoning, particularly in children.

Dosage and administration By intramuscular injection:

Adults: 400 to 800 mg, in divided doses, on the first day.
200 to 400 mg, in divided doses, on second and third days.
100 to 200 mg, in divided doses, on subsequent days.

Within the above dose range, individual dosage should be calculated on a body-weight basis, and will depend upon the severity of symptoms and the causative agent. As a general guide, single doses should not exceed 3 mg/kg; however, in severe acute poisoning, single doses up to 5 mg/kg may be required initially.

Children: Dimercaprol Injection is well tolerated by children and dosage should be calculated on the basis of body-weight, using the same unit dose per kilogram of body-weight as for an adult under similar clinical circumstances.

Precautions: The use of Dimercaprol Injection does not eliminate the need for the general treatment of poisoning due to the particular heavy metal. Any abnormal reaction (e.g. pyrexia) occurring after the initial injection of dimercaprol should be assessed before continuing treatment.

Elderly: There is no specific data on the use of dimercaprol in the elderly but since it is eliminated via the kidney, it should be used with caution in this age group.

Contra-indications, warnings, etc Dimercaprol Injection is contra-indicated in poisoning by iron and cadmium.

Dimercaprol Injection is contra-indicated in the presence of extensive hepatic insufficiency or damage.

Dimercaprol Injection should be used with caution in the hypertensive patient.

Side-effects are relatively frequent, but, at the therapeutic dosage usually employed, are seldom severe enough to warrant cessation of treatment and are almost invariably reversible. There is some evidence to indicate that 30–60 mg of ephedrine sulphate, by mouth, given half an hour before each injection of dimercaprol, will reduce these reactions. Also, a minimum interval of four hours between doses appears to reduce side-effects.

Dimercaprol Injection may cause the following side-effects particularly at the higher dosage levels:

Elevation of blood pressure accompanied by tachycardia; nausea and possibly vomiting; a burning sensation of the lips, mouth, throat and eyes; salivation and lachrymation; conjunctivitis; rhinorrhoea; muscle pain and spasm; abdominal pain; headache; tingling of the hands and other extremities; a feeling of constriction in the chest and throat; sweating of the forehead and hands.

Local pain may occur at the site of injection, and gluteal abscess has occasionally been encountered.

A side-effect apparently peculiar to children is a fever which develops after the second or third injection, and persists until treatment with dimercaprol is terminated.

Dimercaprol Injection may not be effective in cases of concomitant renal failure, e.g. in arsine poisoning and some cases of arsenic poisoning.

Use in pregnancy: Dimercaprol Injection has been used in Wilsons Disease with successful full-term pregnancies, but since there is no other experience of its use in pregnancy, it should be prescribed with caution.

Pharmaceutical precautions Dimercaprol Injection may become cloudy in cold weather; if this occurs, warm slightly before use.

Protect from light.

Legal category POM.

Package quantities 12 ampoules of 2 ml.

Further information Nil.

Product licence number 0014/5509R.

8.5% FREAMINE* III

Presentation A clear solution of synthetic L-form amino acids in combination with selected electrolytes. Sterile and pyrogen-free.

Contents per litre:

L-Isoleucine	5.9 g
L-Leucine	7.7 g
L-Lysine acetate	8.7 g†
L-Methionine	4.5 g
L-Phenylalanine	4.8 g
L-Threonine	3.4 g
L-Tryptophan	1.3 g
L-Valine	5.6 g
L-Arginine	8.1 g
L-Histidine	2.4 g
L-Alanine	6.0 g
Glycine	11.9 g
L-Proline	9.5 g
L-Serine	5.0 g
L-Cysteine HCL.H_2O	<0.2 g

† 6.2 g as free base

Electrolytes:

Sodium	10 mmol
Phosphate	10 mmol
Acetate	72 mmol
Chloride	<3 mmol
Sodium metabisulphite (antioxidant)	<1 g

Providing:

13 g nitrogen (82 g amino acids)
Total energy content 328 kcal (1.4 MJ)

Hypertonic solution
Calculated osmolarity: Approximately 810 mOsmol/l
pH: Approximately 6.5.

Uses 8.5% FreAmine III provides a balanced ratio of L-form essential and non-essential amino acids together with selected electrolytes for use in parenteral nutrition. To ensure optimal utilisation of the infused amino acids, administration of 8.5% FreAmine III should be accompanied by simultaneous infusion of an appropriate energy source, for example Steriflex* or Polyfusor* Dextrose

Injection 20, 40 or 50%. The use of lipid emulsion can be used as an additional energy supplement as well as a source of essential fatty acids.

Dosage and administration
Adult dosage: 500–2000 ml per 24 hours depending on individual requirements.

Infusion rate: Infusion of the completed admixture should be at a rate in accordance with the clinical condition of the patient; wherever possible administration should be at a steady rate over 24 hours.

Children's dosage: at clinician's discretion.

Whenever possible the daily dosage of 8.5% FreAmine III should be based upon the nitrogen requirement of the patient, this best being assessed by means of daily nitrogen balance estimations. In the absence of nitrogen balance measurements, administration of 0.15–0.3 g of nitrogen/kg (total 10.5–21 g of nitrogen in a 70 kg patient) or more may be considered depending on the degree of catabolism present.

In infants and in severely hypercatabolic states, requirements may be higher at 0.30–0.50 g of nitrogen/kg. To ensure adequate utilisation of the infused nitrogen, non-protein energy should be provided at a minimum of 120 kcal (0.5 MJ)/g of nitrogen. Administration of parenteral nutrition regimens should be accompanied by a rigorous programme of clinical and biochemical monitoring particularly where high dose regimens are used.

Where possible, parenteral nutrition regimens should be administered by continuous infusion via a central venous catheter to reduce the incidence of thrombophlebitis. The tip of the catheter should be located in the superior vena cava, using X-ray to verify placement. If practical considerations dictate that a peripheral infusion site be employed, frequent changing of catheter sites will be necessary to avoid thrombophlebitis. Infusion should be over the maximum available time period of 24 hours where administration regimens permit. If the administration rate falls behind the planned schedule, no attempt should be made to 'catch-up' as this may result in overdosage. The giving set used to administer the regimen should be changed every 24 hours.

Contra-indications, warnings, etc
Solution to be used only for aseptic compounding of parenteral nutrition regimens. The container is not designed for direct infusion into patients.

Caution should be exercised when considering the infusion of 8.5% FreAmine III in patients with renal or hepatic impairment of varying degrees. In such patients the use of disease-specific amino acid solutions may be more appropriate.

Parenteral nutrition should be accompanied by frequent clinical evaluation and laboratory determinations as part of a rigorous patient monitoring programme. Studies should include electrolyte estimations, urea, blood sugar, serum protein, renal and liver function tests, haemoglobin, blood gases, serum osmolarities, blood ammonia levels and blood cultures. Frequent monitoring of blood ammonia should be undertaken in infants or if administration in hepatic insufficiency is contemplated. In infants hyperammonaemia appears to be related to a defect in the ability to synthesise urea. Should symptoms of hyperammonaemia develop, administration of amino acids should be discontinued and the patient's clinical status assessed.

Electrolyte and trace element supplementation should be based on and tailored to patient requirements. Vitamin supplementation should also be undertaken, particularly with respect to folic acid as infusion of amino acid mixtures may precipitate folic acid deficiency. Routine vitamin B_{12} supplementation should also be undertaken.

Care should be exercised when instituting parenteral nutrition in patients with cardiovascular disease. In particular circulatory overload should be avoided and caution exercised in the choice of calorie source, as in hypoxia, free fatty acids may not be utilised by the myocardium and glucose becomes the calorie source of choice.

Side-effects: Complications may be associated with the route of administration (e.g. phlebitis, thrombosis, erythema, infection) or the solution itself (e.g. flushing, fever, nausea, hypervolaemia, biochemical imbalances). If adverse effects occur, the infusion should be discontinued, the patient evaluated and appropriate clinical counter-measures instituted where necessary.

Pharmaceutical precautions Solution under vacuum.

Do not administer unless solution is clear, container undamaged and vacuum present.

Protect from freezing. Store below 25°C.

Protect solution and compounded mixtures from light. Compounding should be undertaken in an aseptic environment.

Compounded solutions if not intended for immediate administration should be stored at 2–8°C in a refrigerator and used within 24 hours unless pharmacy indicates otherwise. Pack inserts, data sheets, pharmacy, solution and additive manufacturers may be consulted for advice.

Data on compatibility and stability of levels of permissible admixtures should be sought before compounding is undertaken. Instability of lipid emulsions can arise with compounded admixtures of 8.5% FreAmine III, dextrose, lipid and electrolytes, if recommended regimens are not adhered to.

Legal category POM.

Package quantities Glass bottles of 500 ml and 1000 ml.

Further information For information on the availability of special solutions, pack sizes, compatibility of compounded formulations etc. contact the manufacturer, The Boots Company PLC., Nottingham, England.

Product licence number 0014/0294.

FROBEN*

Presentation Light yellow, sugar-coated tablets containing either 50 mg or 100 mg of flurbiprofen. The 50 mg tablets are overprinted 'F50' in black; the 100 mg tablets are overprinted 'F100', also in black.

Uses Froben is a nonsteroidal anti-inflammatory agent which has significant anti-inflammatory, analgesic and antipyretic properties and is indicated in the treatment of rheumatoid disease, osteoarthritis and ankylosing spondylitis.

Dosage and administration The recommended daily dose is 150–200 mg in divided doses.

In patients with severe symptoms or disease of recent origin, or during acute exacerbations, the total daily dosage may be increased to 300 mg in divided doses.

Although Froben is generally well tolerated in the elderly, some patients, especially with impaired renal function, may eliminate nonsteroidal anti-inflammatory drugs more slowly than normal. In these cases Froben should be used with caution and dosage should be assessed individually.

Contra-indications, warnings, etc As with other nonsteroidal anti-inflammatory drugs Froben should be avoided in patients with peptic ulceration, gastrointestinal haemorrhage and ulcerative colitis.

Fluid retention and oedema have been reported in common with other nonsteroidal anti-inflammatory agents. Froben should be used with caution in patients with a history of cardiac decompensation and hypertension.

Froben should not be given to patients with a history of asthma or to patients who have experienced bronchospasm, anaphylactoid reactions, angioedema or other hypersensitivity type reactions from use of aspirin or other nonsteroidal anti-inflammatory drugs.

As it has been shown that Froben may prolong bleeding time, it should be used with caution in patients with a potential for abnormal bleeding.

Side-effects: Dyspepsia, nausea, vomiting, gastrointestinal haemorrhage, diarrhoea and ulcers of the mouth have been recorded. Occasionally peptic ulceration and perforation have been reported.

Urticaria, angioedema and rashes of varying descriptions have been reported. Photosensitivity has not been a problem.

Very rarely cholestatic jaundice has been reported. It is reversible on withdrawal of the drug.

Thrombocytopenia has been reported. It is usually reversible on withdrawal of the drug.

Very rarely aplastic anaemia and agranulocytosis have been reported in association with the use of Froben.

Toxic nephropathies have been associated with use of nonsteroidal anti-inflammatory agents in general and have occasionally been reported in patients who have received Froben.

Treatment of overdosage: Gastric lavage and, if necessary, correction of serum electrolytes. There is no specific antidote to flurbiprofen.

Use in pregnancy: The safety of Froben during pregnancy or lactation has not been established. Pre-clinical studies have not revealed any teratogenic effects but parturition was delayed and prolonged.

Drug interactions: Special clinical studies have shown that the diuretic response to frusemide can occasionally be reduced by Froben. Similarly, interference with the action of anticoagulants has occasionally been reported.

Other studies have failed to show any interaction between Froben and digoxin, tolbutamide or antacids.

Interference with laboratory tests: There is no evidence so far that flurbiprofen interferes with laboratory tests.

Pharmaceutical precautions No special storage requirements are necessary.

Legal category POM.

Package quantities *50 mg Tablets:* Packs of 100 and 500.
100 mg Tablets: Packs of 100.

Further information Froben is a potent nonsteroidal anti-inflammatory agent which has significant anti-inflammatory, analgesic and antipyretic properties. It is a highly potent inhibitor of prostaglandin synthetase enzymes which are known to be associated with inflammation, pain and fever.

Studies in the treatment of rheumatoid disease, osteoarthritis and ankylosing spondylitis have indicated that Froben is as effective as the more potent of the established nonsteroidal anti-inflammatory agents and, in many patients, better tolerated. Long-term clinical studies have not revealed any evidence of significant effects upon the hepatic, renal or haemopoietic systems.

Because of the flexible dosage range, Froben is available as 50 mg tablets and 100 mg tablets, the higher strength preparation providing a convenient dose-form for those patients requiring 300 mg daily in three divided doses.

Product licence numbers
Froben 50 mg Tablets   0014/0167
Froben 100 mg Tablets   0014/0168

GASTROZEPIN*

Presentation Gastrozepin is pirenzepine dihydrochloride, available as white tablets each containing the equivalent of 50 mg of anhydrous substance. The tablets are scored on one face and impressed with 'G' on one side of the score and '50' on the other. The obverse is impressed with the symbol

Uses Gastrozepin is indicated in the treatment of gastric and duodenal ulcers.

Dosage and administration In most patients Gastrozepin should be given in a dosage of 100 mg daily as one tablet each morning and one at night. Freedom from discomfort is usually achieved with Gastrozepin after a few days but treatment should be continued for a total of 4–6 weeks to allow the condition to be completely healed.

In patients with severe symptoms, the total daily dosage may be increased to 150 mg, one tablet to be taken three times a day.

In patients requiring longer term therapy, Gastrozepin may be given continuously for up to three months.

The tablets are best taken half an hour or more before meals with a little liquid.

Elderly: There is no evidence to suggest that Gastrozepin should not be used at normal therapeutic doses in the elderly.

Contra-indications, warnings, etc At doses sufficient to produce ulcer healing, Gastrozepin does not cross the blood/brain barrier in significant amounts and so central pharmacological effects are likely to be minimal.

In animal studies Gastrozepin had no teratogenic effects in the species tested, even at high dosages. The use of Gastrozepin is not recommended during pregnancy.

Gastrozepin appears in the milk of lactating mothers in minimal amounts after therapeutic doses but is not likely to adversely affect the infant.

Pharmacological interaction between sympathomimetics or monoamine oxidase inhibitors and pirenzepine is a theoretical possibility.

Side Effects: Few side effects are associated with Gastrozepin. Occasionally dry mouth and accommodation difficulties may occur but these are transitory and rarely sufficiently severe to warrant discontinuation of therapy.

Treatment of Overdosage: There is no specific antidote to pirenzepine. The treatment of overdosage is entirely symptomatic.

Pharmaceutical precautions Recommended storage conditions: in a cool dry place.

Legal category POM.

Package quantities Gastrozepin tablets 50 mg – pack of 60.

Further information In animal studies Gastrozepin has been shown to differentiate between muscarinic receptors in different tissues with preferential binding to receptors in the gastric mucosa. This property probably explains the selectivity of clinical activity throughout the normal therapeutic dose range, producing gastric antisecretory effects leading to ulcer healing without marked effects at other peripheral muscarinic receptor sites.

In addition to a reduction in acid secretion, Gastrozepin also reduces the secretion of pepsinogen/pepsin.

Gastrozepin has a mean half-life of approximately 12 hours and therefore provides a continuous therapeutic activity from a twice daily dosage.

Product licence number 0014/0260

HYDRENOX*

Presentation Hydrenox Tablets are Hydroflumethiazide Tablets BP each containing 50 mg of Hydroflumethiazide BP, oral diuretic of the thiazide group.

Uses Hydrenox is indicated in all cases where the reduction of fluid retention by diuresis is required, i.e. oedema of cardiac, renal or hepatic origin; premenstrual, iatrogenic and all other types of oedema. Hydrenox is also indicated in the treatment of hypertension, either used alone or in combination with a hypotensive agent.

Dosage and administration *Diuretic:* 50 to 200 mg daily, depending upon the severity of the oedema, as a single dose in the morning. The daily dose should be given early enough to complete diuresis by bedtime. Doses of 25 to 50 mg on alternate days are usually adequate for maintenance therapy.

Hypotensive: 25 to 50 mg daily; when given as an adjunct to a specific hypotensive agent, the dose of the latter should be halved.

Dosage in children will be at the discretion of the physician; 1 mg per kg of body-weight daily has been suggested as suitable for most cases.

The dosage of thiazide diuretics may need to be reduced in the elderly, particularly when renal function is impaired.

Contra-indications, warnings, etc
Electrolyte imbalance: All thiazide diuretics can produce a degree of electrolyte imbalance, especially in patients with renal or hepatic impairment or when dosage is high or prolonged. Serum electrolyte levels should be checked for abnormalities, particularly hypokalaemia which should be corrected by the addition of a potassium supplement to the regimen. Hydrenox does not contain a potassium supplement.

Digitalis intoxication: Sensitivity to digitalis may be increased by the kaliuretic effect of concurrent hydroflumethiazide. Patients should be observed for signs of digitalis intoxication and, if these appear, the dosage of digitalis reduced and a potassium supplement added to restore stability.

Uric acid retention: Thiazide diuretics may raise serum uric acid levels with consequent exacerbation of gout in susceptible patients.

Diabetes: Thiazide diuretics sometimes lower carbohydrate tolerance and the insulin dosage of the diabetic patient may require adjustment.

Care is necessary when hydroflumethiazide is given to those with a known predisposition to diabetes.

Pregnancy: Thiazides cross the placental barrier; therefore it is reasonable to assume that side-effects occurring in the adult may also appear in the neonate.

Treatment of overdosage: Monitor blood pressure and serum electrolytes. Treatment is symptomatic.

Pharmaceutical precautions Recommended storage conditions, 5° to 20°C.

Legal category POM.

Package quantities Bottle of 100, bottle of 500.

Further information Nil.

Product licence number 0014/5119.

HYDROCORTISTAB* INJECTION

Presentation Hydrocortistab Injection is Hydrocortisone Acetate Injection BP, containing 25 mg of Hydrocortisone Acetate BP per ml.

Uses Hydrocortistab Injection is indicated for the local treatment, by intra-articular or peri-articular injection of arthritic conditions such as rheumatoid arthritis and osteoarthritis when few joints are involved and in traumatic arthritis, except when associated with fractures into the joint. It is also suitable for the symptomatic treatment, by the local injection, of certain non-articular inflammatory conditions such as inflamed tendonsheaths and bursae.

Hydrocortistab Injection is not suitable for the production of systemic effects.

Dosage and administration By intra-articular or peri-articular injection, 5 mg to 50 mg depending upon the size of the joint. Not more than three joints should be treated in one day.

Elderly: Steroids should be used cautiously in the elderly, since adverse effects are enhanced by old age.

Contra-indications, warnings, etc As with all corticosteroids, the administration of Hydrocortistab Injection is contra-indicated when the affected site is infected. It should not be injected directly into tendons, nor should it be injected into spinal or any other than true diarthrodial joints.

Caution: Since joints and tissues injected with corticosteroids have an increased susceptibility to infection, local injections of Hydrocortistab should be carried out with full aseptic precautions.

Side-effects: The principal side-effect encountered with local injections of corticosteroids is a temporary local exacerbation, with increased pain and swelling. This usually subsides after a few hours. In certain circumstances, particularly after high or prolonged local dosage, corticosteroids can be absorbed in amounts sufficient to produce systemic effects.

Treatment of overdosage: Treatment is symptomatic but is unlikely to be required.

Pharmaceutical precautions Store between 15°C to 20°C; protect from light.

Legal category POM.

Package quantities Vial of 5 ml.

Further information Nil.

Product licence number 0014/5510.

KAODENE*

Presentation Kaodene is an aqueous suspension containing Codeine Phosphate BP 10 mg and Light Kaolin BP 3 g in each 10 ml. It is an off-white liquid with the odour and flavour of aniseed.

Uses Kaodene is indicated for the symptomatic relief of simple diarrhoea. It cannot be used as a substitute for rehydration therapy.

Dosage and administration *Adults and Children over 12 years:* 20 ml three or four times daily.

Children from 5 to 12 years: 10 ml three or four times daily.

Kaodene is not recommended for children under 5 years.

The long term administration of Kaodene, particularly in the elderly, is not recommended.

Contra-indications, warnings, etc Kaodene is contra-indicated in patients with pseudomembranous colitis and diverticular disease and must be used with caution in patients with ulcerative colitis and hepatic dysfunction.

Codeine phosphate is a narcotic analgesic and, given in large doses, may induce tolerance and psychological and physical dependence. At the recommended dosage, however, it is unlikely that such effects would be encountered with Kaodene.

Large doses of codeine may cause drowsiness and CNS depression, but this should not be a problem with the recommended doses of Kaodene.

Whilst there is no adequate evidence of safety in human pregnancy, codeine has been widely used without apparent ill-effect for many years and studies in animals have not demonstrated any hazard.

Drug interactions: Kaodene may interfere with the absorption of some drugs from the gastro-intestinal tract.

Interference with laboratory tests: Administration of Kaodene may interfere with laboratory estimations of serum amylase and certain liver function tests.

Treatment of overdosage: Gastric lavage and symptomatic treatment as for codeine phosphate is recommended. Naloxone may be used to counteract CNS depression.

Pharmaceutical precautions *Recommended storage conditions:* 5°–20°C.

Legal category CD (Sch 5), P.

Package quantities Bottle of 250 ml.

Further information Nil.

Product licence number 0014/0233.

LIGNOSTAB*

Presentation Lignostab is injection of lignocaine hydrochloride 2%. It is supplied in glass cartridges designed for use with dental-type cartridge syringes. Each cartridge contains 2.0 ml of solution.

Uses Lignostab is a local anaesthetic. It is mainly for use in dental procedures where the addition of a vasoconstrictor is either contra-indicated or not required. Since Lignostab contains no vasoconstrictor, the local anaesthetic effect is of relatively short duration.

Dosage and administration Lignostab is given by injection, in dental procedures, into the gum. The amount of Lignostab required to produce adequate anaesthesia must be determined on an individual basis, bearing in mind that it is desirable to use the minimal effective dose.

The dosage for Lignostab in the elderly should be individualised for each patient, as advised for other age groups.

Contra-indications, warnings, etc
Contra-indications: Known sensitivity to lignocaine. Injection into inflamed or infected areas is to be avoided.

Caution: Care should be taken to avoid the accidental intravenous injection of Lignostab.

Side-effects: Provided the correct injection technique is used and the lowest effective dose employed, side-effects with Lignostab are extremely rare. However, idiosyncratic reactions to local anaesthetics have been reported in some patients.

Toxic effects: Transient drowsiness and amnesia proceeding to severe central nervous system depression may sometimes occur, but excitation of the central nervous system is uncommon.

Pharmaceutical precautions *Recommended storage conditions:* 2–25°C; protect from light.

Legal category POM.

Package quantities Boxes of 500 cartridges.

Further information Shelf-life of at least two years.

Product licence number 0014/5368.

LIGNOSTAB*-A
LIGNOSTAB*-A100

Presentation Lignostab-A is injection of lignocaine hydrochloride 2% with adrenaline 1:80,000. Lignostab-A100 is injection of lignocaine hydrochloride 2% with adrenaline 1:100,000. Both are supplied in glass cartridges designed for use with dental-type syringes. Each cartridge contains 2.0 ml of solution.

Uses Lignostab-A and Lignostab-A100 are local anaesthetics, mainly for use in dental procedures.

Both these preparations include a vasoconstrictor (adrenaline), the effect of which is to prolong the local anaesthesia by delaying the diffusion of the anaesthetic into the surrounding tissues.

Dosage and administration Lignostab-A and Lignostab-A100, in dental procedures, are injected into the gum. The amount of either preparation needed to provide adequate anaesthesia must be determined on an individual basis, bearing in mind that it is desirable to use the minimal effective dose.

The dosage for Lignostab in the elderly should be individualised for each patient, as advised for other age groups.

Contra-indications, warnings, etc
Contra-indications: Known sensitivity to lignocaine. Lignostab-A and -A100 should not be injected into inflamed or infected areas. Because of their adrenaline content, these preparations should be used with caution in patients with hypertension. Lignostab-A and -A100 are contra-indicated in patients taking antidepressants of the tricyclic group.

Caution: Care should be taken to avoid the accidental intravenous injection of Lignostab-A or -A100. Lignostab-A and -A100 should not be injected into extremities.

Side-effects: Provided the correct injection technique is used and the lowest effective dose employed, side-effects with Lignostab-A and -A100 are extremely rare. However, idiosyncratic reactions to local anaesthetics have been reported in some patients. The injection of excessive amounts of Lignostab-A or -A100 may, due to the adrenaline content, cause ischaemia. This can be followed by a reactive hyperaemia resulting in post-extraction bleeding.

Toxic effects: Transient drowsiness and amnesia proceeding to severe central nervous system depression may occur, but excitation of the central nervous system is uncommon.

Treatment of overdosage: Respiratory failure may need assisted respiration. The circulation can be controlled with electrolyte or plasma infusions. If convulsions develop, these can be controlled by a short-acting barbiturate.

Pharmaceutical precautions *Recommended storage conditions:* 2–25°C. Protect from light.

Legal category POM.

Package quantities Boxes of 500 cartridges.

Further information Shelf-life of at least two years.

Product licence numbers
Lignostab-A   0014/5384
Lignostab-A100   0014/5385

LIGNOSTAB*-N

Presentation Lignostab-N is injection of lignocaine hydrochloride 2% with noradrenaline 1:80,000. It is supplied in glass cartridges designed for use with dental-type cartridge syringes. Each cartridge contains 2.0 ml of solution.

Uses Lignostab-N is a local anaesthetic, mainly for use in dental procedures. Lignostab-N includes the vasoconstrictor noradrenaline, the effect of which is to prolong the local anaesthesia by delaying the diffusion of the anaesthetic into the surrounding tissues.

Lignostab-N provides an alternative to local anaesthetics which contain adrenaline as a vasoconstrictor.

Dosage and administration Lignostab-N is given by injection, in dental procedures, into the gum. The amount required to provide adequate anaesthesia must be determined on an individual basis, bearing in mind that it is desirable to use the minimal effective dose.

The dosage for Lignostab in the elderly should be individualised for each patient, as advised for other age groups.

Contra-indications, warnings, etc
Contra-indications: Known sensitivity to lignocaine. Injection into inflamed or infected areas to be avoided. Because of the noradrenaline content, Lignostab-N should be used with caution in patients with hypertension. Lignostab-N is contra-indicated in patients taking antidepressants of the tricyclic group.

Caution: Care should be taken to avoid the accidental intravenous injection of Lignostab-N.

Side-effects: Provided the correct injection technique is used and the lowest effective dose employed, side-effects are extremely rare with Lignostab-N.

However, idiosyncratic reactions to local anaesthetics have been reported in some patients. The injection of excessive amounts of Lignostab-N may, due to the vasoconstrictor, cause ischaemia. This can be followed by a reactive hyperaemia and result in post-extraction bleeding.

Toxic effects: Transient drowsiness and amnesia proceeding to severe central nervous system depression may sometimes occur, but excitation of the central nervous system is uncommon.

Treatment of overdosage: Respiratory failure may need assisted respiration. The circulation can be maintained with electrolyte or plasma infusions. Should convulsions develop, these can be controlled with a short-acting barbiturate.

Pharmaceutical precautions *Recommended storage conditions:* 2–25°C. Protect from light.

Legal category POM.

Package quantities Boxes of 500 cartridges.

Further information Shelf-life of at least two years.

Product licence number 0014/5386.

MUSTINE HYDROCHLORIDE FOR INJECTION BP

Synonyms: Nitrogen Mustard. Mechlorethamine Hydrochloride USP, Mustargen Hydrochloride, Chlorethazine Hydrochloride, Chlormethine Hydrochloride INN, 'HN$_2$'.

Presentation Mustine hydrochloride is supplied in sterile vials each containing 10 mg of the powder. The injection is prepared by dissolving this in Sodium Chloride Injection BP 0.9% w/v or Water for Injections BP.

Mustine hydrochloride is di (2-chloroethyl) methylamine hydrochloride. It is a white or almost white hygroscopic, vesicant, crystalline powder or mass and is very soluble in water. A 0.2% solution in water has a pH of 3 to 5.

Uses The principal use of mustine hydrochloride is as part of combination treatment for Hodgkin's disease. It is also sometimes used in non-Hodgkin's lymphomas and carcinoma of bronchus, ovary and breast. It may be injected into pleural or peritoneal cavities for the treatment of malignant effusions. It may be applied locally for the treatment of mycosis fungoides.

Dosage and administration *Malignancy:* The normal intravenous dose of mustine hydrochloride is 0.1 mg per kg body-weight daily for three or four days. In selected cases, larger doses of 0.2 to 0.3 mg per kg body-weight daily may be given, but the course should then be limited to two injections. Alternatively, a single treatment using

0.4 mg per kg body-weight (15 mg per square metre body surface area) can be administered. The term 'body-weight' is defined, in this case, as the actual body-weight at the time of treatment except in cases where the weight has been artificially increased by oedema, ascites, or other fluid collections. The weight of the body before the increase is used in such cases.

UNDER NO CIRCUMSTANCES SHOULD MUSTINE BE GIVEN INTRAMUSCULARLY.

A repeat course of mustine therapy should not be undertaken for at least 6 weeks or until the bone-marrow has recovered its haemopoietic activity.

Preparation of intravenous injection: A fresh solution is prepared by dissolving 10 mg of mustine hydrochloride in 10 ml of Sodium Chloride Injection BP 0.9% w/v, or Water for Injections BP. The best method of administration is to set up an intravenous drip of Sodium Chloride Injection BP 0.9% w/v or Dextrose Injection BP 5% w/v; the required dose of mustine prepared as above, is then injected into the tubing. This avoids the hazard of extravasation during injection. The drip rate should be 60 drops per minute and the injection of mustine should be carried out over 2 minutes. The drip should then be reduced to 20 drops per minute.

Alternatively the concentrated solution of mustine hydrochloride is freshly prepared as above and transferred aseptically to 500 ml of Sodium Chloride Injection BP 0.9% w/v.

Pleural effusions: Mustine is sometimes injected into the peritoneal or pleural cavities. There are minor variations in the techniques. Half an hour before the injection a short acting barbiturate such as oral quinalbarbitone 0.2 g, and chlorpromazine 25 mg should be given to reduce the nausea. Most articles advise the use of paracentesis to remove as much fluid as possible. Mustine hydrochloride may be injected into the cavity in a single dose up to 0.4 mg/kg body-weight (15 to 30 mg of mustine in about 100 to 200 ml of normal saline).

The quinalbarbitone and chlorpromazine may be repeated if there is further nausea.

Mycosis fungoides: Mycosis fungoides may be treated by topical application of a dilute solution of mustine hydrochloride. Various strengths of mustine hydrochloride have been used but 20 mg in 100 ml of 0.9% w/v sodium chloride solution or water is frequently recommended. The solution is applied to the affected cutaneous areas using a gauze pad. The person applying the solution should wear polyvinylchloride gloves to give protection. Some patients develop an allergic contact dermatitis after topical application of mustine hydrochloride.

No specific data is available on the use of mustine hydrochloride in the elderly.

Contra-indications, warnings, etc
Warning: To prevent blistering, gloves should be worn when handling mustine hydrochloride, and because of its irritating powers the drug should be kept well away from the nose and eyes. Polyvinylchloride gloves give adequate protection but rubber and polyethylene gloves have been shown to be ineffective. Mustine hydrochloride accidentally spilled on the skin should be washed away immediately with large amounts of water or, if at hand, sodium carbonate solution or an isotonic solution of sodium thiosulphate. If mustine is accidentally splashed into the eye it should be immediately washed out for a long period of time with large amounts of water and, if available, irrigated with isotonic solution of sodium

thiosulphate. The person concerned then should be seen by an ophthalmologist.

After treatment with mustine all apparatus, including PVC gloves, should be washed thoroughly. A 2.5% solution of sodium carbonate is particularly suitable for the lavage.

Adverse reactions and precautions: Nausea and vomiting often occur during the eight hours following injection. The administration of chlorpromazine, either alone or with a suitable barbiturate such as quinalbarbitone, often helps to control this and should be given thirty to sixty minutes before injection, repeated if necessary.

Transient anorexia, occasional diarrhoea and fever may occur. Peptic ulcers have been reported.

Severe haemopoietic depression may follow mustine therapy, with lymphocytopenia, granulocytopenia and occasionally agranulocytosis. It may lead to severe anaemia and thrombocytopenia. Leucocytes and platelet counts in peripheral blood start to fall about one week after treatment with a nadir between 14 and 18 days. During the same period there is a fall in haemoglobin level. Both leucocyte and platelet counts return to normal before the end of the fourth week. Mustine should not be used in patients with severe leucopenia, thrombocytopenia or anaemia and in coexistent or suspected granuloma. Extravasation during injection should be avoided as this may cause severe local reactions and even local tissue necrosis. If extravasation does occur during injection the involved area should be infiltrated with isotonic sodium thiosulphate solution followed by the application of an ice compress intermittently for six to twelve hours.

This product should not normally be administered to patients who are pregnant or to mothers who are breast-feeding.

If considered for use in pregnancy the risk to the foetus should be weighed against the potential benefits to the patient. The drug possesses foetotoxic and teratogenic potential.

Thrombophlebitis and venous thrombosis are potential complications to mustine therapy.

In non-pregnant women delayed menstruation or temporary amenorrhoea may follow the treatment. In males a reduction of active spermatogenesis has been reported. Hyperuricaemia may develop in patients with large tumour masses.

Treatment of overdose: Sodium thiosulphate will neutralise an injection of mustine hydrochloride BUT ONLY IF GIVEN IMMEDIATELY AFTERWARDS. Each 10 mg mustine requires 640 mg sodium thiosulphate given as an isotonic solution. This is equivalent to approximately 1.5 ml of a 50% solution of sodium thiosulphate diluted with 20 ml 0.9% sodium chloride solution or approximately 21 ml of 3% sodium thiosulphate solution.

Stability: An early study of the stability of mustine hydrochloride in saline solution at room temperature, using a colorimetric assay method, showed that the solution lost 7% of alkylating potential per hour. A later study indicated that solutions of mustine hydrochloride stored at room temperature lost approximately 50% of activity in one to two months.

Studies in Boots' laboratories storing 10 mg mustine hydrochloride in 20 ml Water for Injections showed no significant loss of activity over the first 10 days. Thereafter a slow but steady loss of activity occurred until the 40th day resulting in an overall loss of 20%.

Pharmaceutical precautions Store at 2° to 15°C.

Legal category POM.

Package quantities Pack of 10 vials.

Further information Nil.

Product licence number 0014/5512.

NEPHRAMINE*

Presentation Nephramine is a sterile, non-pyrogenic solution containing crystalline essential amino acids. Each 250 ml unit contains the daily requirement of essential amino acids (according to Rose) plus 625 mg of histidine. The total nitrogen content is approximately 1.6 g.

Each 100 ml contains:

Active constituents

L-histidine	250 mg	L-phenylalanine	880 mg
L-isoleucine	560 mg	L-threonine	400 mg
L-leucine	880 mg	L-tryptophan	200 mg
L-lysine acetate	900 mg	L-valine	640 mg
(free base	640 mg)	L-cysteine	
L-methionine	880 mg	HCl H_2O	<20 mg

Non-active constituents
Sodium bisulphate USP (as an antioxidant) <50 mg
pH adjusted with sodium hydroxide as required
pH: approx. 6.5
Total nitrogen: approx. 650 mg/100 ml
Calculated osmolarity: approx. 435 mOsm/litre
Concentration of electrolytes (mEq/litre): sodium 5, acetate 44
Chloride <3

Uses Nephramine is indicated in the management of potentially reversible renal decompensation where adequate nutrition cannot be achieved orally and standard parenteral amino acid solutions are contra-indicated.

Dosage and administration The recommended dosage for adults is 0.25–0.5 litres (1.6–3.2 g nitrogen) per 24 hours, the rate being determined by clinical and biochemical assessment of the patient. When an energy source has been added Nephramine should initially be given at approximately 1–10 drops per minute building up, over a period of 24 to 48 hours, to a maximum rate of 20–25 drops per minute. Although nitrogen requirements may be higher than 3.2 g per day in the acutely uraemic patient, the provision of additional nitrogen may be limited by restricted fluid intake or glucose intolerance. Children should not exceed 0.1 g of nitrogen per kg per day. Dextrose is the preferred source and is available in 500 ml units at 70% strength which, when mixed with 1 unit of Nephramine, gives a calorie to nitrogen ratio of 744:1. Electrolyte supplementation of the infusion may be required.

Administration through a central venous catheter is recommended, the rate being determined by clinical and biochemical assessment of the patient.

Contra-indications, warnings, etc Nephramine is contra-indicated in elderly patients with hyperammonemia, decreased (subcritical) circulating blood volume, severe uncorrected electrolyte and acid/base imbalance or with inborn errors of amino acid metabolism.

Nephramine should not be given to patients with absolute protein intolerance or a progressively deteriorating acid base balance. It does not replace dialysis and supportive therapy in patients with renal failure. The intake of non-essential amino acids should be restricted during Nephramine therapy.

Care must be taken with all additives particularly when phosphate, calcium and magnesium are introduced. The patient's biochemistry should be checked regularly to identify electrolyte imbalance, protein intolerance, acid-base imbalance, hyperglycaemia and rebound hypoglycaemia. Fluid balance must be carefully monitored in patients with renal failure to avoid circulatory overload, particularly in association with cardiac insufficiency.

Pharmaceutical precautions Do not use unless solution is clear and vacuum is present. Protect from excessive heat (above 40°C) and freezing. Protect from light until use.

Legal category POM.

Product licence number 0014/0232.

Nephramine is an American McGaw product from Boots Hospital Products, The Boots Company PLC, Nottingham.

NIVEMYCIN* TABLETS AND ELIXIR

Presentation Nivemycin Tablets are Neomycin Tablets BP each containing 350000 Units (approximately 500 mg) of Neomycin Sulphate BP.

Nivemycin Elixir is Neomycin Elixir BP. Each 1 ml contains 12,500 Units (approximately 20 mg) of Neomycin Sulphate BP.

Uses Nivemycin Tablets and Elixir are indicated for the pre-operative sterilisation of the bowel. Nivemycin is also used in the treatment of impending hepatic coma, including portal systemic encephalopathy.

Dosage and administration Pre-operative sterilisation of the bowel:

Adult: 2 tablets every hour for 4 hours, then 2 tablets every 4 hours for 2 or 3 days before the operation.

Children over 12 years: 2 tablets every 4 hours for 2 or 3 days before the operation.

Children from 6 to 12 years: $\frac{1}{2}$ to 1 tablet every 4 hours for 2 or 3 days before the operation.

Children from 1 to 5 years: 10 to 20 ml of Elixir every 4 hours for 2 or 3 days before the operation.

Children up to 1 year: 2.5 to 10 ml of Elixir every 4 hours for 2 or 3 days before operation.

Elderly: Elderly patients who are prescribed long-term Nivemycin should have a regular assessment made of renal function and hearing.

Contra-indications, warnings, etc Nivemycin Tablets or Elixir should not be given when intestinal obstruction is present.

Caution: Prolonged use of neomycin may result in the overgrowth of non-sensitive organisms; to minimise this risk, treatment should not be extended beyond the periods recommended. Care should be taken when administering Nivemycin to patients with impaired renal function or hearing.

Side-effects: Gastric disturbance is encountered occasionally.

Treatment of overdosage: Monitor renal and auditory function. If these are impaired dialysis is indicated.

Pharmaceutical precautions Nivemycin Tablets: Store below 30°C. Protect from light.

Nivemycin Elixir: Store in a cool place. Protect from light.

Legal category POM.

Package quantities Nivemycin Tablets: Bottle of 100. Nivemycin Elixir: 100 ml bottle.

Further information Nil.

Product licence numbers
Nivemycin Tablets   0014/5069.
Nivemycin Elixir   0014/5742.

OCUSOL* EYE DROPS

Presentation Ocusol Eye drops are a sterile preparation of Sulphacetamide Sodium BP 5% w/v, Zinc Sulphate BP 0.1% w/v and Cetrimide BP 0.01% w/v in an aqueous base of adjusted tonicity, viscosity and pH.

Uses Ocusol Eye drops are indicated in the treatment of superficial eye infections such as blepharitis, conjunctivitis and infections of the cornea. They may also be used as a prophylactic measure against infection following eye injury or the removal of foreign bodies from the eye.

Dosage and administration One drop to be instilled into the affected eye three or four times daily.

There is no evidence to suggest that the dosage of Ocusol should be reduced when treating the elderly.

Contra-indications, warnings, etc There are no known contra-indications to the use of Ocusol; no side-effects associated specifically with Ocusol have been reported.

Warning: Ocusol should not be used later than four weeks after the bottle has been opened.

Treatment of overdosage: There is no toxicological hazard even if the whole bottle is swallowed.

Pharmaceutical precautions None.

Legal category POM.

Package quantities 10 ml dropper-bottle.

Further information The formulation of Ocusol has an antibacterial activity equivalent approximately to that of a 30% solution of sulphacetamide sodium but is much less likely to cause local irritation than the latter more concentrated solution.

Product licence number 0014/5164.

POLYFUSOR* DEXTROSE INJECTIONS

Presentation Polyfusor Dextrose Injections are sterile, pyrogen-free solutions of Anhydrous Dextrose in Water for Injections prepared to British Pharmacopoeial standards. The solutions are enclosed in disposable, semi-rigid containers of pure polyethylene and are available in the following strengths:

Concentration of dextrose w/v (%)	Energy value in calories per litre	Concentration of anhydrous dextrose in grams per litre
2.5	94	25
5.0	188	50
10.0	375	100
20.0	750	200
40.0	1,500	400
50.0	1,875	500

Uses Polyfusor Dextrose Injections are given by intravenous infusion and are indicated in simple dehydration, carbohydrate depletion, hypoglycaemic coma. They can also be used to provide a temporary increase in blood volume in haemorrhage and shock.

Dosage and administration The volume, strength and rate of infusion of dextrose solutions given intravenously will depend upon the requirements of the patient and the judgement of the physician.

Elderly: Care should be taken to avoid circulatory overload, particularly in patients with cardiac and renal insufficiency.

Contra-indications, warnings, etc
Contra-indications: Diabetes, except as a treatment for hypoglycaemia. The intravenous infusion of dextrose solutions may be hazardous in patients with impaired hepatic or renal function.

Precautions: The intravenous infusion of dextrose solutions should not be too rapid or very prolonged. The rapid administration of large volumes of these solutions can cause water intoxication; conversely, infusion over a long period can cause dehydration.

Side-effects: Thrombosis of the chosen vein is always a possibility with intravenous infusion.

Treatment of overdosage: Introduce measures to correct water intoxication or dehydration as appropriate (see 'Precautions').

Pharmaceutical precautions Recommended storage conditions: 2–25°C. The shelf-life of Polyfusor Dextrose Injections is three years.

To prevent gross contamination of the outside surface of the Polyfusor, the outer envelope in which the Polyfusor is supplied should not be opened or removed until immediately before use.

Note: Immediately before use, the intact outer envelope in which the Polyfusor is supplied should be examined for moisture upon the inside surface; if moisture is observed, the integrity of the enclosed Polyfusor is suspect and it must be discarded. Unused solution remaining in a Polyfusor after use must also be discarded.

Legal category POM.

Package quantities Carton of 10 × 500 ml. Carton of 10 × 1,000 ml.

Further information Polyfusor Dextrose Injections provide a range of dextrose solutions designed to meet the many and varied requirements of intravenous carbohydrate therapy. Prepared to an exceptionally high standard, the solutions are supplied in disposable, semi-rigid containers made from a specially developed neutral plastic free from plasticisers, anti-oxidants and other additives likely to leach out and contaminate the enclosed

solution. The intact wall of the Polyfusor is impervious to micro-organisms and virtually impermeable to water vapour, thus ensuring the stability of the contents for very long periods under normal storage conditions (see 'Shelf-life'). Polyfusor Dextrose Injections are part of the Polyfusor range of solutions for intravenous infusion – a range of solutions which, both in quality and extent, can meet the general and specific requirements of modern intravenous therapy.

Product licence numbers
2.5%	0014/5886
5%	0014/5245
10%	0014/5244
20%	0014/5884
40%	0014/5892
50%	0014/5893

POLYFUSOR* GLYCEROL AND SALINE INJECTION

Presentation Polyfusor Glycerol Solution is a sterile pyrogen-free solution of Glycerol and Sodium Chloride in Water for Injections prepared to British Pharmacopoeial standards. The solution contains Glycerol 10 parts (by weight) and Sodium Chloride 0.9% 100 parts (by volume). Approximate ion concentration in millimoles per litre: Sodium 143, Chloride 143.

Uses Polyfusor Glycerol Solution is used in the treatment of acute cerebral oedema.

Dosage and administration The volume and rate of infusion of Glycerol and Saline given intravenously will depend upon the requirements of the patient and the judgement of the physician. Glycerol has been given intravenously as a 10% solution in 0.9% Sodium chloride Solution in a dosage of 1.2 g per kg body weight and every 24 hours for up to six days.

Elderly: Care should be taken to avoid circulatory overload, particularly in patients with cardiac and renal insufficiency.

Contra-indications, warnings, etc
Contra-indications: Cardiac or renal failure.

Precautions: The infusion must be given slowly.

Side-effects: Haemolysis, haemoglobinuria, and renal failure. Local phlebitis may occur.

Treatment of overdosage: Discontinue infusion.

Pharmaceutical precautions *Recommended storage conditions:* 2°C–25°C. The shelf-life of Polyfusor Glycerol and Saline Injection is three years.

To prevent gross contamination of the outside surface of the Polyfusor, the outer envelope in which the Polyfusor is supplied should not be opened before use.

Note: Immediately before use, the intact outer envelope in which the Polyfusor is supplied should be examined for moisture upon the inside surface; if moisture is observed, the integrity of the enclosed Polyfusor is suspect and it must be discarded. Unused solution remaining in a Polyfusor after use must also be discarded.

Legal category POM.

Package quantities Carton of 10 × 500 ml.

Further information Polyfusor Glycerol and Saline Injection is designed to meet the requirements of intravenous therapy. Prepared to an exceptionally high standard, the solution is supplied in disposable, semi-rigid containers made from a specially developed neutral plastic free from plasticisers, antioxidants and other additives likely to leach out and contaminate the enclosed solution. The intact wall of the Polyfusor is impervious to micro-organisms and virtually impermeable to water vapour, thus ensuring the stability of the contents for very long periods under normal storage conditions (see Shelf-life). Polyfusor Glycerol and Saline Injection is part of the Polyfusor range of solutions for intravenous infusion – a range of solutions which, both in quality and extent, can meet the general and specific requirements of modern intravenous therapy.

Product licence number 0014/5853.

POLYFUSOR* HARTMANN'S SOLUTION

Presentation Polyfusor Hartmann's Solution is a sterile pyrogen-free preparation of Compound Sodium Lactate Injection prepared to British Pharmacopoeial standards. The solution is enclosed in disposable semi-rigid containers of pure polyethylene.

Approximate ion concentration in millimoles per litre: Sodium, 131; Chloride, 111; Calcium, 2; Potassium, 5; Bicarbonate (as Lactate) 29.

Uses Polyfusor Hartmann's Solution is administered by intravenous infusion and is used for the treatment of dehydration with acidosis. It may also be used to expand extracellular fluids or restore extracellular electrolyte. Hartmann's Solution may also be used in the treatment of diabetic coma and the fluid and electrolyte losses associated with infantile diarrhoea.

Dosage and administration The volume, strength and rate of infusion of compound sodium lactate solution given by intravenous infusion will depend upon the requirements of the patient and the judgement of the physician. A dosage of 300 ml per hour should not be exceeded.

Elderly: Care should be taken to avoid circulatory overload, particularly in patients with cardiac and renal insufficiency.

Contra-indications, warnings, etc

Contra-indications: Hartmann's Solution should not be administered to patients with severe liver damage who would be unable to convert lactate to bicarbonate.

Precautions: Hartmann's Solution should be used with caution in patients with cardiac failure, hypertension, impaired renal function, peripheral and pulmonary oedema, and in toxaemia of pregnancy.

Side-effects: Thrombosis of the chosen vein is always a possibility with intravenous infusion.

Treatment of overdosage: Administer a suitable diuretic.

Pharmaceutical precautions Recommended storage conditions: 2–25°C. The shelf-life of Polyfusor Hartmann's Solution is three years.

To prevent gross contamination of the outside surface of the Polyfusor, the outer envelope in which the Polyfusor is supplied should not be opened or removed until immediately before use.

Note: Immediately before use, the intact outer envelope in which the Polyfusor is supplied should be examined for moisture upon the inside surface; if moisture is observed, the integrity of the enclosed Polyfusor is suspect and it must be discarded. Unused solution remaining in a Polyfusor after use must also be discarded.

Legal category POM.

Package quantities Carton of 10 × 500 ml. Carton of 10 × 1,000 ml.

Further information Polyfusor Hartmann's Solution is designed to meet the varied requirements of fluid therapy. Prepared to an exceptionally high standard, the solutions are supplied in disposable, semi-rigid containers made from a specially developed neutral plastic free from plasticisers, anti-oxidants and other additives likely to leach out and contaminate the enclosed solution. The intact wall of the Polyfusor is impervious to micro-organisms and virtually impermeable to water vapour, thus ensuring the stability of the contents for very long periods under normal storage conditions (see 'Shelf-life'). Polyfusor Hartmann's Solution is part of the Polyfusor range of solutions for intravenous infusion – a range of solutions which, both in quality and extent, can meet the general and specific requirements of modern intravenous therapy.

Product licence number
Hartmann's Solution 0014/5410.

POLYFUSOR* MANNITOL INJECTIONS

Presentation Polyfusor Mannitol Injections are sterile, pyrogen-free solutions of Mannitol in Water for Injections prepared to British Pharmacopoeial standards. The solutions are enclosed in containers of pure polyethylene. Polyfusor Mannitol Injections are available as solutions of 10% and 20% w/v.

Uses Polyfusor Mannitol Injections are administered by intravenous infusion and are used as an osmotic diuretic alone or to supplement the action of other diuretics in order to promote renal function. Other uses include the treatment of oliguria and to assist the elimination of drugs such as aspirin and barbiturates which are excreted by the kidneys.

Dosage and administration The volume, strength and rate of infusion of mannitol solutions given in intravenous infusion will depend upon the requirements of the patient and the judgement of the physician. A dose of 200 g daily by intravenous infusion should not be exceeded.

Elderly patients are more susceptible to the adverse effects associated with Mannitol. This is due to diminished renal and cardiac reserves. Elderly patients should, therefore, be given a test dose as described below for patients with renal failure.

Contra-indications, warnings, etc Mannitol is contra-indicated in cases of metabolic oedema associated with abnormal capilliary fragility. If renal flow is inadequate, water intoxication is likely in patients receiving intravenous mannitol; therefore, its use in oedematous conditions associated with diminished cardiac reserve should only be considered if the advantages outweigh the risks. Patients with impaired renal function should be given a test dose of 200 mg/kg body weight administered over five minutes and, if 40 ml or more of urine is produced in an hour, mannitol may be given in therapeutic doses.

Solutions of mannitol given in intravenous infusion should be administered slowly and should not be mixed with blood in transfusion apparatus.

Side-effects: Rapid intravenous infusion of mannitol may produce headache, chills or chest pain. It may also depress respiration by altering the acid-base and electrolyte balance of the body fluids. Convulsions have been noted in patients administered excessive doses of mannitol solution.

Treatment of overdosage: Introduce measures to correct water and electrolyte imbalance.

Pharmaceutical precautions Recommended storage conditions: 20–30°C. Exposure to lower temperatures may cause deposition of crystals. Carefully examine the solution for crystals immediately before use. If necessary redissolve by raising the temperature to 60°C. Cool to blood heat before use. The shelf-life of Polyfusor Mannitol Injection is three years. To prevent gross contamination of the outside surface of the Polyfusor, the outer envelope in which the Polyfusor is supplied should not be opened or removed until immediately before use.

Note: Immediately before use the intact outer envelope in which the Polyfusor is supplied should be examined for moisture upon the inside surface; if moisture is observed, the integrity of the enclosed Polyfusor is suspect and it must be discarded. Unused solution remaining in a Polyfusor after use must also be discarded.

Legal category POM.

Package quantities Carton of 10 × 500 ml.

Further information Polyfusor Mannitol Injections are designed to meet the many requirements of intravenous diuretic therapy. Prepared to an exceptionally high standard, the solution is supplied in disposable, semi-rigid containers made from a specially developed neutral plastic free from plasticisers, antioxidants and other additives likely to leach out and contaminate the enclosed solution. The intact wall of Polyfusor is impervious to micro-organisms and virtually impermeable to water-vapour, thus ensuring the stability of the contents for very long periods under normal storage conditions (see 'Shelf-life'). Polyfusor Mannitol Injections are part of the Polyfusor range of solutions for intravenous infusion – a range of solutions which, both in quality and extent, can meet the general and specific requirements of modern intravenous therapy.

Product licence numbers
10% 0014/5359
20% 0014/5360

POLYFUSOR* PAEDIATRIC ELECTROLYTE

Presentation Polyfusor Paediatric Electrolyte Solution is a sterile pyrogen-free solution prepared to British Pharmacopoeial standards. The solution is enclosed in disposable, semi-rigid containers of pure polyethylene.

Uses Polyfusor Paediatric Electrolyte Solution is given by intravenous infusion and is an electrolyte replacement solution for use in the treatment of infants, particularly where there is Potassium loss.

Dosage and administration The volume and rate of infusion of Polyfusor Paediatric Electrolyte Solution given intravenously will depend upon the requirements of the infant and the judgement of the physician.

Contra-indications, warnings, etc
Contra-indications: Severe liver damage, since such patients would be unable to convert lactate to bicarbonate; impaired renal or cardiac function.

Precautions: Because of the high potassium level, this infusion must be given slowly.

Side-effects: Thrombosis of the chosen vein is always a possibility with intravenous infusion.

Treatment of overdosage: Discontinue infusion and treat symptomatically.

Pharmaceutical precautions *Recommended storage conditions:* 2°C–25°C. The shelf-life of Polyfusor Paediatric Electrolyte Solution is one-and-a-half years.

To prevent gross contamination of the outside surface of the Polyfusor, the outer envelope in which the Polyfusor is supplied should not be opened or removed until immediately before use.

Note: Immediately before use, the intact outer envelope in which the Polyfusor is supplied should be examined for moisture upon the inside surface; if moisture is observed, the integrity of the enclosed Polyfusor is suspect and it must be discarded. Unused solution remaining in a Polyfusor after use must also be discarded.

Legal category POM.

Package quantities Carton of 10 × 500 ml.

Further information Polyfusor Paediatric Electrolyte Solution is designed to meet the requirements of intravenous electrolyte replacement therapy. Prepared to an exceptionally high standard, the solution is supplied in disposable, semi-rigid containers made from a specially developed neutral plastic free from plasticisers, antioxidants and other additives likely to leach out and contaminate the enclosed solution. The intact wall of the Polyfusor is impervious to micro-organisms and virtually impermeable to water vapour, thus ensuring the stability of the contents for very long periods under normal storage conditions (see Shelf-life). Polyfusor Paediatric Electrolyte Solution is part of the Polyfusor range of solutions for intravenous infusion – a range of solutions

Polyfusor Paediatric Electrolyte

Concentrations w/v (%)	Energy value in Calories per litre	Approximate ion concentrations in millimoles per litre
Sodium Lactate Molar Solution 1.825		Sodium 38
Potassium Phosphate BPC 1949 0.130		Potassium 35
Sodium Chloride BP 0.117		Chloride 45
Potassium Chloride BP 0.149		Phosphate 7.5
Hydrochloric Acid BP 0.042% v/v		Bicarbonate (as lactate) 18
Anhydrous Dextrose 5	188 Calories provided by 50 g of Anhydrous Dextrose	
Water for Injections BP to 100		

which, both in quality and extent, can meet the general and specific requirements of modern intravenous therapy.

Product licence number 0014/5799.

POLYFUSOR* PHOSPHATES INJECTION

Presentation Polyfusor Phosphates Injection is a sterile, pyrogen-free solution of Sodium Phosphate and Potassium Acid Phosphate in Water for Injections prepared to British Pharmacopoeial standards. The solution is enclosed in disposable, semi-rigid containers of pure polyethylene.

Concentrations w/v (%)	Approximate ion concentrations in millimoles per litre
Sodium Phosphate 2.9 Potassium Acid Phosphate 0.259	Sodium 162 Phosphorus 100 Potassium 19

Uses Polyfusor Phosphates Injection is given by intravenous infusion and is indicated in the treatment of severe hypercalcaemia, particularly that occurring in conjunction with cancer, hyperparathyroidism, hypervitaminosis-D, hyperthyroidism and sarcoidosis.

Dosage and administration The volume of phosphate solution given intravenously will depend upon the requirements of the patient and the physician. No more than 100 millimoles of phosphorus should be given over 24 hours. The infusion must be given slowly.

Elderly: Careful monitoring of elderly patients is essential (see *Precautions*).

Contra-indications, warnings, etc
Contra-indications: Intravenous phosphate therapy should not be used if the serum phosphorus concentration before therapy is raised.

Precautions: The patient must be carefully monitored. Rising blood urea nitrogen, elevation of serum phosphorus persisting more than 24 hours after therapy and normal or low serum calcium levels are among the contraindications to continued phosphate administration. Great caution should be undertaken during phosphate administration to patients with impaired renal function. In such patients 15–30 millimoles of phosphorus can be infused over 24 hours with constant monitoring of serum calcium and phosphorus.

Side-effects: Hypotension, tachycardia, pulmonary oedema, fever, hypocalcaemia and tetany, thrombophlebitis and calcification at infusion site.

Treatment of overdosage: Discontinue infusion and give appropriate supportive treatment depending on electrolyte determination.

Recommended storage conditions: 2°C–25°C. The shelf-life of Polyfusor Phosphates Injection is three years.

To prevent gross contamination of the outside surface of the Polyfusor, the outer envelope in which the Polyfusor is supplied should not be opened or removed until immediately before use.

Note: Immediately before use, the intact outer envelope in which the Polyfusor is supplied should be examined for moisture upon the inside surface; if moisture is observed, the integrity of the enclosed Polyfusor is suspect and it must be discarded. Unused solution remaining in a Polyfusor after use must also be discarded.

Legal category POM.

Package quantities Carton of 10 × 500 ml.

Further information Polyfusor Phosphates Injection is designed to meet the requirements of intravenous phosphate therapy. Prepared to an exceptionally high standard, the solution is supplied in disposable, semi-rigid containers made from a specially developed neutral plastic free from plasticisers, antioxidants and other additives likely to leach out and contaminate the enclosed solution. The intact wall of the Polyfusor is impervious to micro-organisms and virtually impermeable to water vapour, thus ensuring the stability of the contents for very long periods under normal storage conditions (see Shelf-life). Polyfusor Phosphate Injection is part of the Polyfusor range of solutions for intravenous infusion – a range of solutions which, both in quality and extent, can meet the general and specific requirements of modern intravenous therapy.

Product licence number 0014/0203.

POLYFUSOR* POTASSIUM CHLORIDE AND SODIUM CHLORIDE INJECTION

Presentation Polyfusor solution of Potassium Chloride and Sodium Chloride for intravenous infusion is Potassium Chloride 0.3% w/v and Sodium Chloride 0.9% w/v Injection BP in disposable containers of semi-rigid plastic. Each Polyfusor contains 500 ml of solution. Expressed in millimoles per litre, the electrolyte content of this solution is Sodium 150, Potassium 40 and Chloride 190.

Uses Polyfusor Potassium Chloride and Sodium Chloride Injection is given by intravenous infusion for the replacement of potassium loss.

Dosage and administration The amount of potassium administered by intravenous infusion depends upon the needs of the patient and the judgement of the physician; however, there are certain well-established principles concerned with potassium replacement.

1. The intravenous infusion of potassium solutions should be carried out slowly, i.e. at a rate not exceeding 20 millimoles of potassium per hour.
2. The concentration of potassium solutions given by intravenous infusion should not exceed 40 millimoles of potassium per litre.
3. An adult suffering from severe potassium loss may need up to 80 millimoles of intravenous potassium per day.
4. The administration of potassium (not necessarily by intravenous infusion) should be continued for at least three days after plasma potassium levels have returned to within normal levels.

Elderly: Care should be taken to avoid circulatory overload, particularly in patients with cardiac and renal insufficiency. Frequent monitoring of serum potassium is advisable.

Contra-indications, warnings, etc
Contra-indications: Addison's disease, adrenal insufficiency, acute or chronic renal disease, oliguria or anuria would preclude the giving of intravenous potassium.

Precautions: Before administering potassium by the intravenous route, it is essential to ensure that renal output is adequate and, by first giving a non-potassium hydrating solution, to ensure an adequate urine flow.

Side-effects: The adverse effects associated with the intravenous infusion of potassium solutions are almost invariably due to hyperkalaemia; these are listlessness, mental confusion, paraesthesia in extremities, weakness in the legs, hypotension, arrhythmias and, sometimes, cardiac arrest. Thrombosis of the selected vein is always a possibility with intravenous infusion.

Treatment of overdosage: Stop the infusion of potassium and, if there is persistent acidosis, replace with an infusion of sodium lactate or bicarbonate. Hyperkalaemia can be treated with an intravenous injection over a period of 145 minutes of Calcium Gluconate Injection BP.

Pharmaceutical precautions *Recommended storage conditions:* 2–25°C. The shelf-life of this product is 18 months.

To prevent gross contamination of the outside surface of the Polyfusor, the outer envelope in which the Polyfusor is supplied should not be opened or removed until immediately before use.

Note: Immediately before use, the intact outer envelope in which the Polyfusor is supplied should be examined for moisture upon its inside surface; if moisture is observed, the integrity of the enclosed Polyfusor is suspect and it must be discarded.

Legal category POM.

Package quantities Cartons of 10 × 500 ml.

Further information Polyfusor Potassium Chloride and Sodium Chloride Injection provides an immediately available source of intravenous potassium which obviates the inconvenient and somewhat hazardous use of extemporaneously prepared potassium solutions. Other Polyfusor solutions for use in potassium replacement therapy include Potassium Chloride and Dextrose, Darrow's Solution, Hartmann's Solution and Ringer's Solution. These intravenous fluids are part of an extensive range of Polyfusor Solutions for Intravenous Infusion designed to meet almost every requirement in intravenous therapy. Polyfusor solutions are supplied in disposable, semi-rigid containers of a pure polyethylene free from plasticisers, stabilisers or other additives likely to leach out and contaminate the enclosed solution.

Product licence number 0014/5856.

POLYFUSOR* RINGER'S INJECTION

Presentation Polyfusor Ringer's Injection is a sterile, pyrogen free solution of Sodium Chloride. Potassium Chloride and Calcium Chloride in Water for Injections prepared to British Pharmacopoeial standards. The solution is enclosed in disposable, semi-rigid containers of pure polyethylene. The solution contains, in 1 litre, approximately 147 millimoles of sodium ions, 4 millimoles of potassium ions, 2 millimoles of calcium ions and 155 millimoles of chloride ions.

Uses Polyfusor Ringer's Injection is given by intravenous infusion and is used to correct the water and electrolyte depletion associated with dehydration.

Dosage and administration The volume and rate of infusion of Ringer's solution given by intravenous route will depend upon the requirements of the patient and the judgement of the physician.

Elderly: Care should be taken to avoid circulatory overload, particularly in patients with cardiac and renal insufficiency.

Contra-indications, warnings, etc
Contra-indications: Intravenous Ringer's solution may be contra-indicated in patients with impaired renal or cardiac functions

Precautions: Ringer's solution should not be administered rapidly or for prolonged periods. Rapid injection may cause sudden cardiac arrest or circulatory overloading.

Side-effects: Thrombosis of the chosen vein is always a possibility with intravenous infusion.

Treatment of overdosage: Discontinue the infusion. The use of a diuretic may be indicated.

Pharmaceutical precautions *Recommended storage conditions:* 2°C–25°C. The shelf-life of Polyfusor Ringer's Injection is three years.

To prevent gross contamination of the outside surface of the Polyfusor, the outer envelope in which the Polyfusor is supplied should not be opened or removed until immediately before use.

Note: Immediately before use, the intact outer envelope in which the Polyfusor is supplied should be examined for moisture upon the inside surface; if moisture is observed, the integrity of the enclosed Polyfusor is suspect and it must be discarded.

Legal category POM.

Package quantities Carton of 10 × 500 ml.

Further information Polyfusor Ringer's Injection is designed to meet the requirements of intravenous therapy. Prepared to an exceptionally high standard, the solutions are supplied in disposable, semi-rigid containers made from specially developed neutral plastic free from plasticisers, antioxidants and other additives likely to leach out and contaminate the enclosed solution. The intact wall of the Polyfusor is impervious to microorganisms and virtually impermeable to water vapour, thus ensuring the stability of the contents for very long periods under normal storage conditions (see shelf-life). Polyfusor Ringer's Injection is part of the Polyfusor range of solutions for intravenous infusion – a range of solutions which, both in quality and extent, can meet the general and specific requirements of modern intravenous therapy.

Product licence number 0014/5253.

POLYFUSOR* SODIUM CHLORIDE INJECTIONS

Presentation Polyfusor Sodium Chloride Injections are sterile, pyrogen-free solutions of Sodium Chloride in Water for Injections prepared to British Pharmacopoeial standards. The solutions are enclosed in disposable, semi-rigid containers of pure polyethylene and are available in the following strengths:

Concentrations of sodium chloride w/w	Approximate ion concentration in millimoles per litre	
	Sodium	Chloride
0.18%	31	31
0.45%	77	77
0.9%	150	150
1.8%	308	308
2.7%	460	460
5.0%	855	855

Uses Polyfusor Sodium Chloride Injections are administered by intravenous infusion and are used mainly as an immediate measure to correct the water and electrolyte depletion associated with dehydration. Hypertonic solutions are used in the treatment of acute sodium deficiency and of water intoxication. Other uses include maintenance saline therapy in secondary dehydration and in haemorrhage, as a means of temporarily increasing blood volume.

Dosage and administration The volume, strength and rate of infusion of saline solutions given by the intravenous route will depend upon the requirements of the patient and the judgement of the physician. The effect of saline therapy on dehydration can often be assessed from relief of symptoms, observation of blood pressure and measurement of the volume and concentration of urine output.

Elderly: Care should be taken to avoid circulatory overload, particularly in patients with cardiac and renal insufficiency.

Contra-indications, warnings, etc
Contra-indications: Intravenous saline solutions may be contra-indicated in patients with impaired renal or cardiac function.

Precautions: Saline solutions should not be administered rapidly or for prolonged periods particularly in infants and the elderly. A too rapid injection of hypertonic saline may cause sudden cardiac arrest or circulatory overloading.

Side-effects: Thrombosis of the chosen vein is always a possibility with intravenous infusion.

Treatment of overdosage: An excess of sodium may be removed by the injection of a diuretic.

Pharmaceutical precautions Recommended storage conditions: 2–25°C. The shelf-life of Polyfusor Sodium Chloride Injections is three years.

To prevent gross contamination of the outside surface of the Polyfusor, the outer envelope in which the Polyfusor is supplied should not be opened or removed until immediately before use.

Note: Immediately before use, the intact outer envelope in which the Polyfusor is supplied should be examined for moisture upon the inside surface; if moisture is observed, the integrity of the enclosed Polyfusor is suspect and it must be discarded. Unused solution remaining in a Polyfusor after use must be discarded.

Legal category POM.

Package quantities Carton of 10 × 500 ml. Carton of 10 × 1,000 ml.

Further information Polyfusor Sodium Chloride Injections provide a range of saline solutions designed to meet the many and varied requirements of intravenous saline therapy. Prepared to an exceptionally high standard, the solutions are supplied in disposable, semi-rigid containers made from a specially developed neutral plastic free from plasticisers, antioxidants and other additives likely to leach out and contaminate the enclosed solution. The intact wall of the Polyfusor is impervious to micro-organisms and virtually impermeable to water vapour, thus ensuring the stability of the contents for very long periods under normal storage conditions (see 'Shelf-life'). Polyfusor Sodium Chloride Injections are part of the Polyfusor range of solutions for intravenous infusion – a range of solutions which, both in quality and extent, can meet the general and specific requirements of modern intravenous therapy.

Product licence numbers
0.18% 0014/5394
0.45% 0014/5696
0.9% 0014/5395
1.8% 0014/5738
2.7% 0014/5902
5.0% 0014/5906

POLYFUSOR* SODIUM CHLORIDE AND DEXTROSE INJECTION

Presentation Polyfusor solutions of saline and dextrose are sterile, pyrogen-free solutions of Sodium Chloride and Anhydrous Dextrose in Water for Injections prepared to British Pharmacopoeial standards. The solutions are enclosed in disposable semi-rigid containers of pure polyethylene and are available in the following strengths:

Concentrations of saline and dextrose w/v (%)	Energy value in calories per litre	Approximate ion concentration in millimoles per litre		Anhydrous dextrose in grams per litre
		Sodium	Chloride	
Sodium chloride 0.18 and dextrose 4	150	30	30	40
Sodium chloride 0.45 and dextrose 2.5	94	77	77	25
Sodium chloride 0.45 and dextrose 5	188	77	77	50
Sodium chloride 0.9 and dextrose 5	188	154	154	50

Uses Polyfusor Saline and Dextrose Solutions are given by intravenous infusion and are indicated for the treatment of dehydration with carbohydrate loss.

Dosage and administration The volume, strength and rate of infusion of saline and dextrose solutions given by intravenous infusion will depend upon the requirements of the patient and the judgement of the physician.

Elderly: Care should be taken to avoid circulatory overload, particularly in patients with severe cardiac and renal insufficiency.

Contra-indications, warnings, etc
Contra-indications: Intravenous saline and dextrose solutions may be contra-indicated in patients with impaired renal and cardiac function.

Precautions: Saline and dextrose solutions should not be administered rapidly or for prolonged periods – particularly in infants and the elderly.

Side-effects: Thrombosis of the chosen vein is always a possibility with intravenous infusion.

Treatment of overdosage: Injection of a diuretic.

Pharmaceutical precautions Recommended storage conditions 2–25°C. The shelf-life of Polyfusor Sodium Chloride and Dextrose Solutions is 18 months. To prevent gross contamination of the outside surface of the Polyfusor, the outer envelope in which the Polyfusor is supplied should not be opened or removed until immediately before use.

Note: Immediately before use, the intact outer envelope in which the Polyfusor is supplied should be examined for moisture upon the inside surface; if moisture is observed, the integrity of the enclosed Polyfusor is suspect and it must be discarded. Unused solution remaining in a Polyfusor after use must also be discarded.

Legal category POM.

Package quantities Carton of 10 × 500 ml. Carton of 10 × 1,000 ml.

Further information Polyfusor Sodium Chloride and Dextrose Solutions are designed to meet the many and varied requirements of intravenous therapy. Prepared to an exceptionally high standard, the solutions are supplied in disposable, semi-rigid containers made from a specially developed neutral plastic free from plasticisers, anti-oxidants and other additives likely to leach out and contaminate the enclosed solution. The intact wall of the Polyfusor is impervious to micro-organisms and virtually impermeable to water vapour, thus ensuring the stability of the contents for very long periods under normal storage conditions (see 'shelf-life') Polyfusor Sodium Chloride and Dextrose are part of the Polyfusor range of solutions for intravenous infusion – a range of solutions which, both in quality and extent, can meet the general and specific requirements of modern intravenous therapy.

Product licence numbers

Sodium Chloride 0.18% and Dextrose 4%	0014/5252
Sodium Chloride 0.45% and Dextrose 2.5%	0014/5869
Sodium Chloride 0.45% and Dextrose 5%	0014/5251
Sodium Chloride 0.9% and Dextrose 5%	0014/5250

POLYFUSOR* SODIUM LACTATE INJECTION

Presentation Polyfusor Sodium Lactate Injection is a sterile, pyrogen-free solution of Sodium Lactate prepared to British Pharmacopoeial Standards. The solution is enclosed in disposable, semi-rigid containers of pure polyethylene. The injection is one-sixth molar and contains, in 1 litre, approximately 167 millimoles of sodium ions and 167 millimoles of bicarbonate ions (as lactate).

Uses Polyfusor Sodium Lactate Injection is given by intravenous infusion and is used to treat acidosis and to alkalise the urine.

Dosage and administration The volume and rate of infusion of sodium lactate solution given intravenously will depend upon the requirements of the patient. It should be remembered that the conversion of sodium lactate to bicarbonate in the liver takes one to two hours so that for immediate correction of acidosis an injection of sodium bicarbonate should be given. The rate of infusion should not exceed 300 ml/hour.

Contra-indications, warnings, etc
Contra-indications: Intravenous sodium lactate solutions are contra-indicated in patients with severe liver damage.
Precautions: Sodium lactate solutions should not be administered rapidly or for prolonged periods – particularly in infants and the elderly.

Side-effects: Thrombosis of the chosen vein is always a possibility with intravenous infusion.
Treatment of overdosage: Discontinue the infusion and treat symptomatically.

Pharmaceutical precautions *Recommended storage conditions:* 2°C–25°C. The shelf-life of Polyfusor Sodium Lactate Injection is three years.

To prevent gross contamination of the outside surface of the Polyfusor, the outer envelope in which the Polyfusor is supplied should not be opened or removed until immediately before use.

Note: Immediately before use, the intact outer envelope in which the Polyfusor is supplied should be examined for moisture upon the inside surface; if moisture is observed, the integrity of the enclosed Polyfusor is suspect and it must be discarded. Unused solution remaining in a Polyfusor after use must also be discarded.

Legal category POM.

Package quantities Carton of 10 × 500 ml.

Further information Polyfusor Sodium Lactate Injection is designed to meet the requirements of intravenous sodium lactate therapy. Prepared to an exceptionally high standard, the solution is supplied in disposable, semi-rigid containers made from a specially developed neutral plastic free from plasticisers, anti-oxidants and other additives likely to leach out and contaminate the enclosed solution. The intact wall of the Polyfusor is impervious to micro-organisms and virtually impermeable to water vapour, thus ensuring the stability of the contents for very long periods under normal storage conditions (see shelf-life). Polyfusor Sodium Lactate Injection is part of the Polyfusor range of solutions for intravenous infusion – a range of solutions which, both in quality and extent, can meet the general and specific requirements of modern intravenous therapy.

Product licence number 0014/5248.

PROTHIADEN*

Presentation Prothiaden is Dothiepin Hydrochloride BP an antidepressant of the tricyclic group. It is available as sugar-coated tablets, each containing 75 mg of Dothiepin Hydrochloride BP and as hard gelatin capsules, each containing 25 mg of Dothiepin Hydrochloride BP. The tablets are red in colour and bear the overprint 'P75' in white. The capsules are red/brown with the overprint 'P25' in white.

Uses Prothiaden is indicated in the treatment of symptoms of depressive illness especially where an anti-anxiety effect is required.

Dosage and administration
Adults: Initially 75 mg/day in divided doses or as a single dose at night, increasing to 150 mg/day. In certain circumstances, e.g. in hospital use, dosages up to 225 mg daily have been used. Suggested regimens: 25 or 50 mg three times daily or, alternatively, 75 or 150 mg as a single dose at night. Should the regimen of 150 mg as a single night-time dose be adopted, it is better to give a smaller dose for the first few days.

Elderly: 50–75 mg daily initially. As with any antidepressant, the initial dose should be increased with caution under close supervision. Half the normal adult dose may be sufficient to produce a satisfactory clinical response.

Children: Not recommended.

Contra-indications, warnings, etc

Contra-indications: Recent myocardial infarction. Any degree of heart block or other cardiac arrhythmias. Mania. Severe liver disease. During breast-feeding.

Use in pregnancy: Do not use during pregnancy, especially during the first and last trimesters, unless there are compelling reasons. There is no evidence as to the drug safety in human pregnancy nor is there evidence from animal work that it is free from hazard.

Precautions: The elderly are particularly liable to experience adverse reactions to antidepressants, especially agitation, confusion and postural hypotension. Patients posing a high suicidal risk require close supervision. Prothiaden should be given with caution to epileptic patients and to those with cardiovascular disorders.

Avoid if possible in patients with narrow angle glaucoma, symptoms suggestive of prostatic hypertrophy and a history of epilepsy.

Tricyclic antidepressants potentiate the central nervous depressant action of alcohol.

Anaesthetics given during tri/tetracyclic antidepressant therapy may increase the risk of arrythmias and hypotension. If surgery is necessary, the anaesthetist should be informed that a patient is being so treated.

Drug interactions: Prothiaden should not be given concurrently with an MAO Inhibitor nor within fourteen days of ceasing such treatment.

Prothiaden may alter the pharmacological effect of some concurrently administered drugs including CNS depressants such as alcohol and narcotic analgesics; the effect of these will be potentiated as will be the effects of adrenaline and noradrenaline (some local anaesthetics contain these sympathomimetics). The hypotensive activity of certain antihypertensive agents (e.g. bethanidine, debrisoquine, guanethidine) may be reduced by Prothiaden.

It would be advisable to review all antihypertensive therapy during treatment with tricyclic antidepressants.

Barbiturates may decrease and methyl phenidate may increase the serum concentration of dothiepin and thus affect its antidepressant action.

Warning: It may be two to four weeks from the start of treatment before there is an improvement in the patient's depression; the subject should be monitored closely during this period. The anxiolytic effect may be observed within a few days of commencing treatment. Initially, Prothiaden may impair alertness; patients likely to drive vehicles or operate machinery should be warned of this possibility.

Adverse effects: The following adverse effects, although not necessarily all reported with dothiepin have occurred with other tricyclic antidepressants. Atropine-like side-effects including dry mouth, disturbances of accommodation, tachycardia, constipation and hesitancy of micturition are common early in treatment, but usually lessen.

Other adverse effects include drowsiness, sweating, postural hypotension, tremor and skin rashes. Interference with sexual function may occur. Serious adverse effects are rare. These include depression of the bone marrow, agranulocytosis, cholestatic jaundice, hypomania and convulsions. Psychotic manifestations, including mania and paranoid delusions may be exacerbated during treatment with tricyclic antidepressants. Withdrawal symptoms may occur on abrupt cessation of tricyclic therapy and include insomnia, irritability and excessive perspiration. Similar symptoms in neonates whose mothers received tricyclic antidepressants during the third trimester have also been reported, although this has not been observed following treatment with dothiepin.

Cardiac arrhythmias and severe hypotension are likely to occur with high dosage or in deliberate overdosage. They may also occur in patients with pre-existing heart disease taking normal dosage.

Treatment of Overdosage: Gastric lavage; when the patient is unconscious or the cough reflex depressed the lungs should be protected by a cuffed endotracheal tube. Repeated gastric/intestinal aspiration or repeated administration of activated charcoal may remove drug and metabolites excreted into the gut via the bile. Continuous ECG monitoring is advisable. Abnormalities of cardiac rhythm and epileptic convulsions may occur and should be treated accordingly. Forced diuresis is *not* recommended. Bedrest is advisable, even after recovery.

Interference with laboratory tests: There is no evidence so far that dothiepin interferes with laboratory tests.

Pharmaceutical precautions Recommended storage conditions: 5°C to 20°C.

Legal category POM.

Package quantities
Prothiaden Tablets: 75 mg: Calender Pack of 28; Bottle of 500.

Prothiaden Capsules: 25 mg: Bottle of 100, Bottle of 600.

Further information It has been found that, in certain cases of depression, the daily dose of Prothiaden given as a single night-time dose is more effective and even better tolerated than the conventional divided day-time dosage. There is evidence that this single bed-time dose improves the sleep pattern of the depressed patient.

When administered during lactation the results from a study in two patients indicated that dothiepin is not actively secreted into the breast milk. Assuming a daily milk intake of 150 ml/kg/day (2½ oz/lb) on a weight-basis (mg/kg) the baby would ingest 1/650 of the adult dose (mg/kg) of the drug. Other factors to be taken into account include the range of maternal blood levels, the presence of metabolites and the lowered drug metabolising capacity of babies which may result in elevated serum levels of unchanged drug.

Product licence numbers
Prothiaden Capsules   0014/5941
Prothiaden Tablets   0014/0209

QUICKSOL*
MONOPHANE*
TEMPULIN*

Presentation *Quicksol:* Neutral Insulin Injection BP (Highly Purified), a clear, neutral solution of purified bovine insulin.

Monophane: Isophane Insulin Injection BP (Highly Purified), a cloudy neutral suspension of a purified bovine insulin/protamine complex.

Tempulin: Insulin Zinc Suspension Injection BP (Highly Purified), a cloudy neutral suspension of purified bovine insulin consisting of 30% insulin zinc suspension (amorphous) and 70% insulin zinc suspension (crystalline).

All the above insulins are available in a strength of 100 units per ml.

Uses For the management of diabetes mellitus.

Quicksol may also be used in emergencies where a fast acting insulin is required, such as Hyperglycaemic Coma.

Dosage and administration The daily unit dosage of insulin is determined by the physician in accordance with the patient's requirements. The site of each injection should be changed according to a suitable routine.

Quicksol can be given by subcutaneous, intramuscular or intravenous injection, it may also be mixed in the syringe with either Monophane or Tempulin. When Quicksol is injected subcutaneously onset of action occurs within 30-60 minutes, with an overall duration of action of approximately 6-8 hours. Consequently, 2 or 3 injections daily before meals may be appropriate if not used in combination with other, slow acting insulins.

Slow acting insulins such as Monophane and Tempulin should only be given by subcutaneous or intramuscular injection, and not by intravenous injection.

Vials of both Monophane and Tempulin should be inverted several times before use in order to ensure adequate dispersal.

Monophane is normally injected subcutaneously. Onset of action occurs within 2 hours, with an overall duration of action extending to 18-28 hours.

Tempulin is normally injected subcutaneously. Onset of action within 2 hours, with an overall duration of action which may extend to 28-30 hours.

Intramuscular injection of all insulins gives a more rapid onset of action with an overall shorter duration of action than the subcutaneous route.

Transfer from conventional insulin: When patients treated with conventional insulin are transferred to Boots purified bovine insulin, there is no general decrease in dose requirements in the short term. Boots purified bovine insulins may therefore be given in similar unit dosage to the corresponding conventional insulins, without risk of provoking sudden Hypoglycaemia. Nevertheless the patient should be advised to take particular care during the period immediately following the changeover.

Contra-indications, warnings, etc Hypoglycaemia is an absolute contra-indication.

Insulin dosage requirements may change if the species of origin or type of insulin is changed.

Interactions: Insulin requirements may be affected by changes in life-style, diet, pregnancy, infections, other medical conditions or certain drug therapies.

Insulin requirements may be increased by the concomitant use of corticosteroids, oral contraceptives, thyroid hormones, thiazide diuretics and may be decreased by beta-adrenergic blocking agents and monoamine oxidase inhibitors. Since the clinical effects are variable, diabetic patients should be carefully observed initially when any drug therapy is co-prescribed.

Side-effects: The most important side-effect is hypoglycaemia. Reduction of hyperglycaemia in newly diagnosed diabetics may alter visual refraction.

Localised reactions at the injection site may include transient erythema, induration, urticaria and oedema. These usually resolve with continuing usage of insulin.

True generalised hypersensitivity reactions approaching anaphylaxis are very rare. Clinical evidence suggests that purified insulins are unlikely to cause localised lipodystrophy.

Treatment of Overdose: Hypoglycaemia caused by insulin overdose may be treated by intramuscular, subcutaneous or intravenous injection of glucagon. Subcutaneous injection of adrenaline may also be helpful in an emergency. Both these methods are short lived and must be supplemented by freely available carbohydrate as soon as possible.

Pharmaceutical precautions Store at 2°C to 8°C. Do not freeze. Avoid direct sunlight.

Legal category P.

Package quantities 100 units per ml: 10 ml vial.

Further information *Mixing in the Syringe:* Care should be taken to draw the neutral insulin into the syringe first.

Product licence numbers
Tempulin 100 units per ml 0014/0265
Quicksol 100 units per ml 0014/0266
Monophane 100 units per ml 0014/0267

STABILLIN* V-K ELIXIRS AND TABLETS

Presentation Stabilin V-K Elixirs '62.5', '125' and '250' are preparations of dry granules which, when reconstituted with the specified volume of water, provide elixirs (Phenoxymethylpenicillin Elixir BPC) containing respectively the phenoxymethylpenicillin potassium equivalent to 62.5, 125 and 250 mg of phenoxymethylpenicillin in each 5 ml.

Stabillin V-K Tablets are Phenoxymethylpenicillin Tablets BP 250 mg.

Uses Stabilin V-K preparations are indicated in the treatment of mild to moderate infections due to susceptible Gram-positive organisms and to prevent the recurrence of rheumatic fever.

Dosage and administration Phenoxymethylpenicillin should be taken 30 minutes before food.

Adult: 0.5 to 1.5 g daily in divided doses.

Children 6 to 12 years: 250 mg every 6 hours.

Children 1 to 5 years: 125 mg every 6 hours.

Children up to 1 year: 62.5 mg every 6 hours.

As a prophylactic: 1 tablet twice daily for adults; adjust dosage for children.

Elderly: Stabillin should be prescribed cautiously in elderly patients with severe renal impairment.

Contra-indications, warnings, etc Stabilin V-K is contra-indicated in patients with a known sensitivity to penicillin and should be given with caution to those with a history of allergy. Phenoxymethylpenicillin is secreted in the milk and should be used with caution in nursing mothers as it may cause an allergic reaction in the offspring.

Side-effects: Penicillins given by mouth sometimes produce transient diarrhoea and, occasionally, nausea, heartburn and pruritus ani.

Treatment of overdosage: Treatment is symptomatic, but is unlikely to be required.

Pharmaceutical precautions Stabillin V-K Elixir and the reconstituted Elixir should be stored in a cool place; the latter should be used within one week of preparation.

Legal category POM.

Package quantities
Stabillin V-K Elixirs: Bottle of granules to make 100 ml.
Stabillin V-K Tablets: Bottle of 500.

Further information Nil.

Product licence numbers
Stabilin V-K Elixir '62.5': 0014/5341
Stabilin V-K Elixir '125': 0014/5342
Stabilin V-K Elixir '250': 0014/5343
Stabilin V-K Tablets: 0014/5082

STERIFLEX* No. 1

Presentation Steriflex No. 1 is Sodium Chloride
Injection BP and is a sterile, colourless preparation of
normal saline for infusion in a clear, collapsible container.
Sodium Chloride Injection BP contains 9 g sodium
chloride per litre; sodium 150 millimoles per litre; chloride
150 millimoles per litre.

Indications Steriflex No. 1 is used in the treatment of
dehydration to correct water and electrolyte depletion.
It is useful in the treatment of acute sodium deficiency or
water intoxication.

Dosage and administration Intravenous infusions
are preferably administered through a needle inserted
into a superficial vein. However in obese patients or
young children this may prove difficult and then it will be
necessary to cut down to the vein and insert a cannula.
During intravenous infusion the limb should be immobilised, so there is less discomfort to the patient. If a leg
vein is selected this may increase the incidence of
thrombotic complications. Transfusion may be conducted under pressure, using the Martin or other suitable
rotary pump, or by application of pressure to the Steriflex
bag. The rate of administration and volume transfused
will depend on the requirements of the individual patient.
The correction of dehydration may be judged by relief of
symptoms, restoration of blood pressure, reversal of
haemoconcentration and the output of an adequate
volume of urine of normal concentration.

Elderly: Care should be taken to avoid circulatory
overload, particularly in patients with cardiac and renal
insufficiency.

Contra-indications, warnings, etc
Contra-indications: Patients with sodium overload. It is
well known that this may occur with myocardial and
renal damage, but it should also be appreciated that in
the first five or six days after surgery or severe trauma
there may be an inability to excrete unwanted sodium.

Precautions: Steriflex No. 1 is not suitable for protracted
use unless there is heavy continued loss of electrolytes;
even then, it should be used with care. In potassium-
deficient patients administration of normal saline will
increase potassium loss, so that if it is given, potassium
supplements should also be given.

Side-effects: Thrombosis of the chosen vein is always a
possibility with intravenous infusion. If infusion is
protracted then another vein should be selected after
12–24 hours.

Treatment of overdosage: An excess of sodium may be
removed by the injection of a diuretic.

Pharmaceutical precautions *Storage:* Store at 2°C–
25°C. The shelf-life is two years. The outer polythene

bag is not sterilised but simply serves to protect the
steriflex bag. Before use the pack should be inspected
and rejected if it is not clear or if the inner container is
damaged.

Legal category POM.

Package quantities Steriflex is packed in containers
of 10, in volumes of 500 ml and 1,000 ml.

Product licence number 0014/0190.

STERIFLEX* No. 3

Presentation Steriflex No. 3 is a sterile, colourless
preparation of Sodium Chloride and Dextrose Injection
BP containing 5% of anhydrous dextrose in a clear,
collapsible container and is intended for intravenous
infusion. It contains 8 g per litre of sodium chloride,
which represents 154 millimoles sodium and 154
millimoles chloride.
   The anhydrous dextrose in Steriflex No. 3 provides
188 Calories per litre.

Indications Steriflex No. 3 is generally the standard
solution for the correction of dehydration. In many
conditions it is preferable to Sodium Chloride Injection
BP (Steriflex No. 1), since the patient's carbohydrate
store may be depleted. It is also of value in Addisonian
crises and in dehydration with alkalosis.

Dosage and administration Intravenous infusions
are preferably administered through a needle inserted
into a superficial vein. However, in obese patients or
young children this may prove difficult and then it will be
necessary to cut down to the vein and insert a cannula.
During intravenous infusion the limb should be immobilised so there is less discomfort to the patient. If a leg is
selected this may increase the incidence of thrombotic
complications.
   Transfusions may be conducted under pressure, using
the Martin or other rotary pump, or by application of
pressure to the Steriflex bag.
   The rate of administration and volume transfused will
depend on the requirements of the individual patient.
The correction of dehydration may be judged by relief of
symptoms, restoration of blood pressure, reversal of
haemoconcentration and the output of an adequate
volume of urine of normal concentration. Where acidosis
is a feature, correction is indicated by the disappearance
of hyperventilation.

Elderly: Care should be taken to avoid circulatory
overload, particularly in patients with cardiac and renal
insufficiency.

Contra-indications, warnings, etc
Contra-indications: Patients with sodium overload. It is
well known that this may occur with myocardial and
renal damage, but it should also be appreciated that in
the first five or six days after surgery or severe trauma
there may be an inability to excrete unwanted sodium.
Steriflex No. 3 is not suitable for the treatment of insulin
coma.

Precautions: Steriflex No. 3 is not suitable for protracted
use unless there is a heavy continued loss of electrolytes;
even then, it should be used with care. In potassium-
deficient patients administration of normal saline solution
will increase potassium loss, so that if it is given,
potassium should also be given.

Side-effects: Thrombosis of the chosen vein is always a

possibility with intravenous infusion. If infusion is protracted then another vein should be selected after 12–24 hours.

Treatment of overdosage: Injection of a diuretic.

Pharmaceutical precautions *Storage:* Store at 2°C–25°C. The shelf-life is two years. The outer polythene bag is not sterilised but simply serves to protect the Steriflex bag. Before use the pack should be inspected and rejected if it is not clear or if the inner container is damaged.

Legal category POM.

Package quantities Steriflex is packed in containers of 10 in volumes of 500 ml and 1,000 ml.

Product licence number 0014/0191.

STERIFLEX* No. 6
STERIFLEX* No. 7

Presentation Steriflex Nos. 6 and 7 are sterile, colourless preparations of dextrose in water and are Dextrose Injection BP 5% and Dextrose Injection BP 10%, respectively. They are in clear, collapsible containers and are intended for intravenous infusion.

Steriflex No. 6 contains 50 g of anhydrous dextrose per litre providing 188 Calories per litre.

Steriflex No. 7 contains 100 g of anhydrous dextrose per litre, providing 375 Calories per litre.

Indications Steriflex No. 6 is an isotonic solution used for maintenance therapy of dehydration after electrolyte depletion has been corrected. It is also useful as a source of water and carbohydrate for patients who have undergone abdominal surgery and who are not able to take oral fluids. It may be used for the treatment of insulin coma. Steriflex No. 7 has the same uses as Sterilflex No. 6, but it provides more carbohydrate per litre and it is hypertonic.

Dosage and administration Intravenous infusions are preferably administered through a needle inserted into a superficial vein. However, in obese patients or young children this may prove difficult and then it will be necessary to cut down to the vein and insert a cannula. During intravenous infusion the limb should be immobilised, so there is less discomfort to the patient. If a leg vein is selected this may increase the incidence of thrombic complications.

Transfusion may be conducted under pressure, using the Martin or other suitable rotary pump, or by application of pressure to the Steriflex bag. The rate of administration and volume transfused will depend on the requirements of the individual patient.

Elderly: Care should be taken to avoid circulatory overload, particularly in patients with cardiac and renal insufficiency.

Contra-indications, warnings, etc The administration of these solutions in diabetic patients must be conducted with caution.

Precautions: The infusion of these solutions should not be rapid or very prolonged. Large volumes of these solutions given too quickly may cause water intoxication, infusion over a long period can cause dehydration.

Side-effects: Thrombosis of the chosen vein is always a possibility with intravenous infusion. If infusion is

protracted then another vein should be selected after 12–24 hours.

Pharmaceutical precautions *Storage:* Store at 2°C–25°C. The shelf-life is two years. The outer polythene bag is not sterilised but simply serves to protect the Steriflex bag. Before use the pack should be inspected and rejected if it is not clear or if the inner container is damaged.

Legal category POM.

Package quantities Steriflex is packed in containers of 10. Steriflex Nos 6 and 7 are available in volumes of 500 ml and 1,000 ml.

Product licence numbers
No. 6   0014/0193
No. 7   0014/0194

STERIFLEX* No. 9

Presentation Steriflex No. 9 is a sterile, colourless preparation of Ringer's Solution for Injection in clear, collapsible containers. It is intended for intravenous infusion. Each litre contains sodium chloride 8.6 g potassium chloride 0.3 g and calcium chloride 0.48 g; that is sodium 147 millimoles per litre, potassium 4 millimoles per litre, calcium 2 millimoles per litre and chloride 155 millimoles per litre.

Indications Steriflex No. 9 is used as an intravenous infusion when an isotonic solution is needed for the treatment of dehydration with salt depletion and where there has been some loss of intracellular potassium.

Dosage and administration Intravenous infusions are preferably administered through a needle inserted into a superficial vein. However, in obese patients or young children this may prove difficult and then it will be necessary to cut down to the vein and insert a cannula. During intravenous infusion the limb should be immobilised, so there is less discomfort to the patient. If a leg is selected this may increase the incidence of thrombotic complications. Transfusion may be conducted under pressure, using the Martin or other suitable rotary pump, or by application of pressure to the Steriflex bag. The rate of administration and volume transfused will depend on the requirements of the individual patient. The correction of dehydration may be judged by relief of symptoms, restoration of blood pressure, reversal of haemoconcentration and the output of an adequate volume of urine of normal concentration. Where acidosis is a feature, correction is indicated by the disappearance of hyperventilation.

Elderly: Care should be taken to avoid circulatory overload, particularly in patients with cardiac and renal insufficiency.

Contra-indications, warnings, etc
Contra-indications: Patients with sodium overload. It is well known that this may occur with myocardial and renal damage, but it should also be appreciated that in the first five or six days after surgery or severe trauma there may be an inability to excrete unwanted sodium.

Precautions: Although Steriflex No. 9 contains potassium the quantity may be inadequate in the presence of intracellular potassium loss.

Side-effects: Thrombosis of the chosen vein is always a possibility with intravenous infusion. If infusion is protracted then another vein should be selected after 12–24 hours.

Treatment of overdosage: An excess of sodium may be removed by the injection of a diuretic.

Pharmaceutical precautions *Storage:* Store at 2°C–25°C. The shelf-life is two years. The outer polythene bag is not sterilised but simply serves to protect the Steriflex bag. Before use the pack should be inspected and rejected if it is not clear or if the inner container is damaged.

Legal category POM.

Package quantities Steriflex is packed in containers of 10 in volumes of 500 ml and 1,000 ml.

Product licence number 0014/0195.

STERIFLEX* No. 10

Presentation Steriflex No. 10 is a sterile, colourless preparation of Darrow's solution in a clear, collapsible container. It can be administered intravenously. Each litre of Steriflex No. 10 contains sodium chloride 4 g, potassium chloride 2.7 g, molar solution of sodium lactate 53.3 ml. The millimole concentrations per litre are sodium 121, potassium 35, chloride 103, bicarbonate (as lactate) 53.

Indications Metabolic acidosis with potassium deficiency. In cases of dehydration and shock there may be deficiency of intracellular potassium in the presence of normal or high serum potassium values. If dehydration is corrected without potassium supplementation hypokalaemia may occur.

Darrow's solution is frequently employed where acidosis is due to fluid loss from the alimentary tract, e.g. diarrhoea or excessive vomiting, or due to diabetic coma.

Dosage and administration Steriflex No. 10 should be used with caution. As with all solutions containing potassium, administration should be by slow intravenous infusion. Where there is established potassium depletion 3 litres per 24 hours will be required for adults. In infants and children a total of 80 ml per kg per 24 hours is a guide to maximum dosage.

Elderly: Care should be taken to avoid circulatory overload, particularly in patients with cardiac and renal insufficiency. Frequent monitoring of serum potassium is advisable.

Contra-indications, warnings, etc

Contra-indications: Potassium-containing solutions should not usually be given intravenously to correct potassium depletion if potassium can be given by the oral route. Steriflex No. 10 should not be given to patients with cardiac arrhythmias.

Precautions: Particular care should be taken with patients who have oliguria or who have a plasma-sodium level below 120 millimoles per litre.

Side-effects: Untoward effects are likely to be due to hyperkalaemia and the first signs of this are shown in the electrocardiograph with the T wave becoming high and peaked. With increasing hyperkalaemia there is prolonged duration of the PR interval, leading to conduction defects, arrhythmias and possible cardiac arrest. Other symptoms include listlessness and mental confusion, numbness and tingling of the extremities, weakness of

the legs, hypotension and, particularly in oliguric patients, an ascending faccid paralysis.

Treatment of overdosage: When signs of hyperkalaemia are observed the infusion should be stopped and if acidosis persists replaced with a sodium bicarbonate or sodium lactate infusion. Hyperkalaemia may be treated by intravenous injection of 10 ml of calcium gluconate 10% solution with 50 ml or 50% dextrose solution and 10 units of soluble insulin.

Pharmaceutical precautions *Storage:* Store at 2°C–25°C. The shelf-life is two years. The outer polythene bag is not sterilised but simply serves to protect the Steriflex bag. Before use the bag should be inspected and rejected if it is not clear or if the inner container is damaged.

Legal category POM.

Package quantities Steriflex is packed in containers of 10, in volumes of 500 ml and 1,000 ml.

Product licence number 0014/0196.

STERIFLEX* No. 11

Presentation Steriflex No. 11 is a sterile, colourless preparation of Compound Sodium Lactate Injection BP in a clear, collapsible container. It is also known as Hartmann's Solution for Injection and as Ringer-Lactate Solution for Injection. It can be administered intravenously. Each litre of Steriflex No. 11 contains sodium chloride 6.0 g potassium chloride 0.4 g, calcium chloride 0.27 g, sodium lactate equivalent to 2.4 ml lactic acid. The millimole concentrations per litre are sodium 131, potassium 5, calcium 2, chloride 111, and bicarbonate (as lactate) 29.

Indications Steriflex No. 11 is indicated for the treatment of metabolic acidosis and dehydration with acidosis. It may be used to expand extracellular fluids or restore extracellular electrolyte in practically all patients.

The treatment of diabetic coma.

Dosage and administration Intravenous infusions are preferably administered through a needle inserted into a superficial vein. However, in obese patients or young children this may prove difficult and then it will be necessary to cut down to the vein and insert a cannula. During intravenous infusion the limb should be immobilised so there is less discomfort to the patient. If a leg vein is selected this may increase the incidence of thrombotic complications. Transfusion may be conducted under pressure, using the Martin or other suitable rotary pump, or by application of pressure to the Steriflex bag. The rate of administration and volume transfused will depend on the requirements of the individual patient.

Elderly: Care should be taken to avoid circulatory overload, particularly in patients with cardiac and renal insufficiency.

Contra-indications, warnings, etc

Contra-indications: Patients with sodium overload. It is well known that this may occur with myocardial and renal damage, but it should also be appreciated that in the first five or six days after surgery or severe trauma there may be an inability to excrete unwanted sodium.

Lactate-containing solutions are contra-indicated in patients with liver diseases.

Precautions: Although Steriflex No. 11 provides potassium this is only enough to maintain the potassium content of extracellular fluid and would be quite inadequate for patients with severe potassium loss. Under these circumstances potassium supplements must be given. Lactate overdose in patients with heart disease may provoke arrhythmias and heart failure. ECG monitoring is recommended if administering Steriflex No. 11 to such patients.

Side-effects: Thrombosis of the chosen vein is always a possibility with intravenous infusion. If infusion is protracted then another vein should be selected after 12–24 hours.

Treatment of overdosage: Where facilities exist for control of water and electrolyte balance overdosage should not occur. In less than ideal situations accidental over-administration can be treated with intravenous injection of a diuretic.

Pharmaceutical precautions *Storage:* Store at 2°C– 25°C. The shelf-life is two years. The outer polythene bag is not sterilised but simply serves to protect the Steriflex bag. Before use the pack should be inspected and rejected if it is not clear or if the inner container is damaged.

Legal category POM.

Package quantities Steriflex is packed in containers of 10, in volumes of 500 ml and 1,000 ml.

Product licence number 0014/0197.

STERIFLEX* No. 18

Presentation Steriflex No. 18 is Sodium Chloride and Dextrose Injection BP, a sterile, colourless preparation of sodium chloride 0.18% and anhydrous dextrose 4.0% in a clear, collapsible container. Each litre of Steriflex No. 18 contains sodium chloride 1.8 g and anhydrous dextrose 40 g. In each litre there are 30 millimoles of sodium, 30 millimoles of chloride and 150 calories.

Indications Steriflex No. 18 is probably the most generally used isotonic solution for maintenance intravenous fluid replacement. It can be employed for maintenance therapy. It can be used for the treatment of moderate-prolonged dehydration due to water-loss, but in severe cases 1 or 2 litres of Steriflex No. 1 (Sodium Chloride Injection BP) should be given before continuing with Steriflex No. 18.

Dosage and administration Intravenous infusions are preferably administered through a needle inserted into a superficial vein. However, in obese patients or young children this may prove difficult and then it will be necessary to cut down to the vein and insert a cannula. During intravenous infusion the limb should be immobilised, so there is less discomfort to the patient. If a leg vein is selected this may increase the incidence of thrombotic complications. Transfusion may be conducted under pressure, using the Martin or other suitable rotary pump, or by application of pressure to the Steriflex bag. The rate of administration and volume transfused will depend on the requirement of the individual patient.

Elderly: Care should be taken to avoid circulatory overload, particularly in patients with cardiac and renal insufficiency.

Contra-indications, warnings, etc
Contra-indications: Patients with sodium overload. It is well known that this may occur with myocardial and renal damage, but it should also be appreciated that in the first five or six days after surgery or severe trauma there may be an inability to excrete unwanted sodium.

Precautions: In patients with potassium deficiency it may be necessary to add potassium supplements.

It should not be used as initial therapy for patients in diabetic coma.

Side-effects: Thrombosis of the chosen vein is always a possibility with intravenous infusion. If infusion is protracted then another vein should be selected after 12–24 hours.

Treatment of overdosage: Injection of a diuretic.

Pharmaceutical precautions *Storage:* Store at 2°C– 25°C. The shelf-life is two years. The outer polythene bag is not sterilised but simply serves to protect the Steriflex bag. Before use the pack should be inspected and rejected if it is not clear or if the inner container is damaged.

Legal category POM.

Package quantities Steriflex is packed in containers of 10, in volumes of 500 ml and 1,000 ml.

Product licence number 0014/0192.

*Trade Mark

B. Braun Medical Ltd
Evett Close,
Stocklake,
Aylesbury,
Bucks. HP20 1DN

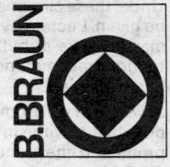

AMINOPLASMAL* L3, L5, L10

Presentation Colourless or faintly yellow coloured solutions for intravenous use, containing pure crystalline amino acids in the physiologically available L-form with added electrolytes. The product is supplied in three strengths and contains the following ingredients in each 1000 ml.

	L3 3%	L5 5%	L10 10%
Amino acids (g/l)			
L-Isoleucine	1.55	2.55	5.10
L-Leucine	2.65	4.45	8.90
L-Lysine . HCl	2.10	3.50	7.00
L-Methionine	1.15	1.90	3.80
L-Phenylalanine	1.55	2.55	5.10
L-Threonine	1.25	2.05	4.10
L-Tryptophane	0.55	0.90	1.80
L-Valine	1.45	2.40	4.80
L-Arginine	2.75	4.60	9.20
L-Histidine	1.55	2.60	5.20
Aminoacetic Acid	2.35	3.95	7.90
L-Alanine	4.10	6.85	13.70
L-Proline	2.65	4.45	8.90
L-Aspartic Acid	0.40	0.65	1.30
L-Asparagine H_2O	1.12	1.86	3.72
L-Cysteine HCl H_2O	0.22	0.36	0.73
L-Glutamic Acid	1.40	2.30	4.60
L-Ornithine HCl	0.95	1.60	3.20
L-Serine	0.70	1.20	2.40
L-Tyrosine	0.30	0.30	0.30
N-Acetyl-L-Tyrosine	0.12	0.43	1.23
Electrolytes mmol/l (mEq/l)			
Sodium	48	48	48
Potassium	25	25	25
Magnesium	2.5	2.5	2.5
Acetate	59	59	59
Chloride	18	31	62
$H_2PO_4^-$	9	9	9
Malate	7.5	7.5	7.5
α-Amino nitrogen (g/l)	3.47	5.78	11.56
Total nitrogen (g/l)	4.82	8.03	16.06

Uses Aminoplasmal L is a physiologically balanced amino acid infusion which also provides in its electrolyte content maintenance requirements of sodium, potassium and magnesium.

Aminoplasmal L can be used in the following conditions:

Parenteral nutrition: Prophylaxis and therapy of protein deficiency resulting from increased protein losses and/or increased protein requirements.

Surgery: In pre- and post-operative or post-traumatic conditions.

After resections in the gastrointestinal area.

Internal medicine for example:
Malabsorption syndromes.
Inflammatory diseases of the G.I. tract.
Persisting diarrhoeas and vomiting.

Nephrology: Kidney insufficiency with only slightly raised residual nitrogen values after dialysis treatment.

Dosage and administration The usual dosage is up to 30 ml per kg body weight per day.

For prophylaxis and therapy of slight protein deficiencies: 0.8–1.6 g amino acids per kg of body weight per day.

For covering protein requirements in pregnant women and in the post-operative phase: 1.6–2.0 g amino acids per kg of body weight per day.

For covering protein requirements of premature and newborn infants and after surgery on new-born infants: 2-3 g amino acids per kg of body weight per day.

For covering protein requirements in cases of kidney insufficiency under observation of the clinical-chemical parameters: 0.4–2 g amino acids per kg of body weight per day.

For balancing of massive protein losses, in particular after traumas, surgery, burns or fractures, higher doses must be administered on an individual basis. In such cases, an additional supply of calories is recommended in the form of fatty emulsions and carbohydrate solutions.

Aminoplasmal L is administered by slow intravenous infusion at an approximate rate of 40–60 drops per minute (120–180 ml per hour).

Contra-indications, warnings, etc

Contra-indications: Aminoplasmal L should not be administered in the following conditions:
Advanced liver disease.
Disturbed protein metabolism.
Manifest cardiac insufficiency.
Renal insufficiency with increased residual nitrogen values.
Acidosis.
Hyperhydration.

Warnings: Aminoplasmal L is not recommended for use in cases of hyperkalaemia.

Amino acid mixtures may precipitate acute folate deficiency and folic acid should be given daily.

Precautions: In order to ensure optimum metabolic utilisation of the amino acids administered the therapy should be supported by an energy supply of 35 kcal (145 kJ) per gram of amino acids.

Water balance, serum-ionogram, blood glucose level and acid base state should be regularly checked.

Side-effects: Providing the contra-indications are observed, side-effects are not to be anticipated.

Pharmaceutical precautions The product may be stored at room temperature. It is not recommended that any additives should be incorporated into Aminoplasmal L solution. They should, in preference, be given in standard carbohydrate or electrolyte solutions. However, if admixture with Aminoplasmal is essential then the compatibility of the additive should be checked before administration.

Legal category POM.

Package quantities 500 ml glass bottles.

Further information Nil.

Product licence numbers

Aminoplasmal L3	4296/0001
Aminoplasmal L5	4296/0002
Aminoplasmal L10	4296/0003

AMINOPLASMAL* PED

Presentation Colourless or faintly yellow coloured sterile solution free from particulate matter with the following composition:

Amino acids (g/l)

L-Isoleucine	1.40
L-Leucine	2.50
L-Lysine Acetate	4.50
L-Methionine	0.80
L-Phenylalanine	1.90
L-Threonine	3.00
L-Tryptophane	0.60
L-Valine	1.60
L-Arginine	2.20
L-Histidine	3.00
Aminoacetic Acid	4.90
L-Alanine	5.80
L-Proline	2.70
L-Aspartic Acid	1.90
L-Asparagine . H_2O	0.91
L-Cysteine . HCl . H_2O	1.46
L-Glutamic Acid	9.80
L-Ornithine . HCl	1.14
L-Serine	1.00
L-Tyrosine	0.30
N-Acetyl-L-Tyrosine	0.86

Electrolytes mmol/l (mEq/l)

Sodium	50
Potassium	25
Magnesium	2.5 (5.0)
Acetate	27
Chloride	15
Total amino acids (g/l)	50
α-Amino nitrogen (g/l)	5.7
Total nitrogen (g/l)	7.4
Caloric value:(kJ/l)	850
(kcal/l)	200

Uses Aminoplasmal Ped is a physiologically balanced

paediatric amino acid i.v. infusion which also provides in its electrolyte content maintenance requirements of sodium, potassium and magnesium.

Aminoplasmal Ped can be used for prophylaxis and therapy of protein deficiency in paediatrics when oral food intake is either contra-indicated or impossible as in cases like:

Premature birth.
Small-for-date syndromes.
Gastro-intestinal diseases and malformations.
Peri-operatively in paediatric surgery.
Intensive care after burns and severe injuries.

Dosage and administration *Premature and newborn infants:* Unless otherwise prescribed 40–60 ml corresponding to 2–3 g amino acids per kg of body weight per day. When administered during the first days of life, dosage should be restricted to 1 g amino acids per kg body weight per day and gradually increased to the above stated standard rate.

Babies: 40–80 ml corresponding to 2–4 g amino acids per kg of body weight per day.

The flow rate should be set in such a manner that the intended amount of solution to be administered is infused within 10–24 hours (preferably with an infusion pump).

Contra-indications, warnings, etc
Contra-indications: Aminoplasmal Ped should not be administered in the following conditions:
Disturbances in protein metabolism.
Renal insufficiency.
Advanced liver insufficiency.
Manifest cardiac insufficiency.

Warnings: Possible hyperhydration, hypotonic dehydration, hypokalaemia, hyponatraemia as well as acidosis have to be treated prior to commencing the infusion.

Amino acid mixtures may precipitate acute folate deficiency and folic acid should be given daily.

Precautions: In order to ensure the best possible economic utilisation of the amino acids administered, a therapy with Aminoplasmal Ped should adequately be supported by an energy supply of 145 kJ (35 kcal) per gram of amino acids.

Water balance, serum-ionogram, blood glucose level and acid base state should be regularly checked.

Side-effects: Providing the contra-indications are observed, side-effects are not to be anticipated.

Pharmaceutical precautions The product may be stored at room temperature. It is not recommended that any additives should be incorporated into Aminoplasmal Ped solution. They should, in preference, be given in the carbohydrate solution. However, if admixture with Aminoplasmal Ped is essential then the compatibility of the additive should be checked before administration.

Legal category POM.

Package quantities 100 ml and 250 ml glass bottles.

Further information Nil.

Product licence number 4296/0004.

*Trade Mark

Bristol-Myers Pharmaceuticals
Division of Bristol-Myers Company Limited
Uxbridge UB 10 8NS

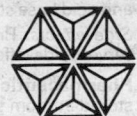

ALPHA KERI* BATH OIL

Presentation Alpha Keri Bath Oil is a clear colourless water dispersible anti-pruritic bath additive.

The product contains the following active ingredients: mineral oil (91.7%) and lanolin oil (3.0%).

Uses Alpha Keri effectively deposits a thin uniform emulsified film of oil over the skin, and thus retards evaporation of moisture, helps to relieve itching, lubricates and softens the skin.

Alpha Keri is valuable as an aid in the management of dry pruritic skin, especially in senile pruritus, ichthyosis and other dermatoses where dermal hydration is an important part of the therapy (as in the prevention of decubitus ulcer).

Alpha Keri Bath Oil is particularly suitable for infant bathing. The preparation also overcomes the problem of cleansing the skin in conditions where the use of soaps, soap substitutes and colloid or oat-meal baths prove irritating.

Dosage and administration Alpha Keri should always be either added to water or rubbed onto wet skin.

Because of its inherent cleansing properties soap should not be used with Alpha Keri.

Bath: Add 1–2 capfuls (10–20 ml) to the bath water. Soak for 10–20 minutes.

Sponge bath: Add 1–2 capfuls (10–20 ml) to a basin of warm water. Apply over entire body with a sponge or flannel.

Infant bath: Add ½ capful (5 ml) to bath water.

Skin cleansing: Rub a small amount onto wet skin, rinse and pat dry.

Shower: Pour a small amount onto a wet sponge or flannel and rub onto wet skin, rinse and pat dry.

Contra-indications, warnings, etc As Alpha Keri deposits a film of oil over the skin, special care should be taken to guard against slipping, especially in the bath or shower.

Alpha Keri contains lanolin oil and is therefore contra-indicated in those patients allergic to this ingredient.

Pharmaceutical precautions Nil.
Expiry date: 3 years from date of manufacture.

Legal category P.

Package quantities Alpha Keri Bath Oil is available in bottles containing 240 ml.

Further information Nil.

Product licence number 0125/0141.

AMIKIN*

Presentation *Amikin Injection:* Each multidose vial contains in 2 ml, amikacin sulphate equivalent to amikacin activity 500 mg (500,000 international units). The vial contains methyl and propyl paraben.

Amikin Paediatric Injection: Each ampoule contains in 2 ml, amikacin sulphate equivalent to amikacin activity 100 mg (100,000 international units). The ampoule contains no preservatives.

Uses AMIKIN is a semi-synthetic, aminoglycoside antibiotic which is active against a broad spectrum of Gram-negative organisms, including pseudomonas and some Gram-positive organisms.

Sensitive Gram-negative organisms include; Pseudomonas spp., *Escherichia coli*, indole-positive and indole-negative Proteus spp., Klebsiella-Enterobacter-Serratia spp., *Citrobacter freundii*, Salmonella, Shigella, Acinetobacter and Providencia spp.

Many strains of these Gram-negative organisms resistant to gentamicin and tobramycin show sensitivity to Amikin *in vitro*.

The principal Gram-positive organism sensitive to Amikin is *Staphylococcus aureus*, including methicillin-resistant strains. Amikin has some activity against other Gram-positive organisms including *Streptococcus pyogenes, Diplococcus pneumoniae*, and certain strains of enterococci.

Amikin is indicated in the short-term treatment of serious infections due to susceptible strains of Gram-negative bacteria, including Pseudomonas species. Although Amikin is not the drug of choice for infections due to staphylococci, at times it may be indicated for the treatment of known or suspected staphylococcal disease. These situations include: the initiation of therapy for severe infections when the organisms suspected are either Gram-negative or staphylococci, patients allergic to other antibiotics, and mixed staphylococcal/Gram-negative infections.

Therapy with Amikin may be instituted prior to obtaining the results of sensitivity testing.

Surgical procedures should be performed where indicated.

Dosage and administration At the recommended dosage level, uncomplicated infections due to sensitive organisms should respond to therapy within 24 to 48 hours.

If clinical response does not occur within three to five days, consideration should be given to alternative therapy.

Intramuscular or intravenous administration: For most infections the intramuscular route is preferred, but in life-threatening infections, or in patients in whom intramuscular injection is not feasible, the intravenous route, either slow bolus (two to three minutes) or infusion (0.25% over 30 minutes) may be used.

If required, suitable diluents for intravenous use are: normal saline, 5% dextrose in water, lactated Ringer's injection and lactated Ringer's injection with 5% dextrose. Once the product has been diluted the solution must be used as soon as possible and NOT STORED.

Adults and Children: 15 mg/kg/day in two equally divided doses (equivalent to 500 mg b.i.d. in adults):

Use of the 100 mg/2 ml strength is recommended for children for the accurate measurement of the appropriate dose.

Neonates and Premature Infants: An initial loading dose of 10 mg/kg followed by 15 mg/kg/day in two equally divided doses.

Sufficient extensive clinical use has not been achieved to enable firm dosage guidelines to be given in premature infants.

Elderly: Amikacin is excreted by the renal route, renal function should be assessed whenever possible and dosage adjusted as described under impaired renal function.

Life-threatening infections and/or those caused by pseudomonas: The adult dose may be increased to 500 mg every eight hours but should neither exceed 1.5 g/day nor be administered for a period longer than 10 days. A maximum total adult dose of 15 g should not be exceeded.

Urinary tract infections: (other than pseudomonal infections): 7.5 mg/kg/day in two equally divided doses (equivalent to 250 mg b.i.d. in adults). As the activity of amikacin is enhanced by increasing the pH, a urinary alkalinising agent may be administered concurrently.

Impaired renal function: In patients with impaired renal function, the daily dose should be reduced and/or the intervals between doses increased to avoid accumulation of the drug. A suggested method for estimating dosage in patients with known or suspected diminished renal function is to multiply the serum creatinine concentration (in mg/100 ml) by 9 and to use the resulting figure as the interval in hours between doses.

Serum Creatinine Concentration (mg/100 ml)		Interval between Amikin doses of 7.5 mg/kg/IM (hours)
1.5		13.5
2.0		18
2.5		22.5
3.0		27
3.5		31.5
4.0	X9 =	36
4.5		40.5
5.0		45
5.5		49.5
6.0		54

As renal function may alter appreciably during therapy, the serum creatinine should be checked frequently and the dosage regimen modified as necessary.

Intraperitoneal use: Following exploration for established peritonitis, or after peritoneal contamination due to faecal spill during surgery, Amikin may be used as an irrigant after recovery from anaesthesia in concentrations of 0.25% (2.5 mg/ml). It may also be instilled into the wound at closure. If instillation is desired in adults, a single dose of 500 mg is diluted in 20 ml of sterile distilled water and may be instilled through a polyethylene catheter sutured into the wound at closure. If possible, instillation should be postponed until the patient has fully recovered from the effects of anaesthesia and muscle-relaxing drugs.

Other routes of administration: Amikin in concentrations of 0.25% (2.5 mg/ml) may be used satisfactorily as an irrigating solution in abscess cavities, the pleural space, the peritoneum and the cerebral ventricles.

Only the paediatric dosage form (which contains no preservatives) should be used for intraventricular administration.

Contra-indications, warnings, etc Patients should be well hydrated during Amikin therapy.

In patients with impaired renal function or diminished glomerular filtration, Amikin should be used cautiously. In such patients, renal function should be assessed by the usual methods prior to therapy and periodically during therapy. Daily doses should be reduced and/or the interval between doses lengthened in accordance with serum creatinine concentrations to avoid accumulation of abnormally high blood levels and to minimise the risk of ototoxicity.

If therapy is expected to last seven days or more in patients with renal impairment, or 10 days in other patients, a pre-treatment audiogram should be obtained and repeated during therapy. Amikin therapy should be stopped if tinnitus or subjective hearing loss develops, or if follow-up audiograms show significant loss of high-frequency response.

As with other aminoglycosides, ototoxicity and/or nephrotoxicity can result from the use of Amikin; precautions on dosage and adequate hydration should be observed.

If signs of renal irritation appear (such as albumin, casts, red or white blood cells), hydration should be increased and a reduction in dosage may be desirable. These findings usually disappear when treatment is completed. However, if azotaemia or a progressive decrease in urine output occurs, treatment should be stopped.

The use of Amikin in patients with a history of allergy to aminoglycosides or in patients who may have subclinical renal or eighth nerve damage induced by prior administration of nephrotoxic and/or ototoxic agents such as streptomycin, dihydrostreptomycin, gentamicin, tobramycin, kanamycin, bekanamycin, neomycin, polymyxin B, colistin, cephaloridine, or viomycin should be considered with caution, as toxicity may be additive. In these patients Amikin should be used only if, in the opinion of the physician, therapeutic advantages outweigh the potential risks.

The risk of ototoxicity is increased when Amikin is used in conjunction with rapidly acting diuretic drugs, particularly when the diuretic is administered intravenously. Such agents include frusemide and ethacrynic acid, which is itself an ototoxic agent. Irreversible deafness may result.

The intraperitoneal use of Amikin is not recommended in young children or in patients under the influence of anaesthetics or muscle-relaxing drugs (including ether, halothane, d-tubocurarine, succinylcholine and decamethonium) as neuromuscular blockade and consequent respiratory depression may occur.

Pregnancy: The safety of Amikin in pregnancy has not yet been established.

Side-effects: When the recommended precautions and dosages are followed the incidence of toxic reactions, such as tinnitus, vertigo, and partial reversible or irreversible deafness, skin rash, drug fever, headache, paraesthesia, nausea and vomiting is low. Urinary signs of renal irritation (albumin, casts, and red or white cells), azotaemia and oliguria have been reported.

Overdosage: In the event of overdosage or toxic reaction, peritoneal dialysis or haemodialysis will aid in the removal of amikacin from the blood.

Pharmaceutical precautions At times, Amikin may be indicated as concurrent therapy with other antibacterial agents in mixed or superinfections. In such instances, Amikin should not be physically mixed with other antibacterial agents in syringes, infusion bottles or any other equipment. Each agent should be administered separately.

AMIKIN, as supplied, is stable at 25°C for a period of three years. At times, the solution may darken from colourless to a pale yellow but this does not indicate a loss in potency.

Expiry Date: 36 months from date of manufacture.

Legal category POM.

Package quantities *Amikin Injection:* 2 ml vials packed in cartons of 5.

Amikin Paediatric Injection: 2 ml ampoules packed in cartons of 5.

Further information Amikin is rapidly absorbed after intramuscular injection. Peak serum levels of approximately 11 mg/l and 23 mg/l are reached one hour after i.m. doses of 250 mg and 500 mg respectively. Levels 10 hours after injection are of the order of 0.3 mg/l and 2.1 mg/l respectively.

Twenty per cent or less is bound to serum protein and serum concentrations remain in the bactericidal range for sensitive organisms for 10 to 12 hours.

Amikin diffuses readily through extracellular fluids and is excreted in the urine unchanged, primarily by glomerular filtration. Half-life in individuals with normal renal functions is two to three hours.

Following intramuscular administration of a 250 mg dose, about 65% is excreted in six hours and 91% within 24 hours. The urinary concentrations average 563 mg/l in the first six hours and 163 mg/l over 6 to 12 hours. Mean urine concentrations after a 500 mg i.m. dose average 832 mg/l in the first six hours.

Single doses of 500 mg administered to normal adults as an intravenous infusion over a period of 30 minutes produce a mean peak serum concentration of 38 mg/l at the end of the infusion. Repeated infusions do not produce drug accumulation.

Amikin has been found in cerebrospinal fluid, pleural fluid, amniotic fluid and in the peritoneal cavity following parenteral administration.

Product licence numbers
Paediatric Injection 100 mg/2 ml   0125/0087
Injection 500 mg/2 ml   0125/0092

BAXAN* ▼

Presentation *Baxan Capsules:* white capsules containing cefadroxil monohydrate equivalent to 500 mg cefadroxil activity.

Baxan Suspension: supplied as a bottle containing powder for reconstitution to provide 125 mg, 250 mg or 500 mg per 5 ml.

Uses Baxan is bactericidal in vitro against a wide range of Gram-positive and Gram-negative micro-organisms.

Sensitive Gram-positive organisms include: penicillinase and non-penicillinase-producing staphylococci, β-haemolytic streptococci, *Streptococcus pneumoniae* and *Streptococcus pyogenes*. Sensitive Gram-negative organisms include *Escherichia coli, Klebsiella pneumoniae*, and some strains of *Proteus mirabilis, Haemophilus influenzae*, Salmonella spp. and Shigella spp.

Baxan is indicated in the treatment of the following infections when due to susceptible micro-organisms

Respiratory tract infections: Tonsillitis, pharyngitis, lobar and bronchopneumonia, acute and chronic bronchitis, pulmonary abscess, empyema, pleurisy, sinusitis, laryngitis, otitis media.

Skin and soft-tissue infections: Lymphadenitis, abscesses, cellulitis, decubitus ulcers, mastitis, furunculosis, erysipelas.

Genitourinary tract infections: Pyelonephritis, cystitis, urethritis, gynaecological infections, including puerperal sepsis.

Other infections: Osteomyelitis, septic arthritis, septicaemia, peritonitis, typhoid.

Dosage and administration
Adults and children weighing more than 40 kg (88 lbs): 500 mg to 1 g twice a day, depending upon the severity of infection.

Alternatively, in skin and soft tissue and uncomplicated urinary tract infections, 1 g once a day.

Children weighing less than 40 kg (88 lbs):
Under 1 year: 25 mg/kg daily in divided doses
1-6 years: 250 mg twice a day
Over 6 years: 500 mg twice a day.

Elderly: Cefadroxil is excreted by the renal route, renal function should be assessed whenever possible and dosage adjusted as described under impaired renal function.

The bioavailability and consequent chemotherapeutic effects of cefadroxil are unaffected by food. It may, therefore, be taken with meals or on an empty stomach.

Note: In patients with renal impairment, the dosage should be adjusted according to creatinine clearance rates to prevent drug accumulation and serum levels should be monitored. A modified dosage schedule is unnecessary in patients with creatinine rates of greater than 50 ml/min. In those patients with creatinine clearance rates of 50 ml/min or less, the following reduced dosage schedule is recommended as a guideline, based upon the creatinine clearance rate (ml/min/1.73m^2).

Patients with renal insufficiency may be treated with an initial dose of 1000 mg of Baxan. Subsequent doses may be administered according to the following table:

Creatinine clearance	Dose	Dose Interval
0-10 ml/min/1.73m^2	1000 mg	36 hrs
11-25 ml/min/1.73m^2	1000 mg	24 hrs
26-50 ml/min/1.73m^2	1000 mg	12 hrs

Contra-indications, warnings, etc Baxan is contra-indicated in patients with a history of hypersensitivity to cephalosporins.

In patients with a history of penicillin allergy, Baxan should be used with caution. There is evidence of partial cross-allergenicity between the penicillins and the cephalosporins. Should an allergic reaction to Baxan occur, the drug should be discontinued and the patient treated with the usual agents (pressor amines, corticosteroids and/or antihistamines), depending on the severity of the reaction.

The safe use of Baxan during pregnancy has not been established.

Precautions: As experience in premature infants and neonates is limited, the use of Baxan in these patients should only be undertaken with caution.

There are not sufficient data available to indicate whether the concurrent use of Baxan and potential nephrotoxic agents such as aminoglycosides causes any alteration in their nephrotoxic effects.

A false-positive Coombs' reaction may occur in some patients receiving Baxan.

Urine from patients treated with Baxan may give a false-positive glycosuria reaction when tested with Benedict's or Fehling's solutions. This does not occur with enzyme based tests.

Adverse reactions: Rash, pruritus, urticaria and angioneurotic oedema may be observed infrequently. Side effects, including nausea, vomiting, diarrhoea, dyspepsia, abdominal discomfort, dizziness, headache, and monilial vaginitis may also occur. Reversible neutropenia may occur rarely, as may leucopenia, and minor elevations in serum transaminase.

Colitis, including rare instances of pseudo-membraneous colitis, has been reported.

Pharmaceutical precautions Expiry date – 36 months from date of manufacture.

Legal category POM.

Package quantities Capsules – Containers of 100. Suspension – Bottles containing 60 ml

Further information Nil.

Product licence numbers
Baxan 500 mg capsules   0125/0107
Baxan 125 mg/5 ml suspension   0125/0110
Baxan 250 mg/5 ml suspension   0125/0111
Baxan 500 mg/5 ml suspension   0125/0112

BiCNU*

Presentation *BiCNU Injection:* each package contains a 30 ml vial containing 100 mg carmustine and a 5 ml vial containing 3 ml sterile ethanol diluent.

Uses BiCNU is indicated as palliative therapy as a single agent or in established combination therapy with other approved chemotherapeutic agents in the following:

1. Brain tumours – Glioblastoma, brainstem glioma, medulloblastoma, astrocytoma, ependymoma, and metastatic brain tumours.
2. Multiple myeloma – In combination with prednisone.
3. Hodgkin's Disease – As secondary therapy in combination with other approved drugs in patients who relapse while being treated with primary therapy, or who fail to respond to primary therapy.
4. Non-Hodgkin's lymphomas – As secondary therapy in combination with other approved drugs in patients who relapse while being treated with primary therapy, or who fail to respond to primary therapy.
5. BiCNU has also been used in the palliative management of other cancers such as malignant melanoma.

Dosage and administration

Intravenous administration: The recommended dose of BiCNU as single agent in previously untreated patients is 200 mg/m^2 intravenously every six weeks. This may be given as a single dose or divided into daily injections such as 100 mg/m^2 on two successive days.

When BiCNU is used in combination with other myelosuppressive drugs or in patients in whom bone marrow reserve is depleted the doses should be adjusted accordingly.

A repeat course of BiCNU should not be given until circulating blood elements have returned to acceptable levels (platelets above 100,000/mm^3; leucocytes above 4,000/mm^3) and this is usually in six weeks. Blood counts should be monitored frequently and repeat courses should not be given before six weeks because of delayed toxicity.

Doses subsequent to the initial dose should be adjusted according to the haematological response of the patient to the preceding dose. The following schedule is suggested as a guide to dosage adjustment.

Nadir after Prior Dose		Percentage of prior dose to be given
Leucocytes (/mm^3)	Platelets (/mm^3)	
>4000	>100,000	100
3000–3999	75,000–99,999	100
2000–2999	25,000–74,999	70
<2000	<25,000	50

Elderly: No dosage adjustment is required on the grounds of age.

Contra-indications, warnings, etc BiCNU should not be given to individuals who have demonstrated a previous hypersensitivity to it.

BiCNU should not be given to individuals with decreased circulating platelets, leucocytes, or erythrocytes either from previous chemotherapy or other causes.

BiCNU should not normally be administered to patients who are pregnant or mothers who are breast-feeding.

Safe use in pregnancy has not been established and therefore the benefit to risk of toxicity must be carefully weighed. BiCNU is embryotoxic and teratogenic in rats and embryotoxic in rabbits at dose levels equivalent to the human dose. BiCNU also affects fertility in male rats at doses somewhat higher than the human dose.

BiCNU is carcinogenic in rats and mice, producing a marked increase in tumour incidence in doses approximating those employed clinically.

BiCNU should be administered by individuals experienced in antineoplastic therapy. Since delayed bone marrow toxicity is the major toxicity, complete blood counts should be monitored frequently for at least six weeks after a dose. Repeat doses of BiCNU should not be given more frequently than every six weeks. The bone marrow toxicity of BiCNU is cumulative and therefore dosage adjustment must be considered on the basis of nadir blood counts from prior dose (see Dosage Adjustment Table under Dosage).

It is recommended that liver function tests also be monitored.

Adverse reactions: Haematological: The most frequent and most serious toxicity of BiCNU is delayed myelosuppression. It usually occurs four to six weeks after drug administration and is dose-related. Platelet nadirs occur at four to five weeks; leucocyte nadirs occur at five to six weeks post therapy. Thrombocytopenia is generally more severe than leucopenia. However both may be dose limiting toxicities. Anaemia also occurs, but is generally less severe.

Gastro-intestinal: Nausea and vomiting after i.v. administration of BiCNU are noted frequently. This reaction appears within two hours of dosing, usually lasting four to six hours and is dose-related. Prior administration of anti-emetics is effective in diminishing and sometimes preventing this side-effect.

Hepatic: When high doses of BiCNU have been employed, a reversible type of hepatic toxicity, manifested by increased transaminase, alkaline phosphatase and bilirubin levels, has been reported in a small percentage of patients.

Local: Burning at the site of injection is common but true thrombosis is rare.

Other: Rapid i.v. infusion of BiCNU may produce intense flushing of the skin and suffusion of the conjunctiva within two hours, lasting about four hours.

Guidelines for the safe handling of antineoplastic agents:
1. Trained personnel should reconstitute the drug.
2. This should be performed in a designated area.
3. Adequate protective gloves should be worn.
4. Precautions should be taken to avoid the drug accidentally coming into contact with the eyes. In the event of contact with the eyes, flush with copious amounts of water and/or saline.
5. The cytotoxic preparation should not be handled by pregnant staff.
6. Adequate care and precaution should be taken in the disposal of items (syringes, needles etc) used to reconstitute cytotoxic drugs. Excess material and body waste may be disposed of by placing in double sealed polythene bags and incinerating at a temperature of 1,000°C. Liquid waste may be flushed with copious amounts of water.
7. The work surface should be covered with disposable plastic-backed absorbent paper.
8. Use Luer-Lock fittings on all syringes and sets. Large bore needles are recommended to minimise pressure and the possible formation of aerosols. The latter may also be reduced by the use of a venting needle.

Pharmaceutical precautions *Preparation of intravenous solution:* Dissolve BiCNU with 3 ml of the supplied sterile diluent (absolute ethanol) and then aseptically add 27 ml of sterile water for injection to the alcohol solution. Each ml of the resulting solution will contain 3.3 mg of BiCNU in 10% ethanol and has a pH of 5.6 to 6.0.

Reconstitution as recommended results in a clear colourless solution which may be further diluted with sodium chloride for injection, or 5% dextrose for injection.

The reconstituted solution must be given intravenously and should be administered by i.v. drip over a one- to two-hour period. Injection of BiCNU over shorter periods of time may produce intense pain and burning at the site of injection.

Important note: The lyophilised dosage formulation contains no preservatives and is not intended as a multiple dose vial.

Stability: Unopened vials of the dry powder must be stored in a refrigerator (2°C–8°C). The recommended storage of unopened vials prevents significant decomposition for at least three years.

After reconstitution as recommended, decomposition of BiCNU at room temperature is linear with time. After three hours, approximately 6% of the solution has decomposed and after six hours, approximately 8%. Refrigeration (4°C) of the reconstituted BiCNU significantly increases the stability of the solution. After 24 hours, when protected from light, there is only 4% decomposition. Further dilution of the reconstituted solution with 500 ml of sodium chloride for injection or 5% dextrose for injection, results in a solution which is stable for 48 hours when protected from light and refrigerated.

Important note: BiCNU has a low melting point (approximately 27°C or 80.6°F). Exposure of the drug to this temperature or above will cause the drug to liquefy and appear as an oil film in the bottom of the vials. This is a sign of decomposition and vials should be discarded.

Legal category POM.

Package quantities BiCNU Injection packed in cartons of 10 units, each unit consisting of one vial of carmustine 100 mg and one vial of sterile absolute alcohol 3 ml.

Further information BiCNU alkylates DNA and RNA and has also been shown to inhibit several enzymes by carbamoylation of amino acids in proteins.

Intravenously administered BiCNU is rapidly degraded, with no intact drug detectable after 15 minutes. However, in studies with C^{14} labelled drug, prolonged levels of the isotope were observed in the plasma and tissue, probably representing radioactive fragments of the parent compound.

It is thought that the antineoplastic and toxic activities of BiCNU may be due to metabolites. Approximately 60 to 70% of a total dose is excreted in the urine in 96 hours and about 10% as respiratory CO_2. The fate of the remainder is undetermined.

Because of the high lipid solubility and the relative lack of ionisation at a physiological pH, BiCNU crosses the blood brain barrier.

Levels of radioactivity in the CSF are at least 50% higher than those measured concurrently in plasma.

Product licence number 0125/0108.

DEFENCIN CP*

Presentation Hard gelatin capsules (No. 4), having a pale pink cap and red body. Each capsule is coded Defencin VS40 and contains the equivalent of 40 mg isoxsuprine, in graded release form.

Uses Cerebral vascular disease including cerebral arteriosclerosis, cerebral vasospasm, and cerebral ischaemia.

Peripheral vascular disease including peripheral arteriosclerosis, Buerger's disease, Raynaud's disease and peripheral vasospasm.

Dosage and administration *Adults:* 1 capsule every 12 hours.

Children: The product is not intended for administration to children.

Elderly: The majority of clinical evidence relates to the use of the product in the older patient. No dosage adjustment is necessary.

Contra-indications, warnings, etc Recent arterial bleeding or immediately post-partum.

Defencin is extremely well tolerated and side-effects are rare. Occasional hypotension, tachycardia, flushing or palpitations have been reported with preparations of isoxsuprine, but these are controlled by a reduction in dose.

Overdosage: Gross overdosages have not been reported; treatment would be gastric lavage, and if necessary, a non-selective beta-blocker may be administered intra-muscularly.

Pharmaceutical precautions To be stored in a cool dry place, at temperatures generally not exceeding 20°C, protected from light.
Expiry date – 36 months from date of manufacture.

Legal category P.

Package quantities Blister strip of 14 capsules with 4 strips to a carton.

Further information Isoxsuprine (Defencin) is a myovascular relaxant which acts directly on vascular smooth muscle.

Product licence number 0125/0074.

KERALYT* GEL

Presentation A clear colourless gel containing 6% salicylic acid.

Uses Keralyt is a topical aid to the removal of excessive keratin in hyperkeratotic skin disorders, including various ichthyoses, keratoses, pityriasis rubra pilaris and psoriasis (including body, scalp, palms and soles).

Dosage and administration Apply thoroughly to the affected area and place under occlusion at night. The skin should be hydrated for at least five minutes prior to application. The medication is washed off in the morning, and if excessive drying and/or irritation is observed, a bland cream or lotion may be applied. Once clearing is apparent, the occasional use of Keralyt will usually maintain the remission. In those areas where occlusion is difficult or impossible, application may be made more frequently, and hydration by wet packs or baths prior to application may enhance the effect. Unless hands are being treated, rinse hands thoroughly following application.

Elderly: No dosage adjustment is necessary.

Contra-indications, warnings, etc Known sensitivity to any of the ingredients.

Precautions: For external use only. Avoid contact with eyes and mucous membranes.
Salicylate poisoning has followed the application of salicylic acid to large areas of skin.
Keep out of reach of children.

Pharmaceutical precautions Nil.
Expiry date: 4 years from date of manufacture.

Legal category P.

Package quantities 55 g

Further information Nil.

Product licence number 0125/0140

KERI* THERAPEUTIC LOTION

Presentation Keri Therapeutic Lotion is a white lotion containing mineral oil, 16%.

Uses Keri Therapeutic Lotion has emollient properties. It is indicated for the symptomatic treatment of dermatitis, eczema, ichthyosis, ammoniacal dermatitis (nappy rash), protection of raw and abraded skin areas, pruritus and related conditions where dry scaly skin is a problem. It is also indicated as an emollient before bathing for dry/eczematous skin, to alleviate drying effects.

Dosage and administration Keri Therapeutic Lotion should be gently massaged into the skin three times daily or as often as required.
Elderly: No dosage adjustment is necessary.

Contra-indications, warnings, etc Keri Therapeutic Lotion contains lanolin oil and is therefore contra-indicated in those patients allergic to this ingredient.

Pharmaceutical precautions Nil.
Expiry date: 3 years from date of manufacture.

Legal category P.

Package quantities Bottles containing 190 ml & 380 ml.

Further information Nil.

Product licence number 0125/0152

MEGACE*

Presentation Megace 40 mg tablets: White, circular, scored tablets, engraved '40' on one face, each tablet containing Megestrol Acetate BP 40 mg.
Megace 160 mg tablets – off-white, oval scored tablets, engraved '160' on one face, each tablet containing Megestrol Acetate BP 160 mg.

Uses Megace is a progestational agent, indicated for the treatment of certain hormone-dependent neoplasms, such as endometrial or breast cancer.

Dosage and administration Oral.
Breast cancer: 160 mg/day (40 mg qid or 160 mg taken once daily).
Endometrial cancer: 40–320 mg/day in divided doses (40–80 mg one to four times daily or one to two 160 mg tablets daily).
At least two months of continuous treatment is considered an adequate period for determining the efficacy of Megace.

Elderly: No dosage adjustment is necessary.

Contra-indications, warnings, etc Megace is contra-indicated in patients who have demonstrated hypersensitivity to the drug.

Precautions: Megace should be used with caution in patients with a history of thrombophlebitis.

Adverse reactions: The major side-effect experienced by patients while taking megestrol acetate, particularly at high doses, is weight gain, which is usually not associated with water retention, but which is secondary to an increased appetite and food intake. A rarely encountered side-effect of prolonged administration of megestrol acetate is urticaria, presumably an idiosyncratic reaction to the drug. An occasionally noted, usually transient, side-effect is nausea. Reports have been received of patients developing carpal tunnel syndrome, deep vein thrombophlebitis and alopecia while taking megestrol acetate. The drug is devoid of the myelosuppressive activity characteristic of many cytotoxic drugs and it causes no significant changes in haematology, blood chemistry or urinalysis.

Overdosage: No serious side effects have resulted from studies involving Megace (megestrol acetate) administered in dosages as high as 800 mg/day.

Pharmaceutical precautions Megace tablets should be stored at room temperature. Shelf-life: 40 mg tablet – 5 years; 160 mg tablet – 3 years.

Legal category POM.

Package quantities 40 mg tablet – units of 100 and 250 tablets.
160 mg tablet – units of 30 tablets.

Further information Nil.

Product licence numbers
40 mg tablet   0125/0144
160 mg tablet   0125/0173

NEOPLATIN*

Presentation *Neoplatin injection:* Vials containing 10 mg and 50 mg cisplatin (cis-diamminedichloroplatinum).

Uses Neoplatin is indicated as palliative therapy to be employed in addition to other modalities, or in established combination therapy with other approved chemotherapeutic agents in the management of neoplastic diseases, especially:

Metastatic Testicular Tumours – In patients who have already received appropriate surgical and/or radiotherapeutic procedures. The combination of Neoplatin, bleomycin and vinblastine has been reported to be highly effective. Other combinations have also been reported to be active.

Metastatic Ovarian Tumours – As secondary therapy in patients refractory to standard chemotherapy.

Dosage and administration
Single agent therapy: The recommended dose of Neoplatin in adults and children is 50–120 mg/m^2 as a single i.v. dose every three to four weeks, or 15–20 mg/m^2 i.v. daily for five days every three to four weeks.

Combination therapy: In general, current multiple drug treatment schedules including Neoplatin employ lower doses ranging from 20 mg/m^2 upwards, administered i.v. every three to four weeks.

Pretreatment hydration with 1–2 litres of fluid infused for 8–12 hours prior to a Neoplatin dose is recommended in order to initiate diuresis.

Reconstitute the 10 mg vial contents with 10 ml, and the 50 mg vial contents with 50 ml of Sterile Water for Injection PhEur. The resulting drug solution is then administered in 2 litres of a suitable diluent such as 0.9% saline, or a dextrose-saline solution. It is recommended that administration should be over a six–eight hour period. Diuresis may be aided by the addition to the infusion solution of 37.5 g mannitol.

Adequate hydration and urinary output must be maintained during the 24 hours following infusion.

A repeat course of Neoplatin should not be given until the serum creatinine is below 1.5 mg/100 ml (130 mcmol/l) and/or the blood urea below 55 mg/100 ml (9 mmol/l). A repeat course should not be given until circulating blood elements are at an acceptable level. Subsequent doses of Neoplatin should not be given until an audiometric analysis indicates that auditory acuity is within normal limits.

Elderly: No specific dosage adjustments but extra care should be taken to evaluate renal function prior to administration.

Contra-indications, warnings, etc Neoplatin induces nephrotoxicity, myelosuppression, neurotoxicity and ototoxicity which may be additive to pre-existing dysfunctions. Consequently, the use of Neoplatin in patients with hearing or renal impairment or depressed bone marrow function may be associated with increased toxicities. Such conditions represent relative contra-indications.

Neoplatin is contra-indicated in patients with a history of hypersensitivity to Neoplatin or other platinum-containing compounds.

Warnings: Neoplatin produces cumulative nephrotoxicity. The serum creatinine, BUN or creatinine clearance should be measured prior to initiating therapy, and prior to each subsequent course.

Anaphylactic-like reactions to Neoplatin have been reported. These reactions have occurred within minutes of administration to patients with prior exposure to Neoplatin and have been alleviated by administration of adrenaline, steroids and antihistamines.

Safe use in pregnancy has not been established. This product should not normally be administered to patients who are pregnant or to mothers who are breast-feeding. Neoplatin is mutagenic in bacteria and produces chromosome aberrations in animal cells in tissue culture. Although carcinogenicity and teratogenicity have not been established, compounds with similar mechanisms of action and mutagenicity have been reported to be carcinogenic.

The influence of Neoplatin on human reproduction has not been determined. Neoplatin therapy might have an anti-fertility effect.

Precautions: Neoplatin should be administered by individuals experienced in the use of antineoplastic therapy.

Neurotoxicity appears to be cumulative. Prior to each course, the absence of symptoms of peripheral neuropathy should be established. (*See* Adverse Reactions.)

Since renal toxicity is cumulative, measurements of BUN, serum creatinine or creatinine clearance should be performed prior to initiating therapy and prior to each subsequent course. At the recommended dosage, Neoplatin should not be given more frequently than once every three to four weeks. (*See* Adverse Reactions.)

Since ototoxicity of Neoplatin is cumulative, audiometric testing should be performed prior to initiating therapy and prior to each subsequent course of the drug. (*See* Adverse Reactions.)

Peripheral blood counts should be monitored weekly. Liver function should be monitored periodically. Neurological examination should also be performed regularly. (*See* Adverse Reactions.)

Adverse reactions: Nephrotoxicity: Renal toxicity has been noted in about one third of patients given a single dose of Neoplatin *when prior hydration has not been employed.* It is first noted during the second week after a dose and is manifested by elevations in BUN and serum creatinine, serum uric acid and/or a decrease in creatinine clearance.

Renal toxicity becomes more prolonged and severe with repeated courses of the drug. Renal function must return to normal before another dose of Neoplatin can be given.

Renal function impairment has been associated with renal tubular damage. The administration of Neoplatin using a six to eight hour infusion with intravenous hydration and mannitol has been used to reduce nephrotoxicity. However, renal toxicity still can occur after utilisation of these procedures.

Neurotoxicity: Neurotoxicity, usually characterised by peripheral neuropathies, has occurred in some patients. Loss of taste and seizures have also been reported. Neuropathies resulting from Neoplatin treatment may occur after prolonged therapy (four to seven months); however, neurological symptoms have been reported to occur after a single dose.

Neoplatin therapy should be discontinued when the symptoms are first observed. Preliminary evidence suggests peripheral neuropathy may be irreversible in some patients.

Ototoxicity: Ototoxicity has been observed in patients treated with a single dose of Neoplatin, 50 mg/m^2, and is manifested by tinnitus and/or hearing loss in the high frequency range (4,000 to 8,000 Hz).

Decreased ability to hear normal conversational tones may occur occasionally. Ototoxic effects may be more severe in children receiving Neoplatin. Hearing loss can be unilateral or bilateral and tends to become more frequent and severe with repeated doses. It is unclear whether Neoplatin-induced ototoxicity is reversible. Careful monitoring by audiometry should be performed prior to initiation of therapy and prior to subsequent doses of Neoplatin.

Haematological: Myelosuppression may occur in patients treated with Neoplatin. The nadirs in circulating platelets and leucocytes occur between days 18 to 23 (range 7.5 to 45) with most patients recovering by day 39 (range 13 to 62). Leucopenia and thrombocytopenia are more pronounced at higher doses. Anaemia (decrease in haemoglobin level by 2 g/100 ml blood) occurs at approximately the same frequency and with the same timing as leucopenia and thrombocytopenia.

Gastro-intestinal: Marked nausea and vomiting occur in almost all patients treated with Neoplatin and are occasionally so severe that the drug must be discontinued. Nausea and vomiting usually begin within one to four hours after treatment and last up to 24 hours. Various degrees of nausea and anorexia may persist for up to one week after treatment.

Other toxicities: Hyperuricaemia: Hyperuricaemia has been reported to occur at approximately the same frequency as the increases in BUN and serum creatinine. It is more pronounced after doses greater than 50 mg/m^2, and peak levels of uric acid generally occur between three to five days after the dose. Allopurinol therapy for hyperuricaemia effectively reduces uric acid levels.

Anaphylactic-like reactions: Anaphylactic-like reactions, possibly secondary to Neoplatin therapy, have been occasionally reported in patients previously exposed to Neoplatin. The reactions consist of facial oedema, wheezing, tachycardia and hypotension within a few minutes of drug administration. All reactions may be controlled by intravenous adrenaline, corticosteroids or antihistamines. Patients receiving Neoplatin should be observed carefully for possible anaphylactic-like reactions and supportive equipment and medication should be available to treat such a complication.

Other toxicities reported to occur infrequently are cardiac abnormalities, anorexia and elevated SGOT.

Guidelines for the safe handling of antineoplastic agents:
1. Trained personnel should reconstitute the drug.
2. This should be performed in a designated area.
3. Adequate protective gloves should be worn.
4. Precautions should be taken to avoid the drug accidentally coming into contact with the eyes. In the event of contact with the eyes, wash with water and/or saline.
5. The cytotoxic preparation should not be handled by pregnant staff.
6. Adequate care and precaution should be taken in the disposal of items (syringes, needles etc) used to reconstitute cytotoxic drugs. Excess material and body waste may be disposed of by placing in double sealed polythene bags and incinerating at a temperature of 1,000°C. Liquid waste may be flushed with copious amounts of water.
7. The work surface should be covered with disposable plastic-backed absorbent paper.
8. Use Luer-Lock fittings on all syringes and sets. Large bore needles are recommended to minimise pressure and the possible formation of aerosols. The latter may also be reduced by the use of a venting needle.

Pharmaceutical precautions Neoplatin injection should be stored at room temperature.

Expiry date: 36 months from date of manufacture.

Preparation of intravenous solution: Reconstitute the 10 mg vial contents with 10 ml, and the 50 mg vial contents with 50 ml of Sterile Water for Injection PhEur. The resulting drug solution is then administered in 2 litres of a suitable diluent, such as 0.9% saline, or a dextrose-saline solution. It is recommended that administration should be over a six to eight hour period. Diuresis may be aided by the addition to the infusion solution of 37.5 g mannitol.

The reconstituted solution should be protected from light, kept at room temperature and is stable for 20 hours. Refrigeration will result in precipitation.

Legal category POM.

Package quantities Neoplatin injection is packed in vials, each vial containing 10 mg or 50 mg lyophilised cisplatin.

Further information Cisplatin has biochemical properties similar to that of bifunctional alkylating agents producing inter-strand and intra-strand crosslinks in DNA. It is apparently cell-cycle non-specific. Following a single i.v. dose, cisplatin concentrates in liver, kidneys, and large and small intestines in animals and humans. Cisplatin apparently has poor penetration into the CNS.

Plasma levels of radioactivity decay in a biphasic manner after an i.v. bolus dose of radioactive cisplatin to patients. The initial plasma half-life is 25 to 49 minutes, and the post-distribution plasma half-life is 58 to 73 hours. During the post-distribution phase, greater than 90% of the radioactivity in the blood is protein-bound. Cisplatin is excreted primarily in the urine. However, urinary excretion is incomplete with only 27 to 43% of the radioactivity being excreted within the first five days post-dose in human beings. There are insufficient data to determine whether biliary or intestinal excretion occurs.

Product licence number 0125/0109.

PARAPLATIN* ▼

Presentation Vials containing 150 mg carboplatin [cis-diammine (1,1-cyclobutanedicarboxylato) platinum].

Uses Paraplatin is indicated for the treatment of:
1. advanced ovarian carcinoma of epithelial origin in:
   (a) first line therapy
   (b) second line therapy, after other treatments have failed.
2. small cell carcinoma of the lung.

Dosage and administration After reconstitution, Paraplatin should be used by the intravenous route only. The recommended dosage of Paraplatin in previously untreated adult patients with normal kidney function is 400 mg/m^2 as a single i.v. dose administered by a short term (15 to 60 minutes) infusion. Therapy should not be repeated until four weeks after the previous Paraplatin course.

Reduction of the initial dosage by 20–25% is recommended for those patients who present with risk factors such as prior myelosuppressive treatment and low performance status (ECOG-Zubrod 2–4 or Karnofsky below 80).

Determination of the haematological nadir by weekly blood counts during the initial courses of treatment with Paraplatin is recommended for future dosage adjustment.

Impaired renal function: The optimal use of Paraplatin in patients presenting with impaired renal function requires adequate dosage adjustments and frequent monitoring of both haematological nadirs and renal function.

Combination therapy: The optimal use of Paraplatin in combination with other myelosuppressive agents requires dosage adjustments according to the regimen and schedule to be adopted.

Paediatrics: Sufficient usage of Paraplatin in paediatrics has not occurred to allow specific dosage recommendations to be made.

Elderly: Dosage adjustment, initially or subsequently, may be necessary dependent on the physical condition of the patient.

Reconstitution: Immediately before use, the content of each vial must be reconstituted with Sterile Water for Injection PhEur, 5% dextrose for injection or 0.9% sodium chloride for injection to a final concentration of 10 mg of Paraplatin per ml, using a diluent volume of 15 ml.

Solutions in 5% Dextrose for Injection BP, or Sodium Chloride for Injection BP, may be further diluted with the same vehicles originally used for reconstitution, to concentrations as low as 0.5 mg/ml (500 mcg/ml), while solutions originally reconstituted with Sterile Water for Injection PhEur may be further diluted with either of these two fluids.

Contra-indications, warnings, etc

Contra-indications: Paraplatin should not be used in patients with severe pre-existing renal impairment (creatinine clearance at or below 20 ml/minute).

Paraplatin should not be employed in severely myelosuppressed patients. Paraplatin is also contra-indicated in patients with a history of severe allergic reactions to Paraplatin, other platinum containing compounds, or mannitol.

Warnings: Paraplatin should be administered by individuals experienced in the use of anti-neoplastic therapy.

Paraplatin myelosuppression is closely related to its renal clearance: patients with abnormal kidney function or receiving concomitant therapy with other drugs with nephrotoxic potential are likely to experience more severe and prolonged myelotoxicity. Renal function parameters should, therefore, be carefully assessed before and during therapy. Paraplatin courses should not be repeated more frequently than monthly under normal circumstances. Thrombocytopenia, leukopenia and anaemia occur after administration of Paraplatin. Frequent monitoring of peripheral blood counts is recommended throughout and following therapy with Paraplatin. Paraplatin combination therapy with other myelosuppressive compounds must be planned very carefully with respect to dosages and timing in order to minimise additive effects. Supportive transfusional therapy may be required in patients who suffer severe myelosuppression.

Paraplatin can cause nausea and vomiting. Premedication with anti-emetics has been reported to be useful in reducing the incidence and intensity of these effects.

Renal function impairment may be encountered with Paraplatin. Although no clinical evidence on compounding nephrotoxicity has been accumulated, it is recommended not to combine Paraplatin with aminoglycosides or other nephrotoxic compounds.

As for other platinum co-ordination compounds, allergic reactions to Paraplatin have been reported. These may occur within minutes of administration and should be managed with appropriate supportive therapy. Anaphylactic-like reactions may also occur as with other platinum co-ordination compounds.

The safe use of Paraplatin during pregnancy has not been established; Paraplatin has been shown to be an embryotoxin and mutagen in several experimental systems.

Its carcinogenic potential has not been studied but compounds with similar mechanisms of action and mutagenicity have been reported to be carcinogenic.

Precautions: Peripheral blood counts and renal function tests should be monitored closely. Blood counts at the beginning of the therapy and weekly to assess haematological nadir for subsequent dose adjustment are recommended. Neurological evaluations should also be performed on a regular basis.

Adverse reactions: Incidences of adverse reactions reported hereunder are based on cumulative data obtained in a large group of patients with various pretreatment prognostic features.

Haematological toxicity: Myelosuppression is the dose-limiting toxicity of Paraplatin. At maximum tolerated dosages of Paraplatin administered as a single agent, thrombocytopenia, with nadir platelet counts of less than 50×10^9/L, occurs in about a third of the patients. The nadir usually occurs between days 14 and 21, with recovery within 35 days from the start of therapy. Leukopenia has also occurred in approximately 20% of patients but its recovery from the day of nadir (day 14–28) may be slower and usually occurs within 42 days from the start of therapy. A haemoglobin decrease may be observed in some patients.

Myelosuppression may be more severe and prolonged in patients with impaired renal function, extensive prior treatment, poor performance status and age above 65. Myelosuppression is also worsened by therapy combining Paraplatin with other compounds that are myelosuppressive.

Myelosuppression is usually reversible and not cumulative when Paraplatin is used as a single agent and at the recommended dosages and frequencies of administration.

Infectious complications have occasionally been reported. Haemorrhagic complications, usually minor, have also been reported.

Nephrotoxicity: Renal toxicity is usually not dose-limiting in patients receiving Paraplatin, nor does it require preventive measures such as high volume fluid hydration or forced diuresis. Nevertheless, increasing blood urea or serum creatinine levels can occur. Renal function impairment, as defined by a decrease in the creatinine clearance below 60 ml/min, may also be observed. The incidence and severity of nephrotoxicity may increase in patients who have impaired kidney function before Paraplatin treatment. It is not clear whether an appropriate hydration programme might overcome such effect, but dosage reduction or discontinuation of therapy is required in the presence of severe alteration of renal function tests.

Decreases in serum electrolytes (magnesium, potassium and, rarely, calcium) have been reported after treatment with Paraplatin but have not been reported to be severe enough to cause the appearance of clinical signs or symptoms.

Gastrointestinal toxicity: Nausea without vomiting occurs in about a quarter of the patients receiving Paraplatin; vomiting has been reported in half of the patients and one-third of these suffer severe emesis. Nausea and vomiting usually disappear within 24 hours after treatment and are usually responsive to (and may be prevented by) anti-emetic medication. A quarter of patients experience no nausea or vomiting.

Allergic reactions: Infrequent allergic reactions to Paraplatin have been reported. These reactions are similar to those observed after administration of other platinum-containing compounds, i.e. erythematous rash, fever with no other apparent cause and pruritus.

Ototoxity: Subclinical decrease in hearing acuity, consisting of high-frequency (4000–8000 Hz) hearing loss determined by audiogram, has been reported in 15% of the patients treated with Paraplatin. However, only 1% of patients present with clinical symptoms, manifested in the majority of cases by tinnitus. In patients who have been previously treated with cisplatin and have developed hearing loss related to such treatment, the hearing impairment may persist, or worsen.

Neurotoxicity: The incidence of peripheral neuropathies after treatment with Paraplatin is 6%. In the majority of the patients neurotoxicity is limited to paraesthesia and decreased deep tendon reflexes. The frequency and intensity of this side effect increases in patients previously treated with cisplatin.

Paraesthesia present before commencing Paraplatin therapy, particularly if related to prior cisplatin treatment, may persist or worsen during treatment with Paraplatin.

Other: Abnormalities of liver function tests (usually mild to moderate) have been reported with Paraplatin in about one-third of the patients with normal baseline values. The alkaline phosphatase level is increased more frequently than SGOT, SGPT or total bilirubin. The majority of these abnormalities regress spontaneously during the course of treatment.

Rare events consisting of taste alteration, alopecia, fever and chills without evidence of infection or allergic reaction have occurred in less than 2% of the patients receiving Paraplatin.

Guidelines for the safe handling of antineoplastic agents:

1. Trained personnel should reconstitute the drug.
2. This should be performed in a designated area.
3. Adequate protective gloves should be worn.
4. Precautions should be taken to avoid the drug accidentally coming into contact with the eyes. In the event of contact with the eyes, wash with water and/or saline.
5. The cytotoxic preparation should not be handled by pregnant staff.
6. Adequate care and precautions should be taken in the disposal of items (syringes, needles etc) used to reconstitute cytotoxic drugs. Excess material and body waste may be disposed of by placing in double sealed polythene bags and incinerating at a temperature of 1,000°C. Liquid waste may be flushed with copious amounts of water.

Reconstitution:

7. The work surface should be covered with disposable plastic-backed absorbent paper.
8. Use Luer-Lock fittings on all syringes and sets. Large bore needles are recommended to minimise pressure and the possible formation of aerosols. The latter may also be reduced by the use of a venting needle.

Pharmaceutical precautions Paraplatin should be stored at room temperature.

Reconstitution: Immediately before use, the content of each vial must be reconstituted with Sterile Water for Injection PhEur, 5% dextrose for injection or 0.9% sodium chloride for injection to a final concentration of 10 mg of Paraplatin per ml, using a diluent volume of 15 ml.

Solutions in 5% Dextrose for Injection BP, or sodium chloride for injection BP, may be further diluted with the same vehicles originally used for reconstitution, to concentrations as low as 0.5 mg/ml (500 mcg/ml), while solutions originally reconstituted with Sterile Water for Injection PhEur may be further diluted with either of these two fluids.

When reconstituted as directed, Paraplatin solutions are stable for eight hours. Since no antibacterial preservatives are contained in the formulation it is recommended that any Paraplatin solution be discarded after eight hours from reconstitution.

Expiry date: 18 months from date of manufacture.

Legal category POM.

It is proposed to make Paraplatin available only on prescription and supplied to centres with experience in the chemotherapy of malignant diseases.

Package quantities Vials containing 150 mg carboplatin.

Further information Paraplatin has biochemical properties similar to that of cisplatin, thus producing predominantly interstrand and intrastrand DNA crosslinks. Following administration of Paraplatin in man, linear relationships exist between dose and plasma concentrations of total and free ultrafilterable platinum. The area under the plasma concentration versus time curve for total platinum also shows a linear relationship with the dose.

Repeated dosing during four consecutive days did not produce an accumulation of platinum in plasma. Following the administration of Paraplatin reported values for the terminal elimination half-lives of free ultrafilterable platinum and Paraplatin in man are approximately 6 hours and 1.5 hours respectively. During the initial phase, most of the free ultrafilterable platinum is present as Paraplatin. The terminal half-life for total plasma platinum is 24 hours. Approximately 87% of plasma platinum is protein bound within 24 hours following administration. Paraplatin is excreted primarily in the urine, with recovery of approximately 70% of the administered platinum within 24 hours. Most of the drug is excreted in the first 6 hours. Total body and renal clearances of free ultrafilterable platinum correlate with the rate of glomerular filtration but not tubular secretion.

Product licence number 0125/0180.

PLATINEX* ▼

Presentation Platinex: vials containing 10, 25 and 50 mg of cisplatin (cis-diamminedichloroplatinum) as a 0.5 mg/ml solution.

Uses Platinex is indicated as palliative therapy to be employed in addition to other modalities, or in established combination therapy with other approved chemotherapeutic agents in the management of neoplastic diseases, especially:

Metastatic Testicular Tumours: in patients who have already received appropriate surgical and/or radiotherapeutic procedures. The combination of Platinex, bleomycin and vinblastine has been reported to be highly effective. Other combinations have also been reported to be active.

Metastatic Ovarian Tumours: as a secondary therapy in patients refractory to standard chemotherapy.

Dosage and administration
Single Agent Therapy: The recommended dose of Platinex in adults and children is 50–120 mg/m² as a single i.v. dose every 3–4 weeks, or 15–20 mg/m² i.v. daily for 5 days every 3–4 weeks.

Combination Therapy: In general, current multiple drug treatment schedules including Platinex employ lower doses ranging from 20 mg/m² upwards, administered i.v. every 3–4 weeks.

Pretreatment hydration with 1–2 litres of fluid infused for 8–12 hours prior to a Platinex dose is recommended in order to initiate diuresis.

The contents of the vial are added to 2 litres of a suitable diluent such as 0.9% saline, or a dextrose-saline solution. It is recommended that administration should be over a 6–8 hour period. Diuresis may be aided by the addition to the infusion of 37.5 g mannitol.

Adequate hydration and urinary output must be maintained during the 24 hours following infusion.

A repeat course of Platinex should not be given until the serum creatinine is below 1.5 mg/100 ml (130 mcmol/l) and/or the blood urea below 55 mg/100 ml (9 mmol/l). A repeat course should not be given until circulating blood elements are at an acceptable level. Subsequent doses of Platinex should not be given until an audiometric analysis indicates that auditory acuity is within normal limits.

Elderly: No specific dosage adjustments but extra care should be taken to evaluate renal function prior to administration.

Contra-indications, warnings, etc Platinex induces nephrotoxicity, myelosuppression, neurotoxicity and ototoxicity which may be additive to pre-existing dysfunctions. Consequently, the use of Platinex in patients with hearing or renal impairment or depressed bone marrow function may be associated with increased

toxicities. Such conditions represent relative contra-indications.

Platinex is contra-indicated in patients with a history of hypersensitivity to Platinex or other platinum-containing compounds.

Warnings: Platinex produces cumulative nephrotoxicity. The serum creatinine, BUN or creatinine clearance should be measured prior to initiating therapy, and prior to each subsequent course.

Anaphylactic-like reactions to Platinex have been reported. These reactions have occurred within minutes of administration to patients with prior exposure to Platinex and have been alleviated by administration of adrenaline, steroids and antihistamines.

Safe use in pregnancy has not been established. This product should not normally be administered to patients who are pregnant or to mothers who are breast feeding. Platinex is mutagenic in bacteria and produces chromosome aberrations in animal cells in tissue culture. Although carcinogenicity and teratogenicity have not been established, compounds with similar mechanisms of action and mutagenicity have been reported to be carcinogenic.

The influence of Platinex on human reproduction has not been determined. Platinex therapy might have an anti-fertility effect.

Precautions: Platinex should be administered by individuals experienced in the use of anti-neoplastic therapy.

Neurotoxicity appears to be cumulative. Prior to each course, the absence of symptoms of peripheral neuropathy should be established. (See *Adverse reactions*).

Since renal toxicity is cumulative, measurements of BUN, serum creatinine or creatinine clearance should be performed prior to initiating therapy and prior to each subsequent course. At the recommended dosage, Platinex should not be given more frequently than once every 3 to 4 weeks. (See *Adverse reactions*).

Since ototoxicity of Platinex is cumulative, audiometric testing should be performed prior to initiating therapy and prior to each subsequent course of the drug. (See *Adverse reactions*).

Peripheral blood counts should be monitored weekly. Liver function should be monitored periodically. Neurological examination should also be performed regularly. (See *Adverse Reactions).*

Adverse reactions:

Nephrotoxicity: Renal toxicity has been noted in about one third of patients given a single dose of Platinex **when prior hydration has not been employed.** It is first noted during the second week after a dose and is manifested by elevations in BUN and serum creatinine, serum uric acid and/or a decrease in creatinine clearance.

Renal toxicity becomes more prolonged and severe with repeated courses of the drug. Renal function must return to normal before another dose of Platinex can be given.

Renal function impairment has been associated with renal tubular damage. The administration of Platinex using a 6–8 hour infusion with intravenous hydration and mannitol has been used to reduce nephrotoxicity. However, renal toxicity still can occur after utilisation of these procedures.

Neurotoxicity: Neurotoxicity, usually characterised by peripheral neuropathies, has occurred in some patients. Loss of taste and seizures have also been reported. Neuropathies resulting from Platinex treatment may occur after prolonged therapy (4 to 7 months); however, neurological symptoms have been reported to occur after a single dose.

Platinex therapy should be discontinued when the symptoms are first observed. Preliminary evidence suggests peripheral neuropathy may be irreversible in some patients.

Ototoxicity: Ototoxicity has been observed in patients treated with a single dose of Platinex, 50 mg/m^2, and is manifested by tinnitus and/or hearing loss in the high frequency range (4,000 to 8,000 Hz).

Decreased ability to hear normal conversational tones may occur occasionally. Ototoxic effects may be more severe in children receiving Platinex. Hearing loss can be unilateral or bilateral and tends to become more frequent and severe with repeated doses. It is unclear whether Platinex-induced ototoxicity is reversible. Careful monitoring by audiometry should be performed prior to initiation of therapy and prior to subsequent doses of Platinex.

Haematological: Myelosuppression may occur in patients treated with Platinex. The nadirs in circulating platelets and leucocytes occur between days 18 to 23 (range 7.5 to 45) with most patients recovering by day 39 (range 13 to 62). Leucopenia and thrombocytopenia are more pronounced at higher doses. Anaemia (decrease in haemoglobin level by 2 g/100 ml blood) occurs at approximately the same frequency and with the same timing as leucopenia and thrombocytopenia.

Gastro-intestinal: Marked nausea and vomiting occur in almost all patients treated with Platinex and are occasionally so severe that the drug must be discontinued. Nausea and vomiting usually begin within one to four hours after treatment and last up to 24 hours. Various degrees of nausea and anorexia may persist for up to one week after treatment.

Other toxicities

Hyperuricaemia: Hyperuricaemia has been reported to occur at approximately the same frequency as the increases in BUN and serum creatinine. It is more pronounced after doses greater than 50 mg/m^2, and peak levels of uric acid generally occur between 3 to 5 days after the dose. Allopurinol therapy for hyperuricaemia effectively reduces uric acid levels.

Anaphylactic-like reactions: Anaphylactic-like reactions, possibly secondary to Platinex therapy, have been occasionally reported in patients previously exposed to Platinex. The reactions consist of facial oedema, wheezing, tachycardia and hypotension within a few minutes of drug administration. All reactions may be controlled by intravenous adrenaline, corticosteroids or antihistamines. Patients receiving Platinex should be observed carefully for possible anaphylactic-like reactions and supportive equipment and medication should be available to treat such a complication.

Other toxicities reported to occur infrequently are cardiac abnormalities, anorexia and elevated SGOT.

Guidelines for the safe handling of antineoplastic agents:
1. Trained personnel should reconstitute the drug.
2. This should be performed in a designated area.
3. Adequate protective gloves should be worn.
4. Precautions should be taken to avoid the drug accidentally coming into contact with the eyes. In the event of contact with the eyes, wash with water and/or saline.
5. The cytotoxic preparation should not be handled by pregnant staff.
6. Adequate care and precaution should be taken in the disposal of items (syringes, needles etc) used to reconstitute cytotoxic drugs. Excess material and body waste may be disposed of by placing in double sealed polythene bags and incinerating at a temperature of 1,000°C. Liquid waste may be flushed with copious amounts of water.
7. The work surface should be covered with disposable plastic-backed absorbent paper.
8. Use Luer-Lock fittings on all syringes and sets. Large bore needles are recommended to minimise pressure and the possible formation of aerosols. The latter may also be reduced by the use of a venting needle.

Pharmaceutical precautions Platinex should be stored at room temperature (maximum 25°C); avoid freezing.

Expiry date: 24 months from date of manufacture.

Preparation of intravenous solution: The contents of the vial should be added to 2 litres of a suitable diluent, such as 0.9% saline, or a dextrose-saline solution. It is recommended that administration should be over a 6–8 hour period. Diuresis may be aided by the addition to the infusion solution of 37.5 g mannitol.

Legal category POM.

Package quantities Each vial contains 10, 25 or 50 mg cisplatin as a 0.5 mg/ml solution.

Further information Cisplatin has biochemical properties similar to that of bifunctional alkylating agents producing inter-strand and intra-strand crosslinks in DNA. It is apparently cell-cycle non-specific. Following a single i.v. dose, cisplatin concentrates in liver, kidneys, and large and small intestines in animals and humans. Cisplatin apparently has poor penetration into the CNS.

Plasma levels of radioactivity decay in a biphasic manner after an i.v. bolus dose of radioactive cisplatin to patients. The initial plasma half-life is 25 to 49 minutes, and the post-distribution phase, greater than 90% of the radioactivity in the blood is protein-bound. Cisplatin is excreted primarily in the urine. However, urinary excretion is incomplete with only 27% to 43% of the radioactivity being excreted within the first 5 days postdose in human beings. There are insufficient data to determine whether biliary or intestinal excretion occurs.

Product licence number 0125/0145

QUESTRAN*

Presentation Questran sachets containing 9 g of orange-flavoured powder. Each sachet supplies 4 g of anhydrous cholestyramine (a basic anion-exchange resin).

Uses Questran is used for:
1. Reduction of plasma cholesterol in hypercholesterolaemia, particularly in those patients who have been diagnosed as Fredrickson's Type II (high plasma cholesterol with normal or slightly elevated triglycerides).
2. Relief of diarrhoea associated with ileal resection, Crohn's disease, vagotomy and diabetic vagal neuropathy.
3. Relief of pruritus associated with partial biliary obstruction.
4. Management of radiation-induced diarrhoea.

Dosage and administration *Adults:* As a precautionary measure, where concurrent drug therapy exists then such drugs should be administered 30 minutes to 1 hour before Questran.

1. To reduce cholesterol: After initial introduction, 3 to 6 Questran sachets per day, administered either as a single daily dose or in divided doses up to four times daily according to dosage requirement and patient acceptability. Dosage may be modified according to response and can be increased to 9 sachets per day if necessary.

2. To relieve diarrhoea: as for reduction of cholesterol, but it may be possible to reduce this dosage.

3. To relieve pruritus: 1 or 2 sachets daily are usually sufficient. Questran may be administered mixed with water, skimmed milk, fruit juice, soups, pulpy fruit, etc.

Children 6–12 years: The initial dose is determined by the following formula:

$$\frac{\text{child's weight in lb} \times \text{adult dose}}{150}$$

Subsequent dosage adjustment may be necessary.

Infants and children under 6 years: The dose has not been established.

Elderly: No dosage adjustment is necessary.

Contra-indications, warnings, etc Questran is contra-indicated in patients with complete biliary obstruction, since Questran cannot be effective where bile is not secreted into the intestine.

Because it sequesters bile acids, Questran may interfere with normal fat absorption and prevent absorption of fat-soluble vitamins such as A, D and K. If Questran is to be administered in high dosage for a prolonged period, fat-soluble vitamins should be given daily in a water-miscible form, or, if preferred, administered parenterally.

Gastro-intestinal side-effects are those most frequently reported. The principal complaint is constipation, which may be controlled with the usual remedies, and frequently disappears on continued usage of Questran.

The use of Questran in pregnancy or lactation or by women of childbearing age requires that the potential benefits of drug therapy be weighed against the possible hazards to the mother and child. The safe use of Questran by pregnant women has not been established.

Overdosage: Overdosage of Questran has not been reported. Should overdosage occur, however, the chief potential harm would be obstruction of the gastro-intestinal tract. The location of such potential obstruction, the degree of obstruction, and the presence or absence of normal gut motility would determine treatment.

Pharmaceutical precautions Questran should not be taken in its dry form. The powder should be prepared immediately prior to administration.

There are no special directions for storage.

Expiry Date – 48 months from date of manufacture.

Legal category POM.

Package quantities Questran is available in packs containing 20 and 160 sachets.

Further information The correlation between high blood cholesterol levels and ischaemic heart conditions has prompted the dietary control of patients who have shown signs or symptoms of coronary artery disease. With Questran it is possible to reduce cholesterol levels without recourse to excessively stringent dietary measures or systemically absorbed drugs.

Questran (cholestyramine) is a basic anion-exchange resin. It is not absorbed in the gut and its affinity for bile acids in the intestinal tract prevents their reabsorption. To compensate for the faecal loss of bile acids, their major precursor, cholesterol, is oxidised at an increased rate in the liver and plasma cholesterol levels are thus lowered.

Product licence number 0125/5009.

SOTACOR*

Presentation *Sotacor tablets:* Sotacor 80 mg tablets – pink, circular, tablets, engraved 'SOTACOR 80' on one face, each tablet containing 80 mg sotalol hydrochloride.

Sotacor 160 mg tablets – blue, circular, tablets, engraved 'SOTACOR 160' on one face, each containing 160 mg sotalol hydrochloride.

Sotacor injection: Ampoules containing sotalol hydrochloride 10 mg in each 5 ml of solution.

Ampoules containing sotalol hydrochloride 100 mg in each 10 ml of solution.

Uses Sotacor, the hydrochloride of 4-(2-isopropylamino-1-hydroxyethyl)-methanesulphonanilide, is a synthetic beta-adrenergic receptor blocking agent. Sotacor exerts a significant antihypertensive effect and additionally protects the heart from undesirable sympathetic drive. It is devoid of intrinsic sympathomimetic and local anaesthetic activity.

1. *Hypertension:* Sotacor produces smooth and gradual reduction of blood pressure on a long-term basis.

2. *Angina pectoris:* Sotacor reduces the frequency and severity of anginal attacks and increases exercise tolerance.

3. *Thyrotoxicosis:* Sotacor relieves the effect of adrenergic over-activity.

4. *Cardiac arrhythmias:* Sotacor tablets may be used prophylactically and as maintenance therapy in the management of cardiac arrhythmias. Sotacor Injection is used in the management of acute cardiac arrhythmias, especially following myocardial infarction, to restore normal rate and rhythm.

5. *Myocardial Infarction:* Sotacor tablets may be used prophylactically to reduce the incidence of infarction following an acute myocardial infarct.

Dosage and administration When administering beta-blocking drugs to previously untreated patients it is desirable to start with a low dose and gradually increase the dose until optimum response has occurred. It is usually undesirable to reduce the heart rate below 55 beats per minute.

Sotacor Tablets: Sotacor may be administered daily in either single or divided doses.

Children: Sotacor is not intended for administration to children.

Adults: 1. *Hypertension:* Initial daily dose should be one 160 mg tablet. The majority of mild to moderate hypertensives will respond to one tablet daily and be adequately controlled at this level.

2. *Angina pectoris:* Initial daily dose should be one 160 mg tablet. The majority of anginal patients will be controlled at this dosage level.

N.B. A gradual transfer of therapy over a two-week period is recommended in patients receiving other anti-anginal therapy.

3. *Thyrotoxicosis:* Initial daily dose should be one 160 mg tablet.

4. *Arrhythmia:* In the management of cardiac arrhythmias, as prophylaxis or maintenance therapy, Sotacor dosage will normally be between 160 mg and 240 mg daily.

N.B. In all these indications dosage may be increased by increments of up to 160 mg per day – the rapidity with which this dosage increase takes place depends upon the patient's tolerance, particularly as measured by the degree of induced bradycardia and the clinical response.

Sotacor Injection should be administered slowly in doses of 20–60 mg intravenously over two to three minutes. Larger doses, up to 100 mg should be injected over three minutes or longer. Continuous ECG monitoring is recommended. Should repeated administrations be necessary, a 10-minute interval between injections is advised, remembering that additive effect and prolongation of effect may ensue.

5. *Myocardial Infarction:* As prophylaxis following an acute myocardial infarction, Sotacor dosage will normally be 320 mg once daily commenced 5–14 days after infarction.

Elderly: As sotalol is renally excreted dosage will need to be adjusted in patients with poor renal function and should be used with caution in patients with poor cardiac reserve.

Contra-indications, warnings, etc Sotacor should not be used where there is evidence of heart block; metabolic acidosis; history of bronchospasm; diabetic ketoacidosis. Beta-blockade may precipitate heart failure in subjects with poor cardiac reserve or may aggravate existing heart failure. Patients whose heart failure is well controlled with digitalis and diuretics may be given Sotacor.

Treated diabetes: Sotacor, like other beta-blocking drugs, may reduce or mask pre-hypoglycaemic warning signs.

Anaesthesia: It is not necessary to discontinue Sotacor prior to most forms of elective surgery, although there is some doubt as to whether beta-receptor blockers should be continued up to the time of surgery involving cardiopulmonary bypass. However, as with other beta-blockers, sudden withdrawal of Sotacor Tablets or Injection might expose the patient to severe angina, arrhythmias, and even myocardial infarction.

If the drug is to be discontinued prior to surgery, especially in patients with ischaemic heart disease, then the drug should be withdrawn over a period of one week. It is usual to discontinue Sotacor Injection 24 to 48 hours prior to elective surgery.

In the presence of Sotacor, anaesthesia may proceed provided that vagal dominance is counteracted by an intravenous injection of atropine sulphate (0.5–2 mg) immediately prior to induction of anaesthesia. Some anaesthetic agents such as ether, cyclopropane, trichloroethylene, methoxyflurane and enflurane appear to cause impairment of myocardial contractility in the presence of beta-receptor blockade. Caution is advised in the use of these agents in patients receiving Sotacor. No evidence of serious interaction has been found between nitrous oxide, halothane or isoflurane and beta-receptor blockers. Raised pCO_2 levels should be avoided in patients receiving Sotacor.

Cases of torsade de pointes (atypical ventricular tachycardia) have been reported infrequently during treatment with Sotacor. Experience indicates that this can occur in hypokalaemic patients and in patients concomitantly treated with drugs which may cause torsade such as antidepressants and Class I antiarrhythmics. Thus, the patient's electrolyte balance, especially potassium levels, should always be checked and any abnormality corrected prior to initiation of Sotacor therapy. It is also important to monitor the electrolyte balance frequently during Sotacor treatment. Patients should be instructed to stop Sotacor therapy during episodes of diarrhoea or when encountering conditions that may result in hypokalaemia. Institution of concurrent therapy with drugs known to prolong the QT interval and/or to be associated with atypical ventricular tachycardia especially quinidine, disopyramide and tricyclic antidepressants should be done under close medical supervision.

Pregnancy: Notice should be taken of current views on the undesirability of administering drugs during pregnancy. Animal studies with sotalol hydrochloride have shown no evidence of teratogenicity or other harmful effects on the foetus.

Side-effects: There have been reports of skin rashes and/or dry eyes associated with the use of beta-adrenergic blocking drugs. The reported incidence is small and in most cases the symptoms have cleared when the treatment was withdrawn. Discontinuance of the drug should be considered if any such reaction is not otherwise explicable. Cessation of therapy with a beta-adrenergic blocker should be gradual.

Sotacor tablets: At the recommended dosage side effects are uncommon. However, minor side effects such as bradycardia, nausea, insomnia, lassitude and diarrhoea have been reported. These are usually transient and can be avoided by gradual introduction of treatment and usually remit on reduction of dosage.

Sotacor Injection is usually well tolerated. Side effects due to beta-blockade, manifested as bradycardia and hypotension, should be treated, if necessary, as for overdosage.

Overdosage: In the rare event of profound cardiovascular effects such as excessive bradycardia or hypotension, atropine sulphate, 0.5–2 mg intravenously, should be administered. It may also be necessary to administer isoprenaline 5 mcg per minute, up to 25 mcg, by slow intravenous injection in order to reverse beta-receptor blockade.

Pharmaceutical precautions Sotacor Tablets should be protected from light.

Expiry Date:

Sotacor 80 mg	36 months from date of manufacture.
Sotacor 160 mg	36 months from date of manufacture.
Sotacor Injection	36 months from date of manufacture.

Legal category POM.

Package quantities Sotacor 80 mg and 160 mg tablets: Units of 28 – blister strips of 14 tablets with 2 strips to a carton and units of 300.
Sotacor Injection is supplied in two strengths – as 10 mg sotalol hydrochloride in 5 ml ampoules and as 100 mg sotalol hydrochloride in 10 ml ampoules, with 5 ampoules per box.

Further information The maximum dose of Sotacor is usually 320 mg daily. Where improved control of hypertension is required the addition of a diuretic will often give a more satisfactory response.

Product licence numbers

Sotacor 80 mg tablets	0125/0076
Sotacor 160 mg tablets	0125/0093
Sotacor Injection: 10 mg/5 ml	0125/0078
100 mg/10 ml	0125/0123

SOTAZIDE*

Presentation *Sotazide tablets:* Pale blue, capsule-shaped, concave tablets containing 160 mg sotalol hydrochloride and 25 mg hydrochlorothiazide.

Uses In the management of mild or moderate hypertension. The combination product may be suitable for use when satisfactory control of arterial blood pressure cannot be obtained with either a diuretic or a beta-adrenoreceptor blocking drug used alone.

Dosage and administration *Initial dose:* One Sotazide tablet daily increasing to two if necessary.

The individual optimal dosage and the rapidity with which dosage increase occurs should be determined from blood pressure and pulse rate readings and by the degree of induced bradycardia.

Following a reduction in blood pressure the dosage should not be increased until the new blood pressure is stable.

A slight reduction in dosage will alleviate symptoms of weakness and dizziness if blood pressure continues to fall after a month or two on the maintenance dose.

Elderly: As sotalol is renally excreted dosage will need to be adjusted in patients with poor renal function and should be used with caution in patients with poor cardiac reserve.

Contra-indications, warnings, etc

Contra-indications: Sotazide should not be used where there is evidence of heart block; history of broncho-spasm; diabetic keto-acidosis; impending or uncontrolled cardiac failure; anaesthesia that produces myocardial depression; hypersensitivity to sotalol, hydrochlorothiazide or sulphonamide derivatives.

Since thiazides appear in breast milk, patients should stop nursing if the use of Sotazide is essential.

Warnings: Pregnancy: In animal studies Sotazide has been shown to have no adverse teratogenic effects in doses up to 25 times the recommended human dose. However, its safe use in human pregnancy has not been fully established.

Treated diabetes: Hypoglycaemic therapy may have to be altered in diabetics; Sotazide may potentiate the insulin hypoglycaemic effects and mask the symptoms of hypoglycaemia.

Hepatic/renal disease: Sotazide should be used with caution in patients with impaired hepatic function, liver disease or severe renal disease, since they are particularly sensitive to alterations of fluid and electrolyte balance, Thiazides may precipitate azotaemia. Cumulative effects of the hydrochlorothiazide may develop in patients with impaired renal function.

Cases of torsade de pointes (atypical ventricular tachycardia) have been reported infrequently during treatment with Sotazide. Experience to date indicates that this can occur in hypokalaemic patients and in patients concomitantly treated with drugs which may cause torsade such as antidepressants and Class I

antiarrhythmics. Thus, the patient's electrolyte balance, especially potassium levels, should always be checked and any abnormality corrected prior to initiation of Sotazide therapy. It is also important to monitor the electrolyte balance frequently during Sotazide treatment. Patients should be instructed to stop Sotazide therapy during episodes of diarrhoea or when encountering conditions that may result in hypokalaemia. Institution of concurrent therapy with drugs known to prolong the QT interval and/or to be associated with atypical ventricular tachycardia especially quinidine, disopyramide and tricyclic antidepressants should be done under close medical supervision.

Anaesthesia: It is not necessary to discontinue Sotazide prior to most forms of elective surgery, although there is some doubt as to whether beta-receptor blockers should be continued up to the time of surgery involving cardiopulmonary bypass. However, sudden withdrawal of Sotazide might expose the patient to severe angina, arrhythmias, and even myocardial infarction.

If the drug is to be discontinued prior to surgery, especially in patients with ischaemic heart disease, then the drug should be withdrawn over a period of one week.

In the presence of Sotazide, anaesthesia may proceed provided that vagal dominance is counteracted by an intravenous injection of atropine sulphate (0.5–2 mg) immediately prior to induction of anaesthesia. Some anaesthetic agents such as ether, cyclopropane, trichloroethylene, methoxyflurane and enflurane appear to cause impairment of myocardial contractility in the presence of beta-receptor blockade. Caution is advised in the use of these agents in patients receiving Sotazide. No evidence of serious interaction has been found between nitrous oxide, halothane, or isoflurane and beta-receptor blockers. Raised pCO_2 levels should be avoided in patients receiving Sotazide.

Precautions: In view of the minimal myocardial depressant effect of sotalol and the lack of myocardial effect of hydrochlorothiazide, Sotazide has only a remote potential for precipitation or exacerbation of cardiac failure. Nevertheless, Sotazide should not be given to patients with cardiac decompensation unless incipient or established heart failure is controlled. At the first sign of impending cardiac failure or the progression of failure, Sotazide dosage should be reduced or discontinued.

The dosage of Sotazide should be decreased or therapy discontinued if the pulse rate falls below 50 beats/minute. Following a reduction in blood pressure, the dosage of Sotazide should not be increased before a stable level of blood pressure is attained.

Institution of concurrent therapy with drugs known to prolong the QT interval and/or to be associated with atypical ventricular tachycardia (AVT, torsade de pointes), especially quinidine, disopyramide, tricyclic antidepressants should be under close medical supervision.

Sudden withdrawal of treatment with beta-blockers in hypertensive patients with angina pectoris has induced severe and continuous angina in some cases. Although this effect has not been observed with Sotazide, should such a reaction occur, Sotazide treatment should be reinstituted and then withdrawn gradually by reducing the dosage over a period of weeks.

All patients receiving hydrochlorothiazide (as in Sotazide) therapy should be checked periodically for clinical signs of fluid or electrolyte imbalance: hyponatraemia, hypochloraemic alkalosis and hypokalaemia. Hypokalaemia can sensitise or exaggerate the response of the heart to the toxic effects of cardiac glycosides. With the lower dose of hydrochlorothiazide present in Sotazide, the possibility of any imbalance becomes less likely.

With the use of hydrochlorothiazide (as in Sotazide), serum protein-bound iodine may decrease without producing symptoms of thyroid disturbance.

Side-effects: The overall incidence of side-effects with Sotazide is low. The few reported adverse reactions were largely the pharmacological effects seen with the use of beta-blocking agents and diuretics. These reactions are mild, or moderate in intensity, most often transitory, and usually do not require interruption or withdrawal of therapy.

Sotalol, when used alone, is generally well tolerated. Dyspnoea, tiredness, dizziness, light-headedness, head-ache, fever and excessive bradycardia have been reported. Most of these side-effects are transient or disappear when the dosage is reduced, e.g. with the use of Sotazide.

There have been reports of skin rashes and/or dry eyes associated with the use of beta-adrenergic blocking drugs. The reported incidence is small and in most cases the symptoms have cleared when the treatment was withdrawn. Discontinuance of the drug should be considered if any such reaction is not otherwise explic-able. Cessation of therapy with a beta-adrenergic blocker should be gradual.

Hyperuricaemia has been observed with thiazides but clinical gout is rare. Other side-effects for thiazides are documented but uncommon. Photosensitivity, anaphy-lactic reactions and depression of the formed elements of the blood have been reported.

The relevance of these observations to Sotazide therapy has not yet been determined.

Overdosage: If excessive bradycardia (and/or hypotension) occurs, atropine 0.5–2.0 mg should be given intravenously, immediately followed, if necessary, by a beta-receptor stimulating agent, such as isoprenaline, intravenously, 5 mcg/minute up to 25 mcg initially.

Pharmaceutical precautions *Expiry date:* Blister strip pack: 36 months from date of manufacture. Units of 300: 24 months from date of manufacture.

Legal category POM.

Package quantities Units of 28 – blister strips of 14 tablets with 2 strips per carton and units of 300.

Further information Sotazide is an effective anti-hypertensive which combines sotalol hydrochloride, a beta-adrenergic blocking agent, and hydrochlorothia-zide, a diuretic/antihypertensive. The concomitant use of these agents frequently produces a more pronounced anti-hypertensive effect than if either is used alone. By using lower doses than would be required if each agent were used alone, side-effects, especially the hypokalae-mia associated with diuretics, are minimised. In hyper-tensive patients, where sodium and water retention is frequently a problem, the diuretic component will help control fluid imbalance.

Product licence number 0125/0113.

TETREX* CAPSULES

Presentation Capsules having a yellow body and orange cap, printed 'BRISTOL/BRISTOL' in green. Each capsule contains tetracycline phosphate compound equivalent to tetracycline activity 250 mg.

Uses The absorption of tetracycline may be inhibited in the presence of calcium ions in the intestinal contents. The phosphate component of Tetrex combines with calcium and leaves more free tetracycline available for absorption.

Tetrex is indicated in the treatment of the following infections when due to sensitive organisms:

Infections of the respiratory tract.
Infections of the gastro-intestinal tract.
Infections of the genito-urinary tract.
Infections of the skin and soft tissues.

Dosage and administration *Adults:* Usual dose 1 g per day in 4 divided doses of 250 mg each or 2 divided doses of 500 mg each.

Higher doses may be required to control acute episodes.

Acute gonococcal urethritis – 500 mg three times daily for one to two days. Female patients require more prolonged therapy.

Children: Usual dose 25 mg/kg/day in 4 divided doses. Children weighing more than 40 kg should be given the recommended adult dose.

Elderly: If renal impairment exists, even usual oral doses of the drug may lead to excess systemic accumulation of tetracycline and possible liver toxicity. Under such conditions lower than usual doses are indicated.

Therapy for most infections should be continued for 24–48 hours after the patient has become asymptomatic or afebrile.

Contra-indications, warnings, etc This drug is contra-indicated in individuals who have shown serious hypersensitivity to tetracycline, unless the need for this therapy necessitates its use with proper safeguards.

If renal impairment exists, even usual oral doses of the drug may lead to excess systemic accumulation of tetracycline and possible liver toxicity. Under such conditions, lower than usual doses are indicated, and if therapy is prolonged, tetracycline serum-level determi-nations may be advisable.

Tetracycline may form a stable calcium complex in any bone-forming tissue with no serious harmful effects reported thus far in humans. However, use of tetracycline during tooth development (last trimester of pregnancy, neonatal period, infancy and early childhood) may cause discoloration of the teeth (yellow-grey-brownish). This effect occurs mostly during long-term therapy, but it has also been observed following short treatment courses.

Enamel hypoplasia has been observed in a few children. If superinfection with non-susceptible organ-isms occurs proper measures should be taken.

Pharmaceutical precautions Expiry date – 36 months from date of manufacture.
There are no special directions for storage.

Legal category POM.

Package quantities Containers of 100 capsules.

Further information Tetracycline phosphate com-pound is absorbed rapidly from the gastro-intestinal tract providing reliable high tetracycline levels in the blood. It is serum bound to a much lesser degree than most other tetracyclines and therefore allows greater concentrations of active antibiotic to reach the site of infection.

Product licence number 0125/0066.

THERADERM* 5 & 10

Presentation Theraderm is a white water based gel containing benzoyl peroxide. It is available in two strengths, Theraderm 5 and Theraderm 10, containing benzoyl peroxide 5% and 10% respectively.

Uses Theraderm is indicated in the topical treatment of acne vulgaris. The active ingredient, benzoyl peroxide, is an established and effective anti-bacterial and mild keratolytic agent.

Theraderm may be applied in conjunction with other topical preparations such as salicylic acid and antibacterials.

Dosage and administration After washing with soap and water, apply once or twice daily to the affected area. The degree of drying and peeling can be adjusted by modification of the dosage schedule.

Should discomfort such as burning, redness or excessive peeling occur at any time discontinue treatment temporarily. As the skin becomes tolerant to Theraderm 5, peeling will diminish. When this occurs, Theraderm 10 should be used.

Contra-indications, warnings, etc Known sensitivity to benzoyl peroxide.

Precautions: For external use only. Avoid contact with eyes and mucous membranes.

Warnings: A mild burning sensation may be noticed on first application and moderate erythema and desquamation appear within a few days. Indiscriminate application may produce a marked erythema. Such conditions will subside if treatment is discontinued temporarily.

May bleach coloured fabrics and rarely hair and eyebrows.

Pharmaceutical precautions Nil.

Expiry date: 36 months from date of manufacture.

Legal category P.

Package quantities 56 g.

Further information Nil.

Product licence numbers
Theraderm 5   0125/0142
Theraderm 10   0125/0143

TOLERZIDE*

Presentation Tolerzide: circular, lilac, tablets containing 80 mg sotalol hydrochloride and 12.5 mg hydrochlorothiazide.

Uses In the management of mild or moderate hypertension particularly where a gradual fall in blood pressure is indicated such as in the elderly.

Dosage and administration Dose: one Tolerzide tablet daily.

Elderly: As sotalol is renally excreted dosage will need to be adjusted in patients with poor renal function and should be used with caution in patients with poor cardiac reserve.

Contra-indications, warnings, etc Tolerzide should not be used where there is evidence of heart block; history of bronchospasm; diabetic keto-acidosis; impending or uncontrolled cardiac failure; anaesthesia that produces myocardial depression; hypersensitivity to sotalol, hydrochlorothiazide or sulphonamide derivatives.

Since thiazides appear in breast milk, patients should stop nursing if the use of Tolerzide is essential.

Warnings:

Pregnancy: In animal studies Tolerzide has been shown to have no adverse teratogenic effects in doses up to 50 times the recommended human dose. However its safe use in human pregnancy has not been fully established.

Treated diabetes: Hypoglycaemic therapy may have to be altered in diabetics; Tolerzide may potentiate insulin hypoglycaemic effects and mask the symptoms of hypoglycaemia.

Hepatic/renal disease: Tolerzide should be used with caution in patients with impaired hepatic function or severe renal disease; such patients are particularly sensitive to alterations in fluid and electrolyte balance. Thiazides may precipitate azotaemia. Cumulative effects of hydrochlorothiazide may develop in patients with impaired renal function.

Anaesthesia: It is not necessary to discontinue Tolerzide prior to most forms of elective surgery, although there is some doubt as to whether beta-receptor blockers should be continued up to the time of surgery involving cardiopulmonary bypass. However, sudden withdrawal of Tolerzide might expose the patient to severe angina, arrhythmias, and even myocardial infarction.

If the drug is to be discontinued prior to surgery, especially in patients with ischaemic heart disease, then the drug should be withdrawn over a period of one week.

In the presence of Tolerzide, anaesthesia may proceed provided that vagal dominance is counteracted by an intravenous injection of atropine sulphate (0.5-2 mg) immediately prior to induction of anaesthesia. Some anaesthetic agents such as ether, cyclopropane, trichloroethylene, methoxyflurane and enflurane appear to cause impairment of myocardial contractility in the presence of beta-receptor blockade. Caution is advised in the use of these agents in patients receiving Tolerzide. No evidence of serious interaction has been found between nitrous oxide, halothane, or isoflurane and beta-receptor blockers. Raised pCO_2 levels should be avoided in patients receiving Tolerzide.

Precautions: In view of the minimal myocardial depressant effect of sotalol and the lack of myocardial effect of hydrochlorothiazide, Tolerzide has only a remote potential for precipitation or exacerbation of cardiac failure. Nevertheless, Tolerzide should not be given to patients with cardiac decompensation unless incipient or established heart failure is controlled. At the first sign of impending cardiac failure or the progression of failure, Tolerzide dosage should be reduced or discontinued.

The dosage of Tolerzide should be decreased or therapy discontinued if the pulse rate falls below 50 beats/minute.

Sudden withdrawal of treatment with beta-blockers in hypertensive patients with angina pectoris has induced severe and continuous angina in some cases. Although this effect has not been observed with Tolerzide, should such a reaction occur, Tolerzide treatment should be reinstituted and then withdrawn gradually by reducing the dosage over a period of weeks.

All patients receiving hydrochlorothiazide (as in Tolerzide) therapy should be checked periodically for clinical signs of fluid or electrolyte imbalance: hyponatraemia, hypochloraemic alkalosis and hypokalaemia. Hypokalaemia can sensitise or exaggerate the response of the heart to the toxic effects of cardiac glycosides. With the lower dose of hydrochlorothiazide present in Tolerzide, the possibility of any imbalance becomes less likely.

With the use of hydrochlorothiazide (as in Tolerzide), serum protein bound iodine may decrease without producing symptoms of thyroid disturbance.

Side effects: The overall incidence of side effects with Tolerzide is low. The few reported adverse reactions are largely the pharmacological effects seen with the use of beta-blocking agents and diuretics. These reactions are mild or moderate in intensity, most often transitory, and usually do not require interruption or withdrawal of therapy.

Sotalol, when used alone, is generally well tolerated. Dyspnoea, tiredness, dizziness, light-headedness, headache, fever and excessive bradycardia have been reported. Most of these side effects are transient or disappear when the dosage is reduced, eg with the use of Tolerzide.

There have been reports of skin rashes and/or dry eyes associated with the use of beta-adrenergic blocking drugs. The reported incidence is small and in most cases the symptoms have cleared when the treatment was withdrawn. Discontinuance of the drug should be considered if any such reaction is not otherwise explicable. Cessation of therapy with a beta-adrenergic blocker should be gradual.

Hyperuricaemia has been observed with thiazides but clinical gout is rare. Other side effects for thiazides are documented but uncommon. Photosensitivity, anaphylactic reactions and depression of the formed elements of the blood have been reported.

The relevance of these observations to Tolerzide therapy has not yet been determined.

Overdosage: If excessive bradycardia (and/or hypotension) occurs atropine 0.5 to 2.0 mg should be given intravenously, immediately followed, if necessary, by a beta-receptor stimulating agent such as isoprenaline, intravenously, 5 mcg/minute up to 25 mcg total dose. Patients experiencing this effect on initial administration of Tolerzide should be removed temporarily from therapy. Tolerzide could be reintroduced at a lower dosage and then gradually increased.

Pharmaceutical precautions Nil.

Expiry Date: 24 months from date of manufacture.

Legal category POM.

Package quantities Tolerzide tablets: units of 28 – blister strips of 14 tablets with 2 strips per carton.

Further information Tolerzide is an effective antihypertensive which combines sotalol hydrochloride, a beta-adrenergic blocking agent, and hydrochlorothiazide, a diuretic/anti-hypertensive. The concomitant use of these agents frequently produces a more pronounced antihypertensive effect than if either is used alone. By using lower doses than would be required if each agent were used alone, side effects, especially the hypokalaemia associated with diuretics, are minimised. In hypertensive patients where sodium and water retention is frequently a problem, the diuretic component will help control fluid imbalance.

Product licence number
Tolerzide tablets: 0125/0133

VEPESID* CAPSULES ▼
VEPESID* INJECTION ▼

Presentation Vepesid Injection-ampoules containing 100 mg etoposide in 5 ml.

Vepesid Capsules-soft gelatin, pale pink capsules containing 50 mg and 100 mg etoposide.

Uses Vepesid is an anti-neoplastic drug for intravenous or oral use, which can be used alone or in combination with other oncolytic drugs.

Present data indicate that Vepesid is applicable in the therapy of: small cell lung cancer, resistant non-seminomatous testicular carcinoma.

Dosage and administration The recommended course of Vepesid Injection is 60–120 mg/m², i.v., daily for five consecutive days. As Vepesid produces myelosuppression, courses may not be repeated more frequently than at 21 day intervals. In any case, repeat courses of Vepesid should not be given until the blood picture has been checked for evidence of myelosuppression and found to be satisfactory

Immediately before administration, the required dose of Vepesid Injection must be diluted with 0.9% saline solution for injection to give a solution concentration of not more than 0.25 mg/ml of etoposide; it should then be given by intravenous infusion over a period of not less than 30 minutes.

Care should be taken to avoid extravasation.

If oral dosing is preferred, twice the relevant i.v. dose should be given daily, for five consecutive days. As Vepesid produces myelosuppression, courses may not be repeated more frequently than at 21 day intervals. In any case, repeat courses of Vepesid should not be given until the blood picture has been checked for evidence of myelosuppression and found to be satisfactory.

Elderly: No dosage adjustment is necessary.

Contra-indications, warnings, etc Vepesid is contra-indicated in patients with severe hepatic dysfunction or in those patients who have demonstrated hypersensitivity to the drug.

Vepesid must not be given by intra-cavity injection.

Warnings: Vepesid should not normally be administered to patients who are pregnant or to mothers who are breast feeding. Safe use in pregnancy has not been established.

Vepesid is teratogenic in rats at dose levels equivalent to those employed clinically.

The influence of Vepesid on human reproduction has not been determined.

In-vitro tests indicate that Vepesid is mutagenic.

Precautions: Vepesid should be administered by individuals experienced in the use of antineoplastic therapy.

When Vepesid is administered intravenously care should be taken to avoid extravasation.

If radiotherapy and/or chemotherapy has been given prior to starting Vepesid treatment, an adequate interval should be allowed to enable the bone marrow to recover. If the leucocyte count falls below 2,000/mm³, treatment should be suspended until the circulating blood elements have returned to acceptable levels (platelets above 100,000 mm³, leucocytes above 4,000/mm³), this is usually within 10 days.

Peripheral blood counts and liver function should be monitored. (See Adverse Reactions.)

Bacterial infections should be brought under control before treatment with Vepesid commences.

Adverse reactions: Haematological: The dose limiting toxicity of Vepesid is myelosuppression, predominantly leucopenia and thrombocytopenia. Anaemia occurs infrequently.

The leucocyte count nadir occurs approximately 21 days after treatment.

Alopecia: Alopecia occurs in approximately 50% of patients and is reversible on cessation of therapy.

Gastrointestinal: Nausea and vomiting are the major gastrointestinal toxicities and occur in approximately 30% of patients. Anti-emetics are useful in controlling these side effects. Abdominal pain, diarrhoea and anorexia occur infrequently.

Other Toxicities: Hypotension may occur following an excessively rapid infusion and may be reversed by slowing the infusion rate.

Anaphylactic-like reactions have been reported rarely following administration of Vepesid. Reactions respond to cessation of therapy and administration of an anti-histamine.

No specific toxic effects have been observed with respect to the cardiovascular system, nervous system, the liver or kidney. However, Vepesid has been shown to reach high concentrations in the latter two organs, thus presenting a potential for accumulation in cases of functional impairment.

Guidelines for the safe handling of antineoplastic agents:
1. Trained personnel should reconstitute the drug.
2. This should be performed in a designated area.
3. Adequate protective gloves should be worn.
4. Precautions should be taken to avoid the drug accidentally coming into contact with the eyes. In the event of contact with the eyes, irrigate with large amounts of water and/or saline.
5. The cytotoxic preparation should not be handled by pregnant staff.
6. Adequate care and precautions should be taken in the disposal of items (syringes, needles etc) used to reconstitute cytotoxic drugs. Excess material and body waste may be disposed of by placing in double sealed polythene bags and incinerating at a temperature of 1,000°C. Liquid waste may be flushed with copious amounts of water.
7. The work surface should be covered with disposable plastic-backed absorbent paper.
8. Use Luer-Lock fittings on all syringes and sets. Large bore needles are recommended to minimise pressure and the possible formation of aerosols. The latter may also be reduced by the use of a venting needle.

Pharmaceutical precautions Vepesid capsules and injection should be stored at room temperature. The injection should be protected from light.

Preparation of intravenous solution: Immediately before administration the required dose of Vepesid Injection must be diluted with 0.9% saline solution for injection to give a solution concentration of not more than 0.25 mg/ml of etoposide; it should then be given by intravenous infusion over a period of not less than 30 minutes. The infusion solution should be kept at room temperature and should be used within six hours of preparation. Solutions of concentration greater than 0.25 mg/ml may show signs of precipitation, and are therefore not recommended. Any solutions showing signs of precipitation should be discarded.

The intravenous solution is suitable for infusion in glass or PVC containers.

Vepesid should not be physically mixed with any other drug.

Expiry date: Vepesid injection: 5 years from date of manufacture. Vepesid capsules: 2 years from date of manufacture.

Legal category POM.

Package quantities Vepesid injection is packed in cartons of 10 ampoules, each ampoule containing 100 mg etoposide in 5 ml of solution.

Vepesid 100 mg capsules are packed in bottles of 10 capsules, each capsule containing 100 mg etoposide.

Vepesid 50 mg capsules are packed in bottles of 20 capsules, each capsule containing 50 mg etoposide.

Further information Etoposide is a semisynthetic derivative of podophyllotoxin.

Experimental data indicate that etoposide arrests the cell cycle in the G_2 phase. Etoposide differs from the vinca alkaloids in that it does not cause an accumulation of cells in metaphase, but prevents cells from entering mitosis or destroys cells in the G_2 phase. The incorporation of thymidine into DNA is inhibited in-vitro by etoposide. Etoposide does not interfere with microtubule assembly. Etoposide is approximately 94% protein-bound in human serum. Plasma decay kinetics follow a bi-exponential curve and correspond to a two compartmental model. The mean volume of distribution is approximately 32% of body weight. Etoposide demonstrates relatively poor penetration into the cerebrospinal fluid. Urinary excretion is approximately 45% of an administered dose, 29% being excreted unchanged in 72 hours.

An information sheet on the storage, preparation and handling of the product is available

Product licence numbers
Vepesid 50 mg Capsules 0125/0153
Vepesid 100 mg Capsules 0125/0124
Vepesid Injection 0125/0121

*Trade Mark

Britannia Pharmaceuticals Limited
Forum House
47–75 Brighton Road
Redhill
Surrey RH1 6YS

ELDEPRYL* ▼
Presentation White, scored, uncoated tablets 6 mm diameter containing 5 mg selegiline hydrochloride.

Uses
Properties: Eldepryl is a selective MAO-B inhibitor which prevents dopamine breakdown in the brain. It also inhibits the re-uptake of dopamine at the pre-synaptic dopamine receptor. These effects potentiate dopaminergic function in the brain and help to even out and prolong the effect of exogenous or endogenous dopamine.

Thus Eldepryl potentiates and prolongs the effect of levodopa in the treatment of Parkinsonism. The addition of Eldepryl to levodopa (with or without decarboxylase inhibitor) therapy helps to alleviate dose related fluctuations and end of dose deterioration. At a later stage in the disease it can also smooth the symptoms of the on/off effect. When Eldepryl is added to such a regimen it is possible to reduce the levodopa dosage by an average of 30 per cent.

Unlike conventional MAO inhibitors, which inhibit both the MAO-A and MAO-B enzyme, Eldepryl is a specific MAO-B inhibitor and can be given safely with levodopa. There are no dietary restrictions associated with Eldepryl treatment, i.e. it does not cause the so called 'cheese effect'.

Indications: Eldepryl is indicated for the treatment of Parkinson's disease, or symptomatic Parkinsonism, which is being treated with levodopa alone or levodopa and peripheral decarboxylase inhibitor.

Dosage and administration Eldepryl should always be given together with existing levodopa therapy.

The initial dose of Eldepryl is 5 mg (1 tablet) in the morning. If little response is achieved with 1 tablet the dose of Eldepryl can be increased to 10 mg (2 tablets) in the morning.

Contra-indications, warnings, etc
Contra-indications: None known.

Precautions: Because Eldepryl potentiates the effects of levodopa the side effects of levodopa might be emphasised, particularly when the patient is on a very high dosage of levodopa. The addition of Eldepryl to maximal doses of levodopa may cause involuntary movement and/or agitation. Such side effects disappear when the levodopa dosage is decreased. Levodopa treatment can be reduced by an average of 30 per cent when Eldepryl is added to the treatment and when an optimal levodopa dose has been established the side effects of the combination have been found to be fewer than for levodopa alone.

Side effects: Hypotension and nausea have been reported as isolated symptoms associated with Eldepryl treatment. Confusion or psychosis have also been reported.

Pharmaceutical precautions Protect from heat, moisture and light.

Legal category POM.

Package quantities 100 tablets.

Further information Eldepryl has a long duration of action allowing a once daily dosage.

Product licence number 4483/0024.

LEJGUAR*
Presentation Each pack contains 250 g of Lejguar, a palatable granule, containing approximately 90% of guar meal flour.

The granules are white to slightly yellow, 0.6–3.5 mm in diameter and have a neutral taste.

Uses
Action: Ingestion of Lejguar results in a reduction of post-prandial glucose levels. This action is probably due to the fact that Lejguar forms a viscous gel in the gastro-intestinal tract resulting in a reduction of the gastric emptying rate and a thickening of the unstirred water layer adjacent to the intestinal villi.
The bulking action of Lejguar helps to reduce energy intake by diminishing appetite.

Indications: Lejguar is indicated for use in diabetics to stabilise post-prandial glucose levels.
This stabilisation facilitates control of the disease and, in appropriate cases, allows the reduction of insulin or oral hypoglycemic dosage levels.

Dosage and administration
Adult dose: 7 g (two scoops) three times a day, during the first six weeks of treatment. After this initial period the dose can usually be reduced to 7 g (two scoops) twice a day.

Children's dose: The products is not recommended for use in children.

Administration: 7 g (two level scoops) of Lejguar should be taken at meal-times. One 3.5 g scoopful before the meal and the other 3.5 g scoopful during the meal.

One level scoopful (3.5 g) of granules should be stirred into a glass containing at least 100 ml of water, or sugar-free fruit juice, then swallowed quickly and washed down with another 100 ml of water or sugar-free fruit juice.

Note: If water is not used the sugar content of the liquid should be taken into account.

Contra-indications, warnings, etc

Precautions: To avoid the risk of oesopageal obstruction or rupture, Lejguar should not be given to patients with a history of oesophageal disease or difficulties in swallowing.

Lejguar should not be ingested as dry granules. For optimum results and to minimise non-compliance, it is essential for the granules to be mixed with water or fruit juice before swallowing; the gel must be washed down with lots of liquid.

During initial therapy and when reducing dosage of Lejguar, blood glucose levels should be carefully monitored and concurrent treatment adjusted where necessary, to minimise the danger of hypoglycemia.

Side-effects: Reported side-effects are a laxative effect and increased flatulence. Occasional excessive laxation is usually transient and normally improves after 1–2 weeks or after temporarily reducing the dosage.

Pharmaceutical precautions Lejguar should be stored in a cool, dry place.

Legal category P.

Package quantities Each carton of Lejguar contains 250 g of granules plus a 3.5 g scoop.

Further information Nil.

Product licence number PL 4483/0027.

RIMSO-50*

Presentation Sterile aqueous solution containing dimethyl sulphoxide 50% w/w.

Uses Indicated only for the symptomatic relief of patients with interstitial cystitis (Hunner's Ulcer).
   For bladder instillation only.
   Not for IM or IV injection.

Dosage and administration Instillation of 50 ml of Rimso-50 (dimethyl sulphoxide) directly into the bladder may be accomplished by catheter or bladder syringe and allowed to remain for 15 minutes. Application of an analgesic lubricant gel such as lignocaine jelly to the urethra is suggested prior to the insertion of the catheter to avoid spasm. The medication is expelled by spontaneous voiding. It is recommended that treatment be repeated every two weeks until maximum symptomatic relief is obtained. Thereafter, time intervals between therapy may be increased appropriately. In selected cases where symptomatic relief is not complete, the bladder may be gently distended by gravity instillation with up to 500 ml of a solution prepared immediately prior to instillation in a glass vial, with one part Rimso-

50 and one part sterile water prior to the instillation of the standard dose of 50 ml of Rimso-50. After retention of Rimso-50 for 15 minutes the medication is again expelled by spontaneous voiding. Administration of oral analgesic medication or suppositories containing belladonna and opium prior to instillation of Rimso-50 can reduce bladder spasm in particularly sensitive patients.

In patients with very sensitive bladders, the treatment should be done under anaesthesia (preferably saddle block type).

Rimso-50 is recommended for bladder instillation only.

Contra-indications, warnings, etc

Contra-indications: None.

Precautions: Changes in the refractive index and lens opacities have been seen in monkeys, dogs and rats given dimethyl sulphoxide chronically. No ophthalmic changes attributable to intravesical instillation of dimethyl sulphoxide have been reported in patients carefully followed for up to 17 months; nevertheless, full eye evaluations, including slit lamp examinations, are recommended prior to and at six months intervals during treatment.

Along with the ophthalmological examinations, patients should be investigated with respect to biochemical parameters, particularly renal and hepatic function, at six month intervals.

Intravesical instillation of Rimso-50 may be harmful to patients with urinary tract malignancy because of dimethyl sulphoxide-induced vasodilation.

Warnings: Dimethyl sulphoxide can initiate the liberation of histamine and there has been an occasional hypersensitivity reaction with topical administration of dimethyl sulphoxide. This hypersensitivity has not occurred in patients receiving intravesical Rimso-50; however, the physician should be cognizant of this possibility in prescribing Rimso-50. If anaphylactoid symptoms develop, appropriate therapy should be instituted. Some data indicated that dimethyl sulphoxide potentiates other concomitantly administered medications.

Use in pregnancy: The safety of dimethyl sulphoxide for the human foetus has not been established, hence it should be given to pregnant women only when the potential benefits to the mother have been weighed against possible hazards to the child.

Pharmaceutical precautions Store in a cool place protected from light.

Legal category POM.

Package quantities Bottles of 50 ml.

Further information Nil.

Product licence number 4047/0001.

*Trade Mark

Brocades Great Britain Limited
Brocades House
Pyrford Road
West Byfleet, Surrey

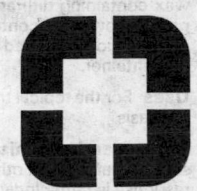

AMFIPEN* CAPSULES
AMFIPEN* SYRUP
AMFIPEN* SYRUP FORTE
AMFIPEN* INJECTION

Presentation Amfipen Capsules (Ampicillin Capsules BP) are presented as grey and red capsules each containing 250 mg or 500 mg Ampicillin BP, imprinted 'Amfipen 250' or 'Amfipen 500'.

Amfipen Syrup (Ampicillin Mixture BPC) and Amfipen Syrup Forte (Strong Ampicillin Mixture BPC) are presented as bottles containing dry powder for the preparation of 100 ml of a pink-coloured suspension. On reconstitution each 5 ml dose contains 125 mg or 250 mg respectively Ampicillin BP.

Amfipen Injections (Ampicillin sodium for injection BP) are presented as vials containing 250 mg or 500 mg ampicillin as Ampicillin Sodium BP.

Uses Amfipen is a broad-spectrum penicillin for the treatment of a wide range of infections caused by ampicillin-sensitive organisms.

Dosage and administration *Usual adult oral dosage:* Ear, nose and throat infections: 250 mg four times a day.

Bronchitis: usually 250 mg four times a day in routine therapy; 1 g four times a day in high-dosage regimes.

Pneumonia: 500 mg four times a day.

Gastro-intestinal infection: 500–750 mg three or four times daily.

Urinary tract infections: 500 mg four times daily.

Enteric fevers: in acute cases 1–2 g four times a day for 14 days; carriers should be treated with this dosage for 4–12 weeks.

In the treatment of gonorrhoea 2 g should be given with 1 g probenecid as a single dose. In the treatment of females repeated doses are recommended.

Usual children's oral dosage: Half of the adult dosage.

The doses above are recommended dosages, only as a guide. In severe infections the dosages may be increased.

Amfipen should be given a half to one hour before meals.

Usual adult parenteral dosage: Septicaemia, endocarditis, osteomyelitis: 500 mg four to six times a day for one to six weeks by intramuscular or intravenous injection.

Meningitis: 2 g six-hourly for two days by intravenous injection, followed by 500 mg to 1 g six-hourly by intramuscular injection.

Usual children's parenteral dosage: Meningitis: 100 mg per kg daily in divided doses by intravenous injections.

The dosages above are recommended dosages only as a guide. In severe infections the dosages may be increased.

Administration: Amfipen may be administered orally as capsules or syrup or syrup forte. Parenteral dosage by means of Amfipen Injection should be administered as follows: For intramuscular injection dissolve 250 mg or 500 mg in 1.5 ml water for injections BP. For intravenous injection dissolve 500 mg in 5 ml water for injections BP and administer by injection over three to five minutes. For intraperitoneal injection and intrapleural injection dissolve 500–1,000 mg in 5–10 ml water for injections BP. For intra-articular injection 500 mg dissolved in up to 5 ml water for injections BP or 0.5% procaine hydrochloride.

Contra-indications, warnings, etc
Contra-indicated in patients with penicillin hypersensitivity and glandular fever.

Side-effects: Skin reactions may occur rarely, and be due to either penicillin hypersensitivity (urticarial rash) or specific ampicillin sensitivity (erythematous rash); treatment should be discontinued if a rash occurs. Occasionally, diarrhoea may occur. As with all ampicillins, Amfipen may reduce the efficacy of oral contraceptives, and patients should be warned accordingly.

Pharmaceutical precautions Amfipen preparations should be stored in a cool dry place. On reconstitution, Amfipen Syrup and Amfipen Syrup Forte should be used within seven days if stored in a cool place.

In order to obtain a homogeneous suspension it is recommended that the bottle be well shaken before reconstitution of the syrup.

Legal category POM.

Package quantities *Amfipen Capsules 250 mg:* Bottles of 250, and packs of 2,500.

Amfipen capsules 500 mg: Bottles of 250, and packs of 1,500.

Amfipen Syrup and Syrup Forte: Bottles for the preparation of 100 ml.

Amfipen Injections 250 mg and 500 mg: Boxes of 10 vials.

Further information Nil.

Product licence numbers
Amfipen Capsules 250 mg	0166/0065
Amfipen Capsules 500 mg	0166/0066
Amfipen Syrup	0166/0067
Amfipen Syrup Forte	0166/0068
Amfipen Injection 250 mg	0166/0069
Amfipen Injection 500 mg	0166/0070

ANTRADERM* MILD
ANTRADERM*
ANTRADERM* FORTE

Presentation *Antraderm Mild*: a pale yellow wax containing dithranol BP 0.5%. *Andraderm*: a pale yellow

wax containing dithranol BP 1.0%. *Antraderm Forte*: a
pale yellow wax containing dithranol BP 2.0%. Each
presentation is packed as 20 ml sticks in a plastic twist-
up container.

Uses For the topical treatment of subacute and chronic
psoriasis.

Dosage and administration Clinical experience has
shown that, as with other methods of treatment, patient
response is rather individualised and therefore it may be
necessary to adjust treatment during the initial period. It
is recommended that treatment be normally started with
the 1.0% concentration. If irritation or stinging occurs
and it persists the problem can often be overcome by
changing to the lower 0.5% strength. If the effect of the
1.0% strength is insufficient or if tolerance develops after
a period of treatment the 2.0% strength will often produce
the required response.

Antraderm is suitable for use in both prolonged-
contact and short-contact therapy. In all cases Antraderm
should be applied directly to the lesions. The tip of the
wax stick is softened by skin temperature enabling a thin
layer of dithranol to be gently applied to the required
areas only. When treating very scaly lesions the debris
should be removed before applying Antraderm. For
prolonged-contact therapy Antraderm should preferably
be applied at bedtime and washed off in the morning.
For short-contact therapy Antraderm may be applied at
any convenient time during the day and then removed
by washing off, usually within an hour of application;
Antraderm 2.0% is particularly suitable for short-contact
therapy.

Treatment should continue until the skin is clear.
Intermittent courses may be required to maintain therapeutic response.

Contra-indications, warnings, etc A small proportion of patients initially experience slight toxic reactions
to dithranol. This reaction is often transient and is usually
seen during the first 2–3 days of treatment. It is more
likely to occur when potent topical steriods have recently
been used. These effects can usually be overcome by:
a) reducing the frequency of treatment for a few days
e.g. applications very 2nd or 3rd night.
b) using a lower concentration of Antraderm. If neither
action overcomes the toxic response, it may be necessary
to stop treatment.

Antraderm must not be used for psoriasis in the acute
phase. Care should be taken to avoid application to
surrounding areas of unaffected skin. Avoid contact with
the eyes.

An excessive quantity should not be applied as this
may cause unnecessary staining of clothing and bed
linen. In the morning a bath will remove any surplus
dithranol.

During treatment the edges of the lesions will gradually
acquire a purplish-brown stain which will completely
disappear after the treatment has finished.

Pharmaceutical precautions Keep in a cool place.
Use within 6 months of breaking the foil outer pack.

Legal category
Antraderm Mild   P.
Antraderm   POM.
Antraderm Forte   POM.

Package quantities All strengths are supplied in 20 ml
sticks.

Further information Antraderm is suitable for home

treatment as its advantages make it easier and more
economic in use than other forms of dithranol. It is
however equally suitable for use in dermatology wards
and clinics as a standard dithranol treatment.

Product licence numbers
Antraderm Mild   0166/0103
Anterderm   0166/0104
Antraderm Forte   0166/0105

BICILLIN* INJECTION

Presentation Bicillin Injection is presented as vials of
dry powder for the preparation of Fortified Procaine
Penicillin Injection BP. Each vial contains 3 mega units
(3 g) procaine penicillin G and 1 mega unit (0.6 g)
sodium penicillin G.

Uses Antibiotic for the treatment of infections due to
penicillin-sensitive organisms, where prolonged release
is desired.

Dosage and administration For intramuscular injection only.
Adults: 400,000 units (300 mg procaine penicillin G and
60 mg sodium penicillin G) 24-hourly or 12-hourly.
Children: Over 25 kg as for adults; under 25 kg proportionally.

Contra-indications, warnings, etc
Contra-indications: Hypersensitivity to penicillin or procaine.
Special precautions: Appropriate treatment for systemic
reactions should be readily available.
Side-effects: Skin reactions may occur but usually
resolve on cessation of therapy; generalised systemic
reactions are rare and usually associated with a history
of allergy or penicillin intolerance.

The safety of Bicillin Injection during pregnancy has
not been established.

Pharmaceutical precautions Store in a cool dry
place. Use within five days after reconstitution if stored
at room temperature or 14 days if stored at 4°C.

Legal category POM.

Package quantities Boxes of 10 vials each containing
4 mega units (3 g procaine penicillin G and 0.6 g sodium
penicillin) per vial.

Further information Upon reconstitution with 7.5 ml
Water for Injections BP, each ml of suspension contains
300,000 units (300 mg) procaine penicillin G and
100,000 units (60 mg) sodium penicillin G.

Product licence number 0166/0073.

BROCADOPA* CAPSULES

Presentation Brocadopa is presented as clear colourless hard gelatine capsules each containing 125 mg,
250 mg or 500 mg Levodopa BP, imprinted 'Brocadopa
125', '250' or '500'. Brocadopa Capsules comply with
the monograph for Levodopa Capsules BP.

Uses Dopaminergic, for the treatment of all forms of
Parkinsonism, except drug-induced (neuroleptic syndrome).

Dosage and administration By oral administration.
Adults: Initially 250 mg daily in divided doses, increasing

by 250 mg every three to four days until optimal response is obtained. This may occur at any level between 1 g and 8 g daily in divided doses after a period of four to six weeks.

Children: As for adults.

Contra-indications, warnings, etc
Contra-indicated in patients receiving monoamine oxidase inhibitors.

Special precautions: Use with caution in patients receiving pyridoxine, hypotensive agents, phenothiazines and butyrophenones, or tricyclic antidepressants, and in patients suffering from heart disease (heart block, myocardial infarct or insufficiency and cardiac arrhythmia), dementia and psychoses, liver disease or pregnancy.

Side-effects: Gastro-intestinal disturbances, such as nausea, vomiting and anorexia, are the commonest side-effects and occur early. They may be diminished by administration after food and by finer fractionation of the daily dose. A non-phenothiazine anti-emetic drug may be given half an hour before each dose.

Hypotension, generally postural in type, may occur, usually unaccompanied by symptoms or change in pulse rate. Smaller dosage increments will reduce the incidence.

Involuntary movements usually occur at higher dosage level, and may be alleviated by a small reduction in dosage of 0.5–1 g daily or by fractionation of dosage.

Psychic manifestations such as restlessness and nervousness may occur with some disturbance of sleep. More rarely, agitation or mania with hallucinations have been reported. Psychiatric side-effects are more likely to occur in patients with a pre-existing psychosis but may be diminished or abolished by reduction or cessation of dosage.

Cardiac distrubances, e.g. paroxysmal tachycardia and arrhythmias, have been reported. It may be advisable to stop dosage and recommence at a lower level.

Overdosage: No reports of overdosage have been received.

Pharmaceutical precautions Normal pharmaceutical storage and handling are indicated.

Legal category POM.

Package quantities *Capsules:* 250 × 125 mg, 100 × 250 mg, 250 × 250 mg, 100 × 500 mg and 250 × 500 mg.

Further information Nil.

Product licence numbers
Capsules 125 mg 0166/5013
Capsules 250 mg 0166/5014
Capsules 500 mg 0166/5015

CYCLOSPASMOL* SUSPENSION

Presentation Cyclospasmol Suspension is presented as a dry powder, ready for reconstitution at the time of dispensing by the addition of 375 ml distilled water. The resulting suspension provides 90 doses each of 5 ml, each 5 ml dose containing 400 mg cyclandelate.

Uses For the treatment of organic vasospastic peripheral and cerebrovascular diseases associated with impaired circulation, especially in the long-term management of chronic insufficiency and in the sequelae of strokes, and

in the improvement of mental function, dementia, confusion etc., and in intermittent claudication, Raynaud's phenomenon, chilblains, night cramps, acrocyanosis, cold hands and feet, etc.

Dosage and administration By oral administration.

Adults: 1,600 mg (20 ml) daily in 2 or 4 divided doses.

Children: A dosage for children has not been established.

Contra-indications, warnings, etc Contra-indicated in the acute phase of a cerebrovascular accident.

Special precautions: None.

Side-effects: At very high dosage, nausea, gastro-intestinal distress or flushing may occur.

Overdosage: Gross overdosages have not been reported; theoretically circulatory collapse could occur and treatment would be gastric lavage and, if necessary, vasopressors.

Pharmaceutical precautions Normal pharmaceutical storage and handling are indicated. Upon reconstitution, Cyclospasmol suspension carries an expiry date of 3 months from the date of reconstitution.

Legal category P.

Package quantities Each bottle, after reconstitution, provides 90 doses each of 400 mg cyclandelate in 5 ml.

Further information Each 5 ml dose contains approximately 500 mg sucrose. For maximum therapeutic effect it is recommended that the daily dose of 1,600 mg be given; maximal therapeutic response may not be seen within the first one or two months of treatment.

Product licence number 0166/0062.

CYCLOSPASMOL* TABLETS
CYCLOSPASMOL* CAPSULES

Presentation Cyclospasmol is presented as pink sugar-coated tablets each containing 400 mg cyclandelate, imprinted 'Cyclospasmol'; and as pink/grey hard gelatine capsules each containing 400 mg cyclandelate, imprinted 'Cyclospasmol'.

Uses For the treatment of organic vasospastic peripheral and cerebrovascular diseases associated with impaired circulation, especially in the long-term management of chronic insufficiency and in the sequelae of strokes, and in the improvement of mental function, dementia, confusion, etc., and in intermittent claudication, Raynaud's phenomenon, chilblains, night cramps, acrocyanosis, cold hands and feet, etc.

Dosage and administration By oral administration.

Adults: 1,600 mg daily in 2 or 4 divided doses.

Children: A dosage for children has not been established.

Contra-indications, warnings, etc
Contra-indicated in the acute phase of a cerebrovascular accident.

Special precautions: None.

Side-effects: At very high dosages, nausea, gastro-intestinal distress or flushing may occur.

Overdosage: Gross overdosages have not been reported; theoretically circulatory collapse could occur and treatment would be gastric lavage and, if necessary, vasopressors.

Pharmaceutical precautions Normal pharmaceutical storage and handling are indicated.

Legal category P.

Package quantities Tablets 250 × 400 mg. Capsules 250 × 400 mg and treatment packs of 112 tablets.

Further information For maximum therapeutic effect, it is recommended that the daily dosage of 1,600 mg be given; maximal therapeutic response may not be seen within the first one or two months of treatment.

Product licence numbers
Cyclospasmol Capsules   0166/0021
Cyclospasmol Tablets   0166/0052

DE-NOLTAB* AND DE-NOL*

Presentation De-Noltab is presented as flat round pink tablets, each tablet containing 120 mg tri-potassium di-citrato bismuthate (calculated as Bi_2O_3). De-Nol is presented as a clear red liquid in a 560 ml bottle containing 120 mg tri-potassium di-citrato bismuthate (calculated as Bi_2O_3) in each 5 ml.

Uses Ulcer healing agent. For the treatment of gastric and duodenal ulcers.

Dosage and administration By oral administration. Each tablet is to be crushed in the mouth and swallowed with a draught of water. Each dose of the liquid presentation is to be diluted with 15 ml of water.

Adults: One tablet or 5 ml four times a day on an empty stomach, half an hour before each of the three main meals and two hours after the last meal of the day. Alternatively, two tablets or two 5 ml spoonfuls twice daily (half an hour before breakfast and half an hour before the evening meal). The treatment course should be taken for the full 28 day period and it is important that a dose is not missed. If necessary, *one* further course of therapy may be given. Maintenance therapy with De-Noltab/De-Nol is not indicated.

Children: As for adults.

Contra-indications, warnings, etc De-Noltab and De-Nol should not be administered to patients with renal disorders, and on theoretical grounds the products are contraindicated in pregnancy.

Special precautions: De-Noltab and De-Nol may inhibit the efficacy of orally administered tetracyclines.

Side effects: Blackening of the stool usually occurs. Darkening of the tongue, nausea and vomiting have been reported.

Overdosage: No reports of overdosage have been received; gastric lavage and, if necessary, supportive therapy would be indicated.

Pharmaceutical precautions Normal pharmaceutical storage and handling are indicated.

Legal category P.

Package quantities
De-Noltab: Foil treatment packs of 112 tablets.
De-Nol: Treatment packs of 560 ml.

Further information Some patients with an associated gastritis may experience an initial discomfort whilst taking De-Nol liquid. Milk should not be drunk by itself during the course of treatment as this can prevent the medicine from working properly. Small quantities of milk on a breakfast cereal or in tea or coffee taken with meals are permissible. Antacids should not be taken for half an hour before or half an hour after taking a dose of De-Noltab/De-Nol as these can interfere with the action of the drug.

Product licence numbers
De-Noltab   0166/0102
De-Nol   0166/5024

DEPOCILLIN* INJECTION

Presentation Depocillin Injection is presented as vials of dry powder for the preparation of Procaine Penicillin Injection BP. Each vial contains 3 mega units (3 g) of procaine penicillin G.

Uses Antibiotic for the treatment of infections due to penicillin-sensitive organisms, where prolonged release is desired.

Dosage and administration For intramuscular injection only.

Adults: 300,000 units (300 mg) 24-hourly or 12-hourly.

Children: Over 25 kg as for adults; under 25 kg proportionally.

Contra-indications, warnings, etc
Contra-indications: Hypersensitivity to penicillin or procaine.

Special precautions: Appropriate treatment for systemic reactions should be readily available.

Side-effects: Skin reactions may occur but usually resolve on cessation of therapy; generalised systemic reactions are rare and usually associated with a history of allergy or penicillin intolerance.

The safety of Depocillin Injection during pregnancy has not been established.

Pharmaceutical precautions Store in a cool dry place. Use within five days after reconstitution if stored at room temperature or 14 days if stored at 4°C.

Legal category POM.

Package quantities Boxes of 10 vials each containing 3 mega units (3 g) per vial.

Further information Upon reconstitution with 8 ml Water for Injections BP each ml of suspension contains 300,000 units (300 mg) of procaine Penicillin G.

Product licence number 0166/0072.

DISIPAL* TABLETS
DISIPAL* INJECTION

Presentation Disipal Tablets are presented as yellow sugar-coated tablets each containing 50 mg Orphenadrine Hydrochloride BP, imprinted 'Disipal'. Disipal Tablets comply with the monograph for Orphenadrine Hydrochloride Tablets BP.

Disipal Injection is presented as a sterile aqueous solution in clear glass 2 ml ampoules each containing 20 mg/ml Orphenadrine Hydrochloride BP.

Uses Anticholinergic, for the treatment of all forms of Parkinsonism, including drug-induced (neuroleptic syndrome).

Dosage and administration *By oral administration:*
Adults: Initially 150 mg daily in divided doses, increasing

by 50 mg every two or three days until maximum benefit is obtained. Optimal dosage is usually 250–300 mg daily in divided doses in idiopathic and post-encephalitic Parkinsonism, 100–150 mg daily in divided doses in arteriosclerotic Parkinsonism, and 150–300 mg daily in divided doses in the neuroleptic syndrome. Maximal dosage, 400 mg daily in divided doses.

Children: As for adults.

By intramuscular injection: Adults: 20–40 mg (1–2 ml) as determined by the physician.

Children: As for adults.

Contra-indications, warnings, etc Contra-indicated in patients with glaucoma or prostatic hypertrophy.

Special precautions: Use with caution in patients with micturition difficulties or in pregnancy.

Side-effects: Occasionally dry mouth, disturbances of visual accommodation and micturition difficulties may occur; these usually disappear spontaneously or may be controlled by a slight reduction in dosage.

Overdosage: Toxic effects are anticholinergic in nature and the treatment is gastric lavage, cholinergics such as carbachol, anticholinesterases such as physostigmine and general non-specific treatment.

Pharmaceutical precautions Normal pharmaceutical storage and handling are indicated.

Legal category POM.

Package quantities *Tablets:* 100 × 50 mg, 250 × 50 mg, 1,000 × 50 mg, 10,000 × 50 mg.
Ampoules: 10 × 40 mg/2 ml.

Further information Although very rarely reported, there may be provocation of dextropropoxyphene side-effects when that drug is administered concurrently with orphenadrine.

Product licence numbers
Tablets   0166/5001
Injection 0166/5005

LOCOID* CREAM
LOCOID* OINTMENT

Presentation Locoid Cream, containing 0.1% hydrocortisone 17-butyrate in a cream base.
Locoid Ointment, containing 0.1% hydrocortisone 17-butyrate in an ointment base.

Uses The products are recommended for clinical use in the treatment of conditions responsive to topical corticosteroids, e.g. eczema, dermatitis and psoriasis.
The products are intended for topical application.

Dosage and administration For adults and children, to be applied to the affected part two to four times a day, or as directed by the physician.
Where necessary, application may be made under an occlusive dressing.

Contra-indications, warnings, etc These preparations are contra-indicated in the presence of viral or fungal infections, tubercular or syphilitic lesions, and in bacterial infections unless used in conjunction with appropriate chemotherapy. Contact with the eye should be avoided.
In pregnant animals, administration of corticosteroids can cause abnormalities of foetal development. The

relevance of this finding to human beings has not been established. However, topical steroids should not be used extensively in pregnancy, i.e. in large amounts or for long periods.
In infants, long-term continuous topical therapy should be avoided. Adrenal suppression can occur, even without occlusion.

Pharmaceutical precautions Store at room temperature (15–25°C).

Legal category POM.

Package quantities *Locoid Cream:* Tubes of 30 g and 100 g.
Locoid Ointment: Tubes of 30 g and 100 g.

Further information Locoid is a non-fluorinated topical steroid. Whilst clinical trials have shown it to be as effective as the potent fluorinated steroids, in clinical practice there is a low incidence of reported clinical side-effects.

Product licence numbers
Locoid Cream   0166/0058
Locoid Ointment   0166/0059

LOCOID LIPOCREAM*

Presentation Locoid Lipocream, containing 0.1% hydrocortisone 17-butyrate in a fatty cream base.

Uses The product is recommended for clinical use in the treatment of conditions responsive to topical corticosteroids, e.g. eczema, dermatitis and psoriasis. The product is intended for topical application.

Dosage and administration For adults and children, to be applied to the affected part two to four times a day, or as directed by the physician. Where necessary, application may be made under an occlusive dressing.

Contra-indications, warnings, etc Topical corticosteroids are contra-indicated in the presence of viral or fungal infections, tubercular or syphilitic lesions, and in bacterial infections unless used in conjunction with appropriate chemotherapy. Contact with the eye should be avoided. In pregnant animals, administration of corticosteroids can cause abnormalities of foetal development. The relevance of this finding to human beings has not been established. However, topical steroids should not be used extensively in pregnancy, i.e. in large amounts or for long periods.
In infants, long-term continuous therapy should be avoided. Adrenal suppression can occur, even without occlusion. Occlusive dressings are not recommended in the presence of infections.

Pharmaceutical precautions Store at room temperature (15–25°C).

Legal category POM.

Package quantities Tubes of 30 g.

Further information Locoid, a non-fluorinated topical steroid has been shown to be as affective as the potent fluorinated steroids, yet in clinical practice there is a low incidence of reported side-effects.
Lipocream is 70% oil, oil in water emulsion. This base promotes both hydration of the stratum corneum and suppleness of dry scaly, excoriated skin, with greater patient acceptability than an ordinary ointment. The

product is particularly suited for use on dry, subacute and chronic lesions or for those patients presenting with mixed lesions.

Product licence number 0166/0112.

LOCOID* C CREAM
LOCOID* C OINTMENT

Presentation Locoid C cream, containing 0.1% hydrocortisone 17-butyrate and 3% chlorquinaldol, in a cream base.

Locoid C ointment, containing 0.1% hydrocortisone 17-butyrate and 3% chlorquinaldol, in an ointment base.

Uses The products are recommended for clinical use in the treatment of conditions responsive to topical corticosteroids, e.g. eczema, dermatitis and psoriasis, where secondary bacterial or fungal infection is present or suspected, or may complicate the condition.

The products are intended for topical application.

Dosage and administration For adults and children, to be applied to the affected part two to four times a day, or as directed by the physician, until the infection has resolved. If the underlying dermatological condition still persists, treatment may be continued with Locoid cream or ointment.

Contra-indications, warnings, etc *Contra-indications:* These preparations are contra-indicated in the presence of viral, tubercular or syphilitic lesions. Contact with the eye should be avoided.

Warnings: In pregnant animals, administration of corticosteroids can cause abnormalities of foetal development. The relevance of this finding to human beings has not been established. However, topical steroids should not be used extensively in pregnancy, i.e. in large amounts or for long periods.

In infants, long-term continuous topical therapy shold be avoided. Adrenal suppression can occur, even without occlusion.

Occlusive dressings are not recommended in the presence of infections.

Locoid C preparations should not be used for longer than 14 days at a time, nor should more than 60 g be applied during this period.

Pharmaceutical precautions Store under normal pharmaceutical conditions of storage.

Legal category POM.

Package quantities *Locoid C cream:* Tubes of 30 g. *Locoid C ointment:* Tubes of 30 g.

Further information Locoid is a non-fluorinated topical steroid. Whilst clinical trials have shown it to be as effective as the potent fluorinated steroids, in clinical practice there is a low incidence of reported side-effects.

Chlorquinaldol is an effective topical antibacterial and antimycotic.

Product licence numbers
Locoid C cream   0166/0056
Locoid C ointment 0166/0057

LOCOID* SCALP LOTION

Presentation Locoid Scalp Lotion contains 0.1% hydrocortisone 17-butyrate in an iso-propyl alcohol/water base, specially formulated for the treatment of skin disorders of the scalp.

Uses In the treatment of steroid-responsive dermatoses of the scalp, including seborrhoea capitis with or without an associated severe dandruff.

Dosage and administration Apply twice daily to the scalp, or as directed.

Contra-indications, warnings, etc These preparations are contra-indicated in the presence of viral or fungal infections, tubercular or syphilitic lesions, and in bacterial infections unless used in conjunction with appropriate chemotherapy. Contact with the eye should be avoided.

In pregnant animals, administration of corticosteroids can cause abnormalities of foetal development. The relevance of this finding to human beings has not been established. However, topical steroids should not be used extensively in pregnancy, i.e. in large amounts or for long periods.

In infants, long-term continuous topical therapy should be avoided. Adrenal suppression can occur, even without occlusion.

Pharmaceutical precautions Store under normal pharmaceutical conditions of storage.

Legal category POM.

Package quantities Plastic squeeze bottles of 30 ml and 100 ml.

Further information Locoid lotion should be kept away from the eyes, and not used near a fire or naked flame.

Product licence number 0166/0060.

LIPOBASE*

Presentation Lipobase is the bland cream base as used in Locoid Lipocream.

Uses For use where it is desired by the physician to reduce gradually the topical dosage of Locoid Lipocream. It may also be used where a continuously alternating application of the active product and the base is required e.g. in prophylactic therapy. Application of the Lipobase is also recommended where it is felt by the physician that the use of a bland emollient base is preferable to the cessation of therapy with the active product. Lipobase may also be used as diluent for the active product in those cases where dilution is regarded as necessary by the prescriber.

Dosage and administration Lipobase may be used either by replacing an application of the active product or alternating the application of the active product and the base, gradually diminishing the application of active product until therapy ceases.

Contra-indications, warnings, etc None.

Pharmaceutical precautions Store at room temperature (15–25°C).

Legal category P.

Package quantities Tubes of 50 g.

Further information Nil.

Product licence number 0166/0125.

LOCOBASE* CREAM, OINTMENT

Presentation Locobase Cream and Locobase Ointment are a bland base cream and base ointment respectively as used in Locoid Cream and Locoid Ointment.

Uses For use where it is desired by the physician to reduce gradually the topical dosage of Locid Cream or Ointment. They may also be used where a continuously alternating application of the active product and the base is required, e.g. in prophylactic therapy. Application of Locobase Cream or Ointment is also recommended where it is felt by the physician that the use of a bland base is preferable to the cessation of therapy with the active product. Locobase Cream or Ointment may also be used as a diluent for the active product in those cases where dilution is regarded as necessary by the prescriber.

Dosage and administration Locobase Cream and Ointment may be used either by replacing an application of the active product, or alternating the application of the active product and the base, gradually diminishing the application of the active product until therapy ceases.

Contra-indications, warnings, etc None.

Pharmaceutical precautions Store at room temperature (15–25°C).

Legal category P.

Package quantities Tubes of 100 g.

Further information Nil.

Product licence number
Locobase Cream   0166/0096
Locobase Ointment   0166/0097

MEDITAR* STICK

Presentation Meditar Stick is presented as a 20 g greenish-brown stick in a twist-up plastic container. The stick consists of a wax base containing 5% coal tar.

Uses Topical treatment of psoriasis and eczema mainly in chronic phases.

Dosage and administration Apply to the affected area once or twice daily or as directed by the physician. When used in conjunction with U.V.B. light, the tar should be removed before exposure to U.V.B. The Meditar Stick softens on contact with skin enabling a thin layer to be applied lightly and accurately to the affected area.

Contra-indications, warnings, etc The use of Meditar is not recommended in generalised pustular psoriasis, infections of the skin or in patients allergic to coal tar.
    Coal tar can sensitise the skin to U.V. light which can lead to sunburn. Coal tar should, therefore, be used cautiously in sunlight.

Pharmaceutical precautions Keep in a cool place.

Legal category P.

Package quantities 20 ml containers.

Further information Nil.

Product licence number 0166/0106.

PIMAFUCIN* CREAM

Presentation Pimafucin Cream is presented as a white cream in 30 g tubes containing 20 mg/g natamycin (2%).

Uses Antifungal antibiotic for the treatment of candidal infections of the anus, genitalia, skin, nails and oral mucosa, and acute fungal skin infections.

Dosage and administration By topical application.
Adults: Apply two to three times a day. (In cases of chronic paronychia and onychia treatment must continue for several months to prevent relapses.)
Children: As for adults.

Contra-indications, warnings, etc
Contra-indications: None.
Special precautions: None.
Side-effects: None have been reported.
Overdosage: Has not been reported.

Pharmaceutical precautions Normal pharmaceutical storage and handling are indicated.

Legal category POM.

Package quantities Tubes 30 g.

Further information Nil.

Product licence number 0166/5009.

PIMAFUCIN* 1% SUSPENSION

Presentation Pimafucin 1% Suspension is presented as a cream-white sterile suspension in ready-to-use 5 ml dropper bottles containing 10 mg/ml natamycin.

Uses Antifungal antibiotic for the treatment of oral thrush (due to *Candida albicans*) and also for mouth ulcers secondarily infected with *Candida albicans*.

Dosage and administration By local oral administration.
Infants: 4 drops under the tongue after every feed.
Children and adults: 10 drops after each meal, preferably directly on to the lesions.

Contra-indications, warnings, etc
Contra-indications: None.
Special precautions: None.
Side-effects: None have been reported.
Overdosage: Has not been reported.

Pharmaceutical precautions Normal pharmaceutical storage and handling are indicated. Store away from light.

Legal category POM.

Package quantities 5 ml dropper/dispenser.

Further information Nil.

Product licence number 0166/0047.

PIMAFUCIN* 2½% SUSPENSION

Presentation Pimafucin 2½% Suspension is presented as a cream-white sterile suspension in a clear glass 20 ml vial, containing 25 mg/ml natamycin (2½%).

Uses Antifungal antibiotic for the treatment of infections of the lungs and respiratory tract caused by fungi and yeasts, particularly Aspergillus spp. and candida albicans.

Dosage and administration By inhalation.

Adults: 2.5 mg natamycin three times a day for four weeks and 2.5 mg twice a day thereafter until a consistently negative sputum culture for the causative organism is obtained. A minimum total treatment period of six weeks is usually necessary. Administration must be made by a power nebuliser. The suspension should be diluted with sterile physiological saline or a sterile mucolytic preparation, and used within 48 hours of preparation.

Children: As for adults.

Contra-indications, warnings, etc
Contra-indications: None.

Special precautions: None.

Side-effects: None have been reported.

Overdosage: Has not been reported.

Pharmaceutical precautions Normal pharmaceutical storage and handling are indicated.

Legal category POM.

Package quantities Vials 20 ml.

Further information Nil.

Product licence number 0166/5010.

PIMAFUCIN* VAGINAL TABLETS

Presentation Pimafucin Vaginal Tablets are presented as creamy-white ovoid vaginal tablets, each containing 25 mg natamycin.

Uses Antifungal antibiotic with antitrichomonal activity, for the treatment of vaginal irritation and discharge whether due to candidal, trichomonal or mixed infections.

Dosage and administration By intravaginal administration.

Candida Albicans: One Tablet should be inserted at night, and one in the morning for a total of ten days. Alternatively, one tablet to be inserted nightly for a total of 20 nights.

Trichomonas Vaginalis: One tablet to be inserted nightly for a total of 20 nights.

Children: Not recommended.

Contra-indications, warnings, etc
Contra-indications: None.

Special precautions: Insert with care during pregnancy.

Side-effects: Occasionally local irritation may occur.

Overdosage: Has not been reported.

Pharmaceutical precautions Normal pharmaceutical storage and handling are indicated.

Legal category POM.

Package quantities Vaginal tablets 20 × 25 mg with applicator.

Further information Nil.

Product licence number 0166/5008.

STAFOXIL* CAPSULES ▼

Presentation Hard gelatin capsule with cream cap and light brown body, inscribed gbr 191 (250 mg capsule) or bgr 192 (500 mg capsule, containing 250 mg or 500 mg flucloxacillin as Flucoxacillin Sodium BP.

Uses Stafoxil is indicated in the treatment of infections caused by flucloxacillin sensitive micro-organisms, in particular penicillinase-producing staphylococci, as in respiratory tract infections, infections of the skin and soft tissues and generalised infections.

Dosage and administration
Adults: In mild to moderately severe infections, usually 250 mg four times daily, half to one hour before food.

Children: 2–12 years, usually half the daily adult dose or 50 mg/kg body weight per 24 hours divided into four doses, half to one hour before food.
   In serious infections the dosages may be doubled.
   In chronic relapsing and severe infections parenteral administration is to be preferred.

Contra-indications, warnings, etc Contra-indicated in penicillin hypersensitivity. There are no contra-indications for the use of Staxofil during pregnancy. Flucloxacillin is secreted in mothers milk and may occasionally cause a sensitisation of the infant. In patients with infectious mononucleosis and lymphatic leukaemia, exanthema is common. Cross-allergy and cross-resistance between the penicillins and cephalosporins may exist.
   Probenecid shows down the excretion of flucloxacillin.
   Gastrointestinal side effects have been reported such as nausea, vomiting and diarrhoea. Although transient and not severe, macular and maculopapular skin reactions may occur. Typical allergic reactions have been observed such as urticaria and purpora. Anaphylaxis has occasionally resulted from the oral use of penicillin or one of its derivatives. With high, chiefly parenteral, doses, neurotoxicity may develop.

Pharmaceutical precautions Store under normal pharmaceutical conditions.

Legal category POM.

Package quantities Both strengths of capsule available in 28s and 100s.

Further information Nil.

Product licence numbers
Stafoxil 250 mg Capsules   0166/0116
Stafoxil 500 mg Capsules   0166/0117

*Trade Mark

Edwin Burgess Limited
Longwick Road
Princes Risborough
Aylesbury
Buckinghamshire
HP17 9RR

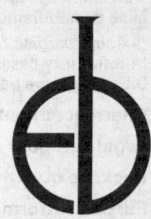

BETIM*

Presentation White, flat circular tablets engraved with '102' on the scored face and with an Assyrian lion on the reverse. Each tablet contains Timolol Maleate BP 10 mg.

Uses *Mode of Action:* Betim is a beta-adrenergic receptor blocking agent. It competitively antagonises the action of adrenergic transmitters on beta receptors and thus blocks beta-sympathomimetic activity in the heart, the bronchi and blood vessels.

Betim is considered to be a highly specific beta-adrenergic blocking drug since it does not block the chronotropic or inotropic effects of calcium, glucagon, theophylline or digitalis. It does not have significant local anaesthetic or direct myocardial depressant activity nor any significant beta-adrenergic stimulant effect.

Betim reduces heart rate, force of myocardial contractions and myocardial oxygen consumption. The modification of the cardiac response to stress or exercise is therapeutically useful in angina pectoris.

Betim is also of therapeutic value in hypertension although the mechanism of action is unclear.

Betim is rapidly absorbed from the gut. Its beta blocking activity is apparent within thirty minutes of administration and has been shown to last for up to 24 hours.

Indications: Betim is indicated in angina pectoris due to ischaemic heart disease and for the treatment of hypertension and to reduce mortality and reinfarction in patients surviving acute myocardial infarction. Betim is also indicated in the prophylactic treatment of patients with common and classic migraine in which it effectively reduces the incidence of attacks.

Dosage and administration *For angina and hypertension:* The recommended dose range is 10–60 mg per day. Therapy should begin with a dose of 10 mg daily increasing, if necessary, in steps of 10 mg at intervals of 3-4 days.

Most hypertensive patients will be controlled by 10–30 mg timolol which can be administered once daily or in divided doses if preferred. The dose of Betim may need adjustment when used in conjunction with other antihypertensive drugs.

In angina, Betim should be administered in divided doses.

After myocardial infarction: Start with 5 mg ($\frac{1}{2}$ tablet) twice daily for two days. If there are no adverse reactions, increase dosage to 10 mg twice daily and maintain at this dose.

For the prophylactic treatment of common and classic migraine: 10 to 20 mg once daily or in two divided doses.

Dosage in the elderly: Initiate treatment with lowest adult dose and thereafter adjust according to response.

Contra-indications, warnings, etc *Contra-indications:* Heart failure, unless adequately controlled. Sinus bradycardia or heart block. Cardiogenic shock. Bronchial asthma, chronic obstructive pulmonary disease. Patients receiving adrenergic augmenting drugs (monoamine oxidase inhibitors and tricyclic antidepressants). Anaesthesia with agents that produce myocardial depression, such as chloroform and ether. Pregnancy.

Precautions: Although Betim has no direct myocardial depressant activity, the continued depression of sympathetic drive through beta-blockade may lead to cardiac failure. All patients should be observed for evidence of cardiac failure, and, if it occurs, digitalisation and diuretic therapy should be considered.

Betim should be administered with caution to patients subject to spontaneous hypoglycaemia or diabetic patients who are on insulin or oral hypoglycaemic agents.

Beta-adrenergic blockers may mask the premonitory signs and symptoms of acute hypoglycaemia.

Caution is recommended when Betim is administered to patients on catecholamine depleting drugs such as reserpine or guanethidine.

Betim should be administered with caution to patients with impaired renal function or impaired hepatic function. Parasthesiae and coldness of the limb extremities have also been reported.

Side-effects: Gastro-intestinal symptoms (e.g. epigastric distress, nausea, vomiting, diarrhoea), dizziness, insomnia, sedation, depression, weakness, dyspnoea, bradycardia, heart block, bronchospasm and heart failure.

Warning: There have been reports of skin rashes, and/or dry eyes associated with the use of beta-adrenergic blocking drugs. The reported incidence is small and in most cases the symptoms have cleared when treatment was withdrawn. Discontinuance of the drug should be considered if any such reaction is not otherwise explicable. Cessation of therapy with the beta-blocker should be gradual.

Overdosage: The most common signs of overdosage are bradycardia, hypotension, bronchospasm, and acute cardiac failure.

Suggested treatments are as follows:

Severe bradycardia: I.V. atropine sulphate 0.25–2 mg. If bradycardia persists, I.V. isoprenaline 25 mcg may be given.

Severe hypotension: I.V. noradrenaline or adrenaline.

Bronchospasm: Isoprenaline hydrochloride, orciprenaline or salbutamol.

Acute cardiac failure: Digitalis, diuretics and oxygen. In refractory cases I.V. aminophylline and I.V. glucagon 0.5–1 mg have been reported useful.

Pharmaceutical precautions Nil.

Legal category POM.

Package quantities Packs of 100 tablets.

Further information Timolol maleate crosses the placenta and appears in breast milk.

Product licence number 0748/0015

CENTYL* TABLETS

Presentation *Tablets 2.5 mg:* Each contains 2.5 mg Bendrofluazide BP, white uncoated tablets, no coding marks.

Tablets 5 mg: Each contains 5 mg Bendrofluazide BP, white uncoated tablets, circular groove embossed on one face and score line on other.

Uses *Mode of Action:* Centyl contains the diuretic bendrofluazide, which is as effective as chlorothiazide at 100th the dose and produces a more prolonged diuresis. The diuresis is usually complete in 12–18 hours. In common with other thiazides, it increases the renal excretion of sodium, chloride and to a lesser extent potassium ions, together with an accompanying volume of water.

Indications: Hypertension: Control of blood pressure in mild and in some cases of moderate hypertension.

Oedema: Oedema of cardiac, hepatic or renal origin. Pre-menstrual oedema. Toxaemia of pregnancy. Oedema induced by use of steroids.

Dosage and administration *Adults and the elderly:* Initially, 5–10 mg bendrofluazide once daily. Maintain with 2.5–10 mg daily. Centyl should be taken in the morning to avoid nocturia.

Children: Pro rata, according to age and body weight.

Contra-indications, warnings, etc *Contra-indications:* Anuria. Centyl should not be used in patients with renal failure or with a history of hypersensitivity to thiazides. As with other diuretics, Centyl should not be administered concurrently with lithium salts. Diuretics can reduce lithium clearance resulting in high serum levels of lithium.

Precautions: Thiazide diuretics should be used with caution in patients with renal or hepatic dysfunction. Fluid and electrolyte levels should be measured in patients undergoing prolonged or intense diuresis as potassium depletion may occur and potassium supplements may be needed. Potassium depletion is a particular danger to digitalised patients or those with hepatic cirrhosis with ascites. Periodic testing for urine glucose is advisable in patients with latent or overt diabetes. The dose of hypoglycaemic agents in diabetic patients may require adjustment. Thiazide diuretics are used to treat hypertension, therefore it may be necessary to reduce the dose of other hypotensive agents e.g. reserpine, hydrallazine, β-blocking agents and ganglion blocking agents when used with Centyl.

Adverse Reactions: Thiazide diuretics may cause excessive depletion of fluid and electrolytes during prolonged or intense use. Symptoms are muscle pain or fatigue, thirst, gastro-intestinal upset and oliguria. Hypokalaemia is most severe in patients already depleted of potassium, as in renal or hepatic insufficiency.

Coma may be precipitated in hepatic cirrhosis.

The thiazide diuretics may induce hyperglycaemia and glycosuria in diabetic and other susceptible patients. This is usually reversible if the treatment is stopped. Hyperuricaemia sometimes occurs but an attack of gout is rare. The thiazide diuretics increase blood urea which is most pronounced in patients with renal disease and pre-existing retention of nitrogen.

Reports of other adverse reactions include skin rashes with associated photosensitivity, necrotising vasculitis, acute pancreatitis, blood dyscrasias and aggravation of pre-existing myopia.

Pregnancy: Thiazide diuretics cross the placenta and are secreted in breast milk.

Overdosage: Symptoms would be those caused by excessive diuresis. Empty stomach by gastric lavage or emesis. General measures should be taken to restore blood volume, maintain blood pressure and correct electrolyte depletion.

Pharmaceutical precautions Nil.

Legal category POM.

Package quantities Bottles of 100 tablets.

Further information Nil.

Product licence numbers
Tablets 2.5 mg   0748/5901
Tablets 5 mg   0748/5902

CENTYL* K

Presentation Each tablet contains Bendrofluazide BP (Centyl) 2.5 mg and Potassium Chloride BP 573 mg (7.7 mmol potassium in a slow-release wax core). Green ovoid tablets. No identification marks.

Uses *Mode of Action:* Centyl K is a combination of the diuretic bendrofluazide with a potassium supplement.

Bendrofluazide is as effective as chlorothiazide at 100th the dose and produces a more prolonged diuresis, which is usually complete in 12–18 hours. In common with other thiazides, it increases the renal excretion of sodium, chloride and, to a lesser extent, potassium ions together with an accompanying volume of water. Potassium depletion is frequently associated with prolonged diuretic therapy; a potassium supplement is therefore included in Centyl K. This should minimise potassium depletion.

Because of the risk of localised high concentrations of potassium salts in the small bowel, potassium is included in an inert wax core, from which it is released slowly over several hours. Bendrofluazide is contained in a shell which surrounds the central core.

Indications: Oedema: Oedema of cardiac, hepatic or renal origin. Toxaemia of pregnancy.

Hypertension: Control of blood pressure in mild and in some cases of moderate hypertension.

Renal calcium stones: Prophylaxis against recurrent renal calcium stones.

Dosage and administration *Adults and the elderly: Oedema and Hypertension:* Initially 2–4 tablets daily.

Maintain with 1–4 tablets daily or on alternate days. Centyl K should be taken in the morning to avoid nocturia.

For renal calcium stones: 2–3 tablets daily.

The tablets should be swallowed whole with at least 100 mls water.

Contra-indications, warnings, etc *Contra-indications:* Anuria. Centyl K should not be used in patients with a history of hypersensitivity to thiazides. As with other diuretics, Centyl K should not be administered concurrently with lithium salts. Diuretics can reduce lithium clearance resulting in high serum levels of lithium.

All solid forms of potassium medication are contra-indicated in the presence of obstructions in the digestive tract (e.g. resulting from compression of the oesophagus due to dilation of the left atrium or from stenosis of the gut).

Precautions: Thiazide diuretics should be used with caution in patients with renal or hepatic dysfunction. Fluid and electrolyte levels should be measured in patients undergoing prolonged or intense diuresis. Even though Centyl K contains a potassium supplement, depletion may occur, which is of particular danger to digitalised patients or those with hepatic cirrhosis with ascites.

Periodic testing for urine glucose is advisable in patients with latent or overt diabetes. The dose of hypoglycaemic agents in diabetic patients may require adjustment. Thiazide diuretics are used to treat hypertension, therefore it may be necessary to reduce the dose of other hypotensive agents, e.g. reserpine, hydrallazine, β–blocking agents and ganglion blocking agents, when used with Centyl K.

Non-specific small bowel lesions characterised by stenosis and possibly accompanied by ulceration have been associated with the oral administration of tablets and capsules containing potassium salts. Symptoms and signs which might indicate ulceration or obstruction of the small bowel in patients taking tablets or capsules containing potassium salts are indications for stopping treatment with such a preparation immediately.

Adverse Reactions: Thiazide diuretics may cause excessive depletion of fluid and electrolytes during prolonged or intense diuresis. Symptoms are muscle pain or fatigue, thirst and dry mouth, gastro-intestinal upset and oliguria. Hypokalaemia is most severe in patients already depleted of potassium, as in renal or hepatic insufficiency. Coma may be precipitated in hepatic cirrhosis. The thiazide diuretics may induce hyperglycaemia and glycosuria in diabetic and other susceptible patients. This is usually reversible if treatment is stopped.

Hyperuricaemia sometimes occurs, but an attack of gout is rare. The thiazide diuretics may increase blood urea, which is most pronounced in patients with renal disease and pre-existing retention of nitrogen.

Reports of other adverse reactions include skin rashes with associated photosensitivity, necrotising vasculitis, acute pancreatitis, blood dyscrasias and aggravation of pre-existent myopia.

Pregnancy: Thiazide diuretics cross the placenta and are secreted in breast milk.

Overdosage: General measures to restore blood volume, maintain blood pressure and correct electrolyte imbalance.

Pharmaceutical precautions Nil.

Legal category POM.

Package quantities Packs of 100, 500 and 1,000 tablets.

Further information Nil.

Product licence number 0748/5903.

HEPARIN (MUCOUS) INJECTION BP

Presentation Heparin (Mucous) Injection BP 1,000 units per ml: each ml contains 1,000 units sodium heparin. (Presented in 5 ml ampoules without preservative, and 5 ml vials with preservative.)

Heparin (Mucous) Injection BP 5,000 units per ml: each ml contains 5,000 units sodium heparin (with preservative).

Heparin (Mucous) Injection BP 25,000 units per ml: each ml contains 25,000 units sodium heparin (with preservative).

Uses *Mode of Action:* Heparin is a naturally occurring anticoagulant which prevents the coagulation of blood in-vivo and in-vitro. It potentiates the inhibition of several activated coagulation factors, including thrombin and factor X.

The anticoagulant properties of heparin are valuable for the prophylaxis and management of intravascular clotting and embolism. It is also used in extra-corporeal circulation i.e. heart-lung and renal dialysis machines and blood transfusions.

In addition to the anticoagulant properties heparin also has some lipaemia-clearing effect which may be utilised in the treatment of fat embolism.

Indications: Treatment of thromboembolic disorders such as: deep vein thrombosis, thrombophlebitis, pulmonary embolism, fat embolism.

Dosage and administration Heparin is usually administered by intravenous injection or subcutaneously. Although the intramuscular route can be used, it is not recommended because of the high incidence of haematomata.

The increase in clotting time provided by heparin becomes apparent immediately after administration and lasts for 4 to 6 hours after intravenous injection and for about eight hours after subcutaneous injection.

Dosage: Intravenous administration: 5,000–10,000 units every 4 hours either by bolus injection or continuous infusion in Sodium Chloride Injection or Dextrose Injection. However, the dose should be monitored with coagulation tests, and varied according to individual response.

Subcutaneous administration: 5,000 units every eight hours.

The treatment period varies from 7–10 days in peri-operative prophylaxis to as much as 6 weeks in the treatment of established thrombosis.

Dosage in the elderly: Elderly women have a greater tendency to bleed and it may be necessary to reduce the dose according to coagulation tests.

Contra-indications, warnings, etc *Contra-indications:* Haemorrhagic disorders and patients with an actual or potential bleeding site, e.g. peptic ulcer.

Precautions: Heparin therapy should be given with caution to patients about to undergo surgery, and those with impaired renal or hepatic function.

Overdosage: The effect of heparin can be reversed immediately by intravenous administration of a 1%

protamine sulphate solution. The quantity of protamine required for neutralisation falls rapidly with the lapse of time after the administration of heparin and can be accurately determined by titration of the patient's plasma, containing heparin, with protamine. If given within 15 minutes of the heparin injection 10 mg of protamine will neutralise 1,000 units of heparin, while 30 minutes after the heparin injection, only 5 mg of protamine per 1,000 units of heparin is needed.

It is important to avoid overdosage of protamine sulphate because protamine itself has anticoagulant properties. A single dose of protamine sulphate should never exceed 50 mg. Intravenous injection of protamine may cause a sudden fall in blood pressure, bradycardia, dyspnoea and transitory flushing, but these may be avoided or diminished by slow and careful administration.

Pharmaceutical precautions Store below 25°C. Admixture of heparin with solutions of other medicinal products may result in precipitation or loss of potency.

Legal category POM.

Package quantities Heparin 1,000 units per ml: 5 ml ampoules (without preservative), 5 ml vials (with preservative). Packs of 5.
Heparin 5,000 units per ml: 5 ml. Packs of 5 vials.
Heparin 25,000 units per ml: 5 ml: 1 vial.

Further information Preservative used: 1,000 units (with preservative) and 5,000 units: 0.5% Chlorbutol. 25,000 units: 0.4% Chlorbutol.

Menstruation and pregnancy are not contra-indications to heparin therapy. Heparin does not cross the placenta or appear in breast milk.

Available for low dose prophylactic use: single dose ampoules containing 5,000 units sodium heparin in 0.2 ml.

Heparin (Mucous) Injection BP is also available in unit dose ampoules without preservative in strengths of 1,000 units in 1 ml, 5,000 units in 1 ml and 25,000 units in 1 ml.

Product licence numbers

1,000 units (with preservative)	0748/0007
1,000 units (without preservative)	0748/0040
5,000 units (with preservative)	0748/0008
25,000 units (with preservative)	0748/0009

HEPARIN (MUCOUS) INJECTION BP

5,000 units in 0.2 ml (25,000 units per ml).

Presentation Single dose ampoules containing sodium heparin 5,000 units in 0.2 ml (no preservative).

Uses *Mode of Action:* Heparin is an anticoagulant which, even in low doses, prevents the formation of thrombin by accelerating the neutralisation of activated factor X by naturally occurring inhibitors.

Indications: Prophylaxis against deep vein thrombosis and thromboembolic events in susceptible patients.

Dosage and administration Administration is by subcutaneous injection. Patients undergoing surgery: 5,000 units in 0.2 ml should be given 2 to 6 hours preoperatively and every 8 hours postoperatively for 10–14 days, or until ambulation, whichever is the longer.

Other patients: 5,000 units in 0.2 ml should be given every 8–12 hours.

Dosage in the elderly: Elderly women have a greater

tendency to bleed but dosage alterations are unlikely for prophylaxis in the elderly.

Contra-indications, warnings, etc Low doses of heparin, administered as recommended above, do not cause alterations in clotting times in most patients, but occasionally local haematomata may occur at injection sites.

Patients with haemorrhagic disorders may experience bleeding, especially from surgical wounds. The relative risks and benefits of heparin administration in these patients should be assessed carefully. Oral anticoagulants or drugs which interfere with platelet function, e.g. aspirin and dextran solutions, should be administered with caution.

Overdosage: If bleeding should occur, the effect of heparin can be reversed immediately by intravenous administration of a 1% protamine sulphate solution. The dose of protamine sulphate required for neutralisation should be determined accurately by titrating with the patient's plasma.

Pharmaceutical precautions Store below 25°C. Admixture of heparin with solutions of other medicinal products may result in precipitation or loss of potency.

Legal category POM.

Package quantities 10 ampoules of 0.2 ml.

Further information Menstruation and pregnancy are not contraindications to heparin therapy. Heparin does not cross the placenta or appear in breast milk.

Heparin (Mucous) Injection BP is also available in 5 ml vials with preservative in strengths of 1,000, 5,000 and 25,000 units per ml and in unit dose ampoules without preservative in strengths of 1,000 units in 1 ml, 5,000 units in 1 ml and 25,000 units in 1 ml. 5 ml ampoules of 1,000 units per ml without preservative are also available.

Product licence number 0748/0043

HEP-FLUSH

Presentation Heparin flush solution, each ml contains 100 units heparin sodium (mucous) injection BP in saline, with 0.5% chlorbutol as preservative. (i.e. 200 units per ampoule).

Uses Heparin is an anticoagulant which prevents the formation of thrombin by accelerating the neutralisation of activated Factor X by naturally occurring inhibitors.

Indications: This strength of heparin is used as a 'heparin flush' every four hours, or as necessary, to keep intravenous lines patent. It is not recommended that this low dose heparin be used therapeutically.

Dosage and administration For routine use, 2 ml containing 200 units of heparin sodium should be administered into the catheter/cannula every 4 to 8 hours.

Contra-indications, warnings, etc When used as recommended the low dose of heparin reaching the blood should have no systemic effects.

Pharmaceutical precautions Store below 25°C.
Hep-flush is compatible with normal saline. Admixture with other drugs may cause inactivation of either the heparin solution or the drugs.

Legal category POM.

Package quantities Packs of 10 × 2 ml ampoules.

Further information Nil.

Product licence number 0748/0010

IMUNOVIR* ▼

Presentation White, ovoid tablets with the number 148 on one side and the letters IMV on the other. Each tablet contains 500 mg inosine pranobex.

Uses Imunovir is an agent demonstrating anti-viral activity and possessing immunopotentiating action in viral diseases.

Indications: Imunovir is indicated in the management of:
(a) Mucocutaneous infections due to herpes simplex virus (type I and/or type II).
(b) Genital warts as adjunctive therapy to podophyllin or carbon dioxide laser.

Dosage and administration
Mucocutaneous herpes simplex: 1 g q.d.s. (4 g daily) for 7–14 days.
Genital warts: 1 g t.d.s. (3 g daily) for 14–28 days as adjunctive therapy to podophyllin or carbon dioxide laser.
Dosage in the elderly: No dosage alterations are necessary in the elderly.

Contra-indications, warnings, etc
Contra-indications: None known.

Warnings: As the inosine component of Imunovir is metabolised to uric acid, it should be used with caution in patients with renal impairment, a history of gout or hyperuricaemia.

Pregnancy: Although animal tests have shown no teratogenic effect, the use of Imunovir in women where pregnancy is suspected or confirmed, should be avoided.

Adverse reactions: Side-effects are rare and usually of a mild and transitory nature. The only commonly associated adverse effects occurring during treatment with Imunovir are elevated serum and urinary concentrations of uric acid. These return to normal once treatment is withdrawn.

Symptoms and treatment of overdosage: There has been no experience of overdosage with Imunovir. However, serious adverse effects, apart from increased levels of uric acid in the body, seem unlikely in view of the animal toxicity studies. Treatment should be restricted to symptomatic and supportive measures.

Pharmaceutical precautions Store below 25°C.

Legal category POM.

Package quantities Available in bottles of 100 tablets.

Further information Nil.

Product licence number 0748/0049.

MINILOK*
Heparin (mucous) Injection BP 10 units per ml

Presentation 2 ml ampoule, each ml containing 10 units sodium heparin in saline (no preservative).

Uses Heparin is an anticoagulant which prevents the formation of thrombin by accelerating the neutralisation of activated Factor X by naturally occurring inhibitors.

Indications: This strength of heparin is used as 'heparin flush' every four hours, or as necessary, to keep intravenous lines patent. It is not recommended that this low dose heparin be used therapeutically.

Dosage and administration For routine use 1–5 ml (10–50 units sodium heparin) should be administered into the catheter/cannula every 4 hours.

Contra-indications, warnings, etc When used as recommended the low dose of heparin reaching the blood should have no systemic effects.

Pharmaceutical precautions Store below 25°C.
Admixture with other drugs may cause inactivation of either the heparin solution or the drugs.

Legal category POM.

Package quantities Packs of 10 × 2 ml ampoules.

Further information Nil.

Product licence number 0748/0046.

NATUDERM*

Presentation Natuderm is a white cream. The cream is a stable ambiphilic emulsion system.

Composition: The lipid component (about 35% of total product) contains approximately:

Free fatty acids	14.26%
Squalene	9.4%
Squalane	1.41%
Waxes	19.97%
Sterol Esters	3.81%
Free Sterols	2.37%
Glycerides	44.27%
Phospholipids	0.48%
dl-α-tocopherol	0.0085%
Butylated Hydroxyanisole	0.0085%
Span 60 Sorbitan Monostearate	2.71%
Phenonip	1.27%

The aqueous component (about 65% of total product) contains approximately:

Glycerol	5.63%
Polyoxyethylene Sorbitan Monostearate	1.64%
De-ionised water	92.2%
Phenonip	0.46%

Uses Natuderm is an emollient and protective cream. It has a lipid component similar in composition to human sebum.
Its uses include conditions where skin film emulsion deficiency is a factor.

Indications: As a moisturising emollient and protective for general dermatological use where the secretion of skin film emulsion is deficient.

Dosage and administration A thin application of the cream should be made to the affected area three times daily or as required. It should be rubbed gently into the skin. When used as a protective cream, Natuderm should be applied sparingly to areas of skin at risk, just before or immediately after exposure to potentially harmful factors.

Contra-indications, warnings, etc For external use only. Natuderm is entirely compatible with skin physiology and does not contain unmodified lanolin.

Contra-indications: Nil.

Side-effects: Hypersensitivity is a rare possibility.

Overdosage: Not applicable.

Pharmaceutical precautions Nil.

Legal category P.

Package quantities Jars of 40 g and 450 g and tubes of 100 g.

Further information Nil.

Product licence number 0748/0001.

PONDOCILLIN* TABLETS
PONDOCILLIN* SUSPENSION
PONDOCILLIN* SACHETS

Presentation *Tablets:* Each tablet contains 500mg pivampicillin – a white film-coated ovoid tablet with the number 128 printed on one side and an Assyrian Lion on the other.

Suspension: Bottles containing powder for the preparation of 50 ml and 100ml suspension. When reconstituted each 5 ml contains 162 mg pivampicillin.

Sachets: Each unit dose sachet contains 162 mg pivampicillin as off-white granules.

Uses Pondocillin (pivampicillin) is the pivaloyloxymethyl ester of ampicillin, and is rapidly hydrolysed in the body to ampicillin by non-specific enzymes present in serum, gastro-intestinal mucosa and other tissues.

After oral administration of Pondocillin, the plasma levels of ampicillin are 2–3 times higher than those obtained with equimolar doses of oral ampicillin. The tablets are formulated to disintegrate readily and produce rapid therapeutic plasma levels. A peak level generally occurs after 1 hour compared to approximately 2 hours with oral ampicillin. These levels are comparable to those obtained with an equimolar dose of intramuscular ampicillin.

Concentrations achieved in the urine are similarly raised. Generally, twice the amount of antibiotic can be recovered after treatment with Pondocillin when compared with equimolar doses of oral ampicillin. Whereas between 30–40% of the administered dose appears in the urine in the first 6 hours after oral administration of ampicillin, 70% can be recovered after an equimolar dose of Pondocillin.

Pondocillin is stable in the presence of gastric acid, and, unlike oral ampicillin, absorption is not affected by the presence of food. Plasma concentrations achieved in the post-prandial state do not differ significantly when compared with the fasting state. Like ampicillin, Pondocillin is destroyed by penicillinase-producing bacteria.

Indications: Like ampicillin, Pondocillin has a broad spectrum of activity against both gram-negative and gram-positive organisms. It is particularly indicated for the treatment of infections caused by susceptible strains of *Shigella, Salmonella, N. gonorrhoea, Esch. coli, H. influenzae, Pr. mirabilis* and is also indicated for pneumococcal, streptococcal and non-penicillinase-producing staphylococcal infections.

Specific infections include:

(a) Acute and chronic bronchitis
(b) Pneumonia
(c) Ear, nose and throat infections
(d) Gynaecological infections
(e) Urinary tract infections
(f) Skin and soft tissue infections
(g) Gonorrhoea

Dosage and administration *Tablets:* Usual dosage for adults: 500 mg pivampicillin to be administered twice daily. Dosage may be doubled in cases of severe infection. Gonorrhoea: 1.5–2 g pivampicillin as a single dose. 1 g probenecid can be given concurrently as desired. The medication may be taken with food or fluids.

Suspension (in bottle): Infants under 1 yr: 40–60 mg/Kg bodyweight per day.

Children aged 1–5 yrs: 10–15 ml per day

Children aged 6–10 yrs: 15–20 ml per day

Adults and children over 10 yrs: 30ml per day.

Sachets (for suspension): Children aged 1–5 years: 2–3 sachets per day.

Children aged 6–10 yrs: 3–4 sachets per day

Adults and children over 10 yrs: 6 sachets per day.

The daily dosage may be given either as 2 or 3 equal divided doses.

Dosage may be doubled where appropriate.

Dosage in the elderly: Renal excretion of ampicillin is delayed in the elderly but significant accumulation of the drug is not likely at the recommended adult dosage of Pondocillin.

Contra-indications, warnings, etc *Contra-indications:* Pondocillin is contra-indicated in any patient with a history of hypersensitivity to any of the penicillins or cephalosporins. Because of the high frequency of exanthemata associated with ampicillin therapy in infectious mononucleosis, treatment with Pondocillin is contra-indicated in this disease.

Pondocillin is also contra-indicated in infections caused by penicillinase producing bacteria.

Precautions: Care should be exercised when treating patients with a history of sensitivity to a variety of allergens, since serious hypersensitivity (anaphylactic) reactions are more likely to occur. If lymphatic leukaemia is treated with Pondocillin then caution is urged because of the frequency of exanthemata associated with ampicillin therapy.

The use of concurrent antacid therapy with Pondocillin is not recommended, since it reduces absorption of the antibiotic, and may cause underdosing.

During long-term therapy it is advisable to carry out routine liver and kidney function tests.

Pregnancy: In keeping with current practice use during the first trimester of pregnancy should be avoided. Ampicillin crosses the placenta and small amounts have been detected in breast milk.

Adverse Reactions: Pondocillin is a compound of low toxicity. Like ampicillin, skin rashes of two types have been noted: a non-specific erythema which usually disappears during treatment, and urticaria which may cause withdrawal of the drug. Anaphylactic reactions have occurred as with other penicillins.

Upper gastro-intestinal disturbances, such as nausea, vomiting, retrosternal pain and flatulence have occurred more frequently when a dose has been given on an empty stomach. Diarrhoea has been reported, but less frequently than with ampicillin. This observation underlines the importance of giving Pondocillin with or just after a meal. None of these effects appear to be dose-related. Other side effects reported are dizziness and pruritis.

Warning: Pondocillin suspension is not recommended for the treatment of *severe* infections in infancy.

Overdosage: There is no experience of overdosage with Pondocillin. However, excessive doses of Pondocillin are likely to induce nausea, vomiting and gastritis. Treatment should be restricted to symptomatic and supportive measures.

Pharmaceutical precautions *Tablets:* Nil.
Suspension: Pondocillin suspension when reconstituted, is stable for 14 days at room temperature or for 4 weeks when kept in a refrigerator.
Sachets: Contain a single dose and when reconstituted, use suspension immediately.

Legal category POM.

Package quantities *Tablets:* Bottles of 500, 100 and 20 tablets.
Suspension: Available in amber bottles making 50 ml or 100 ml suspension when dispensed.
Sachets: Boxes of 10 sachets.

Further information Nil.

Product licence numbers
Tablets   0748/0019
Suspension   0748/0020
Sachets   0748/0057

PUMP-HEP*
Heparin for Continuous Infusion

Presentation Heparin (Mucous) Injection BP 1000 i.u./ml. Single dose 20 ml ampoule containing 1,000 units sodium heparin per ml, in saline, without preservative (i.e. 20,000 units per ampoule).

Uses
Mode of action: Heparin is a naturally occurring anticoagulant which prevents the coagulation of blood in vivo and in vitro. It potentiates the inhibition of several activated coagulation factors, including thrombin and factor X.

The anticoagulant properties of heparin are valuable for the prophylaxis and management of intravascular clotting and embolism. It is also used in extra-corporeal circulation, i.e. heart-lung and renal dialysis machines and blood transfusions.

In addition to the anticoagulant properties heparin also has some lipaemia-clearing effect which may be utilised in the treatment of fat embolism.

Indications: Treatment of thrombo-embolic disorders such as: Deep vein thrombosis, thrombophlebitis, pulmonary embolism, fat embolism.

Dosage and administration Pump-Hep may be used when heparin is being administered intravenously via a continuous infusion pump, as an alternative to diluting heparin taken from multidose vials.

Usually, 20,000–40,000 units of heparin are infused daily. However, the dose should be monitored with coagulation tests and varied according to individual response.

The treatment period varies and can be as long as six weeks in patients with established thrombosis.

Dosage in the elderly: Elderly women have a greater tendency to bleed and it may be necessary to reduce the dose according to coagulation tests.

Contra-indications, warnings, etc
Contra-indications: Haemorrhagic disorders and pa-

tients with an actual or potential bleeding site, e.g. peptic ulcer.
Precautions: Heparin therapy should be given with caution to patients about to undergo surgery and those with impaired renal or hepatic function.
Overdosage: The effect of heparin can be reversed immediately by intravenous administration of a 1% protamine sulphate solution, 1 mg for every 100 units of heparin to be neutralised. The precise dose required may be determined by titration of the patient's plasma with protamine. It is important to avoid overdosage of protamine sulphate because protamine itself has anticoagulant properties. A single dose of protamine sulphate should never exceed 50 mg. Intravenous injection of protamine may cause a sudden fall in blood pressure, bradycardia, dyspnoea and transitory flushing, but these may be avoided or diminished by slow and careful administration.

Pharmaceutical precautions Store below 25°C. Admixture of heparin with solutions of other medicinal products may result in precipitation or loss of potency.

Legal category POM.

Package quantities Packs of 10 × 20 ml ampoules.

Further information Menstruation and pregnancy are not contra-indications to heparin therapy. Heparin does not cross the placenta or appear in breast milk.

Product licence number 0748/0047.

SELEXID* TABLETS
SELEXID* SUSPENSION

Presentation *Tablets:* Each tablet contains 200 mg pivmecillinam hydrochloride – a white film-coated tablet with convex surfaces, an Assyrian lion printed on one side and the number 137 on the other.
Suspension: Unit-dose foil sachets, each containing 100 mg of pivmecillinam as white granules.

Uses Selexid is an orally active antibiotic. Chemically it is the pivaloyloxymethyl ester of the amidino-penicillanic acid, mecillinam. On oral administration, it is well absorbed and subsequently hydrolysed in the body to mecillinam, the active antibacterial agent, by non-specific esterases present in blood, gastro-intestinal mucosa and other tissues. Peak serum levels of mecillinam averaging 5 mcg/ml are reached after one hour following a dose of 10 mg/kg body weight in children and 400 mg in adults.

The serum half-life is 1.2 hours. The protein binding amounts to 5–10%. Approximately 50% of the administered dose is excreted as mecillinam in the urine within the first six hours. Mecillinam is partly excreted with the bile giving rise to biliary concentrations about three times the serum levels. Concurrent administration of probenecid delays the renal excretion of mecillinam, producing more sustained serum levels. The absorption of Selexid is practically unaffected by taking the tablets or suspension with food.

Selexid is highly active against most Enterobacteriaceae, including E. coli, Klebsiella, Proteus, Enterobacter, Serratia, Salmonella, Shigella, and Yersinia.

Selexid is less active against gram-positive bacteria, and organisms such as *Pseudomonas aeruginosa* and *Streptococcus faecalis* are practically resistant to mecillinam.

Whilst Selexid, like the penicillins and cephalosporins, interferes with the biosynthesis of the bacterial cell wall, the target of the inhibition is different. This different mode of action is probably responsible for the synergistic action which has been found, both *in-vitro* and *in-vivo*, between Selexid and various penicillins and cephalosporins.

Indications: Selexid is indicated in the treatment of infections due to mecillinam sensitive organisms, including.

(a) Urinary tract infections.

(b) Salmonellosis.

Preliminary experience in a small number of patients suggests Selexid may be a useful alternative antibiotic in the treatment of acute typhoid fever, and in some carriers of salmonellae when antibiotic treatment is considered essential.

Dosage and administration Both the tablets and suspension should be preferably taken with or immediately after a meal, or with bland fluids such as water or milk.

Suspension: Mix the contents of the sachet in a little water (5–10 mls) and stir before taking. The suspension should be taken immediately.

Dosage for adults and children weighing more than 40 kg:

Urinary tract infections:
Tablets:
　(a) Acute uncomplicated cystitis: 2 tablets stat then 1 tablet 3 times daily to a total of 10 tablets.
　(b) Chronic or recurrent bacteriuria: 2 tablets three to four times daily.
Sachets:
　(a) Acute uncomplicated cystitis: 4 sachets stat then 2 sachets 3 times daily to a total of 20 sachets.
　(b) Chronic or recurrent bacteriuria: 4 sachets three to four times daily.
Salmonellosis:
　1. Enteric fever: 1.2–2.4 g daily for 14 days.
　2. Salmonella carriers: 1.2–2.4 g daily for 2–4 weeks.

Dosage for children weighing less than 40 kg:

Urinary tract infections: 20–40mg/kg body weight, daily, in three to four divided doses.

Salmonellosis: 30–60 mg/kg body weight, daily, in three to four divided doses.

Dosage in the elderly: Renal excretion of mecillinam is delayed in the elderly, but significant accumulation of the drug is not likely at the recommended adult dosage of Selexid.

Contra-indications, warnings, etc

Contra-indications: Penicillin and cephalosporin hypersensitivity.

Precautions: During long term usage, it is advisable to carry out routine liver and kidney function tests.

As with other antibiotics which are excreted mainly by the kidneys, raised blood levels of mecillinam may occur if repeated doses are given to patients with impaired renal function.

Pregnancy: Although tests in two animal species have shown no teratogenic effects, in keeping with current practice, use during the first trimester of pregnancy should be avoided. The drug, as mecillinam, crosses the placenta.

Adverse Reactions: Anaphylactic reactions, though not

yet reported, may occur. Upper gastro-intestinal disturbances such as nausea, vomiting and indigestion have occurred, more frequently when a dose has been given on an empty stomach. Other side effects reported are diarrhoea and urticarial rash.

Overdosage: There has been no experience of overdosage with Selexid. However, excessive doses are likely to induce nausea, vomiting and gastritis. Treatment should be restricted to symptomatic and supportive measures.

Pharmaceutical precautions *Tablets:* Store below 25°C in a dry place. *Suspension:* Store below 15°C. Once reconstituted use the suspension immediately.

Legal category POM.

Package quantities *Tablets:* Bottles of 10 and 100 tablets.
Suspension: Boxes of 20 sachets.

Further information Nil.

Product licence numbers
Tablets　　　0748/0027
Suspension　0748/0028

SELEXIDIN* INJECTION

Presentation Each vial contains either 200 mg or 400 mg mecillinam, a white crystalline powder.

Uses Selexidin is the amidino-penicillanic acid, mecillinam. It may be administered by both intravenous and intramuscular injection.

Peak serum levels averaging 6 mcg/ml and 12 mcg/ml are obtained following intramuscular doses of 200 mg and 400 mg respectively. Intravenous injection produces initially very high concentrations, which rapidly decline as the compound is excreted. The serum half life is 1.2 hours, and the protein binding amounts to 5–10%. Approximately 50–60% of the dose may be recovered in the urine within the first six hours. Mecillinam is partly excreted with the bile giving rise to biliary concentrations about three times the serum level. Concurrent administration of probenecid delays the renal excretion of mecillinam.

Selexidin is highly active against most Enterobacteriaceae, including E. coli, Klebsiella, Proteus, Enterobacter, Serratia, Salmonella, Shigella and Yersinia.

Selexidin is less active against gram-positive bacteria and organisms such as *Pseudomonas aeruginosa* and *Streptococcus faecalis* are practically resistant to mecillinam.

Whilst Selexidin, like the penicillins and cephalosporins, interferes with the biosynthesis of the bacterial cell wall, the target of the inhibition is different. This different mode of action is probably responsible for the synergistic action which has been found, both *in-vivo* and *in-vitro*, between Selexidin and various penicillins and cephalosporins.

Indications: Selexidin injection is indicated in the treatment of serious infections due to mecillinam-sensitive organisms, and in those patients where oral therapy, with Selexid, is considered inappropriate.

Dosage and administration Selexidin should be dissolved in Water for Injections and administered either intramuscularly or by slow intravenous injection (three to four minutes) in the following concentrations:

Intravenous: Dissolve the mecillinam, in sterile water, as a 10% w/v solution, e.g. 400 mg in 4 ml.

Intramuscular: Dissolve 200 mg in 1 ml sterile water. Dissolve 400, 600 or 800 mg in 2 ml sterile water.

Alternatively, mecillinam, following dissolution in Water for Injections BP, may be added to either Sodium Chloride Injection or 5% dextrose and infused over 15–30 minutes. Such solutions should be made immediately before use and not stored. It is not recommended to store aqueous solutions of mecillinam. Mecillinam should not be added to infusion fluids containing other antibiotics.

Dosage: Adults and children.
1. *Urinary tract infections:* 5 mg/kg body weight every six to eight hours.
2. *Severe gram-negative infections due to susceptible organisms:* 10 mg/kg body weight every six hours.
3. *Enteric fever:* 12.5–15.0 mg/kg body weight every six hours. (Probenecid may also be administered.)

In some instances, for example where there was reason to expect a synergistic interaction, mecillinam has been given in combination with a broad-spectrum penicillin or cephalosporin. When combination therapy has been employed, normal dosages of both compounds were given.

Dosage in the elderly: Renal excretion of mecillinam is delayed in the elderly, but significant accumulation of the drug is not likely at the recommended adult dosage of Selexidin.

Contra-indications, warnings, etc

Contra-indications: Penicillin and cephalosporin hypersensitivity.

Precautions: During long-term usage, it is advisable to carry out routine liver and kidney function tests.

As with other antibiotics which are excreted mainly by the kidneys, raised blood levels of mecillinam may occur if repeated doses are given to patients with impaired renal function.

Pregnancy: Although tests in two animal species have shown no teratogenic effects, in keeping with current practice, use during the first trimester of pregnancy should be avoided. The drug, as mecillinam, crosses the placenta.

Adverse reactions: Reported side-effects include urticarial rash, and suspected drug fever in a few patients with enteric fever. Anaphylactic reactions, though not yet reported, may occur. Preliminary experience indicates that intramuscular injections of mecillinam are well tolerated.

Overdosage: There has been no experience of overdosage with Selexidin. Treatment should be restricted to symptomatic and supportive measures.

Pharmaceutical precautions Store below 25°C.

Legal category POM.

Package quantities Boxes of 10 vials.

Further information Nil.

Product licence numbers
0748/0029 (200 mg)
0748/0030 (400 mg)

TENAVOID* TABLETS

Presentation Each tablet contains Bendrofluazide BP 3 mg and Meprobamate BP 200 mg. Orange ovoid coated tablets. No identification marks.

Uses For premenstrual tension in those cases where there is evidence of water retention as well as of emotional problems.

Dosage and administration

Adults: 1 tablet three times daily beginning five to seven days before the expected onset of the period.

Children: Not recommended.

Contra-indications, warnings, etc

Contra-indications: Because of the meprobamate content, Tenavoid should not be used in epileptic patients or in patients in whom habituation to meprobamate has occurred.

As with other diuretics, Tenavoid should not be administered concurrently with lithium salts. Diuretics can reduce lithium clearance resulting in high serum levels of lithium.

Pregnancy and mothers who are breast feeding: There is no evidence as to drug safety in human pregnancy, nor is there evidence from animal work that it is free from hazard.

Tenavoid should not be used in patients with a history of hypersensitivity to the active ingredients and related compounds.

Acute intermittent porphyria.

Patients with a history of alcohol or drug abuse.

Precautions: Because Tenavoid is used intermittently, electrolyte disturbance is uncommon. However, it may be desirable to monitor serum electrolytes particularly serum potassium, in patients undergoing regular Tenavoid therapy. Potassium supplements may be particularly necessary in digitalised patients.

Periodic testing for urine glucose is advisable in patients with latent or overt diabetes.

The dose of hypoglycaemic agents in diabetic patients may need adjustment.

In hepatic or renal insufficiency the concurrent use of other CNS depressant drugs should be avoided.

In epilepsy, meprobamate withdrawal may precipitate convulsions.

The toxicity of meprobamate in overdosage requires that particular caution should be taken in regard to prescribing Tenavoid for patients with depression or others who may be liable to suicidal ideation or intent.

Like barbiturates, meprobamate causes induction of liver enzymes so that the availability and blood levels of drugs given concurrently that are metabolised by the liver may be affected. These include the following: coumarin-type anti-coagulants, systemic steroids (including oral contraceptives), phenytoin, griseofulvin, rifampicin, phenothiazines such as chlorpromazine or tricyclic antidepressants.

Addiction Potential: Barbiturate-type dependence may occur particularly when meprobamate is given in higher than recommended dosages or for long periods. It may also occur on normal therapeutic dosages, particularly in individuals with emotionally unstable personalities or in others prone to alcohol or other drug dependence. Severe withdrawal reactions ranging in severity from tremulousness and insomnia to confusion, delirium tremens, convulsions and occasionally death have occurred.

Adverse reactions: Prolonged courses of thiazides may cause depletion of fluid and electrolytes but these symptoms should normally not occur during the intermittent treatment of pre-menstrual tension.

Coma may be precipitated in hepatic cirrhosis. The thiazide diuretics may induce hyperglycaemia and glycosuria in diabetic and other susceptible patients. This is usually reversible if treatment is stopped. Hyperuricaemia sometimes occurs, but an attack of gout is rare.

Skin rashes with associated photosensitivity, necrotising vasculitis, acute pancreatitis, blood dyscrasias and aggravation of pre-existent myopia have been reported.

Due to the meprobamate content performance at skilled tasks and alertness may be impaired. Patients should be warned of this hazard and advised not to drive or operate machinery during treatment. These effects are potentiated by alcohol.

Drowsiness and sedation are common adverse effects of meprobamate use. Unsteadiness, dizziness, incoordination, nausea, vomiting, diarrhoea, constipation, slurred speech, headache, palpitations, arrhythmia, syncope, paraesthesiae, blurred vision, excitement, euphoria, tachycardia may occur.

Hypersensitivity reactions have been reported in some 2% of patients being treated with meprobamate and may occur after a single tablet in patients not previously exposed to the drug. These may include skin reactions of urticaria, itchy maculopapular or erythematous skin rashes which may be generalised or local. Severe systemic reactions with shaking, chills and fever, nausea, vomiting, hypotension and collapse have occasionally occurred. Blood disorders including thrombocytopenia, non-thrombocytopenic purpura, agranulocytosis, aplastic anaemia and pancytopenia have occurred. Rarely reported hypersensitivity reactions include: hyperpyrexia, angioneurotic oedema, bronchospasm, oliguria and anuria. Also, anaphylaxis, erythema multiforme, exfoliative dermatitis, stomatitis, proctitis, Stevens Johnson syndrome, and bullous dermatitis have been reported.

Overdosage: For bendrofluazide general measures should be taken to restore blood volume, maintain blood pressure and correct electrolyte disturbance.

Acute toxicity from the ingestion of meprobamate may result in loss of consciousness, hypotensive reactions, shock and respiratory depression. Treatment of overdosage involves maintenance of the blood pressure and counteraction of shock. Respiration may have to be assisted. Death has occurred after ingestion of 12 grams meprobamate.

Pharmaceutical precautions Nil.

Legal category CD (Sch 3), POM.

Package quantities Packs of 24 tablets.

Further information Safety and efficacy have not been established beyond short-term use for this combination.

Product licence number 0748/5900R

*Trade Mark

Cabot Limited
Copyground Lane
High Wycombe
Bucks HP 12 3HE

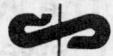

GYNATREN* ▼

Presentation A white sterile suspension for intramuscular injection. Each 0.5 ml ampoule of the vaccine contains 7×10^9 inactivated Lactobacillus acidophilus organisms in isotonic saline with 0.25% w/v of phenol as preservative.

Uses Gynatren is a vaccine that stimulates antibody production against aberrant coccoid forms of lactobacilli associated with trichomoniasis and also, by cross-reaction, against the trichomonads themselves. The normal vaginal flora and acidity is restored.

Indication: Prophylaxis of recurrent trichomoniasis in women.

Dosage and administration Three intramuscular injections of 0.5 ml at an interval of two weeks between each dose. Shake the ampoule before opening.

Contra-indications, warnings, etc
Contra-indications: Gynatren should not be administered during acute febrile infections nor in the presence of significant haematopoietic, renal nor heart disease with decompensation.

Precautions: Although anaphylaxis following Gynatren injections has never been reported, facilities for its management should always be available during vaccination.

Side- and adverse-effects: Local inflammation at the injection site has been reported and fever may occur concurrently.

Use in pregnancy: There is no recorded experience of use during pregnancy or lactation.

Pharmaceutical precautions Gynatren should be stored refrigerated at 4–8°C. Do not freeze.

Legal category POM.

Package quantities In packs of 3×0.5 ml ampoules.

Further information A trichomonacide preparation may be given at the time of first injection.

Product licence number 1317/0001.

SOLCO* HIDA KIT

Presentation A kit contains 5 vials, each vial contains 45.5 mg N-(2,6-diethylphenylcarbamoylmethyl)-imi-nodiacetic acid disodium salt (Etifenin disodium salt, pINN) and 0.18 mg stannous chloride dihydrate. The sterile, pyrogen-free formulation is freeze-dried and sealed under nitrogen.

Uses Addition of sodium pertechnetate (^{99m}Tc) injection to a maximum of 1.1 GBq (30 mCi) labels the reagent for total and regional hepatobiliary function and visualisation scintigraphy.

Dosage and administration The adult dose is 75–150 MBq (2–4 mCi) by intravenous injection and serial scanning is carried out at 5–10 minute intervals for up to 40 minutes. If necessary, later scans of the abdominal region may be taken. Preparation of the Tc-99m SOLCO HIDA injection should use aseptic technique as follows:
1. Wipe the closure of a vial with a sterilising swab, place the vial in a lead shield.
2. Using a 10 ml sterile syringe inject 1–5 ml of sterile, pyrogen-free Tc-99m eluate into the vial. Remove an equal volume of the inert gas from the vial with the syringe to normalise the pressure.
3. Dissolve the contents of the vial by repeated shaking and allow to incubate at room temperature for 5 minutes.

Contra-indications, warnings, etc The radiation dose to the patient, particularly those under 18 and women of child-bearing age, should be considered in the context of the potential diagnostic advantage. The precautions and regulations for handling radioactive materials should be adhered to.

Pharmaceutical precautions Store the SOLCO HIDA Kit at 2–8°C.
Store the prepared injection at room temperature and use within 2 hours.

Legal category POM.

Package quantities Each pack contains 5 vials.

Further information To date, no adverse reactions, or interfering reactions with other drugs have been reported.

Product licence number 4113/0001.

Produce licence holder: Nucletron (Servicing) Ltd., 129a Nantwich Road, Crewe CW2 6DE

*Trade Mark

Calmic Medical Division
The Wellcome Foundation Limited
Crewe Hall
Crewe, Cheshire CW1 1UB

AEROSPORIN*

Presentation Each rubber-capped vial contains 500,000 i.u. of sterile freeze-dried Polymyxin B Sulphate BP, for preparation of parenteral and other sterile solutions.

Uses Bactericidal antibiotic.

In systemic, urinary tract, meningeal, and local infections caused by a wide range of susceptible Gram-negative organisms, particularly *Pseudomonas aeruginosa*. Pulmonary infections due to *Ps. aeruginosa, E. coli,* and *H. influenzae.*

Dosage and administration *Intrathecal administration* (for meningitis).

Adults and children over 2 years: 50,000 to a maximum of 100,000 units once daily.

Children under 2 years: 20,000 to a maximum of 40,000 units once daily. Administer the appropriate dosage in 1–2 ml of 0.9% sterile sodium chloride solution.

Treatment should continue daily until the cerebrospinal fluid is sterile and then on alternate days for 1–3 weeks.

If systemic infection is present, concurrent parenteral therapy is required.

Use in the elderly: No specific studies have been carried out in the elderly, but the drug has been widely used in older people. However, it may be advisable to monitor renal function in these patients and if there is any impairment then serum levels should be monitored.

Intravenous administration – Adults and children: 15,000–25,000 units per kg. bodyweight per day. Total daily dosage must not exceed 2,000,000 units.

No dosage information is available for intravenous administration in neonates.

The total daily dose may be given as a continuous infusion or as 2 infusions per day each for 1–2 hours and given 12 hours apart. 5% Dextrose in water is recommended as the diluent.

Intramuscular administration – Adults and children: 15,000 to 25,000 units per kg bodyweight per day. Total daily dosage must not exceed 2,000,000 units.

Neonates: 15,000–45,000 units per kg bodyweight per day.

The total daily dose should be given in 4 equally divided doses at 6-hourly intervals. 1–2 mls of water for injection, 0.9% sterile sodium chloride or 1% sterile procaine hydrochloride solution should be used as diluent.

Dosage in renal failure:

Creatinine clearance	Dosage (units/kg/day)
Normal or 80% of normal	25,000
80% to 30% of normal	1st day: 25,000
	Daily thereafter 10,000–15,000
25% of normal	1st day: 25,000
	Every 2–3 days thereafter 10,000–15,000
Anuria	1st day: 25,000
	Every 5–7 days thereafter 10,000

Patients with impaired renal function excrete the drug more slowly and an appropriate adjustment in the intravenous or intramuscular dosage should be made. The table above gives guidelines based on creatinine clearance. Additional guidance should be obtained by regular monitoring of serum levels of polymyxin B and renal function. The serum level of polymyxin B should be kept below 10 μg/ml.

Local administration: A solution of 0.1–1% (approximately 10,000–100,000 units/ml) in sterile saline or an ointment or cream of similar strength is recommended. When used as a solution it may be applied either as drops, as a wet dressing, as a spray, by irrigation or as an aerosol.

Inhalation of an aerosol containing Aerosporin is particularly valuable in treating pulmonary infections due to *Ps. aeruginosa, E. coli* and *H. influenzae.* Inhalation of 1–2 ml of solution of 1,000–10,000 i.u. per ml in sterile saline or 5% dextrose in water four to eight times daily is recommended. The total amount given per day should not be more than that used parenterally.

For the treatment of superficial eye infections Aerosporin may be applied in the form of eye drops or by subconjunctival injection:

Eye drops: 3 drops of a 0.1% solution in sterile water or 0.9% sodium chloride solution should be instilled hourly, then less frequently depending on the response.

Subconjunctival injection: Up to 100,000 units per day is recommended, administered in water for injection or sterile 0.9% sodium chloride solution. A concentration of 500,000 units per ml is suggested and not more than 1 ml of diluent should be administered per injection.

Contra-indications, warnings, etc
Contra-indications: Hypersensitivity to polymyxins.

Precautions: Nephropathy and neuropathy may result from the use of this drug. It may therefore be advisable to monitor renal function before and during parenteral therapy. Ototoxicity may occur and Aerosporin should be used with care in patients where the tympanic membrane may be perforated.

The concomitant use of other potentially nephrotoxic drugs should be avoided if possible.

Due to the possibility of neuromuscular blockade leading to respiratory paralysis and apnoea, caution is advised in the administration of other agents with a similar action (eg muscle relaxants, general anaesthetics, antibiotics with muscle relaxant properties). Respiratory distress may rarely occur with aerosol administration.

Side- and adverse effects: Occasionally mild drug fever and a variety of skin eruptions, including urticaria, have been reported after parenteral therapy. Allergic reactions after topical application are rare.

Local pain at the injection site may occur when the drug is given intramuscularly. Subconjunctival injection may also be painful. Intrathecal injection may cause meningeal irritation, particularly in daily doses above 50,000 units and the patient should be observed for reactions.

Polymyxin B may cause nephrotoxicity. This effect is dose-related and rarely a serious clinical problem in patients with adequate renal function receiving recommended doses; it is usually reversible on discontinuation. As with all antibacterial preparations prolonged use may result in the overgrowth of non-susceptible organisms including fungi.

Neurological symptoms of varying intensity may occur. There may be circumoral and peripheral paraesthesia, some dizziness and a feeling of weakness without, however, any objective signs. These effects are transient and disappear within 48 hours of stopping treatment.

Use in pregnancy and lactation: The safety of Aerosporin in pregnancy has not been established. No information is available on its excretion in breast milk, and its use in lactating mothers is not recommended.

Toxicity and treatment of overdosage: Antihistamines may relieve some of the subjective symptoms. If respiratory paralysis occurs, artificial respiration should be instituted. There is some evidence that haemodialysis lowers serum levels of the drug. However, the value of this procedure is open to doubt due to tissue localisation of the antibiotic.

Pharmaceutical precautions Store in a dry place, below 25°C. Protect from light. Use immediately after reconstitution. Aerosporin should not be mixed with solutions containing heparin, prednisolone, protein hydrolysate, or other antibiotics.

Legal category POM.

Package quantities Rubber-capped vial of 500,000 i.u.

Further information It is desirable to continue therapy until the lesions are healed; otherwise infecting organisms may reappear if the antibiotic is withdrawn too soon.

In the strengths recommended, Aerosporin is not irritating to delicate tissues such as the eye, mucous membranes or granulating surfaces.

Product licence number 0003/5006.

ALKERAN* TABLETS AND INJECTION

Presentation *Alkeran Tablets:* 2 mg Melphalan BP coloured pink with a white core and coded Wellcome A2A.

5 mg Melphalan BP coloured pink with a white core and coded Wellcome B2A.

Alkeran Injection: Each vial contains the equivalent of 100 mg sterile anhydrous Melphalan BP. 1 ml ampoule of Wellcome Acid-Alcohol Solvent and 9 ml ampoule of Wellcome Diluent are included in the unit pack.

Uses Cytotoxic agent. Alkylating agent.

Alkeran tablets are indicated in the treatment of multiple myeloma and advanced ovarian adenocarcinoma. Alkeran has a significant therapeutic effect in a proportion of patients suffering from advanced breast cancer and polycythaemia vera. Alkeran has been used as an adjuvant to surgery in the management of breast carcinoma.

Alkeran injection is indicated in the treatment of localised malignant melanoma of the extremities and localised soft tissue sarcoma of the extremities, when treated by regional perfusion.

Dosage and administration

Adults: The absorption of Alkeran after oral administration is variable and in some patients it is poorly absorbed. Dosage may need to be cautiously increased until myelosuppression is seen, in order to ensure that potentially therapeutic levels have been reached.

Use in the elderly: There is no specific information on the use of Alkeran in the elderly. However, caution should be taken where there is renal impairment.

Multiple myeloma: The administration of Alkeran and prednisone is more effective than Alkeran alone. The combination is usually given on an intermittent basis, although the superiority of this technique over continuous therapy is not established. A typical dosage schedule is 0.15 mg/kg bodyweight/day in divided doses for 4 days together with 40 mg prednisone daily for 4 days, repeated at intervals of six weeks. Numerous regimes have been used and the literature should be consulted for details. Prolonging treatment beyond one year in responders does not appear to improve results.

Ovarian adenocarcinoma: The usual regime is 0.2 mg/kg bodyweight/day, given orally in divided doses, three times daily, for 5 days. This is repeated every 4–8 weeks, provided the bone marrow has recovered. Similar results have been reported following a single intravenous infusion of 1 mg/kg bodyweight over 8 hours every 4 weeks.

Advanced carcinoma of the breast: Alkeran may be given orally at a dose of 0.2–0.3 mg/kg bodyweight daily or 6 mg/m² body surface area daily for 4–6 days and repeated every 3–6 weeks.

Malignant melanoma: Regional perfusion with Alkeran has been used as an adjuvant to surgery for early malignant melanoma and as palliative treatment for advanced but localised disease. The literature should be consulted for details of perfusion technique and dosage.

Soft tissue sarcoma: Regional perfusion with Alkeran has been used in the management of all stages of localised soft tissue sarcoma, usually in combination with surgery. Alkeran has frequently been given with actinomycin D and the literature should be consulted for details of dose regimes.

Polycythaemia vera: For remission induction the usual dose is 6–10 mg daily for 7–10 days, the maintenance dose is 2–4 mg daily. During maintenance careful haematological control is essential with dosage adjustment according to the results of frequent blood counts.

Children: Alkeran is very rarely indicated in children and dosage guidelines cannot be stated.

Administration of injection: Alkeran is unstable in infusion fluids. It should not be given in dextrose solutions. Infusions may be given with saline but, at room temperature, the same solution should not be used for more than 2 hours. Alternatively, Alkeran may be injected into the tubing of a fast running infusion.

When using Alkeran injection precautions should be taken to avoid contact with it. It is recommended that the handling of Alkeran injection follows the 'Guidelines for the Handling of Cytotoxic Drugs', issued by the PSCG.

Preparation of Alkeran Melphalan Injection: 1 ml Wellcome Acid-Alcohol Solvent should be added to the vial containing 100 mg anhydrous melphalan. The vial should be shaken at once and the melphalan will dissolve in up to 2 minutes. When it has dissolved, 9 ml Wellcome Diluent should be added to give a resulting solution with a pH of about seven which will remain clear for some time. The solution should be prepared as required and used without delay.

Contra-indications, warnings, etc

Contra-indications: In view of the seriousness of the indications there are no absolute contra-indications.

Precautions: Alkeran is an active cytotoxic agent for use only under the direction of physicians experienced in the administration of such agents.

Careful attention should be paid to the monitoring of blood counts to avoid the possibility of excessive myelosuppression and the risk of irreversible bone marrow aplasia.

The main side-effect of Alkeran treatment is bone marrow depression, leading to leucopenia and thrombocytopenia. Blood counts may continue to fall after treatment is stopped, so at the first sign of an abnormally large fall in leukocyte or platelet counts treatment should be temporarily interrupted.

Alkeran should not be given to patients who have recently received radiotherapy or other cytotoxic agents.

In patients with moderate to severe renal impairment, the initial dose of the intravenous preparation should be reduced by 50%. Subsequent dosage should be determined according to haematological response. Currently available pharmacokinetic data does not justify an absolute recommendation on dosage reduction when administering the oral preparation to these patients, but it may be prudent to use a reduced dose initially.

Patients with renal impairment should be closely observed as they may have uraemic marrow suppression. Temporary significant elevation of the blood urea has been seen in the early stages of Alkeran therapy in myeloma patients with renal damage.

Alkeran is mutagenic in animals and chromosome aberrations have been observed in patients being treated with the drug.

The evidence is growing that Alkeran in common with other alkylating agents may be leukaemogenic in man. There have been reports of acute leukaemia occurring after prolonged Alkeran treatment for diseases such as amyloid, malignant melanoma, macroglobulinaemia, cold agglutinin syndrome and ovarian cancer.

A comparison of patients with ovarian cancer who received alkylating agents with those who did not showed that the use of alkylating agents, including Alkeran, significantly increased the incidence of acute leukaemia. The leukaemogenic risk must be balanced against the potential therapeutic benefit when considering the use of Alkeran.

Alkeran causes suppression of ovarian function in premenopausal women resulting in amenorrhoea in a significant number of patients.

Simultaneous administration of nalidixic acid with Alkeran should be avoided. The combination of high dose Alkeran and cyclosporin is known to cause a deterioration in renal function and can be potentially dangerous.

Side- and adverse effects: The most common side-effect is bone marrow depression.

Gastro-intestinal effects such as nausea and vomiting occur in up to 30 per cent of patients receiving Alkeran. Diarrhoea and stomatitis may occasionally occur. Gastrointestinal disturbance is usually mild and occurs less frequently than with combination cytotoxic therapy.

Alopecia has been reported but is uncommon. Maculopapular rashes and pruritus have occasionally been noted. There have also been case reports of pulmonary fibrosis and haemolytic anaemia occurring after melphalan treatment.

A life-threatening immediate allergic reaction has been reported after intravenous administration.

Use in pregnancy and lactation: Although there are no data available the possibility that melphalan may be teratogenic should be borne in mind because of its similarity to other alkylating agents which are potentially teratogenic.

The use of Alkeran should be avoided whenever possible during pregnancy, particularly during the first trimester. In any individual case the potential hazard to the foetus must be balanced against the expected benefit to the mother.

Mothers receiving Alkeran should not breastfeed.

Toxicity and treatment of overdosage: The principal toxic effect is on the bone marrow and as there is no known antidote the blood picture should be closely monitored for two weeks.

General supportive measures, together with appropriate blood transfusion, should be instituted if necessary.

Pharmaceutical precautions *Alkeran Tablets:* Store below 25°C in a dry place.

Alkeran Injection: Store below 25°C. Protect from light.

Legal category POM.

Package quantities *Tablets 2 mg:* Bottle of 25.

Tablets 5 mg: Bottle of 25.

Unit Pack: 1 vial containing the equivalent of Melphalan BP 100 mg; 1 ampoule of 1 ml Wellcome Acid-Alcohol Solvent for Alkeran; 1 ampoule of 9 ml Wellcome Diluent for Alkeran.

Further information Alkeran has the general pharmacological properties of nitrogen mustard compounds. It is well absorbed by the oral route, both in animals and in man.

Product licence numbers
Tablets 2 mg 0003/5008
Tablets 5 mg 0003/5009
Injection 0003/5010

ANECTINE* INJECTION

Presentation Each ampoule of Anectine contains 100 mg Suxamethonium Chloride Injection BP (succinylcholine chloride) in 2 ml aqueous solution. The pH is adjusted to 3.5 with hydrochloric acid.

Uses Anectine is a short-acting depolarizing neuromuscular blocking agent. It is used in anaesthesia as a muscle relaxant to facilitate endotracheal intubation, mechanical ventilation and a wide range of surgical and obstetric procedures.

It is also used to reduce the intensity of muscular contractions associated with pharmacologically or electrically-induced convulsions.

Dosage and administration The dose of Anectine is dependent on body weight, the degree of muscular relaxation required and the response of individual patients. It ranges between 20–80 mg in an adult. To achieve endotracheal intubation Anectine is usually administered intravenously in a dose of 1 mg/kg. This dose will usually produce muscular relaxation in about 30–60 seconds and has a duration of action of about 2–6 minutes. Larger doses will produce more prolonged muscular relaxation, but doubling the dose does not necessarily double the duration of relaxation.

For prolonged surgical procedures Anectine may be given by intravenous infusion as a 0.1% to 0.2% solution at a rate of 2.5 to 4 mg per minute in an adult, or a proportionately lower dose in children according to weight.

When given by intravenous infusion Anectine should be diluted in a sterile 5% dextrose solution or sterile isotonic saline solution.

Anectine may be given intramuscularly especially to children in doses up to 2.5 mg per kilogram body weight, but not more than 150 mg total dose should be given. Neonates and premature infants may be relatively resistant to Anectine.

Use in the elderly: The elderly may be more susceptible to cardiac arrythmias, especially if digitalis-like drugs are also being taken.

Contra-indications, warnings, etc
Contra-indications: Suxamethonium causes slight transient rise in ocular pressure and therefore should not be used in the presence of open eye injuries or where an increase in intra-ocular pressure is contra-indicated.

Anectine is contra-indicated in patients with personal or family history of malignant hyperthermia. Administration of Anectine (especially in conjunction with halothane) can trigger a sustained myofibrillar contraction resulting in a rapid rise in metabolism and body temperature.

Anectine is contra-indicated in patients known to have an inherited atypical or low serum level of plasma cholinesterase.

Under certain circumstances Anectine may cause a massive increase in serum potassium and cardiac arrest. For this reason Anectine is contra-indicated in:
Any patient with pre-existing hyperkalaemia.
Any patient with a major injury.
Any patient with severe burns.
Any patient with major denervation of muscle (upper and lower motor neurone lesions or a combination thereof, e.g. spinal cord injury).

The potential for potassium release is not seen immediately but begins 5–15 days after injury and persists for 2–3 months with burns and trauma and 3–6 months following neurological lesions.

There are case reports of cardiac arrest following the administration of suxamethonium in patients with congenital cerebral palsy, Duchenne muscular dystrophy and tetanus.

Precautions: Anectine should be administered only by or under close supervision of an anaesthetist familiar with its action, characteristics and hazards, who is skilled in the management of artificial respiration and only where there are adequate facilities for immediate endotracheal intubation with administration of oxygen by intermittent positive pressure ventilation.

Anectine should not be administered to a patient who is not fully anaesthetised.

It is recommended that the patient is fully monitored with a peripheral nerve stimulator during prolonged administration in order to avoid overdosage.

Anectine is rapidly hydrolysed by plasma cholinesterases which thereby limits the intensity and duration of the neuromuscular blockade. In patients with low levels of plasma cholinesterases, or with an abnormal pseudocholinesterase which has a low affinity for succinylcholine, the action of Anectine may be greatly intensified and very prolonged. Low levels of plasma cholinesterases may occur in patients with severe liver disease, severe anaemia, malnutrition, severe dehydration, changes in body temperature, exposure to a neurotoxic insecticide or those receiving antimalarial drugs or cytostatics. Anectine should be administered with extreme care to such patients and dosage should be minimal. Inhibitors of plasma cholinesterases such as neostigmine and phospholine iodide should not be given concurrently with suxamethonium, nor should competitive inhibitors such as intravenous procainamide.

If Anectine is given over a prolonged period, the characteristic depolarising neuromuscular (or Phase I) block may change to one with characteristics of a non-depolarising (or Phase II) block. This may be associated with prolonged respiratory depression and apnoea which may be partially or temporarily reversed by neostigmine preceded by atropine.

Normally, concomitant use of suxamethonium and neostigmine can result in prolonged muscular block and apnoea.

Tachyphylaxis occurs after repeated administration of Anectine.

The use of Anectine is inadvisable in patients exhibiting myotonia, since it may induce generalised myotonia. Use of suxamethonium in myotonia has, in general, been avoided but occasional administration has not resulted in cardiovascular collapse, or marked increase in serum potassium, when this has been measured.

It is inadvisable to administer Anectine to patients with advanced myasthenia gravis. Although these patients are resistant to Anectine they develop a state of dual block more easily which may result in prolonged recovery. Patients with Eaton–Lambert syndrome are more sensitive than normal to Anectine – the dose should be reduced.

Anectine may induce cardiac arrhythmias. The effects of digitalis may be enhanced with increased ventricular irritability.

Halothane, enflurane, diethylether and methoxyflurane have little effect on the usual Phase I block produced by Anectine. After repeated dosage, however, these anaesthetics will enhance so-called Phase II block.

Other drugs which may enhance or prolong the effect of Anectine include propanidid, procainamide, lignocaine, oxytocin, certain non-penicillin antibiotics, beta-adrenergic blockers, trimethaphan, phenelzine, aprotinin, quinidine, promazine, lithium carbonate, magnesium salts, quinine, chloroquine, and cytostatic agents such as cyclophosphamide, thiotepa and azathioprine.

Use in pregnancy and lactation: Although Anectine does not readily cross the placental barrier it should not be administered to pregnant women unless the potential benefit outweighs possible hazards.

Plasma pseudocholinesterase levels are decreased by approximately 25% in pregnancy and for several days postpartum; a high proportion of patients may be expected to show sensitivity or prolonged apnoea during pregnancy and postpartum.

Side- and adverse effects: Muscle pains are frequently experienced after administration of suxamethonium and most commonly occur in ambulatory patients undergoing short surgical procedures under general anaesthesia. There appears to be no direct connection between the degree of visible muscle fasciculation after Anectine administration and the incidence or severity of pain.

The following adverse reactions have been reported after administration of Anectine:

bradycardia, tachycardia, hypertension, hypotension, arrhythmias, prolonged respiratory depression or apnoea, hyperthermia, increased intraocular pressure, muscle fasciculation, post-operative muscle pain, myoglobinaemia, excessive salivation.

Toxicity and treatment of overdosage: Apnoea and prolonged muscle paralysis are the main and serious effects of overdosage. It is essential, therefore, to maintain the airway and adequate ventilation until spontaneous respiration occurs.

The use of neostigmine to reverse a Phase II block is a decision depending on the subject, and the experience and judgement of the clinician. If neostigmine is used its administration should be preceded by that of atropine.

Pharmaceutical precautions Anectine should not be mixed in the same syringe with any other agent, especially thiopentone. Store below 4°C and protect from light. Do not freeze. Do not resterilise.

Legal category POM.

Package quantities Box of 5 × 2 ml ampoules.

Further information Nil.

Product licence number 0003/5203.

CALPOL* INFANT SUSPENSION
CALPOL* SIX PLUS SUSPENSION

Presentation *Calpol Infant Suspension:* Each 5 ml of viscous, pink, strawberry flavoured suspension contains 120 mg Paracetamol BP.

Calpol Six Plus Suspension: Each 5 ml of viscous, orange coloured and orange flavoured suspension contains 250 mg Paracetamol BP.

Uses Calpol products are indicated for the treatment of mild to moderate pain (including teething pain), and as antipyretics.

Dosage and administration *Adults:* The optimal dosage range is 500 mg to 1 g paracetamol, i.e. 10–20 ml Calpol Six Plus Suspension (maximum 1 g), which may be repeated every 4 hours to a maximum of 4 g paracetamol (80 ml Calpol Six Plus Suspension), per day.

	Calpol Infant Suspension	Calpol Six Plus Suspension
Children 6 to 12 years	Use Calpol Six Plus	5 to 10 ml (250 mg–500 mg paracetamol)
1 to under 6 years	5 to 10 ml (120 mg–240 mg paracetamol	2.5 to 5 ml (125 mg–250 mg paracetamol)
3 months to under 1 year	2.5 to 5 ml (60 mg–120 mg paracetamol)	Use Calpol Infant Suspension
Infants under 3 months	NOT RECOMMENDED	

Use in the elderly: In the elderly the rate and extent of paracetamol absorption is normal but plasma half-life is longer and paracetamol clearance is lower than in young adults.

Contra-indications, warnings, etc

Contra-indications: Calpol is contra-indicated in patients with known hypersensitivity to paracetamol.

Precautions: Calpol should be used with caution in severe hepatic or renal dysfunction.

Side- and adverse effects: Paracetamol has been widely used and, when taken at the usual recommended dosage, side-effects are mild and infrequent and reports of adverse reactions are rare. Skin rashes and other allergic reactions occur rarely.

Most reports of adverse reactions to paracetamol relate to overdosage with the drug.

Isolated cases of thrombocytopenic purpura, haemolytic anaemia and agranulocytosis have been recorded.

Chronic hepatic necrosis has been reported in a patient who took daily therapeutic doses of paracetamol for about a year and liver damage has been reported after daily ingestion of excessive amounts for shorter periods. A review of a group of patients with chronic active hepatitis failed to reveal differences in the abnormalities of liver function in those who were long-term users of paracetamol nor was the control of their disease improved after paracetamol withdrawal.

Nephrotoxicity following therapeutic doses of paracetamol is uncommon, but papillary necrosis has been reported after prolonged administration.

Drug interactions: Patients who have taken barbiturates, tricyclic antidepressants and alcohol may show diminished ability to metabolise large doses of paracetamol, the plasma half-life of which can be prolonged.

Alcohol can increase the hepatotoxicity of paracetamol overdosage and may have contributed to the acute pancreatitis reported in one patient who had taken an overdose of paracetamol.

Chronic ingestion of anticonvulsants or oral steroid contraceptives induce liver enzymes and may prevent attainment of therapeutic paracetamol levels by increasing first pass metabolism or clearance.

Use in pregnancy and lactation: Data is not available on the use of Calpol during pregnancy. There is epidemiological evidence of safety of paracetamol in human pregnancy.

A pharmacokinetic study in 12 nursing mothers revealed that less than 1% of the dose ingested by a nursing mother appears in human milk, therefore maternal ingestion of therapeutic doses does not present a risk to the infant.

Toxicity and treatment of overdosage; Pallor, anorexia, nausea and vomiting are frequent early symptoms of paracetamol overdosage. Hepatic necrosis is a dose-related complication of paracetamol overdosage. Hepatic enzymes may become elevated and prothrombin time prolonged within 12–48 hours but clinical symptoms may not be apparent until 1 to 6 days after ingestion. Toxicity is likely in adults who have taken more than 10 g.

To protect the patient against delayed hepatotoxicity, paracetamol overdosage should be treated promptly by gastric lavage followed by intravenous N-acetylcysteine or oral methionine. Additional therapy (further methionine or intravenous cysteamine or intravenous N-acetylcysteine) is normally considered in the light of blood paracetamol content and the time elapsed since ingestion. Fulminant hepatic failure which may follow paracetamol overdosage requires specialised management.

In paracetamol overdosage with liver cell damage paracetamol half life is often prolonged from around 2 hours in normal adults to 4 hours or longer. However liver cell damage has been found in patients with a paracetamol half life less than 4 hours. Diminution in $^{14}CO_2$ excretion after oral ^{14}C-aminopyrine has been reported to correlate better with liver cell damage in paracetamol overdosage than do either plasma paracetamol concentration or half life or conventional liver function test measurements. Concomitant renal failure due to acute tubular necrosis may accompany paracetamol-induced fulminate hepatic failure. The incidence is, however, no more frequent in these patients than in others with fulminant hepatic failure from other causes.

Pharmaceutical precautions Store below 25°C. Protect from light.

Dilution: Calpol suspension should NOT be diluted. Where a dilution of Calpol Six Plus Suspension is prescribed, Calpol Infant Suspension should be dispensed.

Legal category P.

Package quantities *Calpol Infant Suspension:* bottles of 70 ml, 140 ml, and 1 litre.
Calpol Six Plus Suspension: bottles of 100 ml.

Further information The viscous consistency of Calpol Infant Suspension and Calpol Six Plus Suspension helps keep the medicine on the spoon and so makes it easier to administer.

Paracetamol does not cause the gastro-intestinal side-effects often seen after standard doses of aspirin.

Product licence numbers
Calpol Infant Suspension:	0003/5067
Calpol Six Plus Suspension:	0003/0182

CICATRIN* AEROSOL

Presentation Each gram contains:

Neomycin Sulphate BP	16,500 units
Zinc Bacitracin BP	1,250 units
l-Cysteine	12 mg
Glycine	60 mg

Uses Topical broad-spectrum antibacterial. Superficial bacterial infections of skin.

Dosage and administration *Adults:* A thin, uniform spray should be applied to affected areas, as required. This can be obtained from a spray of about one second's duration to the wound surface at a distance of not less than 20 cm. The application of one can of spray daily for a maximum period of 10–12 weeks should not be exceeded in adults. After such a course, treatment should not be repeated for at least three months.

Children: The maximum dosage should be reduced in proportion to body weight.

Use in the elderly: No specific studies have been carried out in the elderly, however, it may be advisable to monitor renal function in these patients and if there is any impairment then caution should be exercised.

Contra-indications, warnings, etc
Contra-indications: Hypersensitivity to bacitracin or the neomycin group of antibiotics.

Precautions: The following statements take into account the possibility that the constituent drugs of Cicatrin Aerosol, particularly neomycin, may be absorbed to a significant degree after topical application.

Ototoxicity and nephrotoxicity have been reported in association with large or prolonged doses of neomycin and nephrotoxicity has also been reported with inappropriate dosing with bacitracin. While these effects are normally reversible on cessation of therapy, the ototoxic effect of neomycin is not.

In cases where there is established partial nerve deafness and where a significant degree of neomycin absorption could occur it might be inappropriate to use any neomycin-containing product and treatment with an antibacterial without an aminoglycoside constituent should be used if possible. In renal impairment the plasma clearance of neomycin is reduced, therefore a reduction in dose should be made that relates to the degree of renal impairment.

The inappropriate use of topical antibiotics has been associated with the emergence of resistant strains of bacteria.

The spray should not be used on large denuded areas (e.g. burns or ulcers) because of the risk of systemic absorption. Patients with hypostatic leg ulcers may have an increased sensitivity to a large number of topically applied drugs, including neomycin.

Concurrent administration of other aminoglycoside antibiotics is not recommended.

As neomycin has a neuromuscular blocking effect, patients concurrently receiving other agents with a similar action should be observed for signs of possible respiratory insufficiency.

Side- and adverse effects: Allergic reactions following the topical application of neomycin have been reported in the literature, but such reactions following the application of zinc bacitracin are rare events. As with all antibacterial preparations prolonged use may result in the overgrowth of non-susceptible organisms including fungi.

Use in pregnancy and lactation: Due to a lack of detailed information, the use of Cicatrin during pregnancy and lactation cannot be recommended in circumstances where significant systemic absorption of the active ingredients may occur.

Toxicity and treatment of overdosage: In the event of signs of toxicity developing following significant systemic absorption of the active ingredients of Cicatrin aerosol the patient's general status, hearing acuity and renal function should be monitored and blood levels of neomycin and zinc bacitracin determined. Serum levels of neomycin can be reduced by haemodialysis.

Pharmaceutical precautions Store below 25°C. Keep away from heat. Do not puncture or incinerate can.

Legal category POM.

Package quantities Pressurised aerosol powder spray. Net content of powder 3 g approx.

Further information Nil.

Product licence number 0003/5083

CICATRIN* POWDER
CICATRIN* CREAM

Presentation Each gram of powder/cream contains:

Neomycin Sulphate BP	3,300 units
Zinc Bacitracin BP	250 units
l-Cysteine	2 mg
Glycine	10 mg
dl-Threonine	1 mg

Uses Topical broad-spectrum antibacterial.
Superficial bacterial infection of skin, such as impetigo, varicose ulcers, pressure sores, trophic ulcers and burns.

Dosage and administration *Adults:* A light dusting of the powder or thin layer of the cream should be applied to the affected skin area up to three times daily. See Contra-indications, warnings, etc.

Children: As for adults.

Use in the elderly: No specific studies have been carried out in the elderly, however, it may be advisable to monitor renal function in these patients and if there is any impairment then caution should be exercised.

Contra-indications, warnings, etc
Contra-indications: Hypersensitivity to bacitracin or the neomycin group of antibiotics.

Precautions: The following statements take into account the possibility that the constituent drugs of Cicatrin Powder/Cream, particularly neomycin, may be absorbed to a significant degree after topical application.
Ototoxicity and nephrotoxicity have been reported in association with large or prolonged doses of neomycin and nephrotoxicity has also been reported with inappropriate dosing with bacitracin. While these effects are normally reversible on cessation of therapy the ototoxic effect of neomycin is not. In consequence, the application of two 30 g tubes of the cream daily for three weeks, or one 50 g puffer pack of the powder daily for four weeks should not be exceeded in adults. After such a course, treatment should not be repeated for at least three months. In children this maximum dosage should be reduced in proportion to body weight.
In renal impairment the plasma clearance of neomycin is reduced, therefore a reduction in dose should be made that relates to the degree of renal impairment.
In cases where there is established partial nerve deafness and where a significant degree of neomycin absorption could occur it might be inappropriate to use any neomycin-containing product and treatment with an antibacterial without an aminoglycoside constituent should be used if possible.
Concurrent administration of other aminoglycoside antibiotics is not recommended.
As neomycin has a neuromuscular blocking effect, patients concurrently receiving other agents with a similar action should be observed for signs of possible respiratory insufficiency.

Patients with hypostatic leg ulcers may have an increased sensitivity to a large number of topically applied drugs, including neomycin.

Side- and adverse effects: Allergic reactions following the topical application of neomycin have been reported in the literature, but such reactions following the application of zinc bacitracin are rare events. As with all antibacterial preparations prolonged use may result in the overgrowth of non-susceptible organisms including fungi.

Use in pregnancy and lactation: Due to a lack of detailed information, the use of Cicatrin during pregnancy and lactation cannot be recommended in circumstances where significant systemic absorption of the active ingredients may occur.

Toxicity and treatment of overdosage: In the event of signs of toxicity developing following significant systemic absorption of the active ingredients of Cicatrin Powder/Cream the patient's general status, hearing acuity and renal function should be monitored and blood levels of neomycin and zinc bacitracin determined. Serum levels of neomycin can be reduced by haemodialysis.

Pharmaceutical precautions Store below 25°C. Keep dry.

Legal category POM.

Package quantities *Cicatrin Powder:* Puffer packs of 15 g and 50 g.
Cicatrin Cream: Tubes of 15 g and 30 g.

Further information Nil.

Product licence numbers
Powder   0003/5081.
Cream   0003/5082.

COPARVAX* ▼

Presentation Each vial contains 7 mg (dry weight of the *Corynebacterium parvum* organisms (inactivated) WFL strain CH 6134) in a freeze-dried form. Thiomersal and glycine are added to concentrations of 0.01% and 2.3% prior to freeze-drying.

Uses Coparvax is indicated for the alleviation of malignant pleural effusions and malignant ascites.

Dosage and administration The recommended dose is 7–14 mg, although some patients have responded to lower doses.
Freeze-dried Coparvax should be reconstituted with 1 ml of physiological saline for injection and diluted in a further volume of 10–20 ml prior to injection into the pleural or peritoneal cavity.
Coparvax is injected into the pleural or peritoneal cavity via the paracentesis needle immediately after the effusion has been aspirated. Instillation of Coparvax may be repeated, if necessary, at intervals of one to four weeks.
The suspension should be administered within 24 hours of reconstitution.

Use in the elderly: No special comment.

Contra-indications, warnings, etc
Contra-indications: There are no specific contra-indications.

Precautions: The incidence and severity of side-effects attributable to Coparvax administered intrapleurally appears to be intensified if given within 10 days of thoracotomy and lung resection probably due to enhanced systemic absorption of Coparvax. It should not be given during the immediate post-operative period.

Following intrapleural or intra-abdominal administration, leakage of Coparvax into subcutaneous tissues may result in local tenderness. Intense fibrinous reaction in the pleural and peritoneal cavities has been observed following local administration of Coparvax. Intestinal obstruction due to the formation of adhesions is a theoretical possibility, although it has not been reported as a complication of Coparvax administration.

Side- and adverse effects: Fever occurs in 10 to 60% of patients following intracavitary injection of Coparvax.

Abdominal pain or mild abdominal discomfort has been reported in some 20% of patients following intraperitoneal injection of Coparvax. Nausea and vomiting may occur in a minority of patients following intracavitary administration of Coparvax.

Use in pregnancy and lactation: Since there is no laboratory or clinical data on mutagenicity or teratogenicity, Coparvax should not be administered during pregnancy or lactation.

Pharmaceutical precautions Store between 2 and 8°C. Do not freeze. Protect from light.

Legal category POM.

Package quantities Single vials of 7 mg.

Further information Nil.

Product licence number 0003/0097.

CYCLIMORPH* 10 INJECTION
CYCLIMORPH* 15 INJECTION

Presentation Cyclimorph 10 Injection contains morphine tartrate 10 mg, cyclizine tartrate 50 mg, in 1 ml.

Cyclimorph 15 Injection contains morphine tartrate 15 mg, cyclizine tartrate 50 mg, in 1 ml.

Uses Cyclimorph Injection is indicated in all medical and surgical conditions where cyclizine is needed in addition to morphine. Cyclimorph contains cyclizine, a non-phenothiazine anti-emetic, which minimises the nausea and vomiting which may be caused by the narcotic. It is particularly useful in the management of myocardial infarction where control of nausea and vomiting is also clearly desirable. Cyclimorph can also be used for the relief of severe pain; left ventricular failure, pulmonary oedema, shock, and post-operative sedation.

Dosage and administration *Adults and children over 12 years:* Usual adult dose – 10–20 mg morphine tartrate subcutaneously, intramuscularly or intravenously.

Children 6–12 years: 5–10 mg morphine tartrate as a maximum single dose.

1–5 years: 2.5–5 mg morphine tartrate as a maximum single dose.

Use in the elderly: Use reduced dosage.

If required, repeat not more often than 4-hourly with not more than 3 doses (representing 150 mg cyclizine tartrate) in any 24-hour period.

Contra-indications, warnings, etc
Contra-indications: Respiratory depression; obstructive airways disease. Concurrent administration with mono-

amine oxidase inhibitors or within 2 weeks of their discontinuation.

Precautions: Use reduced dosage in the elderly, in hypothyroidism and chronic hepatic disease. Administration during labour may cause respiratory depression in the new-born infant.

Side- and adverse effects: Tolerance and dependence may occur. Drowsiness, dry mouth and blurred vision may occur in a small number of patients, due to the cyclizine component.

Use in pregnancy and lactation:
Morphine: There is inadequate evidence of safety in human pregnancy but the drug has been widely used for many years without apparent ill consequence and animal studies have not shown any hazard. No data available on its excretion in breast milk.

Cyclizine: There is some clinical evidence of safety in human pregnancy. No data available on its excretion in breast milk.

Toxicity and treatment of overdosage: These are likely to consist of respiratory depression, hypotension, with circulatory failure and deepening coma.

Naloxone, given intravenously, intramuscularly or subcutaneously, effectively antagonises the toxic effects of morphine. The circulation should be maintained with infusions of dextrose and suitable electrolyte solutions. Assisted respiration may be required.

Note: The use of the specific antidote in addicts tolerant to morphine may produce withdrawal symptoms.

Pharmaceutical precautions Store below 25°C, Protect from light.

Legal category CD (Sch 2), POM.

Package quantities *Cyclimorph 10 Injection;* 1 ml ampoules: Box of 5.
Cyclimorph 15 Injection; 1 ml ampoules: Box of 5.

Further information Nil.

Product licence numbers
Cyclimorph 10   0003/5022.
Cyclimorph 15   0003/5023.

DICONAL* TABLETS

Presentation Each tablet contains 10 mg of Dipipanone Hydrochloride BP and 30 mg of Cyclizine Hydrochloride BP, coloured deep pink, scored and coded 'Wellcome F3A'.

Uses Analgesic with anti-emetic action.

Indicated in those medical and surgical conditions where morphine would normally be used. It also contains cyclizine, an anti-emetic which effectively overcomes the nausea and vomiting which may be caused by the narcotic. Often effective in patients who have ceased to respond to morphine or pethidine.

Dosage and administration *Adults:* In all cases an initial dose of 1 tablet should not be exceeded. The onset of action is within an hour and adequate relief from a single dose will last about six hours. The dose can be repeated every six hours if necessary. Should the initial dose prove inadequate, as in cases of severe intractable pain or where other potent analgesics have been used previously, the dose may be increased subsequently by ½ tablet increments. It will seldom be necessary to exceed a dose of 3 tablets.

Children: Not applicable.

Use in the elderly: Although there is no absolute contra-indication to the use of Diconal in the elderly, opioid drugs may cause confusion in this age group and careful monitoring should be ensured.

Contra-indications, warnings, etc
Contra-indications: Respiratory depression, obstructive airways disease. Concurrent administration with mono-amine oxidase inhibitors or within 2 weeks of their discontinuation.

Precautions: Use with caution in patients with severe liver or kidney diseases.

As with all potent analgesics the possibility of addiction cannot be excluded and the usual precautions should be observed.

Misuse of Diconal has been reported, particularly by young addicts who have previously been dependent on, or have misused other agents, both opiate and non-opiate. Extreme caution is warranted when prescribing Diconal to this group of patients.

As with morphine-type drugs respiratory depression is a hazard. Particular care should therefore be taken when increasing the dosage and when treating patients with impaired respiration. Concurrent administration with other CNS depressants including alcohol may enhance the central effects of Diconal.

Side- and adverse effects: Cyclizine may cause drowsiness, dryness of the mouth and blurred vision in a small number of patients. Diconal may cause confusion in the elderly.

Use in pregnancy and lactation: No data are available on the use of Diconal in human pregnancy nor of the excretion of it or its metabolites in human milk. Its administration to pregnant or lactating mothers is best avoided unless there are compelling reasons for its use.

Administration during labour may cause respiratory distress in the newborn.

Toxicity and treatment of overdosage: The main problem with overdosage is likely to be respiratory depression. Depressed respiration can be counteracted by the administration of naloxone. Gastric lavage. Oxygen and respiratory support if necessary.

Pharmaceutical precautions Store below 25°C. Protect from light. Keep dry.

Legal category CD (Sch 2), POM.

Package quantities Bottle of 100 tablets.

Further information Nil.

Product licence number 0003/5027.

ESBATAL* TABLETS

Presentation Esbatal Tablets containing 10 mg Bethanidine Sulphate BP in each tablet. Peach coloured, scored and coded 'Wellcome P3A'.

Esbatal Tablets containing 50 mg Bethanidine Sulphate BP in each tablet. Peach coloured, scored and coded 'Wellcome T3A'.

Uses Antihypertensive agent.
Esbatal is an adrenergic neurone blocking agent which acts selectively on peripheral sympathetic nerves.

It is indicated for all grades of hypertension. Because of its speed of action, it is of special value in malignant hypertension, hypertensive crises and hypertensive heart disease.

Adrenergic neurone blockade is apparent within two hours, with peak effect two to four hours later, and usually disappears within 10–12 hours. There may be some cumulative effect where renal function is impaired.

Esbatal has been used successfully in combination with other established antihypertensive agents.

Dosage and administration *Adults:* Blood pressure should be recorded when the patient is standing.

Starting dose – one 10 mg tablet three times daily, after meals. Where necessary the dosage should be increased by half a tablet three times daily, at intervals, until effective control is obtained. Doses should not exceed 200 mg daily. Diuretics may be given concurrently. For the elderly and patients with a history of a cerebrovascular accident, half the starting dose is recommended.

Where rapid lowering of blood pressure is urgently needed, an initial dose of 20 mg should be increased by 10–20 mg every four to six hours until control is achieved.

Children: Not applicable.

Use in the elderly: Use half the usual starting dose in the elderly. Use with caution in those with renal, coronary, or cerebral impairment.

Contra-indications, warnings, etc
Contra-indications: Patients become very sensitive to any circulating sympathomimetic agent after adrenergic neurone blockade. Hence Esbatal is contra-indicated for patients with phaeochromocytoma. Adrenaline, amphetamine or any other sympathomimetic such as, for example, appetite suppressants, should not be used in patients on Esbatal except on the very rare occasion that its action requires antagonising.

Precautions: Special care should be taken when treating hypertension in patients with disease of cerebral or coronary vasculature or with severe renal damage. As Esbatal is excreted mainly by the kidneys, reduced doses may suffice in renal impairment.

Tricyclic antidepressants antagonise the activity of Esbatal thus necessitating larger doses. If simultaneously prescribed tricyclic antidepressants are discontinued, a substantial reduction in Esbatal requirements must be anticipated.

Side- and adverse effects: The beneficial effects of Esbatal derive from reduced peripheral vascular resistance and are most marked in the erect posture. Transient symptoms of a further reduction in resistance such as faintness, sweating, muscle fatigue and headache may occur with sudden changes in posture, excessive exercise and extremes of temperature, all of which should be avoided. Regularly repeated symptoms can be managed by reducing the size of the dose preceding their onset or by taking the dose after a meal. Sometimes Esbatal disturbs the normal ejaculation of semen. After omission of one or two doses normal sexual function returns. Nasal stuffiness and disturbed micturition may occur. It rarely causes diarrhoea.

Use in pregnancy and lactation: Esbatal may exacerbate placental insufficiency, and its benefits must be balanced against the risks of its use. There are no data on its use in lactating mothers.

Toxicity and treatment of overdosage: The main problem with overdosage would be severe hypotension. Treatment of overdosage is by means of general supportive measures with intravenous injection of plasma. *Slow* intravenous injection of noradrenaline or phenylephrine may be given under expert supervision.

Pharmaceutical precautions Store below 25°C in a dry place.

Legal category POM.

Package quantities *Tablets 10 mg:* Bottles of 100 and 500 tablets.
Tablets 50 mg: Bottle of 100 tablets.

Further information Nil.

Product licence numbers
Tablets 10 mg 0003/5037.
Tablets 50 mg 0003/5038.

FERROMYN* TABLETS
FERROMYN* ELIXIR

Presentation Ferromyn Tablets each contain 100 mg of Ferrous Succinate BP (equivalent to 35 mg elemental iron). Orange coloured.

Ferromyn Elixir: each 5 ml contains 106 mg Ferrous Succinate BP (equivalent to 37 mg elemental iron). Brown coloured.

Uses For the prevention and treatment of iron-deficiency anaemias.

Dosage and administration *Adults:* 1 tablet three times a day or 5 ml elixir three times a day.
Children: Ferromyn Elixir.
Up to 2 years: Up to 1 ml twice daily.
2–5 years: 2.5 ml three times daily.
5–10 years: 5 ml twice daily.
Over 10 years: As for adults.
Use in the elderly: No special comment.
Ferromyn Elixir may be diluted with Syrup BP.

Contra-indications, warnings, etc
Contra-indications: No special comments.

Precautions: May be less well absorbed if taken with food. Iron absorption may be impaired by magnesium trisilicate and carbonates.

If Ferromyn and oral tetracycline are given concomitantly, absorption and therefore serum levels of the antibiotic will be reduced. As with other conventional iron preparations, Ferromyn should not be given within 2 to 3 hours of an oral dose of tetracycline.

Side- and adverse effects: Rarely, gastrointestinal upset may occur.

Use in pregnancy and lactation: As pregnancy is frequently an indication for iron therapy there is no reason to expect problems with Ferromyn therapy. Iron is excreted in breast milk but not in clinically significant amounts (about 0.5 mg/day).

Toxicity and treatment of overdosage: The initial symptoms of acute overdosage with iron are acute gastric disturbance with epigastric pain, nausea, vomiting and diarrhoea. Haematemesis may occur. These features may be followed by profound cardiovascular collapse and acute encephalopathy.

If serum iron levels exceed 5 mg/l within six hours of dosing, then treatment is a matter of urgency.

Lavage should be carried out using a solution of desferrioxamine (2 g/l of warm water) and 5 g of desferrioxamine (in 50 to 100 ml water) should be left in the stomach. In addition, 1 g should be given twice daily by intramuscular injection. The antidote may be administered by continuous infusion (15 mg/kg/hr) but blood pressure should be monitored to avoid desferrioxamine hypotension.

It is important to maintain an adequate urine flow.

Pharmaceutical precautions *Tablets:* Store below 25°C.
Elixir: Store below 25°C. Protect from light.

Legal category P.

Package quantities *Ferromyn Tablets:* Container of 100 tablets.
Ferromyn Elixir: Bottle of 100 ml.

Further information Nil.

Product licence numbers
Tablets 0003/5086.
Elixir 0003/5088.

FERROMYN* 'B' TABLETS
FERROMYN* 'B' ELIXIR

Presentation Ferromyn 'B' Tablets each contain 106 mg Ferrous Succinate BP (equivalent to 37 mg elemental iron), Thiamine Hydrochloride BP 1 mg, Riboflavin BP 1 mg, Nicotinamide BP 10 mg. Chocolate brown coloured.

Ferromyn 'B' Elixir. Each 5 ml contains 106 mg Ferrous Succinate BP (equivalent to 37 mg elemental iron), Thiamine Hydrochloride BP 1 mg, Riboflavin BP 1 mg, Nicotinamide BP 10 mg. Dark brown coloured.

Uses For the prevention and treatment of iron-deficiency anaemias accompanied by vitamin B deficiency.

Dosage and administration *Adults:* 1 tablet or 5 ml elixir three times a day, between meals.
Children: Ferromyn 'B' Elixir.
Up to 2 years: Up to 1 ml twice daily.
2–5 years: 2.5 ml three times daily.
5–10 years: 5 ml twice daily.
Over 10 years: As for adults.
Use in the elderly: No special comment.

Ferromyn 'B' Elixir may be diluted with Syrup BP.

Contra-indications, warnings, etc
Contra-indications: No special comments.

Precautions: May be less well absorbed if taken with food. Iron absorption may be impaired by magnesium trisilicate and carbonates.

If Ferromyn 'B' and oral tetracycline are given concomitantly, absorption and therefore serum levels of the antibiotic will be reduced. As with other conventional iron preparations, Ferromyn 'B' should not be given within 2 to 3 hours of an oral dose of tetracycline.

Side- and adverse effects: Rarely gastrointestinal upset may occur.

Use in pregnancy and lactation: As pregnancy is frequently an indication for iron therapy there is no reason to expect problems with Ferromyn 'B' therapy. Iron is excreted in breast milk but not in clinically significant amounts (about 0.5 mg/day).

Toxicity and treatment of overdosage: The initial symptoms of acute overdosage with iron are acute gastric disturbance with epigastric pain, nausea, vomiting and diarrhoea. Haematemesis may occur. These features may be followed by profound cardiovascular collapse and acute encephalopathy.

If the serum iron levels exceed 5 mg/l within six hours of dosing, then treatment is a matter of urgency.

Lavage should be carried out using a solution of desferrioxamine (2 g/l of warm water) and 5 g of desferrioxamine (in 50 to 100 ml water) should be left in the stomach. In addition, 1 g should be given twice daily by intramuscular injection. The antidote may be administered by continuous infusion (15 mg/kg/hr) but blood pressure should be monitored to avoid desferrioxamine hypotension.

It is important to maintain an adequate urine flow.

Pharmaceutical precautions *Tablets:* Store below 25°C.

Elixir: Store below 25°C. Protect from light.

Legal category P.

Package quantities *Ferromyn 'B' Tablets:* Container of 100 tablets.
Ferromyn 'B' Elixir: Bottle of 100 ml.

Further information Nil.

Product licence numbers
Tablets   0003/5091.
Elixir   0003/5090.

FERROMYN* 'S' TABLETS

Presentation Ferromyn 'S' Tablets each contain 106 mg Ferrous Succinate BP (equivalent to 37 mg elemental iron) and succinic acid 110 mg. Orange coloured.

Uses For the prevention and treatment of iron-deficiency anaemias.

Dosage and administration *Adults:* 1 tablet three times a day.

Children: Not applicable.

Use in the elderly: No special comment.

Contra-indications, warnings, etc
Contra-indications: No special comments.

Precautions: May be less well absorbed if taken with food. Iron absorption may be impaired by magnesium trisilicate and carbonates.

If Ferromyn 'S' and oral tetracycline are given concomitantly, absorption and therefore serum levels of the antibiotic may be reduced. As with other conventional iron preparations, Ferromyn 'S' should not be given within 2 to 3 hours of an oral dose of tetracycline.

Side- and adverse effects: Rarely, gastrointestinal upset may occur.

Use in pregnancy and lactation: As pregnancy is frequently an indication for iron therapy there is no reason to expect any problems with Ferromyn 'S' therapy. Iron is excreted in breast milk, but not in clinically significant amounts (about 0.5 mg/day).

Toxicity and treatment of overdosage: The initial symptoms of acute overdosage with iron are acute gastric disturbance with epigastric pain, nausea, vomiting and diarrhoea. Haematemesis may occur. These features may be followed by profound cardiovascular collapse and acute encephalopathy.

If the serum iron levels exceed 5 mg/l within six hours of dosing, then treatment is a matter of urgency.

Lavage should be carried out using a solution of desferrioxamine (2 g/l of warm water) and 5 g of desferrioxamine (in 50 to 100 ml water) should be left in the stomach. In addition, 1 g should be given twice daily by intramuscular injection. The antidote may be administered by continuous infusion (15 mg/kg/hr) but blood pressure should be monitored to avoid desferrioxamine hypotension.

It is important to maintain an adequate urine flow.

Pharmaceutical precautions Store below 25°C.

Legal category P.

Package quantities Container of 100 tablets.

Further information Succinic acid is an iron absorption promoter.

Product licence number 0003/5084.

FERROMYN* 'S' FOLIC TABLETS

Presentation Ferromyn 'S' Folic Tablets each contain 106 mg Ferrous Succinate BP (equivalent to 37 mg elemental iron), succinic acid 110 mg and Folic Acid BP 100 mcg. Cerise coloured.

Uses For the prevention and treatment of combined iron and folic acid deficiency states, such as occur in pregnancy.

Dosage and administration *Adults:* 1 tablet three times a day.

Children: Not applicable.

Use in the elderly: No special comment.

Contra-indications, warnings, etc
Contra-indications: No special comments.

Precautions: May be less well absorbed if taken with food. Iron absorption may be impaired by magnesium trisilicate and carbonates.

If Ferromyn 'S' Folic and oral tetracycline are given concomitantly, absorption and therefore serum levels of the antibiotic will be reduced. As with other conventional iron preparations, Ferromyn 'S' Folic should not be given within 2 to 3 hours of an oral dose of tetracycline.

Side- and adverse effects: Rarely, gastrointestinal upset may occur.

Use in pregnancy and lactation: Since pregnancy is frequently an indication for iron and folic acid therapy there is no reason to expect any problems with Ferromyn 'S' Folic therapy. Iron is excreted in breast milk but not in clinically significant amounts (about 0.5 mg/day).

Toxicity and treatment of overdosage: The initial symptoms of acute overdosage with iron are acute gastric disturbance with epigastric pain, nausea, vomiting and diarrhoea. Haematemesis may occur. These features may be followed by profound cardiovascular collapse and acute encephalopathy.

If the serum iron levels exceed 5 mg/l within six hours of dosing, then treatment is a matter of urgency.

Lavage should be carried out using a solution of desferrioxamine (2 g/l of warm water) and 5 g of desferrioxamine (in 50 to 100 ml of water) should be left in the stomach. In addition, 1 g should be given twice daily by intramuscular injection. The antidote may be administered by continuous infusion (15 mg/kg/hr) but blood pressure should be monitored to avoid desferriox-amine hypotension.

It is important to maintain an adequate urine flow.

Pharmaceutical precautions Store below 25°C.

Legal category POM.

Package quantities Container of 100 tablets.

Further information Succinic acid is an iron absorption promoter.

Product licence number 0003/5085.

HYPON* TABLETS

Presentation Each tablet contains:

Acetylsalicylic Acid BP	325 mg
Caffeine BP	10 mg
Codeine Phosphate BP	5 mg

The tablets are yellow and impressed with the word 'HYPON' on one side.

Uses Analgesic and antipyretic.

For symptomatic relief of pain and fever associated with acute and chronic rheumatism, dysmenorrhoea, neuralgia, tonsillitis, influenza, coryza, headaches, and all conditions where an analgesic is indicated.

Dosage and administration *Adults:* 2 tablets every four hours.

Children 6–12 years: 1 tablet every four hours.

A maximum of 12 tablets to be taken in 24 hours.

Use in the elderly: Use with caution in those with renal impairment.

Contra-indications, warnings, etc
Contra-indications: Hypersensitivity to any of the constituents. Contra-indicated in haemophiliacs and in those with active peptic ulcers.

Precautions: Aspirin may prolong labour and contribute to maternal and neonatal bleeding, and is best avoided at term. Aspirin may enhance the effects of oral hypoglycaemics and anticoagulants and inhibit the action of uricosurics. It may precipitate bronchospasm or asthma in susceptible patients. Caution is necessary in renal impairment.

Side- and adverse effects: Occasionally, aspirin may induce hypersensitivity or asthmatic reactions. Gastrointestinal haemorrhages, (occasionally major) have been reported with aspirin. Codeine may sometimes cause constipation.

Use in pregnancy and lactation: No data are available on the use of Hypon in human pregnancy nor on the excretion of it or its metabolites in human milk.

Toxicity and treatment of overdosage: Acute aspirin toxicity would be characterised mainly by vomiting, abdominal pain, tinnitus and hyperventilation. In severe cases, there may be pyrexia and convulsions. Hypoglycaemia and convulsions occur most commonly in children. Respiratory depression from the codeine content may occur.

Treatment comprises gastric aspiration with thorough lavage. Replace fluids and electrolytes as necessary. Forced alkaline diuresis is the treatment of choice for accelerating elimination of absorbed salicylate.

Pharmaceutical precautions Store below 25°C in a dry place.

Legal category CD (Sch 5), P.

Package quantities Strip pack of 12. Drum of 300.

Further information Nil.

Product licence number 0003/0119.

IMURAN* TABLETS AND INJECTION

Presentation Each yellow tablet contains 50 mg Azathioprine BP, is imprinted 'Imuran', and the code 'K7A'. Each vial of injection contains the equivalent of 50 mg Azathioprine BP as its sodium salt, freeze-dried.

Uses Imuran (Tablets and Injection) facilitates the survival and function of organ transplants.

Imuran Tablets have a significant therapeutic effect in a proportion of patients suffering from chronic active hepatitis, severe rheumatoid arthritis, systemic lupus erythematosus (SLE), idiopathic thrombocytopenic purpura, acquired haemolytic anaemia, severe cases of specified dermatological diseases (pemphigus vulgaris, dermatomyositis, polyarteritis nodosa, pyoderma gangrenosa) when these conditions are: (a) refractory to corticosteroids or (b) when corticosteroids are contra-indicated or (c) controlled by corticosteroids in dosages which are producing severe side-effects. In patients with such side-effects, the aim of Imuran medication is to reduce the required maintenance dose of steroids.

In pemphigus and rheumatoid arthritis Imuran has been shown to have significant therapeutic activity when used without corticosteroids.

The risks associated with Imuran therapy should be considered against the severity of the patient's condition and the expected clinical effect.

The use of Imuran in other indications must be regarded as experimental.

Dosage and administration *Adults:* Imuran Tablets are given by mouth, but patients unable to take oral medication may be given Imuran Injection for a short period.

Transplantation: A loading dose of up to 5 mg/kg orally or intravenously is usually given. The dosage during the first three months after transplantation is usually 1.0–4.0 mg/kg body weight per day (median 2.4 mg/kg body weight per day). 1.0–2.5 mg/kg body weight per day may be given intravenously as a maintenance dose, but only if oral therapy is impracticable. Cessation of Imuran therapy, even after a period of years, carries a high risk of rejection within a few weeks.

Other conditions: for the treatment of the conditions listed under *Uses,* except for chronic active hepatitis, the dosage is usually between 2.0 and 2.5 mg/kg body weight per day. For the treatment of chronic active hepatitis the dosage is usually between 1.0 and 1.5 mg/kg body weight per day.

The dosage of Imuran and the duration of treatment may vary according to the condition, its severity and the clinical response obtained. A therapeutic response may not be evident for a few days or even weeks after initiation of Imuran therapy. If no discernible improvement occurs in the patient's condition within three months, consideration should be given to the withdrawal of the drug. Treatment is otherwise undertaken on a long-term basis unless the patient exhibits evidence of intolerance to the drug.

Administration by intravenous injection (in transplantation only): the contents of each vial should be dissolved in not less than 5 ml of sterile pyrogen-free water for injection. The solution is alkaline and very irritant and must, therefore, be given slowly (not less than one minute) and then flushed through with at least 50 ml of physiological saline or glucose saline. The solution should be prepared immediately before use and any remainder discarded. There are no data on the compatibility of Imuran Injection with other intravenous fluids.

Children: As for adults.

Use in the elderly: It is advisable to monitor white cell count, particularly in cases of renal or hepatic insufficiency.

Contra-indications, warnings, etc
Contra-indications: Imuran hypersensitivity will generally be a contra-indication to continued use.

Precautions: There are potential hazards in the use of this preparation. Therefore, it should not be prescribed unless the patient can be adequately monitored for toxic effects throughout the duration of the therapy.

During the first eight weeks of therapy with Imuran complete blood counts, including platelet counts, must be performed at least weekly (and more frequently when higher dosages are used or in the presence of disturbed renal or hepatic function), and with decreasing frequency thereafter.

Imuran may be given long-term unless the patient cannot tolerate the preparation. Withdrawal of an effective dose in certain instances, e.g. SLE with nephritis, may result in a serious relapse of the condition. In other instances, such as rheumatoid arthritis and certain haematological conditions, treatment may be withdrawn after a suitable interval without any ill-effect. Withdrawal should always be a gradual process performed under close supervision.

In the presence of severe renal or hepatic impairment careful monitoring is initially required, since the dosage of Imuran may have to be reduced.

Severe secondary infections, often with uncommon organisms, are a hazard of immunosuppressive therapy. These are seen more frequently in transplant recipients than in patients being treated for other indications.

Imuran is potentially mutagenic and has been shown to cause chromosome damage in man. The clinical significance of these findings is unclear since the damage is apparently reversible on withdrawal of Imuran.

Imuran has no detectable inhibitory effect on either male or female fertility. The depression of fertility accompanying chronic uraemia is generally reversed after transplantation and its accompanying azathioprine treatment.

An increased number of malignant tumours especially lymphoreticular and epithelial has been observed in transplant recipients. The skin tumours that have occurred in transplant patients have been primarily on sun-exposed skin. Patients should be cautioned against undue sun exposure, and the skin should be examined at regular intervals. There is, however, as yet no conclusive evidence of an increased incidence of tumours in other Imuran treated subjects. In such patients the risk may be indistinguishable from that accompanying some of the diseases under treatment.

The few cases reported show a different pattern from that seen in transplantation: tumour occurrence is much less common, has an increased latency, is seen mainly after prolonged continuous therapy, is less exclusively lymphoreticular and tends to occur in those patients also treated with alkylating agents. Use with caution in hypersplenism.

Concomitant Zyloric (allopurinol) therapy: When Imuran and Zyloric are given concomitantly only one quarter of the usual dosage of Imuran should be given since Zyloric has an inhibitory effect on its metabolism.

Concomitant use of cytotoxics: Imuran should be used with caution in patients receiving, or who have recently received, other bone marrow suppressive agents.

Concomitant use of muscle relaxants: There is clinical evidence that Imuran antagonises the effect of non-depolarising muscle relaxants such as curare, d-tubocurarine and pancuronium. Experimental data confirm that Imuran reverses the neuromuscular blockade caused by d-tubocurarine, and show that Imuran potentiates the neuromuscular blockage caused by succinylcholine.

Concomitant use of penicillamine is not recommended.

Side- and adverse effects: The principal side-effect of Imuran is a dose-related, generally reversible, depression of bone marrow function expressed as leucopenia, thrombocytopenia and rarely anaemia.

An additional form of haematological toxicity in patients receiving Imuran is megaloblastic erythropoiesis and macrocytosis.

Haematological toxicity is most frequently noted at the outset of therapy but reports of the late occurrence of leucopenia and anaemia confirm the wisdom of continuing haematological surveillance of patients even on stable long-term treatment.

The reported incidence of gastro-intestinal intolerance to oral administration of Imuran is variable. It is manifested largely as nausea and anorexia with occasional vomiting. In some instances it seems to be a dose-related phenomenon and after a brief interruption administration may often be successfully reinstituted, at a lower dose. Doses should, when possible, be taken with food. Other more serious gastro-intestinal complications of therapy have been recorded. Pancreatitis is seen most commonly in transplant recipients and has also been reported in patients with granulomatous bowel disease treated with Imuran.

Gastro-duodenal ulcer, intestinal haemorrhage and intestinal necrosis and perforation are complications seen only after transplantation and it appears likely that they are due to concomitant steroid therapy.

Imuran may occasionally cause cholestatic, dose-related reversible hepatotoxicity. In such cases it is advisable to withdraw Imuran. A variety of possibly allergic manifestations has been reported. Drug fever, skin rash, myalgia and arthralgia are well documented though uncommon complications. There are also single case reports of possible Imuran-related effects including acute renal insufficiency, haemolytic anaemia, acute restrictive lung disease and unexplained meningitic reactions.

Use in pregnancy and lactation: The potential teratogenicity of Imuran should be borne in mind. Although it has been shown to be teratogenic in laboratory animals clinical evidence suggests that the risk is not appreciable in man. There is no doubt that Imuran and its metabolites cross the placenta. A temporary impairment of immune function has been noted following exposure *in utero* to Imuran combined with prednisone. The long-term consequences of these properties of Imuran are unknown, but many children exposed *in utero* have now completed the first decade of life without reported problems.

It has not been possible to detect Imuran or its metabolites in the breast milk of treated patients.

Toxicity and treatment of overdosage: The most likely side-effect of overdosage is bone marrow depression, which may not reach its maximum until 9–14 days later. A single large dose of Imuran is less likely to have a toxic effect than a chronic minor overdosage on prescription. Although the effects of overdosage may be delayed it is not uncommon for improvement to commence after day 12 provided that the patient has not had high doses during the intervening period. If overdosage occurs the blood picture and hepatic function in particular should be monitored. Imuran is known to be dialysable and dialysis may be used in severe cases.

Pharmaceutical precautions *Tablets:* Store below 25°C. Protect from light.

Injection: Store below 25°C. Protect from light. Keep dry.

Legal category POM.

Package quantities Foil pack of 100 tablets. Single vials.

Further information Nil.

Product licence numbers
Tablets   0003/0036
Injection   0003/5043

LANVIS* TABLETS

Presentation Each pale greenish yellow biconvex tablet, scored and coded Wellcome U3B, contains 40 mg Thioguanine.

Uses Cytotoxic agent.

The main indication is acute myeloblastic leukaemia, but it has also been used in acute lymphoblastic and chronic granulocytic (myelocytic, myeloid, myelogenous) leukaemia.

Cross-resistance exists between Lanvis and Puri-Nethol (6-mercaptopurine) and it is not to be expected that patients who no longer respond to Puri-Nethol will respond to Lanvis or vice versa.

Dosage and administration The dosage and duration of its administration must be carefully adjusted to obtain optimum benefit without undue toxic effects.

Adults: The usual dosage of Lanvis is between 2.0 and 2.5 mg/kg body weight/day, the total daily doses being calculated to the nearest multiple of 20 mg and given at one time. The duration of drug administration will depend on the nature and dosage of other antineoplastic drugs administered with thioguanine, the patient's condition and whether early signs of toxicity occur. For induction therapy thioguanine is usually administered as one of a number of drugs for periods of 5–20 days according to the regimen adopted and the patient's tolerance.

For maintenance therapy, the usual dosage of thioguanine is 2.0 mg/kg body weight/day, but the patient must be monitored for bone-marrow toxicity, particularly if other cytotoxic drugs are given conjointly.

Children: As for adults.

Use in the elderly: No specific studies have been carried out in the elderly, however, it may be advisable to monitor renal or hepatic function and if there is serious impairment then caution should be exercised.

Consult the literature for details of various combination chemotherapy.

Contra-indications, warnings, etc
Contra-indications: In view of the seriousness of the indications there are no absolute contra-indications.

Precautions: Lanvis is an active cytotoxic agent for use only under the direction of physicians experienced in the administration of such agents.

Since Lanvis is strongly myelosuppressive, full blood counts must be taken daily during remission induction. Patients must be carefully monitored during therapy.

The main side-effect of treatment with Lanvis is bone marrow suppression leading to leucopenia and thrombocytopenia. The leucocyte and platelet counts continue to fall after treatment is stopped, so at the first sign of an abnormally large fall in the counts, treatment should be temporarily interrupted. Bone marrow suppression is readily reversible if the drug is withdrawn early enough. During remission induction in acute myelogenous leukaemia the patient may frequently have to survive a period of relative bone marrow aplasia and it is important that adequate supportive facilities are available.

Patients on myelosuppressive chemotherapy are particularly susceptible to a variety of infections.

During remission induction, particularly when rapid cell lysis is occurring, adequate precautions should be taken to avoid hyperuricaemia and/or hyperuricosuria and the risk of uric acid nephropathy.

In view of its action on cellular DNA, Lanvis is potentially mutagenic and carcinogenic, and consideration should be given to the theoretical risk of carcinogenesis when Lanvis therapy is given. It is advised that care be taken when handling or halving these tablets not to contaminate hands or to inspire drug.

Side- and adverse effects: Gastro-intestinal intolerance has been reported. Similar intolerance has been noted with Lanvis but individual patients may tolerate either Lanvis or Puri-Nethol better than the other. At high doses gastro-intestinal symptoms may be more apparent and stomatitis has also been reported. Intestinal necrosis and perforation has been reported in patients who received combination chemotherapy including Lanvis.

Liver function abnormalities and jaundice have been reported during treatment with Lanvis and may be reversible if therapy is withdrawn. There has been a report of veno-occlusive disease of the liver occurring in patients who received combination chemotherapy including Lanvis.

Use in pregnancy and lactation: Lanvis like other cytotoxic agents is potentially teratogenic. Its use should be avoided whenever possible during pregnancy, particularly during the first trimester. In any individual case the potential hazard to the foetus must be balanced against the expected benefit to the mother. There have been isolated cases where men who have received combinations of cytotoxic agents including Lanvis have fathered children with congenital abnormalities and consideration should be given to this potential risk when treating male patients.

Mothers receiving Lanvis should not breast feed.

Toxicity and treatment of overdosage: The principal toxic effect is on the bone marrow and haematological toxicity is likely to be more profound with chronic overdosage than with a single ingestion of Lanvis. As there is no known antidote the blood picture should be closely monitored and general supportive measures instituted together with appropriate blood transfusion if necessary.

Pharmaceutical precautions Store below 25°C. Protect from light. Keep dry.

Legal category POM.

Package quantities Bottle of 25 tablets.

Further information The concomitant use of Zyloric* (allopurinol) to inhibit uric acid formation does not necessitate reduction of the dosage of Lanvis as is necessary with Puri-Nethol* (6-mercaptopurine) and Imuran* (azathioprine).

Product licence number 0003/0083.

LEUKERAN* TABLETS

Presentation *Leukeran Tablets:* 2 mg Chlorambucil BP, coded Wellcome C2A. Coloured yellow with white core.

5 mg Chlorambucil BP, coded Wellcome H2A. Coloured yellow with white core.

Uses Cytotoxic agent.

Leukeran is indicated in the treatment of Hodgkin's disease, certain forms of non-Hodgkin's lymphoma, chronic lymphocytic leukaemia, Waldenstrom's macroglobulinaemia and advanced ovarian adenocarcinoma. Leukeran has a significant therapeutic effect in a proportion of patients with breast cancer.

Dosage and administration *Adults: Hodgkin's disease:* Used as a single agent a typical dosage is 0.2 mg/kg/day for 4–8 weeks. Leukeran is usually included in combination therapy and a number of regimes have been used. Leukeran has been used as an alternative to nitrogen mustard with a reduction in toxicity but similar therapeutic results.

Non-Hodgkin's lymphoma: Used as a single agent the usual dosage is 0.1–0.2 mg/kg/day for 4–8 weeks initially; maintenance therapy is then given either by a reduced daily dosage or intermittent courses of treatment. Leukeran is useful in the management of patients with advanced diffuse lymphocytic lymphoma and those who have relapsed after radiotherapy. There is no significant difference in the overall response rate obtained with chlorambucil as a single agent and combination chemotherapy in patients with advanced non-Hodgkin's lymphocytic lymphoma.

Chronic lymphocytic leukaemia: Treatment with Leukeran is usually started after the patient has developed symptoms or when there is evidence of impaired bone marrow function (but not marrow failure) as indicated by the peripheral blood count. Initially Leukeran is given at a dosage of 0.15 mg/kg/day until the total leucocyte count has fallen to 10,000 per μl. Treatment may be resumed 4 weeks after the end of the first course and continued at a dosage of 0.1 mg/kg/day. In a proportion of patients, usually after about 2 years of treatment, the blood leucocyte count is reduced to the normal range, enlarged spleen and lymph nodes become impalpable and the proportion of lymphocytes in the bone marrow is reduced to less than 20 per cent. Patients with evidence of bone marrow failure should first be treated with prednisolone and evidence of marrow regeneration should be obtained before commencing treatment with Leukeran. Intermittent high dose therapy has been compared with daily Leukeran but no significant difference in therapeutic response or frequency of side effects was observed between the two treatment groups.

Waldenstrom's macroglobulinaemia: Leukeran is the treatment of choice in this indication. Starting doses of 6–12 mg daily until leucopenia occurs are recommended followed by 2–8 mg daily indefinitely.

Ovarian carcinoma: Used as a single agent a typical dosage is 0.2 mg/kg/day for 4–6 weeks. A dosage of 0.3 mg/kg/day has been given until leucopenia had been induced. Maintenance dosage of 0.2 mg/kg/day has been given aiming to keep the total leucocyte count below 4,000/mm³. In practice, maintenance courses tend to last 2–4 weeks with intervals of 2–6 weeks between each course.

Advanced breast cancer: Used as a single agent a typical dosage is 0.2 mg/kg bodyweight per day for 6 weeks. Leukeran may be given in combination with prednisolone at a dose range of 14–20 mg daily, regardless of bodyweight, over 4–6 weeks provided there is no serious haemopoietic depression. Leukeran may be given in combination with methotrexate, 5-fluorouracil, and prednisolone at a dosage of 5 to 7.5 mg/m²/day.

Children: Leukeran may be used in the management of Hodgkin's disease and non-Hodgkin's lymphomas in children. The dosage regimens are similar to those used in adults.

Use in the elderly: No specific studies have been carried out in the elderly, however, it may be advisable to monitor renal or hepatic function and if there is serious impairment then caution should be exercised.

Contra-indications, warnings, etc
Contra-indications: In view of the seriousness of the indications there are no absolute contra-indications.

Precautions: Leukeran is an active cytotoxic agent for use only under the direction of physicians experienced in the administration of such agents.

Since Leukeran is capable of producing irreversible bone marrow suppression, blood counts should be closely monitored in patients under treatment.

At therapeutic dosage Leukeran depresses lymphocytes and has less effect on neutrophil and platelet counts and on haemoglobin levels. Discontinuation of Leukeran is not necessary at the first sign of a fall in neutrophils but it must be remembered that the fall may continue for 10 days or more after the last dose.

Leukeran should not be given to patients who have recently undergone radiotherapy or received other cytotoxic agents.

When lymphocytic infiltration of the bone marrow is present or the bone marrow is hypoplastic, the daily dose should not exceed 0.1 mg/kg body weight.

Patients with evidence of impaired renal function should be carefully monitored as they are prone to additional myelosuppression associated with azotaemia.

The metabolism of Leukeran is still under investigation and consideration should be given to dose reduction in patients with gross hepatic dysfunction.

Leukeran has been shown to cause chromatid or chromosome damage in man. Development of acute leukaemia after Leukeran therapy for chronic lymphocytic leukaemia has been reported. However, it was not clear whether the acute leukaemia was part of the natural history of the disease or if the chemotherapy was the cause.

A comparison of patients with ovarian cancer who received alkylating agents with those who did not, showed that the use of alkylating agents, including Leukeran, significantly increased the incidence of acute leukaemia.

Acute myelogenous leukaemia has been reported in a small proportion of patients receiving Leukeran as long-term adjuvant therapy for breast cancer.

The leukaemogenic risk must be balanced against the potential therapeutic benefit when considering the use of Leukeran.

Chlorambucil may cause suppression of ovarian function and amenorrhoea has been reported following chlorambucil therapy.

Azoospermia has been observed as a result of therapy with Leukeran although it is estimated that a total dose of at least 400 mg is necessary.

Varying degrees of recovery of spermatogenesis have been reported in patients with lymphoma following treatment with Leukeran in total doses of 410–2,600 mg. Patients receiving phenylbutazone may require a reduced dose of Leukeran.

Side- and adverse effects: The most common side-effect is bone marrow suppression. Although this frequently occurs, it is usually reversible if Leukeran is withdrawn early enough. However, irreversible bone marrow failure has been reported.

Gastro-intestinal disturbances such as nausea and vomiting, diarrhoea and oral ulceration occur infrequently. Other side-effects may be encountered but usually only when the therapeutic dosage has been exceeded.

Severe interstitial pulmonary fibrosis has occasionally been reported in patients with chronic lymphocytic leukaemia on long-term Leukeran therapy. However, this may be reversible on withdrawal of Leukeran.

Hepatotoxicity and jaundice have been reported after Leukeran treatment.

Other reported adverse reactions include fever, skin hypersensitivity, peripheral neuropathy, interstitial pneumonia and sterile cystitis.

Seizures have occurred in children with nephrotic syndrome treated with Leukeran and dose-related focal fits in adults have been reported.

Use in pregnancy and lactation: As with other cytotoxic agents Leukeran is potentially teratogenic. The use of Leukeran should be avoided whenever possible during pregnancy, particularly during the first trimester. In any individual case, the potential hazard to the foetus must be balanced against the expected benefit to the mother.

Mothers receiving Leukeran should not breast feed.

Toxicity and treatment of overdosage: Reversible pancytopenia was the main finding of inadvertent overdoses of Leukeran. Neurological toxicity ranging from agitated behaviour and ataxia to multiple grand mal seizures has also occurred. As there is no known antidote the blood picture should be closely monitored and general supportive measures should be instituted, together with appropriate blood transfusion if necessary.

Pharmaceutical precautions Store at 2–8°C in a dry place.

Legal category POM.

Package quantities *2 mg:* Bottle of 25 tablets. *5 mg:* Bottle of 25 tablets.

Further information Leukeran has the pharmacological properties of the nitrogen mustard compounds. The drug is only partly radiomimetic, affecting chiefly the lymphoid tissues. Experimental studies have shown that chlorambucil is well absorbed and well tolerated by the oral route.

Product licence numbers
Tablets 2 mg   0003/5264
Tablets 5 mg   0003/5265

LoAsid* TABLETS ▼

Presentation Off-white dispersible tablets with minty flavour, imprinted 'Wellcome' and coded 'P4C'. Each contains:

Dried Aluminium Hydroxide BP	230 mg
Magnesium Hydroxide BP	230 mg
Simethicone USP	12 mg

Uses Antacid. Indicated for the relief of indigestion, heartburn and flatulence in the treatment of peptic ulcer, hiatus hernia, reflux oesophagitis and gastritis. LoAsid is also used as a mucosal protective when hyperacidity is a regular problem.

Dosage and administration *Adults:* One to two tablets to be taken as required, after or between meals and at bedtime, or as directed by a physician.

Children: There are insufficient data to recommend the use of LoAsid in children.

The tablets may be sucked, chewed, swallowed whole or dispersed and stirred in a quarter full glass of water.

Use in the elderly: Use with caution in renal insufficiency – see also *Precautions*, below.

Contra-indications, warnings, etc
Contra-indications: None known.

Precautions: Use with caution in renal insufficiency with glomerular filtration rate in the range 10–50 ml/min and avoid in patients with glomerular filtration rates less than 10 ml/min because of the risk of hypermagnesaemia.

LoAsid should be used with caution in patients with low dietary phosphate, as aluminium hydroxide is converted to aluminium phosphate in the intestine and can cause a phosphate deficiency syndrome with anorexia, muscular weakness and osteomalacia.

Side- and adverse effects: None reported.

Drug interactions: Concomitant administration of antacids may reduce the absorption of cimetidine, tetracyclines, digoxin and isoniazid, and may increase the absorption of dicoumarol and pseudoephedrine. Quinidine intoxication associated with alkali ingestion has been reported.

Use in pregnancy and lactation: No data are available on the use of LoAsid during pregnancy or on its excretion in human milk.

Toxicity and treatment of overdosage: No special recommendations, as serious symptoms are unlikely following overdosage with LoAsid.

Pharmaceutical precautions Store below 25°C in a dry place. Protect from light.

Legal category P.

Package quantities Blister pack of 1 × 10 tablets.

Further information Nil.

Product licence number 0003/0185.

MYLERAN* TABLETS

Presentation *Myleran Tablets:* 0.5 mg Busulphan BP, coded Wellcome F2A. Coloured white with yellow core.

2.0 mg Busulphan BP, coded Wellcome K2A. Coloured white with yellow core.

Uses Cytotoxic agent. Myleran is indicated for the treatment of chronic granulocytic leukaemia. Myleran has been shown to be superior to splenic irradiation when judged by survival times, control of spleen size and maintenance of haemoglobin levels. Although not curative, Myleran reduces the total granulocyte mass, relieves symptoms of disease, and improves the clinical state of the patient. Myleran is not useful once blast transformation has occurred. Myleran is also effective in producing remission in polycythaemia vera. It is especially useful in cases resistant to radiophosphorous (P³²) therapy and where there is marked thrombocytosis. Myleran may be useful in selected cases of essential thrombocythaemia and myelofibrosis.

Dosage and administration *Adults: Chronic Granulocytic Leukaemia: Remission induction:* The dosage is 0.06 mg/kg daily with a maximum daily dose of 4 mg which may be given as a single dose.

Administration of Myleran should be discontinued when the white blood cell count has fallen to between 20–25,000/cu mm or earlier if the platelet count falls below 100,000/cu mm otherwise there is a considerable risk of causing irreversible bone marrow aplasia since the counts may continue to fall for some time after treatment is stopped. The blood count should be monitored at least weekly during the induction phase and the dose should be increased only if the response after three weeks is inadequate.

Maintenance therapy: Although the white count may be controlled without further therapy for long periods after induction therapy, most clinicians use some form of maintenance treatment.

Dosage is usually between 0.5–2 mg per day but individual requirements may be much less. The aim is to maintain a white blood count of 10–15,000/cu mm and blood counts should be performed at least every four weeks.

Polycythaemia vera and essential thrombocythaemia: Remission induction: The dosage is 4–6 mg daily. The total dose required to produce remission varies so that very careful haematological control is essential. Maintenance therapy: The dosage is approximately half the induction dose but the exact amount must be assessed individually for each patient. Prolonged treatment is necessary, requiring close supervision and frequent blood counts.

Myelofibrosis: The usual dosage is 2–4 mg per day, with a lower dose for maintenance. Very careful haematological control is required because of the great sensitivity of the bone marrow in this condition.

Children: Very rarely indicated.

Use in the elderly: No special comment.

Contra-indications, warnings, etc
Contra-indications: In view of the seriousness of the indications, there are no absolute contra-indications.

Precautions: Careful attention should be paid to the monitoring of blood counts to avoid the possibility of excessive myelosuppression and the risk of irreversible bone marrow aplasia.

The main side-effect of Myleran treatment is bone marrow depression, particularly thrombocytopenia. Special care must be taken when the initial platelet count is low and when the count falls during treatment. Administration of Myleran should be stopped immediately at any stage of treatment if there is a sharp fall in the platelet count or if purpura develops.

Myleran should not be given to patients who have recently received radiotherapy or other cytotoxic drugs.

Hyperuricaemia and/or hyperuricosuria are not uncommon in untreated patients with chronic granulocytic leukaemia and should be corrected before starting therapy with Myloran. During treatment hyperuricaemia and the risk of uric acid nephropathy should be prevented by adequate prophylaxis.

Various chromosome abberations have been noted in cells from patients receiving Myleran. Widespread epithelial dysplasia has been reported.

The possibility that Myleran is carcinogenic should be borne in mind. A number of malignant tumours have been reported in patients receiving busulphan.

Ovarian suppression and amenorrhoea with menopausal symptoms commonly occur in pre-menopausal patients.

Busulphan interferes with spermatogenesis in experimental animals and there have been clinical reports of sterility, azoospermia and testicular atrophy in man.

Side- and adverse effects: The most common side-effect is bone marrow depression. Gastro-intestinal effects such as nausea, vomiting and diarrhoea have been reported rarely. Such intolerance is not a significant problem and can be controlled by giving the daily treatment in divided doses.

Hyperpigmentation is the most common skin reaction and occurs in 5–10% of patients, particularly those with a dark complexion. In a few cases a clinical syndrome resembling adrenal insufficiency and characterised by weakness, severe fatigue, anorexia, weight loss, nausea and vomiting, and hyperpigmentation of the skin has developed after prolonged busulphan therapy. The syndrome has sometimes resolved when busulphan has been withdrawn.

Diffuse pulmonary fibrosis with progressive dyspnoea and a persistent non-productive cough has occurred rarely, usually after prolonged treatment over a number of years. In a single case pulmonary ossification also occurred. The lung pathology may be complicated by superimposed infections. It is possible that subsequent radiotherapy can augment subclinical lung injury caused by Myleran Lens changes, and cataracts which may be bilateral, have been reported during Myleran therapy.

Other reported adverse reactions include urticaria, erythema multiforme, erythema nodosum, alopecia, porphyria cutanea tarda, excessive dryness and fragility of the skin with complete anhydrosis, dryness of the oral mucous membranes and cheilosis, gynaecomastia, cholestatic jaundice, endocardial fibrosis and myasthenia gravis. Most of these are single case reports and in many a clear cause and effect relationship with Myleran has not been demonstrated.

Use in pregnancy and lactation: Myleran is potentially teratogenic and embryotoxic, although there have been a number of reported cases where apparently normal children have been born after busulphan treatment during pregnancy, Myleran should be avoided during pregnancy, particularly during the first trimester. In each case, the potential benefit to the mother must be weighed against the risk to the foetus.

Mothers receiving Myleran should not breast feed.

Toxicity and treatment of overdosage: The principal toxic effect is on the bone marrow. Survival after a single large dose has been reported but haematological toxicity is likely to be more profound with chronic overdosage. As there is no known antidote the blood picture should be closely monitored and general supportive measures, together with appropriate blood transfusion, instituted if necessary.

Pharmaceutical precautions Store below 25°C in a dry place.

Legal category POM.

Package quantities *0.5 mg:* Bottle of 25 tablets. *2.0 mg:* Bottle of 25 tablets.

Further information Myleran is more selective than nitrogen mustard or the folic acid antagonists in its effect on the myeloid cells and may be somewhat safer in use; certain patients have received daily doses of 4 mg for as long as a year.

Product licence numbers
Tablets 0.5 mg   0003/5113
Tablets 2.0 mg   0003/5112

NEOSPORIN* EYE DROPS

Presentation Each ml of the sterile faintly opalescent solution contains:

Polymyxin B Sulphate BP 5,000 units
Neomycin Sulphate BP   1,700 units
Gramicidin USP   25 units

Also contains Thiomersal BP (0.001%) as preservative.

Uses Topical antibacterial agent.
   For the prophylaxis and treatment of external bacterial infections of the eye. Prophylactically, it is useful following removal of foreign bodies, and before and after ophthalmic surgery, to help provide and maintain a sterile field.

Dosage and administration *Adults:* 1 or 2 drops in the affected eye, two to four times daily or more frequently as required. In severe infections, therapy should be started with 1 or 2 drops every 15 to 30 minutes, reducing the frequency of instillation gradually as the infection is controlled.

Children: As for adults.

Use in the elderly: No special comment.

Contra-indications, warnings, etc
Contra-indications: Hypersensitivity to polymyxins, gramicidin or the neomycin group of antibiotics.

Precautions: Neomycin is ototoxic and nephrotoxic if absorbed from open surfaces. Polymyxin B and gramicidin are also nephrotoxic. However, these effects are unlikely with ocular administration.
   Neosporin eye drops should not be used during surgical procedures nor before surgery in circumstances where access of the product to intra-ocular fluids could occur.

Side- and adverse effects: Allergic reactions following the topical application of neomycin have been reported in the literature, but such reactions following the application of polymyxin B and gramicidin are rare events.
   As with all antibacterial preparations prolonged use may result in the overgrowth of non-susceptible organisms including fungi.

Toxicity and treatment of overdosage: Not applicable.

Pharmaceutical precautions Store below 15°C. Keep dry. Protect from light.
   Not suitable for injection. Discard four weeks after opening.

Legal category POM.

Package quantities Special dropper tube of 5 ml.

Further information Neosporin is a non-irritating isotonic solution and is well tolerated by the sensitive structures of the eye.

Product licence number 0003/5108.

OTOSPORIN* EAR DROPS

Presentation Each ml of aqueous vehicle contains:

Polymyxin B Sulphate BP   10,000 units
Neomycin Sulphate BP   3,400 units
Hydrocortisone BP   10 mg

White in colour.

Uses Topical antibacterial and anti-inflammatory.
   In the treatment of bacterial infection and inflammation of the external auditory meatus.

Dosage and administration *Adults:* 3 drops should be instilled into the affected ear three or four times daily. Alternatively, a gauze wick may be introduced into the external auditory canal and kept saturated with the solution; the wick may be left in place for 24 to 48 hours.

Children: As for adults.

The external auditory meatus and canal should be thoroughly cleansed and carefully dried before each application, but soap should not be used as the antibiotics may be inactivated by it.

Use in the elderly: No special comment.

Contra-indications, warnings, etc
Contra-indications: Hypersensitivity to polymyxins or the neomycin group of antibiotics.

Precautions: Delayed progressive ototoxicity has been reported in animals following administration of neomycin and polymyxin B to the middle ear. In patients who may have a perforation of the ear drum, it is recommended that the dosage should be restricted to a maximum of three drops three times daily for 10 days.
   As with all antibacterial preparations prolonged use may result in the overgrowth of non-susceptible organisms including fungi.
   In infants long-term continuous topical steroid therapy should be avoided. Adrenal suppression can occur, even without occlusion.

Side- and adverse effects: Allergic reactions following the topical application of neomycin have been reported in the literature, but such reactions following the application of polymyxin B are rare events.

Use in pregnancy and lactation: Due to a lack of detailed information the use of Otosporin during pregnancy or lactation cannot be recommended in circumstances where significant systemic absorption could occur.

Toxicity and treatment of overdosage: Not applicable.

Pharmaceutical precautions Store below 15°C. Protect from light.

Legal category POM.

Package quantities Plastic drop-dose bottles of 5 ml and 10 ml.

Further information Nil.

Product licence number 0003/5106.

PARAHYPON* TABLETS

Presentation Each tablet contains:

Paracetamol BP	500 mg
Codeine Phosphate BP	5 mg
Caffeine BP	10 mg

The tablets are pink, scored on one side and impressed with the word 'PARA-HYPON' on the other.

Uses Analgesic.

For the relief of pain associated with arthritis, rheumatism and other diseases of the skeletal system, headache, toothache, colds and influenza and other conditions where simple analgesia is required.

Dosage and administration *Adults and children over 12 years:* 2 tablets up to four times daily.

Children 6–12 years: 1 tablet up to four times daily.

Not more than 4 doses should be administered in any 24-hour period; do not repeat dose more frequently than 4-hourly.

Use in the elderly: Use with caution in those with renal or hepatic impairment.

Contra-indications, warnings, etc

Contra-indications: Hypersensitivity to any of the constituents.

Precautions: Use with caution in the presence of renal or hepatic dysfunction.

Drug interactions: In cases of paracetamol overdosage, liver microsomal inducing agents such as barbiturates, tricyclic antidepressants, and alcohol may increase the hepatotoxicity of paracetamol.

Side- and adverse effects: Side-effects with Parahypon are rare in therapeutic doses. Paracetamol has been widely used and reports of adverse reactions are rare, and are generally associated with overdosage. Isolated cases of thrombocytopenic purpura, methaemoglobinaemia, and agranulocytosis have been recorded. Isolated cases of chronic hepatic necrosis, acute pancreatitis and nephrotoxicity have been reported after overdosage or prolonged administration.

Codeine may sometimes cause constipation.

Use in pregnancy and lactation: No data are available on the use of Parahypon in human pregnancy nor on the excretion of it or its metabolites in human milk.

Toxicity and treatment of overdosage: Even in severe cases, initial symptoms are likely to be mild and may comprise pallor, nausea and vomiting. Liver damage may not become apparent for 24 hours to 6 days after ingestion.

Overdosage should therefore be treated promptly by gastric lavage followed by i.v. N-Acetylcysteine or oral methionine. Additional therapy (further methionine, i.v. N-Acetylcysteine or i.v. cysteamine) is normally considered in the light of blood paracetamol content and the time elapsed since ingestion. Such therapy is probably best undertaken in a specialised unit.

Pharmaceutical precautions Store below 25°C. Keep dry. Protect from light.

Legal category CD (Sch 5), P.

Package quantities Strip-pack of 12. Container of 100 tablets.

Further information Nil.

Product licence number 0003/0118.

PHYSEPTONE* INJECTION
PHYSEPTONE* TABLETS
PHYSEPTONE* LINCTUS

Presentation Physeptone Injection contains 10 mg Methadone Hydrochloride BP in each ml.

Physeptone Tablets each contain 5 mg Methadone Hydrochloride BP, scored, coded Wellcome L4A and white in colour.

Physeptone Linctus contains 2 mg Methadone Hydrochloride BP, in each 5 ml and is a clear orange-brown syrup.

Uses 1. *Analgesic:* In conditions where morphine would make a reasonable alternative, particularly for the relief of pain of visceral origin. It is not recommended for use in ambulant patients.

2. *Cough suppressant:* For the control of severe cough where diamorphine linctus would be a reasonable alternative.

Dosage and administration *Analgesic use: Adults:* Usual single dose 5–10 mg by mouth, subcutaneous or intramuscular injection.

Owing to its long plasma half-life caution with repeated dosage should be observed in the very ill or elderly. The usual initial dose should be 5–10 mg, 6–8 hourly, later adjusted to the degree of pain relief obtained.

Children: Not suitable.

Anti-tussive use: Adults: 5 ml every 3–4 hours.

Children: Dilute 1 volume of linctus with 7 volumes Syrup BP. Doses of diluted preparation are:
   Children over 10 years: 10 ml every 4 hours.
   Children under 10 years: 5 ml every 4 hours.
Where the drug is given by mouth for the control of pain associated with a chronic condition it is wise to restrict the dose to the smallest amount which adequately controls the symptoms.

Physeptone has less hypnotic effect than morphine.

If it is necessary to give a patient a potent analgesic for a prolonged period, some increase in dose may be found necessary; in such circumstances it is probably sound practice to change to another drug (codeine, morphine, pethidine) for a time. Physeptone may then be resumed in diminished doses.

Use in the elderly: Use caution with repeated dosage in elderly and ill patients.

Contra-indications, warnings, etc

Contra-indications: Respiratory depression, obstructive airways disease. Concurrent administration with monoamine oxidase inhibitors, or within 2 weeks of discontinuation of treatment with them. Obstetric use is not recommended.

Precautions: Children are very sensitive to the depressant effects.

The possibility of addiction cannot be excluded and patients should be reminded of the necessity of adhering to the prescribed dosage.

Side- and adverse effects: Euphoria, dizziness, drowsiness, vomiting or nausea, and respiratory depression may occur in some patients. In rare cases a hypersensitive subject may react with a sudden transient fall in blood pressure; this is short-lived and self-terminating. Side-effects are more common and more severe in ambulant patients. Nausea and vomiting appear to be more frequent after oral administration than after injection.

In known drug addicts, Physeptone has produced withdrawal symptoms but these are mild. Tolerance and dependence of the morphine type may occur.

Use in pregnancy and lactation: There is no, or inadequate, evidence of safety in human pregnancy but the drug has been widely used for many years without apparent ill-consequence and animal studies have not shown any hazard. From theoretical considerations methadone is likely to be excreted in breast milk.

Toxicity and treatment of overdosage: Toxic doses of methadone cause unconsciousness, pin-point pupils, slow, shallow respiration, cyanosis and weak pulse. Often there is a 2–3 hour delay between ingestion and the appearance of symptoms. Lavage, dialysis and CNS stimulation are contra-indicated. Intravenous naloxone should be given and repeated at 5–10 minute intervals to attain full benefit.

Acidification of the urine will increase the rate of elimination of the drug via the kidney.

Pharmaceutical precautions *Tablets:* Store below 25°C.

Linctus: Store below 25°C, protect from light.

Injection: Store below 25°C, protect from light.

Physeptone Linctus may be diluted with Syrup BP.

Legal category CD (Sch 2), POM.

Package quantities *Physeptone Injection:* 10 mg in 1 ml ampoules. Boxes of 5 and 100 ampoules.

Physeptone Tablets: Bottle of 100 tablets.

Physeptone Linctus. Bottle of 500 ml.

Further information Nil.

Product licence numbers
Injection   0003/5100
Tablets   0003/5099
Linctus   0003/5232

POLYBACTRIN* SOLUBLE GU

Presentation One vial contains, in sterile dry powder:

Polymyxin B Sulphate BP   75,000 units
Neomycin Sulphate BP   20,000 units
Bacitracin BP 1968   1,000 units

Uses Antibacterial for bladder irrigation only.

To treat and prevent bacteriuria and prevent Gram-negative rod bacteraemia associated with the use of indwelling catheters. For temporary retention in the bladder following intermittent catheterisation and following cystoscopy.

Dosage and administration Reconstitute in 10 ml of isotonic saline then transfer to the appropriate volume of isotonic saline and mix. *Adults:* For continuous irrigation of the bladder for periods up to 10 days, a three-way catheter should be used. Two vials of powder dissolved in 500 ml of isotonic saline provide for a slow drip to be delivered over 24 hours. For patients with a urine output exceeding 2 litres per day, it is recommended that the drip rate be doubled.

Following intermittent catheterisation or cystoscopy, 1 vial of powder dissolved in 10–40 ml of isotonic saline may be introduced into the bladder and retained for an hour. This treatment may be used twice daily. See Contra-indications, warnings, etc.

Children: Proportionate reduction in dose according to weight.

Use in the elderly: No specific studies have been carried out in the elderly, however, it may be advisable to monitor renal function in these patients and if there is any impairment then caution should be exercised.

Contra-indications, warnings, etc
Contra-indications: Hypersensitivity to polymyxins, bacitracin or the neomycin group of antibiotics.

Precautions: The following statements take into account the possibility that the constituent drugs of Polybactrin Soluble GU, particularly neomycin, may be absorbed to a significant degree after topical application. There is some evidence that neomycin diffuses across, particularly the denuded, bladder mucosa, hence such factors should be taken into consideration in the use of Polybactrin Soluble GU.

Ototoxicity and nephrotoxicity have been reported in association with large or prolonged doses of neomycin; nephrotoxicity and neurotoxicity with polymyxin B; nephrotoxicity with inappropriate dosing of bacitracin. While these effects are normally reversible on cessation of therapy, the ototoxic effect of neomycin is not.

Due to the fact that if neomycin-related ototoxicity occurs there is a delay in onset of its appearance, it would be unwise to give a further course of Polybactrin Soluble GU before three months have elapsed from the prior course, by which time any such effects would be evident on examination.

In renal impairment the plasma clearance of neomycin is reduced, therefore a reduction in dose should be made that relates to the degree of renal impairment.

In cases where there is established partial nerve deafness and where a significant degree of neomycin absorption could occur it might be inappropriate to use any neomycin-containing product and treatment with an antibacterial without an aminoglycoside constituent should be used if possible.

Concurrent administration of other aminoglycoside antibiotics is not recommended.

As neomycin has a neuromuscular blocking effect, patients concurrently receiving other agents with a similar action should be observed for signs of possible respiratory insufficiency.

Side- and adverse effects: Allergic reactions following the topical application of neomycin have been reported in the literature, but such reactions following the application of polymyxin B and bacitracin are rare events.

Use in pregnancy and lactation: Due to a lack of detailed information the use of Polybactrin Soluble GU during pregnancy and lactation cannot be recommended in circumstances where significant systemic absorption of the active ingredients may occur.

Toxicity and treatment of overdosage: In the event of signs of toxicity developing following significant systemic absorption of the active ingredients of Polybactrin Soluble GU, the patient's general status, hearing acuity, renal function and neuromuscular function should be monitored and blood levels of polymyxin B, neomycin, and bacitracin determined. Serum levels of neomycin can be reduced by haemodialysis.

Pharmaceutical precautions Store below 25°C. Keep dry. Protect from light.

Solutions should be used within 24 hours of their preparation.

Legal category POM.

Package quantities Pack of 5 sterile vials.

Further information Nil.

Product licence number 0003/5055.

POLYBACTRIN* SPRAY

Presentation A sterile powder. Each 115 ml pressurised canister contains:

Polymyxin B Sulphate BP	150,000 units
Neomycin Sulphate BP	495,000 units
Zinc Bacitracin BP	37,500 units

in aerosol propellant.

Uses Topical antibacterial powder.

Prevention of wound infection in surgery. Treatment of infected skin.

Dosage and administration *Adults:* A thin, uniform spray should be applied to affected areas, as required. This can be obtained from a spray of about one second's duration to the wound surface at a distance of not less than 20 cm. The application of one can of spray daily for seven days should not be exceeded. After such a course, treatment should not be repeated for at least three months.

Children: The maximum dosage should be reduced in proportion to body weight.

Use in the elderly: No specific studies have been carried out in the elderly, however, it may be advisable to monitor renal function in these patients and if there is any impairment then caution should be exercised.

Contra-indications, warnings, etc
Contra-indications: Hypersensitivity to polymyxins, bacitracin or the neomycin group of antibiotics.

Precautions: The following statements take into account the possibility that the constituent drugs of Polybactrin Spray, particularly neomycin, may be absorbed to a significant degree after topical application.

Ototoxicity and nephrotoxicity have been reported in association with large or prolonged doses of neomycin; nephrotoxicity and neurotoxicity with polymyxin B; nephrotoxicity with inappropriate dosing of bacitracin. While these effects are normally reversible on cessation of therapy, the ototoxic effect of neomycin is not.

In cases where there is established partial nerve deafness and where a significant degree of neomycin absorption could occur it might be inappropriate to use any neomycin-containing product and treatment with an antibacterial without an aminoglycoside constituent should be used if possible.

In renal impairment the plasma clearance of neomycin is reduced, therefore a reduction in dose should be made that relates to the degree of renal impairment.

The inappropriate use of topical antibiotics has been associated with the emergence of resistant strains of bacteria.

The spray should not be used on large denuded areas (e.g. burns or ulcers) because of the risk of systemic absorption. Patients with hypostatic leg ulcers may have an increased sensitivity to a large number of topically applied drugs, including Neomycin.

Concurrent administration of other aminoglycoside antibiotics is not recommended.

As neomycin has a neuromuscular blocking effect, patients concurrently receiving other agents with a similar action should be observed for signs of possible respiratory insufficiency. As with all antibacterial preparations prolonged use may result in the overgrowth of non-susceptible organisms including fungi.

Side- and adverse effects: Allergic reactions following the topical application of neomycin have been reported in the literature, but such reactions following the application of polymyxin B and bacitracin are rare events.

Use in pregnancy and lactation: Due to a lack of detailed information the use of Polybactrin Spray during pregnancy and lactation cannot be recommended in circumstances where significant systemic absorption of the active ingredients may occur.

Toxicity and treatment of overdosage: In the event of signs of toxicity developing following significant systemic absorption of the active ingredients of Polybactrin Spray, the patient's general status, hearing acuity, renal function and neuromuscular function should be monitored and blood levels of polymyxin B, neomycin, and bacitracin determined. Serum levels of neomycin can be reduced by haemodialysis.

Pharmaceutical precautions Do not expose to temperatures over 25°C. Do not puncture or incinerate even after use. Do not autoclave.

Legal category POM.

Package quantities Pressurised aerosol powder spray, volume 115 ml.

Further information Nil.

Product licence number 0003/5056.

POLYFAX* OINTMENT

Presentation Polyfax Ointment contains 10,000 units of Polymyxin B Sulphate BP and 500 units of Zinc Bacitracin BP per gram, in a stable petrolatum base. The translucent ointment is off-white in colour.

Uses Topical antibacterial agent.

Polyfax Ointment is indicated for the treatment of infected wounds, burns, skin grafts, ulcers, pyoderma, sycosis barbae, impetigo, and in secondarily infected skin lesions of scabies, pediculosis, tinea pedis and contact and allergic dermatitis.

Dosage and administration *Adults:* Polyfax Ointment should be applied thinly over the affected area, which is best left exposed. Two or more applications a day may be necessary, depending on the severity of the condition.

Children: As for adults.

Use in the elderly: No specific studies have been carried out in the elderly, however, it may be advisable to monitor renal function in these patients and if there is any impairment then caution should be exercised.

Contra-indications, warnings, etc
Contra-indications: Hypersensitivity to bacitracin, polymyxins or cross-sensitising substances.

Precautions: The following statements take into account

the possibility that the constituent drugs of Polyfax Ointment may be absorbed to a significant degree after topical application.

Nephrotoxicity may result from the absorption of bacitracin, and nephrotoxicity and neurotoxicity from polymyxin B.

In patients with renal impairment the dosage of polymyxin B should be restricted to 10,000 to 15,000 units/kg/day, which is equivalent to about three tubes of Polyfax Ointment each day for an average adult.

As with all antibacterial preparations prolonged use may result in the overgrowth of non-susceptible organisms including fungi.

Side- and adverse effects: Allergic reactions following topical application of polymyxin B and zinc bacitracin have rarely been reported.

Use in pregnancy and lactation: Due to a lack of detailed information, the use of Polyfax Ointment during pregnancy and lactation cannot be recommended in circumstances where significant systemic absorption of the active ingredients may occur.

Toxicity and treatment of overdosage: In the unlikely event of significant systemic absorption of the active ingredients of Polyfax Ointment occurring, signs of neurotoxicity and nephrotoxicity may be noted. In such an event, the patient's general status and renal function should be monitored and blood levels of polymyxin B and zinc bacitracin determined.

Pharmaceutical precautions Store below 25°C.

Legal category POM.

Package quantities Tube of 20 g.

Further information Nil.

Product licence number 0003/5230.

POLYFAX* OPHTHALMIC OINTMENT

Presentation Polyfax Ophthalmic Ointment contains 10,000 units of Polymyxin B Sulphate BP and 500 units of Zinc Bacitracin BP per gram, in a stable petrolatum base. The ointment is pale yellow in colour.

Uses Topical antibacterial agent.

Polyfax Ophthalmic Ointment is indicated for the treatment of styes, conjunctivitis, keratitis, corneal ulcers and blepharitis. It may also be used prophylactically after the removal of foreign bodies from the eye, and in pre- and post-operative management.

Dosage and administration *Adults:* Polyfax Ophthalmic Ointment should be applied thinly to the affected area or inside the lower eyelid. Two or more applications a day depending on the severity of the condition.

Children: As for adults.

Use in the elderly: No special comment.

Contra-indications, warnings, etc
Contra-indications: Hypersensitivity to bacitracin or polymyxins.

Precautions: Polymyxin B and bacitracin are nephrotoxic if absorbed from open surfaces. However, these effects are unlikely with ocular administration.

Use in pregnancy and lactation: Due to a lack of detailed information, the use of Polyfax Ophthalmic Ointment during pregnancy and lactation cannot be recommended

in circumstances where significant systemic absorption of the active ingredients may occur.

Side- and adverse effects: Allergic reactions following topical application of polymyxin B and zinc bacitracin have rarely been reported.

Toxicity and treatment of overdosage: Not applicable.

Pharmaceutical precautions Store below 25°C.

Legal category POM.

Package quantities Tube of 4 g.

Further information Polyfax Ophthalmic Ointment is bland and non-irritating and is well tolerated by the sensitive structures of the eye.

Product licence number 0003/5229R.

PRO-VENT* ▼

Presentation Each Pro-Vent capsule contains 300 mg of Theophylline BP in specially formulated pellets to provide continuous therapeutic effect for 12 hours. Each capsule has a white opaque cap and a clear colourless body and is coded B7C.

Uses Pro-Vent capsules are indicated for the prevention and treatment of bronchial smooth-muscle constriction in patients with asthma and chronic bronchitis.

Dosage and administration *Adults and children over 12 years:* The usual dose is one capsule (300 mg) 12 hourly.

Children under 12 years: Formulation not applicable.

Theophylline pharmacokinetics are very variable between individuals. Smoking may decrease the duration of action of theophylline and some diseases such as heart or liver failure may increase plasma levels of theophylline. Dosage in an individual should be adjusted according to the response. If inadequate plasma levels are believed to be the cause of the failure to respond, dosage may be modified by the addition of a further 300 mg capsule either night or morning. When such large doses appear to be necessary and when excretion is likely to be delayed, increases should only be made after measurement of plasma theophylline levels.

Use in the elderly: No specific studies have been carried out using Pro-Vent, however, it may be advisable to monitor hepatic function in these patients and if there is impairment or evidence of heart failure, then serum levels shoud be monitored.

Pharmacology: Theophylline inhibits phosphodiesterase, leading to an increase in intracellular cyclic AMP which results in smooth-muscle relaxation.

Contra-indications, warnings, etc
Contra-indications: Theophylline is contra-indicated in patients who are sensitive to theophylline or to other xanthines.

Precautions: Caution should be exercised when prescribing theophylline for patients with heart failure or liver failure or chronic alcoholism. These diseases may reduce the clearance of theophylline and lead to higher than normal serum levels and a greater risk of toxicity. Theophylline should not be used with other preparations containing xanthine derivatives. Caution should be exercised in patients with peptic ulcer, cardiac arrhythmias, other cardiovascular diseases, hyperthyroidism, or hypertension.

Intravenous injections of aminophylline should not be given to patients who are receiving theophylline regularly by mouth. The total daily dose of theophylline may need to be reduced when converting from an immediate release to a sustained-release preparation.

Side- and adverse effects: Nausea, vomiting and anorexia may occur in some patients. Central nervous stimulation, headaches and insomnia are rarely seen unless plasma levels rise above 20 micrograms per ml. Convulsions may occur when blood levels are high. The correct use of a sustained-release preparation means that potentially toxic peaks in theophylline serum levels are avoided.

Drug interactions: Theophylline may interact with other xanthine derivatives or sympathomimetics to produce exaggerated effects. The excretion of lithium carbonate may be increased by theophylline. Increased theophylline plasma levels have been described when erythromycin, clindamycin, lincomycin or cimetidine are administered concurrently.

Use in pregnancy and lactation: No data are available on the use of Pro-Vent in human pregnancy. The excretion of theophylline in human milk is known to occur and care should be exercised in nursing mothers where theophylline therapy is felt to be indicated.

Toxicity and treatment of overdosage: Symptoms are likely to be similar to those described in the side- and adverse effects section above. In gross overdosage, especially in children, convulsions and death may occur without pre-existing signs of toxicity.

If overdosage is quickly discovered, an emetic should be administered. If signs of toxicity have already appeared, an emetic is not likely to be of value and a saline cathartic should be given to hasten transit of the capsule through the gut. If convulsions occur, they may be controlled by diazepam, and general supportive measures should be taken to maintain respiration and circulation.

Pharmaceutical precautions Store below 25°C.

Legal category P.

Package quantities Container of 100 capsules.

Further information The specially formulated pellets in Pro-Vent capsules give both rapid and predictable absorption along with prolonged therapeutic blood levels of theophylline for up to 12 hours.

Product licence number 0003/0167.

PURI-NETHOL* TABLETS

Presentation Each tablet contains 50 mg Mercaptopurine BP, fawn coloured, scored and coded Wellcome 04A.

Uses Cytotoxic agent.

Puri-Nethol is indicated for the treatment of acute leukaemia. It is of value in remission induction and is particularly indicated for maintenance therapy in acute lymphoblastic leukaemia and acute myelogenous leukaemia. Puri-Nethol is used in the treatment of chronic granulocytic leukaemia.

Dosage and administration For adults and children the usual dose is 2.5 mg/kg bodyweight per day, but the dose and duration of administration depend on the nature

and dosage of other cytotoxic agents given in conjunction with Puri-Nethol. The dosage should be carefully adjusted to suit the individual patient. Puri-Nethol has been used in various combination therapy schedules for acute leukaemia and the literature should be consulted for details. Consideration should be given to reducing the dosage in patients with impaired hepatic or renal function. When Zyloric (allopurinol) and mercaptopurine are administered concomitantly it is essential that only a quarter of the usual dose of mercaptopurine is given since Zyloric (allopurinol) decreases the rate of catabolism of mercaptopurine.

Use in the elderly: No specific studies have been carried out in the elderly, however, it is advisable to monitor renal and hepatic function in these patients, and if there is any impairment consideration should be given to reducing the Puri-Nethol dosage.

Contra-indications, warnings, etc
Contra-indications: In view of the seriousness of the indications there are no absolute contra-indications.

Precautions: Puri-Nethol is an active cytotoxic agent for use only under the direction of physicians experienced in the administration of such agents.

Since Puri-Nethol is strongly myelosuppressive full blood counts must be taken daily during remission induction. Patients must be carefully monitored during therapy.

Treatment with Puri-Nethol causes bone marrow suppression leading to leucopenia and thrombocytopenia.

The leucocyte and platelet counts continue to fall after treatment is stopped, so at the first sign of an abnormally large fall in the counts, treatment should be interrupted immediately.

Bone marrow suppression is reversible if Puri-Nethol is withdrawn early enough.

During remission induction in acute myelogenous leukaemia the patient may frequently have to survive a period of relative bone marrow aplasia and it is important that adequate supportive facilities are available.

Puri-Nethol is hepatotoxic and liver function tests should be monitored weekly during treatment. More frequent monitoring may be advisable in those with pre-existing liver disease or receiving other potentially hepatotoxic therapy. The patient should be instructed to discontinue Puri-Nethol immediately if jaundice becomes apparent.

During remission induction when rapid cell lysis is occurring, uric acid levels in blood and urine should be monitored as hyperuricaemia and/or hyperuricosuria may develop, with the risk of uric acid nephropathy.

Puri-Nethol in common with other antimetabolites is potentially mutagenic and chromosome damage has been reported in rats and man.

In view of its action on cellular deoxyribonucleic acid (DNA) mercaptopurine is potentially carcinogenic and consideration should be given to the theoretical risk of carcinogenesis with this treatment.

When Zyloric [allopurinol] and Puri-Nethol are administered concomitantly it is essential that only a quarter of the usual dose of Puri-Nethol is given since Zyloric decreases the rate of catabolism of Puri-Nethol.

Inhibition of the anticoagulant effect of warfarin, when given with Puri-Nethol, has been reported.

It is advised that care be taken when handling or halving these tablets not to contaminate hands or to inspire drug.

Side- and adverse effects: The main side-effect of treatment with Puri-Nethol is bone marrow suppression leading to leucopenia and thrombocytopenia. Puri-Nethol is hepatotoxic in animals and man. The histological findings in man have shown hepatic necrosis and biliary stasis. The incidence of hepatotoxicity varies considerably and can occur with any dose but more frequently when the recommended dose of 2.5 mg/kg bodyweight daily is exceeded. Monitoring of liver function tests may allow early detection of liver toxicity. This is usually reversible if Puri-Nethol therapy is stopped soon enough. However, irreversible liver damage leading to a fatal outcome has occurred.

Anorexia, nausea and vomiting have occasionally been noted.

Oral ulceration has been reported during Puri-Nethol therapy and rarely intestinal ulceration has occurred.

Rare complications are drug fever and skin rash.

Use in pregnancy and lactation: Puri-Nethol is embryotoxic in rats. This effect is dose dependent.

Normal offspring have been born after Puri-Nethol therapy during human pregnancy, but abortion, prematurity and malformation have been reported. The small numbers involved do not allow an evaluation of the degree of risk of Puri-Nethol therapy during pregnancy and the possible hazard to the foetus must be balanced against the expected benefit in individual cases.

Mothers receiving Puri-Nethol should not breast feed.

Toxicity and treatment of overdosage: The principal toxic effect is on the bone marrow and haematological toxicity is likely to be more profound with chronic overdosage than with a single ingestion of Puri-Nethol. The risk of overdosage is also increased when Zyloric is being given concomitantly with Puri-Nethol. As there is no known antidote the blood picture should be closely monitored and general supportive measures, together with appropriate blood transfusion, instituted if necessary.

Pharmaceutical precautions Store below 25°C. Keep dry, protect from light.

Legal category POM.

Package quantities Bottle of 25 tablets.

Further information Puri-Nethol is an analogue of adenine and hypoxanthine, and microbiological studies have shown it to be an antagonist of these; its mode of action differs thus from that of the folic acid antagonists.

Product licence number 0003/5227.

SUDAFED* TABLETS
SUDAFED* ELIXIR

Presentation Each tablet contains 60 mg Pseudoephedrine Hydrochloride BP, and is white in colour and coded 'Wellcome S7A'.

Each 5 ml of deep pink elixir contains 30 mg Pseudoephedrine Hydrochloride BP.

Uses Nasal and sinus decongestant.

Dosage and administration *Adults and children over 12 years:* 1 tablet or 10 ml three times a day.

Children: 6–12 years: 5 ml elixir three times a day.

2–5 years: 2.5 ml elixir three times a day.

Sudafed elixir may be diluted with Syrup BP.

Use in the elderly: No specific studies have been carried out in the elderly, but Sudafed has been widely used in older people. However, it may be advisable to monitor renal and hepatic function, and if there is any impairment then caution should be exercised.

Pharmacology: Pseudoephedrine has direct and indirect sympathomimetic activity and is an orally effective upper respiratory tract decongestant. Pseudoephedrine is substantially less potent than ephedrine in producing both tachycardia and elevation in systolic blood pressure and considerably less potent in causing stimulation of the central nervous system.

Contra-indications, warnings, etc
Contra-indications: Contra-indicated in patients who have previously shown intolerance to pseudoephedrine. It is contra-indicated in persons under treatment with monoamine oxidase inhibitors and within two weeks of stopping such treatment.

Precautions: Sudafed should be used with caution in patients with cardiovascular disorders, including hypertension. The effect of antihypertensive agents which modify sympathetic activity may be partially reversed by Sudafed.

Caution should also be exercised in patients taking other sympathomimetic agents, such as decongestants, appetite suppressants and amphetamine-like psychostimulants. The effects of a single dose on the blood pressure of these patients should be observed before recommending repeated or unsupervised treatment.

As with other sympathomimetic agents, caution should be exercised in patients with prostatic enlargement or bladder dysfunction.

In severe hepatic or renal dysfunction a single dose of Sudafed should be given and the patient's response used as a guide to the dosage requirement for further administration.

The antibacterial agent furazolidone is known to cause a progressive inhibition of monoamine oxidase and although there are no reports of hypertensive crises having occurred, it should not be administered concurrently with Sudafed.

Side- and adverse effects: Side-effects are uncommon. In some patients pseudoephedrine may occasionally cause insomnia. Rarely, sleep disturbances and hallucinations have been reported.

A fixed drug eruption to pseudoephedrine, taking the form of erythematous nummular patches has been reported, but is a rare occurrence.

Urinary retention has been reported in patients in whom prostatic enlargement could have been an important predisposing factor.

Use in pregnancy and lactation: No data are available on the use of Sudafed in human pregnancy. Pseudoephedrine is excreted in breast milk.

Toxicity and treatment of overdosage: As with other sympathomimetic agents, symptoms of overdosage include irritability, convulsions, palpitations, hypertension and difficulty in micturition. Gastric lavage and supportive measures for respiration and circulation should be performed if indicated. Convulsions should be controlled with an anticonvulsant. Catheterisation of the bladder may be necessary. Alpha-adrenergic blockade may be required to treat hypertensive crises and beta-adrenergic blockade for the control of supraventricular dysrhythmias.

If desired, the elimination of pseudoephedrine can be accelerated by acid diuresis or by dialysis.

Pharmaceutical precautions Store below 25°C in a dry place. Elixir should be protected from light.

Legal category P.

Package quantities *Sudafed tablets:* Container of 100 tablets. 12 tablets in blister strips of 6.
Sudafed elixir: Bottles of 100 ml and 1 litre.

Further information Nil.

Product licence numbers
Tablets   0003/5061.
Elixir   0003/5062.

SUDAFED* SA ▼

Presentation Each Sudafed SA capsule has a red cap and a clear colourless body, is marked Sudafed SA, and contains 120 mg Pseudoephedrine Hydrochloride USP in specially formulated pellets designed to provide continuous therapeutic effect for 12 hours.

Uses For the symptomatic relief of allergic rhinitis, vasomotor rhinitis, and congestion associated with the common cold.

Dosage and administration
Adults and children over 12 years: One capsule every 12 hours.
Children 6–12 years: It is recommended that Sudafed Elixir be used.
Use in the elderly: No specific studies have been carried out in the elderly, however, it may be advisable to monitor renal function in these patients and if there is any impairment then caution should be exercised.
Pharmacology: Pseudoephedrine has direct and indirect sympathomimetic activity and is an orally effective upper respiratory tract decongestant.
    Pseudoephedrine is substantially less potent than ephedrine in producing both tachycardia and elevation in systolic blood pressure and considerably less potent in causing central nervous system stimulation.

Contra-indications, warnings, etc
Contra-indications: Contra-indicated in patients who have previously shown intolerance to pseudoephedrine and in persons under treatment with monoamine oxidase inhibitors or within two weeks of stopping such treatment.
Precautions: Although pseudoephedrine has virtually no pressor effect in patients with normal blood pressure, Sudafed SA should be used with caution in patients with cardiovascular disorders, including hypertension. The effect of antihypertensive agents which modify sympathetic activity may be partially reversed with Sudafed SA.
    Caution should be exercised in patients taking other sympathomimetic agents, such as decongestants, appetite suppressants and amphetamine-like psychostimulants. The effects of a single dose on the blood pressure of these patients should be observed before recommending repeated or unsupervised treatment.
    As with other sympathomimetic agents, caution should be exercised in patients with prostatic enlargement or bladder dysfunction.
    In severe hepatic or renal dysfunction a single dose of Sudafed SA should be given and the patient's response used as a guide to the dosage requirement for further administration.

    The antibacterial agent furazolidone is known to cause a progressive inhibition of monoamine oxidase and, although there are no reports of a hypertensive crisis having occurred, it should not be administered concurrently with Sudafed SA.
Side- and adverse effects: Side-effects are uncommon. In some patients pseudoephedrine may occasionally cause insomnia. Rarely, sleep disturbances and hallucinations have been reported. A fixed drug eruption to pseudoephedrine, taking the form of erythematous nummular patches, has been reported, but should be regarded as a rare occurrence.
    Urinary retention has been reported in patients in whom prostatic enlargement could have been an important predisposing factor.
Use in pregnancy and lactation: No data are available on the use of Sudafed SA in human pregnancy. Pseudoephedrine is excreted in breast milk.
Toxicity and treatment of overdosage: As with other sympathomimetic agents, symptoms of overdosage include irritability, convulsions, palpitations, hypertension and difficulty in micturition. Gastric lavage and supportive measures for respiration and circulation should be performed if indicated. Convulsions should be controlled with an anti-convulsant. Catheterization of the bladder may be necessary.
    Alpha adrenergic blockade may be required to treat hypertensive crises and beta adrenergic blockage for the control of supraventricular dysrhythmias. If desired, the elimination of pseudoephedrine can be accelerated by acid diuresis or by dialysis.

Pharmaceutical precautions Store below 25°C in a dry place. Protect from light.

Legal category POM.

Package quantities Container of 100 capsules.

Further information Nil.

Product licence number 0003/0158.

SUDAFED*-CO TABLETS

Presentation White scored tablets coded 'Wellcome A7C' containing 500 mg Paracetamol BP and 60 mg Pseudoephedrine Hydrochloride BP.

Uses For the relief of conditions where upper respiratory congestion is associated with pyrexia or pain. These conditions include the common cold, influenza, sinusitis and nasopharyngitis.

Dosage and administration *Adults and children over 12 years:* One tablet three times a day.
Children 6–12 years: Half a tablet three times a day.
Children under 6 years: Not recommended.
Use in the elderly: No specific studies have been carried out in the elderly, but Sudafed-Co has been widely used in older people. However, it may be advisable to monitor renal and hepatic function, and if there is any impairment then caution should be exercised.
Pharmacology: Pseudoephedrine has direct and indirect sympathomimetic activity and is an orally effective upper respiratory tract decongestant. Pseudoephedrine is substantially less potent than ephedrine in producing both tachycardia and elevation in systolic blood pressure and considerably less potent in causing stimulation of the central nervous system. Paracetamol provides analgesic

and antipyretic activity, probably by antagonising cerebral prostaglandin synthetase.

Contra-indications, warnings, etc

Contra-indications: Contra-indicated in patients with a known hypersensitivity to paracetamol or pseudoephedrine. It is contra-indicated in persons under treatment with monoamine oxidase inhibitors and within two weeks of stopping such treatment.

Precautions: Sudafed-Co should be used with caution in patients with cardiovascular disorders including hypertension. The effect of antihypertensive agents which modify sympathetic activity may be partially reversed by Sudafed-Co.

Also caution should be exercised in patients taking other sympathomimetic agents, such as decongestants, appetite suppressants and amphetamine-like psychostimulants. The effects of a single dose on the blood pressure of these patients should be observed before recommending repeated or unsupervised treatment.

As with other sympathomimetic agents, caution should be exercised in patients with prostatic enlargement or bladder dysfunction.

In severe hepatic or renal dysfunction a single dose of Sudafed-Co should be given and the patient's response used as a guide to the dosage requirement for further administration.

The antibacterial agent furazolidone is known to cause a progressive inhibition of monoamine oxidase and, although there are no reports of a hypertensive crisis having occurred, it should not be administered concurrently with Sudafed-Co.

Drug interactions: In cases of paracetamol overdosage, liver microsomal inducing agents such as barbiturates, tricyclic antidepressants, and alcohol may increase the hepatotoxicity of paracetamol.

Side- and adverse effects: Side-effects are uncommon. In some patients pseudoephedrine may occasionally cause insomnia. Rarely, sleep disturbances and hallucinations have been reported. A fixed drug eruption to pseudoephedrine taking the form of erythematous nummular patches has been reported but is a rare occurrence. Paracetamol has been widely used and reports of adverse reactions are rare, and are generally associated with overdosage.

Isolated cases of chronic hepatic necrosis, acute pancreatitis or nephrotoxicity have been reported, after overdosage or prolonged administration of paracetamol. Isolated cases of thrombocytopenic purpura, methaemoglobinaemia, haemolytic anaemia, and agranulocytosis have been recorded. Nephrotoxic effects are uncommon and have not been reported in association with therapeutic doses, except after prolonged administration.

Urinary retention has been reported in patients in whom prostatic enlargement could have been an important predisposing factor.

Use in pregnancy and lactation: No data are available on the use of Sudafed-Co in human pregnancy. Pseudoephedrine is excreted in breast milk.

Toxicity and treatment of overdosage: Pallor, nausea and vomiting may occur due to the paracetamol component. With pseudoephedrine, symptoms of overdosage may include irritation, convulsions, palpitations, hypertension, and difficulty in micturition. Hepatoxicity may be a complication from the paracetamol content but may not be apparent from 24 hours–6 days after ingestion.

Overdosage should, therefore, be treated promptly by gastric lavage followed by i.v. N-acetylcysteine, or oral methionine. Additional therapy (further methionine or i.v. cysteamine or i.v. N-acetylcysteine) is normally considered in the light of blood paracetamol content and the time elapsed since ingestion. Such therapy is probably best undertaken in a specialised unit. Supportive measures for respiration and circulation should be performed if indicated. Convulsions should be controlled with an anticonvulsant. Catheterisation of the bladder may be necessary. Alpha-adrenergic blockade may be required to treat hypertensive crises and beta-adrenergic blockade for the control of supraventricular dysrhythmias. If desired, the elimination of pseudoephedrine can be accelerated by acid diuresis or by dialysis.

Pharmaceutical precautions Store below 25°C in a dry place. Protect from light.

Legal category P.

Package quantities 12 tablets in blister strips of 6.

Further information Nil.

Product licence number 0003/0157.

SUDAFED* EXPECTORANT

Presentation Each 5 ml of orange red syrup contains 100 mg Guaiphenesin BP and 30 mg Pseudoephedrine Hydrochloride BP.

Uses Conditions where an expectorant and upper respiratory tract decongestant are required.

Dosage and administration *Adults and children over 12 years:* 10 ml three times a day.

6–12 years: 5 ml three times a day.

2–5 years: 2.5 ml three times a day.

May be diluted with Syrup BP.

Use in the elderly: No specific studies have been carried out in the elderly, but Sudafed Expectorant has been widely used in older people. However, it may be advisable to monitor renal and hepatic function, and if there is any impairment then caution should be exercised.

Pharmacology: Pseudoephedrine has direct and indirect sympathomimetic activity and is an orally effective upper respiratory tract decongestant. Pseudoephedrine is substantially less potent than ephedrine in producing both tachycardia and elevation in systolic blood pressure and considerably less potent in causing stimulation of the central nervous system. On the basis of widespread and long established clinical use, guaiphenesin is recognised as an expectorant in bronchitis.

Contra-indications, warnings, etc

Contra-indications: Contra-indicated in patients who have previously shown intolerance to pseudoephedrine or guaiphenesin. Sudafed Expectorant is contra-indicated in persons under treatment with monoamine oxidase inhibitors and within two weeks of stopping such treatment.

Precautions: Although pseudoephedrine has virtually no pressor effect in patients with normal blood pressure, Sudafed Expectorant should be used with caution in patients with cardiovascular disorders, including hypertension. The effect of antihypertensive agents, which modify sympathetic activity may be partially reversed by Sudafed Expectorant.

Also caution should be exercised in patients taking

other sympathomimetic agents, such as decongestants, appetite suppressants and amphetamine-like psychostimulants. The effects of a single dose of Sudafed Expectorant on the blood pressure of these patients should be observed before recommending repeated or unsupervised treatment.

As with other sympathomimetic agents, caution should be exercised in patients with prostatic enlargement or bladder dysfunction.

In severe hepatic or renal dysfunction a single dose of Sudafed Expectorant should be given and the patient's response used as a guide to the dosage requirement for further administration.

The antibacterial agent furazolidone is known to cause a progressive inhibition of monoamine oxidase and, although there are no reports of hypertensive crises having occurred, it should not be administered concurrently with Sudafed Expectorant.

Side- and adverse effects: Side-effects are uncommon. In some patients pseudoephedrine may occasionally cause insomnia. Rarely, sleep disturbances and hallucinations have been reported.

A fixed drug eruption to pseudoephedrine, taking the form of erythematous nummular patches has been reported, but is a rare occurrence.

Use in pregnancy and lactation: No data are available on the use of Sudafed Expectorant in human pregnancy. Pseudoephedrine is excreted in breast milk.

Toxicity and treatment of overdosage: As with other sympathomimetic agents, symptoms of overdosage include irritability, convulsions, palpitations, hypertension and difficulty in micturition. Gastric lavage and supportive measures for respiration and circulation should be performed if indicated. Convulsions should be controlled with an anticonvulsant. Catheterisation of the bladder may be necessary.

Alpha-adrenergic blockade may be required to treat hypertensive crises and beta-adrenergic blockade for the control of supraventricular dysrhythmias. If desired, the elimination of pseudoephedrine can be accelerated by acid diuresis or by dialysis.

Pharmaceutical precautions Store below 25°C. Protect from light. Do not refrigerate.

Legal category P.

Package quantities Bottles of 100 ml and 1 litre.

Further information Nil.

Product licence number 0003/0145.

TRACRIUM* INJECTION ▼

Presentation Tracrium injection contains atracurium besylate, 10 mg per ml, as a clear, faint-yellow solution for intravenous administration. Each 2.5 ml ampoule contains 25 mg atracurium besylate and each 5 ml ampoule contains 50 mg atracurium besylate.

Uses Tracrium is a highly selective, competitive (nondepolarising) neuromuscular blocking agent.

It is used in anaesthesia to relax skeletal muscles during a wide range of surgical procedures and to facilitate controlled ventilation. Tracrium is highly suitable for endotracheal intubation especially where subsequent muscle relaxation is required. Tracrium is suitable for maintenance of muscle relaxation in Caesarian Section.

Tracrium is suitable for administration by continuous infusion to maintain neuromuscular block during long surgical procedures.

Metabolism: Tracrium is degraded spontaneously mainly by a non-enzymatic decomposition process (Hofmann elimination) which occurs at plasma pH and at body temperature and produces breakdown products which are inactive.

Tests with plasma from patients with pseudo-cholinesterase deficiency show that the inactivation of Tracrium proceeds unaffected. It is possible that some decomposition may occur by non-specific plasma esterases.

The termination of the neuromuscular blocking action of Tracrium is not dependent on metabolism and excretion by the liver or kidneys. The duration of action is therefore unlikely to be affected by impaired renal, hepatic or circulatory function.

Dosage and administration Tracrium is administered by intravenous injection.

The dosage range recommended for adults is 0.3–0.6 mg/kg depending on the duration of full block required and will provide relaxation for about 15–35 minutes.

Endotracheal intubation can usually be accomplished within 90 seconds of intravenous injection of 0.5–0.6 mg/kg.

Full block can be prolonged with supplementary doses of 0.1–0.2 mg/kg as required. Successive supplementary dosing does not give rise to accumulation.

The neuromuscular block produced by Tracrium can be rapidly and permanently reversed by standard doses of neostigmine, which should be preceded by the administration of atropine.

Recovery from the end of full block without the use of neostigmine occurs in about 35 minutes as measured by the restoration of the tetanic response to 95% of normal neuromuscular function.

Children: The dosage in children over the age of 1 year is similar to that in adults on a mg/kg basis.

Elderly and high-risk patients: Tracrium may be used at standard dosage in elderly patients and in those with respiratory, renal or hepatic failure.

Continuous infusion: Tracrium is suitable for administration by continuous infusion at rates of 0.005–0.01 mg/kg/minute (0.3–0.6 mg/kg/hour) to maintain neuromuscular block during long surgical procedures. Tracrium maintains acceptable physical and chemical stability in daylight at concentrations of 0.5 mg/ml and above at temperatures of up to 30°C for:
4 hours in Compound Sodium Lactate Intravenous Infusion BP.
8 hours in Ringer's Injection USP; Glucose Intravenous Infusion BP 5% w/v; or 0.18% w/v Sodium Chloride and 4% w/v Glucose Intravenous Infusion BP.
And for up to 24 hours in Sodium Chloride Intravenous Infusion BP.

Tracrium can be administered by infusion during cardiopulmonary bypass surgery, at the recommended infusion rates. Induced hypothermia to a body temperature of 25°C to 26°C reduces the rate of inactivation of atracurium, therefore full neuromuscular block may be maintained by approximately half the original infusion rates at these temperatures.

Contra-indications, warnings, etc
Contra-indications: There are no contra-indications to the use of Tracrium except known hypersensitivity to the drug.

Precautions. In common with all the other neuromuscular blocking agents, Tracrium paralyses the respiratory muscles as well as other skeletal muscles. Therefore it should be administered only by or under the close supervision of an anaesthetist and adequate facilities must be available for endotracheal intubation and artificial ventilation.

Tracrium should be used with caution in patients with myasthenia gravis, other neuromuscular disease and severe electrolyte disorders in which potentiation of other non-depolarising agents has been noted.

Patients with severe cardiovascular disease may be more susceptible to the effects of transient hypotension. In these patients slow intravenous injection in divided doses is recommended.

Drug interactions: The neuromuscular block produced by Tracrium may be increased by the concomitant use of inhalation anaesthetics such as halothane.

Neuromuscular block produced by Tracrium may be increased by the concomitant use of aminoglycosides (such as neomycin) and polypeptide antibiotics (such as polymyxin).

A depolarising muscle relaxant such as suxamethonium chloride should not be administered to prolong the neuromuscular blocking effects of non-depolarising blocking agents such as atracurium, as this may result in a 'mixed block' which is difficult to reverse with anticholinesterase drugs.

Side- and adverse effects: Tracrium does not have significant vagal or ganglionic blocking properties in the recommended dosage range. Consequently, Tracrium will not counteract the bradycardia produced by many anaesthetic agents, and by vagal stimulation during surgery.

In common with most neuromuscular blocking agents the potential exists for histamine release in susceptible patients. Associated with the use of Tracrium there have been reports of skin flushing, and transient hypotension which have been attributed to histamine release. Rarely, bronchospasm and, very rarely, anaphylactoid reactions have also been reported.

Use in pregnancy and obstetrics: Although animal studies have indicated that Tracrium has no adverse effects on foetal development, nevertheless, as with all neuromuscular blocking agents it should be used with caution in pregnant women.

Tracrium may be used to maintain neuromuscular relaxation in Caesarean section as atracurium does not cross the placenta in clinically significant amounts.

Toxicity and treatment of overdosage: In the event of overdosage or delayed recovery, the patient should be given atropine and neostigmine and maintained on artificial ventilation until spontaneous respiration returns.

Pharmaceutical precautions Tracrium must not be mixed in the same syringe with thiopentone or any alkaline agent, as the high pH will inactivate Tracrium.

Where a small vein is selected as the injection site, Tracrium should be flushed through the vein after injection. Where other anaesthetic drugs are administered through the same in-dwelling needle or cannula as Tracrium, it is important that each drug is flushed through with Water for Injections BP or physiological saline.

Store at 2–8°C. Protect from light. Do not freeze. Short periods at temperatures up to 30°C are permissible but only to allow transportation or temporary storage outside a cold store. It is estimated that an 8% loss of potency

would occur if Tracrium Injection was stored at 30°C for one month.

Legal category POM.

Package quantities Box of 5 × 2.5 ml ampoules (each ampoule containing 25 mg atracurium besylate).

Box of 5 × 5 ml ampoules (each ampoule containing 50 mg atracurium besylate).

Further information Tracrium has no effect on the intra-ocular pressure, which makes it suitable for use in ophthalmic surgery.

Variations in the blood pH and body temperature of the patient within the physiological range will not significantly alter the duration of action of Tracrium.

Product licence number 0003/0166.

TUBARINE* INJECTION

Presentation Each ampoule of Tubarine Injection (miscible) contains 15 mg of Tubocurarine Chloride BP in 1.5 ml isotonic solution.

Uses Tubarine is used to relax skeletal muscles to facilitate a wide range of surgical, obstetric, and orthopaedic procedures under general anaesthesia. It is similarly used for investigatory procedures and in the intensive care of patients undergoing mechanical ventilation.

Dosage and administration Tubarine should be administered by intravenous injection over a period of about one minute.

Flaccid paralysis of skeletal muscle develops to reach a maximum within three to five minutes which persists for between twenty and forty minutes. This is followed by a recovery period during which full neuromuscular function progressively returns. The restoration of full neuromuscular function is usually accelerated by the injection of an anticholinesterase agent such as neostigmine (neostigmine is usually preceded by an injection of atropine). Tubarine does not affect the level of consciousness.

Since the dose response to Tubarine varies considerably from one patient to another the physician has to adjust the dose to meet each individual patient's needs.

The average dose for a 70 kg man is between 15 and 25 mg, but in individual patients the effective dose level may be as low as 10 mg or as high as 40 mg. Supplementary doses of 5 mg may be administered for the maintenance of muscle relaxation at intervals of between 25 and 60 minutes as necessary.

The average initial dose of Tubarine in children is between 0.3 and 0.5 mg/kg bodyweight and in neonates 0.25 mg/kg bodyweight. Supplementary doses of 20% of the initial dose may be administered at intervals to maintain muscle relaxation.

Use in the elderly: The hypotension produced by Tubarine is more common in the aged and is potentiated by dose and alveolar concentration of halothane and nitrous oxide. Use with caution in renal impairment.

Contra-indications, warnings, etc Tubarine is contra-indicated in persons who are known to be hypersensitive to d-tubocurarine.

Malignant hyperthermia.

Precautions: Tubarine should be administered only by or under close supervision of an anaesthetist familiar with its action, characteristics and hazards, who is skilled in the management of artificial respiration and only where there are adequate facilities for immediate endotracheal intubation with administration of oxygen by intermittent positive pressure ventilation.

Patients with myasthenia gravis have been shown to be, on average, 5.5 times as sensitive to d-tubocurarine as non-myasthenic subjects. Marked sensitivity to d-tubocurarine has also been shown in patients with myasthenic syndrome complicating bronchial carcinoma, carcinomatous neuropathy, amyotrophic lateral sclerosis and von Recklinghausen's disease. The effect of d-tubocurarine is also prolonged in Duchenne muscular dystrophy.

Use in pregnancy and lactation: Tubarine in normal therapeutic doses does not cross the placental barrier in sufficient amounts to affect the respiration of the infant. It has not been established, however, that Tubarine is free from possible adverse effects on a pregnancy or the foetus. It should not be administered to pregnant women unless the potential benefit outweighs possible hazards.

A case has been reported in which arthrogryposis multiplex congenita followed the use of d-tubocurarine for a 10 day period at the 10th–12th week of pregnancy.

Side- and adverse effects: The most frequent side-effect of Tubarine is hypotension which is usually transient. A rapid intravenous injection of a large dose may cause a precipitous fall in blood pressure. Flushing of the skin of the neck and upper chest is not uncommon. This was unrelated to the degree of hypotension in individual patients. Hypotension is probably due to a combination of factors including peripheral vasodilation resulting from curare-induced release of histamine and diminished venous return from skeletal muscle.

Curare has the capacity to release histamine but signs of histamine release other than hypotension are rarely evoked by the therapeutic doses. Nevertheless Tubarine can provoke bronchospasm and circulatory collapse particularly in patients with a history of allergic disposition; asthma or urticaria have been reported as a rare complication.

The magnitude and/or duration of neuromuscular blockade due to Tubarine may be increased by the following:

1. Inhalation anaesthetics, for example isoflurane and halothane.
2. Various antibiotics including neomycin, streptomycin, dihydrostreptomycin, kanamycin, gentamicin, colistin, polymyxin B, certain tetracyclines and possibly bacitracin, clindamycin and lincomycin.
3. Other neuromuscular blocking agents.
4. Administration of Tubarine during the previous 24 hours.
5. Propranolol and other beta-blockers.
6. Frusemide, and possibly mannitol.
7. Myasthenic conditions such as myasthenia gravis (see Precautions) myasthenic syndrome complicating bronchial carcinoma, carcinomatous neuropathy, amyotrophic lateral sclerosis and multiple neurofibromatosis.
8. Respiratory acidoses.

Cooling decreases the magnitude of the neuromuscular blockade produced by Tubarine. Thus, in patients after operations under hypothermia, prolonged curarisation could occur on rewarming.

Decreased response to Tubarine may occur in patients with hepatic impairment or respiratory alkalosis.

Two cases have been reported in which malignant hyperpyrexia may have been triggered by d-tubocurarine.

Toxicity and treatment of overdosage: The important responses to overdosage are prolonged apnoea, cardiovascular collapse, and the effects of histamine release. The respiratory paralysis should be treated by the continuation of positive pressure artificial respiration with oxygen and maintenance of a patent airway until complete recovery of normal respiration is assured. Recovery may be hastened by the administration of neostigmine methyl sulphate, 2.5 mg to 5 mg. Atropine sulphate, 0.6–1.2 mg should be injected simultaneously or immediately before the neostigmine. Neostigmine antagonises the skeletal muscle blocking action but it may aggravate other side-effects of Tubarine such as hypotension and/or bronchospasm. Sympathomimetic amines may be given to support the blood pressure.

In neonates, one hour after the recommended initial dose, reversal may be obtained with atropine 0.018 mg/kg and neostigmine 0.08 mg/kg.

If neuromuscular blockade cannot be adequately reversed by the use of an anticholinesterase, then measures should be taken to maintain respiration and, if necessary, the circulation until neuromuscular function returns. Sedation may also be required since consciousness is retained.

Pharmaceutical precautions Although not recommended, up to 1 ml of Tubarine (Miscible) Injection may be mixed with not less than 20 ml of 2.5% thiopentone; the solution should be prepared immediately prior to injection and used only if it remains clear. Tubarine (Miscible) Injection should not be mixed with any other anaesthetic agents because differences in pH could cause precipitation or there may be chemical incompatibility.

Store below 25°C. Do not freeze. Protect from light.

Legal category POM.

Package quantities Box of 5 × 1.5 ml ampoules.

Further information Nil.

Product licence number 0003/5065.

VALOID* TABLETS
VALOID* INJECTION

Presentation Valoid Tablets each contain 50 mg Cyclizine Hydrochloride BP, scored, coded 'Wellcome T4A', white in colour.

Valoid Injection contains 50 mg cyclizine lactate in each 1 ml ampoule.

Uses Anti-emetic. In the prevention and treatment of nausea and vomiting and drug-induced vomiting, especially that associated with the administration of narcotic drugs. It has been widely and effectively used in the prophylaxis and treatment of motion sickness, in the symptomatic management of vertigo and labyrinthine disorders (Meniere's syndrome), in postoperative vomiting and in radiation sickness, particularly when this is associated with the treatment of breast cancer.

Dosage and administration *Valoid Tablets: Adults and children over 10 years:* 1 tablet three times daily.
Children 1–10 years: ½ tablet three times daily.
Valoid Injection: Adults: 50 mg intramuscularly or intravenously three times daily.

Use in the elderly: No specific information is available.

For the prevention of postoperative nausea and vomiting, administer the first dose 15–20 minutes before the anticipated end of surgery.

Contra-indications, warnings, etc

Contra-indications: Some animal studies are interpreted as indicating that cyclizine may be teratogenic. The relevance of these studies to the human situation is not known, but in the absence of any certain human data the use of Valoid in pregnancy is not advised.

Precautions: Drowsiness, dryness of the mouth and blurred vision may occur in a small number of patients. It is, therefore, advisable that patients should determine their responses before driving or operating machinery. In some patients the action of Valoid may be potentiated by alcohol and other central sedatives.

Valoid may increase the side-effects of anticholinergic drugs and enhance the soporific effects of pethidine.

Side- and adverse effects: Intravenous cyclizine may increase the incidence of tremors and muscle movements if given before methohexitone anaesthesia.

Although very rare, anaphylaxis of a severe degree has been reported with the co-administration of intravenous cyclizine and propanidid.

Single case reports of fixed drug eruption, generalised chorea and hypersensitivity hepatitis have been reported.

Use in pregnancy and lactation: See contra-indications above. No information is available on the use of cyclizine in lactating mothers.

Toxicity and treatment of overdosage: A child of 3 years is known to have survived taking 8×50 mg tablets. Toxicity may comprise drowsiness, dizziness, convulsions, hyperpyrexia and respiratory depression. Rarely, agitation, ataxia and hallucinations may occur. Gastric lavage and general supportive measures are indicated. Control any convulsions with diazepam injections.

Pharmaceutical precautions *Injection:* Store below 25°C. Protect from light.
Tablets: Store below 25°C.

Legal category Tablets P.
Injection POM.

Package quantities *Valoid Tablets:* Bottle of 100.
Valoid Injection: Box of 5 ampoules.

Further information Nil.

Product licence numbers
Tablets 0003/5213.
Injection 0003/5212.

ZYLORIC* TABLETS
ZYLORIC-300* TABLETS

Presentation Zyloric Tablets each contain 100 mg Allopurinol BP imprinted Zyloric 100 and coded U4A. Creamy white in colour. Zyloric-300 Tablets each contain 300 mg Allopurinol BP imprinted Zyloric 300 and coded C9B. Creamy white in colour.

Uses

1. *Conditions of excess body urate including gout:* Zyloric is used to reduce urate levels in the body when these levels are excessive (serum is theoretically saturated with urate at a concentration between 0.38– 0.42 mmol/l (6.4–7.0 mg%)). The higher levels seen in practice may be accounted for by (a) the formation of supersaturated solutions: (b) protein binding of urate. Excess body urate may be indicated by hyperuricaemia and/or hyperuricosuria. It may lead to deposition of urate in the tissues or it may be present with no obvious signs or symptoms.

The main clinical manifestations of urate deposition are gouty arthritis, skin tophi and/or renal involvement: Excess body urate is frequently of idiopathic origin but may also be found in association with other conditions including the following: neoplastic disease and its treatment; certain enzyme disorders (in particular Lesch-Nyhan syndrome); renal failure; renal calculus formation; diuretic therapy and psoriasis.

2. *Calcium renal lithiasis:* Zyloric is of benefit in the prophylaxis and treatment of calcium renal lithiasis in patients with raised serum or urinary uric acid.

Allopurinol and its major metabolite, oxipurinol, act by inhibiting the enzyme xanthine oxidase which catalyses the end stage of the metabolism of purines to uric acid. Allopurinol and its metabolites are excreted by the kidney but the renal handling is such that allopurinol has a plasma half-life of about one hour whereas that of oxipurinol exceeds 18 hours. Thus therapeutic effect may be achieved by once-a-day dosage.

Dosage and administration *Adults:* The initial dosage should be in the range 100–300 mg per day which may be taken as a single dose. Doses in excess of 300 mg should be administered in divided doses. It has rarely been found necessary to exceed 900 mg per day. The dose should be adjusted by monitoring serum uric acid and/or urinary uric acid levels at appropriate intervals until the desired effect is attained, which may take one to three weeks. The maintenance dose is normally 200– 600 mg per day.

Children: 10–20 mg/kg bodyweight/day.

Use in children is mainly indicated in malignant conditions especially leukaemia, and certain enzyme disorders (e.g. Lesch-Nyhan syndrome).

Initiation of therapy: In early stages of treatment with Zyloric, as with the uricosuric agents, an acute attack of gouty arthritis may be precipitated. Therefore it is advisable to give a prophylactic dose of a suitable anti-inflammatory agent or colchicine for at least one month.

Use in the elderly: The dose should be maintained at the minimum necessary to maintain serum and urinary urate levels normal.

Use with uricosurics: Oxipurinol, the major metabolite of allopurinol and itself therapeutically active, is excreted by the kidney in a similar way to urate. Hence drugs with uricosuric activity such as probenecid or large doses of salicylate may accelerate the excretion of oxipurinol. This may decrease Zyloric's therapeutic effect, but the significance needs to be assessed in each case.

To prevent acute uric acid nephropathy in neoplastic conditions, treatment with Zyloric should precede treatment with cytotoxic drugs (see also sections under *Contra-indications, warnings, etc*).

Dose recommendations in impaired renal function: Since allopurinol and its metabolites are excreted via the kidney, impairment of renal function may lead to retention of the drug and its metabolites with consequent prolongation of action. Thus the amount and frequency of the dosage may require reduction as indicated by monitoring serum uric acid levels. The following schedule is provided for guidance in adults.

If creatinine clearance exceeds 20 ml/minute – give standard dose.

If creatinine clearance is between 20 and 10 ml/ minute – give 100–200 mg/day.

If creatinine clearance is less than 10 ml/minute – give 100 mg/day or at longer intervals.

Dose recommendations in renal dialysis: Allopurinol and its metabolites are removed by renal dialysis. If frequent dialysis is required, an alternative schedule of 300–400 mg Zyloric after each dialysis, with none in the interim, should be considered.

Contra-indications, warnings, etc

Contra-indications: Known intolerance of allopurinol. Zyloric is contra-indicated as a treatment for the acute attack of gout. Prophylactic therapy may be started when the acute attack has completely subsided, provided anti-inflammatory agents are also taken.

Precautions: Treatment with Zyloric should not be started during an attack of gout. When Puri-Nethol* (6-mercaptopurine) or Imuran* (azathioprine) is given concurrently with Zyloric, only one quarter of the usual dose of Puri-Nethol or Imuran should be given because inhibition of xanthine oxidase will prolong their activity. Evidence suggests that the plasma half-life of adenine arabinoside is increased in the presence of allopurinol. When the two products are used concomitantly, extra vigilance is necessary to recognise enhanced toxic effects. There is no unequivocal evidence that Zyloric potentiates the activity of other cytotoxic drugs. A reduction of dosage should be considered in the presence of severe renal or hepatic disorders.

Side- and adverse effects: Adverse reactions in association with Zyloric are usually rare and mostly of a minor nature. The incidence is higher in the presence of renal and/or hepatic disorders.

In the early stages of treatment with Zyloric, as with the uricosuric agents, an acute attack of gouty arthritis may be precipitated. Therefore it is advisable to give a prophylactic dose of a suitable anti-inflammatory agent or colchicine for at least one month.

Although there is no evidence that the interaction between allopurinol and the coumarins seen under experimental conditions has any clinical significance, this possibility should be borne in mind when a patient on anticoagulants is given Zyloric. If Zyloric is given concomitantly with chlorpropamide when renal function is poor, there may be an increased risk of prolonged hypoglycaemic activity.

In conditions where the rate of urate formation is greatly increased (e.g. malignant disease and its treatment; the Lesch–Nyhan syndrome), xanthine deposition may occur in the urinary tract. This risk may be minimised by adequate hydration to achieve optimal urine dilution. Adequate therapy with Zyloric will lead to dissolution of large renal pelvic uric acid stones with the remote possibility of impaction in the ureter.

Skin reactions: These are the most common reactions and may occur at any time during treatment. They may be pruritic, maculopapular, sometimes scaly or purpuric and rarely exfoliative. Zyloric should be withdrawn immediately should such reactions occur. After recovery from mild reactions Zyloric may, if desired, be reintroduced at a low dose (e.g. 50 mg/day) which may be gradually increased. If the rash recurs, Zyloric should be permanently withdrawn.

Generalised hypersensitivity: Skin reactions associated with exfoliation, fever, lymphadenopathy, arthralgia and/or eosinophilia resembling Stevens–Johnson and/or Lyell's syndrome occur rarely. Associated vasculitis and tissue response may be manifested in various ways including hepatitis, interstitial nephritis and, very rarely, epilepsy. If such reactions do occur, it may be at any time during treatment. Zyloric should be withdrawn *immedi-*

ately and permanently. Corticosteroids may be beneficial in overcoming them. When generalised hypersensitivity reactions have occurred, renal and/or hepatic disorder has usually been present particularly when the outcome has been fatal.

Granulomatous hepatitis: Very rarely granulomatous hepatitis, without overt evidence of more generalised hypersensitivity, has been described. It appears to be reversible on withdrawal of Zyloric.

Gastrointestinal disorder: In early clinical studies, nausea and vomiting were reported. Further reports suggest that this reaction is not a significant problem and can be avoided by taking Zyloric after meals.

Recurrent haematemesis has been reported as an extremely rare event, as has steatorrhoea.

Blood and lymphatic system: There have been occasional reports of transient reduction in the numbers of circulating formed elements of the blood, usually in association with renal and/or hepatic disorder. The clinical significance has yet to be demonstrated.

Miscellaneous: Exacerbation of acute gouty attacks may occur in the early stages of hypouricaemic therapy (see section under *Dosage and administration*). In those conditions where the body's miscible urate pool is greatly increased (e.g. malignant disease and its treatment; Lesch-Nyhan syndrome), the rise in the xanthine concentration resulting from the action of Zyloric may lead to tissue deposition of xanthine. Fluid intake should ensure adequate urinary output. Xanthine crystals have been seen in muscle tissue of patients receiving allopurinol, but this appears to have no clinical significance. The following complaints have been reported occasionally, but do not appear to have clear cause and effect relationship with allopurinol; fever, general malaise, asthenia, headache, vertigo, ataxia, somnolence, coma, depression, paralysis, paraesthesiae, neuropathy, visual disorder, cataract, macular changes, taste perversion, stomatitis, changed bowel habit, infertility, impotence, nocturnal emission, diabetes mellitus, hyperlipaemia, furunculosis, alopecia, discoloured hair, angina, hypertension, bradycardia, oedema, uraemia, haematuria.

Use in pregnancy and lactation: High dose intraperitoneal allopurinol in mice has been associated with foetal abnormalities but extensive animal studies with oral allopurinol have shown none. In human pregnancy there is no evidence that Zyloric taken orally causes foetal abnormalities; however, as with all drugs, due caution should be exercised in the use of Zyloric in pregnancy. No data are available on the excretion of allopurinol and its metabolites in human breast milk.

Toxicity and treatment of overdosage: No reports of overdosage or acute intoxication are available. The most likely reaction would be gastro-intestinal intolerance. Massive absorption of Zyloric may lead to considerable inhibition of xanthine oxidase activity, which should have no untoward effects unless Puri-Nethol,* (6-mercaptopurine), adenine arabinoside, and/or Imuran* (azathioprine), is being taken concomitantly. In this case, the risk of increased activity of these drugs must be recognised. Adequate hydration to maintain optimum diuresis facilitates excretion of allopurinol and its metabolites. Dialysis may be resorted to if considered necessary.

Pharmaceutical precautions Store below 25°C. Keep dry.

Legal category POM.

Package quantities *Zyloric Tablets:* bottle of 100 tablets.

Zyloric-300 Tablets: Calendar pack of 2 × 15 tablets.

Further information Zyloric presents definite advantages over uricosuric agents or simple anti-inflammatory drugs, especially in patients with gouty nephropathy, in those who form renal urate stones and those with unusually severe disease. In most patients with extensive tophaceous deposits, progressive formation of tophi has been halted and draining urate sinuses have healed.

Product licence numbers
Zyloric Tablets   0003/5207.
Zyloric-300 Tablets   0003/0092.

*Trade Mark

Care Laboratories Limited
Lindow House
Beech Lane
Wilmslow
Cheshire

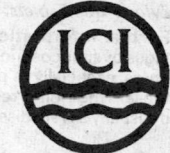

CETAVLEX* CREAM

Presentation A white water-miscible cream containing 0.5% w/w cetrimide (incorporated as Strong Cetrimide Solution BP).

Uses Cetavlex is a general purpose antiseptic cream for application to minor wounds, burns and abrasions, napkin rash and skin disorders.

Dosage and administration Apply liberally to the affected area. In some cases it may be necessary to cover the wound or burn with a clean dressing.

Contra-indications, warnings, etc
Contra-indications: Cetavlex is contra-indicated for patients who have previously shown a hypersensitivity reaction to cetrimide preparations.

Precautions: For topical application only. Keep out of the eyes and avoid contact with the brain, meninges or middle ear. Do not use in body cavities or as an enema.

Side-effects: Irritative skin reactions can occasionally occur and rare hypersensitivity to cetrimide preparations, usually developing after repeated application, has been reported. Clinical appearance of the skin conforms to that of other chemical sensitisation reactions. Should such a reaction occur stop application of the product.

Accidental ingestion: The toxicity of Cetavlex arises from the content of cetrimide. It seems unlikely that systemic toxicity will occur from accidental ingestion of the cream. However, in the event of large quantities being swallowed carry out gastric lavage with milk, egg-white, gelatin or mild soap. Do not induce vomiting. Do not give alcohol in any form. Employ supportive measures as appropriate.

Pharmaceutical precautions Store at room temperature and use undiluted. Cetavlex is incompatible with anionic agents.

Legal category GSL.

Package quantities Tubes of 50 g.

Further information Nil.

Product licence number 0029/5015.

CETAVLON* PC

Presentation A perfumed amber liquid containing 17.5% w/v cetrimide (incorporated as Strong Cetrimide Solution BP).

Uses Cetavlon PC (Pro Capite) is an antiseptic shampoo for the treatment and control of seborrhoea, pityriasis capitis and allied conditions of the scalp.

Dosage and administration *For adults and children:* Dilute 5 ml of Cetavlon PC with 50 ml of water. Wet hair thoroughly, apply the diluted solution to the scalp and massage thoroughly. Rinse and repeat the process. Finally, rinse thoroughly with clean water. Any tendency to matting of the hair can usually be overcome by further washing with Cetavlon PC.

As with similar preparations, keep the solution out of the eyes with a dry towel or face flannel.

Weekly hair washing with Cetavlon PC is generally sufficient, but the preparation may be used more frequently if necessary.

Contra-indications, warnings, etc
Contra-indications: Cetavlon PC is contra-indicated for patients who have previously shown a hypersensitivity reaction to cetrimide preparations.

Precautions: For external use only. Dilute with water before use. Keep out of the eyes and avoid contact with the brain, meninges or middle ear. Do not use in body cavities or as an enema.

Side-effects: Irritative skin reactions can occasionally occur and rare hypersensitivity to cetrimide preparations, usually developing after repeated application, has been reported. There have also been rare reports of severe burn-like reactions to concentrated cetrimide solutions. Should such a reaction occur treat as a chemical burn. In all cases stop application of the product.

Accidental oral or rectal administration: Fatal poisoning may arise even when the only pathological signs are visceral congestion, cloudy swelling, mild pulmonary oedema or varying degrees of gastro-intestinal irritation. Severe CNS depression, sometimes preceded by excitement and convulsions, can cause death from respiratory paralysis.

Specific antidotes: Soap, anionic surfactants.

General measures: Do not give alcohol in any form. If the product is swallowed give large quantities of milk, egg-white, gelatin or mild soap. Avoid vomiting or lavage if it is believed that a concentrated solution has been ingested.

Central paralysis cannot be countered by curare antagonists or CNS stimulants but sympathomimetic drugs have been given.

Mechanically assisted ventilation with oxygen may be necessary. Persistent convulsions may be controlled with cautious doses of a short-acting barbiturate.

Accidental intravenous transfusion: Massive haemolysis can occur which will require blood transfusion.

Accidental intra-uterine administration: Introduction into the uterus can lead to haemolysis and pulmonary embolism.

Pharmaceutical precautions Store at room temperature. Dilute with water. Cetavlon PC is incompatible with anionic agents.

Legal category GSL.

Package quantities Bottles of 125 ml.

Further information Nil.

Product licence number 0029/5055.

HIBITANE* ANTISEPTIC LOZENGES

Presentation A circular, flat, white lozenge with a bevelled edge containing 5 mg Chlorhexidine Hydrochloride BP and 2 mg Benzocaine PhEur.

Uses Hibitane Antiseptic Lozenges provide an antiseptic effect as an adjuvant to therapy in throat and mouth infections. They are also recommended for use after tonsillectomy and dental extraction to help prevent secondary infection.

Dosage and administration One lozenge should be sucked every two hours. For prophylaxis 4 or 5 lozenges a day should prove adequate. These dosages are applicable both to adults and to children.

Contra-indications, warnings, etc
Contra-indications: Hibitane preparations are contraindicated for patients who have previously shown a hypersensitive reaction to chlorhexidine. However, such reactions are extremely rare.

Side-effects: Irritative skin reactions to chlorhexidine preparations can occasionally occur. Generalised allergic reactions to chlorhexidine have also been reported, but are extremely rare.

Overdosage: Overdosage has not been reported. Gastric lavage is probably advisable using milk, egg-white, gelatin or mild soap however, systemic effects are unlikely as Hibitane taken orally is poorly absorbed.

Pharmaceutical precautions Store at room temperature.

Legal category P.

Package quantities Tubes containing 20 lozenges.

Further information Nil.

Product licence number 0029/5021.

LOREXANE* CREAM 1%

Presentation Lorexane Cream 1% contains 1% Lindane BP (gamma benzene hexachloride) in a white vanishing cream base.

Uses Lorexane is a powerful parasiticide with a rapid action against the majority of external parasites, including the burrowing mite *Sarcoptes scabiei var. hominis.*

Lorexane Cream 1% is for the eradication of scabies, and pediculosis of the scalp, body and pubes.

Dosage and administration The following recommendations are applicable to both children and adults.

Scabies: Before treatment, the body should be washed liberally with soap and water and thoroughly dried. Lorexane Cream is then rubbed into the skin over the entire body surface, with the exception of the face and scalp until completely absorbed. The contents of one tube are adequate for the treatment of an adult and

usually, half this quantity will be found sufficient for a single application, with proportionately reduced amounts for children. Special attention should be given to areas between the fingers and toes, also wrists, armpits, genitals and buttocks. Subjective relief from irritation appears within a few hours. A bath should be taken after a period of 24 hours and all patients should be examined after four days to determine if a further application is necessary. Underclothes and bed linen should be washed, but it is generally unnecessary to send blankets, bedding and clothes to be disinfested.

Pediculosis: The affected area should be thoroughly washed with soap and water and dried. Lorexane Cream is then well rubbed into the involved skin and hair, and also adjacent areas. The hair may be combed with a dust comb after 24 hours to remove dead lice but, to ensure that any larvae which may subsequently develop from the nits are destroyed, the patient should be discouraged from washing the hair for a period of 7–10 days. As in scabies a single application usually suffices.

Contra-indications, warnings, etc For external use only.

Lorexane Cream 1% should be used with caution, especially on infants, children and pregnant women. Lindane penetrates human skin and has the potential for CNS toxicity. Studies indicate that potential toxic effects of topically applied Lindane are greater in the young. Seizures have been reported after the use of Lindane, but a cause and effect relationship has not been established. Simultaneous application of creams, ointments or oils may enhance the percutaneous absorption of Lindane.

Side-effects: Isolated incidents of mild skin reaction have been reported.

Overdosage: Accidental ingestion: CNS excitation, hyper-irritability, ataxia, clonic and tonic convulsions can occur. Subsequent CNS depression results in respiratory failure and pulmonary oedema. There is damage to the liver and kidneys. Carry out gastric lavage and administer saline cathartics. (Avoid oil laxatives, adrenaline, morphine, pethidine, atropine, aminophylline and tranquillisers). Give sedatives and 10% calcium gluconate (10 ml intravenously) if convulsions are present.

Give 250 000 i.u. penicillin six-hourly as a prophylactic measure.

The diet should be a low-fat, high-protein and high-carbohydrate diet. No milk or glucose should be given.

Artificial respiration may be indicated to counteract pulmonary failure.

Pharmaceutical precautions Use undiluted. Store at room temperature.

Legal category P.

Package quantities 30 g tubes.

Further information Since *Pediculosis* can spread rapidly, it is important that the entire family be treated when any one member is infested.

Product licence number 0029/5068.

LOREXANE* MEDICATED SHAMPOO

Presentation Lorexane Medicated Shampoo is a cream containing 2% Lindane BP (gamma benzene hexachloride) in a detergent base.

Uses Lorexane is a powerful parasiticide with a rapid

action against the majority of external parasites, including *Pediculus humanus var. capitis*.

Lorexane Medicated Shampoo is for the eradication of head lice.

Dosage and administration The following recommendations are applicable to both children and adults.

Pediculosis: After thoroughly wetting the hair, rub in about 2 inches of Lorexane Medicated Shampoo and work well into the scalp. No lather will be produced at this stage. Rinse well with warm water, apply more Lorexane Medicated Shampoo and work up to a lather. Rinse thoroughly with warm water and then comb to remove any nits remaining. Dry the hair. Repeat the treatment one week later.

Contra-indications, warnings, etc For external use only.

Lorexane Medicated Shampoo should be used on the scalp only and contact with the eyes should be avoided.

Lorexane Medicated Shampoo must be used with water.

Lorexane Medicated Shampoo should be used with caution, especially on infants, children and pregnant women. Lindane penetrates human skin and has the potential for CNS toxicity. Studies indicate that potential toxic effects of topically applied Lindane are greater in the young. Seizures have been reported after the use of Lindane, but a cause and effect relationship has not been established. Simultaneous application of creams, ointments or oils may enhance the percutaneous absorption of Lindane.

Overdosage: Accidental ingestion: CNS excitation, hyper-irritability, ataxia, clonic and tonic convulsions can occur. Subsequent CNS depression results in respiratory failure and pulmonary oedema. There is damage to the liver and kidneys. Carry out gastric lavage and administer saline cathartics (Avoid oil laxatives, adrenaline, morphine, pethidine, atropine, aminophylline and tranquillisers). Give sedatives and 10% calcium gluconate (10 ml intravenously) if convulsions are present.

Give 250 000 i.u. penicillin six-hourly as a prophylactic measure.

The diet should be a low-fat, high-protein and high-carbohydrate diet. No milk or glucose should be given.

Artificial respiration may be indicated to counteract pulmonary failure.

Side-effects: Isolated incidents of mild skin reaction have been reported.

Pharmaceutical precautions Store at room temperature.

Legal category P.

Package quantities 50 g tubes.

Further information Since *Pediculosis* can spread rapidly, it is important that the entire family be treated when any one member is infested.

Lorexane Medicated Shampoo has been formulated to leave the hair in a clean condition, and is therefore more likely to be accepted by family contacts.

Product licence number 0029/5004.

SIOPEL* CREAM

Presentation A white water-repellant barrier cream which contains 0.3% w/w cetrimide (incorporated as Strong Cetrimide Solution BP) and 10% w/w Dimethicone 1,000 BP.

Uses Siopel Cream combines the antiseptic properties of cetrimide with the water-repellant properties of the silicone dimethicone. It is useful whenever the skin needs to be protected from water-soluble irritants. Specific indications are:

Chronic dermatoses – especially useful to doctors, nurses and veterinary surgeons whose skins are sensitive to antibiotics, local anaesthetic and other sensitising agents.

Colostomies, ileostomies, haemorrhoidectomies and other forms of surgery where skin requires protection from body fluids and discharges.

Pruritus ani due to persistent diarrhoea; napkin rash and the effects of incontinence in geriatric patients.

Eczematous and neurodermatitic lesions, and for protecting the intact skin surrounding varicose ulcers.

Dosage and administration Wash and dry the skin. Apply Siopel sparingly and massage well into the skin. Apply three to five times daily for three to four days then once or twice daily. These recommendations apply to both children and adults.

Contra-indications, warnings, etc
Contra-indications: Siopel is contra-indicated for patients who have previously shown a hypersensitive reaction to cetrimide preparations.

Precautions: For topical application only. Keep out of the eyes and avoid contact with the brain, meninges or middle ear. Do not use in body cavities or as an enema. Do not use on skin that is acutely inflamed or weeping, or before the skin has been cleansed of contaminating irritants.

Side-effects: Irritative skin reactions can occasionally occur and hypersensitivity to cetrimide preparations, usually developing after repeated application, has been reported. Should such a reaction occur stop application of the product.

Accidental ingestion: It seems unlikely that systemic toxicity will occur from accidental ingestion of the cream. However, in the event of large quantities being swallowed, carry out gastric lavage with milk, egg-white, gelatin or mild soap and apply supportive measures as appropriate. Do not induce vomiting. Do not give alcohol in any form.

Pharmaceutical precautions Store at room temperature and use undiluted. Siopel is incompatible with anionic agents.

Legal category GSL.

Package quantities Containers of 50 g.

Further information Nil.

Product licence number 0029/5014.

*Trade Mark

G. W. Carnrick Co Ltd.
431 Victoria House
Bloomsbury Square
London WC1B 4EB

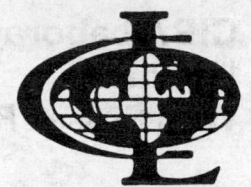

HORMONIN*

Presentation Each pink tablet contains:

Oestriol	0.27 mg
Oestradiol	0.6 mg
Oestrone	1.40 mg

Uses Hormonin has been designed for replacement therapy in oestrogen-deficiency states, particularly those associated with the menopause such as nocturnal sweating, vasomotor disturbances, psychological upsets, atrophic vaginitis and pruritus vulvae. By maintaining the physiological levels of the three naturally occurring human oestrogens, Hormonin helps to prevent these symptoms that are associated with the menopause.

Dosage and administration Hormonin is given by mouth. The dosage for the relief of menopausal symptoms range from 2 tablets per day to $\frac{1}{2}$ tablet per day or 1 tablet on alternate days, depending upon the severity of the symptoms. In general, the maximum dosage is required for not more than two weeks to initiate therapy. Where it is necessary to control irregular cycles in women approaching the menopause, a dosage of 1 tablet daily is usually adequate.

For prophylactic use in post-menopausal women, a dosage of 1 tablet is recommended daily or on alternate days, according to the needs of the individual patient. Cyclic therapy may be used.

Contra-indications, warnings, etc Hormonin is contra-indicated in patients with pre-existing genital cancer or primary cancer of the breast. A very small proportion of women may complain of a sense of fullness or slight pain in the breasts. This is usually controlled by stopping therapy on alternate days, or, in post-menopausal women, for one week each month. Oestrogens should not be administered to women with recurrent mastitis or abnormal mammograms except in instances where the physician feels that treatment is warranted despite the possibility of aggravation of the mastitis or stimulation of undiagnosed oestrogen neoplasia. A complete pre-treatment physical examination should be performed with special reference to the pelvis and breast. Oestrogen-withdrawal bleeding during cyclic therapy of women patients is a natural occurrence. However, irregular uterine bleeding or spotting should always be thoroughly investigated. The physician should be alert to the earliest manifestation of thrombotic disorders. Should this problem occur, discontinue oestrogen therapy immediately. Pre-existing fibromyomata may increase in size while using oestrogen. For this reason, patients should be examined at regular intervals. Prolonged use might increase the risk of the development of endometrial carcinoma.

Pharmaceutical precautions Store in a closed container in a cool dry place.

Legal category POM.

Package quantities Securitainers of 100 tablets.

Further information Nil.

Product licence number 0271/5000.

MIDRID*

Presentation Each scarlet capsule contains:

Isometheptene mucate	65 mg
Dichloralphenazone	100 mg
Paracetamol	325 mg

Uses In the treatment of vascular headaches, including migraine and tension headaches. Midrid contains isometheptene, a cerebral vasoconstrictor, which provides prompt relief of vascular head-pain by reducing the underlying cerebrovascular disturbances. Midrid also contains dichloralphenazone, which is a sedative/tranquilliser.

The addition of paracetamol in Midrid is designed to bring relief to the throbbing head-pain of migraine that is the first consideration of the patient. Acting centrally, it raises the pain threshold between the thalamus and the cortex, in doses that produce few, if any, other central or peripheral effects.

Dosage and administration *Treatment of migraine headache:* 2 capsules at once, followed by 1 capsule every hour until relief is obtained. Up to 5 capsules within a 12-hour period.

Treatment of tension headache: 2 capsules at once, followed by 1 or 2 capsules every four hours. Up to 8 capsules a day. Administration is by the oral route.

Contra-indications, warnings, etc

Contra-indications: Midrid is contra-indicated in severe renal, hepatic or organic heart disease, severe hypertension, glaucoma, and in those patients who are on monoamine-oxidase inhibitor therapy.

Side-effects: Transient dizziness may appear in hypersensitive patients. This can usually be eliminated by reducing the dose.

Overdosage; No specific antidote. Gastric lavage plus appropriate supportive treatment.

Pharmaceutical precautions Store in a closed container in a cool, dry place.

Legal category POM.

Package quantities Securitainers of 100 capsules.

Further information Nil.

Product licence number 0271/5001.

*Trade Mark

CIBA Laboratories
Horsham
West Sussex RH12 4AB

CIBA

APRESOLINE*

Presentation Tablets containing 25 mg hydralazine hydrochloride BP, circular, polished, sugar-coated, pale yellow in colour marked CIBA on one side and the letters GF on the other.

Tablets containing 50 mg hydralazine hydrochloride BP, circular, polished, sugar-coated, violet-red in colour, marked CIBA on one side and the letters HG on the other.

Ampoules for intravenous use containing 20 mg hydralazine hydrochloride, as a white or yellowish lyophilised powder (requiring reconstitution before use – see 'Dosage' below).

Uses

Indications: Hypertension – *Oral:* Moderate to severe hypertension usually as an adjunct to other anti-hypertensive agents. *Intravenous:* Hypertensive emergencies, particularly those associated with pre-eclampsia and toxaemia of pregnancy and in hypertension with renal complications.

Moderate to severe chronic congestive cardiac failure in patients in whom optimal doses of diuretics and cardiac glycosides prove insufficient. In patients with high left ventricular filling pressure, it is advisable to combine Apresoline with a nitrate.

Mode of action: Hydralazine is a direct acting vasodilator which exerts its effects principally on the arterioles. Its precise mode of action is not known. Administration of hydralazine produces a fall in peripheral resistance and a decrease in arterial blood pressure, effects which induce reflex sympathetic cardiovascular responses. The comcomitant use of a beta-blocker will reduce these reflex effects and enhance the anti-hypertensive effect. The changes in vascular resistance which it produces in all vascular beds causes an increase in blood flow which is greatest in the renal and hepatic system. In heart failure cardiac output is improved as a result of the afterload reduction which is induced by hydralazine; tachycardia or hypotension are seldom seen in this group.

Pharmacokinetics: Orally administered Apresoline is rapidly and completely absorbed but is subject to a dose-dependent first pass effect (systemic biovailability: 26–55%) which is dependent upon the individuals acetylator status. Peak plasma concentrations are attained after 0.5 to 1.5 hours. Apresoline appears in the plasma chiefly in the form of a readily hydrolysable conjugate with pyruvic acid. Plasma half-life averages 2–3 hours but is prolonged up to 16 hours in severe renal failure (creatine clearance less than 20 ml/min) and shortened to approximately 45 minutes in rapid acetylators. Apresoline is rapidly distributed in the body and displays a particular affinity for the blood-vessel walls. Plasma protein binding is of the order of 90%. Within 24 hours after an oral dose, the quantity recovered in the urine averages 80% of the dose. The bulk of the dose is excreted as acetylated and hydroxylated metabolites, some of which are conjugated with glucoronic acid.

Dosage and administration SEE 'PRECAUTIONS' BEFORE USE.

Adults

Hypertension: Oral: Initially 25 mg, two or three times daily in combination with a beta-blocker plus thiazide diuretic. Dosage should be increased gradually to the minimum effective dose which should not exceed 200 mg daily. Parenteral: 20 mg by slow intravenous injection or intravenous drip and repeated as necessary after 20–30 minutes. The contents of the vial should be reconstituted by dissolving in 1 ml of Water for Injections BP. This should then be further diluted with 10 ml of Sodium Chloride Injection BP 0.9% and administered by slow intravenous injection. The injection must be given immediately and any remainder discarded. The product reconstituted as for direct iv injection may be added via the infusion container to 500 ml of Sodium Chloride Injection BP 0.9% and given by continuous infusion. The addition should be made immediately before administration and the mixture should not be stored. Apresoline for infusion can also be used with 5% sorbitol solution or isotonic inorganic infusion solutions such as Ringer's solution. It is inadvisable to use dextrose containing solutions as vehicles for the parenteral administration of hydralazine.

Chronic congestive cardiac failure: Initially 25 mg three to four times daily, increasing every second day up to 50–70 mg three to four times daily, depending on clinical response. Occasionally where oral therapy is inappropriate, 20 mg may be given intravenously and repeated at hourly intervals depending upon response.

Children: Not recommended.

Elderly: Clinical evidence would indicate that no special dosage regime is necessary but concurrent hepatic and renal insufficiency should be taken into account.

Use in pregnancy and lactation: Apresoline has been found to be teratogenic in mice producing a small incidence of cleft palate and certain other minor bony malformations, in oral doses ranging from 20–120 mg/kg. Its use should therefore be avoided during the period of organogenesis. Hydralazine crosses the placental barrier.

Since hydralazine passes into the breast milk mothers in whom its use proves unavoidable should refrain from breast feeding their infants.

Contra-indications, warnings, etc

Contra-indications: Tachycardia. Hypersensitivity to hydralazine. Left ventricular heart failure due to severe aortic or mitral stenosis. Constrictive pericarditis.

Precautions: Prolonged treatment with hydralazine (i.e.

usually for more than 6 months) may provoke a lupus erythematosus (LE)-like syndrome, especially where doses exceed 100 mg daily. First symptoms are likely to be arthralgia, sometimes associated with fever and rash and are reversible after withdrawal of the drug. The more severe form resembles acute LE, and in rare cases renal and ocular involvement have been reported. Long-term treatment with corticosteroids may be required to reverse these changes. Since such reactions tend to occur more frequently the higher the dose and the longer its duration, and since they are also more common in slow acetylators, it is recommended that for maintenance therapy the lowest effective dose should be used. If 100 mg daily fails to elicit an adequate clinical effect, the patients acetylator status should be evaluated. Slow acetylators and women run a greater risk of developing the LE-like syndrome and every effort should therefore be made to keep the dosage below 100 mg daily and a careful watch kept for signs and symptoms suggestive of this syndrome. If such symptoms do develop the drug should be gradually withdrawn. Rapid acetylators often respond inadequately even to doses of 100 mg daily and therefore the dose can be raised without significantly increasing the risk of an LE-like syndrome.

During long-term treatment with Apresoline it is advisable to determine the antinuclear factors and conduct urinalysis at intervals of approximately 6 months. In the event of positive findings, the titres should be monitored more frequently. At the first signs or symptoms suggestive of LE the drug should be withdrawn.

Apresoline should be used with caution in patients with coronary artery disease (since it may increase angina) or cerebrovascular disease.

A number of studies designed to determine the carcinogenicity of hydralazine, in which mice and rats were given hydralazine in very high doses for long periods have proved inconclusive. A positive mutagenic finding in bacterial test systems has been observed, but the significance of this is unclear. Thirty years of extensive international use have not implied an association of hydralazine with human cancer.

In severe renal failure the interval between doses should be prolonged to avoid accumulation; also in hepatic dysfunction a reduction in dosage or prolonged dosage interval may be indicated.

Drug interactions: Potentiation of effects: Concurrent treatment with other anti-hypertensives, anaesthetics, minor tranquilisers or drugs exerting a central depressant action.

Reduction in effects: Concomitant treatment with sympathomimetics, tricyclic antidepressants or MAO inhibitors.

Adverse effects: Tachycardia, headache, dizziness, flushing, nasal congestion, anorexia, gastro-intestinal disturbances, fluid retention.

Lupus-like syndrome (see 'Precautions').

Occasional liver damage resembling a hepatitis-like syndrome (reversible upon withdrawal of the drug).

Rare instances of anxiety and depression, skin rash, febrile reactions and changes in blood count (Apresoline should be withdrawn in these cases).

Isolated cases of glomerulonephritis.

Rare cases of peripheral neuritis, causing paraesthesiae, can be reversed by the administration of pyridoxine or the withdrawal of Apresoline.

Overdosage: Symptoms include hypotension, tachycardia, myocardial ischaemia, dysrrhythmias and coma.

Gastric lavage should be instituted as soon as possible.

Supportive measures including intravenous fluids are also indicated. If hypotension is present, an attempt should be made to raise the blood pressure without increasing the tachycardia. Adrenaline should therefore be avoided.

Pharmaceutical precautions The tablets should be protected from heat and moisture. The ampoules should be protected from heat and light.

Legal category POM.

Package quantities
Apresoline tablets: Securitainers of 100.
Apresoline ampoules: Boxes of 5.

Further information Nil.

Product licence numbers
Apresoline Tablets 25 mg   0008/5002R
Apresoline Tablets 50 mg   0008/0029R
Apresoline Ampoules 20 mg   0008/5065R

DESFERAL*

Presentation A sterile, lyophilised powder available in vials containing 500 mg of desferrioxamine mesylate.

Uses A highly specific iron chelating agent recommended for the treatment of acute iron poisoning, chronic iron accumulation, primary haemochromatosis and secondary haemochromatosis (haemosiderosis); for the diagnosis of iron storage disease and certain anaemias; and for the management of corneal rust stains and ocular siderosis.

Dosage and administration When administered parenterally, the drug should be employed in the form of a 10% solution, e.g. by dissolving the contents of one vial (500 mg) in 5 ml of distilled water. If the solution is slightly opalescent, it can still safely be given intramuscularly or subcutaneously. The 10% Desferal solution can be diluted with routinely employed infusion solutions (saline, glucose, dextrose or dextrose-saline). For intravenous infusions, however, only clear solutions should be used.

The dosage recommendations are the same for adults and children.

Treatment of pathological iron overload: As a rule, treatment with Desferal should be continued for at least several months, possibly on an intermittent basis. To assess the response, urinary iron excretion should initially be monitored daily, and later at longer intervals (but not less than once every 2 weeks).

Although Desferal can be given by intramuscular injection, in most cases it exerts a considerably greater effect when administered — preferably with the aid of a portable, light-weight, infusion pump — by continuous intravenous or subcutaneous infusion. Intravenous infusions usually prove somewhat more effective than subcutaneous infusions, which are particularly suitable for ambulant patients.

However, since the iron excretion rates obtained with the above mentioned modes of administration vary from patient to patient, one should first individually determine which of them yields the best results before embarking on long-term medication.

For the purposes of infusion treatment the average daily dose is 1.5–4 g administered intravenously or subcutaneously over a period of approximately 12 hours. In some cases it is possible to achieve a further increase in iron excretion by infusing the same daily dose over a 24-hour period.

For intramuscular treatment the average initial dose is 0.5–1 g daily, given in 1–2 injections. The maintenance dose to be selected will depend on the patient's iron excretion rate.

Treatment of acute iron poisoning: In this indication larger doses, administered both orally and parenterally, are usually required. Speed is essential.

Gastric lavage should be carried out as quickly as possible using, if readily available, 1% sodium bicarbonate solution. This should be followed by the oral administration, by stomach tube if necessary, of 5–10 g (the contents of 10–20 vials) of Desferal in 50–100 ml of fluid. This will chelate any iron remaining in the stomach and prevent any further absorption.

To eliminate the iron that has already been absorbed, 1–2 g Desferal should be injected intramuscularly every 3–12 hours; alternatively, Desferal should be infused either subcutaneously or – particularly if the patient is seriously ill and already in a state of shock – intravenously at a rate of not more than 15 mg/kg/h, the maximum dose in any 24 hours being 80 mg/kg. Duration of treatment will depend on the patient's condition.

Further measures, e.g. sodium bicarbonate, sedatives, oxygen, etc., may be given as necessary. The patient's progress should be checked by serum iron determinations.

It should be noted that the serum iron level may rise sharply when the iron is released from the tissues.

Theoretically 100 mg of Desferal can chelate approximately 8.5 mg of iron, thus 5 g can chelate the iron contained in about 10 tablets of ferrous sulphate or ferrous gluconate.

Desferal test for iron overload: This test is based on the principle that normal subjects do not excrete more than a fraction of a milligram of iron in their urine daily and a standard intramuscular injection of 500 mg of Desferal does not increase this above 1 mg. In iron storage diseases, however, the increase may be well over 1.5 mg.

Procedure:

1. The haemoglobin, serum iron and total iron binding capacity are estimated.
2. 500 mg of Desferal are given intramuscularly and 400 ml of water are drunk.
3. All urine is collected over the next six hours.
4. The urinary iron is estimated in the six hour urine specimen.

An excretion of 1–1.5 mg (18–27 mcmol) of iron during this 6-hour period is suggestive of an iron-storage disease; values of more than 1.5 mg (27 mcmol) can be regarded as definitely pathological. The test yields reliable results only in cases where renal function is normal.

Use in the elderly: No special dosage regime is necessary but concurrent renal insufficiency should be taken into account.

Contra-indications, warnings, etc *Contra-indications:* None.

Precautions: Desferal should only be used with caution in patients with renal dysfunction.

In acute iron poisoning requiring treatment with Desferal in patients suffering from severe renal dysfunction, dialysis might help to eliminate the chelated iron.

Rapid intravenous injections of Desferal may give rise to hypotonic shock. This seems to be due to too rapid injection of the material. It is therefore wiser to adhere to the recommendation to give Desferal by intravenous infusion.

Oral administration of Vitamin C in the standard dosage (150–250 mg daily, given in fractional doses) may serve to enhance excretion of the iron complex in response to Desferal; larger doses of vitamin C fail to produce an additional effect. In patients with severe chronic iron-storage disease undergoing combined treatment with Desferal and high doses of vitamin C (more than 500 mg daily) impairment of cardiac function has been encountered; this proved reversible when the vitamin C was withdrawn. Monitoring of cardiac function is indicated during such combined therapy.

Pregnancy: Desferal should not be given during pregnancy unless, in the judgment of the physician, the expected benefits outweigh the potential risk.

Side-effects; There have been only rare reports of: allergic skin reactions and cardiovascular (e.g. hypotension, shock), neurological (e.g. dizziness, convulsions), and gastro-intestinal disturbances, impairment of hepatic and renal function, as well as changes in the blood picture (e.g. thrombocytopenia). Some of these manifestations, however must be considered as signs and symptoms of the underlying disease. The iron complex excreted under treatment with Desferal may cause reddish-brown discoloration of the urine.

Opacities of the lens have been observed in animal experiments after prolonged administration of very high doses. Patients should therefore have their eyes examined both prior to the institution of long-term treatment with Desferal and also from time to time during medication.

Retinal changes have been described in patients on higher than recommended, intensive Desferal therapy. Initial symptoms include night blindness, loss of colour vision, field defects and blurred vision. If eye symptoms, in any way suggestive of a retinopathy occur, high dose Desferal should be discontinued. In cases where a dose in excess of the recommended one is decided upon, examination of the retina is essential prior to and during the treatment period.

Local pain may occur after intramuscular injection.

Pharmaceutical precautions Desferal should be stored in a cool place.

Legal category POM.

Package quantities Available in packs of 10 vials, each containing 500 mg. Desferal.

Further information Desferal is readily soluble in water so that it can be rapidly administered both orally and parenterally in situations where speed is essential. It is highly specific for trivalent iron and the resulting chelate is stable and non-toxic. The intestinal chelate is not absorbed and that formed systemically as a result of parenteral administration is rapidly excreted via the kidneys without deleterious effects. Desferal mobilises and removes iron from all human organs, tissues and proteins excepting haemoglobin and undesirable effects on erythropoiesis have not been reported.

Method for preparing desferrioxamine eye drops:

1. *Preparation of solvent:* Formula:

Methyl cellulose 4,000 cps	25 mg	0.5%
Benzyl alcohol	50 mg	1.0%
Water for Injection q.s.	5.0 ml	100%

Method: The methyl cellulose is dispersed in water for

injection at 90°C. This is cooled with continuous stirring. When the temperature reaches 35°C, benzyl alcohol is added and the solution diluted to volume with water for injection. The solution should be filtered through a No 1, then No 2 sintered glass filter. 5 ml of this solution are filled into brown/amber eye drop bottles, stoppered and autoclaved at 110°C for 20 minutes.

2. *Preparation of drops:* To be carried out under aseptic conditions.

(a) Remove foil disc from Desferal vial containing 500 mg Desferal.
(b) Unscrew eye drop bottle cap and take up 5 ml of solvent into a sterile syringe; replace cap.
(c) Inject solvent into vial and shake to dissolve the Desferal. Care should be taken to dissolve all the Desferal.
(d) Withdraw the solution into the sterile syringe; remove cap from bottle; transfer solution to bottle and replace cap.

The drops are now ready for use.

Note: Desferal (desferrioxamine mesylate) is unstable in solution and thus the eye drops should be prepared at the time of use. The solution should be discarded at the end of one week from the date of preparation.

Product licence number 0008/5073

ESIDREX*

Presentation Tablets containing 25 mg Hydrochlorothiazide BP, circular, flat, white, with bevelled edges, impressed with the monogram CIBA on one side and the letters CE and a break line on the other.

Tablets containing 50 mg of Hydrochlorothiazide BP, circular, flat, white, with bevelled edges impressed with the monogram CIBA on one side and the letters UT and a break line on the other.

Uses *Mode of action;* Esidrex is a thiazide diuretic which exerts its diuretic effect in inhibiting the reabsorption of sodium, chloride and water, probably at the proximal renal tubules.

Indications: It is indicated for the treatment of oedema associated with acute and chronic heart failure, various hepatic conditions, renal disorders; such as chronic glomerular nephritis and nephrotic syndrome, the premenstrual syndrome and fluid retention associated with obesity, diabetes insipidus or drug therapy (e.g. with corticosteroids.) It is also recommended for the treatment of hypertension, including hypertension occurring during pregnancy. It is also used to potentiate other antihypertensives such as guanethidine and reserpine.

Dosage and administration Esidrex is given orally. The dosage for adults is:

In acute and chronic heart failure – initially 50–100 mg daily, reducing to a maintenance dose of 25–50 mg three or four days weekly.

Chronic glomerular nephritis, nephrotic syndrome, ascites and hepatic cirrhosis, initially 50–75 mg daily. This may be reduced to a maintenance dose of 25–50 mg on alternate days.

Pre-menstrual oedema – 25 mg daily from the onset of symptoms until menstruation begins.

Drug-induced oedema, 25–50 mg on alternate days.

Hypertension – 25 mg increasing gradually to 75 mg daily according to the response.

Hypertension and oedema of pregnancy, mild symptoms, 25–50 mg daily, moderate hypertension – 50–100 mg daily initially and then reducing to a lower dose when control is achieved.

In all indications the total daily dose may be given as a single dose after breakfast. As Esidrex increases salt excretion it is usually possible to relax dietary salt restrictions.

Children: At the discretion of the physician.

Use in the elderly: No special dosage regime is necessary (also see 'Precautions').

Contra-indications, warnings, etc
Side-effects: Side-effects such as mild anorexia, nausea, constipation and diarrhoea, skin rashes and photosensitivity may occur. There have been reports of blood dyscrasias including thrombocytopenia, but these are rare.

Contra-indications: Esidrex, in common with other thiazides is contra-indicated in the presence of precoma associated with hepatic cirrhosis, or Addison's disease or advanced renal failure.

Precautions: In patients with some degree of renal impairment, a rise in blood urea can occur and in extreme cases result in an oliguric crisis. In such cases, either the dose should be reduced or the treatment interrupted temporarily.

Prolonged doses may bring about a decrease in glucose tolerance and precipitate a diabetic condition. In known diabetics the addition of Esidrex to the treatment regime will almost certainly alter the insulin requirement.

In common with other thiazide diuretics hyperuricaemia may be induced by Esidrex. Gout may be exacerbated in patients with a previous history or family history of this condition.

Patients who are being treated with this preparation may require regular monitoring of fluid and electrolyte balance particularly when diuresis is substantial or in patients suffering from renal impairment. Potassium supplements may be required. Particular caution is needed with this preparation in the elderly since electrolyte balance is more likely to be precarious due to bowel or renal dysfunction. Also urinary retention is more likely.

Esidrex should only be used during pregnancy if considered essential by the physician.

The concomitant administration of this preparation with cardiac glycosides or hypotensive agents may necessitate adjustment of the dosage of those drugs.

Drug interactions; The action of tricyclic antidepressants and MAO inhibitors may be potentiated by Esidrex.

Overdosage: Esidrex is self-limiting in its action and toxic effects have not been observed.

Pharmaceutical precautions Esidrex should be protected from moisture and should preferably be dispensed in a moisture-proof container.

Legal category POM.

Package quantities Esidrex 25 mg and 50 mg Tablets are available in Securitainers of 100.

Further information Esidrex has a powerful saluretic and diuretic action, is well tolerated and remains effective when administered for long periods.

Esidrex acts on the renal tubules, inhibiting the reabsorption of sodium and chloride. Low-salt diets may therefore be relaxed during Esidrex therapy.

Esidrex reduces high blood pressure and potentiates

the action of other antihypertensives but has no effect on the blood pressure in normotensive individuals.

Product licence numbers
Esidrex Tablets 25 mg   0008/5045
Esidrex Tablets 50 mg   0008/5046

ESIDREX*-K

Presentation Round white, sugar-coated tablets, 12.1 mm in diameter with a maximum height of 7.7 mm. The inner, slow-release wax core contains 600 mg Potassium Chloride BP (8.06 mEq) and the outer coat contains 12.5 mg Hydrochlorothiazide BP.

Uses *Mode of Action:* Esidrex-K is a thiazide diuretic which exerts its diuretic effect by inhibiting the reabsorption of sodium, chloride and water, probably at the proximal renal tubules.

Indications: It is indicated for the treatment of oedema associated with acute and chronic heart failure; various hepatic conditions; various renal disorders, such as chronic glomerular nephritis and nephrotic syndrome, pre-menstrual syndrome and fluid retention associated with obesity, diabetes insipidus or drug therapy (e.g. with corticosteroids). It is also recommended for the treatment of hypertension, including hypertension occurring during pregnancy. It is also used to potentiate other antihypertensives such as guanethidine and reserpine.

Dosage and administration Esidrex-K is given orally and the tablets should be swallowed whole. The dosage for adults is:

In acute and chronic heart failure – initially 50–100 mg daily (4–8 tablets), reducing to a maintenance dose of 25–50 mg (2–4 tablets) three or four days a week.

Chronic glomerular nephritis, nephrotic syndrome, ascites and hepatic cirrhosis – initially 50–75 mg (4–6 tablets) daily. This may be reduced to a maintenance dose of 25–50 mg (2–4 tablets) on alternate days.

Pre-menstrual oedema: 25 mg daily from the onset of symptoms until menstruation begins.

Drug-induced oedema – 25–50 mg (2–4 tablets) on alternate days.

Hypertension – 25 mg increasing gradually to 75 mg daily according to the response.

Hypertension and oedema of pregnancy, mild symptoms – 25–50 mg daily (2–4 tablets), moderate hypertension – 50–100 mg (4–8 tablets), daily initially, reducing to a lower dose when control is achieved.

In all indications the total daily dose may be given as 1 dose before breakfast, or 2 equally divided doses after breakfast and lunch. As Esidrex-K increases salt excretion, it is usually possible to relax dietary salt restrictions.

Children: At the discretion of the physician.

Use in the elderly: No special dosage regime is necessary (also see 'Precautions').

Contra-indications, warnings, etc
Side-effects: Side-effects such as mild anorexia, nausea, constipation and diarrhoea, skin rashes and photosensitivity may occur as a result of treatment with Esidrex-K. In common with other thiazides, there have been reports of thrombocytopenia, but these are rare.

Esidrex-K tablets are designed to avoid the risks of gastro-intestinal irritation. However, if a patient under treatment with Esidrex-K develops severe vomiting, severe abdominal pains or flatulence or gastro-intestinal

haemorrhage, the preparation should be withdrawn at once, because in the presence of an obstruction it could conceivably give rise to ulceration or perforation.

Contra-indications: Esidrex-K is contra-indicated in the presence of hyperkalaemia or precoma associated with hepatic cirrhosis, Addison's disease or advanced renal failure.

All solid forms of potassium medication are contra-indicated in the presence of obstructions in the digestive tract (e.g. resulting from compression of the oesophagus due to dilation of the left atrium or from stenosis of the gut).

Precautions: In patients with some degree of renal impairment, a rise in blood urea can occur and in extreme cases result in an oliguric crisis. In such cases, either the dose should be reduced or the treatment interrupted temporarily.

Prolonged doses of thiazides may bring about a decrease in glucose tolerance and precipitate a diabetic condition. In known diabetics the addition of Esidrex-K to the treatment regime will almost certainly alter the insulin requirement.

In common with other thiazide diuretics, hyperuricaemia may be induced by Esidrex-K. Gout may be exacerbated in patients with a previous history or family history of this condition.

Patients who are being treated with this preparation may require regular monitoring of fluid and electrolyte balance particularly when diuresis is substantial or in patients suffering from renal impairment. Potassium supplements may be required. Particular caution is needed with this preparation in the elderly since electrolyte balance is more likely to be precarious due to bowel or renal dysfunction. Also urinary retention is more likely.

Esidrex-K should only be used during pregnancy if considered essential by the physician.

The concomitant administration of this preparation with cardiac glycosides or hypotensive agents may necessitate adjustment of the dosage of those drugs.

Drug interactions: The action of tricyclic anti-depressants and MAO inhibitors may be potentiated by Esidrex-K.

Overdosage: Esidrex-K is self-limiting in its action and toxic effects have not been observed.

Pharmaceutical precautions Esidrex-K should be protected from moisture and should preferably be dispensed in a moisture-proof container.

Legal category POM.

Package quantities Esidrex-K Tablets are available in Securitainers of 100.

Further information Esidrex-K has a powerful saluretic and diuretic action, is well tolerated and remains effective when administered for long periods.

Esidrex-K acts on the renal tubules inhibiting the reabsorption of sodium and chloride. Low salt diets should therefore be relaxed during Esidrex-K therapy.

Esidrex-K reduces high blood pressure and potentiates the action of other antihypertensives but has no effect on the blood pressure in normotensive individuals.

Product licence number 0008/5035.

ISMELIN*

Presentation Ismelin Tablets each containing 10 mg Guanethidine Sulphate BP. Circular, flat, white tablets with bevelled edges, impressed with the monogram CIBA on one side and Ismelin 10 on the other.

Ismelin Tablets each containing 25 mg Guanethidine Sulphate BP. Circular, flat pale red tablets, with bevelled edges, impressed with the monogram CIBA on one side and Ismelin 25 on the other.

Ismelin Ampoules each containing 10 mg/ml clear, colourless solution of Guanethidine Sulphate BP in a clear glass 1 ml ampoule. When Ismelin is given by intravenous infusion, the contents of the ampoule should be added to saline or dextrose saline.

Uses *Mode of action:* Ismelin is a peripheral sympathetic blocking drug which lowers blood pressure by inhibiting vasoconstrictive mechanisms.

Recommended for the treatment of all grades of hypertension. The parenteral formulation is intended for control of hypertensive crises and to obtain more rapid blood-pressure control.

Dosage and administration *Adults: oral:* Ismelin has a sustained length of action in excess of 24 hours, and can therefore be given as a single daily dose which has to be titrated to the patient's particular needs. In mild to moderate hypertension, dosage should begin at 20 mg daily, increasing if necessary to 30 mg daily. A daily dose in excess of 30 mg is rarely required in the milder grades of hypertension.

In patients with more severe hypertension, the majority will be adequately controlled and free from hypertensive symptoms on a daily dose of 40 mg or less. Occasionally, a daily dose of up to 100 mg may be required and, in exceptional cases, even more.

Increments in dosage should not exceed 10 mg and an interval of at least one week should be allowed to elapse before a further increase in dosage is introduced.

Frequent adjustment of dosage during the stabilisation period is not necessary, and according to individual assessment the interval between consultations may be up to one month.

Parenteral: In the management of hypertensive crises, including toxaemia of pregnancy, Ismelin should be given by intramuscular injection. One injection of 10–20 mg will generally cause a fall of blood pressure within 30 minutes which reaches a maximum in one to two hours and is maintained for four to six hours. If a further dose of 10–20 mg is deemed necessary, then three hours should be allowed to elapse between doses.

Children: Ismelin has been given to children, but the dosage needs to be established for each individual child.

Use in the elderly: Clinical evidence would indicate that no special dosage regime is necessary but concurrent coronary or cerebral insufficiency should be taken into account.

Contra-indications, warnings, etc *Side-effects:* Side-effects are often an indication of excessive dosage. By adhering to the dosage recommendations, using small increments where necessary at intervals of at least a week, these effects due to excessive hypotension may be avoided. Should faintness occur, despite the patient being advised against rising quickly from the lying or sitting position, the daily dose should be reduced by 10 mg until the next visit.

If diarrhoea proves a problem the following courses of action can be taken: (a) divide the dosage of Ismelin; (b) lower the daily dosage and add a diuretic; (c) add codeine phosphate to the regime.

Failure of ejaculation has been reported. Other side-effects on rare occasions have included breathlessness on exertion, nasal congestion, weakness or paraesthesia, myalgia or muscle weakness and aggravation of intermittent claudication.

Toxic effects have not been reported with Ismelin in prolonged dosage.

Contra-indications: Theoretically, Ismelin is contra-indicated in the presence of phaeochromocytoma; however, in practice, this is a relative contra-indication as there are reports in the literature of successful antihypertensive treatment of patients with phaeochromocytoma by the use of Ismelin.

Precautions: Ismelin should be used with caution in treating patients with renal failure or a raised blood urea. Ismelin may increase the tendency to fluid retention, this is usually readily corrected by the concurrent administration of a diuretic. As is the case with other antihypertensive agents, Ismelin may increase the risk of further clotting by lowering blood pressure in patients with recent cerebral or myocardial infarction.

Caution should be exercised in giving Ismelin to patients with a history of peptic ulceration, as there have been occasional reports of aggravation of this condition.

When patients have to undergo surgery, it is recommended that treatment with Ismelin be withheld on the day of operation. As there is a theoretical risk of cardiac arrest during anaesthesia, it is advisable to premedicate with larger doses of atropine than usual.

N.B. Intravenous injections of Ismelin may provoke a *hyper*tensive response, hence if the i.v. route is preferred it should be by slow i.v. infusion.

Interaction with other drugs: Antagonistic effect: MAO inhibitors, tricyclic antidepressants and the amphetamine group of drugs tend to antagonise the hypotensive actions of Ismelin: this should be borne in mind when treating patients already undergoing therapy with appetite suppressants, antidepressants or stimulants in these classes. The hypotensive action of Ismelin may be enhanced by alcohol or anaesthetic agents.

Additive effects: The thiazide diuretics, reserpine and other Rauwolfia alkaloids may be given in association with Ismelin, bearing in mind that the antihypertensive effects of reserpine and Ismelin are additive and that the thiazides potentiate its action. Smaller doses of Ismelin than normal will be required. When transferring from thiazides or reserpine to Ismelin, a low initial dose of Ismelin, such as 10 mg daily, is advisable for the first week, at the same time gradually withdrawing the previous compounds.

Treatment of overdosage: Overdosage produces orthostatic collapse, which usually requires no treatment other than keeping the patient recumbent. Occasionally pressor agents may be required in severe cases.

Pharmaceutical precautions Ampoules – protect from light. Tablets – protect from moisture.

Legal category POM.

Package quantities Tablets 10 mg and 25 mg of Ismelin in blister packs of 100 (5 modules of 20 tablets). Also ampoules of 1 ml containing 10 mg in boxes of 6.

Further information Ismelin can be relied upon to lower blood pressure in almost all patients with hypertension. It is widely used in those patients whose blood pressure needs lowering more than can be achieved with a diuretic alone. Such patients can be managed on a simple regime of two Navidrex* K and two Ismelin 10 mg tablets daily. Response to Ismelin is usually reliable and predictable for long periods, as tolerance requiring adjustment of dosage is not normally a problem.

Product licence numbers

Ismelin Tablets 10 mg	0008/5006
Ismelin Tablets 25 mg	0008/5007
Ismelin Ampoules	0008/5077

LIORESAL*

Presentation Lioresal tablets each containing 10 mg baclofen; circular, flat, white tablets, uncoated, with bevelled edges, having the monogram CIBA on one side and the letters KJ and a break line on the other.

Lioresal liquid containing 5 mg/5 ml baclofen; clear, very slightly yellow solution with a raspberry flavour.

Uses Lioresal is chemically unrelated to any other antispastic agent and acts at spinal level, reducing spasticity and spasm and thereby improving the activities of daily living.

Lioresal is indicated for the relief of spasticity of voluntary muscle resulting from such disorders as: multiple sclerosis, other spinal lesions e.g. tumours of the spinal cord, syringomyelia, motor neurone disease, transverse myelitis, traumatic partial section of the cord.

Lioresal is also indicated in adults and children for the relief of spasticity of voluntary muscle arising from e.g. cerebrovascular accidents, cerebral palsy, meningitis, traumatic head injury.

Patient selection is important when initiating Lioresal therapy; it is likely to be of most benefit in patients whose spasticity constitutes a handicap to activities and/or physiotherapy. Treatment should not be commenced until the spastic state has become stabilized.

Dosage and administration Lioresal is given orally in either tablet or liquid form. These two formulations are bioequivalent. The liquid may be particularly suitable for children or those adults who are unable to take tablets. Dosage titration can be more precisely managed with the liquid. Before starting treatment with Lioresal it is prudent to realistically assess the overall extent of clinical improvement that the patient may be expected to achieve. Careful titration of dosage is essential (particularly in the elderly) until the patient is stabilised. If too high a dosage is initiated or if dosage is increased too rapidly side-effects may occur. This is particularly relevant if the patient is ambulant, in order to minimise muscle weakness in the unaffected limbs or where spasticity is necessary for support.

Adults: The following gradually increasing dosage regime is suggested but should be adjusted to suit individual patient's requirements.

5 mg three times a day for three days
10 mg three times a day for three days
15 mg three times a day for three days
20 mg three times a day for three days

Satisfactory control of symptoms is usually obtained with doses up to 60 mg daily, but a careful adjustment is often necessary to meet the requirements of each individual patient. The dose may be increased slowly if required, but a maximum daily dose of more than 100 mg is not advised unless the patient is in hospital under careful medical supervision. Small frequent dosage may prove better in some cases than larger spaced doses. Also some patients benefit from the use of Lioresal only at night to counteract painful flexor spasm. Similarly a single dose given approximately 1 hour prior to the performance of specific tasks such as washing, dressing, shaving, physiotherapy, will often improve mobility.

Once the maximum recommended dose has been reached, if the therapeutic effect is not apparent within 6 weeks a decision whether to continue Lioresal should be taken.

Children: In children under eight years of age the starting dose may need to be as low as 5–10 mg daily in three or four divided doses, increasing gradually over a two week period to a maximum of 40 mg daily in divided doses. For children over eight years a starting dose of 10 mg daily in divided doses and a maximum dose of 60 mg daily are recommended.

There have been no reports of tolerance.

Lioresal should be withdrawn gradually.

Use in the elderly: Elderly patients may be more susceptible to side effects, particularly in the early stages of introducing Lioresal. Small doses should therefore be used at the start of treatment, the dose being titrated gradually against the response under careful supervision. There is no evidence that the eventual average maximum dose differs from that in younger patients.

Contra-indications, warnings, etc
Contra-indications: Peptic ulceration.

Side-effects: Nausea, vomiting, daytime sedation and confusion, as well as muscle hypotonia and fatigue, have been observed after treatment with Lioresal. The incidence of these effects may be reduced by lowering the dosage with little or no loss of therapeutic effect. Should nausea persist then it is recommended that Lioresal be ingested with food or a milk beverage.

Abrupt discontinuation of Lioresal has resulted in occasional severe withdrawal symptoms; these have included visual hallucinations, convulsions and cardiac complications.

Precautions: Lioresal should be used with extreme care in patients already receiving antihypertensive therapy.

It should be noted that psychotic states and epileptic manifestations may be exacerbated by treatment with Lioresal.

Use in pregnancy: The customary practice of avoiding drugs during the first three months of pregnancy whenever possible should also apply to Lioresal. Although Lioresal passes into breast milk, the concentrations are so low that the use of therapeutic doses should generally entail no risk for the child.

Treatment of overdosage: In cases of overdosage the induced hypotonia can involve the muscles of respiration. Muscular flaccidity may persist for up to three days following recovery of consciousness.

As Lioresal is principally excreted via the kidneys, it is important to maintain a high urinary output by means of an increased fluid intake and, if necessary, the use of diuretics.

There is no specific antidote to Lioresal. Symptomatic measures should be applied as required.

Pharmaceutical precautions Lioresal tablets should be protected from heat. Lioresal liquid should be protected from heat and light.

Dilution: Lioresal liquid may be diluted with Purified

Water BP and stored at room temperature for up to 14 days.

Legal category POM.

Package quantities Tablets 10 mg: Securitainers of 100. Liquid 5 mg/5 ml: Bottles of 300 ml with child proof closure.

Further information The major benefits of Lioresal stem from its ability to reduce painful flexor or extensor spasms and spontaneous clonus thereby facilitating the mobility of the patient, increasing his independence and helping rehabilitation. General well being is often improved and sedation is less often a problem than with centrally acting drugs.

Lioresal liquid contains no sucrose and is therefore suitable for diabetics and children.

Product licence number
Tablets 10 mg   0008/0053
Liquid 5 mg/5 ml   0008/0195

LUDIOMIL*

Presentation Ludiomil tablets each containing 10 mg maprotiline hydrochloride, pale yellow, circular, film-coated tablets with CIBA on one side and the letters CO on the reverse.

Ludiomil Tablets each containing 25 mg maprotiline hydrochloride, greyish-red, circular, film-coated tablets with CIBA on one side and the letters DP on the reverse.

Ludiomil Tablets each containing 50 mg maprotiline hydrochloride; light orange, circular, film-coated tablets with CIBA on one side and the letters ER on the reverse.

Ludiomil Tablets each containing 75 mg maprotiline hydrochloride; brownish-orange, circular, film-coated tablets with CIBA on one side and the letters FS and a break line on the reverse.

Uses *Indications:* Symptoms of depressive illness especially where sedation is required.

Dosage and administration The optimum dose depends on the severity of the depression and the individual patient response to treatment. The usual dose range is 25–75 mg daily which may be given in one dose at night or in three divided doses.

Clinical evidence suggests that Ludiomil given once daily is effective and well tolerated, especially when given at night. Dosage at night should reduce the need for hypnotics or tranquillisers to be prescribed with Ludiomil.

Pharmacokinetic studies show that virtually the same steady-state blood levels are produced whether Ludiomil is given in once daily or divided doses.

For moderate or severe depression, treatment should start with 75 mg daily, increasing, if necessary, to a maximum of 150 mg daily. Initially the patient should be closely monitored and dosage adjusted after one to two weeks according to the response. Treatment will need to be maintained until remission of the depression permits gradual weaning off Ludiomil or the use of a lower dose for maintenance.

Use in the elderly: It may be advisable in elderly patients, or those who may be sensitive to this type of drug, to start treatment with lower doses such as 30 mg at night or 10 mg three times a day. This should then be adjusted in one to two weeks according to the response. In the majority of cases half the normal dose will be sufficient.

Children: Not recommended.

Contra-indications, warnings, etc
Side-effects: In some patients improvement may not occur for 2–3 weeks. Convulsions have been reported as occurring in patients both with and without a history of epilepsy.

Skin rashes are not uncommon.

In common with all other substances in this therapeutic group, Ludiomil may impair alertness (e.g. driving ability, operating machinery, etc.) to a varying degree, depending on dosage and individual susceptibility. Patients should be warned of this possible hazard.

Anticholinergic side-effects such as dry mouth, disturbances of accommodation, tachycardia, constipation and hesitancy of micturition have been reported less frequently with maprotiline than with standard tricyclic antidepressants.

The following adverse effects, although not necessarily all reported with Ludiomil, have occurred with tri/tetracyclic antidepressants:

Possible adverse effects include drowsiness, dizziness, sweating, postural hypotension, tremor, paraesthesia, vivid dreams and skin rash. Interference with sexual function may occur. The incidence and severity of these side-effects does not prejudice treatment in the majority of patients.

Serious adverse effects are rare and have included depression of the bone marrow, agranulocytosis, cholestatic jaundice, hypomania.

Psychotic manifestations, including mania and paranoid delusions may be exacerbated.

Withdrawal symptoms may occur on abrupt cessation of therapy and include insomnia, irritability and excessive perspiration.

Withdrawal symptoms in neonates whose mothers received tri/tetracyclic antidepressants during the third trimester have also been reported.

Contra-indications: Ludiomil is contra-indicated in mania, severe liver or renal disease, history of epilepsy, narrow angle glaucoma, retention of urine, recent myocardial infarction.

Pregnancy: Do not use during pregnancy especially during the first and last trimesters, or during lactation, unless there are compelling reasons. There is no evidence as to drug safety in human pregnancy, nor is there evidence from animal work that it is free from hazard. Ludiomil is excreted in the breast milk. Nursing mothers should be advised to cease breast feeding.

Precautions: In common with other substances in this therapeutic group, Ludiomil should be used with caution in patients with cardiovascular disease, such as any degree of heart block or other cardiac arrhythmias.

The elderly are particularly liable to experience side-effects, especially agitation, confusion and postural hypotension. The initial dosage should be increased with caution under close supervision (see dosage).

Ludiomil should be administered with caution to patients with symptoms suggestive of bladder neck obstruction.

Patients posing a high suicidal risk require close initial and continuing supervision.

Drug interactions: Ludiomil should not be given concurrently with or within 2 weeks of cessation of therapy with monoamine oxidase inhibitors.

Ludiomil may decrease the antihypertensive effect of guanethidine, debrisoquine, bethanidine and possibly clonidine. It would be advisable to review all antihypertensive therapy during treatment with tri/tetracylic antidepressants.

Ludiomil should be used with caution in patients receiving sympathomimetic agents such as ephedrine, isoprenaline, noradrenaline, phenylephrine and phenylpropanolamine.

Barbiturates may decrease whilst neuroleptics and methylphenidate may increase the plasma levels of Ludiomil.

The effects of alcohol may be potentiated by Ludiomil.

Anaesthetics given during tri/tetracylic antidepressant therapy may increase the risk of arrhythmias and hypotension. If surgery is necessary, the anaesthetist should be informed that a patient is being so treated.

Treatment of overdosage: There is no specific antidote to Ludiomil. Major signs of overdosage include coma, convulsions and cardiovascular disturbances. The stomach should be emptied as quickly as possible by gastric lavage or emesis and unconscious patients should be hospitalised in a unit where full support of vital functions and cardiac monitoring are possible. Treatment is symptomatic.

Pharmaceutical precautions Nil.

Legal category POM.

Package quantities Ludiomil Tablets are available in four strengths, 10 mg, 25 mg and 50 mg in containers of 100 tablets, 75 mg in containers of 28 tablets. All tablets are packed in PVC/foil bubble packs.

Further information Ludiomil is a novel compound with a tetracyclic nucleus belonging to the chemical class of dibenzo-bicyclo-octadienes. It shows a broad spectrum of antidepressant activity, being highly effective in both endogenous and reactive depression. Ludiomil works quickly, some symptoms, such as insomnia, anxiety and mood, begin to improve within three to four days. This, coupled with the good tolerability of once daily dosage, makes Ludiomil a very worthwhile treatment for all forms of depression. The 75 mg tablets of Ludiomil are packed in daily reminder packs of 28 tablets, making it simple for the patient to remember to take them.

Product licence numbers

Ludiomil Tablets 10 mg	0008/0117
Ludiomil Tablets 25 mg	0008/0118
Ludiomil Tablets 50 mg	0008/0119
Ludiomil Tablets 75 mg	0008/0129

METOPIRONE*

Presentation Metopirone Capsules each containing 250 mg metyrapone in an opaque cylindrical soft gelatine capsule, coloured white.

Uses *Mode of action:* Metopirone inhibits the enzyme responsible for the 11 β-hydroxylation stage in the synthesis of hydrocortisone (cortisol) and to a lesser extent aldosterone.

When used as a diagnostic test of anterior pituitary function, one is relying upon its inhibiting effect on cortisol production. The consequent fall in plasma concentration of circulating glucocorticoids stimulates the anterior pituitary to produce more corticotrophin. This in turn stimulates the production of more of the precursors which are then excreted in the urine where they can be measured.

Indications: As a diagnostic aid in:
(a) Investigation of anterior pituitary function in hypopituitarism.
(b) Evaluation of the effect of prolonged corticosteroid therapy upon the hypothalamic pituitary adrenal axis.

For the management of patients with Cushing's syndrome.

In conjunction with glucocorticoids, in the treatment of resistant oedema due to increased aldosterone secretion in patients suffering from cirrhosis, nephrosis and congestive heart failure.

Dosage and administration *Oral dose when used as a diagnostic test:* The urinary 17-oxygenic steroid excretion is determined on complete 24-hour collections for four consecutive days. The first two days serve as a control period. On the third day the subject is given by mouth a total of 6 doses, at four hourly intervals of 3 capsules (750 mg).

Children should be given a smaller amount based upon 6 four-hourly doses of 15 mg per kg, with a minimum dose of 250 mg.

Oral dose for therapeutic treatment: For the treatment of resistant oedema 2.5 g to 4.5 g (10–18 capsules) should be given daily in divided doses.

Use in the elderly: Clinical evidence would indicate that no special dosage regime is necessary.

Contra-indications, warnings, etc *Side-effects:* Metopirone may give rise to nausea and vomiting which can be controlled to some extent by taking a biscuit and milk at the same time as the capsule.

Note: Failure to absorb the drug due either to vomiting or malabsorption may give false results.

Precautions: Metopirone should be used with extreme caution in patients where gross hypopituitarism is suspected because of the risk of precipitating acute adrenal failure.

Because of the risk that Metopirone can impair the biosynthesis of foetal-placental steroids, it would seem unwise to administer it during pregnancy.

Treatment of Overdosage: The clinical picture of acute Metopirone poisoning is characterised by gastro-intestinal symptoms and acute adreno-cortical insufficiency. General measures should be taken to reduce the absorption and increase the elimination of the drug. A large dose of hydrocortisone should be administered, together with i.v. saline and glucose. This should be repeated as necessary in accordance with the patient's clinical condition.

Pharmaceutical precautions The capsules should be protected from heat and moisture.

Legal category POM.

Package quantities 250 mg capsules of Metopirone in Securitainers of 100.

Further information Since the response to Metopirone involves the adrenal cortex, it is necessary to ensure that the adrenal function is adequate (by means of ACTH or 'Synacthen') before ascribing a subnormal response to hypothalamic or pituitary dysfunction. It must be emphasised that this procedure assesses only the feedback control mechanism, and a normal response does not necessarily indicate the ability of the HPA axis to respond to stress.

Product licence number 0008/5078.

MONASPOR* ▼

Presentation Vials containing cefsulodin sodium dry active substance corresponding to 0.5 g, 1 g cefsulodin free acid for intramuscular and intravenous use.

Uses *Mode of action:* Monaspor is a semi-synthetic bactericidal beta-lactam antibiotic for parenteral use which displays marked activity against Pseudomonas aeruginosa. The minimum inhibitory concentrations (MIC) are very low, lying within the range of 0.25–8 mcg/ml for 88% of the Pseudomonas strains investigated.

Monaspor is stable against the majority of relevant beta-lactamases and is also active against most strains of Pseudomonas aeruginosa resistant to carbenicillin and gentamicin.

Indications: Monaspor is indicated for the treatment of infections caused by sensitive strains of Pseudomonas aeruginosa. These include:

Chronic recurrent urinary tract infections e.g. pyelonephritis, infections accompanying obstructions of the urinary tract (e.g. in the presence of neoplasms; calculi of the urinary tract, or following surgery), prostatitis.

Respiratory tract infections e.g. pneumonia, chronic purulent bronchitis and infections associated with mucoviscidosis.

A number of cases of Pseudomonas infection of bone and soft tissue, such as osteomyelitis, and infected wounds and burns have been treated successfully with Monaspor.

Dosage and administration *Adults:* In adults with normal renal function the usual daily dose is 1–4 grams daily in 2–4 fractional doses.

In urinary tract infections, and chronic bronchitis, 1–3 grams daily in 2–4 fractional doses usually suffices.

In critical cases (e.g. severe pneumonia, osteomyelitis) daily doses of 6 grams or more may be necessary.

Children: The recommended daily dose is 20–50 mg/kg bodyweight.

Administration: Intramuscular: The dry powder should be dissolved using 0.5% lignocaine solution before intramuscular administration.

Intravenous: The dry powder should be reconstituted with Water for Injection to a concentration of 1 g in 10 ml and slowly injected either directly into a vein or into the tube of an intravenous drip.

Infusion: Monaspor can be dissolved in the routinely employed solutions e.g. Sodium Chloride Intravenous Infusion BP, Ringer's Injection USP, Dextrose Intravenous Infusion BP, Dextran 40 Intravenous Infusion BP (10%). It must not be mixed with sodium bicarbonate.

When administering an infusion lasting more than 30–60 minutes and in order to obtain high initial blood levels, it is advisable to inject the first dose as a slow bolus injection.

If Monaspor is infused intermittently via a Y-attachment to another infusion, administration of the latter should be interrupted while the Monaspor infusion is in progress.

Monaspor can be administered in combination with other antibiotics such as gentamicin or carbenicillin. They can either be infused together or injected in the same syringe (diluted with Water for Injection to a total volume of 10 ml). Monaspor, however, should not be pre-mixed with tobramycin but they may be administered separately.

Aqueous solutions of the drug take on a yellow colouration. This has no effect on the drug's antibiotic activity.

Solutions displaying clouding or precipitation after admixing of the drug should not be used.

Only freshly prepared Monaspor solutions should be employed. Monaspor infusion solutions should not be used if they have been stored for longer than 24 hours in a refrigerator (5°C) or 12 hours at room temperature (23°C). Mixtures containing Monaspor and other drugs in the same syringe should not be stored for more than 4 hours at room temperature. The stability of Monaspor solutions is greatest between pH 4–7. Solutions with a pH of greater than 7 should be administered immediately after they have been prepared.

Use in the elderly: No specific information on use in the elderly is available. Concurrent renal insufficiency should be taken into account.

Contra-indications, warnings, etc *Contra-indications:* Hypersensitivity to cephalosporins.

Precautions: In chronic infections it is important that the treatment should be of sufficiently long duration to obtain a successful clinical result.

In cases where lengthy treatment with large doses of Monaspor is required, blood counts and tests of renal function should be performed.

As with any type of antibiotic therapy, it is advisable to determine the sensitivity of the causative microorganisms before initiating treatment.

In patients known to be allergic to penicillin, caution should be exercised when employing Monaspor, since cross-sensitivity with cephalosporins may be encountered. If allergic reactions occur, Monaspor should be withdrawn and suitable countermeasures taken.

In patients with renal failure, the priming dose should be the same as in patients without renal disease. Repeat doses, however, must be reduced in size or the interval between them prolonged. The recommendations in the following table may be used as a guide. The elimination of the drug in dialysis fluid is about 45% of the dose and it is suggested that a normal dose be given at the beginning and end of the dialysis period.

Creatinine clearance	Maintenance doses in % of normal doses at following intervals:			
ml/min	6 h	8 h	12 h	24 h
50	90	90	95	—
30	75	80	90	—
20	65	70	80	—
10	55	60	70	—
5	45	55	65	—
2.5	40	45	60	—
0	—	—	—	75

In patients suffering from severe liver damage and in those allergic to local anaesthetics, Monaspor should be given intramuscularly with sterile Water for Injection or intravenously (i.e. without lignocaine).

When determining urinary sugar levels, enzymatic methods should be used because other techniques may yield false positive results.

Pregnancy: As with other drugs, the use of Monaspor during pregnancy is advised only if there are compelling reasons.

Side-effects: Monaspor is generally well tolerated. The following have been observed as rare side effects: nausea, dizziness, allergic skin reactions, and eosinophilia, as well as occasional increases in the values for transaminases, alkaline phosphatase, non-protein nitrogen, and serum creatinine. Intravenous injections of Monaspor are usually painless when administered slowly. Local pain occurring as a reaction to intramuscular injections can be prevented by using 0.5% lignocaine solution.

Pharmaceutical precautions The vials should be stored below 25°C and protected from light.

Legal category POM.

Package quantities Vials containing 0.5 g or 1 g of active substance.

Further information Nil.

Product licence numbers
500 mg vials   0008/0159
1 g   vials   0008/0162

NAVIDREX*

Presentation Navidrex Tablets containing 0.5 mg of cyclopenthiazide BP as white, flat, circular tablets with bevelled edges, bearing the monogram CIBA on one side, and the letters AO on each side of a breakline on the other.

Uses *Mode of action:* Navidrex is a thiazide diuretic which exerts its diuretic effect by inhibiting the reabsorption of sodium, chloride and water, probably at the proximal renal tubules.

Indications: Navidrex is indicated for the treatment of mild to moderate hypertension, in more severe hypertension it may be used in conjunction with other antihypertensive agents. It is also indicated for the treatment of acute and chronic heart failure, oedema associated with renal disease, pre-menstrual tension, liver disease, oedema and hypertension associated with pregnancy.

Dosage and administration *Adults:* Hypertension 0.25 mg to 0.5 mg daily, increasing rarely to a maximum of 1.5 mg. For best results in hypertension doses should be given seven days a week, the entire dose being taken in the morning.

In acute and chronic heart failure, oedema associated with renal or liver disease, an initial dose of 0.5 mg to 1 mg until a satisfactory clinical response is attained. The maximum effective dose is 1.5 mg daily although this is rarely required. When a satisfactory clinical response is achieved a dose of 0.5 mg on alternate days is usually adequate.

Pre-menstrual tension 0.25 mg to 0.5 mg daily from the onset of symptoms until menstruation begins.

Since Navidrex increases salt excretion it is usually possible to relax dietary salt restriction.

Use in the elderly: No special dosage regime is necessary (also see 'Precautions').

Contra-indications, warnings, etc *Side-effects:* Side-effects such as mild anorexia, nausea, constipation and diarrhoea, skin rashes and photosensitivity may

occur. There have been reports of blood dyscrasias including thrombocytopenia, but these are rare.

Contra-indications: Navidrex is contra-indicated in the presence of precoma associated with hepatic cirrhosis or Addison's disease or advanced renal failure.

Precautions: In patients with some degree of renal impairment, a rise in blood urea can occur and in extreme cases result in an oliguric crisis. In such cases, either the dose should be reduced or the treatment interrupted temporarily.

Prolonged doses may bring about a decrease in glucose tolerance and precipitate a diabetic condition. In known diabetics the addition of Navidrex to the treatment regime will almost certainly alter the insulin requirement.

In common with other thiazide diuretics hyperuricaemia may be induced by Navidrex. Gout may be exacerbated in patients with a previous history or family history of this condition.

Patients who are being treated with this preparation may require regular monitoring of fluid and electrolyte balance particularly when diuresis is substantial or in patients suffering from renal impairment. Potassium supplements may be required. Particular caution is needed with this preparation in the elderly since electrolyte balance is more likely to be precarious due to bowel or renal dysfunction. Also urinary retention is more likely.

Navidrex should only be used during pregnancy if considered essential by the physician.

The concomitant administration of this preparation with cardiac glycosides or hypotensive agents may necessitate adjustment of the dosage of those drugs.

Pharmaceutical precautions Protect from heat and moisture.

Legal category POM.

Package quantities Navidrex is available in Securitainers of 100.

Further information After a single oral dose diuresis starts within one or two hours reaching a maximum in four to eight hours, lasting up to 12 hours. If taken in the morning the clearly defined duration of action ensures that the patient can sleep undisturbed at night. It is important that the patient be encouraged to take a potassium rich diet during treatment with Navidrex. For routine use, it is advisable to give supplementary potassium, e.g. 'Slow-K' or alternatively to use 'Navidrex-K' which contains 'Slow-K'.

Product licence number 0008/5047.

NAVIDREX-K*

Presentation Yellow-ochre, polished, sugar coated tablets, about 12 mm in diameter, having an inner slow-release wax core containing Potassium Chloride BP 600 mg (8.06 mEq) and an outer coat containing 0.25 mg cyclopenthiazide BP.

Uses Navidrex-K is a thiazide diuretic, which exerts its diuretic effect by inhibiting the reabsorption of sodium, chloride and water, probably at the proximal renal tubules. It is indicated for the treatment of mild to moderate hypertension. In more severe hypertension it may be used in conjunction with other antihypertensive agents. Navidrex-K is also indicated for the treatment of acute and chronic heart failure, oedema associated with renal disease, pre-menstrual tension, liver disease, oedema and hypertension associated with pregnancy.

Dosage and administration *Adults: Oral:* In hypertension, 0.25–0.5 mg (1 or 2 tablets) daily is usually sufficient. Rarely, 1.5 mg (6 tablets) daily may be required. For best results in hypertension doses should be given seven days a week. In acute and chronic heart failure and oedema associated with renal or liver disease, an initial dose of 0.5–1 mg (2–4 tablets) daily until a satisfactory clinical response is attained.

The maximum effective dose is 1.5 mg (6 tablets) daily, although this is rarely required.

When a satisfactory clinical response is achieved, a maintenance dose of 0.25–0.5 mg (1 or 2 tablets) daily or 0.5 mg (2 tablets) on alternate days is usually adequate.

Pre-menstrual tension, 0.25–0.5 mg (1 or 2 tablets) daily from the onset of symptoms until menstruation begins.

The entire daily dose should be taken in the morning and it is important that the tablet be swallowed whole.

Children: Oral: At the discretion of the physician.

Use in the elderly: No special dosage regime is necessary (also see 'Precautions').

Note: Since Navidrex-K increases salt excretion it is usually possible to relax dietary salt restrictions.

Contra-indications, warnings, etc *Side-effects:* Side-effects such as mild anorexia, nausea, constipation and diarrhoea, skin rashes and photosensitivity may occur as a result of treatment with Navidrex-K. In common with other thiazides, there have been reports of thrombocytopenia, but these are rare.

Navidrex-K tablets are designed to avoid the risks of gastro-intestinal irritation. However, if a patient under treatment with Navidrex-K develops severe vomiting, severe abdominal pains or flatulence or gastro-intestinal haemorrhage, the preparation should be withdrawn at once, because in the presence of an obstruction it could conceivably give rise to ulceration or perforation.

Contra-indications: Navidrex-K is contra-indicated in the presence of hyperkalaemia or precoma associated with hepatic cirrhosis, Addison's disease or advanced renal failure.

All solid forms of potassium medication are contra-indicated in the presence of obstructions in the digestive tract (e.g. resulting from compression of the oesophagus due to dilation of the left atrium or from stenosis of the gut).

Precautions: In patients with some degree of renal impairment, a rise in blood urea can occur and in extreme cases result in an oliguric crisis. In such cases, either the dose should be reduced or the treatment interrupted temporarily.

Prolonged doses of thiazides may bring about a decrease in glucose tolerance and precipitate a diabetic condition. In known diabetics the addition of Navidrex-K to the treatment regime will almost certainly alter the insulin requirement.

In common with other thiazide diuretics, Navidrex-K may precipitate an attack of gout in patients predisposed to this condition.

Patients who are being treated with this preparation may require regular monitoring of fluid and electrolyte balance particularly when diuresis is substantial or in patients suffering from renal impairment. Potassium supplements may be required. Particular caution is needed with this preparation in the elderly since electrolyte balance is more likely to be precarious due to bowel or renal dysfunction. Also urinary retention is more likely.

Navidrex-K should only be used during pregnancy if considered essential by the physician.

The concomitant administration of this preparation with cardiac glycosides or hypotensive agents may necessitate adjustment of the dosage of those drugs.

Pharmaceutical precautions Navidrex-K Tablets should be protected from heat and moisture. The tablets should be dispensed in a moisture-proof container.

Legal category POM.

Package quantities Navidrex-K Tablets are available in Securitainers of 100 and 500.

Further information The low absolute doses required with Navidrex-K, compared to other thiazide diuretics, make it economical in all appropriate indications. After a single dose, diuresis starts within 1–2 hours, reaches a maximum in 4–8 hours and lasts about 12 hours. Thus a morning dose will permit the patient to sleep undisturbed at night. Hypertension is also controlled by a single daily dose. The built-in potassium supplement is based on Slow-K* and compared with other potassium supplements, is less likely to produce an unpalatable taste, gastro-intestinal irritation or inadequate absorption.

Product licence number 0008/5036.

ORIMETEN* ▼

Presentation Tablets containing 250 mg aminoglutethimide. White to yellowish white, round with slightly convex faces and slightly bevelled edges, printed 'CG' on one side and 'GG' with score on the other.

Uses *Mode of action:* Orimeten inhibits several cytochrome P450 mediated hydroxylation steps in the adrenal cortex, including the initial step of cholesterol side chain cleavage to $\Delta 5$ pregnenolone. It further inhibits the extra-adrenal aromatisation of androgens to oestrogens.

The mode of action of Orimeten in prostatic carcinoma is not fully understood, and the concurrent use of a corticosteroid is at present recommended.

Pharmacokinetics: Orimeten is well absorbed and peak plasma levels are attained within 1–2 hours. The drug is 21–25% bound to plasma proteins and during long term therapy plasma half-life averages 7 hours (during the first 7–14 days of therapy auto-induction occurs). Approximately 40% of the dose is excreted in the urine unchanged and up to 25% in the form of N-acetylaminoglutethimide.

Indications: Advanced carcinoma of the breast in postmenopausal or oophorectomised women (especially where the tumours are oestrogen-sensitive), including in particular patients who have previously responded to endocrine therapy or have painful bony metastases.

Advanced carcinoma of the prostate as palliative treatment. Subjective improvement and pain relief have been noted in up to 50% of patients.

Cushing's syndrome due to malignant disease, e.g. adrenocortical carcinoma or ectopic ACTH syndrome, in place of or in conjunction with surgery.

Dosage and administration Orimeten tablets should be administered orally.

Adults:
Advanced carcinoma of the breast and of the prostate:
Starting at one tablet daily the dose should be increased each week by one tablet per day to the maximum tolerated dose, not exceeding 1000 mg daily e.g. Week 1 – 250 mg once daily, Week 2 – 250 mg twice daily, Week 3 – 250 mg three times daily, Week 4 – 250 mg four times daily.

In the majority of patients treated for carcinoma of the prostate the effective dose has not exceeded 750 mg daily.

Supplementary therapy: In order to provide physiological replacement, a glucorticoid should be given in conjunction with Orimeten.

20 mg hydrocortisone twice daily is suitable at all Orimeten dose levels. Orimeten accelerates the metabolism of dexamethasone to a variable extent, therefore individual titration to a relatively high dose (up to 3 mg daily) may be required if this glucocorticoid is used.

Cushings syndrome due to malignant disease: Initially 250 mg daily, increasing gradually according to response up to 1 g daily in divided doses. In some cases, especially ectopic ACTH syndrome, higher dosages (of up to 1.5–2 g daily) may occasionally prove necessary to achieve adequate suppression.

Supplementary therapy: With initial treatment no corticosteroids should be necessary. Plasma cortisol levels should be regularly monitored and dosage adapted accordingly. In some cases, an 'escape' phenomenon may occur, i.e. the plasma cortisol concentration may rise again after a certain time; in other cases – especially in patients with adrenocortical tumours, who possibly respond more sensitively to Orimeten – it may show excessive decrease. Should adrenocortical insufficiency occur supplementary glucocorticoids may be given.

Use in the elderly: There is no evidence to suggest that dosage should be different in the elderly.

Use in children: Dosage not established.

Contra-indications, warnings, etc
Precautions: In some patients the suppression of aldosterone synthesis may lead to hyponatraemia, hyperkalaemia, hypotension and dizziness, in which case a mineralocorticoid (e.g. fludrocortisone 0.1–0.15 mg daily or on alternate days) should be given.

The patients blood count and plasma electrolytes should be checked regularly. If, during treatment with aminoglutethimide, signs of Cushing's Syndrome (due to concomitant glucocorticoid medication) appear, the dosage of the glucocorticoid should be reduced.

Treatment with Orimeten and steroids may impair the adrenal response to stress.

Drug interactions: Orimeten may increase the rate of metabolism and therefore necessitate dosage adjustment of some drugs e.g. coumarin anti-coagulants, oral anti-diabetic agents and synthetic glucocorticoids.

Contra-indications:
Use in pregnancy and lactation: Since foetal abnormalities have been observed in animals and there have been cases of pseudohermaphroditism in newborn infants of women treated with Orimeten, use during pregnancy and lactation is contra-indicated.

Side-effects: The tolerability of Orimeten varies greatly from patient to patient and after the first 6–8 weeks of treatment side-effects diminish or abate completely.

Central nervous side effects, such as dizziness, somnolence and lethargy are not uncommon, but unsteadiness occurs only in the higher dosage range. Gastrointestinal effects such as nausea, vomiting or diarrhoea, are less frequent. All these effects are dose dependent. Drug rash – accompanied sometimes by fever – may develop after 7–14 days; it usually subsides within 7–10 days despite continued treatment, but if it fails to do so, the treatment must be reduced or temporarily withdrawn or the dosage of the concomitant glucocorticoid raised. There have been rare reports of pancytopenia, leucopenia and agranulocytosis.

Occasionally, Orimeten has been found to interfere with thyroid function by inhibiting thyroxine biosynthesis.

Accidental overdosage: Clinical experience with Orimeten in overdose is limited. However, it may reduce the production of steroids from the adrenal cortex to a degree which is clinically relevant. Overdosage may lead to hypotension, central nervous system depression, impaired consciousness, electrolyte disturbances, respiratory depression and hypoventilation.

Removal of the tablets from the gastro-intestinal tract is recommended. Supportive treatment to maintain fluid and electrolyte balance and treatment with iv steroids may be needed. The chemical structure of Orimeten indicates that it may have a great affinity for fatty tissue and symptoms may therefore recur.

Pharmaceutical precautions Protect from heat, light and moisture.

Legal category POM.

Package quantities Securitainers of 100 tablets.

Further information In many cases of carcinoma of the breast, metastases or recurring tumours diminish in size or even disappear during treatment with Orimeten. Such remission may be maintained for several years. Bone metastases attributable to breast cancer respond particularly well, the patient often experiencing marked relief of pain.

In advanced carcinoma of the prostate, patients may also benefit from marked relief of bone pain. Objective tumour regression has been seen in some patients.

Product licence number 0008/0147.

RIMACTANE*

Presentation Rimactane Capsules each containing 150 mg Rifampicin BP. An opaque, two-piece, hard gelatine capsule size 2, reddish-brown in colour, marked with the monogram CIBA on each half and the code JZ 150. The capsule has a diameter of 6.2 mm approx. and is 17.8 mm approx. in length.

Rimactane Capsules each containing 300 mg Rifampicin BP. An opaque, two-piece, hard gelatine capsule size 1, coloured reddish-brown and dark brown, marked with the monogram CIBA on each half and the code CS 300. The capsule is approx. 6.8 mm in diameter and 18.7 mm approx. in length.

Rimactane Syrup: An opaque, red-coloured suspension having the odour and taste of raspberry; each 5 ml contains 100 mg Rifampicin BP.

Uses *Mode of action:* Rimactane is a semi-synthetic antibiotic with bactericidal activity against most groups of mycobacteria. Rimactane is active in vitro at low concentrations against Gram positive organisms and at higher concentrations against Gram negative organisms.

Indications: Rimactane is a major drug in the management of tuberculosis and certain opportunist mycobacterial infections. It is effective in cases resistant to other anti-tuberculous agents and shows no cross-resistance outside the rifamycin group of drugs. It is effective in combination with isoniazid, streptomycin, pyrazinamide, ethambutol and the majority of second-line drugs.

Dosage and administration Rimactane should be given as a single dose, preferably on an empty stomach, at least 30 minutes before breakfast to ensure a high peak serum concentration. Dosage should be adjusted according to body weight of patients.

Adults: Oral: 450–600 mg daily as a single dose (based on approximately 10 mg per kg body weight). (Those patients 50 kg (8 stone) and over should take 600 mg rifampicin daily, whilst patients under 50 kg should take 450 mg).

Children: Oral: Up to 20 mg per kg body weight daily to a maximum of 600 mg as a single dose.

Premature and newborn infants: Oral: 10 mg/kg once daily. Do not exceed this dosage. These infants, in whom the liver enzyme system is not yet fully developed, should be given Rimactane only in grave emergencies.

Rimactane must always be given in association with at least one and preferably two other anti-tuberculosis drugs, to prevent the emergence of resistant strains. Especially good results have been reported when Rimactane has been used in combination with isoniazid and ethambutol. Whilst it is not generally recommended that rifampicin be used in combination with PAS, if for any reason this regimen is used, the drugs should be given not less than eight hours apart to ensure satisfactory blood levels.

Use in the elderly: No special dosage regime is necessary but concurrent hepatic insufficiency should be taken into account.

Use in pregnancy and lactation: Rifampicin has been shown to have teratogenic effects in animals on very high doses, therefore during pregnancy the use of Rimactane should, if possible, be avoided. Particularly during the first 3 months of pregnancy, the drug's possible risks for the foetus must be carefully weighed against its therapeutic benefits for the mother.

When administered during the last few weeks of pregnancy, Rimactane can cause post-natal haemorrhages in mother and infant, for which treatment with vitamin K may be indicated.

Rifampicin is excreted in breast milk. Mothers in whom its use proves unavoidable should refrain from breast-feeding their infants.

Contra-indications, warnings, etc *Contra-indications:* Rimactane is contra-indicated in patients with jaundice or where there is known hypersensitivity to rifamycins.

Precautions: As Rimactane is excreted principally by the biliary tract, caution should be exercised in treating patients with hepatic disorders. Such patients should have liver function monitored during treatment.

In the presence of complete renal failure rifampicin is excreted entirely in the bile, provided hepatic function is not impaired the dosage of rifampicin need not be adjusted.

The occurrence of liver function abnormalities is more common when rifampicin and isoniazid are used in combination, special care is therefore required in patients

with pre-existing liver impairment, or in the elderly, malnourished or very young patient.

When resuming treatment with Rimactane after a temporary or a prolonged interval, the drug should be given in small, gradually increasing doses. In adults an initial dose of 75 mg daily should be administered raised subsequently by 75 mg per day until the desired dosage level is attained. If, as may happen in exceptional cases the patient develops renal failure, thrombocytopenia, purpura or haemolytic anaemia, treatment with Rimactane should be stopped at once and not re-instituted at a later date.

Microbiological techniques for assaying the serum concentrations of folic acid and vitamin B_{12} are not suitable for use during treatment with rifampicin.

Drug interactions: Rifampicin is a potent inducer of liver enzymes which may increase the metabolism of concomitantly administered drugs such as corticosteroids, oral contraceptives, oral anti-coagulants, oral anti-diabetic agents, dapsone, phenytoin, some digitalis preparations, quinidine and methadone. The dosage of these drugs may need considerable review when Rimactane is being prescribed, larger doses usually being needed when Rimactane is introduced and a reduction on withdrawal.

In women receiving treatment with rifampicin it has been found that the contraceptive activity of oral contraceptives may be impaired. In such cases, additional non-hormonal methods should be employed.

Side-effects: Occasionally, gastrointestinal disturbances and skin rashes have been reported after treatment with Rimactane.

Side-effects to rifampicin, probably of immunological/allergic origin have been reported, particularly in connection with intermittent, interrupted or repeated treatment; e.g. influenza-like symptoms and rarely skin rashes, fever and dyspnoea have occurred. If serious complications arise such as thrombocytopenia, purpura, renal failure or haemolytic anaemia, rifampicin should be stopped at once and never restarted.

There may be an elevation of serum bilirubin levels, SGOT and SGPT levels and more rarely alkaline phosphatase during the early stages of treatment. In patients with previously normal liver function these changes are transient and usually revert towards normal pre-treatment levels in about two weeks even when Rimactane is continued. Routine liver function tests during treatment are unnecessary unless the patient becomes unwell or exhibits frank jaundice. The occurrence of jaundice may call for temporary cessation of treatment however in most patients it is possible to resume therapy. (See Precautions).

In common with other antibiotics, mild leucopenia and eosinophilia have been reported in a few patients, but appear to be of no particular clinical significance and no causal relationship has been established.

Treatment of overdosage: There is no specific antidote to Rimactane. In cases of severe overdosage gastric lavage may be undertaken and general supportive treatment administered.

Pharmaceutical precautions This product should be protected from heat and moisture.

The syrup to be stored below 25°C.

Legal category POM.

Package quantities Capsules of 150 mg Rimactane (red) and 300 mg Rimactane (red and brown) in securitainers of 100.

Syrup containing 100 mg in 5 ml; in bottles of 100 ml.

Further information Rimactane is orally active, very well tolerated and its activity is comparable with that of isoniazid. In combination, these two agents are commonly used as first-line therapy and offer the greatest chance of rapid eradication of the infection. It is usual, however, to employ a third drug during the first two months of treatment or at least until the results of sensitivity tests are known. The orange-red colour imparted to the urine, sputum and tears by rifampicin is a valuable guide to adherence to the drug regime. Rifampicin may also permanently discolour soft contact lenses.

Product licence numbers
Rimactane Capsules 150 mg   0008/5080
Rimactane Capsules 300 mg   0008/5081
Rimactane Syrup   0008/0106

RIMACTANE* INFUSION

Presentation 10 ml vial containing 300 mg Rifampicin BP (red lyophilised powder) with an accompanying 5 ml ampoule of clear colourless solvent solution (Water for Injection BP + polysorbate 81).

Uses Rimactane is active in vitro at low concentrations against gram-positive organisms and at higher concentrations against gram-negative organisms. Rimactane Infusion is indicated in patients with all forms of tuberculosis who are unable to tolerate oral therapy, e.g. post operative or comatose patients or patients in whom gastro-intestinal absorption is impaired.

Dosage and administration *Treatment of tuberculosis* with Rimactane Infusion should concurrently include the use of other effective anti-tuberculous drugs to prevent the emergence of rifampicin-resistant strains of Mycobacteria.

Adults: In tuberculosis daily adminstration of 600 mg when given in an intravenous drip over two to three hours has been found to be effective and well tolerated for the majority of adult patients. Serum concentrations following this dosage regimen are similar to those obtained after 600 mg by mouth. Lower doses are recommended for small, or frail and elderly patients. A daily dose of 8 mg/kg bodyweight should not be exceeded in patients with impaired liver function.

Transfer to oral therapy: When patients are able to accept oral medication, they should be transferred to Rimactane capsules or syrup. Oral dosage would be expected to be the same as that used with the infusion (see oral Rimactane data sheet).

Children: Paediatric usage has not yet been established. However, the following regimens are suggested:

In tuberculosis, a single daily dose of up to 20 mg/kg bodyweight is recommended, although total daily dose should not usually exceed 600 mg.

Use in the elderly: No special dosage regime is necessary but concurrent hepatic insufficiency should be taken into account.

Preparation of Infusion: Rimactane Infusion is prepared for use by aseptically adding the solvent to the vial of rifampicin powder and shaking vigorously and continuously for about 30 seconds.

When the powder has completely dissolved, the solution should be immediately diluted in 250 ml of 5% glucose solution or other suitable infusion fluid (see

Pharmaceutical Precautions). It is suggested that the infusion is administered over a period of 2–3 hours. The preparation should be used within 6 hours.

Contra-indications, warnings, etc
Contra-indications: Hypersensitivity to rifamycins.

Although not recommended for use in patients with jaundice, the therapeutic benefit of Rimactane Infusion should be weighed against the possible risks.

During pregnancy the use of Rimactane should if possible be avoided. Particularly during the first 3 months of pregnancy the drug's possible risks for the foetus must be carefully weighed against its therapeutic benefits for the mother.

When administered during the last few weeks of pregnancy, Rimactane can cause post-natal haemorrhages in the mother and infant, for which treatment with vitamin K may be indicated.

Rimactane passes into the breast milk. Mothers in whom its use proves unavoidable should refrain from breast-feeding their infants.

Precautions: As rifampicin is excreted principally by the biliary tract, caution should be exercised in treating patients with hepatic disorders. Such patients should have liver function monitored during treatment and lower doses of Rimactane Infusion may be necessary.

The occurrence of liver function abnormalities is more common when rifampicin and isoniazid are used in combination and special care is therefore required when these are used in patients with pre-existing liver impairment or in the elderly, malnourished or very young patients.

Rifampicin is a potent inducer of liver enzymes which may increase the metabolism of concomitantly administered drugs such as corticosteroids, oral contraceptives, oral anticoagulants, oral antidiabetic agents, dapsone, digitalis preparations, quinidine, and methadone. The dosage of these drugs may need considerable review when rifampicin is being prescribed, larger doses usually being needed when rifampicin is introduced and a reduction when it is withdrawn.

Women taking oral contraceptives should use additional non-hormonal means of contraception.

When resuming treatment with rifampicin after a prolonged interval, renal function should be closely monitored. If, as may happen in exceptional cases, the patient develops renal failure, thrombocytopenia, purpura, or haemolytic anaemia, treatment with rifampicin should be stopped at once and not re-instituted at a later date.

Notes: In the presence of complete renal failure, rifampicin is excreted entirely in the bile; provided hepatic function is not impaired the dosage of rifampicin need not be adjusted.

Microbiological techniques for assaying the serum concentrations of folic acid and Vitamin B_{12} are not suitable for use during treatment with rifampicin.

Side-effects: Rimactane Infusion is generally very well tolerated and accepted by patients, although hypersensitivity reactions have been described, and occasionally patients have experienced fever, skin rashes and nausea/vomiting. A few cases of broncho-spasm, occurring mainly in chronic asthmatics, have been reported; no causal relationship has been established.

Local tolerability: occasional instances of phlebitis and pain at the infusion site have been reported.

Side-effects to rifampicin, probably of immunological/allergic origin have been reported, particularly in connection with intermittent, interrupted or repeated treatment; for example, influenza-like symptoms, and, rarely skin rashes, fever and dyspnoea have occurred. If serious complications arise such as thrombocytopenia, purpura, renal failure or haemolytic anaemia, rifampicin should be stopped at once and never restarted.

In patients with previously normal liver function, experience has shown that in many cases changes in liver function are transient and usually revert towards normal pre-treatment levels in about two weeks, even when rifampicin is continued. Routine liver function tests during treatment are unnecessary unless the patient becomes unwell or exhibits frank jaundice. An isolated report showing a moderate rise in the serum bilirubin and/or transaminase or more rarely alkaline phosphatase level is not usually itself an indication for interrupting treatment. The decision should be made after repeating the tests, noting the trends in the levels and considering them in conjunction with the patient's clinical condition. It has been possible in most patients in whom alterations to liver function caused interruption of Rimactane Infusion therapy, to carefully reinstate the drug.

In common with other antibiotics, mild leucopenia, and eosinophilia have been reported in a few patients, but appear to be of no particular clinical significance and no causal relationship has been established.

Rifampicin may produce a reddish discolouration of the urine, sputum and tears; soft contact lenses may also be discoloured.

Pharmaceutical precautions Rimactane Infusion should be freshly prepared. The vials should be protected from heat and light.

Compatibility: Rimactane Infusion is compatible with the following infusion solutions for up to 6 hours: Mannitol 10% and 20%. Macrodex with saline solution, Macrodex with glucose solution, Rheomacrodex, sodium bicarbonate 1.4%, laevulose 5% and 10%, Ringer lactate, Ringer acetate, dextrose 5% and 10%, saline solution.

Incompatibility: Rimactane Infusion is incompatible with the following: Perfudex, sodium bicarbonate 5%, sodium lactate 0.167M, Ringer acetate with dextrose.

Rimactane Infusion should not be mixed with other drugs as precipitation may occur; concurrent intravenous therapy should be administered via a different site of injection.

Legal category POM.

Package quantities
Rimactane Infusion 300 mg: Combined pack of 1 vial + 1 × 5 ml solvent ampoule.

Product licence number
Rimactane Infusion 300 mg   0008/0151

RIMACTAZID* COMBINED TABLETS

Presentation Rimactazid 150 Tablets each containing 150 mg Rifampicin BP (Rimactane*) and 100 mg Isoniazid BP, pink, round, bi-convex, sugar-coated tablets, marked with the monogram CG on one side and the letters EI on the other.

Rimactazid 300 Tablets each containing 300 mg Rifampicin BP (Rimactane*) and 150 mg Isoniazid BP; brownish orange, capsule-shaped, bi-convex, sugar-coated tablets, marked with the monogram CG on one side and the letters DH on the other.

Uses *Mode of action:* Rimactazid contains the semi-synthetic antibiotic Rimactane, which has bactericidal activity against most groups of Mycobacteria, and isoniazid, which is an effective anti-bacterial agent against Mycobacterium tuberculosis.

Indications: Rimactane and isoniazid are both major drugs in the management of tuberculosis and in certain opportunist mycobacterial infections. This combination has been shown to eradicate tuberculosis infection faster and more effectively than any previous regimen. Extensive UK experience has led to the routine use of Rimactane and isoniazid as basic therapy supported in the first six to eight weeks, or until cultures are negative, by a third drug, e.g. streptomycin, pyrazinamide, ethambutol and the majority of second-line drugs. Whilst it is not generally recommended that rifampicin be used in combination with PAS, if for any reason this regimen is used, the drugs should be given not less than eight hours apart to ensure satisfactory blood levels. Rifampicin is effective in cases resistant to other anti-tuberculous agents and shows no cross-resistance outside the rifamycin group of drugs.

Dosage and administration Rimactazid should be given as a single dose, preferably on an empty stomach, if possible 30 minutes before breakfast to ensure a high peak serum concentration. Dosage should be adjusted according to body weight of patients.

Adults: Oral: The combined tablets of Rimactazid provide Rimactane and isoniazid in the accepted ratios to provide the currently recommended adult dose of these two drugs. Thus, 2 tablets daily of Rimactazid 300 are recommended for patients of 50 kg (8 stone) and over and 3 tablets daily of Rimactazid 150 for patients under 50 kg (i.e. the usual daily dosage of 600 mg or 450 mg Rimactane, each with 300 mg isoniazid).

Use in the elderly: No special dosage regime is necessary but concurrent hepatic insufficiency should be taken into account.

Use in pregnancy and lactation: Rifampicin has been shown to have teratogenic effects in animals on very high doses, therefore during pregnancy the use of Rimactazid should, if possible, be avoided. Particularly during the first 3 months of pregnancy the drug's possible risks to the foetus must be carefully weighed against its therapeutic benefits for the mother.

When administered during the last few weeks of pregnancy, Rimactane can cause post-natal haemorrhages in mother and infant, for which treatment with vitamin K may be indicated.

Rifampicin is excreted in breast milk. Mothers in whom its use proves unavoidable should refrain from breast-feeding their infants.

Contra-indications, warnings, etc *Contra-indications:* Rimactazid is contra-indicated in patients with jaundice or where there is known hypersensitivity to rifamycins and/or isoniazid. The causative agent should be replaced by another antituberculous drug in combination therapy.

Psychotic states characterised by mania and hypomania are contra-indications for isoniazid.

Precautions: As Rimactane and isoniazid are metabolised in the liver, patients with impaired liver function should be treated with caution. Such patients should have liver function monitored during treatment. Any deterioration in liver function in these patients is an indication for stopping treatment.

The occurrence of liver function abnormalities is more

common when rifampicin and isoniazid are used in combination and special care is therefore required in patients with pre-existing liver impairment or in the elderly, malnourished or very young patients.

In the presence of complete renal failure rifampicin is excreted entirely in the bile, provided hepatic function is not impaired the dosage of rifampicin need not be adjusted.

When resuming treatment with rifampicin after a temporary interruption or a prolonged interval, the drug should be given in small gradually increasing doses. For this purpose, rifampicin and isoniazid should temporarily be administered in free combination. In adults an initial dose of rifampicin 75 mg daily should be administered, raised subsequently by 75 mg per day until the desired dosage level is attained. During this period, renal function should be closely monitored. If as may happen in exceptional cases the patient develops renal failure, thrombocytopenia, purpura or haemolytic anaemia, treatment with rifampicin should be stopped at once and not re-instituted at a later date. Normal dosage of isoniazid should be continued over this period.

Microbiological techniques for assaying the serum concentrations of folic acid and Vitamin B_{12} are not suitable for use during treatment with rifampicin.

Care should be taken in giving isoniazid to patients suffering from convulsive disorders, chronic alcoholism or impaired liver or kidney function. Pyridoxine may be useful in preventing the occurrence of peripheral neuritis.

Drug Interactions: Rifampicin is a potent inducer of liver enzymes which may increase the metabolism of concomitantly administered drugs such as corticosteroids, oral contraceptives, oral anti-coagulants, oral anti-diabetic agents, dapsone, some digitalis preparations, quinidine and methadone. The dosage of these drugs may need considerable review when Rimactazid or Rimactane is being prescribed, larger doses being needed when Rimactazid or Rimactane is introduced and a reduction when either is withdrawn.

In women receiving treatment with rifampicin it has been found that the contraceptive activity of oral contraceptives may be impaired. In such cases, additional non-hormonal methods should be employed.

In patients under treatment with phenytoin, the dosage of this drug should be individually readjusted, because isoniazid raises, and rifampicin lowers its plasma concentration.

It is not advisable to administer isoniazid concomitantly with disulphiram, although the mechanism of this interaction is unclear.

Side effects: Associated with Rimactane. Occasionally gastrointestinal disturbance and drug rashes have been reported after treatment with Rimactane.

There may be an elevation of serum bilirubin levels, SGOT and SGPT levels and more rarely alkaline phosphatase during the early stages of treatment.

In patients with previously normal liver function these changes are transient and usually revert towards normal pre-treatment levels in about two weeks even when Rimactane is continued. Routine liver function tests during treatment are unnecessary unless the patient becomes unwell or exhibits frank jaundice. The occurrence of jaundice may call for temporary cessation of treatment however in most patients it is possible to resume therapy. (See Precautions).

In common with other antibiotics, mild leucopenia and eosinophilia have been reported in a few patients, but appear to be of no particular clinical significance and no causal relationship has been established.

Associated with isoniazid: Side-effects with isoniazid are not common, but hypersensitivity reactions characterised by fever, rash and lymphadenopathy do occur. Isoniazid can cause a mood elevating effect in high dosage which can result in more severe manic disturbances. Occasionally peripheral neuritis has been described, also liver function disturbances, blood dyscrasias, rheumatic syndrome and lupus erythematosis – like signs and symptoms. Hyperglycaemia and gynaecomastia have also been associated with isoniazid treatment.

Treatment of overdosage: There is no specific antidote to Rimactane. In cases of severe overdosage gastric lavage may be undertaken and general supportive treatment administered.

Severe overdosage of isoniazid has been treated with phenobarbitone given intravenously, pyridoxine and oxygen. Peritoneal dialysis has also been used.

Pharmaceutical precautions Rimactazid Tablets should be protected from heat and moisture. The combined tablets have a shelf-life of four years.

Legal category POM.

Package quantities Rimactazid 150 Tablets (pink) and Rimactazid 300 Tablets (brownish orange) in securitainers of 100. Rimactazid 150 tablets – blister packs of 84. Rimactazid 300 tablets blister packs of 56.

Further information Rimactane is orally active, very well tolerated and its activity is comparable with that of isoniazid. In combination, these two agents are commonly used as first-line therapy and offer the greatest chance of rapid eradication of the infection. It is usual, however, to employ a third drug during the first two months of treatment or at least until the results of sensitivity tests are known. Continuation therapy with rifampicin and isoniazid has been shown to eradicate the infection in almost all patients faster and with a lower relapse rate than any alternative regime. The combined tablets of Rimactazid thus make the most effective combination simpler to take. The orange-red colour imparted to the urine, sputum and tears by rifampicin is a valuable guide to drug adherence; rifampicin may also permanently discolour soft contact lenses.

Product licence numbers

Rimactazid 150 mg	0008/0121
Rimactazid 300 mg	0008/0120

ROGITINE*

Presentation Clear glass ampoules each containing 50 mg phentolamine mesylate presented as a colourless to pale yellow solution in 5 ml water for injection. Each box contains 5 × 5 ml ampoules. Also available as ampoules containing 10 mg phentolamine mesylate in 1 ml water for injection. Each box contains 6 × 1 ml ampoules.

Uses *Mode of Action:* Acute, severe cardiac insufficiency is often characterised by a high degree of sympathico-adrenergic stimulation which leads to a pronounced increase in the myocardial oxygen requirement. Marked peripheral vasoconstriction and a rise in left-ventricular filling pressure, accompanied by pulmonary congestion or pulmonary oedema, are usually also present.

In patients with acute, severe cardiac insufficiency, particularly when due to recent myocardial infarction, parenteral administration of Rogitine elicits a prompt improvement in the clinical picture. By acting directly on vascular smooth muscle, by blocking the alpha-receptors, and by indirectly stimulating the beta-receptors, Rogitine exerts a rapid and potent vasodilator effect which also extends to the venous system. Systemic and pulmonary vascular resistance, as well as left-ventricular filling pressure, are reduced. The work load on the heart is thus diminished – alternatively the level of cardiac performance attained at a given work load is improved. Stroke volume and cardiac output are increased, which has the effect of limiting the fall in blood pressure.

Moreover, the positive inotropic activity of Rogitine also helps to enhance cardiac performance. Rogitine, however, does not unduly accelerate the heart rate; on the contrary, the net result of its various effects is a marked easing of the strain on the heart. Besides its direct haemodynamic effect, the drug also stimulates secretion of insulin, which is reduced in the presence of severe cardiac insufficiency; this stimulant action tends to have a favourable influence on myocardial metabolism. The anti-arrhythmic properties possessed by Rogitine may diminish the occurrence of ventricular or supraventricular extra systoles.

Indications: Acute left ventricular failure (cardiogenic shock) particularly following myocardial infarction.

Paroxysmal hypertension associated with phaeochromocytoma or interaction of foodstuffs with MAOI's; and as prophylactic treatment (in combination with a beta-blocker) before and during surgical removal of phaeochromocytoma.

As a diagnostic agent in cases of suspected phaeochromocytoma.

Dosage and administration *Cardiogenic Shock:* The dosage should be individually adapted to the patient's requirements and will depend on the severity of the cardiac insufficiency and on the blood pressure.

Rogitine should be administered in the form of an intravenous infusion in 5% sterile glucose, saline or dextrose saline solution. A dose of 5–60 mg Rogitine should be given over a period of 10–30 minutes at an infusion rate of 0.1–2 mg per minute. If necessary, especially in cases where the systemic arterial blood pressure is elevated, the infusion rate during the first minute can be raised up to 5 mg per minute.

Systolic blood pressure should be carefully monitored during the infusion and a fall below 100 mm Hg is an indication for reducing the infusion rate (see Precautions).

Depending on the patient's response, the treatment can either be continued for several hours or repeated at intervals.

Paroxysmal hypertension: 5–10 mg intramuscularly or intravenously to be repeated if necessary. When used prior to surgical removal of phaeochromocytoma, administer the injection 2 hours before surgery and repeat if necessary during the operation. In children during surgery for the removal of phaeochromocytoma, the dosage is 1 to 5 mg given intravenously according to age.

As a diagnostic test for phaeochromocytoma: This test is based upon the fact that Rogitine produces a fall in blood pressure when it is caused by excess circulating adren-

aline and/or noradrenaline, so it is of value only in the hypertensive phase of the paroxysmal type of case. False positives may result from patients suffering from uraemia, or who have received sedatives or narcotics during the twenty-four hours prior to the test.

The initial step in the test is to determine the basal blood pressure of the patient – this is essential for the correct interpretation of the test. An intravenous injection of 5 mg of Rogitine (1 mg in children) is then administered. As the insertion of the needle may involve a pressor response the blood pressure should be allowed to drop back to within 3 to 4 mm of the basal level before injecting Rogitine.

In the event of a positive response the blood pressure will fall rapidly, and quickly return to basal levels. The blood pressure must be measured at 30 second intervals for 3 minutes after injections, and then every 60 seconds for 7 more minutes.

An immediate marked drop in both systolic and diastolic blood pressure is the typical positive response in patients having a phaeochromocytoma which is discharging adrenaline or noradrenaline at the time of the test. The maximum depressor effect usually occurs within two minutes and usually involves a fall in systolic pressure of about 60 mm and the diastolic fall usually exceeds 25 mm. The blood pressure remains low for only a relatively short time and may return to pre-injection levels within 10–15 minutes. Positive results should be confirmed by either estimation of catecholamines in the urine or by another diagnostic procedure.

False positive results may be seen in patients with uraemia and those having taken sedatives prior to the test.

Whilst false negative results may be seen:

(a) if at the time of injection the tumour is not discharging sufficient adrenaline or noradrenaline to elevate the blood pressure significantly;
(b) when a phaeochromocytoma is present in a patient also having essential hypertension, the test may not cause such a marked fall in blood pressure.

The other clinical findings and tests would usually assist in interpreting such results.

The intravenous administration of Rogitine may cause tachycardia in rare instances, weakness, dizziness or flushing, but are not considered serious in relation to the test.

Further details available on request from CIBA Laboratories, Horsham, West Sussex.

Use in the elderly: Clinical evidence would indicate that no special dosage regime is necessary, but concurrent coronary insufficiency should be taken into account.

Contra-indications, warnings, etc *Contra-indication:* Severe hypotension.

Precautions: Monitoring of the patient's blood pressure, heart rate, and clinical condition is necessary not only to ensure correct selection of cases suitable for treatment with Rogitine but also to decide upon the appropriate dosage and duration of parenteral therapy. As a general rule, a *systolic* pressure of 80 mmHg should be regarded as the lowest limit at which the drug can still be employed.

Side-effects: When administered in the recommended dosages, Rogitine is generally well tolerated. Hypotension, tachycardia and dizziness may occur, particularly if the drug is given parenterally. Nausea, diarrhoea, and nasal congestion have been reported in response to fairly high doses, but they subside again following discontinuation of the infusion.

Treatment of Overdosage: In the event of overdosage (as evidenced by an excessive fall in blood pressure, or by tachycardia) it is usually sufficient simply to discontinue the infusion; if necessary, the effect of Rogitine can be attenuated by giving noradrenaline.

Pharmaceutical precautions Protect from heat and light.

Legal category POM.

Package quantities
(a) Ampoules each containing 50 mg Rogitine in 5 ml Water for Injection. Boxes of 5.
(b) Ampoules each containing 10 mg Rogitine in 1 ml Water for Injection. Boxes of 6.

Further information Nil.

Product licence numbers
Rogitine Ampoules 50 mg/5 ml   0008/0145
Rogitine Ampoules 10 mg/1 ml   0008/5070.

SLOW-K*

Presentation Pale orange, polished, sugar-coated tablets about 12 mm in diameter, printed with the name Slow-K, containing 600 mg (8.06 mEq) of Potassium Chloride BP.

Uses *Mode of Action:* The potassium chloride in Slow-K is finely distributed in a neutral wax base, from which it is gradually released over a period of 3–6 hours during its passage through the digestive tract. This special form of potassium substitution therapy is designed to avoid high localised concentrations of potassium chloride which might irritate or damage the mucosa. The potassium chloride present in Slow-K is completely absorbed in the intestinal tract.

Indications: For the treatment and specific prevention of hypokalaemia especially in cases of the following kinds.

Where protracted or intensive diuretic medication is being given as treatment for hypertension or cardiac failure, and where diuretics have been prescribed to resolve massive oedema. Potassium substitution is of particular importance in patients undergoing concomitant digitalisation because hypokalaemia may cause hypersensitivity to digitalis.

Renal disease associated with increased potassium excretion e.g. nephrotic syndrome.

Liver cirrhosis, especially during diuretic therapy.

Gastro-intestinal disorders accompanied by potassium depletion e.g. chronic diarrhoea, repeated vomiting, ulcerative colitis, status post ileostomy.

Hypochloraemic alkalosis, cases in which a low salt diet or prolonged fasting have been imposed and patients receiving an unbalanced diet deficient in potassium.

Protracted or intensive treatment with corticosteroids, ACTH or carbenoxolone, primary or secondary hyperaldosteronism and Cushing's syndrome.

Initial treatment for megaloblastic anaemia.

In these conditions Slow-K is particularly indicated if a diet rich in potassium cannot be guaranteed.

Dosage and administration *Adults:* The dosage of Slow-K should be adapted to the cause, degree and duration of potassium depletion. 2–6 tablets are usually an adequate supplement. It is important that the tablets should be swallowed whole with fluid during meals.

In states of severe potassium deficiency, a higher dose of 9–12 tablets daily may be needed. According to the dosage of diuretic used and the needs of the individual patient, a dose ratio of one Slow-K tablet with each tablet of thiazide diuretic will usually suffice when administered as a potassium supplement. However, when the more potent diuretics such as frusemide are used, larger doses of Slow-K may be required. Where intermittent diuretic therapy is being used it is probably best to continue the Slow-K on the days between the diuretic administration.

Children: At the discretion of the physician.

Use in the elderly: No special dosage adjustment is usually necessary, but concurrent renal insufficiency should be taken into account (also see 'Precautions').

Contra-indications, warnings, etc *Side-effects:* Side-effects are rare with Slow-K, as any excess potassium is rapidly excreted in the urine.

In rare cases, oral potassium preparations may provoke gastro-intestinal disturbances (nausea, vomiting, abdominal pains, diarrhoea) necessitating either a reduction in dosage or withdrawal of medication (see Precautions).

Contra-indications: Advanced renal failure, untreated Addison's disease, acute dehydration, hyperkalaemia and conditions involving extensive cell destruction (e.g. severe burns).

All solid forms of potassium medication are contra-indicated in the presence of obstructions in the digestive tract (e.g. resulting from compression of the oesophagus due to dilation of the left atrium or from stenosis of the gut).

In cases of metabolic acidosis, the hypokalaemia should be treated not with potassium chloride but with an alkaline potassium salt (e.g. potassium bicarbonate).

Precautions: If a patient under treatment with Slow-K develops severe vomiting, severe abdominal pains or flatulence, or gastro-intestinal haemorrhage, the preparation should be withdrawn at once, because in the presence of an obstruction it could conceivably give rise to ulceration or perforation.

Oral potassium preparations should be prescribed with particular caution in patients with a history of peptic ulcer.

Caution should be exercised when prescribing solid oral potassium preparations, particularly in high dosage, in patients concurrently receiving anticholinergics because of their potential to slow gastrointestinal motility.

In patients suffering from impaired renal function, special care should be exercised when prescribing potassium salts owing to the risk of their producing hyperkalaemia. Monitoring of the serum electrolytes is particularly necessary in patients with diseases of the heart or kidneys.

To guard against the risk of hyperkalaemia, one should also refrain from administering potassium salts together with potassium-sparing diuretics such as aldosterone antagonists or triamterene.

Use in pregnancy: Because of gastro-intestinal hypomotility associated with pregnancy, solid forms of oral potassium preparations should be given to pregnant women only if clearly needed.

Overdosage
Signs and symptoms: Mainly cardiovascular (hypotension, shock, ventricular arrhythmias, bundle-branch block, ventricular fibrillation leading possibly to cardiac arrest) and neuromuscular (paraesthesiae, convulsions,

areflexia, flaccid paralysis of striated muscle leading possibly to respiratory paralysis). Beside elevation of serum potassium concentration, typical ECG changes are also encountered (increasing amplitude and peaking of T waves, disappearance of P wave, widening of QRS complex and S-T depression).

Treatment: Gastric lavage, administration of cation-exchange agents, infusion of glucose and insulin, forced diuresis and possibly peritoneal dialysis or haemodialysis.

Pharmaceutical precautions Slow-K Tablets should be protected from heat and moisture. The tablets should be dispensed in moisture-proof containers.

Legal category GSL.

Package quantities Slow-K Tablets (600 mg Potassium Chloride BP in a special slow-release core, equivalent to 8.06mEq K⁺) Securitainers of 500 and containers of 5000.

Further information The potassium chloride in Slow-K has been shown to be completely absorbed, but occasionally patients may notice 'ghost' tablet cores in the faeces, these have been shown not to contain any potassium. The administration of Slow-K does not obviate the need to encourage the patient to take an adequate potassium-containing diet.

Slow-K has been successfully used in those patients who cannot tolerate liquid potassium chloride preparations or who find their taste unacceptable.

Product licence number 0008/5039.

SLOW-TRASICOR*

Presentation Slow-Trasicor Tablets each containing 160 mg Oxprenolol Hydrochloride BP in a special sustained-release formulation. Circular, slightly bi-convex, white film-coated tablets, having the monogram CIBA impressed on one side and Slow-Trasicor on the other.

Uses *Mode of action:* Slow-Trasicor Tablets release oxprenolol hydrochloride (a non-selective beta-adrenergic receptor blocking drug) gradually from a special sustained release formulation, thus prolonging the pharmacological action.

Slow-Trasicor protects the heart and cardiovascular system against excessive adrenergic stimulation caused by either physical or emotional activity. Accordingly, under conditions of sympathetic drive, heart rate, force of contraction and output are reduced, leading to a fall of myocardial work and oxygen consumption. The extra-cardiac effect of Slow-Trasicor include attenuation of both renin and free fatty acid release.

Slow-Trasicor has partial agonist activity (PAA) also known as intrinsic sympathomimetic activity (ISA). This property means that some degree of stimulation of the beta receptors is maintained. Under conditions of rest, this tends to counterbalance the reduction in heart rate and force of contraction.

Indications: Hypertension: All grades of hypertension in once-daily dosage. The concomitant use of a thiazide diuretic will enhance the antihypertensive effect of Slow-Trasicor, resulting in better control from reduced dosage.

Angina pectoris: For continuous prophylaxis in once-daily dosage to improve exercise tolerance and reduce the frequency and severity of anginal attacks.

Anxiety: For the control of anxiety and anxiety tachycardia.

Dosage and administration Slow-Trasicor Tablets release oxprenolol gradually from a special sustained-release formulation. This provides a considerably longer pharmacological action from a given dose, thus allowing once-daily dosage.

Adults: Hypertension: Initially one tablet daily, given in the morning. If necessary, this dose can be raised to two or more tablets, usually given once daily until satisfactory blood pressure control is achieved. However, when used as monotherapy, dosage should not exceed 3 tablets daily, i.e. 480 mg Slow-Trasicor, since experience has shown that hardly any increase in the response can be achieved by this means. The addition of a diuretic will often give a quicker and more satisfactory response. Usually, patients respond to a dose of one or two tablets of Slow-Trasicor in combination with a diuretic and most of the antihypertensive effect is achieved within 2–3 days. The addition of a vasodilator will often enable control to be achieved in the minority of patients who might otherwise fail to respond.

Angina pectoris: Initially one tablet daily, given in the morning. This can be increased to two or three tablets, usually given once daily depending on patient response. An evening dose may be beneficial in nocturnal angina. Increased dosage is related to increased exercise tolerance, but doses higher than three tablets should not normally be required. Slow-Trasicor is compatible with glyceryl trinitrate and the two drugs are complementary since they reduce heart work by different mechanisms. It may be possible, however, to reduce the use of glyceryl trinitrate when the patient has become established on Slow-Trasicor.

As with other beta-blocking drugs, sudden withdrawal of treatment may induce severe and continuous angina. Patients should, therefore, be advised to avoid interruption of established therapy and if withdrawal becomes necessary it should be done gradually.

Anxiety states: One tablet daily. Although no evidence of habituation or tolerance has been observed with Trasicor its effectiveness in the long term treatment of anxiety has not been established. In the treatment of transient situational anxiety it may be appropriate to prescribe a single dose of 40–80 mg conventional Trasicor. Trasicor can be administered concurrently with benzodiazepines. When withdrawal of pre-existing anxiolytic therapy is indicated this should take place gradually.

Use in the elderly: No special dosage regime is necessary but concurrent hepatic insufficiency should be taken into account.

Contra-indications, warnings, etc *Side-effects:* Slow-Trasicor is well tolerated. However, dizziness, drowsiness, headache, insomnia, excitement and gastro-intestinal disturbance may occur particularly at the start of treatment. Like other beta-blockers, isolated cases of excessive bradycardia and thrombocytopenia have been reported. As with other beta-blockers, bronchospasm and heart failure may occasionally be precipitated in susceptible patients (see Precautions) and exertional tiredness and feelings of coldness in the extremities have been reported on rare occasions. However, the incidence of these side-effects is low, possibly due to the partial protection afforded by the sympathomimetic effect of Slow-Trasicor.

Slow-Trasicor possess antihypertensive effects but these are unlikely to be noted in normotensive subjects.

There have been reports of skin rashes and/or dry eyes associated with the use of beta-adrenergic blocking drugs. The reported incidence is small, and in most cases the symptoms have cleared when the treatment was withdrawn. Discontinuance of the drug should be considered if any such reaction is not otherwise explicable. Cessation of therapy with a beta-adrenergic blocker should be gradual.

Contra-indications: Slow-Trasicor is contra-indicated in patients with atrio-ventricular block, marked bradycardia, uncontrolled heart failure and cardiogenic shock.

Precautions: If there is evidence of cardiac failure this must be controlled by digitalis and/or diuretics before and during Slow-Trasicor therapy. Should the pulse rate fall before 50 per minute, then treatment should be restarted at a lower dose. Caution should be observed when treating asthmatics, chronic bronchitics or other individuals where bronchospasm may be provoked. Slow-Trasicor should be given cautiously to patients with metabolic acidosis, or anaesthesia with ether or chloroform. For anaesthesia the agent selected should be one exhibiting as little negative inotropic activity as possible e.g. halothane, nitrous oxide. Treatment with a beta-blocker is liable to mask symptoms of hypoglycaemia and also to affect carbohydrate metabolism. In patients with labile or insulin dependent diabetes in particular, it may therefore be necessary to readjust the dosage of anti-diabetic medication. Like other beta-blockers, Slow Trasicor should not be given in combination with calcium antagonists of the verapamil type because their concomitant use may result in bradycardia, hypotension or even cardiac arrest.

Pregnancy: Beta-blockers may cause bradycardia in the fetus which can also persist after birth. During pregnancy, in the course of labour and during lactation beta-blockers should only be employed after the needs of the mother have been weighed against the possible risks to the fetus.

Treatment of overdosage: Overdosage with Slow-Trasicor may lead to excessive bradycardia, hypotension, coma and convulsions. It should also be noted that severe toxicity may develop rapidly and that there may be severe hypotension and bradycardia despite a normal ECG. For sinus bradycardia and hypotension 0.5–2.0 mg of atropine should be slowly administered by intravenous infusion. If this does not raise the heart rate sufficiently isoprenaline may be necessary. The dose of isoprenaline needs to be sufficient to reverse the blockade and should be assessed by the clinical response. A reasonable starting dose would be 25 mcg of isoprenaline hydrochloride.

In severe cardiogenic shock the treatment of choice appears to be glucagon. The initial dose should be 5–10 mg intravenously, further boluses or an infusion can be used according to the patient's condition. Transvenous pacing has been used, sometimes with success. If bronchospasm develops bronchodilators should be used. Patients should be monitored for several days as the beta-blocking effects of Slow-Trasicor exceed its plasma half-life.

Pharmaceutical precautions The tablets have no special storage requirements.

Legal category POM.

Package quantities Cartons of 28 Slow-Trasicor Tablets consisting of two reminder calendar foils of 14. (Each carton of 28 represents 2–4 weeks' treatment, depending on whether storage is one or two tablets daily).

Further information Slow-Trasicor is a sustained release preparation of Trasicor* (oxprenolol hydrochloride) designed to release oxprenolol so that maximal response is obtained within 1–2 hours (as with plain Trasicor tablets), whilst the pharmacological action is sustained for 24 hours. Thus Slow-Trasicor produces a smoother absorption of Trasicor and by levelling out peak serum concentrations, avoids 'wastage' and minimises unwanted effects of beta-blockade. Accordingly, there is greater utilisation of Trasicor (oxprenolol) mg for mg (i.e. greater distance walked by an anginal patient before the onset of pain) with Slow-Trasicor.

Trasicor protects the cardiovascular system from excess adrenergic discharge and the resulting elevation of catecholamine levels which are a known risk factor in coronary heart disease and which in the long term, may contribute to the secondary effects of hypertension.

Trasicor prevents emotional tachycardia during environmental stress. In anxiety, Trasicor does not produce sedation or cause dependence. The best response is seen in patients who have not previously received benzodiazepines.

Slow-Trasicor is presented in day-of-the week calendar packs to improve patient compliance.

Product licence number 0008/0130.

SYNACTHEN*

Presentation A clear, colourless, sterile solution containing 0.25 mg tetracosactrin per ml. This preparation is available in 1 ml ampoules.

Uses Mode of action: Synacthen is a synthetic polypeptide with corticotrophic activity and a short duration of action. Synacthen consists of the first 24 amino acids occurring in natural adrenocorticotrophin.

Indications: Since Synacthen has all the properties of natural ACTH it can be used in all situations where a short acting ACTH preparation is indicated but only if other therapeutic measures have failed and under strict medical supervision. Also as a diagnostic test for the investigation of adrenocortical insufficiency.

Dosage and administration Synacthen may be given by intravenous or intramuscular or subcutaneous injection.

Adult dosage for therapeutic use: Intravenously 0.25 mg of Synacthen in 500 ml of infusion fluid (isotonic dextrose or other electrolyte solution) over a six-hour period. By intramuscular injection 0.25 mg every three to four hours.

As a diagnostic aid: Withdraw 5–8 ml of venous blood into a heparinised tube, then inject intramuscularly 0.25 mg of Synacthen. After 30 minutes withdraw a further 5–8 ml into a heparinised tube, centrifuge the blood specimen, measure plasma hydroxycorticoids and interpret the results. (The Mattingly method is suitable.)

For a normal test the initial level of plasma cortisol should be greater than 5 mcg/100 ml (138 nmol/l), provided that the patient has not received a glucocorticoid within the previous 12 hours. The plasma cortisol level 30 minutes after the injection of Synacthen should be greater than 18 mcg/100 ml (500 nmol/l) irrespective of the initial level, and should have risen by at least 7 mcg/100 ml (200 nmol/l).

Synacthen should not be added to blood or plasma transfusions as it is liable to be inactivated by the enzymes.

When administering Synacthen for a therapeutic effect the route of choice is by intravenous infusion in isotonic dextrose or electrolyte solution. The rate of infusion is important. It is suggested that 500 ml containing 0.25 mg of Synacthen should be given over six hours at the rate of approximately 24 drops per minute. When given intravenously 1 mg of Synacthen is equivalent in activity to approximately 100 units of corticotrophin.

Use in the elderly: No specific information on use in the elderly available but no evidence to suggest that an alteration in dosage is required.

Contra-indications, warnings, etc *Contra-indications:* In rare cases, particularly in patients subject to asthma and/or other forms of allergy, severe anaphylactic shock reactions may occur. Such reactions usually start within 30 minutes after administration of Synacthen and should be considered an absolute contra-indication to further treatment with this polypeptide. In view of this Synacthen should not be used for the treatment of asthma or other allergic disorders.

Milder reactions of an allergic or hypersensitive nature should also be considered as an indication that the course of treatment should be stopped and not restarted, since a trivial reaction may be followed by a more serious event if further injections are given. These milder reactions include urticaria, pruritis, flushing and faintness and dyspnoea. Since some reactions have occurred without warning wherever possible patients should remain at the hospital or doctor's surgery for a recovery period following an injection.

As with any treatment that may carry an allergic risk, injections of Synacthen should be administered under medical supervision and in the event of a severe anaphylactic reaction occurring despite these precautions, the following measures are recommended: administer 0.5 mg adrenaline s.c. or i.m. as well as a large i.v. dose of corticosteroid for example 50–100 mg prednisolone as prednisolone sodium phosphate BP, repeating the dose if necessary.

The doctor should routinely enquire about possible previous reactions to Synacthen or drugs in general and about a past history of allergic disorders.

Synacthen is contra-indicated in patients allergic or sensitive to Synacthen Depot; in acute psychoses, in the presence of systemic infections without specific anti-infective therapy, in Cushing's syndrome and in patients with peptic ulcer and heart failure. Synacthen is also contra-indicated during pregnancy.

Precautions: Synacthen should be used cautiously in patients hypersensitive to ACTH of animal origin; and in patients suffering from diabetes mellitus or hypertension, where the dosage of concomitant medication may need adjustment.

Patients who have an allergic disorder, especially asthma, in addition to the condition being treated should only be given Synacthen if other therapeutic measures have failed to elicit the desired response and if the condition is severe enough to warrant such medication.

Side-effects: When employed as a therapeutic agent, Synacthen is liable to give rise to side-effects which are due to the drugs hormonal activity e.g. sodium and water retention, raised blood pressure, hypokalaemia, hyper-

glycaemia, increased susceptibility to infection, Cushings syndrome, hyperpigmentation and psychological disturbances. The more serious side-effects usually associated with steroids, peptic ulcer, osteoporosis, retarded wound healing and myopathy are less frequent. Troublesome side-effects are often an indication of overdosage.

Pharmaceutical precautions Synacthen should be protected from light and stored in a refrigerator (2–8°C).

Legal category POM.

Package quantities Synacthen Ampoules 0.25 mg per ml in boxes of 6.

Further information Nil.

Product licence number 0008/0034.

SYNACTHEN* DEPOT

Presentation Tetracosactrin Acetate BP with zinc injection. A sterile white suspension, which settles on standing, containing 1 mg of Synacthen per ml. The preparation is intended for intra-muscular injection, and is available in 1 ml ampoules and 2 ml multi-dose vials.

Uses *Mode of action:* Synacthen is a synthetic polypeptide consisting of the first 24 amino acids of the naturally occurring anterior pituitary hormone ACTH. These 24 amino acids are the ones responsible for the corticotrophic activity. Those numbering 25 to 39, some of which vary from one species to another, but which do not appear necessary for corticotrophic activity, are omitted. Synacthen thus has the same biological action as natural human ACTH. Synacthen is a hexa-acetate. In the depot form it is adsorbed on to a zinc phosphate complex, to prolong its action.

Indications: For the treatment of rheumatoid arthritis and other allied rheumatic conditions, including juvenile rheumatoid diseases and rheumatic fever, acute gout, psoriatic arthropathy, dermatomyositis, chronic skin disorders such as pemphigus, generalised bullous or exfoliative dermatitis, dermatitis herpetiformis and erythroderma, nephrotic syndrome, ulcerative colitis, Crohn's Disease, acute neurological conditions such as exacerbations of multiple sclerosis, Guillain-Barré syndrome, Bell's paralysis, optic neuritis, systemic lupus erythematosis, hypsarrhythmia and peri-arteritis nodosa. To transfer or wean patients from corticosteroid therapy.

Dosage and administration Synacthen Depot should be given intramuscularly, preferably into the buttock.

Adults: Usually 0.5–1 mg twice a week (sometimes less or at longer intervals according to response). For best results the dosage regime should be tailored to individual requirements.

In acute cases, 1 mg i.m. daily for three days. A maintenance regime should be adopted as soon as an adequate response is obtained. The cortisol response is rapid and lasts about 28 hours, the clinical response usually lasts longer.

Infants: Initially 0.25 mg daily by i.m. injection. Maintenance dose 0.25 mg every two to eight days.

Small children: Initially 0.25–0.5 mg daily by i.m. injection. Maintenance dose 0.25–0.5 mg every two to eight days.

Children of school age: Initially 0.25–1 mg daily by i.m.

injection. Maintenance dose 0.25–1 mg every two to eight days.

If secondary adrenocortical atrophy has occurred, Synacthen Depot can restore adrenal responsiveness over three or four days. This effect may be utilised in weaning patients from corticosteroid therapy. 1 mg of Synacthen Depot being given daily for three days, the steroid dosage being reduced by a quarter each day. If desired the adrenal responsiveness may be checked, using the 30-minute Synacthen test. A further course of Synacthen Depot may be given if necessary.

Use in the elderly: No specific information on use in the elderly available but no evidence to suggest that an alteration in dosage is required.

Contra-indications, warnings, etc
Contra-indications: In rare cases, particularly in patients subject to asthma and/or other forms of allergy, severe anaphylactic shock reactions may occur. Such reactions usually start within 30 minutes after administration of Synacthen Depot and should be considered an absolute contra-indication to further treatment with this polypeptide. In view of this Synacthen Depot should not be used for the treatment of asthma or other allergic disorders. Milder reactions of an allergic or hypersensitive nature should also be considered as an indication that the course of treatment should be stopped and not restarted, since a trivial reaction may be followed by a more serious event if further injections are given. These milder reactions include urticaria, pruritus, flushing and faintness and dyspnoea. Since some reactions have occurred without warning wherever possible patients should remain at the hospital or doctor's surgery for a recovery period following an injection. As with any treatment that may carry an allergic risk, injections of Synacthen Depot should be administered under medical supervision and in the event of a severe anaphylactic reaction occurring despite these precautions, the following measures are recommended: administer 0.5 mg adrenaline s.c. or i.m. as well as a large i.v. dose of corticosteroid for example 50–100 mg prednisolone as Prednisolone Sodium Phosphate BP, repeating the dose if necessary.

The doctor should routinely enquire about possible previous reactions to Synacthen Depot or drugs in general and about a past history of allergic disorders.

Synacthen Depot is also contra-indicated in acute psychoses, in the presence of systemic infections without specific anti-infective therapy, in Cushings Syndrome, in patients with peptic ulcer, heart failure and during pregnancy. Synacthen Depot is contra-indicated for use by the intravenous route.

Side-effects: Glucocorticoid effects such as 'moon face', raised blood sugar, psychological disturbances and decreased resistance to infection may occur with Synacthen Depot. Mineralocorticoid and androgenic effects such as hypertension, water retention, and weight gain, acne, hirsuitism, skin pigmentation and disturbances of the menstrual cycle can sometimes be troublesome. On the other hand the more serious side-effects usually associated with steroids – such as gastric pain and ulcer formation, skin atrophy, bruising, retarded wound healing, osteoporosis and myopathy – are less frequent. Troublesome side-effects are often an indication of overdosage.

Provided the dosage is carefully individualised, Synacthen Depot is unlikely to inhibit growth in children. Nevertheless in children undergoing long-term treatment, growth should be monitored.

Precautions: Synacthen Depot should be used cautiously in patients hypersensitive to ACTH of animal origin and in patients suffering from diabetes mellitus or hypertension, where the dosage of concomitant treatment may need adjustment.

Patients who have an allergic disorder, especially asthma, in addition to the condition being treated should only be given Synacthen Depot if other therapeutic measures have failed to elicit the desired response and if the condition is severe enough to warrant such medication.

Overdosage: Overdosage may temporarily lead to fluid retention and signs of excessive adrenocorticotrophic activity (Cushing's Syndrome). In such cases the interval between injections should be extended or dosage reduced as necessary. An oral diuretic may be given, but it is wise to give a potassium supplement, e.g. 'Slow-K'.

Pharmaceutical precautions Synacthen Depot should be stored in a refrigerator (2–6°C) and protected from light. Before administration, it should be well shaken.

Legal category POM.

Package quantities Ampoules of 1 mg in 1 ml packed in boxes of 10.

Multi-dose vials of 2 mg in 2 ml, packed singly.

Further information Synacthen Depot is a free-flowing, fine suspension which can be easily injected using a fine needle.

Since it contains a shorter chain molecule which is not 'foreign' to the human species it may often be well tolerated by patients who are sensitive to animal-extracted ACTH.

The Depot formulation, an inorganic complex, is much longer acting than the gel or CMC forms of ACTH. Thus injections of Synacthen Depot can be more widely spaced. The therapeutic effect far outlasts the cortisol response.

Long-term treatment with Synacthen Depot does not cause adrenal suppression. In fact Synacthen Depot is frequently used to wean patients off steroids. Many cases have been reported where it has eventually been possible to withdraw the Synacthen Depot also, even in patients who initially showed evidence of considerable adrenal atrophy.

Product licence numbers

Ampoules 1 mg	0008/5071
Vials 2 mg	0008/5072

TRANSIDERM*-NITRO 5 and 10 ▼

Presentation Transiderm-Nitro is a transdermal drug delivery system, comprising a self-adhesive, pink coloured patch, containing a drug reservoir of glyceryl trinitrate.

For each Transiderm-Nitro 5, the average amount of glyceryl trinitrate absorbed per patch in 24 hours is 5 mg. Each patch has a contact surface measuring 10 cm², and a glyceryl trinitrate content of 25 mg.

For Transiderm-Nitro 10, the average amount of glyceryl trinitrate absorbed per patch in 24 hours is 10 mg. Each patch has a contact surface measuring 20 cm², and a glyceryl trinitrate content of 50 mg.

Uses *Indication:* Prophylactic treatment of attacks of angina pectoris, as monotherapy or in combination with other anti-anginal agents.

Mode of action: Transiderm-Nitro is a novel drug delivery system designed to achieve a prolonged and constant release of glyceryl trinitrate. Glyceryl trinitrate acts by venous and arterial vasodilatation and redistribution of myocardial blood flow.

Following the application of Transiderm-Nitro the plasma level of glyceryl trinitrate reaches a constant plateau within two hours, which is maintained for at least 24 hours. During the first hour after removal of the patch the plasma level falls rapidly.

Dosage and administration One Transiderm-Nitro 5 patch is to be applied every 24 hours. If a higher dose is required a Transiderm-Nitro 10 patch may be substituted. It is recommended that the patch is applied to the lateral chest wall. The patch should be removed after 24 hours, and the replacement patch applied to a new area of skin. Allow several days to elapse before applying a fresh patch to the same area of skin.

If acute attacks of angina pectoris occur, rapidly acting nitrates may be required.

Use in the elderly: No specific information on use in the elderly available but no evidence to suggest that an alteration in dose is required.

Contra-indications, warnings, etc
Side-effects: Headache may occur and usually regresses after a few days. Reflex tachycardia can be controlled by concomitant treatment with a beta-blocker. Postural hypotension, nausea and dizziness occur rarely. Allergic skin reactions, a local mild itching or burning sensation may occasionally occur. Upon removal of the patch, any slight reddening of the skin will usually disappear in a few hours.

Precautions: In recent myocardial infarction or acute heart failure, Transiderm-Nitro should be employed only under careful clinical surveillance.

As with all anti-anginal nitrate preparations, withdrawal of treatment should be gradual, by replacement with decreasing doses of long-acting oral nitrates.

The system should be removed before cardioversion or DC defibrillation is attempted. This is to avoid the possibility of arcing between the patch and the electrodes.

Contra-indications: Transiderm-Nitro should not be prescribed to patients hypersensitive to nitrates, or in severe hypotension.

Marked anaemia, increased intraocular pressure or intracranial pressure.

Pregnancy: As with all drugs, Transiderm-Nitro should not be prescribed during pregnancy, particularly during the first trimester, unless there are compelling reasons for doing so.

Treatment of overdosage: High doses of glyceryl trinitrate are known to cause pronounced systemic side-effects, e.g. a marked fall in blood pressure or collapse. However, with Transiderm-Nitro, the rate controlling membrane will reduce the likelihood of overdosage occurring. In contrast to long-acting oral nitrate preparations, the effect of Transiderm-Nitro can be rapidly terminated simply by removing the system. Any fall in blood pressure or signs of collapse that may occur, may be managed by resuscitative measures.

Pharmaceutical precautions Store below 25°C.

Legal category P.

Package quantities Boxes of 30 patches.

Further information Transiderm-Nitro gives a controlled release of glyceryl trinitrate over at least 24 hours, and thereby avoids high peaks of blood levels, minimising the incidence of side-effects.

Although glyceryl trinitrate is volatile, resulting, in the case of most products, in loss of the drug after relatively short storage, the design of the Transiderm-Nitro patch ensures that the dosage to the patient is maintained even after 2 years' storage.

Product licence numbers
Transiderm-Nitro 5   0001/0094
Transiderm-Nitro 10 0001/0095

TRASICOR*

Presentation Trasicor Tablets each containing 20 mg Oxprenolol Hydrochloride BP. Circular, flat, white, film-coated tablets with bevelled edges, having the monogram CIBA impressed on one side and Trasicor 20 on the other.

Trasicor Tablets each containing 40 mg Oxprenolol Hydrochloride BP. Circular, flat, white, film-coated tablets with bevelled edges, having the monogram CIBA impressed on one side and Trasicor 40 on the other.

Trasicor Tablets each containing 80 mg Oxprenolol Hydrochloride BP. Circular, pale yellow, slightly bi-convex, film-coated tablets having the monogram CIBA impressed on one side and Trasicor 80 on the other.

Trasicor Tablets each containing 160 mg Oxprenolol Hydrochloride BP. Circular, pale orange, slightly bi-convex, film-coated tablets, having the monogram CIBA impressed on one side and Trasicor 160 on the other.

Trasicor Ampoules each containing 2 mg Oxprenolol Hydrochloride BP. A white lyophilised mass supplied in a clear glass 2 ml size ampoule.

Uses *Mode of action:* Trasicor is a beta-adrenergic receptor blocking drug. Its principal effects are seen on the heart where the rate is slowed (negative chronotropic effect) with consequent reduction in heart work and myocardial oxygen consumption.

Trasicor provides effective prophylactic control of angina throughout the day in the majority of patients. The frequency and severity of anginal attacks are reduced, whether precipitated by exercise or emotional stress, and exercise tolerance is improved. ST segment depression seen on exercise is also reduced.

Trasicor has partial agonist activity (PAA) also known as intrinsic sympathomimetic activity (ISA). This property means that some degree of stimulation of beta receptors is maintained. Under conditions of rest this tends to balance the negative chronotropic and negative inotropic effects. Trasicor blocks the effects of excessive catecholamine stimulation resulting from stress.

The mechanism of the antihypertensive effect of Trasicor is not clearly understood. Whilst haemodynamic effects on cardiac output and peripheral resistance appear to be factors, effects on plasma renin and/or the central nervous system may be of significance.

Indications: For the treatment of angina pectoris, all grades of hypertension and sympathetically induced cardiac arrhythmias. For the control of anxiety and anxiety tachycardia. Subsidiary indications include functional heart disorders, hypertrophic obstructive cardiomyopathy, as an adjunct to the treatment of thyrotoxicosis and dysrhythmias associated with anaesthesia.

Dosage and administration *Adults: Angina pectoris:*

Most patients respond to 40–160 mg three times daily. Individual patients may require more, but only rarely are doses above 480 mg daily required.

Trasicor is compatible with glyceryl trinitrate and they are complementary since they reduce heart work by different mechanisms. It is usually possible, however, to reduce or even discontinue the use of glyceryl trinitrate when the patient has become established on Trasicor.

As with other beta-blocking drugs, sudden withdrawal of treatment with Trasicor may induce severe and continuous angina. Patients should, therefore, be advised to avoid interruption of established therapy and if withdrawal becomes necessary it should be done gradually.

Hypertension: Initially 80 mg twice daily. If necessary, this daily dose can be increased at convenient intervals (e.g. weekly or fortnightly) until satisfactory blood-pressure control is achieved. When used as monotherapy, doses of 480 mg/day should not be exceeded, since experience has shown that hardly any increase in the response can be achieved by this means. The addition of a diuretic will often give a quicker and more satisfactory response. Usually, patients respond to a dose of 80–320 mg Trasicor in combination with a diuretic and most of the antihypertensive effect is achieved within 2–3 days. The addition of a vasodilator will often enable control to be achieved in the minority of patients who might otherwise fail to respond.

Cardiac arrhythmias: Initial dose 20–40 mg three times daily. This may be increased if necessary to achieve the desired effect.

Trasicor Ampoules 2 mg for parenteral use. Trasicor may be given intramuscularly or intravenously for the emergency treatment of severe cardiac arrhythmias. The recommended starting dose is 2 mg dissolved in 10 ml Water for Injection BP or Injection of Sodium Chloride BP and given slowly, i.e. over 30 seconds, by intravenous injection. If there has been no adequate response within 5 minutes, additional doses of 2 mg, followed by 4 mg, then 8 mg can be given at 5-minute intervals, giving a maximum cumulative dosage of 16 mg in cases of persistent atrial arrhythmias.

N.B. Parenteral administration should be restricted to patients in hospital, preferably under ECG control.

Anxiety states: The majority of patients will respond to a total daily dose of 160 mg. Although no evidence of habituation or tolerance has been observed with Trasicor, its effectiveness in the long term treatment of anxiety has not been established. In the treatment of transient situational anxiety a single dose of 40–80 mg of Trasicor may be prescribed. Trasicor can be administered concurrently with benzodiazepines. When withdrawal of pre-existing anxiolytic therapy is indicated, this should take place gradually.

Hyperthyroidism: 40–120 mg daily in 2 or 3 divided doses.

Pre-operatively: Patients with thyrotoxicosis and phaeochromocytoma may be managed on 60 mg daily in three divided doses. Atropine must always be used pre-operatively.

Anaesthesia: 2 mg ampoules. For the management of prophylaxis of anaesthetic arrhythmias up to 2 mg should be given by slow intravenous injection. Patients should be fully atropinized. Further doses of up to 2 mg at a time may be administered cautiously as required for the management of resistant cases or to maintain the effect.

In patients undergoing elective surgery, it may be considered desirable to employ a beta-blocker as pre-medication, by shielding the heart against the effects of stress, the beta-blocker may serve to guard against excessive sympathetic stimulation, which is liable to provoke such cardiac disturbances as arrhythmia or acute coronary insufficiency. In a patient under beta-blockade, the anaesthetic selected should be one exhibiting as little negative inotropic activity as possible, e.g. halothane, nitrous oxide. If, on the other hand, inhibition of sympathetic tone during the operation is regarded as undesirable, the beta blocker can be withdrawn gradually prior to surgery.

Children: Occasionally Trasicor has been given to children and infants to control arrhythmias. No dosage scheme has been worked out but oral Trasicor has been given empirically on a body-weight basis of approximately 1 mg/kg.

Use in the elderly: No special dosage regime is necessary but concurrent hepatic insufficiency should be taken into account.

Contra-indications, warnings, etc *Side-effects:* Trasicor is well tolerated. However dizziness, drowsiness, headache, insomnia, excitement and gastro-intestinal disturbance may occur particularly at the start of treatment. Isolated cases of excessive bradycardia and thrombocytopenia have been reported.

As with other beta-blockers, bronchospasm and heart failure may occasionally be precipitated in susceptible patients (see 'Precautions') and exertional tiredness and feelings of coldness in the extremities have been reported on rare occasions. However, the incidence of these side-effects is low, possibly due to the partial protection afforded by the sympathomimetic effect of Trasicor.

Trasicor possesses antihypertensive effects, but these are unlikely to be noted in normotensive subjects.

There have been reports of skin rashes and/or dry eyes associated with the use of beta-adrenergic blocking drugs. The reported incidence is small, and in most cases the symptoms have cleared when the treatment was withdrawn. Discontinuance of the drug should be considered if any such reaction is not otherwise explicable. Cessation of therapy with a beta-adrenergic blocker should be gradual.

Contra-indications: Trasicor is contra-indicated in patients with atrioventricular block, marked bradycardia, uncontrolled heart failure and cardiogenic shock.

Precautions: If there is evidence of cardiac failure, this must be controlled by digitalis and/or diuretics before and during Trasicor therapy. Should the pulse rate fall much below 50 per minute, then treatment should be withdrawn and re-started at a lower dose. Caution should be observed when treating asthmatics, chronic bronchitics or other individuals where bronchospasm may be provoked. Trasicor should be given cautiously to patients with metabolic acidosis or anaesthesia with ether or chloroform (see Dosage and Administration). Treatment with a beta-blocker is liable to mask symptoms of hypoglycaemia and also to affect carbohydrate metabolism. In patients with labile or insulin dependent diabetes in particular, it may therefore be necessary to readjust the dosage of anti-diabetic medication. Like other beta-blockers, Trasicor should not be given in combination with calcium antagonists of the verapamil type, because their concomitant use may result in bradycardia, hypotension or even cardiac arrest.

Beta-blockers may cause bradycardia in the fetus which can also persist after birth. During pregnancy and in the course of labour and during lactation beta-blockers should only be employed after the needs of the mother have been weighed against the possible risks to the fetus.

Treatment of overdosage: Overdosage with Trasicor may lead to excessive bradycardia, hypotension, coma and convulsions. It should also be noted that severe toxicity may develop rapidly and that there may be severe hypotension and bradycardia despite a normal ECG. For sinus bradycardia and hypotension 0.5–2.0 mg of atropine should be administered slowly by intravenous infusion.

If this does not raise the heart rate sufficiently isoprenaline may be necessary. The dose of isoprenaline needs to be sufficient to reverse the blockade and should be assessed by the clinical response. A reasonable starting dose would be 25 mcg of isoprenaline hydrochloride.

In severe cardiogenic shock the treatment of choice appears to be glucagon. The initial dose should be 5–10 mg intravenously, further boluses or an infusion can be used according to the patient's condition. Transvenous pacing has been used, sometimes with success. If bronchospasm develops bronchodilators should be used. Patients should be monitored for several days as the beta-blocking effects of Trasicor exceed its plasma half-life.

Pharmaceutical precautions The ampoules should be protected from light; the tablets should be protected from moisture.

Legal category POM.

Package quantities
20 mg Tablets: 100s.
40 mg Tablets: 100s.
80 mg Tablets: 100s.
160 mg Tablets: 100s.
All Trasicor Tablets are in blister packs.
Ampoules 2 mg: Boxes of 5.

Further information In hypertension, Trasicor blocks only the beta-receptors and does not share the problems usually associated with other antihypertensive therapy, e.g. postural effects, failure of ejaculation, diarrhoea. Mental and physical lethargy is not a problem with Trasicor, many patients reporting an increased sense of well-being.

Trasicor protects the cardiovascular system from excess adrenergic discharge and the resulting elevation of catecholamine levels, which are a known risk factor in coronary heart disease and which, in the long term, may contribute to the secondary effects of hypertension.

Trasicor prevents emotional tachycardia during environmental stress. In anxiety, Trasicor does not produce sedation or cause dependence. The best response is seen in patients who have not previously received benzodiazepines.

Product licence numbers
Trasicor Tablets 20 mg   0008/0124
Trasicor Tablets 40 mg   0008/0125
Trasicor Tablets 80 mg   0008/0122
Trasicor Tablets 160 mg   0008/0123
Trasicor Ampoules 2 mg   0008/5068

TRASIDREX

Presentation Trasidrex tablets each contain 160 mg Oxprenolol Hydrochloride BP in a sustained release core and 0.25 mg Cyclopenthiazide BP in the coat. The tablets are circular, with a red sugar coat, and printed CIBA on one side and TRASIDREX on the other, both words in black.

Uses *Mode of action:* Trasicor* (oxprenolol) is a non-selective beta-adrenergic receptor blocking drug with antihypertensive properties. It exerts a competitive and reversible blockade of the beta-adrenergic receptors, thereby protecting the cardiovascular system against excessive adrenergic stimuli, such as those produced by emotional stress and environmental factors. Oxprenolol also has partial agonist activity (PAA) also known as intrinsic sympathomimetic activity (ISA). This property means that some degree of stimulation of the beta receptors is maintained. Under conditions of rest this tends to counter-balance the negative chronotropic and negative inotropic effects of beta-blockade.

The gradual release of oxprenolol from a special sustained release core in Trasidrex prolongs its pharmacological action to 24 hours.

Navidrex* (cyclopenthiazide) is a thiazide diuretic with sustained antihypertensive activity.

The combination of cyclopenthiazide and a slow-release formulation of oxprenolol in a single tablet has a number of advantages:

1. Since oxprenolol and cyclopenthiazide have different modes of antihypertensive activity their therapeutic actions are complementary.
2. Once daily dosage with the combination improves patient compliance.
3. Trasicor inhibits the rise in renin caused by diuretics alone. Conversely Navidrex may be expected to improve the response in low renin hypertensives.
4. The addition of Navidrex to Trasicor further reduces the minimal risk of cardiac failure.

Indications: In the treatment of mild and moderate hypertension.

Dosage and administration *Adults:* Initially 1 tablet daily, usually given in the morning. Most of the antihypertensive effect of the combination is achieved within two to three days. If necessary, the dose can be increased to 2 or more tablets given once daily, until satisfactory blood pressure control is achieved. Most patients should respond to 1 or 2 tablets.

Trasidrex can be successfully combined with other single antihypertensive drugs having a different pharmacological effect. In particular, a free combination with a vasodilator will often be beneficial.

Use in the elderly: No special dosage regime is necessary but concurrent hepatic insufficiency should be taken into account (also see 'Precautions').

Contra-indications, warnings, etc *Side-effects:* Trasidrex is well tolerated. However dizziness, drowsiness, headache, insomnia, excitement and gastrointestinal disturbances may occur, particularly at the start of treatment. Like other beta-blockers, there have been isolated reports of bradycardia and thrombocytopenia.

As with other beta-blockers, bronchospasm, and heart failure may occasionally be precipitated in susceptible patients (see precautions) and exertional tiredness and feelings of coldness in the extremities have been reported on rare occasions. However, the incidence of these side-effects is low, possibly due to the partial protection afforded by the sympathomimetic effect of Trasicor.

There have been reports of skin rashes and/or dry eyes associated with the use of beta-adrenergic blocking drugs. The reported incidence is small, and in most cases the symptoms have cleared when the treatment was withdrawn. Discontinuance of the drug should be considered if any such reaction is not otherwise explicable. Cessation of therapy with a beta-adrenergic blocker should be gradual.

Like other diuretics with a similar mode of action, cyclopenthiazide may cause latent gout or latent diabetes mellitus to become manifest. In a few cases, allergic skin reactions, mild anorexia, nausea, constipation and diarrhoea have been reported. In common with other thiazides, there have been isolated reports of thrombocytopenia.

In contrast with other antihypertensive agents, Trasidrex does not cause postural hypotension, sedation or interference with sexual function.

Contra-indications: Trasidrex is contra-indicated in patients with atrio-ventricular block, marked bradycardia, uncontrolled heart failure and cardiogenic shock. Because of the cyclopenthiazide content, it is contra-indicated in patients with marked renal insufficiency.

An antidiuretic effect has been reported following concomitant treatment with thiazide diuretics and lithium. As with all products which contain thiazide diuretics Trasidrex is contra-indicated during lithium treatment.

Pregnancy: Beta-blockers may cause bradycardia in the fetus, which can also persist after birth. During pregnancy, in the course of labour and during lactation beta-blockers should only be employed after the needs of the mother have been weighed against the possible risks to the fetus.

Precautions: If there is evidence of cardiac failure, this must be controlled by digitalis before and during Trasidrex therapy. Should the pulse rate fall below 50 per minute, treatment should be re-started at a lower dose, if feasible. Particular caution should be observed when treating asthmatics, chronic bronchitics or other individuals where bronchospasm may be provoked.

Trasidrex should be given cautiously to patients with metabolic acidosis or anaesthesia with ether or chloroform. For anaesthesia the agent selected should be one exhibiting as little negative inotropic activity as possible e.g. halothane, nitrous oxide.

Treatment with a beta-blocker is liable to mask the symptoms of hypoglycaemia and also to affect carbohydrate metabolism. In patients with labile or insulin-dependent diabetes in particular, it may therefore be necessary to readjust the dosage of anti-diabetic medication. Navidrex, a thiazide diuretic, may also decrease glucose tolerance.

Like other beta-blockers, Trasidrex should not be given in combination with calcium-antagonists of the verapamil type, because their concomitant use may result in bradycardia, hypotension or even cardiac arrest.

As with other beta-blocking drugs, sudden withdrawal of treatment with Trasidrex may induce severe and continuous angina. Patients should, therefore, be advised to avoid interruption of established therapy and if withdrawal becomes necessary it should be done gradually.

Because of its Navidrex content, Trasidrex should be used with care in patients with some degree of renal impairment, as a rise in blood urea can occur and in extreme cases result in an oliguric crisis.

During long-term treatment with Trasidrex, salt restriction is unnecessary.

The potassium sparing action of Trasicor may obviate the necessity of giving potassium supplements to counter the effects of the thiazide.

Treatment of overdosage: Overdosage with Trasidrex may lead to excessive bradycardia, hypotension, coma and convulsions. It should also be noted that severe toxicity may develop rapidly and that there may be severe hypotension and bradycardia despite a normal ECG. For sinus bradycardia and hypotension 0.5–2.0 mg of atropine should be administered slowly by intravenous infusion. If this does not raise the heart rate sufficiently isoprenaline may be necessary. The dose of isoprenaline needs to be sufficient to reverse the blockade and should be assessed by the clinical response. A reasonable starting dose would be 25 mcg of isoprenaline hydrochloride.

In severe cardiogenic shock the treatment of choice appears to be glucagon. The initial dose should be 5–10 mg intravenously, further boluses or an infusion can be used according to the patient's condition. Transvenous pacing has been used, sometimes with success. If bronchospasm develops bronchodilators should be used. Patients should be monitored for several days as the beta-blocking effects of Trasidrex exceed its plasma half-life. Because Trasidrex is a slow-release formulation, it is likely that the effects of overdosage will be more persistent than following conventional oxprenolol. Further information may be obtained from CIBA Laboratories, Horsham.

Pharmaceutical precautions The tablets should be protected from heat, light and moisture.

Legal category POM.

Package quantities Cartons of 28 tablets consisting of two reminder calendar foils of 14 tablets (each carton of 28 represents two to four weeks' treatment depending on whether dosage is 1 or 2 tablets daily).

Further information By combining a beta-blocker (Trasicor*) and a thiazide diuretic (Navidrex*) in a single tablet in a calendar pack, the management of hypertension can be greatly simplified for the majority of patients. Compliance will be improved and many of the pharmacological actions of the two components produce beneficial complementary effects.

Product licence number 0008/0138.

*Trade Mark

Consolidated Chemicals Limited
The Industrial Estate
Wrexham
Clwyd LL 13 9PS

APP* STOMACH POWDER AND TABLETS

Presentation Available as a white powder and a plain flat tablet 12 mm in diameter.

Powder: Contains in 100 g:

Calcium Carbonate BP	37.82%
Magnesium Carbonate BP	37.50%
Magnesium Trisilicate BP	19.48%
Bismuth Carbonate BP	2.00%
Gel. Alum. Hydrox. BP	3.00%
Papaverine Hyd. BP	0.10%
Homatropine Methyl Bromide USP	0.10%

Tablets: Each tablet contains:

Calcium Carbonate BP	180.5 mg
Magnesium Carbonate BP	195.0 mg
Magnesium Trisilicate BP	92.5 mg
Bismuth Carbonate BP	12.5 mg
Gel. Alum. Hydrox. BP	15.0 mg
Papaverine Hyd. BP	3.0 mg
Homatropine Methyl Bromide USP	1.5 mg

Uses Dyspepsia, excess acidity, gastric and intestinal spasms, symptomatic treatment of gastric and duodenal ulcer.

Dosage and administration *Powder:* 1 × 5 ml (teaspoonful) in water or milk three or four times a day.

Tablets: 1-2 tablets three or four times daily after meals.

Contra-indications, warnings, etc APP is contra-indicated in glaucoma, myasthenia gravis, because of anticholinergic effects of homatropine.

Pharmaceutical precautions None.

Legal category POM.

Package quantities *Powder:* Cartons 100 g.
Tablets: Cartons of 50 and 250.

Further information Nil.

Product licence numbers
Powder   0183/5033
Tablets   0183/5013

CARDIACAP*

Presentation Slow-release capsules. Each capsule contains pentaerythritol tetranitrate (PETN) 30 mg. Blue/yellow capsule SC21 size 2 containing white and cream granules.

Uses Sustained relief in angina pectoris.

Dosage and administration One capsule to be taken every 12 hours.

Contra-indications, warnings, etc Cardiacap is contra-indicated in glaucoma, cerebral haemorrhage, acute myocardial infarction.

Pharmaceutical precautions None.

Overdosage: Treat by gastric lavage.

Legal category P.

Package quantities 30 and 200 capsules.

Further information Cardiacap is presented as a diffusion release preparation of microencapsulated PETN, which will provide therapeutic activity for 12 hours.

Product licence number 0183/5018.

DEANASE* DC TABLETS

Presentation White, oval, enteric-coated tablet containing 10 mg of delta-chymotrypsin.

Uses Control and reduction of acute inflammatory oedematous conditions such as in surgical or accidental trauma. Deanase also effectively reduces the viscosity of mucous and sputum in bronchitis and other respiratory disorders.

Dosage and administration Two tablets twice daily for three days and 1 tablet twice daily as maintenance dose.

Contra-indications, warnings, etc No known reaction reported, but protein sensitisation similar to pollen allergy cannot be entirely disregarded.

Pharmaceutical precautions Store in a cool place.

Legal category P.

Package quantities 16 and 200 tablets.

Further information Delta-chymotrypsin has approximately 50% greater activity than the more common alpha-chymotrypsin and therefore is markedly more effective in its anti-inflammatory action.

Product licence number 0183/5010.

ENTEROMIDE* TABLETS

Presentation White tablet containing 500 mg of Calcium N-[p-[(3 hydroxy methyl ureido) sulphonyl] phenyl] phthalamate. The approved name is calcium sulphaloxate. A round, flat tablet 12 mm in diameter.

Uses Diarrhoea in children and adults, bacterial dysentery, enteritis, colitis, food poisoning, pre-operative bowel sterilisation, 'Tourist Tummy', prophylactic against intestinal infections in tropical countries.

Dosage and administration *Adults and teenager:* 3 × 2 tablets daily.

Children: 3 × 1 tablet daily.

Infants: 3 × ½ tablet daily.

In serious infections these doses can be doubled.

Contra-indications, warnings, etc Sulphonamide sensitivity. If administration is prolonged, white blood cell count must be checked.

Overdosage: Gastric lavage. High fluid intake.

Pharmaceutical precautions None.

Legal category POM.

Package quantities 25 and 200 tablets.

Further information Enteromide exerts both a bactericidal and bacteriostatic action. Approximately 95% of the ingested Enteromide remains unabsorbed in the intestine, thus exerting maximum concentration at the site of the infection and reducing systemic side-effects.

Product licence number 0183/5008.

FERROCAP* CAPSULES

Presentation Capsules containing time-release granules. Each capsule contains:

Ferrous fumarate   330 mg
  (equiv. 110 mg elemental iron)

Green/orange capsule size 0 containing brown and white granules.

Uses Ferrocap Capsules are recommended for treatment of anaemia from iron deficiency or blood loss (especially chronic haemorrhages, such as bleeding ulcers, haemorrhoids and some gynaecological disorders), and in all cases where dietary iron supplementation is desired.

Dosage and administration One capsule daily.

Contra-indications, warnings, etc None known.

Overdosage: Induce vomiting; gastric lavage. Parenteral administration of desferrioxamine mesylate 2 g and then leave 5 g of desferrioxamine in 100 ml of fluid in the stomach.

Pharmaceutical precautions None.

Legal category P.

Package quantities 20 and 200 capsules.

Further information Ferrocap releases its active principle by diffusion rather than disintegration. This patent process ensures constant release over four hours and is independent of pH, enzymatic activity and agitation.

Product licence number 0183/5014.

FERROCAP*-F 350 CAPSULES

Presentation Capsules containing time release granules. Each capsule contains:

Ferrous fumarate
  (equivalent 110 mg
  elemental iron)   330 mg
Folic acid   350 mcg

Standard pink capsule size 0 containing brown, white and yellow granules.

Uses Ferrocap-F 350 Capsules are recommended in the management of anaemia in pregnancy. For folate deficiency and where iron intolerance is a factor.

Dosage and administration One capsule daily.

Contra-indications, warnings, etc None known.

Overdosage: Induce vomiting; gastric lavage. Parenteral administration or desferrioxamine mesylate 2 g and then leave 5 g of desferrioxamine in 100 ml of fluid in the stomach.

Pharmaceutical precautions None.

Legal category POM.

Package quantities 30 and 200 capsules.

Further information Ferrocap-F 350 releases its active principle by diffusion rather than disintegration. This patent process ensures constant release over four hours and is independent of pH, enzymatic activity and agitation.

Product licence number 0183/5017.

FOSFOR* SYRUP

Presentation Phosphorylcolamine 5% w/v in a pink, raspberry-flavoured, sugar syrup.

Uses As a tonic and appetite stimulant in convalescence after illness or surgery, or in depressive states.

Dosage and administration *Adults:* 4 × 5 ml dose (1 tablespoonful). Three times daily.

Children: 2 × 5 ml doses (1 dessertspoonful). Three times daily.

Contra-indications, warnings, etc None known.

Pharmaceutical precautions None.

Legal category P.

Package quantities Bottles of 200 ml and 5 litres.

Further information Phosphorylcolamine is an amino acid with a high phosphorus content, easily assimilated, present as a natural product of cellular metabolism.

Product licence number 0183/5006.

FOSFOR* INJECTION

Presentation 10 ml ampoule, 25% w/v sodium phosphorylcolamine.

Uses Addition to parenteral drip in preventing postoperative body weight loss and enhancing the recovery of general well-being after surgery.

Dosage and administration Single doses 20 ml (i.e. 5 gm) by intravenous injection. The injection to be administered daily or every other day for a period of two to three weeks, a course of 10-20 injections.

Contra-indications, warnings, etc None known.

Pharmaceutical precautions Solutions of Calcium/magnesium salt can cause precipitation.

Legal category POM.

Package quantities Boxes 5 × 10 ml ampoules.
Boxes 50 × 10 ml ampoules.

Further information Phosphorylcolamine is an aminoacid with a high phosphorus content.

Product licence number 0183/5027.

GELOFUSINE*

Presentation Sterile 4% w/v succinylated Gelatin (Modified Fluid Gelatin) in Saline.

Av. Mw.	30,000
Av. Mn.	22,600
Gelatin (MFG)	40 gm/litre
Sodium	154 mmol/litre
Potassium	0.4 mmol/litre
Magnesium	0.4 mmol/litre
Calcium	0.4 mmol/litre
Chloride	125 mmol/litre
Relative Viscosity at 37°C.	1.9
Iso-electric point	pH 4.5 ± 0.3
pH	7.4 ± 0.3
Colloid Osmotic pressure (at 37°C.)	465 mm H_2O
Gel point	0°C.

Uses
Indications: Gelofusine increases and maintains the circulating blood volume for several hours in cases of acute blood and fluid losses. The duration of its effect suffices in most cases to allow normal homeostatic mechanisms to operate. The gelatin is excreted through the kidneys. Gelofusine has no antigenic properties; it is non-toxic and does not interfere with blood clotting factors. It may be given to restore plasma volume following gastro-intestinal fluid losses, in burns and cases of hypovolaemia due to extravascular extravasation of plasma (e.g. venous thrombo-embolism).

Dosage and administration Gelofusine is given by drip infusion and the rate of administration can be increased by the application of pressure to the container or by the giving set pump. When given rapidly it should be warmed to 37–40°C if possible. In severe acute blood loss, Gelofusine may be given rapidly (one unit in 5–10 minutes) until signs of hypovalaemia are relieved. Two litres for an adult (30 ml/kg in children) should only be exceeded if blood is unavailable.

Contra-indications, warnings, etc There are no contra-indications to the use of Gelofusine to restore acute losses of blood or plasma. Anaphylactoid reactions are exceedingly rare but may be likely to occur if Gelofusine is given rapidly to normovolaemic patients in common with other plasma substitutes. It should not be used to prevent falls in arterial pressure consequent on spinal or epidural analgesia.

Pharmaceutical precautions Gelofusine is stable for eight years and can be stored at room temperature. Only clear solution should be used; it contains no preservative and any unused Gelofusine should be discarded once the seal has been opened. Although water soluble drugs can be given in Gelofusine, this is not recommended. If essential, they may be given through the giving set, close to the intravenous cannula. The small calcium content of Gelofusine does not give rise to clotting in the giving set when citrated blood precedes or follows its administration.

Legal category POM.

Package quantities Plastic infusion containers of 500 ml. Packs of 10.

Further information Nil.

Product licence number 0183/5025.

HEPACON* B FORTE INJECTION

Presentation 2 ml ampoules liver extract 15 mcgm B_{12}, vitamin B, pyrophosphate 50 mg, folic acid 2.5 mg.

Uses Defective formation and maturation of red cells. Pernicious anaemia. etc.

Dosage and administration General tonic 2 ml every four days until red blood count is maintained. Anaemia intramuscular injection of 2 ml every day for the first week, then decreasing doses every two weeks for several months. Permanent maintenance treatment is needed in pernicious anaemia.

Contra-indications, warnings, etc Sensitivity to protein.

Pharmaceutical precautions Store in cool place.

Legal category POM.

Package quantities Boxes 50 × 2 ml and 6 × 2 ml.

Further information Nil.

Product licence number 0183/5023.

HEPACON* B_{12}

Presentation 1 ml ampoules of vitamin B_{12}, 50, 100, 500 or 1,000 mcg per 1 ml.

Uses Pernicious anaemia, (Addisonian) anaemia, macrocytic anaemia of sprue (tropical and non-tropical), macrocytic nutritional anaemia, megaloblastic anaemia of infancy (certain cases), neurological symptoms of pernicious anaemia and neuropathies.

Dosage and administration *In anaemia:* Therapy is initiated with injections of 15-30 mcg once or twice per week, depending upon the nature and severity of the case and the response of the patient. For maintenance, injections of 15-30 mcg may be given at intervals of 15–30 days, or as indicated.

In neurological disturbances: 1,000 mcg, daily decreasing as improvement is noted, or as determined by the physician.

Contra-indications, warnings, etc None.

Pharmaceutical precautions Store in a cool place.

Legal category POM.

Package quantities
3 × 1 ml 50, 100, 500 or 1,000 mcg.
6 × 1 ml 50, 100, 500 or 1,000 mcg.

Further information Nil.

Product licence number 0183/5022.

HEPACON* LIVER EXTRACT

Presentation Ampoules 2 ml in strengths of 100 or 1,000 mcg B_{12}.

Uses Pernicious anaemia, tropical sprue, pellagra, tropical macrocytic anaemia, anaemia of pregnancy, fish tapeworm anaemia, gastric carcinoma or resection, hepatitis cirrhosis and chronic intestinal disease with protracted diarrhoea.

Dosage and administration 1–2 ampoules administered intramuscularly.

Contra-indications, warnings, etc Possible protein sensitivity.

Pharmaceutical precautions Store in cool place.

Legal category POM.

Package quantities Boxes 50 × 2 ml and 6 × 2 ml.

Further information Nil.

Product licence number 0183/5019.

HEPACON*-PLEX VITAMIN B COMPLEX

Presentation Ampoules 2 ml

Vitamin B₁	100 mg
Vitamin B₂	2 mg
Vitamin B₆	5 mg
Vitamin B₁₂	8 mcg
Nicotinamide	150 mg
Calcium pantothenate	10 mg

Uses Vitamin B complex deficiencies, neuropsychiatric diseases, gastro-intestinal diseases, cutaneous diseases of nutritional origin, etc.

Dosage and administration 1–2 ampoules intramuscularly as required.

Contra-indications, warnings, etc None.

Pharmaceutical precautions Store in cool place.

Legal category POM.

Package quantities Boxes 50 × 2 ml and 6 × 2 ml.

Further information Nil.

Product licence number 0183/5021.

MINAMINO* COMPOUND SYRUP

Presentation Pleasant palatable syrup. Each 100 ml contains:

Biologicals:

Liver extract from	70 g fresh liver
Spleen extract from	15 g fresh spleen
Gastric mucosa extract from	7 g fresh gastric mucosa

Vitamins:

Vitamin B₁	300 mg
Vitamin B₂	40 mg
Vitamin B₆	35 mg
Vitamin PP	400 mg
Vitamin B₁₂	100 mcg

Amino acids: 2,000 mg of which the following are present. Typical analysis: histidine 175 mg, Arginine 140 mg, methionine 73 mg, tryptophane 84 mg; threonine 136 mg, tyrosine 150 mg, glutamic acid 207 mg, aspartic acid 46 mg, proline 14 mg, glycine 53 mg; alanine 85 mg, valine 102 mg, phenylalanine 153 mg, isoleucine 74 mg, leucine 306 mg, lysine 194 mg.

Minerals:

Iron citrate	410 mg
Manganese sulphate	1.7 mg
Copper sulphate	2.8 mg
Flavoured excipient to	100 ml

Uses As a vitamin and mineral supplement.

Dosage and administration *Children:* 2 × 5 ml in water three times daily.

Adults: 4 × 5 ml three times daily.

Contra-indications, warnings, etc None known.

Pharmaceutical precautions None.

Legal category POM.

Package quantities Bottles of 100 ml and 500 ml.

Further information Nil.

Product licence number 0183/5003.

NU-K*

Presentation Pale Blue opaque hard gelatin capsule size 0 containing 600 mg potassium chloride BP equiv. to 315 mg K or approx. 8 mEq of K^+, in slow release granules.

Uses Treatment or prevention of potassium depletion or hypokalaemia from any cause eg. prolonged treatment with diuretics (especially thiazides or frusemide) or corticosteroids, cirrhosis, malabsorption, conditions associated with chronic diarrhoea.

Dosage and administration Dosage depends on the degree of potassium depletion. In most patients one to six capsules per day, preferably one at a time after food. It should be remembered that the degree of depletion of tissue potassium is not accurately reflected by the serum potassium level.

Where oesophageal transit may be delayed, the outer hard gelatin capsule should be opened and the enclosed micro-encapsulated granules swallowed with a draught of fluid.

The same procedure can be applied whenever a patient experiences difficulty in swallowing the capsules. The Nu-K capsule should be opened and the contents can then be taken on a spoonful of honey or jam, or taken with a draught of fluid.

Contra-indications, warnings, etc Obstruction of the alimentary tract, advanced renal failure and conditions associated with hyperkalaemia, such as untreated Addison's disease, are all contra-indications. The risk of gastro-intestinal irritation or ulceration inherent in oral administration of potassium preparations is minimised by the mode of action of the time release granules, but the occurence of symptoms of obstruction or ulceration indicates withdrawal of oral potassium preparations. In the presence of impaired renal function, or when potassium-sparing diuretics are used, the serum potassium level should be monitored to adjust dosage.

Overdosage: Treatment should be directed to the removal of ingested material by induced emesis or gastric lavage as appropriate. Fluid intake and output should be monitored and measures directed to the restoration of fluid and electrolyte balance. Measures to combat hypotension should be taken if required.

Pharmaceutical precautions Store in a cool place.

Legal category P.

Package quantities 100 capsules and 500 capsules.

Further information Nil.

Product licence number 0183/0018.

OTOTRIPS* EAR DROPS

Presentation Vial with dropper containing:

Polymixin B sulphate	16,000 i.u.
Bacitracin	20,000 i.u.
Crystalline trypsin	25,000 NF. units
Sodium chloride	27 mg
Gelatin	15 mg

One ampoule distilled water

Uses All forms of bacterial ear infections. Acute inflammatory conditions of middle and external ear.

Dosage and administration Three to four drops instilled into ear three times daily.

Contra-indications, warnings, etc Allergy to Polymixin or Bacitracin

Pharmaceutical precautions Store in cool place.

Legal category POM.

Package quantities One box with vial, dropper and ampoule solvent.

Further information Nil.

Product licence number 0183/5000.

TACHOSTYPTAN* HAEMOSTAT

Presentation Each 5 ml ampoule of cream coloured colloidal solution contains 2% w/v standardised thromboplastin extracted from brain tissue.

Uses Tachostypan is indicated in the treatment and the prophylaxis of haemorrhage arising from many medical and surgical conditions. It is of particular value before and after operations associated with oozing surfaces.

Dosage and administration The optimal therapeutic effect is obtained by slow intravenous injection. The haemostatic effect begins after several minutes and decreases gradually after four to five hours. Tachostyptan can also be injected locally into the tissue (e.g. tonsillectomy) or administered locally by swab in easily accessible wounds. Especially advantageous is the combined simultaneous dosage by parenteral and local administration. In general 1–2 × 5 ml ampoules are injected at intervals of three to four hours up to 12 ampoules. In severe haemorrhage the administration in an intravenous drip has been successful, 12 ampoules in 1,000 ml normal saline over a period of six hours. As a prophylactic measure in patients in whom post-operative bleeding is suspected 1–2 ampoules should be given prior to surgery.

Contra-indications, warnings, etc None known.

Pharmaceutical precautions None.

Legal category POM.

Package quantities Boxes of 6 × 5 ml ampoules. Hospital packs of 50 × 5 ml ampoules.

Further information The arrest of bleeding (haemostasis) is a complex physiochemical process which depends on two main factors: 1) clotting of the blood: 2) capillary retraction.

Tachostyptan shortens clotting time only at the point of haemorrhage, and also appears to have a local action on capillaries by inducing retraction and reducing permeability.

Product licence number 0183/5029.

UROMIDE* DRAGEES

Presentation A specifically synthesised sulphonamide for urinary tract infections, with an anaesthetic for the relief of pain. Each dragee of Uromide contains:

Sulphacarbamide	500 mg
Phenazopyridine hydrochloride	50 mg

Uses Infections of the descending urinary tract accompanied by pain, urethral burning or micturition difficulties (urethritis, cystitis, cystopyelitis). Infection prophylaxis in cases of instrumentation (catheterisation, cystoscopy). Follow-up treatment after urological operations.

Dosage and administration *Adults and teenagers:* 2 dragees (tablets) three times daily.

Children: 1 dragee (tablet) three times daily.

Infants: ½ dragee three times daily.

The unique shaped dragee is placed in the mouth and swallowed with a little water.

Contra-indications, warnings, etc The phenazopyridine hydrochloride content of the product demands that a daily dose of ten dragees should not be exceeded. Sulphonamide sensitivity. (Side effects common to all sulphonamides, i.e. nausea, depression, headaches, skinrashes.)

Pharmaceutical precautions None.

Overdosage: Wash out stomach. Maintain high fluid intake for four days, and give potassium citrate.

Legal category POM.

Package quantities 25 and 200 dragees.

Further information The rapid resorption and high renal clearance of sulphacarbamide account for the fact that about half the quantity resorbed will be present in the urine after periods of less than two to three hours. Due to its exceptionally good solubility in any pH range crystallisation in the lower urinary tract is avoided, and increased intake of liquid or pH adjustment are not necessary.

Product licence number 0183/5012.

*Trade Mark

Cox Pharmaceuticals
A. H. Cox & Co. Limited
Whiddon Valley
Barnstaple
North Devon EX32 8NS

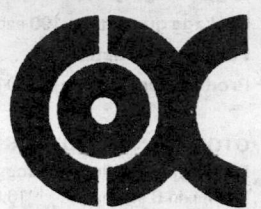

ANTOIN*

Presentation White, uncoated, dispersible, aspirin compound tablets, impressed one side 'Antoin' and a division line on the reverse, each tablet containing:

Codeine Phosphate BP	5 mg
Aspirin BP	400 mg
Caffeine Citrate BPC 1959	15 mg
Calcium Carbonate BP	130 mg
Anhydrous Citric Acid BP	40 mg

Uses Antoin has analgesic and anti-inflammatory actions. It is indicated for all mild to moderate pain conditions such as headache, dental pain and that resulting from dysmenorrhoea.

Dosage and administration *Adults:* 1–2 tablets dissolved in water, three to four times a day; maximum daily dose is 10 tablets.

Children: Not recommended for children.

Contra-indications, warnings, etc Antoin should not be given to patients with a known idiosyncrasy to aspirin or those suffering from active peptic ulceration or haemophilia.

Special precautions: There is clinical and epidemiological evidence of the safety of aspirin in pregnancy, but it may prolong labour and contribute to maternal and neonatal bleeding and is best avoided at term.

Warnings and adverse effects: Aspirin may precipitate bronchospasm, and induce attacks of asthma in susceptible subjects; it may also induce gastro-intestinal haemorrhage, occasionally major.

Aspirin may enhance the activity of coumarin anticoagulants and oral hypoglycaemic agents. The activity of methotrexate may be markedly enhanced and its toxicity increased. The toxicity of sulphonamides may also be increased. Aspirin diminishes the effects of uricosuric agents such as probenecid and sulphinpyrazone.

Codeine may sometimes cause constipation.

Overdosage: Normal procedures for overdosage with aspirin and codeine should be followed. Gastric lavage and forced alkaline diuresis should be used if appropriate.

Pharmaceutical precautions Antoin tablets should be stored in a tightly-closed container, in a cool dry place and protected from the light.

Legal category CD (Sch 5), P.

Package quantities Antoin is available in containers of 50 and 250.

Further information Nil.

Product licence number 0142/0184.

ASPAV*

Presentation Buff-coloured, circular, flat bevelled-edge tablets, which disperse in water to give a fine suspension containing the equivalent of Aspirin BP 500 mg and Papaveretum BPC 10 mg.

Uses Analgesic. For the relief of moderate to severe pain in post-operative states and the relief of chronic pain associated with inoperable carcinoma.

Dosage and administration
Adults (not recommended for children under 12 years); One or two tablets dispersed in water every 4–6 hours. (Not more than eight tablets in any 24 hour period).

Contra-indications, warnings, etc
Contra-indications: Should not be administered to patients with known idiosyncrasy to aspirin or papaveretum. Aspav should not be given to patients with respiratory depression, or obstructive airways disease and should not be given to patients receiving concurrent therapy with monoamine oxidase inhibitors, or within two weeks of their withdrawal.

Warnings and adverse effects: Papaveretum is an analgesic with CNS depressant properties; these properties may be enhanced when Aspav is taken in combination with other CNS depressants and/or alcohol. Aspirin may give rise to hypersensitivity reactions, asthma and may induce gastro-intestinal haemorrhage (occasionally major).

Precautions: Aspav should be given with care to patients known to have a lesion of the gastric mucosa. Aspirin may enhance the activity of coumarin anticoagulants and oral hypoglycaemic agents. The activity of methotrexate may be markedly enhanced and its toxicity increased; the toxicity of sulphonamides may also be increased. Aspirin diminishes the effect of uricosuric agents such as probenecid and sulphinpyrazone. Aspirin may precipitate bronchospasm and may induce attacks of asthma in susceptible subjects.

Reduced dosage is advised in elderly and debilitated patients, hypothyroid patients and those with head injuries or chronic hepatic disease. As with all narcotics, patients taking Aspav should avoid alcohol.

Aspav may also modify patients' reactions and they should be advised against driving or performing other complex manual tasks.

Use in pregnancy: There is clinical and epidemiological evidence of the safety of aspirin in the human pregnancy. Animal studies with papaveretum have shown no apparent hazard and papaveretum has been widely used for many years without noticeable ill consequences. Nevertheless, the safety of the combination has not been established in pregnancy, and therefore, the established principle of using only essential drugs in the early months of pregnancy should be observed. Aspirin may prolong labour and contribute to maternal and neonatal bleeding; its use is best avoided at term.

Tolerance: Repeated administration of Aspav may give rise to tolerance and dependence of the morphine-type.

Side-effects: These include nausea, vomiting, constipation and confusion.

Effects of overdosage: Side-effects of overdosage are similar to those with morphine, but occur to a lesser extent; they may include pin-point pupils, depressed respiration and coma. In severe poisoning there may be dilatation of the pupils, shock, severe respiratory depression and pulmonary oedema.

Gastric lavage should be performed soon after ingestion, and oxygen, intravenous fluids and other intensive supportive therapy carried out, as necessary. Levallorphan tartrate 1–2 mg IV, naloxone, or nalorphine are antidotes for papaveretum.

Pharmaceutical precautions Aspav Tablets should be stored in a cool dry place, in a tightly closed container, and protected from light.

Legal category POM

Package quantities Securitainers of 100 tablets.

Further information Aspav has advantages over morphine combinations, as papaveretum has intrinsic spasmolytic activity in addition to its analgesic properties. Aspav is not subject to the prescribing regulations of the Misuse of Drugs Act.

Product licence number 0142/5597.

COBADEX*

Presentation Cobadex Cream is available in two strengths containing Hydrocortisone BP 0.5% w/w or Hydrocortisone BP 1.0% w/w; and Dimethicone 350 BPC 20% w/w.

Uses Cobadex Cream is formulated to include volatile and skin-penetrating solvents. This enables the hydrocortisone to be carried into the skin by the organic solvent vehicle, and at the same time evaporation of water will take place from the external surface of the cream, leaving a water-repellent silicone film in contact with the air. Cobadex is indicated, therefore, in all steroid responsive dermatoses wherever water, soap, chemicals, etc. cause irritation, e.g. contact dermatitis (especially of hands and body), pruritus ani and pruritus vulvae.

Dosage and administration A thin layer of cream should be applied to the affected area two or three times daily.

Contra-indications, warnings, etc The cream should not be used on raw, weeping surfaces because it tends to hold back any exudate. The area of skin around the eye should be avoided.

Long-term continuous topical steroid therapy should be avoided in infants, since adrenal suppression may occur, even without occlusion.

Special precautions: Topical administration of corticosteroids to pregnant animals can cause abnormalities of foetal development. The relevance of this finding to human beings has not been established. However, topical steroids should not be used extensively in pregnancy, i.e. in large amounts or for prolonged periods.

Adverse reactions: Discontinue treatment should sensitisation occur.

Pharmaceutical precautions Cobadex should be stored in a cool dry place; avoid freezing.

Legal category POM.

Package quantities Both strengths of Cobadex are available in 20 g tubes.

Further information Nil.

Product licence numbers
0.5% cream   1866/5004
1% cream   1866/5005

CO-PROXAMOL

Presentation White film-coated oval tablets impressed with the word COX on one face and the letters CC on the reverse. Each tablet contains Dextropropoxyphene Hydrochloride BP 32.5 mg, and Paracetamol BP 325 mg.

Uses Analgesic. For the relief of mild to moderate pain.

Dosage and administration Two tablets, three or four times daily.

Dosage in the elderly: Initial dosage of one tablet, two or three times daily.

Children: Not recommended for children.

Contra-indications, warnings, etc
Contra-indications: Hypersensitivity to dextropropoxyphene or paracetamol.

Use in pregnancy: The safety of dextropropoxyphene has not been established in pregnancy.

Precautions: Co-proxamol should be administered with caution to patients with severe renal or hepatic impairment as delayed elimination or elevated serum levels may result.

Isolated reports suggest that dextropropoxyphene may inhibit the metabolism of some concurrently administered drugs. Patients receiving anticonvulsants, antidepressants or warfarin-like drugs should be monitored during therapy.

Warnings and adverse effects: Because co-proxamol is an analgesic with CNS depressing properties, it should be used with great caution in patients taking other CNS depressants, including alcohol.

The patient should be advised that alcohol should be avoided when taking co-proxamol.

Care should be exercised in prescribing co-proxamol for patients with a psychological or personality disorder.

An overdosage of paracetamol can cause hepatic necrosis.

Dextropropoxyphene may impair the mental and/or the physical abilities required for the performance of potentially hazardous tasks such as driving a car or operating machinery.

Tolerance: Psychological and physical dependence may occur rarely.

Side-effects: Dizziness, drowsiness, headache, nausea and vomiting are all possible side-effects and appear to be more likely to occur in ambulatory than in non-ambulatory patients, therefore alleviation of these side-effects can be sometimes produced by lying down after taking the tablets.

Other reported side-effects are constipation, abdominal pain, skin rashes, euphoria, lightheadedness and minor visual disturbances.

Overdosage: A chronic ingestion of dextropropoxyphene in doses exceeding 720 mg as base (equivalent to 780 mg as hydrochloride) per day has caused toxic psychoses and convulsions.

The symptoms of acute toxicity may be rapid in onset with the danger of respiratory arrest. Symptoms exhibited are similar to those experienced with morphine and other narcotics. These are respiratory depression, (a decrease in respiratory rate and/or tidal volume) Cheyne-Stokes respiration, cyanosis, extreme somnolence (progressing to stupor or coma), constriction of pupil, circulatory collapse and other characteristic symptoms of narcotic poisoning. Cardiac arrhythmias and pulmonary oedema have been reported.

Fatalities due to apnoea and cardiac arrest have occurred on rare occasions.

Treatment of overdosage: Firstly, adequate respiratory exchange should be re-established by provision of an adequate airway and assisted or controlled ventilation.

The narcotic antagonist naloxone is a specific antidote against the respiratory depression produced by dextropropoxyphene. An initial dose of 0.4–2 mg should be administered intravenously with simultaneous efforts at respiratory resuscitation. If the desired degree of improvement is not obtained, the dose should be repeated at two to three minute intervals. Subsequent doses of naloxone may be necessary for up to 24 hours due to the slow elimination of dextropropoxyphene. Naloxone may also be administered by infusion.

In addition to the use of a narcotic antagonist, the patient may require careful titration with an anticonvulsant to control seizures. Analeptic drugs (e.g. caffeine or amphetamines) should not be used because of their tendency to precipitate convulsions.

Early assessment of the severity of paracetamol poisoning by measurement of plasma paracetamol levels is essential if treatment, which should be instituted within ten hours of ingestion, is to be effective. Present evidence suggests that cysteamine, methionine or N-acetylcysteine given within this period are effective in greatly reducing the toxic effects of paracetamol. Oxygen, intravenous fluids, vasopressors and other supportive measures should be employed as indicated.

Gastric lavage may be helpful. Activated charcoal can adsorb a significant amount of ingested dextropropoxyphene.

Pharmaceutical precautions No special requirements. Advisable to store in a cool, dry place.

Legal category CD (Sch 5), POM.

Package quantities Cartons of 100 tablets containing 10 blisters of 10 tablets.

Further information Nil.

Product licence number 0142/0187.

CYCLOGEST*

Presentation White suppositories, suitable for vaginal or rectal insertion. Each 1.85 g suppository contains either 200 mg or 400 mg Progesterone BP.

Uses Treatment of premenstrual syndrome, including premenstrual tension and depression, treatment of puerperal depression.

Dosage and administration 200 mg daily to 400 mg twice a day, by vaginal or rectal insertion. For premenstrual syndrome commence treatment on day 14 of menstrual cycle and continue treatment until onset of menstruation. If symptoms are present at ovulation commence treatment on day 12.

Contra-indications, warnings, etc
Contra-indications: There are no known contra-indications.

Warnings: Use rectally if barrier methods of contraception are used.

Precautions: Use vaginally if patients suffer from colitis or faecal incontinence. Use rectally if patients suffer from vaginal infection (especially moniliasis) or recurrent cystitis.

Side-effects: Menstruation may occur earlier than expected, or, more rarely, menstruation may be delayed. Soreness, diarrhoea and flatulence may occur with rectal administration.

Overdosage: There is a wide margin of safety with Cyclogest suppositories, but overdosage may produce euphoria or dysmenorrhoea.

Pharmaceutical precautions Store in a cool, dry place.

Legal category POM.

Package quantities
Packs of 12 Suppositories   200 mg
Packs of 12 Suppositories   400 mg

Further information Nil.

Product licence numbers
Cyclogest Suppositories 200 mg   2343/0001
Cyclogest Suppositories 400 mg   2343/0002

Product Licence Holder: L. D. Collins & Co Ltd. Sunray House, 9 Plantagenet Road, New Barnet, Herts. EN5 5JG.

DOXATET*

Presentation Green film-coated oval tablets impressed with the word COX on one face and the letters DX on the reverse. Each tablet contains Doxycycline Hydrochloride BP equivalent to 100 mg doxycycline.

Uses *Mode of Action:* Doxycycline is believed to exert bacteriostatic antimicrobial action by inhibition of protein synthesis. Doxycycline is active against a wide range of Gram-negative and Gram-positive organisms and is stable in normal serum. It has a high lipid solubility and a low affinity for calcium. After oral administration doxycycline is almost completely absorbed, and absorption is virtually unaffected by food or milk.

Doxycycline has been found effective for the treatment of infections caused by a wide range of susceptible micro-organisms.

Respiratory tract infections: Pharyngitis; tonsillitis; otitis media; bronchitis and sinusitis caused by susceptible strains of beta-haemolytic Streptococci, Staphylococci, Pneumococci and *H. influenzae.*

Pneumonia: Single and multilobe pneumonia and bronchopneumonia due to susceptible strains of Pneumococci; Streptococci; Staphylococci; *H. influenzae,*

Klebsiella pneumoniae and *Mycoplasma pneumoniae* (Eaton agent PPLO).

Genito-urinary tract infections: Pyelonephritis; cystitis; urethritis; caused by susceptible strains of the Klebsiella-Aerobacter groups; *E. coli,* Enterococci, Staphylococci, Streptococci, *Neisseria gonorrhoeae,* and *Chlamydia trachomatis.* Acute gonococcal anterior urethritis in the adult male has been effectively treated with a single large dose of doxycycline. Longer term therapy improves the cure rates obtained.

Soft-tissue infections: Impetigo; furunculosis; cellulitis; abscess; infected traumatic and post-operative wounds; paronychia caused by susceptible strains of *Staphylococcus aureus* and *albus*; Streptococci; *E. coli* and the Klebsiella-Aerobacter group. In the treatment of soft-tissue infections, indicated surgical procedures should be carried out in conjunction with Doxatet treatment.

Opthalmic infections: Due to susceptible strains of Gonococci, Staphylococci, *H. influenzae.* Doxatet is indicated in the treatment of trachoma, although the infectious agent is not always eliminated, as judged by immuno-fluorescence. Inclusion conjunctivitis may be treated with oral Doxatet alone or in combination with topical agents.

Gastro-intestinal infections: Due to susceptible strains of such organisms as *E. histolytica,* pathogenic *E. coli* and species of Shigella and Salmonella.

Miscellaneous: Psittacosis. Prostatitis and trigonitis due to Proteus or Pseudomonas; other infections due to susceptible strains of Bacteroides; Pasteurella; Brucella (in combination with streptomycin). Listeria; Rickettsia; *H. pertussis; B. anthracis; C. welchii; N. meningitidis;* spirochaetes (Treponema); *Donovania granulomatis.*

Doxatet may be useful in the treatment of acne vulgaris and acne conglobata.

Dosage and administration *Adults: Initially:* 200 mg (two tablets) as a single dose or divided into two 100 mg (one tablet) doses with a 12 hour interval.

Maintenance: 100 mg (one tablet) per day.

For severe infections, particularly urinary tract infections, the maintenance dose should be increased to 200mg daily.

Increased side-effects may occur at dose levels above the recommended dosage. Therapy should continue for 24 to 48 hours after symptoms have subsided. Therapy should be maintained for 10 days when treating Streptococcal infections to prevent rheumatic fever or glomerulonephritis developing.

Acute gonococcal anterior urethritis: Adult males: A single dose of 300 mg or 100 mg at 12 hour intervals for two to four days. The dose should be given with food including milk or carbonated drinks.

Acute gonococcal infections: Adult females: 100 mg at 12 hour intervals until infection is cured.

Primary and Secondary Syphilis: 300 mg (3 tablets) daily in divided doses for at least 10 days.

If Doxatet causes gastric irritation, administration should be accompanied by food or milk. Unlike other tetracyclines, the absorption of doxycycline is not markedly influenced by food or milk.

Contra-indications, warnings, etc
Warnings: Tetracycline drugs may cause permanent tooth discolouration (yellow-grey-brown) if administered during tooth development (last half of pregnancy,

infancy up to twelve years of age). Enamel hypoplasia has also been reported.

Photo-erythema has been observed in some patients taking tetracyclines. Patients exposed to direct sunlight or ultraviolet light should be advised to discontinue treatment if any skin reaction occurs. Studies with doxycycline indicate that the increase in BUN, caused by other tetracyclines in renally impaired patients, does not occur.

Preparations containing magnesium, aluminium, calcium or iron may impair absorption and should not be given to patients receiving therapy with Doxatet. The plasma half-life and blood concentrations of Doxatet may be decreased when administered concurrently with anticonvulsants such as barbiturates, phenytoin and carbamazepine.

Absorption of tetracyclines may be impaired when concurrently administered with gastric-acid secretion inhibitors (e.g. Cimetidine, Ranitidine).

Pregnancy: Doxatet should not be used during pregnancy unless essential to the patient's welfare. Tetracyclines cross the placenta and may have toxic effects on foetal tissues particularly on skeletal development.

(*See* Warnings on tooth development).

Tetracyclines are also found in the milk of lactating women receiving therapy.

Use in children: Doxycycline forms a stable calcium complex in bone-forming tissue and may decrease the growth-rate of bone. The decrease in growth-rate is reversed when therapy is withdrawn.

Precautions: Occasional overgrowth of non-susceptible organisms may occur with any antibiotic therapy. If overgrowth occurs, Doxatet therapy should be withdrawn and appropriate therapy commenced.

When treating gonorrhoea, where co-existent syphilis is suspected, proper diagnostic procedures, including dark-field examinations, should be utilised. In all such cases, monthly serological tests should be made for at least four months.

A minimum of 10 days therapy should be used to treat Group A beta-haemolytic streptococcal infections.

Patients receiving anticoagulant therapy may require downward adjustment when receiving Doxatet due to depression of plasma prothrombin activity.

Doxatet may interfere with the bactericidal effect of penicillins. Patients taking Doxatet should not therefore receive simultaneous therapy with penicillins.

Adverse reactions: Gastro-intestinal side-effects are rare. The following adverse reactions have been reported in patients receiving tetracycline therapy:

Skin: Maculopapular and erythematous rashes. Exfoliative dermatitis has been reported, but is uncommon. Photosensitivity is discussed in the 'Warnings' section.

Hypersensitivity reactions: Urticaria; angioneurotic oedema; anaphylaxis; anaphylactoid purpura; pericarditis and exacerbation of systemic lupus erythematosus.

Bulging fontanelles have been reported in young infants following full therapeutic dose. This sign disappeared rapidly when the drug was discontinued.

Blood: Haemolytic anaemia; thrombocytopenia; neutropenia and eosinophilia have been reported with tetracyclines.

When given over prolonged periods, tetracyclines have been reported to produce brown-black microscopic discoloration of thyroid glands. No abnormalities of thyroid function are known to occur.

Gastro-intestinal: Anorexia; nausea; vomiting; diarrhoea; glossitis; dysphagia; entercolitis and inflammatory lesions (with monilial overgrowth) in the anogenital region. These reactions have been caused by both the oral and parenteral administration of tetracyclines.

Overdose and toxic effects: Acute overdosage with antibiotics is rare. Toxic effects are usually due to hypersensitivity reactions and should be treated as such.

Pharmaceutical precautions Store in a cool place protected from light.

Legal category POM.

Package quantities Doxatet 100 mg: film-coated tablets in blister packs of 10.

Further information Doxycycline is a semi-synthetic tetracycline derived from oxytetracycline or methacycline.

Studies have shown that doxycycline given at the normal dose levels does not accumulate in patients with renal impairment. The normal serum half-life of doxycycline (18 to 22 hours) is unaffected by haemodialysis routines.

Doxatet is highly stable in normal human serum. Doxatet will not degrade into an epianhydro form.

Product licence number 0142/0186.

KLOREF*

Presentation White, effervescent, lemon and lime flavoured tablets: each tablet contains Potassium Bicarbonate BPC, Potassium Chloride BP, Potassium Benzoate and Betaine Hydrochloride BPC 1949, which provide 6.7 mmol potassium (K^+) and 6.7 mmol chloride (Cl^-) (equivalent to 500 mg potassium chloride) when dissolved in water.

Uses Kloref is indicated in all cases of potassium depletion resulting from intensive or prolonged diuretic therapy, an inadequate potassium dietary intake, and those receiving digitalis – here the elderly population are a special risk. A lack of cellular potassium in the latter can increase the toxic effect of digitalis.

Other indications are corticosteroid therapy, use of carbenoxolone sodium, advanced hepatic cirrhosis, chronic renal disease, Cushing's syndrome, diabetic ketosis, patients on a low-salt diet and in conditions requiring potassium supplementation due to prolonged or chronic diarrhoea or vomiting.

Dosage and administration *Adults:* In most cases 1–2 tablets three times daily (20–40 mmol K^+ and Cl^-). A few patients may need considerably bigger doses. Each tablet should be fully dissolved in at least 100 ml of cold or refrigerated water before drinking.

The tablets themselves should not be swallowed.

Children and pregnant women: Treatment should only be initiated under close medical observation in hospital, with frequent monitoring of serum electrolytes.

Elderly: The elderly also require monitoring of serum electrolytes.

Contra-indications, warnings, etc Contra-indicated in hyperchloraemia; renal tubular or metabolic acidosis.

Special precautions: Cautious administration required in cases of chronic renal disease.

Overdosage: Hyperkalaemia. Poisoning is usually minimal below 6.5 mmol/l, moderate between 6.5 and 8 mmol/l and severe above that level. The absolute toxicity is governed by both pH and associated sodium levels. Hyperkalaemic symptoms and particularly the ECG effects, may be transiently controlled by calcium gluconate, administration of glucose or glucose and insulin, sodium bicarbonate or hypertonic sodium infusions, cation exchange resins or by haemodialysis and peritoneal dialysis. Caution should be exercised in patients who are digitalised and who may experience acute digitalis intoxication in the course of potassium removal.

Pharmaceutical precautions Kloref Tablets should be stored in a tightly closed container in a cool dry place. Avoid storing at temperatures in excess of 25°C.

Legal category P.

Package quantities Kloref is available in packs of 50, also available in containers of 1,000 for supply to hospitals only.

Further information The addition of each tablet to water brings about a reaction between the betaine hydrochloride and potassium bicarbonate; effervescence results from the liberation of carbon dioxide.

Betaine is a naturally occurring substance found in beet, and is metabolised by the body.

Product licence number 1866/5009.

KLOREF-S*

Presentation Kloref-S is presented as lemon and lime flavoured effervescent granules in individual sachets: each sachet contains Potassium Bicarbonate BPC, Potassium Chloride BP and Betaine Hydrochloride BPC 1949, which provide 20 mmol potassium (K^+) and 20 mmol chloride (Cl^-) (equivalent to 1.5 g potassium chloride) when dissolved in water.

Uses Kloref-S is indicated in all cases of potassium depletion resulting from intensive or prolonged diuretic therapy, an inadequate potassium dietary intake, and those receiving digitalis – here the elderly population are a special risk. A lack of cellular potassium in the latter can increase the toxic effect of digitalis.

Other indications are corticosteroid therapy, use of carbenoxolone sodium, advanced hepatic cirrhosis, chronic renal disease, Cushing's syndrome, diabetic ketosis, patients on a low-salt diet and in conditions requiring potassium supplementation due to prolonged or chronic diarrhoea or vomiting.

Dosage and administration *Adults:* In most cases 1 or 2 sachets daily (20–40 mmol K^+ and Cl^-) preferably after meals. A few patients may need considerably bigger doses. Each sachet should be dissolved in at least 200 ml of cold water.

Children and pregnant women: Treatment should only be initiated under close medical observation in hospital, with frequent monitoring of serum electrolytes.

Elderly: The elderly also require monitoring of electrolytes.

Contra-indications, warnings, etc Contra-indicated in hyperchloraemia, renal tubular or metabolic acidosis.

Special precautions: Cautious administration required in cases of chronic renal disease.

Overdosage: Hyperkalaemia. Poisoning is usually minimal below 6.5 mmol/l, moderate between 6.5 and 8 mmol/l and severe above that level. The absolute toxicity is governed by both pH and associated sodium levels. Hyperkalaemic symptoms and particularly the ECG effects, may be transiently controlled by calcium gluconate, administration of glucose or glucose and insulin, sodium bicarbonate or hypertonic sodium infusions, cation exchange resins or by haemodialysis and peritoneal dialysis. Caution should be exercised in patients who are digitalised and who may experience acute digitalis intoxication in the course of potassium removal.

Pharmaceutical precautions Kloref-S Sachets should be stored in a cool dry place. Avoid storing at temperatures in excess of 25°C.

Legal category P.

Package quantities Kloref-S is available in boxes of 30 sachets.

Further information The addition of each sachet to water brings about a reaction between the betaine hydrochloride and potassium bicarbonate; effervescence results from the liberation of carbon dioxide.

Betaine is a naturally occurring substance found in beet, and is metabolised by the body.

Product licence number 1866/0001.

MYOLGIN*

Presentation White, uncoated, dispersible, aspirin, paracetamol and codeine tablets impressed one side 'Myolgin' and a division line on the reverse, each tablet containing:

Codeine Phosphate BP	5 mg
Aspirin BP	200 mg
Paracetamol BP	200 mg
Citric Acid BP	15 mg
Calcium Carbonate BP	60 mg
Caffeine Citrate BPC 1959	15 mg

Uses Myolgin has analgesic and anti-inflammatory actions. It is indicated for all mild to moderate pain conditions such as headache, dental pain and that resulting from dysmenorrhoea.

Dosage and administration One or two tablets dissolved in water, three to four times a day; maximum daily dose is 16 tablets. Myolgin should not be given to children.

Contra-indications, warnings, etc Myolgin should not be given to patients with a known idiosyncrasy to either aspirin or paracetamol; or those suffering from active peptic ulceration or haemophilia.

Special precautions: There is clinical and epidemiological evidence of the safety of aspirin in pregnancy, but it may prolong labour and contribute to maternal and neonatal bleeding, and is best avoided at term.

Warnings and adverse effects: Aspirin may precipitate bronchospasm, and induce attacks of asthma in susceptible subjects; it may also induce gastro-intestinal haemorrhage, occasionally major.

Aspirin may enhance the activity of coumarin anticoagulants and oral hypoglycaemic agents. The activity of methotrexate may be markedly enhanced and its toxicity

increased. The toxicity of sulphonamides may also be increased.

Aspirin diminishes the effect of uricosuric agents such as probenecid and sulphinpyrazone. An overdose can cause hepatic necrosis.

Codeine may sometimes cause constipation.

Overdosage: Normal procedures for overdosage with aspirin, paracetamol and codeine should be followed. Gastric lavage may be helpful. Early assessment of the severity of paracetamol poisoning by measurement of plasma paracetamol levels is essential if treatment, which should be instituted within ten hours of ingestion, is to be effective. Present evidence suggests that cysteamine, methionine or N-acetylcysteine given within this period are effective in greatly reducing the toxic effects of paracetamol. Oxygen, intravenous fluids, vasopressors and other supportive measures should be employed as indicated.

Pharmaceutical precautions Myolgin tablets should be stored in a tightly-closed container, in a cool dry place and protected from the light.

Legal category CD (Sch 5), P.

Package quantities Myolgin is available in packs of 20 and 250.

Further information Nil.

Product licence number 0142/0185.

NYBADEX* (Cobadex–Nystatin*)

Presentation Nybadex is a pale yellow ointment containing Nystatin BP 100,000 i.u./g, Hydrocortisone BP 1% w/w, Dimethicone 350 BPC 20% w/w, Benzalkonium Chloride BP 0.2% w/w.

Uses Nybadex is indicated in all steroid responsive dermatoses, including eczema, intertrigo, seborrhoeic dermatitis, household and industrial dermatitis, pruritus ani and vulvae, and in all other skin irritations requiring steroid therapy in which *Candida albicans* is a factor.

Dosage and administration A thin layer of ointment sufficient to cover the affected area should be applied two or three times daily until the lesion is healed.

Contra-indications, warnings, etc
Contra-indications: The ointment should not be used on raw, weeping surfaces because it tends to hold back any exudate. The area of skin around the eye should be avoided.

Long-term continuous topical steroid therapy should be avoided in infants, since adrenal suppression may occur, even without occlusion.

Special precautions: Topical administration of corticosteroids to pregnant animals can cause abnormalities of foetal development. The relevance of this finding to human beings has not been established. However, topical steroids should not be used extensively in pregnancy, i.e. in large amounts or for prolonged periods.

Adverse reactions: Discontinue treatment should sensitisation occur.

Pharmaceutical precautions Nybadex should be stored in a cool dry place; avoid freezing.

Legal category POM.

Package quantities Tubes of 20 g.

Further information Nil.

Product licence number 1866/0005.

*Trade Mark

CP Pharmaceuticals Limited
Incorporating Weddel Pharmaceuticals
Red Willow Road
Wrexham Industrial Estate
Wrexham
Clwyd LL 13 9PX

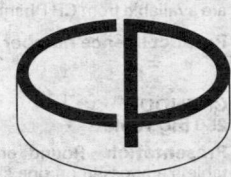

ANTABUSE 200

Presentation White scored tablet marked $\frac{ANT}{200}$ on one side and CP on reverse. Each tablet contains 200 mg Disulfiram BP.

Uses Anti-alcoholic agent. Antabuse 200 is indicated as an adjuvant in the treatment of co-operative chronic alcoholics but its use should be supported by appropriate psychiatric treatment.

Dosage and administration It is recommended that treatment with Antabuse 200 should be initiated only in a hospital or specialised clinic and by physicians experienced in its use. Before initiation of therapy, suitable patients should not have ingested alcohol for at least 12 hours and must be warned of the potential dangers of an Antabuse-alcohol reaction.

On the first day of treatment, the patient should be given at least 4 tablets of Antabuse 200 in one dose (800 mg). The next day the patient should take 3 tablets followed on the third day by 2 tablets and on the fourth and fifth days by 1 tablet. Subsequently, daily dosing should continue at 1 tablet or half a tablet daily until, in the opinion of the physician, the patient is restored to the social order. Dosage may be continued for up to 12 months.

After the fifth day of dosage, challenge doses of alcohol may be given but due to the potential severity of an Antabuse-alcohol reaction, alcohol challenges should only be performed in units with full resuscitation facilities.

Contra-indications, warnings, etc

Warnings: Great care should be taken when challenging patients taking Antabuse 200 with alcohol. The extent of the reaction is very variable; it may not appear at all on the first challenge or alternatively, it may be severe. Further information is available from CP Pharmaceuticals.

Patients should not ingest alcohol at all unless as a challenge dose in a suitable unit. Deaths have been reported following the drinking of large volumes of alcohol by patients receiving Antabuse 200.

Many liquid medicines and tonics contain sufficient alcohol to elicit an Antabuse-alcohol reaction and patients should be made aware of this.

Patients must be warned of the unpredictable and potentially severe nature of an Antabuse-alcohol reaction.

All personnel involved in the administration of Antabuse to the patient must know that disulfiram should *not* be given during a drinking episode.

Contra-indications, precautions: Antabuse 200 is con-tra-indicated in the presence of cardiac failure, coronary artery disease, pregnancy, psychosis and drug addiction. Caution should be exercised in the presence of renal failure, hepatic or respiratory disease, diabetes mellitus and epilepsy.

Drug interactions: Antabuse 200 may potentiate the toxic effects of warfarin, antipyrine, phenytoin, chlordi-azepoxide and diazepam by inhibiting their metabolism. Animal studies have indicated similar inhibition of metabolism of pethidine, morphine and amphetamines. A few case reports of increase in confusion and changes in affect behaviour have been noted with the concurrent administration of metronidazole, isoniazid or paralde-hyde. Potentiation of organic brain syndrome with amitriptyline and choreoathetosis following pimozide have occurred very rarely. The intensity of the Antabuse-alcohol reaction may be increased by chlorpromazine and amitriptyline and decreased by diazepam and certain components decreased by chloropromazine.

Side-effects: During initial treatment, drowsiness and fatigue may occur. Nausea, vomiting, halitosis and reduction in libido have been reported. if side-effects are marked the dosage may be reduced.

Psychotic reactions, including depression, paranoia, schizophrenia and mania occur rarely in patients receiv-ing Antabuse 200. There are occasional reports of allergic dermatitis, peripheral neuritis and hepatic cell damage.

Treatment of Antabuse-alcohol reaction: Antabuse 200 blocks the metabolism of alcohol and leads to an accumulation of acetaldehyde in the blood stream. The Antabuse-alcohol reaction can occur within 10 minutes of ingestion of alcohol and may last several hours. It is characterised by violent flushing, dyspnoea, headache, palpitations, tachycardia, nausea and vomiting.

Intensive supportive therapy should be available in the event of severe reaction to alcohol. Oxygen should be available and supportive measures may be necessary to counteract hypotension. Severe vomiting may occur and may require administration of intravenous fluids.

Treatment of Antabuse overdose: Antabuse alone has low toxicity, gastric lavage and observation are recom-mended.

Pharmaceutical precautions Keep tightly closed, protect from light.

Legal category POM.

Package quantities Pack of 50 Tablets.

Further information Antabuse 200 is rapidly ab-sorbed from the gastro-intestinal tract but is very slowly eliminated and may be detected in body fluids up to seven days after cessation of administration.

Patient information booklets and patient warning cards are available from CP Pharmaceuticals on request.

Product licence number 0495/5900.

CHENDOL*
250 mg Tablet ▼

Presentation Round orange-coloured, film-coated tablets embossed on one surface with 'CHENDOL' and on the reverse with '250'. The reverse side is scored. Each tablet contains 250 mg chenodeoxycholic acid.

Uses For dissolution of radiolucent cholesterol-rich gallstones in functioning gallbladders. Cholesterol stones coated with calcium, or stones composed of bile pigments are not dissolved by chenodeoxycholic acid. It has a particular place in the treatment of patients in whom surgery is contra-indicated or who are anxious to avoid surgery.

Pharmacology: Chenodeoxycholic acid is a normal constituent of human bile. It is known as a primary bile acid since it is one of the main acids synthesised by the liver. Its possible main mechanism of action is that it reduces the output of cholesterol secreted into the bile by inhibiting the enzyme HMG CoA reductase. A secondary mechanism of action is the expansion in the bile acid pool which accompanies taking exogenous chenodeoxycholic acid.

Dosage and administration The present clinical evidence suggests that optimum results will be obtained on a dose level of 10–15 mg per kg body weight daily, either as a single night-time dose or in divided doses.

Duration of treatment appears to be correlated with size of stone. Generally speaking the smaller the stones, the shorter the treatment – dissolution may occur after only three months. On the other hand, larger stones may require up to two years treatment. It is recommended that treatment continues for three months after dissolution.

Elderly patients: No current evidence for alteration of the recommended dose.

Contra-indications, warnings, etc Chendol should not be administered to patients with radio-opaque calcified gallstones nor to patients with non-functioning gallbladders.

Chendol should not be administered to women who may become pregnant, nor to patients with chronic liver disease, nor with inflammatory diseases of the small intestine and colon.

Chendol is generally well tolerated; the only side-effects reported to date are diarrhoea and pruritis. It has been found that after a slight reduction in dose for a few days, diarrhoea ceases and the dose can then gradually be increased to the former level.

The clinician's discretion should be applied to the necessity, in individual cases, for laboratory monitoring.

Chenodeoxycholic acid given in long-term studies at doses of 600 mg/kg/day to rats and 1000 mg/kg/day to mice, induced malignant liver cell tumours in female rats and benign liver cell tumours in female rats and male mice. The clinical significance of these findings is not known.

Pharmaceutical precautions Store in a well closed container.

Legal category POM.

Package quantities 50.

Further information Nil.

Product licence number 0495/0026.

CHENDOL*

Presentation Each orange and pearl capsule contains 125 mg of chenodeoxycholic acid.

Uses
1. *Indications:* For dissolution of radiolucent cholesterol-rich gallstones in functioning gallbladders. Cholesterol stones coated with calcium, or stones composed of bile pigments are not dissolved by chenodeoxycholic acid. It has a particular place in the treatment of patients in whom surgery is contra-indicated or who are anxious to avoid surgery.
2. *Pharmacology:* Chenodeoxycholic acid is a normal constituent of human bile. It is known as a primary bile acid since it is one of the two main bile acids synthesised by the liver. Its possible main mechanism of action is that it reduces the output of cholesterol secreted into the bile by inhibiting the enzyme HMG CoA reductase. A secondary mechanism of action is the expansion in the bile acid pool which accompanies taking exogenous chenodeoxycholic acid.

Dosage and administration The present clinical evidence suggests that optimum results will be obtained on a dose level of 10–15 mg per kg body weight daily either as a single night time dose or in divided doses.

Elderly patients: No current evidence for alteration of the recommended dose.

Duration of treatment appears to be correlated with size of stone. Generally speaking the smaller the stones, the shorter the treatment – dissolution may occur after only three months. On the other hand, larger stones may require up to two years' treatment. It is recommended that treatment continues for three months after dissolution.

Contra-indications, warnings, etc Chendol should not be administered to patients with radio-opaque calcified gallstones nor to patients with non-functioning gallbladders. In addition, Chendol should not be administered to women who may become pregnant, nor to patients with chronic liver disease, nor with inflammatory diseases of the small intestine and colon.

Chendol is generally well tolerated; the only side-effects reported to date are diarrhoea and pruritus.

It has been found that after a slight reduction in dose for a few days, diarrhoea ceases and the dose can then gradually be increased to the former level. The clinician's discretion should be applied to the necessity, in individual cases, for laboratory monitoring.

Pharmaceutical precautions Store in a well closed container.

Legal category POM.

Package quantities 100 and 500.

Further information Nil.

Product licence number 0495/0003.

DEXTRAVEN* 110 IN SALINE

Presentation Dextraven 110 in Saline: a clear, almost colourless slightly viscous liquid. Dextran 110 Injection BP in 0.9% sodium chloride. A sterile solution containing 6% w/v dextrans of weight average molecular weight 110,000 in Sodium Chloride Injection BP.

Uses For the restoration and maintenance of blood volume where this has been reduced as a result of haemorrhage, extravasation of blood or plasma, accidental or surgical wounds, and in burns. Prophylactically, in major surgery to maintain blood volume and pressure during prolonged operations.

Dosage and administration
Haemorrhage: In moderate blood loss 500 ml are infused rapidly, taking 15 minutes. A further 500 ml are given more slowly, taking 30–45 minutes. In severe haemorrhage, 1000 ml are infused as rapidly as possible. A further 500 ml may be given more slowly, depending on the clinical condition of the patient and the availability of cross-matched blood.

Crush injuries: The loss of plasma proteins into injured tissues and the consequent attraction of water out of the circulation may be combated by the infusion of 500–1,500 ml of Dextraven 110. The rate of infusion is dictated by the degree of shock. Where this is severe, rapid infusion is necessary.

Burns: As a guiding principle up to 3,000 ml of Dextraven 110 may be given in the first 36–48 hours. Electrolytes, dextrose and possibly blood will also be required according to the clinical situation.

Prophylaxis: Prior to major surgery a Dextraven 110 drip at the rate of 10–20 drops a minute is set up as soon as the patient is anaesthetised. The drip rate may be adjusted to maintain the blood pressure during the operation. It is seldom necessary to continue the infusion after the operation is complete.

Elderly patients: No current evidence for alteration of the recommended dose schedules.

Contra-indications, warnings, etc Anaphylactoid reactions occur rarely. They are more common and may be more severe in patients with a history of asthma.

The most frequently observed signs of such reactions are hypotension and bronchospasm, progressing on very rare occasions to cardiac arrest. In addition, skin manifestations such as erythema and urticaria may be seen.

In view of the above it is essential to observe patients closely throughout the infusion, particularly during the first few minutes. If there is any suspicion of an anaphylactoid reaction, treatment with Dextraven should be discontinued *immediately* and appropriate resuscitative measures instituted.

In continuing haemorrhage, whole blood or packed cells may be indicated after 1,000–1,500 ml of Dextraven 110 have been infused. This prevents over-dilution of clotting factors and maintains oxygen-carrying capacity. Where clotting factors are already reduced (e.g. in hypofibrinogenaemia or thrombocytopenia) correction of this condition must be undertaken prior to or concomitantly with the Dextraven infusion.

Pharmaceutical precautions Do not store in excess of 25°C or expose to undue fluctuations in temperature. Do not use if cloudy or if a deposit is present. Discard any unused solution.

Legal category POM.

Package quantity 500 ml.

Further information If blood samples are required for grouping and cross-matching, they should be taken when possible before infusion.

Product licence number 0113/5059.
Product Licence held by Fisons plc, Loughborough.

ELYZOL*

Presentation *Suppositories:* Each containing 500 mg or 1 g Metronidazole BP. *Infusion:* A sterile, clear, colourless to pale-yellowish solution containing 500 mg Metronidazole BP per 100 ml.

Uses Metronidazole is active against a broad spectrum of obligate anaerobic bacteria including *Bacteroides, Fusobacterium, Clostridium* and various anaerobic cocci. Its action is bactericidal.

Elyzol may be used in the treatment of infections in which anaerobic bacteria have been identified or are suspected as pathogens. Elyzol may also be used in the prevention of post-operative infections due to anaerobic bacteria, particularly following gynaecological and gastro-intestinal surgery.

Dosage and administration
1. TREATMENT OF ANAEROBIC INFECTIONS: Generally, metronidazole treatment should be given for at least 7 days:

(a) Rectal administration: Adults and children over 12 years of age: 1 suppository of 1 g Elyzol rectally every 8 hours for the first 3 days of treatment; thereafter the suppositories should be administered every 12 hours.

Children under 12 years: 1 suppository of 500 mg Elyzol according to the time-schedule for adults above.

(b) Intravenous administration: Elyzol intravenous infusion is available for use in patients with severe anaerobic infections for whom oral or rectal administration is not possible or is contra-indicated.

Adults and children over 12 years of age: 500 mg (100 ml) every 8 hours.

Children under 12 years of age: 7 mg/kg body weight every 8 hours.

Elyzol intravenous infusion may be given alone or in conjunction (but separately) with other parenteral antibacterial agents.

It should be infused at the rate of 5 ml per minute (100 ml over 20 minutes). It may be given together with sodium chloride injection (0.9%) or Ringers solution.

2. PREVENTION OF ANAEROBIC INFECTIONS: Generally, metronidazole prophylaxis should be given for 7 days.

(a) Elective surgery e.g. hysterectomy and colonic surgery:
Pre-operatively: Adults and children over 12 years of age: on the last pre-operative day 1 g oral metronidazole followed by 500 mg orally until pre-operative starvation.

Children under 12 years: 7 mg/kg body weight orally every 8 hours.

With pre-medication: Adults and children over 12 years of age: one Elyzol 1 g suppository rectally or 500 mg Elyzol (100 ml) intravenous infusion.

Children less than 12 years of age: one Elyzol 500 mg suppository rectally or 7 mg/kg Elyzol intravenous infusion.

Operative and post-operative periods: Adults and children over 12 years of age: one Elyzol 1 g suppository rectally 8 hourly for the first three days and 12 hourly thereafter *or* 500 mg (100 ml) Elyzol intravenous infusion at intervals of 8 hours.

Children less than 12 years of age: One Elyzol 500 mg suppository rectally for the first three days and 12 hourly thereafter *or* 7 mg/kg Elyzol intravenous infusion at intervals of 8 hours.

Oral medication may be substituted as soon as feasible.

(b) Acute surgery e.g. appendicectomy, gastro-intestinal perforation:

Adults and children over 12 years of age: 500 mg (100 ml) Elyzol intravenous infusion immediately before, during or after surgery followed by the same dose 8 hourly until medication can be given by another route.

Children under 12 years of age: 7 mg/kg body weight Elyzol intravenous infusion every 8 hours until medication can be given by another route.

Contra-indications, warnings, etc
Contra-indications: A history of known allergy to metronidazole.

Warnings and adverse effects: Regular clinical and biological surveillance are advised if administration of Elyzol for more than 10 days is considered necessary. Serious adverse reactions occur very rarely. Side effects of metronidazole are usually mild and may include gastro-intestinal disturbances, nausea, unpleasant taste in the mouth, coated tongue, headache and skin rashes. There have been occasional reports of urticaria and angioedema. Anaphylaxis may occur rarely. Drowsiness, dizziness, depression and darkening of the urine have been reported.

During intensive and/or prolonged metronidazole therapy, peripheral neuropathy has been reported. A temporary decrease in white cell count has been reported in some patients.

Elderly patients: No current evidence for alteration of the recommended adult dose.

Precautions: Metronidazole should not be used in patients with blood dyscrasias or with active non-infectious disease of the central nervous system.

Metronidazole should not be given during the first trimester of pregnancy or lactation unless the physician considers it essential.

High doses of metronidazole may mask the presence of syphilis.

Drug interactions: Occasionally metronidazole may provoke a disulfiram-like reaction with alcohol. Patients receiving metronidazole should be advised not to take alcoholic drinks. Metronidazole and disulfiram taken concurrently may cause a confusional condition.

Metronidazole enhances the activity of warfarin. Anticoagulant therapy should be closely monitored in patients receiving metronidazole concurrently.

Metronidazole has exhibited synergism with several agents active against anaerobes, for instance clindamycin, erythromycin, rifampicin and nalidixic acid.

Phenobarbitone increases the metabolism of metronidazole, reducing the half-life to approximately 3 hours.

Pharmaceutical precautions Store below 25° and protect from light.

Legal category POM.

Package quantities Suppositories: Packs of 10 × 500 mg and 10 × 1 g suppositories. Infusion: Packs of 10 × 100 ml 5 mg/ml infusion.

Further information Nil.

Product licence numbers
Infusion 4543/0187
Suppositories 500 mg 4543/0184
Suppositories 1 mg 4543/0185

HEPARIN INJECTION BP (Multiparin*/Monoparin*)

Presentation A clear, colourless or straw-coloured pyrogen-free solution of Heparin Sodium (Mucous) in Water for Injections BP adjusted to a pH of 5 to 8. It is supplied in 5 ml multidose vials (Multiparin), containing 1,000, 5,000 and 25,000 units heparin per ml, with 0.15% chlorocresol. In addition, preservative free single-dose ampoules (Monoparin), containing 1,000, 5,000 and 25,000 units heparin per ml (1 ml) and 1,000 units per ml (5 ml) and 5,000 units in 0.2 ml are available.

Uses Heparin is an anticoagulant. It is believed to act by enhancing the effects of antithrombin III, thereby inactivating several activated clotting factors including activated factor X (Xa).

The chief use of heparin is in the treatment of arterial and venous thrombosis. It may also be used as a prophylaxis against postoperative venous thrombosis; in extra-corporeal circulation (heart-lung and dialysis machines); in blood transfusions; and in coronary thrombosis as a cover for the first 36–48 hours of oral anticoagulant therapy.

Dosage and administration *Adults:* An initial intravenous injection of 12,500 units may be given, followed by maintenance doses of about 6,000 to 12,000 units every 4 hours. The dose should, however, be adjusted to individual response, monitored by anticoagulation tests. For continuous infusion, 10,000 to 20,000 units are given in Dextrose Injection or Sodium Chloride Injection over 12 hours. In an emergency, heparin may be given subcutaneously, in doses of 10,000 to 12,500 units at 6 to 12 hour intervals. The intramuscular route of administration is not recommended.

In prophylaxis of postoperative venous thrombosis, the usual dose is 5,000 units subcutaneously 2 hours before surgery and then every 12 hours for about 10 days after surgery.

Elderly patients: No current evidence for alteration of the recommended adult dose.
Children: The initial dose is 50 units per kg body weight by intravenous infusion, increased to about 100 units per kg every 4 hours.

Contra-indications, warnings, etc Heparin is contra-indicated in surgery of the brain, spinal cord and eye, because of the special hazard of post-operative haemorrhage in these patients which could cause significant disability.

The relative risks and benefits of heparin therapy should be carefully assessed in patients with a bleeding tendency (e.g. haemophilia, purpura, severe hypertension or scurvy), or those patients with an actual or potential bleeding site (e.g. peptic ulcer, visceral carcinoma, postoperative oozing of blood, subacute bacterial endocarditis, suspected intracranial haemorrhage, cerebral thrombosis or threatened abortion). Neither menstruation nor pregnancy is a contra-indication.

Heparin does not cross the placenta or appear in the milk.

In patients with advanced renal or hepatic disease, a reduction in dosage may be necessary. Although heparin hypersensitivity is rare, it is advisable to give a trial dose of 1,000 units in patients with a history of allergy.

Drugs that interfere with platelet aggregation, such as aspirin, may prolong the anticoagulant action of heparin.

The chief danger of heparin therapy is haemorrhage, but this is usually due to overdosage and is minimised by strict laboratory control. Slight haemorrhage can usually be treated by withdrawing the drug. Overdosage is treated by intravenous injection of Protamine Sulphate, 1 mg for every 100 units of heparin to be neutralised.

Rare side effects include acute, reversible thrombocytopenia, alopecia and osteoporosis with spontaneous fractures (after prolonged therapy).

Pharmaceutical precautions Heparin should be stored at a temperature not exceeding 25°C, when it can be expected to retain its potency for at least 3 years after the date of manufacture. Heparin is incompatible in aqueous solution with certain substances e.g. antibiotics, hydrocortisone, phenothiazines and antihistamines.

Legal category POM.

Package quantities Vials: Packs of ten. Ampoules: Packs of ten.

Further information Nil.

Product licence numbers

1,000 units/ml with preservative	0495/5001
5,000 units/ml with preservative	0495/5002
25,000 units/ml with preservative	0495/5003
1,000 units/ml without preservative	0495/5015
5,000 units/ml without preservative	0495/0028
25,000 units/ml without preservative	0495/0009

HEPSAL*

Presentation A sterile, pyrogen-free, clear, colourless solution, of Heparin Sodium (Mucous) BP in Sodium Chloride Injection BP adjusted to pH 5 to 8. The solution is preservative free. Each 5 ml ampoule contains 50 units Heparin Sodium (10 units per ml).

Uses Heparin is an anticoagulant. It is believed to act by enhancing the effects of antithrombin III, thereby inactivating several activated clotting factors, including activated Factor X (Xa).

Hepsal is indicated in any clinical circumstances in which it is desired to maintain the patency of indwelling, intravascular catheters/cannulae, attendant lines or heparin locks.

Hepsal is not recommended for systemic use.

Dosage and administration Flush with 5 mls (50 units) every 4 hours or as required.

Elderly patients: No current evidence for alteration of the recommended adult dose.

Contra-indications, warnings, etc The very rare occurrence of established hypersensitivity to heparin is the only contra-indication to Hepsal.

Used as directed, it is extremely unlikely that the low levels of heparin reaching the blood will have any systemic effect.

Rigorous aseptic technique should be observed at all times in its use.

Pharmaceutical precautions Heparin may be incompatible with solutions of certain other drugs. Hepsal should be stored at a temperature not exceeding 25°C when it can be expected to retain its potency for at least three years after the date of manufacture.

Legal category POM.

Package quantities Packs of 10 × 5 ml Ampoules.

Further information Nil.

Product licence number 0495/0014.

HYALASE*

Presentation A white, fluffy, odourless powder. Each ampoule contains 1,500 international units of Hyaluronidase BP (Ovine).

Uses Hyaluronidase has a temporary and reversible depolymerising action on the polysaccharide hyaluronic acid which is present in the intra-cellular matrix of connective tissue. This action allows the rapid dispersal and absorption of substances given by subcutaneous or intra-muscular injection. Hyaluronidase also facilitates the dispersal of extravasated fluid and haematomatous swellings.

Dosage and administration *Adults:* In hypodermoclysis – a two-way subcutaneous infusion set is required with the fluid container supported about one metre above the patient. Suitable hypodermic needles are attached to the connecting tubes after any contained air has been expelled. The needles are then inserted into the subcutaneous tissues at selected sites and the fluid allowed to run in by gravity. The contents of one ampoule of Hyalase (1,500 international units), dissolved in one ml of water for injections, are injected through the rubber tubing about 2 cm from each needle, at the beginning of the infusion.

When this method is employed, approximately 200 ml of fluid can be administered in 20 minutes.

Repeated infusions may be given as required, but it is advisable to change the site of injection.

Injection may alternatively be given from a syringe directly into a site into which one ml water for injections containing 1,500 international units of Hyalase has previously been injected. The needle should be maintained in the site adopted throughout the procedure which, in this case, should not be unduly prolonged.

It is not advisable to raise the temperature of the fluid prior to infusion since this has been observed to reduce the rate of absorption.

Site of injection: The possible sites of administration are numerous, irrespective of the position of the patient. Choice may be made, for example, from the axillae pectoral regions, subscapular and trunk areas, thighs and calves.

In general 1,500 international units of Hyalase are sufficient for the administration of 500–1,000 ml of most fluids. In the case of whole blood, however, 3,000 units may be required.

Obstetric anaesthesia: The anaesthetic mixture is prepared as follows:
Hyalase 1,500 international units.
Adrenaline hydrochloride 0.5 ml of 1:1,000 dilution.
Procaine hydrochloride 30 ml of 1% solution.

Heins' method is as follows: 'The needle is passed horizontally to the ischial spine, and 5 ml of the solution is deposited here to anaesthetise the pudendal nerve as it enters Alcock's canal. Next, 5 ml of the mixture is infiltrated in the superior portion of the labia minora to anaesthetise the perineal branches of the ilioinguinal nerve. The same procedure is carried out on both sides of the perineum.'

Prevention of post partum haemorrhage: 1,500 international units of Hyalase are dissolved in one ml of a solution containing 0.5 mg ergometrine for intramuscular injection. The injection is given in the thigh at the moment of crowning or delivery of the foetal head. When ergometrine is given with Hyalase in this way, the oxytocic effect is apparent 3–4 minutes earlier than when ergometrine is given alone and the effect is approximately that of intravenous ergometrine.

As an aid to local anaesthesia in ophthalmology: The solution employed consists of a 2% solution of procaine hydrochloride and 0.4% potassium sulphate. One drop of adrenaline hydrochloride (1:1,000) and approximately 150 international units of Hyalase are added to each 5 ml of the solution.

Two further drops of adrenaline are added for cone injections if this is not contra-indicated.

As an aid to local anaesthesia in fracture reduction
For Colles fracture: 20 ml of 1% procaine are mixed with 1,500 international units of Hyalase. Two injections are made: the bulk of the solution is put directly into the fracture haematoma from the extensor aspect of the forearm, and 2–3 ml are infiltrated around the ulnar styloid process. The anaesthetic solution diffuses rapidly all around the injured area and the fracture can be manipulated as soon as the needle is withdrawn.

For Potts fracture: 40 ml of 1% procaine are mixed with 1,500 international units of Hyalase.

Radiography: The contents of one ampoule of Hyalase are dissolved in one ml water for injections (a fresh solution must be prepared on each occasion).

Half a millilitre of Hyalase solution is then added to 5.0 ml of 35 per cent diodone solution and made up to 15.0 ml with water for injections.

Fifteen millilitres of the mixture are injected subcutaneously in the scapular region and are followed immediately by a further 15.0 ml at another site, e.g. the contralateral scapular region.

The area of injection is massaged vigorously to aid dispersion. Normally renal secretion commences five minutes after injection; adequate concentration is obtained in 24–25 minutes and is equal to that obtained by the intravenous method.

Note – The volumes stated are also applicable to children aged from a few weeks to five years and to elderly patients provided that renal function is not grossly impaired.

Contra-indications, warnings, etc
Contra-indications: Not to be used to reduce the swelling of bites or stings, or at sites where infection or malignancy is present. Not to be used for intravenous injections.

Pharmaceutical precautions Store in a cool, dry place. Solutions of Hyalase rapidly lose activity and should be used within 12–24 hours of preparation.

Legal category POM.

Package quantities Boxes of 10 ampoules.

Further information Nil.

Product licence number 0113/5021.
Product Licence held by Fisons plc, Loughborough.

HYPURIN NEUTRAL*
HYPURIN ISOPHANE*
HYPURIN LENTE*
HYPURIN PROTAMINE ZINC*

Presentation *Hypurin Neutral:* Complies with the requirements of the British Pharmacopoeia for Neutral Insulin Injection. It is a clear, neutral solution of highly purified bovine insulin.

Hypurin Isophane: Complies with the requirements of both the British Pharmacopoeia for Isophane Insulin Injection and the European Pharmacopoeia for Isophane Protamine Insulin Injection. It is a white, neutral suspension of highly purified bovine insulin complexed with protamine.

Hypurin Lente: Complies with the requirements of both the British and European Pharmacopoeias for Insulin Zinc Suspension (Mixed). It is a white, neutral suspension of highly purified bovine insulin with zinc chloride; consisting of 30% insulin zinc suspension (amorphous) and 70% insulin zinc suspension (crystalline).

Hypurin Protamine Zinc: Complies with the requirements of both the British and European Pharmacopoeias for Protamine Zinc Insulin Injection. It is a white, neutral suspension of highly purified bovine insulin complexed with an excess of protamine.

Uses The treatment of insulin dependent diabetes mellitus.

Hypurin Neutral: May be used for diabetics who require an insulin of prompt onset and short duration. It is a suitable preparation for admixture with longer acting insulins. It is particularly useful where intermittent, short term or emergency therapy is required, during initial stabilisation and in the treatment of labile diabetes.

Hypurin Isophane: May be used for diabetics requiring a depot insulin of medium duration. Where a more rapid, intense onset is desirable it may be mixed with Hypurin Neutral.

Hypurin Lente: May be used for diabetics requiring a depot insulin of medium to extended duration. Where a more rapid, intense onset is desirable it may be mixed with Hypurin Neutral.

Hypurin Protamine Zinc: May be used for diabetics requiring a depot insulin of extended duration. It is characteristically slow in onset and is commonly used in conjunction with Hypurin Neutral.

Dosage and administration The dosage is determined by the physician according to the needs of the patient.

Hypurin Neutral: Is usually administered subcutaneously but, where necessary it may be given intramuscularly or for very rapid effect intravenously. Onset of action occurs within 30–60 minutes after subcutaneous injection with an overall duration of 6–8 hours. Maximum effect is exerted over the mid range.

Hypurin Isophane: It is usually administered subcutaneously but where necessary it may be given intramuscularly in which case onset is more rapid and overall duration shorter. It should not be given intravenously. Onset of action occurs within 2 hours after subcutaneous injection with an overall duration of 18–24 hours.

Maximum effect is exerted between the sixth and twelfth hours.

Hypurin Lente: Is usually administered subcutaneously but where necessary it may be given intramuscularly in which case onset is more rapid and overall duration shorter. It should not be given intravenously. Onset of action occurs approximately 2 hours after subcutaneous injection with an overall duration extending towards 30 hours. Maximum effect is exerted between the eighth and twelfth hours.

Hypurin Protamine Zinc: Is administered subcutaneously, it is not recommended for intramuscular use and should not be given intravenously. Onset of action occurs after 4–6 hours with an overall duration of 24–36 hours. Maximum effect is exerted between the tenth and twentieth hours.

Contra-indications, warnings, etc Hypurin Isophane, Hypurin Lente and Hypurin Protamine Zinc should be shaken gently before the dose is withdrawn. In no circumstances should they be given intravenously. Hypurin Isophane or Hypurin Lente may be mixed with Hypurin Neutral in the syringe, in which case Hypurin Neutral should be the first dose to be withdrawn. The mixing of Hypurin Protamine Zinc and Hypurin Neutral in the syringe is inadvisable. Injections should be made immediately. Insulin requirements may increase during illness, puberty, pregnancy, emotional upsets or if drugs with hyperglycaemic activity are being taken. Insulin requirements may decrease during periods of increased activity in liver or kidney diseases or when drugs with hypoglycaemic activity are being taken. Insulin is contraindicated in hypoglycaemia. Overdosage causes hypoglycaemia. The patient should take sugar and rest. If the patient is comatose, then Strong Dextrose Injection BPC should be given intravenously. Patients transferred to Hypurin insulins from other commercially available preparations may require dosage adjustment.

Pharmaceutical precautions Hypurins should be stored between 2 and 8°C. They should not be frozen.

Legal category P.

Package quantities 10 × 10 ml vials each containing 100 i.u./ml.

Further information Nil.

Product licence numbers

	100 i.u.
Hypurin Neutral	0495/0022
Hypurin Isophane	0495/0023
Hypurin Lente	0495/0042
Hypurin Protamine Zinc	0495/0025

HYPURIN* SOLUBLE

Presentation A sterile, clear, colourless, isotonic, aqueous solution of highly purified crystalline insulin (bovine), adjusted to a pH of 3.0 to 3.5. Insulin Injection is supplied in 10 ml multidose glass vials containing 100 units per ml. Hypurin Soluble complies with the requirements of the British Pharmacopoeia and European Pharmacopoeia for Insulin Injection.

Uses Insulin is used in juvenile-onset diabetes mellitus, and in maturity-onset diabetes mellitus unresponsive to diet or oral hypoglycaemic agents.

Insulin Injection is particularly useful in diabetic coma and ketoacidosis, pregnancy, trauma and infection.

Dosage and administration The dose depends on the individual requirements of the patient and should be determined empirically.

Insulin Injection has a rapid onset of action (about 30 minutes); its effects last for 6 to 8 hours. It may be used in conjunction with a longer-acting insulin.

Insulin Injection is normally administered subcutaneously. Suitable sites are the upper arm, upper thigh, buttocks and lower abdomen. Whenever possible, the patient should be taught to give the injection. The same injection site should not be used more than about once a month. Care should be taken to ensure that a blood vessel has not been entered. The Injection site should not be massaged.

Insulin Injection may be given intramuscularly or, for very rapid effect, intravenously.

Contra-indications, warnings, etc When Insulin Injection is mixed with Isophane Insulin in the same syringe, Insulin Injection should be drawn into the syringe first, to prevent contamination with the longer-acting preparation. The mixing of Insulin Injection and Protamine Zinc Insulin Injection in the same syringe is not recommended, as the excess protamine in the latter preparation reacts with the Insulin Injection, reducing its immediate effect. Because of pharmaceutical incompatibility, Insulin Injection should not be mixed with Insulin Zinc Suspension.

Care should be taken if patients are changed from one insulin to another of a different animal source as the dosage required may differ.

Development of insulin antibodies may occasionally lead to a gradual increase in dosage requirement. Insulin requirements may also increase during illness (especially infection), pregnancy, puberty, emotional upsets, and concomitant administration of oral contraceptives, adrenaline, thiazide diuretics and other hyperglycaemic agents. Insulin requirements may decrease during periods of increased activity, liver or kidney disease, and concomitant administration of alcohol, monoamine oxidase inhibitors, propranolol, aspirin and other hypoglycaemic agents.

New patients often experience minor skin reactions, which generally cease spontaneously. Insulin may sometimes cause local lipo-atrophy.

Insulin overdosage causes hypoglycaemia. The early warning signs are weakness, giddiness, pallor, sweating, palpitations, trembling etc. Later symptoms are depression or euphoria, inability to concentrate, drowsiness, amnesia etc. In children, headache, nausea and vomiting are common. Treatment of hypoglycaemia is sugar ingestion, and rest. If untreated, hypoglycaemia leads to convulsions and coma. A comatose patient should be treated intravenously with up to 50 ml of a 50% solution of dextrose.

Pharmaceutical precautions Insulin Injection should be stored in a refrigerator (between 2°C and 8°C), when it may be expected to retain its potency for at least two years after the date of manufacture. It should not be frozen.

Legal category P.

Package quantities Packs of 10 vials.

Further information Nil.

Product licence number 100 units/ml   0495/0045

LITAREX*

Presentation Oval, white, biconvex, controlled-release tablets of diameter 16 mm and 8 mm. Each tablet contains lithium citrate 564 mg equivalent to 6 mmol lithium.

Uses Litarex is a source of lithium ions in a controlled-release dosage form. Lithium may act by competing with sodium ions at various sites in the body. It changes the electrolyte composition of body fluids and increases the intracellular and total body water volume. The mechanism of action in affective disorders is not known. It is used for the treatment of acute mania and for the prophylaxis of recurrent affective disorders.

Dosage and administration Prophylactic long term treatment with Litarex should be started with a low dosage and then increased step-wise over a period of several weeks. Treatment is managed by measuring serum lithium concentration and monitoring clinical symptoms.

The initial dose is one tablet (6 mmol Li^+) each morning and evening. Estimation of plasma-lithium concentration should be carried out after 48 hours and then at weekly intervals, and the dosage adjusted to produce a concentration of 0.80 to 1.00 mmol/litre. In some patients effective serum lithium levels may lie within the wider range 0.5 to 1.3 mmol/litre. Toxic symptoms are usually associated with serum lithium levels exceeding 1.5 mmol/litre. When the dosage is stabilised plasma-lithium estimations should be carried out weekly for one month and thereafter at monthly intervals.

Blood samples for estimation of lithium should be taken exactly 12 hours after the evening dose.

There is considerable biological variation in renal lithium clearance and thus the number of Litarex tablets required by individual patients to reach their particular effective plasma concentration is variable. Tablets should be taken in two or three divided doses. Treatment of acute mania should be initiated in hospital. The required initial dose may be high, for example, 48 mmol lithium daily in four divided doses and access to immediate examination of plasma-lithium level is necessary. Lithium concentrations should not exceed 1.5 mmol/litre.

Use in elderly: Elderly patients may require smaller doses. Toxic symptoms are likely with serum concentrations above 1.0 mmol/litre.

Use in children: Not recommended.

Contra-indications, warnings, etc *Contra-indications:* Lithium is contra-indicated in patients with renal disease, cardiovascular disease or Addison's disease, and in women who are breast feeding.

Precautions: Lithium therapy should not be initiated unless adequate facilities for monitoring serum concentrations are available.

The use of lithium for long-term prophylactic treatment requires careful supervision. Serum lithium concentration should be monitored regularly and determined from a blood sample drawn 12 hours after the last dose. Frequent monitoring is advisable after a change in dose; during an intercurrent illness provoking fluid loss; after starting a slimming diet; in the treatment of elderly patients; if signs of lithium toxicity or of mania or depressive relapse occur.

As bioavailability varies from product to product, a change of product should be regarded as initiation of new treatment. Blood levels should therefore be monitored weekly until restabilisation is achieved.

ECG, renal function and thyroid function should be determined prior to treatment. Patients should be euthyroid before starting treatment.

Use in pregnancy: The lithium ion crosses the placenta. It is, therefore, advisable that a pregnancy test should be carried out prior to treatment; and that women treated with lithium should adopt adequate contraceptive methods; and that treatment should be withdrawn for the first trimester of pregnancy. Treatment with lithium throughout pregnancy is associated with an incidence of congenital abnormality greater than that for the general population. Lithium dosage requirements may vary during pregnancy and after delivery; serum lithium concentrations should be monitored closely.

Lithium is excreted in breast milk, and therefore lithium treated patients should not breast feed.

Drug interactions: Lithium should be given with great care to patients taking diuretics as lithium clearance is reduced. A low sodium intake facilitates lithium reabsorption in the renal tubules and may lead to lithium accumulation.

Raised plasma levels of ADH may occur during treatment.

Symptoms of nephrogenic diabetes are particularly prevalent in patients receiving concurrent treatment with tri/tetracyclic antidepressants.

Serum lithium concentrations may increase during concomitant therapy with indomethacin or tetracycline.

Long-term treatment with lithium may result in permanent changes in the kidney and impairment of renal function. High serum concentrations of lithium, including episodes of acute lithium toxicity may enhance these changes. The minimum clinically effective dose of lithium should always be used. Patients should be maintained on lithium after 3–5 years only if, on assessment, benefit persists.

Renal function should be routinely monitored in patients with polyuria and polydypsia. Clear instructions regarding the symptoms of impending toxicity should be given by the doctor to all patients receiving long-term lithium therapy. Patients should also be warned to report if polyuria or polydypsia develop. Episodes of nausea and vomiting or other conditions leading to salt/water depletion should also be reported. Patients should be advised to maintain their usual salt and fluid intake.

Overdosage: Symptoms of severe lithium poisoning include hyper-reflexia, attacks of hyper-extension of the limbs, epileptic seizures, toxic psychosis, syncope, oliguria, circulatory failure and coma. Deaths have been reported. Gross overdosage with serum concentration of 3 mmol per litre is managed by haemodialysis or peritoneal dialysis.

Side-effects: Thirst and polyuria, fine tremor of the hands, muscular weakness, nausea and loose stools are the commonest side-effects during the first days or weeks of treatment. These often subside as treatment progresses.

During maintenance therapy fine hand tremor, weight gain, oedema, polyuria, hypothyroidism and goitre may occur.

More serious side-effects which may signal imminent lithium toxicity include loss of appetite, slurred speech, drowsiness, coarse hand tremor, vomiting, diarrhoea, fasiculation, vertigo and confusion.

Mild cognitive impairment may occur during long-term use.

Hypercalcaemia, hypermagnesaemia, hyperparathyroidism and an increase in antinuclear antibodies have also been reported.

Exacerbation of psoriasis may occur.

Pharmaceutical precautions: Tablets should be swallowed whole.

Legal category POM.

Package quantities Containers of 100.

Further information The lithium citrate in Litarex tablets is distributed in a plastic/lipid matrix from which the lithium salt is released over a period of four to five hours during passage through the gastro-intestinal tract. The tablets are formulated in such a way as to give absorption which is slow and even, so that rapid increases and high peak levels in serum lithium concentrations are avoided.

Product licence number 0495/0024.

LOMODEX* 40 IN DEXTROSE
LOMODEX* 40 IN SALINE

Presentation *Lomodex 40 in Dextrose:* a clear, almost colourless, slightly viscous liquid. Dextran 40 Injection BP in 5% dextrose. A sterile solution containing 10% w/v dextrans of weight average molecular weight 40,000 in 5% w/v Dextrose Injection BP.

Lomodex 40 in Saline: a clear, almost colourless, slightly viscous liquid. Dextran 40 Injection BP in 0.9% sodium chloride. A sterile solution containing 10% w/v dextrans of weight average molecular weight 40,000 in Sodium Chloride Injection BP.

Uses Lomodex 40 solutions are given by intravenous infusion for the prevention and treatment of intravascular 'sludging'.
1. In the management of the crush syndrome, fat embolism, severe burns and mesenteric infarction.
2. In vascular surgery.
3. In extra-corporeal circulation procedures.
4. Before angiography.
5. In plastic surgery e.g. skin grafts.
6. Vascular insufficiency.
7. Peripheral vascular disorders.
8. Short-term plasma expander in shock.

Dosage and administration *Crush syndrome, fat embolism, severe burns and mesenteric infarction:* 1st day: 500–1,000 ml Lomodex 40 should be given by IV infusion, followed by a further 1,000–2,000 ml given slowly over the next 24 hours. 2nd day: 1,000–2,000 ml by slow infusion. 3rd day: 500–1,000 ml by slow infusion (N.B. larger doses may be required in burns).

Vascular surgery: Before surgery: 500 ml by continuous infusion. During surgery: a further 500 ml. After surgery: 500 ml daily for at least three days.

Extra-corporeal circulation procedures: Lomodex 40 is added to the perfusion fluid (not more than 20 ml Lomodex 40/kg body weight).

Before angiography: e.g. aortography: 10–15 ml Lomodex 40/kg body weight is administered by intravenous infusion over 30 minutes.

Plastic surgery and vascular insufficiency: The rate of infusion and dosage will depend on clinical circumstances, bearing in mind the precautions indicated below.

Peripheral vascular disorders: 500 ml are given every 12 hours until 2,000 ml have been infused. Repeat infusions are required two to four times a year.

Shock: A rapid infusion of 500 ml followed by a further 500–1,000 ml over the next three to five hours, depending on the degree of shock.

Elderly patients: No current evidence for alteration of the recommended adult dose.

Contra-indications, warnings, etc Anaphylactoid reactions occur rarely. They are more common and may be more severe in patients with a history of asthma.

The most frequently observed signs of such reactions are hypotension and bronchospasm, progressing on very rare occasions to cardiac arrest. In addition, skin manifestations such as erythema and urticaria may be seen.

In view of the above, it is essential to observe patients closely throughout the infusion, particularly during the first few minutes. If there is any suspicion of an anaphylactoid reaction, treatment with Lomodex should be discontinued *immediately* and appropriate resuscitative measures instituted.

Lomodex 40 should not be used in patients with renal failure, with blood urea levels above 10 mmol/litre (60 mg/100 ml) or whose urine output cannot be maintained above 1,500 ml/day.

Renal function should be monitored, especially when treatment is prolonged for more than two to three days consecutively. Lomodex 40 should be withdrawn if the specific gravity of the urine rises above 1.045 or if there is a reduced output of urine. If oliguria occurs, urine output should be stimulated with diuretics and intravenous fluids as appropriate.

Dehydration should preferably be corrected prior to, or at least concomitantly with, the infusion of Lomodex 40. Until dehydration is corrected, the infusion rate should not exceed 500 ml/hour.

In surgery, dosage for any one infusion should not exceed 20 ml Lomodex 40/kg body weight because of the risk of capillary oozing. When clotting factors are already reduced (e.g. in hypofibrinogenaemia or thrombocytopenia) correction of the condition must be undertaken prior to, or concomitantly with, infusion of Lomodex 40.

With Lomodex 40 there is no necessity to take blood for cross-matching prior to infusion as there is no interference if a sample is subsequently required.

Pharmaceutical precautions Do not store in excess of 25°C or expose to undue fluctuations in temperature. Do not use if cloudy or if a deposit is present. Discard any unused solution.

Legal category POM.

Package quantity Bags of 500 ml.

Further information Nil.

Product licence numbers
Lomodex 40 in Dextrose   0113/5062
Lomodex 40 in Saline   0113/5063
Product licences held by Fisons plc.

LOMODEX* 70 IN DEXTROSE
LOMODEX* 70 IN SALINE

Presentation *Lomodex 70 in Dextrose:* a clear, almost colourless, slightly viscous liquid. Dextran 70 Injection BP in 5% Dextrose. A sterile solution containing 6% w/v dextrans of weight average molecular weight, 70,000 in 5% w/v Dextrose Injection BP.

Lomodex 70 in Saline: a clear, almost colourless, slightly viscous liquid. Dextran 70 Injection BP in 0.9% sodium chloride. A sterile solution containing 6% w/v dextrans of weight average molecular weight 70,000 in Sodium Chloride Injection BP.

Uses 1. Prevention of post-operative deep vein thrombosis.
2. Short-term blood volume expansion.

Dosage and administration
Prevention of post-operative deep vein thrombosis: Continuous infusion before, during and after surgery. A total infusion of 1,000 ml over a period of six hours.

Short-term blood volume expansion: Haemorrhage: In moderate blood loss 500 ml are infused rapidly, taking 15 minutes. A further 500 ml are given more slowly taking 30–45 minutes. In severe haemorrhage 1,000 ml are infused as rapidly as possible. A further 500 ml may be given more slowly, depending on the clinical condition of the patient and the availability of cross-matched blood.

Crush injuries: The loss of plasma proteins into injured tissues and the consequent attraction of water out of the circulation may be combated by the infusion of 500–1,500 ml of Lomodex 70. The rate of infusion is dictated by the degree of shock. Where this is severe, rapid infusion is necessary.

Burns: As a guiding principle, up to 3,000 ml of Lomodex 70 may be given in the first 36–48 hours. Electrolytes, dextrose and possibly blood will also be required according to the clinical situation.

Elderly patients: No current evidence for alteration of the recommended adult dose.

Contra-indications, warnings, etc Anaphylactoid reactions occur rarely. They are more common and may be more severe in patients with a history of asthma. The most frequently observed signs of such reactions are hypotension and bronchospasm, progressing on very rare occasions to cardiac arrest. In addition, skin manifestations such as erythrema and urticaria may be seen.

In view of the above, it is essential to observe the patients closely throughout the infusion, particularly during the first few minutes. If there is any suspicion of an anaphylactoid reaction, treatment with Lomodex should be discontinued *immediately* and appropriate resuscitative measures instituted.

In continuing haemorrhage, whole blood or packed cells may be indicated after 1,000–1,500 ml of Lomodex 70 have been infused. This prevents over-dilution of clotting factors and maintains oxygen-carrying capacity. Where clotting factors are already reduced (e.g. in hypofibrinogenaemia or thrombocytopenia) correction of this condition must be undertaken prior to or concomitantly with the infusion.

Pharmaceutical precautions Do not store in excess of 25°C or expose to undue fluctuations in temperature. Do not use if cloudy or if a deposit is present. Discard any unused solution.

Legal category POM.

Package quantity Bags of 500 ml.

Further information Nil.

Product licence numbers
Lomodex 70 in Dextrose   0013/5060
Lomodex 70 in Saline   0113/5061
Product licence held by Fisons plc, Loughborough.

PROTAMINE SULPHATE INJECTION BP

Presentation A sterile, pyrogen-free, clear, colourless 1% solution of Protamine Sulphate (Salmine) in Sodium Chloride Intravenous Infusion BP (0.9% w/v) adjusted to a pH of 2.5 to 3.5 and supplied in 5 ml glass ampoules.

Uses Protamine is a basic protein which combines with heparin to form a stable, inactive complex. It is used to counteract the anticoagulant effect of heparin; before surgery; after renal dialysis; after open-heart surgery; if excessive bleeding occurs and when an overdose has inadvertently been given.

Dosage and administration Protamine Sulphate Injection should be administered by slow intravenous injection over a period of about 10 minutes. The dose is dependent on the amount of heparin to be neutralised. 1 mg of Protamine Sulphate will usually neutralise at least 100 international units of mucous heparin or 80 units of lung heparin. Since heparin is being continuously excreted the dose of Protamine Sulphate should be reduced if more than 15 minutes have elapsed since the heparin injection. Ideally, the dose required to neutralise the action of heparin should be calculated from the results of determinations of the amount required to produce an acceptable blood clotting time in the patient. In gross excess, protamine itself acts as an anticoagulant.

Contra-indications, warnings, etc Not more than 50 mg Protamine Sulphate (5 ml) should be given at any one time. Protamine is not suitable for reversing the effect of oral anticoagulants.

A sudden fall in blood pressure, bradycardia, dyspnoea, transitory flushing and a feeling of warmth have been observed following injection of Protamine Sulphate.

Pharmaceutical precautions Store between 15°C and 25°C.

Legal category POM.

Package quantities 1% – 5 ml × 10 ampoules.

Further information Nil.

Product licence number 0495/5000.

STESOLID INJECTION*

Presentation Amber ampoules each containing 10 mg/2 ml or 20 mg/4 ml of a clear, colourless to yellow solution of diazepam 5 mg/ml.

Uses Diazepam has anticonvulsant, sedative and muscle relaxant properties. It is used in the treatment of anxiety and tension states, as a sedative and premedicant, in the control of muscle spasm and in the management of alcohol withdrawal symptoms.

Dosage and administration In severe anxiety or acute muscle spasm, diazepam 10 mg may be given intravenously or intramuscularly and repeated after 4 hours. Patients with tetanus may be given 100 to 300 mcg per kg body-weight intravenously and repeated every 1 to 4 hours: alternatively, a continuous infusion of 3 to 10 mg per kg every 24 hours may be used or similar doses may be given by nasoduodenal tube. In status epilepticus 150 to 250 mcg per kg is given by intramuscular or intravenous injection and repeated if required after 30 to 60 minutes. Once the patient is controlled, recurrence of seizures may be prevented by a slow infusion providing 3 mg per kg over 24 hours. The usual dose in minor surgical procedures and dentistry is 200 mcg per kg by injection adjusted to the patient's requirements.

Children: A suggested initial dose is 100 to 200 mcg per kg body weight daily by mouth, but up to 800 mcg per kg daily has been given. If either intramuscular or intravenous injection is required Stesolid up to 200 mcg per kg may be given.

Stesolid injection is not recommended for premature infants.

Elderly patients: Doses should not exceed half those normally recommended.

In order to reduce the likelihood of untoward effects during intravenous sedation the injection should be given slowly (1.0 ml solution per minute).

Intravenous injections should be given into a large vein of the antcubital fossa. It is advisable to keep the patient supine for at least an hour after administration.

Where continuous intravenous infusion is necessary it is suggested that 2 ml Stesolid Injection is mixed with at least 200 ml of infusion fluid such as Sodium Chloride Injection or Dextrose Injection and that such solutions should be used immediately. There is evidence that diazepam is absorbed onto plastic infusion bags and giving sets. It is therefore recommended that glass bottles should be used for the administration of diazepam by intravenous infusion.

Contra-indications, warnings, etc Known sensitivity to diazepam.

Acute pulmonary insufficiency; respiratory depression.

Use in pregnancy. There is no evidence as to drug safety in human pregnancy, nor is there evidence from animal work that it is free from hazard. Do not use during pregnancy, especially during the first and last trimesters unless there are compelling reasons.

Precautions: Stesolid should be used with caution in patients with renal or hepatic dysfunction, chronic pulmonary insufficiency, closed-angle glaucoma or organic brain changes, particularly arteriosclerosis.

Elderly or debilitated patients are particularly susceptible to side-effects and may require lower doses.

Alertness and performance at skilled tasks may be impaired. Patients should be warned not to drive or operate machinery. Alcohol may potentiate these effects.

Alcohol may alter the response to diazepam.

In labour, high single doses or repeated low doses have been reported to produce hypotonia, poor suckling and hypothermia in the neonate and irregularities in the foetal heart.

Diazepam is excreted in breast milk and therefore its use during lactation should be avoided.

Drug interactions: If diazepam is combined with centrally-acting drugs such as neuroleptics, antidepressants, hypnotics, analgesics and anaesthetics the sedative effect may be intensified.

Furthermore, if such centrally-acting depressant drugs are given parenterally in conjunction with intravenous diazepam, severe respiratory and cardiovascular depression may occur.

When intravenous diazepam is to be administered concurrently with a narcotic analgesic agent, e.g. in dentistry, it is recommended that diazepam be given after the analgesic and that the dose be carefully titrated to meet the patient's needs.

Diazepam may potentiate the effect of phenytoin when taken concurrently. Valproate displaces protein bound diazepam and inhibits its metabolism. Occasionally diazepam has been reported to antagonise the effect of levodopa. Cimetidine may potentiate the effect of diazepam because of decreased hepatic metabolism.

Adverse effects: Intravenous injection may be associated with local reactions and thrombophlebitis and venous thrombosis may occur.

The most common side-effects are drowsiness, lightheadedness, unsteadiness and ataxia.

Elderly patients are particularly susceptible to these effects.

Other rare side-effects include hypotension, gastrointestinal and visual disturbances, skin rashes, urinary retention, headaches, confusion, vertigo, changes in libido, blood dyscrasias and jaundice.

Paradoxical reactions to benzodiazepines have been reported, provoking excitement instead of sedation.

Pharmaceutical precautions The recommended maximum storage temperature is 30°. Protect from light. Stesolid injection should not be mixed with other drugs in the same infusion solution or in the same syringe.

Legal category CD (Sch 4), POM.

Package quantities Ampoules in boxes of ten 2 ml or 4 ml.

Further information As with a number of other medicaments, intramuscular injection of diazepam (but not intravenous administration) can lead to a rise in serum creatine phosphokinase activity, with a maximum between 12 and 24 hours after the injection. This fact should be taken into account in the differential diagnosis of myocardial infarction.

Diazepam is a long-acting benzodiazepine, it is one of the main metabolites of medazepam and is itself metabolised to active metabolites n-desmethyl-diazepam and oxazepam. Repeated doses will lead to cumulation of the whole drug and its metabolites. It may take 2 weeks for N-desmethyldiazepam to reach steady state and the concentration after chronic administration may exceed that of diazepam.

Product licence number 4543/0179.

STESOLID RECTAL TUBES*

Presentation White, polyethylene rectal tubes containing a clear, colourless to slightly yellowish solution of 2 mg/ml or 4 mg/ml diazepam. Approximately 2.5 ml can be squeezed from each tube, giving an individual dose of 5 mg or 10 mg diazepam.

Uses Diazepam has anticonvulsant, sedative and muscle relaxant properties. It is used in the treatment of anxiety and tension states, as a sedative and premedicant, in the control of muscle spasm and in the management of alcohol withdrawal symptoms.

Stesolid rectal tubes may be used in acute anxiety and agitation, epileptic and febrile convulsions, tetanus, as a sedative in minor surgical and dental procedures or other circumstances in which a rapid effect is required but where intravenous injection is impracticable or undesirable.

Stesolid rectal tubes may be of particular value for the immediate treatment of convulsions in infants and children.

Dosage and administration Sensitivity to diazepam varies with age.

Children: 1 to 3 years of age – one 5 mg tube. Over 3 years of age – one 10 mg tube.

Adults: One 10 mg tube.

Elderly patients: one 5 mg tube.

Higher doses may be required in some patients. If no effect is seen after five minutes, one further tube (5 mg or 10 mg diazepam respectively) can be administered. Further doses of Stesolid rectal tubes should be administered only after consultation with a physician.

If convulsions are still not controlled, then other anticonvulsive measures should be instituted.

Contra-indications, warnings, etc Known sensitivity to diazepam. Acute pulmonary insufficiency.

Precautions: Stesolid should be used with caution in patients with renal or hepatic dysfunction, chronic pulmonary insufficiency or closed-angle glaucoma.

Elderly or debilitated patients are particularly susceptible to side-effects and may require lower doses.

Alertness and performance at skilled tasks may be impaired. Patients should be warned not to drive or operate machinery. Alcohol may potentiate these effects.

Diazepam may enhance the effects of other CNS depressants. Their concurrent use should be avoided.

Alcohol may alter the response to diazepam.

There is no evidence as to the safety of diazepam in human pregnancy. It should not be used, especially during the first and last trimesters, unless the benefit is considered to outweight the potential risk.

In labour, high single doses or repeated low doses have been reported to produce hypotonia, poor sucking and hypothermia in the neonate and irregularities in the foetal heart.

Diazepam is excreted in breast milk and therefore its use during lactation should be avoided.

Side-effects: The side-effects of diazepam are usually mild and infrequent.

The most common side-effects are drowsiness, light-headedness, unsteadiness and ataxia.

Elderly patients are particularly susceptible to these effects.

Other rare side-effects include hypotension, gastro-intestinal and visual disturbances, skin rashes, urinary retention, headache, confusion, vertigo, changes in libido, blood dyscrasias and jaundice.

Paradoxical reactions to benzodiazepines have been reported, provoking excitement instead of sedation.

Pharmaceutical precautions Stesolid rectal tubes should be stored in a cool place.

Legal category CD (Sch 4), POM.

Package quantities Packs of 5 tubes.

Further information Nil.

Product licence numbers
  5 mg rectal tube   4543/0180
10 mg rectal tube   4543/0181

UNIPARIN*

Presentation A sterile pyrogen-free, clear, colourless or slightly straw coloured solution of Heparin Sodium in Water for Injections BP adjusted to a pH of 5 to 8.

It is available in pre-filled sterile unit-dose syringes containing 5,000 i.u. in 0.2 ml.

Uses Heparin is an anticoagulant and acts by inhibiting thrombin and by potentiating the naturally occurring inhibitors of activated factor X (Xa). It is used in large doses (e.g. 10,000 i.u. six-hourly intravenously) in the treatment of arterial and venous thrombosis. Low blood levels of heparin produced by subcutaneous injections (5,000 i.u. twelve-hourly) exert an anti-thrombotic effect by inactivating factor Xa.

Uniparin is used in the prophylaxis of venous thrombosis and thromboembolism in surgical patients. Uniparin may also be considered in prophylaxis of thromboembolism in other situations, medical or obstetrical, in which there is considered to be increased risk of thromboembolism.

Dosage and administration Prophylactic administration of Uniparin consists of the subcutaneous injection of 5,000 i.u. every 12 hours. In the case of prophylactic administration to surgical patients, the first dose should be given 2 hours before operation and continued for at least 10 days post-operatively.

Uniparin should be injected into the subcutaneous tissue of the lateral abdominal wall inserting the needle vertically into a pinched-up fold of skin.

Contra-indications, warnings, etc Heparin is contra-indicated in surgery of the brain, spinal cord and eye, because of the special hazard of post-operative haemorrhage in these patients which could cause significant disability.

The relative risks and benefits of heparin should be carefully assessed in patients with a bleeding tendency or those patients with an actual or potential bleeding site, e.g. hiatus hernia, peptic ulcer, neoplasm, bacterial endocarditis, retinopathy, bleeding haemorrhoids. Neither menstruation nor pregnancy is a contra-indication. Heparin does not cross the placenta or appear in the milk.

In most patients the recommended low-dose regimen produces no alteration in clotting time. However, patients show an individual response to heparin and it is therefore essential that the effect of therapy on coagulation time should be monitored in patients undergoing major surgery. Drugs that interfere with platelet aggregation, e.g. aspirin, dextran solutions, should be used with care.

Although the Uniparin syringe is specifically designed to minimise the risk of overdosage, bleeding can occur and, under these circumstances, clotting time and platelet count should be determined. Prolonged clotting time will indicate the presence of an anticoagulant effect requiring neutralisation by protamine sulphate, and the dose should be calculated by titration of the individual patient's requirements.

Thrombocytopenia has been observed occasionally. There is some evidence that prolonged dosing with heparin (i.e. for many months) may cause alopecia and osteoporosis. Hyper-sensitivity reactions occur but are extremely rare.

Pharmaceutical precautions Uniparin should be stored at a temperature not exceeding 25°C when it can be expected to maintain its potency for at least three years after date of manufacture. Store protected from light.

Legal category POM.

Package quantities Packs of 50 pre-filled sterile disposable syringes.

Further information Nil.

Product licence number 0495/0009.

*Trade Mark

Davis+Geck
(A Division of Cyanamid of Great Britain Limited)
Fareham Road
Gosport, Hampshire PO13 0AS

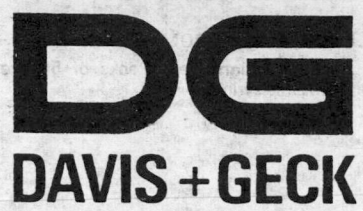

DAVIS + GECK

DEXON* 'S'
DEXON* PLUS

Presentation Dexon 'S' and Dexon Plus sutures are Synthetic Absorbable Sutures made of polyglycolic acid. Dexon Plus sutures are coated with Poloxamer 188, an absorbable surfactant which is inert, non-collagenous, non-antigenic and non-pyrogenic. Dexon 'S' and Dexon Plus are available undyed, with a natural beige colour, or coloured green to enhance visibility in tissues.

Uses Dexon 'S' or Dexon Plus may be used for suturing surgical and traumatic wounds and for ligating blood vessels.

Polyglycolic acid is a synthetic absorbable material which provokes minimal tissue reaction and may therefore be used where an absorbable suture is indicated.

Absorption characteristics: Absorption studies of Dexon 'S' and Dexon Plus in rabbits revealed minimal absorption at 7 to 15 days, significant absorption at 30 days and essentially complete absorption in 60–90 days. There have been occasional reports of its persistence within tissues for a longer period.

Dosage and administration As indicated in the surgical procedure.

Contra-indications, warnings, etc
Contra-indications: Dexon 'S' and Dexon Plus are contra-indicated where a non-absorbable suture is needed to provide prolonged wound support. The safe use of Dexon 'S' and Dexon Plus in neural tissue and in cardiovascular surgery has not been established.

Precautions: When tying Dexon 'S' special care is needed in placing the first knot.

Dexon Plus sutures are coated to enhance surface smoothness and may therefore require additional knot throws if indicated by surgical circumstances and the experience of the surgeon.

Adverse reactions: Although there have been a few reports of foreign body giant cell reactions, these are not considered to be specific to Dexon 'S' or Dexon Plus. As with all suture materials, inflammation at the site of absorption can occur although its incidence is less than with catgut. Wound dehiscence and bleeding have occasionally occurred.

Pharmaceutical precautions Discard opened, unused sutures. Do not re-sterilise.

Legal category P.

Package quantities Sealed envelopes containing sterile sutures in size 9.0 USP (0.3 metric) to 2 USP (5 metric), either as non-needled pre-cut lengths or attached to needles of varying types and sizes. These envelopes are sealed within a clear peel-apart secondary envelope, with the interspace being sterile. The sales unit is boxes of 1 dozen or 3 dozen envelopes.

Further information Radioisotope studies show that less than 3% of the coating of Dexon Plus sutures remains on the suture or within 1 gram of the surrounding tissue at 7 hours after implantation. Absorption studies in rabbits have shown that 80% to 97% of the coating was excreted in the urine during the first three days following implantation, with the remainder being excreted within 40 days.

Product licence numbers

Dexon 'S' (undyed beige)	0095/5092
Dexon 'S' (dyed green)	0095/0023
Dexon Plus (undyed beige)	0095/0082
Dexon Plus (dyed green)	0095/0083

HISTOACRYL*

Presentation The tissue adhesive Histoacryl is a butyl 2-cyanoacrylate monomer, which is supplied as a sterile liquid in sealed plastic vials. Histoacryl contains a blue dye to indicate clearly the thickness of the adhesive film applied. The plastic vials are packed in cylindrical plastic tubes.

Uses Histoacryl is a tissue adhesive for wound closure when established techniques, e.g. sutures, are inconvenient or inappropriate. Histoacryl may be used to bond tissue without sutures in surgical and traumatic wounds or in combination with sutures to provide additional security and to seal off the suture tracks.

Dosage and administration Histoacryl tissue adhesive must always be applied as a very thin film as otherwise its adhesive quality will be greatly impaired. Before Histoacryl is applied the tissue must be swabbed dry as much as possible. If larger surfaces have to be joined together Histoacryl must be applied to small patches of the total area only. After accurate adaptation the tissue surfaces to be bonded must be pressed together for one minute, however, caution must be taken to adapt the tissue exactly, because polymerization time is only 10 seconds and mistakes cannot be corrected later.

Contra-indications, warnings, etc As is the case with all cyanoacrylates, Histoacryl is contra-indicated where direct contact to nerve tissue takes place, e.g. for use on brain surface or parts of the central nervous system, since cell necrosis and scar tissue formation can be a consequence.

Contact of Histoacryl with parts of the major vascular

system is contra-indicated. Blood in contact with Histoacryl polymers form thrombi. Histoacryl must not come into contact with the conjunctival sac since conglutination may occur.

It must be pointed out that the polymerisation of Histoacryl produces heat. This is insignificant as long as Histoacryl is applied as a very thin film only. An injuring degree of heat on the surrounding tissue does not occur if the adhesive is applied in such a thin layer.

Pharmaceutical precautions The adhesive should be stored in the refrigerator or freezer, and must be protected from the light if removed from the packing for any length of time.

Care must be taken that no instruments, cloths, swabs or gloves come in contact with the adhesive. In that case they stick to the tissue. Instruments which have been contaminated with adhesive can be cleaned with dimethyl formamide or acetone.

Opened vials must be discarded. Histoacryl must not be resterilised.

Legal category P.

Package quantities 1 Box of Histoacryl contains 5 vials. Each vial contains 0.5 g of monomer.

Further information Nil.

Product licence number 3551/0001.

KIEL BONE GRAFT

Presentation Kiel Bone Graft, prepared by the method of Maatz and Bauermeister, is a mineral and collagenous matrix specially processed from calf bone, purified and gamma-ray-sterilised. According to the nature of the materials selected, Kiel Bone Graft consists of spongy or cortical tissue or a combination of both in various proportions. The grafts are packed in sterile double plastic bags in an outer box.

Uses The usual indications for Kiel Bone Graft are replacement of bone cysts, intervertebral locking, reparation of bone surface defects and the use as osteotomy wedges.

Dosage and administration As indicated in the surgical procedure.

Contra-indications, warnings, etc Kiel Bone Graft should not be implanted into a potentially infected host site. If the nature of the implant bed precludes the resorption process and the ingrowth of new bone, Kiel Bone Graft should not be used.

Pharmaceutical precautions Store in a dry place at room temperature. Opened and unused packages should be discarded and Kiel Bone Graft should not be resterilised.

Legal category P.

Package quantities Kiel Bone Graft is available in various sizes and types. Boxes contain 1 to 33 packages.

Further information Nil.

Product licence number 3551/5900.

LYODURA*

Presentation Lyodura is a sterile transplant material consisting of a mesh-like texture of collagenous fibres,

which is developed from homologous human dura mater cerebri by special processing, lyophilised and gamma-ray sterilised. Lyodura is supplied in sterile double peel pouches in several sizes.

Uses Lyodura is a patch material which is substituted after implantation by connective tissue. Lyodura is used in the repair of defects, lesions and as a reinforcement of body tissue, e.g. for covering and sealing defects and for sheathing and securing sutures, in neuro-thoracic and general surgery.

Dosage and administration As indicated in the surgical procedure. Lyodura must be rehydrated before use.

Contra-indications, warnings, etc The use of Lyodura in an infected operating region is contra-indicated since the healing-in of Lyodura cannot be expected in such a case. The use of Lyodura as a replacement for parts of the arterial system of the heart wall must be considered as being contra-indicated.

Degenerative changes in scarred wall replacement can cause aneurisms and calcification.

Pharmaceutical precautions Store in dry place at room temperature. Opened and unused packages should be discarded and material must not be resterilised.

Legal category P.

Package quantities Lyodura is available in various sizes and types. Boxes contain 1 to 5 pieces.

Further information Nil.

Product licence number 3551/0004.

SOFTGUT*

Presentation Uniform, firmly twisted strands of collagen prepared from healthy mammals, purified, softened, dry packed and sterilised. Available as both plain and chromic sutures.

Uses Softgut is sterile catgut used for suturing surgical and traumatic wounds and for ligating blood vessels. It may be used in practically all tissues. Softgut Plain is relatively rapidly absorbed and should therefore be used only where short term wound support is required. It is generally considered advisable to use Softgut Chromic where somewhat more prolonged wound support is desired.

Dosage and administration As indicated in the surgical procedure.

Contra-indications, warnings, etc Softgut is contra-indicated in situations where a non-absorbable suture is needed.

Adverse reactions may include tissue reaction or inflammation.

Wound dehiscence and bleeding may occasionally occur.

Pharmaceutical precautions Discard opened unused sutures. Do not re-sterilise. Store at room temperature.

Legal category P.

Package quantities Sutures are available in varying sizes, in non-needled pre-cut lengths or swaged to needles of varying types and sizes in packages of one dozen and/or two dozen and/or three dozen sutures.

Further information Nil.

Product licence numbers
Softgut Plain	0095/0096
Softgut Chromic	0095/0097

STERILISED SURGICAL CATGUT

Presentation 1. *Plain:* Uniform, firmly twisted strands of collagen prepared from healthy mammals, purified and sterilised. Available in sizes of 6/0 to 3 (i.e. 1 to 7 metric).

2. *Mild Chromic:* Black, uniform, firmly twisted strands of collagen (treated with chromicising agent) from healthy mammals, purified and sterilised. Available in sizes 7/0 to 4/0 (i.e. 0.5 to 2 metric).

3. *Chromic:* Uniform, firmly twisted strands of collagen (treated with chromicising agent) from healthy mammals, purified and sterilised. Available in sizes 5/0 to 3 (i.e. 1.5 to 7 metric).

Uses Sterilised Surgical Catgut may be used for suturing surgical and traumatic wounds and for ligating blood vessels. It may be used in practically all tissues. Catgut is relatively rapidly absorbed and should therefore be used only where short-term wound support is required. It is generally considered advisable to use Chromic Catgut where somewhat more prolonged wound support is desired.

Dosage and administration As indicated in the surgical procedure.

Contra-indications, warnings, etc Sterilised Surgical Catgut is contra-indicated where a non-absorbable suture is needed to provide prolonged wound support.

Opened and unused sutures should be discarded and material must not be re-sterilised. Adverse reactions may include tissue reaction or inflammation. Wound dehiscence and bleeding may occasionally occur.

Pharmaceutical precautions Store in a cool dry place. Discard opened unused sutures.

Legal category P.

Package quantities Sutures are available in varying sizes (Plain 6/0 to 3; Mild Chromic 7/0 to 4/0; and Chromic 5/0 to 3) in non-needled pre-cut lengths or swaged to Atraumatic* carbon steel needles of varying types and sizes in three dozen packages (N.B. certain ophthalmic sutures are available in one dozen packages).

Further information Nil.

Product licence numbers
Sterilised Surgical Catgut (Plain)	0095/5090
Sterilised Surgical Catgut (Mild Chromic)	0095/5091
Sterilised Surgical Catgut (Chromic)	0095/5091

*Trade Mark

Delandale Laboratories Limited
Delandale House
37 Old Dover Road
Canterbury, Kent, CT1 3JF

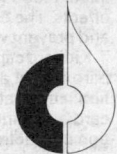

DICYNENE*

Presentation *Dicynene Tablets 500 mg.* Each oval white, bi-convex tablet, engraved 'DICYNENE' one side, '500' on the other, contains 500 mg ethamsylate.

Dicynene Tablets 250 mg: Each circular, white bi-convex tablet, engraved 'DICYNENE' on one side, contains 250 mg ethamsylate.

Dicynene 1000 Injection: Each clear glass 2 ml ampoule printed 'DICYNENE 1000' contains 1 g ethamsylate.

Dicynene Injection: Each clear glass 2 ml ampoule printed 'DICYNENE' contains 250 mg ethamsylate.

Uses Dicynene is a synthetic non-hormonal agent, used orally or parenterally to reduce excessive capillary blood loss. Dicynene acts principally by maintaining capillary integrity probably by promoting polymerisation of mucopolysaccharide in vessel walls.

Following systemic administration of Dicynene, the mean bleeding time is significantly reduced without any effect on cell counts, fibrinolysis, plasma protein levels, prothrombin time or clotting time. Dicynene does not have a vasoconstricting action nor does it have any effect on hepatic or renal function.

Dicynene is used clinically for the prophylaxis and treatment of small-vessel haemorrhage, including the following indications.

Gynaecology: Non hormonal control of menorrhagia and control of bleeding during gynaecological surgery.

Paediatrics: Limiting or preventing periventricular haemorrhage in low birth weight babies.

Urology: Control of haemorrhage during and after prostatectomy. Symptomatic control of urinary tract haemorrhage of unknown aetiology.

Oral and dental surgery: Control of haemorrhage following oral surgery and dental extractions.

Ophthalmology: Control of surgical haemorrhage and retinal bleeding.

ENT: Epistaxis and control of surgical haemorrhage e.g. tonsillectomy, adenoidectomy, middle ear surgery.

General surgery: Control of haemorrhage occurring during or after surgery.

General medicine: The prophylaxis and treatment of small vessel haemorrhage occurring in the gastro-intestinal or respiratory tract; the control of haemorrhage during anticoagulant therapy.

Dosage and administration *Adult dosage: Menorrhagia:* One 500 mg tablet four times a day from the start of bleeding until menstruation ceases.

Pre-surgical prophylaxis: 1 g from Dicynene 1000 Injection (or Dicynene Injection) either intramuscularly with the premedication or intravenously at induction of anaesthesia.

Haemorrhagic emergency: 1 g from Dicynene 1000 Injection intravenously. When used in conjunction with high molecular weight plasma volume expanders Dicynene is more effective if administered first.

Maintenance therapy: 500 mg intravenously, intramuscularly or orally every four to six hours.

Paediatric dosage: 250–750 mg parenterally for the control of haemorrhage; 250 mg orally or parenterally every four to six hours for maintenance therapy.

Neonatal dosage: 12.5 mg/kg intravenously or intramuscularly six hourly.

Contra-indications, warnings, etc There are no known contra-indications. Dicynene is well tolerated even in high dosage or during prolonged treatment.

Following intravenous injection there may be a transient fall in blood pressure of the order of 30 mm Hg, lasting four to five minutes. No major side-effects have been reported, but occasional headache or skin rashes may occur which usually disappear on reduced dosage. A few patients may experience nausea, however this can be overcome by administering the dose after food.

Pharmaceutical precautions *Tablets:* Protect from light and moisture. Dispense in airtight containers.

Ampoules: Protect from light. Discard if solution is coloured.

Legal category POM.

Package quantities

Tablets 500 mg:	Securitainers of 100
Tablets 250 mg:	Securitainers of 100
Injection:	10 × 2 ml ampoules
1000 Injection:	10 × 2 ml ampoules

Further information Dicynene is excreted unchanged largely by the urinary route. Studies in animals have revealed no teratogenic effect.

Product licence numbers

Tablets 500 mg	0357/5003
Tablets 250 mg	0357/5002
Dicynene Injection	0357/5001
Dicynene 1000 Injection	0357/0013

KIDITARD*

Presentation Hard gelatin capsules, size 0, with clear light blue and clear dark blue shell. Each capsule contains 250 mg quinidine bisulphate (equivalent to 200 mg quinidine sulphate) in the form of sustained release micro-pellets.

Uses Sustained release quinidine therapy. The active ingredient is absorbed from the gastro-intestinal tract over a 12 hour period. An even pattern of release of the drug is established which prevents excessively high initial blood levels and therefore limits undesirable side effects. The capsules permit a twice daily dosage regime and prevent wide fluctuation in plasma quinidine levels.

Kiditard capsules are used clinically for: extra-systoles; paroxysmal atrial tachycardia; nodal tachycardia; atrial fibrillation; atrial flutter; paroxysmal ventricular tachycardia; maintenance of sinus rhythm following restoration by electro-conversion.

Dosage and administration Kiditard dosage should be individually adapted to each patient. As a rule, treatment should commence with two capsules every 10–12 hours, after a test dose of 1 capsule to test for patient sensitivity.

Kiditard capsules are not recommended for use in children.

Contra-indications, warnings, etc Acute infections, atrio-ventricular block and idiosyncrasy to quinidine form absolute contra-indications to Kiditard therapy. Special care must be taken with heavily digitalised patients and in patients with congestive heart failure, hypotension or ventricular tachycardia due to possible overdosage with quinidine. Special care is also needed in patients on prolonged anti-coagulant treatment since cases of quinidine-induced hypoprothrombinaemic haemorrhage have been recorded. Patients should be carefully observed for their reactions to the first dose of the drug since idiosyncrasy is a possible response to quinidine. The following allergic reactions to quinidine have been reported: urticaria, purpura, asthma, thrombocytopaenia. Gastro-intestinal upset, commonly associated with quinidine therapy, is largely avoided through the use of Kiditard. There are reports of hepatitis due to quinidine; none has been fatal and signs and symptoms disappear on withdrawal. Cardiotoxic side-effects (ventricular extra systole, A-V block, increased QRS complex above 50%, ventricular tachycardia) may occur; repeated high doses may lead to cinchonism.

If overdosage occurs treatment should be as for quinidine. Gastric lavage and a saline purgative should be employed. Promote excretion by acidifying urine with ammonium chloride. Maintain fluid balance and blood pressure. Assist respiration and monitor cardiac rhythm.

Pharmaceutical precautions Protect from light and moisture.

Legal category POM.

Package quantities Containers of 100 capsules.

Further information Nil.

Product licence number 0357/0012.

PRIADEL*

Presentation Controlled release lithium carbonate tablets. White, circular, bi-convex tablets engraved PRIADEL one side, scored on the other side. Each containing 400 mg Lithium Carbonate PhEur in a controlled release dosage form.

Uses 1. Treatment of mania and hypomania.
2. Lithium may also be tried in the treatment of some patients with recurrent bipolar depression, where treatment with other antidepressants has been unsuccessful.
3. Prophylactic treatment of recurrent affective disorders.

Dosage and administration A simple treatment schedule has been evolved which except for some minor variations should be followed whether using Priadel therapeutically or prophylactically. The minor variations to this schedule depend on the elements of the illness being treated and these are described later.

1. In patients of average weight (70 kg) an initial dose of 1–3 tablets (400–1,200 mg) of Priadel may be given as a single daily dose in the morning or on retiring. Alternatively, the dose may be divided and given morning and evening. The tablets should not be crushed, chewed or swallowed with hot liquids. When changing from other lithium preparations serum lithium levels should first be checked, then Priadel therapy commenced at a daily dose as close as possible to the dose of the other form of lithium. As bioavailability varies from product to product (particularly with regard to retard or slow release preparations) a change of product should be regarded as initiation of new treatment.

2. Four to five days after starting treatment (and never longer than one week) a blood sample should be taken for the estimation of serum lithium level.

3. The objective is to adjust the Priadel dose so as to maintain the serum lithium level permanently within the diurnal range of 0.5–1.5 mmol/l. In practice, the blood sample should be taken between 12 and 24 hours after the previous dose of Priadel. 'Target' serum lithium concentrations at 12 and 24 hours are shown in the table below.

	'Target' serum lithium concentration (mmol/l)	
	At 12 hours	At 24 hours
Once daily dosage	0.7–1.0	0.5–0.8
Twice daily dosage	0.5–0.8	

Priadel tablets are scored, therefore they can be divided accurately to provide dosage adjustments of 200 mg. Serum lithium levels should be monitored weekly until stabilisation is achieved.

4. Lithium therapy should not be initiated unless adequate facilities for routine monitoring of serum concentrations are available. Following stabilisation of serum lithium levels, the period between subsequent estimations can be increased gradually but should not normally exceed three months. Additional measurements should be made following alteration of dosage, on development of intercurrent disease, signs of manic or depressive relapse, following significant change in sodium or fluid intake, or if signs of lithium toxicity occur.

5. Whilst a high proportion of acutely ill patients may respond within three to seven days of the commencement of Priadel therapy, Priadel should be continued through any recurrence of the affective disturbance. This is important as the full prophylactic effect may not occur for 6 to 12 months after the initiation of therapy.

6. In patients who show a positive response to Priadel therapy, treatment is likely to be long term. Careful clinical appraisal of the patient should be exercised throughout medication (see Precautions).

Prophylactic treatment of recurrent affective disorders: It is recommended that the described treatment schedule is followed.

Treatment of acute mania, hypomania and recurrent bipolar depression: It is likely that a higher than normal Priadel intake may be necessary during an acute phase and divided doses would be required here. Therefore as soon as control of mania or depression is achieved, the serum lithium level should be determined and it may be necessary, dependent on the results, to lower the dose of Priadel and re-stabilise serum lithium levels. In all other details the described treatment schedule is recommended.

Use in elderly: In elderly patients or those below 50 kg in weight, it is recommended that the starting dose be one tablet (400 mg). Elderly patients may be more sensitive to undesirable effects of lithium and also may require lower doses in order to maintain normal serum lithium levels. It follows therefore that long term patients often require a reduction in dosage over a period of years.

Use in children and adolescents: Not recommended.

Contra-indications, warnings, etc

Contra-indications. Renal insufficiency, cardiovascular insufficiency, Addison's disease and untreated hypothyroidism are all contra-indications to lithium therapy.

Use in pregnancy: There is epidemiological evidence that lithium may be harmful to the foetus in human pregnancy.

Total no. 'lithium babies' reported	Malformed infants	Ebstein's anomaly and other major cardiovascular malformations
225	25 (11%)	18 (8%)

It is strongly recommended that lithium be discontinued before a planned pregnancy. If it is considered essential to maintain Priadel treatment during pregnancy, serum lithium levels should be monitored closely since renal function changes gradually during pregnancy and suddenly at parturition, requiring dosage adjustments. It is recommended that lithium be discontinued shortly before delivery and recommenced a few days postpartum.

Babies may show signs of lithium toxicity necessitating fluid therapy in the neonatal period. Babies born with low serum lithium concentrations may have a flaccid appearance which returns to normal without any treatment. Lithium is secreted in breast milk, therefore bottle feeding is recommended.

Precautions: When considering Priadel therapy, it is necessary to ascertain whether patients are receiving lithium in any other form. If so, check serum levels before proceeding. It is important to ensure that renal function is normal – if necessary a creatinine clearance test or other renal function test should be performed. Cardiac and thyroid function should be assessed before commencing lithium treatment. Patients should be euthyroid before the initiation of lithium therapy. Renal function, cardiac function and thyroid function should be reassessed periodically.

Clear instructions regarding the symptoms of impending toxicity should be given by the doctor to all patients receiving long term lithium therapy (see Toxic effects). Patients should also be warned to report if polyuria or polydipsia develop. Episodes of nausea and vomiting or other conditions leading to salt/water depletion (including severe dieting) should also be reported. Elderly patients are particularly liable to lithium toxicity.

Caution should be exercised to ensure that diet and fluid intake are normal thus maintaining a stable electrolyte balance. This may be of special importance in very

hot weather or work environment. Infectious diseases including colds, influenza, gastro-enteritis and urinary infections may alter fluid balance and thus affect serum lithium levels. Treatment should be discontinued during any intercurrent infection and should only be reinstituted after the patient's physical health has returned to normal.

Drug interactions: Concurrent use of lithium and diuretics may cause reduced lithium clearance, leading to intoxication. If a diuretic has to be prescribed for a lithium patient, the lithium dosage should first be lowered and the patient re-stabilised with frequent monitoring. Similar precautions should be exercised on diuretic withdrawal. Other drugs affecting electrolyte balance e.g. steroids, may alter lithium excretion and should be avoided in patients on lithium. If other psychotrophic drugs are used they should be initiated at a lower dosage than usual, as their side effects may be potentiated by the use of lithium. This has been shown to be of particular importance for the concurrent use of lithium and haloperidol or flupenthixol.

There have been isolated reports of possible interactions between lithium and diazepam (resulting in hypothermia), methyldopa, tetracyclines, phenytoin, carbamazepine, indomethacin and other prostaglandin-synthetase inhibitors.

Warnings and adverse effects: Side effects are usually related to serum lithium concentrations and are infrequent at levels below 1.0 mmol/l.

Mild gastrointestinal effects, nausea, vertigo, muscle weakness and a dazed feeling may occur initially, but frequently disappear after stabilisation. Fine hand tremors, polyuria and mild thirst may persist. Weight gain or oedema may present in some patients but should not be treated with diuretics.

Hypercalcaemia, hypermagnesaemia and hyperparathyroidism have been reported. Skin conditions including acne, psoriasis, generalised pustular psoriasis, rashes and leg ulcers have occasionally been reported as being aggravated by lithium treatment.

Long term treatment with lithium may be associated with disturbances of thyroid function, including goitre, hypothyroidism and thyrotoxicosis. Lithium-induced hypothyroidism may be managed successfully with concurrent thyroxine.

Memory impairment may occur during long term use.

Nephrotoxicity: Up to one third of patients on lithium may develop polyuria with a urinary output of up to three litres per day. This is usually due to lithium blocking the effect of ADH and is reversible on lithium withdrawal. However, long term treatment with lithium may also result in permanent changes in kidney histology and impairment of renal function. High serum concentrations of lithium including episodes of acute lithium toxicity may aggravate these changes. The minimum clinically effective dose of lithium should always be used. In patients who develop polyuria or polydipsia, renal function should be monitored, e.g. with measurement of blood urea, serum creatinine and urinary protein levels in addition to the routine serum lithium estimations.

After a period lasting 3–5 years, patients should be carefully assessed to ensure that benefit persists.

Toxic effects: Such effects are indicative of impending lithium intoxication and fall into two groups:

1. Gastro-intestinal: increasing anorexia, diarrhoea and vomiting.
2. Central nervous system: muscle weakness, lack of co-ordination, drowsiness or lethargy progressing to

giddiness with ataxia, tinnitus, blurred vision, dysarthria, coarse tremor and muscle twitching.

At blood levels above 2–3 mmol/l there may be a large output of dilute urine, with increasing disorientation, seizures, coma and death.

Patients should be instructed to stop taking their tablets if toxic symptoms appear and to report immediately for a serum lithium estimation.

Lithium intoxication: There is no specific antidote to lithium poisoning. In the event of accumulation, lithium should be stopped and serum estimations should be carried out every six hours.

Under no circumstances should a diuretic be used. Osmotic diuresis (mannitol or urea infusion) or alkalinisation of the urine (sodium lactate or sodium bicarbonate infusion) should be initiated.

If the serum lithium level is over 4.0 mmol/l, if there is a deterioration in the patient's condition, or if the serum lithium concentration is not falling at a rate corresponding

to a half-life of under 30 hours, peritoneal or haemodialysis should be instituted promptly. This should be continued until there is no lithium in the serum or dialysis fluid. Serum lithium levels should be monitored for at least a further week to take account of any possible rebound in serum lithium levels as a result of delayed diffusion from body tissues.

Pharmaceutical precautions Store in a cool, dry place. Dispense in airtight containers.

Legal category POM.

Package quantities Securitainers of 100 and 1,000 tablets and Hospital Packs of 100 tablets.

Further information Nil.

Product licence number 0357/5000R.

*Trade Mark

Dental Health Promotion Ltd
51 Greencroft Gardens
London NW6 3LL

FLUOR-A-DAY* LAC

Presentation Round, biconvex, buff coloured tablets, embossed with NaF on one side and a break-line on the reverse. They have a slightly sweet taste. Each tablet contains 2.2 mg sodium fluoride BP equivalent to 1.00 mg available fluorine.

Uses For the prevention of dental caries especially in children. The protective action is thought to be due to one or more of the following properties:

1. By reducing the solubility of enamel formed during exposure to fluoride, probably due to the conversion of some hydroxyapatite to less soluble fluoropetite.
2. Remineralisation of enamel.
3. An antibacterial action.

Dosage and administration For oral administration.

From birth – 2 years of age: Half a tablet daily or 1 tablet every two days.

From 2 years until teeth are fully developed: 1 tablet daily. There is evidence that keeping the tablet in the mouth may provide extra benefit particularly after a meal. Thus as soon as the child is old enough he or she should be encouraged to suck the tablet allowing it to dissolve slowly in the mouth.

For babies half a tablet should be dissolved in a small quantity of boiled and cooled water and added to the milk.

The value of taking fluoride may extend until the age of 20 years but the benefits fall off quite sharply from birth onwards so it is most important that an early start should be made.

Contra-indications, warnings, etc There are no known contra-indications.

No allergy to fluoride has ever been established but the lactose base in the tablets may cause a slight reaction in some children who are allergic to this ingredient.

There are very few reports of dental fluorosis even when children have taken tablets in fluoridated areas. Those cases that have occurred are so slight that the condition can generally only be detected by dentists.

Precautions: Tablets are not recommended in those areas where the water supply is fluoridated to levels of 1 p.p.m.

Overdosage: Treatment is by aspiration and lavage with Calcium Hydroxide Solution BP, or a solution of Calcium Chloride or other Calcium salt. Convulsions may be controlled by intravenous injection of 10 ml Solution of Calcium Gluconate 10%, repeated every 4–6 hours if necessary. Injections of pethidine or morphine may be used to control colic. Respiration may require assistance, and the circulation should be maintained with infusions of suitable electrolyte solutions. Haemodialysis has been used.

The manufacturer will supply details of local concentrations of fluoride as far as possible but there is considerable variation from area to area. Local Dentists generally know the fluoride levels, also the Area Dental Officer and Pharmacists are kept informed to some extent.

Pharmaceutical precautions Store tablets in cool dry place.

Legal category P.

Package quantities Packs of 200.

Further information The best results are obtained when the mother takes Fluor-a-day Lac during the last six months of pregnancy whether the local water supply is fluoridated or not. One tablet a day is all that is required. Fluoride does not pass into the mothers milk so in order to maintain benefit babies should be given fluoride as above.

Product licence number 0111/5001.

*Trade Mark

Dermal Laboratories Limited

Tatmore Place
Gosmore,　Hitchin
Herts, SG4 7QR

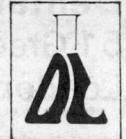

ANHYDROL FORTE*

Presentation Colourless evaporative solution containing 20% w/v Aluminium Chloride Hexahydrate.

Uses For the topical treatment of hyperhidrosis specifically involving axillae, hands or feet.

Dosage and administration Apply to the affected sites at night, as required, and allow to dry. Wash off in the morning.

Contra-indications, warnings, etc Care should be taken to restrict the application to the affected sites only. Do not bathe immediately before use and, if the axillae are treated, do not shave or use depilatories on this area within 12 hours before or after use.
Keep away from the eyes.
    Care should be taken to avoid Anhydrol Forte coming into direct contact with clothing, polished surfaces, jewellery or metal.
    Sensitivity to any of the ingredients.

Pharmaceutical precautions Store upright in a cool place away from flames. Replace cap tightly after use.

Legal category POM.

Package quantity Anhydrol Forte is supplied in a glass roll-on bottle containing 10 ml.

Further information The formulation of Anhydrol Forte has been tested in widespread clinical practice, and has been shown to be effective when used in accordance with the recommended instructions. Should irritation occur, reduce the frequency of application and if necessary apply mild hydrocortisone cream.

Ingredients: Aluminium Chloride Hexahydrate; Industrial Methylated Spirit BP.

Product licence number 0173/0030.

CALLUSOLVE*

Presentation Amber coloured paint containing 25% Benzalkonium Chloride Bromine.

Uses For topical use in the treatment of warts, especially multiple or mosaic warts.

Dosage and administration Gently rub the surface of the wart with a piece of pumice stone or manicure emery board, or pare down any hard skin. Using the applicator provided, carefully apply a few drops of the paint to the wart, taking care to localise the application to the affected area. Allow each drop to dry before the next is applied. Cover with an adhesive plaster and leave for 24 hours. On subsequent days, remove the plaster and repeat the above instructions.

Contra-indications, warnings, etc Keep away from the eyes and mucous membranes. Not to be used on the face, anal or perineal region. Avoid spreading onto surrounding uninvolved skin. If the treated area becomes inflamed or painful, treatment should be suspended until the inflammation resolves.
    Sensitivity to any of the ingredients.

Pharmaceutical precautions Store upright in a cool place. Replace cap tightly after use. Avoid spillage.

Legal category P.

Package quantity Callusolve is supplied in an amber glass bottle containing 10 ml, incorporating a spatula for ease of application.

Further information Benzalkonium chloride bromine is an adduct of benzalkonium chloride with bromine, which is dissolved in a non-aqueous volatile solvent. When applied to the wart, a slow release of bromine attacks the immature keratin, fragmenting the lesion and killing the virus.

Ingredients: Benzalkonium Chloride Bromine; Liquid Paraffin BP; Chloroform (ethanol-free).

Product licence number 0173/5005.

DIODERM*

Presentation White aqueous cream containing 0.1% Hydrocortisone BP.

Uses Topical treatment of eczema, dermatitis and all types of inflammatory, pruritic and allergic skin conditions. In view of its relative safety, Dioderm is particularly suitable for children.

Dosage and administration Rub well into the affected areas twice daily. Frequency of application may be modified according to individual patient response.

Contra-indications, warnings, etc As with all topical steroids, Dioderm is contra-indicated in the presence of viral or fungal infections, tubercular or syphilitic lesions and in bacterial infections, unless used in conjunction with appropriate chemotherapy. It should not be applied extensively in pregnancy, i.e. in large amounts or for prolonged periods. In infants, long term or continuous topical therapy should be avoided, as adrenal suppression can occur even without occlusion.
    Sensitivity to any of the ingredients.

Pharmaceutical precautions Store in a cool place. Replace cap after use.

Legal category POM.

Package quantity Dioderm is supplied in a collapsible tube containing 30 g.

Further information Dioderm represents a significant advance in the formulation of a topical hydrocortisone preparation. It has been shown to be clinically effective, and significantly more active than other hydrocortisone preparations, including those containing urea.

Ingredients: Hydrocortisone BP; Citric Acid BP; Emulsifying Ointment BP; Propylene Glycol BP; Water BP.

Product licence number 0173/0018.

DITHROCREAM*

Presentation Dithrocream is presented as a pale yellow aqueous cream containing 0.1%, 0.25%, 0.5% (Forte) or 1.0% (HP) Dithranol BP, supplied in a collapsible tube containing 50 g.

Uses Dithrocream is recommended for the topical treatment of sub-acute and chronic psoriasis, including psoriasis of the scalp. Dithrocream Forte (0.5%) and Dithrocream HP (1.0%) should only be used for those patients who have failed to respond to lower strengths of dithranol. Dithrocream HP (1.0%) should normally only be applied for 'short contact' periods.

Dosage and administration Where the response to Dithrocream has not previously been established, always commence treatment with Dithrocream 0.1%, continuing for at least one week and then, if necessary, increase to the 0.25% followed by the 0.5% (Forte), and finally the 1.0% (HP) strength. Dithrocream Forte and Dithrocream HP should always be used under medical supervision.

To open the tube, unscrew the cap and invert to pierce membrane.

Dithrocream should be applied once every 24 hours, at any convenient time of the day or evening, and then removed by washing off, usually no more than one hour after application. Alternatively, it may be applied at night before retiring and washed off in the morning.

Dithrocream should be applied sparingly, only to the affected areas. Rub the cream gently and carefully into the skin until completely absorbed. It is most important to avoid applying an excessive amount of the cream, which may cause unnecessary soiling and staining of clothing and/or bed linen. After each period of treatment, a bath/shower should be taken to remove any residual cream. To prevent the possibility of discolouration, particularly where Dithrocream HP (1.0%) has been used, always rinse the bath/shower with hot water immediately after washing/showering and then use a suitable cleanser to remove any deposit on the surface of the bath or shower.

Always wash the hands after use.

For use on the scalp, first comb the hair to remove scalar debris and, after suitably parting, rub the cream well into the affected areas.

Treatment should be continued until the skin is entirely clear, i.e. when there is nothing to feel with the fingers and the texture is normal.

Contra-indications, warnings, etc Acute or pustular psoriasis.

If the initial treatment produces excessive soreness, or if the lesions spread, reduce frequency of application, and, in extreme cases, stop treatment. Use with care on the face and intertriginous areas. Keep away from the eyes and mucous membranes.

Contact with fabrics, plastics and other materials may cause staining and should be avoided.

Use in pregnancy: Although there is no experimental evidence to support the safety of the drug in pregnancy, no adverse effects have been reported.

Use in children: No evidence of any adverse effects. However, use cautiously with regular supervision.

Accidental ingestion: Dithranol is a cathartic and if accidentally swallowed should be removed by gastric lavage.

Sensitivity to any of the ingredients.

Pharmaceutical precautions Store in a cool place. Replace cap tightly after use.

Legal category P.

Package quantities All strengths of Dithrocream are supplied in collapsible tubes containing 50 g.

Further information Dithrocream has been developed as a cream formulation of dithranol for particular convenience for home treatment, and is especially suitable for the exposed surfaces and hairy regions of the body, including psoriasis of the scalp.

Ingredients: Dithranol BP; White Soft Paraffin BP; Salicylic Acid BP; Cetostearyl Alcohol BP; Chlorocresol BP; Ascorbic Acid BP; Sodium Lauryl Sulphate BP; Water BP.

Product licence numbers

Dithrocream 0.1%	0173/0029
Dithrocream 0.25%	0173/0028
Dithrocream Forte (0.5%)	0173/0027
Dithrocream HP (1.0%)	0173/0039

DITHROLAN*

Presentation Stiff yellow ointment containing 0.5% Dithranol BP, 0.5% Salicylic Acid BP, in equal quantities of hard and soft paraffin.

Uses For the topical treatment of quiescent psoriasis.

Dosage and administration Apply accurately to the psoriatic lesions, commencing treatment on a few of the thicker lesions. Aim for a localised feeling of warmth; a sensation of burning can be controlled by varying the quantity and frequency of application.

At first, the ointment should only be left in contact with the skin for a few hours, e.g. during the evening whilst watching television, before removal by bathing. The duration of contact can later be extended to intensify the response. As resting aids the response to treatment, the ointment may conveniently be applied before retiring to bed and removed by bathing the next morning.

Bathing is necessary to remove residual ointment, and to control the reaction to treatment by preventing a build-up of dithranol in the skin.

The lesions will reduce in thickness as a red-brown stain develops. This is indicative of an effective response. No attempt should be made to remove the stain, which will disappear completely following cessation of treatment. In view of the staining of clothing and bed linen which can occur as part of dithranol therapy, it is advisable to utilise old pyjamas, under garments, bed linen and towels.

In the treatment of thinner lesions and flexures, a smaller amount of ointment should be applied accurately once or twice weekly.

Treatment should be continued until the skin is entirely clear, i.e. when there is nothing to feel with the fingers and the texture is normal. When in doubt, continue treatment for a further week, leaving the ointment on the skin for shorter periods.

During treatment, the ointment may be stored in a warm place to reduce stiffness and assist ease of application.

Contra-indications, warnings, etc In view of the rebound effect which may be experienced, after the use of potent topical steroids it is recommended that patients be treated with a bland emollient preparation for approximately two weeks. Treatment may then be commenced, using Dithrolan diluted with four parts of yellow soft paraffin, reducing the dilution as tolerance develops.

If the initial treatment produces soreness, or if the lesions spread (particularly when potent topical steroids have recently been used), reduce frequency of application and, in extreme cases, stop treatment. Cautiously resume treatment, commencing with a few of the thicker lesions, alternating application of the ointment with yellow soft paraffin.

Not to be used for acute psoriasis. Keep away from the eyes. Wash hands after use.

Sensitivity to any of the ingredients.

Pharmaceutical precautions Store in a dark place. Do not expose to direct heat. Replace cap after use.

Legal category P.

Package quantity Dithrolan is supplied in an amber glass jar containing 90 g.

Further information Dithrolan provides the clinical efficacy of the dithranol paste which has been established as part of the Ingram regime. It is, however, easier to apply and remove, whilst retaining adequate stiffness.

Ingredients: Dithranol BP; Salicylic Acid BP; Hard Paraffin BP; White Soft Paraffin BP.

Product licence number 0173/0024.

EMULSIDERM*

Presentation Pale blue/green liquid emulsion containing 0.5% Benzalkonium Chloride BP, 25.0% Liquid Paraffin BP, 25.0% Isopropyl Myristate BPC.

Uses An aid in the treatment of dry skin conditions, especially those associated with eczema, ichthyosis or xeroderma. It permits re-hydration of the keratin by replacing lost lipids, and its antiseptic properties assist in overcoming secondary infection.

Dosage and administration Shake bottle before use.
For use in the bath: Add 2–3 capfuls to a 6–8 inch bath of warm water. For infant bathing use 1–2 capfuls. Soak for 5–10 minutes. Pat dry.

For application to the skin: Rub a small amount of undiluted emollient into the dry areas of skin until absorbed.

Contra-indications, warnings, etc Keep away from the eyes. Take care to avoid slipping in the bath.

Sensitivity to any of the ingredients.

Pharmaceutical precautions Store in a cool place. Replace cap after use.

Legal category P.

Package quantities Emulsiderm is supplied in poly-thene bottles containing 250 ml, with a 10 ml measuring cap and 1 litre, with a 30 ml measure.

Further information Emulsiderm contains the anti-septic benzalkonium chloride in an emulsion system which permits rapid dispersion of its oil content in the bathwater.

Ingredients. Benzalkonium Chloride BP; Liquid Paraffin BP; Isopropyl Myristate BPC; Sorbitan Monostearate 60 BP (Span 60); Polysorbate 60 BP (Tween 60); Brilliant Green BP; Industrial Methylated Spirit BP; Ascorbic Acid BP; Water BP.

Product licence number 0173/0036.

EXOLAN* CREAM

Presentation Pale yellow aqueous cream containing 1% 1, 8, 9 Triacetoxyanthracene.

Uses For the topical treatment of sub-acute and chronic psoriasis, including psoriasis of the scalp.

Dosage and administration Gently rub the cream into the lesions until completely absorbed, taking care to localise the application to the affected areas. The following morning, a bath should be taken to remove any residue of the cream.

For use on the scalp, shampoo to remove scalar debris and any previous application. Dry the hair and, after suitably parting, rub the cream well into the lesions.

Contra-indications, warnings, etc Acute psoriasis. Keep away from the eyes. Wash hands after use.

Sensitivity to any of the ingredients.

Pharmaceutical precautions Store in a cool place. Replace cap tightly after use.

Legal category P.

Package quantity Exolan Cream is supplied in a collapsible tube containing 50 g.

Further information Triacetoxyanthracene has a similar mode of action to dithranol whilst minimising the problems of irritation and staining.

Ingredients: 1,8,9-Triacetoxyanthracene; Emulsifying Wax BP; White Soft Paraffin BP; Chlorocresol BP; Water BP.

Product licence number 0173/5004.

EXTEROL*

Presentation Viscous solution containing 5% w/w Urea Hydrogen Peroxide.

Uses An aid in the removal of hardened ear wax.

Dosage and administration Remove the protective cap, invert the pipette above the opening of the affected ear and, with the head tilted sideways, gently squeeze 5–10 drops into the ear. Retain drops in ear for several minutes by keeping head tilted and then wipe away any surplus.

Repeat once or twice daily for at least 3–4 days, or as required.

Contra-indications, warnings, etc Keep away from the eyes. Do not use if eardrum is known or suspected to be perforated. Stop usage if irritation or pain occurs.

Sensitivity to any of the ingredients.

Pharmaceutical precautions Store in a cool place, but do not refrigerate. Replace cap after use, and return bottle to carton.

Legal category P.

Package quantity Exterol is supplied in an amber glass bottle containing 12 ml, incorporating a specially designed pipette enclosed in a protective cap.

Further information After insertion of the drops into the ear, the urea hydrogen peroxide liberates oxygen which acts to break up the hardened wax. Subsequently, the glycerol and urea assist in the softening of the wax in order that it may more easily be removed from the ear, either with or without syringing. Due to the release of oxygen, patients may experience a mild, temporary effervescence in the ear.

Ingredients: Urea Hydrogen Peroxide; 8-Hydroxyquinoline BP; Glycerol BP.

Product licence number 0173/0037.

GLUTAROL*

Presentation Colourless evaporative solution containing 10% w/v Glutaraldehyde.

Uses For the topical treatment of warts, especially plantar warts.

Dosage and administration Gently rub the surface of the wart with a piece of pumice stone or manicure emery board, or pare down any hard skin. Using the applicator provided, carefully apply a few drops of the paint to the wart, taking care to localise the application to the affected area. Allow each drop to dry before the next is applied. Repeat twice daily. On subsequent days, repeat the above instructions. It is not necessary to cover the treated wart(s) with an adhesive plaster.

Contra-indications, warnings, etc Keep away from the eyes and mucous membranes. Not to be used on the face, anal or perineal region. Avoid spreading onto surrounding uninvolved skin.
  Sensitivity to any of the ingredients.

Pharmaceutical precautions Store in a cool place away from flames. Replace cap tightly after use. Avoid spillage.

Legal category P.

Package quantity Glutarol is supplied in an amber glass bottle containing 10 ml, incorporating a specially designed spatula, for ease of application.

Further information Glutaraldehyde is virucidal and thus inactivates the wart virus. On the skin, it also acts as an anhidrotic, drying the warts and surrounding skin, thus reducing the spread of lesions and simplifying the removal of persistent warts by curettage.
  As glutaraldehyde stains the outer layers of the skin brown, treatment can be seen to be carried out. This stain soon disappears after cessation of treatment.

Ingredients: Glutaraldehyde; Bitrex; Industrial Methylated Spirit BP; Water BP.

Product licence number 0173/0022.

PSORIDERM* BATH EMULSION

Presentation Buff-coloured liquid emulsion containing 40% special coal tar extract.

Uses An aid in the treatment of sub-acute and chronic psoriasis.

Dosage and administration Add 30 ml of the emulsion to a standard bath of warm water. Soak for 5 minutes, pat dry.

Contra-indications, warnings, etc Keep away from the eyes.
  Sensitivity to any of the ingredients.

Pharmaceutical precautions Store in a cool, dark place. Replace cap after use.

Legal category P.

Package quantity Psoriderm Bath Emulsion is supplied in an amber glass bottle containing 200 ml.

Further information The use of coal tar has long been advocated as a therapeutic agent in the management of psoriasis. Psoriderm Bath Emulsion conveniently provides a coal tar bath which may be used alone, or as part of a more extensive treatment regime.

Ingredients: Special Coal Tar Fraction; Polysorbate 20 BP; Triethanolamine BP; Water BP.

Product licence number 0173/5003.

PSORIDERM* CREAM

Presentation Buff coloured aqueous cream containing 6% special coal tar extract, 0.4% lecithin.

Uses For the topical treatment of sub-acute and chronic psoriasis, including psoriasis of the scalp and flexures.

Dosage and administration Apply to the affected areas twice daily, or as required.

Contra-indications, warnings, etc Acute psoriasis. Keep away from the eyes and mucous membranes. Wash hands after use.
  Sensitivity to any of the ingredients.

Pharmaceutical precautions Store in a cool, dark place. Replace cap after use.

Legal category P.

Package quantity Psoriderm cream is supplied in an amber glass jar containing 225 ml.

Further information The use of coal tar has long been advocated as a therapeutic agent in the management of psoriasis. Psoriderm Cream may be used alone, or as part of a more extensive treatment regime, and is particularly suitable for treating the hair bearing areas of the body and the flexures.

Ingredients: Lecithin; Special Coal Tar Fraction; Stearic Acid BPC; Isopropyl Palmitate; Polyethylene Glycol 400 Monostearate; Methyl-4-Hydroxybenzoate BP; Propylene Glycol BP; Triethanolamine BPC; Water BP.

Product licence number 0173/5000.

PSORIDERM* SCALP LOTION

Presentation Amber coloured foaming shampoo containing 2.5% special coal tar extract, 0.3% lecithin.

Uses For the topical treatment of psoriasis of the scalp.

Dosage and administration Wet the hair thoroughly. Apply a small amount of the shampoo to the scalp, and massage gently until a rich lather has been generated. Retain on the scalp for a few minutes. Remove excess lather with the hands, before rinsing with warm water. Repeat the above procedure.

Contra-indications, warnings, etc Keep away from the eyes and mucous membranes.
Sensitivity to any of the ingredients.

Pharmaceutical precautions Store in a cool, dark place. Replace cap after use.

Legal category P.

Package quantities Psoriderm Scalp Lotion is supplied in polythene bottles containing 112 ml and 250 ml.

Further information The use of coal tar has long been advocated as a therapeutic agent in the management of psoriasis. Psoriderm Scalp Lotion may be used alone as a coal tar shampoo, or as part of a more extensive treatment regime.

Ingredients: Lecithin; Special Coal Tar Fraction; Triethanolamine Lauryl Sulphate (Empicol TLR); Lauric Acid Diethanolamide (Loramine DL 203); Disodium Edetate BP; Sodium Chloride BP; Water BP.

Product licence number 0173/5001.

SALACTOL*

Presentation Colourless evaporative paint containing 16.7% w/w Salicylic Acid BP, 16.7% w/w Lactic Acid BP, 66.6% w/w Flexible Collodion BP.

Uses For the topical treatment of warts, especially plantar warts.

Dosage and administration Soak the wart and pat dry. Gently rub the surface of the wart with a pumice stone or manicure emery board to remove any hard skin. Using the applicator provided, carefully apply a few drops of the paint to the wart, taking care to localise the application to the affected area. Cover with an adhesive plaster, if a plantar wart. Leave for 24 hours. Repeat this procedure daily, removing old Collodion on each occasion.

Contra-indications, warnings, etc Keep away from the eyes and mucous membranes. Not to be used on the face, anal or perineal region. Avoid spreading onto surrounding uninvolved skin.
If the treated area becomes inflamed or painful, treatment should be suspended until the inflammation resolves.
Sensitivity to any of the ingredients.

Pharmaceutical precautions Inflammable. Store in a cool place, away from flames. Replace cap tightly after use. Avoid spillage.

Legal category P.

Package quantity Salactol is supplied in an amber glass bottle containing 10 ml, incorporating a specially designed spatula for ease of application.

Further information Salactol is formulated to provide keratolytic and antiviral activity. In a clinical study on 76 patients with plantar warts, 84% of warts resolved at 12 weeks, without any reported side-effects.

Ingredients: Salicylic Acid BP; Lactic Acid BP; Flexible Collodion BP.

Product licence number 0173/5006.

VARICLENE*

Presentation Green aqueous gel containing 0.5% w/w Brilliant Green BP, 0.5% w/w Lactic Acid BP.

Uses An aid in the topical treatment of venous and other types of skin ulcers.

Dosage and administration Ensure that the area of skin to be treated is as clean and dry as possible. Using a disposable applicator (e.g. cotton wool bud, wooden spatula or gauze pad), gently apply and smooth the Variclene gel over the affected area, until the ulcer site is completely covered. For extensive ulceration, the gel may be spread initially over a sterile dressing, which is then applied to the affected area. Minimise spreading onto surrounding skin and avoid direct contact between the nozzle of the tube and the ulcer.
The treated area should then be dressed using an impregnated paste bandage such as Viscopaste* PB7 or Quinaband*, followed by stockinette or, in the case of a venous ulcer, pressure bandaging. This allows a clean granulating bed to develop.
If the dressings become soaked in exudate, a layer of cotton wool, or lint or gamgee may be 'sandwiched' between the paste and stockinette/pressure bandaging to absorb exudate.
The dressing should be changed at regular intervals (usually 48 to 72 hours) and not left longer than 7 days.

Contra-indications, warnings, etc Avoid contact with clothing and linen. Some patients may experience transient stinging on application. In cases of arterial or extensive, painful venous ulceration, this may be prolonged, when treatment should be discontinued until greater tolerance has been achieved.
Keep away from the eyes.
Sensitivity to any of the ingredients.

Pharmaceutical precautions Store in a cool place. Always replace cap after use.

Legal category P.

Package quantity Variclene is supplied in a collapsible tube containing 50 g.

Further information As with all open wounds, care should be taken to keep the affected area clean and, as far as possible, free from contamination.
Where appropriate, Variclene should be used in conjunction with a treatment regime involving the use of pressure bandaging.

Ingredients: Lactic Acid BP; Brilliant Green BP; Methyl Cellulose 10,000 (Celacol); Industrial Methylated Spirit BP; Water BP.

Product licence number 0173/0015.

*Trade Mark

Dista Products Limited
Kingsclere Road,
Basingstoke,
Hants. RG21 2XA

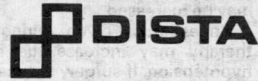

ALLEGRON*

Presentation Tablets each containing the equivalent of 25 mg nortriptyline (as the hydrochloride). The tablets are orange, scored and have a diameter of 8 mm. They are marked 'DISTA'.

Tablets each containing the equivalent of 10 mg nortriptyline (as the hydrochloride). The tablets are white, unscored and have a diameter of 5.5 mm. They are marked 'DISTA'.

Uses Allegron is indicated for the relief of symptoms of depression. It may also be used for the treatment of some cases of nocturnal enuresis.

Dosage and administration For oral administration.

Adults: The usual adult dose is 20–40 mg daily in divided doses, increasing to 100 mg daily where necessary. The usual maintenance dose is 30–75 mg/day.

The elderly: Initial dosage should be 10 mg three times a day. This may be increased with caution under close supervision. Half the normal maintenance dose may be sufficient to produce a satisfactory clinical response.

Children: (for nocturnal enuresis only)

Age (years)	Weight		Dose (mg)
	kg	lbs	
6–7	20–25	44–55	10
8–11	25–35	55–77	10–20
>11	35–54	77–119	25–35

The dose should be administered thirty minutes before bedtime.

The maximum period of treatment should not exceed three months. A further course of treatment should not be started until a full physical examination, including an ECG, has been made.

Contra-indications, warnings, etc

Contra-indications: Hypersensitivity to nortriptyline.

Recent myocardial infarction, any degree of heart block or other cardiac arrhythmias.

Severe liver disease. Mania.

Nortriptyline is contra-indicated for the nursing mother and for children under the age of six years.

Warnings: As improvement may not occur during the initial weeks of therapy, patients, especially those posing a high suicidal risk, should be closely monitored during this period.

Withdrawal symptoms, including insomnia, irritability and excessive perspiration, may occur on abrupt cessation of therapy.

The use of nortriptyline in schizophrenic patients may result in an exacerbation of the psychosis or may activate latent schizophrenic symptoms. If administered to over-active or agitated patients, increased anxiety and agitation may occur. In manic-depressive patients, nortriptyline may cause symptoms of the manic phase to emerge.

Cross sensitivity between nortriptyline and other tricyclic antidepressants is a possibility.

Patients with cardiovascular disease should be given nortriptyline only under close supervision because of the tendency of the drug to produce sinus tachycardia and to prolong the conduction time. Myocardial infarction, arrhythmia and strokes have occurred. Great care is required if nortriptyline is administered to hyperthyroid patients or to those receiving thyroid medication, since cardiac arrhythmias may develop.

Nortriptyline may impair the mental and/or physical abilities required for the performance of hazardous tasks, such as operating machinery or driving a car; therefore the patient should be warned accordingly.

Drug interactions: Under no circumstances should nortriptyline be given concurrently with, or within two weeks of cessation of, therapy with monoamine oxidase inhibitors. Hyperpyretic crises, severe convulsions and fatalities have occurred when similar tricyclic anti-depressants were used in such combinations.

Nortriptyline should not be given with sympatho-mimetic agents such as adrenaline, ephedrine, isoprenaline, noradrenaline, phenylephrine and phenylpropanolamine.

Nortriptyline may decrease the antihypertensive effect of guanethidine, debrisoquine, bethanidine and possibly clonidine. Concurrent administration of reserpine has been shown to produce a 'stimulating' effect in some depressed patients. It would be advisable to review all antihypertensive therapy during treatment with tricyclic antidepressants.

Barbiturates may increase the rate of metabolism of nortriptyline.

Usage in pregnancy: The safety of nortriptyline for use during pregnancy has not been established, nor is there evidence from animal studies that it is free from hazard; therefore the drug should not be administered to pregnant patients or women of childbearing age unless the potential benefits clearly outweigh any potential risk.

Precautions: The elderly are particularly liable to experience adverse reactions, especially agitation, confusion and postural hypotension.

Behavioural changes may occur in children receiving therapy for nocturnal enuresis.

If possible, the use of nortriptyline should be avoided in patients with narrow angle glaucoma, symptoms suggestive of prostatic hypertrophy or a history of epilepsy.

When it is essential, nortriptyline may be administered

with electroconvulsive therapy, although the hazards may be increased.

Anaesthetics given during tricyclic antidepressant therapy may increase the risk of arrhythmias and hypotension. If surgery is necessary, the drug should be discontinued, if possible, for several days prior to the procedure, or the anaesthetist should be informed if the patient is still receiving therapy.

Tricyclic antidepressants may potentiate the CNS depressant effect of alcohol.

Both elevation and lowering of blood sugar levels have been reported.

Side-effects: Cardiac arrhythmias and severe hypotension are likely to occur with high dosage, or in patients with pre-existing heart disease taking normal dosage.

Other common side-effects include drowsiness, sweating, postural hypotension, tremor and skin rashes.

The following are seen occasionally: dizziness, confusion, restlessness, weakness, impotence and blurred vision. Side-effects rarely noted are epigastric distress, nausea and vomiting, dysgeusia, excessive weight gain, excessive weight loss, fatigue, insomnia, headache, paraesthesiae and pruritus.

The following adverse effects, although not necessarily all reported with nortriptyline, have occurred with other tricyclic antidepressants: atropine-like side-effects including dry mouth, disturbances of accommodation, tachycardia, constipation and hesitancy of micturition are common early in treatment, but usually lessen.

Serious adverse effects are rare; the following have been reported: depression of the bone marrow including agranulocytosis, cholestatic jaundice, hypomania, convulsions and peripheral neuropathy.

Adverse effects such as withdrawal symptoms, respiratory depression and agitation have been reported in neonates whose mothers had taken tricyclic antidepressants during the last trimester of pregnancy.

Overdose: Toxic overdosage may result in confusion, restlessness, agitation, vomiting, hyperpyrexia, muscle rigidity, hyperactive reflexes, tachycardia, cardiac arrhythmias, ECG evidence of impaired conduction, shock, congestive heart failure, severe hypotension, stupor, coma and CNS stimulation with convulsions followed by respiratory depression. Deaths have occurred following overdosage with drugs of this class.

Treatment: No specific antidote is known. General supportive measures are indicated, with gastric lavage. Activated charcoal adsorbs tricyclic antidepressants very effectively. Respiratory assistance is apparently the most effective measure when indicated. The use of CNS depressants may worsen the prognosis.

Intramuscular paraldehyde or diazepam provides anticonvulsant activity with less respiratory depression than the barbiturates.

The use of digitalis and/or pyridostigmine may be considered in the event of serious cardiovascular abnormalities or cardiac failure.

The value of dialysis has not been established.

Pharmaceutical precautions Store in a cool (6°–15°C), dry place.

Legal category POM.

Package quantities
Tablets 25 mg: Bottles of 100 and 500.
Tablets 10 mg: Bottles of 100 and 500.

Further information Nil.

Product licence numbers
Tablets 25 mg   0006/5003
Tablets 10 mg   0006/5002

CAPASTAT*

Presentation Capreomycin sulphate as sterile white powder for intramuscular injection, in sealed vials each containing 1,000,000 Units (approximately equivalent to 1 g capreomycin base).

Uses For the treatment of pulmonary infections caused by capreomycin-susceptible strains of *M. tuberculosis* when the primary agents (isoniazid, rifampicin, streptomycin and ethambutol) have been ineffective or cannot be used because of toxicity or the presence of resistant tubercle bacilli.

Dosage and administration The usual dose is 1 g daily (not to exceed 20 mg/kg/day) given intramuscularly for 60 to 120 days, followed by 1 g intramuscularly two or three times a week. Capreomycin sulphate should be dissolved in 2 ml of 0.9% Sodium Chloride Intravenous Infusion BP or Water for Injections PhEur. Two or three minutes should be allowed for complete solution. For administration of a 1 g dose, the entire contents of the vial should be given.

The elderly: As for adults. Reduce dosage if renal function is impaired.

Contra-indications, warnings, etc
Contra-indication: Hypersensitivity to the drug.

Warnings: The use of capreomycin in patients with renal insufficiency or pre-existing auditory impairment must be undertaken with great caution, and the risk of additional eighth cranial nerve impairment or renal injury should be weighed against the benefits to be derived from therapy.

Simultaneous administration of other antituberculous agents (e.g. streptomycin, viomycin) which also have ototoxic and nephrotoxic potential is not recommended.

Use with non-antituberculous drugs (polymyxin, colistin sulphate, gentamicin, tobramycin, vancomycin, kanamycin and neomycin) having ototoxic or nephrotoxic potential should also be undertaken only with great caution.

Usage in pregnancy: The safety of capreomycin for use during pregnancy has not been established.

The safety of capreomycin for use in infants and children has not been established.

Precautions: Audiometric measurements and assessment of vestibular function should be performed prior to initiation of therapy with capreomycin and at regular intervals during treatment.

Regular tests of renal function should be made throughout the period of treatment, and reduced dosage should be employed in patients with known or suspected renal impairment. It is advisable to monitor drug serum levels at regular intervals in such patients.

Since hypokalaemia may occur during capreomycin therapy, serum potassium levels should be determined frequently. Periodic determinations of liver function are recommended.

Capreomycin should be administered cautiously to patients with a history of drug allergy.

Side-effects: Renal – Elevation of serum creatinine or blood urea and abnormal urine sediment have been observed.

Hepatic – A decrease in bromsulphthalein excretion without change in serum enzymes has been noted in the presence of pre-existing liver disease. Abnormal results in liver function tests have occurred in many patients receiving capreomycin in combination with other antituberculous agents which are also known to cause changes in hepatic function.

Haematological – Leucocytosis and leucopenia have been observed. There is a high incidence of eosinophilia in patients receiving daily injections of capreomycin.

Hypersensitivity – Urticaria and maculopapular skin rashes associated in some cases with febrile reactions have been reported when capreomycin and other antituberculous drugs were given concomitantly.

Ototoxicity – Clinical and subclinical auditory loss has been noted. Some audiometric changes are reversible, and others with permanent loss are not progressive following withdrawal of capreomycin. Tinnitus and vertigo have occurred.

Pain and induration at the injection sites have been observed. Excessive bleeding at the injection site has been reported. Sterile abscesses have been noted.

Loss of visual acuity has been reported rarely.

Pharmaceutical precautions *Dry powder:* Store in a cool (6°–15°C), dry place. *When reconstituted:* The solution should be stored in a refrigerator (0°–6°C) and be used within 14 days. At room temperature (15°–25°C) it should be used within 48 hours.

Legal category POM.

Package quantities Vials of 1,000,000 Units (1 g base approximately). Individual vials.

Further information Must be used only in conjunction with adequate doses of other antituberculous drugs. The use of Capastat alone allows the rapid development of strains resistant to it. Frequent cross-resistance occurs between capreomycin and viomycin. Varying degrees of cross-resistance between capreomycin and kanamycin or neomycin have been reported. No cross-resistance has been observed between capreomycin and isoniazid, para-aminosalicylic acid, cycloserine, streptomycin, ethionamide or ethambutol.

Product licence number 0006/5005.

DISTACLOR*

Presentation Capsules (violet and white, printed Distaclor 250) containing 250 mg cefaclor.

Granules (pink) for suspension containing 125 mg cefaclor/5 ml.

Granules (pink) for suspension containing 250 mg cefaclor/5 ml.

Uses Distaclor is indicated for the treatment of the following infections due to susceptible micro-organisms:

Respiratory tract infections, including pneumonia, bronchitis, exacerbations of chronic bronchitis, pharyngitis and tonsillitis, and as part of the management of sinusitis.

Otitis media.

Skin and soft tissue infections.

Urinary tract infections, including pyelonephritis and cystitis.

Distaclor has been found to be effective in both acute and chronic urinary tract infections.

Cefaclor is active against the following organisms *in vitro:*

Alpha- and beta-haemolytic streptococci

Staphylococci; including coagulase-positive, coagulase-negative and penicillinase-producing strains

Streptococcus pneumoniae

Escherichia coli

Proteus mirabilis

Klebsiella species

Haemophilus influenzae, including ampicillin-resistant strains.

Cefaclor has no activity against *Pseudomonas* species.

Cefaclor is not active against most strains of enterococci *(Str. faecalis), Enterobacter,* indole-positive *Proteus* and *Serratia* species. Some rare strains of staphylococci are resistant to cefaclor.

Dosage and administration Distaclor is administered orally.

Adults: The usual adult dosage is 250 mg every eight hours. For more severe infections or those caused by less susceptible organisms, doses may be doubled. Doses of 4 g per day have been administered safely to normal subjects for 28 days, but the total daily dosage should not exceed this amount.

Distaclor may be administered in the presence of impaired renal function. Under such conditions dosage is unchanged (see *Precautions*).

Patients undergoing haemodialysis: Haemodialysis shortens serum half-life by 25–30%. In patients undergoing regular haemodialysis, a loading dose of 250 mg–1 g administered prior to dialysis and a therapeutic dose of 250–500 mg every six to eight hours maintained during interdialytic periods is recommended.

The elderly: As for adults.

Children: The usual recommended daily dosage for children is 20 mg/kg/day in divided doses every eight hours, as indicated.

Distaclor suspension

	125 mg/5 ml	250 mg/5 ml
< 1 year	2.5 ml tid	
1–5 years	5.0 ml tid	
Over 5 years		5.0 ml tid

In more serious infections, otitis media, sinusitis and infections caused by less susceptible organisms, 40 mg/kg/day is recommended, up to a daily maximum of 1 g.

In the treatment of beta-haemolytic streptococcal infections, therapy should be continued for at least 10 days.

Contra-indications, warnings, etc

Contra-indication: Hypersensitivity to cephalosporins.

Warnings: Cephalosporins should be given cautiously to patients with known penicillin sensitivity, as there is evidence of partial cross-allergenicity between the penicillins and cephalosporins. Severe reactions (including anaphylaxis) have been reported occasionally in patients receiving penicillins or cephalosporins.

Usage in pregnancy: Although laboratory studies and clinical experience have shown no evidence of teratogenicity, caution should be exercised when prescribing for the pregnant patient.

Precautions: If an allergic reaction to cefaclor occurs the drug should be discontinued and the patient treated with the appropriate agents.

Cefaclor should be administered with caution in the presence of markedly impaired renal function. Under such conditions, safe dosage may be lower than that usually recommended.

Prolonged use of cefaclor may result in the overgrowth of non-susceptible organisms. If superinfection occurs during therapy, appropriate measures should be taken.

Positive direct Coombs' tests have been reported during treatment with the cephalosporin antibiotics. In haematological studies or in transfusion cross-matching procedures when anti-globulin tests are performed on the minor side, or in Coombs' testing of newborns whose mothers have received cephalosporin antibiotics before parturition, it should be recognised that a positive Coombs' test may be due to the drug.

A false-positive reaction for glucose in the urine may occur with Benedict's or Fehling's solutions or with copper sulphate test tablets, but not with Tes-Tape* (urine sugar analysis paper, Lilly).

Side-effects: Gastro-intestinal – The most frequent side-effect has been diarrhoea. It is rarely severe enough to warrant cessation of therapy. Colitis, including rare instances of pseudomembranous colitis, has been reported. Nausea and vomiting have also occurred.

Hypersensitivity – Allergic reactions, such as urticaria, morbilliform eruptions and pruritus, have been observed. These reactions usually subsided upon discontinuation of therapy. Serum sickness-like reactions, including the above skin manifestations, fever and arthralgia/arthritis, have been reported. Anaphylaxis has also occurred.

Liver – Slight elevations in AST and ALT have been reported.

Miscellaneous – Eosinophilia, positive Coombs' tests and genital pruritus and vaginitis have occurred.

Overdosage: There are no well documented reports of overdosage. Symptoms of nausea, vomiting and diarrhoea would be anticipated.

Treatment: General management may consist of supportive therapy.

Pharmaceutical precautions Store at room temperature (15°–25°C). Keep containers tightly closed and protect from light. After reconstitution, the suspension should be stored in a refrigerator (0°–6°C) and be used within 14 days. When dilution is unavoidable, Syrup BP should be used after the suspension has been prepared according to the manufacturer's instructions.

Legal category POM.

Package quantities
Capsules 250 mg: Bottles of 20 and 100.
Suspension 125 mg/5 ml: Bottles of 100 ml.
Suspension 250 mg/5 ml: Bottles of 100 ml.

Further information Nil.

Product licence numbers
Capsules 250 mg   0006/0118
Suspension 125 mg/5 ml   0006/0120
Suspension 250 mg/5 ml   0006/0121

DISTALGESIC*
Approved name: Co-proxamol

Presentation Tablets each containing 32.5 mg Dextropropoxyphene Hydrochloride BP (equivalent to approximately 30 mg dextropropoxyphene base) with 325 mg Paracetamol PhEur. The tablets are white, pillow-shaped, film coated, 14 mm in length and marked 'DG'.

Uses Analgesic: For the management of mild to moderate pain.

Dosage and administration For oral administration to adults only.

Dosage: The usual dose is 2 tablets three or four times daily and should not normally be exceeded.

The elderly: As for adults. Reduce dosage if renal or hepatic function is impaired.

Contra-indications, warnings, etc
Contra-indication: Hypersensitivity to dextropropoxyphene or paracetamol.

Warnings: Dextropropoxyphene is an analgesic with CNS depressant properties and should be used with caution in patients who are receiving other CNS depressant drugs, as an additive effect may occur. Patients should be warned to avoid alcohol.

As with other drugs which affect the CNS, care should be taken when prescribing for patients with personality or other psychological disorders. Tolerance, psychological and physical dependence may rarely occur.

Like other centrally acting drugs, dextropropoxyphene may impair patients' mental and physical reactions in the performance of potentially hazardous tasks (e.g. driving ability, operation of machinery, etc.) to a varying extent, depending on dosage and individual susceptibility.

Overdosage of paracetamol may damage the liver, due to the accumulation of intermediate metabolites which cause hepatic necrosis.

Use in pregnancy: The safety of Distalgesic for use during pregnancy has not been established.

Precautions: Distalgesic should be administered with caution to patients with severe renal or hepatic impairment as delayed elimination or elevated serum levels may result.

Isolated reports suggest that dextropropoxyphene may inhibit the metabolism of some concurrently administered drugs. Patients receiving anticonvulsants, antidepressants or warfarin-like drugs should be monitored during therapy.

Side-effects: Side-effects such as dizziness, sedation, nausea and vomiting seem to be more prominent in ambulatory than in non-ambulatory patients, and some of these side-effects may be alleviated if the patient lies down.

Other reported side-effects include constipation, abdominal pain, skin rashes, lightheadedness, headache, weakness, euphoria, dysphoria and minor visual disturbances.

Overdosage: The chronic ingestion of dextropropoxyphene in doses exceeding 720 mg (as base) per day has caused toxic psychoses and convulsions.

Symptoms of acute toxicity may be rapid in onset, with the danger of respiratory arrest. Other recognised manifestations include respiratory depression, coma, circulatory collapse, pulmonary oedema, convulsions and cardiac arrhythmias.

Deterioration may be rapid, with fatal outcome.

Paracetamol overdosage is associated with nausea and vomiting and frequently with abdominal pain. Subsequent evidence of liver dysfunction may be apparent after 24 hours, and if severe, may lead to irreversible hepatic necrosis and death.

Treatment: Primary attention should be given to the re-establishment of adequate respiratory exchange through provision of a patent airway and institution of assisted or controlled ventilation. The narcotic antagonist naloxone is a specific antidote against the respiratory depression produced by dextropropoxyphene. An initial dose of 0.4–2 mg should be administered intravenously with simultaneous efforts at respiratory resuscitation. If the desired degree of improvement is not obtained, the dose should be repeated at two to three minute intervals. Subsequent doses of naloxone may be necessary for up to 24 hours due to the slow elimination of dextropropoxyphene. Naloxone may also be administered by infusion. The rate of infusion should be such as to maximise the reversal of CNS depression.

In addition to the use of a narcotic antagonist, the patient may require careful titration with an anticonvulsant to control seizures. Analeptic drugs (for example, caffeine or amphetamine) should not be used because of their tendency to precipitate convulsions.

Early assessment of the severity of paracetamol poisoning by measurement of plasma paracetamol levels is essential if treatment, which should be instituted within 10 hours of ingestion, is to be effective. Present evidence suggests that cysteamine, methionine or N-acetylcysteine given within this period are effective in greatly reducing the toxic effects of paracetamol.

Oxygen, intravenous fluids, vasopressors and other supportive measures should be employed as indicated. Gastric lavage may be helpful. Activated charcoal can adsorb a significant amount of ingested dextropropoxyphene.

Pharmaceutical precautions Store in a cool (6°–15°C), dry place.

Legal category CD (Sch 5), POM.

Package quantities
Distalgesic tablets: Blister packs of 100 (10 strips of 10 tablets).

Further information Nil.

Product licence number
Distalgesic tablets 0006/5000.

DISTAMINE*

Presentation Tablets each containing 50 mg, 125 mg or 250 mg D-penicillamine base. The 50 mg tablets are white, coated, scored and have a diameter of 5.5 mm. The 125 mg tablets are white, coated and have a diameter of 8 mm. They are marked 'DS' on one face and '125' on the other. The 250 mg tablets are white, coated and have a diameter of 10 mm. They are marked 'DM' on one face and '250' on the other.

Uses
(a) Severe active rheumatoid arthritis, including juvenile forms.
(b) Wilson's disease (hepatolenticular degeneration).
(c) Cystinuria – Dissolution and prevention of cystine stones.
(d) Lead poisoning.
(e) Primary biliary cirrhosis.
(f) Chronic active hepatitis.

Dosage and administration For oral administration.
(a) Rheumatoid arthritis: Adults: 125–250 mg daily for the first month. Increase by the same amount every 4 to 12 weeks until remission occurs. The minimum maintenance dose to achieve suppression of symptoms should be used and treatment should be discontinued if no benefit is obtained within twelve months. Improvement may not occur for some months.

The usual maintenance dose is 500–750 mg daily. Up to 1.5 g daily may be required. If possible, penicillamine should be taken at least half an hour before meals, or on retiring.

If remission is established and has been sustained for six months, gradual reduction by 125–250 mg amounts every 12 weeks may be attempted.

The elderly: Increased toxicity has been observed in this patient population regardless of renal function. Initial dose should not exceed 50–125 mg daily for the first month, increasing by similar increments every 4 to 12 weeks until the minimum maintenance dose to suppress symptoms is reached. Daily dosage should not exceed 1 g.

Children: 15–20 mg/kg/day as a maintenance dose, starting with 50 mg daily for one month and increasing at four-weekly intervals.

(b) Wilson's disease: Adults: 1.5–2 g daily in divided doses 30 minutes before food. Dose may be reduced to 750 mg–1 g daily when control of the disease is achieved. Patients must be maintained in negative copper balance and the minimum dosage of penicillamine required to achieve this should be given.

It is advisable that a dose of 2 g/day should not be continued for more than a year.

The elderly: 20 mg/kg/day in divided doses. Adjust dosage to control disease and maintain negative copper balance.

Children: Up to 20 mg/kg/day in divided doses before food. Minimum dose 500 mg/day.

(c) Cystinuria: Ideally, establish the lowest effective dose by quantitative amino acid chromatography of urine.
    (i) *Dissolution of cystine stones: Adults:* 1–3 g daily in divided doses 30 minutes before food, where possible. Urine cystine levels of not more than 200 mg/l should be maintained.
    (ii) *Prevention of cystine stones: Adults:* 500 mg–1 g on retiring. Fluid intake should be not less than 3 litres/day. Urine cystine levels of not more than 300 mg/l should be maintained.

The elderly: Use the minimum dose to maintain urinary cystine levels below 200 mg/l.

Children: No dose range established, but urinary cystine levels must be kept below 200 mg/l. The minimum dose of penicillamine required to achieve this should be given.

(d) Lead poisoning: Adults: 1–1.5 g daily in divided doses before food until urinary lead is stabilised at less than 0.5 mg/day.

The elderly: 20 mg/kg/day in divided doses until urinary lead is stabilised at less than 0.5 mg/day.

Children: 20 mg/kg/day.

(e) Primary biliary cirrhosis: Adults: An initial dose of 250 mg daily, increasing weekly to the maintenance dose of 750 mg–1 g daily, in divided doses. Most patients will have elevated levels of copper in the liver; penicillamine causes copper concentrations to decrease, hence a lower maintenance dose should be considered for patients whose liver-copper concentrations return within

the normal range. Penicillamine should be administered with caution to patients with portal hypertension, and is not recommended for patients with a history of bleeding from varices or of hepatic encephalopathy.

The elderly: Not recommended.

(f) Chronic active hepatitis: Adults: For maintenance treatment after the disease process has been brought under control with corticosteroids. The initial dosage of 500 mg daily, in divided doses, should be increased gradually over three months to a maintenance dose of 1.25 g daily. During this period, the dosage of corticosteroids should be phased out. Throughout therapy, liver function tests should be carried out periodically to assess the disease status.

The elderly: Not recommended.

(g) Desensitisation: No fixed dose regimen. An initial dose of 25 mg daily is suggested, this to be gradually increased in accordance with the response of the patient. Higher initial doses have been employed in cystinuric patients.

Contra-indications, warnings, etc

Contra-indications: Hypersensitivity to penicillamine, except in a life-threatening situation, when desensitisation should be attempted (see Dosage and Administration). Agranulocytosis or severe thrombocytopenia due to penicillamine. Lupus erythematosus.

Warnings and adverse effects
Usage in pregnancy: The safety of penicillamine for use during pregnancy has not been established. It has been shown to be teratogenic in rats when given in doses several times higher than those recommended for human use.

Wilson's disease: There has been one case reported of reversible cutis laxa in an infant born to a mother taking 1.5 g penicillamine daily throughout pregnancy. Although there have been no controlled studies on the use of penicillamine during pregnancy, two retrospective studies have reported the successful delivery of 43 normal infants to 28 women receiving between 0.5 g and 2 g of penicillamine daily.

Cystinuria: There have been reports of patients delivered of normal infants, and one report of a severe connective tissue abnormality in the infant of a mother who received 2 g penicillamine daily throughout pregnancy. Whenever possible, penicillamine should be withheld during pregnancy, but if stones continue to form, the benefit of resuming treatment must be weighed against the possible risk to the fetus.

Rheumatoid arthritis, primary biliary cirrhosis, chronic active hepatitis: Penicillamine should not be administered to patients who are pregnant, and therapy should be stopped when pregnancy is diagnosed or suspected, unless considered to be absolutely essential by the physician.

NB: The incidence and severity of some of the adverse reactions, noted below, varies according to the dosage and nature of the disease under treatment.

Nausea, anorexia, fever and rash may occur early in therapy, especially when full doses are given from the start. Antihistamines, steroid cover, or temporary reduction of dose will control urticarial reactions.

Reversible loss of taste may occur. Mineral supplements to overcome this are not recommended.

Thrombocytopenia occurs commonly and neutropenia less often. These reactions may occur at any time during treatment and are usually reversible. Deaths from agranulocytosis and aplastic anaemia have occurred. Full blood counts should be carried out weekly or fortnightly during the first eight weeks of therapy, in the week after any increase in dose, and otherwise monthly thereafter. In cystinuria or Wilson's disease, longer intervals may be adequate.

Withdrawal of treatment should be considered if platelets fall below 120,000 or white blood cells below 2,500/mm³, or if three successive falls are noted within the normal range. Treatment may be restarted at a reduced dosage when counts return to normal, but should be permanently withdrawn on recurrence of neutropenia or thrombocytopenia.

Proteinuria occurs in up to 30 per cent of patients and is partially dose-related. Urine should be tested weekly at first and after each increase in dose, then monthly, though again longer intervals may be adequate with cystinuria and Wilson's disease. Increasing proteinuria may necessitate withdrawal of treatment.

Haematuria is rare, but if it occurs in the absence of renal stones or other known cause, treatment should be stopped immediately.

Other complications have included haemolytic anaemia, nephrotic syndrome, drug induced lupus erythematosus, and conditions closely resembling myasthenia gravis, pemphigus, Goodpasture's syndrome, Stevens-Johnson syndrome and rheumatoid arthritis.

A late rash, described as acquired epidermolysis bullosa and penicillamine dermopathy, may occur after several months or years of therapy. This may necessitate a reduction in dosage.

Precautions: Full blood and platelet counts should be performed and renal function should be assessed prior to treatment with penicillamine. Monitoring of blood and platelet counts should be carried out at appropriate intervals, together with urinalysis for detection of haematuria and proteinuria.

If concomitant oral iron therapy is indicated, this should not be given within two hours of taking penicillamine.

Caution should be observed when anti-inflammatory or other drugs with known propensity for causing marrow injury are taken concurrently with penicillamine.

Care should be exercised in patients with renal insufficiency; modification of dosage may be necessary.

Treatment of overdosage: No instances of adverse reactions to an overdose of penicillamine have been recorded and no specific measures are indicated.

Further information Nil.

Pharmaceutical precautions Store in a dry place below 25°C. Keep containers tightly closed.

Legal category POM.

Package quantities Tablets 50 mg: Bottles of 100
Tablets 125 mg: Bottles of 100
Tablets 250 mg: Bottles of 100

Product licence numbers
Tablets 50 mg 0006/0105
Tablets 125 mg 0006/0090
Tablets 250 mg 0006/5008

DISTAQUAINE* V-K

Presentation *Phenoxymethylpenicillin Potassium Tablets BP:* containing the equivalent of 125 mg or 250 mg phenoxymethylpenicillin. The 125 mg tablets are white, scored, 8 mm in diameter and marked 'DD VK'. The 250 mg tablets are white, scored, 10.5 mm in diameter and marked 'DD KF'.

Syrup: granules for the preparation of Phenoxymethylpenicillin Elixir BP, 125 mg/5 ml or 250 mg/5 ml. The granules are pale pink, converting to orange liquid on reconstitution.

Elixir: granules for the preparation of Phenoxymethylpenicillin Elixir BP, 62.5 mg/5 ml. The granules are pale pink, converting to orange liquid on reconstitution.

Uses Penicillin exerts high activity *in vitro* against staphylococci (except penicillinase-producing strains), streptococci (groups A, C, G, H, L and M), pneumococci, *Corynebacterium diphtheriae, Bacillus anthracis, Actinomyces bovis, Streptobacillus moniliformis, Listeria monocytogenes, Neisseria gonorrhoeae, Treponema pallidum, Clostridium* species and Leptospira.

Phenoxymethylpenicillin and potassium phenoxymethylpenicillin are indicated in the treatment of mild to moderately severe infections associated with microorganisms whose susceptibility to penicillin is within the range of serum levels attained with these dosage forms.

The following infections will usually respond to adequate doses:

Streptococcal infections (without bacteraemia) – mild to moderate infections of the upper respiratory tract, scarlet fever and mild erysipelas.

Pneumococcal infections – mild to moderately severe infections of the respiratory tract.

Staphylococcal infections sensitive to penicillin – mild infections of the skin and soft tissues.

Fusospirochaetosis (Vincent's gingivitis and pharyngitis) – mild to moderately severe infections of the oropharynx usually respond to therapy with oral penicillin.

Prophylactic use – Prophylaxis with oral penicillin has proved effective in preventing recurrence of rheumatic fever and chorea.

Patients with a past history of rheumatic fever receiving continuous prophylaxis may harbour penicillin-resistant organisms. In these patients, the use of another prophylactic agent should be considered.

Dosage and administration For oral administration.

Adults: 125 mg or 250 mg every four to six hours depending on the severity of the condition.

The elderly: As for adults. Reduce dosage if renal function is markedly impaired.

Children over 5 years: The adult dose.

Children 5 years or less: 125 mg every six hours.

Infants (up to 1 year): 62.5 mg every six hours.

In all but the most serious cases, the last dose of the day may be doubled to avoid disturbing sleep. Ideally, each dose should be given half an hour before (or at least three hours after) a meal.

Prophylactic use: 125 mg twice daily is recommended for long term prophylaxis of rheumatic fever.

Contra-indications, warnings, etc

Contra-indications: A previous hypersensitivity reaction to any penicillin.

Warnings: All degrees of hypersensitivity including fatal anaphylaxis have been observed with oral penicillin. These reactions are more likely to occur in individuals with a history of sensitivity to multiple allergens, and

inquiry should be made for such a history before therapy is begun. If an allergic reaction occurs, the drug should be discontinued and the patient treated with the usual agents (e.g. adrenaline and other pressor amines, antihistamines and corticosteroids).

Usage in pregnancy: Although laboratory and clinical studies have shown no evidence of teratogenicity, caution should be exercised when prescribing for the pregnant patient.

Precautions: Penicillin should be used with caution in individuals with histories of significant allergies and/or asthma.

Oral therapy should not be relied upon in patients with severe illness, or with nausea, vomiting, gastric dilatation, cardiospasm or intestinal hypermotility.

Occasionally patients do not absorb therapeutic amounts of orally administered penicillin.

Administer with caution in the presence of markedly impaired renal function, as safe dosage may be lower than that usually recommended.

Streptococcal infections should be treated for a minimum of 10 days, and post-therapy cultures should be performed to confirm the eradication of the organisms.

Prolonged use of antibiotics may promote the overgrowth of non-susceptible organisms, including fungi. If superinfection occurs, appropriate measures should be taken.

Adverse reactions: Gastro-intestinal: The most common reactions to oral penicillin are nausea, vomiting, epigastric distress and diarrhoea.

Hypersensitivity: Skin eruptions, urticaria, reactions resembling serum sickness (chills, fever, oedema, arthralgia, prostration), laryngeal oedema and anaphylaxis. Fever and eosinophilia may frequently be the only reactions observed.

Haemolytic anaemia, leucopenia, thrombocytopenia, neuropathy and nephropathy are infrequent reactions and are usually associated with high doses of parenteral penicillin.

Overdosage: Symptoms: nausea, vomiting and diarrhoea.

Treatment: General management may consist of supportive therapy.

Pharmaceutical precautions *Tablets:* Store in a cool (6°–15°C), dry place. Protect from moisture.

Syrup and Elixir: Store in a cool place and protect from moisture. Reconstituted preparations may be stored for seven days at room temperature (15°–25°C) or 14 days in a refrigerator (0°–6°C).

Legal category POM.

Package quantities
Tablets 125 mg: Bottles of 100 and 500.
Tablets 250 mg: Bottles of 100, 500 and 1,000.
Syrup Granules 125 mg/5 ml: Bottles of 100 ml.
Syrup Granules 250 mg/5 ml: Bottles of 100 ml.
Elixir Granules 62.5 mg/5 ml: Bottles of 100 ml.

Further information Nil.

Product licence numbers
Tablets 125 mg   0006/5031
Tablets 250 mg   0006/5032
Syrup 125 mg/5 ml   0006/5121

Syrup 250 mg/5 ml   0006/5122
Elixir 62.5 mg/5 ml   0006/5119

FENOPRON* 300
FENOPRON* 600

Presentation Fenoprofen Calcium Tablets BP, each containing fenoprofen calcium equivalent to 300 mg or 600 mg fenoprofen.

Fenopron 300 tablets are orange, elliptical, 14 mm long and marked DISTA 4019.

Fenopron 600 tablets are orange, para-capsule, scored, 20 mm long and marked DISTA 4021.

Uses For the treatment of osteoarthritis, rheumatoid arthritis and ankylosing spondylitis.

For the relief of mild/moderate pain.

Dosage and administration For oral administration to adults only, and not recommended for administration to children.

Dosage: 300–600 mg three or four times per day.

Fenopron 300: Recommended initial dosage is 2 tablets three times per day, then adjusted to the needs of the patient.

Fenopron 600: Recommended initial dosage is 1 tablet three times per day, plus one at night if necessitated by a more severe condition. The dosage may then be adjusted to the needs of the patient.

The maximum daily dose should not exceed 3 g.

Gastro-intestinal intolerance can be minimised by taking Fenopron with milk or at meal times.

The elderly: There is no difference in the metabolism or pharmacokinetics of fenoprofen in the elderly. However, it may be advisable to start therapy with a low dose, as side-effects of non-steroidal anti-inflammatory drugs are more pronounced in this patient population.

Contra-indications, warnings, etc

Contra-indications: Hypersensitivity to the drug. Active peptic ulceration.

Warnings: Adverse effects may include gastro-intestinal intolerance and episodes of bleeding. Although fenoprofen has been associated with less gastro-intestinal microbleeding than aspirin, patients with a history of peptic ulcer or gastro-intestinal bleeding should be closely supervised during fenoprofen therapy.

Bronchospasm may be precipitated in patients suffering from, or with a previous history of, bronchial asthma or allergic disease.

Although cross-sensitivity has not been established, the drug should not be given to patients in whom salicylates induce the syndrome of asthma, rhinitis or urticaria.

Usage in pregnancy: The safety of fenoprofen for use during pregnancy or lactation has not been established therefore it should not be administered to pregnant women or nursing mothers unless the potential benefits clearly outweigh any potential risk. Animal studies showed prolongation of parturition, but no evidence of teratogenicity.

Precautions: Because of its affinity for albumin, fenoprofen may displace other drugs from their binding sites, and this may lead to drug interaction. In patients receiving coumarin-type anticoagulants, the addition of fenoprofen could prolong the prothrombin time. Patients receiving hydantoins or sulphonylureas should be carefully monitored.

When aspirin and fenoprofen are administered concurrently, plasma concentrations of fenoprofen are reduced. It may be advisable to discontinue the concomitant use of aspirin to maximise the beneficial effects of fenoprofen. However, single or intermittent doses of aspirin may be administered if they are indicated.

Since fenoprofen is eliminated primarily by the kidneys, the drug should not be administered to patients with significantly impaired renal function, and patients likely to have compromised renal function should be monitored periodically.

Patients with initial low haemoglobin values who are receiving long-term therapy should be monitored, as transient reduction of haemoglobin and haematocrit values due to fenoprofen have been reported.

Elevation of AST, LDH and ALP levels have been reported occasionally, and it is therefore recommended that fenoprofen be discontinued if any significant liver abnormalities occur.

Side-effects:

Gastro-intestinal – These are the most commonly observed side-effects and include dyspepsia, constipation, diarrhoea, ulceration of the buccal mucosa, nausea, vomiting, anorexia and occult blood in the stool. Cases of peptic ulceration, including some complicated by bleeding, have occurred.

Renal – Rare cases of acute renal insufficiency, in association with interstitial nephritis, nephrotic syndrome or papillary necrosis, have been reported. As a general rule, these are reversible on withdrawal of the drug. Episodes of dysuria, cystitis and haematuria have occurred.

Hepatic – Severe hepatic reactions, including jaundice and fatal hepatitis, have been reported rarely.

Haematological – Various syndromes involving the bone marrow have been reported rarely; thrombocytopenia, pancytopenia and aplastic anaemia have occurred.

Allergic – Pruritus, rash, urticaria, Stevens-Johnson syndrome and angioneurotic oedema have been reported.

Neurological – Reactions reported include headache, somnolence, dizziness, tremor, confusion and insomnia.

Miscellaneous – Tinnitus, hearing decrease, amblyopia, blurred vision, palpitations, increased sweating, nervousness and peripheral oedema have been reported.

Overdosage: Information on intentional overdosage is limited. Symptoms of nephrotoxicity include dysuria, haematuria, proteinuria and oliguria. Gastro-intestinal symptoms may include nausea and vomiting, progressing to abdominal pain, distension and ileus. Circulatory collapse and hypotension may occur; one patient suffered a fatal cardiac arrest. Loss of consciousness, headache and tinnitus have also been reported.

Treatment: Standard therapy to evacuate gastric contents and to support vital functions should be employed. Since fenoprofen is acidic and is excreted in the urine, it would seem theoretically beneficial to try forced alkaline diuresis.

Pharmaceutical precautions Store in a cool (6°–15°C), dry place.

Legal category POM.

Package quantities
Fenopron 300   Bottles of 100 tablets
Fenopron 600   Bottles of 100 tablets

Further information Nil.

Product licence numbers
Fenopron 300   0006/0101
Fenopron 600   0006/0104

HAELAN*
HAELAN-X*

Presentation *Haelan:* Collapsible tubes containing 0.0125% flurandrenolone in cream or ointment base. The cream is white in colour and the ointment is translucent.

Haelan-X: Collapsible tubes containing 0.05% flurandrenolone in cream or ointment base. The cream is white in colour and the ointment is translucent.

Uses Topical steroid. For the topical management of those dermatological disorders which may be expected to respond to corticosteroids and, in the case of Haelan, those which may require prolonged application.

Dosage and administration *Cream:* For moist weeping lesions the cream should be applied gently to the affected area two or three times daily.

Ointment: For dry, scaly lesions, the ointment should be applied as a thin film to the affected area two or three times daily.

The elderly: As the skin is likely to be thin, apply sparingly to avoid development of atrophy.

Dilution is not recommended, but if considered necessary Aqueous Cream BP may be used for the creams and White Soft Paraffin BP for the ointments.

Contra-indications, warnings, etc
Contra-indication: Not to be used in the presence of tuberculosis of the skin.

Warnings: Preparations of Haelan are not intended for ophthalmic use.

A few individuals may be sensitive to Haelan. If any reaction indicating sensitisation is observed, discontinue the use of the products.

In infants, long-term continuous topical steroid therapy should be avoided. Adrenal suppression can occur even without occlusion.

Usage in pregnancy: Topical administration of corticosteroids to pregnant animals can cause abnormalities of fetal development. The relevance of these findings to human beings has not been established; however, topical steroids should not be used extensively in pregnancy, i.e. in large amounts or for prolonged periods.

Side-effects: Neither local nor systemic side-effects have been reported so far from the use of either Haelan Cream or Ointment. Evidence of absorption of the steroid has been observed only when a much higher concentration has been used under an occlusive dressing.

Pharmaceutical precautions No special pharmaceutical precautions. See 'Administration' for diluents.

Legal category POM.

Package quantities
Haelan Cream (0.0125% flurandrenolone): Tubes of 60 g.
Haelan Ointment (0.0125% flurandrenolone): Tubes of 60 g.
Haelan-X Cream (0.05% flurandrenolone): Tubes of 15 g.
Haelan-X Ointment (0.05% flurandrenolone): Tubes of 15 g.

Further information As with all topical steroids the activity can be enhanced by the use of occlusive dressings. Preparations of Haelan are recommended only as a supplement to, and not as a substitute for, preparations (lotions, wet dressings, etc.) used in the conventional management of skin lesions.

Haelan and Haelan-X preparations do not contain parahydroxybenzoates or lanolin.

Product licence numbers
Haelan Cream   0006/5012
Haelan Ointment   0006/5011
Haelan-X Cream   0006/5020
Haelan-X Ointment   0006/5039

HAELAN-C*

Presentation Collapsible tubes containing 0.0125% flurandrenolone with the addition of 3% Clioquinol BP in cream or ointment base. The cream is white in colour and the ointment is translucent.

Uses Topical steroid with antibacterial added. For the topical management of those dermatological disorders complicated by bacterial or fungal infection and which may be expected to respond to corticosteroids, particularly those requiring prolonged application.

Dosage and administration *Cream:* For moist weeping lesions, the cream should be applied gently to the affected area two or three times a day.

Ointment: For dry, scaly lesions, the ointment should be applied as a thin film to the affected area two or three times a day.

The elderly: As the skin is likely to be thin, apply sparingly to avoid development of atrophy.

Dilution is not recommended, but if considered necessary Aqueous Cream BP may be used for the creams and White Soft Paraffin BP for the ointments.

Contra-indications, warnings, etc
Contra-indication: Not to be used in the presence of tuberculosis of the skin.

Warnings: Preparations of Haelan-C are not intended for ophthalmic use.

A few individuals may be sensitive to Haelan-C. If any reaction indicating sensitisation is observed, discontinue the use of the product.

In infants, long-term continuous topical steroid therapy should be avoided. Adrenal suppression can occur even without occlusion.

Usage in pregnancy: Topical administration of corticosteroids to pregnant animals can cause abnormalities of fetal development. The relevance of these findings to human beings has not been established; however, topical steroids should not be used extensively in pregnancy, i.e. in large amounts or for prolonged periods.

Haelan-C may cause staining of the hair, clothing and many fabrics.

Side-effects: Neither local nor systemic side-effects have been reported so far from the use of either Haelan-C Cream or Ointment. Evidence of absorption of the steroid has been observed only when a much higher concentration has been used under an occlusive dressing.

Pharmaceutical precautions No special pharmaceutical precautions. See 'Administration' for diluents.

Legal category POM.

Package quantities
Haelan-C Cream (0.0125% flurandrenolone with 3% Clioquinol BP): Tubes of 30 g.
Haelan-C Ointment (0.0125% flurandrenolone with 3% Clioquinol BP): Tubes of 30 g.

Further information When secondary bacterial and fungal infection of the skin is present or suspected in an otherwise steroid responsive skin condition, Haelan-C should be used and treatment resumed with Haelan after the infection has been controlled. Such patients must be under constant medical observation.

Product licence numbers
Haelan-C Cream   0006/5018
Haelan-C Ointment   0006/5021

HAELAN* Tape

Presentation A translucent, polythene adhesive film impregnated with 4 mcg flurandrenolone per square centimetre and protected by a removable paper liner.

Uses Occlusive topical steroid. Adjunctive therapy for chronic recalcitrant dermatoses that may respond to topical corticosteroids, and particularly dry, scaling and localised lesions.

Dosage and administration For application to the skin, which should be clean, dry and shorn of hair. In most instances the tape need only remain in place for 12 out of 24 hours.
   Cosmetics may be applied over the tape.

Application: The tape is cut so as to cover the lesion and a ¼ inch margin of normal skin. Corners should be rounded off. After removing the lining paper, the tape is applied to the centre of the lesion with gentle pressure and worked to the edges, avoiding excessive tension of the skin. If longer strips of tape are to be applied, the lining paper should be removed progressively.

Contra-indications, warnings, etc
Contra-indications: Chicken pox, vaccinia, tuberculosis of the skin and hypersensitivity to any of the components.

Warnings: Not advocated for acute and weeping dermatoses.

Usage in pregnancy: Topical administration of corticosteroids to pregnant animals can cause abnormalities of fetal development. The relevance of these findings to human beings has not been established; however, topical steroids should not be used extensively in pregnancy, i.e. in large amounts or for prolonged periods.

Side-effects: Irritation, itching, dryness and folliculitis may be troublesome. Maceration of the skin, secondary infection, skin atrophy, striae and miliaria are more likely to occur under occlusion. In their presence, the use of the tape should be discontinued. If extensive areas are treated there may be undue systemic absorption, especially in infants, where long-term continuous use should be avoided.

Pharmaceutical precautions Store in a dry place, below 25°C.

Legal category POM.

Package quantities
Single rolls of tape, 7.5 cm wide, 50 cm long.
Single rolls of tape, 7.5 cm wide, 200 cm long.

Further information Nil.

Product licence number 0006/5158.

ILOSONE*

Presentation Capsules each containing the equivalent of 250 mg erythromycin base as Erythromycin Estolate BP. The capsules are ivory/red, marked 'DISTA' and are 2.1 cm long.
   Tablets each containing the equivalent of 500 mg erythromycin base as Erythromycin Estolate BP. The tablets are pink, para-capsule shaped, 1.9 cm long and coded DISTA DI.
   Ready-mixed suspension, each 5 ml containing the equivalent of 125 mg erythromycin base as Erythromycin Estolate BP. The suspension is orange coloured.
   Ready-mixed suspension forte, each 5 ml containing the equivalent of 250 mg erythromycin base as Erythromycin Estolate BP. The suspension is orange coloured.

Uses Antibiotic. Erythromycin is indicated in the treatment of conditions associated with the following micro-organisms:

Streptococcus pyogenes (group A beta-haemolytic): Upper and lower respiratory tract, skin, and soft tissue infections of mild to moderate severity.

Alpha-haemolytic streptococci (viridans group): Short term prophylaxis against bacterial endocarditis prior to dental or other operative procedures in patients with a history of rheumatic fever or congenital heart disease who are hypersensitive to penicillin.

Staphylococcus aureus: Acute infections of skin and soft tissue which are mild to moderately severe. Resistance may develop during treatment.

Streptococcus pneumoniae: Upper and lower respiratory tract infections of mild to moderate severity.

Mycoplasma pneumoniae: Primary atypical pneumonia when due to this organism.

Bordetella pertussis: When given early after exposure to whooping cough, erythromycin may reduce the risk of development of classical symptoms.

Treponema pallidum: Erythromycin is an alternative choice of treatment for syphilis in penicillin-allergic patients.

Corynebacterium diphtheriae: As an adjunct to antitoxin, to prevent establishment of carriers, and to eradicate the organism in carriers.

Corynebacterium minutissimum: In the treatment of erythrasma.

Entamoeba histolytica: In the treatment of intestinal amoebiasis only. Extra-enteric amoebiasis requires treatment with other agents.

Listeria monocytogenes: Infections due to this organism.

Legionnaires' disease: Although no controlled clinical studies have been conducted, *in vitro* and limited preliminary clinical data suggest that erythromycin may be effective in treating Legionnaires' disease.

Dosage and administration For oral administration.
Adults: The usual dose is 250 mg every six hours. This may be increased up to 4 g per day according to the severity of the infection.
The elderly: As for adults.
Children: Age, weight, and severity of the infection are

important factors in determining the correct dosage. The usual range is 20–50 mg/kg/day in divided doses.

For mild to moderate infections

Body weight	Total daily dose
10 kg or less	250 mg
10–18 kg	375 mg
18–25 kg	500 mg
25–36 kg	750 mg
More than 36 kg	1000 mg (adult dose)

For more severe infections these dosages may be doubled.

If administration on a twice daily schedule is desirable, one-half of the total daily dose may be given every 12 hours.

Streptococcal infections: In the treatment of group A beta-haemolytic streptococcal infections, a therapeutic dosage of erythromycin should be administered for at least 10 days. In continuous prophylaxis of streptococcal infections in persons with a history of rheumatic heart disease, the dosage is 250 mg twice daily.

When Ilosone is used prior to surgery to prevent endocarditis caused by alpha-haemolytic streptococci (viridans group) a recommended schedule for adults is 1 g pre-operatively and 500 mg every six hours for eight doses post-operatively: for children, 30–50 mg/kg/day divided into three or four evenly spaced doses.

Pertussis: Doses of erythromycin estolate utilised in reported clinical studies were 40–50 mg/kg/day, given in divided doses for five to 14 days.

Syphilis: A regimen of 20 g of erythromycin estolate in divided doses over a period of 10 days has been shown to be effective.

Amoebic dysentery: Dosage for adults is 250 mg four times daily for 10 to 14 days: for children, 30–50 mg/kg/day in divided doses for 10 to 14 days.

Legionnaires' disease: Although optimum regimens have not been established, 1–4 g daily in divided doses has been utilised in reported clinical studies.

Contra-indications, warnings, etc

Contra-indications: Hypersensitivity to erythromycin.

Patients who have previously developed jaundice or who have pre-existing liver disease or dysfunction.

Warnings: The administration of erythromycin estolate has been associated with the infrequent occurrence of reversible cholestatic hepatitis. Hepatic dysfunction with or without jaundice has occurred, chiefly in adults. It may be accompanied by malaise, nausea, vomiting, abdominal colic and fever. In some instances severe abdominal pain may simulate the pain of biliary colic, pancreatitis, perforated ulcer, or an acute abdominal surgical problem. In other instances, clinical symptoms and results of liver function tests have resembled findings in extrahepatic obstructive jaundice. Laboratory findings have been characterised by abnormal hepatic function test values, peripheral eosinophilia and leucocytosis. If the above findings occur, discontinue Ilosone promptly.

Initial symptoms have developed in some cases after a few days of treatment, but generally have followed one or two weeks of continuous therapy. Symptoms reappear promptly, usually within 48 hours, after the drug is re-administered to sensitive patients. The syndrome seems to result from a form of sensitisation, occurs chiefly in adults, and has been reversible when medication is discontinued.

Usage in pregnancy: Clinical and laboratory studies have

shown no evidence of teratogenicity or toxicity. However, caution should be exercised when prescribing for the pregnant patient. Erythromycin is readily excreted in breast milk.

Precautions: The use of erythromycin in patients who are receiving concomitant high doses of theophylline may be associated with an increase in serum theophylline levels and potential theophylline toxicity. If symptoms of toxicity develop, the dose of theophylline should be reduced.

During prolonged or repeated therapy, there is a possibility of overgrowth of non-susceptible bacteria or fungi. If such infections arise, the drug should be discontinued and appropriate therapy instituted.

Side-effects: The most frequent side-effects of erythromycin preparations are gastro-intestinal (e.g. abdominal cramping and discomfort) and are dose-related. Nausea, vomiting and diarrhoea occur infrequently with usual oral doses.

Mild allergic reactions, such as urticaria and other skin rashes, have occurred. Serious allergic reactions, including anaphylaxis, have been reported.

Overdosage: Symptoms – nausea, vomiting and diarrhoea.

Treatment: General management may consist of supportive therapy.

Pharmaceutical precautions Capsules and tablets: Keep container tightly closed and store in a cool place (6°–15°C).

Suspensions: Keep container tightly closed and protect from light. Store in a cool place. Shake well before use. For dilution, use Syrup BP, and when diluted use within 14 days.

Legal category POM.

Package quantities
Capsules 250 mg   Bottles of 100 and 500
Tablets 500 mg   Bottles of 12
Ready-mixed Suspension 125 mg/5 ml: Bottles of 100 ml
Ready-mixed Suspension 250 mg/5 ml: Bottles of 100 ml

Strengths expressed are base equivalent as Erythromycin Estolate BP.

Further information Nil.

Product licence numbers
Capsules 250 mg	0006/5022
Tablets 500 mg	0006/5015
Suspension 125 mg/5 ml	0006/5023
Suspension 250 mg/5 ml	0006/5024

KEFADOL*

Presentation 10 ml vials containing cefamandole nafate for injection equivalent to 500 mg or 1 g cefamandole.

100 ml vials containing cefamandole nafate for injection equivalent to 2 g cefamandole.

The vials also contain 63 mg Sodium Carbonate USP per gram of cefamandole.

Uses Cefamandole is indicated in the treatment of infections of the respiratory tract, genito-urinary tract, bones and joints, bloodstream (septicaemia), skin and soft tissue, gall bladder and peritoneum, and pelvic inflammatory disease in women, when due to susceptible micro-organisms.

Prophylactic use: Perioperative administration of cefamandole may reduce the incidence of postoperative infections in patients undergoing contaminated or potentially contaminated surgical procedures associated with a high risk of infection, or where the occurrence of a postoperative infection could be especially serious.

Cefamandole is usually active against most strains of the following organisms:

Beta-haemolytic and other streptococci (many strains of enterococci, e.g., *Streptococcus faecalis,* are relatively resistant)

Staphylococci, including coagulase-positive, coagulase-negative (e.g., *Staphylococcus epidermidis*), penicillinase-producing and most methicillin-resistant strains

Streptococcus pneumoniae

Haemophilus influenzae (including ampicillin-resistant strains)

Escherichia coli and other coliform bacteria

Klebsiella spp.

Proteus mirabilis

Proteus spp. (indole-positive, including *Pr. rettgeri* and *Pr. vulgaris*)

Morganella morganii

Enterobacter spp.

Salmonella spp., including *S. typhi*

Serratia spp. (many strains are relatively resistant).

Pseudomonas species are resistant to cefamandole.

Cefamandole has demonstrated *in vitro* activity against the following anaerobic bacteria: Anaerobic streptococci, *Peptococcus* and *Peptostreptococcus* spp., *Bacteroides* spp. and *Clostridium* spp.

Cefamandole is resistant to degradation by beta-lactamases from *Staph. aureus* and certain members of the *Enterobacteriaceae.*

Dosage and administration Cefamandole nafate may be given intravenously or by deep intramuscular injection.

Adults and the elderly: The dosage range for cefamandole is 500 mg to 2 g every four to eight hours, depending on the severity and site of infection.

Impaired renal function: When renal function is impaired, a reduced dosage must be employed and serum concentrations should be monitored when feasible. After an initial dose of 1 to 2 g (depending on the severity of infection), a maintenance dosage schedule should be followed (see table). Continued dosage should be determined by degree of renal impairment, severity of infection and susceptibility of the causative organism.

Maintenance dosage of cefamandole in patients with impaired renal function

Creatinine clearance ml/min/1.73 m²	Life threatening infections	Severe infections	Less severe infections
50-80	2 g q 6 h	1.5 g q 6 h	0.75 g q 6 h
25-50	2 g q 8 h	1.5 g q 8 h	0.75 g q 8 h
10-25	1.25 g q 8 h	0.75 g q 8 h	0.5 g q 8 h
2-10	1 g q 12 h	0.75 g q 12 h	0.5 g q 12 h
<2	0.75 g q 12 h	0.5 g q 12 h	0.25 g q 12 h

Intramuscular administration: Cefamandole should be reconstituted with Water for Injections PhEur or Sodium Chloride Intravenous Infusion BP. Shake well until dissolved.

Intravenous administration:

1. *For direct intermittent intravenous administration,* add 10 ml of Water for Injections PhEur, 5% Dextrose Intravenous Infusion BP, or Sodium Chloride Intravenous Infusion BP per gram of cefamandole. Slowly inject directly into the vein over a period of three to five minutes or give through the tubing of an administration set while the patient is also receiving one of the following intravenous fluids:

Sodium Chloride Intravenous Infusion BP

5% Dextrose Intravenous Infusion BP

10% Dextrose Intravenous Infusion BP

5% Dextrose and 0.9% Sodium Chloride Intravenous Infusion BP

5% Dextrose and 0.45% Sodium Chloride Intravenous Infusion BP

Sodium Lactate Intravenous Infusion BP

2. *Intermittent intravenous infusion with a Y-type administration set or volume control set* can also be accomplished while any of the above mentioned intravenous fluids are being infused. However, during infusion of the solution containing cefamandole, it is desirable to discontinue the other solution. When this technique is employed, careful attention should be paid to the volume of the solution containing cefamandole so that the calculated dose will be infused. When a Y-tube connection is used, 100 ml of an appropriate diluent should be added to the 2 g (100 ml) vial. If Water for Injections PhEur is used as the diluent, reconstitute with approximately 20 ml per g to avoid a hypotonic solution.

3. *For continuous intravenous infusion,* each gram of cefamandole should be diluted with 10 ml of Water for Injections PhEur. An appropriate quantity of the resulting solution may be added to an i.v. bottle containing one of the previously mentioned intravenous fluids.

If combination therapy with cefamandole and an aminoglycoside is indicated, each of these should be administered at separate sites.

Infants and children: Administration of 50 to 100 mg/kg/day in equally divided doses every four to eight hours has been effective for most infections susceptible to cefamandole. This may be increased to a total daily dose of 150 mg/kg (not to exceed the maximum adult dose) for serious infections. Kefadol has been safely administered to infants under the age of thirty days. Accumulation of cephalosporins (with resulting prolongation of drug half-life) has been reported in neonates.

Prophylactic use:

The following schedules are recommended for perioperative use:

Adults and the elderly: 1 or 2 g intravenously or intramuscularly one-half to one hour prior to surgical incision, followed by 1 or 2 g every six hours for 24 hours.

For patients undergoing procedures involving implantation of prosthetic devices, administration for up to 72 hours is recommended.

Children (more than three months of age): 50–100 mg/kg/day in equally divided doses by the same routes and schedule designated for adults.

If signs of infection occur, cultures should be obtained and appropriate therapy instituted.

Contra-indications, warnings, etc

Contra-indication: Cefamandole is contra-indicated in

patients with known allergy to the cephalosporin group of antibiotics.

Warnings: This product should be given cautiously to penicillin-sensitive patients. There is some evidence of partial cross-allergenicity of the penicillins and the cephalosporins. Patients have been reported to have had severe reactions to both classes of drugs. Antibiotics should be administered with caution to any patient who has demonstrated some form of allergy, particularly to drugs.

Usage in pregnancy: The safety of this product for use during pregnancy has not been established. Animal studies have shown no evidence of teratogenicity or toxicity.

Precautions: Although cefamandole rarely produces alteration in kidney function, evaluation of renal status is recommended, especially in seriously ill patients receiving maximum doses, or those receiving concurrent aminoglycoside therapy. Patients with impaired renal function should be placed on the dosage schedule recommended under **Dosage and administration.** Usual doses in such individuals may result in excessive serum concentrations.

As with other broad-spectrum antibiotics, hypoprothrombinaemia, with or without bleeding, has been reported rarely, but it has been promptly reversed by administration of vitamin K. Such episodes usually have occurred in elderly, debilitated or otherwise compromised patients with deficient stores of vitamin K. Prophylactic administration of vitamin K may be indicated in such patients, especially when intestinal sterilisation and surgical procedures are performed.

In a few patients receiving cefamandole, nausea, vomiting and vasomotor instability with hypotension and peripheral vasodilatation occurred following the ingestion of alcohol.

Prolonged use of cefamandole may result in the overgrowth of non-susceptible organisms. Careful observation of the patient is essential. If superinfection occurs during therapy, appropriate measures should be taken.

A false positive reaction for glucose in the urine may occur with Benedict's or Fehling's solutions or with Clinitest tablets but not with 'Tes-Tape' (urine sugar analysis paper, Lilly). A false positive test for proteinuria may occur with acid and denaturisation precipitation tests.

The results of experimental studies in animals suggest that the concurrent use of potent diuretics such as frusemide or ethacrynic acid may increase the risk of renal toxicity with cephalosporin antibiotics.

Side-effects: Hypersensitivity: Maculopapular rash, urticaria, eosinophilia and drug fever have been reported. These reactions are more likely to occur in patients with a history of allergy, particularly to penicillin.

Blood: Neutropenia and thrombocytopenia have been reported rarely. Some individuals have developed positive direct Coombs' tests during treatment with the cephalosporin antibiotics.

Liver: Transient rise in AST, ALT and ALP levels have been noted.

Kidney: Rise in blood urea and decreased creatinine clearance have been reported, particularly in patients with prior renal impairment. The rôle of cefamandole in renal changes is difficult to assess, because other factors predisposing to pre-renal azotaemia or to acute renal failure usually have been present.

Gastro-intestinal: Nausea and vomiting occur infrequently. Colitis, including rare instances of pseudomembranous colitis, has been reported.

Local reactions: Pain on intramuscular injection is infrequent. Thrombophlebitis occurs rarely.

Overdosage: In the event of serious overdosage, general supportive care is recommended, with monitoring of haematological, renal and hepatic functions, and coagulation status, until the patient is stable.

Pharmaceutical precautions *Unreconstituted vials:* Store at room temperature (15°–25°C). Protect from light.

It is good practice to reconstitute immediately before use. If this is not feasible, reconstituted solutions may be stored in a refrigerator (0°–6°C) and used within 96 hours. If kept at room temperature (15°–25°C), use within 24 hours. During storage at room temperature, carbon dioxide develops inside the vial after reconstitution. This pressure may be dissipated prior to withdrawal of the vial contents, or it may be used to aid withdrawal if the vial is inverted over the syringe needle and the contents are allowed to flow into the syringe.

Do not mix an aminoglycoside with cefamandole in the same intravenous fluid container.

Legal category POM.

Package quantities

Vials 500 mg	Individual vials in packs of 10.
Vials 1 g	Individual vials in packs of 10.
Vials 2 g	Individual vials.

Further information Solutions of cefamandole range from light yellow to amber, depending upon a variety of factors, including concentration and the diluent used.

Product licence number 0006/0111.

*Trade Mark

Dome/Hollister-Stier
Strawberry Hill
Newbury
Berkshire RG13 1JA

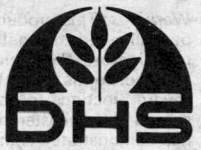

ALLPYRAL* ALLERGEN EXTRACTS

Presentation *Ingredients:* An Allpyral Allergen Extract is a sterile, pyridine-extracted, alum-precipitated antigen complex suspended in an aqueous solution of 0.9% saline containing 0.4% phenol as a preservative. Allpyral Allergen Extracts are standardised on a protein nitrogen unit (PNU) basis.

Allpyral Allergen Extracts are prepared *either* according to the specific sensitivities of individual patients (these Extracts are designated Allpyral-Specific), *or* as standard extracts of pollens of five common grasses (these Extracts are designated Allpyral-G).

Allpyral-Specific Allergen Extracts are prepared from one or more of the following source materials (subject to conditions given in Notes 1–6):

Pollens

Grass mix (see Note 1)
Oil seed rape
Plantain
Mugwort
Nettle
Flower mix compositae
  (see Note 2)
Beech
Hazel
Alder
Willow
Sycamore

Ash ⎫
Birch ⎪ Tree mix (see
Elm ⎬ Note 3)
Oak ⎪
Plane ⎭

Other inhalants

⎧ D. pteronyssinus
⎨ Mite Fortified house dust
⎩ (see Note 4)
House dust
Cat
Cow
Dog

Feather mix (see
  Note 5)
Rye flour
Wheat flour
Horse
Rabbit
Sheep wool

Moulds

Botrytis cinerea
Dry rot (Merulius lacrymans)
Phoma betae
Sporobolomyces roseus
Candida albicans
Fusarium oxysporum
Helminthosporium sativum
Mucor racemosus
Alternaria tenuis ⎫
Aspergillus fumigatus ⎪ Mould mix (see
Cladosporium herbarum ⎬ Note 3)
Penicillium notatum ⎭
Pullularia pullulans
Rhizopus nigricans

Stinging insects (see Note 6)

Wasp   Bee

Note 1. Grass mix contains extracts of the pollens of cocksfoot, meadow fescue, perennial rye, timothy, and Yorkshire fog.

These extracts are available *only* as constituents of Allpyral-Specific (grass mix) and *not* as individual extracts.

Note 2. Flower mix compositae contains extracts of the pollens of golden rod, aster, Michaelmas daisy, dahlia and chrysanthemum.

These extracts are available *only* as constituents of Allpyral-Specific (flower mix) and *not* as individual extracts.

Note 3. Those individual tree pollens and moulds underlined are available *either* individually *or* as constituents of tree mix and mould mix.

Note 4. D.pteronyssinus and Mite Fortified house dust are available *only* as individual extracts and not mixed with any other extract.

Note 5. Feather mix contains extracts of the feathers used in bedding and soft furnishing. These are available *only* as constituents of Allpyral-Specific (feather mix) and not as individual extracts.

Note 6. The stinging insect extracts of wasp and bee are available *either* individually *or* as a wasp/bee mixture, but *not* mixed with any other allergens.

Allpyral-G Allergen Extract contains extracts of the pollens of cocksfoot, meadow fescue, perennial rye, timothy, and Yorkshire fog. Allpyral-G is recommended for the treatment of classical hay fever and/or grass pollen asthma. (This is a standard item available immediately from stock.)

Form and appearance: The colour of Allpyral Allergen Extracts depends upon the type of allergens used and the strength of extract in each vial. Grass pollen extracts range from pale to olive green, extracts of house dust and mite fortified house dust range from grey to black, mould extracts range from clear to pale brown, epithelial extracts range from clear to milky white, tree pollen extracts range from olive to dark green, and D. pteronyssinus extracts range from clear to milky white. Allpyral Allergen Extracts are available in three types of treatment set:

1. Initial Treatment Sets consist of 3 colour-coded, graduated-strength vials.
Vial No. 1 (Green Label) contains extract of 100 PNU/ml strength.
Vial No. 2 (Blue Label) contains extract of 1,000 PNU/ml strength.
Vial No. 3 (Black Label) contains extract of 10,000 PNU/ml strength.
2. Special Dilution Treatment Sets consist of 1 vial containing extract of 10 PNU/ml strength. This treatment set may be required for use *before* the Initial Treatment Set in certain cases (see 'Dosage and administration'

below), and will be supplied on *request* with the Initial Treatment Set.

3. Maintenance Treatment Sets consist of 1 vial (Black Label) containing extract of 10,000 PNU/ml strength (see 'Dosage and administration' below).

All treatment sets are supplied complete with sufficient sterile disposable syringes and needles for the course ordered.

Uses Indications

Allpyral-Specific: For immunotherapy of patients whose allergies have been determined by case history and confirmed by skin testing. To ensure conformity between the results of skin-testing and subsequent treatment, it is recommended that DHS Glycerinated Skin Testing Solutions are used. There is a DHS Glycerinated Skin Testing Solution for each of the Allpyral Allergen Extracts listed above with the exception of bee and wasp extracts; the diagnostic solutions and the treatment extracts are prepared from common source materials.

Allpyral-G: For immunotherapy of patients known to suffer from classical hay fever and/or grass pollen asthma.

Dosage and administration Allpyral Allergen Extracts should be administered only by subcutaneous injection. Patients sensitive to seasonal allergens should be treated *pre-seasonally*, in order to ensure that treatment is completed before the seasonal allergen becomes airborne.

Patients sensitive only to perennial, i.e. non-seasonal, allergens may be treated at any time of the year.

Each Allpyral-Specific Treatment Set is supplied with a dosage schedule with complete instructions on administration prepared from the information given on the Allpyral Order Form by the prescribing physician.

SEASONAL ALLERGENS

Initial treatment: Each year's treatment with Allpyral Allergen Extracts *should always commence with an Initial Treatment Set.*

Initial treatment on a pre-seasonal basis consists of a course of 10 subcutaneous injections from the Allpyral-G or Allpyral-Specific Initial Treatment Set.

This course should be completed not less than three weeks before the particular allergen becomes airborne. Clinical evidence suggests that best results are obtained if the pre-seasonal course is timed to end approximately three weeks before pollination.

It is recommended that children under 14 in the first year of treatment should be treated according to the 'Extremely Sensitive' dosage schedule. For extremely sensitive patients a Special Dilution Treatment Set can be supplied *on request*. This should *precede* administration of the Initial Treatment Set.

Increasingly, clinical experience indicates that if pre-seasonal immunotherapy is repeated for three consecutive years, long-lasting relief may be expected, rendering treatment in subsequent years unnecessary. *For each year of treatment an Initial Treatment Set will be required.*

Maintenance treatment: Maintenance treatment is advisable in cases where pre-seasonal initial treatment has been completed long before the onset of pollination, e.g. in the case of grass pollen, if the course has finished in February (the grass pollen season usually starts in late May). Treatment with an Allpyral Maintenance Set involves repeat injections of the top dose achieved on the preceding initial treatment course, given at four to six weekly intervals until three weeks before the onset of pollination.

Not more than six weeks should elapse between the last injection of the initial treatment course and the first maintenance injection, or between subsequent maintenance injections. If more than six weeks elapse, then the dosage should be reduced accordingly.

PERENNIAL ALLERGENS

Initial treatment: Treatment with Allpyral Allergen Extracts *should always commence with an Initial Treatment Set.*

Initial treatment consists of 10 subcutaneous injections from the Allpyral-Specific Initial Treatment Set. Where only perennial or non-seasonal allergens are involved, treatment with Allpyral-Specific may be started at any time of the year. It is recommended that children under 14 in the first course of treatment should be treated according to the 'Extremely Sensitive' dosage schedule. For extremely sensitive patients a Special Dilution Treatment Set can be supplied *on request*. This should *precede* administration of the Initial Treatment Set.

Maintenance treatment: Maintenance treatment is intended to maintain the protection afforded by the initial treatment course and should only be given where an initial treatment course has previously been completed. Maintenance treatment consists of repeat injections of the top dose achieved on the initial treatment course, given every four to six weeks.

Not more than six weeks should elapse between the final injection of the initial treatment course and the first maintenance injection, or between subsequent maintenance injections. If more than six weeks elapse, then the dosage should be reduced accordingly.

Other advice on the administration of Allpyral Allergen Extracts is as follows:

1. Observe the usual sterile techniques.
2. Do not inject intravenously.
3. Shake the vial before withdrawing the dose.

Where two different courses are being given concurrently the two extracts must *never* be mixed within the same syringe. Injections of the two extracts may be given at the same visit, but in opposite arms.

Alternatively, the normal weekly interval between injections may be increased to two weeks, so that the two courses can be given on alternate weeks (i.e. one course on weeks 1, 3, 5, 7, etc., the other course on weeks 2, 4, 6, 8, etc.).

For recommendations concerning dilution see 'Pharmaceutical precautions' below.

Contra-indications, warnings, etc

Contra-indications: Whilst no adverse reactions have been reported, it is not considered advisable to administer Allpyral Allergen Extracts during pregnancy.

Precautions: Patients should be detained in the surgery for 30 minutes following each injection, and should be advised not to take any strenuous exercise for some hours.

Adrenaline Injection BP should always be available when administering immunotherapy.

Overdosage: See 'Main side-effects/adverse reactions' below.

Main side-effects/adverse reactions: As with all forms of immunotherapy the possibility of reactions in very sensitive individuals cannot be ruled out. This risk is considerably reduced in the case of Allpyral Allergen Extracts, since the antigens are slowly released from the site of injection.

Small local reactions (i.e. swelling at injection site up to

2.5 cm in diameter): If a small local reaction occurs at the injection site consisting of a swelling less than 2.5 cm in diameter, proceed to the next dose on the dosage schedule.

Large local reaction (i.e. swelling at injection site greater than 2.5 cm in diameter): If a large local reaction occurs at the injection site consisting of a swelling greater than 2.5 cm in diameter the next injection should be reduced to that previously tolerated and subsequent injections increased cautiously thereafter. Discontinue injections if reaction size increases.

Mild systemic reactions: If a mild systemic side-effect occurs such as mild itching of the eyes, nose, throat or skin, or localised urticaria, reduce the next dose to that previously tolerated. If necessary give an antihistamine.

Severe systemic reactions: A severe systemic side-effect may require treatment with 0.5 ml Adrenaline Injection BP and antihistamines. If bronchospasm is severe Isoprenaline Sulphate BP by inhalation may be of value. A parenteral steroid such as Hydrocortisone Sodium Succinate BP intravenously, after adrenaline has been given, may help to prevent prolonged reactions. Further treatment with Allpyral should be discontinued.

Pharmaceutical precautions *Storage:* Store between 2°C and 8°C. Do not freeze.

Dilution: Allpyral Allergen Extracts are supplied ready for use. It is important that, in the event of a pharmacist or physician wishing to dilute an Allpyral Allergen Extract, only diluent supplied for this purpose by Dome/Hollister-Stier should be used. Failure to observe this recommendation may adversely affect the integrity of the Allpyral Allergen Extract, thereby reducing its safety.

Legal category POM.

Package quantities Initial Treatment Sets consist of three colour-coded, graduated-strength vials.
Special Dilution Courses consist of 1 vial.
Maintenance Treatment Sets consist of 1 (top-strength) vial. For details of PNU strengths please see 'Presentation – Form and appearance' above.
All Allpyral Allergen Extracts are supplied complete with the appropriate dosage schedule and a sufficient quantity of sterile, disposable syringes and needles for the course.

Further information Allpyral Allergen Extracts are prepared by a process which minimises residual free allergen, and allows slow absorption from the site of injection. Thus fewer severe reactions, both local and systemic, are experienced than with aqueous extracts, and fewer injections are required.
Treatment with Allpyral Allergen Extracts reduces the patient's hypersensitivity, thereby dealing with the cause of his allergic symptoms. Thus Allpyral Allergen Extracts provide prophylactic rather than palliative therapy.

Product licence number 0055/5001.

CONJUVAC*
Presentation Conjuvac Initial Treatment Set contains 12 colour coded unit dose vials of allergen extracts which have been dialysed and chemically conjugated to alginate and then freeze dried.

Strengths
4 Green vials   10 units/ml (when reconstituted)
4 Gold vials   100 units/ml (when reconstituted)
3 Blue vials   500 units/ml (when reconstituted)
1 Red vial   1000 units/ml (when reconstituted)
12 × 2 ml ampoules of Water for Injections BP are supplied for reconstitution of the unit dose vials of Conjuvac.
Conjuvac is prepared from the following source materials and is available as the standard mixtures described below.

Grass pollens: Two Grass Mix of cocksfoot (*Dactylis glomerata*) and timothy (*Phleum pratense*).

Other inhalants: D. pteronyssinus.

Uses Immunotherapy of patients sensitive to specific allergens. There is an equivalent diagnostic solution (Alpha-Test) for each Conjuvac allergen extract. The diagnostic solutions and the treatment extracts are prepared from common source materials.

Dosage and administration Immunotherapy with Conjuvac should begin with an Initial Treatment Set and be continued with Maintenance Treatment Sets. It is recommended that treatment is given for 3 consecutive years.
The initial course consists of 11 deep subcutaneous injections given at weekly intervals. If more than 2 weeks have elapsed since the previous injection, repeat the same dose or reduce it depending on the interval involved.

Dosage schedule

Vial colour	Vial no.	Units Dose	Volume injected (ml)
Green	1	1	0.10
(10 units/ml)	2	2	0.20
	3	4	0.40
	4	8	0.80
Gold	5	15	0.15
(100 units/ml)	6	30	0.30
	7	60	0.60
	Spare vial		
Blue	8	100	0.20
(500 units/ml)	9	200	0.40
	10	400	0.80
Red	11	800†	0.80
(1000 units/ml)			

† Top dose and maintenance dose

Seasonal Allergies: Seasonal allergies should be treated pre-seasonally. An Initial Treatment Set is required for each year of therapy, which should start in December or January. If treatment is started after the end of February, it is unlikely that there will be sufficient time to complete the full course.
Injections should not be given during the grass pollen season.
Should the initial course be completed well before the pollen season, maintenance injections should begin 2 weeks after the top dose of initial therapy and the second maintenance injection given 2 weeks later. This is followed by an injection every 4–6 weeks until 2 weeks before pollination.

Perennial allergies: Initial injections of perennial allergens can begin at any time of year and should be followed by maintenance injections.

After initial therapy, maintenance treatment should continue after 2 weeks and the second maintenance injection 2 weeks later. This is then followed by an injection every 4 to 6 weeks for the remainder of treatment.

If a reaction occurs please refer to the information under main side effects/adverse reactions.

Reconstitution: Conjuvac is reconstituted by adding 1.0 ml of Water for Injections BP to the vial using a sterile syringe. Swirl or rock the container to dissolve the extract completely. *Do not shake,* since this leads to foaming which can cause denaturation (inactivation) of the protein.

Contra-indications, warnings, etc Animal studies have shown no teratogenic potential. However, it is not considered advisable to administer Conjuvac during pregnancy. Conjuvac should not be administered during an asthmatic attack, nor during a febrile illness.

Precautions
1. Do not inject intravenously.
2. Adrenaline Injection BP should always be available when administering any immunotherapy.
3. Patients should be detained in the surgery for at least 30 minutes following each injection and should be advised not to take strenuous exercise, hot baths, sauna nor to apply any form of heat locally to the injection site for the remainder of the day.
4. Always determine whether any reaction occurred after the previous injection before administering the next one.

Main side-effects/adverse reactions: As with all forms of immunotherapy local reactions or systemic reactions may occur. Injections of Conjuvac are often associated with some itching and redness at the injection site. Reactions may be classified as follows:
1. Small local reactions (i.e. swelling at injection site up to 5 cm in diameter): If a small local reaction occurs at the injection site consisting of a swelling less than 5 cm in diameter, proceed to the next dose on the dosage schedule.
2. Large local reaction (i.e. swelling at injection site greater than 5 cm in diameter): If a large local reaction occurs at the injection site consisting of a swelling greater than 5 cm in diameter the next injection should be reduced to that previously tolerated and subsequent injections increased cautiously thereafter. Discontinue injections if reaction size increases.

3. Mild systemic reactions: If a mild systemic side-effect occurs such as mild itching of the eyes, nose, throat or skin, or localised urticaria, reduce the next dose to that previously tolerated. If necessary give an anti-histamine.
4. Severe systemic reactions: A severe systemic side-effect may require treatment with 0.5 ml Adrenaline Injection BP and antihistamines. If bronchospasm is severe Isoprenaline Sulphate BP by Inhalation may be of value. A parenteral steroid such as Hydrocortisone Sodium Succinate BP intravenously, after adrenaline has been given, may help to prevent prolonged reactions. Further treatment with Conjuvac should be discontinued.

Overdosage: See *Main side-effects/adverse reactions.*

Pharmaceutical precautions
1. Proper aseptic precautions should be taken during reconstitution and subsequent withdrawal including swabbing of bungs with a suitable antiseptic.
2. Unreconstituted lyophilised material does not require refrigeration but should be stored in a cool dry place.
3. Vigorous shaking or handling during reconstitution may result in foaming.
4. *Once reconstituted Conjuvac must be used within 12 hours.*

Legal category POM.

Package quantities Initial treatment sets consist of 12 colour coded vials of graduated strengths, 12 ampoules of Water for Injections BP and full instructions for use.

Maintenance Treatment Sets for seasonal allergies consist of 4 top strength vials, 4 ampoules of Water for Injections BP and full instructions for use.

Maintenance Treatment Sets for perennial allergies consist of 10 top strength vials, 10 ampoules of Water for Injections BP and full instructions for use.

Further information Conjuvac consists of dialysed aqueous allergen extract which has been chemically conjugated to Sodium Alginate BPC and has been standardised by the inhibition radioallergosorbent test (RAST) against a reference allergen.

Product licence numbers
Conjuvac   0055/0051
Water for Injections BP   2848/5924

*Trade Mark

Duncan, Flockhart & Co. Limited
700 Oldfield Lane North
Greenford, Middlesex UB6 0HD

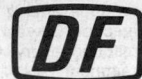

ACEPRIL* TABLETS ▼

Presentation Acepril Tablets 12.5 mg: round, white, biconvex tablets, half-scored on one side, containing 12.5 mg of captopril.

Acepril Tablets 25 mg: round, white, biconvex tablets, engraved ACE 25 on one side and quarter-scored on the reverse side for identification only, containing 25 mg of captopril.

Acepril Tablets 50 mg: round, white, biconvex tablets, engraved ACE 50 on one side and half-scored on the reverse side, containing 50 mg of captopril.

Uses
Actions: Captopril, 1-[(2S)-3 mercapto-2-methyl-propionyl]-L-proline, is a highly specific competitive inhibitor of angiotensin I-converting enzyme, the enzyme responsible for the conversion of angiotensin I to angiotensin II.

Until further experience has been obtained in the treatment of acute hypertensive crises, the use of Acepril should be avoided in these patients.

Indications:

Mild-to-moderate hypertension: As an adjunct to thiazide therapy in patients who have not responded effectively to thiazide treatment alone.

Severe hypertension: Where standard therapy has failed.

Congestive heart failure: Acepril is indicated for the treatment of severe, treatment-refractory congestive heart failure. The drug should be used together with diuretics and, where appropriate, digitalis but only after these agents have failed to produce a satisfactory response.

Dosage and administration
Adults

Hypertension: Treatment with Acepril should be at the lowest effective dose, which should be titrated according to the needs of the patient.

Mild-to-moderate hypertension: In mild-to-moderate hypertension, Acepril should be used as an adjunct to thiazide therapy.

The initial dose is 12.5 mg twice daily. The usual maintenance dose is 25 mg twice daily which can be increased incrementally, at two to four week intervals, until a satisfactory response is achieved, to a maximum of 50 mg twice daily.

Severe hypertension: In severe hypertension the starting dose is 12.5 mg b.d. The dosage may be increased incrementally to a maximum of 50 mg t.i.d. Acepril can be used together with other antihypertensive agents but the dose of these should be individually titrated. A daily dose of 150 mg of Acepril should not normally be exceeded.

Heart failure: Acepril therapy must be started under close medical supervision. The usual dose is 25 mg three times a day. A starting dose of 6.25 or 12.5 mg may minimise a transient hypotensive effect. The usual maximum dose is 150 mg daily. Further increases in dosage should be delayed for at least two weeks to determine if a satisfactory response has occurred.

Acepril should be used in conjunction with a diuretic and where appropriate digitalis.

Elderly
The dose should be titrated against the blood pressure response and kept as low as possible to achieve adequate blood pressure control. Since elderly patients may have reduced renal function and other organ dysfunctions, it is suggested that a low dose of captopril be used initially.

Children
Captopril is not recommended for the treatment of mild-to-moderate hypertension in children.

Safety and effectiveness in children have not been established.

Experience in neonates and premature infants is limited.

The starting dose should be 0.3 mg/kg bodyweight up to a maximum of 6 mg/kg bodyweight in divided daily doses. The dose should be individualised according to the response and may be given two or three times daily.

Patients with renal impairment
Acepril is not recommended in patients with renal impairment. Where it is clinically indicated in severely hypertensive patients with impaired renal function, the dose should be kept as low as possible to maintain adequate blood pressure control. The dose can be titrated against the response but adequate time should be allowed between dosage adjustments.

In these patients a loop-diuretic rather than a thiazide should be the diuretic of choice.

Acepril is readily eliminated by haemodialysis.

Contra-indications, warnings, etc
Contra-indications: A history of previous hypersensitivity to captopril.

Pregnancy: Acepril has been shown to be lethal to rabbit and sheep fetuses. There were no fetotoxic effects in hamster or rat fetuses.

Acepril is contra-indicated in pregnancy and should not be used in women of child-bearing potential unless protected by effective contraception.

Precautions: Evaluation of the hypertensive patient should include assessment of renal function before Acepril therapy is started. Patients with renal impairment should not normally be treated with Acepril.

Acepril should not be used in patients with aortic stenosis or outflow tract obstruction.

Warnings: The incidence of adverse reactions to captopril is principally associated with renal function since the drug is excreted primarily by the kidney. The dose should not exceed that necessary for adequate blood pressure control and should be reduced in patients with impaired renal function.

Haematological: Neutropenia/agranulocytosis, thrombocytopenia and anaemia have been reported in patients receiving Acepril.

In patients with normal renal function and no other complicating factors, neutropenia occurs rarely.

Acepril should not be routinely used in patients with pre-existing impaired renal function, collagen vascular disease, immunosuppressant therapy, treatment with allopurinol or procainamide, or a combination of these complicating factors, because neutropenia has been limited almost exclusively to this group. Some of these patients developed serious infections which in a few instances did not respond to intensive antibiotic therapy. If Acepril is used in such patients, it is advised that white blood cell count and differential counts should be performed prior to therapy, every two weeks during the first three months of Acepril therapy, and periodically thereafter.

During treatment, all patients should be instructed to report any sign of infection (e.g., sore throat, fever), when a differential white blood cell count should be performed. Acepril and other concomitant medication should be withdrawn if neutropenia (neutrophils less than 1000/mm³) is detected or suspected. In most patients neutrophil counts rapidly returned to normal upon discontinuing Acepril.

Renal: Proteinuria in patients with prior normal renal function is rare. Where proteinuria has occurred it has usually been in patients with severe hypertension and evidence of prior renal disease. Nephrotic syndrome occurred in some of these patients. In patients with evidence of prior renal disease, monthly urinary protein estimations (dip stick) are recommended for the first nine months of therapy. If repeated determinations show increasing amounts of urinary protein, a 24-hour quantitative determination should be obtained, and if this exceeds 1 g/day, the benefits and risks of continuing Acepril should be evaluated.

Although membranous glomerulopathy was found in biopsies taken from some proteinuric patients, a causal relationship to Acepril has not been established.

Some patients with renal disease, particularly those with bilateral renal artery stenosis or unilateral renal artery stenosis in a single functioning kidney, have developed increased concentrations of blood urea and serum creatinine. Acepril dosage reduction and/or discontinuation of diuretic may be required. For some of these patients it may not be possible to normalise blood pressure and maintain adequate renal perfusion.

Hypotension: With the first one or two doses some patients may experience symptomatic hypotension. In most instances, symptoms are relieved simply by the patient lying down.

In patients with severe and renin-dependent hypertension (e.g. renovascular hypertension) or severe congestive heart failure who are receiving large doses of diuretic, exaggerated hypotensive responses have occurred usually within one hour of the initial dose of Acepril. In these patients, by discontinuing diuretic therapy or significantly reducing the diuretic dose for four to seven days prior to initiating Acepril the possibility of this occurrence is reduced. By commencing Acepril therapy with small doses (6.25 or 12.5 mg) the duration of any hypotensive

effect is lessened. Some patients may benefit from an infusion of saline.

The occurrence of first-dose hypotension does not preclude subsequent dose titration with Acepril.

Serum potassium: Since Acepril decreases aldosterone production, serum potassium is usually maintained in patients on diuretics. Potassium-sparing diuretics or potassium supplements should not therefore be used routinely. In patients with marked renal impairment a significant elevation of serum potassium may occur.

Nursing mothers: Because captopril is excreted in breast milk, Acepril should not be used in nursing mothers.

Surgery/Anaesthesia: In patients undergoing major surgery, or during anaesthesia with agents which produce hypotension, captopril will block angiotensin II formation secondary to compensatory renin release. This may lead to hypotension which can be corrected by volume expansion.

Clinical chemistry: Acepril may cause a false-positive urine test for acetone.

Side-effects

Haematological: Neutropenia, anaemia and thrombocytopenia (see 'Warnings').

Renal: Proteinuria, elevated blood urea and creatinine, elevated serum potassium and acidosis (see 'Warnings').

Cardiovascular: Hypotension (see 'Warnings'), tachycardia.

Skin: Rashes, usually pruritic, may occur. They are usually mild transient and maculopapular, rarely urticarial. In a few cases the rash has been associated with fever and some patients have developed angio-neurotic oedema. Pruritus, flushing, vesicular rash, and photosensitivity have been reported.

Gastro-intestinal: Reversible and usually self-limiting taste impairment has been reported. Weight loss may be associated with the loss of taste. Stomatitis resembling aphthous ulcers, has been reported. Elevation of liver enzymes has been noted in a few patients. Rare cases of hepato-cellular injury and cholestatic jaundice have been reported. Gastric irritation and abdominal pain may occur.

Other: Paraesthesias of the hands, serum sickness, cough, bronchospasm, and lymphadenopathy have been reported.

Overdosage: In the event of overdosage, blood pressure should be monitored and if hypotension develops volume expansion is the treatment of choice. Acepril is removed by dialysis.

Drug interactions

Diuretics: Diuretics potentiate the antihypertensive effectiveness of Acepril.

Potassium-sparing diuretics (triamterene, amiloride and spironolactone), or potassium supplements may cause significant increases in serum potassium.

Indomethacin: A reduction of antihypertensive effectiveness may occur. This is probably also the case with other non-steroidal anti-inflammatory drugs.

Vasodilators: Acepril has been reported to act synergistically with peripheral vasodilators such as minoxidil. Awareness of this interaction may avert an initial hypotensive response.

Clonidine: It has been suggested that the antihypertensive effect of Acepril can be delayed when patients treated with clonidine are changed to Acepril.

Allopurinol and procainamide: There have been reports of neutropenia and/or Stevens-Johnson syndrome in patients on Acepril plus either allopurinol or procainamide. Although a causal relationship has not been established, these combinations should only be used with caution, especially in patients with impaired renal function.

Immunosuppressants: Azathioprine and cyclophosphamide have been associated with blood dyscrasias in patients with renal failure who were also taking Acepril.

Probenecid: The renal clearance of Acepril is reduced in the presence of probenecid.

Pharmaceutical precautions Store at room temperature.

Legal category POM.

Package quantities Acepril Tablets 12.5 mg are available in bottles of 100 tablets.

Acepril Tablets 25 mg and 50 mg are each available in bottles of 100 tablets and in calendar blister packs of 56 tablets.

Further information None.

Product licence numbers
Acepril Tablets 12.5 mg   0021/0024
Acepril Tablets 25 mg   0021/0022
Acepril Tablets 50 mg   0021/0023

AIRBRON*

Presentation Airbron is a clear, colourless, sterile aqueous solution of 20% w/v Acetylcysteine BP (N-acetyl-3-mercapto-alanine) adjusted to pH 7.0 with sodium hydroxide.

Uses Acetylcysteine, a derivative of the naturally occurring amino acid L-cysteine, is neither an enzyme nor a detergent.

Airbron dramatically reduces the viscosity and tenacity of sputum, its liquefying action being due to the presence in acetylcysteine of a free sulphydryl group which opens up disulphide bonds present in mucus. The high viscosity of secretions in various pulmonary conditions is dependent primarily on their content of mucoprotein and, when an acute infection is involved, of deoxyribonucleic acid. The mucolytic activity of acetylcysteine is unaffected by the presence of deoxyribonucleic acid and it is, therefore, equally effective against purulent and non-purulent mucus.

Airbron facilitates the removal of mucus in broncho-pulmonary diseases:

In general medicine: Chronic bronchitis with or without emphysema, Bronchiectasis, Lung abscesses.

In anaesthetics: During general anaesthesia. Post-operative care. Pulmonary complications of heart or lung surgery. Intensive care (including routine cleansing of tracheostomies).

Dosage and administration Airbron is administered topically by nebulisation, direct instillation or, occasionally, by percutaneous intratracheal catheter. Apparatus should be of plastic or glass. Metals (particularly iron, copper and nickel) and rubber should be avoided as they react with the drug. Airbron is rapidly inactivated by high concentrations of oxygen.

By nebulisation: 1 to 10 ml Airbron may be given into a face mask, mouthpiece, tracheostomy tube or opening every two to six hours. Usually 2 to 5 ml three or four times a day are sufficient for most cases.

If given into a tent, sufficient Airbron should be used to maintain a heavy mist for the duration of the treatment period and up to 250 ml may be administered.

By direct instillation: 1 to 2 ml Airbron may be given every one to four hours.

Contra-indications, warnings, etc Studies in various animal species have shown that acetylcysteine is virtually non-toxic and no contra-indications have been reported.

Precautions: As Airbron loosens large volumes of mucus, patients who cannot cough it up may require mechanical suction to maintain an open airway.

Care should be exercised in administering Airbron to asthmatic patients, as cases of bronchospasm have been reported. If bronchospasm occurs, Airbron should be replaced by a sympathomimetic agent, such as salbutamol, in aerosol form.

Side-effects: Side-effects due to Airbron are slight and infrequent. Stomatitis, nausea and vomiting, coughing and irritation have occasionally been reported. During nebulisation the patient may at first notice a slightly disagreeable odour, but this usually disappears. With a face mask, there may be stickiness on the face which can easily be removed by washing with warm water.

Pharmaceutical precautions Airbron should be stored in a cool place. If only a portion of a vial is used, the remainder should be stored in a refrigerator and used within 96 hours.

Legal category POM.

Package quantities Airbron is supplied in ampoules of 2 ml in containers of 25, and in multidose vials of 10 ml in containers of 3.

Further information Airbron is not suitable for use with an ordinary hand nebuliser as pressure of between 6 and 10 lbs per square inch should be used to produce a particle size of 10 microns or less.

Product licence number 0021/5026.

ANCOLOXIN* TABLETS

Presentation White tablets engraved DF/AR, each tablet containing:

Meclozine Hydrochloride BP	25 mg
Pyridoxine Hydrochloride BP	50 mg

Uses Meclozine hydrochloride is an anti-histamine of the piperazine group with marked anti-emetic properties and a duration of action of 12 to 24 hours. Its toxicity is low and it has been widely investigated for possible teratogenic effects in man. Pyridoxine hydrochloride (vitamin B_6) complements the action of meclozine. It forms, with other vitamins of the B group, part of an enzyme system concerned with the metabolism of amino acids. Severe vomiting is sometimes associated with a specific deficiency of pyridoxine and administration of this vitamin is of value in the treatment of such cases. Ancoloxin is indicated for the prevention and treatment of most forms of nausea and vomiting.

Dosage and administration *Radiation sickness:* 1 or 2 tablets two or three times a day.

Post-operative vomiting: 2 tablets not less than four hours before surgery.

Severe nausea and vomiting of pregnancy: 2 tablets at night; an additional tablet may be taken in the morning (see *Warnings, Pregnancy*).

Nausea and vomiting in other conditions: 1 or 2 tablets two or three times daily, according to the severity of the symptoms.

The Elderly: As elderly patients may have hepatic insufficiency, it is suggested that the dose of Ancoloxin is reduced.

Ancoloxin is not recommended for children.

Contra-indications, warnings, etc There are no contra-indications.

Pregnancy: Teratogenic effects have been reported in animals. Epidemiological studies in pregnant women do not indicate that meclozine increases the risk of fetal abnormalities, nevertheless, Ancoloxin should not be used in pregnancy unless considered medically essential.

Side-effects: Like other antihistamines, Ancoloxin occasionally gives rise to drowsiness. Patients should be advised not to drive a car or operate machinery if they feel sleepy and warned that drowsiness is more likely to occur if alcohol is taken.

Overdosage: Gastric aspiration and lavage with 1% sodium bicarbonate solution and general supportive measures.

Pharmaceutical precautions Ancoloxin Tablets should be stored in well closed containers.

Legal category POM.

Package quantities Ancoloxin Tablets are available in containers of 50 and 250.

Further information Nil.

Product licence number 0021/5060.

BETA-CARDONE*

Presentation *Beta-Cardone Tablets 200 mg:* White, circular, scored tablets engraved DF/BC20, each containing sotalol hydrochloride 200 mg.

80 mg: Red, circular, scored tablets engraved DF/BC8, each containing sotalol hydrochloride 80 mg.

40 mg: Green, circular, scored tablets engraved DF/BC4, each containing sotalol hydrochloride 40 mg.

Uses Beta-Cardone is a β-adrenoceptor blocking agent which is devoid of intrinsic sympathomimetic and local anaesthetic activity. Its major therapeutic effect is to protect the heart from undesirable sympathetic activity. Beta-Cardone reduces the rate and force of contraction of the heart; cardiac work and oxygen consumption are diminished.

In angina pectoris: Beta-Cardone reduces the frequency and severity of anginal attacks and increases exercise tolerance.

In hypertension: Beta-Cardone reduces blood pressure without the side-effects usually associated with peripherally acting hypotensive drugs.

In cardiac arrhythmias: Beta-Cardone is used to restore normal rate and rhythm or to reduce the rate of ventricular contraction, particularly in arrhythmias of supraventricular origin.

In thyrotoxicosis: Beta-Cardone is recommended for short-term symptomatic relief of sympathetic overactivity as an adjunct to specific anti-thyroid therapy.

Dosage and administration *Oral administration in adults:*

General instructions: When administering Beta-Cardone to a patient for the first time, it is desirable to start with a low dose and gradually increase the dose until the desired response is obtained; as a general rule the heart rate should not be reduced to less than 55 beats per minute.

No special precautions, other than the observance of the contra-indications listed below, are required when transferring patients to Beta-Cardone from other β-blockers. Beta-Cardone can be administered in conjunction with diuretic agents (see *'Warnings'*), digitalis, lignocaine and specific anti-thyroid drugs such as carbimazole. The following are guide lines for oral administration.

The Elderly: Since elderly patients may have renal insufficiency, a low initial dose and cautious titration of the effects of incremental doses are recommended.

Dosage in angina pectoris: The optimum dosage is usually found to be between 200 mg and 600 mg per day in a single or divided dose.

Treatment should be initiated with 80 mg twice daily for the first 7 to 10 days. The patient may then be given 200 mg once daily, preferably on rising in the morning. Further increments of 200 mg may thereafter be given, if necessary, at intervals of two or more weeks but, in angina pectoris, it is rarely found necessary to administer more than 400 mg per day.

Dosage in hypertension: The optimum dosage is usually found to be between 200 mg and 600 mg per day in a single or divided dose.

Again treatment should be initiated with 80 mg twice daily for the first 7 to 10 days. The patient may then be given 200 mg once daily, preferably on rising in the morning. Further increments of 200 mg may thereafter be given, if necessary, at intervals of two or more weeks and, in hypertension, there have been occasional reports of up to 4,000 mg being administered daily in divided doses.

Dosage in cardiac arrhythmia: The optimum dosage is usually found to be between 120 mg and 240 mg per day in a single or divided dose.

Dosage in Thyrotoxicosis: In most cases it has been found that a dosage of between 120 mg and 240 mg per day, in a single or divided dose, will reduce sympathetic overactivity.

In cardiac arrhythmia and thyrotoxicosis, treatment should be commenced with a dose of 40 mg, three times daily for the first 7 to 10 days. Once the maintenance phase is reached a single dose of 200 mg daily, preferably on rising in the morning, may be adequate.

Contra-indications, warnings, etc
Heart block and bronchospasm: Beta-Cardone should not be given to patients suffering from heart block or who have a history of bronchospasm.

In patients with poor cardiac reserve β-blockade can precipitate heart failure; in such cases, Beta-Cardone therapy should not be commenced until the patient has been controlled by cardiac glycosides and, if necessary, diuretic therapy.

Warning: There have been reports of skin rashes and/or dry eyes associated with the use of β-adrenoceptor-blocking drugs. The reported incidence is small and in most cases the symptoms have cleared when the treatment was withdrawn. Discontinuance of the drug should be considered if any such reaction is not otherwise explicable. Cessation of therapy with a β-blocker should be gradual.

Diabetic keto-acidosis and metabolic acidosis: Beta-Cardone should not be given to patients suffering from diabetic keto-acidosis or metabolic acidosis; therapy with Beta-Cardone can be commenced or resumed when the metabolic condition has been corrected.

Treated diabetes: Beta-Cardone, like other β-blocking agents, may reduce or mask the usual pre-hypoglycaemic warning signs. It may be necessary to adjust the dose of antidiabetic therapy.

General anaesthesia: If desired, Beta-Cardone may be stopped four days prior to surgery. However, where sudden withdrawal might expose the patient to severe angina or arrhythmias, anaesthesia can proceed provided that the following precautions are taken.

1. Vagal dominance is counteracted by premedication with atropine sulphate (0.25 to 2.0 mg) administered intravenously.

2. Ether, chloroform, cyclopropane and trichlorethylene are not used.

Pregnancy: Animal studies with sotalol hydrochloride have shown no evidence of teratogenicity or other harmful effects to the fetus, nevertheless its use throughout pregnancy should be avoided unless it is absolutely necessary. It crosses the placenta and may cause fetal bradycardia.

Breast milk: Infants should not be fed with breast milk from mothers being treated with Beta-Cardone.

Alcoholism: β-adrenoceptor blocking drugs may precipitate cardiac failure in alcoholic patients.

Renal insufficiency: Since Beta-Cardone is mainly excreted unchanged in the urine, accumulation may be avoided by reduction in dosage.

Serum sotalol levels increase in renal insufficiency and correlate with prolongation of the Q-Tc interval (see *Overdosage* below).

Upper respiratory infections: In these conditions patients without a history of airways obstruction may suffer bronchospasm from β-blockade.

Hypokalaemia: Avoid use with potassium-losing diuretics or in gastroenteritis: ventricular tachyarrhythmia has been reported.

Side-effects: Beta-Cardone is usually well tolerated. Bronchoconstriction has been reported in a few sensitive individuals; it may be controlled by the intravenous administration of atropine sulphate (0.25 to 2.0 mg) and/or by inhalation of a selective β-adrenoceptor stimulant such as salbutamol.

Interactions: In combined therapy clonidine should not be discontinued until several days after withdrawal of Beta-Cardone. Use with great caution with drugs that also prolong QT interval. Care should be taken in the concomitant use of sotalol and either Class I antiarrhythmic agents or calcium antagonists of the verapamil type.

Overdosage: Overdosage causes excessive bradycardia and hypotension; to counteract this atropine sulphate (0.25 to 2.0 mg) should be administered intravenously and, if need be, isoprenaline (about 5 micrograms per minute) by slow intravenous injection.

In severe overdose, intravenous glucagon may be preferred: an initial bolus dose of 5 to 10 mg in dextrose or saline should be followed by an intravenous infusion of 4 mg/hour or as sufficient to maintain cardiac output.

Prolongation of the Q-Tc interval has been reported. Transvenous pacing may be required.

Pharmaceutical precautions Beta-Cardone Tablets should be protected from light.

Legal category POM.

Package quantities *Beta-Cardone Tablets 200 mg* are available in containers of 30 tablets.

Beta-Cardone Tablets 80 mg are available in containers of 100 and 500 tablets.

Beta-Cardone Tablets 40 mg are available in containers of 100 and 500 tablets.

Further information Beta-Cardone is not metabolised and, in the main, is excreted in the urine. After oral administration the plasma half life has been shown to be 17 hours; the lipid solubility is very low.

Product licence numbers
Beta-Cardone Tablets 200 mg   0021/0056
Beta-Cardone Tablets 80 mg   0021/0055
Beta-Cardone Tablets 40 mg   0021/0054

CYTACON* LIQUID AND TABLETS

Presentation Cytacon Tablets are white, film-coated and engraved 'Cytacon' on one side. Each contains 50 micrograms cyanocobalamin.

Cytacon Liquid is red coloured and contains 35 micrograms cyanocobalamin in each 5 ml.

Uses *Post-gastrectomy deficiency:* As many as 50% of patients who have had a partial gastrectomy are likely to develop abnormally low serum vitamin B_{12} levels within five years of the operation unless supplementary vitamin B_{12} is given. Megaloblastic anaemia is not uncommon and subacute degeneration of the cord has been reported. After total gastrectomy, it is better to administer vitamin B_{12} by injection (as Neo-Cytamen* or Cytamen*) rather than orally. Diseases of the alimentary tract, such as 'blind-loop' syndrome and small bowel diverticula, may also be associated with vitamin B_{12} deficiency.

Nutritional deficiency: Low serum vitamin B_{12} levels may occur in strict vegetarians and in old people subsisting on limited diets. The diagnosis of pernicious anaemia should be excluded before administering oral vitamin B_{12}.

Tropical sprue: Both folic acid and vitamin B_{12} may be needed: in some cases oral vitamin B_{12} may be sufficiently well absorbed to avoid the need for injections.

Pernicious anaemia: If injections of vitamin B_{12} (Neo-Cytamen or Cytamen) cannot be used, large daily oral doses may be substituted (see Dosage below) but the blood must be examined at least every three months.

Dosage and administration *Adults:* 1 to 3 tablets or more daily at the discretion of the physician. Alternatively, one or two 5 ml spoonfuls Cytacon Liquid 2 or 3 times daily or at the discretion of the physician. In pernicious anaemia at least 300 micrograms should be given daily.

Children: One 5 ml spoonful Cytacon Liquid 2 to 3 times daily or at the discretion of the physician.

Where possible, doses should be taken between meals.

Contra-indications, warnings, etc

Contra-indications: Hypersensitivity to oral cyanocobalamin.

Precautions: In pernicious anaemia, an adequate dose must be used and the blood picture must be examined regularly at least every three months.

Doses in excess of 10 micrograms daily may produce a haematological response in patients with folate deficiency. Indiscriminate administration may mask precise diagnosis.

Pregnancy: Cytacon should not be used for the treatment of megaloblastic anaemia of pregnancy.

Side-effects: Sensitisation to cyanocobalamin is rare but it may present as an itching exanthema, and exceptionally as anaphylactic shock. Acneiform and bullous eruptions have been reported rarely.

Persons who have become sensitised to cyanocobalamin by injection are often able to take it by the oral route without trouble.

Interactions: Absorption of Cytacon may be reduced by para-aminosalicylic acid, colchicine, biguanides, neomycin, cholestyramine, potassium chloride, methyldopa and cimetidine. Chloramphenicol treated patients may respond poorly to Cytacon. Serum concentrations of cyanocobalamin may be lowered by oral contraceptives.

Overdosage: Treatment is unlikely to be needed in cases of overdosage.

Pharmaceutical precautions Protect from light. Store in well closed containers.

Legal category P.

Package quantities *Tablets:* packs of 50.
Liquid: bottles of 200 ml and 2 litres.

Further information Nil.

Product licence numbers

Cytacon Tablets	0021/5909
Cytacon Liquid	0021/5908

CYTAMEN* (Cyanocobalamin Injection BP)

Presentation Cytamen '1000' is a clear, red solution containing 1,000 micrograms cyanocobalamin per millilitre.

Cytamen complies with the specification for Cyanocobalamin Injection BP.

Uses Addisonian pernicious anaemia. Prophylaxis and treatment of other macrocytic anaemias associated with vitamin B_{12} deficiency. Schilling test.

Dosage and administration The following dosage schemes are suitable for adults and children.

Addisonian pernicious anaemia and other macrocytic anaemias without neurological involvement: Initially: 250 to 1,000 micrograms intramuscularly on alternate days for one to two weeks, then 250 micrograms weekly until the blood count is normal.

Maintenance: 1,000 micrograms monthly.

Addisonian pernicious anaemia and other macrocytic anaemias, anaemias with neurological complications: Initially: 1,000 micrograms intramuscularly on alternate days as long as improvement is occurring.

Maintenance: 1,000 micrograms monthly.

Prophylaxis of macrocytic anaemia associated with vitamin B_{12} deficiency resulting from gastrectomy, some

malabsorption syndromes and strict vegetarianism: 250 to 1,000 micrograms monthly.

Schilling test: An intramuscular injection of 1,000 micrograms cyanocobalamin is an essential part of this test.

Contra-indications, warnings, etc

Contra-indications: Hypersensitivity to cyanocobalamin.

Not indicated for treatment of toxic amblyopias – use Neo-Cytamen.

Precautions: The dosage schemes given above are usually satisfactory, but regular examination of the blood is advisable. If megaloblastic anaemia fails to respond to Cytamen, folate metabolism should be investigated.

Doses in excess of 10 micrograms daily may produce a haematological response in patients with folate deficiency. Indiscriminate administration may mask the true diagnosis. Cardiac arrhythmias secondary to hypokalaemia during initial therapy have been reported. Plasma potassium should therefore be monitored during this period.

Pregnancy: Cytamen should not be used for the treatment of megaloblastic anaemia of pregnancy.

Side-effects: Sensitisation to cyanocobalamin is rare but it may present as an itching exanthema, and exceptionally as anaphylactic shock. Acneiform and bullous eruptions have been reported rarely.

Interactions: Chloramphenicol-treated patients may respond poorly to Cytamen. Serum concentrations of cyanocobalamin may be lowered by oral contraceptives.

Overdosage: Treatment is unlikely to be needed in cases of overdosage.

Pharmaceutical precautions Protect from light.

Legal category POM.

Package quantities Ampoules of 1 ml in boxes of 5.

Further information Nil.

Product licence numbers

Cytamen '1000'	0021/0118

DF 118* (Dihydrocodeine Tartrate BP)

Presentation *DF 118 Tablets:* White tablets engraved DF 118. Each tablet contains Dihydrocodeine Tartrate BP 30 mg.

Elixir DF 118: A brown syrup. Each 5 ml contains Dihydrocodeine Tartrate BP 10 mg.

DF 118 Injection: A colourless solution. Each ampoule contains in 1 ml Dihydrocodeine Tartrate BP 50 mg.

Uses Relief of moderate to severe pain. 30 mg given parenterally has been shown to have an analgesic potency equivalent to that of 10 mg of morphine; in a study of oral analgesics for the relief of chronic pain, the same dose was found to be equivalent to 100 mg of pethidine. In both these trials dihydrocodeine was found to have a lower incidence of side-effects than either morphine or pethidine.

In the recommended doses sedative or hypnotic effects are rare and it causes little or no respiratory depression; in addition to being a potent analgesic the compound also exhibits well-defined antitussive activity.

DF 118 is indicated in all painful conditions where an alert patient is desired, viz. sciatica, osteoarthritis, chronic rheumatoid arthritis, arthritis of the spine, peripheral vascular disease, post-herpetic neuralgia, Paget's disease, malignant disease, post-operative pain.

Because DF 118, in the recommended doses, causes little or no respiratory depression, its use in the treatment of post-operative pain may reduce the risk of chest complications.

Dosage and administration *General information:* The oral route is to be preferred whenever possible. The analgesic effect of DF 118 is not materially enhanced by increasing the dose above that recommended below; in severe cases the interval between doses should be reduced to obtain the requisite analgesic cover.

DF 118 is best administered with or after food. It is not recommended for administration to children under 4 years.

Elixir DF 118 is a pleasant tasting liquid suitable for administration to patients who may have difficulty swallowing the tablets.

Dosage – Analgesia.

Adults: DF 118 Tablets: 1 tablet (30 mg) every four to six hours or at the discretion of the physician.

Elixir DF 118: One to three 5 ml spoonfuls (10 to 30 mg) every four to six hours or at the discretion of the physician.

DF 118 Injection: Patients who, for one reason or another are unable to be treated with the tablets or elixir may be given up to 50 mg by intramuscular or deep subcutaneous injection.

Children aged 4 to 12 years: 0.5 to 1 mg/kg body weight every 4 to 6 hours. The Elixir is to be preferred.

Dosage – Antitussive.

Adults: Elixir DF 118: One 5 ml spoonful (10 mg) every four to six hours or at the discretion of the physician.
Children aged 4 to 12 years: 200 micrograms/kg body weight every 4 to 6 hours. The Elixir is to be preferred.

Contra-indications, warnings, etc Respiratory depression; obstructive airways disease.

Precautions: As dihydrocodeine may bring about histamine-release, DF 118 should not be given during an attack of asthma and it should be administered with due care to persons liable to such attacks.

Dosage should be reduced in the elderly, in hypothyroidism, in chronic hepatic disease and in renal insufficiency. Alcohol should be avoided whilst under treatment with DF 118.

There is no, or inadequate evidence of safety in human pregnancy but the drug has been used for many years without apparent ill consequence.

Side-effects: Constipation, nausea, vomiting, headache and vertigo occur and are relatively more common when the dose is increased above 30 mg. If constipation occurs it can be treated with a gentle laxative.

Overdosage: Conservative management is recommended; gastric lavage should be carried out. Severe respiratory depression can be treated with naloxone hydrochloride 0.4 to 2 mg subcutaneously, repeated as required at 2 or 3 minute intervals.

Pharmaceutical precautions The recommended diluent of the Elixir is Unpreserved Syrup BP, or syrup preserved with *p*-hydroxybenzoic acid. The resulting dilution will keep for 14 days at room temperature.

DF 118 preparations should be protected from light.

Legal category DF 118 Tablets   CD (Sch 5), POM.
                              Elixir DF 118   CD (Sch 5), POM.
                              DF 118 Injection   CD (Sch 2), POM.

Package quantities DF 118 Tablets are available in packs of 100 and 500.

Elixir DF 118 is available in bottles of 150 ml and 1 litre.

DF 118 Injection is available in boxes of 5 ampoules of 1.1 ml.

Further information In patients already habituated to a drug such as pethidine, the substitution of dihydrocodeine in equi-analgesic doses has led to the appearance of abstinence symptoms. This suggests that dihydrocodeine, despite its effectiveness as an analgesic, has a low addiction potential and can be administered more frequently than the more potent narcotic drugs and for longer periods.

Product licence numbers
DF 118 Tablets   0021/5063R
Elixir DF 118   0021/0053R
DF 118 Injection   0021/5028R

DINDEVAN* TABLETS

Presentation *Dindevan Tablets 10 mg:* White tablets engraved DF/D10, each tablet containing Phenindione BP 10 mg.

Dindevan Tablets 25 mg: Green tablets engraved DF/D25, each tablet containing Phenindione BP 25 mg.

Dindevan Tablets 50 mg: White tablets engraved DF/D50, each tablet containing Phenindione BP 50 mg.

Uses Dindevan (Phenindione BP) is a synthetic anticoagulant which acts by interfering with the formation of certain clotting factors. It produces its effect in 36 to 48 hours after the initial dose; the effect wanes over a period of 48 to 72 hours after Dindevan is stopped.

Coronary occlusion; deep vein thrombosis; pulmonary embolism; peripheral vascular thromboembolic states; mesenteric and retinal thromboembolism. In emergencies, such as the conditions listed above, anticoagulant therapy should be initiated with heparin and Dindevan together. Where there is less urgency, as in patients at special risk of thromboembolism, anticoagulant therapy may be initiated with Dindevan alone.

Appropriate indications include predisposition to thromboembolism following surgery, during pregnancy and the puerperium, and chronic embolic pulmonary hypertensive disease.

Dosage and administration *Initial loading dose:* Usually 200 mg, followed on the second day with a dose of 100 mg.

Maintenance therapy: Dosage must be adjusted, from the third day, in accordance with the results of appropriate coagulation tests. Concomitant heparin therapy affects the results of control tests and should be discontinued at least six hours before the first test is carried out.

Control tests must be made at regular intervals and the dosage further adjusted according to the results obtained. As a general guide, a maintenance dosage of between 50 to 150 mg per day will prove satisfactory in most cases. Occasionally, a resistant patient may need 200 mg or more per day; on the other hand a sensitive patient may need less than 50 mg per day.

Contra-indications, warnings, etc

Contra-indications: Dindevan should not be given in the presence of severe hepatic or renal disease, actual or potential haemorrhagic conditions, or to patients with uncontrolled hypertension. Its use within 24 hours following surgery or labour should be undertaken with caution, if at all.

Precautions: The following factors may exaggerate the effects of Dindevan and necessitate a reduction in dosage; loss of weight; elderly subject; acute illness; deficient renal function; decreased dietary intake of vitamin K; administration of a number of drugs, including salicylates, quinidine, broad-spectrum antibiotics, phenformin, tolbutamide, phenylbutazone, sulphinpyrazone, cimetidine, azapropazone, clofibrate, ACTH and corticosteroids and all potentially hepato-toxic drugs.

Factors which may call for an increase in maintenance dosage include weight gain, gastro-intestinal upset, increased intake of vitamin K, fats and oils, and administration of drugs (e.g. phenobarbitone) that increase liver enzyme activity.

Oral anticoagulants should not be used in pregnancy unless there are firm indications. In particular, because of possible teratogenicity, they should not be used for the remainder of the first trimester following diagnosis. In addition the risk of fetal haemorrhage is increased when they are used near term. It is therefore suggested that heparin (which does not cross the placenta) be used during the first trimester and after 37 weeks' gestation. However, the use of heparin in pregnancy is not absolutely safe and specialist guidance is advisable for those who are pregnant and who need anti-coagulant therapy. Women of child-bearing age who are receiving treatment with Dindevan should be cautioned about the possible complications of pregnancy. Infants should not be fed with breast milk from mothers being treated with Dindevan.

Side-effects: The following effects have been reported: skin rashes of various kinds, skin necrosis, fever, leucopenia and agranulocytosis, diarrhoea, hepatitis and renal damage with tubular necrosis. If any of these are observed administration of Dindevan should stop immediately and full investigations of blood and of liver and kidney function should be carried out. Possible sensitivity to other drugs should be considered. Other anticoagulants, such as Marevan*, are usually tolerated by patients sensitive to Dindevan. If therapy is controlled as recommended then bleeding due to overdosage of anticoagulant is rare. An episode of bleeding occurring during anticoagulant therapy must, therefore, be investigated fully and not regarded automatically as a manifestation of overdosage.

N.B. The metabolites of Dindevan often colour the urine pink or orange. This may be distinguished from discoloration caused by haemoglobin by the addition of a few drops of dilute acetic acid to the urine. If the colour is due to Dindevan it will disappear immediately.

Overdosage: If haemorrhage occurs or a potential bleeding state arises, excessive depression of the coagulation activity can be corrected by temporary withdrawal of Dindevan accompanied, if necessary, by administration of vitamin K_1, in oral doses of 2 to 20 mg; rarely it may be necessary to give vitamin K_1 intravenously, or to infuse fresh whole blood.

Pharmaceutical precautions No special requirements or precautions.

Legal category POM.

Package quantities Dindevan Tablets 10 mg and Dindevan Tablets 50 mg are each available in containers of 100 and 500 tablets. Dindevan Tablets 25 mg are available in containers of 100 tablets.

Further information Nil.

Product licence numbers
Dindevan Tablets 10 mg   0021/5064
Dindevan Tablets 25 mg   0021/5065
Dindevan Tablets 50 mg   0021/5066

FERSADAY* TABLETS

Presentation Fersaday Tablets are ochre, film-coated tablets engraved 'Fersaday' on one side. Each tablet contains Ferrous Fumarate BP equivalent to 100 mg ferrous iron.

These tablets comply with the specification for Ferrous Fumarate Tablets BP.

Uses Prophylaxis and treatment of iron deficiency states.

Dosage and administration The usual adult dose is one tablet daily. (The foil enclosing the tablets is printed with the days of the week in sequence.) In severe or refractory iron deficiency one Fersaday Tablet may be given twice daily.

This presentation of ferrous fumarate is not intended for the treatment of children.

Contra-indications, warnings, etc

Contra-indications: There are no known contra-indications.

Precautions: Some post-gastrectomy patients show poor absorption of iron. Care is needed when treating patients with peptic ulceration. Fersaday Tablets should be kept out of the reach of children.

Pregnancy: Administration of Fersaday during the first trimester of pregnancy may be undesirable.

Side-effects: Gastro-intestinal disorders have been reported.

Interactions: Absorption of both iron and antibiotic may be reduced if Fersaday is given with a tetracycline.

Concurrent administration of antacids may reduce absorption of iron.

Overdosage: Ingestion of an overdose of iron orally requires emergency treatment along the following lines. Vomiting should be induced immediately, followed as soon as possible by parenteral injection of desferrioxamine mesylate and then gastric lavage. In the meantime it is helpful to give milk and/or 5% sodium bicarbonate solution by mouth.

Dissolve 2 grams desferrioxamine mesylate in 2 or 3 ml of Water for Injections and give intramuscularly. A solution of 5 grams desferrioxamine in 50 to 100 ml of fluid may be left in the stomach. If desferrioxamine is not available, leave 300 ml of 1% to 5% sodium bicarbonate solution in the stomach. Fluid replacement is essential.

Pharmaceutical precautions Protect from light.

Legal category P.

Package quantities Calendar wallet of 28 tablets.

Further information Nil.

Product licence number 0021/5912.

FERSAMAL* TABLETS AND SYRUP

Presentation Fersamal Tablets are small, light brown tablets engraved 'Fersamal' on one side. Each tablet contains Ferrous Fumarate BP equivalent to 65 mg ferrous iron. These tablets comply with the specification for Ferrous Fumarate Tablets BP.

Fersamal Syrup is a brown aqueous suspension containing Ferrous Fumarate BP equivalent to 45 mg ferrous iron per 5 ml.

Uses Prophylaxis and treatment of iron-deficiency states.

For prophylaxis during pregnancy, a combination of iron and folic acid is usually recommended, e.g. Prega-day* Tablets.

Dosage and administration *Adults:* 1 tablet three times a day or two 5 ml spoonfuls of syrup twice a day. The dose may be doubled if required. The tablets are easily swallowed but may also be crushed or chewed being almost tasteless.

Full term infants and young children: Half to one 5 ml spoonful of syrup twice a day.

Premature infants: The usual dosage is 0.6 ml/kg/day but some may require 2.4 ml/kg/day.

Contra-indications, warnings, etc
Contra-indications: There are no known contra-indications.

Precautions: Some post-gastrectomy patients show poor absorption of iron. Care is needed when treating patients with peptic ulceration. Fersamal should be kept out of the reach of children.

Pregnancy: Administration of Fersamal during the first trimester of pregnancy may be undesirable.

Side-effects: Gastro-intestinal disorders have been reported.

Interactions: Absorption of both iron and antibiotic may be reduced if Fersamal is given with a tetracycline.

Concurrent administration of antacids may reduce absorption of iron.

Overdosage: Ingestion of an overdose of iron orally requires emergency treatment along the following lines. Vomiting should be induced immediately, followed as soon as possible by parenteral injection of desferrioxamine mesylate, and then gastric lavage. In the meantime, it is helpful to give milk and/or 5% sodium bicarbonate solution by mouth.

Dissolve 2 grams desferrioxamine mesylate in 2 to 3 ml of Water for Injections and give intramuscularly. A solution of 5 grams desferrioxamine in 50 to 100 ml of fluid may be left in the stomach. If desferrioxamine is not available, leave 300 ml of 1% to 5% sodium bicarbonate solution in the stomach. Fluid replacement is essential.

Pharmaceutical precautions Protect from light.

Legal category P.

Package quantities Tablets: packs of 100 and 1,000. Syrup: bottles of 200 ml.

Further information Fersamal Syrup may be diluted with Syrup BP at the time of dispensing if required.

Product licence numbers
Fersamal Tablets: 0021/5910
Fersamal Syrup: 0021/5911

ILUBE* EYE DROPS ▼

Presentation Ilube Eye Drops: a clear, colourless, sterile solution containing Acetylcysteine BP 5% w/v and Hypromellose 0.35% w/v, preserved with benzalkonium chloride 0.01% w/v. It is presented in a 15 ml glass bottle with a separate glass dropper.

Uses Ilube Eye Drops are artificial tears with mucolytic and lubricant properties, suitable for the relief of dry eye syndromes associated with deficient tear secretion, impaired or abnormal mucous production.

Acetylcysteine has marked mucolytic properties which reduce the viscosity and tenacity of mucus in the eyes. This, combined with the emollient properties of hypromellose, ensures lubrication and soothing relief for dry eye syndromes.

Dosage and administration The usual dosage is one or two drops instilled into the affected eye three or four times daily.

Contra-indications, warnings, etc
Contra-indications: Known hypersensitivity to any component is a contra-indication to the use of Ilube Eye Drops.

Precautions: Ilube eye drops contain benzalkonium chloride as preservative and therefore should not be used to treat patients who wear soft contact lenses.

Discontinue use if discomfort, increased reddening or irritation occurs and persists.

Pharmaceutical precautions Store below 25°C. Protect from light. Avoid touching tip of dropper to prevent contamination. The contents should be discarded 4 weeks after first opening the bottle.

Legal category POM.

Package quantities Amber glass bottle containing 15 ml with separate glass dropper.

Further information Nil.

Product licence number 0021/0116.

JEXIN*

Presentation Jexin is Tubocurarine Injection BP and is a clear colourless, or faintly coloured sterile solution containing Tubocurarine Chloride BP 10 mg per ml.

Uses Jexin produces paralysis of voluntary muscle by interfering with transmission across the neuromuscular junction. It acts by competitive blockade of motor endplates. Paralysis appears in the muscles of the face and neck, of the limbs and of the abdomen, in that order, the intercostal muscles and diaphragm being affected last. The paralysis reaches its maximum two to five minutes after intravenous injection and lasts for about 30 minutes. There is, however, a residual action lasting for as long as 24 hours, and during this time smaller doses are required to reproduce the effect of the initial dose.

Jexin is mainly indicated as an adjunct to anaesthesia to secure muscular relaxation in surgery and obstetrics. It can also be used in tetanus.

Dosage and administration *Adults:* Dosage should

be based on the response to an initial intravenous injection of 10 to 15 mg. A test dose of 5 mg in the unanaesthetised patient may be administered before giving the full initial dose. Supplementary doses of 5 mg are adequate, if required for lengthy operations. A total of 40 mg for a single operation should not be exceeded.

Children: The initial dose is of the order of 0.32 mg per kg of body weight.

Contra-indications, warnings, etc

Contra-indications: Jexin is contra-indicated in patients with respiratory insufficiency or in the presence of renal or hepatic impairment.

Precautions: In patients with myasthenia gravis or myasthenic syndrome, Jexin should be administered in very small doses and with extreme caution; a reduction in dosage is also advisable in cases of gross obesity, myopathy and after poliomyelitis. Patients with asthma or those susceptible to bronchospasm require especial care as Jexin is known to cause the release of histamine. In such patients the prophylactic administration of an anti-histamine may be advisable.

Care is necessary if Jexin has to be given to a patient on two occasions within 24 hours. Administration of Jexin either with or before a depolarising relaxant, such as suxamethonium, may cause a muscle relaxation which is irreversible by neostigmine. The effects of Jexin are enhanced by ether; the hypotension produced by halothane anaesthesia is increased by Jexin and a reduced dose of Jexin should be used. This caution should also be noted in the elderly.

Jexin may be potentiated by diazepam and by clindamycin, colistin, kanamycin, neomycin, polymyxins, streptomycin, tobramycin, framycetin, amikacin, gentamicin and other amino-glycoside antibiotics and by quinidine.

Pregnancy: The drug should not be administered to pregnant women unless the potential benefit outweighs the possible hazard.

Side-effects: The dosage recommended produces few side-effects; a transient fall in blood pressure may sometimes occur.

Overdosage: Intravenous neostigmine with atropine sulphate. Oxygen and assisted respiration may be required.

Pharmaceutical precautions No special requirements or precautions.

Legal category POM.

Package quantities Jexin is supplied in 1.5 ml ampoules in boxes of 5.

Further information Although Jexin should not normally be mixed with thiopentone, this can be done if prepared immediately prior to injection and used only if the solution remains perfectly clear.

Product licence number 0021/5025.

LOCAN* CREAM

Presentation Locan Cream, a smooth, white cream, contains:

Amylocaine	1%
Amethocaine	0.8%
Cinchocaine BPC	0.4%

in a non-greasy base which does not soil or stain the clothing.

Uses The combination of the lipid-soluble free bases of amethocaine, amylocaine and cinchocaine provides rapid, yet sustained, relief from pruritic and painful conditions.

Locan Cream is of particular value in the treatment of pruritus ani, pruritus vulvae, external haemorrhoids and anal fissure; it should also be found useful in relieving the pain of cracked or sore nipples, minor burns, chilblains and athlete's foot. The analgesic effect may also be found useful in alleviating localised muscular pain arising from conditions which do not need prolonged treatment.

Administration A thin layer of Locan Cream should be applied over the affected area and massaged in gently until absorption is complete. The application may be renewed as required.

Contra-indications, warnings, etc

Contra-indications: Known sensitivity to local analgesics.

Precautions: Sensitisation may occur to the local analgesics contained in Locan Cream. This should be suspected, and application stopped, if increased irritation or reddening occurs.

Side-effects: No other side-effects are likely to be encountered.

Overdosage: Not applicable.

Pharmaceutical precautions No special requirements or precautions.

Legal category P.

Package quantities Locan Cream is available in tubes of 30 g.

Further information Nil.

Product licence number 0021/5010.

MAREVAN* TABLETS

Presentation Marevan Tablets are Warfarin Tablets BP.

Marevan Tablets 1 mg: Brown tablets engraved DF/M1, each tablet containing Warfarin Sodium BP 1 mg.

Marevan Tablets 3 mg: Blue tablets engraved DF/M3, each tablet containing Warfarin Sodium BP 3 mg.

Marevan Tablets 5 mg: Pink tablets engraved DF/M5, each tablet containing Warfarin Sodium BP 5 mg.

Uses Marevan is a synthetic anticoagulant of the coumarin series and acts by inhibiting the formation of certain clotting factors. An effect on prothrombin time is produced in 24 to 36 hours after the initial dose. This reaches a maximum in 36 to 48 hours and is maintained for 48 hours or more after administration is stopped.

Coronary occlusion; deep vein thrombosis; pulmonary embolism; peripheral vascular thromboembolic states; mesenteric and retinal thromboembolism.

In emergencies, such as the conditions listed above, anticoagulant therapy should be initiated with heparin and Marevan together. Where there is less urgency, as in patients disposed to or at special risk of thromboembolism, anticoagulant therapy may be initiated with Marevan alone. Appropriate indications include predisposition to thromboembolism following surgery, during pregnancy and the puerperium and chronic embolic pulmonary hypertensive disease.

Dosage and administration 10 to 15 mg daily, according to age and body weight, and adjusted with relation to the results of daily control tests until the desired level of anticoagulant activity is achieved – usually three to six days after the initiation of treatment.

Concomitant heparin therapy affects the results of control tests and should be discontinued at least six hours before the first test is carried out.

Control tests should be made at regular intervals and Marevan maintenance dosage further adjusted according to the results obtained.

Contra-indications, warnings, etc
Contra-indications: Marevan should not be given in the presence of severe hepatic or renal disease, actual or potential haemorrhagic conditions, or to patients with uncontrolled hypertension. Its use within 24 hours following surgery or labour should be undertaken with caution if at all.

Precautions: The following factors may exaggerate the effects of Marevan and necessitate a reduction in dosage: loss of weight; elderly patient; acute illness; deficient renal function; decreased dietary intake of vitamin K; administration of a number of drugs, including salicylates, sulphinpyrazone, cimetidine, azapropazone, quinidine, broad spectrum antibiotics, phenformin, tolbutamide, phenylbutazone, clofibrate, ACTH and corticosteroids and all potentially hepatotoxic drugs. Factors which may call for an increase in maintenance dosage include weight gain, gastro-intestinal upset, increased intake of vitamin K, fats and oils, and administration of drugs (e.g. phenobarbitone) that increase liver enzyme activity.

Oral anticoagulants should not be used in pregnancy unless there are firm indications. In particular, because of possible teratogenicity, they should not be used for the remainder of the first trimester following diagnosis. In addition the risk of fetal haemorrhage is increased when they are used near term. It is therefore suggested that heparin (which does not cross the placenta) be used during the first trimester and after 37 weeks' gestation. However, the use of heparin in pregnancy is not absolutely safe and specialist guidance is advisable for those who are pregnant and who need anticoagulant therapy. Women of child-bearing age who are receiving treatment with Marevan should be cautioned about the possible complications of pregnancy.

Side-effects: Side-effects from Marevan are uncommon. A few instances of alopecia, skin rashes of various kinds, diarrhoea and an unexplained drop in haematocrit have been reported, and a 'purple toes' syndrome has been described. If any of these are observed administration of Marevan should cease and a change be made to another anticoagulant. It may be advisable to avoid other coumarin preparations when a suitable alternative could be Dindevan*.

Skin necrosis within a few days of starting treatment has been infrequently reported. Most subjects are obese, elderly women. The first sign is an erythematous swollen patch. Administration of vitamin K_1 at this stage may prevent the development of ecchymosis and infarction.

Possible sensitivity to other drugs used should be considered. Bleeding due to anticoagulant overdosage is uncommon and unlikely to occur if the recommended method and degree of control is practised and the patient is maintained stable within the therapeutic range. An episode of bleeding occurring during anticoagulant therapy must, therefore, be investigated fully and not regarded simply as a manifestation of overdosage.

Overdosage: If haemorrhage occurs or a potential bleeding state arises, excessive depression of the coagulation activity can be corrected by temporary withdrawal of Marevan accompanied, if necessary, by administration of vitamin K_1, in oral doses of 2 to 20 mg; rarely it may be necessary to give vitamin K_1 intravenously, or to infuse fresh whole blood.

Pharmaceutical precautions Replace cap securely and protect from light.

Legal category POM.

Package quantities Marevan Tablets 1 mg are available in containers of 100 and 500.

Marevan Tablets 3 mg are available in containers of 100 and 500.

Marevan Tablets 5 mg are available in containers of 100 and 500.

Further information Nil.

Product licence numbers
Marevan Tablets 1 mg　0021/5071R
Marevan Tablets 3 mg　0021/5072R
Marevan Tablets 5 mg　0021/5073R

MULTIVITE* PELLETS

Presentation A dark brown, sugar-coated pellet. Each Multivite Pellet contains:

Vitamin A　2,500 i.u.
Vitamin B_1　0.5 mg
Vitamin C　12.5 mg
Vitamin D　250 i.u.

Uses Vitamins A, B_1, C and D are essential to health and vitality. Although these vitamins occur naturally in various foods, adequate nutrition is not always attainable for all. Even if balanced diets are achieved the vitamin content may be reduced or even completely destroyed by cooking. Patients with diminished appetites, restricted diets or inadequate meals, especially during childhood, pregnancy, illness and old age, often develop vitamin deficiencies. Multivite will help to correct a vitamin deficiency, and to build resistance against infection.

Dosage and administration *Adults:* 2 Multivite daily.

Children: 1 Multivite daily.

Multivite Pellets are pleasant tasting and may be chewed or swallowed whole, according to preference.

Contra-indications, warnings, etc There are no contra-indications.

Precautions: Excessive prolonged dosage of vitamins A and D may lead to hypervitaminosis.

Side-effects: None in the absence of overdosage.

Overdosage: No emergency treatment is necessary.

Pharmaceutical precautions To be stored in a cool place and protected from light.

Legal category P.

Package quantities Multivite Pellets are available in containers of 50, 150 and 500.

Further information Nil.

Product licence number 0021/5081.

NEO-CYTAMEN* (Hydroxocobalamin Injection BP)

Presentation Ampoules containing a clear, red solution which provides either 250 micrograms (Neo-Cytamen '250') or 1,000 micrograms (Neo-Cytamen '1000') of hydroxocobalamin per millilitre. Neo-Cytamen Injection complies with the specification for Hydroxocobalamin Injection BP.

Uses Addisonian pernicious anaemia. Prophylaxis and treatment of other macrocytic anaemias associated with vitamin B_{12} deficiency. Tobacco amblyopia and Leber's optic atrophy.

Dosage and administration The following dosage schemes are suitable for adults and children.

Addisonian pernicious anaemia and other macrocytic anaemias without neurological involvement: Initially: 250 to 1,000 micrograms intramuscularly on alternate days for one to two weeks, then 250 micrograms weekly until the blood count is normal.

Maintenance: 1,000 micrograms every two or three months.

Addisonian pernicious anaemia and other macrocytic anaemias with neurological involvement: Initially: 1,000 micrograms on alternate days as long as improvement is occurring.

Maintenance: 1,000 micrograms every two months.

Prophylaxis of macrocytic anaemia associated with vitamin B_{12} deficiency resulting from gastrectomy, some malabsorption syndromes and strict vegetarianism: 1,000 micrograms every two or three months.

Tobacco amblyopia and Leber's optic atrophy: Initially: 1,000 micrograms or more daily by intramuscular injection for two weeks then twice weekly as long as improvement is occurring.

Maintenance: 1,000 micrograms monthly.

Contra-indications, warnings, etc

Contra-indications: Hypersensitivity to hydroxocobalamin.

Precautions: The dosage schemes given above are usually satisfactory, but regular examination of the blood is advisable. If megaloblastic anaemia fails to respond to Neo-Cytamen, folate metabolism should be investigated. Doses in excess of 10 micrograms daily may produce a haematological response in patients with folate deficiency. Indiscriminate administration may mask the true diagnosis.

Cardiac arrhythmias secondary to hypokalaemia during initial therapy have been reported. Plasma potassium should therefore be monitored during this period.

Pregnancy: Neo-Cytamen should not be used for the treatment of megaloblastic anaemia of pregnancy.

Side-effects: Sensitisation to hydroxocobalamin is rare but may manifest itself as itching exanthema, and exceptionally, anaphylaxis. Acneiform and bullous eruptions have been reported rarely.

Interactions: Chloramphenicol-treated patients may respond poorly to Neo-Cytamen. Serum concentrations of hydroxocobalamin may be lowered by oral contraceptives.

Overdosage: Treatment is unlikely to be needed in cases of overdosage.

Pharmaceutical precautions Protect from light.

Legal category POM.

Package quantities Ampoules of 1 ml in boxes of 5.

Further information An intramuscular injection of hydroxocobalamin produces higher serum levels than the same dose of cyanocobalamin, and these levels are well maintained.

Product licence numbers
Neo-Cytamen '250'   0021/0120
Neo-Cytamen '1000'   0021/0121

NEO-NACLEX*

Presentation Small white tablets engraved 'Neo-NaClex' on one side and scored on the reverse. Each tablet contains 5 mg bendrofluazide and complies with the specification for Bendrofluazide Tablets BP.

Uses *Oedema:* Neo-NaClex inhibits the renal tubular absorption of salt and water. Sodium and chloride ions are excreted in equivalent proportions, and there is little or no disturbance of the acid/base equilibrium. There is no important effect upon carbonic anhydrase. Neo-NaClex causes a steady diuresis lasting for about 12 hours. It is indicated in the treatment of oedema associated with conditions such as: congestive heart failure, nephrotic syndrome, cirrhosis of the liver, and pre-menstrual tension.

Suppression of unwanted lactation: Neo-NaClex can inhibit lactation as effectively as the oestrogens, but without early engorgement of the breast or other hormonal effects.

Essential hypertension: The mechanism whereby the thiazides exert their antihypertensive effect has not been clearly established. In non-oedematous patients there may be little noticeable diuretic effect. Neo-NaClex may be used as the sole antihypertensive agent, or as an adjunct to other drugs whose action it potentiates.

Dosage and administration *Oedema:* In adults 5 mg given orally once daily in the morning usually produces the desired effect, but this dose can be increased to 10 mg if required. During the first few days of treatment there is usually a large increase in urinary volume, which diminishes as treatment continues.

Maintenance: Many patients will respond adequately to a daily dose of 2.5 mg or 5 mg on only two or three days in the week: sometimes a single dose once a week may be sufficient. The intervals allow opportunity for replenishment of any potassium loss. Appropriately smaller doses should be used for children.

Essential hypertension: 2.5 to 10 mg once daily, alone or in conjunction with other antihypertensive agents.

Pre-menstrual tension: 2.5 mg taken each morning for seven days before the period is due is usually adequate.

Suppression of lactation: A suitable dosage is 5 mg (or 10 mg) on rising in the morning and 5 mg about noon. A course of five days' treatment is usually adequate.

Contra-indications, warnings, etc

Contra-indications: Severe renal insufficiency, hypercalcaemia. Neo-NaClex should not be administered concurrently with lithium carbonate.

Precautions: Neo-NaClex may impair control of diabetes in patients receiving sulphonylureas.

Thiazide diuretics are secreted in mothers' milk, hence breast feeding should be avoided.

When treatment with Neo-NaClex is intensive or continuous, some loss of potassium may occur, and in these circumstances potassium chloride supplements are recommended. If the patient is elderly or vomiting, has diarrhoea or is suffering from an acute febrile or chronic illness (especially cirrhosis of the liver or heart failure) supplementary potassium may be particularly important. Supplementary potassium is strongly recommended if patients receiving digitalis require prolonged diuretic treatment. Concurrent therapy with carbenoxolone may also necessitate potassium supplements.

Potassium depletion may cause polyuria, malaise, muscle weakness or cramp, decreased tendon reflexes, anorexia, dizziness, nausea or vomiting. Also, sensitivity to digitalis may increase and signs of over-dosage appear. Prolonged potassium deficiency may induce chronic pyelonephritis. Potassium supplements should not be given in renal insufficiency complicated by hyperkalaemia.

Side-effects: Impotence may occur and is usually reversible within a few weeks of stopping Neo-NaClex therapy. Mild anorexia or indigestion may occur occasionally, but it can be avoided or reduced by taking the dose during or immediately after a meal.

Skin reactions have been reported in a few patients and blood dyscrasias have occurred rarely. Expectant mothers who receive thiazide diuretics may be at increased risk from acute haemorrhagic pancreatitis; thrombocytopenia has been reported in newborn infants following antepartum use of thiazides. Such cases are very rare, and should not prevent the use of thiazide diuretics when indicated in pregnancy. Thiazides may aggravate existing diabetes mellitus, and cause symptoms in patients with latent disease. Serum uric acid levels may be raised, with or without gout, in some patients.

Overdosage: Treatment should be symptomatic and directed at fluid and electrolyte replacement. In the case of recent ingestion gastric lavage should be carried out.

Pharmaceutical precautions Protect from light.

Legal category POM.

Package quantities Containers of 100 and 500 tablets.

Further information Nil.

Product licence number 0021/5906.

NEO-NACLEX*-K

Presentation Neo-NaClex-K is a film-coated, two-layer tablet containing bendrofluazide in the white layer and potassium chloride in the pink layer. The white side is engraved 'Neo-NaClex-K'. The potassium chloride is in a special matrix which provides gradual release of the electrolytes, so minimising gastro-intestinal irritation. Each tablet contains 2.5 mg bendrofluazide and 630 mg potassium chloride, providing 330 mg elemental potassium (8.4 mEq).

Uses *Essential hypertension:* The mechanism whereby the thiazides exert their antihypertensive effect has not been clearly established. In non-oedematous patients there may be little noticeable diuretic effect. Neo-NaClex-K may be used as the sole antihypertensive agent, or as an adjunct to other drugs whose action it potentiates. When Neo-NaClex-K is used alone in hypertension, the fall in diastolic blood pressure is often between 10 and 20 mm Hg.

When Neo-NaClex-K is added to other antihypertensive drugs, the dosage of the latter can usually be reduced gradually as the Neo-NaClex-K takes effect.

The potassium chloride contained in Neo-NaClex-K provides a useful supplement to offset the potassium-losing effect of bendrofluazide.

Oedema: Neo-NaClex-K is particularly suitable for the treatment of chronic oedema.

Dosage and administration *Essential hypertension: Adults:* 1 to 4 tablets once daily, alone or in conjunction with other antihypertensive agents.

Oedema: In adults: 2 tablets given orally once daily in the morning usually produce the desired effect, but this dose can be increased to 4 tablets if required. During the first few days of treatment there is usually a large increase in urinary volume, which diminishes as treatment continues.

Maintenance: Many patients will respond adequately to a daily dose of 1 or 2 tablets on only two or three days in the week, sometimes a single dose once a week may be sufficient.

Appropriately smaller doses should be used for oedema in children.

Contra-indications, warnings, etc
Contra-indications: Gross impairment of renal function; hypercalcaemia, hyperkalaemia, Addison's Disease. Neo-NaClex-K should not be administered concurrently with lithium carbonate.

Precautions: Thiazide diuretics are secreted in mothers' milk, hence breast feeding should be avoided.

When treatment is prolonged and intensive, potassium depletion can develop insidiously particularly in the elderly or in the presence of diarrhoea or vomiting. Neo-NaClex-K Tablets usually provide sufficient potassium to maintain the serum concentration in hypertension, but in oedema it is sometimes advisable to give potassium chloride in addition to that contained in Neo-NaClex-K. Potassium deficiency increases the activity of digitalis and signs of overdosage may appear.

Neo-NaClex-K may impair control of diabetes in patients receiving sulphonylureas.

Side-effects: Impotence may occur and is usually reversible within a few weeks of stopping Neo-NaClex-K therapy. Mild anorexia or indigestion may occur occasionally, but it can be avoided or reduced by taking the dose during or immediately after a meal. If abdominal pain, distension, nausea, vomiting or gastro-intestinal bleeding occur during the administration of tablets containing potassium salts, administration should be discontinued immediately. Small bowel lesions are usually associated with enteric-coated tablets, and are less likely to occur with Neo-NaClex-K.

Skin reactions have been reported in a few patients and blood dyscrasias have occurred rarely. Expectant mothers who receive thiazide diuretics may be at increased risk from acute haemorrhagic pancreatitis; thrombocytopenia has been reported in newborn infants following ante-partum use of thiazides. Such cases are very rare and should not prevent the use of thiazide diuretics when indicated in pregnancy. Thiazides may aggravate existing diabetes mellitus, and cause symptoms in patients with latent disease. Serum uric acid levels may be raised, with or without gout, in some patients.

Overdosage: Treatment should be symptomatic and

directed at fluid and electrolytic replacement. In the case of recent ingestion gastric lavage should be carried out.

Severe hyperkalaemia following overdose with potassium-containing thiazide combinations is rare. ECG monitoring is required and treatment depends on the plasma potassium levels. When this is less than 6.5 mEq/L, fluid replacement with intravenous glucose/saline is usually sufficient. For levels between 6.5 and 8 mEq/L, administer oral sodium polystyrene sulphonate 30 g in 150 to 200 ml of water.

If the plasma potassium concentration exceeds 8 mEq/L, an intravenous injection of 10 to 30 ml calcium gluconate 10% should be given.

Pharmaceutical precautions None.

Legal category POM.

Package quantities Containers of 100 and 500 tablets.

Further information Nil.

Product licence number 0021/5907.

PARAMOL* TABLETS (Co-dydramol— Dihydrocodeine and Paracetamol Tablets)

Presentation A white tablet engraved Paramol, each tablet containing:

Paracetamol BP	500 mg
Dihydrocodeine Tartrate BP	10 mg

Uses Paracetamol is an effective analgesic possessing a remarkably low level of side-effects. Its broad clinical utility has been extensively reported, and it now largely replaces aspirin for routine use. Paracetamol is well tolerated; having a bland effect on gastric mucosa, unlike aspirin, it neither exacerbates symptoms of peptic ulcer nor precipitates bleeding. Dihydrocodeine tartrate has been widely used for a number of years as a powerful analgesic; 30 mg of dihydrocodeine has been reported to have analgesic potency equal to 60 to 120 mg codeine.

In addition the compound exhibits well-defined antitussive activity.

By fortifying paracetamol with 10 mg dihydrocodeine, Paramol provides an effective combination of drugs for the treatment of mild to moderate pain and as an antipyretic.

Dosage and administration Paramol Tablets should, if possible, be taken during or after meals.

Adults and children over 12 years: Analgesia: 1 tablet every four hours. This may be increased to 2 tablets four times a day if necessary.

Antitussive: 1 tablet every four hours.

Paramol is not recommended for children under 12 years.

Contra-indications, warnings, etc Respiratory depression, obstructive airways disease.

Precautions: Additive CNS depression may occur with alcohol.

Paramol should be given with caution to patients with allergic disorders and should not be given during an attack of asthma. Caution should also be observed if there is marked impairment of liver function or advanced kidney disease.

Dosage should be reduced in the elderly, in hypothy-roidism and in chronic hepatic disease. An overdose can cause hepatic necrosis.

There is no, or inadequate evidence of safety in human pregnancy but the drug has been used for many years without apparent ill consequence.

Side-effects: Constipation, if it occurs, is readily treated with a mild laxative. Nausea, headache, vertigo and giddiness may occur in a few patients.

Overdosage: Conservative management is recommended; gastric lavage should be carried out. Severe respiratory depression can be treated with naloxone hydrochloride 0.4 to 2 mg subcutaneously, repeated as required at 2 or 3 minute intervals. Treatment for paracetamol overdosage should be commenced as soon as possible after ingestion using preferably acetylcysteine or cysteamine or methionine.

Pharmaceutical precautions No special requirements or precautions.

Legal category CD (Sch 5), POM.

Package quantities Paramol Tablets are available in containers of 100 and 500.

Further information Nil.

Product licence number 0021/5056R.

PARVOLEX*

Presentation Parvolex is a clear, colourless, sterile, pyrogen-free, aqueous solution of 20% w/v Acetylcysteine BP (N-acetyl-3-mercapto-alanine) adjusted to pH 7.0 with sodium hydroxide. Parvolex contains 200 mg acetylcysteine in each ml i.e., each 10 ml ampoule contains 2 g.

Uses Acetylcysteine is a derivative of the naturally-occurring amino acid L-cysteine.

In paracetamol overdosage the observed hepatotoxicity is due to the formation of a toxic metabolite which is thought to cause liver cell damage and necrosis. Hepatic-reduced glutathione inactivates the toxic metabolite by conjugation but glutathione stores are rapidly depleted with hepatotoxic doses of paracetamol. Acetylcysteine, being a sulphydryl (SH) group donor, protects the liver possibly by restoring depleted hepatic-reduced glutathione or by acting as an alternative substrate for the toxic paracetamol metabolite.

Indications: Paracetamol overdosage.

Dosage and administration An initial dose of 150 mg/kg body weight of acetylcysteine is infused in 200 ml of 5% dextrose intravenously over 15 minutes, followed by an intravenous infusion of 50 mg/kg body weight in 500 ml of 5% dextrose over the next four hours, and 100 mg/kg body weight in 1 litre of 5% dextrose over the next 16 hours. (This gives a total dose of 300 mg/kg body weight of acetylcysteine in 20 hours.)

NOTE: Parvolex contains 200 mg acetylcysteine per ml; i.e., each 10 ml ampoule contains 2 g.

Children: The quantity of intravenous fluid used in children should be modified to take into account age and weight.

Critical times: Parvolex is very effective when administered up to eight hours after paracetamol overdosage. The protective effect falls off slowly between eight and ten hours, more rapidly after ten hours and increasingly between twelve and fifteen hours. Parvolex is ineffective after fifteen hours and its use after this time may be associated with harmful effects.

Contra-indications, warnings, etc No contra-indications have been reported.

Precautions: Administer with caution in asthma or a history of same. Acetylcysteine is not compatible with rubber and metals, particularly, iron, copper and nickel. Silicone rubber and plastic are satisfactory for use with Parvolex.

Side-effects: Rash and anaphylaxis have been reported. These have occurred between fifteen minutes and one hour after the start of the infusion.

Hypokalaemia and ECG changes have been noted in patients with paracetamol poisoning irrespective of the treatment given. Monitoring of plasma potassium concentration is therefore recommended. The safety of Parvolex in pregnancy has not been established.

Overdosage: There is a theoretical risk of hepatic encephalopathy. There is no specific treatment and general supportive measures should be carried out.

Pharmaceutical precautions Parvolex should be stored in a cool place.

Legal category POM.

Package quantities Parvolex is supplied in ampoules of 10 ml. 10 × 10 ml ampoules are packed in printed cartons.

Further information Nil.

Product licence number 0021/0086.

PERNIVIT* TABLETS

Presentation Salmon-pink, sugar-coated tablets, each tablet containing:

Acetomenaphthone BP   7 mg
Nicotinic Acid BP   25 mg

Uses The action of Pernivit is based principally on the vasodilating effect of nicotinic acid while aceto-menaphthone (vitamin K analogue) is also known to alleviate symptoms. A combination of these two substances, Pernivit has long been recognised as a simple and useful preparation for the prophylaxis and treatment of chilblains.

Dosage and administration *Adults:* 2 to 3 tablets three times a day after meals.

Children: 1 to 2 tablets three times a day after meals. For prophylactic treatment half the recommended dose should be taken.

Patients with advanced atherosclerosis may not obtain the maximum benefit from Pernivit.

Contra-indications, warnings, etc
Contra-indications: Patients who are undergoing anti-coagulant therapy.

Precautions: Pernivit should be given cautiously to patients with a history of peptic ulceration, and to those receiving antihypertensive agents.

Allergic reactions to Pernivit have been reported on rare occasions and treatment should be stopped if a rash appears.

The Elderly: The dose range should be reduced to 1 to 2 tablets three times a day after meals.

Pregnancy: Notice should be taken of current views that

any drug should be prescribed with caution during pregnancy.

Side-effects: A flushing of the face is sometimes associated with the tablets, but this is normally transient.

Overdosage: The toxic effects normally subside without treatment.

Pharmaceutical precautions There are no special requirements or precautions.

Legal category P.

Package quantities Pernivit Tablets are available in containers of 100.

Further information Nil.

Product licence number 0021/5083.

PREGADAY* TABLETS

Presentation Pregaday Tablets are reddish brown, film-coated tablets engraved 'Pregaday' on one face. Each tablet contains Ferrous Fumarate BP equivalent to 100 mg ferrous iron and 350 micrograms (0.35 mg) anhydrous folic acid.

Uses There is evidence that a daily intake of 100 mg of elemental iron in the ferrous form is adequate to prevent development of iron deficiency in expectant mothers. If a mild iron deficiency is present when Pregaday administration is started, this will be corrected by increased absorption of iron. The daily folate requirement rises steeply during the final trimester of pregnancy, and evidence of maternal depletion may be found. To ensure normal tissue folate levels in the mother after delivery, a daily supplement of about 300 micrograms is required during the second and third trimester of pregnancy. This dose does not obscure the blood picture of Addisonian pernicious anaemia. Pregaday is indicated during the second and third trimester of pregnancy for prophylaxis against iron deficiency and megaloblastic anaemia of pregnancy. Pregaday is not intended as a treatment for established megaloblastic anaemia of pregnancy.

Dosage and administration It is usual to begin therapy with Pregaday about the thirteenth week of pregnancy (see Precautions) either as routine prophylaxis or selectively if the haemoglobin concentration is less than 11 grams/100 ml (less than 75% of normal).

One tablet daily by mouth (the foil enclosing the tablets is printed with the days of the week in sequence). When necessary, one tablet may be given twice daily.

Contra-indications, warnings, etc
Contra-indications: Vitamin B_{12} deficiency.

Precautions: Administration of Pregaday during the first trimester of pregnancy may be undesirable.

A minority of pregnant women are not protected by physiological doses of folic acid. The development of anaemia despite prophylaxis with Pregaday calls for investigation. Some post-gastrectomy patients show poor absorption of iron. Care is needed when treating patients with peptic ulceration. Pregaday Tablets should be kept out of the reach of children.

Side-effects: Gastro-intestinal disorders and allergic reactions have been reported.

Interactions: Absorption of both iron and antibiotic may be reduced if Pregaday is given with a tetracycline.

Concurrent administration of antacids may reduce absorption of iron.

Co-trimoxazole may inhibit megaloblastic haemopoiesis.

Serum anticonvulsant levels may be reduced by administration of folate.

Overdosage: Ingestion of an overdose of iron orally requires emergency treatment along the following lines. Vomiting should be induced immediately, followed as soon as possible by parenteral injection of desferrioxamine mesylate, and then gastric lavage. In the meantime, it is helpful to give milk and/or 5% sodium bicarbonate solution by mouth.

Dissolve 2 grams desferrioxamine mesylate in 2 to 3 ml of Water for Injections and give intramuscularly. A solution of 5 grams desferrioxamine in 50 to 100 ml of fluid may be left in the stomach. If desferrioxamine is not available, leave 300 ml of 1% to 5% sodium bicarbonate solution in the stomach. Fluid replacement is essential.

Pharmaceutical precautions Protect from light.

Legal category POM.

Package quantities Calendar wallet of 28 tablets.

Further information Nil.

Product licence number 0021/0119.

PROSPAROL* EMULSION

Presentation A white emulsion containing 50% Arachis Oil BP in water and providing 4.5 calories per ml (1.9 MJ per 100 ml).

Uses The special homogenising process used in the manufacture of Prosparol produces exceptionally fine particles of approximately 1 to 2 microns in diameter which have little tendency to separate out. The resulting emulsion is palatable and better tolerated than natural fats.

In radiology (cholecystography): Prosparol fulfils all the essentials of a satisfactory gall-bladder contraction medium – quick absorption, reliable visualisation, speedy examination.

In dietetics: Prosparol is indicated in trauma, illness, in a ketogenic diet in the management of epilepsy and convalescence, whenever a high calorie intake will minimise tissue destruction and favour recovery. Calorie intake following trauma, or in preparation for surgery, should provide an adequate margin over the basal requirement to correct possible deficits: 3,000 calories for total nourishment and 2,000 calories as supplement would permit steady weight gain.

Dosage and administration *Cholecystography:* 30 to 60 ml.

Dietetics: Up to 500 ml (2,250 calories) per day may generally be administered without any digestive disturbance. It is best given in frequent small doses 20 to 40 ml at a time.

Prosparol may be taken neat, or diluted with milk or fruit juice; some patients prefer it chilled. It can be given orally or by nasogastric tube. 1 oz (28.3 g) Prosparol mixed with 1 oz sugar in ½ pint (284 ml) water can be used as a non-protein milk substitute in tea, coffee or made into custard or instant whip.

Easily prepared supplemental and total diets containing Prosparol have been recommended in conjunction with milk, lactose and finely divided protein with the addition of electrolytes as needed.

Infants with sugar intolerance can be fed initially with a low-fat preparation and then, when they begin to thrive, to increase the fat intake gradually by adding Prosparol to the feeds. Prosparol is a valuable calorific supplement to Aminogran* (Allen & Hanburys), and other amino-acid preparations used in the management of phenylketonuria.

For the dietetic treatment of patients with anorexia nervosa, a liquid diet has been suggested containing Prosparol, a liquid food substitute, and glucose suitably flavoured with instant coffee or cocoa.

Contra-indications, warnings, etc There are no contra-indications.

Precautions: Prosparol should only be given to diabetic patients as part of their diet.

Patients with liver or gall-bladder disorders are unlikely to tolerate appreciable quantities of Prosparol.

Side-effects: Occasional fat intolerance may be encountered.

Overdosage: An overdosage will produce intolerance and no special treatment is necessary.

Pharmaceutical precautions Prosparol should be stored in a cool place but must not be frozen.

Legal category P.

Package quantities Prosparol is available in containers of 1 litre.

Further information Fat contains considerably less bulk per calorie than does protein or carbohydrate and there is over 90% absorption.

Unlike protein, fat is not wasted by 'spill-over' through the kidneys and the small rise in blood sugar following fat ingestion causes less interference to appetite than do carbohydrates.

Prosparol contains 0.1% w/v Sodium Benzoate (6.9 milliequivalents of sodium per litre); it does not contain potassium.

Product licence number 0021/5009.

SCOLINE*

Presentation A clear, colourless, sterile solution containing Suxamethonium Chloride (succinylcholine chloride) BP 50 mg per ml. This is equivalent to 36.5 mg of active cation.

Uses Scoline is a depolarising, short-acting neuromuscular blocking agent for intravenous administration. It is suitable for brief procedures in which profound muscular relaxation is required such as tracheal intubation, short operations, orthopaedic manipulations, electroconvulsive therapy and closure of the peritoneum. Prolonged muscular relaxation in surgery can be attained by means of repeated injections of the drug or by continuous intravenous drip.

Dosage and administration Scoline must not be administered to the conscious patient. It is given intravenously after anaesthesia has been induced (e.g. after thiopentone and from a different syringe) and should be accompanied by assisted respiration. The dosage for children and adults depends on body weight and the degree of muscular relaxation required. It ranges from 20 mg (0.4 ml) to 100 mg (2 ml) according to the body weight of the patient and the degree of muscular relaxation required. In adults the dosage for intubation is from 50mg (1 ml) to 80 mg (1.6 ml), for electroconvulsive therapy 40 mg (0.8 ml) to 75 mg (1.5 ml) and for manipulation 80 mg (1.6 ml). For administration by continuous intravenous drip, a 0.1% solution may be prepared by mixing 10 ml injection of Scoline with 500 ml of 5% glucose or isotonic sodium chloride. The adult dose ranges from 2 to 5 mg per minute.

Contra-indications, warnings, etc

Contra-indications: Scoline should not be used in patients known to have atypical serum pseudocholinesterase or low serum levels of pseudocholinesterase. Deficiency of this serum enzyme may occur as a very rare inherited characteristic or result from liver disease, severe anaemia, malnutrition or poisoning with an organo-phosphorus insecticide.

Patients with myasthenia gravis are resistant to Scoline and a state of dual block may develop rapidly.

Patients with the myasthenic (Eaton-Lambert) syndrome are relatively sensitive to Scoline and the dose should be reduced.

If eye drops containing long-acting cholinesterase inhibitor drugs, such as ecothiopate iodide (Phospholine iodide* Ayerst Laboratories Ltd) or demecarium bromide (Tosmilen* Sinclair), are used within a period of one month prior to an operation, then decreased plasma cholinesterase levels may preclude the use of Scoline.

Scoline should not be used in ophthalmic cases when the anterior chamber of the eye is open. Nor must it be used in cases of hyperkalaemia.

Precautions: Neostigmine and other anticholinesterase drugs are not antidotes to Scoline but would normally have the effect of intensifying the depolarisation effect. However, in some cases of prolonged apnoea following Scoline, a state of 'dual block' may be responsible. In dual block the muscle relaxation is due to non-depolarising blockade and is reversible with neostigmine. To investigate this possibility the short-acting anticholinesterase drug, edrophonium, should be given and a transitory return of muscle power confirms the presence of dual block, which can then be reversed with neostigmine. In seriously burnt children Scoline can precipitate gross cardiac arrhythmias and cardiac arrest. This can be prevented by the administration of tubocurarine 6 mg five minutes before giving Scoline. Sinus tachycardia and rise in blood pressure has occurred after the continuous infusion of suxamethonium chloride. Care should be taken with patients currently receiving systemic antibiotics such as streptomycin, neomycin, kanamycin, tobramycin, framycetin, amikacin, gentamicin, colistin and the polymyxins, as they can potentiate the action of Scoline.

Since the initial contractions caused by Scoline are painful, Scoline should not be administered until the anaesthetic has taken full effect. Suxamethonium chloride is fairly quickly hydrolysed by thiopentone therefore, when this anaesthetic is used, Scoline should be injected after thiopentone using a different syringe.

The Elderly: Caution is required because of the possible cardiovascular effects of depolarising agents.

Pregnancy: The drug should not be administered to pregnant women unless the potential benefit outweighs the possible hazard.

Side-effects: Muscle pain (particularly in the muscles of the chest, abdomen and shoulder girdle) can occur following the use of Scoline. It occurs most frequently in patients who are ambulant in the early post-operative period and can be avoided by the prior administration of any of the non-depolarising muscle relaxants.

Malignant hyperpyrexia is a rare, possibly fatal, complication in patients anaesthetised with general anaesthetic agents and has been increasingly associated with concomitant administration of suxamethonium chloride. It occurs in apparently healthy individuals genetically predisposed to this syndrome.

Myoglobinuria has been reported, either alone or associated with malignant hyperpyrexia.

Other side-effects which have been reported include hypertension, fever, hypersensitivity reactions and bronchospasm.

Suxamethonium chloride causes a transient rise in intra-ocular pressure and salivary gland enlargement. There may be some increase in bowel movements and in gastric and salivary secretions due to the muscarinic action of suxamethonium chloride.

Overdosage: Because Scoline is usually administered by an anaesthetist, overdosage is unlikely. However, the unsuspected presence of low pseudocholinesterase levels in the serum, or this being replaced by the atypical enzyme, or the occurrence of dual block, can lead to a similar situation: prolonged apnoea. Management first consists of maintaining light anaesthesia and continued mechanical respiration to ensure an adequate supply of oxygen whilst the cause is determined. Dual block can be recognised by the response to edrophonium, and treatment then consists of reversal with neostigmine. Subsequently, the patient should remain under observation as the dual block may outlast the duration of action of neostigmine (at least 20 minutes) and if apnoea recurs a further dose of neostigmine is indicated. Apnoea due to atypical or low serum cholinesterase levels can be corrected by intravenous administration of a highly concentrated preparation of pseudocholinesterase or transfusion of plasma or whole blood.

Pharmaceutical precautions Scoline should be stored at as low a temperature as possible above its freezing point and not exceeding 4°C; under these conditions it may be expected to retain its potency for at least two years from the date of preparation.

Scoline Injection should not be re-sterilised.

Legal category POM.

Package quantities Scoline is available in boxes of five 2 ml ampoules and in 10 ml multidose vials.

Further information Nil.

Product licence number 0021/5024.

TRANDATE* INJECTION

Presentation Trandate Injection: 20 ml ampoules each containing 100 mg (5 mg/ml) labetalol hydrochloride in an aqueous colourless solution.

Labetalol hydrochloride is 2-hydroxy-5-[1-hydroxy-2-(1-methyl-3-phenyl-propylamino) ethyl] benzamide hydrochloride.

Uses *Indications:* Trandate Injection is indicated when rapid control of blood pressure is essential in severely hypertensive patients including severe hypertension of pregnancy and for use in anaesthesia where a hypotensive technique is indicated.

It is also indicated in hypertensive episodes following acute myocardial infarction.

Mode of action: Trandate lowers the blood pressure primarily by blocking alpha-adrenoceptors in peripheral arterioles and thereby reducing the peripheral resistance. Concurrent beta-blockade protects the heart from reflex sympathetic drive normally induced by peripheral vasodilatation. Cardiac output is not significantly reduced at rest or after moderate exercise. Increases in systolic pressure during exercise are, however, reduced after Trandate; corresponding changes in diastolic pressure are essentially normal. All these effects would be expected to benefit hypertensive patients.

Dosage and administration *Adults:* Trandate Injection is intended for intravenous use in hospitalised patients. The plasma concentrations achieved after intravenous doses of Trandate in severe hypertension are substantially greater than those following oral administration of the drug and provide the greater degree of blockade of alpha-adrenoceptors necessary to control the more severe disease. Patients should, therefore, always receive the drug whilst in the supine or left lateral position. Raising the patient into the upright position, within three hours of intravenous Trandate administration, should be avoided since excessive postural hypotension may occur. If it is essential to reduce the blood pressure quickly, as, for example, in hypertensive encephalopathy, a dose of 50 mg of Trandate should be given by intravenous injection over a period of at least one minute. If necessary, doses of 50 mg may be repeated at five minute intervals until a satisfactory response occurs. The total dose should not exceed 200 mg. After bolus injection, the maximum effect usually occurs within five minutes and the effective duration of action is usually about six hours but may be as long as eighteen hours. An alternative method for administering Trandate is intravenous infusion of a solution made by diluting the contents of two ampoules (200 mg) to 200 ml with Sodium Chloride and Dextrose Injection BP or 5% Dextrose Intravenous Infusion BP. The resultant infusion solution contains 1 mg/ml of Trandate. It should be administered using a paediatric giving set fitted with a 50 ml graduated burette to facilitate dosage.

In the hypertensions of pregnancy, the infusion can be started at the rate of 20 mg per hour and this dose may be doubled every thirty minutes until a satisfactory reduction in blood pressure has been obtained or a dosage of 160 mg per hour is reached. Occasionally, higher doses may be necessary.

In hypertensive episodes following acute myocardial infarction, infusion should be commenced at 15 mg per hour and gradually increased to a maximum of 120 mg per hour, depending on the control of blood pressure.

In hypertension due to other causes the rate of infusion of Trandate should be about 2 mg (2 ml of infusion solution) per minute, until a satisfactory response is obtained; the infusion should then be stopped. The effective dose is usually in the range of 50 to 200 mg, depending on the severity of the hypertension. For most patients it is unnecessary to administer more than 200 mg but larger doses may be required especially in patients with phaeochromocytoma. The rate of infusion may be adjusted according to the response, at the discretion of the physician. The blood pressure and pulse rate should be monitored throughout the infusion. It is desirable to monitor the heart rate after injection and during infusion. In most patients, there is a small decrease in the heart rate; severe bradycardia is unusual but may be controlled by injecting atropine 1 to 2 mg intravenously. Respiratory

function should be observed particularly in patients with any known impairment.

Once the blood pressure has been adequately reduced, maintenance therapy with Trandate Tablets should be instituted with a starting dose of one 200 mg tablet twice daily. (See Trandate Tablets Data Sheet for further details.) Trandate Injection has been administered to patients with uncontrolled hypertension already receiving other hypotensive agents, including beta-blocking drugs, without adverse effects.

In hypotensive anaesthesia induction should be with standard agents (e.g. sodium thiopentone) and anaesthesia maintained with nitrous oxide and oxygen with or without halothane. The recommended starting dose of Trandate Injection is 10 to 20 mg intravenously depending on the age and condition of the patient. Patients for whom halothane is contra-indicated usually require a higher initial dose of Trandate (25 to 30 mg). If satisfactory hypotension is not achieved after five minutes, increments of 5 to 10 mg should be given until the desired level of blood pressure is attained.

Halothane and Trandate act synergistically therefore the halothane concentration should not exceed 1 to 1.5% as profound falls in blood pressure may be precipitated. Following Trandate Injection the blood pressure can be quickly and easily adjusted by altering the halothane concentration and/or adjusting table tilt. The mean duration of hypotension following 20 to 25 mg of Trandate is fifty minutes.

Hypotension induced by Trandate Injection is readily reversed by atropine 0.6 mg and discontinuation of halothane.

Tubocurarine and pancuronium may be used when assisted or controlled ventilation is required. IPPV may further increase the hypotension resulting from Trandate Injection and/or halothane.

Children: Not applicable.

Contra-indications, warnings, etc *Contra-indications:* Where peripheral vasoconstriction suggests low cardiac output, the use of Trandate Injection to control hypertensive episodes following acute myocardial infarction is contra-indicated.

There are no other known absolute contra-indications to the use of Trandate Injection.

Precautions: Trandate Injection should not normally be given to patients with digitalis-resistant heart failure or atrioventricular block.

Caution must be observed if Trandate is used to treat asthmatic patients or individuals prone to bronchospasm. Any resultant bronchospasm may be controlled by an inhaled selectively-acting bronchodilator such as salbutamol; the required dose may be greater than the normal anti-asthmatic dose. If further treatment is required, intravenous atropine 1 mg should be given.

It is not necessary to discontinue Trandate therapy in patients requiring anaesthesia but they should be given intravenous atropine prior to induction; the effect of halothane on blood pressure may be enhanced by Trandate. During anaesthesia Trandate may mask the compensatory physiological responses to sudden haemorrhage (tachycardia and vasoconstriction). Close attention must therefore be paid to blood loss and the blood volume maintained.

Care should be taken in the concomitant use of labetalol and either Class I antiarrhythmic agents or calcium antagonists of the verapamil type.

Although no teratogenic effects have been demonstrated in animals the unnecessary use of Trandate during the first trimester of pregnancy is undesirable. Trandate crosses the placental barrier and the possibility of the consequences of alpha- and beta-adrenoceptor blockade in the fetus and neonate (e.g. bradycardia and hypoglycaemia) should be borne in mind. Experience has shown this to have been an exceptionally rare occurrence. Trandate is excreted in breast milk. No adverse effects in breast feeding infants have been reported.

Side-effects: Trandate Injection is usually well tolerated. Excessive postural hypotension may occur if patients are allowed to assume the upright position within three hours of receiving Trandate Injection.

Overdosage: Overdosage with Trandate causes excessive hypotension, which is posture sensitive, and sometimes excessive bradycardia. Patients should be laid supine and their legs raised if necessary to improve the blood supply to the brain. Atropine 3 mg should be given intravenously to relieve bradycardia.

Massive overdosage with Trandate in man has not been reported, but profound cardiovascular effects are to be expected. Atropine at least 3 mg intravenously should always be given. If further measures are required to obtain adequate circulatory function, intravenous noradrenaline may be preferable to isoprenaline, the established pharmacological treatment for excessive cardiac beta-blockade. The recommended starting dose of noradrenaline in patients is 5 to 10 micrograms by intravenous injection repeated as required according to the response.

Alternatively, noradrenaline may be infused at a rate of 5 micrograms per minute until a satisfactory response is achieved.

Pharmaceutical precautions Protect from light.

Legal category POM.

Package quantities *Trandate Injection 20 ml ampoules:* Boxes of 5.

Further information Trandate does not adversely affect renal function and is a particularly suitable drug for use in hypertensive patients with renal disease. The metabolites of Trandate are excreted in the faeces as well as in the urine and so the drug is unlikely to accumulate in the body even in renal failure.

In non-pregnant patients the half-life of Trandate in plasma is about four hours and somewhat less in pregnancy. Only about 50% of Trandate in the blood is protein bound. Trandate fluoresces in alkaline solution at an excitation wavelength of 334 nm and a fluorescence wavelength of 412 nm and may therefore interfere with the assays of certain fluorescent substances.

Product licence number 0045/0104.

TRANDATE* TABLETS   50 mg
TRANDATE* TABLETS 100 mg
TRANDATE* TABLETS 200 mg
TRANDATE* TABLETS 400 mg

Presentation *Trandate Tablets 50 mg:* Circular, orange coloured, film-coated biconvex tablets, each containing labetalol hydrochloride 50 mg, marked TRANDATE 50 on one face.
Trandate Tablets 100 mg: Circular, orange coloured, film-coated biconvex tablets, each containing labetalol hydrochloride 100 mg, marked TRANDATE 100 on one face.
Trandate Tablets 200 mg: Circular, orange coloured, film-coated biconvex tablets, each containing labetalol hydrochloride 200 mg, marked TRANDATE 200 on one face.
Trandate Tablets 400 mg: Circular, orange coloured, film-coated biconvex tablets, each containing labetalol hydrochloride 400 mg, marked TRANDATE 400 on one face.

Labetalol hydrochloride is 2-hydroxy-5-[1-hydroxy-2-(1-methyl-3-phenyl-propylamino) ethyl]benzamide hydrochloride.

Uses *Indications:* Trandate Tablets are indicated for the treatment of all forms of hypertension, including the hypertensions of pregnancy, and all grades of hypertension (mild, moderate and severe) when oral antihypertensive therapy is desirable.

Trandate Tablets are also indicated for the treatment of patients with angina pectoris coexisting with hypertension.

Mode of action: Trandate lowers the blood pressure primarily by blocking alpha-adrenoceptors in peripheral arterioles and thereby reducing the peripheral resistance. Concurrent beta-blockade protects the heart from the reflex sympathetic drive normally induced by peripheral vasodilatation. Cardiac output is not significantly reduced at rest or after moderate exercise. Increases in systolic pressure during exercise are, however, reduced after Trandate; corresponding changes in the diastolic pressure are essentially normal. In patients with coexisting angina the reduced peripheral resistance leads to a decreased left ventricular afterload and, hence, reduced myocardial oxygen demand. All these effects would be expected to benefit hypertensive patients and those with coexisting angina.

Dosage and administration *Adults:* Treatment may start with one 200 mg tablet twice daily but in some patients, including those already being treated with antihypertensive drugs and those of low bodyweight, one 100 mg tablet twice daily is more appropriate.

If the blood pressure is not controlled by the initial dosage, increases should be made at intervals of about 14 days. By prescribing tablets of increasing strength, the dose can be maintained at one tablet twice daily until a total daily dose of 800 mg is reached. Daily doses of up to 2,400 mg have been given in the treatment of severe and refractory hypertension. In such patients it is preferable to administer Trandate three or four times daily.

Satisfactory control of blood pressure will be obtained in many patients at a total daily dosage of 400 mg (one 200 mg tablet twice daily).

In severe hypertension, particularly that of pregnancy, the dosage may be increased on a daily basis until adequate control of blood pressure is obtained.

Tablets should be taken with food.

For hospital in-patients daily increases in dosage may be made if the need to reduce blood pressure is urgent. If it is necessary to reduce the blood pressure rapidly in very severe hypertension, Trandate Injection is indicated (see Data Sheet for Trandate Injection).

Patients who have received Trandate Injection to control hypertensive episodes following acute myocardial infarction (see Trandate Injection Data Sheet) may receive Trandate Tablets, if long-term control of hypertension is required; oral therapy should be commenced with the usual starting dose. In hypertensive patients with angina, the dose of Trandate will be that required to control the hypertension.

Elderly: In elderly patients, an initial dose of 50 mg twice daily is recommended. This has provided satisfactory control in some cases.

Children: Not applicable.

Use with other agents: Hypertension is usually controlled by Trandate alone. Diuretic therapy is not usually necessary in patients receiving Trandate Tablets, but may be introduced or continued if required. Diuretics usually increase the antihypertensive action of Trandate.

If Trandate Tablets are prescribed together with another antihypertensive drug, such as methyldopa or clonidine, an additive effect may be expected in patients who are responsive to both drugs. When transferring patients from other drugs, Trandate Tablets should be introduced as recommended above and the dosage of the existing therapy progressively decreased.

Abrupt withdrawal of clonidine or beta-adrenoceptor blockers is undesirable.

Contra-indications, warnings, etc

Contra-indications: There are no known absolute contra-indications to the use of Trandate Tablets.

Warnings: There have been reports of skin rashes and/or dry eyes associated with the use of beta-adrenoceptor blocking drugs. The reported incidence is small and in most cases the symptoms have cleared when the treatment was withdrawn. Discontinuance of the drug should be considered if any such reaction is not otherwise explicable. On rare occasions labetalol has been associated with jaundice (both hepatic and cholestatic). It is therefore recommended that treatment with labetalol should be discontinued should a patient develop jaundice, since the latter has been shown to be reversible on stopping the drug.

Precautions: Heart failure should be controlled with digitalis and diuretic therapy before treatment is initiated. Trandate should not normally be given to patients with digitalis-resistant heart failure or atrio-ventricular block. Patients with severe liver damage may have higher than normal plasma concentrations of labetalol due to reduced metabolism. Consequently, patients with liver disease may require lower than the usual doses of Trandate to control their blood pressure.

Caution must be observed if Trandate is used to treat asthmatic patients or individuals prone to bronchospasm. Any resultant bronchospasm may be controlled by an inhaled selectively-acting bronchodilator such as salbutamol; the required dose may be greater than the normal anti-asthmatic dose. If further treatment is required, intravenous atropine 1 mg should be given.

It is not necessary to discontinue Trandate Tablets in patients requiring anaesthesia but they should be given intravenous atropine prior to induction; the effect of halothane on blood pressure may be enhanced by Trandate.

Care should be taken in the concomitant use of labetalol and either Class 1 antiarrhythmic agents or calcium antagonists of the verapamil type. Although no teratogenic effects have been demonstrated in animals the unnecessary use of Trandate during the first trimester of pregnancy is undesirable.

Trandate crosses the placental barrier and the possibility of the consequences of alpha- and beta-adrenoceptor blockade in the fetus and neonate (e.g. bradycardia and hypoglycaemia) should be borne in mind. Experience has shown this to have been an exceptionally rare occurrence.

Trandate is excreted in breast milk. No adverse effects in breast feeding infants have been reported.

Side-effects: Where side-effects to Trandate have occurred they have usually done so during the first weeks of treatment and have been transient. Symptoms tend to have been similar in nature to those often observed in untreated hypertensive patients and have included headache, tiredness, dizziness, depressed mood and lethargy. If the initial dosage is too high, or the dose increased too rapidly, symptoms of postural hypotension may occur. These are uncommon, except at very high doses, if the drug is used as recommended.

In a few patients certain other side-effects have occurred which appear to be more directly related to Trandate treatment. These include difficulty in micturition, epigastric pain, nausea and vomiting.

Again, in a few patients a tingling sensation in the scalp associated with Trandate treatment has been reported. It usually occurs early in the treatment and tends to be transient in nature.

In a very small number of patients a lichenoid rash has appeared during Trandate treatment but has disappeared on withdrawing treatment. Other skin rashes not necessarily induced by Trandate treatment have been reported. Blurring of vision, eye irritation and cramps have also been reported but have been difficult to relate directly to Trandate treatment.

Interactions: Concomitant use of tricyclic antidepressants may increase the incidence of tremor.

Cimetidine may increase the bioavailability of labetalol and care is required in oral dosing of the latter.

Overdosage: Overdosage with Trandate causes excessive hypotension, which is posture sensitive and sometimes, excessive bradycardia. Patients should be laid supine and their legs raised if necessary to improve the blood supply to the brain. Atropine 3 mg should be given intravenously to relieve bradycardia. Massive overdosage with Trandate in man has not been reported but profound cardiovascular effects are to be expected. Atropine at least 3 mg intravenously should always be given. Gastric lavage or induced emesis is warranted for a few hours after oral ingestion of the drug. If further measures are required to obtain adequate circulatory function, intravenous noradrenaline may be preferable to isoprenaline, the established pharmacological treatment for excessive cardiac beta-blockade. The recommended starting dose of noradrenaline in patients is 5 to 10 micrograms by intravenous injection repeated as required according to the response. Alternatively, noradrenaline may be infused at a rate of 5 micrograms per minute until a satisfactory response is achieved.

Pharmaceutical precautions No special storage precautions are required.

Legal category POM.

Package quantities Trandate Tablets 100 mg and 200 mg are available in containers of 250. Trandate Tablets 400 mg in containers of 50 and 250. Trandate Tablets 50 mg, 100 mg and 200 mg are also available in calendar blister packs of 56 tablets.

Further information Trandate does not adversely affect renal function and is a particularly suitable drug for use in hypertensive patients with renal disease. The metabolites of Trandate are excreted in the faeces as well as the urine and so the drug is unlikely to accumulate in the body even in renal failure.

In non-pregnant patients the half-life of Trandate in plasma is about four hours and somewhat less in pregnancy. Only about 50% of Trandate in the blood is protein bound. Trandate fluoresces in alkaline solution at an excitation wavelength of 334 nm and a fluorescence wavelength of 412 nm and may therefore interfere with the assays of certain fluorescent substances.

Product licence numbers

Trandate Tablets	50 mg	0045/0111
Trandate Tablets	100 mg	0045/0106
Trandate Tablets	200 mg	0045/0107
Trandate Tablets	400 mg	0045/0109

*Trade Mark

Duphar Laboratories Limited
Gaters Hill
West End
Southampton SO3 3JD

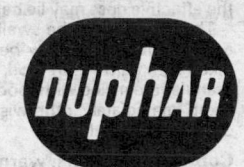

ALGESAL*

Presentation Off white, lavender-scented cream containing diethylamine salicylate 10% w/w in a vanishing cream base.

Uses An analgesic cream for the symptomatic relief of rheumatic and minor musculo-skeletal conditions including, lumbago, fibrositis, sciatica, bruises and sprains.

Dosage and administration
Adults and children over 6 years: Apply three times daily to the affected area, massaging until cream is fully absorbed.

Children under 6 years: Not recommended.

Contra-indications, warnings, etc Algesal should not be used if the surface of the skin is broken. This product contains a salicylate which is related to aspirin.

Treatment of overdosage: Adverse systemic effects are unlikely even after accidental oral ingestion. No special measures are necessary.

Pharmaceutical precautions Store at room temperature.

Legal category P.

Package quantities Tube containing 50 g.

Further information Nil.

Product licence number 0512/0066.

COLOFAC*

Presentation 1. White sugar-coated tablets each containing 135 mg mebeverine hydrochloride.
2. Yellow, banana-flavoured, sugar-free suspension containing mebeverine pamoate equivalent to 50 mg mebeverine hydrochloride per 5 ml.

Uses Mebeverine is a musculotropic antispasmodic with a direct action on the smooth muscle of the gastro-intestinal tract, relieving spasm without affecting normal gut motility. Since this action is not mediated by the autonomic nervous system, the usual anticholinergic side-effects are absent. Mebeverine is suitable for patients with prostatic hypertrophy and glaucoma.

Indications:
1. Irritable bowel syndrome and other conditions usually included in this grouping such as: chronic irritable colon, spastic constipation, mucous colitis, spastic colitis. Colofac is effectively used to treat the symptoms of these conditions, such as: abdominal pain and cramps, persistent, non-specific diarrhoea (with or without alternating constipation) and flatulence.
2. Gastro-intestinal spasm secondary to organic diseases.

Dosage and administration Tablets: *Adults and children 10 years and over:* One tablet three times a day preferably 20 minutes before meals.
Suspension: *Adults and children 10 years and over:* 15 ml (150 mg) three times a day preferably 20 minutes before meals.
After a period of several weeks when the desired effect has been obtained, the dosage may be gradually reduced.

Children under 10 years: Not applicable.

Use in the elderly: The same dosage may be used in the elderly as in the general population.

Contra-indications, warnings, etc
Contra-indications: None known.

Warnings: Animal experiments have failed to show any teratogenic effects. However, the usual precautions concerning the administration of any drug during pregnancy should be observed.

Treatment of overdosage: On theoretical grounds it may be predicted that CNS excitability will occur in cases of overdosage. No specific antidote is known; gastric lavage and symptomatic treatment is recommended.

Pharmaceutical precautions Tablets: Store in a dry place, at room temperature, protected from light.
Suspension: Store at room temperature. Shake well before use. The recommended diluent is water. The diluted product is stable for up to 14 days.

Legal category POM.

Package quantities Tablets: Available in packs of 100 (5 strips of 20 blister-packed tablets).
Suspension: Available in bottles of 300 ml.

Further information Mebeverine does not produce false positive reactions in standard diagnostic urine tests.

Product licence numbers
Tablets   0512/0044
Suspension   0512/0061

CREON*

Presentation Brown/yellow hard gelatin capsules containing buff coloured enteric coated granules of pancreatin, equivalent to:
8,000 BP units of lipase
9,000 BP units of amylase
210 BP units of protease

Uses Replacement therapy in pancreatic enzyme deficiency states.

Indications: Pancreatic exocrine insufficiency.

Dosage and administration *Adults and children:* Initially one to two capsules with meals, then adjust according to response. Clinical experience indicates that the effective dose may lie between 5–15 capsules daily. *

The capsules can be swallowed whole, or for ease of administration they may be opened and the granules taken with fluid or soft food, but without chewing. If the granules are mixed with food it is important that they are taken immediately, otherwise dissolution of the enteric coating may result.

Contra-indications, warnings, etc

Contra-indications: Substitution with pancreatic enzymes is contra-indicated in the early stages of acute pancreatitis.

Warnings:

Use in pregnancy: There is inadequate evidence of safety in use during pregnancy.

The product is of porcine origin.

Rarely cases of hyper-uricosuria and hyper-uricaemia have been reported with very high doses of pancreatin.

Overdosage could precipitate meconium ileus equivalent.

Perianal irritation could occur, and rarely, inflammation when large doses are used.

Pharmaceutical precautions Store at room temperature.

Legal category P.

Package quantities Available in packs of 100 capsules.

Further information Nil.

Product licence number 5727/0001.

Product licence holder: Kali Chemie Pharma GmbH, Postfach 220, D-3000, Hannover 1, West Germany.

DUPHALAC*

Presentation A colourless to pale yellow solution containing lactulose 3.35 g/5 ml. Also contains lactose 0.3 g/5 ml, galactose 0.55 g/5 ml. The product complies with the specification for Lactulose Solution BP.

Uses The action of Duphalac in treating constipation depends on the inability of the enzymes in the small intestine to hydrolyse the synthetic disaccharide, lactulose, into its component molecules of fructose and galactose. Therefore, as lactulose is virtually unabsorbed, it passes into the large bowel chemically unchanged and forms a substrate for commensal saccharolytic bacteria.

The resulting breakdown products, simple organic compounds like lactic and acetic acid, give rise to increased intra-colonic osmotic pressure, with consequent increased faecal bulk, and stimulate peristalsis. The growth of saccharolytic bacteria is favoured and the normal colonic flora restored.

A soft stool is formed, and normal bowel action encouraged without irritation or direct interference with the gut mucosa.

In patients with hepatic encephalopathy larger doses of Duphalac are used; a significant reduction in the pH of the colonic contents results, which reduces markedly the formation and absorption of ammonium ions and other nitrogenous toxins into the portal circulation. Rapid decrements in blood ammonia concentration have been reported following Duphalac treatment.

Indications: 1. Constipation.

2. Hepatic encephalopathy (Portal systemic encephalopathy): hepatic coma.

Dosage and administration *Constipation:* Initially Duphalac may be given twice daily. In due course the dose should be adjusted to the needs of the individual, but the following serves as a guide.

Starting dose

Adults	15 ml twice daily
Children 5 to 10 years	10 ml twice daily
Children under 5 years	5 ml twice daily
Babies	2.5 ml twice daily

Each dose of Duphalac may, if necessary, be taken with water or fruit juices, etc.

Use in the elderly: Duphalac has been shown to be a suitable laxative for use in the elderly.

Hepatic encephalopathy: Initially 30–50 ml. (6–10 × 5 ml spoonfuls) three times a day. Subsequently adjust the dose to produce two or three soft stools each day.

Contra-indications, warnings, etc

Contra-indications: Galactosaemia. In common with other preparations used for the treatment of constipation, Duphalac should not be used when there is evidence of gastro-intestinal obstruction.

Precaution: Lactose intolerance.

Pharmaceutical precautions Store below 20°C. Do not freeze. Dilution and subsequent storage not recommended.

Legal category P.

Package quantities Available in bottles of 300 ml, 1 litre and plastic containers of 5 litres.

Further information Because of Duphalac's physiological mode of action it may take up to 48 hours before effects are obtained. However, clinical experience has shown that this medicament does exhibit a 'carry-over' effect which may enable the patient to reduce the effective dose gradually over a period of time.

A maintenance dose of 15 ml per day provides only 58 kJ (14 kcals), and is therefore, unlikely to adversely affect diabetics.

Product licence number 0512/5001.

DUPHASTON*

Presentation White, flat, round tablet scored on one side with the imprint '155' on each half of the tablet and imprinted 'DUPHAR' on the reverse, each containing 10 mg Dydrogesterone BP.

Uses Dydrogesterone is an orally active progestogen which produces a complete secretory endometrium in an oestrogen-primed uterus. It is indicated in all cases of endogenous progesterone deficiency.

Indications: Dysmenorrhoea, endometriosis, threatened and habitual abortion (associated with proven progesterone deficiency), infertility, irregular cycles, functional bleeding (with added oestrogen), secondary amenorrhoea (with added oestrogen), premenstrual syndrome, conditions of progesterone deficiency and to counteract the effects of unopposed oestrogen in Hormone Replacement Therapy.

Dosage and administration *Adults: Dysmenorrhoea:* 10 mg twice daily from day 5 to 25 of the cycle.

Endometriosis: 10 mg two to three times daily from day 5 to 25 of the cycle, or continuously.

Threatened abortion: 40 mg at once then 10 mg every

eight hours until symptoms remit. If symptoms persist or return during treatment the dose can be increased by one tablet every eight hours. The effective dose must be maintained for a week after symptoms have ceased and can then be gradually decreased unless symptoms return.

Habitual abortion: Treatment should be started as early as possible, preferably before conception. 10 mg should be given twice daily from day 11 to day 25 of the cycle until conception and then continuously (10 mg twice daily) until the twentieth week of pregnancy, then dosage may be gradually reduced.

Infertility or irregular cycles: 10 mg twice daily from day 11 to day 25 of the cycle. Treatment should be maintained for at least six consecutive cycles. If the patient conceives, it is advisable to continue treatment for the first few months of pregnancy as described under 'habitual abortion'.

Functional bleeding – to arrest bleeding: 10 mg twice daily together with an oestrogen once daily for five to seven days.

Functional bleeding – to prevent bleeding: 10 mg twice daily together with an oestrogen once daily from day 11 to 25 of the cycle.

Amenorrhoea: An oestrogen once daily from day 1 to 25 of the cycle, together with 10 mg dydrogesterone twice daily from day 11 to 25 of the cycle.

Premenstrual syndrome: 10 mg twice daily from day 12 to 26 of the cycle. The dosage may be increased if necessary.

Hormone replacement therapy: If continuous oestrogen is given, 10 mg dydrogesterone twice daily for the first 12–14 days of each calendar month. If cyclical oestrogen is given, 10 mg dydrogesterone twice daily for the last 12–14 days of each treatment cycle.

Children: Not applicable.

Contra-indications, warnings, etc
Contra-indications: None known.

Warning: Breakthrough bleeding may occur in a few patients. It can, however, be prevented by increasing the dosage.

Treatment of overdosage: No reports of ill effects from overdosage have been recorded and remedial action is generally unnecessary. If a large overdosage is discovered within 2–3 hours and treatment seems desirable, gastric lavage is recommended. There are no special antidotes and treatment should be symptomatic.

Pharmaceutical precautions
Store in a dry place, at room temperature, protected from light.

Legal category POM.

Package quantities
Available in packs of 40 (4 strips of 10 blister-packed tablets).

Further information
Duphaston is non-androgenic, non-oestrogenic, non-thermogenic, non-corticoid, non-anabolic and is not excreted as pregnanediol.

Dydrogesterone does not produce false positive reactions in standard diagnostic urine tests.

Product licence number 0512/5004R.

DUVADILAN*

Presentation 1. Round, pink tablets imprinted with the name 'Duvadilan' on one face, scored on the reverse, each tablet containing 20 mg isoxsuprine hydrochloride.

2. 2 ml ampoules containing a clear, colourless solution of isoxsuprine hydrochloride 5 mg/ml.

Uses Duvadilan (isoxsuprine hydrochloride) is a vaso-relaxant which acts through stimulation of the beta-receptors situated in the walls of blood vessels. In high doses it also relaxes skin vessel walls, where alpha-sympathetic receptors predominate. Duvadilan also lowers blood viscosity. In addition, Duvadilan has a stimulating action on the beta-adreno-receptors of the myometrium with a resulting inhibition of uterine contractions. In high doses, it also has a direct papaverine-like action on the smooth muscle of the uterus.

Indications: Peripheral vascular disorders: arteriosclerosis, Buerger's disease, Raynaud's syndrome, ischaemic and vasospastic symptoms (e.g. intermittent claudication, night cramps, pain in limbs, paraesthesia, cold extremities, ulcers).
Pre-term labour.

Dosage and administration *Peripheral vascular disease:* 1. Intravenous infusion: 20 mg (2 × 2 ml amps) diluted in 100 ml of recommended infusion fluid, twice daily at a rate of 300 micrograms (1.5 ml) per minute for a maximum of 67 minutes.

2. Intramuscular injection: Duvadilan Injection (10 mg in 2 ml) may be given by the intramuscular route up to four times daily.

3. Oral: Tablets, 20 mg isoxsuprine hydrochloride, four times daily. Capsules, equivalent of 40 mg isoxsuprine hydrochloride in a sustained release formulation, morning and evening (see Duvadilan Retard).

Pre-term labour:
1. Intravenous infusion: To be administered at the onset of pre-term labour and continued until control is obtained.

Infusion solution: Duvadilan 100 mg in 500 ml infusion fluid. The recommended infusion fluid is dextrose.

Infusion rate: 1.0–1.5 ml/min (200–300 micrograms/min) increasing up to 2.5 ml/min (500 micrograms/min) until control is obtained.

Blood pressure and heart rate should be checked regularly during intravenous infusion. Adjustment of the drip rate should be made according to the result and possible side-effects such as a serious drop in blood pressure.

2. Intra-muscular injection: When labour is arrested: Duvadilan 10 mg (1 × 2 ml ampoule) three hourly for 24 hours, then four to six-hourly for a further 48 hours.

3. Oral: When contractions have ceased for 48 hours Duvadilan 1 × 20 mg tablet four times a day.

Use in the elderly: The same dosage may be used in the elderly as in the general population.

Contra-indications, warnings, etc
Contra-indications: Recent arterial haemorrhage, parenteral use in patients with known heart disease, premature detachment of placenta, and severe anaemia.

Precaution: Use of large volumes of fluid is not recommended as this may cause fluid overloading. A dextrose solution is preferred to isotonic saline. Patients in pre-term labour should be maintained in the left lateral position during infusion. Blood pressure and heart rate should be recorded regularly during infusion. If a prolonged fall in blood pressure occurs the rate of infusion should be reduced or the infusion discontinued.

Side-effects: Hypotension (see Precautions): transient tachycardia, mild flushing, nausea and vomiting have been noted. If it is necessary to reverse the cardiovascular effects, treatment with a non-selective beta-blocker should be considered.

Treatment of overdosage: Gross overdosages have not been reported, treatment would be gastric lavage, and if necessary, a non-selective beta-blocker may be administered intramuscularly.

Pharmaceutical precautions Injections should be stored above 0°C but below 20°C, protected from light. The infusion may be prepared with dextrose, isotonic saline or Hartmanns solution.

Legal category
Tablets P.
Injection POM.

Package quantities Ampoules containing isoxsuprine hydrochloride 5 mg/ml in packs of 6 × 2 ml.

Tablets containing 20 mg isoxsuprine hydrochloride, in packs of 100 (5 strips of 20 blister packed tablets).

Further information Isoxsuprine does not produce false positive reactions in standard diagnostic urine tests.

Product licence numbers
Duvadilan Tablets   0512/5002
Duvadilan Injection   0512/5003

DUVADILAN* RETARD

Presentation Isoxsuprine in a graded release formulation. Red/opaque white, hard gelatine capsules, imprinted 'DUPHAR 133'. Each capsule contains isoxsuprine (equivalent to 40 mg of the hydrochloride) complexed with a sulphonated polystyrene resin.

Uses The active ingredient is isoxsuprine, which has a direct vasorelaxant effect on the vascular wall and has also viscosity lowering properties. Its vasodilating action is more marked on the arteries and arterioles where the beta-sympathetic receptors predominate.

Indications: Peripheral arteriosclerosis; peripheral vasospasm; acute vascular occlusion; Buerger's disease; acrocyanosis; thrombophlebitis; Raynaud's disease.

Dosage and administration *Adults:* 1 capsule morning and evening.

The product is not intended for administration to children.

Use in the elderly: The same dosage may be used in the elderly as in the general population.

Contra-indications, warnings, etc
Contra-indication: Recent arterial haemorrhage.

Side-effects: Side-effects in the form of flushing or palpitations are rare and transient.

Treatment of overdosage: Gross overdosages have not been reported; treatment would be gastric lavage, and if necessary, a non-selective beta-blocker may be administered intramuscularly.

Pharmaceutical precautions Store in a dry place at a temperature below 20°C.

Legal category P.

Package quantities Compliance pack of 56 capsules (4 strips of 14 blister packed capsules).

Further information Duvadilan Retard can be given to patients with hypertension, diabetes, coronary insufficiency, peptic ulcer and glaucoma. Duvadilan Retard may also be given with the commonly used diuretics, corticosteroids and antihypertensive drugs.

Isoxsuprine does not produce false positive reactions in standard diagnostic urine tests.

Product licence number 0512/0030.

INFLUVAC* SUB-UNIT

Presentation A colourless, opalescent suspension of inactivated Influenza Vaccine (Surface Antigen) BP containing the purified haemagglutinin and neuraminidase antigens prepared from influenza virus. The product contains appropriate quantities of the A and B strains currently recommended by the WHO.

Uses Prophylaxis of influenza. Particularly recommended in:

1. Chronic pulmonary disease, e.g. chronic bronchitis and emphysema, asthma, bronchiectasis, pulmonary tuberculosis and fibrosis.
2. Chronic heart disease, e.g. valvular and hypertensive heart disease.
3. Chronic renal disease, e.g. chronic nephritis, including patients with renal disease on immunosuppressive drugs.
4. Diabetes and possibly other less common endocrine disorders.
5. Elderly people.
6. Key personnel.
7. Chronic furunculosis or other chronic staphylococcal infections.
8. Persons living in residential establishments in which rapid spread is likely following the introduction of infection.

Dosage and administration
Adults and children (over 13 years): 0.5 ml.

Children (4–13 years): 0.5 ml, followed by a second injection of 0.5 ml after an interval of 4–6 weeks, unless previously primed with a trivalent influenza vaccine in the past 4 years, in which case one dose of 0.5 ml is sufficient.

To be given by intramuscular or deep subcutaneous injection after allowing the vaccine to reach room temperature. It is recommended that the contents of multi-dose vials are used within 4 hours of opening.

Contra-indications, warnings, etc
Contra-indications: Persons with hypersensitivity to eggs, chicken proteins or feathers and influenza viral proteins should not be vaccinated.

Immunisation should be postponed in patients with febrile illness.

Warnings: Side-effects: Local effects such as transient erythema and swelling at the site of injection may occur. Systemic effects such as pyrexia, fatigue and headache may also be experienced. Reactions of both types can be expected to occur only rarely and less frequently than those associated with the administration of whole virus vaccine.

Precautions: Neurological disorders such as encephalomyelitis and neuritis after influenza vaccination have rarely been reported. An association has not been demonstrated except in the case of the Guillain Barré Syndrome (USA mass vaccination programme 1976).

The vaccine may contain a maximum per dose of 0.00625 Units polymyxin and 0.00625 mcg neomycin. Use with caution in patients hypersensitive to these antibiotics.

Treatment of overdosage: Not applicable.

Pharmaceutical precautions Store at 2–10°C, protected from light. Do not freeze.

Legal category POM.

Package quantities Single-dose (0.5 ml) disposable syringes, 10 dose (5 ml) and 50 dose (25 ml) vials.

Further information Non-essential viral components have been removed thus decreasing the reactogenicity. Studies have shown that the purified haemagglutinin and neuraminidase antigens contained in Influvac Sub-Unit produce a protective antibody level in a high percentage of patients.

Product licence number 0512/0056.

MONOTRIM*

Presentation Tablets – white, flat, round, with bevelled edges, imprinted with the manufacturer's symbol Ⓐ on one face, with a single break bar and coded on the reverse.

100 mg tablets coded $\dfrac{AE}{2}$.

200 mg tablets coded $\dfrac{DE}{5}$.

Suspension – white, sugar free, aniseed flavoured suspension containing 50 mg trimethoprim per 5 ml.

Uses Trimethoprim is active *in-vitro* against most Gram-positive and Gram-negative aerobic organisms. The antimicrobial activity is due to selective inhibition of bacterial dihydrofolate reductase.

Indications: Treatment of susceptible infections caused by trimethoprim-sensitive organisms including urinary and respiratory tract infections.

Dosage and administration *Acute infections:*

Tablets:
Adults and children over 12 years: 200 mg twice daily
Children 6 years to 12 years: 100 mg twice daily
Children 6 months to 5 years: 50 mg twice daily

Suspension:
Adults and children over 12 years: 200 mg (20 ml) twice daily
Children 6 years to 12 years: 100 mg (10 ml) twice daily
Children 6 months to 5 years: 50 mg (5 ml) twice daily
Children 6 weeks to 5 months: 25 mg (2.5 ml) twice daily
Treatment should continue for at least one week. The first dose can be doubled. The approximate dosage in children is 8 mg trimethoprim per kg body weight per day.

Long-term treatment and prophylactic therapy:
Tablets:
Adults and children over 12 years: 100 mg at night
Children 6 years to 12 years: 50 mg at night

Suspension:
Adults and children over 12 years: 100 mg (10 ml) at night
Children 6 years to 12 years: 50 mg (5 ml) at night

Children 6 months to 5 years: 25 mg (2.5 ml) at night
The approximate dosage in children is 2 mg trimethoprim per kg body weight per day.

Dosage advised where there is reduced kidney function:

Creatinine clearance (ml/sec)	Plasma creatinine (micromol/l)		Dosage advised
Over 0.45	men women	<250 <175	normal
0.25–0.45	men women	250–600 175–400	normal for 3 days then half dose
Under 0.25	men women	>600 >400	half the normal dose

Contra-indications, warnings, etc
Contra-indications: Pregnancy, trimethoprim hypersensitivity, blood dyscrasias, severe renal insufficiency where blood levels cannot be monitored.

Precautions: Caution should be exercised in the administration of trimethoprim to patients with actual or potential folate deficiency and administration of folate supplement should be considered. Although an effect on folic acid metabolism is possible, interference with haematopoiesis rarely occurs at the recommended dose. If any such change is seen, folinic acid should reverse the effect. Elderly people may be more susceptible and a lower dose may be advisable. In neonates, trimethoprim should be used under careful medical supervision.

In patients with impairment of renal function, care should be taken to avoid accumulation.

Although trimethoprim is excreted in breast milk it is not a contra-indication for short-term therapy in lactating mothers.

Side-effects: Skin rashes, nausea and vomiting have been reported in rare instances.

Treatment of overdosage: Symptomatic treatment, gastric lavage and forced diuresis can be used. Depression of haematopoiesis by trimethoprim can be counteracted by intramuscular administration of calcium folinate.

Pharmaceutical precautions Monotrim suspension should be stored below 25°C. It may be diluted with water or sorbitol solution BP. The diluted suspension is stable for 14 days.

Legal category POM.

Package quantities
Tablets: 200 mg containers of 100 and 500 tablets
100 mg containers of 100 and 500 tablets
Suspension: Bottle of 100 ml.

Further information Trimethoprim is effective *in-vitro* against most Gram-positive and Gram-negative aerobic organisms, including *enterobacteria – E. coli, Proteus, Klebsiella pneumoniae; Streptococcus faecalis; Streptococcus pneumoniae; Haemophilus influenzae;* and *Staphylococcus aureus.*

It is not active against *Mycobacterium tuberculosis, Neisseria gonorrhoeae, Pseudomonas aeruginosa, Treponema pallidum,* or anaerobic bacteria.

Product licence numbers
Tablets: 200 mg 4012/0003
Tablets: 100 mg 4012/0001
Suspension: 100 ml 4012/0002

Product licence holder: GEA Limited, DK-2000, Copenhagen F, Denmark.

MONOTRIM* INJECTION

Presentation Ampoules containing a sterile, clear, colourless, aqueous solution (pH=4.0), containing trimethoprim lactate equivalent to 20 mg trimethoprim base per ml. Each ampoule contains 5 ml corresponding to 100 mg of trimethoprim base.

Uses Trimethoprim is active *in-vitro* against most Grampositive and Gram-negative aerobic organisms. The antimicrobial activity is due to selective inhibition of bacterial dihydrofolate reductase.

Indications: Treatment of susceptible infections caused by trimethoprim-sensitive organisms, particularly Gram-negative infections.

Dosage and administration *Dosage:* Adults and children over 12 years: 200 mg every 12 hours.

Children under 12 years: The approximate dosage in children is 8 mg trimethoprim per kg body weight per day, divided into two or three equal doses.

In severely ill patients, the initial doses may be higher or given more frequently.

Dosage advised where there is reduced kidney function:

Creatinine clearance (ml/sec)	Plasma creatinine (micromol/l)		Dosage advised
Over 0.45	men	<250	normal
	women	<175	
0.25–0.45	men	250–600	normal for 3 days
	women	175–400	then half dose
Under 0.25	men	>600	half the normal dose
	women	>400	

Administration: Monotrim Injection may be administered:

1. By direct intravenous injection, or
2. Via the tubing of an established intravenous infusion.

It is compatible with the following commonly used infusion fluids:

Dextran 40 Injection BP 10% w/v in normal saline
Dextran 70 Injection BP 6% w/v in normal saline
Dextrose Injection BP 5% w/v
Laevulose Injection BP 5% w/v
Ringer's Injection USP
Sodium Chloride Injection BP 0.9% w/v
Sodium Chloride 0.45% w/v and Dextrose 2.5% w/v Injection BP
Sodium Lactate Injection BP
Compound Sodium Lactate Injection BP

Contra-indications, warnings, etc

Contra-indications: Pregnancy, trimethoprim hypersensitivity, blood dyscrasias, severe renal insufficiency where blood levels cannot be monitored.

Precautions: Caution should be exercised in the administration of trimethoprim to patients with actual or potential folate deficiency and administration of folate supplement should be considered. Although an effect on folic acid metabolism is possible, interference with haematopoiesis rarely occurs at the recommended dose.

If any such change is seen, folinic acid should reverse the effect. Elderly people may be more susceptible and a lower dose may be advisable.

In patients with impairment of renal function, care should be taken to avoid accumulation.

Although trimethoprim is excreted in breast milk, it is not a contra-indication for short term therapy in lactating mothers.

Side effects: Skin rashes, nausea and vomiting have been reported in rare instances.

Treatment of overdosage: Symptomatic treatment, gastric lavage and forced diuresis can be used. Depression of haematopoiesis by trimethoprim can be counteracted by intramuscular administration of calcium folinate.

Pharmaceutical precautions Store below 25°C, protected from light.

Monotrim Injection is incompatible with solutions of sulphonamides and should not be mixed with such preparations.

Legal category POM.

Package quantities Boxes of 5 × 5 ml ampoules.

Further information Trimethoprim is effective *in-vitro* against most Gram-positive and Gram-negative aerobic organisms, including *enterobacteria – E. coli, Proteus, Klebsiella pneumoniae; Streptococcus faecalis; Streptococcus pneumoniae; Haemophilus influenzae;* and *Staphylococcus aureus.*

It is not active against *Mycobacterium tuberculosis, Neisseria gonorrhoeae, Pseudomonas aeruginosa, Treponema pallidum,* or anaerobic bacteria.

Monotrim Injection may be given in conjunction with, but separately from, other parenterally administered antibacterials, for example, aminoglycosides, metronidazole or sulphonamides whenever such a combination seems suitable.

Product licence number 4012/0008.

Product licence holder: GEA Limited, DK-2000, Copenhagen F, Denmark.

SERC*

Presentation A white, flat, round tablet, imprinted '256' on one side and 'DUPHAR' on the reverse, each tablet containing 8 mg betahistine dihydrochloride.

Uses Betahistine is an orally effective treatment for Ménière's syndrome, which appears to exert its effect by reducing endolymphatic pressure. It is a histamine analogue which was developed following the successful parenteral use of histamine in patients with Ménière's syndrome. Animal studies have confirmed its specific effect. Clinical experience has demonstrated the efficacy of betahistine on all the principal symptoms of Ménière's syndrome, not only reducing vertiginous episodes and tinnitus but also arresting hearing loss.

Indications: Vertigo, tinnitus and hearing loss associated with Ménière's syndrome.

Dosage and administration *Adults:* Initially two tablets three times daily, taken preferably with meals. Maintenance doses are generally in the range 3–6 tablets daily.

Children: No dosage recommendations are made for children.

Use in the elderly: The same dosage may be used in the elderly as in the general population.

Contra-indications, warnings, etc
Contra-indication: Phaeochromocytoma.

Precautions: Clinical intolerance to Serc in bronchial asthma patients has not been shown, but caution should be exercised when administering this histamine analogue to bronchial asthma patients.

High-dosage animal tests have shown no teratogenic properties, but the usual precautions should be observed when administering Serc to patients during pregnancy.

Though an antagonism between Serc and anti-histamines could be expected on a theoretical basis, no such interactions have been reported.

Side-effects: There have been a small number of reports of gastric upset.

Pharmaceutical precautions As Serc Tablets are hygroscopic they should be stored and dispensed in the original unopened pack or an airtight container which should be kept in a cool dry place.

Legal category POM.

Package quantities Available in packs of 120 tablets (8 strips of 15 blister packed tablets).

Further information Betahistine does not produce false positive reactions in standard diagnostic urine tests.

Product licence number 0512/0076.

TACHYROL*

Presentation A white, round, slightly biconvex tablet, imprinted 'DHT' on one face, and with a scoreline on the reverse. Each tablet contains 0.2 mg dihydrotachysterol₂ USP. XX.

Uses Dihydrotachysterol is a synthetic analogue of vitamin D. Like vitamin D and its active metabolites, dihydrotachysterol raises plasma calcium and promotes mineralisation of bone by its actions on intestinal transport of calcium and phosphate and possibly on other target tissues such as bone, kidney and the parathyroid glands. Dihydrotachysterol requires transformation by the liver (25-hydroxylation) to exert maximal biological effects but, unlike vitamin D, it does not require further metabolism by the kidney (1α-hydroxylation) for its activity.

Several disorders of mineral metabolism are known to be due in part to defective renal metabolism of vitamin D, including renal osteodystrophy, hypoparathyroidism and pseudohypoparathyroidism, and some forms of osteomalacia or rickets resistant to physiological doses of vitamin D. The use of dihydrotachysterol bypasses this metabolic block: moreover the onset and offset of action of dihydrotachysterol are more rapid than vitamin D, which facilitates titration of dose and reduces the risk of hypercalcaemia. Thus accidental hypercalcaemia can be rapidly reversed by stopping treatment.

Indications: Rickets, osteomalacia, post-operative hypoparathyroidism, idiopathic hypoparathyroidism, renal osteodystrophy and other conditions where Vitamin D therapy may be indicated.

Dosage and administration *Adults:* Initially 0.2 mg (1 tablet) daily. This dosage should be adjusted according to the requirements of individual patients as indicated by blood calcium levels (determined initially after two weeks, or earlier, then at least at monthly intervals), and appropriate clinical response.

Children: Dosage is adjusted to the requirements of individual patients as indicated by blood calcium levels.

Contra-indications, warnings, etc
Contra-indication: Hypercalcaemia.

Precautions: Overdosage is likely to cause hypercalcaemia which may be symptomless; symptoms which can occur include anorexia, nausea, vomiting, griping, polyuria and polydipsia. Chronic hypercalcaemia may lead to calcium deposition in soft tissues such as the kidney. In renal disease, hyperphosphataemia contributes to the tendency to extraskeletal calcium deposition, and should therefore be controlled if necessary by phosphate binding agents.

In patients with renal osteodystrophy, overdosage may increase the rate of deterioration of renal function.

Concurrent administration of barbiturates has been reported to influence vitamin D metabolism, and increased doses of dihydrotachysterol may therefore be required in patients taking barbiturates or anti-convulsant drugs.

Like all vitamin D analogues, dihydrotachysterol is excreted in breast milk. Animal experiments in rats show evidence of calcification in suckling neonatal rats, therefore it seems prudent, until human evidence is obtained to the contrary, to recommend that mothers receiving dihydrotachysterol do not nurse their infants.

Treatment of Overdosage: It is important to monitor plasma calcium, phosphate and creatinine levels, especially in patients with chronic renal failure.

There is no specific antidote to the effects of Tachyrol. As the drug is excreted rapidly from the patient, withdrawal should be sufficient in cases of overdosage.

Calcium supplements, if given, should also be stopped. Severe hypercalcaemia may be additionally treated using corticosteroids, 'loop diuretics' and i/v fluids. Hyperphosphataemia should be controlled if necessary by phosphate binding agents.

Pharmaceutical precautions Tachyrol tablets should be stored and dispensed in the original unopened pack or an airtight container. The product has a shelf-life of three years from the date of manufacture, if kept at temperatures below 20°C. Protect from light.

Legal category P.

Package quantities Available in bottles of 75 tablets.

Further information Nil.

Product licence number 0512/0037.

YUTOPAR*

Presentation *Tablets* – Round, buff, with the inscription 'Yutopar' on one face; breakline on the reverse. Each tablet contains 10 mg ritodrine hydrochloride.

Injection – Clear, aqueous solution containing 10 mg/ml of ritodrine hydrochloride.

Uses Yutopar is a betamimetic drug developed for obstetric use. It mainly stimulates the beta₂-receptors, thereby decreasing uterine contractility. However, some chronotropic cardiac effect and peripheral vasodilation are also seen at therapeutic doses. Yutopar is active after oral, intramuscular and intravenous administration, and inhibits frequency and intensity of uterine contractions.

Indications:

The management of:

Uncomplicated pre-term labour.

Fetal Asphyxia in labour where it is desired to obtain uterine relaxation.

Dosage and administration *Pre-term labour: I/V:* To be administered as early as possible at the onset of pre-term labour. Initial dose 50 micrograms per minute to be gradually increased according to the response by 50 micrograms/minute every 10 minutes until the desired result is obtained, or the maternal heart rate reaches 140 beats per minute. The effective dosage usually lies between 150 micrograms and 350 micrograms/minute. The infusion should be continued for 12 to 48 hours after the uterine contractions have ceased.

The recommended infusion fluid is dextrose.

I/M: If intravenous administration is considered to be inappropriate, intramuscular administration may be substituted, giving 10 mg intramuscularly every three to eight hours. The intramuscular regime should be continued for 12–48 hours following arrest of labour.

Oral: One tablet (10 mg) may be given approximately 30 minutes before the termination of intravenous therapy. The usual dosage schedule for the first 24 hours of oral maintenance is one tablet (10 mg) every two hours. Thereafter, the usual dose is one or two tablets (10–20 mg) every four to six hours depending on uterine activity and unwanted effects.

The total daily dose of oral ritodrine should not exceed 120 mg. The treatment may be continued as long as the physician considers it desirable to prolong pregnancy.

Fetal asphyxia: I/V: This treatment scheme is only recommended as a means of improving the condition of the fetus, so that intervention may be carried out under better conditions for the baby.

The recommended starting dose is 50 micrograms per minute by intravenous infusion rapidly increasing the infusion rate until the uterine activity is suppressed, or the maternal heart rate reaches 140 beats per minute. The required dose is unlikely to exceed 350 micrograms per minute. Whilst the infusion is given preparations should be made for the assisted delivery of the baby. Fifteen to 20 minutes after starting the infusion a fetal scalp blood sample should be taken. If the fetal scalp pH has not improved during the 15–20 minutes of infusion then the planned assisted delivery should be carried out. If the pH has significantly risen, the obstetrician may decide to continue the infusion for a further 15–30 minutes, with continued careful observation before proceeding with the delivery.

Contra-indications, warnings, etc

Contra-indications:

1. Antepartum haemorrhage which demands immediate delivery.
2. Eclampsia and severe pre-eclampsia.
3. Intra-uterine fetal death.
4. Chorioamnionitis.
5. Maternal cardiac disease.
6. Cord compression.

Precautions: Maternal pulmonary oedema has been reported in patients treated concomitantly with betamimetics and corticosteroids. Therefore, close monitoring of the patients state of hydration is advised and if pulmonary oedema develops during administration treatment should be discontinued.

Careful monitoring is required in patients with suspected heart disease, or those receiving other drugs, in particular those which could interact with ritodrine such as monoamine oxidase inhibitors, tricyclic antidepressants, corticosteroids, sympathomimetic amines, beta-adrenergic blocking drugs, anaesthetics used in surgery and potassium-depleting diuretics, as intravenous administration of Yutopar has been shown to decrease plasma potassium levels.

Experiments in animals have shown that even in high dosage Yutopar has no teratogenic properties. Nevertheless, in view of the limited available information from human studies, the administration of Yutopar is not recommended during the first 16 weeks of pregnancy.

In diabetic patients, glucose levels should be closely monitored and insulin requirements adjusted accordingly during intravenous treatment. On oral treatment no alterations have been reported. It is also advisable to screen patients with potential cardiac risk before deciding on ritodrine treatment.

The drug should not be administered to patients with mild to moderate pre-eclampsia, hypertension or hyperthyroidism unless the attending physician considers that the benefits clearly outweigh the risks.

Side-effects: In appropriate dosage Yutopar is well tolerated. In particular no hypotension occurs if the recommended administration schedule is followed and the patient is maintained in the left lateral position. It is only rarely that side-effects call for discontinuation of the treatment. The maternal pulse rate may progressively increase, usually to a moderate degree. This may lead to palpitations.

Any pronounced tachycardia that may arise during an intravenous infusion of Yutopar disappears shortly after decreasing the dosage or after the infusion is stopped. Whether the maternal tachycardia is considered acceptable must be determined from case to case, but it is recommended that, in healthy patients, a heart rate of more than 140/min should be avoided.

Flushing, sweating, tremor, nausea and vomiting have been reported in a few cases. In cases of overdosage of Yutopar, a non-selective beta-sympatholytic agent may be given as an antidote.

Pharmaceutical precautions *Tablets:* Store in a cool dry place, protected from light.

Injection: Store in a cool place, protected from light. Do not use if solution is discoloured or contains a precipitate.

Legal category POM.

Package quantities *Tablets* – Packs of 40 tablets each containing 10 mg ritodrine hydrochloride.

Injection – Boxes of 10 × 5 ml ampoules containing ritodrine hydrochloride 10 mg/ml.

Further information Less effect can be expected if the membranes are ruptured or the dilation of the cervix exceeds 4 cm.

Ritodrine does not produce false positive reactions in standard diagnostic urine tests.

Product licence numbers

Tablets　　　0512/0018

Injection　　　0512/0020R

*Trade Mark

Du Pont (UK) Limited
Pharmaceuticals
Wedgwood Way
Stevenage
Herts SG1 4QN

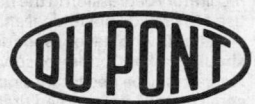

NARCAN*
NARCAN* NEONATAL

Presentation A sterile, clear, colourless solution of naloxone hydrochloride in clear, colourless ampoules.

Narcan (1 ml ampoules and 10 ml vials): each 1 ml of solution contains 0.4 mg naloxone hydrochloride.

Narcan Neonatal (2 ml ampoules): each 1 ml of solution contains 0.02 mg naloxone hydrochloride.

Uses Narcan may be used for the complete or partial reversal of opioid depression, including mild to severe respiratory depression induced by natural and synthetic opioids, the agonist/antagonists nalbuphine and pentazocine, or dextropropoxyphene. It may also be used for the diagnosis of suspected acute opioid overdosage. Narcan Neonatal may be used to counteract respiratory and other CNS depression in the new-born resulting from the administration of analgesics to the mother during childbirth.

Dosage and administration Narcan is for intravenous, intramuscular or subcutaneous injection or intravenous infusion.

Intravenous infusion: Narcan may be diluted for intravenous infusion in normal saline (0.9%) or 5% dextrose in water or saline: the addition of 2 mg of Narcan in 500 ml of either solution provides a concentration of 0.004 mg/ml. Mixtures should be used within 24 hours. After 24 hours, the remaining unused solution must be discarded. The rate of administration should be titrated in accordance with the patient's response to both the Narcan infusion and to any previous bolus doses administered.

Parenteral drug products should be inspected visually for particulate matter and discolouration prior to administration whenever solution and container permit. Narcan should not be mixed with preparations containing bisulphite, metabisulphite, long-chain or high molecular weight anions or any solution having an alkaline pH. No drug or chemical agent should be added to Narcan unless its effect on the chemical and physical stability of the solution has first been established.

Opioid overdosage (known or suspected): Adults: An initial dose of 0.4 mg to 2 mg of Narcan may be administered intravenously. If the desired degree of counteraction and improvement in respiratory function is not obtained it may be repeated at 2 to 3 minute intervals. If no response is observed after 10 mg of Narcan have been administered the diagnosis of opioid-induced or partial opioid-induced toxicity should be questioned. Intramuscular or subcutaneous administration may be necessary if dosing by the intravenous route is not feasible.

N.B. The duration of action of certain opioids can outlast that of an IV bolus of Narcan, e.g. dextropropoxyphene (present in commonly prescribed analgesics which in over-dosage have been associated with suicide), dihydrocodeine and methadone. In situations where one of these opioids is known or suspected it is recommended that an infusion of Narcan (see above) be used to produce sustained antagonism to the opioid without repeated injection.

Post-operative use: When Narcan is used post-operatively, the dose should be titrated for each patient in order to obtain optimum respiratory response while maintaining adequate analgesia. Intravenous doses of 0.1–0.2 mg (1.5–3 micrograms/kg body weight) are usually sufficient, but a full two minutes should be allowed between each 0.1 mg increment of Narcan administered. Further intramuscular doses may be needed within one to two hours, depending on the interval since the last opioid administration and the amount and type (i.e. long or short-acting) of drug used. Alternatively Narcan may be administered as an intravenous infusion (see above).

Children: The usual initial dose in children is 0.01 mg (10 micrograms) per kg body weight given IV. If this dose does not result in the desired degree of clinical improvement, a subsequent dose of 0.1 mg (100 micrograms) per kg of body weight may be administered. Narcan may be required by infusion as described above. If an IV route of administration is not feasible, Narcan may be administered IM or SC in divided doses.

Neonatal use: An adequate airway should be established in the apnoeic infant before Narcan is administered. The usual dose for opioid-induced depression is 0.01 mg/kg (10 micrograms/kg) body weight administered IV, IM or SC. If the desired degree of counteraction and improvement in respiratory function is not obtained it may be repeated at 2 to 3 minute intervals. Alternatively, a single dose of 0.2 mg (200 micrograms or approximately 60 micrograms/kg body weight) may be given intramuscularly at birth. It should, however, be noted that onset of action is slower following IM injection.

Contra-indications, warnings, etc Narcan should not be given to patients who are known to be hypersensitive to it. It should be administered cautiously to patients who have received large doses of opioids or to those physically dependent on opioids since too rapid reversal of opioid effects by Narcan may precipitate an acute withdrawal syndrome in such patients. The same caution is needed when giving Narcan to neonates delivered of such patients.

Although animal reproduction studies have not demonstrated any teratogenic or embryotoxic effects, Narcan should, like all drugs, be used with caution during pregnancy. However, Narcan may be administered to the mother during the second stage of labour to correct respiratory depression in the new-born caused by opioids used to provide obstetrical analgesia.

Patients who have responded satisfactorily to Narcan should be kept under observation. Repeated doses of Narcan may be necessary since the duration of action of some opioids may exceed that of Narcan.

Narcan is not effective against respiratory depression caused by non-opioid drugs.

Two patients with ventricular irritability have developed tachycardia or fibrillation following the administration of naloxone. Although a direct relationship has not been established, it is suggested that Narcan be used with caution in patients with cardiac irritability.

Adverse effects: Occasionally, nausea and vomiting have been reported in post-operative patients who have received Narcan in doses higher than those recommended; however, a cause and effect relationship has not been established.

Overdosage: There have been no reports of acute overdosage with Narcan. Single doses of 10 mg intravenously and subcutaneous doses of 15 mg every four hours for two weeks have been administered without producing either respiratory depression or psychotomimetic effects.

Pharmaceutical precautions Protect from light.

Legal category POM.

Package quantities Narcan ampoules each containing 1 ml are supplied in boxes of 3 or 10 ampoules.

Narcan vials each containing 10 ml are supplied individually packed.

Narcan Neonatal ampoules each containing 2 ml are supplied in boxes of 10 ampoules.

Further information Nil.

Product Licence Numbers
Narcan ampoule   4524/0001
Narcan vial   4524/0001
Narcan Neonatal   4524/0002

NUBAIN* ▼

Presentation Ampoules containing a clear colourless sterile aqueous solution of 20 mg nalbuphine hydrochloride in 2 ml or 10 mg nalbuphine hydrochloride in 1 ml.

Uses Nubain injection is indicated for the relief of moderate to severe pain. It can also be used as a premedication, for pre- and post-operative analgesia, and as a component of balanced anaesthesia. It can also be used in the management of pain due to suspected myocardial infarction.

Dosage and administration Nubain injection may be administered subcutaneously, intramuscularly or intravenously. It may also be administered by patient-controlled on demand intravenous infusion, using a delivery system which is appropriately calibrated and does not interact with the drug.

The usual recommended dosage is 10 mg–20 mg for a 70 kg individual. The dosage should be adjusted according to the severity of pain, physical status of the patient and other medications the patient may be receiving.

Balanced anaesthesia
Induction: 0.3 mg/kg to 1 mg/kg I.V. over a 10–15 minute period.
Maintenance: 0.25–0.5 mg/kg at 30 minute intervals.
Premedication: 0.1–0.2 mg/kg.

Suspected myocardial infarction: Usual dose 20 mg by slow intravenous injection. Some patients may be successfully managed on 10 mg while others may need to have the dose increased to 30 mg. In the absence of pain relief a repeat dose of 20 mg may be given within 30 minutes.

Contra-indications, warnings, etc
Contra-indications: Nubain should not be administered to patients who are hypersensitive to it.

Warnings: Drug dependence: Nubain has low abuse potential. However, caution should be observed in prescribing it for emotionally unstable patients or for patients with a history of opioid abuse.

When Nubain is selected for the control of chronic pain, its suggested prolonged activity may delay the need for larger or more frequent doses.

Abrupt discontinuation of Nubain following prolonged use has been followed by symptoms of opioid withdrawal.

Use in ambulatory patients: Nubain may impair the mental or physical abilities required by the performance of potentially dangerous tasks such as driving a car or operating machinery. Therefore, Nubain should be administered with caution to ambulatory patients who should be warned to avoid such hazards.

Use in children: Because clinical experience in children under the age of 12 is limited, the administration of Nubain in this age group is not recommended.

Use in pregnancy: Safe use of Nubain in pregnancy (including labour) has not been established.

Although animal studies have not revealed teratogenic or embryotoxic effects, nalbuphine should only be administered to pregnant women when, in the judgement of the physician, the potential benefits outweigh the possible hazards.

Nubain should be used to provide analgesia in patients with head injury and increased intracranial pressure only when essential, and then should be administered with extreme caution.

Patients receiving an opioid analgesic, general anaesthetic, phenothiazine or other tranquillizer, sedative, hypnotic or other CNS depressant (including alcohol) concomitantly with Nubain may exhibit an additive effect. When such combined therapy is contemplated, the dose of one or both agents should be reduced.

Precautions: Nubain used as a premedication causes some respiratory depression. Caution should be observed in administering the drug to patients with impaired respiration, or with other medications which produce respiratory depression.

In the presence of bronchial asthma, uraemia, severe infection, cyanosis or respiratory obstruction, Nubain should be administered with caution and in reduced doses.

Nubain should be used with caution and administered in reduced amounts in patients with impaired renal or hepatic function.

Adverse effects: The most frequently seen reaction to Nubain is sedation. Less frequent are sweating, nausea, vomiting, dizziness, dry mouth, vertigo and headache. Rarely seen are CNS effects such as nervousness, depression, confusion and dysphoria. Also reported have been hyper- and hypotension, bradycardia, tachycardia, urticaria, speech difficulty, blurred vision and flushing.

Management of overdosage: The immediate intravenous administration of Narcan* (naloxone hydrochloride) is a specific antidote. Oxygen, intravenous fluids, vasopressors and other supportive measures should be used as indicated.

Pharmaceutical precautions Protect from light. Store at room temperature (15–30°C).

Legal category POM.

Package quantities
Nubain 2 ml ampoules are supplied in boxes of 3 or 10.
Nubain 1 ml ampoules are supplied in boxes of 10.

Further information Nubain is compatible with 0.9% sodium chloride, 5% dextrose, 4.3% dextrose/0.18% saline and Hartmann's solution used in glass, PVC and polyethylene infusion containers.

Product licence number 4524/0003.

*Trade Mark

Ethicon Limited
PO Box 408
Bankhead Avenue
Edinburgh EH11 4HE

ABSELE* STERILE ABSORBABLE BONE SEALANT

Presentation A paste of putty-like consistency, sterilised by gamma irradiation and composed of:

Stabilised bovine fibrin	17.5% w/w
Solubilised bovine collagen	17.5% w/w
Dextran 70	8.0% w/w
Glycerol	30.0% w/w
Water	to 100

Physically it is a yellowish brown to brown, slightly sticky paste having a distinct honey-like odour. It is malleable and adheres to wet cut bone surfaces. Complete absorption of the paste has been shown experimentally in rats in two to three weeks.

Uses The paste is used to control bleeding from the divided, drilled or chipped edges of bone by physically plugging the osseous canals which contain the bleeding capillaries. It is suitable for use in neurosurgery, cardiothoracic surgery and orthopaedic surgery.

Dosage and administration Implantation by application to bone as required to control haemorrhage.

Contra-indications, warnings, etc To date there have been no contra-indications to the use of this product.

Pharmaceutical precautions The product remains in optimum condition when stored at low temperatures. The shelf-life is two years when stored at 15°C, but storage under refrigeration will extend the expected shelf-life. Exposure to temperatures in excess of 30°C may cause irreversible adverse changes to the product.

Legal category P.

Package quantities Flat discs of approximately 2 grams in weight are packaged in a sealed inner aluminium foil pack. This pack is contained in a peel-apart secondary pack. The unit of sale is 12 packs contained in a film wrapped drawer-style carton.

Further information Absorbable bone sealant will harden if left exposed to the atmosphere for long periods, particularly under the heat of operating lights. The package should, therefore, only be opened immediately before use. The package will be damaged by caustics, chlorides and mercurials.

Product licence number 0508/0006.

BIETHIUM* STERILE ABSORBABLE OX FIBRIN PROSTHESIS

Presentation Moulded pliable implants in various shapes and sizes, sterilised by gamma irradiation and contained in a sealed foil sachet, which is in turn contained in a sterilised overwrap. The implant is composed of 65% heat treated bovine fibrin and 35% glycerol. Physically, it is a yellowish brown translucent product with a distinctive honey-like odour. It is pliable and resilient and has a specific gravity of 1.2. Absorption of the implant as observed experimentally in rats is approximately six weeks. However, if the implant is treated with a buffered formaldehyde solution prior to gamma irradiation, the absorption period can be extended for up to five months.

Uses
1. A bean-shaped prosthesis is used for the surgical correction of female stress incontinence. The bean is placed surgically at the urethro-vesical junction to reconstruct the normal angle of exit of the urethra from the bladder.
2. The buffer is rectangular and, used in pairs, effectively compresses the liver substance, following biopsy or liver resection, again by broadening the surface area of pressure of the ligating suture.
3. The rod shaped prosthesis provides support for exteriorising the loop of large bowel during a defunctioning colostomy.

Dosage and administration One bean only is required in stress incontinence, one rod for a defunctioning colostomy, while the liver buffers are used in pairs. Administration is by implant at a surgical procedure.

Contra-indications, warnings, etc Biethium is supplied sterile and should not be resterilised.

Pharmaceutical precautions Store under normal shelf conditions. Observe expiry date.

Legal category P.

Package quantities One bean per foil pack, with five foil packs per box. Two buffers per foil pack, with five foil packs per box. One rod per foil pack with five foil packs per box. Each foil pack is overwrapped in a peel-open container. The boxes containing the foil packs are film overwrapped.

Further information *Storage:* Two years' shelf life. Avoid storing beside caustics, chlorides and mercurials which could damage the aluminium foil pack.

Product licence number 0508/0003.

Coated VICRYL* (Polyglactin 910)
Sterilised Absorbable Synthetic Suture

Presentation The basic Vicryl (Polyglactin 910) Suture is prepared from a copolymer of glycolide and lactide. The substances are derived respectively from glycolic and lactic acids. The empirical formula of the copolymer is $(C_2H_2O_2)m(C_3H_4O2)n$.

Coated Vicryl (polyglactin 910) Sutures are obtained by coating the braided suture material with a mixture composed of a copolymer of glycolide and lactide and an equal amount of calcium stearate. This coating does not affect the biological properties of the suture.

Vicryl (Polyglactin 910) Sutures are coloured by adding D & C Violet No 2 during polymerisation of the lactide and glycolide. Sutures may also be manufactured in the undyed form.

These sutures are relatively inert, nonantigenic, non-pyrogenic and elicit only a mild tissue reaction during absorption.

Two important characteristics describe the in vivo behaviour of absorbable sutures. The first of these is tensile strength retention and the second absorption rate or loss of mass.

Subcutaneous tissue implantation studies of Coated Vicryl Suture in rats show at two weeks post-implantation approximately 55% of its original tensile strength remains, while at three weeks approximately 20% of its original strength is retained.

Intramuscular implantation studies in rats show that the absorption of these sutures is minimal until about the 40th post-implantation day. Absorption is essentially complete between the 60th and 90th days.

Uses Coated Vicryl synthetic absorbable sutures are intended for use where an absorbable suture or ligature is indicated.

Dosage and administration By implantation.

Contra-indications, warnings, etc These sutures, being absorbable, should not be used where extended approximation of tissues under stress is required.

Sutures placed in skin and conjunctiva may cause localised irritation if left in place for longer than 7 days and should be removed as indicated.

At the discretion of the surgeon, appropriate non-absorbable sutures may be used to provide additional wound support when coated Vicryl sutures are used in ophthalmic procedures.

The safety and effectiveness of Vicryl (Polyglactin 910) and Coated Vicryl Sutures in neural tissue and in cardiovascular tissue have not been established.

Pharmaceutical precautions Do not re-sterilise.

Legal category Pharmacy medicine sold to surgeons and hospitals through surgical dealers.

Package quantities Various lengths of material packaged in sealed aluminium foil sachets. This primary pack is contained in a peel-apart secondary pack. The unit of sale is 12 packs contained in a film wrapped drawer style carton.

Further information No suture related adverse reactions were reported during clinical trials, although a number of minor reactions were classified as being of unknown cause.

Product licence number 0508/0009

PDS* (Polydioxanone)
Sterilised Absorbable Synthetic Suture

Presentation PDS (Polydioxanone) Monofilament Synthetic Absorbable Suture is prepared from the polyester poly (p-dioxanone). The empirical molecular formula of the polymer is $(C_4H_6O_3)n$. PDS (Polydioxanone) sutures are coloured by adding either D & C Blue No 6 (gauges Metric 0.2 and 0.3, 10/0 and 9/0) or D & C Violet No 2 (gauges metric 0.4 to 5.0, 8/0 to 2) during polymerisation. These sutures may also be manufactured undyed (clear).

PDS (Polydioxanone) sutures are relatively inert, non-antigenic, non-pyrogenic and elicit only a mild tissue reaction during absorption.

Action: Two important characteristics describe the in vivo behaviour of absorbable sutures. The first of these is tensile strength retention and the second absorption rate or loss of mass.

Data obtained from implantation studies in rats show that, at two weeks post implantation, approximately 70% of the suture strength is retained whilst at four weeks the strength retention is approximately 50%. At eight weeks approximately 14% of the original strength remains. *This indicates a significantly longer period of wound support than previously available with an absorbable suture.*

The absorption or loss of mass is minimal until about the 90th post implantation day and is essentially complete within six months.

Uses PDS (Polydioxanone) monofilament sutures are intended for use where an absorbable suture or ligature is indicated. They may have particular application where longer wound support is required. See strength retention data above.

Dosage and administration By implantation.

Contra-indications, warnings, etc These sutures, being absorbable, should not be used where extended approximation of tissues under stress is required.

As with all monofilament synthetic sutures, care should be taken to ensure proper knot security.

Conjunctival, cuticular and vaginal epithelium sutures could cause localised irritation if left in place for longer than 10 days. Superficial placement of subcuticular sutures may also be associated with enythema and reaction during the course of absorption.

The safety and effectiveness of PDS (Polydioxanone) sutures in neural and cardiac tissue have not been established.

Pharmaceutical precautions Do not re-sterilise.

Legal category P.
Pharmacy medicine sold to surgeons and hospitals through surgical dealers.

Package quantities The gauge range initially available will be 0.2 metric (10/0) to 5 metric (2). Various lengths of material attached to non traumatic stainless steel needles are packaged in sealed aluminium foil sachets.

This primary pack is contained in a peel-apart secondary pack. The unit of sale is 12 or 24 packs contained in a film wrapped drawer style carton.

Further information No suture related adverse reactions were reported during clinical trials, although a number of minor reactions were classified as being of unknown cause.

Product licence number 0508/0011
0508/0012

POLYTEF* PASTE FOR INJECTION

Presentation A sterile, white, injectable paste in tin tubes within a see-through, peel-apart overwrap. Polytef Paste contains 50% of polytetrafluoroethylene powder (which has been pyrolised to purify it) in Glycerin USP containing polyoxyethylene sorbitan monolaurate (Tween 20)

Uses Polytef Paste for Injection is used for intravocal cord injection of the paralysed vocal cord. It is administered by injection directly into the cord.

Dosage and administration By injection. Dose varies according to size of cord, but should not exceed 0.6 cc per site of injection.

Contra-indications, warnings, etc Contra-indicated until at least six months have elapsed following the onset of paralysis, and/or until an intensive trial of rehabilitation by voice therapy has been given since many patients are capable of overcoming their vocal disability.

In bilateral laryngeal paralysis. In vocal disorders of psychogenic origin. In the presence of foreign bodies in the larynx (e.g. fragments of shells or bullets).

In the presence of an acute inflammation, infection or inadequately controlled malignancy, or a rapidly advancing disease, especially when these are in the laryngeal or upper respiratory tract area.

Warnings: Intra-cordal injection is a delicate procedure and should be conducted with precision and great caution. This product should be used only by trained ENT surgeons.

General anaesthesia is not advisable. Over-sedation may lead to an unco-operative patient and difficult airway problems. Intravascular injections must be avoided. Likewise, over-injection should be avoided.

It is safer to under-inject the involved cord than to over-inject because treatment may be repeated at a later time. If the procedure is followed by upper respiratory tract inflammatory changes in excess of the reaction expected at the site of injection, diagnostic and therapeutic procedures should be implemented. In acute fulminating reactions, steroid and antibiotic therapy may be indicated. This therapy should be at the discretion of the surgeon.

Pharmaceutical precautions Store in a cool place.

Legal category POM.

Package quantities Polytef Paste for Injection is packaged in tin tubes containing 7 cc and contained in a peel-apart overwrap.

Further information Nil.

Product licence number 0508/0002.

STERILISED FASCIA LATA

Presentation Straw-coloured strip 20 cm × 6 mm consisting of bovine connective tissue from below the hide. Fascia Lata is packaged in a tubing fluid containing isopropanol and water.

Uses In surgical operations upon the human body as a substitute for human fascia.

Dosage and administration By implantation.

Contra-indications, warnings, etc There are no contra-indications or warnings.

It is recommended that Fascia Lata is rinsed in sterile water or sterile saline solution to remove tubing fluid before use.

Pharmaceutical precautions Do not subject to heat. Store in a cool place.

Legal category P.

Package quantities Three heat-sealed foil packs overwrapped and placed in a film-wrapped plastic suture box.

Further information Individual unopened packs which have been removed from the overwrap may be re-sterilised by immersion in a solution of 1% w/v formaldehyde in 93% isopropanol q.s. water. Avoid contact with caustics, chlorides and mercurials which could cause damage to the aluminium foil pack.

Product licence number 0508/5004.

STERILISED SURGICAL BONE WAX

Presentation Solid wax. A white solid, somewhat translucent when in thin layers. Comprises: Refined white beeswax 90%; isopropyl palmitate 10%.

Uses For controlling haemorrhaging in osseous surgery and the control of the escape of fluids from osseous tissues.

Dosage and administration By implantation and application to bone as required to control haemorrhage.

Contra-indications, warnings, etc Bone wax should not be used where rapid osseous regeneration and fusion are desired.

Bone wax may inhibit osteogenesis and may act as a physical barrier to the reparative process. Bone wax should not be re-sterilised or subjected to excessive heat.

Pharmaceutical precautions The package containing Ethicon bone wax should be opened just prior to use to minimise the possibility of contamination and excessive drying.

Bone wax should be used immediately after removal from the package and, using an aseptic technique, warmed to the desired consistency by manipulation with the fingers. Bone wax should be used sparingly and any excess removed from the operative site.

Bone wax should be stored under normal warehouse conditions.

Legal category P.

Package quantities Slabs (5 × 2 × 0.13 cm) of approximately 2.5 g in weight packed in a paper slide and sleeve which is overwrapped packed. The overwraps are presented in a filmwrapped cardboard box containing one dozen.

Further information Mild inflammatory reactions have been reported in tissue immediately adjacent to the site of implantation. Studies have suggested that Bone Wax as a foreign body may impair the ability of cancellous bone to clear bacteria (Johnson, Peter, and Fronn, David, Effects of Bone Wax on Bacterial Clearance. *Surgery* 89(2), 1981). In animal models, the local accumulation of foreign body giant cells has been observed and histological examination has revealed the appearance of macrophages and occasionally polymorphonuclear leucocytes and lymphocytes.

Product licence number 0508/5001R.

STERILISED SURGICAL CATGUT BP – ETHICON* BRAND

Presentation An absorbable strand, with or without a needle attached, consisting of collagen derived from the intestinal tract or gut of healthy mammals uniformly twisted to produce virtually a monofilament strand with a diameter conforming to the requirements set out in the British Pharmacopoeia.

It is capable of being absorbed by living mammalian tissue but may be treated to modify its resistance to absorption.

Plain catgut is Sterilised Surgical Catgut which has not been treated to prolong its resistance to digestion. It is straw coloured.

Chromic catgut is material which has been hardened by treatment with chromium salts in trivalent form and with oxidised pyrogallol (oxidised pyrogallic acid) to prolong its resistance to absorption. It is brown coloured.

Extra chromic catgut is chromic catgut which has been treated to prolong its resistance slightly further.

Plain and chromic catgut may be dyed with a blue (indigo) dye.

Sterilised Surgical Catgut is packed in tubing fluid containing isopropanol and water.

Uses Sterilised Surgical Catgut is used in surgical operations upon the human body.

Dosage and administration By implantation.

Contra-indications, warnings, etc Should not be used in situations where a non-absorbable suture would normally be used.

Pharmaceutical precautions Do not subject absorbable surgical suture to heat. Do not rinse or soak in fluids other than the tubing fluid. Store in a cool place.

Legal category P.

Package quantities Various lengths (40 cm to 1.5 m) in heat-sealed foil packs. The foil packs are contained in a peel-open overwrap and packed into film-wrapped boxes containing one dozen sutures.

Further information Individual unopened packs which have been removed from the overwrap may be re-sterilised by immersion in a solution of 1% w/v formaldehyde in 93% isopropanol q.s. water. Avoid contact with caustics, chlorides and mercurials which could cause damage to the aluminium foil pack.

Product licence number 0508/5002R.

STERILISED SURGICAL COLLAGEN

Presentation An absorbable strand of re-constituted collagen with a needle attached. Available plain or chromicised. Sterilised Surgical Collagen is packed in tubing fluid containing isopropanol and water.

Uses Used in surgical operations upon the human body.

Dosage and administration By implantation.

Contra-indications, warnings, etc Should not be used in situations where a non-absorbable suture would normally be used.

Pharmaceutical precautions Do not subject absorbable surgical suture to heat. Do not rinse or soak in fluids other than the tubing fluid. Store in a cool place.

Legal category P.

Package quantities Various lengths in heat-sealed foil packs. The foil pack is contained in a peel-open overwrap and packed into film-wrapped boxes which hold one dozen sutures.

Further information Individual unopened packs which have been removed from the overwrap may be re-sterilised by immersion in a solution of 1% w/v formaldehyde in 93% isopropanol q.s. water. Avoid contact with caustics, chlorides and mercurials which could cause damage to the aluminium foil pack.

Product licence number 0508/5008R.

ZENODERM* CORIUM IMPLANT

Presentation A white biscuit-like matrix of enzyme treated, glutaraldehyde cross-linked, lyophilised or air dried porcine dermis. All non-collagenous elements are removed by immersion in a proteolytic enzyme whilst glutaraldehyde treatment crosslinks the collagen for strength. Individual sheets are cut to various sizes and thicknesses depending upon their ultimate clinical application.

Uses As a biological implant for tissue replacement in areas where tissue is weak, deficient or absent, e.g. in: Dural Replacement, Fascia Lata Substitute, Bladder Sling, Oro Antral Fistulae, Senile Entropion, Repair of Herniae, Perforations of the Tympanic Membrane.

Dosage and administration By implantation.

Contra-indications, warnings, etc No situation has presented, to date, in the areas listed above, where the use of the material is contra-indicated. Supplied sterile, Zenoderm Corium Implant should not be resterilised. Open unused Zenoderm implant should be discarded.

Pharmaceutical precautions Under normal storage conditions, a shelf life of 5 years is recommended for Zenoderm Corium Implant. It should be stored in a cool place and not subjected to heat.

Legal category Not applicable.

Package quantities Supplied sterile in double peel apart overwrap envelopes (foil backing transparent fronts), Zenoderm Corium Implant is available in the following sizes, packaged 5 sheets per box.

25 cm × 12 cm × 0.6 mm	(ZD 6251)
10 cm × 10 cm × 0.3 mm	(ZD 3101)
30 cm × 2 cm × 0.6 mm	(ZD 6301)
20 cm × 1.5 cm × 0.6 mm	(ZD 6201)

10 cm ×	5 cm × 0.6 mm	(ZD 6101)
14 cm ×	7 cm × 0.3 mm	(ZD 3143)
3 cm ×	3 cm × 0.3 mm	(ZD 3033)
2 cm ×	2 cm × 0.1 mm	(ZD 1021)

Further information Zenoderm Corium Implant is crosslinked in a buffered solution of glutaraldehyde then freeze or air dried before sterilisation by gamma irradiation. After implantation into the human body Zenoderm is gradually replaced by host tissue.

Product licence number 0508/0007.

Trade Mark

Evans Medical Limited
318 High Street North
Dunstable
Beds LU6 1BE

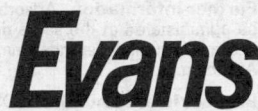

ADSORBED DIPHTHERIA AND TETANUS VACCINE BP (DT/Vac/Ads)

Presentation Adsorbed Diphtheria and Tetanus Vaccine is a mixture of diphtheria formol toxoid and tetanus formol toxoid adsorbed on aluminium hydroxide; each 0.5 ml dose contains not less than 30 i.u. of diphtheria toxoid and not less than 40 i.u. of tetanus toxoid.

Uses Active immunisation against diphtheria and tetanus in infants and children. Reinforcement of immunity to diphtheria and tetanus in children under the age of 10 years.

Dosage and administration *Children under 10 years:* A dose of 0.5 ml of vaccine should be administered by deep subcutaneous or intramuscular injection. The container should be shaken before withdrawing the prescribed dose.

Basic course: The course consists of three doses with an interval of 6–8 weeks between the first and second dose and 4–6 months between the second and third dose.

Reinforcing doses: Children under the age of 10 years immunised in infancy with adsorbed diphtheria and tetanus vaccine or diphtheria, tetanus and pertussis vaccine should receive a reinforcing dose of diphtheria and tetanus vaccine at 5 years of age.

Contra-indications, warnings, etc
Contra-indications: Presence of acute infectious disease.

Warnings: A sterile syringe and Adrenaline Injection BP should be ready for use in case the need arises for emergency treatment of an allergic reaction.
   Not for intradermal use.

Adverse effects: Transient pyrexia, headache, malaise, local swelling, redness and tenderness may occur. A small painless nodule may form at the injection site. Severe anaphylactoid reactions are rare. Neurological symptoms have been reported occasionally.

Pharmaceutical precautions Protect from light. Store in a refrigerator between 2°C and 8°C (36°F and 46°F). Do not freeze.
   Partly used multidose containers should be discarded within three hours of withdrawal of the first dose.

Legal category POM.

Package quantities Carton of 10 × 0.5 ml ampoules and vial of 5 ml.

Further information Nil.

Product licence number 0039/0114.

ADSORBED TETANUS VACCINE BP (Tet/Vac/Ads)

Presentation Adsorbed Tetanus Vaccine BP is a suspension of purified formol toxoid, prepared by formalin detoxification of *Clostridium tetani* exotoxin, adsorbed on aluminium hydroxide. Each 0.5 ml dose contains not less than 40 i.u. of tetanus toxoid.

Uses Active immunisation against tetanus. Reinforcement of immunity to tetanus.

Dosage and administration The vaccine should be administered by deep subcutaneous or intramuscular injection. The container should be shaken before withdrawing the prescribed dose.

Primary immunisation: The course consists of 3 doses each of 0.5 ml; the second dose is administered after an interval of 6–8 weeks and the third dose after a further interval of four to six months.

Reinforcing doses: A reinforcing dose of 0.5 ml should be given 5 years after the basic course, and another 5 to 15 years later should provide a satisfactory degree of protection.
   After a basic course has been given, a single reinforcing dose will provide protection in the event of an injury which is considered might give rise to tetanus. Reinforcing doses should not be given at too frequent intervals as they may provoke hypersensitivity reactions.
   Tetanus vaccine should not routinely be given to any patient who has received a booster dose in the preceding 5 years, unless the wound is regarded as carrying an unusually high risk of tetanus, and even then vaccine is not necessary if a booster has been given during the preceding year.

Contra-indications, warnings, etc
Contra-indications: Acute infection is a contra-indication to routine tetanus immunisation, except in the presence of a tetanus-prone wound.

Warnings: A sterile syringe and Adrenaline Injection BP should be ready for use, in case the need arises for emergency treatment of an allergic reaction.
   Not for intradermal use.

Side-effects: Transient pyrexia, headache, malaise, local swelling, redness and tenderness may occur. A small painless nodule may form at the injection site. Severe anaphylactoid reactions are rare. Neurological symptoms have been reported occasionally.

Pharmaceutical precautions Protect from light. Store in a refrigerator between 2°C and 8°C (36°F and 46°F). Do not freeze. Partly used multi-dose containers should be discarded within 3 hours of withdrawal of the first dose.

Legal category POM.

Package quantities Carton of 10 × 0.5 ml ampoules and vial of 5 ml.

Further information Adsorbed tetanus vaccine may be administered at the same time as, but at a different site from Human Tetanus Immunoglobulin or Tetanus Antitoxin.

Product licence number 0039/0115.

BCG VACCINE (INTRADERMAL)

Presentation Multidose ampoules containing a white freeze-dried pellet which easily disperses to form an opalescent liquid on reconstitution. This vaccine is a suspension containing living Bacillus Calmette-Guérin, a strain of tubercle bacillus which has been attenuated by growth on a special medium.

Development of special culture conditions by Glaxo research has resulted in a vaccine which, in the dry state, resists the effects of heat. Even after exposure to a temperature of 37°C for four weeks, sufficient activity remained to give 100% tuberculin conversion after reconstitution (Wright et al, Tubercle 53, 92, (1972)).

This vaccine complies with the specifications for Bacillus Calmette-Guérin Vaccine BP, and Vaccinum Tuberculosis (BCG) Cryodesiccatum (Ph Eur), and is of standardised potency.

It also complies with WHO Requirements for Dried BCG Vaccine – Revised 1978.

Uses BCG Vaccine (Intradermal) induces active immunity to tuberculosis. Vaccinated persons normally become Mantoux-positive after a period of eight weeks has elapsed but sometimes up to 14 weeks are needed.

Dosage and administration *Adults and children over three months of age:* 0.1 ml strictly by **intradermal** injection (subcutaneous injection should be avoided).

Neonates: 0.05 ml by **intradermal** injection.

The inoculation should be given in the arm, over the insertion of the deltoid muscle. Administration in the leg has been associated with more severe reactions in neonates and should be avoided.

No special precautions are necessary when opening the ampoule to avoid dispersal of the vaccine, despite the ampoule being sealed under reduced pressure, as the dextran content produces a solid plug. The vaccine must not be contaminated with any antiseptic or detergent. If alcohol is used to swab the skin, it must be allowed to evaporate before the vaccine is injected.

The vaccine suspension is prepared by adding 1 ml of Water for Injections or Sodium Chloride Injection BP (sterile isotonic saline) to the 1 ml multidose ampoule. When using the 5 ml multidose ampoule, 5 ml of Sodium Chloride Injection BP (not Water for Injections) should be added. Do NOT shake as this causes frothing. Allow to stand for one minute, then draw it into the syringe once or twice to ensure homogeneity. Once the liquid vaccine has been prepared, it should be used in the same session, i.e. within 4 hours.

The injection site is best left uncovered to facilitate healing.

Contra-indications, warnings, etc
Contra-indications: Unless specifically indicated, BCG Vaccine should not be given to patients suffering from generalised eczema, infective dermatoses, hypogammaglobulinaemia, or to those with a history of deficient immunity, particularly to bacterial infections. The same applies to patients being treated with antimetabolites, irradiation, systemic corticosteroids, or any substance that depresses the immune response. The effect of Intradermal BCG vaccine may be exaggerated in these patients, and a more generalised infection is possible.

Intradermal BCG vaccine should not be given to patients who are receiving prophylactic doses of anti-tuberculous drugs.

Tuberculin-positive persons, i.e. those with induration of 6 mm or greater in diameter in the Mantoux test, or those in Heaf grades 2 to 4, do not require the vaccine. Its administration to these persons may result in an accelerated local reaction of larger size.

Pregnancy: When there is a risk of tuberculous infection, the importance of vaccination may outweigh the possible risk of BCG to the fetus.

Warnings: BCG Vaccine may be given at the same time as oral poliomyelitis vaccine. With other live vaccines it is preferable to allow an interval of three weeks between administration of BCG and the other vaccine, but the interval can be reduced to 10 days if a longer period is not available. In neonates concomitant administration of BCG and smallpox vaccines is effective, but different arms must be used. This could result in vaccination lesions in both arms.

Any prepared vaccine remaining at the end of the session (maximum 4 hours) should be discarded, and preferably incinerated or treated with a disinfectant such as strong hypochlorite solution.

Side-effects: Occasionally an excessive response to BCG Vaccine results in a discharging ulcer. Frequently this is attributable to inadvertent subcutaneous injection, or to excessive dosage. The ulcer should be encouraged to dry and abrasion avoided, e.g. by tight clothes. Waterproof dressings should not be used. If the ulcer persists, it can be treated by application of a cream containing neomycin and a corticosteroid, or by local application of isoniazid powder.

In the rare cases of severe local reactions with abscess formation, aspiration should be carried out, perhaps with streptomycin replacement. Enlargement of axillary lymph glands is unlikely, except occasionally in young infants.

Overdosage: If gross overdosage occurs, and there is reason to suspect the development of a more generalised infection with BCG, systemic treatment with isoniazid or any other suitable anti-tuberculous drug, should be given.

Pharmaceutical precautions Protect from light and store in a refrigerator between 2°C and 8°C (36°F and 46°F) but avoid freezing ampoules of diluent. Refrigeration during actual delivery is not essential but the vaccine should be kept as cool as possible.

Legal category POM.

Package quantities Carton of 10 × 1 ml multidose ampoules.

Composite pack of five 1 ml multidose ampoules with five 1 ml ampoules of Water for Injections.

Composite pack of 5 × 5 ml multidose ampoules with 5 × 5 ml ampoules of Sodium Chloride Injection BP.

All packs are available to United Kingdom Health Authorities and hospitals through Department of Health and Social Security contract.

Further information No batch of vaccine is released until it has been shown to resist a temperature of 37°C for 28 days.

Measles or rubella infection can cause tuberculin positive patients to revert temporarily to tuberculin negative.

The intradermal administration of BCG Vaccine (Intradermal) should preferably be carried out with a syringe fitted with a short bevel gauge 25 needle.

If other apparatus is used, e.g. a jet injector, it is essential to ensure that the vaccine is still deposited strictly intradermally and in the correct dosage.

Isoniazid Resistant BCG Vaccine (Intradermal) is available on request direct from Evans Medical (Sales Administration Department).

Product licence number 0039/0110R.

BCG VACCINE (PERCUTANEOUS)

Presentation Multidose ampoules containing a white freeze-dried pellet which easily disperses to form an opalescent suspension on reconstitution. This vaccine contains dextran and living Bacillus Calmette-Guérin (BCG) with a higher viable bacterial count than BCG Vaccine (Intradermal). The BCG is an attenuated form of a strain of tubercle bacillus. This vaccine complies with the specification for Percutaneous BCG Vaccine BP, and is of standardised potency.

Uses BCG Vaccine (Percutaneous) induces active immunity to tuberculosis. Vaccinated persons normally become Mantoux-positive after a period of eight weeks has elapsed, but sometimes up to 14 weeks are needed.

Dosage and administration Percutaneous BCG Vaccine is used with a multiple puncture apparatus equipped with not less than 20 needles giving reliable penetration of the skin to a depth of 2 mm. Ethyl or isopropyl alcohol may be used to prepare the skin, which must be dry before the vaccine is used.

With a dry syringe add 0.3 ml of Water for Injections or Sodium Chloride Injection to the ampoule of BCG, and allow to stand for about one minute to allow a suspension to form. Do NOT shake, as this causes frothing. A small amount (about 0.03 ml) is transferred onto the skin by means of a glass rod, platinum loop or spatula. The treated area of skin is then immediately punctured with the multiple puncture apparatus.

Once the liquid vaccine has been prepared, it should be used in the same session i.e. within 4 hours.

The injection site is best left uncovered; waterproof dressings are particularly undesirable. The multiple puncture apparatus should be sterilised according to the maker's instructions. Any alcohol or ether used should be burnt off before the apparatus is used, and IT MUST BE ALLOWED TO COOL before use. Detergents or antiseptics should not be used.

Contra-indications, warnings, etc

Contra-indications: Unless specifically indicated, Percutaneous BCG Vaccine should not be given to patients suffering from generalised eczema, infective dermatoses, hypogammaglobulinaemia or a history of deficient immunity, especially to bacterial infections. This vaccine is also contra-indicated in patients treated with antimetabolites, irradiation, systemic corticosteroids, or any substance which depresses the immune response.

This vaccine should not be given to patients who are receiving prophylactic doses of anti-tuberculous drugs.

Tuberculin positive persons, i.e., those with induration of 6 mm or greater in diameter with the Mantoux test or those in Heaf grades 2 to 4 do not require BCG

vaccination and slightly enhanced local reactions may be seen if they are vaccinated.

Pregnancy: When there is a risk of tuberculous infection, the importance of vaccination may outweigh the possible risks of BCG to the fetus.

Warnings: Percutaneous BCG Vaccine must NOT be given by intradermal injection.

BCG Vaccine may be given at the same time as oral poliomyelitis vaccine. With other live vaccines it is preferable to allow an interval of three weeks between administration of BCG and the other vaccine, but the interval can be reduced to 10 days if a longer period is not available.

Any prepared vaccine remaining at the end of the session (maximum 4 hours) should be discarded, and incinerated or treated with a disinfectant such as stong hypochlorite solution.

Side-effects: Occasionally an excessive response to percutaneous BCG vaccine results in a discharging ulcer. This should be encouraged to dry and abrasion avoided, e.g. by tight clothes. Waterproof dressings should not be used. If the ulcer persists, it can be treated by application of a cream containing a corticosteroid, with neomycin to prevent secondary infection, or by local application of isoniazid powder.

In the rare cases of severe local reactions with abscess formation, aspiration should be carried out, perhaps with streptomycin replacement. Enlargement of axillary lymph glands is unlikely, except occasionally in young infants.

Overdosage: If there is reason to suspect the development of a generalised infection with BCG, systemic treatment with isoniazid or any other suitable anti-tuberculous drug should be given.

Pharmaceutical precautions Protect from light and store in a refrigerator between 2°C and 8°C (36°F and 46°F). Refrigeration during actual delivery is not essential, but the vaccine should be kept as cool as possible.

Legal category POM.

Package quantities Carton of 10 multidose ampoules.

Further information Infections such as measles or rubella may cause tuberculin-positive patients to revert temporarily to tuberculin-negative.

Product licence number 0039/0112R.

FLUVIRIN*

Presentation Fluvirin is Inactivated Influenza Vaccine (Surface Antigen) BP containing highly purified haemagglutinin and neuraminidase antigens prepared from those strains of influenza virus currently recommended by the WHO.

Uses Protection against influenza in those groups regarded as being at special risk, especially the elderly, which include those suffering from the following conditions:

Chronic pulmonary disease, e.g. chronic bronchitis and emphysema, asthma, bronchiectasis, pulmonary tuberculosis and fibrosis.

Chronic heart disease, e.g. valvular and hypertensive heart disease.

Chronic renal disease, e.g. chronic nephritis; patients with renal disease on immunosuppressive drugs.

Diabetes and possibly other less common endocrine disorders.

Patients who are being actively considered for immunosuppressive therapy.

Immunisation against influenza is also recommended in:

School children over four years of age and in elderly persons living in residential establishments, in which rapid spread is likely to follow the introduction of infection.

Doctors, nurses, ambulance men, and others at special risk of infection by reason of their contacts with persons suffering from influenza.

Dosage and administration *Adults and children aged 4 and over:* 0.5 ml by deep subcutaneous or intramuscular injection. Young children who may not have been previously infected, or who have not received trivalent influenza vaccine in the past four years may require two doses of vaccine given at an interval of 4–6 weeks, to ensure a protective antibody response.

The vaccine must be allowed to reach room temperature before use: the container should be well shaken immediately before making the injection.

Contra-indications, warnings, etc
Contra-indications: Fluvirin is contra-indicated in persons sensitive to egg, chicken or influenzal viral protein. Immunisation should be delayed if there is active or suspected infection.

Pregnancy: There is no evidence that Fluvirin causes damage to the foetus. It would however be prudent, as with other drug preparations in pregnancy, particularly the first trimester, to restrict administration to patients where there is an indication for its use.

Warnings: Because the vaccine contains highly purified haemagglutinin and neuraminidase antigens the total viral content of the vaccine has been reduced to about one tenth of that of whole virus vaccines. Even so, a sterile syringe and Adrenaline Injection BP should be ready for use, in case the need arises for emergency treatment of an allergic reaction.

Spirit should not be allowed to come in contact with the vaccine.

Side-effects: Local effects such as redness and soreness at the site of injection may occur.

Systemic effects, such as headache, pyrexia and a feeling of malaise may occur.

Both local and systemic side effects are less frequent with Fluvirin than with Inactivated Influenza Vaccine (Split Virus) BP.

Overdosage: Not applicable.

Pharmaceutical precautions Fluvirin should be protected from light and stored in a refrigerator between 2°C and 8°C (36°F and 46°F). Do not freeze. Though limited exposure to light and higher temperatures has no adverse effect on the vaccine, temperatures above 20°C (68°F) should be avoided.

Legal category POM.

Package quantities Fluvirin is available in 0.5 ml disposable syringe packs only.

Further information Studies with surface antigen influenza vaccine have shown that the purified haemagglutinin and neuraminidase antigens contained in a single dose of Fluvirin will produce a protective antibody response in up to 90% of patients for up to nine months.

Product licence number 0039/0127.

MEVILIN*-L
Measles Vaccine (Live Attenuated) BP
(Schwarz strain) Meas/Vac (Live)

Presentation Mevilin-L is a freeze-dried preparation of living attenuated virus of the Schwarz strain. It must be reconstituted with Water for Injections BP immediately prior to injection; the reconstituted vaccine may vary in colour from pale straw to pink – this variation is not indicative of deterioration.

Uses General prophylaxis against measles and within 3 days of exposure to measles.

Dosage and administration One dose by deep subcutaneous or intramuscular injection (contains not less than 1,000 $TCID_{50}$ of measles virus). Mevilin-L should be administered to infants at about 12 to 15 months. There is no upper age limit for measles vaccination.

To reconstitute Mevilin-L inject 0.5 ml of Water for Injections BP from the ampoule provided into the vial containing the freeze-dried vaccine, allow to stand for about a minute then mix the suspension by withdrawing it into the syringe and expelling it back into the vial. The use of a 2 ml disposable syringe is recommended. The dose of the reconstituted vaccine is 0.5 ml.

Contra-indications, warnings, etc
Contra-indications: Mevilin-L should not be given to children below the age of one year unless at special risk of contracting measles. If this is the case, a second dose should be given at a later date as interference from maternally derived antibody may cause a failure to respond.

Any active or suspected infection is reason for delaying vaccination.

Mevilin-L should not be given to children suffering from leukaemia, Hodgkin's disease or other malignant conditions or hypogammaglobulinaemia. Also those with impaired immune responsiveness, whether occurring naturally or as a result of treatment with steroids, radiotherapy, cytotoxic drugs or other agents.

Pregnancy is a contra-indication. Also hypersensitivity to neomycin and polymyxin.

Allergy to hens' eggs is no longer considered to be a contra-indication to the vaccine except in patients with severe hypersensitivity. Individuals with a history of anaphylactoid reactions to egg ingestion should not be given measles vaccine. Persons who have allergies to egg that are not of an anaphylactoid nature and those with allergies to chicken feathers may be vaccinated in the usual manner.

Children with the following conditions should be given measles vaccine but only with the simultaneous administration of specially DILUTED normal immunoglobulin for use with measles vaccine.

1. Personal history of convulsions.
2. History of idiopathic epilepsy in parents or siblings.
3. Chronic disease of the heart or lungs.
4. Seriously underdeveloped.

The DILUTE immunoglobulin contains 8–16 International Units (ius) measles antibody in 1.8 ml, and the recommended dose is 0.4 to 0.8 iu of measles antibody/kg body weight.

A separate syringe should be used for injecting the immunoglobulin into the contralateral arm. It is important not to exceed the dose as overdosage can prevent the development of immunity.

The attenuated vaccine virus is not excreted after vaccination and thus there is no risk of infection from vaccine recipients.

Management of measles outbreaks: Human NORMAL immunoglobulin is available for individuals for whom the live vaccine is contra-indicated. Children under the age of one year and those who are immunosuppressed should be given human normal immunoglobulin, with a specific content of measles antibody, if they have been in contact with measles infection. Dose: Under 1 year 0.25 g; 1–2 years 0.5 g; over 3 years 1.5 g.

Precautions: Attenuated measles vaccine is quickly killed by ether, alcohol and detergents: these agents should not be used for sterilising syringes prior to immunisation. Liquids used for cleansing the skin prior to injection should be allowed to dry before the vaccine is given.

Warnings: A sterile syringe and Adrenaline Injection BP should be ready for use, in case the need arises for emergency treatment of an allergic reaction.

Mevilin-L must not be given intravenously and should not normally be given within 3 months of a transfusion of blood or human plasma or treatment with Human Immunoglobulin except as previously specified. If any of these substances have been used near to the time of vaccination a test for the presence of measles antibody should be made at a later date.

The vaccine should not normally be given less than 3 weeks before or after immunisation with other live virus vaccines.

Measles vaccine may depress tuberculin skin sensitivity for 4 weeks or longer.

Adverse effects: When adverse reactions occur they usually appear about the eighth day. The symptoms are usually mild and may include malaise, cough, coryza, rash, pharyngitis, pyrexia and headache. Convulsions may accompany the fever.

Severe reactions are uncommon and encephalitis has been reported on rare occasions.

Pharmaceutical precautions Mevilin-L should be protected from light and stored in a refrigerator between 2°C and 8°C (36°F and 46°F). Do not freeze.

The reconstituted vaccine should be used as soon as possible and certainly within one hour.

Neomycin and polymyxin are used in the tissue culture medium employed during manufacture and traces of these antibiotics may be present in the final vaccine.

Legal category POM.

Package quantities Single dose vial with 0.5 ml ampoule of Water for Injections BP.

Further information It is important to recognise that children with chronic conditions affecting physical development (e.g. cystic fibrosis, congenital heart disease), and those in residential or day care over the age of one year are at special risk of contracting measles.

Human NORMAL immunoglobulin is available from Regional Transfusion centres in England and Blood Transfusion centres in Scotland and Wales. Specially DILUTED human normal immunoglobulin with a specific content of measles antibody is obtainable from The Blood Products Laboratory, Elstree (Tel 01 953 6191)

Product licence number 0039/0144.

NEPENTHE* INJECTION

Presentation A clear, colourless, sterile solution containing the equivalent of 0.84% w/v (4.2 mg in 0.5 ml) anhydrous morphine of which 0.05% w/v is derived from Papaveretum BPC and 0.79% w/v from Morphine Hydrochloride BP.

Uses To relieve severe pain, especially when it causes anxiety and/or sleeplessness.

Dosage and administration Not to be used for children under 6 years of age, since this would necessitate administering less than 0.5 ml.

6–12 years: Maximum single dose 0.5–1.0 ml.

Adults: Usual single dose 1–2 ml but not to be repeated more often than four hourly.

Nepenthe Injection should be administered by the subcutaneous or intramuscular routes using a syringe graduated in 1/100ths of a ml. It must not be given intravenously.

When fractional doses of a ml are prescribed special care should be taken in view of the small volumes involved.

Contra-indications, warnings, etc Nepenthe Injection should not be given concurrently with other opiates, with monoamine oxidase inhibitors, nor within two weeks of discontinuation of treatment with them.

Nepenthe Injection is contra-indicated in respiratory depression and obstructive airways disease. Use with care in the elderly. Safety in pregnancy has not been established. Use with caution in myxoedema and chronic hepatic disease. Administration in labour may cause respiratory depression in the new born infant.

Tolerance and dependence may occur and nausea and vomiting may be troublesome.

Effects of overdosage and their treatment: Signs of morphine overdosage include pin-point pupils, depressed respiration and coma. In severe poisoning there may be dilation of the pupils, shock, severe respiratory depression and pulmonary oedema.

Naloxone, nalorphine or levallorphan tartrate may be given as an antidote.

Pharmaceutical precautions Protect from light.

Legal category POM: MDA.

Package quantities Carton of 5 × 0.5 ml ampoules.

Further information Nil.

Product licence number 0039/0063R.

NEPENTHE* ORAL SOLUTION

Presentation A brown, bright solution with characteristic odour containing 0.84% w/v anhydrous morphine of which 0.79% w/v is derived from Morphine alkaloid and 0.05% w/v from Tincture of Opium BP. 1 ml contains 8.4 mg anhydrous morphine.

Uses To relieve severe pain, especially when it causes anxiety and/or sleeplessness.

Dosage and administration Nepenthe Oral Solution is for use as an ingredient in the preparation of narcotic analgesic mixtures. The recommended diluent is Syrup BP.

This product must always be diluted when being dispensed by the pharmacist and the dosage expressed in units of 5 ml.

Children under 1 year: not recommended.
 1–5 years: maximum single dose 0.25–0.5 ml.
 6–12 years: maximum single dose 0.5–1.0 ml.
Adults: Usual single dose 1–2 ml, not to be repeated more often than four hourly.

Contra-indications, warnings, etc

Nepenthe Oral Solution should not be given concurrently with other opiates, with monoamine oxidase inhibitors, nor within two weeks of discontinuation of treatment with them.

Nepenthe Oral Solution is contra-indicated in respiratory depression and obstructive airways disease. Use with care in the elderly. Safety in pregnancy has not been established. Use with caution in myxoedema and chronic hepatic disease. Administration in labour may cause respiratory depression in the new born infant.

Tolerance and dependence may occur and nausea and vomiting may be troublesome.

Effects of overdosage and their treatment: Signs of morphine overdosage include pin-point pupils, depressed respiration and coma. In severe poisoning there may be dilation of the pupils, shock, severe respiratory depression and pulmonary oedema.

Gastric lavage should be performed as soon as possible after ingestion and intensive supportive therapy carried out.

Naloxone, nalorphine or levallorphan tartrate may be given as an antidote.

Pharmaceutical precautions Nepenthe Oral Solution should be diluted with Syrup BP. Any diluted portion not used within four weeks should be discarded. Protect from light. Nepenthe Oral Solution is compatible with Ethanol BP, Chloroform Spirit BP and Glycerol BP. It is incompatible with alkalis.

Because of the volatile nature of the solvent, Nepenthe Oral Solution should be stored in a cool place and the bottle should be tightly closed. If evaporation is thought to have occurred during storage, the solution must not be used.

Legal category CD (Sch 2), POM.

Package quantities Bottle of 100 ml.

Further information Nil.

Product licence number 0039/0062R.

STREPTOMYCIN SULPHATE BP

Presentation Streptomycin sulphate is presented as a white sterile powder for preparation of Streptomycin Sulphate Injection BP.

Uses Streptomycin has antibacterial activity particularly against *Mycobacterium tuberculosis, Klebsiella pneumoniae* and *Escherichia coli.*

Streptomycin may be used in the treatment of: tuberculosis; non-tuberculous infections, including chronic respiratory infections, septicaemia and bacterial endocarditis (usually in conjunction with penicillin); pneumonia due to *Klebsiella pneumoniae*; infections with *Escherichia coli*, particularly of the urinary tract; tularaemia and plague; brucellosis (normally in conjunction with a tetracycline).

Dosage and administration *Tuberculosis: Adults:* Commonly 1 g daily, but in patients over 40 years of age, 0.75 g daily by intramuscular injection may be appropri-

ate. Streptomycin is given in conjunction with other antituberculosis drugs. The injection should be given deeply into muscle, and the site changed for each injection. A 1 g dose is usually dissolved in 2 or 3 ml of Water for Injections.

Children: Usually 30 mg/kg (13.6 mg/lb) body weight daily up to 1 g a day by intramuscular injection.

Tuberculous meningitis: Intramuscular dosage 30–40 mg/kg (13.6–18 mg/lb) body weight up to 1 g a day. In addition to this streptomycin may be given intrathecally: adults, 50 mg a day; infants and children, 1 mg per kilogram body weight daily. The antibiotic is dissolved in Sodium Chloride Injection, using 5 ml for infants and 10 ml or more for children and adults. The concentration of streptomycin in the injection must not exceed 5 mg/ml. After withdrawal of an equal volume of cerebrospinal fluid, the solution is injected slowly, taking at least 10 minutes. An injection may be given once a day for 10 days, perhaps followed by a dose on three alternate days.

Use of a sterile disposable membrane filter of 0.45 micron pore size is convenient to ensure clarity of the solution.

Non-tuberculous infections. Adults: Usually 1 g a day by intramuscular injection for three to seven days.

Children: 22–40 mg/kg (10–18 mg/lb) body weight daily. Divided doses are often used.

N.B. In urinary-tract infections the urine should be kept alkaline.

Contra-indications, warnings, etc

Contra-indications: Allergy to streptomycin.

Diseases of the ear, particularly suppurative otitis media and labyrinthine disturbances.

Precautions: In the presence of actual or suspected renal insufficiency, treatment of non-tuberculous infections may start with a dose of 250–500 mg streptomycin. No further dose should be given until the blood level has fallen to 20 mcg/ml or less (*Brit. Med. J.* 1963, **1**, 1393).

In tuberculous patients over 60 years of age, the serum level of streptomycin 24 hours after injection should not exceed 1 mcg/ml. It is important to repeat this estimation several times in the early weeks of treatment (*Brit. Med. J.* 1963, **1**, 1527).

Skin sensitisation may occur in persons handling the antibiotic and care should be taken to avoid contact with the substance. Use of rubber gloves is recommended.

Side-effects: Ototoxicity: Some impairment of vestibular function (less often of auditory function) can occur, particularly with prolonged or intensive therapy, in the presence of renal dysfunction, and in the elderly patient. Prolonged streptomycin therapy given during pregnancy can cause deafness and vestibular dysfunction in the child.

Sensitivity: Occasional allergic-type reaction, rarely severe, often responding to antihistamine treatment. Anaphylactic reaction is rarely reported.

Overdosage: Streptomycin can be removed from the body by haemodialysis.

Pharmaceutical precautions Sterile solutions of streptomycin should be used as soon as possible but they can be kept for up to 28 days in a refrigerator (below 4°C). Limited storage (up to seven days) is permissible in a cool place (below 20°C) if protected from light.

Although solutions may discolour slightly on keeping, potency is not decreased.

Legal category POM.

Package quantities Carton of 10 vials each containing 1 g Streptomycin base as sulphate.

Further information To obtain fractional doses:

Volume of water to be added to 1 g vial	Streptomycin per ml of solution
4.2 ml	200 mg
3.2 ml	250 mg
1.2 ml	500 mg

1 g streptomycin in solution displaces 0.82 ml.

Product licence number 0039/6002.

TUBERCULIN PURIFIED PROTEIN DERIVATIVE (PPD) BP

Presentation Sterile aqueous solutions for intradermal injection containing Tuberculin PPD BP are prepared from human strains of *Mycobacterium tuberculosis*.

Use As a diagnostic test for hypersensitivity to tubercle bacilli.

Dosage and administration

1. *Mantoux Test:* The Mantoux test enables an estimate to be obtained of the degree of hypersensitivity of a particular patient. It consists of injecting intradermally ready diluted Tuberculin PPD.

First, clean the skin of the volar surface of the left forearm with alcohol. Then using a disposable syringe inject 0.1 ml intradermally so that a weal 7 mm in diameter is raised.

The following doses are given, the second and subsequent injections being given only if a negative reaction is obtained from the previous injection.

1. 0.1 ml of 10 units per ml Tuberculin dilution (1 unit).
2. 0.1 ml of 100 units per ml Tuberculin dilution (10 units).
3. 0.1 ml of 1,000 units per ml Tuberculin dilution (100 units).

An interval of two days is allowed between the injections. A further injection of 0.1 ml containing 1,000 units may be given if no reaction has been obtained to the third injection. Children are given one half of the above dose but the 1,000 units in 0.1 ml is not usually given. A positive reaction is characterised by an area of 6 mm or greater of palpable induration, which may sometimes be surrounded by erythema and the results should be read after 72 hours but usually a valid reading can be obtained up to 96 hours.

This test may be carried out and at the same time the control solution may be used to assess individual patients response to the vehicle used.

2. *Heaf test:* This test is performed using undiluted Tuberculin PPD at a strength of 100,000 units per ml.

Clean the skin as for the Mantoux test and allow to dry, then transfer undiluted tuberculin using a syringe needle or loop and smooth over a circular area of about 1 cm in diameter. Using the Heaf multiple puncture apparatus set the apparatus to give a puncture of 1 mm for children under the age of two years or 2 mm for older children and adults. Holding the apparatus at right angles to the skin, place the end plate firmly and evenly in the centre of the film of tuberculin and press the handle to release the needles. No dressing need be applied and the gun should be sterilised after each application or a disposable end plate should be used.

The test should be read at 3 to 10 days. A positive result should be recorded only when there is palpable induration around at least four puncture points. The induration is best felt by passing the finger lightly over the punctures, and if no resistance is felt, a negative result should be recorded.

Four grades of positive response are recognised.

Grade 1 – at least 4 small indurated papules.

Grade 2 – an indurated ring formed by confluent papules.

Grade 3 – a solid induration 5 to 10 mm wide.

Grade 4 – induration over 10 mm wide.

Contra-indications, warnings, etc Temporary diminution of skin sensitivity to tuberculin may occur after ultra-violet light treatment, during treatment with corticosteroids or immunosuppressive agents, and for 4 weeks or longer following measles or measles vaccination.

Tuberculin can cause a severe acute local reaction in some individuals if the solution is allowed to come into contact with open cuts, the eyes and the mouth.

The affected area should be washed with copious quantities of water followed, if necessary, by local corticosteroids.

The potency of tuberculins may be affected if they are diluted with diluents which differ in composition from the vehicle used in their preparation.

Pharmaceutical precautions The BP directs that Tuberculin presentations should be stored in a refrigerator between 2°C and 8°C. Data is available however which shows that the potency remains unaffected even after storage at temperatures up to 37°C for one month.

Use contents of ampoule at once or within one hour of opening, provided adequate aseptic precautions are taken. Any unused solution should be disposed of by flushing away to waste with copious water. Care should be taken to avoid contamination of the ampoule contents.

Legal category POM.

Package quantities *Undiluted:* – Carton of 5 × 1 ml ampoules.

Dilutions: Carton of 5 × 1 ml ampoules.

Control solution: Carton of 5 × 1 ml ampoules for Mantoux test.

Tuberculin undiluted and Tuberculin 100 units per ml (dilution 1 in 1,000), 5 × 1 ml ampoule packs are available to United Kingdom Health Authorities and hospitals through Department of Health & Social Security contract.

Further information 1 ml of each dilution is sufficient for 6 to 8 Mantoux tests, while 1 ml of undiluted Tuberculin should be sufficient for 50 to 100 Heaf tests.

Product licence numbers
Tuberculin PPD BP undiluted 100,000 units per ml for Heaf Multiple Puncture Test 0039/5975R
Tuberculin PPD BP dilutions for Mantoux Test

10 units per ml	1/10,000 dilution	0039/5976R
100 units per ml	1/1,000 dilution	0039/5977R
1,000 units per ml	1/100 dilution	0039/5978R
Control Solution for Mantoux Test		0039/5984R

*Trade Mark

Farmitalia Carlo Erba Limited
Italia House
23 Grosvenor Road,
St Albans,
Hertfordshire AL1 3AW

ADRIAMYCIN*

Presentation Sterile, pyrogen-free, orange-red, freeze-dried powder in vials of 10 mg and 50 mg of doxorubicin hydrochloride with lactose.

Uses Antimitotic and cytotoxic. Adriamycin has been used successfully to produce regression in a wide range of neoplastic conditions including acute leukaemias, lymphomas, soft-tissue and osteogenic sarcomas, paediatric malignancies and adult solid tumours, in particular breast and lung carcinomas.

Adriamycin is frequently used in combination chemotherapy regimens involving other cytotoxic drugs.

Dosage and administration For reconstitution the contents of the 10 mg vial may be dissolved in 5 ml Water for Injections or Sodium Chloride Injection and those of the 50 mg vial in 25 ml of the same solvents.

After adding the diluent, the vial should be shaken and the contents allowed to dissolve. The approximate displacement value of the contents of a 50 ml vial of Adriamycin (50 mg Adriamycin and 250 mg of lactose), after 25 ml of solvent have been added, is 0.15 ml.

Intravenous administration: This is the most frequently used route of administration. The reconstituted solution is given via the tubing of a freely-running intravenous infusion, taking two to three minutes over the injection. This technique minimises the risk of thrombosis or perivenous extravasation which can lead to severe cellulitis and vesication. Commonly used acceptable solutions are Sodium Chloride Injection, Dextrose Injection 5% or Sodium Chloride and Dextrose Injection.

Dosage is usually calculated on the basis of body surface area. On this basis, 60–75 mg/m² may be given every three weeks when Adriamycin is used alone. If it is used in combination with other antitumour agents having overlapping toxicity, the dosage of Adriamycin may need to be reduced to 30–40 mg/m² every three weeks. If dosage is to be calculated on the basis of body weight, 1.2–2.4 mg/kg should be given as a single dose every three weeks.

It has been shown that giving Adriamycin as a single dose every three weeks greatly reduces the distressing toxic effect, mucositis; however, there are still some who believe that dividing the dose over three successive days (0.4–0.8 mg/kg or 20–25 mg/m² on each day) gives greater effectiveness even though at the cost of higher toxicity.

Dosage may need to be reduced for patients who have had prior treatment with other cytotoxics and for the elderly.

If hepatic function is impaired, Adriamycin dosage should be reduced according to the following table:

Serum bilirubin levels	BSP retention	Recommended dose
1.2–3.0 mg/100 ml	9–15%	50% normal dose
>3.0 mg/100 ml	>15%	25% normal dose

Intra-arterial administration: More recently, intra-arterial injection has been used in attempts to produce intense local activity while keeping the total dose low and therefore reducing general toxicity. It should be emphasised that this technique is potentially extremely hazardous and can lead to widespread necrosis of the perfused tissues unless due precautions are taken. Intra-arterial injection should only be attempted by those fully conversant with this technique.

Intravesicular administration: Adriamycin is being increasingly used by intravesical administration for the treatment of transitional cell carcinoma, papillary bladder tumours and carcinoma-in-situ. It should not be employed in this way for the treatment of invasive tumours which have penetrated the bladder wall. It has also been found useful to instil Adriamycin into the bladder at intervals after transurethral resection of a tumour in order to reduce the probability of recurrence. While at present many regimens are in use, making interpretation difficult, the following may be helpful guides:

The concentration of Adriamycin in the bladder should be 50 mg per 50 ml.

To avoid undue dilution with urine, the patient should be instructed not to drink any fluid in the 12 hours prior to instillation. This should limit urine production to approximately 50 ml per hour. The patient should be rotated a quarter turn every 15 minutes while the drug is in situ.

Exposure to the drug solution for one hour is generally adequate and the patient should be instructed to void at the end of this time.

Contra-indications, warnings, etc Adriamycin is intended for use under the direction of those experienced in cytotoxic therapy.

Dosage should not be repeated in the presence of bone-marrow depression or buccal ulceration. The latter may be preceded by premonitory buccal burning sensations and repetition in the presence of this symptom is not advised.

Haematological monitoring should be undertaken regularly in both haematological and non-haematological conditions, because of the possibility of bone-marrow depression which may become evident around ten days from the time of administration.

Cardiotoxicity may be manifested in tachycardia and ECG changes. Routine ECG monitoring is recommended and caution should be exercised in patients with impaired cardiac function.

A cumulative dose of 550 mg/m² should only be exceeded with extreme caution. Above this level, the risk of irreversible congestive cardiac failure increases greatly. The total dose of Adriamycin administered to the individual patient should also take account of any previous or concomitant therapy with other potentially cardiotoxic agents such as high-dose IV cyclophosphamide, mediastinal irradiation or related anthracycline compounds such as daunorubicin. It should be noted that cardiac failure may also occur several weeks after administration and may not respond to treatment.

Baseline and follow-up ECGs during and immediately after drug administration are advisable. Transient ECG changes, such as T-wave flattening, S-T segment depression and arrhythmias, are not considered indications for the suspension of Adriamycin therapy. A reduction of the QRS wave is considered more indicative of cardiac toxicity. If this change occurs, the benefit of continued therapy must be carefully evaluated against the risk of producing irreversible cardiac damage.

Severe cardiac failure may occur suddenly, without premonitory ECG changes.

Adriamycin may impart a red colour to the urine, particularly to the first specimen passed after the injection, and patients should be advised that this is no cause for alarm.

Alopecia occurs frequently, including the interruption of beard-growth, but all hair growth normally resumes after treatment is stopped.

Nausea, vomiting and diarrhoea may also occur.

The risk of thrombophlebitis at the injection site may be minimised by following the procedure for administration recommended above. A stinging or burning sensation at the site of administration signifies a small degree of extravasation and the infusion should be stopped and re-started in another vein.

There is no conclusive information as to whether Adriamycin may adversely affect human fertility or cause teratogenesis. Experimental data, however, suggest that Adriamycin may harm the foetus and should, therefore, not be administered to pregnant women or to mothers who are breast-feeding.

Accidental contact with the skin or eyes should be treated immediately by copious lavage, with water or soap and water, or if available sodium bicarbonate solution.

Overdosage: Single doses of 250 mg and 500 mg of Adriamycin have proved fatal. Such doses may cause acute myocardial degeneration within 24 hours and severe myelosuppression, the effects of which are greatest between 10 and 15 days after administration. Treatment should aim to support the patient during this period and should utilise such measures as blood transfusions and reverse barrier nursing. Delayed cardiac failure may occur up to six months after the overdose. Patients should be observed carefully and should signs of cardiac failure arise, be treated along conventional lines.

Pharmaceutical precautions The vial contents are under a negative pressure to minimise aerosol formation during reconstitution: care should be taken when the needle is inserted. Reconstitution has occasionally resulted in the formation of a gelatinous mass which will completely dissolve on further shaking. It is recommended that personnel handling Adriamycin should wear protective gloves. Care should be taken to avoid the inhalation of any aerosol produced during reconstitution.

The reconstituted solution may be stored for up to 24 hours at room temperature or 48 hours at 4°C without significant deterioration. Discard any unused solution.

Exposure to sunlight can result in degradation. Prolonged contact with any solution of an alkaline pH should be avoided as it will result in hydrolysis of the drug. Adriamycin should not be mixed with heparin as a precipitate may form and it is not recommended that Adriamycin be mixed with other drugs.

Spillage or leakage should be treated with dilute sodium hypochlorite (1% available chlorine) solution, preferably soaking overnight, and then water. All cleaning materials should be placed in high-risk, waste-disposal bags for incineration.

Legal category POM.

Package quantities 10 mg and 50 mg vials for injection.

Further information Nil.

Product licence number 3433/0025.

CISPLATIN

Presentation Cisplatin for injection. Yellowish-white freeze-dried cake in vials containing 10 mg, 25 mg and 50 mg cisplatin (cis-diamminedichloroplatinum). The formulation also contains sodium chloride and mannitol.

Uses Cisplatin has antitumour activity either as a single agent or in combination chemotherapy particularly in the treatment of testicular and metastatic ovarian tumours, also cervical tumours, lung carcinoma and bladder cancer.

Dosage and administration Cisplatin should be dissolved in Water for Injections such that the reconstituted solution contains 1 mg/ml of cisplatin. This solution should then be diluted in 2 litres of 0.9% saline or a dextrose/saline solution (to which 37.5 g of mannitol may be added) and administration should be over a 6–8 hour period.

Single agent therapy

Adults and children: The usual dose regimen given as a single agent is 50–120 mg/m² by infusion once every 3 to 4 weeks or 15–20 mg/m² by infusion daily for five consecutive days, every 3 to 4 weeks.

Combination chemotherapy

Dosage may be adjusted if the drug is used in combination with other anti-tumour chemotherapy.

With multiple drug treatment schedules cisplatin is usually given in doses from 20 mg/m² upward every 3 to 4 weeks.

Dosage should be reduced for patients with renal impairment or depressed bone marrow function (see Contra-indications, Warnings etc).

Pretreatment hydration with 1 to 2 litres of fluid infused for 8 to 12 hours prior to the cisplatin will initiate diuresis. Adequate subsequent hydration should maintain diuresis during the 24 hours following administration.

Contra-indications, warnings, etc

Contra-indications: Cisplatin is contra-indicated in patients who have had previous allergic reactions to cisplatin or other platinum compounds as anaphylactic-like reactions have been reported. Relative contra-indications are pre-existing renal impairment, hearing disorders and depressed bone marrow function which may increase toxicity (see Warnings).

Warnings: This agent should only be administered under the direction of physicians experienced in cancer chemotherapy.

Nephrotoxicity of cisplatin is cumulative and serum creatinine, BUN and creatinine clearance should be measured before starting each course of therapy. Repeat courses of cisplatin should not be given unless levels of serum creatinine are below 1.5 mg/100 ml (100 mcmol/l) or blood urea below 55 mg/100 ml (9 mmol/l) and circulating blood elements are at an acceptable level.

Diuresis should be controlled and serum electrolyte levels monitored regularly. Adequate pre-treatment and 'during treatment' hydration should be ensured and such agents as mannitol given to minimise hazards of renal toxicity. In addition, adequate post-treatment hydration and urinary output should be monitored. Concomitant use of nephrotoxic drugs may seriously impair kidney function.

Ototoxicity is cumulative and occurs with high dose regimens. Hearing function should be evaluated before, and regularly during, therapy (see Adverse Reactions).

Haematologic toxicity is dose-related and may be cumulative, RBC, WBC and platelet counts should be monitored.

The nephrotoxicity, ototoxicity and myelosuppression induced by cisplatin will be additive to existing impairment or to the similar toxicity of agents such as cephaloridine, frusemide, aminoglycosides, etc. administered concurrently.

Anaphylactic-like reactions to cisplatin have been observed. These reactions can be controlled by administration of antihistamines, adrenaline and/or glucocorticoids.

Neurotoxicity secondary to cisplatin administration has been reported and therefore neurological examinations are recommended (see Adverse Reactions). Cisplatin has been shown to be mutagenic. It may also have an anti-fertility effect. Other anti-neoplastic substances have been shown to be carcinogenic and this possibility should be borne in mind in long term use of cisplatin.

Cisplatin has been shown to be teratogenic and embryotoxic in animals. The use of the drug should be avoided in pregnant or nursing women if possible.

Adverse reactions:
Nephrotoxicity: Immediate renal toxicity is greatly reduced when extensive saline hydration is used but cumulative toxicity may remain a problem and requires careful monitoring when repeat courses of cisplatin are administered.

Renal function impairment is evidenced by an increase in blood urea nitrogen, creatinine and serum uric acid levels and by a decreased creatinine clearance.

Cisplatin induces pathological lesions in the distal renal tubules and the collecting ducts.

Gastrointestinal toxicity: Nausea and vomiting occur in the majority of patients, usually starting within 1 hour of treatment and lasting up to 24 hours. Anorexia, nausea and occasional vomiting may persist for up to a week.

Myelosuppression: Cisplatin can cause suppression of all three blood elements.

Leucopenia is dose-related, possibly cumulative, usually reversible. The onset of leucopenia occurs usually between days 6 and 26 and the time of recovery ranges from 21 to 45 days. Thrombocytopenia is also a dose-limiting effect of cisplatin but is usually reversible. The onset of thrombocytopenia is usually from days 10 to 26 and the time of recovery ranges from about 28 to 45 days.

The incidence of cisplatin-induced anaemia (haemoglobin drop of 2 g/100 ml) ranges from 9% to 40%, although this is a difficult toxic effect to assess because it may have a complex aetiology in cancer patients.

Ototoxicity: Unilateral or bilateral tinnitus, which is usually reversible, and/or hearing loss in the high frequency range may occur.

The overall incidence of audiogram abnormalities is 24%, but large variations exist. These abnormalities usually appear within 4 days after drug administration and consist of at least a 15 decibel loss in pure tone threshold. The damage seems to be cumulative and is not reversible. The audiogram abnormalities are most common in the 4000–8000 Hz frequencies.

Neurotoxicity: Peripheral neuropathies with parasthaesia in both upper and lower extremities, tremor and loss of taste have been observed in some patients, generally those treated with repeated courses.

Anaphylactic-like reactions: Anaphylactic-like reactions such as flushing, facial oedema, wheezing, tachycardia and hypotension may occur within a few minutes after intravenous administration. Antihistamines, adrenaline and/or glucocorticoids control all these reactions.

Hyperuricaemia: Hyperuricaemia occurring with cisplatin is more pronounced with doses greater than 50 mg/m². Allopurinol effectively reduces uric acid levels.

Hypomagnesaemia: Asymptomatic hypomagnesaemia has been documented in a certain number of patients treated with cisplatin, symptomatic hypomagnesaemia has been observed in a limited number of cases.

Pharmaceutical precautions The unopened vials should be stored at room temperature protected from light. The reconstituted solution must not be cooled or refrigerated as cooling may result in precipitation; it should be stored at room temperature protected from light and used within 20 hours. It is recommended that diluted infusion solutions of cisplatin be protected from light during administration.

Any unused solution should be discarded.

Cisplatin is degraded on contact with aluminium. Aluminium containing equipment should not be used for administration of cisplatin.

It is recommended that personnel handling cisplatin wear protective gloves. Spillage or leakage should be mopped up wearing protective gloves and all cleaning materials should be placed in high-risk, waste-disposal bags and then incinerated. Contaminated surfaces should be washed with copious amounts of water.

Legal category POM.

Package quantities 10 mg, 25 mg and 50 mg vials for injection.

Further information Nil.

Product licence numbers

Cisplatin 10	3433/0061
Cisplatin 25	3433/0062
Cisplatin 50	3433/0063

CYCLOPHOSPHAMIDE

Presentation White, biconvex, sugar-coated tablets containing 53.5 mg Cyclophosphamide BP (equivalent to 50 mg anhydrous cyclophosphamide). Cyclophosphamide for injection is a sterile white powder in clear glass vials, with rubber caps and aluminium seals, containing 107 mg, 214 mg, 535 mg or 1070 mg Cyclophosphamide BP (equivalent to 100 mg, 200 mg, 500 mg or 1000 mg anhydrous cyclophosphamide) with sodium chloride.

Uses Alkylating, antineoplastic agent. Cyclophosphamide has been used successfully to induce and maintain regressions in a wide range of neoplastic conditions, including leukaemias, lymphomas, soft tissue and osteogenic sarcomas, paediatric malignancies and adult solid tumours; in particular, breast and lung carcinomas.

Cyclophosphamide is frequently used in combination chemotherapy regimens involving other cytotoxic drugs.

Dosage and administration The dosage regimen should be tailored to the individual requirements of the patient, depending on his general condition, concurrent therapy, the type and state of tumour, and the patient's response. Three sample regimens may serve as guides:

Low dose — 80 to 240 mg/m² (2 to 6 mg/kg) as a single dose weekly i.v., or in divided doses orally.

Medium dose — 400 to 600 mg/m² (10 to 15 mg/kg) as a single dose weekly i.v.

High dose — 800 to 1,600 mg/m² (20 to 40 mg/kg) as a single dose i.v. at 10–20 day intervals.

Higher doses should be used only at the discretion of a physician experienced in cytotoxic chemotherapy.

It is recommended that the calculated dose of cyclophosphamide be reduced when it is given in combination with other anti-neoplastic agents or radiotherapy, and in patients with bone marrow depression.

Cyclophosphamide tablets should be swallowed whole, preferably on an empty stomach, but if gastric irritation is severe, they may be taken with meals.

Cyclophosphamide injection should be reconstituted with Water for Injections, 5 ml for each 100 mg of anhydrous cyclophosphamide. After reconstitution the solution will remain stable at room temperature for 2–3 hours. It should be given by slow intravenous injection over a period of 2–3 minutes or into the tubing of a freely running intravenous infusion over a period of 2–3 minutes.

Contra-indications, warnings, etc Cyclophosphamide should be used only under the direction of physicians experienced in cytotoxic or immunosuppressant therapy.

Contra-indications: Hypersensitivity and haemorrhagic cystitis.

Warnings: Cyclophosphamide should be withheld in the presence of severe bone marrow depression and reduced doses should be used in the presence of lesser degrees of bone marrow depression. Single doses will produce a leucopenia which may be severe but usually returns to normal within 21 days. Regular blood counts should be performed in patients receiving cyclophosphamide. This product should not normally be administered to patients who are pregnant or to mothers who are breast-feeding. It should not normally be given to patients with severe infections and should be withdrawn if such infections become life-threatening.

Cyclophosphamide should be used with caution in debilitated patients and those with renal and/or hepatic failure. In all such cases, dosage should be reduced. Oral hypoglycaemic agents may be potentiated by cyclophosphamide.

Amenorrhoea and azoospermia often occur during treatment with cyclophosphamide but in most cases are reversible. Alkylating agents, including cyclophosphamide, have been shown to possess mutagenic, teratogenic and carcinogenic potential. Pregnancy should therefore be avoided during cyclophosphamide therapy and for three months thereafter.

Cyclophosphamide is excreted mainly in the urine, largely in the form of active metabolites. These may give rise to a chemical cystitis which may be haemorrhagic. Because of this, a high fluid intake should be maintained with frequent emptying of the bladder. However, cyclophosphamide may give rise to fluid retention with subsequent water intoxication. Should this arise, a diuretic may be given. Cyclophosphamide may cause myocardial toxicity, especially at high dosage.

Cyclophosphamide may induce permanent sterility in children.

Adverse reactions: In addition to those noted above, the following may accompany cyclophosphamide therapy: hair loss, which may be total, although generally reversible; mucosal ulceration, anorexia, nausea and vomiting, pigmentation typically affecting the palms and nails of the hands and the soles of the feet, and interstitial pulmonary fibrosis.

Overdosage: Myelosuppression (particularly granulocytopenia) and haemorrhagic cystitis are the most serious consequences of overdosage. Recovery from myelosuppression will occur by the 21st day after the overdose in the great majority of patients (at doses up to 200 mg/kg iv) while granulocytopenia is usually seen by day 6 and lasts for a mean period of 12 days (up to 18 days). A broad spectrum antibiotic may be administered until recovery occurs. Transfusion of whole-blood, platelets or white cells and reverse barrier nursing may be necessary.

If the drug has been taken in the form of tablets, early gastric lavage may reduce the amount of drug absorbed. During the first 24 hours and possibly up to 48 hours after overdosage, iv mesna may be beneficial in ameliorating damage to the urinary system. Normal supportive measures such as analgesics and maintenance of fluid balance should be instituted. If the cystitis does not resolve, more intensive treatment may be necessary. No further courses should be given until the patient has fully recovered.

Pharmaceutical precautions *Tablets:* Store in a cool dry place and protect from light.
Injection: Store in a cool place and protect from light. If heated above 32°C, cyclophosphamide may decompose to a damp-looking gel. It is, therefore, recommended that this product is never stored where heat build-up may occur such as near radiators, etc.

Legal category POM.

Package quantities
Tablets: Containers of 100 and 250 tablets of 50 mg.
Injection:
Vials of 100 mg in packs of 6 and 24.
Vials of 200 mg in packs of 6 and 24.
Vials of 500 mg in packs of 6.
Vials of 1,000 mg in packs of 6.
Each vial contains dry powder for reconstitution.

Further information Nil.

Product licence numbers
Cyclophosphamide Tablets 50 mg   3433/0036
Cyclophosphamide Injection 100 mg   3433/0037

Cyclophosphamide Injection 200 mg 3433/0038
Cyclophosphamide Injection 500 mg 3433/0039
Cyclophosphamide Injection 1,000 mg 3433/0040

FARLUTAL*

Presentation *Injection* – White, sterile suspension for i.m. injection, which settles on standing and readily disperses on shaking, containing 500 mg of medroxyprogesterone acetate in 2.5 ml, or 1000 mg in 5.0 ml.

Tablets: White, uncoated, round, biconvex, scored tablets, diameter 9 mm (100 mg) or 11 mm (250 mg), stamped '100' or '250' diametrically and containing 100 mg or 250 mg of medroxyprogesterone acetate, respectively.

White, uncoated, capsule-shaped tablets, measuring about 22 mm × 7 mm, scored on both faces and stamped 'FCE' and '500' on one face, containing 500 mg of medroxyprogesterone acetate.

Uses Palliative treatment of hormone-sensitive malignancies. Farlutal has been successfully used to produce regressions in breast, endometrial, prostatic and renal cell carcinoma. High dose Farlutal therapy has proved especially useful in breast carcinoma and in achieving subjective improvements in terminally ill patients, notably pain relief and improved performance status.

Dosage and administration Suggested dosage schemes are as follows:

Breast carcinoma
Initial dose 500–1000 mg/day i.m. for 4 weeks.
Maintenance 500 mg i.m. twice a week.
Alternatively, 1000–1500 mg daily, orally, is recommended, although doses of up to 2000 mg daily have been used. Daily oral administration, to be effective, must be at least 2–3 times the recommended i.m. dosage.

Endometrial carcinoma
Initial dose 500 mg i.m. twice weekly for 3 months.
Maintenance 500 mg i.m. weekly.
Alternatively 100–500 mg/day orally.

Renal adenocarcinoma
Initial dose 500 mg i.m. on alternate days for 30 days.
Maintenance 500 mg i.m. twice weekly until 60th day, then 250 mg i.m. weekly.
Alternatively 100–500 mg/day orally.

Prostatic adenocarcinoma
Initial dose 500 mg i.m. twice weekly.
Maintenance 500 mg i.m. weekly.
Alternatively 100–500 mg/day orally.

Intramuscular administration should be by deep injection into alternate gluteal muscles using a long wide-bore needle such as 21 G × 1½" (8/10 40 mm). Narrow-bore or short needles must not be used.

Large tablets, and in this case particularly Farlutal 500, should be taken while sitting or standing and with copious amounts of liquid. The tablets may be broken in half before administration, if necessary.

Contra-indications, warnings, etc

Contra-indications: Thrombophlebitis, thrombo-embolic disorders, severe hepatic insufficiency and hypercalcaemia as may occur in patients with osseous metastases; also, suspected or early breast carcinoma, missed abortion, metrorrhagia, pregnancy and known hypersensitivity to medroxyprogesterone acetate or, for

the injectable formulation, hydroxybenzoates (excipients).

Warnings: Farlutal should be used under the direction of those experienced in cancer chemotherapy.

Since medroxyprogesterone acetate appears to enhance blood clotting potential, treatment should be discontinued upon the appearance of thrombo-embolic episodes, migraine or associated ocular problems such as sudden partial or total loss of vision, diplopia or vascular lesions of the retina.

In the event of vaginal bleeding occurring, an accurate diagnosis should be made. If a histological examination is indicated, the laboratory should be informed that the patient has been receiving a progestogen.

Precautions: Animal studies have shown that medroxyprogesterone acetate possesses adrenocorticoid activity and this effect has also been observed in humans. Patients treated with high doses continuously over long periods should be carefully observed for signs normally associated with adrenocorticoid therapy, such as hypertension, sodium retention, oedema, etc, and care is needed in treating patients with diabetes and/or arterial hypertension.

Farlutal may raise plasma calcium levels; some cases of hypercalcaemia have been reported in the treatment of breast carcinoma.

Administration of progesterone during the first months of pregnancy may possibly be associated with the occurrence of congenital cardiac malformations in the neonate. In addition, instances of masculinisation of female foetuses have been reported following high dose therapy during pregnancy. For these reasons, Farlutal is contra-indicated during pregnancy.

It should be noted that long term administration of medroxyprogesterone acetate to beagle dogs has resulted in the development of mammary nodules which were occasionally found to be malignant. The relevance of these findings to humans has, however, not been established.

Adverse reactions: As is generally found after intramuscular administration of large volumes of suspension, the i.m. preparation may cause local lesions at the injection site, such as sterile abscesses or inflammatory infiltrates. The suspension should, therefore, be well shaken before use and injected deeply into healthy gluteal muscle.

In common with other progestogens, Farlutal may cause mastodynia, galactorrhoea, vaginal bleeding, changes in menstrual flow, amenorrhoea, cervical erosions and modifications of cervical secretions. Farlutal also exerts a corticoid-like effect which may lead to facies lunaris, Cushingoid syndrome and weight changes; and an adrenergic-like action which may result in fine hand tremors, sweating and cramps in the calves at night. Cholestatic jaundice has occasionally been reported.

Pharmaceutical precautions The vials for injection should be well shaken before use and the contents should not be mixed with other agents. The vials are for single dose administration only, should be stored between 15°–30°C and should not be frozen.

The tablets should be stored in a dry place.

Package quantities
Farlutal 100 Cartons containing 100 tablets
Farlutal 250 Cartons containing 50 tablets
Farlutal 500 Cartons containing 56 tablets
Farlutal 500
for Injection Vials in individual cartons

Farlutal 1000
  for Injection   Vials in individual cartons

Legal category POM.

Further information Analysis of the various i.m. dosage schedules so far employed indicates that higher response rates may be obtained by attainment and maintenance of high plasma levels. The intramuscular injection of Farlutal as a 20% suspension of medroxyprogesterone acetate, enables these levels to be achieved while minimising the local ˜side effects associated with high dose therapy using formulations of lower concentrations.

  After oral administration of medoxyprogesterone acetate, absorption is rapid. The plasma half life is of the order of 2 days and with repeated dosing once daily a steady state concentration is reached in about 10 days. Plasma concentrations are usually proportional to the administered dose, but considerable individual variation occurs. In general, to obtain concentrations comparable to those achieved after 4 weeks i.m. administration, at least twice the daily i.m. dose should be given.

Product licence numbers

Farlutal 100	3433/0056
Farlutal 250	3433/0058
Farlutal 500	3433/0080
Farlutal 500 for Injection and	
Farlutal 1000 for Injection	3433/0045

KELFIZINE W*

Presentation White, uncoated tablets each containing sulfametopyrazine 2 g stamped 'Kelfizine' on the face, and 'Weekly Dose' on the obverse.

Uses The treatment of infections due to sulphonamide-sensitive organisms. It has been used in the management of: chronic bronchitis (including prophylaxis); urinary tract infections; ear, nose and throat infections; bacillary dysentery; meningitis.

Dosage and administration Adults: 2 g once weekly by mouth. Children: Not recommended.
  The tablet should be stirred into half a tumblerful of water or orange squash.

Contra-indications, warnings, etc
Contra-indications: Not to be taken by persons sensitive to sulphonamides. The use of Kelfizine W is not recommended for infants under one year of age; it is therefore, also not recommended for use in breast-feeding mothers. Sulfametopyrazine should be used with caution in patients with renal or hepatic dysfunction, dehydration, or blood dyscrasias. Sulphonamides should not be used during the last few weeks of pregnancy unless considered essential by the physician.

Overdosage: Doses up to 8 g have been taken over 36 hours without evidence of ill effects. To increase excretion a high fluid intake should be maintained for seven days and the urine rendered alkaline with Potassium Citrate mixture BP or Sodium Bicarbonate. The sulphonamide will then be retained in the urine in higher concentrations in the form of the alkali metal salt.

Legal category POM.

Package quantities Pack of 5 tablets individually foil wrapped.

Further information Sulfametopyrazine has a long half-life. This is due not to a high degree of serum protein binding (which is only 60%) but to a high degree of renal tubular re-absorption coupled with a low rate of hepatic metabolism of the drug.

Product licence number 3433/5916.

KEMICETINE* SUCCINATE

Presentation Individual glass vials of chloramphenicol sodium succinate for injection containing the equivalent of 1 g of chloramphenicol.

Uses Kemicetine (chloramphenicol) is a broad-spectrum antibiotic and is active against many gram-positive and gram-negative organisms, spirillae and rickettsia. Kemicetine should not be used for trivial infections due to the possibility of severe blood dyscrasias, which may prove fatal.
  Kemicetine succinate is indicated for typhoid, paratyphoid, meningitis caused by *H. influenzae* infections and other serious infections. It is also indicated wherever chloramphenicol is deemed the antibiotic of choice and oral administration is not possible, or higher than usual blood concentrations are required.

Dosage and administration
In order to ensure rapid attainment of high blood levels, Kemicetine succinate is best administered by i.v. injection. Where this is not possible, however, intramuscular administration may be used, although it should be borne in mind that absorption may be slow and unpredictable.
  The injection should be reconstituted with Water for Injections, Sodium Chloride Injection, or Dextrose Injection 5%. The following dilution table may be useful for the administration of a proportion of the contents of a vial:

Concen-tration	Solution strength	Volume of diluent to be added	Total volume after dilution
40%	400 mg/ml	1.7 ml	2.5 ml
25%	250 mg/ml	3.2 ml	4.0 ml
20%	200 mg/ml	4.2 ml	5.0 ml
10%	100 mg/ml	9.2 ml	10.0 ml

The dose administered and the concentration used is dependent on the severity of the infection. The recommended standard dosage is as follows:

Adults: The equivalent of 1 g chloramphenicol every 6–8 hours.

Children: The equivalent of 50 mg/kg chloramphenicol, according to body weight, daily in divided doses every 6 hours (this dose should not be exceeded). The patient should be carefully observed for signs of toxicity.

Neonates and premature infants: 25 mg/kg in divided doses.
  Certain infections, such as meningitis or septicaemia, may require substantially higher doses.
  The 10% solution should be given by intravenous injection over a period of about a minute, or in a larger volume of fluid, by slow intravenous infusion.

Contra-indications, warnings, etc Kemicetine is to be administered only under the direction of a medical practitioner. Chloramphenicol may cause severe bone marrow depression which may lead to agranulocytosis, thrombocytopenic purpura or aplastic anaemia. These effects on the haemopoietic system are usually associated with a high dose, prolonged administration, or repeated courses, but they may occur at relatively low doses. Chloramphenicol should not, therefore, be used in the treatment of any infection for which a less toxic antibiotic is available. It is also advisable to perform blood tests in the case of prolonged or repeated administration. Evidence of any detrimental effect on blood elements is an indication to discontinue therapy immediately.

Other adverse reactions which may become apparent after chloramphenicol treatment are: dryness of the mouth, nausea and vomiting, diarrhoea, urticaria, optic neuritis and blurring, or temporary loss of vision. Superinfection by fungi, e.g. *C. albicans* in the gastro-intestinal tract, or vagina, may also occur due to the disturbance of normal bacterial flora.

Chloramphenicol has been shown to interact with, and enhance the effects of, coumarin anticoagulants, some hypoglycaemic agents (e.g. tolbutamide) and phenytoin. When given concurrently, a dose reduction of these agents may, therefore, be necessary. Chloramphenicol may also impede the development of immunity and should therefore not be given during active immunisation.

The drug should be used with great caution in patients with impairment of hepatic or renal function. 'The Grey Syndrome' may occur after administration, in patients with immature hepatic metabolic capacity, i.e. infants and neonates, usually in those treated with doses substantially in excess of those recommended.

Pharmaceutical precautions Any Kemicetine succinate solution remaining in the vial after use should be discarded, as chloramphenicol sodium succinate is not bactericidal or bacteristatic.

Legal category POM.

Package quantities Cartons containing 20 individual vials.

Further information Nil.

Product licence number 3433/5903

LEVIUS*

Presentation Uncoated, controlled-release tablets each containing aspirin 500 mg microencapsulated with ethylcellulose.

Uses Analgesic, anti-inflammatory. For use as an alternative to Aspirin Tablets BP in chronic painful conditions such as rheumatoid arthritis, osteoarthritis and chronic rheumatic conditions where prolonged treatment may be needed.

Dosage and administration *Adults:* One or two tablets every four hours or as prescribed by the physician. The maximum daily dose should generally not exceed 4 g except in the treatment of acute rheumatism for which 4–8 g in divided doses is recommended.

Elderly: While limited study does not indicate a need for specific dose adjustment it is wise to prescribe with caution in the elderly, who tend to experience more adverse reactions than younger patients.

Children (10–12 years of age): One tablet every four hours up to 4 doses in 24 hours, or as prescribed.

Contra-indications, warnings, etc

Contra-indications: Active peptic ulceration, haemophilia and hypersensitivity to aspirin or salicylates.

Use in pregnancy: Clinical and epidemiological experience has produced no evidence that aspirin constitutes a hazard when used during pregnancy, but caution should be exercised when prescribing for pregnant patients. Aspirin may prolong labour and contribute to maternal and neonatal bleeding and is best avoided at term.

Precautions: Aspirin may enhance the effect of anticoagulants and inhibit the action of uricosurics. It may precipitate bronchospasm or induce attacks of asthma in susceptible subjects.

Warnings and adverse effects: Levius may induce 'aspirin-type' hypersensitivity, asthma or gastro-intestinal haemorrhage which may occasionally be severe.

Overdosage: The fatal dose varies, 10–30 g have caused death but much larger doses have been ingested without fatal outcome. The symptoms of overdosage include headache, epigastric pain, dizziness, tinnitus, sweating, nausea, vomiting, confusion and hyperventilation. More serious signs of toxicity include fever, ketosis, respiratory alkalosis and metabolic acidosis. Depression of the CNS may lead to coma, cardiovascular collapse and respiratory failure. Treatment is largely symptomatic and the patient should be hospitalised. Absorption from the G.I. tract may be reduced by emesis, gastric lavage and/or administration of activated charcoal. In severe poisoning, extra-renal measures such as exchange transfusion, peritoneal dialysis, haemodialysis and haemoperfusion are the most effective measures available for the removal of salicylate, while electrolyte imbalance may need constant monitoring and i.v. infusion correction.

Pharmaceutical precautions Store in a cool dry place.

Legal category P.

Package quantities Amber, child-resistant containers of 30 tablets and Securitainers of 500 tablets.

Further information Aspirin is released from the microcapsules by a process of dialysis over a period of about one hour. As this process is steady and progressive, no part of the alimentary tract receives the full irritant effect of all the aspirin contained in the tablet. Moreover, the analgesia resulting from the aspirin is more prolonged than from a conventional tablet.

Product licence number 3433/0018R.

MAXTREX*

Presentation *Maxtrex tablets:* Round, uncoated, convex tablets diameter 6 mm, containing 2.5 mg (pale yellow tablets marked 'M2.5' on one side and 'F' on the other) and 10 mg (deep yellow tablets marked 'M10' on one side and scored on the other) methotrexate.

Maxtrex 5 solution for injection: Clear light yellow liquid. Vials containing 2 ml of a 2.5 mg/ml solution of methotrexate as the sodium salt and sodium chloride at pH 8.5.

Maxtrex 50, 500, 1000, and 5000 solution for injection: Clear light yellow liquid. Vials containing 2 ml, 20 ml, 40 ml or 200 ml of a 25 mg/ml solution of methotrexate as the sodium salt and sodium chloride at pH 8.5.

Maxtrex solutions for injection do not contain preservatives.

Uses Methotrexate is a folic acid antagonist and is classified as an antimetabolite cytotoxic agent.

Methotrexate has been used to produce regression in a wide range of neoplastic conditions including acute leukaemias, non-Hodgkin's lymphoma, soft-tissue and osteogenic sarcomas, and solid tumours particularly breast, lung, head and neck, bladder, cervical, ovarian, and testicular carcinoma.

Methotrexate has also been used in the treatment of severe, uncontrolled psoriasis which is not responsive to other therapy.

Dosage and administration There are three usual methods of administration:
- (a) small doses, either orally, i.v. or i.m.
- (b) large doses as i.v. bolus injection or infusion.
- (c) intrathecal or intraventricular injection.

Oral administration: Single doses, not exceeding 30 mg/m^2, on not more than 5 successive days. A rest period of at least two weeks is recommended between treatments, in order to allow the bone marrow to return to normal.

Intravenous administration: The solutions should be given over two to three minutes preferably via the tubing of a freely-running intravenous infusion. Doses in excess of 100 mg are usually given by intravenous infusion over a period of not more than 24 hours, although part of the dose may initially be given as a bolus injection. Doses in excess of 70 mg/m^2 should not be administered without leucovorin rescue (folinic acid rescue) or assay of the serum methotrexate levels 24–48 hours after dosing.

Methotrexate has been used both alone and in combination chemotherapy with radiotherapy and surgery. Dosage regimens may therefore vary considerably. Intermittent high-dose therapy with leucovorin (folinic acid) rescue has also been used. Leucovorin rescue regimens are discussed briefly under 'Further information'.

Examples of dosages which have been used in individual indications are as follows:

12 mg/m^2 up to 15 mg: meningeal leukaemia in children (intrathecally) at weekly intervals.

5 mg/m^2 up to 60 mg: choriocarcinoma (i.m. every 2 days for 4 courses).

Up to 1000 mg/m^2: breast, lung, head and neck and bladder carcinoma, osteosarcoma, non-Hodgkin's lymphoma.

1 g/m^2 to 5 g/m^2: lung carcinoma and osteosarcoma.

5 g/m^2 to 14 g/m^2: osteosarcoma.

The above regimens are usually used cyclically, often in combination with other agents.

If methotrexate is administered in combination chemotherapy regimens, the dosage should be reduced, taking into consideration any overlapping toxicity of the other drug components.

Dosage for psoriasis: For the treatment of severe psoriasis 10–25 mg orally, once weekly, is recommended. Dosage should be adjusted according to the patient's response and the haematological toxicity.

Contra-indications, warnings, etc Maxtrex is usually intended for use under the direction of those experienced in cytotoxic therapy.

Contra-indications: Methotrexate is contra-indicated in the presence of severe renal or hepatic impairment and serious anaemia, leucopenia or thrombocytopenia.

Warnings: Methotrexate should be used with extreme caution in patients with haematological depression, renal impairment, diarrhoea, ulcerative disorders of the G.I.

tract and psychiatric disorders and in the elderly and very young. Hepatic toxicity has been observed. Renal lesions may develop if the urinary flow is impeded and urinary pH is low, especially if large doses have been administered.

The administration of low doses of methotrexate for prolonged periods may give rise, in particular, to hepatic toxicity. Liver function tests should be periodically carried out and abnormalities are an indication for discontinuing treatment for at least a period of 2 weeks.

Particular care and possible cessation of treatment are indicated if stomatitis or G.I. toxicity occurs as haemorrhagic enteritis and intestinal perforation may result.

After intrathecal administration, leucoencephalopathies have been observed, especially with concomitant cerebral radiotherapy.

Reversible eosinophilic pulmonary reactions and treatment-resistant, interstitial fibrosis may occur, particularly after long-term treatment. Methotrexate is teratogenic and should not ordinarily be administered to patients who are pregnant or to mothers who are breast-feeding. The drug affects spermatogenesis and oogenesis and may therefore decrease fertility. The effect appears to be reversible after discontinuation of therapy. Conception should be prevented for at least 6 months after administration has ceased.

There are isolated reports in the literature of tumours occurring in patients following treatment with methotrexate, and in some studies in animals. However controlled animal studies and human epidemiological surveys have not demonstrated carcinogenicity. Nevertheless, the possibility of such an effect should be borne in mind when designing long-term management. Methotrexate is immunosuppressive and may therefore reduce immunological response to concurrent vaccination. Severe antigenic reactions may occur if a live vaccine is given concurrently.

Precautions: Before, during and after treatment with methotrexate a complete haematological analysis should be performed, together with renal and hepatic function tests. Haemopoietic depression may occur suddenly even with low doses. A severe reduction of any blood element requires immediate cessation of treatment and suitable supportive measures such as blood transfusion and reverse barrier nursing. During therapy urine should be kept alkaline, if necessary, by giving oral or i.v. sodium bicarbonate, to prevent crystal deposition.

The disappearance of methotrexate from plasma should be monitored, if possible. This is recommended in particular when high, or very high doses are administered, in order to permit calculation of an adequate dose of leucovorin rescue. (See under 'Further information'.)

Radiotherapy to the CNS should not be given concomitantly with intrathecally administered methotrexate.

After intrathecal administration the drug is transported into the general circulation and may therefore still give rise to systemic toxicity, particularly myelosuppression.

Drug interactions: Methotrexate is extensively protein bound and may displace, or be displaced by, other acidic drugs. The concurrent administration of agents such as aminobenzoic acid, chloramphenicol, phenytoin, propionic acid anti-inflammatory agents, salicylates, sulphonamides, tetracyclines, thiazide diuretics, probenecid or sulphinpyrazone will decrease the methotrexate transport function of renal tubules, thereby reducing excretion and almost certainly increasing methotrexate toxicity.

Side-effects: Common side-effects are leucopenia and

thrombocytopenia (which are usually reversible), nausea and vomiting, diarrhoea and stomatitis. Other side-effects include G.I. ulceration, alopecia, erythematous skin reactions and suppression of ovarian and testicular function.

Megaloblastic anaemia has been reported. Renal and hopatic damage may occur, particularly after high doses or prolonged administration, respectively. Reversible, eosinophilic pulmonary reactions and treatment-resistant interstitial fibrosis have been recorded.

CNS side-effects that may follow intrathecal or intraventricular use are headache, drowsiness, blurred vision, ataxia and, rarely, dementia and convulsions.

Overdosage: Leucovorin is a specific antidote for methotrexate and, following accidental overdosage, should be administered within one hour at a dosage equal to, or greater than, the methotrexate dose. It may be administered by i.v. bolus or infusion. Further doses may be required. The patient should be observed carefully and blood transfusions, renal dialysis and reverse barrier nursing may be necessary.

Pharmaceutical precautions Maxtrex should be stored at room temperature protected from light. All solutions are stable for at least 24 hours when diluted in the common infusion solutions such as Sodium Chloride, Dextrose or Sodium Chloride and Dextrose.

Maxtrex solutions for injection do not contain preservatives. Any unused solutions should be destroyed.

Methotrexate solutions should not be mixed with other drugs because of possible incompatibility. In particular, absorption spectrum changes have been seen when methotrexate is mixed with 5-fluorouracil, prednisolone sodium phosphate, and cytarabine.

Legal category POM.

Package quantities
Maxtrex 2.5 tablets: Bottles of 100.
Maxtrex 10 tablets: Bottles of 100.
Maxtrex 5 solution for injection: Vials of 5 mg in packs of 10.
Maxtrex 50 solution for injection: Vials of 50 mg in packs of 10.
Maxtrex 500 solution for injection: Individual vial of 500 mg.
Maxtrex 1000 solution for injection: Individual vial of 1000 mg.
Maxtrex 5000 solution for injection: Individual vial of 5000 mg.

Further information Methotrexate is a folic acid antagonist and its major site of action is the enzyme dihydrofolate reductase. Its main effect is inhibition of DNA synthesis, but it also acts directly both on RNA and protein synthesis. Methotrexate is a phase specific substance, the main effect being directed during the S-phase of cell division.

The inhibition of dihydrofolate reductase can be circumvented by the use of leucovorin (folinic acid; citrovorum factor) and protection of normal tissues can be carried out by properly timed administration of leucovorin calcium. Dosage regimens for leucovorin rescue vary, depending on the dose of methotrexate administered. Up to 120 mg are generally given (as the calcium salt), usually in divided doses over 12–24 hours, by i.m., or i.v. bolus, or intravenous infusion in normal saline. This is followed by 12–15 mg i.m. or 15 mg orally every 6 hours for 48 hours.

Product licence numbers
Maxtrex 2.5   3433/0071
Maxtrex 10   3433/0072
Maxtrex 5 solution for injection   3433/0087
Maxtrex 50, 500, 1000 and 5000
solution for injection   3433/0088

MINODIAB*

Presentation Minodiab is available as white, biconvex, 8 mm tablets containing 2.5 or 5 mg of glipizide. The 5 mg tablets are scored.

Uses Minodiab is an orally active hypoglycaemic sulphonylurea and has been shown to be effective in the treatment of diabetes mellitus Type II. In certain patients receiving insulin, the concurrent use of Minodiab allows a reduction in the daily dose of insulin.

Dosage and administration The usual dose range of Minodiab is 2.5–30 mg daily but if control is not achieved within this range then it may be increased to a total daily dose of 40 mg, although the additional proportion of patients responding to this higher dosage may not be large.

Patients previously untreated: The initial dose is 2.5–5 mg daily. Doses of 2.5 mg daily should be taken as a single dose before breakfast. Doses of 5 mg daily may be taken as a single dose before breakfast or as two doses; one in the morning and one in the evening before meals.

Patients changing from other oral antidiabetics: The recommended starting dose is 5 mg daily taken as a single dose or in two divided doses.

Dosage adjustments in all patients, either upwards or downwards, should be in 2.5–5 mg steps at weekly intervals until good control is achieved. The maximum recommended single dose is 15 mg. Doses above 15 mg should ordinarily be taken in 2 divided doses before meals. Multiple divided doses (2 or 3 daily) are recommended for patients who experience particularly high post-prandial blood glucose peaks.

Concomitant food intake may delay absorption and administration should therefore be 15–20 minutes before a main meal: therapeutic effects are usually seen within 30 minutes and peak at about 60 minutes. Glipizide is rapidly metabolised and excreted mainly in the urine and therefore it is unlikely that delayed hypoglycaemic episodes will occur.

When administered in divided daily doses glipizide can be considered as having a physiological action as its peak effect coincides with post-prandial peak blood-sugar levels.

A biguanide may be added to the treatment if control is not achieved with Minodiab.

Contra-indications, warnings, etc
Contra-indications: Minodiab is contra-indicated in pregnancy, juvenile diabetes, diabetic ketoacidosis, diabetic coma, severe renal or hepatic insufficiency, infections and febrile conditions, gangrene and in severe trauma and major surgical procedures.

Warnings: Concurrent use of MAOIs, phenylbutazone, β-blockers, sulphonamides, coumarin derivatives or salicylates may enhance the hypoglycaemic effect. Conversely the effect may be diminished in the presence of adrenaline, corticosteroids, oral contraceptives and thiazide diuretics.

Patients should be instructed to take their meals regularly and not to exercise excessively without additional calorie intake. Failure to do so may result in a hypoglycaemic episode. The hypoglycaemia is controlled by giving carbohydrates.

Adverse reactions: Side-effects are not common with Minodiab. Those that do occur are associated with the gastro-intestinal tract, and include nausea, vomiting, anorexia, gastric pain, etc. Skin reactions have been reported, e.g. rash, urticaria, pruritus, etc. Other reactions include headache, dizziness and vertigo.

Overdosage: Gastric lavage should be performed as soon as possible. Hypoglycaemia should be treated as it occurs with appropriate measures including oral or i.v. glucose.

Pharmaceutical precautions None.

Legal category POM.

Package quantities Cartons containing 60 tablets.

Further information Glipizide is almost completely absorbed from the GI tract and appears to act by stimulating insulin secretion from pancreatic β cells, but may also act by potentiating peripheral insulin action. Peak concentrations in blood are achieved within 60 minutes and the half-life is approximately $3\frac{1}{2}$ hours.

Product licence numbers
Minodiab 2.5   3433/0022.
Minodiab 5   3433/0023.

NAXOGIN* 500

Presentation Naxogin 500 is available as white or slightly yellow bi-convex tablets scored on one side and plain on the other. Each tablet contains 500 mg nimorazole.

Uses Naxogin is a trichomonacidal agent. It is indicated for the systemic treatment of trichomonal vaginitis. Sexual partners should also be treated even if they are free of symptoms.

Naxogin is also effective against other protozoa and may be used for the treatment of giardiasis, amoebiasis and acute ulcerative gingivitis.

Dosage and administration *For the treatment of trichomoniasis:* 2 g (4 tablets) to be taken together as a single dose with a main meal. This may be repeated if there is no clinical improvement.

For acute ulcerative gingivitis: 500 mg twice daily for two days.

For giardiasis or amoebiasis: Adults: 500 mg twice daily for five days.
   Children (over 10 kg body weight): 500 mg daily for five days.
   Children (under 10 kg body weight): 250 mg daily for five days.

Contra-indications, warnings, etc Like all nitroimidazoles, Naxogin 500 is contra-indicated for nursing mothers as it is excreted in breast milk and the effect on the neonate is unknown. Also this group of drugs should not be given in the presence of active CNS disease. Treatment should be discontinued if ataxia or other CNS symptoms appear.

Naxogin 500 should be given with caution during pregnancy although there is no known teratogenicity. Clinical studies have been carried out during pregnancy and no untoward effects of any kind have been associated with this drug.

As Naxogin 500 is excreted principally via the kidneys, overt renal insufficiency is also a contra-indication.

Unwanted effects are rare and may comprise transient gastro-intestinal effects such as nausea and vomiting. No blood dyscrasias have been reported. Intolerance to alcohol, similar to that induced by disulfiram, has been observed with the nitroimidazoles but is rarely troublesome with nimorazole.

Overdosage: There is no specific treatment but gastric lavage should be performed as soon as possible. Supportive measures should be instituted as required and a high fluid intake maintained.

Pharmaceutical precautions None.

Legal category P.

Package quantities Bottles of 8 and 100 tablets.

Further information Naxogin 500 is well absorbed after oral administration, achieving blood levels of 32 mcg/ml within two hours and 1.9 mcg/ml at 24 hours. The metabolites of the drug are trichomonacidal and are excreted mainly by the kidney so that there are high urinary concentrations. Concentrations are high in vaginal and salivary secretions.

Naxogin 500 is also recommended for the treatment of acute ulcerative gingivitis in patients hypersensitive to penicillin.

Product licence number 3433/5914.

PHARMIDONE*

Presentation Yellow, scored, tablets each containing:

Codeine Phosphate Ph Eur	10 mg
Diphenhydramine Hydrochloride BP	5 mg
Paracetamol Ph Eur	400 mg
Caffeine Ph Eur	50 mg

Uses Analgesic, in the treatment of headache, migraine, muscular pain and nerve pain.

Dosage and administration *For adults and children over 12 years of age:* One or two tablets orally every four hours, up to a maximum of ten tablets in 24 hours.

Contra-indications, warnings, etc Pharmidone may cause drowsiness, and if affected, the patient should not drive or operate machinery. The effect of alcohol and other sedatives may be potentiated.

Pharmidone should not be given to patients with known liver or renal impairment.

Pharmidone should not be administered to children.

Safety in pregnancy has not been established.

Overdosage: The effects of overdosage are predominantly those of paracetamol; vomiting, gastrointestinal haemorrhage, liver damage, cerebral oedema and renal tubular necrosis may occur. Gastric lavage should be carried out and haemodialysis may be necessary if renal failure occurs.

Pharmaceutical precautions None.

Legal category CD (Sch 5), P.

Package quantities Boxes of 12 and containers of 100 tablets.

Further information Nil.

Product licence number 3433/0042.

PHARMORUBICIN* ▼

Presentation Sterile, pyrogen-free, red, freeze-dried powder in vials containing 10 mg, 20 mg and 50 mg of epirubicin hydrochloride with lactose.

Uses Antimitotic and cytotoxic.

Pharmorubicin as a single agent has produced regression in a wide range of neoplastic conditions, including breast, ovarian, gastric and colorectal carcinomas, lymphomas, leukaemias and multiple myeloma. Pharmorubicin may be used in combination chemotherapy regimens involving other cytotoxic drugs. Comparative studies on the effects of Pharmorubicin with doxorubicin in inducing remission and estimating cardiotoxicity have only been performed in breast cancer.

Dosage and administration For reconstitution the contents of the 10 mg vial should be dissolved in 5 ml of Water for Injections, the 20 mg vial in 10 ml of Water for Injections and the 50 mg vial in 25 ml of Water for Injections.

Pharmorubicin should be administered only by the intravenous route and the reconstituted solution should be given via the tubing of a freely running intravenous infusion of Sodium Chloride Injection taking 3–5 minutes over the injection. This technique minimises the risk of thrombosis or perivenous extravasation which can lead to severe cellulitis and necrosis. Venous sclerosis may result from injection into small veins or repeated injections into the same vein.

Dosage is usually calculated on the basis of body surface.

Single agent: The dose range most commonly used in clinical trials has been 75–90 mg/m^2.

The dose should be repeated at 21-day intervals; the total dose for the cycle may be divided over two successive days. The dosage schedule should however, take into account the haematological status of the patient. In particular, a lower dose is recommended for patients whose bone marrow function has been impaired by previous chemotherapy or radiotherapy and in the elderly.

Combination chemotherapy: When Pharmorubicin is used in combination with other antitumour agents the dosage should be reduced. A comparative combination study in advanced breast carcinoma has shown that the combination FEC (5-FU, epirubicin, cyclophosphamide) is as efficacious as FAC (5-FU, Adriamycin, cyclophosphamide) when the Pharmorubicin (epirubicin) and Adriamycin components are both given at 50 mg/m^2.

Since the major excretory route is the hepatobiliary system the dosage should also be reduced in patients with impaired liver function to avoid an increase of overall toxicity. Moderate liver impairment (bilirubin 1.2–3 mg/100 ml or BSP retention 9–15%), requires a dose reduction of the order of 50%, while severe impairment (bilirubin >3 mg/100 ml or BSP retention >15%) necessitates a dose reduction of the order of 75%.

Contra-indications, warnings, etc Pharmorubicin is intended for use under the direction of those experienced in cytotoxic therapy.

The drug should not be given to patients with marked myelosuppression induced by previous drug therapy or radiotherapy. Administration is normally contra-indicated in patients with a current or previous history of cardiac impairment and in patients already treated with maximum cumulative doses of other anthracyclines such as doxorubicin or daunorubicin.

During the first cycles of treatment with Pharmorubicin patients must be carefully and frequently monitored.

Haematological monitoring should be undertaken regularly in both haematological and non-haematological conditions in view of the possibility of bone-marrow depression. Leucopenia is usually transient with the recommended dosage schedules, reaching a nadir between 10 and 14 days after administration. A return to normal blood values usually occurs within 21 days from administration.

Before starting treatment, and if possible during therapy, liver function should be evaluated [SGOT (AST), SGPT (ALT), alkaline phosphatase, bilirubin, BSP].

The data obtained in different animal species and the results of clinical trials have consistently indicated that Pharmorubicin is less cardiotoxic than doxorubicin. There is objective evidence that cardiac toxicity may occur when the cumulative dose exceeds 700 mg/m^2.

Although uncommon, left ventricular failure can occur, particularly in patients who have received a cumulative dose that exceeds 1000 mg/m^2, or a lower cumulative dose in patients who have received radiotherapy to the mediastinal area. The total dose of Pharmorubicin administered should also take into account prior or concomitant therapy with related anthracycline compounds such as doxorubicin or daunorubicin, or anthracene derivatives. In particular, patients who have received prior cumulative doses of more than 450 mg/m^2 of doxorubicin or daunorubicin are at a high risk of developing congestive heart failure (CHF). CHF and/or cardiomyopathy may occur several weeks after discontinuation of Pharmorubicin therapy.

Cardiac function should be carefully monitored during treatment in order to minimise the risk of cardiac failure of the type described for other anthracycline compounds. It is recommended that an ECG, be taken before and after each treatment cycle. Alterations of the ECG, such as flattening or inversion of the T wave, depression of the S-T segment, or the onset of arrhythmias, are generally transient and reversible and need not necessarily indicate that treatment should be stopped. Cardiomyopathy induced by anthracyclines, and by doxorubicin in particular, is associated with persistent QRS voltage reduction, prolongation beyond normal limits of the systolic interval (PEP/LVET) and a reduction of the ejection fraction. It is also advisable to assess cardiac function by non-invasive techniques such as ECG, echocardiography and, if necessary, measurement of the ejection fraction by radionuclide angiography.

Early clinical diagnosis of drug induced heart failure appears to be essential for successful treatment with digitalis, diuretics, peripheral vasodilators, a low salt diet and bed rest.

Alopecia is common and nausea, vomiting and diarrhoea may occur. Alopecia and lack of beard growth in males are usually reversible. Mucositis may appear 5–10 days after starting treatment and usually involves stomatitis with painful erosions, often along the sides of the tongue and on the sublingual mucosa. The frequency and severity of these side-effects is, however, lower than that described with other anthracycline compounds, such as doxorubicin.

The risk of thrombophlebitis at the injection site may be minimised by following the recommended procedure for administration.

Pharmorubicin may impart a red colour to the urine and patients should be advised that this is no cause for alarm.

There is no conclusive information as to whether Pharmorubicin may adversely affect human fertility, or cause teratogenesis. Experimental data, however, suggest that Pharmorubicin may harm the foetus. This product should not normally be administered to patients who are pregnant or to mothers who are breast-feeding. Like most other anticancer agents, Pharmorubicin has shown mutagenic and carcinogenic properties in animals.

Accidental contact with the skin or eyes should be treated immediately by copious lavage with soap and water. The conjunctiva should be washed with saline solution.

Overdosage: Very high single doses of Pharmorubicin may be expected to cause acute myocardial degeneration within 24 hours and severe myelosuppression within 10–14 days. Treatment should aim to support the patient during this period and should utilise such measures as blood transfusions and reverse barrier nursing. Delayed cardiac failure has been seen with the anthracyclines up to 6 months after the overdose. Patients should be observed carefully and should, if signs of cardiac failure arise, be treated along conventional lines.

Pharmaceutical precautions The vial contents are under a negative pressure to minimise aerosol formation during reconstitution: care should be taken when the needle is inserted. During reconstitution a gelatinous mass may form which will completely dissolve on further shaking. The reconstituted solution is chemically stable for up to 48 hours at 2°–8°C or 24 hours at room temperature; however, it is recommended that, in line with good pharmaceutical practice, the solution should not normally be stored for longer than 24 hours at 2°–8°C. Avoid exposure of the product to sunlight or direct light.

Prolonged contact with any solution of an alkaline pH should be avoided as it may result in hydrolysis of the drug. Pharmorubicin should not be mixed with heparin as a precipitate may form and it is not recommended that Pharmorubicin be directly mixed with other drugs when given in combination.

Discard any unused solution.

It is recommended that personnel handling Pharmorubicin should wear protective gloves. Care should be taken to avoid the inhalation of any aerosol produced during reconstitution. Spillage or leakage should be treated with dilute sodium hypochlorite solution and then water. All cleaning materials should be placed in high-risk, waste-disposal bags and incinerated.

Legal category POM.

Package quantities 10 mg, 20 mg and 50 mg vials for injection.

Further information In patients with normal hepatic and renal function plasma levels, after i.v. injection of 75–90 mg/m^2 of the drug, follow a tri-exponential decrease with a very fast first phase and a slow terminal phase corresponding to a half-life of about 40 hours. Plasma levels of the main metabolite, the 13-OH derivative, are constantly lower and virtually parallel those of the unchanged drug. Pharmorubicin is mainly eliminated via the hepatobiliary system; high plasma clearance values (0.9 l/min) indicate that the slow elimination is due to extensive tissue distribution. Pharmorubicin does not cross the blood–brain barrier.

Product licence number 3433/0082

REFOLINON*

Presentation Clear, pale yellow liquid for injection containing leucovorin 3 mg/ml (as the calcium salt) in ampoules of 2 ml and 10 ml.

Pale yellow, round, convex, scored, uncoated tablet; diameter 9 mm containing 15 mg leucovorin (as the calcium salt).

Uses Leucovorin (folinic acid) is the formyl derivative of tetrahydrofolic acid and is an intermediate product of the metabolism of folic acid. Leucovorin is used in cytotoxic therapy as an antidote to folic acid antagonists such as methotrexate. Leucovorin is effective in the treatment of megaloblastic anaemia due to folate deficiency.

Dosage and administration (Adults and children)

Leucovorin rescue: Depending upon the dose of methotrexate administered, dosage regimens of leucovorin calcium vary. Up to 120 mg leucovorin calcium are generally given, usually in divided doses over 12–24 hours by intramuscular injection, bolus intravenous injection or intravenous infusion in normal saline. This is followed by 12–15 mg intramuscularly or 15 mg orally every 6 hours for 48 hours. Rescue therapy is usually started 24 hours after the commencement of methotrexate administration.

If overdosage of methotrexate is suspected, the dose of leucovorin calcium should be equal to or greater than the dose of methotrexate and should be administered within one hour of the methotrexate administration.

Megaloblastic anaemia (folate deficiency): 15 mg (one tablet) leucovorin per day.

Contra-indications, warnings, etc Calcium folinate should not be used for the treatment of pernicious anaemia or other megaloblastic anaemia where vitamin B12 is deficient.

Leucovorin should not be given simultaneously with a folic acid antagonist, for the purpose of reducing or preventing clinical toxicity, as the therapeutic effect of the antagonist may be nullified.

High-dose methotrexate therapy together with leucovorin rescue should only be carried out under the direction of physicians experienced in antitumour chemotherapy.

Adverse reactions to leucovorin calcium are rare, but following parenteral administration occasional pyrexial reactions have been reported.

Pharmaceutical precautions Protect from light.

Refolinon for injection has been shown to be compatible with 0.9% sodium chloride solution. Under normal light conditions and at room temperature solutions of calcium folinate in 0.9% sodium chloride have been shown to be stable for 24 hours.

Legal category POM.

Package quantities

Refolinon for Injection	10 × 2 ml ampoules
	10 × 10 ml ampoules
Refolinon Tablets	Containers of 30 tablets

Further information Nil.

Product licence numbers
Refolinon for Injection 3433/0079
Refolinon Tablets 3433/0078

SINTISONE*

Presentation White, scored tablets each containing 6.65 mg of prednisolone steaglate, therapeutically equivalent to prednisolone 5 mg.

Uses Sintisone is a synthetic glucocorticoid and is indicated in all conditions that respond to corticosteroid treatment, such as: rheumatoid arthritis, rheumatic fever, asthma, ulcerative colitis, pemphigus, sarcoidosis, systemic lupus erythematosus, nephrotic syndrome, scleritis, skin conditions and polyarteritis nodosa.
Sintisone may also be used in cancer chemotherapy when a corticosteroid is indicated.

Dosage and administration *Adults:* The average initial dose for adults is 2–4 tablets, orally, twice daily, gradually reducing this to a maintenance dose of 1–3 tablets daily.
Children: Initial dose: 0.6–2 mg/kg body weight, orally in divided doses. Maintenance dose: 1 mg/kg body weight, orally in divided doses.
Treatment may be given in short (6–10 day) courses for the alleviation of the symptoms of acute inflammatory episodes.
Alternate-day corticosteroid therapy is known to reduce the incidence of unwanted effects. Sintisone may be used with advantage in this manner by giving twice the normal daily dose every other day.
Treatment with corticosteroids should not terminate abruptly but should be withdrawn gradually.

Contra-indications, warnings, etc The contra-indications are those common to other corticosteroids: active tuberculosis, peptic ulcer, acute psychosis, Cushing's disease, osteoporosis, hypertension, diabetes mellitus and a tendency to thromboembolic episodes. Corticosteroids are usually also contra-indicated in the presence of acute bacterial or viral infections.
Patients receiving corticosteroids or who have been prescribed them during the preceding two years should be given supplementary corticosteroids for one to two days before surgery, and continued until stress has ceased before tapering off the dose.
Corticosteroids should be used with caution in pregnancy, especially during the first trimester.
Overdosage: There is no specific treatment but gastric lavage should be performed as soon as possible. Supportive measures should be instituted as required.

Pharmaceutical precautions Store in airtight containers and protect from light.

Legal category POM.

Package quantities Bottles of 100 tablets.

Further information Sintisone is a lipid soluble ester of prednisolone which is absorbed intact from the gut more completely than prednisolone. It circulates in the blood as the ester and is slowly metabolised to prednisolone. These properties confer on Sintisone a reduced tendency to the side-effects associated with corticosteroid therapy such as suppression of the pituitary/adrenal axis (Metyrapone test), salt and water retention, calcium loss and raised intraocular pressure.

Product licence number 3433/5906.

TAMOXIFEN

Presentation Tamoxifen 10: White, round, convex, uncoated tablet, diameter 6 mm containing 15.2 mg tamoxifen citrate equivalent to 10 mg tamoxifen, marked with an 'F' on one side and '10' on the other.
Tamoxifen 20: White, round, convex, uncoated tablet, diameter 9 mm containing 30.4 mg tamoxifen citrate equivalent to 20 mg tamoxifen, marked with an 'F' on one side and '20' on the other.

Uses Breast carcinoma, particularly in oestrogen receptor positive patients.

Dosage and administration *Adults:* The recommended daily dose is 20–40 mg tamoxifen orally in two divided doses. A response to therapy is usual only after 1–3 months' treatment.
Elderly: The adult dosage range has been used in elderly patients with breast cancer.
Children: Not applicable.

Contra-indications, warnings, etc
Contra-indications: The use of tamoxifen is contra-indicated in pregnancy. Pre-menopausal patients should have pregnancy excluded before treatment is commenced.
Warnings: Tamoxifen should be used under the direction of those experienced in hormonal cancer chemotherapy.
Precautions: Blurred vision caused by retinal changes has been reported in some patients who have received continuous therapy with 12–16 times the normal recommended lower dose or with lower doses for a very long time.
Side-effects: Compared to androgen and oestrogen therapy the side-effects caused by tamoxifen are more rare and more mild, very occasionally they have led to discontinuation of treatment.
Due to the anti-oestrogenic effect the most common side-effects are of the climacteric type: hot flushes, vaginal bleeding, fluid retention and pruritus. In addition, abdominal pain, GI intolerance, tumour pain and dizziness have been reported.
The tendency towards thrombophlebitis may increase and transient thrombocytopenia may occur. In some patients with bone metastases hypercalcaemia has been observed at the start of treatment.
Menstruation is completely inhibited when tamoxifen is given to premenopausal patients.
Reversible oedema of the ovaries has occasionally been observed with a dose of 40 mg twice daily. When side-effects are severe, a reduction in dosage may be adequate to reduce them to tolerable levels while still maintaining control of the disease.
Overdosage: Animal experiments have indicated that an excessive overdose (100–200 times the daily dose) may give rise to oestrogenic effects and not the expected anti-oestrogenic effects.

Pharmaceutical precautions Protect from heat and light.

Legal category POM.

Package quantities Packs. of 30 or 250 tablets, containing aluminium blister strips of 10 tablets.

Further information Tamoxifen is a non-steroidal, anti-oestrogen. It is specifically bound to oestrogen receptors in the cytoplasm and competes for the receptor sites with oestrogen. The tamoxifen receptor complex however, has no DNA synthesising effect on the nucleus, thus cellular replication is prevented. Peak concentrations in serum are achieved 4–7 hours after oral dosing. The half-life of the distribution phase is about 11 hours. The slow terminal half-life is around 7 days.

Tamoxifen is mainly eliminated as conjugates in the faeces. The main metabolite in serum is N-desmethyl tamoxifen.

Product licence numbers
Tamoxifen 10   3433/0083
Tamoxifen 20   3433/0089

TEMAZEPAM

Presentation
Temazepam capsules 10 mg: Green, soft gelatin capsules marked "10" in white, containing temazepam 10 mg in solution.

Temazepam capsules 15 mg: Green, soft gelatin capsules marked "15" in white, containing temazepam 15 mg in solution.

Temazepam capsules 20 mg: Green, soft gelatin capsules marked "20" in white, containing temazepam 20 mg in solution.

Temazepam capsules 30 mg: Green, soft gelatin capsules marked "30" in white, containing temazepam 30 mg in solution.

Temazepam elixir: A clear, green, lemon-mint flavoured elixir containing 10 mg temazepam per 5 ml.

Uses Temazepam capsules 10, 15, 20, 30 mg and Temazepam elixir are indicated for the short-term treatment of sleep disturbances. These products are especially useful in those patients for whom the persistance of hypnotic effect after rising would be undesirable.

Temazepam elixir is indicated particularly where a liquid formulation is preferable.

Products in the temazepam range are particularly suitable for patients with transient sleep disorders in whom the re-establishment of normal sleep patterns is expected following the resolution of precipitating factors.

They are also indicated for pre-medication for minor surgical and investigative procedures, especially in the case of out-patients.

Dosage and administration
Adults: Temazepam capsules 10 mg – *Insomnia:* One to three capsules on retiring. A dose of two capsules will be found satisfactory for most patients. This may be increased to four or six capsules in patients who do not respond to the lower dose. *Premedication:* 2 to 4 capsules from half an hour to one hour prior to surgery or investigative procedures.

Temazepam capsules 15 mg – *Insomnia:* One to two capsules on retiring. *Premedication:* 1 to 2 capsules from half an hour to one hour prior to surgery or investigative procedures.

Temazepam capsules 20 mg – *Insomnia:* For those patients resistant to low hypnotic dosage, two or three capsules before retiring. *Premedication:* 1 to 2 capsules from half an hour to one hour prior to surgery or investigative procedures.

Temazepam capsules 30 mg – *Insomnia:* For those patients resistant to low hypnotic dosage 1 or 2 capsules before retiring. *Premedication:* 1 capsule from half an hour to one hour prior to surgery or investigative procedures.

Temazepam elixir – *Insomnia:* Each 5 ml spoonful of temazepam elixir is equivalent to 10 mg temazepam. The usual dose is 5–15 ml orally on retiring; a dose of 10 ml will be found to be satisfactory for most patients and is equivalent to 20 mg temazepam in capsule form. This may be increased to 20 or 30 ml (40–60 mg temazepam) in patients who do not respond to the lower dose. *Premedication:* 10 to 20 ml from half an hour to one hour prior to surgery or investigative procedures.

Elderly: Elderly patients or those suffering from cerebral vascular changes such as arteriosclerosis are likely to respond to smaller doses. Half the normal dose may be sufficient for a therapeutic response.

Children: Not recommended.

Contra-indications, warnings, etc
Contra-indications: Known sensitivity to benzodiazepines. Acute pulmonary insufficiency.

Warnings: Although hangover effect is uncommon, patients should be warned against driving or operating dangerous machinery if so affected. Doses of 30 mg and above of temazepam are more likely to cause hangover effects to persist into the following day than lower doses, particularly in patients unused to hypnotics and in the elderly. As with all compounds which have an effect on the CNS, patients should be advised not to consume alcohol whilst taking Temazepam.

Use in pregnancy: There is no evidence as to drug safety in human pregnancy, nor is there evidence from animal work that the drug is free from hazard. Do not use during pregnancy, especially during the first and last trimesters unless there are compelling reasons.

Adverse effects: Common adverse effects of benzodiazepines include drowsiness, sedation, blurring of vision and unsteadiness and ataxia. These symptoms are liable to be potentiated by alcohol. The elderly are more liable to experience such effects. (See also under Dependence potential and withdrawal symptoms.) Abnormal psychological reactions to benzodiazepines have been reported. Rare behavioural adverse effects include paradoxical aggressive outbursts, excitement, confusion and the uncovering of depression with suicidal tendencies.

Other rare adverse effects, including hypotension, gastro-intestinal and visual disturbances, skin rashes, urinary retention, headache, vertigo, changes in libido, blood dyscrasias and jaundice have been reported.

Precautions: Give with caution to patients with chronic pulmonary insufficiency, or renal or hepatic dysfunction. Avoid benzodiazepines if possible during lactation.

The concurrent use of other CNS depressants such as alcohol, general anaesthetics, narcotic analgesics, monoamine oxidase inhibitors and antidepressants should be avoided as it will result in an accentuation of their effects.

Where Temazepam is used as medication before surgical or investigative procedures, patients should be accompanied home.

Dependence potential and withdrawal symptoms: In general, the dependence potential of benzodiazepines is low, but this increases when high dosage is used, especially when given over long periods. This is particularly so in patients with a history of alcoholism, drug abuse or in patients with marked personality disorders. Regular monitoring of treatment in such patients is essential, and routine repeat prescriptions should be avoided.

Treatment in all patients should be withdrawn gradually as symptoms such as depression, nervousness, rebound insomnia, irritability, sweating and diarrhoea have been reported following abrupt cessation of treatment with benzodiazepines in patients receiving even normal therapeutic doses for short periods of time.

Abrupt withdrawal following excessive dosage may produce confusion, toxic psychosis, convulsions or a condition resembling delirium tremens.

Overdosage: Doses substantially in excess of those recommended, have been taken without ill effect. As with other benzodiazepines, treatment of overdosage should be symptomatic with general supportive measures as required. Although temazepam in this formulation is rapidly absorbed, gastric lavage may be useful if performed shortly after ingestion.

Pharmaceutical precautions
Temazepam capsules 10, 15, 20 and 30 mg: Dispense in glass or plastic containers.

Temazepam elixir: Store below 25°C and protect from direct light.

Temazepam elixir is sugar-free being based on a glycerol vehicle. If dilution of the elixir is required, glycerol BP is a suitable diluent.

Legal category CD (Sch 4), POM.

Package quantities
Temazepam capsules 10 mg: Containers of 30, 60, 500 and 1000 capsules.

Temazepam capsules 15 mg: Containers of 30 and 60 capsules.

Temazepam capsules 20 mg: Containers of 30, 60, 250 and 500 capsules.

Temazepam capsules 30 mg: Containers of 30 and 60 capsules.

Temazepam elixir: Bottles of 300 ml.

Further information The formulation of temazepam as a solution in soft gelatin capsules or as an elixir ensures rapid and complete absorption which, with its short half life and lack of active metabolites, results in prompt induction of sleep and a low incidence of hangover effects.

Temazepam is a short-acting benzodiazepine. As accumulation tends not to occur, patients are less likely to experience excessive drowsiness or impairment in the performance of skilled tasks. The short half-life of this drug may offer advantages in the treatment of the elderly, in patients with impaired renal or liver function, and in situations where day-time alertness is desirable.

Product licence numbers
Temazepam capsules 10 mg   3433/0094
Temazepam capsules 15 mg   3433/0105
Temazepam capsules 20 mg   3433/0095
Temazepam capsules 30 mg   3433/0106
Temazepam elixir   3433/0054

TETRALYSAL*

Presentation Tetralysal is available as white, hard gelatin capsules marked Farmitalia Carlo Erba containing 204 mg of Lymecycline BP, equivalent to 150 mg tetracycline base.

Uses Tetralysal is a broad spectrum antibiotic and is recommended for the treatment of all infections caused by tetracycline-sensitive organisms and may be utilised in all conditions where tetracycline therapy is indicated. In common with other tetracyclines, it is also indicated in penicillin-sensitive patients for the treatment of staphylococcal infections.

Typical indications include: Ear, nose and throat infections; acute and chronic bronchitis (including prophylaxis); infections of the gastro-intestinal and urinary tracts; non-gonoccocal urethritis of chlamydial origin and other chlamydial infections such as trachoma; acne; rickettsial fevers; soft tissue infections.

Dosage and administration The usual recommended dose is 2 capsules b.d. If higher doses are required, 6–8 capsules may be given over 24 hours. Lower doses may be given for prophylaxis and for the chronic treatment of acne; in such cases treatment should be continued for at least 8 weeks. In the management of sexually transmitted disease both partners should be treated.

Contra-indications, warnings, etc Tetracyclines are selectively absorbed by developing bones and teeth and may cause dental staining and enamel hypoplasia. In addition, these compounds readily cross the placental barrier and therefore Tetralysal should not be administered to pregnant women or children below the age of 8 years.

As Tetralysal is mainly excreted by the kidneys, it should not be administered to patients with overt renal insufficiency.

Its use is also contra-indicated in patients hypersensitive to tetracyclines.

The absorption of tetracyclines may be affected by the simultaneous administration of antacids and iron preparations.

It should also be borne in mind that the prolonged use of broad spectrum antibiotics may result in the appearance of resistant organisms and superinfection.

Overdosage: There is no specific treatment, but gastric lavage should be performed as soon as possible. Supportive measures should be instituted as required and a high fluid intake maintained.

Pharmaceutical precautions The capsules should be stored in air-tight containers in a cool place protected from light.

Legal category POM.

Package quantities Bottles of 16 and 100 capsules.

Further information Tetralysal (lymecycline) is tetracycline chemically bonded to the amino-acid L-lysine. It has been estimated that 204 mg of lymecycline (containing the equivalent of 150 mg tetracycline base) is equivalent in its action to 250 mg of tetracycline hydrochloride. Lymecycline is approximately 5000 times more soluble than tetracycline base and unlike tetracycline hydrochloride it is soluble at all physiological pH values (a 5% aqueous solution does not precipitate in the presence of serum).

Product licence number 3433/5909.

TETRALYSAL* 300

Presentation Tetralysal 300 is available as white, hard gelatin capsules marked Farmitalia Carlo Erba containing

408 mg of Lymecycline BP, equivalent to 300 mg tetracycline base.

Uses Tetralysal 300 is a broad spectrum antibiotic and is recommended for the treatment of all infections caused by tetracycline-sensitive organisms and may be utilised in all conditions where tetracycline therapy is indicated. In common with other tetracyclines, it is indicated in penicillin-sensitive patients for the treatment of staphylococcal infections.

Typical indications include: Ear, nose and throat infections; acute and chronic bronchitis (including prophylaxis); infections of the gastro-intestinal and urinary tracts; non-gonoccocal urethritis of chlamydial origin and other chlamydial infections such as trachoma; acne; rickettsial fevers; soft tissue infections.

Dosage and administration The usual recommended dose is 1 capsule b.d. If higher doses are required, 3–4 capsules may be given over 24 hours. Lower doses may be given for prophylaxis and for the chronic treatment of acne: in such cases treatment should be continued for at least 8 weeks. In the management of sexually transmitted disease both partners should be treated.

Contra-indications, warnings, etc Tetracyclines are selectively absorbed by developing bones and teeth and may cause dental staining and enamel hypoplasia. In addition, these compounds readily cross the placental barrier and therefore Tetralysal 300 should not be administered to pregnant women or children below the age of 8 years.

As Tetralysal 300 is mainly excreted by the kidneys, it should not be administered to patients with overt renal insufficiency.

Its use is also contra-indicated in patients hypersensitive to tetracyclines.

The absorption of tetracyclines may be affected by the simultaneous administration of antacids and iron preparations.

It should also be borne in mind that the prolonged use of broad spectrum antibiotics may result in the appearance of resistant organisms and superinfection.

Overdosage: There is no specific treatment, but gastric lavage should be performed as soon as possible. Supportive measures should be instituted as required and a high fluid intake maintained.

Pharmaceutical precautions The capsules should be stored in air-tight containers in a cool place protected from light.

Legal category POM.

Package quantities Bottles of 20 and 100 capsules.

Further information Tetralysal 300 (lymecycline) is tetracycline chemically bonded to the amino-acid L-lysine. It has been estimated that 408 mg of lymecycline (containing the equivalent of 300 mg of tetracycline base) is equivalent in its action to 500 mg of tetracycline hydrochloride. Lymecycline is approximately 5000 times more soluble than tetracycline base and unlike tetracycline hydrochloride it is soluble at all physiological pH values (a 5% aqueous solution does not precipitate in the presence of serum).

Product licence number 3433/0044

*Trade Mark

Fisons plc
Pharmaceutical Division
12 Derby Road
Loughborough, Leics LE11 0BB

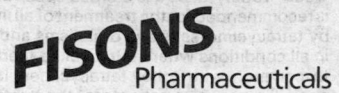

ACNIL*

Presentation A smooth, soft, brownish-pink cream containing:

Precipitated Sulphur BP	3.0% w/w
Resorcinol BP	0.5% w/w
Cetrimide BP	0.5% w/w

Uses Acnil is a mild antiseptic and keratolytic for the treatment of acne vulgaris.

Dosage and administration *Adults:* Spread sparingly over the affected area only, twice daily until the spots disappear.

Children: At the discretion of the physician.

Elderly: No current evidence for alteration of the adult dose.

Contra-indications, warnings, etc
Contra-indication: Rosacea.

Pharmaceutical precautions Nil.

Legal category P.

Package quantities Tube of 25 g.

Further information Nil.

Product licence number 0113/5000.

AURALGICIN*

Presentation A pale yellow, viscous liquid containing:

Benzocaine BP	1.4% w/v
Ephedrine Hydrochloride BP	1.0% w/v
Phenazone BPC	5.5% w/v
Chlorbutol BP	1.0% w/v
Potassium Hydroxyquinoline Sulphate BPC	0.1% w/v
Glycerol BP	to 100%

Uses Antibacterial, analgesic ear drops for the treatment of acute and subacute otitis media.

Dosage and administration *Adults and children:*
1. The patient should be lying on his side – affected ear uppermost.
2. Pour the ear drops from the bottle into the affected ear until the ear is filled. (The patient will find it more soothing if the ear drops are warmed before placing them in the ear. This can be achieved by placing a teaspoon in warm water and then pouring the drops onto the dried warm spoon. The drops can now be applied to the ear from the spoon.)
3. Wait a few minutes before placing a plug of cotton wool into the ear.
4. Repeat the treatment hourly until no further pain is felt.

5. Thereafter the treatment should be repeated three-hourly for a period of 24 hours or until the doctor advises that no further treatment is necessary.

Note: If pain and inflammation persist after 24 hours the doctor should be consulted again.

Elderly: No current evidence for alteration of the adult dose.

Contra-indications, warnings, etc
Contra-indications: Hypersensitivity to benzocaine or other ingredients. Not recommended for use in patients with perforated ear drums.

Pharmaceutical precautions *Important:* Replace the cap immediately after use. Do not use if cloudy as the effectiveness will be reduced.
For external use only.

Legal category P.

Package quantities Bottle of 12 ml.

Further information Appropriate systemic therapy may also be required.

Product licence number 0113/5003.

BARQUINOL* HC

Presentation Smooth, buff cream containing:

Hydrocortisone Acetate BP	0.5% w/w
Clioquinol BP	3.0% w/w

Uses Exudative or secondarily infected eczema (including infantile, nummular, allergic or stasis type), dermatitis (seborrhoeic, atopic or contact) and anogenital intertrigo.

Dosage and administration Apply directly to the affected area as a smear or as a spread on a dressing.

Adults and children: Apply two or three times daily for up to 14 days or up to 7 days on the face.

Infants: Apply sparingly for short courses up to 7 days (occlusion should not be used).

Elderly: No current evidence for alteration of the dose.

Contra-indications, warnings, etc
Contra-indications: Acne rosacea, primary skin infections (e.g. Herpes simplex and impetigo) and secondary infections which are infected with yeasts.

Precautions:
Use in pregnancy: There is inadequate evidence of safety in human pregnancy and there may be a very small risk of cleft palate and intrauterine growth retardation in the foetus. There is evidence of harmful effects in pregnancy in animals, therefore the benefits of using steroid

preparations during pregnancy should be weighed against the possible risks to mother and foetus.

Use in lactating women: Steroids are known to be excreted in milk and therefore mothers using large doses of topical steroids should be advised not to breast-feed their infants.

Use in infants: Long-term continuous topical therapy should be avoided. Adrenal suppression can occur even without occlusion.

If no improvement is noted after 14 days of the normal recommended dose, then cultural investigation of the causative organisms should be undertaken to identify the specific infective agent.

Side-effects: Clioquinol may occasionally cause severe irritation. Long-term use of topical corticosteroids may cause changes in the skin, particularly on the face, including striae, thinning and telangiectasia, particularly when occlusive dressings are used.

Pharmaceutical precautions Nil.

Legal category POM.

Package quantities Tube of 15 g.

Further information Nil.

Product licence number 0113/5004.

DIMYRIL* LINCTUS
Approved name: Isoaminile cough linctus

Presentation Faintly opalescent, red liquid, each 5 ml of which contains 40 mg isoaminile citrate.

Uses For the treatment of cough associated with acute and chronic bronchitis, influenza, common cold, laryngitis and measles.

Dosage and administration *Oral: Adults:* 5 ml three to five times per day.

Children: 2.5–5 ml three to five times per day.

Infants: As recommended by the physician.

Elderly: No current evidence for alteration of the adult dose.

Contra-indications, warnings, etc *Side-effects:* Dizziness, nausea and constipation occur rarely.

Overdosage: Symptoms: Hallucinations and mania. Treatment: Withdrawal of drug; induction of vomiting/gastric lavage if large quantities taken; medical observation and supportive measures as necessary.

Pharmaceutical precautions Nil.

Legal category POM.

Package quantities Bottle of 150 ml.

Further information Dimyril contains a single active ingredient and hence is reimbursible under the NHS if prescribed generically as Isoaminile Cough Linctus.

Product licence number 0113/5012.

FRAMYCORT* EYE AND EAR DROPS
Presentation Clear, very pale fawn coloured supernatant fluid with a fine white deposit which readily disperses on shaking. Contains:

Framycetin Sulphate BP	0.5% w/v
Hydrocortisone Acetate BP	0.5% w/v

Uses Treatment of superficial bacterial eye infections, conjunctivitis, blepharitis, marginal corneal ulceration and otitis externa.

Dosage and administration Direct application to the eye or into the auditory canal, 1–4 drops three to four times daily, or as directed by the physician.

Contra-indications, warnings, etc
Contra-indications: Viral infections. Known hypersensitivity to framycetin or benzalkonium chloride.

Precautions: In pregnant animals, administration of corticosteroids can cause abnormalities of foetal development. The relevance of this finding to human beings has not been established. However, topical steroids should not be used extensively in pregnancy, i.e. in large amounts or for long periods.

In infants, long-term continuous topical therapy should be avoided. Adrenal suppression can occur even without occlusion.

Cross sensitivity can occur in neomycin sensitive patients.

Pharmaceutical precautions Store in a cool place. Protect from freezing. Shake well before use. Discard two weeks after first opening container.

Legal category POM.

Package quantities Dropper bottle of 5 ml.

Further information Nil.

Product licence number 0113/5089.

FRAMYCORT* EYE OINTMENT
Presentation Smooth, pale yellow ointment containing:

Framycetin Sulphate BP	0.5% w/w
Hydrocortisone Acetate BP	0.5% w/w

Uses The treatment of superficial bacterial eye infections, conjunctivitis, blepharitis, marginal corneal ulceration.

Elderly: No current evidence for alteration of the dose.

Dosage and administration To be applied to the eye two or three times daily.

Contra-indications, warnings, etc
Contra-indications: Viral infections. Known hypersensitivity to framycetin.

Precautions: In pregnant animals, administration of corticosteroids can cause abnormalities of foetal development. The relevance of this finding to human beings has not been established. However, topical steroids should not be used extensively in pregnancy, i.e. in large amounts or for long periods.

In infants, long-term continuous topical therapy should be avoided. Adrenal suppression can occur even without occlusion.

Cross sensitivity can occur in neomycin sensitive patients.

Pharmaceutical precautions Store in a cool place.

Legal category POM.

Package quantities Tube of 3.5 g.

Further information Nil.

Product licence number 0113/5065.

FRAMYCORT* OINTMENT

Presentation Off-white ointment containing:

Framycetin Sulphate BP 0.5% w/w
Hydrocortisone Acetate BP 0.5% w/w

Uses Subacute and chronic eczema-dermatitis complicated by secondary infection, seborrhoeic dermatitis, anogenital pruritus.

Dosage and administration *Topical application:* Rub in gently and thoroughly two to three times daily, leaving a light surface layer over the affected area. Cover with a light dressing.

Adults and children: Apply for up to 14 days or up to 7 days on the face.

Infants: Apply sparingly for short courses up to 7 days (occlusion should not be used).

Elderly: No current evidence for alteration of the dose.

Contra-indications, warnings, etc
Contra-indications: Known sensitivity to framycetin.
   Cross-sensitivity can occur in patients sensitised to other aminoglycoside antibiotics.

Precautions:
Use in pregnancy: There is inadequate evidence of safety in human pregnancy and there may be a very small risk of cleft palate and intrauterine growth retardation in the foetus. There is evidence of harmful effects in pregnancy in animals, therefore the benefits of using steroid preparations during pregnancy should be weighed against the possible risks to mother and foetus.

Use in lactating women: Steroids are known to be excreted in milk and therefore mothers using large doses of topical steroids should be advised not to breast-feed their infants.

Use in infants: Long-term continuous topical therapy should be avoided. Adrenal suppression can occur even without occlusion.

Use in elderly patients: Patients with impaired renal function may be at risk of ototoxicity when the ointment is applied to extensive areas.

Warnings: Prolonged or recurrent use may cause sensitisation. Long-term use may cause changes in the skin, particularly on the face, including striae, thinning and telangiectasia, particularly when occlusive dressings are used.

Pharmaceutical precautions Store in a cool place.

Legal category POM.

Package quantities Tube of 15 g.

Further information Nil.

Product licence number 0113/5067.

FRAMYGEN* CREAM

Presentation Smooth, white cream containing Framycetin Sulphate BP 0.5% w/w.

Uses All uncomplicated bacterial skin infections including: sycosis barbae, impetigo and other pyogenic infections.

Dosage and administration Topical application smeared directly on to lesions or as a spread on a dressing two to three times a day.

Elderly: No current evidence for alteration of the dose.

Contra-indications, warnings, etc
Contra-indications: Known hypersensitivity to framycetin.

Warnings: Cross sensitivity can occur in neomycin sensitive patients.

Pharmaceutical precautions Store in a cool place.

Legal category POM.

Package quantities Tube of 15 g.

Further information Nil.

Product licence number 0113/5068.

FRAMYGEN* EYE AND EAR DROPS

Presentation A clear, very pale fawn coloured fluid containing Framycetin Sulphate BP 0.5% w/w.

Uses *In ophthalmology:* Treatment of styes, blepharitis, conjunctivitis and other superficial eye infections, corneal abrasions.

In otology: Otitis externa.

Dosage and administration To be applied to the eye or into the auditory canal, 1–4 drops three to four times daily, or as directed by the physician.

Elderly: No current evidence for alteration of the dose.

Contra-indications, warnings, etc
Contra-indications: Known hypersensitivity to framycetin or benzalkonium chloride.

Warnings: Cross sensitivity can occur in neomycin sensitive patients.

Pharmaceutical precautions Store in a cool place. Protect from freezing. Discard four weeks after first opening container.

Legal category POM.

Package quantities Dropper bottle of 5 ml.

Further information Nil.

Product licence number 0113/5090.

FRAMYGEN* EYE OINTMENT

Presentation A smooth, pale yellow ointment containing Framycetin Sulphate BP 0.5% w/w.

Uses The treatment of blepharitis and styes, blepharoconjunctivitis, infected conjunctivitis and infected corneal abrasions.

Elderly: No current evidence for alteration of the dose.

Dosage and administration Direct application to the eye four to six times daily.

Contra-indications, warnings, etc
Contra-indications: Known hypersensitivity to framycetin.

Warnings: Cross sensitivity can occur in neomycin sensitive patients.

Pharmaceutical precautions Store in a cool place.

Legal category POM.

Package quantities Tube of 3.5 g.

Further information Nil.

Product licence number 0113/5069.

GENISOL*

Presentation A clear, golden-yellow liquid containing sodium sulphosuccinated undecylenic monoalkolamide 1% w/v, purified coal-tar fractions 0.25% w/v designed to be therapeutically equivalent to 2% Prepared Coal Tar BP and comprising:

Phenol	8% w/w	o-Cresol	8% w/w
Quinoline	4% w/w	Pyridine	2% w/w
α-Picoline	2% w/w	Toluene	16% w/w
Xylene	8% w/w	Phenanthrene	32% w/w
Carbazole	20% w/w		

Uses Seborrhoeic dermatitis of the scalp (dandruff) and psoriasis of the scalp.

Dosage and administration To be used once per week or more frequently if required, in the manner of a shampoo. Stir about 10 ml of Genisol into half a tumblerful of warm water. Wet the hair thoroughly, apply half the solution and work into the scalp with the fingers. Rinse and repeat the application. Finally, rinse the hair thoroughly in clean water.

Elderly: No current evidence for alteration of the dose.

Contra-indications, warnings, etc When washing the hair, care should be taken to keep the solution away from the eyes.

Pharmaceutical precautions Nil.

Legal category P.

Package quantities Bottles of 58 ml, 250 ml and 600 ml.

Further information Nil.

Product licence number 0113/5020.

IMFERON*

Presentation Imferon is dark brown, slightly viscous, sterile liquid complex of ferric hydroxide and low molecular weight dextran in a 0.9% sodium chloride solution for injection. It contains the equivalent of 50 mg elemental iron (as iron dextran) per ml.

Uses Imferon is indicated for the parenteral treatment of proven severe iron deficiency anaemia. Imferon is administered by intramuscular injection for patients who cannot tolerate, or do not respond to oral iron. If essential, it may also be given by intravenous injection or total dose infusion: such use must be confined to the hospital treatment of patients for whom the intramuscular route or other forms of therapy such as blood transfusion are inappropriate or are not available.

Dosage and administration *Dosage: Adults:* The dose of Imferon is determined by the haemoglobin level, bodyweight and sex of the patient. The following table provides a convenient means of determining the dose. This dose is intended to provide sufficient iron to restore haemoglobin levels to a normal level (14.8 g/dl) and to replenish depleted iron stores. The table takes account of the higher iron stores in men. In pregnancy, a further 10 ml should be added to the dose.

Alternatively the total dose required may be calculated. If the patient's bodyweight in kilograms is W and the haemoglobin level is H g/dl.

Dose of Imferon in ml required for women =
$$[0.0476 \times W \times (14.8 - H)] + 6$$
Dose of Imferon in ml required for men =
$$[0.0476 \times W \times (14.8 - H)] + 14.0$$

The dose may also be calculated if the bodyweight in kilograms (W) and the percentage haemoglobin deficit (D) are known.

Dose of Imferon in ml required for women =
$$0.00705 \times W \times D + 6$$
Dose of Imferon in ml required for men =
$$0.00705 \times W \times D + 14.$$

Children up to 15 years: A separate entry is provided in the dosage table for children up to 15 years of age which takes account of lower iron stores. Imferon should not normally be given in the first four months of life. Alternatively the total dose may be calculated. If the child's bodyweight in kilograms is W and the haemoglobin level is H g/dl:

Dose of Imferon required in ml = $0.0476 \times W \times (14.8 - H)$.

The dose may also be calculated if the bodyweight in kilograms (W) and the percentage haemoglobin deficit (D) are known.

Dose of Imferon in ml required = $0.00705 \times W \times D$.

Administration: Imferon may be given intramuscularly or intravenously. The intramuscular route is to be used unless there are valid reasons for intravenous administration. The intravenous administration of Imferon by the Total Dose Infusion method should be restricted to hospital usage only.

Intramuscular administration: The total amount of Imferon required is determined either from the dosage table or by calculation. It is administered as a series of injections: the volume of each is ordinarily determined by the patient's bodyweight. Infants below 10 lb (5 kg) should receive 0.5 ml; children below 20 lb (9 kg) 1.0 ml; adults normally 2.0 ml up to a maximum of 5.0 ml. If the patient is moderately active, injections may be given daily into alternate buttocks. In inactive or bed-ridden patients, the frequency of injections should be reduced to once or twice weekly.

Imferon must be given by deep intramuscular injection to minimise the risk of subcutaneous staining. It should be injected only into the muscle mass of the upper outer quadrant of the buttock – never into the arm or other exposed areas. A 20–21 gauge needle at least 50 mm long should be used for normal adults. For obese patients the length should be 80–100 mm, while for children and small adults a shorter and smaller needle (23 gauge × 32 mm) is used. The patient should be lying in the lateral position with the injection site uppermost, or standing bearing their weight on the leg opposite the injection site. To avoid injection or leakage into the subcutaneous tissue, a Z-track technique (displacement of the skin laterally prior to injection) is recommended. Imferon is injected slowly and smoothly. It is important to wait for a few seconds before withdrawing the needle to allow the muscle mass to accommodate the injection volume. To minimise leakage up the injection track the patient shoud be encouraged not to rub the injection site.

Intravenous administration: Imferon may be adminis-

Total dose of Imferon in millilitres

Observed haemoglobin levels

Bodyweight kg	lb	3.0 g/dl 20% Man	Woman	Child	4.4 g/dl 30% Man	Woman	Child	5.9 g/dl 40% Man	Woman	Child	7.4 g/dl 50% Man	Woman	Child	8.9 g/dl 60% Man	Woman	Child	10.4 g/dl 70% Man	Woman	Child
5	11	—	—	3	—	—	2	—	—	2	—	—	2	—	—	1	—	—	1
10	22	—	—	6	—	—	5	—	—	4	—	—	4	—	—	3	—	—	2
15	33	—	—	8	—	—	7	—	—	6	—	—	6	—	—	4	—	—	3
20	44	—	—	11	—	—	10	—	—	8	—	—	8	—	—	6	—	—	4
25	55	—	—	14	—	—	12	—	—	11	—	—	11	—	—	7	—	—	5
30	66	31	23	17	29	21	15	27	19	13	25	17	13	22	14	8	20	12	6
35	77	34	26	20	31	23	17	29	21	15	26	18	14	24	16	10	21	13	7
40	88	37	29	23	34	26	20	31	23	17	28	20	17	25	17	11	22	14	8
45	99	39	31	25	36	28	22	33	25	19	30	22	19	27	19	13	24	16	10
50	110	42	34	28	39	31	25	35	27	21	31	23	21	28	20	14	25	17	11
55	121	45	37	31	41	33	27	37	29	23	33	25	23	30	22	16	26	18	12
60	132	48	40	34	44	36	30	39	31	25	35	27	25	31	23	17	27	19	13
65	143	51	43	—	46	38	—	41	33	—	37	29	—	32	24	—	28	20	—
70	154	53	45	—	49	41	—	44	36	—	39	31	—	34	26	—	29	21	—
75	165	56	48	—	51	43	—	46	38	—	40	32	—	35	27	—	30	22	—
80	176	59	51	—	53	45	—	48	40	—	42	34	—	37	29	—	31	23	—
85	187	62	54	—	56	48	—	50	42	—	44	36	—	38	30	—	32	24	—
90	198	65	57	—	58	50	—	52	44	—	46	38	—	39	31	—	33	25	—
95	209	68	60	—	61	53	—	54	46	—	47	39	—	41	33	—	34	26	—
100	220	70	62	—	63	55	—	56	48	—	49	41	—	42	34	—	35	27	—
105	231	73	65	—	66	58	—	58	50	—	51	43	—	44	36	—	36	28	—
110	242	76	68	—	68	60	—	61	53	—	53	45	—	45	37	—	37	29	—
115	253	79	71	—	71	63	—	63	55	—	55	47	—	46	38	—	38	30	—
120	264	82	74	—	73	65	—	65	57	—	56	48	—	47	39	—	39	31	—

tered in large volumes intravenously, either diluted as in the Total Dose Infusion technique or undiluted, for the hospital treatment of patients for whom the intramuscular route or other forms of therapy are inappropriate or are not available.

Whenever Imferon is given intravenously, it is *essential* that one of the test-dose procedures described below is followed in full. Anaphylactoid reactions to Imferon are usually evident within a few minutes, and close observation is necessary to ensure early recognition. *If at any time during the intravenous administration of Imferon, any signs of a hypersensitivity reaction or intolerance are detected, administration must be stopped immediately.* Resuscitative equipment should be available, and anaphylactoid reactions should be treated with 0.5 ml of aqueous adrenaline 1:1000 given subcutaneously with general supportive measures. This should be followed by either oral or parenteral antihistamines and/or corticosteroids.

The intravenous route should not be used for patients with a history of asthma. If it is judged necessary to use the intravenous route for patients with a history of allergy, effective antihistamine cover should be given before administration of Imferon.

1. *Total Dose Infusion (TDI) Technique:* The total amount of Imferon required, determined from the dosage table or by calculation, is added aseptically immediately before administration to the required volume, usually 500 ml, of sterile normal saline or 5% dextrose solution. *The initial rate of infusion must not exceed 5 drops per minute for 10 minutes* and the patient must be kept under close medical supervision during this period. If the test dose is well tolerated, the rate of infusion may be increased *progressively* to 45–60 drops per minute. Patients should be observed carefully during the infusion and for at least one hour after it is completed.

2. *Undiluted Imferon Administration:* The total amount of Imferon is determined from the dosage table or by calculation: it may be given as a single dose or divided and given as a series of two or more intravenous injections. Before receiving the therapeutic dose of Imferon, *all patients must be given a slowly-administered test dose of 0.5 ml Imferon* diluted with 4–5 ml or more of the patient's own blood. The patient should then be observed carefully for at least 30 minutes and the therapeutic dose given only if the test dose is well tolerated. The therapeutic dose should be given as a slow intravenous injection: *the rate must not exceed 1 ml per minute* and the patient must be under strict medical supervision throughout the injection. Careful observation should continue for at least one hour thereafter.

Contra-indications, warnings, etc
Contra-indications: Imferon is contra-indicated in patients who have shown hypersensitivity to iron dextran. It should not be used during the acute phase of infectious kidney disease. It should not be given intravenously to patients with a history of asthma.

Warnings: The use of Imferon, as with the parenteral use of other iron-carbohydrate complexes, carries a risk of immediate and potentially severe anaphylactoid reactions. Patients should be closely observed during and immediately after administration. Resuscitative equipment, adrenaline, antihistamines and corticosteroids should be available for immediate treatment of reactions.

Imferon should be used with extreme care in patients with serious impairment of liver function. Caution should

be used when Imferon is given to patients suffering from an acute infection, or with a history of allergy or chronic infection. The intramuscular route should be used, and a graded series of injections is strongly recommended, starting with 0.5 ml, 1.0 ml, then 2.0 ml. Should it be judged necessary to use the intravenous route for patients with a history of allergy, effective antihistamine cover should be given before administration of Imferon.

An increased incidence of sepsis, primarily due to E.coli, has been reported when Imferon is given to neonates in Polynesian populations. The association with Imferon remains unclear. Iron supplementation is rarely necessary in the first four months of life and Imferon should not normally be given during this period.

A high incidence of post-infusion arthralgia has been reported in patients with rheumatoid arthritis treated by the intravenous route. This route should be used *only* when all other methods of treatment have been shown to be unsuccessful in these patients.

The intramuscular and subcutaneous injection of iron-carbohydrate complexes in very large doses under experimental conditions in animals produced sarcoma in rats, mice, rabbits, possibly hamsters but not in guinea-pigs. Cumulative information and independent assessment indicate that the risk of sarcoma formation in man is minimal.

Overdosage: Overdosage with Imferon is unlikely and is not known to be associated with any acute manifestations. Excessive doses beyond the requirements for haemoglobin restoration and replenishment of iron stores may lead to haemosiderosis. Such iron overload is more likely to occur in patients with haemoglobinopathies and other refractory anaemias which might erroneously be diagnosed as iron deficiency anaemia. Periodic monitoring of serum ferritin levels should be helpful in recognising a deleterious progressive accumulation of iron.

Adverse effects: Anaphylactoid reactions occur rarely with both intravenous and intramuscular administration. They may be severe, and fatalities have been reported. They occur usually within the first few minutes of administration, and are generally characterised by the sudden onset of respiratory difficulty and/or cardiovascular collapse. Other manifestations of immediate hypersensitivity include urticaria, rashes, itching, nausea and shivering. Administration must be stopped *immediately* when signs of an anaphylactoid reaction are seen.

Delayed reactions are well described and may be severe. These reactions, of unknown aetiology, are seen more frequently when large doses are given intravenously. They are characterised by arthralgia, myalgia and sometimes fever. The onset varies from several hours up to four days after administration. Symptoms usually last two to four days and settle spontaneously or following the use of simple analgesics.

Other reactions reported include: soreness and inflammation at or near injection site, sterile abscess (IM); brown skin discoloration (IM); local phlebitic reaction (IV); peripheral vascular flushing and hypotension (IV); lymphadenopathy; exacerbation of joint pain in rheumatoid arthritis.

Use in pregnancy: Imferon has been shown to be teratogenic and embryocidal in non-anaemic pregnant animals at high single doses above 2.5 ml/kg. The highest dose in clinical use is approximately 1 ml/kg. Iron deficiency anaemia occurring in the first trimester of pregnancy can normally be adequately treated with oral iron. If the benefit of Imferon treatment is judged to outweigh the potential risk to the foetus, it is recommended that treatment should be confined to the second and third trimester.

There is no information available on the excretion of iron dextran in human breast milk.

Pharmaceutical precautions Protect from heat: do not freeze. Intravenous infusions containing Imferon should be prepared immediately before use. Solutions of Imferon in 5% dextrose must not be autoclaved, because precipitation may occur. Other agents should not be added to Imferon infusions, nor is it recommended that Imferon is added to blood for transfusion.

Imferon has a particle size of 2–3 nm and will pass through the usual particulate filters. It does not cross the membranes commonly used in haemodialysis.

Legal category POM.

Package quantities
Ampoules of 2 ml (100 mg Fe) in boxes of 10 and 100.

Ampoules of 5 ml (250 mg Fe) in boxes of 5 and 50.

Ampoules of 20 ml for Total Dose Infusion (hospital use only) in boxes of 5.

Further information After intramuscular injection, iron dextran is taken up into the capillaries and the lymphatic system. Circulating iron dextran is gradually removed from the plasma by the reticuloendothelial cells, primarily of the liver and spleen. The complex is split into its components of iron and dextran, and the iron is immediately bound to the available protein moieties to form haemosiderin or ferritin and to a lesser extent transferrin. This iron, which is subject to physiological control, replenishes haemoglobin and depleted iron stores.

Laboratory Investigations: Evidence of a therapeutic response can be seen within a few days of administration of Imferon as an increase in the reticulocyte count. Serum ferritin levels usually provide a good guide to the replenishment of iron stores. In renal dialysis patients receiving Imferon, this correlation may not be valid.

Caution should be used in interpreting the results of serum iron determinations for up to 3 weeks after the administration of large doses of Imferon intravenously. Brown discoloration of serum has been reported after intravenous doses of 5 ml or more. Bone scans with radiolabelled technetium diphosphonate (^{99M}Tc) have been reported to show a dense crescentic area of activity in the buttocks visualised 1–6 days after intramuscular injection of Imferon.

Product licence number 0113/5073.

INTAL*

Presentation Intal is a presentation for inhalation of Sodium Cromoglycate BP 20 mg in micronised powder form. It is presented in a yellow/colourless, transparent, hard gelatin cartridge, bearing the overprint 'FISONS INTAL P'.

Uses Intal is indicated for the preventive treatment of bronchial asthma which may be due to allergy, exercise, cold air or chemical and occupational irritants. Sodium cromoglycate inhibits the release from sensitised mast cells of histamine, SRS-A and chemotactic factors which mediate the allergic reaction. In the lung this inhibition of mediator release prevents both the immediate and late asthmatic response (i.e. Type I and Type III responses) to immunological stimuli. Sodium cromoglycate also prevents the bronchoconstriction caused by exercise, cold air and chemical irritants.

Dosage and administration Intal is presented in a single dose cartridge, the 'Spincap', for use in either the 'Spinhaler' or the 'Halermatic'. Inhalation of the drug is controlled by the patient's inspiratory effort. Intal is not effective if the 'Spincap' is swallowed because the prevention of the asthmatic attack depends upon local application to the lung.

Dosage: Since Intal therapy is essentially preventive, it is important that the patient is instructed to maintain regular dosage, as distinct from inhaling the drug intermittently to relieve symptoms.

Adults and children: The normal dose is one 'Spincap' four times daily, i.e. one night and morning and at intervals of 3–6 hours in between. It may be necessary to increase this to 6–8 times daily in more severe cases or during periods of severe antigen challenge. Additional doses may be taken before exertion to prevent exercise induced asthma or before exposure to other trigger factors.

When the asthmatic condition is stabilised, it may be possible to reduce the dosage provided that adequate control of the asthma is maintained.

Elderly: No current evidence for alteration of the adult dose.

Concomitant steroid therapy: In patients currently treated with steroids, the addition of Intal to the regime may make it possible to reduce the maintenance dose or to discontinue steroids completely. The patient must be carefully supervised while steroid dose is reduced; a rate of reduction of 10% weekly is suggested. An increase in steroid dosage may be necessary if symptoms increase and at times of infection, severe antigen challenge or stress. If reduction in steroid dosage has been possible Intal should not be withdrawn until steroid cover has been re-instituted.

Concomitant bronchodilator therapy: If bronchodilators are used concomitantly patients may find that the frequency of bronchodilator usage can be reduced as their asthma is stabilised with Intal.

Contra-indications, warnings, etc
Contra-indications: There are no specific contra-indications.

Side-effects: Occasional throat irritation or coughing may occur in some patients sensitive to the inhalation of a dry powder. These can usually be overcome by changing to Intal Compound. In rare cases, severe bronchospasm has been reported, usually at the beginning of treatment, necessitating withdrawal of the drug.

Overdosage: No action other than medical observation should be necessary.

Withdrawal of Intal therapy: Since Intal acts prophylactically, it is important to continue treatment in those patients who benefit. If it is necessary to withdraw Intal, this should be done progressively over a period of one week. Symptoms of asthma may recur.

Use in pregnancy: As with all medications, particular caution must be exercised during the first trimester of pregnancy.

Pharmaceutical precautions Store in a moisture-proof container in a cool, dry place protected from light.

Legal category POM.

Package quantities Containers of 50 'Spincap' cartridges are available in packs of two. 'Spinhaler' and 'Halermatic' Insufflators are supplied in individual containers. Instructions for use are supplied with each pack.

Further information Nil.

Product licence number 0113/5022R.

INTAL* COMPOUND

Presentation Intal Compound is a presentation for inhalation of Sodium Cromoglycate BP 20 mg (micronised) and Isoprenaline Sulphate BP 0.1 mg in powder form. It is presented in an orange/colourless, transparent, hard gelatin cartridge bearing the overprint 'FISONS INTAL PC'.

Uses Intal Compound is indicated for the preventive treatment of bronchial asthma which may be due to allergy, exercise, cold air or chemical and occupational irritants. Sodium cromoglycate inhibits the release from sensitised mast cells of histamine, SRS-A and chemotactic factors which mediate the allergic reaction. In the lung this inhibition of mediator release prevents both the immediate and late asthmatic response (i.e. Type I and Type III responses) to immunological stimuli. Sodium cromoglycate also prevents the bronchoconstriction caused by exercise, cold air and chemical irritants. Isoprenaline sulphate is included to offset the transient bronchospasm which occurs in some patients on inhalation of a fine dry powder.

Dosage and administration Intal Compound is presented in a single dose cartridge, the 'Spincap', for use in either the 'Spinhaler' or the 'Halermatic'. Inhalation of the drug is controlled by the patient's inspiratory effort. Intal Compound is not effective if the 'Spincap' is swallowed because prevention of the asthmatic attack depends upon local application to the lung.

Dosage: Since Intal Compound therapy is essentially preventive, it is important that the patient is instructed to maintain regular dosage, as distinct from inhaling the drug intermittently to relieve symptoms.

Adults and children: The normal dose is one 'Spincap' four times daily, i.e. one night and morning and at intervals of 3–6 hours in between. It may be necessary to increase this to 6–8 times daily in more severe cases or during periods of severe antigen challenge. Additional doses may be taken before exertion to prevent exercise induced asthma or before exposure to other trigger factors.

When the asthmatic condition is stabilised, it may be possible to reduce the dosage provided that adequate control of the asthma is maintained.

Elderly: No current evidence for alteration of the adult dose.

Concomitant steroid therapy: In patients currently treated with steroids, the addition of Intal Compound to the regime may make it possible to reduce the maintenance dose or discontinue steroids completely. The patient must be carefully supervised while the steroid dose is reduced: a rate of reduction of 10% weekly is suggested. An increase in steroid dosage may be necessary if symptoms increase and at times of infection, severe antigen challenge or stress.

If reduction of steroid dosage has been possible Intal Compound should not be withdrawn until steroid cover has been re-instituted.

Concomitant bronchodilator therapy: If additional bronchodilators are used concomitantly, patients may find that the frequency of bronchodilator usage can be reduced as their asthma is stabilised with Intal Compound.

Contra-indications, warnings, etc
Contra-indications: There are no specific contra-indications.

Side-effects: Occasional irritation of the throat and trachea may occur. In rare cases severe bronchospasm has been reported, usually at the beginning of treatment, necessitating withdrawal of the drug.

Precautions: The precautions normally applying to isoprenaline should be observed. Where concomitant bronchodilator therapy is prescribed, the possibility of isoprenaline overdosage should be remembered.

Overdosage: No action other than medical observation should be necessary.

Withdrawal of Intal Compound therapy: Since Intal Compound acts prophylactically, it is important to continue treatment in those patients who benefit. If it is necessary to withdraw Intal Compound, this should be done progressively over a period of one week. Symptoms of asthma may recur.

Use in pregnancy: As with all medications, particular caution must be exercised during the first trimester of pregnancy.

Pharmaceutical precautions Store in a moisture-proof container in a cool, dry place protected from light.

Legal category POM.

Package quantities Containers of 50 'Spincap' cartridges are available in packs of two. 'Spinhaler' and 'Halermatic' Insufflators are supplied in individual containers. Instructions for use are supplied with each pack.

Further information Nil.

Product licence number 0113/5023R.

INTAL* INHALER ▼

Presentation Metered dose pressurised aerosol delivering 200 inhalations each containing a total of 1.0 mg Sodium Cromoglycate, BP.

Uses Intal Inhaler is indicated for the treatment of bronchial asthma, including the prevention of exercise-induced asthma.

Dosage and administration Since Intal Inhaler therapy is essentially preventative it is important that the patient is instructed to maintain regular dosage, as distinct from inhaling the drug intermittently to relieve symptoms.

Adults and Children: Two inhalations of the inhaler four times daily for routine prevention of asthma. The dose may be increased to two inhalations six or eight times daily in more severe cases or during periods of severe antigen challenge. Additional doses before exercise may also be taken.

Elderly: No current evidence for alteration of the adult dose.

Contra-indications, warnings, etc
Contra-indications: There are no specific contra-indications.

Side-effects: No significant side-effects have been reported. Although it has not been reported with Intal Inhaler, where Intal Spincaps have been administered via the Spinhaler, rare cases involving severe bronchospasm have been reported.

Overdosage: No action other than medical observation should be necessary.

Withdrawal of Intal Inhaler Therapy: Since the therapy is essentially prophylactic it is important to continue therapy in those patients who benefit. If it is necessary to withdraw this treatment, it should be done progressively over a period of one week. Symptoms of asthma may recur.

Use in pregnancy: As with all medication particular caution must be exercised during the first trimester of pregnancy.

Pharmaceutical precautions Store the inhaler in a cool place. The Intal Inhaler canister is pressurised. The canister should be protected from direct sunlight and must not be punctured or burnt, even when empty.

Legal category POM.

Package quantities Each pack contains a canister delivering 200 metered inhalations of sodium cromoglycate and a plastic mouthpiece. Instructions for use are supplied with each pack.

Further information
Concomitant bronchodilator therapy: Where a concomitant aerosol bronchodilator is prescribed, it is recommended that this be administered prior to the Intal Inhaler.

Concomitant steroid therapy: In patients currently treated with steroids the addition of Intal Inhaler to the regimen may make it possible to reduce the maintenance dose or to discontinue steroids completely. The patient must be carefully supervised while the steroid dose is reduced; a rate of reduction of 10% weekly is suggested.

   If reduction of steroid dosage has been possible Intal Inhaler should not be withdrawn until steroid cover has been re-instituted.

Product licence number 0113/0080.

INTAL* 5 INHALER

Presentation Metered dose pressurised aerosol delivering 112 inhalations each containing a total of 5.0 mg Sodium Cromoglycate BP.

Uses Intal 5 Inhaler is indicated for the treatment of bronchial asthma, including the prevention of exercise-induced asthma.

Dosage and administration Since Intal 5 Inhaler therapy is essentially preventative it is important that the patient is instructed to maintain regular dosage, as distinct from inhaling the drug intermittently to relieve symptoms.

Adults and children: Initial dose is two inhalations of the aerosol four times daily. Once adequate control of symptoms has been achieved it may be possible to reduce to a maintenance dose of one inhalation four times daily. However, the dose may be increased to two inhalations six or eight times daily in more severe cases

or during periods of severe antigen challenge. Additional doses before exercise may also be taken.

Elderly patients: No current evidence for alteration of the recommended adult dosage.

Contra-indications, warnings, etc
Contra-indications: There are no specific contra-indications.

Side-effects: No significant side-effects have been reported. Although it has not been reported with Intal 5 Inhaler, when Intal Spincaps have been administered via the Sphinhaler, rare cases involving severe bronchospasm have been reported.

Overdosage: No action other than medical observation should be necessary.

Withdrawal of Intal 5 Inhaler therapy: Since the therapy is essentially prophylactic it is important to continue therapy in those patients who benefit. If it is necessary to withdraw this treatment, it should be done progressively over a period of one week. Symptoms of asthma may recur.

Use in pregnancy: As with all medication particular caution must be exercised during the first trimester of pregnancy.

Pharmaceutical precautions Store the inhaler in a cool place. The aerosol inhaler canister is pressurised. The canister should be protected from direct sunlight and must not be punctured or burnt, even when empty.

Legal category POM.

Package quantities Each pack contains a canister delivering 112 metered inhalations of sodium cromoglycate and a plastic mouthpiece. Instructions for use are supplied with each pack.

Further information Intal Inhaler delivering 1 mg/shot is also available. Intal 5 provides a higher dose of sodium cromoglycate by pressurised aerosol for those patients who require it for greater prophylactic control of asthma symptoms.

Concomitant bronchodilator therapy: Where a concomitant aerosol bronchodilator is prescribed, it is recommended that this be administered prior to the Intal 5 Inhaler.

Concomitant steroid therapy: In patients currently treated with steroids the addition of Intal 5 Inhaler to the regimen may make it possible to reduce the maintenance dose or to discontinue steroids completely. The patient must be carefully supervised while the steroid dose is reduced; a rate of reduction of 10% weekly is suggested.

   If reduction of a steriod dosage has been possible Intal 5 Inhaler should not be withdrawn until steroid cover has been re-instituted.

Product licence number 0113/0109.

INTAL* NEBULISER SOLUTION

Presentation Intal Nebuliser Solution is presented in ampoules containing Sodium Cromoglycate BP 20 mg in 2 ml of a clear colourless sterile aqueous solution.

Uses Intal Nebuliser Solution is indicated for the preventive treatment of bronchial asthma which may be due to allergy, exercise, cold air or chemical and occupational irritants. Sodium cromoglycate inhibits the release from sensitised mast cells of histamine, SRS-A and chemotactic factors which mediate the allergic reaction. In the lung this inhibition of mediator release prevents both the immediate and late asthmatic response (i.e. Type I and Type III responses) to immunological stimuli. Sodium cromoglycate also prevents the broncho-constriction caused by exercise, cold air and chemical irritants.

Dosage and administration Intal Nebuliser Solution should be administered from a power-operated nebuliser at an adequate flow rate, *via* a face mask or mouthpiece. Information on suitable power operated nebulisers is available on request. Hand operated nebulisers are not suitable for the administration of Intal Nebuliser Solution.

Dosage: Since Intal Nebuliser Solution therapy is essentially preventive, it is important that regular dosage is maintained, as distinct from intermittent use to relieve symptoms.

Adults and children: The contents of one ampoule are administered by nebulisation four times a day, i.e. night and morning and at intervals of 3–6 hours. In severe cases frequency of administration may be increased to 5 or 6 times daily.

Elderly: No current evidence for alteration of the adult dose.

Concomitant steroid therapy: In patients currently treated with steroids the addition of Intal Nebuliser solution to the regime may make it possible to reduce the maintenance dose or discontinue steroids completely. The patient must be carefully supervised while the steroid dose is reduced; a rate of reduction of 10% weekly is suggested. An increase in steroid dosage may be necessary if symptoms increase and at times of infection, severe antigen challenge or stress.

If reduction of steroid dosage has been possible, Intal Nebuliser Solution should not be withdrawn until steroid cover has been re-instituted.

Concomitant bronchodilator therapy: If bronchodilators are used concomitantly, patients may find that the frequency of bronchodilator usage can be reduced as their asthma is stabilised with Intal Nebuliser Solution.

Contra-indications, warnings, etc
Contra-indications: There are no specific contra-indications. Intal Nebuliser Solution must not be given by injection.

Side-effects: Occasional irritation of the throat and trachea, and in rare cases severe bronchospasm, have been reported with powder forms of sodium cromoglycate.

Overdosage: No action other than medical observation should be necessary.

Withdrawal of Intal Nebuliser Solution therapy: Since sodium cromoglycate acts prophylactically, it is important to continue treatment in those patients who benefit. If it is necessary to withdraw Intal Nebuliser Solution this should be done progressively over a period of one week. Symptoms of asthma may recur.

Use in pregnancy: As with all medication, particular caution must be exercised during the first trimester of pregnancy.

Pharmaceutical precautions Store in a cool place protected from sunlight. Should the physician decide to mix Intal Nebuliser Solution with other agents, the mixture should be prepared just prior to use and discarded if any turbidity develops. Any unused solution should be

discarded immediately and the chamber of the nebuliser thoroughly cleaned.

Legal category POM.

Package quantities Box containing 48×2 ml ampoules.

Further information Nil.

Product licence number 0113/0068R.

NALCROM*

Presentation Nalcrom is a presentation of sodium cromoglycate for oral use. It is presented in clear/clear hard gelatin capsules printed Fisons 101 in black. Each capsule contains 100 mg sodium cromoglycate as a white powder.

Uses Food allergy (where adequate investigations have been performed to determine sensitivity to one or more ingested allergens) in conjunction with restriction of main causative allergens.

Sodium Cromoglycate inhibits the release from mast cells of histamine, SRS-A and chemotactic factors which mediate the allergic reaction. In gastro-intestinal disease the release of mediators causes a local inflammation which can either result in gastrointestinal symptoms or may allow absorption of antigenic material leading to systemic allergic reactions.

Dosage and administration
Initial dose: Adults: 2 capsules four times daily before meals.

Children: From 2–14 years: 1 capsule four times daily before meals.

For adults and children if satisfactory control is not achieved within two to three weeks the dosage may be doubled but should not exceed 40 mg/kg/day.

Maintenance dose: Once a therapeutic response has been achieved the dose may be reduced to the minimum required to maintain the patient free of symptoms.

Patients who are unable to avoid allergenic foods under certain circumstances (e.g. school meals, restaurants) may be able to protect themselves against the effect of these foods by taking a single dose of Nalcrom 15 minutes before the meal. The optimum dosage will need to be determined for each patient and a suitable starting dose would be 200 mg in adults and 100 mg in children.

Elderly: No current evidence for alteration of the adult dose.

Administration: The capsules may be swallowed whole or the powder contents may be dissolved in a small quantity of very hot water and diluted with cold water to drink. Administration as a solution in water is probably the method of choice.

Contra-indications, warnings, etc
Contra-indications: There are no specific contra-indications.

Warnings: The safety of Nalcrom in pregnancy and for the treatment of children under two years has not yet been established.

Side-effects: Nausea, skin rashes and joint pains have been reported in a few cases.

Overdosage: As Nalcrom is absorbed only to a very limited extent, no action other than medical observation should be necessary.

Pharmaceutical precautions Store in a dry place. Reclose the container tightly after use.

Legal category POM.

Package quantities Containers of 100 capsules.

Further information If oral steroid therapy is to be reduced or withdrawn this should be done cautiously and not more rapidly than 10% per week.

Product licence number 0113/0073.

OPTICROM* EYE DROPS

Presentation A clear colourless aqueous solution of Sodium Cromoglycate BP 2% w/v, with benzalkonium chloride 0.01% w/v.

Uses For the relief and treatment of acute allergic conjunctivitis such as hay fever, chronic allergic conjunctivitis and vernal kerato conjunctivitis. Sodium cromoglycate inhibits the release from sensitised mast cells of histamine, SRS-A and chemotactic factors which mediate the allergic reaction.

Dosage and administration One or two drops into each eye four times daily.

Elderly: No current evidence for alteration of the dose.

Contra-indications, warnings, etc Known hypersensitivity to benzalkonium chloride.

Pharmaceutical precautions Store below 30°C. Protect from direct sunlight.

Legal category POM.

Package quantities 10 ml.

Further information Discard any remaining contents four weeks after opening the bottle. As with other ophthalmic solutions containing benzalkonium chloride, soft contact lenses should not be worn during the treatment period.

Product licence number 0113/0039R.

OPTICROM* EYE OINTMENT

Presentation Opticrom Eye Ointment is a cream coloured opaque sterile ointment containing 4% w/w Sodium Cromoglycate BP.

Uses For the relief and treatment of allergic conjunctivitis such as hay fever, chronic allergic conjunctivitis and vernal kerato conjunctivitis. Sodium cromoglycate inhibits the release from sensitised mast cells of histamine, SRS-A and chemotatic factors which mediate the allergic reaction.

Dosage and administration *Adults and children:* To be applied to the eye two to three times daily.

Care should be taken to avoid direct contact between the eye and the tube nozzle.

Contra-indications, warnings, etc
Contra-indications: nil.
Warnings: As with other ophthalmic ointments, transient blurring of vision may occur.

Pharmaceutical precautions Store below 25°C. Protect from direct sunlight. It is desirable that the contents should be discarded four weeks after opening.

Legal category POM.

Package quantities 5 g.

Further information Patients may prefer to use Opticrom Eye Drops during the day and Opticrom Ointment at night.

Product licence number 0113/0103.

PARACODOL*
Approved name: Co-codamol Eff

Presentation Large, white, soluble, effervescent tablets each containing:

Paracetamol BP	500 mg
Codeine Phosphate BP	8 mg

Uses For the treatment of pain, including muscular and rheumatic pains, headache, migraine, neuralgia, toothache, sore throat, period pains, aches and pains. Discomfort associated with influenza, feverishness and feverish colds.

Dosage and administration The tablets are to be dissolved in water before oral administration.

Adults: 1–2 tablets, which may be repeated every four to six hours with a maximum of 8 in 24 hrs.

Children: Aged 6–12 years: $\frac{1}{2}$–1 tablet. Not more than 4 doses to be taken in 24 hours. The tablets are not scored and care should be taken to halve them accurately. Discard the unused half of the tablet.

Under 6 years: Not recommended.

Elderly: No current evidence for alteration of the adult dose except where there is impaired hepatic function when dosage reduction may be necessary.

Contra-indications, warnings, etc *Precautions:* The tablet base is designed to be equivalent to 1.5 g Sodium Citrate BP equivalent to 352 mg or 15.3 millimole Na$^+$. It should therefore be prescribed with caution in long term treatment of patients in whom a restricted salt intake is indicated.

Preparations containing paracetamol should be given with care to patients with impaired liver function.

Overdosage: It is unlikely that a toxic dose of large, effervescent tablets would be ingested. In the event of an overdose, the toxic effects of codeine may be reversed by the administration of naloxone injection. Symptoms of paracetamol overdose are often delayed for at least 24 hours but to prevent hepatic damage, treatment should be given as soon as possible and within 10 hours of ingestion. Treatment is by the administration of oral methionine, oral or intravenous acetylcysteine.

Pharmaceutical precautions Store in a cool dry place.

Legal category CD (Sch 5), P.

Package quantities Boxes of 10 or 100 tablets.

Further information Under the limited list regulations, NHS prescriptions for Paracodol will not be reimbursed. However, Paracodol complies with the specification for Co-codamol dispersible or effervescent tablets and if supplied against generic prescriptions is eligible for reimbursement under the NHS.

Product licence number 0113/5076R.

RYNACROM*

Presentation *Nasal Spray:* A metered dose presentation of a clear aqueous solution of sodium cromoglycate 2% w/v. The pack contains a bottle of solution and pump, ready assembled.

Nasal Drops: a plastic dropper bottle containing a clear, aqueous solution of Sodium Cromoglycate BP, 2.0% w/v.

Cartridges: pink, transparent hard gelatin cartridges, each bearing the overprint 'RYNACROM'. Each cartridge contains 10 mg Sodium Cromoglycate BP in powder form for nasal insufflation.

Uses Rynacrom is indicated for the preventive treatment of allergic rhinitis (seasonal and perennial). Sodium cromoglycate inhibits the release from sensitised mast cells of histamine, SRS-A and chemotactic factors which mediate the allergic reaction. In the nose this inhibition of mediator release prevents the symptoms of rhinitis.

Dosage and administration Since therapy with Rynacrom is essentially preventive, it is important that the patient is instructed to maintain regular dosage, as distinct from using the drug intermittently to relieve symptoms.

Adults and children: Rynacrom Nasal Spray – 1 squeeze to each nostril four or six times daily.

One squeeze delivers approximately 2.6 mg of sodium cromoglycate from the metered dose device.

Rynacrom Nasal Drops: Instil 2 drops into each nostril six times daily.

Rynacrom Cartridges: The contents of one cartridge are insufflated into each nostril up to four times daily. The first dose should be insufflated on rising and the last one immediately before retiring.

Elderly: No current evidence for alteration of the adult dose.

Contra-indications, warnings, etc There are no specific contra-indications.

Side-effects: Occasional irritation of the nasal mucosa may occur during the first days of use. In rare cases wheezing or tightness of the chest have been reported by patients.

Overdosage: No action other than medical supervision should be necessary.

Pharmaceutical precautions Store below 30°C. Rynacrom Nasal Spray and Nasal Drops should be protected from direct sunlight. Rynacrom Cartridges should be protected from light and kept dry.

Legal category P.

Package quantities Rynacrom Nasal Spray: 26 ml bottle with pump.
Rynacrom Nasal Drops: bottle of 15 ml.
Rynacrom Cartridges: containers of 100 cartridges.
Rynacrom Insufflators are supplied in separate containers. Instructions for use are supplied with each pack.

Further information A reduction in concomitant antihistamine therapy will often be possible.

Product licence numbers
Rynacrom Nasal Spray: 0113/0066
Rynacrom Nasal Drops: 0113/0040
Rynacrom Cartridges: 0113/5032

RYNACROM* COMPOUND ▼

Presentation A metered-dose presentation of a clear aqueous solution of Sodium Cromoglycate BP 2% w/v and Xylometazoline Hydrochloride BP 0.025% w/v. The pack contains a bottle of solution and a pump unit ready assembled.

Uses Rynacrom Compound is indicated for the treatment of allergic rhinitis (such as hayfever and perennial rhinitis) where this is accompanied by nasal congestion.

Sodium cromoglycate inhibits the release of mediators of the allergic reaction from sensitised mast cells. In the nose, this inhibition of mediator release prevents the symptoms of rhinitis.

Xylometazoline hydrochloride is a sympathomimetic agent with alpha-adrenergic activity. It produces vasoconstriction thus reducing nasal congestion.

Dosage and administration *Adults and children:* One squeeze to each nostril four times daily.

One squeeze delivers approximately 2.6 mg of sodium cromoglycate and 0.0325 mg of xylometazoline hydrochloride from the metered-dose device.

Elderly: No current evidence for alteration of the adult dose.

Contra-indications, warnings, etc
Contra-indications: There are no specific contra-indications.

Side-effects: No serious side effects have been reported. Occasional irritation of the nasal mucosa may occur during the first days of use. In rare cases with sodium cromoglycate solutions alone wheezing and tightness of the chest have been reported. Because a lower dose of xylometazoline is employed in this presentation than in other formulations, the side-effects usually attributed to this drug are expected to be minimal or absent.

Exposure to higher doses of xylometazoline than are likely with the correct use of Rynacrom Compound are reported to cause mild side-effects such as nasal irritation, dryness of the nose, sneezing, headache, insomnia, drowsiness and palpitations.

Precautions: The prolonged use or abuse of decongestants in general may lead to rebound congestion or drug induced rhinitis. This is reported to be less likely with xylometazoline.

Use in pregnancy: As with all medicines, caution should be exercised during pregnancy, especially in the first trimester.

Overdosage: Adults: Generally no action other than medical supervision should be necessary.

Infants and children: Overdosage of decongestants may cause sedation; uneventful recovery is usual, although medical supervision is recommended. Should accidental overdosage lead to convulsions or respiratory depression, gastric lavage and symptomatic therapy should be instituted.

Pharmaceutical precautions Store below 30°C. Protect from direct sunlight.

Legal category P.

Package quantities Bottle of 26 ml and pump unit.

Further information Nil.

Product licence number 0113/0097.

THEO-DUR* ▼

Presentation A slow release tablet containing Theophylline BP (anhydrous), designed to give therapeutic blood levels over 8–12 hours.

200 mg Tablet: Off-white mottled flat elliptical scored tablet.

300 mg Tablet: Off-white mottled bi-convex oblong scored tablet.

Uses As a bronchodilator in the symptomatic or prophylactic treatment of bronchospasm associated with chronic obstructive airways disease including asthma & chronic bronchitis.

Dosage and administration

Standard dosing:

Adults: the usual maintenance dose is one 300 mg tablet 12 hourly.

Children: <35 kg body weight: 100 mg ($\frac{1}{2}$ 200 mg tablet) 12 hourly. >35 kg body weight: 200 mg 12 hourly.

Elderly: No current evidence for alteration of the recommended adult dose unless there is hepatic failure or other conditions which decrease theophylline clearance. In such cases individual dosing should be adopted. See below.

Individual dosing:

If sufficient therapeutic effect is not achieved or if side effects occur, the dose of Theo-Dur may be increased or decreased by 100 mg ($\frac{1}{2}$ 200 mg tablet) or 150 mg ($\frac{1}{2}$ 300 mg tablet) stages. If doses higher than the usual maintenance doses are to be given, it is recommended that the patient's serum theophylline level is determined and the dose adjusted to maintain this level between 10–20 mcg/ml (55–110 μmol/l). The following procedure is recommended.

Adults: 150 mg ($\frac{1}{2}$ 300 mg tablet) 12 hourly for 4–7 days then 300 mg 12 hourly for 7–10 days.

Children: <35 kg body weight: 100 mg ($\frac{1}{2}$ 200 mg tablet) 12 hourly for 7–14 days. >35 kg body weight: 100 mg ($\frac{1}{2}$ 200 mg tablet) 12 hourly for 4–7 days then 200 mg 12 hourly for 7–10 days.

Blood for theophylline assay should be taken 3–8 hours after a dose when there has been no dosage adjustment for at least 4 days and no doses have been missed for 48 hours. The dose of Theo-Dur may be adjusted as follows:

Peak serum theophylline level	Dosage adjustment
<7.9 mcg/ml	Increase dose by 50%*.
8–9.9 mcg/ml	Increase dose by 20% to the nearest 50 mg.
10–13.9 mcg/ml	If the patient's symptoms persist, increase the dose by 10% to the nearest 50 mg.
14–19.9 mcg/ml	Do not adjust the dose unless side-effects occur in which case a 10% decrease, to the nearest 50 mg, may be necessary.
20–24.9 mcg/ml	Decrease dose by 10% to the nearest 50 mg.
25–29.9 mcg/ml	Miss next dose and decrease maintenance dose by 25%*.
>30 mcg/ml	Miss next two doses and decrease maintenance dose by 50%.

* With patients falling into these categories it is advisable to re-check the serum theophylline concentration 3–5 days after dosage adjustment.

Note:

1. The tablet must not be crushed or chewed but swallowed whole or as a half.
2. Any previous theophylline or aminophylline therapy should be discontinued.
3. If a patient has not previously been treated with theophylline or aminophylline, it is advisable to give half the maintenance dose of Theo-Dur (100 mg or 150 mg) for the first 4–7 days of treatment. This procedure should reduce the incidence of caffeine-like side effects.

Contra-indications, warnings, etc
Contra-indications: None.

Side effects: Side effects of theophylline depend to a great extent on serum concentration and are frequent only at theophylline concentrations exceeding 20 mcg/ml. The Theo-Dur slow release formulation reduces fluctuation in serum levels of theophylline, thereby reducing the incidence of side effects.

Most common side effects are gastro-intestinal disturbances (nausea, vomiting and anorexia) which, in most cases, disappear on reducing the dose.

Severe side effects (cramps, convulsions and supraventricular tachycardia) may appear at very high serum concentration, in which case the medication should be discontinued.

Treatment of overdosage: Gastric lavage and symptomatic treatment to maintain fluid and electrolyte balance. Give oxygen as necessary. Monitor serum theophylline levels. Oral activated Charcoal may reduce serum theophylline concentration. In severe cases charcoal haemoperfusion may be required. Tablets in the intestine may continue to release theophylline for several hours.

Pregnancy and lactation: No influence on the reproduction process is reported. Only small amounts of theophylline pass out to maternal milk. In therapeutic dose there is no risk of influence on the child.

Pharmaceutical precautions Nil.

Legal category P.

Package quantities 100 tablets.

Further information
1. Theopylline clearance is increased in cigarette

smokers and such patients may require increased doses of Theo-Dur to achieve a therapeutic effect.

2. Theophylline clearance is decreased in patients with hepatic cirrhosis, congestive heart failure, acute pulmonary oedema, acute febrile illness, concomitant administration of erythromycin, cimetidine or influenza vaccine; in these circumstances, patients may require a reduced dose of Theo-Dur to avoid the occurrence of side-effects.

3. If a patient taking an oral theophylline preparation develops severe acute asthma, intravenous amino-phylline should not be administered unless the serum theophylline level is known.

4. In patients with congestive heart failure associated with chronic obstructive airways disease, theophylline treatment may be of additional benefit because of its cardiac stimulant effect.

Product licence numbers 0113/0081 200 mg
0113/0082 300 mg

*Trade Mark

Geigy Pharmaceuticals
Horsham
West Sussex
RH12 4AB

ANAFRANIL
ANAFRANIL SR*

Presentation The active ingredient, clomipramine hydrochloride, is presented as:

Pink, film coated tablets, round, slightly biconvex with slightly bevelled edges, imprinted 'GEIGY' on one face and GD on the other, diameter approximately 8 mm, thickness approximately 4.3 mm, each containing 75 mg in a sustained release formulation.

Two-tone blue/caramel-coloured capsules, hard gelatin size No. 4, imprinted GEIGY, each containing 50 mg.

Two-tone orange/caramel-coloured capsules, hard gelatin size No. 4, imprinted GEIGY, each containing 25 mg.

Two-tone yellow/caramel-coloured capsules, hard gelatin size No. 4, imprinted GEIGY, each containing 10 mg.

Orange flavoured and coloured syrup containing the equivalent of 25 mg clomipramine hydrochloride in 5 ml.

Ampoules of clear glass containing 25 mg clomipramine hydrochloride in 2 ml.

Uses *Antidepressant:* Symptoms of depressive illness especially where sedation is required. Obsessive and phobic states. Cataplexy associated with narcolepsy.

Dosage and administration

Dosage: Adults: Oral – 10 mg/day initially, increasing gradually to 30–150 mg/day, if required, in divided doses throughout the day or as a single dose at bedtime. Many patients will be adequately maintained on 30–50 mg/day. Higher doses may be needed in some patients, particularly those suffering from obsessional or phobic disorders. Where a higher dosage is required, the 75 mg S.R. formulation may be preferable.

Elderly: 10 mg/day initially. The initial dose should be increased with caution under close supervision to 30–75 mg daily. Half the normal maintenance dose may be sufficient to produce a satisfactory clinical response.

Children: not recommended.

Intramuscular administration: Treatment may be commenced with intramuscular injections of up to 6 × 25 mg ampoules daily. Once therapy has started to be effective, a change to oral dosing should be made as soon as possible.

Dosage: Intravenous infusion: Any standard giving set may be used but a cannula or fine needle with a flange which can be strapped in position should be chosen. Anafranil ampoules may be diluted with either physiological saline or 5% Dextrose BP. The required dose of Anafranil should be introduced into the infusion fluid with a sterile syringe and the contents should be agitated to ensure even distribution of the drug before infusion is commenced, into a forearm vein.

In the first instance a small dose of Anafranil (25 mg or 50 mg) should be diluted in 200–500 ml of infusion fluid and infused over a period of two hours to assess tolerance. If satisfactory, the dose may be increased by 25 mg daily until an optimum therapeutic dose has been achieved. At the same time the bulk of fluid may be reduced (to a minimum of 125 ml) and the duration of infusion decreased (to a minimum of 45 minutes).

On average the optimum therapeutic dose will be in the region of 100 mg but higher doses may be required in more severe depressions or in obsessional and phobic states.

Length of treatment: Infusions should be given only to patients who are unable to take the drug orally. Oral therapy should be substituted once therapy has started to be effective, usually after 7–10 days.

Changeover to oral therapy: Following a satisfactory response to infusion, the quantity of intravenous Anafranil should be gradually reduced and oral therapy substituted. It is advisable to give double the maximum intravenous dosage orally until the patient's response is assured. Thereafter, a suitable maintenance dose, if considered necessary, can be selected.

Monitoring during treatment: During the course of infusion, patients should be carefully monitored for adverse effects. Particular attention should be paid to blood pressure recording, especially if there are any changes of position after conclusion of the infusion, as hypotension may occur. Patients often feel pleasantly drowsy during treatment and not infrequently fall asleep.

Contra-indications, warnings, etc

Contra-indications: Recent myocardial infarction, cardiac failure, any degree of heart block or other cardiac arrhythmias. Severe liver disease. Concurrent administration with monoamine oxidase inhibitors. Narrow angle glaucoma. Retention of urine. Mania.

Precautions: The elderly are particularly liable to experience adverse effects, especially agitation, confusion and postural hypotension. (See dosage).

Avoid if possible in patients with a history of epilepsy or with symptoms of bladder neck obstruction, e.g. prostatic hypertrophy.

Patients posing a high suicide risk require close initial supervision.

Tricyclic antidepressants potentiate the central nervous depressant action of alcohol.

Anaesthetics given during tri/tetracyclic antidepressant therapy may increase the risk of arrhythmias and hypotension. If surgery is necessary, the anaesthetist should be informed that a patient is being so treated.

As improvement may not occur during the first 2–4 weeks of treatment, patients should be closely monitored during this period.

Clomipramine may initially impair alertness. Patients

should be warned of the possible hazard when driving or operating machinery.

Use in pregnancy and lactation: Do not use during pregnancy, especially during the first and last trimesters, unless there are compelling reasons. There is no evidence as to drug safety in human pregnancy; animal work has not shown clomipramine to be free from hazard.

Anafranil is excreted in breast milk. Do not use during lactation unless considered essential; in this case nursing mothers should be advised to cease breast feeding.

Withdrawal symptoms in neonates whose mothers receive tri/tetracyclic antidepressants during the third trimester have also been reported and include respiratory depression, convulsions and jitteriness.

Drug interactions: Clomipramine should not be given concurrently, or within 3 weeks of cessation of therapy, with monoamine oxidase inhibitors.

Clomipramine may decrease the antihypertensive effect of guanethidine, debrisoquine, bethanidine and possibly clonidine, and methyldopa. It would be advisable to review all antihypertensive therapy during treatment with tricyclic antidepressants.

Clomipramine should not be given with sympathomimetic agents such as adrenaline, ephedrine, isoprenaline, noradrenaline, phenylephrine and phenylpropanolamine.

Barbiturates may decrease and methylphenidate and neuroleptics may increase the plasma level of clomipramine.

Side-effects: The following adverse effects, although not necessarily all reported with Anafranil have occurred with other tri/tetracyclic antidepressants:

Atropine-like side effects including dry mouth, disturbances of accommodation, tachycardia, constipation and hesitancy of micturition may occur early in treatment, but usually lessen.

Other possible adverse effects include nausea, drowsiness, sweating, postural hypotension, hypomania, tremor, paraesthesia, ataxia and, rarely, skin rashes.

Male patients may occasionally experience ejaculation disorders and, more rarely, impotence. Women occasionally experience orgasmic impotence.

Epileptiform convulsions have been experienced in a small number of patients.

Serious adverse effects are rare; these include impaired liver function and jaundice, bone marrow depression, including leucopenia, eosinophilia and thrombocytopenia. Agranulocytosis has occasionally occurred in patients receiving tricyclic antidepressants. It is advisable to perform blood counts during treatment with Anafranil especially if the patient develops fever, sore throat or other signs of infection. Cardiac arrhythmias and severe hypotension are likely to occur with high dosage or in deliberate overdosage. They may also occur in patients with pre-existing heart disease taking normal dosage.

Although not indicative of addiction, withdrawal symptoms may occur on abrupt cessation of therapy and include insomnia, irritability and excessive perspiration.

Psychotic manifestations, including mania and paranoid delusions, may be exacerbated during treatment with tricyclic antidepressants.

Accidental overdosage: Major symptoms of overdosage include coma, convulsions, cardiovascular disturbances. Gastric lavage should be performed immediately and patients removed to an intensive care unit where cardiac monitoring is possible. Although there is no specific antidote, slow intravenous injection of physostigmine

has yielded particularly good results in the presence of central nervous disturbances (coma, myoclonia, athetoid movements); physostigimine may possibly also exert a favourable effect on cardiac arrhythmias. The single dosage, which must be adapted to the patient's requirements and can, if necessary, be repeated several times, is 1–4 mg for adults and 0·5 mg for children.

Pharmaceutical precautions *Storage: Tablets* – protect from moisture. *Capsules* – protect from heat and moisture. *Syrup* – protect from heat. Keep containers tightly closed. *Ampoules* – protect from heat and light.

Dilutions: Syrup – dilutions down to 15 mg/5 ml can be prepared with boiled, distilled or de-ionised water. For dilutions below 15 mg/5 ml the recommended diluent is equal parts simple Syrup BP and freshly prepared Tragacanth mucilage BPC 1973. After dilution the solution should be used within a few days.

Legal category POM.

Package quantities
Tablets 75 mg SR.: Blister packs of 100.
Capsules 50 mg: Blister packs of 100.
Capsules 25 mg: Blister packs of 100.
Capsules 10 mg: Blister packs of 100.
Syrup 25 mg/5 ml: Bottles of 150 ml.
Ampoules 25 mg/2 ml: Boxes of 10.

Further information Nil.

Product licence numbers

Tablets 75 mg S.R.	0001/0087
Capsules 50 mg	0001/0068
Capsules 25 mg	0001/5000
Capsules 10 mg	0001/0037
Syrup 25 mg/5 ml	0001/5001
Ampoules 25 mg/2 ml	0001/5036

ANDURSIL*

Presentation *Andursil suspension:* White slightly thixotropic suspension odour and flavour of mint, containing the active ingredients

Aluminium hydroxide gel	$\equiv Al_2O_3$	200 mg
Magnesium hydroxide		200 mg
Aluminium hydroxide/magnesium carbonate co-dried gel		200 mg
Activated polymethylsiloxane		150 mg in each 5 ml

Andursil tablets: White, bevelled-edge, round tablets with 'ANDURSIL' impressed on either side, diameter approximately 2.1 cm, containing the active ingredients:

Aluminium hydroxide/magnesium carbonate co-dried gel	750 mg
Activated polymethylsiloxane	250 mg in each tablet

Uses *Antacid/antiflatulent:* Symptomatic relief of pain, discomfort, abdominal distension, heartburn (including heartburn of pregnancy), flatulence and vomiting associated with peptic ulceration, hiatus hernia, gastritis, functional gastro-intestinal disorders.

Dosage and administration Andursil is taken orally in either suspension or tablet form.

Andursil Suspension: 5–10 ml three or four times a day and at bedtime or when necessary.

Andursil Tablets: 1 or 2 tablets three or four times a day and at bedtime or when necessary.

Contra-indications, warnings, etc

Contra-indications: With the exception of hypophosphataemia, there are no known contra-indications to Andursil.

Precautions: As with other drugs, the administration of Andursil during the first three months of pregnancy is only advised if there are compelling reasons for so doing.

Side-effects: Side-effects are unlikely to occur in the recommended dosage.

Overdosage: No cases of overdosage are known at present. The various components of Andursil, namely aluminium hydroxide/magnesium carbonate (dry gel) and activated polymethylsiloxane, are not expected to cause either local or systemic signs of poisoning, even in cases of extreme oral overdosage.

Pharmaceutical precautions *Storage:* Protect from heat.

Legal category GSL.

Package quantities *Suspension:* Bottles of 100 ml and 300 ml.

Tablets: Carton of 100 tablets containing 5 packs of 20 tablets.

Further information *In vitro* tests on Andursil Suspension and Tablets have shown that the optimum buffering pH of between pH 3.0 and pH 5.0 is reached very quickly and is prolonged without producing a systemic alkalosis. Andursil is non-constipating and is not a laxative.

Product licence numbers
Andursil Suspension   0001/0049
Andursil Tablets   0001/0060

ANTURAN*

Presentation Tablets containing 200 mg Sulphinpyrazone BP, light yellow, sugar coated, round, biconvex, approximately 10.6 mm diameter printed GEIGY on one side. Tablets containing 100 mg Sulphinpyrazone BP, pale yellow, sugar coated, round, biconvex, approximately 8.5 mm diameter printed GEIGY on one side.

Uses *Mode of action:* Anturan lowers serum urate levels by blocking tubular reabsorption, thereby increasing renal excretion of uric acid. As a result of increased excretion, serum urate deposits are mobilised and tophi are no longer formed.

Indication: Chronic, including tophaceous gout; recurrent gouty arthritis; hyperuricaemia.

Dosage and administration Anturan is administered orally in tablet form with meals or milk.

Dosage: Adults: 100–200 mg daily increasing gradually (over the first two or three weeks) to 600 mg daily, and maintained until the serum urate level has fallen within the normal range. Subsequent dosage should be reduced, to the lowest level which maintains serum urate within the normal range. Maintenance dose may be as low as 200 mg daily. Reduced dose required in renal impairment. Not to be used in severe renal impairment.

Children: Paediatric usage not established.

Contra-indications, warnings, etc

Contra-indications: Active peptic ulcer. Sensitivity to phenylbutazone or other pyrazole derivatives. Severe hepatic disease.

In the treatment of chronic gout salicylates antagonise the action of Anturan and should not be given concurrently.

Precautions: Use with caution in patients with impaired renal function, and with healed peptic ulcer as well as in those in whom attacks of asthma have been precipitated by acetylsalicylic acid or by other drugs with prostaglandin synthesis inhibiting activity.

In patients with an elevated plasma uric acid level and/or with a history of nephrolithiasis or renal colic, and also when resuming treatment after interruption of the medication, a cautious incremental dosage schedule should be adopted. As with any form of long-term uricosuric medication, renal function tests should be performed regularly, particularly in cases where there is pre-existing evidence of renal failure.

Since Anturan may lead to sodium and water retention caution is indicated in patients with latent heart failure.

Since Anturan may potentiate the action of coumarin-type anticoagulants, frequent estimation of prothrombin time should be undertaken when these drugs are given concurrently, and the dosage of anticoagulant adjusted accordingly.

Anturan may also potentiate the action of other plasma protein binding drugs such as hypoglycaemic agents and sulphonamides, which may necessitate a modification in dosage.

Anturan should be used with caution in pregnant women, weighing the potential risk against the possible benefits.

Warnings and side-effects: During the early stages of treatment in patients with hyperuricaemia or gout, acute attacks of gout may be precipitated. To help prevent episodes of urolithiasis or renal colic, ensure adequate fluid intake and alkalinisation of the urine during initial stages of therapy.

Gastro-intestinal bleeding has been reported; transient gastro-intestinal side-effects may occur and are usually of a mild nature.

Impairment of renal function may occur, with changes in the electrolyte balance; as a rule the respective values revert to normal after the drug has been withdrawn; occasional cases of renal failure have also been reported, although no clear-cut causal relationship has been established. Rash or blood dyscrasias may occur, and are contra-indications to further treatment; onset may be sudden or gradual, and occur after small doses or after long periods of treatment.

For the early detection of a haematological abnormality, careful clinical supervision and full blood count should be done before and at regular intervals during treatment.

Accidental overdosage: There is no antidote to Anturan, and treatment is symptomatic. Immediate treatment consists of forced emesis to recover undigested tablets. This is followed by gastric lavage preferably with mild alkaline solution such as sodium bicarbonate solution and supportive therapy as indicated.

Pharmaceutical precautions *Storage:* Protect from heat and moisture.

Legal category POM.

Package quantities Tablets 100 mg: Containers of 100. Tablets 200 mg: Cartons of 112 consisting of 4 calendar reminder foils of 28.

Product licence numbers

Tablets 100 mg   0001/5002
Tablets 200 mg   0001/0080

BUTACOTE*

Presentation The active ingredient, Phenylbutazone BP is presented as: sugar-coated, enteric tablets, bi-convex, approximately 7.6 mm in diameter, pale violet coloured and imprinted GEIGY on one side, each tablet containing 100 mg.

Sugar-coated, enteric tablets, bi-convex, approximately 10.7 mm in diameter, pale violet coloured and imprinted GEIGY on one side, each tablet containing 200 mg.

Uses Ankylosing spondylitis. Butacote should only be used where other therapies have been found unsuitable.

Dosage and administration The dosage selected should be as low as possible, and duration of treatment should be as short as possible; when long term treatment is unavoidable, special precautions should be taken (see Precautions), and the dosage should be adjusted to the needs of the patient's age and general condition.

Butacote tablets should be swallowed whole with a meal together with liquid.

Adults: For the initial 48 hr 400–600 mg daily in divided doses. Thereafter, reduce to the minimum amount necessary, usually 200–300 mg daily in divided doses.

Elderly: In the elderly, always use the minimum effective dose (see Precautions).

Children: Not recommended for children under 14 years.

Contra-indications, warnings, etc

Contra-indications: History, however remote, of peptic ulcer, gastrointestinal haemorrhage, or blood dyscrasia. Haemorrhagic diathesis (thrombocytopenia, disorders of blood coagulation), severe cardiac, hepatic or renal insufficiency, oedema or hypertension, where there is danger of cardiac decompensation, thyroid disease, Sjogren's syndrome and previous adverse reactions to pyrazoles.

Like other non-steroidal anti-inflammatory agents, Butacote is also contra-indicated in asthmatic patients in whom attacks of asthma, urticaria or acute rhinitis are precipitated by acetylsalicylic acid or other drugs with prostaglandin synthetase inhibiting activity.

Last trimester of pregnancy.

Precautions and warnings: Like all potent drugs, Butacote should be used only under close medical supervision.

In elderly patients who are generally more prone to side-effects, particular caution should be exercised.

History of dyspepsia.

As blood dyscrasias may occur suddenly after a small dose, or insidiously after prolonged therapy, particularly in the elderly, blood counts should be monitored before and regularly during therapy, if it is anticipated that treatment may continue for more than one week. If significant changes occur e.g. decrease in leucocyte and/or platelet count or in the haematocrit, the drug should be withdrawn. Therapy should also be stopped if symptoms suggestive of these complications arise (e.g. bruising, fever, sore throat, rash, mouth ulceration) and patients should be advised accordingly.

Sodium retention and oedema may occur, and this should be considered in patients with cardiovascular disease.

Butacote may aggravate or acutely exacerbate systemic lupus erythematosus. If allergic reactions, fever, sore throat, salivary gland swelling or jaundice occur, or if blood appears in the stools, the medication should be discontinued at once.

Butacote should not be administered during the last 3 months of pregnancy, as it may lead to premature closure of the ductus arteriosus in the fetus. During the first six months of pregnancy, Butacote should be used with caution, especially in the first trimester, weighing the potential risks against the possible benefits. Since phenylbutazone passes into breast milk, albeit in small quantities, nursing mothers taking Butacote should not breast feed their infants.

Side-effects: Allergic reactions, rash and gastro-intestinal disorders (dyspepsia, epigastric pain, bleeding, recurrence of peptic ulcer) may occur. There have also been very occasional reports of headache, muzziness, nausea, vomiting, oedema due to sodium retention, stomatitis, salivary gland swelling, disturbances of vision, goitre, hepatitis, pancreatitis, and nephritis, and as rare complications, Stevens-Johnson syndrome, Lyells syndrome, leucopenia, thrombocytopenia, agranulocytosis and aplastic anaemia.

Isolated occurrences of an 'acute pulmonary syndrome' – marked by dyspnoea, fever, shadows in radiographs of the lungs and sometimes also by eosinophilia – have been reported. Although a causal relationship has not been proven, the drug should be withdrawn at first signs of this potentially serious syndrome, for the treatment of which corticosteroids and supportive cardiotherapy may be necessary.

Drug interactions: By competitively displacing them from their serum-protein binding sites, phenylbutazone may increase the activity and duration of effects of other drugs, e.g. other anti-inflammatory agents, oral anticoagulants, oral antidiabetic drugs, phenytoin and sulphonamides. Phenylbutazone may also accelerate the metabolism of dicoumarol, digitoxin and cortisone by inducing hepatic microsomal enzymes. Conversely it may inhibit the metabolic degradation of phenytoin and potentiate the effect of insulin. In patients previously treated with drugs which activate the hepatic microsomal enzyme system, e.g. barbiturates, chlorpheniramine, rifampicin, promethazine and corticosteroids (e.g. prednisone) the elimination half life of phenylbutazone is shortened. When phenylbutazone is given together with methylphenidate the serum concentration of metabolite oxyphenbutazone rises and the elimination half life of phenylbutazone is prolonged.

During concomitant administration of anabolic steroids and phenylbutazone, the serum concentration of metabolite oxyphenbutazone rises.

Since phenylbutazone may potentiate the effect of methotrexate, caution is indicated in cases where the two drugs are given concomitantly. Concomitant administration of cholestyramine reduces the enteral absorption of phenylbutazone. Phenylbutazone displaces thyroid hormone from its serum protein-binding sites and may thus make it more difficult to interpret tests of thyroid function.

When given together with lithium preparations, phenylbutazone causes increased tubular reabsorption of lithium, thereby raising the latter's serum concentration.

Overdosage: Where the recommended dosage has been appreciably exceeded, the following are the chief complications liable to be encountered: nausea, retching, gastro-intestinal pains or ulceration, respiratory depression, hypotension, coma, convulsions, hepatic and renal failure, thrombocytopenia, leucopenia and elevated transaminase values.

Treatment: Evacuation of the stomach (induction of vomiting, gastric lavage), and activated charcoal. If necessary, saline purgatives, artificial respiration, measures to support the circulation, anticonvulsants (e.g. diazepam iv) and haemodialysis. Haemoperfusion may be useful.

Pharmaceutical precautions Tablets 100 and 200 mg: Protect from heat and moisture.

Legal category POM.

Package quantities
Tablets 100 mg: Containers of 100 and 500
Tablets 200 mg: Containers of 100.

Further information Butacote tablets are available through hospitals only.

Product licence numbers
Tablets 100 mg   0001/0024.
Tablets 200 mg   0001/0056.

BUTAZOLIDIN*

Presentation The active ingredient, Phenylbutazone BP, is presented as: red, sugar-coated tablets, bi-convex, approximately 7.6 mm diameter and imprinted GEIGY on one side, each containing 100 mg; and white sugar-coated tablets, bi-convex, approximately 10 mm diameter and imprinted GEIGY on one side, each containing 200 mg.

Uses Ankylosing spondylitis. Butazolidin should only be used where other therapies have been found unsuitable.

Dosage and administration The dosage selected should be as low as possible, and duration of treatment should be as short as possible; when long term treatment is unavoidable, special precautions should be taken (see Precautions), and the dosage should be adjusted to the needs of the patient's age and general condition.

Butazolidin tablets should be swallowed whole with a meal together with liquid. Patients with sensitive stomachs should be given a sodium-free antacid at the same time.

Adults: For the initial 48 hr 400–600 mg daily in divided doses. Thereafter, reduce to the minimum amount necessary, usually 200–300 mg daily in divided doses.

Elderly: In the elderly, always use the minimum effective dose (see Precautions).

Children: Not recommended for children under 14 years.

Contra-indications, warnings, etc
Contra-indications: History, however remote, of peptic ulcer, gastrointestinal haemorrhage, or blood dyscrasia. Haemorrhagic diathesis (thrombocytopenia, disorders of blood coagulation), severe cardiac, hepatic or renal insufficiency, oedema or hypertension where there is danger of cardiac decompensation, thyroid disease, Sjogren's syndrome and previous adverse reactions to pyrazoles.

Like other non-steroidal anti-inflammatory agents, Butazolidin is also contra-indicated in asthmatic patients in whom attacks of asthma, urticaria or acute rhinitis are precipitated by acetylsalicyclic acid or other drugs with prostaglandin synthetase inhibiting activity.

Last trimester of pregnancy.

Precautions and warnings: Like all potent drugs, Butazolidin should be used only under close medical supervision.

In elderly patients who are generally more prone to side effects, particular caution should be exercised.

History of dyspepsia.

As blood dyscrasias may occur suddenly after a small dose, or insidiously after prolonged therapy, particularly in the elderly, blood counts should be monitored before and regularly during therapy, if it is anticipated that treatment may continue for more than one week. If significant changes occur e.g. decrease in leucocyte and/or platelet count or in the haematocrit, the drug should be withdrawn. Therapy should also be stopped if symptoms suggestive of these complications arise (e.g. bruising, fever, sore throat, rash, mouth ulceration) and patients should be advised accordingly.

Sodium retention and oedema may occur, and this should be considered in patients with cardiovascular disease.

Butazolidin may aggravate or acutely exacerbate systemic lupus erythematosus. If allergic reactions, fever, sore throat, salivary gland swelling or jaundice occur, or if blood appears in the stools, the medication should be discontinued at once.

Butazolidin should not be administered during the last 3 months of pregnancy, as it may lead to premature closure of the ductus arteriosus in the fetus. During the first six months of pregnancy, Butazolidin should be used with caution, especially in the first trimester, weighing the potential risks against the possible benefits. Since phenylbutazone passes into breast milk, albeit in small quantities, nursing mothers taking Butazolidin should not breast feed their infants.

Side-effects: Allergic reactions, rash and gastro-intestinal disorders (dyspepsia, epigastric pain, bleeding, recurrences of peptic ulcer) may occur. There have also been very occasional reports of headache, muzziness, nausea, vomiting, oedema due to sodium retention, stomatitis, salivary gland swelling, disturbances of vision, goitre, hepatitis, pancreatitis, and nephritis, and as rare complications, Stevens-Johnson syndrome, Lyells syndrome, leucopenia, thrombocytopenia, agranulocytosis and aplastic anaemia.

Isolated occurrences of an 'acute pulmonary syndrome' – marked by dyspnoea, fever, shadows in radiographs of the lungs and sometimes also by eosinophilia – have been reported. Although a causal relationship has not been proven, the drug should be withdrawn at first signs of this potentially serious syndrome, for the treatment of which corticosteroids and supportive cardiotherapy may be necessary.

Drug interactions: By competitively displacing them from their serum-protein binding sites, phenylbutazone may increase the activity and duration of effects of other drugs, e.g. other anti-inflammatory agents, oral anticoagulants, oral antidiabetic drugs, phenytoin and sulphonamides. Phenylbutazone may also accelerate the metabolism of dicoumarol, digitoxin and cortisone by inducing hepatic microsomal enzymes. Conversely it may inhibit the metabolic degradation of phenytoin and potentiate the effect of insulin. In patients previously treated with drugs which activate the hepatic microsomal enzyme system, e.g. barbiturates, chlorpheniramine, rifampicin, promethazine and corticosteroids (e.g. prednisone) the elimination half life of phenylbutazone is shortened. When phenylbutazone is given together with methylphenidate the serum concentration of metabolite oxyphenbutazone rises and the elimination half life of phenylbutazone is prolonged.

During concomitant administration of anabolic steroids and phenylbutazone, the serum concentration of metabolite oxyphenbutazone rises.

Since phenylbutazone may potentiate the effect of methotrexate, caution is indicated in cases where the two drugs are given concomitantly. Concomitant administration of cholestyramine reduces the enteral absorption of phenylbutazone. Phenylbutazone displaces thyroid hormone from its serum protein-binding sites and may thus make it more difficult to interpret tests of thyroid function.

When given together with lithium preparations, phenylbutazone causes increased tubular reabsorption of lithium, thereby raising the latter's serum concentration.

Overdosage: Where the recommended dosage has been appreciably exceeded, the following are the chief complications liable to be encountered: nausea, retching, gastro-intestinal pains or ulceration, respiratory depression, hypotension, coma, convulsions, hepatic and renal failure, thrombocytopenia, leucopenia and elevated transaminase values.

Treatment: Evacuation of the stomach (induction of vomiting, gastric lavage), and activated charcoal. If necessary, saline purgatives, artificial respiration, measures to support the circulation, anticonvulsants (e.g. diazepam iv) and haemodialysis. Haemoperfusion may be useful.

Pharmaceutical precautions Tablets 100 and 200 mg: Protect from moisture.

Legal category POM.

Package quantities
Tablets 100 mg: Containers of 100 and 1000
Tablets 200 mg: Containers of 100 and 500.

Further information Butazolidin tablets are available through hospitals only.

Product licence numbers
Tablets 100 mg 0001/5004.
Tablets 200 mg 0001/5005.

EURAX*

Presentation The active ingredient, Crotamiton BP, is presented as: white to cream coloured, non-staining ointment with an odour of perfume, containing 10% crotamiton. Also as a white to yellowish-white non-staining emulsion, with an odour of perfume, containing 10% crotamiton.

Uses *Antipruritic/sarcopticide:* Neurodermatitis; anogenital, senile pruritus. Pruritus associated with dermatoses. Pruritus as a symptom of systemic disease; allergic pruritus in the presence of diabetes mellitus or jaundice; pruritus due to drug hypersensitivity. Scabies.

Dosage and administration Eurax is applied externally in either ointment or lotion form.

Method of use: Pruritus: Eurax Ointment or Lotion should be massaged into the affected areas as frequently as required to prevent itching. Treatment can be expected to remain effective for 6 to 10 hours after each application.

Scabies: The patient should take a hot bath, using soap and flannel, and dry himself on a towel. Eurax should then be applied to the body from the chin down, with particular attention to the interdigital spaces, the flexor surfaces of the wrists, the inner and outer aspects of the elbows, the axillae, the under surface of the breasts, the umbilicus, the buttocks, and the inner aspects of the thighs. To ensure complete eradication, a second application 24 hours later is advisable, but a bath should not be taken until the day after, to wash off the application. The clothes should then be changed and sheets sent to the laundry.

Contra-indications, warnings, etc
Contra-indications: Acute exudative dermatoses.

Eurax should not be used near the eyes since contact with the eyelids may give rise to conjunctival inflammation.

Pharmaceutical precautions *Storage:* Ointment and Lotion – protect from heat.

Dilutions: Diluents or other additives to these formulations are not recommended.

Legal category P.

Package quantities
Ointment: Tubes of 30 g and 100 g.
Lotion: Bottles of 150 ml and 1 litre.

Further information Nil.

Product licence numbers
Ointment 0001/5008
Lotion 0001/5009

EURAX* – HYDROCORTISONE

Presentation The active ingredients, Crotamiton BP and Hydrocortisone BP, are presented as: white to cream coloured soft cream with a faint odour of perfume, containing Crotamiton BP 10% and Hydrocortisone BP 0.25%.

Uses *Antipruritic/anti-inflammatory:* Eurax-Hydrocortisone is useful in the symptomatic treatment of many types of itching dermatoses, since it combines a distinctive antipruritic action with bacteriostatic, anti-inflammatory and anti-allergic properties.

Pruritus ani, pruritus vulvae, pruritus scroti, senile pruritus.

Dermatoses with associated pruritus.

Seborrhoeic dermatitis, eczema, contact dermatitis, lichen simplex, dermatitis herpetiformis, neurodermatitis, pityriasis rosea, varicose eczema, urticaria.

Allergic pruritus; pruritus in the presence of diabetes mellitus or jaundice; pruritus due to drug hypersensitivity.

Dosage and administration Eurax-Hydrocortisone is applied externally.

Method of application: A thin layer of Eurax-Hydrocortisone Cream should be applied to the affected area two to three times a day.

Use in the elderly: Clinical evidence would indicate that no special dosage regime is necessary.

Contra-indications, warnings, etc
Contra-indications: Hypersensitivity to crotamiton.

Chickenpox, skin eruptions following vaccination, tuberculosis of the skin, and syphilitic skin affections.

Eurax-Hydrocortisone should not be used in the presence of acute exudative dermatoses.

Precautions: It has been shown that corticosteroids can be absorbed by eczematous skin. Long-term administration of Eurax-Hydrocortisone to large areas should, therefore, be avoided if possible, regardless of whether occlusion is used. If such administration is unavoidable, precautions similar to those taken with patients receiving small doses of oral steroids should be used. Topical administration of corticosteroids to pregnant animals can cause abnormalities of foetal development. The relevance of this finding to human beings has not been established; however, topical steroids should not be used extensively in pregnancy, i.e. in large amounts or for prolonged periods.

In infants, long-term continuous topical therapy should be avoided. Adrenal suppression can occur even without occlusion.

Eurax-Hydrocrotisone should not be allowed to come into contact with the conjunctiva.

Side-effects: Eurax-Hydrocortisone is generally well tolerated. Only in exceptional cases may the crotamiton component give rise to skin sensitisation; in such cases, the preparation should be withdrawn.

Pharmaceutical precautions *Storage:* Protect from heat.

Dilutions: Diluents and additives to this formulation are not recommended.

Legal category POM.

Package quantities Tubes of 30 g.

Further information Crotamiton is effective against all common forms of pruritus. The relief it affords sets in rapidly and lasts for approximately 6 hours. Crotamiton minimises the risk of secondary skin infection by relieving itching and thus preventing damage to the skin caused by scratching. In addition, crotamiton exerts a bacteriostatic action on streptococci and staphylococci. Hydrocortisone possesses anti-inflammatory, anti-allergic, anti-exudative, and anti-pruritic activity. The therapeutic properties of crotamiton and hydrocortisone complement one another, the combined preparation being particularly effective in the treatment of eczema and pruritus.

Product licence number 0001/5010.

HYGROTON*

Presentation Pale yellow compressed tablets, containing 50 mg Chlorthalidone BP, approximately 7 mm diameter, flat with bevelled edge and impressed GEIGY on one side, breakline and ZA on the other.

White compressed tablets, containing 100 mg Chlorthalidone BP, 7 mm diameter, flat with bevelled edge and impressed GEIGY on one side, breakline and BA on the other.

Uses Hygroton has been shown to have two separate therapeutic actions:

Diuretic: Following a single oral dose a marked salt and water diuresis is evident within two hours and a maximum effect within 12 hours. This natriuretic activity of Hygroton persists for 48–72 hours.

Antihypertensive: In hypertensive subjects Hygroton lowers both systolic and diastolic pressure, the degree of reduction depending on the original blood pressure of the patient. In general, the higher the blood pressure the greater the fall brought about by Hygroton.

Hygroton is indicated for: Hypertension. Oedema due to cardiac failure, hepatic cirrhosis, nephrosis. Pathological oedema of pregnancy. Diabetes insipidus.

Dosage and administration Hygroton is given orally in tablet form.

Hygroton tablets should be taken orally as a single daily dose at breakfast time.

Hypertension: In mild to moderate hypertension, 25 mg of Hygroton at breakfast time, increasing to 50 mg if necessary.

In more severe cases Hygroton may be combined with other antihypertensive agents in order to increase their hypotensive effects or to allow the use of a lower dose of the latter where side-effects are becoming troublesome.

Oedema: 1 to 2 × 100 mg tablets on alternate days. If preferred the 50 mg tablets may be given on a daily basis. In severe cases of oedema, a single loading dose of 4 × 100 mg Hygroton tablets may be required.

The maintenance dose should be the minimum amount needed to keep the patient free from oedema and may be as low as 100 mg twice weekly.

Pathological oedema of pregnancy: The dose of Hygroton used in the treatment of oedema in pregnancy is similar to that in other forms of oedema.

Diabetes insipidus: Hygroton, when used in the treatment of diabetes insipidus can be used either alone or as an adjunct to treatment with antidiuretic hormone. In either case the usual starting dose is 100 mg twice daily, reducing where possible to a maintenance dose of 50 mg daily.

Potassium supplementation: Potassium supplements may be required in digitalised patients, severe cases of oedema, hepatic cirrhosis and in long-term therapy. In digitalised patients, the dose of digoxin may need to be reduced.

Routine supplementation with potassium is not necessary in patients with uncomplicated hypertension.

Paediatric dosage: The recommended dosage for babies up to 10 kg (22 lb) in weight is 5 mg/kg on alternate days. In older children the recommended dose is 50 mg on alternate days for children up to the age of five years, and 50–100 mg on alternate days for children over the age of five years.

Use in the elderly: Chlorthalidone may be excreted more slowly in the elderly and therefore a reduction in the recommended adult dosage may be necessary.

Contra-indications, warnings, etc
Contra-indications: Hypersensitivity to chlorthalidone. Severe renal or hepatic insufficiency. Concomitant lithium therapy.

Side-effects: In the majority of patients Hygroton is well tolerated. Side-effects are infrequent and generally mild. Gastro-intestinal disturbances may occasionally occur. In rare cases, especially at the start of treatment, patients may complain of slight dizziness and tiredness, which generally resolves spontaneously or following a temporary reduction in the dosage.

There have also been occasional reports of the occurrence of cardiac arrhythmias, disturbances of vision, allergic skin reactions, neutropenia and thrombocytopenia.

Precautions: As with the use of other sulphonamide-type oral diuretics decreased glucose tolerance, as shown by hyperglycaemia and glycosuria, may occur. Hygroton may occasionally aggravate diabetes mellitus or precipitate diabetes in patients who have not previously displayed symptoms. This condition is usually reversible on cessation of therapy. During prolonged Hygroton therapy regular tests for glycosuria should be carried out and any unexpected polyuria investigated.

Hyperuricaemia may occasionally occur and acute attacks of gout may be precipitated. In cases where prolonged elevation of serum uric acid occurs, the concurrent use of a uricosuric agent will reverse the hyperuricaemia without loss of therapeutic effect.

Hypokalaemia may occur, but in most patients this appears to be of little clinical significance. Muscle weakness, cramps, lassitude and ECG changes are signs of significant potassium depletion which may be remedied by the use of oral potassium supplements (16–40 mEq/day). Supplementary potassium medication is indicated in the presence of an underlying disease (hepatic cirrhosis) associated with increased potassium excretion or in patients receiving concomitant treatment with digitalis, glucocorticoids or ACTH.

As with all antihypertensive agents a cautious dosage schedule is indicated in patients with severe coronary or cerebral arteriosclerosis. In cases where renal function is impaired, creatinine clearance and the electrolyte balance should be monitored. The marked loss of fluid and electrolytes occurring during long-term treatment with large doses of diuretics may aggravate signs of renal failure.

In patients under treatment with lithium, diuretics should be prescribed with caution, because they diminish the excretion of lithium and thus raise the blood lithium levels. Where lithium has induced polyuria, ingestion of diuretics has been observed to exert a paradoxical anti-diuretic effect.

Caution is needed with this preparation in the elderly since electrolyte balance is likely to be precarious due to bowel or renal dysfunction. Also urinary retention (in the male) is more likely.

Pregnancy and lactation: Since Hygroton, like other diuretics, is liable during pregnancy to reduce plasma volume as well as the blood supply to the uterus and placenta, its use in pregnant women calls for careful consideration. Diuretics should not be prescribed as treatment for eclampsia or pre-eclampsia or non-pathological oedema occurring during pregnancy.

Chlorthalidone passes into the breast milk and thus mothers taking Hygroton should refrain from breast-feeding their infants.

Accidental overdosage: Symptoms of overdosage include nausea, weakness, dizziness and disturbances of electrolyte balance. There is no specific antidote, but gastric lavage has been recommended. Supportive treatment aimed at maintaining normal fluid and electrolyte balance is essential.

Pharmaceutical precautions *Storage:* None.

Legal category POM.

Package quantities *Tablets 50 mg:* Containers of 100 and 500.
Tablets 100 mg: Containers of 100 and 500.

Further information Nil.

Product licence numbers
Tablets 50 mg   0001/5011
Tablets 100 mg   0001/5012

HYGROTON*–K

Presentation Round, red, sugar coated tablets of approximately 11.3 mm diameter and imprinted GEIGY on one side, containing 25 mg chlorthalidone BP and 500 mg potassium chloride BP–6.7 mEqK (controlled release).

Uses Hygroton has been shown to have two separate therapeutic actions.

Diuretic: Following a single oral dose, a marked salt and water diuresis is evident within two hours and a maximum effect within 12 hours. The natriuretic activity of Hygroton persists for 48–72 hours.

Antihypertensive: In hypertensive subjects Hygroton lowers both systolic and diastolic pressure, the degree of reduction depending on the original blood pressure of the patient. In general the higher the blood pressure the greater the fall brought about by Hygroton.

Potassium supplementation: Hygroton–K contains 500 mg controlled release potassium chloride providing 6.7 mEqK.

Hygroton–K is indicated for the same conditions as for Hygroton but particularly where the physician believes that potassium supplementation is indicated, as in the long-term treatment of hypertension, oedema due to cardiac failure, hepatic cirrhosis, nephrosis, pathological oedema of pregnancy, diabetes insipidus and patients receiving concomitant medication with digitalis, glucocorticoids or ACTH.

Dosage and administration Hygroton–K tablets should be swallowed whole with meals and not chewed.

Hypertension: In mild to moderate hypertension, 1 tablet of Hygroton–K at breakfast time, increasing to 2 tablets if necessary.

In more severe cases Hygroton–K may be combined with other antihypertensive agents in order to increase their hypotensive effect, or to allow the use of a lower dose of the latter, where side-effects are becoming troublesome.

Oedema: 1 or 2 tablets of Hygroton–K once or twice daily. The maintenance dose should be the minimum amount needed to keep the patient free from oedema.

Pathological oedema of pregnancy: The dosage of Hygroton–K is similar to that used in other forms of oedema.

Diabetes insipidus: When Hygroton is indicated for maintenance or as an adjunct to maintenance with antidiuretic hormone the determined dose of Hygroton may be given as Hygroton–K if potassium supplementation is desired.

Where possible the maintenance dose of Hygroton–K should be 2 tablets daily.

Paediatric dosage: Hygroton–K tablets must be swallowed whole and not crushed. Consequently this dosage form of Hygroton is not convenient for paediatric use.

Use in the elderly: Chlorthalidone may be excreted more slowly in the elderly and therefore a reduction in the recommended adult dosage may be necessary.

Contra-indications, warnings, etc
Contra-indications: Hypersensitivity to chlorthalidone. Hyperkalaemia. Severe renal or hepatic failure. Concomitant lithium therapy.

All solid dosage forms of potassium salts are contra-indicated in patients suffering from obstructions in the digestive tract (e.g. oesophageal compression due to enlargement of the left atrium, stenosis of the gut).

Side-effects: In the majority of patients Hygroton–K is well tolerated. Side-effects are infrequent and generally mild. Gastro-intestinal disturbances may occasionally occur. In rare cases, especially at the start of treatment, patients may complain of slight dizziness and tiredness, which generally resolves spontaneously or following a temporary reduction in the dosage.

There have also been the occasional reports of the occurence of cardiac arrhythmias, disturbances of vision, allergic skin reactions, neutropenia and thrombocytopenia.

Hygroton–K tablets are designed to minimise gastrointestinal irritation. However, complaints of abdominal pain, distension, nausea, vomiting or gastro-intestinal bleeding are indications for stopping treatment with potassium containing preparations immediately.

Precautions: As with the use of other sulphonamide type diuretics, decreased glucose tolerance as shown by hyperglycaemia and glycosuria may occur. Hygroton may occasionally aggravate diabetes mellitus or precipitate diabetes in patients who have not previously displayed symptoms. This condition is usually reversible on cessation of therapy. During prolonged Hygroton therapy regular tests for glycosuria should be carried out and any unexpected polyuria investigated.

Hyperuricaemia may occasionally occur and acute attacks of gout may be precipitated. In cases where prolonged elevation of serum uric acid occurs the concurrent use of a uricosuric agent will reverse the hyperuricaemia without loss of therapeutic effect.

Muscle weakness, cramps, lassitude and ECG changes are signs of significant potassium depletion which may be remedied by adding additional oral potassium supplements.

When Hygroton–K is used particular care should be taken not to combine it with potassium sparing diuretics.

As with all antihypertensive agents a cautious dosage schedule is indicated in patients with severe coronary or cerebral arteriosclerosis.

In cases where renal function is impaired, creatinine clearance and the electrolyte balance should be monitored. The marked loss of fluid and electrolytes occurring during long-term treatment with large doses of diuretics may aggravate signs of renal failure.

In patients under treatment with lithium, diuretics should only be prescribed with caution, because they diminish the excretion of lithium and thus raise the blood lithium levels. Where lithium has induced polyuria, ingestion of diuretics has been observed to exert a paradoxical anti-diuretic effect.

Caution is needed with this preparation in the elderly since electrolyte balance is likely to be precarious due to bowel or renal dysfunction. Also urinary retention (in the male) is more likely.

Pregnancy and lactation: Since chlorthalidone, like other diuretics, is liable during pregnancy to reduce plasma volume as well as the blood supply to the uterus and placenta, its use in pregnant women calls for careful consideration. Diuretics should not be prescribed as treatment for eclampsia or pre-eclampsia, or non-pathological oedema occurring during pregnancy.

As chlorthalidone passes into the breast-milk, mothers taking Hygroton–K should refrain from breast-feeding their infants.

Accidental overdosage: Symptoms of Hygroton overdosage include nausea, weakness, dizziness and disturbances of electrolyte balance. There is no specific antidote but gastric lavage has been recommended.

Supportive treatment aimed at maintaining normal fluid and electrolyte balance is essential. Particular care should be taken to prevent serum potassium levels from exceeding normal values.

Pharmaceutical precautions Protect from heat and moisture.

Legal category POM.

Package quantities Containers of 100 and 250 tablets.

Further information *Note* – Hygroton–K alone is not considered to be effective therapy for hypokalaemia from any cause.

Product licence number 0001/0059.

LAMPRENE*

Presentation The active ingredient, clofazimine, is presented as: red-brown, soft gelatin capsules, containing 100 mg clofazimine in each capsule.

Uses Antileprotic agent:

Prevention of the development of *M. leprae* resistant to sulphones, in patients with lepromatous and borderline leprosy.

Prevention of lepra reactions in patients with lepromatous and borderline leprosy.

Treatment for lepromatous and borderline forms of leprosy resistant to sulphones.

Treatment of lepra reactions e.g. Erythema nodosum leprosum (ENL).

Treatment of *M. ulcerans* infection (Buruli ulcer).

Dosage and administration For the treatment of leprosy, Lamprene should be employed in combination with other suitable anti-leprosy agents.

The capsules should preferably be taken during meals or together with milk. The dosage of Lamprene must be adapted to the patient's body weight and to the state of activity of the disease.

For the prevention of resistance to sulphones and for the prevention of lepra reactions in cases of lepromatous and borderline leprosy: 50–100 mg Lamprene daily or 100 mg 3 times weekly, during the first 4–6 months of long-term treatment with dapsone (50–100 mg daily).

In cases resistant to sulphones: Long-term treatment with Lamprene in a dosage of 100 mg daily, combined during the first 2–3 months with rifampicin 600 mg daily.

In lepra reactions: If lepra reactions (e.g. ENL) occur, the basic therapy given hitherto should be continued. To suppress the lepra reactions, Lamprene should be administered under surveillance in relatively large, individually determined doses. The dosage generally recommended is one of 300 mg daily for 3 months. As soon as the lepra reaction has been brought under control, the dosage should be gradually lowered to a level at which its suppressant effect is still just sufficient.

Use in the elderly: Clinical evidence would indicate that no special dosage regime is necessary but concurrent renal or hepatic insufficiency should be taken into account.

Contra-indications, warnings, etc

Contra-indications: There are no known conditions in which Lamprene would be contra-indicated.

Precautions: Treatment with Lamprene should be given only under medical supervision. Daily doses of 300 mg or more should not be administered for longer than 3 months.

If gastro-intestinal symptoms develop during treatment with Lamprene, the dosage should be reduced or the interval between doses prolonged. In the event of persistent diarrhoea or vomiting, the patient should be hospitalised.

During long-term medication with Lamprene, as well as in patients with a history of liver or kidney disease, it is advisable to perform clinical examinations and hepatic or renal tests every 3 months. The use of Lamprene in patients complaining of recurrent abdominal pains, or suffering from damage to the liver or kidneys, should wherever possible be avoided.

Pregnancy: For general medical reasons, it is not advisable to prescribe Lamprene during the first three months of pregnancy unless the drug's use is urgently indicated. The active substance of Lamprene crosses the placental barrier; newborn infants of women under treatment with the drug may therefore show relatively pronounced discolouration.

Side-effects: Lamprene is generally well tolerated. The side-effects occasionally met with are mostly of a mild nature and disappear after the daily dose has been reduced or the medication withdrawn.

The following side-effects have been observed:

Red to brownish-black discolouration of the skin and of the leprous lesions in lighter-skinned patients at sites exposed to light; discolouration of the hair, the conjunctiva, and the lacrimal fluid, as well as discolouration of sweat, sputum, urine and faeces.

Dryness of the skin, ichthyosis, pruritus, photosensitivity, acneform eruptions and non-specific skin rashes. Nausea, vomiting, abdominal pains, diarrhoea, anorexia, and loss of weight are sometimes encountered. These occur mainly in the presence of accompanying gastrointestinal disease (e.g. amoebiasis or bacterial infections of the gut) or in cases where large daily doses (>300 mg) have been given for a prolonged period (>3 months).

Accidental overdosage: There is no specific antidote for Lamprene and treatment is symptomatic.

Pharmaceutical precautions *Storage:* Protect from heat and moisture.

Legal category POM.

Package quantities *Capsules:* Containers of 100.

Further information Lamprene (clofazimine) is a highly active preparation which exerts a potent inhibitory effect on the growth of *Mycobacterium leprae* (Hansen's bacillus) and which almost invariably also elicits good effects in patients intolerant of, or resistant to, other anti-leprosy drugs. During long-term treatment with sulphone preparations, Lamprene serves to guard against the development of resistance. No cross-resistance between Lamprene and either dapsone or rifampicin has been reported.

Lamprene also possesses anti-inflammatory properties and is suitable for treating lepra reactions occurring in the course of treatment with other drugs. Not only can such reactions be suppressed by administering Lam-prene, but in patients previously requiring corticosteroid therapy it is possible to reduce the dosage of corticosteroids gradually and finally to withdraw them completely. During treatment with sulphone preparations, concomitant administration of Lamprene reduces the frequency of lepra reactions.

In rare cases where lepra reactions also occur under treatment with Lamprene, they can be combated by temporarily increasing the dosage.

Product licence number 0001/5041.

LOPRESOR* ▼

Presentation The active ingredient metoprolol tartrate is presented as: pale red, round, slightly biconvex, film-coated tablets with slightly bevelled edges: approximately 9 mm diameter, engraved GEIGY on one side and scored on the other side. Each tablet contains 50 mg.

Lopresor is also available as: light blue, round, slightly biconvex, film-coated tablets with slightly bevelled edges: approximately 10 mm diameter, engraved GEIGY on one side and scored on the other. Each tablet contains 100 mg.

Uses Beta-adrenergic receptor blocking agent.

Indications: Hypertension and angina pectoris, cardiac arrhythmias, especially supraventricular tachyarrhythmias.

Adjunct to treatment of thyrotoxicosis.

Early intervention with Lopresor in acute myocardial infarction reduces infarct size and the incidence of ventricular fibrillation. Pain relief may also decrease the need for opiate analgesics.

Lopresor has been shown to reduce mortality when administered to patients with acute myocardial infarction.

Prophylaxis of migraine.

Dosage and administration *Administration:* Lopresor tablets should be administered orally.

Dosage: Hypertension: Initially a dose of 100 mg in the morning should be prescribed.

Depending upon the response the dosage may be increased to 400 mg daily given in single or divided doses. Over the dosage range most patients may be expected to respond rapidly and satisfactorily. A further reduction in blood pressure may be achieved if Lopresor is used in conjunction with an antihypertensive diuretic such as chlorthalidone or a vasodilator such as hydralazine.

Lopresor may be administered with benefit both to previously untreated patients with hypertension and to those in whom the response to previous therapy is inadequate. In the latter type of patient the previous therapy may be continued and Lopresor added in to the regime with adjustment of the previous therapy if necessary.

Angina pectoris: 50–100 mg, twice or three times daily.

In general a significant improvement in exercise tolerance and reduction of anginal attacks may be expected with a dose of 50–100 mg twice daily.

Cardiac arrhythmias: A dosage of 50 mg two or three times daily is usually sufficient. If necessary the dose can be increased up to 300 mg per day administered in divided doses.

Following the treatment of an acute arrhythmia with Lopresor Injection (see separate Data Sheet) continuation therapy with Lopresor tablets should be initiated 4–

6 hours later. In such cases, the initial oral dose should not exceed 50 mg three times daily.

Thyrotoxicosis: 50 mg four times daily.

If it becomes necessary to discontinue treatment with a beta-blocker, one should withdraw the drug gradually, i.e. over a period of 8–10 days, because abrupt interruption of the medication – particularly in cases of ischaemic heart disease – may be followed by an acute deterioration in the patient's condition.

Myocardial infarction: Early intervention.

To achieve optimal benefits from intravenous Lopresor suitable patients should present within 12 hours of the onset of chest pain. Therapy should commence with 5 mg iv every 2 minutes to a maximum of 15 mg total as determined by blood pressure and heart rate. Oral therapy should commence 15 minutes after the injection, with 50 mg every 6 hours for 48 hours. Patients who fail to tolerate the full intravenous dose should be given half the suggested oral dose.

Maintenance: The usual maintenance dose is 200 mg daily.

Prophylaxis of migraine: 100–200 mg daily, given in divided doses (morning and evening).

Use in the elderly: There is no evidence to suggest that dosage requirements are different in the elderly.

Contra-indications, warnings, etc

Contra-indications: Atrioventricular block of second or third degree, uncontrolled heart failure, severe bradycardia and cardiogenic shock.

Precautions: Metoprolol has proved safe in a large number of asthmatic patients: although it is a selective beta-blocker it is prudent to exercise care in the treatment of patients with chronic obstructive pulmonary disease. Therapy with a β_2-stimulant may become necessary or current therapy require adjustment.

Lopresor must not be used in patients with untreated heart failure, but may be administered when the failure has been brought under control.

Lopresor should be given cautiously to patients with metabolic acidosis.

Lopresor may mask some of the symptoms of hypoglycaemia. Since treatment with a beta-blocker may affect carbohydrate metabolism, it may be necessary to adjust the dose of the hypoglycaemic agent in labile and insulin dependent diabetics.

Lopresor therapy should be brought to the attention of the anaesthetist prior to general anaesthesia. In a patient under beta-blockade, the anaesthetic selected should be one exhibiting as little negative inotropic activity as possible (halothane/nitrous oxide).

Like other beta-blockers, Lopresor should not be given in combination with antiarrhythmic agents of the verapamil type because their concomitant use may result in bradycardia, hypotension or even cardiac arrest.

There have been reports of skin rashes and/or dry eyes associated with the use of beta-adrenoceptor blocking drugs. The reported incidence is small and in most cases the symptoms have cleared when treatment was withdrawn. Discontinuance of the beta-adrenoceptor blocking drug should be considered if any such reaction is not otherwise explicable. Cessation of therapy with a beta-blocker should be gradual.

Pregnancy: The administration of Lopresor during pregnancy, as with other drugs is advised only if there are compelling reasons. If Lopresor is used during pregnancy and lactation special attention should be paid to the foetus, neonate and breast fed infant for undesirable effects of the drug's beta-blocking action (e.g. slowing of heart rate).

Side-effects: Gastro-intestinal upsets; sleep disturbances and exertional tiredness may occasionally occur. In most cases these effects have been transient or have disappeared after a reduction in dosage. In rare cases, feelings of coldness in the extremities may occur. As with other beta-blockers excessive bradycardia may occasionally occur; bronchospasm and heart failure may occasionally be precipitated in susceptible patients.

Accidental overdosage: The symptoms of overdosage will be marked bradycardia and possible hypotension. Bradycardia may be overcome by the administration of intravenous atropine sulphate metaraminol or noradrenaline should be employed.

These drugs have a pressor effect which may also help to overcome hypotension. The positive inotropic and chronotropic properties of glucagon may be useful when it is given in doses of 1–5 mg (max. 10 mg).

Pharmaceutical precautions *Storage:* Protect from heat, light and moisture.

Legal category POM.

Package quantities *Lopresor 50 mg:* Containers of 100 tablets.
Lopresor 100 mg: Containers of 100 tablets. Calendar packs of 56 tablets.

Further information Lopresor is a cardioselective beta-adrenergic blocking agent. It has a relatively greater blocking effect on beta$_1$-receptors (i.e. those mediating adrenergic stimulation of heart rate and contractility and release of free fatty acids from fat stores) than on beta$_2$-receptors, which are chiefly involved in broncho- and vasodilation.

Lopresor therefore possesses the therapeutically desirable effects of shielding the heart and blood vessels from the harmful effects of excessive adrenergic challenge during stress or exercise with minimal interference with respiratory function or vascular tone.

In hypertension Lopresor is effective during the first few days of treatment and reaches its full effect in a few weeks. No orthostatic hypotension or tendency to collapse has been observed even with fairly high doses.

In angina pectoris Lopresor diminishes the elevation of pulse rate and blood pressure in response to exercise or stress so permitting more efficient use of the oxygen supply to the myocardium. Ischaemic ECG changes are usually prevented or normalised and the patient's capacity for exercise is increased.

Because of its cardioselectivity, Lopresor can be administered even to patients with obstructive respiratory disorders, provided that adequate precautions are taken.

Product licence numbers
Tablets 50 mg   0001/0065
Tablets 100 mg   0001/0066

LOPRESOR* INJECTION ▼

Presentation Lopresor ampoules each containing 5 mg metoprolol tartrate in a clear, colourless solution of 5 ml volume.

Uses *Mode of action:* Lopresor is a cardioselective β_1-

receptor blocker exhibiting no intrinsic sympathomimetic activity.

Indications: Beta-adrenergic receptor blocking agent: Disturbances of cardiac rhythm, especially supraventricular tachyarrhythmias.

In acute myocardial infarction early intervention with Lopresor reduces infarct size and the incidence of ventricular fibrillation. Pain relief may also reduce the need for opiate analgesics.

Dosage and administration Initially up to 5 mg, injected i.v. (1–2 mg/minute). The injection can be repeated at 5 minute intervals until a satisfactory response has been obtained. A total dose of 10–15 mg generally proves sufficient; raising the dose to 20 mg or more does not usually yield better results.

During anaesthesia: 2–4 mg injected slowly i.v. at induction is usually sufficient to prevent the development of dysrhythmias during anaesthesia. The same dosage can also be used to control dysrhythmias developing during anaesthesia. Further injections of 2 mg may be given as required to a maximum overall dose of 10 mg.

Myocardial Infarction: Early intervention.

To achieve optimal benefits from intravenous Lopresor suitable patients should present within 12 hours of the onset of chest pain. Therapy should commence with 5 mg iv every 2 minutes to a maximum of 15 mg total as determined by blood pressure and heart rate. Oral therapy should commence 15 minutes after the injection, with 50 mg every 6 hours for 48 hours. Patients who fail to tolerate the full intravenous dose should be given half the suggested oral dose.

Use in the elderly: There is no evidence to suggest that dosage requirements are different in the elderly.

The active substance of Lopresor has a plasma half-life of 3–5 hours. The duration of its beta-blocking effect is dose-dependent: 4 hours after intravenous administration of 20 mg Lopresor, for example, its beta-blocking effect in healthy subjects is reduced by one-half.

Contra-indications, warnings, etc

Contra-indications: Atrioventricular block of second or third degree, uncontrolled heart failure, severe bradycardia or cardiogenic shock.

Precautions: Intravenous injections of Lopresor are suitable only for acute administration in hospitalised patients and should be given only if facilities are available for monitoring the electrocardiogram and blood pressure.

The i.v. administration of Lopresor to patients with a systolic blood pressure below 100 mm Hg (13.3 kPa) should only be made with special care as it can result in a further significant decrease of blood pressure.

In a patient under beta-blockade, the anaesthetic selected should be one exhibiting as little negative inotropic activity as possible (e.g. halothane/nitrous oxide).

Metoprolol has proved safe in a large number of asthmatic patients, although it is a selective beta-blocker it is prudent to exercise care in the treatment of patients with chronic obstructive pulmonary disease. Therapy with a β_2 stimulant may become necessary or current therapy require adjustment.

Lopresor must not be used in patients with untreated heart failure, but may be administered when the failure has been brought under control. Where heart failure appears during treatment with Lopresor the drug may be temporarily withdrawn until the failure has been controlled.

Lopresor may mask some of the symptoms of hypoglycaemia. Since treatment with a beta-blocker may affect carbohydrate metabolism, it may be necessary to adjust the dose of the hypoglycaemic agent in labile and insulin dependent diabetics.

Lopresor should be given cautiously to patients with metabolic acidosis.

Like other beta-blockers, Lopresor should not be given in combination with antiarrhythmic agents of the verapamil type, because their concomitant use may result in bradycardia, hypotension, or even cardiac arrest.

There have been reports of skin rashes and/or dry eyes associated with the use of beta-adrenoceptor blocking drugs. The reported incidence is small and in most cases the symptoms have cleared when treatment was withdrawn. Discontinuance of the beta-adrenoceptor blocking drug should be considered if any such reaction is not otherwise explicable. Cessation of therapy with a beta-blocker should be gradual.

Pregnancy: The administration of Lopresor during pregnancy as with other drugs is advised only if there are compelling reasons. If Lopresor is used during pregnancy and lactation special attention should be paid to the foetus, neonate and breast fed infants for undesirable effects of the drug's beta-blocking action (e.g. slowing of heart rate).

Side-effects: As with other beta-blockers, a marked fall in blood pressure may sometimes occur following intravenous injection of Lopresor.

Excessive bradycardia may also occasionally occur and bronchospasm and heart failure may occasionally be precipitated in susceptible patients.

Overdosage: The symptoms of overdosage will be marked bradycardia and possible hypotension. Bradycardia may be overcome by the administration of intravenous atropine sulphate (0.25–2.0 mg) which will decrease vagal tone. If bradycardia persists – sympathomimetic drugs such as metaraminol or noradrenaline should be employed. These drugs have a pressor effect which may also help to overcome hypotension. The positive inotropic and chronotropic properties of glucagon may be useful when it is given in doses of 1–5 mg (max. 10 mg).

Pharmaceutical precautions *Storage:* Protect from light.

Legal category POM.

Package quantities Packs of 10 ampoules.

Further information In patients with paroxysmal atrial tachycardia, use of Lopresor often enables normal sinus rhythm to be re-established or the ventricular rate to be reduced. Similarly, in cases of atrial fibrillation or flutter, Lopresor is not only capable of lowering the ventricular rate but, in some instances, may, also restore sinus rhythm. In addition, it diminishes the number of ventricular extrasystoles. When given in therapeutic doses, Lopresor exerts less influence on peripheral blood vessels and bronchial muscle than non-cardioselective beta-blockers. Provided adequate caution is observed, it can therefore also be administered in the presence of obstructive pulmonary diseases. When employed in higher dosage ranges, however, Lopresor may in rare cases increase airways resistance in the same manner as other selective beta-blockers.

Product licence number 0001/0086.

LOPRESOR* SR

Presentation The active ingredient metoprolol tartrate is presented as pale yellow, round, film-coated tablets with slightly convex faces; approximately 10.1 mm diameter, imprinted GEIGY on one side and CDC on the other. Each tablet contains 200 mg metoprolol tartrate in a sustained release formulation.

Uses Selective beta-adrenergic receptor blocking agent.

Indications: Hypertension and angina pectoris. Prophylaxis of migraine.

Dosage and administration *Administration:* Lopresor SR tablets should be administered orally.

Dosage: Hypertension: Initially one Lopresor SR tablet should be given in the morning. Most patients may be expected to respond satisfactorily within 14 days to one or two tablets once daily. Further antihypertensive effect may be achieved by the addition of a diuretic such as chlorthalidone or a vasodilator such as hydralazine.

Lopresor SR may be administered with benefit to both previously untreated patients with hypertension and to those in whom the response to previous therapy is inadequate. In the latter type of patient therapy may be continued and Lopresor SR added to the regime with adjustment of previous therapy if necessary.

Angina pectoris: Initially, one Lopresor SR tablet daily. The dose may be increased to two tablets once daily if required. In general a significant improvement in exercise tolerance and a reduction of anginal attacks may be expected with a dose of one Lopresor SR tablet daily.

Prophylaxis of migraine: One tablet daily given in the morning.

Use in the elderly: There is no evidence to suggest that dosage requirements are different in the elderly.

Contra-indications, warnings, etc
Contra-indications: Atrioventricular block of second or third degree, uncontrolled heart failure, severe bradycardia and cardiogenic shock.

Precautions: Metoprolol has proved safe in a large number of asthmatic patients, although it is a selective beta-blocker it is prudent to exercise care in the treatment of patients with chronic obstructive pulmonary disease. Therapy with a β_2 stimulant may become necessary or current therapy require adjustment.

Lopresor SR must not be used in patients with untreated heart failure, but may be administered when the failure has been brought under control. Where heart failure appears during treatment with Lopresor SR the drug may be temporarily withdrawn until the failure has been controlled.

Lopresor SR may mask some of the symptoms of hypoglycaemia. Since treatment with a beta-blocker may affect carbohydrate metabolism, it may be necessary to adjust the dose of the hypoglycaemic agent in labile and insulin dependent diabetics.

Lopresor SR should be given cautiously to patients with metabolic acidosis.

Lopresor SR therapy should be brought to the attention of the anaesthetist prior to general anaesthesia. In a patient under beta-blockade, the anaesthetic selected should be one exhibiting as little negative inotropic activity as possible, (e.g. halothane/nitrous oxide).

There have been reports of skin rash and/or dry eyes associated with the use of beta-adrenergic blocking drugs. The reported incidence is small and in most cases the symptoms have cleared when treatment was withdrawn. Discontinuance of the beta-adrenoceptor blocking drug should be considered if any such reaction is not otherwise explicable. Cessation of therapy with a beta-blocker should be gradual.

Like other beta-blockers, Lopresor SR should not be given in combination with antiarrhythmic agents of the verapamil type because their concomitant use may result in bradycardia, hypotension or even cardiac arrest.

If it becomes necessary to discontinue treatment with a beta-blocker, one should withdraw the drug gradually i.e. over a period of 8–10 days, because abrupt interruption of the medication – particularly in cases of ischaemic heart disease – may be followed by an acute deterioration in the patient's condition.

Pregnancy: The administration of Lopresor SR during pregnancy as with other drugs is advised only if there are compelling reasons. If Lopresor SR is used during pregnancy and lactation special attention should be paid to the foetus, neonate and breast fed infant for undesirable effects of the drug's beta-blocking action (e.g. slowing of heart rate).

Side-effects: Gastro-intestinal upsets, sleep disturbances and exertional tiredness may occasionally occur. In most cases these effects have been transient or have disappeared after a reduction in dosage. In rare cases, feelings of coldness in the extremities may occur.

As with other beta-blockers excessive bradycardia may occasionally occur, bronchospasm and heart failure may occasionally be precipitated in susceptible patients.

Overdosage: The symptoms of overdosage will be marked bradycardia and possible hypotension.

Bradycardia may be overcome by the administration of intravenous atropine sulphate (0.25–2.0 mg) which will decrease vagal tone. If bradycardia persists, sympathomimetic drugs such as metaraminol or noradrenaline should be employed. These drugs have a pressor effect which may also help to overcome hypotension. The positive inotropic and chronotropic properties of glucagon may be useful when it is given in doses of 1–5 mg (maximum 10 mg).

Pharmaceutical precautions No special precautions.

Legal category POM.

Package quantities Lopresor SR packs of 28 tablets (2 × 14 calendar pack foils).

Further information Lopresor SR is a sustained release preparation of Lopresor (metoprolol tartrate) designed to release this selective beta-adrenergic receptor blocking drug so that maximal response is obtained within 4–6 hours while the pharmacological action is sustained for 24 hours. This formulation reduces peak serum concentration which, in turn, minimises unwanted side-effects of beta-blockade.

Lopresor SR is a cardioselective beta-adrenergic blocking agent. It has relatively greater blocking effects on β_1 receptors (i.e. those mediating adrenergic stimulation of heart rate and contractility and release of free fatty acids from fat stores) than on β_2 receptors which are chiefly involved in broncho- and vasodilation.

Lopresor SR therefore possesses the therapeutically desirable effect of shielding the heart and blood vessels from the harmful effects of extensive adrenergic challenge during stress or exercise with minimal interference with respiratory function or vascular tone.

In hypertension, Lopresor SR is effective during the first few days of treatment and reaches its full effect in fourteen days. No orthostatic hypotension or tendency has been observed even with fairly high doses.

Because of its cardioselectivity, Lopresor SR may be administered even to patients with obstructive respiratory disorders, provided that adequate precautions are taken.

Product licence number 0001/0081.

LOPRESORETIC*

Presentation Off-white, round, bi-convex film-coated tablets with slightly bevelled edges, approximately 10 mm diameter, with a breakline on one face and GEIGY impressed on the other. Each tablet contains metoprolol tartrate (active ingredient of Lopresor*) 100 mg and chlorthalidone BP (active ingredient of Hygroton*) 12.5 mg.

Uses Antihypertensive agent.

Principal therapeutic actions: Lopresor (metoprolol tartrate) is a beta-adrenergic receptor blocking agent which is relatively more selective for beta-1-receptors which mediate heart rate and force of contraction, free fatty acid release and renin production, than for beta-2-receptors which mediate bronchodilation and peripheral vascular dilation. Consequently Lopresor protects the heart and cardiovascular system from excessive sympathetic stimulation caused by either physical or emotional activity while having relatively little effect on the airways or on peripheral vascular responses. The attenuation of the effects of excessive sympathetic drive on the heart result in a fall in myocardial work and oxygen consumption. Systolic pressure is reduced and this is most noticeable in hypertensive subjects, in whom the diastolic pressure is also reduced significantly.

Hygroton (chlorthalidone BP) is a long acting diuretic which lowers both systolic and diastolic pressures in hypertensive patients. In general the higher the initial blood pressure, the greater the fall brought about by Hygroton. The addition of Hygroton enhances the antihypertensive effect of the selective beta-blocker thus resulting in a better control in a higher proportion of patients. This is probably the result of the two active ingredients having different sites of action, Lopresor acting on the heart and possibly also centrally while Hygroton reduces peripheral resistance.

Indications: In the treatment of mild and moderate hypertension.

Dosage and administration *Dosage:* Lopresoretic tablets should be administered orally. Initial starting dose, one tablet in the morning. However, in patients who have not been successfully controlled by a diuretic or beta-blocking drug used alone, a dose of two tablets in the morning would be appropriate. Most patients may be expected to respond within 14 days.

Occasionally the response may be unsatisfactory in which case it may be found beneficial to raise the dosage to 3–4 tablets given in single or divided doses and/or to add a vasodilator such as hydralazine at an initial dose of 25 mg twice daily, increasing as necessary.

Use in the elderly: No specific information available.

Contra-indications, warnings, etc
Contra-indications: Atrioventricular block of second or third degree, uncontrolled heart failure, severe bradycardia, cardiogenic shock and marked renal insufficiency. Anti-diuretic effect has been reported following concom-

itant treatment with diuretics and lithium. As with all products which contain diuretics, Lopresoretic tablets are contra-indicated during lithium therapy.

Precautions: Metoprolol has proved safe in a large number of asthmatic patients, although it is a selective beta-blocker it is prudent to exercise care in the treatment of patients with chronic obstructive pulmonary disease. Therapy with a β_2 stimulant may become necessary or current therapy require adjustment.

As with other preparations containing beta-blockers, Lopresoretic tablets must not be used in patients with untreated heart failure, but may be administered when the failure has been brought under control. Where heart failure appears during treatment with Lopresoretic the drug may be temporarily withdrawn until the failure has been controlled.

Lopresoretic may mask some of the symptoms of hypoglycaemia. Since treatment with a beta-blocker may affect carbohydrate metabolism, it may be necessary to adjust the dose of the hypoglycaemic agent in labile and insulin dependent diabetics. Chlorthalidone may also decrease glucose tolerance.

Hyperuricaemia may occasionally occur and acute attacks of gout may be precipitated. Where prolonged elevation of serum uric acid occurs the concurrent use of a uricosuric agent will reverse the hyperuricaemia without loss of therapeutic effect.

Lopresoretic tablets should be given cautiously to patients with metabolic acidosis.

Lopresoretic therapy should be brought to the attention of the anaesthetist prior to general anaesthesia. In a patient under beta-blockade, the anaesthetic selected should be one exhibiting as little negative inotropic activity as possible, (e.g. halothane/nitrous oxide).

If it becomes necessary to discontinue treatment with a beta-blocker one should withdraw the drug gradually i.e. over a period of 8–10 days, because abrupt interruption of the medication – particularly in cases of ischaemic heart disease – may be followed by an acute deterioration in the patient's condition.

Like other beta-blockers, Lopresoretic should not be given in combination with antiarrhythmic agents of the verapamil type because their concomitant use may result in bradycardia, hypotension or even cardiac arrest.

There have been reports of skin rashes and/or dry eyes associated with the use of beta-adrenoceptor blocking drugs. The reported incidence is small and in most cases the symptoms have cleared when treatment was withdrawn. Discontinuance of the beta-adrenoceptor blocking drug should be considered if any such reaction is not otherwise explicable. Cessation of therapy with a beta-blocker should be gradual.

Because of their chlorthalidone content, Lopresoretic tablets should be used with care in patients with some degree of renal impairment.

Pregnancy: The administration of Lopresoretic during pregnancy as with other drugs is advised only if there are compelling reasons. If Lopresoretic is used during pregnancy and lactation special attention should be paid to the foetus, neonate and breast fed infant for undesirable effects of the drug's beta-blocking action (e.g. slowing of the heart).

Side-effects: Gastro-intestinal upsets; sleep disturbances and exertional tiredness may occasionally occur. In most cases these effects have been transient or have disappeared after a reduction in dosage. In rare cases, feelings of coldness in the extremities may occur.

As with other beta-blockers excessive bradycardia

may occasionally occur; bronchospasm and heart failure may occasionally be precipitated in susceptible patients.

Like other diuretics with a similar mode of action, chlorthalidone may cause latent gout or latent diabetes mellitus to become manifest. In a few cases, allergic skin reactions, mild anorexia, nausea, constipation and diarrhoea have been reported. There have been isolated reports of leucopenia, but these are rare.

Overdosage: The symptoms of overdosage will be marked bradycardia and possible hypotension. Bradycardia may be overcome by the administration of intravenous atropine sulphate (0.25–2.0 mg) which will decrease vagal tone. If bradycardia persists – sympathomimetic drugs such as metaraminol or noradrenaline should be employed. These drugs have a pressor effect which may also help to overcome hypotension. The positive ino-tropic and chronotropic properties of glucagon may be useful when it is given in doses of 1–5 mg (max. 10 mg). Supportive treatment aimed at maintaining normal fluid and electrolyte balance is essential.

Pharmaceutical precautions   Protect from moisture.

Legal category   POM.

Package quantities   Cartons of 56 tablets consisting of blister pack modules each containing 14 tablets (each carton represents 2–8 weeks treatment depending on the dose).

Further information   Lopresoretic tablets simplify the management of hypertension since they combine two effective antihypertensive agents which act together in a complementary manner. In addition to the two modes of action already described, the Lopresor component prevents the increase in plasma renin which occurs as a result of diuretic therapy.

Lopresoretic tablets contain a selective beta-blocker and thus can be administered to patients with obstructive respiratory disease provided they have access to a beta-2-stimulant bronchodilator; being a selective agent, Lopresoretic is less likely to interfere with the action of beta-2-stimulants.

Product licence number   0001/0085.

PERTOFRAN*

Presentation   The active ingredient, Desipramine Hydrochloride BP, is presented as: pale apricot-pink, sugar-coated tablets, bi-convex, 5.6 mm diameter and imprinted GEIGY on one side. Containing 25 mg Desipramine Hydrochloride BP in each tablet.

Uses   *Antidepressant:* Symptoms of depressive illness.

Dosage and administration   Pertofran is given orally in tablet form.

Adult dosage: 1 × 25 mg tablet three times a day for the first three days, increasing to 2 tablets three or four times daily. It will often be possible for the daily dose to be given as a single dose at night.

Elderly: Patients over 60 years of age may respond to lower doses of Pertofran than those recommended, usually 25 mg daily initially. The initial dose should be increased with caution under close supervision.

Children: Not recommended.

Contra-indications, warnings, etc
Contra-indications: Recent myocardial infarction. Any degree of heart block or other cardiac arrhythmias. Mania. Severe liver disease. Narrow angle glaucoma. Retention of urine.

Precautions: The elderly are particularly liable to experience adverse reactions, especially agitation, confusion and postural hypotension. Avoid if possible in patients with a history of epilepsy or with symptoms of bladder neck obstruction e.g. prostatic hypertrophy. Patients posing a high suicide risk require close initial supervision. Tricyclic anti-depressants potentiate the central nervous depressant action of alcohol.

Anaesthetics given during tri/tetracyclic antidepressant therapy may increase the risk of arrhythmias and hypotension. If surgery is necessary, the anaesthetist should be informed that a patient is being so treated.

As improvement in depression may not occur during the first four weeks of treatment, patients should be closely monitored during this period.

Pertofran may cause drowsiness. Patients should be warned of the possible hazard when driving or operating machinery.

Cardiac arrhythmias and severe hypotension are likely to occur with high dosage or in deliberate overdosage. They may also occur in patients with pre-existing heart disease taking normal dosage.

Do not use during pregnancy, especially during the first and last trimesters, unless there are compelling reasons. There is no evidence as to drug safety in humans; evidence from animal work has shown that desipramine is not totally free from hazard.

Pertofran is excreted in breast milk. Do not use during lactation unless essential; nursing mothers should be advised to cease breast feeding.

Drug interactions: Pertofran should not be given concurrently with, or within 2 weeks of cessation of therapy with monoamine oxidase inhibitors.

Pertofran may decrease the antihypertensive effect of guanethidine, debrisoquine, bethanidine and possibly clonidine. It would be advisable to review all antihypertensive therapy during treatment with tricyclic antidepressants.

Pertofran should not be given with sympathomimetic agents such as adrenaline, ephedrine, isoprenaline, noradrenaline, phenylephrine and phenylpropanolamine.

Barbiturates may decrease and neuroleptics and methylphenidate may increase respectively the plasma level of tricyclic antidepressants. Such changes may alter the clinical response to tricyclic antidepressants but clinical data on this is inconclusive.

Side-effects: The following adverse effects, although not necessarily all reported with Pertofran, have occurred with other tricyclic antidepressants:

Atropine-like side effects including dry mouth, disturbances of accommodation, tachycardia, constipation and hesitancy of micturition are common early in treatment, but usually lessen.

Serious adverse effects are rare; the following have been reported: Impaired liver function and jaundice, hypomania, epileptiform convulsions. Bone marrow depression, including leucopenia, eosinophilia and thrombocytopenia. Agranulocytosis has occasionally occurred in patients receiving tricyclic antidepressants. It is advisable to perform blood counts during treatment with tri/tetracyclic antidepressants, especially if the patient develops fever, sore throat or other signs of infection.

Other possible adverse effects include sweating,

postural hypotension, tremor and skin rashes. Interference with sexual function may occur.

Psychotic manifestations, including mania and paranoid delusion, may be exacerbated during treatment with tricyclic antidepressants.

Although not indicative of addiction, withdrawal symptoms may occur on abrupt cessation of therapy and include insomnia, irritability and excessive perspiration.

Adverse effects such as withdrawal symptoms, respiratory depression and agitation have been reported in neonates whose mothers had taken Pertofran during the last trimester of pregnancy.

Accidental overdosage: Major symptoms of overdosage include coma, convulsions and cardiovascular disturbances. Gastric lavage should be performed immediately and patients removed to an intensive care unit where cardiac monitoring is possible. Although there is no specific antidote, slow intravenous injection of physostigmine has yielded particularly good results in the presence of central nervous disturbances (coma, myoclonia, athetoid movements); physostigmine may possibly also exert a favourable effect on cardiac arrhythmias. The single dose, which must be individually adapted to the patient's requirements and can, if necessary, be repeated several times, is 1–4 mg for adults and 0.5 mg for children.

Pharmaceutical precautions *Storage:* Protect from moisture.

Legal category POM.

Package quantities Blister packs of 100 tablets.

Further information Nil.

Product licence number 0001/5019.

SINTHROME*

Presentation The active ingredient, Nicoumalone BP, is presented as white, compressed, scored tablets, approx. 7 mm diameter, impressed GEIGY on one side containing 4 mg in each tablet.

Pink, compressed tablets, approx. 5 mm diameter, containing 1 mg in each tablet.

Uses Oral anticoagulant. Arterial thrombosis and embolism, venous thrombosis and embolism, thrombophlebitis. Myocardial infarction, coronary thrombosis. For prophylaxis whenever thromboembolic complications may be anticipated and particularly in rheumatic heart disease with atrial fibrillation.

Dosage and administration Sinthrome is given orally in tablet form.

Sinthrome is available as 1 mg and 4 mg tablets and the use of both tablets in combination enables control of oral anticoagulant therapy with a single daily dose.

Initial therapy: If the prothrombin time is within the normal range, the following daily dosage schedule is suggested:

First day   8–12 mg
Second day   4–8 mg

Maintenance therapy: Maintenance dosage of Sinthrome varies from patient to patient and must be determined on the basis of regular laboratory estimations of the clotting time of the patient's blood as determined by Quick's one-stage test – prothrombin time. The daily maintenance dosage will vary also depending upon the intensity of treatment indicated and any other drugs that the patient may be taking. In general, however, this will lie between 1 mg and 8 mg daily. In practice the upper dosage limits are seldom required and only rarely need to be exceeded, when Sinthrome is the only drug administered (see 'Precautions').

The aim of therapy is to keep the prothrombin time between the limits of a predetermined therapeutic range. As an indication of the degree of anticoagulation, the prothrombin time itself is not of much help to the practising physician unless he knows also the range of prothrombin time which reflects a satisfactory response. This range varies between different laboratories according to the sensitivity of the thromboplastin used in the test.

A uniform system of testing and reporting has been proposed and is widely used. This is based on the use of a standardised thromboplastin, the British (Manchester) Comparative Thromboplastin (BCT). The control prothrombin time for this reagent is 12 seconds and the therapeutic range for adequate anticoagulation is 22–36 seconds. The ratio of patient's prothrombin time (using the BCT) to control is termed the British Ratio (BR), the therapeutic range for which is 1.8–3.0. A patient on Sinthrome, therefore, with a British Ratio of less than 1.8 would need an increase in dosage, whilst a BR over 3.0 would require a reduction in dosage.

Not all hospitals use the BCT and in these cases control prothrombin times and therapeutic ranges will possibly differ from those referred to above. If in doubt it is best to contact the laboratory concerned.

Sometimes the result may be expressed as percentage prothrombin activity or coagulation valency. This is an indication of the prothrombin content of the patient's blood relative to a normal control of 100%. In view of the variability of thromboplastin from different sources it is difficult to give precise therapeutic ranges using this system.

However, the usually accepted therapeutic range using Quick's one-stage test, expressed as a percentage activity and using a saline dilution curve, would be 25–20% if human brain thromboplastin is used.

The administration of daily requirements of Sinthrome and the taking of blood specimens for laboratory purposes should occur at the same time of day, but not after a heavy meal or a meal rich in fats.

Withdrawal of Sinthrome entails no additional risk of thromboembolism; hence, at the end of treatment, it is not necessary to give gradually diminishing doses.

Use in the elderly: A dose lower than the recommended adult dose may be sufficient in elderly patients.

Contra-indications, warnings, etc
Contra-indications: Sinthrome is contra-indicated in all haemorrhagic conditions, including peptic ulceration and occult risks implied by severe hypertension, subacute bacterial endocarditis and surgical procedures. This is absolute in operations on the central nervous system. Sinthrome is also contra-indicated in severe liver disease. Similarly in pregnancy and parturition the use of Sinthrome is contra-indicated.

Precautions: Administration with other drugs.

1. Potentiation of anticoagulant effect: Sinthrome is transported in plasma, the major proportion being as an inactive complex with plasma proteins. Many drugs will compete with Sinthrome for these protein binding sites, the consequence being displacement of Sinthrome into the plasma and an increase in anticoagulant activity. This

phenomenon has been reported with such commonly used drugs as clofibrate, indomethacin, oxyphenbutazone, paracetamol and phenylbutazone. In addition to this effect, aspirin and the salicylates have a direct anticoagulant action through an effect on platelet adhesiveness. Patients taking Sinthrome who also require treatment with these or any other drugs with similar affinity for protein-binding sites may need a reduction of their anticoagulant dosage.

Administration of broad-spectrum antibiotics may decrease the requirements for Sinthrome and potentiate its effects due to interference with the synthesis of vitamin K.

2. Inhibition of anticoagulant effect. Barbiturates, chloral hydrate, glutethimide, cardiac glycosides, carbamazepine and other drugs which are metabolised in the liver may increase the metabolism of Sinthrome by stimulation of liver microsomal enzyme systems. Diuretics can reduce anticoagulant activity by altering the concentration of plasma clotting factors. During combined therapy with these drugs it is likely that anticoagulant requirements will be increased, whilst cessation of treatment will necessitate a reduction in the dosage of Sinthrome.

Intramuscular injections during anticoagulant therapy may leave haematomata. Care is also necessary when subcutaneous injection is contemplated, but intravenous injections may be given without danger.

Side-effects: Sinthrome is well tolerated and side-effects such as nausea, loss of appetite, headache or giddiness are rarely encountered. Like other anticoagulants, Sinthrome may rarely cause skin necrosis, particularly after childbirth and during the menopause.

Accidental overdosage: Where slight bleeding occurs a temporary reduction or withdrawal of Sinthrome dosage will usually result in control being re-established. Transfusions of fresh whole blood are also effective. Where these measures are inadequate to control haemorrhage, the administration of vitamin K is the best measure for treating Sinthrome overdosage. However, this should normally be reserved for serious haemorrhages since, after administration of vitamin K, the patient remains resistant to anticoagulant therapy for some time.

Pharmaceutical precautions Sinthrome is light-sensitive. Store and dispense in the original or a dark container.

Legal category POM.

Package quantities *Tablets 1 mg:* Containers of 500 and 200.
Tablets 4 mg: Containers of 500 and 100.

Further information *Laboratory controls:* The patient's prothrombin time should be determined before anticoagulant therapy is begun. Should the initial level be abnormal, treatment should be instituted with caution.

During the early stages of anticoagulant therapy, or when any of the patient's drugs are changed (see Precautions), daily determination of prothrombin time should be made. The frequency of laboratory evaluation can be reduced when the patient's response to Sinthrome has been established.

Product licence numbers
Tablets 1 mg   0001/5021
Tablets 4 mg   0001/5022

SYMMETREL* CAPSULES

Presentation The active ingredient, amantadine hydrochloride, is presented as: brownish-red hard gelatin capsules, imprinted GEIGY in white on both cap and body, each containing 100 mg amantadine hydrochloride.

Uses Parkinson's disease. Herpes zoster. Prophylaxis and treatment of A₂, A/NJ/1/76, A/Moscow/77, A/Hong Kong/77, A/Brazil/11/78 and A/Alaska/78 influenza.

Note: Herpes zoster: It is recommended that the drug be given to elderly or debilitated patients in whom the physician suspects that a severe and painful rash could occur.

A₂ Influenza: It is suggested that Symmetrel be given to patients suffering from clinical influenza in whom complications might be expected to occur. In addition, Symmetrel is recommended prophylactically in cases particularly at risk, for example those with chronic respiratory disease or debilitating conditions, the elderly, those living in crowded conditions and for individuals in families where influenza has already been diagnosed, or those in essential services who are unvaccinated.

Dosage and administration *Parkinson's disease:* Initially one capsule daily for the first week, increasing to one capsule twice daily. In combination therapy, Symmetrel may be administered at these same doses. In many cases it will be possible after a few days to reduce the dosage of the other anti-Parkinson drug without loss of benefit.

Herpes zoster: Treatment should be started as soon as possible after the diagnosis has been made. The dosage is 1 capsule twice daily for 14 days. If post-herpetic pain persists after this period it is recommended that treatment be continued for a further 14 days.

Treatment of A₂ influenza: Adults: 1 capsule to be taken twice daily for five to seven days or at the discretion of the physician.

Prophylaxis of A₂ influenza: Adults: 1 capsule twice daily for as long as protection from influenza infection is required. In most instances this is expected to be for 7–10 days.

Treatment and prophylaxis in children: 10–15 years: 1 capsule every morning for the recommended period or at the discretion of the physician.

Below 10 years: As a reduced dosage is unavailable, it is not recommended that the drug be prescribed for this age group.

It is not recommended that the dosage be increased above that stated.

It may be found convenient to administer the drug at about 8 a.m. and 4 p.m.

Use in the elderly: No special dose regime is necessary but concurrent cardiovascular, renal or hepatic insufficiency should be taken into account.

Contra-indications, warnings, etc
Contra-indications: It is not recommended that Symmetrel be used to treat individuals who are subject to convulsions, or who have a history of gastric ulceration.

Symmetrel should not be used in patients with severe renal disease.

Although there are no specific contra-indications to the drug being administered to a person who has received a recent dose of influenza vaccine, such administration would be considered unnecessary.

Precautions: Symmetrel should be used with caution in patients with confusional or hallucinatory states.

As Symmetrel is excreted by the kidneys a cautious dosage scheme is recommended in the presence of impaired renal function. Care should be exercised when administering Symmetrel to patients with liver disease.

Patients who note central nervous system effects or blurring of vision should be advised to avoid situations where alertness is essential.

When employing Symmetrel in combination with other anti-Parkinson drugs, a watch should be kept for the latter's side-effects. Symmetrel may aggravate central nervous, gastro-intestinal or other side-effects provoked by anticholinergic drugs or L-dopa.

Although no incompatibilities with other drugs have become known, caution should be exercised if dextro-amphetamine or other central nervous stimulants are used during Symmetrel therapy.

Peripheral oedema thought to be due to an alteration in the responsiveness of peripheral vessels may occur in some patients during treatment with Symmetrel. This should be considered when the drug is prescribed for those with congestive heart failure.

Use in pregnancy: Symmetrel has not been studied in pregnant women. The use of this drug in women of child-bearing age should be undertaken only after weighing the possible risks to the foetus against benefit to the patient. Symmetrel has been reported to be embryotoxic and teratogenic in rats at 50 mg/kg/day, about 12 times the recommended human dose, but not at 37 mg/kg/day. Embryotoxic and teratogenic effects were not seen in rabbits which received up to 25 times the usual recommended adult human dose.

Side-effects: Symmetrel is well tolerated. Nevertheless, side-effects may occur in some patients. Livedo reticularis and peripheral oedema have been noted. In addition central nervous system effects such as nervousness, insomnia, dizziness and convulsions or psychic reactions such as hallucinations, or feeling of detachment have occurred. Skin rash has occurred rarely in patients sensitive to the drug.

Accidental overdosage: There is no specific antidote to Symmetrel. Supportive therapeutic measures aimed at those symtoms arising from excessive central stimulation should be instituted.

Pharmaceutical precautions *Storage:* Protect from heat and light.

Legal category POM.

Package quantities *Capsules 100 mg:* Containers of 100.

Further information Symmetrel warrants serious consideration in the management of herpes zoster. This has been confirmed by a large double-blind study involving 100 patients which showed that Symmetrel can significantly reduce the proportion of patients experiencing pain of long duration.

Symmetrel has been shown to have an antiviral activity predominantly against A_2 influenza. When administered as a treatment to patients with clinical influenza, it results in a reduction of the duration of fever and symptoms of the infection. Used prophylactically, Symmetrel will provide rapid cover against influenza infection which will last for as long as therapy is continued.

The majority of studies have shown that Symmetrel does not interfere with normal antibody production.

Product licence number 0001/0006.

SYMMETREL* SYRUP

Presentation A clear, citrus flavoured syrup containing 50 mg/5 ml of the active ingredient amantadine hydrochloride.

Uses Parkinson's disease. Herpes zoster.

Note: Herpes zoster: It is recommended that the drug be given to elderly or debilitated patients in whom the physician suspects that a severe and painful rash could occur.

Dosage and administration *Parkinson's disease:* Initially 100 mg daily for the first week, increasing to 100 mg twice daily. In combination therapy, Symmetrel may be administered at these same doses. In many cases it will be possible after a few days to reduce the dosage of the other anti-Parkinson drug without loss of benefit.

Herpes zoster: The treatment should be started as soon as possible after the diagnosis has been made. The dosage is 100 mg Symmetrel twice daily for 14 days. If post-herpetic pain persists after this period it is recommended that treatment be continued for a further 14 days.

It is not recommended that the dosage be increased above that stated.

It may be found convenient to administer the drug at about 8 a.m. and 4 p.m.

Use in the elderly: No special dose regime is necessary but concurrent cardiovascular, renal or hepatic insufficiency should be taken into account.

Contra-indications, warnings, etc

Contra-indications: It is not recommended that Symmetrel be used to treat individuals who are subject to convulsions, or who have a history of gastric ulceration.

Symmetrel should not be used in patients with severe renal disease.

Precautions: Symmetrel should be used with caution in patients with confusional or hallucinatory states.

As Symmetrel is excreted by the kidneys a cautious dosage scheme is recommended in the presence of impaired renal function. Care should be exercised when administering Symmetrel to patients with liver disease.

Patients who note central nervous system effects or blurring of vision should be advised to avoid situations where alertness is essential.

When employing Symmetrel in combination with other anti-Parkinson drugs, a watch should be kept for the latter's side-effects. Symmetrel may aggravate central nervous, gastro-intestinal or other side-effects provoked by anticholinergic drugs or L-dopa.

Although no incompatibilities with other drugs have become known, caution should be exercised if dextroamphetamine or other central nervous stimulants are used during Symmetrel therapy.

Peripheral oedema thought to be due to an alteration in the responsiveness of peripheral vessels may occur in some patients during treatment with Symmetrel. This should be considered when the drug is prescribed for those with congestive heart failure.

Use in pregnancy: Symmetrel has not been studied in pregnant women. The use of this drug in women of child-bearing age should be undertaken only after weighing the possible risks to the foetus against benefit to the patient. Symmetrel has been reported to be embryotoxic and teratogenic in rats at 50 mg/kg/day, about 12 times the recommended human dose, but not at 37 mg/kg/day. Embryotoxic and teratogenic effects were not seen in rabbits which received up to 25 times the usual recommended adult human dose.

Side-effects: Symmetrel is well tolerated. Nevertheless, side-effects may occur in some patients. Livedo reticularis and peripheral oedema have been noted. In addition central nervous system effects such as nervousness, insomnia, dizziness and convulsions or psychic reactions such as hallucinations, or feeling of detachment have occurred. Skin rash has occurred rarely in patients sensitive to the drug.

Accidental overdosage: There is no specific antidote to Symmetrel. Supportive therapeutic measures aimed at those symptoms arising from excessive central stimulation should be instituted.

Pharmaceutical precautions *Storage:* Protect from heat and light.

Legal category POM.

Package quantities 150 ml bottles.

Further information Symmetrel warrants serious consideration in the management of herpes zoster. This has been confirmed by a large double-blind study involving 100 patients which showed that Symmetrel can significantly reduce the proportion of patients experiencing pain of long duration.

Product licence number 0001/0067.

TEGRETOL*

Presentation The active ingredient, Carbamazepine BP, is presented as: 100 mg white, compressed tablets, 7mm diameter, impressed TEGRETOL 100 on one side, breakline on the other.

200 mg white, scored, compressed tablets, 9 mm diameter impressed TEGRETOL 200 on one side.

400 mg white, rod shaped, flat faced tablets with bevelled edges, 17 mm long, 5.5 mm wide and 5.3 mm thick, impressed GEIGY/GEIGY on one face with breakline. Other face impressed TEGRETOL with breakline.

White liquid with a flavour of caramel, containing 100 mg/5ml Carbamazepine BP.

Uses *Anticonvulsant and analgesic:* Epilepsy – generalised tonic – clonic and partial seizures. The paroxysmal pain of trigeminal neuralgia.

Dosage and administration Tegretol is given orally in either tablet or liquid form.

Epilepsy: It is advised that a gradually increasing dosage scheme is used and this should be adjusted to suit the needs of the individual patient.

Adults: Initially: 100–200 mg once or twice a day, followed by a slow increase until the best response is obtained, often 800–1,200 mg daily. In some instances, 1,600 mg daily may be necessary.

Children: Usual dosage 10–20 mg/kg bodyweight daily in divided doses.

Age up to 1 year: 1–2 × 100 mg tablets or 5–10 ml liquid per day.

1–5 years: 2–4 × 100 mg tablets or 10–20 ml liquid per day.

5–10 years: 2–3 × 200 mg tablets or 20–30 ml liquid per day.

10–15 years: 3–5 × 200 mg tablets or 30–50 ml liquid per day.

It is usually possible to maintain control with Tegretol as sole drug therapy, but in patients already receiving other therapy the same incremental dosage pattern should be followed as above.

It may be helpful to monitor the plasma concentration of Tegretol to ensure adequate therapeutic levels. In most cases the optimum therapeutic plasma level for Tegretol ranges from 3–10 mcg/ml (13–42 mc moles/l).

Trigeminal neuralgia: The individual dosage requirements of Tegretol vary considerably, depending on the age and weight of the patient. It is recommended that the initial dose be small, particularly in the frail and elderly, and that 100 mg tablets or liquid are used in the first instance.

The dose may be increased gradually until a satisfactory clinical response is obtained, which in some instances necessitates 1,600 mg Tegretol daily. It has been found that in the majority of patients a dosage of 200 mg three or four times a day is sufficient to maintain a pain-free state. It is suggested that Tegretol is taken only during acute stage of the condition and not as a prophylactic measure.

Contra-indications, warnings, etc

Contra-indications: Previous drug sensitivity to Tegretol.

Because Tegretol depresses AV-conduction, it is inadvisable to administer this drug to patients with atrioventricular conduction abnormalities unless paced.

Precautions: Use in pregnancy: If pregnancy occurs in a woman receiving Tegretol, or if the problem of initiating treatment with Tegretol arises during pregnancy, the drug's potential benefits must be carefully weighed against its possible hazards for the unborn child. This applies particularly to the first 3 months of pregnancy.

Induction of hepatic enzymes in response to Tegretol may have the effect of diminishing the activity of certain drugs that are metabolised in the liver. In patients receiving oral anticoagulant medication, it may be necessary to adjust the dosage when Tegretol is prescribed.

Tegretol may also reduce the activity of those hormones contained in the combined oral contraceptive pill. This may present clinically as breakthrough bleeding or spotting. We would recommend that patients taking Tegretol and requiring oral contraception should receive a preparation containing not less than 50 mcg of oestrogen or use some alternative non-hormonal method of contraception.

Tegretol should not be administered with, or within two weeks of cessation of MAOI therapy.

In rats treated with carbamazepine for two years, the incidence of tumours of the liver was found to be increased. There is, however, no evidence to indicate that this observation has any significant bearing on the therapeutic use of the drug.

Certain drugs have been shown to elevate carbamazepine levels including macrolide antibiotics (e.g. erythromycin) and isoniazid.

Note: In keeping with current opinion it is suggested that the level of serum folic acid is observed during anticonvulsant therapy.

Side-effects: Dizziness may occur, but this is much less likely to be noted if the gradually increasing dosage which has been recommended is followed.

Diplopia may occur and is usually dose dependent. Drowsiness, dry mouth, diarrhoea, nausea and vomiting have also occurred amongst some patients, but these symptoms are less frequent and seldom severe.

Hyponatraemia has been reported in a few patients on higher doses of Tegretol. Similarly oedema has occasionally been noted. Both are reversible upon reduction in dosage.

A generalised erythematous rash, in some cases severe, has been reported in about 3% of patients. This has been found to disappear leaving no sequelae on stopping therapy. Isolated occurrences of exfoliative dermatitis, leucopenia, thrombocytopenia, agranulocytosis, aplastic anaemia, cholestatic jaundice and acute renal failure have been reported.

It is suggested that blood count is checked at regular intervals during the early stages of treatment.

Accidental overdosage: There is no specific antidote. Signs of overdosage include somnolence increasing to unconsciousness, hyporeflexia and convulsions. Treatment recommended:

1. Simple aspiration of gastric contents.
2. Maintenance of airway, initially by means of pharyngeal airway. If necessary, pass endotracheal tube or perform a tracheotomy.
3. Routine temperature, pulse, respiration and blood pressure readings.
4. Administration of oxygen.
5. Curarisation and artificial ventilation have been successfully employed in one case of toxic overdosage which developed convulsions.

Pharmaceutical precautions *Storage:* Liquid – Protect from heat, keep container tightly closed.

Dilutions: Tragacanth mucilage BPC 1973 is suitable when used in a 1 : 1 ratio with Tegretol Liquid.

After dilution the liquid should be used within 14 days.

Legal category POM.

Package quantities *Tablets 100 mg:* Blister packs of 100 and containers of 500.
Tablets 200 mg: Blister packs of 100 and containers of 500.
Tablets 400 mg: Containers of 100.
Liquid 100 mg/5 ml: Bottles of 300 ml.

Further information Tegretol liquid contains no sucrose and is therefore suitable for diabetics and children.

Product licence numbers
Tablets 100 mg 0001/5027
Tablets 200 mg 0001/5028
Tablets 400 mg 0001/0088
Liquid 100 mg/5 ml 0001/0050

TOFRANIL*

Presentation The active ingredient, imipramine hydrochloride BP, is presented as: red-brown, sugar-coated tablets, bi-convex, 5.6 mm diameter, imprinted GEIGY on one side, each containing 25 mg.

Red-brown, sugar-coated, triangular-shaped tablets, 5.6 mm diameter, imprinted GEIGY on one side, each containing 10 mg.

Syrup – white, with a cream flavour, containing the equivalent to 25 mg/5 ml imipramine hydrochloride BP.

Uses Symptoms of depressive illness. Relief of nocturnal enuresis in children.

Dosage and administration
Adults: 1 × 25 mg three times daily for the first three days increasing to 2 × 25 mg three or four times daily. It will often be possible for the daily dose of 75 mg or 150 mg to be given as a single dose, usually at night. In hospitalised patients, or in patients under close medical supervision, it is sometimes necessary to give doses up to 225 mg or more in cases of severe depression.

Elderly: Patients over 60 years of age may respond to lower doses of Tofranil than those recommended, usually 10 mg at night initially, increasing to 10–25 mg three times daily. The initial dose should be increased with caution and under close supervision.

Children (for nocturnal enuresis only)
Not for use in children under 6 years.
6–7 years (weight 20–25 kg or 44–55 lbs) 25 mg
8–11 years (weight 25–35 kg or 55–77 lbs) 25–50 mg
Over 11 years (weight 35–54 kg or 77–119 lbs) 50–75 mg
The dose should not exceed 75 mg. The dose should be taken just before bedtime.

The maximum period of treatment should not exceed three months, and withdrawal should be gradual. Should a relapse occur, a further course of treatment should not be started until a full physical examination has been made.

Contra-indications, warnings, etc
Contra-indications: Recent myocardial infarction. Any degree of heart block or other cardiac arrhythmias. Mania. Severe liver disease. Narrow angle glaucoma. Infants and children under 6 years. Retention of urine.

Precautions: The elderly are particularly liable to experience adverse reactions, especially agitation, confusion and postural hypotension (see Dosage). Behavioural changes may occur in children receiving Tofranil for the treatment of nocturnal enuresis. Avoid if possible in patients with a history of epilepsy or with symptoms of bladder neck obstruction e.g. prostatic hypertrophy. Patients posing a high suicide risk require close initial supervision. Tricyclic antidepressants potentiate the central nervous depressant action of alcohol.

Anaesthetics given during tri/tetracyclic antidepressant therapy may increase the risk of arrhythmias and hypotension. If surgery is necessary, the anaesthetist should be informed that a patient is being so treated.

As improvement in depression may not occur during the first two to four weeks treatment, patients should be closely monitored during this period.

Tofranil may initially impair alertness. Patients should be warned of the possible hazard when driving or operating machinery.

Use in pregnancy: Do not use during pregnancy, especially during the first and last trimesters, unless there are compelling reasons. There is no, or inadequate, evidence of safety of the drug in human pregnancy; there is evidence of harmful effects in pregnancy in animals, when given in exceptionally high doses.

Tofranil is excreted in breast milk. Do not use during lactation unless considered essential; in this case nursing mothers should be advised to cease breast feeding.

Drug interactions: Tofranil should not be given concurrently with, or within 2 weeks of cessation of therapy with monoamine oxidase inhibitors.

Tofranil may decrease the antihypertensive effect of guanethidine, debrisoquine, bethanidine and possibly clonidine. It would be advisable to review all antihypertensive therapy during treatment with tricyclic antidepressants.

Tofranil should not be given with sympathomimetic agents such as adrenaline, ephedrine, isoprenaline, noradrenaline, phenylephrine and phenylpropanolamine.

Barbiturates may decrease and methylphenidate and neuroleptics may increase respectively the plasma level of Tofranil.

Side-effects: Atropine-like side-effects including dry mouth, disturbances of accommodation, tachycardia, constipation and hesitancy of micturition are common early in treatment, but usually lessen.

Other possible adverse effects include drowsiness, sweating, postural hypotension, tremor and skin rashes. Interference with sexual function may occur.

Serious adverse effects are rare; the following have been reported: Impaired liver function and jaundice, hypomania, epileptiform convulsions, bone marrow depression, including leucopenia, eosinophilia and thrombocytopenia. Agranulocytosis has occasionally occurred in patients receiving tricyclic antidepressants. It is advisable to perform blood counts during treatment with tri/tetracyclic antidepressants, especially if the patient develops fever, sore throat or other signs of infection.

Cardiac arrhythmias and severe hypotension are likely to occur with high dosage or in deliberate overdosage. They may also occur in patients with pre-existing heart disease taking normal dosage.

Psychotic manifestations, including mania and paranoid delusion, may be exacerbated during treatment with tricyclic antidepressants.

Although not indicative of addiction, withdrawal symptoms may occur on abrupt cessation of therapy and include insomnia, irritability and excessive perspiration.

Adverse effects such as withdrawal symptoms, respiratory depression and agitation have been reported in neonates whose mothers had taken imipramine during the last trimester of pregnancy.

Accidental overdosage: There is no specific antidote to Tofranil. Signs of overdose include anticholinergic effects, disturbances in cardiac rate and rhythm, central nervous system and respiratory depression, convulsions, disturbances in temperature regulation and reduced renal function and possible disturbance of acid/base balance. Treatment may include removal from the gastro-intestinal tract. Respiratory insufficiency may need intubation and ventilation, and convulsions can be controlled by i.v. diazepam. Any serious overdose requires continuous cardiac monitoring for at least 48 hours, and dysrhythmias treated on an individual basis.

Pharmaceutical precautions *Storage:* Syrup – protect from heat; keep containers tightly closed. Tablets – protect from moisture.

Dilutions: Syrup – for dilutions down to 15 mg/5 ml, boiled distilled or de-ionised water can be used. For dilutions below 15 mg/5 ml, the recommended diluent is equal parts simple Syrup BP and freshly prepared Tragacanth mucilage BPC 1973. After dilution the solution should be used within a few days.

Legal category POM.

Package quantities *Tablets 25 mg:* Blister packs of 100.
Tablets 10 mg: Blister packs of 100.
Syrup 25 mg/5 ml: Bottles of 150 ml.

Further information Nil.

Product licence numbers
Tablets 25 mg	0001/5029
Tablets 10 mg	0001/5030
Syrup 25 mg/5 ml	0001/5032

VOLTAROL/VOLTAROL RETARD

Presentation Tablets containing 25 mg diclofenac sodium, slightly biconvex with bevelled edges, yellow enteric coated, approximately 7 mm diameter, imprinted GEIGY on one side and Voltarol 25 on the other.

Tablets containing 50 mg diclofenac sodium, circular, slightly biconvex with bevelled edges, light brown enteric coated, approximately 8 mm diameter, imprinted GEIGY on one side and Voltarol 50 on the other.

Retard tablets containing 100 mg diclofenac sodium in a slow release formulation, circular, slightly biconvex, pale red, approximately 9 mm diameter, imprinted VOLTAROL R on one side, GEIGY on the other side.

Suppositories containing 100 mg diclofenac sodium in a yellowish-white, torpedo shaped, waxy base, weighing approximately 2.00 g.

Suppositories containing 12.5 mg diclofenac sodium in an off-white, torpedo shaped, waxy base, weighing approximately 900 mg.

Ampoules for intramuscular injection containing 75 mg/3 ml diclofenac sodium.

Uses
Indications: Tablets and suppositories.

Adults: Rheumatoid arthritis; osteoarthrosis; low back pain; acute musculo-skeletal disorders, such as periarthritis (especially frozen shoulder), tendinitis, tenosynovitis, bursitis, sprains, strains and dislocations; ankylosing spondylitis; acute gout; control of pain and inflammation in orthopaedic, dental and other minor surgery.

Children: Juvenile chronic arthritis.

Ampoules for injection: Acute exacerbations of rheumatoid arthritis and osteoarthrosis; acute back pain; acute gout; post-operative pain.

Mode of action: Voltarol is a non-steroidal agent with marked analgesic/anti-inflammatory and antipyretic properties. It is an inhibitor of prostaglandin synthetase (cyclo-oxygenase).

Pharmacokinetics: Diclofenac sodium is rapidly absorbed from the gut and is subject to first-pass metabolism. Tablets give peak plasma concentrations after 1–4 hours, suppositories within 1 hour and ampoules within half an hour. The active substance is 99.7% protein bound and plasma half-life for the terminal elimination phase is 1–2 hours. Approximately 60% of the administered dose is excreted via the kidneys in the form of metabolites and less than 1% in unchanged form. About 30% of the dose is excreted via the bile in metabolised form.

Dosage and administration
Adults: Tablets 25 and 50 mg: 75–150 mg daily in two or three divided doses.

Voltarol Retard: One tablet daily, preferably with food.

Suppositories: One 100 mg suppository daily, usually administered at night. In more severe cases, combined therapy with 25 or 50 mg tablets is recommended. The total daily dose should not exceed 150 mg.

Injection: One ampoule once or (in severe cases) twice daily intramuscularly by deep intragluteal injection into the upper outer quadrant. If two injections daily are required it is advised that the alternate buttock be used for the second injection. Voltarol ampoules should not be given for more than a few days; if necessary, treatment can be continued with tablets or suppositories. Voltarol should not be administered by intravenous injection.

Children (1 year or over). 1–3 mg/kg per day in divided doses.

Elderly: The pharmacokinetics of Voltarol are not impaired in elderly patients and the standard adult dose may be used (also see 'Precautions').

Nonsteroidal anti-inflammatory drugs should be used with particular caution in older patients who generally are more prone to adverse reactions.

Contra-indications, warnings, etc

Use in pregnancy and lactation: Voltarol should not be prescribed during pregnancy, unless there are compelling reasons for doing so. Use of prostaglandin synthetase inhibitors may result in premature closure of the ductus arteriosus if given in the last trimester of pregnancy.

Following oral doses of 150 mg daily, traces of active substance have been detected in breast milk.

Contra-indications: Active or suspected peptic ulcer or gastro-intestinal bleeding. Previous sensitivity to Voltarol.

Asthmatic patients in whom attacks of asthma, urticaria or acute rhinitis are precipitated by aspirin or other non-steroidal anti-inflammatory agents. Use of Voltarol suppositories in ulcerative or acute inflammatory conditions of the anus, rectum and sigmoid colon.

Precautions: History of gastro-intestinal ulceration, haematemesis or melaena, ulcerative colitis, Crohn's disease, bleeding diathesis or haematological abnormalities. Patients with severe hepatic, cardiac or renal insufficiency or the elderly should be kept under close surveillance.

All patients who are receiving long-term treatment with non-steroidal anti-inflammatory agents should be monitored as a precautionary measure (e.g. renal, hepatic function and blood counts).

Drug interactions: Voltarol may increase plasma concentrations of lithium and digoxin.

Pharmacodynamic studies have shown no potentiation of oral hypoglycaemic and anticoagulant drugs, but caution and adequate monitoring are nevertheless advised.

Voltarol has been reported to depress salicylate levels and vice versa. The clinical relevance of this phenomenon is not yet clear.

The natriuretic effect of frusemide type diuretics has been reported to be inhibited by some non-steroidal anti-inflammatory drugs.

Side-effects: Initially, some patients may complain of epigastric pain, eructation, nausea and diarrhoea, headache or slight dizziness. These side-effects are usually of a mild nature. Central nervous side effects, such as tiredness, insomnia or irritability, have occurred in rare instances.

Occasionally skin reactions, fluid retention and abnormalities of serum transaminases have been reported.

There have been reports of gastro-intestinal ulceration, haematemesis and melaena. Jaundice, hepatitis, renal failure and nephrotic syndrome have also been documented. If these occur Voltarol should be withdrawn.

In the course of extensive clinical usage, very rarely blood dyshaemopoiesis (leucopenia, thrombocytopenia, aplastic anaemia) have been reported.

There have been isolated reports of anaphylactoid/anaphylactic reactions, bronchospasm and erythema multiforme.

Suppository: local reactions include itching, burning and increased frequency of bowel movement.

Injection: local reactions may include pain and induration. In isolated instances, abscesses and local necrosis have occurred, particularly in elderly diabetics.

Overdosage: There is no specific antidote to Voltarol and the treatment is symptomatic. Symptomatology of overdose with Voltarol is not well defined; gastro-intestinal, renal and hepatic effects are possible.

Immediate treatment consists of forced emesis to recover undigested tablets.

Pharmaceutical precautions Tablets 25 and 50 mg – protect from heat and moisture. Voltarol Retard tablets 100 mg – protect from moisture. Suppositories 12.5 mg and 100 mg – protect from heat. Ampoules for injection – protect from heat and light.

Legal category POM.

Package quantities
Tablets: Blister packs of 100.
Voltarol Retard tablets: Blister packs of 28.
Suppositories 12.5 mg and 100 mg: packs of 10.
Injection: packs of 10 ampoules.

Further information Nil

Product licence numbers

Tablets 25 mg	0001/0036
Tablets 50 mg	0001/0082
Suppositories 100 mg	0001/0083
Suppositories 12.5 mg	0001/0102
Ampoules for injection 75 mg/3 ml	0001/0091
Voltarol Retard 100 mg	0001/0101

*Trade Mark

Geistlich Sons Limited
Newton Bank
Long Lane
Chester CH2 3QZ

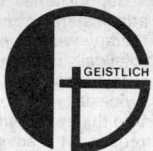

AMINOPLEX* 5

Presentation A solution of synthetic L-form amino acids in combination with calorie supplement. Sterile and pyrogen-free.

Active ingredients per litre: Synthetic-L-form amino acids:

L-Isoleucine	1.53 g
L-Leucine	2.33 g
L-Lysine HCl	2.74 g*
L-Methionine	1.93 g
L-Phenylalanine	2.77 g
L-Threonine	1.29 g
L-Tryptophan	0.56 g
L-Valine	1.80 g
L-Arginine	3.70 g
L-Histidine	0.89 g
L-Alanine	4.03 g
L-Glutamic acid	0.80 g
Glycine	1.77 g
L-Proline	4.83 g
L-Ornithine-L-Aspartate	0.80 g
L-Serine	0.97 g

(*2.19 g as base)

Calorie source:

Sorbitol	125 g
Ethanol	50 g

Electrolytes:

Sodium	35 mmol
Potassium	28 mmol
Magnesium	4 mmol
Chloride	43 mmol
Acetate	28 mmol

Additional nutrient:

L-Malic acid	1.85 g

Providing: 5 g/l of utilisable nitrogen, 4.2 MJ (1000 kcal). Total energy content, 3.6 MJ (868 kcal) non-nitrogen energy content.

Hypertonic solution pH 7.4 ± 0.2
Osmolality approximately 2415 mosmol/kg.

Uses For intravenous feeding, providing in a utilisable form, basic body requirements for amino acids, calories and certain electrolytes in one solution. This provides a simple regime for short-term total intravenous feeding, or alternatively a basis for more complex nutritional programmes tailored to specific clinical requirements.

Indications are clinical situations when oral feeding is impossible or contra-indicated. Alternatively Aminoplex 5 infusion would be appropriate pre- or post-operatively or in gastro-intestinal disturbances such as malabsorptive states, where adequate nutrition cannot be achieved orally.

Dosage and administration *Adult Dose (70 kg bodyweight):* Generally 1000–3000 ml in 24 hours by central intravenous injection. Maximum 40 ml/kg/day.

Infusion Rate: Maximum 40 to 50 drops per minute corresponding to an infusion time of 8 hours per litre.

Children's dosage at physicians' discretion.

Infusion rate should be tailored to patient body weight and should be commenced slowly at 20 ml/kg/day on the first day. For the second day and thereafter the infusion rate may be increased to a maximum of 40 ml/kg/day; the aim should be to maintain a constant infusion rate over the full 24 hours of each day.

Utilisable nitrogen is provided as synthetic L-form amino acids, 1 g of nitrogen being administered with each 175 non-nitrogen kcal. In cases with greatly increased requirements, e.g. sepsis or complications of surgery where glucose may be a more appropriate energy source, patients may benefit from an alternative regimen of Aminoplex 12 plus GluCoplex (with or without insulin).

Contra-indications, warnings, etc Before commencing infusion with Aminoplex 5, it is important to exclude conditions which may promote the risk of acidosis; for this reason, certain patient selection criteria should be applied during regimen planning – these are:–

(a) Adequate circulating volume.
(b) Adequate liver function.
(c) Adequate renal function.
(d) Absence of acidosis or hypoxaemia.

Patients not conforming to these criteria may have elevated lactate levels; for patients in this category or where the requirement for nitrogen and calories cannot be met within the maximum recommended infusion rate of 40 ml/kg/day, a regimen of Aminoplex 12 and GluCoplex will be more appropriate.

Depending on the patients clinical state and electrolyte balance, there may be a need for supplementary electrolyte replacement based on biochemical monitoring. Routine supplementation with vitamins and trace elements should also be undertaken as and when necessary. Of special importance is folic acid as amino acid mixtures may precipitate acute folate deficiency; accordingly folic acid should be given daily together with B vitamins. As Aminoplex 5 contains ethanol and sorbitol, care should be taken when considering the administration of drugs which interfere with their pathways of metabolism.

Pharmaceutical precautions Check that the solution is clear, and the container undamaged. Discard if not fully used at one injection.

Store below 25°C.

Keep away from light.

Data on compatibility and levels of permissible additions of vitamins and trace elements are available from the manufacturers.

The addition of drugs to amino acid solutions should be avoided.

Legal category POM.

Package quantities Glass bottles of 1000 ml.

Further information Due to optical sensitivity of the ingredients, some colour variation of the solution may be anticipated.

Product licence number 0184/0036.

AMINOPLEX* 12

Presentation A concentrated solution of synthetic L-form amino acids. Sterile and pyrogen-free.

Active ingredients per litre: Synthetic L-form amino acids:

L-Isoleucine	3.80 g
L-Leucine	5.80 g
L-Lysine HCl*	6.80 g
L-Methionine	4.80 g
L-Phenylalanine	6.88 g
L-Threonine	3.20 g
L-Tryptophan	1.40 g
L-Valine	4.48 g
L-Arginine	9.20 g
L-Histidine	2.20 g
L-Alanine	10.00 g
L-Glutamic acid	2.00 g
Glycine	4.40 g
L-Proline	12.00 g
L-Ornithine-L-Aspartate	2.00 g
L-Serine	2.40 g
(*5.44 g as base)	

Electrolytes:

Sodium	35 mmol
Potassium	30 mmol
Magnesium	2.5 mmol
Chloride	67 mmol
Acetate	5 mmol

Additional nutrient: L-Malic acid 4.6 g.

Providing: 12.44 g/l of utilisable nitrogen. Total energy content 315 kcal (1.3MJ).

Hypertonic solution pH 7.4 ± 0.2
Osmolality approximately 830 mosmol/kg.

Uses A synthetic L-form amino acid and electrolyte mixture for intravenous administration in intravenous feeding when a high level intake of protein amino acids is required in low fluid volume and also situations where flexibility of choice of calorific substrate is preferred.

In cases with greatly increased requirements, eg sepsis or complications of surgery and trauma, glucose is considered the appropriate energy source, and patients may benefit from a regimen of Aminoplex 12 plus GluCoplex (with or without insulin). Administration of Aminoplex 12 should always be accompanied by concurrent administration of a suitable energy source, for example, GluCoplex.

Dosage and administration *Adult Dose (70 kg bodyweight):* Generally 500–2000 ml in 24 hours by central intravenous injection.

Infusion Rate: Approx. 40–50 drops per minute corresponding to an infusion time of 8 hours per litre.

Children's dosage at physicians' discretion.

Contra-indications, warnings, etc Caution should be exercised when administering Aminoplex 12 to patients with irreversible liver damage.

Moderate liver damage and uraemic states where facilities for dialysis exist are not contra-indications for the use of Aminoplex 12.

Amino acid mixtures may precipitate acute folate deficiency and folic acid should be given daily. Vitamin B_{12} status should be checked and prophylaxis given if necessary.

Pharmaceutical precautions Check that the solution is clear, and the container undamaged. Discard if not fully used at one injection.

Store below 25°C.

Keep away from light.

Data on compatibility and levels of permissible additions of lipid emulsions, vitamins and trace elements are available from the manufacturers.

The addition of drugs to amino acid solutions should be avoided.

Legal category POM.

Package quantities Glass bottles of 500 ml and 1000 ml.

Further information Due to optical sensitivity of the ingredients, some colour variation of the solution may be anticipated.

Product licence number 0184/0030.

AMINOPLEX* 14

Presentation A concentrated solution of synthetic L-form amino acids. Sterile and pyrogen-free.

Active ingredients per litre: Synthetic L-form amino acids:

L-Isoleucine	3.20 g
L-Leucine	4.40 g
L-Lysine HCl	8.49 g
L-Methionine	6.40 g
L-Phenylalanine	4.40 g
L-Threonine	3.20 g
L-Tryptophan	1.60 g
L-Valine	5.20 g
L-Arginine	9.20 g
L-Histidine	2.80 g
L-Alanine	14.80 g
Glycine	12.00 g
L-Proline	4.00 g
L-Ornithine-L-Aspartate	2.00 g

Electrolytes:

Sodium	35 mmol
Potassium	30 mmol
Chloride	79 mmol

Additional nutrients:

Vitamin B_6 HCl	0.03 g
Nicotinamide	0.05 g
L-Malic acid	5.36 g

Providing: 13.4 g/l of utilisable nitrogen. Total energy content 340 kcal (1.4MJ).

Hypertonic solution pH 7.4 ± 0.2
Osmolality approximately 875 mosmol/kg.

Uses A synthetic L-form amino acid and electrolyte mixture for intravenous administration in intravenous feeding when a high level intake of protein amino acids is required in low fluid volume and also situations where flexibility of choice of calorific substrate is preferred.

In cases with greatly increased requirements, eg. sepsis or complications of surgery and trauma, glucose is considered the appropriate energy source, and patients may benefit from a regimen of Aminoplex 14 plus GluCoplex (with or without insulin). Administration of Aminoplex 14 should always be accompanied by concurrent administration of a suitable energy source, for example, GluCoplex.

Dosage and administration *Adult Dose (70 kg bodyweight):* Generally 500–2000 ml in 24 hours by central intravenous injection.

Infusion Rate: Approx. 40–50 drops per minute corresponding to an infusion time of 8 hours per litre.

Children's dosage at physician's discretion.

Contra-indications, warnings, etc Caution should be exercised when administering Aminoplex 14 to patients with irreversible liver damage.

Moderate liver damage and uraemic states where facilities exist for dialysis are not contra-indications for the use of Aminoplex 14. Amino acid mixtures may precipitate acute folate deficiency and folic acid should be given daily. Vitamin B_{12} status should be checked and prophylaxis given if necessary.

Pharmaceutical precautions Check that solution is clear and the container undamaged. Discard if not fully used at one injection.

Store below 25°C.

Keep away from light.

The addition of drugs to amino acid solutions should be avoided.

Legal category POM.

Package quantities Glass bottles of 500 ml.

Further information Due to optical sensitivity of the ingredients some colour variation of the solution may be anticipated.

Product licence number 0184/5002.

AMINOPLEX* 24

Presentation A concentrated solution of synthetic L-form amino acids. Sterile and pyrogen-free.

Active ingredients per litre: Synthetic L-form amino acids:

L-Isoleucine	7.60 g
L-Leucine	11.60 g
L-Lysine HCl	6.80 g }
L-Lysine-L-Malate	10.44 g } *
L-Methionine	9.60 g
L-Phenylalanine	13.76 g
L-Threonine	6.40 g
L-Tryptophan	2.80 g
L-Valine	8.96 g
L-Arginine	18.40 g
L-Histidine	4.40 g
L-Alanine	20.00 g
L-Glutamic Acid	4.00 g
Glycine	8.80 g
L-Proline	24.00 g
L-Ornithine-L-Aspartate	4.00 g
L-Serine	4.80 g
(*10.88 g as base)	

Electrolytes:

Sodium	35 mmol
Potassium	30 mmol
Magnesium	2.5 mmol
Chloride	67 mmol
Acetate	5 mmol

Additional nutrient:

L-Malic acid	4.50 g

Providing: 24.9 g/l of utilisable nitrogen. Total energy content 630 kcal (2.6 MJ).

Hypertonic solution pH 7.4 ± 0.2. Osmolality approximately 1570 mosmol/kg.

Uses Aminoplex 24 is an intravenous feeding solution comprising amino acids and electrolytes at physiological neutral pH, for maintenance and repair of body tissues. Aminoplex 24 should be used in patients requiring a high nitrogen load and/or a low infusion volume, whether prophylactically or therapeutically, in conditions leading to protein breakdown.

In order to obtain an optimum metabolic effect and promote positive nitrogen balance, additional calories such as glucose, with or without insulin and/or lipid emulsion, should be administered concurrently. Approximately 75–250 calories/g nitrogen are required depending on the clinical state.

Aminoplex 24 complements GluCoplex 1000 and GluCoplex 1600 (glucose solutions in combination with sodium, potassium, magnesium, phosphate and zinc) to provide balanced intravenous nutrition.

Indications: Surgical: Preoperative malnourished patients; postoperative patients where gastrointestinal function is impaired; post-trauma as a counterpoise to the catabolic state; following resection of the absorptive area of the gut.

Medical: Malabsorption; inflammatory bowel disease; neurological or mechanical dysphagia.

If amino acid therapy is indicated in cases of renal and liver failure, the low fluid volume of Aminoplex 24 may be advantageous. In such circumstances caution should be exercised – see Contraindications, Warnings etc.

Dosage and administration

Adult dose (70 kg bodyweight): Generally 250–1000 ml in 24 hours by slow, central intravenous infusion over the full 24-hour period where possible.

Infusion rate: Maximum 20–25 drops per minutes.

The usual nitrogen load for patients requiring simple protein replacement is 0.15 g nitrogen/kg/day. In catabolic postoperative and post-trauma patients about 0.25 g nitrogen/kg/day are needed. In severely catabolic, and, glucose intolerant patients, especially in the early stages of recovery, 0.35 g nitrogen/kg/day may be preferred but nitrogen requirements must be determined on an individual basis by clinical assessment and biochemical monitoring. Adequate supplements of essential elements and vitamins should also be given as dictated by the results of biochemical monitoring.

Children's dosage at physician's discretion.

Contra-indications, warnings, etc Aminoplex 24 should not be administered in: Irreversible liver-disease; advanced renal disease – if dialysis facilities are not available; inherited disorders of amino acid metabolism.

Care is required in administration to patients with: Hyperkalaemia; overhydration; acidosis; cardiac failure.

Water balance, essential elements, acid-base status and blood glucose levels should be checked regularly. Potassium replacement therapy should be used with extreme caution in patients with cardiac disease, renal dysfunction, digitalization and hepatic insufficiency. Where potassium replacement therapy is critical, plasma electrolyte levels should be carefully monitored, especially in patients with pre-existing imbalances, in renal failure or in hepatic disease. Plasma levels may not be directly related to tissue levels.

Abnormalities of liver function tests and cholestasis have been observed in patients receiving total intravenous nutrition.

Central venous catheters for intravenous feeding should be placed using strict aseptic technique, with proper fixation and dressing and X-ray confirmation where possible. Asepsis should be maintained during changes of tubing and dressing, and use of the catheter should be confined to intravenous feeding alone. Care should be taken to avoid nonmetabolic complications such as air embolism, central venous thrombosis, catheter-linked sepsis and infusion thrombophlebitis.

Amino acid mixtures may precipitate acute folate deficiency and folic acid should be given daily. Vitamin B_{12} status should be checked and prophylaxis given if necessary.

Pharmaceutical precautions Check that the solution is clear, and the container undamaged. Discard if not fully used at one injection. Store at 15–25°C. Keep away from light. Data on compatibility and levels of permissible additions of lipid emulsions, vitamins and trace elements are available from the manufacturers. The addition of drugs to amino acid solutions should be avoided.

Legal category POM.

Package quantities Glass bottles of 250 ml and 500 ml.

Further information Due to optical sensitivity of the ingredients, some colour variation of the solution may be anticipated. Slight deposition of amino acids may occur if inadvertently stored below 15°C, and will dissolve on shaking the container.

Product licence number 0184/0042.

ANAFLEX* AEROSOL

Presentation Antibacterial and antifungal spray containing Polynoxylin 2% for the control of localised infection by external application.

Uses Anaflex Aerosol is indicated for the treatment of athlete's foot, nappy rash, pressure sores, pruritus ani, pruritus vulvae, boils, infective dermatitis, intertrigo, minor wounds.

It is of benefit for colostomy and ileostomy control and for general use in casualty.

Dosage and administration Apply freely to the site of infection or of potential infection.

Contra-indications, warnings, etc For external application only. Caution when spraying near the eyes. Not for intubation nor inhalation.

Pharmaceutical precautions The aerosol can should be stored away from direct heat. The container should not be punctured or destroyed by burning, even when empty.

Legal category P.

Package quantities Aerosol canisters of 100 g.

Further information Contains talc.

Product licence number 0184/5008.

ANAFLEX* CREAM

Presentation A smooth white water-miscible cream with a pleasant odour containing 10% Polynoxylin.

Uses An antibacterial and antifungal preparation for use in a wide variety of dermatological conditions including athlete's foot, nappy rash, pressure sores, boils, stasis ulcers, pruritus ani, pruritus vulvae.

The product has proved of value in promoting wound healing and for the control of tissue reaction following radiotherapy.

Anaflex Cream is indicated also for the treatment of a wide range of aural and nasal infections including otitis externa.

Dosage and administration By application to the affected site once or twice daily.

For the treatment of infected ears the cream should be applied daily by means of a $\frac{1}{2}$-inch ribbon gauze wick.

Contra-indications, warnings, etc Nil.

Pharmaceutical precautions Store below 25°C.

Legal category P.

Package quantities Tubes of 50 g.

Further information Anaflex Cream may be applied direct in the treatment of stasis ulcers. Any surrounding eczema will benefit by the application of Anaflex Paste.

Product licence number 0184/5006.

ANAFLEX* LOZENGES

Presentation Flat, white, circular lozenges with a bevelled edge and embossed 'GEISTLICH' on each face. Each lozenge contains 30 mg Polynoxylin in a citrus-flavoured base.

Uses An antibacterial, antifungal preparation having an anti-inflammatory action and ideally suited for the treatment of mouth and throat infections in tonsillitis, oral thrush, mouth ulcers.

Dosage and administration In most conditions 6–10 lozenges per day will be found suitable. Minor throat infections usually respond in two to three days. More difficult infections (eg Candida) will take longer to respond and treatment can be continued if necessary for four to six weeks.

The lozenges do not contain local anaesthetic and sensitisation will not occur when given over a period of time.

Contra-indications, warnings, etc *Accidental overdosage:* No instance of adverse reaction to an overdosage of Anaflex Lozenges has been recorded and no specific measures are indicated.

Pharmaceutical precautions Store below 25°C.

Legal category P.

Package quantities Containers of 50 lozenges.

Further information Nil.

Product licence number 0184/5007.

ANAFLEX* PASTE

Presentation A smooth white paste containing Poly-noxylin 10%.

Uses Anaflex Paste is beneficial for the control of external infections of bacterial and fungal origin in body areas where moisture is present.

It is indicated for use in athlete's foot, nappy rash, intertrigo, colostomy and ileostomy control, infective dermatitis, boils and stasis ulcers.

Dosage and administration Application to the area for treatment once or twice daily.

Colostomy and ileostomy control: Anaflex Paste gently massaged into the surrounding area will control and effectively treat excoriated tissue present. It will be noted that a colostomy bag will adhere to a surface treated with Anaflex Paste.

Stasis ulcers: Anaflex Cream may be applied direct to the ulcer. Any surrounding eczema will benefit by the application of Anaflex Paste.

Contra-indications, warnings, etc Nil.

Pharmaceutical precautions Store below 25°C.

Legal category P.

Package quantities Tubes of 20 g.

Further information Anaflex Paste may be used in conjunction with Anaflex Cream in the treatment of stasis ulcers.

Product licence number 0184/5005.

ANAFLEX* POWDER

Presentation A white powder with antibacterial, antifungal and anti-inflammatory properties containing Polynoxylin 10%.

Uses For the control of infection on the body surface including athlete's foot, nappy rash, pressure sores, minor wounds, stasis ulcers and in casualty.

Anaflex Powder is indicated also for the treatment of a wide range of aural and nasal infections including otitis externa.

Dosage and administration Apply freely to infected area or area of potential infection by means of the sprinkler pack.

Contra-indications, warnings, etc For external application only. Exclude perforated ear drum.

Pharmaceutical precautions Store below 25°C.

Legal category P.

Package quantities Sprinkler pack of 30 g.

Further information Contains talc.

Product licence number 0184/5003.

GLUCOPLEX* 1000

Presentation A clear solution of 24% glucose premixed with electrolytes and trace elements. Sterile and pyro-gen-free.

Active ingredients per litre:

Sodium	50.0 mmol
Potassium	30.0 mmol
Magnesium	2.5 mmol
Zinc	45.6 mcmol
Dihydrogen phosphate	18.0 mmol
Chloride	67.0 mmol
Anhydrous glucose	240.0 g

Providing: 4.2 MJ (1000 kcal) per litre.
Hypertonic solution
Osmolality approximately 1750 mosmol/kg.

Uses A solution of glucose calories, electrolytes and trace elements for use in intravenous feeding; it is intended for use in combination with a nitrogen source, for example, Aminoplex 12 or Aminoplex 24.

Dosage and administration *Adult Dose (70 kg bodyweight):* Generally 1000–3000 ml in 24 hours by intravenous injection.

Infusion Rate: Maximum 40 to 50 drops per minute corresponding to an infusion time of 8 hours per litre.
Children's dosage at physicians' discretion.'

Contra-indications, warnings, etc Special precautions to be taken in diabetes mellitus, diabetes insipidus, hyperosmotic coma, hyperkalaemia, renal insufficiency, water intoxication, liver disease, myocardial insufficiency and patients with glucose/galactose malabsorption syndrome. Where shock, metabolic acidosis or severe dehydration is present, the condition should be stabilised before the commencement of intravenous feeding.

Administration must be continuous to avoid osmotic and hence volume overload leading to cardiac failure. Rapid infusion may invoke hyperglycaemia, hyperosmolar states, osmotic diuresis and resultant dehydration if used in inappropriately high doses or in patients with impaired glucose metabolism.

Because GluCoplex contains potassium, hyperkalaemia may be exacerbated or induced on rapid infusion. Where potassium therapy is critical it must be guided by electrocardiography. Plasma levels may not be directly related to tissue levels and potassium replacement should be used with extreme caution in patients with cardiac disease, renal dysfunction, digitalisation or hepatic insufficiency. Administration of potassium chloride in glucose solutions will yield lower levels of serum potassium than if given without glucose.

If glucose solutions are given at a rate which exceeds their metabolism a hyper-osmolar condition with a rising serum sodium may occur. In such cases there may be hypernatraemia and a rise in the MCV which must be differentiated from iatrogenic sodium overload. Alternatively the respiratory quotient (RQ) may rise above one giving a high CO_2 production. These complications are more common in severely ill patients. The appropriate glucose load for the patient may be judged from patient clinical state, biochemical response to glucose or by assessment of resting metabolic expenditure.

Hypertonic glucose can induce thrombophlebitis which may occur depending upon the nature and duration of the infusion administered. Central venous feeding catheters should be placed using strict aseptic technique with proper fixation and dressing and X-ray confirmation where possible. Asepsis should be maintained during changes of tubing and dressing and use of the catheter should be confined to intravenous feeding alone.

Administration of intravenous feeding regimens should only be carried out under specialist surveillance with comprehensive biochemical monitoring e.g. fluid balance and plasma electrolyte levela – particularly in patients with pre existing imbalances, renal failure or hepatic disease.

Pharmaceutical precautions Check that the solution is clear and the container undamaged. Discard if not fully used at one injection. Store below 25°C. Keep away from light.

Data on compatibility and levels of permissible additions of lipid emulsions, vitamins and trace elements are available from the manufacturers.

Legal category POM.

Package quantities Clear glass bottles of 500 ml and 1000 ml.

Further information Nil.

Product licence number 0184/0032.

GLUCOPLEX* 1600

Presentation A clear solution of 40% glucose premixed with electrolytes and trace elements. Sterile and pyrogen-free.

Active ingredients per litre:

Sodium	50.0 mmol
Potassium	30.0 mmol
Magnesium	2.5 mmol
Zinc	45.6 mcmol
Dihydrogen phosphate	18.0 mmol
Chloride	67.0 mmol
Anhydrous glucose	400.0 g

Providing: 6.72 MJ (1600 kcal) per litre.
Hypertonic solution
Osmolality approximately 2900 mosmol/kg.

Uses A solution of glucose calories, electrolytes and trace elements for use in intravenous feeding; it is intended for use in combination with a suitable nitrogen source, for example, Aminoplex 12 or Aminoplex 24.

Dosage and administration *Adult Dose (70 kg bodyweight):* Generally 1000–3000 ml in 24 hours by intravenous injection.

Infusion Rate: Maximum 40 to 50 drops per minute corresponding to an infusion time of 8 hours per litre.

Children's dosage at physicians' discretion.

Contra-indications, warnings, etc Special precautions to be taken in diabetes mellitus, diabetes insipidus, hyperosmotic coma, hyperkalaemia, renal insufficiency, water intoxication, liver disease, myocardial insufficiency and patients with glucose/galactose malabsorption syndrome. Where shock, metabolic acidosis or severe dehydration is present, the condition should be stabilised before the commencement of intravenous feeding.

Administration must be continuous to avoid osmotic and hence volume overload leading to cardiac failure. Rapid infusion may invoke hyperglycaemia, hyperosmolar states, osmotic diuresis and resultant dehydration if used in inappropriately high doses or in patients with impaired glucose metabolism.

Because GluCoplex contains potassium, hyperkalaemia may be exacerbated or induced on rapid infusion. Where potassium therapy is critical it must be guided by electrocardiography. Plasma levels may not be directly related to tissue levels and potassium replacement should be used with extreme caution in patients with cardiac disease, renal dysfunction, digitalisation or hepatic insufficiency. Administration of potassium chloride in glucose solution will yield lower levels of serum potassium than if given without glucose.

If glucose solutions are given at a rate which exceeds their metabolism a hyper-osmolar condition with a rising serum sodium may occur. In such cases there may be hypernatraemia and a rise in the MCV which must be differentiated from iatrogenic sodium overload. Alternatively the respiratory quotient (RQ) may rise above one giving a high CO_2 production. These complications are more common in severely ill patients. The appropriate glucose load for the patient may be judged from patient clinical state, biochemical response to glucose or by assessment of resting metabolic expenditure.

Hypertonic glucose can induce thrombophlebitis which may occur depending upon the nature and duration of the infusion administered. Central venous feeding catheters should be placed using strict aseptic technique with proper fixation and dressing and X-ray confirmation where possible. Asepsis should be maintained during changes of tubing and dressing and use of the catheter should be confined to intravenous feeding alone.

Administration of intravenous feeding regimens should only be carried out under specialist surveillance with comprehensive biochemical monitoring e.g. fluid balance and plasma electrolyte levels – particularly in patients with pre-existing imbalances, renal failure or hepatic disease.

Pharmaceutical precautions Check that the solution is clear and the container undamaged. Discard if not fully used at one injection. Store below 25°C. Keep away from light.

Data on compatibility and levels of permissible additions of lipid emulsions, vitamins and trace elements are available from the manufacturers.

Legal category POM.

Package quantities Clear glass bottles of 500 ml and 1000 ml.

Further information Nil.

Product licence number 0184/0033.

KAY-CEE-L* SYRUP

Presentation A clear red cherry flavoured sugar-free syrup containing Potassium Chloride BP 7.50% w/v providing Potassium – 1 mmol per ml.

Uses Indicated in all situations where oral potassium supplementation is required. Typical examples—diuretic therapy, Cushing's syndrome, megaloblastic anaemia, diabetic ketosis; during intensive steroid, corticotrophin and carbenoxolone therapy. Primary aldosteronism, metabolic alkalosis.

Dosage and administration *Adults:* 10–50 ml per day at clinician's discretion.

Children: At clinician's discretion.

Doses should be given in divided amounts, after food.

Contra-indications, warnings, etc Impaired renal function, dehydration, and hyperkalaemia.

High doses taken inadvertently will act as an emetic.

Pharmaceutical precautions Store below 25°C.

Legal category P.

Package quantities Bottles of 500 ml.

Further information Potassium chloride in an oral syrup form has recently been cited as potentially more effective than tablets because of its rapid absorption from the stomach. The syrup is also without risk of causing small bowel haemorrhage, ulceration, and stricture formation. It is important to recognise the use of the chloride salt of potassium, due to the effect of the chloride moiety in controlling metabolic alkalosis. Contains Sorbitol.

Product licence number 0184/0031.

NOXYFLEX* 'S'

Presentation A white crystalline powder containing 2.5 g Noxythiolin.

Uses Noxythiolin has a wide spectrum of antifungal and antibacterial activity for the prevention and eradication of infection from the body surface and specified accessible cavities. Intraperitoneally, it is an effective anti-endotoxin and anti-adhesion agent.

Dosage and administration Noxyflex 'S' Solution is most commonly used at concentrations of 1%, 2.5% and 5%.

When possible pre-warm the Solution to 37°C prior to instillation/irrigation and ensure contact of the Solution on the body surface or in specified body cavities for at least 30 minutes.

Duration of treatment will vary according to the clinical/bacteriological situation, but will normally be 3 to 7 days. Thereafter clinical/bacteriological assessments should be undertaken and the prescribed treatment regimen either repeated or modified accordingly.

Intermittent catheterisation: 100 ml of a 2.5% Solution is pre-warmed to 37°C and slowly instilled into the bladder. The catheter is clamped and the Solution allowed to remain in situ for 30–60 minutes before draining. The procedure is repeated at each catheterisation.

Indwelling catheterisation:
Prophylaxis: 100 ml of a 2.5% Solution is pre-warmed to 37°C and slowly instilled into the bladder. The catheter is clamped and the Solution allowed to remain in situ for 30–60 minutes before draining. The procedure should be carried out 2–3 times per week, although for patients with a past history of recurrent infection daily instillations are preferable.

Treatment of existing infection: 100 ml of a 2.5% Solution is pre-warmed to 37°C and slowly instilled into the bladder. The catheter is clamped and the Solution allowed to remain in situ for 30–60 minutes before draining. This procedure should be carried out twice daily.

In cases of particularly heavy infections, perhaps with associated catheter obstruction, the two instillations should be consecutive. Here, the first instillation is allowed to remain in situ for a minimum of 40 minutes; drainage is immediately followed by the second instillation which is retained for a further 40 minutes.

Whichever treatment regimen is chosen, the duration of therapy should be 5–7 days, following which routine clinical/microbiological assessments should be carried out and the prescribed regimen either repeated or modified accordingly.

If infection is slow to clear:
Check concentration of Noxyflex 'S' Solution used is correct.

Check that Noxyflex 'S' Solution is allowed to remain in the bladder for the correct length of time.

Check for systemic involvement; if present, supplement Noxyflex 'S' instillations with an appropriate course of systemic therapy.

Peritonitis
Noxyflex 'S' is used locally in the peritoneal cavity as an adjunct to the routine treatment of peritonitis and its accompanying shock.

Treatment is based on the following five principles:
– Removal of the cause of peritoneal soiling by surgical exploration.
– Mechanical cleansing of the peritoneal cavity by irrigation with saline.
– Treatment of systemic infection by appropriate antibiotics, such as an aminoglycoside or third generation cephalosporin plus metronidazole.
– Supportive therapy with blood transfusion, intravenous electrolyte solutions and steroids if required to combat shock.
– Intraperitoneal instillation of Noxyflex 'S':
As a single instillation at the time of laparotomy in straightforward bacterial infection. As a repeated instillation or by per- and postoperative irrigation in severe peritonitis, *or* where it is anticipated there may be an accumulation of toxic products such as blood or pus, *or* continuing soiling of the peritoneum.

Technique of single instillation: Following laparotomy and toilet of the peritoneum, the wound is closed after instillation of 5.0 g of Noxyflex 'S' in 200 ml of Water for Injections BP or saline, at the site of maximum contamination. If a drain is left in situ it should be clamped for two hours to prevent drainage of the Noxyflex 'S' Solution.

Technique of repeated instillation: At laparotomy a fine No 9 umbilical catheter is inserted through a stab wound in the upper abdomen to lie in relation to the right lobe of the liver. A tube drain down to the site of maximum contamination is brought out through a stab wound in the lower abdomen. 5.0 g of Noxyflex 'S' in 200 ml of Water for Injections BP or saline is instilled into the abdomen before closing the wound. Thereafter, 2.5 mg Noxyflex 'S' in 100 ml of Water for Injections BP or saline is injected twice daily through the umbilical catheter for five days postoperatively. The lower drain should be clamped for two hours after each instillation.

Technique of per- and postoperative irrigation: At laparotomy the peritoneal cavity is lavaged with 5.0 g of Noxyflex 'S' in 500 ml of Water for Injections BP or saline until the returning fluid is clear. In severe contamination a second 500 ml aliquot is used. Following conclusion of the operative procedure, a Ryles tube is inserted via a stab wound into the peritoneal cavity to lie in relation to the site of maximum contamination. Two corrugated drains are introduced by separate stab incisions to permit free egress of the drainage fluid. The Ryles tube is connected to a conventional drip arrangement, and 5.0 g of Noxyflex 'S' in 500 ml of Water for Injections BP or saline is dripped in continuously every 12 hours for one to three days depending on the estimated degree of contamination.

Empyema
Acute: 100 ml of a 1% or 2.5% Solution instilled daily for a minimum of five days leaving the intercostal drain clamped for a minimum period of 30 minutes.

Chronic: Begin with four-hourly irrigations of 100 ml of

1% Solution and after 12–24 hours alternate these with one or more four-hourly cycles of normal saline.

Infected wounds and fistulae: Irrigate with a 1%–2.5% Solution twice daily for five days.

Infected burns: 1%–2.5% Solution as a wet dressing twice daily.

Abscess cavities: Irrigate with a 2.5% Solution via polythene tube, twice daily.

Radiotherapy (Ca Bladder): 50 ml of 2.5% Solution instilled via catheter during planning.

Contra-indications, warnings, etc The use of Noxyflex 'S' in conjunction with other pharmaceutical agents for combined irrigation/instillation therapy is not recommended and Solution preparation should be carried out as stated under 'Pharmaceutical preparation'. The normal daily usage of Noxyflex 'S' in adults should not exceed 10 g for either accumulative (ie. repeated) instillation regimens or continuous irrigation regimens. Solutions are not intended for intravenous use.

Pharmaceutical precautions *Storage of powder:* The powder vials should be stored below 25°C.

Storage of Solution: Solution should be kept at 2–10°C and used within 7 days. Containers of prepared Solution are intended for single use only.

Solution Preparation (20 ml vial): The powder should be dissolved completely in a sufficient quantity of Water for Injections BP or Sodium Chloride Intravenous Infusion BP (0.9 per cent w/v) by an aseptic technique. Slight difficulty may be experienced in preparing Solutions.

To make a 2.5% Solution: Add contents of one vial (2.5 g) to 100 ml of Water for Injections BP or Sodium Chloride Intravenous Infusion BP (0.9 per cent w/v) and shake for a half to two minutes.

To make a 1% Solution: Add contents of one vial (2.5 g) to 250 ml of Water for Injections BP or Sodium Chloride Intravenous Infusion BP (0.9 per cent w/v) and shake for a half to two minutes.

Solution preparation (100 ml vial): Reconstitution procedure to produce 100 ml Noxyflex 'S' Solution (e.g. 2.5%):

Materials: Transfer needle; 100 ml of Water for Injections BP or Sodium Chloride Intravenous Infusion BP (0.9% w/v); Alcohol Swabs; IVA additive seal.

Procedure:
1. Using aseptic technique, expose rubber stoppers of Noxyflex 'S' 100 ml vial and diluent vial. Swab exposed surfaces.
2. Remove transfer needle set from wrapping.
3. Remove protective sheath from one end of transfer set and insert spike *fully* into stopper of Noxyflex 'S' vial.
4. Remove protective sheath from other end of transfer set and insert spike *fully* into stopper of diluent vial.
5. Invert assembly so that the vial of diluent is uppermost and allow fluid to drain into Noxyflex 'S' vial. (Briefly shake assembly if flow is reluctant to start.)
6. Withdraw transfer spike from Noxyflex 'S' vial.
7. Swab stopper of Noxyflex 'S' vial.
8. Remove protective backing from IVA seal and apply IVA seal to stopper of Noxyflex 'S' vial.
9. Ensure Noxyflex 'S' has completely dissolved; if necessary, shake vial until solution is clear.

Legal category POM.

Package quantities 20 ml vials containing 2.5 g: Boxes of 10 vials.

100 ml vials containing 2.5 g: Boxes of 8 vials with transfer-needle sets and additive seals.

Further information Where desirable, the discretionary use of a suitable local anaesthetic may be used. Noxyflex (ie with amethocaine hydrochloride) may therefore be more appropriate for urological use, or when a degree of pain might be expected. Noxyflex 'S' can be used concurrently with the administration of systemic drugs.

Product licence number 0184/5012

NOXYFLEX*

Presentation A white crystalline powder containing 2.5 g Noxythiolin and 10 mg Amethocaine Hydrochloride BP.

Uses Noxythiolin has a wide spectrum of antifungal and antibacterial activity. It is intended for the prevention and eradication of infection from the body surface and specified accessible cavities, particularly for urological use, or when a degree of pain might be expected.

Dosage and administration Noxyflex Solution is most commonly used at concentrations of 1%, 2.5% and 5%.

When possible, pre-warm the Solution to 37°C prior to instillation/irrigation and ensure contact of the Solution on the body surface or in specified body cavities for at least 30 minutes.

Duration of treatment will vary according to the clinical/bacteriological situation, but will normally be 3 or 7 days. Thereafter clinical/bacteriological assessments should be undertaken and the prescribed treatment regimen either repeated or modified accordingly.

Intermittent catheterisation: 100 ml of a 2.5% Solution is pre-warmed to 37°C and slowly instilled into the bladder. The catheter is clamped and the Solution allowed to remain in situ for 30–60 minutes before draining. The procedure is repeated at each catheterisation.

Indwelling catheterisation:
Prophylaxis: 100 ml of a 2.5% Solution is pre-warmed to 37°C and slowly instilled into the bladder. The catheter is clamped and the Solution allowed to remain in situ for 30–60 minutes before draining. The procedure should be carried out 2–3 times per week, although for patients with a past history of recurrent infection daily instillations are preferable.

Treatment of existing infections: 100 ml of a 2.5% Solution is pre-warmed to 37°C and slowly instilled into the bladder. The catheter is clamped and the Solution allowed to remain in situ for 30–60 minutes before draining. This procedure should be carried out twice daily.

In cases of particularly heavy infections, perhaps with associated catheter obstruction, the two instillations should be consecutive. Here, the first instillation is allowed to remain in situ for a minimum of 40 minutes; drainage is immediately followed by the second instillation which is retained for a further 40 minutes.

Whichever treatment regimen is chosen, the duration of therapy should be 5–7 days, following which routine clinical/microbiological assessments should be carried out and the prescribed regimen either repeated or modified accordingly.

If infection is slow to clear:

Check concentration of Noxyflex Solution used is correct.

Check that Noxyflex Solution is allowed to remain in the bladder for the correct length of time.

Check for systemic involvement; if present, supplement Noxyflex instillations with an appropriate course of systemic therapy.

Infected wounds and fistulae: Irrigate with a 1%–2.5% Solution twice daily for five days.

Infected burns: 1%-2.5% Solution as a wet dressing twice daily.

Abscess cavities: Irrigate with a 2.5% Solution via polythene tube, twice daily.

Radiotherapy (Ca Bladder): 50 ml of 2.5% Solution instilled via catheter during planning.

Contra-indications, warnings, etc The use of Noxyflex in conjunction with other pharmaceutical agents for combined irrigation/instillation therapy is not recommended and Solution preparation should be carried out as stated under 'Pharmaceutical preparation'. The normal daily usage of Noxyflex in adults should not exceed 10 g for either accumulative (ie. repeated) instillation regimens or continuous irrigation regimens. Solutions are not intended for intravenous use.

Pharmaceutical precautions *Storage of powder:* The powder vials should be stored below 25°C.

Storage of Solution: Solution should be kept at 2–10°C and used within 7 days. Containers of prepared Solution are intended for single use only.

Solution Preparation (20 ml vial): The powder should be dissolved completely in a sufficient quantity of Water for Injections BP or Sodium Chloride Intravenous Infusion BP (0.9 per cent w/v) by an aseptic technique. Slight difficulty may be experienced in preparing Solutions.

To make a 2.5% Solution: Add contents of one vial (2.5 g) to 100 ml of Water for Injections BP or Sodium Chloride Intravenous Infusion BP (0.9 per cent w/v) and shake for a half to two minutes.

To make a 1% Solution: Add contents of one vial (2.5 g) to 250 ml of Water for Injections BP or Sodium Chloride Intravenous Infusion BP (0.9 per cent w/v) and shake for a half to two minutes.

Solution preparation (100 ml vial): Reconstitution procedure to produce 100 ml Noxyflex solution (e.g. 2.5%):

Materials: Transfer needle; 100 ml of Water for Injections BP or Sodium Chloride Intravenous Infusion BP (0.9% w/v); Alcohol Swabs; IVA additive seal.

Procedure:

1. Using aseptic technique, expose rubber stoppers of Noxyflex 100 ml vial and diluent vial. Swab exposed surfaces.

2. Remove transfer needle set from wrapping.

3. Remove protective sheath from one end of transfer set and insert spike *fully* into stopper of Noxyflex vial.

4. Remove protective sheath from other end of transfer set and insert spike *fully* into stopper of diluent vial.

5. Invert assembly so that the vial of diluent is uppermost and allow fluid to drain into Noxyflex vial. (Briefly shake assembly if flow is reluctant to start).

6. Withdraw transfer spike from Noxyflex vial.

7. Swab stopper of Noxyflex vial.

8. Remove protective backing from IVA seal and apply IVA seal to stopper of Noxyflex vial.

9. Ensure Noxyflex has completely dissolved; if necessary, shake vial until solution is clear.

Legal category POM.

Package quantities 20 ml vials containing 2.5 g: Boxes of 10 vials.

100 ml vials containing 2.5 g: Boxes of 8 vials with transfer-needle sets and additive seals.

Further information In those situations where the inclusion of local anaesthetic is undesirable or unnecessary, Noxyflex 'S' should be used. Noxyflex can be used concurrently with the administration of systemic drugs.

Product licence number 0184/5013.

*Trade Mark

Glaxo Laboratories Limited
Greenford
Middlesex UB6 0HE

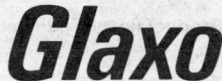

BETNELAN* TABLETS

Presentation Small white tablets engraved 'Betnelan Glaxo' on one side and scored on the reverse. Each tablet contains 500 mcg (0.5 mg) betamethasone.

The product complies with the specification for Betamethasone Tablets BP.

Uses Betamethasone is a glucocorticosteroid which is about eight to ten times as active as prednisolone on a weight-for-weight basis.

A wide variety of diseases may sometimes require corticosteroid therapy. Some of the principal indications are: asthma, severe allergic disturbances, leukaemia, rheumatoid arthritis, collagen diseases and various inflammatory skin diseases. Other indications are the nephrotic syndrome, ulcerative colitis, regional ileitis (Crohn's disease), pemphigus, sarcoidosis (especially with hypercalcaemia), rheumatic carditis and various blood dyscrasias, including selected cases of haemolytic anaemia, agranulocytosis and thrombocytopenic purpura.

Dosage and administration The lowest dosage that will produce an acceptable result should be used; when it is possible to reduce the dosage, this must be accomplished by stages. During prolonged therapy, dosage may need to be increased temporarily during periods of stress or in exacerbations of illness.

Adults: The dose used will depend upon the disease, its severity and the clinical response obtained. The following regimens are for guidance only. Divided dosage is usually employed.

Short-term treatment: 2 to 3 mg daily for the first few days, subsequently reducing the daily dosage by 250 or 500 mcg (0.25 or 0.5 mg) every two to five days, depending upon the response.

Rheumatoid arthritis: 500 mcg (0.5 mg) to 2 mg daily. For maintenance therapy the lowest effective dosage is used.

Most other conditions: 1.5 to 5 mg daily for one to three weeks, then reducing to the minimum effective dosage.

Larger doses may be needed for collagen diseases and ulcerative colitis.

Children: Fractions of the adult dosage may be used (e.g. 75% at 12 years, 50% at seven years and 25% at 1 year), but clinical factors must be given due weight.

Contra-indications, warnings, etc
Contra-indications: Systemic infections, unless specific anti-infective therapy is employed.

Live virus immunisation. Hypersensitivity to any component of the tablet.

Precautions: Administration of corticosteroids may impair the ability to resist and counteract infection; in addition clinical signs and symptoms of infection are suppressed.

Corticosteroid treatment is likely to reduce the response of the pituitary-adrenal axis to stress, and relative insufficiency may persist for up to a year after withdrawal of prolonged therapy.

Because of the possibility of fluid retention, care must be taken when corticosteroids are administered to patients with congestive heart failure.

In pregnant animals, systemic administration of corticosteroids can cause abnormalities of fetal development. The relevance of this finding to humans has not been established.

Depression of hormone levels has been described in pregnancy but the significance of this finding is not clear.

Corticosteroids may worsen diabetes mellitus.

Since corticosteroids are secreted in the breast milk, the advisability of breast feeding should be considered in women on high dosage.

Steroids may reduce the effects of anticholinesterases in myasthenia gravis, cholecystographic X-ray media and salicylates.

The effect of steroids may be reduced by phenytoin, phenobarbitone, ephedrine and rifampicin.

The dosage of concomitantly administered anti-coagulants may have to be altered (usually decreased).

In patients with liver failure, blood levels of corticosteroid may be increased, as with other drugs which are metabolised in the liver.

Side-effects: Prolonged treatment with corticosteroids in high dosage is occasionally associated with subcapsular cataract or glaucoma. In addition, any of the features of hypercorticism, such as osteoporosis, may occur. Aseptic osteonecrosis, particularly of the femoral head, may occur after prolonged corticosteroid therapy, or after repeated short courses involving high dosage. Peptic ulceration may develop, or be aggravated. In children, prolonged therapy may retard growth.

In patients on long-term therapy, fluid and electrolyte balance may be altered. Other rare side effects which have been reported include benign intracranial hypertension and psychic instability.

Drug interactions: Steroids may reduce the effects of anticholinesterases in myasthenia gravis, cholecystographic X-ray media and non-steroidal anti-inflammatory agents. It should also be remembered that the effects of steroids may be reduced by phenytoin, phenobarbitone, ephedrine and rifampicin.

Overdosage: Treatment is unlikely to be needed in cases of acute overdosage.

Pharmaceutical precautions Protect from light.

Legal category POM.

Package quantities Bottles of 100 or 500 tablets.

Further information Betnelan does not normally cause retention of salt and water, and the risk of inducing oedema and hypertension is almost negligible.

Product licence number 0004/5134.

BETNESOL* EYE, EAR AND NOSE PREPARATIONS

Presentation Betnesol Drops contain betamethasone sodium phosphate 0.1% w/v, and benzalkonium chloride 0.02% w/v in a clear and colourless aqueous solution that is sterile until the bottle is opened. This product complies with the BPC specification for Betamethasone Eye Drops.

Betnesol Eye Ointment contains betamethasone sodium phosphate 0.1% w/w in a bland, soft paraffin base of white, translucent appearance. Sterile until opened.

Uses Non-infected inflammatory conditions of the eye, ear or nose.

Dosage and administration *Eyes:* 1 or 2 drops instilled into the eye every one or two hours until control is achieved, when the frequency may be reduced. An extrusion of the ointment about ¼ inch long may be introduced beneath the lower lid two or three times daily and/or at night.

Ears: 2 or 3 drops instilled into the ear every two or three hours until control is achieved, when the frequency may be reduced.

Nose: 2 or 3 drops instilled into each nostril two or three times daily.

Contra-indications, warnings, etc
Contra-indications: Viral, fungal, tuberculous or purulent conditions. Use in the eye is contra-indicated if glaucoma is present or where herpetic keratitis (dendritic ulcer) is considered a possibility. Inadvertent use of topical steroids in the latter condition can lead to the enlargement of the ulcer and marked visual deterioration.

Hypersensitivity to any component of the preparation. Betnesol Eye Drops contain benzalkonium chloride as a preservative and therefore should not be used to treat patients who wear soft contact lenses.

Precautions: Topical administration of corticosteroids to pregnant animals can cause abnormalities of fetal development. The relevance of this finding to human beings has not been established; however, topical steroids should not be used extensively in pregnancy, i.e. in large amounts or for prolonged periods.

Side-effects: Eye drops containing corticosteroids cause a serious rise in intra-ocular pressure in a small percentage of the population, including most of those with a family history of glaucoma. A milder rise may be experienced by a larger proportion of subjects if treatment is continued for longer than a few weeks. Thinning of the cornea leading to perforation, has occurred with use of topical corticosteroids. Cataract is reported to have occurred after unduly prolonged treatment with topical corticosteroids.

Pharmaceutical precautions It is desirable that the contents should not be used more than four weeks after first opening the bottle or tube.

Legal category POM.

Package quantities *Betnesol Drops:* Plastic dropper bottles containing 5 ml or 10 ml.

Betnesol Eye Ointment: Narrow-nozzle tubes containing 3 g.

Further information Nil.

Product licence numbers
Betnesol Drops   0004/5135
Betnesol Eye Ointment   0004/5137R

BETNESOL*-N EYE, EAR AND NOSE PREPARATIONS

Presentation Betnesol-N Drops contain betamethasone sodium phosphate 0.1% w/v, neomycin sulphate 0.5% w/v and thiomersal 0.005% w/v in a clear and colourless aqueous solution. Sterile until opened.

Betnesol-N Eye Ointment contains betamethasone sodium phosphate 0.1% w/w and neomycin sulphate 0.5% w/w in a bland, soft paraffin base of white translucent appearance. Sterile until opened.

Uses Betamethasone has topical corticosteroid activity. The presence of neomycin should prevent the development of bacterial infection.

Eye: Non-infected inflammatory conditions where development of bacterial infection is likely.

Ear: Otitis externa and other inflammatory conditions where bacterial infection is present or suspected (see 'Contra-indications').

Nose: Inflammatory conditions where infection is present or suspected.

Dosage and administration *Eyes:* 1 or 2 drops instilled into the eye every one or two hours until control is achieved, when the frequency may be reduced. An extrusion of the ointment about ¼ inch long may be introduced beneath the lower lid two or three times daily and/or at night.

Ears: 2 or 3 drops instilled into the ear every two or three hours until control is achieved, when the frequency can be reduced.

Nose: 2 or 3 drops instilled into each nostril two or three times daily.

Contra-indications, warnings, etc
Contra-indications: Viral, fungal or tuberculous conditions; use in the eye is contra-indicated if purulent infection or glaucoma is present.

Inadvertent use in herpetic keratitis (dendritic ulcer) can lead to enlargement of the ulcer and marked visual deterioration.

Hypersensitivity to any component of the preparation.

Because of the risk of ototoxicity, preparations containing neomycin should not be used until an intact tympanic membrane has been visualised.

Precautions: Topical administration of corticosteroids to pregnant animals can cause abnormalities of fetal development. The relevance of this finding to human beings has not been established; however, topical steroids should not be used extensively in pregnancy, i.e. in large amounts or for prolonged periods.

The unnecessary topical use of neomycin containing products should be avoided in order to minimise the occurrence of neomycin-resistant organisms (and organisms cross-resistant to other aminoglycosides.

Side-effects: Eye drops containing corticosteroids cause

a serious rise in intra-ocular pressure in a small percentage of the population, including most of those with a family history of glaucoma. A milder rise may be experienced by a larger proportion of subjects if treatment is continued for longer than a few weeks. Thinning of the cornea leading to perforation has occurred with use of topical corticosteroids.

Acute sensitisation to neomycin is a rare event but can occur after topical application to the eye or ear.

Cataract is reported to have occurred after unduly prolonged treatment of eye conditions with topical corticosteroids.

Pharmaceutical precautions It is desirable that the contents should not be used more than four weeks after first opening the bottle or tube.

Legal category POM.

Package quantities *Betnesol-N Drops:* Plastic dropper bottles containing 5 ml or 10 ml.

Betnesol-N Eye Ointment: Tubes containing 3 g.

Further information Nil.

Product licence numbers
Betnesol-N Drops   0004/5136
Betnesol-N Eye Ointment   0004/5138R

BETNESOL* INJECTION

Presentation Each ampoule of ready-prepared Betnesol Injection contains 4 mg betamethasone as the sodium phosphate ester in 1 ml of sterile aqueous solution. The injection is clear and colourless or pale yellow, and complies with the specification for Betamethasone Sodium Phosphate Injection BP.

Uses Betamethasone is a glucocorticosteroid which is about eight to ten times as active as prednisolone on a weight-for-weight basis. It may be indicated in the following conditions:

Status asthmaticus and acute allergic reactions, in anaphylactic reaction to drugs. Betnesol Injection supplements the action of adrenaline.

Severe shock arising from surgical or accidental trauma or overwhelming infection.

Adrenal crisis precipitated by abnormal stress in Addison's disease, Simmonds' disease, following adrenalectomy, and when adrenocortical function has been suppressed by prolonged corticosteroid therapy.

Soft tissue lesions such as tennis elbow and periarthritis of the shoulder joint (by local injection).

N.B. Betnesol Injection does not replace other forms of therapy for the treatment of shock and status asthmaticus.

Dosage and administration *Systemic therapy in adults:* 4 to 20 mg betamethasone (1 to 5 ml) administered by intravenous injection over half to one minute. This dose can be repeated three or four times in 24 hours, or as required, depending upon the condition being treated and the patient's response. Alternatively, Betnesol Injection may be given in an intravenous infusion. The same dose can be given by intramuscular injection, but the response is likely to be less rapid, especially in shock.

Systemic therapy in children: Infants up to 1 year may be given 1 mg betamethasone intravenously; children aged 1 to 5 years, 2 mg; 6 to 12 years, 4 mg (1 ml).

Other routes: Local injections of 4 to 8 mg Betnesol may be used when treating soft tissue lesions in adults; children may require smaller doses.

Betnesol Injection has also been administered subconjunctivally as a single injection of 0.5 to 1 ml.

Intrathecal use is not recommended.

Contra-indications, warnings, etc
Contra-indications: Systemic infections, unless specific anti-infective therapy is employed. Live virus immunisation. Hypersensitivity to any component of the injection.

Betnesol Injection should not be injected directly into tendons.

Precautions: Administration of corticosteroids may impair the ability to resist and counteract infection; in addition clinical signs and symptoms of infection are suppressed.

In pregnant animals, systemic administration of corticosteroids can cause abnormalities of fetal development. The relevance of this finding to humans has not been established.

Steroids may reduce the effects of anticholinesterases in myasthenia gravis, cholecystographic X-ray media and salicylates.

The effect of steroids may be reduced by phenytoin, phenobarbitone, ephedrine and rifampicin.

Side-effects: In the short term, high dosage of betamethasone involves little risk of adverse reactions, except that peptic ulceration may occur, or be aggravated. With continued use, signs of hypercorticism may become apparent.

Pharmaceutical precautions Protect from light.

Legal category POM.

Package quantities 1 ml ampoules in box of 5.

Further information Nil.

Product licence number 0004/5139.

BETNESOL* TABLETS

Presentation Small, soluble pink tablets engraved 'Betnesol Glaxo' on one side and scored on the reverse. Each tablet contains 500 mcg (0.5 mg) betamethasone as the sodium phosphate ester.

The tablets comply with the specification for Betamethasone Sodium Phosphate Tablets BP.

Uses Betamethasone is a glucocorticosteroid which is about eight to ten times as active as prednisolone on a weight-for-weight basis.

Betamethasone sodium phosphate is very soluble in water, and is therefore less likely to cause local gastric irritation than corticosteroids which are only slightly soluble. This is important when high dosages are required, as in immunosuppressive therapy.

Betnesol does not normally cause retention of salt and water, and the risk of inducing oedema and hypertension is almost negligible.

A wide variety of diseases may sometimes require corticosteroid therapy. Some of the principal indications are: asthma, severe allergic disturbances, leukaemia, rheumatoid arthritis, collagen diseases, and various inflammatory skin diseases. Other indications are the nephrotic syndrome, ulcerative colitis, regional ileitis (Crohn's disease), pemphigus, sarcoidosis (especially with hypercalcaemia), rheumatic carditis and various blood dyscrasias, including selected cases of haemolytic anaemia, agranulocytosis and thrombocytopenic purpura.

Dosage and administration Betnesol Tablets are best taken dissolved in water, but they can be swallowed whole without difficulty. The lowest dosage that will produce an acceptable result should be used; when it is possible to reduce the dosage, this must be accomplished by stages. During prolonged therapy, dosage may need to be increased temporarily during periods of stress or in exacerbations of illness.

Adults: The dose used will depend upon the disease, its severity and the clinical response obtained. The following regimens are for guidance only. Divided dosage is usually employed.

Short-term treatment: 2 to 3 mg daily for the first few days, subsequently reducing the daily dosage by 250 or 500 mcg (0.25 or 0.5 mg) every two to five days, depending upon the response.

Rheumatoid arthritis: 500 mcg (0.5 mg) to 2 mg daily. For maintenance therapy the lowest effective dosage is used.

Most other conditions: 1.5 to 5 mg daily for one to three weeks, then reducing to the minimum effective dosage.

Larger doses may be needed for collagen diseases and ulcerative colitis.

Children: Fractions of the adult dosage may be used (e.g. 75% at 12 years, 50% at seven years and 25% at 1 year), but clinical factors must be given due weight.

Contra-indications, warnings, etc
Contra-indications: Systemic infections, unless specific anti-infective therapy is employed. Live virus immunisation. Hypersensitivity to any component of the tablets.

Precautions: Administration of corticosteroids may impair the ability to resist and counteract infection; in addition clinical signs and symptoms of infection are suppressed.

Corticosteroid treatment is likely to reduce the response of the pituitary-adrenal axis to stress, and relative insufficiency may persist for up to a year after withdrawal of prolonged therapy.

Because of the possibility of fluid retention, care must be taken when corticosteroids are administered to patients with congestive heart failure.

In pregnant animals, systemic administration of corticosteroids can cause abnormalities of fetal development. The relevance of this finding to humans has not been established.

Depression of hormone levels has been described in pregnancy but the significance of this finding is not clear.

Corticosteroids may worsen diabetes mellitus.

Since corticosteroids are secreted in the breast milk, the advisability of breast feeding should be considered in women on high dosage.

Steroids may reduce the effects of anticholinesterases in myasthenia gravis, cholecystographic X-ray media and salicylates.

The effect of steroids may be reduced by phenytoin, phenobarbitone, ephedrine and rifampicin.

The dosage of concomitantly administered anti-coagulants may have to be altered (usually decreased).

In patients with liver failure, blood levels of corticosteroid may be increased, as with other drugs which are metabolised in the liver.

Side-effects: Prolonged treatment with corticosteroids in high dosage is occasionally associated with subcap-

sular cataract or glaucoma. In addition, any of the features of hypercorticism, such as osteoporosis, may occur. Aseptic osteonecrosis, particularly of the femoral head, may occur after prolonged corticosteroid therapy, or after repeated short courses involving high dosage. Peptic ulceration may develop, or be aggravated. In children, prolonged therapy may retard growth.

In patients on long-term therapy, fluid and electrolyte balance may be altered. Other rare side effects which have been reported include benign intracranial hypertension and psychic instability.

Drug interactions: Steroids may reduce the effects of anticholinesterases in myasthenia gravis, cholecystographic X-ray media and non-steroidal anti-inflammatory agents. It should also be remembered that the effects of steroids may be reduced by phenytoin, phenobarbitone, ephedrine and rifampicin.

Overdosage: Treatment is unlikely to be needed in cases of acute overdosage.

Pharmaceutical precautions Nil.

Legal category POM.

Package quantities The tablets are strip-packed in cartons of 100.

Further information Betnesol Tablets do not contain carbohydrates.

Product licence number 0004/5140.

BETNOVATE* RECTAL PREPARATIONS

Presentation Betnovate Rectal Ointment is a white, translucent preparation containing 0.05% w/w betamethasone valerate, 0.1% w/w phenylephrine hydrochloride, and 2.5% w/w lignocaine hydrochloride.

Betnovate Compound Suppositories are white and opaque, and each contains 0.5 mg betamethasone valerate, 2 mg phenylephrine hydrochloride and 40 mg lignocaine hydrochloride.

Uses The clinical effectiveness of the Betnovate rectal preparations is attributable to the marked local anti-inflammatory property of the corticosteroid betamethasone valerate, the analgesic effect of lignocaine, and the vasoconstrictor effect of phenylephrine.

Betnovate Rectal Ointment or Suppositories are indicated for: pain and bleeding associated with anal fissures and internal or external haemorrhoids; post-haemorrhoidectomy pain; minor degrees of proctitis.

Dosage and administration *Ointment:* Apply a small amount of ointment two or three times a day initially, using the applicator if internal administration is required. When inflammation is subsiding, once-daily application is sufficient in most cases. One tube should provide treatment for at least a week.

Suppositories: Insert a suppository night and morning after defaecation.

Contra-indications, warnings, etc
Contra-indications: Corticosteroids should not be used in the presence of infection unless effective chemotherapy is also employed. Hypersensitivity to any component of the preparations.

Precautions: Topical administration of corticosteroids to pregnant animals can cause abnormalities of fetal development. The relevance of this finding to human beings has not been established; however, topical steroids should not be used extensively in pregnancy, i.e. in large amounts or for prolonged periods.

Side-effects: As with all topical corticosteroids, if the Betnovate preparations are used for prolonged periods, the consequences of systemic absorption should be considered, especially in children.

Prolonged and intensive treatment with active corticosteroid preparations may cause local atrophic changes in the skin.

Pharmaceutical precautions Nil.

Legal category POM.

Package quantities *Betnovate Compound Suppositories:* Box of 10.

Betnovate Rectal Ointment: Tube of 25 g with applicator nozzle.

Further information Nil.

Product licence numbers
Betnovate Compound Suppositories   0004/5129
Betnovate Rectal Ointment   0004/5128

BETNOVATE* SCALP APPLICATION

Presentation Betnovate Scalp Application is a transparent, slightly gelled solution containing 0.1% w/w betamethasone as valerate. The vehicle contains 50% of isopropyl alcohol, which has antibacterial activity. This preparation complies with the specification for Betamethasone Valerate Scalp Application, BP.

Uses Steroid-responsive dermatoses of the scalp, such as psoriasis, seborrhoea capitis and the inflammation associated with severe dandruff.

Dosage and administration A small quantity of Betnovate Scalp Application should be applied to the scalp night and morning until improvement is noticeable. It may then be possible to sustain improvement by applying once a day, or less frequently.

Contra-indications, warnings, etc
Contra-indications: Infections of the scalp. Hypersensitivity to the preparation.

Precautions: Care must be taken to keep the preparation away from the eyes. Do not use near a naked flame.

Long-term continuous topical therapy should be avoided where possible, particularly in infants and children, as adrenal suppression can occur even without occlusion.

Development of secondary infection requires withdrawal of topical corticosteroid therapy and commencement of appropriate systemic antimicrobial therapy.

Topical administration of corticosteroids to pregnant animals can cause abnormalities of fetal development. The relevance of this finding to human beings has not been established; however, topical steroids should not be used extensively in pregnancy, i.e. in large amounts or for prolonged periods.

Side-effects: Betnovate preparations are usually well tolerated, but if signs of hypersensitivity appear, application should be stopped immediately.

As with other topical corticosteroids, when extensive areas are treated, sufficient systemic absorption may occur to produce the features of hypercorticism. This effect is more likely to result in infants and children, and if occlusive dressings are used, or if treatment is prolonged. Local atrophy may occur after prolonged treatment under occlusion.

In rare instances, treatment of psoriasis with corticosteroids (or its withdrawal) is thought to have provoked the pustular form of the disease.

Pharmaceutical precautions Nil.

Legal category POM.

Package quantities Plastic squeeze bottles of 30 and 100 ml.

Further information The least potent corticosteroid which will control the disease should be selected. The viscosity of the scalp application has been adjusted so that the preparation spreads easily without being too fluid. The specially-designed bottle and nozzle allow easy application direct to the scalp through the hair.

Product licence number 0004/5133.

BETNOVATE* SKIN PREPARATIONS

Presentation The Betnovate skin preparations contain 0.1% betamethasone as the valerate ester. The Betnovate R.D. (Ready Diluted) skin preparations contain 0.025% betamethasone as the valerate ester.

Betnovate Cream is a smooth, white, water-miscible preparation. It complies with the specifications for Betamethasone Valerate Cream BP. Betnovate Ointment is a white preparation based on soft paraffin. It complies with the specification for Betamethasone Valerate Ointment BP. Betnovate Lotion is a white, translucent, aqueous fluid. It complies with the specification for Betamethasone Valerate Lotion BP. Betnovate R.D. Cream and Ointment are ready-diluted 1 in 4 preparations.

Uses Betamethasone valerate is an active topical corticosteroid which produces a rapid response in those inflammatory dermatoses that are normally responsive to topical corticosteroid therapy, and is often effective in the less responsive conditions such as psoriasis.

Betnovate preparations are indicated for the treatment of: eczema, including atopic, infantile and discoid eczemas, prurigo, psoriasis, neurodermatoses, including lichen simplex, lichen planus, seborrhoeic dermatitis, intertrigo, contact sensitivity reactions, discoid lupus erythematosus and they may be used as an adjunct to systemic steroid therapy in generalised erythroderma.

Betnovate can also be used in the management of insect bites, sunburn and prickly heat.

Betnovate R.D. preparations are indicated for maintenance treatment when control has been achieved with Betnovate.

Dosage and administration A small quantity of Betnovate should be applied to the affected area two or three times daily until improvement occurs. It may then be possible to maintain improvement by applying once a day, or even less often, or by using the appropriate ready-diluted (1 in 4) preparation Betnovate R.D.

Betnovate and Betnovate R.D. Creams are especially appropriate for moist or weeping surfaces and Betnovate and Betnovate R.D. Ointments for dry, lichenified or scaly lesions, but this is not invariably so. Betnovate Lotion is particularly suitable when a minimal application to a large area is required.

In the more resistant lesions, such as the thickened plaques of psoriasis on elbows and knees, the effect of

Betnovate can be enhanced, if necessary, by occluding the treatment area with polythene film. Overnight occlusion only is usually adequate to bring about a satisfactory response in such lesions; thereafter, improvement can usually be maintained by regular application without occlusion.

Contra-indications, warnings, etc

Contra-indications: Rosacea, acne and peri-oral dermatitis.

Skin lesions caused by infection with viruses (e.g., herpes simplex, chickenpox), fungi (e.g., candidiasis; tinea) or bacteria (e.g., impetigo).

Hypersensitivity to the preparation.

Precautions: Long-term continuous topical therapy should be avoided where possible, particularly in infants and children, as adrenal suppression can occur even without occlusion. The face, more than other areas of the body, may exhibit atrophic changes after prolonged treatment with potent topical corticosteroids. This must be borne in mind when treating such conditions as psoriasis, discoid lupus erythematosus and severe eczema. If applied to the eyelids, care is needed to ensure that the preparation does not enter the eye, as glaucoma might result.

Appropriate antimicrobial therapy should be used whenever treating inflammatory lesions which have become infected. Any spread of infection requires withdrawal of topical corticosteroid therapy and systemic administration of antimicrobial agents. Bacterial infection is encouraged by the warm, moist conditions induced by occlusive dressings, and so the skin should be cleansed before a fresh dressing is applied.

Topical administration of corticosteroids to pregnant animals can cause abnormalities of fetal development. The relevance of this finding to human beings has not been established; however, topical steroids should not be used extensively in pregnancy, i.e., in large amounts or for prolonged periods.

Side-effects: Prolonged and intensive treatment with highly active corticosteroid preparations may cause local atrophic changes in the skin such as striae, thinning and dilatation of the superficial blood vessels, particularly when occlusive dressings are used or when skin folds are involved.

As with other topical corticosteroids, prolonged use of large amounts, or treatment of extensive areas, can result in sufficient systemic absorption to produce the features of hypercorticism. This effect is more likely to occur in infants and children, and if occlusive dressings are used. In infants, the napkin may act as an occlusive dressing.

In rare instances, treatment of psoriasis with corticosteroids (or its withdrawal) is thought to have provoked the pustular form of the disease.

The Betnovate and Betnovate R.D. preparations are usually well tolerated, but if signs of hypersensitivity appear, application should stop immediately.

Pharmaceutical precautions Nil.

Legal category POM.

Package quantities Betnovate Cream and Ointment
are supplied in 15, 30 and 100 g tubes.

Betnovate R.D. Cream and Ointment are supplied in 100 g tubes.

Betnovate Lotion is supplied in 20 ml bottles.

Further information The least potent corticosteroid
which will control the disease should be selected. None of these preparations contain lanolin. Betnovate Cream and Ointment and the corresponding R.D. preparations, do not contain parabens. Betnovate Lotion contains parabens.

Product licence numbers

Betnovate Cream	0004/5121
Betnovate Ointment	0004/5124
Betnovate R.D. Cream	0004/0277
Betnovate R.D. Ointment	0004/0278
Betnovate Lotion	0004/5130

BETNOVATE*-C SKIN PREPARATIONS

Presentation The Betnovate-C skin preparations contain 0.1% betamethasone as the valerate ester and 3% clioquinol.

Betnovate-C Cream is a smooth, straw-coloured water-miscible cream.

Betnovate-C Ointment is a white or pale straw-coloured paraffin-based ointment.

Uses Betamethasone valerate is an active topical corticosteroid which produces a rapid response in those inflammatory dermatoses that are normally responsive to topical corticosteroid therapy, and is often effective in the less responsive conditions such as psoriasis.

Clioquinol is an anti-infective agent which has both antibacterial and anticandidal activity.

Betnovate-C preparations are indicated for the treatment of the following conditions where secondary bacterial and/or fungal infection is present, suspected, or likely to occur: eczema, including atopic, infantile and discoid eczemas, and prurigo; psoriasis; neurodermatoses, including lichen simplex; lichen planus; seborrhoeic dermatitis; intertrigo; contact sensitivity reactions; discoid lupus erythematosus; and they may be used as an adjunct to systemic steroid therapy in generalised erythroderma.

Betnovate-C can also be used in the management of insect bites, sunburn, prickly heat, anal and vulval pruritus, and otitis externa.

Dosage and administration A small quantity should be applied gently to the affected area two or three times daily until improvement occurs. It may then be possible to maintain improvement by applying once a day or even less often. Betnovate-C Cream is often appropriate for moist or weeping surfaces, and Betnovate-C Ointment for dry, lichenified or scaly lesions, but this is not invariably so.

In the more resistant lesions, such as the thickened plaques of psoriasis on elbows and knees, the effect of Betnovate-C can be enhanced, if necessary, by occluding the treatment area with polythene film. Overnight occlusion only is usually adequate to bring about a satisfactory response in such cases, thereafter improvement can usually be maintained by regular application without occlusion.

Contra-indications, warnings, etc

Contra-indications: Rosacea, acne and peri-oral dermatitis.

Skin lesions caused by infection with viruses (e.g., herpes simplex, chickenpox), fungi (e.g., candidiasis; tinea) or bacteria (e.g., impetigo).

Hypersensitivity to the preparation.

Precautions: Long-term continuous topical therapy should be avoided where possible, particularly in infants and children, as adrenal suppression can occur even without occlusion.

The face, more than other areas of the body, may exhibit atrophic changes after prolonged treatment with potent topical corticosteroids. This must be borne in mind when treating such conditions as psoriasis, discoid lupus erythematosus and severe eczema with Betnovate. If applied to the eyelids, care is needed to ensure that the preparation does not enter the eye, as glaucoma might result.

If infection persists, systemic chemotherapy is required. Any spread of infection requires withdrawal of topical corticosteroid therapy. Bacterial infection is encouraged by the warm, moist conditions induced by occlusive dressings, and the skin should be cleansed before a fresh dressing is applied.

Topical administration of corticosteroids to pregnant animals can cause abnormalities of fetal development. The relevance of this finding to human beings has not been established; however, topical steroids should not be used extensively in pregnancy, i.e., in large amounts or for prolonged periods. Betnovate-C may stain hair, skin or fabric, and the application should be covered with a dressing to protect clothing.

Side-effects: Prolonged and intensive treatment with highly active corticosteroid preparations may cause local atrophic changes in the skin such as striae, thinning, and dilatation of the superficial blood vessels, particularly when occlusive dressings are used or when skin folds are involved.

As with other topical corticosteroids, prolonged use of large amounts, or treatment of extensive areas, can result in sufficient systemic absorption to produce the features of hypercorticism. This effect is more likely to occur in infants and children, and if occlusive dressings are used. In infants, the napkin may act as an occlusive dressing.

In rare instances, treatment of psoriasis with corticosteroids (or its withdrawal) is thought to have provoked the pustular form of the disease.

The Betnovate preparations are usually well tolerated, but if signs of hypersensitivity appear, application should stop immediately.

Pharmaceutical precautions Nil.

Legal category POM.

Package quantities Betnovate-C Cream and Ointment are supplied in 15 and 30 g tubes.

Further information The least potent corticosteroid which will control the disease should be selected. These preparations do not contain lanolin or parabens.

Product licence numbers
Betnovate-C Cream   0004/5122
Betnovate-C Ointment 0004/5126

BETNOVATE*-N SKIN PREPARATIONS

Presentation The Betnovate-N skin preparations contain 0.1% betamethasone as the valerate ester and 0.5% neomycin sulphate (3,500 units per gram or per millilitre).

Betnovate-N Cream is a smooth, white, water-miscible cream.

Betnovate-N Ointment is a white, paraffin-based ointment.

Betnovate-N Lotion is a white, aqueous translucent fluid.

Uses Betamethasone valerate is an active topical corticosteroid which produces a rapid response in those inflammatory dermatoses that are normally responsive to topical corticosteroid therapy, and is often effective in the less responsive conditions such as psoriasis.

Neomycin sulphate is a broad-spectrum, bactericidal antibiotic effective against the majority of bacteria commonly associated with skin infections.

Betnovate-N preparations are indicated for the treatment of the following conditions where secondary bacterial infection is present, suspected, or likely to occur: Eczema, including atopic, infantile and discoid eczemas; prurigo; psoriasis; neurodermatoses, including lichen simplex; lichen planus; seborrhoeic dermatitis; intertrigo; contact sensitivity reactions; discoid lupus erythematosus; and they may be used as an adjunct to systemic steroid therapy in generalised erythroderma.

Betnovate-N preparations can also be used in the management of insect bites, sunburn, prickly heat, anal and vulval pruritus, and otitis externa (see 'Contra-indications').

Dosage and administration A small quantity should be applied to the affected area two or three times daily until improvement occurs. It may then be possible to maintain improvement by applying once a day or even less often. Betnovate-N Cream is especially appropriate for moist or weeping surfaces, and Betnovate-N Ointment for dry, lichenified or scaly lesions, but this is not invariably so. Betnovate-N Lotion is particularly suitable when a minimal application to a large area is required.

In the more resistant lesions, such as the thickened plaques of psoriasis on elbows and knees, the effect of Betnovate-N can be enhanced, if necessary, by occluding the treatment area with polythene film. Overnight occlusion only is usually adequate to bring about a satisfactory response in such cases, thereafter improvement can usually be maintained by regular application without occlusion.

Contra-indications, warnings, etc
Contra-indications: Rosacea, acne and peri-oral dermatitis.

Skin lesions caused by infection with viruses (e.g., herpes simplex, chickenpox), fungi (e.g., candidiasis; tinea) or bacteria (e.g., impetigo).

Preparations containing neomycin should not be used for the treatment of otitis externa when the ear drum is perforated, because of the risk of ototoxicity.

Hypersensitivity to the preparations.

Precautions: Long-term continuous topical therapy should be avoided where possible, particularly in infants and children, as adrenal suppression can occur even without occlusion.

The face, more than other areas of the body, may exhibit atrophic changes after prolonged treatment with potent topical corticosteroids. This must be borne in mind when treating such conditions as psoriasis, discoid lupus erythematosus and severe eczema with Betnovate. If applied to the eyelids, care is needed to ensure that the preparation does not enter the eye, as glaucoma might result.

If bacterial infection persists, systemic chemotherapy is required. Any spread of infection requires withdrawal of topical corticosteroid therapy. Bacterial infection is encouraged by the warm, moist conditions induced by occlusive dressings, and the skin should be cleansed before a fresh dressing is applied.

Topical administration of corticosteroids to pregnant

animals can cause abnormalities of fetal development. The relevance of this finding to human beings has not been established; however, topical steroids should not be used extensively in pregnancy, i.e. in large amounts or for prolonged periods.

Side-effects: Prolonged and intensive treatment with highly active corticosteroid preparations may cause local atrophic changes in the skin such as striae, thinning and dilatation of the superficial blood vessels, particularly when occlusive dressings are used or when skin folds are involved.

As with other topical corticosteroids, prolonged use of large amounts, or treatment of extensive areas, can result in sufficient systemic absorption to produce the features of hypercorticism. This effect is more likely to occur in infants and children, and if occlusive dressings are used. In infants, the napkin may act as an occlusive dressing.

The Betnovate preparations are usually well tolerated, but if signs of hypersensitivity appear, application should stop immediately.

In rare instances, treatment of psoriasis with corticosteroids (or its withdrawal) is thought to have provoked the pustular form of the disease.

Pharmaceutical precautions Nil.

Legal category POM.

Package quantities Betnovate-N Cream and Ointment are supplied in 15, 30 and 100 g tubes.
Betnovate-N Lotion is supplied in 20 ml bottles.

Further information The least potent corticosteroid which will control the disease should be selected. These preparations do not contain lanolin. Betnovate-N Cream and Betnovate-N Ointment do not contain parabens. Betnovate-N Lotion contains parabens.

Product licence numbers
Betnovate-N Cream   0004/5123
Betnovate-N Ointment   0004/5127
Betnovate-N Lotion   0004/5131

BEXTASOL* INHALER

Presentation Bextasol Inhaler is a pressurised aerosol containing a suspension of betamethasone valerate in propellants. One canister delivers 200 metered puffs, each providing 100 micrograms of betamethasone valerate.

Uses *Rationale:* Betamethasone valerate is a corticosteroid which possesses high topical activity relative to its systemic activity. Inhalation of this steroid in a low dose that is delivered direct to the respiratory tract can thus provide a considerable local therapeutic effect without causing depression of hypothalamic-pituitary-adrenal function when used in the recommended dosage. There is also evidence that the growth of asthmatic children is not retarded by Bextasol therapy.

Bextasol is a prophylactic treatment for asthma and it is important that patients understand that regular daily administration is necessary – a dose cannot give immediate relief. The full effect of Bextasol usually develops within three days, but occasionally a longer period is needed.

Bextasol is indicated for the treatment of extrinsic and intrinsic asthma in children and adults.

Unlike bronchodilators and sodium cromoglycate, Bextasol has a marked anti-inflammatory effect on the respiratory tract, so that it can often control asthma which is not fully controlled by bronchodilators or sodium cromoglycate as a result of local inflammation of the respiratory tract. Additionally, Bextasol can usually replace previous systemic corticosteroid therapy either entirely or in part.

Dosage and administration The recommended initial dosage of Bextasol Inhaler for treatment of asthma in both adults and children is 800 micrograms daily, usually taken as 2 puffs four times each day, in addition to any other therapy that the patient is receiving. The container should be shaken before each puff. Where asthma is complicated by hypersecretion of mucus, Bextasol may not reach the mucosa in effective amounts. A short intensive course of systemic corticosteroid therapy will usually clear the bronchi and enable Bextasol to be fully effective.

Provided the asthma is fully controlled, the dosage of ancillary drugs such as bronchodilators and sodium cromoglycate can often be reduced slowly over a period of a few weeks. It is recommended that the daily dosage of Bextasol should then be reduced to the minimum necessary to control the asthma.

Where severe asthma has required maintenance treatment with systemic corticosteroids or ACTH, it is generally possible to reduce the dosage of these compounds, and often they can be withdrawn eventually, but great care is necessary in case of pituitary or adrenal hypofunction. The systemic steroid should be withdrawn slowly, e.g. by reducing the daily dosage by the equivalent of 1 mg prednisolone at weekly or monthly intervals. Corticosteroid withdrawal symptoms, including anorexia, nausea, vomiting and muscle and joint pains, may occur. Furthermore, atopic conditions such as rhinitis and eczema, which were suppressed by systemic corticosteroid, may be unmasked and require therapy.

Contra-indications, warnings, etc
Contra-indications: Hypersensitivity to betamethasone valerate.

Precautions: Caution should be exercised in the presence of bacterial, mycobacterial, viral or fungal infections of the respiratory tract.

Hypothalamic-pituitary-adrenal function recovers only gradually after systemic corticosteroid therapy has been terminated, depending upon the dosage used and the duration of systemic therapy. The possibility that stress may precipitate acute adrenal insufficiency can remain for a year or longer.

Should stress arise, systemic steroid therapy should be reinstated or the existing dosage increased if there is doubt about the ability of the hypothalamic-pituitary-adrenal system to respond adequately. It may also be advisable to increase the dosage of Bextasol temporarily, where this has been reduced.

It is advisable for the patient to have a reserve supply of corticosteroid tablets, so that if the asthma deteriorates, or infection occurs, doses can be taken pending instructions from his physician.

In pregnant animals, administration of corticosteroids can cause abnormalities of fetal development. The relevance of this finding to human beings has not been established.

Side-effects: Some patients have reported hoarseness. Occasionally localised colonisation by *Candida albicans* occurs in the mouth and throat, and this usually requires topical antifungal therapy. If the response is unsatisfactory, a temporary reduction in the dosage of Bextasol will often speed resolution.

Overdosage: Treatment is unlikely to be needed in cases of acute overdosage.

Pharmaceutical precautions Store below 25°C away from sunlight. Do not puncture or burn the can.

Legal category POM.

Package quantities Single canisters.

Further information Each pack contains an illustrated leaflet describing how the asthmatic patient should use Bextasol.

Product licence number 0004/0142.

CEPOREX*

Presentation Ceporex Tablets are pink, film-coated tablets, each containing 250 mg or 500 mg cephalexin. They are engraved 'Ceporex 250' or 'Ceporex 500' respectively on one side and 'Glaxo' on the reverse. They comply with the BP specification for Cephalexin Tablets.

Ceporex Capsules are caramel and grey, hard gelatine capsules, each containing 250 mg or 500 mg cephalexin. They are marked 'Ceporex 250' or 'Ceporex 500' respectively, and 'Glaxo'. They comply with the BP specification for Cephalexin Capsules.

Ceporex Syrups are prepared by adding water to the granules to give orange-flavoured and coloured suspensions containing 125 mg, 250 mg or 500 mg cephalexin in each 5 ml. All strengths comply with the BP specification for Cephalexin Mixture.

Ceporex Paediatric Drops are prepared by adding water to give 10 ml of orange-flavoured and coloured suspension containing 125 mg cephalexin in each 1.25 ml. The dropper is calibrated at 125 mg and 62.5 mg.

Ceporex Suspension is a ready-prepared, yellow, banana-flavoured suspension of cephalexin in vegetable oil. Each 5 ml contains 125 mg or 250 mg cephalexin.

Uses Ceporex is a bactericidal antibiotic of the cephalosporin group which is active against a wide range of Gram-positive and Gram-negative organisms. It is indicated for treatment of the following conditions, when caused by susceptible bacteria.

Respiratory tract infections: acute and chronic bronchitis and infected bronchiectasis.

Ear, nose and throat infections: otitis media; mastoiditis; sinusitis; follicular tonsillitis and pharyngitis.

Urinary tract infections: acute and chronic pyelonephritis, cystitis and prostatitis. Prophylaxis of recurrent urinary tract infection.

Gynaecological and obstetric infections.

Skin, soft-tissue and bone infections.

Gonorrhoea and syphilis (when Penicillin is unsuitable).

Dental procedures: temporary replacement of penicillin prophylaxis in patients with heart disease who are undergoing dental treatment.

Dosage and administration Many infections in adults will respond to oral dosage of 1 gram to 2 grams per day in divided doses; however, for most infections, the following simple dosage scheme will be found satisfactory:

Adults and children over 12 years	500 mg t.d.s.
Children 5 to 12 years	250 mg t.d.s.
Children 1 to 5 years	125 mg t.d.s.

Children under 1 year	125 mg b.d.

To aid compliance, especially in ambulatory patients, the daily dosage may be given in two equal doses, e.g., 1 g twice daily in adults with urinary tract infections.

The following additional information should also be considered:

Adults: For severe or deep-seated infections, especially when less sensitive organisms are involved, the dosage should be increased to 1 g t.d.s. or 1.5 g q.d.s.

For prophylaxis of recurrent urinary tract infections in adults, a dose of 125 mg each night is recommended and may be continued for several months. (The 125 mg/5 ml Suspension is suitable for this purpose.)

Children: Ideally, dosage should be calculated on a body-weight basis, particularly in infants. The following dosage recommendations for children are derived from a normal dosage of 25 to 60 mg/kg/day. For chronic, severe or deep-seated infections, this should be increased to 100 mg/kg/day (maximum 4 g/day).

0 to 3 months: 62.5 to 125 mg twice daily.

4 months to 2 years: 62.5 to 125 mg four times daily or 125 to 250 mg twice daily.

3 to 6 years: 125 to 250 mg four times daily or 250 to 500 mg twice daily.

7 to 12 years: 250 to 500 mg four times daily or 500 mg to 1 g twice daily.

Notes: For most acute infections, treatment should continue for at least two days after signs have returned to normal and symptoms have subsided, but in chronic, recurrent or complicated urinary tract infections and syphilis, treatment for two weeks (giving 500 mg four times daily) is recommended. For gonorrhoea, a single dose of 3 g with 1 g probenecid for males or 2 g with 0.5 g probenecid for females is usually effective. Concurrent administration of probenecid delays excretion of cephalexin and raises the serum levels by 50 to 100%.

Ceporex has not been shown to have a toxic effect on the kidney, but as with other antibiotics which are excreted mainly by the kidneys, unnecessary accumulation may occur in the body when renal function is below about half of normal. Therefore the maximum recommended dosages (i.e., adults 6 g/day, children 4 g/day) should be reduced proportionately in these patients.

In elderly patients the possibility of renal impairment should be considered.

Adult patients receiving intermittent dialysis should be given an additional 500 mg Ceporex after each dialysis, i.e., a total dosage of up to 1 g on that day. Children should receive an additional 8 mg per kg.

Contra-indications, warnings, etc *Contra-indications:* Hypersensitivity to cephalosporins.

Precautions: Ceporex is usually well tolerated by patients allergic to penicillin, but cross-reaction has been encountered rarely. As with other antibiotics that are excreted mainly by the kidneys, when renal function is poor, dosage of Ceporex should be suitably reduced (see 'Dosage and administration'). Laboratory experiments and clinical experience show no evidence of teratogenicity, but it would be wise to proceed with caution during the early months of pregnancy, as with all drugs.

In patients receiving Ceporex, a false-positive reaction for glucose in the urine may be given, with Benedict's or Fehling's solution, or with 'Clinitest' tablets, but not with enzyme-based tests.

Ceporex can interfere with the alkaline picrate assay

for creatinine, giving a falsely high reading, but the degree of elevation is unlikely to be of clinical importance.

Side-effects: A small proportion of patients receiving Ceporex experience gastro-intestinal disturbances such as nausea, vomiting and diarrhoea. As with other antibiotics, prolonged use may result in the overgrowth of non-susceptible organisms, e.g., Candida. This may present as vulvo-vaginitis.

Reversible neutropenia has occurred in a few patients, but is very rare. Drug rashes – both urticarial and maculopapular – are uncommon.

Overdosage: Serum levels of cephalexin can be reduced greatly by peritoneal dialysis or haemodialysis.

Pharmaceutical precautions Ceporex Tablets and Capsules should be protected from light. Ceporex Suspension should not be refrigerated.

The reconstituted syrups retain their potency for 10 days when kept in a cool place, preferably a refrigerator. The reconstituted syrups may be diluted with water (not Syrup BP), after which they should be used within seven days. Ceporex Suspension must not be diluted with water or syrup.

Legal category POM.

Package quantities *Tablets 250 mg and 500 mg:* Bottles of 20, 100 and 500.

Capsules 250 mg and 500 mg: Bottles of 20, 100 and 500.

Syrup 125 mg/5 ml, 250 mg/5 ml and 500 mg/5 ml: Bottles of 100 ml.

Paediatric Drops 125 mg/1.25 ml: Bottles of 10 ml.

Suspension 125 mg/5 ml and 250 mg/5 ml: Bottles of 100 ml.

Further information Ceporex is resistant to the action of staphylococcal penicillinase, and is therefore active against strains of *Staph. aureus* that are insensitive to penicillin (or ampicillin) through production of that enzyme. Ceporex is also active against the majority of ampicillin-resistant *E. coli.*

Absorption of Ceporex is almost complete, even in the presence of food, and is not adversely affected by coeliac disease, partial gastrectomy, achlorhydria, jaundice or diverticulosis (duodenal or jejunal). Ceporex is excreted in the urine in high concentration.

The serum half-life is normally about one hour, but is longer in the newborn (see 'Dosage and administration'). Ceporex has a wide margin of safety.

Product licence numbers

Ceporex Tablets 250 mg	0004/5046
Ceporex Tablets 500 mg	0004/5047
Ceporex Capsules 250 mg	0004/5041
Ceporex Capsules 500 mg	0004/5042
Ceporex Syrup 125 mg	0004/5043
Ceporex Syrup 250 mg	0004/5044
Ceporex Syrup 500 mg Ceporex Paediatric Drops }	0004/5045
Ceporex Suspension 125 mg	0004/0268
Ceporex Suspension 250 mg	0004/0269

CORLAN* PELLETS

Presentation Small white pellets engraved 'Corlan Glaxo' on one side. Each pellet contains 2.5 mg hydrocortisone in the form of the water-soluble ester hydrocortisone sodium succinate. The pellets comply with the specification for Hydrocortisone Lozenges BPC.

Uses Local use in aphthous ulceration of the mouth, whether simple or occurring as a complication in diseases such as sprue, idiopathic steatorrhoea and ulcerative colitis.

Dosage and administration *Adults and children:* Corlan Pellets should not be sucked, but be kept in the mouth and allowed to dissolve slowly in close proximity to the ulcers. One pellet should be used in this way four times a day. When ulcers recur quickly after withdrawal of treatment, maintenance therapy with reduced dosage is desirable for a period.

Contra-indications, warnings, etc
Contra-indications: Corlan Pellets should not be used in the presence of oral infection unless effective chemotherapy is also employed. Hypersensitivity to any component of the product.

Precautions: In pregnant animals, systemic administration of corticosteroids can cause abnormalities of fetal development. The relevance of this finding to humans has not been established.

Side-effects: Corticosteroids may worsen diabetes.

Overdosage: Treatment is unlikely to be needed in cases of acute overdosage.

Pharmaceutical precautions Replace cap firmly after use.

Legal category POM.

Package quantities Vial of 20 pellets.

Further information Nil.

Product licence number 0004/5077.

CORTELAN* TABLETS

Presentation White tablets engraved 'Cortelan Glaxo' on one side and scored on the reverse. Each tablet contains 25 mg cortisone acetate, and complies with the specification for Cortisone Tablets BP.

Uses Replacement therapy in Addison's disease and following adrenalectomy.

Dosage and administration In adults with Addison's disease, 25 to 40 mg daily are usually needed, divided into 2 doses. In replacement therapy after adrenalectomy, the dosage required may be slightly higher.

During intercurrent infection, dosage requirements may be increased to between 75 and 100 mg a day.

Children may require lower dosage.

Contra-indications, warnings, etc
Contra-indications: Systemic infections, unless specific anti-infective therapy is employed. Hypersensitivity to any component of the tablet.

Precautions: In infections (including latent tuberculosis), effective chemotherapy should be given. In pregnant animals, systemic administration of corticosteroids can cause abnormalities of fetal development. The relevance of this finding to humans has not been established.

Side-effects: Long term treatment in high dosage may cause any of the features associated with hypercorticism.

Overdosage: Treatment is unlikely to be needed in cases of acute overdosage.

Pharmaceutical precautions Protect from light.

Legal category POM.

Package quantities Bottles of 100 tablets.

Further information Nil.

Product licence number 0004/5078.

CRYSTAPEN* INJECTION

Presentation Vials containing sodium benzylpenicillin (penicillin G) as a white, crystalline, water-soluble powder. Also vials containing sodium benzylpenicillin with 4.5% sodium citrate as a buffer (5 and 10 mega unit vials only). For preparation of Benzylpenicillin Injection BP.

Ampoules of Crystapen Intrathecal containing freeze-dried sodium benzylpenicillin.

Uses Crystapen has bactericidal activity in infections due to penicillin-sensitive organisms, particularly streptococci, pneumococci *(Streptococcus pneumoniae),* meningococci, gonococci and staphylococci (excluding penicillinase-producing strains). Crystapen is indicated for most wound infections, pyogenic infections of the skin, soft tissue infections and infections of the nose, throat, nasal sinuses, respiratory tract and middle ear, etc.

Generalised infections, septicaemia and pyaemia from susceptible bacteria. Acute and chronic osteomyelitis, subacute bacterial endocarditis, and meningitis caused by susceptible organisms. Gonorrhoea.

Dosage and administration The following dosages apply to both intramuscular and intravenous injection.

Adults: Usually 600 to 1,200 mg (1 to 2 mega units) daily, divided into 2 to 4 doses. In bacterial endocarditis, 8 mega units or more may be given daily in divided doses by the intravenous route, often by infusion. Intravenous doses in excess of 1.2 g (2 mega units) should be given slowly, taking at least one minute for each 300 mg (0.5 mega unit) to avoid high levels causing irritation of the central nervous system. High dosage of sodium benzyl-penicillin may result in hypernatraemia and hypokalaemia unless the sodium content is taken into account.

Children aged 1 month to 12 years: 10 to 20 mg (17,000 to 34,000 units) per kilogram body weight in 24 hours, usually divided into 4 doses. In meningitis the dosage may be doubled.

Newborn infants: 30 mg/kg/day (50,000 units) in divided doses, usually twice daily in the first few days of life, then three or four times a day. In meningitis the systemic dosage may be increased to 60 to 90 mg/kg/day (100,000 to 150,000 units) divided into 3 or 4 doses.

PREPARATION OF SOLUTIONS

Intramuscular injection: A 600 mg (1 mega unit) dose is usually dissolved in 1.6 to 2.0 ml of Water for Injections.

Intravenous injection: A suitable concentration is 600 mg (1 mega unit) dissolved in 4 to 10 ml of Water for Injections.

Intravenous infusion: It is recommended that 600 mg (1 mega unit) should be dissolved in at least 10 ml of Sodium Chloride Injection or other transfusion solution.

OTHER ROUTES OF ADMINISTRATION

These usually supplement systemic dosage.

Subconjunctival injection: 300 or 600 mg dissolved in 0.5 to 1 ml of Water for Injections.

Intrathecal injection: For adults, 6 mg (10,000 units) dissolved in 10 ml of Sodium Chloride Injection BP, or in 10 ml of the patient's own cerebrospinal fluid. Maximum dose, 12 mg (20,000 units). For infants and children, 0.1 mg/kg (170 units/kg) is suitable. The concentration of penicillin in the injection should not exceed 0.6 mg/ml (1,000 units/ml). Only freshly prepared solutions should be used. **Overdosage is dangerous**.

If the special freeze-dried Crystapen (intended for intrathecal use) is not available, a disposable membrane filter of 0.45 micron pore size should be used to ensure clarity of the solution.

Contra-indications, warnings, etc

Contra-indications: Allergy to penicillins.

Precautions: Massive doses of sodium penicillin can cause hypokalaemia and sometimes hypernatraemia. Use of a potassium-sparing diuretic may be helpful.

If renal function is very poor, large doses of penicillin (e.g. 12 mega units or more) can cause cerebral irritation and fits.

Skin sensitisation may occur in persons handling the antibiotic, and care should be taken to avoid contact with the substance.

It should be recognised that any patient with a history of allergy, especially to drugs, is more likely to develop a hypersensitivity reaction to penicillin.

Side-effects: Occasionally hypersensitivity to penicillin, in the form of urticarial rash, may occur; it may be treated with antihistamine drugs. More rarely, anaphylactic reactions have been reported.

Haemolytic anaemia (sometimes with leucopenia) can be induced by high dosage of penicillin.

Overdosage: Excessive blood levels of penicillin G can be corrected by haemodialysis.

Pharmaceutical precautions Solutions of penicillin should be used promptly although unbuffered solutions will retain satisfactory potency for up to seven days if refrigerated.

Buffered solutions retain satisfactory potency for up to three days at temperatures not exceeding 25°C (77°F), and for up to fourteen days if refrigerated at 2 to 10°C. For intrathecal injection only freshly prepared solutions should be used.

Legal category POM.

Package quantities *Ampoules:* 12 mg (20,000 units) unbuffered for intrathecal injection, box of 3.

Vials: 300 mg (500,000 units) unbuffered, box of 10, 0.6 g (1,000,000 units) unbuffered, box of 10.

Bottles: 3 g (5 mega units) buffered and 6 g (10 mega units) buffered.

Further information 600 mg Crystapen in solution displaces 0.4 ml. Each mega unit of unbuffered Crystapen represents 1.68 mmol of sodium; the figure for buffered Crystapen is 2.08 mmol.

Product licence numbers

Crystapen 12 mg	0004/5074
Crystapen 300 mg	0004/5069
Crystapen 0.6 g	0004/5070
Crystapen 3.0 g	0004/5072
Crystapen 6.0 g	0004/5073

CRYSTAPEN* V PREPARATIONS

Presentation Crystapen V Tablets are orange, film-coated tablets each containing 250 mg penicillin V as the potassium salt and engraved 'Crystapen V' on one side and 'Glaxo' on the reverse. The product complies with the specification for Penicillin V-K Tablets BP.

Crystapen V Syrups are prepared by adding water to the granules to produce a red, pleasant-flavoured, clear syrup. Each 5 ml syrup contains 125 mg or 250 mg penicillin V as the potassium salt. The products comply with the specification for Penicillin V Elixir BP.

Uses Crystapen V has bactericidal activity in infections due to penicillin-susceptible organisms, e.g., those due to beta-haemolytic streptococci, pneumococci and some staphylococci. Prophylaxis before and after surgery and dental extractions to prevent subacute bacterial endocarditis in patients with congenital or rheumatic heart disease.

Dosage and administration *Infants:* 62.5 to 125 mg.
Children: 125 to 250mg.
Adults: 250 to 500 mg.

All given four times a day, preferably before meals. Higher or more frequent dosage may sometimes be indicated.

N.B. In serious and overwhelming infections when rapid control is essential, injections of sodium penicillin G are necessary initially.

In patients with beta-haemolytic streptococcal infection it is advisable to continue treatment for 10 days to prevent bacteriological relapse and complications such as rheumatic fever or acute nephritis.

Contra-indications, warnings, etc
Contra-indications: Allergy to penicillins.

Precautions: It should be recognised that any patient with a history of allergy, especially to drugs, is more likely to develop a hypersensitivity reaction to penicillin V.

Side-effects: Occasionally patients experience diarrhoea. Sensitivity reactions such as urticarial rash are uncommon, and anaphylaxis is very rare.

Overdosage: Toxic blood levels are unlikely to occur following oral administration. However, if they do, treatment should be symptomatic.

Pharmaceutical precautions Crystapen V Syrups, when reconstituted, should be used within seven days if kept below 20°C, or within 14 days if kept in a refrigerator.

Crystapen V Syrups can be diluted with Syrup BP if required.

Legal category POM.

Package quantities *Crystapen V Tablets:* Bottles of 500 and 1,000.

Crystapen V Syrups: Granules to produce 100 ml of syrup in each bottle when reconstituted with 51 ml water for 250 mg Syrup, or 60 ml water for 125 mg Syrup.

Further information Nil.

Product licence numbers
Crystapen V Tablets   0004/5059
Crystapen V Syrup 125 mg   0004/5057
Crystapen V Syrup 250 mg   0004/5058

DERMOVATE* CREAM AND OINTMENT

Presentation Dermovate Cream and Ointment each contain 0.05% w/w clobetasol propionate. The water-miscible cream and the paraffin-based ointment are both white in appearance.

Uses Clobetasol propionate is a very active topical corticosteroid which is of particular value when used in short courses for the treatment of more resistant dermatoses such as psoriasis, recalcitrant eczemas, lichen planus, discoid lupus erythematosus, and other conditions which do not respond satisfactorily to less-active steroids.

Dosage and administration Apply sparingly to the affected area once or twice daily until improvement occurs. As with other highly-active topical steroid preparations, therapy should be discontinued when control is achieved. In the more responsive conditions this may be within a few days. If a longer course is necessary, it is recommended that treatment should not be continued for more than four weeks without the patient's condition being reviewed. Repeated short courses of Dermovate may be used to control exacerbations. If continuous steroid treatment is necessary, a less potent preparation should be used.

In very resistant lesions, especially where there is hyperkeratosis, the anti-inflammatory effect of Dermovate can be enhanced, if necessary, by occluding the treatment area with polythene film. Overnight occlusion only is usually adequate to bring about a satisfactory response. Thereafter improvement can usually be maintained by application without occlusion.

Contra-indications, warnings, etc
Contra-indications: Rosacea, acne and peri-oral dermatitis.

Skin lesions caused by infection with viruses (e.g., herpes simplex, chickenpox), fungi (e.g., candidiasis, tinea) or bacteria (e.g., impetigo).

Hypersensitivity to the preparation.

Precautions: Long-term continuous therapy with Dermovate should be avoided, particularly in infants and children, in whom adrenal suppression occurs readily. If Dermovate is required for use in children, it is recommended that the treatment should be reviewed weekly. It should be noted that the infant's napkin may act as an occlusive dressing.

The face, more than other areas of the body, may exhibit atrophic changes after prolonged treatment with potent topical corticosteroids. This must be borne in mind when treating facial conditions which warrant use of Dermovate, and frequent observation of the patient is important. If applied to the eyelids, care is needed to ensure that the preparation does not enter the eye, as glaucoma might result.

Appropriate antimicrobial therapy should be used whenever treating inflammatory lesions which have become infected. Any spread of infection requires withdrawal of topical corticosteroid therapy and institution of suitable systemic chemotherapy.

Bacterial infection is encouraged by the warm, moist conditions induced by occlusive dressings, and the skin should be cleansed before a fresh dressing is applied.

Topical administration of corticosteroids to pregnant animals can cause abnormalities of fetal development. The relevance of this finding to human beings has not been established; however, topical steroids should not be used extensively in pregnancy, i.e., in large amounts or for prolonged periods.

Side-effects: Provided the weekly dosage is less than 50 g in adults, any pituitary-adrenal suppression is likely to be transient with a rapid return to normal values once the short course of steroid therapy has ceased. The same applies to children given proportionate dosage. Use of occlusive dressings increases the absorption of topical corticosteroids.

Prolonged and intensive treatment with highly-active corticosteroid preparations may cause atrophic changes, such as striae, thinning of the skin, and dilatation of the superficial blood vessels, particularly when occlusive dressings are used, or where skin folds are involved.

In rare instances, treatment of psoriasis with corticosteroids (or its withdrawal) is thought to have provoked the pustular form of the disease.

Dermovate is usually well tolerated, but if signs of hypersensitivity appear, application should be stopped immediately.

Pharmaceutical precautions None.

Legal category POM.

Package quantities Tubes of 25 and 100 g.

Further information The least potent corticosteroid which will control the disease should be selected. Dermovate preparations do not contain lanolin or parabens.

Product licence numbers
Dermovate Ointment 0004/0220
Dermovate Cream 0004/0219

DERMOVATE* SCALP APPLICATION

Presentation Dermovate Scalp Application is a transparent, slightly gelled solution containing 0.05% w/w clobetasol propionate. The vehicle contains 50% isopropyl alcohol, which has antibacterial activity.

Uses Psoriasis and recalcitrant eczemas of the scalp. Clobetasol propionate is a highly-active topical corticosteroid which is indicated for use in short courses for conditions which do not respond satisfactorily to less active steroids.

Dosage and administration Apply sparingly to the scalp night and morning until improvement occurs. As with other highly-active topical steroid preparations, therapy should be discontinued when control is achieved. Repeated short courses of Dermovate Scalp Application may be used to control exacerbations. If continuous steroid treatment is necessary, a less potent preparation should be used.

Contra-indications, warnings, etc
Contra-indications: Infections of the scalp.
Hypersensitivity to the preparation.
Precautions: Care must be taken to keep the preparation away from the eyes. Do not use near a naked flame.

Long-term continuous therapy with Dermovate Scalp Application should be avoided, particularly in infants and children, in whom adrenal suppression occurs readily.

Development of secondary infection requires withdrawal of topical corticosteroid therapy and commencement of appropriate systemic antimicrobial therapy.

Topical administration of corticosteroids to pregnant animals can cause abnormalities of fetal development. The relevance of this finding to human beings has not been established; however, topical steroids should not be used extensively in pregnancy, i.e., in large amounts or for prolonged periods.

Side-effects: Dermovate preparations are usually well tolerated, but if signs of hypersensitivity appear, application should be stopped immediately.

As with other topical corticosteroids, local atrophy may result from prolonged treatment, particularly if occlusive dressings are used.

When extensive areas are treated, sufficient systemic absorption may occur to produce the features of hypercorticism, especially in infants and children. This effect is more likely to occur after prolonged treatment, particularly if occlusive dressings are used.

In rare instances, treatment of psoriasis with corticosteroids (or its withdrawal) is thought to have provoked the pustular form of the disease.

Pharmaceutical precautions None.

Legal category POM.

Package quantities Plastic squeeze bottle with elongated nozzle containing 25 or 100 ml.

Further information The least potent corticosteroid which will control the disease should be selected. The viscosity of the scalp application has been adjusted so that the preparation spreads easily without being too fluid. The specially-designed bottle and nozzle allow easy application direct to the scalp through the hair.

Product licence number 0004/0242.

DERMOVATE*-NN SKIN PREPARATIONS

Presentation Dermovate-NN skin preparations contain clobetasol propionate 0.05% w/w, neomycin sulphate 0.5% and nystatin 100,000 units per gram.

Dermovate-NN Ointment is a buff paraffin-based ointment.

Dermovate-NN Cream is buff in colour.

Uses Clobetasol propionate is a highly active topical corticosteroid which is of particular value when used in short courses for the treatment of recalcitrant eczemas, neurodermatoses, and other conditions which do not respond satisfactorily to less active steroids.

Dermovate-NN is indicated in those dermatoses where secondary bacterial or candidal infection is present, suspected, or likely to occur, as when using occlusive dressings in conditions such as psoriasis.

Dosage and administration Apply sparingly to the affected area once or twice daily until improvement occurs. As with other highly-active topical steroid preparations therapy should be discontinued when control is achieved. In the more responsive conditions this may be within a few days. If a longer course is necessary, it is recommended that treatment should not be continued for more than four weeks without the patient's condition being reviewed. Repeated short courses of Dermovate-NN may be used to control exacerbations. If continuous steroid treatment is necessary, a less potent preparation should be used.

In very resistant lesions, especially where there is hyperkeratosis, the anti-inflammatory effect of Dermovate-NN can be enhanced, if necessary, by occluding the treatment area with polythene. Overnight occlusion only is usually adequate to bring about a satisfactory response, thereafter improvement can usually be maintained by application without occlusion.

Contra-indications, warnings, etc

Contra-indications: Rosacea, acne and peri-oral dermatitis.

Skin lesions caused by infection with viruses (e.g., herpes simplex, chickenpox), fungi (e.g., candidiasis, tinea) or bacteria (e.g., impetigo).

Preparations containing neomycin should not be used for the treatment of otitis externa when the ear drum is perforated, because of the risk of ototoxicity.

Hypersensitivity to the preparations.

Precautions: Long-term continuous therapy with Dermovate-NN should be avoided, particularly in infants and children, in whom adrenal suppression occurs readily. If Dermovate-NN is required for use in children, it is recommended that the treatment should be reviewed weekly. It should be noted that the infant's napkin may act as an occlusive dressing.

The face, more than other areas of the body, may exhibit atrophic changes after prolonged treatment with potent topical corticosteroids. This must be borne in mind when treating facial conditions which warrant use of Dermovate-NN, and frequent observation of the patient is important. If applied to the eyelids, care is needed to ensure that the preparation does not enter the eye, as glaucoma might result.

If infection persists, systemic chemotherapy is required. Any spread of infection requires withdrawal of topical corticosteroid therapy. Bacterial infection is encouraged by the warm, moist conditions induced by occlusive dressings, and the skin should be cleansed before a fresh dressing is applied.

Topical administration of corticosteroids to pregnant animals can cause abnormalities of fetal development. The relevance of this finding to human beings has not been established; however, topical steroids should not be used extensively in pregnancy, i.e., in large amounts or for prolonged periods.

Side-effects: Provided the weekly dosage is less than 50 g in adults, any pituitary adrenal suppression is likely to be transient with a rapid return to normal values once the short course of steroid therapy has ceased. The same applies to children given proportionate dosage. Use of occlusive dressings increases the absorption of topical corticosteroids.

Prolonged and intensive treatment with highly-active corticosteroid preparations may cause atrophic changes such as striae, thinning of the skin, and dilatation of the superficial blood vessels, particularly when occlusive dressings are used, or where skin folds are involved.

Dermovate-NN is usually well tolerated, but if signs of hypersensitivity appear, application should be stopped immediately.

In rare instances, treatment of psoriasis with corticosteroids (or its withdrawal) is thought to have provoked the pustular form of the disease.

Pharmaceutical precautions None.

Legal category POM.

Package quantities Tubes of 25 g.

Further information The least potent corticosteroid which will control the disease should be selected. Dermovate-NN preparations contain neither lanolin nor parabens.

Product licence numbers

Dermovate-NN Ointment 0004/0237
Dermovate-NN Cream 0004/0255

DIONOSIL* SUSPENSIONS

Presentation Dionosil Aqueous Suspension contains 50% w/v propyliodone. It complies with the BP specification for Propyliodone Suspension.

Dionosil Oily Suspension contains 60% w/v propyliodone in arachis oil. It complies with the BP specification for Propyliodone Oily Suspension.

Uses Radiographic visualisation of the bronchial tree. Propyliodone is distributed on the mucosal surfaces of the bronchi without filling the lumen. Thus, if coughing occurs, alveolar filling is unlikely. Shadows remain well defined for at least 30 minutes; any contrast agent remaining in the lungs usually disappears within three days, but may persist longer in bronchiectatic cavities. It is excreted by the kidneys.

Dosage and administration The volume of Dionosil required is normally 0.75 to 1 ml for each year of age up to a maximum of 18 ml for an adult. The contrast medium is best administered into the trachea, but can be given by the cricothyroid route. The 'over the tongue' route is best avoided with Dionosil Aqueous.

Before use, it is essential to shake the vial vigorously until the propyliodone is completely suspended. This normally takes about half a minute.

The temperature of the suspension should be not lower than room temperature, nor higher than body temperature at the time of instillation. If Dionosil Aqueous is used in an all-glass syringe, it is advisable to lubricate the piston to avoid the slight risk of jamming. Arachis oil is a suitable lubricant.

Contra-indications, warnings, etc

Contra-indications: No absolute contra-indication is known.

Warning: Patients sensitive to iodine may also be sensitive to propyliodone, and the risk involved must be balanced against the importance of the information required. Caution should be exercised in all patients with a history of allergy or hypersensitivity to drugs.

Precautions: As with all bronchographic contrast media, if Dionosil is introduced too rapidly, or the volume is excessive, occlusion of the smaller bronchi can cause lung collapse. Where respiratory function is reduced, as in asthmatics, special care should be taken; if bilateral bronchography is necessary in such patients, it is wise to allow an interval of several days between the investigation of each side. Where respiratory function is normal, it is advisable to allow at least 15 minutes between right-sided and left-sided bronchography in case an immediate hypersensitivity reaction occurs.

Adequate anaesthesia, local and/or general, must be employed in order to suppress the cough reflex. In children under general anaesthesia, Dionosil should be removed from one lung before the other is examined. If inadvertently injected into the tissues, Dionosil is non-irritant, but may be rather persistent.

Administration of iodine-containing media may invalidate PBI determination for 3 to 12 months.

Side-effects: Hypersensitivity reactions are uncommon, but may cause respiratory dysfunction and skin eruptions. Following bronchography with Dionosil there may occur a transient pyrexia sometimes associated with malaise and aching of the joints. The cause is unknown. It has been noted following the use of all bronchographic media but is more common with aqueous than with oily preparations. The symptoms usually subside spontaneously within 48 hours and require no specific treatment. Alveolarisation and atelectasis have been reported.

Overdosage: Remove the Dionosil by postural drainage and/or a bronchoscope. Systemic use of corticosteroids and potent diuretics may be needed if there is excessive effusion of fluid.

Pharmaceutical precautions Protect from light.

Legal category POM.

Package quantities 20 ml vial.

Further information Nil.

Product licence numbers
Dionosil Aqueous Suspension 0004/5097
Dionosil Oily Suspension 0004/5098

EFCORTELAN* SKIN PREPARATIONS

Presentation Efcortelan Cream contains 0.5%, 1% or 2.5% hydrocortisone in a smooth, white, water-miscible cream base.

Efcortelan Ointment contains 0.5%, 1% or 2.5% hydrocortisone in an off-white paraffin-based ointment.

Efcortelan Lotion contains 1% hydrocortisone in a white, aqueous, translucent fluid.

Efcortelan Cream 1% complies with the specification for Hydrocortisone Cream BPC.

Efcortelan Ointments comply with the specification for Hydrocortisone Ointment BP.

Efcortelan Lotion complies with the specification for Hydrocortisone Lotion BPC.

Uses Hydrocortisone has topical anti-inflammatory activity of value in the treatment of a wide variety of dermatological conditions, including the following: eczema, including atopic, infantile, discoid and stasis eczemas; prurigo, neurodermatoses, including lichen simplex, seborrhoeic dermatitis, intertrigo, contact sensitivity reactions; discoid lupus erythematosus, generalised erythroderma.

Efcortelan preparations can also be used in the management of insect bites, sunburn, prickly heat, and otitis externa.

Dosage and administration A small quantity should be applied to the affected area two or three times daily.

Efcortelan Cream is often appropriate for moist or weeping surfaces, and Efcortelan Ointment for dry, lichenified or scaly lesions, but this is not invariably so. Efcortelan Lotion is particularly suitable when a minimal application to a large area is required.

Contra-indications, warnings, etc
Contra-indications: Skin lesions caused by infection with viruses (e.g. herpes simplex, chickenpox), fungi (e.g. candidiasis, tinea) or bacteria (e.g. impetigo). Hypersensitivity to the preparations.

Precautions: In infants and children, long-term continuous topical therapy should be avoided where possible, as adrenal suppression can occur even without occlusion. In infants, the napkin may act as an occlusive dressing, and increase absorption.

Appropriate antimicrobial therapy should be used whenever treating inflammatory lesions which have become infected. Any spread of infection requires withdrawal of topical corticosteroid therapy, and systemic administration of antimicrobial agents.

As with all corticosteroids, prolonged application to the face is undesirable.

Topical administration of corticosteroids to pregnant animals can cause abnormalities of fetal development. The relevance of this finding to human beings has not been established; however, topical steroids should not be used extensively in pregnancy, i.e., in large amounts or for prolonged periods.

Side-effects: Efcortelan preparations are usually well tolerated, but if signs of hypersensitivity appear, application should stop immediately.

Local atrophic changes may occur where skin folds are involved, or in areas such as the nappy area in small children, where constant moist conditions favour the absorption of hydrocortisone. Sufficient systemic absorption may also occur in such sites to produce the features of hypercorticism after prolonged treatment. This effect is more likely to occur in infants and children, and if occlusive dressings are used.

Pharmaceutical precautions None.

Legal category POM.

Package quantities Efcortelan Cream and Ointment 1% are supplied in 15 and 50 g tubes.

Efcortelan Cream and Ointment 0.5% and 2.5% are supplied in 15 g tubes.

Efcortelan Lotion is supplied in 20 ml bottles.

Further information The least potent corticosteroid which will control the disease should be selected. None of these preparations contain lanolin. Efcortelan Cream and Efcortelan Ointment are free from parabens. Efcortelan Lotion contains parabens.

Product licence numbers
Efcortelan Cream 0.5%	0004/5080
Efcortelan Cream 1%	0004/5081
Efcortelan Cream 2.5%	0004/5082
Efcortelan Ointment 0.5%	0004/5085
Efcortelan Ointment 1%	0004/5086
Efcortelan Ointment 2.5%	0004/5087
Efcortelan Lotion 1%	0004/5084

EFCORTELAN* SOLUBLE

Presentation Vials of Efcortelan Soluble contain freeze-dried hydrocortisone sodium succinate as a white plug. Each vial contains 100 mg hydrocortisone as the sodium succinate ester; this readily dissolves in the 2 ml ampoule of Water for Injections supplied with the vial. When prepared as directed, this preparation complies with the specification for Hydrocortisone Sodium Succinate Injection BP.

Uses Status asthmaticus and acute allergic reactions, including anaphylactic reaction to drugs. Efcortelan Soluble supplements the action of adrenaline.

Severe shock arising from surgical or accidental trauma or overwhelming infection.

Adrenal crisis precipitated by abnormal stress in Addison's disease, Simmonds' disease, following adrenalectomy, and when adrenocortical function has been suppressed by prolonged corticosteroid therapy.

Intrathecal injection and adjunctive treatment in tuberculous meningitis and other meningitides.

Note: Efcortelan Soluble does not replace other forms of therapy for the treatment of shock and status asthmaticus.

Dosage and administration For intravenous injection, 100 mg Efcortelan Soluble may be dissolved in 2 ml Water for Injections immediately before administration. Efcortelan Soluble may also be given as an intravenous infusion.

A clinical effect is seen in two to four hours, and it persists for up to eight hours after intravenous injection.

Efcortelan Soluble can be given by intramuscular injection, but the response is likely to be less rapid, especially in shock.

Systemic therapy in adults: 100 to 500 mg administered by slow intravenous injection taking half to one minute. This dose can be repeated three or four times in 24 hours, or as required, depending upon the condition being treated and the patient's response.

Systemic therapy in children: Infants up to 1 year may be given 25 mg hydrocortisone intravenously; children 1 to 5 years, 50 mg; 6 to 12 years, 100 mg.

Other uses: Intrathecal injection. For children, intrathecal doses between 10 and 20 mg, according to age, have been used. A 20 mg dose is suitable for adults. Intrathecal injections may be given daily for a few days if required; then the interval between injections is usually increased. Use of a disposable membrane filter of 0.45 micron pore size is convenient for ensuring clarity of the solution.

Local treatment of soft tissue lesions – up to 200 mg of Efcortelan Soluble can be used.

Contra-indications, warnings, etc
Contra-indications: Systemic infections, unless specific anti-infective therapy is employed. Live virus immunisation. Hypersensitivity to any component of the injection.

Efcortelan Soluble should not be injected directly into tendons.

Precautions: Administration of corticosteroids may impair the ability to resist and counteract infection; in addition, clinical signs and symptoms of infection are suppressed.

In pregnant animals, systemic administration of corticosteroids can cause abnormalities of fetal development. The relevance of this finding to humans has not been established.

Steroids may reduce the effects of anticholinesterases in myasthenia gravis, cholecystographic X-ray media and salicylates.

The effect of steroids may be reduced by phenytoin, phenobarbitone, ephedrine and rifampicin.

Side-effects: In the short term, high levels of hydrocortisone involve little risk of adverse reactions, except that peptic ulceration may occur, or be aggravated. With continued use, signs of hypercorticism may become apparent.

Pharmaceutical precautions Protect from light.

Legal category POM.

Package quantities Vials of 100 mg hydrocortisone with a 2 ml ampoule of Water for Injections.

Further information Each vial provides 8.5 mg (0.37 mmol) of sodium and 0.45 mmol of phosphate (PO_4).

Product licence number 0004/5088.

EFCORTESOL* INJECTION

Presentation Ampoules of Efcortesol Injection contain an aqueous, ready-prepared buffered solution of hydrocortisone sodium phosphate. Each millilitre contains 100 mg hydrocortisone as the sodium phosphate ester. The solution is clear and colourless or pale yellow. Efcortesol Injection complies with the specification for Hydrocortisone Sodium Phosphate Injection BP.

Uses This presentation permits rapid use in emergency situations involving the following conditions.

Status asthmaticus and acute allergic reactions, including anaphylactic reaction to drugs. Efcortesol supplements the action of adrenaline.

Severe shock arising from surgical or accidental trauma or overwhelming infection.

Adrenal crisis precipitated by abnormal stress in Addison's disease, Simmonds' disease, following adrenalectomy, and when adrenocortical function has been suppressed by prolonged corticosteroid therapy.

Soft tissue lesions.

Note: Efcortesol does not replace other forms of therapy for the treatment of shock and status asthmaticus.

Dosage and administration *Systemic therapy in adults:* 100 to 500 mg hydrocortisone (1 to 5 ml) administered by slow intravenous injection, taking at least half to one minute. This dose can be repeated three or four times in 24 hours, or as required, depending upon the condition being treated and the patient's response. Alternatively, Efcortesol injection may be given as an intravenous infusion. A clinical effect is seen in two to four hours, and it persists for up to eight hours after intravenous injection. The same dose can be given by intramuscular injection, but the response is likely to be less rapid, especially in shock.

Systemic therapy in children: As a guide, infants up to 1 year may be given 25 mg hydrocortisone intravenously; children 1 to 5 years, 50 mg; 6 to 12 years, 100 mg (1 ml).

Other uses: Local treatment of soft tissue lesions – 100 to 200 mg.

Efcortesol Injection is not recommended for intrathecal use.

Contra-indications, warnings, etc
Contra-indications: Systemic infections, unless specific anti-infective therapy is employed. Live virus immunisation. Hypersensitivity to any component.

Efcortesol Injection should not be injected directly into tendons.

Precautions: Administration of corticosteroids may impair the ability to resist and counteract infection; in addition clinical signs and symptoms of infection are suppressed. In pregnant animals, systemic administration of corticosteroids can cause abnormalities of fetal development. The relevance of this finding to humans has not been established.

Steroids may reduce the effects of anticholinesterases in myasthenia gravis, cholecystographic X-ray media and salicylates.

The effect of steroids may be reduced by phenytoin, phenobarbitone, ephedrine and rifampicin.

Side-effects: On receiving a bolus dose by intravenous injection, some patients have experienced paraesthesia, often localised in the genital area. The unpleasant sensation usually passes off within a few minutes, and no sequelae have been reported. This effect has not been reported after use of Betnesol Injection or Efcortelan Soluble Injection.

In the short term, high dosage of hydrocortisone involves little risk of adverse reactions, except that peptic ulceration may occur, or be aggravated. With continued use, signs of hypercorticism may become apparent.

Pharmaceutical precautions Protect from light.

Legal category POM.

Package quantities Ampoules 1 ml (100 mg) in box of 5.

Ampoules 5 ml (500 mg) in box of 10.

Further information It should be noted that 10 ml Efcortesol Injection contains 152 mg (6.6 mmol) sodium and 298 mg (28.2 mmol) phosphate (PO_4).

Product licence number 0004/5089.

ELTROXIN* TABLETS

Presentation Small white tablets engraved 'Eltroxin 50 Glaxo' or 'Eltroxin 100 Glaxo' containing 50 micrograms (0.05 mg) or 100 micrograms (0.1 mg) anhydrous thyroxine sodium respectively. The lower-strength tablets are scored. Eltroxin Tablets comply with the specification for Thyroxine Tablets BP.

Uses Hypothyroidism.

Dosage and administration *Adults:* Initially 50 to 100 micrograms daily, preferably taken before breakfast, and adjusted at three to four week intervals by 50 micrograms until normal metabolism is steadily maintained; this may require doses of 150 to 300 micrograms daily. With patients aged over 50 years, it is not advisable to exceed 50 micrograms a day initially, and where there is cardiac disease, 25 micrograms daily, or 50 micrograms on alternate days, is more suitable. In this condition the daily dosage may be increased by 25 micrograms at intervals of perhaps four weeks.

In younger patients, and in the absence of heart disease, a serum thyroxine (T4) level of about 70 to 160 nanomols per litre, or a serum thyrotrophin level of less than 5 milli-units per litre, should be aimed at. In those aged over 50, and/or in the presence of heart disease, clinical response is probably a more acceptable criterion of dosage than serum levels.

A pre-therapy ECG is valuable, as changes induced by hypothyroidism may be confused with ECG evidence of ischaemia. If too rapid an increase of metabolism is produced (causing diarrhoea, nervousness, rapid pulse, insomnia, tremors and sometimes anginal pain where there is latent myocardial ischaemia) dosage must be reduced or withheld for a day or two, then begun again at a lower level.

Cretinism and juvenile myxoedema: The largest dose consistent with freedom from toxic effects should be given. Clinically, normal pulse rate and absence of diarrhoea or constipation are the most useful indications. For cretinous infants, a suitable starting dose is 25 micrograms Eltroxin daily, with increments of 25 micrograms every two to four weeks until mild toxic symptoms appear. Dosage is then slightly reduced. The same applies to juvenile myxoedema, except that the starting dose for children older than one year may be 2.5 to 5 micrograms/kg/day.

Contra-indications, warnings, etc
Contra-indications: Thyrotoxicosis. Hypersensitivity to any component.

Precautions: Patients with panhypopituitarism or other causes predisposing to adrenal insufficiency may react unfavourably to thyroxine treatment, and it is advisable to initiate corticosteroid therapy before giving thyroxine in these cases.

Especial care is needed when there are symptoms of myocardial insufficiency or ECG evidence of myocardial infarction.

Side-effects: The following effects are indicative of excessive dosage, and usually disappear on reduction of dosage or withdrawal of treatment for a few days. Anginal pain, cardiac arrhythmias, palpitation, and cramps in skeletal muscle; also tachycardia, diarrhoea, restlessness, excitability, headache, flushing, sweating, excessive loss of weight and muscular weakness.

Overdosage: Gastric lavage or emesis is required if the patient is seen within several hours of taking the dose. The appearance of clinical hyperthyroidism may be delayed for up to five days. Treatment is symptomatic, and tachycardia has been controlled in an adult by 40 mg doses of propranolol given every six hours.

Pharmaceutical precautions Protect from light.

Legal category POM.

Package quantities Bottles of 100 and 1,000 tablets.

Further information 100 micrograms thyroxine is equivalent in activity to 20 to 30 micrograms liothyronine or 60 mg Thyroid BP.

Product licence numbers
Tablets 50 micrograms   0004/5018
Tablets 100 micrograms   0004/5019

EUMOVATE* CREAM AND OINTMENT

Presentation Eumovate Cream and Ointment contain 0.05% clobetasone butyrate, and are white in appearance. The emollient cream is water-miscible, whilst the ointment has a paraffin base.

Uses Clobetasone butyrate is a topically active corticosteroid which provides an exceptional combination of activity and safety. When formulated as Eumovate it is more effective in the treatment of eczemas than 1% hydrocortisone, or the less-active synthetic steroid preparations that are in common use, yet has little effect on hypothalamic-pituitary-adrenal function. This has been so even when Eumovate was applied to adults in large amounts under whole-body occlusion. All topical corticosteroids can cause cutaneous atrophy if grossly misused. However, studies in animal and human models indicate that Eumovate and hydrocortisone cause less thinning of the epidermis than the other topical steroids tested.

Eumovate is suitable for treating the milder forms of eczema, seborrhoeic dermatitis, and other steroid responsive skin conditions, e.g., sunburn, which do not require the use of a more active topical corticosteroid. In the more resistant dermatoses, Eumovate may be used as maintenance therapy between courses of one of the more active topical steroids.

Use of Eumovate is particularly appropriate when treating infants and young children, who are more liable to experience undesirable effects after prolonged application of steroid preparations than are older patients. Eumovate may be used as the standard corticosteroid treatment for napkin rash, seborrhoeic dermatitis and atopic eczema, reserving the more potent preparations for use in short courses on resistant areas.

Dosage and administration Eumovate should be applied to the affected area up to four times a day until improvement occurs, when the frequency of application may be reduced.

Contra-indications, warnings, etc
Contra-indications: Skin lesions caused by infection with viruses (e.g., herpes simplex, chickenpox), fungi (e.g., candidiasis, tinea) or bacteria (e.g., impetigo). Hypersensitivity to the preparations.

Precautions: In infants and children, long-term continuous topical corticosteroid therapy should be avoided where possible, as adrenal suppression can occur even without occlusion. In infants, the napkin may act as an occlusive dressing, and increase absorption.

Appropriate antimicrobial therapy should be used whenever treating inflammatory lesions which have become infected. Any spread of infection requires withdrawal of topical corticosteroid therapy, and systemic administration of antimicrobial agents.

As with all corticosteroids, prolonged application to the face is undesirable.

Topical administration of corticosteroids to pregnant animals can cause abnormalities of fetal development. The relevance of this finding to human beings has not been established; however, topical steroids should not be used extensively in pregnancy, i.e., in large amounts or for prolonged periods.

Side-effects: In the unlikely event of signs of hypersensitivity appearing, application should stop immediately. When large areas of the body are being treated with Eumovate it is possible that some patients will absorb sufficient steroid to cause transient adrenal depression despite the low degree of systemic activity associated with clobetasone butyrate.

Local atrophic changes could possibly occur in situations where moisture increases absorption of clobetasone butyrate, but only after prolonged use.

Pharmaceutical precautions None.

Legal category POM.

Package quantities Tubes of 25 and 100 g.

Further information The least potent corticosteroid which will control the disease should be selected. Neither of these preparations contain lanolin or parabens.

Product licence numbers
Eumovate Cream   0004/0233
Eumovate Ointment   0004/0254

EUMOVATE* EYE DROPS ▼

Presentation Eumovate Drops contain clobetasone 17-butyrate 0.1% w/v, with benzalkonium chloride 0.01% w/v as a preservative, as an off-white suspension that is sterile until the bottle is opened.

Uses Eumovate Eye Drops are indicated for the treatment of non-infected inflammatory conditions of the eye including diseases of the external eye and of the anterior segments. In these conditions it has been shown

to have comparable anti-inflammatory activity to Betamethasone Sodium Phosphate Eye Drops.

Eumovate Eye Drops have less adverse effect on intraocular pressure than hydrocortisone (1%), betamethasone sodium phosphate (0.1%), prednisolone sodium phosphate (0.5%), or dexamethasone (0.1%) eye drops.

Dosage and administration The usual dosage is one or two drops four times a day; for severe inflammatory conditions one or two drops should be instilled into the eye every one or two hours until signs of improvement are apparent, when the frequency may be reduced.

Contra-indications, warnings, etc
Contra-indications: Viral, fungal, tuberculous, or purulent conditions. Use in the eye is contra-indicated if glaucoma is present or where herpetic keratitis (dendritic ulcer) is considered a possibility. Inadvertent use of topical steroids in the latter condition can lead to the enlargement of the ulcer and marked visual deterioration. Hypersensitivity to the preparation.

Eumovate Eye Drops contain benzalkonium chloride as a preservative and therefore should not be used to treat patients who wear soft contact lenses.

Precautions: Although Eumovate Eye Drops have been shown to have little adverse effect on intra-ocular pressure in most patients, those patients receiving long term treatment should have their intra-ocular pressure monitored frequently.

Cataract is reported to have occurred after unduly prolonged treatment with some topical corticosteroids and in those diseases which cause thinning of the cornea, perforation has been known to occur.

Topical administration of corticosteroids to pregnant animals can cause abnormalities of fetal development. The relevance of this finding to human beings has not been established; however, topical steroids should not be used extensively in pregnancy, i.e. in large amounts or for prolonged periods.

Side-effects: Rises in intra-ocular pressure have been reported in susceptible patients but these are generally much less than with other corticosteroid eye preparations, including hydrocortisone.

Pharmaceutical precautions The contents should not be used more than four weeks after first opening the bottle.

Legal category POM.

Package quantities Plastic dropper bottles containing 5 or 10 ml.

Further information Nil.

Product licence number 0004/0260.

EUMOVATE*-N EYE DROPS ▼

Presentation Eumovate-N Drops contain clobetasone 17-butyrate 0.1%, and neomycin sulphate 0.5% w/v, with benzalkonium chloride 0.01% w/v as a preservative, as an off-white suspension that is sterile until the bottle is opened.

Uses Eumovate-N Eye Drops are indicated for the treatment of inflammatory conditions of the eye where secondary bacterial infection is likely to occur. In these conditions it has been shown to have comparable anti-inflammatory activity to Betamethasone Sodium Phosphate with Neomycin Eye Drops.

Eumovate-N Eye Drops have less adverse effect on intra-ocular pressure than hydrocortisone (1%), betamethasone sodium phosphate (0.1%), prednisolone sodium phosphate (0.5%), or dexamethasone (0.1%) eye drops.

Dosage and administration The usual dosage is one or two drops four times a day; for severe inflammatory conditions one or two drops should be instilled into the eye every one or two hours until signs of improvement are apparent, when the frequency may be reduced.

Contra-indications, warnings, etc
Contra-indications: Viral, fungal or tuberculous conditions; use in the eye is contra-indicated if purulent infection or glaucoma is present. Inadvertent use in herpetic keratitis (dendritic ulcer) can lead to the enlargement of the ulcer and marked visual deterioration. Hypersensitivity to any component of the preparation.

Eumovate-N Eye Drops contain benzalkonium chloride as a preservative and therefore should not be used to treat patients who wear soft contact lenses.

Precautions: Although Eumovate-N Eye Drops have been shown to have little adverse effect on intra-ocular pressure in most patients, those patients receiving long term treatment should have their intra-ocular pressure monitored frequently.

Cataract is reported to have occurred after unduly prolonged treatment with some topical corticosteroids and in those diseases which cause thinning of the cornea, perforation has been known to occur.

Topical administration of corticosteroids to pregnant animals can cause abnormalities of fetal development. The relevance of this finding to human beings has not been established; however, topical steroids should not be used extensively in pregnancy, i.e. in large amounts or for prolonged periods.

The unnecessary topical use of neomycin containing products should be avoided in order to minimise the occurrence of neomycin-resistant organisms (and organisms cross-resistant to other aminoglycosides).

Side-effects: Rises in intra-ocular pressure have been reported in susceptible patients but these are generally much less than with other corticosteroid eye preparations, including hydrocortisone.

Acute sensitisation to neomycin is a rare event but can occur after topical application to the eye.

Pharmaceutical precautions The contents should not be used more than four weeks after first opening the bottle.

Legal category POM.

Package quantities Plastic dropper bottles containing 5 or 10 ml.

Further information Nil.

Product licence number 0004/0276.

FORTUM FOR INJECTION ▼

Presentation Fortum for Injection is supplied as a white to faintly yellow powder in vials containing 250 mg, 500 mg, 1 g and 2 g ceftazidime (as pentahydrate) with sodium carbonate (118 mg per gram of ceftazidime). On the addition of Water for Injections, Fortum for Injection dissolves with effervescence to produce a solution for injection.

Fortum for Injection contains approximately 52 mg

(2.3 mmol) of sodium per gram of ceftazidime. 116 mg ceftazidime pentahydrate is equivalent to 100 mg ceftazidime free acid. For laboratory tests associated with ceftazidime administration, use ceftazidime pentahydrate obtainable on request from Glaxo.

Uses Ceftazidime is a bactericidal cephalosporin antibiotic which is resistant to most beta-lactamases and is active against a wide range of Gram-positive and Gram-negative bacteria.

It is indicated for the treatment of single infections and for mixed infections caused by two or more susceptible organisms.

Ceftazidime, because of its broad antibacterial spectrum, may be used alone as first choice drug, pending sensitivity test results.

In meningitis it is recommended that the results of a sensitivity test are known before treatment with ceftazidime as a single agent. It may be used for infections caused by organisms resistant to other antibiotics including aminoglycosides and many cephalosporins. When appropriate, however, it may be used safely in combination with an aminoglycoside or other beta-lactam antibiotic, for example in the presence of severe neutropenia, or with an antibiotic active against anaerobes when the presence of *Bacteroides fragilis* is suspected (see Pharmaceutical precautions).
Indications include:
Severe infections in general: for example, septicaemia, bacteraemia, peritonitis, meningitis, infections in immunosuppressed patients with haematological or solid malignancies, and in patients in intensive care units with specific problems, e.g., infected burns.
Respiratory tract infections: for example, pneumonia, bronchopneumonia, infected pleurisy, empyema, lung abscess, infected bronchiectasis and bronchitis and in lung infections in patients with cystic fibrosis.
Ear, nose and throat infections: for example, otitis media, malignant otitis externa, mastoiditis, sinusitis and other severe ear and throat infections.
Urinary tract infections: for example, acute and chronic pyelonephritis, pyelitis, prostatitis, cystitis, urethritis (bacterial only), renal abscess, and infections associated with bladder and renal stones.
Skin and soft tissue infections: for example, erysipelas, abscesses, cellulitis, infected burns and wounds, mastitis, skin ulcers.
Gastrointestinal, biliary and abdominal infections: for example, cholangitis, cholecystitis, empyema of gall bladder, intra-abdominal abscesses, peritonitis, diverticulitis, enterocolitis, post-partum and pelvic inflammatory conditions.
Bone and joint infections: for example, osteitis, osteomyelitis, septic arthritis, infected bursitis.
Dialysis: infections associated with haemo- and peritoneal dialysis and with continuous ambulatory peritoneal dialysis (CAPD).
Bacteriology:
Ceftazidime is bactericidal in action, exerting its effect on target cell wall proteins and causing inhibition of cell wall synthesis. A wide range of pathogenic strains and isolates associated with hospital-acquired infections are susceptible to ceftazidime *in vitro*, including strains resistant to gentamicin and other aminoglycosides. It is highly stable to most clinically important beta-lactamases produced by both Gram-positive and Gram-negative organisms and consequently is active against many ampicillin- and cephalothin-resistant strains. Ceftazidime has high intrinsic activity *in vitro* and acts within

a narrow MIC range for most genera with minimal changes in MIC at varied inoculum levels. Ceftazidime has been shown to have *in vitro* activity against the following organisms:

Gram-negative:
Pseudomonas aeruginosa, Pseudomonas spp. (other), *Klebsiella pneumoniac,* Klebsiella spp. (other), *Proteus mirabilis, Proteus vulgaris, Morganella morganii* (formerly *Proteus morganii), Proteus rettgeri,* Providencia spp., *Escherichia coli,* Enterobacter spp., Citrobacter spp., Serratia spp., Salmonella spp., Shigella spp., *Yersinia enterocolitica, Pasteurella multocida,* Acinetobacter spp., *Neisseria gonorrhoeae, Neisseria meningitidis, Haemophilus influenzae* (including ampicillin-resistant strains), *Haemophilus parainfluenzae* (including ampicillin-resistant strains).

Gram-positive:
Staphylococcus aureus (methicillin-sensitive strains), *Staphylococcus epidermidis* (methicillin-sensitive strains), Micrococcus spp., *Streptococcus pyogenes,* Streptococcus Group B, *Streptococcus pneumoniae, Streptococcus mitis,* Streptococcus spp. (excluding *Streptococcus faecalis*).

Anaerobic strains:
Peptococcus spp., Peptostreptococcus spp., Streptococcus spp., Propionibacterium spp., *Clostridium perfringens,* Fusobacterium spp., Bacteroides spp. (many strains of *Bact. fragilis* are resistant). Ceftazidime is not active *in vitro* against methicillin-resistant staphylococci, *Streptococcus faecalis* and many other Enterococci, *Listeria monocytogenes,* Campylobacter spp. or *Clostridium difficile.*

In vitro the activities of ceftazidime and aminoglycoside antibiotics in combination have been shown to be at least additive; there is evidence of synergy in some strains tested. This property may be important in the treatment of febrile neutropenic patients.

Dosage and administration *General dosage recommendations:* Ceftazidime is to be used by the parenteral route, the dosage depending upon the severity, sensitivity and type of infection and the age, weight and renal function of the patient.

Adults: The adult dosage range for ceftazidime is 1 to 6 g per day: for instance, 500 mg, 1 g or 2 g given 12 or 8-hourly by i.v. or i.m. injection. In urinary tract infections and in many less serious infections, 500 mg or 1 g 12-hourly is usually adequate. In the majority of infections, 1 g 8-hourly or 2 g 12-hourly should be given. In very severe infections, especially in immunocompromised patients, including those with neutropenia, 2 g 8 or 12-hourly should be administered.

Cystic fibrosis: In fibrocystic adults with normal renal function who have pseudomonal lung infections, high doses of 100 to 150 mg/kg/day as three divided doses should be used. In adults with normal renal function 9 g/day has been used safely.

Infants and children: The usual dosage range for children aged over two months is 30 to 100 mg/kg/day, given as two or three divided doses.

The dosage for children aged over 2 months but under 1 year is generally 25 to 50 mg/kg twice daily. Doses up to 50 mg/kg three times per day, to a maximum of 6 g daily, may be given to infected immunocompromised or fibrocystic children or to children with meningitis.

Neonates and children up to 2 months of age: Whilst clinical experience is limited, a dose of 25 to 60 mg/kg/day given as two divided doses has proved to be effective. In the neonate the serum half-life of ceftazidime can be three to four times that in adults.

Recommended maintenance doses of ceftazidime in renal insufficiency

Creatinine clearance ml/min	Approx. Serum creatinine* μmol/l (mg/dl)	Recommended Unit dose of ceftazidime g	Frequency of dosing hourly
50–31	150–200 (1.7–2.3)	1.0	12
30–16	200–350 (2.3–4.0)	1.0	24
15–6	350–500 (4.0–5.6)	0.5	24
⩽5	>500 (5.6)	0.5	48

*These values are guide-lines and may not accurately predict renal function in all patients especially in the elderly in whom the serum creatinine concentration may overestimate renal function.

Dosage in impaired renal function: Ceftazidime is excreted by the kidneys almost exclusively by glomerular filtration. Therefore, in patients with impaired renal function it is recommended that the dosage of ceftazidime should be reduced to compensate for its slower excretion, except in mild impairment, i.e., glomerular filtration rate (GFR) greater than 50 ml/min. In patients with suspected renal insufficiency, an initial loading dose of 1 g of ceftazidime may be given. An estimate of GFR should be made to determine the appropriate maintenance dose.

Recommended maintenance doses are shown above.

In patients with severe infections, especially in neutropenics, who would normally receive 6 g of ceftazidime daily were it not for renal insufficiency, the unit dose given in the table above may be increased by 50% or the dosing frequency increased appropriately. In such patients it is recommended that ceftazidime serum levels should be monitored and trough levels should not exceed 40 mg/litre.

When only serum creatinine is available, the following formula (Cockcroft's equation) may be used to estimate creatinine clearance. The serum creatinine should represent a steady state of renal function:

Males:

$$\text{Creatinine clearance (ml/min)} = \frac{\text{Weight (kg)} \times (140 - \text{age in years})}{72 \times \text{serum creatinine (mg/dl)}}$$

Females:
0.85 × above value.
To convert serum creatinine in μmol/litre into mg/dl divide by 88.4.

In children the creatinine clearance should be adjusted for body surface area or lean body mass and the dosing frequency reduced in cases of renal insufficiency as for adults.

The serum half-life of ceftazidime during haemodialysis ranges from 3 to 5 hours. The appropriate maintenance dose of ceftazidime should be repeated following each haemodialysis period.

Dosage in peritoneal dialysis: Ceftazidime may also be used in peritoneal dialysis and continuous ambulatory

Table   Preparation of Solution

Vial Size		Amount of Diluent to be added (ml)	Approximate Concentration (mg/ml)
250 mg	intramuscular	1.0 ml	200
250 mg	intravenous	2.5 ml	90
500 mg	intramuscular	1.5 ml	250
500 mg	intravenous	5 ml	90
1 g	intramuscular	3 ml	250
1 g	intravenous	10 ml	90
2 g	intravenous bolus	10 ml	170
2 g	intravenous infusion	50 ml*	40

*NOTE: Addition should be in two stages (see text).

peritoneal dialysis (CAPD). As well as using ceftazidime intravenously, it can be incorporated into the dialysis fluid (usually 125 to 250 mg for 2 L of dialysis fluid).

Administration: Ceftazidime may be given intravenously or by deep intramuscular injection into a large muscle mass such as the upper outer quadrant of the gluteus maximus or lateral part of the thigh.

Instructions for reconstitution: See table for addition volumes and solution concentrations, which may be useful when fractional doses are required.

All sizes of vials as supplied are under reduced pressure. As the product dissolves, carbon dioxide is released and a positive pressure develops. For ease of use, it is recommended that the following techniques of reconstitution are adopted.

250 mg i.m./i.v., 500 mg i.m./i.v., 1 g i.m./i.v. and 2 g i.v. bolus vials:

1. Insert the syringe needle through the vial closure and inject the recommended volume of diluent. The vacuum may assist entry of the diluent. Remove the syringe needle.
2. Shake to dissolve: carbon dioxide is released and a clear solution obtained in about 1 to 2 minutes.
3. Invert the vial. With the syringe plunger fully depressed, insert the needle through the vial closure and withdraw the total volume of solution into the syringe (the pressure in the vial may aid withdrawal). Ensure that the needle remains within the solution and does not enter the headspace. The withdrawn solution may contain small bubbles of carbon dioxide; they may be disregarded.

2 g i.v. infusion vial:

This vial may be reconstituted for short intravenous infusion (e.g., up to 30 minutes) as follows:

1. Insert the syringe needle through the vial closure and inject 10 ml of diluent. The vacuum may assist entry of the diluent. Remove the syringe needle.
2. Shake to dissolve; carbon dioxide is released and a clear solution obtained in about 1 to 2 minutes.
3. Insert a gas relief needle through the vial closure to relieve the internal pressure and, with the gas relief in position, add a further 40 ml of diluent. Remove the gas relief needle and syringe needle; shake the vial and set up for infusion use in the normal way.

NOTE: To preserve product sterility, it is important that a gas relief needle is *not* inserted through the vial closure before the product has dissolved.

These solutions may be given directly into the vein or introduced into the tubing of a giving set if the patient is receiving parenteral fluids. Ceftazidime is compatible with the most commonly used intravenous fluids (see Pharmaceutical precautions).

Contra-indications Ceftazidime is contra-indicated in patients with known hypersensitivity to cephalosporin antibiotics.

Warnings: As with other beta-lactam antibiotics, before therapy with ceftazidime is instituted, careful inquiry should be made for a history of hypersensitivity reactions to ceftazidime, cephalosporins, penicillins, or other drugs. Ceftazidime should be given only with special caution to patients with type I or immediate hypersensitivity reactions to penicillin. If an allergic reaction to ceftazidime occurs, discontinue the drug. Serious hypersensitivity reactions may require epinephrine (adrenaline), hydrocortisone, antihistamine or other emergency measures.

Precautions Cephalosporin antibiotics at high dosage should be given with caution to patients receiving concurrent treatment with nephrotoxic drugs, e.g., aminoglycoside antibiotics, or potent diuretics such as frusemide, as these combinations are suspected of affecting renal function adversely. Clinical experience with ceftazidime has shown that this is not likely to be a problem at the recommended dose levels. There is no evidence that ceftazidime adversely affects renal function at normal therapeutic doses: however, as for all antibiotics eliminated via the kidneys, it is necessary to reduce the dosage according to the degree of reduction in renal function (see Dosage in Impaired Renal Function).

There is no experimental evidence of embryopathic or teratogenic effects attributable to ceftazidime but, as with all drugs, it should be administered with caution during the early months of pregnancy and in early infancy. Use in pregnancy requires that the anticipated benefit be weighed against the possible risks. Ceftazidime is excreted in human milk in low concentrations and consequently caution should be exercised when ceftazidime is administered to a nursing mother.

Ceftazidime does not interfere with enzyme-based tests for glycosuria. Slight interference with copper reduction methods (Benedict's, Fehling's, Clinitest) may be observed. Ceftazidime does not interfere in the alkaline picrate assay for creatinine.

The development of a positive Coombs' test associated with the use of ceftazidime in about 5% of patients may interfere with the cross-matching of blood.

As with other broad spectrum antibiotics, prolonged use of ceftazidime may result in the overgrowth of non-susceptible organisms (e.g., Candida, Enterococci) which may require interruption of treatment or adoption of appropriate measures. Repeated evaluation of the patient's condition is essential.

Side effects: Clinical trial experience has shown that ceftazidime is generally well tolerated.

Adverse reactions are infrequent and include:

Local: phlebitis or thrombophlebitis with i.v. administration; pain and/or inflammation after i.m. injection.

Hypersensitivity: maculopapular or urticarial rash, fever, pruritus, and very rarely angioedema and anaphylaxis (bronchospasm and/or hypotension).

Gastrointestinal: diarrhoea, nausea, vomiting, abdominal pain, and very rarely oral thrush or colitis.

Other adverse events which may be related to ceftazidime therapy or of uncertain aetiology include:

Genito-urinary: candidosis, vaginitis.
Central Nervous System: headache, dizziness, paraesthesiae and bad taste.

Laboratory test changes noted transiently during ceftazidime therapy include: eosinophilia, positive Coombs' test without haemolysis, thrombocytosis and slight elevations in one or more of the hepatic enzymes, ALT (SGPT), AST (SGOT), LDH, GGT and alkaline phosphatase. As with some other cephalosporins, transient elevations of blood urea, blood urea nitrogen and/or serum creatinine have been observed occasionally. Very rarely, transient leucopenia, neutropenia, thrombocytopenia and lymphocytosis have been seen.

Overdosage: Serum levels of ceftazidime are reduced by dialysis.

Pharmaceutical precautions Vials of Fortum for Injection as supplied are under reduced pressure; a positive pressure is produced on reconstitution due to the release of carbon dioxide. See Administration section above for recommended techniques of reconstitution.

Vials of Fortum for Injection should be stored at a temperature below 25°C. Occasional storage at temperatures not higher than 30°C for up to 2 months is not detrimental to the product.

Vials of Fortum for Injection do not contain any preservatives and should be used as single-dose preparations.

In keeping with good pharmaceutical practice it is preferable to use freshly constituted solutions of Fortum for Injection. If this is not practicable, satisfactory potency is retained for 18 hours at room temperature (below 25°C) when prepared in Water for Injections BP or any of the injections listed below.

At ceftazidime concentrations between 1 mg/ml and 40 mg/ml in:
0.9% Sodium Chloride Injection BP
M/6 Sodium Lactate Injection BP
Compound Sodium Lactate Injection BP (Hartmann's Solution)
5% Dextrose Injection BP
0.225% Sodium Chloride and 5% Dextrose Injection BP
0.45% Sodium Chloride and 5% Dextrose Injection BP
0.9% Sodium Chloride and 5% Dextrose Injection BP
0.18% Sodium Chloride and 4% Dextrose Injection BP
10% Dextrose Injection BP
Dextran 40 Injection BP 10% in 0.9% Sodium Chloride Injection BP
Dextran 40 Injection BP 10% in 5% Dextrose Injection BP
Dextran 70 Injection BP 6% in 0.9% Sodium Chloride Injection BP
Dextran 70 Injection BP 6% in 5% Dextrose Injection BP
(Ceftazidime is less stable in Sodium Bicarbonate Injection than in other intravenous fluids. It is not recommended as a diluent.)

At concentrations of between 0.05 mg/ml and 0.25 mg/ml in Intraperitoneal Dialysis Fluid (Lactate) BPC 1973.

When reconstituted for intramuscular use with 0.5% or 1% Lignocaine Hydrochloride Injection BP

When admixed at 4 mg/ml with: (both components retain satisfactory potency)
Hydrocortisone (hydrocortisone sodium phosphate)

1 mg/ml in 0.9% Sodium Chloride Injection BP or 5% Dextrose Injection BP
Cefuroxime (cefuroxime sodium) 3 mg/ml in 0.9% Sodium Chloride Injection BP
Cloxacillin (cloxacillin sodium) 4 mg/ml in 0.9% Sodium Chloride Injection BP
Heparin 10 u/ml or 50 u/ml in 0.9% Sodium Chloride Injection BP
Potassium Chloride 10 mEq/l or 40 mEq/l in 0.9% Sodium Chloride Injection BP

The contents of a 500 mg vial of Fortum for Injection, reconstituted with 1.5 ml Water for Injections, may be added to metronidazole injection (500 mg in 100 ml) and both retain their activity. Ceftazidime and aminoglycosides should not be mixed in the same giving set or syringe.

Solutions range from light yellow to amber depending on concentration, diluent and storage conditions used. Within the stated recommendations, product potency is not adversely affected by such colour variations.

Legal category POM.

Package quantities Individually cartoned vials containing 250 mg, 500 mg or 1 g ceftazidime (as pentahydrate) for intramuscular or intravenous use in packs of 5.

Individually cartoned vials containing 2 g ceftazidime (as pentahydrate) for intravenous injection in packs of 5.

Individually cartoned vials containing 2 g ceftazidime (as pentahydrate) for intravenous infusion in packs of 5.

Further information Ceftazidime administered by the parenteral route reaches high and prolonged serum levels. In man after intramuscular administration of 500 mg and 1 g, serum mean peak levels of 18 and 37 mg/litre respectively are rapidly achieved. Five minutes after an intravenous bolus injection of 500 mg, 1 g or 2 g, serum mean levels are respectively 46, 87 and 170 mg/litre.

Therapeutically effective concentrations are still found in the serum 8 to 12 hours after both intravenous and intramuscular administration. The serum half-life is about 1.8 hours in normal volunteers and about 2.2 hours in patients with apparently normal renal function. The serum protein binding of ceftazidime is low at about 10%.

Ceftazidime is not metabolised in the body and is excreted unchanged in the active form into the urine by glomerular filtration. Approximately 80 to 90% of the dose is recovered in the urine within 24 hours. Less than 1% is excreted via the bile, significantly limiting the amount entering the bowel.

Concentrations of ceftazidime in excess of the minimum inhibitory levels for common pathogens can be achieved in tissues such as bone, heart, bile, sputum, aqueous humour, synovial and pleural and peritoneal fluids. Transplacental transfer of the antibiotic readily occurs. Ceftazidime penetrates the intact blood brain barrier poorly and low levels are achieved in the CSF in the absence of inflammation. Therapeutic levels of 4 to 20 mg/litre or more are achieved in the CSF when the meninges are inflamed.

Product licence numbers
250 mg vials   0004/0304
500 mg vials   0004/0292

1 gram vials   0004/0293
2 gram vials   0004/0294

GRISOVIN* TABLETS

Presentation Grisovin Tablets contain 125 mg or 500 mg of the antibiotic griseofulvin in fine particle form. Both are white, film-coated, bi-convex tablets engraved 'Grisovin 125' or 'Grisovin 500' on one side as appropriate and 'Glaxo' on the other. They comply with the specification for Griseofulvin Tablets BP.

Uses The treatment of fungal infections of the skin, scalp, hair or nails where topical therapy is considered inappropriate or has failed. When griseofulvin is given orally for systemic treatment of ringworm infections, it enables newly formed keratin of the skin, hair and nails to resist attack by the fungi. As the new keratin extends, the old infected keratin is shed.

Grisovin is effective against the dermatophytes causing ringworm (tinea), including *Microsporum canis, Trichophyton rubrum* and *T. verrucosum.*

Grisovin is not effective in infections caused by *Candida albicans* (monilia), Aspergilli, *Malassezia furfur (Pityriasis versicolor)* and Nocardia species.

Dosage and administration Doses should be taken after meals, otherwise absorption is likely to be inadequate.

Adults: Normally 500 to 1,000 mg daily, but not less than 10 mg/kg body weight daily. A single dose daily is often satisfactory, but divided doses may be more effective in patients who respond poorly.

Children: Usually 10 mg per kg (5 mg/lb) body weight daily in divided doses.

Duration of treatment: This depends upon the thickness of keratin at the site of infection. For hair or skin at least four weeks' treatment is required, whereas toe or finger nails may need six to twelve months' treatment. Therapy should be continued for at least two weeks after all signs of infection have disappeared.

Contra-indications, warnings, etc
Contra-indications: Porphyria or severe liver disease. Griseofulvin may cause liver disease to deteriorate, and liver function should be monitored in such conditions.

Systemic lupus erythematosus: Griseofulvin has been reported to exacerbate the condition.

Precautions: Griseofulvin may decrease the effect of the coumarin anticoagulants.

Griseofulvin has also been reported as interfering with the efficacy of oral contraceptives.

Absorption of griseofulvin is inhibited when phenobarbitone is taken concurrently. The blood level, and hence efficacy, of griseofulvin may also be impaired as the result of concurrent administration of substances such as phenylbutazone and sedative and hypnotic drugs which induce metabolising enzymes.

Photosensitivity reactions can occur on exposure to intense natural or artificial sunlight.

In those rare cases where individuals are affected by drowsiness whilst taking griseofulvin, they should not drive vehicles or operate machinery. Patients should be warned that an enhancement of the effects of alcohol by griseofulvin has been reported.

Griseofulvin administered at high dosages to rats during pregnancy has been associated with fetotoxicity and tail deformities. There is no evidence of its safety in human pregnancy and therefore griseofulvin should not be used in pregnancy.

Long-term administration of high doses of griseofulvin with food has been reported to induce hepatomas in mice and thyroid tumours in rats but not hamsters. The clinical significance of these findings is not known. In view of these data, griseofulvin tablets should not be used prophylactically.

No additional precautions are necessary in the elderly.

Side-effects: Headache and gastric discomfort sometimes occur, but usually disappear as treatment continues. On rare occasions urticarial reactions, erythematous rashes and precipitation of systemic lupus erythematosus have been reported.

Overdosage: Treatment is unlikely to be required in cases of acute overdosage.

Pharmaceutical precautions None.

Legal category POM.

Package quantities *125 mg tablets:* Bottles of 100 tablets.
500 mg tablets: Bottles of 100 tablets.

Further information Customary hygienic measures should be adopted to minimise the risk of re-infection, and concurrent use of a topical fungicide may be helpful to minimise any spread of infective material.

Product licence numbers
Grisovin Tablets 125 mg   0004/5060
Grisovin Tablets 500 mg   0004/5061

MYODIL*

Presentation Ampoules containing Iophendylate Injection BP, a colourless to pale yellow viscous liquid which darkens on exposure to light. It contains 30% of organically combined iodine, has a density of approximately 1.26 g/ml, and is immiscible with cerebrospinal fluid.

Uses Myelography.
Ventriculography; Visualisation of the third and fourth ventricles and the aqueduct of Sylvius.
Intra-uterine use; To outline the fetus prior to intra-uterine blood transfusion.

Dosage and administration *Myelography:* In general, sufficient Myodil is introduced into the spinal subarachnoid space to allow all the structures under suspicion to be outlined by simple posturing of the patient. Usually 6 to 9 ml are ample, and if complete block is present, a smaller volume is adequate. Occasionally up to 18 ml are necessary if the subarachnoid space is wide. The material should be removed by aspiration after the examination unless it is required for further study.

Ventriculography: Good visualisation of the third and fourth ventricles and the aqueduct of Sylvius can be obtained by use of Myodil. The amount injected into the selected lateral ventricle is usually 1 to 1.6 ml, but the dose can range from 0.5 ml to 2 ml according to circumstances.

Intra-uterine use: 9 ml of Myodil has been injected into the amniotic sac to outline the fetus prior to intra-uterine blood transfusion.

Contra-indications, warnings, etc
Contra-indications: As for simple lumbar puncture,

Myodil should not be used when there is a history of reaction to iophendylate or to iodine. The procedure should be postponed if there is blood or bilirubin in the spinal fluid.

Warnings: Myodil should NOT be emulsified with cerebrospinal fluid, as this is reported to increase the frequency of toxic reactions. If Myodil enters the blood stream, it can cause shock and violent coughing.

When myelography has to be performed during pregnancy, the raised maternal iodine levels may result in congenital goitre and hypothyroidism in the fetus. Patients with nodular goitre may become thyrotoxic.

Ideally, all-glass syringes should be used, as Myodil may dissolve substances from some plastic syringes and/or their rubber plungers. If a plastic syringe is used, the Myodil should be drawn into it immediately prior to injection to minimise contact with the syringe.

The risk of induced arachnoiditis and aseptic meningitis has been reported to be enhanced in patients with multiple sclerosis.

Precautions: If possible, 10 to 14 days should elapse between lumbar puncture and subsequent myelography. As much Myodil as possible should be removed after the procedure, but when only small amounts are involved, most consider it reasonable not to aspirate if this requires another lumbar puncture. Retention of Myodil may cause prolonged elevation of the serum protein-bound iodine, thus invalidating diagnostic PBI estimations.

Side-effects: Myodil is usually well-tolerated, and provided a suitable technique of injection is used, preferably with video control, serious effects are rare. Myodil usually causes a slight increase in the white cell count and protein of the CSF, and diagnostic examination should therefore precede use of this contrast agent.

Hypersensitivity reactions, probably anaphylactic in type, are rare, but may be severe or even fatal. Immediate withdrawal of the Myodil should be performed if there is indication of such a process. Emergency drugs should always be available to deal with crises. As with simple lumbar puncture, headache is frequent, and after myelography it is sometimes severe, with vomiting and photophobia.

Pyrexia and stiff neck can occur, usually soon after myelography; rarely, they appear some weeks after the examination. Low back pain is not uncommon, and previous symptoms such as sciatica may be exacerbated. Symptoms normally resolve within several days, but if they persist, any residual Myodil should be removed, and where warranted, a suitable dose of hydrocortisone sodium succinate injected intrathecally.

Post-myelography arachnoiditis, which may be severe, occurs in some patients, and adhesions and fibrous exudate may be found on operation in patients who had at some time undergone myelography with iophendylate. This emphasises the importance of removing as much Myodil as possible at the time of investigation.

Overdosage: Aspirate the Myodil.

Pharmaceutical precautions Protect from light; do not use if discoloured.

Legal category POM.

Package quantities Box of three 3 ml ampoules.

Further information Nil.

Product licence number 0004/5099.

PREDNESOL* TABLETS

Presentation Small, pink, soluble tablets engraved 'Prednesol Glaxo' on one side and scored on the reverse. Each tablet contains 5 mg prednisolone as the sodium phosphate ester.

Uses Prednisolone is a glucocorticosteroid which is about four times as active as hydrocortisone on a weight-for-weight basis.

Prednisolone sodium phosphate is very soluble in water, and is therefore less likely to cause local gastric irritation than prednisolone alcohol, which is only slightly soluble. This is important when high dosages are required, as in immunosuppressive therapy.

A wide variety of diseases may sometimes require corticosteroid therapy. Some of the principal indications are: asthma, severe allergic disturbances, leukaemia, rheumatoid arthritis, collagen diseases, and various inflammatory skin diseases. Other indications are the nephrotic syndrome, ulcerative colitis, regional ileitis (Crohn's disease), pemphigus, sarcoidosis (especially with hypercalcaemia), rheumatic carditis and various blood dyscrasias, including selected cases of haemolytic anaemia, agranulocytosis and thrombocytopenic purpura.

Dosage and administration Prednesol Tablets are best taken dissolved in water, but they can be swallowed whole without difficulty.

The lowest dosage that will produce an acceptable result should be used; when it is possible to reduce the dosage, this must be accomplished by stages. During prolonged therapy, dosage may need to be increased temporarily during periods of stress or in exacerbations of illness.

Adults: The dose used will depend upon the disease, its severity, and the clinical response obtained. The following regimens are for guidance only. Divided dosage is usually employed.

Short-term treatment: 20 to 30 mg daily for the first few days, subsequently reducing the daily dosage by 2.5 or 5 mg every two to five days, depending upon the response.

Rheumatoid arthritis: 7.5 to 10 mg daily. For maintenance therapy the lowest effective dosage is used.

Most other conditions: 10 to 100 mg daily for one to three weeks, then reducing to the minimum effective dosage.

Children: Fractions of the adult dosage may be used (e.g., 75% at 12 years, 50% at 7 years and 25% at 1 year), but clinical factors must be given due weight.

Contra-indications, warnings, etc
Contra-indications: Systemic infections, unless specific anti-infective therapy is employed. Live virus immunisation. Hypersensitivity to any component of the tablet.

Precautions: Administration of corticosteroids may impair the ability to resist and counteract infection; in addition clinical signs and symptoms of infection are suppressed.

Corticosteroid treatment is likely to reduce the response of the pituitary-adrenal axis to stress, and relative insufficiency may persist for up to a year after withdrawal of prolonged therapy.

Because of the possibility of fluid retention, care must be taken when corticosteroids are administered to patients with congestive heart failure.

In pregnant animals, systemic administration of corticosteroids can cause abnormalities of fetal development. The relevance of this finding to humans has not been established.

Depression of hormone levels has been described in pregnancy but the significance of this finding is not clear.

Corticosteroids may worsen diabetes mellitus.

Since corticosteroids are secreted in the breast milk, the advisability of breast feeding should be considered in women on high dosage.

Steroids may reduce the effects of anticholinesterases in myasthenia gravis, cholecystographic X-ray media and salicylates.

The effect of steroids may be reduced by phenytoin, phenobarbitone, ephedrine and rifampicin.

The dosage of concomitantly administered anti-coagulants may have to be altered (usually decreased).

In patients with liver failure, blood levels of corticosteroid may be increased, as with other drugs which are metabolised in the liver.

Side-effects: Prolonged treatment with corticosteroids in high dosage is occasionally associated with subcapsular cataract and glaucoma. In addition, any of the features of hypercorticism, such as osteoporosis, may occur. Aseptic osteonecrosis, particularly of the femoral head, may occur after prolonged corticosteroid therapy, or after repeated short courses involving high dosage. Peptic ulceration may develop, or be aggravated.

In children, prolonged therapy may retard growth.

In patients on long-term therapy, fluid and electrolyte balance may be altered. Other rare side effects which have been reported include benign intracranial hypertension and psychic instability.

Drug interactions: Steroids may reduce the effects of anticholinesterases in myasthenia gravis, cholecystographic X-ray media and non-steroidal anti-inflammatory agents. It should also be remembered that the effects of steroids may be reduced by phenytoin, phenobarbitone, ephedrine and rifampicin.

Overdosage: Treatment is unlikely to be needed in cases of acute overdosage.

Pharmaceutical precautions None.

Legal category POM.

Package quantities The tablets are strip-packed in cartons of 100.

Further information Prednesol Tablets do not contain carbohydrates.

Product licence number 0004/5091.

PREDSOL* DROPS FOR EYE AND EAR

Presentation Predsol Drops contain prednisolone sodium phosphate 0.5% w/v and benzalkonium chloride 0.02% w/v in a sterilised clear and colourless aqueous solution. The product complies with the specification for Prednisolone Sodium Phosphate Eye Drops BPC.

Uses Non-infected inflammatory conditions of the eye and ear.

Dosage and administration *Eyes:* 1 or 2 drops instilled into the eye every one or two hours until control is achieved, when the frequency may be reduced.

Ears: 2 or 3 drops instilled into the ear every two or three hours until control is achieved, when the frequency can be reduced.

Contra-indications, warnings, etc

Contra-indications: Viral, fungal, tuberculous or purulent conditions. Use in the eye is contra-indicated if glaucoma is present or where herpetic keratitis (dendritic ulcer) is considered a possibility. Inadvertent use of topical steroids in the latter condition can lead to the enlargement of the ulcer and marked visual deterioration.

Hypersensitivity to any component of the preparation.

Predsol Eye Drops contain benzalkonium chloride as a preservative and therefore should not be used to treat patients who wear soft contact lenses.

Precautions: Topical administration of corticosteroids to pregnant animals can cause abnormalities of fetal development. The relevance of this finding to human beings has not been established; however, topical steroids should not be used extensively in pregnancy, i.e. in large amounts or for prolonged periods.

Side-effects: Eye Drops containing corticosteroids cause a serious rise in intra-ocular pressure in a small percentage of the population, which includes most of those with a family history of glaucoma. A milder rise may be experienced by a larger proportion of subjects if treatment is continued for longer than a few weeks. Thinning of the cornea leading to perforation has occurred with use of topical corticosteroids. Cataract is reported to have occurred after unduly prolonged treatment of eye conditions with topical corticosteroids.

Pharmaceutical precautions It is desirable that the contents should not be used more than four weeks after first opening the bottle.

Legal category POM.

Package quantities Plastic dropper bottles containing 5 ml or 10 ml.

Further information Nil.

Product licence number 0004/5092.

PREDSOL*-N DROPS FOR EYE OR EAR

Presentation Predsol-N Drops contain prednisolone sodium phosphate 0.5% w/v, neomycin sulphate 0.5% w/v and thiomersal 0.005% w/v in a clear, colourless aqueous solution. Sterile until opened.

Uses *Eye:* Non-infected inflammatory conditions where development of bacterial infection is a possibility.

Ear: Otitis externa (see 'Contra-indications') and other inflammatory conditions where bacterial infection is present or suspected (see 'Contra-indications').

Dosage and administration *Eyes:* 1 or 2 drops instilled into the eye every one or two hours until control is achieved, when the frequency may be reduced.

Ears: 2 or 3 drops instilled into the ear every two or three hours until control is achieved, when the frequency may be reduced.

Contra-indications, warnings, etc

Contra-indications: Viral, fungal or tuberculous conditions; use in the eye is contra-indicated if purulent infection or glaucoma is present.

Inadvertent use in herpetic keratitis (dendritic ulcer) can lead to enlargement of the ulcer and marked visual deterioration.

Hypersensitivity to any component of the preparation.

Because of the risk of ototoxicity, preparations containing neomycin should not be used until an intact tympanic membrane has been visualised.

Precautions: Topical administration of corticosteroids to pregnant animals can cause abnormalities of fetal development. The relevance of this finding to human beings has not been established; however, topical steroids should not be used extensively in pregnancy, i.e., in large amounts or for prolonged periods.

The unnecessary topical use of neomycin containing products should be avoided in order to minimise the occurrence of neomycin-resistant organisms (and organisms cross-resistant to other aminoglycosides).

Side-effects: Eye drops containing corticosteroids cause a serious rise in intra-ocular pressure in a small percentage of the population, which includes most of those with a family history of glaucoma. A milder rise may be experienced by a larger proportion of subjects if treatment is continued for longer than a few weeks. Thinning of the cornea leading to perforation has occurred with use of topical corticosteroids.

Acute sensitisation to neomycin is a rare event but can occur after topical application to the eye or ear.

Cataract is reported to have occurred after unduly prolonged treatment of eye conditions with topical corticosteroids.

Sensitivity to neomycin is uncommon, but if it occurs, avoid further use of the antibiotic.

Pharmaceutical precautions It is desirable that the contents should not be used more than four weeks after first opening the bottle.

Legal category POM.

Package quantities Plastic dropper bottles containing 5 ml or 10 ml.

Further information Nil.

Product licence number 0004/5093.

PREDSOL* RETENTION ENEMA

Presentation 100 ml disposable plastic bags, each containing 20 mg prednisolone as the sodium phosphate ester in a buffered solution. The product complies with the specification for Prednisolone Sodium Phosphate Enema BPC.

Uses Predsol Retention Enema provides local corticosteroid activity to the lower part of the colon. It is indicated in the treatment of ulcerative colitis.

Dosage and administration *Adults:* 1 enema used nightly, for two to four weeks. Treatment may be continued in patients showing progressive improvement, but it should not be persisted with if the response has been inadequate. Some patients may relapse after an interval but are likely to respond equally well to a repeated course of treatment.

Predsol Retention Enema as packed is not suitable for use in children.

The enema is used each night on retiring. It may be warmed before administration by placing the bag in a vessel of hot water for a few minutes. When in bed and lying on the left side with knees drawn up, the patient should remove the stopper from the bag, lubricate the nozzle with petroleum jelly and gently insert about half the length of the nozzle into the rectum. The bag should then be slowly rolled up like a tube of toothpaste until it is emptied, taking a minute or two to do so. The nozzle should then be removed, with the bag still rolled up, and the whole unit discarded. The patient should then roll over to lie face down for three to five minutes but may sleep in any comfortable position.

Contra-indications, warnings, etc
Contra indications: Corticosteroids should not be used in the presence of infection unless effective chemotherapy is also employed.

Precautions: Topical administration of corticosteroids to pregnant animals can cause abnormalities of fetal development. The relevance of this finding to human beings has not been established; however, topical steroids should not be used extensively in pregnancy, i.e., in large amounts or for prolonged periods.

Side-effects: The consequences of systemic absorption should be considered if Predsol Retention Enema is used over long periods or in high dosage.

Pharmaceutical precautions Protect from light.

Legal category POM.

Package quantities Boxes of seven 100 ml disposable bags (instructions to patients enclosed).

Further information The volume of the enema is considered to be the optimum to ensure maximum coverage of the affected area.

Product licence number 0004/5094.

PREDSOL* SUPPOSITORIES

Presentation Predsol Suppositories are white and opaque. Each suppository contains 5 mg prednisolone as the sodium phosphate ester.

Uses Prednisolone is a glucocorticosteroid which is about four times as potent as hydrocortisone on a weight-for-weight basis.

Predsol Suppositories are indicated for the treatment of haemorrhagic and granular proctitis and the anal complications of Crohn's disease.

Dosage and administration One suppository inserted at night and one in the morning after defaecation for adults or children. When the response is good, treatment is usually continued for some months. If symptoms recur later, treatment should be resumed.

Contra-indications, warnings, etc
Contra-indications: Corticosteroids should not be used in the presence of infection unless effective chemotherapy is also employed.

Precautions: Topical administration of corticosteroids to pregnant animals can cause abnormalities of fetal development. The relevance of this finding to human beings has not been established; however, topical steroids should not be used extensively in pregnancy, i.e., in large amounts or for prolonged periods.

Side-effects: As with all topical corticosteroids, if Predsol Suppositories are used for prolonged periods the consequences of systemic absorption should be considered, especially in children.

Pharmaceutical precautions Nil.

Legal category POM.

Package quantities Cartoned plastic moulds each containing 10 suppositories.

Further information Nil.

Product licence number 0004/5095.

TERTROXIN* TABLETS

Presentation Small, white, uncoated tablets engraved 'Tertroxin Glaxo' on one side and scored on the other. Each tablet contains 20 micrograms (0.02 mg) liothyronine sodium and complies with the specification for Liothyronine Tablets BP.

Uses Liothyronine (L-triiodothyronine) sodium is a naturally occurring thyroid hormone. Its biological action is qualitatively similar to that of thyroxine, but the effect develops in a few hours and disappears within 24 to 48 hours of stopping treatment.

Tertroxin is particularly suitable for treating severe and acute hypothyroid states because of its rapid, intensive and short-lived effect.

It is indicated in the treatment of: coma due to myxoedema; management of severe chronic thyroid deficiency; hypothyroid states arising in treatment of thyrotoxicosis.

Tertroxin is also used therapeutically in thyrotoxicosis as an adjunct to carbimazole. After six months of this treatment it may be possible to distinguish drug-responsive patients from relapse-prone patients who are better treated with radioiodine or surgery.

Large doses of liothyronine normally suppress the uptake of iodine by the thyroid, but not in thyrotoxicosis, and this forms the basis of a routine test for thyrotoxicosis.

Dosage and administration *Thyroid deficiency:* Treatment of adults may be begun with 10 or 20 micrograms daily, increasing by increments of 10 micrograms daily every seven days to a total daily dosage of 80 to 100 micrograms.

For children and elderly patients it is suggested that the initial dosage should be 5 micrograms daily. (To obtain small doses, tablets may be crushed and triturated with lactose for administration as a powder.)

Tertroxin should be given in divided doses two or three times daily.

Myxoedema coma: Initially, 60 micrograms may be given by stomach tube, then 20 micrograms every eight hours.

Thyrotoxicosis: As a diagnostic test in adults, 80 micrograms or more of liothyronine are given daily for seven or eight days. The daily amount should be divided into 3 or 4 doses. Radioiodine is then administered, and uptake by the thyroid can be estimated about 20 minutes later. Failure to suppress the uptake of radioiodine is indicative of thyrotoxicosis.

As therapy for thyrotoxicosis with carbimazole: In adults, 80 micrograms of liothyronine daily. In some patients it is possible to discontinue the carbimazole after about a year without subsequent relapse.

Contra-indications, warnings, etc
Contra-indications: Tertroxin is contra-indicated in patients with angina of effort or cardiovascular disorders.

Precautions: In myxoedema, care must be taken to avoid imposing excessive burden on cardiac muscle affected by prolonged severe thyroid depletion.

Side-effects: The following effects are indicative of excessive dosage, and usually disappear on reduction of dosage or withdrawal of treatment for a day or two. Anginal pain, cardiac arrhythmias, palpitation, and cramps in skeletal muscle; also tachycardia, diarrhoea,

restlessness, excitability, headache, flushing, sweating, excessive loss of weight and muscular weakness.

Overdosage: Gastric lavage or emesis is required if the patient is seen within several hours of taking the dose. Treatment is symptomatic; tachycardia has been controlled in an adult by 40 mg doses of propranolol given every six hours.

Pharmaceutical precautions Protect from light.

Legal category POM.

Package quantities Bottles of 100 tablets.

Further information 20 micrograms liothyronine is equivalent in activity to 60 to 100 micrograms thyroxine or to 60 mg Thyroid BP.

Product licence number 0004/5032.

TRIIODOTHYRONINE INJECTION

Presentation A freeze-dried sterile white plug containing 20 micrograms sodium triiodothyronine (Liothyronine Sodium, BP) with dextran. The plug is dissolved in Water for Injections for preparation of an intravenous injection.

Uses Treatment of myxoedema coma, usually in conjunction with other measures, including intravenous injection of a corticosteroid. For lesser degrees of myxoedema and for maintenance therapy, orally administered thyroxine should be used.

Dosage and administration Triiodothyronine injection is usually given by the intravenous route, as the alkalinity of the solution might cause irritation of the tissues if given by deep intramuscular injection. The solution is prepared by adding 1 ml or 2 ml of Water for Injections and shaking the ampoule gently until the substance has dissolved.

The dosage may be 5 to 20 micrograms given by slow intravenous injection and repeated at intervals of 12 hours, or sometimes more frequently. The minimum interval between doses is four hours. Some authorities have advocated an initial dose of 50 micrograms intravenously, followed by further intravenous injections of 25 micrograms every eight hours until improvement occurs. The dosage may then be reduced to 25 micrograms intravenously twice daily.

Contra-indications, warnings, etc
Contra-indications: No absolute contra-indication is known.

Precautions: Triiodothyronine must be given with extreme caution in myxoedema coma, as too large a dose can precipitate heart failure, especially in elderly patients and in those with ischaemic heart disease. Electrocardiographic monitoring can give a useful indication of impending ischaemia, but the ST changes of hypothyroidism may be confused with ECG evidence of ischaemia.

Use of sedatives may cause respiratory depression.

Side-effects: The following effects are indicative of excessive dosage, and usually disappear on reduction of dosage or withdrawal of treatment for a day or two. Anginal pain, cardiac arrhythmias, palpitation, and/or cramps in skeletal muscle. Also tachycardia, diarrhoea, restlessness, excitability, headache, flushing, sweating and muscular weakness.

Overdosage: Treatment of overdosage is symptomatic;

tachycardia has been controlled in an adult by 40 mg doses of propranolol given every six hours.

Pharmaceutical precautions Protect from light.

Legal category POM.

Package quantities Ampoules containing 20 micrograms sterile Liothyronine Sodium BP. Boxes of 3 ampoules.

Further information 20 micrograms liothyronine are equivalent in activity to 60 to 100 micrograms thyroxine.

Product licence number 0004/5033.

TRIMOVATE* CREAM

Presentation Trimovate Cream is a yellow water-miscible cream, containing clobetasone butyrate 0.05% w/w, oxytetracycline 3.0% w/w as calcium oxytetracycline and nystatin 100,000 units per gram.

Uses Clobetasone butyrate is a topically active corticosteroid which provides an exceptional combination of activity and safety. Topical formulations have been shown to be more effective in the treatment of eczemas than 1% hydrocortisone, yet to have little effect on hypothalamic-pituitary-adrenal function.

The combination of the topically active antibiotics, nystatin and oxytetracycline, provides a broad spectrum of antibacterial and anticandidal activity against many of the organisms associated with infected dermatoses.

Trimovate is indicated for the treatment and management of steroid-responsive dermatoses where candidal or bacterial infection is present, suspected, or likely to occur, and the use of a more potent topical corticosteroid is not required. These include infected eczemas, intertrigo, napkin rash, anogenital pruritus and seborrhoeic dermatitis.

Dosage and administration Apply to the affected area up to four times a day.

Suitable for treating infants, children and adults.

Contra-indications, warnings, etc Viral (e.g., herpes simplex) and dermatophyte (tinea/ringworm) infections of the skin, and tuberculous lesions.

Hypersensitivity to the preparation.

Precautions: In infants and children, long-term continuous topical steroid therapy should be avoided where possible, as adrenal suppression can occur even without occlusion. In infants, the napkin may act as an occlusive dressing, and increase absorption.

Any spread of infection requires withdrawal of topical corticosteroid therapy and institution of appropriate systemic chemotherapy.

With all corticosteroids, prolonged application to the face is undesirable.

Topical administration of corticosteroids to pregnant animals can cause abnormalities of fetal development. The relevance of this finding to human beings has not been established; however, topical steroids should not be used extensively in pregnancy, i.e., in large amounts or for prolonged periods.

Trimovate may cause slight staining of hair, skin or fabric, but this can be removed by washing. The application may be covered with a simple dressing to protect clothing.

Side-effects: In the unlikely event of signs of hypersensitivity appearing, application should stop immediately.

If large areas of the body were to be treated with Trimovate, it is possible that some patients would absorb sufficient steroid to cause transient adrenal depression despite the low degree of systemic activity associated with clobetasone butyrate.

Local atrophic changes could possibly occur in situations where moisture increases absorption of clobetasone butyrate, but only after prolonged use.

Pharmaceutical precautions Nil.

Legal category POM.

Package quantities Tubes of 25 grams.

Further information The least potent corticosteroid which will control the disease should be selected. Trimovate Cream does not contain lanolin or parabens.

The low systemic activity of clobetasone butyrate has been demonstrated in adults under conditions of whole body occlusion. In animal and human models, preparations of clobetasone butyrate and of hydrocortisone caused less thinning of the epidermis than the other topical corticosteroids tested.

Product licence number 0004/0266.

TRIMOVATE* OINTMENT

Presentation Trimovate Ointment is a yellow ointment containing clobetasone butyrate 0.05% w/w, chlortetracycline hydrochloride 3.0% w/w and nystatin 100,000 units per gram in soft paraffin base.

Uses Clobetasone butyrate is a topically active corticosteroid which provides an exceptional combination of activity and safety. Topical formulations have been shown to be more effective in the treatment of eczemas than 1% hydrocortisone, yet to have little effect on hypothalamic-pituitary-adrenal function.

The combination of the topically active antibiotics, nystatin and chlortetracycline hydrochloride, provides a broad spectrum of antibacterial and anticandidal activity against many of the organisms associated with infected dermatoses. Trimovate is indicated for the treatment and management of steroid responsive dermatoses where candidal or bacterial infection is present, suspected or likely to occur and the use of a more potent topical corticosteroid is not required. These include infected eczemas, intertrigo, napkin rash, anogenital pruritus and seborrhoeic dermatitis.

Dosage and administration Apply to the affected area up to four times a day.

Suitable for treating infants, children and adults.

Contra-indications, warnings, etc Viral (e.g., herpes simplex) and dermatophyte (tinea/ringworm) infections of the skin and tuberculous lesions.

Hypersensitivity to the preparation.

Precautions: In infants and children, long-term continuous topical steroid therapy should be avoided where possible, as adrenal suppression can occur even without occlusion. In infants, the napkin may act as an occlusive dressing, and increase absorption. Any spread of infection requires withdrawal of topical corticosteroid therapy and institution of appropriate systemic chemotherapy.

With all corticosteroids, prolonged application to the face is undesirable.

Topical administration of corticosteroids to pregnant animals can cause abnormalities of fetal development. The relevance of this finding to human beings has not been established; however, topical steroids should not be used extensively in pregnancy, i.e., in large amounts or for prolonged periods.

Trimovate may cause slight staining of hair, skin or fabric, but this can be removed by washing. The application may be covered with a simple dressing to protect clothing.

Side-effects: In the unlikely event of signs of hypersensitivity appearing, application should stop immediately.

If large areas of the body were to be treated with Trimovate, it is possible that some patients would absorb sufficient steroid to cause transient adrenal depression despite the low degree of systemic activity associated with clobetasone butyrate.

Local atrophic changes could possibly occur in situations where moisture increases absorption of clobetasone butyrate, but only after prolonged use.

Pharmaceutical precautions Nil.

Legal category POM.

Package quantities Tubes of 25 grams.

Further information The least potent corticosteroid which will control the disease should be selected. Trimovate Ointment does not contain lanolin or parabens.

The low systemic activity of clobetasone butyrate has been demonstrated in adults under conditions of whole body occlusion. In animal and human models, preparations of clobetasone butyrate and of hydrocortisone caused less thinning of the epidermis than the other topical corticosteroids tested.

Product licence number 0004/0265.

TRIPLOPEN*

Presentation Each single-dose vial contains a white, sterile powder consisting of:

Benethamine penicillin	475 mg (500,000 units)
Procaine penicillin	250 mg (250,000 units)
Sodium penicillin	300 mg (500,000 units)

A suspension for intramuscular injection (Benethamine Penicillin Injection Fortified, BPC) is formed on addition of Water for Injections.

Uses The dose of sodium penicillin gives a prompt, high blood level which supplements the lower but more prolonged level of the procaine penicillin. The therapeutic level is further maintained by the benethamine penicillin. Altogether, the effect lasts for two or three days.

Triplopen is of value in the following infections: acute localised infections such as boils, carbuncles and cellulitis; many infections caused by the more sensitive bacteria, e.g., haemolytic streptococci and pneumococci; prophylaxis against infections after accident or surgery; gonorrhoea and syphilis.

Dosage and administration To prepare the suspension for intramuscular administration, inject 1.3 ml Water for Injections into the inverted vial. On shaking, a very fluid suspension is formed which may be injected with a 23 SWG needle.

General infections in adults: Effective treatment can be carried out conveniently by a single injection of Triplopen, which can be repeated every two or three days. Triplopen is given only by deep intramuscular injection, preferably into the thigh or buttocks.

Gonorrhoea: Two vials as a single injection given once.

Syphilis: One vial daily for a week.

General infections in infants and children: Age 0 to 6 years: A quarter vial, *7 to 12 years:* A half vial. *13 years and over:* One vial.

Any suspension remaining after giving a fractional dose should be discarded unless it can be used promptly.

Contra-indications, warnings, etc
Contra-indications: Hypersensitivity to penicillins.

Precautions: Inadvertent injection into a blood vessel can cause serious reactions. The risk can usually be avoided by attempting to aspirate blood before injecting the antibiotics.

It should be recognised that a patient with a history of allergy, especially to drugs, is more likely to develop a hypersensitivity reaction.

Side-effects: Penicillin hypersensitivity usually takes the form of an urticarial rash which can be treated with systemic antihistamine drugs. Occasionally anaphylactic reactions to penicillin occur, and resuscitative measures, including subcutaneous injection of adrenaline and use of an intravenous corticosteroid should be employed.

Skin sensitisation may occur in persons handling penicillin, and appropriate protective measures should be taken to avoid contact with the substance.

Overdosage: Excessive blood levels of penicillin G can be corrected by haemodialysis.

Pharmaceutical precautions As this product does not contain a bacteriostat, it should be used without undue delay after reconstitution.

Legal category POM.

Package quantities Single-dose vial in box of 10.

Further information If 1.3 ml of water are used to suspend Triplopen, the total volume will be 2.27 ml, but the full amounts of antibiotics are contained in 2 ml of suspension. Each vial contains 27 mg sodium (1.2 mmol).

Product licence number 0004/5076.

ZANTAC* INJECTION ▼

Presentation Zantac Injection: 2 ml ampoules each containing 50 mg ranitidine (as hydrochloride) in 2 ml aqueous solution for intravenous or intramuscular administration.

2 ml Zantac Injection contains 2.82 mg (0.122 mmol) sodium.

Uses *Indications:* Zantac Injection is indicated for the treatment of duodenal ulcer, benign gastric ulcer, post-operative ulcer, reflux oesophagitis, Zollinger-Ellison syndrome, and the following conditions where reduction of gastric secretion and acid output is desirable: the prophylaxis of gastrointestinal haemorrhage from stress ulceration in seriously ill patients, the prophylaxis of recurrent haemorrhage in patients with bleeding peptic ulcers and before general anaesthesia in patients considered to be at risk of acid aspiration, particularly obstetric patients during labour (Mendelson's syndrome).

For appropriate cases, Zantac Tablets are also available (see separate Data Sheet).

Mode of action: Zantac is a specific, rapidly acting histamine H_2-antagonist. It inhibits basal and stimulated secretion of gastric acid, reducing both the volume and the acid and pepsin content of the secretion.

Dosage and administration *Adults:* Zantac Injection may be given either as a slow (over one minute) intravenous injection of 50 mg, which may be repeated every six to eight hours; or as an intermittent intravenous infusion at a rate of 25 mg per hour for two hours; the infusion may be repeated at six to eight hour intervals; or as an intramuscular injection of 50 mg (2 ml) every six to eight hours.

In the prophylaxis of haemorrhage from stress ulceration in seriously ill patients or the prophylaxis of recurrent haemorrhage in patients bleeding from peptic ulceration, parenteral administration may be continued until oral feeding commences. Patients considered to be still at risk may then be treated with Zantac Tablets 150 mg twice daily (see separate Data Sheet).

In patients considered to be at risk of developing acid aspiration syndrome Zantac Injection 50 mg may be given intramuscularly or by slow intravenous injection (over one minute) 45 to 60 minutes before induction of general anaesthesia.

Children: The use of Zantac Injection in children has not been evaluated.

Contra-indications, warnings, etc
Contra-indications: Ranitidine is contra-indicated for patients known to have hypersensitivity to the drug.

Precautions: Treatment with a histamine H_2-antagonist may mask the symptoms associated with carcinoma of the stomach and therefore may delay diagnosis of the condition. Accordingly, where gastric ulcer is suspected the possibility of malignancy should be excluded before therapy with Zantac is instituted.

Ranitidine is excreted via the kidney and in the presence of severe renal impairment, plasma levels of ranitidine are increased. Accordingly, it is recommended in such patients that Zantac be administered in doses of 25 mg.

It has been reported that use of higher than recommended doses of intravenous H_2-antagonists has been associated with rises in liver enzymes when treatment has been extended beyond five days.

Zantac crosses the placenta but therapeutic doses administered to obstetric patients in labour or undergoing caesarean section have been without any adverse effect on labour, delivery or subsequent neonatal progress. Zantac is also excreted in human breast milk. Like other drugs, Zantac should be used during pregnancy only if considered essential.

Side-effects: The following have been reported as events in clinical trials or in the routine management of patients treated with ranitidine. The relationship to ranitidine therapy has not been established in many cases.

Transient and reversible changes in liver function tests can occur. There have been occasional reports of reversible hepatitis (hepatocellular, hepatocanalicular or mixed) with or without jaundice.

Leucopaenia and thrombocytopaenia have occurred rarely in patients and have reversed on drug withdrawal.

Hypersensitivity reactions (urticaria, angioneurotic oedema, bronchospasm, hypotension) have been seen rarely following the parenteral and oral administration of ranitidine. These reactions have occasionally occurred after a single dose.

Rare reports have occurred of bradycardia.

Headache, sometimes severe, and dizziness have been reported in a very small proportion of patients. Rare cases of reversible mental confusion have been reported, predominantly in severely ill and elderly patients.

Skin rash has been rarely reported.

No clinically significant interference with endocrine or gonadal function has been reported. There have been a few reports of breast symptoms (swelling and/or discomfort) in men taking ranitidine; most cases have resolved on continued ranitidine treatment. Discontinuation of therapy may be necessary in order to establish the underlying cause.

Overdosage: Zantac is very specific in its action and accordingly no particular problems are expected following overdosage with the drug. Symptomatic and supportive therapy should be given as appropriate. If need be, the drug may be removed from the plasma by haemodialysis.

Pharmaceutical precautions Zantac Injection has been shown to be compatible with the following intravenous infusion fluids: 0.9% Sodium Chloride BP, 5% Dextrose BP, 0.18% Sodium Chloride and 4% Dextrose BP, 4.2% Sodium Bicarbonate BP and Hartmann's Solution. Although compatibility studies have only been undertaken in polyvinyl chloride infusion bags (in glass for Sodium Bicarbonate BP) and a polyvinyl chloride administration set it is considered that adequate stability would be conferred by the use of a polyethylene infusion bag. All unused admixtures of Zantac Injection with infusion fluids should be discarded 24 hours after preparation.

Store below 30°C (86°F). Protect from light. Zantac Injection should not be autoclaved.

Legal category POM.

Package quantities Zantac Injection: 2 ml ampoules, boxes of five.

Further information *Drug interactions:* Ranitidine does not inhibit the hepatic cytochrome P450-linked mixed function oxygenase enzyme system. Accordingly, ranitidine does not potentiate the action of drugs which are oxidised or inactivated by this enzyme; these include diazepam, lignocaine, phenytoin, propranolol, theophylline and warfarin.

Pharmacokinetics: Absorption of ranitidine after intramuscular injection is rapid and peak plasma concentrations are usually achieved within 15 minutes of administration. The elimination half-life of ranitidine is approximately two hours. Ranitidine is excreted via the kidneys mainly as the free drug and in minor amounts as metabolites. Its major metabolite is an N-oxide and there are smaller quantities of S-oxide and desmethyl ranitidine. The 24-hour urinary recovery of free ranitidine and its metabolites is about 75% after intravenous administration.

Use in renal transplants: Zantac has been used without adverse effects in patients with renal transplants.

Product licence number 0004/0289.

ZANTAC* TABLETS ▼

Presentation Zantac Tablets 150 mg: white, round, film-coated tablet, engraved ZANTAC 150 on one face and GLAXO on the other. Each Tablet contains ranitidine 150 mg (as hydrochloride).

Zantac Tablets 300 mg: white, capsule-shaped, film-coated tablet, engraved ZANTAC 300 on one face and GLAXO on the other. Each Tablet contains ranitidine 300 mg (as hydrochloride).

Zantac Dispersible Tablets: white, capsule-shaped,

film-coated tablet with GLAXO engraved on one face and a breakline on the other. Each Tablet contains ranitidine 150 mg (as hydrochloride).

Uses *Indications:* Zantac Tablets are indicated for the treatment of duodenal ulcer, benign gastric ulcer, post-operative ulcer, reflux oesophagitis, Zollinger-Ellison syndrome, and the following conditions where reduction of gastric secretion and acid output is desirable: the prophylaxis of gastrointestinal haemorrhage from stress ulceration in seriously ill patients, the prophylaxis of recurrent haemorrhage in patients with bleeding peptic ulcers and before general anaesthesia in patients considered to be at risk of acid aspiration (Mendelson's syndrome), particularly obstetric patients during labour.

For appropriate cases, Zantac Injection is also available (see separate Data Sheet).

Mode of action: Zantac is a specific, rapidly acting histamine H_2-antagonist. It inhibits basal and stimulated secretion of gastric acid, reducing both the volume and the acid and pepsin content of the secretion. Zantac has a relatively long duration of action and so a single 150 mg dose effectively suppresses gastric acid secretion for twelve hours.

Dosage and administration Zantac Dispersible Tablets should be placed in half a glass of water (minimum 75 ml) and stirred until dispersed before swallowing.

Adults: The usual dosage is one 150 mg tablet twice daily, taken in the morning and evening. Alternatively, patients with duodenal or gastric ulceration may be treated with a single bedtime dose of 300 mg. It is not necessary to time the dose in relation to meals. In most cases of duodenal ulcer, benign gastric ulcer and post-operative ulcer, healing occurs in four weeks. Healing usually occurs after a further four weeks of treatment in those patients whose ulcers have not fully healed after the initial course of therapy. Maintenance treatment at a reduced dosage of one 150 mg tablet at bedtime is recommended for patients who have responded to short-term therapy, particularly those with a history of recurrent ulcer. In the management of reflux oesophagitis, the recommended course of treatment is one 150 mg tablet twice daily for up to 8 weeks.

In patients with Zollinger-Ellison syndrome, the starting dose is 150 mg three times daily and this may be increased, as necessary. Patients with this syndrome have been given increasing doses up to 6 grams per day and these doses have been well tolerated.

In the prophylaxis of haemorrhage from stress ulceration in seriously ill patients or the prophylaxis of recurrent haemorrhage in patients bleeding from peptic ulceration, treatment with Zantac Tablets 150 mg twice daily may be substituted for Zantac Injection (see separate Data Sheet) once oral feeding commences in patients considered to be still at risk from these conditions.

In patients thought to be at risk of acid aspiration syndrome an oral dose of 150 mg can be given 2 hours before induction of general anaesthesia, and preferably also a 150 mg tablet the previous evening. Alternatively, Zantac Injection for intravenous and intramuscular use is also available (see separate Data Sheet).

In obstetric patients at commencement of labour, an oral dose of 150 mg may be given followed by 150 mg at six hourly intervals. It is recommended that since gastric emptying and drug absorption are delayed during labour, any patient requiring emergency general anaesthesia should be given, in addition, a non-particulate antacid (e.g. sodium citrate) prior to induction of

anaesthesia. The usual precautions to avoid acid aspiration should also be taken.

Children: Experience with Zantac Tablets in children is limited and such use has not been fully evaluated in clinical studies. It has however been used successfully in children aged 8 to 18 years in doses up to 150 mg twice daily without adverse effect.

Contra-indications, warnings, etc

Contra-indications: Ranitidine is contra-indicated for patients known to have hypersensitivity to the drug.

Precautions: Treatment with a histamine H_2-antagonist may mask symptoms associated with carcinoma of the stomach and may therefore delay diagnosis of the condition. Accordingly, where gastric ulcer is suspected the possibility of malignancy should be excluded before therapy with Zantac Tablets is instituted.

Ranitidine is excreted via the kidney and so plasma levels of the drug are increased in patients with severe renal failure. Accordingly, it is recommended that the therapeutic regimen for Zantac in such patients be 150 mg at night for 4 to 8 weeks. The same dose should be used for maintenance treatment should this be deemed necessary. If an ulcer has not healed after treatment the standard dosage regimen of 150 mg twice daily should be instituted, followed, if need be, by maintenance treatment at 150 mg at night.

Zantac crosses the placenta but therapeutic doses administered to obstetric patients in labour or undergoing caesarean section have been without any adverse effect on labour, delivery or subsequent neonatal progress. Zantac is also excreted in human breast milk. Like other drugs, Zantac should only be used during pregnancy and nursing if considered essential.

Side-effects: The following have been reported as events in clinical trials or in the routine management of patients treated with ranitidine. The relationship to ranitidine therapy has not been established in many cases.

Transient and reversible changes in liver function tests can occur. There have been occasional reports of reversible hepatitis (hepatocellular, hepatocanalicular or mixed) with or without jaundice.

Leucopaenia and thrombocytopaenia have occurred rarely in patients and have reversed on drug withdrawal.

Hypersensitivity reactions (urticaria, angioneurotic oedema, bronchospasm, hypotension) have been seen rarely following the parenteral and oral administration of ranitidine. These reactions have occasionally occurred after a single dose.

Rare reports have occurred of bradycardia.

Headache, sometimes severe, and dizziness have been reported in a very small proportion of patients. Rare cases of reversible mental confusion have been reported, predominantly in severely ill and elderly patients.

Skin rash has been rarely reported.

No clinically significant interference with endocrine or gonadal function has been reported. There have been a few reports of breast symptoms (swelling and/or discomfort) in men taking ranitidine; most cases have resolved on continued ranitidine treatment. Discontinuation of therapy may be necessary in order to establish the underlying cause.

Use in elderly patients: Rates of healing of ulcers in clinical trial patients aged 65 and over have not been found to differ from those in younger patients. Additionally, there was no difference in the incidence of adverse effects.

Overdosage: Zantac is very specific in action and

accordingly no particular problems are expected following overdosage with the drug. Symptomatic and supportive therapy should be given as appropriate. If need be, the drug may be removed from the plasma by haemodialysis.

Pharmaceutical precautions No special storage conditions are necessary.

Legal category POM.

Package quantities Zantac Tablets (150 mg): Carton of 60 tablets, foil-wrapped.
Zantac Tablets (300 mg): Carton of 30 tablets, foil-wrapped.
Zantac Dispersible Tablets (150 mg): Carton of 60 tablets, foil-wrapped.

Further information *Drug interactions:* Ranitidine does not inhibit the hepatic cytochrome P450-linked mixed function oxygenase system. Accordingly, ranitidine does not potentiate the actions of drugs which are inactivated by this enzyme; these include diazepam, lignocaine, phenytoin, propranolol, theophylline and warfarin.

Pharmacokinetics: Absorption of ranitidine after oral administration is rapid and peak plasma concentrations are usually achieved within two hours of administration. Absorption is not significantly impaired by food or antacids. The elimination half-life of ranitidine is approximately two hours. Ranitidine is excreted via the kidneys mainly as the free drug and in minor amounts as metabolites. Its major metabolite is an N-oxide and there are smaller quantities of S-oxide and desmethyl ranitidine. The 24-hour urinary recovery of free ranitidine and its metabolites is about 40% with orally administered drug.

Use in renal transplants: Zantac has been used without adverse effect in patients with renal transplants.

Product licence numbers
Zantac Tablets (150 mg): 0004/0279
Zantac Tablets (300 mg): 0004/0302
Zantac Dispersible Tablets (150 mg): 0004/0298

ZINACEF*

Presentation Vials containing 250 mg, 750 mg or 1.5 g cefuroxime as cefuroxime sodium.
Cefuroxime is a white to faintly yellow powder to which appropriate amounts of water are added to prepare an off-white suspension for intramuscular use or a yellowish solution for intravenous administration. Variations in the intensity of this colour do not indicate any change in either the efficacy or safety of the product.

Uses Zinacef is a bactericidal cephalosporin antibiotic which is resistant to most β-lactamases and is active against a wide range of Gram-positive and Gram-negative organisms. It is indicated for the treatment of infections before the infecting organism has been identified or when caused by sensitive bacteria. In addition, it is an effective prophylactic against post-operative infection in a variety of operations. Usually Zinacef will be effective alone, but when appropriate it may be used in combination with an aminoglycoside antibiotic, or in conjunction with metronidazole (orally or by suppository or injection), especially for prophylaxis in colonic surgery (see Pharmaceutical precautions).

Indications include:
Respiratory tract infections for example, acute and chronic bronchitis, infected bronchiectasis, bacterial pneumonia, lung abscess and post-operative chest infections.
Ear, nose and throat infections for example, sinusitis, tonsillitis and pharyngitis.
Urinary tract infections for example, acute and chronic pyelonephritis, cystitis and asymptomatic bacteriuria.
Soft-tissue infections for example, cellulitis, erysipelas, peritonitis and wound infections.
Bone and joint infections for example, osteomyelitis and septic arthritis.
Obstetric and gynaecological infections pelvic inflammatory diseases.
Gonorrhoea particularly when penicillin is unsuitable.
Other infections including septicaemia and meningitis.
Prophylaxis against infection in abdominal, pelvic, orthopaedic, cardiac, pulmonary, oesophageal and vascular surgery where there is increased risk from infection.
Bacteriology: Zinacef is highly active against *Staphylococcus aureus,* including strains which are resistant to penicillin (but not the rare methicillin resistant strains), *Staph. epidermidis, Haemophilus influenzae,* Klebsiella spp., Enterobacter spp., *Streptococcus pyogenes, Escherichia coli, Str. mitis* (viridans group), Clostridium spp., *Proteus mirabilis, Pr. rettgeri, Salmonella typhi, S. typhimurium* and other Salmonella spp. Shigella spp., Neisseria spp. (including β-lactamase producing strains of *N. gonorrhoeae*) and *Bordetella pertussis.* It is also moderately active against strains of *Pr. vulgaris, Pr. morganii* and *Bacteroides fragilis.*
In vitro the activities of Zinacef and aminoglycoside antibiotics in combination have been shown to be at least additive with occasional evidence of synergy.

Dosage and administration *General dosage recommendations: Adults:* Many infections will respond to 750 mg t.i.d. by i.m. or i.v. injection. For more severe infections, this dose should be increased to 1.5 g t.i.d. i.v. The frequency of i.m. or i.v. injections can be increased to six-hourly if necessary, giving total doses of 3 g to 6 g daily.
Infants and children: Doses of 30 to 100 mg/kg/day, given as three or four divided doses. A dose of 60 mg/kg/day will be appropriate for most infections.
Neonates: Doses of 30 to 100 mg/kg/day, given as two or three divided doses. In the first weeks of life the serum half-life of cefuroxime can be three to five times that in adults.
Other recommendations: Gonorrhoea: 1.5 g should be given as a single dose. This may be given as 2 × 750 mg injections into different sites, e.g., each buttock.
Meningitis: Zinacef is suitable for sole therapy of bacterial meningitis due to sensitive strains. The following dosages are recommended.
Infants and children: 200 to 240 mg/kg/day i.v. in three or four divided doses. This dosage may be reduced to 100 mg/kg/day i.v. after three days or when clinical improvement occurs.
Neonates: The initial dosage should be 100 mg/kg/day i.v. A reduction to 50 mg/kg/day i.v. may be made when clinically indicated.
Adults: 3 g i.v. every eight hours. Data are not yet sufficient to recommend a dose for intrathecal administration.

Prophylaxis: The usual dose is 1.5 g i.v. with induction of anaesthesia for abdominal, pelvic and orthopaedic operations, but may be supplemented with two 750 mg i.m. doses eight and sixteen hours later. In cardiac, pulmonary, oesophageal and vascular operations, the usual dose is 1.5 g i.v. with induction of anaesthesia continuing with 750 mg i.m. t.i.d. for a further 24 to 48 hours.

In total joint replacement, 1.5 g cefuroxime powder may be mixed dry with each pack of methyl methacrylate cement polymer before adding the liquid monomer.

Dosage in impaired renal function: Cefuroxime is excreted by the kidneys. Therefore, as with all such antibiotics, in patients with impaired renal function it is recommended that the dosage of Zinacef should be reduced to compensate for its slower excretion. However, it is not necessary to reduce the dose until the creatinine clearance falls below 20 ml/min. In adults with marked impairment (creatinine clearance 10 to 20 ml/min) 750 mg b.d. is recommended and with severe impairment (creatinine clearance < 10 ml/min) 750 mg once daily is adequate. For patients on dialysis a further 750 mg dose should be given at the end of each dialysis. When continuous peritoneal dialysis is being used, a suitable dosage is usually 750 mg twice daily.

Administration: Intramuscular: Add 1 ml Water for Injections to 250 mg Zinacef or 3 ml Water for Injections to 750 mg Zinacef. Shake gently to produce an opaque suspension.

Intravenous: Dissolve Zinacef in Water for Injections using at least 2 ml for 250 mg, at least 6 ml for 750 mg, or 15 ml for 1.5 g. For short intravenous infusion (e.g., up to 30 minutes), 1.5 g may be dissolved in 50 ml Water for Injections. These solutions may be given directly into the vein or introduced into the tubing of the giving set if the patient is receiving parenteral fluids.

Zinacef is compatible with the more commonly used intravenous fluids. (See Pharmaceutical precautions.)

Contra-indications, warnings, etc

Contra-indications: Hypersensitivity to cephalosporin antibiotics.

Precautions: Cephalosporin antibiotics may in general be given safely to patients who are hypersensitive to penicillins, although cross-reactions have been reported. Especial care is indicated in patients who have experienced an anaphylactic reaction to penicillin.

Cephalosporin antibiotics at high dosage should be given with caution to patients receiving concurrent treatment with potent diuretics such as frusemide, as these combinations are suspected of adversely affecting renal function. Clinical experience with Zinacef has shown that this is not likely to be a problem at the recommended dose levels.

There is no experimental evidence of embryopathic or teratogenic effects attributable to Zinacef but, as with all drugs, it should be administered with caution during the early months of pregnancy.

Zinacef does not interfere in enzyme-based tests for glycosuria. Slight interference with copper reduction methods (Benedict's, Fehling's, Clinitest) may be observed. However, this should not lead to false-positive results, as may be experienced with some other cephalosporins.

It is recommended that either the glucose oxidase or hexokinase methods are used to determine blood/plasma glucose levels in patients receiving Zinacef. This anti-biotic does not interfere in the alkaline picrate assay for creatinine.

Side-effects: Adverse reactions to Zinacef have occurred relatively infrequently and have been generally mild and transient in nature. Effects reported include rashes and gastro-intestinal disturbance. As with other antibiotics, prolonged use may result in the overgrowth of non-susceptible organisms, e.g., Candida.

The principal changes in haematological parameters seen in some patients have been of decreased haemoglobin concentration and of eosinophilia. A positive Coombs' test has been found in some patients treated with cefuroxime – this phenomenon can interfere with the cross-matching of blood.

Although there are sometimes transient rises in serum liver enzymes or serum bilirubin, particularly in patients with pre-existing liver disease, there is no evidence of hepatic involvement.

There may also be some variation in the results of biochemical tests of renal function, but these do not appear to be of clinical importance. As a precaution, renal function should be monitored if this is already impaired.

Transient pain may be experienced at the site of intramuscular injection. This is more likely to occur with higher doses. However, it is unlikely to be a cause for discontinuation of treatment.

Overdosage: Serum levels of cefuroxime are reduced by dialysis.

Pharmaceutical precautions Protect from light.

Zinacef should not be mixed in the syringe with aminoglycoside antibiotics.

Suspensions of Zinacef for intramuscular injection and aqueous solutions for direct intravenous injection retain their potency for five hours if kept below 25°C and for 48 hours if refrigerated. More dilute solutions, i.e., 1.5 g plus 50 ml Water for Injections, retain satisfactory potency for 24 hours if kept below 25°C and for 72 hours if refrigerated.

Some increase in the colour of prepared solutions and suspensions of Zinacef may occur on storage.

1.5 g Zinacef constituted with 15 ml Water for Injections may be added to metronidazole injection (500 mg/ 100 ml) and both retain their activity for up to 24 hours below 25°C. 1.5 g Zinacef is compatible with azlocillin 1 g (in 15 ml) or 5 g (in 50 ml) for up to 24 hours at 4°C or 6 hours below 25°C.

Zinacef (5 mg/ml) in 5% w/v or 10% w/v xylitol injection may be stored for up to 24 hours at 25°C.

Zinacef is compatible with the more commonly used intravenous infusion fluids. It will retain potency for up to 24 hours at room temperature in Sodium Chloride Injection BP 0.9% w/v, 5% Dextrose Injection BP, 0.18% w/v Sodium Chloride plus 4% Dextrose Injection BP, and Compound Sodium Lactate Injection BP (Hartmann's solution). The pH of 2.74% w/v Sodium Bicarbonate Injection BP considerably affects the colour of the solution and therefore this solution is not recommended for the dilution of Zinacef. However, if required, for patients receiving Sodium Bicarbonate Injection by infusion the Zinacef may be introduced into the tube of the giving set. The stability of Zinacef in Sodium Chloride Injection BP 0.9% w/v and in 5% Dextrose Injection is not affected by the presence of hydrocortisone sodium phosphate.

Zinacef is also compatible with aqueous solutions containing up to 1% lignocaine hydrochloride.

Legal category POM.

Package quantities Vials containing 250 mg or 750 mg cefuroxime as the sodium salt (for use by intramuscular or intravenous injection) in packs of 5.

Vials containing 1.5 g cefuroxime as the sodium salt (for use by intravenous injection), packed singly.

Vials containing 1.5 g cefuroxime as the sodium salt (for use by intravenous infusion), packed singly.

Further information Peak levels of cefuroxime are achieved within 30 to 45 minutes after intramuscular administration. The serum half-life after either intramuscular or intravenous injection is approximately 70 minutes. Concurrent administration of probenecid prolongs the excretion of the antibiotic and produces an elevated peak serum level. There is almost complete recovery of unchanged cefuroxime in the urine within 24 hours of administration, the major part being eliminated in the first six hours. Approximately 50% is excreted through the renal tubules and approximately 50% by glomerular filtration. Concentrations of cefuroxime in excess of the minimum inhibitory levels for common pathogens can be achieved in bone, synovial fluid and aqueous humour. Cefuroxime passes the blood-brain barrier when the meninges are inflamed.

Each 750 mg vial contains 42 mg sodium (1.8 mmol). When dissolved, the contents of a 750 mg vial displace 0.53 ml on average.

Product licence number 0004/0263.

*Trade Mark

Glenwood Laboratories Ltd
19 Wincheap
Canterbury
Kent

MYOTONINE*

Presentation Bethanechol chloride tablets: 10 mg – pale blue, scored; 25 mg – pale blue, cross scored.

Uses
Mode of Action: Myotonine is a choline ester which produces the effects of stimulation of the parasympathetic nervous system. Myotonine is not hydrolysed by cholinesterase. The muscarinic effects are exerted mainly on the urinary bladder, the gastro-intestinal tract and the eye. The pharmacological effect is usually apparent within 30 to 90 minutes of administration and lasts about an hour.

Indications: Reflux oesophagitis. Urinary retention (post operative, postpartum and neurogenic). Adynamic ileus. Gastric atony and retention. Megacolon.

Dosage and administration
Adults: The therapeutic dose of Myotonine should be individualised by titrating the dose to the response of the patient. In many cases a satisfactory response can be obtained with 10 mg to 25 mg Myotonine, three or four times a day. Occasionally it may be felt necessary to initiate therapy with a 50 mg dose. Myotonine tablets should be administered when the stomach is empty as nausea and vomiting may occur when they are taken soon after eating.

Children: Experience with Myotonine tablets in children is limited. The dose of Myotonine should be adjusted on a weight basis.

Contra-indications, warnings, etc Parasympathomimetic or cholinergic drugs are contraindicated in patients with asthma or susceptibility to asthmatic attacks, hyperthyroid states, marked vagotonia, pronounced vasomotor instability, severe bradycardia and hypotension, recent myocardial infarction, epilepsy, parkinsonism or during pregnancy. Parasympathomimetic or cholinergic drugs should not be used in patients with urinary or gastro-intestinal obstruction or where increased muscular activity of the urinary bladder or gastro-intestinal tract may prove harmful.

Side effects: Untoward reactions are rare following oral administration of therapeutic doses of bethanechol chloride. Nausea and vomiting may occur if the drug is taken immediately after the ingestion of food. Reported side effects include frequency of micturition, lower abdominal cramps, blurred vision.

Antidote: The pharmacological effects of bethanechol chloride can be promptly abolished by the administration of atropine sulphate.

Pharmaceutical precautions No special storage conditions are necessary. For oral use only.

Legal category POM.

Package quantities Myotonine tablets 10 mg 100 tablets. Myotonine tablets 25 mg 100 tablets.

Further information Nil.

Product licence number 0245/5009.

POTABA*

Presentation Potaba is pure potassium para-aminobenzoate. It is available in the following presentations:
Potaba envules. Single dose sachets, each containing 3 g Potaba.
Potaba tablets – White concave tablets each containing 500 mg Potaba.
Potaba capsules – Red/white capsules each containing 500 mg Potaba.

Uses
Mode of Action: Potaba is an antifibrosis agent. It has been suggested that the antifibrosis activity of Potaba is brought about by the drug increasing oxygen uptake at the tissue level. Fibrosis is believed to occur from either too much serotonin or too little monoamine oxidase activity over a period of time. The activity of monoamine oxidase is dependent upon an adequate oxygen supply. By increasing oxygen supply at the tissue level Potaba enhances monoamine oxidase activity thereby preventing or bringing about regression of fibrosis.

Indications: Scleroderma. Peyronie's disease (Induratio penis plastica).

Dosage and administration The usual dose of Potaba is 3 g, four times a day. This dosage is best achieved by the administration of one Potaba Envule four times a day taken with food. The contents of the envule is dissolved in any desired drink. Citrus juices are excellent vehicles. Alternatively, six Potaba tablets or capsules may be taken four times a day with food.

Contra-indications, warnings, etc Potaba should not be administered to patients taking sulphonamides, as it will inactivate this medication.

Precautions: Treatment with Potaba should be interrupted during periods of low food intake (eg, during fasting, anorexia, nausea). This is to avoid the possible development of hypoglycaemia.
Potaba should be given cautiously to patients with renal impairment.
Potaba treatment should be discontinued if a hypersensitivity reaction occurs.

Side effects: No serious adverse effects have been reported in patients treated with Potaba. Anorexia, nausea, fever and rash occur infrequently and subside with omission of the drug. Desensitisation can often be accomplished and treatment with Potaba resumed.

Overdose: No particular problems are expected following overdosage with Potaba. Symptomatic and supportive therapy should be given as appropriate.

Pharmaceutical precautions Potaba preparations should be stored in a cool place.

Legal category POM.

Package quantities Potaba Envules – Box of 40 envules. Potaba tablets – Containers of 120 and 1000 tablets. Potaba capsules – Containers of 240 and 1000 capsules.

Further information It is necessary to continue treatment with Potaba at the full recommended dose (12 g daily) for up to twelve months or longer to effect regression of the fibrous plaque in the penis. Patients should be instructed not to interrupt treatment, except during periods of low food intake (see precautions above).

p–Aminobenzoate is considered to be a member of the vitamin B complex. Small amounts are found in yeast, cereal, eggs, milk and meats. Detectable amounts are normally present in human blood and other biological fluids.

Product licence number 0245/5000–2.

*Trade Mark

Gold Cross Pharmaceuticals
Division of G. D. Searle & Company Limited
PO Box 53
Lane End Road
High Wycombe
Bucks HP 12 4HL

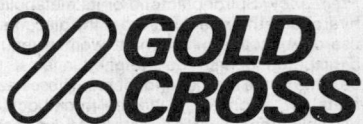

ALDACTIDE* 50
ALDACTIDE* 25

Presentation

Aldactide 50: Buff, film-coated tablets engraved 'SEARLE 180' on one side containing Spironolactone B.P. 50 mg and Hydroflumethiazide B.P. 50 mg.

Aldactide 25: Buff, film-coated tablets engraved 'SEARLE 101' on one side containing Spironolactone B.P. 25 mg and Hydroflumethiazide B.P. 25 mg.

Uses Aldactide is a potassium-conserving diuretic with antihypertensive activity. It is recommended for the treatment of essential hypertension and for the control of oedema in congestive cardiac failure.

Dosage and administration Food has been reported to increase the bioavailability of spironolactone and thiazides. It is recommended that tablets are taken with meals.

Adults

Essential hypertension: Aldactide 50 – one to two tablets with breakfast or the first main meal of the day. Aldactide 25 – one to four tablets with breakfast or the first main meal of the day.

Congestive cardiac failure: Most patients will require an initial dosage of four tablets Aldactide 25 or two tablets Aldactide 50 daily. The dosage should be adjusted as necessary and may range from one tablet Aldactide 25 to eight tablets Aldactide 25 or four tablets Aldactide 50 daily.

Elderly: It is recommended that treatment is started with the lowest dose and titrated upwards as required to achieve maximum benefit. Care should be taken in severe hepatic and renal impairment which may alter drug metabolism and excretion.

Children: Although clinical trials using Aldactide have not been carried out in children, as a guide, a daily dosage providing 1.5 to 3 mg of spironolactone per kilogram body weight, given in divided doses, may be employed.

Contra-indications, warnings, etc

Contra-indications: Aldactide is contra-indicated in patients with anuria, acute renal insufficiency, rapidly deteriorating or severe impairment of renal function, hyperkalaemia, Addison's disease and in patients who are hypersensitive to spironolactone, thiazide diuretics or to other sulphonamide derived drugs.

Aldactide should not be administered concurrently with other potassium-conserving diuretics and potassium supplements should not be given routinely with Aldactide as hyperkalaemia may be induced.

Warnings: Carcinogenicity: Spironolactone has been shown to produce tumours in rats when administered at high doses over a long period of time. The significance of these findings with respect to clinical use is not certain. However, the long term use of spironolactone in young patients requires careful consideration of the benefits and the potential hazard involved.

Sulphonamide derivatives, including thiazides, have been reported to exacerbate or activate systemic lupus erythematosus.

Precautions: Fluid and electrolyte balance: Fluid and electrolyte status should be regularly monitored, particularly in the elderly and in those with initial mild renal impairment.

Hyperkalaemia may occur in patients with impaired renal function or excessive potassium intake and can cause cardiac irregularities which may be fatal. Should hyperkalaemia develop Aldactide should be discontinued, and if necessary, active measures taken to reduce the serum potassium to normal.

Hypokalaemia may develop as a result of profound diuresis, particularly when Aldactide is used concomitantly with loop diuretics, glucocorticoids or ACTH.

Hyponatraemia may be induced, especially when Aldactide is administered in combination with other diuretics.

Hepatic impairment: Caution should be observed in patients with acute or severe liver impairment as vigorous diuretic therapy may precipitate encephalopathy in susceptible patients. Regular estimation of serum electrolytes is essential in such patients.

Reversible hyperchloraemic metabolic acidosis usually in association with hyperkalaemia has been reported to occur in some patients with decompensated hepatic cirrhosis, even in the presence of normal renal function.

Urea and uric acid: Reversible increases in blood urea have been reported, particularly accompanying vigorous diuresis or in the presence of impaired renal function.

Thiazides may cause hyperuricaemia and precipitate attacks of gout in some patients.

Diabetes mellitus: Thiazides may aggravate existing diabetes and the insulin requirements may alter. Diabetes mellitus which has been latent may become manifest during thiazide administration.

Drug interactions: Potentiation of the effect of other antihypertensive drugs occurs and their dosage may need to be reduced when Aldactide is added to the treatment regime, and then adjusted as necessary.

As carbenoxolone may cause sodium retention and

thus decrease the effectiveness of Aldactide, concurrent use should be avoided.

Spironolactone reduces vascular responsiveness to noradrenaline. Caution should be exercised in the management of patients subjected to regional or general anaesthesia while they are being treated with Aldactide.

Pregnancy. Spironolactone or its metabolites may, and hydroflumethiazide does, cross the placental barrier. The use of Aldactide in pregnant women requires that the anticipated benefit be weighed against the possible hazards to the mother and foetus. These hazards include foetal or neonatal jaundice, thrombocytopenia, and possibly other adverse effects that have been reported in adults.

Nursing mothers: Canrenone, a metabolite of spironolactone, and hydroflumethiazide appear in breast milk. If use of Aldactide is considered essential, an alternative method of infant feeding should be instituted.

Adverse effects: Gynaecomastia may develop in association with the use of spironolactone. Development appears to be related to both dosage level and duration of therapy and is normally reversible when the drug is discontinued. In rare instances some breast enlargement may persist. Other adverse reactions reported in association with spironolactone include: gastrointestinal intolerance, drowsiness, lethargy, headache, mental confusion, ataxia, drug fever, skin rashes, menstrual irregularities, impotence and mild androgenic effects.

Adverse reactions reported in association with thiazides include: gastrointestinal upset, skin rashes, photosensitivity, blood dyscrasias, aplastic anaemia, purpura, muscle cramps, weakness, restlessness, headache, dizziness, vertigo, jaundice, orthostatic hypotension, impotence, paraesthesia, and rarely pancreatitis, necrotising vasculitis and xanthopsia. Rarely hypercalcaemia has been reported in association with thiazides, usually in patients with pre-existing metabolic bone disease or parathyroid dysfunction.

Overdosage: Acute overdosage may be manifested by drowsiness, mental confusion, nausea, vomiting, dizziness or diarrhoea. Hyponatraemia, hypokalaemia or hyperkalaemia may be induced, or hepatic coma may be precipitated in patients with severe liver disease, but these effects are unlikely to be associated with acute overdosage. Symptoms of hyperkalaemia may manifest as paraesthesia, weakness, flaccid paralysis or muscle spasm and may be difficult to distinguish clinically from hypokalaemia. Electrocardiographic changes are the earliest specific signs of potassium disturbances. No specific antidote has been identified. Improvement may be expected after withdrawal of the drug. General supportive measures including replacement of fluids and electrolytes may be indicated.

Pharmaceutical precautions Store below 30°C (86°F).

Legal category POM.

Package quantities Aldactide 50: Calendar pack of 28 tablets and bottles containing 100 and 500 tablets. Aldactide 25: Bottles containing 100 and 500 tablets.

Further information Hydroflumethiazide induces diuresis usually within two hours, which lasts for 12–18 hours.

Spironolactone, as a competitive aldosterone antagonist, increases sodium excretion whilst reducing potassium loss at the distal renal tubule. It has a gradual and prolonged action, maximum response being usually attained after 2–3 days' treatment.

Product licence numbers
Aldactide 50 0020/0082
Aldactide 25 0020/5001

CONOVA* 30

Presentation White, film-coated tablets engraved 'SEARLE 930' on one side containing Ethynodiol Diacetate BP 2 mg and Ethinyloestradiol PhEur 30 mcg.

Uses Oral contraception.

Dosage and administration One tablet daily for 21 days, starting on Day 5 of the menstrual cycle (where Day 1 is the first day of bleeding). The next course of tablets should be started after seven tablet free days. This 'three weeks on, one week off' regimen is continued for as long as contraception is required. Women should be advised to use an additional form of contraception (a sheath or a cap plus spermicide) for the first 14 days of the first pack.

Women switching from another combined oral contraceptive should start Conova 30 seven days after finishing their current pack.

After pregnancy oral contraception is usually started as soon as spontaneous menstruation has been resumed. However, if thought appropriate, oral contraception can be started within 7–12 days of vaginal delivery provided the woman is ambulant and there are no puerperal complications. An additional form of contraception (a sheath or a cap plus spermicide) should be used for the first 14 days of the first pack.

Missed tablets: Women who miss a single tablet should be instructed to take the missed tablet as soon as they remember, even though this may mean taking two tablets on one single day. The regular tablet for that day should be taken at the usual time. An additional method of contraception (a sheath or a cap plus spermicide) should be used for the remainder of the cycle. If two consecutive tablets are missed, women should be instructed to take two tablets each day for the next two days and use an additional method of contraception for the rest of the cycle. Those who miss more than two tablets should resume as soon as they remember, ignoring those tablets they have missed, and should use additional contraceptive precautions for the rest of the cycle.

Vomiting or diarrhoea: Vomiting or diarrhoea may reduce the effectiveness of the tablets, particularly if this should occur at or around the time of ovulation. The woman should be advised to use an additional form of contraception for the rest of the cycle when an episode of vomiting and/or diarrhoea occurs.

Contra-indications, warnings, etc
Contra-indications: The contra-indications for combined oral contraceptives are: thrombophlebitis, thromboembolic disorders, cerebral vascular disease, myocardial infarction, coronary artery disease, or a past history of these conditions; known, suspected or a past history of breast, genital or hormone dependent cancer; past or present, benign or malignant liver tumours; impaired liver function; active liver disease; history during pregnancy of idiopathic jaundice or severe pruritus; disorders of lipid metabolism; haemoglobinopathies; undiagnosed abnormal vaginal bleeding or amenorrhoea; known or suspected pregnancy.

Warnings: Combined oral contraceptives have been associated with an increase in the risk of thromboembolic and thrombotic disease including cerebral and myocardial infarction, subarachnoid haemorrhage, pulmonary embolism, deep vein thrombosis and transient ischaemic attacks. Risk has been reported to be related to both oestrogenic and progestogenic activity. The risk of arterial thrombosis associated with combined oral contraceptives increases with age, and this risk is aggravated by cigarette smoking. The use of combined oral contraceptives by women in the older age group, especially those who are cigarette smokers, should therefore be discouraged, and alternative methods advised.

Certain factors may predispose to the development of coronary artery disease, e.g. smoking, obesity, diabetes, hypertension, hypercholesterolaemia, history of pre-eclamptic toxaemia, regardless of whether or not oral contraceptives are used. The suitability of a combined oral contraceptive should be judged according to the severity of such conditions in the individual case and should be discussed with the woman before she decides to take it.

An increase in blood pressure has been reported in women receiving oral contraceptives. The amount of increase may correlate directly with increasing progestogenic activity.

Persistence of risk after discontinuation of oral contraceptives has been reported for circulatory disease including non-rheumatic heart disease and cerebrovascular disease such as subarachnoid haemorrhage, cerebral thrombosis and transient ischaemic attacks.

Conova 30 should be discontinued at least six weeks before elective surgery or during periods of prolonged immobilisation. It would be reasonable to resume oral contraceptives two or three weeks after surgery provided the woman is ambulant. Every woman however, should be considered individually with regard to the nature of the operation, the extent of immobilisation, the presence of additional risk factors and the chance of unwanted conception.

Conova 30 should be discontinued if there is a gradual or sudden, partial or complete loss of vision or any evidence of ocular changes, onset or aggravation of migraine or development of headache of a new kind which is recurrent, persistent or severe, suspicion of thrombosis or infarction, significant rise in blood pressure or if jaundice occurs.

Oestrogens have been reported to increase the risk of endometrial carcinoma. Although some epidemiological studies have suggested an increased risk of breast cancer or of cervical dysplasia, erosion and carcinoma in long-term pill users, cause and effect has not been established.

Precautions: Women receiving treatment with oestrogen or progestogen or both, should be kept under regular surveillance.

Caution should be exercised where there is the possibility of an interaction between a pre-existing disorder and a known or suspected side-effect. The use of Conova 30 in women suffering from epilepsy, or with a history of migraine, or cardiac or renal dysfunction may result in exacerbation of these disorders, because of fluid retention. Caution should also be observed in women who wear contact lenses, women with impaired carbohydrate tolerance, hypertension, asthma, depression, gallstones, chloasma, varicose veins, or any disease that is prone to worsen during pregnancy, and in young women in whom the growth period has not yet ended.

Drug interactions: Conova 30 may be rendered less effective and increased incidence of breakthrough bleeding may occur by virtue of drug interactions. At present, drugs suspected to interact in this way include rifampicin, anticonvulsants and antibiotics. Vitamin C may enhance the effect of contraceptive steroids by increasing the bioavailability of ethinyloestradiol.

Pregnancy: Several reports suggest an association between foetal exposure to female sex hormones, including oral contraceptives, and congenital anomalies. Pregnancy should be excluded before continuing treatment in women who have missed two consecutive periods.

Nursing mothers: Active ingredients of oral contraceptives have been detected in the milk of mothers taking such drugs. The effect of Conova 30 on breast-fed infants has not been determined. Oral contraceptives may diminish lactation when given immediately postpartum.

Adverse effects: In addition to those mentioned under Warnings and Precautions other known or suspected side effects of oral contraceptives include nausea, vomiting, other gastro-intestinal symptoms (e.g., abdominal cramps and bloating), irregular vaginal bleeding, amenorrhoea, dysmenorrhoea, increase in size of uterine myofibromata, change in cervical erosion and secretion, endocervical hyperplasia, vaginal candidiasis, skin disorders including chloasma, breast and weight changes, ocular changes, headache, hypertension, Raynaud's disease, migraine, depression, change in libido and appetite, fluid retention, infertility after discontinuation, and changes in carbohydrate, lipid and vitamin metabolism.

The use of oral contraceptives has also been associated with a possible increased incidence of gallbladder disease.

Benign hepatic adenomas, although rare, have been reported with long term use of oral contraceptives. The adenoma may present as an abdominal mass, intra-abdominal bleeding and/or with signs and symptoms of acute abdomen.

Tests of endocrine, hepatic and thyroid function, as well as coagulation tests, may be affected by this preparation.

There is evidence of an association between the use of oral contraceptives and mesenteric thrombosis, Budd–Chiari syndrome, neuro-ocular lesions (e.g., retinal thrombosis and optic neuritis), although confirmatory studies have not been done.

Haemolytic uraemic syndrome has been reported in users of oral contraceptives.

Overdosage: Serious ill-effects have not been reported following acute ingestion of large doses of oral contraceptives by young children. Nausea and vomiting may occur and vaginal withdrawal bleeding may present in pre-pubertal girls. In general, treatment of overdosage is not necessary. However if thought appropriate, as there is no specific antidote, treatment should be symptomatic.

Pharmaceutical precautions Store below 30°C (86°F).

Legal category POM.

Package quantities Carton containing one strip of 21 tablets, with instructions.

Further information Nil.

Product licence number 0020/0066.

DIATENSEC*

Presentation Off-white, film coated tablets engraved SEARLE 916. Each tablet contains Spironolactone BP 50 mg.

Uses Essential hypertension and hypertension associated with diabetes.

Dosage and administration Food has been reported to increase the bioavailability of Diatensec. It is recommended that tablets are taken with meals.

Adults: Usual dose – 50–100 mg/day, which for difficult or severe cases may be gradually increased at two weekly intervals up to 200 mg/day. Treatment should be continued for two weeks or longer since an adequate response may not occur before this time. Dosage should subsequently be adjusted according to the response of the patient.

Elderly: It is recommended that treatment is started with the lowest dose and titrated upwards as required to achieve maximum benefit. Care should be taken in severe hepatic and renal impairment which may alter drug metabolism and excretion.

Children: Initial daily dosage should provide 3 mg of spironolactone per kilogram body weight, given in divided doses. Dosage should be adjusted on the basis of response and tolerance. If necessary a suspension may be prepared by crushing Diatensec tablets. A suitable suspending vehicle is methylcellulose mixture '450' (900 mg/10 ml) [Cologel*] 20% v/v, purified water to 100%. Such a suspension is chemically stable for one month when refrigerated.

Contra-indications, warnings, etc

Contra-indications: Diatensec is contra-indicated in patients with anuria, acute renal insufficiency, rapidly deteriorating or severe impairment of renal function, hyperkalaemia, Addison's disease and in patients who are hypersensitive to spironolactone. Diatensec should not be administered concurrently with other potassium-conserving diuretics and potassium supplements should not be given routinely with Diatensec as hyperkalaemia may be induced.

Warnings: Carcinogenicity: Spironolactone has been shown to produce tumours in rats when administered at high doses over a long period of time. The significance of these findings with respect to clinical use is not certain. However, the long term use of spironolactone in young patients requires careful consideration of the benefits and the potential hazard involved.

Precautions: Fluid and electrolyte balance: Fluid and electrolyte status should be regularly monitored, particularly in the elderly and those with significant renal impairment.

Hyperkalaemia may occur in patients with impaired renal function or excessive potassium intake and can cause cardiac irregularities which may be fatal. Should hyperkalaemia develop, Diatensec should be discontinued, and if necessary, active measures taken to reduce the serum potassium to normal.

Hyponatraemia may be induced, especially when Diatensec is administered in combination with other diuretics.

Urea: Reversible increases in blood urea have been reported in association with Diatensec therapy, particularly in the presence of impaired renal function.

Drug interactions: Potentiation of the effect of other antihypertensive drugs occurs and their dosage may need to be reduced when Diatensec is added to the treatment regime, and then adjusted as necessary.

As carbenoxolone may cause sodium retention and thus decrease the effectiveness of spironolactone, concurrent use should be avoided.

Spironolactone reduces vascular responsiveness to noradrenaline. Caution should be exercised in the management of patients subjected to regional or general anaesthesia while they are being treated with Diatensec.

Pregnancy: Spironolactone or its metabolites may cross the placental barrier. The use of Diatensec in pregnant women requires that the anticipated benefit be weighed against the possible hazards to the mother and foetus.

Nursing mothers: Canrenone, a metabolite of spironolactone, appears in breast milk. If use of Diatensec is considered essential, an alternative method of infant feeding should be instituted.

Adverse effects: Gynaecomastia may develop in association with the use of spironolactone. Development appears to be related to both dosage level and duration of therapy and is normally reversible when spironolactone is discontinued. In rare instances some breast enlargement may persist. Other adverse reactions reported in association with spironolactone include: gastrointestinal intolerance, drowsiness, lethargy, headache, mental confusion, ataxia, drug fever, skin rashes, menstrual irregularities, impotence and mild androgenic effects.

Overdosage: Acute overdosage may be manifested by drowsiness, mental confusion, nausea, vomiting, dizziness or diarrhoea. Hyponatraemia or hyperkalaemia may be induced but these effects are unlikely to be associated with acute overdosage. Symptoms of hyperkalaemia may manifest as paraesthesia, weakness, flaccid paralysis or muscle spasm and may be difficult to distinguish clinically from hypokalaemia. Electrocardiographic changes are the earliest specific signs of potassium disturbances. No specific antidote has been identified. Improvement may be expected after withdrawal of the drug. General supportive measures including replacement of fluids and electrolytes may be indicated. For hyperkalaemia, reduce potassium intake, administer potassium-excreting diuretics, intravenous glucose with regular insulin, or oral ion-exchange resins.

Pharmaceutical precautions Store below 30°C (86°F).

Legal category POM.

Package quantities Bottles containing 100 tablets.

Further information Diatensec as a competitive aldosterone antagonist increases sodium excretion whilst reducing potassium loss at the distal renal tubule. It has a gradual and prolonged action, maximum response being usually attained after 2–3 days' treatment. Combination of Diatensec with a conventional, more proximally acting diuretic usually enhances diuresis without excessive potassium loss.

Product licence number 0020/0089.

FEMULEN

Presentation White tablets engraved 'SEARLE' on both sides, containing Ethynodiol Diacetate BP 500 mcg.

Uses Oral contraception.

Dosage and administration Starting on the first day of menstruation, one tablet every day without a break in medication for as long as contraception is required. Additional contraceptive precautions (a sheath or a cap plus spermicide) should be taken for the first 14 days of the first pack. Tablets should be taken at the same time each day.

Missed tablets: If the woman misses one tablet or takes it later than the usual time, contraceptive efficacy may be reduced and additional contraceptive precautions (a sheath or a cap plus spermicide) should be used until the next period occurs. Women who miss a single tablet should be instructed to take the missed tablet as soon as they remember, even though this may mean taking two tablets on one single day. The regular tablet for that day should be taken at the usual time. If two or more consecutive tablets are missed Femulen should be discontinued and alternative contraceptive measures should be taken until menstruation occurs and the possibility of pregnancy is excluded.

Vomiting or diarrhoea: Vomiting or diarrhoea may reduce the effectiveness of Femulen, particularly if this should occur at or around the time of ovulation. If an episode of vomiting and/or diarrhoea occurs the woman should be advised to use an additional form of contraception (a sheath or a cap plus spermicide) until the next menstrual period occurs.

Contra-indications, warnings, etc
Contra-indications: The contra-indications for progestogen-only oral contraceptives are: known, suspected, or a past history of breast, genital or hormone dependent cancer; past or present, benign or malignant liver tumours; impaired liver function; active liver disease; history during pregnancy of idiopathic jaundice or severe pruritus; disorders of lipid metabolism; undiagnosed abnormal vaginal bleeding or amenorrhoea; known or suspected pregnancy.

Combined oestrogen/progestogen preparations have been associated with an increase in the risk of thromboembolic and thrombotic disease. Risk has been reported to be related to both oestrogenic and progestogenic activity. In the absence of long term epidemiological studies with progestogen-only oral contraceptives, it is required that the existence or history of thrombophlebitis, thromboembolic disorders, cerebral vascular disease, myocardial infarction, coronary artery disease, or a haemoglobinopathy be described as a contra-indication to Femulen as it is to oestrogen containing oral contraceptives.

Warnings: Femulen should be discontinued if there is a gradual or sudden, partial or complete loss of vision or any evidence of ocular changes, onset or aggravation of migraine or development of headache of a new kind which is recurrent, persistent or severe, suspicion of thrombosis or infarction, significant rise in blood pressure or if jaundice occurs.

Progestogen-only oral contraceptives may offer less protection against ectopic pregnancy, than against intrauterine pregnancy.

Precautions: Women receiving treatment with Femulen should be kept under regular medical surveillance.

Femulen should be discontinued at least 6 weeks before elective surgery or during periods of prolonged immobilisation. It would be reasonable to resume Femulen two or three weeks after surgery provided the woman is ambulant. Every woman, however, should be considered individually with regard to the nature of the operation, the extent of immobilisation, the presence of additional risk factors and the chance of unwanted conception.

Caution should be exercised where there is the possibility of an interaction between a pre-existing disorder and a known or suspected side-effect. The use of Femulen in women suffering from epilepsy, or with a history of migraine or cardiac or renal dysfunction may result in exacerbation of these disorders because of fluid retention. Caution should also be observed in women who wear contact lenses, women with impaired carbohydrate tolerance, depression, gallstones, varicose veins, hypertension, asthma or any disease that is prone to worsen during pregnancy.

Pregnancy: Several reports suggest an association between foetal exposure to female sex hormones, including oral contraceptives, and congenital anomalies.

If a woman does not have a menstrual period within 45 days of her last menstrual period, the possibility of pregnancy should be excluded.

Drug interactions: Femulen may be rendered less effective and increased incidence of breakthrough bleeding may occur by virtue of drug interaction. At present, drugs suspected to interact in this way include rifampicin, barbiturates, anticonvulsants, and antibiotics.

Nursing mothers: There is no evidence that progestogen-only oral contraceptives diminish the yield of breast milk. In a study of nursing mothers taking Femulen, the median percentage of norethisterone, the principal metabolite of ethynodiol diacetate given to the mother which was ingested by the infant was 0.02%. No adverse effect of the drug on the infants was noted.

Adverse effects: Women taking progestogen-only oral contraceptives for the first time may initially experience menstrual irregularity. This may include amenorrhoea, prolonged bleeding and/or spotting and should decrease with time. Clinical investigations with Femulen indicate that side-effects are infrequent and tend to decrease as treatment continues. Known or suspected side-effects of progestogen-only oral contraceptives include nausea, vomiting, other gastrointestinal symptoms, skin disorders including chloasma, breast and weight changes, ocular changes, headache, migraine, depression, change in libido, and appetite, increase in size of uterine myofibromata, and changes in carbohydrate, lipid or vitamin metabolism.

The use of oral contraceptives has also been associated with a possible increased incidence of gallbladder disease.

Benign hepatic adenomas, although rare, have been reported with long-term use of oral contraceptives. The adenoma may present as an abdominal mass, intra-abdominal bleeding and/or with signs and symptoms of acute abdomen.

Tests of endocrine, hepatic and thyroid function, as well as coagulation tests may be affected by this preparation.

Overdosage: Serious ill-effects have not been reported following acute ingestion of large doses of oral contraceptives by young children. Nausea and vomiting may occur and vaginal withdrawal bleeding may present in pre-pubertal girls. In general, treatment of overdosage is not necessary. However, if thought appropriate, as there is no specific antidote, treatment should be symptomatic.

Pharmaceutical precautions Store below 30°C (86°F).

Legal category POM.

Package quantities Carton of 28 tablets with instructions.

Further information Femulen does not necessarily inhibit ovulation but it is believed to discourage implantation of the fertilised ovum by altering the endometrium. Cervical mucus viscosity is also changed which may render the passage of sperm less likely.

Product licence number 0020/0054.

GRAVIGARD*
MINI-GRAVIGARD*

Presentation Two sizes of Gravigard intrauterine device are available.

Gravigard – Transverse arm 26 mm; vertical arm 36 mm.

Mini-Gravigard – Transverse arm 22 mm; vertical arm 28 mm

Each device consists of pure electrolytic copper wire, surface area approximately 200 mm², wound onto the vertical arm of a plastic carrier which approximates the shape of the number 7. The plastic carrier is composed of polypropylene homopolymer impregnated with barium sulphate to render it radio-opaque, with a monofilament thread attached to the base of the vertical arm. Each device is presented partially loaded in its inserter tube and instructions for use are included with each sterile pack.

Uses Intrauterine contraception.

Dosage and administration Gravigard is recommended for women with a uterine size measurement from external os to fundus greater than 6.5 cm. Mini-Gravigard is recommended for women with a uterine size measurement from external os to fundus of 5.5 to 6.5 cm. Gravigard and Mini-Gravigard should be replaced every two years. The procedure for insertion is fully detailed in the instructions for use leaflet included with each sterile pack. Insertion is not recommended if uterine size from external os to fundus measures less than 5.5 cm.

Although IUCDs may be inserted at any time during the menstrual cycle, insertion during or shortly after the menstrual period reduces the possibility of an existing undiagnosed pregnancy. Postpartum insertion is usually delayed until involution of the uterus is complete. The benefits of immediate post abortion insertion should be weighed against the risks due to the relatively soft structure of the uterus.

Contra-indications, warnings, etc

Contra-indications: Contra-indications are pregnancy; history of ectopic pregnancy; postpartum endometritis or septic abortion within the past three months; abnormalities of the uterine cavity including developmental abnormalities; large or multiple fibroids; acute pelvic inflammatory disease; a history of repeated, recent or severe pelvic inflammatory disease; acute cervicitis; cervical dysplasia; endometrial disease such as hyperplasia or uterine polyps; suspected or proven malignancy of the genital organs, including unresolved abnormal Papanicolaou smear; severe dysmenorrhoea; menorrhagia and/or intermenstrual bleeding, significant anaemia; heart disease; leukaemia; use of corticosteroid therapy because of the increased susceptibility to infection with certain micro-organisms which may possibly be introduced at the time of an IUCD insertion; Wilson's disease or a hypersensitivity to copper.

Medical diathermy to the abdominal and sacral regions is contra-indicated in Gravigard or Mini-Gravigard users because of the possibility of heat injury to the surrounding tissue.

Warnings: An increased incidence of pelvic inflammatory disease and menorrhagia associated with the use of IUCDs has been reported. Pelvic infection may result in future infertility. Women with certain known or suspected heart diseases are more susceptible to development of subacute bacterial endocarditis. Use of an IUCD in these women may represent a potential source of septic emboli. Appropriate precautions including administration of antibiotics should be observed when inserting an IUCD in such cases.

Syncope or bradycardia may occur in some women during insertion or removal of an IUCD. In the event of early signs of vasovagal attack, insertion may need to be abandoned or the device removed. The women should be kept supine, the head lowered and the legs elevated to the vertical position if necessary in order to restore cerebral blood flow. A clear airway must be maintained; an airway should always be at hand. Persistent bradycardia may be controlled with intravenous atropine in a dose of 0.6 mg. If oxygen is available it may be administered by using an Ambu bag. In the very rare emergency situation where the woman fails to regain consciousness she should be transferred to hospital intensive care.

Post-insertion cramps are usually of only a few minutes duration, but some women may experience cramps for several hours or days. Spotting, intermenstrual bleeding or increased menstrual flow may occur. If heavy or persistent bleeding or persistent abdominal cramps occur, removal of the device may be indicated.

Gravigard or Mini-Gravigard should be removed in the event of partial expulsion and a new device inserted. If perforation of the uterus or cervix is suspected, the device should be removed as soon as medically feasible. Adhesions, foreign body reactions and intestinal obstruction may result if an IUCD is left within the peritoneal cavity. Removal is also indicated in cases of pelvic infection resistant to treatment, menorrhagia producing significant anaemia, or intractable pain.

Precautions: A complete gynaecological examination, including measurement of the uterus, should precede insertion of the device. Ideally the woman should be re-examined within the first three months after insertion and annually thereafter. After insertion the woman should be taught to examine herself to ascertain the continued presence of the retrieval thread. Advise her to consult her doctor if pregnancy is suspected.

Intrauterine devices should be used with caution in women with anaemia, menorrhagia, hypermenorrhoea, a history of a previous uterine incision or perforation of the uterus and those receiving anticoagulants, steroid therapy or having a coagulopathy.

The possibility of a seizure being precipitated in an epileptic at or shortly after the insertion of an IUCD should also be borne in mind.

It has been reported that IUCDs may be less effective in insulin-dependent diabetics.

Lost threads: If the retrieval thread is not visible at the cervix on follow-up examination, it may have been drawn up into the uterus or cervical canal and may reappear during the next menstrual period. The thread may usually be located by gently probing with a suitable instrument.

If it cannot be found, it may have broken off, or the device may have been expelled. Ultrasound or X-ray may be used to locate the device.

Pregnancy: The risk of ectopic pregnancy is reported to be greater in women who conceive with an IUCD in situ than in those without an IUCD. Therefore, if a woman becomes pregnant with an IUCD in situ, she should be carefully evaluated for possible ectopic pregnancy.

There have been reports of an increased incidence of septic abortion, associated in some instances with septicaemia, septic shock and death in women who become pregnant with an IUCD in situ. Women who are pregnant with an IUCD in situ should be closely observed and told to report immediately all abnormal symptoms such as 'flu-like symptoms, fever, cramp-like pain, bleeding or excessive discharge, as the onset of septicaemia associated with septic abortion may be insidious with general symptoms rather than initial signs of spontaneous abortion. Also, the incidence of spontaneous abortion appears to be increased over that in unprotected women when conception occurs with an IUCD in situ. If pregnancy occurs with an IUCD in situ and the thread is visible then the device should be removed. If the thread is not visible or device removal would be difficult, the IUCD may be left in situ until the pregnancy goes to term or until a decision is made to terminate the pregnancy. If the woman elects to continue the pregnancy, careful observation is required. The long term effects of intrauterine copper on the foetus are unknown.

Adverse effects: Uterine or cervical perforation, vaginal discharge, embedment and allergic reactions have been reported.

Pharmaceutical precautions Gravigard and Mini-Gravigard are supplied in sterile packs which should not be opened until required for insertion. Each device should be handled with aseptic precautions and should not be left folded in its inserter tube for more than two minutes, as this may prevent the transverse arm from reassuming its correct position.

Care should be taken not to damage the sterile package which should be stored below 30°C (86°F).

Legal category POM.

Package quantities
Gravigard: Pack containing one sterile device.
　　　　　　Outer containing five packs.
　　　　　　Pack containing ten sterile devices.
Mini-Gravigard: Pack containing one sterile device.
　　　　　　Outer containing five packs.
　　　　　　Pack containing ten sterile devices.

Further information The average amount of copper eluted from copper IUCDs is well below the daily dietary intake of copper. Small increases of endometrial copper levels have been noted in the presence of copper IUCDs, but these are not cumulative. No changes in blood levels of copper have been detected.

Product licence numbers
Gravigard: 　　　0020/0062
Mini-Gravigard: 　0020/0085

LOMOTIL* TABLETS
LOMOTIL* LIQUID

Presentation *Lomotil Tablets:* White tablets engraved SEARLE on one side. Each tablet contains Diphenoxylate

Hydrochloride BP 2.5 mg with Atropine Sulphate PhEur 25 mcg.

Lomotil Liquid: Red, cherry flavoured liquid. Each 5 ml measure contains Diphenoxylate Hydrochloride BP 2.5 mg with Atropine Sulphate PhEur 25 mcg.

Uses Adjunctive therapy to appropriate rehydration in acute and chronic diarrhoea.

Control of stool formation after colostomy or ileostomy.
Relief of symptoms in ulcerative colitis (see Warnings)

Dosage and administration *Caution:* The recommended dosage should not be exceeded. Once satisfactory control is achieved, dosage should be reduced to suit the requirements of the individual patient.

Adults: The recommended starting dose is four tablets, or four 5 ml measures, followed by two tablets or two 5 ml measures every six hours.

Elderly: Consideration should be given to the presence of other disease and concomitant drug therapy (see *Precautions*).

Children: Recommended dosage guide:
Under 2 years: Not recommended.
2-3 years: 　1 tablet or one 5 ml measure twice daily.
4-8 years: 　1 tablet or one 5 ml measure three times daily.
9-12 years: 　1 tablet or one 5 ml measure four times daily.
13-16 years: 2 tablets or two 5 ml measures three times daily.

Contra-indications, warnings, etc Lomotil is contra-indicated in patients with a known hypersensitivity to diphenoxylate hydrochloride or atropine, in patients with jaundice or intestinal obstruction, and in the treatment of diarrhoea associated with pseudomembranous enterocolitis.

Appropriate fluid and electrolyte therapy should be given to protect against dehydration. If severe dehydration or electrolyte imbalance is present, Lomotil should be withheld until appropriate corrective therapy has been initiated.

In some patients with acute ulcerative colitis, agents which inhibit intestinal motility or delay intestinal transit time have been reported to induce toxic megacolon. Patients with acute ulcerative colitis should be observed carefully and Lomotil therapy should be discontinued promptly if abdominal distension or other untoward symptoms develop.

Lomotil should be used with extreme caution in patients with advanced hepatorenal disease and in all patients with abnormal liver function since hepatic coma may be precipitated.

Precautions: Because a subtherapeutic dose of atropine is added to Lomotil, atropinic effects may occur in susceptible individuals or in overdosage. Individuals with Down's syndrome appear to have an increased susceptibility to the actions of atropine.

Drug interactions: Since the chemical structure of diphenoxylate hydrochloride resembles that of meperidine hydrochloride, concurrent use with MAO inhibitors could precipitate hypertensive crisis. Close observation is required when these medications are given concomitantly with diphenoxylate hydrochloride.

Diphenoxylate hydrochloride may potentiate the action of central nervous system depressants such as barbiturates, tranquillisers and alcohol.

Pregnancy: The safety of Lomotil in pregnancy has not

been established. Animal teratology and reproduction studies have demonstrated no adverse effects. The benefits of therapy must be weighed against the possible hazards to the mother and foetus.

Nursing mothers: Diphenoxylate hydrochloride and atropine sulphate may be excreted in human milk. If a nursing mother is taking Lomotil, the infant may exhibit some effects of the drug.

Adverse effects:

Adverse reactions reported include: *Central nervous system:* malaise/lethargy/sedation/somnolence, confusion, dizziness, restlessness, depression, euphoria, hallucinations, headache.

Allergic: anaphylaxis, angioedema, urticaria, pruritus.

Gastrointestinal system: paralytic ileus, toxic megacolon, gastrointestinal intolerance such as nausea and vomiting, anorexia, abdominal discomfort.

Atropine effects, such as flushing, dryness of skin and mucous membranes, tachycardia, hyperthermia and urinary retention may occur, especially in children.

Overdosage: Accidental overdosage may produce narcosis with respiratory depression or atropine poisoning or both, particularly in children. Symptoms of overdosage include dryness of the skin and mucous membranes, flushing, hyperthermia and tachycardia, nystagmus, pinpoint pupils, hypotonic reflexes, lethargy, coma and severe respiratory depression. The onset of symptoms of overdosage may be considerably delayed and respiratory depression may not become evident until as late as 12 to 30 hours after ingestion, and may recur in spite of an initial response to narcotic antagonists. Continuous observation should be maintained for at least 48 hours.

If respiratory depression develops, naloxone, a specific antidote, should be administered. The duration of action of naloxone hydrochloride is considerably shorter than that of diphenoxylate hydrochloride and repeated injections of the antidote may be required. Establishment of a patent airway and artificial ventilation may be needed. If the patient is not comatose gastric lavage and administration of a slurry of activated charcoal may be indicated.

Pharmaceutical precautions Store below 30°C (86°F).

Legal category POM.

Package quantities

Lomotil Tablets: Pack of 100 containing 5 blister strips of 20 tablets. Bottles containing 500 and 1,000 tablets.

Lomotil Liquid: Bottles containing 100 ml (with 5 ml measure) and 500 ml.

Further information Nil.

Product licence numbers
Lomotil Tablets: 0020/5014
Lomotil Liquid: 0020/5015

NOVAGARD*

Presentation Novagard is an intrauterine device consisting of pure copper wire with a silver core, surface area approximately 200 mm², wound onto the vertical arm of a T-shaped plastic carrier. The plastic carrier is composed of polyethylene impregnated with barium sulphate to render it radio-opaque, with a polyethylene thread attached to the base of the vertical arm. The device is presented partially loaded in its inserter tube and instructions for use are included with each sterile pack.

Novagard dimensions – Transverse arms 32 mm; vertical arm 32 mm.

Uses Intrauterine contraception.

Dosage and administration Novagard is recommended for women with a uterine size measurement from external os to fundus greater than 5.5 cm.

Novagard should be replaced at least every five years. The procedure for insertion is fully detailed in the instructions for use leaflet included with each sterile pack.

Although IUCDs may be inserted at any time during the menstrual cycle, insertion during or shortly after the menstrual period reduces the possibility of an existing undiagnosed pregnancy. Postpartum insertion is usually delayed until involution of the uterus is complete. The benefits of immediate post abortion insertion should be weighed against the risks due to the relatively soft structure of the uterus.

Contra-indications, warnings, etc

Contra-indications: Contra-indications are pregnancy; history of ectopic pregnancy; postpartum endometritis or septic abortion within the past three months; abnormalities of the uterine cavity including developmental abnormalities; large or multiple fibroids; acute pelvic inflammatory disease; a history of repeated, recent or severe pelvic inflammatory disease; acute cervicitis; cervical dysplasia; endometrial disease such as hyperplasia or uterine polyps; suspected or proven malignancy of the genital organs, including unresolved abnormal Papanicolaou smear; severe dysmenorrhoea; menorrhagia and/or intermenstrual bleeding; significant anaemia; heart disease; leukaemia; use of chronic corticosteroid therapy because of the increased susceptibility to infection with certain micro-organisms which may possibly be introduced at the time of an IUCD insertion; Wilson's disease or a hypersensitivity to copper.

Medical diathermy to the abdominal and sacral regions is contra-indicated in Novagard users because of the possibility of heat injury to the surrounding tissues.

Warnings: An increased incidence of pelvic inflammatory disease and menorrhagia associated with the use of IUCDs has been reported. Pelvic infection may result in future infertility. Women with certain known or suspected heart diseases are more susceptible to development of subacute bacterial endocarditis. Use of an IUCD in these women may represent a potential source of septic emboli. Appropriate precautions including administration of antibiotics should be observed when inserting an IUCD in such cases.

Syncope or bradycardia may occur in some women during insertion or removal of an IUCD. In the event of early signs of vasovagal attack, insertion may need to be abandoned or the device removed. The woman should be kept supine, the head lowered and the legs elevated to the vertical position if necessary in order to restore cerebral blood flow. A clear airway must be maintained; an airway should always be at hand. Persistent bradycardia may be controlled with intravenous atropine in a dose of 0.6 mg. If oxygen is available it may be administered by using an Ambu bag. In the very rare emergency situation where the woman fails to regain consciousness she should be transferred to hospital intensive care.

Post-insertion cramps are usually of only a few minutes duration, but some women may experience cramps for several hours or days. Spotting, intermenstrual bleeding or increased menstrual flow may occur. If heavy or persistent bleeding or persistent abdominal cramps occur, removal of the device may be indicated.

Novagard should be removed in the event of partial expulsion and a new device inserted. If perforation of the uterus or cervix is suspected, the device should be removed as soon as medically feasible. Adhesions, foreign body reactions and intestinal obstruction may result if an IUCD is left within the peritoneal cavity. Removal is also indicated in cases of pelvic infection resistant to treatment, menorrhagia producing significant anaemia, or intractable pain.

Precautions: A complete gynaecological examination, including measurement of the uterus, should precede insertion of the device. Ideally the woman should be re-examined within the first three months after insertion and annually thereafter. After insertion the woman should be taught to examine herself to ascertain the continued presence of the retrieval thread. Advise her to consult her doctor if pregnancy is suspected.

Intrauterine devices should be used with caution in women with anaemia, menorrhagia, hypermenorrhoea, a history of a previous uterine incision or perforation of the uterus and those receiving anticoagulants, steroid therapy or having a coagulopathy.

The possibility of a seizure being precipitated in an epileptic, at or shortly after the insertion of an IUCD should also be borne in mind.

It has been reported that IUCDs may be less effective in insulin-dependent diabetics.

Lost threads: If the retrieval thread is not visible at the cervix on follow-up examination, it may have been drawn up into the uterus or cervical canal and may reappear during the next menstrual period. The thread may usually be located by gently probing with a suitable instrument. If it cannot be found, it may have broken off, or the device may have been expelled. Ultrasound or X-ray may be used to locate the device.

Pregnancy: The risk of ectopic pregnancy is reported to be greater in women who conceive with an IUCD in situ than in those without an IUCD. Therefore, if a woman becomes pregnant with an IUCD in situ, she should be carefully evaluated for possible ectopic pregnancy.

There have been reports of an increased incidence of septic abortion, associated in some instances with septicaemia, septic shock and death, in women who became pregnant with an IUCD in situ. Women who are pregnant with an IUCD in situ should be closely observed and told to report immediately all abnormal symptoms such as 'flu-like symptoms, fever, cramp-like pain, bleeding or excessive discharge, as the onset of septicaemia associated with septic abortion may be insidious with general symptoms rather than initial signs of spontaneous abortion. Also, the incidence of spontaneous abortion appears to be increased over that in unprotected women when conception occurs with an IUCD in situ. If pregnancy occurs with an IUCD in situ and the thread is visible then the device should be removed. If the thread is not visible or device removal would be difficult, the IUCD may be left in situ until the pregnancy goes to term or until a decision is made to terminate the pregnancy. If the woman elects to continue the pregnancy, careful observation is required. The long term effects of intrauterine copper on the foetus are unknown.

Adverse-effects: Uterine or cervical perforation, vaginal discharge, embedment and allergic reactions have been reported.

Pharmaceutical precautions Novagard is supplied in a sterile pack which should not be opened until required for insertion. Each device should be handled with aseptic precautions and it is advisable that the folded device in the inserter tube should not be left for more than two minutes, as this may prevent the transverse arms from reassuming the correct position.

Care should be taken not to damage the sterile package which should be stored below 30°C (86°F).

Legal category POM.

Package quantities
Pack containing one sterile device.
Outer containing five packs of one sterile device.
Pack containing ten sterile devices.

Further information The average amount of copper eluted from copper IUCDs is well below the daily dietary intake of copper. Small increases of endometrial copper levels have been noted in the presence of copper IUCDs, but these are not cumulative. No changes in blood levels of copper have been detected.

Product licence number 0022/0046.
The product licence is held by Kabi Vitrum.

PRO-BANTHINE*

Presentation Pink, sugar coated, biconvex tablets, printed SEARLE on one side. Each tablet contains Propantheline Bromide BP 15 mg.

Uses *Gastrointestinal:* Peptic ulcer, acute pancreatitis.

Genitourinary: Enuresis.

Miscellaneous: Diagnostic radiological procedures, hyperhidrosis.

Dosage and administration *Caution:* Food has been reported to reduce the bioavailability of Pro-Banthine. Tablets should be taken at least one hour before meals.

Adults: Peptic ulcer: The recommended initial starting dose is one tablet before each meal, and two tablets at bedtime. Subsequently, dosage should be adjusted according to the patient's individual response and tolerance.

Diagnostic radiological procedures: Two tablets should be given 45 minutes prior to the diagnostic procedure.

Other indications: A dosage of up to eight tablets daily may be required.

Elderly: Consideration should be given to the presence of other disease and concomitant drug therapy (see *Contra-indications, warnings, etc.*). Elderly patients may be more susceptible to anticholinergic side-effects.

Children: For enuresis the usual dosage is one to three tablets taken at bedtime. Although clinical trials using Pro-Banthine tablets for other indications have not been conducted in children, as a guide the total daily dosage should not exceed 2 mg per kilogram body weight, and should be given in divided doses.

Contra-indications, warnings, etc Pro-Banthine is contra-indicated in patients with obstructive diseases of the gastrointestinal or urinary tract, pyloric stenosis, intestinal atony, severe ulcerative colitis or toxic megacolon, hiatus hernia associated with reflux oesophagitis, unstable cardiovascular adjustment in acute haemorrhage, myasthenia gravis, glaucoma and in patients who are hypersensitive to propantheline bromide.

In some patients, especially those with ileostomy or colostomy, diarrhoea may be a symptom of incomplete intestinal obstruction. Pro-Banthine therapy should be avoided in such patients.

Patients with severe heart disease in whom an increase in heart rate is undesirable should be observed closely if Pro-Banthine is administered.

Pro-Banthine may produce drowsiness or blurred vision. Patients should not drive or operate machinery if affected in this way.

Precautions: Patients with prostatic hypertrophy may experience some urinary hesitancy. This may be minimised if such patients are advised to micturate at the time the medication is taken.

Patients with ulcerative colitis should be treated with caution, since Pro-Banthine may suppress intestinal motility to the point of producing paralytic ileus, thus precipitating or aggravating toxic megacolon.

Pro-Banthine should be used with caution in the elderly and in all patients with autonomic neuropathy, hepatic or renal disease, hyperthyroidism, coronary heart disease, congestive heart failure, cardiac arrhythmias or hypertension.

Drug interactions: Concurrent use of Pro-Banthine with slow-dissolving tablets of digoxin may cause increased serum digoxin levels.

Since anticholinergics tend to delay gastric emptying they may alter the absorption of other medication given concomitantly.

Excessive cholinergic blockade may occur if Pro-Banthine is given concomitantly with belladonna alkaloids or synthetic and semisynthetic anticholinergic agents.

Pregnancy: Animal reproduction and teratology studies have not been performed. The use of Pro-Banthine in pregnant women requires that the anticipated benefit be weighed against the possible hazards to mother and foetus.

Nursing mothers: Whether propantheline bromide is excreted in human breast milk is unknown. No animal studies have been conducted. If use of the drug is considered essential the anticipated benefit should be weighed against the possible hazards to mother and child.

Adverse effects: Varying degrees of drying of salivary secretion may occur, as well as mydriasis, blurred vision and heat stroke. Other adverse reactions reported include: nervousness, drowsiness, dizziness, insomnia, headache, tachycardia, loss of the sense of taste, nausea, vomiting, constipation, urinary hesitancy and retention, impotence, allergic dermatitis and anaphylaxis.

Overdosage: Intensification of the usual side effects may occur. Severe intoxication may result in disturbances of the central nervous system (from restlessness and excitement to psychotic behaviour), circulatory changes (flushing, fall in blood pressure, circulatory failure), respiratory failure, paralysis and coma.

In the event of overdosage, empty the stomach by aspiration or lavage. Physostigmine salicylate 0.5 to 2 mg should be injected intravenously to control the central and peripheral effects of propantheline bromide. Since it has a brief duration of action of about 1 to 2 hours, it may be necessary to repeat injections up to a total dose of 5 mg.

Excitement may be controlled by small doses of a short-acting barbiturate such as thiopentone sodium 100 mg.

Supportive therapy may require oxygen and assisted respiration, ice bags or alcohol sponges for hyperpyrexia, especially in children, bladder catheterisation and the administration of fluids.

Pharmaceutical precautions Store below 30°C (86°F).

Legal category POM.

Package quantities Bottles containing 100 and 1,000 tablets.

Further information Propantheline bromide is extensively metabolised in man. Some enzymic hydrolysis of the drug may occur in the gastrointestinal tract prior to its absorption.

Studies in healthy men demonstrated that peak plasma levels of unchanged drug were reached within 2 hours of a single, oral dose of propantheline bromide. Following single oral dosing the plasma elimination half-life was about 2–3 hours and some 1–10% of propantheline bromide was excreted in urine as unchanged drug.

In healthy men studies have shown onset of anticholinergic effects within 1 hour of oral administration. Effects persisted for up to 6 hours after oral dosing.

Product licence number 0020/5026

REGULAN*

Presentation Premeasured, single-dose sachet containing 6.4 g of beige rough ground powder. Active ingredient – 3.6 g Ispaghula Husk BP.

Uses For the treatment of constipation and patients requiring a high fibre regimen.

Dosage and administration
1. Pour measured dosage into a glass.
2. Slowly add 150 ml ($\frac{1}{4}$ pint) COOL water.
3. Drink entire contents immediately. An additional glass of liquid may be taken if needed. Adequate fluid intake should be maintained.

Adults and Children over 12 years: The usual dosage is the entire contents of one sachet taken one to three times daily.

Elderly: See *Precautions.*

Children: A reduced dosage based upon the age and size of the child should be given.

6–12 years: $\frac{1}{2}$–1 level 5 ml teaspoonful one to three times daily.

Contra-indications, warnings, etc Regulan should not be given to patients with intestinal obstruction, faecal impaction or hypersensitivity to ispaghula.

Regulan should always be taken as a liquid suspension and should be drunk immediately after mixing.

Precautions: It may be advisable to supervise treatment in the elderly or debilitated and patients with intestinal narrowing or decreased motility, as rare instances of gastrointestinal obstruction have been reported with mucilloid preparations when taken with insufficient liquid, contrary to the administration instructions.

The sucrose content of each 6.4 g dose has a calorific value of approximately 3.5 kilocalories, this should be considered when taken by diabetics.

Pregnancy and Lactation: The benefits of therapy should be weighed against any possible hazards if used during pregnancy and lactation.

Adverse effects: Allergy, gastrointestinal obstruction or impaction have been reported with hydrophilic mucilloid preparations.

Overdosage: No instances of true overdosage have been reported. If overdosage should occur there is no specific treatment and symptomatic measures should be employed.

Pharmaceutical precautions Store below 30°C (86°F).

Legal category GSL.

Package quantities Box of 30 sachets.

Further information Regulan is gluten-free. Each sachet of Regulan contains 0.23 mmol sodium.

Product licence number 0020/0087.

*Trade Mark

GX Limited
The Old Post House
London End
Beaconsfield
Bucks HP9 2JH

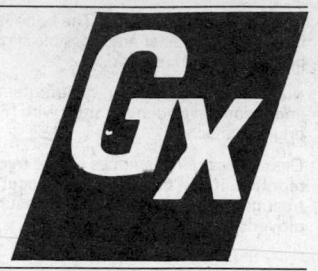

GX* ALLOPURINOL TABLETS

Presentation Round, biconvex, creamy white, un-coated tablets engraved on one face with GX logo and on reverse with strength and code number on either side of breakline i.e. 100 mg–100/238 and 300 mg–300/239. Each tablet contains 100 mg or 300 mg of allopurinol.

Allopurinol is a white, odourless, tasteless micro-crystalline powder.

Uses 1. Treatment of excess body urate including gout.
2. Prophalaxis of uric acid and calcium oxalate stones.

Dosage and administration The initial dose should be 100–200 mg daily. The maintenance dose is 200–600 mg daily. Doses in excess of 300 mg should be taken in divided doses. It has rarely been found necessary to exceed 900 mg per day.

The dose should be adjusted by monitoring serum uric acid and/or urinary uric acid levels at appropriate intervals until the desired effect is attained. This may take one to three weeks.

Children: 10–20 mg/kg body weight per day. Use in children is mainly indicated in malignant conditions, especially leukaemia and certain enzyme disorders (e.g. Lesch-Nyhan syndrome).

Initiation of therapy: in early stages of treatment with allopurinol, as with the uricosuric agents, an acute attack of gouty arthritis may be precipitated. It is therefore advisable to give, for at least one month, a prophylactic dose of colchicine or other suitable anti-inflammatory agent.

Use with uricosurics: Allopurinol does not interfere with the action of uricosuric agents. They may, therefore, be given concurrently. When changing from uricosuric therapy to allopurinol 1–3 weeks overlap is recommended to ensure continuous hypouricaemic effect.

Use in neoplastic conditions: It is advisable to start treatment with allopurinol before cytotoxic therapy when allopurinol is being given to prevent uric acid nephro-pathy in these conditions.

Dose recommendations in impaired renal function: As allopurinol and its metabolites are excreted via the kidney, impaired renal function may cause retention of allopurinol and its metabolites with consequent prolon-gation of action. Serum uric acid levels should be monitored in such patients as the amount or frequency of dosage might require reduction:

If creatinine clearance exceeds 20 ml/minute, give standard dose.

If creatinine clearance is between 20 and 10 ml/minute, give 100–200 mg/day.

If creatinine clearance is less than 10 ml/minute give 100 mg/day or at longer intervals.

Dose recommendations in renal dialysis: As allopurinol and its metabolites are removed by renal dialysis, if frequent dialysis is required, an alternative schedule of 300–400 mg allopurinol after each dialysis (with none in the interim) should be considered.

Contra-indications, warnings, etc Acute gout. Known intolerance to allopurinol. Treatment should not be started during or immediately after an acute attack of gout. When 6-mercaptopurine or azathioprine is given concurrently with allopurinol, only one quarter of the usual dose of the cytotoxic should be given because inhibition of xanthine oxidase will prolong its activity. Because of an increase in the plasma half life of adenine arabinoside in the presence of allopurinol, extra vigilance is necessary to recognise enhanced toxic effects. There is no unequivocal evidence that allopurinol potentiates the activity of other cytotoxic drugs. A reduction in dosage should be considered in the presence of renal and/or hepatic disorders.

Adverse reactions are rare and mostly of a minor nature. The incidence is higher in the presence of renal and/or hepatic disorders. When a patient on chlorpro-pamide is given allopurinol there may be a risk of prolonged hypoglycaemic activity if renal function is poor.

The possible potentiation of anticoagulant action should be borne in mind when a patient on anticoagulants is given allopurinol.

Skin reactions: These are the most common reactions and may occur at any time during treatment. They may be pruritic, maculopapular, sometimes scaly or purpuric and rarely exfoliative. Should such reactions occur, allopurinol should be withdrawn immediately. After recovery from mild reactions, allopurinol can be re-introduced at a low dose (e.g. 50 mg/day) which may be gradually increased. If the rash recurs, allopurinol should be withdrawn.

Generalised hypersensitivity: If exfoliative skin reactions associated with other signs of hypersensitivity including fever, lymphadenopathy, arthralgia and eosinophilia occur (although this is rare), allopurinol should be withdrawn immediately and permanently. Corticoste-roids may be beneficial in overcoming these reactions. Patients manifesting generalised hypersensitivity reac-tions usually have pre-existing renal and/or hepatic disorders.

Gastro-intestinal disorder: Nausea and vomiting have

been reported – these may be avoided by prescribing allopurinol to be taken after meals.

Blood and lymphatic system: There have been occasional reports of transient reduction in the numbers of circulating formed elements of the blood. These are usually in association with pre-existing renal and/or hepatic disorders. Any clinical significance has yet to be demonstrated.

Miscellaneous: Exacerbation of acute gouty attacks can occur in the early stages of hypouricaemic therapy. In conditions where the body's miscible urate pool is increased (e.g. malignant disease and its treatment, Lesch-Nyhan syndrome), the rise in xanthine concentration resulting from allopurinol action may lead to deposition of xanthine in tissue. The risk of this deposition in the kidney will be reduced by adequate hydration and fluid intake should ensure urinary output. Xanthine crystals have been observed in muscle tissue of patients taking allopurinol but this does not appear to have any clinical significance.

The following complaints have been occasionally reported: fever, general malaise, headache, vertigo, somnolence, taste perversion, hepatic necrosis, granulomatous hepatitis, abnormal liver function tests, hyperlipaemia, visual disorder, cataracts, macular changes, neurophathy, impotence, diebetes mellitus, furunculosis, alopecia, hypertension, haematuria, oedema.

However, the above do not appear to have a clear cause and effect relationship with allopurinol.

Treatment of overdosage: No reports of overdosage or acute intoxication have been published.

Pharmaceutical precautions Store below 25°C. Keep dry.

Legal category POM.

Package quantities
GX Allopurinol Tablets 100 mg: containers of 100.
GX Allopurinol Tablets 300 mg: containers of 30.

Further information Nil.

Product licence numbers
GX Allopurinol Tablets 100 mg   6502/0013
GX Allopurinol Tablets 300 mg   6502/0014

GX* AMITRIPTYLINE TABLETS

Presentation Round, biconvex, coloured, film-coated tablets engraved on one face with GX logo and on reverse with strength and code number. 25 mg – yellow coded 25/103. The tablets contain the stated weight of amitriptyline hydrochloride.

Uses Symptoms of depressive illness where sedation is required.

Dosage and administration *Adults:* Therapy should be started with an initial low dosage of 75 mg per day in divided doses or a single dose at night and increased gradually up to 200 mg per day according to clinical response and any evidence of intolerance. Maintenance dosage is 50–100 mg at night. Maintenance therapy should continue for at least 3 months to lessen chances of relapse.

Elderly patients and adolescents: Often respond to lower dosage (10 50 mg daily).

Not recommended for children under 12 years.

Contra-indications, warnings, etc Recent myocardial infarction, arrhythmias, heart block of any degree, congestive cardiac failure, coronary artery insufficiency, mania, severe liver disease, hypersensitivity to tricyclic antidepressants. Co-administration with monoamine oxidase inhibitors.

Use in pregnancy should be avoided unless there are compelling reasons – the safety of amitriptyline in pregnancy and nursing mothers has not been established.

The elderly are particularly liable to experience side effects especially agitation, confusion, postural hypotension.

Patients with severe depression should be closely monitored (particularly during early stages of therapy) when partial response may increase risk of suicide.

Amitriptyline may enhance the response to alcohol, barbiturates and other CNS depressants. Barbiturates may decrease the antidepressant action of amitriptyline.

Because of its atropine-like action, caution should be exercised when treating patients with a history of narrow-angle glaucoma, urinary retention or increased intra-ocular pressure. Similarly epilepsy or recent convulsions, hepatic insufficiency, hyperthyroidism, cardiovascular disorders or blood dyscrasias or symptoms suggestive of prostatic hypertrophy.

Anaesthetics given during therapy may increase risk of arrhythmias and hypotension – should surgery be necessary, the anaesthetist should be informed that the patient is being treated with GX Amitriptyline.

Drug interactions: At least 2 weeks should elapse after treatment with monoamine oxidase inhibitors before amitriptyline treatment is commenced. Even then amitriptyline treatment should be cautious – commencing with low dosage and slow increments.

It is advisable to review all antihypertensive therapy during tricyclic antidepressant treatment – amitriptyline may decrease the effect of guanethidine, debrisoquine, bethanidine and clonidine.

Amitriptyline should not be given with directly acting sympathomimetic agents such as adrenaline, ephedrine, isoprenaline, noradrenaline, phenylephrine and phenylpropanolamine. Caution should be exercised when administering GX Amitriptyline in combination with ethclorvynol or any drugs having an anticholinergic action.

Amitriptyline may enhance response to alcohol, barbiturates and other CNS depressants. Barbiturates may, in turn, increase the antidepressant action of amitriptyline.

Thyroid hormone medication may need to be reduced when given concurrently with amitriptyline.

Patients should be closely monitored during the first month of therapy as improvement may not occur.

Amitriptyline may impair alertness in some patients who should be warned not to drive vehicles or operate machinery.

Confusion may occur at high doses or in elderly patients. Cardiac arrhythmias and severe hypotension are likely to occur with high dosage. These may also occur in patients with pre-existing heart disease taking normal dosage.

The following adverse effects have been reported with tricyclic antidepressants. Essentially those associated with the tricyclic group of antidepressants and may take 2–4 weeks to become apparent. Thus side effects may be: *Cardiovascular* mainly hypotension or tachycardia; *CNS* mainly confusional states; *Anticholinergic* mainly dry mouth, blurred vision, constipation, urinary retention; *Allergic* mainly skin rashes, oedema of face and tongue;

Haematological mainly bone marrow depression; *Gastro-intestinal* mainly nausea, vomiting, diarrhoea, anorexia; *Endocrine* mainly breast enlargement, testicular swelling, increased or decreased libido.

Other side effects include dizziness, fatigue, headache, weakness, increased perspiration, increased appetite, urinary frequency, mydriasis, alopecia.

Abrupt withdrawal after prolonged administration can cause nausea, headache and malaise. This is not indicative of addiction.

Overdosage: There is no specific antidote for tricyclic antidepressant poisoning. Treatment should be symptomatic and based on cardiac and respiratory support.

The stomach should be emptied by aspiration and lavage. Intravenous diazepam or intramuscular paraldehyde should be given to control convulsions. Parenteral neostigmine has been used to correct cardiac irregularities. Fluid intake should be maintained by infusion of electrolyte solutions. Respiration may need to be assisted and corticosteroids administered.

Pharmaceutical precautions Store below 25°C in a dry place.

Legal category POM

Package quantities 25 mg tablets in Securitainers of 100.

Further information Nil.

Product licence number 6502/0029.

GX* AMPICILLIN CAPSULES

Presentation Capsules containing ampicillin trihydrate, equivalent to the stated strength in terms of ampicillin. 1.15 g Ampicillin trihydrate is approximately equivalent to 1 g of ampicillin. Grey/red capsules overprinted with GX logo, strength and code number i.e. 250 mg (GX 250/232) and 500 mg (GX 500/233).

Uses Treatment of infections of the respiratory tract such as pneumonia and bronchitis and especially when *H. influenzae* is the causative organism. Treatment of infections of the urinary tract and of gonorrhoea.

Dosage and administration Dose for adults: 1 g to 8 g daily in divided doses.

Contra-indications, warnings, etc Should not be prescribed for penicillin hypersensitive patients and with caution for patients with known history of allergy.

If a rash is reported, treatment with ampicillin should be discontinued.

Suppression of intestinal bacteria by ampicillin has been blamed for a number of cases of failure of oral contraceptives.

Allergic reactions occur in hypersensitive patients. These can be severe with anaphylactic shock, collapse and sometimes death occurring within a few minutes. Skin reactions are the most common side effect and are of two types – urticarial and typical of penicillin hypersensitivity and maculopapular characteristic of ampicillin hypersensitivity often appearing about 5 days after treatment has finished.

Most patients with infectious mononucleosis (glandular fever) develop a skin rash when treated with ampicillin.

Diarrhoea, nausea and vomiting also occur in some patients.

Small amounts of ampicillin excreted in milk may provoke allergic reactions in breast-fed infants.

At the first sign of immediate allergic reaction, 0.3 ml to 1 ml adrenalin injection should be given intramuscularly followed by a further dose if no improvement occurs.

Cutaneous reactions usually subside spontaneously within a few hours or days, or control may be effected by oral administration of antihistamines.

Pharmaceutical precautions Store below 30°C. Keep well closed.

Legal category POM.

Package quantities
GX Ampicillin capsules 250 mg: Containers of 100.
GX Ampicillin capsules 500 mg: Containers of 100.

Further information Nil.

Product licence numbers
GX Ampicillin capsules 250 mg: 6502/0015
GX Ampicillin capsules 500 mg: 6502/0016

GX* AMPICILLIN SYRUP

Presentation Syrups containing ampicillin trihydrate, equivalent to the stated strength in terms of ampicillin. 1.15 g Ampicillin trihydrate is approximately equivalent to 1 g of ampicillin. Pleasantly flavoured granules to which water is added to produce 100 mls of cream coloured suspension. Two strengths: 125 mg/5 ml and 250 mg/5 ml.

Uses Treatment of infections of the respiratory tract such as pneumonia and bronchitis and especially where *H. influenzae* is the causative organism. Treatment of infections of the urinary tract and gonorrhoea.

Dosage and administration *Adults:* 1 g to 8 g daily in divided doses.

Children: Up to 1 year 62.5 mg to 125 mg every six hours.

1–5 years: 125 mg to 187.5 mg every six hours.
6–12 years: 187.5 mg to 250 mg every six hours.

Contra-indications, warnings, etc Should not be prescribed for penicillin hypersensitive patients and with caution for patients with known history of allergy.

If a rash is reported, treatment with ampicillin should be discontinued.

Suppression of intestinal bacteria by ampicillin has been blamed for a number of cases of failure of oral contraceptives.

Allergic reactions occur in hyper-sensitive patients. These can be severe with anaphylactic shock, collapse and sometimes death occurring within a few minutes.

Skin reactions are the most common side effect and are of two types – urticarial and typical of penicillin hypersensitivity and maculopapular characteristic of ampicillin hypersensitivity often appearing about 5 days after treatment has finished.

Most patients with infectious mononucleosis (glandular fever) develop a skin rash when treated with ampicillin. Diarrhoea, nausea and vomiting also occur in some patients. Small amounts of ampicillin excreted in milk may provoke allergic reactions in breast-fed infants.

At the first sign of immediate allergic reaction, 0.3 ml to 1 ml of adrenalin injection should be given intramuscularly followed by a further dose if no improvement occurs.

Cutaneous reactions usually subside spontaneously

within a few hours or days, or control may be effected by oral administration of antihistamines.

Pharmaceutical precautions Store below 15°C in a dry place. When dispensed ampicillin syrup should be stored in a cool place (preferably in a refrigerator) and used within 7 days. When a dose of less than 5 ml is prescribed, the ampicillin syrup should be diluted to 5 ml with Syrup BP.

Legal category POM.

Package quantities
GX Ampicillin Syrup 125 mg/5 ml in 100 ml bottles.
GX Ampicillin Syrup 250 mg/5 ml in 100 ml bottles.

Product licence numbers
GX Ampicillin Syrup 125 mg/5 ml   6502/0017
GX Ampicillin Syrup 250 mg/5 ml   6502/0018

GX* CHLORPROPAMIDE TABLETS

Presentation GX Chlorpropamide tablets are round, white, biconvex, uncoated tablets each containing chlorpropamide either 100 mg or 250 mg engraved with the GX logo on one side and on the reverse 100/236 or 250/237.

Uses As a potent oral hypoglycaemic agent in treatment of mild or moderately severe, non-ketotic, uncomplicated maturity-onset diebetes mellitus unresponsive to diet alone.

It may also be useful in controlling patients who have shown inadequate response or failure to other sulphonylurea agents or patients requiring high or frequent doses of another oral agent.

The hypoglycaemic effect of chlorpropamide occurs only when the β cells of the islet tissue in the pancreas retain some functional capacity. Chlorpropamide has no effect on glucose tolerance.

The appropriate biguanide data sheet should be consulted for details of patient selection, indications, warnings and dose, when chlorpropamide is being used concurrently with biguanide (metformin).

Dosage and administration The total daily dose is generally taken as a single dose with breakfast. Gastrointestinal intolerance may be removed by dividing the dose. In complicated maturity-onset diabetes, the initial dose is 250 mg daily. The maximum dose taken as two 250 mg tablets, is 500 mg, this should be reduced to maintenance level as soon as possible. As three days are necessary for blood levels of chlorpropamide to become stable at a particular dosage, changes should not be made at shorter intervals and should be in steps of 50–100 mg. Most patients are stabilised on a dosage of 100–375 mg daily.

Several weeks may be required to achieve a correct dosage level and the patient's blood sugar should be monitored throughout where possible and the urine tested for glycosuria at least four times daily in all cases.

Elderly patients should be started on half the usual dosage since they are often very sensitive to the sulphonylureas and may develop hypoglycaemia if given full dosage.

In the treatment of diabetes insipidus, daily dosage has been in the range of 100–500 mg daily for older children and adults. Because of the risk of hypoglycaemia that can develop in these individuals, it is desirable to start therapy at the lower range, gradually adjusting the dose as indicated. Chlorpropamide should be discontin-

ued if hypoglycaemia develops. When physicians are considering chlorpropamide for the treatment of diabetes insipidus, it is essential that they read the following paragraphs relating to precautions and adverse reactions.

No transition period is necessary when transferring patients from other oral hypoglycaemic agents to chlorpropamide or in patients who take less than 40 units of insulin daily. For patients requiring more than 40 units of insulin daily therapy with chlorpropamide may be initiated with a 50% reduction in insulin for the first few days, followed by further reductions dependent on response.

Chloropropamide/metformin dosage: The dosage of chlorpropamide should be maintained at or increased to 500 mg. If control is still inadequate, metformin may be added at a dosage of 0.5 g twice daily, increasing by 0.5 to 1.0 g every one to two weeks to a maximum of 3 g daily.

If adequate control is obtained without side-effects, reduction in dosage of both chlorpropamide and metformin should be undertaken slowly (reducing the dosage of one drug at a time) in an attempt to maintain control with the least possible medication.

Contra-indications, warnings, etc GX Chlorpropamide is contra-indicated in: Hypersensitivity to chlorpropamide; juvenile or growth-onset diabetes mellitus; severe or unstable 'brittle' diabetes; diabetes complicated by ketosis and acidosis, diabetic coma, major surgery, severe infection, or severe trauma; patients with serious impairment of hepatic, renal or thyroid function; pregnancy.

Barbiturates should be employed with caution. Similarly cautious use in patients with Addison's disease is recommended.

Chlorpropamide is contra-indicated in diabetic ketosis, diabetes complicated by fever trauma or gangrene and in patients with impaired renal, hepatic or thyroid function.

Patients taking chlorpropamide may become intolerant of alcohol, a reaction like the disulfiram alcohol reaction being produced. Patients should be warned of this possibility.

The hypoglycaemic effect of chlorpropamide may be increased by coumarin derivatives, MAO inhibitors, salicylates and propranolol.

Diminution of hypoglycaemic action of chlorpropamide may occur with aggravation of the diabetic state with the concomitant administration of thiazide diuretics, ethacrynic acid, frusemide, oestrogens and corticosteroids.

Diabetic control may be altered in patients also treated with cyclophosphamide.

Because of the possibility of blood dyscrasia a white cell count should be performed and should be repeated in five days should an infection or symptoms of infection appear.

Chlorpropamide should not be used as a substitute for dietary treatment.

Gastric and intestinal disturbance, jaundice, headache, tinnitus, weakness, parasthesia and skin rashes have been reported. Blood dyscrasias have been reported and include agranulocytosis, leucopenia and thrombocytopenia. A prolonged hypoglycaemia may very occasionally be produced by chlorpropamide.

Treatment of overdosage: To treat hypoglycaemia, which can occur up to 5 days after an overdose, glucose or 3 or 4 lumps of sugar should be taken at once with water and may be repeated in 10 to 15 minutes if needed. If coma occurs, up to 50 ml of a 50% solution of glucose should be given intravenously, or glucose or sucrose may be given by stomach tube.

Pharmaceutical precautions Store in a cool, dry place.

Legal category POM.

Package quantities
100 mg tablets in Securitainers of 100.
250 mg tablets in Securitainers of 100.

Further information Nil.

Product licence numbers
100 mg   6502/0026
250 mg   6502/0027

GX* CO-TRIMOXAZOLE TABLETS

Presentation GX Co-trimoxazole tablets (Co-trimoxazole Tablets BP) containing 80 mg Trimethoprim BP, 400 mg Sulphamethoxazole BP. Round, white, biconvex, uncoated tablets with a breakline on one face.

Uses GX Co-trimoxazole is effective against a wide range of Gram positive and Gram negative organisms. The addition of the folic acid antagonist trimethoprim to sulphamethoxazole increases the activity of the latter against Gram negative bacteria except pseudomonas.
Clinical indications: Respiratory tract infections: Acute and chronic bronchitis, bronchiectasis, lung abscess, pneumonia, sinusitis and otitis media.
    Genito-urinary tract: Cystitis, urethritis, pyelitis, pyelonephritis, prostatitis and gonorrhoea.
    Gastro-intestinal tract: Typhoid and paratyphoid fevers, invasive salmonella infections, cholera and shigellosis.
    Skin and soft tissue infections: Pyoderma, abscesses and wound infections.
    Other bacterial infections: Brucellosis, osteomyelitis, and septicaemias.

Dosage and administration *Adults:* 2 tablets twice daily. In the case of severe infections 2 tablets three times daily.
Children over 12 years: 2 tablets twice daily. In the case of severe infections 2 tablets three times daily.
Children 6–12 years: 1 tablet twice daily.
Gonorrhoea: In uncomplicated gonorrhoea 4 tablets every 12 hours for two days or 5 tablets followed 8 hours later by a further dose of 5 tablets.

Contra-indications, warnings, etc GX Co-trimoxazole is contra-indicated in pregnancy, renal or hepatic failure, jaundice and blood disorders and in patients with a history of trimethoprim or sulphonamide sensitivity.
    GX Co-trimoxazole should not be given to neonates during the first 6 weeks.
    Patients on prolonged treatment should have blood counts at monthly intervals.
Drug interactions: Care should be exercised when giving co-trimoxazole to patients receiving sulphonylurea, hypoglycaemics, oral anticoagulants of the coumarin group or phenytoin as the action of these agents may be increased.
    In common with all sulphonamides there is a possibility of blood dyscrasias more especially in elderly patients.
    In long term therapy rare cases of megaloblastic

changes have been reported. These cases can be reversed by treatment with folic acid therapy.
Side effects: Nausea, vomiting, rashes, erythema multiforme bullosa, epidermal necrolysis.
    A number of serious side effects i.e. aplastic anaemia, pancytopenia are reported as occurring more frequently in the elderly. Accordingly co-trimoxazole should not be prescribed in elderly patients unless the benefits are thought to exceed these serious side effects.
Overdosage: Symptoms of acute overdosage are likely to be nausea, vomiting, abdominal pain, dizziness and confusion. Treatment should consist of gastric lavage if within 1 hour of ingestion. Increased fluid intake will increase the elimination of sulphamethoxazole, but decrease that of trimethoprim. Calcium folinate 3 to 6 mg given orally or intramuscularly for 5 to 7 days should counteract any bone marrow effects of trimethoprim. General supportive methods are recommended.

Pharmaceutical precautions Store below 25°C and protect from light.

Legal category POM.

Package quantities GX Co-trimoxazole packs of 30 and 100.

Further information Absorption by oral route is rapid – within 1 hour significant plasma levels are obtained, between 2 and 4 hours peak levels are reached. Peak levels are maintained over a 12 hour period.
    Eradication of group A beta-haemolytic streptococci from the oro-pharynx in the treatment of tonsillopharyngitis is not as rapid as some alternative antibiotics.
    Trimethoprim may cause an apparent rise in serum creatinine levels.
    Co-trimoxazole may cause a fall in circulating thyroid hormone levels (although clinical significance requires confirmation).

Product licence number 6502/0051.

GX* FRUSEMIDE TABLETS

Presentation Round, white, flat, bevel-edged, uncoated tablets each containing 40 mg frusemide, engraved with GX logo on one side and strength above and code number below breakline on reverse (40/147).

Uses Frusemide is a loop diuretic which inhibits resorption of electrolytes from the ascending loop of Henle in the renal tubule of the kidney. GX Frusemide is rapidly absorbed when given by mouth provoking an intense diuresis lasting 4 to 6 hours.
    All indications when prompt and effective diuresis is required e.g. cardiac, pulmonary, hepatic and renal oedema, peripheral oedema due to mechanical obstruction or changes in the walls of veins, ascites, toxaemia of pregnancy, hypertension and miscellaneous conditions such as acute barbiturate poisoning.

Dosage and administration The usual initial dosage is 40 mg daily which may then be adjusted according to patient requirements ranging from 20 mg on alternative days to 120 mg daily.
Children: From 1 to 3 mg per kg body weight daily.

Contra-indications, warnings, etc Patients with prostatic hypertrophy or impairment of micturition have an increased risk of developing acute retention.
    Dosage of concurrently administered cardiac glyco-

sides or antihypertensive agents may require adjustments.

Nephrotoxicity of cephaloridine and aminoglycoside antibiotics may be increased by concomitant administration of potent diuretics such as frusemide.

Latent diabetes may become manifest or insulin requirements of diabetic patients may increase.

In common with other diuretics, serum lithium levels may be increased when lithium is given concomitantly with frusemide necessitating adjustment of the lithium dosage.

Certain non-steroidal anti-inflammatory agents have been shown to antagonise the action of diuretics such as frusemide.

There is clinical evidence of the safety of frusemide in the third trimester of pregnancy but not evidence of its safety in early pregnancy.

As frusemide may inhibit lactation, it should be used with caution in nursing mothers.

Pharmaceutical precautions Store in a dry place below 25°C.

Legal category POM.

Package quantities 40 mg tablets in Securitainers of 60 and 250.

Further information Nil.

Product licence number 6502/0009.

GX* GLIBENCLAMIDE TABLETS

Presentation White circular tablets with a breakline marked 2.5/259 on one side and GX on the reverse containing 2.5 mg Glibenclamide BP. White eliptical tablets with a breakline marked 5/261 on one side and GX on the reverse containing 5 mg Glibenclamide BP.

Uses Glibenclamide is an oral hypoglycaemic agent which is used in treatment of non-insulin dependent diabetics who do not respond adequately to only dietary measures.

Dosage and administration *Treatment of previously untreated diabetes:* Therapy should be started with 5 mg per day (taken during or straight after breakfast). If control is inadequate, the daily dose may be increased (not more frequently than weekly) in increments of usually 2.5 mg (5 mg maximum) daily to a maximum dose of 15 mg per day. This is normally given in a single dose. Consideration should be given to the patient's dietary habits and daily activity in apportioning the dosage.

Elderly: If a patient is elderly or debilitated, it is wise to start at a lower dose (2.5 mg).

Change-over from other oral anti-diabetics: Changeover to GX Glibenclamide from other drugs with a similar mode of action can be carried out without any break in therapy. Treatment should start with one 5 mg tablet daily and be adjusted by steps of 2.5–5 mg to gain control. Patients not adequately controlled on other oral agents should be started on the equivalent dose of GX Glibenclamide (although not exceeding an initial dose of 10 mg). The dose can be raised in increments to 15 mg daily if response is inadequate.

One 5 mg GX Glibenclamide tablet is approximately equivalent to: tolbutamide 1 g; glymidine 1 g; acetohexamide 500 mg; tolazamide 250 mg; chlorpropamide 250 mg; glibonuride 25 mg; glipizide 5 mg.

Change-over from biguanides such as metformin: Glibenclamide treatment should begin with 2.5 mg glibenclamide and the biguanide withdrawn. Dosage should then be adjusted by increments of 2.5 mg to achieve control (but not greater than 15 mg per day).

Combination therapy with biguanides: If adequate control is not possible with 15 mg GX Glibenclamide and diet, a combination of GX Glibenclamide and a biguanide derivative may re-establish control.

Change-over from insulin: A few patients with very low daily insulin requirements may remain stabilised if transferred to GX Glibenclamide. They should be treated as new patients.

Children: Juvenile-onset diabetes is usually insulin-dependent. Consequently, GX Glibenclamide is not suitable for use in children.

Contra-indications, warnings, etc Patients suffering from or with a history of diebetic keto-acidosis. Patients with serious impairment of function to the kidneys, liver or adrenal glands. Patients undergoing surgery. Pregnancy when insulin treatment is normally preferred.

Warnings: The hypoglycaemic effect of GX Glibenclamide may be enhanced by: Coumarin anticoagulants; monoamine oxidase inhibitors; beta-adrenergic blocking agents; sulphonamides; phenylbutazone; chloramphenicol; cyclophosphamide; salicylates e.g. aspirin.

The hypoglycaemic effect of GX Glibenclamide may be diminished by: sympathomimetic agents e.g. adrenalin; steroids including oral contraceptives; thiazide diuretics.

Precautions: Special care must be exercised when using GX Glibenclamide in elderly or debilitated patients (they are more likely to suffer from hypoglycaemia) and pregnancy and lactation.

In patients suffering from intercurrent infections or trauma, the dosage of GX Glibenclamide may need to be increased. If complications are severe, diabetic control may be lost necessitating withdrawal of GX Glibenclamide and maintenance of diabetic control with insulin. GX Glibenclamide should be re-introduced when the patient has recovered from the infection or trauma.

Side-effects: GX Glibenclamide is well tolerated and serious side effects are uncommon. Gastro-intestinal symptoms (nausea, anorexia and diarrhoea) and allergic skin conditions are uncommon. Reversible leucopenia and thrombocytopenia are rare (these are reversible when treatment stops). Transient changes in liver function have been observed during treatment but are not known to be directly attributable to glibenclamide.

As with all oral hypoglycaemic agents an over response to treatment might occur especially in unexpected heavy exercise. These attacks are not long and should be managed as for overdosage.

Overdosage: Hypoglycaemia in the conscious patient should be treated by administration of glucose or 3–4 lumps of sugar with water repeated as necessary.

In a comatose patient, glucose should be given as an intravenous infusion. Bolus glucose injections are not advised because of the possibility of rebound hypoglycaemia. 1 mg of glucagon may be administered subcutaneously or intramuscularly to restore consciousness.

Pharmaceutical precautions Store below 25°C. Protect from light.

Legal category POM.

Package quantities 2.5 mg and 5 mg tablets in Securitainers of 100.

Further information Nil.

Product licence numbers
GX Glibenclamide Tablets 2.5 mg 6502/0038
GX Glibenclamide Tablets 5 mg 6502/0039

GX* IBUPROFEN TABLETS

Presentation Round, pink, sugar-coated tablets containing ibuprofen 200 mg and 400 mg.

Uses GX Ibuprofen (isobutylphenylpropionic acid) has analgesic, anti-inflammatory and antipyretic actions. It is absorbed from the gastrointestinal tract producing a peak plasma concentration about $1\frac{1}{2}$ hours after ingestion. (If taken on an empty stomach, this time may be reduced by half.)

Treatment of rheumatoid arthritis, ankylosing spondylitis, osteoarthritis and other non-rheumatoid (seronegative) arthropathies.

In the treatment of non articular rheumatic conditions, GX Ibuprofen is indicated in periarticular conditions such as frozen shoulder (capsulitis), bursitis, tendinitis, tenosynovitis and low back pain. It can also be used for soft tissue injuries such as sprains and strains.

Dosage and administration *Adults:* 1.2 g daily in divided doses. After 2 to 4 weeks, a maintenance dose could be anywhere between 600 mg and 1.2 g daily in divided doses.

Children: 20 mg per kg body weight for children weighing more than 30 kg. A maximum recommended dose of 400 mg per day for children weighing between 20 kg–30 kg. GX Ibuprofen is not recommended for children weighing below 20 kg.

Contra-indications, warnings, etc Ibuprofen should not be given to patients with severe or active peptic ulceration. Whilst no teratogenic effects have been demonstrated in animal experiments, the use of ibuprofen during pregnancy should, if possible, be avoided. Ibuprofen should be prescribed with caution for those with asthma and especially for patients who have developed bronchospasm with other non-steroidal agents, and for patients with renal or hepatic impairment.

Adverse effects reported include dyspepsia, gastrointestinal intolerance and bleeding and skin rashes. Less frequently, thrombocytopenia has occurred. Toxic amblyopia has occurred very rarely, but in those cases recovery occurred on cessation of treatment.

Other side effects include headache, dizziness, nervousness, oedema, tinnitus and blurred vision.

Overdosage: In case of overdosage the stomach should be emptied by aspiration and lavage and blood electrolytes corrected if necessary. There is no specific antidote to ibuprofen.

Pharmaceutical precautions Store below 25°C. Keep well closed.

Legal category POM.

Package quantities 200 mg and 400 mg tablets in containers of 100.

Further information Nil.

Product licence numbers
GX Ibuprofen 200 mg tablets 6502/0049
GX Ibuprofen 400 mg tablets 6502/0050

GX* INDOMETHACIN CAPSULES

Presentation Pale yellow Indomethacin Capsules BP 25 mg and 50 mg.

Uses As a non-steroidal anti-inflammatory agent with analgesic properties to relieve the painful symptoms of: rheumatoid arthritis; osteoarthritis; ankylosing spondylitis; gout; degenerative joint disease of the hip; acute periarticular disorders (bursitis, tendinitis, synovitis and capsulitis of the shoulder); low back pain ('lumbago'); inflammation, pain and oedema following orthopaedic procedures.

Dosage and administration Gastro-intestinal side effects may be minimised if patients take indomethacin capsules, with food, milk or antacids.

Adults: 75–150 mg daily in divided doses.

Dosage should be carefully adjusted to suit the needs of the individual patient starting with low dosage, increasing gradually to achieve best results with minimal side effects.

Children: A paediatric dose is not yet established.

Contra-indications, warnings, etc Indomethacin should not be used in cases of active peptic ulcers or where a history of recurrent gastro-intestinal lesions exist, and in patients with renal or hepatic dysfunction. Rare cases of hepatitis have been reported.

Elderly patients seem to be specially susceptible to side effects of indomethacin.

Patients driving or operating machinery should be advised of possible relevant side effects of indomethacin.

Bronchospasm may be precipitated in patients suffering from, or with a previous history of, bronchial asthma or allergic disease.

Indomethacin should be used carefully in patients with psychiatric disorders, epilepsy or Parkinsonism as it may aggravate these conditions.

Safety of indomethacin in pregnancy and lactation has not been established and so precautions should be taken.

Indomethacin may potentiate the action of oral anticoagulants and reduce the effect of anti-hypertensive drugs.

Treatment of overdosage: In case of overdosage, gastric lavage should be performed if ingestion is recent. Otherwise therapy is supportive. Antacids may be useful in relation to possible gastro-intestinal ulceration and haemorrhage.

Headache and dizziness occur frequently at beginning of treatment. Anorexia, nausea, vomiting, dyspepsia and diarrhoea may occur. Peptic ulceration possibly with gastro-intestinal haemorrhage can also occur. Other side effects reported include blood dyscrasias, particularly thrombocytopenia, haematuria, oedema and hypertension, angioneurotic oedema, skin rashes, alopecia, drowsiness, confusion, psychotic reactions and convulsions, dyspnoea, tinnitus, corneal deposits and retinal disturbances.

Pharmaceutical precautions Store at room temperature. Protect from light.

Legal category POM.

Package quantities
25 mg GX Indomethacin Capsules: Securitainers of 100 and 250 capsules.
50 mg GX Indomethacin Capsules: Securitainers of 100 capsules.

Product licence numbers
GX Indomethacin Capsules 25 mg   6502/0033
GX Indomethacin Capsules 50 mg   6502/0034

GX* INDOMETHACIN SUPPOSITORIES

Presentation Creamy white Indomethacin Suppositories BP 100 mg.

Uses As a non-steroidal anti-inflammatory agent with analgesic properties to relieve the painful symptoms of ankylosing spondylitis, osteoarthritis and to relieve the pain and swelling in gout, rheumatoid arthritis and acute musculoskeletal disorders.

Also to relieve inflammation, pain and oedema following orthopaedic procedures.

Suppositories may be used when night pain and morning stiffness are prominent or when gastro-intestinal side effects from oral indomethacin therapy are severe. Use per rectum will certainly reduce, if not entirely eliminate gastro-intestinal problems in all patients.

Dosage and administration GX Indomethacin Suppositories should be administered singly, one in the morning and, if necessary, one at night.

Children: A paediatric dose is not yet established.

Contra-indications, warnings, etc Elderly patients seem to be specially susceptible to side effects of indomethacin.

Patients driving vehicles or operating machinery should be advised of possible relevant side effects of indomethacin.

Indomethacin should be used cautiously in patients with psychiatric disorders, epilepsy or Parkinsonism as it may aggravate these conditions.

Safety of indomethacin in pregnancy and lactation has not been established.

Indomethacin may potentiate the action of oral anticoagulants and reduce the effect of antihypertensive drugs.

Indomethacin should not be used in cases of active peptic ulcers or where a history of recurrent gastro-intestinal lesions exist, and in patients with renal or hepatic dysfunction. Rare cases of hepatitis have been reported.

Treatment of overdosage: In case of overdosage, gastric lavage should be performed if ingestion is recent. Otherwise therapy is supportive. Antacids may be useful in relation to possible gastro-intestinal ulceration and haemorrhage.

Warnings and adverse effects: Headache and dizziness occur frequently at beginning of treatment. Anorexia, nausea, vomiting, dyspepsia and diarrhoea may occur. Peptic ulceration possibly with gastro-intestinal haemorrhage can also occur. Other side effects reported include blood dyscrasias, haematuria, oedema and hypertension, angioneurotic oedema, skin rashes, alopecia, drowsiness, confusion, psychotic reactions and convulsions, dyspnoea, tinnitus, corneal deposits and retinal disturbances.

Use of indomethacin suppositories has been associated with tenesmus, proctitis, rectal bleeding, burning pain, discomfort and itching.

Pharmaceutical precautions Store in a cool dry place. Protect from light.

Legal category POM.

Package quantities Plastic strip of 10 suppositories (100 mg) inside carton.

Further information Nil.

Product licence number 6502/0032.

GX* METHYLDOPA TABLETS

Presentation Round, biconvex, yellow, film-coated tablets each containing 125 mg, 250 mg or 500 mg of methyldopa.

Uses An antihypertensive agent which may act centrally by stimulating alpha-adrenergic receptors. It inhibits decarboxylation of dopa to dopamine but this action does not appear to be responsible for its hypotensive effect. It is suggested that a metabolite, alphamethylnoradrenaline, may act as a false transmitter in the CNS. GX Methyldopa reduces tissue concentrations of dopamine, noradrenaline, adrenaline and serotonin.

Its effects may appear after about 2 hours reaching a maximum in 6 to 8 hours but this may be delayed for up to 48 hours.

Methyldopa is used in the treatment of hypertension.

Dosage and administration *Adults:* The usual initial dose is 250 mg two or three times a day, for two days. This dose is then adjusted at intervals of not less than two days until an adequate response is achieved. The maximum recommended daily dose is 3 g.

When methyldopa is given to patients on other antihypertensives the dose of these agents may need to be adjusted.

Use in the elderly: Syncope in older patients may be related to an increased sensitivity and advanced arteriosclerotic vascular disease. This may be avoided by lower doses.

Children: The initial starting dose is 10 mg/kg daily in 2–4 divided doses increased as required to a maximum of 65 mg/kg daily or 3.0 g daily whichever is less.

Contra-indications, warnings, etc Methyldopa should not be given to patients with active hepatic disease, (such as acute hepatitis and active cirrhosis), hypersensitivity to the drug or phaeochromocytoma.

Methyldopa should be used with caution in patients with impaired renal or hepatic function or with a history of hepatic disease or mental depression.

When methyldopa is used with other antihypertensive agents, potentiation of antihypertensive action may occur. Therapy with methyldopa may be initiated in most patients already on treatment with other antihypertensive agents by terminating these antihypertensive medications gradually if required (see manufacturer's recommendations on stopping these drugs). Following such previous antihypertensive therapy, methyldopa should be limited to an initial dose of not more than 500 mg daily and increased as required at intervals of not less than two days.

Patients may require reduced doses of anaesthetics when on methyldopa. If hypotension does occur during anaesthesia, it can usually be controlled by vasopressors.

Withdrawal of methyldopa is followed by return of hypertension, usually within 48 hours. This is not complicated generally by an overshoot of blood pressure.

Dialysis removes methyldopa; therefore, hypertension may recur after this procedure.

The hypotensive effects of methyldopa may be diminished by sympathomimetics, tricyclic antidepressants, phenothiazine derivatives and monoamine oxidase inhibitors. The effects may be enhanced by thiazide diuretics and levodopa.

The development of a positive direct Coombs' test occurs in 10–20% of patients and is dose related. It develops rarely in the first six months of treatment and if not encountered within 12 months is unlikely to occur. Special care must be taken when transfusion of a patient with a positive result Coombs' test is being considered and a haematologist should be consulted.

It is recommended that total and differential white blood cell counts and liver function tests be performed in the first 6–12 weeks of treatment or if an unexplained fever develops. If fever, abnormal liver function tests or jaundice occur, methyldopa should be discontinued. If related to methyldopa, the temperature and abnormalities in liver function will then return to normal. Methyldopa should not be used again in these patients.

Interference with laboratory tests: Methyldopa may interfere with the measurement of urinary uric acid by the phosphotungstate method, serum creatinine by the alkaline picrate method, and SGOT by colorimetric method. Interference with spectrophotometric methods for SGOT analysis has not been reported.

As methyldopa fluoresces at the same wavelengths as catecholamines, spuriously high amounts of urinary catecholamines may be reported interfering with a diagnosis of phaeochromocytoma. It is important to recognise this phenomenon before a patient with a possible phaeochromocytoma is subjected to surgery. Methyldopa does not interfere with measurement of VMA (vanillymandelic acid) by those methods which convert VMA to vanillin. Methyldopa is not recommended for the treatment of patients with phaeochromocytoma.

Methyldopa has been used for the treatment of hypertension during pregnancy with close medical supervision. Methyldopa crosses the placental barrier and appears in cord blood and breast milk. Although no obvious teratogenic effects have been reported, the possibility of foetal injury cannot be excluded and the use of the drug in women who are, or may become, pregnant or who are nursing their newborn infant requires that anticipated benefits be weighed against possible risks.

Side-effects: Sedation is the most frequent side-effect. It usually wears off after an effective maintenance dose has been established. Depression may occur. Other minor side effects are headache with a feeling of weakness, these also wear off with time. Symptoms of cerebrovascular insufficiency may occur and include dizziness, faintness and light headedness, if such symptoms occur, dosage should be reduced. Symptoms of postural hypotension and exercise hypotension have been reported, if such symptoms occur dosage should be reduced. Occasionally bradycardia, prolonged carotid sinus hypertension, aggravation of angina pectoris, nasal stuffiness, mild dryness of the mouth and gastrointestinal symptoms of varying types may occur. These are generally relieved by reducing the dosage. Vomiting has been reported and sore or black tongue has been observed rarely. Weight gain and oedema occur infrequently and are usually relieved by administering a thiazide diuretic. If oedema becomes progressive or other

signs of heart failure occur, methyldopa should be withdrawn. On rare occasions breast enlargement, hyperprolactinaemia, amenorrhoea, lactation, impotence, skin rash, mild arthralgia, myalgia, parasthesias, Parkinsonism, psychic disturbances – including nightmares and reversible mild psychosis have been reported. Positive tests for anti-nuclear antibody, LE cells and rheumatoid factor have been reported. A rise in blood urea has been found in some cases. Methyldopa may occasionally cause urine to darken because of the breakdown of the drug or its metabolites.

Haemolytic anaemia has occurred rarely in association with methyldopa. Should symptoms suggest the possibility of haemolytic anaemia, the appropriate investigations should be carried out. If haemolytic anaemia is present, methyldopa should be discontinued.

Thrombocytopenia, leucopenia and granulocytopenia have also been reported but are usually reversible on withdrawal of the drug.

Fever in the first few weeks has been reported occasionally and has sometimes been associated with eosinophilia or abnormalities in one or more liver function tests.

Jaundice, with or without fever may occur, usually within the first 8–12 weeks of treatment. In some cases, the findings have been consistent with cholestasis. Rare cases of fatal hepatic necrosis have been reported.

Rarely, involuntary choreoathetotic movements have been observed during treatment with methyldopa in patients with severe bilateral cerebrovascular disease. Should these movements occur, therapy should be discontinued.

Overdosage: If overdosage occurs the stomach should be emptied by aspiration and lavage. Treatment is largely symptomatic but if necessary intravenous infusion may be given to promote urinary excretion and pressor agents given cautiously. Methyldopa is dialysable.

Pharmaceutical precautions Store below 25°C. Protect from light.

Legal category POM.

Package quantities
Tablets 125 mg containers of 100.
Tablets 250 mg containers of 100 and 500.
Tablets 500 mg containers of 100.

Further information Nil.

Product licence numbers
GX Methyldopa tablets 125 mg   6502/0010
GX Methyldopa tablets 250 mg   6502/0011
GX Methyldopa tablets 500 mg   6502/0012

GX* OXPRENOLOL TABLETS

Presentation Round, film-coated tablets containing Oxprenolol Hydrochloride BP engraved with the GX logo on one side and on the reverse with strength and code number.

GX Oxprenolol 20 mg tablet: coloured white and engraved '20 over 249'.

GX Oxprenolol 40 mg tablet: coloured white and engraved '40 over 251'.

GX Oxprenolol 80 mg tablet: coloured yellow and engraved '80 over 252'.

GX Oxprenolol 160 mg tablet: coloured orange and engraved '160 over 253'.

Uses Oxprenolol is a beta-adrenoceptor blocking agent

or antagonist and, like all other such drugs, is a competitive inhibitor of the effects of catecholamines at beta adrenergic receptor sites in the heart, peripheral vasculature, bronchi, pancreas and liver.

Oxprenolol possesses partial agonist activity (PAA) or intrinsic sympathomimetic activity (ISA) which means it has the capacity to stimulate as well as to block adrenergic receptors. As a result it tends to cause less bradycardia and less coldness of the extremities than do some other beta-blockers.

The principal effects of oxprenolol are seen on the heart where the rate is slowed with consequent reduction in heart work and myocardial oxygen consumption. The anti-hypertensive effect of oxprenolol appears to be associated with haemodynamic effects on cardiac output, and peripheral resistance, but effects on plasma renin and/or CNS may also be of significance. By reducing the rate and force of contraction of the heart and decreasing the rate of conduction of impulses through the conducting system the response of the heart to stress and exercise is reduced.

Oxprenolol, like all beta-blockers, also has an antithyroid action and in appropriate dosage can render a patient clinically euthyroid within 4 days.

Treatment of hypertension alone or concurrently with a thiazide diuretic.

Treatment of cardiac arrhythmias and to improve tolerance to exercise in patients with angina of effort.

Since oxprenolol reduces responses to the beta-adrenoreceptor stimulating effects of adrenaline, it is used (in conjunction with an alpha-adrenoreceptor blocking agent such as phenyoxybenzamine) in the management of phaeochromocytoma. It is also used for the symptomatic relief of catecholamine provoked tremor in conditions such as anxiety or hyperthyroidism. Oxprenolol can often be effective in alleviating the palpitations and diarrhoea which accompany anxiety and apprehension.

Oxyprenolol is compatible with glyceryl trinitrate and they are complimentary since they reduce heart work by different mechanisms.

Dosage and administration *Adults:*

Hypertension: Initially 80 mg twice daily increased at convenient intervals until satisfactory blood pressure control is achieved.

Cardiac arrhythmias: Initially 20 to 40 mg three times daily, increased as necessary.

Pre-operatively: Patients with thyrotoxicosis and phaeochromocytoma may be managed on 20 mg three times daily.

Anxiety states: The majority of patients will respond to a total daily dose of 160 mg.

Angina pectoris: 40 to 160 mg three times daily.

Children: There is no recommended dosage for children but in the management of arrhythmias a dose of 1 mg per kg body weight has been used.

Contra-indications, warnings, etc Oxprenolol should not be given to patients with bronchial asthma or bronchospasm, hypoglycaemia, metabolic acidosis (e.g. in some diabetics), sinus bradycardia, partial heart block. Treatment with oxprenolol should be avoided during pregnancy and lactation.

Great care should be exercised in giving oxprenolol to patients undergoing anaesthesia and myocardial depressants such as chloroform and ether must be avoided.

Side-effects: Oxprenolol is usually well tolerated. Minor side effects such as cold extremities, nausea, vomiting, insomnia, lassitude and diarrhoea usually resolve on withdrawal of the drug.

Paraesthesia of hands, skin rashes and dry eyes have also been reported. Bronchospasm may occur particularly in susceptible individuals. Bradycardia, congestive heart failure, heart block and hypotension have occurred in patients intolerant to oxprenolol.

Treatment of overdosage: bradycardia and severe hypotension – immediate treatment with 1–2 mg intravenous atropine followed, if necessary, by a beta receptor stimulant such as 25 mcg isoprenaline or 500 mcg orciprenaline by slow intravenous injection.

Bronchospasm – intravenous aminophylline or isoprenaline.

Heart failure – digitalis and diuretic therapy.

Pharmaceutical precautions GX Oxprenolol tablets should be stored below 25°C.

Legal category POM.

Package quantities Securitainers of 100 tablets.

Product licence numbers

GX Oxprenolol Tablets 20 mg	6502/0001
GX Oxprenolol Tablets 40 mg	6502/0002
GX Oxprenolol Tablets 80 mg	6502/0003
GX Oxprenolol Tablets 160 mg	6502/0004

GX* PROPRANOLOL TABLETS

Presentation Round, biconvex, pink-coloured film-coated tablets containing Propranolol Hydrochloride BP 10 mg, 40 mg, 80 mg, 160 mg respectively. The tablets are engraved on one face with the GX logo and on reverse with strength and code number over a break line i.e. 10/217, 40/218, 80/219, 160/221 respectively.

Uses Propranolol is a beta-adrenergic receptor blocking agent. The principal effect is to reduce cardiac activity. By reducing rate and force of contraction of the heart and decreasing the rate of conduction of impulses through the conduction system, the response of the heart to stress and exercise is reduced.

Propranolol also has an antihypertensive effect but the mode of action has not been fully established.

Treatment of hypertension, alone or concurrently with a thiazide diuretic. Treatment of cardiac arrhythmias.

To improve tolerance to exercise in patients with angina of effort. In the surgical treatment of phaeochromocytoma together with an adrenergic alpha-receptor blocking agent such as phenoxybenzamine.

Dosage and administration Best taken before meals.

Dosage is determined largely by the response of the patients so, in most conditions, treatment should begin with a small dose which should be increased gradually.

Usual daily dosage:

Hypertension	160 mg–320 mg
Angina	120 mg–320 mg
Arrhythmias	30 mg–160 mg
Phaeochromocytoma for 3 days	60 mg

BP Dosage: 20 mg to 320 mg daily in divided doses, the initial daily dose not exceeding 40 mg.

Contra-indications, warnings, etc Propranolol should not be given to patients with bronchial asthma or bronchospasm, hypoglycaemia, metabolic acidosis (e.g. in some diabetics), sinus bradycardia, partial heart block. Treatment with propranolol should be avoided during pregnancy and lactation.

Great care should be exercised in giving propranolol to patients undergoing anaesthesia and myocardial depressants such as chloroform and ether must be avoided.

Propranolol is usually well tolerated. Minor side effects such as cold extremities, nausea, vomiting, insomnia, lassitude and diarrhoea usually resolve on withdrawal of the drug. Paraesthesia of hands, skin rashes and dry eyes have also been reported. Bronchospasm may occur particularly in susceptible individuals. Bradycardia, congestive heart failure, heart block and hypotension have occurred in patients intolerant to propranolol.

Treatment of overdosage: bradycardia and severe hypotension immediate treatment with 1 mg–2 mg intravenous atropine followed if necessary by a beta receptor stimulant such as 25 mcg isoprenaline or 500 mcg orciprenaline by slow intravenous injection.

Bronchospasm: intravenous aminophylline or isoprenaline.

Heart failure: digitalis and diuretic therapy.

Pharmaceutical precautions GX Propranolol tablets should be stored below 25°C. Protect from light.

Legal category POM.

Package quantities
Tablets 10 mg: containers of 100.
Tablets 40 mg: containers of 100, 250.
Tablets 80 mg: containers of 100.
Tablets 160 mg: containers of 100.

Further information The action of propranolol has been reported to be potentiated in patients concurrently taking cimetidine because of interference in the hepatic enzyme system.

Product licence numbers
GX Propranolol tablets 10 mg   6502/0005
GX Propranolol tablets 40 mg   6502/0006
GX Propranolol tablets 80 mg   6502/0007
GX Propranolol tablets 160 mg   6502/0008

GX* SALBUTAMOL INHALER

Presentation Metered-dose aerosol delivering 100 micrograms Salbutamol BP per actuation, with a specially designed actuator.

Uses Salbutamol BP is a beta-adrenergic stimulant which has a highly selective action on the receptors in bronchial muscle and, in therapeutic dosage, little or no action on the cardiac receptors.

Salbutamol is also highly active in preventing antigen-induced release of histamine and slow-reacting substance of anaphylaxis, SRS(A), from mast cells in human lung sensitised with 1gE antibody. Such Type 1 hypersensitivity reactions are generally considered to be the primary triggers of the allergic asthma syndrome.

GX Salbutamol Inhaler is, therefore, indicated both for the treatment and prophylaxis of bronchial asthma, and also for the treatment of other conditions, such as bronchitis and emphysema, with associated reversible airways obstruction. Because GX Salbutamol Inhaler is long-acting it is ideally suited for routine maintenance therapy in chronic asthma and chronic bronchitis. The inhaler drug-delivery system, using salbutamol in microgram dosage, avoids the skeletal muscle tremor sometimes associated with oral therapy.

GX Salbutamol Inhaler acts rapidly and may be used when necessary to relieve attacks of acute dyspnoea.

Doses may be taken prophylactically before exertion or to prevent exercise-induced asthma.

Because of the selective action on the bronchi and its lack of effects on the cardiovascular system, GX Salbutamol Inhaler is suitable for treating bronchospasm in patients with coexisting heart disease or hypertension, including those taking beta-blocking drugs which often impair respiratory function.

Dosage and administration *Adults:* For the relief of acute bronchospasm and for managing intermittent episodes of asthma, one or two inhalations may be administered as a single dose. The recommended dose for chronic maintenance or prophylactic therapy is two inhalations three or four times a day.

To prevent exercise-induced bronchospasm, two inhalations should be taken before exertion.

Children: One inhalation is the recommended dose for the relief of acute bronchospasm, in the management of episodic asthma or before exercise.

One inhalation should be administered three or four times a day for routine maintenance or prophylactic therapy. These doses may be increased to two inhalations, if necessary.

For optimum results, in most patients, GX Salbutamol Inhaler should be used regularly.

The bronchodilator effect of each administration of inhaled GX Salbutamol lasts for at least four hours, except in patients whose asthma is becoming worse. Such patients should be warned not to increase their usage of inhaler but should seek medical advice in case treatment with an inhaled and/or systemic glucocorticosteroid is indicated.

Contra-indications, warnings, etc
Contra-indications: Although salbutamol is occasionally used to prevent premature labour GX Salbutamol preparations should not be used for threatened abortion during the first or second trimesters.

In the event of a previously effective dose of GX Salbutamol Inhaler failing to give relief for at least three hours, the patient should be advised to seek medical advice in order that any necessary additional steps may be taken. GX Salbutamol should be administered cautiously to patients suffering from thyrotoxicosis.

Unnecessary administration of drugs during the first trimester of pregnancy is undesirable.

Side-effects: No important side-effects have been reported following GX Salbutamol Inhaler therapy.

Overdosage: The preferred antidote for overdosage with GX Salbutamol Inhaler is a cardioselective beta-blocking agent, but beta-blocking drugs should be used with caution in patients with a history of bronchospasm.

Pharmaceutical precautions GX Salbutamol Inhaler should be stored in a cool place, protected from frost and direct sunlight. The canister should not be broken, punctured or burnt, even when apparently empty.

Legal category POM.

Package quantities GX Salbutamol Inhaler is a metered-dose aerosol with a specially designed actuator. Each canister provides 200 inhalations.

Further information GX Salbutamol does not cause difficulty in micturition because, unlike sympathomimetic drugs such as ephedrine, it does not stimulate alpha-adrenoreceptors. GX Salbutamol is not contra-indicated in patients under treatment with monoamine oxidase inhibitors (MAOIs).

Product licence number 6502/0035.

GX* SALBUTAMOL TABLETS

Presentation GX Salbutamol Tablets 2 mg – pink tablets each containing Salbutamol BP 2 mg as sulphate. Engraved GX one side and 2 over 269 on the reverse. GX Salbutamol Tablets 4 mg – pink tablets each containing Salbutamol BP 4 mg as sulphate. Engraved GX on one side and 4 over 271 on the reverse.

Uses GX Salbutamol is a beta-adrenergic stimulant which has a highly selective action on the receptors in bronchial muscle and, in therapeutic dosage, little or no action on the cardiac receptors.

Tablets 2 mg and 4 mg are indicated for the relief of bronchospasm in bronchial asthma of all types, chronic bronchitis and emphysema.

Because of their selective action on the bronchi and their lack of effects on the cardiovascular system, oral preparations are suitable for treating bronchospasm in patients with coexisting heart disease or hypertension.

Dosage and administration *Adults:* The usual effective dose is 4 mg three or four times per day. If adequate bronchodilation is not obtained each single dose may be gradually increased to as much as 8 mg.

However, it has been established that some patients obtain adequate relief with 2 mg three or four times daily. In elderly patients or in those known to be unusually sensitive to beta-adrenergic stimulant drugs, it is advisable to initiate treatment with 2 mg three or four times per day.

Children: The following doses should be administered three or four times daily:
2–6 years: 1–2 mg
6–12 years: 2 mg
Over 12 years: 2–4 mg
The drug is well tolerated by children so that, if necessary, these doses may be cautiously increased.

In the management of premature labour, after uterine contractions have been controlled by intravenous infusion of salbutamol and the infusion has been withdrawn, maintenance therapy can be continued with oral GX Salbutamol. The usual dosage is 4 mg three or four times daily.

Contra-indications, warnings, etc GX Salbutamol tablets and beta-blocking drugs, such as propranolol should not usually be prescribed together.

GX Salbutamol should be administered cautiously to patients suffering from thyrotoxicosis.

Unnecessary administration of drugs during the first trimester of pregnancy is undesirable.

Side-effects: The only side-effect of significance with oral GX Salbutamol is a fine tremor of skeletal muscle which occurs in some patients, usually the hands are most obviously affected. This effect is dose related and is common to all beta-adrenergic stimulants. With doses of GX Salbutamol higher than those recommended or in patients who are unusually sensitive to beta-adrenergic stimulants peripheral vasodilatation and a compensatory small increase in heart rate may occur. Occasionally headaches have been reported.

Overdosage: The preferred antidote for overdosage with GX Salbutamol is a cardioselective beta-blocking agent, but beta-blocking drugs should be used with caution in patients with a history of bronchospasm.

Pharmaceutical precautions Store at a temperature not exceeding 30°C. Keep well closed.

Legal category POM.

Package quantities 2 mg and 4 mg tablets in containers of 100 and 250.

Further information GX Salbutamol does not cause difficulty in micturition because, unlike sympathomimetic drugs such as ephedrine, it does not stimulate alpha-adrenoceptors. GX Salbutamol is not contra-indicated in patients under treatment with monoamine oxidase inhibitors (MAOIs).

Product licence numbers
GX Salbutamol Tablets 2 mg   6502/0036
GX Salbutamol Tablets 4 mg   6502/0037

GX* SPIRONOLACTONE TABLETS

Presentation GX Spironolactone tablets are available in two strengths containing Spironolactone BP 25 mg and 100 mg. Round, biconvex, buff-coloured, film-coated tablets engraved on one face with GX logo and on reverse with strength and code number. 25 mg–25/246, 100 mg–100 over 247.25 mg tablets have a break-line.

Uses Spironolactone is a steroid with a structure resembling that of the natural adrenocortical hormone, aldosterone, to which it acts as a competitive inhibitor. Thus it increases sodium excretion and reduces potassium excretion in the distal renal tubules. The action is slow and prolonged – maximum response after about 3 days of treatment with action continuing for 2–3 days after discontinuation of treatment.

Spironolactone is used in the treatment of:
1. Congestive heart failure.
2. Diagnosis and treatment of primary aldosteronism.
3. Cirrhosis with ascites and oedema.
4. Malignant ascites.
5. Nephrotic syndrome.

Dosage and administration *Adults:* Usually between 50 mg and 200 mg daily in divided doses. This can be increased up to 300 mg to 400 mg daily and an initial dose of up to 400 mg daily may be used where necessary.

In diagnosis of primary aldosteronism, daily dosage of 400 mg is administered. Correction of hypokalaemia and hypertension provides presumptive evidence for diagnosis of primary hyperaldosteronism. Treatment is then by daily dosage of 100 mg – 400 mg prior to surgery.

Children: A dose of 3 mg per kilogram body weight daily in divided doses. Dosage should be adjusted on the basis of response and tolerance.

Contra-indications, warnings, etc Spironolactone is contra-indicated in patients with anuria, acute renal insufficiency, rapidly progressing impairment of renal function, hyperkalaemia and in patients hypersensitive to spironolactone.

Side-effects: Headache and gastric disturbance, occasional skin rashes, drowsiness, mental confusion, impotence and mild androgenic effect. Numerous other side effects including hyperkalaemia reported infrequently.

Gynaecomastia may develop in association with the use of spironolactone. Development appears to be related to both dosage level and duration of therapy and is normally reversible when spironolactone is discontinued.

Pharmaceutical precautions GX Spironolactone tablets should be stored below 25°C. Protect from light.

Legal category POM.

Package quantities
GX Spironolactone 25 mg: Securitainers containing 60 and 250 tablets.
GX Spironolactone 100 mg: Securitainers containing 30 and 100 tablets.

Further information Nil.

Product licence numbers
GX Spironolactone tablets   25 mg   6502/0019
GX Spironolactone tablets 100 mg   6502/0020

GX* TAMOXIFEN TABLETS

Presentation White, circular, film-coated tablets engraved on one face with GX logo and on reverse with strength and code number i.e. 10 mg – 10 over 272 and 20 mg – 20 over 273. Each tablet contains respectively Tamoxifen Citrate BP equivalent to 10 mg and 20 mg tamoxifen.

Uses Tamoxifen has an anti-oestrogen activity and binds to oestrogen receptors preventing the uptake of oestrogen.
Tamoxifen is indicated in the treatment of
1. Breast cancer.
2. Anovulatory infertility.

Dosage and administration
1. *Breast cancer:* 20 mg to 40 mg daily (usually given twice a day) in divided doses.
2. *Anovulatory infertility:* In women with regular menstruation but with anovular cycles treatment should commence with 20 mg daily in either one or two doses administered on the second, third, fourth and fifth days of the menstrual cycle. In unsuccessful cases further courses may be given during subsequent menstrual periods, increasing the dosage to 20 mg then 40 mg twice daily.
In women with irregular menstruation the commencement of treatment may take place on any day. If this initial course is not successful then a further course may be initiated after an interval of 45 days with the higher dosage level (30 mg to 40 mg twice daily). If a patient responds with menstruation then the next course of treatment should be initiated on the second day of the cycle.

Contra-indications, warnings, etc
Contra-indications: Pregnancy.

Precautions: The possibility of pregnancy must be excluded before administration of Tamoxifen to premenopausal women.

Adverse effects: The following side effects have been reported: hot flushes, skin rash, pruritus vulvae, gastrointestinal disturbances, nausea and fluid retention. Tumour pain has occasionally been reported.
Transient thrombocytopenia with platelet counts usually between 80,000 – 90,000 have been reported which revert to normal without cessation of treatment.
Deep vein thromboses have occurred at high dose levels and rare cases of visual disturbance such as retinopathy and corneal changes have been reported where exceptionally high doses have been employed over long periods of time.
Suppression of menstruation will occur in a number of premenopausal women treated for breast cancer and reversible cystic ovarian swelling has been reported in patients treated with 80 mg Tamoxifen daily for short periods.
Adverse reactions can occasionally be controlled by reducing the dosage without loss of therapeutic effect. Severe and persistent side effects may necessitate the discontinuation of treatment.

Overdosage: Overdosage may cause an increase in anti-oestrogenic effects. Animal studies have demonstrated that extremely high dosage (greater than 100 times the recommended daily dose) have caused oestrogenic effects. Treatment of overdosage should be carried out symptomatically.

Pharmaceutical precautions Protect from light and moisture. Store below 25°C.

Legal category POM.

Package quantities GX Tamoxifen is packed in containers of 30 and 250 (10 mg) and 30 (20 mg).

Further information Tamoxifen is light sensitive with the possible formation of the oestrogenic cis form of the isomer where the product is in contact with light. GX Tamoxifen tablets are film coated to give extra protection and eliminate this problem.

Product licence numbers
GX Tamoxifen tablets 10 mg   6502/0021
GX Tamoxifen tablets 20 mg   6502/0022

*Trade Mark

Hoechst/Albert

Hoechst UK Limited
Pharmaceutical Division
Hoechst House, Salisbury Road
Hounslow, Middlesex TW4 6JH

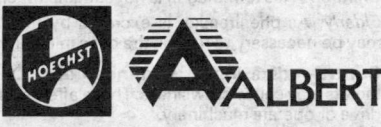

ARELIX* CAPSULES ▼

Presentation Arelix Capsules each contain 6 mg piretanide in a sustained release formulation. The capsules have a light green body and an orange cap.

Uses Arelix is a diuretic for the treatment of mild to moderate hypertension.

Dosage and administration One or two capsules daily. The capsules should be taken with food as a single dose in the morning.

Children: There is at present insufficient experience of the use of this product in children to enable dosage recommendations to be made.

Elderly: Piretanide may be excreted more slowly in the elderly.

Contra-indications, warnings, etc
Contra-indications: Arelix is contra-indicated in patients with severe electrolyte imbalance or hypovolaemia.

Warnings: Patients with impaired micturition or prostatic hypertrophy may develop retention of urine after Arelix administration.

Cephalosporin nephrotoxicity and aminoglycoside ototoxicity have been reported to be increased by the concomitant administration of intravenous or large oral doses of diuretics.

In common with all thiazide and loop diuretics, Arelix can cause hypokalaemia. In patients with severe liver disease, Arelix may precipitate hepatic coma; the use of potassium-sparing diuretics may be preferable in the first instance in these patients.

There have been reports that diuretics may cause latent diabetes to become manifest or may necessitate adjustment of the dosage of concurrently administered hypoglycaemic agents.

The dosage of concurrently administered anti-hypertensive agents, cardiac glycosides and agents used in the treatment of gout may require adjustment.

In common with other diuretics, serum lithium levels may be increased when lithium is given concomitantly with Arelix, necessitating adjustment of the lithium dosage.

Certain non-steroidal anti-inflammatory agents have been shown to antagonise the action of diuretics such as Arelix.

Precautions: Arelix is not known to have been used in the first trimester of pregnancy; however, there is no evidence of an adverse effect from animal studies.

Serum electrolytes should be regularly monitored in patients with severely impaired renal function or pre-comatose states associated with liver cirrhosis.

Caution should be observed in patients liable to electrolyte imbalance; the levels of serum potassium should be monitored where cardiac glycosides or corticosteroids are to be administered and in patients with liver disease.

Nursing mothers: Arelix may inhibit lactation in nursing mothers; piretanide and its metabolites appear in the breast milk of animals.

Overdosage: In cases of overdose there is a danger of dehydration and electrolyte depletion due to excessive diuresis. Treatment should therefore be aimed at fluid replacement and correction of the electrolyte imbalance.

Side-effects: Arelix is generally well tolerated. Reactions such as gastro-intestinal upset (nausea, vomiting or diarrhoea) or allergic reactions such as skin rashes are very rare.

Side-effects associated with increased excretion of water and electrolytes may occur, particularly following prolonged treatment with high doses; circulatory disturbance due to fluid loss may occur, especially in the elderly.

In isolated instances, serum creatinine, urea and uric acid concentrations may rise during Arelix treatment.

Muscle cramps have been reported following the administration of high doses of Arelix but not when used within the dose range recommended for the treatment of hypertension.

Pharmaceutical precautions Arelix should be stored in a cool dry place, protected from light, in containers similar to those of the manufacturer.

Legal category POM.

Package quantities Arelix capsules are supplied in calendar packs containing 28 capsules.

Further information The diuretic effect of Arelix capsules begins about two hours after administration and lasts for about eight hours. The diuretic effect is gradual and exhibits no marked peak effect.

Product licence number 0086/0092.

DANERAL* SA TABLETS

Presentation Daneral SA Tablets each contain 75 mg Pheniramine Maleate BP in a sustained release formulation. Daneral SA is presented as unmarked pink, sugar-coated tablets 10.3 mm in diameter.

Uses All allergic conditions. Examples of its use include hay fever, vasomotor rhinitis, acute rhinitis, urticaria, allergic dermatoses, pruritus.

Dosage and administration One tablet at bedtime will be sufficient for most patients. In more severe cases two tablets may be taken at night or one tablet night and morning. The tablet should be swallowed whole and not sucked or chewed.

Children: This formulation is not suitable for children.

Elderly: As pheniramine is excreted by the kidneys, it may be necessary to reduce the dose in elderly patients.

Contra-indications, warnings, etc Daneral SA tablets may cause drowsiness. Those affected should not drive or operate machinery.

In common with all antihistamines, the sedative effect of other central nervous system depressant agents, e.g. alcohol may be potentiated.

In infants and children antihistamines may act as central stimulants.

Overdosage: The primary symptom is sedation. Following doses of 300–1,800 mg cerebral stimulation, convulsions and hyperpyrexia may occur. If an overdose has been taken recently by mouth the stomach should be emptied by aspiration and lavage. Peritoneal dialysis is not effective. The patient should be kept quiet, diazepam i.v. may be given to prevent paroxysms and excessive hyperkinesia.

Precautions: There is little evidence of the safety of Daneral SA in human or animal pregnancy, although the drug has been in wide, general use for many years without apparent ill consequence.

Pharmaceutical precautions Daneral SA Tablets should be stored in a cool dry place, protected from light, in containers similar to those of the manufacturer.

Legal category P.

Package quantities Daneral SA Tablets are available in packs of 50.

Further information Nil.

Product licence number 0086/5001.

DAONIL* TABLETS
SEMI-DAONIL* TABLETS

Presentation Daonil Tablets each contain 5 mg Glibenclamide BP. Daonil is presented as white oblong tablets, scored in the middle, one half bearing the Hoechst insignia, the other bearing the letters LDI. The tablet is 10 mm in length and 5 mm wide.

Semi-Daonil Tablets each contain 2.5 mg Glibenclamide BP. Semi-Daonil is presented as white circular biplanar tablets, 6 mm in diameter, one side bearing the Hoechst insignia, the other scored and bearing the letters LBG on either side of the score mark.

Uses Daonil is a hypoglycaemic agent, indicated for the oral treatment of patients with non-insulin dependent diabetes who respond inadequately to dietary measures alone.

Dosage and administration

1. *Treatment of previously untreated diabetics:* Stabilisation can be started with one 5 mg tablet of Daonil daily. The dose should be taken by mouth, with or immediately after breakfast or the first main meal. Where control is satisfactory, 1 tablet is continued as the maintenance dose. If control is unsatisfactory, the dose can be adjusted by increments of 2.5 or 5 mg at weekly intervals. The total daily dosage rarely exceeds 15 mg and increasing the daily dosage above this does not generally produce any additional effect. The total daily requirement

should normally be administered as a single dose at breakfast, or with the first main meal; due consideration should be given to the patient's dietary habits and daily activity in apportioning the dosage.

Elderly: In debilitated or aged patients, who may be more liable to hypoglycaemia, treatment should be initiated with one Semi-Daonil tablet daily.

2. *Change-over from other oral anti-diabetics:* The change over to Daonil from other drugs with a similar mode of action can be carried out without any break in therapy.

Daonil treatment should be started with one 5 mg tablet daily and adjusted by increments of 2.5–5 mg to achieve control. For patients not adequately controlled on other oral agents, treatment is commenced with the equivalent dose of Daonil, without exceeding an initial dose of 10 mg. If response is inadequate, the dose can be raised in a stepwise fashion to 15 mg daily. One 5 mg tablet of Daonil is approximately equivalent to 1 g tolbutamide or glymidine, 250 mg chlorpropamide or tolazamide, 500 mg acetohexamide, 25 mg glibornuride or 5 mg glipizide.

3. *Change-over from biguanides:* Daonil treatment should be started with 1 tablet of Semi-Daonil (2.5 mg) and the biguanide withdrawn. The dosage should then be adjusted by increments of 2.5 mg to achieve control.

Combination with biguanides: If adequate control is not possible with diet and 15 mg of Daonil, control can often be re-established by combined administration of Daonil and a biguanide derivative.

4. *Change-over from insulin:* While it is appreciated that most patients who are on insulin therapy will continue to need it, there may be a few patients, particularly those on low daily doses, who will remain stablilised if transferred from insulin to Daonil.

The tablets should always be taken with, or immediately after, the first main meal.

Children: As non-insulin dependent diabetes is not usually a disease of childhood, Daonil is not recommended for use in children.

Contra-indications, warnings, etc

Contra-indications: Daonil should not be used in patients who have or have ever had diabetic ketoacidosis or those who have insulin-dependent diabetes mellitus, serious impairment of renal, hepatic or adrenocortical function, in patients who are hypersensitive to glibenclamide, or in circumstances of unusual stress, e.g. surgical operations or during pregnancy, when dietary treatment and insulin are essential.

Warnings: The hypoglycaemic effect of glibenclamide may be enhanced by dicoumarol, monoamine oxidase inhibitors, beta-adrenergic blocking agents, sulphonamides, phenylbutazone, chloramphenicol, cyclophosphamide, benzafibrate, clofibrate, fenfluramine, pentoxifylline (high dose, parenteral), sulphinpyrazone, tetracycline compounds and salicylates or diminished by adrenaline, corticosteroids, oral contraceptives, phenothiazine derivatives, thyroid hormones, nicotinic acid (high dose), thiazide diuretics and abuse of laxatives.

There is no information on the use of Daonil in human pregnancy but it has been in wide, general use for many years without apparent ill consequence. Animal studies have shown no hazard.

Nursing mothers: It has not yet been established whether glibenclamide is transferred to human milk. However, other sulphonylureas have been found in milk and there is no evidence to suggest that glibenclamide differs from the group in this respect.

Overdosage: Hypoglycaemia may be treated in the conscious patient by the administration of glucose, or three to four lumps of table sugar with water. This may be repeated as necessary.

If the patient is comatose, glucose should be administered as an intravenous infusion. Bolus glucose injections are not recommended because of the possibility of rebound hypoglycaemia. Alternatively, glucagon may be administered in a dose of 1 mg subcutaneously or intramuscularly to restore consciousness.

Side-effects: Adverse reactions serious enough to warrant discontinuation of treatment are uncommon, but mild gastro-intestinal or allergic skin reactions have occurred. Reversible leucopenia and thrombocytopenia have been reported but are rare. Transient changes in liver function tests have been observed during treatment with Daonil, but are not known to be directly attributable to the drug. Hypoglycaemic symptoms have occasionally been reported when the dose has been administered without due regard to the patients' dietary habits.

Pharmaceutical precautions Daonil Tablets should be stored in a cool, dry place protected from light and in containers similar to those of the manufacturer.

Legal category POM.

Package quantities Daonil and Semi-Daonil Tablets are available in blister packs of 100.

Further information Orally administered Daonil is rapidly absorbed. It is substantially metabolised prior to its excretion in urine and bile. Some of the metabolites have hypoglycaemic activity, markedly reduced in comparison with the parent compound and usually without clinical significance.

Product licence numbers
Daonil Tablets 5 mg	0086/5002
Semi-Daonil Tablets 2.5 mg	0086/0068

FERTIRAL* ▼

Presentation Fertiral contains Gonadorelin BP (luteinising hormone releasing hormone) 500 micrograms in 1 ml aqueous solution presented as a 2 ml ampoule containing 1000 micrograms.

Uses Amenorrhoea and infertility associated with:
1. Hypogonadotrophic hypogonadism.
2. Multifollicular ovaries: where this finding implies that pulse frequency and amplitude of endogenous LHRH are abnormal, e.g. in patients in whom weight related amenorrhoea has been corrected.

Dosage and administration Gonadorelin is given by means of an intermittent pulsatile pump, a pulse being delivered every 90 minutes over the entire 24 hour period. Treatment should be initiated by subcutaneous infusion but in some patients intravenous therapy may be required. Dosage should be determined individually but a starting dose of 10–20 micrograms given over 1 minute every 90 minutes is recommended. Treatment should be continued until conception occurs, or for a maximum of 6 months. Ultrasound of ovary or oestradiol or urinary oestrogen levels or basal body temperature measurements may be used to monitor treatment. (*See also Pharmaceutical Precautions*).

Contra-indications, warnings, etc Gonadorelin should not be used in patients with endometriotic cysts or polycystic disease of the ovaries. Treatment with gonadorelin should not be started in women with weight related amenorrhoea until the weight has been corrected and the ponderal index is above 19.5. Gonadorelin may be discontinued once evidence of conception has been obtained.

Side-effects: Side-effects are very rare. A skin rash has been reported at the infusion site. The following reactions have been reported after treatment with the high dose diagnostic preparation of gonadorelin: Abdominal pain, nausea, headache and increased menstrual bleeding.

Overdosage: No symptoms have been reported after overdosage with LHRH although some patients have received very large doses.

Pharmaceutical precautions Gonadorelin should be infused using a pulsatile pump e.g. Graseby MS 27 with an infusion set of minimum volume e.g. Butterfly 25 or Butterfly 19 cannulae (Abbott). For intravenous administration heparin is added to the gonadorelin solution at a concentration of 150 IU/ml.

Store in a cool dark place. Use normal saline to dilute if necessary; use immediately after dilution. The solution is stable in the pump, at about body temperature, for 4 days.

Fertiral contains benzyl alcohol 1% as a preservative.

Legal category POM.

Package quantities Fertiral is available in packs of 5 × 2 ml ampoules.

Further information Results from clinical studies show a rate of multiple pregnancy very similar to that of the normal population.

Product licence number 0086/0093.

FIBROGAMMIN P*

Presentation Fibrogammin P, heat treated Factor XIII Concentrate, is presented in clear glass vials, each containing approximately 85 mg lyophilised concentrate, having Factor XIII activity equivalent to at least 250 ml fresh pooled citrated plasma. Each vial is provided with an ampoule containing 4 ml Water for Injections for reconstitution of the lyophilisate.

Uses Factor XIII Concentrate is indicated for replacement therapy in congenital Factor XIII deficiency.

Dosage and administration The contents of one vial should be dissolved in 4 ml of Water for Injections and the solution should be administered by slow intravenous injection.

When reconstituted, the dosage for congenital Factor XIII deficiency is as follows:

1. For substitution therapy, the normal adult dose is 8 ml (about 170 mg) intravenously every four weeks. The interval between doses should be decreased if spontaneous bleeding occurs.
2. For prophylaxis prior to surgery, 8–16 ml (about 170–340 mg) i.v. in the immediate pre-operative period followed by 8–12 ml (about 170–255 mg) i.v. on each of the following five days.
3. For therapy in severe bleeding or massive haematomata 8–16 ml (about 170–340 mg) i.v. daily until the bleeding stops.

Children: In children under the age of 14 years, the dose is normally half the adult dose.

Contra-indications, warnings, etc Factor XIII Concentrate is contra-indicated for patients with fresh thrombosis because of its fibrin-stabilising effect.

No side effects have been observed.

Pharmaceutical precautions Factor XIII Concentrate should be stored at 4°C. Prepared solutions of Factor XIII Concentrate should be used immediately and any remainder discarded. No additives or diluents should be used other than pyrogen-free Water for Injections.

Legal category POM.

Package quantities The product is supplied as single vials each with an ampoule containing Water for Injections.

Further information Fibrogammin P, a heat treated Factor XIII Concentrate, is a purified standardised and concentrated preparation of human coagulation factor XIII, fibrin-stabilising factor. The method of production of Factor XIII Concentrate has been shown to remove experimental artificial contamination with Australia Antigen; thus, there is little risk of transmission of hepatitis from the concentrate. In addition, every batch is routinely tested for freedom from HB_sAg.

Product licence number 0086/0047.

FRISIUM*

Presentation Frisium capsules each contain 10 mg clobazam. Frisium is presented as hard gelatin capsules coloured powder blue opaque with 'Frisium' printed on both cap and body.

Uses Frisium is a 1,5-benzodiazepine indicated for the relief of acute or chronic anxiety, tension and agitation. Physical symptoms associated with an underlying anxiety state, phobias and psychosomatic disorders may all respond to treatment with Frisium as may symptoms of anxiety associated with underlying organic disease. Frisium may be used together with antidepressants in the treatment of anxiety associated with depression. Frisium has also been shown to have a beneficial effect in the treatment of sleep disturbances associated with anxiety. Frisium may be used as adjunctive therapy in epilepsy.

Dosage and administration The usual anxiolytic dose for adults is 20–30 mg daily in divided doses or as a single dose given at night. Doses of up to 60 mg daily have been used in the treatment of adult in-patients with severe anxiety.

Epilepsy: In epilepsy a starting dose of 20–30 mg/day is recommended, increasing as necessary up to a maximum of 60 mg daily. A break in therapy may be beneficial if drug exhaustion develops, recommencing therapy at a low dose.

Elderly: Doses of 20 mg daily in anxiety may be used in the elderly, who are more sensitive to the effects of psychoactive agents.

Children: When prescribed for children over three years of age, dosage should not exceed half the recommended adult dose. There is insufficient experience of the use of Frisium in children under three years of age to enable any dosage recommendation to be made.

Contra-indications, warnings, etc *Contra-indica-*

tions: Frisium should not be used in patients known to be hypersensitive to benzodiazepines.

Precautions, warnings: Frisium is a benzodiazepine derivative and, in common with other members of this group, may potentiate the effects of central nervous system depressant drugs, such as alcohol, analgesics, hypnotics and neuroleptics.

Addition of Frisium to established anticonvulsant medication may cause a change in plasma levels of these drugs.

The ability to drive or operate machinery may be impaired in individuals who are particularly sensitive to the effects of Frisium or in patients taking high doses.

Frisium should be used in reduced doses in patients with impaired renal or hepatic function.

There is little information on the use of Frisium in early pregnancy but no untoward effects have been found in animal studies. However, there are reports of a possible association between malformations in infants and the administration of other benzodiazepines in early pregnancy.

Nursing mothers: Clobazam has been detected in the breast milk of nursing mothers, but the effect on the neonate is not known.

Overdosage: Muscle weakness, ataxia, drowsiness and sedation may occur and, after very high doses, the patient may lose consciousness. The treatment of overdosage is symptomatic. The stomach should be emptied as soon as possible by gastric lavage and general supportive measures should be undertaken as necessary.

Side-effects: Frisium is generally well tolerated. Side-effects such as drowsiness, dizziness or dryness of the mouth have been reported. These are more likely to occur at the beginning of treatment and often disappear with continued treatment or a reduction in dose.

Pharmaceutical precautions Frisium capsules should be stored in a cool, dry place in the original containers or in containers similar to those of the manufacturer.

Legal category CD (Sch 4), POM.

Package quantities Frisium is available as 10 mg capsules packed in blister packs of 100 capsules.

Further information Experimental evidence shows that, in general, when given as a single dose of up to 20 mg or in divided doses of up to 30 mg Frisium does not affect psychomotor function. However, individuals who are sensitive to the effects of Frisium may be adversely affected, particularly at the beginning of treatment.

Clobazam may be supplied at NHS expense if prescribed for epilepsy and prescription is endorsed 'S3B' (or 'S2B' in Scotland).

Product licence number 0086/0065.

HAEMACCEL* INFUSION SOLUTION

Presentation 3.5% colloidal infusion solution for plasma substitution.

Composition:

Haemaccel contains	Per 500 ml bottle	Per 1,000 ml
Polygeline (degraded and modified gelatin of average molecular weight 35,000)	17.50 g	35.00 g

Cations		
Na^+	72.50 mmol	145.00 mmol
K^+	2.55 mmol	5.10 mmol
Ca^{++}	3.13 mmol	6.25 mmol

Anions		
Cl^-	72.50 mmol	145.00 mmol
PO_4^{---} and SO_4^{--}	traces	traces

Isoionic equilibrium is made up by the polypeptides. There are no preservatives.

Physico-Chemical Properties:

Electrophoretic mobility	$\alpha_2 - \beta$
Viscosity ratio	1.7–1.8
Dynamic viscosity (at 38°C)	1.15–1.20 kPa.s (cP)
The iso-electric point is at	pH 4.7 ± 0.3
pH of the infusion solution	7.2–7.3
Colloid osmotic pressure (at 37°C)	3.432–3.824 kPa (350–390 mmH_2O)
Gel point	below $+3$°C
Appearance	straw-coloured
Nitrogen equivalent of polygeline	3.15 g

Uses

1. As a plasma volume substitute in hypovolaemic shock due to:
(a) Haemorrhage (visible or concealed)
(b) Burns, peritonitis, pancreatitis, crush injuries
(c) Water and electrolyte loss from persistent vomiting and diarrhoea, diseases of the kidneys and adrenals, portal vein thrombosis, ileus, diabetic coma.
2. Fluid replacement in plasma exchange.
3. Extra-corporeal circulation.
4. Isolated organ perfusion.
5. As a carrier solution for insulin.

Dosage and administration Haemaccel should be administered intravenously in a volume approximately equal to the estimated blood loss.

In common with all intravenous infusion solutions, Haemaccel should, if possible, be warmed to body temperature before use. However, in emergencies, it may be infused at ambient temperatures.

Infusion rate: The rate of infusion is determined by the condition of the patient. Normally 500 ml will be infused in not less than 60 minutes, but in emergencies Haemaccel can be rapidly infused. Losses of up to 25% of the blood volume can be replaced by Haemaccel alone.

Plastic infusion bottle: It is advisable to disinfect the bottle top then pull out the plastic ring. A hole will be exposed through which the piercing needle of an infusion set can be pushed. There is no need to disinfect the cap further.

Hypovolaemic shock: 500–1,000 ml Haemaccel should be infused intravenously initially. Up to 1,500 ml blood loss can be replaced entirely by Haemaccel. For between

1,500 ml and 4,000 ml blood loss, fluid replacement should be with equal volumes of Haemaccel and blood, given separately (see Pharmaceutical precautions). For losses over 4,000 ml the separate infusions should be in the ratio of two parts blood to one part Haemaccel. The haematocrit should not be allowed to fall below 25%.

Burns: It is suggested that at least 1 ml Haemaccel be infused per kg body weight, multiplied by the % of body surface burned for each 24 hours for two days, e.g. if a 70 kg person has burns covering 10% of body surface, then the dosage of Haemaccel should be at least 1 (ml) $\times$ 70 (kg) $\times$ 10(%) = 700 ml/24 hours. Additional crystalloid solutions should be given to cover the normal fluid loss, i.e. about 2,000 ml per 24 hours. In severe burns, additional protein and vitamin therapy may be required. The volume of colloid and crystalloid given should be varied according to the clinical response of the patient, the urine volume, its specific gravity and osmolality, etc.

Plasma exchange: Haemaccel should be given either alone or in combination with other replacement fluids in a volume adequate to replace the plasma removed. Up to 2 litres have been given as sole replacement fluid.

Contra-indications, warnings, etc There are no absolute contra-indications to the use of Haemaccel. However, caution should be used in infusing Haemaccel in any patient likely to develop circulatory overloading (e.g. severe congestive cardiac failure). Inappropriately rapid administration of Haemaccel, especially to normo-volaemic patients, may cause the release of vasoactive substances. The exact mechanism of such histamine release has not been clearly defined. Histamine release may be especially hazardous in patients with known allergic conditions such as asthma. In the event of histamine release, the infusion should be discontinued and appropriate action taken with antihistamines, etc. Haemaccel contains calcium ions and caution should be observed in patients being treated with cardiac glycosides.

Pharmaceutical precautions There are no special storage requirements. Haemaccel will gel below 3°C; however, warming will reverse this. Freezing does not alter its physico-chemical characteristics in any way. Haemaccel contains no preservatives; any unused fluid should be discarded once a bottle has been opened.

Haemaccel may be mixed with other infusion solutions (e.g. saline, dextrose, Ringer's solution, etc.) or with heparinised blood. Sterility must be maintained. Compatible water-soluble drugs may be infused in Haemaccel, e.g. insulin, streptokinase, etc. Any additive should be injected into the bottle through the small hole located next to the pull-ring.

Citrated blood should *not* be mixed with Haemaccel since the calcium ions present in Haemaccel may cause recalcification. However, citrated blood may be infused before or after Haemaccel provided that there is adequate flushing of the infusion set.

Do not use Haemaccel if the seal has been broken or if the contents are cloudy.

Haemaccel has a shelf life of five years.

Legal category POM.

Package quantities Available in 500 ml plastic bottles.

Further information Haemaccel is of particular value as a volume replacement as it promotes a demonstrable osmotic diuresis, thereby protecting the kidneys. Provided that the recipient's red cells are suspended in saline rather than serum it does not interfere with subsequent blood grouping and cross matching, nor does it interfere with the coagulation system. It is non-immunogenic and does not induce antibody formation.

Product licence number 0086/0040.

LASIKAL* TABLETS ▼

Presentation Lasikal Tablets each contain 20 mg Frusemide BP and 750 mg (10 mmol K^+) slow-release potassium chloride. They are presented as film-coated, biconvex, twin-layered tablets, 12.5 mm in diameter, marked 'LK' on one side. The frusemide layer is white and the slow-release potassium chloride layer is yellow.

Uses Lasikal contains a short-acting diuretic and a slow-release potassium supplement. It is intended for the treatment of oedema in patients who require potassium supplementation.

Dosage and administration The recommended initial adult dose is 2 tablets (40 mg frusemide and 20 mmol K^+) to be taken each morning. This may be increased to four tablets daily, to be taken as 2 tablets each morning and evening, or may be decreased to 1 tablet each morning, according to clinical response.

Lasikal tablets must be swallowed whole.

Children: Lasikal tablets cannot be sub-divided and are unsuitable for paediatric use.

Elderly: Frusemide and potassium may both be excreted more slowly in the elderly.

Contra-indications, warnings, etc

Contra-indications: Lasikal is contra-indicated in hyperkalaemia, precomatose states associated with liver cirrhosis, Addison's disease and in patients taking potassium-sparing diuretics. Hypersensitivity to sulphonamides is also a contra-indication.

Warnings: Patients with prostatic hypertrophy or impairment of micturition have an increased risk of developing acute retention.

Where indicated, steps should be taken to correct hypotension or hypovolaemia before commencing therapy.

The dosage of concurrently administered cardiac glycosides or antihypertensive agents may require adjustment.

Cephaloridine nephrotoxicity may be increased by concomitant administration of potent diuretics such as frusemide.

Latent diabetes may become manifest or the insulin requirements of diabetic patients may increase.

Care should be exercised when treating patients with renal insufficiency because of the risk of hyperkalaemia.

In common with other diuretics, serum lithium levels may be increased when lithium is given concomitantly with frusemide, necessitating adjustment of the lithium dosage.

Certain non-steroidal anti-inflammatory agents have been shown to antagonise the action of diuretics such as frusemide. Salicylates may also have this effect.

The effects of curariform muscle relaxants may be enhanced by frusemide. Interactions have also been reported with ototoxic antibiotics. Glucocorticoids may cause sodium retention and exacerbate potassium loss.

Precautions: Results of animal work, in general, show no hazardous effect of Lasix in pregnancy. There is clinical evidence of safety of the drug in the third trimester of

human pregnancy; however, Lasix should be used in pregnancy only if strictly indicated and for short term treatment.

Nursing mothers: As Lasix may inhibit lactation, it should be used with caution in nursing mothers.

Overdosage: In cases of overdose there is a danger of dehydration and electrolyte depletion due to excessive diuresis. Treatment should therefore be aimed at fluid replacement and correction of the electrolyte imbalance.

Side-effects: Lasikal is generally well tolerated. Side-effects of a minor nature such as nausea, malaise or gastric upset may occur but are not usually severe enough to necessitate withdrawal of treatment.

Calcium depletion may occur. Nephrocalcinosis has been reported in premature infants.

Auditory disorders and acute pancreatitis have been reported with high dose parenteral frusemide.

As with other diuretics a transient rise in creatinine and urea levels has also been reported with frusemide.

The incidence of allergic reactions, such as skin rashes, is very low, but when these occur treatment should be withdrawn.

In common with other sulphonamide-based diuretics, hyperuricaemia may occur and, in rare cases, clinical gout may be precipitated.

Bone marrow depression has been reported as a rare complication and necessitates withdrawal of treatment.

There may be an aggravation of metabolic alkalosis.

Reduced mental alertness may impair ability to drive or operate dangerous machinery.

Pharmaceutical precautions Lasikal should be stored in a cool dry place, protected from light, in the original containers or in containers similar to those of the manufacturer. Lasikal tablets should be dispensed in moisture-tight containers which offer protection from light.

Legal category POM.

Package quantities Lasikal is available in containers of 100 and 250 tablets.

Further information Lasix produces a prompt and effective diuresis which lasts for approximately four hours following oral administration. The potassium chloride in Lasikal tablets is contained in an inert matrix which allows slow release of potassium ions, thereby helping to avoid high local K^+ ion concentrations in the intestine.

Ghost tablets may appear in the patient's faeces.

Product licence number 0086/0060.

LASILACTONE* CAPSULES ▼

Presentation Lasilactone Capsules each contain 20 mg of Frusemide BP and 50 mg Spironolactone BP. They are presented as hard gelatin capsules with a light blue opaque cap and white opaque body.

Uses Lasilactone contains a short-acting diuretic and a long-acting aldosterone antagonist. It is indicated in the treatment of resistant oedema where this is associated with secondary hyperaldosteronism; conditions include chronic congestive cardiac failure and hepatic cirrhosis.

Treatment with Lasilactone should be reserved for cases refractory to a diuretic alone at conventional dosage.

This fixed ratio combination should only be used if

titration with the component drugs separately indicates that this product is appropriate.

The use of Lasilactone in the management of essential hypertension should be restricted to patients with demonstrated hyperaldosteronism. It is recommended that in these patients also, this combination should only be used if titration with the component drugs separately indicates that this product is appropriate.

Dosage and administration In accordance with the recommendations on usage given above the dosage of Lasilactone will normally be in the range of 1 to 4 capsules daily (20–80 mg Lasix and 50–200 mg spironolactone).

Children: The product is not suitable for use in children.

Elderly: Frusemide and spironolactone may both be excreted more slowly in the elderly.

Contra-indications, warnings, etc
Contra-indications: Lasilactone should not be given in acute renal insufficiency, anuric states, hyperkalaemia or Addison's disease. Hypersensitivity to sulphonamides.

Warnings: Patients with prostatic hypertrophy or impairment of micturition have an increased risk of developing acute retention. Caution should also be exercised in the presence of liver disease as hepatic coma may be precipitated in susceptible cases. Administration of Lasilactone should be avoided in the presence of a raised serum potassium. Concomitant administration of triamterene, amiloride or potassium supplements is not recommended as hyperkalaemia may result. Where indicated, steps shoud be taken to correct hypotension and hypovalaemia before starting therapy.

The dosage of concurrently administered cardiac glycosides or hypotensive agents may require adjustment.

Cephaloridine nephrotoxicity may be potentiated by concurrent administration of potent diuretics such as frusemide.

Latent diabetes may become manifest; the insulin requirements of diabetic patients may increase.

In common with other diuretics, serum lithium levels may be increased when lithium is given concomitantly with frusemide, necessitating adjustment of the lithium dosage.

Certain non-steroidal anti-inflammatory agents have been shown to antagonise the action of diuretics such as frusemide. Salicylates may also have this effect. The effects of curariform muscle relaxants may be enhanced by frusemide. Interaction has also been reported with carbenoxolone.

Carcinogenicity: Spironolactone has been shown to produce tumours in rats when administered at high doses over a long period of time. The significance of these findings with respect to clinical use is not certain. However, the long-term use of spironolactone in young patients requires careful consideration of the benefits and the potential hazard involved.

Precautions: Caution should be observed in patients liable to electrolyte deficiency.

Results of animal work, in general, show no hazardous effect of frusemide in pregnancy. There is clinical evidence of the safety of the drug in the third trimester of human pregnancy; however, Lasix should be used in pregnancy only if strictly indicated and for short term treatment.

Spironolactone or its metabolites may cross the placental barrier.

Nursing mothers: As frusemide may inhibit lactation it should be used with caution in nursing mothers. Canrenone, a metabolite of spironolactone appears in breast milk. If use of spironolactone is considered essential, an alternative method of infant feeding should be instituted.

Overdosage: In cases of overdosage with Lasilactone there is a danger of severe electrolyte disturbance and dehydration due to excessive diuresis. Signs of overdosage may include drowsiness, mental confusion, nausea, vomiting, dizziness or diarrhoea. Electrolyte disturbances such as hyperkalaemia, hypokalaemia and hyponatraemia may be induced. Hyperkalaemia may be manifested clinically by paraesthesia, weakness, flaccid paralysis or muscle spasm and may be difficult to distinguish from hypokalaemia. Electrocardiographic changes may be the earliest signs of potassium disturbances.

Treatment should be aimed at the replacement of fluid and the correction of any electrolyte imbalance.

Side-effects: Lasix is generally well tolerated. Side-effects of a minor nature such as nausea, malaise or gastric upset may occur but are not usually severe enough to necessitate withdrawal of treatment.

The incidence of allergic reactions, such as skin rashes, is very low, but when these occur treatment should be withdrawn.

Auditory disorders and acute pancreatitis have been reported with high dose parenteral frusemide.

Nephrocalcinosis has been reported in premature infants. A transient rise in creatinine and urea levels has also been reported.

In common with other sulphonamide-based diuretics, the administration of Lasix may induce a rise in serum uric acid; in rare cases, clinical gout may be precipitated.

Certain non-steroidal anti-inflammatory agents have been shown to antagonise the action of diuretics such as frusemide. Salicylates may also have this effect.

Bone marrow depression has been reported as a rare complication of Lasix therapy and necessitates withdrawal of treatment.

Spironolactone has been reported to induce gastrointestinal intolerance and also drowsiness, headache, ataxia and mental confusion. Mastodynia and reversible gynaecomastia may occur. Maculopapular or erythematous cutaneous eruptions have been reported rarely, as have mild androgenic manifestations such as hirsutism and menstrual irregularities.

Reduced mental alertness may impair the ability to drive or operate dangerous machinery.

Pharmaceutical precautions Lasilactone should be stored in a cool dry place, protected from light, in the original container or in containers similar to those of the manufacturer.

Legal category POM.

Package quantities Lasilactone is available in blister strips packed in cartons of 50 capsules.

Further information Lasix is an effective short-acting diuretic; diuresis usually commences within one hour and lasts for four to six hours.

Spironolactone is a competitive inhibitor of aldosterone and thus increases sodium excretion whilst reducing potassium loss at the distal renal tubule. It has a slow and prolonged action, maximum response being usually attained after 2-3 days' treatment.

Product licence number 0086/0039.

LASIPRESSIN* ▼

Presentation Lasipressin Tablets each contain 20 mg Frusemide BP and 40 mg penbutolol sulphate. They are presented as yellowish-white, oblong, film-coated tablets, with a score mark on both sides.

Uses In the management of mild or moderate hypotension.

Dosage and administration The normal dose is one tablet each morning. This can be increased, if necessary, to one tablet twice daily.

Children: Lasipressin is not suitable for use in children.

Elderly: Frusemide may be excreted more slowly in the elderly. Penbutolol undergoes metabolism in the liver and is predominantly excreted by the kidney.

Contra-indications, warnings, etc
Contra-indications: Severe bradycardia, conduction defects (2nd and 3rd degree AV block, sinoatrial block, sick-sinus syndrome), digitalis refractory heart failure, cardiogenic shock, metabolic acidosis, bronchial asthma, chronic obstructive pulmonary disease, peripheral circulatory disorders, concurrent administration of general anaesthetics with myocardial depressant activity, hepatic coma, uncompensated hypokalaemia, hyponatraemia and hypovolaemia, the terminal stages of renal failure, phaeochromocytoma not treated with alpha-adrenergic receptor blockers, hypersensitivity to sulphonamides.

Warnings: Cessation of therapy with all beta-blockers should be gradual. Close observation is recommended when Lasipressin is administered to patients receiving catecholamine-depleting drugs such as reserpine and guanethidine or other negatively inotropic drugs. The dosage of concurrently administered cardiac glycosides or antihypertensive agents may require adjustment. Simultaneous administration of anti-arrhythmic agents and calcium antagonists of the verapamil type increases the risk of conduction disorders of the heart.

Patients with diabetes or a predisposition to diabetes should be carefully monitored. Frusemide may cause latent diabetes to become manifest or the insulin requirements of diabetics to increase. Penbutolol may mask the symptoms of hypoglycaemia.

Patients with prostatic hypertrophy or impairment of micturition have an increased risk of developing acute retention when taking frusemide.

Serum lithium levels may be increased when lithium is given concomitantly with frusemide, necessitating adjustment of the lithium dosage.

Certain non-steroidal anti-inflammatory agents have been shown to antagonise the action of diuretics such as frusemide. Salicylates may also have this effect.

Precautions: Caution should be observed in patients liable to or sensitive to electrolyte deficiency.

Pregnancy: Studies in animals with the component drugs have not shown any evidence of teratogenicity. However, it is recommended that Lasipressin should not be given in pregnancy.

Nursing mothers: As frusemide may inhibit lactation Lasipressin should be used with caution in nursing mothers.

Overdosage: Excessive bradycardia or hypotension may be counteracted with 1–2 mg atropine intravenously followed, if necessary, by a beta-receptor stimulant such as isoprenaline 25 micrograms intravenously. Excessive diuresis may cause dehydration and electrolyte (sodium, potassium and calcium) depletion, treatment should be aimed at fluid replacement and the correction of electrolyte imbalance.

Side-effects: Penbutolol: There have been occasional reports of dizziness, drowsiness, headache, cold extremities, insomnia and gastro-intestinal disturbance and, rare isolated cases of bradycardia observed.

As with other beta-blocking agents, penbutolol may precipitate bronchospasm and heart failure in susceptible patients. However, the incidence of these side-effects is low, possibly due to the partial protection afforded by the intrinsic sympathomimetic effect of penbutolol. Anginal attacks may be aggravated and triggered in Prinzmetal angina. The incidence of skin rash and/or dry eyes associated with the use of beta-blockers is small, and, in most cases, symptoms have cleared when treatment was withdrawn. Discontinuation of the drug should be considered if there is no adequate explanation for such a reaction.

Impairment of potency may occur.

Frusemide: Generally well tolerated. Side-effects of a minor nature such as nausea, malaise or gastric upset may occur but are not usually severe enough to necessitate withdrawal of treatment.

Auditory disorders and acute pancreatitis have been reported with high dose parenteral frusemide. As with other diuretics a transient rise in creatinine and urea levels has also been reported with frusemide.

The incidence of allergic reactions, such as skin rashes, is very low, but when these occur treatment should be withdrawn. Hyperuricaemia may occur and, in rare cases, clinical gout may be precipitated.

Bone marrow depression has been reported as a rare complication with Lasix and necessitates withdrawal of treatment.

Reduced mental alertness may impair ability to drive or operate dangerous machinery.

Pharmaceutical precautions Lasipressin tablets should be stored in a cool, dry place in containers similar to those of the manufacturer.

Legal category POM.

Package quantities Lasipressin tablets are available in blister packs of 30.

Further information Nil.

Product licence number 0086/0087.

LASIX* TABLETS 20 mg
LASIX* TABLETS 40 mg

Presentation Lasix Tablets 20 mg each contain 20 mg Frusemide BP. They are presented as white, circular, biplanar tablets, 6 mm in diameter, one side bearing the Hoechst insignia, the other side scored and bearing the letters DLF on either side of the score mark.

Lasix Tablets 40 mg each contain 40 mg Frusemide BP. They are presented as white, circular, biplanar tablets, 8 mm in diameter, one side bearing the Hoechst insignia, the other scored and bearing the letters DLI on one side of the score mark and '40' on the other.

Uses Lasix is a diuretic recommended for use in all indications when a prompt and effective diuresis is required. Indications for Lasix Tablets 40 mg include cardiac, pulmonary, hepatic and renal oedema, peripheral oedema due to mechanical obstruction or venous insufficiency and hypertension.

Lasix Tablets 20 mg are indicated for the maintenance therapy of mild oedema of any origin.

Dosage and administration Lasix has an exceptionally wide therapeutic range, the effect being proportional to the dosage. Lasix is best given as a single dose either daily or on alternate days.

The usual initial daily dose is 40 mg. This may require adjustment until the effective dose is achieved. In mild cases, 20 mg daily or 40 mg on alternate days may be sufficient, whereas in cases of resistant oedema, daily doses of 80 mg and above may be used.

Children: Oral doses for children range from 1 to 3 mg/kg body weight daily.

Elderly: In the elderly, frusemide is generally eliminated more slowly. Dosage should be titrated until the required response is achieved.

Contra-indications, warnings, etc
Contra-indications: Lasix is contra-indicated in electrolyte deficiency and pre-comatose states associated with liver cirrhosis. Hypersensitivity to sulphonamides.

Warnings: Patients with prostatic hypertrophy or impairment of micturition have an increased risk of developing acute retention.

Where indicated, steps should be taken to correct hypotension or hypovolaemia before commencing therapy.

The dosage of concurrently administered cardiac glycosides or anti-hypertensive agents may require adjustment.

Cephaloridine nephrotoxicity may be increased by concomitant administration of potent diuretics such as frusemide.

Latent diabetes may become manifest or the insulin requirements of diabetic patients may increase.

In common with other diuretics, serum lithium levels may be increased when lithium is given concomitantly with frusemide, necessitating adjustment of the lithium dosage.

Certain non-steroidal anti-inflammatory agents have been shown to antagonise the action of diuretics such as frusemide. Salicylates may also have this effect.

The effects of curariform muscle relaxants may be enhanced by frusemide.

Interactions have also been reported with ototoxic antibiotics. Glucocorticoids may cause sodium retention and exacerbate potassium loss.

Precautions: Caution should be observed in patients liable to electrolyte deficiency.

Results of animal work, in general, show no hazardous effect of Lasix in pregnancy. There is clinical evidence of safety of the drug in the third trimester of human pregnancy; however, Lasix should be used in pregnancy only if strictly indicated and for short term treatment.

Nursing mothers: As Lasix may inhibit lactation it should be used with caution in nursing mothers.

Overdosage: In cases of overdose there is a danger of dehydration and electrolyte depletion due to excessive diuresis. Treatment should therefore be aimed at fluid replacement and correction of the electrolyte imbalance.

Side-effects: Lasix is generally well tolerated. Side-effects of a minor nature such as nausea, malaise or gastric upset may occur but are not usually severe enough to necessitate withdrawal of treatment.

Calcium depletion may occur. Nephrocalcinosis has been reported in premature infants.

Auditory disorders and acute pancreatitis have been reported with high dose parenteral frusemide.

As with other diuretics a transient rise in creatinine and urea levels has also been reported with frusemide.

The incidence of allergic reactions, such as skin rashes, is very low, but when these occur treatment should be withdrawn.

In common with other sulphonamide-based diuretics, hyperuricaemia may occur and, in rare cases, clinical gout may be precipitated.

Bone marrow depression has been reported as a rare complication and necessitates withdrawal of treatment.

There may be an aggravation of metabolic acidosis.

Reduced mental alertness may impair ability to drive or operate dangerous machinery.

Pharmaceutical precautions Lasix tablets should be stored in a cool dry place, protected from light, in containers similar to those of the manufacturer.

Legal category POM.

Package quantities Lasix Tablets 20 mg are available in packs of 60 and 600. Lasix Tablets 40 mg are available in packs of 250 and 1,000.

Further information Lasix produces a prompt and effective diuresis which lasts for approximately four hours following oral administration. Therefore the time of administration can be adjusted to suit the patient's requirements.

Product licence numbers
Lasix Tablets 20 mg   0086/0017
Lasix Tablets 40 mg   0086/5011

LASIX* INJECTION 20 mg/2 ml
LASIX* INJECTION 50 mg/5 ml ▼

Presentation Lasix Injection 20 mg contains 20 mg Frusemide BP in 2 ml. Lasix Injection 50 mg contains 50 mg Frusemide BP in 5 ml.

Uses Lasix is a diuretic recommended for use when a prompt and effective diuresis is required. The intravenous formulation is appropriate for use in emergencies or when oral therapy is precluded. Indications include cardiac, pulmonary, hepatic and renal oedema.

Dosage and administration Lasix injection *must* always be given slowly. The diuretic effect of Lasix is proportional to the dosage. Doses of 20–50 mg intramuscularly or intravenously may be given initially. If larger doses are required, they should be given by slow infusion and titrated according to the response. In such cases the use of Lasix 250 mg ampoules should be considered.

Children: Parenteral doses for children range from 0.5–1.5 mg/kg body weight daily.

Elderly: In the elderly, frusemide is generally eliminated more slowly. Dosage should be titrated until the required response is achieved.

Contra-indications, warnings, etc Intravenous injections of Lasix *must* always be given slowly, i.e. at a rate not exceeding 4 mg/minute.

Contra-indications: Lasix is contra-indicated in electrolyte deficiency and pre-comatose states associated with liver cirrhosis. Hypersensitivity to sulphonamides.

Warnings: Patients with prostatic hypertrophy or impairment of micturition have an increased risk of developing acute retention.

Where indicated, steps should be taken to correct hypotension or hypovalaemia before commencing therapy.

The dosage of concurrently administered cardiac glycosides or antihypertensive agents may require adjustment.

Cephaloridine nephrotoxicity may be increased by concomitant administration of potent diuretics such as frusemide.

Latent diabetes may become manifest or the insulin requirements of diabetic patients may increase.

In common with other diuretics, serum lithium levels may be increased when lithium is given concomitantly with frusemide, necessitating adjustment of the lithium dosage.

Certain non-steroidal anti-inflammatory agents have been shown to antagonise the action of diuretics such as frusemide. Salicylates may also have this effect.

The effects of curariform muscle relaxants may be enhanced by frusemide.

Interactions have also been reported with ototoxic antibiotics and parenteral cisplatin. Glucocorticoids may cause sodium retention and exacerbate potassium loss.

Precautions: Caution should be observed in patients liable to electrolyte deficiency.

Results of animal work, in general, show no hazardous effect of Lasix in pregnancy. There is clinical evidence of safety of the drug in the third trimester of human pregnancy; however, Lasix should be used in pregnancy only if strictly indicated and for short term treatment.

Nursing mothers: As Lasix may inhibit lactation it should be used with caution in nursing mothers.

Overdosage: In cases of overdose there is a danger of dehydration and electrolyte depletion due to excessive diuresis. Treatment should therefore be aimed at fluid replacement and correction of the electrolyte imbalance.

Side-effects: Lasix is generally well tolerated. Side-effects of a minor nature such as nausea, malaise or gastric upset may occur but are not usually severe enough to necessitate withdrawal of treatment. Calcium depletion may occur. Nephrocalcinosis has been reported in premature infants.

The incidence of allergic reactions, such as skin rashes, is very low but, when these occur, treatment should be withdrawn.

Auditory disorders and acute pancreatisis have been reported with high dose parenteral frusemide.

As with other diuretics a transient rise in creatinine and urea levels has been reported with frusemide.

In common with other sulphonamide-based diuretics hyperuricaemia may occur and, in rare cases, clinical gout may be precipitated.

Bone marrow depression has been reported as a rare complication and necessitates withdrawal of treatment.

There may be an aggravation of metabolic acidosis.

Reduced mental alertness may impair ability to drive or operate dangerous machinery.

Pharmaceutical precautions Lasix injections should be stored in a cool dry place, protected from light. Injections of Lasix should not be mixed with any other preparations. Opened ampoules should be used immediately and any remainder discarded.

Legal category POM.

Package quantities Lasix ampoules 20 mg are available in packs of 25×2 ml. Lasix ampoules 50 mg are available in packs of 5×5 ml.

Further information Lasix 20 mg and 50 mg injections contain approximately 0.14 mmol Na^+/ml.

Product licence numbers
Lasix injection 20 mg   0086/5012
Lasix injection 50 mg   0086/0054

LASIX* TABLETS 500 mg

Presentation Lasix Tablets 500 mg each contain 500 mg of Frusemide BP. They are presented as yellow, circular, biplanar, uncoated tablets, 13 mm in diameter, one side bearing the Hoechst insignia; the other is quarter-scored bearing the letters DLX, one in each of three of the four quarters.

Uses Lasix 500 mg is a diuretic for the management of oliguria due to acute or chronic renal insufficiency with a GFR below 20 ml/minute.

Dosage and administration In patients with chronic renal insufficiency, an initial daily dose of 250 mg ($\frac{1}{2}$ tablet) is employed. If a satisfactory diuresis is not produced then the dose may be increased in steps of 250 mg at four to six hourly intervals up to a maximum dose of 2,000 mg (4 tablets) as a single dose.

In cases of acute renal failure which have been initially controlled using Lasix Injection 250 mg, oral therapy may be substituted for parenteral therapy, regarding one 500 mg tablet as approximately equal to one 250 mg ampoule. Appropriate dosage adjustments may then be made according to the observed clinical response.

Children: Lasix Tablets 500 mg are unlikely to be suitable for use in children.

Elderly: In the elderly, frusemide is generally eliminated more slowly. Dosage should be titrated until the required response is achieved.

Contra-indications, warnings, etc During treatment with high-dosage forms of Lasix, fluid balance should be carefully controlled. In the particular case of patients with shock, steps should be taken to correct the blood pressure and circulating blood volume before commencing therapy. Regular checks of plasma electrolytes, particularly sodium, potassium, chloride and bicarbonate, should be carried out and electrolyte replacement therapy instituted accordingly.

Contra-indications: Lasix Tablets 500 mg are contra-indicated in renal failure as a result of poisoning by nephrotoxic or hepatotoxic agents and in renal failure associated with hepatic coma.

Hypersensitivity to sulphonamides is also a contra-indication.

Lasix tablets 500 mg should not be given to patients with normal renal function.

Warnings: The dosage of concurrently administered cardiac glycosides or antihypertensive agents may require adjustment.

Cephaloridine nephrotoxicity may be increased by concomitant administration of potent diuretics such as frusemide.

Latent diabetes may become manifest or the insulin requirements of diabetic patients may increase.

In common with other diuretics, serum lithium levels may be increased when lithium is given concomitantly with frusemide, necessitating adjustment of the lithium dosage.

Certain non-steroidal anti-inflammatory agents have been shown to antagonise the action of diuretics such as frusemide. Salicylates may also have this effect.

The effects of curariform muscle relaxants may be enhanced by frusemide.

Interactions have also been reported with ototoxic antibiotics and parenteral cisplatin. Glucocorticoids may cause sodium retention and exacerbate potassium loss.

Precautions: There is little evidence of safety of high-dose Lasix in human pregnancy, although the results of animal work, in general, show no hazardous effects. However, Lasix should be used in pregnancy only if strictly indicated and for short term treatment.

Nursing mothers: As Lasix may inhibit lactation it should be used with caution in nursing mothers.

Overdosage: In cases of overdosage there is a danger of dehydration and electrolyte depletion due to excessive diuresis. Treatment should therefore be aimed at fluid replacement and correction of the electrolyte imbalance.

Side-effects: Lasix Tablets 500 mg are generally well tolerated. Side-effects of a minor nature such as nausea, malaise or gastric upset may occur but are not usually severe enough to necessitate withdrawal of treatment.

The incidence of allergic reactions, such as skin rashes, is very low but, when these occur, treatment should be withdrawn.

Calcium depletion may occur. Nephrocalcinosis has been reported in premature infants.

As with other diuretics a transient rise in creatinine and urea levels has also been reported with frusemide.

Auditory disorders and acute pancreatitis have been reported with high-dose parenteral frusemide.

In common with other sulphonamide-based diuretics, hyperuricaemia may occur and, in rare cases, clinical gout may be precipitated.

Bone marrow depression has been reported as a rare complication and necessitates withdrawal of treatment.

There may be an aggravation of metabolic acidosis.

Reduced mental alertness may impair ability to drive or operate dangerous machinery.

Pharmaceutical precautions Lasix tablets should be stored in a cool dry place, protected from light, in the original containers or in containers similar to those of the manufacturer.

Legal category POM.

Package quantities Lasix Tablets 500 mg are available in packs of 100.

Further information Diuresis commences within one hour of taking the tablets and the effect lasts for approximately four hours.

Product licence number 0086/5013.

LASIX* INJECTION 250 mg/25 ml

Presentation Lasix 250 mg ampoules contain 250 mg Frusemide BP in 25 ml.

Uses Lasix Injection 250 mg is a diuretic for the management of oliguria due to acute or chronic renal insufficiency with a GFR below 20 ml/minute.

Dosage and administration Lasix 250 mg should be administered by intravenous injection at a rate not exceeding 4 mg/minute.

The recommended initial dose is one 25 ml ampoule (250 mg) diluted in approximately 225 ml Sodium Chloride Injection BP or Ringer's Solution for Injection administered over one hour. This gives an approximate drip rate of 80 drops/minute, ensuring that the infusion is at the level of 4 mg/minute.

If a satisfactory increase in urine output, such as 40–50 ml/hour, is not attained within the next hour, a second infusion of two 25 ml ampoules (500 mg) in an appropriate infusion fluid should be given, the total volume of the infusion being governed by the patient's state of hydration. If a satisfactory output is still not achieved within one hour of the end of the second infusion, a third infusion consisting of four 25 ml ampoules (1,000 mg) can be given. The rate of infusion should not exceed 4 mg/minute.

If the third infusion using the maximum intravenous dose of 1,000 mg over four hours is not effective, then dialysis will probably be required.

In oliguric or anuric patients with significant fluid overload, it may not be practicable to administer high-dose Lasix injection by the method suggested above. Under these circumstances, the use of a constant-rate infusion pump (e.g. Sage pump) with micrometer screw-gauge adjustment may be considered for direct administration of the injection into the vein. The rate of administration should not exceed 4 mg/minute.

If the Lasix infusion produces a satisfactory response of 40–50 ml/hour, then the effective dose (up to 1,000 mg) can be repeated every 24 hours. Alternatively, maintenance therapy can be continued with oral Lasix 500 mg Tablets when one 500 mg tablet may be regarded as being approximately equal to one 250 mg ampoule. Appropriate dosage adjustments may then be made according to the observed clinical response.

Children: Doses for children can only be determined on the basis of the severity of the renal insufficiency and clinical response to initial doses.

Elderly: In the elderly, frusemide is generally eliminated more slowly. Dosage should be titrated until the required response is achieved.

Contra-indications, warnings, etc During treatment with high-dosage forms of Lasix, fluid balance should be carefully controlled. In the particular case of patients with shock, steps should be taken to correct the blood pressure and circulating blood volume before commencing therapy. Regular checks of plasma electrolytes, particularly sodium, potassium, chloride and bicarbonate, should be carried out, and electrolyte replacement therapy instituted accordingly.

Intravenous injections of Lasix *must* be given slowly.

If the recommended infusion rate of 4 mg/minute is exceeded, transient deafness may occur.

Contra-indications: Lasix Injection 250 mg is contra-indicated in renal failure as a result of poisoning by nephrotoxic or hepatotoxic agents and in renal failure associated with hepatic coma.

Hypersensitivity to sulphonamides is also a contra-indication.

Lasix Injection 250 mg should not be given to patients with normal renal function.

Warnings: The dosage of concurrently administered cardiac glycosides or antihypertensive agents may require adjustment.

Cephaloridine nephrotoxicity may be increased by

concomitant administration of potent diuretics such as frusemide.

Latent diabetes may become manifest or the insulin requirements of diabetic patients may increase.

In common with other diuretics, serum lithium levels may be increased when lithium is given concomitantly with frusemide, necessitating adjustment of the lithium dosage.

Certain non-steroidal anti-inflammatory agents have been shown to antagonise the action of diuretics such as frusemide. Salicylates may also have this effect.

The effects of curariform muscle relaxants may be enhanced by frusemide.

Interactions have also been reported with ototoxic antibiotics and parenteral cisplatin. Glucocorticoids may cause sodium retention and exacerbate potassium loss.

Precautions: There is little evidence of safety of high-dose Lasix in human pregnancy although the results of animal work, in general, show no hazardous effects. However, Lasix should be used in pregnancy only if strictly indicated and for short term treatment.

Nursing mothers: As Lasix may inhibit lactation it should be used with caution in nursing mothers.

Overdosage: In cases of overdose there is a danger of dehydration and electrolyte depletion due to excessive diuresis. Treatment should therefore be aimed at fluid replacement and correction of the electrolyte imbalance.

Side-effects: Lasix injection 250 mg is generally well tolerated. Side-effects of a minor nature such as nausea, malaise or gastric upset may occur but are not usually severe enough to necessitate withdrawal of treatment.

Calcium depletion may occur. Nephrocalcinosis has been reported in premature infants.

The incidence of allergic reactions, such as skin rashes, is very low but, when these occur, treatment should be withdrawn.

Acute pancreatitis has been reported.

In common with other sulphonamide-based diuretics, hyperuricaemia may occur and, in rare cases, clinical gout may be precipitated.

As with other diuretics a transient rise in creatinine and urea levels has also been reported with frusemide.

Bone marrow depression has been reported as a rare complication and necessitates withdrawal of treatment.

Transient ototoxicity has also been reported; it is generally only associated with rapid intravenous administration.

There may be an aggravation of metabolic acidosis.

Reduced mental alertness may impair ability to drive or operate dangerous machinery.

Pharmaceutical precautions Lasix Injection 250 mg should be stored in a cool place protected from light. Frusemide may precipitate in solutions of low pH and therefore dextrose solutions are not suitable infusion fluids for Lasix injections. The injection solution should not be mixed with other drugs in the infusion bottle.

Opened ampoules should be used immediately and any remainder of either the ampoule content or the prepared infusion solution should be discarded.

Legal category POM.

Package quantities Lasix Injections 250 mg are available in packs of 10 × 25 ml.

Further information Diuresis should commence within a few minutes and last for approximately two hours. A diuretic effect is seen during the infusion and its duration is related to the infusion time.

Lasix Injection 250 mg contains approximately 0.04 mmol Na$^+$/ml.

Product licence number 0086/5014.

LASIX* + K COMBINATION PACK

Presentation Lasix Tablets 40 mg each contain 40 mg of Frusemide BP. They are presented as white, circular, biplanar tablets measuring 8 mm in diameter. On one side they bear the Hoechst insignia. The other side is scored and bears the letters DLI on one side of the score mark and '40' on the other.

The potassium chloride slow-release tablets each contain 750 mg (10 mmol) of potassium chloride. They are presented as yellow, circular, biconvex tablets, 12 mm in diameter, and have no superficial markings.

These tablets are presented together in a calendar pack as Lasix + K.

Uses Lasix + K contains a short-acting diuretic and a slow-release potassium supplement. The calendar pack is designed for patients who require a fixed dose comprising 40 mg of Lasix (1 tablet) and 20 mmol of potassium (2 tablets) each day. It is not intended for patients who require individual titration of dosage.

Dosage and administration Lasix + K is supplied in calendar packs bearing directions for use. The instructions state that the Lasix 40 mg tablet is taken in the morning, that one potassium chloride tablet is taken at noon, and one in the evening. This ensures that the release of the latter occurs outside the diuretic phase, at a time when conditions are optimal for absorption and retention.

Children: Lasix + K is not suitable for paediatric use.

Elderly: Frusemide and potassium may both be excreted more slowly in the elderly.

Contra-indications, warnings, etc

Contra-indications: Lasix + K is contra-indicated in hyperkalaemia, precomatose states associated with liver cirrhosis and Addison's disease, and in patients taking potassium-sparing diuretics. Hypersensitivity to sulphonamides.

Warnings: Patients with prostatic hypertrophy or impairment of micturition have an increased risk of developing acute retention.

Where indicated, steps should be taken to correct hypotension or hypovolaemia before commencing therapy.

The dosage of concurrently administered cardiac glycosides or antihypertensive agents may require adjustment.

Cephaloridine nephrotoxicity may be increased by concomitant administration of potent diuretics such as frusemide.

Latent diabetes may become manifest or the insulin requirements of diabetic patients may increase.

Care should be exercised when treating patients with renal insufficiency because of the risk of hyperkalaemia.

In common with other diuretics, serum lithium levels may be increased when lithium is given concomitantly with frusemide, necessitating adjustment of the lithium dosage.

Certain non-steroidal anti-inflammatory agents have

been shown to antagonise the action of diuretics such as frusemide. Salicylates may also have this effect.

The effects of curariform muscle relaxants may be enhanced by frusemide.

Interactions have also been reported with ototoxic antibiotics. Glucocorticoids may cause sodium retention and exacerbate potassium loss.

Precautions: Results of animal work, in general, show no hazardous effect of Lasix in pregnancy. There is clinical evidence of safety of the drug in the third trimester of human pregnancy; however, Lasix should be used in pregnancy only if strictly indicated and for short-term treatment.

Nursing mothers: As Lasix may inhibit lactation it should be used with caution in nursing mothers.

Overdosage: In cases of overdose there is a danger of dehydration and electrolyte depletion due to excessive diuresis. Treatment should therefore be aimed at fluid replacement and correction of the electrolyte imbalance.

Side-effects: Lasix+K is generally well tolerated. Side-effects of a minor nature such as nausea, malaise or gastric upset may occur but are not usually severe enough to necessitate withdrawal of treatment.

Calcium depletion may occur. Nephrocalcinosis has been reported in premature infants.

Auditory disorders and acute pancreatitis have been reported with high dose parenteral frusemide.

As with other diuretics a transient rise in creatinine and urea levels has been reported with frusemide.

The incidence of allergic reactions, such as skin rashes, is very low, but when these occur treatment should be withdrawn.

In common with other sulphonamide-based diuretics hyperuricaemia may occur and, in rare cases, clinical gout may be precipitated.

Bone marrow depression has been reported as a rare complication and necessitates withdrawal of treatment.

There may be an aggravation of metabolic acidosis.

Reduced mental alertness may impair ability to drive or operate dangerous machinery.

Pharmaceutical precautions Lasix+K should be stored in a cool dry place, protected from light, in the original container or in containers similar to those of the manufacturer.

Legal category POM.

Package quantities Lasix+K is packed in blister strips, each containing 10 Lasix tablets and 20 potassium chloride tablets. It is supplied in boxes of three blister strips.

Further information Lasix produces a prompt and effective diuresis which lasts for approximately four hours following oral administration. The potassium chloride is contained in an inert matrix allowing sustained release over a period of six to eight hours.

If the prescribing instructions are followed, this ensures potassium release outside the diuretic phase at a time when conditions are optimal for absorption and retention.

Ghost tablets may appear in the patient's faeces.

Product licence number 0086/0037.

LASIX* PAEDIATRIC LIQUID ▼

Presentation Lasix Paediatric Liquid is presented as a granulate for reconstitution. The granulate is reconsti-

tuted with distilled water to produce a solution containing 1 mg/ml Frusemide BP in a volume of 150 ml.

Uses Lasix Paediatric Liquid is a diuretic which is indicated for the treatment of oedema in children. It may also be used in elderly patients or other patients unable to take solid oral dose forms of Lasix.

Dosage and administration The recommended daily dose of Lasix Paediatric Liquid for children is 1–3 mg/kg body weight (1–3 ml/kg as the reconstituted liquid).

When Lasix Paediatric Liquid is used as a substitute for tablet therapy in adults, the normal dose range is 20–80 mg (20–80 ml) daily (see 'Side-effects' section).

Elderly: In the elderly, frusemide is generally eliminated more slowly. Dosage should be titrated until the required response is achieved.

Reconstitution: Lasix Paediatric Liquid is supplied in a 150 ml bottle containing granules for reconstitution. The granules are reconstituted by the addition of 142 ml distilled water to the bottle which is then shaken vigorously to dissolve the granulate before oral administration. Tap water should not be used.

Contra-indications, warnings, etc

Contra-indications: Lasix Paediatric Liquid is contra-indicated in electrolyte deficiency and pre-comatose states associated with liver cirrhosis. Hypersensitivity to sulphonamides.

Warnings: Lasix Paediatric Liquid contains sorbitol and may cause flatulence, abdominal distension or diarrhoea if given in large quantities to adults who are unable to take solid oral dose forms of Lasix.

Patients with prostatic hypertrophy or impairment of micturition have an increased risk of developing acute retention.

Where indicated, steps should be taken to correct hypotension or hypovolaemia before commencing therapy.

The dosage of concurrently administered cardiac glycosides or hypotensive agents may require adjustment.

Cephaloridine nephrotoxicity may be increased by concomitant administration of potent diuretics such as frusemide.

Latent diabetes may become manifest or the insulin requirements of diabetic patients may increase.

In common with other diuretics, serum lithium levels may be increased when lithium is given concomitantly with frusemide, necessitating adjustment of the lithium dosage.

Certain non-steroidal anti-inflammatory agents have been shown to antagonise the action of diuretics such as frusemide. Salicylates may also have this effect.

The effects of curariform muscle relaxants may be enhanced by frusemide.

Interactions have also been reported with ototoxic antibiotics. Glucocorticoids may cause sodium retention and exacerbate potassium loss.

Precautions: Caution should be exercised in patients liable to electrolyte deficiency.

Results of animal work, in general, show no hazardous effect of Lasix in pregnancy. There is clinical evidence of safety of the drug in the third trimester of human pregnancy; however, Lasix should be used in pregnancy only if strictly indicated and for short term treatment.

Nursing mothers: As Lasix may inhibit lactation it should be used with caution in nursing mothers.

Overdosage: In cases of overdose there is a danger of dehydration and electrolyte depletion due to excessive diuresis. Treatment should therefore be aimed at fluid replacement and correction of the electrolyte imbalance.

Side-effects: Lasix is generally well tolerated. Side-effects of a minor nature such as nausea, malaise or gastric upset may occur but are not usually severe enough to necessitate withdrawal of treatment.

Flatulence, abdominal distension or diarrhoea may occur following the ingestion of large quantities of Lasix Paediatric Liquid, due to its sorbitol content.

Calcium depletion may occur. Nephrocalcinosis has been reported in premature infants.

Auditory disorders and acute pancreatitis have been reported with high dose parenteral frusemide.

As with other diuretics a transient rise in creatinine and urea levels has been reported with frusemide.

The incidence of allergic reactions, such as skin rashes, is very low but, when these occur, treatment should be withdrawn.

In common with other sulphonamide-based diuretics, hyperuricaemia may occur and, in rare cases, clinical gout may be precipitated.

Bone marrow depression has been reported as a rare complication and necessitates withdrawal of treatment.

There may be an aggravation of metabolic acidosis.

Reduced mental alertness may impair ability to drive or operate dangerous machinery.

Pharmaceutical precautions Lasix Paediatric Liquid granulate should be stored in a cool dry place, protected from light, in the original container.

The granulate should be reconstituted only with 142 ml of distilled water. When reconstituted the liquid should be stored in a cool place, preferably in a refrigerator at 5°C, protected from light.

Under these conditions, reconstituted Lasix Paediatric Liquid may be used for up to 30 days, after which any remaining solution must be discarded.

The shelf-life of the granulate prior to reconstitution is three years. The use of sterile distilled water is recommended when the product is intended for administration to neonates.

Legal category POM.

Package quantities Lasix Paediatric Liquid is available in 150 ml bottles.

Further information Lasix produces a prompt and effective diuresis which lasts for approximately four hours following oral administration. Therefore, the time of administration can be adjusted to suit the patient's requirements. Lasix Paediatric Liquid does not contain sucrose.

Product licence number 0086/0063.

METENIX* 5 TABLETS

Presentation Metenix 5 Tablets each contain 5 mg metolazone. They are presented as blue flat uncoated round tablets, 7 mm in diameter, marked with a figure '5' on one side and the Hoechst insignia on the other side.

Uses Metenix 5 is a diuretic for use in the treatment of mild and moderate hypertension. Metenix 5 may be used in conjunction with non-diuretic antihypertensive agents and, in these circumstances, it is usually possible to achieve satisfactory control of blood pressure with a reduced dose of the non-diuretic agent. Patients who have become resistant to therapy with these agents may respond to the addition of Metenix 5 to their antihypertensive regimen.

Metenix 5 may also be used for the treatment of cardiac, renal and hepatic oedema, ascites or toxaemia of pregnancy.

Dosage and administration

Hypertension: The recommended initial dose in mild and moderate hypertension is 5 mg daily. After three to four weeks, the dose may be reduced if necessary to 5 mg on alternate days as maintenance therapy.

Oedema: In oedematous conditions, the normal recommended dose is 5–10 mg daily, given as a single dose. In resistant conditions, this may be increased to 20 mg daily or above. However, no more than 80 mg should be given in any 24-hour period.

Children: There is insufficient knowledge of the effects of Metenix 5 in children for any dosage recommendations to be made.

Elderly: Metolazone may be excreted more slowly in the elderly.

Contra-indications, warnings, etc

Contra-indications: Metenix 5 is contra-indicated in electrolyte deficiency states, anuria, coma or pre-comatose states associated with liver cirrhosis; also in patients with known allergy or hypersensitivity to metolazone.

Warnings: The dosage of concurrently administered cardiac glycosides may require adjustment. Metenix 5 may aggravate the increased potassium excretion associated with steroid therapy or diseases such as cirrhosis or severe ischaemic heart disease.

Latent diabetes may become manifest or the insulin requirements of diabetic patients may increase.

Precautions: Because of the antihypertensive effects of metolazone the dosage of concurrently administered non-diuretic antihypertensive agents may need to be reduced.

Caution should be exercised during Metenix 5 therapy in patients liable to electrolyte deficiency.

Fluid and electrolyte balance should be carefully monitored during therapy especially if Metenix 5 is used concurrently with other diuretics. In particular, Metenix 5 may potentiate the diuresis produced by frusemide and, if the two agents are used concurrently, patients should be carefully monitored. This combination of drugs has been used in the treatment of resistant oedema.

Prolonged therapy with Metenix 5 may result in hypokalaemia. Serum potassium levels should be determined at regular intervals and, if necessary, potassium supplementation should be instituted.

Chloride deficit, hyponatraemia and a low salt syndrome may also occur, particularly when the patient is also on a diet with restricted salt intake. Hypomagnesaemia has been reported as a consequence of prolonged diuretic therapy.

There is little evidence of safety of the drug in human pregnancy, but it has been in wide, general use for many years without apparent ill consequence, animal studies having shown no hazard.

Nursing mothers: If Metenix 5 is given to nursing mothers, metolazone may be present in the breast milk.

Overdosage: In cases of overdose there is a danger of dehydration and electrolyte depletion. Treatment should therefore be aimed at fluid replacement and correction of the electrolyte imbalance.

Side-effects: Metenix 5 is generally well tolerated. There have been occasional reports of headache, anorexia, vomiting, abdominal discomfort, muscle cramps and dizziness. There have been isolated reports of urticaria, leucopenia, tachycardia, chills and chest pain.

Hyperuricaemia or azotaemia may occur during treatment with Metenix 5, particularly in patients with impaired renal function. On rare occasions, clinical gout has been reported.

Pharmaceutical precautions Metenix 5 Tablets should be stored in a cool dry place, protected from light, in the original containers or in containers similar to those of the manufacturer.

Legal category POM.

Package quantities Metenix 5 Tablets are available in blister strips packed in cartons of 100 tablets.

Further information Metolazone is a substituted quinazolinone diuretic.

Diuresis and saluresis begin within one hour of administration of Metenix 5 Tablets, reaching a maximum in two hours and continuing for 12–24 hours according to dosage.

Product licence number 0086/0056.

RASTINON* TABLETS 500 mg

Presentation Rastinon Tablets each contain 500 mg Tolbutamide BP. They are presented as uncoated white, circular, scored tablets, 13 mm in diameter, one side bearing the Hoechst insignia, the other bearing the marks 'Rastinon' and '0.5' on either side of the score mark.

Uses Rastinon is a hypoglycaemic agent, indicated for the oral treatment of patients with non-insulin dependent diabetes who respond inadequately to dietary treatment alone. Rastinon is particularly suitable for elderly patients.

Dosage and administration

1. *Treatment of previously untreated diabetics:* Stabilisation can be achieved by commencing with 2 tablets daily. The subsequent dosage must depend on the patient's individual response. The average daily dose is 1–3 tablets which can be taken as a single or divided dose as required. Generally, patients who do not respond to 4 tablets (2 g) daily will not respond to higher doses.

2. *Change-over from other oral antidiabetics:* The change-over to Rastinon, from other drugs with a similar mode of action, can be carried out without any break in therapy, even with chlorpropamide despite the long persistence of this agent in the body.

Stabilisation can be achieved by commencing with 2 tablets daily, subsequent dosage depending on the patient's individual response.

3. *Combination with biguanides:* If adequate control is not possible with diet and 4 tablets of Rastinon daily, control can often be re-established by combined administration of Rastinon and a biguanide derivative.

4. *Change-over from insulin:* Some cases of non-insulin dependent diabetes, previously treated with insulin, can be changed to Rastinon. Low insulin doses (less than 20 units) can be replaced immediately. With higher doses a gradual change is advisable by giving insulin and Rastinon concurrently and reducing the dose of insulin.

The tablets may be taken by mouth as a single dose with or immediately after the first main meal of the day, or as a divided dose.

Children: As non-insulin dependent diabetes is not usually a disease of childhood, Rastinon is not recommended for use in children.

Elderly: Rastinon is particularly suitable for elderly patients.

Contra-indications, warnings, etc

Contra-indications: Rastinon should not be used in patients who have or have ever had diabetic ketoacidosis, who have insulin-dependent diabetes mellitus, serious impairment of renal, hepatic, adrenocortical or thyroid function or in circumstances of unusual stress, e.g. surgical operations or during pregnancy, when dietary treatment and insulin are essential.

Rastinon should not be used during the first trimester of pregnancy. There is some evidence of harmful effects in pregnancy in animals and isolated reports which suggest a hazard in human pregnancy.

Nursing mothers: Tolbutamide has been detected in breast milk in small quantities; the effect of this low dose on the neonate is unknown.

Warnings: Debilitated or aged patients may be more liable to hypoglycaemia. The hypoglycaemic effect of tolbutamide may be enhanced by dicoumarol, monoamine oxidase inhibitors, beta-adrenergic blocking agents, sulphonamides, phenylbutazone, chloramphenicol, cyclophosphamide and salicylates, or diminished by adrenaline, corticosteroids, oral contraceptives or thiazide diuretics.

Overdosage: Hypoglycaemia may be treated in the conscious patient by the administration of glucose or 3–4 lumps of table sugar with water. This may be repeated as necessary.

If the patient is comatose, glucose should be administered as an intravenous infusion. Bolus glucose injections are not recommended because of the possibility of rebound hypoglycaemia. Alternatively, glucagon may be administered in a dose of 1 mg subcutaneously or intramuscularly to produce consciousness.

Side-effects: Adverse reactions serious enough to warrant discontinuation of treatment are uncommon but mild gastro-intestinal and allergic skin reactions have occurred. There have been reports of anaemia, pancytopenia and transient changes in liver enzyme concentrations and liver function tests during treatment with tolbutamide, but these effects are not known to be directly attributable to the drug. Hypoglycaemic symptoms have occasionally been reported when the dose has been administered without due regard to the patient's dietary habits.

Pharmaceutical precautions Rastinon tablets should be stored in a cool dry place, protected from light, in the original containers or in containers similar to those of the manufacturer.

Legal category POM.

Package quantities Rastinon tablets are available as loose tablets packed in tubs of 100 and 500.

Further information Orally administered Rastinon is rapidly absorbed. It is extensively metabolised in the liver prior to excretion in the urine. Both of its metabolites possess some hypoglycaemic activity; this, however, is less pronounced than that of the parent compound.

Product licence number 0086/5016.

RELEFACT* LH-RH INJECTION ▼

Presentation Each ampoule contains 100 mcg Gonadorelin BP (luteinizing hormone releasing hormone) in 1 ml aqueous solution.

Uses Intravenous injection of Relefact LH-RH causes release of LH (luteinizing hormone) and FSH (follicle-stimulating hormone) from the pituitary gland. It provides a means of assessing the reserve of LH and FSH in the pituitary glands of patients with suspected pituitary impairment. In addition, Relefact LH-RH may be of value in the differential diagnosis of delayed puberty and hypogonadism.

Dosage and administration Relefact LH-RH should be administered intravenously to adults or children as a single dose of 100 mcg. The test is based upon the pituitary response to this dose measured as serum LH and FSH levels. Qualitative data may be obtained from a single test but each laboratory must establish its own normal range for values of serum LH and FSH to obtain quantitative assessment of pituitary reserve.

Test procedure:

1. Obtain venous blood sample for control value of LH and, if facilities are available for its measurement, FSH.
2. Rapid intravenous injection of 100 mcg Relefact LH-RH.
3. Obtain venous blood sample 20 minutes after injection for measurement of LH/FSH response.

Interpretation of results:

1. *Normal response:* Following the administration of Relefact LH-RH there is a rise in serum LH within two minutes of injection; the response is dose-dependent. Peak levels are achieved 20–30 minutes after injection and baseline levels are approached six hours after a dose of 100 mcg. The FSH response is similar but of lesser magnitude (except (a) prior to puberty when, in girls, the FSH response is higher than the LH response and (b) in some patients with hypothalamic-pituitary dysfunction, e.g. anorexia nervosa). The normal female response to Relefact LH-RH shows cyclical variation, the response in the luteal phase being about twice that seen in the early follicular phase.

It is important for each laboratory to establish its own normal ranges of LH and FSH according to the time of the menstrual cycle before attempting to obtain quantitative results.

2. *Assessment of pituitary function:* Relefact LH-RH is a very sensitive index of pituitary function. Consequently, many patients with pituitary tumours, who do not respond to other dynamic tests of pituitary function (such as the growth hormone response to hypoglycaemia), will show a normal response to Relefact LH-RH; others will show an impaired or absent response. A normal response to the Relefact LH-RH test in clinically hypogonadal patients with pituitary abnormalities indicates that their pituitary glands are capable of producing LH and FSH in response to therapy. Similar responses may be seen in patients with hypothalamic tumours such as craniopharyngiomas.

3. *Assessment of primary and secondary hypogonadism:* Patients with primary hypogonadism resulting from gonadal failure or gonadal dysgenesis will have an exaggerated response to Relefact LH-RH. The majority of these patients will also have elevated basal values.

The test is of particular value in those cases where basal levels are normal.

The majority of patients with congenital hypogonadotrophic hypogonadism with or without hyposmia (Kallman's syndrome) show a normal or impaired response to single doses of Relefact LH-RH.

These results indicate that, in most cases of isolated pituitary gonadotrophin deficiency, there is a reduced output of hypothalamic hormone releasing factor. An absent response to a single injection, however, is not necessarily indicative of pituitary failure, as more than one injection may be required in order to produce a response.

4. *Assessment of delayed puberty:* In simple delayed puberty the LH and FSH responses are within the normal range, whereas patients with hypogonadotrophic hypogonadism or hypopituitarism have an absent or impaired response. Patients with primary gonadal failure will have an exaggerated response.

Contra-indications, warnings, etc Relefact LH-RH should not be administered in pregnancy. There is a theoretical possibility of induction of ovulation following the administration of LH-RH.

Side-effects: Side-effects of any description are rare, but the following reactions have been reported in isolated cases in healthy women: abdominal pain, nausea, headache and increased menstrual bleeding.

Overdosage: Overdosage with Relefact LH-RH has never been reported and is unlikely to be a problem.

Pharmaceutical precautions Store in a cool dark place. Do not dilute or administer with any additive.

Legal category POM.

Package quantities Relefact LH-RH is available in packs of 10 ampoules.

Further information Relefact LH-RH (luteinizing hormone-releasing hormone) is a synthetic decapeptide. It has also been referred to in the literature as LRF (luteinizing hormone/releasing factor), as LH/FSH-RH (luteinizing hormone/follicle stimulating hormone-releasing hormone) and as luliberin.

Product licence number 0086/0019.

RELEFACT* LH-RH/TRH INJECTION ▼

Presentation Each ampoule contains 100 mcg Gonadorelin BP (luteinizing hormone-releasing hormone) and 200 mcg protirelin (thyrotrophin-releasing hormone) in 1 ml aqueous solution.

Uses Intravenous injection of Relefact LH-RH/TRH causes the release of LH (luteinizing hormone), FSH (follicle-stimulating hormone) and TSH (thyroid-stimulating hormone) from the pituitary gland. In addition, TRH is also known to cause the release of prolactin.

The use of a combined releasing hormone preparation provides a means of simultaneous assessment of anterior pituitary reserve of these hormones in patients with suspected pituitary impairment.

Dosage and administration The contents of 1 ampoule of LH-RH/TRH should be administered intravenously to adults and children as a single dose (100 mcg LH-RH and 200 mcg TRH). The test is based upon the pituitary response to this dose measured as serum TSH, LH and FSH levels. Qualitative data may be obtained from a single combined test but each laboratory must establish its own normal range for the serum level of these hormones to obtain a quantitative assessment of pituitary function.

Test procedure:

1. Obtain venous blood sample for control measurements of TSH, LH and, if required, FSH.
2. Rapid intravenous injection of one ampoule LH-RH/TRH.
3. Obtain venous blood sample 20 minutes after injection to give peak LH, FSH and TSH values.
4. A further venous blood sample may be taken at 60 or 90 minutes to detect a delayed or prolonged response.

Interpretation of results:

LH-RH

1. *Normal response:* Following the administration of LH-RH there is a rise of serum LH within two minutes of injection; the response is dose-dependent. Peak levels are achieved 20–30 minutes after injection and baseline levels are approached six hours after a dose of 100 mcg. The FSH response is similar but of lesser magnitude (except (a) prior to puberty when, in girls, the FSH response is higher than the LH response and (b) in some patients with hypothalamic-pituitary dysfunction, e.g. anorexia nervosa). The normal female response to LH-RH shows cyclical variation, the response in the luteal phase being about twice that seen in the early follicular phase.

It is important for each laboratory to establish its own normal ranges of LH and FSH according to the time of the menstrual cycle before attempting to obtain quantitative results.

2. *Assessment of pituitary function:* LH-RH response is a very sensitive index of pituitary function. Consequently, many patients with pituitary tumours who do not respond to other dynamic tests of pituitary function (such as the growth hormone response to hypoglycaemia) will show a normal response to LH-RH; others will show an impaired or absent response. A normal response to the LH-RH test in clinically hypogonadal patients with pituitary abnormalities indicates that their pituitary glands are capable of producing LH and FSH in response to therapy. Similar response may be seen in patients with hypothalamic tumours such as craniopharyngiomas.

3. *Assessment of primary and secondary hypogonadism:* Patients with primary hypogonadism resulting from gonadal failure or gonadal dysgenesis will have an exaggerated response to LH-RH. Most of these patients will also have elevated basal values. The test is of particular value in those cases where basal levels are normal.

The majority of patients with congenital hypogonadotrophic hypogonadism with or without hyposmia (Kallman's syndrome) show a normal or impaired response to single doses of LH-RH.

These results indicate that, in most cases of isolated pituitary gonadotrophin deficiency, there is a reduced output of hypothalamic hormone-releasing factor. An absent response to a single injection, however, is not necessarily indicative of pituitary failure, as more than one injection may be required in order to produce a response.

4. *Assessment of delayed puberty:* In simple delayed puberty the LH and FSH responses are within the normal range, whereas patients with hypogonadotrophic hypogonadism or hypopituitarism have an absent or

impaired response. Patients with primary gonadal failure will have an exaggerated response.

TRH

1. *Normal response:* In normal subjects, intravenous injection of TRH causes a prompt rise (within five minutes) in serum TSH. This increases to a maximum at about 20 minutes and is declining at 60 minutes. Basal levels are reached about four hours after TRH administration.

2. *Thyroid disease:* **Hyperthyroidism.** Diagnosis is based upon the measurement of two parameters.

(a) the increase in TSH values from basal levels, 20 minutes after TRH administration ($\triangle$TSH).
(b) the ratio of 20 minute TSH value to its basal value (TSH_{20}/TSH_0).

The usual hyperthyroid response is as follows:

(a) increase in TSH 20 minutes after injection will be less than 2 mcU/ml ($\triangle$TSH < 2).
(b) the ratio of 20 minute TSH to its basal value will be equal to or less than 1.5 ($TSH_{20}/TSH_0 \leqslant 1.5$).

Primary hypothyroidism. Primary hypothyroidism is characterised by a high basal TSH level and an exaggerated and prolonged rise in serum TSH following the administration of TRH.

3. *Hypothalamic or pituitary disease:* **Pituitary disease.** An absent or impaired TSH response indicates a reduction in pituitary reserve (although failure to respond to TRH is also found in patients with hyperthyroidism, this will not usually cause diagnostic difficulty).

Hypothalamic disease. Patients with hypothyroidism caused by hypothalamic disease may have a normal TSH response to TRH. However, more usually, a delayed response is found.

Note: The administration of TRH together with LH-RH may cause slightly greater FSH release in males than that caused by LH-RH alone.

Contra-indications, warnings, etc Relefact LH-RH/TRH should not be used in patients with bronchial asthma or obstructive airways disease. Care should be exercised in patients with myocardial ischaemia.

LH-RH/TRH should not be administered in pregnancy; there is a theoretical possibility of induction of ovulation following the administration of LH-RH/TRH.

Side-effects: The following minor transient side-effects have been reported in patients given TRH: desire to micturate, sensation of heat, slight dizziness and a peculiar taste. There have been isolated reports of transient amaurosis, severe headache, unconsciousness, convulsions and hypotension.

LH-RH administration has been associated with the following reactions in isolated cases in healthy women: abdominal pain, nausea, headache and increased menstrual bleeding.

Overdosage: Overdosage with LH-RH/TRH should be treated symptomatically.

Pharmaceutical precautions Store in a cool dark place; do not dilute or administer with any additive.

Legal category POM.

Package quantity Relefact LH-RH/TRH is available in packs of 10 ampoules.

Further information LH-RH, TRH and insulin have been administered at the same time for a full and rapid assessment of anterior pituitary function. Such combined administration does not appreciably affect the various hormone responses (LH, FSH, TSH, growth hormone, ACTH, corticosteroids and prolactin).

Note: The mixing of insulin and LH-RH/TRH in the same syringe is not recommended.

Product licence number 0086/0059.

STREPTASE* INJECTION

Presentation Streptase is presented as a freeze-dried powder in vials containing 100,000 Units, 250,000 Units and 750,000 Units of purified streptokinase.

Uses Streptase is a fibrinolytic agent which will produce intravascular dissolution of thrombi and emboli in:

extensive deep venous thrombosis
pulmonary embolism
acute occlusion of peripheral arteries

also in:

rethrombosis after vascular surgery
thrombosis of vascular prostheses
clotting in external arteriovenous shunts of patients on
haemodialysis
renal vein thrombosis
central retinal venous or arterial thrombosis

Dosage and administration Streptase should be given by intravascular infusion in physiological saline or Haemaccel.

Loading dose: Since human exposure to streptococci is common, antibodies to streptokinase (streptokinase resistance) are found normally. Thus, a loading dose of Streptase sufficient to neutralize the resistance is required. A dose of 250,000 Units of Streptase infused into a peripheral vein over 30 minutes has been found appropriate in over 90% of patients.

Maintenance dose: A maintenance dose infusion of 100,000 Units/hour is given following the loading dose. Administer the maintenance dose of 100,000 Units per hour for 72 hours for the treatment of deep vein thrombosis, for 24 hours for the treatment of pulmonary embolism (up to 72 hours if concurrent deep vein thrombosis is suspected) and for 24–72 hours for the treatment of arterial thrombosis. If the thrombin time or any other parameter of lysis after 4 hours of therapy is less than approximately $1\frac{1}{2}$ times the normal control value, discontinue Streptase as excessive resistance to streptokinase is present.

Children: In children, in whom it is always advisable to estimate the initial dose by means of the streptokinase resistance test (see 'Warnings' section), the correct maintenance dose per hour is 20 Units/ml blood volume.

Patient monitoring: Before commencing thrombolytic therapy, it is desirable to obtain a thrombin time (TT), pro-thrombin time (PT), haematocrit and platelet count to obtain the haemostatic status of the patient. If heparin has been given it should be discontinued, and the TT should be less than twice the normal control value before thrombolytic therapy is started.

During the infusion, decreases in the plasminogen and fibrinogen level and an increase in the level of fibrin degradation products (FDP) (the latter two serving to

*A variable dosage of Streptase and frequent laboratory monitoring have been recommended. However, since experience shows that these do not seem to increase the efficacy or safety of Streptase therapy, they are no longer recommended.

prolong the clotting times of coagulation tests) will generally confirm the existence of a lytic state. Therefore, therapy can be monitored by performing the TT or PT approximately 4 hours after initiation of therapy.

Following the infusion, before (re-)instituting heparin, the TT should be less than twice the normal control value.

Anticoagulation after terminating intravenous streptokinase treatment: At the end of Streptase therapy, treatment with heparin by continuous intravenous infusion is recommended to prevent recurrent thrombosis. Heparin treatment (without a loading dose) should not begin until the thrombin time has decreased to less than twice the normal control value (approximately 3 to 4 hours). (See manufacturer's prescribing information for proper use of heparin.) This should be followed by oral anticoagulation in the conventional manner.

Contra-indications, warnings, etc

Contra-indications: Manifest or recent haemorrhage, haemorrhagic diathesis (with the exception of consumption coagulopathy), severe hypertension, streptococcal infections and subacute bacterial endocarditis are contra-indications to Streptase therapy.

Drug-induced coagulation defects represent a temporary contra-indication. The effect of heparin can be rapidly neutralised with protamine sulphate or protamine chloride. In patients who have been receiving coumarin drugs, the time at which Streptase therapy may be commenced must be decided in the light of the coagulation status. It is advisable to carry out the appropriate tests at shorter intervals than usual.

Drugs affecting platelet function, such as acetylsalicylic acid, phenylbutazone and dipyridamole should be discontinued at least 3 days before Streptase therapy commences because of a possible increased risk of bleeding.

Recent surgery is a relative contra-indication to Streptase therapy. However, in cases of embolism, the indication for treatment may be very strong. After careful consideration of all the risks, Streptase may be given 6 days after the operation. The danger of bleeding from the operative area must, of course, be taken into account. In cases of severe pulmonary embolism, the use of Streptase might be considered earlier; the risks, however, should be weighed against the benefits.

Warnings: Caution is necessary in patients with recent cavitating tuberculous lesions of the lungs, gastrointestinal ulceration or serious liver disease accompanied by a bleeding tendency.

Precautions: The use of Streptase before the sixteenth week of pregnancy and again, immediately post-partum, involves a risk which should be carefully assessed before therapy is instituted. If the patient has just recovered from a streptococcal infection or if it is urgently necessary to give a further course of Streptase within three months of the first course, the streptokinase resistance test must be used to estimate the correct initial dose and corticosteroid cover is essential.

Treatment with streptokinase causes a marked increase in the level of streptokinase antibodies. This normally precludes repeated therapy within 3 months.

Titrated initial dose: The determination of the initial dose by the streptokinase resistance test is recommended in the following circumstances:

(a) in children
(b) when there is a history of recent streptococcal infection

(c) when the patient has previously received streptokinase therapy.

However low the titre determined, the initial dose must not be less than 100,000 Units of Streptase.

As streptokinase is an antigen it is advisable to cover the initial dose of Streptase by prophylactic administration of a corticosteroid, e.g. hydrocortisone hemisuccinate 100 mg i.v., so as to preclude any possibility of allergic reactions.

Side-effects: A mild rise in temperature, usually of short duration, may be noted in some cases. With the prophylactic administration of a corticosteroid before commencing treatment, pyrexia should not be encountered. Allergic-anaphylactic reactions are possible but very rare. Such reactions are more liable to occur if Streptase is injected too rapidly. Should a major reaction be encountered, discontinue Streptase and initiate therapy with adrenaline, corticosteroids and antihistamines as appropriate.

Overdose: Haemorrhage, considered the main potential complication of streptokinase therapy, is uncommon with the recommended dosage technique. Bleeding episodes are usually confined to oozing from sites of venepuncture and do not require the discontinuation of therapy. Intramuscular therapy can cause formation of local haematomas.

Should serious haemorrhage occur, Streptase therapy should be stopped and tranexamic acid (10 mg/kg) should be administered by slow intravenous injection. The use of tranexamic acid is not advised during pregnancy when aprotinin should be administered. In only a very few cases will substitution therapy with fibrinogen be necessary.

A transient increase in serum enzymes has been reported following Streptase therapy. This is due to a stimulation of the kallikrein system and not to a hepatotoxic effect.

Pharmaceutical precautions Streptase is stable for at least 3 years when stored at room temperature (<25 °C).

Solutions prepared for infusion but left over or not used should be discarded.

Legal category POM.

Package quantities Available in vials in the following packs:

1 × 100,000 Units and 10 × 100,000 Units
1 × 250,000 Units and 10 × 250,000 Units
1 × 750,000 Units and 10 × 750,000 Units

Streptase for diagnostic use is also supplied in packs of 4 × 5,000 Units.

Further information Streptase activates the intrinsic fibrinolytic system by the formation of a linkage compound between streptokinase and the proactivator-plasminogen molecule. This complex possesses activator properties and brings about the conversion of plasminogen into the fibrinolytic enzyme plasmin. Plasminogen adsorbed on the fibrin clot is also activated, therefore lysis can take place internally as well as externally.

Product licence numbers

Streptase 100,000 Units	0086/5018
Streptase 250,000 Units	0086/5020
Streptase 750,000 Units	0086/5021

SUPREFACT* INJECTION ▼
SUPREFACT* NASAL SPRAY ▼

Presentation Suprefact injection contains 1.00 mg buserelin as buserelin acetate in 1 ml aqueous solution containing benzyl alcohol as preservative.

Suprefact nasal spray contains 100 micrograms buserelin as buserelin acetate in one spray dose (100 mg) of aqueous solution containing benzyl alcohol as preservative.

1.00 mg buserelin is equivalent to 1.05 mg buserelin acetate.

Uses For the treatment of advanced prostatic carcinoma (stage C or stage D according to the classification of Murphy et al. in Cancer, 45, p 1889–95, 1980) in which suppression of testosterone is indicated. Buserelin acts by blockade and subsequent down-regulation of pituitary LHRH receptor synthesis. Gonadotrophin release is consequently inhibited. As a result of this inhibition there is reduced stimulation of testosterone secretion and serum testosterone levels fall to the castration range. Before inhibition occurs there is a brief stimulatory phase during which testosterone levels may rise.

Dosage and administration

1. Initiation of therapy: is most conveniently carried out in hospital; 0.5 ml Suprefact injection should be injected subcutaneously at 8 hourly intervals for 7 days.

2. Maintenance therapy: on the 8th day of treatment the patient is changed to intranasal administration of Suprefact. One spray dose is introduced into each nostril 6 times a day according to the following schedule:

1st dose before breakfast
2nd dose after breakfast
3rd and 4th doses before and after midday meal
5th and 6th doses before and after evening meal.

This dosage regimen is to ensure adequate absorption of the material and to distribute the dose throughout the day.

Contra-indications, warnings, etc

Contra-indications: Suprefact should not be used if the tumour if found to be insensitive to hormone manipulation or after surgical removal of the testes. It is contra-indicated in cases of known hypersensitivity to benzyl alcohol or buserelin.

Precautions and warnings: Monitoring of the clinical effect of Suprefact is carried out by the methods generally used in prostatic carcinoma. Initially serum testosterone levels rise and a clinical effect will not be seen until levels start to fall into the therapeutic (castration) range. Disease flare (temporary deterioration of patient's condition) has been reported at the beginning of treatment. The incidence is variable, but of the order of 10%. Symptoms are usually confined to transient increase in pain, but the exact nature depends on the site of the lesions. Neurological sequelae have been reported where secondary deposits impinge upon the spinal cord or CNS. Disease flare is prevented by the prophylactic use of an anti-androgen, e.g. cyproterone acetate, 300 mg daily. It is recommended that treatment should be started at least 3 days before the first dose of Suprefact and continued for at least 3 weeks after commencement of Suprefact therapy.

Once testosterone levels have started to fall below their baseline concentration clinical improvement should start to become apparent. If testosterone levels do not reach the therapeutic range within 4 weeks (6 weeks at the latest) the dose schedule should be checked to be sure that it is being followed exactly. It is unlikely that a patient who is taking the full dose will not show a suppression of testosterone to the therapeutic range. If this is the case, alternative therapy should be considered.

A proportion of patients will have tumours which are not sensitive to hormone manipulation. Absence of clinical Improvement in the face of adequate testosterone suppression is diagnostic of this condition, which will not benefit from further therapy with buserelin.

Side-effects: Suprefact is generally well tolerated. Side-effects consequent upon the suppression of testosterone secretion are hot flushes and loss of potency and libido. These occur in most patients. Transient nasal irritation has been reported after nasal application but is rare.

Pharmaceutical precautions Store at room temperature. The spray solution should last for 1 week of treatment. Any residual material after this time should be discarded.

Legal category POM.

Package quantities
Suprefact for Injection: Box of 2 × 5.5 ml multidose vials each containing 1.05 mg buserelin acetate per 1 ml, corresponding to 1.00 mg buserelin per 1 ml.
Suprefact Nasal Spray: Box of 4 bottles each containing 10 g solution, and 4 spray pumps.

Further information The therapeutic effect of Suprefact can only be achieved if the dosage is conscientiously adhered to. It is, therefore, advisable to administer Suprefact nasal spray before and after meals. It can also be used at other times provided uniform intervals are maintained between doses.

If used correctly, reliable absorption of the active substance takes place via the nasal mucous membrane. Suprefact nasal is absorbed even if the patient has a cold.

Product licence numbers
0086/0101
0086/0102

SYNADRIN* TABLETS 60 mg

Presentation Synadrin tablets each contain 76 mg Prenylamine Lactate BP, equivalent to 60 mg free base. They are presented as bi-convex, pink, sugar-coated tablets having a diameter of 11 mm.

Uses Synadrin is a catecholamine-depleting agent indicated in the long-term management of angina pectoris.

Dosage and administration One tablet three times daily is adequate for the majority of patients. This can be increased to 1 tablet four or five times daily in patients who do not respond within fourteen days. Reduction in the frequency of anginal attacks should be observed within two weeks, after which a lower maintenance dose, adjusted to individual requirements, is sufficient. The tablet should be swallowed whole.

Children: Synadrin is not suitable for use in children.

Elderly: In elderly patients where there is serious impairment of hepatic or renal function, Synadrin is not recommended.

Contra-indications, warnings, etc Synadrin is contra-indicated where serious impairment of hepatic or renal function, defects of cardiac conduction or severe uncompensated heart failure are present.

Synadrin may have a slight hypotensive action and the dosage of concurrently administered hypotensive agents may require adjustment.

Synadrin should not be administered concurrently with negative inotropic drugs, e.g. beta-adrenergic receptor blocking agents, quinidine, procainamide, amiodarone or lignocaine. Reports indicate that such combinations are capable of producing paroxysmal ventricular tachycardia or fibrillation. Synadrin should be used with caution in combination with diuretics, laxatives or other drugs likely to cause potassium deficiency. It is recommended that serum potassium concentrations be determined at regular intervals and, if necessary, potassium supplementation should be instituted. If the ECG shows a marked increase in the duration of the QS or QT interval above the rate-adjusted norm, it is recommended that Synadrin treatment be withdrawn.

Some caution should be observed in patients requiring the administration of cardio-depressive inhalation anaesthetics, as there is a theoretical risk of some potentiation of their negative inotropic effects.

There is no information on the use of Synadrin in pregnancy but no untoward effects have been found in animal studies.

Nursing mothers: There is no information on the use of Synadrin in nursing mothers.

Overdosage: In cases of overdosage gastric lavage is indicated, even after some considerable time, as there is a delay in absorption of large doses of Synadrin due to its relative insolubility. Treatment is symptomatic: if convulsions occur i.v. diazepam should be considered. Muscle relaxants may also be given, and artificial respiration may be necessary. If there is a severe fall in blood pressure (collapse) an i.v. drip may be set up. *Avoid* giving adrenaline, noradrenaline or isoprenaline because of the risk of ventricular fibrillation.

Side-effects: Synadrin is well tolerated. Gastro-intestinal upsets have been reported infrequently. Some degree of sedation has been reported following the administration of high doses. In susceptible patients, catecholamine depletion can lead to the onset of extrapyramidal signs. Isolated cases of mild intention tremor have been reported. Hypersensitivity reactions such as skin rashes have occurred.

Pharmaceutical precautions Synadrin tablets should be stored in a cool dry place in the original containers or in containers similar to those of the manufacturer.

Legal category POM.

Package quantities Synadrin tablets are available in blister packs of 100 and loose in tubs of 500.

Further information Synadrin depletes myocardial catecholamine stores and slows calcium transport through the endoplasmic reticulum, thus reducing myocardial oxygen demand in stress situations and thereby reducing the incidence of anginal attacks.

Product licence number 0086/5019.

TRENTAL* INJECTION 100 mg/5 ml

Presentation Trental Injection contains 100 mg oxpentifylline in 5 ml aqueous solution.

Uses Trental Injection is indicated in the treatment of peripheral vascular disease.

Dosage and administration Depending upon the

condition being treated, Trental may be given orally, as a combined oral/parenteral treatment or as a parenteral treatment alone.

The preferred parenteral route is by infusion.

Parenteral administration: Intravenous infusion: It is recommended that an initial dose of 100 mg in 250–500 ml of fluid be infused intravenously over 90–180 minutes. This dose may be increased by 50 mg per day up to a maximum daily dosage of 400 mg. Trental is compatible with 0.9% sodium chloride, 5% laevulose or glucose infusion solutions.

Intra-arterial infusion: 100–300 mg (1–3 ampoules) daily intra-arterially in 20–50 ml of 0.9% sodium chloride infused over 10–30 minutes.

Intravenous injection: This can be used for the initial therapy of peripheral vascular disorders; the recommended dose is 100 mg i.v. The injection must be given slowly with the patient lying down. It is best to start a course of intravenous injections with a preliminary dose of 50 mg to 100 mg diluted in 5 ml of 0.9% sodium chloride and injected over several minutes.

Larger doses can be given by intravenous infusion.

Children: Trental is not suitable for use in children.

Contra-indications, warnings, etc

Contra-indications: Trental is contra-indicated in cases where there is known hypersensitivity to the active constituent oxpentifylline.

Warnings: In diabetic patients stabilised on insulin or oral antidiabetic agents, high dose parenteral administration of Trental may intensify the hypoglycaemic activity of the antidiabetic agent concerned. In such cases the dose of insulin or oral antidiabetic agent should be reduced.

Trental may potentiate the effect of anti-hypertensive agents and the dosage of the latter may need to be reduced.

In patients with hypotension or severe coronary artery disease, Trental should be used with caution, as a transient hypotensive effect is possible and, in isolated cases, might result in a reduction in coronary artery perfusion.

In patients with a creatinine clearance of less than 10 ml/min it may be necessary to adjust the daily dose of oxpentifylline to avoid accumulation.

Precautions: There is no information on the use of Trental in pregnancy but no untoward effects have been found in animal studies.

Nursing mothers: There is no information on the use of Trental in nursing mothers.

Overdosage: The treatment of overdosage should be symptomatic.

Side-effects: Trental is generally well tolerated. Nausea, malaise, gastric upset, vertigo and flushing may occur but these are generally mild and transient.

Pharmaceutical precautions Trental should be stored in a cool dry place.

Legal category POM.

Package quantities Trental injection is available in packs of 5 × 5 ml.

Further information Investigations have shown that Trental has no effect on the bleeding or clotting time of blood. No interaction with anticoagulants has been reported. Trental injection is compatible with 0.9%

sodium chloride, 5% laevulose or glucose infusion solutions. Trental injection contains 0.12 mmol Na$^+$ per ml of solution.

Product licence number 0086/0022.

TRENTAL* 400

Presentation Trental 400 Tablets each contain 400 mg oxpentifylline in a slow-release formulation. They are presented as oblong, pink, sugar-coated tablets, 17.5 mm long, 8.75 mm wide and 6 mm thick.

Uses Trental is indicated in the treatment of peripheral vascular disease, including intermittent claudication and rest pain.

Dosage and administration The recommended initial dose is 1 tablet (400 mg) three times daily; two tablets daily may prove sufficient in some patients, particularly for maintenance therapy.

Children: Trental 400 is not suitable for use in children.

Contra-indications, warnings, etc

Contra-indications: Trental 400 is contra-indicated in cases where there is known hypersensitivity to the active constituent, oxpentifylline.

Warnings: High doses of Trental injection have been shown, in rare cases, to intensify the hypoglycaemic action of insulin and oral hypoglycaemic agents. However, no effect on insulin release has been observed with Trental following oral administration.

Trental 400 may potentiate the effect of anti-hypertensive agents and the dosage of the latter may need to be reduced.

In patients with hypotension or severe coronary artery disease, Trental 400 should be used with caution, as a transient hypotensive effect is possible and, in isolated cases, might result in a reduction in coronary artery perfusion.

In patients with a creatinine clearance of less than 10 ml/min it may be necessary to adjust the daily dose of oxpentifylline to avoid accumulation.

Precautions: There is no information on the use of Trental in pregnancy but no untoward effects have been found in animal studies.

Nursing mothers: There is no information on the use of Trental 400 in nursing mothers.

Overdosage: The treatment of overdosage should be symptomatic.

Side-effects: Trental 400 is generally well tolerated. Nausea, malaise, gastric upset, vertigo and flushing may occur but these are generally mild and transient. In cases where gastric upset does occur, Trental 400 should be given with or immediately after food.

Pharmaceutical precautions Trental 400 should be stored in a cool dry place in the original containers or in containers similar to those of the manufacturer.

Legal category POM.

Package quantities Trental 400 tablets are available in packs of 100 and 250.

Further information Investigations have shown that Trental has no effect on the bleeding or clotting time of blood. No interaction with anticoagulants has been reported.

Product licence number 0086/0058.

*Trade Mark

Hough, Hoseason & Company Limited
Chapel Street
Levenshulme
Manchester M19 3PT

MANUSEPT*

Presentation A clear, blue coloured solution containing 70% v/v Isopropyl Alcohol BP, 0.5% w/v Triclosan.

Uses For the disinfection of intact skin.
(i) For preoperative disinfection of physically clean hands.
(ii) For skin disinfection prior to surgery, injection or venepuncture.

Dosage and administration
(i) For the disinfection of physically clean hands: Dispense approximately 5 ml of Manusept into the palm of one hand. Rub both hands, wrists and forearms together vigorously, paying particular attention to the area around the fingernails. Continue rubbing until dry. Repeat this procedure once more.
(ii) For the disinfection of intact skin before surgery, injection or venepuncture: Apply a quantity of Manusept with a sterile swab. Rub vigorously until dry. Repeat this procedure once more.

Contra-indications, warnings, etc *Treatment of overdosage:* If swallowed, gastric aspiration and lavage avoiding pulmonary aspiration. Apomorphine should not be used.
Avoid contact with eyes. For external use only.

Pharmaceutical precautions Store at or below normal ambient temperatures. Do not use in the vicinity of naked flames.

Legal category GSL.

Package quantities 500 ml, 250 ml and 5 Litre.

Further information Triclosan is compatible with soap, which can be used to obtain physically clean hands.

Product licence number 0423/0008.

STER-ZAC* BATH CONCENTRATE

Presentation A clear solution containing 2% Triclosan.

Uses Ster-zac Bath Concentrate has an antibacterial effect in bath water.
For the prevention of cross-infection and secondary infection.

Dosage and administration *Baths:* Add 28.5 ml of Ster-zac Bath Concentrate to a bathful of water (approx. 140 litres) immediately prior to the patient entering the water.
For washing: Add 1 ml of Ster-zac Bath Concentrate to 5 litres of water prior to use.

Contra-indications, warnings, etc Avoid contact with the eyes. For external use only.

Pharmaceutical precautions For external use only. Store in a cool dry place.

Legal category P.

Package quantities 28.5 ml, 500 ml and 2 litres.

Further information Nil.

Product licence number 0423/5001.

STER-ZAC* DC SKIN CLEANSER

Presentation A white cream. Contains 3% Hexachlorophane BP.

Uses Ster-Zac DC has an antibacterial effect and is used for the pre-operative preparation of the hands.

Indications For the pre-operative disinfection of the hands of surgical personnel.

Dosage and administration For external use only. Apply 3 ml to 5 ml to pre-moistened hands and wash for up to three minutes. Rinse and repeat.

Contra-indications To be administered to children under two years of age on medical advice only. Do not use for whole body bathing. Do not apply to burns or badly damaged skin. For external use only.

Pharmaceutical precautions No special requirements.

Legal category POM.

Package quantities 150 ml 4.5 litres.

Further information Ster-Zac DC skin cleanser is resistant to contamination in use.

Product licence number 0423/0007.

STER-ZAC* POWDER

Presentation An antibacterial powder containing hexachlorophane in a sterilised powder base.

Hexachlorophane BPC	0.33%
Zinc Oxide BP	3.00%
Sterilised Purified Talc BPC	88.67%
Starch BP sterilised	8.00%

Uses For the prevention of neo-natal staphylococcal cross infection.
As an adjunct for the treatment of furunculosis.
For the routine treatment of cord stumps and for ward use in maternity hospitals and in domiciliary midwifery.

Dosage and administration For the prevention of

neo-natal staphylococcal cross infection – immediately after ligature, dust the cord and surrounding area and apply the powder to the perineum, buttocks and axillae. Repeat at each napkin change.

For the treatment of furunculosis – dust the affected area and surrounds regularly.

Contra-indications, warnings, etc This product is to be administered to children under two years of age on medical advice only. For external use only.

Pharmaceutical precautions No special requirements.

Legal category P.

Package quantities Sprinkler tins of 30 g and 225 g.

Further information Nil.

Product licence number 0423/5000.

TERPOIN*

Presentation A yellow, clear, syrupy, solution with a predominant menthol odour and taste. Each 5 ml contains:

Codeine Phosphate BP	15.0 mg
Guaiphenesin	50.0 mg
Terpin Hydrate BPC	9.15 mg
Eucalyptol BPC	4.15 mg
Menthol BP	18.3 mg

Uses Terpoin is an antitussive preparation designed specifically to control unproductive cough.

Indications Terpoin is indicated in the treatment of persistent cough. Chronic bronchitis.

Dosage and administration *Adults:* 5 to 10 ml in a little water (if necessary) every three hours.

Children: Up to 5 ml, according to age.

Contra-indications, warnings, etc Severe respiratory depression.

Treatment for overdosage: Empty the stomach by aspiration and lavage. Use a saline purgative such as sodium sulphate 30 g in 250 ml of water to aid peristalsis. If consciousness is impaired and respiration is depressed nalorphine hydrobromide may be given intravenously in doses of 5 to 10 mg, repeated in 15 minutes if necessary up to a total of 40 mg.

Pharmaceutical precautions No special requirements.

Legal category CD (Sch 5), POM.

Package quantities Plastic bottles of 225 ml and 2.25 litres.

Further information Nil.

Product licence number 0423/5005.

*Trade Mark

ICI Pharmaceuticals (UK)
Alderley House
Alderley Park
Macclesfield, Cheshire SK 10 4TF

ATROMID*-S

Presentation Atromid-S is presented as red, soft gelatine capsules, each containing 500 mg Clofibrate BP.

Uses

Atromid-S is indicated in the treatment of severe hyperlipoproteinaemia where full investigation has been performed to define the abnormality. It should be used in conjunction with appropriate dietary measures and after diet alone has failed to produce an adequate response. Other risk factors such as hypertension and smoking should be dealt with. Examples of abnormal lipid patterns are:

Frederickson type	Lipoprotein elevated	Major lipid elevations
1 (very rare)	Chylomicrons	Triglycerides
11a	β(LDL)	Cholesterol
11b	pre-β+β (LDL+VLDL)	Cholesterol + Triglycerides
111 (rare)	abnormal β(LDL)	Chol. + TG
IV	pre-β(VLDL)	Triglycerides
V (rare)	Chylomicrons + pre-β(VLDL)	Triglycerides + Cholesterol

Atromid-S is effective in patients with Type III hyperlipidaemia and in patients with severe hypertriglyceridaemia found in some patients in Types IIb, IV and V.

Dosage and administration A dose of 20–30 mg/kg body weight is given daily. This should be divided into 2 or 3 doses after meals. The effective dose level must be maintained. Examples of dosage:

Patients over 65 kg: 2 g daily (4 × 500 mg capsules).

Patients 50–65 kg: 1.5 g daily (3 × 500 mg capsules).

The biochemical response to clofibrate is variable, and it is not always possible to predict from the lipoprotein type or other factors which patients will obtain favourable results. It is essential that lipid levels be measured and that the drug be discontinued in any patient in whom lipids do not show significant improvement within three months of initiating therapy.

Elderly patients: There are no special dosage recommendations for the elderly, but it may be advisable to monitor elderly patients so that optimum dosage can be individually determined.

Contra-indications, warnings, etc Due to its action on cholesterol metabolism, Atromid-S may increase the lithogenicity of bile and there is an increased frequency of gall stones. Accordingly, clofibrate should not be used in patients with a history of, or existent gallbladder disease, or stones.

Also, it is contra-indicated in patients with impairment of renal or hepatic function (e.g. biliary cirrhosis).

In patients with low serum albumin levels, for example those with nephrotic syndrome, high levels of unbound drug may give rise to myalgia with raised serum creatinine kinase levels. Caution is advised in treating such patients.

Patients taking anticoagulants and Atromid-S together should have their dose of anticoagulant halved and adjusted later as necessary.

Atromid-S may also displace other acidic drugs such as phenytoin or tolbutamide and this possibility should be borne in mind when treating patients with either of these drugs and Atromid-S.

Clofibrate has been shown to produce liver tumours in rats and mice. The liver changes found in rodents have not been seen in other species, including sub-human primates and man. The relevance of this finding to man has not been established.

Pregnancy: It is considered advisable on theoretical grounds not to give Atromid-S during pregnancy.

Side-effects: Atromid-S has been in clinical use since 1963 and has been subjected to many long-term studies. Side-effects are seldom seen but include transient slight upper abdominal discomfort, nausea and looseness of the bowels and impotence. It is usually unnecessary to discontinue treatment. Very occasionally myalgia has been reported. Due to its action on bile there is an increased incidence of gallstones (see 'Contra-indications and warnings' above).

Liver function: At therapeutic doses Atromid-S does not enter the liver cell. In some cases slight and usually transient increases in serum transaminase levels have been observed. It is considered that these reflect adaptive responses of the liver. In large, long-term studies, even transient increases in transaminase levels have seldom been reported. Atromid-S has not been shown to affect serum bilirubin or bromosulphthalein tests. Serial liver biopsy studies in patients undergoing long-term treatment have confirmed the absence of hepatotoxicity in man.

Cardiovascular system: There has been a published report of venticular arrhythmia associated with Atromid-S treatment. However, the patient had an unstable rhythm prior to treatment.

Blood: Atromid-S normally has no effect on the blood picture. Isolated cases of adverse effects include slight fluctuation in haemoglobin values and occasional reduction in white cell counts. There is no evidence of marrow toxicity, but one case of agranulocytosis has been reported in a patient undergoing multiple drug therapy which included Atromid-S.

Overdosage: No adverse biochemical or clinical effects have been observed upon overdosage with Atromid-S, but should these occur, symptomatic treatment should be administered.

One case of a 15-year-old boy has been recorded who took 12.25 g of Atromid-S with no resulting adverse effects.

Pharmaceutical precautions Store at room temperature, protected from light and moisture.

Legal category POM.

Package quantities Containers of 50, 250 and 500 capsules.

Further information Nil.

Product licence number 0029/5022.

AVLOCLOR*

Presentation Avloclor is presented as white, bi-convex tablets, each with a bisecting line and bearing the ICI roundel. The tablets each contain 250 mg Chloroquine Phosphate BP, equivalent to 155 mg chloroquine base.

Uses Avloclor is an antimalarial agent highly active against the erythrocytic forms of Plasmodium falciparum, Plasmodium vivax and Plasmodium malariae. It also possesses amoebicidal properties and is useful in treating chronic discoid and systemic lupus erythematosus and rheumatoid arthritis.

It is indicated for treatment and suppression of malaria, and the treatment of amoebic hepatitis and abscess, lupus erythematosus and rheumatoid arthritis.

Dosage and administration
Treatment of malaria:
Children:

Age (years)	Initial dose	Second dose 6 hrs after first	Dose on each of the two subsequent days
1–4	1 tablet	½ tablet	½ tablet
4–8	2 tablets	1 tablet	1 tablet
8–12	3 tablets	1½ tablets	1½ tablets

Adults: A three-day course is sufficient to effect disappearance of symptoms and parasitaemia as follows: initial dose 4 Avloclor tablets, followed by 2 tablets six hours later, then 2 tablets a day for two days.

Overt attacks of Vivax and Quartan malaria are treated with a single dose consisting of 4 Avloclor tablets, followed by a course of treatment with Primaquine Phosphate BP (15 mg of base daily for 14 days).

Prophylaxis and suppression of malaria:
Children: A dose appropriate to the age group (see below) should be taken once a week, on the same day each week, during exposure to risk and continued for 6 weeks after leaving the malarious area.

1–4 years: ½ tablet.

4–8 years: 1 tablet.

8–12 years: 1½ tablets.

Children over 12 years are dosed as described for adults.

Adults: A dose of 2 Avloclor tablets should be taken once a week, on the same day each week, during exposure to risk and continued for 6 weeks after leaving the malarious area.

Amoebic hepatitis: The initial dose is 4 Avloclor tablets daily for two days followed by 1 tablet twice daily for two or three weeks.

lupus erythematosus: The initial dose is 1 tablet of Avloclor twice daily for one to two weeks followed by a maintenance dose of 1 tablet daily.

Rheumatoid arthritis: The usual dose is 1 tablet of Avloclor daily, at bedtime.

Elderly patients: There are no special dosage recommendations for the elderly, but it may be advisable to monitor elderly patients so that optimum dosage can be individually determined.

Contra-indications, warnings, etc Caution is necessary when giving Avloclor to patients with porphyria who also have hepatic dysfunction or cirrhosis as the drug may precipitate severe constitutional symptoms and an increase in the amount of porphyrins excreted in the urine. This reaction is especially apparent in alcoholics.

The most serious toxic hazard of prolonged therapy with high doses is the occasional development of irreversible retinal damage. For this reason considerable caution is needed in the use of Avloclor for long-term high dosage therapy and such use should only be considered when no other drug is available.

Patients receiving Avloclor continuously at higher dose levels for periods longer than 12 months should undergo ophthalmic examination at three monthly intervals. This also applies to patients receiving Avloclor at weekly intervals for a period of more than 3 years as a prophylactic against malarial attacks, or if the total consumption exceeds 1.6 g/kg.

Defects in visual accommodation may occur on first taking Avloclor and patients should be warned regarding driving or operating machinery.

Pregnancy: As with all drugs, the use of Avloclor during pregnancy should be avoided if possible, unless in the case of life threatening infections, in the judgement of the physician, potential benefit outweighs the risk. There is evidence to suggest that Avloclor given to women in high doses throughout pregnancy can give rise to foetal cochlear damage.

In any locality where drug resistant malaria is known or suspected, it is essential to take local medical advice on what prophylactic regimen is appropriate.

Side-effects: When used at the standard dosage regimes recommended for the control of malaria, Avloclor is well tolerated, and side-effects such as headache and gastro-intestinal disturbances which may occur are not of a serious nature. Where prolonged high dosage is required side-effects can be of greater severity and patients may develop skin eruptions, occasional depigmentation or loss of hair, difficulty in accommodation, blurring of vision, corneal opacities and less often, retinal degeneration. Corneal opacities disappear completely when the drug is stopped. Rarely thrombocytopenia, agranulocytosis and aplastic anaemia have been reported.

Overdosage: In the event of gross overdosage with Avloclor prompt measures will be required to counteract the depressant effect of the drug on the cardiovascular and respiratory systems. Vomiting should be induced or gastric lavage carried out as soon as possible, followed by appropriate resuscitative measures, such as tracheal intubation with artificial respiration and the administration of vasopressor agents or intravenous fluids. Intravenous molar sodium lactate solution 30–50 ml has been used to counteract the quinidine-like action of chloroquine on the myocardium. To promote excretion of the drug, the administration of enteric-coated ammonium chloride tablets 0.5 g every eight hours is also recommended.

Pharmaceutical precautions Store at room temperature. When in plastic containers, protect from light and moisture.

Legal category POM.
P. for prevention of malaria.

Package quantities Containers of 20 and 100 tablets.

Further information Nil.

Product licence number 0029/5053.

CETAVLON* SOLUTION 40%
(Strong Cetrimide Solution BP)

Presentation A colourless to pale straw coloured aqueous solution containing 40% w/v cetrimide.

Uses Cetavlon is a potent antimicrobial agent with useful detergent properties. It is used in wound and burn therapy, skin disinfection, removing ointment, scabs, crusts, etc, in skin diseases, and seborrhoeic dermatitis.

Dosage and administration Dilute and use as follows:

Wound and burn therapy: A 0.1% aqueous solution of Cetavlon is used. In cases involving contamination with dirt or grease a 0.5–1.0% solution may be used.

Such solutions should be sterilised by autoclaving at 115–116°C for 30 minutes or 121–123°C for 15 minutes.

Skin disinfection: A rapid and prolonged disinfection of the skin is produced by swabbing with Cetavlon 0.5% solution in 70% alcohol.

Skin diseases: A 1% aqueous solution of Cetavlon may be used to clean the skin of scabs, crusts, etc, and remove ointments.

Dandruff: In the treatment of seborrhoea of the scalp, Cetavlon is used at strengths of 1–3% in water, the solution being applied to the wet hair to form a lather which is finally removed by rinsing with clean water.

Contra-indications, warnings, etc
Contra-indications: Cetavlon is contra-indicated for patients who have previously shown a hypersensitivity reaction to cetrimide preparations.

Precautions: For external use only. Dilute before use. Keep out of the eyes and avoid contact with the brain, meninges or middle ear. Do not use in body cavities or as an enema.

Solutions applied to wounds, burns or broken skin must be sterilised in accordance with BPC recommendations.

Side-effects: Irritative skin reactions can occasionally occur and rare hypersensitivity to cetrimide preparations usually developing after repeated application, has been reported. There have also been rare reports of severe burn-like reactions to concentrated cetrimide solutions. Should such a reaction occur treat as a chemical burn. In all cases stop application of the product.

Accidental oral or rectal administration: Fatal poisoning may arise even when the only pathological signs are visceral congestion, cloudy swelling, mild pulmonary oedema or varying degrees of gastro-intestinal irritation. Severe CNS depression, sometimes preceded by excitement and convulsions, can cause death from respiratory paralysis.

Specific antidotes: Soap, anionic surfactants.

General measures: Do not give alcohol in any form. If the product is swallowed give large quantities of milk, egg-white, gelatin or mild soap. Avoid vomiting or lavage if it is believed that a concentrated solution has been ingested.

Central paralysis cannot be countered by curare antagonists or CNS stimulants but sympathomimetic drugs have been given.

Mechanically assisted ventilation with oxygen may be necessary. Persistent convulsions may be controlled with cautious doses of a short-acting barbiturate.

Accidental intravenous transfusion: Massive haemolysis can occur which will require blood transfusion.

Intra-uterine administration: Introduction into the uterus can lead to haemolysis and pulmonary embolism.

Pharmaceutical precautions Dilute with freshly distilled water or alcohol (ethanol, Industrial Methylated Spirit or isopropanol). Add diluent slowly to prevent excessive foaming.

As a precaution against bacterial contamination, aqueous stock solutions should contain at least 4% v/v of isopropanol or 7% v/v of ethanol which may be denatured (i.e. Industrial Methylated Spirit).

As cork may protect certain Gram-negative organisms from the action of antiseptics, Cetavlon solutions must be stored in glass-, plastic-, or rubber-stoppered bottles.

Incompatible with anionic agents.

Store at room temperature. Cetavlon Solution 40% must be stored in the manufacturer's original container, or in glass or plastic containers which comply with British Standard No 1679. The container should be kept tightly closed.

Legal category P.

Package quantities Cetavlon Solution 40% – bottles of 1 litre and 5 litres.

Further information Nil.

Product licence number 0029/0169.

CORSODYL* DENTAL GEL

Presentation A clear red gel containing 1% w/w chlorhexidine gluconate (equivalent to 5% v/w Chlorhexidine Gluconate Solution BP).

Uses Corsodyl Gel inhibits the formation of dental plaque. It is indicated as an aid in the treatment and prevention of gingivitis and in the maintenance of oral hygiene.

Dosage and administration Brush the teeth thoroughly with 1 inch of gel on a moistened toothbrush, once or twice daily for about one minute. For the treatment of gingivitis, a course of about one month is advisable.

Corsodyl is incompatible with anionic agents which are usually present in conventional dentifrices. These should therefore be used before Corsodyl (rinsing the mouth *and* toothbrush between applications) or at a different time of day.

Contra-indications, warnings, etc
Contra-indications: Corsodyl is contra-indicated for patients who have previously shown a hypersensitivity reaction to chlorhexidine. However, such reactions are extremely rare.

Precautions: For oral use only, keep out of the eyes.

Side-effects: Irritative skin reactions to chlorhexidine preparations can occasionally occur. Generalised allergic reactions to chlorhexidine have also been reported but are extremely rare.

A superficial discolouration of the tongue may occur, this disappears after treatment is discontinued. Discolouration of the teeth and silicate or composite restorations may also occur. This stain is not permanent and can largely be prevented by brushing with a conventional toothpaste daily before using the gel. However, in certain cases, a dental prophylaxis may be necessary to remove this stain completely.

Transient disturbances of taste sensation and a burning sensation of the tongue may occur on initial use. These usually diminish with continued use.

Overdosage: This has not been reported.

Accidental ingestion: Chlorhexidine taken orally is poorly absorbed. Systemic effects are unlikely even if large amounts are ingested. However, gastric lavage may be advisable using milk, egg-white, gelatin or mild soap. Employ supportive measures as appropriate.

Hypochlorite bleaches may cause brown stains to develop in fabrics which have previously been in contact with chlorhexidine preparations. Detailed literature is available on request.

Pharmaceutical precautions Store at room temperature.

Legal category P.

Package quantities Tubes of 50 g.

Further information Corsodyl Dental Gel has an antiplaque action. The effect on gingivitis is maximal after removal of subgingival deposits by scaling.

Product licence number 0029/0080.

CORSODYL* MOUTHWASH

Presentation A clear pink solution containing 0.2% w/v chlorhexidine gluconate (equivalent to 1% v/v Chlorhexidine Gluconate Solution BP).

Uses Corsodyl Mouthwash is an antibacterial solution which inhibits the formation of dental plaque. It is indicated as an aid in the treatment and prevention of gingivitis, and in the maintenance of oral hygiene, particularly in situations where toothbrushing cannot be adequately employed (e.g. following oral surgery or in physically-handicapped patients). It may also be used in a post-periodontal surgery regime to promote gingival healing. It is of value in the management of aphthous ulceration and oral candidal infections, (e.g. denture stomatitis and thrush).

Dosage and administration Thoroughly rinse the mouth for about one minute with 10 ml twice daily.

Corsodyl is incompatible with anionic agents which are usually present in conventional dentifrices. These should therefore be used before Corsodyl (rinsing the mouth between applications) or at a different time of day.

For the treatment of gingivitis, a course of about a month is advisable although some variation in response is to be expected. In the case of aphthous ulceration and oral candidal infections, treatment should be continued for 48 hours after clinical resolution. For the treatment of denture stomatitis the dentures should be cleansed and soaked in the solution for 15 minutes twice daily.

Contra-indications, warnings, etc

Contra-indications: Corsodyl is contra-indicated for patients who have previously shown a hypersensitivity reaction to chlorhexidine. However, such reactions are extremely rare.

Precautions: For oral use only, keep out of the eyes.

Side-effects: Irritative skin reactions to chlorhexidine preparations can occasionally occur. Generalised allergic reactions to chlorhexidine have also been reported but are extremely rare.

A superficial discolouration of the dorsum of the tongue may occur, this disappears after treatment is discontinued. Discolouration of the teeth and silicate or composite restorations may also occur. This stain is not permanent and can largely be prevented by brushing with a conventional toothpaste daily before using the mouthwash, or in the case of dentures, cleaning with a conventional denture cleanser. However, in certain cases, a dental prophylaxis may be required to remove this stain completely. Similarly where normal toothbrushing is not possible, as for example with intermaxillary fixation, or with extensive orthodontic appliances, a dental prophylaxis may be required once the underlying condition has resolved.

Transient disturbances of taste sensation and a burning sensation of the tongue may occur on initial use of the mouthwash. These effects usually diminish with continued use.

In cases where oral desquamation occurs, dilution of the mouthwash (5 ml mouthwash with 5 ml tap water freshly mixed) and instructions to rinse less vigorously will often allow continued use of the mouthwash.

Very occasionally, swelling of the parotid glands during use of chlorhexidine mouthwash has been reported. In all cases spontaneous resolution has occurred on discontinuing treatment.

Overdosage: This has not been reported.

Accidental ingestion: Chlorhexidine taken orally is poorly absorbed. Systemic effects are unlikely even if large volumes are ingested. However, gastric lavage may be advisable using milk, egg-white, gelatin or mild soap. Employ supportive measures as appropriate.

Pharmaceutical precautions Hypochlorite bleaches may cause brown stains to develop in fabrics which have previously been in contact with chlorhexidine solutions. Detailed literature is available on request.

Store at room temperature.

Legal category P.

Package quantities 250 ml bottle.

Further information Nil.

Product licence number 0029/0124,

DIPRIVAN* ▼

Presentation White, aqueous and isotonic emulsion for intravenous injection containing 10 mg propofol per 1 ml. The vehicle contains soybean oil and purified egg phosphatide.

Uses Diprivan is a short-acting intravenous anaesthetic agent suitable for induction and maintenance of general anaesthesia for surgical procedures which generally do not exceed one hour in duration.

Dosage and administration In unpremedicated and in premedicated patients, it is recommended that Diprivan should be titrated (approximately 4 ml every 10 seconds in an average healthy adult) against the response of the patient until the clinical signs show the onset of anaesthesia. Most adult patients aged less than 55 years are likely to require 2.0 to 2.5 mg/kg of Diprivan. Over this age, the requirement will generally be less. In patients of ASA Grades 3 and 4, lower rates of administration should be used (approximately 2 ml every 10 seconds).

Anaesthesia can be maintained by administering Diprivan to prevent the clinical signs of light anaesthesia. The average rate of administration varies considerably between patients but rates in the region of 0.1 to 0.2 mg/kg/min (6 to 12 mg/kg/hr) usually maintain satisfactory anaesthesia. When Diprivan is given by continuous infusion, slightly higher rates of administration may be required for 10 to 20 minutes after induction of anaesthesia. Alternatively, if a technique involving repeat bolus injections is used, increments of 25 mg (2.5 ml) to 50 mg (5.0 ml) may be given. Experience in procedures lasting more than one hour is limited. Supplementary analgesic agents are generally required in addition to Diprivan.

Diprivan has been used in association with spinal and epidural anaesthesia and with commonly used premedicants, neuromuscular blocking drugs, inhalational agents and analgesic agents; no pharmacological incompatibility has been encountered.

This formulation should not be mixed prior to administration with other therapeutic agents or infusion fluids. Diprivan may be administered via a Y-piece close to the injection site, into infusions of Dextrose 5% (Intravenous Infusion BP), Sodium Chloride 0.9% (Intravenous Infusion BP), or Dextrose 4% with Sodium Chloride 0.18% (Intravenous Infusion BP).

Elderly patients: Diprivan should be titrated against the response of the patient. Patients over the age of about 55 years may require lower doses of Diprivan for induction of anaesthesia (approximately 20% less).

Paediatric usage: At this stage, there is no experience of Diprivan in children.

Contra-indications, warnings, etc
Contra-indications: There are no absolute contra-indications to the use of Diprivan.

Precautions: During induction of anaesthesia, mild hypotension and transient apnoea, similar to effects with other intravenous anaesthetic agents, may occur depending on the dose and use of premedicants and other agents. Diprivan should be given by those trained in anaesthesia and facilities for maintenance of a patent airway, artificial ventilation, and oxygen enrichment should be available.

As with other intravenous anaesthetic agents, caution should be applied in patients with cardiac, respiratory, renal or hepatic impairment or in hypovolaemic or debilitated patients. Appropriate care should be applied in patients with disorders of fat metabolism and in other conditions where lipid emulsions must be used cautiously.

Pregnancy: On general principles, Diprivan should not be used in pregnancy. Diprivan has been used, however, during termination of pregnancy.

Side effects: General. Side effects during induction,

maintenance and recovery occur uncommonly, although bradycardia responsive to atropine has been reported. Induction is generally smooth with minimal evidence of excitation. During the recovery phase nausea, vomiting and headache occur in only a small proportion of patients.

Local. The local pain which may occur during intravenous injection of Diprivan can be minimised when the larger veins of the forearm and antecubital fossa are used. Venous sequelae are rare. Accidental clinical extravasation and animal studies showed minimal tissue reaction. Intra-arterial injection in animals did not induce local tissue effects.

Overdosage: Accidental overdosage is likely to cause cardiorespiratory depression. Respiratory depression should be treated by artificial ventilation with oxygen. Cardiovascular depression would require lowering of the patient's head and, if severe, use of plasma expanders and pressor agents.

Pharmaceutical precautions
Storage precautions: The emulsion should be stored at room temperature; it must not be frozen.

In-use precautions: Each ampoule should be shaken before use.

Any portion of the contents remaining after use should be discarded.

The emulsion should not be mixed prior to administration with other therapeutic agents or infusion fluids.

Legal category POM.

Package quantities Ampoules of 20 ml in boxes of 5.

Further information Diprivan is distributed rapidly with a half-life between 1.8 and 8.3 minutes. Diprivan is metabolised by conjugation in the liver (half-life between 34 and 64 minutes) and this facilitates control of anaesthetic depth during maintenance as well as promoting rapid, clear-headed recovery. Inactive metabolites are excreted by the kidney. Under the usual maintenance regimens, significant accumulation of propofol does not occur.

In vitro studies have shown that Diprivan, at the concentrations likely to occur clinically, does not inhibit the synthesis of adrenocortical hormones.

Product licence number 0029/0190.

EPODYL*

Presentation Epodyl, a tumour inhibitor of the bis-epoxide group, is a clear, colourless, slightly viscous liquid presented in ampoules of 1 ml (containing 1.13 gramme ethoglucid). It is miscible in all proportions with water, giving neutral solutions.

Uses For intracavitary instillation in multiple papillomatosis of the bladder – diluted to a 1 or 2% solution.

Dosage and administration *Note:* (i) Epodyl must be diluted before administration and only fresh, aseptically prepared solutions should be used.

(ii) Glass irrigation syringes are preferred for the administration of Epodyl because some plastic materials interact with ethoglucid even in aqueous dilution. However, polypropylene and PVC irrigation sets which do not contain latex rubber components may also be used with the diluted solution.

(iii) See Pharmaceutical Precautions section for

guidelines on the safe handling and disposal of Epodyl solutions.

Intracavitary instillation in the treatment of bladder tumours: A freshly prepared 1–2% v/v solution of Epodyl in sterile water or physiological saline should be instilled into the bladder and retained there for as long as possible.

Treatment may be repeated daily for two weeks and then at less frequent intervals.

Elderly patients: There are no special dosage recommendations for the elderly.

Contra-indications, warnings, etc Epodyl must not be administered undiluted.

Pregnancy: This product should not normally be administered to patients who are pregnant, or to mothers who are breast-feeding.

Side-effects: Intracavitary administration into the bladder has produced no severe haematological changes although a fall in leucoyte count has been noted in a few patients. Local side-effects from bladder administration are dysuria and frequency. Chemical cystitis and mucosal changes have also been observed.

Overdosage: There is no specific antidote and treatment is symptomatic.

Pharmaceutical precautions The ampoule should be opened and the dilution prepared under aseptic conditions immediately before use. Water for Injection PhEur and Sodium Chloride Injection BP are suitable diluents.

Plastic disposable syringes may not be suitable for use with Epodyl and only glass syringes are recommended to be used.

The ampoules should be stored at room temperature.

Some plastic materials interact with ethoglucid and therefore glass syringes are recommended for the preparation of Epodyl solutions.

Epodyl solutions may be stored for up to twenty-four hours at room temperature in glass, PVC or polypropylene containers which do not have latex rubber components.

When preparing or disposing of Epodyl solutions, the following should be considered:

1. Trained personnel should prepare Epodyl solutions.
2. This should be performed in a designated area.
3. Adequate protective gloves should be worn.
4. The work surface should be covered with disposable plastic-backed absorbent paper.
5. Use Luer-lock fittings on all syringes and sets. Large bore needles are recommended to minimise pressure and the possible formation of aerosols. The latter may also be reduced by the use of a venting needle.
6. Precautions should be taken to avoid Epodyl accidentally coming into contact with the eyes. In case of contact with eyes, irrigate with copious amounts of water and seek medical advice.
7. Epodyl should not be handled by pregnant staff.
8. Adequate care and precautions should be taken in the disposal of items (syringes, needles, etc) used to prepare Epodyl solutions.
9. If Epodyl comes into contact with the skin or mucous membranes it must be washed off immediately with water.
10. Diluted solutions of Epodyl may be rendered harmless by adding one volume of concentrated hydrochloric acid to three volumes of Epodyl solution with stirring in a fume cupboard. After allowing to stand for 30 minutes, the solution should be neutralised with 10% sodium hydroxide and washed down a sink or drain.

11. Undiluted Epodyl may be disposed of by adding an equal volume of 10% hydrochloric acid with stirring in a fume cupboard. The mixture should then be neutralised as described above (Wilson, S.J., *J. Clin. Hosp. Pharm.* 1983 **8** 295–299).

Legal category POM.

Package quantities 1 ml ampoules in boxes of five.

Further information Following repeated intracavity use in multiple papillomatosis of the bladder, a partial or complete response may be expected in over 80% of patients without the risk of systemic side-effects (*British Journal of Urology* (1971) **43**, 181–4).

Product licence number 0029/5010.

ERALDIN* INJECTION

Presentation Eraldin is presented as an injectable solution in 5 ml ampoules which each contain 10 mg of Practolol BP in 5 ml of a buffered aqueous solution.

Uses Eraldin is a beta-adrenoceptor blocking drug which is cardioselective. However, treatment with practolol is now known to produce serious adverse effects (the practolol oculomucocutaneous syndrome) in some patients. This syndrome has arisen only on oral treatment (after a mean duration of treatment of approximately 24 months) and oral dosage forms have been withdrawn. It has not been reported after short-term intravenous therapy.

Eraldin Injection remains available for emergency use and should only be used for the control of cardiac dysrhythmias caused or maintained by excessive sympathetic activity in association with organic disease, particularly post-infarction dysrhythmias, and during anaesthesia, where clinical benefit cannot be obtained with alternative forms of treatment. A most careful assessment of the necessity for treatment with Eraldin should be made before treatment is undertaken.

This preparation is available solely for emergency use in life threatening situations and Eraldin Injection should not be considered for other use. Fuller information on the serious adverse effects associated with practolol may be obtained from the manufacturers.

Dosage and administration *Cardiac dysrhythmias: Intravenous:* 5 mg (2.5 ml, i.e. half an ampoule) is given slowly, and if no response occurs may be repeated. Doses of more than 20 mg (10 ml) are not normally required.

Elderly patients: A reduction in dosage may be required, especially in patients with impaired renal function.

Contra-indications, warnings, etc *Contra-indications:* 1. Eraldin should not be used in the presence of second or third degree heart block.
2. Eraldin is contra-indicated in the presence of metabolic acidosis.

Precautions: Eraldin need not necessarily be withheld from patients with signs of heart failure. For such patients, however, myocardial contractility must be maintained and signs of failure controlled with digitalis and diuretics.

One of the pharmacological actions of beta-adrenoceptor blocking drugs is to reduce heart rate. In the rare instance when symptoms may be attributable to the slow heart rate, the dose may be reduced.

Eraldin modifies the tachycardia of hypoglycaemia.

Eraldin may be used with caution in patients with chronic obstructive airways disease. However, occasionally some increase in airways resistance may occur in asthmatic patients.

Care should be taken in prescribing a beta-adrenoceptor blocking drug with Class 1 antidysrhythmic agents such as disopyramide.

Beta-adrenoceptor blocking agents should be used with caution in combination with verapamil in patients with impaired ventricular function. The combination should not be given to patients with conduction abnormalities. Neither drug should be administered intravenously within 48 hours of discontinuing the other.

Caution should be exercised when transferring patients from clonidine to beta-adrenoceptor blocking drugs. If beta-adrenoceptor blocking drugs and clonidine are given concurrently, clonidine should not be discontinued until several days after withdrawal of the beta-adrenoceptor blocking drug (see also prescribing information on clonidine).

Anaesthesia: Eraldin is compatible with light anaesthesia using Fluothane* (halothane). Ether, chloroform, cyclopropane and possibly trichloroethylene depend for their safety on increased circulating levels of endogenous catecholamines and it is probable that they are therapeutically incompatible with beta-adrenoceptor blocking drugs. Vagal dominance, if it occurs, may be countered with atropine (1–2 mg intravenously).

Pregnancy: As with all other drugs, Eraldin should not be given in pregnancy unless its use is essential. There is no evidence of teratogenicity with Eraldin.

Side-effects: Apart from the severe practolol oculomucocutaneous syndrome (see above), there have been occasional reports of nausea, sleep disturbance, paraesthesia and also of constipation.

In the rare event of intolerance manifested as bradycardia and hypotension, the drug should be withdrawn and if necessary, treatment for overdosage instituted.

Overdosage: Excessive bradycardia can be countered with atropine 1–2 mg intravenously, followed, if necessary, by a beta-adrenoceptor stimulant such as isoprenaline 25 micrograms initially, or orciprenaline 0.5 mg, given by slow intravenous injection. Care must be taken to ensure that the blood pressure does not fall too low if the dose of the beta-adrenoceptor agonist has to be increased. Glucagon has been reported to be useful as a cardiac stimulant in a dose of 10 mg intravenously.

Pharmaceutical precautions Store at room temperature, protected from light.

Legal category POM.

Sale and supply restricted to hospitals, clinics and nursing homes.

Package quantities The ampoules (10 mg in 5 ml) are packed in boxes of 10.

Further information The physical compatibility of Eraldin injection with the following intravenous infusion solutions has been investigated over a period of 48 hours immediately following addition of the drug solution to the respective infusion bag. In each case 6 mg Eraldin was added to 100 ml infusion fluid.

0.9% sodium chloride and 5% dextrose
0.3% potassium chloride and 0.9% sodium chloride
0.3% potassium chloride and 5% dextrose

No signs of incompatibility were seen. As these tests were done over 48 hours and long-term stability has not been investigated, it is recommended that mixtures of Eraldin with intravenous fluids should be used within 24 hours of preparation.

Product licence number 0029/5056.

EXELDERM* CREAM

Presentation Exelderm is a white to off-white cream containing 1% w/w sulconazole nitrate.

Uses Exelderm Cream is designed for topical application and contains an imidazole antimycotic with a broad spectrum of activity against the causative organisms of tinea pedis, tinea corporis and tinea cruris, pityriasis versicolor and candidiasis.

Dosage and administration Exelderm Cream should be gently massaged into the affected and surrounding skin areas twice daily (morning and evening). For less severe cases once daily administration may be sufficient.

Often clinical improvement with relief of symptoms occurs within one week. However, treatment should be continued for 2 to 3 weeks after clinical cure to prevent relapse.

Contra-indications, warnings, etc Exelderm is contra-indicated in patients with hypersensitivity to the formulated product or imidazoles.

Precautions: The treatment should be discontinued if a reaction suggesting sensitivity or irritation occurs. If the patient shows no clinical improvement after 4 weeks of treatment the diagnosis should be reviewed. Avoid the introduction of Exelderm into the eyes. Lens changes were seen in one animal species following very high repeated oral doses.

Pregnancy: Reproductive toxicology studies produced no evidence of teratogenicity in laboratory animals, although some more general toxicological effects were seen in the dams and foetuses in these studies. Therefore this product should not be used in pregnancy unless considered essential to the welfare of the patient.

Side-effects: Occasional itching, burning, erythema, stinging and blistering have been reported.

Accidental ingestion: The 30 g tube of Exelderm contains 300 mg of sulconazole nitrate. Toxic effects are very unlikely even if the full contents are ingested but if they occur symptomatic treatment should be given.

Pharmaceutical precautions Store at room temperature.

Legal category POM.

Package quantities Exelderm Cream is supplied in 30 g tubes.

Further information Nil.

Product licence number 0029/0185.

FLUOTHANE*

Presentation Fluothane is a colourless, volatile liquid, non-explosive and non-flammable in the concentrations usually used. Chemically it is 2-bromo-2-chloro-1,1,1-trifluoroethane stabilised with thymol 0.01% w/w (Halothane PhEur).

Uses Fluothane is a volatile anaesthetic which is

suitable for the induction and maintenance of anaesthesia for all types of surgery and in patients of all ages.

Dosage and administration A number of anaesthetic vaporisers specially designed for use with Fluothane are available. Open, semi-open, semi-closed and closed circuit systems have all been used with good results.

For induction of anaesthesia in the adult patient a concentration of 2–4% Fluothane in oxygen or oxygen/nitrous oxide may be used. In children a concentration of 1.5–2% Fluothane in oxygen or oxygen/nitrous oxide is used. A concentration of 0.5–2% is usually adequate for maintenance of anaesthesia in both adults and children. The lower concentration is usually most suitable for elderly patients.

Contra-indications, warnings, etc As Fluothane causes relaxation of the uterine muscle it is advisable that anaesthesia should be maintained in the lightest plane possible during obstetric operations.

The use of moderate hyperventilation during neurosurgery is recommended to counteract the rise in cerebrospinal fluid pressure which may occur with Fluothane.

Caution should be exercised during the administration of adrenaline to patients anaesthetised with Fluothane as dysrhythmias may be precipitated. For this reason the dose of adrenaline should be restricted and beta-receptor antagonists administered if necessary.

The role of Fluothane in the liver damage occasionally observed after anaesthesia has not been definitely established. However, as such cases appear more frequently after repeated anaesthetic administration, the appearance of unexplained jaundice following exposure to Fluothane should be regarded as a contra-indication to its later use. It has been suggested that repeated exposure to any anaesthetic within a period of four weeks should be avoided where possible, and as with all anaesthetics, consideration should be given to the frequency of usage.

Malignant hyperpyrexia has been reported in some patients receiving Fluothane. This syndrome occurs with other anaesthetic agents, and may respond to intravenous dantrolene sodium.

It is advisable to ensure adequate room ventilation when Fluothane is being used.

During the induction of Fluothane anaesthesia a moderate fall in blood pressure commonly occurs. The pressure tends to rise when the vapour concentration is reduced to maintenance levels, but it usually remains steady below the pre-operative level. This hypotensive effect is useful in providing a clear operating field and a reduction in haemorrhage. However, if necessary, intravenous doses of methoxamine (5 mg are usually adequate) can be given to counteract the fall in blood pressure.

Cardiac arrhythmias have been reported during anaesthesia.

Fluothane augments the action of non-depolarising muscle relaxants.

Pregnancy: Although the data from experimental investigations in animals cannot be directly related to man, it would be prudent to avoid general anaesthesia with inhalation agents during early pregnancy, except where such use is essential.

Accidental ingestion: Cases of ingestion must be treated symptomatically.

Pharmaceutical precautions Bottles of Fluothane

must be securely closed and stored at room temperature, protected from light. Fluothane must be kept in the original container until immediately prior to its use.

Whilst in the liquid phase, Fluothane must not be diluted or contaminated; however, in the vapour phase it may be administered together with oxygen or a mixture of nitrous oxide and oxygen.

Legal category P.

Package quantities Fluothane is supplied in bottles of 250 ml.

Further information Nil.

Product licence number 0029/5058.

FULCIN* 500 TABLETS
FULCIN* 125 TABLETS
FULCIN* ORAL SUSPENSION

Presentation Fulcin is griseofulvin in a fine-particle form designed to give optimal absorption when taken orally.

Fulcin 500 is presented as white, film-coated, bi-convex tablets, one side plain, the obverse marked with the ICI roundel. Each contains 500 mg Griseofulvin Ph. Eur. Fulcin 125 Tablets are white, bi-convex, one side bisected, the obverse marked with the ICI roundel. Each contains 125 mg Griseofulvin PhEur.

Fulcin Oral Suspension is a brown aqueous suspension which contains 2.5% w/v Griseofulvin PhEur.

Uses Fulcin is an antifungal agent which when taken orally is active against a number of dermatophytes including: *M. audouinii, M. canis, M. distortum, M. ferrugineum, M. fulvum, M. gypseum, E. floccosum, T. equinum, T. mentagrophytes, T. rubrum, T. schoenleinii, T. soudanense, T. tonsurans, T. verrucosum, T. violaceum.*

Fulcin is indicated in fungal infections of the skin, hair and nails when topical therapy has failed or is considered inappropriate. These may be known as: Tinea capitis, Tinea corporis, Tinea cruris, Tinea pedis, Tinea unguium, Tinea imbricata, Tinea barbae, Favus.

Dosage and administration The adult dosage is normally 500 mg daily, but in severe conditions up to twice this amount may be given, reducing to the lower level when a clinical response has occurred. The normal dosage may be given as one 125 mg tablet or 5 ml of suspension four times a day, or as one 500 mg tablet once daily after food.

For children the most suitable form is the pleasantly flavoured Fulcin Oral Suspension. The daily dosage is 10 mg griseofulvin per kg body weight daily, i.e. 5 ml of suspension for every 12.5 kg in single or divided doses. If dilution is required Syrup BP is suitable.

Elderly patients: There are no special dosage recommendations for the elderly, but it may be advisable to monitor elderly patients so that optimum dosage can be individually determined.

The duration of treatment depends on the type of infection and the time required for normal replacement of infected tissues.

For complete eradication of the infection, Fulcin treatment should be combined with general measures of care and hygiene. Reservoirs of infection may include clothing, footwear and bedding as well as the patient's hair.

Contra-indications, warnings, etc Fulcin should

not be administered to patients who have established porphyria or hepatocellular failure or to patients with systemic lupus erythematosus. Fulcin should not be used for prophylaxis.

Fulcin may decrease the response to coumarin anticoagulants administered concomitantly and both barbiturates and anticoagulants may reduce the effectiveness of Fulcin therapy.

Breakthrough bleeding, amenorrhoea and failure of contraceptive therapy have been reported in patients taking griseofulvin and oral contraceptive steroids.

In those rare cases when individuals are affected by drowsiness whilst taking Fulcin, they should not drive a vehicle, nor operate machinery and should also avoid alcoholic drink.

Pregnancy: Griseofulvin administered to rats during pregnancy has been associated with foetotoxicity and tail deformities at high dosages. There is no evidence of its safety with use in human pregnancy and therefore griseofulvin should not be used in pregnancy.

Long-term administration of high doses of griseofulvin with food has been reported to induce hepatomas in mice and thyroid tumours in rats but not in hamsters. The clinical significance of this finding for man is not known.

Side-effects: Fulcin is generally well tolerated. Urticarial reactions and erythematous rashes have been noted in a few cases. There have been occasional complaints of thirst, headache and gastric discomfort which, in most cases, have regressed during treatment. Photosensitivity associated with griseofulvin therapy has been recorded and there have been rare reports of aggravation or precipitation of systemic lupus erythematosus.

Overdosage: Treatment of overdosage should be symptomatic.

Pharmaceutical precautions Store at room temperature, protected from light.

Legal category POM.

Package quantities *Fulcin 500 tablets:* Containers of 25, 100 and 250 tablets.
Fulcin 125 Tablets: Containers of 100 and 1,000 tablets.
Fulcin Oral Suspension: Bottles of 100 ml.

Further information A suitable diluent for Fulcin Oral Suspension is Syrup BP.

Product licence numbers
Fulcin 500 Tablets   0029/5061
Fulcin 125 Tablets   0029/5060
Fulcin Oral Suspension   0029/5059

HIBIDIL*

Presentation A pink aqueous solution containing 0.05% w/v chlorhexidine gluconate (equivalent to 0.25% Chlorhexidine Gluconate Solution BP). A ready-to-use solution in sachets and bottles sterilised by autoclaving.

Uses Hibidil is a potent antibacterial agent active against a wide range of organisms. It is recommended for swabbing wounds and burns and in obstetrics.

Dosage and administration Apply to treatment area without further dilution.

Contra-indications, warnings, etc
Contra-indications: Hibidil is contra-indicated for patients who have previously shown a hypersensitivity

reaction to chlorhexidine. However, such reactions are extremely rare.

Precautions: For external use only. Keep out of the eyes and avoid contact with brain, meninges or middle ear. Do not inject. Do not use in body cavities.

Side-effects: Irritative skin reactions can occasionally occur. Generalised allergic reactions to chlorhexidine have also been reported but are extremely rare.

Accidental ingestion. Chlorhexidine taken orally is poorly absorbed. Treat with a gastric lavage using milk, egg white, gelatin or mild soap. Employ supportive measures as appropriate.

Accidental intravenous transfusion: Blood transfusion may be necessary to counteract haemolysis.

Pharmaceutical precautions Store at room temperature.

Use contents immediately after opening – do not keep any surplus solution. Hypochlorite bleaches may cause brown stains to develop in fabrics which have previously been in contact with chlorhexidine solutions. Detailed literature is available on request.

Hibidil is incompatible with anionic agents.

Legal category P.

Package quantities Packs of 250 × 25 ml and 60 × 100 ml individual sachets. Bottles of 500 ml and 1,000 ml.

Further information The British Pharmaceutical Codex (1973) recommends that antiseptics applied to broken skin should be sterile. The use of Hibidil complies with this recommendation.

Product licence number 0029/0143.

HIBISCRUB*

Presentation A red detergent solution containing 4% w/v chlorhexidine gluconate (equivalent to 20% v/v Chlorhexidine Gluconate Solution BP).

Uses Hibiscrub is a potent antiseptic skin-cleansing solution for pre-operative surgical hand disinfection, antiseptic handwashing on the ward and pre-operative skin preparation for patients undergoing elective surgery.

Dosage and administration *Pre-operative surgical hand preparation:* Wet the hands and forearms, apply 5 ml of Hibiscrub and wash for one minute cleaning the fingernails with a brush or scraper. Rinse, apply a further 5 ml of Hibiscrub and continue washing for a further two minutes. Rinse thoroughly and dry.

Antiseptic handwash on the ward: Wet the hands and forearms, apply 5 ml of Hibiscrub and wash for one minute. Rinse thoroughly and dry.

Pre-operative skin preparation for the patient: The patient washes his whole body in the bath or shower on at least two occasions, usually the day before and the day of operation as follows:

The day before the operation, the patient washes with 25 ml of Hibiscrub beginning with the face and working downwards paying particular attention to areas around the nose, axillae umbilicus, groin and perineum. The body is then rinsed and the wash repeated with a further 25 ml, this time including the hair. Finally the patient rinses his entire body thoroughly and dries on a clean towel. This procedure should be repeated the following day. Bedridden patients can be washed with Hibiscrub using a standard bed-bath technique.

Conventional disinfection of the operation site will then be performed when the patient is in theatre.

Contra-indications, warnings, etc
Contra-indications: Hibiscrub is contra-indicated for persons who have previously shown a hypersensitivity reaction to chlorhexidine. However, such reactions are extremely rare.

Precautions: For external use only. Keep out of the eyes and avoid contact with brain, meninges or middle ear. In patients with head or spinal injuries or perforated ear drum, the benefit of use in pre-operative preparation should be evaluated against the risk of contact.

Side-effects: Irritative skin reactions can occasionally occur. Generalised allergic reactions to chlorhexidine have also been reported but are extremely rare.

Accidental ingestion: Chlorhexidine taken orally is poorly absorbed. Treat with gastric lavage using milk, egg-white, gelatin or mild soap. Employ supportive measures as appropriate.

Pharmaceutical precautions Store at room temperature protected from light.

Hypochlorite bleaches may cause brown stains to develop in fabrics which have previously been in contact with chlorhexidine preparations. Detailed literature is available on request.

Hibiscrub is incompatible with anionic agents.

Legal category GSL.

Package quantities Containers of 100 ml, 250 ml, 500 ml, 5 litres. Elbow operated dispensers are available.

Further information Nil.

Product licence number 0029/0127.

HIBISOL*

Presentation A blue alcoholic solution containing 0.5% w/v chlorhexidine gluconate (equivalent to 2.5% v/v Chlorhexidine Gluconate Solution BP) in 70% w/w Isopropyl Alcohol BP with emollients.

Uses Hibisol is a potent, rapid-acting antiseptic solution for the disinfection of clean intact skin. It is used for pre-operative surgical hand disinfection, hand disinfection on the ward prior to aseptic procedures or after handling contaminated material, and for disinfection of patients' skin prior to surgery or other invasive procedures.

Dosage and administration
Pre-operative surgical hand disinfection: Dispense 5 ml of Hibisol and spread thoroughly over both hands and forearms, rubbing vigorously. When dry apply a further 5 ml and repeat the procedure.

NB. Before the first operation on a list or subsequently when hands are soiled the hands should be cleansed and disinfected with an effective antiseptic/detergent hand-wash (e.g. Hibiscrub).

Antiseptic hand disinfection on the ward: Dispense 3 ml of Hibisol and spread thoroughly over the hands and wrists rubbing vigorously until dry.

NB. If the hands are soiled, cleanse and *dry* before using Hibisol or alternatively use an effective antiseptic/detergent handwash (e.g. Hibiscrub).

Disinfection of patients' skin: Prior to surgery, apply

Hibisol to a sterile swab and rub vigorously over the operation site for a minimum of two minutes. Hibisol is also used for preparation of the skin prior to invasive procedures such as venepuncture.

Contra-indications, warnings, etc
Contra-indications: Hibisol is contra-indicated for persons who have previously shown a hypersensitivity reaction to chlorhexidine. However, such reactions are extremely rare.

Precautions: For external use only. Keep out of the eyes and avoid contact with brain, meninges or middle ear. Do not inject. Do not use in body cavities.

Side-effects: Irritative skin reactions can occasionally occur. Generalised allergic reactions to chlorhexidine have also been reported but are extremely rare.

Accidental ingestion: Chlorhexidine taken orally is poorly absorbed. Treat with gastric lavage using milk, egg-white, gelatin or mild soap avoiding pulmonary aspiration. Do not use apomorphine. Assist respiration if necessary and keep patient warm. Intravenous laevulose can accelerate alcohol metabolism. In severe cases, haemodialysis or peritoneal dialysis.

Pharmaceutical precautions Flammable. Store at room temperature.

Hypochlorite bleaches may cause brown stains to develop in fabrics which have previously been in contact with chlorhexidine solutions. Detailed literature is available on request.

Hibisol is incompatible with anionic agents.

Legal category GSL.

Package quantities Containers of 250 ml, 500 ml, and 5 L.

Further information A suitable antiseptic-detergent preparation which is compatible with Hibisol is Hibiscrub.

Product licence number 0029/0134.

HIBITANE* ACETATE
(Chlorhexidine Acetate BP)

Presentation A white, microcrystalline powder soluble in water (up to 1.9%), alcohol (up to 5%), glycerol, polyethylene glycols and propylene glycol.

Uses Hibitane Acetate is a potent antibacterial agent for general antiseptic purposes. This presentation, when diluted, allows Hibitane solutions to be used on body tissues where other antiseptics may prove too irritant. It also enables delicate instruments such as cystoscopes to be chemically disinfected.

Dosage and administration Dilute and use as follows:

Concentration of active constituent	Use
1 in 5,000 (0.02%) aqueous	Bladder irrigation† Pleural or peritoneal irrigation,† Cystoscopy medium†
1 in 2,000 (0.05%) aqueous	Patient use – Eye irrigation† Dip bowls† Inanimates – Clean instrument disinfection including endoscopes (30 minutes immersion) Storage of sterile instruments.
1 in 2000 (0.05%) in glycerine. (Sterile Hibitane Acetate and sterile glycerin mixed aseptically)‡	Urethral disinfection Catheter lubrication
1 in 200 (0.5%) in 70% alcohol.	Patient use – Pre-operative skin preparation Inanimates – Emergency disinfection of clean instruments. (2 minutes immersion)

† Sterilise the solution by autoclaving at 115–116°C for 30 minutes or 121–123°C for 15 minutes.
‡ See product literature for details.

Contra-indications, warnings, etc
Contra-indications: Hibitane preparations are contra-indicated for patients who have previously shown a hypersensitivity reaction to chlorhexidine. However, such reactions are extremely rare.

Precautions: Dilute before use. Avoid contact with the brain, meninges or middle ear. Do not inject.

Syringes and needles which have been immersed in Hibitane solutions should be thoroughly rinsed in sterile water or saline before use.

Solutions introduced into body cavities, eyes, or on to broken skin must be sterilised in accordance with BPC recommendations.

After immersion in alcohol solutions rinse instruments with sterile water or aqueous 0.02% Hibitane before use.

Side-effects: Irritative skin reactions can occasionally occur. Generalised allergic reactions to chlorhexidine have also been reported but are extremely rare.

Accidental ingestion: Chlorhexidine taken orally is poorly absorbed. Treat with gastric lavage using milk, egg-white, gelatin or mild soap. Employ supportive measures as appropriate.

Accidental intravenous transfusion: Blood transfusion may be necessary to counteract haemolysis.

Pharmaceutical precautions Dilute with freshly distilled water, alcohol (ethanol, Industrial Methylated Spirit, or isopropanol) or glycerin.

As a precaution against bacterial contamination, aqueous stock solutions should contain at least 4% v/v of isopropanol or 7% v/v ethanol which may be de-natured (i.e. Industrial Methylated Spirit).

Aqueous dilutions of Hibitane used for instrument storage should contain 0.1% sodium nitrite to inhibit metal corrosion. Such solutions must be changed every 7 days.

As cork may protect certain Gram-negative organisms from the action of antiseptics, Hibitane solutions must be stored in glass, plastic, or rubber-stoppered bottles.

Store at room temperature.

Hypochlorite bleaches may cause brown stains to develop in fabrics which have previously been in contact with Hibitane solutions. Detailed literature is available on request.

Hibitane is incompatible with anionic agents.

Legal category GSL.

Package quantities Containers of 500 g are available.

Further information Nil.

Product licence number 0029/5029

HIBITANE* ANTISEPTIC CREAM

Presentation A white water-miscible cream containing 1% w/w chlorhexidine gluconate (equivalent to 5% v/w Chlorhexidine Gluconate Solution BP).

Uses Hibitane Antiseptic Cream is a powerful antibacterial designed for application to broken skin surfaces. It may also be applied to the hands of nurses, surgeons and other hospital staff as a barrier against bacterial infection.

Dosage and administration Applied liberally to the wound and surrounding skin, or to the hands.

Contra-indications, warnings, etc
Contra-indications: Hibitane Antiseptic Cream is contra-indicated for patients who have previously shown a hypersensitivity reaction to chlorhexidine. However, such reactions are extremely rare.

Precautions: For topical application only. Keep out of the eyes and avoid contact with the brain, meninges or middle ear.

Side-effects: Irritative skin reactions can occasionally occur. Generalised allergic reactions to chlorhexidine have also been reported but are extremely rare.

Accidental ingestion: Chlorhexidine taken orally is poorly absorbed. Treat with gastric lavage using milk, egg-white, gelatin or mild soap. Employ supportive measures as appropriate.

Pharmaceutical precautions Store at room temperature and use undiluted.

Hypochlorite bleaches may cause brown stains to develop in fabrics which have previously been in contact with chlorhexidine preparations. Detailed literature is available on request.

Legal category GSL.

Package quantities Tubes of 50 g.

Further information Nil.

Product licence number 0029/5020.

HIBITANE* OBSTETRIC CREAM

Presentation A pourable, water-miscible cream containing 1% w/w chlorhexidine gluconate (equivalent to 5% v/w Chlorhexidine Gluconate Solution BP).

Uses Hibitane Obstetric Cream is a powerful antibacterial for use as a general antiseptic in obstetric and gynaecological practice.

Dosage and administration Applied liberally to the skin around the vulva and perineum of the patient, and to the hands of the midwife. It may also be smeared over gloved hands to facilitate vaginal examination.

Contra-indications, warnings, etc
Contra-indications: Hibitane Obstetric Cream is contra-indicated for patients who have previously shown a hypersensitivity reaction to chlorhexidine. However, such reactions are extremely rare.

Precautions: For topical application only. Keep out of the eyes and avoid contact with the brain, meninges or middle ear.

Side-effects: Irritative skin reactions can occasionally occur. Generalised allergic reactions to chlorhexidine have also been reported but are extremely rare.

Accidental ingestion: Chlorhexidine taken orally is poorly absorbed. Treat with gastric lavage using milk, egg-white, gelatin or mild soap. Employ supportive measures as appropriate.

Pharmaceutical precautions Store at room temperature and use undiluted.

Hypochlorite bleaches may cause brown stains to develop in fabrics which have previously been in contact with chlorhexidine preparations. Detailed literature is available on request.

Legal category GSL.

Package quantities Polythene dispenser pack 250 ml.

Further information Nil.

Product licence number 0029/5019.

HIBITANE TINCTURE*

Presentation A colourless alcoholic solution 0.5% w/v chlorhexidine gluconate (equivalent to 2.5% v/v Chlorhexidine Gluconate Solution BP) in 70% w/w Isopropyl Alcohol BP. An alcoholic solution of red dye is provided to colour the solution as required.

Uses Hibitane Tincture is a rapid acting antiseptic solution for disinfection of clean intact skin at the operation site, immediately prior to surgery. It may be used colourless or as a staining tincture to demark the treated area. Hibitane Tincture can also be used for emergency disinfection of clean surgical instruments either as a colourless solution or tinted pink for identification purposes.

Dosage and administration The tincture is for topical use only and should be used undiluted.

Pre-operative skin disinfection: using sterile swabs rub Hibitane Tincture vigorously onto the skin of the operation site and surrounding area for a minimum of 2 minutes.

Emergency disinfection of clean instruments: When terminal sterilisation is not feasible, immerse in the solution for a minimum of 2 minutes.

Preparation of coloured solutions:
1. Tinted – pour about $\frac{1}{2}$ of the red dye solution (Edicol carmoisine) from the small bottle and mix well by shaking.
2. Staining – pour all of the red dye solution (edicol carmoisine) from the small bottle directly into the large bottle and mix well by shaking. The concentration of dye in this final solution is 0.05%.

Contra-indications, warnings, etc
Contra-indications: Hibitane Tincture is contra-indicated for patients who have previously shown a hypersensitivity reaction to chlorhexidine. However, such reactions are extremely rare.

Precautions: For external use only. Keep out of the eyes and avoid contact with brain, meninges or middle ear. Not for injection. Do not use in body cavities. This preparation contains alcohol and is flammable. When use is to be followed by diathermy do not allow pooling of the fluid to occur, and ensure that the skin and surrounding drapes are dry.

Hibitane Tincture is not sporidical. Where sterilisation of instruments is required, other methods, such as autoclaving, should be used.

Syringes and needles which have been immersed in Hibitane Tincture should be thoroughly rinsed in sterile water or saline before use.

Side-effects: Irritative skin reactions can occasionally occur. Generalised allergic reactions to chlorhexidine have also been reported but are extremely rare. Should such a reaction occur stop application of the product.

Accidental ingestion: Hibitane taken orally is poorly absorbed. Treat with gastric lavage using milk, egg-white, gelatin or mild soap avoiding pulmonary aspiration. Do not use apomorphine. Assist respiration if necessary and keep patient warm. Intravenous laevulose can accelerate alcohol metabolism. In severe cases, haemodialysis or peritoneal dialysis may be necessary.

Pharmaceutical precautions Flammable. Store at room temperature.

The staining solution should be used within 8 days of preparation in order to avoid the problem of precipitation.

Hypochlorite bleaches may cause brown stains to develop in fabrics which have previously been in contact with chlorhexidine solutions. Detailed literature is available on request.

Chlorhexidine is incompatible with anionic agents.

Legal category GSL.

Package quantities Containers of 490 ml + 10 ml dye solution.

Further information Nil.

Product licence number 0029/0187.

HIBITANE* 5% CONCENTRATE

Presentation A red aqueous solution containing 5% w/v chlorhexidine gluconate (equivalent to 25% v/v Chlorhexidine Gluconate Solution BP).

Uses Hibitane 5% Concentrate is a potent antibacterial agent for general antiseptic purposes. A surface active agent is present to inhibit precipitation when dilutions are made with hard water.

Dosage and administration

Mode of preparation	Concentration of active ingredient required (chlorhexidine gluconate)	Use
10 ml made up to 1 litre with water (1 in 100)	1 in 2,000 (0.05%) Aqueous	*Patient use –* swabbing in obstetrics, wounds and burns† *Inanimates –* storage of sterile instruments
10 ml with 15 ml water made up to 100 ml with 95% alcohol (1 in 10)	1 in 200 (0.5%) in 70% Alcohol	*Patient use –* pre-operative skin disinfection. *Inanimates –* emergency instrument disinfection (2 minutes' immersion). (Excluding endoscopes containing cemented glass components)

† Sterilise the dilution by autoclaving at 115–116°C for 30 minutes or 121–123°C for 15 minutes.

Contra-indications, warnings, etc

Contra-indications: Hibitane preparations are contra-indicated for patients who have previously shown a hypersensitivity reaction to chlorhexidine. However, such reactions are extremely rare.

Precautions: For external use only. Dilute before use. Keep out of the eyes and avoid contact with brain, meninges or middle ear. Do not inject. Do not use in body cavities.

Syringes and needles which have been immersed in Hibitane solutions should be thoroughly rinsed in sterile water or saline before use.

Solutions applied to wounds, burns or broken skin must be sterilised in accordance with BPC recommendations.

After immersion in alcoholic solutions rinse instruments with sterile water or aqueous 0.02% Hibitane before use.

Side-effects: Irritative skin reactions can occasionally occur. Generalised allergic reactions to chlorhexidine have also been reported but are extremely rare.

Accidental ingestion: Chlorhexidine taken orally is poorly absorbed. Treat with gastric lavage using milk, egg-white, gelatin or mild soap. Employ supportive measures as appropriate.

Accidental intravenous transfusion: Blood transfusion may be necessary to counteract haemolysis.

Pharmaceutical precautions Dilute with freshly distilled water, tap water of an acceptable bacteriological standard or alcohol (ethanol, Industrial Methylated Spirit or isopropanol).

As a precaution against bacterial contamination, stock aqueous solutions should contain at least 4% v/v of isopropanol or 7% v/v of ethanol, which may be denatured (for example, Industrial Methylated Spirit).

Aqueous dilutions of Hibitane used for instrument storage should contain 0.1% sodium nitrite to inhibit metal corrosion. Such solutions must be changed every 7 days.

Instruments containing cemented glass components should not be disinfected with solutions prepared from Hibitane 5% Concentrate.

As cork may protect certain Gram-negative organisms from the action of antiseptics, Hibitane solutions must be stored in glass-, plastic- or rubber-stoppered bottles.

Store at room temperature.

Hypochlorite bleaches may cause brown stains to develop in fabrics which have previously been in contact with Hibitane solutions. Detailed literature is available on request.

Hibitane is incompatible with anionic agents.

Legal category GSL.

Package quantities Containers of 500 ml and 5 litres are available, as are 10 ml sachets in packs of 50. Dispensers to fit 5L are available.

Further information Nil.

Product licence number 0029/5032.

HIBITANE* GLUCONATE 20% SOLUTION (Chlorhexidine Gluconate Solution BP)

Presentation An aqueous solution containing 20% w/v chlorhexidine gluconate.

Uses Hibitane Gluconate is a potent antibacterial agent for general antiseptic purposes. This presentation is an aqueous solution without additives which, when diluted allows use on body tissues where other antiseptics may prove too irritant. It also enables delicate instruments such as cystoscopes to be chemically disinfected.

Dosage and administration

Mode of preparation	Concentration of active ingredient required (chlorhexidine gluconate)	Use
1.0 ml made up to 1 litre with water (1 in 1,000)	1 in 5,000 (0.02%) Aqueous	Bladder irrigation† Pleural or peritoneal irrigation† Cystoscopy medium†
2.5 ml made up to 1 litre with water (1 in 400)	1 in 2000 (0.05%) Aqueous	*Patient use –* eye irrigation† dip bowls† *Inanimates –* clean instrument disinfection including endoscopes (30 minutes' immersion)
2.5 ml of sterile solution made up to 1 litre with sterile glycerine and mixed aseptically (1 in 400)‡	1 in 2,000 (0.05%) in glycerine	Urethral disinfection and catheter lubrication
25 ml with 225 ml water made up to 1 litre with 95% alcohol (1 in 40)	1 in 200 (0.5%) in 70% alcohol	Emergency disinfection of clean instruments (2 minutes' immersion)

† Sterilise the dilution by autoclaving at 115°–116°C for 30 minutes or 121°–123°C for 15 minutes.
‡ See Product literature for full details.

Contra-indications, warnings, etc
Contra-indications: Hibitane preparations are contra-indicated for patients who have previously shown a hypersensitivity reaction to chlorhexidine. However, such reactions are extremely rare.

Precautions: Dilute before use. Avoid contact with the brain, meninges or middle ear. Do not inject.

Syringes and needles which have been immersed in Hibitane solutions should be thoroughly rinsed in sterile water or saline before use.

Solutions introduced into body cavities, eyes, or on to broken skin must be sterilised in accordance with BPC recommendations.

After immersion in alcoholic solutions rinse instruments with sterile water or aqueous 0.02% Hibitane before use.

Side-effects: Irritative skin reactions can occasionally occur. Generalised allergic reactions to chlorhexidine have also been reported but are extremely rare.

Accidental ingestion: Chlorhexidine taken orally is poorly absorbed. Treat with gastric lavage using milk, egg-white, gelatin or mild soap. Employ supportive measures as appropriate.

Accidental intravenous transfusion: Blood transfusion may be necessary to counteract haemolysis.

Pharmaceutical precautions Dilute with freshly distilled water, alcohol (ethanol, Industrial Methylated Spirit, or isopropanol) or glycerine. Mix well before use.

As a precaution against bacterial contamination, aqueous stock solution should contain at least 4% v/v of isopropanol or 7% v/v of ethanol which may be denatured (i.e. Industrial Methylated Spirit).

Aqueous dilutions of Hibitane used for instrument storage should contain 0.1% sodium nitrite to inhibit metal corrosion. Such solutions must be changed every 7 days.

As cork may protect certain Gram-negative organisms from the action of antiseptics, Hibitane solutions must be stored in glass-, plastic- or rubber-stoppered bottles.

Store at room temperature.

Hypochlorite bleaches may cause brown stains to develop in fabrics which have previously been in contact with Hibitane solutions. Detailed literature is available on request.

Hibitane is incompatible with anionic agents.

Legal category GSL.

Package quantities Containers of 500 ml and 5 litres are available. Dispensers to fit 5L are available.

Further information Nil.

Product licence number 0029/5031.

IMPERACIN* TABLETS

Presentation Yellow, biconvex, film-coated tablets marked with IMPERACIN on one side. Each tablet contains 250 mg of Oxytetracycline Dihydrate PhEur.

Uses Imperacin is a bacteriostatic broad-spectrum antibiotic well absorbed after oral administration. It is active against a variety of Gram-positive and Gram-negative bacteria, spirochaetes, certain mycoplasma species, rickettsiae, protozoa and the psittacosislympho-granuloma-venereum-trachoma group (Chlamydia). It is indicated in the treatment of the folllwing conditions when they are caused by susceptible organisms.

The acute exacerbations of chronic bronchitis.

Venereal diseases, including penicillin-resistant gonorrhoea, non-gonococcal urethritis and lymphogranuloma verereum.

Brucellosis, typhus, amoebic dysentery and psittacosis.

Tetracyclines are of value in the treatment of stapylococcal and streptococcal infections in penicillin-sensitive patients where tetracycline resistance is not a problem.

Dosage and administration
Adults: 250 to 500 mg four times daily.

Children: 25 to 50 mg/kg bodyweight daily, divided into four equal doses.

Elderly patients: There are no special dosage recommendations for the elderly, but it may be advisable to monitor elderly patients so that optimum dosage can be individually determined.

Doses are best given either 1 hour before or 2 hours after food.

Therapy should be continued for at least 24 to 48 hours after symptoms and fever have subsided.

In the treatment of streptococcal infections, a therapeutic dose should be administered for at least 10 days.

Contra-indications, warnings, etc Imperacin is contra-indicated in persons who have previously shown hypersensitivity to any of the tetracyclines.

Imperacin is contraindicated in chronic renal failure.

In the presence of renal impairment, normal doses may lead to excessive systemic accumulation of the drug and possible liver toxicity. Under such circumstances, lower than usual total doses are indicated and, if therapy is prolonged, serum level determinations of the drug may be advisable.

Imperacin should be used with caution in the presence of hepatic dysfunction.

The use of tetracyclines during tooth development (last half of pregnancy, infancy and childhood to the age of eight years) may cause permanent discolouration of the teeth. This adverse reaction is more common during long term use but has been observed following repeated short term courses. Enamel hypoplasia has also been reported. Tetracycline drugs, therefore, should not be used in this age group unless other drugs are not likely to be effective or are contra-indicated.

As with other antibiotic preparations, Imperacin may result in overgrowth of non-susceptible organisms. If superinfection occurs, appropriate measures should be taken.

Antacids containing aluminium, calcium or magnesium impair absorption and should not be given to patients taking Imperacin.

Food and some dairy products also interfere with absorption.

Tetracyclines have been shown occasionally to depress plasma prothombin activity and patients who are on anticoagulant therapy may require an adjustment of their anticoagulant dosage.

Since bacteriostatic drugs may interfere with the bactericidal action of penicillin, it is advisable to avoid giving Imperacin in conjunction with penicillin.

Tetracylines have been shown in very rare instances to cause pseudomembranous colitis.

Photosensitivity, manifested by an exaggerated sunburn reaction has been observed in some patients taking tetracyclines.

Hypersensitivity reactions and anaphylaxis are rarely seen during treatment with Imperacin. Treatment of anaphylaxis includes the immediate administration of adrenaline (0.5 ml Adrenaline Injection BP subcutaneously), oxygen and artificial respiration.

Treatment of dyspnoea includes administration of aminophylline, calcium and antihistamines. General measures include administration of plasma, blood vasopressor drugs (noradrenaline) and hydrocortisone (100 mg i.v.).

Pregnancy: It is known that tetracyclines cross the placental barrier and may have a toxic effect on the foetus. Special care should be exercised if administered during pregnancy.

Side-effects: These are uncommon in the recommended dosage, but nausea, diarrhoea and morbilliform skin reactions have been reported. Overgrowth with resistant organisms, e.g. Candida, may occur and cause glossitis, rectal and vaginal irritation. Similarly, resistant staphylococci may cause enterocolitis.

Overdosage: Serious symptoms are unlikely. Gastric lavage might be beneficial in the first hours after ingestion followed by conservative management. Milk will reduce absorption.

Pharmaceutical precautions Store at room temperature, protected from light and moisture.

Legal category POM.

Package quantities *Tablets:* Containers of 100 and 1,000.

Further information Nil

Product licence number
Imperacin Tablets   0029/5087.

INDERAL* TABLETS AND INJECTION

Presentation

1. Tablets each containing 10 mg Propranolol Hydrochloride BP. Pink, round, bi-convex, film coated tablets, impressed with the legend 'INDERAL' 10 on one face and ICI on the obverse. The impressions are highlighted in white.

2. Tablets each containing 40 mg Propranolol Hydrochloride BP. Pink, round, bi-convex, film coated tablets, impressed with the legend 'INDERAL' 40 on one face and ICI on the obverse. The impressions are highlighted in white.

3. Tablets each containing 80 mg Propranolol Hydrochloride BP. Pink, round, bi-convex, film coated tablets, impressed with the legend 'INDERAL' 80 on one face and ICI on the obverse. The impressions are highlighted in white.

4. Tablets each containing 160 mg Propranolol Hydrochloride BP. Pink, round, bi-convex, film coated

tablets, impressed with the legend 'INDERAL' 160 on one face and ICI on the obverse. The impressions are highlighted in white.

5. Injection – a solution containing Propranolol Hydrochloride BP. 1 mg per 1 ml in printed glass ampoules of 1 ml.

Uses Inderal, a beta-adrenoceptor blocking drug, is indicated in:

(a)   the control of essential and renal hypertension
(b)   the management of angina pectoris
(c)   the long term prophylaxis after recovery from acute myocardial infarction
(d)   the control of most forms of cardiac dysrhythmias
(e)   the prophylaxis of migraine
(f)   management of essential tremor
(g)   the control of anxiety and anxiety tachycardia
(h)   the adjunctive management of thyrotoxicosis and thyrotoxic crisis
(i)   management of hypertrophic obstructive cardiomyopathy
(j)   management of phaeochromocytoma (with an alpha blocker)

Dosage and administration *Adults: Oral: Hypertension:* A starting dose of 80 mg twice a day may be increased at weekly intervals according to response. The usual dose range is 160–320 mg per day. With concurrent diuretic or other antihypertensive drugs a further reduction of blood pressure is obtained.

Angina, anxiety, migraine and essential tremor: A starting dose of 40 mg two or three times daily may be increased by the same amount at weekly intervals according to patient response. An adequate response in anxiety, migraine and essential tremor is usually seen in the range 80–160 mg/day and in angina in the range 120–240 mg/day.

Dysrhythmias, anxiety tachycardia, hypertrophic obstructive cardiomyopathy and thyrotoxicosis: A dosage range of 10–40 mg three or four times a day usually achieves the required response.

Post myocardial infarction: Treatment should start between days 5 and 21 after myocardial infarction, with an initial dose of 40 mg four times a day for 2 or 3 days. In order to improve compliance the total daily dosage may thereafter be given as 80 mg twice a day.

Phaeochromocytoma: (Used only with an alpha-receptor blocking drug). Pre-operative: 60 mg daily for three days is recommended. Non-operable malignant cases: 30 mg daily.

Intravenous; Before injecting Inderal, atropine 1–2 mg should be given intravenously. The initial dose of Inderal is 1 mg (1 ml) injected over one minute. This may be repeated at two-minute intervals until a response is observed or to a maximum dose of 10 mg in conscious patients or 5 mg in patients under anaesthesia.

Children: Dysrhythmias, phaeochromocytoma, thyrotoxicosis; The dose of Inderal should be determined according to the cardiac status of the patient and the circumstances necessitating treatment. These doses are only a guide: *Oral:* 0.25–0.5 mg/kg three or four times daily as required. *Intravenous:* 0.025–0.05 mg/kg injected slowly under ECG control and repeated three or four times daily as required.

Migraine: Oral: Under the age of 12: 20 mg two or three times daily.

Over the age of 12: the adult dose.

Fallot's Tetralogy: The value of Inderal in this condition is confined mainly to the relief of right-ventricular outflow tract shut-down. It is also useful for treatment of associated dysrhythmias and angina. Dosage should be individually determined according to circumstances and the following is only a guide: *Oral:* Up to 1mg/kg repeated three or four times daily as required. *Intravenous:* Up to 0.1mg/kg injected slowly under ECG control, repeated three or four times daily as required.

Elderly patients: Evidence concerning the relation between blood level and age is conflicting. With regard to the elderly, the optimum dose should be individually determined according to clinical response.

Contra-indications, warnings, etc
Inderal should not be used:

1. In the presence of second or third degree heart block.
2. If there is a history of bronchospasm.
3. After prolonged fasting.
4. In metabolic acidosis (e.g. in some diabetics).

The intravenous injection is intended for the emergency treatment of cardiac dysrhythmias and thyrotoxic crisis only.

Special care should be taken with patients whose cardiac reserve is poor. Heart failure following myocardial infarction must have been controlled before treatment with Inderal is started. Heart failure due to thyrotoxicosis often responds to Inderal alone, but if other adverse factors co-exist myocardial contractility must be maintained and signs of failure controlled with digitalis and diuretics.

One of the pharmacological actions of Inderal is to reduce heart rate. In the rare instance when symptoms may be attributable to the slow heart rate, the dose may be reduced.

Inderal modifies the tachycardia of hypoglycaemia.

In patients suffering from ischaemic heart disease, as with other beta-blocking agents, treatment should not be discontinued abruptly. Either the equivalent dosage of another beta-blocker may be substituted or the withdrawal of Inderal should be gradual.

Caution should be exercised when transferring patients from clonidine to beta-adrenoceptor blocking drugs. If beta-adrenoceptor blocking drugs and clonidine are given concurrently, clonidine should not be discontinued until several days after withdrawal of the beta-adrenoceptor blocking drug (see also prescribing information on clonidine).

Care should be taken in prescribing a beta-adrenoceptor blocking drug with Class 1 antidysrhythmic agents such as disopyramide.

Beta-adrenoceptor blocking drugs should be used with caution in combination with verapamil in patients with impaired ventricular function. The combination should not be given to patients with conduction abnormalities. Neither drug should be administered intravenously within 48 hours of discontinuing the other.

Anaesthesia: As with all other beta-adrenoceptor blocking drugs, it may be decided to withdraw Inderal before surgery. In this case, 24 hours should be allowed to elapse between the last dose and anaesthesia. If treatment is continued, care should be taken when using anaesthetic agents such as ether, cyclopropane and trichloroethylene. Vagal dominance, if it occurs, may be corrected with atropine (1–2 mg i.v.).

Pregnancy: As with all other drugs, Inderal should not be given in pregnancy unless its use is essential. There is no evidence of teratogenicity with Inderal.

Side-effects: Inderal is usually well tolerated. Minor side-effects such as cold extremities, nausea, insomnia, lassitude and diarrhoea are usually transient. Isolated cases of paraesthesia of the hands have been reported.

There have been reports of skin rashes and/or dry eyes associated with the use of beta-adrenergic blocking drugs. The reported incidence is small and in most cases the symptoms have cleared when treatment was withdrawn. Discontinuance of the drug should be considered if any such reaction is not otherwise explicable. Cessation of therapy with a beta-adrenergic blocker should be gradual. In the rare event of intolerance, manifested as bradycardia and hypotension, the drug should be withdrawn and, if necessary, treatment for overdosage instituted.

Overdosage: Excessive bradycardia may be countered with atropine 1–2 mg intravenously, followed, if necessary by a beta-adrenoceptor stimulant such as isoprenaline 25 micrograms initially or orciprenaline 0.5 mg given by slow intravenous injection. Glucagon has also been reported to be useful as a cardiac stimulant in a dose of 10 mg intravenously.

Pharmaceutical precautions All Inderal preparations should be stored at room temperature, protected from light.

Compatibility with intravenous injection fluids: Inderal Injection is compatible with 0.9% w/v sodium chloride and 5% w/v dextrose.

Details of a suitable formula for the extemporaneous preparation of a paediatric oral suspension of Inderal are available on request to the manufacturer.

Legal category POM.

Package quantities *Tablets 10 mg:* Containers of 100 and 1,000.
Tablets 40 mg: Containers of 100 and 1,000.
Tablets 80 mg: Containers of 60 and 500.
Tablets 160 mg: Containers of 60 and 250.
Injection: 1 ml ampoules in boxes of 10.

Further information Nil.

Product licence numbers
Inderal Tablets 10 mg   0029/5063
Inderal Tablets 40 mg   0029/5064
Inderal Tablets 80 mg   0029/5065
Inderal Tablets 160 mg   0029/0103
Inderal Injection   0029/5062

INDERAL* LA
HALF-INDERAL* LA

Presentation Inderal LA and Half-Inderal LA capsules contain spheroids of the beta-adrenoceptor blocking drug propranolol hydrochloride which have a sustained release coating to provide long action.

Inderal LA capsules each contain 160 mg Propranolol Hydrochloride BP. Inderal LA is presented as size 1 gelatin capsules with a clear pink body and opaque, lavender cap bearing the ICI Roundel and marked Inderal LA in white ink.

Half-Inderal LA capsules each contain 80 mg Propranolol Hydrochloride BP. Half-Inderal LA is presented as size 3 gelatin capsules with a clear pink body and opaque, pale lavender cap bearing the ICI Roundel and marked Half-Inderal LA in black ink.

Uses *Inderal LA and Half-Inderal LA* are indicated in the management of angina, anxiety and essential tremor, the adjunctive management of thyrotoxicosis, and the prophylaxis of migraine.

Inderal LA is indicated in the control of hypertension.

One Half-Inderal LA capsule daily is unlikely on its own to be sufficient to treat hypertension, but it may be used as a starting dose in appropriate patients (e.g. the elderly) or to provide a convenient method of gradual dosage alteration.

Dosage and administration *Adults: Hypertension:* The usual starting dose is one 160 mg Inderal LA capsule daily, taken either morning or evening. An adequate response is seen in most patients at this dosage. If necessary, it can be increased in Half-Inderal LA increments until an adequate response is achieved. A further reduction in BP can be attained if a diuretic or other antihypertensive agent is given in addition to Inderal LA and Half-Inderal LA.

Angina, anxiety, essential tremor, thyrotoxicosis and the prophylaxis of migraine: One 80 mg Half-Inderal LA capsule daily taken either morning or evening may be sufficient to provide adequate control in many patients. If necessary the dose may be increased to one 160 mg Inderal LA capsule per day and an additional 80 mg Half-Inderal LA increment may be given.

Patients who are already established on equivalent daily doses of Inderal tablets should be transferred to the equivalent doses of 80 mg Half-Inderal LA or 160 mg Inderal LA daily taken either morning or evening.

Children: Inderal LA and Half-Inderal LA are not intended for use in children.

Elderly patients: Evidence concerning the relation between blood level and age is conflicting. It is suggested that treatment should start with one Half-Inderal LA capsule once a day. The dose may be increased to one Inderal LA capsule daily or higher as appropriate.

Contra-indications, warnings, etc Inderal LA and Half-Inderal LA should not be used:

1. In the presence of second or third degree heart block.
2. If there is a history of bronchospasm.
3. After prolonged fasting.
4. In metabolic acidosis (e.g. in some diabetics).

Special care should be taken with patients whose cardiac reserve is poor. Myocardial contractility must be maintained and signs of failure controlled with digitalis and diuretics. One of the pharmacological actions of Inderal LA or Half-Inderal LA is to reduce the heart rate. In the rare instance when symptoms may be attributable to the slow heart rate the dose may be reduced.

Inderal LA and Half-Inderal LA modify the tachycardia of hypoglycaemia.

In patients suffering from ischaemic heart disease, as with other beta-blocking agents, treatment should not be discontinued abruptly. Either the equivalent dosage of another beta-blocker may be substituted or the withdrawal should be gradual. This can be achieved by first substituting the daily Inderal LA dose by the equivalent in Half-Inderal LA capsules and then gradually reducing the number of capsules.

Caution should be exercised when transferring patients from clonidine to beta-adrenoceptor blocking drugs. If beta-adrenoceptor blocking drugs and clonidine are given concurrently, clonidine should not be discontinued until several days after withdrawal of the beta-adrenoceptor blocking drug (see also prescribing information on clonidine).

Care should be taken in prescribing a beta-adrenoceptor blocking drug with Class 1 antidysrhythmic agents such as disopyramide.

Beta-adrenoceptor blocking drugs should be used with caution in combination with verapamil in patients with impaired ventricular function. The combination should not be given to patients with conduction abnormalities. Neither drug should be administered intravenously within 48 hours of discontinuing the other.

Anaesthesia: As with all beta-adrenoceptor blocking drugs it may be decided to withdraw Inderal LA or Half-Inderal LA before surgery. In this case 48 hours should be allowed to elapse between the last dose and anaesthesia. If treatment is continued care should be taken when using anaesthetic agents such as ether, cyclopropane and trichloroethylene. Vagal dominance, if it occurs, may be corrected with atropine (1–2 mg i.v.).

Pregnancy: As with all other drugs, neither Inderal LA nor Half-Inderal LA should be given in pregnancy unless their use is essential. There is no evidence of teratogenicity with Inderal.

Side-effects: Inderal LA and Half-Inderal LA are usually well tolerated. Minor side-effects, such as cold extremities, nausea, insomnia, lassitude and diarrhoea are usually transient. Isolated cases of paraesthesia of the hands have been reported. There have been reports of skin rashes and/or dry eyes associated with the use of beta-adrenergic blocking drugs. The reported incidence is small and in most cases the symptoms have cleared when treatment was withdrawn. Discontinuance of the drug should be considered if any such reaction is not otherwise explicable. Cessation of therapy with a beta-adrenergic blocker should be gradual. In the rare event of intolerance, manifested as bradycardia and hypotension, the drug should be withdrawn and, if necessary, treatment for overdosage instituted.

Overdosage: Excessive bradycardia can be countered with atropine 1–2 mg intravenously, followed, if necessary, by a beta-receptor stimulant such as isoprenaline 25 micrograms initially, or orciprenaline 0.5 mg given by slow intravenous injection. Glucagon has been reported to be useful as a cardiac stimulant in a dose of 10 mg intravenously.

Pharmaceutical precautions Store at room temperature, protected from light and moisture.

Legal category POM.

Package quantities Patient Calendar Pack of 28 capsules.

Further information Inderal LA and Half-Inderal LA capsules provide controlled release of propranolol hydrochloride such that blood levels are maintained for over 24 hours following a single oral dose and, unlike therapy with conventional tablets, irregular peaks and troughs of blood level are avoided.

Product licence numbers
Inderal LA   0029/0128.
Half-Inderal LA   0029/0173

INDERETIC*

Presentation White, opaque capsules, printed with Inderetic and the ICI Roundel. Each capsule contains

80 mg Propranolol Hydrochloride BP and 2.5 mg Bendrofluazide BP.

Uses The management of hypertension. Inderal, propranolol hydrochloride, is a beta-adrenergic blocking drug, and bendrofluazide is a thiazide diuretic. Inderetic presents both these components in a single preparation for the treatment of mild to moderate hypertension.

Dosage and administration *Adults:* One capsule twice daily should prove effective in most cases.

For new patients a maximum response is achieved usually within two weeks. If a greater antihypertensive effect is desired, Inderetic is compatible with most other antihypertensives which may be added (see *Warnings* below).

In those patients being transferred from a combination of treatments, which includes a beta-blocker, this treatment should be withdrawn gradually as Inderetic is introduced.

Children: There is no specific experience with Inderetic and for this reason it is not recommended for children.

Elderly patients: Evidence concerning the relation between blood level and age is conflicting. With regard to the elderly, the optimum dose should be individually determined using conventional Inderal and bendrofluazide tablets according to clinical response. This dose may then be achieved with the appropriate number of Inderetic capsules.

Contra-indications, warnings, etc Inderetic should not be used:

1. In the presence of second or third degree heart block.
2. If there is a history of bronchospasm.
3. In patients with anuria, renal failure, or with a history of sensitivity to thiazides.
4. After prolonged fasting.
5. In patients with metabolic acidosis (e.g. in some diabetics).

Special care should be taken with patients whose cardiac reserve is poor, although the concurrent diuretic therapy is likely to be beneficial in such cases.

Normally, cardiac failure is considered a contraindication to beta-blockade, unless or until signs of failure are controlled with digitalis or diuretics.

One of the pharmacological actions of beta-adrenoceptor blocking drugs is to reduce heart rate. In the rare instance when symptoms may be attributable to the slow heart rate, the dose may be reduced.

Inderetic modifies the tachycardia of hypoglycaemia.

In patients suffering from ischaemic heart disease, as with other beta-blocking agents, treatment should not be discontinued abruptly. Either the equivalent dosage of another beta-blocker may be substituted or the withdrawal of Inderetic should be gradual.

Caution should be exercised when transferring patients from clonidine to beta-adrenoceptor blocking drugs. If beta-adrenoceptor blocking drugs and clonidine are given concurrently, clonidine should not be discontinued until several days after withdrawal of the beta-adrenoceptor blocking drug (see also prescribing information on Clonidine).

Care should be taken in prescribing a beta-adrenoceptor blocking drug with Class 1 antidysrhythmic agents such as disopyramide.

Beta-adrenoceptor blocking drugs should be used with caution in combination with verapamil in patients with impaired ventricular function. The combination should not be given to patients with conduction abnormalities. Neither drug should be administered intravenously within 48 hours of discontinuing the other.

Inderetic contains a thiazide diuretic which may decrease glucose tolerance. Care is necessary when Inderetic is administered to patients with a known predisposition to diabetes.

As with other combinations of beta-adrenoceptor blocking drugs and diuretics, Inderetic may be associated with minor changes in potassium status. Potassium depletion may be dangerous in patients receiving digitalis or those with hepatic cirrhosis with ascites.

Preparations containing lithium generally should not be given with diuretics because they may reduce its renal clearance.

Anaesthesia: As with all beta-adrenoceptor blocking drugs, it may be decided to withdraw Inderetic before surgery. In this case, 24 hours should be allowed to elapse between the last dose and anaesthesia. If treatment is continued, care should be taken when using anaesthetic agents such as ether, cyclopropane and trichloroethylene. Vagal dominance, if it occurs, may be corrected with atropine (1–2 mg i.v.).

Pregnancy: Although there is no evidence of teratogenicity, both constituents cross the placental barrier and Inderetic is, therefore, considered to be unsuitable for pregnant patients.

Side-effects: Propranolol hydrochloride is usually well tolerated. Minor side-effects, such as cold extremities, nausea, insomnia, lassitude and diarrhoea are usually transient. Isolated cases of paraesthesia of the hands have been reported. There have been reports of skin rashes and/or dry eyes associated with the use of beta-adrenergic blocking drugs. The reported incidence is small and in most cases the symptoms have cleared when treatment was withdrawn. Discontinuance of the drug should be considered if any such reaction is not otherwise explicable. Cessation of therapy with a beta-adrenergic blocker should be gradual. In the rare event of intolerance to the propranolol hydrochloride in Inderetic, manifested as bradycardia and hypotension, the drug should be withdrawn and, if necessary, treatment for overdosage instituted.

Adverse effects of bendrofluazide are very uncommon in the small dose contained in Inderetic. Hypokalaemia, usually manifest as muscular weakness, is most severe in patients already depleted of potassium, as in renal or hepatic insufficiency. Potassium depletion is dangerous in patients receiving digitalis. Coma may be precipitated in hepatic cirrhosis. Hyperuricaemia sometimes occurs, but an attack of gout is rare. The thiazide diuretics increase blood urea, which is most pronounced in patients with renal disease and pre-existing retention of nitrogen. Reports of other adverse reactions to thiazides are rare. They include skin rashes with associated photosensitivity, necrotising vasculitis, acute pancreatitis, blood dyscrasias and aggravation of pre-existing myopia.

Overdosage: Excessive bradycardia can be countered with atropine 1–2 mg intravenously, followed, if necessary, by a beta-adrenoceptor stimulant such as isoprenaline 25 micrograms initially, or orciprenaline 0.5 mg given by slow intravenous injection. Glucagon has also been reported to be useful as a cardiac stimulant in a dose of 10 mg intravenously. Excessive diuresis should be countered by maintaining normal fluid and electrolyte balance.

Pharmaceutical precautions Store at room temperature, protected from light and moisture.

Legal category POM.

Package quantities Containers of 100 capsules.

Further information Inderetic is designed to aid drug compliance by providing a convenient presentation of the standard beta-adrenoceptor blocking drug Inderal, propranolol hydrochloride, with the diuretic bendrofluazide for the treatment of mild to moderate hypertension. Concurrent use of propranolol and bendrofluazide produces a more pronounced and consistent antihypertensive response than when either component is used alone.

Product licence number 0029/0138.

INDEREX*

Presentation Capsules, having opaque pink caps and opaque grey bodies printed with the name Inderex and the ICI Roundel. Each capsule contains 160 mg Propranolol Hydrochloride BP in the form of spheroids having a sustained release coating to provide long action, and 5 mg Bendrofluazide BP.

Uses The management of mild to moderate hypertension. Inderal, propranolol hydrochloride, is a beta-adrenergic blocking drug, and bendrofluazide is a thiazide diuretic. Inderex presents both these components in a single preparation.

Dosage and administration *Adults:* One capsule daily should prove effective in most cases.

For new patients a maximum response is achieved usually within one week. If a greater antihypertensive effect is desired, Inderex is compatible with most other antihypertensives which may be added (see Warnings below). In those patients being transferred from a combination of treatments, which includes a beta-blocker, these treatments should be withdrawn gradually as Inderex is introduced.

Children: There is no paediatric experience with Inderex and for this reason is not recommended for children.

Elderly patients: Evidence concerning the relation between blood level and age is conflicting. With regard to the elderly, the optimum dose should be individually determined using conventional Inderal and bendrofluazide tablets according to clinical response. This dose may then be achieved with the appropriate number of Inderex capsules once daily.

Contra-indications, warnings, etc Inderex should not be used:

1. In the presence of second or third degree heart block.
2. If there is a history of bronchospasm.
3. In patients with anuria, renal failure, or with a history of sensitivity to thiazides.
4. After prolonged fasting.
5. In patients with metabolic acidosis (e.g. in some diabetics).

One of the pharmacological effects of beta-blockade is a reduction in heart rate; if this falls much below 50–55 beats/minute, the dose should not be increased further.

Special care should be taken with patients whose cardiac reserve is poor, although the concurrent diuretic therapy is likely to be beneficial in such cases.

Normally, cardiac failure is considered a contra-indication to beta-blockade, unless or until signs of failure are controlled with digitalis or diuretics.

Inderex modifies the tachycardia of hypoglycaemia.

In patients with ischaemic heart disease, it is important that treatment with a beta-blocking agent is not discontinued abruptly. Either the equivalent dosage of another beta-blocker may be substituted or the withdrawal of Inderex should be gradual. This can be achieved by first substituting the Inderex by the equivalent in 40 mg Inderal tablets plus bendrofluazide tablets spread throughout the day and then gradually reducing the dose of both agents.

Caution should be exercised when transferring patients from clonidine to beta-adrenoceptor blocking drugs. If beta-adrenoceptor blocking drugs and clonidine are given concurrently, clonidine should not be discontinued until several days after withdrawal of the beta-adrenoceptor blocking drug (see also prescribing information on Clonidine).

Care should be taken in prescribing a beta-adrenoceptor blocking drug with Class 1 antidysrhythmic agents such as disopyramide.

Beta-adrenoceptor blocking drugs should be used with caution in combination with verapamil in patients with impaired ventricular function. The combination should not be given to patients with conduction abnormalities. Neither drug should be administered intravenously within 48 hours of discontinuing the other.

Inderex contains a thiazide diuretic which may decrease glucose tolerance. Care is necessary when Inderex is administered to patients with a known predisposition to diabetes.

As with other combinations of beta-adrenoceptor blocking drugs and diuretics, Inderex may be associated with minor changes in potassium status. Potassium depletion may be dangerous in patients receiving digitalis or those with hepatic cirrhosis with ascites.

Preparations containing lithium generally should not be given with diuretics because they may reduce its renal clearance.

Anaesthesia: As with all beta-adrenoceptor blocking drugs, it may be decided to withdraw Inderex before surgery. In this case, 48 hours should be allowed to elapse between the last dose and anaesthesia. If treatment is continued, care should be taken when using anaesthetic agents such as ether, cyclopropane and trichloroethylene. Vagal dominance, if it occurs, may be corrected with atropine (1–2 mg i.v.).

Pregnancy: Although there is no evidence of teratogenicity, both constituents cross the placental barrier and Inderex is, therefore, considered to be unsuitable for pregnant patients.

Side-effects: Propranolol hydrochloride is usually well tolerated. Minor side effects, such as cold extremities, nausea, insomnia, lassitude and diarrhoea are usually transient. Isolated cases of paraesthesia of the hands have been reported. There have been reports of skin rashes and/or dry eyes associated with the use of beta-adrenergic blocking drugs. The reported incidence is small and in most cases the symptoms have cleared when treatment was withdrawn. Discontinuance of the drug should be considered if any such reaction is not otherwise explicable. Cessation of therapy with a beta-adrenergic blocker should be gradual. In the rare event of intolerance to the propranolol hydrochloride in Inderex, manifested as bradycardia and hypotension, the drug should be withdrawn and, if necessary, treatment for overdosage instituted.

Adverse effects of bendrofluazide are very uncommon in the dose contained in Inderex. Hypokalaemia, usually manifest as muscular weakness, is most severe in patients already depleted of potassium, as in renal or hepatic insufficiency. Potassium depletion is dangerous in patients receiving digitalis. Coma may be precipitated in hepatic cirrhosis. Hyperuricaemia sometimes occurs, but an attack of gout is rare. The thiazide diuretics increase blood urea, which is most pronounced in patients with renal disease and pre-existing retention of nitrogen. Reports of other adverse reactions to thiazides are rare. They include skin rashes with associated photosensitivity, necrotising vasculitis, acute pancreatitis, blood dyscrasias and aggravation of pre-existing myopia.

Overdosage: Excessive bradycardia can be countered with atropine 1–2 mg intravenously, followed, if necessary, by a beta-adrenoceptor stimulant, such as isoprenaline 25 micrograms initially, or orciprenaline 0.5 mg given by slow intravenous injection. Glucagon has also been reported to be useful as a cardiac stimulant in a dose of 10 mg intravenously. Excessive diuresis should be countered by maintaining normal fluid and electrolyte balance.

Pharmaceutical precautions Store at room temperature, protected from light and moisture.

Legal category POM.

Package quantities Patient calendar pack of 28 capsules.

Further information Inderex is designed to aid drug compliance by providing a convenient presentation of a sustained release formulation of propranolol hydrochloride with the diuretic bendrofluazide for the treatment of mild to moderate hypertension. Concurrent use of propranolol and bendrofluazide produces a more pronounced and consistent antihypertensive response than when either component is used alone.

Product licence number 0029/0157.

MYSOLINE* TABLETS
MYSOLINE* ORAL SUSPENSION

Presentation Mysoline tablets are round, white, biconvex, marked with a parallel line on each side of the bisecting line on one face and the ICI roundel on the obverse, and contain 250 mg Primidone BP.

Mysoline Oral Suspension is a white, pleasantly flavoured aqueous suspension which contains 250 mg Primidone BP per 5 ml.

Uses Mysoline is indicated in the management of grand mal and psychomotor (temporal lobe) epilepsy. It is also of value in the management of focal or Jacksonian seizures, petit mal, myoclonic jerks and akinetic attacks.

Dosage and administration Mysoline is given by mouth. Treatment must always be planned on an individual basis. In many patients it will be possible to use Mysoline alone, but in some, Mysoline will need to be combined with other anticonvulsants or with supporting therapy.

Begin with ½ tablet once daily late in the evening. Every three days increase the daily dosage by ½ tablet until the patient is receiving 2 tablets daily. Thereafter, every three days increase the daily dosage by 1 tablet in adults or ½ tablet in children under 9 years – until control is obtained or the maximum tolerated dosage is being

given. This may be as much as 6 tablets a day in adults; 4 tablets a day in children.

Average daily maintenance doses:

	Tablets (250 mg) or 5 ml measures of suspension (250 mg/5 ml)	Milligrams
Adults and children over 9 years	3–6	750–1,500
Children 6–9 years	3–4	750–1,000
Children 2–5 years	2–3	500–750
Children up to 2 years	1–2	250–500

The total daily dose is usually best divided and given in two equal amounts, one in the morning and the other in the evening. In certain patients, it may be considered advisable to give a larger dose when the seizures are more frequent. For instance: 1) if the attacks are nocturnal then all or most of the day's dose may be given in the evening; 2) if the attacks are associated with some particular event such as menstruation, a slight increase in the appropriate dose is often beneficial.

When it is necessary to give 125 mg of Mysoline Suspension to a small child, it is advisable to dilute the suspension and administer a 5 ml dose.
A suitable diluent is:

Sodium carboxymethyl cellulose (50 cp)	1% w/v
Sucrose	20%
Methylhydroxybenzoate	0.15%
Propylhydroxybenzoate	0.015%
Water	to 100%

Elderly patients: It is advisable to monitor elderly patients with reduced renal function who are receiving primidone.

Patients on other Anticonvulsants: Where a patient's attacks are not sufficiently well controlled with other anticonvulsants, or disturbing side effects have arisen, 'Mysoline' may be used to augment or replace existing treatment. First add 'Mysoline' to the current anticonvulsant treatment by the method of gradual introduction described previously. When a worthwhile effect has been achieved and the amount of 'Mysoline' being given has been built up to at least half the estimated requirement, withdrawal of the previous treatment can then be attempted. This should be done gradually over a period of two weeks, during which time it may be necessary to increase the 'Mysoline' dosage to maintain control. Withdrawal of previous treatment should not be too rapid or status epilepticus may occur. Where phenobarbitone formed the major part of the previous treatment, however, both its withdrawal and 'Mysoline' substitution should be made earlier, so as to prevent excessive drowsiness from interfering with accurate assessment of the optimun dosage of 'Mysoline'.

Contra-indications, warnings, etc Primidone should not be administered to patients with acute intermittent porphyria. The drug should be given with caution and may be required in reduced dosage in children, the elderly, debilitated patients or those with impaired renal, hepatic or respiratory function.

Patients who exhibit hypersensitivity or an allergic reaction to primidone should not receive the drug.

Primidone is a potent CNS depressant and is partially metabolised to phenobarbitone. After prolonged administration there is a potential for tolerance, dependence and a withdrawal reaction on abrupt cessation of treatment.

During breast feeding the baby should be monitored for sedation.

Both primidone and its major metabolite phenobarbitone induce liver enzyme activity. This may lead to altered pharmacokinetics in concomitantly administered drugs including other anticonvulsants such as phenytoin and coumarin anticoagulants.

The effects of other CNS depressants such as alcohol and barbiturates may be enhanced by the administration of primidone.

Pregnancy: There is some evidence of a higher than average incidence of congenital abnormalities in infants born of epileptic mothers. The precise factors influencing this are unknown, but the possibility that anticonvulsant therapy may be involved and the very slight risk of an abnormal foetus must be weighed against the risks of withholding treatment during pregnancy.

As with most other anticonvulsants, patients who drive vehicles or operate machinery should be aware of the possibility of impaired reaction time.

Long-term anticonvulsant therapy can be associated with decreased serum folate levels. As folic acid requirements are also increased during pregnancy, regular screening of patients at risk is advised, and treatment with folic acid and vitamin B_{12}, although controversial, should be considered.

Anticonvulsant therapy in pregnancy has occasionally been associated with coagulation disorders in the neonates. For this reason pregnant patients should be given vitamin K_1 through the last month of pregnancy up to the time of delivery. In the absence of such pretreatment then 10 mg vitamin K_1 may be given to the mother at the time of delivery, and 1 mg should be given immediately to the neonate at risk.

Breakthrough bleeding and failure of contraceptive therapy have been noted in patients taking anticonvulsant drugs and oral contraceptive steroids. This is usually assumed to be due to induction of liver enzymes by the anticonvulsant with accelerated breakdown of the hormones.

Side-effects: If side-effects do appear they are generally confined to the early stages of treatment when patients frequently feel drowsy and listless.

Symptoms of neurotoxicity such as visual disturbances, nausea, headache, vomiting, nystagmus and ataxia have been reported but are usually transient even when pronounced. On occasions an idiosyncratic reaction may occur which involves these symptoms in an acute and severe form necessitating withdrawal of treatment. Dermatological reactions are infrequent and usually occur at the onset of therapy. Rarely personality changes, which may include psychotic reactions have been reported.

Other rare side-effects include oedema of the legs, thirst and polyuria and impairment of sexual potency. Exceptionally, as with phenytoin and phenobarbitone, megaloblastic anaemia may develop requiring discontinuation of primidone. This condition may respond to treatment with folic acid and/or Vitamin B_{12}. There have been isolated reports of other blood dyscrasias.

Overdosage: Primidone is metabolised extensively to phenobarbitone and overdosage leads to varying degrees of CNS depression which, depending on the dose ingested, may include ataxia, loss of consciousness, respiratory depression and coma. Treatment should

include aspiration of stomach contents and general supportive measures. There is no specific antidote.

Pharmaceutical precautions Store at room temperature.

Legal category POM.

Package quantities *Tablets 250 mg:* Containers of 100 and 1,000.
Suspension (250 mg/5 ml): Bottles of 250 ml and 2 litres.

Further information Nil.

Product licence numbers
Mysoline Tablets   0029/5074
Mysoline Oral Suspension   0029/5072

NASEPTIN*

Presentation A non-greasy, white, water-miscible cream containing 0.1% w/w Chlorhexidine Hydrochloride BP and 0.5% w/w Neomycin Sulphate PhEur.

Uses Naseptin is an antiseptic cream, intended for application to the nares. It can be used for: (1) Treatment of staphylococcal infections in general practice (e.g. removing the source of infections which cause recurrent boils, styes etc); (2) prophylaxis against nasal-carriage of staphylococci by hospital staff, patients and newborn infants.

Dosage and administration The following recommendations apply both to adults and children. A small amount of Naseptin, about the size of a match-head, is placed on the little finger and applied to the inside of each nostril. By squeezing the nares the cream is then spread forward into the vestibule. A smooth glass rod or swab may be used for application to infants or patients who are very ill.

For prophylaxis: Naseptin is applied as above, twice daily, to prevent patients from becoming carriers and to inhibit the dispersion of staphylococci.

For eradication of infection: Naseptin is applied four times daily for 10 days to eliminate organisms from the nares.

Contra-indications, warnings, etc
Contra-indications: Naseptin is contra-indicated for patients who have previously shown a hypersensitivity reaction to either chlorhexidine or neomycin. However, such reactions are extremely rare.

Precautions: For nasal application only. Keep out of the eyes and ears.

Prolonged use of neomycin preparations can lead to skin sensitisation, ototoxicity and nephrotoxicity.

Side-effects: Irritative skin reactions and hypersensitivity can occasionally occur. Generalised allergic reactions to chlorhexidine have also been reported but are extremely rare. In such cases the use of Naseptin must be discontinued and if necessary symptomatic treatment given.

Accidental ingestion: Accidental ingestion of the contents of a Naseptin tube is not likely to have any adverse effect on the patient; neomycin is routinely taken orally, and chlorhexidine hydrochloride is poorly absorbed by this route.

Pharmaceutical precautions Store at room temperature and use undiluted.

Chlorhexidine is incompatible with anionic agents.

Hypochlorite bleaches may cause brown stains to develop in fabrics which have previously been in contact with chlorhexidine preparations.

Legal category POM.

Package quantities Tubes of 5 g.

Further information Nil.

Product licence number 0029/5009.

NOLVADEX*

Presentation White, round, bi-convex tablets, marked with Nolvadex 10 on one face and ICI on the reverse. Each tablet contains Tamoxifen Citrate BP equivalent to 10 mg of tamoxifen.

Uses At the recommended doses Nolvadex has anti-oestrogenic properties and competes with oestrogen for binding sites in target organs. It does not have androgenic properties.

Nolvadex is indicated for:

1. The treatment of breast cancer. The proportion of patients with breast cancer who respond to Nolvadex is similar to that seen with oestrogens or androgens. However, because Nolvadex produces fewer serious side-effects it is more acceptable to the patient.

2. The treatment of anovulatory infertility.

Dosage and administration

1. *Breast cancer:* The dose range is 20 to 40 mg given as either 10 mg or 20 mg twice daily.

2. *Infertility:* Before commencing any course of treatment, whether initial or subsequent, the possibility of pregnancy must be excluded. In women who are menstruating regularly, but with anovular cycles the initial course of treatment consists of twice-daily doses of 10 mg (1 tablet) of Nolvadex given on the second, third, fourth and fifth days of the menstrual cycle. If unsatisfactory basal temperature records or poor pre-ovulatory cervical mucus indicate that this initial course of treatment has been unsuccessful, further courses may be given during subsequent menstrual periods, increasing the dosage to 20 mg and then to 40 mg twice daily.

In women who are not menstruating regularly the initial course may begin on any day. If no signs of ovulation are demonstrated then a subsequent course of treatment may start 45 days later with dosage increased as above. If a patient responds with menstruation then the next course of treatment is commenced on the second day of the cycle.

Elderly patients: Similar dosing regimes of Nolvadex have been used in elderly patients with breast cancer and in some of these patients it has been used as sole therapy.

Contra-indications, warnings, etc *Pregnancy:* Nolvadex must not be given during pregnancy. Pre-menopausal patients must be carefully examined before treatment for breast cancer or infertility to exclude the possibility of pregnancy.

Menstruation is suppressed in a proportion of pre-menopausal women receiving Nolvadex for the treatment of breast cancer. Reversible cystic ovarian swelling has very occasionally been observed when such women have been treated with 40 mg Nolvadex twice daily for short periods.

A small number of patients with bony metastases have developed hypercalcaemia on initiation of therapy.

Side-effects: During long-term treatment side-effects are not as numerous or as serious with Nolvadex as with the androgens and oestrogens which are also used to treat breast cancer. Those that have been reported can be classified as either due to the anti-oestrogenic action of the drug, e.g. hot flushes, vaginal bleeding, and pruritus vulvae, or as more general effects, e.g. gastro-intestinal intolerance, tumour flare, light-headedness and, occasionally, fluid retention.

When side-effects are severe it is sometimes possible to control them by a simple reduction of dosage without loss of control of the disease. If side-effects do not respond to this measure, it may be necessary to stop the treatment.

Transient falls in platelet count, usually only to 80 000–90 000 but occasionally lower, have been reported in patients taking Nolvadex for breast cancer. No haemorrhagic tendency has been reported and the platelet counts have recovered even though treatment with Nolvadex has continued.

A small number of cases of visual disturbance, corneal changes and/or retinopathy have been described, mainly in patients treated with exceptionally high doses for long periods of time.

There have been infrequent reports of thromboembolic events occurring during Nolvadex therapy. As an increased incidence of these events is known to occur in patients with malignant disease, a causal relationship with Nolvadex has not been established.

Overdosage: On theoretical grounds an overdosage would be expected to cause enhancement of the anti-oestrogenic side-effects mentioned above. Observations in animals show that extreme overdosage (100–200 × recommended daily dose) may produce oestrogenic effects.

There is no specific antidote to overdosage, and treatment must be symptomatic.

Pharmaceutical precautions Store at room temperature protected from light.

Legal category POM.

Package quantities Nolvadex is packed in containers of 30 and 250 tablets.

Further information Nil.

Product licence number 0029/0064.

NOLVADEX*-D

Presentation White, octagonal, biconvex tablets, marked with 'Nolvadex D' on one face and ICI on the obverse. The tablets are formulated for once daily dosing. Each tablet contains Tamoxifen Citrate BP equivalent to 20 mg of tamoxifen.

Uses At the recommended doses Nolvadex-D has anti-oestrogenic properties, and it competes with oestrogen for binding sites in target organs. It does not have androgenic properties.

Nolvadex-D is indicated for:

1. The treatment of breast cancer. The proportion of patients with breast cancer who respond to Nolvadex-D is similar to that seen with oestrogens or androgens. However, because Nolvadex-D produces fewer serious side-effects it is more acceptable to the patient.

2. The treatment of anovulatory infertility.

Dosage and administration

1. *Breast Cancer:* The dose range is 20 to 40 mg given as either 20 or 40 mg once daily.

2. *Infertility:* Before commencing any course of treatment, whether initial or subsequent, the possibility of pregnancy must be excluded. In women who are menstruating regularly but with anovular cycles the initial course of treatment consists of once daily doses of 20 mg (1 tablet) of Nolvadex-D given on the second, third, fourth and fifth days of the menstrual cycle. If unsatisfactory basal temperature records or poor preovulatory cervical mucus indicate that this initial course of treatment has been unsuccessful, further courses may be given during subsequent menstrual periods, increasing the dosage to 40 mg and then to 80 mg daily.

In women who are not menstruating regularly the initial course may begin on any day. If no signs of ovulation are demonstrable then a subsequent course of treatment may start 45 days later with dosage increased as above. If a patient responds with menstruation then the next course of treatment is commenced on the second day of the cycle.

Elderly patients: Similar dosing regimes of Nolvadex have been used in elderly patients with breast cancer and in some of these patients it has been used as sole therapy.

Contra-indications, warnings, etc Nolvadex-D must not be given during pregnancy. Pre-menopausal patients must be carefully examined before treatment for breast cancer or infertility to exclude the possibility of pregnancy.

Menstruation is suppressed in a proportion of pre-menopausal women receiving Nolvadex-D for the treatment of breast cancer. Reversible cystic ovarian swellings have very occasionally been observed when such women have been treated with 40 mg twice daily for short periods.

A small number of patients with bony metastases have developed hypercalcaemia on initiation of therapy.

Side-effects: During long-term treatment side-effects are not as numerous or as serious with Nolvadex-D as with the androgens and oestrogens which are also used to treat breast cancer. Those that have been reported can be classified as either due to the anti-oestrogenic action of the drug, e.g. hot flushes, vaginal bleeding, and pruritus vulvae, or as more general effects, e.g. gastro-intestinal intolerance, tumour flare, light-headedness and, occasionally, fluid retention.

When side-effects are severe it is sometimes possible to control them by a simple reduction of dosage without loss of control of the disease. If side-effects do not respond to this measure, it may be necessary to stop the treatment.

Transient falls in platelet count, usually only to 80,000–90,000 but occasionally lower, have been reported in patients taking tamoxifen for breast cancer. No haemorrhagic tendency has been reported and the platelet counts have recovered even though treatment with the drug has continued.

A small number of cases of visual disturbance corneal changes and/or retinopathy, have been described, mainly in patients treated with exceptionally high doses for long periods of time.

There have been infrequent reports of thromboembolic events occurring during Nolvadex therapy. As an increased incidence of these events is known to occur in patients with malignant disease, a causal relationship with Nolvadex has not been established.

Overdosage: On theoretical grounds an overdosage would be expected to cause enhancement of the anti-oestrogenic side-effects mentioned above. Observations in animals show that extreme overdosage (100–$200 \times$ recommended daily dose) may produce oestrogenic effects.

There is no specific antidote to overdosage, and treatment must be symptomatic.

Pharmaceutical precautions Store at room temperature protected from light.

Legal category POM.

Package quantities Nolvadex-D is packed in containers of 30 and 250 tablets.

Further information Nil.

Product licence number 0029/0155.

NOLVADEX*-FORTE

Presentation White, elongated, octagonal tablets marked with Nolvadex-Forte on one side and bisected on the other side with the letters ICI in each segment. Each tablet contains Tamoxifen Citrate BP equivalent to 40 mg of tamoxifen.

Uses At the recommended dosage Nolvadex-Forte has anti-oestrogenic properties and it competes with oestrogen for binding sites in target organs. It does not have androgenic properties.

Nolvadex-Forte is indicated for:

1. The treatment of breast cancer. The proportion of patients with breast cancer who respond to Nolvadex-Forte is similar to that seen with oestrogens or androgens. However, because Nolvadex-Forte produces fewer serious side effects, it is more acceptable to the patient.

2. The treatment of anovulatory infertility.

Dosage and administration

1. *Breast Cancer:* The daily dose is 20 to 40 mg given as a single dose.

2. *Infertility:* Before commencing any course of treatment, whether initial or subsequent, the possibility of pregnancy must be excluded. In women who are menstruating regularly, but with anovular cycles, the initial course of treatment consists of 20 mg given daily on the second, third, fourth and fifth days of the menstrual cycle. If unsatisfactory basal temperature records or poor pre-ovulatory cervical mucus indicate that this initial course of treatment has been unsuccessful, further courses may be given during subsequent menstrual periods, increasing the dosage to 40 mg and then to 80 mg daily.

In women who are not menstruating regularly, the initial course may begin on any day. If no signs of ovulation are demonstrable, then a subsequent course of treatment may start 45 days later, with dosage increased as above. If a patient responds with menstruation, then the next course of treatment is commenced on the second day of the cycle.

Elderly patients: Similar dosing regimes of Nolvadex have been used in elderly patients with breast cancer and in some of these patients it has been used as sole therapy.

Contra-indications, warnings, etc
Pregnancy: Nolvadex-Forte must not be given during pregnancy. Premenopausal patients must be carefully examined before treatment for breast cancer or infertility to exclude the possibility of pregnancy.

Menstruation is suppressed in a proportion of premenopausal women receiving Nolvadex-Forte for the treatment of breast cancer. Reversible cystic ovarian swellings have very occasionally been observed when such women have been treated with 40 mg twice daily for short periods.

A small number of patients with bony metastases have developed hypercalcaemia on initiation of therapy.

Side-effects: During long-term treatment, side-effects are not as numerous or as serious as with the androgens and oestrogens which are also used to treat breast cancer. Those that have been reported can be classified as either due to the anti-oestrogenic action of the drug, e.g. hot flushes, vaginal bleeding, and pruritus vulvae, or as more general effects, e.g. gastro-intestinal intolerance, tumour flare, lightheadedness and, occasionally, fluid retention. When side-effects are severe, it is sometimes possible to control them by a simple reduction of dosage without loss of control of the disease. If side-effects do not respond to this measure, it may be necessary to stop the treatment.

Transient falls in platelet count, usually only to 80,000–90,000 but occasionally lower, have been reported in patients taking tamoxifen for breast cancer. No haemorrhagic tendency has been reported and the platelet counts have recovered even though treatment with the drug has continued.

A small number of cases of visual disturbance, corneal changes and/or retinopathy have been described, mainly in patients treated with exceptionally high doses for long periods of time.

There have been infrequent reports of thromboembolic events occurring during Nolvadex therapy. As an increased incidence of these events is known to occur in patients with malignant disease, a causal relationship with Nolvadex has not been established.

Overdosage: On theoretical grounds, an overdosage would be expected to cause enhancement of the anti-oestrogenic side effects mentioned above. Observations in animals show that extreme overdosage (100–200 times recommended daily dose) may produce oestrogenic effects.

There is no specific antidote to overdosage, and treatment must be symptomatic.

Pharmaceutical precautions Store at room temperature protected from light.

Legal category POM.

Package quantities Nolvadex-Forte is packed in containers of 30 tablets.

Further information Nil.

Product licence number 0029/0176.

PALUDRINE* TABLETS
Presentation White, bi-convex tablets marked with the ICI roundel on one side and bisected on the other

side with a letter P in each segment. Each tablet contains 100 mg of Proguanil Hydrochloride BP.

Uses Paludrine is an effective antimalarial agent. It is recommended for the prevention and suppression of malaria.

Dosage and administration *Adults:* The standard dosage is 1 tablet of 100 mg daily. In highly endemic areas this dose may be safely increased to 2 tablets daily. The daily dose is best taken with water after food. Non-immune subjects entering a malarious region are advised to begin treatment with Paludrine 24 hours before arrival. A daily dose of Paludrine should be continued for six weeks after leaving the area.

Children: Under 1 year: $\frac{1}{4}$ tablet (25 mg) daily.

   1–4 years: $\frac{1}{2}$ tablet (50 mg) daily.

   5–8 years: $\frac{3}{4}$ tablet (75 mg) daily.

   9–12 years: 1 tablet (100 mg) daily.

   Over 12 years: Adult dose daily.

Provided the tablet fragment gives the minimum amount specified precise accuracy in children's dosage is not essential, since the drug possesses a wide safety margin. For a young child, the dose may be administered crushed and mixed with milk, honey or jam.

Elderly patients: There are no special dosage recommendations for the elderly, but it may be advisable to monitor elderly patients so that optimum dosage can be individually determined.

Contra-indications, warnings, etc Paludrine should be used with caution in patients with severe renal failure.

Pregnancy: It is generally accepted that all drug treatment should be avoided if possible during the first trimester of pregnancy and medical advice sought. Paludrine has been widely used for over 30 years and a causal connection between its use and any adverse effect on mother or foetus has never been established.

Side-effects: At normal dosage levels the side-effect most commonly encountered is mild gastric intolerance. This usually subsides as treatment is continued.

Overdosage: The following effects have been reported in cases of overdosage: haematuria, renal irritation, epigastric discomfort and vomiting.

There is no specific antidote, and symptoms should be treated as they arise.

Pharmaceutical precautions Store at room temperature.

Legal category P.

Package quantities Containers of 100 and 1,000.

Further information In any locality where drug-resistant malaria is known or suspected, it is essential to take local medical advice on what prophylactic regimen is appropriate.

Product licence number 0029/5079.

PEPTAVLON*
Presentation Peptavlon (Pentagastrin Injection BP) is a clear, colourless, sterile, isotonic solution containing 250 mcg/ml of Pentagastrin BP. It is packed in neutral, clear glass ampoules which each contain 500 mcg of Pentagastrin BP in 2 ml of solution.

Uses Peptavlon is an analogue of the C-terminal

tetrapeptide sequence of the hormone gastrin which stimulates gastric secretion. It exhibits all the physiological effects of the natural hormone. Peptavlon is used for the diagnostic testing of gastric secretion.

Dosage and administration The following procedure is adopted for testing gastric secretion with Peptavlon.

The patient receives no medication (e.g. antacids, etc.) that might affect the results of the tests for 24 hours and no food for 12 hours before the test. On the morning of the test a radio-opaque tube (Leven No. 7 or Ryle's 12-16Fr) is passed into the patient's stomach by way of the nose. Radiological observation is used to ensure that the tube is correctly positioned in the lower part of the body of the stomach.

The tube is securely fastened to the patient's nose and forehead with adhesive tape to ensure that it is not displaced. The patient lies on his left side.

The gastric juices are then collected by applying continuous suction (at 30–50 mm Hg below atmospheric pressure) to this tube, supplemented by manual suction. The patient takes occasional deep breaths to improve collection. The basal secretion is obtained by collecting samples at 15 minute intervals over an hour.

Peptavlon is then given, either at a dose of (a) 6 mcg/kg body weight subcutaneously, or (b) 0.6 mcg/kg/hour as a continuous intravenous infusion. A Tuberculin syringe is used to give a dose correct to 0.01 ml.

Specimens of the gastric juice are again collected, over periods of 10 or 15 minutes. The volume of the sample is measured and it is immediately filtered through gauze into a bottle. The acidity of each sample is determined by titration. The same doses and method may be used in both adults and children. If dilution is required normal saline may be used.

Contra-indications, warnings, etc When the patient has previously shown a severe idiosyncratic response to the drug, Peptavlon should not be administered.

Pregnancy: Peptavlon should not be administered during pregnancy.

Side-effects: At the recommended dosage the incidence of side-effects is extremely small, although very occasionally an individual may respond with hypotension and associated faintness. Other unwanted effects reported are mild abdominal discomfort, abdominal cramps, nausea, vomiting, flushing, sweating, headaches, drowsiness or exhaustion, heaviness or weakness of the legs, allergic reactions, bradycardia, tachycardia. These effects disappear once administration of Peptavlon has ceased.

Overdosage; The form of presentation makes it unlikely that overdosage will occur, and no such occurrence has been reported. As maximal secretory response is produced by the normal dosage, increased dosage would be expected to have no sequel other than an accentuation of the known side-effects.

Pharmaceutical precautions Peptavlon ampoules must be kept below 4°C but above freezing point and protected from light. If dilution is required Sodium Chloride Injection BP may be used. This solution should be prepared immediately before it is required for use.

Legal category POM.

Package quantities Ampoules containing 2 ml Peptavlon, supplied in boxes of 5.

Further information Nil.

Product licence number 0029/5013.

PRIMAQUINE PHOSPHATE TABLETS

Presentation Primaquine phosphate is presented as brown, bi-convex, sugar-coated tablets, which each contain 13.2 mg of Primaquine Phosphate BP (equivalent to 7.5 mg of base).

Uses Primaquine phosphate is an antimalarial drug belonging to the 8-aminoquinoline group. It is indicated for the radical cure of vivax and quartan malaria.

Dosage and administration *Adults:* A daily dose of 2 tablets is given for 10–14 days.

Children: The following dosage scheme has been found satisfactory:

up to 15 lb body weight: 1 mg daily for 14 days.

16–60 lb body weight: 2–4 mg daily for 14 days.

61–90 lb body weight: 5–7.5 mg daily for 14 days.

Over 90 lb body weight: As for adult dosage.

Elderly patients: There are no special dosage recommendations for the elderly, but it may be advisable to monitor elderly patients so that optimum dosage can be individually determined.

Contra-indications, warnings, etc To terminate overt attacks of malaria a schizonticidal drug such as Avloclor* (chloroquine phosphate) should be given.

Caution is necessary when giving primaquine to non-Caucasian patients since from 5% to 10% of these have a genetic deficiency which makes them liable to develop blood dyscrasias on taking the drug. Initially only low doses of primaquine should be given to non-Caucasian patients. Further increments are then made to reach the therapeutic dose. During this period frequent blood examinations should be made to detect the possible occurrence of haemolytic anaemia or methaemoglobinaemia.

Pregnancy; If vivax malaria occurs during pregnancy a curative course of chloroquine should be given and radical cure with primaquine delayed until after delivery.

Side-effects: When used within the recommended dosage range, toxic effects need not be expected in lightly pigmented races. However, in deeply pigmented patients the same doses may occasionally produce haemolytic anaemia. If blood dyscrasias develop (haemolytic anaemia or methaemoglobinaemia) treatment should be stopped.

Overdosage; The symptoms of overdosage include anorexia, nausea, epigastric distress, abdominal cramps, occasional vomiting, weakness, cyanosis, haemolytic anaemia and jaundice, bone marrow depression and methaemoglobinaemia.

There is no specific antidote and treatment must therefore be symptomatic.

Pharmaceutical precautions Store at room temperature, protected from light and moisture.

Legal category P.

Package quantities Containers of 1,000 tablets.

Further information Nil.

Product licence number 0029/5081.

RAZOXIN* ▼

Presentation Razoxin Tablets, each containing 125 mg razoxane, are white to pale cream, and marked on one side with the ICI roundel and a bisection line on the other.

Uses In contrast to most anti-cancer agents Razoxin interferes with cell division at the G_2M phase of the cycle.

Razoxin in combination with radiotherapy may be used for all forms of soft-tissue, chondro- and osteo-sarcomas. In comparison with radiotherapy alone, this combination may increase the response rate and reduce recurrence. Razoxin can produce remissions in previous radio-resistant lesions.

Razoxin may be useful alone or in combination with other antimitotic agents in the treatment of malignant lymphomas, including mycosis fungoides, acute leukaemias, especially the acute blast cell-crisis of chronic myeloid leukaemia, and Kaposi's sarcoma. Experience to date has been in open studies which indicated that the product is of value in patients in whom previous therapies have been unsuccessful.

Dosage and administration *Note:* Because of an association between administration of Razoxin and the development of acute myeloid leukaemia or skin epitheliomata, the drug should only be used in the above malignant conditions and then when its administration is essential such as when other treatments have failed.

Adults and children: Razoxin is administered orally. The following guidelines are based on the regimens with which responses have been obtained. In all regimens, if unacceptable degrees of leucopenia thrombocytopenia or gastrointestinal disturbance occur, the dosage of Razoxin should be reduced or temporarily withdrawn to allow recovery.

Soft-tissue, Osteo- and Chondro-sarcomata: 125 mg (1 tablet) twice daily 3 days before the start of radiotherapy, continued throughout that therapy. On days when radiation is given, 1 tablet of Razoxin should be taken 1–4 hours before radiotherapy; the other tablet in the evening. The dosage of radiation should be selected and administered using normal criteria.

Malignant lymphomas (including mycosis fungoides): 0.5 to 1.5g/m²/week should be administered orally as long as a remission is maintained. For example the dosage can be given as:

(a) 125 mg (1 tablet) twice daily on 3–5 days/week or
(b) three doses of 375 mg (3 tablets) given eight hours apart and repeated weekly

If an inadequate response is obtained the dosage may be increased, provided that the white cell count permits.

Acute leukaemias (including blast cell crisis of chronic myeloid leukaemia): 150–500 mg/m²/day for 3–5 days. Treatment should be repeated at 14–28 day intervals, depending on the peripheral blood count. Allopurinol may also be given to prevent uric acid deposition.

Kaposi's sarcoma: 333 mg/m² three times daily for 3 days every 3 weeks, and adjusted as necessary according to peripheral blood count.

Elderly patients: There are no special dosage recommendations for the elderly, but it may be advisable to monitor elderly patients so that optimum dosage can be individually determined.

Contra-indications, warnings, etc Razoxin is contra-indicated in the treatment of non-malignant conditions such as psoriasis.

Mice and rats developed tumours following long term intraperitoneal administration of Razoxin. There is an association between the development of acute myeloid leukaemia or skin epitheliomata and the administration of Razoxin in man.

Razoxin is contra-indicated in pregnancy because of its action on cell division. Animal studies have revealed abnormalities of foetal development. It should not normally be administered to mothers who are breast feeding.

The peripheral blood count should be monitored throughout Razoxin therapy. Unacceptable degrees of leucopenia or thrombocytopenia are quickly reversed on cessation of treatment. Unacceptable degrees of myelo-suppression are more likely to occur in patients who have received extensive chemotherapy previously.

Side-effects: The principal reported side-effects include leucopenia, thrombocytopenia, nausea, vomiting, diarrhoea, skin reactions and alopecia. Early skin reactions in patients receiving Razoxin plus radiotherapy may be more marked than those expected from radiotherapy alone. Severe late subcutaneous fibrosis has been reported in some patients receiving the combined therapy. There appears to be an increased likelihood of oesophagitis and pneumonitis in patients who require radiotherapy for thoracic lesions.

Overdosage: In cases of overdosage, signs and symptoms are likely to be qualitatively similar to side-effects; there is no specific antidote and treatment must be symptomatic.

Pharmaceutical precautions Store at room temperature, protected from light and moisture.

It is recommended that adequate protective gloves be worn when handling Razoxin Tablets and that Razoxin tablets should not be handled by pregnant staff.

Legal category POM.

Package quantities Containers of 30 tablets.

Further information In contrast to most anti-cancer agents, Razoxin interferes with cell division at the G_2M phase of the cell cycle and in multiple-drug chemotherapy regimens, it is logical to combine razoxane with agents acting at the other phases in the cell cycle.

Product licence number 0029/0065.

SAVLOCLENS*

Presentation An amber yellow aqueous solution containing 0.05% w/v chlorhexidine gluconate (equivalent to 0.25% v/v Chlorhexidine Gluconate Solution BP) and 0.5% cetrimide (incorporated as Strong Cetrimide Solution BP). A ready-to-use solution in sachets and bottles sterilised by autoclaving.

Uses A broad spectrum antiseptic with added detergent properties. Savloclens is used for cleansing and disinfecting physically contaminated wounds and burns.

Dosage and administration Apply to treatment area without further dilution.

Contra-indications, warnings, etc
Contra-indications: Savloclens is contra-indicated for patients who have previously shown a hypersensitivity

reaction to either chlorhexidine or cetrimide. However, such reactions are extremely rare.

Precautions: For external use only. Keep out of the eyes and avoid contact with the brain, meninges or middle ear.

Do not inject. Do not use in body cavities or as an enema.

Side-effects: Irritative skin reactions can occasionally occur and rare hypersensitivity to cetrimide preparations, usually developing after repeated application, has been reported. Generalised allergic reactions to chlorhexidine have also been reported but are extremely rare.

Accidental ingestion: Do not give alcohol in any form. Carry out a gastric lavage with milk, egg-white, gelatin or mild soap. Do not induce vomiting. Employ supportive measures as appropriate.

Accidental intravenous transfusion: Blood transfusion may be necessary to counteract haemolysis.

Pharmaceutical precautions Store at room temperature. Use contents immediately after opening – do not keep any surplus solution.

Hypochlorite bleaches may cause brown stains to develop in fabrics which have previously been in contact with chlorhexidine solutions. Detailed literature is available on request.

Savloclens is incompatible with anionic agents.

Legal category P.

Package quantities Packs of 60 × 100 ml individual sachets.

Further information The British Pharmaceutical Codex (1973) recommends that antiseptics applied to broken skin should be sterile. The use of Savloclens complies with this recommendation.

Product licence number 0029/0142.

SAVLODIL*

Presentation A clear yellow aqueous solution containing 0.015% w/v chlorhexidine gluconate (equivalent to 0.075% v/v Chlorhexidine Gluconate Solution BP) and 0.15% w/v cetrimide (incorporated as Strong Cetrimide Solution BP). A ready to use solution in sachets and bottles sterilised by autoclaving.

Uses Savlodil is a broad-spectrum antiseptic with detergent properties for swabbing in obstetrics and during dressing changes. For disinfecting and cleansing traumatic and surgical wounds and burns.

Dosage and administration Apply to treatment area without further dilution.

Contra-indications, warnings, etc
Contra-indications: Savlodil is contra-indicated for patients who have previously shown a hypersensitivity reaction to either chlorhexidine or cetrimide. However, such reactions are extremely rare.

Precautions: For external use only. Keep out of the eyes and avoid contact with the brain, meninges or middle ear. Do not inject. Do not use in body cavities or as an enema.

Side-effects: Irritative skin reactions can occasionally occur and rare hypersensitivity to cetrimide preparations, usually developing after repeated application, has been reported. Generalised allergic reactions to chlorhexidine

have also been reported but are extremely rare. In all cases stop application of the product.

Accidental ingestion: Do not give alcohol in any form. Carry out gastric lavage with milk, egg-white, gelatin or mild soap. Do not induce vomiting. Employ supportive measures as appropriate.

Accidental intravenous transfusion: Blood transfusion may be necessary to counteract haemolysis.

Pharmaceutical precautions Store at room temperature. Use contents immediately after opening – do not keep any surplus solution.

Hypochlorite bleaches may cause brown stains to develop in fabrics which have previously been in contact with chlorhexidine solutions. Detailed literature is available on request.

Savlodil is incompatible with anionic agents.

Legal category P.

Package quantities Packs of 250 × 25 ml and 60 × 100 ml individual sachets. Bottles of 500 ml and 1,000 ml.

Further information The British Pharmaceutical Codex (1973) recommends that antiseptic applied to broken skin should be sterile. The use of Savlodil complies with this recommendation.

Product licence number 0029/0114.

SAVLON* HOSPITAL CONCENTRATE

Presentation A deep orange aqueous solution containing 1.5% w/v chlorhexidine gluconate (equivalent to 7.5% v/v Chlorhexidine Gluconate Solution BP) and 15% w/v cetrimide (incorporated as Strong Cetrimide Solution BP).

Uses Savlon Hospital Concentrate is a potent antimicrobial agent for general antiseptic purposes. Activity against a wide range of organisms is combined with useful cleansing properties.

Dosage and administration

Mode of preparation	Dilution rate	Use
10 ml made up to 1 litre with water	1 in 100 (1%) Aqueous	*Patient use –* Cleansing/disinfection of post-operative and casualty wounds.† Antiseptic treatment of burns.† Swabbing in obstetrics, gynaecology and urology. *Inanimates‡ –* Cleansing/disinfectant soak for used metal instruments. Clean instruments disinfection (30 minutes' immersion). Cleansing/disinfection of equipment, furniture and fittings in the vicinity of the patient. Storage of clinical thermometers and sterile instruments.

Mode of preparation	Dilution rate	Use
35 ml made up to 1 litre with water	1 in 30 (approx) Aqueous	*Patient use* Cleansing/disinfection of post-operative woundst and casualty wounds where extra detergency/antimicrobial effects are indicated.† Antiseptic treatment of burns† where this higher strength is indicated. *Inanimates‡ –* Cleansing/disinfectant soak for used items which are normally contaminated with adherent substances, e.g. catheters, rubber appliances, etc.
35 ml with 200 ml water made up to 1 litre with 95% alcohol	1 in 30 (approx) in 70% Alcohol	*Patient use* Skin disinfection before pre-operative and other invasive procedures. *Inanimates‡ –* Disinfection of clean instruments and equipment (two minutes immersion). Disinfection of clinical thermometers.

NB. Savlon Hospital Concentrate is also supplied in 25 ml sachets for addition to patients bath water as a measure to prevent cross infection in hospital.

† Sterilise the dilution by autoclaving at 115–116°C for 30 minutes or 121–123°C for 15 minutes.

‡ Endoscopes should not be introduced into solutions of Savlon.

Contra-indications, warnings, etc

Contra-indications: Savlon solutions are contra-indicated for patients who have previously shown a hypersensitivity reaction to chlorhexidine or cetrimide. However, such reactions are extremely rare.

Precautions: For external use. Dilute before use. Keep out of the eyes and avoid contact with brain, meninges or middle ear. Do not inject. Do not use in body cavities or as an enema.

Syringes and needles which have been immersed in Savlon solutions should be thoroughly rinsed in sterile water or saline before use.

Solutions applied to wounds, burns or broken skin must be sterilised in accordance with BPC recommendations.

After immersion in alcoholic solutions rinse instruments with sterile water or aqueous 0.02% Hibitane before use.

Side-effects: Irritative skin reactions can occasionally occur and rare hypersensitivity to cetrimide preparations, usually developing after repeated application, has been reported. There have been rare reports of severe burn-like reactions to concentrated cetrimide solutions. Should such a reaction occur treat as a chemical burn. Generalised allergic reactions to chlorhexidine have also been reported but are extremely rare. In all cases stop application of the product.

Accidental oral or rectal administration: Fatal poisioning may arise due to the presence of cetrimide when the only pathological signs are visceral congestion, cloudy swelling, mild pulmonary oedema or varying degrees of gastro-intestinal irritation. Severe CNS depression,

sometimes preceded by excitement and convulsions can cause death from respiratory paralysis.

Specific antidotes: Soap, anionic surfactants.

General measures: Do not give alcohol in any form. If the product is swallowed give large quantities of milk, egg-white, gelatin or mild soap. Avoid vomiting or lavage if it is believed that a concentrated solution has been ingested.

Central paralysis cannot be countered by curare antagonists or CNS stimulants but sympathomimetic drugs have been given.

Mechanically assisted ventilation with oxygen may be necessary. Persistent convulsions may be controlled with cautious doses of a short-acting barbiturate.

Accidental intravenous infusion: Massive haemolysis can occur which will require blood transfusion.

Accidental intra-uterine administration: Introduction into the uterus can lead to haemolysis and pulmonary embolism.

Pharmaceutical precautions Dilute with tap water of an acceptable bacteriological standard or alcohol (ethanol, Industrial Methylated Spirit or isopropanol). Add diluent slowly to prevent excessive foaming.

As a precaution against bacterial contamination, aqueous stock solutions should contain at least 4% v/v of isopropanol or 7% v/v of ethanol which may be denatured (i.e. Industrial Methylated Spirit).

Savlon solutions used for instrument storage should contain 0.4% sodium nitrite to inhibit metal corrosion. Such solutions must be changed every 7 days. Prolonged immersion of rubber appliances in Savlon solutions is undesirable.

As cork may protect certain Gram-negative organisms from the action of antiseptics, Savlon solutions must be stored in glass-, plastic- or rubber-stoppered bottles.

Store at room temperature.

Hypochlorite bleaches may cause brown stains to develop in fabrics which have previously been in contact with chlorhexidine. Detailed literature is available on request.

Solutions of Savlon are incompatible with anionic agents.

Legal category GSL.

Package quantities Containers of 1 litre and 5 litres. Laminated foil sachets of 50 × 10 ml and 25 × 25 ml. Dispensers to fit 5L packs are also available.

Further information Nil.

Product licence number 0029/5012.

SULPHAMEZATHINE* INJECTION

Presentation A pale straw-coloured, sterile, aqueous solution containing 1 g Sulphadimidine Sodium BP in 3 ml.

Uses Sulphamezathine is a broad-spectrum bacteriostatic antimicrobial particularly effective in meningococcal meningitis and urinary tract infections.

Dosage and administration Sulphamezathine injection can be given intramuscularly or intravenously. Intramuscular injections should be given deeply because the solution is irritant. The solution should be given intravenously by slow injection into the drip tubing every six hours.

The doses below represent averages and can be modified to suit inidividual needs. In very severe infections both initial and maintenance doses can safely be increased by one third.

	Initial	Maintenance
Adults and children	9 ml	3–4.5 ml (1–1.5 g)
over 16 years:	(3 g)	every six hours
Children	1.5 ml	0.75 ml (0.25 g)
up to 6 months	(0.5 g)	every six hours
6 months–4 years	3 ml	1.5 ml (0.5 g)
	(1 g)	every six hours
4–8 years	4.5 ml	2.25 ml (0.75 g)
	(1.5 g)	every six hours
8–12 years	6 ml	2.25–3.0 ml (0.75–
	(2 g)	1.0 g)
		every six hours
12–16 years	7.5 ml	3–3.75 ml (1–1.25 g)
	(2.5 g)	every six hours

Elderly patients: There are no special dosage recommendations for the elderly, but it may be advisable to monitor elderly patients so that optimum dosage can be individually determined.

Contra-indications, warnings, etc Sulphamezathine is contra-indicated in patients who have previously shown hypersensitivity to sulphonamides. Sulphamezathine must not be administered intrathecally.

Pregnancy: On theoretical grounds all sulphonamides, including 'Sulphamezathine' are contra-indicated in pregnant women and premature infants.

Side-effects: Sulphamezathine is one of the best tolerated and least toxic sulphonamides. Side-effects are infrequent, but may include nausea, vomiting, cyanosis, drug fever, rashes and leucopenia. Isolated reports have been received of crystalluria, haematuria and short-lasting anuria.

Overdosage: Give sodium bicarbonate 10 g every hour orally, or continuous intravenous infusion of one-sixth molar sodium lactate (1.87%). Ensure a high fluid intake to produce at least 1.5 litres of urine daily.

Pharmaceutical precautions Protect from light.

Legal category POM.

Package quantities Ampoules 3 ml. Boxes of 25.

Further information Nil.

Product licence number 0029/5033.

SYNALAR* CREAM
SYNALAR* OINTMENT
SYNANDONE* CREAM
SYNANDONE* OINTMENT
SYNALAR* FORTE CREAM

Presentation Synalar and Synandone are presented as white, water-miscible creams and greasy ointments. Synalar Forte is presented as a white, water-miscible cream.

Synalar, Synandone and Synalar Forte (referred to as Synalar Preparations below) are presentations of the steroid Fluocinolone Acetonide BP.

The following percentages of this corticosteroid are contained in the three preparations:

Synandone   0.01% w/w fluocinolone acetonide

Synalar   0.025% w/w fluocinolone acetonide
Synalar Forte   0.2% w/w fluocinolone acetonide

Uses Synalar preparations contain an effective topical corticosteroid, and are suitable for treating a wide variety of local inflammatory, pruritic and allergic disorders of the skin. Synalar is particularly suitable for topical application in:

Eczema and dermatitis; atopic eczema, seborrhoeic eczema, discoid eczema, pompholyx, otitis externa, contact dermatitis, neurodermatitis, intertrigo.

Non-specific ano-genital pruritis; prurigo.

Psoriasis. Lichen planus. Discoid lupus erythematosus.

Synandone is indicated for milder forms of these conditions; for maintenance therapy when control has been achieved with Synalar; for use under occlusive dressings; and for paediatric dermatology, e.g. infantile eczema.

Synalar Forte is a more concentrated preparation and is useful in intractable skin conditions, particularly: mycosis fungoides, chronic discoid lupus erythematosus and localised conditions, e.g. pretibial myxoedema, necrobiosis lipoidica diabeticorum and granuloma annulare.

Dosage and administration A small quantity of the Synalar preparation is applied lightly to the affected area two or three times a day, and massaged gently and thoroughly into the skin. When an occlusive dressing is required, the affected area should first be thoroughly cleansed, the Synalar preparation is then applied and covered with a suitable plastic dressing.

In some cases the application of hot, moist compresses may be an advantage. The creams are particularly suitable for moist or weeping surfaces and for flexures of the body. The ointments are suitable for dry, scaly lesions.

These recommendations apply to both children and adults.

Contra-indications, warnings, etc Synalar preparations are contra-indicated in primary infections of the skin caused by bacteria, fungi or viruses and in rosacea, acne and perioral dermatitis.

Long-term continuous topical steroid therapy can produce local atrophic skin changes. Particular care should therefore be taken if applying steroids to the face. Prolonged use of topical steroids or treatment of extensive areas, even without occlusion, can result in sufficient absorption of the steroid to produce the features of adrenal suppression, especially in infants and children. When there is an infection associated with an inflammatory skin condition, Synalar preparations should only be administered if adequate anti-infective cover is given.

The amount of Synalar Forte used under occlusion should be restricted to 2 g per day.

Treatment should be discontinued if unfavourable reactions are seen.

Pregnancy: Topical administration of corticosteroids to pregnant animals has been shown to cause abnormalities of foetal development. Although the relevance of this finding to human application has not been established, when topical steroid treatment is considered necessary during pregnancy both the amount applied and the length of treatment should be minimised.

Side-effects: With Synalar preparations, side-effects are extremely rare, but, as with all topical corticosteroids, the occasional patient may show an adverse reaction such as hypersensitivity. Extensive treatment can result in both local atrophic changes, such as striae, skin thinning and telangiectasia and systemic effects such as adrenal suppression.

The use of topical steroids on infected lesions, without the addition of appropriate anti-infective therapy, can result in the spread of opportunist infections.

Accidental ingestion: The 50 g tube of Synalar contains 12.5 mg of the steroid, other tubes containing proportionately less. No toxic effects are likely to occur even if the full contents of a 50 g tube are ingested. Similarly the ingredients of the base are unlikely to have any toxic effect in the quantities in which they occur. Therefore no remedial action is required in the event of accidental ingestion.

Pharmaceutical precautions Store at room temperature and use undiluted.

Legal category POM.

Package quantities

	Dispensing packs – tubes			Hospital pack only
	15 g	30 g	50 g	500 g
Synalar	†	†	†	†
Synandone		†		
Synalar Forte	†			

Further information Nil.

Product licence numbers

Synalar Cream	0029/5037
Synalar Ointment	0029/5041
Synandone Cream	0029/5047
Synandone Ointment	0029/5049
Synalar Forte	0029/5038

SYNALAR* CREAM 1 IN 4 DILUTION
SYNALAR* CREAM 1 IN 10 DILUTION

Presentation Synalar Cream in dilutions of 1 in 4 and 1 in 10 are presented as white, water-miscible creams which contain 0.00625% and 0.0025% w/w Fluocinolone Acetonide BP respectively.

Uses Synalar Cream dilutions contain an effective topical corticosteroid and are suitable for treating the milder forms of a wide variety of local inflammatory, pruritic and allergic disorders of the skin. Synalar Cream dilutions are particularly suitable for topical application in:

Eczema and dermatitis: atopic eczema, seborrhoeic eczema, discoid eczema, pompholyx, otitis externa, contact dermatitis, neurodermatitis, intertrigo.
Non-specific ano-genital pruritus; prurigo.
Psoriasis. Lichen planus.

Synalar Cream dilutions are indicated for milder forms of these conditions; for maintenance therapy when control has been achieved with Synalar; for use under occlusive dressings; and for paediatric dermatology, e.g.: infantile eczema.

Dosage and administration A small quantity of Synalar Cream dilution is applied lightly to the affected area two or three times a day, and massaged gently and thoroughly into the skin. When an occlusive dressing is required, the affected area should first be thoroughly cleansed; Synalar Cream dilution is then applied and

covered with a suitable plastic dressing. Synalar Cream dilutions are particularly suitable for moist or weeping surfaces and for flexures of the body.

These recommendations apply to both children and adults.

Contra-indications, warnings, etc Synalar Cream dilutions are contra-indicated in primary infections of the skin caused by bacteria, fungi or viruses and in rosacea, acne and peri-oral dermatitis.

Long-term continuous topical steroid therapy can produce local atrophic skin changes. Particular care should therefore be taken if applying steroids to the face. Prolonged use of topical steroids or treatment of extensive areas, even without occlusion, can result in sufficient absorption of the steroid to produce the features of adrenal suppression, especially in infants and children. When there is an infection associated with an inflammatory skin condition, Synalar preparations should only be administered if adequate anti-infective cover is given.

Treatment should be discontinued if unfavourable reactions are seen.

Pregnancy: Topical administration of corticosteroids to pregnant animals has been shown to cause abnormalities of foetal development. Although the relevance of this finding to human application has not been established, when topical steroid treatment is considered necessary during pregnancy both the amount applied and the length of treatment should be minimised.

Side-effects: With Synalar Cream dilutions, side-effects are extremely rare, but, as with all topical corticosteroids, the occasional patient may show an adverse reaction such as hypersensitivity. Extensive treatment can result in both local atrophic changes, such as striae, skin thinning and teleangiectasia and systemic effects such as adrenal suppression.

The use of topical steroids on infected lesions, without the addition of appropriate anti-infective therapy, can result in the spread of opportunist infections.

Accidental ingestion: Toxic effects are not likely to occur following accidental ingestion of the contents of a 50 g tube. If greater quantities are ingested and toxicity develops, symptomatic treatment should be given.

Pharmaceutical precautions Store at room temperature and use undiluted.

Legal category POM.

Package quantities Synalar Cream dilutions 1 in 4 and 1 in 10 are supplied 50 g tubes.

Further information Nil.

Product licence numbers
Synalar Cream 1 in 4 dilution   0029/0151
Synalar Cream 1 in 10 dilution   0029/0152

SYNALAR* GEL

Presentation Synalar Gel consists of Fluocinolone Acetonide BP 0.025% w/w, presented as a clear, water-miscible gel.

Uses Synalar Gel is an effective topical corticosteroid formulated as a clear, non-greasy gel. It is designed for application to the scalp and other hairy regions, but can equally well be applied elsewhere on the body. Specific indications for Synalar Gel are seborrhoea, seborrhoeic dermatitis and psoriasis of the scalp, but it may be applied satisfactorily to inflammatory dermatoses on other parts of the body.

Dosage and administration A small quantity of Synalar Gel is massaged into the scalp night and morning using the finger tips. For maintenance therapy, treatment should be repeated once or twice weekly.

These recommendations apply to both children and adults.

Contra-indications, warnings, etc Synalar Gel is contra-indicated in primary infections of the skin caused by bacteria, fungi or viruses and in rosacea, acne and peri-oral dermatitis.

Long-term continuous topical steroid therapy can produce local atrophic skin changes. Particular care should therefore be taken if applying steroids to the face. Prolonged use of topical steroids or treatment of extensive areas, even without occlusion, can result in sufficient absorption of the steroid to produce the features of adrenal suppression, especially in infants and children. Where there is an infection associated with an inflammatory skin condition, Synalar preparations should only be administered if adequate anti-infective cover is given.

Treatment should be discontinued if unfavourable reactions are seen.

Pregnancy: Topical administration of corticosteroids to pregnant animals can cause abnormalities of foetal development. Although the relevance of this finding to human application has not been established, when topical steroid treatment is considered necessary during pregnancy both the amount applied and the length of treatment should be minimised.

Side-effects: With Synalar preparations, side-effects are extremely rare, but, as with all topical corticosteroids, the occasional patient may show an adverse reaction such as hypersensitivity. Extensive treatment can result in both local atrophic changes, such as striae, skin thinning and telangiectasia and systemic effects such as adrenal suppression.

The use of topical steroids on infected lesions, without the addition of appropriate anti-infective therapy, can result in the spread of opportunist infections.

Accidental ingestion: The 30 g tube of Synalar Gel contains 7.5 mg of the steroid. No toxic effects are likely to occur, even if the full contents of a 30 g tube are ingested. Similarly the ingredients of the base are unlikely to have any toxic effects in the quantities in which they occur. Therefore no remedial action is required in the event of ingestion.

Pharmaceutical precautions Store at room temperature and use undiluted.

Legal category POM.

Package quantities Synalar Gel is supplied in 30 g tubes.

Further information Nil.

Product licence number 0029/5039.

SYNALAR* C CREAM AND OINTMENT

Presentation These products contain 0.025% w/w of the steroid Fluocinolone Acetonide BP and 3% w/w of Clioquinol BP (chinoform, iodochlorhydroxyquinoline). Synalar C is presented as an off-white, water-miscible cream and as a greasy ointment.

Uses Synalar C combines the effective topical corticosteroid Synalar with the effective antibacterial and antifungal agent Clioquinol BP.

It is indicated for inflammatory dermatoses – including eczema, dermatitis, seborrhoea, psoriasis, sycosis barbae, intertrigo and ano-genital pruritus – where secondary bacterial and/or fungal infection is present or is likely to occur.

Dosage and administration A small quantity of the Synalar C preparation is applied lightly to the affected area two or three times a day, and massaged gently and thoroughly into the skin. If an occlusive dressing is indicated, the affected area is first thoroughly cleansed, the Synalar C preparation is then applied and covered with a suitable plastic dressing. Synalar C Cream is particularly suitable for very inflamed or weeping surfaces and for flexures of the body; whilst Synalar C Ointment is more suitable for dry scaly lesions. These recommendations apply to both children and adults.

Contra-indications, warnings, etc Synalar C preparations are contra-indicated in primary infections of the skin caused by bacteria, fungi or viruses and in rosacea, acne and peri-oral dermatitis.

Long-term continuous topical steroid therapy can produce local atrophic skin changes. Particular care should therefore be taken if applying steroids to the face. Prolonged use of topical steroids or treatment of extensive areas, even without occlusion, can result in sufficient absorption of the steroid to produce the features of adrenal suppression, especially in infants and children.

In the presence of a viral infection, the use of an appropriate agent should be instituted. If a favourable response does not occur promptly Synalar C should be discontinued until the infection has been adequately controlled.

Treatment should be discontinued if unfavourable reactions are seen.

Pregnancy: Topical administration of corticosteroids to pregnant animals can cause abnormalities of foetal development. Although the relevance of this finding to human application has not been established, when topical steroid treatment is considered necessary during pregnancy, both the amount applied and the length of treatment should be minimised.

Side-effects: With Synalar preparations, side-effects are extremely rare, but, as with all topical corticosteroids, the occasional patient may show an adverse reaction such as hypersensitivity. Extensive treatment can result in both local atrophic changes, such as striae, skin thinning and telangiectasia and systemic effects such as adrenal suppression.

Local application of clioquinol in creams or ointments may occasionally cause severe irritation, which may be less marked because of the fluocinolone acetonide.

Staining may occur due to breakdown of the clioquinol. A protective covering may be placed over the application to prevent staining of clothing or linen.

Accidental ingestion: The 15 g tube of Synalar C contains 3.75 mg of steroid and 0.45 g of Clioquinol BP. No toxic effects are likely to occur, even if the full contents of a tube are ingested. Similarly the ingredients of the base are unlikely to have any toxic effects in the quantities in which they occur. Therefore no remedial action is required in the event of ingestion.

Pharmaceutical precautions Store at room temperature and use undiluted.

Legal category POM.

Package quantities Synalar C Cream and Ointment are available in tubes of 15 g.

Further information Nil.

Product licence numbers
Synalar C Ointment   0029/5043
Synalar C Cream   0029/5042

SYNALAR* N CREAM AND OINTMENT

Presentation These products contain 0.025% w/w of the steroid Fluocinolone Acetonide BP and 0.5% w/w of Neomycin Sulphate PhEur. Synalar N is presented as a white, water-miscible cream and a greasy ointment.

Uses Synalar N combines the effective topical corticosteroid Synalar with an effective antibacterial agent. Neomycin Sulphate PhEur.

It is indicated for inflammatory dermatoses – including eczema, dermatitis, seborrhoea, psoriasis, intertrigo and ano-genital pruritus – where secondary bacterial infection is present or is likely to occur.

Dosage and administration A small quantity of the Synalar N preparation is applied lightly to the affected area two or three times a day, and massaged gently and thoroughly into the skin. If an occlusive dressing is indicated, the affected area is first thoroughly cleansed, the Synalar N preparation is then applied and covered with a suitable plastic dressing. Synalar N Cream is particularly suitable for very inflamed or weeping surfaces and for flexures of the body, whilst Synalar N Ointment is more suitable for dry, scaly lesions.

These recommendations apply to both children and adults.

Contra-indications, warnings, etc Synalar N preparations are contra-indicated in primary infections of the skin caused by bacteria, fungi or viruses and in rosacea, acne and peri-oral dermatitis. Synalar N is contra-indicated in those patients with a history of hypersensitivity to neomycin. Topical neomycin preparations should not be applied to the external auditory canal of patients with perforated eardrums

Long-term continuous topical steroid therapy can produce local atrophic skin changes. Particular care should therefore be taken if applying steroids to the face. Prolonged use of topical steroids or treatment of extensive areas, even without occlusion, can result in sufficient absorption of the steroid to produce the features of adrenal suppression, especially in infants and children.

In the presence of a viral or fungal infection, the use of an appropriate agent should be instituted. If a favourable response does not occur promptly, Synalar N should be discontinued until the infection has been adequately controlled.

Because of the potential hazard of nephrotoxicity and ototoxicity associated with neomycin, prolonged use or use of large amounts of the product should be avoided in conditions where absorption of neomycin is possible.

These preparations are not for ophthalmic use.

Treatment should be discontinued if unfavourable reactions are seen.

Pregnancy: Topical administration of corticosteroids to pregnant animals can cause abnormalities of foetal development. Although the relevance of this finding to human application has not been established, when topical steroid treatment is considered necessary during pregnancy, both the amount applied and the length of treatment should be minimised.

Side-effects: With Synalar preparations, side-effects are extremely rare, but, as with all topical corticosteroids, the occasional patient may show an adverse reaction such as hypersensitivity. Extensive treatment can result in both local atrophic changes, such as striae, skin thinning and telangiectasia and systemic effects such as adrenal suppression.

Accidental ingestion: The 30 g tube of Synalar N contains 7.5 mg of steroid and 150 mg of neomycin. No toxic effects are likely to occur, even if the full contents of a 30 g tube are ingested. Similarly the ingredients of the base are not likely to have any toxic effects in the quantities in which they occur. Therefore no remedial action is required in the event of ingestion.

Pharmaceutical precautions Store at room temperature and use undiluted.

Legal category POM.

Package quantities Synalar N Cream and Ointment are available in tubes of 15 g and 30 g.

Further information Nil.

Product licence numbers
Synalar N Cream   0029/5044
Synalar N Ointment   0029/5046

TETMOSOL* SOAP

Presentation Tetmosol Soap is a yellow perfumed soap tablet containing 5% w/w Monosulfiram BP (Sulfiram INN).

Uses Tetmosol is a parasiticide, active against the burrowing mite *Sarcoptes scabiei*. It is indicated for the treatment and prophylaxis of scabies. The soap is especially useful for prophylaxis in hospitals and schools, etc.

Application Tetmosol Soap is used in place of ordinary toilet soap for the prophylaxis of scabies. Ideally, the person should bathe in hot water and soap themselves liberally with Tetmosol Soap paying particular attention to the folded areas of the skin. After bathing, the body should be allowed to dry naturally or dried with a towel using a 'blotting' action. Tetmosol Soap should be used daily for as long as the danger of infection remains.

Contra-indications, warnings, etc Tetmosol is contra-indicated when the patient has previously shown an idiosyncratic response to its application.

Side-effects: Very few side-effects occur with Tetmosol. A few cases of erythematous rash have been reported, but these are rare enough to be considered as idiosyncratic responses of the patients concerned.

Overdosage: Over application is unlikely to have any adverse effect. In the event of the soap being ingested, symptomatic treatment should be given.

Legal category P.

Pharmaceutical precautions Tetmosol Soap must be stored in the manufacturer's original wrapper, at room temperature.

Package quantities 75 g (2.6 oz).

Further information Nil.

Product licence number 0029/5006.

TETMOSOL* SOLUTION

Presentation Tetmosol Solution is a clear, brown liquid, forming a fine suspension when diluted with water. It contains Monosulfiram BP (Sulfiram INN) as a 25% w/w solution in industrial methylated spirit.

Uses Tetmosol Solution is a parasiticide active against the burrowing mite *Sarcoptes scabiei*. It is indicated for the treatment and prophylaxis of scabies.

Dosage and administration Before application Tetmosol Solution should be diluted with two to three parts of water. The patient's body should be liberally washed with soap and water and thoroughly dried. Apart from the face and scalp, the entire body should be painted with the dilute solution, which is rubbed well in and left to dry. About ten minutes is allowed for the skin to dry naturally and the patient then dresses. Application is suitable for use in clinics dealing with children. In difficult cases this routine may be repeated successively for two or three days. These instructions are applicable to adults and children.

Contra-indications, warnings, etc Tetmosol Solution is contra-indicated when the patient has previously shown an idiosyncratic response to its application. The solution is flammable and should not be applied near a naked flame. Because of the close chemical relationship between monosulfiram and disulfiram, it is considered advisable to abstain from alcohol before and for at least 48 hours after the application of Tetmosol.

Side-effects; Very few side-effects occur with Tetmosol Solution, even in cases of undiluted application. A few cases of erythematous rash have been reported, but these are rare enough to be considered as idiosyncratic responses of the patients concerned.

Overdosage: The solution contains alcohol and monosulfiram, and if ingested this combination will produce a severe reaction, with flushing, dyspnoea, headache, dizziness, nausea, vomiting, drowsiness or sleep. Tachycardia and hypotension may also occur and the resultant myocardial ischaemia may be fatal.

Symptomatic measures are required – oxygen, if dyspnoea is excessive, and control of the blood pressure. Other treatment which has been found useful includes cardiac stimulants, intravenous iron, ascorbic acid and nicotinamide, adenine and intravenous sodium thiosulphate.

Pharmaceutical precautions Tetmosol Solution should not be stored in a cold place as this causes deposition of crystals. These can be redissolved by immersing the bottle in warm water. The solution is flammable and should not be kept near a naked flame. Water is a suitable diluent for Tetmosol.

Legal category P.

Package quantities Bottles of 100 ml and 2 litres.

Further information Nil.

Product licence number 0029/5011.

TOPAL*

Presentation Round, pale cream tablets with a fragrant odour and sweet, slightly gelatinous taste. Dried Aluminium Hydroxide Gel 30 mg, Light Magnesium Carbonate 40 mg, Alginic Acid 200 mg, plus excipients to 1.65 g.

Uses Relief of discomfort due to gastic reflux or mucosal irritation in conditions such as heartburn, reflux oesophagitis, hiatus hernia, gastritis, acid dyspepsia.

Dosage and administration One to three tablets chewed four times a day after meals and at bedtime.

Contra-indications, warnings, etc No specific contra-indications, but care should be observed if used by diabetics because of the sugar content (see 'Further information').

Antacids may interfere with the absorption of some drugs, especially tetracyclines.

Pharmaceutical precautions Store at room temperature protected from moisture.

Legal category GSL.

Package quantities Blister packs of 42 tablets.

Further information Each tablet also contains 880 mg of Sucrose, 220mg Lactose, but no added colouring.

Product licence number 0603/0021.

Product licence holder: Concept Pharmaceuticals Ltd.

TRILENE*

Presentation Trilene is Trichloroethylene PhEur. It is a clear blue, volatile liquid, non-explosive and non-flammable in the concentration usually used. It resembles chloroform in odour but is distinguished by the inclusion of an inert blue dye.

Trilene consists of trichloroethylene stabilised with thymol 0.01% w/w.

Uses Trilene is a volatile anaesthetic, which is suitable for the induction and maintenance of anaesthesia for all types of surgery and in patients of all ages. Trilene can be used for the production of analgesia without loss of consciousness.

Dosage and administration A number of special Trilene vaporisers are available for administration.

The vapour concentration should be minimal at all times (0.5–2% by volume) and it is never necessary to bubble the carrier gas through the liquid. Trilene may be used alone with air or oxygen, but it is more commonly used as an adjunct to nitrous oxide/oxygen anaesthesia.

For the production of analgesia without loss of consciousness, Trilene should be administered in low concentrations (0.35–0.5%), from draw-over units using room air as carrier gas. Several vaporisers capable of delivering Trilene in analgesic concentrations are available.

The above dosages are suitable for both adults and children. The lower concentration is usually most suitable for elderly patients.

Trilene should be withdrawn before the completion of surgery to facilitate recovery.

Contra-indications, warnings, etc Trilene must never be used in closed circuit systems with soda lime.

Profound muscular relaxation cannot be achieved with unsupplemented Trilene anaesthesia, and if tachypnoea and cardiac arrhythmias are to be avoided, no attempt should be made to deepen anaesthesia by using Trilene concentrations in excess of 2.5%.

The concurrent administration of adrenaline and Trilene is inadvisable. Trichloroethylene anaesthesia in the presence of high grade beta-blockade may result in dangerous reductions of cardiac output.

Pregnancy: It is prudent to avoid general anaesthesia with inhalation agents during early pregnancy except where such use is essential.

Side-effects: Post-operative nausea, vomiting and headache occur rarely. Cardiac arrhythmias may occur if attempts to deepen anaesthesia are made.

Overdosage: Ingestion cases should be treated by gastric emptying and supportive treatment.

Pharmaceutical precautions Trilene and its vapour are not flammable, but they must not come into contact with hot surfaces as toxic decomposition products are thereby produced. Trilene must be stored in closed containers and protected from light and air.

Trilene should be kept in its original container until immediately prior to use.

It is not advisable to retain Trilene in an inhaler or anaesthetic machine for any length of time after use, and to avoid possible oxidation it is recommended that a fresh supply is placed in the vaporiser every few days.

Whilst in the liquid phase Trilene must not be diluted or contaminated; however, in the vapour phase it may be administered with air, oxygen or nitrous oxide/oxygen.

Legal category P.

Package quantities Bottles of 500 ml.

Further information Trilene allows a smooth, simple induction of anaesthesia without the patient coughing or struggling. Absence of capillary oozing is particularly appreciated with Trilene, and the non-flammable nature of the vapour avoids the risk of fire, or explosion from lights, cauteries, etc. In addition Trilene provides a marked degree of post-operative analgesia, which contributes greatly to the comfort of the patient.

Product licence number 0029/5083.

VIVALAN*

Presentation 1. Tablets each containing viloxazine hydrochloride equivalent to 50 mg viloxazine. Round, bi-convex, yellow, film-coated tablets marked VIVALAN on one face.

2. Tablets each containing viloxazine hydrochloride equivalent to 100 mg viloxazine. Round, bi-convex, yellow, film-coated tablets marked $\frac{\wedge}{\vee}$ on one face and ICI on the reverse.

Uses Symptoms of depressive illness, especially where sedation is not required.

Dosage and administration *Adults:* Most patients respond to 300 mg/day preferably taken as 200 mg in the morning and 100 mg at lunchtime. Total daily dose should not exceed 400 mg and the last dose of the day should not be taken later than 6.00 pm.

Elderly: 100mg/day initially. The initial dose should be increased with caution under close supervision. Half the normal maintenance dose may be sufficient to produce a satisfactory clinical response.

Children: Vivalan is not recommended in children under 14 years of age.

Contra-indications, warnings, etc

Contra-indications: Mania, severe liver disease, history of peptic ulcer, recent myocardial infarction, during breast feeding.

Pregnancy: There is no evidence as to the drug's safety in human pregnancy; do not use during pregnancy, especially during the first and third trimesters, unless there are compelling reasons.

Precautions: Vivalan should be used with caution in patients with ischaemic heart disease and congestive cardiac failure, or any degree of heart block.

Caution is advised when administering Vivalan to patients with epilepsy, especially those receiving phenytoin (see below).

Patients posing a high suicidal risk require close initial supervision.

If surgery is necessary during therapy, the anaesthetist should be informed that the patient has received Vivalan.

Drug interactions: Vivalan should not be given concurrently with, or within two weeks of cessation of therapy with monoamine oxidase inhibitors.

Vivalan may decrease the antihypertensive effect of guanethidine, debrisoquine, bethanidine, and possibly clonidine.

Caution is advised when administering Vivalan to patients taking phenytoin. The dose of phenytoin may need reducing to prevent toxic blood levels occurring.

On theoretical grounds, caution is advised when patients receiving L-DOPA are treated with Vivalan.

Most antidepressants have been shown to potentiate the central nervous depressant action of alcohol, and, therefore, patients should be advised of the risks involved in drinking alcohol whilst on antidepressant medication.

Warnings and adverse effects: Nausea is frequently observed, but may be transient. Headache and vomiting may also occur.

As improvement may not occur during the first two weeks of treatment, patients should be closely monitored during this period.

Vivalan initially may impair alertness, and patients should be advised of the possible hazard when driving or operating machinery.

Anticholinergic side-effects, such as dry mouth, disturbance of accommodation, tachycardia, constipation and hesitancy of micturition have been reported less frequently with viloxazine than with tricyclic antidepressants.

Cardiac arrhythmias and severe hypotension are less likely to occur with viloxazine than with tricyclic antidepressants in high dosage or in deliberate overdosage.

Adverse effects which have been reported rarely with viloxazine include exacerbation of anxiety and agitation, drowsiness, confusion, ataxia, dizziness, insomnia, tremor, paraesthesia, sweating, musculo-skeletal pain, mild hypertension and skin rashes.

Psychotic manifestations, including hypomania and aggressive behaviour may be exacerbated.

Two serious adverse effects possibly associated with Vivalan have been reported:

(a) jaundice with elevated transaminases
(b) convulsions

Withdrawal symptoms are rare, but may include malaise, headache and vomiting.

Overdosage: Vivalan is rapidly absorbed and gastric lavage should be carried out with minimum delay. Overdosage should be treated on general principles with careful monitoring of vital functions, together with intensive supportive therapy where necessary. As the drug is almost exclusively excreted in urine, forced diuresis may be performed to reduce blood levels. There is no specific antidote.

Pharmaceutical precautions Store at room temperature.

Package quantities Tablets 50 mg: Containers of 100. Tablets 100 mg: Containers of 84 and 250.

Further information Vivalan is an oxazine and is chemically distinct from the tri- and tetracyclic antidepressants, while retaining the biogenic amine reuptake inhibitory properties in the central nervous system. Pharmacologically, it differs from these drugs in its decreased sedative and anticholinergic properties, and its lesser effect on the cardiovascular system.

Legal category POM.

Product licence numbers
Vivalan Tablets   50 mg   0029/0074
Vivalan Tablets 100 mg   0029/0191

*Trade Mark

Immuno Ltd
Arctic House, Rye Lane
Dunton Green, Nr. Sevenoaks,
Kent, TN14 5HB

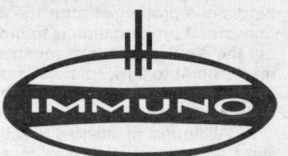

FEIBA IMMUNO* HEAT TREATED ▼
Factor VIII Inhibitor By-passing – Fraction Human

Presentation Feiba Immuno in its lyophilised form is an amorphous powder. After reconstitution with Water for Injections BP it is a clear yellowish solution. It is prepared from the plasma of suitable human donors as described in the British Pharmacopoeia 1980 Vol. II under Albumin, whose donations are shown by RIA to be free from HBsAg. Pooled plasma and the final product are also tested for freedom from HBsAg.

During production Feiba Immuno is heated for 10 hours at 80°C to reduce the risk of transmission of infectious agents.

It is presented in vials each containing 500 or 1000 Feiba units; 1 Feiba unit being defined as the Feib activity which shortens the activated partial thromboplastin time of a high titre Factor VIII Inhibitor Reference Plasma to 50% of the blank value.

A separate vial containing Water for Injections BP is provided for reconstitution.

Uses Feiba Immuno is mainly used to control bleeding episodes in haemophilia A patients with Factor VIII Inhibitors and also in patients with acquired Factor VIII Inhibitors.

Dosage and administration Feiba Immuno should only be administered intravenously.

On the basis of available clinical trial results obtained in the treatment of Factor VIII inhibitor patients it is possible that Feiba's effectiveness may vary between patients, this may be due to varying inhibitor titres and other, as yet unknown, factors. As a result larger doses may be necessary if the inhibitor titres are high, but this is not a general rule.

The determination of the whole blood clotting time (WBCT) according to Lee White and/or the calculation of the r-value in the thromboelastogram (TEG) help to determine the most effective dose and to check the success of therapy.

Care must be taken to distinguish between the following indications.

Spontaneous bleeding episodes: A dosage of 50 to 100 units per kg bodyweight administered in 8- to 12-hourly intervals is recommended and should be continued until clear signs of therapeutic improvement appear. This means, in the case of exterior bleeding, healing of the bleeding site, or in the case of internal bleeding, a lessening of pain, reduction in swelling or mobilisation of the joint. If there are no signs of therapeutic improvement despite the administration of 100 units of Feiba per kg given 8-hourly, combined therapy with 40 units per kg of a Factor VIII concentrate (Kryobulin* or Factor VIII Concentrate Human Immuno) is recom-

mended. The Factor VIII must be administered after each individual dose of Feiba Immuno.

In home treatment of bleeding complications up to 150 u/kg bodyweight have been administered, the effective dose very likely depending on the extent of bleeding. In some cases a kind of maintenance prophylaxis was successfully undertaken in home treatment with three applications weekly of approximately 30 units of Feiba Immuno per kg bodyweight followed by approximately 60 units of Factor VIII concentrate per kg.

Minor surgery: Basically, the same kind of therapy should be followed as in the case of spontaneous bleeding episodes. It is, however, necessary to check the substitution effect before the operation and, if necessary, increase the dose or give consideration to combined treatment with Factor VIII concentrate (40 units per kg).

For checking effectiveness, the following tests should be carried out: whole blood clotting time (WBCT) according to Lee White; r-value of the thromboelastogram (TEG).

When combination therapy with Factor VIII concentrate is used the activated partial thromboplastin time (APTT) may be shortened to normal values.

Since disseminated intravascular coagulation (DIC) cannot be totally excluded in the course of this treatment, it is advisable to carry out repeated tests on platelets, fibrinogen and FDP.

Use in the elderly: No specific precautions have to be taken into account when using the drug in the elderly, attention is, however, drawn to the fact that in patients with a tentative or definitive diagnosis of coronary heart disease the use of Feiba Immuno is only indicated in life-threatening bleeding events.

Use in pregnancy: Animal reproduction studies have not been conducted with Feiba Immuno. It is also not known, whether Feiba Immuno can cause fetal harm when administered to a pregnant woman or can affect reproduction capacity. Feiba Immuno should only be given to a pregnant woman if clearly needed.

Contra-indications, warnings, etc
Contra-indications: Presence of disseminated intravascular coagulation (DIC).

Precautions and warnings:
1. Before each individual application of Feiba Immuno with Factor VIII inhibitor patients it is advisable to count the patient's platelets, since some investigators have found that Feiba's effectiveness depends on the presence of a normal number of platelets. If the number of platelets is below 100,000/mm³ this should be normalised by giving platelet-concentrate before administering Feiba Immuno. In this connection special attention must be drawn to the platelet drop which follows the use of animal AHG, which may render Feiba Immuno ineffective.

2. Caution is also necessary if the APTT or prothrombin time is prolonged after the administration of Feiba Immuno. If prolongation is found, it is essential to carry out the 3 obligatory tests mentioned above. Should the results point to DIC, (platelet drop, fibrinogen decrease, FDP increase), the administration of Feiba Immuno must be interrupted.

3. All forms of allergic reaction ranging from mild short term urticarial rashes to anaphylactic shock are possible following the administration of human plasma derivatives. If such reactions occur, the administration of Feiba Immuno must be immediately discontinued. Allergic reactions should be treated with antihistamines. Shock should be treated in the usual way.

4. Despite the measures taken to reduce the risk, the transmission of viral hepatitis or other viral infections cannot be ruled out.

5. The occurrence of an anamnestic reaction giving a raised inhibitor titre cannot be totally excluded after administration of Feiba Immuno. Experience shows, however, that some patients treated with Feiba Immuno show lowered inhibitor titres whilst in the majority of patients, the titre remains unchanged.

Treatment of overdosage: Extremely high doses of Feiba Immuno may cause laboratory and/or clinical signs and symptoms of disseminated intra-vascular coagulation. In these cases treatment with Feiba Immuno should be discontinued promptly.

Pharmaceutical precautions Feiba Immuno must be stored between $+2°$ and $+8°C$ when it will have a shelf life of 2 years.

Legal category POM.

Package quantities Feiba Immuno is supplied in packs containing 500 and 1000 Feiba units together with a separate vial containing 20 ml Water for Injections BP as solvent. All packs contain sufficient equipment for reconstitution and administration.

Further information
(1) *Effect on laboratory tests:* Inherent in its mechanism of action Feiba Immuno causes a shortening of the following clotting times: activated partial thromboplastin time (APTT), whole blood clotting time (WBCT), activated clotting time (ACT), thromboelastogram (TEG).

Coagulation tests measuring the extrinsic coagulation system such as the prothrombin time, which is usually normal in haemophiliacs, remained unchanged after treatment with Feiba Immuno. Overdosage of the product may result in laboratory signs of DIC; as are the presence of fibrinopeptide A, fibrin/fibrinogen degradation products, a fall in fibrinogen, a prolonged APTT, thrombin time and prothrombin time.

(2) Feiba Immuno is only available to Haemophilia Treatment Centres.

Product licence number 0215/0021-22.

GAMMABULIN*
Normal Immunoglobulin Injection BP.

Presentation Gammabulin is a concentrate of antibodies present in the IgG fraction of human plasma and is available in liquid or lyophilised forms. It is produced from pooled human plasma obtained from suitable human

donors† whose donations are shown by RIA to be free from HBsAg. Pooled plasma and the final product are also tested for freedom from HBsAg.

Gammabulin liquid is a clear solution varying in colour from pale yellow to light brown. It has a protein content of 16% of which at least 90% is gamma globulin. Glycine is added at a strength of 2.25% as a stabiliser and Merthiolate at a strength of 0.01% as a preservative. Gammabulin lyophilised is a white to slightly yellowish powder or solid friable mass completely soluble in Water for Injections BP.

When the lyophilised powder is reconstituted with the amount of Water for Injections BP indicated on the label, it has a protein content of 16% of which at least 90% is gamma globulin. Glycine is added at a strength of 6% as a stabiliser and Merthiolate at a strength of 0.01% as a preservative.

Uses Gammabulin is used in the treatment of:
Antibody deficiency syndrome and recurring bacterial infections in dys-, hypo- and agammaglobulinaemia.
Hepatitis A prophylaxis.
Prevention or modification of measles infection.
Treatment of susceptible pregnant women exposed to Rubella infection in whom continuing pregnancy places the fetus at risk.

Dosage and administration Gammabulin must be administered by the intramuscular route.

All recommendations and doses given below refer to the 16% solution and are expressed in ml.

Antibody deficiency syndrome in dys-, hypo- and agammaglobulinaemia: By intramuscular administration of Gammabulin antibody concentrate the frequency and severity of recurring bacterial infections can be reduced. For treatment of gamma globulin deficiency, it is necessary to achieve and maintain a gamma globulin level of approximately 200 mg per 100 ml serum.

Initial dosage: 1.8 ml per kg bodyweight e.g. in three single administrations of 0.6 ml/kg bodyweight each at intervals of 24 hours.

Maintenance dose: 0.6 ml per kg bodyweight, monthly.

Hepatitis A: Gammabulin is an efficient agent for the prevention or modification of hepatitis A. It must be pointed out that after gamma globulin administration an anicteric course of hepatitis has been observed. Because of this, regular monitoring of transaminase levels may be warranted.

Dosage for children: 0.02–0.04 ml per kg bodyweight. If exposure continues, repeat the dose after 4–6 months.

Dosage for adults:

(a) for a short period of exposure of less than 2 months: 0.02 to 0.04 ml per kg bodyweight.

(b) for longer periods of exposure 0.08 to 0.12 ml per kg bodyweight. If exposure continues, repeat the dose after 4 to 6 months

Note: No benefit may be expected if administered after the onset of clinical symptoms.

Measles: Gammabulin should be given as soon as possible at a dose of 0.25 ml/kg to prevent or modify measles in a susceptible person exposed less than six days previously. Gammabulin may be especially indicated for susceptible household contacts of measles

† Human donors as described in the British Pharmacopoeia 1980 Vol. II under Albumin.

patients, particularly with children under one year of age or children who are immunosuppressed or have an immune deficiency disease and should not receive measles vaccine or any other live viral vaccine.

Prophylaxis: 0.2 ml per kg bodyweight with continued or repeated exposure repeat after 3 weeks.

Mitigation without influence on the immunising effect: 0.04 ml per kg bodyweight.

Rubella: (German Measles) The routine use of Gammabulin prophylaxis of Rubella in early pregnancy is of dubious value and cannot be justified. Some studies suggest that the use of Gammabulin in exposed, susceptible women can lessen the likelihood of infection and fetal damage, therefore, 20 ml of Gammabulin may benefit those women in whom continuing pregnancy places the fetus at risk.

Use in the elderly: In older people, the elimination of parenterally administered homologous proteins (e.g. gammaglobulin) may be increased. Therefore, the upper limits given in the dosage recommendations should always be taken as a basis (or, in special cases, even be exceeded).

Use in pregnancy: After application of gammaglobulin, a broad spectrum of antibodies (e.g. measles and rubella) appear in the serum, which must be taken into consideration in case of vaccination with live viruses (e.g. rubella). Such vaccinations should only be given after an interval of three months after administration of immunoglobulin. This interval is absolutely necessary for the vaccination to be successful (interaction). According to present knowledge, no influence of gammaglobulin administrations in temporal connection with Rh_0-prophylaxis with anti-D gammaglobulin can be proved. The diaplacental passage of i.m. gammaglobulin (IgG) into the fetus may be assumed.

Contra-indications, warnings, etc Gammabulin is generally well tolerated without reactions. On very rare occasions (e.g. in special forms of a- or hypogammaglobulinaemia) anaphylactoid reactions may occur in patients who have antibodies against Immune Globulin A (IgA) or who have shown atypical reaction after blood transfusion or following administration of blood derivatives.

Gammabulin must not be administered intravenously.

Treatment of overdosage: Gammabulin is a homologous protein the antibody spectrum and protein structure of which corresponds qualitatively to that of an average donor population. Overdosage need not be expected to lead to more frequent or more severe adverse reactions than the recommended dose.

Pharmaceutical precautions Gammabulin liquid should be stored between $+2°$ and $+8°C$ when it will have a shelf life of 3 years.

Gammabulin lyophilised should be stored at room temperature ($+2°$ to $+25°C$) when it will have a shelf life of 5 years.

Both preparations should be protected from the light.

Legal category POM.

Package quantities *Gammabulin liquid:* Rubber capped vials containing 2 ml, 5 ml or 10 ml.

Gammabulin lyophilised: Rubber capped vial containing 320 mg lyophilised powder. A 2 ml ampoule of Water for Injections BP is also enclosed.

Further information *Effect on laboratory tests:* Laboratory tests as far as antibody determinations are concerned are influenced inasmuch as the application of Gammabulin may lead to an increased or new appearance of types of antibodies (e.g. antibacterial, antiviral or antitoxic antibodies). In case of very high doses, determinations of serum complement may give reduced values (consumption). Phagocytosis (phagocytosis index) may be increased.

Product licence numbers liquid   0215/0018
lyophilised 0215/0019.

HEPARIN – INJECT 5,000 BP IMMUNO

Presentation Heparin-Inject 5,000 BP is a sterile solution of 5,000 i.u. Heparin Sodium (mucous) dissolved in 0.3 ml Water for Injections BP. It is a clear liquid varying from colourless to straw coloured. Each pre-loaded syringe contains 2.7 mg of Sodium Chloride in 0.3 ml of injection.

Uses Prevention of thrombosis following surgery and for prophylactic treatment of other patients at risk from thromboembolic events.

Dosage and administration Heparin – Inject 5,000 BP must be administered by the subcutaneous route preferably through the adipose tissue of the abdominal wall. The following dosage is recommended:

Pre-operative administration: 1 pre-loaded syringe containing Heparin – Inject 5,000 BP to be given two hours before surgery.

Post-operative administration: 1 pre-loaded syringe containing Heparin – Inject 5,000 BP to be given at intervals of 8–12 hours up to the 7th–12th day.

Other patients: 1 pre-loaded syringe containing Heparin – Inject 5,000 BP to be given at intervals of 8–12 hours.

Use in the elderly: No specific precautions or side effects have to be taken into account in the elderly.

Use in pregnancy: Heparin Inject 5000 BP has been used in pregnancy for prophylaxis of deep venous thrombosis particularly in patients with a history of thrombo-embolic events, when given in a dose of 5000 i.u. every 8 to 12 hours.

Contra-indications, warnings, etc Heparin should not be used in patients with the following conditions:

1. Heparin allergy.
2. Surgery carried out on the central nervous system and the eye.
3. Haemorrhagic diatheses including haemophilia, thrombocytopenia and when linked with endocarditis.
4. Advanced stages of kidney, liver or pancreatic disease.
5. Post-operative seeping haemorrhage.

Precautions are necessary in patients with potential bleeding sites such as peptic ulcer and ulcerative colitis. Also in pregnancy and in patients with persistent hypertension or cerebral thrombosis; and during simultaneous administration of Warfarin, Aspirin, other salicylates or other medicaments having an impact on blood coagulation. Experience indicates that Heparin can be used with very little risk in the prophylaxis of thrombosis. If, however, bleeding complications occur during or after an operation, the patient's thrombin time or partial thromboplastin time should be determined. If the results of these tests are within the normal range it is unlikely that heparinisation is the cause.

It must, however, be borne in mind that on very rare occasions Heparin can cause thrombocytopenia and could therefore be the cause of the haemorrhage.

Treatment of overdosage: Slight haemorrhage caused by overdosage can usually be controlled by withdrawing the drug. In case of severe bleeding neutralisation of heparin by administration of protamine sulphate is recommended. Protamine Sulphate Injection BP (10 mg in 1 ml) must be given by slow (10 min) intravenous injection. Ideally, the dose required should be accurately determined by titration. If there is insufficient time to titrate the dose, the following dosage scale is recommended:

Time interval following dose of 5,000 i.u. Heparin	Dose of Protamine Sulphate injection 10 mg in 1 ml
Immediately after	5.0 ml
Half an hour after	2.5 ml
One hour after	1.25 ml

Pharmaceutical precautions It should be stored at a temperature not exceeding 25°C when it will have a shelf life of three years.

Legal category POM.

Package quantities Pre-loaded syringes containing 0.3 ml solution of 5,000 i.u. Heparin Sodium supplied in packs of 10 and 100 pre-loaded syringes.

Further information An increased tendency towards haemorrhage must be carefully avoided during the operation period and any error of dosage excluded.

Heparin – Inject 5,000 BP is packed in a pre-loaded syringe which enables an accurate dose to be administered. The hazard of overdosage can therefore be avoided.

Effect on laboratory tests: Heparin causes a dose-dependent prolongation of the following clotting times: thrombin time; activated PTT (partial thromboplastin time); to some extent also the prothrombin time; whole blood clotting time. High dose heparin treatment may result in decreased AT III values.

Product licence number 0215/0017.

HUMAN ALBUMIN 20% BP IMMUNO

Presentation Human Albumin 20% BP Immuno is a solution in water of human albumin containing a low proportion of salt and is described as Salt Poor Albumin. It is a clear liquid varying in colour from amber to orange-brown and is presented as a solution for intravenous injection or infusion to human beings. It is prepared from the plasma of suitable human donors† whose donations are shown by RIA to be free from HBsAg. Pooled plasma and the final product are also tested by RIA for freedom from HBsAg. It contains 20% protein of which at least 96% is albumin, the rest being thermostable alpha and beta globulins.

It is stabilised with 16 mmol/L Sodium Caprylate and 16 mmol/L Sodium Acetyltryptophanate.

† Human donors as described in the British Pharmacopoeia 1980 Vol II under Albumin.

There is no preservative added to the solution.

Uses Human Albumin 20% BP 'Immuno' is administered as an injection or an infusion in the treatment of acute oedema; hypoalbuminaemia; pre-eclampsia; hyperbilirubinaemia; shock with a high haematocrit due to loss of fluid into the extravascular compartment. For the treatment of the acute phase of burns or haemorrhagic shock, Human Albumin 20% BP 'Immuno' is diluted with 3 parts of dextrose, fructrose or electrolyte solutions and the resulting 5% solution administered by infusion.

Dosage and administration *Acute oedema:* There is an increased tendency for oedema to occur in patients with hypoalbuminaemia. Attempts should be made to bring about diuresis using the appropriate dose of Human Albumin 20% BP 'Immuno'. A reduction in oedema may then result.

Adults: 100 ml Human Albumin 20% BP 'Immuno' (20 g).

Children: 2 ml Human Albumin 20% BP 'Immuno' (0.4 g) per kg bodyweight.

Hypoalbuminaemia: In debilitated patients stabilisation of the protein balance with Human Albumin 20% BP 'Immuno' may considerably improve the pre-operative condition of the patient. Following surgery on the gastro-intestinal tract, albumin catabolism can be severely disturbed and hypoalbuminaemia may result. Albumin breakdown can also be increased in certain pathological conditions leading to hypoalbuminaemia and the administration of Human Albumin 20% BP 'Immuno' can be valuable in such cases.

Adults 100–200 ml Human Albumin 20% BP 'Immuno' (20–40 g) daily in concentrated or diluted form depending on the serum albumin level and plasma volume of the patient.

Children 1.5–3 ml Human Albumin 20% B.P. 'Immuno' (0.3–0.6 g) per kg bodyweight daily in concentrated or diluted form.

Other hypoalbuminaemia: In Hepatic cirrhosis a loss of parenchyma results in decreased albumin synthesis and associated hypoalbuminaemia giving increased risk of ascites and oedema. Treatment with albumin will remove the oedema and reduce ascites.

Adults 100–200 ml Human Albumin 20% BP 'Immuno' (20–40 g) daily.

Children 1.5–3 ml Human Albumin 20% BP 'Immuno' (0.3–0.6 g) per kg bodyweight.

In cases of nephrotic syndrome especially with patients who give minimal or no response to diuretics, administration of Human Albumin 20% BP 'Immuno' will reduce the oedema by inducing diuresis.

Adults 200–400 ml Human Albumin 20% BP 'Immuno' (40–80 g) daily.

Children 3–6 ml Human Albumin 20% BP 'Immuno' (0.6–1.2 g) per kg bodyweight infused over a period of 60–90 minutes.

Pre-eclampsia: Pre-eclamptic symptoms may occur in pregnancy due to fluid balance disturbance associated with increased vascular permeability. The danger of eclampsia can be lessened by reversal of the circulatory disorder by administration of Human Albumin 20% BP 'Immuno'.

Adults 50 ml Human Albumin 20% BP 'Immuno' (10 g) daily.

Hyperbilirubinaemia: 5–10 ml Human Albumin 20% BP 'Immuno' can be injected or transfused into the newborn or added to a blood transfusion if exchange is being carried out.

Shock: In the treatment of acute shock, distinction must be drawn between (a) restoration of normal blood volume in the case of severe blood loss by the administration of iso-oncotic fluids and (b) the return of fluid from the extravascular compartment to the circulation.

Restoration of normal blood volume following severe blood loss: Shock due to blood loss should be treated with Human Albumin 20% BP 'Immuno' diluted with electrolyte and/or dextrose or fructose solutions.

Adults 50–200 ml Human Albumin 20% BP 'Immuno' (10–40 g) diluted 1:4 with electrolyte and/or dextrose solution corresponding to 200–800 ml of a 5% solution.

Children 1–2 ml Human Albumin 20% BP 'Immuno' (0.2–0.4 g) per kg bodyweight diluted 1:4 corresponding to 4–8 ml/kg bodyweight of a 5% solution.

With severe blood loss an initial dose of 400 ml of the 5% solution should be infused rapidly and repeated if shock is uncontrolled.

In burns with associated hypoalbuminaemia the return of fluid from the extravascular compartment to the circulation must be ensured.

Shock associated with a high haematocrit due to loss of fluid to the extravascular compartment: In these cases return of fluid to the circulation is essential and Human Albumin 20% BP 'Immuno' should be infused undiluted.

Adults 50–200 ml Human Albumin 20% BP 'Immuno' (10–40 g).

Children 1–2 ml Human Albumin 20% BP 'Immuno' (0.2–0.4 g) per kg bodyweight.

The initial dose should be infused over a period of 5–15 minutes.

Burns: In the acute phase of extensive and severe burns Human Albumin 20% BP 'Immuno' is diluted with dextrose, fructose or electrolyte solutions to provide a 5% solution.

Recommended initial doses: Adults 200–400 ml Human Albumin 20% BP 'Immuno' (40–80 g) diluted 1:4 corresponding to 800–1600 ml of a 5% solution.

Children 4 ml Human Albumin 20% BP 'Immuno' (0.8 g) per kg bodyweight diluted 1:4 corresponding to 16 ml of a 5% solution.

The total dose in the first 24 hours should be in accordance with the formula 2 ml × bodyweight in kg × percentage of surface burned + 1500 ml. After the acute phase has passed, any subsequent hypoalbuminaemia can be corrected by the following dosage:

Adults 50 ml Human Albumin 20% BP 'Immuno' (10 g) twice a day.

Children 1 ml Human Albumin 20% BP 'Immuno' (0.2 g) per kg bodyweight twice a day.

Use in the elderly: In elderly patients careful haemodynamic and respiratory monitoring is essential throughout the administration of Human Albumin 20% BP 'Immuno' as a circulatory overload may lead to decompensation of the haemodynamic system.

In dehydrated patients only low concentrated protein solutions (up to 5% protein content) should be administered.

Use in pregnancy: As some patients show renal insufficiency during pregnancy concentrated human albumin should be administered only when absolutely indicated and with utmost caution. Based on a persisting hypertension careful haemodynamic monitoring is essential to avoid an overloading syndrome which may lead to cardiac decompensation.

Contra-indications, warnings, etc Human Albumin 20% BP 'Immuno' must only be used if the solution is clear. Once the cap has been pierced by a needle, the contents must be used within 4 hours.

Caution is indicated in the administration of Human Albumin 20% BP 'Immuno' to patients suffering from hypertension or in cases of latent or manifest cardiac insufficiency. The single doses should be reduced to relatively small amounts and the infusion given slowly. A careful watch must be kept for the possible development of pulmonary oedema. If pulmonary oedema occurs the infusion must be stopped immediately.

In all cases of considerable blood loss, whole blood or packed red cells must be given in addition to Human Albumin 20% BP 'Immuno'. Careful selection and testing of donors and donations and the inclusion of filtration and heating at 60°C for 10 hours in the preparation of the product have virtually eliminated the risk of serum hepatitis. As with all blood products, however, this risk cannot be absolutely excluded. Intolerance reactions are extremely rare with Human Albumin 20% BP Immuno.

Treatment of overdosage: Interrupt infusion immediately and carefully watch the patient's haemodynamic parameters.

The half life of human albumin in the tissue is approximately 16–18 days. The disappearance rate of intravascular albumin depends on the permeability of the vascular system and on the catabolic rate.

Pharmaceutical precautions Human Albumin 20% BP Immuno should be stored between +2°C and +25°C. It must be protected from light. The shelf life is 3 years.

Legal category POM.

Package quantities Human Albumin 20% BP 'Immuno' is supplied in rubber capped vials of 10 ml, 50 ml and 100 ml.

Further information Human Albumin 20% BP 'Immuno' is processed in such a way that removal of all antibodies, particularly isoagglutinins, is achieved. It can therefore be given to patients regardless of their blood group or rhesus factor. It will not interfere with subsequent blood investigations.

Effect on laboratory tests: As a consequence of haemodilution patients' blood samples taken during or shortly after infusion show lower laboratory test results (e.g. haematocrit) corresponding to the amount of Human Albumin 20% BP 'Immuno' administered to the patient (calculation based on isotonic solutions).

Human Albumin 20% BP 'Immuno' does not interfere with the determination of patients' Rh-factors nor is there any adverse effect on thrombocyte function or blood coagulation.

Product licence number 0215/0009.

KRYOBULIN* HEAT TREATED ▼

Presentation Dried Factor VIII Fraction BP is a white to yellowish amorphous powder or friable solid without any characteristic odour.

It is prepared from the plasma of suitable human

donors† whose donations are shown by RIA to be free from HBsAg. Pooled plasma and the final product are also tested for freedom from HBsAg.

The product has been heat treated at 60°C for 10 hours. This step has been introduced to reduce the risk of transmission of infectious agents.

It is packed in vials each containing approximately 250, 500 or 1,000 International Units of Factor VIII. Separate vials of Water for Injections BP are provided for reconstitution.

1 International Unit (i.u.) of Factor VIII (based on the corresponding international WHO standard) corresponds to the Factor VIII activity in 1 ml of fresh normal plasma.

Uses Kryobulin corrects Factor VIII deficiency, and is used in the treatment of bleeding due to such deficiency in:

Haemophilia A
von Willebrand's disease
Haemophilia complicated by Factor VIII inhibitors.

Dosage and administration Frequent tests of the patient's plasma level of Factor VIII must be made to allow correction of the deficiency by administration of Kryobulin, but for guidance an estimation of the required dosage can be made by the following calculation:

To achieve an increase of Factor VIII concentration of 1% it is necessary to administer 1 i.u. of Kryobulin per kg bodyweight, both for adults and children.

Initial treatment requires doses to be given at shorter intervals than in maintenance therapy, to provide an initial high level of activity and to replenish the extravascular compartment.

Bleeding from skin, nose and oral mucous membrane: Initial dose should be 10 i.u./kg at intervals of 6 to 12 hours.

Haemarthrosis: The initial dose should be approximately 10 i.u./kg and the maintenance dose 5 to 10 i.u. per kg at intervals of 6 to 12 hours. Combined with immobilisation of the affected joint for several days, the treatment should be sufficient to restore function.

Bruising: In most cases a single dose of 10 i.u./kg is sufficient. For widespread bruising, repeated administration of 5 to 10 i.u./kg at intervals of 6 to 12 hours may be required.

Heavy bleeding into muscles: Immediate treatment is required to prevent permanent deformity and loss of function, and initial immobilisation of the affected area is important. An initial dose of 15 to 20 i.u./kg should be given, the maintenance dose to be 10 i.u./kg at intervals of 6 hours from the first to the second day, and at intervals of 12 hours from the third to the fifth day.

Haematuria: The initial dose should be 15 to 20 i.u./kg, and the maintenance dose 10 i.u./kg at intervals of 12 hours.

Major surgery on haemophilic patients: The initial dose should be at least 25 to 50 i.u./kg, and the maintenance dose 20 to 40 i.u./kg at intervals of 4 hours from the first to the fourth day, of 8 hours from the fifth to the eighth day, and of 12 hours until all wounds are healed.

The effect of treatment must be checked daily. Factor VIII activity should not be allowed to fall below 50% of the normal 100% average value. It is important that

† Human donors as described in the British Pharmacopoeia 1980 Vol II under Albumin.

treatment be continued until all wounds have healed completely, as the risk of haemorrhage persists till then.

In addition to monitoring Factor VIII activity, tests for the development of Factor VIII inhibitors should also be made.

Dental extractions: The required dosage depends on the number and type of teeth to be extracted, and on the severity of the haemophilia. If *one or two teeth* are to be extracted from a patient with severe haemophilia, an initial dose of 10 to 20 i.u./kg should be given.

Maintenance treatment with this dosage at intervals of 6 hours from the first to the third day, and 8 hours from the fourth to the eighth day after extraction, should be given. If *more than two teeth are to be extracted from patients with severe haemophilia* a minimum initial dose of 20 to 30 i.u./kg should be given, and a maintenance dose of 10 to 20 i.u./kg at intervals of 6 hours from the first to the third day, and of 8 hours for twelve more days. The plasma concentration of Factor VIII should not be allowed to fall below 10% of the normal 100% average value.

Factor VIII assays should be used to monitor the effectiveness of treatment, as partial thromboplastin time gives a less accurate value when large quantities of Kryobulin are being used.

Solutions of Kryobulin must be administered intravenously, at a rate not exceeding 10 ml in 3 minutes.

Use in the elderly: No specific precautions or side effects have to be taken into account in the elderly.

Use in pregnancy: The use of Kryobulin need not be restricted during pregnancy.

Contra-indications, warnings, etc Although the danger of volume overload is small with Kryobulin, during major surgery monitoring of the patient's central venous pressure and blood pressure, and serial chest X-rays, may be advisable.

In disseminated intravascular coagulation associated with low Factor VIII levels, Heparin should be given to interrupt intravascular coagulation before therapy with Kryobulin is started.

A low incidence of adverse reactions is experienced with Kryobulin, but the following may occur:

1. All forms of allergic reaction from mild and transient urticaria to severe anaphylactic shock are possible when human plasma derivatives are administered. If such reactions occur, treatment with Kryobulin must be interrupted at once. Allergic reactions should be controlled with antihistamines and corticosteroids and routine treatment given for anaphylactic shock.

Monitoring of pulse rate and blood pressure is essential. If the pulse rate increases and/or blood pressure falls transfusion of 5% Dextrose should be started.

2. Despite the measures taken to reduce the risk, the transmission of viral hepatitis or other viral infections cannot be ruled out.

3. The appearance of a circulating Factor VIII inhibitor is possible. Its appearance cannot be predicted as it does not relate to the amount of Kryobulin administered, nor to the frequency of administration. As far as is known neither corticosteroids nor immunosuppressive agents significantly influence the formation of inhibitors.

Treatment of overdosage: No specific side effects have been reported with the overdosage of Kryobulin (Factor VIII-activity above 120%). The half life of about 12 hours will rapidly normalise Factor VIII-activity in the patient.

Pharmaceutical precautions Kryobulin must be

stored between +2°C and +6°C, and protected from the light. It then has a shelf-life of two years. When stored between +20°C and +30°C it has a life of six months.

Legal category POM.

Package quantities
Kryobulin Home Treatment Pack
Each pack contains:
1 rubber capped vial containing 250 or 500 i.u. Dried Factor VIII Fraction BP
1 rubber capped vial containing Water for Injections BP
This pack also contains a syringe, I/V needles, winged adaptor needle, filter needle, venting needle and swabs.

Kryobulin Hospital Pack
Each pack contains:
1 rubber capped vial containing 1,000 i.u. Dried Factor VIII Fraction BP
1 rubber capped vial containing Water for Injections BP.
The pack also contains a filter needle and venting needle.

Further information Kryobulin is especially suitable for Home Treatment. Packs contain all requirements and can be stored in a domestic refrigerator for two years and for up to six months at room temperatures not exceeding 30°C.

Effect on laboratory tests: Laboratory tests influenced in patients treated with Kryobulin are: Factor VIII assays; activated PTT; fibrinogen determination according to Clauss.

Product licence number 0215/0003.

PLASMA PROTEIN FRACTION BP 4.3% IMMUNO (Human Albumin Fraction Saline)

Presentation Plasma Protein Fraction BP 4.3% 'Immuno' is a clear amber liquid, presented as a solution for intravenous administration to human beings. It is prepared from the plasma of suitable human donors† whose donations are shown by RIA to be free from HBsAg. Pooled plasma and the final product are also tested by RIA for freedom from HBsAg.

Plasma Protein Fraction BP 4.3% 'Immuno' contains 4.3% protein of which at least 96% is albumin, the rest being heat stable alpha – and beta – globulins. As stabilisers sodium caprylate and sodium acetyltryptophanate have been added, both at a concentration of 3.44 mmol/L.

Uses Plasma Protein Fraction BP 4.3% 'Immuno' is indicated for volume replacement in hypovolaemic shock (e.g. following crush injury, severe trauma, surgery, burns and abdominal emergency) and for use whenever a predominant loss of plasma fluid has occurred.

Dosage and administration Adult dosage of Plasma Protein Fraction BP 4.3% 'Immuno' for hypovolaemic shock is in the range of 250 to 500 ml. A flow rate of up to 16 ml/min (1 litre/hr) has been well tolerated in adults. The rate of infusion, which can be increased in emergency treatment, depends on response. In hypoproteinaemia the usual dosage range is 1,500 to 2,000 ml daily (equivalent to 65 to 85 g plasma protein), but larger amounts can be given in severe hypoproteinaemia with

† Human donors as described in the British Pharmacopoeia 1980 Vol II under Albumin.

continuing loss. The flow rate should not exceed 5 to 8 ml/min.

Dosage for infants and young children in whom Plasma Protein Fraction BP 4.3% 'Immuno' is indicated for shock due to dehydration or infection, should be in the range of 20 to 30 ml/kg bodyweight, infused at a rate of 10 ml/min. The infusion rate should be adjusted in accordance with the clinical response. Administration is by intravenous infusion. A site should be chosen away from the area of injury or infection.

Use in the elderly: In elderly patients careful haemodynamic and respiratory monitoring is essential throughout the administration of Plasma Protein Fraction BP 4.3% 'Immuno' as a circulatory overload may lead to decompensation of the haemodynamic system.

In dehydrated patients only low concentrated protein solutions (up to 5% protein content) should be administered.

Use in pregnancy: As some patients show renal insufficiency during pregnancy concentrated human albumin should be administered only when absolutely indicated and with utmost caution. Based on a persisting hypertension careful haemodynamic monitoring is essential to avoid an overloading syndrome which may lead to cardiac decompensation.

Contra-indications, warnings, etc Careful monitoring of the patient's clinical condition is necessary so that hypervolaemia is not caused. Signs to be watched for are dyspnoea, pulmonary oedema, rise of blood pressure and central venous pressure.

Careful selection of donors and the inclusion of filtration and heating at 60°C for 10 hours in the preparation of the product have virtually eliminated the risk of Serum Hepatitis. As with all blood products, however, this risk cannot be absolutely excluded.

A turbid solution must not be given. Once set up, the entire contents of the infusion bottle should be administered within 4 hours.

Treatment of overdosage: Interrupt infusion immediately and carefully watch the patient's haemodynamic parameters.

The half life of human albumin in the tissue is approximately 16–18 days. The disappearance rate of intravascular albumin depends on the permeability of the vascular system and on the catabolic rate.

Pharmaceutical precautions Plasma Protein Fraction BP 4.3% 'Immuno' should be stored at +2°C to +25°C. It must be protected from light. The shelf life is 5 years.

Legal category POM.

Package quantities Plasma Protein Fraction BP 4.3% 'Immuno' is supplied in 50 ml, 100 ml, 250 ml, and 400 ml infusion bottles.

Further information Plasma Protein Fraction BP 4.3% 'Immuno' is processed in such a way that removal of all isoagglutinins and other antibodies is achieved. It can therefore be given without restriction to patients, regardless of blood group. It will not interfere with subsequent blood investigations.

Effects on laboratory tests: As a consequence of haemodilution patients' blood samples taken during or shortly after infusion show lower laboratory test results (e.g. haematocrit) corresponding to the amount of Plasma Protein Fraction BP 4.3% 'Immuno' administered to the patient (calculation based on isotonic solutions).

Plasma Protein Fraction BP 4.3% 'Immuno' does not interfere with the determination of patients' Rh-factors nor is there any adverse effect on thrombocyte function or blood coagulation.

Product licence number 0215/0002.

PROTHROMPLEX* Partial Prothrombin Complex (Human)

Presentation Prothromplex contains coagulation Factors II, IX and X and is a white, amorphous freeze-dried powder or friable solid without any characteristic odour. It is packed in rubber-capped vials containing 200 units or 500 units each of Factor II, IX & X.

It is prepared from the plasma of suitable human donors† whose donations are shown by RIA to be free from HB$_s$Ag. Pooled plasma and the final product are also tested by RIA for freedom from HB$_s$Ag. Prothromplex is also tested to discount the likelihood of causing disseminated intravascular coagulation.

Uses Treatment of cases of Factor IX deficiency (Haemophilia B).

By administering an appropriate dose of Prothromplex, it is possible to achieve a prompt and sufficient rise of Factor IX in the patient's plasma.

The effectiveness of treatment can be checked by simple laboratory tests. The activity of Factor IX is assayed through determination of the Partial Thromboplastin Time (PTT), however the most reliable results are obtained by quantitative activity assays of Factor IX.

Dosage and administration Immediately before use Prothromplex must be dissolved in 10 ml of the solvent provided.

After sterilising the cap of the solvent bottle remove 10 ml using the disposable syringe and one of the needles provided. Next sterilise the cap of the Prothromplex bottle and introduce the solvent using the second disposable needle. Reconstitute by gently shaking to and fro, thus avoiding frothing. Withdraw the reconstituted Prothromplex, then remove the syringe from the needle and attach the third disposable needle.

Prothromplex is now ready for slow intravenous injection taking about ten minutes.

Only general directions can be given for the dosage of Prothromplex. It is dependent upon the severity of the coagulation defect and the degree of the traumatic and haemorrhagic tissue damage. The suggested dosage for the treatment of Factor IX deficiency is given in the guide below.

Dosage guide for the treatment of severe and semisevere cases of Factor IX deficiency: Formula for the calculation of the necessary quantity of Factor IX:

One unit of Factor IX/kg bodyweight = 1% increase of Factor IX in the patient's plasma.

† Human donors as described in the British Pharmacopoeia 1980 Vol II under Albumin.

Prothromplex dosage table (Factor IX)

Clinical Manifestation	Minimum Factor IX level required	Initial dose in units Factor IX per kg bodyweight	Maintenance dose at intervals of 6 to 12 (24) hours in units per kg bodyweight
Surface haemorrhage from the skin and mucosae Superficial or deep haematoma Haemarthroses Slight bleeding following injuries Uncomplicated dental extractions Severe muscle haematoma	5–10%	15 U	7–15 U
Moderate bleeding following injuries Gastric and intestinal haemorrhages Bone fractures Cerebral bleeding Haematuria Complicated dental extractions Minor surgery	15–30%	20–30 U	15–30 U
Major surgery	more than 50%	75 U	50–75 U

It is suggested that a high initial dosage be chosen to ensure a rapid and sufficient increase of Factor IX thus achieving a reliable cessation of bleeding. Here, as well as with the subsequent maintenance therapy the initial short half-life of the coagulation factors has to be considered. Depending on the in-vivo half-life of Factor IX, which is approx 12–30 hours, a successful result will be achieved by repeated administration of Prothromplex at intervals of 6–12 hours. To assure absolute control of treatment, determination of the PTT should be made and, where possible, quantitative assays of Factor IX activity. Treatment should be maintained up to the resorption of the tissue haemorrhage or until the wounds have healed completely, thus ensuring a complication-free postoperative course. The special advantage of Prothromplex lies in the fact that by application of small volumes of fluid and a low amount of protein a high concentration of circulating coagulation Factor IX is achieved. The danger of volume or protein overloading of the patient is avoided even with the administration of high doses.

Use in the elderly: No specific precautions or side effects have to be taken into account in the elderly.

Use in pregnancy: The use of Prothromplex need not be restricted during pregnancy.

Contra-indications, warnings, etc With patients suffering from disseminated intravascular coagulation, (DIC), Prothromplex should not be given unless consumption of the coagulation factors has been previously interrupted by Heparin.

Side-effects are rarely observed during treatment with Prothromplex though the following reactions may occur:

1. *Allergic reactions:* All forms of allergic reactions from mild and temporary urticarial rashes to severe anaphylactic shock are possible when human plasma derivatives are administered. If these occur, treatment with Prothromplex must be interrupted at once. Allergic reactions should be controlled with antihistamines and

glucocorticoids and routine shock-treatment given for anaphylactic shock. Careful and frequent recording of pulse rate and blood pressure is essential. If the pulse rate increases and/or the blood pressure falls a transfusion of 5% Dextrose should be started.

2. Despite the precautions taken in the checking of donors, donations and the final product, the transmission of hepatitis cannot be entirely excluded following the administration of coagulation factors. This should be taken into account before using Prothromplex to control haemorrhage in non life saving situations in liver disease patients and those undergoing anticoagulant therapy.

3. During every type of therapy involving blood or coagulation factor concentrates, the occurrence of a circulating coagulation factor inhibitor is a possibility. The time at which such an inhibitor is produced cannot be predicted and depends neither on the amount of the plasma preparation administered nor on the frequency of the administration. As far as is known neither corticosteroids nor immunosuppressive agents significantly influence the formation of inhibitors.

Treatment of overdosage: Overdosage of Prothromplex must be avoided, since even so-called non activated Prothrombin Complex Concentrates (PCC) may in high doses cause thromboembolic complications. In case thrombosis or DIC (Disseminated Intravascular Coagulation) occur, specific therapy with Heparin and/or Antithrombin III should be initiated.

Pharmaceutical precautions Prothromplex has a

shelf life of two years when stored between +2°C and +6°C, and should be protected from light.

Legal category POM.

Package quantities 200 units or 500 units of Factors II, IX and X in each container.

1 rubber-capped vial containing lyophilised Prothromplex.

1 rubber-capped vial containing 10 ml Water for Injections BP.

1 10 ml disposable syringe.

3 disposable needles.

Further information Prothromplex can be stored in a domestic refrigerator, and can therefore be kept available for home treatment.

Prothromplex can be given in small volume injections, and is therefore suitable for home treatment.

Prothromplex can be moved in insulated containers to a refrigerator at some other location, giving a patient a greater degree of mobility.

Effect on laboratory tests: Laboratory tests influenced in patients treated with Prothromplex are: clotting assays for Factors II, IX, X; activated PTT; prothrombin time (PT).

Product licence numbers 0215/0006 – 200 U
0215/0007 – 500 U

*Trade Mark

International Laboratories Limited
Charwell House
Wilsom Road
Alton, Hampshire GU34 2TJ

MIGRALEVE*

Presentation *Pink Migraleve:* Blister-packed, pink, capsule-shaped, film-coated tablets, engraved 'MGE' on one face, each containing:

Buclizine hydrochloride	6.25 mg
Paracetamol BP	500 mg
Codeine Phosphate BP	8 mg
Dioctyl Sodium Sulphosuccinate (Docusate Sodium INN) BPC 1973	10 mg

Yellow Migraleve: Blister-packed, yellow, capsule-shaped, film-coated tablets, engraved 'MGE' on one face, each containing:

Paracetamol BP	500 mg
Codeine Phosphate BP	8 mg
Dioctyl Sodium Sulphosuccinate (Docusate Sodium INN) BPC 1973	20 mg

Uses Symptomatic and prophylactic treatment of classical and non-classical migraine and variants, including migrainous neuralgia (cluster headache), facial and ophthalmoplegic migraine and 'sick' headache. Paracetamol and codeine phosphate are analgesics. Buclizine hydrochloride is an antihistamine which is included for its antinauseant properties. These three in combination appear to act synergistically in preventing and/or aborting migraine attacks. The surface active agent docusate sodium prevents codeine constipation.

Dosage and administration *Adult: Treatment:* 2 Pink Migraleve immediately or prior to the attack if warning symptoms are apparent. If symptoms persist, 2 Yellow Migraleve every three or four hours. Maximum 8 tablets (2 Pink and 6 Yellow) in 24 hours.

Prophylaxis: 2 Pink tablets at night during periods of impending attacks.

Children: Normally 1 tablet of the appropriate colour where 2 are indicated for adults.

Contra-indications, warnings, etc *Side-effects:* Drowsiness is an occasional feature of migraine attacks. It may, theoretically, also be caused by the small antihistamine content of Pink Migraleve, but this has never been apparent from clinical observations.

Precautions: Migrainous patients suffering from high blood pressure should first be treated for this condition independently. Individuals with a history of renal disease should be treated cautiously as with any long-term analgesic therapy. Because of the possibility of drowsiness, consideration should be given to patients involved in hazardous occupations.

Treatment of overdosage: If more than 10 tablets have been taken, stomach washout. Correct electrolyte imbalance. Early alkaline diuresis may be valuable. Seek advice from specialised treatment centre

Pharmaceutical precautions Nil.

Legal category P.

Package quantities 24 (16 Pink and 8 Yellow) tablets. Also continuation packs of 24 Pink and 24 Yellow tablets.

Further information *Treatment:* Migraleve does not contain ergotamine, making it particularly suitable for those patients in whom ergotamine induces nausea and vomiting or potentiates any nausea and/or vomiting already present as symptoms. Clinical trials have shown an appreciable reduction in nausea and vomiting with Migraleve.

Migraleve does not compromise the peripheral circulation and no significant side-effects have been reported.

Prophylaxis: Migraleve is particularly valuable for prophylactic treatment, its use not being restricted to attacks of any single aetiology. Again, no significant side-effects have been reported with prophylactic treatment and it can be used for those patients in whom depression is present.

Product licence number 0232/5008.

SULEO-C* LOTION

Presentation A clear blue alcohol-based lotion containing carbaryl 0.5% w/v.

Uses Eradicates head lice infestation.

Dosage and administration Rub the lotion gently into the scalp until all hair and scalp is thoroughly moistened. Allow to dry naturally in a well ventilated room. Do not use hair dryer or other artificial heat. After 2 hours shampoo in normal manner. Rinse and comb the hair while wet to remove the dead lice.

In the event of early re-infestation Suleo-C lotion may be applied again provided seven days have elapsed since the first application.

Contra-indications, warnings, etc Avoid contact with the eyes.

It is advisable that nursing staff should wear gloves when carrying out treatment.

Not to be used on children under 6 months of age except under medical supervision.

Suleo-C lotion is for external use only and should be kept out of reach of children.

Keep away from naked flame during use and until hair is dry.

Accidental ingestion: Gastric lavage, assisted respiration and, if necessary, administration of atropine.

Pharmaceutical precautions Store in a cool dry place, below 25°C. Protect from sunlight.

Legal category P.

Package quantities Bottles of 55 ml.

Further information Suleo-C lotion is lethal to both lice and their eggs. Residual protective effect is variable and of short duration and should not be relied upon.

Local health authorities have a policy of using insecticides in sequence to discourage resistance. It is advisable to check on local current policy.

Product licence number 0232/0054.

SULEO-C* SHAMPOO

Presentation A clear green shampoo containing carbaryl 0.5% w/w.

Uses Eradicates head lice infestation.

Dosage and administration Wet hair thoroughly with tepid (not hot) water and massage Suleo into the scalp (the same quantity as used for ordinary shampoo). Rinse out thoroughly. Apply a second measure of Suleo and work into a rich lather. Allow it to remain on the head for at least 5 minutes and then rinse off with clean water. Comb out hair with a fine-toothed comb. Allow to dry naturally without heat. Do not use hair dryer. Apply as directed at 3 day intervals for a total of 3 applications.

Contra-indications, warnings, etc As with all shampoos, avoid contact with the eyes.

It is advisable that nursing staff should wear gloves when carrying out treatment.

Not to be used on children under 6 months of age except under medical supervision.

Suleo-C Shampoo is for external use only and should be kept out of the reach of children.

Accidental ingestion: Gastric lavage, assisted respiration and, if necessary, administration of atropine.

Pharmaceutical precautions Store in carton in a cool place. Protect from sunlight.

Legal category P.

Package quantities Bottles of 75 ml.

Further information Carbaryl is a carbamate insecticide which is lethal to both lice and their eggs. Residual protective effect is variable and of short duration and should not be relied upon.

Local health authorities have a policy of using insecticides in sequence to discourage resistance. It is advisable to check on local current policy.

Product licence number 0232/0049.

SULEO-M* LOTION

Presentation A clear colourless alcohol-based lotion containing malathion 0.5% w/v.

Uses Eradicates head lice infestation.

Dosage and administration Rub the lotion gently into the scalp until all hair and scalp is thoroughly moistened. Allow to dry naturally in a well ventilated room. Do not use hair dryer or other artificial heat. After 2 hours, shampoo in normal manner. Rinse and comb the hair while wet to remove the dead lice.

In the event of early re-infestation, Suleo-M lotion may be applied again provided seven days have elapsed since the first application.

Contra-indications, warnings, etc Avoid contact with the eyes.

It is advisable that nursing staff should wear gloves when carrying out treatment.

Not to be used on children under 6 months of age except under medical supervision.

Suleo-M lotion is for external use only and should be kept out of reach of children.

Keep away from naked flame during use and until hair is dry.

Accidental ingestion: Gastric lavage, assisted respiration and, if necessary, administration of atropine.

Pharmaceutical precautions Store in a cool dry place, below 25°C. Protect from sunlight.

Legal category P.

Package quantities Bottles of 55 ml.

Further information Suleo-M lotion is lethal to both lice and their eggs. Residual protective effect is variable and of short duration and should not be relied upon.

Local health authorities have a policy of using insecticides in sequence to discourage resistance. It is advisable to check on local current policy.

Product licence number 0232/0055.

*Trade Mark

Janssen Pharmaceutical Limited
Grove
Wantage
Oxfordshire OX12 0DQ

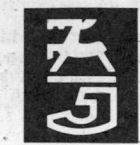

ANQUIL*

Presentation White, uncoated tablets marked 'JANS-SEN' on one side and 'A' above '0.25' on the reverse. Each tablet contains 0.25 mg benperidol.

Uses Anquil is a neuroleptic for the control of deviant and anti-social sexual behaviour.

Dosage and administration Anquil is intended for oral administration to adults only. The recommended daily dose is 0.25–1.5 mg in divided doses. Dosage is best initiated and adjusted under close clinical supervision, as individual response to neuroleptic drugs is variable.

In determining dosage, consideration should be given to the patient's age, severity of symptoms and previous response to other neuroleptic drugs.

Use in elderly: Patients who are elderly or debilitated, or those with previously reported adverse reactions to neuroleptic drugs, may require less Anquil, and half the normal starting dose may be sufficient for therapeutic response.

Contra-indications, warnings, etc

Contra-indications: Comatose states; patients with extra-pyramidal symptoms.

Use in pregnancy: The safety of Anquil in pregnancy has not been established, although studies in animals have not demonstrated teratogenic effects. As with other drugs, it is not advisable to administer Anquil in pregnancy.

Warnings: In common with all neuroleptics, Anquil can increase the central nervous system depression produced by other CNS-depressant drugs, including alcohol, hypnotics, sedatives, or strong analgesics, and may antagonise the action of adrenaline and other sympathomimetic agents.

Anquil may impair the anti-Parkinson effects of levodopa. The dosage of anti-convulsants may need to be increased to take account of the lowered seizure threshold.

Enhanced CNS effect, when combined with methyldopa, has been reported for some butyrophenones.

Acute withdrawal symptoms, including nausea, vomiting and insomnia, have very rarely been described after abrupt cessation of high doses of anti-psychotic drugs. Relapse may also occur and gradual withdrawal is advisable.

Precautions: Butyrophenones are excreted in breast milk and are not recommended during lactation. If the use of Anquil is considered essential, breast-feeding should be discontinued.

Where prolonged treatment with Anquil is envisaged, it would be a reasonable precaution to carry out regular blood counts and tests of liver function.

Caution is advised in patients with liver disease, renal failure, Parkinson's disease, epilepsy, and conditions predisposing to epilepsy or convulsions.

Adverse effects: Some degree of sedation or impairment of alertness may occur, particularly with higher doses, and at the start of treatment, and may be potentiated by alcohol. Patients should be advised not to drive or operate machinery during treatment, until their susceptibility is known.

In common with all neuroleptics, extrapyramidal symptoms may occur. Acute dystonias may occur early in treatment. Parkinsonian rigidity, tremor and akathisia tend to appear less rapidly. Oculogyric crises and laryngeal dystonias have been reported.

Anti-Parkinson agents should only be given, as required; they should not be prescribed routinely because of the possible risk of impairing Anquil's therapeutic efficacy.

Tardive dyskinesia may occur during administration or after withdrawal of neuroleptic drugs, including Anquil. The syndrome is common among patients treated with moderate to high doses of anti-psychotic drugs for prolonged periods of time and may prove irreversible, particularly in patients over the age of 50.

It is unlikely to occur in the short-term when low or moderate doses of Anquil are used as recommended, but since its occurrence may be related to duration of treatment as well as daily dose, Anquil should be given in the minimal effective dose for the minimum possible time.

The potential seriousness and unpredictability of tardive dyskinesia and the fact that it has occasionally been reported to occur when neuroleptic anti-psychotic drugs have been prescribed for relatively short periods in low dosage, means that the prescribing of such agents requires especially careful assessments of risks versus benefit. Tardive dyskinesia can be precipitated or aggravated by anti-Parkinson drugs. Short-lived dyskinesias may occur after abrupt drug withdrawal.

Gastrointestinal symptoms, nausea, loss of appetite and dyspepsia have been reported.

Hormonal effects of anti-psychotic neuroleptic drugs include hyper-prolactinaemia, which may cause galactorrhoea, gynaecomastia and oligo- or amenorrhoea.

Weight changes may occur.

Dose-related hypotension is uncommon, but can occur, particularly in the elderly, who are more susceptible to the sedative and hypotensive effects.

Anquil, even in low dosage in susceptible (especially non-psychotic) individuals, may cause unpleasant subjective feelings of being mentally dulled or slowed down, dizziness, headache, or paradoxical effects of excitement, agitation or insomnia.

Jaundice or transient abnormalities of liver function in the absence of jaundice have been reported.

The following effects have been reported rarely: Oedema, skin rashes or reactions, confusional or agitated states, epileptic fits.

Blood dyscrasias, including granulocytopenia have been reported very rarely.

Overdosage: There have been no serious toxic effects attributed to Anquil and fatal overdosage has not been reported. Treatment of overdosage consists of supportive measures combined with sedative or anti-Parkinsonian drugs, as required.

Pharmaceutical precautions Protect from light.

Legal category POM.

Package quantities Anquil Tablets, each containing 0.25 mg benperidol, are supplied in packs of 100.

Further information Nil.

Product licence number 0242/0014R.

CLINIUM*

Presentation White, flat, uncoated tablets marked 'Janssen' on one side and 'C/120' on the reverse. Each tablet contains lidoflazine 120 mg.

Uses Clinium is indicated in ambulant patients with ischaemic heart disease for the long term management of angina pectoris. Clinium increases exercise tolerance and allows greater cardiac work to be done without altering the maximal heart rate achieved and with the resting heart rate virtually unchanged. As a result the amount of external work possible before the onset of anginal pain is increased.

Clinium has no β adrenergic blocking activity, no significant effect on blood pressure and no autonomic activity. It has no negative inotropic effects on the heart.

The response to Clinium therapy develops gradually and is usually apparent after 6–8 weeks of treatment. In some cases up to six months will be needed for maximum clinical benefit.

Dosage and administration Clinium is for oral administration and should be taken with or after meals.

The usual daily dose is 360 mg (120 mg three times daily).

Side effects are minimised by gradual achievement of this dose and the following schedule is recommended:

Week 1 (initial) | 120 mg once daily
Week 2 | 120 mg twice daily
Week 3 and subsequently | 120 mg three times daily

Use in elderly: As above but with careful monitoring.

Contra-indications, warnings, etc
Contra-indications: Clinium should not be given to women unless pregnancy has been excluded.

Warnings: Clinium may cause prolongation of the QT interval of the ECG in some patients. In common with other drugs which affect repolarisation Clinium may precipitate ventricular tachycardia in some patients already susceptible to this arrhythmia. Patients with severe ischaemia, with conduction defects or with clinically significant arrhythmia have potential for developing ventricular tachycardia which may, in a small proportion of cases, be aggravated by Clinium.

Overdosage: In the event of accidental overdosage supportive measures including gastric lavage should be employed. Continuous ECG monitoring is recommended.

Forced diuresis may be of benefit since 33% of Clinium excretion is renal.

Side effects: Gastric upset or transient dizziness, tinnitus and headaches have all been observed occasionally. More rarely disturbing dreams or hallucinations have been reported. These usually occur in the initial phase of treatment and may normally be avoided by the gradual dosage increment regime recommended.

Pharmaceutical precautions Nil.

Legal category POM.

Package quantities Clinium is supplied in packs of 100 tablets.

Product licence number 0242/0002.

DAKTACORT*

Presentation *Cream:* White, non-staining, water-miscible cream containing Miconazole Nitrate BP 2% w/w and hydrocortisone 1% w/w.

Uses Daktacort is indicated for the topical treatment of skin conditions where inflammation and infection by susceptible organisms coexist e.g. infected eczema, intertrigo.

Miconazole nitrate is a potent, broad spectrum antifungal and antibacterial agent with marked activity against dermatophytes, pathogenic yeasts (e.g. Candida spp) and many Gram-positive bacteria including most strains of streptococcus and staphylococcus.

Hydrocortisone is a widely used topical anti-inflammatory of value in the treatment of inflammatory skin conditions including atopic and infantile eczema, contact sensitivity reactions and intertrigo.

Daktacort's properties indicate it particularly for the initial stages of treatment. Once the inflammatory symptoms have disappeared, treatment can be continued with miconazole cream.

Dosage and administration Daktacort should be applied to the affected area two or three times daily. Occlusive dressing is usually only necessary in the case of nail lesions.

Use in elderly: Natural thinning of the skin occurs in the elderly, hence corticosteroids should be used sparingly and for short periods of time.

Contra-indications, warnings, etc
Contra-indications; True hypersensitivity to any of the ingredients. Tubercular or viral infections of the skin or those caused by Gram negative bacteria.

Precautions: As with any topical corticosteroid, care is advised with infants and children when Daktacort is to be applied to extensive surface areas or under occlusive dressings including baby napkins; similarly application to the face shoud be avoided.

Warning: In infants, long term continuous topical corticosteroid therapy should be avoided. Adrenal suppression can occur even without occlusion.

Use in pregnancy: Administration of corticosteroids to pregnant animals can cause abnormalities of foetal development. The relevance of this finding to humans has not been established. However, topical steroids should not be used extensively in pregnancy.

Side-effects: Rarely, local sensitivity may occur requiring discontinuation of treatment.

Overdosage: Topically applied corticosteroids can be

absorbed in sufficient amounts to produce systemic effects.

Pharmaceutical precautions Store in a cool place.

Legal category POM.

Package quantities Daktacort cream is supplied in 30 g tubes.

Further information Nil.

Product licence number 0242/0042.

DAKTARIN* CREAM AND TWIN PACK

Presentation *Cream:* White, non-staining, water-miscible cream containing miconazole nitrate 2% w/w.

Twin pack: White, non-staining, water-miscible cream containing miconazole nitrate 2% w/w *plus* white, non-staining powder containing miconazole nitrate 2% w/w.

Uses Daktarin exhibits potent antifungal activity and antibacterial activity against Gram-positive organisms. It is used for the topical treatment of fungal infections of the skin and nails and super-infection due to Gram-positive bacteria.

Dosage and administration Both Daktarin cream and powder are applied topically.

Skin infections: Daktarin cream should be applied to the lesions in the mornings and in the evenings. Daktarin powder should be applied to the lesions simultaneously and dusted inside articles of clothing in contact with the affected areas. To prevent relapse treatment should be continued for ten days after all lesions have disappeared.

Nail infections: Daktarin cream should be applied thinly to the infected nail once daily and the nail should be covered with an occlusive dressing. Treatment should continue uninterrupted *until the growth of the new nail is established.*

Use in elderly: As above.

Contra-indications, warnings, etc
Contra-indications: None known.

Side-effects: Occasionally, irritation has been reported. Rarely, local sensitisation may occur, requiring discontinuation of treatment.

Overdosage: Not applicable.

Pharmaceutical precautions Store away from direct heat.

Legal category P.

Package quantities *Cream:* Daktarin cream, 30 g tube.

Twin Pack: Daktarin cream 30 g tube *plus* Daktarin powder 30 g 'puffer' pack.

Further information Daktarin twin pack is particularly indicated for those infections involving moist areas of the body especially Athlete's Foot.

A leaflet outlining to the patient the hygiene routines to be observed and the correct method of application of Daktarin is included in each pack of cream and in the twin pack.

Product licence numbers

Daktarin Cream	0242/0016
Daktarin Twin Pack	0242/0016
	0242/0017

DAKTARIN* ORAL GEL

Presentation Sugar-free orange flavoured oral gel containing miconazole base 2% w/w (25 mg/ml).

Uses Miconazole is a synthetic imidazole anti-fungal substance with a broad spectrum of activity against pathogenic fungi (including yeast and dermatophytes) and Gram-positive bacteria (staph. and strep. spp.).

Miconazole is incompletely absorbed from the gastro-intestinal tract. Blood levels of up to 1 mcg/ml can be achieved following ingestion of 1 gram per day of miconazole base.

Daktarin oral gel is indicated for the treatment of fungal infection of the oropharynx and gastrointestinal tract. This includes oral candidosis in adults and children; also for the eradication of fungi from gut reservoirs when necessary (such as an adjunct to local treatment of vulvo-vaginitis).

Dosage and administration Daktarin oral gel should be taken after meals (one 5 ml spoonful contains 125 mg miconazole).

Adults: One to two spoonsful (5–10 ml) of gel four times daily.

Children Aged over 6: One spoonful (5 ml) of gel four times daily.

Aged 2–6: One spoonful (5 ml) of gel twice daily.

Infants under 2 years of age: Half spoonful (2.5 ml) of gel twice daily.

Treatment should be continued for two days after symptoms have cleared.

For best results in the treatment of oral lesions, miconazole should be kept in contact with the affected area as long as possible. This can be achieved by retaining the gel in the mouth for the maximum time possible.

Use in elderly: As for adults.

Contra-indications, warnings, etc
Contra-indications: There are no known contra-indications to the use of miconazole.

Warnings: Systemic miconazole may potentiate the activity of anticoagulants, antiepileptics or hypoglycaemic drugs, the dosage of which may require adjustment.

Use in pregnancy: Although teratogenic effects have not been observed in animals, the safety of oral miconazole in pregnancy has not been definitely established. Its use during pregnancy is therefore not recommended.

Side effects: No major side effects have been recorded from the use of Daktarin oral gel. Mild gastrointestinal disturbances have occasionally been reported.

Overdosage: No cases of overdosage have been reported. Gastric lavage is recommended.

Pharmaceutical precautions Nil.

Legal category P.

Package quantities Daktarin oral gel is supplied in a 40 g tube provided with a 5 ml plastic spoon, marked with a 2.5 ml graduation.

Further information Oral miconazole is also available as Daktarin oral tablets, supplied in blister packs of 20 tablets each containing miconazole base 250 mg. For details of dosage and administration refer to separate data sheet.

Product licence number
Daktarin Oral Gel   0242/0048

DAKTARIN* ORAL TABLETS

Presentation White, cross-scored tablets containing miconazole base 250 mg.

Uses Miconazole is a synthetic imidazole anti-fungal substance with a broad spectrum of activity against pathogenic fungi (including yeasts and dermatophytes) and Gram-positive bacteria (staph. and strep. spp.).

Miconazole is incompletely absorbed from the gastrointestinal tract. Blood levels of up to 1 mcg/ml can be achieved following ingestion of 1 gram per day of miconazole base.

Daktarin oral tablets are for the treatment (including prophylaxis) of fungal infections of the oropharynx and gastrointestinal tract.

Daktarin oral tablets may be used prophylactically in the management of patients at high risk from opportunistic fungal infection. Patients likely to benefit from this treatment include those who are immuno-suppressed such as transplant patients, cancer patients (particularly those undergoing cyto-toxic therapy) and patients suffering from congenital immunological abnormalities. Daktarin oral tablets may also be used for the eradication of fungi from gut reservoirs when necessary (such as prior to relevant surgery).

Dosage and administration Daktarin oral tablets should be taken after meals.

Dosage is based on 15 mg/kg/day.

Adults: One 250 mg tablet four times/day for 10 days or for up to 2 days after the symptoms have cleared.

Use in elderly: As for adults.

Topical treatment of the oropharynx may be achieved by sucking the tablet, allowing it to dissolve slowly in the mouth.

Contra-indications, warnings, etc
Contra-indications: There are no known contra-indications to the use of miconazole.

Warnings: Systemic miconazole may potentiate the activity of anticoagulants, anti-epileptics or hypoglycaemic drugs, the dosage of which may require adjustment.

Use in pregnancy: Although teratogenic effects have not been observed in animals, the safety of oral miconazole in pregnancy has not been definitely established. Its use during pregnancy is therefore not recommended.

Side effects: No major side effects have been recorded from the use of Daktarin oral tablets. Mild gastrointestinal disturbances have occasionally been reported.

Overdosage: No cases of overdosage have been reported. Gastric lavage is recommended.

Pharmaceutical precautions Nil.

Legal category POM.

Package quantities Daktarin oral tablets are supplied in blister packs of 20.

Further information Oral miconazole is also available as a sugar-free orange flavoured gel containing miconazole base 2% w/w (25 mg/ml). Daktarin Oral Gel is supplied in a 40 g tube provided with a 5 ml plastic spoon. For details of dosage and administration refer to separate data sheet.

Product licence number
Daktarin Oral Tablets   0242/0047

DAKTARIN* INTRAVENOUS SOLUTION

Presentation Clear glass ampoules (20 ml), each containing a sterile solution of miconazole (base) 200 mg (10% of polyethyoxylated castor oil is included as solvent).

Uses *Indications:* Daktarin intravenous solution is indicated for the treatment of systemic mycoses, such as systemic candidosis, aspergillosis, coccidioidomycosis, cryptococcosis, blastomycosis.

Actions: Miconazole, a synthetic imidazole compound, has a broad spectrum of *in vitro* activity against fungi, yeasts and Gram-positive bacteria, including *Candida albicans, Candida tropicalis, Candida parapsilosis. Aspergillus fumigatus, Aspergillus niger, Cryptococcus neoformans, Coccidioides immitis, Paracoccidioides brasiliensis,* and a range of other less commonly occurring pathogens.

Intravenous infusion of doses above 9 mg/kg produces effective peak blood levels in excess of 1 mcg/ml. The drug is rapidly metabolised. The pharmacokinetics are unaffected in patients with renal insufficiency, including those on haemodialysis. Plasma levels, however, may be somewhat elevated. Clinical use has revealed no evidence of serious renal or hepatic toxicity associated with intravenous miconazole.

Dosage and administration Daktarin intravenous solution must be diluted with either physiological saline (Sodium Chloride Injection BP) or 5% Dextrose Injection BP and administered slowly *by intravenous infusion* over a period of at least 30 minutes. The usual adult dose is 600 mg (3 ampoules) three times daily; as an infusion of 200–500 ml infusion fluid. The incidence of side effects or the sensitivity of the fungal strain involved may require individual adjustment of this dose.

As a guide, clinically effective daily doses have ranged as low as 600 mg/day, in a few patients, as high as 3,600 mg/day.

In children a daily dose of about 40 mg/kg is recommended. A dose of 15 mg/kg per infusion should not be exceeded.

Duration of treatment is dictated by the rate of response of the infection to miconazole rather than an arbitrary number of days. Treatment should be continued until mycological evidence of remission or cure is obtained. Daktarin intravenous solution has been used without major side-effects or toxicity for periods of over 20 weeks.

Use in elderly: As for adults – the incidence of side effects may require individual adjustment of the dose.

Contra-indications, warnings, etc
Contra-indications: Patients who are hypersensitive to Daktarin intravenous solution, since in animal studies polyethoxylated castor oil has been shown to produce adverse effects associated with histamine release; and

similar anaphylactoid reactions have been observed in rare cases following Daktarin i.v.

Warnings: Rapid injection of a bolus of undiluted drug can produce transient tachycardia and cardiac arrhythmias. These, if not spontaneously reversible, usually respond promptly to lignocaine. Daktarin intravenous solution is well tolerated (including patients with pre-existing cardiovascular disorders) if given by intravenous infusion.

Systemic miconazole may potentiate the activity of anti-coagulant, anti-epileptic or hypoglycaemic drugs, the dosage of which may require adjustment. Antagonism of the in vitro activity of miconazole by amphotericin B has been reported.

Use in pregnancy: The safety of Daktarin intravenous solution in pregnancy has not been established and its use in pregnant women should be avoided if possible.

Side-effects: Haematological and biochemical controls are recommended since the infusion of Daktarin intravenous solution in large volumes of fluid may produce a decrease in haemoglobin, haematocrit and serum sodium. When cremophor (polyethoxylated castor oil) is given to patients over a period of several days, it may cause hyperlipidemia and an abnormal plasma lipoprotein electro-phoretic pattern, aggregation of erythrocytes or rouleaux formation on blood smears. These effects are reversible on discontinuation of treatment and are not usually sufficiently severe to warrant discontinuation of intravenous miconazole.

The adverse reactions reported during clinical investigations of Daktarin intravenous solution are phlebitis, pruritus, nausea and vomiting, febrile reactions, rash, drowsiness, diarrhoea, anorexia and flushes. Using a subclavian catheter or changing the sites of infusion every 48–72 hours reduces the incidence and severity of phlebitis. Nausea and vomiting can be prevented by giving an antiemetic drug before infusion, by reducing the dose, by slowing the rate of infusion or by avoiding mealtime administration.

Overdosage: In the case of overdosage, the following symptoms may occur, vomiting, diarrhoea, convulsions or cardiac rhythm disorders.

Pharmaceutical precautions Storage should be at room temperature. Shelf life is five years. Daktarin intravenous solution should be mixed only with the recommended diluents, Sodium Chloride Injection BP or 5% Dextrose Injection BP.

Legal category POM.

Package quantities Daktarin intravenous solution is supplied in 20 ml glass ampoules, packed in boxes of ten. Each ampoule contains miconazole (base) 200 mg.

Further information Miconazole's broad spectrum of antifungal activity and its lack of serious toxicity suggest that Daktarin intravenous solution may be considered for treatment in cases of life-threatening systemic fungal infection.

Product licence number 0242/0052.

DROLEPTAN*

Presentation *Injection:* Clear, colourless, aqueous injection in 2 ml ampoules. Each millilitre contains 5 mg droperidol.
Tablets: Yellow uncoated, scored tablets marked 'JANS-SEN' on one side and D above 10 on the reverse. Each tablet contains 10 mg droperidol.
Liquid: Clear, colourless, odourless liquid containing 1 mg droperidol/ml for oral administration.

Uses Droleptan is a major tranquilliser of the butyrophenone series with the following indications:
1. In anaesthesia:
   (a) in conjunction with a narcotic analgesic in the technique of neuroleptanalgesia;
   (b) either alone or in combination with a narcotic analgesic for premedication;
   (c) for post-operative nausea and vomiting.
2. For treatment of chemotherapy-induced nausea and vomiting.
3. In psychiatry for rapidly calming the manic, agitated patient.

Dosage and administration
Neuroleptanalgesia
Adults: 5–15 mg iv at induction of anaesthesia with a narcotic analgesic.
Children: 0.2–0.3 mg/kg iv.

Premedication in anaesthesia
Adults: Up to 10 mg im or oral.
Children: 0.2–0.5 mg/kg im or 0.3–0.6 mg/kg oral.

Anti-emetic
Adults: Post-operative 5 mg iv or im; in cancer chemotherapy – a loading dose of 5–10 mg should be given 30 minutes before commencement of therapy, followed either by a continuous infusion of 1–3 mg/hr or 1–5 mg im or iv every 1–4 hours as required. The dosage must be individually determined according to the needs and status of the patient.
Children: Doses used have ranged between 0.02–0.075 mg/kg im or iv dependent on emetic stimulus.

In psychiatry
Adults: 5–15 mg iv; up to 10 mg im; 5–20 mg oral. The dosage may be repeated at intervals of 4–6 hours (im or iv) or 4–8 hours (oral).
Children: 0.5–1 mg/day im or oral adjusted according to response.

In pyschiatry, dosage should be individually determined and is best initiated and titrated under close clinical supervision. To determine the initial dose, consideration should be given to the patient's age, severity of symptoms, and previous response to other neuroleptic drugs.

Patients who are elderly or debilitated or those with previously reported adverse reactions to neuroleptic drugs, may require less Droleptan and half the normal starting dose in psychiatry may be sufficient for therapeutic response. The optimal response in such patients is usually obtained with more gradual titration and at lower dose levels. In adolescents a lower starting dose may be advisable.

Contra-indications, warnings, etc
Contra-indications: Comatose states, severe depression.

Use in pregnancy: The safety of Droleptan in pregnancy has not been established, although studies in animals have not demonstrated teratogenic effects. As with other drugs, it is not advisable to administer Droleptan in pregnancy.

Precautions: Butyrophenones are excreted in breast milk and are not recommended during lactation. If the use of Droleptan is essential, breast feeding should be discontinued.

Caution is advised in patients with liver disease, renal failure, Parkinson's disease, epilepsy, and conditions predisposing to epilepsy or convulsions.

In anaesthesia intravenous induction agents will generally be required in lower dosage where Droleptan is used as part of the anaesthetic technique, and the effects of heavy sedative premedication may be potentiated. When using Droleptan at induction of anaesthesia provision should be made for rapid infusion of intravenous fluid to correct any large fall in blood pressure, which, if it occurs, is due to relative hypovolaemia and is more common in the elderly or untreated hypertensives.

Warnings: In common with all neuroleptics Droleptan can increase the central nervous system depression produced by other CNS-depressant drugs, including alcohol, hypnotics, sedatives or strong analgesics; and may antagonise the action of adrenaline and other sympathomimetic agents.

Droleptan may impair the anti-Parkinson effects of levodopa. The dosage of anti-convulsants may need to be increased to take account of the lowered seizure threshold.

Enhanced CNS effects, when combined with methyldopa, has been reported for some butyrophenones.

Acute withdrawal symptoms, including nausea, vomiting and insomnia, have very rarely been described after abrupt cessation of high doses of anti-psychotic drugs. Relapse may also occur and gradual withdrawal is advisable.

Adverse effects: Some degree of sedation or impairment of alertness may occur, particularly with higher doses and at the start of treatment and may be potentiated by alcohol. Patients should be advised not to drive or operate machinery during treatment until their susceptibility is known, or on the day following administration if early discharge is envisaged.

In common with all neuroleptics, extrapyramidal symptoms may occur. Acute dystonias may occur early in treatment. Parkinsonian rigidity, tremor and akathisia tend to appear less rapidly. Oculogyric crises and laryngeal dystonias have been reported. Extrapyramidal symptoms are less common at the low single doses used in anaesthesia, or as an anti-emetic.

Anti-Parkinson agents should only be given as required; they should not be prescribed routinely because of the possible risk of impairing the therapeutic efficacy of Droleptan.

Tardive dyskinesia may occur during administration or after withdrawal of neuroleptic drugs, including Droleptan, and can be precipitated or aggravated by anti-Parkinson drugs; Tardive dyskinesia has not been reported following anti-emetic or anaesthetic uses of Droleptan.

The syndrome is unlikely to occur in the short-term when low or moderate doses of Droleptan are used as recommended, but since its occurrence may be related to duration of treatment, as well as daily dose, Droleptan should be given in the minimum effective dose for the minimum possible time.

The potential seriousness and unpredictability of tardive dyskinesia, and the fact that it has occasionally been reported to occur when neuroleptic anti-psychotic drugs have been prescribed for relatively short periods in low doses, means that the prescribing of such agents requires especially careful assessment of risks versus benefits.

Gastrointestinal symptoms, nausea, loss of apetite and dyspepsia, have been reported.

Hormonal effects of anti-psychotic neuroleptic drugs include hyper-prolactinaemia, which may cause galactorrhoea, gynaecomastia and oligo- or amenorrhoea.

Dose-related hypotension is uncommon, but can occur, particularly in the elderly, who are more susceptible to the sedative and hypotensive effects.

Droleptan, even in low dosage in susceptible (especially non-psychotic) individuals, may cause unpleasant subjective feelings of being mentally dulled or slowed down, dizziness, headache, or paradoxical effects of excitement, agitation or insomnia.

The following effects have been reported rarely: oedema, various skin rashes and reactions, hypertensivity, jaundice or transient abnormalities or liver function in the absence of jaundice; anxiety or confusional states or epileptic fits, vision disturbances, sweating.

Blood dyscrasias have been reported very rarely.

Overdosage: There have been no serious toxic effects attributed to Droleptan and fatal over-dosage has not been reported. Treatment of overdosage consists of supportive measures combined with sedative or anti-Parkinsonian drugs, as required.

Pharmaceutical precautions Droperidol preparations should be protected from light.

If desired, Droleptan injection can be mixed with intravenous infusion solutions and with most agents commonly used in anaesthesia, but it is chemically incompatible with the induction agents thiopentone, propanidid and methohexitone, because of the wide difference in pH.

Legal category POM.

Package quantities Droleptan injection is supplied in 2 ml ampoules (5 mg/ml) in packs of 10.

Droleptan tablets each containing 10 mg droperidol are supplied in packs of 50.

Droleptan liquid is supplied in amber glass bottles of 100 ml (1 mg/ml).

Further information Nil.

Product licence numbers
Droleptan injection 0242/5003R
Droleptan tablets 0242/5004R
Droleptan liquid 0242/0080R

GYNO-DAKTARIN*

Presentation *Intravaginal Cream:* White, non-staining, water-miscible cream containing miconazole nitrate 2% w/w.

Pessary: White, non-staining pessaries each containing 100 mg miconazole nitrate.

Combi-pack: White, non-staining pessaries each containing 100 mg miconazole nitrate plus white, non-staining, water miscible topical cream containing miconazole nitrate 2% w/w.

Tampon: Tampons, each coated with 100 mg miconazole nitrate.

Uses Miconazole is a synthetic imidazole antifungal agent with a broad spectrum of activity against pathogenic fungi (including yeasts and dermatophytes) and Gram-positive bacteria (staph. and strep. spp.).

Gyno-Daktarin is for the local treatment of vulvovaginal candidosis and super infection due to susceptible Gram-positive bacteria.

Gyno-Daktarin cream may also be used for treatment of mycotic balanitis.

Dosage and administration Gyno-Daktarin may be used in both adults and children.

Vaginitis: 10 g of the cream, or two pessaries should be inserted at night high into the vagina. Disposable applicators are provided for insertion of the cream.

This procedure should be repeated for 7 days, even though symptomatic cure of the pruritis and leukorrhea will have been noted within a few days of commencing therapy.

Alternatively, one tampon should be inserted high into the vagina twice daily (morning and evening) for 5 days.

Vulvitis or balanitis: The cream should be applied topically twice daily.

Use in elderly: As above.

Contra-indications, warnings, etc
Contra-indications: None known.

Side-effects: Occasionally, irritation has been reported. Rarely, local sensitisation may occur requiring discontinuation of treatment.

Overdosage: Not applicable.

Pharmaceutical precautions Store in a cool place.

Legal category POM.

Package quantities *Cream:* Gyno-Daktarin intravaginal cream is supplied in 78 g tubes with disposable applicators – seven days' treatment.

Pessary: Gyno-Daktarin pessaries are supplied in packs each containing 14 pessaries – seven days' treatment.

Combi-pack: Gyno-Daktarin combi-pack consists of 14 pessaries plus 15 g topical cream.

Tampons: Gyno-Daktarin tampons are supplied in packs each containing 10 tampons.

Further information Gyno-Daktarin may be used in 'problem vaginitis' as seen in diabetic patients and in women using oral contraceptives.

A leaflet instructing the patient on the correct use is included in each package of Gyno-Daktarin.

Product licence numbers

Gyno-Daktarin Cream	0242/0015
Gyno-Daktarin Pessaries	0242/0037
Gyno-Daktarin Combi-Pack	{ 0242/0015 { 0242/0037
Gyno-Daktarin Tampons	0242/0056

HALDOL*

Presentation Pale blue scored uncoated tablets marked Janssen on one side and H/5* on the reverse, containing 5.0 mg Haloperidol BP.

Yellow scored uncoated tablets marked Janssen on one side and H/10* on the reverse, containing 10 mg Haloperidol BP.

Clear glass ampoules containing 5 mg Haloperidol BP in 1 ml aqueous solution for injection.

Clear glass ampoules containing 10 mg Haloperidol BP in 2 ml aqueous solution for injection.

Clear colourless, odourless liquid containing 2 mg Haloperidol BP per ml for oral administration.

Clear, colourless, odourless liquid containing 10 mg Haloperidol BP per ml for oral administration following dilution (see Package insert).

Uses Haldol is a highly effective neuroleptic butyrophenone drug, with a wide range of actions. Haldol is recommended for the rapid control of the symptoms of hostility, aggression, hyperactivity, disruptive and violent behaviour, confusion, emotional withdrawal, hallucinations and delusions associated with acute and chronic schizophrenia, mania and hypomania, organic brain syndrome, alcohol withdrawal syndrome and delirium tremens, childhood behavioural disorders. Haldol is also indicated for the treatment of motor tics, stuttering and persistent hiccoughs, nausea and vomiting, anxiety states and as pre-anaesthetic medication.

Dosage and administration *Adults:* As with all neuroleptic drugs it is vitally important to titrate the dose of Haldol to the needs of each patient. Titration should be carried out as rapidly as practicable to achieve optimum therapeutic control. To determine the initial dose, consideration should be given to the patient's age, severity of symptoms and previous response to other neuroleptic drugs. It is important to increase dosage progressively until maximum control of symptoms has been achieved. Thereafter, dosage may be reduced gradually to the lowest effective maintenance level.

Patients who are elderly or debilitated or those with previous adverse reactions to neuroleptic drugs may require less Haldol. The optimal response in such patients is usually obtained with more gradual titration and at lower dose levels. In adolescents a lower dose may be advisable.

1. Oral administration-initial dosage: General
Moderate symptomatology 0.5–2.0 mg b.i.d. or t.i.d.
Severe symptomatology 3.0–5.0 mg b.i.d. or t.i.d.
To achieve prompt control, higher doses may be required in some cases.
Geriatric or debilitated patients 0.5–2.0 mg b.i.d. or t.i.d.

Resistant patients:
Chronic or resistant patients 3.0–5.0 mg b.i.d. or t.i.d.
Patients who remain severely disturbed or inadequately controlled may occasionally require further titration of dosage. Daily dosages up to 100 mg may be necessary to achieve an optimal response. Haldol (haloperidol) has been used in doses of 200 mg for severely resistant patients.

Maintenance dosage: Upon achieving a satisfactory therapeutic response, dosage should be gradually reduced to the lowest effective maintenance level, often as low as 5–10 mg/day. Too rapid dosage reduction should be avoided.

Anxiety states: 0.5 mg twice daily. At this dosage level no interaction with moderate amounts of alcohol nor any deleterious effect on intellectual or psychomotor (including driving) abilities has been demonstrated.

Tics, choreiform movements, stuttering: Haldol administered orally in doses of 0.5–1.5 mg t.d.s. significantly reduces the degree of stuttering in most but not all stutterers. Tics, choreiform movements and dyskinesias have all been treated with Haldol. In Gilles de la Tourette syndrome daily maintenance doses of 10 mg and higher may be required.

2. Parenteral administration: Parenteral medication administered intramuscularly in initial doses of 2–10 mg is utilised for prompt control of the acutely agitated patient with moderate symptoms. Very severely disturbed patients may require an initial dose of up to 30 mg. Depending on the response of the patient subsequent doses of 5 mg may be given as often as every hour if necessary, although 4–8 hour intervals may be satisfactory to achieve control. Oral treatment should succeed intramuscular administration as soon as practicable.

Haldol can also be parenterally administered by the intravenous route.

For pre-anaesthetic medication: a single intravenous or i.m. dose of 1–5 mg effectively reduces the incidence of postoperative nausea and vomiting, and also controls apprehension and nervousness before surgery.

Haldol administered parenterally by intramuscular injection 2–5 mg every 4–6 hours for up to 24 hours effectively controls anxiety, irritability, insomnia, anorexia and nausea in the *Alcohol withdrawal syndrome.*

Children – Oral administration
Childhood behavioural disorders: Orally administered Haldol provides useful adjunctive therapy in controlling overactivity, destructiveness, resentment and aggressiveness in disturbed and schizophrenic children, in total daily maintenance doses of 0.05 mg/kg/day, half the total dose given in the morning and the other half in the evening.

Gilles de la Tourette disease: The sudden involuntary movements and utterances of this syndrome can be controlled with oral maintenance doses of up to 10 mg per day in most cases.

Stuttering: Oral doses of 0.05 mg/kg/day have proved useful adjunct therapy in the treatment of stuttering.

Use in elderly: Patients who are elderly or debilitated or those with previously reported adverse reactions to neuroleptic drugs may require less Haldol, and half the normal starting dose may be sufficient for therapeutic response. The optimal response in such patients is usually obtained with more gradual titration and at lower dose levels.

Contra-indications, warnings, etc

Contra-indications: Comatose states.

Use in pregnancy and lactation: The safety of Haldol in pregnancy has not been established. There is some evidence of harmful effects in some but not all animal studies; human experience suggests that there may be teratogenic effects, although a causal relationship has not been established. Haldol is excreted in breast milk and is not recommended during lactation: if the use of Haldol is considered essential, breast feeding should be discontinued.

Warnings: In common with all neuroleptics extrapyramidal symptoms may occur. Acute dystonias may occur early in treatment. Parkinsonian rigidity, tremor and akathisia tend to appear less rapidly. Oculogyric crisis and laryngeal dystonias have been reported.

Anti-Parkinson agents should not be prescribed routinely, but only be given as required, because of the possible risk of impairing the efficacy of Haldol.

Tardive dyskinesia may occur during administration or after withdrawal of neuroleptic drugs, including Haldol, and can be precipitated or aggravated by anti-Parkinson drugs. The syndrome is unlikely to occur in the short term when low or moderate doses of Haldol are used as recommended. However since its occurrence may be related to duration of treatment, as well as daily dose, Haldol should be given in the minimum effective dose for the minimum possible time, unless it is established that long term administration for the treatment of schizophrenia is required.

The potential seriousness and unpredictability of tardive dyskinesia, and the fact that it has occasionally been reported to occur when neuroleptic antipsychotic drugs have been prescribed for relatively short periods in low doses, means that the prescribing of such agents requires especially careful assessment of risks versus benefit.

In common with other antipsychotic drugs, haloperidol has been associated with rare cases of neuroleptic malignant syndrome, an idiosyncratic response characterised by hyperthermia, muscle rigidity, autonomic instability, altered consciousness and coma. Signs of autonomic dysfunction such as tachycardia, labile arterial pressure and sweating may precede the onset of hyperthermia, acting as early warning signs. Recovery usually occurs within five to seven days of antipsychotic withdrawal. Affected patients should be carefully monitored.

Gastrointestinal symptoms, nausea, loss of appetite and dyspepsia have been reported.

Hormonal effects of antipsychotic neuroleptic drugs include hyperprolactinaemia, which may cause galactorrhoea, gynaecomastia and oligo- or amenorrhoea.

Weight changes may occur.

Dose related hypotension is uncommon, but can occur, particularly in the elderly, who are more susceptible to the sedative and hypotensive effects.

Haldol, even in low dosage in susceptible (especially non-psychotic) individuals, may cause unpleasant subjective feelings of being mentally dulled or slowed down, dizziness, headache or paradoxical effects of excitement, agitation or insomnia. The following effects have been reported rarely: oedema, various skin rashes and reactions, including exfoliative dermatitis and erythema multiforme; jaundice or transient abnormalities of liver function in the absence of jaundice; confusional states or epileptic fits; impairment of sexual function, including erection and ejaculation.

The following have been reported very rarely: blood dyscrasias, including agranulocytosis and transient leucopenia, and photosensitive skin reactions.

Caution is advised in patients with liver disease, renal failure, Parkinsons disease, phaeochromocytoma, thyrotoxicosis, epilepsy and conditions predisposing to epilepsy or convulsions.

Acute withdrawal symptoms including nausea, vomiting and insomnia have very rarely been described after abrupt cessation of high doses of antipsychotic drugs. Relapse may also occur and gradual withdrawal is advisable.

Precautions: In common with all neuroleptics Haldol can increase the central nervous system depression produced by other CNS-depressant drugs, including alcohol, hypnotics, sedatives or strong analgesics; and may antagonise the action of adrenaline and other sympathomimetic agents.

Haldol may impair the anti-Parkinson effects of levodopa. The dosage of anti-convulsants may need to be increased to take account of the lowered seizure threshold. Enhanced CNS effect when combined with methyldopa has been reported. Neurotoxic reactions during combined treatment with lithium and Haldol have been reported, but the mechanism for this effect is undetermined. In schizophrenia the response to antipsychotic drug treatment may be delayed. If drugs are withdrawn, recurrence of symptoms may not become apparent for several weeks or months.

Some degree of sedation or impairment of alertness may occur, particularly with higher doses and at the start of treatment and may be potentiated by alcohol. Patients should be advised not to drive or operate machinery during treatment, until their susceptibility is known.

Overdose: There have been no serious toxic effects attributed to Haldol and fatal overdosage has not been reported. Treatment of overdosage consists of supportive measures combined with sedative or anti-Parkinsonian drugs, as required.

Pharmaceutical precautions Store tablets in a cool dry place. Haldol liquid and ampoules should be protected from light and Haldol liquid from cold.

Legal category POM.

Package quantities

5.0 mg Tablet: 100.
10.0 mg Tablet: 100 in canisters.
5 mg/ml Injectable Solution: 5 × 1 ml ampoules.
10 mg/2 ml Injectable Solution: 5 × 2 ml ampoules.
2 mg/ml Oral Liquid: 100 ml amber glass bottles, with calibrated pipette.
10 mg per ml Oral Liquid: 100 ml amber glass bottles with leaflet insert.

Further information Haldol is well absorbed following oral administration of either the tablet or the oral liquid. Plasma levels and areas under the plasma level–time curve are essentially the same for the tablet and oral liquid, thus bioavailability of Haldol tablets is the same as that of an oral solution.

Dilution instructions Haldol Oral Liquid Concentrate 10 mg/ml should normally be diluted with purified water to meet individual patient requirements. Following dilution it is advised that the solution be used as soon as possible. If a more prolonged shelf life is required, dilution with an aqueous solution of methyl paraben (0.5 mg/ml) and propyl paraben (0.05 mg/ml) is recommended, thus maintaining the original concentration of preservatives. Further information is to be found in the package insert leaflet.

Product licence numbers

5.0 mg tablet	0242/0031
10.0 mg tablet	0242/0039
5 mg/ml injectable solution	0242/0036
10 mg/2 ml injectable solution	0242/0036
2 mg/ml oral liquid	0242/0035
10 mg/ml oral liquid	0242/0049

HALDOL* DECANOATE ▼

Presentation Straw coloured, viscous solution presented in 1 ml brown glass ampoules equivalent to 100 mg/ml haloperidol (as decanoate ester) and in 1 ml brown glass ampoules containing haloperidol 50 mg/ml (as decanoate ester).

Uses Haldol decanoate is an ester of the potent butyrophenone neuroleptic, haloperidol. The active agent is slowly released from an intramuscular depot injection of Haldol decanoate. Haldol decanoate is indicated where long term maintenance treatment with a neuroleptic is required; for example in schizophrenia, other psychoses (especially paranoid), and other mental or behavioural problems where maintenance treatment is clearly indicated.

Dosage and administration Haldol decanoate is for use in adults only and has been formulated to provide one month's therapy for most patients following a single deep intramuscular injection in the gluteal region.

Since individual response to neuroleptic drugs is variable, dosage should be individually determined and is best initiated and titrated under close clinical supervision.

In mild symptomatology and in the elderly up to 100 mg every 4 weeks, in moderate symptomatology 100–200 mg every 4 weeks, and in severe cases 200–300 mg or more every 4 weeks.

As with other depot preparations lumps or irritation at the site of injection can be avoided by injecting haloperidol decanoate deep intramuscularly with a 2–2.5 inch needle of at least 21 gauge.

Contra-indications, warnings, etc *Contra-indications:* Haldol is excreted in breast milk and is not recommended during lactation: if the use of haloperidol is considered essential, breast feeding should be discontinued.

Use in pregnancy: The safety of haloperidol in pregnancy has not been established. There is some evidence of harmful effects in some but not all animal studies. Human experience suggests that there may be teratogenic effects, although a causal relationship has not been established.

Precautions: Caution is advised in patients with liver disease, renal failure, Parkinson's disease, phaeochromocytoma, thyrotoxicosis, epilepsy and conditions predisposing to epilepsy (e.g. alcohol withdrawal and brain damage).

In common with all neuroleptics haloperidol can increase the central nervous system depression produced by other CNS-depressant drugs, including alcohol, hypnotics, sedatives or strong analgesics.

Haloperidol may antagonise the action of adrenaline and other sympathomimetic agents and reverses the blood-pressure-lowering effects of adrenergic-blocking agents such as guanethedine.

Haloperidol may impair the metabolism of tricyclic anti-depressants (clinical significance unknown) and the anti-Parkinson effects of levodopa. The dosage of anti-convulsants may need to be increased to take account of the lowered seizure threshold.

Antagonism of the effect of phenindione has been reported.

Enhanced CNS effect, when combined with methyldopa, has been reported.

Neurotoxic reactions to combined treatment with lithium and Haloperidol have been reported, but the mechanism for this effect is undetermined.

Warnings and adverse effects: Some degree of sedation or impairment of alertness may occur, particularly with higher doses and at the start of treatment. Patients should be advised not to drive or operate machinery during treatment, until their susceptibility is known.

In common with all neuroleptics, extra-pyramidal symptoms may occur. Acute dystonias may occur early in treatment. Parkinsonian rigidity, tremor and akathisia tend to appear less rapidly. Oculogyric crises and laryngeal dystonias have been reported.

Anti-Parkinson agents should only be given as required; they should not be prescribed routinely because of the possible risk of impairing haloperidol's therapeutic efficacy. Preliminary results suggest that withdrawal of anti-Parkinson medication may be attempted following transfer from oral to monthly depot injections of Haldol* decanoate.

Tardive dyskinesia is common among patients treated with moderate to high doses of antipsychotic drugs for prolonged periods of time and may prove irreversible, particularly in patients over 50 years.

The potential seriousness and unpredictability of tardive dyskinesia and the fact that it has occasionally been reported to occur when neuroleptic antipsychotic drugs have been prescribed for relatively short periods in low dosage means that the prescribing of such agents requires especially careful assessment of risk versus benefit. Tardive dyskinesia can be precipitated or aggravated by anti-Parkinson drugs. Short-term dyskinesias may occur after abrupt drug withdrawal.

In schizophrenia, the response to antipsychotic drug treatment may be delayed. If drugs are withdrawn, recurrence of symptoms may not become apparent for several weeks or months.

Haloperidol, even in low dosage in susceptible (especially non-psychotic) individuals, may cause unpleasant subjective feelings of being mentally dulled or slowed down, dizziness, headache or paradoxical effects of excitement, agitation or insomnia.

Gastro-intestinal symptoms, nausea, loss of appetite and dyspepsia have been reported.

Hormonal effects of antipsychotic neuroleptic drugs include hyper-prolactinaemia, which may cause galactorrhoea, gynaecomastia and oligo- or amenorrhoea.

Weight changes may occur.

Dose-related hypotension is uncommon, but can occur, particularly in the elderly.

Autonomic effects, such as blurring of vision and tachycardia, are uncommon.

The following effects have been reported rarely: oedema; various skin rashes and reactions, including exfoliative dermatitis and erythema multiforma; jaundice or transient abnormalities of liver function in the absence of jaundice; confusional states or epileptic fits; impairment of sexual function, including erection and ejaculation. The elderly are more susceptible to the sedative and hypotensive effects.

The following effects have been reported very rarely: blood dyscrasias, including agranulocytosis and transient leucopenia, and photosensitive skin reactions. Occasional local reactions such as erythema, swelling or tender lumps have been reported in common with other antipsychotics.

In common with other antipsychotics, haloperidol has been associated with rare cases of neuroleptic malignant syndrome, an idiosyncratic response characterised by hyperthermia, muscle rigidity, autonomic instability, altered consciousness and coma. Signs of autonomic dysfunction such as tachycardia, labile arterial pressure and sweating may precede the onset of hyperthermia, acting as early warning signs. Recovery usually occurs within five to seven days of antipsychotic withdrawal. Affected patients should be carefully monitored.

Overdosage: There have been no serious toxic effects attributed to Haldol decanoate and fatal overdosage has not been reported. Treatment of overdosage consists of supportive measures combined with sedative or anti-Parkinsonian drugs, as required.

Pharmaceutical precautions Haldol decanoate should be protected from light and stored at room temperature. In common with other depot neuroleptics, if stored for long periods in the cold, precipitation may occur which may clear on storage at room temperature.

If precipitate does not clear, the contents of the ampoule should be discarded. Do not store below room temperature.

Further information Haloperidol is a butyrophenone. Its pharmacological profile of activity includes a low incidence of autonomic side effects, such as hypotension, and a capacity to induce extrapyramidal reactions.

Legal category POM.

Package quantities 100 mg/ml ampoules: 1 ml ampoules in packs of 5. 50 mg/ml ampoules: 1 ml in packs of 5.

Product licence numbers
50 mg/ml   0242/0094
100 mg/ml   0242/0095

HISMANAL* ▼

Presentation White, biconvex, half-scored, uncoated tablets. Each tablet is marked 'Janssen' on one side and 'Ast/10' on the reverse, and contains astemizole 10 mg.

Uses Hismanal is a potent and long acting histamine H_1-antagonist with no central sedative or anti-cholinergic effects.

Hismanal is indicated for allergic rhinitis and conjunctivitis and other conditions normally responsive to antihistamines, including allergic skin reactions (urticaria).

Dosage and administration For optimal absorption, Hismanal should be taken an hour before food or on an empty stomach.

Adults and children over 12 years: Usually 10 mg daily. When necessary, up to 30 mg once daily may be given for up to 7 days, then 10 mg daily.

Children 6–12 years: Half a tablet daily (5 mg). When necessary, up to 1½ tablets (15 mg) once daily may be given for up to 7 days, then ½ tablet daily.

Use in elderly: There have been no specific studies in the elderly.

Contra-indications, warnings, etc
Contra-indications: Hismanal is contra-indicated in women who are pregnant.

Precautions: Adequate contraceptive precautions should be taken by women of childbearing potential during therapy, and, in view of the prolonged half-life, for several weeks after stopping.

Specific studies of possible liver enzyme induction have been carried out with negative results. There is, therefore, no reason to suggest any modification of oral contraceptive dosages in users of Hismanal.

Like many other antihistamines, Hismanal has been associated with adverse effects on the maintenance of pregnancy in rats. No teratogenic effects were observed in animal studies with Hismanal. The safety of Hismanal in human pregnancy has not been established.

There have been no specific studies of Hismanal in children under 6 years.

Adverse reactions: Hismanal has no sedative or anti-cholinergic activity. Other adverse reactions are infrequent during Hismanal therapy. Weight gain has been reported.

Overdosage: In the event of overdosage cases should be treated symptomatically with supportive measures or gastric lavage, as necessary.

Pharmaceutical precautions Nil.

Legal category POM.

Package quantities Supplied in packs of 30 tablets.

Further information Hismanal has no known interaction with CNS-depressant drugs including alcohol. Controlled clinical trials with placebo and reference antihistamines have demonstrated that Hismanal is non-sedative, and does not interfere with activities requiring mental alertness, for example, driving or operating machinery.

Product licence number 0242/0086.

HYPNOMIDATE*

Presentation Clear, colourless solution containing 2 mg/ml etomidate. The aqueous vehicle contains 35% propylene glycol.

Uses Hypnomidate is an intravenous induction agent.

Dosage and administration In adults and children a dose of 0.3 mg/kg given intravenously at induction of anaesthesia gives sleep lasting from 6 to 10 minutes.

Since Hypnomidate has no analgesic action, appropriate analgesics should be used in procedures involving painful stimuli. Hypnomidate is pharmacologically compatible with the muscle relaxants, premedicant drugs and inhalation anaesthetics in current clinical use.

Use in elderly: As for adults.

Contra-indications, warnings, etc

Warnings: Reduced serum cortisol levels unresponsive to ACTH injections, have been reported in some patients during maintenance of anaesthesia with etomidate; for this reason etomidate should not be used for maintenance. However, when etomidate is used for induction, the post-operative rise in serum cortisol which has been observed after thiopentone induction is delayed for approximately 3–6 hours.

Hypnomidate should not be administered to patients with evidence or suggestion of, reduced adrenal cortical function. Convulsions may occur in unpremedicated patients.

Side-effects: The use of narcotic analgesics as premedication and during surgery will reduce the uncontrolled spontaneous muscle movements shown by some patients after Hypnomidate administration.

Pain can occur after injection into the small veins of the dorsum of the hand. Use of larger veins reduces pain on injection.

Other side-effects are rare.

Precautions: Hypnomidate by injection should be given slowly.

Animal experiments have shown no evidence of teratogenicity but Hypnomidate should be used with caution in pregnancy.

Pharmaceutical precautions Store at room temperature. Combinations with pancuronium bromide may show a very slight opalescence; for this reason the two should not be mixed together.

Legal category POM.

Package quantities Hypnomidate is supplied as 10 ml ampoules in packs of 10.

Further information Hypnomidate is rapidly metabolised and eliminated and recovery of consciousness from a single dose is rapid and complete.

Product licence number 0242/0019.

HYPNOMIDATE* CONCENTRATE ▼

Presentation Concentrate for dilution: Clear, colourless liquid presented in 1 ml ampoules. Each millilitre contains etomidate hydrochloride equivalent to 125 mg etomidate base. One ampoule should be sufficient for 4–5 inductions.

Uses Hypnomidate is a short-acting intravenous hypnotic drug which may be used for induction of anaesthesia.

Dosage and administration

In adults (including the elderly): The contents of the ampoule should be withdrawn into a glass syringe and immediately added to a 50 ml glass bottle, containing Sodium Chloride or Dextrose Intravenous Infusion BP, and the contents thoroughy mixed. 8–10 ml of the solution should then be withdrawn for use as a bolus injection (approx dose 0.3 mg/kg).

Following withdrawal of the concentrate from the ampoule, the entire contents shold be added to the diluent immediately. The diluted solution should be used within 12 hours.

In high risk patients, slow induction may be desirable, in which case, anaesthesia may be induced by up to 0.1 mg/kg/minute until anaesthesia is obtained. The patient should fall asleep after about 3 minutes. Some loss of activity can occur through infusion sets but the clinical response should be used to determine the rate of infusion and thus the dose of the drug required by the individual patient.

Since Hypnomidate has no analgesic action, appropriate analgesics shoud be used in procedures involving painful stimuli. Hypnomidate is pharmacologically compatible with the muscle relaxants, premedicant drugs and inhalation anaesthetics in current clinical use.

Use in children: Not recommended.

Contra-indications, warnings, etc

Contra-indications: There are no absolute contra-indications to the use of Hypnomidate.

Use in pregnancy: Safety in human pregnancy has not been established although studies in animals have not demonstrated teratogenic effects. As with other drugs, the risk should be weighed against potential benefit to the patient.

Warnings: The concentrate must be diluted before use. Hypnomidate should be given slowly.

Reduced serum cortisol levels, unresponsive to ACTH injections, have been reported in some patients during maintenance of anaesthesia with etomidate; for this reason etomidate should not be used for maintenance. However, when etomidate is used for induction, the post-operative rise in serum cortisol which has been observed after thiopentone induction is delayed for approximately 3–6 hours.

Hypnomidate should not be administered to patients with evidence, or suggestion, of reduced adrenal cortical function. Convulsions may occur in the unpremedicated patient.

Side-effects: The use of narcotic analgesics as premedication and during surgery will reduce the uncontrolled spontaneous muscle movement shown by some patients after Hypnomidate administration.

Pain can occur after administration into the small veins of the dorsum of the hand. Use of larger veins reduces pain on injection; venous irritation has also been occasionally reported following Hypnomidate infusions. Other side effects are rare.

Pharmaceutical precautions Store at room temperature. Hartmann's Solution is not recommended for use with Hypnomidate. Combinations with pancuronium bromide may show a very slight opalescence; for this reason the combination is not to be recommended. A pharmaceutical overfill of 0.1 ml is included in each 1 ml ampoule of the concentrate.

Since an interaction between Hypnomidate concentrate and syringes containing styrene/acrylonitrile copolymer has been reported, plastic syringes should not be used for withdrawal of the contents of the ampoule.

Only glass syringes should be used.

Once opened, the entire contents of the ampoule should be diluted immediately and once diluted, the solution should be used within 12 hours.

Legal category POM.

Package quantities Pack of 10 ampoules.

Further information Nil.

Product licence number 0242/0123.

IMODIUM*

Presentation *Capsules:* Hard gelatin capsules with a dark green, opaque cap and a standard grey opaque body. Each capsule contains loperamide hydrochloride 2 mg.

Syrup: Red, fruity flavoured syrup containing loperamide hydrochloride 1 mg in 5 ml.

Uses Imodium is indicated for the symptomatic control of acute and chronic diarrhoea of any aetiology. Since persistent diarrhoea can be an indicator of potentially more serious conditions, Imodium should not be used for prolonged periods until the underlying cause of the diarrhoea has been investigated.

Dosage and administration Imodium capsules and Imodium syrup are for oral administration.

Acute diarrhoea: Adults: Two capsules initially, followed by 1 capsule after every loose stool.

The usual dosage is 3 to 4 capsules a day; the maximum daily dose should not exceed 8 capsules.

Children: 4–8 years: Syrup 5 ml four times daily until diarrhoea is controlled. In children under 8 years, further investigation may be necessary if diarrhoea has not responded to three days' treatment.

9–12 years: Syrup 10 ml (or 1 capsule) four times daily until diarrhoea is controlled.

Chronic diarrhoea: Adults: Studies have shown that patients may need widely differing amounts of Imodium. The starting dosage should be between 2 and 4 capsules per day in divided doses, depending on severity. If required, this dose can be adjusted according to response.

Having established the patient's daily maintenance dose, the capsules may be administered on a twice daily regimen. Tolerance has not been observed and therefore subsequent dosage adjustment should be unnecessary.

Use of Imodium syrup: 10 ml is equivalent to 1 capsule.

Use in elderly: As for adults.

Contra-indications, warnings, etc There are no specific contra-indications to Imodium.

Use in pregnancy: Safety in human pregnancy has not been established although studies in animals have not demonstrated any teratogenic effects. As with other drugs it is not advisable to administer Imodium in pregnancy.

Side-effects: In trials no side-effects have been reported that can be reliably distinguished from the symptoms of the gastrointestinal disorder being treated.

Overdosage: No instances of overdosage have been reported. Overdosage will result in constipation; gastric lavage or induced emesis and/or enema or laxatives may be recommended.

Pharmaceutical precautions No special storage requirements.

Legal category POM.

Package quantities Imodium is supplied in packs of 30 capsules. Imodium syrup is supplied in bottles of 100 ml.

Further information Water is a satisfactory diluent for Imodium syrup; dilutions are stable for at least two weeks at 20°C.

Imodium syrup is sugar-free

No drugs are known to be incompatible with Imodium.

Product licence numbers
Capsules   0242/0028
Syrup   0242/0040

MOTILIUM* ▼

Presentation *Suspension:* Sweet tasting, sugar free, white suspension containing domperidone 1 mg/ml.

Tablets: Small, white, film coated tablets marked Mm/10 each containing domperidone maleate equivalent to 10 mg domperidone base.

Suppositories: White suppositories each containing domperidone 30 mg.

Uses Motilium is indicated for the symptomatic relief of acute nausea and vomiting in adults, from any cause, and in Parkinson's disease for the treatment of nausea and vomiting caused by L-dopa and bromocriptine.

Motilium is not recommended for use in children unless indicated for the management of nausea and vomiting following cancer chemotherapy or irradiation.

Motilium is not recommended for chronic administration.

Dosage and administration Dose, route and frequency of administration should be adjusted according to severity and duration of symptoms. For treatment of the nausea and vomiting induced by L-dopa or bromocriptine the maximum duration of treatment is 12 weeks.

Adults: 10–20 mg by mouth or 2 suppositories, at 4–8 hourly intervals.

Children: 0.2–0.4 mg/kg by mouth at 4–8 hourly intervals.

Children aged 2–12 years: 1–4 suppositories per day, depending on body weight (approx. 4 mg/kg).

Use in elderly: As for adults.

Contra-indications, warnings, etc No specific contra-indications.

Use in pregnancy: Safe use in pregnant women has not been established, although studies in animals have not demonstrated teratogenic effects. It is therefore not advisable to administer Motilium in pregnancy.

Side-effects: In common with other dopamine blocking agents Motilium produces a rise in serum prolactin, which may be associated with galactorrhoea and less frequently with gynaecomastia.

Motilium does not cross the normally functioning blood brain barrier and therefore does not interfere with central dopaminergic systems.

Overdosage: No case has been reported. There is no specific antidote to Motilium but in the event of overdosage, gastric lavage may be useful.

Pharmaceutical precautions Motilium suppositories should be stored in a cool place.

Legal category POM.

Package quantities Suspension – bottles of 200 ml (1 mg/ml).
Tablets – packs of 30 tablets.
Suppositories – packs of 10 suppositories.

Further information Nil.

Product licence numbers
Suspension   0242/0077
Tablets   0242/0100
Suppositories 0242/0075

NIZORAL* ▼

Presentation White, flat, half-scored uncoated tablets. Each tablet is marked 'Janssen' on one side and K/200 on the reverse. Each tablet contains ketoconazole 200 mg. Pink, cherry flavoured suspension in 100 ml amber glass bottles containing 20 mg ketoconazole per ml. The suspension contains sucrose and saccharin.

Uses Nizoral is an imidazole-dioxolane antimycotic which is effective after oral administration and has a broad spectrum of activity against dermatophytes, yeasts and other pathogenic fungi.

The indications for Nizoral are:

In adults and children
1. Systemic mycoses, e.g. systemic candidosis, paracoccidioidomycosis, coccidioidomycosis, histoplasmosis.
2. Serious chronic mucocutaneous candidosis (including exceptionally disabling paronychia) not responsive to other therapy or when the organism is resistant to other therapy.
3. Serious mycoses of the gastrointestinal tract not responsive to other therapy or when organisms are resistant to other therapy.
4. Chronic vaginal candidosis not responsive to other therapy.
5. Prophylactic treatment to prevent mycotic infection in patients with reduced immune responses, e.g. in cancer, during treatment with immunosuppressive medication, or with burns.
6. Culturally determined dermatophyte infections of skin or finger nails which have failed to respond to adequate dose regimes of conventional anti-dermatophyte agents (excluding fungus infection of toe nails).

Nizoral is not indicated for Pityriasis versicolor, usually an asymptomatic skin rash.

Dosage and administration Nizoral is for oral administration and should always be taken with meals.

As the risk of hepatitis (see 'Warnings') may increase in relation to the duration of treatment, if therapy is continued for more than 14 days the benefits must be weighed against the possible risks.

In adults
Mycoses and dermatophyte infections (except vaginal candidosis):
1. One tablet or two teaspoonsful of suspension (200 mg) once daily usually for 14 days.
2. If an adequate response has not been achieved after 14 days' treatment can be continued until at least one week after symptoms have cleared and cultures have become negative. The dose may also be increased to 400 mg once daily.

As nail infections always require long term therapy they should only be treated when a clinical rather than a purely cosmetic problem exists and only after alternative treatment has failed.

Prophylaxis and maintenance treatment: One tablet or 2 teaspoonsful of suspension (200 mg) once daily.

Chronic vaginal candidosis: Two tablets or 4 teaspoonsful of suspension (400 mg) once daily for 5 days.

In Children: Dosage should be reduced to 50 or 100 mg depending on bodyweight (i.e. approximately 3 mg/kg), for example:

Age 1– 4 years— 50 mg
Age 5–12 years—100 mg

Use in elderly:
In the absence of specific data, chronic vaginal candidosis – as for adults; all other indications – 200 mg daily.

Contra-indications, warnings, etc
Contra-indications: Nizoral should not be used in patients with a known hypersensitivity to ketoconazole or to any other imidazole antifungal.

Since it cannot be excluded that patients with pre-existing liver disease may be at greater risk of developing hepatic damage, ketoconazole treatment is contraindicated in these patients.

In patients suspected of having pre-existing liver disease, liver function tests should be performed prior to treatment and ketoconazole should not be used if significant abnormalities are observed.

When administered in high doses (>80 mg/kg) to pregnant rats, Nizoral has been shown to cause abnormalities of foetal development. The relevance of this finding to humans has not been established and consequently Nizoral is contra-indicated in pregnancy.

Warnings: Hepatitis has been reported. The risk of developing hepatitis is greater in patients on long term treatment (>14 days). In patients receiving long term treatment, the benefits must be weighed against possible risks.

In patients in whom long term treatment (i.e.: >14 days) with ketoconazole is indicated, LFT's should be performed prior to starting treatment.

Asymptomatic elevations in serum transaminase can occur early during treatment with ketoconazole. These may either be insignificant and transient, or can represent early evidence of hepatotoxicity. Patients should therefore be monitored clinically and biochemically with serum transaminase determinations after the first 2 weeks of treatment, at 4 weeks and at monthly intervals thereafter. If significantly elevated levels are observed, liver function tests (LFT's) should be performed at weekly intervals until transaminase levels return to normal. If significant progressive elevation occurs or the patient develops symptoms of hepatitis (malaise, dark urine, pale stools or jaundice), treatment with ketoconazole should be stopped immediately. The patient should then be monitored both clinically and biochemically for at least 2 months or until enzyme levels return to normal. Patients should also be told to consult their doctor if any of the above symptoms develop.

Hepatic damage has usually been reversible on discontinuation of treatment. Rarely, however, fatalities have been reported following ketoconazole treatment, usually where therapy has been continued despite development of symptoms of hepatitis.

Precautions: Absorption of Nizoral is maximal when taken during a meal, as it depends on stomach acidity. Concomitant treatment with agents that reduce gastric secretion (anti-cholinergic drugs, antacids, H_2 blockers) should be avoided and, if indicated, such drugs should be taken not less than two hours after Nizoral.

Ketoconazole is extensively bound to plasma proteins.

Imidazole compounds like ketoconazole, may enhance the anticoagulant effect of coumarin-like drugs, thus if concomitant use is envisaged, the anti-coagulant effect should be carefully monitored and titrated.

Concomitant use of rifampicin with ketoconazole may reduce the blood levels of both drugs so if this combination is to be used, plasma levels should be carefully monitored.

Concomitant use of ketoconazole and phenytoin may alter the metabolism of one or both drugs.

Ketoconazole, when given together with cyclosporin A can result in increased blood levels of cyclosporin A. It is therefore important that blood levels of cyclosporin A are carefully monitored if the two drugs are to be given concomitantly.

Side-effects: Alterations in liver function tests have occurred in patients on ketoconazole; these changes may be transient. Cases of hepatitis have been reported (see 'Warnings' section).

In rare cases, anaphylactoid reactions have been reported after the first dose. Hypersensitivity reactions including urticaria and angio-oedema have also been reported. The most commonly observed side-effects are gastric upsets (nausea, vomiting, abdominal pain), rash, urticaria, pruritis and headache. Thrombocytopenia has been reported rarely.

Ketoconazole, 200 mg once daily, produces a transient decrease in plasma levels of testosterone during the first 4–6 hours after intake of the drug. During long term therapy at this dose, testosterone levels are usually not significantly different from controls. In rare instances, gynaecomastia has been reported. A few cases of menstrual irregularities associated with the oral contraceptive pill have been reported. Although impaired response of plasma cortisol to ACTH has been described, it is unlikely to occur at the recommended dosage. No symptoms of adrenal insufficiency have been reported.

Overdosage: In the event of overdosage, cases should be treated symptomatically with supportive measures or gastric lavage as necessary.

Pharmaceutical precautions Nil.

Legal category POM.

Package quantities Nizoral is supplied in packs of 30 tablets, and in 100 ml bottles of suspension.

Further information Nil.

Product licence numbers
Nizoral tablets 0242/0083
Nizoral suspension 0242/0101

NIZORAL* CREAM ▼

Presentation White, non-staining, water miscible cream containing ketoconazole 2% w/w.

Uses Nizoral has a potent antimycotic activity against dermatophytes and yeasts. Nizoral cream acts rapidly on pruritis which is commonly seen in dermatophyte and yeast infections. This symptomatic improvement often occurs before the first signs of healing are observed.

After *topical* application Nizoral is not systemically absorbed and does not produce detectable blood levels.

Nizoral cream is indicated for topical application in the treatment of dermatophyte infections of the skin: tinea corporis, tinea cruris, tinea manus and tinea pedis infections due to *Trichophyton rubrum, Trichophyton mentagrophytes, Microsporum canis* and *Epidermophyton floccosum,* as well as in the treatment of cutaneous candidosis (including external application in vulvitis) and tinea (pityriasis) versicolor.

Dosage and administration Nizoral cream should be applied to the affected areas once or twice daily, depending on the severity of the infection.

Treatment should be continued for a sufficient period, at least until a few days after disappearance of all symptoms. The diagnosis should be reconsidered if no clinical improvement is noted after 4 weeks of treatment. General measures in regard to hygiene should be observed to control sources of infection or reinfection. The usual duration of treatment is: tinea versicolor 2–3 weeks, tinea corporis 3–4 weeks, tinea pedis 4–6 weeks.

Contra-indications, warnings, etc
Contra-indicated in patients who have shown hypersensivity to any of the ingredients (propylene glycol, cetyl alcohol, stearyl alcohol, sorbitan monostearate, polysorbates 60 and 80, sodium sulphite. Isopropyl myristate).

Warnings: Not for ophthalmic use.

Side-effects: A few instances of irritation, dermatitis, and burning sensation have been observed during treatment with Nizoral cream.

Pharmaceutical precautions Store away from direct heat.

Legal category POM.

Package quantities 15 g tubes.

Further information Nil.

Product licence number 0242/0107.

OPERIDINE*

Presentation Clear colourless aqueous injection presented in 2 ml and 10 ml ampoules. Each millilitre contains 1 mg phenoperidine hydrochloride.

Uses Operidine is a narcotic analgesic. It is used:
(a) as an analgesic.

(b) in conjunction with a neuroleptic in neuro-leptanalgesia.

(c) as a respiratory depressant/analgesic in patients requiring prolonged assisted ventilation in intensive care.

Dosage and administration Operidine, by the intravenous route, can be administered to both adults and children according to the following dosage regimen:

	Adults		
	initial	supple-mental	Children
Spontaneous respiration	Up to 1 mg	0.5 mg	0.03–0.05 mg/kg
Assisted ventilation	2–5 mg	1.0 mg	0.1–0.15 mg/kg

Depending on the degree of pain stimulus and/or the depth of respiratory depression required, supplemental doses should be administered at intervals of 40–60 minutes.

In intensive care, Operidine may be administered by the intramuscular route at the above dosages.

Use in elderly: It is wise to reduce the dosage in the elderly.

Contra-indications, warnings, etc
Contra-indications: Obstructive airways disease; respiratory depression if not electively ventilating.

Concomitant administration with monoamine oxidase inhibitors or within 2 weeks of their discontinuation.

Warnings: Significant respiratory depression will occur following administration of phenoperidine in doses in excess of 1 mg. This and the other pharmacological effects of Operidine can be reversed with naloxone 0.1–0.2 mg i.m. or i.v. (to be repeated as required).

Bradycardia may occur and this may be antagonised with atropine. Muscular rigidity (morphine-like effect) may occur, in which case muscle relaxants have been found helpful.

If other narcotic or CNS depressant drugs are used concomitantly with Operidine, the effects of the drugs can be expected to be additive.

Precautions: It is wise to reduce the dosage in the elderly, in hypothyroidism and chronic liver disease.

As with other narcotic analgesics, administration in labour may cause respiratory depression in the newborn infant.

As with all potent opioids, profound analgesia is accompanied by marked respiratory depression, which may persist into or recur in the early post-operative period. Care should be taken after infusions or large doses of phenoperidine to ensure that adequate spontaneous breathing has been established and maintained before discharging the patient from the recovery area. Hyperventilation during anaesthesia may alter the patients' response to CO_2, thus affecting respiration postoperatively. Use of opioid premedication may enhance or prolong the respiratory depressant effects of phenoperidine.

Side-effects: Tolerance and dependence may occur. Nausea and vomiting may be troublesome. A few cases of jaundice have been reported.

Use in Pregnancy: Little human usage but no evidence of adverse effect in animals.

Overdosage: Overdosage should be treated with the antidotes mentioned above.

Pharmaceutical precautions If desired Operidine can be mixed with 5% dextrose or 0.9% saline solutions for infusion and with most agents commonly used in anaesthesia, but the product is chemically incompatible with the induction agents thiopentone, propanidid, and methohexitone because of the wide difference in pH.

Legal category CD (Sch 2), POM.

Package quantities Operidine is supplied in 2 ml ampoules (1 mg/ml) in packs of 10 and in 10 ml ampoules (1 mg/ml) in packs of 5.

Further information Operidine does not contain preservatives.

Product licence number 0242/5000R.

ORAP*

Presentation White, scored, uncoated tablets marked 'JANSSEN' on one side and $\frac{2}{2}$ on the other, each contains 2 mg pimozide.

Pale green, scored, uncoated tablets marked 'JANSSEN' on one side and $\frac{4}{4}$ on the other, each contains 4 mg pimozide.

White, scored, uncoated tablets marked 'JANSSEN' on one side and $\frac{0}{10}$ on the other, each contains 10 mg pimozide.

Uses Orap is an anti-psychotic of the diphenyl butyl-piperidine series and is indicated in:

Acute and chronic schizophrenia, for the treatment of symptoms and prevention of relapse.

Other psychoses, especially paranoid and monosymptomatic hypochondriacal psychosis (e.g. delusional parasitosis).

Mania and hypomania.

As an adjunct to the short-term management of anxiety, moderate to severe psychomotor agitation and excitement.

Dosage and administration Orap is intended for once daily oral administration in adults and children over 12 years of age. Clinical experience in younger children is limited and Orap should be used at the physician's discretion in children under 12.

Since individual response to anti-psychotic drugs is variable, dosage should be individually determined and is best initiated and titrated under close clinical supervision.

In schizophrenia, paranoid psychoses: In the acute phase, the starting dose is 20 mg. Up to 60 mg daily has been used. For prevention of relapse, dosage ranges between 2–20 mg daily, with 8 mg as a starting dose which may be varied according to response and tolerance to achieve an optimum maintenance dose.

Monosymptomatic hypochondriacal psychosis (MHP): An initial dose of 4 mg/day may be adjusted according to response to a maximum of 16 mg/day.

Anxiety: 2–4 mg daily.

Mania, hypomania, psychomotor agitation and excitement: An initial dose of 20 mg adjusted according to response to a maximum of 60 mg daily.

Use in elderly: Elderly patients require half the normal starting dose of Orap.

Contra-indications, warnings, etc
Contra-indications: None.

Precautions: Preliminary reports suggest Orap is excreted in breast milk and is not recommended during lactation. If the use of Orap is considered essential, breast feeding should be discontinued.

Caution is advised in patients with epilepsy and conditions predisposing to epilepsy (e.g. alcohol withdrawal and brain damage), and in Parkinson's disease, renal failure and liver disease.

Warnings: As with all neuroleptics, Orap may increase the central nervous system depression produced by other CNS depressant drugs, including alcohol, hypnotics, sedatives, or strong analgesics. It may impair the anti-Parkinson effects of levo-dopa. The dosage of anti-convulsants may need to be increased to take account of the lowered seizure threshold.

In schizophrenia, the response to anti-psychotic drug treatment may be delayed. If drugs are withdrawn recurrence of symptoms may not become apparent for several weeks or months.

Acute withdrawal symptoms, including nausea, vomiting and insomnia, have very rarely been described after abrupt cessation of high doses of anti-psychotic drugs. Gradual withdrawal is advisable. Orap is slowly eliminated from plasma with a half life of the order of two days.

Use in pregnancy: The safety of Orap in human pregnancy has not been established, although studies in animals have not demonstrated teratogenic effects. As with other drugs, it is not advisable to administer Orap in pregnancy.

Side-effects: Dose-related side-effects, including drowsiness, insomnia, anxiety, and gastrointestinal symptoms, such as nausea, constipation or dyspepsia may occur. Dry mouth and hypotension have been reported, but autonomic symptoms are infrequent.

Orap may impair alertness, especially at the start of treatment. These effects may be potentiated by alcohol. Patients should be warned of the risks of sedation and advised not to drive or operate machinery during treatment until their susceptibility is known.

Anti-Parkinson agents should not be prescribed routinely. They should only be given as required.

Tardive dyskinesia is common among patients treated with moderate to high doses of antipyschotic drugs for prolonged periods of time and may prove irreversible, particularly in patients over 50 years.

The potential seriousness and unpredictability of tardive dyskinesia and the fact that it has occasionally been reported to occur when neuroleptic antipsychotic drugs have been prescribed for relatively short periods in low dosage means that the prescribing of such agents requires especially careful assessment of risk versus benefit. Tardive dyskinesia can be precipitated or aggravated by anti-Parkinson drugs. Short-term dyskinesias may occur after abrupt drug withdrawal.

Epileptic fits have been reported even in low dosage. The elderly may be more liable to experience adverse effects.

Hormonal effects of anti-psychotic neuroleptic drugs include hyperprolactinaemia, which may cause galactorrhoea, gynaecomastia and oligo-or amenorrhoea.

Glycosuria has been reported.

Skin rashes have rarely been reported.

Overdosage: There is no specific antidote to an overdose of pimozide. Cases should be treated symptomatically.

Cases of overdosage have been reported at doses up to 200 mg with no serious side-effects other than extrapyramidal symptoms.

Pharmaceutical precautions Nil.

Legal category POM.

Package quantities Orap tablets each containing 2 mg pimozide are supplied in packs of 100.

Orap tablets each containing 4 mg pimozide are supplied in a pack of 100.

Orap tablets each containing 10 mg pimozide are supplied in a pack of 100.

Further information Pimozide is an anti-psychotic neuroleptic of the diphenylbutylpiperidine group. Its pharmacological profile of activity includes a relative lack of autonomic effects or sedative action, with a moderate tendency to induce extrapyramidal reactions.

Product licence numbers
Orap 2 mg 0242/5010R
Orap 4 mg 0242/0038R
Orap 10 mg 0242/0069R

RAPIFEN* ▼

Presentation Clear, colourless, aqueous injection presented in 2 ml and 10 ml ampoules. Each millilitre contains 500 mcg of alfentanil as the hydrochloride.

Uses Rapifen is a potent, narcotic analgesic with a very rapid and short-lived action. This makes it especially suitable for use as an adjunct to anaesthesia in short operative procedures and out-patient surgery, requiring spontaneous respiration.

Rapifen may also be administered to ventilated patients undergoing longer operative procedures, either as a bolus followed by i.v. increments or infusion, or as an i.v. infusion throughout.

Dosage: Rapifen by the intravenous route can be administered to both adults and children according to the following dosage regimen:

	Initial	Supplemental
Adults		
Spontaneous respiration	up to 500 mcg (1 ml)	250 mcg (0.5 ml)
Assisted ventilation	30–50 mcg/kg	15 mcg/kg
Children		
Assisted ventilation	30–50 mcg/kg	15 mcg/kg

Children may require higher or more frequent dosing owing to a shorter half life of Rapifen in this age group.

Use in elderly: The elderly may require lower or less frequent dosing owing to a longer half life.

In spontaneously breathing patients, the initial bolus dose should be given slowly over about 30 seconds (dilution may be helpful).

After intravenous administration in unpremedicated adult patients, 1 ml Rapifen may be expected to have a peak effect in 90 seconds and to provide analgesia for 5–10 minutes. Periods of more painful stimuli may be overcome by the use of small increments of Rapifen. For procedures of longer duration additional increments will be required.

In ventilated patients, the last dose of alfentanil should not be given later than about 10 minutes before the end of surgery to avoid the continuation of respiratory depression after surgery is complete.

In ventilated patients undergoing longer procedures, Rapifen may be infused at a rate of 0.5–1 mcg/kg/minute. Adequate plasma concentrations of alfentanil will only be achieved rapidly if this infusion is preceded by a loading dose of 50–100 mcg/kg given as a bolus or fast infusion over 10 minutes. Even lower doses may be adequate, for example, in geriatric patients or where anaesthesia is being supplemented by other agents. The infusion should be discontinued up to 30 minutes before the anticipated end of surgery. Increasing the infusion rate may prolong recovery and supplementation of the anaesthetic if required is best managed by extra bolus doses of Rapifen (1–2 ml) or low concentrations of a volatile agent for brief periods.

The exact dose always depends on the length and type of surgery and on the individual patient.

Contra-indications, warnings, etc

Contra-indications: Obstructive airways disease or respiratory depression if not ventilating.

Concurrent administration with monoamine oxidase inhibitors or within 2 weeks of their discontinuation.

Administration in labour or before clamping of the cord during Caesarian section due to the possibility of respiratory depression in the newborn infant.

Warnings: Following administration of Rapifen, a transient fall in blood pressure may occur.

Significant respiratory depression will occur following administration of alfentanil in doses in excess of 1000 mcg (2 ml). This and the other pharmacological effects of Rapifen are usually of short duration and can be reversed with naloxone 0.1–0.2 mg i.v. or i.m.

Like other opioids, alfentanil may cause bradycardia, an effect that may be marked and rapid in onset but which can be antagonised by atropine. Bradycardia may be more pronounced when alfentanil is combined with other anaesthetic agents which depress the heart or increase vagal activity. Heart rate should therefore be monitored carefully. As asystole has been reported on very rare occasions in non-atropinised patients it is advisable to be prepared to administer an anticholinergic drug if the heart rate is considered low.

If other narcotic or CNS depressant drugs are used concurrently with alfentanil, the effects of the drugs can be expected to be additive.

Precautions: It is wise to reduce the dosage in the elderly, in hypothyroidism and in chronic liver disease.

As with all potent opioids, profound analgesia is accompanied by marked respiratory depression, which may persist into or recur in the early postoperative period. Care should be taken after infusions or large doses of alfentanil to ensure that adequate spontaneous breathing has been established and maintained in the absence of stimulation before discharging the patient from the recovery area. Hyperventilation during anaesthesia may alter the patient's response to CO_2, thus affecting respiration postoperatively. Use of opioid premedication may enhance or prolong the respiratory depressant effects of alfentanil.

Side-effects: Nausea and vomiting and dizziness have been reported.

Use in pregnancy: Safety in human pregnancy has not been established although studies in animals have not demonstrated teratogenic effects. As with other drugs, risk should be weighed against potential benefit to the patient.

Overdosage: Symptoms and treatment are as follows:
Bradycardia: atropine.
Hypoventilation or apnoea: O_2 administration, assisted or controlled respiration may be required.
Muscle rigidity: intravenous neuromuscular blocking agent may be given.
Body temperature and adequate fluid intake should be maintained and the patient observed for 24 hours.

A specific narcotic antagonist (e.g. naloxone) should be available to treat respiratory depression.

Pharmaceutical precautions If desired, Rapifen can be mixed with sodium chloride intravenous infusion BP, glucose intravenous infusion BP or Compound Sodium Lactate Intravenous infusion BP (Hartmann's solution). Such dilutions are compatible with plastic bags and giving sets.

Legal category CD (Sch 2), POM.

Package quantities Rapifen is supplied in 2 ml ampoules (0.5 mg/ml) in packs of 10 and in 10 ml ampoules (0.5 mg/ml) in packs of 10.

Further information The analgesic potency of Rapifen is one quarter that of fentanyl. The duration of action of Rapifen is one third that of an equianalgesic dose of fentanyl and is clearly dose-related. Its depressant effects on respiratory rate and alveolar ventilation are also of shorter duration than those of fentanyl and in most cases the analgesic effect lasts longer than the respiratory depression.

The onset of action of Rapifen is 4 times more rapid than that of an equianalgesic dose of fentanyl. The peak analgesic and respiratory depressant effects occur within 90 seconds.

Product licence number 0242/0091.

STUGERON* FORTE 75 mg

Presentation Hard gelatin capsules (No. 4) with an orange cap and cream body; each capsule contains cinnarizine 75 mg.

Uses Cinnarizine protects arterial smooth muscle from the effects of vasospastic agents including angiotensin, bradykinin, serotonin and noradrenaline. Cinnarizine has been shown to reduce the viscosity of whole blood in arteriosclerotic patients.

Stugeron Forte is indicated for the long term management of peripheral arterial disease, including intermittent claudication, rest pain, muscular cramps and vasospastic disorders, e.g. Raynaud's disease.

Dosage and administration Stugeron Forte is for oral administration to adults.

The recommended starting dose is 1 capsule three times daily. Maintenance dose is 1 capsule, two or three times daily according to response.

Peripheral arterial disease is slow to improve with any form of drug treatment. Maximum benefit with Stugeron Forte will not be seen until after several weeks of continuous treatment although significant improvement in blood flow has frequently been demonstrated after one month.

Use in elderly: As above.

Contra-indications, warnings, etc

Contra-indications: There are no specific contra-indications. Stugeron Forte has not been found to decrease blood pressure significantly. However, the drug should be used with reasonable caution in hypotensive patients.

Use in pregnancy: The safety of Stugeron Forte in human pregnancy has not been established although studies in animals have not demonstrated teratogenic effects. As with other drugs, it is not advisable to administer Stugeron Forte in pregnancy.

Warnings: Stugeron Forte may cause drowsiness; patients affected in this way should not drive or operate machinery. Avoid alcoholic drink.

Overdosage: There is no specific antidote to Stugeron Forte and, in the event of overdosage, gastric lavage is recommended.

Side-effects: Allergic skin reactions and fatigue have been reported on rare occasions.

Pharmaceutical precautions Nil.

Legal category P.

Package quantities Stugeron Forte is supplied in packs of 100 capsules.

Further information No drug interactions have been seen with Stugeron Forte when administered concomitantly with antihypertensives, diuretics, anticoagulants or hypoglycaemics.

Animal studies have shown that cinnarizine protects the arterial wall from arteriosclerotic degeneration due to hypertension.

Product licence number 0242/0008.

STUGERON*

Presentation White, uncoated, scored tablets marked 'JANSSEN' on one side and S above 15 on the reverse. Each tablet contains 15 mg cinnarizine.

Uses Stugeron is used for the control of vestibular disorders such as vertigo, tinnitus, nausea and vomiting as seen in Ménière's disease. Stugeron is also effective in the control of motion sickness.

Dosage and administration Stugeron is for oral administration to both adults and children according to the following dosage regimen:

Vestibular symptoms: Adults and children over 12: 2 tablets three times a day.

Children 5–12 years: One half the adult dose.

Motion sickness: Adults and children over 12: 2 tablets 2 hours before you travel and 1 tablet every 8 hours during your journey.

Children 5–12 years: One half the adult dose.

Use in elderly: As for adults.

Contra-indications, warnings, etc

Contra-indications: None.

Use in pregnancy: The safety of Stugeron in human pregnancy has not been established although studies in animals have not demonstrated teratogenic effects. As with other drugs, it is not advisable to administer Stugeron in pregnancy.

Warnings: Stugeron may cause drowsiness; patients affected in this way should not drive or operate machinery. Avoid alcoholic drink.

Overdosage: There is no specific antidote to Stugeron and, in the event of overdosage, gastric lavage is recommended.

Side-effects: Rarely, allergic skin reactions have been reported which have responded to discontinuation of therapy.

Pharmaceutical precautions Nil.

Legal category P.

Package quantities Stugeron tablets each containing 15 mg cinnarizine are supplied in packs of 100 tablets.

Further information Nil.

Product licence number 0242/5009.

SUBLIMAZE*

Presentation Clear, colourless, aqueous injection presented in 2 ml and 10 ml ampoules. Each millilitre contains 50 mcg fentanyl.

Uses Sublimaze is a narcotic analgesic. It is used in low doses to provide analgesia during short surgical procedures. In larger doses it is used as an analgesic/respiratory depressant in patients requiring assisted ventilation. In combination with a neuroleptic, Sublimaze is used in the technique of neuroleptanalgesia.

Dosage and administration Sublimaze, by the intravenous route, can be administered to both adults and children according to the following dosage regimen.

	Adults		Children	
	Initial	Supplemental	Initial	Supplemental
	mcg	mcg	mcg/kg	mcg/kg
Spontaneous respiration	50–200	50	3–5	1
Assisted ventilation	300–3500	100–200	15	1–3

Doses in excess of 200 mcg are for use in anaesthesia only. As a premedicant, 1–2 ml Sublimaze may be given intramuscularly 45 minutes before induction of anaesthesia.

After intravenous administration in unpremedicated adult patients 2 ml Sublimaze may be expected to provide sufficient analgesia for 10–20 minutes in surgical procedures involving low pain intensity. 10 ml Sublimaze injected as a bolus gives analgesia lasting about one hour. The analgesia produced is sufficient for surgery involving moderately painful procedures. Giving a dose of 50 mcg/kg Sublimaze will provide intense analgesia for some four to six hours, for intensely stimulating surgery. When judging the dose it is important to assess the likely degree of surgical stimulation, the effect of premedicant drugs, and the duration of the procedure.

Use in elderly: It is wise to reduce the dosage in the elderly.

Contra-indications, warnings, etc Respiratory depression: Obstructive airways disease.

Concurrent administration with monoamine oxidase inhibitors, or within two weeks of their discontinuation.

Warnings: Following intravenous administration of fentanyl, a transient fall in blood pressure may occur.

Significant respiratory depression will occur following

the administration of fentanyl in doses in excess of 0.2 mg. This, and the other pharmacological effects of fentanyl, can be reversed with naloxone 0.1–0.2 mg.

Bradycardia may occur and this can be antagonised by atropine. Muscular rigidity (morphine-like effect) may occur, in which case muscle relaxants have been found helpful.

If other narcotics or CNS depressant drugs are used concomitantly with fentanyl, the effects of the drugs can be expected to be additive. Tolerance and dependence may occur. Nausea and vomiting may be troublesome.

Precautions: As with all narcotic analgesics, care should be observed when administering fentanyl to patients with myasthenia gravis.

It is wise to reduce dosage in the elderly, in hypothyroidism, and chronic hepatic disease.

Administration in labour may cause respiratory depression in the new born infant.

As with all potent opioids, profound analgesia is accompanied by marked respiratory depression, which may persist into or recur in the early post-operative period. Care should be taken after large doses or infusions of fentanyl to ensure that adequate spontaneous breathing has been established and maintained before discharging the patient from the recovery area. Hyperventilation during anaesthesia may alter the patients' response to CO_2, thus affecting respiration post operatively. Use of opioid premedication may enhance or prolong the respiratory depressant effects of fentanyl.

Use in pregnancy: Little human usage but no adverse animal evidence.

Overdosage: Overdosage should be treated with the antidotes mentioned above.

Pharmaceutical precautions If desired Sublimaze can be mixed with i.v. infusion solutions and with most agents commonly used in anaesthesia, but the product is chemically incompatible with the induction agents thiopentone and methohexitone because of the wide differences in pH.

Legal category CD (Sch 2), POM.

Package quantities Sublimaze is supplied in 2 ml ampoules (0.05 mg/ml) in packs of 10 and in 10 ml ampoules (0.05 mg/ml) in packs of 10.

Further information Nil.

Product licence number 0242/5001 R.

THALAMONAL*

Presentation Clear, colourless, aqueous injection presented in 2 ml ampoules. Each millilitre contains 50 mcg fentanyl and 2.5 mg droperidol.

Uses Thalamonal is a combination of a major tranquilliser and narcotic analgesic. It is used in the technique of neuroleptanalgesia or as a premedication. It can be used as an adjunct to general and regional anaesthesia in major, minor and diagnostic surgical procedures. Thalamonal can also be used in intractable labyrinthine vertigo, e.g. Ménière's disease, where rapid relief of symptoms can be expected.

Dosage and administration Thalamonal can be administered intravenously to adults or intramuscularly to both adults and children. The following dosage regimen is recommended:

Neuroleptanalgesia/Premedication:
Route: Intramuscular.
Adults: 1–2 ml.
Children: 0.03–0.045 ml/kg (approx 0.4–1.5 ml).
5–45 minutes pre-operatively.

At induction of anaesthesia:
Route: Intravenous.
Adults: 6–8 ml.
Followed by assisted ventilation.

Maintenance of anaesthesia:
Route: Intravenous.
Adults: 1–2 ml.
When signs of lightening of anaesthesia are observed.

Intractable labyrinthine vertigo:
Route: Intravenous.
Adults: 1–2 ml.
By slow injection.

Use in elderly: It is wise to reduce the dosage in the elderly.

Contra-indications, warnings, etc
Contra-indications: Severe depression, obstructive airways disease; respiratory depression if not ventilating.

Concurrent administration with monoamine oxidase inhibitors or within two weeks of discontinuation of them.

Warnings: Significant respiratory depression will occur following the administration of Thalamonal in doses in excess of 4 ml (200 mcg fentanyl). This may be reversed with naloxone 0.1–0.2 mg i.v.

Intravenous induction agents will generally be required in lower dosages where Thalamonal is used as part of the anaesthetic technique, and the effects of heavy sedative premedication may be potentiated. When using Thalamonal at induction of anaesthesia, provision should be made for rapid infusion of intravenous fluid to correct any large fall in blood pressure, which, if it occurs, is due to relative hypovolaemia and is more common in the elderly or untreated hypertensives.

Bradycardia may occur and this may be antagonised by atropine. Muscular rigidity (morphine-like effect) may occur in which case muscle relaxants have been found helpful.

Extra-pyramidal effects have been seen and may be reversed by anti-Parkinson drugs.

If other narcotic or CSN depressant drugs are used concomitantly with Thalamonal, the effects can be expected to be additive.

Precautions: It is wise to reduce the dosage in the elderly, who are more sensitive to the sedative and hypotensive effects, in hypo-thyroidism and severe hepatic disease. Administration in labour may cause respiratory depression in the newborn infant.

Caution is advised in patients with liver disease, renal failure, Parkinson's disease, epilepsy, and conditions predisposing to epilepsy or convulsions.

As with all potent opioids, profound analgesia is accompanied by marked respiratory depression, which may persist into or recur in the early post-operative period. Care should be taken after infusions or large doses of Thalamonal to ensure that adequate spontaneous breathing has been established and maintained without stimulation before discharging the patient from the recovery area. Hyperventilation during anaesthesia may alter the patient's response to CO_2, thus affecting respiration post-operatively. Use of opioid premedication may enhance or prolong the respiratory depressant effects of Thalamonal.

Minor central effects can, in some instances, persist for up to 48 hours after administration. Hence where early discharge is envisaged, patients should be advised not to drive or operate machinery on the day following administration.

Use in pregnancy: The safety of Thalamonal in pregnancy has not been established, although studies in animals have not demonstrated teratogenic effects.

Side-effects: Tolerance and dependence may occur.

Overdosage: Overdosage should be treated with the antidotes mentioned above.

Pharmaceutical precautions Thalamonal should be protected from light. Thalamonal can be mixed with intravenous infusion solutions (sodium chloride intravenous infusion BP, glucose intravenous infusion BP, or compound sodium lactate intravenous infusion BP (Hartmann's Solution)) where slow administration is desired.

This product is chemically incompatible with thiopentone and methohexitone because of the wide difference in pH.

Legal category CD (Sch 2), POM.

Package quantities Thalamonal is supplied in 2 ml ampoules in packs of 10.

Further information Nil.

Product licence number 0242/5002R.

TINSET* ▼

Presentation White biconvex scored tablets marked 'JANSSEN' on one side and OX/30 on the reverse; containing oxatomide 30 mg.

Uses Oxatomide is indicated for the symptomatic control of allergic rhinitis, conjunctivitis and urticaria and other conditions responsive to drugs with anti-histaminic properties. Food allergy.

Dosage and administration Twice daily oral administration (morning and evening after meals):

Adults and children over 14: 30 mg b.d. which may be increased to 60 mg b.d. if required (i.e. 1–2 tablets, twice daily).

Children aged 5–14: 15–30 mg b.d. ($\frac{1}{2}$–1 tablet, twice daily).

Use in elderly: 30 mg b.d.

Contra-indications, warnings, etc There are no specific contra-indications to the use of oxatomide.

Use in pregnancy: Although no teratogenic effects have been observed in experimental animals, the safety of oxatomide in pregnancy has not yet been established.

Side-Effects: Oxatomide may cause drowsiness in some patients, who, if affected, should not drive or operate machinery. Avoid alcoholic drink. Increased appetite leading to weight gain has been occasionally reported in patients at higher dosage levels (above 60 mg b.d.), but is rare at the recommended dosage. This effect is reversible on discontinuation of treatment.

Overdosage: In event of accidental overdosage supportive measures and/or gastric lavage are recommended.

Pharmaceutical precautions Nil.

Legal category POM.

Package quantities Packs of 25 tablets.

Further information Nil.

Product licence number 0242/0064.

VERMOX*

Presentation *Vermox tablets:* Pale pink, flat, scored, chewable tablets, approximately 10 mm in diameter, marked 'JANSSEN' on one side and Me/100 on the reverse. Each tablet contains mebendazole 100 mg.

Vermox suspension: White, banana flavoured suspension of mebendazole 2% w/v. Each 5 ml contains mebendazole 100 mg.

Uses Vermox is a broad spectrum anthelmintic indicated for the treatment of:

Enterobius vermicularis ⎫ Oxyuris vermicularis ⎬	(Threadworm/Pinworm)
Trichuris trichiura	(Whipworm)
Ascaris lumbricoides	(Large Roundworm)
Ancylostoma duodenale	(Common Hookworm)
Necator americanus	(American Hookworm)

in single or mixed infestations.

Dosage and administration Vermox tablets and suspension are for oral administration. The tablets are orange flavoured and may be chewed or swallowed whole. Vermox suspension provides an alternative liquid formulation.

The same dosage applies to adults and children aged two years and above. No special procedures such as purging, use of laxatives and/or dietary changes are required.

(a) Threadworm *(Enterobius vermicularis)*
A single dose of one tablet, or 5 ml suspension. Care should be taken to avoid reinfection and it is strongly recommended that all members of the family are treated simultaneously.

(b) Whipworm *(Trichuris trichiura)*
Large Roundworm *(Ascaris lumbricoides)*
Common Hookworm *(Ancylostoma duodenale)*
American Hookworm *(Necator americanus)*
One tablet or 5 ml suspension twice daily (morning and evening) for three consecutive days.

Use in elderly: As above.

Contra-indications, warnings, etc *Pregnancy:* Vermox has shown embryotoxic and teratogenic activity in rats at single oral doses. No such findings have been reported in the rabbit, dog, sheep, or horse. Since there is a risk that Vermox could produce foetal damage if administered during pregnancy, *it is contra-indicated in pregnant women.*

Use in infants: Vermox has not been studied extensively in children under two years of age – for this reason it is not currently recommended in the treatment of children under two years.

Side effects reported for Vermox have been minor. Transient abdominal pain and diarrhoea have been reported, only rarely, in cases of massive infestation and expulsion of worms.

No case of overdose has so far been reported for Vermox. In the event of overdosage, gastric lavage is recommended.

Pharmaceutical precautions Vermox suspension has

a shelf-life of 5 years under normal storage conditions. Vermox suspension should be shaken before use.

Legal category POM.

Package quantities
Tablets: Blister pack of 6 tablets.
Suspension: 30 ml bottle.

Further information The efficacy of Vermox in threadworm *(Enterobius vermicularis)* infestations is such that treatment failures will be rare. However, the possibility of re-infection means that some patients may require a second treatment after two or three weeks.

Product licence numbers
Tablets   0242/0011
Suspension   0242/0050

*Trade Mark

KabiVitrum Limited
KabiVitrum House
Riverside Way
Uxbridge
Middlesex UB8 2YF

ADDAMEL*

Presentation A straw coloured solution containing electrolytes and trace elements for addition to the Vamin amino acid solutions in the intravenous nutrition of adults. Addamel corresponds to the following formula:

Calcium chloride $2H_2O$	73.5 mg
Magnesium chloride $6H_2O$	30.42 mg
Ferric chloride $6H_2O$	1.35 mg
Zinc chloride	0.27 mg
Manganese chloride $4H_2O$	0.79 mg
Copper chloride $2H_2O$	85 mcg
Sodium fluoride	0.21 mg
Potassium iodide	17 mcg
Sorbitol	0.3 g
Water for injections to 1 ml	
pH 2.5	

One ampoule (10 ml of Addamel) contains the following amounts of electrolytes and trace elements:

Ca^{2+}	5 mmol
Mg^{2+}	1.5 mmol
Fe^{3+}	50 micromol
Zn^{2+}	20 micromol
Mn^{2+}	40 micromol
Cu^{2+}	5 micromol
F^-	50 micromol
I^-	1 micromol
Cl^-	13.3 mmol

One ampoule of Addamel contains less than 1 mmol of both potassium and sodium.

Uses Addamel is an integral part of a complete intravenous nutrition regimen. It should be used in conjunction with a Vamin solution, Intralipid and a suitable phosphate preparation containing potassium. This will provide the patient's basal requirements for electrolytes and trace elements. As the requirements for electrolytes and trace elements may vary in different clinical conditions these substances may have to be added as appropriate in the individual patient.

Dosage and administration *Recommended dosage for adults:* 1 ampoule (10 ml) of Addamel is added to 500 ml or 1,000 ml of a solution listed in the following table. In this way the normal daily requirements of Ca, Mg, Fe, Zn, Mn, Cu, F, I and Cl can be supplied. Where higher amounts of trace elements are considered necessary, 2 ampoules of Addamel may be added to 1,000 ml of solution.

Recommended dosage for infants: For infants the electrolyte solution Pedel should be used.

The requirements of potassium and sodium vary with different patient conditions. Addamel is not intended to meet these requirements. Potassium and sodium salts should be added as appropriate to the individual patient. (Vamin 9, Vamin 9 Glucose and Vamin 14 contain potassium and sodium. See appropriate data sheet.)

Contra-indications, warnings, etc Should not be given undiluted. Care should be taken in the administration of Addamel to patients with impaired renal function.

One ampoule of Addamel contains 3 g sorbitol which is metabolised to fructose, and should therefore be given with caution to patients with fructose intolerance.

Pharmaceutical precautions Addition of other drugs to be avoided due to the risk of precipitation.

1. Store at below 25°C protected from light.
2. A cloudy solution or one containing a precipitate must not be used.
3. The following mixtures containing Vamin should be infused at an appropriate rate for the amino acid solution. One ampoule of Addamel should be infused over a minimum of 2–3 hours in patients with normal renal function so as to minimise renal losses.

Infusion solution	Volume to which 10 ml Addamel may be added (ml)	Infusion of admixture must be completed within: (hours)
Vamin 9	500	12
Vamin 9	1000	24
Vamin 9 Glucose	500	24
Vamin 9 Glucose	1000	48
Vamin 14	500–1000	48
Vamin 14 Electrolyte-Free	500–1000	48
Glucose 5–60%	250–1000	48

Addamel should only be added to solutions where compatibility is known.

4. The addition of Addamel should be performed aseptically immediately before the start of the infusion and the mixtures infused before the time shown in the table. See under 'Dosage and administration'.

Legal category POM.

Package quantities Boxes of 10 × 10 ampoules.

Further information The manufacturer can be consulted for full information on complete and balanced intravenous nutrition regimens.

Product licence number 0022/0034.

ADDIPHOS* ▼

Presentation Sterile colourless solution containing phosphate, potassium and sodium for addition to infusion fluids. Addiphos corresponds to the following formula:

Monobasic potassium phosphate	170.1 mg
Sodium phosphate 2H$_2$O	133.5 mg
Potassium hydroxide	14.0 mg
Sorbitol	1.0 mg
Water for injections to 1 ml	

pH: 6.3–6.4

One vial (20 ml Addiphos) provides the following:

Phosphate	40 mmol
Potassium	30 mmol
Sodium	30 mmol

Uses Addiphos may be added to infusion solutions such as Vamin solutions and glucose solutions to provide phosphate during complete intravenous nutrition. This also provides potassium and sodium. For precise details on compatibility with individual infusion solutions see Pharmaceutical Precautions section.

Dosage and administration *Recommended dosage for adults:* A daily requirement for phosphate during complete intravenous nutrition would normally be within the range 10–40 mmol. This can be met by using 5–20 ml of Addiphos. 5–20 ml Addiphos also provides 7.5–30 mmol each of potassium and sodium. The infusion should be given intravenously at a rate corresponding to not more than 10 mmol K$^+$ per hour so as to avoid hyperkalaemia and also within the maximum infusion rate for the Vamin.

Recommended dosage for infants: Dosage should be reduced appropriately according to age and weight.

Contra-indications, warnings, etc This preparation must not be administered undiluted. For information on rate of infusion see dosage recommendations above. Addiphos should not be used in patients with hyperkalaemia such as is associated with adrenal insufficiency or severe renal insufficiency, nor should it be given in the presence of dehydration without fluid replacement.

Precautions: Care should be exercised in patients with cardiac disease, diabetes mellitus, renal dysfunction or hepatic insufficiency. Infusion of potassium may depress cardiac function and counteract the effects of digitalis. Simultaneous infusion of potassium and glucose will lower the serum potassium levels attained. Plasma levels and clinical signs suggesting hyperkalaemia require discontinuation.

Pharmaceutical precautions
1. Store at 5° to 25°C.
2. The addition of Addiphos should be performed aseptically immediately before the start of the infusion and should be used within 24 hours unless the mixture is refrigerated when it may be used within 48 hours of preparation.

Compatibility has been demonstrated with the following solutions up to the maximum levels indicated:

Infusion solution (500 ml volume)	Maximum volume of Addiphos which may be added to 500 ml of infusion solution
Vamin 9	30 ml
Vamin 9 Glucose	30 ml
Vamin 14	20 ml
Vamin 14 Electrolyte-Free	30 ml
Vamin 18 Electrolyte-Free	30 ml
Glucose 5–60%	30 ml

Addiphos must not be added to the foregoing undiluted solutions in the presence of Addamel.
3. Addiphos must only be added to solutions where compatibility is known.
4. Each vial is for single use only. It should be mixed well immediately after addition to the infusion solution.
5. A cloudy solution or one containing a precipitate must not be used.

Legal category POM.

Package quantities Boxes of 10 × 20 ml vials.

Further information In regimens including Intralipid, it should be noted that 500 ml Intralipid provides approximately 7.5 mmol organic phosphate. The manufacturer can be consulted for full information on complete and balanced intravenous nutrition regimens.

Product licence number 0022/0050.

CETIPRIN*

Presentation *Cetiprin Tablets 100 mg:* White, coated and slightly bulged tablets of 10 mm diameter, marked (CT) on one side. Each tablet contains 100 mg emepronium bromide.

Uses *Main pharmacological action:* Emepronium bromide is a quaternary ammonium anticholinergic drug which blocks peripheral cholinergic nerves and ganglionic transmission. In man, it increases bladder capacity, delays the first desire to void and decreases voiding pressure.

Indications:
1. Urinary frequency and incontinence in old people.
2. Nocturnal frequency.
3. After bladder surgery, prostatectomy or bladder radiotherapy.

In order to obtain an optimal response the treatment should continue for at least three to four weeks.

Dosage and administration *Route of administration:* By mouth with an adequate amount of fluid (minimum 100 ml).

Cetiprin tablets should always be taken with the patient sitting or standing and the patient should not lie down within 10–15 minutes following ingestion.

Recommended dosage:
1. *Urinary frequency and incontinence in old people:* up to 200 mg (2 × 100 mg tablets) three times daily dependant on response.
2. *Nocturnal frequency:* 200–400 mg at bedtime.
3. *After bladder surgery, prostatectomy or bladder radiotherapy:* 200 mg (2 × 100 mg tablets) three times daily in most cases.

Contra-indications, warnings, etc Cetiprin is contra-indicated in the following:
1. In patients with symptoms or signs of oesophageal obstruction.
2. In patients with pre-existing oesophagitis.
3. In patients with prostatic enlargement associated with large amounts of residual urine and flaccid bladder.

Precautions: Caution should be observed in patients with glaucoma or gastric retention.

Pregnancy: No teratogenic effect has been observed but the usual precautions in early pregnancy should be observed.

Side-effects: Rarely, dryness of the mouth. Ulceration of

the gums and mouth has been reported, particularly in geriatric patients who hold the tablets in their mouths for long periods. There have also been instances of oesophageal ulceration when the tablets have not been swallowed with an adequate amount of fluid. See dosage recommendations above.

Overdosage: Treat as for atropine: Gastric lavage. In normal therapeutic dosage emepronium bromide does not cross the blood brain barrier. In massive, acute overdosage confusion, neuromuscular blockade and breathing difficulties have been reported.

Pharmaceutical precautions Nil.

Legal category POM.

Package quantities Bottles of 50, 250 and 500 tablets.

Further information Nil.

Product licence number
100 mg tablets 0022/5001

CYKLOKAPRON*

Presentation *Cyklokapron tablets:* White, film-coated, oblong tablets, 8 × 18 mm, engraved CY with an arc above and below the lettering. Each tablet containing Tranexamic Acid BP 500 mg.

Cyklokapron syrup: A colourless or slightly yellow syrup containing Tranexamic Acid BP 500 mg in each 5 ml.

Cyklokapron solution for injection: Ampoules of 5 ml of colourless solution containing Tranexamic Acid BP 100 mg/ml.

Uses *Action:* Tranexamic acid is an antifibrinolytic agent which competitively inhibits the activation of plasminogen to plasmin.

Indications: Short-term use for haemorrhage or risk of haemorrhage in increased fibrinolysis or fibrinogenolysis.

1. Local fibrinolysis as occurs in the following conditions:

(a) Prostatectomy and bladder surgery.
(b) Menorrhagia.
(c) Epistaxis.
(d) Conisation of the cervix.
(e) Traumatic hyphaema.

2. Hereditary angioneurotic oedema.
3. Management of dental extraction in haemophiliacs.
4. General fibrinolysis, as in prostatic and pancreatic cancer; after thoracic and other major surgery in obstetrical complications such as abruptio placentae and post-partum haemorrhage, and in connection with thrombolytic therapy.

Dosage and administration *Local fibrinolysis:* The recommended standard dose is 5–10 ml by slow intravenous injection at a rate of 1 ml/minute or 2–3 tablets or 10–15 ml syrup, two to three times daily. For the indications listed below the following doses may be used:

1a. Prostatectomy and bladder operations: 1.0 g (2 ampoules of 5 ml) by slow intravenous injection every eight hours (the first injection being given during the operation) for the first three days after surgery; thereafter 2 tablets or 10 ml syrup, three to four times daily until macroscopic haematuria is no longer present. As a bladder washout, 1 g (2 ampoules) is added to 1,000 ml

of normal saline daily. The bladder is then irrigated at a rate of 1 ml/minute, for 2–5 days following surgery.

1b. Menorrhagia: 2–3 tablets or 10–15 ml syrup three to four times daily for three to four days. Cyklokapron therapy is initiated only after heavy bleeding has started and its use should be restricted to not more than three menstrual cycles.

1c. Epistaxis: Cyklokapron solution for injection may be applied topically to the nasal mucosa of patients suffering from epistaxis. This can be done either using a spray or by soaking a gauze strip in the solution, and then packing the nasal cavity. Where recurrent bleeding is anticipated oral therapy (2 tablets or 10 ml syrup three times a day) should be administered for seven days.

1d. Conisation of the cervix: 1.5 g (3 tablets or 15 ml syrup or 3 ampoules) three times a day.

1e. Traumatic hyphaema: 2–3 tablets or 10–15 ml syrup three times daily. The dose is based on 25 mg/kg three times a day.

2. *Hereditary angioneurotic oedema:* Some patients are aware of the onset of the illness, a suitable treatment for these patients is intermittently 2–3 tablets or 10–15 ml syrup two to three times daily for some days. Other patients are treated continuously at this dosage.

3. *Haemophilia:* 1.0–1.5 g (2–3 tablets or 10–15 ml syrup) every eight hours in the management of dental extractions. The dose is based on 25 mg/kg.

4. *General fibrinolysis:* 1.0 g (2 ampoules of 5 ml) by slow intravenous injection every six to eight hours (15 mg/kg). Alternatively, 20–25 mg/kg orally, two to three times daily.

Children's dosage: This should be calculated according to body weight, at 25 mg/kg/dose orally and 10 mg/kg dose intravenously.

Contra-indications, warnings, etc Cyklokapron is contra-indicated in patients with thromboembolic disease.

Precautions:

1. In patients with renal insufficiency, because of the risk of accumulation. The dose should be reduced according to the following table:

Serum creatinine	Dose i.v.	Dose frequency
120–250 micromol/l	10 mg/kg	twice daily
250–500 micromol/l	10 mg/kg	every 24th hour
>500 micromol/l	5 mg/kg	every 24th hour

2. In massive haematuria from the upper urinary tract (especially in haemophilia) since, in a few cases, ureteric obstruction has been reported.

3. In patients with a recent history of a thromboembolic episode.

4. In the long-term treatment of patients with hereditary angioneurotic oedema regular eye examination (e.g. visual acuity, slit lamp, intra-ocular pressure, visual fields) and liver function tests should be performed.

Pregnancy: Although there is no evidence from animal studies of a teratogenic effect, the usual caution with use of drugs in pregnancy should be observed.

Lactation: Tranexamic acid passes into breast milk to a concentration of approximately one hundredth of the concentration in the maternal blood. An antifibrinolytic effect in the infant is unlikely.

Elderly patients: No reduction in dosage is necessary unless there is evidence of renal failure (see guidelines above).

Side-effects: Gastro-intestinal disorders (nausea, vomiting, diarrhoea) may occur but disappear when the dosage is reduced. Rare instances of giddiness have been reported when intravenous injection is given too rapidly.

Antidote: In case of overdosage stomach lavage and maintain high fluid intake.

Pharmaceutical precautions The solution for injection may be mixed with the following solutions:

Isotonic sodium chloride
Isotonic glucose
20% fructose
10% invertose
Dextran 40
Dextran 70
Ringer's solution
Cyklokapron solution for injection may be mixed with heparin.
Cyklokapron syrup may be diluted with Syrup BP, and the resulting solution may be stored for up to 14 days.
Cyklokapron solution for injection should NOT be added to blood for transfusion or to injections containing penicillin.

Legal category POM.

Package quantities Bottle of 50 tablets. Bottle of 300 ml syrup. Boxes of 10 × 5 ml ampoules.

Further information Nil.

Product licence numbers
Tablets 500 mg   0022/0003
Syrup   0022/0044
Solution for injection   0022/0004

DIAZEMULS* ▼

Presentation Ampoules of a white, opaque emulsion containing Diazepam BP 10 mg in 2 ml.

Uses *Action:* Diazepam is a potent anxiolytic, anticonvulsant and central muscle relaxant mediating its effects mainly via the limbic system as well as the polysynaptic spinal reflexes. The formulation of diazepam in an oil-in-water emulsion similar to Intralipid reduces the incidence of local pain and thrombophlebitis after injection.

Indications:

1. As a premedication before major or minor surgery or dental procedures, endoscopy, cardiac catheterization.
2. In the control of acute muscle spasms such as tetanus, status epilepticus and convulsions due to poisoning.
3. In the management of severe acute anxiety or agitation including delirium tremens.

Dosage and administration Diazemuls may be administered by slow intravenous injection (1 ml per min), or by infusion. Diazemuls should be drawn up into the syringe immediately prior to injection.

1. *Premedication:* 0.1–0.2 mg diazepam/kg body weight by i.v. injection.
2. *Status epilepticus:* An initial dose of 0.15 – 0.25 mg/kg by i.v. injection repeated in 30 to 60 minutes if required, and followed if necessary by infusion (see below) of up to 3 mg/kg over 24 hours.
3. *Tetanus:* 0.1–0.3 mg diazepam/kg body weight by i.v. injection and repeated every 1 to 4 hours as required.

Alternatively, a continuous infusion (see below) of 3–10 mg/kg body weight every 24 hours may be used.

4. *Anxiety and tension, acute muscle spasms, acute states of excitation, delirium tremens:* The usual dose is 10 mg repeated at intervals of 4 hours as required.

Elderly or debilitated patients: Elderly and debilitated patients are particularly sensitive to the benzodiazepines. Dosage should initially be reduced to one half of the normal recommendations.

If a continuous infusion is required Diazemuls may be added to dextrose solution 5% or 10% to achieve a final diazepam concentration within the range 0.1–0.4 mg/ml (i.e. 2–8 ml Diazemuls per 100 ml dextrose solution). A dextrose solution containing added Diazemuls should be used within 6 hours of the admixture. Diazemuls can also be mixed in the container with Intralipid 10% or 20% but not with saline solutions. It can be injected into the infusion tube during an ongoing infusion of isotonic saline or dextrose solution 5% or 10%. As with other diazepam injections, adsorption may occur to plastic infusion equipment. This adsorption occurs to a lesser degree with Diazemuls than with aqueous diazepam injection preparations when mixed with dextrose solutions.

Contra-indications, warnings, etc Concomitant use of central nervous system depressants, e.g. alcohol, general anaesthetics, narcotic analgesics, or antidepressants, including MAOI's will result in accentuation of their effects. Treatment with diazepam may cause drowsiness and increase the patient's reaction time. This should be considered in situations where alertness is required, e.g. driving a car. As with any benzodiazepine, excessive or prolonged use may result in the development of some psychological dependence with withdrawal symptoms on discontinuation. Use with caution in patients with impairment of renal or hepatic function.

Pregnancy: Diazepam crosses the placenta and should not be used during pregnancy unless considered essential, for example in treatment of pre-eclampsia. Large maternal doses administered during delivery may produce clinical effects in the newborn, for example hypotonia and hypothermia.

Lactation: Diazepam can be transmitted in breast milk and clinical effects may occur in the breast-fed infant.

Side-effects: This formulation may rarely cause local pain or thrombophlebitis in the vein used for administration.

Rare instances have been reported of a local painless erythematous rash around the site of injection, which has resolved in 1–2 days. Urticaria and, rarely, anaphylaxis have been reported following the injection of Diazemuls.

Overdosage: CNS depression and coma. Treatment symptomatic.

Pharmaceutical precautions For full information on admixture see dosage and administration. Diazemuls should only be mixed in the same container or syringe with dextrose solution 5% or 10% or Intralipid 10% or 20%. The contents of the ampoule should not be mixed with any drugs other than the infusion solutions mentioned above. Store at room temperature. Do not freeze.

Legal category CD (Sch 4), POM.

Package quantities Boxes of 10 × 2 ml ampoules.

Further information Nil.

Product licence number 0022/0043.

INTRALIPID* 10%
INTRALIPID* 20%

Presentation A white, oil in water emulsion containing:

	Intralipid 10%	Intralipid 20%
Fractionated soybean oil	50 g	100 g
Fractionated egg phospho-lipids	6 g	6 g
Glycerol	11 g	11 g
Water for injections to 500 ml		
pH 7.		

The emulsion is sterile and pyrogen free.

Uses *Action:*
1. Intralipid is a concentrated source of energy for complete intravenous nutrition. Provision of a sufficient amount of energy in the form of carbohydrate is often restricted by such considerations as hypertonicity, hypervolaemia, tendency to thrombophlebitis and the limit beyond which further carbohydrate cannot be utilised. By the use of Intralipid it is possible to provide a high energy intake in a relatively small volume. One litre of Intralipid 20% provides 2,000 kcal (8.4 MJ) and one litre of Intralipid 10% 1,100 kcal (4.6 MJ).
2. Intralipid is a rich source of the essential fatty acids; linoleic and linolenic acids.
3. Intralipid has a protein-sparing effect when given in conjunction with amino acid and carbohydrate solutions.
4. Intralipid 20% has an osmolality of ~350 mosmol per kg water.

Intralipid 10% has an osmolality of ~300 mosmol per kg water. (Plasma ~290).

Therefore both these preparations are suitable for infusion into peripheral veins.

Indications: Intralipid should be used as part of a balanced intravenous feeding regimen in patients who are unable to receive sufficient amounts of nutrients enterally. Intralipid is especially valuable in providing a high energy intake to compensate for increased energy expenditure following trauma, infections, severe burns, etc.

Dosage and administration The dosage administered should be within the ranges recommended below and should be governed by the patient's ability to utilise fat.

Electrolyte, fluid, acid-base imbalance and shock should be corrected prior to commencement of intravenous nutrition. In the metabolic and nutritional management of the seriously ill patient, specific preliminary investigations and continuous monitoring are essential, particularly of electrolyte levels. Monitoring of vitamin and trace element levels should be included, especially in patients receiving long-term intravenous nutrition.

To achieve optimal nutritional support Intralipid should be given with amino acids (Vamin) and glucose, together with electrolytes (Addiphos), trace elements (Addamel or Ped-el) and vitamins (Solivito and Vitlipid).

As with all infusions, care should be taken to avoid complications of catheterisation including air embolism and central venous thrombosis. The risk of serious thoracic complications can be avoided by the use of a peripheral catheter. The provision of intravenous nutrition via a peripheral catheter is facilitated by the near isotonicity of Intralipid. Strict asepsis should be maintained especially in the immunosuppressed patient. For safe administration of intravenous fluids from non-collapsible containers, a giving set with an integral airway is recommended.

Recommended dosage for adults: Intralipid 20%: 500–1000 ml per 24 hrs in conjunction with intravenous administration of amino acid and carbohydrate solutions. For lesser energy requirements Intralipid 10% 500–1500 ml per 24 hrs in conjunction with amino acid and carbohydrate solutions.

Intralipid 10% and 20% are administered by slow intravenous infusion. During the first 10 minutes the drip should be adjusted to 20 drops per minute and then gradually increased to a final rate after half an hour of 25–40 drops per minute for Intralipid 20% and 40–60 drops per minute for Intralipid 10%. 500 ml of Intralipid 20% should be given over a period of not less than five hours. 500 ml of Intralipid 10% should be given over a period of not less than three hours. On the first day of infusion it is advisable to administer 5 ml Intralipid 20% per kg body weight or 10 ml Intralipid 10% per kg body weight. Subsequently the dose is usually doubled and when a larger intake is indicated the dosage may be increased to 3 g fat per kg body weight per 24 hrs.

Recommended dosage for infants: Dosage is governed by the maturity and birth-weight of the infant. In mature infants dosage scheme 1. should be used. In small for gestational age and low birth-weight infants where ability to handle fat may be impaired, dosage scheme 2. should be utilised.

In all cases the infant's ability to eliminate infused fat from the circulation should be checked daily as described in the fat elimination test in the precautions section. If lipaemia is present re-testing should be carried out after an interval of four hours.

When administered to infants Intralipid should, if possible, be infused continuously over twenty-four hours and to maintain a constant rate of infusion it is essential that an appropriate pump is used.
1. *Infants:* 0.5–4 g fat per kg body weight in 24 hrs. In practice 0.02–0.17 g/kg body weight should be administered each hour. The equivalent volumes of Intralipid are 10% 0.21–1.70 ml/kg/hr; 20% 0.10–0.85 ml/kg/hr. The dosage should be gradually increased during the first week of administration.
2. In small for gestational age and low birthweight infants with impaired capacity to handle fat, commencing dosage should be 0.5 g fat per kg body weight in 24 hrs. In the absence of measurement of serum triglycerides the dosage should not exceed 2 g fat per kg body weight in 24 hrs.

The rates given are maximum rates and no attempt should be made to exceed these in order to compensate for missed doses.

Contra-indications, warnings, etc Intralipid may be contraindicated in severe disorders of fat metabolism such as in severe liver damage and acute shock.

Precautions: Fat metabolism may be disturbed in conditions such as renal insufficiency, uncompensated diabetes, certain forms of liver insufficiency, metabolic disorders and sepsis. If intravenous administration of fat is considered in patients with the above mentioned disorders, the elimination of fat should be checked daily. In newborns with neonatal hyperbilirubinaemia Intralipid should be used with caution, especially in low birth weight infants, because of the risk of free fatty acids displacing bilirubin from albumin. Intralipid should be administered with caution to infants with known or suspected pulmonary hypertension.

Animal reproduction studies have not been carried out with Intralipid. There are, however, published reports of its successful and safe administration during pregnancy in the human.

Caution: Interference with certain laboratory measurements may occur if blood samples are taken before fat has been adequately cleared from the bloodstream.

Fat elimination test: In order to prevent the development of cumulative lipaemia the patient's capacity of fat elimination can be tested in the following manner. In the morning following the first day's infusion, a citrated blood sample is drawn, preferably when the patient is still in a fasting state. The blood sample is centrifuged at 1,200–1,500 rpm. If the plasma is found to be opalescent or milky, further infusion should be postponed. This test should be repeated at weekly intervals in patients in stable metabolic conditions. In the majority of patients, the plasma is completely clear 12 hours after the conclusion of an infusion of 2 g fat per kg body weight (corresponding to 10 ml of Intralipid 20% or 20 ml of Intralipid 10% per kg body weight). In patients with diagnosed or suspected metabolic disturbances (see precautions) the fat elimination capacity should be checked daily.

Side effects: In rare instances, initial administration of Intralipid has produced a rise in temperature with shivering. Infusion of Intralipid should be discontinued in such cases. Increased levels of transaminases, alkaline phosphatases and bilirubin have been observed in patients receiving intravenous nutrition. If the dosage is reduced values usually return to normal. Cholestasis has been reported in patients receiving intravenous nutrition.

The infusion of Intralipid has been associated with an altered lipoprotein profile. The significance of these changes is not known.

Pharmaceutical precautions Store at below 25°C. Do not freeze. After long periods of storage the bottle of Intralipid should be gently inverted two or three times before use.

Do not use if the bottle is leaking.

Discard any unused contents.

Additives may only be added to Intralipid where compatibility is known. The following additions can be recommended:

1. Vitlipid Adult or Vitlipid Infant.
2. Solivito (see Solivito data sheet for details on reconstitution).
3. Diazemuls.
4. Heparin.

Legal category POM.

Package quantities Intralipid 10% and 20%: 100 or 500 ml.

Further information Intralipid and Vamin solutions can be infused simultaneously, centrally or peripherally when the mixture reaches the vein through the same cannula. Intralipid can be mixed with other solutions in a single container (e.g. 3-litre bag). Such mixing must follow defined formulae and mixing techniques, details of which are available on request. The manufacturer can be consulted for full information on complete and balanced intravenous nutrition regimens.

Product licence numbers
Intralipid 10%   0022/0027R
Intralipid 20%   0022/0028R

KABIGLOBULIN*

Presentation Ampoules containing Human Normal Immunoglobulin solution 16%, a clear pale straw colour. The active constituent is gamma globulin.

Uses *Main pharmacological action:* The immunoglobulins present in Kabiglobulin may be used prophylactically and therapeutically to provide passive immunity against infectious diseases.

Indications: Prophylaxis against infectious hepatitis (Hepatitis A). Prophylaxis against Rubella following exposure during pregnancy. Prevention, or modification of symptoms, following measles exposure in susceptible individuals. Antibody deficiency syndromes; to reduce the incidence and severity of infections in agammaglobulinaemia, hypogammaglobulinaemia and dysgammaglobulinaemia. Following burns injury.

Dosage and administration *Route of administration:* By intramuscular injection only.

Recommended dosage: Infectious hepatitis (Hepatitis A): for prophylaxis against infectious hepatitis for up to 3 months, in adults and children, 0.02–0.04 ml per kg body weight is recommended by WHO. In massive exposure, e.g. to people visiting highly endemic areas, 0.06–0.12 ml per kg body weight is recommended. The effect of the larger injection lasts for a period of at least four months.

Rubella in pregnancy: 20 ml is administered as soon as possible following exposure. The effect of an injection lasts about 3 weeks and therefore the dosage should be repeated after this time in the case of renewed exposure to the disease.

Measles prevention: 0.2 ml per kg body weight is injected within five days of exposure. The preventive effect of an injection normally lasts three weeks. The dosage should therefore be repeated after that period of time in the case of renewed exposure to the disease.

Measles modification: 0.04 ml per kg body weight is injected within five days of exposure.

Antibody deficiency syndromes: agammaglobulinaemia, hypogammaglobulinaemia, dysgammaglobulinaemia. As an initial dosage, 1.3 ml per kg body weight (maximum 60 ml) injected in divided doses over 48 hours. Half this dosage, 0.65 ml per kg (maximum 30 ml), is then given every three to four weeks.

Burns injury: during the first week following the trauma a total of about 50 g gamma globulin in the form of Kabiglobulin should be given in addition to plasma and blood. From the third up to the tenth day, 15–30 ml (2.5–5.0 g gamma globulin) per day is administered.

Contra-indications, warnings, etc Kabiglobulin should not be given at the same time as live vaccines, such as measles, mumps, rubella and oral polio vaccines. If Kabiglobulin (2 ml) has been administered these vaccines should not be given for 3 months. This period should be increased to 4 months for the 5 ml injection. Following administration of live vaccines a period of 2–3 weeks should elapse before giving Kabiglobulin. Kabiglobulin may be given at the same time as tetanus, typhus, diphtheria, polio (the inactivated form) and yellow fever.

Side-effects: In exceptional cases, intramuscular injections of gamma globulin may give rise to adverse reactions of the following type:

Local reactions: at the site of injection such as erythema, swelling, tenderness and induration, which generally subside within a few days after the injection.

General reactions: such as fever (38–40°C), chills and general malaise. These symptoms have appeared 6–8 hours after the injection and have generally subsided by the following day.

Hypersensitivity reactions: such as exanthema and pruritus. Flush, tachycardia and shock are rare. The reactions are more frequent in patients with hypogammaglobulinaemia or dysgammaglobulinaemia and may be delayed for some hours following administration.

Pharmaceutical precautions Store between 2°C and 8°C.

Legal category POM.

Package quantities Ampoules of 2.0 and 5.0 ml.

Further information The IgA content of Kabiglobulin does not exceed 0.01% of the total protein content. Kabiglobulin contains no preservative agents.

Product licence number 0022/5009.

KABIKINASE*

Presentation Vials containing a straw coloured lyophilised powder. Three preparations are available, vials of 100,000 iu, 250,000 iu and 600,000 iu of streptokinase. Human albumin and buffering agents are present as stabilisers.

Uses *Action:* By activating the fibrinolytic system streptokinase induces dissolution of intravascular thrombi and emboli.

Indications: Thrombolytic therapy by intravenous Kabikinase infusion is indicated in the treatment of deep vein thrombosis, acute major pulmonary embolism, acute arterial thromboembolism.

Additionally, thrombolytic therapy by local streptokinase administration is indicated in the treatment of myocardial infarction (see b, below) and in the clearance of clotted haemodialysis shunts (see c, below).

Dosage and administration *Routes of administration:* By intravascular infusion; intracoronary infusion.

Recommended dosage for adults:
(a) Standard intravenous infusion regimen: The standard intravenous dosage scheme includes a loading dose sufficient to neutralise circulating streptococcal antibody, followed by a maintenance dose to maintain an appropriate degree of fibrinolysis.
Loading dose: Streptokinase 600,000 iu is infused via a peripheral vein over a period of 30–60 minutes.
Maintenance dose: Streptokinase 100,000 iu/hour is infused for 72 hr. If further treatment is considered necessary it should be continued for not more than a further 3 days.
(b) Intracoronary administration in myocardial infarction: Intracoronary thrombolysis is performed using standard techniques for selective coronary angiography by either the brachial or femoral approach. Early inter-

vention is recommended, ideally within 6 hours following onset of chest pain.

Using a standard 7 or 8 French catheter, angiography is used to identify the presence and location of the thrombus. Nitroglycerin (100–400 mcg) is administered into the involved vessel, to relieve coronary artery spasm. Initially a bolus dose of streptokinase 10,000–25,000 iu is administered followed by a continuous infusion of 4,000 iu/minute, which is continued until vessel patency is restored, or for 60–75 minutes (total dose 240,000–300,000 iu). If reperfusion is achieved prior to this time then the infusion rate may be reduced when patency is restored, and infusion should continue for an additional 30–60 minutes (80,000–100,000 iu streptokinase) in order to lyse any remaining residual thrombus.

Subsequent anticoagulant treatment with heparin is necessary in order to prevent rethrombosis in the infarct-related coronary artery. However, in the majority of patients intracoronary streptokinase administration produces significant fibrinogen (and plasminogen) depletion. Additionally, circulating fibrin/fibrinogen degradation products exert an anticoagulant effect. Accordingly heparin should be administered incrementally and judiciously during the first 24 hr following treatment. The partial thromboplastin time should be monitored at regular intervals, and the heparin dosage adjusted to maintain the former within the range 2–2.5 times normal.

(c) Local application in occluded haemodialysis shunts: Kabikinase 100,000 iu is dissolved in normal saline 100 ml. 10,000–25,000 iu (10–25 ml) is deposited in the clotted portion of the shunt, which is then sealed on the venous side with forceps. A sterile single-dose syringe is attached on the arterial side to form an air cushion against which the artery can pulsate. If required, the treatment may be repeated after 30–45 minutes.

Recommended dosage for infants: Although the standard dosage scheme may be reduced proportionally to circulating volume, it may be preferable to titrate the initial dose followed by a maintenance dose of 1300–1400 iu/kg body weight/hr for 3 days. Response normally occurs within this period but if further therapy is considered it should not be for more than an additional 3 days.

Preparation of solution: The contents of a vial of Kabikinase are dissolved at room temperature in 5 ml water for injections carefully avoiding the formation of a foam. The concentrated solution thus obtained is transferred asceptically into an infusion bottle of glucose or saline of suitable volume, according to the needs of the patient. The rate of infusion is then adjusted to give the required dosage rate.
Standard intravenous infusion regimen: For the loading dose; a vial of 600,000 iu Kabikinase is made up in 100 ml 5% glucose or physiological saline and is administered over 30 minutes.
For the maintenance dose; a vial of 600,000 iu made up in 500 ml 5% glucose or physiological saline, and is administered at a rate of 80 ml per hr (100,000 iu hourly). If desired, smaller volumes can be employed, to enable the use of a syringe pump.
Intracoronary administration: The contents of a reconstituted vial are added to a volume of 5% glucose or physiological saline in order to achieve a final streptokinase concentration of not less than 1,000 iu/ml.

Control of therapy (standard intravenous infusion regimen): Therapy is controlled by the thrombin clotting time performed at intervals and should be within the limits of two to four times the normal value.

Contra-indications, warnings, etc

Contra-indications: Kabikinase should not be administered intramuscularly. Since thrombolytic therapy increases the risk of bleeding, Kabikinase is contraindicated in the following:

1. Surgery within the last 10 days.
2. Invasive procedures during the last 10 days.
3. Gastrointestinal bleeding within the last six months.
4. Thrombocytopenia or other evidence of defective haemostasis.
5. Liver or kidney disease.
6. Cerebrovascular accident.
7. Severe hypertension treated and untreated.
8. Parturition (within the last 10 days).
9. Ulcerative colitis.
10. Visceral carcinoma.
11. Menstrual bleeding.
12. During the first 18 weeks of pregnancy (see note below).
13. Sub-active bacterial endocarditis.

Precautions and warnings: Following 7–10 days' treatment with streptokinase, the patient's streptokinase antibody titre increases considerably, and returns to normal only after 3–6 months. Normally, a second treatment with streptokinase should not be considered within 3 months of the first. If a second treatment is considered necessary within 3–6 months then the initial loading dose should be individually determined. The titrated initial dose may be calculated following determination of the smallest quantity of Kabikinase required to lyse a clot, formed from 1.0 ml of the patient's blood within 10 minutes.

If heparin or oral anticoagulants have been given before commencing Kabikinase thrombolytic therapy, further administration should cease (it is not advisable to give Kabikinase and heparin simultaneously). The Kabikinase infusion can then be started after 4 hours. If immediate Kabikinase therapy is required the heparin in the blood should be neutralised with protamine sulphate.

On termination of Kabikinase treatment, the patient should be given anticoagulants in an attempt to prevent rethrombosis. Preferably heparin should be used, starting four hours after the end of thrombolysis, and then oral anticoagulants may be introduced in the usual manner. Drugs which affect blood platelet function, such as salicyclic acid preparations, pyrazolone, or indole derivatives, should not be administered concurrently with Kabikinase since the risk of bleeding will be increased.

Pregnancy: Thrombolytic therapy with Kabikinase during the first 18 weeks of pregnancy should be avoided, since there may be a risk of placental separation.

Negligible amounts of streptokinase cross the placenta. The foetal blood concentration reaches about one thousandth of the maternal blood concentration. Fibrinolytic effects in the foetus are unlikely.

Elderly patients: The incidence of cerebral haemorrhage resulting from thrombolytic therapy is increased in elderly patients. Therapy should be restricted to those patients in whom the benefit of treatment outweighs this additional hazard.

Side-effects: Kabikinase therapy may be accompanied by a slight to moderate elevation in body temperature. Mild allergic reactions such as urticaria occur uncommonly. Anaphylaxis occurs extremely rarely. These reactions may be controlled by the prior administration

of corticosteroids (25 mg prednisolone or a corresponding amount of another glucocorticoid). Minor oozing or bleeding occurring at injection sites may be controlled by applying local pressure.

Exceptionally there may be severe haemorrhage, in which case administration of Kabikinase must be discontinued. If necessary, the antifibrinolytic agent Cylokapron (tranexamic acid 10 mg/kg body weight) should be given immediately by slow intravenous injection. Cryoprecipitate may be used to correct haemostatic deficiency.

Antidote: Tranexamic acid 10 mg/kg body weight by slow intravenous injection.

Pharmaceutical precautions Vials of Kabikinase should be stored below 25°C before reconstitution. Reconstituted vials may be stored for up to 24 hr when kept in a refrigerator. Kabikinase solutions diluted for infusion should be used within 12 hours of preparation.

Legal category POM.

Package quantities Vials of: 100,000 iu; 250,000 iu; 600,000 iu.

Further information Kabikinase is a highly purified streptokinase preparation. It is prepared from beta-haemolytic streptococci culture filtrates. Subsequent purification ensures that Kabikinase is virtually free from streptodornase, streptolysin, hyaluronidase and other enzymes. Kabikinase is soluble in water, is non-toxic and is non-pyrogenic, but is weakly antigenic. Kabikinase is stabilised with sterile human albumin and this imparts a faint straw colour to the preparation. The activity of Kabikinase is measured in Christensen units.

Product licence numbers
100,000 iu   0022/5013
250,000 iu   0022/5012
600,000 iu   0022/5006.

PED-EL*

Presentation A straw-coloured solution containing electrolytes and trace elements for addition to the Vamin 9 Glucose or Vamin 9 amino acid solutions in the intravenous nutrition of neonates and infants. Ped-el corresponds to the following formula:

Calcium chloride $2H_2O$	22.06 mg
Magnesium chloride $6H_2O$	5.08 mg
Ferric chloride $6H_2O$	135 mcg
Zinc chloride	20.4 mcg
Manganese chloride $4H_2O$	49.5 mcg
Copper chloride $2H_2O$	12.8 mcg
Sodium fluoride	31.5 mcg
Potassium iodide	1.7 mcg
Phosphoric acid	8.65 mg
Sorbitol	0.3 g
Water for injections to 1 ml	
pH 2.0	

1 ml of Ped-el contains the following amounts of electrolytes and trace elements:

Ca^{2+}	0.15 mmol
Mg^{2+}	25 micromol
Fe^{3+}	0.5 micromol
Zn^{2+}	0.15 micromol
Mn^{2+}	0.25 micromol
Cu^{2+}	0.075 micromol
F^-	0.75 micromol

I⁻	0.01 micromol
P	75 micromol
Cl⁻	0.35 mmol

I^- 0.01 micromol
P 75 micromol
Cl^- 0.35 mmol

1 vial of Ped-el contains less than 1 micromol potassium and less than 1.5 mmol sodium.

Uses Ped-el is an integral part of the complete intravenous nutrition of neonates and infants. It should be used in conjunction with Vamin 9 Glucose or Vamin 9, Intralipid and a suitable phosphate preparation containing potassium. This will provide the infant's basal requirement of electrolytes and trace elements. As the requirements of electrolytes and trace elements may vary in different clinical conditions, these substances may have to be added as appropriate in the individual patient. Ped-el administration should not be started until kidney function is established – usually during the second day of life.

Dosage and administration *Recommended dosage for neonates and infants:* As part of a complete intravenous nutritional regimen 4 ml of Ped-el per kg body weight per day will cover the basal requirements of neonates and infants for electrolytes and trace elements and should be added to Vamin 9 Glucose or Vamin 9. This infusion should be given at a very slow rate and is best done with an appropriate infusion pump or an automatic drop rate counter. The requirements of potassium and sodium vary with different patient conditions. Ped-el is not intended to meet these requirements.

Contra-indications, warnings, etc Should not be given undiluted.

Care should be taken in the administration of Ped-el to patients with impaired renal function.

Ped-el contains sorbitol which is metabolised to fructose and should therefore be given with caution to patients with fructose intolerance.

Pharmaceutical precautions Addition of other drugs to be avoided due to the risk of precipitation.

Store at 8° to 15°C.

A cloudy solution or one containing a precipitate must not be used.

The addition of Ped-el should be performed aseptically immediately before the start of the infusion and should be used within 24 hours unless the mixture is refrigerated when it may be used within 48 hours of preparation.

Legal category POM.

Package quantities Boxes of 10 × 20 ml vials.

Further information The manufacturer can be consulted for full information on complete and balanced intravenous nutrition regimens.

Product licence number 0022/0037.

SOLIVITO*

Presentation A yellow lyophilised mixture of water-soluble vitamins to be added, after reconstitution, to glucose solution or Intralipid for intravenous infusion. (pH of Solivito reconstituted in water is 5.6). One vial of Solivito corresponds to the following formula:

Thiamine mononitrate (B_1)	1.24 mg
Sodium riboflavine phosphate (B_2)	2.47 mg
Nicotinamide	10 mg
Pyridoxine hydrochloride (B_6)	2.43 mg
Sodium pantothenate	11 mg
Biotin	0.3 mg
Folic acid	0.2 mg
Cyanocobalamin (B_{12})	2 mcg
Sodium ascorbate	34 mg
Glycine	100 mg
Sodium edetate	0.5 mg
Methyl hydroxybenzoate	0.5 mg

One vial of Solivito contains the following quantities of water-soluble vitamins:

Vitamin B_1	1.2 mg
Vitamin B_2	1.8 mg
Nicotinamide	10 mg
Vitamin B_6	2 mg
Pantothenic acid	10 mg
Biotin	0.3 mg
Folic acid	0.2 mg
Vitamin B_{12}	2 mcg
Vitamin C	30 mg

Uses Solivito is intended as a supplement in intravenous nutrition in order to cover the daily requirements of the water-soluble vitamins in both adults and infants.

Dosage and administration

Recommended dosage for adults: The contents of 1 vial of Solivito are dissolved by the addition of 10 ml of one of the following:

(i) Vitlipid Adult
(ii) Intralipid (10% or 20%)
(iii) Glucose solution (5–50%)
(iv) Water for injections

The reconstituted mixtures (i) or (ii) should be aseptically transferred to 500 ml Intralipid (10% or 20%) for infusion. The reconstituted mixtures (iii) or (iv) should be added to either 500 ml glucose solution (5–50%) or 500 ml Intralipid (10% or 20%). In this way, the basal requirements of the water-soluble vitamins are provided.

Recommended dosage for infants: The contents of one vial are dissolved by the addition of 10 ml of one of the following:

(i) Intralipid (10% or 20%)
(ii) Glucose solution (5–20%)
(iii) Water for injections

The basal requirements of water-soluble vitamins in infants are provided by 1.0 ml of this reconstituted mixture per kg body weight. The reconstituted mixture (i) should be aseptically transferred to Intralipid (10% or 20%) for infusion. The reconstituted mixtures (ii) and (iii) should be added to either glucose solution (5–20%) or to Intralipid (10% or 20%).

For infants weighing 4 kg or less, 10 ml Vitlipid Infant may be used to dissolve 1 vial Solivito. The daily dosage of this mixture is as above, but should not exceed 4 ml.

1 vial of Solivito should be infused over a minimum of 2–3 hours in patients with normal renal function so as to minimise renal losses.

Contra-indications, warnings, etc Intravenous administration of vitamin B_1 can in exceptional cases cause hypersensitivity reactions, as can methyl-hydroxybenzoate.

Pharmaceutical precautions

1. Store the lyophilised powder before reconstitution at 6 to 15°C, protected from light.
2. The addition of Solivito should be performed aseptically before the start of the infusion and should be used within 24 hours of preparation.

3. Solutions containing Solivito should be protected from light, e.g. with a red plastic sleeve, which allows the level of the solution to be viewed directly, or with aluminium foil.

Legal category POM.

Package quantities Boxes of 10 vials.

Further information The manufacturer can be consulted for full information on complete and balanced intravenous nutrition regimens.

Product licence number 0022/0035.

SOMATONORM* 4 IU ▼

Presentation A vial of sterile lyophilised powder of somatrem corresponding to 4 iu of human somatotropin (also containing aminoacetic acid and sodium phosphate as stabilisers) and supplied with a 2 ml ampoule of water for injections for use in the reconstitution of the injection.

Uses The treatment of short stature caused by decreased or absent secretion of pituitary growth hormone. The diagnosis should be verified by appropriate investigations of pituitary function by a specialist medical practitioner.

Dosage and administration *Route of administration:* By intramuscular injection.

Recommended dosage: The dosage should be calculated according to the patient's body weight. Generally a dose of 0.5 iu/kg body weight per week is recommended. This weekly dose should be divided into 2 or 3 intramuscular injections.

Preparation of solution: The solution is prepared by adding 2 ml of water for injections to the lyophilised substance in the vial. Gently dissolve the drug with a slow swirling motion. Do not shake vigorously as this may cause denaturation of the active ingredient.

Contra-indications, warnings, etc Only patients with unfused epiphyses should be treated. Diabetes mellitus.

Precautions: Patients treated with Somatonorm should be regularly assessed by a specialist in child growth. This assessment should include accurate determination of growth response and endocrinological status, as relative deficiencies of other pituitary hormones may be exposed or exacerbated by an adequate growth response.

Overdosage: Acute overdosage is unlikely and does not represent a hazard to the patient. The consequences of long term administration of doses above the normal therapeutic range are unknown.

Side-effects: Clinical experience with Somatonorm is limited and recipients may develop antibody to growth hormone and E. coli protein. However, as with pituitary derived hormone, only in very rare instances has growth retardation occurred. No other adverse reactions have been noted.

Pharmaceutical precautions Store at 2–8°C. Reconstituted Somatonorm may be stored in the refrigerator for 24 hours before use.

Legal category POM.

Package quantities Combined package containing one vial of somatrem 4 iu and one ampoule of 2 ml water for injections.

Further information Somatonorm is produced using recombinant DNA technology. Somatrem is the British Approved Name for methionyl human somatotropin.

Product licence number 0022/0060.

VAMIN* 9

Presentation A clear, colourless to straw-coloured solution of amino acids in the physiological L-form together with electrolytes for intravenous nutrition:

L-Alanine	3.0 g	
L-Arginine	3.3 g	
L-Aspartic acid	4.1 g	
L-Cysteine/cystine	1.4 g	
L-Glutamic acid	9.0 g	
Glycine	2.1 g	
L-Histidine	2.4 g	
L-Isoleucine	3.9 g	
L-Leucine	5.3 g	70.2 g
L-Lysine	3.9 g	
L-Methionine	1.9 g	
L-Phenylalanine	5.5 g	
L-Proline	8.1 g	
L-Serine	7.5 g	
L-Threonine	3.0 g	
L-Tryptophan	1.0 g	
L-Tyrosine	0.5 g	
L-Valine	4.3 g	
Sodium	50 mmol	
Potassium	20 mmol	
Calcium	2.5 mmol	
Magnesium	1.5 mmol	
Chloride	55 mmol	

in each 1,000 ml. pH 5.2. Free from antioxidant additives.

Osmolality: 700 mosmol per kg water.

Nitrogen per litre: 9.4 g corresponding to about 60 g of first-class protein.

Energy content per litre: 250 kcal (1.0 MJ).

Uses Vamin 9 provides a balanced mixture of all essential and non-essential amino acids. Electrolytes are present, but may need supplementing according to patient needs. Vamin 9 is indicated in conditions of protein depletion where sufficient enteral nutrition is impossible or impracticable.

Dosage and administration Electrolyte, fluid, acid-base imbalance and shock should be corrected prior to commencement of intravenous nutrition. In the metabolic and nutritional management of the seriously ill patient, specific preliminary investigations and continuous monitoring are essential, particularly of electrolyte levels. Monitoring of vitamin and trace element levels should be included, especially in patients receiving long-term intravenous nutrition.

To achieve an optimal utilisation of administered amino acids, adequate energy sources, e.g. glucose solutions and fat emulsions (Intralipid) should be provided, together with electrolytes, trace elements (Addamel) and vitamins (Solivito and Vitlipid).

Hypertonic preparations such as amino acid solutions and concentrated glucose solutions are commonly infused into a central vein. As with all infusions, care should be taken to avoid complications of catheterisation including air embolism and central venous thrombosis.

The risk of serious thoracic complications can be avoided by the use of a peripheral catheter if Vamin 9 is given simultaneously with Intralipid through the same cannula, since the reduced osmolality of the overall mixture may reduce the risk of thrombophlebitis.

Strict asepsis should be maintained especially in the immunosuppressed patient. For safe administration of intravenous fluids from non-collapsible containers, a giving set with an integral airway is recommended.

Recommended dosage for adults: Depending upon patient requirements 0.5–2.0 litres intravenously per 24 hours.

Vamin 9 is administered by slow intravenous infusion at approx. 40–55 drops per minute (2.1–2.8 ml/min) corresponding to an infusion time of six to eight hours per litre.

Recommended dosage for infants: 30 ml per kg body weight in 24 hours to be achieved gradually during first week of administration.

Contra-indications, warnings, etc Vamin 9 is contra-indicated in patients with irreversible liver damage and in severe uraemia when dialysis facilities are not available. It should not be given to patients with hyperkalaemia – Vamin 14 Electrolyte-Free and Vamin 18 Electrolyte-Free may be suitable alternatives.

Care must be exercised in the administration of large volume infusion fluids to patients with cardiac insufficiency. Amino acid infusions must also be administered with caution to patients with disturbances in protein metabolism.

Precautions: Hyperkalaemia, hypernatraemia, and acidosis should be corrected prior to commencement of intravenous nutrition. Serum electrolytes, blood glucose levels and acid-base balance should be regularly monitored. Fluid balance should also be monitored since hypertonic dehydration may occur. Amino acid solutions may precipitate acute folate deficiency and folic acid should be given daily.

Vamin 9 should be given with caution to patients with electrolyte retention e.g. impaired renal function and to those with cardiac disease requiring electrolyte restriction or drug therapy e.g. Digitalis. Vamin 14 Electrolyte-Free or Vamin 18 Electrolyte-Free may be suitable in such patients. In particular, potassium replacement therapy should be carefully controlled as plasma potassium levels may not be directly related to tissue levels.

Animal reproduction studies have not been carried out with Vamin 9. There are, however, published reports on the successful and safe infusion of amino acid solutions during pregnancy in the human.

Side-effects: Vamin 9 is well tolerated. In exceptional cases, nausea may occur. As with all hypertonic infusion solutions, thrombophlebitis may occur when peripheral veins are used. The incidence could be reduced by the simultaneous infusion of Intralipid as described above.

Vomiting, flushing and sweating may occur if the recommended rate of infusion is exceeded. Abnormal liver function tests have been observed during intravenous nutrition but all values return to normal on cessation of artificial feeding. Cholestasis has been reported in some patients receiving intravenous nutrition.

Pharmaceutical precautions
1. Store at 5 to 25°C.
2. Do not use if the bottle is leaking or if the solution is cloudy or contains a precipitate.
3. Discard any unused contents.

4. For long-term feeding (i.e. a period of longer than one week) or in short-term feeding if a deficiency of trace elements exists, a trace element solution should be added. Addamel and Ped-el have been specifically designed for this purpose and are compatible with Vamin 9 when used in the recommended proportions.

Additives may only be added to Vamin 9 where compatibility is known.

Legal category POM.

Package quantities Bottles of 500 ml and 1000 ml.

Further information The manufacturer can be consulted for full information on complete and balanced intravenous nutrition regimens.

Product licence number 0022/0031.

VAMIN* 9 GLUCOSE

Presentation A clear, pale yellow to yellow solution of amino acids in the physiological L-form together with glucose and electrolytes for intravenous nutrition:

L-Alanine	3.0 g	
L-Arginine	3.3 g	
L-Aspartic acid	4.1 g	
L-Cysteine/cystine	1.4 g	
L-Glutamic acid	9.0 g	
Glycine	2.1 g	
L-Histidine	2.4 g	
L-Isoleucine	3.9 g	
L-Leucine	5.3 g	
L-Lysine	3.9 g	70.2 g
L-Methionine	1.9 g	
L-Phenylalanine	5.5 g	
L-Proline	8.1 g	
L-Serine	7.5 g	
L-Threonine	3.0 g	
L-Tryptophan	1.0 g	
L-Tyrosine	0.5 g	
L-Valine	4.3 g	
Glucose anhydrous	100 g	
Sodium	50 mmol	
Potassium	20 mmol	
Calcium	2.5 mmol	
Magnesium	1.5 mmol	
Chloride	55 mmol	

in each 1,000 ml. pH 5.2. Free from antioxidant additives.

Osmolality: 1350 mosmol per kg water.

Nitrogen per litre: 9.4 g corresponding to about 60 g of first-class protein of which 400 kcal (1.7 MJ) are provided by the glucose.

Energy content per litre: 650 kcal (2.7 MJ).

Uses Vamin 9 Glucose provides a balanced mixture of all essential and non-essential amino acids. Glucose is included to meet part of the carbohydrate requirements. Electrolytes are present, but may need supplementing according to patient needs. Vamin 9 Glucose is indicated in conditions of protein depletion where sufficient enteral nutrition is impossible or impracticable.

Dosage and administration Electrolyte, fluid, acid-base imbalance and shock should be corrected prior to commencement of intravenous nutrition. In the metabolic and nutritional management of the seriously ill patient, specific preliminary investigations and continuous monitoring are essential, particularly of electrolyte levels. Monitoring of vitamin and trace element levels should be included, especially in patients receiving long-term intravenous nutrition.

To achieve an optimal utilisation of administered amino acids, adequate energy sources, e.g. glucose solutions and fat emulsions (Intralipid) should be provided, together with electrolytes, trace elements (Addamel) and vitamins (Solivito and Vitlipid).

Hypertonic preparations such as amino acid solutions and concentrated glucose solutions are commonly infused into a central vein. As with all infusions, care should be taken to avoid complications of catheterisation including air embolism and central venous thrombosis. The risk of serious thoracic complications can be avoided by the use of a peripheral catheter if Vamin 9 Glucose is given simultaneously with Intralipid through the same cannula, since the reduced osmolality of the overall mixture may reduce the risk of thrombophlebitis.

Strict asepsis should be maintained especially in the immunosuppressed patient. For safe administration of intravenous fluids from non-collapsible containers, a giving set with an integral airway is recommended.

Recommended dosage for adults: Depending upon patient requirements 0.5–2.0 litres intravenously per 24 hours.

Vamin 9 Glucose is administered by slow intravenous infusion at approx. 40–55 drops per minute (2.1–2.8 ml/min) corresponding to an infusion time of six to eight hours per litre.

Recommended dosage for infants: 30 ml per kg body weight in 24 hours to be achieved gradually during first week of administration.

Contra-indications, warnings, etc Vamin 9 Glucose is contra-indicated in patients with irreversible liver damage and in severe uraemia when dialysis facilities are not available. It should not be given to patients with hyperkalaemia – Vamin 14 Electrolyte-Free and Vamin 18 Electrolyte-Free may be suitable alternatives.

Care must be exercised in the administration of large volume infusion fluids to patients with cardiac insufficiency. Amino acid infusions must also be administered with caution to patients with disturbances in protein metabolism.

Precautions: Hyperkalaemia, hypernatraemia, and acidosis should be corrected prior to commencement of intravenous nutrition. Serum electrolytes, blood glucose levels and acid-base balance should be regularly monitored. Fluid balance should also be monitored since hypertonic dehydration may occur. Amino acid solutions may precipitate acute folate deficiency and folic acid should be given daily.

Vamin 9 Glucose should be given with caution to patients with electrolyte retention e.g. impaired renal function and to those with cardiac disease requiring electrolyte restriction or drug therapy e.g. Digitalis. Vamin 14 Electrolyte-Free or Vamin 18 Electrolyte-Free may be suitable in such patients. In particular, potassium replacement therapy should be carefully controlled as plasma potassium levels may not be directly related to tissue levels.

Animal reproduction studies have not been carried out with Vamin 9 Glucose. There are, however, published reports on the successful and safe infusion of amino acid solutions during pregnancy in the human.

Side-effects: Vamin 9 Glucose is well tolerated. In exceptional cases, nausea may occur. As with all hypertonic infusion solutions, thrombophlebitis may occur when peripheral veins are used. The incidence could be reduced by the simultaneous infusion of Intralipid as described above.

Vomiting, flushing and sweating may occur if the recommended rate of infusion is exceeded. Abnormal liver function tests have been observed during intravenous nutrition but all values return to normal on cessation of artificial feeding. Cholestasis has been reported in some patients receiving intravenous nutrition.

Pharmaceutical precautions
1. Store at 5 to 25°C.
2. Do not use if the bottle is leaking or if the solution is cloudy or contains a precipitate.
3. Discard any unused contents.
4. For long-term feeding (i.e. a period of longer than one week) or in short-term feeding if a deficiency of trace elements exists, a trace element solution should be added. Addamel and Ped-el have been specifically designed for this purpose and are compatible with Vamin 9 Glucose when used in the recommended proportions.

Additives may only be added to Vamin 9 Glucose where compatibility is known.

Legal category POM.

Package quantities Bottles of 100 ml, 500 ml and 1,000 ml.

Further information The manufacturer can be consulted for full information on complete and balanced intravenous nutrition regimens.

Product licence number 0022/0030.

VAMIN* 14 ▼

Presentation A clear, colourless to slightly yellow solution of amino acids in the physiological L-form with electrolytes, for intravenous nutrition:

L-Alanine	12.0 g	
L-Arginine	8.4 g	
L-Aspartic acid	2.5 g	
L-Cysteine/cystine	420 mg	
L-Glutamic acid	4.2 g	
Glycine	5.9 g	
L-Histidine	5.1 g	
L-Isoleucine	4.2 g	
L-Leucine	5.9 g	85 g
L-Lysine	6.8 g	
L-Methionine	4.2 g	
L-Phenylalanine	5.9 g	
L-Proline	5.1 g	
L-Serine	3.4 g	
L-Threonine	4.2 g	
L-Tryptophan	1.4 g	
L-Tyrosine	170 mg	
L-Valine	5.5 g	
Sodium	100 mmol	
Potassium	50 mmol	
Calcium	5 mmol	
Magnesium	8 mmol	
Chloride	100 mmol	
Sulphate	8 mmol	
Acetate	135 mmol	

in each 1,000 ml. pH 5.6. Free from antioxidant additives.
Osmolality: 1145 mosmol per kg water.

Nitrogen per litre: 13.5 g corresponding to about 84 g of protein.

Energy content per litre: 350 kcal (1.4 MJ).

Uses Vamin 14 provides a concentrated and balanced mixture of all essential and non-essential amino acids. Electrolytes are present, but may need supplementing according to patient needs. See under Dosage and Administration for information on compatibility. Vamin 14 is indicated for the prophylaxis or therapeutic treatment of protein depletion, where sufficient enteral nutrition is impossible or impracticable. It is particularly suited to meet moderately increased requirements for nitrogen in patients in whom fluid intake is a limiting factor.

Dosage and administration Electrolyte, fluid, acid-base imbalance and shock should be corrected prior to commencement of intravenous nutrition. In the metabolic and nutritional management of the seriously ill patient specific preliminary investigations and continuous monitoring are essential, particularly of electrolyte levels. Monitoring of vitamin and trace element levels should be included, especially in patients receiving long-term intravenous nutrition.

To achieve an optional utilisation of administered amino acids, adequate energy sources, e.g. glucose solutions and fat emulsions (Intralipid) should be provided, together with electrolytes, trace elements (Addamel) and vitamins (Solivito and Vitlipid Adult).

Hypertonic preparations such as amino acid solutions and concentrated glucose solutions are commonly infused into a central vein. As with all infusions, care should be taken to avoid complications of catheterisation including air embolism and central venous thrombosis. The risk of serious thoracic complications can be avoided by the use of a peripheral catheter if Vamin 14 is given simultaneously with Intralipid through the same cannula, since the reduced osmolality of the overall mixture may reduce the risk of thrombophlebitis.

Strict asepsis should be maintained especially in the immuno-suppressed patient. For safe administration of intravenous fluids from non-collapsible containers, a giving set with an integral airway is recommended.

Recommended dosage for adults: Depending upon patient requirements, up to 1 litre intravenously per 24 hours. In severe catabolism, Vamin 18 Electrolyte-Free may be used. Vamin 14 is administered by slow intravenous infusion at a rate not exceeding 2 ml per minute corresponding to approximately 40 drops per minute or to an infusion time of at least 8 hours per litre.

Infant dosage: Can be administered at the physician's discretion. An amino acid solution containing larger amounts of cysteine/cystine and tyrosine may be considered more appropriate in infants.

Contra-indications, warnings, etc Vamin 14 is contra-indicated in patients with irreversible liver damage and in severe uraemia when dialysis facilities are not available. It should not be given to patients with hyperkalaemia – Vamin 14 Electrolyte-Free is a suitable alternative.

Care must be exercised in the administration of large volume infusion fluids to patients with cardiac insufficiency. Amino acid infusions must also be administered with caution to patients with disturbances in protein metabolism.

Precautions: Hyperkalaemia, hypernatraemia, and acidosis should be corrected prior to commencement of intravenous nutrition. Serum electrolytes, blood glucose levels and acid-base balance should be regularly monitored. Fluid balance should also be monitored since hypertonic dehydration may occur. Amino acid solutions may precipitate acute folate deficiency and folic acid should be given daily.

Vamin 14 should be given with caution to patients with electrolyte retention, e.g. impaired renal function and to those with cardiac disease requiring electrolyte restriction or drug therapy, e.g. Digitalis. Vamin 14 Electrolyte-Free is recommended in such patients. In particular, potassium replacement therapy should be carefully controlled as plasma potassium levels may not be directly related to tissue levels.

Animal reproduction studies have not been carried out with Vamin 14. There are, however, published reports on the successful and safe infusion of amino acid solutions during pregnancy in the human.

Side-effects: Vamin 14 is well tolerated. Rarely, nausea may occur. As with all hypertonic infusion solutions, thrombophlebitis may occur when peripheral veins are used. The incidence could be reduced by the simultaneous infusion of Intralipid as described above. Vomiting, flushing and sweating may occur if the recommended rate of infusion is exceeded. Abnormal liver function tests have been observed during intravenous nutrition but all values return to normal on cessation of artificial feeding. Cholestasis has been reported in some patients receiving intravenous nutrition.

Pharmaceutical precautions
1. Do not use if the bottle is leaking or if the solution is cloudy or contains a precipitate.
2. Discard any unused contents.
3. Vamin 14 contains electrolytes, but additional electrolytes and trace elements may be required according to patient needs. Up to 20 ml Addamel can be added to one litre Vamin 14 without risk of precipitation. Phosphate may be added to one litre Vamin 14 as up to 40 ml Addiphos (containing 80 mmol phosphate, 60 mmol Na^+ and 60 mmol K^+) provided Addamel is not present. All additions should be performed aseptically immediately before the start of the infusion and should be used within 24 hours unless the mixture is refrigerated when it may be used within 48 hours of preparation.

Additives may only be added to Vamin 14 where compatibility is known.

Legal category POM.

Package quantities Bottles of 500 ml and 1000 ml.

Further information The manufacturer can be consulted for full information on complete and balanced intravenous nutrition regimens.

Product licence number 0022/0053.

VAMIN* 14 ELECTROLYTE-FREE ▼

Presentation A clear, colourless to slightly yellow solution of amino acids in the physiological L-form for intravenous nutrition:

L-Alanine	12.0 g	
L-Arginine	8.4 g	
L-Aspartic acid	2.5 g	
L-Cysteine/cystine	420 mg	
L-Glutamic acid	4.2 g	
Glycine	5.9 g	
L-Histidine	5.1 g	
L-Isoleucine	4.2 g	
L-Leucine	5.9 g	
L-Lysine	6.8 g	85 g
L-Methionine	4.2 g	
L-Phenylalanine	5.9 g	
L-Proline	5.1 g	
L-Serine	3.4 g	
L-Threonine	4.2 g	
L-Tryptophan	1.4 g	
L-Tyrosine	170 mg	
L-Valine	5.5 g	

in each 1,000 ml. pH 5.6. Free from antioxidant additives.

Osmolality: 810 mosmol per kg water.

Nitrogen per litre: 13.5 g corresponding to about 84 g of protein.

Energy content per litre: 350 kcal (1.4 MJ).

Uses Vamin 14 Electrolyte-Free provides a concentrated and balanced mixture of all essential and non-essential amino acids. It is free from chlorides and other inorganic electrolytes, and electrolyte requirements can therefore be met by the addition of individually adjusted doses. See under Dosage and Administration for information on compatibility. Vamin 14 Electrolyte-Free is indicated for the prophylaxis or therapeutic treatment of protein depletion, where sufficient enteral nutrition is impossible or impracticable. It is particularly suited to meet moderately increased requirements for nitrogen in patients in whom fluid intake is a limiting factor.

Dosage and administration Electrolyte, fluid, acid-base imbalance and shock should be corrected prior to commencement of intravenous nutrition. In the metabolic and nutritional management of the seriously ill patient, specific preliminary investigations and continuous monitoring are essential, particularly of electrolyte levels. Monitoring of vitamin and trace element levels should be included, especially in patients receiving long-term intravenous nutrition.

To achieve an optimal utilisation of administered amino acids, adequate energy sources, e.g. glucose solutions and fat emulsions (Intralipid) should be provided, together with electrolytes, trace elements (Addamel) and vitamins (Solivito and Vitlipid Adult).

Hypertonic preparations such as amino acid solutions and concentrated glucose solutions are commonly infused into a central vein. As with all infusions, care should be taken to avoid complications of catheterisation including air embolism and central venous thrombosis. The risk of serious thoracic complications can be avoided by the use of a peripheral catheter if Vamin 14 Electrolyte-Free is given simultaneously with Intralipid through the same cannula, since the reduced osmolality of the overall mixture may reduce the risk of thrombophlebitis.

Strict asepsis should be maintained especially in the immunosuppressed patient. For safe administration of intravenous fluids from non-collapsible containers, a giving set with an integral airway is recommended.

Recommended dosage for adults: Depending upon patient requirements, up to 1 litre intravenously per 24 hours. In severe catabolism, Vamin 18 Electrolyte-Free

may be used. Vamin 14 Electrolyte-Free is administered by slow intravenous infusion at a rate not exceeding 2 ml per minute corresponding to approximately 40 drops per minute or an infusion time of at least 8 hours per litre.

Recommended dosage for infants: Can be administered at the physician's discretion. An amino acid solution containing larger amounts of cysteine/cystine and tyrosine may be considered more appropriate in infants.

Contra-indications, warnings, etc Vamin 14 Electrolyte-Free is contra-indicated in patients with irreversible liver damage and in severe uraemia when dialysis facilities are not available.

Care must be exercised in the administration of large volume infusion fluids to patients with cardiac insufficiency. Amino acid infusions must also be administered with caution to patients with disturbances in protein metabolism.

Precautions: Hyperkalaemia, hypernatraemia and acidosis should be corrected prior to commencement of intravenous nutrition. Serum electrolytes, blood glucose levels and acid-base balance should be regularly monitored. Fluid balance should also be monitored since hypertonic dehydration may occur. Amino acid solutions may precipitate acute folate deficiency and folic acid should be given daily.

Animal reproduction studies have not been carried out with Vamin 14 Electrolyte-Free. There are, however, published reports on the successful and safe infusion of amino acid solutions during pregnancy in the human.

Side-effects: Vamin 14 Electrolyte-Free is well tolerated. Rarely, nausea may occur. As with all hypertonic infusion solutions, thrombophlebitis may occur when peripheral veins are used. The incidence could be reduced by the simultaneous infusion of Intralipid as described above. Vomiting, flushing and sweating may occur if the recommended rate of infusion is exceeded. Abnormal liver function tests have been observed during intravenous nutrition but all values return to normal on cessation of artificial feeding. Cholestasis has been reported in some patients receiving intravenous nutrition.

Pharmaceutical precautions
1. Do not use if the bottle is leaking or if the solution is cloudy or contains a precipitate.
2. Discard any unused contents.
3. Vamin 14 Electrolyte-Free contains no electrolytes. Electrolyte and trace element requirements can be met by the addition of individually adjusted doses. Laboratory studies have shown that the maximum levels of electrolytes which are compatible with 1 litre of Vamin 14 Electrolyte-Free are as follows: 20 ml Addamel, 480 mmol Na^+ (as NaCl), 480 mmol K^+ (as KCl), 24 mmol Ca^{2+} (as calcium glubionate) and 48 mmol Mg^{2+} (as $MgSO_4$) which can be added either singly or in any combination. Phosphate may be added to 1 litre Vamin 14 Electrolyte-Free as up to 60 ml Addiphos (containing 120 mmol phosphate, 90 mmol Na^+ and 90 mmol K^+) with or without addition of up to 480 mmol Na^+ and 480 mmol K^+ as chlorides and 48 mmol Mg^{2+} as sulphate, provided Addamel is not present. All additions should be performed aseptically immediately before the start of the infusion and should be used within 24 hours unless the mixture is refrigerated when it may be used within 48 hours of preparation.

Additives may only be added to Vamin 14 Electrolyte-Free where compatibility is known.

Legal category POM.

Package quantities Bottles of 500 ml and 1000 ml.

Further information The manufacturer can be consulted for full information on complete and balanced intravenous nutrition regimens.

Product licence number 0022/0052.

VAMIN* 18 ELECTROLYTE-FREE ▼

Presentation A clear, colourless to slightly yellow solution of amino acids in the physiological L-form for intravenous nutrition:

L-Alanine	16.0 g	
L-Arginine	11.3 g	
L-Aspartic acid	3.4 g	
L-Cysteine/cystine	560 mg	
L-Glutamic acid	5.6 g	
Glycine	7.9 g	
L-Histidine	6.8 g	
L-Isoleucine	5.6 g	
L-Leucine	7.9 g	114 g
L-Lysine	9.0 g	
L-Methionine	5.6 g	
L-Phenylalanine	7.9 g	
L-Proline	6.8 g	
L-Serine	4.5 g	
L-Threonine	5.6 g	
L-Tryptophan	1.9 g	
L-Tyrosine	230 mg	
L-Valine	7.3 g	

in each 1,000ml. pH 5.6. Free from antioxidant additives.

Osmolality: 1130 mosmol per kg water.

Nitrogen per litre: 18.0 g corresponding to 112 g of protein.

Energy content per litre: 460 kcal (1.9 MJ).

Uses Vamin 18 Electrolyte-Free provides a concentrated and balanced mixture of all essential and non-essential amino acids. It is free from chlorides and other inorganic electrolytes, and electrolyte requirements can therefore be met by the addition of individually adjusted doses. See under Dosage and Administration for information on compatibility.

Vamin 18 Electrolyte-Free is indicated for the prophylaxis or therapeutic treatment of protein depletion, where sufficient enteral nutrition is impossible or impracticable. It is particularly suited to meet increased requirements for nitrogen in patients in whom fluid intake is a limiting factor.

Dosage and administration Electrolyte, fluid, acid-base imbalance and shock should be corrected prior to commencement of intravenous nutrition. In the metabolic and nutritional management of the seriously ill patient, specific preliminary investigations and continuous monitoring are essential, particularly of electrolyte levels. Monitoring of vitamin and trace element levels should be included, especially in patients receiving long-term intravenous nutrition.

To achieve an optimal utilisation of administered amino acids, adequate energy sources, e.g. glucose solutions and fat emulsions (Intralipid) should be provided, together with electrolytes, trace elements (Addamel) and vitamins (Solivito and Vitlipid Adult).

Hypertonic preparations such as amino acid solutions and concentrated glucose solutions are commonly infused into a central vein. As with all infusions, care

should be taken to avoid complications of catheterisation including air embolism and central venous thrombosis. The risk of serious thoracic complications can be avoided by the use of a peripheral catheter if Vamin 18 Electrolyte-Free is given simultaneously with Intralipid through the same cannula, since the reduced osmolality of the overall mixture may reduce the risk of thrombophlebitis.

Strict asepsis should be maintained especially in the immunosuppressed patient. For safe administration of intravenous fluids from non-collapsible containers, a giving set with an integral airway is recommended.

Recommended dosage for adults: Depending upon patient requirements, up to 1 litre intravenously per 24 hours. Vamin 18 Electrolyte-Free is administered by slow intravenous infusion at a rate not exceeding 2 ml per minute corresponding to approximately 40 drops per minute or an infusion time of at least 8 hours per litre.

Recommended dosage for infants: Can be administered at the physician's discretion. An amino acid solution containing larger amounts of cysteine/cystine and tyrosine may be considered more appropriate in infants.

Contra-indications, warnings, etc Vamin 18 Electrolyte-Free is contra-indicated in patients with irreversible liver damage and in severe uraemia when dialysis facilities are not available.

Care must be exercised in the administration of large volume infusion fluids to patients with cardiac insufficiency. Amino acid solutions must also be administered with caution to patients with disturbances in protein metabolism.

Precautions: Hyperkalaemia, hypernatraemia and acidosis should be corrected prior to commencement of intravenous nutrition. Serum electrolytes, blood glucose levels and acid-base balance should be regularly monitored. Fluid balance should also be monitored since hypertonic dehydration may occur. Amino acid solutions may precipitate acute folate deficiency and folic acid should be given daily.

Animal reproduction studies have not been carried out with Vamin 18 Electrolyte-Free. There are, however, published reports on the successful and safe administration of amino acid solutions during pregnancy in the human.

Side-effects: Vamin 18 Electrolyte-Free is well tolerated. Rarely, nausea may occur. As with all hypertonic infusion solutions, thrombophlebitis may occur when peripheral veins are used. The incidence could be reduced by the simultaneous infusion of Intralipid as described above. Vomiting, flushing and sweating may occur if the recommended rate of infusion is exceeded. Abnormal liver function tests have been observed during intravenous nutrition but all values return to normal on cessation of artificial feeding. Cholestasis has been reported in some patients receiving intravenous nutrition.

Pharmaceutical precautions
1. Do not use if the bottle is leaking or if the solution is cloudy or contains a precipitate.
2. Discard any unused contents.
3. Vamin 18 Electrolyte-Free contains no electrolytes. Electrolyte requirements can be met by the addition of individually adjusted doses. Laboratory studies have shown that the maximum levels of electrolytes which are compatible with 1 litre of Vamin 18 Electrolyte-Free are as follows: 480 mmol Na^+ (as NaCl), 480 mmol K^+ (as KCl), 24 mmol Ca^{2+} (as calcium glubionate) and 48 mmol Mg^{2+} (as $MgSO_4$) which can be added either

singly or in any combination. Phosphate may be added to 1 litre Vamin 18 Electrolyte-Free as up to 60 ml Addiphos (containing 120 mmol phosphate, 90 mmol Na^+ and 90 mmol K^+) with or without addition of up to 480 mmol Na^+, and 480 mmol K^+ as chlorides and 48 mmol Mg^{2+} as sulphate. Addamel should not be added to Vamin 18 Electrolyte-Free. All additions should be performed aseptically immediately before the start of the infusion and should be used within 24 hours unless the mixture is refrigerated when it may be used within 48 hours of preparation.

Additives may only be added to Vamin 18 Electrolyte-Free where compatibility is known.

Legal category POM.

Package quantities Bottles of 500 ml and 1000 ml.

Further information The manufacturer can be consulted for full information on complete and balanced intravenous nutrition regimens.

Product licence number 0022/0054.

VITLIPID ADULT*

Presentation A white, oil in water emulsion containing the fat soluble vitamins A, D_2 and K_1, in the oil phase of the emulsion with a composition corresponding to that of Intralipid 10%. Vitlipid Adult is intended for addition to Intralipid 10% or 20% and for use in adults on intravenous nutrition. One ampoule of Vitlipid Adult contains:

Retinol palmitate	
corresponding to retinol	750 mcg (2,500 i.u.)
Calciferol	3 mcg (120 i.u.)
Phytomenadione	150 mcg
Fractionated soybean oil	1 g
Fractionated egg	
phospholipids	120 mg
Glycerol	225 mg
Water for injections to 10 ml	

Uses Vitlipid Adult is indicated as a supplement to Intralipid 10% or 20% in intravenous nutrition of adults in order to cover the daily requirements of the fat soluble vitamins A, D_2 and K_1.

Dosage and administration *Recommended dosage for adults:* One ampoule (10 ml) of Vitlipid Adult is added to 500 ml of Intralipid 10% or 20%. After gentle shaking, the emulsion is infused as described for Intralipid. The daily maintenance dosages of the vitamins A, D_2 and K_1 are thereby supplied.

Recommended dosage for infants: For infants the preparation Vitlipid Infant should be used.

Contra-indications, warnings, etc Should not be given undiluted.

Pharmaceutical precautions Store at 2 to 8°C protected from light. Do not freeze.

The addition of Vitlipid Adult should be performed aseptically immediately before the start of the infusion and should be used within 24 hours unless the mixture is refrigerated when it may be used within 48 hours of preparation.

Legal category POM.

Package quantities Boxes of 10 × 10 ml ampoules.

Further information Vitlipid Adult is specially formulated for addition to either Intralipid 10% or 20%. It may be used for the reconstitution of Solivito before addition to Intralipid (see Solivito data sheet for details).

The manufacturer can be consulted for full information on complete and balanced intravenous nutrition regimens.

Product licence number 0022/0036.

VITLIPID INFANT*

Presentation A white, oil in water emulsion containing the fat soluble vitamins A, D_2 and K_1, in the oil phase of the emulsion with a composition corresponding to that of Intralipid 10%. Vitlipid Infant is intended for addition to Intralipid 10% or 20% and for use in infants on intravenous nutrition. One ml contains:

Retinol palmitate	
corresponding to retinol	100 mcg (333 i.u.)
Calciferol	2.5 mcg (100 i.u.)
Phytomenadione	50 mcg
Fractionated soybean oil	100 mg
Fractionated egg	
phospholipids	12 mg
Glycerol	22.5 mg
Water for injections to 1 ml	

Uses Vitlipid Infant is indicated as a supplement to Intralipid 10% or 20% in intravenous nutrition of infants in order to cover the daily requirements of the fat soluble vitamins A, D_2 and K_1.

Dosage and administration *Recommended dosage for infants:* Vitlipid Infant in a dosage of 1 ml per kg body weight per day is added to Intralipid 10% or 20%. The daily dosage must not exceed 4 ml. After gentle shaking the emulsion is infused as stated for Intralipid.

Recommended dosage for adults: For adults the preparation Vitlipid Adult should be used.

Contra-indications, warnings, etc Should not be given undiluted.

Pharmaceutical precautions Store at 2 to 8°C protected from light. Do not freeze.

The addition of Vitlipid Infant should be performed aseptically immediately before the start of the infusion and should be used within 24 hours unless the mixture is refrigerated when it may be used within 48 hours of preparation.

Legal category POM.

Package quantities Boxes of 10 × 10 ml ampoules.

Further information Vitlipid Infant is specially formulated for addition to either Intralipid 10% or 20%. It may be used for the reconstitution of Solivito before addition to Intralipid (see Solivito data sheet for details).

The manufacturer can be consulted for full information on complete and balanced intravenous nutrition regimens.

Product licence number 0022/0038.

*Trade Mark

Kirby-Warrick Pharmaceuticals Ltd
Mildenhall
Bury St Edmunds
Suffolk IP28 7AX

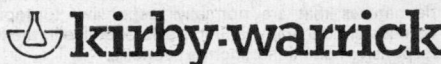

ACNEGEL*
ACNEGEL* FORTE

Presentation Acnegel contains 5% benzoyl peroxide in a gel base formulated with colloidal magnesium aluminium silicate, hydroxypropylmethyl-cellulose, ethyl alcohol, polyoxyethylene lauryl ether, citric acid and purified water.

Acnegel Forte contains 10% benzoyl peroxide in a gel base formulated as above.

Uses Acnegel and Acnegel Forte are indicated for the treatment of acne.

Benzoyl peroxide exerts an antibacterial effect and provides a drying and desquamative action. Penetration is enhanced by the gel base, which is invisible on the skin.

Dosage and administration Treatment should normally commence with Acnegel. Apply the gel to the affected areas once daily. Washing with soap and water prior to application greatly enhances the efficacy of the preparation.

The reaction of the skin to benzoyl peroxide differs in individual patients and for this reason the higher percentage of benzoyl peroxide in Acnegel Forte may be required in order to provide a satisfactory drying and desquamative action.

Contra-indications, warnings, etc Patients with a known sensitivity to benzoyl peroxide should not use these products. For external use only. Take care to keep the product away from contact with the mouth, the eyes and other mucous membranes to avoid irritation. The product should only be applied to other sensitive areas, such as the skin of the neck, with caution.

In normal use a mild burning sensation will probably be felt on first application and a moderate reddening and peeling of the skin will occur within a few days. During the first few weeks of treatment a sudden increase in peeling will occur in most patients; this is not harmful and will subside within a day or two if treatment is temporarily discontinued. If discomfort such as burning, redness or excess peeling occurs, discontinue treatment temporarily or consult a doctor. Keep away from children. The product may bleach dyed clothing and fabrics.

Pharmaceutical precautions Store in a cool place.

Legal category P.

Package quantities Acnegel and Acnegel Forte are supplied in tubes each containing 50 g.

Further information Nil.

Product licence numbers
Acnegel 3478/0029
Acnegel Forte 3478/0030

DIPROBASE* ▼

Presentation Diprobase Cream is a smooth, uniform white cream containing chlorocresol (0.1% w/w) as preservative. Diprobase Ointment is a smooth white preservative-free ointment, containing 5% w/w Liquid Paraffin BP and 95% White Soft Paraffin BP.

Diprobase presentations, because of their emollient and soothing properties, are particularly suitable for the care of the skin. They are also exceptionally well tolerated.

Uses Diprobase Cream and Ointment are emollients, with moisturizing and protective properties, indicated for follow-up treatment with topical steroids or in spacing such treatment. They may also be used as diluents for topical steroids. Diprobase products are recommended for the symptomatic relief of red inflamed, damaged, dry or chapped skin, the protection of raw skin areas and as a pre-bathing emollient for dry/eczematous skin to alleviate drying effects.

Dosage and administration The Cream or Ointment should be thinly applied to cover the affected area completely massaging gently and thoroughly into the skin. Frequency of application should be established by the physician. Generally, Diprobase Cream and Ointment can be used as often as required.

Contra-indications, warnings, etc Hypersensitivity to any of the components of the Cream or Ointment is a contraindication to their use.

Side-effects: No side-effects have been reported.

Pharmaceutical precautions Store in a cool place.

Legal category P.

Package quantities Diprobase Cream is supplied in 50 g tubes and 500 g dispensers. Diprobase Ointment is supplied in 50 g tubes.

Further information Nil.

Product licence numbers
Cream 3478/0059
Ointment 3478/0064

DIPROSALIC* ▼

Presentation Diprosalic Ointment contains 0.05% betamethasone as the diprofrionate ester and 3% salicylic acid. It is a smooth white, preservative-free ointment.

Diprosalic Lotion contains 0.05% betamethasone as

the dipropionate ester and 2% salicylic acid in a preservative-free isopropyl alcohol base. It is formulated to spread easily without adherence to the hair.

Uses Betamethasone dipropionate is a synthetic fluorinated corticosteroid. It is active topically and produces a rapid and sustained response in those inflammatory dermatoses that are normally responsive to topical corticosteroid therapy, and it is also effective in the less responsive conditions, such as psoriasis.

Topical salicylic acid softens keratin, loosens cornified epithelium and desquamates the epidermis.

Diprosalic presentations are therefore indicated for the treatment of hyperkeratotic and dry corticosteroid-responsive dermatoses where the cornified epithelium may resist penetration of the steroid. The salicyclic acid constituent of Diprosalic preparations, as a result of its descaling action, allows access of the corticosteroid to the underlying diseased areas of the dermis more rapidly than by applying steroid alone.

Dosage and administration Once to twice daily.

Diprosalic Ointment: In most cases a thin film should be applied to cover the affected area once or twice daily.

Diprosalic Lotion: In most cases a few drops should be applied to the affected areas once or twice daily and massaged gently and thoroughly into the skin.

For some patients adequate maintenance therapy may be achieved with less frequent application.

It is recommended that Diprosalic preparations are prescribed for 2 weeks, and that treatment is reviewed at that time. The maximum weekly dose should not exceed 60 g.

Contra-indications, warnings, etc Rosacea, acne and peri-oral dermatitis. Hypersensitivity to any of the ingredients of the Diprosalic presentations contraindicates their use as do tuberculous and most viral lesions of the skin, particularly herpes simplex, vaccinia, varicella. Diprosalic Ointment and Lotion should not be used in fungal or bacterial skin infections without suitable concomitant anti-infective therapy.

Occlusion must not be used, since under these circumstances the keratolytic action of salicylic acid may lead to enhanced absorption of the steroid.

Warnings: As with all fluorinated topical corticosteroids long term continuous therapy should be avoided where possible, particularly in infants and children as adrenal suppression can occur even without occlusion. Prolonged treatment with topical steroids may result in atrophic striae, this may be exhibited on the face more than other areas of the body.

It is dangerous if Diprosalic presentations come into contact with the eyes. Avoid contact with eyes and mucous membranes.

The safety of using Diprosalic Ointment and Lotion in pregnant women has not yet been established and so should not be used on pregnant women in large amounts for prolonged periods of time.

The systemic absorption of betamethasone dipropionate and salicylic acid may be increased if extensive body surface areas or skin folds are treated for prolonged periods or with excessive amounts of steroids. Suitable precautions should be taken in these circumstances, particularly with infants and children.

Side-effects: Diprosalic skin preparations are generally well tolerated and side-effects are rare. Continuous application without interruption may result in local atrophy of the skin, striae and superficial vascular dilation,

particularly on the face. In addition prolonged use of salicylic acid preparations may cause dermatitis.

Overdosage: Excessive prolonged use of topical corticosteroids can suppress pituitary-adrenal functions resulting in secondary adrenal insufficiency which is usually reversible. In such cases appropriate symptomatic treatment is indicated.

With topical preparations containing salicylic acid excessive prolonged use may result in symptoms of salicylism. Treatment is symptomatic.

The steroid and salicyclic acid content of each tube is so low as to have little or no toxic effect in the unlikely event of accidental oral ingestion.

Pharmaceutical precautions Nil.

Legal category POM.

Package quantities Diprosalic Ointment is supplied in 30 g and 100 g tubes. Diprosalic Lotion is supplied in 30 ml and 100 ml bottles.

Further information Diprosalic Ointment and Lotion are formulated to avoid the problems of incompatibility normally experienced between steroids and salicyclic acid.

Product licence numbers
Diprosalic Ointment   3478/0066
Diprosalic Lotion   3478/0067

DIPROSONE* ▼

Presentation The Diprosone skin preparations contain 0.05% betamethasone as the dipropionate ester.

Diprosone Cream is a smooth white cream. It contains chlorocresol as the preservative.

Diprosone Ointment is a smooth white preservative free ointment.

Diprosone Scalp Application is a slightly gelled solution containing isopropyl alcohol, which has antibacterial activity. It is formulated to spread without adherence to hair.

Uses Betamethasone dipropionate is a synthetic fluorinated corticosteroid. It is active topically and produces a rapid and sustained response in those inflammatory dermatoses that are normally responsive to topical corticosteroid therapy, and is often effective in the less responsive conditions such as psoriasis.

Diprosone Scalp Application is indicated for serious steroid responsive dermatoses of the scalp.

Dosage and administration Once to twice daily. In most cases a thin film of Diprosone Cream or Ointment should be applied to cover the affected area once or twice daily. For some patients adequate maintenance therapy may be achieved with less frequent application.

Diprosone Cream is especially appropriate for moist or weeping surfaces and the ointment for dry, lichenified or scaly lesions but this is not invariably so.

Control over the dosage regimen may be achieved during intermittent and maintenance therapy by using Diprobase Cream or Ointment (PL 3478/0059 and 3478/0064) the base vehicles of Diprosone Cream and Ointment. Such control may be necessary in mild and improving dry skin conditions requiring low dose steroid treatment.

A few drops of Diprosone Scalp Application should be applied to the affected areas twice daily and massaged gently and thoroughly into the scalp. For some patients adequate maintenance therapy may be achieved with less frequent application.

Contra-indications, warnings, etc Rosacea, acne and peri-oral dermatitis. Hypersensitivity to any of the ingredients. Tuberculosis and most viral lesions of the skin, particularly herpes simplex, vaccina, varicella. Diprosone should not be used in fungal or bacterial skin infections without suitable concomitant anti-infective therapy.

Warnings: As with all fluorinated topical steroids long term continuous therapy should be avoided where possible, particularly in infants and children as adrenal suppression may occur even without occlusion. The face more than other areas of the body may exhibit atrophic changes after prolonged treatment with potent topical corticosteroids.

Topical administration of corticosteroids to pregnant animals can cause abnormalities of foetal development. The relevance of this finding to human beings has not been established; however, topical steroids should not be used extensively in pregnancy i.e. in large amounts or for prolonged periods.

Diprosone skin preparations are generally very well tolerated and side effects are rare. Systemic absorption of topical corticosteroids will be increased if extensive body surface areas or skin folds are treated for prolonged periods of time. This effect is more likely to occur in the elderly or in infants and children in which case the napkin may act as an occlusive dressing.

Side-effects: Continuous application without interruption may result in local atrophy of the skin, stria and superficial vascular dilation, particularly on the face.

Overdosage: Excessive prolonged use of topical corticosteroids can result in suppression of pituitary-adrenal function resulting in secondary adrenal insufficiency which is usually reversible. In such cases appropriate symptomatic treatment is indicated.

The steroid content of each tube is so low as to have little or no toxic effect in the unlikely event of accidental oral ingestion.

Pharmaceutical precautions Store in a cool place.

Legal category POM.

Package quantities Diprosone Cream and Ointment are supplied in 30 g and 100 g tubes.

Diprosone Scalp Application is supplied in 30 ml and 100 ml plastic bottles.

Further information These preparations do not contain lanolin or parabens. The high potency of the dipropionate ester enables use of betamethasone in low concentrations.

Product licence numbers

Cream	3478/0003
Ointment	3478/0004
Scalp Application	3478/0065

GARAMYCIN* EYE/EAR DROPS
GARAMYCIN* EYE OINTMENT ▼

Presentation Each ml of Garamycin Eye/Ear Drops contains gentamicin sulphate equivalent to 3.0 mg of gentamicin base in a sterile, aqueous isotonic solution. Benzalkonium chloride is included as a preservative. Each gram of the sterile Garamycin Eye Ointment contains gentamicin sulphate, equivalent

to 3.0 mg of gentamicin base, liquid paraffin, white soft paraffin and methylhydroxybenzoate and propylhydroxybenzoate as preservatives.

Uses Gentamicin is a bactericidal antibiotic active against a wide variety of pathogenic Gram-negative and Gram-positive bacteria. Garamycin Eye/Ear Drops and the Eye Ointment are indicated in the topical treatment of infections of the external structures of the eye and its adnexa caused by susceptible bacteria. Such infections include conjunctivitis, keratitis and kerato-conjunctivitis, corneal ulcers, blepharitis and blepharo-conjunctivitis, acute meibomianitis, episcleritis and dacryocystitis. Garamycin may be used for the prevention of ocular infection after: removal of a foreign body, burns or lacerations of the conjunctiva; damage from chemical or physical agents and after ocular surgery.

Garamycin Eye/Ear Drops are also indicated for the topical treatment of otitis externa caused by susceptible bacteria.

Dosage and administration For Adults and Children.

Eye: Instill 1–2 drops Garamycin Eye/Ear drops in affected eye every four hours as required.

Apply a sufficient amount of Garamycin Eye Ointment two or four times a day.

Ear: The ear canal should be cleaned thoroughly and 3–4 drops instilled three to four times a day.

After a favourable response is obtained, the dosage may be reduced and discontinued as cure is achieved.

Contra-indications, warnings, etc Garamycin Eye/Ear Drops and Garamycin Eye Ointment are contraindicated in patients with known hypersensitivity to any of the components of these preparations. Fungal and viral infections are contraindications to the use of these products. Prolonged use of topical antibiotics may give rise to overgrowth of non-susceptible organisms. If this occurs, appropriate therapy is indicated. Cross-allerginicity among aminoglycosides has been demonstrated. Transient eye irritation has been reported.

The safety of these products has not been established in children less than six years old or in pregnant women.

Ophthalmic ointments may retard corneal healing.

Overdosage: A single overdosage of gentamicin would not be expected to produce symptoms.

Pharmaceutical precautions Store at room temperature.

Legal category POM.

Package quantities Garamycin Eye/Ear Drops are available in natural polyethylene dropper bottles containing 10 ml Garamycin Eye/Ear Drops. Garamycin Eye Ointment is available in 3 g tubes.

Further information Nil.

Product licence numbers

Garamycin Eye/Ear Drops	3478/0028
Garamycin Eye Ointment	3478/0027

GARAMYCIN* INJECTION

Presentation Garamycin for parenteral use is available as: Garamycin Injection in 2 ml ampoules, or 2 ml multiple-dose vials each containing the equivalent of 80 mg gentamicin base as the sulphate.

Uses Garamycin is gentamicin, an aminoglycoside antibiotic produced by the fermentation of Micromonospora purpurea. Gentamicin is active against a wide variety of pathogenic Gram-negative and Gram-positive bacteria, e.g. *Pseudomonas aeruginosa, Proteus* species, *Escherichia coli, Klebsiella – Enterobacter – Serratia* species, *Staphylococcus* species (including penicillin- and methicillin-resistant strains). It is also active against clinical isolates of bacteria resistant to other aminoglycoside antibiotics (kanamycin, neomycin, paromomycin and tobramycin).

Garamycin Injection is indicated in: kidney and genitourinary tract infections, respiratory tract infections, septicaemia, serious infections of the central nervous system (meningitis), gastro-intestinal tract infections, infected wounds, bone and soft tissue infections including peritonitis, septic abortion and burns complicated by sepsis, where susceptible organisms are involved or suspected.

Dosage and administration *Adult patients with normal renal function:* The recommended dosage of Garamycin Injection for adult patients with serious infections is 3 mg/kg/day administered intramuscularly eight-hourly for 7–10 days. For patients with life-threatening infections in the absence of impaired renal function, dosages up to 5 mg/kg/day in equally divided doses six or eight hourly are given. This dosage should be reduced to 3 mg/kg/day as soon as clinically indicated. When systemic or urinary tract infections are of moderate severity and the causative organism is likely to be highly responsive, a dosage of 2 mg/kg/day given 12 hourly should be considered. However, if prompt clinical response is not apparent, dosage should be increased to 3 mg/kg/day given eight hourly.

Adult patients with impaired renal function: Approximate dosage guidelines for Garamycin Injection in adult patients based on renal function, are given in the table below.

In patients undergoing 14 hour haemodialysis twice weekly, the recommended dosage is 1 to 1.7 mg/kg of gentamicin at the end of each dialysis period depending on the severity of the infection.

Routes of administration: Gentamicin may be administered intramuscularly or intravenously. The recommended dosage and precautions for intramuscular and intravenous administration are identical.

Intravenous administration:

Direct intravenous injection: A single dose of Garamycin may be given over a period of two to three minutes either directly into the vein or directly into i.v. tubing.

Infusion: A single dose is diluted into sterile isotonic saline or 5% dextrose solution and may be infused over a period of up to two hours.

Contra-indications, warnings, etc A history of hypersensitivity to gentamicin is a contra-indication to its use. Safety for use in pregnancy has not been established. Patients with impaired renal function treated with gentamicin injection may be exposed to an increased risk of ototoxicity. In these patients, renal, auditory and vestibular functions should be monitored. When feasible, gentamicin serum levels should be monitored; prolonged concentration above 12 mcg/ml and trough concentrations of above 2 mcg/ml should also be avoided. The concurrent use of gentamicin with potent diuretics such as ethacrynic acid and frusemide should be avoided since these diuretics may by themselves cause ototoxicity. Concurrent use of other neurotoxic and/or nephrotoxic drugs, particularly streptomycin, neomycin, kanamycin, cephaloridine, viomycin, polymyxin B, and polymyxin E (colistin), should be avoided. Neuromuscular blockade and respiratory paralysis may occur with gentamicin especially if it is administered to patients receiving neuromuscular blocking agents, such as succinylcholine or tubocurarine, or massive transfusions of citrate – anticoagulated blood. If blockade occurs, calcium salts may reverse it. In some patients with impaired renal function, there has been reported a rise in BUN and NPN, serum creatinine and oliguria. Monitoring of renal and eighth cranial nerve functions is recommended during therapy, particularly for patients with reduced renal function.

When carbenicillin is used concurrently with gentamicin each should be injected at a separate site.

Patients should be well hydrated during treatment.

Overdosage: haemodialysis or peritoneal dialysis will aid the removal of gentamicin from the blood.

Pharmaceutical precautions Store at room temperature. Do not freeze. Each pack is clearly marked with an expiry date.

Legal category POM.

Package quantities 2 ml vials and ampoules in packs of 25.

Further information Nil.

Product licence number 3478/0005.

Renal function tests

Body weight of adult patient	Dose	Creatinine clearance rate (ml/ min)	Serum creatinine level		Blood urea nitrogen		Frequency of administration
			mg/100 ml	S.I. Units μmol/l	mg/100 ml	S.I. Units mmol/1	
Over 60 kg (132 lb)	80 mg (2 ml)	Over 70	Less than 1.4	123.76	Less than 18	6.42	Every 8 hrs
		35–70	1.4–1.9	123.76–167.96	18–29	6.42–10.35	Every 12 hrs
		24–34	2.0–2.8	176.80–247.52	30–39	10.71–13.92	Every 18 hrs
		16–23	2.9–3.7	256.36–327.09	40–49	14.28–17.49	Every 24 hrs
		10–15	3.8–5.3	335.93–468.53	50–74	17.84–26.41	Every 36 hrs
		5–9	5.4–7.2	477.37–630.49	75–100	26.77–35.69	Every 48 hrs
60 kg or less (132 lb)	60 mg (1.5 ml)			(Same as above)			

GARAMYCIN* PAEDIATRIC INJECTION

Presentation Garamycin for parenteral use in paediatrics is available as Garamycin Paediatric Injection in 2 ml multiple-dose vials each containing the equivalent of 20 mg gentamicin base as the sulphate.

Uses Garamycin is gentamicin, an aminoglycoside antibiotic produced by the fermentation of Micromonospora purpurea. Gentamicin is active against a wide variety of pathogenic Gram-negative, and Gram-positive bacteria. *Pseudomonas aeruginosa, Proteus* species, *Escherichia coli, Klebsiella – Enterobacter – Serratia* species, *staphylococcus* species (including penicillin- and methicillin-resistant strains). It is also active against clinical isolates of bacteria resistant to other aminoglycoside antibiotics (kanamycin, neomycin, paromomycin and tobramycin).

Gentamicin injection is indicated in: kidney and genito-urinary tract infections, septicaemia, serious infection of the central nervous system (meningitis), gastro-intestinal tract infections, infected wounds, bone and soft tissue infections (including burns), where susceptible organisms are involved or suspected.

Dosage and administration *Children with moderate or severe infections:* 6–7.5 mg/kg/day in three equally divided doses. Neonates (premature or full term) require a dosage of 5–6 mg/kg/day given 12 hourly. Infants older than one week may be administered gentamicin 7.5 mg/kg/day in two equal doses 12 hourly or three equal doses eight hourly. The usual duration of treatment for children, infants and neonates is 7–10 days.

Peak concentrations should be in the range of 4–6 mcg/ml. Determination of an adequate serum level should take into consideration susceptibility of the causative micro-organism, severity of infection, and status of patient's host-defence mechanisms.

Patients with impaired renal function: Dosage frequency should be reduced in accordance with gentamicin serum levels. The serum half-life (in hours) may be estimated by multiplying the serum creatinine (expressed in mg %) by four. The interval between doses, in hours, may be approximated by doubling the serum half-life or by multiplying serum creatinine (expressed in mg %) by eight.

In children undergoing 14 hour haemodialysis twice weekly, the recommended dosage is 1–1.7 mg/kg of gentamicin intramuscularly or intravenously at the end of each dialysis period depending on the severity of the infection.

Routes of administration: Gentamicin may be administered intramuscularly or intravenously. The recommended dosage and precautions for intramuscular and intravenous administration are identical.

Intravenous administration:
  Direct intravenous injection: A single dose of Garamycin may be given over a period of two to three minutes either directly into the vein or directly into i.v. tubing.

  Infusion: A single dose is diluted into sterile isotonic saline or 5% dextrose solution and may be infused over a period of up to two hours.

Contra-indications, warnings, etc A history of hypersensitivity to gentamicin is a contra-indication to its use. Patients with impaired renal function treated with gentamicin injection may be exposed to an increased risk of ototoxicity. In these patients, renal, auditory and vestibular functions should be monitored. When feasible, gentamicin serum levels should be monitored; prolonged concentration above 12 mcg/ml and trough concentrations of above 2 mcg/ml should also be avoided. The concurrent use of gentamicin with potent diuretics such as ethacrynic acid and frusemide should be avoided since these diuretics may by themselves cause ototoxicity. Concurrent use of other neurotoxic and/or nephrotoxic drugs, particularly streptomycin, neomycin, kanamycin, cephaloridine, viomycin, polymixin B, and polymixin E (colistin), should be avoided. Neuromuscular blockade and respiratory paralysis may occur with gentamicin especially if it is administered to patients receiving neuromuscular blocking agents, such as succinylcholine, or tubocurarine, or massive transfusions of citrate – anticoagulated blood. If blockade occurs, calcium salts may reverse it. In some patients with impaired renal function, there has been reported a rise in BUN and NPN, serum creatinine and oliguria. Monitoring of renal and eighth cranial nerve functions is recommended during therapy, particularly for patients with reduced renal function.

When carbenicillin is used concurrently with gentamicin each should be injected at a separate site.

Patients should be well hydrated during treatment.

Overdosage: Haemodialysis or peritoneal dialysis will aid the removal of gentamicin from the blood.

Pharmaceutical precautions Store at room temperature. Do not freeze. Each pack is clearly marked with an expiry date.

Legal category POM.

Package quantities 2 ml vials in packs of 5.

Further information Nil.

Product licence number 3478/0006.

MODRASONE* CREAM AND OINTMENT ▼

Presentation Modrasone Cream contains 0.05% alclometasone dipropionate in a smooth white emollient cream base. It contains chlorocresol as the preservative.

Modrasone Ointment contains 0.05% alclometasone dipropionate in a preservative-free ointment base.

Uses Alclometasone dipropionate is a non-fluorinated, topically active synthetic corticosteroid.

Modrasone cream or ointment is indicated for the treatment of inflammatory and pruritic manifestations of corticosteroid responsive dermatoses.

Dosage and administration For adults and children, a thin film of Modrasone Cream or Ointment should be applied to the affected skin area two or three times daily or as directed by the physician. Massage gently into the skin until the medication disappears.

Contra-indications: Hypersensitivity to any of the ingredients. Rosacea, acne and peri-oral dermatitis. Tuberculous and viral lesions of the skin, particularly herpes simplex, vaccina, varicella. Modrasone should not be used in fungal or bacterial skin infections.

Warnings: As with all topical steroids, long term continuous therapy should be avoided where possible, particularly in infants and children as adrenal suppression may occur even without occlusion. In infants the napkin may act as an occlusive dressing and thus increase absorption.

Topical administration of corticosteroids to pregnant animals can cause abnormalities to foetal development. The relevance of this finding to human beings has not been established; however, topical steroids should not be used extensively in pregnancy, i.e. in large amounts or for long periods.

Side-effects: Excessive prolonged use may result in local atrophy of the skin, striae and superficial vascular dilatation, particularly on the face.

Overdosage: Excessive prolonged use of topical corticosteroids may result in suppression of pituitary-adrenal function resulting in secondary adrenal insufficiency which is usually reversible. In such cases appropriate symptomatic treatment is indicated.

The total steroid content of each tube is low and is unlikely to have any toxic effect in the unlikely event of accidental oral ingestion.

Pharmaceutical precautions Store in a cool place.

The dilution of Modrasone Cream and Ointment is not recommended.

Legal category POM.

Package quantities Modrasone Cream or Ointment are supplied in 30 g and 100 g tubes.

Further information Nil.

Product licence numbers
Cream   0201/0060
Ointment   0201/0061

NETILLIN* Injection ▼

Presentation Netillin Injection for parenteral use is an aqueous solution of netilmicin sulphate. Each millilitre contains netilmicin sulphate equivalent to 100 mg, 50 mg or 10 mg of netilmicin base, and is available in ampoules.

Uses Netilmicin sulphate is a semi-synthetic, water-soluble antibiotic of the aminoglycoside group. It is a rapidly acting bactericidal antibiotic which probably acts by inhibiting normal protein synthesis in susceptible organisms. It is active at low concentrations against many strains of a wide variety of pathogenic bacteria including *Escherichia coli, Klebsiella-Enterobacter-Serratia* species, *Citrobacter* species, *Proteus* species (indole-positive and indole-negative), including *Proteus mirabilis, Proteus morganii, Proteus rettgeri, Proteus vulgaris; Pseudomonas aeruginosa,* and *Staphylococcus* species (coagulase-positive and coagulase-negative, including penicillin and methicillin-resistant strains).

Netillin Injection is indicated in: bacteraemia, septicaemia (including neonatal sepsis), serious infections of the respiratory tract, kidney and genitourinary tract infections, skin and soft tissue infections, bone and joint infections, burns, wounds and peri-operative infections, intra-abdominal infections (including peritonitis) and infections of the gastro-intestinal tract.

Netillin Injection is recommended for prophylactic use.

Netillin Injection has also been effective in the treatment of infections caused by organisms resistant to other aminoglycosides, such as kanamycin, gentamicin, tobramycin and amikacin.

Dosage and administration The recommended dosage for intramuscular and intravenous administration is identical.

Patients with normal renal function:

Adults: The recommended dosage of Netillin Injection for patients with urinary tract or systemic infections with normal renal function is 4.0–6.0 mg/kg/day given in two equal doses every 12 hours. It may also be given in three equal doses every eight hours. In general, within this dose range, lower dosage will be used for urinary tract infections and higher dosage for systemic infections. For both uses, dosage should be adjusted depending on severity of infection and patient condition.

For adults weighing 50–90 kg, a dose of 150 mg may be given every twelve hours or 100 mg every eight hours. For adults smaller or larger than the above range, dosage should be calculated in mg/kg of lean body weight.

For patients with life-threatening infections, dosages up to 7.5 mg/kg/day may be administered in three equal doses every eight hours. This dosage should be reduced to 6 mg/kg/day or less as soon as clinically indicated, usually within 48 hours.

Children: 6.0–7.5 mg/kg/day (2.0 to 2.5 mg/kg administered every eight hours).

Infants and neonates over one week of age: 7.5 to 9.0 mg/kg/day (2.5 to 3.0 mg/kg administered every eight hours).

Premature or Full Term Neonates One Week of Age or Less: 6 mg/kg/day (3.0 mg/kg administered every 12 hours).

The usual duration of treatment is seven to fourteen days. Longer courses have been well tolerated but it is important that patients treated beyond the usual period be carefully monitored for changes in renal, auditory and vestibular function. Dosage should be reduced if clinically indicated. Netillin should usually be administered intramuscularly, or be injected directly into a vein or I.V. tubing slowly over a period of 3 to 5 minutes.

Infusion: In adults a single dose of Netillin injection may be diluted in 50 to 200 ml of sterile normal saline or in a sterile solution of dextrose 5% in water; in infants and children the volume of diluent should be dependent on the patient's fluid requirements. The solution may be infused over a period of one half to two hours.

Netillin Injection should not be physically pre-mixed with other drugs, but should be administered separately in accordance with the recommended route of administration and dosage schedule.

Netillin Injection is physically compatible with the following parenteral solutions: Sterile Water for Injections, Normal Saline, 5% and 10% Dextrose in Water.

Patients with impaired renal function:

Dosage must be adjusted and should be individualised on an eight hourly mg/kg basis as follows. The standard daily dose should be given at eight hourly intervals on the first day (loading dose). Serum creatinine or creatinine clearance rate should then be measured and the dosage of netilmicin adjusted according to the table below. Monitor netilmicin serum concentrations and serum creatinine or creatinine clearance rates at regular intervals.

Haemodialysis: The recommended dose at the end of each dialysis period is 2 mg/kg. In children a dose of 2 to 2.5 mg/kg may be administered, depending upon the severity of infection.

Dosages recommended above for patients with normal and impaired renal function should not be reduced when netilmicin is administered concomitantly with other antibiotics.

Contra-indications, warnings, etc Hypersensitivity to netilmicin contra-indicates its use. A history of hypersensitivity or serious toxic reactions to other aminoglycosides may also be a contra-indication.

Dosage adjustment guide for patients with renal function impairment

Loading Dose Administer initial standard daily dose as follows	Approx. creatinine clearance rate (ml/min/ 1.73 sq m)	Serum creatinine level		Percent of loading dose adjusted according to serum creatinine level
		mg/100 ml	S.I. Units μmol./l	
1. Adults with urinary tract and systemic infections 4–6 mg/kg/day	100	1.0	80	100
	71–100	1.1–1.3	100–120	80
2. Adults with life threatening infections 7.5 mg/kg/day	56–70	1.4–1.6	130–150	65
	46–55	1.7–1.9	160–175	55
3. Children 6–7.5 mg/kg/day	41–45	2.0–2.2	180–190	50
4. Infants & neonates over 1 week of age 7.5–9.0 mg/kg/ day	36–40	2.3–2.5	210–220	40
	31–35	2.6–3.0	230–260	35
5. Premature or full-term neonates one week of age or less 6 mg/kg/day	26–30	3.1–3.5	270–310	30
	21–25	3.6–4.0	320–360	25
	16–20	4.1–5.1	365–450	20
	10–15	5.2–6.6	460–580	15
	< 10	6.7–8.0	600–700	10

Patients treated with aminoglycosides should be under close clinical observation because of the potential toxicity associated with their use. Monitoring of renal and eighth cranial nerve functions is desirable during therapy, particularly for patients with known or suspected reduced renal function.

Evidence of ototoxicity requires dosage adjustment or discontinuance of the drug.

Serum concentration assays of aminoglycosides are of value to assure adequate levels and to avoid potentially toxic levels. At the recommended dosage, peak levels will generally not exceed 12 mcg/ml. Prolonged levels above 16 mcg/ml should be avoided. If trough levels are monitored (just prior to next dose) they will usually be 3 mcg/ml or less with the recommended dosage. Increasing trough concentrations above 4 mcg/ml should be avoided.

Concurrent and/or sequential systemic or topical use of other potentially neurotoxic and/or nephrotoxic drugs, such as polymyxin B, colistin, cephaloridine, kanamycin, gentamicin, amikacin, tobramycin, neomycin, streptomycin and vancomycin should be avoided. Advanced age and dehydration may also increase the risk of toxicity.

The concurrent use of netilmicin with potent diuretics, such as ethacrynic acid or frusemide, should be avoided since these diuretics by themselves may cause ototoxicity. In addition, when administered intravenously, diuretics may enhance aminoglycoside toxicity by altering the antibiotic concentrations in serum and tissue.

Neurotoxic or nephrotoxic antibiotics may be absorbed from body surfaces after local irrigation or application. The potential toxic effect of such antibiotics administered in this fashion should be considered.

Increased nephrotoxicity has been reported following concomitant administration of aminoglycoside antibiotics and cephalothin.

Although neuromuscular blockade has been reported in animals receiving netilmicin at doses considerably above those clinically recommended, the possibility of this phenomenon occurring in man should be considered, particularly if aminoglycosides are administered to patients receiving anaesthetics, neuromuscular blocking agents (such as succinylcholine or tubocurarine), or massive transfusions of citrate-anticoagulated blood. If blockade occurs, calcium salts may reverse it.

Aminoglycosides should be used with caution in patients with neuromuscular disorders, such as myasthenia gravis or parkinsonism, since these drugs theoretically may aggravate muscle weakness because of their potential curare-like effects on the neuromuscular junction.

Elderly patients may have reduced renal function which might not be evident by routine screening tests, such as BUN or serum creatinine. A creatinine clearance determination may be more useful. Monitoring of renal function during netilmicin treatment, as with other aminoglycosides, is particularly important in these patients.

Cross-allergenicity among aminoglycosides has been demonstrated. Patients should be well hydrated during treatment.

Although the *in vitro* mixing of netilmicin and carbenicillin results in a rapid and significant inactivation of netilmicin, this interaction has not been demonstrated in patients with normal renal function who received both drugs by different routes of administration. In patients with severe renal impairment receiving carbenicillin concomitantly with an aminoglycoside, a reduction in aminoglycoside serum half-life has been reported.

Treatment with netilmicin may result in overgrowth of non-susceptible organisms. If this occurs, appropriate therapy is indicated.

Netilmicin is not intended for intrathecal use.

Side-effects: Adverse renal effects, generally mild in nature, have been reported infrequently after netilmicin administration. They occur more frequently in patients with a history of renal impairment, in patients treated with larger than the recommended dosage, and are most often reversible. While eighth cranial nerve toxicity has been reported with netilmicin, the incidence is lower and the severity appears milder than with other aminoglycosides. Some clinical studies indicate that at therapeutic dosage, netilmicin may have less effect than other aminoglycosides on eighth cranial nerve function. Adverse effects on both the vestibular and auditory branches of the eighth cranial nerve occur primarily in patients with renal impairment and in patients on high doses and/or prolonged therapy. Symptoms which are often transient may include dizziness, vertigo, tinnitus, roaring in the ears and hearing loss. The latter is usually manifested by diminution of high-tone acuity. Total deafness has not been reported.

Some patients who have had previous ototoxic reactions to other aminoglycosides have been treated safely with Netillin Injection.

Other rarely reported adverse reactions possibly related to netilmicin include: headache, malaise, visual disturbances, disorientation, tachycardia, paraesthesia, rash, chills, fever, fluid retention, vomiting and diarrhoea.

Laboratory abnormalities possibly related to netilmicin include: increased blood sugar, increased alkaline phosphatase, increased SGOT or SGPT; other abnormal liver function studies; decreased haemoglobin, WBCs, and platelets; eosinophilia and increase in prothrombin time.

While local tolerance of Netillin Injection is generally excellent, there has been an occasional report of pain at the injection site or local reaction.

Safety for use in pregnancy has not been established.

Overdosage: In the event of overdose or toxic reaction, haemodialysis or peritoneal dialysis will aid the removal of netilmicin from the blood.

Pharmaceutical precautions Netillin Injection should be stored at 2°C to 30°C (35.6°F to 86°F). Protect from freezing.

Netillin Injections should not be physically premixed with other drugs, but should be administered separately in accordance with the recommended route of administration and dosage schedule.

Legal category POM.

Package quantities All the presentations of Netillin are colour coded on both cartons and the containers. The 100 mg/ml strength is available in 2 ml (colour coded red), 1.5 ml (orange) and 1 ml (yellow) ampoules. The 50 mg/ml and 10 mg/ml strengths are available in 1 ml (green) and 1.5 ml (blue) ampoules respectively. All ampoules are supplied in packs of ten.

Further information Nil.

Product licence numbers
Netillin Injection 100 mg/ml   3478/0041
Netillin Injection 50 mg/ml   3478/0040
Netillin Injection 10 mg/ml   3478/0039

OPTIMINE*

Presentation *Optimine Tablets:* Each white tablet, with score mark on one side and Schering Corporation USA Trademark on the other, contains 1.0 mg Azatadine Maleate USP.

Optimine Syrup: Each 5 ml of Syrup, which is a clear, colourless solution with a characteristic odour and flavour of blackcurrant, contains 0.5 mg of azatadine maleate USP.

Indications Optimine Tablets and Syrup are indicated for the symptomatic relief of allergic conditions such as hayfever, vasomotor rhinitis, urticaria, pruritus of allergic origin and allergic reactions associated with insect bites and stings.

Dosage and administration *Adults, the elderly and children over 12 years of age:* In most conditions, 1 mg of azatadine maleate (1 tablet or 10 ml of syrup) in the morning and evening is recommended in the majority of patients. In refractory or more severe cases, 2 mg twice daily may be used.

Children 6–12 years of age: 0.5 to 1.0 mg of azatadine maleate ($\frac{1}{2}$ to 1 tablet or 5 to 10 ml of syrup) twice daily.

Children 1–6 years of age: 0.25 mg azatadine maleate (2.5 ml of syrup) twice daily.

Optimine Syrup may be diluted with Syrup BP.

Contra-indications, warnings, etc Until the safety of azatadine maleate concerning adverse effects on human foetal development has been established, the drug is not recommended for use in pregnant or lactating women.

Patients taking azatadine maleate should be cautioned against ingestion of alcohol. The drug may potentiate central nervous system depressants.

Although drowsiness is infrequent and impairment of psychomotor function is not manifested at the recommended dosage, patients should be cautioned against engaging in mechanical operations requiring mental alertness until individual response to azatadine maleate has been determined.

Due to the anticholinergic effect of azatadine maleate, the drug should be used with caution in patients with prostatic hypertrophy, urinary retention, glaucoma, stenosing peptic ulcer or pyloroduodenal obstructions.

Mono-amine oxidase inhibitors, which are known to intensify or prolong the anticholinergic and sedative action of drugs, should not be used concomitantly with azatadine maleate.

Side Effects: Azatadine maleate is well tolerated and side-effects are generally dose-related and transient. Among these are: weakness, nervousness, dry mouth, increased appetite, anorexia, nausea, headache, drowsiness, dysuria and blurring of vision.

Overdosage: Symptoms may vary from central nervous system depression to stimulation, the latter is particularly likely in children. Atropine-like symptoms may also occur. If vomiting has not occured spontaneously the patient should be induced to vomit. If unsuccessful the stomach should be emptied by aspiration and lavage. Stimulants should not be used and vasopressors may be used to treat hypotension.

Pharmaceutical precautions There are no pharmaceutical precautions for Optimine tablets or syrup.

Legal category P.

Package quantities Optimine tablets are supplied in bottles containing 250 tablets and cartons of blister packs containing 10 tablets. Optimine syrup is supplied in a 120 ml bottle.

Further information Azatadine maleate possesses potent antihistamine and antiserotonin activity. It has an inherently long action which enables effective and sustained control of symptoms from twice a day administration.

Product licence numbers
Optimine Tablets   3478/0024
Optimine Syrup   3478/0025

PALACOS* R

Presentation Palacos R is a radiopaque rapidly setting bone cement formed from the mixture of two separate pre-measured sterilised components.

One component is supplied in a polyethylene coated paper packet and consists of 40 g of a powder (polymer) with the following composition:

Methyl methacrylate –
methylacrylate copolymer	33.80 g
Benzoyl peroxide	0.20 g
Zirconium dioxide	6.00 g
Chlorophyll	0.001 g

The other component is supplied in an amber ampoule and consists of 20 ml of a liquid (monomer) with the following composition:

Methyl methacrylate (stabilised with hydroquinone)	18.40 g
N,N-Dimethyl-p-toluidine	0.40 g
Chlorophyll	0.0004 g

The liquid monomer is sterile filtered and the powder is sterilised by ethylene oxide. The polyethylene coated paper packet containing the powder as well as the exterior of the ampoule containing the liquid are also sterilised with ethylene oxide. Palacos R is pigmented light green in order to make it clearly visible in the operative field.

Note: Palacos R powder is double packaged. The outer aluminium protective foil which is NON-STERILE contains two polyethylene peel-packs. Each peel pack encloses a STERILE polyethylene paper coated packet of Palacos R Powder.

The ampoule containing the liquid monomer is packaged in a protective plastic blister pack.

When the powder (polymer) and the liquid (monomer) are mixed, the dimethyl-p-toluidine in the liquid activates the benzoyl peroxide catalyst in the powder. This initiates the polymerisation of the monomer which then binds together granules of polymer. As polymerisation proceeds, a dough-like mass is formed which, over a period of five to six minutes, hardens into a mechanically uniform solid. Polymerisation is an exothermic reaction with temperatures rising to as high as 80°C. Although the spontaneous generation of heat accelerates the reaction, the polymerisation of this self-curing resin occurs even if the temperature is reduced by irrigation with a cool physiologic saline solution.

Action Palacos R is a radiopaque cement-like substance which allows seating and fixation of prostheses to bone.

Indications Palacos R bone cement is indicated for fixation of prostheses to bone in partial or total arthroplastic procedures of the hip, knee or other joints.

Contra-indications, warnings, etc
Contra-indications: Palacos R is contra-indicated in patients allergic to any of its components.

Warnings: Prior to using Palacos R, surgeons should be thoroughly familiar with its properties, handling characteristics and application to arthroplasty. (See Presentation, Precautions, and Dosage and Preparation.) It is advisable for the surgeon to go through the entire mixing, handling and setting process before using the material in an actual surgical procedure.

The liquid monomer is highly volatile and flammable; therefore, appropriate precaution should be taken particularly with its use in the operating room. It is also a potent lipid solvent and should not be allowed to come into direct contact with the body. Contact of the liquid monomer, with rubber, including surgical rubber gloves, should also be avoided.

Care should be exercised during the mixing of the two components to prevent excessive exposure to the concentrated vapours of the monomer. These may irritate the respiratory tract and eyes, and may possibly be harmful to the liver. Skin reactions apparently resulting from contact with the monomer have been reported.

Long-term durability, wearability and stability of the polymerised bone cement in situ are unknown. This should be considered in light of the expected longevity of the patients for whom the substance will be used. The long-term effects of this preparation are unknown. Thus the physician should decide whether the benefits expected from its use outweigh any possible long-term adverse effects.

Precautions: Blood pressure, pulse and respiration should be carefully monitored during and immediately after implantation of the bone cement. Any significant alteration in these vital signs should be corrected with appropriate measures.

When Palacos R is used in total hip replacements, care should be taken to clean and aspirate the proximal portion of the femoral medullary canal just prior to insertion of the bone cement.

Adverse reactions: Transient fall in blood pressure immediately after implantation of the bone cement and endo-prosthesis is frequently observed. Rare cases have been reported in which the hypotension was associated with cardiac arrest and sudden death.

The following additional adverse reactions have been reported with the use of the methylmethacrylate bone cements:

Thrombophlebitis	Superficial wound infection
Pulmonary embolism	
Haemorrhage and haematoma	Deep wound infection
	Trochanteric bursitis
Loosening or displacement of the prosthesis	Trochanteric separation

Others which have been observed:

Heterotopic new bone	Myocardial infarction
Short-term irregularities in cardiac conduction	Cerebrovascular accident

Dosage and preparation A dose is prepared by mixing the entire contents of one packet of powder (40 g polymer) with one ampoule of liquid (20 ml monomer). One or two doses will usually suffice, although this will depend upon the specific surgical procedure and the techniques employed. (At least one extra unit of Palacos R should be available before starting a surgical procedure.) Each dose is prepared separately. The following are required for preparation of the bone cement:

Sterile working area

Sterile porcelain or stainless steel bowls

Sterile porcelain or stainless steel mixing spoons or spatulas.

The polyethylene package and the blister pack are opened by a circulating nurse or assistant and the sterile paper packet and ampoule are aseptically placed on a sterile table. The paper packet and the ampoule are opened under sterile conditions. *The liquid is poured into a bowl and the powder is added.* The mixture is then stirred vigorously, but carefully, for 30–40 seconds until a dough-like mass is formed which does not adhere to rubber gloves. At this stage, the mass is kneadable and will remain so for about four to five minutes. The ideal working consistency of the Palacos R for application to bone is best determined by the surgeon's experience in using the preparation. When the desired consistency is obtained, the preparation may be applied to bone and prosthesis as required. To assure adequate fixation, the prosthesis should be held securely in place without movement until the bone cement has fully hardened. Generally, this occurs seven to eight minutes after the onset of mixing the powder with the liquid. Excessive cement must be removed while it is still soft. The above doughing, working and setting times apply at approximately 23°C (73°F). Higher temperatures will shorten these times. Conversely, lowering of the ambient temperature or that of the material below 23°C will increase doughing, working and setting times. If, during the surgical procedure, additional cement is required, another packet of powder and ampoule of liquid may be mixed as described above. The resulting kneadable mass may be applied to previously hardened bone cement.

Since each packet of powder contains a premeasured quantity of polymer to react with a premeasured quantity of monomer, care should be taken to mix the entire contents of one packet with the entire contents of one ampoule.

The mixing and subsequent kneading of the polymerising mass should be thorough and at least four (4) minutes in duration. Because of the volatile nature of the monomer, the above procedure may assist in causing its evaporation and thereby reduce the amount to which the patient is exposed. On the other hand, if the kneading process is extended too long, the polymerisation may proceed to a point where the mass is no longer soft and pliable, making manipulation and application to bone difficult.

The completion of polymerisation occurs in the patient and is associated with the liberation of heat. The long-term effects of this heat on the tissues surrounding the bone cement are not known. To more rapidly dissipate the heat, the polymerising cement may be irrigated with a cool physiologic saline solution.

Pharmaceutical precautions Do not store the liquid component above 30°C (86°F) or in direct sunlight to prevent premature polymerisation. Sterilisation shall only be performed by the manufacturer and is only guaranteed if the containers are undamaged. Resterilisation of any of the components should not be attempted under any circumstances.

Legal category POM.

Package quantities Carton consisting of: 2 packets, each containing 40 g sterilised powder (polymer); 2 ampoules, each containing 20 ml of sterilised liquid (monomer).

Further information Nil.

Product licence number 3478/0008.

PALACOS* R WITH GENTAMICIN
PALACOS* R-20 WITH GENTAMICIN

Presentation Palacos R with gentamicin and Palacos R-20 with gentamicin is a radiopaque rapidly-setting bone cement containing the antibiotic gentamicin, it is formed from the mixture of two separate pre-measured sterilised components.

One component is supplied in a polyethylene coated paper packet consisting of powder (polymer) with the following composition.

	Palacos R with gentamicin	Palacos R-20 with gentamicin
Methyl methacrylate – methyl acrylate co-polymer	33.80 g	16.9 g
Benzoyl peroxide	0.20 g	0.10 g
Zirconium dioxide	6.00 g	3.00 g
Chlorophyll with	0.001 g	0.0005 g
Gentamicin (as the sulphate)	0.50 g	0.25 g

The other component is supplied in an amber ampoule and consists of a liquid (monomer) with the following composition.

	Palacos R with gentamicin	Palacos R-20 with gentamicin
Methyl-methacrylate (stabilised with hydroquinone)	18.40 g	9.20 g
N,N-Dimethyl-p-toluidine	0.40 g	0.20 g
Chlorophyll	0.0004 g	0.0002 g

The liquid monomer is sterile filtered and the powder polymer and gentamicin mixture is sterilised by ethylene oxide. The polyethylene coated paper packet containing the powder as well as the exterior of the ampoule containing the liquid are also sterilised with ethylene oxide.

Palacos R with gentamicin and Palacos R-20 with gentamicin are pigmented light green in order to make them clearly visible in the operative field.

Note: The powder polymer plus gentamicin is double packaged. The outer aluminium protective foil which is NON-STERILE contains two polyethylene peel-packs. Each peel-pack encloses a STERILE polyethylene paper coated packet of powder polymer plus gentamicin.

The ampoule containing the liquid monomer is packaged in a protective plastic blister pack.

When the powder (polymer) and liquid (monomer) are mixed, the dimethyl-p-toluidine in the liquid activates the benzoyl peroxide polymerisation catalyst in the powder. This initiates the polymerisation of the monomer which then binds together granules of polymer. As polymerisation proceeds, a dough-like mass is formed which subsequently, over a period of five to six minutes, hardens into a mechanically uniform solid. Polymerisation is an exothermic reaction with temperatures rising as high as 80°C. Although the spontaneous generation of heat accelerates the reaction, the polymerisation of this self-curing resin occurs even if the temperature is reduced by irrigation with a cool physiologic saline solution.

Gentamicin is a broad spectrum bactericidal aminoglycoside antibiotic having activity against Gram-negative and Gram-positive bacteria. It is water soluble and heat stable. *In vitro*, gentamicin has been shown to be released in active form from the bone cement complex for periods of greater than one year. After implantation in animals, the antibiotic is detected in the blood as well as in fluid removed from the site of implantation. In man, following total hip replacement in which Palacos R with gentamicin was used as a bone cement, the antibiotic was found in joint fluid, blood and urine. Concentrations in the urine have been detected for up to three weeks after surgery, suggesting good release of antibiotic.

Uses Palacos R with gentamicin and Palacos R-20 with gentamicin bone cement is indicated for fixation of prostheses to bone in partial or total arthroplastic procedures of the hip, knee or other joints in which infection by gentamicin-sensitive organisms is confirmed or suspected.

Contra-indications, warnings, etc
Contra-indications: Palacos R with gentamicin and Palacos R-20 with gentamicin is contra-indicated in patients allergic to any of its components.

Warnings: Prior to using Palacos R with gentamicin and Palacos R-20 with gentamicin surgeons should be thoroughly familiar with its properties; handling characteristics and application to arthroplasty (see Presentation, Precautions and Dosage and Preparation). It is advisable for the surgeon to go through the entire mixing, handling and setting process before using the materials in an actual surgical procedure.

The liquid monomer is highly volatile and flammable, therefore appropriate precautions should be taken particularly with its use in the operating room. It is also a potent lipid solvent and should not be allowed to come into direct contact with the body. Contact of the liquid monomer with rubber, including surgical gloves, should also be avoided.

Care should be exercised during the mixing of the two components to prevent excessive exposure to the concentrated vapours of the monomer. These may irritate the respiratory tract and eyes, and may possibly be harmful to the liver. Skin reactions apparently resulting from contact with the monomer have been reported.

Long term durability, wearability and stability of the polymerised bone cement *in situ* are unknown. This should be considered in light of the expected longevity of the patients for whom the substance will be used. The long-term effects of this preparation are unknown. Thus the physician should decide whether the benefits from its use outweigh any possible long-term adverse effects.

Precautions: Blood pressure, pulse and respiration should be carefully monitored during and immediately after implantation of the bone cement. Any significant alteration in these vital signs should be corrected with appropriate measures.

When Palacos R with gentamicin is used in total hip replacements, care should be taken to clean and aspirate the proximal portion of the femoral medullary canal just prior to insertion of the bone cement.

Adverse Reactions: Transient fall in blood pressure immediately after implantation of the bone cement and endo-prosthesis is frequently observed. Rare cases have been reported in which the hypotension was associated with cardiac arrest and sudden death.

The following additional adverse reactions have been reported with the use of methyl methacrylate bone cements:

Thrombophlebitis	Superficial wound
Pulmonary embolism	infection
Haemorrhage and	Deep wound infection
haematoma	Trochanteric bursitis
Loosening or	Trochanteric separation
displacement of the	
prosthesis	

Others which have been observed:

Heterotopic new bone	Myocardial infarction
Short-term irregularities in	Cerebrovascular accident
cardiac conduction	

Since the concentration of gentamicin reaching the VIII nerve and the kidney will be quite low, ototoxic and nephrotoxic reactions are very unlikely to result from the use of Palacos R with gentamicin and Palacos R-20 with gentamicin. Hypersensitivity to gentamicin is rare.

Dosage and preparation: A dose is prepared by mixing the entire contents of one packet of powder with one ampoule of liquid (40 g polymer plus 0.5 g gentamicin and 20 ml monomer *OR* 20 g polymer plus 0.25 g gentamicin and 10 ml monomer). The number of doses and pack size required will depend upon the specific surgical procedure and technique employed. (At least one extra unit of the desired pack size should be available before starting a surgical procedure).

Each dose is prepared separately.

The following are required for preparation of the bone cement: sterile working area; sterile porcelain or stainless steel bowls; sterile porcelain or stainless steel mixing spoons or spatulas.

The polyethylene package and the blister pack are opened by a circulating nurse or assistant and the sterile paper packet and ampoule are aseptically placed on a sterile table. The paper packet and the ampoule are opened under sterile conditions. *The liquid is poured into a bowl and the powder is added.* The mixture is then stirred vigorously, but carefully, for 30–40 seconds until a dough-like mass is formed which does not adhere to rubber gloves. At this stage, the mass is kneadable and will remain so for about four to five minutes. The ideal working consistency of the Palacos R with gentamicin and Palacos R-20 with gentamicin for application to bone is best determined by the surgeon's experience in using the preparation. When the desired consistency is obtained the preparation may be applied to bone and prosthesis as required. To assure adequate fixation, the prosthesis should be held securely in place without movement until the bone cement has fully hardened. Generally, this occurs seven to eight minutes after the onset of mixing the powder with the liquid. Excessive cement must be removed while it is still soft. The above doughing, working and setting times apply at approximately 23°C (73°F). Higher temperatures will shorten these times. Conversely, lowering of the ambient temperature or that of the material below 23°C will increase doughing, working and setting times.

If, during the surgical procedure, additional cement is required, another packet of powder and ampoule of liquid may be mixed as described above. The resulting kneadable mass may be applied to previously hardened bone cement.

Since each packet of powder contains a premeasured quantity of polymer to react with a premeasured quantity of monomer, care should be taken to mix the entire contents of one packet with the entire contents of one ampoule.

The mixing and subsequent kneading of the polymerising mass should be thorough and at least four (4) minutes in duration.

Because of the volatile nature of the monomer, the above procedure may assist in causing its evaporation and thereby reducing the amount to which the patient is exposed. On the other hand, if the kneading process is extended too long, the polymerisation may proceed to a point where the mass is no longer soft and pliable, making manipulation and application to bone difficult.

The completion of polymerisation occurs in the patient and is associated with the liberation of heat. The long-term effects of this heat on the tissues surrounding the bone cement are not known. To more rapidly dissipate the heat, the polymerising cement may be irrigated with a cool physiologic saline solution.

Pharmaceutical precautions Do not store components above 30°C (86°F) or in direct sunlight to prevent premature polymerisation. Sterilisation shall only be performed by the manufacturer and is only guaranteed if the containers are undamaged. Resterilisation of any of the components should not be attempted under any circumstances.

Legal category POM.

Package quantities Palacos R with gentamicin is supplied in white cartons consisting of 2 packets each containing 40 g sterilised powder (polymer) with 0.5 g gentamicin (as the sulphate); 2 ampoules each containing 20 ml of sterilised liquid (monomer).

Palacos R-20 with gentamicin is supplied in blue cartons consisting of 2 packets each containing 20 g sterilised powder (polymer) with 0.25 g gentamicin (as the sulphate); 2 ampoules each containing 10 ml of sterilised liquid (monomer).

Further information Nil

Product licence number 3478/0009

TINADERM*-M CREAM

Presentation Each gram of Tinaderm-M Cream contains 10 mg of tolnaftate and 100,000 units of Nystatin in a white, water-washable, vanishing cream base.

Uses Tinaderm-M Cream is recommended for the topical treatment of cutaneous mycotic infections such as Tinea pedis, Tinea cruris, Tinea corporis, Tinea barbae and Tinea manuum due to Trichophyton rubrum, T. mentagrophytes, T. tonsurans, Microsporum canis, M. audouinii, Epidermophyton floccosum, Candida (monilia) albicans and Tinea versicolor (Malassezia furfur).

If Candida albicans is the primary cause of infections, such conditions as 'Athlete's foot' (dermatophytosis), perleche, paronychia, intertrigo, 'nappy rash' and other cutaneous lesions can be successfully treated with Tinaderm-M.

Tinaderm-M is particularly recommended for the treatment of fungal infections localised in intertriginous and other moist areas of the skin where Candida infections are present or likely to develop.

Dosage and administration A sufficient quantity of Tinaderm-M should be applied to completely cover the affected area two or three times daily until healing is complete. Lesions generally begin to clear during the first treatment week and disappear completely after two to three weeks of treatment. If thickening of skin has occurred, treatment for as long as 4–6 weeks may be required. The concomitant use of a mild keratolytic agent may be indicated in areas where the skin has become hyperkeratotic. Use of wet compresses prior to application of Tinaderm-M aids in the healing of exudative lesions and does not interfere with the fungicidal action of the medication. Surgical debridement of dead skin and treatment of calluses is advised when necessary.

If after four weeks of therapy there has not been a progressive improvement, diagnosis should be reconfirmed. Mycosis complicated by bacterial infections may require additional antibiotic treatment.

Contra-indications, warnings, etc Tinaderm-M should not be administered to patients with known hypersensitivity to any ingredients. Should sensitivity occur, discontinue use.

Keep away from eyes and mucous membranes. In mixed infections caused by non-susceptible bacteria or fungi, supplementary topical or systemic anti-infective therapy is indicated.

Tinaderm-M is for dermatological use only.

Side-effects: A few cases of mild irritation and sensitization have been reported.

Pharmaceutical precautions There are no pharmaceutical precautions for Tinaderm-M.

Legal category POM.

Package quantities Tinaderm-M is available in 20 g tubes.

Further information Tolnaftate is a highly active, nonsensitising, fungicidal agent that is very effective in the treatment of superficial fungal infections of the skin. Nystatin, an antibiotic with antifungal activity, provides specific therapy for all localised forms of moniliasis.

Tinaderm-M Cream does not ordinarily sting or irritate intact or broken skin and is inactive systemically. Tinaderm-M Cream will not stain or discolour skin, hair, nails or clothing.

Product licence number 3478/0020

*Trade Mark

Knoll Limited
The Brow
Burgess Hill
West Sussex RH15 9NE

knoll

SECURON* ▼

Presentation Securon tablets containing 40 mg Verapamil Hydrochloride BP are white, film coated tablets impressed with 40 on one side and the Knoll logo on the other.

Securon tablets containing 80 mg Verapamil Hydrochloride BP are white, film coated tablets impressed with SECURON 80 on one side and KNOLL above the score-line on the other.

Securon tablets containing 120 mg Verapamil Hydrochloride BP are white, film coated tablets impressed with SECURON 120 on one side and KNOLL above the score-line on the other.

Uses Securon is a calcium antagonist which blocks the inward movement of calcium in cardiac muscle cells, in smooth muscle cells of the coronary and systemic arteries and in the cells of the intracardiac conduction system. Securon lowers peripheral vascular resistance with little or no reflex tachycardia. Its efficacy in reducing both raised systolic and diastolic blood pressure is thought to be primarily due to this mode of action.

The decrease in systemic and coronary vascular resistance and the sparing effect on intracellular oxygen consumption appear to explain the anti-anginal properties of the product.

Because of its effect on the movement of calcium in the intracardiac conduction system, it reduces automaticity, decreases conduction velocity and increases the refractory period.

Securon is indicated for:

(1) the treatment of mild to moderate hypertension and of renal hypertension, used alone or in conjunction with other antihypertensive therapy.

(2) the treatment and prophylaxis of all forms of angina pectoris.

(3) the treatment and prophylaxis of supraventricular tachycardia (paroxysmal tachycardia, premature supraventricular contractions, atrial fibrillation and flutter) and paroxysmal supraventricular tachycardia of the reciprocating type, associated with the Wolff-Parkinson-White syndrome.

Dosage and administration

Hypertension: Adults: Initially 120 mg b.d. increasing to 160 mg b.d. where necessary. In some cases dosages of up to 480 mg daily, in divided doses, have been used. A further reduction in blood pressure may be obtained by combining Securon with other antihypertensive agents, e.g. thiazide diuretics. For concomitant administration with β-blockers see precautions. *Children:* A suitable dose of Securon for children has not been established.

Angina: Adults: 120 mg t.d.s. is recommended. 80 mg t.d.s. can be completely satisfactory in some patients with angina of effort. Less than 120 mg t.d.s. is not likely to be effective in angina at rest and variant angina.

Supraventricular tachycardias: Adults: 40–120 mg t.d.s. according to the severity of the condition.

Children: Up to 2 years: 20 mg, 2–3 times a day. 2 years and above: 40–120 mg, 2–3 times a day, according to age and effectiveness.

Contra-indications, warnings, etc

Contra-indications: Hypotension associated with cardiogenic shock; acute myocardial infarction complicated by bradycardia, hypotension, left ventricular failure; second or third degree atrioventricular block; sick sinus syndrome; uncompensated heart failure; marked bradycardia (less than 50 beats/minute).

Precautions: Securon may affect impulse conduction and should be used with caution in patients with first degree atrioventricular block. The effects of Securon and beta blockers may be additive both with respect to conduction and contraction, therefore care must be exercised when these are administered concurrently or closely together.

Securon may affect left ventricular contractility as a result of its mode of action. This effect is small and normally not important but cardiac failure may be precipitated or aggravated if it exists. In cases with poor ventricular function therefore Securon should only be given after appropriate therapy for cardiac failure such as digitalis, etc.

Patients with atrial flutter/fibrillation and an accessory pathway (e.g. WPW-syndrome) may develop increased conduction across the anomalous pathway and ventricular tachycardia may be precipitated.

Verapamil hydrochloride has been shown to increase the serum concentration of digoxin and caution should be exercised with regard to digitalis toxicity.

In patients with impaired liver function, particular attention should be paid to the dosage because of reduced drug metabolism.

Although animal studies have not shown any teratogenic effect, Securon should not be given during the first trimester of pregnancy unless, in the clinician's judgement, it is essential for the welfare of the patient.

Side-effects: Securon is generally well-tolerated. Constipation may occur, flushing is observed occasionally, headaches, nausea and vomiting rarely. Allergic reactions are only very rarely seen.

On very rare occasions a reversible impairment of liver function characterised by an increase in transaminases and/or alkaline phosphatase may occur during verapamil treatment and is most probably a hypersensitivity reaction.

Overdosage: The specific antidote is calcium, e.g. 10–20 ml of 10% calcium gluconate solution i.v. (2.25–4.5 mmol), if necessary by repeated injection or continuous infusion (e.g. 5 mmol/hr). Usual emergency measures for acute cardiovascular side-effects should be applied, e.g.: In the case of cardiac arrest, heart massage, mechanical respiration, followed by appropriate intensive care; in the case of second and third degree AV block, atropine, isoprenaline and, if required, pace-maker therapy; in the case of signs of myocardial insufficiency, dopamine, dobutamine, cardiac glycosides or calcium gluconate (10–20 ml of a 10% solution); in the case of hypotension, appropriate positioning of patient, dopamine, dobutamine, noradrenaline.

Pharmaceutical precautions Store at room temperature under dry conditions. Shelf life 3 years.

Legal category POM.

Package quantities Securon: 28 day calendar pack of 56 × 120 mg tablets.

Securon 40 mg, 80 mg, 120 mg: 100 tablets in plastic containers.

Further information Nil.

Product licence numbers
Securon Tablets 40 mg   0169/0003
Securon Tablets 80 mg   0169/0004
Securon Tablets 120 mg   0169/0005

*Trade Mark

Labaz
Floats Road
Wythenshawe
Manchester, M23 9NF

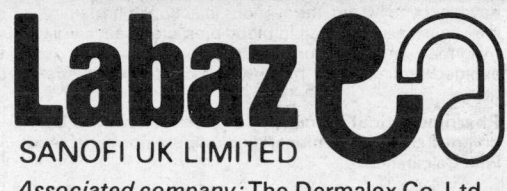

Labaz
SANOFI UK LIMITED
Associated company: The Dermalex Co. Ltd.

CALCIPARINE*

Presentation Sterile, clear, pyrogen-free solution for subcutaneous injection containing Heparin Calcium dissolved in Water for Injections BP.

Contains no preservatives.

Calciparine is available in unit dose disposable syringes and ampoules.

One Calciparine unit dose disposable syringe contains 5,000 international units heparin in 0.2 ml.

Calciparine ampoules contain 12,500 international units heparin in 0.5 ml, or 20,000 international units heparin in 0.8 ml.

Uses As an anticoagulant for the prophylaxis and treatment of thromboembolic phenomena, especially myocardial infarction, acute arterial embolism or thrombosis, deep vein thrombosis, thrombophlebitis or pulmonary embolism.

Dosage and administration

Administration: Calciparine should be given by subcutaneous injection, using a 25-gauge needle. The best site is the subcutaneous tissue of the lateral abdominal wall. The needle should be inserted perpendicularly into a pinched-up fold of skin and held gently but firmly within the skinfold until injection has been completed.

Standard prophylactic dosage: In patients over 40 years of age undergoing major elective surgery 5,000 iu 2 hours before operation, followed by 5,000 iu every 8 hours for 7 days. In patients still confined to bed at the end of this period, the dosage should be continued until they are ambulant.

Following myocardial infarction 5,000 iu twice daily for 10 days or until the patient is mobile. In other medical conditions in which there is an associated increased risk of thromboembolic phenomena, the same dosage is recommended. These standard prophylactic regimens do not require routine control but see below.

Treatment dosage: For existing thrombosis the standard dose is 0.1 ml Calciparine (2,500 iu) per 10 kg body weight 12 hourly. To enable dosage to be individually adjusted to maintain a coagulation time twice that of control it is recommended that the thrombin clotting time, whole blood clotting time or the activated partial thromboplastin time be measured on blood withdrawn 4 hours after the first injection and then at intervals until the patient is stabilised. During long-term therapy, the test should be repeated at least once each week.

Considerations for dosage: For both prophylaxis and treatment, higher doses are likely to be required in patients of abnormally high body weight and in those suffering from cancer, diabetes mellitus or other diseases associated with marked hypercoagulability. Lower doses are usually indicated in the elderly and those with low serum albumin or impaired renal or hepatic function. In such patients, coagulation times should be checked frequently and dosage adjusted accordingly.

Children: treatment dosage: Dosage should be individually adjusted according to changes in whole blood clotting time and/or thrombin clotting time and/or APTT. The initial dose should be 0.1 ml Calciparine (2,500 iu) per 10 kg of body weight. The usual interval between doses is 12 hours, but this also may require individual adjustment.

Prophylactic dosage in pregnancy: There is clinical evidence that heparin does not cause foetal damage and may be the anticoagulant of choice when anticoagulation is indicated during pregnancy. However, the risk of maternal bleeding may be increased. Individual control is essential and the aim should be to maintain plasma heparin levels between 0.1 and 0.4 units/ml, as assessed by the Anti-Xa assay, and a whole blood clotting time of 15 to 20 minutes.

A prophylactic dosage of 5,000 iu every 8 hours is a suitable starting dose in the first 3 or 4 months of pregnancy but higher doses are needed as pregnancy progresses, 10,000 iu two or three times daily being usual in the last trimester. Dosage must be reduced during labour and standard prophylactic dosage is suitable post-partum.

Contra-indications, warnings, etc Calciparine is contra-indicated in patients hypersensitive to heparin. Calciparine is contra-indicated in patients with a condition in which there is an increased danger of haemorrhage. Such conditions include haemophilia, thrombocytopenia and other haemorrhagic diatheses; gastric and duodenal ulcer; sub-acute bacterial endocarditis; threatened abortion and major surgery involving the brain, spinal cord and eye.

Calciparine should not be used in patients with advanced renal or hepatic dysfunction, in severe hypertension or patients in shock.

Care should be used in patients receiving salicylates or any drug likely to prolong coagulation.

Special care should be taken when elderly patients and pregnant women are involved.

Side-effects: Hypersensitivity reactions may occur, but are rare. Acute reversible thrombocytopenia has been reported but is rare. Osteoporosis and alopecia have occurred in patients treated over many months.

Treatment of overdosage: If bleeding should occur, the effect of heparin can be reversed immediately by intravenous administration of a 1% protamine sulphate solution. The dose of protamine sulphate required for neutralisation should be determined accurately by titrating the patient's plasma.

It is important to avoid overdosage of protamine sulphate because protamine itself has anticoagulant properties. A single dose of protamine sulphate should never exceed 50 mg. Intravenous injection of protamine may cause a sudden fall in blood pressure, bradycardia, dyspnoea and transitory flushing, but these may be avoided or diminished by slow and careful administration.

Pharmaceutical precautions Store below 25°C but do not freeze. Other preparations should not be mixed with Calciparine.

Legal category POM.

Package quantities Calciparine unit dose disposable syringes sterilised ready for use (5,000 iu) are supplied in cartons of 10. Calciparine ampoules (12,500 iu or 20,000 iu) are supplied in 10 individual packs each containing an ampoule and sterile disposable syringe and needle.

Further information Nil.

Product licence number 0623/0010.

CORDARONE* X ▼

Presentation
1. Cordarone X 200 Tablets: White to off-white scored round biconvex tablets marked with the action potential symbol and 200, approximately 10.5 mm in diameter, each containing 200 mg amiodarone hydrochloride.

2. Cordarone X 100 Tablets: White to off-white scored round biconvex tablets marked with the action potential symbol and 100, approximately 9.0 mm in diameter, each containing 100 mg amiodarone hydrochloride.

3. Cordarone X Intravenous: Ampoules for intravenous injection: clear, pale yellow solution containing 150 mg amiodarone hydrochloride in 3 ml.

Uses Treatment should be initiated only under hospital or specialist supervision.

Tablets: Tachyarrhythmias associated with Wolff-Parkinson-White syndrome.

Atrial flutter and fibrillation when other drugs cannot be used.

All types of tachyarrhythmias of paroxysmal nature including: supraventricular, nodal and ventricular tachycardias, ventricular fibrillation; when other drugs cannot be used.

Tablets are used for stabilisation and long-term treatment.

Injection for intravenous use: Tachyarrhythmias associated with Wolff-Parkinson-White syndrome. All types of tachyarrhythmias including: supraventricular, nodal and ventricular tachycardias; atrial flutter and fibrillation; ventricular fibrillation; when other drugs cannot be used.

The injection is to be used where a rapid response is required.

Dosage and administration
Tablets: It is particularly important that the minimum effective dose be used. In all cases the patient's management must be judged on the individual response and well being. The following dosage regimen is generally effective.

Initial stabilisation: Treatment should be started with 200 mg, 3 times a day and may be continued for 1 week. The dosage should then be reduced to 200 mg, twice daily for a further week.

Maintenance: After the initial period the dosage should be reduced to 200 mg daily, or less if appropriate. Rarely, the patient may require a higher maintenance dose. The

scored 100 mg tablet should be used to titrate the minimum dosage required to maintain control of the arrhythmia. The maintenance dose should be regularly reviewed, especially where this exceeds 200 mg daily.

General considerations: The high initial dose is necessary because of the slow onset of action whilst the necessary tissue levels of amiodarone are achieved. Cordarone X has a low acute toxicity and in this initial treatment period serious problems have not been reported. However, excessive dosage during maintenance therapy can cause side effects which are believed to be related to excessive tissue retention of amiodarone and/or its metabolites. Side effects slowly disappear as the tissue levels fall after the dosage is reduced or the drug withdrawn.

If the drug is withdrawn, residual tissue-bound amiodarone may protect the patient for up to 3 months, but the likelihood of recurrence of cardiac arrhythmias during this period should be a consideration. The important factor is that the patient requires monitoring regularly to ensure that clinical features of excessive dosage are detected and the dosage adjusted accordingly.

It is particularly important that the minimum effective dose be used.

Intravenous injection: Cordarone X Intravenous should only be used when facilities exist for cardiac monitoring and defibrillation, should the need arise.

The standard recommended dose is 5 mg/kg bodyweight given by intravenous infusion over a period of 20 minutes to 2 hours. Where possible this should be administered as a dilute solution in 250 ml 5% dextrose. This may be followed by repeat infusions up to 1200 mg, i.e. (approximately 15 mg/kg bodyweight) in up to 500 ml 5% dextrose per 24 hours, the rate of infusion being adjusted on the basis of clinical response. In extreme clinical emergency the drug may, at the discretion of the clinician, be given as a slow injection of 150–300 mg in 10–20 ml 5% dextrose over 1–2 minutes. Patients treated in this way must be closely monitored, e.g. in an intensive care unit.

When given by infusion Cordarone X may reduce drop size and if appropriate, adjustments should be made to the rate of infusion.

Oral therapy should be initiated as soon as possible after an adequate response is obtained and the intravenous therapy gradually phased out. Repeated or continuous infusion via the peripheral veins may lead to local discomfort and inflammation. When repeated or continuous infusion is anticipated, administration by a central venous catheter is recommended.

Use in the elderly: As with all patients it is important that the minimum effective dose is used. Whilst there is no evidence that dosage requirements are different for this group of patients they may be more susceptible to bradycardia and conduction defects if too high a dose is employed. Particular attention should be paid to monitoring of thyroid function. See Contra-indications, warnings, etc.

Contra-indications, warnings, etc In patients in whom bradycardia or AV block is sufficient to cause syncope, Cordarone X should only be used in conjunction with a pacemaker.

Cordarone X is contra-indicated in patients with evidence or history of thyroid dysfunction.

Too high a dosage may lead to severe bradycardia and to conduction disturbances with the appearance of an idioventricular rhythm, particularly in elderly patients or during digitalis therapy. In these circumstances, Cordarone X treatment should be withdrawn. If necessary beta-adrenostimulants or glucagon may be given.

Oral Cordarone X is not contra-indicated in patients with latent or manifest heart failure, but caution should be exercised as, occasionally, existing heart failure may be worsened. In this case, Cordarone X should be associated with the usual cardiotonic and diuretic treatment.

Cordarone X Intravenous is contra-indicated in circulatory collapse or severe arterial hypotension and may cause moderate and transient reduction in blood pressure. Circulatory collapse may be precipitated by too rapid an administration or overdosage (atropine has been used successfully in such patients presenting with bradycardia).

U-waves and deformed T-waves may occur in the ECG because of the fixing of Cordarone X in myocardial tissues. These are not signs of intoxication and administration may be continued.

Side effects: Because some side effects may arise only after long-term treatment patients should be regularly monitored.

Ophthalmological: Patients on continuous therapy may develop microdeposits in the cornea. The deposits are usually discernible only by slit-lamp examination and very rarely give rise to symptoms such as visual haloes. They regress with reduction of dose or termination of treatment and are considered essentially benign in nature. During long-term administration regular ophthalmological examination is recommended.

Dermatological: Cordarone X may induce photosensitisation in some patients; this can usually be alleviated by the use of total sun block barrier creams and other protective measures. Rarely a slate grey or bluish discolouration of the skin has been reported.

Thyroid: Both hyper and hypothyroidism have occurred during, or soon after, treatment with Cordarone X. Simple monitoring of the usual biochemical tests is confusing because some (PBI and ^{131}I uptake) are invalidated and others (T_4, T_3 and FTI) may be altered where the patient is clearly euthyroid. Clinical monitoring is therefore recommended and should be continued for some months after discontinuation of Cordarone X treatment. This is particularly important in the elderly.

Clinical features of hyperthyroidism such as weight loss, asthenia, restlessness, increase in heart rate or a recurrence of the cardiac dysrhythmia, should alert the clinician. The diagnosis may be supported by the finding of an elevated serum tri-iodothyronine (T_3), a low level of thyroid stimulating hormone (TSH) and a reduced TSH response to thyrotrophin releasing hormone (TRH). Elevation of reverse T_3 (r.T_3) may also be found.

The clinical features of hypothyroidism such as weight gain and reduced activity should alert the clinician. The onset may be abrupt. The diagnosis may be supported by the presence of an elevated serum TSH level and an exaggerated TSH response to TRH. The thyroxine (T_4), T_3 and free thyroxine index (FTI) may be low.

Courses of anti-thyroid drugs have been used for the treatment of thyroid hyperactivity; large doses may be required initially.

Thyroid hypofunction may be treated cautiously with L-thyroxine.

Pulmonary: Diffuse pulmonary alveolitis has been reported, sometimes presenting as unexplained or disproportionate dyspnoea. Patients developing dyspnoea without signs of cardiac failure or loss of control of arrhythmias should be carefully evaluated clinically and chest X-ray and lung function tests should be performed. Pulmonary alveolitis has usually been reversible with corticosteroid therapy and/or reduction or withdrawal of Cordarone X therapy.

Hepatic: Elevations of liver enzymes may occur from time to time during therapy and are usually transient or respond to reduction in dosage.

There have been reports of hepatotoxicity with Cordarone X and it is important to be aware of this possibility. This has usually responded to withdrawal of the drug, but despite this, very rarely the condition has progressed to irreversible liver damage. The histology has been variable and has included cirrhosis.

It is advisable to monitor liver function before treatment and periodically thereafter.

Patients with abnormal liver function tests should be reassessed clinically and tests of liver function should be monitored closely until they return to normal.

If patients present with abnormal liver function tests, dosage reduction should be considered. If liver function test values continue to rise despite reduction in dosage or in situations where dosage reduction is not feasible, discontinuation of the drug should be considered. The patient's clinical condition should be carefully monitored both as regards the hepatic condition and control of the arrhythmias.

Neurological: Peripheral neuropathy has been reported in some patients. This has usually been ultimately reversible on withdrawing the drug. Nightmares, vertigo, headaches and sleeplessness may also occur. Tremor and ataxia have also infrequently been reported usually with complete regression after reduction of dose or withdrawal of the drug.

Other: Other unwanted effects occasionally reported include nausea, vomiting, fatigue and metallic taste. There have been reports of epididymo-orchitis.

Drug interactions: Administration of Cordarone X to a patient already receiving digoxin may bring about an increase in the plasma digoxin concentration and thus precipitate symptoms and signs associated with high digoxin levels.

It may potentiate oral anticoagulant therapy. Consideration should be given to the possibility that Cordarone X may alter the plasma concentrations of other drugs particularly those which are highly protein-bound e.g. phenytoin.

Cordarone X should be used with caution in combination with beta-blocking agents or calcium antagonists, as any tendency to produce bradycardia may be potentiated.

Women of child-bearing age: Although no teratogenic effects have been observed in animals, there are insufficient data on the use of Cordarone X during pregnancy in humans to judge any possible toxicity.

Breast-feeding: Cordarone X is present in the breast milk in significant quantities and breast-feeding is contra-indicated.

Treatment of overdosage: Animal studies indicate that Cordarone X has a high LD_{50}, hence it is most unlikely that a patient will ingest an acute toxic dose. In such an event gastric lavage may be employed to reduce absorption in addition to general supportive measures. The patient should be monitored and if bradycardia ensues beta-adrenostimulants or glucagon may be given.

Pharmaceutical precautions Tablets and ampoules

should be protected from light. Cordarone X Intravenous is incompatible with saline and should be administered solely in 5% Dextrose solution.

Legal category POM.

Package quantities *Tablets:* carton of 30 tablets (in blister pack of 10 tablets).
Intravenous injection: carton of 10 ampoules.

Further information Cordarone X Intravenous may be used prior to DC cardioversion. It has been used to treat successfully atrial, junctional and ventricular tachy-arrhythmias. It may be used where a rapid response is required, such as following a myocardial infarction.

Cordarone X is strongly protein-bound and the plasma half-life is usually of the order of 50 days. However there may be considerable inter-patient variation; in individual patients a half-life of less than 20 days and a half-life of more than 100 days has been reported. High doses of Cordarone X, for example 600 mg/day, should be given initially to achieve effective tissue levels as rapidly as possible. Owing to the long half-life of the drug, a maintenance dose of only 200 mg/day, or less is usually necessary. Sufficient time must be allowed for a new distribution equilibrium to be achieved between adjustments of dose.

The long half-life is a valuable safeguard for patients with potentially lethal arrhythmias as omission of occasional doses does not significantly influence the protection afforded by Cordarone X.

Product licence numbers
Cordarone X 100   0623/0017
Cordarone X 200   0623/0007
Cordarone X Intravenous   0623/0012

DERMALEX* SKIN LOTION

Presentation A white oil-in-water emulsion containing Cosbiol (Squalane) 3.0%, hexachlorophane 0.5%, allantoin 0.25%.

Uses Prevention of pressure sores. Prevention and treatment of incontinence rash and non-specific rashes. Skin antiseptic for preparation of split-skin donor areas. As a hand cream for medical and surgical staff to reduce the risk of cross infection.

Dosage and administration Apply sparingly as a routine procedure every 4 to 6 hours and after washing.

Only a thin film is needed on the skin for good results. Over generous application can occasionally cause redness.

It is important to ensure that no barrier creams are used on a patient using Dermalex skin lotion.

Contra-indications, warnings, etc Dermalex skin lotion should not be applied to broken skin, open pressure sores, seriously burnt skin or mucous membranes. During regular use in the treatment of pressure areas it is inadvisable to apply to areas of the skin in excess of half of the total body surface area.

Dermalex should not be administered except on medical advice to children under two years of age.

Pharmaceutical precautions No special storage requirements.

Legal category P.

Package quantities 100 mls: Community nursing pack: 'I patient for 4 weeks'. 250 mls: Ward pack '10 patients for 7 days' (Pump action dispenser available for this size).

Further information Dermalex is a deep penetrating lotion effective against a wide range of organisms and with a long allergy free history. It maintains its deep antiseptic activity in the skin for at least six hours, and in addition Cosbiol provides a beneficial effect for patients with dry skin.

Product licence number 1983/5000.

EPILIM*

Presentation
1. *Epilim 200 Enteric-Coated:* A lilac-coloured enteric-coated tablet containing 200 mg sodium valproate.
2. *Epilim 500 Enteric-Coated:* A lilac-coloured enteric-coated tablet containing 500 mg sodium valproate.
3. *Epilim 100 mg Crushable Tablets:* A white scored tablet containing 100 mg sodium valproate.
4. *Epilim Syrup:* A red, cherry-flavoured syrup containing 200 mg sodium valproate per 5 ml.
5. *Epilim Liquid:* A red, cherry-flavoured, sugar-free liquid containing 200 mg sodium valproate per 5 ml.

Uses In the treatment of generalised, partial or other epilepsy. In women of childbearing age Epilim should be used only in severe cases or in those resistant to other treatment.

Dosage and administration Daily dosage requirements vary according to age and body weight.

Monotherapy: Usual requirements are as follows:

Adults: Dosage should start at 600 mg daily increasing by 200 mg at three day intervals until control is achieved. This is generally within the dosage range 1000 mg to 2000 mg per day, i.e. 20–30 mg/kg body weight. Where adequate control is not achieved within this range the dose may be further increased to 2500 mg per day.

Children over 20 kg: Initial dosage should be 400 mg/day (irrespective of weight) with spaced increases until control is achieved; this is usually within the range 20–30 mg/kg body weight per day. Where adequate control is not achieved within this range the dose may be increased to 35 mg/kg body weight per day.

Children under 20 kg: 20 mg/kg of body weight per day; in severe cases this may be increased up to 40 mg/kg/day but increases above this should be undertaken only in patients in whom plasma valproic acid levels, clinical chemistry and haematological parameters can be monitored.

Use in the elderly: Although the pharmacokinetics of Epilim are modified in the elderly, they have limited clinical significance and dosage should be determined by seizure control. The volume of distribution is increased in the elderly and because of decreased serum albumin, the proportion of free drug is increased. This will affect the clinical interpretation of plasma valproic acid levels.

Administration: Epilim tablets, syrup and liquid may be given twice daily. Uncoated tablets may be crushed if necessary.

Combined therapy: In certain cases it may be necessary to raise the dose by 5 to 10 mg/kg/day when used in combination with anticonvulsants which induce liver enzyme activity, e.g. phenytoin, phenobarbitone, and carbamazepine. Once known enzyme inducers have been withdrawn it may be possible to maintain seizure control on a reduced dose of Epilim. When barbiturates are being administered concomitantly the dosage of barbiturate should be reduced should sedation be observed.

General considerations: Optimum dosage is mainly determined by seizure control and routine measurement of plasma levels is unnecessary. However, a method for measurement of plasma levels is available and may be helpful where there is poor control or side-effects are suspected, see Further Information.

Contra-indications, warnings, etc
Contra-indication: Active liver disease.

Side-effects
Hepatic: Liver dysfunction, including hepatic failure resulting in fatalities, has occurred in patients whose treatment included valproic acid or sodium valproate. The incidents mainly occurred during the first six months of therapy, the period of maximum risk being 2–12 weeks.

Clinical symptoms are more helpful than laboratory investigations in the early stages of hepatic failure. The onset of an acute illness, especially within the first six months, which may include symptoms of vomiting, lethargy or weakness, drowsiness, anorexia, jaundice or loss of seizure control, is an indication for immediate withdrawal of the drug. Patients should be instructed to report any such signs to the clinician should they occur. Available evidence to date does not establish which, if any, investigation could predict this possible adverse effect. However, routine measurement of liver function should be undertaken in the first six months of therapy in those who seem most at risk, e.g. patients with a prior history of liver disease, children with severe epilepsy associated with mental retardation or structural brain damage or metabolic disorder, and such patients should have close clinical supervision. Raised liver enzymes are not uncommon during treatment with Epilim and are usually transient or respond to reduction in dosage of Epilim. Patients with such biochemical abnormalities should be reassessed clinically and tests of liver function should be monitored until they return to normal.

Metabolic: Hyperammonaemia without hepatic damage can occur in patients during treatment with valproic acid or sodium valproate. This is usually transient, but may occasionally present clinically as vomiting, ataxia and increasing clouding of consciousness. Should these symptoms occur Epilim should be discontinued. Oedema has been rarely reported.

Pancreatic: There have been reports of pancreatitis occurring in patients receiving valproic acid or sodium valproate, usually within the first six months of therapy. Patients experiencing acute abdominal pain should have the serum amylase estimated; if these levels are elevated treatment should be discontinued.

Haematological: Valproic acid inhibits the second stage of platelet aggregation. Reversible prolongation of bleeding time and thrombocytopenia have been reported, but are usually associated with doses above those recommended. Spontaneous bruising or bleeding is an indication for withdrawal of medication pending investigations; it is recommended that patients receiving Epilim be monitored for platelet function before major surgery. Red cell hypoplasia and leucopenia have been rarely reported; the blood picture returned to normal when the drug was discontinued.

Neurological: Ataxia and tremor have been occasionally reported and appear to be dose related effects.

Sedation has been reported occasionally, usually when used in combination with other anticonvulsants. In Epilim monotherapy it occurred early in treatment on rare occasions and is usually transient. Rare cases of lethargy and confusion occasionally progressing to stupor, sometimes with associated hallucinations have been reported. Coma has very rarely been observed. These cases have usually been in association with other anticonvulsants, notably phenobarbitone, and have been reversible on withdrawal of treatment.

An increase in alertness may occur; this is generally beneficial but occasionally aggression, hyperactivity and behavioural deterioration have been reported.

Gastro-intestinal: Increase in appetite may occur and an increase in weight is not uncommon. Minor gastric irritation and, less frequently, nausea have been observed in some patients at the start of treatment, but these problems can usually be overcome by administering Enteric Coated Epilim or administering Epilim with or after food.

Dermatological: Transient hair loss has been noted in some patients. This effect does not appear to be dose-related and regrowth normally begins within six months, although the hair may become more curly than previously. Rashes have been rarely reported.

Endocrine: There have been isolated reports of amenorrhoea.

Drug interactions: Like many other drugs, Epilim may potentiate the effect of monoamine oxidase inhibitors and other anti-depressants. The enzyme inducing effect of valproate is appreciably less than that of certain other anti-convulsants and loss of efficacy of oral contraceptive agents does not appear to be a problem.

Dosage of Epilim may require adjustment when used in combination with other anti-convulsants. See Dosage, Combined Therapy Section.

Diabetic patients: Epilim is eliminated mainly through the kidneys, partly in the form of ketone bodies; this may give false positives in the urine testing of possible diabetics. In addition, care should be taken when treating diabetic patients with Epilim Syrup, as this contains 3.6 g sucrose per 5 ml; Epilim Liquid is, however, sugar-free.

Women of childbearing age: Valproic acid and sodium valproate, like certain other anti-convulsants, have been shown to be teratogenic in animals. In women of childbearing age, the benefits of these compounds should be weighed against the possible hazard suggested by these findings and their pregnancies should be carefully monitored.

Breast feeding: The concentration of valproic acid found in the breast milk is very low, between 1% and 10% of total maternal plasma levels. There are no known contra-indications to breast feeding by patients on Epilim. The decision to allow the patients to breast feed should be taken with regard to all the known facts.

Overdosage: Cases of accidental and suicidal overdosage have been reported. At plasma concentrations of up to 5 to 6 times the maximum therapeutic levels, there are unlikely to be any symptoms other than nausea, vomiting and dizziness.

In massive overdose, i.e. with plasma concentrations 10 to 20 times maximum therapeutic levels there may be serious CNS depression and respiration may be impaired. Full recovery is usual following treatment including induced vomiting, gastric lavage, assisted ventilation, and other supportive measures.

Pharmaceutical precautions Epilim tablets are hygroscopic and must be kept in their protective foil until taken; they should be stored in a dry place. Epilim Syrup and Epilim Liquid should be kept cool and away from direct sunlight.

Dilutions: If it is necessary to dilute Epilim Syrup, the recommended diluent is Syrup BP; but syrup containing SO_2 as a preservative should not be used. The diluted product will have a 14 day shelf life. Epilim Liquid should not be diluted.

Legal category POM.

Package quantities Epilim 200 Enteric-Coated, Epilim 500 Enteric-Coated tablets and Epilim 100 mg crushable tablets are packed in foil, in cartons of 100 tablets. Epilim Syrup and Epilim Liquid are packed in 200 ml bottles.

Further information The beneficial effects of Epilim may not be clearly correlated with the total plasma valproic acid levels. The reported effective range is usually between 40–100 mg/litre (278–694 micro mol/litre) depending on time of sampling and presence of co-medication.

The percentage of free drug then is usually between 6% and 15% of the total levels. Above this range an increased incidence of adverse effects may occur.

The half-life of sodium valproate is usually reported to be within the range of 8–20 hours.

Product licence numbers

Epilim Syrup	0623/0004
Epilim 500 Enteric-Coated	0623/0005
Epilim 200 Enteric-Coated	0623/0006
Epilim 100 mg crushable tablets	0623/0015
Epilim Liquid	0623/0016

OSSOPAN*

Presentation The active ingredient of Ossopan preparations is microcrystalline hydroxyapatite compound (MCHC), which provides calcium, phosphorus and essential trace elements in a protein base.

Ossopan 800 tablets are pale buff, film-coated. Each tablet contains 830 mg MCHC, providing 178 mg calcium and 83 mg phosphorus.

Ossopan powder is pale brown, granular, with an aromatic odour. Each gram contains 820 mg MCHC, providing 176 mg calcium and 82 mg phosphorus. One level 5 ml spoonful contains approximately 4 grams.

Uses Provision of calcium and phosphorus in osteoporosis, rickets and osteomalacia.

Dosage and administration
Ossopan 800: 4–8 tablets to be taken daily in divided doses, before meals.

Ossopan powder: One to two level 5 ml spoonfuls daily in divided doses with or before food.

Use in the elderly: There are no special dosage recommendations.

Contra-indications, warnings, etc
Contra-indications: Hypercalcaemia, hypercalciuria.

Precautions: Care should be exercised in patients with severe immobilisation, e.g. paraplegia, and in patients with a history of renal calcium stone formation.

Treatment of overdosage: No cases of intoxication with Ossopan due to deliberate or accidental overdosage have been reported to the Company. It is considered that overdosage is unlikely to be a problem.

Pharmaceutical precautions Store in a cool, dry place.

Legal category P.

Package quantities
Ossopan 800: packs of 50 tablets.
Ossopan powder: jars containing 50 grams.

Further information Hydroxyapatite is the complex biological calcium salt which forms the basis of skeletal structure; its overall formula is $Ca_{10}(PO_4)_6(OH)_2$. MCHC contains about 50 per cent hydroxyapatite and X-ray diffraction studies have confirmed the presence and microcrystalline nature of the salt. It also contains many essential trace elements together with natural skeletal protein (collagen), substituent amino acids and glycosaminoglycans. Clinical studies suggest that MCHC may be more readily assimilable than synthetic calcium supplements.

Product licence numbers

Ossopan 800 tablets	0376/0001
Ossopan powder	0376/5001

TRIFYBA* ▼

Presentation Trifyba is a light brown fibrous powder, derived from the husk of wheat (Testa Triticum Tricum). The fibre consists of hemicellulose, cellulose, lignin and pectin. It is presented as single dose sachets containing 3.5 g or as bulk packs containing 250 g.

Uses Colonic and gastro-intestinal disorders where a high-fibre regimen is indicated including simple constipation, uncomplicated diverticular disease, irritable colon, haemorrhoidal disorders and fissures and other conditions where straining at stool should be avoided.

Dosage and administration
Adults: One sachet or 25 ml measure two to three times daily.

Children: Half to one sachet or a half to a full 25 ml measure once or twice daily depending on age and size.

Trifyba should be taken mixed with food or liquids. For maximum effect adequate fluids should be taken.

Use in the elderly: There are no special dosage recommendations for the elderly except that it is most important to ensure that their fluid intake is adequate.

Contra-indications, warnings, etc Trifyba is contra-indicated in cases of intestinal obstruction. Some patients may experience transient abdominal distention and flatulence, but this rapidly diminishes and usually disappears within two weeks.

Treatment of overdosage: Due to the nature of the preparation, overdosage is unlikely. If it does occur, it should be treated conservatively and the patient given copious fluids by mouth.

Pharmaceutical precautions Nil.

Legal category GSL.

Package quantities Cartons containing 30 sachets and bulk packs containing 250 g.

Further information Trifyba is a highly concentrated source of fibre with approximately 40% hemicellulose, 20% cellulose, 15% lignin, 5% pectin and other dietary fibres. Trifyba contains clinically insignificant levels of phytic acid and does not interfere with mineral absorption from the gastro-intestinal tract. Trifyba is free from sugar and other additives, contains no starch and can be used for diabetics and others on a calorie restricted diet. Trifyba contains negligible amounts of sodium, a factor of importance in the treatment of patients with cardiac or renal disease.

Product licence number 5287/0001.

Trade Mark

Laboratories for Applied Biology Limited
91 Amhurst Park
London N16 5DR

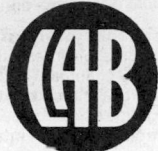

CERUMOL* EAR DROPS

Presentation A clear oily preparation containing p-Dichlorobenzene BPC (1949) 2% Chlorbutol BP 5%, Ol. Terebinth BP 10%.

Uses Occlusion or partial occlusion of external auditory meatus by either a collection of soft wax or a harder wax plug.

Dosage and administration *At home:* With the head inclined, 5 drops are put into the ear. This may cause a harmless tingling sensation. A plug of cotton wool moistened with Cerumol should then be applied to retain the liquid. One hour later, or the next morning, the plug is removed. The procedure is repeated twice a day for three days; the loosened wax may then come out on its own making syringing unnecessary. If any wax remains the doctor should be consulted so that syringing of the softened residue may be carried out.

At the surgery: If there has been no prior treatment with Cerumol, 5 drops are instilled as described above and left for at least 20 minutes. Then syringing or a probe tipped with cotton wool may be employed.

Contra-indications, warnings, etc Otitis externa, seborrhoeic dermatitis and eczema affecting the external ear.

Overdosage: Accidental ingestion should not give rise to any clinical disturbance. The amounts of the various ingredients in the 11 ml bottle are too small to give rise to toxic effects.

Pharmaceutical precautions No special storage precautions.

Legal category P

Package quantities 11 ml vial with separate dropper. 55 ml (for hospital use only).

Further information Nil.

Product licence number 0118/0013.

DUROMORPH*

Presentation A long-acting aqueous suspension of morphine in microcrystalline form presented in ampoules each containing 64 mg morphine in 1 ml 1.3% sodium chloride solution. The ampoules are light amber marked 1 ml Duromorph 64 mg morphine in 1 ml. For subcutaneous or intramuscular injection LAB LTD London.

Uses Duromorph is indicated for relief of severe pain in malignant conditions and for post operative analgesia. Sedative, narcotic and analgesic effects are produced within 10–30 minutes and last for up to nine hours.

Dosage and administration The standard dose is 1 ml of Duromorph (64 mg of morphine base). This can safely be increased to 96 mg where necessary. Administration is by subcutaneous or intramuscular injection (Needle gauge 21 g). Before opening the ampoule ensure thorough mixing by up-ending the ampoule and flicking finger against base. Good mixing is essential and will not be achieved by shaking.

Not intended for administration to children.

Contra-indications, warnings, etc Because of the effect on respiration, caution should be exercised where there is likelihood of hypoxia due to respiratory or cardiac disease, or postoperative ventilation difficulty. Also, alcohol, hypnotics, phenothiazines and especially mono-amine oxidase inhibitors intensify the depressant effects of morphine on the respiratory centre. As with regular morphine, reduction in dosage must be considered in the elderly, in hyperthyroidism and in liver and renal disease; a suitable precaution would be to give half the normal dose and carefully assess the response. Nausea and vomiting may occur.

Overdosage: Treatment is as for morphine, i.e. to maintain respiration and circulation. Oxygen should be administered and assisted ventilation may be necessary. The effective antidote is naloxone hydrochloride 0.4 mg–2 mg given intravenously which could be repeated at intervals of 2–3 minutes if necessary. In view of the prolonged action of Duromorph such treatment is better sustained with a naloxone infusion: 0.4 mg–2 mg per hour according to response.

Pharmaceutical precautions Protect from heat and light.

Legal category CD (Sch 2) POM.

Package quantities 10 ampoules containing 1 ml Duromorph (64 mg morphine) per box.

Further information Nil.

Product licence number 0118/5001.

EMESIDE* CAPSULES AND SYRUP

Presentation Soft orange gelatin capsules each containing 250 mg of Ethosuximide BP.

Blackcurrant or orange-flavoured syrup containing 250 mg of Ethosuximide BP per 5 ml.

Uses Emeside gives selective control of petit-mal either alone or when complicated by grand-mal. The reduction of seizure frequency is thought to be achieved by depression of the motor cortex and elevation of the threshold to convulsive stimuli as seen by the suppression of the characteristic spike and wave EEG pattern. Emeside may be prescribed together with other anticonvulsants such as phenobarbitone, phenytoin, primidone or sodium valproate where grandmal or other forms of epilepsy may require additional treatment.

Dosage and administration *Adults and children over 6 years:* Start with a small dose – 500 mg daily with increments of 250 mg every five to seven days until control is achieved usually with 1,000–1,500 mg (4–6 capsules) daily. Occasionally 2,000 mg daily in divided dose may be necessary.

The half life of ethosuximide in the plasma is about 60 hours in adults but the daily dose if large is more comfortably divided between morning and evening.

If Emeside is being substituted for another anti-epileptic drug the latter must not be withdrawn abruptly but the replacement made gradually with overlap of the preparations otherwise petit mal may break through; the slow withdrawal applies to Emeside when another drug is to replace it.

Children and infants under six years: Begin with a daily dose of 250 mg (5 ml syrup) and increase the dose gradually by small increments every few days until control is achieved, the maximum dose should be 1,000 mg.

Peak concentrations occur in plasma 1–7 hours after injection and the plasma half life is about 30 hours in children and 60 hours in adults. Plasma levels of ethosuximide to be effective lie between 40 and 85 mcg per ml but the clinical response should be the criterion for regulation of dosage. Because young children metabolise ethosuximide more rapidly than adults higher and more frequent doses may be necessary.

Contra-indications, warnings, etc Plasma concentrations are not accurately predictable and since compliance is variable, monitoring of plasma concentrations can be of value in unresponsive cases. Known hypersensitivity to succinimides. Exercise caution with regular appropriate tests in patients with hepatic or renal disease and monitor drug plasma concentrations. Porphyrias. Ethosuximide may be excreted into breast milk. Mothers receiving the drug should not breastfeed. There is a recognised small increase in the incidence of congenital malformations in children born to mothers receiving anticonvulsants. For women planning pregnancy or who are already pregnant the risk should be weighed carefully against the benefit of treatment.

As with all syrups it is advisable to brush the teeth or rinse the mouth after taking Emeside syrup.

Side Effects: Nausea, vomiting, anorexia and epigastric pain are common at first and generally subside. High dosage may cause sedation or confusion. Unusual symptoms are headache, fatigue, drowsiness, dizziness, ataxia, dyskinesia, hiccough, photophobia, depression and skin rash. Isolated reports have been made of erythema nodosum, erythema multiforme, agranulocytosis, aplastic anaemia and systemic lupus. In some instances, patients who become leucopenic on other anticonvulsant therapy have been treated satisfactorily with ethosuximide.

Drug Interaction: The plasma concentrations of ethosuximide are reduced by carbamazepine and increased by isoniazid, phenytoin and sodium valproate.

Overdosage: Where more than 2 g has been thought to be ingested gastric lavage may be employed, if the time lapse is less than four hours.

Routine observation of respiration and circulation will indicate the need for supportive measures.

Pharmaceutical precautions Store in a cool dry place.

Legal category POM.

Package quantities *Capsules:* 100 and 500. *Syrup (blackcurrant or orange flavour):* Bottles of 200 ml and 1,000 ml.

Further information As with all syrups it is advisable to brush the teeth or rinse the mouth after taking Emeside syrup.

Product licence numbers
Emeside Capsules   0118/5002
Emeside Syrup orange   0118/5003
Emeside Syrup blackcurrant   0118/5004.

HALYCITROL* VITAMIN EMULSION ▼

Presentation Orange flavoured emulsion containing 27,600 mcg (92,000 iu)/100 ml Vitamin A and 190 mcg (7,600 iu) Vitamin D per 100 ml. This is equivalent to 1,380 mcg (4,600 iu) of Vitamin A and 9.5 mcg (380 iu) of Vitamin D in a 5 ml daily dose.

Uses For prevention of vitamin A and D deficiency.

Dosage and administration *Adults and children above 6 months:* 5 ml daily.

Infants up to six months: 2 ml daily.

Contra-indications, warnings, etc Prolonged excessive ingestion of vitamins A and D can lead to hypervitaminosis states.

Hypervitaminosis A: Symptoms include dry rough skin, painful joint swellings, anorexia and vomiting.

Hypervitaminosis D: Infants already receiving vitamin D from such sources as vitaminised margarine and cereals can develop infantile hypercalcaemia from excessive vitamin D intake.

In children and adults the symptoms of hypercalcaemia are weakness, anorexia, abdominal pain, constipation, thirst and polyuria with the development of nephrocalcinosis, renal stones and renal failure. Individuals with renal disease and Sarcoidosis are particularly susceptible.

Pharmaceutical precautions Store in a cool place.

Legal category GSL.

Package quantities Bottles of 114 ml.

Further information This is a preparation of fish oil devoid of any fish odour or taste.

Product licence number 0118/0015.

LABITON* TONIC

Presentation A brown liquid containing vitamin B_1 0.75 mg, dried extract of kola nuts 6.05 mg, alcohol 2.8 ml, caffeine (total) 7 mg per 10 ml.

Uses The kola nut contains complex catechine-caffeinates which give central stimulation, increase muscular performance and reduce fatiguability. Vitamin B_1 is included to make up deficiency resulting from recent illness or anorexia. Labiton is indicated for use as a tonic for fatigue, anorexia and debility in convalescence after infections such as influenza and after operations.

Dosage and administration 10–20 ml twice daily, before or after meals, with or without water.

Not intended for administration to children.

Contra-indications, warnings, etc Undesirable in cases of hepatitis and patients taking sedatives. Car drivers should be made aware of the presence of alcohol and should be advised not to exceed the recommended dosage, especially if taking tranquillisers or remedies for allergies that have sedative side effects.

Drug interactions: With correct dosage, the alcohol content should give no interaction. With excessive dosage there could be potentiation of CNS depressants and potentiation of the hypoglycaemic effect of insulin.

Overdosage: Treatment is that for alcohol with correction of dehydration, attendance to the airway and other supportive measures for coma.

Pharmaceutical precautions Store in a cool place. Use within nine months of opening.

Legal category GSL.

Package quantities Supplied in bottles of 200 ml and 1 litre.

Further information Nil.

Product licence number 0118/5005.

LABOPRIN*

Presentation A round, scored tablet, white with brown flecks, containing 300 mg aspirin and 245 mg lysine.

Uses For the relief of headache, musculo-skeletal pains, arthralgia, pain and inflammation due to rheumatoid and other forms of arthritis.

Dosage and administration 1–3 tablets every 4–6 hours as necessary; maximum 12 tablets daily.

Not suitable for children under 1 year.

Children 1–2 years, $\frac{1}{4}$–$\frac{1}{2}$ tablet every 6 hours; 3–5 years, $\frac{1}{2}$–1 tablet every 8 hours; 6–12 years, 1–1$\frac{1}{2}$ tablets every 6 hours.

Contra-indications, warnings, etc Peptic ulcer, dyspepsia, allergy to aspirin such as asthma, haemophilia, concurrent anticoagulant therapy.

Precautions: Use with care in patients with chronic renal insufficiency or hepatic disorder and in pregnancy, particularly avoiding large doses in late pregnancy and in lactation. There is an added risk of erosive gastritis if taken with alcohol, corticosteroids and nonsteroidal anti-inflammatory drugs.

Drug interaction: The activity of coumarin anticoagulants, heparin and hypoglycaemic agents is increased. The effects of other drugs may be altered, particularly uricosuric agents, methotrexate, spironolactone and corticosteroids. There is potentiation by metoclopramide and phenytoin is potentiated by aspirin.

Overdosage: Treatment is that of salicylate poisoning; gastric aspiration and lavage (gastric lavage is worthwhile even if there is delay in treating aspirin self-poisoning), correction of dehydration and of hypokalaemia; cautious use of sodium bicarbonate for the acidosis; intravenous vitamin K. If salicylate level exceeds 500 mg/l administer forced alkaline diuresis but if greater than 900 mg/l consider haemoperfusion and haemodialysis. Self-poisoning has been successfully treated by resin or charcoal haemoperfusion.

The above notes apply to all forms of oral aspirin.

Pharmaceutical precautions Laboprin tablets are extremely hygroscopic. They should be kept in the manufacturer's original container. The inner seal and screw cap should be replaced immediately after use. If discoloration or swelling takes place, the tablets should not be used.

Legal category GSL.

Package quantities 20 tablets per bottle.

Further information Nil.

Product licence number 0118/5006.

LABOSEPT* PASTILLES

Presentation Hexagonal red pastilles each containing Dequalinium Chloride BP 0.25 mg in a slow dissolving gelatine base.

Uses For bacterial and fungal infections of the mouth and throat.

Dosage and administration *Adults and children:* To be sucked slowly every three or four hours. For maximum benefit pastilles should be lodged comfortably between gum and cheek rather than be chewed. The daily dose should not exceed eight pastilles.

Contra-indications, warnings, etc Side effects and ill-effects from overdosage have not been reported.

Pharmaceutical precautions No special precautions.

Legal category P.

Package quantities Carton containing 20 pastilles.

Further information Contains no sugar.

Product licence number 0118/0012.

MONPHYTOL*

Presentation A colourless, rapidly drying, non-greasy paint containing boric acid 2%, chlorbutol 3%, undecenoic acid (as methyl and propylesters) 5%, salicylic acid (free and methyl ester) 31%.

Uses Monphytol is indicated for chronic paronychia, intertrigo, erosio interdigitalis, tinea pedis, tinea circinata, tinea unguium.

Dosage and administration Twice daily (4 times daily for fingers). Moisten brush with Monphytol and apply to the affected parts, reaching gently into the folds of the skin. Treatment should be repeated from time to time after the condition has subsided to prevent reinfection.

Contra-indications, warnings, etc Monphytol may sting sensitive weeping areas of acutely inflamed skin. Other treatment (to reduce inflammation and exudation) may first be necessary. Although there is only a small amount of boric acid present, caution is advised in the repeated application of Monphytol to extensive areas of the skin.

Pharmaceutical precautions Store away from heat.

Legal category P.

Package quantities Bottles containing 18 ml.

Further information Nil.

Product licence number 0118/5010.

PERNOMOL* CHILBLAIN PAINT

Presentation A quick-drying, colourless solution contained in a small pencil-shaped glass vial with a narrow opening to permit direct application. The solution contains per 100 ml: Chlorbutol BP 2 g, Phenol BP 0.95 g, Camphor BP 10 g, Tannic Acid BP 2.2 g.

Uses Pernomol is indicated for the treatment of chilblains. The different substances promote vasodilatation and give an anaesthetising and soothing effect. Being readily absorbed below the skin surface, Pernomol gives immediate relief of irritation and rapid reduction of the inflammatory swelling.

Dosage and administration Pernomol is applied directly from its container to the affected areas three to four times daily. Pernomol may be applied to chilblains at any stage, including broken chilblains. Early treatment will prevent this complication.

Contra-indications, warnings, etc None known.

Pharmaceutical precautions Protect from light.

Legal category GSL.

Package quantities Glass vial containing $2\frac{1}{2}$ ml in tube.

Further information Nil.

Product licence number 0118/5011.

VOLITAL*

Presentation Round white, bi-convex tablets scored and marked P9 and containing 20 mg pemoline.

Uses For treatment of tiredness, lassitude due to stress, or in convalescence after illness or surgery. To combat drowsiness induced by drugs. In association with amantadine in extra pyramidal disorders and for treatment of hyperkinesia in children.

Dosage and administration *Adults:* 1 tablet Volital (20 mg) in the morning. This can be increased to 60 mg daily given as 2 tablets in the morning and 1 in the afternoon up to a maximum of 120 mg daily.

Children over 6 years also elderly patients: $\frac{1}{2}$–1 tablet morning and again in the afternoon.

Contra-indications, warnings, etc Glaucoma, extrapyramidal disorders, hyperexcitable states (thyrotoxicosis). Nervousness and tachycardia may result from large doses.

Precautions: The drug should not be given in the evening, otherwise insomnia is likely to occur.

The safe use of pemoline during pregnancy has not been established and therefore the physician must use his judgement in prescribing it.

Interactions: With monoamine oxidase inhibitors can enhance CNS stimulation and cause a hypertensive crisis.

Side Effects: With prolonged use in children, anorexia and loss of weight have been reported. Other symptoms such as dizziness or headache seem to have been just as common as the placebo in reported trials.

Overdosage: There are reports of mania, chorea, Gilles de la Tourette syndrome. Acute accidental overdosage has been reported in a child who became overactive and had choreiform movements. Pulse rate and blood pressure were unaffected and recovery took place in 48 hours.

Gastric lavage may be undertaken up to 4 hours after ingestion. Treatment with diazepam and intravenous fluids should be given.

Pharmaceutical precautions To be kept cool and dry.

Legal category POM.

Package quantities Tubes containing 25 tablets. Plastic bottles containing 500 tablets.

Further information Nil.

Product licence number 0118/5012.

*Trade Mark

Lagap Pharmaceuticals Ltd
Woolmer Way
Bordon
Hants GU35 9QE

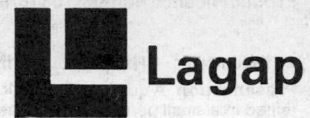

BENDOGEN*

Presentation Tablets containing 10 mg and 50 mg Bethanidine Sulphate BP.

Uses All grades of hypertension. Bethanidine tablets are effective within a few hours after administration and are therefore of special value in patients with hypertensive heart disease, hypertensive crises and malignant hypertension. Bethanidine tablets may be used in combination with diuretics and other established antihypertensive agents.

Dosage and administration

Adults: The usual initial dose is 5–10 mg thrice daily. Each dose should then be gradually increased by 5–10 mg thrice daily until effective control is obtained. Blood pressure should be recorded when the patient is standing.

Daily maintenance dosage averages 100–200 mg. When diuretics, alpha-methyldopa or beta-blocking agents are used concurrently, a reduced dose of Bethanidine tablets should be used.

Where rapid control of blood pressure is urgently needed an initial dose of 20 mg should be given and increased by 10–20 mg every 4–6 hours until effective control is achieved.

Children: Dosage not established.

Contra-indications, warnings, etc Phaeochromocytoma, as the adrenergic neurone blockade leads to increased sensitivity to any circulating sympathomimetic agents. Bethanidine should not be given to patients treated with monoamine oxidase inhibitors.

Precautions: Special care should be taken in patients with renal, cerebral or coronary insufficiency, or with a history of peptic ulceration. In renal impairment reduced doses may suffice.

Patients taking Bethanidine are extremely sensitive to adrenaline, amphetamine, most appetite-suppressants and other sympathomimetic preparations. Such drugs should therefore not be taken unless a need to antagonise the effect of Bethanidine arises, and even then with caution.

The antihypertensive effect of Bethanidine is inhibited by tricyclic antidepressants thus necessitating larger doses.

Pharmaceutical precautions Store in a cool dry place, protect from light.

Legal category POM.

Package quantities Bendogen 10 mg Tablets: Packs of 100, 500. Bendogen 50 mg Tablets: Packs of 100.

Further information Nil.

Product licence numbers
Bendogen 10 mg Tablets   4012/0006
Bendogen 50 mg Tablets   4012/0007

CARBO CORT* 0.25% CREAM

Presentation
Active ingredients:
Hydrocortisone PhEur 0.25%
Coal Tar Solution BP 3.0%

Form and appearance: Carbo Cort 0.25% Cream is a buff-coloured cream containing the active ingredients in a water-miscible, Acid Mantle base which is buffered to the pH range of normal skin.

Uses
Actions: Carbo Cort 0.25% Cream combines the antiinflammatory and antipruritic effects of hydrocortisone with the keratoplastic and antipruritic actions of coal tar.

Indications: When inflammation and irritation are present in a wide variety of subacute and chronic dermatoses, such as: Eczema (Atopic, contact, medicamentosa, infantile, nummular); lichen planus; urticaria.

Dosage and administration For topical application only. Apply to affected areas two or three times daily. This dosage is recommended for both children and adults.

Contra-indications, warnings, etc
Contra-indications: Tuberculous lesions of the skin. Known sensitivity to any of the ingredients.

Precautions: For external use only. Keep away from eyes.

In infants, long-term continuous topical steroid therapy should be avoided. Adrenal suppression can occur even without occlusion. As with other topical corticosteroids, systemic absorption may occur when extensive areas are treated, particularly under occlusion. Topical administration of corticosteroids to pregnant animals can cause abnormalities of fetal development. The relevance of this finding to humans has not been established: however, topical steroids should not be used extensively in the first trimester of pregnancy – i.e. in large amounts or for prolonged periods. However, the unproven theoretical tetrogenic hazard must be placed in perspective against the need to maintain the health of the patient.

Overdosage: Not applicable.

Main side-effects/adverse reactions: None reported.

Pharmaceutical precautions *Storage:* Store in a cool place.

Legal category P.

Package quantities 30 g tubes.

Further information If sensitivity occurs, or if infection appears, discontinue use and institute appropriate therapy.

The micronisation and microdispersion of the hydrocortisone in Carbo Cort 0.25% Cream ensure that the dispersal of this active ingredient over the affected area is as uniform as possible.

Carbo Cort 0.25% Cream is a non-staining preparation of coal tar.

Product licence number 0055/5012.

Carbo Cort is a trade mark of Miles Laboratories Inc, USA.

CARBO DOME* CREAM

Presentation
Active ingredients: Coal Tar Solution USP 10% w/w.

Form and appearance: Carbo Dome Cream is a buff-coloured cream containing the active ingredient in a water-miscible base which is adjusted to the pH range of normal skin.

Uses
Actions: The coal tar solution in Carbo Dome Cream has a keratoplastic and antipruritic effect in psoriasis.

Indications: Psoriasis.

Dosage and administration For topical application only. Apply to the affected areas two or three times daily. This dosage is recommended for both children and adults.

Contra-indications, warnings, etc
Contra-indications: Known sensitivity to any of the ingredients.

Precautions: For external use only. Keep away from eyes.

Overdosage: Not applicable.

Main side-effects/adverse reactions: None reported.

Pharmaceutical precautions *Storage:* Store in a cool place.

Legal category P.

Package quantities 30 g and 100 g tubes.

Further information If sensitivity occurs, or if infection appears, discontinue use and institute appropriate therapy.

Carbo Dome Cream is a non-staining preparation of coal tar.

Product licence number 4416/0106.

Carbo Dome is a trade mark of Miles Laboratories Inc, USA.

DOME ACNE* CREAM
DOME ACNE* LOTION

Presentation
Active ingredients:
Colloidal sulphur 4.0% w/w.
Resorcinol Monoacetate NF (Acetoxyphenol NF) 3.0% w/w.

Form and appearance: Dome Acne Cream is a salmon-coloured, opaque cream containing the active ingredients in a water-miscible base. Dome Acne Lotion is a light cream emulsion containing the active ingredients in a lotion base.

Uses
Actions: Dome Acne Cream and Lotion encourage drying and peeling of lesions in acne vulgaris. They also have a mild antiseptic action.

Indications: Acne Vulgaris and related conditions.

Dosage and administration For topical application only. Dome Acne Cream or Lotion should be used in more severe cases of acne vulgaris after skin cleansing with Dome Acne Medicated Cleanser.

Dome Acne Cream and Lotion should be applied to lesions in the morning and at night, after washing or (in the more severe cases) after cleansing with Dome Acne Medicated Cleanser. The lotion should be shaken well before use. These dosage recommendations apply both to children and adults.

Contra-indications, warnings, etc
Contra-indications: Known sensitivity to any of the ingredients. Resorcinol is contra-indicated in myxoedema.

Precautions: For external use only. Keep out of eyes. If excessive drying or irritation occurs, discontinue use.

Overdosage; Not applicable.

Main side-effects/adverse reactions: None reported.

Pharmaceutical precautions *Storage:* Store in a cool place.

Legal category P.

Package quantities Dome Acne Cream 30 g tubes. Dome Acne Lotion 50 g bottle.

Further information If sensitivity occurs, or if infection appears, discontinue use and institute appropriate therapy.

Product licence numbers
Dome Acne Cream   0055/5015
Dome Acne Lotion   0055/5014

Dome Acne is a trade mark of Miles Laboratories Inc, USA.

DOME ACNE* MEDICATED CLEANSER

Presentation
Active ingredients:
Colloidal sulphur 2.0% w/w
Salicylic acid 2.0% w/w

Form and appearance: Dome Acne Medicated Cleanser is a cream/buff coloured, semi-solid preparation containing the active ingredients in a detergent base.

Uses
Actions: Dome Acne Medicated Cleanser removes dirt, debris and excess sebaceous secretions from the skin surface, exerts a mild antiseptic action, and encourages drying or peeling of the skin.

Indications: Acne vulgaris and related conditions.

Dosage and administration For topical application only.

In mild cases, Dome Acne Medicated Cleanser alone may be sufficient. In more severe cases, Dome Acne Medicated Cleanser should be followed by either Dome Acne Cream or Lotion.

Apply Dome Acne Medicated Cleanser with the moistened sponge applicator to the affected area, having first wet the skin. Lather and massage into the skin for five minutes, and then rinse thoroughly. Use night and morning.

These dosage recommendations apply to both children and adults.

Contra-indications, warnings, etc
Contra-indications: Known sensitivity to any of the ingredients.

Precautions: For external use only. Keep out of eyes. If excessive drying or irritation occurs, discontinue use.

Overdosage: Not applicable.

Main side-effects/adverse reactions: None reported.

Pharmaceutical precautions *Storage:* Store in a cool place.

Legal category P.

Package quantities 100 g Dispensajar with sponge applicator.

Further information If sensitivity occurs, or if infection appears, discontinue use and institute appropriate therapy.

Product licence number 0055/5013.

Dome Acne is a trade mark of Miles Laboratories Inc, USA.

DOME CORT* 0.125% CREAM

Presentation
Active ingredients: Hydrocortisone Alcohol PhEur 0.125% w/w.

Form and appearance: Dome Cort 0.125% Cream is a white cream containing the active ingredient in a water-miscible base which is buffered to the pH range of normal skin.

Uses
Actions: Hydrocortisone exercises a vasoconstrictive effect, thus reducing inflammation and oedema, and also has an antipruritic effect.

Indications: Where anti-inflammatory action for suppressing topical oedema, hyperaemia and pruritis is required, as for example in non-infected eczema.

Also for maintenance therapy after a condition has been brought under control by a more potent topical corticosteroid.

Dosage and administration For topical application only.

Apply liberally to the affected area 2–3 times daily. In cases where there is frequent or repeated exposure to irritants, the number of applications should be increased. This dosage is recommended for both children and adults.

Contra-indications, warnings, etc
Contra-indications: Tuberculous lesions of the skin. Infected skin conditions. Known sensitivity to any of the ingredients.

Precautions: For external use only. Keep away from eyes.

In infants, long-term continous topical steroid therapy should be avoided. Adrenal suppression can occur even without occlusion. As with other topical corticosteroids systemic absorption may occur when extensive areas are treated, particularly under occlusion. Topical administration of corticosteroids to pregnant animals can cause abnormalities of fetal development. The relevance of this finding to humans has not been established; however topical steroids should not be used extensively in the first trimester of pregnancy, i.e. in large amounts or for prolonged periods. However, the unproven theoretical teratogenic hazard must be placed in perspective against the need to maintain the health of the patient.

Overdosage: Not applicable.

Main side-effects/adverse reactions: None reported.

Pharmaceutical precautions *Storage:* Store in a cool place.

Legal category POM.

Package quantities 100 g tubes.

Further information If sensitivity occurs, or if infection appears, discontinue use and institute appropriate therapy.

The micronisation and microdispersion of the hydrocortisone in Dome Cort 0.125% Cream ensures that the dispersal of this active ingredient over the affected area is as uniform as possible.

Product licence number 0055/5012.

Dome Cort is a trade mark of Miles Laboratories Inc, USA.

DOXYLAR*

Presentation Capsules containing Doxycycline Hydrochloride BP equivalent to 100 mg Doxycycline.

Uses Doxylar is clinically useful in treatment of a variety of infections caused by susceptible strains of Gram-positive and Gram-negative bacteria. These include pneumonia and other respiratory tract infections including acute and chronic bronchitis, genito-urinary infections and soft tissue infections caused by susceptible strains of *Staph aureus* and *albus*, Streptococcus, *E. coli* and the Klebsiella-Aerobacter group.

As a member of the tetracycline group of antibiotics Doxylar may be expected to be useful in the treatment of infections which respond to other tetracyclines e.g. ophthalmic and gastrointestinal infections and a wide range of other infections such as psittacosis, prostatitis and trigonitis due to Proteus or Pseudomonas and infections due to susceptible strains of Bacteroides, Pasteurella, *Brucella* (in combination with streptomycin). Listeria, Rickettsia, *H. pertussis, B. anthracis, C. welshii, N. meningitis* spirochaetes, Donovaria granulomatis.

It may also be useful in treatment of acne vulgaris and acne conglobata.

Dosage and administration
Adults: 200 mg first day followed by maintenance dose of 100 mg/day. For more severe infections 200 mg should be given throughout treatment.

Children: Over 50 kg normal adult dose should be given. Not recommended for children weighing 50 kg or less.

Acute gonococcal anterior urethritis in males: Single dose of 300 mg or 100 mg b.i.d. 4 days (administered with food).

Acute gonococcal infections in the adult female: 100 mg b.i.d.

Primary and secondary syphilis: 300 mg a day in divided doses for at least 10 days.

If gastric irritation occurs Doxylar should be given with food or milk.

Concomitant therapy: antacids containing aluminium,

calcium or magnesium impair absorption and should therefore not be given to patients taking Doxylar.

Administration of Doxycycline does not lead to excessive accumulation of the antibiotic in patients with renal impairment.

Contra-indications, warnings, etc Doxylar should not be administered to patients who have shown hypersensitivity to tetracyclines.

The use of drugs of the tretracycline class during tooth development (last half of pregnancy, infancy and childhood to the age of eight years) may cause permanent discolouration of the teeth (yellow-grey-brown). This adverse reaction is more common during long-term use of the drugs but has been observed following repeated short-term courses. Enamel hypoplasia has also been reported. Patients likely to be exposed to direct sunlight or ultraviolet light should be advised that an exaggerated sunburn reaction can occur with tetracycline drugs and treatment should be discontinued at the first evidence of skin erythema.

The antianabolic action of the tetracyclines may cause an increase in BUN. Studies to date indicate that this does not occur with the use of Doxycycline in patients with impaired renal function.

Doxylar should not normally be used in pregnant women.

Use in children: (See Precaution section about use during tooth development).

As with other tetracyclines, Doxycycline forms a stable calcium complex in any bone-forming tissue. A decrease in the fibula growth rate has been observed in prematures given oral tetracycline in doses of 25 mg/kg every six hours. This reaction was shown to be reversible when the drug was discontinued.

Tetracyclines are present in the milk of lactating women who are taking a drug of this class.

Penicillins: Since Bacteriostatic drugs may interfere with the bacteriocidal action of penicillin, Doxylar should not be administered in conjunction with penicillins.

Pharmaceutical precautions Store in a cool dry place, protect from light.

Legal category POM.

Package quantities Packs of 10 and 50 capsules.

Further information Nil.

Product licence number 4416/0007.

INDOLAR* SR

Presentation Blue/colourless capsules containing white sustained release beads. Each capsule containing 75 mg Indomethacin BP.

Uses Non-steroidal analgesic and anti-inflammatory agent indicated in active rheumatoid arthritis, osteoarthritis, ankylosing spondylitis. Also indicated in periarticular disorders such as bursitis, tendinitis, synovitis, tenosynovitis and capsulitis. Also indicated in inflammation, pain and oedema following orthopaedic procedures.

Dosage and administration Indolar SR Capsules should always be given with food or milk to reduce the chance of gastro-intestinal disturbance.

Adults: Dose one capsule once or twice daily, depending on patient needs and response.

Not to be administered to children less than 14.

Contra-indications, warnings, etc Not to be used in children aged under 14.

It is not known if indomethacin is safe to use in children or in pregnancy or during lactation and it should not be given to such patients.

Active peptic ulcer, a history of recurrent gastrointestinal lesions, sensitivity to indomethacin or to aspirin are also contra-indications.

It must be expected that about 20% of patients will complain of side-effects, but starting treatment at a low dosage and increasing it gradually until symptomatic relief is obtained will minimise their incidence.

The most common side-effects are headache, dizziness and dyspepsia. If headache persists, even after dosage reduction, indomethacin should be withdrawn.

Other CNS side-effects which may occur include mental confusion, depression, convulsions, coma, depersonalisation and tinnitus. These are often transient and disappear with time or on reduction of dosage.

Indomethacin may aggravate psychiatric disorders, epilepsy and Parkinsonism.

Gastro-intestinal disorders which occur most frequently are nausea, anorexia, vomiting, epigastric distress, abdominal pain and diarrhoea. Giving indomethacin with food, milk or antacids, lowers the incidence of these side-effects. Ulceration of the oesophagus, stomach or duodenum may also occur, accompanied by haemorrhage and perforation (a few fatalities have been reported). Gastro-intestinal bleeding without obvious ulceration may also occur. If this happens, indomethacin treatment should be discontinued.

Blood dyscrasias, particularly thrombocytopenia, have been reported.

Blurred vision and orbital and peri-orbital pain are seen infrequently. Corneal deposits and retinal disturbances have been reported in some patients with rheumatoid arthritis on prolonged therapy with indomethacin, and ophthalmic examinations are desirable in patients given prolonged treatment.

Oedema and increased blood pressure also sometimes occur, as does haematuria.

Hypersensitivity reactions include pruritus, urticaria, angiitis, erythema nodusum. Skin rash and hair loss may also occur.

Acute respiratory distress, including sudden dyspnoea and asthma, have been reported on rare occasions. Bronchospasm may be precipitated in patients suffering from, or with a previous history of, bronchial asthma or allergic disease.

Indomethacin should be used with caution in patients with hepatic or renal dysfunction. Hepatitis and jaundice have been reported rarely.

Patients should be warned not to drive, or operate machinery, if they become dizzy.

In common with other anti-inflammatory analgesic antipyretic agents, indomethacin may mask the signs and symptoms of infectious disease and this should be borne in mind in order to avoid delay in starting treatment for infection.

Indomethacin should be used with caution in patients with an existing, albeit controlled infection.

Particular care should be taken with older patients who are more susceptible to side-effects from indomethacin.

Pharmaceutical precautions Store in a cool, dry place.

Legal category POM.

Package quantities 100 capsules.

Further information Nil.

Product licence number 4416/0066.

LARATRIM*

Presentation Laratrim Tablets containing 80 mg Trimethoprim BP, 400 mg Sulphamethoxazole BP.

Laratrim Forte Tablets containing 160 mg Trimethoprim BP, 800 mg Sulphamethoxazole BP.

Laratrim Paediatric Suspension containing 40 mg Trimethoprim BP, 200 mg Sulphamethoxazole BP in each 5 ml of suspension.

Laratrim Adult Suspension containing 80 mg Trimethoprim BP, 400 mg Sulphamethoxazole BP in each 5 ml of suspension.

Uses Antibacterial agent. Laratrim is effective against a wide range of Gram positive and Gram negative organisms.

Laratrim is of value in the treatment of the following:

Respiratory tract: Acute and chronic bronchitis, bronchiectasis, empyema, lung abscess, lobar and bronchopneumonia, pneumonitis, otitis media and sinusitis.

Genito-urinary tract: Urethritis, cystitis, pyelitis, pyelonephritis, and prostatitis. Male and female gonorrhoea.

Gastro-intestinal tract: Typhoid and paratyphoid fevers, salmonella typhi and paratyphi, cholera and shigellosis.

Skin infections: Abscesses and wound infections.

Other bacterial infections: Acute and chronic osteomyelitis, acute brucellosis, septicaemias.

Dosage and administration
Laratrim Tablets
Adults: 2 tablets twice daily. Maximum dosage (for severe infections) 3 twice daily.
Children over 12 years: As for adults.
6–12 years: 1 tablet twice daily.

Laratrim Forte Tablets:
Adults: 1 tablet twice daily. Maximum dosage (for severe infections) 1½ twice daily.
Children over 12 years: As for adults.
Under 12 years: Not to be used.

Laratrim Paediatric Suspension
Adults: 20 ml twice daily. Maximum dosage (for severe infections) 35 ml twice daily. For long term treatment, minimum dosage 10 ml twice daily.
Children 6–12 years: 10 ml twice daily.
6 months to 6 years: 5 ml twice daily.
6 weeks to 6 months: 2.5 ml twice daily.

Laratrim Adult Suspension:
Adults: 10 ml twice daily. For severe infections: 15 ml twice daily. For long-term treatment (more than 14 days): 5 ml twice daily.
Children over 12 years: As for adults.

Dosage in Gonorrhoea: In uncomplicated gonorrhoea 4 Laratrim tablets every 12 hours for two days or 5 tablets followed 8 hours later by a further dose of 5 tablets.

In treatment of pneumocystis carinii pneumonitis dosage is 20 mg trimethoprim/100 mg sulphamethoxazole per day in 2 divided doses for 2 weeks. Treatment should normally only be carried out when facilities for regular estimation of the sulphamethoxazole component are available.

Contra-indications, warnings, etc Laratrim should not be given to patients with a history of sulphonamide or cotrimoxazole sensitivity.

Contra-indicated in patients showing marked liver parenchymal damage or blood dyscrasias.

Contra-indicated in renal insufficiency where repeated measurements of the plasma concentrations cannot be measured.

Laratrim should not be given to infants during first 6 weeks of life. The product should not be given in pregnancy.

If Laratrim treatment is prolonged it is suggested that complete blood counts including thrombocytes should be performed at least monthly. Nausea, vomiting and skin sensitivity reactions have been reported.

Laratrim contains a sulphonamide and the possibility of blood dyscrasias like those associated with sulphonamide should be borne in mind. These are more likely in elderly patients.

During long term therapy isolated cases of megaloblastic changes have been reported: these are reversible by folinic acid therapy.

Sulphamethoxazole is strongly bound to proteins. Patients receiving anticoagulants of the coumarin group should therefore be carefully monitored.

Cotrimoxazole has been shown to increase the hypoglycaemic action of sulphonylureas in diabetic patients.

Pharmaceutical precautions *Tablets and Suspension:* Store below 25° and protect from light.

Legal category POM.

Package quantities *Laratrim Tablets:* Packs of 100 and 500.
Laratrim Forte Tablets: Packs of 100.
Laratrim Paediatric Suspension: 100 ml bottles.
Laratrim Adult Suspension: 100 ml bottles.

Further information Nil.

Product licence numbers
Laratrim Tablets	4416/0020
Laratrim Forte Tablets	4416/0021
Laratrim Paediatric Suspension	4416/0019
Laratrim Adult Suspension	4416/0077

MALIX*

Presentation Malix tablets containing 2.5 and 5 mg Glibenclamide BP.

Uses Malix (glibenclamide) is an oral hypoglycaemic agent of the sulphonylurea type.

Glibenclamide is indicated for the treatment of maturity-onset diabetes which is not adequately controlled by dietary measures alone.

Dosage and administration Malix should be taken with or immediately after food. The total daily dosage is preferably given as a single dose at breakfast or with the first main meal, but due consideration should be given to the patient's meal habits and daily activity when apportioning dosage.

1. New diabetics: In maturity-onset diabetes of mild to moderate severity, treatment should be started with 5 mg daily or 2.5 mg in debilitated or elderly patients. If this dosage is not sufficient for proper control it should be increased by 2.5 mg at intervals of one week, or as directed by the clinician. The total daily dose of glibenclamide rarely exceeds 15 mg. Increasing dosage beyond this level is unlikely to produce further response.

2. Transfer from other oral sulphonylureas: Transfer to Malix can usually be carried out without any break in therapy.

Glibenclamide treatment should be started with 5 mg daily and, if necessary, adjusted in steps of 2.5 or 5 mg. A dose of 5 mg glibenclamide is approximately equivalent to 1,000 mg tolbutamide, 250 mg chlorpropamide, 25 mg glibornuride or 5 mg glipizide.

3. Changeover from biguanides: Glibenclamide treatment should be started with 2.5 mg of glibenclamide and the biguanide withdrawn. Dosage should then be adjusted by increments of 2.5 mg to achieve control.

Combination with biguanides: If adequate control is not possible with diet and 15 mg of glibenclamide, control can often be re-established by a combination of glibenclamide and a biguanide derivative.

4. Glibenclamide and insulin: While it is appreciated that most patients who are on insulin therapy will continue to need it, there may be a few patients, particularly those on low daily dosages, who will remain stabilised if transferred to glibenclamide.

No dosage recommendations can be made for the administration of glibenclamide to children.

Contra-indications, warnings, etc Glibenclamide is contra-indicated in:
1. The treatment of juvenile or unstable diabetes.
2. Patients who have had serious metabolic decompensation with ketosis and, in particular, diabetic pre-coma and coma.
3. Serious impairment of renal, hepatic, thyroid or adrenocortical function.
4. Pregnancy. After delivery glibenclamide therapy can be started or resumed.

Precautions: Debilitated or aged patients may be more liable to hypoglycaemia.

The hypoglycaemic action of oral anti-diabetic agents including glibenclamide may be enhanced by sulphonamides, salicylates, phenylbutazone, coumarin derivatives, beta-blocking agents, monoamine oxidase inhibitors, cyclophosphamide, chloramphenicol and tuberculostatics.

Conversely, thiazide diuretics, frusemide, ethacrynic acid, oral contraceptives containing oestrogens, and corticosteroids may diminish hypoglycaemic activity.

In patients suffering from intercurrent infections or trauma, the dosage of glibenclamide may need to be increased. If such complications are severe, diabetic control may be lost necessitating withdrawal of glibenclamide and maintenance of diabetic control with insulin. Glibenclamide should be re-introduced when the patient has recovered from the infection or trauma.

Pharmaceutical precautions Store in a cool dry place, protect from light.

Legal category POM.

Package quantities Malix 2.5 mg tablets are supplied in packs of 100 tablets, Malix 5 mg tablets are supplied in packs of 100 and 1000 tablets.

Further information Nil.

Product licence numbers

Malix 2.5 mg tablets	4416/0063
Malix 5 mg tablets	4416/0058

METROLYL*

Presentation *Metrolyl Tablets* containing 200 mg and 400 mg Metronidazole BP.

Metrolyl Suppositories containing 500 mg Metronidazole BP and 1 g Metronidazole BP.

Metrolyl Injection (for intravenous infusion) 0.5 per cent w/v in 100 ml bottles or Steriflex* minibags (500 mg metronidazole per 100 ml).

Uses 1. Treatment of infections in which bacteria have been identified or are suspected as pathogens, particularly *Bacteroides fragilis* and other species of bacteroides and including other species for which metronidazole is bactericidal e.g. fusobacteria, eubacteria, clostridia and anaerobic cocci.

Metrolyl can be used in septicaemia, bacteraemia, brain abscess, necrotising pneumonia, osteomyelitis, puerperal sepsis, pelvic abscess, peritonitis and post operative wound infection from which one or more of these anaerobes have been isolated.
2. Prevention of post operative infections due to anaerobic bacteria.
3. Use in treatment of acute ulcerative gingivitis and acute dental, pericoronitis and apical infections.
4. Trichomonas infections.
5. Amoebiasis.
6. Giardiasis.

Dosage and administration Seven days treatment should be satisfactory for most patients. Prolonged treatment can be used if the physician considers it to be necessary.

1. Treatment of anaerobic infections
  A. Oral medication: Metrolyl tablets may be given alone or in association with other appropriate bactericidal agents. Adults and children over 12 years: 400 mg three times daily. Children under 12 years: 7.5 mg per kg body weight three times daily.

B. Rectal medication: Rectal administration using Metrolyl Suppositories can be used in patients for whom oral medication is not possible or is contra-indicated. The suppositories may be administered alone or concurrently with other bacteriologically appropriate antibacterial agents.

Treatment of anaerobic infections: Adults and children over 12 years: 1 gram suppository inserted into the rectum eight-hourly for three days. If rectal medication must be continued for more than three days the suppositories should be inserted at 12-hourly intervals. In any event, treatment should not be continued for more than seven days. Children (5 to 12 years): As for adults but with 500 mg suppositories three times daily. Infants and children under five years: As for children of 5 to 12 years but with appropriate reduction in dosage of suppositories (one-half of a 500 mg suppository for one to five years and one-quarter of a 500 mg suppository for under one year).

C. Intravenous medication: Intravenous medication can be used in patients with severe anaerobic infections for whom oral medication is not possible: it is particularly useful in emergencies and is indicated in patients needing surgery who:

Have anaerobic sepsis such as septicaemia, peritonitis, subphrenic or pelvic abscesses.

At operation shown signs of established or impending anaerobic sepsis.

Undergo operations in which contamination occurs with anaerobes from the gastro intestinal or female genital tract or the oropharynx.

In infants and other patients maintained on intravenous fluids, Metrolyl Injection may be diluted with appropriate volumes of normal saline, dextrose-saline, dextrose 5% w/v or potassium chloride injections (20 mmol and 40 mmol.)

Treatment: Adults and children over 12 years: 100 ml by intravenous injection eight hourly. Injection should be infused intravenously at the rate of 5 ml per minute but may be administered alone or concurrently (but separately) with other antibacterial agents in parenteral dosage forms. Oral medication (400 mg 3 times daily) should be substituted as soon as possible.

Children under 12 years: As for adults but single dose is based on 1.5 ml (7.5 mg metronidazole) per kg body weight and the oral dose on 7.5 mg per kg body weight.

2. *Prevention of anaerobic infections*
   A. *Oral medication:*
   (a) Gynaecological surgery: Adults: 1 gram orally as a single dose followed by 200 mg orally 3 times daily until pre-operative witholding of solids and liquids by mouth becomes necessary. Oral medication with 200 mg 3 times daily should be resumed after the operation and for up to 7 days.
   (b) Pre-operative medication for elective colonic surgery: Adults: 200 mg orally six hourly co-administered with an aminoglycoside antibiotic for 3 days before surgery; or 400 mg orally 8 hourly with phthalylsulphathiazole (2.5 g six hourly) for 4 days before surgery.

B. *Rectal medication:* In appendicectomy: Adults and children over 12 years: 1 gram suppository inserted into the rectum two hours before surgery and repeated at eight-hourly intervals. If rectal medication is necessary after the third post-operative day, the frequency of administration should be reduced to 12-hourly.

Children (5 to 12 years): 500 mg suppositories administered as for adults.

C. *Intravenous medication:* Adults and children over 12 years: 100 ml by intravenous infusion immediately before, during or after operation, followed by the same dose eight hourly until oral medication (200 to 400 mg 3 times daily) can be given to complete a seven day course.

Children under 12 years: As for adults but the single intravenous dose is based on 1.5 ml (7.5 mg metronidazole) per kg body weight and the oral dose on 3.7 to 75 mg per kg body weight.

3. *Treatment of acute ulcerative gingivitis:* Adults and children over 12 years – 200 mg orally 3 times daily for 3 days or 400 mg orally morning and evening for 3 days.

4. *Treatment of acute dental infections:* Adults and children over 12 years – 200 mg orally 3 or 4 times daily for 3 to 5 days.

5. *Treatment of trichomonas infections* (To prevent re-infection the consort should receive a similar course of treatment concurrently): Adults and children over 12 years – Either 200 mg three times daily for seven days, or 800 mg morning and 1.2 g evening for 2 days.

6. *Treatment of amoebic infections:* Adults and children over 12 years – 400–800 mg three times daily for 5 to 10 days.

7. *Treatment of giardiasis:* Adults and children over 12 years – 2 g once daily for 3 days.

Contra-indications, warnings, etc There are no known absolute contra-indications for the use of Metrolyl. However, known sensitivity to metronidazole is an absolute contra-indication.

Precautions: Recommended doses are given as a guideline based on experience. Regular clinical and biological surveillance are advised if administration of Metrolyl for more than 10 days is considered necessary.

Clinicians considering continuous therapy for relief of chronic conditions are advised to consider the therapeutic benefit against risk of peripheral neuropathy.

Patients with various degrees of renal impairment appear to handle metronidazole like patients having normal renal function.

Alcohol should not be consumed during Metrolyl therapy.

Metronidazole enhances the activity of Warfarin. Dosage of this or other oral anticoagulants should be recalibrated.

Metronidazole has no activity against aerobic or facultative anaerobic bacteria.

Metrolyl should not be given during pregnancy.

Pharmaceutical precautions Store in a cool place, protect from light. The injection is not intended for multi-dose use.

Legal category POM.

Package quantities 200 mg tablets – packs of 250. 400 mg tablets – packs of 100. 500 mg suppository – packs of 10. 1 g suppository – packs of 10. 100 ml bottle or Steriflex minibag containing 500 mg metronidazole BP.

Product licence numbers

Metrolyl 200 mg Tablets	4416/0060
Metrolyl 400 mg Tablets	4416/0061
Metrolyl 500 mg suppository	4416/0053
Metrolyl 1 g suppository	4416/0054
Metrolyl Injection 500 mg/100 ml	4416/0010

PARMID*

Presentation *Tablets:* White tablet with a single break line on reverse. Each tablet contains 10 mg Metoclopramide Monohydrochloride BP.

Syrup: Each 5 ml contains 5 mg Metoclopramide Monohydrochloride BP.

Injection: Each 2 ml ampoule contains 10 mg Metoclopramide Monohydrochloride BP.

Uses Digestive disorders: Metoclopramide restores normal co-ordination and tone to the upper digestive tract and relieves upper gastro-intestinal symptoms including heartburn, flatulence, dyspepsia and sickness pain. Regurgitation of bile associated with such conditions as: peptic ulcer, reflux oesophagitis, gastritis, duodenitis, hiatus hernia, cholelithiasis and post cholecystectomy dyspepsia.

Nausea and vomiting: Parmid is indicated for treatment of nausea and vomiting associated with gastrointestinal disorders (above) cyclical vomiting intolerance to essential drugs including digitalis, antibacterial and cytotoxic drugs. Congestive heart failure, deep X-ray or cobalt therapy. Post anaesthetic vomiting.

Migraine: Metoclopramide relieves symptoms of nausea, vomiting gastric stasis associated with attacks of migraine. Gastric emptying assists in absorption of oral analgesics employed in migraine therapy.

Post-operative conditions: Post-operative hypotonia, Post-operative syndrome.

Diagnosis: To facilitate barium meal examinations where barium meal studies are held up by spasm of the duodenal cap and to facilitate examination of the hypotonic stomach with delayed emptying, gastric stasis and pyloric channel syndrome.

To facilitate duodenal intubation procedures.

Dosage and administration Daily dose level of Parmid is based upon 0.5 mg/kg body weight in divided doses. This should in normal circumstances be regarded as the maximum dose especially for children and young adults.

General therapeutic dosage (Oral)
Adults: 10 mg three times daily.

Young adults: 15–20 years 5–10 mg three times daily, commencing at the lower dosage.

Children: Parmid should only be used after careful examination to avoid masking an underlying disorder, e.g. cerebral irritation. The following dosage recommendations should be strictly adhered to if side-effects of the dystonic type are to be avoided.

Accurate dosage is facilitated by the use of the syrup. Tablets should not be used in children under the age of 15.

5–14 years	2½–5 mg three times daily
3–5 years	2 mg two or three times daily
1–3 years	1 mg two to three times daily
under 1 year	1 mg twice daily

Treatment of children should commence at the lower dosage.

IM or IV: Parmid may be administered at the dosages stated above.

Diagnostic indications: A single dose of Parmid may be given 5–10 minutes before the examination.

Adults (over 15 years)	10–20 mg
5–14 years	2½–5 mg
3–5 years	2 mg
Under 3 years	1 mg

Contra-indications, warnings, etc There are no absolute contra-indications to the use of Metoclopramide.

If vomiting persists the patient should be re-assessed to exclude the possibility of an underlying disorder, e.g. cerebral irritation.

Various extra-pyramidal reactions to metoclopramide usually of the dystonic type, have been reported. The incidence of these reactions in children and young adults may be increased if daily dosages higher than 0.5 mg/kg body weight are administered.

Reactions reported include: Facial muscle spasm, trismus, rhythmic protusion of the tongue, bulbar type of speech, spasm of extra-ocular muscles, unnatural positioning of head and shoulders, tetanic spasms (opisthotonos).

Reactions usually occur within 36 hours of commencement of treatment. Effects disappear within 24 hours of discontinuation of therapy. An anticholinergic anti-Parkinsonian drug or a benzodiazepine may be used to treat reaction where required.

Both metoclopramide and the phenothiazines can cause extra pyramidal symptoms. Care should therefore be taken when both drugs are presented concurrently.

Raised serum prolactin levels have been observed during metoclopramide therapy.

The action of Parmid on the gastro-intestinal tract is antagonised by anticholinergics.

Parmid should not be used in pregnancy.

Parmid should not be used following operations such as pyloroplasty or gut anastomosis until 3–4 days have elapsed, since vigorous muscular contractions may impair healing.

Pharmaceutical precautions Store in a cool place. Protect from light.

Legal category POM.

Package quantities
Tablets: Containers of 100 and 500
Syrup: Bottles of 100 ml 1 litre
Ampoules: Boxes of 10 × 2 ml.

Further information Parmid has the unique action of normalising the hypomotile stomach and small intestine and also possesses a powerful antiemetic effect.

Product licence numbers
Parmid Tablets	4416/0018
Parmid Syrup	4416/0040
Parmid Injection	4416/0036

PHASAL*

Presentation White sustained-release tablets marked on one side with 'P' inside a hexagon. Each Phasal tablet contains 300 mg Lithium Carbonate BP.

Uses Lithium is an antimanic agent, it can also exert a stabilising influence on recurrent affective disorders.

Recommended uses: 1. Treatment of acute manic or hypnomanic episodes. 2. Prophylaxis in manic-depressive disorders, recurrent depression.

Dosage and administration Dosage may be adjusted in the individual patient according to clinical condition and the results of regular blood lithium determinations.

1. Acute episode: Initially 2 tablets b.d. Increase by 1 or 2 tablets per day if no response. Maintain blood lithium levels in the range 0.5–1.5 mmol. Dosage should be reduced rapidly once the initial attack subsides.

2. Prophylaxis: Usually 600–1,200 mg/day given in divided doses. Clinical improvement is usually associated with serum concentrations of 0.5 mmol or above. Toxic symptoms are usually associated with concentrations exceeding 1.5 mmol.

When starting directly on prophylactic therapy administer 2 tablets daily initially, with subsequent increments of 1 tablet until therapeutic blood levels are achieved.

Use in elderly: 500–1,000 mg/day given in divided doses. Toxic symptoms are likely with serum concentrations above 1.0 mmol.

Use in children: The use of lithium in children is not recommended.

Measurement of serum lithium concentrations: Lithium therapy should not be initiated unless adequate facilities for routine monitoring of serum concentrations are available. On initiation of therapy, serum concentrations should be measured weekly until stabilisation is achieved, then weekly for one month and at monthly intervals thereafter. Additional measurements should be made if signs of lithium toxicity occur (see below), on dosage alteration, development of significant intercurrent disease, signs of manic or depressive relapse and if significant change in sodium or fluid intake occurs. More frequent monitoring is required if patients are receiving diuretics. With Phasal maximum blood levels normally occur within two to four hours of dosing.

As bioavailability varies from product to product (particularly with regard to substained-release preparations) a change of product should be regarded as initiation of new treatment. Blood levels should therefore be monitored weekly until re-estabilisation is achieved. **Tablets must be swallowed whole, not chewed.**

Contra-indications, warnings, etc

Contra-indications: Renal or cardiovascular disease, Addison's disease, hypothyroidism, sodium depletion or conditions requiring low sodium intake. Lithium should not be given to mothers who are breast feeding a child.

Use in pregnancy: There is epidemiological evidence that the drug may be harmful in human pregnancy. Should the use of lithium be unavoidable, close monitoring of serum concentrations should be made throughout the pregnancy and during parturition.

Precautions: Pre-treatment and periodic routine clinical monitoring is essential. This should include assessment of renal function, urine analysis, assessment of thyroid function and cardiac function, especially in patients with cardiovascular disease. Patients should be euthyroid before the initiation of lithium therapy. Clear instructions regarding the symptoms of impending toxicity should be given by the doctor to all patients receiving long-term lithium therapy (see Warnings and Adverse Effects). Patients should also be warned to report if polyuria or polydypsia develop. Episodes of nausea and vomiting or other conditions leading to salt/water depletion (including severe dieting) should also be reported. Patients should be advised to maintain their usual salt and fluid intake. Elderly patients are particularly liable to lithium toxicity.

Drug interactions: Lithium should only be given with great care to patients taking diuretics. Lower doses of lithium may be needed during diuretic therapy as lithium clearance is reduced. In some cases, a paradoxical antidiuretic effect leading to water retention has been reported following the use of diuretics during treatment with lithium salts. There is a possibility of water intoxication and lithium intoxication where diuretics and lithium salts are co-prescribed.

Raised plasma levels of the ADH may occur during lithium therapy. Symptoms of nephrotoxic diabetes are particularly prevalent in patients receiving concurrent treatment with tri/tetracyclic antidepressants. Serum lithium concentrations may increase during concomitant therapy with indomethacin or tetracycline.

Warnings and adverse effects: Long-term treatment with lithium may result in permanent changes in the kidney and impairment of renal function. High serum concentrations of lithium, including episodes of acute lithium toxicity may enhance these changes. The minimum clinically effective dose of lithium should always be used. Patients should be maintained on lithium after 3–5 years only if, on assessment, benefit persists.

Renal function should be routinely monitored in patients with polyuria and polydypsia.

Side-effects are usually related to serum lithium concentrations and are infrequent at levels below 1.0 mmol.

Mild gastrointestinal effects, nausea, vertigo, muscle weakness and a dazed feeling may occur, but frequently disappear after stabilisation. Fine hand tremors, polyuria and mild thirst may persist.

Long term treatment with lithium is frequently associated with disturbances of thyroid function including goitre, hypothyroidism and thyrotoxicosis.

Mild cognitive impairment may occur during long term use.

Hypercalcaemia, hypermagnesaemia, hyperparathyroidism and an increase in antinuclear antibodies have also been reported.

Exacerbation of psoriasis may occur.

Signs of impending toxicity: Appearance or aggravation of gastrointestinal symptoms, muscle weakness, lack of co-ordination, drowsiness or lethargy may be early signs of intoxication. With increasing toxicity there is ataxia, giddiness, tinnitus, blurred vision, coarse tremor, muscle twitching and a large output of dilute urine. At blood levels above 2–3 mmol/l, there is increasing disorientation, seizures, coma and death.

Overdosage: Early signs of toxicity usually respond to reduction or cessation of dosage.

There is no specific antidote for lithium poisoning. Treatment comprises general supportive measures and maintenance of electrolyte balance. Elimination of lithium may be facilitated by infusion of sodium bicarbonate, acetazolamide, urea or mannitol.

Prolonged continuous peritoneal dialysis may be more effective than haemodialysis.

Pharmaceutical precautions Store in a cool dry place.

Legal category POM.

Package quantities Securitainers of 60 tablets.

Further information Phasal is a sustained release preparation designed to facilitate control of blood lithium levels within the optimum range. The smaller diurnal variation provided by the use of a sustained release tablet: (i) reduces the risk of rapid and excessive absorption of lithium and thereby improves safety; (ii) maintains the desired blood levels and so provides continuous protection against relapse; (iii) improves convenience of dosing for the patient.

Product licence number 4416/0076

TRIDESILON*

Presentation
Active ingredient: Desonide 0.05% w/w.

Form and appearance: Tridesilon 0.05% Cream is a white cream containing the active ingredient in an aqueous cream base which is buffered to the pH range of normal skin.

Tridesilon 0.05% Ointment is a white, translucent ointment, which contains the active ingredients in a white soft paraffin base.

Uses
Actions: Desonide exerts an anti-inflammatory action, controlling pruritus, erythema and swelling.

Indications: Tridesilon 0.05% Cream and Ointment are indicated in the treatment of those dermatoses known to respond to topical steroid therapy such as eczema, contact allergic eczema, atopic eczema, discoid eczema, seborrhoeic eczema, pompholyx, lichen simplex and psoriasis.

Tridesilon 0.05% Ointment is useful where a lubricating and softening effect is desirable, e.g. dry hyperkeratotic lesions.

Dosage and administration For topical application only.

Lightly massage a thin film into the affected area two or three times daily. This dosage is recommended for both children and adults but may be increased in the treatment of refractory cases.

Contra-indications, warnings, etc

Contra-indications: Tubercular and viral infections of the skin including herpes simplex. Known sensitivity to any of the ingredients.

Precautions: For external use only. Keep out of eyes.

In infants long term continuous topical steroid therapy should be avoided. Adrenal suppression can occur even without occlusion. As with other topical corticosteroids, systemic absorption may occur when extensive area are treated particularly under occlusion. Topical administration of corticosteroids to pregnant animals can cause abnormalities of fetal development. The relevance of this finding to humans has not been established; however, topical steroids should not be used extensively in the first trimester of pregnancy, i.e. in large amounts or for prolonged periods. However, the unproven theoretical teratogenic hazard must be placed in perspective against the need to maintain the health of the patient.

Overdosage: Not applicable.

Main side-effects/adverse reactions: None reported.

Pharmaceutical precautions *Storage:* Store in a cool place.

Dilution: Tridesilon 0.05% Cream may be diluted with Cetamacrogol Cream (A or B) BPC or Aqueous Cream BP. Diluted material should be used within two to three months.

Tridesilon 0.05% Ointment may be diluted with white soft paraffin BP. Diluted material should be used within two to three months.

Legal category POM.

Package quantities Tridesilon 0.05% Cream 15 g and 30 g tubes.
Tridesilon 0.05% Ointment 30 g tubes.

Further information Since the activity of all the other previously available potent topical steroids was potentiated by one or more halogen radicals, it was assumed that halogenation was synonymous with potency.

Clinical studies with Tridesilon 0.05% Cream and Ointment, which contain the topically potent, non-halogenated steroid desonide, have now shown that the equation of halogenation with potency is not valid.

Product licence numbers
Tridesilon 0.05% Cream   0055/0040
Tridesilon 0.05% Ointment   0055/0043

Tridesilon is a trade mark of Miles Laboratories Inc, USA.

TRIPERIDOL*

Presentation Tablets 0.5 mg: White uncoated, scored, marked T above 0.5 on one side, plain on reverse. Each tablet contains 0.5 mg trifluperidol.
Tablets 1 mg: White uncoated, scored, marked T above 1 on one side, plain on reverse. Each tablet contains 1 mg trifluperidol.

Uses Triperidol is a potent antipsychotic used in the treatment of acute and chronic schizophrenia. It is particularly useful in the manic phase of the disease.

Dosage and administration Triperidol tablets are for oral administration to both adults and children.

The following dosage regimen is recommended.

Adults: Initially 0.5 mg daily, increasing by 0.5 mg every three or four days to a maximum of 6–8 mg daily. A large dose, e.g. 3 mg can be administered initially and adjusted up or down according to response. However, in such cases anti-Parkinson medication should be used routinely from the start.

Children: 5–12 years: Initially 0.25 mg per day, increasing as necessary to a maximum of 2 mg per day. In general a maintenance dose of 1 mg per day will be required.

Contra-indications, warnings, etc

Contra-indications: Triperidol is contra-indicated in neurological disorders accompanied by pyramidal or extra-pyramidal symptoms, and the drug should not be administered during pregnancy.

Precautions: Care is required in patients receiving barbiturates or morphine because of possible potentiating effects.

Where prolonged treatment with Triperidol is envisaged it would be a reasonable precaution to carry out regular blood counts and tests of liver function.

Overdosage: In the event of severe overdosage there is no specific antidote other than the use of anti-Parkinson medication and gastric lavage.

Side effects: Extrapyramidal side-effects may occur which are generally controlled with anti-Parkinson drugs. Rarely, severe muscle spasms or neuro-dysleptic crises may occur in which case chlorpromazine (25–50 mg) or prothipendyl (40–80 mg) intramuscularly may be required.

Pharmaceutical precautions Triperidol Tablets should be protected from light.

Legal category POM.

Package quantities *Triperidol Tablets 0.5 mg* are supplied in packs of 100.
Triperidol Tablets 1 mg are supplied in packs of 50 and 250.

Further information Nil.

Product licence numbers
Triperidol Tablets 0.5 mg   0242/5006
Triperidol Tablets 1 mg   0242/5007

* Trade Mark

Lederle Laboratories
(A Division of Cyanamid of Great Britain Limited) Fareham Road Gosport, Hants PO13 0AS

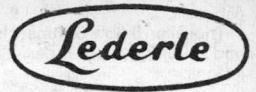

ACHROMYCIN* (ORAL PREPARATIONS)

Presentation *Capsules 250 mg:* Each opaque, orange capsule printed 'Lederle 4874' contains 250 mg tetracycline hydrochloride.

Tablets 250 mg: Each orange tablet printed 'Lederle 4745' contains 250 mg tetracycline hydrochloride.

Syrup 125 mg/5 ml: Each 5 ml of cherry-red suspension contains tetracycline equivalent to tetracycline hydrochloride 125 mg.

Powder 25 g: Each bottle contains 25 g tetracycline hydrochloride.

Uses Achromycin is a broad-spectrum antibiotic used for the treatment of infections caused by tetracycline-sensitive organisms. Typical indications include: Ear, nose and throat infections. Acute and chronic bronchitis. Pneumonia. Venereal Diseases. Non-Gonococcal Urethritis. Gastro-intestinal Infections. Urinary tract infections. Soft tissue infections. Acne. Typhus fever. Psittacosis. Other infections due to Achromycin-sensitive organisms. Achromycin is also indicated for prophylaxis before or after surgical and dental procedures.

Dosage and administration *Adults: (tablets, capsules):* 1 tablet or capsule four times a day. This may be increased to 6 or 8 tablets or capsules daily in severe infections. *Syrup:* 10 ml four times a day.

Children: Not recommended for children under 8 years of age. Information on dosage is available on request where specifically indicated.

Elderly: Achromycin should be used with caution in the treatment of elderly patients where accumulation is a possibility.

Administration: Achromycin should be taken an hour before or two hours after meals and therapy should be continued for up to three days after characteristic symptoms of the infection have subsided.

Contra-indications, warnings, etc
Contra-indications: A history of hypersensitivity to tetracyclines. Overt renal insufficiency. Systemic lupus erythematosus.

Warnings: Tetracyclines may cause a yellow to brown discoloration of the teeth in the developing foetus or child and therefore Achromycin should only be administered if considered essential to pregnant women and young children under eight years of age. Achromycin should be used with caution in patients with renal or hepatic dysfunction, or in conjunction with other potentially hepatotoxic drugs. Cross-resistance between tetracyclines may develop in micro-organisms and cross-sensitisation in patients.

Precautions: Absorption of Achromycin is impaired by the concomitant administration of calcium, magnesium, iron and particularly aluminium salts commonly used as antacids. Tetracyclines depress plasma prothrombin activity therefore reduced dosages of concurrent anticoagulants may be required. Lower doses are indicated in cases of renal impairment to avoid excessive systemic accumulation, and if therapy is prolonged, serum level determinations are advisable.

Side-effects: Gastro-intestinal disturbances may occur and as with all antibiotics overgrowth of resistant organisms may cause glossitis, stomatitis, vaginitis, or staphylococcal enterocolitis. Photosensitivity and dermatological reactions are rare. Occurrences of enamel hypoplasia have been reported. Rarely increased intracranial pressure with bulging fontanelles, has been observed in infants which disappears rapidly upon cessation of treatment.

Overdosage: No specific antidote. Gastric lavage plus oral administration of milk or antacids.

Pharmaceutical precautions The products should be stored at room temperature (except Achromycin syrup which should be stored in a cool place) in either the original pack or in containers which prevent access of light and moisture.

Achromycin Syrup may be diluted with Syrup BP, provided the dilution is freshly prepared and not used after more than two weeks.

Legal category POM.

Package quantities *Capsules 250 mg:* Bottles of 100 and 1,000.

Tablets 250 mg: Bottles of 100 and 1,000.

Syrup 125 mg/5 ml: Bottles of 100 ml and 500 ml.

Powder: Bottle of 25 g.

Further information Achromycin Syrup contains 0.181 millimoles of sodium per 5 ml

Product licence numbers
Capsules 250 mg   0095/0041
Tablets 250 mg   0095/5026
Syrup 125 mg/5 ml   0095/5027
Powder   0095/5037

ACHROMYCIN* (TOPICAL PREPARATIONS)

Presentation *Achromycin Ointment 3%:* Each gram of yellow ointment contains tetracycline hydrochloride 30 mg, methylparaben 2.4%, propylparaben 0.6%, in a white soft paraffin and wool-fat base.

Achromycin Eye and Ear Ointment 1%: Each gram of yellow ointment contains 10 mg tetracycline hydrochloride in a white soft paraffin and wool-fat base.

Achromycin Ophthalmic Oil Suspension 1%: Each millilitre of yellow oily suspension contains 10 mg tetracycline hydrochloride in a vehicle of sesame oil.

Uses Achromycin is a broad-spectrum antibiotic.

Achromycin Ointment 3% is indicated for the treatment of superficial pyogenic infections of the skin and for the prevention of infection in wounds, abrasions and after surgery. It is indicated for local infections caused by both Gram-positive and Gram-negative organisms including Streptococci, Staphylococci and the Coli-aerogenes group.

Achromycin Eye and Ear Ointment and Achromycin Ophthalmic Oil Suspension are indicated for the treatment of susceptible ocular infections caused by Staphylococci, Pneumococci, H. influenzae, Diplococcus of Morax-Axenfeld *(H. lacunatus)*, Streptococci, *A. aerogenes, Proteus vulgaris, Proteus morganii, E. coli, Alcaligenes faecalis* and *Pseudomonas aeruginosa.*

Achromycin Eye and Ear Ointment is also indicated in the treatment of external otitis due to tetracycline-susceptible organisms.

Dosage and administration *Adults and children: Achromycin Ointment 3%:* Apply the ointment directly to the involved area, preferably on sterile gauze once or more daily as the condition indicates. In severe local infections, local treatment should be supplemented by oral therapy.

Achromycin Eye and Ear Ointment 1%: Apply directly to the affected area every two hours. Severe ocular infections may require treatment for many days, and may also require oral therapy.

Achromycin Ophthalmic Oil Suspension 1%: In most bacterial infections gently squeeze the plastic dropper bottle to instil 1 or 2 drops in the affected eye, two to four times daily, or more often if the severity of the infection merits this. Chronic trachoma may require extensive treatment (one to two months).

Contra-indications, warnings, etc
Contra-indications: Achromycin Ointment, Achromycin Eye and Ear Ointment, and Achromycin Ophthalmic Oil Suspension are contra-indicated in patients with a history of hypersensitivity to tetracycline hydrochloride or any other ingredient.

Precautions: The use of antibiotics may result in overgrowth of non-susceptible organisms. Constant observation of the patient is essential. If new infections appear during therapy, appropriate measures should be taken.

Side-effects: Some patients may be allergic to any of the components.

If adverse reaction or idiosyncrasy occurs, discontinue medication.

Pharmaceutical precautions The products should be stored in a cool place in the original pack. Dilution is not recommended.

Achromycin Ointment may cause a yellow staining of clothes. Following extended use a similar local staining of the skin may occur which disappears on cessation of treatment.

Legal category POM.

Package quantities *Achromycin Ointment 3%:* Tubes of 30 g.

Achromycin Eye and Ear Ointment 1%: Tubes of 3.5 g.

Achromycin Ophthalmic Oil Suspension 1%: Plastic dropper bottle containing 6 ml.

Further information Nil.

Product licence numbers

Achromycin Ointment 3%	0095/5031
Achromycin Eye and Ear Ointment	0095/5032
Achromycin Ophthalmic Oil Suspension	0095/5030

ACHROMYCIN* INTRAMUSCULAR

Presentation Achromycin Intramuscular 100 mg. Each vial contains:

Tetracycline hydrochloride	100 mg
Procaine hydrochloride	40 mg
Magnesium chloride	46.84 mg
Ascorbic acid	250 mg

Uses Achromycin is a broad spectrum antibiotic indicated alone or adjunctively in the treatment of infections caused by tetracycline-sensitive organisms, and for prophylaxis before or after dental and surgical procedures.

For example, Achromycin is highly effective in the treatment of infections caused by *Borrellia recurrentis* (relapsing fever), *Calymmatobacterium granulinatis* (granuloma inguinale), *Chlamydia* species (psittacosis, lymphogranuloma venereum, trachoma, inclusion conjunctivitis), *Francisella tularensis* (tularaemia), *Haemophilus ducreyi* (chancroid), *Leptospira* (meningitis, jaundice), *Mycoplasma pneumoniae* (non-gonococcal urethritis), *Pseudomonas mallei* and *pseudomallei* (glanders and melioidosis), *Rickettsiae* (typhus fever, Q fever, rocky mountain spotted fever), *Vibrio* species (cholera). It is also highly effective alone or in combination with streptomycin, in the treatment of infections due to *Brucella* species (brucellosis), and *Yersinia pestis* (bubonic plague).

Other sensitive organisms include: *Actinomyces israelii, Bacillus anthracis* (pneumonia), *Bordetella pertussis* (whooping cough), *Clostridium* species (gas gangrene, tetanus), *Entamoeba histolytica* (dysentery), *Haemophilus influenzae* (pharyngitis, otitis media), *Listeria monocytogenes* (bacteraemia), *Neisseria gonorrhoeae, Shigella* species (acute gastroenteritis), *Streptococcus pyogenes, pneumoniae* and anaerobic species, *Treponema pallidum* and *pertenue* (syphilis and yaws).

Dosage and administration *Adults:* By intramuscular injection only.

100 mg two or three times a day. In severe infections 100 mg every four to six hours.

Children: 10 mg per kg of body weight per day, in divided doses, by intramuscular injection.

Elderly: Achromycin should be used with caution in the treatment of elderly patients where accumulation is a possibility.

Administration: Dissolve the contents of each vial, immediately before use, by the addition of 2 ml of Water for Injection. The appropriate dose of the resulting solution (50 mg/ml) should be injected deeply into the gluteal region.

Oral Achromycin medication should replace parenteral as soon as practical, and be continued for up to three days after characteristic symptoms of the infection have subsided. Streptococcal infections should be treated for 10 days to prevent the development of rheumatic fever or glomerulonephritis, and acute staphylococcal infections for 10–14 days.

Contra-indications, warnings, etc

Contra-indications: Known hypersensitivity to tetracyclines or procaine hydrochloride. Overt renal insufficiency. Systemic lupus erythematosus.

Precautions: Achromycin may cause a yellow to brown discoloration of the teeth in the developing foetus or child and therefore should only be administered if considered essential to pregnant women and young children under eight years of age. Achromycin should be used with caution in patients with renal or hepatic dysfunction or in conjunction with other potentially hepatotoxic drugs. Lower doses are indicated in cases of renal impairment to avoid excessive systemic accumulation, and, if therapy is prolonged, serum level determinations are advisable. Patients who are pregnant or who have known liver disease should not receive more than 1 g daily. Tetracyclines depress plasma prothrombin activity therefore reduced dosages of concurrent anticoagulants may be required. Concurrent use with the anaesthetic methoxyflurane increases the risk of kidney failure.

Warnings and adverse effects: As with all antibiotics, overgrowth of resistant or non-susceptible organisms may occur. Excessive systemic accumulation, due to renal impairment or other reasons, will cause a rise in blood urea nitrogen leading to uraemia, hyperphosphataemia and acidosis. Rarely, increased intracranial pressure with bulging fontanelles has been observed in infants which disappears rapidly upon cessation of treatment. Enamel hypoplasia has been reported.

Cross-resistance between tetracyclines may develop in micro-organisms, and cross-sensitisation in patients.

Overdosage: No specific antidote. Use appropriate supportive treatment.

Pharmaceutical precautions No special handling or storage requirements are necessary. The increase in injection volume, caused by displacement, during dissolution of the powder with 2 ml of Water for Injection, is clinically insignificant when calculating dosage and volume to be injected. The brown appearance of the vial is produced when the injection is sterilised by irradiation and does not indicate any degradation.

Legal category POM.

Package quantities 6 × 100 mg vials.

Further information Nil.

Product licence number 0095/5033.

ACHROMYCIN* INTRAVENOUS/INTRA-PLEURAL

Presentation Achromycin Intravenous 250 mg and 500 mg. Each vial contains tetracycline hydrochloride 250 mg or 500 mg buffered with 625 mg or 1,250 mg of ascorbic acid respectively.

Uses

1. Achromycin is a broad spectrum antibiotic indicated alone or adjunctively in the treatment of infections caused by tetracycline-sensitive organisms, and for prophylaxis before or after dental and surgical procedures.

For example, Achromycin is highly effective in the treatment of infections caused by *Borrellia recurrentis* (relapsing fever), *Calymmatobacterium granulinatis* (granuloma inguinale), *Chlamydia* species (psittacosis,

lymphogranuloma venereum, trachoma, inclusion conjunctivitis), *Francisella tularensis* (tularaemia), *Haemophilus ducreyi* (chancroid), *Leptospira* (meningitis, jaundice), *Mycoplasma pneumoniae* (non-gonococcal urethritis), *Pseudomonas mallei* and *pseudomallei* (glanders and melioidosis), *Rickettsiae* (typhus fever, Q fever, rocky mountain spotted fever), *Vibrio* species (cholera). It is also highly effective, alone or in combination with streptomycin, in the treatment of infections due to *Brucella* species (brucellosis), and *Yersinia pestis* (bubonic plague).

Other sensitive organisms include: *Actinomyces israelii, Bacillus* anthracis (pneumonia), *Bordetella pertussis* (whooping cough), *Clostridium* species (gas gangrene, tetanus), *Entamoeba histolytica* (dysentery), *Haemophilus influenzae* (pharyngitis, otitis media), *Listeria monocytogenes* (bacteraemia), *Neisseria gonorrhoeae, Shigella* species (acute gastroenteritis), *Streptococcus pyogenes, pneumoniae,* and anaerobic species, *Treponema pallidum* and *pertenue* (syphilis and yaws).

2. The treatment of recurrent pleural effusions, secondary to neoplastic disease or end stage cirrhosis, by intrapleural administration.

Dosage and administration

1. *For Antibiotic use by Intravenous Infusion: Adults:* 500 mg every 12 hours by intravenous infusion. Maximum daily dosage should not exceed 2 g.

Children: Up to 10 mg/kg body weight per day in divided doses by intravenous infusion.

Elderly: Achromycin should be used with caution in the treatment of elderly patients where accumulation is a possibility.

Administration: Achromycin should be reconstituted and diluted immediately before administration by intravenous infusion. The use of a terminal filter (suitable pore size 0.22 micron) in-line with the IV Giving Set is recommended. Reconstitute the injection by adding 5 ml of Water for Injection to the 250 mg vial (or 10 ml of Water for Injection to the 500 mg vial) and then dilute the resulting solution (50 mg/ml) to at least 100 ml (up to 1,000 ml) with any of the following diluents immediately before administration by intravenous infusion at a rate not exceeding 100 ml in five minutes: Sodium Chloride Intravenous Infusion BP 0.9%, Glucose Intravenous Infusion BP, Sodium Chloride and Glucose Intravenous Infusion BP, Compound Sodium Lactate Intravenous Infusion BP.

Oral Achromycin medication should replace parenteral as soon as practical, and be continued for up to three days after characteristic symptoms of the infection have subsided. Streptococcal infections should be treated for 10 days, to prevent the development of rheumatic fever or glomerulonephritis, and acute staphylococcal infections for 10–14 days.

2. *For Pleural Effusions by Intrapleural Administration: Adults:* A single dose of 500 mg by intrapleural administration.

Administration: The pleural space should first be completely drained with a thoracostomy tube which should be positioned to give optimum drainage. 500 mg of Achromycin in 30–50 ml of sterile saline is then instilled through the tube into the pleural space followed by flushing of the thoracostomy tube with more saline. The patient's position must then be altered frequently to ensure contact of the Achromycin with both the visceral and parietal pleural surfaces. It is recommended that initially the patient should be rotated to the left and right lateral decubitus, prone and supine positions for intervals of 2–3 minutes and then left in each of these positions for 30 minutes with the tube clamped. The thoracostomy tube should then be reconnected to negative pressure and the tube removed when drainage is complete or minimal. This can take up to 48–72 hours.

This procedure has been reported to produce pleural symphysis in up to 90% of cases.

Contra-indications, warnings, etc
Contra-indications: Known hypersensitivity to tetracyclines. Overt renal insufficiency. Systemic lupus erythematosus.

Precautions: Achromycin may cause a yellow to brown discoloration of the teeth in the developing foetus or child and therefore should only be administered if considered essential to pregnant women and young children under eight years of age. The treatment period should be as short as feasible and repeated courses should be avoided. Achromycin should be administered with great caution in patients with hepatic insufficiency or in conjunction with other potentially hepatotoxic drugs. Parenteral administration, particularly during pregnancy or in cases of renal dysfunction may lead to severe hepatic damage. Patients who are pregnant or who have known liver disease should not receive more than 1 g daily and careful monitoring of dosage by serum levels is necessary. Lower doses are indicated in cases of renal impairment to avoid excessive systemic accumulation, and, if therapy is prolonged, serum level determinations are advisable. Tetracyclines depress plasma prothrombin activity therefore reduced dosages of concurrent anticoagulants may be required. Concurrent use with the anaesthetic methoxyflurane increases the risk of kidney failure.

Warnings and adverse effects: As with all antibiotics, overgrowth of resistant or non-susceptible organisms may occur. Excessive systemic accumulation, due to renal impairment or other reasons, will cause a rise in blood urea nitrogen leading to uraemia, hyperphosphataemia and acidosis. Rarely, increased intracranial pressure with bulging fontanelles has been observed in infants which disappears rapidly upon cessation of treatment. Enamel hypoplasia has been reported. Cross-resistance between tetracyclines may develop in micro-organisms, and cross-sensitisation in patients. Thrombophlebitis may occur at sites of injection. Photosensitivity and dermatological reactions are rare.

Intrapleural administration may be associated with transient local pain (which can be controlled by analgesics) and/or pyrexia.

Overdosage: No specific antidote. Use appropriate supportive treatment.

Pharmaceutical precautions
No special handling or storage requirements are necessary. The increase in injection volume, caused by displacement, during dissolution of the powder with Water for Injection, is clinically insignificant when calculating dosage and volume to be injected. The brown appearance of the vial is produced when the injection is sterilised by irradiation and does not indicate any degradation.

The following substances are incompatible in solution with Achromycin Intravenous, and should not be administered in the same drip:

Aminophylline, amphotericin, barbiturates, cephalothin, chloramphenicol, chlorothiazide, chlorpromazine, cyanocobalamin, dimenhydrinate, erythromycin, heparin, hydrocortisone, methicillin, methohexitone, methyl-

dopa, nitrofurantoin, novobiocin, penicillins, phenytoin, polymyxin B, prochlorperazine, riboflavine, sodium bicarbonate, sulphadiazine, sulphafurazole, thiopentone sodium, vitamin B complex, warfarin, various inorganic ions (Ca, Mg, Al, Mn, Fe) and donor blood.

Note: The use of solutions containing calcium should be avoided as these tend to form precipitates (especially in neutral to alkaline solution) and therefore should not be used unless necessary. However, Compound Sodium Lactate Intravenous Infusion BP may be used with caution since the calcium ion content in this diluent does not normally precipitate tetracycline in an acid medium.

Legal category POM.

Package quantities *Achromycin Intravenous 250 mg:* 6 × 250 mg vials.
Achromycin Intravenous 500 mg: 6 × 500 mg vials.

Further information Nil.

Product licence numbers
Achromycin Intravenous 250 mg   0095/5034
Achromycin Intravenous 500 mg   0095/5035

ACHROMYCIN* V
Presentation *Capsules 250 mg:* Each pink capsule, printed 'Lederle 4885', contains tetracycline equivalent to 250 mg of tetracycline hydrochloride buffered with sodium metaphosphate.

Uses Achromycin V is a broad-spectrum antibiotic used for the treatment of infections caused by tetracycline-sensitive organisms. Typical indications include: Ear, nose and throat infections. Acute and chronic bronchitis. Pneumonia. Venereal Diseases. Non-Gonococcal Urethritis. Gastro-intestinal Infections. Urinary tract infections. Soft tissue infections. Acne. Typhus fever. Psittacosis. Other infections due to Achromycin-sensitive organisms. Achromycin V is also indicated for prophylaxis before or after surgical and dental procedures.

Dosage and administration *Adults:* One capsule four times a day. This may be increased to 6 or 8 capsules daily in severe infections.

Children: Not recommended for children under 8 years of age. Information on dosage is available on request where specifically indicated.

Elderly: Achromycin V should be used with caution in the treatment of elderly patients where accumulation is a possibility.

Administration: Achromycin V should be taken an hour before or two hours after meals and therapy should be continued for up to three days after characteristic symptoms of the infection have subsided.

Contra-indications, warnings, etc
Contra-indications: A history of hypersensitivity to tetracyclines. Overt renal insufficiency. Systemic lupus erythematosus.

Warnings: Tetracyclines may cause a yellow to brown discoloration of the teeth in the developing foetus or child and therefore Achromycin V should only be administered if considered essential to pregnant women and young children under eight years of age. Achromycin V should be used with caution in patients with renal or hepatic dysfunction, or in conjunction with other potentially hepatotoxic drugs. Cross-resistance between tetracyclines may develop in micro-organisms and cross-sensitisation in patients.

Precautions: Absorption of Achromycin V is impaired by the concomitant administration of calcium, magnesium, iron and particularly aluminium salts commonly used as antacids. Tetracyclines depress plasma prothrombin activity therefore reduced dosages of concurrent anti-coagulants may be required. Lower doses are indicated in cases of renal impairment to avoid excessive systemic accumulation, and if therapy is prolonged, serum level determinations are advisable.

Side-effects: Gastro-intestinal disturbances may occur and as with all antibiotics overgrowth of resistant organisms may cause glossitis, stomatitis, vaginitis, or staphylococcal enterocolitis. Photosensitivity and der-matological reactions are rare. Occurrences of enamel hypoplasia have been reported. Rarely increased intra-cranial pressure with bulging fontanelles has been observed in infants which disappears rapidly upon cessation of treatment.

Overdosage: No specific antidote. Gastric lavage plus oral administration of milk or antacids.

Pharmaceutical precautions Achromycin V capsules should be stored at room temperature.

Legal category POM.

Package quantities Bottles of 100 and 500.

Further information Nil.

Product licence number
Capsules 250 mg   0095/0061

ARTANE* TABLETS

Presentation *Tablets 2 mg:* Each white scored tablet coded 'Lederle 4434' contains benzhexol hydrochloride 2 mg.

Tablets 5 mg: Each white scored tablet coded 'Lederle 4436' contains benzhexol hydrochloride 5 mg.

Uses Artane is an antispasmodic drug which exerts a direct inhibitory effect on the parasympathetic nervous system. It also has a relaxing effect on smooth muscle.

It is indicated in all forms of Parkinsonism – post-encephalitic, arteriosclerotic and idiopathic – as well as to prevent and control extrapyramidal disorders due to central nervous system drugs such as reserpine and the phenothiazines. These disorders include tremor, rigidity and increased salivation as commonly encountered in Parkinson's disease; akathisia manifested by extreme restlessness; and dyskinesia characterised by spastic contractions and involuntary movements.

Artane is especially effective in reducing the rigidity of muscle spasm and is useful in relieving the depression and mental inertia characteristic of this syndrome. It decreases sialorrhoea and is a particularly valuable adjunct in the treatment of arteriosclerotic Parkinsonism.

Dosage and administration *Adults only:* Optimal dosage should always be determined empirically, usually by initiating therapy at a relatively low level and by subsequent graduated increments.

Normal dosage for Parkinsonism is 6–10 mg per day, although some patients chiefly in the post-encephalitic group may require an average total dose of 12–15 mg daily. It should be given orally either three or four times a day at mealtimes. The total daily milligram dose may be replaced by the slow release Artane Sustets.

Normal dosage for drug-induced Parkinsonism is usually between 5 mg and 15 mg per day, although some cases have been controlled by 1 mg daily.

In all cases, Artane dosage should be increased or decreased only by small increments over a period of several days. In initial therapy the dose should be 1 mg the first day, 2 mg the second day with further increases of 2 mg per day at three to five-day intervals until the optimum dose is reached.

If patients are already being treated with other parasympathetic inhibitors, Artane should be substituted as part of the therapy.

Artane may be taken before or after meals according to the way the patient reacts. If Artane tends to dry the mouth excessively, it may be better to take it before meals, unless it causes nausea. If taken after meals, induced thirst can be allayed by peppermint, chewing gum or water.

Elderly: Patients over 65 years of age tend to be relatively more sensitive and require smaller amounts of the drug.

Contra-indications, warnings, etc
Precautions: Since the use of Artane must, of necessity, continue indefinitely, the patient should be under careful observation over the long term. It should be administered with care to avoid allergic or other untoward reactions.

Incipient glaucoma may be precipitated by para-sympatholytic drugs such as Artane.

Hypertension, cardiac, liver or kidney disorders are not contra-indications, but such patients should be followed closely.

Artane should be used with caution in patients with glaucoma, obstructive disease of the gastro-intestinal or genito-urinary tracts, and in elderly males with possible prostatic hypertrophy.

Side-effects: Minor side-effects such as dryness of mouth, blurring of vision, dizziness, mild nausea or nervousness will be experienced by 30–50% of all patients. These reactions tend to become less pro-nounced as treatment continues.

Patients with arteriosclerosis or with a history of other drug idiosyncrasies may exhibit reactions of mental confusion, agitation, or nausea and vomiting. Such patients should be allowed to develop a tolerance using the smaller initial dose, with gradual increases until the effective level is reached.

Overdosage: No specific antidote. Gastric lavage, emetic, high enema. Usual general treatment plus cold com-presses and forcing of fluid are mandatory. Atropine antagonists may be useful.

Pharmaceutical precautions The products should be stored at room temperature in either the original pack or in containers which prevent the access of moisture.

Legal category POM.

Package quantities *Artane Tablets 2 mg:* Bottles of 100, 1,000 and 5,000.

Artane Tablets 5 mg: Bottles of 100, 1,000 and 2,500.

Further information Nil.

Product licence numbers
Artane Tablets 2 mg   0095/5041
Artane Tablets 5 mg   0095/5042

ARTANE* SUSTETS*

Presentation Each aquamarine, transparent ovoid gelatine capsule, printed 'A9L', contains benzhexol hydrochloride 5 mg in a sustained release formulation. The preparation has been specially compounded to release 1.25 mg of benzhexol hydrochloride immediately and the remaining 3.75 mg gradually over a period of 6–8 hours.

Uses Artane is an antispasmodic drug which exerts a direct inhibitory effect on the parasympathetic nervous system. It also has a relaxing effect on smooth muscle.

It is indicated in all forms of Parkinsonism – post-encephalitic, arteriosclerotic and idiopathic – as well as to prevent and control extrapyramidal disorders due to central nervous system drugs such as reserpine and the phenothiazines. These disorders include tremor, rigidity and increased salivation as commonly encountered in Parkinson's disease; akathisia manifested by extreme restlessness; and dyskinesia characterised by spastic contractions and involuntary movements.

Artane is especially effective in reducing the rigidity of muscle spasm and is useful in relieving the depression and mental inertia characteristic of this syndrome. It decreases sialorrhoea and is a particularly valuable adjunct in the treatment of arteriosclerotic Parkinsonism.

Dosage and administration *Adults only:* One to three capsules daily as a single dose in the morning, or in divided doses, depending upon the stabilising dose required.

The stabilising dose may be determined by treatment with Artane Tablets, whose dosage should be increased or decreased only by small increments over a period of several days. In initial therapy the dose should be 1 mg the first day, 2 mg the second day with further increases of 2 mg per day at three to five-day intervals until the optimum dose is reached.

The optimum daily dose can then be administered in a once daily dosage regime with Sustets.

If patients are already being treated with other para-sympathetic inhibitors, Artane should be substituted as part of the therapy. Artane may be taken before or after meals according to the way the patient reacts. If Artane tends to dry the mouth excessively, it may be better to take it before meals, unless it causes nausea. If taken after meals, induced thirst can be allayed by peppermint, chewing gum or water.

Elderly: Patients over 65 years of age tend to be relatively more sensitive and require smaller amounts of drug.

Contra-indications, warnings, etc *Precautions:* Since the use of Artane Sustets must, of necessity, continue indefinitely, the patient should be under careful observation over the long term. It should be administered with care to avoid allergic or other untoward reactions.

Incipient glaucoma may be precipitated by para-sympatholytic drugs such as Artane Sustets.

Hypertension, cardiac, liver or kidney disorders are not contra-indications, but such patients should be followed closely.

Artane Sustets should be used with caution in patients with glaucoma, obstructive disease of the gastro-intestinal or genito-urinary tracts, and in elderly males with possible prostatic hypertrophy.

Side-effects: Minor side-effects such as dryness of mouth, blurring of vision, dizziness, mild nausea or nervousness will be experienced by 30–50% of all patients. These reactions tend to become less pronounced as treatment continues.

Patients with arteriosclerosis or with a history of other drug idiosyncrasies may exhibit reactions of mental confusion, agitation, or nausea and vomiting. Such patients should be allowed to develop a tolerance using the smaller initial dose, with gradual increases until the effective level is reached.

Overdosage: No specific antidote. Gastric lavage, emetic, high enema. Usual general treatment plus cold compresses and forcing of fluid are mandatory. Atropine antagonists may be useful.

Pharmaceutical precautions Nil.

Legal category POM.

Package quantities Bottles of 100.

Further information Artane tablets are available as scored, white tablets containing 2 mg or 5 mg of benzhexol hydrochloride in bottles of 100, 1,000 and 5,000.

Product licence number 0095/5050.

AUDICORT*

Presentation Ear drops. Each millilitre contains:
Triamcinolone acetonide 1.0 mg
Neomycin undecylenate equivalent to:
    3.5 mg neomycin base and
    7.0 mg undecylenic acid
Benzocaine 50 mg

Uses Audicort is an anti-inflammatory, antibacterial, and antifungal preparation.

It is indicated in the treatment of acute and chronic otitis externa due to or complicated by bacterial or fungal infection; for eczematous or seborrhoeic dermatitis of the external auditory meatus; as an adjunct to systemic therapy in chronic otitis media and for the treatment of cavities after mastoidectomy and fenestration operations.

Dosage and administration *Adults and children:* After careful cleansing or the ear, Audicort is administered in doses of 2–5 drops, usually three or four times daily. If desired, the drops may be used to saturate a gauze or cotton wick placed in the ear. Excessive heating of the solution should be avoided.

Contra-indications, warnings, etc
Contra-indications: Audicort is contra-indicated in tuberculosis of the skin, viral exanthemata, herpes simplex, smallpox vaccination reactions, and in patients with a history of hypersensitivity to any of the ingredients.

It should not be used in the eyes.

Precautions: Use of an antibiotic may occasionally result in an overgrowth of non-susceptible micro-organisms, while the presence of an anti-inflammatory steroid may encourage their spread. If superinfection does occur, the drug should be stopped and appropriate therapy instituted.

Topical administration of corticosteroids to pregnant animals can cause abnormalities of foetal development. The relevance of this finding to human beings has not been established; however, topical steroids should not be used extensively in early pregnancy i.e. in large amounts for long periods.

In infants, long term continuous topical steroid therapy

should be avoided. Adrenal suppression can occur even without occlusion.

In the adjunctive treatment of otitis media, the benefit expected from the use of Audicort in patients with a perforated eardrum should outweigh the risk of neomycin ototoxicity.

Side-effects: Adverse local effects from triamcinolone acetonide are rare, but neomycin and benzocaine have occasionally been responsible for localised skin sensitisation. If local reactions occur, such as irritation, erythema and oedema, discontinue medication.

Pharmaceutical precautions Audicort should be stored at room temperature in the original pack.

Audicort should not be diluted.

Legal category POM.

Package quantities 10 ml of sterile solution in plastic dropper bottle.

Further information Nil.

Product licence number 0095/5069.

AUREOCORT* CREAM
AUREOCORT* OINTMENT
AUREOCORT* AEROSOL SPRAY

Presentation *Ointment:* Each gram of yellow ointment contains:

Chlortetracycline hydrochloride	30 mg
Triamcinolone acetonide	1 mg

in a greasy base of anhydrous wool fat and white soft paraffin, with 0.16% methylparaben and 0.04% propylparaben as preservative.

Cream: Each gram of yellow cream contains:

Chlortetracycline equivalent to	
chlortetracyline hydrochloride	30 mg
Triamcinolone acetonide	1 mg

in a smooth yellow water-miscible cream, with 0.2% chlorocresol as preservative.

Aerosol Spray: Each can contains:

Chlortetracycline hydrochloride	600 mg
Triamcinolone acetonide	15 mg

in a vehicle/propellant of isopropyl myristate and fluorinated hydrocarbons.

Uses Aureocort combines the anti-inflammatory action of triamcinolone acetonide with the anti-infective properties of chlortetracycline.

It is indicated in the treatment of atopic dermatitis, contact dermatitis, eczema, infected wounds and ulcers, neurodermatitis, otitis externa, seborrhoeic dermatitis, septic types of contact dermatitis, varicose eczema, vesiculo-pustular dermatitis. It may also be used in the treatment of infection and inflammation associated with burns, abrasions, lacerations, contact dermatoses, industrial dermatoses, insect bites, etc.

Dosage and administration *Adults and children:* Aureocort Ointment should be applied sparingly to the affected area either directly or on sterile gauze two or three times daily.

In varicose ulcers the ointment should be applied to the ulcer on sterile gauze, and the surrounding skin edges smeared thinly prior to dressing and pressure bandaging.

Aureocort Cream should be applied sparingly to the affected areas two or three times daily.

Aureocort Spray should be applied sparingly to the affected area two or three times daily. Hold the nozzle four to six inches from the affected area and depress the button for one to three seconds.

Contra-indications, warnings, etc
Contra-indications: The use of Aureocort is contra-indicated in tuberculous, fungal or viral lesions of the skin (herpes simplex, vaccinia and varicella).

Precautions: The use of antibiotics topically may result in overgrowth of non-susceptible organisms; if new infections appear during therapy appropriate measures should be taken.

The use of corticosteroids on infected areas should be continuously and carefully observed, bearing in mind the potential spreading of infection by anti-inflammatory corticosteroids (caused by organisms not sensitive to chlortetracycline) and the possible advisability of discontinuing corticosteroid therapy and/or initiating alternative antibacterial measures. Generalised dermatological conditions may require systemic corticosteroid therapy.

Topical administration of corticosteroids to pregnant animals can cause abnormalities of foetal development. The relevance of this finding to human beings has not been established; however, topical steroids should not be used extensively in early pregnancy, i.e. in large amounts or for long periods.

In infants, long term continuous topical steroid therapy should be avoided. Adrenal suppression can occur even without occlusion.

Side-effects: A few patients may be allergic to any of the components. If adverse reaction or idiosyncrasy occurs discontinue medication.

The use of corticosteroids over extensive body areas, with or without occlusive non-permeable dressings, may result in systemic absorption of the corticosteroid, and the physician should be aware of such possible absorption and take appropriate precautions. When occlusive non-permeable dressings are used, miliaria, folliculitis and pyoderma may sometimes develop beneath the occlusive material. Localised atrophy and striae have been reported with the use of corticosteroids by the occlusive technique.

Pharmaceutical precautions Aureocort Cream should be stored in a cool place. Dilution of Aureocort Ointment and Cream is not recommended as it will affect the stability of the product.

Aureocort Cream and Ointment may cause a yellow staining of clothes. Following extended use a similar local staining of the skin may occur which disappears on cessation of treatment.

Legal category POM.

Package quantities *Aureocort Ointment:* Tubes of 15 g.

Aureocort Cream: Tubes of 15 g.

Aureocort Aerosol Spray: Spray can of 60 g.

Further information Nil.

Product licence numbers

Aureocort Ointment	0095/5076
Aureocort Cream	0095/0019
Aureocort Aerosol Spray	0095/5077

AUREOMYCIN* CAPSULES
AUREOMYCIN* POWDER

Presentation *Capsules 250 mg:* Each yellow capsule, printed 'Lederle 4739' contains chlortetracycline hydrochloride 250 mg.

Powder 25 g: Each bottle contains 25 g of chlortetracycline hydrochloride as a micropulverised yellow powder.

Uses Aureomycin is a broad-spectrum antibiotic used for the treatment of infections caused by chlortetracycline-sensitive organisms. Typical indications include:

Ear, nose and throat infections. Acute and chronic bronchitis. Pneumonia. Gastro-intestinal infections. Amoebic Hepatitis. Urinary tract infections. Soft tissue infections. Venereal diseases. Acne. Typhus fever.

Other infections due to Aureomycin-sensitive organisms.

Aureomycin is also indicated for prophylaxis before or after surgical and dental procedures.

Dosage and administration *Dosage: Adults:* 1 capsule four times a day. This may be increased to 6 or 8 capsules daily in severe infections.

In the treatment of amoebiasis, at least 2 capsules four times daily for 10–14 days is recommended.

Elderly: Aureomycin should be used with caution in the treatment of elderly patients where accumulation is a possibility.

Administration: Aureomycin should be taken an hour before or two hours after meals and therapy should be continued for up to three days after characteristic symptoms of the infection have subsided.

Contra-indications, warnings, etc
Contra-indications: A history of hypersensitivity to tetracyclines. Systemic lupus erythematosus.

Warnings: Tetracyclines may cause a yellow to brown discoloration of the teeth in the developing foetus or child and therefore Aureomycin should only be administered if considered essential to pregnant women and young children under eight years of age. Aureomycin should be used with caution in patients with renal or hepatic dysfunction, or in conjunction with other potentially hepatotoxic drugs. Cross-resistance beween tetracyclines may develop in micro-organisms and cross-sensitisation in patients.

Precautions: Absorption of Aureomycin is impaired by the concomitant administration of calcium, magnesium, iron and particularly aluminium salts commonly used as antacids. Tetracyclines depress plasma prothrombin activity therefore reduced dosages of concurrent anticoagulants may be required. Lower doses may be required in cases of renal impairment to avoid excessive systemic accumulation, although this is unlikely due to the high biliary excretion of Aureomycin. If therapy in such cases, is prolonged, serum level determinations are advisable.

Side-effects: Gastro-intestinal disturbances may occur and as with all antibiotics overgrowth of resistant organisms may cause glossitis, stomatitis, vaginitis, or staphylococcal enterocolitis. Photosensitivity and dermatological reactions are rare. Occurrences of enamel hypoplasia have been reported. Rarely, increased intracranial pressure with bulging fontanelles has been observed in infants which disappears rapidly upon cessation of treatment.

Overdosage: No specific antidote. Gastric lavage plus oral administration of milk or antacids.

Pharmaceutical precautions Nil.

Legal category POM.

Package quantities *Capsules:* Bottles of 100.

Powder: Bottles containing 25 g.

Further information Nil.

Product licence numbers
Capsules 250 mg   0095/0051
Powder 25 g   0095/5022

AUREOMYCIN* OINTMENT
AUREOMYCIN* CREAM
AUREOMYCIN* OPHTHALMIC OINTMENT

Presentation *Aureomycin Ointment 3%:* Each gram of yellow ointment contains Chlortetracycline hydrochloride 30 mg in a greasy base of anhydrous wool fat and white soft paraffin with 2.4% methylparaben and 0.6% propylparaben as preservatives.

Aureomycin Cream 3%: Each gram of yellow cream contains Chlortetracycline equivalent to chlortetracycline hydrochloride 30 mg in a smooth yellow water-miscible cream, with 0.2% chlorocresol as preservative.

Aureomycin Ophthalmic Ointment 1%: Each gram of yellow ointment contains Chlortetracycline hydrochloride 10 mg in a greasy base of anhydrous wool fat and white soft paraffin.

Uses Aureomycin is a broad-spectrum antibiotic.

Aureomycin Ointment 3% and Aureomycin Cream 3%: Aureomycin topical preparations are indicated for the treatment of superficial pyogenic infections of the skin. They are effective against Gram-positive cocci (Streptococci, Staphylococci and Pneumococci) and Gram-negative bacteria (Coli-aerogenes group).

Aureomycin Ophthalmic Ointment 1%: Aureomycin Ophthalmic Ointment 1% is indicated in the treatment of susceptible ocular infections caused by Staphylococci, Pneumococci, *Haemophilus influenzae,* Diplococcus of Morax-Axenfeld, the Friedlander bacillus, Streptococci, *Aerobacter aerogenes, Proteus vulgaris, Proteus morganii, Escherichia coli, Alcaligenes faecalis, Pseudomonas aeruginosa,* and in the treatment of trachoma (in conjunction with oral therapy).

Dosage and administration *Adults and children: Aureomycin Ointment 3% and Cream 3%:* In the treatment of local skin infections, apply the preparation directly to the involved area, preferably on sterile gauze, one or more times daily as the condition warrants. In severe local infection, topical application should be supplemented by oral administration.

Aureomycin Ophthalmic Ointment 1%: Aureomycin Ophthalmic Ointment should be applied to the infected eye every two hours or more often as the condition warrants and response indicates. Severe or stubborn infections may require treatment for many days or oral administration in addition to local treatment. Mild infections may respond in as little as 48 hours.

Contra-indications, warnings, etc
Contra-indications: Aureomycin topical preparations are contra-indicated in patients with a history of hypersensitivity to chlortetracycline hydrochloride or any other ingredient.

Precautions: The use of antibiotics may result in the overgrowth of non-susceptible organisms. If new infections appear during therapy appropriate measures should be taken.

Side-effects: A few patients may be allergic to any of the components. If adverse reaction or idiosyncrasy occurs, discontinue medication.

Pharmaceutical precautions *Aureomycin Ointment 3%:* The product should be stored in a cool place. The ointment may be diluted with a base of 10% wool-fat in white soft paraffin.

Aureomycin Cream 3%: The product should be stored in a cool place. Dilution is not recommended.

Aureomycin Ophthalmic Ointment: The product should be stored in a cool place. Dilution of Aureomycin Ophthalmic Ointment is not recommended.

Aureomycin Cream and Ointment may cause a yellow staining of clothes. Following extended use a similar local staining of the skin may occur which disappears on cessation of treatment.

Legal category POM.

Package quantities *Aureomycin Ointment 3%:* Tubes of 30 g.

Aureomycin Ophthalmic Ointment 1%: Tubes of 3.5 g.

Aureomycin Cream 3%: Tubes of 30 g.

Further information Nil.

Product licence numbers
Aureomycin Ointment 3% 0095/5019
Aureomycin Ophthalmic Ointment 1% 0095/5020
Aureomycin Cream 3% 0095/0018

CALCIUM LEUCOVORIN

Presentation *Injection 3 mg in 1 ml:* Ampoules containing 3 mg/ml folinic acid as the calcium salt.

Powder for Injection 15 mg and 30 mg: Vials containing a lyophilised powder of 15 mg or 30 mg folinic acid as the calcium salt.

Tablets 15 mg: Each yellowish-white scored tablet contains 15 mg folinic acid as the calcium salt.

Uses Calcium Leucovorin is the calcium salt of a formyl derivative of tetrahydrofolic acid, the metabolite of folic acid, and an essential coenzyme for nucleic acid synthesis. Calcium Leucovorin is used therefore to diminish the toxicity and counteract the action of folic acid antagonists such as Methotrexate in cytotoxic therapy. This procedure is commonly known as Calcium Leucovorin Rescue.

Calcium Leucovorin has also been demonstrated to be effective in producing amelioration of the blood picture in a number of megaloblastic anaemias due to folate deficiency.

Dosage and administration *Calcium Leucovorin Rescue: Adults and children:* Dosage regimes vary, depending upon the dose of Methotrexate administered. In general, up to 120 mg are usually given in divided doses, over 12–24 hours, by intramuscular injection, bolus intravenous injection, or intravenous infusion followed by intramuscularly or 15 mg (1 tablet) orally, every 6 hours for the next 48 hours. Rescue therapy is usually started following a delay of up to 8–24 hours, after the beginning of the Methotrexate infusion. One tablet (15 mg) of Calcium Leucovorin every 6 hours for 48–72 hours may be sufficient when lower doses (less than 100 mg) of Methotrexate have been given. Where overdosage of Methotrexate is suspected, the dose of Calcium Leucovorin should be equal to or higher than the offending dose of Methotrexate, and should be administered within the first hour.

Treatment of Folate Deficiency:

Children up to 12 years of age: 0.25 mg/kg/day.

Adults: 10–20 mg daily. Oral therapy with one tablet of Calcium Leucovorin daily is more usual.

Contra-indications, warnings, etc
Contra-indications: None.

Precautions: Calcium Leucovorin should not be given simultaneously with an anti-neoplastic folic acid antagonist, e.g. Methotrexate to modify or abort clinical toxicity, as the therapeutic effect of the antagonist may be nullified. Concomitant Calcium Leucovorin will not however inhibit the antibacterial activity of other folic acid antagonists such as trimethoprim and pyrimethamine.

Calcium Leucovorin should not be used for the treatment of pernicious anaemia or other megaloblastic anaemias where vitamin B_{12} is deficient.

Side-effects: Adverse reactions to Calcium Leucovorin are rare, but occasional pyrexial reactions have been reported following parenteral administration.

Overdosage: Does not apply.

Pharmaceutical precautions Store at room temperature.

Each vial of Powder for Injection 15 mg and 30 mg should be reconstituted with 3 ml of Water for Injection to produce a solution for intramuscular or intravenous injection. Calcium Leucovorin is stable for at least 24 hours at room temperature when diluted with the following intravenous infusion fluids: Sodium Chloride 0.9%; Glucose 10%; Sodium Chloride 0.9% and Glucose 10%; Compound Sodium Lactate.

As the Powder for Injection does not contain an antimicrobial preservative, solutions of Calcium Leucovorin powder for injection should be used or discarded within 24 hours of preparation.

Legal category POM.

Package quantities *Injection 3 mg in 1 ml:* 10 × 1 ml ampoules.

Powder for Injection 15 mg and 30 mg: Boxes of one vial.

Tablets 15 mg: Bottles of 10 tablets.

Further information Further information, particularly on high-dosage regimes in conjunction with methotrexate, is available on request.

Product licence numbers
Injection 3 mg in 1 ml 0095/5053
Powder for Injection 15 mg and 30 mg 0095/0087
Tablets 15 mg 0095/0033

CISPLATIN* INJECTION
CISPLATIN* POWDER FOR INJECTION

Presentation *Cisplatin Injection 10 mg, 25 mg and 50 mg:* Each vial contains 10 mg, 25 mg or 50 mg of Cisplatin in solution at a concentration of 1 mg Cisplatin in 1 ml.

Cisplatin Powder for Injection 10 mg, 50 mg: Each vial of lyophilised powder contains 10 mg or 50 mg Cisplatin.

Uses Cisplatin is indicated for use alone, or in addition to other modalities, or in established combination therapy with other chemotherapeutic agents in the management of neoplastic disease, especially:

Metastatic testicular tumours – In patients who have already received appropriate surgical and/or radiotherapeutic procedures. The combination of Cisplatin, bleomycin and vinblastine has been reported to be highly effective.

Metastatic ovarian tumours – As secondary therapy in patients refractory to standard chemotherapy.

Dosage and administration

Adults and children:

Single agent therapy: 50–120 mg/m² as a single IV dose every three to four weeks, or 15–20 mg/m² IV daily for five days every three to four weeks.

Combination therapy: In general, current multiple drug treatment schedules including Cisplatin employ lower doses ranging from 20 mg/m² upwards, administered IV every three to four weeks.

Directions for use: Pre-treatment hydration with 1–2 litres of fluid infused for 8–12 hours prior to a Cisplatin dose is recommended in order to initiate diuresis.

Cisplatin should be added to 2 litres of an intravenous infusion fluid prior to administration; either 0.9% Sodium Chloride or Sodium Chloride and Glucose are suitable.

For Cisplatin Powder for Injection, reconstitute the 10 mg vial with 10 ml, and the 50 mg vial contents with 50 ml of Water for Injection, before adding to the infusion fluid.

Cisplatin Injection should be added directly into the infusion fluid.

It is recommended that administration should be over a 6–8 hour period. Diuresis may be aided by the addition to the infusion solution of 37.5 g mannitol.

Adequate hydration and urinary output must be maintained during the 24 hours following infusion.

A repeat course of Cisplatin should not be given until the serum creatinine is below 1.5 mg/100 ml (130 µmol/L) and/or the blood urea below 55 mg/100 ml (9 mmol/L). A repeat course should not be given until circulating blood elements are at an acceptable level.

Subsequent doses of Cisplatin should not be given until an audiometric analysis indicates that auditory acuity is within normal limits.

Contra-indications, warnings, etc

Contra-indications: Cisplatin induces nephrotoxicity, myelosuppression, neurotoxicity and ototoxicity which may be additive to pre-existing dysfunctions. Consequently, the use of Cisplatin in patients with hearing or renal impairment, or depressed bone marrow function, may be associated with increased toxicities. Such conditions represent relative contra-indications.

Cisplatin is contra-indicated in patients with dehydration.

Cisplatin is contra-indicated in patients with a history of hypersensitivity to Cisplatin or other platinum-containing compounds.

Warnings: Cisplatin produces cumulative nephrotoxicity. The serum creatinine, BUN or creatinine clearance should be measured prior to initiating therapy and prior to each subsequent course.

Anaphylactic-like reactions to Cisplatin have been reported. These reactions have occurred within minutes of administration to patients with prior exposure to Cisplatin and have been alleviated by administration of adrenaline, steroids and antihistamines.

Safe use in pregnancy has not been established. Cisplatin should not be administered to patients who are pregnant or to mothers who are breast-feeding. In mice, high doses and doses approaching the maximum therapeutic dose for Cisplatin when used alone have been reported to be embryotoxic. The data concerning its teratogenic potential are inconclusive.

The influence of Cisplatin on human reproduction has not been determined. Cisplatin therapy might have an anti-fertility effect.

The carcinogenic potential in humans is unknown. The possibility of a carcinogenic effect should be kept in mind when planning long term therapy. When evaluated at high doses in mice by repeated intraperitoneal administration, Cisplatin increased the incidence of lung tumours. Cisplatin has been reported to be mutagenic in bacteria and produces chromosomal damage in animal and human cells in tissue culture.

Cisplatin causes immunosuppression. Concomitant use of live vaccines may lead to a generalised systemic reaction.

Precautions: Cisplatin should be administered by individuals experienced in the use of cancer chemotherapeutic agents with adequate facilities available for patient monitoring. Since anaphylactic reactions may occur, appropriate supportive equipment should be available to control such reactions.

Neurotoxicity appears to be cumulative. Prior to each course, the absence of symptoms of peripheral neuropathy should be established. (See Adverse Reactions).

Since renal toxicity is cumulative, measurements of BUN, serum creatinine or creatinine clearance, should be performed prior to initiating therapy and prior to each subsequent course. At the recommended dosage Cisplatin should not be given more frequently than once every three to four weeks (see Adverse Reactions).

Since ototoxicity of Cisplatin is cumulative, audiometric testing should be performed prior to initiating therapy and prior to each subsequent course of the drug (see Adverse Reactions).

Concomitant administration of aminoglycoside antibiotics, cephaloridine or frusemide may result in increased ototoxicity or nephrotoxicity.

Peripheral blood counts should be monitored weekly. Liver function should be monitored periodically. Neurological examinations should also be performed regularly (see Adverse Reactions).

Adverse reactions

Nephrotoxicity: Renal toxicity has been noted in about one third of patients given a single dose of Cisplatin *when prior hydration has not been employed.* It is first noted during the second week after a dose and is manifested by elevations in BUN and serum creatinine, serum uric acid and/or a decrease in creatinine clearance.

Renal toxicity becomes more prolonged and severe with repeated courses of the drug. Renal function must return to normal before another dose of Cisplatin can be given. Renal function impairment has been associated with renal tubular damage. The administration of Cisplatin using a six to eight hour infusion with intravenous hydration and mannitol have been used to reduce nephrotoxicity. However, renal toxicity can still occur after utilisation of these procedures.

Neurotoxicity: Neurotoxicity, usually characterised by peripheral neuropathies, has occurred in some patients. Loss of taste and seizures have also been reported. Neuropathies resulting from Cisplatin treatment may occur after prolonged therapy (four to seven months); however, neurological symptoms have been reported to occur after a single dose.

Cisplatin therapy should be discontinued when the symptoms are first observed. Preliminary evidence suggests peripheral neuropathy may be irreversible in some patients.

Ototoxicity: Ototoxicity has been observed in patients treated with a single dose of Cisplatin, 50 mg/m^2 and is manifested by tinnitus and/or hearing loss in the high frequency range (4000 to 8000 Hz).

Decreased ability to hear normal conversational tones may occur occasionally. Ototoxic effects may be more severe in children receiving Cisplatin. Hearing loss can be unilateral or bilateral and tends to become more frequent and severe with repeated doses. It is unclear whether Cisplatin induced ototoxicity is reversible. Careful monitoring by audiometry should be performed prior to initiation of therapy and prior to subsequent doses of Cisplatin.

Haematological: Myelosuppression may occur in patients treated with Cisplatin. The nadirs in circulating platelets and leucocytes occur between days 18–23 (range 7.5–45) with most patients recovering by day 39 (13–62). Leucopenia and thrombocytopenia are more pronounced at higher doses. Anaemia (decrease in haemoglobin level by 2g/100ml blood) occurs at approximately the same frequency and with the same timing as leucopenia and thrombocytopenia.

Gastro-intestinal: Marked nausea and vomiting occur in almost all patients treated with Cisplatin and are occasionally so severe that the drug must be discontinued. Nausea and vomiting usually begin within one to four hours after treatment and last up to 24 hours. Various degrees of nausea and anorexia may persist for up to one week after treatment.

Other toxicities

Hyperuricaemia: Hyperuricaemia has been reported to occur at approximately the same frequency as the increases in BUN and serum creatinine. It is more pronounced after doses greater than 50 mg/m^2, and peak levels of uric acid generally occur between three to five days after the dose. Allopurinol therapy for hyperuricaemia effectively reduces uric acid levels.

Anaphylactic-like reactions: Anaphylactic-like reactions, possibly secondary to Cisplatin therapy, have been occasionally reported in patients previously exposed to Cisplatin. The reactions consist of facial oedema, wheezing, tachycardia and hypotension within a few minutes of drug administration. All reactions may be controlled by intravenous adrenaline, corticosteroids or antihistamines. Patients receiving Cisplatin should be observed carefully for possible anaphylactic-like reactions and supportive equipment and medication should be available to treat such a complication.

Other toxicities reported to occur infrequently are cardiac abnormalities (including conduction defects and congestive heart failure), anorexia and elevated SGOT.

Hypomagnesaemia: Asymptomatic hypomagnesaemia has been reported in a certain number of patients treated with Cisplatin; symptomatic hypomagnesaemia has been observed in a limited number of patients.

Pharmaceutical precautions

Storage: Cisplatin Injection and Cisplatin Powder for Injection should be stored at room temperature and protected from light.

Do not refrigerate Cisplatin Injection, or the reconstituted solution from Cisplatin Powder for Injection, as refrigeration will result in precipitation.

Preparations of intravenous injection: Cisplatin should be added to 2 litres of an intravenous infusion fluid prior to administration; either 0.9% Sodium Chloride or Sodium Chloride and Glucose are suitable.

For Cisplatin Powder for Injection, reconstitute the 10 mg vial contents with 10 ml, and the 50 mg vial contents with 50 ml of Water for Injection, before adding to the infusion fluid. The reconstituted solution is stable for 20 hours at room temperature.

Cisplatin Injection should be added directly into the infusion fluid.

It is recommended that administration should be over a six to eight hour period. Diuresis may be added by the addition to the infusion solution of 37.5 g mannitol.

Cisplatin interacts with aluminium. Administration sets, cannulae and syringes containing aluminium must not be used with the product.

Legal category POM.

Package quantities *Cisplatin Injection:*
10 mg in 10 ml: single vials
25 mg in 25 ml: single vials
50 mg in 50 ml: single vials

Cisplatin Powder for Injection:
10 mg vial: single vials
50 mg vial: single vials

Further information Cisplatin has biochemical properties similar to that of bifunctional alkylating agents producing inter-strand and intra-strand crosslinks in DNA. It is apparently cell-cycle non-specific. Following a single IV dose, Cisplatin concentrates in liver, kidneys and large and small intestine in animals and humans. Cisplatin apparently has poor penetration into CNS.

Plasma levels of radioactivity decay in a biphasic manner after an IV bolus dose of radioactive Cisplatin to patients. The initial plasma half-life is 25–49 minutes, and the post-distribution plasma half-life is 58–73 hours. During the post-distribution phase, greater than 90% of the radioactivity in the blood is protein-bound. Cisplatin is excreted primarily in the urine. However, urinary excretion is incomplete with only 27–43% of the radioactivity being excreted within the first 5 days post-dose in human beings. There are insufficient data to determine whether biliary or intestinal excretion occurs.

Product licence numbers

Cisplatin Injection	0095/0098
Cisplatin Powder for Injection	0095/0090

DETECLO* TABLETS

Presentation *Tablets 300 mg:* Each blue, film-coated tablet, printed 'Lederle 5422' contains:

Tetracycline hydrochloride	115.4 mg
Chlortetracycline hydrochloride	115.4 mg
Demeclocycline hydrochloride	69.2 mg

Uses For the treatment of infections caused by tetracycline-sensitive organisms. Typical indications include: Ear, nose and throat infections. Acute and chronic bronchitis. Pneumonia. Venereal Diseases. Non-Gonococcal Urethritis. Gastro-intestinal infections. Urinary tract infections. Soft tissue infections. Acne. Typhus fever. Psittacosis. Other infections due to Deteclo-sensitive organisms.

Deteclo is also indicated for prophylaxis before or after surgical and dental procedures.

Dosage and administration *Dosage: Adults:* One tablet every 12 hours.

This may be increased to 3 or 4 tablets daily for short periods in more severe infections.

Gonorrhoea: 1,200 mg (4 tablets) followed by a similar dose six hours later.

Non-gonococcal urethritis: One tablet twice daily for 10–21 days.

Children: Not recommended for children under 8 years of age. Information on dosage is available on request where specifically indicated.

Elderly: Deteclo should be used with caution in the treatment of elderly patients where accumulation is a possibility.

Administration: Deteclo should be taken an hour before or two hours after meals and therapy should be continued for up to three days after characteristic symptoms of the infection have subsided.

Contra-indications, warnings, etc
Contra-indications: A history of hypersensitivity to tetracyclines. Overt renal insufficiency. Systemic lupus erythematosus.

Warnings: Tetracycline may cause a yellow to brown discoloration of the teeth in the developing foetus or child and therefore Deteclo should only be administered if considered essential to pregnant women and young children under eight years of age. Deteclo should be used with caution in patients with renal or hepatic dysfunction, or in conjunction with other potentially hepatotoxic drugs. Cross-resistance between tetracyclines may develop in micro-organisms and cross-sensitisation in patients.

Precautions: Absorption of Deteclo is impaired by the concomitant administration of calcium, magnesium, iron and particularly aluminium salts commonly used as antacids. Tetracyclines depress plasma prothrombin activity. Therefore reduced dosages of concurrent anti-coagulants may be required. Lower doses are indicated in cases of renal impairment to avoid excessive systemic accumulation, and, if therapy is prolonged, serum level determinations are advisable.

Side-effects: Nausea, diarrhoea and dermatitis may occur and, as with all antibiotics, overgrowth of resistant organisms may cause glossitis, stomatitis, vaginitis, or staphylococcal enterocolitis. Photoallergic reactions may occur in hypersensitive persons and such patients should be warned to avoid direct exposure to natural or artificial sunlight and to discontinue treatment at the first sign of skin discomfort. Rarely, increased intracranial pressure with bulging fontanelles has been observed in infants which disappears rapidly upon cessation of treatment.

Overdosage: No specific antidote. Gastric lavage plus oral administration of milk or antacids.

Pharmaceutical precautions Nil.

Legal category POM.

Package quantities Bottles of 100 and 500.

Further information Deteclo is a unique combination of three effective tetracycline broad-spectrum anti-biotics. The ratio of the different tetracyclines has been carefully chosen to ensure that high therapeutic blood levels are rapidly realised and maintained with a reduced potential for side-effects, on a twice daily dosage regime,

because of their different rates of absorption and excretion.

Product licence number
Tablets   0095/5070

DIAMOX*

Presentation *Tablets 250 mg:* Each white scored tablet coded 'Lederle 4395' contains acetazolamide 250 mg.

Sodium Parenteral 500 mg: Each vial contains 500 mg of acetazolamide as the sodium salt with sodium hydroxide to adjust the pH to approximately 9.2.

Uses Diamox is an enzyme inhibitor and acts specifically on carbonic anhydrase. It is indicated in the treatment of:

1. *Glaucoma:* It is felt that Diamox is useful in glaucoma, because it acts on inflow, decreasing the amount of aqueous secretion.

2. *Abnormal retention of fluid:* Diamox is a diuretic whose action is due to the effect on the reversible hydration of carbon dioxide and dehydration of the carbonic acid reaction in the kidney. The result is renal loss of HCO_3-ion which carries out sodium, water and potassium.

Diamox is therefore indicated in the treatment of toxaemia and oedema of pregnancy, pre-menstrual tension, drug-induced oedema, obesity, and congestive heart failure in each case where fluid retention is a problem.

3. *Epilepsy:* Best results with Diamox have been seen in petit mal in children. Good results, however, have been seen in patients, both children and adults, with other types of seizures such as grand mal, mixed seizure patterns, myoclonic jerk patterns, etc.

4. *Other fields:* Certain patients with Ménière's disease have shown a good response, but this is probably limited to those patients who have a component of oedema in the labyrinth mechanism of the inner ear.

Similarly, there have been varying reports on the use of Diamox in hydrocephalus in the infant.

Dosage and administration *Tablets:*
1. *Glaucoma (acute congestive and secondary):* *Adults:* 250–1,000 mg (1–4 tablets) per 24 hours, usually in divided doses for amounts over 250 mg daily.

Children: 125–750 mg ($\frac{1}{2}$–3 tablets) daily in divided doses.

Elderly: See Contra-indications and warnings.

Diamox should be used as an adjunct to the usual therapy.

2. *Abnormal retention of fluid:* Congestive heart failure, toxaemia and oedema of pregnancy, drug-induced oedema. (Adults only.)

For diuresis, the starting dose is usually 1–1½ tablets (250–375 mg) once daily in the morning. If, after an initial response, the patient fails to continue to lose oedema fluid, do not increase the dose but allow for kidney recovery by omitting a day. Best results are often obtained on a regime of 1–1½ tablets daily for two days, rest a day, and repeat, or merely giving the Diamox every other day. The use of Diamox does not eliminate the need for other therapy, e.g. digitalis, bed rest and salt restriction in congestive heart failure and proper supplementation with elements such as potassium in drug-induced oedema.

For cases of pre-menstrual tension where fluid retention is a problem a daily dose (single) of 125–375 mg is suggested beginning 5–10 days prior to onset of menstruation, or at onset of symptoms. Therapy may be alternated with days of rest.

For obesity the recommended dosage is 250–375 mg daily. For some patients therapy may be on an alternate week basis. Diamox is not intended for use in curbing appetite.

3. *Epilepsy: Adults:* 250–1,000 mg daily in divided doses.

Children: 125–750 mg daily in divided doses.

The change from other medication to Diamox should be gradual.

Sodium Parenteral: Intravenous or intramuscular administration may be employed in the same dosage as indicated for oral use. The direct intravenous route is preferred as the intramuscular use is limited by the alkaline pH of the solution.

Each vial should be reconstituted with at least 5 ml of Water for Injection prior to use.

Contra-indications, warnings, etc

Contra-indications: Since Diamox may induce a mild acidosis, its use is contra-indicated in idiopathic renal hyperchloraemic acidosis. Because of the nature of its action, Diamox may be contra-indicated in conditions in which there is a known depletion of sodium and potassium at least until after successful preliminary medication with sodium and potassium salts. It is also contra-indicated in Addison's disease or all types of suprarenal gland failure, precoma associated with hepatic cirrhosis, and renal insufficiency.

Long-term administration is contra-indicated in patients with chronic congestive angle-closure glaucoma since it may permit organic closure of the angle to occur while the worsening glaucoma is masked by lowered intra-ocular pressure. Diamox should not be used in patients hypersensitive to sulphonamides.

Precautions: Patients who are being treated with Diamox require regular supervision with monitoring of fluid and electrolyte state. Increasing the dose does not increase the diuresis but may increase the incidence of drowsiness and/or paraesthesia. Less commonly, fatigue, excitement, gastro-intestinal upsets and increased polyuria have been reported. Disorientation has been observed in a few patients with oedema due to hepatic cirrhosis. Such cases should be under close supervision.

When Diamox is prescribed for long-term therapy, special precautions are advisable. The patient should be cautioned to report any unusual skin rash. Periodic blood cell counts are recommended. A precipitous drop in formed blood cell elements or the appearance of toxic skin manifestations should call for diminution or cessation of Diamox therapy. The transitory loss of hearing calls for immediate cessation of medication. Diamox should only be used with particular caution in elderly patients or those with potential obstruction in the urinary tract, or with disorders rendering their electrolyte balance precarious or with liver dysfunction. It should only be used during pregnancy if considered essential by the physician. The concomitant administration of this preparation with cardiac glycosides or hypotensive agents may necessitate adjustment of the dosage of these drugs.

Side-effects: Instances of flushing, thirst, headache, drowsiness, dizziness, fatigue, irritability, excitement, polydipsia and polyuria, paraesthesia of extremities and face, ataxia, hyperpnoea, and gastro-intestinal upsets such as anorexia and vomiting have been reported. These side-effects have normally disappeared during continued medication or upon diminution or cessation of Diamox therapy.

However, Diamox is a sulphonamide derivative and therefore some side-effects similar to those caused by sulphonamides have occasionally been reported. These include fever, agranulocytosis, thrombocytopenia, thrombocytic purpura, leukopenia, and aplastic anaemia, skin toxicity, crystalluria, calculus formation, renal and ureteral colic, and renal lesions.

Transient myopia has been reported. This condition invariably subsides upon diminution or cessation of the medication.

Drug interactions: Possible potentiation of the effects of folic acid antagonists, hypoglycaemics and oral anticoagulants.

Overdosage: No specific antidote. Supportive measures with correction of electrolyte and fluid balance. Force fluids.

Pharmaceutical precautions The products should be stored at room temperature in either the original pack or in containers which prevent access of moisture.

Reconstituted solutions of Diamox Sodium Parenteral contain no preservative and should be used or discarded within 24 hours.

Legal category POM.

Package quantities *Diamox Tablets 250 mg:* Bottles of 100 and 1,000.

Diamox Sodium Parenteral: Vials, 500 mg.

Further information Diamox Sodium Parenteral contains 2.36 millimoles of sodium per vial.

Product licence numbers
Diamox Tablets 250 mg   0095/5075
Diamox Sodium Parenteral   0095/5073

DIAMOX* SUSTETS*

Presentation Each orange transparent capsule contains acetazolamide 500 mg formulated to release 125 mg immediately and 375 mg gradually over a six to eight hour period.

Uses Diamox is an enzyme inhibitor and acts specifically on carbonic anhydrase which affects the reversible hydration of carbon dioxide and dehydration of carbonic acid in the kidney and other sites. The result is renal loss of HCO_3-ion which carries out sodium, water and potassium.

Indications Glaucoma.

Dosage and administration *Adults:* One Capsule at night and in the morning. The product is not intended for administration to children.

Elderly: See contra-indications and warnings.

Contra-indications, warnings, etc

Contra-indications: Since Diamox Sustets may induce a mild acidosis, its use is contra-indicated in idiopathic renal hyperchloraemic acidosis. Because of the nature of its action, Diamox Sustets may be contra-indicated in conditions in which there is a known depletion of sodium and potassium at least until after successful preliminary medication with sodium and potassium salts. It is also contra-indicated in Addison's disease or all types of suprarenal gland failure, pre-coma associated with hepatic cirrhosis, and renal insufficiency.

Long-term administration is contra-indicated in patients with chronic congestive angle-closure glaucoma since it may permit organic closure of the angle to occur while the worsening glaucoma is masked by lowered intra-ocular pressure. Diamox should not be used in patients hypersensitive to sulphonamides.

Precautions: Patients who are being treated with Diamox require regular supervision with monitoring of fluid and electrolyte state. Increasing the dose does not increase the diuresis and may increase the incidence of drowsiness and/or paraesthesia. Less commonly, fatigue, excitement, gastro-intestinal upsets and increased polyuria have been reported. Disorientation has been observed in a few patients with oedema due to hepatic cirrhosis. Such cases should be under close supervision.

When Diamox Sustets are prescribed for long-term therapy, special precautions are advisable. The patient should be cautioned to report any unusual skin rash. Periodic blood cell counts are recommended. A precipitous drop in formed blood cell elements or the appearance of toxic skin manifestations should call for diminution or cessation of Diamox Sustets therapy. The transitory loss of hearing calls for immediate cessation of medication. Diamox should only be used with particular caution in elderly patients or those with potential obstruction in the urinary tract, or with disorders rendering their electrolyte balance precarious or with liver dysfunction. It should only be used during pregnancy if considered essential by the physician. The concomitant administration of this preparation with cardiac glycosides or hypotensive agents may necessitate adjustment of the dosage of these drugs.

Side-effects: Instances of flushing, thirst, headache, drowsiness, dizziness, fatigue, irritability, excitement, polydipsia and polyuria, paraesthesia of extremities and face, ataxia, hyperpnoea, and gastro-intestinal upsets such as anorexia and vomiting have been reported. These side-effects have normally disappeared during continued medication or upon diminution or cessation of Diamox Sustets therapy.

However, Diamox is a sulphonamide derivative and therefore some side-effects similar to those caused by sulphonamides have occasionally been reported. These include fever, agranulocytosis, thrombocytopenia, thrombocytic purpura, leukopenia, and aplastic anaemia, skin toxicity, crystalluria, calculus formation, renal and ureteral colic, and renal lesions.

Transient myopia has been reported. This condition invariably subsides upon diminution or cessation of the medication.

Drug interactions: Possible potentiation of the effects of folic acid antagonists, hypoglycaemics and oral anticoagulants.

Overdosage: No specific antidote. Supportive measures with correction of electrolyte and fluid balance. Force fluids.

Pharmaceutical precautions Nil.

Legal category POM.

Package quantities Bottles of 30, 100 and 500.

Further information Nil.

Product licence number 0095/5074.

GEVRAL*

Presentation Each brown gelatine capsule coded 'Lederle 4981' contains:

Vitamin A (acetate)	5,000 i.u.
Vitamin D (as calciferol and yeast)	500 i.u.
Vitamin B_1 (as thiamine mononitrate)	5.0 mg
Vitamin B_2 (riboflavine)	5.0 mg
Vitamin B_6 (pyridoxine hydrochloride)	0.5 mg
Vitamin B_{12}	1 mcg
Vitamin C (ascorbic acid)	50.0 mg
Vitamin E (*d*-α-tocopheryl acetate)	10 i.u.
Niacinamide	15.0 mg
Calcium pantothenate	5.0 mg
Calcium (as dibasic calcium phosphate)	145.0 mg
Phosphorus (as dibasic calcium phosphate)	110.0 mg
Elemental iron (as ferrous fumarate)	10.0 mg
Magnesium (as magnesium oxide)	1.0 mg
Potassium (as potassium sulphate)	5.0 mg
Iodine (as potassium iodide)	0.1 mg
Copper (as copper oxide)	1.0 mg
Manganese (as manganese dioxide)	1.0 mg
Zinc (as zinc oxide)	0.5 mg
Inositol	50.0 mg
l – Lysine monohydrochloride	25.0 mg
Choline bitartrate	50.0 mg

Uses Gevral is indicated for the prevention of deficiencies of the vitamins and minerals contained.

Dosage and administration *Adults and children:* One capsule daily, preferably after a meal, or as prescribed by the physician.

Contra-indications, warnings, etc There are no contra-indications, side-effects or adverse reactions. Overdosage does not apply.

Pharmaceutical precautions The product should be stored at room temperature in either the original pack or in containers which prevent access of moisture.

Legal category P.

Package quantities Packs of 30.

Further information Gevral Capsules contain 0.129 millimole of potassium per capsule.

Product licence number 0095/5078.

LEDERCORT* CREAM AND OINTMENT

Presentation *Ledercort Cream 0.1%:* Each gram of white cream contains triamcinolone acetonide 1.0 mg in a water-miscible base with methylparaben 0.16% and propylparaben 0.04% as preservatives.

Ledercort Ointment 0.1%: Each gram of pale yellow ointment contains triamcinolone acetonide 1.0 mg in a greasy base with methylparaben 0.16% and propylparaben 0.04% as preservatives.

Uses Triamcinolone acetonide is a corticosteroid with anti-inflammatory, antipruritis and anti-allergic effects.

Ledercort Cream 0.1% and Ledercort Ointment 0.1% are indicated in the treatment of inflammatory skin conditions such as atopic dermatitis; contact dermatitis; eczematous psoriasis; eczematous dermatitis; generalised erythrodermia; neurodermatitis; nummular eczema; otitis externa; pruritus ani; pruritus vulvae, and seborrhoeic dermatitis.

Dosage and administration *Adults and children:* Apply in small quantities to the affected areas three or four times daily; the cream or ointment may be rubbed in or applied as a thin film.

Some cases of psoriasis may be treated more effectively by application under an occlusive non-permeable dressing.

Contra-indications, warnings, etc

Contra-indications: The use of Ledercort Cream 0.1% and Ledercort Ointment 0.1% is contra-indicated in tuberculous, fungal or viral lesions of the skin (herpes simplex, vaccinia and varicella).

Precautions: In infants, long-term continuous topical steroid therapy should be avoided. Adrenal suppression can occur even without occlusion.

The use of corticosteroids on infected areas should be cautious and carefully observed, bearing in mind the potential spreading of infection by anti-inflammatory corticosteroids and the possible advisability of discontinuing corticosteroid therapy and/or initiating antibacterial measures. Generalised dermatological conditions may require systemic corticosteroid therapy. If infection of the tissues is present, the use of a broad-spectrum systemic antibiotic may be desirable.

Topical administration of corticosteroids to pregnant animals can cause abnormalities of foetal development. The relevance of this finding to human beings has not been established; however, topical steroids should not be used extensively in early pregnancy, i.e. in large amounts or for prolonged periods.

Side-effects: A few patients may be allergic to any of the components. If adverse reaction or idiosyncrasy occurs, discontinue medication.

Side-effects are not ordinarily encountered with topical application of corticosteroids; but as with all drugs some patients react unfavourably under certain conditions. The use of corticosteroids over extensive body areas, with or without occlusive non-permeable dressings, may result in systemic absorption of the corticosteroid being used, and the physician should be aware of such possible absorption and take appropriate precautions. When occlusive non-permeable dressings are used, miliaria, folliculitis and pyoderma may sometimes develop beneath the occlusive material. Localised atrophy and striae have been reported with the use of corticosteroids by the occlusive technique.

Pharmaceutical precautions *Ledercort Cream 0.1%:* Ledercort Cream should be stored in a cool place, in either the original pack or in containers with complete closure.

The cream may be diluted, taking hygienic precautions, with aqueous cream. The diluted cream must be freshly prepared and not used more than one month after issue.

Ledercort Ointment 0.1%: Ledercort Ointment should be stored in a cool place, in either the original pack or in containers which prevent access of moisture. The ointment may be diluted with a basis consisting of 1 part wool fat and 9 parts white soft paraffin.

Legal category POM.

Package quantities *Ledercort Cream 0.1%:* 15 g tube and 250 g jar.

Ledercort Ointment 0.1%: 15 g tube and 250 g jar.

Further information Nil.

Product licence numbers
Ledercort Cream 0.1%   0095/5004
Ledercort Ointment 0.1%   0095/5005

LEDERCORT* TABLETS

Presentation *Tablets 2 mg:* Each blue, oblong tablet coded 'LLII' contains triamcinolone 2 mg.

Tablets 4 mg: Each white, oblong tablet coded 'LL4406' contains triamcinolone 4 mg.

Uses Ledercort is a potent glucocorticoid indicated in the treatment of rheumatoid arthritis; rheumatic fever; disseminated lupus erythematosus and other collagen diseases; nephrotic syndrome; bronchial asthma and respiratory allergy; pulmonary emphysema and fibrosis; allergic and inflammatory dermatoses, and haemolytic diseases.

Dosage and administration

1. *General. Adults and children:* Ledercort is administered orally in a wide range of dosages. The doctor should individualise the dosage according to the condition. In adults and children over 75 lb (34 kg) body weight, the usual initial dose ranges from 8 mg to 16 mg per day in single or divided doses. For children under 75 lb (34 kg) the range is from 4 to 12 mg.

When a satisfactory response is obtained the initial dosage should be reduced gradually by 2 mg every two to three days until the smallest dosage is achieved which will adequately maintain the patient.

Elderly: Steroids should be used with caution in elderly patients.

2. *Dosage in specific conditions:*

(a) *Rheumatoid arthritis:* The initial suppressive dose usually ranges from 8 to 16 mg per day, although an occasional patient may require larger doses to suppress the disease adequately. Once the acute manifestations of the disease have subsided (usually within two to seven days) the dosage should gradually be reduced until the smallest maintenance dose is achieved. The daily maintenance dose has ranged from 2 to 16 mg per day, although an occasional patient may require more.

(b) *Rheumatic fever:* The initial dose is 16–20 mg daily; maintenance dosage is 6–20 mg daily. Dosage varies considerably according to the severity of the carditis and its complications.

(c) *Disseminated lupus erythematosus:* The initial suppressive dose in collagen diseases should be 20–30 mg daily, reducing gradually to maintenance levels when the desired response is noted. Maintenance dosage varies from 3 to 30 mg daily. In severely ill patients, larger doses may be necessary to control the disease.

(d) *Nephrotic syndrome:* 16–20 mg daily should be administered until diuresis occurs, usually by the fourteenth day. After diuresis begins it is advisable to continue treatment until maximum or complete chemical and clinical remission occurs; then dosage should be reduced gradually and finally discontinued.

(e) *Bronchial asthma and respiratory allergy, pulmonary emphysema and fibrosis:* In acute bronchial asthma, initial suppressive doses of 8–16 mg should be given to bring the disease under control within 24–48 hours. Rarely, more than 16 mg may be necessary.

The initial suppressive dose for pulmonary emphysema and pulmonary fibrosis is 8–12 mg daily; the maintenance dose varies and may be as little as 2–4 mg daily.

(f) *Dermatoses:* The initial suppressive dosage should be 8–16 mg daily, or higher in the rare case. The maintenance dose can be as little as 1–2 mg daily.

(g) *Haemolytic diseases:* Where steroid therapy is indicated in haemolytic diseases, the average initial dose of Ledercort is 12–24 mg daily.

3. *Change in maintenance from other glucocorticoids:* Because the variation in response to each glucocorticoid varies considerably with each type of disease, the following schedule should be adjusted according to individual response – 4 mg Ledercort for each:

25 mg cortisone
20 mg hydrocortisone
5 mg prednisone or prednisolone
4 mg methylprednisolone
0.75 mg dexamethasone
0.60 mg betamethasone

4. *Short-term therapy in asthma:* Ledercort can control exacerbations of asthma via a short-term dosage regimen that reduces as it progresses.

Short-term courses of either ten or four days duration may be prescribed, in the following schedules (using the 4 mg tablet):

| | Number of tablets | |
	Ten-day course	Four-day course
1st day	4	4
2nd day	4	3
3rd day	4	2
4th day	3	1
5th day	3	
6th day	3	
7th day	2	
8th day	2	
9th day	1	
10th day	1	

Contra-indications, warnings, etc

Contra-indications: Tuberculosis and herpes simplex are usually considered to be absolute contra-indications. Active peptic ulcer, acute glomerulonephritis, myasthenia gravis, osteoporosis, fresh intestinal anastomoses, diverticulitis, thrombophlebitis, psychic disturbances, pregnancy and local or systemic infections, including fungal and exanthematous diseases, are relative contra-indications.

Precautions: General precautions common to all corticosteroid therapy should be observed. Daily doses over 32 mg are seldom indicated. Patients should be kept under careful observation because a few may react with side-effects under certain conditions; in such an event, the drug should be discontinued.

Since adrenal cortical function may be suppressed by glucocorticoids, it is important that therapy be withdrawn gradually after long-term treatment. Adequate supporting measures, ACTH supplementation or increase in dosage, are indicated when undue stress, such as anaesthesia and surgical procedures, occurs during or after Ledercort therapy. Ledercort is not the treatment of choice in adrenocortical insufficiency.

The possibility of development of infectious disease during glucocorticoid therapy requires careful observation of the patient, because initial signs of the infection may be obscured. Appropriate antibiotic therapy should be instituted in such cases. Concurrent administration of barbiturates, phenytoin, phenylbutazone may increase corticosteroid levels, while if anticoagulants are given with corticosteroids, adjustment of dosage of the former is usually necessary. The use of corticosteroids in the presence of other disorders or drugs with specific actions (e.g., hypoglycaemics) impinging on the effects of corticosteroids will result in imbalance of control. Withdrawal may result in acute rebound exacerbation of disease, acute adrenocortical insufficiency, polyarteritis.

Side-effects: Ledercort may produce the side-effects common to all cortisone-like drugs: moon face, striae, acne, buffalo hump, osteoporosis, spontaneous fractures, amenorrhoea, aggravation of infection, psychic disturbances, thrombo-embolism, peptic ulcer, gastro-intestinal haemorrhage, hyperglycaemia, increased intracranial pressure, headache, insomnia, fatigue, purpura, hirsutism, vertigo and leucopenia, diminished lymphoid tissue and immune response may also occur. Caution is recommended during prolonged use in children because of the possibility of growth suppression. Subcapsular cataracts may be formed on high dosage for long periods. Flushing of the face may occur. Necrotising angiitis is a rare possibility. Ulcerative oesophagitis and acute pancreatitis have occurred during corticosteroid therapy and may be related to its administration.

The long-term administration of all anti-inflammatory steroids results in definite catabolic effects, as indicated by negative protein and calcium balance. This catabolic effect, coupled with anorexia, may produce weight loss, which is undesirable in some patients. A steroid myopathy with advanced muscle weakness may involve muscles of the thighs, pelvis and low back.

The effect of Ledercort on fluid and electrolyte balance differs from that of older corticosteroids in that it promotes mild sodium excretion. Patients with sodium retention and oedema, from underlying disease or from previous therapy with other corticosteroids, will frequently lose weight and show increased urinary output associated with sodium diuresis during the first three to seven days of therapy. This effect will not be seen in patients with decreased glomerular filtration.

Potassium balance is not affected under ordinary dosage circumstances, and potassium supplementation is not ordinarily necessary unless prolonged and/or high dosage is prescribed. Since hypertension and oedema are not commonly observed with Ledercort they should not be used as indications of overdosage.

Overdosage: No specific antidote. Symptomatic treatment with electrolyte supplements.

Pharmaceutical precautions The product should be stored at room temperature in either the original pack or in containers which prevent access of moisture.

Legal category POM.

Package quantities *Tablets 2 mg:* Bottles of 100 and 500.

Tablets 4 mg: Bottles of 30, 100 and 500.

Further information Nil.

Product licence numbers
Ledercort Tablets 2 mg   0095/5006
Ledercort Tablets 4 mg   0095/5007

LEDERFEN*

Presentation

300 mg tablets: Light blue, film coated, capsule shaped tablets each containing 300 mg of fenbufen and engraved 'Lederfen'.

300 mg capsules: Dark blue capsules, each containing 300 mg of fenbufen and printed 'Lederfen' on both the cap and body.

450 mg tablets: Light blue, film coated, lozenge shaped tablets each containing 450 mg of fenbufen and engraved 'Lederfen' on one face and '450' on the other.

Uses Lederfen is a potent non-steroidal anti-inflammatory and analgesic agent indicated for the symptomatic treatment of rheumatoid arthritis, osteoarthritis, ankylosing spondylitis and actual musculoskeletal disorders.

Dosage and administration *Adults: 300 mg:* One in the morning and two at night. *450 mg:* One in the morning and one at night.

Elderly: Lederfen may be used at the normal recommended dosage in elderly patients in whom renal impairment commonly occurs.

Children: Not recommended for administration to children under the age of 14.

Contra-indications, warnings, etc

Contra-indications: Hypersensitivity to propionic acid anti-inflammatory drugs, or aspirin.

Precautions: As with other non-steroidal anti-inflammatory agents, Lederfen should be used with great caution in patients with a history or evidence of active peptic or intestinal ulceration, and only when considered essential in pregnant and nursing women.

Warnings and adverse effects: Skin rashes are the most commonly encountered adverse reactions. Serious reactions such as erythema multiforme have occasionally been reported. Lederfen treatment should be discontinued immediately on appearance of a rash. Other side effects reported include gastrointestinal intolerance such as dyspepsia and nausea. Slight decreases in blood leucocytes, haemoglobin and haematocrit, as well as slight increases in prothrombin time and eosinophils, have occasionally been recorded. Transient elevations in values of liver function tests have occurred in some patients.

Drug interactions: When single doses of aspirin 900 mg and Lederfen 500 mg are administered together, serum concentrations of Lederfen and its metabolites are reduced by 10–20%. Concomitant use of aspirin may require adjustment of dosage of Lederfen.

Lederfen is strongly protein bound. Although no clinically significant interactions have been noted as yet, practitioners should be alert to this possibility.

Overdosage: There is no experience with overdosage, consequently the signs, symptoms and treatment have not been identified. There is no specific antidote.

Pharmaceutical precautions None.

Legal category POM.

Package quantities

300 mg tablets and capsules: Blister calendar packs of 84 designated Lederfen CP.

450 mg tablets: Bottles of 56 designated Lederfen 450.

Further information Fenbufen is a pro-drug.

Product licence numbers

Lederfen 300 mg tablets	0095/0081
Lederfen 300 mg capsules	0095/0043
Lederfen 450 mg tablets	0095/0092

LEDERMIX*

Presentation Ledermix combination kit consists of a package containing 4 units.

1. *Ledermix paste.* Each gram contains: Demeclocycline Calcium equivalent to Demeclocycline hydrochloride 30 mg. Triamcinolone acetonide 10 mg.

2. *Ledermix cement.* Each gram contains: Demeclocycline hydrochloride 20 mg. Triamcinolone acetonide 6.7 mg in combination with zinc oxide and calcium hydroxide.

3. *Hardener 'F' (fast setting time).* 85% w/w Eugenol USP in rectified turpentine oil.

4. *Hardener 'S' (slow setting time).* 85% w/w Eugenol USP and 10% w/w polyethylene glycol 4000 USP in rectified turpentine oil.

Uses Ledermix is a dental treatment which combines the antibiotic action of demeclocycline with the anti-inflammatory action of triamcinolone acetonide.

Ledermix is indicated in pulpitis, periodontitis, and hypersensitive dentine.

Dosage and administration *Adults and Children: Pulpitis:* In all instances of exposed pulp and in acute pulpitis (except total purulent pulpitis) Ledermix Paste is applied with a small cotton pledget to the dentine adjacent to the pulp or to the exposed pulp. The cavity is then closed with a temporary filling such as zinc oxide-eugenol. Approximately 3 to 6 days later the vitality of the tooth is determined, the cavity is reopened, and the cotton pledget is removed. The dentine close to the pulp, or the wound in the pulp, is covered with Ledermix Cement prepared in the following manner: To one drop of the Hardener (no more) add sufficient Ledermix Cement powder to obtain a homogeneous mixture of cream-like consistency. This cement, which hardens rapidly, may be applied with an amalgam plugger or blunt probe.

In small cavities with small areas of pulp exposure, Ledermix Cement suffices as a base. In larger cavities or more extensive pulp exposure, it is advisable to use Ledermix Cement as a lining cement only and then to cover it with a layer of zinc oxyphosphate cement before inserting the permanent amalgam filling. In certain instances of hyperaemia and partial serous pulpitis with closed pulp cavity, the use of Ledermix Paste may be eliminated and Ledermix Cement (mixed with the Hardener) applied in the first treatment period. However, as a general rule, and particularly in acute pulpitis and in teeth where the pulp is exposed, the prepared Ledermix Cement should *NOT* be applied without previous treatment with Ledermix Paste.

Periodontitis: In primary acute periodontitis and acute exacerbations of chronic periodontitis, the canal may be prepared to the apex at the first sitting. After irrigation, the canal may be filled completely with Ledermix Paste and sealed. This treatment can be repeated if necessary on the follow-up visit about one week later, or the canal may be irrigated to remove the paste and further treatment carried out according to one of the generally accepted methods. If an alveolar abscess is present, drainage should be effected before beginning treatment with Ledermix.

Hypersensitive Dentine: In instances of hypersensitive dentine following cavity or crown preparations, Ledermix Cement plus Hardener may be used as a lining for deep cavities.

Preparation of the cement: Ledermix Cement belongs to the class of zinc oxide-eugenol dental cements. The setting time of all such cements is greatly affected by temperature and humidity conditions and by the technique of the individual operator. Vigorous and prolonged mixing, or spreading the mix thinly over the slab leads to accelerated setting whilst lowering the temperature of the mixing slab will prolong the setting time. Under any given set of conditions, however, the operator may obtain a faster or slower setting of the paste by using the appropriate hardener. In general it will be found that the time required for the mixture to set, obtained by the use of Hardener "S", will be approximately 3 to 4 times that obtained with Hardener "F".

Under conditions of high temperature and humidity, care should be taken to blend rapidly a small amount of Ledermix Cement powder (taking no more than 10 to 15 seconds) into 1 drop of Hardener with 2 or 3 strokes of the spatula. All of the resultant mix should then be taken up at once on the spatula blade.

Contra-indications, warnings, etc

Contra-indications: Ledermix is contra-indicated in instances of *total* purulent pulpitis or in patients hypersensitive to any of the active ingredients.

Precautions: The suppression of the inflammatory process by the use of a corticosteroid may result in a temporary reduction of the resistance of the pulp to infection and reduced healing capacity. Prolonged or repeated use of an anti-infective may result in superinfection or development of resistant micro-organisms. Therefore, Ledermix Paste should not be in contact with the exposed pulp for too long. If the application of this water-soluble preparation is uncontrolled, or if the temporary filling fits loosely, the danger exists that the pulp may not survive. The tip of the Ledermix Paste tube should always be kept clean and tightly closed after use.

The Ledermix Cement Vial must be kept tightly closed after use.

If severe reactions or idiosyncrasies are encountered the filling should be removed and appropriate measures instituted. Although limited there is a possibility of systemic absorption of the anti-infective and corticosteroid resulting in the side effects associated with each component.

Side-effects: Since Ledermix is only administered locally, and the various constituents are drained from the site in minute amounts over a long period of time, the possibility of systemic side-effects is remote. Local side reactions are limited to paradental effects.

Pharmaceutical precautions The product should be stored in a cool place in the original pack. Each container must be kept tightly closed.

Legal category POM.

Package quantities *Ledermix Combination Kit:* 2 g bottle of cement powder.

5.0 ml bottle with separate dropper of Hardener 'F' (fast setting time).

5.0 ml bottle with separate dropper of Hardener 'S' (slow setting time).

3 g tube of Ledermix Paste.

Ledermix Refill Kit No. II:
5 g Ledermix Paste.

Ledermix Refill Kit No. III:
3 g Ledermix Powder.

Ledermix Refill Kit No. IV:
5 ml bottle with separate dropper of Hardener 'F'.

Ledermix Refill Kit No. V:
5 ml bottle with separate dropper of Hardener 'S'.

Further information Nil.

Product licence number 0095/5014.

LEDERMYCIN*

Presentation *Capsules 150 mg:* Each two-piece dark red/pale red hard shell capsule printed Lederle 9123 contains 150 mg of demeclocycline hydrochloride.

Tablets 300 mg: Each red, film-coated tablet printed Lederle 9157 contains 300 mg of demeclocycline hydrochloride.

Uses

1. A broad-spectrum antibiotic indicated for the treatment of infective conditions due to demeclocycline-sensitive organisms. Typical indications include: Ear, nose and throat infection. Acute and chronic bronchitis. Pneumonia. Venereal diseases. Non-gonococcal urethritis. Gastro-intestinal infections. Urinary tract infections. Soft tissue infections. Acne. Pre- and post-operative prophylaxis of infection, and other infections caused by Ledermycin-sensitive organisms.

2. For the treatment of chronic hyponatraemia associated with the syndrome of inappropriate secretion of antidiuretic hormone (SIADH), where water restriction is ineffective.

Dosage and administration

1. *For antibiotic use: Adults (Capsules, Tablets):* 600 mg daily in two or four divided doses. For primary atypical pneumonia the average daily dose is 900 mg in 3 divided doses for six days.

Elderly: Use with caution in elderly patients. See contra-indications and warnings.

Children: Not recommended for children under 8 years of age. Information on dosage is available on request where specifically indicated.

2. *For the treatment of chronic hyponatraemia due to SIADH. (Adults only):* Initially: 900–1,200 mg daily in divided doses. Maintenance dose: 600–900 mg daily in divided doses.

Ledermycin should be taken an hour before or two hours after meals and antibiotic therapy should be continued for one to three days after characteristic symptoms or fever have subsided. The incidence of rheumatic fever or glomerulonephritis following streptococcal infections suggests that therapy of a streptococcal infection should be continued for eight full days even though symptoms have subsided.

Ledermycin therapy in the treatment of chronic hyponatraemia due to SIADH should not be withdrawn without commencing other methods of control.

Contra-indications, warnings, etc

Contra-indications: A history of hypersensitivity to tetracyclines. Overt renal insufficiency. Systemic lupus erythematosus.

Warnings: Tetracyclines may cause a yellow to brown discolouration of the teeth in the developing foetus or child and therefore Ledermycin should only be administered if considered essential to pregnant women and young children under eight years of age. Ledermycin should be used with caution in patients with renal or hepatic dysfunction, or in conjunction with other potentially hepatotoxic drugs. Cross-resistance between tetracyclines may develop in micro-organisms and cross-sensitisation in patients. The treatment of chronic hyponatraemia may necessitate the administration of high doses of Ledermycin for prolonged periods, so increasing the potential for nephrotoxicity (manifested by rises in plasma urea and creatinine) and photo-allergic reactions.

Precautions: Absorption of Ledermycin is impaired by the concomitant administration of calcium, magnesium, iron and particularly aluminium salts commonly used as antacids. Tetracyclines depress plasma prothrombin activity therefore reduced dosages of concurrent anticoagulants may be required. Lower doses are indicated in cases of renal impairment to avoid excessive systemic accumulation, and if therapy is prolonged, serum level determinations are advisable.

Side-effects: Nausea, diarrhoea and dermatitis may occur, and, as with all antibiotics, overgrowth of resistant organisms may cause glossitis, stomatitis, vaginitis or staphylococcal enterocolitis. Ledermycin has the greatest potential of the tetracycline analogues for causing photo-allergic reactions in hypersensitive persons. Such patients should be warned to avoid direct exposure to natural or artificial sunlight and to discontinue therapy at the first sign of skin discomfort. Occurrences of enamel hypoplasia have been reported. Rarely, increased intracranial pressure with bulging fontanelles has been observed in infants which disappears rapidly upon cessation of treatment. Rare cases of anaphylactoid reactions have been reported.

Overdosage: No specific antidote. Gastric lavage plus oral administration of milk or antacids.

Pharmaceutical precautions Ledermycin Capsules and Tablets should be stored at room temperature.

Legal category POM.

Package quantities *Capsules 150 mg:* Bottles of 100. *Tablets 300 mg:* Bottles of 100.

Further information Nil.

Product licence numbers
Capsules 150 mg	0095/0052
Tablets 300 mg	0095/5044

LEDERSPAN* INJECTION 20 mg/ml
LEDERSPAN* INJECTION 5 mg/ml

Presentation *Suspension 20 mg/ml:* Vials containing a sterile suspension of 20 mg or 100 mg of micronised triamcinolone hexacetonide in 1 ml or 5 ml respectively of an aqueous vehicle with 0.9% benzyl alcohol as a preservative.

Suspension 5 mg/ml: Vials containing a sterile suspension of 25 mg of micronised triamcinolone hexacetonide in 5 ml of an aqueous vehicle with 0.9% benzyl alcohol as a preservative.

Uses Triamcinolone hexacetonide is a relatively insoluble corticosteroid (0.0003% at 25°C in water). It has a prolonged effect on tissue at the local injection site, the duration usually ranging from a few weeks to several months.

Lederspan 20 mg/ml *(for intra-articular and intrasynovial administration)* is indicated in the treatment of rheumatoid arthritis; osteoarthritis; traumatic arthritis; gouty arthritis; synovitis and bursitis; fibrositis, tendinitis, and epicondylitis; intermittent hydrarthrosis; and other subacute or chronic diseases where glucocorticoids can be expected to be useful.

Lederspan 5 mg/ml *(for intralesional and sublesional administration)* is indicated in the treatment of cystic acne; alopecia areata, nummular and dyshidrotic eczema; granuloma annulare; keloids; lichen planus; discoid lupus erythematosus; localised neurodermatitis; prurigo nodularis; and psoriasis of the nails.

Dosage and administration *Adults and children:* For intra-articular and intrasynovial use, 2–30 mg (0.1–1.5 ml), depending on the size of the joint (or synovial space) to be injected, the degree of inflammation and the amount of fluid present. In general, large joints (such as knee, hips, shoulder), require 10–30 mg whereas small joints (such as interphalangeal, metacarpophalangeal) require 2–6 mg. When much synovial fluid is present, aspiration may be performed before administering Lederspan. Subsequent dosage and frequency of injection can best be judged by clinical response. Since Lederspan provides prolonged activity, injections into a single joint or synovial space more frequently than every three to four weeks are not recommended. Repeated intra-articular injections should be as infrequent as possible, consistent with adequate patient care.

For intralesional and sublesional use, the dosage is 0.5 mg or less per square inch of affected skin.

Strict asepsis is mandatory during administration. Topical ethyl chloride spray may be used locally before injection. Since micronised triamcinolone hexacetonide has been designed for ease of administration, a small-bore needle (including 24 gauge needles) may be used. The vial should be gently agitated to achieve uniform suspension before each use.

The optimum dilution (see under 'Pharmaceutical precautions') should be determined according to the nature of the lesion, its size, the depth of the injection, the volume needed, and the location of the lesion. In general, more superficial injections should be accomplished with more dilution. Certain conditions, such as keloids, require a less dilute suspension. Subsequent dose, dilution and frequency of injection should be determined on the basis of the clinical response. With the 20 mg/ml suspension, concentrations stronger than 1:4 should not be used intralesionally, since local subcutaneous atrophy may result.

Lederspan may be administered by Dermojet and the Porton Injector.

Elderly: Steroids should be used with caution in elderly patients.

Contra-indications, warnings, etc
Contra-indications: Although active, latent or questionably healed tuberculosis, ocular herpes simplex and acute psychosis are generally considered to be absolute contra-indications to glucocorticoid therapy, the minimal systemic activity of triamcinolone hexacetonide after local injection might permit cautious use when indicated. The drug should not be used when there is history of hypersensitivity to any of the components of the formulation or when previous injections have produced

local atrophy. Infected joints should not be injected with corticosteroids.

As with other glucocorticoid agents, relative contra-indications are active peptic ulcer, acute glomerulonephritis, myasthenia gravis, osteoporosis, fresh intestinal anastomoses, diverticulitis, thrombophlebitis, psychic disturbances, pregnancy, diabetes mellitus, hyperthyroidism, acute coronary artery disease, hypertension, limited cardiac reserve and local or systemic infections, including fungal and exanthematous diseases. The minimal systemic activity of this preparation, however, reduces the risks involved in its use in the presence of these conditions.

Precautions and side-effects: As with all glucocorticoids, an exacerbation of symptoms or 'flare-up' may occur following intra-articular or intrasynovial injections. Local atrophy, burning, flushing, pain and swelling may occur. In addition, prolonged and repeated use in weight-bearing joints may result in further joint degeneration. This is probably related to premature use of still-diseased joints following relief of pain and other symptoms. Not more than two or three large joints should be treated simultaneously in the same patient.

In treating conditions such as tendinitis or tenosynovitis care should be taken that Lederspan is injected into the space between tendon sheath and tendon and not into the tendon itself.

Overdosage or excessive frequency of intralesional injections into the same site may produce local subcutaneous atrophy. If this occurs, recovery may be delayed for several months because of the prolonged action of the drug. Other local effects include abscess, erythema, pain, swelling and necrosis at the injection site.

Systemic effects are rare with Lederspan due to its slow release from the injection site. In addition to those common to all glucocorticoids, some effects particularly associated with triamcinolone therapy are anorexia, myopathy and depression of mood.

If severe reactions occur or an acute infection develops during therapy, use of the drug should be discontinued and appropriate measures taken.

Pharmaceutical precautions Lederspan should be stored at room temperature. Do not freeze.

It may be diluted with Water for Injections BP, Sodium Chloride Intravenous Infusion BP, Sodium Chloride and Glucose Intravenous Infusion BP, Lignocaine Hydrochloride Injection BP, immediately prior to injection.

Fluids containing methyl or propyl hydroxybenzoates or phenol should be avoided since these tend to cause flocculation of the steroid.

Legal category POM.

Package quantities *20 mg/ml:* Single vials containing 20 mg in 1 ml or 100 mg in 5 ml.

5 mg/ml: Single vials containing 25 mg in 5 ml.

Further information Nil.

Product licence numbers
Lederspan 20 mg/ml 0095/0008
Lederspan 5 mg/ml 0095/0009

LEUCOVORIN – see Calcium Leucovorin.

METHOTREXATE TABLETS
METHOTREXATE INJECTION
METHOTREXATE POWDER FOR INJECTION

Presentation *Tablets 2.5 mg:* Round, convex, scored, uncoated, yellow tablets embossed 'LL' and 'M1' and containing 2.5 mg of Methotrexate per tablet.

Tablets 10 mg: Round, convex, scored, uncoated, large, yellow tablets embossed 'LL' and 'M11' and containing 10 mg of Methotrexate per tablet.

Injection: A clear, yellow, sterile, aqueous, isotonic solution containing Methotrexate Sodium equivalent to 2.5 mg (ampoule), 5 mg, 25 mg, 50 mg, 100 mg, 200 mg, 500 mg, 1 g, or 5 g of methotrexate per vial together with sodium chloride and sodium hydroxide to adjust the pH to approximately 8.5. The Injection does not contain an antimicrobial preservative.

Powder for Injection 500 mg and 1 g: Vials containing a yellow, lyophilised powder of Methotrexate sodium equivalent to 500 mg or 1 g of Methotrexate, which is reconstituted before use with 10 ml or 20 ml of Water for Injection respectively. The Powder for Injection does not contain an antimicrobial preservative.

Uses *Properties:* Methotrexate, a derivative of folic acid, belongs to the class of cytotoxic agents known as antimetabolites. It acts principally during the 'S' phase of cell division, by the competitive inhibition of the enzyme dihydrofolate reductase, thus preventing the reduction of dihydrofolate to tetrahydrofolate, a necessary step in the process of DNA synthesis and cellular replication.

Indications: The treatment of neoplastic disease. The treatment of severe cases of uncontrolled psoriasis, unresponsive to conventional therapy.

Dosage and administration *Adults and children:* Methotrexate may be given by oral, intramuscular, intravenous (bolus injection or infusion) intrathecal, intra-arterial and intraventricular routes of administration. Dosages are based on the patient's body weight or surface area except in the case of intrathecal or intraventricular administration when a maximum dose of 15 mg is recommended. Doses should be reduced in cases of haematological deficiency and hepatic or renal impairment. Larger doses (greater than 100 mg) are usually given by intravenous infusion over periods not exceeding 24 hours. Part of the dose may be given as an initial rapid intravenous injection.

All parenteral Methotrexate preparations are stable for 24 hours when diluted with the following intravenous infusion fluids:—0.9% Sodium Chloride. Glucose. Sodium Chloride and Glucose. Compound Sodium Chloride (Ringers Injection). Compound Sodium Lactate (Lactated Ringers Injection).

Methotrexate has been used with beneficial effects in a wide variety of neoplastic diseases, alone and in combination with other cytotoxic agents, hormones, immunotherapy, radiotherapy or surgery. Dosage schedules therefore vary considerably, depending on the clinical use, particularly when intermittent high-dose regimes are followed by the administration of Calcium Leucovorin (calcium folinate) in order to rescue normal cells from toxic effects.

Dosage regimes for Calcium Leucovorin rescue are discussed under Further Information.

Examples of doses of Methotrexate that have been used for particular indications are given below.

Choriocarcinoma and other trophoblastic tumours: Non-metastatic gestational trophoblastic neoplasms have been treated successfully with 0.25–1 mg/kg up to a maximum of 60 mg intramuscularly every 48 hours for four doses, followed by Calcium Leucovorin rescue. This course of treatment is repeated at seven day intervals until levels of urinary chorionic gonadotrophin hormone return to normal. Not less than four courses of treatment are usually necessary. Patients with complications, such as extensive metastases, may be treated with Methotrexate in combination with other cytotoxic drugs.

Methotrexate has also been used in similar doses for the treatment of hydatidiform mole and chorio-adenoma destruens.

Leukaemia in children: Remissions in acute lymphocytic leukaemia are usually best induced with a combination of corticosteroids and other cytotoxic agents.

Methotrexate 15 mg/m^2, given parenterally or orally once weekly, in combination with other drugs appears to be the treatment of choice for the maintenance of drug-induced remissions.

Meningeal leukaemia in children: The cerebro-spinal fluid (CSF) should be examined in all leukaemic patients in order to diagnose leukaemic invasion of the central nervous system. Doses up to 15 mg, intrathecally, at weekly intervals, until the CSF appears normal (usually 2–3 weeks), have been found useful for the treatment of meningeal leukaemia. It is now common practice because of the frequency of meningeal leukaemia to administer Methotrexate intrathecally, in similar doses, as prophylaxis in all cases of lymphocytic leukaemia.

Although intravenous doses of the order of 50 mg of Methotrexate do not appreciably penetrate the CSF, larger doses of the order of 500 mg/m^2 do produce cytotoxic levels of Methotrexate in the CSF. This type of therapy has been used in short courses, followed by administration of Calcium Leucovorin, as initial maintenance therapy to prevent leukaemic invasion of the central nervous system in children with poor prognosis lymphocytic leukaemia.

Lymphoma: Non-Hodgkin's lymphoma, e.g. childhood lymphosarcoma has recently been treated with 3–30 mg/kg (approximately 90–900 mg/m^2) of Methotrexate given by intravenous injection and infusion followed by administration of Calcium Leucovorin with the higher doses. Some cases of Burkitt's lymphoma, when treated in the early stages with courses of 15 mg/m^2 daily for five days have shown prolonged remissions. Combination chemotherapy is also commonly used in all stages of the disease and a course of 15 mg/day of Methotrexate intrathecally for four days has been found useful for controlling episodes of invasion of the central nervous system.

Breast cancer: Methotrexate, in intravenous doses of 10–60 mg/m^2, is commonly included in cyclical combination regimes with other cytotoxic drugs in the treatment of advanced breast cancer. Similar regimes have also been used as adjuvant therapy in early cases following mastectomy and/or radiotherapy.

Osteogenic sarcoma: The use of Methotrexate alone and in cyclical combination regimes has recently been introduced as an adjuvant therapy to the primary treatment of osteogenic sarcoma by amputation with or without prosthetic bone replacement. This has involved the use of intravenous infusions of 20–300 mg/kg (approximately 600–9,000 mg/m^2) of Methotrexate followed by Calcium Leucovorin rescue. Methotrexate has also been used as the sole treatment in metastatic cases of osteogenic sarcoma.

Bronchogenic carcinoma: Intravenous infusions of 20–100 mg/m^2 of Methotrexate have been included in cyclical combination regimes for the treatment of advanced tumours. High doses with Calcium Leucovorin rescue have also been employed as the sole treatment.

Head and neck cancer: Intravenous infusions of 240–1,080 mg/m^2 with Calcium Leucovorin rescue have been used recently with encouraging results both as pre-operative adjuvant therapy and in the treatment of advanced tumours. Intra-arterial infusions of Methotrexate are indicated for certain head and neck cancers although this route of administration is not now used extensively.

Bladder carcinoma: Intravenous injections or infusions of Methotrexate in doses up to 100 mg every one to two weeks have been used in the treatment of bladder carcinoma with promising results, varying from only symptomatic relief to complete though unsustained regressions. Diuretics and hydration are employed in an attempt to reduce the excessive drug toxicity that has occurred in cases with renal impairment. The use of higher doses of Methotrexate with Calcium Leucovorin rescue is currently being evaluated.

Psoriasis: In cases of severe uncontrolled psoriasis, unresponsive to conventional therapy, 10–25 mg orally once a week and adjusted by the patient's response is recommended.

Particular attention should be given to the appearance of liver toxicity by carrying out liver function tests before starting Methotrexate treatment and repeating these at two to four month intervals during therapy. Treatment should not be instituted or should be discontinued if any abnormality of liver function tests, or liver biopsy, is present or develops during therapy.

Such abnormalities should return to normal within two weeks after which treatment may be recommenced at the discretion of the physician.

The use of Methotrexate may permit the return to conventional topical therapy which should be encouraged.

Contra-indications, warnings, etc

Contra-indications: Profound impairment of renal or hepatic function. Serious cases of anaemia, leucopenia, or thrombocytopenia. Pregnancy.

Warnings: Methotrexate should not normally be administered to patients who are pregnant or to mothers who are breast-feeding. Methotrexate has been shown to be teratogenic. Methotrexate should be used with extreme caution in patients with haematological depression, renal impairment, peptic ulcer, ulcerative colitis, ulcerative stomatitis, diarrhoea, debility and in extreme youth or old age.

Symptoms of gastro-intestinal toxicity, usually first manifested by stomatitis, indicates interruption of therapy otherwise haemorrhagic enteritis and death from intestinal perforation may occur.

Methotrexate affects spermatogenesis and oogenesis during the period of its administration which may result in decreased fertility. To date this effect appears to be reversible on discontinuing therapy. Conception should be avoided for at least six months after treatment with Methotrexate has ceased. Patients receiving Methotrexate and their partners should be advised appropriately.

Methotrexate has some immunosuppressive activity and therefore the immunological response to concurrent vaccination may be decreased. In addition, concomitant use of a live vaccine could cause a severe antigenic reaction.

Precautions: Methotrexate should only be used by clinicians who are familiar with the various characteristics of the drug and its established clinical usage. It is essential that the following laboratory tests are included as part of the clinical evaluation and monitoring of patients receiving Methotrexate: complete haematological analysis, urinalysis, renal function tests, liver function tests and, when high doses are administered, determination of plasma levels of Methotrexate. These tests should be performed prior to, during and after termination of each course of therapy.

Haemopoietic suppression caused by Methotrexate may occur abruptly and with apparently safe dosages. Any profound drop in white-cell or platelet counts indicates immediate withdrawal of the drug and appropriate supportive therapy.

It should be noted that intrathecal doses are transported into the cardiovascular system and may give rise to unexpected systemic toxicity, as can the use of Methotrexate in patients with renal dysfunction, ascites, or other effusions due to a longer serum half-life.

High doses may cause the precipitation of Methotrexate or its metabolites in the renal tubules. Alkalinisation of the urine to pH 6.5–7.0 by the oral or intravenous administration of sodium bicarbonate (5×625 mg tablets every three hours) or Diamox (500 mg orally four times a day) is recommended as a preventative measure.

Drug interactions: Methotrexate is extensively protein bound and may be displaced by certain drugs such as salicylates, sulphonamides, diuretics, hypoglycaemics, diphenylhydantoins, tetracyclines, chloramphenicol, p-aminobenzoic acid, and the acidic anti-inflammatory agents, so causing a potential for increased toxicity when used concurrently. Concomitant use of other drugs with nephrotoxic or hepatotoxic potential (including alcohol) should be avoided.

Side-effects: These occur as a result of cytotoxic activity on rapidly reproducing normal cells of the haemopoietic system, gastro-intestinal tract, and sometimes skin. Consequently common adverse reactions are bone-marrow depression, leucopenia, anaemia, thrombocytopenia, nausea, vomiting, diarrhoea and ulcerative stomatitis. Upon prolonged treatment erythematous rashes, hepatic cirrhosis, acute liver atrophy and genitourinary toxicity manifested by renal failure, severe nephropathy, defective oogenesis or spermatogenesis may occur.

Adverse effects upon the central nervous system that may occur following intrathecal or intraventricular administration are headache, drowsiness, blurred vision, transient paresis, ataxia, and rarely, dementia and major convulsions. Other reactions such as pneumonitis, osteoporotic effects and photosensitivity have been attributed to the use of Methotrexate.

Overdosage: Calcium Leucovorin is the antidote for neutralising the immediate toxic effects of Methotrexate on the haemopoietic system. It may be administered orally, intramuscularly, or by an intravenous bolus injection or infusion. In cases of accidental overdosage, a dose of Calcium Leucovorin equal to or higher than the offending dose of Methotrexate should be administered within one hour and further doses as required. Other supporting therapy such as a blood transfusion and renal dialysis may be required.

Pharmaceutical precautions Methotrexate Powder

for Injection 500 mg and 1 g should be reconstituted immediately before use with 10 ml or 20 ml Water for Injection respectively. The appropriate dose of the resulting solution (50 mg/ml) is then diluted for administration by intravenous infusion over periods not exceeding 24 hours. Part of the dose may be given by an initial bolus intravenous injection.

Parenteral Methotrexate preparations do not contain an antimicrobial preservative; any unused injection or reconstituted solution from Powder for Injection should be discarded.

Parenteral Methotrexate preparations are stable for 24 hours when diluted with the following intravenous infusion fluids:—0.9% Sodium Chloride. Glucose. Sodium Chloride and Glucose. Compound Sodium Chloride (Ringers Injection). Compound Sodium Lactate (Lactated Ringers Injection).

Methotrexate preparations should be protected from direct sunlight. Other drugs should not be mixed with Methotrexate in the same infusion container.

Legal category POM.

Package quantities

Tablets 2.5 mg: Bottles of 100.

Tablets 10 mg: Bottles of 50.

Injection 2.5 mg in 1 ml: Boxes of 10 ampoules.

Injection 5 mg in 2 ml: Boxes of 5 vials.

Injection 25 mg in 1 ml: Boxes of 1 vial.

Injection 50 mg in 2 ml: Boxes of 1 vial.

Injection 100 mg in 4 ml: Boxes of 1 vial.

Injection 200 mg in 8 ml: Boxes of 1 vial.

Injection 500 mg in 20 ml: Boxes of 1 vial.

Injection 1 g in 40 ml: Boxes of 1 vial.

Injection 5 g in 200 ml: Boxes of 1 vial.

Powder for Injection 500 mg: Boxes of 1 vial.

Powder for Injection 1 g: Boxes of 1 vial.

Further information Dosage regimes for Calcium Leucovorin rescue vary, depending upon the dose of Methotrexate administered. In general, up to 120 mg are usually given in divided doses, over 12–24 hours, by intramuscular injection, bolus intravenous injection or intravenous infusion in normal saline, followed by 12–15 mg intramuscularly, or 15 mg (1 tablet) orally, every six hours for the next 48 hours. Rescue therapy is usually started following a delay, of up to 24 hours, from the beginning of the Methotrexate infusion. One tablet (15 mg) of Calcium Leucovorin every six hours for 48–72 hours may be sufficient when lower doses (less than 100 mg) of Methotrexate have been given.

Calcium Leucovorin is available as an injection (3 mg/ml) in 1 ml ampoules, as a vial of powder for injection (15 mg and 30 mg) and as tablets (15 mg) in bottles of 10.

The clinical use of high doses of Methotrexate with Calcium Leucovorin rescue in the treatment of a wide variety of previously resistant tumours remains the subject of intense research. Further information on other formulations of Methotrexate, on results with particular cyclical regimes of combinations of cytotoxic drugs and any other aspects of cancer chemotherapy with Methotrexate is available on request.

Product licence numbers

Tablets 2.5 mg	0095/5079
Tablets 10 mg	0095/0060

Injection 2.5 mg/ml	0095/0015
Injection 25 mg/ml	0095/0016
Powder for Injection 500 mg	0095/0054
Powder for Injection 1 g	0095/0055

MINOCIN* 50 and 100

Presentation *Tablets 100 mg:* Each orange, film-coated tablet, embossed LL on one face and M/100 on the reverse face, contains Minocycline hydrochloride equivalent to 100 mg Minocycline base.

Tablets 50 mg: Each beige film-coated tablet, embossed LL on one face and M/50 on the reverse face, contains Minocycline hydrochloride equivalent to 50 mg Minocycline base.

Uses Minocycline is a broad spectrum antibiotic used for the treatment of infections caused by tetracycline-sensitive organisms. Some tetracycline-resistant strains of Staphylococci are also sensitive.

Typical indications include: Gonorrhoea. Non-gono-coccal urethritis. Prostatitis. Acne. Acute and chronic bronchitis. Bronchiectasis. Lung abscess. Pneumonia. Ear nose and throat infections. Urinary tract infections. Salpingitis. Skin and soft tissue infections. Ophthalmological infections. Nocardiosis. Prophylactic treatment of asymptomatic meningococcal carriers. Pre- and postoperative prophylaxis of infection.

Dosage and administration *Adults:*
1. Routine antibiotic use: 200 mg initially followed by 200 mg daily in divided doses.
2. Acne: Initially 100–200 mg daily in single or divided doses. Average Maintenance Dose: 50 mg twice daily.
3. Gonorrhoea: In adult males, 300 mg as a single dose. Adult females may require more prolonged therapy.
4. Prophylaxis of asymptomatic meningococcal carriers: 100 mg b.i.d. for five days, usually followed by a course of rifampicin.

Elderly: Minocin may be used at the normal recommended dosage in elderly patients even with mild to moderate renal impairment.

Children: Safety for use in children under 13 years of age has not been established.

Administration: Unlike earlier tetracyclines, absorption of Minocin is not significantly impaired by food or moderate amounts of milk. A normal course of treatment for acute bacterial infections is four days. In more severe infections, treatment should be continued for up to three days after characteristic symptoms of the infection have subsided. Because of the incidence of rheumatic fever or glomerulonephritis following streptococcal infection, therapy should be continued for 10 days even though symptoms have subsided.

Treatment of acne should be continued for a minimum of six weeks.

Contra-indications, warnings, etc
Contra-indications: Known hypersensitivity to tetracyclines. Systemic lupus erythematosus.

Warnings: Tetracyclines may cause a yellow to brown discoloration of the teeth and enamel hypoplasia in the developing foetus or child and therefore Minocin should only be administered if considered essential to pregnant or lactating women and to children under eight years of age.

Minocin should be used with caution in patients with hepatic dysfunction and in conjunction with alcohol or other potentially hepatotoxic drugs. Cross-resistance between tetracyclines may develop in micro-organisms and cross-sensitisation in patients.

Precautions: Clinical studies have shown that there is no significant drug accumulation in patients with renal impairment when they are treated with Minocin in the recommended doses. In cases of extreme renal insufficiency, reduction of dosage and monitoring of renal function may be required.

Tetracyclines depress plasma prothrombin activity and reduced doses of concomitant anticoagulants may be necessary.

Absorption of Minocin is impaired by the concomitant administration of iron salts and by antacids containing calcium, magnesium and aluminium salts.

Side-effects: Gastro-intestinal disturbances may occur and as with all antibiotics overgrowth of resistant organisms may cause glossitis, stomatitis, vaginitis or staphylococcal enteritis. Photo-sensitivity and dermatological reactions are rare.

Lightheadedness, dizziness and vertigo have occurred with Minocin and patients should be warned about the possible hazards of driving or operating machinery during treatment.

Overdosage: No specific antidote. Gastric lavage plus appropriate supportive treatment.

Pharmaceutical precautions The product should be stored under normal room temperature conditions in the original pack or in containers which prevent access of moisture.

Legal category POM.

Package quantities *100 mg Tablets:* Bottles of 20 and 50.

50 mg Tablets: Blister packs of 84.

Further information Nil.

Product licence numbers
100 mg Tablets   0095/0006
50 mg Tablets   0095/0062

MYAMBUTOL*

Presentation *Tablets 100 mg:* Each yellow, coated tablet contains 100 mg ethambutol hydrochloride.

Tablets 400 mg: Each grey, coated tablet contains 400 mg ethambutol hydrochloride.

Powder: Each bottle contains 50 g ethambutol hydrochloride.

Uses The primary treatment and re-treatment of tuberculosis and for prophylaxis in cases of inactive tuberculosis or large tuberculin-positive reaction. Myambutol should only be used in conjunction with other antituberculous drugs to which the patient's organisms are susceptible.

Dosage and administration The dosage of Myambutol must be adjusted according to the body weight of the patient.

Adults: For primary treatment and prophylaxis: Myambutol should be administered in a single daily oral dose of 15 mg/kg, concomitant drugs being used at their recommended dosage levels.

For re-treatment: For the first 60 days of treatment, Myambutol should be administered in a single daily oral dose of 25 mg/kg. Thereafter the dosage should be reduced to 15 mg/kg, concomitant drugs being maintained at their recommended dosage levels.

Children: For primary treatment and re-treatment: For the first 60 days of treatment, a single daily oral dose of 25 mg/kg. Thereafter the dosage should be reduced to 15 mg/kg, concomitant drugs being maintained at their recommended dosage levels.

For prophylaxis: A single daily oral dose of 15 mg/kg, concomitant drugs being used at their recommended dosage levels.

Elderly: Because of potential toxicity Myambutol should be used with extreme caution in elderly patients. See contra-indications and warnings.

Administration: In order to obtain maximum effect due to high serum levels, drug administration should be once daily. Absorption of Myambutol is not significantly altered by administration with food.

Paediatric doses can be given using an extemporaneously prepared syrup (see Further Information).

A table of dosages is given in the next column.

Contra-indications, warnings, etc

Contra-indications: Myambutol is contra-indicated in patients who are known to be hypersensitive to the drug. It is also contra-indicated in patients with known optic neuritis unless clinical judgement determines that it may be used.

Precautions: Patients with decreased renal function may need to have the dosage adjusted as determined by blood levels of Myambutol. Animal studies with Myambutol have not demonstrated any teratogenic potential and there have been several reports of the drug having been administered during pregnancy without untoward effect. Nevertheless, it is recommended that the possibility of such effects should be kept in mind when treating women of child-bearing age.

Because this drug has a unique effect on the eye, it is recommended that patients undergo a full ophthalmic examination before starting treatment. This should include visual acuity, colour vision, perimetry and ophthalmoscopy. Many physicians consider that routine ophthalmological examination for adults is not thereafter necessary, but patients should be informed of the importance of reporting any change in vision. However, routine ophthalmological examinations may be considered desirable when treating young children.

Side-effects: Myambutol may produce a unique type of visual impairment which is generally reversible and which appears to be due to optic neuritis and to be related to dose and duration of treatment. Less than 1% of patients undergoing treatment with the higher dose regimen of 25 mg/kg/day for two months, and 15 mg/kg/day thereafter, have exhibited decrease in visual acuity. The change may be unilateral or bilateral and hence both eyes must be tested individually. The effects are generally reversible when administration of the drug is discontinued promptly. In rare cases recovery may be delayed for up to one year or more and the effect may possibly be irreversible in these cases.

Recovery of visual acuity has usually occurred over a period of weeks to months after the drug was discontinued, and patients have then received Myambutol at lower dosages without toxicity. Test patients receiving Myambutol as sole therapy did not have gastro-intestinal disturbances (e.g. anorexia, nausea, vomiting, diarrhoea), transient impairment of liver function or allergic

Dosage of Myambutol

15 mg/kg (7 mg/lb) schedule:

Weight range	kg	Total daily dose (mg)	Number of tablets		
				100 mg	400 mg
Children	8	120			
	17	255			
	25	375			
	33	495			
Adults					
lb	kg			100 mg	400 mg
85–94.5	38–42.5	600	2	+	1
95–109.5	43–49.5	700	3	+	1
110–124.5	50–56.5	800			2
125–139.5	57–63.5	900	1	+	2
140–154.5	64–70.5	1,000	2	+	2
155–169.5	71–78.5	1,100	3	+	2
170–184.5	79–83.5	1,200			3
185–199.5	84–89.5	1,300	1	+	3
200–214.5	90–96.5	1,400	2	+	3
215 and over	97 and over	1,500	3	+	3

25 mg/kg (11 mg/lb) schedule:

Weight range	kg	Total daily dose (mg)	Number of tablets		
				100 mg	400 mg
Children	5	125			
	10	250			
	15	375			
	20	500			
	25	625			
	30	750			
	35	875			
Adults					
lb	kg			100 mg	400 mg
85–92.5	38–41.5	1,000	2	+	2
93–101.5	42–44.5	1,100	3	+	2
102–109.5	45–49.5	1,200			3
110–118.5	50–53.5	1,300	1	+	3
119–128.5	54–57.5	1,400	2	+	3
129–136.5	58–61.5	1,500	3	+	3
137–146.5	62–66.5	1,600			4
147–155.5	67–70.5	1,700	1	+	4
156–164.5	71–74.5	1,800	2	+	4
165–173.5	75–78.5	1,900	3	+	4
174–182.5	79–82.5	2,000			5
183–191.5	83–86.5	2,100	1	+	5
192–199.5	87–90.5	2,200	2	+	5
200–209.5	91–94.5	2,300	3	+	5
210–218.5	95–98.5	2,400			6
219 and over	99 and over	2,500	1	+	6

reactions, although these have been noted during multiple-drug antituberculous therapy in which Myambutol was employed. Numbness and paraesthesia of the extremities have been reported.

Overdosage: No specific antidote, but gastric lavage should be employed if necessary.

Pharmaceutical precautions Myambutol should be stored at room temperature in either the original pack or in containers which prevent access of moisture.

Legal category POM.

Package quantities *Myambutol 100 mg:* Bottles of 100 and 500.

Myambutol 400 mg: Bottles of 100 and 500.

Powder: Bottles of 50 g.

Further information Details of a formulation for

ethambutol syrup suitable for paediatric use are available on request from the Medical Information Department. A mixture of ethambutol syrup and isoniazid elixir BPC should not be prepared as isoniazid is unstable in the presence of sugars.

Product licence numbers
Myambutol 100 mg   0095/0002
Myambutol 400 mg   0095/0003
Myambutol Powder 50 g   0095/5083

MYNAH*

Presentation *Mynah 200:* Each white tablet coded 'Lederle 5033' contains 200 mg ethambutol hydrochloride plus 100 mg isoniazid.

Mynah 250: Each yellow tablet coded 'Lederle 5133' contains 250 mg ethambutol hydrochloride plus 100 mg isoniazid.

Mynah 300: Each orange tablet coded 'Lederle 5137' contains 300 mg ethambutol hydrochloride plus 100 mg isoniazid.

Mynah 365: Each pink tablet coded 'Lederle 5134' contains 365 mg ethambutol hydrochloride plus 100 mg isoniazid.

Uses The primary treatment and re-treatment of tuberculosis and for prophylaxis in cases of inactive tuberculosis or large tuberculin-positive reaction.

Dosage and administration *Adults:* Dosage of Mynah is gauged according to the patient's body weight, which governs the included amount of ethambutol; the dosage of isoniazid is standardised at 100 mg per tablet.

For primary treatment and prophylaxis: Mynah should be administered in a single daily oral dose such that the patient receives 15 mg/kg of ethambutol plus 300 mg isoniazid, concomitant drugs being used at their recommended dosage levels.

For re-treatment: For the first 60 days of treatment Mynah should be administered in a single daily oral dose such that the patient receives 25 mg/kg of ethambutol plus 300 mg of isoniazid, concomitant drugs being used at their recommended dosage levels. Thereafter proceed as in 'Primary treatment' above.

Children: The quantities and proportions of the component drugs make Mynah tablets unsuitable for most children. (See Further Information).

Elderly: Because of potential toxicity Mynah should be used with extreme caution in elderly patients. See Contra-indications, warnings, etc.

Administration: In order to obtain maximum effect due to high serum levels, drug administration should be once daily. As absorption of isoniazid but not ethambutol is significantly reduced by administration with food, it is recommended that Mynah be taken on an empty stomach.

A table of dosages is given on the next page.

Contra-indications, warnings, etc
Contra-indications: Mynah is contra-indicated in patients who are known to be hypersensitive to ethambutol or isoniazid. It is also contra-indicated in patients with known optic neuritis unless clinical judgement determines that it may be used. Although no absolute contra-indications to the administration of isoniazid have been reported, care should be exercised in the administration of Mynah to epileptic patients since it may induce convulsions, or in psychotic states characterised by mania and hypomania, or in the presence of impaired renal function.

Precautions: Patients with decreased renal function may need to have the dosage adjusted as determined by blood levels of ethambutol. Animal studies with ethambutol have not demonstrated any teratogenic potential and there have been several reports of isoniazid or ethambutol having been administered during pregnancy without untoward effect. Nevertheless, it is recom-

Dosage of Mynah:

Table 1   Mynah tablets weight/dose schedule 15 mg/kg (7 mg/lb)

Body weight		Ingredients		
lb	kg	INH mg	Ethambutol mg	Daily dose
77–98	35–44.5	300	600	3 tablets Mynah 200
99–120	45–54.5	300	750	3 tablets Mynah 250
121–142	55–64.5	300	900	3 tablets Mynah 300
143–175	65–79.5	300	1095	3 tablets Mynah 365

Table 2   Mynah tablets weight/dose schedule 25 mg/kg (11 mg/lb)

Body weight		Ingredients		Daily dose	
lb	kg	INH mg	Ethambutol mg	Mynah	Myambutol
Under 77	Under 35	300	750	3 × 250	
77–83	35–37.8	300	900	3 × 300	
83.5–107	37.9–47	300	1095	3 × 365	
108–125	48–55	300	1300	3 × 300	+ 1 × 400 mg
126–143	56–63	300	1495	3 × 365	+ 1 × 400 mg
144–161	64–71	300	1700	3 × 365	+ 2 × 400 mg
162–180	72–79	300	1895	3 × 365	+ 2 × 400 mg
181–198	80–87	300	2100	3 × 300	+ 3 × 400 mg
199–216	88–94	300	2295	3 × 365	+ 3 × 400 mg
217–234	95–103	300	2500	3 × 300	+ 4 × 400 mg

mended that the possibility of such effects should be kept in mind when treating women of childbearing age.

Because ethambutol has a unique effect on the eye, it is recommended that patients undergo a full ophthalmic examination before starting treatment. This should include visual acuity, colour vision, perimetry and ophthalmoscopy. Many physicians consider that routine ophthalmological examination is not thereafter necessary, but patients should be informed of the importance of reporting any change in vision.

Side-effects: For ethambutol: Ethambutol may produce a unique type of visual impairment which is generally reversible and which appears to be due to optic neuritis and to be related to dose and duration of treatment. Less than 1% of patients undergoing treatment with the higher dose regimen of 25 mg/kg/day for two months and 15 mg/kg/day thereafter, have exhibited decrease in visual acuity. The change may be unilateral or bilateral and hence both eyes must be tested individually. The effects are generally reversible when administration of the drug is discontinued promptly. In rare cases recovery may be delayed for up to one year or more and the effect may possibly be irreversible in these cases.

Recovery of visual acuity has usually occurred over a period of weeks to months after the drug is discontinued, and patients have then received ethambutol at lower dosages without toxicity. Test patients receiving ethambutol as sole therapy did not have gastro-intestinal disturbances (e.g. anorexia, nausea, vomiting, diarrhoea), transient impairment of liver function or allergic reactions, although these have been noted during multiple-drug antituberculous therapy in which ethambutol was employed. Numbness and paraesthesia of the extremities has been reported.

For isoniazid: Side-effects are infrequently encountered and are rarely serious. Peripheral neuritis is most often observed, and correlation exists between the dosage level and this reaction. When the dosage is 3 mg/kg/day, the incidence is approximately 1%; at 10 mg/kg/day, it rises to 15% or higher. Pyridoxine (vitamin B_6) has been used successfully for prophylaxis and treatment of isoniazid-induced peripheral neuritis.

Severe and sometimes fatal hepatitis associated with isoniazid therapy may occur and may develop even after many months of treatment. The risk of developing hepatitis is age related and is increased with daily consumption of alcohol.

CNS effects (insomnia, headache, restlessness, mental confusion, toxic psychoses, increased reflexes, muscle twitching, paraesthesia) may be encountered. Optic neuritis and optic atrophy have been reported. Ophthalmological examinations should be carried out wherever visual complaints occur, since the optic lesions are likely to be reversible if isoniazid is discontinued promptly. Extremely high dosages have produced convulsions in apparently normal individuals.

Urinary disturbances in the male (prostatic obstruction syndrome), constipation and dryness of the mouth have been reported. Allergic reactions occur infrequently. Agranulocytosis and exfoliative dermatitis have occasionally been reported.

Overdosage: No specific antidote, but gastric lavage should be employed if necessary.

Pharmaceutical precautions Mynah Tablets should be stored at room temperature, in either the original pack or in containers which prevent access of moisture.

Legal category POM.

Package quantities *Mynah 200:* Bottles of 84.
Mynah 250: Bottles of 84.
Mynah 300: Bottles of 84.
Mynah 365: Bottles of 84.

Further information The quantities and proportions of the component drugs make Mynah tablets unsuitable for most children. Details of a formulation of ethambutol syrup suitable for paediatric use are available on request from the Medical Information Department. A mixture of ethambutol syrup and isoniazid elixir BPC should not be prepared as isoniazid is unstable in the presence of sugars.

Product licence numbers
Mynah 200   0095/0044
Mynah 250   0095/0045
Mynah 300   0095/0046
Mynah 365   0095/0047

NOLTAM*

Presentation White, round, biconvex film-coated tablets, containing Tamoxifen Citrate BP equivalent to 10 mg and 20 mg of Tamoxifen. 10 mg tablets are marked 'LL' on one face and 'T4' on the reverse face. 20 mg tablets are marked 'LL' on one face and 'T' and '5' either side of a score line of the reverse face.

Uses At the recommended dosage, Noltam has anti-oestrogenic properties, probably because it competes with oestrogen for binding sites in target organs. It does not have androgenic properties.

Noltam is indicated for:

1. The treatment of breast cancer. The proportion of patients with breast cancer who respond to Noltam is similar to that seen with oestrogens or androgens. However, because Noltam produces fewer serious side effects, it is more acceptable to the patient.

2. The treatment of anovulatory infertility.

Dosage and administration

1. *Breast cancer:* The recommended initial dose of Noltam is 20 mg daily in single or divided doses. If no response is seen within one month, dosage should be increased to 40 mg daily in single or divided doses.

2. *Infertility:* Before commencing any course of treatment, whether initial or subsequent, the possibility of pregnancy must be excluded. In women who are menstruating regularly, but with anovular cycles, the initial course of treatment consists of 20 mg daily in single or divided doses given on the second, third, fourth and fifth days of the menstrual cycle. If unsatisfactory basal temperature records or poor pre-ovulatory cervical mucus indicate that this initial course of treatment has been unsuccessful, further courses may be given during subsequent menstrual periods, increasing the dosage to 40 mg and then to 80 mg daily in single or divided doses.

In women who are not menstruating regularly, the initial course may begin on any day. If no signs of ovulation are demonstrable, then a subsequent course of treatment may start 45 days later with dosage increased as above. If a patient responds with menstruation, then the next course of treatment is commenced on the second day of the cycle.

Contra-indications, warnings, etc Noltam must not be given during pregnancy. Pre-menopausal patients must be carefully examined before treatment for breast cancer or infertility to exclude the possibility of pregnancy.

Menstruation is suppressed in a proportion of premenopausal women receiving Noltam for the treatment of breast cancer. Reversible cystic ovarian swelling has very occasionally been observed when such women have been treated with 40 mg Noltam twice daily for short periods.

A small number of patients with bony metastases have developed hypercalcaemia on initiation of therapy.

During long-term treatment, side effects are not as numerous or as serious with Noltam as with the androgens and oestrogens which are also used to treat breast cancer. Those that have been reported can be classified as either due to the anti-oestrogenic action of the drug, e.g. hot flushes, vaginal bleeding, and pruritis vulvae, or as more general effects, e.g. gastro-intestinal intolerance, tumour pain, light-headedness and, occasionally, fluid retention.

When side effects are severe, it is sometimes possible to control them by a simple reduction of dosage without loss of control of the disease. If side effects do not respond to this measure, it may be necessary to stop the treatment.

Transient falls in platelet count, usually only to 80,000–90,000 but occasionally lower, have been reported in patients taking Noltam for breast cancer. No haemorrhagic tendency has been reported and the platelet counts have recovered even though treatment with Noltam has continued.

Overdosage: On theoretical grounds an overdosage would be expected to cause enhancement of the anti-oestrogenic side effects mentioned above. Observations in animals show that extreme overdosage (100–200 × recommended daily dose) may produce oestrogenic effects.

Corneal and macular changes resulting in blurred vision have been described in a small number of cases treated continuously with 12–16 times the recommended starting dose for periods in excess of 17 months.

There is no specific antidote to overdosage, and treatment must be symptomatic.

Pharmaceutical precautions Protect from light.

Legal category POM.

Package quantities Noltam is packed in containers of 30 and 250 tablets.

Further information Nil.

Product licence numbers
10 mg tablets   0095/0094
20 mg tablets   0095/0095

NOVANTRONE* INJECTION ▼

Presentation Novantrone injection (2 mg/ml): Glass vials containing a sterile, dark blue aqueous isotonic solution of mitozantrone hydrochloride equivalent to 20 mg, 25 mg and 30 mg mitozantrone, together with sodium chloride and a buffer of sodium acetate and acetic acid to approximately pH3.

Uses Novantrone is an antineoplastic agent. Novantrone is indicated for the treatment of advanced breast cancer, non-Hodgkin's lymphoma and adult acute non-lymphocytic leukaemia in relapse.

Dosage and administration
1. Advanced breast cancer and non-Hodgkin's lymphoma:

(a) Single agent dosage – The recommended initial dosage of Novantrone used as a single agent is 14 mg/m^2 of body surface area, given as a single intravenous dose which may be repeated at 21-day intervals. A lower initial dosage (12 mg/m^2 or less) is recommended in patients with inadequate bone marrow reserves, e.g. due to prior chemotherapy or poor general condition.

Dosage modification and the timing of subsequent dosing should be determined by clinical judgement depending on the degree and duration of myelosuppression. For subsequent courses the prior dose can usually be repeated if white blood cell and platelet counts have returned to normal levels after 21 days.

The following table is suggested as a guide to dosage adjustment, in the treatment of advanced breast cancer and non-Hodgkin's lymphoma according to haematological nadir, (which usually occurs about 10 days after dosing):

Nadir after prior Dose			
WBC (per mm^3)	Platelets (per mm^3)	Time to recovery	Subsequent dose after adequate haematological recovery
> 1,500 and	> 50,000	≤ 21 days	Repeat prior dose after recovery, or increase by 2 mg/m^2 if myelosuppression is not considered adequate.
> 1,500 and	> 50,000	> 21 days	Withhold until recovery then repeat prior dose
< 1,500 or	< 50,000	Any duration	Decrease by 2 mg/m^2 from prior dose after recovery.
< 1,000 or	< 25,000	Any duration	Decrease by 4 mg/m^2 from prior dose after recovery.

(b) Combination therapy – Novantrone has been given as a part of combination therapy for the treatment of breast cancer and lymphomas. As data on combination therapy is presently limited, dosage recommendations cannot be given. Novantrone should be used with caution in combination therapy until wider experience is available.

As a guide, when Novantrone is used in combination chemotherapy with another myelosuppressive agent, the initial dose of Novantrone should be reduced by 2–4 mg/m^2 below the doses recommended above for single agent usage; subsequent dosing, as outlined in the table above, depends on the degree and duration of myelosuppression.

2. Acute non-lymphocytic leukaemia in relapse

(a) Single agent dosage – The recommended dosage for remission induction is 12 mg/m^2 of body surface area, given as a single intravenous dose daily for five consecutive days (total of 60 mg/m^2).

In clinical studies with a dosage of 12 mg/m^2 daily for 5 days, patients who achieved a complete remission did so as a result of the first induction course.

(b) Combination therapy – Novantrone has been given as part of combination therapy in the treatment of ANLL. As data on combination therapy is currently limited dosage recommendations cannot be given. Novantrone should be used with caution in combination therapy until wider experience is available.

(c) Paediatric leukaemia – As experience with Novan-

tronc in paediatric leukaemia is limited, dosage recommendations in this patient population cannot at present be given.

Method of intravenous administration: Care should be taken to avoid contact of Novantrone with the skin, mucous membranes, or eyes; see *Pharmaceutical Precautions* for further directions on handling.

Dilute the required volume of Novantrone injection to at least 50 ml in either of the following intravenous infusions: Sodium Chloride 0.9%, Glucose 5%, or Sodium Chloride 0.18% and Glucose 4%. Administer the resulting solution over not less than 3 minutes via the tubing of a freely running intravenous infusion of the above fluids. Novantrone should not be mixed with other drugs in the same infusion.

If extravasation occurs the administration should be stopped immediately and restarted in another vein. The nonvesicant properties of Novantrone minimize the possibility of severe local reaction following extravasation.

Contra-indications, warnings, etc

Contra-indications: Demonstrated hypersensitivity to the drug.

Warnings: Novantrone should be used with caution in patients with myelosuppression (*see Dosage Section*) or poor general condition.

Cases of functional cardiac changes, including congestive heart failure and decreases in left ventricular ejection fraction have been reported. The majority of these cardiac events have occurred in patients who have had prior treatment with anthracyclines, prior mediastinal/thoracic radiotherapy, or with pre-existing heart disease. It is recommended that patients in these categories are treated with Novantrone at full cytotoxic dosage and schedule. However, added caution is required in these patients and careful regular cardiac examinations are recommended from the initiation of treatment.

As experience of prolonged treatment with Novantrone is presently limited, it is suggested that cardiac examinations also be performed in patients without identifiable risk factors during therapy exceeding a cumulative dose of 160 mg/m^2.

Careful supervision is recommended when treating patients with severe hepatic insufficiency.

The effects of Novantrone on human fertility or pregnancy have not been established. As with other antineoplastic agents, patients and their partners should be advised to avoid conception for at least six months after cessation of therapy. Novantrone should not normally be administered to patients who are pregnant or to mothers who are breast feeding.

Novantrone is mutagenic in vitro and in vivo in the rat. In the same species there was a possible association between administration of the drug and development of malignant neoplasia. The carcinogenic potential in man is unknown.

There is no experience with the administration of Novantrone other than by the intravenous route. Safety for intrathecal use has not been established.

Precautions: Novantrone is an active cytotoxic drug which should be used by clinicians familiar with the use of antineoplastic agents, and having the facilities for regular monitoring of clinical, haematological and biochemical parameters during and after treatment. Full blood counts should be undertaken serially during a course of treatment. Dosage adjustments may be necessary based on these counts (*see Dosage Section*).

Side-effects: Novantrone is clinically well tolerated demonstrating a low overall incidence of adverse events particularly those of a severe, irreversible, or life-threatening nature. Some degree of leucopenia is to be expected following recommended doses of Novantrone. However, suppression of WBC count below 1000/mm^3 is infrequent; leucopenia is usually transient, reaching its nadir at about 10 days after dosing with recovery usually occurring by the 21st day. Thrombocytopenia can occur and anaemia occurs less frequently. Myelosuppression may be more severe and prolonged in patients having had extensive prior chemotherapy or radiotherapy or in debilitated patients.

When Novantrone is used as a single injection given every 21 days in the treatment of advanced breast cancer and lymphomas, the most commonly encountered side-effects are nausea and vomiting, although in the majority of cases these are mild and transient. Alopecia may occur, but is most frequently of minimal severity and reversible on cessation of therapy.

Other side-effects which have occasionally been reported include amenorrhoea, anorexia, constipation, diarrhoea, dyspnoea, fatigue and weakness, fever, gastrointestinal bleeding, stomatitis/mucositis and non-specific neurological side-effects.

Tissue necrosis following extravasation has been reported rarely. In patients with leukaemia, the pattern of side-effects is generally similar, although there is an increase in both frequency and severity, particularly of stomatitis and mucositis.

Changes in laboratory test values have been observed infrequently e.g. elevated serum creatinine and blood urea nitrogen levels, increased liver enzyme levels (with occasional reports of severe impairment of hepatic function in patients with leukaemia).

Cardiovascular effects, which have only occasionally been of clinical significance, include decreased left ventricular ejection fraction, ECG changes and acute arrhythmia. Congestive heart failure has been reported and has generally responded well to treatment with digitalis and/or diuretics. In patients with leukaemia an increase in the frequency of adverse cardiac events has been observed; the direct role of Novantrone in these cases is difficult to assess as most patients had received prior therapy with anthracyclines and since the clinical course in leukaemic patients is often complicated by anaemia, fever, sepsis and intravenous fluid therapy.

Novantrone may impart a blue-green colouration to the urine for 24 hours after administration and patients should be advised that this is to be expected. A reversible blue colouration of the sclerae may be seen very rarely.

Overdosage: There is no known specific antidote for Novantrone. Haemopoietic, gastrointestinal, hepatic or renal toxicity may be seen depending on dosage given and the physical condition of the patient. In cases of overdosage the patient should be monitored closely and management should be symptomatic and supportive.

Pharmaceutical precautions Store at room temperature. Do not freeze.

Care should be taken to avoid contact of Novantrone with the skin, mucous membranes, or eyes. The use of goggles, gloves and protective gowns is recommended during preparation and administration. Aerosol generation should be minimised. Novantrone can cause staining. Skin accidentally exposed to Novantrone should be rinsed copiously with warm water and if the eyes are involved standard irrigation techniques should be used.

Novantrone injection does not contain an antimicrobial preservative. Therefore, in accordance with normal practice, dilutions for infusion should be used or discarded within 24 hours. Novantrone dilutions will maintain potency for 24 hours at room temperature in PVC or glass containers.

Novantrone must not be mixed in the same infusion as heparin since a precipitate may form. Because specific compatibility data are not available it is recommended that Novantrone should not be mixed in the same infusion with other drugs.

Equipment and spills on environmental surfaces may be cleaned up using 15 ml of a 40% aqueous solution of hypochlorite (calcium or sodium) for every 1 ml of Novantrone Injection; e.g. 150 ml of 40% hypochlorite would be needed to deactivate a spillage of 10 ml Novantrone Injection. More hypochlorite may be required if the blue colour has not been fully discharged. Absorb the resulting solution with gauze or towels and dispose of these in a safe manner. Appropriate safety equipment such as goggles and gloves should be worn while working with hypochlorite and Novantrone solutions.

Legal category POM.

Package quantities Novantrone injection is a sterile aqueous solution of mitozantrone hydrochloride, equivalent to 2 mg/ml mitozantrone. It is available in the following vial sizes:

20 mg in 10 ml – packs of 1 vial
25 mg in 12.5 ml – packs of 1 vial
30 mg in 15 ml – packs of 1 vial

Further information Although its mechanism of action has not been determined, Novantrone is a DNA-reactive agent. It has a cytocidal effect on proliferating and non-proliferating cultured human cells, suggesting activity against rapidly proliferating and slow-growing neoplasms.

Pharmacokinetic studies in patients following intravenous administration of Novantrone demonstrated a triphasic plasma clearance. Distribution to tissues is rapid and extensive. Elimination of the drug is slow with a mean half-life of 12 days (range 5–18) and persistent tissue concentrations. Similar estimates of half-life were obtained from patients receiving a single dose of Novantrone every 21 days and patients dosed on 5 consecutive days every 21 days.

Novantrone is excreted via the renal and hepatobiliary systems. Only 20–32% of the administered dose was excreted within the first five days after dosing (urine 6–11%, faeces 13–25%). Of the material recovered in the urine 65% was unchanged mitozantrone and the remaining 35% is primarily comprised of two inactive metabolites and their glucuronide conjugates. Approximately two thirds of the excretion occurred during the first day.

Animal pharmacokinetic studies in rats, dogs and monkeys given radiolabelled Novantrone indicate rapid, extensive dose proportional distribution into most tissues. Novantrone does not cross the blood-brain barrier to any appreciable extent. Distribution into testes is relatively low. In pregnant rats the placenta is an effective barrier. Plasma concentrations decrease rapidly during the first two hours and slowly thereafter. Animal data established biliary excretion as the major route of elimination. In rats, tissue elimination half-life of radio-

activity ranged from 20 days to 25 days as compared with plasma half-life of 12 days.

Novantrone is not absorbed significantly in animals following oral administration.

Product licence number 0095/0088.

PARFENAC*

Presentation Smooth white cream containing Bufexamac 5% in an aqueous base consisting of cetyl alcohol, glycerin, sodium lauryl sulphate, methyl paraben as a preservative.

Uses Parfenac is a synthetic non-steroidal anti-inflammatory agent for topical application.

It is intended for external use only in the treatment of various mild dermatoses such as contact dermatitis, atopic dermatitis, radiodermatitis (caused by sunburn and radiotherapy) and eczema.

Dosage and administration

Adults and children: Parfenac cream should be applied in small quantities to the affected areas two or three times daily and rubbed in gently until it disappears.

The cream is water-based and stains on clothing may be easily washed off.

Contra-indications, warnings, etc Parfenac is contra-indicated in patients with a history of hypersensitivity to any of its components.

If an infection is present an appropriate anti-infective agent should be prescribed. Parfenac should not be applied to broken skin. It should not be used on infants.

Local intolerance to Parfenac cream is manifested by burning and irritation which is rare and is attributable to the components of the cream vehicle. Bufexamac itself has not been found to have a sensitivity potential. If such a reaction occurs, the use of Parfenac should be discontinued.

Pharmaceutical precautions The product should be stored in a dry, cool place. It is not recommended that the product be diluted as this may affect its stability.

Legal category POM.

Package quantities 15 g and 30 g.

Further information Nil.

Product licence number 0095/0010R.

PIPRIL* INJECTION ▼

Presentation Vials containing 1 g or 2 g of piperacillin as piperacillin sodium.

Infusion bottles containing 4 g of piperacillin as piperacillin sodium.

Infusion pack containing a 4 g piperacillin infusion bottle, a bottle of Water for Injections BP 50 ml and a sterile pyrogen free transfer needle.

Each gram of Pipril contains 1.94 mEq (44.5 mg) of sodium.

Uses Pipril is a broad spectrum bactericidal penicillin antibiotic indicated for the treatment of infections caused by sensitive organisms, and for peri-operative prophylaxis for example in patients undergoing abdominal surgery, vaginal hysterectomy, caesarian section.

Pipril is highly active against the following clinically important bacteria:

Gram-Negative:

Acinetobacter species	Neisseria gonorrhoeae
Citrobacter species	Neisseria meningitidis
Enterobacter species	Proteus sp. (indole
Escherichia coli	positive and negative)
Haemophilus influenzae	Providencia species
Klebsiella pneumoniae and	Pseudomonas aeruginosa
other species	and other species
	Serratia marcescens and
	other species
	Shigella species

Anaerobes:

Bacteroides fragilis	Fusobacterium species
Bacteroides species	Peptococcus species
Clostridium species	Peptostreptococcus species
	Veillonella species

Gram-Positive:

Enterococci	Streptococcus
Staphylococcus species	(Diplococcus) pneu-
(non-β-lactamase-	moniae
producing)	Streptococcus pyogenes
	Other Streptococcus species

Because of its broad spectrum of activity, Pipril is indicated for the treatment of the following systemic and/or local infections in which one or more susceptible organisms have been detected or are suspected.

Systemic infections including bacterial septicaemia and endocarditis.

Urogenital tract infections including gonorrhoea.

Respiratory tract infections.

Ear, nose and throat and oral cavity infections.

Intra-abdominal infections including those of the biliary tract.

Gynaecological and obstetric infections.

Skin and soft tissue infections including infected wounds and burns.

Bone and joint infections.

Proven or suspected infections in patients with impaired or suppressed immunological status.

Peri-operative prophylaxis.

Pipril acts synergistically with aminoglycosides. Concurrent therapy with both drugs given in full therapeutic doses may be used in the treatment of life-threatening infections or in patients with impaired immune status. Pipril and aminoglycosides should not, however, be mixed in the same solution but administered separately.

Pipril may be used in combination with β-lactamase resistant penicillins in proven or suspected mixed infections involving β-lactamase producing Staphylococcus aureus.

Pipril may be administered (separately) with metronidazole in the treatment of mixed aerobic/anaerobic infections.

Cefoxitin should not be given with Pipril when Pseudomonas infections are suspected or confirmed as in vitro data have shown possible antagonism. However, Pipril may be administered concomitantly with other β-lactam antibiotics provided that an additive or synergistic antibacterial action is first ascertained through in vitro tests where appropriate.

Dosage and administration Pipril may be given by slow intravenous injection, by intravenous infusion or by intramuscular injection.

Intravenous Injection: Each gram of Pipril should be reconstituted with at least 5 ml of Water for Injection

Renal function	Creatinine clearance (ml/min)	Maximum daily dosage (in divided doses)	Dose schedule
Mild Impairment	40–80	16 grams	4 g q 6h
Moderate Impairment	20–40	12 grams	4 g q 8h
Severe Impairment	< 20	8 grams	4 g q 12h
Patients on Haemodialysis*		6 grams	2 g q 8 h

* Haemodialysis removes 30% to 50% of the drug in four hours; 1 g of Pipril should be administered following each dialysis period.

and given by slow intravenous injection over three to five minutes.

Intravenous Infusion: Each gram of Pipril should be reconstituted with at least 5 ml Water for Injection. The total dose should then be further diluted to at least 50 ml before infusion over 20–40 minutes. Suitable diluents are listed under Pharmaceutical Precautions.

Intramuscular Injection: Each gram of Pipril should be reconstituted with at least 2 ml of Water for Injection or 0.5–1% lignocaine. Administration should be by deep intramuscular injection. A single dose in adults should not exceed 2 g. A single dose in children should not exceed 0.5 g.

Adult dosage: Patients with normal renal function: Serious and complicated infections: 200–300 mg/kg/day. The usual dose is therefore 4 g every six or eight hours by IV administration. In life-threatening infections, particularly those caused by Pseudomonas and Klebsiella species a dosage of not less than 16 g/day is recommended.

Mild and uncomplicated infections: 100–150 mg/kg/day. The usual dose is therefore 2 g IV every six or eight hours; 4 g IV every twelve hours or 2 g IM every eight or twelve hours.

For peri-operative prophylaxis: 2 g just prior to surgery (or in caesarian section when the umbilical cord is clamped) followed by at least two doses of 2 g at four or six hour intervals.

Acute gonorrhoea: a single dose of 2 g IM.

Patients with renal insufficiency: In adults with renal impairment, intravenous or intramuscular dosage should be adjusted. Given below are the recommended maximum daily dosages of Pipril according to the degree of renal impairment as assessed by the physician.

Duration of Therapy: Pipril treatment in acute infections should be continued for three to four days after the disappearance of clinical signs and symptoms of the disease. However, the duration of treatment should be determined by the physician on the basis of the clinical course of infection.

Elderly: Pipril may be used at the same dose levels as adults except in cases of renal impairment when the dosage should be reduced.

Paediatric dosage: Children: Two months to twelve years of age: 100–300 mg/kg daily in three or four divided doses.

Neonates and Infants: Under two months of age: 100–300 mg/kg daily in two equally divided doses.

Contra-indications, warnings, etc

Contra-indications: Penicillin hypersensitivity or severe cephalosporin hypersensitivity.

Precautions: Safety for use in pregnant or lactating women has not yet been established. Use with caution in patients with infectious mononucleosis.

Warnings and side-effects: In common with other penicillins anaphylactic reactions have occasionally been reported in patients receiving piperacillin.

Side effects are uncommon and typical of other injectable penicillins.

Gastro-intestinal disturbances have been reported and transient leucopenia, neutropenia and/or eosinophilia can occur.

In vitro, Pipril can be inactivated by β-lactamases produced by some strains of gram-negative and gram-positive bacteria.

Pain after intramuscular injections (rarely accompanied by induration) has been observed infrequently. This can be minimised by reconstituting Pipril with 0.5–1.0% lignocaine.

Overdosage: Other than general supportive treatment, no specific antidote is known. Excessive serum levels of piperacillin may be reduced by dialysis. Neuromuscular excitability or convulsions have been known to occur following large intravenous doses of penicillins. General supportive measures, including administration of appropriate anticonvulsant drugs, such as diazepam or barbiturates, may be indicated. Daily doses of piperacillin of 24 grams and above have been administered in man without observation of adverse effects.

Pharmaceutical precautions Pipril should be stored in a dry place at room temperature. Pipril should be freshly prepared prior to administration, any unused solution being discarded.

Pipril may be administered in all commonly used infusion fluids including:

Glucose 5%; Sodium Chloride 0.9%; Sodium Chloride 0.9% and Glucose 5%; Compound Sodium Lactate (Lactated Ringer's Injection). The above fluids admixed with 40 mEq Potassium Chloride and/or 30 mEq Sodium Bicarbonate. Dextran 6% in Sodium Chloride 0.9%, Glucose 30%, Mannitol 20%.

Pipril solutions are stable for at least 24 hours at room temperature or 48 hours at 4°C.

Because of chemical instability, Pipril should not be diluted with solutions containing only sodium bicarbonate.

Pipril should not be added to blood products or protein hydrolysates.

Pipril has also been shown to be compatible over 24 hours at room temperature when mixed with cephazolin sodium, flucloxacillin sodium, cefamandole nafate, or cefoxitin sodium in either Sodium Chloride 0.9% and Glucose 5% or Compound Sodium Lactate (Lactated Ringer's) Intravenous Infusion.

Pipril should not be mixed in the same solution with aminoglycosides and should be administered separately from any other drugs unless compatibility is proven.

Legal category POM.

Package quantities Vials containing 1 g or 2 g Pipril, boxed singly. Infusion bottles containing 4 g Pipril, boxed singly. Pipril 4 g Infusion Packs containing a 4 g infusion bottle, a 50 ml bottle of Water for Injections BP and transfer needle.

Further information Pipril shows a pronounced activity against many clinically significant organisms resistant to other penicillins (including the acylureido group), cephalosporins and aminoglycosides. Some ampicillin-resistant *Escherichia coli* and *Proteus* and carbenicillin-resistant *Citrobacter, Klebsiella, Pseudomonas, Proteus* and *Serratia* are sensitive to piperacillin. Many ticarcillin resistant *Pseudomonas, Klebsiella* and *Serratia;* cephalothin-resistant *Enterobacteriaceae* and many strains of *Pseudomonas* resistant to amikacin, gentamicin or tobramycin are susceptible to Pipril.

Pipril is widely distributed following parenteral administration into human tissues and body fluids, particularly bile. Pipril penetrates into cerebrospinal fluid in the presence of meningitis. It is not absorbed when given orally. As with other penicillins, Pipril is rapidly excreted, unchanged, by glomerular filtration and tubular secretion achieving high urinary concentrations for up to 12 hours after dosing. The binding of piperacillin to human serum protein is low (16%).

Product licence number 0095/0073.

THIOTEPA

Presentation Vials of dry, white, sterile powder, requiring refrigeration (2–8°C). Each vial contains:

Thiotepa	15 mg
Sodium chloride	80 mg
Sodium bicarbonate	50 mg

Uses Thiotepa (triethylenethiophosphoramide) is a polyfunctional alkylating agent used alone or in combination with other cytotoxic drugs, hormones, radiotherapy or surgery in the treatment of neoplastic diseases. It is believed to exert its cytotoxic effects by alkylation of DNA.

Dosage and administration Thiotepa (15 mg) should be reconstituted with 1.5 ml water for injection immediately prior to use. Occasionally on reconstitution a precipitate may form. In this event the solution should be discarded.

Thiotepa may be given by intravenous, intramuscular and intrathecal routes of injection; it may be given directly into pleural, pericardial or peritoneal cavities and as a bladder instillation.

Adults: For intramuscular injection, bladder and intracavitary instillations: Up to 60 mg in single or divided doses. Doses should be reduced in cases of leucopenia as indicated in Table 1. Single dose administration of 90 mg Thiotepa as a bladder instillation is described under 'Bladder Cancer'.

Table 1

WBC Count	Dose of Thiotepa Adults and Children over 12 years
6000	60 mg
5000–6000	45 mg
4500–5000	30 mg
4000–4500	20 mg
3500–4000	10 mg
3000–3500	5 mg
below 3000	omit dose

Intravenous injection: Half of the above adult doses.

Children under 12 years of age: Half of the above adult doses.

Intrathecal injection: Up to a maximum of 10 mg.

It is essential that a full WBC count should be performed 12–24 hours before each dose of Thiotepa.

Dosage schedules of Thiotepa vary widely according to the route of administration and the indication.

Examples of dosage schedules used according to specific tumour types are given below:

Breast cancer: Patients with advanced breast cancer have been treated with Thiotepa, as part of a combination regime, given intramuscularly in divided doses of 15–30 mg three times weekly for two weeks; this representing one course of treatment. An interval of six to eight weeks is recommended between courses to allow bone marrow recovery.

An alternative schedule employs Thiotepa as part of a combination regime, given as an initial priming dose of 15 mg intramuscularly each day for four days. This may be followed in three weeks by maintenance doses of 15 mg I.M. every 14–21 days.

Bladder cancer: Instillations of Thiotepa have been used to treat multiple superficial tumours of the bladder, resulting in a complete clinical response in about one third of patients. Patients are dehydrated for 8–12 hours prior to treatment. Up to 60 mg Thiotepa dissolved in 60 ml sterile water is instilled into the bladder by catheter once a week for four weeks. During removal of the catheter following instillation, Thiotepa injection is continued to ensure bathing of the prostatic and pendulous urethra. The solution should be retained for up to two hours and the patient should be frequently repositioned to ensure maximum contact with the urothelium.

Patients are generally cystoscoped two weeks after a course of four instillations. If a response is observed a second course of four Thiotepa instillations may be given, generally at reduced dosage, e.g. 15–60 mg, with intervals of one to two weeks between instillations.

Instillations of Thiotepa have been used prophylactically as an adjunct to surgical resection of superficial tumours of the bladder, resulting in a marked decrease in the recurrence rate. It is recommended that there should be a minimum interval of one week between tumour resection and the commencement of prophylactic instillations of Thiotepa. 30–60 mg Thiotepa dissolved in 60 ml sterile water is instilled into the bladder for two hours and repeated at intervals of one to two weeks for a total of 4–8 instillations. This initial course may be followed by instillations of Thiotepa, 30–60 mg every four to six weeks for one year or longer.

Single dose Thiotepa instillations have been used prophylactically as an adjunct to surgical resection in the treatment of superficial tumours of the bladder. 90 mg Thiotepa dissolved in 100 ml sterile water is instilled into the bladder with the patient in the left lateral position. After 15 minutes the patient is transferred to the right lateral position and after a further 15 minutes the bladder is emptied. It is felt that such single dose administration decreases the incidence of systemic toxicity by decreasing the extent of systemic absorption of the drug.

Note: Patients who have had previous radiotherapy to the bladder are at increased risk of drug toxicity.

Malignant meningeal disease: Intrathecal injections of Thiotepa have been used to treat carcinomatous, lymphomatous and leukaemic meningeal disease. Thiotepa, at a concentration of 1 mg/ml in sterile water, is administered by intrathecal injection, in doses up to 10 mg, on alternate days, until there is a complete disappearance of abnormal mononuclear cells from the cerebrospinal fluid (CSF). It is recommended that intrathecal injections be given on alternate days for no more than four injections. However, if a CSF specimen taken before the third Thiotepa dose indicates stable or progressive disease, treatment with Thiotepa should be stopped and therapy changed. As with other routes of administration of Thiotepa each dose should be preceded by a full WBC count.

Patients who achieve a complete remission may receive maintenance Thiotepa consisting of two intrathecal doses spaced one week apart, and reducing to one dose per month thereafter.

Ovarian cancer: Ovarian cancer has been treated with Thiotepa as a single agent or as part of a combination regime in a variety of schedules. For example, 15 mg Thiotepa IV or IM may be given daily for four days initially and then continued with single doses administered at weekly or two weekly intervals.

Intracavitary instillation of Thiotepa: Instillations of Thiotepa have been used to treat malignant pleural effusions and abdominal ascites. The procedure recommended is first to aspirate as much fluid as possible and then to instil the dose of Thiotepa, 10–30 mg in 20–60 ml sterile water. This may be repeated at weekly or two weekly intervals.

Prevention of recurrence of Pterygium: A 1:2,000 solution of Thiotepa in sterile Ringer's solution (i.e. 15 mg powder in 30 ml Ringer's) applied topically as eye drops at three hourly intervals daily for up to six weeks after surgical removal of the pterygium, is effective in reducing the recurrence rate following surgery.

Condyloma Acuminata: Thiotepa applied topically or instilled intraurethrally in a gel has been successfully used to eradicate condyloma acuminata. The drug may be administered by first reconstituting 60 mg Thiotepa with 5 ml sterile water. This is diluted to 15 ml using a sterile mixture of water and lubricating jelly made to a consistency viscous enough to remain in the urethra and fluid enough to allow easy injection. This therapy may be repeated at weekly intervals.

Contra-indications, warnings, etc Thiotepa administration is contra-indicated in patients with a WBC count below 3,000 and/or a platelet count below 100,000. Thiotepa should not normally be administered to patients who are pregnant or to mothers who are breast feeding. In addition, the drug has been shown to interfere with spermatogenesis and ovarian function.

Precautions: Thiotepa should only be used by clinicians who are familiar with the various characteristics of cytotoxic drugs and their clinical toxicity. WBC and platelet counts are recommended 12–24 hours before each dose of Thiotepa regardless of route of administration, except when used topically as eye drops or in the treatment of condyloma acuminata. Dosage should be reduced as indicated above in the presence of a compromised bone marrow as manifested by a reduced WBC count.

Side-effects: The most serious side-effect is upon the blood forming elements and is a direct consequence of the cytotoxic action of the drug. In addition, Thiotepa may occasionally cause vomiting, headache and anorexia. Alopecia has been reported as a rare complication of therapy with Thiotepa. Local irritation, comparable to a mild radiation cystitis, may follow bladder instillations of Thiotepa, while haemorrhagic cystitis is rare.

Overdosage: There is no specific antidote. Gastric lavage, forced fluids and general supportive measures are recommended. Blood counts should be carried out to estimate damage to the haematopoietic system and blood transfusions should be given as required.

Pharmaceutical precautions Thiotepa must be stored in a refrigerator (2–8°C). The occurrence of a precipitate on reconstitution (with 1.5 ml of water for injection) indicates that polymerisation has occurred with the formation of less active constituents and the injection must be discarded.

Reconstituted solutions may be stored in a refrigerator (2–8°C) for up to five days.

Thiotepa may be mixed in the same syringe with Procaine Hydrochloride 2% or with adrenaline 1 in 1,000 or with both.

Legal category POM.

Package quantities Boxes of one vial.

Further information Thiotepa contains 1.97 millimoles of sodium per vial.

Product licence number 0095/5060.

TUBERCULIN, OLD, TINE TEST*
(ROSENTHAL)

Presentation Each Tuberculin Tine Test unit consists of a stainless steel disc with four tines or prongs attached to a plastic handle. The tines have been dipped in Old Tuberculin, stabilised and dried. The entire unit has been sterilised. The reactivity of the Tuberculin Tine Test is comparable to the intermediate strength Mantoux test (5 T.U. or 0.0001 mg PPD).

Uses Tuberculin Tine Test is an intradermal test for the detection of tuberculin sensitivity, and is used for screening for tuberculosis. Tuberculin testing may be done during the first year of life. Frequency of repeated tuberculin tests depends on risk of exposure of the child and on the prevalence of tuberculosis in the population group; tuberculin testing may be repeated at intervals of a year or less.

Dosage and administration *Adults and children: Site:* for accurate, standardised tuberculin testing, the volar surface of the mid-forearm is the preferred site. The skin must be clean and dry. It may be cleansed with alcohol, acetone, ether, or soap and water. On other skin areas reactions are less reliable, and quantitatively do not bear the same significance to the standardised test. Hairy areas and areas without adequate subcutaneous tissue, such as concavities over a tendon or bone, should be avoided.

Method of application: Remove the Tuberculin Tine Test unit by levering or snapping the handle from the base of the container. Grasp the patient's arm firmly with one hand, stretching the skin of the forearm tightly, and apply the disc with the other hand. Hold for one second and withdraw. Sufficient pressure should be exerted to produce four visible puncture sites and a circular depression of the skin from the plastic base. The Tine Test should *never* be re-used. Local care of the skin site is not necessary.

Reading the reaction: Tests should be read at 48–72 hours. Induration is the only criterion. It is important to measure it exactly, by examining under adequate light and by thoroughly palpating the area. Identification of the application site is usually easy because of the distinct four-point pattern. A reaction of 2 mm or more of palpable induration around one or more puncture sites is clinically comparable to a zone of induration of 5 mm or more by the intermediate strength PPD (0.0001 mg PPD) Mantoux test. Recently, the interpretation of tuberculin test reactions as recommended by the National Tuberculosis and Respiratory Disease Association has been revised. Their recommendations for interpretation of the tine test are as follows:

5 mm or more of induration Positive Reaction.

The significance of the test and the management of the individual is the same as that for one who reacts with 10 mm or more of induration to the standard Mantoux test.

2 mm through 4 mm of induration Doubtful Reaction.

Even though such reactions may be due to M. tuberculosis, a significant proportion of them may not be confirmed by a positive standard Mantoux test. Therefore, a Mantoux test should be done on all individuals in this group, and management should be based on Mantoux reactions.

Less than 2 mm of induration Negative Reaction.

There is no need for retesting unless the individual is a contact to a case of tuberculosis or there is suggestive clinical evidence of the disease.

Contra-indications, warnings, etc
Contra-indications: None.

Precautions: Tuberculin testing should be done with caution in persons with active tuberculosis. However, activation of quiescent lesions is rare.

Although clinical allergy to acacia is very rare, Tine Test contains some acacia as a stabiliser and should be used with caution in patients with known allergy to this component.

Reactivity to the test may be suppressed in patients who are receiving corticosteroids or immunosuppressive agents, or those who have recently been vaccinated with live virus vaccine such as measles.

With a *large* positive reaction to the Tine Test, further diagnostic procedures must be considered. These may include X-ray of the chest, microbiological examinations of sputa and other specimens and confirmation of the positive Tine Test using the Mantoux method. Antituberculous therapy should not be instituted solely on the basis of a single positive Tine Test.

Side-effects: Vesiculation, ulceration, or necrosis may occur at the test site in highly sensitive persons. Pain, pruritus and discomfort at the test site may be relieved by cold packs or by a topical glucocorticoid ointment or cream. Transient bleeding may be observed at a puncture site and is of no significance.

Overdosage: Does not apply.

Pharmaceutical precautions Tuberculin Tine Test should be stored at room temperature in the original pack. DO NOT REFRIGERATE.

Legal category POM.

Package quantities Container of 25 tests.

Further information Nil.

Product licence number 0095/5002.

VARIDASE* TOPICAL

Presentation Each vial of dry, sterile powder which requires storage under refrigeration (2–8°C) contains; Streptokinase 100,000 units and Streptodornase 25,000 units with thiomersal 2 mg as preservative.

The combi-pack contains a vial of Varidase Topical, a 20 ml vial of sterile Sodium Chloride 0.9% Solution BP (physiological saline) and a sterile transfer needle.

Uses Streptokinase acts indirectly upon a substrate of fibrin or fibrinogen by activating a fibrinolytic enzyme in human serum. Upon application of streptokinase in situ, the activation of this fibrinolytic system brings about rapid dissolution of blood clots and the fibrinous portion of exudates. Streptodornase liquefies the viscous nucleoprotein of dead cells or pus. Thus the action of the enzymes results in the liquefaction of the two main viscous substances resulting from inflammatory or infectious processes thereby facilitating cleansing and desloughing of wounds.

Varidase Topical has no effect on living cells.

Indications: Varidase Topical is indicated wherever clotted blood, fibrinous or purulent accumulations are undesirably present, following trauma or infectious processes which have led to ulceration or abscess formation.

It is indicated in the treatment of suppurative surface lesions such as ulcers, pressure sores, amputation stumps, diabetic gangrene, radiation necrosis, infected wounds, and surgical incisions. It is also indicated in the treatment of burns and may be used prior to skin grafting.

Varidase Topical can be used to dissolve clots in the bladder or in urinary catheters.

Dosage and administration

Adults and children: Directions for use in the cleansing of necrotic and infected wounds, Reconstitution: The contents of each vial should be gently mixed with 20 ml of sterile physiological saline. Care should be taken to control the rate of addition of saline to the vial to avoid frothing. The resulting clear solution can then be withdrawn into a syringe.

Reconstituted solutions are stable for two weeks at room temperature.

Standard methods of application: Pre-soak gauze with Varidase Topical solution then apply to the wound.

Following application a semi-occlusive dressing is necessary to prevent drying-out of the wound, e.g. a polythene film taped on two sides.

Alternatively the wound may be packed with dry gauze which is then soaked with Varidase Topical solution and dressed with a semi-occlusive dressing.

Alternative method of application: Where wounds are covered by a thick dry slough or eschar it is usually necessary to cross hatch the slough into approximately 3–5 mm squares and to a sufficient depth to allow the access of the enzymes to the underlying fibrinous and purulent material. Alternatively, Varidase Topical may be injected under the eschar, taking care that the solution enters only the cavity beneath and that the volume is not sufficient to cause pain through increased pressure. Injection of Varidase Topical in this way often results in the eschar becoming partly detached thus facilitating its mechanical removal.

Special technique of application: Varidase Topical may be applied in jelly form. This can be prepared by dissolving the contents of one vial in 5 ml of sterile water and mixing the resulting solution thoroughly but gently, with 15 ml of inert jelly, such as K–Y^R or carboxymethylcellulose (CMC) jelly. This method can be particularly useful in cases of burns where dressings are not employed.

Frequency of application: Varidase Topical treatment should be repeated once or twice a day. Care should be taken to irrigate the lesion thoroughly with physiological saline and remove loosened material prior to the next application.

Duration of treatment: Treatment should be continued until healthy granulations are present and re-epithelialisation has begun, usually within one to two weeks, although it can be administered until wound healing is complete.

Contra-indications, warnings, etc

Contra-indications: Active haemorrhage.

Precautions: Varidase Topical is intended for local use only. It should not be used intramuscularly or intravenously.

In order to avoid cross-infection the contents of one vial of Varidase Topical and a separate sterile syringe and needle should be used for each individual patient.

Side-effects: Allergic reactions to the topical application of Varidase Topical are infrequent and may be minimised by careful and frequent removal of exudate followed by thorough irrigation using physiological saline prior to retreatment with Varidase Topical.

Pharmaceutical precautions Varidase Topical must be stored in a refrigerator (2–8°C) and should be reconstituted in 20 ml of sterile physiological saline or if unavailable Water for Injection. If the reconstituting fluid has a high calcium content, the solution becomes opalescent, but this does not affect the potency of the enzymes.

Reconstituted solutions may be stored for two weeks at room temperature.

The preparation is buffered to physiological pH. The enzymes of Varidase Topical can be denatured by the concomitant use of other preparations of an acidic or alkaline pH. Varidase Topical is compatible with tetracyclines and other antibiotics such as penicillin and streptomycin.

Legal category POM.

Package quantities Single vials or combi-pack.

Further information Information on the intracavitary use of Varidase Topical in the treatment of, for example, haemothorax or thoracic empyema is available on request to the Medical Information Department.

Product licence number 0095/5038.

VARIDASE* TABLETS

Presentation *Oral Tablets:* Each peach-coloured tablet contains 10,000 units of Streptokinase and at least 2,500 units of Streptodornase. Each tablet is printed 'Lederle 2209'.

Uses Varidase Tablets have a generalised anti-inflammatory effect thereby relieving the symptoms of inflammation; pain; swelling; tenderness; erythema and resolution of the discoloration caused by extravasated blood. Varidase Tablets are therefore indicated for the management of oedema associated with infection or trauma in such conditions as acute and chronic thrombophlebitis; cellulitis; abscesses; sinusitis; haematoma;

contusions; chronic bronchiectasis and chronic bronchitis; arteriosclerotic, varicose and stasis ulcers; sprains and fractures.

They are also indicated for the control of oedema and resorption of local haemorrhage into tissue in certain dental conditions such as extractions involving local surgical trauma, pericoronitis, and wherever the inflammatory process is involved.

The use of Varidase in these conditions should be considered as an adjunct to the usual appropriate therapeutic measures including surgical procedures. In the presence of infection, simultaneous administration of an appropriate antibiotic is recommended.

Dosage and administration *Adults and children:* The usual dose is 1 tablet (10,000 units of Streptokinase) four times daily. In acute situations, more frequent dosage on the first day may be advisable. Usually treatment is continued for four to six days.

Contra-indications, warnings, etc
Contra-indications: Varidase Oral Tablets are contraindicated in patients with reduced plasminogen or fibrinogen. They do not act upon fibrous tissues, mucoproteins or collagen, and therefore are less effective if extensive scarring or organisation of exudate or blood clots has occurred.

Precautions: Where infection is present or suspected, the simultaneous administration of a broad-spectrum antibiotic is recommended. Allergic reactions have not been reported in trials over an extended period. Patients with a history of collagen diseases should be treated with caution. Varidase should be administered with caution when the possibility exists that a defect in blood coagulation or depression of liver function may prolong coagulation.

Side-effects: Side-effects are not common and are usually minor and all have responded promptly to discontinuation of the medication. There have been no serious side-effects. Allergic manifestations have been reported on rare occasions consisting primarily of urticaria and rashes.

Overdosage: No specific antidote. Transfusion, in case of haemorrhage.

Pharmaceutical precautions The product should be stored in a cool dry place in either the original pack or in containers which prevent the access of light and moisture.

Legal category POM.

Package quantities Bottles of 12.

Further information Varidase Oral Tablets contain 0.014 millimole of sodium per tablet.

Product licence number 0095/5072.

VINBLASTINE INJECTION BP 10 mg

Presentation A combination package consisting of (i) one vial of lyophilised powder consisting of 10 mg of Vinblastine sulphate for reconstitution before use with (ii) one ampoule of Diluting Solution, i.e. 10 ml of sodium chloride 0.9% with 2% benzyl alcohol as an antimicrobial preservative.

Uses The treatment of neoplastic disease.

Dosage and administration
Adults and Children: The dosage of Vinblastine must always be adjusted individually because of individual variations in the degree of leucopenia. Vinblastine is administered intravenously at intervals no more frequently than once a week, and has been used alone and in combination or sequence with other cytotoxic agents, radiotherapy or surgery in a wide variety of neoplastic diseases e.g. lymphomas including Hodgkin's disease, breast cancer unresponsive to appropriate endocrine, surgical, and hormonal therapy, testicular cancer, Methotrexate-resistant choriocarcinoma, reticulum cell sarcoma, mycosis fungoides, neuroblastoma and histiocytosis X (Letterer-Siwe disease).

Initial dosage is calculated by body weight or body surface area and varies according to the disease. However, in general, 0.1–0.2 mg/kg is given. Rarely, up to 0.5 mg/kg may be necessary. It is important to monitor the patients white blood cell count before each dose and the dose can be increased by increments of 0.05 mg/kg each week until an objective response is obtained or a nadir in the white cell count of approximately 3,000 cells/mm^3 is observed. A dose one increment smaller than this can then be administered at weekly or longer intervals for maintenance. It should be emphasised that, even if seven days have elapsed, the next dose of Vinblastine should not be given until the white cell count has returned to at least 4,000 cells/mm^3.

Administration: Vinblastine is irritant, particularly to the eyes and skin and it is recommended that goggles and gloves are worn during reconstitution and administration of the product. Following reconstitution, the calculated dose of Vinblastine is withdrawn from the vial and should only be injected either directly into a vein or into the tubing of a fast running intravenous infusion of Sodium Chloride 0.9%.

When reconstituted with the Diluting Solution provided, Vinblastine Injection may be stored in a refrigerator for 30 days without significant loss of potency.

Severe local pain and tissue damage will occur if Vinblastine injection extravasates during intravenous administration. The injection should be discontinued immediately and any remaining portion of the dose should then be introduced into another vein. Local injection of hyaluronidase and the application of moderate heat to the area of leakage help to disperse the drug and are thought to minimise discomfort and the possibility of cellulitis.

Care must be taken to avoid contamination of the eye with concentrations of Vinblastine used clinically. If accidental contamination occurs, severe irritation (or if the drug was delivered under pressure, even corneal ulceration) may result. The eye should be washed with water thoroughly and immediately.

Contra-indications, warnings, etc
Contra-indications: Vinblastine should not normally be administered to patients who are pregnant or to mothers who are breast-feeding. Leucopenia. Concurrent untreated infection. Intrathecal administration. Use in elderly cachectic patients.

Precautions: Vinblastine should be administered under the direction of a specialist oncology service having the facilities for regular monitoring of clinical, biochemical and haematological effects during and after administration.

The use of small amounts of Vinblastine daily for long periods is not advised. Little or no added therapeutic benefit compared with intermittent dosing has been demonstrated and convulsions, severe and permanent central nervous system damage and even death have occurred. If leucopenia with less than 2,000 white blood cells/mm³ occurs following a dose of Vinblastine, the patient should be watched carefully for evidence of infection until the white blood cell count has returned to a safe level.

When cachexia or ulcerated areas of the skin surface are present, there may be a more profound leucopenic response to the drug. Its use should be avoided in older persons suffering from either of these conditions. In patients with malignant-cell infiltration of the bone marrow, the leucocyte and platelet counts have sometimes fallen precipitously after moderate doses of Vinblastine. Further use of the drug in such patients is inadvisable.

Vinblastine has been shown to be teratogenic. However, only limited information is available concerning the effect of Vinblastine on spermatogenesis. Although no abnormalities of the human foetus have been reported thus far, animal studies with Vinblastine would suggest that teratogenic effects may occur. Patients receiving Vinblastine and their partners should be advised to avoid conception.

There is a possibility that Vinblastine may exert a carcinogenic effect with long-term therapy, although to date no positive evidence is available.

Side-effects: Clinically, leucopenia is an expected effect of Vinblastine and the level of the leucocyte count is an important guide of treatment. Following therapy with Vinblastine, the nadir in the white blood cell count may be expected to occur five to ten days after the last day of drug administration, with complete recovery within another seven to fourteen days.

The effect of Vinblastine upon the thrombocyte count and/or red blood cell count is usually insignificant when other treatment does not complicate the picture.

Nausea and vomiting are common but are usually readily controlled by anti-emetic agents.

Stomatitis, constipation, diarrhoea, ileus, anorexia, abdominal pain, rectal bleeding, pharyngitis, bleeding from an old peptic ulcer and, rarely, haemorrhagic enterocolitis have also been observed.

Alopecia is uncommon and is frequently not total. Regrowth may occur during maintenance treatment.

Neurological side effects such as numbness, paraesthesiae, peripheral neuritis, mental depression, loss of deep tendon reflexes, headache or convulsions can occur but are much less common than with Vincristine.

Other adverse reactions that have been reported are malaise, weakness, dizziness, pain in the tumour site and vesiculation of the skin.

Toxicity is increased in patients with obstructive jaundice.

Overdosage: Side-effects following the use of Vinblastine are dose related. Therefore, following administration of more than the recommended dose, patients can be expected to experience these effects in an exaggerated fashion.

In addition, neurotoxicity similar to that seen with vincristine sulphate may be observed.

Treatment: Supportive care should include: (1) prevention of the side effects that result from the syndrome of inappropriate secretion of antidiuretic hormone. This includes restriction of fluid intake and perhaps the use of a diuretic acting on the loop of Henle and distal tubule function; (2) administration of an anticonvulsant; (3) prevention and treatment of ileus; (4) monitoring the

patient's cardiovascular system; and (5) daily blood counts for guidance in transfusion requirement.

The major effect of excessive doses of Vinblastine will be on granulocytopoeisis, and this may be life-threatening.

Pharmaceutical precautions Vinblastine should be stored in a refrigerator (2–8°C). Injections reconstituted with the Diluting Solution provided contain an antimicrobial preservative and may be kept in a refrigerator for 30 days without significant loss of potency. Goggles and gloves should be worn during reconstitution and administration of Vinblastine.

Legal category POM.

Package quantities Combination package consisting of one vial of Vinblastine 10 mg and one ampoule of Diluting Solution.

Further information Nil.

Product licence number 0095/0067.

VINCRISTINE INJECTION BP, 1 mg, 2 mg, 5 mg

Presentation A combination package consisting of (i) one vial of lyophilised powder consisting of 1 mg, 2 mg or 5 mg of Vincristine sulphate with 10 mg, 20 mg or 50 mg of lactose respectively, for reconstitution before use with (ii) one ampoule of Diluting Solution, i.e. 10 ml of sodium chloride 0.9% with 2% benzyl alcohol as an antimicrobial preservative.

Uses The treatment of neoplastic disease.

Dosage and administration
Adults and Children: The dosage must always be adjusted individually because of the narrow range between therapeutic and toxic levels and individual variations in response. Extreme care must be used in calculating and administering doses of Vincristine since overdosage may have a very serious or fatal outcome.

Vincristine is administered intravenously, usually at weekly or longer intervals and has been used alone and in combination or sequence with other cytotoxic agents, radiotherapy and/or surgery in a wide variety of neoplastic diseases, e.g. acute leukaemias, malignant lymphomas including Hodgkin's disease, sarcomas, neuroblastoma, Wilms's tumour and rhabdomyosarcoma. Vincristine may also be considered in the treatment of breast cancer, bronchial carcinoma, and gastro-intestinal cancer. Initial dosage is calculated by body surface area or body weight and varies according to the disease. However; in general, 1.0–2.0 mg/m² is given with a normal maximum weekly adult dose of 2 mg.

In children, remissions from acute leukaemia have been induced with weekly doses of 0.05–0.15 mg/kg of body weight.

In acute leukaemia of children the following incremental approach to dosage may be employed:
First dose: 0.05 mg/kg
Second dose: 0.075 mg/kg
Third dose: 0.1 mg/kg
and Fourth dose: 0.125 mg/kg up to a maximum of 0.15 mg/kg.

There is no need to advance the dosage beyond that level which produces therapeutic benefit. After remission has been obtained, the dosage may be reduced in some cases to a maintenance level of 0.05 to 0.075 mg/kg/week.

In adult leukaemia the suggested dosage is 0.025–0.075 mg/kg of body weight per weekly dose.

For malignancies other than leukaemia, a suggested dosage for Vincristine is 0.025 mg/kg/week intravenously until some beneficial effect is seen. Thereafter much smaller weekly doses in the range of 0.005–0.01 mg/kg may be employed for maintenance therapy for so long as an anti-tumour effect can be maintained.

Administration: Vincristine is irritant, particularly to the eyes and skin, and it is recommended that goggles and gloves are worn during reconstitution and administration of the product. Following reconstitution, the calculated dose of Vincristine is withdrawn from the vial and should only be injected either directly into a vein or into the tubing of a fast running intravenous infusion of Sodium Chloride 0.9%.

When reconstituted with the Diluting Solution provided, Vincristine Injection may be stored in a refrigerator for 14 days without significant loss of potency.

Severe local pain and tissue damage will occur if Vincristine injection extravasates during intravenous administration. The injection should be discontinued immediately and any remaining portion of the dose should then be introduced into another vein. Local injection of hyaluronidase and the application of moderate heat to the area of leakage help to disperse the drug and are thought to minimise discomfort and the possibility of cellulitis.

Care must be taken to avoid contamination of the eye with concentrations of Vincristine used clinically. If accidental contamination occurs, severe irritation (or if the drug was delivered under pressure, even corneal ulceration) may result. The eye should be washed with water thoroughly and immediately.

Contra-indications, warnings, etc

Contra-indications: Vincristine should not normally be administered to patients who are pregnant or to mothers who are breast-feeding.
Intrathecal administration.
Use in the presence of untreated infection.

Precautions: Vincristine should only be administered under the direction of a specialist oncology service having the facilities for regular monitoring of clinical, biochemical and haematological effects during and after administration.

Effective Vincristine therapy does not normally result in leucopenia. Neuromuscular rather than bone-marrow toxicity is usually the dose-limiting factor. However, because of the possibility of leucopenia both physician and patient should remain alert for signs of any complicating infection. Although pre-existing leucopenia does not necessarily contra-indicate the administration of Vincristine the appearance of leucopenia during treatment warrants careful consideration before giving the next dose. Similarly, Vincristine should only be used with caution in patients with malignant infiltration of bone marrow.

Acute uric acid nephropathy has occurred following Vincristine treatment.

Vincristine has been shown to be teratogenic. However, no data are available concerning the effect of Vincristine on spermatogenesis. Patients receiving Vincristine and their partners should be advised to avoid conception.

Routine use of laxatives and enemas is recommended to ensure regular bowel function.

As Vincristine is excreted principally by the liver it may be necessary to reduce initial doses in the presence of significantly impaired hepatic or biliary function.

When chemotherapy is being given in conjunction with radiation therapy through portals which include the liver, the use of Vincristine should be delayed until radiation therapy has been completed.

If central nervous system leukaemia is diagnosed, additional therapy, such as intrathecal Methotrexate, may be required, since Vincristine does not appear to cross the blood-brain barrier in adequate amounts. There is a possibility that Vincristine may exert a carcinogenic effect with long-term therapy, although to date no positive evidence is available.

Side-effects: In general, adverse reactions are reversible and are related to dosage. The most common side-effect is some degree of alopecia.

The main toxicity of Vincristine is neuropathy which may take any form but usually presents as a sensory motor peripheral neuropathy with paraesthesia, loss of tendon reflexes, muscle wasting and muscular weakness.

Frequently, there appears to be a sequence in the development of neuromuscular side-effects, in that initially sensory impairment and paraesthesia develop followed later by neuritic pain and motor difficulties. With single weekly doses, neuritic pain and difficulty in walking are usually of short duration (i.e. less than seven days). Other side-effects, such as sensory loss, paraesthesia, slapping gait, loss of deep tendon reflexes, and muscle wasting do not reverse so rapidly but persist for at least as long as treatment is continued. In most instances, these side-effects have disappeared by about the sixth week after discontinuing treatment, but in some patients neuromuscular difficulties may persist for prolonged periods.

No reports have yet been made of any agent that can reverse the neuromuscular manifestations of Vincristine. Discontinuation of treatment should be considered if neuromuscular effects continue to be a problem.

Vincristine commonly causes constipation which usually responds well to measures such as enemas and laxatives. Constipation may take the form of upper colon impaction and the rectum may be found to be empty on physical examination. Colicky abdominal pain, coupled with an empty rectum, may mislead the physician. A flat film of the abdomen is useful in demonstrating this condition. A routine prophylactic regimen against constipation is recommended for all patients receiving Vincristine.

On rare occasions intestinal necrosis and/or perforation have been reported when Vincristine is used in combination with a steroid.

Convulsions, frequently with hypertension, have been reported in a few patients receiving Vincristine.

Rare occurrences of the syndrome of inappropriate secretion of antidiuretic hormone have also been observed. With fluid deprivation, improvement occurs in the hyponatraemia and in the renal loss of sodium.

Other reported adverse reactions include abdominal cramps, ataxia, foot drop, weight loss, fever, cranial nerve manifestations, paraesthesiae and numbness of the digits, polyuria, dysuria, oral ulceration, headache, vomiting and diarrhoea.

Vincristine does not appear to have any constant or significant effect upon the platelets or the red blood cells. If thrombocytopenia is present when treatment with Vincristine is begun, it may actually improve before the appearance of marrow remission.

Overdosage: Side-effects following the use of Vincristine

are dose related. Therefore, following administration of more than the recommended dose, patients can be expected to experience these effects in an exaggerated fashion.

Treatment: Supportive care should include: (a) prevention of side-effects that result from the syndrome of inappropriate secretion of antidiuretic hormone. This includes restriction of fluid intake and perhaps the use of a diuretic acting on the loop of Henle and distal tubule function; (b) administration of an anticonvulsant; (c) use of cathartics to prevent ileus; (d) monitoring the patients' cardiovascular system; and (e) daily blood counts for guidance in transfusion requirement. Animal studies indicate that folinic acid is effective in the treatment of overdosage. A suggested schedule is to administer 15 mg of folinic acid intravenously every 3 hours for 24 hours and then every 6 hours for at least 48 hours.

Pharmaceutical precautions Vincristine should be stored in a refrigerator (2–8°C). Injections, reconstituted with the Diluting Solution provided, contain an antimicrobial preservative and may be kept in a refrigerator for 14 days without significant loss of potency. Goggles and gloves should be worn during reconstitution and administration of Vincristine.

Legal category POM.

Package quantities Combination packages consisting of one vial of Vincristine 1 mg, 2 mg or 5 mg and one ampoule of Diluting Solution.

Further information Nil.

Product licence numbers
Vincristine Injection BP 1 mg and 2 mg   0095/0065
Vincristine Injection BP 5 mg   0095/0066

ZADSTAT*

Presentation *Tablets 200 mg:* Each white, flat-faced, scored, uncoated tablet, embossed 'M200' on one side and 'LL' on the other side, contains 200 mg of metronidazole BP.

Suppositories 500 mg and 1 g: Each suppository, containing 500 mg or 1 g of metronidazole BP, is sealed in individual plastic suppository moulds.

Injection 500 mg in 100 ml: Each injection (for intravenous infusion) contains 500 mg of metronidazole BP in a 100 ml Steriflex Minipack* container.

Uses Zadstat metronidazole is indicated for:
1. The treatment of infections due to anaerobic bacteria.
2. The prevention of post-operative infections due to anaerobic bacteria.
3. Urogenital trichomoniasis in the female (trichomonal vaginitis) and in the male. Sexual partners should be treated concurrently.
4. All forms of amoebiasis such as acute amoebic dysentery and amoebic liver abscess, and to eradicate cysts from asymptomatic cyst passers.
5. Giardiasis.
6. Acute ulcerative gingivitis.
7. Acute dental infections (e.g. acute pericoronitis and acute apical infections).
8. The treatment of anaerobically-infected leg ulcers and pressure sores.

Dosage and administration Zadstat metronidazole tablets should be taken with or after meals. The recommended dosage regimes (oral, rectal, intravenous) for the treatment and prevention of anaerobic infections are listed below. Oral dosage regimes used for all other indications are given in the table on following page.

1. Treatment of anaerobic infections: Treatment for seven days should be satisfactory for most patients. However, the duration of treatment should be determined by the physician on the basis of the clinical course of infection.

Oral therapy may be substituted for rectal or intravenous medication as soon as this becomes feasible.

A. Oral medication: Adults and children over 10 years: Two tablets (400 mg) three times daily.

Children and infants: 7.5 mg/kg body weight three times daily.

B. Rectal medication: The following doses should be given rectally every eight hours for three days, then every 12 hours therafter.

Adults and children over 10 years: 1 g

Children 5–10 years: 500 mg

Children 1–5 years: 250 mg

Children under 1 year: 125 mg
250 mg and 125 mg suppositories can be prepared by melting 500 mg suppositories and pouring into 1 g or 500 mg suppository moulds respectively.

C. Intravenous medication: Adults and children over 10 years: 100 ml (500 mg metronidazole) by intravenous infusion every eight hours.

Children under 10 years: 1.5 ml (7.5 mg metronidazole) per kg bodyweight every eight hours.
Zadstat metronidazole injection should be infused intravenously at the rate of 5 ml per minute and may be administered alone or concurrently (but separately) with other appropriate parenteral anti-bacterial agents.

2. Prevention of anaerobic infections: Oral and rectal therapy with Zadstat metronidazole is indicated both pre- and post-operatively for the prevention of post-operative infections due to anaerobic bacteria, for example in patients undergoing gynaecological surgery, elective colonic surgery, appendicectomy.

Intravenous medication with Zadstat metronidazole can be used in patients for whom oral or rectal therapy is inappropriate and is particularly indicated in emergencies, for example, in patients needing surgery who:
– have or are believed to have anaerobic sepsis such as septicaemia, peritonitis, subphrenic or pelvic abscesses;
– at operation show signs of established or impending anaerobic sepsis;
– undergo operation in which contamination occurs with anaerobes from the gastro-intestinal or female genital tracts or the oropharynx.
Oral therapy may be substituted for rectal or intravenous medication post-operatively as soon as this becomes feasible to complete a seven-day course.

A. Oral and rectal medication:
(i) *In gynaecological surgery in adults,* a single oral dose of 1 g followed by one tablet (200 mg) eight-hourly both before preoperative starvation, if possible, and soon as possible postoperatively for up to seven days.
ii) *In elective colonic surgery in adults,* three regimes have been used sucessfully, i.e.:
(a) One tablet (200 mg) six-hourly with kanamycin

Oral dosage regimes for Zadstat tablets 200 mg

Indication	Adults and children over 10 years	7–10 years	Children 3–7 years	1–3 years
Urogenital trichomoniasis Sexual partners should be treated concurrently	1 tablet three times daily for seven days OR 4 tablets in the morning and 6 at night for two days OR 10 tablets as a single dose	$\frac{1}{2}$ tablet three times daily for seven days	$\frac{1}{2}$ tablet twice daily for seven days	$\frac{1}{4}$ tablet three times daily for seven days
Amoebiasis (a)　Invasive intestinal disease in susceptible subjects	4 tablets three times daily for five days	2 tablets three times daily for five days	1 tablet four times daily for five days	1 tablet three times daily for five days
(b)　Intestinal disease in susceptible subjects and 'chronic' amoebic hepatitis	2 tablets three times daily for five to ten days	1 tablet three times daily for five to ten days	$\frac{1}{2}$ tablet four times daily for five to ten days	$\frac{1}{2}$ tablet three times daily for five to ten days.
(c)　Amoebic liver abscess and other forms of extra-intestinal amoebiasis	2 tablets three times daily for five days	1 tablet three times daily for five days	$\frac{1}{2}$ tablet four times daily for five days	$\frac{1}{2}$ tablet three times daily for five days
(d)　Eradication of cysts from asymptomatic cyst passers	2 to 4 tablets three times daily for five to ten days	1 to 2 tablets three times daily for five to ten days	$\frac{1}{2}$ to 1 tablet four times daily for five to ten days	$\frac{1}{2}$ to 1 tablet three times daily for five to ten days
Giardiasis	10 tablets once daily for three days	5 tablets once daily for three days	3 to 4 tablets once daily for three days	500 mg once daily for three days
Acute ulcerative gingivitis	1 tablet three times daily for three days	$\frac{1}{2}$ tablet three times daily for three days	$\frac{1}{2}$ tablet twice daily for three days	$\frac{1}{4}$ tablet three times daily for three days
Acute dental infections	1 tablet three times daily for three to seven days			
Leg ulcers and pressure sores	2 tablets three times daily for seven days			

Immature children and babies weighing less than 10 kg should receive proportionately smaller dosages.

(1 g orally six-hourly) for three days before surgery (without further medication).

(*b*)　Two tablets (400 mg) eight-hourly with phthalylsulphathiazole (2.5 g orally six-hourly) for four days before surgery (without further medication).

(*c*)　A single dose of 1 g and one tablet (200 mg) eight-hourly during the 24-hours period before pre-operative starvation followed by a 1 g suppository rectally two hours before surgery and post-operatively every eight hours for three days, and thereafter every twelve hours to complete a seven day course. Oral medication (200–400 mg three times daily) may be substituted as soon as feasible.

(iii)　*In elective colonic surgery in children pre-operative medication:*

	Oral metronidazole (8-hourly for 48 hours)	Oral neomycin (6-hourly for 3 days)
5–10 years	100 mg	500 mg
1–5 years	5 mg/kg	250 mg
Under 1 year	5 mg/kg	125 mg

post-operative medication:

	Metronidazole per rectum or via colostomy (8-hourly for 48 hours)
5–10 years	500 mg
1–5 years	250 mg
Under 1 year	125 mg

250 mg and 125 mg suppositories may be prepared by melting the 500 mg suppositories and pouring in 1g or 500 mg suppository moulds, respectively.

(iv)　*In appendicectomy:* Adults and children over 10 years: a 1 g suppository rectally two hours before surgery and post-operatively every eight hours for three days and thereafter every 12 hours to complete a seven-day course. Oral medication (200–400 mg three times daily) may be substituted as soon as feasible. Children (5 to 10 years): 500 mg suppositories administered as for adults. Oral medication (3.7–7.5 mg/kg body weight three times daily) may be susbstituted as soon as feasible.

B.　*Intravenous medication: Adults and children over 10 years:* 100 ml (500 mg metronidazole) by intravenous infusion immediately before, during or after operation and repeated eight-hourly until oral medication (200–

400 mg three times daily) can be given to complete a seven-day course.

Children under 10 years: 1.5 ml (7.5 mg metronidazole) per kg body weight administered as for adults until oral medication (3.7 to 7.5 mg/kg bodyweight three times daily) can be given to complete a seven-day course.

Zadstat injection should be infused intravenously at the rate of 5 ml per minute and may be administered alone or concurrently (but separately) with other appropriate parenteral anti-bacterial agents.

Elderly: Zadstat may be used at the normal recommended dosage in elderly patients even with mild to moderate renal impairment. Regular monitoring should occur during long term treatment.

Contra-indications, warnings, etc
Contra-indications: A history of known allergy to metronidazole.

Precautions: The recommended dosages, frequencies of administration and duration of medication have been found effective and well tolerated in nearly all cases. However, regular clinical and biological surveillance are advised if administration of metronidazole for more than 10 days is considered to be necessary.

Clinicians who contemplate continuous therapy, for the relief of chronic conditions, for periods longer than those recommended are advised to consider the possible therapeutic benefit against the risks of peripheral neuropathy.

Patients should be advised to avoid alcohol during therapy. Metronidazole may potentiate the action of anticoagulants and their activity should be routinely monitored. Metronidazole passes rapidly into the foetal circulation and into breast milk although no adverse effects on the new-born have been reported. As with all medicines, metronidazole should be used during pregnancy or lactation only when considered essential. In these circumstances the short high dosage regimens are not recommended.

Patients with limited degrees of renal impairment need no alteration in recommended dosage. Patients on haemodialysis should be dosed immediately following this procedure.

Side-effects; There have been occasional reports of an unpleasant taste, furred tongue, nausea, urticaria and angio-oedema, and very rarely vomiting, drowsiness, dizziness, headache, ataxia, skin rashes, pruritis, inco-ordination of movement and darkening of the urine (due to a metronidazole metabolite). Anaphylaxis may occur rarely.

A few instances of peripheral neuropathy or transient epileptiform seizures have been reported during intensive and/or prolonged therapy. In most cases neuropathy resolved on withdrawing therapy or reducing dosage. Moderate transient leucopenia has also been reported.

Overdosage: There is no specific treatment but early gastric lavage is recommended following overdosage by mouth. Uneventful recovery has followed attempts at suicide with oral doses up to 12 g. Metronidazole is readily removed from plasma by haemodialysis.

Pharmaceutical precautions Protect from light. Zadstat metronidazole injection does not contain a preservative and is therefore not intended for multi-dose use. Zadstat metronidazole injection, if necessary, may be added to Sodium Chloride Infusion 0.9%; Sodium Chloride 0.18% and Glucose 4% Infusion; Glucose Injection BP 5%; Potassium Chloride Injection (20 mmol or 40 mmol).

Metronidazole injection is incompatible with Dextrose Injection 10%, Hartmann's solution (compound sodium lactate injection); protein hydrolysates, amino acid infusion or alkaline solutions.

Legal category POM.

Package quantities *Tablets:* Bottles of 21 and 250. *Suppositories:* Boxes of 10 × 500 mg and 10 × 1 g. *Injection:* Boxes containing 2 × 100 ml Steriflex Mini-packs in sales packs of 5 boxes.

Further information Nil.

Product licence numbers
Tablets 200 mg	0095/0048
Suppositories 500 mg	0095/0084
Suppositories 1 g	0095/0085
Injection 500 mg in 100 ml	0095/0086.

*Trade Mark

Leo Laboratories Limited
Longwick Road
Princes Risborough
Aylesbury
Bucks. HP17 9RR

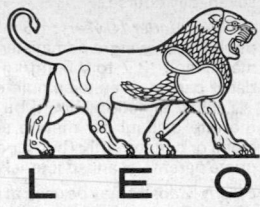

BURINEX* TABLETS
BURINEX* INJECTION
BURINEX* LIQUID

Presentation *Tablets 1 mg:* Each tablet contains 1 mg bumetanide – a yellow, flat, circular, uncoated tablet marked with a score line and '1 mg' on one face.

Tablets 5 mg: Each tablet contains 5 mg bumetanide – a white, flat, circular, uncoated, bevelled-edge tablet, marked with a score line and '5 mg' on one face.

Liquid: An opalescent, pale green, viscous, aqueous solution for oral administration containing 1 mg bumetanide in 5 ml (0.2 mg per ml).

Injection: A solution containing 0.5 mg bumetanide per ml in amber glass ampoules of 2 ml, 4 ml and 10 ml, each ampoule containing 1 mg, 2 mg and 5 mg bumetanide respectively.

Uses *Mode of action:* Burinex (bumetanide) is a potent high ceiling diuretic with a rapid onset and a short duration of action. After oral administration of 1 mg Burinex, diuresis begins within 30 minutes with a peak effect between one and two hours. The diuretic effect is virtually complete in three hours after a 1 mg dose.

After intravenous injection, diuresis usually starts within a few minutes and ceases in about two hours.

In most patients 1 mg of Burinex produces a similar diuretic effect to 40 mg of frusemide.

Burinex is well absorbed after oral administration. Burinex excretion in the urine shows a good correlation with the diuretic response. In patients with chronic renal failure, the liver takes more importance as an excretory pathway, although the duration of action in such patients is not markedly prolonged.

Indications: Burinex is indicated whenever diuretic therapy is required in the treatment of oedema, e.g. that associated with congestive heart failure, cirrhosis of the liver and renal disease including the nephrotic syndrome.

In oedema of cardiac or renal origin where high doses of a potent, short acting diuretic are required, Burinex 5 mg tablets may be used.

For those oedematous conditions where a prompt diuresis is required, Burinex Injection may be used, e.g. acute pulmonary oedema, acute and chronic renal failure, salicylate or barbiturate poisoning. Burinex Injection can be given intravenously or intramuscularly to those patients who are unable to take Burinex tablets or who fail to respond satisfactorily to oral therapy. Burinex liquid may be more appropriate in patients who have difficulty swallowing tablets.

Dosage and administration *Oral dosage: Burinex 1 mg tablets:* Most patients require a daily dose of 1 mg which can be given as a single morning or early evening dose. Depending on the patient's response, a second dose can be given six to eight hours later. In refractory cases, the dose can be increased until a satisfactory diuretic response is obtained, or infusions of Burinex can be given.

Burinex liquid: Usually 1 mg (5 ml) as a single oral dose given morning or early evening. The dosage should be adjusted according to the patient's response.

Burinex 5 mg tablets: The dose should be carefully titrated in each patient according to the patient's response and the required therapeutic activity. As a general rule, in patients not controlled on lower doses, dosage should be started at 5 mg daily, and then increased by 5 mg increments every 12–24 hours until the required response is obtained or side-effects appear. Consideration should be given to a twice daily dosage, rather than once daily. Direct substitution of Burinex for frusemide in a 1:40 ratio at high doses should be avoided. Treatment should be initiated at a lower equivalent dose and gradually increased in 5 mg increments.

Children: Not recommended for children under 12 years of age.

Dosage in the elderly: Adjust dosage according to response; a dose of 0.5 mg bumetanide per day may be sufficient in some elderly patients.

Parenteral dosage: Pulmonary oedema: Initially 1–2 mg by intravenous injection. This can be repeated, if necessary, 20 minutes later.

In those conditions in which an infusion is appropriate, 2–5 mg may be given in 500 ml infusion fluid over 30–60 minutes. (See pharmaceutical precautions.)

When intramuscular administration is considered appropriate, a dose of 1 mg should be given initially and the dose then adjusted according to diuretic response.

Contra-indications, warnings, etc
Contra-indications: Although Burinex can be used to induce diuresis in renal insufficiency, any marked increase in blood urea or the development of oliguria or anuria during treatment of severe progressing renal disease are indications for stopping treatment with Burinex.

Burinex is contra-indicated in hepatic coma and care should be taken in states of severe electrolyte depletion.

As with other diuretics, Burinex should not be administered concurrently with lithium salts. Diuretics can reduce lithium clearance resulting in high serum levels of lithium.

Precautions: Excessively rapid mobilisation of oedema particularly in elderly patients, may give rise to sudden changes in cardiovascular pressure-flow relationships with circulatory collapse. This should be borne in mind when Burinex is given in high doses intravenously or orally. Electrolyte disturbances may occur, particularly in those patients taking a low-salt diet. Regular checks of serum electrolytes, in particular sodium, potassium, chloride and bicarbonate should be performed and replacement therapy instituted where indicated.

Like other diuretics, Burinex shows a tendency to increase the excretion of potassium which can lead to an increase in the sensitivity of the myocardium to the toxic effects of digitalis. Thus the dose may need adjustment when given in conjunction with cardiac glycosides.

Burinex may potentiate the effects of antihypertensive drugs. Therefore, the dose of the latter may need adjustment when Burinex is used to treat oedema in hypertensive patients.

As with other diuretics, Burinex may cause an increase in blood uric acid. Periodic checks on urine and blood glucose should be made in diabetics and patients suspected of latent diabetes.

Patients with chronic renal failure on high doses of Burinex should remain under constant hospital supervision.

Pregnancy: Although tests in four animal species have shown no teratogenic effects, the ordinary precaution of avoiding use of Burinex in the first trimester of pregnancy should at present be observed.

Adverse Reactions: Reported reactions include skin rashes and muscular cramps in the legs, abdominal discomfort, thrombocytopenia and gynaecomastia.

High Dose Therapy: In patients with severe chronic renal failure given high doses of Burinex, there have been reports of severe, generalised, musculoskeletal pain sometimes associated with muscle spasm, occurring one to two hours after administration and lasting up to 12 hours. The lowest reported dose causing this type of adverse reaction was 5 mg by intravenous injection and the highest was 75 mg orally in a single dose. All patients recovered fully and there was no deterioration in their renal function.

The cause of this pain is uncertain but it may be a result of varying electrolyte gradients at the cell membrane level.

Experience suggests that the incidence of such reactions is reduced by initiating treatment at 5–10 mg daily and titrating upwards using a twice daily dosage regimen at doses of 20 mg per day or more.

Overdosage: Symptoms would be those caused by excessive diuresis. Empty stomach by gastric lavage or emesis. General measures should be taken to restore blood volume, maintain blood pressure and correct electrolyte disturbance.

Pharmaceutical precautions Burinex is presented in amber glass containers to protect against deterioration due to exposure to light.

When an intravenous infusion is required, Burinex Injection may be added to Dextrose Injection BP, Sodium Chloride Injection BP or Sodium Chloride and Dextrose Injection BP.

When 25 mg bumetanide (as Burinex Injection) was added to 1 litre of these infusion fluids, no evidence of precipitation was observed over a period of 72 hours. Higher concentrations of Burinex in these infusion fluids may cause precipitation. It is good practice to inspect all infusion fluids containing Burinex from time to time. Should cloudiness appear, the infusion should be discarded.

Burinex Liquid: Do not refrigerate.

Legal category POM.

Package quantities *1 mg Tablets:* Bottles of 100 and 1,000.
5 mg tablets: Bottles of 100.
Liquid: Bottles of 150 ml. A measure-spoon graduated at 2.5 ml and 5 ml is supplied.
Injection: Packs of 5 × 2 ml, 5 × 4 ml and 5 × 10 ml.

Further information Burinex is also available as Burinex K tablets, each containing 0.5 mg bumetanide and 573 mg potassium chloride in a slow release core. Burinex 1 mg tablets contain tartrazine as a colouring agent.

Product licence numbers

Burinex 1 mg	0043/0021
Burinex 5 mg	0043/0043
Burinex Injection	0043/0060
Burinex Liquid	0043/0075

BURINEX* K

Presentation White, ovoid, unmarked tablets each containing 0.5 mg bumetanide (Burinex) and 573 mg Potassium chloride BP (7.7 mmol potassium in a slow release wax core).

Uses *Mode of Action:* Burinex K combines the very potent high-ceiling diuretic bumetanide, with a slow-release potassium chloride supplement. Bumetanide has a rapid onset and a short duration of action. As with most diuretics, long-term therapy may be associated with potassium depletion.

The potassium supplement in Burinex K should help to maintain normal levels of potassium, especially in those patients whose dietary intake of potassium is inadequate.

The formulation of Burinex K presents the following advantages. The diuretic is coated around the tablet, from which it is rapidly released. The diuretic and saluretic effects begin within 30 minutes after oral administration, peak at one to two hours, and are largely complete within three hours. In contrast, the potassium chloride, which is included in an inert wax core, is released only slowly over a period of six hours after oral ingestion. This slow-release minimises the risk of gastro-intestinal intolerance as well as that of ulceration and stenosis resulting from localised high concentrations of potassium salts in the small bowel.

Indications: Burinex K is indicated for the treatment of oedema where a potassium supplement is necessary. Low serum potassium levels are, for example, known to increase the toxic effects of the cardiac glycosides; Burinex K may therefore be of particular value in those patients being treated with digitalis.

Dosage and administration For initial therapy, most patients will be treated with Burinex 1 mg tablets alone. The dose required will be adjusted to the patient's response, but is likely to vary between 0.5 and 2 mg ($\frac{1}{2}$–2 tablets of Burinex). For maintenance therapy Burinex K is more convenient than Burinex. In many patients, 2 tablets daily (1.0 mg Burinex and 15.4 mmol potassium) which may be given as a single morning or early evening dose should prove adequate.

For some patients, however, this maintenance dose may be inadequate. Larger doses should preferably be given in divided doses. If a daily dosage of more than 4 tablets of Burinex K is required, then Burinex itself should be substituted and potassium chloride given separately, in divided doses, as a slow-release preparation (such as Leo K).

Burinex K tablets must be swallowed whole and never chewed.

The tablets should be swallowed with at least 100 mls water.

Dosage in the elderly: Adjust dosage according to response; a dose of 1 tablet per day may be sufficient in some elderly patients.

Contra-indications, warnings, etc

Contra-indications: Burinex K should not be used with potassium-sparing diuretics (e.g. spironolactone, triamterene or amiloride) or in patients with renal insufficiency.

As with other diuretics, Burinex K should not be administered concurrently with lithium salts. Diuretics can reduce lithium clearance resulting in high serum levels of lithium.

All solid forms of potassium medication are contra-indicated in the presence of obstruction in the digestive tract (e.g. resulting from compression of the oesophagus due to dilation of the left atrium or from stenosis of the gut).

Precautions: The 15.4 mmol of potassium included in the usual dose of Burinex K (2 tablets daily) should help to prevent hypokalaemia in many patients. Certain patients, however – as, for example, those with hepatic ascites or those on a very low potassium diet – may require considerably more potassium than this. Periodic checks should therefore be made on the serum potassium level in patients on long-term therapy.

The diuretic in Burinex K may potentiate the effect of antihypertensive drugs, increase blood uric acid and (though rarely) affect carbohydrate metabolism.

Non-specific small bowel lesions characterised by stenosis and possibly accompanied by ulceration have been associated with the oral administration of tablets and capsules containing potassium salts. Symptoms and signs which indicate ulceration or obstruction of the small bowel in patients taking tablets or capsules containing potassium salts are indications for stopping treatment with such preparations immediately.

Adverse reactions: Reported reactions include skin rashes and muscular cramps in the legs, abdominal discomfort, thrombocytopenia and gynaecomastia.

Pregnancy: Although tests in four animal species have shown no teratogenic effects, the ordinary precaution of avoiding use of Burinex in the first trimester of pregnancy should at present be observed.

Overdosage: General methods should be taken to restore blood volume and maintain blood pressure.

Pharmaceutical precautions   Nil.

Legal category   POM.

Package quantities   Packs of 100, 500 and 1,000 tablets.

Further information   Nil.

Product licence number   0043/0027.

FUCIDIN* TABLETS
FUCIDIN* SUSPENSION
FUCIDIN* FOR INTRAVENOUS INFUSION

Presentation   *Fucidin Tablets:* Each white, ovoid enteric-coated tablet contains 250 mg Sodium Fusidate BP.

Fucidin Suspension: Each 5 ml of pale orange, banana-flavoured aqueous suspension contains 250 mg Fusidic Acid BP (therapeutically equivalent to 175 mg Sodium Fusidate BP).

Fucidin for Intravenous Infusion: A pack of 2 vials. One vial contains Diethanolamine Fusidate BPC 1968, 580 mg (equivalent to 500 mg sodium fusidate) as a dry powder. The second vial contains 50 ml sterile phosphate-citrate buffer solution (pH 7.4–7.6).

Sodium fusidate is the sodium salt of fusidic acid.

Uses   *Mode of Action:* Fucidin and its salts are potent antistaphylococcal agents with unusual ability to penetrate tissue. Bactericidal levels have been assayed in bone and necrotic tissue. Blood levels are cumulative, reaching concentrations of 50–100 mcg/ml after oral administration of 1.5 g daily for three to four days. Concentrations of 0.03–0.12 mcg/ml inhibit nearly all strains of *Staphylococcus aureus*.

Fucidin is excreted mainly in the bile, little or none being excreted in the urine.

Indications: Fucidin is indicated in the treatment of all staphylococcal infections such as: osteomyelitis; pneumonia; septicaemia; wound infections; endocarditis; superinfected cystic fibrosis; cutaneous infections.

Fucidin should be administered intravenously whenever oral therapy is inappropriate which includes cases where absorption from the gastro-intestinal tract is unpredictable.

Dosage and administration   *For Fucidin tablets: Adults: Standard dose:* 500 mg three times daily. In severe or fulminating infections, this dosage may be doubled or appropriate combined therapy may be used.

For Fucidin Suspension: Adult dose: 15 ml three times daily.

Children: 0–1 year: 1 ml/kg body weight daily divided into 3 equal doses.

1–5 years: 5 ml three times daily.

5–12 years: 10 ml three times daily.

Intravenous therapy: Adults weighing more than 50 kg: 580 mg diethanolamine fusidate three times daily.

Children and adults weighing less than 50 kg: 6 to 7 mg diethanolamine fusidate per kg body weight, three times daily.

Recommended procedure: Dissolve 580 mg diethanolamine fusidate powder (1 vial) in the 50 ml buffer provided. The enclosed needle may be used for this purpose.

1. For adults weighing more than 50 kg: Add the fusidate/buffer solution to 500 ml of infusion fluid and infuse slowly over a period of not less than six hours.

2. For children and adults weighing less than 50 kg: Each dose corresponds to approximately 0.6 ml of the fusidate/buffer solution per kg body weight. This volume should be further diluted, at least tenfold, with the appropriate infusion fluid, and infused slowly over a period of not less than six hours.

Since Fucidin is excreted in the bile, no dosage modifications are needed in renal impairment.

The dosage in patients undergoing haemodialysis needs no adjustment as Fucidin is not significantly dialysed.

Dosage in the elderly: No dosage alterations are necessary in the elderly.

Contra-indications, warnings, etc   *Intravenous Fu-*

cidin: Contra-indications: Fucidin should not be infused with amino-acid solutions or in whole blood. Due to local tissue injury, Fucidin should not be administered intramuscularly or subcutaneously.

Precautions: Caution should be exercised with other antibiotics which have similar biliary excretion pathways, e.g. lincomycin and rifampicin.

Periodic liver function tests should be carried out when high oral doses are used, when the drug is given for prolonged periods and in patients with liver dysfunction.

Fucidin displaces bilirubin from its albumin binding site in vitro. The clinical significance of this finding is uncertain and kernicterus has not been observed in neonates receiving Fucidin. However, this observation should be borne in mind when the drug is given to preterm, jaundiced, acidotic or seriously ill neonates.

Pregnancy: Fucidin is detected in breast milk and it can cross the placenta.

Intravenous Fucidin: In most cases Sodium Chloride Injection is used as an infusion fluid. It has also been given in plasma and occasionally in 5% dextrose, 40% dextrose, 20% fructose, and in Sodium Chloride and Dextrose Injection. Opalescence may be encountered with more acidic samples of dextrose, when the solution should be discarded. Infusion should be made into a wide bore vein with a good blood flow.

Each 50 ml of phosphate/citrate buffer for intravenous infusion contains 980 mg disodium hydrogen phosphate (equivalent to 5.5 mmols phosphate). Doses of I.V. Fucidin in excess of the recommended dose may result in hypocalcaemia due to the large amount of phosphate/citrate buffer administered. If more than the recommended dose is given for prolonged periods, the serum calcium should be closely monitored. Any hypocalcaemia occurring may be reversed by reducing the dosage of I.V. Fucidin to recommended levels and administering I.V. calcium gluconate.

Adverse reactions: In some patients given Fucidin, a reversible jaundice has been reported, most frequently in patients receiving intravenous Fucidin in high dosage, or where the drug has been infused too rapidly or at too high a concentration in the infusion fluid. In some instances, instituting oral therapy may be beneficial. If the jaundice persists, Fucidin should be withdrawn, following which the serum bilirubin will invariably return to normal.

Overdosage: There has been no experience of overdosage with Fucidin. Treatment should be restricted to symptomatic and supportive measures. Dialysis is of no benefit, since the drug is not significantly dialysed.

Pharmaceutical precautions *Fucidin tablets:* Nil.

Fucidin Suspension: Protect from direct sunlight and heat. The Suspension should be shaken before use and dilution is not recommended.

Fucidin Infusion: Fucidin dry powder is stable for 3 years when stored below 25°C. When the buffer solution is transferred to the powder vial, this vial should be regarded as a unit dose. Although the Fucidin/buffer solution can be kept up to 24 hours, the required amount of solution should be taken once only and any unused portion discarded.

Legal category POM.

Package quantities *Tablets:* Bottles of 100.
Suspension: Bottles of 50 ml.

Infusion: Pack containing a single pair of vials, with transfer needle.

Further information Fucidin should be administered intravenously into a wide bore vein with a good blood flow. Excessive doses may cause venospasm, thrombophlebitis and haemolysis of erythrocytes.

Both oral and intravenous Fucidin have been given in combination with other antibiotics e.g. Cloxacillin, flucloxacillin, ampicillin, methicillin and erythromycin.

Product licence numbers
Tablets: 0043/5000
Suspension: 0043/5014
Infusion: 0043/5003

FUCIDIN* OINTMENT
FUCIDIN* GEL
FUCIDIN* CAVIJECT
FUCIDIN* INTERTULLE
FUCIDIN* CREAM

Presentation *Fucidin Ointment* contains Sodium Fusidate BP 2% in an ointment base (no preservative).

Fucidin Gel contains Fusidic Acid BP 2% in a water-miscible base; methylparaben 0.27% and propylparaben 0.03% as preservative.

Fucidin Caviject is a sterile, single-dose preparation containing Fusidic Acid BP 2% in a water-miscible base (Fucidin gel), methylparaben 0.27% and propylparaben 0.03% as preservative, fitted with an elongated flexible nozzle.

Fucidin Intertulle: Sterile gauze squares each impregnated with Sodium Fusidate BP 2% (Fucidin Ointment) in an ointment base and enclosed between two leaves of sterile parchment in a sealed foil pack.

Fucidin Cream contains Fusidic Acid BP 2% in a cream base; potassium sorbate 0.27% as preservative.

Uses *Mode of Action:* Sodium fusidate is the sodium salt of fusidic acid.

1 g Fucidin Ointment contains 20,000 mcg of Sodium Fusidate BP and 1 g Fucidin Gel or Fucidin Cream contains approx. 20,000 mcg Fusidic Acid BP.

Fucidin is a potent topical antibacterial agent. Fusidic acid and its salts show fat and water solubility and strong surface activity and exhibit unusual ability to penetrate intact skin. Concentrations of 0.03–0.12 mcg/ml inhibit nearly all strains of *Staphylococcus aureus*. Local concentrations with topical Fucidin are also effective against Streptococci, Corynebacteria, Neisseria and certain Clostridia.

Indications: Indicated, either alone or in combination with systemic therapy, in the treatment of skin infections caused by Gram-positive organisms, particularly the Staphylococcus, e.g. abscesses, boils, carbuncles, impetigo, eczema, varicose ulcers, skin grafts, wounds, burns.

Dosage and administration *Fucidin Gel, Fucidin Ointment and Fucidin Cream: Adults and children:* Uncovered lesions – apply gently, three or four times daily. Covered lesions – less frequent applications may be adequate.

Fucidin Caviject: The abscess should be incised and carefully curetted. The cavity is filled by injecting Fucidin Caviject and a dressing applied. The caviject container should be used once only and then discarded.

Fucidin Intertulle: Usually, once a day application but

frequency of application will vary with clinical circumstances.

Contra-indications, warnings, etc
Contra-indications: Infection caused by non-susceptible organisms, in particular, *Pseudomonas aeruginosa.*

Precautions: The sodium salt of fusidic acid has been shown to cause conjunctival irritation. The Ointment and Intertulle should not be used in or near the eye.

Fusidic acid does not appear to cause conjunctival irritation in experimental animals. Caution should, however, still be exercised when using Fucidin Gel, Caviject or Cream near the eye.

Adverse reactions: Hypersensitivity may occur.

Overdosage: Not applicable.

Pharmaceutical precautions *Fucidin Ointment and Cream:* Nil.

Fucidin Gel and Caviject: Store below 25°C but do not freeze.

Fucidin Intertulle: Store below 25°C.

Legal category POM.

Package quantities *Ointment, Cream and Gel:* Tubes of 15 g and 30 g.
Caviject: Tubes of 7 g.
Intertulle: Box of 10 foil packs, each containing one tulle piece (10 cm × 10 cm).

Further information The gel base is non-staining and contains no lanolin or other fatty constituents.
The cream base is a vanishing base and contains no lanolin.

Product licence numbers

Ointment	0043/5005
Gel and Caviject	0043/5018
Intertulle	0043/5007
Cream	0043/0065

FUCIDIN H* OINTMENT
FUCIDIN H* GEL

Presentation Fucidin H Ointment contains Sodium Fusidate BP 2% and Hydrocortisone Acetate BP 1% in an ointment base (no preservative).

Fucidin H Gel contains Fusidic Acid BP 2% and Hydrocortisone Acetate BP 1% in a water-miscible gel base; methylparaben 0.27% and propylparaben 0.03% as preservative.

Sodium fusidate is the sodium salt of fusidic acid.

Uses *Mode of Action:* Fucidin H Ointment and Fucidin H Gel combine the potent topical antibacterial action of fusidic acid with the anti-inflammatory and antipruritic effects of hydrocortisone. Concentrations of 0.03–0.12 mcg per ml inhibit nearly all strains of *Staphylococcus aureus.* Topical Fucidin is also effective against Streptococci, Corynebacteria, Neisseria and certain Clostridia.

Indications: It is indicated in inflammatory dermatoses, including dermatitis; seborrhoeic dermatitis; allergic, infantile and infected eczema and infected acne, where bacterial infection is present or likely to occur.

Dosage and administration *Adults and children:* Uncovered lesions – apply gently, three or four times daily. Covered lesions – less frequent applications may be adequate.

Contra-indications, warnings, etc
Contra-indications: As with other topical corticosteroid preparations, Fucidin H Gel and Fucidin H Ointment are contra-indicated in tuberculous, viral and fungal skin infections.

Precautions: Fucidin H Ointment should not be used in or near the eye, as sodium fusidate causes conjunctival irritation.

Fusidic acid does not appear to cause conjunctival irritation in experimental animals. Caution should still be exercised, however, when Fucidin H Gel is used near the eye.

Pregnancy: Topical administration of any corticosteroid to pregnant animals can cause abnormalities of foetal development. The relevance of this finding to human beings has not been established; however, topical steroids should not be used extensively in pregnancy, i.e. in large amounts or for prolonged periods.

In infants, long-term continuous topical therapy with corticosteroids should be avoided. Adrenal suppression can occur even without occlusion.

Adverse reactions: Hypersensitivity may occur.

Overdosage: Not applicable.

Pharmaceutical precautions *Fucidin H Gel:* Store below 25°C but do not freeze.

Fucidin H Ointment: Nil.

Legal category POM.

Package quantities Tubes of 15 g and 30 g.

Further information The gel base is non-staining and contains no lanolin or other fatty constituents.

Product licence numbers

Fucidin H Gel	0043/0024
Fucidin H Ointment	0043/5012

FUCIDIN* H CREAM

Presentation Fucidin H cream contains Fusidic Acid BP 2% and Hydrocortisone Acetate BP 1% in a cream base; potassium sorbate 0.27% as preservative.

Uses *Mode of Action:* Fucidin H Cream combines the potent topical antibacterial action of fusidic acid with the anti-inflammatory and antipruritic effects of hydrocortisone. Concentrations of 0.03–0.12 mcg per ml inhibit nearly all strains of *Staphylococcus aureus.* Topical Fucidin is also effective against Streptococci, Corynebacteria, Neisseria and certain Clostridia.

Indications: The treatment of eczematous dermatoses including atopic eczema, infantile eczema, discoid eczema, stasis eczema, contact eczema and seborrhoeic eczema when secondary bacterial infection is confirmed or suspected.

Dosage and administration *Adults and children:* Uncovered lesions – apply gently, three or four times daily. Covered lesions – less frequent applications may be adequate.

Contra-indications, warnings, etc
Contra-indications: As with other topical corticosteroid preparations, Fucidin H Cream is contra-indicated in tuberculous, viral and fungal skin infections.

Fusidic acid does not appear to cause conjunctival irritation in experimental animals. Caution should still be exercised, however, when Fucidin H Cream is used near the eye.

Pregnancy: Topical administration of any corticosteroid to pregnant animals can cause abnormalities of foetal development. The relevance of this finding to human beings has not been established; however, topical steroids should not be used extensively in pregnancy i.e. in large amounts or for prolonged periods.

In infants, long-term continuous topical therapy with corticosteroids should be avoided. Adrenal suppression can occur even without occlusion.

Adverse reactions: Hypersensitivity may occur.

Overdosage: Not applicable.

Pharmaceutical precautions Nil.

Legal category POM.

Package quantities Tubes of 15 g and 30 g.

Further information The cream base is a vanishing base and contains no lanolin.

Product licence number 0043/0093.

FUCIBET* CREAM

Presentation Fucibet cream contains betamethasone 0.1% (as the valerate ester) and Fusidic Acid BP 2% in a smooth white to off-white water miscible base; chlorocresol 0.1% as preservative.

Uses Fucibet combines the well-known anti-inflammatory and antipruritic effects of betamethasone with the potent topical antibacterial action of fusidic acid.

Betamethasone valerate is a topical steroid rapidly effective in those inflammatory dermatoses which normally respond to this form of therapy. More refractory conditions can often be treated successfully.

When applied topically, fusidic acid is effective against *Staphylococcus aureus*, Streptococci, Corynebacteria, Neisseria and certain Clostridia and Bacteroides. Concentrations of 0.03 to 0.12 mcg per ml inhibit nearly all strains of *S. aureus*. The antibacterial activity of fusidic acid is not diminished in the presence of betamethasone.

Indications: Fucibet is indicated for the treatment of eczematous dermatoses including atopic eczema, infantile eczema, discoid eczema, stasis eczema, contact eczema and seborrhoeic eczema when secondary bacterial infection is confirmed or suspected.

Dosage and administration A small quantity should be applied to the affected area two or three times daily until a satisfactory response is obtained. It may then be possible to maintain improvement by less frequent application or by the use of a less potent topical steroid/antibacterial preparation such as Fucidin H Ointment or Fucidin H Gel.

In the more resistant lesions the effect of Fucibet can be enhanced by occlusion with polythene film. Overnight occlusion is usually adequate.

Contra-indications, warnings, etc
Contra-indications: Acne rosacea and peri-oral dermatitis. Skin lesions of viral, fungal or bacterial origin. Hypersensitivity to the preparation.

Precautions: Long-term continuous topical therapy should be avoided, particularly in infants and children. Adrenal suppression can occur even without occlusion. Atrophic changes may occur on the face and to a lesser degree in other parts of the body, after prolonged treatment with potent topical steroids.

Caution should be exercised if Fucibet is used near the eye. Glaucoma might result if the preparation enters the eye. Systemic chemotherapy is required if bacterial infection persists.

Pregnancy: Topical administration of any corticosteroid to pregnant animals can cause abnormalities of foetal development. The relevance of this finding to human beings has not been established; however, topical steroids should not be used extensively in pregnancy, i.e. in large amounts or for prolonged periods.

Adverse reactions: Prolonged and intensive treatment with potent corticosteroids may cause local atrophic changes in the skin, including striae, thinning and dilation of superficial blood vessels, particularly when applied to the flexures or when occlusion is employed.

As with other topical corticosteroids sufficient systemic absorption to produce hypercorticism can occur with prolonged or extensive use. Infants and children are at particular risk, more so if occlusive dressings are used. A napkin may act as an occlusive dressing in infants.

Hypersensitivity reactions to fusidic acid are rare and Fucibet does not contain lanolin. However, if signs of hypersensitivity occur, treatment should be withdrawn.

Overdosage: Not applicable.

Pharmaceutical precautions Nil.

Legal category POM.

Package quantities Tubes of 15 g and 30 g.

Further information The least potent corticosteroid, which controls the disease, should be used.

Product licence number 0043/0091.

HEPARIN (MUCOUS) INJECTION BP

Presentation Heparin (Mucous) Injection BP 1,000 units per ml: each ml contains 1,000 units sodium heparin. (Presented in 5 ml ampoules without preservative, and 5 ml vials with preservative.)

Heparin (Mucous) Injection BP 5,000 units per ml: each ml contains 5,000 units sodium heparin (with preservative).

Heparin (Mucous) Injection BP 25,000 units per ml: each ml contains 25,000 units sodium heparin (with preservative).

Uses *Mode of Action:* Heparin is a naturally occurring anticoagulant which prevents the coagulation of blood *in-vivo* and *in-vitro*. It potentiates the inhibition of several activated coagulation factors, including thrombin and factor X.

The anticoagulant properties of heparin are valuable for the prophylaxis and management of intravascular clotting and embolism. It is also used in extra-corporeal circulation, i.e. heart-lung and renal dialysis machines and blood transfusions.

In addition to the anticoagulant properties heparin also has some lipaemia-clearing effect which may be utilised in the treatment of fat embolism.

Indications: Treatment of thrombo-embolic disorders such as: Deep vein thrombosis, Thrombophlebitis, Pulmonary embolism, Fat embolism.

Dosage and administration Heparin is usually administered by intravenous injection or subcutaneously.

Although the intramuscular route can be used, it is not recommended because of the high incidence of haematomata.

The increase in clotting time provided by heparin becomes apparent immediately after administration and lasts for four to six hours after intravenous injection and for about eight hours after subcutaneous injection.

Dosage: Intravenous administration: 5,000–10,000 units every four hours either by bolus injection or continuous infusion in Sodium Chloride Injection or Dextrose Injection. However, the dose should be monitored with coagulation tests, and varied according to individual response.

Subcutaneous administration: 5,000 units every eight hours.

The treatment period varies from 7–10 days in peri-operative prophylaxis to as much as six weeks in the treatment of established thrombosis.

Dosage in the elderly: Elderly women have a greater tendency to bleed and it may be necessary to reduce the dose according to coagulation tests.

Contra-indications, warnings, etc
Contra-indications: Haemorrhagic disorders and patients with an actual or potential bleeding site e.g. peptic ulcer.

Precautions: Heparin therapy should be given with caution to patients about to undergo surgery, and those with impaired renal or hepatic function.

Overdosage: The effect of heparin can be reversed immediately by intravenous administration of a 1% protamine sulphate solution. The quantity of protamine required for neutralisation falls rapidly with the lapse of time after the administration of heparin and can be accurately determined by titration of the patient's plasma, containing heparin, with protamine. If given within 15 minutes of the heparin injection 10 mg of protamine will neutralise 1,000 units of heparin, while 30 minutes after the heparin injection, only 5 mg of protamine per 1,000 units of heparin is needed. It is important to avoid overdosage of protamine sulphate because protamine itself has anticoagulant properties. A single dose of protamine sulphate should never exceed 50 mg. Intravenous injection of protamine may cause a sudden fall in blood pressure, bradycardia, dyspnoea and transitory flushing, but these may be avoided or diminished by slow and careful administration.

Pharmaceutical precautions Store below 25°C. Admixture of heparin with solutions of other medicinal products may result in precipitation or loss of potency.

Legal category POM.

Package quantities *Heparin 1,000 units per ml:* 5 ml ampoules (without preservative), 5 ml vials (with preservative): Packs of 5.
Heparin 5,000 units per ml: 5 ml: Packs of 5 vials.
Heparin 25,000 units per ml: 5 ml: 1 vial.

Further information *Preservative used:* 1,000 units (with preservative) and 5,000 units: 0.5% Chlorbutol. 25,000 Units: 0.4% Chlorbutol.

Available for low dose prophylactic use: Minihep: Single dose ampoules containing 5,000 units sodium heparin in 0.2 ml and
Minihep calcium: Single dose ampoules containing 5,000 units calcium heparin in 0.2 ml.

Heparin (Mucous) Injection BP is also available in 1 ml single dose ampoules without preservative: Unihep Leo 1,000 (1,000 units per ml), Unihep Leo 5,000 (5,000 units per ml), Unihep Leo 10,000 (10,000 units per ml) and Unihep Leo 25,000 (25,000 units per ml).

Menstruation and pregnancy are not contra-indications to heparin therapy. Heparin does not cross the placenta or appear in breast milk.

Product licence numbers

1,000 units (with preservative)	0043/0041
1,000 units (without preservative)	0043/0085
5,000 units (with preservative)	0043/0038
25,000 units (with preservative)	0043/0039

HEPLOK*
Heparin (mucous) Injection BP 10 units per ml

Presentation 5 ml ampoule, each ml containing 10 units sodium heparin in saline (no preservative).

Uses Heparin is an anticoagulant which prevents the formation of thrombin by accelerating the neutralisation of activated Factor X by naturally occurring inhibitors.

Indications: This strength of heparin is used as a 'heparin flush' every four hours, or as necessary, to keep intravenous lines patent. It is not recommended that this low dose heparin be used therapeutically.

Dosage and administration For routine use 1–5 ml (10–50 units sodium heparin) should be administered into the catheter/cannula every 4 hours.

Contra-indications, warnings, etc When used as recommended the low dose of heparin reaching the blood should have no systemic effects.

Pharmaceutical precautions Store below 25°C.
Admixture with other drugs may cause inactivation of either the heparin solution or the drugs.

Legal category POM.

Package quantities Packs of 10 × 5 ml ampoules.

Further information Nil.

Product licence number 0043/0092

LEO* K TABLETS
Presentation Potassium Chloride BP 600 mg (8 mmol potassium in a slow-release wax core). White film-coated, ovoid tablets with no superficial markings.

Uses *Mode of Action:* Potassium depletion can occur insidiously, as the symptoms often resemble those of the underlying condition and may be easily overlooked. It is difficult to assess potassium depletion from serum potassium levels because there is no correlation between intracellular and extracellular potassium concentrations.

Intake of dietary potassium may not be adequate to restore normal levels in patients who already have low cellular potassium. These patients require potassium supplements.

Because of the risk of localised high concentrations of potassium salts in the small bowel, the potassium of Leo K is included in an inert wax core, from which it is released slowly over at least six hours.

Indications: As a potassium supplement, to reduce the risk of potassium depletion which may be associated with prolonged use of diuretics, and corticosteroids; congestive heart failure; primary or secondary aldosteronism; renal tubular acidosis; malabsorption syndrome, ulcerative colitis, liver cirrhosis and other conditions where potassium loss may be severe.

Dosage and administration 3–5 tablets daily in divided doses (24–40 mmol potassium) are often adequate. A smaller dose may be adequate in those patients with a more satisfactory dietary intake of potassium, but some patients, particularly those with hepatic or renal insufficiency, may require considerably more potassium chloride.

The tablets should be swallowed whole with at least 100 mls water.

Dosage in the elderly: Serum potassium levels should be monitored and dosage adjusted according to response.

Contra-indications, warnings, etc
Contra-indications: All solid forms of potassium medication are contra-indicated in the presence of obstructions in the digestive tract (e.g. resulting from compression of the oesophagus due to dilation of the left atrium or from stenosis of the gut).

Precautions: To avoid hyperkalaemia, a potassium supplement should be used with great caution in renal insufficiency or with the potassium-sparing diuretics like spironolactone, triamterene or amiloride. Some patients may develop potassium depletion despite the use of potassium supplements. This is a particular danger to digitalised patients or those with hepatic ascites.

Non-specific small bowel lesions, characterised by stenosis and possibly accompanied by ulceration have been associated with the oral administration of tablets and capsules containing potassium salts. Symptoms and signs which might indicate ulceration or obstruction of the small bowel in patients taking tablets or capsules containing potassium salts are indications for stopping treatment with such a preparation immediately.

Overdosage: Symptoms of overdosage include asthenia, hypotension, mental confusion, parasthesia, and cardiac arrhythmias.

Characteristic ECG changes also occur. Hyperkalaemia should be treated with an intravenous infusion of sodium bicarbonate or by intravenous injection of calcium chloride or calcium gluconate (10–20 ml of a 1% solution).

Pharmaceutical precautions Nil.

Legal category GSL.

Package quantities Packs of 100 and 1,000 tablets.

Further information Nil.

Product licence number 0043/5006.

MINIHEP*
MINIHEP* CALCIUM
MINIHEP* DARTS*
MINIHEP* CALCIUM DARTS*

Presentation *Minihep:* Heparin (Mucous) Injection BP. Single dose ampoules containing Sodium Heparin 5,000 units in 0.2 ml (no preservative).

Minihep calcium: Calcium Heparin Injection (Mucous). Single dose ampoules containing Calcium Heparin 5,000 units in 0.2 ml (no preservative).

Minihep DARTS: Heparin (Mucous) Injection BP. Single dose DARTS, automatic injector system, containing Sodium Heparin 5,000 units in 0.5 ml (no preservative).

Minihep Calcium DARTS: Calcium Heparin Injection (Mucous). Single dose DARTS, automatic injector system, containing Calcium Heparin 5000 units in 0.5 ml (no preservative).

Uses *Mode of Action:* Heparin is an anticoagulant which, even in low doses, prevents the formation of thrombin by accelerating the neutralisation of activated coagulation factors by naturally occurring inhibitors.

Indications: Prophylaxis against deep vein thrombosis and thromboembolic events in susceptible patients.

Dosage and administration Administration is by subcutaneous injection.

Patients undergoing surgery: 5,000 units in 0.2 ml or 0.5 ml should be given two to six hours pre-operatively and every eight hours post-operatively for 10–14 days, or until ambulation, whichever is the longer.

Other patients: 5,000 units in 0.2 ml or 0.5 ml should be given every 8–12 hours.

Dosage in the elderly: Elderly women have a greater tendency to bleed but dosage alterations are unlikely for prophylaxis in the elderly.

Contra-indications, warnings, etc Low doses of heparin, administered as recommended above, do not cause alterations in clotting times in most patients, but occasionally local haematomata may occur at injection sites.

Patients with haemorrhagic disorders may experience bleeding, especially from surgical wounds. The relative risks and benefits of heparin administration in these patients should be assessed carefully. Oral anticoagulants or drugs which interfere with platelet function e.g. aspirin and dextran solutions, should be administered with caution.

Overdosage: If bleeding should occur, the effect of heparin can be reversed immediately by intravenous administration of a 1% protamine sulphate solution. The dose of protamine sulphate required for neutralisation should be determined accurately by titrating with the patient's plasma.

Pharmaceutical precautions Store below 25°C. Admixture of heparin with solutions of other medicinal products may result in precipitation or loss of potency.

Legal category POM.

Package quantities *Minihep and Minihep Calcium:* 10 ampoules of 0.2 ml. *Minihep DARTS and Minihep Calcium DARTS:* 50 DARTS of 0.5 ml

Further information Menstruation and pregnancy are not contra-indications to heparin therapy. Heparin does not cross the placenta or appear in breast milk.

Heparin (Mucous) Injection BP is also available in 5 ml vials with preservative in strengths of 1,000, 5,000 and 25,000 units per ml and in 1 ml single dose ampoules without preservative: Unihep Leo 1,000 (1,000 units per ml), Unihep Leo 5,000 (5,000 units per ml), Unihep Leo 10,000 (10,000 units per ml) and Unihep Leo 25,000 (25,000 units per ml). 5 ml ampoules of 1,000 units per ml without preservative are also available.

Product licence numbers
Minihep   0043/0088
Minihep Calcium   0043/0051

Minihep DARTS   0043/0081
Minihep Calcium DARTS   0043/0094

MIRAXID* TABLETS ▼
MIRAXID* PAEDIATRIC SUSPENSION ▼

Presentation *Tablets:* White, film coated tablets, each containing: Pivampicillin 125 mg and Pivmecillinam hydrochloride 100 mg.

Suspension: Unit dose foil sachets, each containing: Pivampicillin 62.5 mg and Pivmecillinam 46.2 mg.

Uses Miraxid contains the orally active derivatives of mecillinam and ampicillin – pivmecillinam hydrochloride and pivampicillin respectively. Following oral administration, Miraxid is absorbed rapidly and pivmecillinam and pivampicillin are hydrolysed in the body by non-specific enzymes present in blood and other tissues liberating mecillinam and ampicillin. Both drugs produce maximum plasma levels at $\frac{1}{4}$–1 hour after administration. Mecillinam and ampicillin are both mainly excreted unchanged in the urine within the first 8 hours of administration. Smaller amounts of both compounds are excreted with the bile. Miraxid shows high anti-bacterial activity against most commonly occurring Gram-negative and Gram-positive pathogens. Sensitive organisms include: Gram-positive: penicillin-sensitive *Staph. aureus, Strep. pyogenes, Strep. faecalis, Strep. viridans, Strep. pneumoniae* and Clostridia species. Gram negative: *Neisseria meningitidis, Neisseria gonorrhoeae, Haemophilus influenzae, Escherichia coli, Proteus mirabilis, Proteus vulgaris, Klebsiella pneumoniae,* Enterobacter and Citrobacter species, *Salmonella typhi, Salmonella paratyphi,* other Salmonella species and species of Serratia, Shigella and Yersinia.

The anti-bacterial effect of Miraxid is further enhanced by the synergistic action of mecillinam and ampicillin which has been demonstrated with many of the Gram-negative organisms.

Penicillinase-producing staphylococci and *Pseudomonas aeruginosa* are resistant to Miraxid.

Indications: Miraxid is indicated for the treatment of acute bronchitis, pneumonia, acute exacerbations of chronic bronchitis, otitis media, sinusitis, tonsillitis, tracheitis, laryngitis, pharyngitis and urinary tract infections due to organisms sensitive to the combination.

Dosage and administration Both the tablets and suspension should preferably be taken with or immediately after a meal or with bland fluids such as water or milk (up to 100 ml for tablets).

Suspension: Mix the contents of the sachet in a little water (5–10 mls) and stir before taking. The suspension should be taken immediately.

For acute uncomplicated infections
Adults and children over 10 years: Two Miraxid tablets twice daily.

Children aged 6–10 years: One Miraxid tablet or 2 sachets of Miraxid Paediatric Suspension twice daily.

Children under 6 years: One sachet of Miraxid Paediatric Suspension twice daily.

For severe infections
Adults and children over 10 years: Three Miraxid tablets twice daily.

Dosages of up to 4 Miraxid tablets, twice daily, have been gvien to adults.

Children aged 6–10 years: Three sachets of Miraxid Paediatric Suspension twice daily.

Children under 6 years: Two sachets of Miraxid Paediatric Suspension twice daily.

Dosage in the elderly: Renal excretion of mecillinam and ampicillin is delayed in the elderly but significant accumulation of the drug is not likely at the recommended adult dosage.

Contra-indications, warnings, etc
Contra-indications: Penicillin and cephalosporin hypersensitivity. Because of the high frequency of exanthemata associated with ampicillin therapy in infectious mononucleosis, treatment with Miraxid is contra-indicated in this disease.

Precautions: During long term usage, it is advisable to carry out routine liver and kidney function tests. As with other antibiotics which are excreted mainly by the kidneys, raised blood levels of mecillinam and ampicillin may occur if repeated doses are given to patients with impaired renal function.

Caution is urged if patients with lymphatic leukaemia are treated with Miraxid because of the frequency of exanthemata associated with ampicillin therapy.

Pregnancy: Although tests in two animal species have shown no teratogenic effect, in keeping with current practice, use during the first trimester of pregnancy should be avoided. The drug, as mecillinam and ampicillin, crosses the placenta. Ampicillin has been detected in breast milk.

Adverse reactions: Side-effects are rare and usually of a mild and transitory nature. Urticaria, erythematous rash and pruritis may occur. Upper gastro-intestinal disturbances in the form of dyspepsia, nausea and vomiting have been observed but can generally be avoided by administration with meals. Diarrhoea has been reported infrequently. Anaphylactic reactions, though not yet reported, may occur.

Overdosage: There has been no experience of overdosage with Miraxid. However, excessive doses are likely to induce nausea, vomiting and gastritis. Treatment should be restricted to symptomatic and supportive measures.

Pharmaceutical precautions Miraxid tablets: Nil. Miraxid suspension: Store below 15°C. Once reconstituted use the suspension immediately.

Legal category POM.

Package quantities Miraxid tablets: Bottles of 100 tablets. Miraxid Paediatric Suspension: Boxes of 10 sachets.

Further information Nil.

Product licence numbers
Miraxid Tablets   0043/0069
Miraxid Paediatric Suspension   0043/0098

ONE-ALPHA* CAPSULES
ONE-ALPHA* DROPS
DILUENT FOR ONE-ALPHA* DROPS

Presentation *One-Alpha Capsules:* Each capsule contains either 1 microgram (brown) or 0.25 microgram (white) Alfacalcidol (1α-hydroxyvitamin D_3).

One-Alpha drops: A clear or slightly opalescent, colourless solution.

One ml of solution contains 5 microgram Alfacalcidol, corresponding to 0.25 microgram per drop.

Diluent for One-Alpha Drops: A clear or slightly opalescent, colourless solution.

Uses Alfacalcidol (1α-OHD_3) is converted rapidly in the liver to 1,25-dihydroxyvitamin D_3 ($1,25$-$(OH)_2D_3$), the metabolite through which vitamin D is considered to express most of its effects on calcium and phosphorus metabolism. Impaired endogenous production of 1,25-$(OH)_2D_3$ by the kidney appears to contribute to the disturbances in mineral metabolism found in several disorders including renal bone disease, hypoparathyroidism and pseudodeficiency rickets. These disorders, termed 'vitamin D-resistant' since they usually require high doses of vitamin D for their correction, respond to small 'physiological' doses of 1α-OHD_3.

Because 1α-OHD_3 is metabolised rapidly to 1,25-$(OH)_2D_3$, the clinical effects of these agents are very similar. Patients taking barbiturates or other anticonvulsant drugs may need higher doses of 1α-OHD_3 than otherwise, due possibly to interference with the hepatic conversion of 1α-OHD_3 to 1,25-$(OH)_2D_3$ or to target-organ resistance to the actions of 1,25-$(OH)_2D_3$.

In treating 'vitamin D-resistant' disorders with vitamin D itself, the delay in achieving a response and the high doses required make dosage adjustments difficult. Unpredictable hypercalcaemia, once induced, may take several weeks or months to reverse. The major advantage of 1α-OHD_3 resides in the rapidity with which it increases calcium absorption and plasma calcium, and the speed with which these effects can be reversed after stopping treatment, thus allowing dose requirements to be rapidly titrated. Should inadvertent hypercalcaemia occur, it can be reversed within days of stopping treatment.

Indications: One-Alpha drops should be administered whenever the patient is incapable of swallowing the capsules. One-Alpha is indicated in Renal bone disease, Hypoparathyroidism, Hyperparathyroidism (with bone disease), Hypophosphataemic vitamin D-resistant and Pseudo-deficiency (D-dependent) rickets and osteomalacia, Nutritional and Malabsorptive rickets and osteomalacia and Neonatal hypocalcaemia.

Dosage and administration To obtain accurate dosage of the One-Alpha drops the bottle should be held in a vertical position upside down. If the drops do not flow immediately, the bottle should be tapped gently.

If dilution is required the Diluent for One-Alpha drops should be used. The dilution should be performed in the Diluent bottle and then dispensed in this bottle.

Initial dose for all indications: *Adults:* 1 microgram daily.

Children over 20 kg bodyweight: 1 microgram daily.

Children under 20 kg bodyweight: 0.05 microgram/kg/day.

For neonates and premature infants: See neonatal hypocalcaemia.

Dosage in the elderly: A daily dose of 0.5 microgram may be sufficient in some elderly patients.

It is important to adjust dosage thereafter according to the biochemical responses and to avoid hypercalcaemia. Indices of response include levels of plasma calcium, alkaline phosphatase, parathyroid hormone, urinary calcium excretion as well as radiographic and histological investigations. Patients with marked bone disease (other than those with renal failure) may tolerate a higher dose without developing hypercalcaemia. However, failure of the plasma calcium to rise promptly in osteomalacic patients does not necessarily mean that a higher dose is required since calcium from increased intestinal calcium absorption may be incorporated into demineralised bone. Most patients respond eventually to doses between 1–3 microgram daily.

The dose requirements generally decrease in bone disorders at a time when there is biochemical or radiographic evidence of bone healing, and in hypoparathyroid patients after normal plasma calcium levels have been attained. Maintenance doses are generally in the range 0.25–1 microgram daily.

Renal bone disease: Most patients with osteitis fibrosa and osteomalacia show a rapid symptomatic, and a gradual biochemical, radiographic and histological improvement. In these, the only unwanted effect of 1α-OHD_3 appears to be hypercalcaemia which is more likely when there is evidence of bone healing.

Patients with relatively high initial plasma calcium levels may have autonomous hyperparathyroidism which is often unresponsive to 1α-OHD_3; other therapeutic measures may be indicated.

Before and during treatment with 1α-OHD_3, phosphate-binding agents should be considered to prevent hyperphosphataemia, which, especially when associated with hypercalcaemia, is known to increase the risk of metastatic calcification. Because prolonged hypercalcaemia may aggravate the decline in renal function, it is particularly important to make frequent plasma calcium estimations in patients with chronic renal failure.

Early hypercalcaemia is more likely in patients with autonomous hyperparathyroidism, those with histologically 'pure' osteomalacia related possibly to phosphate depletion or aluminium intoxication, and those dialysed against a high dialysate calcium concentration.

Hypoparathyroidism: In contrast to the response to vitamin D, low plasma calcium levels are restored to normal relatively quickly with 1α-OHD_3. Severe hypocalcaemia (e.g. after extensive neck surgery) is corrected and symptoms abolished even more rapidly with higher doses of 1α-OHD_3 (e.g. 3–5 microgram) and calcium supplements. Normocalcaemia may be maintained with smaller doses within a relatively narrow dose range.

Hyperparathyroidism: Following parathyroidectomy, patients with primary or tertiary hyperparathyroidism and bone disease often require large doses of vitamin D and intravenous calcium to avoid severe hypocalcaemia. Preliminary studies suggest that pre-operative treatment with 1α-OHD_3 for two to three weeks alleviates bone pain and myopathy when present without aggravating pre-operative hypercalcaemia. Continued post-operative treatment decreases post-operative hypocalcaemia and should be continued until the plasma alkaline phosphatase levels fall to normal or hypercalcaemia occurs.

Hypophosphataemic vitamin D-resistant rickets and osteomalacia is characterised by hypophosphataemia due to defective renal tubular reabsorption and intestinal absorption of phosphorus. Neither large doses of vitamin D nor phosphate supplements are entirely satisfactory, the latter tending to produce hypocalcaemia and hyperparathyroidism. Treatment of children and adults with 1α-OHD_3 rapidly relieves myopathy when present, increases calcium and phosphorus retention and promotes bone healing. Phosphate supplements may also be required in some patients.

Pseudo-deficiency (D-dependent) rickets requires large doses of vitamin D, probably because of an inherited defect in the production of $1,25-(OH)_2D_3$. In contrast, effective doses of $1\alpha-OHD_3$ are similar to those required to heal nutritional vitamin D deficiency rickets.

Nutritional and malabsorptive rickets and osteomalacia: Nutritional rickets and osteomalacia can be rapidly cured with 'physiological' doses of 1α OHD$_3$. Limited experience suggests that patients with malabsorptive osteomalacia, responding only to large doses of vitamin D given parenterally, respond to small oral doses of $1\alpha-OHD_3$.

Neonatal hypocalcaemia: The normal starting dose of $1\alpha-OHD_3$ is 0.05–0.1 microgram/kg/day. Adjustment of the dose thereafter is by careful titration (but in severe cases doses up to 2 microgram/kg/day may be required). Whilst ionised serum calcium levels may provide a guide to response, measurement of plasma alkaline phosphatase activity may be more useful. Levels of plasma alkaline phosphatase may be markedly raised in the preterm low birthweight infant. Whilst levels of 5 times the normal adult laboratory value may be usual in this group alkaline phosphatase levels above $7\frac{1}{2}$ times the adult range indicate active disease. A dose of $1\alpha-OHD_3$ of 0.1 microgram/kg/day has proved effective as prophylaxis against early neonatal hypocalcaemia in premature neonates.

Contra-indications, warnings, etc *Precautions and side-effects:* If hypercalcaemia is induced by $1\alpha-OHD_3$, it can be rapidly corrected by stopping treatment. Throughout treatment, regular plasma calcium determinations are essential. Indeed, $1\alpha-OHD_3$ should only be used by those with facilities to monitor plasma calcium and other appropriate biochemical parameters on a regular basis. If hypercalcaemia occurs, $1\alpha-OHD_3$ should be stopped until the plasma calcium returns to normal (in about one week) and then restarted at half the dose.

The risk of hypercalcaemia depends on such factors as the degree of any mineralisation defect, renal function, and the dose of $1\alpha-OHD_3$ used. Thus hypercalcaemia is less likely in osteomalacia and more likely in renal failure.

Hypercalcaemia will occur when there is biochemical evidence of bone healing (e.g. a return towards normal in the level of plasma alkaline phosphatase) and the dose of $1\alpha-OHD_3$ is not reduced appropriately. Prolonged hypercalcaemia should be avoided, particularly in chronic renal failure.

Frequency of monitoring: Plasma calcium levels should be measured at weekly to monthly intervals depending on the progress of the patient. Frequent estimations are necessary in the early stages of treatment (particularly when the plasma calcium is already relatively high) and later when there is evidence of bone healing. Plasma calcium levels should also be estimated regularly during the initial treatment of disorders without significant bone involvement, e.g. hypoparathyroidism.

Patients concurrently taking barbiturates and other anticonvulsant drugs may require larger doses of $1\alpha-OHD_3$ to produce the desired effect.

Pregnancy: $1\alpha-OHD_3$ should only be used during pregnancy or lactation if considered essential by the physician.

Overdosage: Hypercalcaemia is treated by stopping $1\alpha-OHD_3$. Severe hypercalcaemia may be treated additionally with a 'loop' diuretic and intravenous fluids, or with corticosteroids.

Pharmaceutical precautions *One Alpha capsules:* Protect from direct sunlight. *One Alpha drops and*

diluted drops: Protect from direct sunlight and store in a cool place (below 15°C).

Legal category
One-Alpha Capsules and Drops: POM
Diluent for One-Alpha Drops: GSL

Package quantities *Capsules:* Bottles of 100 capsules. *Drops:* Amber glass bottle of 10 ml.
Diluent: Packs of 10 amber glass bottles of 100 ml.

Further information Nil.

Product licence numbers

Capsules 1 microgram	0043/0050
Capsules 0.25 microgram	0043/0052
Drops	0043/0071
Diluent	0043/0083

PRESTIM* TABLETS
PRESTIM* FORTE TABLETS ▼

Presentation *Prestim:* White, flat, petal-shaped tablets engraved with 132 on the scored face and with an Assyrian lion on the reverse. Each tablet contains Timolol Maleate BP 10 mg and Bendrofluazide BP 2.5 mg.

Prestim Forte: White, flat, petal-shaped tablets engraved with 146 on the scored face and with an Assyrian lion on the reverse. Each tablet contains Timolol Maleate BP 20 mg and Bendrofluazide BP 5 mg.

Uses *Mode of Action:* Bendrofluazide, a thiazide diuretic, has an established action in the treatment of hypertension.

Timolol maleate is a beta-adrenergic receptor blocking agent with marked hypotensive activity lasting up to 24 hours.

It has been shown that the combination of a beta-blocking agent with a thiazide diuretic gives an enhanced antihypertensive effect. This means that a relatively lower dose of the beta-blocker is required.

Indications: For the treatment of mild to moderate hypertension.

Dosage and administration The recommended dosage range is:

For Prestim Tablets: 1–4 tablets daily. Most patients are controlled on 1 or 2 tablets.

For Prestim Forte Tablets: $\frac{1}{2}$–2 tablets daily.

The dosage can be taken in the morning or in two divided doses, morning and evening.

If blood pressure control is not achieved on 4 tablets Prestim daily or 2 tablets Prestim Forte daily, consideration should be given to titrating timolol and bendrofluazide separately or adding another agent with hypotensive activity.

Dosage in the elderly: Initiate treatment with 1 tablet Prestim or $\frac{1}{2}$ tablet Prestim Forte daily and thereafter adjust according to response.

Contra-indications, warnings, etc
Contra-indications: Anuria. Prestim should not be used in patients with renal failure or with a history of hypersensitivity to the thiazides.

Uncontrolled heart failure, bradycardia, cardiogenic shock, bronchial asthma, chronic obstructive pulmonary disease, patients receiving adrenergic augmenting drugs (monoamine oxidase inhibitors and tricyclic antidepressants).

Anaesthesia with agents that produce myocardial depression, such as chloroform and ether.

Pregnancy.

As with other diuretics, Prestim should not be administered concurrently with lithium salts. Diuretics can reduce lithium clearance resulting in high serum levels of lithium.

Precautions: The continued depression of sympathetic drive through beta blockade may lead to cardiac failure, and, if it occurs, digitalisation should be considered.

Caution should be exercised in patients with diabetes mellitus, spontaneous hypoglycaemia, impaired renal or hepatic function and in patients receiving catecholamine depleting drugs, such as reserpine or guanethidine.

Adverse Reactions: Side-effects associated with beta blockade, e.g. gastro-intestinal symptoms, dizziness, insomnia, sedation, depression, weakness, dyspnoea, bradycardia, heart block, bronchospasm and heart failure.

Thiazide diuretics may cause excessive depletion of fluid and electrolytes during prolonged or intense use. Symptoms are muscle pain or fatigue, thirst and oliguria. With thiazide diuretics hypokalaemia is more severe in patients already depleted of potassium, as in renal or hepatic insufficiency. Coma may be precipitated in hepatic cirrhosis.

The thiazides may induce hyperglycaemia and glycosuria in diabetic and other susceptible patients. The thiazides increase blood urea, which is most pronounced in patients with renal disease and pre-existing retention of nitrogen. Hyperuricaemia sometimes can occur.

Reports of other adverse reactions to the thiazides include skin rashes with associated photosensitivity, necrotising vasculitis, acute pancreatitis, blood dyscrasias and aggravation of pre-existing myopia.

Warning: There have been reports of skin rashes and/or dry eyes associated with the use of beta-adrenergic blocking drugs. The reported incidence is small and in most cases the symptoms have cleared when treatment was withdrawn. Discontinuance of the drug should be considered if any such reaction is not otherwise explicable. Cessation of therapy with the beta-blocker should be gradual.

Overdosage: The most common signs of overdosage are bradycardia, hypotension, bronchospasm and acute cardiac failure. Suggested treatments are as follows:

Severe bradycardia: I.V. atropine sulphate 0.25–2 mg. If bradycardia persists, I.V. isoprenaline 25 mcg may be given.

Severe hypotension: I.V. noradrenaline or adrenaline.

Bronchospasm: Isoprenaline hydrochloride, orciprenaline or salbutamol.

Acute cardiac failure: Digitalis, diuretics and oxygen. In refractory cases I.V. aminophylline and I.V. glucagon 0.5–1 mg have been reported useful.

General measures should be taken to restore blood volume, maintain blood pressure and correct electrolyte imbalance.

Pharmaceutical precautions Nil.

Legal category POM.

Package quantities Prestim: Glass bottles of 100 and 500 tablets.

Prestim Forte: Glass bottles of 100 tablets.

Further information Both constituents cross the placenta and appear in breast milk.

Product licence numbers
Prestim   0043/0047
Prestim Forte   0043/0084

TREOSULFAN* CAPSULES
TREOSULFAN* INJECTION

Presentation *Capsules:* White opaque capsules each containing 250 mg L-threitol 1,4 dimethane sulfonate.

Injection: Infusion bottles containing 5 g L-threitol 1,4 dimethane sulfonate, a white crystalline powder.

Uses Treosulfan is a bifunctional alkylating agent which has been shown to possess anti-neoplastic activity in the animal tumour screen and in clinical trials. The activity of Treosulfan is due to the formation of epoxide compounds in vivo.

Indications: For the treatment of all types of ovarian cancer, either supplementary to surgery or palliatively. Some uncontrolled studies have suggested activity in a wider range of neoplasms.

Because of a lack of cross-resistance reported between Treosulfan and other cytotoxic agents Treosulfan may be useful in any neoplasm refractive to conventional therapy.

Treosulfan has been used in combination regimens in conjunction with vincristine, methotrexate, 5-FU and procarbazine.

Dosage and administration *Capsules:* The following dosage regimens have been indicated. All regimens indicate that a total dose of 21–28 g of treosulfan should be given in the initial 8 weeks of treatment.

Regimen A: 1 g daily, given in four divided doses for four weeks followed by four weeks off therapy.

Regimen B: 1 g daily, given in four divided doses for two weeks, followed by two weeks off therapy.

Regimen C: 1.5 g daily, given in three divided doses for one week only, followed by three weeks off therapy. If no evidence of haematological toxicity at this dose in Regimen C, increase to 2 g daily in four divided doses for one week for the second and subsequent courses.

These cycles should be repeated with the dose being adjusted if necessary, as outlined below, according to the effect on the peripheral blood counts.

The capsules should be swallowed whole and not allowed to disintegrate within the mouth.

Dose modification (All regimens): For excessive haematological toxicity (white blood cell count less than 3,000/mcl or thrombocyte count less than 100,000/mcl) a repeat blood count should be made after 1–2 weeks interval and treatment restarted if haematological parameters are satisfactory, reducing dose as follows:

Regimen A: 1 g daily × 28 to 0.75 g daily × 28 (and to 0.5 g daily × 28 if necessary).

Regimen B: 1 g daily × 14 to 0.75 g daily × 14 (and to 0.5 g daily × 14 if necessary).

Regimen C: 2 g daily × 7 to 1.5 g daily × 7 (and to 1 g daily × 7 if necessary).

Present evidence, whilst not definitive, suggests that Regimens B and C are less myelosuppressive than Regimen A, whilst retaining maximum cytotoxic efficacy.

Injection: 5–15 g i.v. every 1–3 weeks depending on blood count and concurrent chemotherapy. Single injections of up to 15 g have been given with no serious adverse effects. Doses of up to 3 g have been given intraperitoneally. Doses up to 5 g Treosulfan may be given as a bolus injection. Larger doses should be administered as an i.v. infusion at a rate of 5 g every 5–10 minutes. The contents of each infusion bottle should be dissolved in 100 mls Water for Injection, a transfer needle may be used for this purpose. The resulting solution should be used immediately and any contents not used at once should be discarded.

Treatment should not be given if the white blood cell count is less than 3,000/mcl or the thrombocyte count less than 100,000/mcl. A repeat blood count should be made after a weeks interval, when treatment may be restarted if haematological parameters are satisfactory. Lower doses of Treosulfan should be used if other cytotoxic drugs or radiotherapy are being given concurrently. Treatment is initiated as soon as possible after diagnosis.

Care should be taken in administration of the injection to avoid extravasation into tissues since this will cause local pain and tissue damage. If extravasation occurs, the injection should be discontinued immediately and any remaining portion of the dose should be introduced into another vein.

Dosage in the elderly: Treosulfan is renally excreted. Blood counts should be carefully monitored in the elderly and dosage adjusted accordingly.

Contra-indications, warnings, etc

Warning: This product should not normally be administered to patients who are pregnant or to mothers who are breast feeding.

Adverse reactions: The major side-effect of Treosulfan is one of bone marrow depression and, in common with other alkylating agents, there have been reports of patients who have developed acute myeloid leukaemia. Reduction in white blood cell and thrombocyte counts occur during treatment and minimal levels may not occur until two or three weeks after discontinuing treatment. These counts usually return to normal within four weeks of cessation of therapy.

Patients showing marked bone marrow depression in the first course of treatment often respond similarly during subsequent courses. In all cases blood cell counts should be monitored regularly. Other adverse reactions include gastro-intestinal complaints such as nausea, vomiting and abdominal pain, mild allergic reactions in the form of exanthema and skin pigmentation. Alopecia may occur. Stomatitis may occur if the capsules are chewed; the capsules should be swallowed whole. Parenteral therapy has shown no local side-effects (unless extravasation is allowed to occur) and no systemic side-effects apart from the expected bone marrow depression.

Overdosage: Although there is no experience of acute overdosage with Treosulfan, nausea, vomiting and gastritis may occur.

Prolonged or excessive therapeutic doses may result in bone marrow depression which has occasionally been irreversible. The drug should be withdrawn, a blood transfusion given and general supportive measures given.

Pharmaceutical precautions Once brought into solution the injection should be used immediately.

Legal category POM.

Package quantities *Capsules:* Amber glass bottles of 100 capsules.
Injection: Boxes of 5 × 100 ml infusion bottles, each containing 5 g Treosulfan, complete with 5 transfer needles and 5 plastic bottle holders.

Further information All centres using Treosulfan have reported noteworthy improvements in the general condition of patients responding to treatment, particularly in regard to reduction or disappearance of ascites. Treosulfan is remarkably well tolerated allowing many patients to become fully ambulatory and return to their normal day to day work.

Product licence numbers
Capsules   0043/0040
Injection   0043/0072.

UNIHEP LEO* 1,000
UNIHEP LEO* 5,000
UNIHEP LEO* 10,000
UNIHEP LEO* 25,000

Presentation Unihep Leo 1,000: Heparin (Mucous) Injection BP 1,000 i.u. per ml. Single dose ampoules containing Sodium Heparin 1,000 i.u. in 1 ml (no preservative).

Unihep Leo 5,000: Heparin (Mucous) Injection BP 5,000 i.u. per ml. Single dose ampoules containing Sodium Heparin 5,000 i.u. in 1 ml (no preservative).

Unihep Leo 10,000: Heparin (Mucous) Injection BP 10,000 i.u. per ml. Single dose ampoules containing Sodium Heparin 10,000 i.u. in 1 ml (no preservative).

Unihep Leo 25,000: Heparin (Mucous) Injection BP 25,000 i.u. per ml. Single dose ampoules containing Sodium Heparin 25,000 i.u. in 1 ml (no preservative).

Uses *Mode of action:* Heparin is a naturally occurring anticoagulant which prevents the coagulation of blood in-vivo and in-vitro. It potentiates the inhibition of several activated coagulation factors, including thrombin and factor X.

The anticoagulant properties of heparin are valuable for the prophylaxis and management of intravascular clotting and embolism. It is also used in extra-corporeal circulation i.e. heart-lung and renal dialysis machines and blood transfusions.

In addition to the anticoagulant properties heparin also has some lipaemia-clearing effect which may be utilised in the treatment of fat embolism.

Indications: Treatment of thromboembolic disorders such as: deep vein thrombosis, thrombophlebitis, pulmonary embolism, fat embolism.

Dosage and administration Heparin is usually administered by intravenous injection or subcutaneously. Although the intramuscular route can be used, it is not recommended because of the high incidence of haematomata.

The increase in clotting time provided by heparin becomes apparent immediately after administration and lasts for four to six hours after intravenous injection and for about eight hours after subcutaneous injection.

Dosage: Intravenous administration: 5,000–10,000 i.u. every four hours either by bolus injection or continuous infusion in Sodium Chloride Injection or Dextrose Injection. However, the dose should be monitored with coagulation tests and varied according to individual response.

Subcutaneous administration: 5,000 i.u. every eight hours.

The treatment period varies from 7–10 days in peri-operative prophylaxis to as much as six weeks in the treatment of established thrombosis.

Dosage in the elderly: Elderly women have a greater tendency to bleed and it may be necessary to reduce the dose according to coagulation tests.

Contra-indications, warnings, etc

Contra-indications: Haemorrhagic disorders and patients with an actual or potential bleeding site, e.g. peptic ulcer.

Precautions: Heparin therapy should be given with caution to patients about to undergo surgery, and those with impaired renal or hepatic function.

Overdosage: The effect of heparin can be reversed immediately by intravenous administration of a 1% protamine sulphate solution. The quantity of protamine required for neutralisation falls rapidly with the lapse of time after the administration of heparin and can be accurately determined by titration of the patient's plasma, containing heparin, with protamine. If given within 15 minutes of the heparin injection 10 mg of protamine will neutralise 1,000 i.u. of heparin, while 30 minutes after the heparin injection, only 5 mg of protamine per 1,000 i.u. of heparin is needed.

It is important to avoid overdosage of protamine sulphate because protamine itself has anticoagulant properties. A single dose of protamine sulphate should never exceed 50 mg. Intravenous injection of protamine may cause a sudden fall in blood pressure, bradycardia, dyspnoea and transitory flushing, but these may be avoided or diminished by slow and careful administration.

Pharmaceutical precautions Store below 25°C. Admixture of heparin with solutions of other medicinal products may result in precipitation or loss of potency.

Legal category POM.

Package quantities Unihep Leo 1,000: Packs of 5 × 10 ampoules
Unihep Leo 5,000: Packs of 5 × 10 ampoules
Unihep Leo 10,000: Packs of 10 ampoules
Unihep Leo 25,000: Packs of 10 ampoules

Further information Menstruation and pregnancy are not contra-indications to heparin therapy. Heparin does not cross the placenta or appear in breast milk.

Product licence numbers
Unihep Leo 1,000   0043/0085
Unihep Leo 5,000   0043/0086
Unihep Leo 10,000   0043/0064
Unihep Leo 25,000   0043/0087

UROKINASE

Presentation Single ampoules of Urokinase as a sterile, white lyophilised powder. Ampoules of 5,000 and 25,000 Ploug units (1 Ploug unit is equivalent to 1.49 international units and is approximately equivalent to 1.43 CTA units) (see Further information section).

Uses Urokinase is an enzyme prepared from the urine of adult males.

It activates the process of fibrinolysis as described below. Its prime advantage over other activators is that, being of human origin, it is free from antigenic properties in man and free from inherent toxicity.

Mode of Action: Digestion of a fibrin thrombus is brought about by the proteolytic enzyme, plasmin. This is normally present in the blood as an inactive precursor plasminogen and conversion of this substance to plasmin is provoked physiologically by plasminogen-activator. Urokinase activates plasminogen directly, in contrast to Streptokinase which appears to act indirectly on a proactivator in the plasma to form activator.

Indications: Urokinase can be used locally in the treatment of the following conditions: secondary hyphaema, vitreous haemorrhage, and for the unblocking of clotted arteriovenous shunts and intravenous cannulae.

Urokinase (labelled with technetium) may also be used to detect and localise deep vein thrombosis.

Other indications: Urokinase has been used experimentally in pulmonary embolism, deep vein thrombosis, coronary thrombosis, intra-uterine transfusion, meningitis and ventriculitis. It should in theory also be of value in the treatment of retinal vessel thrombosis, peripheral arterial thrombosis and cerebral vascular occlusion, but little clinical evidence is available.

Dosage and administration *Hyphaema:* The following technique is generally used: 5,000 units of Urokinase are dissolved in 2 ml of sterile saline. An anterior chamber or lachrymal irrigator is inserted through a 3 mm incision, made just within the temporal limbus. The irrigator tip is turned towards the inner surface of the cornea, avoiding the pupillary space, and the chamber is irrigated with Urokinase solution using minimum pressure. The clot begins to loosen and may float free, small fragments being either sucked up by the syringe or forced out through the incision.

If a 5,000 unit dose proves ineffective, the dose may be increased to 10,000 or 25,000 units.

Vitreous haemorrhage: 5–25,000 units of Urokinase dissolved in 0.2–1.5 ml of sterile water. The most usual dosage used is 25,000 units dissolved in 0.3 ml sterile water.

Clotted arterio-venous shunts: Generally, 5–25,000 units of Urokinase in 5 ml of saline have been instilled into the affected limb of the shunt, which is then clamped off for two to four hours.

In one study, a concentration of 5,000 units per ml was used, up to a total local dose of 25,000–50,000 units. In some refractory cases, using this dosage, continued improvement has been noted after 6 consecutive doses over a period of three days.

To establish or maintain a state of systemic fibrinolysis, very much larger quantities of Urokinase are used. To detect deep vein thrombosis Urokinase is radio-labelled with technetium.

Dosage in the elderly: No initial dosage alterations are necessary but thereafter dosage should be adjusted according to response.

Contra-indications, warnings, etc

Contra-indications: Any evidence of bleeding constitutes a contra-indication to fibrinolytic therapy, except in 'closed' situations. Post-operative therapy with high doses of Urokinase is generally inadvisable within 48–72 hours.

High dose Urokinase therapy carries the risk of inducing haemorrhage, particularly cerebral haemorrhage, in patients with severe hypertension.

Pregnancy: Contra-indicated during pregnancy and suspected pregnancy.

Precautions: Previous preparations contained a small degree of thromboplastic activity, but the present formulation has been purified to the standard required by the Committee on Thombolytic Agents (CTA) in America.

Use with caution in patients who have had active cardiopulmonary resuscitation with multiple intravascular and intracardiac punctures, and in patients with known gastro-intestinal lesions.

Adverse Reactions: Large doses of 0.5–1 million units have been infused intravenously without untoward effects. Repeated application to the anterior chamber of the eye has not produced any evidence of irritation. Nor have there been any reports of antigenicity associated with its use.

Overdosage: Infusion of Urokinase should be stopped if bleeding occurs. Administration of compatible whole blood may be necessary for patients treated with large doses of Urokinase. Epsilon aminocaproic acid (EACA), Trasylol (aprotinin for injection) and fibrinogen should also be readily available.

Pharmaceutical precautions Lyophilised Urokinase is extremely stable. It should be stored at 4°C and can be kept for at least five years at this temperature. Aqueous solutions at 4°C retain their activity for three to four days and have a high degree of stability over a wide pH range.

Legal category POM.

Package quantities Single ampoules: 5,000 and 25,000 Ploug units.

Further information The activity of Urokinase is expressed in arbitrary Ploug units. There is a difference between the American and British dosage standards. In the US, activity is expressed as an arbitrary unit determined by the Committee on Thrombolytic Agents (CTA). One CTA unit is approximately equivalent to 0.7 Ploug units. More recently, an International Reference preparation has been established: 1 Ploug unit is equal to 1.49 international units.

Product licence numbers
5,000 Ploug units   0043/5011
25,000 Ploug units   0043/5024

*Trade Mark

Eli Lilly & Company Limited
Kingsclere Road
Basingstoke
Hants RG21 2XA

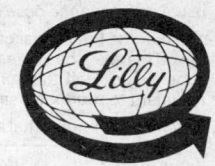

AMYTAL*

Presentation Tablets (white, coded T40) containing 15 mg Amylobarbitone BP.

Tablets (white, coded T56) containing 30 mg Amylobarbitone BP.

Tablets (white, coded T37) containing 50 mg Amylobarbitone BP.

Tablets (white, coded T32) containing 100 mg Amylobarbitone BP.

Tablets (white, scored, coded U13) containing 200 mg Amylobarbitone BP.

Uses For the treatment of severe, intractable insomnia.

Dosage and administration For oral administration to adults only. Normal dosage is 100–200 mg. Occasionally a larger dose may be necessary.

The effects should become apparent between 30 and 60 minutes after administration.

The elderly: See 'Contra-indications' section.

Contra-indications, warnings, etc
Contra-indications: Hypersensitivity to barbiturates, a history of porphyria or the presence of uncontrolled pain.

Barbiturates should not be administered to children, young adults, patients with a history of drug or alcohol abuse, the elderly and the debilitated.

Usage in pregnancy: Barbiturates are contra-indicated during pregnancy and for the nursing mother.

Warnings: Performance and alertness may be impaired during the first week of therapy. Patients should be warned of the possible hazards when driving, or operating machinery. These effects may be potentiated by alcohol.

Drug interactions: Barbiturates cause induction of the liver enzymes responsible for metabolising many other drugs; in particular they should not be administered concurrently with coumarin-type anticoagulants. They may also affect the metabolism of systemic steroids (including oral contraceptives), phenytoin, griseofulvin, rifampicin, tricyclic antidepressants and phenothiazines such as chlorpromazine.

Precautions: A reduction in dosage may be required in patients with decreased hepatic or renal function.

Adverse reactions: Common adverse reactions include drowsiness, sedation, ataxia and vertigo.

Hypersensitive skin reactions may occur in some patients, especially those with asthma, urticaria or angioneurotic oedema.

Other idiosyncratic reactions include a hangover effect, paradoxical excitement, pain, confusion and memory defects.

Overdosage: Symptoms include respiratory depression, depression of superficial and deep reflexes, constriction of the pupils to a slight degree (although in severe poisoning they may dilate), decreased urine formation, hypothermia and coma.

Treatment: General management should consist of symptomatic and supportive therapy, including gastric lavage, administration of intravenous fluids, and maintenance of blood pressure, body temperature and adequate respiratory exchange. Haemodialysis will increase the rate of removal of barbiturates from the body fluids.

Pharmaceutical precautions Nil.

Legal category CD (Sch 3) POM.

Package quantities Tablets 15 mg: Bottles of 500.
Tablets 30 mg: Bottles of 500.
Tablets 50 mg: Bottles of 500.
Tablets 100 mg: Bottles of 100 and 500.
Tablets 200 mg: Bottles of 100.

Further information *Addiction potential:* Barbiturates have a high addiction potential. Long-term use, or use of high dosage for short periods, may lead to tolerance and subsequently to physical and psychological dependence. Symptoms of dependence include confusion, defective judgement and loss of emotional control. Withdrawal symptoms occur after long-term normal use (and particularly after abuse) on rapid cessation of barbiturate treatment. Symptoms include nightmares, irritability and insomnia, and in severe cases, tremors, delirium, convulsions and death. Withdrawal symptoms have been reported in neonates after barbiturate treatment during pregnancy and labour.

Product licence numbers
Tablets 15 mg   0006/5057
Tablets 30 mg   0006/5058
Tablets 50 mg   0006/5059
Tablets 100 mg   0006/5060
Tablets 200 mg   0006/5061

AVENTYL*

Presentation Capsules (yellow and white, coded H17) each containing Nortriptyline Hydrochloride BP equivalent to 10 mg nortriptyline.

Capsules (yellow and white, coded H19) each containing Nortriptyline Hydrochloride BP equivalent to 25 mg nortriptyline.

Liquid (colourless) containing Nortriptyline Hydrochloride BP, equivalent to 10 mg nortriptyline per 5 ml.

Uses Aventyl is indicated for the relief of symptoms of depression. It may also be used for the treatment of some cases of nocturnal enuresis.

Dosage and administration For oral administration.

Adults: The usual adult dose is 20–40 mg daily in divided

doses, increasing to 100 mg daily where necessary. The usual maintenance dose is 30–75 mg/day.

The elderly: Initial dosage should be 10 mg three times a day. This may be increased with caution under close supervision. Half the normal maintenance dose may be sufficient to produce a satisfactory clinical response.

Children: (for nocturnal enuresis only).

Age (years)	Weight		Dose (mg)
	kg	lbs	
6–7	20–25	44–55	10
8–11	25–35	55–77	10–20
> 11	35–54	77–119	25–35

The dose should be administered thirty minutes before bedtime.

The maximum period of treatment should not exceed three months. A further course of treatment should not be started until a full physical examination, including an ECG, has been made.

Contra-indications, warnings, etc

Contra-indications: Hypersensitivity to nortriptyline. Recent myocardial infarction, any degree of heart block or other cardiac arrhythmias. Severe liver disease. Mania. Nortriptyline is contra-indicated for the nursing mother and for children under the age of six years.

Warnings: As improvement may not occur during the initial weeks of therapy, patients, especially those posing a high suicidal risk, should be closely monitored during this period.

Withdrawal symptoms, including insomnia, irritability and excessive perspiration may occur on abrupt cessation of therapy.

The use of nortriptyline in schizophrenic patients may result in an exacerbation of the psychosis or may activate latent schizophrenic symptoms. If administered to overactive or agitated patients, increased anxiety and agitation may occur. In manic-depressive patients, nortriptyline may cause symptoms of the manic phase to emerge.

Cross sensitivity between nortriptyline and other tricyclic antidepressants is a possibility.

Patients with cardiovascular disease should be given nortriptyline only under close supervision because of the tendency of the drug to produce sinus tachycardia and to prolong the conduction time. Myocardial infarction, arrhythmia and strokes have occurred. Great care is required if nortriptyline is administered to hyperthyroid patients or to those receiving thyroid medication, since cardiac arrhythmias may develop.

Nortriptyline may impair the mental and/or physical abilities required for the performance of hazardous tasks, such as operating machinery or driving a car; therefore the patient should be warned accordingly.

Drug interactions: Under no circumstances should nortriptyline be given concurrently with, or within two weeks of cessation of, therapy with monoamine oxidase inhibitors. Hyperpyretic crises, severe convulsions and fatalities have occurred when similar tricyclic antidepressants were used in such combinations.

Nortriptyline should not be given with sympathomimetic agents such as adrenaline, ephedrine, isoprenaline, noradrenaline, phenylephrine and phenylpropanolamine.

Nortriptyline may decrease the antihypertensive effect of guanethidine, debrisoquine, bethanidine and possibly clonidine. Concurrent administration of reserpine has been shown to produce a 'stimulating' effect in some depressed patients. It would be advisable to review all antihypertensive therapy during treatment with tricyclic antidepressants.

Barbiturates may increase the rate of metabolism of nortriptyline.

Usage in pregnancy: The safety of nortriptyline for use during pregnancy has not been established, nor is there evidence from animal studies that it is free from hazard; therefore the drug should not be administered to pregnant patients or women of childbearing age unless the potential benefits clearly outweigh any potential risk.

Precautions: The elderly are particularly liable to experience adverse reactions, especially agitation, confusion and postural hypotension.

Behavioural changes may occur in children receiving therapy for nocturnal enuresis.

If possible, the use of nortriptyline should be avoided in patients with narrow angle glaucoma, symptoms suggestive of prostatic hypertrophy or a history of epilepsy.

When it is essential, nortriptyline may be administered with electro-convulsive therapy, although the hazards may be increased.

Anaesthetics given during tricyclic antidepressant therapy may increase the risk of arrhythmias and hypotension. If surgery is necessary, the drug should be discontinued, if possible, for several days prior to the procedure, or the anaesthetist should be informed if the patient is still receiving therapy.

Tricyclic antidepressants may potentiate the CNS depressant effect of alcohol.

Both elevation and lowering of blood sugar levels have been reported.

Side-effects: Cardiac arrhythmias and severe hypotension are likely to occur with high dosage, or in patients with pre-existing heart disease taking normal dosage.

Other common side-effects include drowsiness, sweating, postural hypotension, tremor and skin rashes.

The following are seen occasionally: dizziness, confusion, restlessness, weakness, impotence and blurred vision. Side-effects rarely noted are epigastric distress, nausea and vomiting, dysgeusia, excessive weight gain, excessive weight loss, fatigue, insomnia, headache, paraesthesiae and pruritus.

The following adverse effects, although not necessarily all reported with nortriptyline, have occurred with other tricyclic antidepressants: atropine-like side-effects including dry mouth, disturbances of accommodation, tachycardia, constipation and hesitancy of micturition are common early in treatment, but usually lessen.

Serious adverse effects are rare; the following have been reported: depression of the bone marrow including agranulocytosis, cholestatic jaundice, hypomania, convulsions and peripheral neuropathy.

Adverse effects such as withdrawal symptoms, respiratory depression and agitation have been reported in neonates whose mothers had taken tricyclic antidepressants during the last trimester of pregnancy.

Overdose: Toxic overdosage may result in confusion, restlessness, agitation, vomiting, hyperpyrexia, muscle rigidity, hyperactive reflexes, tachycardia, cardiac arrhythmias, ECG evidence of impaired conduction, shock, congestive heart failure, severe hypotension, stupor, coma and CNS stimulation with convulsions followed by respiratory depression. Deaths have occurred following overdosage with drugs of this class.

Treatment of overdose: No specific antidote is known. General supportive measures are indicated, with gastric lavage. Activated charcoal adsorbs tricyclic antidepressants very effectively. Respiratory assistance is apparently the most effective measure when indicated. The use of CNS depressants may worsen the prognosis.

Intramuscular paraldehyde or diazepam provides anticonvulsant activity with less respiratory depression than the barbiturates.

The use of digitalis and/or pyridostigmine may be considered in the event of serious cardiovascular abnormalities or cardiac failure.

The value of dialysis has not been established.

Pharmaceutical precautions Keep containers tightly closed and protect from light. Store below 25°C.

Legal category POM.

Package quantities
Capsules 10 mg: Bottles of 100 and 500.
Capsules 25 mg: Bottles of 100 and 500.
Liquid 10 mg/5 ml: Bottles of 120 ml and 500 ml.

Further information Nil.

Product licence numbers
Capsules 10 mg   0006/5054
Capsules 25 mg   0006/5055
Liquid 10 mg/5 ml   0006/5053

BRIETAL* Sodium

Presentation Brietal Sodium (methohexitone sodium for injection), in crystalline form, is supplied as follows:

100 mg (with anhydrous Sodium Carbonate BP 6 mg) in 10 ml rubber-stoppered vials.

500 mg (with anhydrous Sodium Carbonate BP 30 mg) in 50 ml rubber-stoppered vials.

2.5 g (with anhydrous Sodium Carbonate BP 150 mg) in 250 ml rubber-stoppered vials.

Uses Brietal Sodium is used as an intravenous anaesthetic agent for short surgical procedures, for the induction of anaesthesia, and in conjunction with other agents for more prolonged anaesthesia.

Dosage and administration Pre-anaesthetic medication is generally advisable. Brietal Sodium may be used with any recognised pre-anaesthetic medications, but the phenothiazines are less satisfactory than the combination of an opiate and a belladonna derivative.

Brietal Sodium is administered intravenously, usually in a 1% solution (10 mg per ml).

Adults: As an initial guide a rate of 1 ml of a 1% solution (10 mg) in five seconds may be used – although a faster rate than this is preferred by some anaesthetists. The dose usually ranges between 5 and 12 ml (50–120 mg), but it must be adjusted to the needs of the individual patient. The induction dose maintains unconsciousness for about five to seven minutes.

The elderly: Onset of anaesthesia may be slow due to sluggish circulation, therefore methohexitone should be injected slowly.

Children: The dose should be adjusted for age and/or weight.

Maintenance: Brietal Sodium is best used simply as an induction agent. If further injection for maintenance is needed the dose must be individualised; but, as a guide, 2–4 ml of a 1% solution every four to seven minutes may be used.

Preparation of solutions: The recommended diluent for Brietal Sodium is Water for Injections PhEur. Solutions may also be prepared in Sodium Chloride Intravenous Infusion BP or 5% Dextrose Intravenous Infusion BP. These solutions are not stable for more than twenty-four hours. Brietal Sodium is not compatible with Compound Sodium Lactate Intravenous Infusion BP.

For a 1% solution (10 mg per ml) vial contents should be diluted as follows:

100 mg: add 10 ml diluent.
500 mg: add 50 ml diluent.
2.5 g/250 ml: add 250 ml diluent.

Contra-indications, warnings, etc
Contra-indications: Hypersensitivity to barbiturates. When general anaesthesia is contra-indicated, Brietal Sodium should not be used. Patients with a history of porphyria should not receive barbiturates in any form. Barbiturates may stimulate the enzymes responsible for metabolising many other drugs; in particular they should not be administered concurrently with coumarin-type anticoagulants. They may also affect the metabolism of endogenous steroids.

Warnings: May be habit-forming.

Usage in pregnancy: The safety of methohexitone sodium for use during pregnancy has not been established. Brietal Sodium should not be used in the pregnant patient unless in the opinion of the clinician, the expected benefit outweighs the possible risk. Animal studies have shown no evidence of teratogenicity.

Precautions: Brietal Sodium should be administered only by persons who are experienced in anaesthesia and who have appropriate equipment on hand for the prevention and treatment of anaesthetic emergencies. The dosage must be adjusted to each patient as response is variable and respiratory depression, apnoea or hypotension may occur. It is essential that a free airway be maintained at all times. As with any potent anaesthetic agent, pulmonary ventilation should be maintained if prolonged apnoea occurs. Repeated or continuous injection may cause cumulative effects resulting in respiratory and circulatory depression.

The patient's stomach should be empty. The usual pre-anaesthetic medications may be administered for the production of sedation and inhibition of secretions. If increased muscular relaxation is required for the performance of certain surgical procedures, it may be accomplished by the concomitant use of Brietal Sodium and skeletal muscle relaxants.

Extravasation of the solution may cause tissue reaction. Should it occur, moist heat may be applied to the infiltrated area. Special care should be taken to avoid accidental intra-arterial injection.

Caution should be exercised in debilitated patients or in those with impaired function of respiratory, circulatory, renal, hepatic or endocrine systems. Methohexitone sodium should be used with extreme caution in patients in status asthmaticus.

The central nervous system depressant effect of methohexitone sodium may be additive with that of other CNS depressants, including alcohol.

Side-effects: During the induction, especially if it is too rapid, transitory apnoea may occur. This is easily treated by maintaining pulmonary ventilation for a short time until spontaneous respiration is resumed.

Too rapid induction, inadequate dosage, or insufficient or unsuitable pre-anaesthetic medication may result in skeletal muscle activity, laryngospasm, cough, sneezing or hiccups.

Pain at the site of injection and a burning sensation along the course of the vein have occasionally been reported. Extravascular injection may cause pain, swelling, ulceration and necrosis. Intra-arterial injection is dangerous and may produce gangrene of an extremity.

Other reported side-effects include: circulatory or respiratory depression; injury to nerves adjacent to injection site, headache, salivation, nausea, emesis, thrombophlebitis, bronchospasm and emergence delirium have been reported on rare occasions.

Acute allergic reactions, such as rash, erythema, urticaria, pruritus, rhinitis, dyspnoea, hypotension, restlessness, anxiety, abdominal pain and peripheral vascular collapse, have been reported with the use of Brietal Sodium.

Pharmaceutical precautions Owing to differences in pH, solutions of Brietal Sodium should not be mixed with acid solutions such as atropine sulphate, tubocurarine and succinylcholine chloride.

Do not use solvents containing bacteriostats as these may cause precipitation.

Solutions of Brietal Sodium should not be stored in contact with rubber stoppers or parts of disposable syringes that have been treated with silicone as, under these conditions, they are incompatible.

Vials of Brietal Sodium should be stored below 25°C.

After reconstitution: Solutions should be used within 24 hours.

Legal category POM.

Package quantities 100 mg in 10 ml vial: Pack of 10 vials.
500 mg in 50 ml vial: Single vials.
2.5 g in 250 ml vial: Single vials.

Further information Nil.

Product licence numbers
100 mg   0006/5050
500 mg   0006/5051
2.5 g/250 ml   0006/5049

CESAMET* ▼

Presentation Capsules (blue and white, coded Lilly 3101) containing 1 mg nabilone.

Uses Nabilone is indicated for the control of nausea and vomiting caused by chemotherapeutic agents used in the treatment of cancer.

Dosage and administration Nabilone is for oral administration to adults only. It is not recommended for use in children as safety and efficacy have not been established.

The usual adult dosage is 1 mg or 2 mg twice a day. The first dose should be administered the night before initiation of chemotherapy, and the second dose should be given one to three hours before the first dose of the oncolytic agent is administered.

The maximum daily dose should not exceed 6 mg.

Nabilone may be administered throughout each cycle of chemotherapy and, if necessary, for 24 hours after the last dose of each cycle.

The elderly: As for adults.

Contra-indications, warnings, etc
Contra-indication: Nabilone is contra-indicated in patients with a known allergy to cannabinoid agents.

Warnings: As nabilone is excreted primarily by the biliary route, the drug is not recommended for use in patients with severe liver dysfunction.

Nabilone may impair the mental and/or physical abilities required for the performance of potentially hazardous tasks such as operating machinery or driving a car; therefore the patient should be advised accordingly.

Usage in pregnancy: Although laboratory studies have so far shown no evidence of teratogenicity, the safety of this product for use during pregnancy has not been established.

Precautions: Nabilone should be administered with caution to patients who are taking other CNS depressants, including alcohol and narcotic analgesics, or to those with a history of psychosis.

Side-effects: Neurological: The most common side-effect has been drowsiness. The following have also been reported: confusion, disorientation, euphoria, hallucinations, psychosis, depression, headache, decreased concentration, blurred vision, decreased co-ordination, tremors.

Cardiovascular: Postural hypotension, tachycardia.

Miscellaneous: Dry mouth, decreased appetite, abdominal cramps.

Overdosage: No cases of overdosage with nabilone (more than 10 mg/day) have been reported during clinical trials. Signs and symptoms to be anticipated are psychotic episodes, including hallucinations and anxiety reactions, respiratory depression and coma.

Treatment: For severe psychotic episodes, it would seem theoretically beneficial to administer a neuroleptic agent, e.g. haloperidol. General management for respiratory depression and coma should consist of symptomatic and supportive therapy. Particular attention should be paid to the occurrence of hypothermia.

Pharmaceutical precautions Keep containers tightly closed. Store at room temperature (15°–25° C).

Legal category POM.

Package quantities Bottles of 20.

Further information Nil.

Product licence number 0006/0155.

CINOBAC*

Presentation Capsules (green and orange, coded 3056) containing 500 mg cinoxacin.

Uses Cinoxacin is indicated for acute, recurrent and chronic upper and lower urinary tract infections (including cystitis, pyelonephritis or pyelitis and asymptomatic bacteriuria) caused by susceptible micro-organisms.

A single dose of 500 mg taken at bedtime has been shown to be effective as preventive therapy in reducing the number of episodes of infection in patients subject to recurrent urinary tract infections.

Cinoxacin is active against most strains of the following

ELI LILLY & COMPANY LIMITED 791

organisms: *Citrobacter* spp., *Enterobacter* spp. (including *Ent. aerogenes, Ent. cloacae* and *Ent. hafniae), Escherichia coli, Klebsiella* spp., *Morganella morganii, Proteus mirabilis, Pr. vulgaris.*

Cinoxacin is also active against approximately 50 per cent of strains of *Pr. rettgeri, Providencia* and *Serratia* species.

Dosage and administration The usual adult dose is 1 g daily administered orally as 500 mg b.d. for seven to fourteen days.

For prophylactic use, a single dose of 500 mg daily, taken at bedtime.

Not recommended for use in children.

The elderly: As for adults, unless renal function is impaired (see precautions).

Contra-indications, warnings, etc
Contra-indication: Hypersensitivity to cinoxacin.

Warnings: Since cinoxacin, like other drugs in its class, causes arthropathy in immature animals, its use during pregnancy or for pre-pubertal children is not recommended.

Usage in pregnancy: Cinoxacin should not be administered during pregnancy or to the nursing mother as safety has not been established. Animal studies showed no evidence of teratogenicity or toxicity.

Precautions: Since cinoxacin is eliminated primarily by the kidney, it should be used with caution in patients with reduced renal function. Administration of cinoxacin is not recommended for patients with severely impaired renal function.

Adverse reactions: Gastro-intestinal – nausea, anorexia, vomiting, abdominal cramps and diarrhoea have been reported.

Hypersensitivity – rash, itching, urticaria and peripheral and oral oedema have occurred.

Other adverse reactions possibly related to cinoxacin include dizziness, headache, insomnia, tingling sensation, perineal burning, photophobia and tinnitus.

Transient changes in AST, ALT, blood urea, ALP, and creatinine clearance have been observed occasionally.

Overdosage: No cases of overdosage have been reported. Animal studies indicate that symptoms of nausea, vomiting, anorexia, lethargy and CNS excitation could occur.

Treatment: Gastric lavage should be undertaken within two hours of ingestion. Subsequent treatment should ensure increased fluid intake and monitoring of kidney, liver and CNS functions.

Pharmaceutical precautions Store at room temperature (15°–25°C).

Legal category POM.

Package quantities Capsules 500 mg: Blister pack of 14.

Further information Nil.

Product licence number 0006/0124

COLOGEL*
Presentation An aromatised solution each 100 ml containing 9 g methylcellulose in a lemon-flavoured vehicle, with alcohol 5%.

Uses Cologel is a liquid bulk laxative, which does not irritate the intestinal mucosa or interfere with the absorption of foods or vitamins. It is indicated for the treatment of chronic or acute constipation.

Dosage and administration For oral administration.
Adults: 5–15 ml (1–3 teaspoonfuls) with a full glass of water three times daily after meals.

Maintenance dosage: 5–15 ml with a full glass of water once daily. In severe cases, up to 30 ml with a full glass of water may be administered once daily.

Children: The dosage should be scaled down in proportion to size.

The elderly: As for adults.

Contra-indications, warnings, etc
Contra-indications: Cologel should not be given to children who are dehydrated. It should not be used in patients with intestinal obstruction or faecal impaction.

Warnings: Intestinal obstruction has been reported after the administration of bulk laxatives, therefore it is essential that an adequate quantity of water be taken with each dose.

Usage in pregnancy: This product is not absorbed from the gastro-intestinal tract and is therefore considered to be safe for use during pregnancy.

Pharmaceutical precautions Exposure to high temperatures may cause this product to gel. If this occurs, place in a refrigerator. Cologel should not be frozen.

Legal category GSL.

Package quantities Bottles of 500 ml.

Further information Nil.

Product licence number 0006/5047.

CYCLOSERINE
Presentation Capsules (red and grey) containing 125 mg Cycloserine BP, coded H39.

Capsules (red and grey) containing 250 mg Cycloserine BP, coded F04.

Uses Cycloserine inhibits cell wall synthesis in susceptible strains of Gram-positive and Gram-negative bacteria and in *Mycobacterium tuberculosis.*

Cycloserine is indicated in the treatment of active pulmonary and extra-pulmonary tuberculosis (including renal disease) when the organisms are susceptible to this drug and after failure of adequate treatment with the primary medications. Like all anti-tuberculous drugs, cycloserine should be administered in conjunction with other effective chemotherapy and not as the sole therapeutic agent.

Cycloserine may be effective in the treatment of acute urinary tract infections caused by susceptible strains of Gram-positive and Gram-negative bacteria, especially *Klebsiella/Enterobacter* species and *Escherichia coli.* It is generally no more and may be less effective than other antimicrobial agents in the treatment of urinary tract infections caused by bacteria other than mycobacteria. Use of cycloserine in these infections should be considered only when the more conventional therapy has failed and when the organism has been demonstrated to be sensitive to the drug.

Dosage and administration For oral administration. The usual dosage is 500 mg to 1 g daily in divided doses, monitored by blood levels. The initial adult dosage most frequently given is 250 mg twice daily at 12-hour intervals for the first two weeks. The daily dosage of 1 g should not be exceeded.

Children: the usual starting dose is 10 mg/kg/day, then adjusted according to blood levels obtained and therapeutic response.

The elderly: As for adults. Reduce dosage if renal function is impaired.

Contra-indications, warnings, etc

Contra-indications: Administration is contra-indicated in patients with any of the following: Hypersensitivity; epilepsy; depression, severe anxiety or psychosis; severe renal insufficiency; alcohol abuse.

Warnings: Administration of cycloserine should be discontinued or the dosage reduced if the patient develops allergic dermatitis or symptoms of central nervous system toxicity such as convulsions, psychoses, somnolence, depression, confusion, hyper-reflexia, headache, tremor, vertigo, paresis or dysarthria.

Toxicity is usually associated with blood levels of greater than 30 mg/l, which may be the result of high dosage or inadequate renal clearance. The therapeutic index for this drug is low.

Patients should be monitored by haematological, renal excretion, blood level and liver function studies.

Drug interactions: The effects of alcohol may be potentiated. Cycloserine impairs the metabolism of phenytoin, thereby increasing the risk of phenytoin intoxication. Patients receiving cycloserine and isoniazid should be monitored for signs of CNS toxicity, as these drugs have a combined toxic action on the CNS.

Usage in pregnancy: There is no information on the use of cycloserine to treat tuberculosis during pregnancy, and inadequate evidence of safety in the treatment of urinary tract infections. Cycloserine readily crosses the placenta and is excreted in breast milk. Animal studies have shown no evidence of teratogenicity.

Precautions: Before treatment with cycloserine is begun, cultures should be taken and the susceptibility of the organism to the drug should be established. In tuberculous infections, sensitivity to the other anti-tuberculous agents in the regimen should also be demonstrated.

Blood levels should be determined at least weekly for patients having reduced renal function, for individuals receiving a daily dosage of more than 500 mg, and for those showing signs and symptoms suggestive of toxicity. The dosage should be adjusted to keep the blood level below 30 mg/l.

Anticonvulsant drugs or sedatives may be effective in controlling symptoms of central nervous system toxicity, such as convulsion, anxiety and tremor. Patients receiving more than 500 mg of cycloserine daily should be closely observed for such symptoms. The value of pyridoxine in preventing CNS toxicity from cycloserine has not been proved.

Administration of cycloserine and other anti-tuberculous drugs has been associated in a few instances with vitamin B_{12} and/or folic acid deficiency, megaloblastic anaemia and sideroblastic anaemia. If evidence of anaemia develops during treatment, appropriate studies and therapy should be instituted.

Overdosage: Symptoms – CNS depression with accompanying drowsiness, somnolence, dizziness, hyper-reflexia, mental confusion, convulsions and allergic dermatitis.

Treatment – pyridoxine, 300 mg or more daily, and anticonvulsants may be given to relieve convulsions. General management may include symptomatic and supportive therapy such as gastric lavage, oxygen, artificial respiration, intravenous fluids, standard measures for management of circulatory shock and maintenance of body temperature.

Side-effects: Most adverse reactions occurring during therapy with cycloserine involve the nervous system or are manifestations of drug hypersensitivity. The following side-effects have been observed:

Nervous system symptoms (which appear to be related to higher dosages of drug, i.e. more than 500 mg daily): convulsions, drowsiness and somnolence, headache, tremor, dysarthria, vertigo, confusion and disorientation with loss of memory, psychoses, possibly with suicidal tendencies, hyper-irritability, aggression, paresis, hyper-reflexia, paraesthesiae, major and minor (localised) clonic seizures, coma.

Allergic (apparently not related to dosage): skin rash.

Miscellaneous: megaloblastic anaemia, elevated serum aminotransferases, especially in patients with pre-existing liver disease.

Pharmaceutical precautions Keep containers tightly closed. Store below 25°C. Protect from moisture.

Legal category POM.

Package quantities Capsules 125 mg: Bottles of 100. Capsules 250 mg: Bottles of 40 and 100.

Further information Nil.

Product licence numbers
Capsules 125 mg   0006/5044
Capsules 250 mg   0006/5045

DIMELOR*

Presentation Tablets (yellow, scored, coded U07) each containing 500 mg Acetohexamide USP.

Uses For the treatment of diabetes mellitus of the stable type (without such complications as ketosis or acidosis), variously described as type II, relatively mild adult, maturity-onset, or non-ketotic type.

Dosage and administration The daily dose may range from 250 mg to 1.5 g. Many patients are controlled on a single daily dose of 500 mg. Divided dosage may be advantageous where the daily requirements are higher. Patients who do not respond to 1.5 g daily are unlikely to benefit from a higher dose.

Use in children is not recommended.

Moderate diabetes: A loading dose technique can be used in cases which are fairly severe. New patients usually respond to 3 tablets (1.5 g) on the first day, 2 tablets on the second day and 1 tablet on subsequent days. Patients should be re-examined within a week for possible adjustment of dosage.

Mild diabetes: In the mild stable diabetic a loading dose is not necessary. Treatment can start with one-half tablet (250 mg) daily before breakfast. The dose can be increased by 250–500 mg every five to seven days as needed.

Elderly patients: Because some elderly patients are unusually responsive, patients in this group should be started with a single daily dose of one-half tablet (250 mg) before breakfast, and have their blood and/or urine sugar monitored after 24 hours. If satisfactory, this dose may then be continued or gradually increased if control is inadequate. Any tendency towards hypoglycaemia is an indication for reduction of dosage or for discontinuing the drug.

Transfer from other oral agents: Patients who have been maintained on other oral agents may be transferred directly to acetohexamide. It should be remembered that acetohexamide is intermediate in potency between tolbutamide and chlorpropamide, and the first dose of acetohexamide should be only half the previous tolbutamide dose. When the transfer is from chlorpropamide an eventual increase may be necessary.

Transfer from insulin: In general, patients who have been previously maintained on insulin in small dosage, 10 or 20 units per day, may be transferred to acetohexamide directly. During the period of insulin withdrawal, the patient should test his urine for sugar and acetone frequently, so that the appropriate adjustments can be made. Especial care should be observed in the elderly patient. Some cases mey need to be treated in hospital during the transition period. Acetohexamide may be used with biguanides.

Contra-indications, warnings, etc

Contra-indications: Patients with hyperglycaemia and glycosuria which may be associated with primary renal disease. If reduction of the blood sugar becomes essential in these cases, insulin is indicated. Patients with sulphonylurea or sulphonamide intolerance.

Warnings: Acetohexamide is of no value in diabetes complicated by acidosis and coma. These conditions require insulin.

In times of stress to the patient, such as fever of any cause, trauma, infection or surgical procedures, it may be necessary to return the patient to insulin therapy or to use insulin in addition to acetohexamide.

In patients with impaired hepatic and/or renal function and in debilitated or malnourished individuals, careful observation of the patient and adjustment of dosage are mandatory to prevent the occurrence of hypoglycaemia.

Hypoglycaemia may also occur in those patients who do not eat regularly or who exercise without caloric supplementation. It is most likely to appear during the period of transition from insulin.

Drug interactions: Thiazide-type diuretics may aggravate the diabetic state and alter the dosage of acetohexamide required.

Preparations containing phenylbutazone interfere with the excretion of the active metabolite hydroxyhexamide; as a result, increased sulphonylurea levels depress the blood glucose. This may also be true of probenecid, sulphinpyrazone and the absorbed sulphonamides.

Sulphonylurea compounds, like sulphonamides and barbiturates, may aggravate hepatic porphyria.

Patients receiving sulphonylureas may experience a 'disulfiram reaction' following the ingestion of alcohol. Symptoms may include flushing, nausea and vomiting, headache, and hypotension.

Usage in pregnancy and lactation: The safety of acetohexamide for use during pregnancy and lactation has not been established. Acetohexamide is not recommended for the management of the pregnant diabetic; control with insulin is preferable. Acetohexamide is not recommended for mothers who are breast feeding.

Precautions: Secondary failures and the spontaneous tendency of diabetes to fluctuate in severity may occur. Therefore, patients should be seen by their physicians at regular intervals and their diabetes evaluated in order to avoid hyperglycaemic and hypoglycaemic episodes.

Side-effects: These consist mainly of gastro-intestinal disturbances (nausea, epigastric fullness, heartburn) and headache. Both appear to be dose-related, and may disappear when dosage is reduced.

Allergic skin manifestations (pruritus, erythema, urticaria, morbilliform or maculopapular eruptions) occur but are usually transient and may disappear with continued dosage. If the skin reactions persist, the drug should be stopped. Photosensitivity reactions may be noted. Jaundice of both the cholestatic and mixed hepatic types have been observed.

As with other sulphonylurea drugs, leucopenia, thrombocytopenia, pancytopenia, agranulocytosis, aplastic anaemia and haemolytic anaemia may occur.

Pharmaceutical precautions Keep containers tightly closed.

Legal category POM.

Package quantities Bottles of 100 and 500.

Further information Nil.

Product licence number 0006/5069.

DOBUTREX*

Presentation Dobutrex (dobutamine hydrochloride for injection) is supplied in a sterile lyophilised form in 250 mg vials, together with 250 mg Mannitol BP.

Uses *Actions:* The primary action of dobutamine is to augment cardiac contractility by stimulating the β_1 receptors of the heart. It is a direct-acting agent.

Indications: Dobutrex is indicated for adults who require inotropic support in the treatment of heart failure associated with myocardial infarction, open heart surgery, cardiomyopathies, septic shock and cardiogenic shock.

Dosage and administration For intravenous administration only. Dobutrex may be reconstituted with Water for Injections PhEur or 5% Dextrose Intravenous Infusion BP. To dissolve, add 10 ml of diluent to the vial. If the material does not completely dissolve, add an additional 10 ml of diluent. Reconstituted Dobutrex must be diluted further by injecting aseptically the contents of one vial into a 250 ml or 500 ml container of one of the following intravenous solutions:

Sodium Chloride Intravenous Infusion BP
5% Dextrose Intravenous Infusion BP
5% Dextrose + 0.9% Sodium Chloride Intravenous Infusion BP
5% Dextrose + 0.45% Sodium Chloride Intravenous Infusion BP
Sodium Lactate Intravenous Infusion BP

These dilutions will give a concentration for administration as follows:

250 ml contains 1,000 mcg/ml of dobutamine
500 ml contains 500 mcg/ml of dobutamine

These prepared solutions should be used within 24 hours.

Administration: After dilution, Dobutrex should be administered intravenously through an intravenous needle or catheter. An i.v. drip chamber or other suitable metering device is essential for controlling the rate of flow in drops per minute.

Recommended dosage for adults and the elderly: Most patients will respond satisfactorily to doses ranging from 2.5 to 10 mcg/kg/minute. Occasionally, however, a dose as low as 0.5 mcg/kg/minute will elicit a response. Rarely, a dose as high as 40 mcg/kg/minute is required.

The rate of administration and the duration of therapy should be adjusted according to the patient's response as determined by heart rate, blood pressure, urine flow, and, if possible, measurement of cardiac output.

Rather than abruptly discontinuing therapy with Dobutrex, it is often advisable to decrease the dosage gradually.

Side-effects, which are dose-related, are infrequent when Dobutrex is administered at rates below 10 mcg/kg/minute. Rates as high as 40 mcg/kg/minute have been used occasionally without significant adverse effects.

The final volume administered should be determined by the fluid requirements of the patient. Concentrations as high as 5,000 mcg/ml have been used in patients on a restricted fluid intake. High concentrations of dobutamine should only be given with an infusion pump, to ensure accurate dosage.

Contra-indications, warnings, etc

Contra-indications: None.

Warnings: If an undue increase in heart rate or systolic blood pressure occurs or if an arrhythmia is precipitated, the dose of dobutamine should be reduced or the drug should be discontinued temporarily.

Particular care should be exercised when dobutamine is used in patients with acute myocardial infarction because any significant increases in heart rate that occur may intensify ischaemia and cause anginal pain and ST segment elevation.

Dobutamine should be used with great caution in patients with idiopathic hypertrophic subaortic stenosis since positive inotropic agents may increase outlet obstruction in these patients.

No improvement may be observed in the presence of marked mechanical obstruction such as severe valvular aortic stenosis.

Minimal vasoconstriction has occasionally been observed, most notably in patients recently treated with a β-blocking drug. Because the inotropic effect of dobutamine stems from stimulation of cardiac β_1 receptors this effect is, of course, prevented by β-blocking drugs. However, dobutamine has been shown to counteract the cardiodepressive effects of β-adrenergic receptor blocking drugs.

Dobutamine should be used with caution in the presence of severe hypotension complicating cardiogenic shock (mean arterial pressure less than 70 mm Hg).

Usage in pregnancy: Reproduction studies performed in rats and rabbits have revealed no evidence of impaired fertility or harm to the fetus due to dobutamine. To date, the drug has not been administered to pregnant women and safety in this situation remains to be determined.

Paediatric use: The safety and efficacy of dobutamine for use in children have not been established.

Precautions: Hypovolaemia should be corrected when necessary with whole blood or plasma before dobutamine is administered.

Adverse reactions: A 10 to 20 mm rise in systolic blood pressure has been observed in most patients. Those with pre-existing hypertension may exhibit an exaggerated pressor response. An increase in heart rate of five to ten beats per minute may occur. In some instances, patients have developed excessive tachycardia or ectopic beats. Dobutamine may also increase the ventricular rate in patients with pre-existing atrial fibrillation. Temporary discontinuation of the infusion or a reduction in dosage will usually reverse these conditions.

The following side-effects have been reported rarely: nausea, headache, anginal pain, nonspecific chest pain, palpitations or shortness of breath.

No abnormal laboratory values attributable to dobutamine have been observed.

Overdosage: In the event of overdosage, as evidenced by excessive change in blood pressure or tachycardia, reduce the rate of administration or temporarily discontinue dobutamine until the patient's condition stabilises. Because the duration of action of dobutamine is short, any adverse effects are also short-lived.

Pharmaceutical precautions *Unreconstituted vials:* Store at room temperature (15°–25°C). *Reconstituted solutions (in 10 ml):* The vials may be stored under refrigeration (0°–6°C) for 48 hours or at room temperature (15°–25°C) for six hours. The pH of the reconstituted solution is between 2.5 and 5.5.

Prepared intravenous solutions are stable for 24 hours at room temperature.

Do not add Dobutrex to 5% Sodium Bicarbonate Intravenous Infusion BP or to any other strongly alkaline solutions. When Dobutrex is used in conjunction with other agents or diluents, the solution for infusion should not contain final concentrations of more than 0.02% of any bisulphite salt or more than 0.5% ethanol.

Solutions containing Dobutrex may turn pink; the colour may intensify with time. This colour change is due to slight oxidation of the drug, but there is no significant loss of potency during the recommended storage periods.

Legal category POM.

Package quantities 25 ml vials containing 250 mg dobutamine as the hydrochloride.

Further information Nil.

Product licence number 0006/0134.

DOLASAN*

Presentation Tablets (orange, elliptical, coded C54) each containing: Dextropropoxyphene Napsylate BP 100 mg (equivalent to approximately 65 mg dextropropoxyphene hydrochloride or 60 mg dextropropoxyphene base).

Aspirin PhEur 325 mg.

Uses For the relief of mild to moderate pain.

Dosage and administration For oral administration to adults only. The usual dose, which should not normally be exceeded, is 1 tablet taken three or four times daily.

The elderly: As for adults. Reduce dosage if renal or hepatic function is impaired.

Contra-indications, warnings, etc

Contra-indications: Hypersensitivity to dextropropoxyphene or aspirin, active peptic ulceration and haemophilia.

Warnings: Dextropropoxyphene is an analgesic with CNS depressant properties and should be used with caution in patients who are receiving other CNS depressant drugs, as an additive effect may occur. Patients should be warned to avoid alcohol.

As with other drugs which affect the CNS, care should be taken when prescribing for patients with personality or other psychological disorders. Tolerance, psychological and physical dependence may rarely occur.

Like other centrally acting drugs, dextropropoxyphene may impair patients' mental and physical reactions in the performance of potentially hazardous tasks (e.g. in driving ability, operation of machinery, etc.) to a varying extent, depending on dosage and individual susceptibility.

Salicylates should be used with caution in patients with asthma or coagulation abnormalities. They may also induce gastro-intestinal haemorrhage, occasionally major.

Use in pregnancy: The safety of Dolasan for use during pregnancy has not been established. Aspirin may prolong labour and contribute to maternal and neonatal bleeding, and is best avoided at term.

Precautions: Dolasan should be administered with caution to patients with severe renal or hepatic impairment as delayed elimination or elevated serum levels may result.

Isolated reports suggest that dextropropoxyphene may inhibit the metabolism of some concurrently administered drugs. Patients receiving anticonvulsants, antidepressants or warfarin-like drugs should be monitored during therapy.

Aspirin may enhance the effect of anticoagulants, inhibit the action of uricosuric agents, precipitate bronchospasm or induce attacks of asthma in susceptible individuals.

Side-effects: Side-effects such as dizziness, sedation, nausea and vomiting seem to be more prominent in ambulatory than in non-ambulatory patients, and some of these side-effects may be alleviated if the patient lies down.

Other reported side-effects include constipation, abdominal pain, skin rashes, lightheadedness, headache, weakness, euphoria, dysphoria and minor visual disturbances.

Overdosage: The chronic ingestion of dextropropoxyphene in doses exceeding 720 mg (as base) per day has caused toxic psychoses and convulsions.

Symptoms of acute toxicity may be rapid in onset, with the danger of respiratory arrest. Other recognised manifestations include respiratory depression, coma, circulatory collapse, pulmonary oedema, convulsions and cardiac arrhythmias.

Deterioration may be rapid, with fatal outcome.

The clinical picture may be complicated by salicylism.

Treatment: Primary attention should be given to the re-establishment of adequate respiratory exchange through provision of a patent airway and institution of assisted or controlled ventilation. The narcotic antagonist naloxone is a specific antidote against the respiratory depression produced by dextropropoxyphene. An initial dose of 0.4–2 mg should be administered intravenously with simultaneous efforts at respiratory resuscitation. If the desired degree of improvement is not obtained, the dose should be repeated at two to three minute intervals. Subsequent doses of naloxone may be necessary for up to 24 hours due to the slow elimination of dextropropoxyphene. Naloxone may also be administered by infusion. The rate of infusion should be such as to maximise the reversal of CNS depression. In addition to the use of a narcotic antagonist, the patient may require careful titration with an anticonvulsant to control seizures. Analeptic drugs (for example, caffeine or amphetamine) should not be used because of their tendency to precipitate convulsions. Oxygen, intravenous fluids, vasopressors and other supportive measures should be employed as indicated.

Gastric lavage may be helpful. Activated charcoal can adsorb a significant amount of ingested dextropropoxyphene. Dialysis is of little value in poisoning by dextropropoxyphene alone. Salicylates are dialysable.

Pharmaceutical precautions Nil.

Legal category CD (Sch 5), POM.

Package quantities Blister packs of 100 (10 strips of 10 tablets).

Further information Nil.

Product licence number 0006/0077.

DOLOXENE*

Presentation Capsules (opaque orange, coded H64) containing approximately 100 mg Dextropropoxyphene Napsylate BP (equivalent to approximately 65 mg dextropropoxyphene hydrochloride or 60 mg dextropropoxyphene base).

Uses For the relief of mild to moderate pain.

Dosage and administration For oral administration to adults only. The usual dose is one capsule three or four times daily, and should not normally be exceeded.

The elderly: As for adults. Reduce dosage if renal or hepatic function is impaired.

Contra-indications, warnings, etc
Contra-indications: Hypersensitivity to dextropropoxyphene.

Warnings: Dextropropoxyphene is an analgesic with CNS depressant properties and should be used with caution in patients who are receiving other CNS depressant drugs, as an additive effect may occur. Patients should be warned to avoid alcohol.

As with other drugs which affect the CNS, care should be taken when prescribing for patients with personality or other psychological disorders. Tolerance, psychological and physical dependence may rarely occur.

Like other centrally acting drugs, dextropropoxyphene may impair patients' mental and physical reactions in the performance of potentially hazardous tasks (e.g. driving ability, operation of machinery, etc.) to a varying extent, depending on dosage and individual susceptibility.

Use in pregnancy: The safety of Doloxene for use during pregnancy has not been established.

Precautions: Doloxene should be administered with caution to patients with severe renal or hepatic impairment as delayed elimination or elevated serum levels may result.

Isolated reports suggest that dextropropoxyphene may inhibit the metabolism of some concurrently administered drugs. Patients receiving anticonvulsants, antidepressants or warfarin-like drugs shoud be monitored during therapy.

Side-effects: Side-effects such as dizziness, sedation, nausea and vomiting seem to be more prominent in ambulatory than in non-ambulatory patients, and some of these side-effects may be alleviated if the patient lies down.

Other reported side-effects include constipation, abdominal pain, skin rashes, lightheadedness, headache, weakness, euphoria, dysphoria and minor visual disturbances.

Overdosage: The chronic ingestion of dextropropoxyphene in doses exceeding 720 mg (as base) per day has caused toxic psychoses and convulsions.

Symptoms of acute toxicity may be rapid in onset, with the danger of respiratory arrest. Other recognised manifestations include respiratory depression, coma, circulatory collapse, pulmonary oedema, convulsions and cardiac arrhythmias.

Deterioration may be rapid, with fatal outcome.

Treatment: Primary attention should be given to the re-establishment of adequate respiratory exchange through provision of a patent airway and institution of assisted or controlled ventilation. The narcotic antagonist naloxone is a specific antidote against the respiratory depression produced by dextropropoxyphene. An initial dose of 0.4–2 mg should be administered intravenously with simultaneous efforts at respiratory resuscitation. If the desired degree of improvement is not obtained, the dose should be repeated at two to three minute intervals. Subsequent doses of naloxone may be necessary for up to 24 hours due to the slow elimination of dextropropoxyphene. Naloxone may also be administered by infusion. The rate of infusion should be such as to maximise the reversal of CNS depression.

In addition to the use of a narcotic antagonist, the patient may require careful titration with an anticonvulsant to control seizures. Analeptic drugs (for example, caffeine or amphetamine) should not be used because of their tendency to precipitate convulsions.

Oxygen, intravenous fluids, vasopressors and other supportive measures should be employed as indicated.

Gastric lavage may be helpful. Activated charcoal can adsorb a significant amount of ingested dextropropoxyphene. Dialysis is of little value in poisoning by dextropropoxyphene alone.

Pharmaceutical precautions Store below 25°C.

Legal category CD (Sch 5), POM.

Package quantities Blister packs of 100 (10 strips of 10 capsules).

Further information Nil.

Product licence number 0006/5068.

DOLOXENE* Compound

Presentation Doloxene Compound is presented as hard gelatin capsules (light grey opaque cap, red opaque body) coded H91, each containing: Dextropropoxyphene Napsylate BP 100 mg (equivalent to approximately 65 mg dextropropoxyphene hydrochloride or 60 mg dextropropoxyphene base).

Aspirin PhEur   375 mg
Caffeine PhEur   30 mg

Uses For the relief of mild to moderate pain.

Dosage and administration For oral administration to adults only. The usual dose is one capsule three or four times daily, and should not normally be exceeded.

The elderly: As for adults. Reduce dosage if renal or hepatic function is impaired.

Contra-indications, warnings, etc
Contra-indications: Hypersensitivity to any of the constituents, active peptic ulceration and haemophilia.

Warnings: Dextropropoxyphene is an analgesic with CNS depressant properties and should be used with caution in patients who are receiving other CNS depressant drugs, as an additive effect may occur. Patients should be warned to avoid alcohol.

As with other drugs which affect the CNS, care should be taken when prescribing for patients with personality or other psychological disorders. Tolerance, psychological and physical dependence may rarely occur.

Like other centrally acting drugs, dextropropoxyphene may impair patients' mental and physical reactions in the performance of potentially hazardous tasks (e.g. in driving ability, operation of machinery, etc.) to a varying extent, depending on dosage and individual susceptibility.

Salicylates should be used with caution in patients with asthma or coagulation abnormalities. They may also induce gastro-intestinal haemorrhage, occasionally major.

High doses of caffeine may cause tremors and palpitations.

Use in pregnancy: The safety of Doloxene Compound for use during pregnancy has not been established. Aspirin may prolong labour and contribute to maternal and neonatal bleeding, and is best avoided at term.

Precautions: Doloxene Compound should be administered with caution to patients with severe renal or hepatic impairment as delayed elimination or elevated serum levels may result.

Isolated reports suggest that dextropropoxyphene may inhibit the metabolism of some concurrently administered drugs. Patients receiving anticonvulsants, antidepressants or warfarin-like drugs should be monitored during therapy.

Aspirin may enhance the effect of anticoagulants, inhibit the action of uricosuric agents, precipitate bronchospasm or induce attacks of asthma in susceptible individuals.

Side-effects: Side-effects such as dizziness, sedation, nausea and vomiting seem to be more prominent in ambulatory than in non-ambulatory patients, and some of these side-effects may be alleviated if the patient lies down.

Other reported side-effects include constipation, abdominal pain, skin rashes, lightheadedness, headache, weakness, euphoria, dysphoria and minor visual disturbances.

Overdosage: The chronic ingestion of dextropropoxyphene in doses exceeding 720 mg (as base) per day has caused toxic psychoses and convulsions.

Symptoms of acute toxicity may be rapid in onset, with the danger of respiratory arrest. Other recognised manifestations include respiratory depression, coma, circulatory collapse, pulmonary oedema, convulsions and cardiac arrhythmias.

Deterioration may be rapid, with fatal outcome.

The clinical picture may be complicated by salicylism.

Treatment: Primary attention should be given to the re-establishment of adequate respiratory exchange through provision of a patent airway, and institution of assisted or controlled ventilation. The narcotic antagonist naloxone is a specific antidote against the respiratory depression produced by dextropropoxyphene. An initial dose of 0.4–2 mg should be administered intravenously with simultaneous efforts at respiratory resuscitation. If the desired degree of improvement is not obtained, the dose should be repeated at two to three minute intervals. Subsequent doses of naloxone may be necessary for up to 24 hours due to the slow elimination of dextropropoxyphene. Naloxone may also be administered by infusion. The rate of infusion should be such as to maximise the reversal of CNS depression.

In addition to the use of a narcotic antagonist, the patient may require careful titration with an anticonvulsant to control seizures. Analeptic drugs (for example, caffeine or amphetamine) should not be used because of their tendency to precipitate convulsions.

Oxygen, intravenous fluids, vasopressors and other supportive measures should be employed as indicated.

Gastric lavage may be helpful. Activated charcoal can adsorb a significant amount of ingested dextropropoxyphene. Dialysis is of little value in poisoning by dextropropoxyphene alone. Salicylates are dialysable.

Pharmaceutical precautions Store below 25°C.

Legal category CD (Sch 5), POM.

Package quantities Blister packs of 100 (10 strips of 10 capsules).

Further information Nil.

Product licence number 0006/0091.

ELDISINE*

Presentation Vials containing 5 mg Eldisine (vindesine sulphate for injection) and 25 mg Mannitol BP. (Supplied in a combination package with an accompanying vial of diluting solution, 5 ml, containing 45 mg Sodium Chloride PhEur with 2% Benzyl Alcohol BP as a preservative.)

Uses Eldisine is an anti-neoplastic drug for intravenous use which can be used alone or in combination with other oncolytic drugs. Information available at present suggests that Eldisine as a single agent may be useful for the treatment of: acute lymphoblastic leukaemia of childhood resistant to other drugs; blastic crises of chronic myeloid leukaemia; malignant melanoma unresponsive to other forms of therapy; advanced carcinoma of the breast, unresponsive to appropriate endocrine surgery and/or hormonal therapy.

Dosage and administration Extreme care must be used in calculating and administering the dose of Eldisine, since overdosage may have a very serious or fatal outcome.

It is recommended that the drug be administered intravenously in a single bolus injection at weekly intervals. The size of the dose is determined by body surface area. In adults and the elderly, the recommended starting dose is 3 mg/m^2, and children may be started at 4 mg/m^2. Thereafter, granulocyte counts should be made prior to each subsequent dose to determine the patient's sensitivity to the drug. Provided there is no granulocytopenia or other toxicity (see adverse reactions) the dosage may be increased in 0.5 mg/m^2 steps at weekly intervals.

The dose should not be increased after that dose which: (i) reduces the granulocyte count to below 1500 cells/mm^3; or on rare occasions, (ii) reduces the platelet count to below 100,000/mm^3, (iii) causes acute abdominal pain (see under precautions).

On each of the above occasions there should be full recovery before administering the next dose, which should be reduced from the one causing the adverse reaction. For most patients, however, the weekly dosage will prove to be in the range of 3.0 to 4.0 mg/m^2 in adults and 4.0 to 5.0 mg/m^2 in children. (A nomogram for calculation of body surface area is available on request.)

The use of small amounts of Eldisine daily for long periods is not advised, even though the resulting total weekly dosage may be similar to that recommended. Little or no added therapeutic advantage has been demonstrated when such regimens have been used, and side-effects are increased. Strict adherence to the recommended dosage schedule is very important.

To prepare a solution containing 1 mg/ml add the 5 ml of accompanying diluting solution to the 5 mg of Eldisine in the sterile vial. The drug dissolves rapidly to give a clear solution.

The dose of Eldisine solution (calculated to provide the desired number of milligrams per square metre of the patient's surface area) may be injected either into the tubing of a running intravenous infusion (*compatible infusions are 5% Dextrose Intravenous Infusion BP, Sodium Chloride Intravenous Infusion BP and dextrose/saline infusions*), or directly into a vein.

The latter procedure is readily adaptable to outpatient therapy. In either case, the injection should be completed in 1 to 3 minutes. If care is taken to ensure that the needle is securely within the vein and that no solution containing Eldisine is spilled extravascularly, cellulitis and/or phlebitis is unlikely to occur.

Because of the enhanced possibility of thrombosis, it is considered inadvisable to inject a solution of Eldisine into an extremity in which the circulation is impaired, or potentially impaired, by such conditions as compressing or invading neoplasm, phlebitis or varicosity.

Caution: If leakage into surrounding tissue should occur during intravenous administration of Eldisine, it may cause considerable irritation. The injection should be discontinued immediately, and any remaining portion of the dose should be introduced into another vein. Local injection of hyaluronidase or hydrocortisone and the application of moderate heat to the area of leakage help to disperse the drug, and are thought to minimise discomfort and the possibility of cellulitis.

Care must be taken to avoid contamination of the eye with concentrations of Eldisine used clinically. If accidental contamination occurs, severe irritation (or if the drug was delivered under pressure, even corneal ulceration) may result. The eye should be washed thoroughly and immediately with water.

Contra-indications, warnings, etc
Contra-indications: Intrathecal administration.

Use in patients who are granulocytopenic (less than 1500 granulocytes per mm^3) unless the granulocytopenia is a result of the disease affecting the bone marrow. Eldisine should not be used in the presence of bacterial infection. Such infections must be brought under control with antiseptics or antibiotics before using Eldisine.

Warning – Usage in pregnancy: This product should not normally be administered to patients who are pregnant or to mothers who are breast feeding. Although no abnormalities of the human fetus have been reported thus far, animal studies with Eldisine suggest that teratogenic effects may occur.

Precautions: Clinically, the dose-limiting toxicity of Eldisine is granulocytopenia, although, in general, oncolytic activity is obtained at doses causing little or no effect on the granulocytes.

When granulocytopenia occurs, the nadir in the granulocyte count may be expected to occur 3–5 days after the last day of drug administration. Recovery of the granulocyte count is rapid thereafter and is usually complete within 6–8 days after the last dose.

The thrombocyte count is usually either unaffected or increased by weekly therapy with Eldisine. However, significant thrombocytopenia has occurred occasionally, particularly when doses are given more frequently than once a week. It is probably more likely to occur when patients are thrombocytopenic (less than 100,000 cells/mm³) prior to therapy with Eldisine.

The effect of Eldisine upon the red blood cell count and haemoglobin concentration is usually insignificant when other treatment does not complicate the picture. It should be remembered, however, that patients with malignant disease may exhibit anaemia even in the absence of any treatment.

If granulocytopenia with less than 1000 granulocytes/mm³ occurs following a dose of Eldisine, the patient should be watched carefully for evidence of infection until the granulocyte count has returned to a safe level.

Whilst the neurotoxicity is not usually dose-limiting, particular attention should be given to dosage and neurological side-effects if Eldisine is administered to patients with pre-existing neuromuscular disease, and also when other drugs with neurotoxic potential are being used. The neurotoxicity associated with Eldisine therapy may be additive.

Care should be exercised when Eldisine has been the cause of acute abdominal pain, as paralytic ileus may be a significant risk if further doses of Eldisine are given, particularly if the dose is increased.

As Eldisine is excreted principally by the liver, it may be necessary to reduce initial doses in the presence of significantly impaired hepatic or biliary function.

When chemotherapy is being given in conjunction with radiation therapy through portals which include the liver, the use of Eldisine should be delayed until radiation therapy has been completed.

Acute shortness of breath and severe bronchospasm have been reported following the administration of Eldisine. These reactions have been encountered most frequently when Eldisine was used in combination with mitomycin-C. The onset may be within minutes, or several hours after the drug is injected.

Adverse reactions: The incidence of side-effects appears to be related not only to the size of dose employed but also to the total accumulated dose given. Acute toxicity is more likely to occur if doses above 4 mg/m² are employed, and symptoms usually persist for no longer than 24 hours. The onset of peripheral neuropathy appears to be more related to the total accumulated dose given.

The following are manifestations which have been reported as adverse reactions:

Gastro-intestinal – dysphagia, anorexia, nausea, vomiting, dyspepsia, perforated duodenal ulcer, abdominal pain, ileus, diarrhoea, constipation.

Neurological – numbness, paraesthesiae, peripheral neuritis, loss of deep tendon reflexes, myalgia, jaw pain, foot-drop, convulsions.

Cutaneous – maculopapular rashes, mouth ulceration, cellulitis with extravasation, alopecia from mild to total. Alopecia is the commonest side-effect. Regrowth of hair may occur while still on therapy.

Haematological – granulocytopenia (the dose-limiting factor), thrombocytosis, thrombocytopenia, mild anaemia.

Miscellaneous – malaise, spikes of fever, rigors.

In preliminary assessments, neurotoxicity induced by Eldisine is generally less severe and less progressive in nature compared to effects observed with Oncovin (vincristine sulphate).

Overdosage: Side-effects following the use of Eldisine are dose related. Therefore, following administration of more than the recommended dose, patients can be expected to experience these effects in an exaggerated fashion.

Treatment: Supportive care should include: (1) daily blood counts for guidance in transfusion requirement. (2) prevention of the side-effects that result from the syndrome of inappropriate secretion of antidiuretic hormone. This includes restriction of fluid intake and perhaps the use of a diuretic drug acting on the loop of Henle and distal tubule function. (3) use of cathartics to prevent ileus. (4) administration of an anticonvulsant. (5) monitoring the patient's cardiovascular system. Animal studies indicate that folinic acid is effective in the treatment of vinca alkaloid overdosage. A suggested schedule is to administer 15 mg of folinic acid intravenously every 3 hours for 24 hours and then every 6 hours for at least 48 hours.

Clinical experience of Eldisine overdosage is extremely limited, with only one published case.

Pharmaceutical precautions Vials of Eldisine should be stored in a refrigerator between 0° and 6°C.

After reconstitution: After a portion of the solution has been removed from a vial, the remainder of the contents of the vial may be stored in a refrigerator for future use for 30 days without significant loss of potency. When the reconstituted vial of Eldisine is to be stored for more than 48 hours, it is essential to use the accompanying diluting solution or a diluent which contains a preservative.

Eldisine should never be mixed with any other drug.

Legal category POM.

Package quantities Vials 5 mg: Single vials.

Further information Nil.

Product licence numbers
Vials 5 mg   0006/0137
Diluent   0006/5174

FOLIC ACID

Presentation Folic acid is an orange-yellow, almost odourless and tasteless micro-crystalline powder. It is presented as tablets each containing 5 mg Folic Acid BP (coded J66).

Uses Folic acid is a member of the B group of vitamins. It is necessary for the normal production and maturation of red blood cells. Folic acid produces a haemopoietic response in nutritional macrocytic anaemia, megaloblastic anaemia of infancy and the anaemias of pregnancy, pellagra and sprue, the anaemia following gastrectomy, and in pernicious anaemia.

Dosage and administration For oral administration.

Adults and the elderly: In the treatment of megaloblastic anaemia, an initial dose of 10–20 mg daily may be given for 14 days, or until a haemopoietic response is obtained. Daily maintenance dose 2.5–10 mg.

Children: 5–15 mg daily.

Contra-indications, warnings, etc *Contra-indications:* None.

Warnings: Folic acid should not be given for the treatment of pernicious anaemia without adequate amounts of cyanocobalamin, because folic acid alone will not prevent the development of sub-acute combined degeneration of the spinal cord.

Folic acid will not correct folate deficiency due to dihydrofolate reductase inhibitors.

Drug interactions: Folic acid may lower the serum concentrations of phenytoin, phenobarbitone and primidone, but this has seldom been reported to increase the frequency of fits. Concurrent administration with co-trimoxazole, chloramphenicol or sulphasalazine may interfere with folate metabolism.

Side-effects: Folic acid is usually well tolerated, but anorexia, nausea, abdominal distension and flatulence have been reported in association with its use.

Pharmaceutical precautions Folic Acid tablets should be stored in airtight containers, protected from light.

Legal category POM.

Package quantities Bottles of 100 and 1,000 tablets.

Further information Nil.

Product licence number 0006/5113.

GLUCAGON

Presentation The product is in lyophilised form and is supplied with an accompanying diluting solution.

Vials containing 1 unit (1.09 mg) of glucagon as the hydrochloride with 49 mg Lactose PhEur. (Diluting solution, 1 ml, containing Glycerol PhEur, 1.6%, with phenol, 0.2%, as a preservative. Sodium hydroxide and/or hydrochloric acid may have been added during manufacture to adjust the pH).

Crystalline glucagon is a white powder containing less than 0.01% zinc. It is relatively insoluble in water but is soluble at a pH of less than 3 or more than 9.5.

Uses *Actions:* Glucagon causes an increase in blood glucose concentrations and is used in the treatment of hypoglycaemic states. It is effective in small doses. Glucagon acts only on liver glycogen, converting it to glucose, and is therefore helpful only if liver glycogen is available. It is of little or no help in states of starvation, adrenal insufficiency or chronic hypoglycaemia. The patient with juvenile-type diabetes does not have as great a response in blood glucose levels as does the adult-type stable diabetic, therefore supplementary carbohydrate should be given as soon as possible, especially to juvenile patients.

Parenteral administration of glucagon produces relaxation of the smooth muscle of the stomach, duodenum, small bowel and colon.

Indications: Glucagon is indicated for counteracting severe hypoglycaemic reactions in diabetic patients or resulting from insulin shock therapy in psychiatric patients.

Glucagon is indicated as a diagnostic aid in the radiological examination of the stomach, duodenum, small bowel and colon, when a hypotonic state would be advantageous.

Glucagon is as effective for this examination as the anticholinergic drugs, but it has fewer side-effects. When glucagon is administered concomitantly with an anticholinergic agent, the response is not significantly greater than when either drug is used alone. However, the addition of the anticholinergic agent results in increased side-effects.

Dosage and administration The diluent is provided for use only in the preparation of glucagon for intermittent parenteral injection and for no other use.

Glucagon may be given by subcutaneous, intramuscular or intravenous injection. Administration as a continuous infusion for long periods is not recommended.

Dosage in the elderly: As for adults.

Directions for the use of glucagon in hypoglycaemia:

1. Dissolve the lyophilised glucagon in the accompanying diluent.
2. Give 0.5–1 unit of glucagon by subcutaneous, intramuscular or intravenous injection. These doses are equally suitable for adults and children.
3. The patient will normally awaken in 5–20 minutes. If the response is delayed, there is no contra-indication to the administration of 1 or 2 additional doses of glucagon: however, in view of the deleterious effects of cerebral hypoglycaemia and depending on the duration and depth of coma, the use of parenteral glucose must be considered.
4. Intravenous glucose *must* be given if the patient fails to respond to glucagon.
5. When the patient responds, give supplementary carbohydrate to restore the liver glycogen and prevent secondary hypoglycaemia.

Reversal of insulin shock therapy: Dissolve the lyophilised glucagon in the accompanying diluent. After one hour of coma, inject 0.5–1 unit of glucagon by the subcutaneous, intramuscular or intravenous route. Larger doses may be employed if desired. The patient will normally awaken in 10–25 minutes. If no response occurs within the desired interval, the dose may be repeated. Upon awakening, the patient should be fed orally as soon as possible, and the usual dietary regimen followed.

In very deep states of coma, such as Stage IV or Stage V of Himwich, intravenous glucose should be given in addition to glucagon for a more immediate response. Glucagon and glucose may be used together without decreasing the efficacy of glucose administration.

For use as a diagnostic aid: Dissolve the lyophilised glucagon in the accompanying diluting solution.

The following doses may be administered for relaxation of the stomach, duodenum and small bowel, depending on the time of onset of action and the duration of effect required for the examination. Since the stomach is less sensitive to the effect of glucagon, $\frac{1}{2}$ unit i.v. or 2 units i.m. are recommended.

Dose (units)	Route of administration	Time of onset of action (min)	Approximate duration of effect (min)
0.25–0.5	i.v.	1	9–17
1	i.m.	8–10	12–27
2†	i.v.	1	22–25
2†	i.m.	4–7	21–32

†2-unit doses are associated with a higher incidence of nausea and vomiting than the lower doses.

For examination of the colon, it is recommended that a 2-unit dose be administered intramuscularly approximately 10 minutes prior to initiation of the procedure. Relaxation of the colon and reduction of discomfort to the patient will allow the radiologist to perform a more satisfactory examination.

Contra-indications, warnings, etc
Contra-indications: None.

Warnings: Since glucagon is a protein, hypersensitivity is a possibility.

Glucagon should not be administered to patients with known or suspected insulinoma and/or phaeochromocytoma. In patients with insulinoma, intravenous administration of glucagon will, produce an initial increase in blood glucose, but, because of its insulin-releasing effect, may subsequently cause severe hypoglycaemia. Exogenous glucagon also stimulates the release of catecholamines, which can cause a marked increase in blood pressure in patients with phaeochromocytoma.

Glucagon may enhance the anticoagulant effect of warfarin.

Precautions: In the treatment of hypoglycaemic shock with glucagon, liver glycogen must be available. Glucose by the intravenous route or by gavage should be considered in the hypoglycaemic patient.

Glucagon should be used with caution as a diagnostic aid in diabetic patients.

Side-effects: Glucagon is relatively free of adverse reactions, except for occasional nausea and vomiting, which may also occur with hypoglycaemia. Diarrhoea and hypokalaemia have rarely been reported.

Pharmaceutical precautions Glucagon is stable in lyophilised form at room temperature (15°–25°C). *After reconstitution:* Solutions should be used immediately.

Legal category POM.

Package quantities Vials No. 666, 1 unit (1.09 mg) glucagon as the hydrochloride accompanied by Vials No. 667 containing 1 ml of diluent.

Further information Nil.

Product licence numbers
Vials 1 unit   0006/5110
Vials Diluting Solution   0006/5112

HUMULIN* S   ▼
HUMULIN* I   ▼
HUMULIN* Zn   ▼
HUMULIN* M1   ▼
HUMULIN* M2   ▼

Presentation *Humulin S (Soluble):* A sterile, clear, colourless, aqueous solution of human insulin (crb) adjusted to a pH of 6.6–8.0.

Humulin I (Isophane): A sterile suspension of a white, crystalline precipitate of isophane human insulin (crb) in an isotonic phosphate buffer adjusted to a pH of 6.9–7.5.

Humulin Zn (Zinc suspension): A sterile, white suspension of crystalline human insulin (crb) zinc suspension, adjusted to a pH of 6.9–7.5.

Humulin M1: A sterile suspension of human insulin (crb) in the proportion of 10% soluble insulin and 90% isophane insulin.

Humulin M2: A sterile suspension of human insulin (crb) in the proportion of 20% soluble insulin and 80% isophane insulin.
Each presentation contains 100 IU/ml.

Uses For the treatment of insulin-dependent diabetes mellitus.

Humulin S may also be of value during preparation of a diabetic patient for surgery, or in hyperglycaemic coma, trauma or severe infection.

Dosage and administration The dosage should be determined by the physician, according to the requirements of the patient.

Humulin S may be administered by subcutaneous, intramuscular or intravenous injection. Onset of action occurs at approximately 30 minutes, with a duration of 5 to 7 hours and peak activity at 1 to 3 hours.

Humulin I, Humulin Zn, Humulin M1 and Humulin M2 should be administered by subcutaneous or intramuscular injection only.

Humulin I: Onset of action occurs at approximately 1 hour, with a duration of 18 to 20 hours and peak activity at 2 to 8 hours.

Humulin Zn: Onset of action occurs at approximately 3 hours, with an overall duration of activity extending to 20–24 hours and peak activity at 6–14 hours.

Humulin M1: Onset of action occurs at approximately 30 minutes. Total duration of activity is 16 to 18 hours, with peak activity being achieved within 1½ to 2 hours and maintained for 5–7 hours.

Humulin M2: Onset of action occurs at approximately 30 minutes. Total duration of activity is 14 to 16 hours, with peak activity being achieved within 1 to 1½ hours and maintained for 6–8 hours.

Humulin S may be administered in combination with Humulin I as required, and usually as a twice daily regimen.

Humulin I may be given as a single daily dose before breakfast, but some patients may require concurrent administration of Humulin S.

Humulin Zn is administered once, or more usually, twice, a day and may be used in combination with Humulin S as required.

Humulin M1 and Humulin M2 should normally be administered twice daily, usually with two thirds of the daily requirement being given in the morning and the remainder in the evening. For any one injection the dose should not exceed 50 IU.

The effects of mixing with insulins of animal origin have not been studied and this practice is not recommended.

Subcutaneous administration, preferably by the patient, should be in the upper arms, thighs, buttocks or abdomen. Use of injection sites should be rotated so that the same site is not used more than approximately once a month.

Care should be taken to ensure that a blood vessel has

not been entered. The injection site should not be massaged.

Contra-indications, warnings, etc
Contra-indications: Hypoglycaemia. Under no circumstances should Humulin I, Humulin Zn, Humulin M1 or Humulin M2 be given intravenously.

Precautions
Usage in pregnancy: It is essential to maintain good control of the insulin-dependent diabetic patient throughout pregnancy. Insulin requirements usually fall during the first trimester and increase during the second and third trimesters.

Transferring from other insulins: A small number of patients transferring from insulins of animal origin may require a reduced dosage and/or a change in the ratio of soluble to intermediate preparations, especially if they are very tightly controlled and bordering on hypoglycaemia. The dosage reduction may occur immediately after transfer or be a gradual process lasting for several weeks. There is a risk of hypoglycaemia if insulin requirement is decreased, and both the physician and the patient should be aware of this possibility. The risk can be considered minimal if the daily dosage is less than 40 IU. Insulin-resistant patients receiving more than 100 IU daily should be referred to hospital for transfer.

Insulin requirements may be increased during illness or emotional disturbances, or by concurrent administration of drugs with hyperglycaemic activity, e.g. oral contraceptives, corticosteroids or thyroid hormone replacement therapy.

Insulin requirements may be reduced in the presence of renal or hepatic impairment, or by the concurrent administration of drugs with hypoglycaemic activity e.g. monoamine oxidase inhibitors and beta-adrenergic blockers.

Side-effects: Lipodystrophy, insulin resistance and hypersensitivity reactions are among the side-effects associated with insulins of animal origin. The use of Humulin preparations should minimise the incidence of side-effects; thus far such reactions have rarely been reported.

Overdosage: Overdosage causes hypoglycaemia, with accompanying symptoms which may include listlessness, confusion, palpitations, sweating and vomiting.

Treatment: Mild hypoglycaemic episodes will respond to oral administration of glucose or sugar, and rest.

Correction of moderately severe hypoglycaemia can be accomplished by intramuscular or subcutaneous administration of glucagon.

If the patient is comatose, Strong Dextrose Injection BPC should be given intravenously.

Pharmaceutical precautions Humulin preparations should be stored in a refrigerator between 2° and 8°C. They should not be frozen or exposed to excessive heat or sunlight. Under these conditions, potency should be maintained for 2 years from the date of manufacture.

Humulin I, Zn, M1 and M2: The vial should be rotated in palms of hands immediately before use to re-suspend.

Mixing of insulins: The shorter-acting insulin should be drawn into the syringe first, to prevent contamination of the vial by the longer-acting preparation. It is advisable to inject immediately after mixing.

Legal category P.

Package quantities 10 ml glass vials in packs of 5.

Further information Nil.

Product licence numbers

Humulin S	0006/0165
Humulin I	0006/0168
Humulin Zn	0006/0179
Humulin M1	0006/0199
Humulin M2	0006/0200

ILOTYCIN*

Presentation Tablets (special coated, red, coded C03), containing 250 mg Erythromycin BP.

Uses Antibiotic. Erythromycin is indicated in the treatment of conditions associated with the following micro-organisms:

Streptococcus pyogenes (group A beta-haemolytic) – Upper and lower respiratory tract, skin and soft tissue infections of mild to moderate severity.

Alpha-haemolytic streptococci (viridans group) – Short-term prophylaxis against bacterial endocarditis prior to dental or other operative procedures in patients with a history of rheumatic fever or congenital heart disease who are hypersensitive to penicillin.

Str. pneumoniae – Infections of the upper and lower respiratory tract of mild to moderate severity.

Staphylococcus aureus – Acute infections of skin and soft tissue which are mild to moderately severe. Resistance may develop during treatment.

Mycoplasma pneumoniae – Primary atypical pneumonia due to this organism.

Treponema pallidum – Erythromycin is an alternative choice of treatment for syphilis in penicillin-allergic patients.

Corynebacterium diphtheriae – As an adjunct to anti-toxin, to prevent establishment of carriers, and to eradicate the organism in carriers.

C. minutissimum – In the treatment of erythrasma.

Entamoeba histolytica – In the treatment of intestinal amoebiasis only. Extra-enteric amoebiasis requires treatment with other agents.

Listeria monocytogenes – Infections due to this organism.

Bordetella pertussis – When given early after exposure to whooping cough, erythromycin may reduce the risk of development of classical symptoms.

Legionnaires' disease – Although no controlled clinical efficacy studies have been conducted, *in vitro* and limited preliminary clinical data suggest that erythromycin may be effective in treating Legionnaires' disease.

Dosage and administration For oral administration. Optimum blood levels are obtained when doses are given on an empty stomach.

Adults: The usual dosage is 250 mg every six hours. This may be increased up to 4 g per day according to the severity of the infection.

The elderly: As for adults.

Children: Age, weight, and severity of the infection are important factors in determining the correct dosage. The usual regimen is 30–50 mg/kg/day in divided doses. For more severe infections, this dosage may be doubled.

If administration on a twice daily schedule is desirable in either adults or children, one-half of the total daily dose may be given every 12 hours, one hour before meals.

Streptococcal infections: In the treatment of group A beta-haemolytic streptococcal infections, a therapeutic dosage of erythromycin should be administered for at least 10 days.

Prophylaxis: In continuous prophylaxis of streptococcal infections in persons with a history of rheumatic heart disease, the dosage is 250 mg twice daily. When Ilotycin is used prior to surgery to prevent endocarditis caused by alpha-haemolytic streptococci, a recommended schedule for adults is 1 g 1.5–2 hours pre-operatively and 500 mg every six hours for eight doses post-operatively; for children, 20 mg/kg 1.5–2 hours pre-operatively and 10 mg/kg every six hours for eight doses post-operatively.

Syphilis: 30–40 g given in divided doses over a period of 10 to 15 days.

Amoebic dysentery: 250 mg four times daily for 10 to 14 days for adults; 30–50 mg/kg/day in divided doses for 10 to 14 days for children.

Pertussis: Although optimum dosage and duration of treatment have not been established, doses of erythromycin utilised in reported clinical studies were 40–50 mg/kg/day, given in divided doses for 5 to 14 days.

Legionnaires' disease: Although optimum doses have not been established, doses utilised in reported clinical data were 1–4 g erythromycin base daily in divided doses.

Contra-indications, warnings, etc

Contra-indication: Hypersensitivity to erythromycin.

Warnings: Since erythromycin is excreted principally by the liver, caution should be exercised in administering the antibiotic to patients with impaired hepatic function. There have been reports of hepatic dysfunction, with or without jaundice, occurring in patients taking oral erythromycin products.

Usage in pregnancy: Clinical and laboratory studies have shown no evidence of teratogenicity or toxicity. However, caution should be exercised when prescribing for the pregnant patient. Erythromycin is readily excreted in breast milk.

Precautions: Drug Interactions: The use of erythromycin in patients who are receiving concomitant high doses of theophylline may be associated with an increase in serum theophylline levels and potential theophylline toxicity. If symptoms of toxicity develop, the dose of theophylline should be reduced.

During prolonged or repeated therapy, there is a possibility of overgrowth of non-susceptible bacteria or fungi. If such infections arise, the drug should be discontinued and appropriate therapy instituted.

Side-effects: The most frequent side-effects of erythromycin preparations are gastro-intestinal (e.g. abdominal cramping and discomfort) and are dose-related. Nausea, vomiting and diarrhoea occur infrequently with usual oral doses.

Mild allergic reactions, such as urticaria and other skin rashes, have occurred. Serious allergic reactions, including anaphylaxis, have been reported.

Overdosage: Symptoms are mainly confined to nausea, vomiting and diarrhoea.

Treatment: General management may consist of supportive therapy.

Pharmaceutical precautions
Store in a cool place (6°–15°C). Keep containers tightly closed.

Legal category POM.

Package quantities Bottles of 100, 500 and 1,000.

Further information Nil.

Product licence number 0006/5105.

KEFLEX*

Presentation Tablets (pillow shaped, 16 mm long, scored, peach, marked Lilly U49) containing 500 mg Cephalexin BP.

Tablets (9.5 mm diameter, peach, marked Lilly U57) containing 250 mg Cephalexin BP.

Capsules (pale green and dark green, coded H71) containing 500 mg Cephalexin BP.

Capsules (green and white, coded H69) containing 250 mg Cephalexin BP.

Suspension (pink granules) containing 125 mg Cephalexin BP per 5 ml.

Suspension (orange granules) containing 250 mg Cephalexin BP per 5 ml.

Keflex-C

Chewable tablets (pillow shaped, pale yellow, coded Lilly 4091) containing 250 mg Cephalexin BP.

Chewable tablets (pillow shaped, pale yellow, coded Lilly 4090) containing 125 mg Cephalexin BP.

Uses Cephalexin is indicated in the treatment of the following infections due to susceptible micro-organisms: respiratory tract infections; otitis media; skin and soft tissue infections; bone and joint infections; genito-urinary infections, including acute prostatitis; dental infections.

Cephalexin is active against the following organisms *in vitro*: Beta-haemolytic streptococci; staphylococci, including coagulase-positive, coagulase-negative and penicillinase-producing strains; *Streptococcus pneumoniae; Escherichia coli; Proteus mirabilis; Klebsiella species; Haemophilus influenzae; Branhamella catarrhalis.*

Most strains of enterococci (*Streptococcus faecalis*) and a few strains of staphylococci are resistant to cephalexin. It is not active against most strains of *Enterobacter* species, *Morganella morganii* and *Pr. vulgaris.* It has no activity against *Pseudomonas* or *Herellea* species. When tested by *in vitro* methods, staphylococci exhibit cross-resistance between cephalexin and methicillin-type antibiotics.

Dosage and administration Keflex is administered orally. Keflex-C tablets should be chewed thoroughly before swallowing.

Adults: The adult dosage ranges from 1–4 g daily in divided doses; most infections will respond to a dosage of 500 mg every 8 hours. For skin and soft tissue infections, streptococcal pharyngitis and mild, uncomplicated urinary tract infections, the usual dosage is 250 mg every 6 hours, or 500 mg every 12 hours. For more severe infections or those caused by less susceptible organisms, larger doses may be needed. If daily doses of Keflex greater than 4 g are required, parenteral cephalosporins, in appropriate doses, should be considered.

The elderly: As for adults. Reduce dosage if renal function is markedly impaired.

Children: The usual recommended daily dosage for children is 25–50 mg/kg (10–20 mg/lb) in divided doses.

For skin and soft tissue infections, streptococcal pharyngitis and mild, uncomplicated urinary tract infections, the total daily dose may be divided and administered every 12 hours. For most infections the following schedule is suggested:

Children under 5 years: 125 mg every 8 hours.

Children 5 years and over: 250 mg every 8 hours.

In severe infections, the dosage may be doubled. In the therapy of otitis media, clinical studies have shown that a dosage of 75–100 mg/kg/day in 4 divided doses is required.

In the treatment of beta-haemolytic streptococcal infections, a therapeutic dose should be administered for at least 10 days.

Contra-indications, warnings, etc

Contra-indication: Cephalexin is contra-indicated in patients with known allergy to the cephalosporin group of antibiotics.

Warnings: Cephalexin should be given cautiously to patients who have shown hypersensitivity to other drugs. Cephalosporins should be given with caution to penicillin-sensitive patients, as there is some evidence of partial cross-allergenicity between the penicillins and the cephalosporins. Patients have had severe reactions (including anaphylaxis) to both drugs.

Usage in pregnancy: Although laboratory and clinical studies have shown no evidence of teratogenicity, caution should be exercised when prescribing for the pregnant patient.

Precautions: If an allergic reaction to cephalexin occurs the drug should be discontinued and the patient treated with the appropriate agents. Prolonged use of cephalexin may result in the overgrowth of non-susceptible organisms.

Cephalexin should be administered with caution in the presence of markedly impaired renal function. Careful clinical and laboratory studies should be made because safe dosage may be lower than that usually recommended.

A false positive reaction for glucose in the urine may occur with Benedict's or Fehling's solutions or with copper sulphate test tablets, but not with Tes-Tape* (urine sugar analysis paper, Lilly).

Side-effects: Gastro-intestinal – Nausea, vomiting, dyspepsia, and abdominal pain have occurred. Diarrhoea has been reported infrequently. It is rarely severe enough to warrant cessation of therapy. Colitis, including rare instances of pseudomembranous colitis, has been reported.

Hypersensitivity – Allergies (in the form of rash, urticaria and angio-oedema) have been observed. These reactions usually subside upon discontinuation of the drug. Anaphylaxis has also been reported.

Haematological – Eosinophilia, neutropenia and positive Coombs' tests have been reported.

Hepatic – Slight elevations of AST and ALT have been observed.

Miscellaneous – Other reactions have included genital and anal pruritus, genital moniliasis, vaginitis and vaginal discharge, dizziness, fatigue and headache.

Treatment of overdosage – Serum levels can be considerably reduced by haemodialysis or peritoneal dialysis.

Pharmaceutical precautions

Capsules and tablets: Keep containers tightly closed.

Suspensions: After mixing, Keflex suspensions should be stored in a cool place (6°–15°C) or in a refrigerator (0°–6°C) and be used within 10 days. Where dilution is unavoidable, Syrup BP should be used after the suspension has been prepared according to the manufacturer's instructions.

Chewable tablets: Store below 25°C. Protect from light.

Legal category POM.

Package quantities
Tablets 500 mg: Bottles of 20, 100 and 500.
Tablets 250 mg: Bottles of 20, 100 and 500.
Capsules 500 mg: Bottles of 20, 100 and 500.
Capsules 250 mg: Bottles of 20, 100 and 500.
Suspension 125 mg/5 ml: Bottles of 100 ml.
Suspension 250 mg/5 ml: Bottles of 100 ml.
Chewable tablets 250 mg: Foil-wrapped packs of 15.
Chewable tablets 125 mg: Foil-wrapped packs of 15.

Further information Nil.

Product licence numbers

Tablets 500 mg	0006/5096
Tablets 250 mg	0006/0073
Capsules 500 mg	0006/0076
Capsules 250 mg	0006/5103
Suspension 125 mg/5 ml	0006/5097
Suspension 250 mg/5 ml	0006/5098
Chewable tablets 250 mg	0006/0204
Chewable tablets 125 mg	0006/0203

KEFLIN*

Presentation Vials containing the equivalent of 1 g cephalothin as the sodium salt.

Uses Keflin is indicated in the treatment of serious infections of the respiratory tract, genito-urinary tract, soft tissue and skin, gastro-intestinal tract, bones and joints, blood stream and cardiovascular system when due to susceptible organisms. It has also been effective in cases of peritonitis and septic abortion.

Cases of staphylococcal and pneumococcal meningitis have also responded to treatment. However, as only low levels of cephalothin are found in the cerebrospinal fluid, the drug is not reliable for the treatment of this condition and should only be considered when other more reliably effective antibiotics cannot be used.

Prophylactic Use: Perioperative administration has been beneficial in reducing the incidence of postoperative infection in patients undergoing contaminated or potentially contaminated surgical procedures associated with a high risk of infection, in surgical patients with reduced host resistance to bacterial infection, or when the occurrence of a postoperative infection could be especially serious. The best results are observed if cephalothin is administered immediately prior to the operative procedure, thus providing adequate antibiotic concentration in the tissues before bacterial contamination occurs.

Cephalothin is usually active against the following organisms *in vitro:* Staphylococci, including coagulase-positive, coagulase-negative and penicillinase-producing strains; Clostridia, *Streptococcus pneumoniae*, *Haemophilus influenzae,*
Escherichia coli and other coliform bacteria,
Klebsiella species,
Proteus mirabilis,
Salmonella species,
Shigella species.

Beta-haemolytic and other streptococci (many strains of enterococci e.g. *Streptococcus faecalis,* are relatively resistant).

Pseudomonas species are resistant to cephalothin, as are most indole-positive *Proteus* and motile *Enterobacter* species.

Dosage and administration

Adults and the elderly: The usual dosage range in severe or life-threatening infections is 6–12 g per day. In milder infections a dose of 1 g every four to six hours may be indicated. Limit the dose to a maximum of 6 g daily in patients with oliguria or blood urea elevation above 17.8 mmol/l (107 mg/100 ml).

Infants and children: The dosage should be proportionately less in accordance with age, weight and severity of infection. Daily administration of 100 mg/kg (80–160 mg/kg) in divided doses has been found effective for most infections.

Antibiotic therapy for beta-haemolytic streptococcal infections should continue for at least 10 days.

Prophylactic use: The following dosages are recommended for perioperative use:

1 g prior to surgical incision, followed by
1 g during surgery and
1 g every 6 hours for 24 hours postoperatively.

Postoperative administration of cephalothin should be discontinued after twenty-four hours unless signs of infection are present, in which case cultures should be performed and appropriate therapy instituted. Longer courses of preventive antibiotic therapy may be considered necessary when surgical procedures involve implantation of prosthetic devices.

Dosage and renal impairment: In patients with moderately severe oliguria or a blood urea above 17.8 mmol/l (107 mg/100 ml), a maximum dose of 6 g per day is generally adequate. In cases of anuria, after an intravenous loading dose (up to 6 g over the first 24 hours), total daily amounts of 1–3 g may be given in divided doses every 12–24 hours (or every 8–12 hours if dialysis is performed).

Cephalothin is best given intravenously.

For direct intravenous administration: A solution containing 1 g cephalothin in 5 ml of diluent may be slowly injected directly into the vein over a period of three to five minutes, or may be given through the tubing when the patient is receiving parenteral solutions. The cephalothin solution may be further diluted to a larger volume if desired to facilitate measurement of the rate of injection.

Cephalothin may be administered in one of the following intravenous fluids:

Water for Injections PhEur
Sodium Chloride Intravenous Infusion BP
Dextrose Intravenous Infusion BP
Sodium Lactate Intravenous Infusion BP
Compound Sodium Lactate Intravenous Infusion BP
Sodium Chloride and Dextrose Intravenous Infusion BP.

Intra-peritoneal administration: In peritoneal dialysis procedures, cephalothin has been added to dialysis fluid in concentrations up to 6 mg/100 ml and instilled into the peritoneal space throughout an entire dialysis (16–30 hours). Careful assay procedures have shown that 44% of the administered drug was absorbed into the blood stream. Serum levels of 10 mg/l were reported, with no evidence of accumulation and no untoward or systemic reaction.

Contra-indications, warnings, etc

Contra-indication: Hypersensitivity to cephalosporin antibiotics.

Warnings: Before cephalothin therapy is instituted careful enquiry should be made concerning previous hypersensitivity reactions to cephalosporins and penicillin. Cephalosporin C derivatives should be given cautiously to penicillin-sensitive patients.

There is some clinical and laboratory evidence of partial cross-allergenicity of the penicillins and the cephalosporins. Patients have been reported to have had severe reactions (including anaphylaxis) to both drugs.

Antibiotics should be administered with caution to any patient who has demonstrated some form of allergy, particularly to drugs.

Usage in pregnancy: Although clinical and laboratory studies have shown no evidence of teratogenicity, caution should be exercised when prescribing for the pregnant patient.

Precautions: If an allergic reaction to cephalothin occurs the drug should be discontinued.

Prolonged use of cephalothin may result in the overgrowth of non-susceptible organisms.

A false-positive reaction for glucose in the urine may occur with Benedict's or Fehling's solutions or with copper sulphate test tablets, but not with Tes-Tape* (urine sugar analysis paper, Lilly).

Side-effects: Hypersensitivity – Maculopapular rash, urticaria, reactions resembling serum sickness and anaphylaxis have been reported. Eosinophilia and drug fever have been observed to be associated with other allergic reactions. These reactions are most likely to occur in patients with a history of allergy, particularly to penicillin.

Haematological – Neutropenia, leucopenia, granulocytopenia, thrombocytopenia and haemolytic anaemia have been reported. Some individuals, particularly those with uraemia, have developed positive direct Coombs' tests during cephalothin therapy.

Hepatic – Transient rise in AST and alkaline phosphatase has been noted. Toxic intrahepatic cholestasis has been reported.

Renal – Rises in blood urea and decreased creatinine clearances have been reported, particularly in patients with prior renal impairment. Proteinuria has been observed.

Injection site reactions – Pain, induration, tenderness and elevation of temperature have been reported following repeated intramuscular injections. Thrombophlebitis has occurred, and is usually associated with daily doses of over 6 g given by infusion for more than three days.

Overdosage: In the event of serious overdosage, general supportive care is recommended, with monitoring of haematological, renal and hepatic functions, and coagulation status, until the patient is stable.

Pharmaceutical precautions *Unreconstituted vials:* Store in a cool place (6°–15°C). *After reconstitution:* When stored under refrigeration (0°–6°C), the solution has a satisfactory potency for 48 hours. Solutions may precipitate; they can be re-dissolved by being warmed.

The concentrated solution will darken, especially at room temperature.

Legal category POM.

Package quantities 1 g vials: single vials in packs of 10.

Further information Nil.

Product licence number 0006/5099.

KEFZOL*

Presentation Kefzol is supplied in rubber-stoppered vials containing the equivalent of 500 mg and 1 g cephazolin as the sodium salt. The sodium content is 48.3 mg per g of cephazolin sodium.

Uses Kefzol is indicated in the treatment of the following infections due to susceptible micro-organisms:

Respiratory tract infections
Genito-urinary tract infections
Skin and soft tissue infections
Bone and joint infections
Septicaemia
Endocarditis

Kefzol may also be used as antibiotic cover during surgery on the biliary tract and for the treatment of biliary tract infections.

Cephazolin is active against the following organisms *in vitro: Staphylococcus aureus* (penicillin-sensitive and penicillin-resistant) Group A beta-haemolytic streptococci and other strains of streptococci (many strains of enterococci are resistant) – *Streptococcus pneumoniae, Escherichia coli, Klebsiella* species, *Proteus mirabilis, Haemophilus influenzae, Enterobacter aerogenes.*

Most strains of *Enterobacter cloacae, Morganella morganii* and indole-positive *Proteus (Pr. vulgaris, Pr. rettgeri)* are resistant. Methicillin-resistant staphylococci, *Serratia, Pseudomonas, Mima* and *Herellea* species are almost uniformly resistant to cephazolin.

Dosage and administration After reconstitution, Kefzol may be administered intramuscularly or intravenously.

Intramuscular administration: Reconstitute with Water for Injections PhEur, or 0.9% Sodium Chloride Intravenous Infusion BP according to Table 1. Shake well until dissolved. Kefzol should be injected into a large muscle mass.

Table 1. Dilution table

Vial size	Diluent to be added	Approximate available volume	Approximate average concentration
500 mg	4.0 ml	4.1 ml	125 mg/ml
500 mg	2.0 ml	2.2 ml	225 mg/ml
1 g†	2.5 ml	3.0 ml	330 mg/ml

†The 1 g vial should be reconstituted only with Water for Injections PhEur.

Intravenous administration: Kefzol may be administered by intravenous injection or by continuous or intermittent infusion. Total daily dosages are the same as for intramuscular injection.

Intermittent intravenous infusion: Kefzol may be administered along with primary intravenous fluid management programmes in a volume control set or in a separate secondary i.v. bottle. Reconstituted 500 mg or 1 g of Kefzol may be diluted in 50 to 100 ml Water for Injections PhEur or one of the following intravenous solutions:

0.9% Sodium Chloride Intravenous Infusion BP.
5% or 10% Dextrose Intravenous Infusion BP.
5% Dextrose in Compound Sodium Lactate Intravenous Infusion BP.
0.9% Sodium Chloride and 5% Dextrose Intravenous Infusion BP.

Table 2. Usual adult dosage

Type of infection	Dose	Frequency
Pneumococcal pneumonia	500 mg	q 12 h
Mild infections caused by susceptible Gram-positive cocci	500 mg	q 8 h
Acute uncomplicated urinary tract infections	500 mg to 1 g	q 12 h
Moderate to severe infections	500 mg to 1 g	q 6 to 8 h

Table 3. Maintenance dosage of Kefzol in adults with reduced renal function

Renal function	Blood urea†		Creatinine clearance ml/min	Serum Creatinine†		Dosage		Serum half-life (hours)
	mg/100 ml	mmol/l		mg/100 ml	mcmol/l	Mild to moderate infection	Moderate to severe infection	
Mild impairment	42–74	7.0–12.3	70–40	1.3–2.0	114.9–176.8	250–500 mg q 12 h	500 mg–1.25 g q 12 h	3–5
Moderate impairment	75–105	12.5–17.5	40–20	2.1–3.5	185.6–309.4	125–250 mg q 12 h	250–600 mg q 12 h	6–12
Severe impairment	106–160	17.7–26 7	20–5	3.6–7.0	318.2–618.8	75–150 mg q 24 h	150–400 mg q 24 h	15–30
Essentially no function	> 160	> 26.7	< 5	> 7.0	> 618.8	37.5–75 mg q 24 h	75–200 mg q 24 h	30–40

† If used to estimate degree of renal impairment, elevated blood urea and serum creatinine concentrations should reflect a steady state of renal azotaemia.

0.45% Sodium Chloride and 5% Dextrose Intravenous Infusion BP.
Compound Sodium Lactate Intravenous Infusion BP.
5% or 10% Invert Sugar in Water for Injections PhEur.

Direct intravenous injection: Dilute 500 mg or 1 g of reconstituted Kefzol in a minimum of 10 ml of Water for Injections PhEur and inject solution slowly over a period of three to five minutes. The injection may be made directly into a vein or, for patients receiving the above parenteral fluids, through the tubing.

Dosage: The usual adult dosages are given in Table 2.

In adults with renal impairment, cephazolin is not readily excreted. After a loading dose of 500 mg, the following recommendations for maintenance dosage (Table 3) may be used as a guide.

Cephazolin is not readily removed by haemodialysis or peritoneal dialysis.

The elderly: As for adults.

Paediatric dosage: In children, a total daily dosage of 25 to 50 mg/kg of body weight, divided into three or four equal doses, is effective for most mild to moderately severe infections (Table 4). Total daily dosage may be increased to 100 mg/kg of body weight for severe infections.

In children with mild to moderate renal impairment (creatinine clearance of 70–40 ml/min), 60% of the normal daily dose given in divided doses q 12 h should be sufficient. In children with moderate impairment (creatinine clearance of 40–20 ml/min), 25% of the normal daily dose in divided doses q 12 h should be adequate. In children with marked impairment (creatinine clearance of 20–5 ml/min), 10% of the normal daily dose given q 24 h should be sufficient. All dosage recommendations apply after an initial loading dose.

Table 4. Paediatric dosage guide

Weight kg	25 mg/kg/day divided into 3 doses		25 mg/kg/day divided into 4 doses	
	Approximate single dose (q 8h)	Vol. needed with dilution of 125 mg/ml	Approximate single dose (q 6 h)	Vol. needed with dilution of 125 mg/ml
4.5	40 mg	0.35 ml	30 mg	0.25 ml
9.0	75 mg	0.6 ml	55 mg	0.45 ml
13.5	115 mg	0.9 ml	85 mg	0.7 ml
18.0	150 mg	1.2 ml	115 mg	0.9 ml
22.5	190 mg	1.5 ml	140 mg	1.1 ml

Weight kg	50 mg/kg/day divided into 3 doses		50 mg/kg/day divided into 4 doses	
	Approximate single dose (q 8 h)	Vol. needed with dilution of 225 mg/ml	Approximate single dose (q 6 h)	Vol. needed with dilution of 225 mg/ml
4.5	75 mg	0.35 ml	55 mg	0.25 ml
9.0	150 mg	0.7 ml	110 mg	0.5 ml
13.5	225 mg	1.0 ml	170 mg	0.75 ml
18.0	300 mg	1.35 ml	225 mg	1.0 ml
22.5	375 mg	1.7 ml	285 mg	1.25 ml

Contra-indications, warnings, etc

Contra-indication: Cephazolin is contra-indicated in patients with known allergy to the cephalosporin group of antibiotics.

Warnings: Before instituting therapy with cephazolin, every attempt should be made to determine if the patient has had previous hypersensitivity reactions to the cephalosporins, penicillins, or other drugs, in which case this product should be given cautiously.

There is some evidence of partial cross-allergenicity between the penicillins and the cephalosporins. Patients have been reported to have had severe reactions (including anaphylaxis) to both drugs.

The results of experimental studies in animals given cephalosporins suggest that the concurrent use of potent diuretics, such as frusemide or ethacrynic acid, may increase the risk of renal toxicity.

Usage in pregnancy: Although clinical and laboratory studies have shown no evidence of teratogenicity, caution should be exercised when prescribing for the pregnant patient.

Usage in neonates: The safety of this product for use in prematures and infants under one month of age has not been established.

Precautions: If an allergic reaction to cephazolin occurs, the drug should be discontinued and the patient treated with the usual agents (e.g. adrenaline or other pressor amines, antihistamines, or corticosteroids).

Prolonged use of cephazolin may result in the overgrowth of non-susceptible organisms. Careful observation of the patient is essential. If superinfection occurs during therapy, appropriate measures should be taken.

When cephazolin is administered to patients with impaired renal function, the daily dose should be reduced to avoid toxicity (see 'Dosage and administration').

A false positive reaction for glucose in the urine may occur with Benedict's or Fehling's solutions or with copper sulphate test tablets, but not with Tes-Tape* (urine sugar analysis paper, Lilly).

Side-effects: The following side-effects have been reported:

Gastro-intestinal – Nausea, anorexia, vomiting, and diarrhoea.

Hypersensitivity – Drug fever, rash.

Haematological – Neutropenia, leucopenia, eosinophilia, thrombocythaemia and positive direct and indirect Coombs' tests.

Neurological – Convulsions have occasionally been reported, especially after administration of high doses to patients with marked renal impairment.

Transient rise in AST, ALT, ALP and blood urea levels without clinical evidence of hepatic or renal impairment.

Up to 6% of patients have complained of pain, some with induration, following intramuscular injection. Rarely, phlebitis has been encountered upon intravenous injection.

Other side-effects have included genital and anal pruritus, genital and oral moniliasis, and vaginitis.

Overdosage: In the event of serious overdosage, general supportive care is recommended, with monitoring of haematological, renal and hepatic functions, and coagulation status, until the patient is stable.

Pharmaceutical precautions Extemporaneous mixtures with other antibiotics (including aminoglycosides) are not recommended.

Unreconstituted vials: Protect from light.

Stability: Reconstituted Kefzol and dilutions of Kefzol in the recommended intravenous fluids are stable for 24 hours at room temperature (15–25°C) and for 96 hours if stored under refrigeration (0–6°C).

Legal category POM.

Package quantities
500 mg vials (No. 767): Single vials in packs of 10.
1 g vials (No. 768): Single vials in packs of 10.

Further information Nil.

Product licence number 0006/0078.

MOXALACTAM* ▼
Approved name Latamoxef disodium.

Presentation 10 ml vials containing 500 mg or 1 g Moxalactam.
20 ml vials containing 2 g Moxalactam.

The vials also contain 150 mg mannitol per g of Moxalactam activity. The total sodium content is approximately 88 mg per g of Moxalactam activity.

Uses Moxalactam is indicated in the treatment of the following infections when due to susceptible microorganisms:

Lower respiratory tract infections, including pneumonia.

Urinary tract infections.

Intra-abdominal infections such as peritonitis and biliary tract infections.

Gynaecological infections, including endometritis, pelvic cellulitis, and pelvic inflammatory disease.

Septicaemia.

Skin and soft tissue infections.

Bone and joint infections.

Meningitis (except neonatal meningitis due to Group B streptococci).

Moxalactam is usually active against the following organisms *in vitro*:

Beta-haemolytic and other streptococci (strains of enterococci, e.g., *Streptococcus faecalis*, are resistant). Staphylococci, including penicillin-sensitive and penicillin-resistant strains (susceptibility of *Staphylococcus epidermidis* is variable and methicillin-resistant staphylococci are resistant). *Streptococcus pneumoniae. Haemophilus influenzae* (including ampicillin-resistant strains). *Escherichia coli. Klebsiella* species. *Proteus mirabilis. Proteus* species (indole-positive, including *Pr. rettgeri* and *Pr. vulgaris*) *Morganella morganii. Enterobacter* species. *Salmonella* species, including *S. typhi. Providencia* species. *Shigella* species. *Serratia* species. *Acinetobacter* species (many strains are relatively resistant). *Pseudomonas aeruginosa* (some strains are resistant). *Neisseria gonorrhoeae. N. meningitidis.* Anaerobic bacteria, including *Peptococcus, Peptostreptococcus* and *Veillonella* species. *Clostridium* species. *Bacteroides* species, including *B. fragilis. Fusobacterium* species. Moxalactam is resistant to degradation by beta-lactamases from most members of the *Enterobacteriaceae* (including *Enterobacter cloacae, Ent. aerogenes, M. morganii, Pr. rettgeri, Pr. vulgaris* and *Serratia marcescens*), *Ps. aeruginosa* and *B. fragilis.*

Dosage and administration Moxalactam may be given intravenously or by deep intramuscular injection.

Adults: The usual dose is 500 mg to 4 g per day, depending on the severity and site of the infection and the susceptibility of the causative organism.

Moxalactam may be administered as a twice daily regimen, but in life-threatening infections or infections

due to less susceptible organisms, doses of up to 4 g every eight hours (i.e. a maximum of 12 g per day) may be required (but see *Warnings*).

Impaired renal function: When renal function is impaired, a reduced dose must be employed. After an initial dose of 1 to 2 g (depending on the severity of the infection), a maintenance dosage schedule should be followed. Continued dosage should be determined by degree of renal impairment, severity of infection, and susceptibility of the causative organism.

Maintenance dosage guide for patients with renal impairment:

Creatinine clearance ml/min/1.73 m²	Renal function	Usual dosage	Maximum dosage
>80	Normal	0.25–2 g q 8–12 h	4 g q 8 h
50–80	Mild impairment	0.25–1 g q 8 h	3 g q 8 h
25–50	Moderate impairment	0.25–1 g q 12 h	2 g q 8 h OR 3 g q 12 h
2–25	Severe impairment	0.25–0.5 g q 8 h	1 g q 8 h OR 1.25 g q 12 h
<2	Nil	0.25–0.5 g q 12 h	1 g q 24 h

Maintenance doses of Moxalactam should be repeated following regular haemodialysis. The serum half-life during dialysis has ranged from 2 to 5 hours.

If combination therapy with Moxalactam and an aminoglycoside is indicated, the recommended doses of both antibiotics should be administered at separate sites. Do not mix the two antibiotics in the same intravenous fluid container. Under these conditions renal function should be carefully monitored.

Intramuscular administration: Moxalactam should be reconstituted with Water for Injections PhEur, 0.9% Sodium Chloride Intravenous Infusion BP or 0.5% Lignocaine Hydrochloride Injection BP. Shake well until dissolved.

Intravenous administration: The intravenous route may be preferable for patients with septicaemia, meningitis, peritonitis or other severe or life-threatening infections.

1. *For direct intermittent intravenous administration,* add 10 ml of Water for Injections PhEur, 5% Dextrose Intravenous Infusion BP or 0.9% Sodium Chloride Intravenous Infusion BP per g of Moxalactam. Slowly inject directly into the vein over a period of three to five minutes or give through the tubing of an administration set while the patient is also receiving one of the following intravenous fluids:

0.9% Sodium Chloride Intravenous Infusion BP.

5% Dextrose Intravenous Infusion BP.

0.9% Sodium Chloride and 5% Dextrose Intravenous Infusion BP.

0.45% Sodium Chloride and 5% Dextrose Intravenous Infusion BP.

0.15% Potassium Chloride and 5% Dextrose Intravenous Infusion BP.

Sodium Lactate Intravenous Infusion BP.

Compound Sodium Lactate Intravenous Infusion BP.

2. *Intermittent intravenous infusion with a volume control set* can also be accomplished while any of the above-mentioned intravenous fluids are being infused. However, during infusion of the solution containing Moxalactam, it is desirable to discontinue the other

solution. When this technique is employed, careful attention should be paid to the volume of the solution containing Moxalactam so that the calculated dose will be infused. If Water for Injections PhEur is used as the diluent, reconstitute with approximately 20 ml per g to avoid a hypotonic solution.

The elderly: As for adults.

Paediatrics: The following dosage schedule is recommended:

Neonates

0–1 week of age	25 mg/kg q 12 h
1–4 weeks of age	25 mg/kg q 8 h
Infants and children	50 mg/kg q 12 h

For more serious infections the dosage may be doubled. For children, the maximum daily dose should not exceed the maximum adult dose.

Contra-indications, warnings, etc

Contra-indications: Moxalactam is contra-indicated in patients with known allergy to the drug, and those receiving concomitant therapy with high-dose heparin or oral anticoagulants.

Warnings: Moxalactam should be given cautiously to patients sensitive to beta-lactam antibiotics. Antibiotics should be administered with caution to any patient who has demonstrated some form of allergy, particularly to drugs, and corticosteroids should be available for immediate administration, if necessary, after the first dose. Serious acute hypersensitivity reactions may require adrenaline and other emergency measures.

Coagulopathy: Moxalactam can interfere with haemostasis through three different mechanisms: hypoprothrombinaemia, inhibition of platelet function and, very rarely, immune-mediated thrombocytopenia.

Hypoprothrombinaemia, with or without bleeding, has been reported, but can be prevented by the administration of vitamin K. It is recommended that all patients be given prophylactic vitamin K, 10 mg per week.

Inhibition of platelet function is dose-dependent and can usually be avoided by limiting the dose to 4 g per day. It is recommended that bleeding time should be monitored in patients receiving more than 4 g per day for more than three days, and in all patients with significantly impaired renal function.

If the bleeding time becomes unduly prolonged, Moxalactam should be discontinued.

If bleeding occurs and if the prothrombin time is prolonged, vitamin K should be given.

Administration of fresh, frozen plasma, packed red cells and platelet concentrates may also be indicated. Moxalactam should be discontinued if bleeding is due to platelet dysfunction.

Concurrent administration of aspirin or other non-steroidal anti-inflammatory drugs which can affect haemostasis may increase the risk of bleeding.

Usage in pregnancy: The safety of this product for use during pregnancy or for the nursing mother has not been established.

Precautions: Renal function should be carefully monitored in patients with renal impairment, particularly if they are receiving concomitant therapy with other potentially nephrotoxic drugs such as aminoglycosides.

In normal volunteers and a few patients receiving Moxalactam, nausea, vomiting and vasomotor instability with hypotension and peripheral vasodilatation occurred following the ingestion of alcohol. This syndrome has been reported only when alcohol ingestion followed the administration of Moxalactam, and has been observed as late as 48 hours after the last dose of the drug.

Prolonged use of Moxalactam may result in the overgrowth of non-susceptible organisms. Careful observation of the patient is essential. If superinfection occurs during therapy, appropriate measures should be taken.

Side-effects: Hypersensitivity: Morbilliform eruptions, positive Coombs' tests, and drug fever and anaphylaxis have been reported.

Haematological: Eosinophilia, reversible leucopenia and neutropenia, thrombocytopenia, increased bleeding time, and disturbances in vitamin K-dependent clotting function (decreased prothrombin) have occurred.

Gastro-intestinal: The most common symptom has been diarrhoea. Pseudomembranous colitis, with varying degrees of severity, may appear either during or after therapy. Nausea and vomiting have been reported rarely.

Hepatic: Transient rise in AST, ALT, and ALP levels have been noted.

Renal: Elevated blood urea, serum creatinine, pyuria and haematuria, all of unknown aetiology, have been reported rarely.

Miscellaneous: Pain or phlebitis at the site of injection occurs infrequently.

Pharmaceutical precautions *Unreconstituted vials:* Store at room temperature (15°–25° C).

Stability: It is good practice to reconstitute immediately prior to use. If this is not feasible, Moxalactam is stable for 96 hours after reconstitution if stored in a refrigerator (0–6° C) or for 12 hours at room temperature (15–25° C). The pH of freshly reconstituted solutions usually ranges from 5.5 to 6.5.

Legal category POM.

Package quantities 500 mg vials: Single vials in packs of 10.
1 g vials: Single vials in packs of 10.
2 g vials: Single vials in packs of 10.

Further information Moxalactam is the first of a new class of beta-lactam antibiotics, designated as an oxa-beta-lactam. It has been synthesised by substituting the sulphur atom in the cephem nucleus with an oxygen atom. The beta-lactam nucleus, common to the penicillins and cephalosporins, remains unaltered.

Product licence number 0006/0152.

NEBCIN*

Presentation Nebcin is presented in vials in the following strengths: 1 ml vials containing tobramycin sulphate equivalent to 40 mg tobramycin base.

2 ml vials containing tobramycin sulphate equivalent to 80 mg tobramycin base.

2 ml vials containing tobramycin sulphate equivalent to 20 mg tobramycin base.

Also containing 0.5% w/v Phenol BP with sodium bisulphite and Disodium Edetate BP.

Uses Nebcin is indicated for the treatment of the following infections caused by susceptible micro-organisms:

central nervous system infections, including meningitis septicaemia and neonatal sepsis

gastro-intestinal infections, including peritonitis and other significant infections such as:
complicated and recurrent urinary tract infections, including pyelonephritis and cystitis
lower respiratory tract infections, including pneumonia, bronchopneumonia and acute bronchitis
skin, bone and soft tissue infections, including burns.

Nebcin may be considered in serious staphylococcal infections for which penicillin or other less potentially toxic drugs are contra-indicated and when bacterial susceptibility testing and clinical judgement indicate its use.

Tobramycin is usually active against most strains of the following organisms:

Pseudomonas aeruginosa
Proteus species (indole-positive and indole-negative), including *Pr. mirabilis, Pr. rettgeri* and *Pr. vulgaris; Morganella morganii, Escherichia coli, Klebsiella-Enterobacter-Serratia* species, *Citrobacter* species, *Providencia* species, Staphylococci including *Staphylococcus aureus* (coagulase-positive and coagulase-negative).

Some strains of group D streptococci are susceptible *in vivo* although most strains of enterococci demonstrate resistance.

The combination of tobramycin and carbenicillin is synergistic *in vitro* against most strains of *Ps. aeruginosa*. Other Gram-negative organisms may be affected synergistically by the combination of tobramycin and a cephalosporin.

Dosage and administration Nebcin may be given intramuscularly or intravenously. The patient's pretreatment body weight should be obtained for calculation of correct dosage.

The intramuscular dose is the same as the intravenous dose.

Patients with normal renal function:

Adults: The usual recommended dosage for adults with serious infections is 3 mg/kg/day, administered in three equal doses every eight hours (see Table 1). For life-threatening infections, dosages up to 5 mg/kg/day may be administered in three or four equal doses. The dosage should be reduced to 3 mg/kg/day as soon as clinically indicated. To prevent increased toxicity due to excessive blood levels, dosage should not exceed 5 mg/kg/day unless serum levels are monitored.

Table 1.   Dosage schedule guide for adults with normal renal function
(Dosage at 8–hour intervals)

Patient weight kg	Usual dose for serious infections 1 mg/kg q 8 h (Total 3 mg/kg/day)		Maximum dose for life-threatening infections (Reduce as soon as possible) 1.66 mg/kg q 8 h (Total 5 mg/kg/day unless monitored)	
	mg/dose	ml/dose†	mg/dose	ml/dose†
120	120	3.0	200	5.0
100	100	2.5	166	4.0
80	80	2.0	133	3.0
60	60	1.5	100	2.5
40	40	1.0	66	1.6

† Applicable to 40 mg/ml product forms.

Mild to moderate infections of the urinary tract have responded to a dosage of 2–3 mg/kg/day administered as a single intramuscular injection.

The elderly: As for adults, but see recommendations for patients with impaired renal function.

Children: The recommended dosage is 6–7.5 mg/kg/day, administered in three or four equally divided doses. In some patients it may be necessary to administer higher doses.

Premature or full-term neonates (one week of age or less): Dosages of up to 4 mg/kg/day may be administered in two equal doses every 12 hours.

The usual duration of treatment is 7 to 10 days. A longer course of therapy may be necessary in difficult and complicated infections. In such cases, monitoring of renal, auditory and vestibular functions is advised, because neurotoxicity is more likely to occur when treatment is extended for longer than 10 days.

It is recommended that blood levels should be determined whenever possible to ensure the correct dosage is given. Blood levels should always be determined in patients with chronic infections such as cystic fibrosis, or where longer duration of treatment may be necessary, or in patients with decreased renal function.

Patients with impaired renal function: Following a loading dose of 1 mg/kg, subsequent dosage in these patients must be adjusted, either with lower doses administered at eight-hour intervals or with normal doses at prolonged intervals (see Table 2). Both of these regimens are suggested as guides to be used when serum levels of tobramycin cannot be measured directly. They are based on either the creatinine clearance or the serum creatinine of the patient, because these values correlate with the half-life of tobramycin. Neither regimen should be used when dialysis is being performed.

Reduced dosage at eight-hour intervals (Regimen I): An appropriately reduced dosage range can be found in the accompanying table for any patient for whom the blood urea, creatinine clearance or serum creatinine values are known. The choice of dose within the indicated range should be based on the severity of the infection, the sensitivity of the pathogen, and individual patient considerations, especially renal function. An alternative rough guide for determining reduced dosage at eight-hour intervals (for patients whose steady-state serum creatinine values are known) is to divide the normally recommended dose by the patient's serum creatinine value (mg/100 ml).

Normal dosage at prolonged intervals (Regimen II): Recommended intervals between doses are given in the accompanying table. As a general rule, the dosage frequency in hours can be determined by multiplying the patient's serum creatinine level (mg/100 ml) by six.

The dosage schedules derived from either method should be used in conjunction with careful clinical and laboratory observations of the patient and should be modified as necessary.

Intramuscular administration: Nebcin may be administered by withdrawing the appropriate dose directly from the vial.

Intravenous administration: Nebcin may be given by intravenous infusion or by direct intravenous injection. When given by infusion, the usual volume of diluent (0.9% Sodium Chloride Intravenous Infusion BP or 5% Dextrose Intravenous Infusion BP) for adult doses is 50–100 ml. For children, the volume of diluent should be

Table 2. Two maintenance regimens based on renal function and body weight following an initial dose of 1 mg/kg†

Renal function‡					Regimen I	or	Regimen II
					Adjusted doses at 8-hour intervals		Normal dosage at prolonged intervals
Blood urea		Serum creatinine		Creatinine clearance	Weight		Weight/Dose 50–60 kg:60 mg 60–80 kg:80 mg
mg/100 ml	mmol/l	mg/100 ml	mcmol/l	ml/min	50–60 kg	60–80 kg	
Normal:							
≤42	≤7.0	≤1.3	≤114.9	≥70	60 mg	80 mg	q 8 h
42–74	7.0–12.3	1.4–1.9	123.8–168	69–40	30–60 mg	50–80 mg	q 12 h
75–105	12.5–17.5	2.0–3.3	176.8–291.7	39–20	20–25 mg	30–45 mg	q 18 h
106–140	17.7–23.3	3.4–5.3	300.6–468.5	19–10	10–18 mg	15–24 mg	q 24 h
141–160	23.5–26.7	5.4–7.5	477.4–663	9–5	5–9 mg	7–12 mg	q 36 h
>160	>26.7	≥7.6	≥671.8	≤4	2.5–4.5 mg	3.5–6 mg	q 48 h§

†For life-threatening infections, dosages 50% above those normally recommended may be used. The dosages should be reduced as soon as possible when improvement is noted.

‡If used to estimate degree of renal impairment, blood urea and serum creatinine concentrations should reflect a steady state of renal azotaemia.

§When dialysis is not being performed.

proportionately less than for adults. The diluted solution should be infused over a period of 20–60 minutes. Nebcin may be administered by direct intravenous injection or into the tubing of a drip set. When given in this way, serum levels may exceed 12 mg/l for a short time (see Contra-indications, warnings, etc.).

Contra-indications, warnings, etc

Contra-indications: Hypersensitivity to tobramycin sulphate. Intrathecal administration.

Warnings: Patients treated with Nebcin should be under close observation because tobramycin and other aminoglycoside antibiotics have an inherent potential for causing nephrotoxicity and ototoxicity.

Both vestibular and auditory ototoxicity can occur. Eighth cranial nerve impairment may develop in patients with pre-existing renal damage and if Nebcin is administered for longer periods or in higher doses than those recommended. Therefore, renal and eighth cranial nerve function should be closely monitored in patients with known or suspected renal impairment and also in those whose renal function is initially normal but who develop signs of renal dysfunction during therapy. Evidence of impairment in renal, vestibular and/or auditory function requires discontinuation of the drug or dosage adjustment.

Serum concentrations should be monitored when feasible, and prolonged concentrations above 12 mg/l should be avoided. Urine should be examined for increased excretion of protein, cells and casts.

The risk of toxic reactions is low in patients with normal renal function who do not receive Nebcin in higher doses or for longer periods of time than those recommended.

Concurrent and sequential use of other neurotoxic and/or nephrotoxic antibiotics, particularly streptomycin, neomycin, kanamycin, gentamicin, cephaloridine, paromomycin, viomycin, polymyxin B, colistin, vancomycin and amikacin, should be avoided.

Nebcin should not be given concurrently with potent diuretics. Some diuretics themselves cause ototoxicity, and intravenously administered diuretics enhance aminoglycoside toxicity by altering antibiotic concentrations in serum and tissue.

Usage in pregnancy: Tobramycin crosses the placenta and accumulates in the fetal kidney. Therefore it should not be administered to the pregnant patient unless the potential benefits clearly outweigh any potential risk. Tobramycin is excreted in the breast milk.

Precautions: Usage in neonates: Nebcin should be used with caution in premature and neonatal infants because of their renal immaturity and the resulting prolongation of serum half-life of the drug.

Neuromuscular blockade and respiratory paralysis have been reported in cats receiving very high doses of tobramycin (40 mg/kg). The possibility that prolonged secondary apnoea may occur should be considered if tobramycin is administered to anaesthetised patients who are also receiving neuromuscular blocking agents such as succinylcholine or tubocurarine. If neuromuscular blockade occurs, it may be reversed by the administration of calcium salts.

The inactivation of tobramycin by carbenicillin has been demonstrated *in vitro* and in patients with severe renal impairment. Such inactivation has not been found in patients with normal renal function if the drugs are administered by separate routes.

Cross-allergenicity among aminoglycosides has been known to occur.

If overgrowth of non-susceptible organisms occurs, appropriate therapy should be initiated.

Side-effects: Renal function changes, as shown by rising blood urea, non-protein nitrogen and serum creatinine and by oliguria, cylindruria and increased proteinuria, have been reported, especially in patients with a history of renal impairment who are treated for longer periods or with higher doses than those recommended. These changes can occur in patients with initially normal renal function.

Side-effects on both vestibular and auditory branches of the eighth cranial nerve have been reported, especially in patients receiving high doses or prolonged therapy. Symptoms include dizziness, vertigo, tinnitus, roaring in the ears and hearing loss.

Other reported side-effects, possibly related to tobramycin, include increased AST, ALT, and increased serum bilirubin; anaemia, granulocytopenia and thrombocytopenia; and fever, rash, itching, urticaria, nausea, vomiting, headache and lethargy.

Treatment of overdosage: In the event of overdosage or toxic reactions, haemodialysis or peritoneal dialysis will help remove tobramycin from the blood. Between 25%–70% of the administered dose may be removed, depending on the duration and type of dialysis employed; haemodialysis is the more effective method.

Pharmaceutical precautions Undiluted vials: Store at room temperature (15°–25°C). Nebcin should not be physically premixed with other drugs but should be administered separately according to the recommended dose and route.

Legal category POM.

Package quantities Boxes of 10 rubber-stoppered injection vials.

Further information Nil.

Product licence numbers
40 mg per 1 ml 0006/0084
10 mg per 1 ml 0006/0085

NU-SEALS* Aspirin

Presentation Enteric sealed tablets of aspirin. Nu-Seals Aspirin is available in two sizes containing 300 mg (coded B01) and 600 mg (coded B06) Acetylsalicylic Acid PhEur covered in a special coating, red in colour.

Uses Aspirin has analgesic, antipyretic and anti-inflammatory actions. Nu-Seals Aspirin is indicated wherever high and prolonged dosage of aspirin is required. The special coating resists dissolution in gastric juice, but will dissolve readily in the relatively less acid environment of the duodenum. Owing to the delay that the coating imposes on the release of the active ingredient, Nu-Seals Aspirin is unsuitable for the short-term relief of pain.

Dosage and administration Nu-Seals Aspirin is for oral administration. The usual adult dose of aspirin is 300–900 mg repeated three to four times daily according to clinical needs. In acute rheumatic disorders the dose is in the range of 4–8 g daily, taken in divided doses. Nu-Seals Aspirin should not be given to children under the age of 5 years, as the usually recommended maximum single dose is less than that provided by the smaller size tablet. Children aged 6–12 years may be given 300 mg up to four times daily.

The elderly: As for adults. The elderly are more likely to experience gastric side-effects and tinnitus.

Contra-indications, warnings, etc
Contra-indications: Hypersensitivity to aspirin. Hypoprothrombinaemia, haemophilia and active peptic ulceration.

Warnings: Salicylates should be used with caution in patients with a history of peptic ulceration or coagulation abnormalities. They may also induce gastro-intestinal haemorrhage, occasionally major.

In large doses, salicylates may also decrease insulin requirements.

Usage in pregnancy: Although clinical and epidemiological evidence would suggest the safety of aspirin for use during pregnancy, caution should be exercised when prescribing for pregnant patients. Aspirin may prolong labour and contribute to maternal and neonatal bleeding, and is best avoided at term.

Precautions: Salicylates may enhance the effect of anticoagulants and inhibit the uricosuric effect of probenecid. They may also precipitate bronchospasm or induce attacks of asthma in susceptible subjects.

Side-effects: Salicylates may induce hypersensitivity, asthma, urate kidney stones, chronic gastro-intestinal blood loss, tinnitus, nausea and vomiting. The special coating of Nu-Seals Aspirin helps to reduce the incidence of side-effects resulting from gastric irritation.

Overdose: Overdosage produces dizziness, tinnitus, sweating, nausea and vomiting, confusion and hyperventilation. Gross overdosage may lead to CNS depression with coma, cardiovascular collapse and respiratory depression. If overdosage is suspected, the patient should be kept under observation for at least 24 hours, as symptoms and salicylate blood levels may not become apparent for several hours. Treatment of overdosage consists of gastric lavage and forced alkaline diuresis. Haemodialysis may be necessary in severe cases.

Pharmaceutical precautions Keep containers tightly closed.

Legal category P.

Package quantities Bottles of 100 and 500.

Further information Nil.

Product licence numbers
Tablets 300 mg 0006/5093
Tablets 600 mg 0006/5094

ONCOVIN*

Presentation Oncovin Vials containing 1 mg Oncovin (Vincristine Sulphate BP) and 10 mg Lactose PhEur.
Vials containing 2 mg Oncovin (Vincristine Sulphate BP) and 20 mg Lactose PhEur.
Vials containing 5 mg Oncovin (Vincristine Sulphate BP) and 50 mg Lactose PhEur.
Oncovin is supplied in a combination package with an accompanying vial of diluting solution, 10 ml containing 90 mg Sodium Chloride PhEur with 2% Benzyl Alcohol BP as a preservative.
Oncovin Solution: 1 ml vials containing 1 mg Oncovin (Vincristine Sulphate BP) and 100 mg Mannitol BP.
2 ml vials containing 2 mg Oncovin (Vincristine Sulphate BP) and 200 mg Mannitol BP.
The vials also contain 1.8 mg per 1 ml Methyl Hydroxybenzoate PhEur and 0.2 mg per 1 ml Propyl Hydroxybenzoate PhEur as preservatives.

Uses Oncovin is an anti-neoplastic drug for intravenous use.
Information available at present suggests that Oncovin may be useful either alone or in conjunction with other oncolytic drugs for the treatment of:
1. Acute leukaemias.
2. Malignant lymphomas, including Hodgkin's disease, lymphosarcoma and reticulum cell sarcoma.
3. Other neoplasms, e.g. neuroblastoma, Wilms' tumour and rhabdomyosarcoma.

Dosage and administration Extreme care must be used in calculating and administering the dose of Oncovin since overdosage may have a very serious or fatal outcome.
The drug is administered intravenously at weekly intervals. The size of the dose is determined by body weight. In children, remissions from acute leukaemia

have been induced with weekly doses of 0.05–0.15 mg/kg of body weight.

In acute leukaemia of children the following incremental approach to dosage may be employed:

First dose 0.05 mg/kg
Second dose 0.075 mg/kg
Third dose 0.1 mg/kg, and
Fourth dose 0.125 mg/kg up to a maximum of 0.15 mg/kg

There is no need to advance the dosage beyond that level which produces therapeutic benefit. After remission has been obtained, the dosage may be reduced in some cases to a maintenance level of 0.05 to 0.075 mg/kg/week.

In adult leukaemia the suggested dosage is 0.025–0.075 mg/kg of body weight per weekly dose.

Oncovin has also been used successfully either in sequence or in combination with other available agents effective in the treatment of leukaemia.

For malignancies other than leukaemia, a suggested dosage for Oncovin is 0.025 mg/kg/week intravenously until some beneficial effect is seen. Thereafter much smaller weekly doses in the range of 0.005–0.010 mg/kg may be employed for maintenance therapy for so long as an antitumour effect can be maintained.

The elderly: As for adults.

The dosage must always be adjusted individually because of the narrow range between therapeutic and toxic levels, and individual variations in response.

Solutions of Oncovin ranging from 0.01 mg to 1 mg/ml have been administered with equally satisfactory results. With these concentrations, there have been no reports of phlebitis or cellulitis at the site of injection unless extravasation occurred. Various solvents have been employed for the drug, including Water for Injections PhEur and Sodium Chloride Intravenous Infusion BP. Both of the latter appear to be equally satisfactory.

To prepare a solution containing 1 mg/ml add 1 ml of the accompanying diluting solution to the 1 mg vial, 2 ml to the 2 mg vial, or 5 ml to the 5 mg vial. The drug dissolves rapidly to give a clear solution. The calculated dose of the resulting solution or the solution for injection is drawn up into a syringe and injected either directly into a vein or into the tubing of a running intravenous infusion, whichever is more suitable for the patient.

Oncovin solution: The concentration of vincristine is 1 mg/ml. Do not add extra fluid to the vial prior to removal of the dose. Withdraw the solution of Oncovin into an accurate dry syringe, measuring the dose of Oncovin carefully. Do not add extra fluid to the vial in an attempt to empty it completely.

Care should be taken to avoid infiltration of subcutaneous tissues. Injection of Oncovin may be completed in about one minute.

Caution: If leakage into surrounding tissue should occur during intravenous administration of Oncovin, it may cause considerable irritation. The injection should be discontinued immediately and any remaining portion of the dose should then be. introduced into another vein. Local injection of hyaluronidase or hydrocortisone and the application of moderate heat to the area of leakage help to disperse the drug and are thought to minimise discomfort and the possibility of cellulitis.

It is important to avoid contamination of the eyes with concentrations of Oncovin used clinically. If accidental contamination occurs, severe irritation (or if the drug was delivered under pressure, even corneal ulceration) may result. The eye should be washed with water thoroughly and immediately.

Contra-indications, warnings, etc
Contra-indications: The intrathecal administration of Oncovin is usually fatal. Patients with the demyelinating form of Charcot–Marie–Tooth Syndrome should not be given Oncovin.

Warning: Usage in pregnancy: Caution is necessary with the use of all oncolytic drugs during pregnancy. Information on the use of Oncovin during pregnancy is very limited. Although no abnormalities of the human fetus have been reported thus far, animal studies with Oncovin have shown evidence of teratogenicity.

This product should not normally be administered to patients who are pregnant or to mothers who are breast feeding, unless the potential benefits clearly outweigh the risks.

Precautions: Effective therapy with Oncovin is less likely to be followed by granulocytopenia than is the case with Velbe (vinblastine sulphate) and other oncolytic agents. A study of the side-effects of Oncovin in all age groups reveals that it is usually neuromuscular rather than bone marrow toxicity that limits dosage. However, because of the possibility of granulocytopenia both clinician and patient should remain alert for signs of any complicating infection. Although pre-existing granulocytopenia does not necessarily contra-indicate the administration of Oncovin, the appearance of granulocytopenia during treatment warrants careful consideration before giving the next dose. Acute uric acid nephropathy, which may occur after administration of oncolytic agents, has also been reported with Oncovin.

As Oncovin is excreted principally by the liver, it may be necessary to reduce initial doses in the presence of significantly impaired hepatic or biliary function.

When chemotherapy is being given in conjunction with radiation therapy through portals which include the liver, the use of Oncovin should be delayed until radiation therapy has been completed.

Acute shortness of breath and severe bronchospasm have been reported following the administration of the vinca alkaloids. These reactions have been encountered most frequently when using combination therapy with mitomycin-C. The onset may be within minutes, or several hours after the drug is injected.

Adverse reactions: The use of small amounts of Oncovin daily for long periods is not advised as this leads to the prolongation of otherwise short term side-effects (i.e. those lasting less than 7 days).

The incidence of side-effects appears to be related not only to the size of dose employed, but also to the total accumulated dosage given, particularly in the case of neurotoxicity.

Neuromuscular (often dose limiting)–neuritic pain, sensory loss, paraesthesiae, difficulty in walking, slapping gait, loss of deep tendon reflexes, muscle wasting, ataxia, foot drop and cranial nerve palsies. Frequently, there appears to be a sequence in the development of neuromuscular side-effects. Initially, one may encounter only sensory impairment and paraesthesiae. With continued treatment, neuritic pain may appear and later, motor difficulties. No reports have yet been made of any agent that can reverse the neuromuscular manifestations of Oncovin.

Haematological – granulocytopenia; Oncovin does not appear to have any constant or significant effect upon the platelets or the red blood cells. If thrombocytopenia is present when treatment with Oncovin is begun, it may actually improve before the appearance of marrow remission.

Gastro-intestinal – constipation, abdominal cramps, paralytic ileus, vomiting and diarrhoea. The constipation which may be encountered responds well to such usual measures as enemas and laxatives. Constipation may take the form of upper colon impaction and the rectum may be found to be empty on physical examination. Colicky abdominal pain, coupled with an empty rectum, may mislead the clinician. A flat film of the abdomen is useful in demonstrating this condition. A routine prophylactic regimen against constipation is recommended for all patients receiving Oncovin.

Cutaneous – alopecia, oral ulceration.

Miscellaneous – weight loss, fever, polyuria, dysuria, headache, optic atrophy with blindness and transient cortical blindness. Convulsions, frequently with hypertension, have been reported in a few patients receiving Oncovin. Rare occurrences of the syndrome attributed to disorder of antidiuretic hormone secretion have also been observed. This syndrome has been described in association with several disease states. There is high urinary sodium excretion in the presence of hyponatraemia. Renal or adrenal disease, hypotension, dehydration, uraemia and clinical oedema are absent. With fluid deprivation, improvement occurs in the hyponatraemia and in the renal loss of sodium.

With single weekly doses, granulocytopenia, neuritic pain, constipation and difficulty in walking are usually of short duration (i.e. less than seven days). When subsequent dosage is reduced these side-effects may lessen or disappear. Other side-effects, such as alopecia, sensory loss, paraesthesiae, slapping gait, loss of deep tendon reflexes and muscle wasting, do not reverse so rapidly but persist for at least as long as treatment is continued. In most instances, these side-effects have disappeared by about the sixth week after discontinuing treatment, but in some patients neuromuscular difficulties may persist for prolonged periods.

Overdosage: Side-effects following the use of Oncovin are dose related. Therefore, following administration of more than the recommended dose, patients can be expected to experience these effects in an exaggerated fashion.

Treatment: Supportive care should include: (a) prevention of side-effects that result from the syndrome of inappropriate secretion of antidiuretic hormone. This includes restriction of fluid intake and perhaps the use of a diuretic acting on the loop of Henle and distal tubule function; (b) administration of an anticonvulsant; (c) use of cathartics to prevent ileus; (d) monitoring the patient's cardiovascular system; and (e) daily blood counts for guidance in transfusion requirement. Animal studies indicate that folinic acid is effective in the treatment of overdosage. A suggested schedule is to administer 15 mg of folinic acid intravenously every 3 hours for 24 hours and then every 6 hours for at least 48 hours.

Pharmaceutical precautions Vials of Oncovin should be stored in a refrigerator between 0° and 6°C.

After reconstitution: After a portion of the solution has been removed from a vial, the remainder of the contents of the vial may be stored in a refrigerator for further use for 14 days without significant loss of potency. When the reconstituted vial of Oncovin is to be stored for more than 48 hours, it is essential to use the accompanying diluting solution or a diluent which contains a preservative.

Oncovin Solution: Store in a refrigerator between 0° and 6°C. Protect from light.

Oncovin should never be mixed with any other drug.

Legal category POM.

Package quantities
Vials 1 mg: Single vials.
Vials 2 mg: Single vials.
Vials 5 mg: Single vials.
Vials 1 mg/1 ml: Single vials.
Vials 2 mg/2 ml: Single vials.

Further information The use of Oncovin either alone or in combination with other oncolytic drugs in the treatment of malignant conditions other than leukaemia has been investigated and reported by various workers. The clinician is referred to the medical literature. A nomogram dosage card is available on request for the guidance of clinicians who prefer to relate dosage to body surface area. In acute leukaemia a dose of 1.5–2 mg/m^2 weekly has been employed.

If central nervous system leukaemia is diagnosed, additional agents and routes of administration will be required, since Oncovin does not cross the blood brain barrier in therapeutic amounts.

Product licence numbers
Vials 1 mg	0006/5070
Vials 2 mg	0006/5070
Vials 5 mg	0006/5071
Diluent	0006/5174
Vials 1 mg/1 ml	0006/0169
Vials 2 mg/2 ml	0006/0169

PROGESIC*

Presentation Tablets each containing fenoprofen calcium equivalent to 200 mg of fenoprofen. The tablets are round, yellow, 9.5 mm in diameter and marked Lilly 4015.

Uses Analgesic. For the relief of mild/moderate pain. Pyrexia.

Dosage and administration For oral administration to adults only, and not recommended for administration to children.

Dosage: 200 mg three or four times a day; in more intractable pain the dose may be doubled. The maximum daily dose should not exceed 3 g.

The elderly: There is no difference in the metabolism or pharmacokinetics of fenoprofen in the elderly, but side-effects of non-steroidal anti-inflammatory drugs are more pronounced in this patient population.

Contra-indications, warnings, etc
Contra-indications: Hypersensitivity to the drug. Active peptic ulceration.

Warnings: Adverse effects may include gastro-intestinal intolerance and episodes of bleeding. Although fenoprofen has been associated with less gastro-intestinal microbleeding than aspirin, patients with a history of peptic ulcer or gastro-intestinal bleeding should be closely supervised during fenoprofen therapy.
Bronchospasm may be precipitated in patients suffering

from, or with a previous history of, bronchial asthma or allergic disease.

Although cross-sensitivity has not been established, the drug should not be given to patients in whom salicylates induce the syndrome of asthma, rhinitis or urticaria.

Usage in pregnancy: The safety of fenoprofen for use during pregnancy or lactation has not been established; therefore it should not be administered to pregnant women or nursing mothers unless the potential benefits clearly outweigh any potential risk. Animal studies showed prolongation of parturition, but no evidence of teratogenicity.

Precautions: Because of its affinity for albumin, fenoprofen may displace other drugs from their binding sites, and this may lead to drug interaction. In patients receiving coumarin-type anticoagulants, the addition of fenoprofen could prolong the prothrombin time. Patients receiving hydantoins or sulphonylureas should be carefully monitored.

When aspirin and fenoprofen are administered concurrently, plasma concentrations of fenoprofen are reduced. It may be advisable to discontinue the concomitant use of aspirin to maximise the beneficial effects of fenoprofen. However, single or intermittent doses of aspirin may be administered if they are indicated.

Since fenoprofen is eliminated primarily by the kidney, the drug should not be administered to patients with significantly impaired renal function, and patients likely to have compromised renal function should be monitored periodically.

Patients with initial low haemoglobin values who are receiving long-term therapy should be monitored, as transient reduction of haemoglobin and haematocrit values due to fenoprofen have been reported.

Elevation of AST, LDH and ALP levels have been reported occasionally, and it is therefore recommended that fenoprofen be discontinued if any significant liver abnormalities occur.

Side-effects: Gastro-intestinal – These are the most commonly observed side-effects and include dyspepsia, constipation, diarrhoea, ulceration of the buccal mucosa, nausea, vomiting, anorexia and occult blood in the stool. Cases of peptic ulceration, including some complicated by bleeding, have occurred.

Renal – Rare cases of acute renal insufficiency, in association with interstitial nephritis, nephrotic syndrome or papillary necrosis, have been reported. As a general rule, these are reversible on withdrawal of the drug. Episodes of dysuria, cystitis and haematuria have occurred.

Hepatic – Severe hepatic reactions, including jaundice and fatal hepatitis, have been reported rarely.

Haematological – Various syndromes involving the bone marrow have been reported rarely; thrombocytopenia, pancytopenia and aplastic anaemia have occurred.

Allergic – Pruritus, rash, urticaria, Stevens-Johnson syndrome and angioneurotic oedema have been reported.

Neurological – Reactions reported include headache, somnolence, dizziness, tremor, confusion and insomnia.

Miscellaneous – Tinnitus, hearing decrease, amblyopia, blurred vision, palpitations, increased sweating, nervousness and peripheral oedema have been reported.

Overdosage: Information on intentional overdosage is limited. Symptoms of nephrotoxicity include dysuria, haematuria, proteinuria and oliguria. Gastro-intestinal symptoms may include nausea and vomiting, progressing to abdominal pain, distention and ileus. Circulatory collapse and hypotension may occur; one patient suffered a fatal cardiac arrest. Loss of consciousness, headache and tinnitus have also been reported.

Treatment: Standard therapy to evacuate gastric contents and to support vital functions should be employed. Since fenoprofen is acidic and is excreted in the urine, it would seem theoretically beneficial to try forced alkaline diuresis.

Pharmaceutical precautions Store at room temperature (15°–25°C).

Legal category POM.

Package quantities Tablets 200 mg. Blister packs of 100 tablets.

Further information Nil.

Product licence number
Tablets 200 mg　0006/0141.

SECONAL* SODIUM

Presentation Capsules (orange, coded F42) containing 50 mg Secobarbital Sodium BP. Capsules (orange, coded F40) containing 100 mg Secobarbital Sodium BP.

Uses For the treatment of severe, intractable insomnia.

Dosage and administration For oral administration to adults only. Normal dosage is 50–100 mg. Occasionally as much as 200 mg may be required.

The effects should become apparent between 15 and 30 minutes after administration.

Contra-indications, warnings, etc
Contra-indications: Hypersensitivity to barbiturates, a history of porphyria or the presence of uncontrolled pain.

Barbiturates should not be administered to children, young adults, patients with a history of drug or alcohol abuse, the elderly and the debilitated.

Usage in pregnancy: Barbiturates are contra-indicated during pregnancy and for the nursing mother.

Warnings: Performance and alertness may be impaired during the first week of therapy. Patients should be warned of the possible hazards when driving, or operating machinery. These effects may be potentiated by alcohol.

Drug interactions: Barbiturates cause induction of the liver enzymes responsible for metabolising many other drugs; in particular they should not be administered concurrently with coumarin-type anticoagulants. They may also affect the metabolism of systemic steroids (including oral contraceptives), phenytoin, griseofulvin, rifampicin, tricyclic antidepressants and phenothiazines such as chlorpromazine.

Precautions: A reduction in dosage may be required in patients with decreased hepatic or renal function.

Adverse reactions: Common adverse reactions include drowsiness, sedation, ataxia and vertigo.

Hypersensitive skin reactions may occur in some patients, especially those with asthma, urticaria or angioneurotic oedema.

Other idiosyncratic reactions include a hangover effect, paradoxical excitement, pain, confusion and memory defects.

Overdosage: Symptoms include respiratory depression, depression of superficial and deep reflexes, constriction of the pupils to a slight degree (although in severe poisoning they may dilate), decreased urine formation, hypothermia and coma.

Treatment: General management should consist of symptomatic and supportive therapy, including gastric lavage, administration of intravenous fluids, and maintenance of blood pressure, body temperature and adequate respiratory exchange. Haemodialysis will increase the rate of removal of barbiturates from the body fluids.

Pharmaceutical precautions Keep containers tightly closed. Store below 25°C.

Legal category CD (Sch 3) POM.

Package quantities Capsules 50 mg: Bottles of 100. Capsules 100 mg: Bottles of 100 and 500.

Further information *Addiction potential:* Barbiturates have a high addiction potential. Long-term use, or use of high dosage for short periods, may lead to tolerance and subsequently to physical and psychological dependence. Symptoms of dependence include confusion, defective judgement and loss of emotional control. Withdrawal symptoms occur after long-term normal use (and particularly after abuse) on rapid cessation of barbiturate treatment. Symptoms include nightmares, irritability and insomnia, and in severe cases, tremors, delirium, convulsions and death. Withdrawal symptoms have been reported in neonates after barbiturate treatment during pregnancy and labour.

Product licence numbers
Capsules 50 mg 0006/5065
Capsules 100 mg 0006/5066

SODIUM AMYTAL* CAPSULES
SODIUM AMYTAL* TABLETS

Presentation Capsules (blue, coded F23) each containing 60 mg Amylobarbitone Sodium PhEur.

Capsules (blue, coded F33) each containing 200 mg Amylobarbitone Sodium PhEur.

Tablets (uncoated, white, coded U43) each containing 60 mg Amylobarbitone Sodium PhEur.

Tablets (uncoated, white, coded U16) each containing 200 mg Amylobarbitone Sodium PhEur.

Uses For the treatment of severe, intractable insomnia.

Dosage and administration For oral administration to adults only. Normal dosage is 60–200 mg. Occasionally a larger dose may be necessary.

The effects should become apparent between 30 and 45 minutes after administration.

Contra-indications, warnings, etc
Contra-indications: Hypersensitivity to barbiturates, a history of porphyria or the presence of uncontrolled pain.

Barbiturates should not be administered to children, young adults, patients with a history of drug or alcohol abuse, the elderly and the debilitated.

Usage in pregnancy: Barbiturates are contra-indicated during pregnancy and for the nursing mother.

Warnings: Performance and alertness may be impaired during the first week of therapy. Patients should be warned of the possible hazards when driving, or operating machinery. These effects may be potentiated by alcohol.

Drug interactions: Barbiturates cause induction of the liver enzymes responsible for metabolising many other drugs; in particular they should not be administered concurrently with coumarin-type anticoagulants. They may also affect the metabolism of systemic steroids (including oral contraceptives), phenytoin, griseofulvin, rifampicin, tricyclic antidepressants and phenothiazines such as chlorpromazine.

Precautions: A reduction in dosage may be required in patients with decreased hepatic or renal function.

Adverse reactions: Common adverse reactions include drowsiness, sedation, ataxia and vertigo.

Hypersensitive skin reactions may occur in some patients, especially those with asthma, urticaria or angioneurotic oedema.

Other idiosyncratic reactions include a hangover effect, paradoxical excitement, pain, confusion and memory defects.

Overdosage: Symptoms include respiratory depression, depression of superficial and deep reflexes, constriction of the pupils to a slight degree (although in severe poisoning they may dilate), decreased urine formation, hypothermia and coma.

Treatment: General management should consist of symptomatic and supportive therapy, including gastric lavage, administration of intravenous fluids and maintenance of blood pressure, body temperature and adequate respiratory exchange. Haemodialysis will increase the rate of removal of barbiturates from the body fluids.

Pharmaceutical precautions Capsules and tablets: Keep containers tightly closed. Store below 25°C.

Legal category CD (Sch 3) POM.

Package quantities
Capsules 60 mg: Bottles of 100 and 500
Capsules 200 mg: Bottles of 100 and 500
Tablets 60 mg: Bottles of 100 and 1000
Tablets 200 mg: Bottles of 100 and 1000

Further information *Addiction potential:* Barbiturates have a high addiction potential. Long term use, or use of high dosage for short periods, may lead to tolerance and subsequently to physical and psychological dependence. Symptoms of dependence include confusion, defective judgement and loss of emotional control. Withdrawal symptoms occur after long-term normal use (and particularly after abuse) on rapid cessation of barbiturate treatment. Symptoms include nightmares, irritability and insomnia, and in severe cases, tremors, delirium, convulsions and death. Withdrawal symptoms have been reported in neonates after barbiturate treatment during pregnancy and labour.

Product licence numbers
Capsules 60 mg   0006/5084
Capsules 200 mg   0006/5085
Tablets 60 mg   0006/5080
Tablets 200 mg   0006/5082

SODIUM AMYTAL* INJECTION

Presentation Vials for injection, containing 250 mg or 500 mg Amylobarbitone Sodium PhEur.

Uses Sodium Amytal may be used parenterally to control status epilepticus, but it is not the barbiturate of choice in the routine treatment of grand mal epilepsy.

Dosage and administration

Adults: The usual adult dose is in the range of 250 mg–1 g. The maximum single dose should not exceed 1 g and the maximum intramuscular dose should not exceed 500 mg.

The elderly: As for adults, unless renal or hepatic function is impaired (see Precautions).

Children: Because of their higher metabolic rate, children tolerate comparatively larger doses. The final dosage is determined to a great extent by the patient's reaction to the slow administration of the drug. Usually, 65 mg to 500 mg may be given to a child 6 to 12 years of age.

Solutions should be made up aseptically with Water for Injections PhEur. The accompanying table will aid in preparing solutions of various concentrations; ordinarily, a 10% solution is used. After Water for Injections PhEur is added, the vial should be rotated to facilitate solution of the powder. Do not shake the vial.

Quantity of Water for Injections PhEur to be added to the vial contents to obtain a solution of a desired percentage. Solutions derived will be in weight/volume.

Vial Content	1%	2.5%	5%	10%	20%
250 mg	25 ml	10 ml	5 ml	2.5 ml	1.25 ml
500 mg	50 ml	20 ml	10 ml	5 ml	2.5 ml

Intramuscular use: No more than 5 ml should be injected at any one site. Injections should be made deeply into large muscles, such as the gluteus maximus. Superficial intramuscular or subcutaneous injections may be painful and may produce sterile abscesses or sloughing.

If it is desirable to reduce the dosage volume, a 20% solution may be used.

Intravenous use: For intravenous use, the contents of the vial should be diluted.

The rate of intravenous injection should not exceed 1 ml per minute. When the 10% solution is used faster rates of administration may precipitate serious respiratory depression. This is more likely to occur if other central nervous system agents have been used concurrently.

Caution: The intravenous administration of Sodium Amytal carries with it the potential dangers inherent in the intravenous use of any potent hypnotic.

Contra-indications, warnings, etc

Contra-indications: Hypersensitivity to barbiturates, a history of porphyria or the presence of uncontrolled pain.

Warnings

Drug interactions: Barbiturates cause induction of the liver enzymes responsible for metabolising many other drugs; in particular they should not be administered concurrently with coumarin-type anticoagulants. They may also affect the metabolism of systemic steroids (including oral contraceptives), phenytoin, griseofulvin, rifampicin, tricyclic antidepressants and phenothiazines such as chlorpromazine. Sodium Amytal should not be administered to patients who are receiving monoamine oxidase inhibitors or who have received these within the previous 14 days, as they prolong the duration of action of barbiturates.

Usage in pregnancy: This product should not be administered during pregnancy or for the lactating mother unless considered to be essential by the physician.

Precautions: The central nervous system depressant effect of barbiturates may be additive with that of other CNS depressants, including alcohol. The patient should be warned about the possibility of drowsiness if he must operate dangerous machinery or drive a vehicle.

Sodium Amytal should be used with caution in patients with decreased liver function, since a prolongation of effect may occur. A reduced dosage may be required in patients with decreased hepatic or renal function.

If the condition of the patient justifies the intravenous administration of Sodium Amytal, close hospital supervision is also indicated.

Dosage and rate of administration should be selected with great care in patients with hypertension, hypotension or pulmonary or cardiovascular diseases.

Sodium Amytal is not recommended as an anaesthetic agent, but if a patient develops physical signs of severe depression, he should be treated as though deeply anaesthetised. Pulmonary oedema may complicate long periods of unconsciousness.

Adverse reactions: Common adverse reactions include drowsiness, sedation, ataxia and vertigo.

Hypersensitive skin reactions may occur in some patients, especially those with asthma, urticaria or angioneurotic oedema.

Other idiosyncratic reactions include a hangover effect, paradoxical excitement, pain, confusion and memory defects.

Overdosage: Symptoms include respiratory depression, depression of superficial and deep reflexes, constriction of the pupils to a slight degree (although in severe poisoning they may dilate), decreased urine formation, hypothermia and coma.

Treatment: General management should consist of symptomatic and supportive therapy, including gastric lavage, administration of intravenous fluids and maintenance of blood pressure, body temperature and adequate respiratory exchange. Haemodialysis will increase the rate of removal of barbiturates from the body fluids.

Pharmaceutical precautions *Unreconstituted vials:* Store at room temperature (15°–25°C).

A few minutes may be required for the drug to dissolve completely, but under no circumstances should a solution be injected if it has not become absolutely clear within five minutes. Also, a solution that forms a precipitate after clearing should not be used. Sodium Amytal hydrolyses in solution or upon exposure to air.

Legal category CD (Sch 3) POM.

Package quantities
Vials 250 mg: Packs of 25
Vials 500 mg: Packs of 25

Further information Nil.

Product licence numbers
Vials 250 mg   0006/5086
Vials 500 mg   0006/5087

TUINAL*

Presentation Capsules (orange and blue, coded F65) containing 100 mg Tuinal (50 mg Secobarbital Sodium BP and 50 mg Amylobarbitone Sodium PhEur).

Uses Tuinal combines the short onset of action of Seconal Sodium with the more prolonged effect of Sodium Amytal and is indicated whenever prompt and moderately sustained hypnosis is required. Not suitable for continuous daytime sedation.

Dosage and administration *For adults only:* 100–200 mg at bedtime.

The elderly: Oral barbiturates are contra-indicated in the elderly.

Contra-indications, warnings, etc Hypersensitivity to either constituent. Patients with a history of porphyria should not receive barbiturates in any form. Barbiturates may stimulate the enzymes responsible for metabolising many other drugs; in particular they should not be administered concurrently with coumarin-type anticoagulants. They may also affect the metabolism of endogenous steroids. Barbiturates should not be administered in the presence of uncontrolled pain, because excitement may be produced.

Warning: May be habit-forming.

Precautions: Tuinal should be used with caution in patients with decreased liver function, since a prolongation of effect may occur. The central nervous system depressant effect of Tuinal may be additive with that of other CNS depressants, including alcohol.

Except in emergencies, barbiturates should not be given to persons who are known to be, or are likely to become, dependent on sedative or hypnotic drugs. The repeated prescribing of any barbiturate drug for the same patient calls for careful consideration by the physician.

Usage in pregnancy: the safety of Tuinal for use during pregnancy or for the nursing mother has not been established.

Adverse reactions: Idiosyncrasy, manifested as excitement, hangover or pain, may occur. Hypersensitivity reactions occur in some patients, especially in those with asthma, urticaria or angioneurotic oedema.

Overdosage: Symptoms include respiratory depression, depression of superficial and deep reflexes, constriction of the pupils to a slight degree (although in severe poisoning they may dilate) decreased urine formation, hypothermia and coma.

Treatment: General management should consist of symptomatic and supportive therapy, including gastric lavage, administration of intravenous fluids and maintenance of blood pressure, body temperature and adequate respiratory exchange. Haemodialysis will increase the rate of removal of barbiturates from the body fluids.

Pharmaceutical precautions Keep containers tightly closed. Store below 25°C.

Legal category CD (Sch 3) POM.

Package quantities
Capsules 100 mg: Bottles of 100 and 500.

Further information Nil.

Product licence number
Capsules 100 mg   0006/5077

V-CIL-K*
PENICILLIN V POTASSIUM
Presentation *V-Cil-K:*

1. Phenoxymethylpenicillin Potassium Capsules BP (pink, coded H37) containing the equivalent of 250 mg phenoxymethylpenicillin.
2. Phenoxymethylpenicillin Potassium Tablets BP (white, coded C29) containing the equivalent of 250 mg phenoxymethylpenicillin.
3. Phenoxymethylpenicillin Potassium Tablets BP (white, coded C27) containing the equivalent of 125 mg phenoxymethylpenicillin.
4. Syrup: pink/white granules for the preparation of Phenoxymethylpenicillin Elixir BP. Each 5 ml contains the equivalent of 250 mg Phenoxymethylpenicillin PhEur.
5. Paediatric syrup: orange/pink granules for the preparation of Phenoxymethylpenicillin Elixir BP. Each 5 ml contains the equivalent of 125 mg Phenoxymethylpenicillin PhEur.

Penicillin V Potassium:
Paediatric Syrup: orange/pink granules for the preparation of Phenoxymethylpenicillin Elixir BP. Each 5 ml contains the equivalent of 62.5 mg Phenoxymethylpenicillin PhEur.

Uses Penicillin exerts high activity *in vitro* against: staphylococci (except penicillinase-producing strains), streptococci (groups A, C, G, H, L and M), pneumococci, *Corynebacterium diphtheriae, Bacillus anthracis, Actinomyces bovis, Streptobacillus moniliformis, Listeria monocytogenes, Neisseria gonorrhoeae, Treponema pallidum, Clostridium* species and Leptospira.

Phenoxymethylpenicillin and potassium phenoxymethylpenicillin are indicated in the treatment of mild to moderately severe infections associated with microorganisms whose susceptibility to penicillin is within the range of serum levels attained with these dosage forms.

The following infections will normally respond to adequate doses: *Streptococcal infections (without bacteraemia):* Mild to moderate infections of the upper respiratory tract, scarlet fever and mild erysipelas.

Pneumococcal infections: Mild to moderately severe infections of the respiratory tract.

Staphylococcal infections sensitive to penicillin: Mild infections of the skin and soft tissues.

Fusospirochaetosis (Vincent's gingivitis and pharyngitis): Mild to moderately severe infections of the oropharynx usually respond to therapy with oral penicillin.

Prophylactic use: Prophylaxis with oral penicillin has proved effective in preventing recurrence of rheumatic fever and chorea.

Patients with a past history of rheumatic fever receiving continuous prophylaxis may harbour penicillin-resistant organisms. In these patients, the use of another prophylactic agent should be considered.

Dosage and administration For oral administration.

Adults: 125 mg or 250 mg every four to six hours depending on the severity of the condition.

The elderly: As for adults. Reduce dosage if renal function is markedly impaired.

Children over 5 years: The adult dose.

Children 5 years or less: 125 mg every six hours.

Infants (up to 1 year): 62.5 mg every six hours.

In all but the most serious cases, the last dose of the day may be doubled to avoid disturbing sleep. Ideally, each dose should be given half an hour before (or at least three hours after) a meal.

Prophylactic use: 125 mg twice daily is recommended for long term prophylaxis of rheumatic fever.

Contra-indications, warnings, etc
Contra-indication: A previous hypersensitivity reaction to any penicillin.

Warnings: All degrees of hypersensitivity including fatal anaphylaxis have been observed with oral penicillin. These reactions are more likely to occur in individuals with a history of sensitivity to multiple allergens, and enquiry should be made for such a history before therapy is begun. If an allergic reaction occurs, the drug should be discontinued and the patient treated with the usual agents (e.g. adrenaline and other pressor amines, antihistamines and corticosteroids).

Usage in pregnancy: Although laboratory and clinical studies have shown no evidence of teratogenicity, caution should be exercised when prescribing for the pregnant patient.

Precautions: Penicillin should be used with caution in individuals with histories of significant allergies and/or asthma.

Oral therapy should not be relied upon in patients with severe illness, or with nausea, vomiting, gastric dilatation, cardiospasm or intestinal hypermotility. Occasionally patients do not absorb therapeutic amounts of orally administered penicillin.

Administer with caution in the presence of markedly impaired renal function, as safe dosage may be lower than that usually recommended.

Streptococcal infections should be treated for a minimum of 10 days, and post-therapy cultures should be performed to confirm the eradication of the organisms.

Prolonged use of antibiotics may promote the overgrowth of non-susceptible organisms, including fungi. If superinfection occurs, appropriate measures should be taken.

Adverse reactions: Gastro-intestinal: The most common reactions to oral penicillin are nausea, vomiting, epigastric distress, and diarrhoea.
Hypersensitivity: Skin eruptions, urticaria, reactions resembling serum sickness (chills, fever, oedema, arthralgia, prostration), laryngeal oedema and anaphylaxis. Fever and eosinophilia may frequently be the only reactions observed.

Haemolytic anaemia, leucopenia, thrombocytopenia, neuropathy and nephropathy are infrequent reactions and are usually associated with high doses of parenteral penicillin.

Overdosage: Symptoms: nausea, vomiting and diarrhoea.

Treatment: General management may consist of supportive therapy.

Pharmaceutical precautions Keep containers tightly closed.
Capsules: Store below 25°C.
Tablets: Store in a cool place (6°–15°C).
Syrup: After mixing, syrup can be stored for seven days at room temperature (15°–25°C) or fourteen days in a refrigerator (0°–6°C).

Legal category POM.

Package quantities V-Cil-K:
Capsules 250 mg: Bottles of 100, 500 and 1,000.
Tablets 250 mg: Bottles of 100, 500 and 1,000.
Tablets 125 mg: Bottles of 100, 500 and 1,000.
Syrup 250 mg/5 ml: Bottles of 100 ml.
Paediatric syrup 125 mg/5 ml: Bottles of 100 ml.

Penicillin V Potassium:
Paediatric syrup 62.5 mg/5 ml: Bottles of 100 ml.

Further information Nil.

Product licence numbers

Capsules 250 mg	0006/5126
Tablets 250 mg	0006/5164
Tablets 125 mg	0006/5163
Syrup 250 mg/5 ml	0006/5129
Paediatric syrup 125 mg/5 ml	0006/5128
Paediatric syrup 62.5 mg/5 ml	0006/5162

VANCOCIN* INJECTION

Presentation Rubber-stoppered 10 ml vials each containing Vancomycin Injection BP, 500,000 IU, equivalent to 500 mg vancomycin, as a lyophilised plug.

Uses Vancomycin is a glycopeptide antibiotic derived from *Streptomyces* orientalis, and is active against many Gram-positive bacteria including *Staphylococcus aureus*, *Staph. epidermidis*, α and β haemolytic streptococci, group D streptococci, corynebacteria and clostridia.

Vancomycin is indicated in potentially life-threatening infections which cannot be treated with other effective, less toxic antimicrobial drugs, including the penicillins and cephalosporins.

Vancomycin is useful in the therapy of severe staphylococcal infections in patients who cannot receive or who have failed to respond to the penicillins and cephalosporins, or who have infections with staphylococci resistant to other antibiotics.

Vancomycin is used in the treatment of endocarditis and as prophylaxis against endocarditis in patients at risk from dental or surgical procedures.

Its effectiveness has been documented in other infections due to staphylococci, including osteomyelitis, pneumonia, septicaemia and soft tissue infections.

Vancomycin may be used orally for the treatment of staphylococcal enterocolitis and pseudomembranous colitis due to *Clostridium difficile*. Vancomycin is not absorbed from the gastro-intestinal tract and is therefore not effective by the oral route for other types of infection; parenteral administration may be used concomitantly if required.

Dosage and administration For intravenous use only and not for intramuscular administration.

Intravenous use
Adults: The usual intravenous dose is 500 mg (in Sodium Chloride Intravenous Infusion BP or 5% Dextrose Intravenous Infusion BP) every six hours or 1 g every 12 hours. The majority of patients with infections caused by organisms sensitive to the antibiotic show a therapeutic response within 48–72 hours. The total duration of therapy is determined by the type and severity of the infection and the clinical response of the patient. In staphylococcal endocarditis, treatment for three weeks or longer is recommended.

The elderly: As for adults. Reduce dosage if renal function is impaired. Monitor auditory function – see warnings and precautions.

Children: The total daily dosage, calculated on the basis of 44 mg/kg of body weight, can be administered in divided doses in the child's 24-hour requirement of fluid.

Patients with impaired renal function: Dosage adjustments must be made to avoid toxic serum levels. Regular monitoring of serum levels is advised in such patients, as accumulation has been reported, especially after prolonged therapy. The following nomogram, based on creatinine clearance values, is provided:

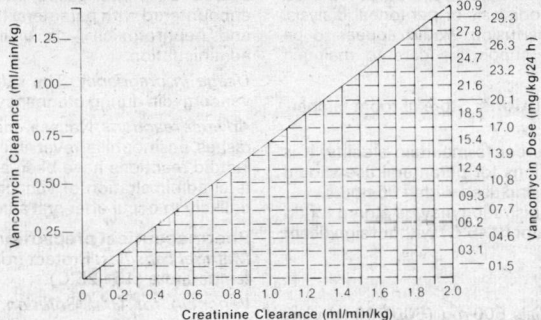

Dosage Nomogram for Vancomycin in Patients with Impaired Renal Function

The nomogram is not valid for functionally anephric patients on dialysis. For such patients, a loading dose of 15 mg/kg body weight should be given to achieve therapeutic serum levels promptly, and the dose required to maintain stable levels is 1.9 mg/kg/24 hours.

Preparation of solution: At the time of use, add 10 ml of Water for Injections PhEur to the vial.

Further dilution is required. Read instructions which follow:

1. Intermittent infusion (the preferred method of administration). The above solution (containing 500 mg vancomycin) can be added to 100–200 ml Sodium Chloride Intravenous Infusion BP or 5% Dextrose Intravenous Infusion BP. The intravenous infusion should be given over a period of at least 60 minutes every six hours. If administered over a shorter period of time or in higher concentrations, there is the possibility of inducing marked hypotension in addition to thrombophlebitis. Rapid administration may also produce flushing and a transient rash over the neck and shoulders.

2. Continuous infusion (should be used only when intermittent infusion is not feasible). Two to four vials (1–2 g) can be added to a sufficiently large volume of Sodium Chloride Intravenous Infusion BP or 5% Dextrose Intravenous Infusion BP to permit the desired daily dose to be administered slowly by intravenous drip over a 24-hour period.

Oral administration

Adults and the elderly: The usual daily dose given is 500 mg–1 g in divided doses. Each dose may be reconstituted in 30 ml water and either given to the patient to drink, or administered by nasogastric tube.

Children: The dose should be adjusted for age and body weight.

Either the oral preparation or the contents of the 500 mg vial for parenteral administration may be used.

Contra-indications, warnings, etc

Contra-indication: Hypersensitivity to vancomycin.

Warnings: Since vancomycin is not significantly absorbed from the gastro-intestinal tract, the toxicity encountered with parenteral therapy is unlikely to occur after oral administration.

Because of its ototoxicity and nephrotoxicity, vancomycin should be used with care in patients with renal insufficiency and the dose should be reduced according to the degree of renal impairment. The risk of toxicity is appreciably increased by high blood concentrations or prolonged therapy. Blood levels should be monitored and renal function tests should be performed regularly.

Vancomycin should also be avoided in patients with previous hearing loss. If it is used in such patients, the dose should be regulated, if possible, by periodic determination of the drug level in the blood. Deafness may be preceded by tinnitus. The elderly are more susceptible to auditory damage. Experience with other antibiotics suggests that deafness may be progressive despite cessation of treatment.

Concurrent and sequential use of other neurotoxic and/or nephrotoxic antibiotics, particularly streptomycin, neomycin, kanamycin, gentamicin, cephaloridine, paromomycin, viomycin, polymyxin B, colistin and tobramycin, should be avoided.

Usage in pregnancy: Animal studies indicate that vancomycin crosses the placental barrier and is excreted in milk.

There is only one documented case of administration during human pregnancy. A patient received 28 days' therapy during the second trimester and no congenital abnormalities were detected in the infant. If it is necessary to prescribe vancomycin during pregnancy, blood levels should be monitored carefully to minimise the risk of fetal toxicity.

Precautions: Patients with borderline renal function and individuals over the age of 60 should be given serial tests of auditory function and of vancomycin blood levels. All patients receiving the drug should have periodic haematological studies, urine analysis, and liver and renal function tests.

Vancomycin is very irritating to tissue, and causes necrosis when injected intramuscularly; it must be injected intravenously. Pain and thrombophlebitis occur in many patients receiving vancomycin and are occasionally severe.

The frequency and severity of thrombophlebitis can be minimised if the drug is administered in a volume of at least 200 ml of a recommended diluent and if the sites of injection are regularly changed.

The use of vancomycin may result in overgrowth of non-susceptible organisms. If new infections due to bacteria or fungi appear during treatment, appropriate measures should be taken.

Adverse reactions: Nausea, chills, fever, urticaria and macular rashes have been associated with the administration of vancomycin. Eosinophilia, reversible neutropenia and anaphylactoid reactions have also been reported.

Treatment of overdosage: Vancomycin is not removed from the blood by haemodialysis or peritoneal dialysis. Amberlite resin haemoperfusion would appear to be effective, together with supportive care to maintain glomerular filtration rate.

Pharmaceutical precautions Store at room temperature (15°–25°C).

After reconstitution: In order to maintain sterility, it is recommended that solutions for parenteral use should be stored in a refrigerator and used within 96 hours.

Solutions for oral administration may be stored for up to two weeks in a refrigerator (0°–6°C) without significant loss of potency.

Legal category POM.

Package quantities Vials 500 mg (500,000 IU vancomycin). Single vials.

Further information Following multiple intravenous doses of 1 g every 12 hours, therapeutic peak levels of 25–40 mg/l and trough levels of 3–10 mg/l are achieved. Ototoxicity has been associated with serum drug levels of 80–100 mg/l, but this is rarely seen when serum levels are kept at or below 30 mg/l.

Product licence number 0006/5076.

VANCOCIN* MATRIGEL CAPSULES
VANCOCIN* FOR ORAL SOLUTION

Presentation Matrigel capsules (dark blue and grey, coded Lilly 3126) containing 250 mg Vancomycin Hydrochloride BP. Matrigel capsules (dark blue and peach, coded Lilly 3125) containing 125 mg Vancomycin Hydrochloride BP.

Screw cap containers each containing Vancomycin Hydrochloride for Oral Solution USP, 10,000,000 IU, equivalent to 10 g vancomycin.

These preparations are for oral use only. If parenteral vancomycin therapy is desired, use Vancocin (Sterile Vancomycin Hydrochloride BP) Injection, and consult literature accompanying that preparation.

Uses Vancomycin may be used orally for the treatment of staphylococcal enterocolitis and pseudomembranous colitis due to *Clostridium difficile.*

Vancomycin is not absorbed from the gastro-intestinal tract and is therefore not effective by the oral route for other types of infection; parenteral administration may be used concomitantly if required.

Dosage and administration For oral administration.

Adults and the elderly: The usual daily dose is 500 mg–1 g in divided doses.

Children: The dose should be adjusted for age and body weight.

Vancocin for Oral Solution: Each dose may be reconstituted in 30 ml water and either given to the patient to drink, or administered by nasogastric tube. The contents of the container may be mixed with distilled or deionized water (115 ml) for oral administration. When mixed with 115 ml of water, each 6 ml provides approximately 500 mg of vancomycin. Mix thoroughly to dissolve.

Either the oral preparations or the contents of the 500 mg vial for parenteral administration may be used.

Contra-indications, warnings, etc
Contra-indication: Hypersensitivity to vancomycin.

Warnings: Since vancomycin is not significantly absorbed from the gastro-intestinal tract, the toxicity encountered with parenteral therapy (mainly ototoxicity and nephrotoxicity) is unlikely to occur after oral administration.

Usage in pregnancy: The safety of orally administered vancomycin during pregnancy has not been established.

Adverse reactions: Nausea, chills, fever, urticaria, macular rashes, eosinophilia, reversible neutropenia, and anaphylactoid reactions have been associated with the parenteral administration of vancomycin. Such reactions are unlikely to occur after oral administration.

Pharmaceutical precautions
Matrigel capsules: Protect from moisture. Store at room temperature (15°–25°C).

Vancocin for Oral Solution: Keep containers tightly closed.

After reconstitution, solutions may be stored for up to two weeks in a refrigerator (0°–6°C) without significant loss of potency.

Legal category POM.

Package quantities *Matrigel capsules:* Blister packs of 20 (2 strips of 10 capsules).

Vancocin for Oral Solution: Single containers of 10 g.

Further information The bitter taste of vancomycin can be avoided by the use of the matrigel capsules. Vancomycin powder should be used when the patient is unable to swallow the capsules.

Product licence numbers
Matrigel Capsules 250 mg 0006/0194
Matrigel Capsules 125 mg 0006/0193
Containers 10 g   0006/0081

VELBE*

Presentation Vials containing 10 mg Velbe (Vinblastine Sulphate BP) in the form of a lyophilised plug.

Velbe is supplied in a combination package with an accompanying vial of diluting solution, 10 ml containing 90 mg Sodium Chloride PhEur, with 2% Benzyl Alcohol BP as a preservative.

Uses Velbe is an anti-neoplastic drug for intravenous use.

Information available at present suggests that Velbe may be useful, either alone or in combination with other oncolytic drugs for the treatment of: Generalised Hodgkin's disease (Stages III and IV). Lymphosarcoma. Reticulum cell sarcoma. Mycosis fungoides. Neuroblastoma. Histiocytosis X (Letterer-Siwe disease). Seminoma and embryonal tumours of the testis. Carcinoma of the breast, unresponsive to appropriate endocrine surgery and hormonal therapy. Some carcinomas of the skin and mucosa. Methotrexate-resistant choriocarcinoma.

Other neoplasms occasionally show a marked response to Velbe, but less frequently than the more susceptible conditions listed above.

Dosage and administration There are variations in the depth of the granulocytopenic response to Velbe. For this reason, it is recommended that the drug be given no more frequently than once every seven days. It is wise to begin therapy with a single intravenous dose of 0.1 mg/kg. A nomogram dosage card is available on request for the guidance of clinicians who prefer to relate dosage to body surface area. Thereafter, granulocyte counts should be made to determine the patient's sensitivity to the drug. A simplified and conservative incremental approach to dosage at weekly intervals may be outlined as follows:

First dose	0.1 mg/kg
Second dose	0.15 mg/kg
Third dose	0.2 mg/kg
Fourth dose	0.25 mg/kg
Fifth dose	0.3 mg/kg

The same increases may be used until a maximum dose (not exceeding 0.5 mg/kg) is reached. *This schedule applies to adults, children and the elderly.* The dose should not be increased after that dose which reduces the granulocyte count to approximately 1,500 cells/mm^3. In some patients, 0.1 mg/kg may produce this granulocytopenia, others may require more than 0.3 mg/kg and very rarely as much as 0.5 mg/kg may be necessary. For most patients, however, the weekly dosage will prove to be in the range of 0.15–0.2 mg/kg.

When the dose of Velbe which will produce the above degree of granulocytopenia has been established, a dose *one increment smaller* than this should be administered at weekly intervals for maintenance. Thus, the patient is receiving the maximum dose that does not cause granulocytopenia. It should be emphasised that, even though seven days have elapsed, the next dose of Velbe should not be given until the granulocyte count has returned to at least 2000/mm^3. In some cases, oncolytic activity may be encountered before granulocytopenic effect. When this occurs there is no need to increase the size of subsequent doses. Maintenance therapy of indefinite duration should consist of the maximum dose than can be administered regularly on an outpatient basis every seven to fourteen days without reducing the granulocyte count to a dangerous level.

Many authorities in recent years have investigated and reported good results with the use of Velbe in combination with other cancer chemotherapeutic agents.

To prepare a solution containing 1 mg/ml add 10 ml of the accompanying diluting solution to the 10 mg vial. The drug dissolves rapidly to give a clear solution.

The dose of Velbe solution (calculated to provide the desired number of milligrams per kilogram of the patient's weight) may be injected either into the tubing of a running intravenous infusion of sodium chloride 0.9% or directly into a vein. The latter procedure is readily adaptable to outpatient therapy. In either case, the injection may be completed in about one minute. If care is taken to ensure that the needle is securely within the vein and that no solution containing Velbe is spilled extravascularly, cellulitis and/or phlebitis will not occur.

Because of the enhanced possibility of thrombosis, it is considered inadvisable to inject a solution of Velbe into an extremity in which the circulation is impaired, or potentially impaired, by such conditions as compressing or invading neoplasm, phlebitis or varicosity.

Caution: If leakage into surrounding tissue should occur during intravenous administration of Velbe, it may cause considerable irritation. The injection should be discontinued immediately, and any remaining portion of the dose should then be introduced into another vein. Local injection of hyaluronidase or hydrocortisone and the application of moderate heat to the area of leakage help to disperse the drug, and are thought to minimise discomfort and the possibility of cellulitis.

It is important to avoid contamination of the eyes with concentrations of Velbe used clinically. If accidental contamination occurs, severe irritation (or if the drug was delivered under pressure, even corneal ulceration) may result. The eye should be washed with water thoroughly and immediately.

Contra-indications, warnings, etc

Contra-indications: Intrathecal administration. Velbe is contra-indicated in patients who are granulocytopenic. It should not be used in the presence of bacterial infection. Such infections must be brought under control with antiseptics or antibiotics before using Velbe.

Warning – Usage in pregnancy: Caution is necessary with the use of all oncolytic drugs during pregnancy. Information on the use of Velbe during pregnancy is very limited. Although no abnormalities of the human fetus have been reported thus far, animal studies with Velbe have shown evidence of teratogenicity.

This product should not normally be administered to patients who are pregnant or to mothers who are breast feeding, unless the potential benefits clearly outweigh the risks.

Precautions: Clinically, granulocytopenia is an expected effect of Velbe, and the level of the granulocyte count is an important guide to treatment. In general, the larger the dose employed, the more profound and longer lasting the granulocytopenia will be. The fact that the granulocyte count returns to normal levels after drug-induced granulocytopenia is an indication that the granulocyte-producing mechanism is not permanently depressed. Usually, the granulocyte count has completely returned to normal after the virtual disappearance of granulocytes from the peripheral blood.

Following therapy with Velbe, the nadir in the granulocyte count may be expected to occur five to ten days after the last day of drug administration. Recovery of the granulocyte count is fairly rapid thereafter and is usually complete within another seven to fourteen days. With the smaller doses employed for maintenance, granulocytopenia may not be a problem.

Although the thrombocyte count is not usually significantly lowered by therapy with Velbe, patients whose bone marrow has been recently impaired by prior therapy with radiation or with other oncolytic drugs may show thrombocytopenia (less than 150,000 platelets/mm^3). When other chemotherapy or radiation has not been employed previously, thrombocyte reduction below the level of 150,000/mm^3 is rarely encountered, even when Velbe may be causing significant granulocytopenia. Rapid recovery from thrombocytopenia within a few days is the rule.

The effect of Velbe upon the red blood cell count and haemoglobin is usually insignificant when other treatment does not complicate the picture. It should be remembered, however, that patients with malignant disease may exhibit anaemia even in the absence of any treatment.

If granulocytopenia with less than 1,000 granulocytes/mm^3 occurs following a dose of Velbe, the patient should be watched carefully for evidence of infection until the granulocyte count has returned to a safe level.

When cachexia or ulcerated areas of the skin surface are present, there may be a more profound granulocytopenic response to the drug. Its use should be avoided in older persons suffering from either of these conditions.

In patients with malignant-cell infiltration of the bone marrow, the granulocyte and platelet counts have sometimes fallen drastically after moderate doses of Velbe. Further use of the drug in such patients is inadvisable.

The use of small amounts of Velbe daily for long

periods is not advised, even though the resulting total weekly dosage may be similar to that recommended. Little or no added therapeutic effect has been demonstrated when such regimens have been used. Strict adherence to the recommended dosage schedule is very important. When amounts equal to several times the recommended weekly dosage were given in seven daily instalments for long periods, convulsions, severe and permanent central nervous system damage, and even death occurred.

As Velbe is excreted principally by the liver, it may be necessary to reduce initial doses in the presence of significantly impaired hepatic or biliary function.

When chemotherapy is being given in conjunction with radiation therapy through portals which include the liver, the use of Velbe should be delayed until radiation therapy has been completed.

Acute shortness of breath and severe bronchospasm have been reported following the administration of the vinca alkaloids. These reactions have been encountered most frequently when using combination therapy with mitomycin-C. The onset may be within minutes, or several hours after the drug is injected.

Adverse reactions: In general, the incidence of side-effects attending the use of Velbe appears to be related to the size of dosage employed. With the exception of alopecia and granulocytopenia, adverse reactions have not usually persisted for longer than 24 hours. Granulocytopenia, the most common adverse reaction, is usually the dose-limiting factor.

Gastro-intestinal – nausea, vomiting, constipation, ileus, diarrhoea, anorexia, abdominal pain, rectal bleeding, pharyngitis, haemorrhagic enterocolitis, bleeding from an old peptic ulcer.

Neurological – numbness, paraesthesiae, peripheral neuritis, mental depression, loss of deep tendon reflexes, headache, convulsions.

Cutaneous – ulceration of the mouth and skin, and alopecia. When alopecia develops it is frequently not total, and, in some cases, hair regrows while maintenance therapy continues.

Miscellaneous – malaise, weakness, dizziness and pain in tumour site. Inappropriate ADH secretion has been reported rarely.

Overdosage: Side-effects following the use of Velbe are dose related. Therefore, following administration of more than the recommended dose patients can be expected to experience these effects in an exaggerated fashion.

In addition, neurotoxicity similar to that seen with Oncovin (vincristine sulphate) may be observed.

Treatment: Supportive care should include: 1) prevention of the side-effects that result from the syndrome of inappropriate secretion of antidiuretic hormone. This includes restriction of fluid intake and perhaps the use of a diuretic acting on the loop of Henle and distal tubule function; 2) administration of an anticonvulsant; 3) prevention and treatment of ileus; 4) monitoring the patient's cardiovascular system; and 5) daily blood counts for guidance in transfusion requirement.

The major effect of excessive doses of Velbe will be on granulocytopoeisis, and this may be life-threatening.

Pharmaceutical precautions Vials of Velbe should be stored in a refrigerator between 0° and 6°C.

After reconstitution: After a portion of the solution has been removed from a vial, the remainder of the contents of the vial may be stored in a refrigerator for further use for 30 days without significant loss of potency. When the reconstituted vial of Velbe is to be stored for more than 48 hours, it is essential to use the accompanying diluting solution or a diluent which contains a preservative. Velbe should never be mixed with any other drug.

Legal category POM.

Package quantities Vials 10 mg: Single vials.

Further information Nil.

Product licence numbers
Vials 10 mg:　　0006/5073
Diluent:　　　　0006/5174

*Trade Mark

Lipha Pharmaceuticals Limited
Harrier House, High Street
Yiewsley
West Drayton
Middlesex UB7 7QG

ARGOTONE*

Presentation Brown liquid containing the following active ingredients:

Ephedrine Hydrochloride BP	0.9%
Mild Silver Protein BPC 1968	1.0%

Uses Nasal decongestant.

Dosage and administration *Argotone Nasal Drops:* 4–6 drops in each nostril three to five times daily.
Argotone Ready Spray: 2–3 sprays in each nostril four to five times daily.

Contra-indications, warnings, etc As with all sympathomimetic amines, prolonged use may cause rebound congestion, although we have not received reports of this caused by Argotone. Concurrent administration with monoamine oxidase inhibitors is contra-indicated.
Side-effects: Either incorrect or excessive usage could cause skin discolouration.
Overdosage – Signs and Symptoms: Argyria – a bluish-black discolouration of the skin would indicate ingestion. The signs and symptoms of toxicity would be those of ephedrine overdosage. Features such as anxiety, insomnia, irritability, giddiness, headache, nausea and vomiting, palpitations, tachycardia, hypertension and difficulty in micturition may occur. In very large doses paranoid psychosis and hallucinations may be prominent. Theoretically, in excessive use sufficient ephedrine could be absorbed via the nasal mucosa, particularly in infants, to produce these symptoms. However, at the present time, we have received no such reports.
Overdosage – Treatment: Since severe overdosage is considered to be so unlikely, treatment should consist mainly of careful monitoring of the patient, particularly respiration and circulation. Methods directed at prevention of further absorption of the ingredients such as emesis or gastric lavage generally are considered inappropriate.

Pharmaceutical precautions Argotone should be protected from light. The shelf-life is 5 years.

Legal category P.

Package quantities *Argotone Nasal Drops:* Glass bottle containing 20 ml.
Argotone Ready Spray: Plastic atomiser containing 15 ml.

Further information Argotone has a rapid effect against all organisms commonly infecting the naso-pharynx. Argotone relieves the congestion of mucous membranes but does not inhibit nasal cilia.

Product licence number 0161/5005.

GLUCOPHAGE*

Presentation White, film-coated tablets, marked 'GL 500', containing 500 mg Metformin Hydrochloride BP.
White, film-coated tablets, marked 'GL 850', containing 850 mg Metformin Hydrochloride BP.

Uses *Indications:* Non-insulin dependent diabetes where diet has failed and especially if the patient is overweight. Glucophage can be given alone as initial therapy, or can be administered in combination with a sulphonylurea.
In insulin-dependent diabetes, Glucophage may be given as an adjuvant to patients whose symptoms are poorly controlled.
Pharmacology: Glucophage is a biguanide oral anti-hyperglycaemic agent. Its mode of action is thought to be multifactorial and includes delayed uptake of glucose from the gastro-intestinal tract, increased peripheral glucose utilisation mediated by increased insulin sensitivity and inhibition of increased hepatic and renal gluconeogenesis.

Dosage and administration
Adults: Initially, one 850 mg tablet twice a day or one 500 mg tablet three times a day, taken after meals. Good diabetic control may be achieved within a few days, but it is not unusual for the full effect to be delayed for up to two weeks. If control is incomplete a cautious increase in dosage to a maximum of 3 g daily is justified. Once control has been obtained it may be possible to reduce the dosage of Glucophage.
Children: Glucophage is not recommended for use in children.
Elderly patients: Renal function may be reduced in some elderly patients and Glucophage should therefore be used with caution.

Contra-indications, warnings, etc
Contra-indications: Diabetic coma and ketoacidosis, impairment of renal function, chronic liver disease, cardiac failure, recent myocardial infarction, alcoholism (acute or chronic), conditions associated with hypoxaemia, states associated with lactic acidosis such as shock or pulmonary insufficiency, history of lactic acidosis.
Precautions: Glucophage is excreted by the kidney and should be used with care in patients with decreased

renal function. Regular monitoring of renal functions is advised in all diabetic patients.

The use of Glucophage is not advised during pregnancy or lactation, in conditions which may cause dehydration, or in patients suffering from serious infections or trauma. Glucophage therapy should be stopped 2–3 days before surgery and clinical investigations such as intravenous urography and intravenous angiography and reinstated only after control of renal function has been regained.

It is recommended that patients receiving continuous Glucophage therapy should have an annual estimation of Vitamin B_{12} levels because of reports of decreased Vitamin B_{12} absorption.

During concomitant therapy with a sulphonylurea, blood glucose should be monitored because combined therapy may cause hypoglycaemia. It is recommended that stabilisation of diabetic patients with Glucophage and insulin should be carried out in hospital because of the possibility of hypoglycaemia until the correct ratio of the two drugs has been obtained.

As with a number of drugs, an interaction between Glucophage and anticoagulants is a possibility and dosage of the latter may need adjustment.

Side-effects: Glucophage is normally well tolerated but gastro-intestinal disturbances sometimes occur. These are usually minor and can often be avoided by taking Glucophage with meals but occasionally a temporary lowering of the dose may be needed. It is important that Glucophage treatment is not abandoned at the first sign of intolerance, since this has been found to resolve spontaneously.

Lactic acidosis has been associated with Glucophage but, in the few cases reported, has occurred in patients with contra-indications to therapy. In patients with a metabolic acidosis lacking evidence of ketoacidosis (ketonuria and ketonaemia), lactic acidosis should be suspected and Glucophage therapy should be stopped. Lactic acidosis is a medical emergency which must be treated in hospital immediately.

Overdosage – Signs and Symptoms: Hypoglycaemia does not occur with Glucophage monotherapy (fifty tablets have been ingested with no untoward effects on blood glucose levels). However, it can occur when Glucophage is given concomitantly with a sulphonylurea, insulin or alcohol.

In excessive dosage, and particularly if there is a possibility of accumulation, lactic acidosis may develop.

Overdosage – Treatment: Intensive supportive therapy is recommended which should be particularly directed at correcting fluid loss and metabolic disturbance.

Pharmaceutical precautions No special storage requirements. The shelf-life is 5 years.

Legal category POM.

Package quantities *500 mg:* Securitainers containing 100 or 500 tablets.
850 mg: Securitainers containing 60 or 300 tablets.

Further information Glucophage does not lower blood glucose levels in non-diabetics, and does not cause hypoglycaemia in diabetics when used as monotherapy. Weight loss often occurs during therapy and levels of plasma cholesterol, triglycerides and prebetalipoproteins may be lowered. Glucophage has been shown to improve peripheral glucose metabolism.

Product licence numbers
Glucophage 500 mg   3759/0012
Glucophage 850 mg   3759/0013

IONAMIN*

Presentation *Ionamin 15:* Grey and yellow opaque capsule containing cationic exchange resin complex equivalent to 15 mg phentermine.
Ionamin 30: Yellow opaque capsule containing cationic exchange resin complex equivalent to 30 mg phentermine.

Uses Ionamin is an anorectic agent intended for short term use as an adjunct to the treatment of patients with moderate to severe obesity for whom close support and supervision are also to be provided.

Dosage and administration 15 or 30 mg as a sustained release capsule daily before breakfast or 10 to 14 hours before retiring. The recommended dose should not be exceeded in an attempt to increase the anorectic effect. In non-responsive cases, the drug should be discontinued.

Ionamin is not recommended for use in the very elderly or in children.

Several clinical studies have indicated that an intermittent dosage regime consisting of treatment for up to 4 weeks followed by a similar period without medication may be as effective as continuous treatment.

The efficacy and safety of Ionamin in long term intermittent use (more than 6 months) have not been established. The possibility of dependence with continuous use should be considered.

Contra-indications, warnings, etc
Contra-indications: Severe hypertension, thyrotoxicosis, patients with a history of psychiatric illness or drug or alcohol abuse, emotionally unstable or vulnerable personalities, concurrent or recent use of MAOI's, concurrent use of other appetite suppressant drugs and patients with a known hypersensitivity to sympathomimetic agents.

Use in pregnancy and nursing mothers: There is inadequate evidence of safety of Ionamin in human pregnancy; there is evidence of harmful effects in animals with amphetamines. As with amphetamines, treatment should cease during pregnancy. Excretion of phentermine into breast milk: No information is available.

Precautions: Ionamin should be used with caution in patients being treated with psychotropic drugs including sympathomimetic agents, antihypertensive medication, and in those receiving anti-diabetic drugs. Additionally, the insulin requirements of the latter group may become altered in association with the use of Ionamin and concomitant dietary regimes.

Warnings: Phentermine is structurally and pharmacologically related to the amphetamines, drugs which have been extensively abused for euphoriant effect, and are capable of inducing physical dependence. Experience has shown that generally neither of these are problems, although dependence has been reported in a few cases.

Phentermine may produce mild CNS excitation and there is a theoretical risk of sedation on withdrawal of the drug: if the patient is affected, his ability to drive or operate machinery may be impaired. Phentermine may enhance the response to alcohol.

Adverse effects: When these occur they may include

dryness of mouth, restlessness, nervousness, insomnia, palpitations, constipation, nausea, vomiting, rashes, euphoria and agitation. There is a theoretical possibility of raised blood pressure.

Overdosage: Manifestations of acute overdosage may include signs of CNS stimulation such as restlessness, agitation, euphoria, hallucinations and tremor; usually followed by fatigue and depression. Cardiovascular effects include arrhythmias, hypertension and circulatory collapse. Gastrointestinal effects include nausea, vomiting, diarrhoea and abdominal cramps.

Management of acute phentermine intoxication is largely symptomatic and includes lavage and sedation with diazepam.

Pharmaceutical precautions No special storage precautions are required. The shelf-life is 3 years.

Legal category CD (Sch 3), POM.

Package quantities Available in packs of 100.

Further information Nil.

Product licence numbers
Ionamin 15 mg 3759/0007
Ionamin 30 mg 3759/0008

KELOCYANOR*

Presentation Clear 20 ml ampoules filled with a sterile aqueous rose-coloured solution containing 300 mg dicobalt edetate (15 mg/ml).

Uses
Indications: Kelocyanor is a specific antidote for acute cyanide poisoning. In view of the difficulty of certain diagnosis in emergency situations, it is recommended that Kelocyanor only be given when the patient is tending to lose, or has lost, consciousness. The product should not be used as a precautionary measure (see warnings section).

Dosage and administration Cyanide poisoning must be treated as quickly as possible.

Adults: One ampoule of Kelocyanor should be given intravenously over approximately one minute. If the patient shows inadequate response, a second ampoule of Kelocyanor may be given. If there is no response after a further five minutes, a third ampoule may be administered.

Each ampoule of Kelocyanor may be followed immediately by 50 ml Dextrose Intravenous Infusion BP 500 g/l.

When the patient's condition is less severe but, in the physician's judgement, still warrants the use of Kelocyanor, the period over which the injection is given should be extended to 5 minutes.

Children: There is no clinical experience of the use of Kelocyanor in children. It is suggested that the dosage of Kelocyanor should be adjusted according to body-weight and response.

Elderly patients: There is no clinical experience of the use of Kelocyanor in the elderly, but there is no reason to believe that the dosage schedule should be different from that for adults.

Contra-indications, warnings, etc
Warnings: There is a reciprocal antidote action between cyanide and cobalt. Thus in the absence of cyanide, Kelocyanor is itself toxic. It is therefore essential that the

product only be used in cases of cyanide poisoning. When the patient is fully conscious, it is unlikely that the extent of poisoning warrants the use of Kelocyanor. However, when cyanide is ingested in solid form, it is possible for the appearance of signs of poisoning to be delayed. In this circumstance, when cyanide ingestion is certain, Kelocyanor can be used.

Side-effects: The initial effects of Kelocyanor are vomiting, a fall in blood pressure, and compensatory tachycardia. After this the patient should recover.

Overdosage – signs and symptoms: These may be due to cobalt toxicity or to an anaphylactic type reaction, which may be dramatic. Symptoms such as oedema (particularly of the face and neck), vomiting, chest pain, sweating, hypotension, cardiac irregularities, and rashes have been reported.

Overdosage – treatment: Intensive supportive therapy followed by careful monitoring for at least 48 hours is required.

Pharmaceutical precautions Store below 25°C. The shelf-life is 3 years.

Legal category POM.

Package quantities Carton containing 6 × 20 ml ampoules.

Further information Nil.

Product licence number 3759/5901.

NITROLINGUAL* SPRAY ▼

Presentation A metered-dose aerosol which delivers 0.4 mg glyceryl trinitrate per spray emission. This presentation provides for very rapid buccal absorption from the spray droplets producing an almost immediate effect.

Uses *Indications:* For the treatment and prophylaxis of angina pectoris and the treatment of variant angina.

Pharmacology: Glyceryl trinitrate relieves angina pectoris by reduction of cardiac work and dilation of the coronary arteries. In this way, not only is there a lessening in arterial oxygen requirement, but the amount of oxygenated blood reaching the ischaemic heart is increased.

Dosage and administration
Dosage: Adults: At the onset of an attack: one or two metered-doses to be sprayed onto the oral mucosa. No more than three metered-doses are generally recommended at any one time. For the prevention of exercise-induced angina or in other precipitating conditions: one or two metered-doses to be sprayed onto the oral mucosa immediately prior to the event.

Children: The spray is not recommended.

Administration: During application the patient should rest, ideally in the sitting position. The canister should be held vertically with the valve head uppermost and the spray orifice as close to the mouth as possible. The dose should preferably be sprayed under the tongue and the mouth should be closed immediately after each dose. THE SPRAY SHOULD NOT BE INHALED. Patients should be instructed to familiarize themselves with the position of the spray orifice, which can be identified by the finger rest on top of the valve, in order to facilitate orientation for administration at night.

Contra-indications, warnings, etc

Contra-indications: As with all nitrates: marked anaemia; shock and hypotension; cerebral haemorrhage and brain trauma; mitral stenosis and angina caused by hypertrophic obstructive cardiomyopathy; hypersensitivity to nitrates.

Precautions: The spray is not recommended for use during pregnancy. As with other nitrates tolerance to this drug and cross tolerance to other nitrates may occur. The hypotensive effect may be enhanced by alcohol.

Adverse Reactions: These are common to all nitrates used for the treatment of angina pectoris. Cutaneous vasodilatation with flushing, tachycardia and occasionally unexplained bradycardia. Headache may occur but can usually be controlled by reducing the dose, or the administration of analgesics.

Postural hypotension which may cause cerebral ischaemia and present as transient episodes of dizziness and weakness.

Overdosage – Signs and Symptoms: As with all nitrates large doses may cause flushing of the face, severe headache, a feeling of suffocation, hypotension and fainting. Rarely cyanosis and methaemoglobinaemia may occur. In a few patients there may be a reaction comparable to shock with nausea, vomiting, weakness, sweating and syncope.

Overdosage – Treatment: Recovery often occurs without special treatment. Hypotension may be corrected by elevation of the legs to promote venous return. Methaemoglobinaemia should be treated by intravenous methylene blue.

In the event of more serious overdosage symptomatic treatment should be given for respiratory and circulatory defects.

Pharmaceutical precautions Nitrolingual Spray should be stored in a cool place, protected from frost and direct heat or sunlight. The canister should not be broken, punctured or burnt, even when apparently empty. Only empty canisters should be discarded. The shelf-life is 3 years.

Legal category P.

Package quantities Canisters containing 200 metered-doses.

Further information Unlike glyceryl trinitrate sublingual tablets, Nitrolingual Spray does not deteriorate on storage. No loss of potency occurs throughout the 3 year shelf-life of the product.

Glyceryl trinitrate is also known as nitroglycerin, trinitroglycerin and trinitrin.

Product licence number 3759/0010.

NITRONAL* ▼

Presentation 5 ml and 25 ml amber glass ampoules and 50 ml clear glass vials containing 1 mg/ml glyceryl trinitrate in isotonic aqueous solution.

Uses

Indications:

1. Unresponsive congestive heart failure, including that secondary to acute myocardial infarction.
2. Refractory unstable angina pectoris and coronary insufficiency, including Prinzmetal's angina.

3. Control of hypertensive episodes and/or myocardial ischaemia during and after cardiac surgery. For the induction of controlled hypotension for surgery.

Pharmacology: Glyceryl trinitrate exerts a spasmolytic action on smooth muscle, particularly in the vascular system. The predominant effect is an increase in venous capacitance resulting in marked diminution of both the left ventricular filling pressure and volume (preload). There is also a reduction in afterload due to moderate dilation of the arteriolar resistance vessels. These haemodynamic changes lower the myocardial oxygen demand. By direct action and through the reduction of myocardial wall tension, glyceryl trinitrate also lowers the resistance to flow in the coronary collateral channels and allows re-distribution of blood flow to ischaemic areas of the myocardium.

Administration of Nitronal by intravenous infusion to patients with congestive heart failure results in a marked improvement in haemodynamics, reduction of elevated left ventricular filling pressure and systolic wall tension, and an increase in the depressed cardiac output. It reduces the imbalance that exists between myocardial oxygen demand and delivery, thereby diminishing myocardial ischaemia and controlling ischaemia-induced ventricular arrhythmias.

Dosage and administration

Dosage: Adults – The dose should be titrated against the individual clinical response.

1. Unresponsive congestive heart failure. The normal dose range is 10–100 µg/minute administered as a continuous intravenous infusion with frequent monitoring of blood pressure and heart rate. The infusion should be started at the lower rate and increased cautiously until the desired clinical response is achieved. Other haemodynamic measurements are extremely important in monitoring response to the drug: these may include pulmonary capillary wedge pressure, cardiac output and precordial electrocardiogram depending on the clinical picture. Under these conditions infusion may be continued for several days.
2. Refractory unstable angina pectoris. An initial infusion rate of 10–15 µg/minute is recommended; this may be increased cautiously in increments of 5–10 µg until either relief of angina is achieved, headache prevents further increase in dose, or the mean arterial pressure falls by more than 20 mm Hg.
3. Use in surgery. An initial infusion rate of 25 µg/minute is recommended; this should be increased gradually until the desired systolic arterial pressure is attained. The usual dose is 25–200 µg/minute.

Children – There is no recommended dose for children.

Administration
Undiluted: Nitronal need not be diluted before use.

Diluted: Nitronal can be diluted with Dextrose Injection BP, Sodium Chloride and Dextrose Injection BP, 0.9% Sodium Chloride Injection BP or other protein-free infusion solution, if required.

Infusion: The solution, whether or not diluted, should be infused *slowly* (see dosage section) and *not* given by bolus injection.

To ensure a constant infusion rate of glyceryl trinitrate, it is recommended that Nitronal be administered by means of a syringe pump or polyethylene infusion bag with a counter, with a glass or rigid polyethylene syringe and polyethylene tubing. Systems made of polyvinylchloride may adsorb up to 50% of the glyceryl trinitrate from the solution, thus reducing the efficacy of the infusion. If the recommended type of system is unavailable, a 1:10 dilution of Nitronal should be used and the infusion rate modified according to the haemodynamic response of the patient, until the required parameters are attained.

Contra-indications, warnings, etc

Contra-indications: Hypotensive shock, known hypersensitivity to nitrates, marked anaemia, severe cerebral haemorrhage, arterial hypoxaemia, uncorrected hypovolaemia, angina caused by hypertrophic obstructive cardiomyopathy.

Precautions: As with other nitrates, caution should be exercised in patients with severe liver or renal disease, hypothermia or hypothyroidism. Safety during pregnancy and lactation has not been established. Glyceryl trinitrate may potentiate the action of other hypotensive drugs, and the hypotensive and anticholinergic effects of tricyclic anti-depressants; it may also slow the metabolism of morphine-like analgesics.

Adverse reactions: Nitronal is generally very well tolerated because a minimum dose is administered in unit time. Flushing of the face, reversible hypotension and tachycardia, dizziness and headache may be encountered, particularly if the infusion is administered too rapidly. Headache may be treated with analgesics if required. Other side effects common to all nitrates which may occur are nausea, diaphoresis, restlessness, retrosternal discomfort, abdominal pain or paradoxical bradycardia. These symptoms should be readily reversible on reducing the rate of infusion or, if necessary, discontinuing treatment.

Overdosage – signs and symptoms: Vomiting, restlessness, hypotension, syncope, cyanosis, coldness of the skin, impairment of respiration, bradycardia and psychosis.

Overdosage – treatment: The symptoms may be readily reversed by discontinuing treatment; if hypotension persists intravenous methoxamine or phenylephrine is recommended. Oxygen and assisted respiration may be required. In severe cases, intravenous administration of methoxamine or phenylephrine is recommended.

Pharmaceutical precautions Store in a cool place away from light. The vial is for single dose use only, and should be stored in the carton until ready for use.

The diluted solution should not be stored and should be administered as soon after dilution as possible; it is stable for up to 24 hours in the recommended infusion system.

Legal category POM.

Package quantities 5 ml ampoules available in cartons of 10 ampoules; 25 ml ampoules available in cartons of 10 ampoules; 50 ml vials available in individual cartons.

Further information Nitronal is available to hospitals only. Glyceryl trinitrate is also known as nitroglycerin, trinitroglycerin and trinitrin.

Product licence number 3759/0025.

NYDRANE*

Presentation White, uncoated tablets engraved 'Nydrane' on one side and a break line on the reverse, containing 500 mg Beclamide INN.

Uses Behaviour disorders, in epileptic or non-epileptic patients, particularly where instability is marked and aggressiveness a feature. Grand mal and psychomotor epilepsy.

Dosage and administration

1. *Behaviour disorders*
Adults: Initially 6 tablets (sometimes up to 8 tablets) of Nydrane daily in divided doses. Maintenance dosage will vary according to patient response. This will usually be from 3 to 6 tablets of Nydrane daily, but occasionally more may be required.

Children 5–10: 3 tablets daily in divided doses.

Children under 5: $1\frac{1}{2}$–2 tablets daily in divided doses.

2. *Epilepsy*
Caution – do not attempt immediate replacement of existing therapy.

Adults: Initially 6 tablets (sometimes up to 8 tablets) of Nydrane daily in divided doses. It is essential to delay reducing previous therapy until the maximum therapeutic effect of Nydrane has been obtained, which may take up to four weeks. Then existing medication may be reduced slowly and cautiously while maintaining control.

Children 5–10: 3 tablets daily in divided doses.

Children under 5: $1\frac{1}{2}$–2 tablets daily in divided doses.

Contra-indications, warnings, etc

Precautions: In epileptics it is essential to delay reducing previous therapy until the maximum therapeutic effect of Nydrane has been obtained, which may take up to four weeks. Caution is particularly essential in patients with a tendency to develop status epilepticus, or with a history of previous attacks.

Although no teratogenic effects have been reported during many years of use, in common with the majority of drugs the use of Nydrane during pregnancy should be avoided if possible. Secretion into breast milk; no information is available.

Side effects: The very few side effects reported have been of a mild and transient nature and include leucopenia, renal disturbance, loss of weight, dizziness, gastro-intestinal symptoms, skin irritation and rash.

Overdosage–Signs and Symptoms: Vertigo and vomiting are thought most likely to occur. Nystagmus has been reported. Theoretically there is a possibility of increased drowsiness leading to coma.

Overdosage – Treatment: Symptomatic treatment is recommended and neurological and biochemical monitoring for at least 48 hours. Patients have recovered from overdoses without special treatment. This information is based on two reported cases only.

Pharmaceutical precautions No special storage requirements. The shelf-life is 5 years.

Legal category POM.

Package quantities Securitainers containing 100 or 500 tablets.

Further information Free from side-effects commonly associated with anticonvulsant drugs, including gum hypertrophy and somnolence. Specific action in behaviour disorders, particularly if instability is marked and aggressiveness a feature.

Product licence number 3759/5900.

PRAXILENE*

Presentation Pale pink capsules overprinted PRAXI-LENE-Lipha each containing 100 mg of naftidrofuryl oxalate.

Uses *Indications:* Peripheral vascular disorders – intermittent claudication, night cramps, rest pain, incipient gangrene, trophic ulcers, Raynaud's syndrome, diabetic arteriopathy and acrocyanosis.

Cerebral vascular disorders – cerebral insufficiency and cerebral atherosclerosis, particularly where these manifest themselves as mental deterioration and confusion in the elderly.

Pharmacology: Praxilene has been shown to exert a direct effect on intracellular metabolism. Thus it has been demonstrated in animals and man that it produces an increase of ATP levels and a decrease of lactic acid levels in ischaemic conditions, evidence for an enhancement of cellular oxidative capacity. Furthermore Praxilene is a powerful spasmolytic agent.

Dosage and administration Peripheral vascular disorders: 1 to 2 capsules three times daily for a minimum of three months, or at the discretion of the Physician.

Cerebral vascular disorders: 1 capsule three times daily for a minimum of three months, or at the discretion of the Physician.

Contra-indications, warnings, etc
Contra-indications: Praxilene is contra-indicated in those patients who show a hypersensitivity to it.

Side-effects: Praxilene is normally well tolerated in the dosage recommended. Occasionally nausea and epigastric pain have been noted.

Overdosage: When this occurs, gastric lavage should be employed. Following overdosage, there may be depression of cardiac conduction, and, in severe cases, treatment with isoprenaline injection or electrical pacemaking should be considered. Convulsive crises may also be observed and these may be managed by diazepam.

Pharmaceutical precautions Store in a cool place away from light. The shelf-life is 3 years.

Legal category POM.

Package quantities Packs of 100 and 500 × 100 mg capsules.

Further information For the treatment of peripheral vascular disorders when symptoms of gross ischaemia, rest pain, or incipient gangrene are present, parenteral treatment with Praxilene Forte should be given in conjunction with oral therapy. The recommended dosing schedule is one 200 mg (10 ml) Praxilene Forte ampoule twice daily, given by infusion, for 7 to 10 days, together with 1 to 2 capsules three times daily.

Product licence number 3759/0002.

PRAXILENE FORTE*

Presentation Clear, colourless, 10 ml ampoules imprinted 'PRAXILENE FORTE', each containing 200 mg of naftidrofuryl oxalate (20 mg/ml).

Uses *Indications:* For the treatment of peripheral vascular disease when symptoms of gross ischaemia, rest pain or incipient gangrene are present.

Pharmacology: Praxilene has been shown to exert a direct effect on intracellular metabolism. Thus, it has been demonstrated in animals that it produces an increase of ATP levels and a decrease of lactic acid levels in ischaemic conditions, evidence for an enhancement of cellular oxidative capacity. Furthermore, Praxilene is a powerful spasmolytic agent.

Dosage and administration One 10 ml ampoule twice daily administered by intravenous or intra-arterial infusion in 250–500 ml of saline, dextrose or low molecular weight dextran, over a minimum of 90 minutes, for a period of 7 to 10 days. Praxilene Forte must NOT be given by bolus injection.

Contra-indications, warnings, etc
Contra-indications: Praxilene Forte should not be given to patients with atrioventricular block, or to those who show a hypersensitivity to the drug.

Precautions: Care should be exercised in patients with severe cardiac insufficiency and conduction disorders. The possibility of an additive effect occurring between Praxilene Forte and antiarrhythmic and beta-adrenergic blocking drugs should be considered.

Side-effects: Praxilene Forte is normally well tolerated in the dosage recommended; however, nausea has been occasionally noted.

Overdosage: When this occurs, there may be depression of cardiac conduction and, in severe cases, treatment with isoprenaline injection or electrical pacemaking should be considered. Convulsive crises may also be observed and these may be managed by diazepam.

Pharmaceutical precautions Store in a cool place away from light. The shelf-life is 3 years.

Praxilene Forte should not be given in solutions containing calcium ions.

Legal category POM.

Package quantities Packs of 10 ampoules.

Further information Praxilene capsules containing 100 mg of naftidrofuryl oxalate should be given together with the infusion therapy at a dosage of 1 or 2 capsules three times daily. On completion of the infusion therapy, the patient should continue on oral treatment, 1 or 2 capsules three times daily for a minimum of three months, or at the discretion of the Physician.

Product licence number 3759/0004.

SLO-PHYLLIN*

Presentation Capsules containing Theophylline BP (anhydrous) in a timed release formulation which provides a prolonged therapeutic effect over 12 hours.

60 mg: Size 2 opaque white capsule with a clear colourless cap, filled with white pellets. Each capsule contains 60 mg Theophylline BP (anhydrous).

125 mg: Size 1 opaque dark brown capsule with a clear colourless cap, filled with a mixture of brown and white pellets. Each capsule contains 125 mg Theophylline BP (anhydrous).

250 mg: Size 0 opaque blue capsule with a clear colourless cap, filled with a mixture of blue and white pellets. Each capsule contains 250 mg Theophylline BP (anhydrous).

Uses
Indications: As a bronchodilator in the symptomatic and

prophylactic treatment of asthma and for reversible bronchoconstriction associated with chronic bronchitis, bronchial asthma and emphysema.

Pharmacology: Theophylline inhibits the enzyme phosphodiesterase. This leads to an increase in intracellular concentrations of cyclic adenosine monophosphate (AMP) resulting in the relaxation of the bronchiolar smooth muscle and relief of bronchospasm.

Dosage and administration

Adults and children over 12 years: 250–500 mg twice daily.
Children 6–12 years (20–35 kg): 125–250 mg twice daily.
Children 2–6 years (10–20 kg): 60–120 mg twice daily.

Initially the lowest dosage suggested for each age group is recommended. This may be increased gradually if optimal bronchodilator effects are not achieved. Generally the total dosage should not exceed 24 mg/kg body weight in 24 hours for children under 9 years and 13 mg/kg body weight for adults. If a higher dosage is required it is strongly recommended that plasma theophylline concentrations should be monitored, since significant variations in the rate of drug elimination can occur among individuals.

Patients should be instructed not to chew or suck the capsules or pellets as this destroys the sustained release properties. However the contents of a capsule may be sprinkled onto a spoonful of soft food such as yoghurt for children who experience difficulty in swallowing the capsules.

Contra-indications, warnings, etc

Precautions: Careful monitoring is recommended for patients with congestive heart failure, chronic alcoholism or hepatic dysfunction as they may have lower total clearance of theophylline which could lead to higher than normal plasma levels.

Caution should be exercised in patients with peptic ulcers, cardiovascular disease (especially if cardiac arrhythmias are present), or with severe hypertension.

Slo-Phyllin should not be used concurrently with other preparations containing xanthine derivatives. If it is necessary to administer aminophylline to a patient who is already receiving Slo-Phyllin, plasma theophylline concentrations should be monitored.

Slo-Phyllin is not recommended during pregnancy since theophylline is known to cross the placenta and its safety in pregnancy has not been established. Theophylline is distributed in breast milk and therefore Slo-Phyllin should be used with caution in nursing mothers.

Side-effects: These usually occur when theophylline blood levels exceed 20 mcg/ml and include gastric irritation, nausea, vomiting, abdominal discomfort, palpitations, a fall in blood pressure, headache, occasional diarrhoea and insomnia. CNS stimulation and diuresis may also occur, especially in children.

Overdosage – signs and symptoms: These include nausea, vomiting, haematemesis, diuresis, restlessness, irritability possibly leading to tremors, convulsions, drowsiness and coma. However, in gross overdosage the first symptom of toxicity could be a convulsion and there may be a latent period before any symptoms appear.

Overdosage – treatment: Intensive therapy is required to maintain respiration and circulation and correct fluid loss and electrolyte imbalance.

Gastric lavage should only be considered after careful assessment of the patient's condition; in particular, the level of consciousness. Oral activated charcoal may provide a useful alternative treatment and charcoal-column haemoperfusion is also effective in cases of severe poisoning. If convulsions occur, they may be controlled with diazepam. It is essential to monitor the patient carefully for two or three days.

Drug interactions: Interactions with theophylline have been reported for phenytoin, cimetidine, diazepam, lithium carbonate, propanolol, frusemide, hexamethonium, digoxin, reserpine, chlordiazepoxide, ephedrine and erythromycin. However the clinical significance of some of these interactions remains uncertain. Probably the most important are those involving cimetidine, erythromycin and frusemide which may result in impaired theophylline elimination and hence an increase in plasma theophylline levels.

Pharmaceutical precautions The containers should be kept tightly closed and stored in a cool, dry place. The shelf-life is 3 years.

Legal category P.

Package quantities Securitainers containing 100 capsules.

Further information The elimination of theophylline and therefore the dosage requirement may be increased in smokers.

Product licence numbers
Slo-Phyllin 60 mg   0161/0021
Slo-Phyllin 125 mg   0161/0019
Slo-Phyllin 250 mg   0161/0020

SONI-SLO* ▼

Presentation Capsules containing Isosorbide Dinitrate INN in a timed release formulation which provides a prolonged therapeutic effect.

20 mg Capsules: Size No. 3 transparent pink capsules with a clear colourless cap, filled with off-white almost spherical pellets. Each capsule contains 20 mg Isosorbide Dinitrate INN.

40 mg Capsules: Size No. 2 transparent red capsule with a clear colourless cap, filled with off-white almost spherical pellets. Each capsule contains 40 mg Isosorbide Dinitrate INN.

Uses For the prophylactic treatment of angina pectoris.

Dosage and administration Dosage should be adjusted according to the response obtained by the individual patient and the severity of the anginal pain.

Adults: 40–120 mg daily in divided doses, generally morning and evening. Eight hourly administration may be found necessary in severe cases.

Initially the lowest dose is generally recommended. This should be increased gradually until the maximum therapeutic effect is achieved. Severe cases may require 120 mg daily. Gradual reduction of dosage after long-term therapy is recommended whenever possible.

Children: There is no recommended dose for children.

Contra-indications, warnings, etc
Contra-indications: Hypersensitivity to this drug, shock, marked hypotension, angina caused by hypertrophic obstructive cardiomyopathy, (nitrates may exaggerate outflow obstruction), marked anaemia.

Precautions: Not recommended during pregnancy or for

nursing mothers. As with other nitrates, tolerance to this drug and cross-tolerance to other nitrates/nitrites may occur. The hypotensive effect may be enhanced by alcohol.

Adverse Reactions: These are common to all nitrates used for the treatment of angina pectoris. Cutaneous vasodilatation with flushing, tachycardia and occasionally unexplained bradycardia. Headache may occur initially, but is less likely if the dose is increased gradually. Analgesics may be useful. Postural hypotension which may cause cerebral ischaemia and present as transient episodes of dizziness and weakness.

This drug can act as a physiological antagonist to noradrenaline, acetylcholine, histamine and many other agents.

Overdosage – Signs and Symptoms: As with all nitrates large doses may cause flushing of the face, severe headache, a feeling of suffocation, hypotension and fainting. Rarely, cyanosis and methaemoglobinaemia may occur. In a few patients there may be a reaction comparable to shock, with nausea, vomiting, weakness, sweating and syncope.

Overdosage – treatment: Recovery often occurs without special treatment. Hypotension may be corrected by elevation of the legs to promote venous return.

In the event of more severe overdosage symptomatic treatment is required. Gastric lavage may be required but should only be considered after careful assessment of the patient's condition, in particular the level of consciousness, and the time since ingestion which should be no more than four hours.

Pharmaceutical precautions Store in a cool dry place protected from light. Keep tightly closed. The shelf-life is 3 years.

Legal category P.

Package quantities Securitainers containing 100 capsules.

Further information Nil.

Product licence numbers
Soni-Slo 20 mg   3759/0020
Soni-Slo 40 mg   3759/0021.

*Trade Mark

Lorex Pharmaceuticals Ltd
Old Bank House
39 High Street
High Wycombe
Buckinghamshire HP11 2AG

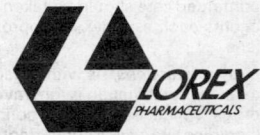

KERLONE* ▼

Presentation White, biconvex, film-coated tablets engraved KE20 on one side with breakline on reverse. Each tablet contains betaxolol hydrochloride 20 mg.

Uses

Actions: Kerlone (betaxolol hydrochloride) is a beta-adrenoceptor blocking agent which is cardio-selective, i.e. acts preferentially on beta$_1$-adrenergic receptors in the heart. It has prolonged activity, permitting once-daily administration which aids patient compliance. Its principal effects are to lower heart rate, especially on exercise, and to lower systolic and diastolic blood pressure in hypertensive subjects. It is devoid of intrinsic sympathomimetic activity and has little membrane stabilising activity. As with other beta-blockers, its mechanism of action in the treatment of hypertension is unclear. Absorption from the gastro-intestinal tract is complete and not affected by food. There is little first-pass extraction in the liver. This results in blood levels which vary little within and between subjects and a reproducible bioavailability of 80–90%.

Its long elimination half-life of 16–20 hours results in protection from excessive or inappropriate sympathetic activity throughout the 24 hours after administration of a once daily dose.

Indications: Management of hypertension.

Dosage and administration

Adults: The usual adult dose is one tablet (20 mg) daily. The single daily dose may be increased to two tablets (40 mg) if response is inadequate.

Elderly patients or those with a history of bronchospasm: A starting dose of half tablet (10 mg) daily is recommended.

Impaired renal function: An adjustment of dose is usually unnecessary in patients with renal insufficiency where creatinine clearance is greater than 20 ml/min. However, clinical surveillance is recommended at the start of treatment until steady state blood levels are attained (4 days on average).

For patients on haemo- or peritoneal dialysis the initial recommended dose is 10 mg daily independent of the dialysis schedule.

Hepatic insufficiency: Adjustment of dosage is usually unnecessary in patients with hepatic insufficiency. However, clinical surveillance is recommended at the start of treatment.

Children: Paediatric experience with Kerlone is limited and for this reason it is not currently recommended for use in children.

Most of the reduction of blood pressure is seen during the first 3 hours following the initial dose, permitting an early evaluation of the anti-hypertensive effect. Little further reduction is seen after seven days of treatment and the response is undiminished in subsequent months. If a further reduction in blood pressure is required, this may be achieved by combining Kerlone with another antihypertensive agent such as a diuretic. However, in a large series of controlled clinical trials, 70–80% of patients responded to betaxolol alone.

Patients can be transferred to Kerlone from other anti-hypertensive treatments with the exception of clonidine (see precautions below).

Contra-indications, warnings, etc

Contra-indications: Kerlone is contra-indicated in cardiogenic shock, in patients with uncontrolled congestive cardiac failure and in second or third degree AV block if no pacemaker is present and in patients with marked bradycardia (heart rate less than 50 beats per minute).

Warnings: Concomitant administration of Kerlone and a myocardial depressant or inhibitor of AV conduction, such as the calcium antagonists of the verapamil type, should be carried out only under close supervision, especially in the case of intravenous administration.

Precautions: Secondary sympathetic hyperactivity has sometimes been reported following discontinuation of treatment with other beta-blockers. Even though Kerlone blood levels decrease slowly, care should be exercised if treatment is withdrawn, especially in patients with ischaemic heart disease.

Patients with a history of cardiac failure, cardiomyopathy, or cardiomegaly should be monitored carefully during treatment with a beta-blocker as sympathetic stimulation may be essential to their circulatory function.

Although Kerlone is beta$_1$-selective it should be used with caution in patients with broncho-obstructive disorders such as chronic bronchitis with bronchospasm, and asthma. It is recommended that Kerlone treatment is started at the dose of 10 mg daily in these conditions. If any increase in airway resistance is provoked, it can be relieved by beta$_2$-mimetics whose effect is not inhibited.

Use with caution where the PR conduction interval is prolonged.

Studies in normal subjects have shown that, unlike non-selective beta-blockers, Kerlone does not inhibit the recovery from insulin-induced hypoglycaemia, nor does it mask the cardiovascular response. Due to its beta$_1$ selectivity, Kerlone is unlikely to interfere with glucose metabolism in insulin-treated diabetics. However, caution is advised when treating such patients.

Anaesthesia: In the event of surgical intervention, the anaesthetist should be advised in advance that the patient is receiving Kerlone. In patients with severe ischaemic heart disease the risk/benefits of continuation of treatment have to be evaluated. If treatment is continued care should be taken when using anaesthetic agents such as ether, cyclopropane and trichloroethylene.

Drug interactions: As with other beta-blockers, use with care in combination with myocardial depressants or drugs which depress AV conduction. If Kerlone and clonidine are given concurrently, clonidine should not be discontinued until several days after withdrawal of the beta-blocker.

Pregnancy: No teratogenic effects have been demonstrated in animal studies but the safety of Kerlone during human pregnancy has not been established. Like other beta-blockers, Kerlone crosses the placental barrier and its use in pregnant women requires that the anticipated benefit be weighed against the possible hazards to the mother and foetus.

Nursing mothers: Kerlone is excreted in human breast milk and the possibility of bradycardic and hypotensive effects on the new-born should therefore be considered if Kerlone is given to nursing mothers.

Side effects: Kerlone is generally well tolerated. The side effects are usually those due to its pharmacological actions and rarely require discontinuation of treatment. Minor side effects include lassitude at the start of treatment, exacerbation of Raynaud's disease or intermittent claudication, and paraesthesia of the extremities. Possible side effects include marked bradycardia and hypotension, AV block, cardiac insufficiency and bronchospasm. There have been reports of rashes and dry eyes associated with the use of all beta-blockers but in most cases the signs and symptoms have cleared when treatment was withdrawn. Nevertheless, the drug should be discontinued if any such reaction is suspected.

Overdosage: Excessive bradycardia can usually be corrected with atropine. If there is no response isoprenaline may be administered with caution. Cardiac failure should be managed with digitalisation and diuretics. Hypotension may be managed with vasopressors such as adrenaline.

Pharmaceutical precautions No special precautions are indicated for Kerlone.

Legal category POM.

Package quantities Calendar pack of 28 tablets (2 × 14).

Further information Kerlone is unique in having high bioavailability, long blood half-life and high selectivity for cardiac beta$_1$-receptors. Unlike most other cardioselective beta-blockers it has high lipid solubility. This may facilitate rapid arrival of the drug at the receptor, but does not induce an increased incidence of side effects.

These characteristics and the rapidity of response increase patient compliance by virtue of the drug's acceptability, the simple dose regimen and narrow dose range.

The only active metabolite is cardio-selective and does not contribute to the clinical effect. Kerlone does not modify the hypoglycaemic response to insulin nor mask the cardiovascular response. It can be used in patients with respiratory disease, and is compatible with most other hypotensive agents.

Product licence number 4969/0001.

TILDIEM* ▼

Presentation Off-white biconvex tablets, engraved Tildiem 60. Each tablet contains 60 mg of diltiazem hydrochloride in a modified release formulation.

Uses
Actions: Tildiem (diltiazem hydrochloride) is a calcium antagonist. It restricts the slow channel entry of calcium into the cell and so reduces the liberation of calcium from stores in the sarcoplasmic reticulum. This results in a reduction of the amount of available intracellular calcium, reducing myocardial oxygen consumption. It increases exercise capacity and improves all indices of myocardial ischaemia in the angina patient.

Tildiem relaxes large and small coronary arteries and relieves the spasm of vasospastic (Prinzmetal's) angina and the response to catecholamines, but has little effect on the peripheral vasculature. There is therefore no possibility of reflex tachycardia.

A small reduction in heart rate occurs which is accompanied by an increase in cardiac output, improved myocardial perfusion and reduction of ventricular work. In animal studies Tildiem protects the myocardium against the effects of ischaemia and reduces the damage produced by excessive entry of calcium into the myocardial cell during reperfusion.

Indications: Angina pectoris.

Dosage and administration
General: The usual dose is one tablet (60 mg) three times daily. However, patient responses may vary and dosage requirements can differ significantly between individual patients. If necessary the divided dose may be increased to 360 mg/day. Higher doses up to 480 mg/day have been used with benefit in some patients especially in unstable angina. There is no evidence of any decrease in efficacy at these high doses. Tildiem has not been reported to precipitate angina.

Elderly and patients with impaired hepatic or renal function: The recommended starting dose is one tablet (60 mg) twice daily. The heart rate should be measured regularly in these groups of patients and the dose should not be increased if the heart rate falls below 50 beats per minute.

Contra-indications, warnings, etc
Contra-indications: Tildiem is contra-indicated in: pregnant women or those of child-bearing potential; patients with sick sinus syndrome; patients with second or third degree AV block; and patients with severe bradycardia.

Warnings and precautions: Patients with mild bradycardia or a prolonged PR interval should be observed closely. Tildiem does not have a significant myocardial depressant effect and is well tolerated in patients with poor left ventricular function.

Drug interactions: Tildiem is effective in most patients as monotherapy. If a beta-blocker is given at the same time as Tildiem the dose of both drugs should be moderated and the heart rate should be closely observed at the initiation of treatment. Patients with pre-existing conduction defects should not receive this combination. Tildiem may increase the blood levels of beta-blockers having a low bioavailability, e.g. propranolol.

In the presence of Tildiem, small increases in plasma levels of digitalis glycosides have sometimes been observed.

The absorption of Tildiem is not affected by the concomitant administration of antacids or aspirin. Tildiem treatment has been continued without problem during anaesthesia, but the anaesthetist should be made aware of the treatment regimen.

Side effects: Tildiem produces few side effects and these are usually mild. Bradycardia and first degree heart block have been seen in a few cases, especially in patients with pre-existing sino-atrial node disease. Ankle oedema may occur, and there have been occasional reports of nausea, headache, finger swelling and skin rash.

Overdosage: Experience of overdosage in man is limited and spontaneous recovery has been seen in reported cases. However, observation in a coronary care unit is advisable with corrective measures for possible hypotension and conduction disturbances available.

Pharmaceutical precautions Store at room temperature, protected from excessive heat and moisture.

Legal category POM.

Package quantities Securitainers of 100 tablets.

Further information Tildiem is effective in angina, protecting the heart against ischaemia and reducing myocardial oxygen requirements. It is well tolerated and does not normally give rise to the side effects associated with peripheral vasodilators, nor cause significant myocardial depression. It protects against excessive catecholamine stimulation but is free of the side effects seen with beta-blockade. Although it tends to lower blood pressure in hypertensive patients, Tildiem is not currently recommended for this indication. Tildiem does not appear to interfere with glucose metabolism.

Product licence number 4969/0005.

*Trade Mark

Luitpold-Werk
Medical & Scientific Office in UK
Hayes Gate House
27 Uxbridge Road
Hayes, Middlesex UB4 0JN

Product licences held by
Farillon Limited
Bryant Avenue
Romford
Essex, RM3 0PJ

LUITPOLD

ANACAL* SUPPOSITORIES
ANACAL* RECTAL OINTMENT
Presentation

	Anacal Suppository (torpedo-shaped, off-white colour) (g%)	Anacal Rectal Ointment (a white odourless, soft ointment) (g%)
Mucopolysaccharide polysulphuric acid ester (Heparinoid)	0.2	0.2
Prednisolone	0.05	0.15
Oxypolyethoxydodecane (Lauromacrogol-400)	2.5	5.0
Hexachlorophane	0.25	0.5

Uses *Pharmacology:* Mucopolysaccharide polysulphuric acid ester stimulates the metabolism of connective tissue, helps to break up microthrombi in the capillaries of the submucous tissue and has anti-exudative properties. Prednisolone is anti-inflammatory, anti-exudative and anti-allergic. Oxypolyethoxydodecane has local analgesic properties, thus relieving acute pain and itching. Hexachlorophane is strongly bactericidal, prevents growth of pathogenic micro-organisms and eradicates infection.

Indications: Haemorrhoids (including perianal haematomas), perianal eczema, pruritus, anal fissure, proctitis, periproctitis and after-care of haemorrhoids treated by surgery or injection.

Dosage and administration *Anacal Suppositories:* 1 suppository to be inserted once or twice daily.

Anacal Rectal Ointment: To be applied one to four times daily, as required. (Nozzle supplied for internal application.)

Contra-indications, warnings, etc
Not intended for administration to children below the age of 7 years.

Pharmaceutical precautions Store suppositories in a cool place.

Legal category POM.

Package quantities *Anacal Suppositories:* Packs of 10 (2 g ea.).
Anacal Rectal Ointment: Tubes of 30 g.

Further information Chronic constipation, faulty dietary habits and alcohol may worsen haemorrhoids. These factors should be taken into account and, if possible, avoided.

Product licence numbers
Anacal Suppositories 0542/5004
Anacal Rectal Ointment 0542/5005

HIRUDOID* CREAM
HIRUDOID* GEL

Presentation Hirudoid Cream contains Organo-heparinoid 'Luitpold' 0.3 g (25,000 units) in 100 g of a white vanishing-cream base.

Hirudoid Gel contains the same active constituent in a colourless gel base.

Uses *Pharmacology:* The active constituent of Hirudoid speedily penetrates the skin, acting uniformly and persistently on diseased tissue. Hirudoid inhibits proteolysis and the spreading of hyaluronidase. It thus counteracts inflammation of traumatic, infective, toxic or allergic origin. It promotes the absorption of traumatic and inflammatory oedema, inhibits the formation and further growth of thrombi, assists in dissolving thrombi, regulates blood and lymph flow, stimulates metabolism and regeneration of damaged connective tissue, and quickly relieves pain from tissue tension.

Indications: Superficial thrombophlebitis, varicose veins and their concomitant symptoms, superficial soft-tissue injuries.

Dosage and administration *Hirudoid Cream:* Two to six inches (5–15 cm) to be applied up to four times daily to the affected area and gently massaged into the skin. If the area is tender to touch or if there is evidence of thrombosis, Hirudoid Cream should be applied thickly to the skin and covered with gauze or lint. In such cases it may be massaged very gently into the skin surrounding the affected area.

Hirudoid Gel: To be applied as a thin layer up to four times daily. Recommended when its cooling effect and rapid action are especially required (e.g. tired, aching legs and sports injuries).

Contra-indications, warnings, etc *Hirudoid Cream:* None.

Hirudoid Gel: The gel contains an alcohol and therefore should not be brought into direct contact with open wounds or mucous membranes.

Pharmaceutical precautions Nil.

Legal category P.

Package quantities *Hirudoid Cream or Gel:* Tubes of 40 g.

Further information Nil.

Product licence numbers
Hirudoid Cream   0542/5000
Hirudoid Gel   0542/0005

MOVELAT* CREAM
MOVELAT* GEL

Presentation Movelat Cream contains mucopolysaccharide polysulphuric acid ester (Heparinoid) 0.2 g, adrenocortical extract 1.0 g (equivalent to 20 mg of corticosteroids), and salicylic acid 2.0 g in a white vanishing-cream base to 100 g.
    Movelat Gel contains the same active constituents in a colourless gel base.

Uses *Pharmacology:* The standardised adrenocortical extract is anti-inflammatory and anti-exudative. Mucopolysaccharide polysulphuric acid ester arrests proteolysis and hyaluronidase activity, so that the anti-inflammatory and anti-exudative effects of the adrenocortical extract are enhanced. Salicylic acid facilitates penetration of the skin by the other active constituents and acts as a powerful analgesic.

Indications: Rheumatic disorders: osteo-arthritis, fibros-

itis. Non-rheumatic disorders of the locomotor apparatus: sprains, muscular strains and spasms, soft tissue injuries.

Dosage and administration *Movelat Cream:* Two to six inches (5–15 cm) to be massaged into the affected area up to four times daily. The Cream may also be used as a dressing, when it should be applied thickly.

Movelat Gel: To be applied gently to the affected area up to four times daily.

Contra-indications, warnings, etc *Movelat Cream:* None.

Movelat Gel: The gel contains an alcohol and therefore should not be brought into direct contact with open wounds or mucous membranes.

Pharmaceutical precautions Nil.

Legal category POM.

Package quantities *Movelat Cream or Gel:* Tubes of 50 g and 100 g.

Further information Nil.

Product licence numbers
Movelat Cream   0542/5001
Movelat Gel   0542/0006

*Trade Mark

Lundbeck Limited
Lundbeck House
Hastings Street
Luton   Bedfordshire LU1 5BE

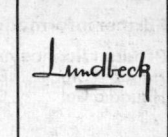

BLEOMYCIN INJECTION

Presentation Bleomycin Lundbeck Injection is a whitish-yellow freeze-dried plug of bleomycin sulphate equivalent to 15 mg bleomycin (standard NIHJ) in clear glass ampoule.

Active ingredients: 15 mg bleomycin per ampoule, as the sulphate.

Uses *Pharmacology:* Bleomycin is a basic water-soluble glycopeptide with cytotoxic activity. The mechanism of action of bleomycin is believed to involve single-strand scission of DNA, leading to inhibition of cell division, of growth and of DNA synthesis in tumour cells.

Apart from its antibacterial and antitumour properties, bleomycin is relatively free from biological activity. When injected intravenously it may have a histamine-like effect on blood pressure and may cause a rise in body temperature. Blood concentrations of bleomycin in patients indicate that the drug is excreted more rapidly after intravenous than after intramuscular injection and that up to one third of the dose is excreted unchanged in the urine within 24 hours.

Indications:

1. Squamous cell carcinoma affecting the mouth, nasopharynx and paranasal sinuses, larynx, oesophagus, external genitalia, cervix or skin. Well-differentiated tumours usually respond better than anaplastic ones.
2. Hodgkin's disease and other malignant lymphomas, including mycosis fungoides.
3. Testicular teratoma.
4. Malignant effusions of serous cavities.
5. Secondary indications in which bleomycin has been shown to be of some value (alone or in combination with other drugs) include metastatic malignant melanoma, carcinoma of the thyroid, lung and bladder.

Dosage and administration *Adults:* Bleomycin is usually administered intramuscularly but may be given intravenously (bolus or drip), intra-arterially, intrapleurally or intraperitoneally as a solution in physiological saline. Local injection directly into the tumour may occasionally be indicated.

1. *Squamous cell carcinoma and testicular teratoma:* The following dosage schedules are recommended for adults:

Age in years	Total dose (mg)	Dose per week (mg)
80 and over	100	15
70–79	150–200	30
60–69	200–300	30–60
Under 60	500	30–60

These doses may need to be adjusted when bleomycin is used in combination therapy.

A total dose of 500 mg should not normally be exceeded, but young men with testicular tumours have frequently tolerated twice this amount.

Used alone normal dose frequency is 15 mg three times a week or 30 mg twice a week, either intramuscularly or intravenously until the total dose indicated in the above table is administered. Continuous intravenous infusion at a rate of 15 mg/24 hours for up to 10 days, or 30 mg/24 hours for up to five days may produce a therapeutic effect more rapidly. The development of stomatitis is the most useful guide to the determination of individual tolerance of maximum therapeutic dose.

2. *Malignant lymphomas:* Used alone the recommended dosage regimen is 15 mg once or twice a week, intramuscularly, to a total dose of 225 mg. For patients 60 years and over, 75% of the dosage recommended in 1 above should be used. These doses may need to be adjusted when bleomycin is used in combination chemotherapy.

3. *Malignant effusions (particularly those associated with carcinoma of breast):* After drainage of the serous cavity affected 60 mg bleomycin dissolved in 100 ml physiological saline is introduced via the drainage needle or cannula, which is then withdrawn.

Bleomycin is commonly used in conjunction with radiotherapy, particularly in the treatment of cancer of the head and neck region. Such a combination may enhance mucosal reactions if full doses of both forms of treatment are used and bleomycin dosage may require reduction, e.g. to 5 mg at the time of each radiotherapy fraction five days a week. Bleomycin is frequently used as one of the drugs in multiple chemotherapy regimens (e.g. in squamous cell carcinoma, testicular teratoma, lymphoma). The mucosal toxicity of bleomycin should be borne in mind in the selection and dosage of drugs with similar toxic potential used in such combinations.

Children: Until further data are available, administration of bleomycin to children should take place only under exceptional circumstances and in special centres. The dosage should be based on that recommended for adults and adjusted to body surface area or body weight.

Reduced kidney function: With serum creatinine values of 2–4 mg%, half the above individual dosage is recommended. With serum creatinine above 4 mg%, a further reduction in dose is indicated.

Preparation of solutions: For intramuscular injections the required dose is dissolved in up to 5 ml of a suitable solvent such as physiological saline. If pain occurs at the site of injection a 1% solution of lignocaine may be used as a solvent.

For intravenous injections the dose required is dissolved in 5–200 ml of physiological saline and injected slowly or added to the reservoir of a running intravenous infusion. For intra-arterial administration a slow infusion in physiological saline is used. For intra-cavitary injection 60 mg is dissolved in 100 ml normal saline.

For local injections bleomycin is dissolved in physiological saline to make a 1–3 mg/ml solution.

Contra-indications, warnings, etc This product should not normally be administered to patients who are pregnant or to mothers who are breast feeding. It is also contra-indicated in patients with acute pulmonary infection or greatly reduced lung function.

Adverse reactions: Like most cytotoxic agents bleomycin can give rise both to immediate and to delayed toxic effects. The most immediate effect is fever on the day of injection. Anorexia, tiredness or nausea also may occur. Pain at the injection site, or in the region of the tumour, has occasionally been reported, and other rare adverse effects are hypotension and local thrombophlebitis after intravenous administration. A few cases of acute fulminant reactions have been observed after intravenous injections of doses higher than those recommended. Hypotension, hyperpyrexia and drug related deaths have been reported rarely following intracavitary injection.

The most serious delayed effect is interstitial pneumonia, which may develop during, or occasionally after, a course of treatment. This condition may sometimes develop into fatal pulmonary fibrosis, although such an occurrence is rare on recommended doses. Previous or concurrent radiotherapy to the chest is an important factor in increasing the incidence and severity of lung toxicity. It has been suggested that those patients who have received bleomycin preoperatively are at a greater risk of developing pulmonary toxicity, and a reduction in inspired oxygen concentration during the operation and post-operatively is recommended.

The majority of patients who receive a full course of bleomycin develop lesions of the skin or oral mucosa. Induration, hyperkeratosis, reddening, tenderness, and swelling of the tips of the fingers, ridging of the nails, bulla formation over pressure points such as elbows, loss of hair and stomatitis are rarely serious and usually disappear soon after completion of the course.

Precautions: Patients undergoing treatment with bleomycin should have chest X-rays weekly. These should continue to be taken for up to four weeks after completion of the course. If breathlessness or infiltrates, not obviously attributable to tumour or to co-existent lung disease, appear, administration of the drug must be stopped immediately and patients should be treated with a corticosteroid (e.g. hydrocortisone 100 mg i.m. as the sodium succinate daily for five days, followed by oral prednisone 10 mg twice daily) and a broad-spectrum antibiotic. No specific clinical incompatibilities with other drugs or food have been encountered.

Overdosage: No specific antidote. The acute reaction to an overdosage with bleomycin would probably include hypotension, fever, rapid pulse and general symptoms of shock. Treatment is purely symptomatic. In the event of respiratory complications, the patient should be treated with a corticosteroid and a broad-spectrum antibiotic.

Pharmaceutical precautions Freeze-dried bleomycin has a shelf life of three years from the date of manufacture when stored at room temperature. Bleomycin should be administered as a freshly prepared solution.

Because of possible skin changes, direct contact of bleomycin with the skin should be avoided.

Pharmaceutical incompatibilities: Bleomycin solutions should not be mixed with solutions of essential amino acids, riboflavine, ascorbic acid, dexamethasone, aminophylline or frusemide.

Legal category POM.

The supply of bleomycin is restricted to centres with special experience in the chemotherapy of malignant diseases and is available on prescription only.

Package quantities Boxes of 10×15 mg ampoules.

Further information Bleomycin has little or no toxic effect on the bone marrow, and has no immunosuppressive action.

Product licence number 0458/0009.

CCNU LUNDBECK CAPSULES

Presentation Blue/white gelatin capsules containing 10 mg lomustine, and blue gelatin capsules containing 40 mg lomustine.

Active ingredient: 10 mg and 40 mg lomustine (CCNU; 1-(2-chloroethyl)-3-cyclohexyl-1-nitrosourea).

Uses The mechanism of action is believed to be partly as an alkylating agent and partly by inhibition of several vital enzymatic processes. Cross-resistance with other nitrosoureas is usual but cross-resistance with conventional alkylating agents is unusual.

Indications: As palliative or supplementary treatment, usually in combination with radiotherapy and/or surgery or as part of multiple drug regimens in:

brain tumours (primary or metastatic);
lung tumours (especially oat-cell carcinoma);
Hodgkin's disease (resistant to conventional combination chemotherapy);
malignant melanoma (metastatic).

CCNU may also be of value as second-line treatment in non-Hodgkin's lymphoma, myelomatosis, gastrointestinal tumours, carcinoma of the kidney, the testis, the ovary, the cervix uteri and the breast.

Dosage and administration *Adults:* CCNU is given by mouth. The recommended dose in patients with normally functioning bone marrow receiving CCNU as their only chemotherapy is 120–130 mg/m^2 as a single dose every six to eight weeks (or as a divided dose over three days, e.g. 40 mg/m^2/day).

Dosage is reduced if:

(a) CCNU is being given as part of a drug regimen which includes other marrow-depressant drugs, and
(b) in the presence of leucopenia below 3,000/mm^3 or thrombocytopenia below 75,000/mm^3.

Marrow depression after CCNU is longer sustained than after nitrogen mustards and recovery of white cell and platelet counts may not occur for six weeks or more. Blood elements depressed below the above levels should be allowed to recover to 4,000/mm^3 (WBC) and 100,000/mm^3 (platelets) before repeating CCNU dosage.

Administration to children: Until further data are available administration of CCNU to children with malignancies other than brain tumours should be restricted to specialised centres and exceptional situations. Dosage in children, like that in adults, is based on body surface area (120–130 mg/m^2 every six to eight weeks, with the same qualifications as apply to adults).

Contra-indications, warnings, etc This product should not normally be administered to patients who are pregnant or to mothers who are breast feeding. Other contra-indications are: 1. Previous hypersensitivity to nitrosoureas; 2. Previous failure of the tumour to respond to other nitrosoureas; 3. Severe bone marrow depression.

Precautions: Patients receiving CCNU chemotherapy should be under the care of doctors experienced in cancer treatment. Blood counts should be carried out before starting the drug and at frequent intervals (preferably weekly) during treatment. Treatment and dosage is governed principally by the haemoglobin, white cell count and platelet count. Liver function should also be assessed periodically.

Adverse effects: Haematological: The principal adverse effect is marrow toxicity of a delayed or prolonged nature. Thrombocytopenia appears about four weeks after a dose of CCNU and lasts one to two weeks at a level around 80–100,000/mm³; leucopenia appears after six weeks and persists for one to two weeks at about 4–5,000/mm³. The haematological toxicity may be cumulative, leading to successively lower white cell and platelet counts with successive doses of the drug.

Gastrointestinal: Nausea and vomiting usually occur four to six hours after a full single dose of CCNU and last for 24–48 hours, followed by anorexia for two to three days. The effects are less troublesome if the six-weekly dose is divided into three doses and given on each of the first three days of the six-week period. Gastrointestinal tolerance is usually good, however, if prophylactic antinauseants are given (e.g. metoclopramide or chlorpromazine). Transient elevation of liver enzymes (SGOT, SGPT, LDH or alkaline phosphatase) are occasionally observed. More rarely patients are troubled by stomatitis.

Other side-effects: Loss of scalp hair has been reported infrequently.

Overdosage: There is no specific antidote. In the event of dangerously low red cell, white cell or platelet counts, cross-matched whole blood should be given as necessary.

Pharmaceutical precautions The capsules should be stored in the original container and protected from light and moisture. The preparation has a shelf life of two years from the date of manufacture, when stored at room temperature.

Legal category POM.
The supply of CCNU capsules is restricted to centres with special experience in the chemotherapy of malignant disease. CCNU capsules are available on prescription only.

Package quantities Bottles of 20 capsules each containing 10 mg or 40 mg lomustine.

Further information Nil.

Product licence number 0458/0018.
                                  0458/0024

CLOPIXOL* INJECTION

Presentation Clopixol Injection is a 20% sterile almost colourless to straw-coloured solution of zuclopenthixol decanoate in thin vegetable oil. It is presented in a clear glass ampoule (1 ml) and vials (10 ml).

Active ingredient: Zuclopenthixol decanoate 200 mg per 1 ml.

Uses *Pharmacology:* Clopenthixol is a potent neuroleptic of the thioxanthene group. In addition to its pronounced antipsychotic effect, it possesses a marked specific calming effect and a non-specific sedative action. Clopenthixol itself is relatively short-acting, but Clopixol Injection, its decanoic acid ester dissolved in thin vegetable oil, provides a predictable slow release depot preparation of the active constituent. Pharmacokinetic studies in humans show that peak serum levels are attained towards the end of the first week and gradually decline over a period of three to four weeks after intramuscular injection. Clinical experience correlates well with the pharmacokinetic findings, using a dosage interval of two to four weeks.

Indications: Clopixol Injection is a depot neuroleptic preparation designed for the treatment of psychoses, especially schizophrenia and particularly for patients with features of agitation or aggression.

Dosage and administration *Adults:* Clopixol Injection is administered by deep intramuscular injection into the upper, outer buttock or lateral thigh in doses of 200–400 mg (1–2 ml) every two to four weeks. A few patients may require higher doses or shorter intervals between doses. The maximum recommended dose is 600 mg (3 ml) a week. Doses greater than 400 mg (2 ml) should be distributed between two injection sites. Treatment is usually started with 100 mg. One week later, or when symptoms recur (but not more than four weeks later) a second injection of 100–200 mg or more is given.

Note: As with all oily injections it is important to ensure by aspiration before injection, that inadvertent intravascular entry does not occur.

Children: Clopixol Injection should not be administered to children.

Transfer of patients to Clopixol Injection:
1. Those not previously treated with a long-acting antipsychotic injection should start with an initial dose of 100 mg intramuscularly and the patient's response and the appearance of extrapyramidal side-effects monitored carefully. Oral neuroleptic therapy should be gradually phased out.
2. Patients being transferred from phenothiazine depot injections should receive a dose in the ratio of 200 mg Clopixol Injection equivalent to 25 mg fluphenazine decanoate.
3. Patients whose schizophrenic symptoms may have been treated with flupenthixol decanoate (Depixol Injection) because of features such as anergia or withdrawal at the time of starting depot neuroleptic treatment may pass to a phase of their psychosis in which features such as agitation or aggression predominate. Such a change in the clinical picture would warrant consideration of a change of treatment to Clopixol Injection, using a comparable antipsychotic dose (200 mg Clopixol Injection ≡ 40 mg Depixol Injection).

Contra-indications, warnings, etc
Contra-indications and precautions: Clopixol Injection is contra-indicated in acute alcohol, barbiturate or opiate poisoning.
Clopixol is unsuitable for patients whose psychoses are accompanied by features of apathy or withdrawal, for those who do not tolerate oral neuroleptic drugs, or for those with Parkinsonism; severe arteriosclerosis; senile confusional states; or advanced renal, hepatic or cardiovascular disease. In common with other therapies it is recommended that Clopixol Injection should not be

administered during pregnancy, particularly the first trimester, unless the importance of control of psychotic symptoms outweighs the theoretical hazard of foetal malformations.

Warning: Ability to drive a car or operate machinery may be affected. Therefore, caution should be exercised initially, until the individual reaction to the treatment is known.

Adverse reactions: Extrapyramidal side-effects may occur, especially during the first few days after injection and during the early phase of treatment. In most cases these side-effects can be satisfactorily controlled by anti-Parkinson drugs though their routine use is not recommended. Initial drowsiness has been reported and in a few patients slight changes in weight. Occasional local reactions such as erythema, swelling or tender fibrous nodules have been reported. Tardive dyskinesia, galactorrhoea and amenorrhoea are adverse effects of the general group of neuroleptic drugs. They have not been reported in patients treated with Clopixol Injection, but the theoretical hazard should be borne in mind.

Overdosage: Overdosage should be treated:

1. By anticholinergic anti-Parkinson drugs if extrapyramidal symptoms occur.
2. By sedation (with benzodiazepines) if akathisia occurs, or in the unlikely event of agitation, excitement or convulsions.
3. By noradrenaline in saline intravenous drip if the patient is in shock. Otherwise observation and symptomatic management should be adequate.

Pharmaceutical precautions Store at room temperature. Under these conditions the preparation has a shelf life of two years from the date of manufacture.

In accordance with normal practice partially used vials should be discarded at the end of each session.

Legal category POM.

Clopixol is available through hospitals, clinics and on prescription only through registered pharmacies for patients whose treatment has been initiated by a psychiatrist.

Package quantities Boxes of 10 × 200 mg (1 ml) ampoules.
Boxes of 1 × 10 ml vials.

Further information Nil.

Product licence number 0458/0017.

CLOPIXOL*-CONC. INJECTION ▼

Presentation Clopixol-Conc. Injection is a sterile, straw-coloured solution of 50% zuclopenthixol decanoate in thin vegetable oil. It is presented in clear glass ampoules (1 ml = 500 mg).

Uses Clopixol-Conc. Injection is a depot neuroleptic preparation for the maintenance treatment of schizophrenia and paranoid psychosis, especially where compliance with oral medication is a problem.

Dosage and administration *Adults:* Clopixol-Conc. Injection is administered by deep intramuscular injection into the upper, outer buttock or lateral thigh in doses of 250–500 mg ($\frac{1}{2}$ ml–1 ml) every 1–4 weeks depending on the response.

Note: As with all oily injections it is important to ensure,

by aspiration before injection, that inadvertent intravascular entry does not occur.

Elderly: In accordance with standard medical practice the dose may need to be reduced in the frail and elderly. Clopixol Injection (20%) may be more suitable in such patients.

Children: Clopixol-Conc. Injection should not be administered to children.

Contra-indications, warnings, etc
Contra-indications: Comatose states.

Precautions: Caution should be exercised in patients having: Liver disease; cardiac disease, or arrhythmias; severe respiratory disease; renal failure; epilepsy (and conditions predisposing to epilepsy, e.g. alcohol withdrawal or brain damage); Parkinson's disease; patients who have shown hypersensitivity to other neuroleptics. The general caution for the use of neuroleptics in hypothyroidism, thyrotoxicosis, myasthenia gravis, phaeochromocytoma or prostatic hypertrophy should be observed, but there is no evidence to suggest that Clopixol gives rise to any particular problem in such conditions. Care should also be taken in the elderly, particularly if frail or at risk of hypothermia, and in patients with personal or family history of narrow angle glaucoma.

As there is no unequivocal evidence as to the safety of Clopixol in human pregnancy, use during pregnancy, especially the first and last trimesters, should be avoided. Clopenthixol is excreted in small amounts in breast milk. It is recommended that mothers receiving Clopixol should not breast feed.

Drug interactions: Clopixol may increase the central depressant effect of alcohol, hypnotics and sedatives and may impair the metabolism of tricyclic antidepressants, the antiparkinson effect of levodopa and the effect of anticonvulsants. The possibility of interaction with lithium should also be borne in mind.

Neuroleptics may interact with sympathomimetic, hypoglycaemic, anti-arrhythmic drugs, but no instances of such drug interactions have been reported relating to patients receiving Clopixol.

Warnings and adverse effects: Drowsiness, sedation, dry mouth and nasal stuffiness may occur, particularly with high dosage and at the start of treatment. Postural hypotension may occur, particularly in the elderly. Other anticholinergic type side effects that should be borne in mind include blurring of vision, tachycardia, constipation and urinary hesitancy or retention.

Because Clopixol may impair alertness, especially at the start of treatment or following the consumption of alcohol, patients should be warned of this risk and advised not to drive or operate machinery, until their susceptibility is known.

Extrapyramidal reactions in the form of acute dystonias (including oculogyric crisis), Parkinsonian rigidity, tremor, akinesia and akathisia have been reported and may occur even at low dosage in susceptible patients. Such effects would usually be encountered early in treatment, but delayed reactions may also occur. Antiparkinson agents should not be prescribed routinely because of possible risk of causing anticholinergic side effects, precipitating toxic-confusional states or impairing therapeutic efficacy. They should only be given if required and their requirement reassessed at regular intervals. Tardive dyskinesia is an adverse effect of the general group of neuroleptic drugs. It has been observed occasionally in patients receiving Clopixol. The concurrent use of anticholinergic antiparkinson drugs may exacerbate this effect.

Confusional states or epileptic fits can occur. The hormonal effects of antipsychotic neuroleptic drugs include hyperprolactinaemia, which may be associated with galactorrhoea, gynaecomastia, oligomenorrhoea or amenorrhoea.

Neuroleptics have been reported to affect cardiac conduction, but no specific reports have been received relating to patients receiving clopenthixol.

Sexual function including libido, erection and ejaculation is rarely impaired. Weight changes have occurred. Occasional local reactions such as erythema, swelling or tender fibrous nodules have been reported.

Body temperature regulation, especially in the elderly, may possibly be compromised. Hypothermia has been reported rarely.

Jaundice and other liver abnormalities have been reported rarely.

Overdosage: Overdosage should be treated: (a) by anticholinergic antiparkinson drugs if extrapyramidal symptoms occur; (b) by sedation (with benzodiazepines) if akathisia occurs, or in the unlikely event of agitation, excitement or convulsions; (c) by noradrenaline in saline intravenous drip if the patient is in shock. Otherwise observation and symptomatic management should be adequate.

Pharmaceutical precautions Store at room temperature and protect from light. Under these conditions the preparation has a shelf life of 2 years from the date of manufacture.

Legal category POM.

Package quantities Boxes of 5 × 500 mg (1 ml ampoules).

Further information Clopenthixol is a potent neuroleptic of the thioxanthene series with a piperazine sidechain. Clopixol-Conc. Injection contains the decanoic ester of clopenthixol in a vegetable oil (Viscoleo*). The decanoic ester is slowly released from the oil depot and is rapidly hydrolysed to release clopenthixol. Whereas clopenthixol itself is relatively short acting, the decanoic ester in oil provides a predictable slow release depot preparation of the active constituent.

Product licence number 0458/0041.

CLOPIXOL* TABLETS ▼

Presentation Clopixol tablets contain zuclopenthixol 2 mg, 10 mg or 25 mg as the dihydrochloride. The tablets are biconvex and film coated. The 2 mg tablets are pink with a diameter of 5 mm, the 10 mg tablets are light brown with a diameter of 6 mm and the 25 mg tablets are brown with a diameter of 7 mm.

Uses The treatment of psychoses, especially schizophrenia and particularly in patients who are agitated, aggressive or hostile.

Dosage and administration *Adults:* The usual initial dose is 20–30 mg/day, increasing as necessary to a maximum of 150 mg/day, in divided doses. The usual maintenance dose in chronic schizophrenia is 20–50 mg/day in divided doses. Lower doses may be appropriate depending on individual patient response.

Children: Not recommended.

Contra-indications, warnings, etc As with other neuroleptics Clopixol may potentiate the effects of other central nervous system depressants and is therefore contra-indicated in acute alcohol, barbiturate or opiate poisoning. Clopixol should not be prescribed for patients who have previously been shown to be intolerant of thioxanthenes. Clopixol is unsuitable for those patients whose psychoses are accompanied by features of apathy or withdrawal. It should be used with caution in patients with extrapyramidal disorders, severe arteriosclerosis, senile confusional states or advanced renal, hepatic or cardiovascular disease. In common with other therapies it is recommended that Clopixol should not be administered during pregnancy, particularly the first trimester, unless the importance of control of psychotic symptoms outweighs the theoretical hazard of foetal malformation.

Warning: The ability to drive a car or to operate machinery may be affected. Therefore caution should be exercised initially, until the individual's reaction to treatment is known.

Adverse reactions: Extrapyramidal side-effects may occur, especially during the early phase of treatment. In most cases these side-effects can be satisfactorily controlled by antiparkinson drugs. Initial drowsiness may occur and weight change has been reported in a few patients. Tardive dyskinesia, galactorrhoea and amenorrhoea are adverse effects of the general group of neuroleptic drugs and occasional instances of these have been encountered in patients receiving Clopixol.

Overdosage: Overdosage should be treated by gastric lavage.

Pharmaceutical precautions The tablets should be stored at room temperature in their original containers, protected from light and moisture. Under these conditions the preparation has a shelf life of three years from date of manufacture.

Legal category POM.

Package quantities Clopixol tablets 2 mg, 10 mg and 25 mg are packed in bottles containing 100 tablets.

Further information Nil.

Product licence numbers

	2 mg	0458/0027
	10 mg	0458/0028
	25 mg	0458/0029

DEPIXOL* INJECTION

Presentation Depixol Injection is a 2% sterile, straw-coloured solution of cis(Z)-flupenthixol decanoate in thin vegetable oil. It is presented in clear glass ampoules, syringes (1 ml and 2 ml) and vials (10 ml).

Active ingredient: cis(Z)-flupenthixol decanoate 20 mg per ml.

Uses *Pharmacology:* Flupenthixol is a potent, non-sedating, neuroleptic drug of the thioxanthene series. In addition to a marked antipsychotic action it has been shown to possess activating, alerting, and anxiolytic effects and, in low doses, antidepressant activity. Flupenthixol itself is relatively short-acting, but Depixol Injection, its decanoic acid ester dissolved in thin vegetable oil, provides a predictable, slow-release depot preparation of the active constituent. Pharmacological studies in animals indicate a duration of action of two to four weeks after intramuscular injection. This has been confirmed in man by pharmacokinetic studies using radioimmunoassay of flupenthixol, which indicate a slow release of active substance after intramuscular injection giving a maximal blood concentration about four to seven days after injection and a plateau lasting from two to three weeks. Further corroboration of this absorption pattern is provided by clinical studies where Depixol Injection has been successfully used by administration at intervals of two to four weeks.

Indications: Depixol Injection is a depot neuroleptic preparation and is indicated in the treatment and maintenance of schizophrenic patients, especially those who are unreliable in taking oral medicines prescribed for them. Features of the illness most likely to benefit are apathy, inertia, withdrawal, anxiety, hallucinations and paranoid delusions.

Dosage and administration *Adults:* Depixol Injection is administered by deep intramuscular injection into the upper, outer buttock or lateral thigh in doses of 20–40 mg (1–2 ml) at intervals of two to four weeks depending on the response. Some patients may need larger doses, or need them at shorter intervals. Doses greater than 40 mg (2 ml) should be distributed between two injection sites.

Note: As with all oily injections it is important to ensure, by aspiration before injection, that inadvertent intravascular entry does not occur.

Children: Depixol Injection should not be administered to children.

Transfer of patients to Depixol Injection:

1. Those not previously treated with long-acting antipsychotic injections should start with a test dose of 20 mg (1 ml) and the patient's response and the appearance of extra-pyramidal symptoms carefully studied during the following 5–10 days. Oral neuroleptic drugs should be continued, but in diminishing dosage.

2. Patients being transferred from phenothiazine depot injections should receive a dose in the ratio of 40 mg Depixol Injection equivalent to 25 mg fluphenazine decanoate.

3. Patients whose psychotic symptoms may have been treated with cis(Z)-clopenthixol decanoate (Clopixol Injection) because of features such as agitation or aggression at the time of starting depot neuroleptic therapy may pass to a phase in their psychoses in which features such as anergia or withdrawal predominate. Such a change in the clinical picture would warrant consideration of a change of treatment to Depixol Injection, using a comparable antipsychotic dose (40 mg Depixol Injection ≡ 200 mg Clopixol Injection).

Two to four weeks later a second dose of 40 mg (2 ml) or more is then given, depending on the response and appearance of unwanted effects. This part of the treatment should normally be given in hospital. Subsequently the dose and frequency of administration should be adjusted for each individual patient so as to achieve maximum control of psychotic symptoms with a minimum of side-effects.

Contra-indications, warnings, etc Depixol Injection is not recommended for excitable or overactive patients since its activating effect may lead to exaggeration of these characteristics. It is also unsuitable for patients who do not tolerate oral neuroleptic drugs, or for those with Parkinsonism, severe arteriosclerosis, senile confusional states, or advanced renal, hepatic or cardiovascular disease. Depixol should be avoided in pregnancy. However teratological studies in three animal species have failed to reveal any specific effect of flupenthixol or its decanoate on foetal anatomy. Therefore, it is reasonable, particularly after the first trimester, to persevere with treatment in a previously unrecognised pregnancy if psychiatric indications outweigh the theoretical hazard of foetal malformation.

Adverse reactions: The commonest unwanted effect is the appearance of extrapyramidal symptoms, both hypo–kinetic and hyperkinetic. When these appear, they generally do so one to three days after injection and last for about five days. The incidence seems to be greater after the first few injections, and to diminish thereafter. Routine anti-Parkinson drug treatment is not recommended. Tardive dyskinesia has been observed very occasionally: these rare cases have been almost exclusively in patients taking concurrent anticholinergic anti-Parkinson drugs. No specific clinical incompatibilities with other drugs or food have been encountered. However on theoretical pharmacodynamic grounds it may be wise to allow an interval of not less than seven days between completion of MAOI treatment and the initiation of Depixol therapy. Occasional depressive reactions have been reported after administration of Depixol Injection, but they appear to be less frequent than after other depot neuroleptics. Occasional local reactions such as erythema, swelling or tender fibrous nodules have been reported. Amenorrhoea has occurred in patients receiving high doses. Galactorrhoea is a rare side-effect of the drug which may be severe enough to warrant reduction of dosage or withdrawal of neuroleptic treatment. No anticholinergic, hepatic, renal, haematological or cardiovascular (e.g. hypotension) side-effects have been confirmed, nor have flupenthixol-induced photosensitivity or alterations in the cornea or lens been reported.

Overdosage: Overdosage should be treated:

1. By anticholinergic anti-Parkinson drugs if extrapyramidal symptoms occur.
2. By sedation (with benzodiazepines) in the unlikely event of agitation or excitement.
3. By noradrenaline in saline intravenous drip if the patient is in shock. Otherwise observation and symptomatic management should be adequate.

Pharmaceutical precautions Store at room temperature and protect from light, Under those conditions the preparation has a shelf life of two years from date of manufacture.

In accordance with normal practice partially used vials should be discarded at the end of each session.

Legal category POM.

For use in hospitals and hospital clinics and from registered pharmacies for dispensing prescriptions in respect of patients stabilised on Depixol. Depixol is available on prescription only.

Package quantities Boxes of 10 × 20 mg (1 ml) ampoules and syringes.
Boxes of 10 × 40 mg (2 ml) ampoules and syringes.
Boxes of 1 × 10 ml vials.

Further information Nil.

Product licence number 0458/0007.

DEPIXOL*-CONC. INJECTION

Presentation Depixol-Conc. Injection is a 10% sterile, straw-coloured solution of cis(Z)-flupenthixol decanoate in thin vegetable oil. It is presented in glass ampoules (1 ml) and vials (5 ml).

Active ingredient: cis(Z)-flupenthixol decanoate 100 mg per ml.

Uses *Pharmacology:* Flupenthixol is a potent, non-sedating neuroleptic drug of the thioxanthene series. In addition to a marked antipsychotic action it has been shown to possess activating, alerting and anxiolytic effects and, in low doses, antidepressant activity. Flupenthixol itself is relatively short-acting, but its decanoic acid ester dissolved in thin vegetable oil, provides a predictable, slow-release depot preparation of the active constituent. Pharmacological studies in animals indicate a duration of action of two to four weeks after intramuscular injection. This has been confirmed in man by pharmacokinetic studies using radioimmunoassay of flupenthixol which indicate a slow release of active substance after intramuscular injection, giving a maximal blood concentration about four to seven days after injection and a plateau lasting from two to three weeks. Further corroboration of this absorption pattern is provided by clinical studies where Depixol-Conc. Injection has been successfully used by administration at intervals of two to four weeks.

Indications: Depixol-Conc. Injection is a depot neuroleptic preparation and is indicated for the treatment of moderate to severe schizophrenia and allied psychoses. Patients for whom the drug is especially appropriate are:

1. Those believed by the Physician to be unreliable in taking oral medication.
2. Patients who are already receiving treatment with Depixol Injection at high dose levels and who may experience discomfort as a result of the large injection volume.
3. Patients who hitherto could not receive effective treatment with depot neuroleptics because of the high doses, and hence large volumes, required to achieve satisfactory therapeutic blood levels.

Features of the illness most likely to benefit are hallucinations, paranoid delusions, apathy, inertia, withdrawal and anxiety.

Dosage and administration Depixol-Conc. Injection is a solution of flupenthixol decanoate five times more concentrated than Depixol (standard) Injection and Depixol-Conc. Injection is therefore appropriate for the treatment of patients requiring single doses of 100 mg or more of the drug. Doses greater than 200 mg (2 ml) should be distributed between two injection sites.

Adults: Depixol-Conc. is administered by deep intramuscular injection into the upper, outer buttock or lateral thigh, usually in doses of 100–200 mg (1–2 ml) every two to four weeks. Individual dosage and intervals between injection should be adjusted according to therapeutic response. Dosage for most patients falls between 100 mg (1 ml) every four weeks and 300 mg (3 ml) every two weeks but some, especially during an exacerbation or acute relapse of the disease, may require single injections of as much as 400 mg (4 ml) fortnightly or even weekly. Adequate control of severe symptoms by Depixol-Conc. Injection is usually achieved in four to six months and this may justify return to lower dose maintenance with standard Depixol 2% injections.

Note: As with all oily injections it is important to ensure, by aspiration before injection, that inadvertent intravascular entry does not occur.

Children: Depixol-Conc. Injection should not be administered to children.

Transfer of patients to Depixol-Conc. Injection:

1. From Depixol Injection. Patients should be transferred on the basis of 1 ml Depixol-Conc. equivalent to 5 ml of Depixol Injection. Control of severe symptoms by Depixol-Conc. Injection (usually achieved within four to six months) may justify a return to low dose maintenance with Depixol Injection. Extrapyramidal effects may occur in a minority of patients, their incidence and severity being of the same order as are encountered in patients treated with Depixol Injection.

2. Patients being transferred from phenothiazine depot injections should start with an equivalent or higher dose in the ratio of 100 mg Depixol-Conc. Injection equivalent to 62.5 mg fluphenazine decanoate.

3. Those not previously treated with long-acting antipsychotic injections should start with a small test dose of Depixol Injection 20 mg (1 ml), (see Depixol Injection Data Sheet), and the response and possible emergence of extrapyramidal symptoms observed over the following 5–10 days. During this period oral medication should be gradually withdrawn. This part of the treatment should normally be given in hospital.

Contra-indications, warnings, etc Depixol-Conc. Injection is not recommended for patients who do not tolerate oral neuroleptic drugs, or for those with Parkinsonism, severe arteriosclerosis, senile confusional states, or advanced renal, hepatic or cardiovascular disease. Depixol-Conc. should be avoided in pregnancy. However teratological studies in three animal species have failed to reveal any specific effect of flupenthixol or its decanoate on foetal anatomy. Therefore, it is reasonable, particularly after the first trimester, to persevere with treatment in previously unrecognised pregnancy if psychiatric indications outweigh the theoretical hazard of foetal malformation.

Adverse reactions: The commonest side-effect is the appearance of extrapyramidal symptoms, both hypokinetic and hyperkinetic. When these appear they generally do so one to three days after injection and last for about five days. The incidence seems to be greater after the first few injections and to diminish thereafter. The incidence and severity of extrapyramidal side-effects is no greater with flupenthixol doses in the higher range (for which Depixol-Conc. Injection is appropriate) than with lower doses (for which Depixol standard injection solution is more appropriate) and routine anti-Parkinson drug treatment is not recommended. Tardive dyskinesia has been observed very occasionally: these rare cases have been almost exclusively in patients taking concurrent anticholinergic anti-Parkinson drugs. No specific clinical incompatibilities with other drugs or food have been encountered. However on theoretical pharmacodynamic grounds it may be wise to allow an interval of not less than seven days between completion of MAOI treatment and the initiation of Depixol therapy.

Occasional depressive reactions have been reported after administration of Depixol-Conc. Injection, but they appear to be less frequent than after other neuroleptics. Occasional local reactions such as erythema, swelling or tender fibrous nodules have been reported. Amenorrhoea has occurred in patients receiving high doses. Galactorrhoea is a rare side-effect of the drug which may be severe enough to warrant reduction of dosage or withdrawal of neuroleptic treatment. Blood dyscrasias have been observed on rare occasions in patients treated with high-dose neuroleptics. It is, therefore, prudent to carry out periodical blood counts in patients receiving high doses of Depixol-Conc. Injection. No anticholinergic, hepatic, renal or cardiovascular (e.g. hypotension) side-effects have been confirmed nor have flupenthixol-induced photosensitivity or alterations in the cornea or lens been reported.

Overdosage: Overdosage should be treated:

1. By anticholinergic anti-Parkinson drugs if extrapyramidal symptoms occur.
2. By sedation (with benzodiazepines) in the unlikely event of agitation or excitement.
3. By noradrenaline in saline intravenous drip if the patient is in shock. Otherwise observation and symptomatic management should be adequate.

Pharmaceutical precautions Store at room temperature and protect from light. Under these conditions the preparation has a shelf life of two years from date of manufacture.

In accordance with normal practice partially used vials should be discarded at the end of each session.

Legal category POM.

For use in hospitals and hospital clinics and from registered pharmacies on prescription only.

Package quantities Boxes of 10×100 mg (1 ml) ampoules.
Boxes of 1×5 ml vials.

Further information Nil.

Product licence number 0458/0015.

DEPIXOL* TABLETS 3 mg

Presentation Depixol Tablets 3 mg contain flupenthixol 3 mg as the dihydrochloride. The tablets are round, biconvex, yellow sugar-coated, with a diameter of about 9 mm. The Lundbeck logo is printed in black on one face.

Uses *Pharmacology:* Flupenthixol is a potent neuroleptic with a rapid onset of antipsychotic, alerting and anxiolytic effects. It is rapidly metabolised and excreted and is relatively short-acting. When sustained action is required, a depot intramuscular injection of Depixol Injection or Depixol-Conc. Injection in the form of flupenthixol decanoate will provide a therapeutic effect for two to four weeks (see Depixol Injection and Depixol Conc. Injection data sheets).

Indications: Depixol Tablets 3 mg are indicated in the treatment of schizophrenia and other psychoses. Its alerting effect makes Depixol particularly useful in patients who are withdrawn, apathetic, anergic or depressed, or in whom neuroleptics with a marked sedative effect cause fatigue or drowsiness.

Dosage and administration *Adults:* 1–3 tablets twice daily, to a maximum of 18 mg [6 tablets] per day. Doses should be reduced in patients with intercurrent disease.

Children: Until further clinical evidence is available it is recommended that this product should not be administered to children.

Contra-indications, warnings, etc Depixol Tablets should be used with caution in patients with Parkinsonism, severe arteriosclerosis, senile confusional states, or advanced renal, hepatic or cardiovascular disease. They are not recommended for excitable or overactive patients in doses below 6 mg daily since the activating effect may

lead to exaggeration of these characteristics. Depixol should be avoided in pregnancy. However teratological studies in three animal species have failed to reveal any specific effect of flupenthixol on foetal anatomy. Therefore, it is reasonable, particularly after the first trimester, to persevere with treatment in previously unrecognised pregnancy if psychiatric indications outweigh the theroetical hazard of foetal malformation.

Adverse reactions: Extrapyramidal symptoms occur in approximately 25% of patients but are usually mild and controllable by dose reduction or concurrent anti-Parkinson (anticholinergic) drugs. Routine anti-Parkinson drug treatment is not recommended. At high dosage a sedative effect may occur in the occasional patient. No adverse interactions have been reported between Depixol Tablets and tricyclic antidepressants and no specific clinical incompatibilities with other drugs or food have been encountered. However on theoretical pharmacodynamic grounds it may be wise to allow an interval of not less than seven days between completion of MAOI treatment and the initiation of Depixol therapy. Amenorrhoea may occur in patients receiving high doses. Tardive dyskinesia and galactorrhoea are adverse effects of the general group of neuroleptic drugs.

Overdosage: Overdosage should be treated by gastric lavage.

Pharmaceutical precautions The tablets should be stored in their original container, protected from light and moisture. Under these conditions, the preparation has a shelf life of five years from date of manufacture.

Legal category POM.

Package quantities Bottles of 100 tablets of 3 mg.

Further information Nil.

Product licence number 0458/0013.

ESTRACYT* CAPSULES

Presentation Off-white gelatin capsules each containing 140 mg estramustine phosphate as the disodium salt.

Active ingredient: 140 mg estramustine phosphate – oestra-1,3,5(10)-triene-3,17β-diol-3-bis-(2-chloroethyl) carbamate-17-disodium phosphate.

Uses *Pharmacology:* Estracyt is a chemical compound of oestradiol and normustine and has both oestrogenic and cytotoxic activity. Its oestrogenic effect is weaker than that of oestradiol and this is reflected by the lower incidence of gynaecomastia and other feminising side-effects in patients treated with Estracyt for prostatic carcinoma. Estracyt also has antioestrogenic activity in that it antagonises the uterotrophic effect of oestrone in juvenile mice, antigonadotrophic activity in that it causes atrophy of the testes and accessory sex organs in rats, and anti-androgenic activity in that it inhibits testosterone-induced growth of the ventral prostate of castrated animals.

Estracyt's cytotoxic activity is weaker than that of conventional alkylating agents. It is concentrated ten times more efficiently than oestradiol in prostatic tissue and has a greater affinity for prostatic than for other tissue. Though active against experimental animal tumours (rat DMBA-induced mammary tumour and hepatoma AH130), Estracyt has weak general cytostatic effects and causes little or no marrow depression at conventional therapeutic dosage. It has no immunosuppressant effect.

Estracyt appears to lose its phosphate moiety in the gut, liver and in phosphatase-rich human tissue, and following breakage of the carbamate linkage the steroid and alkylating moieties are excreted independently. Absorption of Estracyt from the gut is about 75% complete.

Indications Carcinoma of the prostate, especially in cases unresponsive to, or relapsing after, treatment by conventional oestrogens (stilboestrol, polyoestradiol phosphate (Estradurin), etc) or by orchidectomy. The response rate to Estracyt in such oestrogen-resistant cases is about 30% to 50%.

Dosage and administration *Adults:* Dosage range may be from 1 to 10 capsules a day by mouth with meals. The capsules should not be taken with milk or milk products. Standard starting dosage is 4–8 capsules a day in divided doses with later adjustment according to response and gastrointestinal tolerance.

Children: Adenocarcinoma of the prostate is almost unknown in young boys and no relevant clinical studies of Estracyt have been carried out. Estracyt should not be administered to children.

Contra-indications, warnings, etc Peptic ulceration, severe liver disease and severe cardiac disease.

Precautions: Caution should be exercised in administering Estracyt to patients with moderate to severe bone marrow depression.

Adverse reactions: Adverse effects which may be encountered in treatment are gastrointestinal upset (most commonly transient nausea, but occasionally vomiting, and rarely diarrhoea); disturbance of liver function has been reported; rarely thrombocytopenia below 100,000 mm³; gynaecomastia (seen in less than 5% of patients); cardiovascular (with an incidence of angina no greater than that encountered in patients treated with conventional oestrogens, but including rare drug-related deaths from myocardial infarction); and allergy (manifest as a rash and/or fever).

Overdosage: There is no specific antidote. In the event of dangerously low levels of red cell, white cell or platelet counts; cross-matched whole blood should be given as necessary. It may also be advisable to monitor liver function.

Pharmaceutical precautions Store at room temperature. The preparation has a shelf life of three years from the date of manufacture.

Legal category POM.

For use in hospitals and hospital clinics, and supplied to retail pharmacies for dispensing prescriptions for patients whose treatment has been initiated in hospital practice. Estracyt capsules are available on prescription only.

Package quantities Bottles of 100 capsules each containing 140 mg estramustine phosphate as the sodium salt.

Further information Nil.

Product licence number 0458/0016.

ESTRADURIN* INJECTION

Presentation Estradurin Injection contains 40 mg or 80 mg polyoestradiol phosphate per vial, for reconstitution with water for injection.

Estradurin 40 mg vial:

Polyoestradiol phosphate	40 mg
Mepivacaine	5 mg
Nicotinamide	25 mg

Estradurin 80 mg vial:

Polyoestradiol phosphate	80 mg
Mepivacaine	5 mg
Nicotinamide	40 mg

Uses *Pharmacology:* Estradurin is a water-soluble polymer in which molecules of oestradiol-17β alternate with phosphate groups. After intramuscular injection it acts primarily as a long-acting form of oestradiol, but it also has an inhibitory action on acid and alkaline phosphatases.

The prolonged action of Estradurin is attributed to the slow progressive breakdown of the polymer by phosphatases *in vivo*. Since Estradurin has an inhibiting effect on phosphatases this breakdown is very slow, providing sustained oestrogen activity for up to four weeks after a single injection.

Indications: The treatment of oestrogen-responsive carcinoma of the prostate, particularly in men suspected of unreliability in the taking of conventional oral oestrogen.

Dosage and administration *Adults:* The recommended starting dose is 80–160 mg every four weeks for two to three months. Thereafter the dose may be reduced, in accordance with the patient's clinical and biochemical progress, to 40–80 mg every four weeks.

NB. Estradurin must be administered by *deep* intramuscular injection.

Children: Estradurin should not be administered to children.

Contra-indications, warnings, etc There are no contra-indications for Estradurin, but it should be used with caution in patients with serious liver impairment or thromboembolic cardiovascular disease.

Adverse reactions: Certain characteristic oestrogenic side-effects occur (e.g. gynaecomastia, feminisation), but their incidence and severity are considerably less than those encountered in patients receiving conventional stilboestrol therapy. Gastrointestinal disturbances have not been reported during treatment with Estradurin.

Overdosage: There is no specific antidote. Treatment should be purely symptomatic.

Pharmaceutical precautions Store at room temperature.

The product has a shelf life of five years from the date of manufacture. Estradurin solution is prepared by adding 2 ml water for injection to the vial and shaking until solution is complete.

It is recommended that solutions of Estradurin be prepared immediately before use.

Legal category POM.

Package quantities
10 × 40 mg vials: (with 10 × 2 ml ampoules water for injection.
10 × 80 mg vials: (with 10 × 2 ml ampoules water for injection).

Further information Mepivacaine, a local anaesthetic, is included to minimise discomfort at the site of injection.

Nicotinamide is included to enhance solubility of the polymer.

Product licence numbers
Estradurin 40 mg 0458/5000
Estradurin 80 mg 0458/5001

FLUANXOL* TABLETS

Presentation Fluanxol tablets contain flupenthixol as the dihydrochloride. The tablets are red, round, biconvex and sugar-coated, with 'Lundbeck' printed on one face. The 0.5 mg tablet has a diameter of 6 mm and 'Lundbeck' printed in black on one face. The 1 mg tablet has a diameter of 8 mm and 'Lundbeck' printed in white on one face.

Uses Fluanxol tablets are indicated in the short-term symptomatic treatment of depression of mild to moderate severity (with or without anxiety) or where treatment with other antidepressants has failed.

Dosage and administration *Adults:* Standard initial dosage is 1 mg as a single morning dose. After one week the dose may be increased to 2 mg if there is inadequate clinical response. Daily dosage of more than 2 mg should be in divided doses up to a maximum 3 mg. In view of the activating properties of Fluanxol it is advisable to give the last dose of the day no later than 4.00 p.m.

Patients often respond to Fluanxol within two or three days. If no effect has been observed within one week at maximum dosage the drug should be withdrawn.

Elderly: Standard initial dosage is 0.5 mg as a single morning dose. After one week, if response is inadequate, dosage may be increased to 1 mg once a day. Caution should be exercised in further increasing the dosage but occasional patients may require up to a maximum of 2 mg a day which should be given in divided doses (1 mg at breakfast time and 1 mg at about 4.00 pm).

Children: Not recommended for children.

Contra-indications, warnings, etc Fluanxol is not recommended for the treatment of severe depression requiring ECT and/or hospitalisation. It is not recommended in states of excitement or overactivity (including mania).

Precautions: Fluanxol should be used with caution in patients with Parkinson's disease, severe arteriosclerosis, senile confusional state or severe hepatic, renal or cardiovascular disease.

Warnings and adverse effects: precipitation of hypomania has been occasionally reported. Restlessness or insomnia are occasional side-effects. Others more rarely reported include, dizziness, tremor, visual disturbances, headache, migraine and hyperprolactinaemia. Extrapyramidal symptoms, such as akinesia, may occur rarely at the recommended dose and if they do occur treatment with Fluanxol should be withdrawn. Late onset movement disorders, including tardive dyskinesia, have occasionally been reported in patients receiving flupenthixol but no cases have been reported in patients treated with Fluanxol within the data sheet recommendations. Fluanxol may initially cause drowsiness. Patients should be warned of this possibility if driving or operating machinery. Alcohol may potentiate this effect.

Recurrence of depressive symptoms on abrupt withdrawal is rare. However gradual reduction of dosage is advisable. Dependence has not been reported.

Pregnancy: As there is no unequivocal evidence as to the safety of Fluanxol in human pregnancy, use during pregnancy, especially the first and last trimesters, should be avoided.

Treatment of overdose: Overdosage should be treated by gastric lavage and supportive therapy. The toxic hazard is less than with overdosage of tricyclic antidepressants.

Further information Clinical trials have shown that symptoms of apathy, lowered mood, asthenia, despondency, lack of initiative, or inertia are likely to respond well to Fluanxol. Its high therapeutic index is an advantage in view of the suicide risk associated with depressive illness.

No adverse interactions have been reported between Fluanxol and benzodiazepines or tricyclic antidepressants.

Flupenthixol is available in higher doses as Depixol tablets. These are indicated only in the treatment of functional psychotic disorders.

Pharmaceutical precautions The tablets should be stored in their original container, protected from light and moisture. Under these conditions the 0.5 mg tablet and 1.0 mg tablet have a shelf life of five and three years respectively.

Legal category POM.

Package quantities 0.5 mg tablets in bottles of 100 tablets.
1.0 mg tablets in packs of 60, as 6 × 10 blister strips.

Product licence numbers 0458/0011
0458/0037

MEDICOAL*

Presentation Medicoal is a granular formulation of activated charcoal that effervesces in water to form a suspension. The suspension is tasteless and suitable for conventional oral administration or for gastric lavage.

Active ingredient: Each sachet of Medicoal contains 5 g of activated charcoal.

Uses Emergency treatment of acute poisoning or drug overdosage. Medicoal has high adsorptive capacity for a wide range of plant and inorganic poisons and most drugs used in medicine, including those most commonly taken in accidental or deliberate overdosage, e.g. salicylates, barbiturates and tricyclic anti-depressants.

Indications: In the alimentary tract, Medicoal adsorbs (and thus reduces or prevents systemic absorption of) most inorganic and organic compounds of low or high molecular weight. It is indicated, preferably after emptying of the stomach contents by emesis or gastric washout, in cases of poisoning or drug overdosage with:

Vegetable poisons

aconite	hemlock	quinine
belladonna	ipecacuanha	*salicylates*
cocaine	morphine	stramonium
delphinine	muscarine	strychnine
digitalis	nicotine	veratrine
elaterin	opium	

Drugs

amphetamine	chlorpromazine	phenobarbi-
antipyrine	(and related	tone (and
aspirin	phenothiazines)	other *barbi-*
atropine	dextroamphetamine	*turates*)
chlorpheniramine	digoxin	phenytoin
(and related anti-	nortriptyline (and	propoxyphene
histamines)	other *tricyclic*	penicillin
	anti-depressants)	

Inorganic compounds and elements

antimony	silver	mercuric chloride
arsenic	tin	
iodine	titanium	
phosphorus		

Dosage and administration

1. *Conventional oral administration:* Medicoal should be given orally as a suspension in water (one sachet in about 100 ml) as soon as possible after ingestion or suspected ingestion of the potential poison, or after induced emesis or stomach wash-out. The rate and degree of adsorption to activated charcoal varies from substance to substance according to ionisation, pH and molecular size. Many drugs require more than double their dose of charcoal for complete adsorption.

When the dose of drug or poison is known the standard dose of Medicoal is 5–10 times that dose. This is given as an initial dose of one or two sachets, followed by a similar dose 20 minutes later, repeated at 15–20 minute intervals until the appropriate total dose has been given. Higher or more frequent dosage of Medicoal may induce vomiting of the suspension. When the dose of ingested drug or poison is unknown a similar treatment schedule is followed to a maximum Medicoal dose of 10 sachets (50 g activated charcoal).

Medicoal may be effective even several hours after ingestion of the drug or poison in cases where the compound ingested is:

(a) an anticholinergic, slowing gastric emptying.
(b) absorbed and excreted in the bile;
    or where fear or nausea inhibits gastrointestinal motility.

2. *Gastric lavage:* Medicoal is added to the irrigation water in a dose of 30–50 g in ½–1 litre. Subsequent conventional oral dosage of Medicoal is governed by the proportion of dose or suspected dose of drug or poison ingested that is retrieved by stomach wash-out.

Children: The dose of Medicoal is related more to the dose or suspected dose of poison or drug than to the age, weight or surface area of the child, but the volume of the suspension at each administration may need to be reduced.

Contra-indications, warnings, etc

Contra-indications: Medicoal is valueless and contra-indicated in poisoning by strong acids or alkalis. Its adsorptive capacity for the following poisons and drugs is too low to be useful and other more specific forms of treatment should be used:

ferrous sulphate (and	cyanides
other iron salts)	
malathion	tolbutamide (and other
DDT	sulphonylureas)

Warnings: Activated charcoal should not be used simultaneously with systemically acting oral emetics such as ipecacuanha, since it adsorbs the drug, rendering it unavailable for systemic absorption and emetic activity.

If an emetic is required it should be used to induce vomiting before giving Medicoal.

Medicoal is appropriate for the treatment of paracetamol poisoning, either alone or in conjunction with parenteral antidotes such as N-acetylcysteine or cysteamine. However, should a specific oral antidote such as methionine be used, Medicoal is contra-indicated since it will adsorb methionine in the gastrointestinal tract.

Precautions: Although the adsorption of dietary factors such as vitamins and minerals by Medicoal is of no consequence in the treatment of acute poisoning, it should be remembered that concurrent medication, for example for shock or associated infection, should be given parenterally since orally administered drugs may be partly or totally adsorbed and retained in the gut.

Adverse effects: No adverse effects are attributable to activated charcoal, but the release of carbon dioxide from the effervescent suspension may cause belching or vomiting of the dose administered if this is excessive.

Pharmaceutical precautions Medicoal should remain sealed in the sachets until required. The effervescent and dispersive properties of the granules are adversely affected by moisture. The product has a shelf life of five years from the date of manufacture.

Legal category P.

Package quantities Cartons of 5 and 30 sachets, each containing activated charcoal 5 g, as granules.

Further information Care should be exercised in the preparation and administration of Medicoal Suspension, since it may stain if spilt on clothing.

Product licence number 0458/0019.

NICORETTE* ▼

Presentation Square pieces of chewing gum containing 2 mg or 4 mg nicotine.

Active ingredient: 2 mg or 4 mg nicotine as the resin in a chewing gum base.

Uses Nicotine replacement. When Nicorette is chewed, nicotine is slowly released into the mouth and is absorbed through the buccal mucosa. A proportion, by the swallowing of nicotine-containing saliva, reaches the stomach and intestine and any nicotine absorbed by this route is inactivated.

Indications: Nicorette is intended to help smokers who want to give up smoking, but experience great difficulty in doing so because of their nicotine dependence.

Dosage and administration *Adults:* The strength of gum to be used depends upon the smoking habits of the individual. It is recommended that patients beginning treatment should always start with Nicorette 2 mg to determine its acceptability. If more than 15 × 2 mg Nicorette per day are required, transfer to the 4 mg gum may be considered.

Nicorette should be chewed slowly, when there is an urge to smoke, up to a maximum of 15 × 4 mg pieces per day; however the patient's individual need may be considerably less than this number. Most patients require about 10 pieces of 2 mg per day initially.

All available nicotine is released from a piece of gum after about 30 minutes chewing. Since effective absorption is through the buccal mucosa, the rate of chewing should be adjusted to minimise the swallowing and inactivation of nicotine contained in saliva.

After 3 months ad libitum dosage Nicorette should be gradually withdrawn.

Children: Not to be administered to children.

Contra-indications, warnings, etc Nicotine in any form is contra-indicated in pregnancy. Smokers who wear dentures may experience difficulty in chewing Nicorette. Dependence is a rare side-effect and is both less harmful and easier to break than smoking dependence.

Precautions:

1. Swallowed nicotine may exacerbate symptoms in patients suffering from gastritis or peptic ulcer.

2. Nicotine's cardiovascular effects may be deleterious to patients with angina or a history of coronary artery disease. Nicorette presents a lesser hazard, however, than smoking which introduces carbon monoxide as an additional toxic factor.

Adverse effects: Nicorette in the recommended dose has not been found to cause any serious adverse effects. Nicotine from the gum may sometimes cause a slight irritation of the throat at the start of treatment, and may also cause increased salivation. Excessive swallowing of dissolved nicotine may, at first, cause hicupping. Those with a tendency to indigestion may suffer initially from minor degrees of indigestion or heartburn if the 4 mg gum is used; slower chewing and the use of the 2 mg gum (if necessary more frequently) will usually overcome this problem.

Excessive consumption of Nicorette by patients who have not been in the habit of inhaling tobacco smoke could possibly lead to nausea, faintness or headaches (as may be experienced by such patients if tobacco smoke is inhaled).

Overdosage: Overdosage of Nicorette can occur only if many pieces are chewed simultaneously. The fatal acute dose of nicotine in man is probably about 60 mg. Risk of overdosage with Nicorette is, however, small since nausea or vomiting usually occurs at an early stage.

Risk of poisoning by swallowing the gum is also small, since the release of nicotine from the gum is slow. Therefore very little nicotine is absorbed from the stomach or intestine and any that is will be inactivated in the liver. Nicotine is excreted in acid urine four times as rapidly as in alkaline urine.

Treatment of overdosage: In the event of overdosage vomiting should be induced with syrup of ipecacuanha or gastric lavage carried out (wide bore tube). A suspension of activated charcoal (Medicoal) should then be passed through the tube and left in the stomach. Artificial respiration with oxygen should be instituted if needed and continued for as long as necessary. Other therapy, including treatment of shock, is purely symptomatic.

Pharmaceutical precautions No special storage conditions are necessary. The preparation has a shelf life at room temperature of 2 years from the date of manufacture.

Legal category POM.

Package quantities Package of 105 pieces, in the form of 7 blister-packed strips each containing 15 pieces (2 mg or 4 mg).

Further information Nicorette should be chewed slowly. Sufficient nicotine may be released from the gum by chewing intermittently and leaving the gum under the lip or in the corner of the mouth between chews.

Nicorette is sugar-free.

Product licence numbers
2 mg: 0458/0020
4 mg: 0458/0021

*Trade Mark

Martindale Pharmaceuticals Limited
Chesham House
Chesham Close
Romford, Essex RM1 4JX

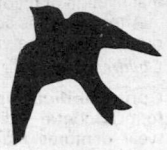

ELECTROSOL*

Presentation Electrosol is presented as a free-flowing powder for reconstitution in individual dose sachets containing:

Sodium Chloride PhEur	200 mg
Sodium Bicarbonate PhEur	300 mg
Potassium Chloride PhEur	300 mg
Glucose BP	8.0 g

When reconstituted as directed with 200 ml of water the solution provides the following electrolytes in a palatable, orange-flavoured vehicle formulated so as to be isotonic with plasma.

Sodium	35 mmol/l
Potassium	20 mmol/l
Chloride	37 mmol/l
Bicarbonate	18 mmol/l
Glucose	200 mmol/l

Uses For oral replacement of fluids and electrolytes in the treatment of dehydration especially when due to diarrhoea. Its lightly flavoured basis makes it particularly suitable for use in children.

Dosage and administration *Reconstitution:* For infants over 3 months and young children the contents of one sachet should be dissolved in sufficient boiled and cooled water to produce 200 ml. (Most infant feeding bottles are now calibrated for this volume.)

For older children and adults, freshly drawn tap water may be substituted for the boiled water.

The usual hygienic precautions including the sterilisation of bottles, teats, etc., should be adopted in the preparation of solutions intended for use in infants. The reconstituted solution is best used immediately but may be stored for up to 12 hours if kept refrigerated. On no account should the reconstituted solution be boiled.

Dosage: Electrosol is for oral administration only. The volume of solution required depends on the weight and condition of the patient. The aim of the therapy is to maintain an adequate level of hydration by replacing lost fluids with an equal volume of Electrosol solution.

Infants: 150–200 ml of solution per kilogram bodyweight (70–90 ml/lb) given in divided doses per 24 hours, depending on the severity of the condition up to a maximum of 1.5 litres in any 24 hours. In very young infants and especially where vomiting is a problem, it is preferable to give Electrosol in very frequent small doses.

During treatment, breast feeding, where practised, may continue but milk or other foods may be briefly withdrawn, if necessary, with early re-introduction encouraged as the appetite returns.

Electrosol should not be mixed with anything other than water, eg, not with milk or milk formulas.

Adults and children: Should be encouraged to take regular drinks sufficient to quench their thirst. Generally 1–3 litres in any 24-hour period is satisfactory.

Contra-indications, warnings, etc Electrosol is not suitable for use in babies of less than 3 months of age except under medical supervision. If symptoms become worse or persist for more than 48 hours, particularly in infants, further investigation and therapy may be warranted. Electrosol should be reconstituted as directed especially in the case of solutions for use by infants where the usual hygienic precautions should be taken. Electrosol should not be mixed with milk or milk formulas.

Caution is required in treating patients with reduced renal function with Electrosol and diabetic patients should be made aware of its carbohydrate content.

Pharmaceutical precautions Store the sachets in a cool dry place. If necessary the reconstituted solution may be stored for 12 hours if kept refrigerated.

Legal category P.

Package quantities Cartons of 24 unit dose sachets.

Further information Each sachet contains glucose 8 g and provides approximately 30 calories. Electrosol is a brand of Compound Sodium Chloride and Dextrose Oral Powder BP.

Electrosol contains no colouring matter.

Product licence number 0156/0028.

E.S.T.P.*
Ether Soluble Tar Paste

Presentation E.S.T.P. is a light tan-coloured, non staining and emollient Ether Soluble Tar Paste containing:

Ether soluble tar distillate	1.5%
Zinc oxide BP	14.0%
Starch BP (Maize)	12.0%
Emollient base to	100%

Uses E.S.T.P. is indicated for the treatment of mild to moderate Eczema and Psoriasis and other skin conditions.

Dosage and administration Apply to the affected areas three or four times daily or as directed by the Physician.

Contra-indications, warnings, etc Known sensitivity to tar extracts.

Pharmaceutical precautions Protect from heat.

Legal category P.

Package quantities E.S.T.P. is available in jars of 500g.

Further information Nil.

Product licence number 0542/5006

GTN 300 mcg

Presentation Plain white uncoated tablets each containing Glyceryl Trinitrate BP 300 micrograms.

Uses As a short acting vasodilator in the prophylaxis and treatment of attacks of angina pectoris.

Dosage and administration One tablet is allowed to dissolve slowly under the tongue; the treatment may be repeated as required.

Contra-indications, warnings, etc As with all glyceryl trinitrate preparations the tablets should not be used in patients with marked anaemia, incipient glaucoma or those with head trauma or cerebral haemorrhage.
Side effects reported include headaches and facial flushing.
Toxic effects include vomiting, restlessness, hypotension, syncope, cyanosis and methaemoglobinaemia. Severe poisoning may result in bradycardia, respiratory depression and psychosis.
Treatment of toxic effects: To minimise the effects of hypotension, the patient is treated in the recumbent position with the head lowered. The stomach should be emptied to prevent further absorption and general supportive measures such as oxygen, assisted respiration, plasma expanders, employed as necessary. Methaemoglobinaemia may be treated with methylene blue intravenously 1–4 mg/kg.

Pharmaceutical precautions Store in a cool dry place with cap tightly closed.

Legal category P.

Package quantities Bottles of 100 tablets.

Further information Nil.

Product licence number 1883/5958.

MEDILAVE* GEL

Presentation Pale buff-coloured gel. Contains Benzocaine PhEur. 1.0% and Cetylpyridinium Chloride BP 0.01% in a specially formulated water-immiscible protective base.

Uses For the relief of pain from abrasions and ulcers of the gums, palate, cheek, tongue and lips, including soreness due to teething.

Dosage and administration Cover the affected area 3 to 4 times daily with a thin film as required, filling the depression in the ulcer, particularly before meals. Do not rub in.

Contra-indications, warnings, etc Not to be used in infants under 6 months of age. In cases of dental abrasion, care should be taken to remove the underlying cause of the lesion. Consult doctor or dentist if symptoms persist. Some individuals may be hypersensitive to Benzocaine. If so, cease treatment immediately.

Pharmaceutical precautions No special precautions required.

Legal category P.

Package quantities Tube of 10 g.

Further information Nil.

Product licence number 0156/0014.

MITOMYCIN-C KYOWA*

Presentation Purple crystalline powder for intravenous injection containing Mitomycin C Kyowa 2 mg with 48 mg sodium chloride, 10 mg with 240 mg sodium chloride, 20 mg with 480 mg sodium chloride for dissolving in water for injections using the volume recommended for each strength.

Uses *Action:* Mitomycin C Kyowa is an antitumour antibiotic that is activated in the tissues to an alkylating agent which disrupts deoxyribonucleic acid (DNA) in cancer cells by forming a complex with DNA and also acts by inhibiting division of cancer cells by interfering with the biosynthesis of DNA. In vivo, Mitomycin C Kyowa is rapidly cleared from the serum after intravenous administration. The time required to reduce the serum concentration by 50% after a 30 mg bolus injection is 17 minutes. After injection of 30 mg, 20 mg, or 10 mg I.V., the maximal serum concentrations were 2.4 mcg/ml, 1.7 mcg/ml and 0.52 mcg/ml respectively. Clearance is effected primarily by metabolism in the liver, but metabolism occurs in other tissues as well. The rate of clearance is inversely proportional to the maximal serum concentration because, it is thought, of saturation of the degradative pathways. Approximately 10% of a dose of Mitomycin C Kyowa is excreted unchanged in the urine. Since metabolic pathways are saturated at relatively low doses, the percentage dose excreted in the urine increases with increasing the dose. In children, excretion of intravenously administered Mitomycin C Kyowa is similar to that in adults.

Indications: Antimitotic and Cytotoxic. Mitomycin C Kyowa is recommended for certain types of cancer, either in combination with other drugs or after primary therapy has failed. In particular, Mitomycin C Kyowa has been successfully used to improve subjective and objective symptoms in a wide range of neoplastic conditions including carcinomas of the stomach, pancreas, breast and uterus; adenocarcinoma of the lung; peritonitis carcinomatosa; colonic, bladder, rectal and skin cancer. In addition, Mitomycin C Kyowa may also be of some value in sarcomas, hepatic cancer, acute and chronic leukaemias and Hodgkin's disease.

Dosage and administration For systemic administration, Mitomycin C Kyowa should be given intravenously using great care to avoid extravasation. The usual dosage is in the range 4–10 mg (0.06–0.15 mg/kg) at 1–6 weekly intervals, depending on whether other drugs are given in combination and on bone marrow recovery. In a number of combination schedules, the dose of Mitomycin C Kyowa per treatment course is 10 mg/m^2 of body surface area, the course being repeated at intervals for as long as required. A dosage course ranging from 40–80 mg (0.58–1.2 mg/kg) is often required for a satisfactory response both when Mitomycin C Kyowa is used alone or as part of a combination. A higher dosage course may be given when Mitomycin C Kyowa is used alone or as part of particular combination schedules and total cumulative doses exceeding 2 mg/kg have been given.
For reconstitution, the contents of the 2 mg vial should be dissolved in 5 ml water for injections, or 20% dextrose solution. The 10 mg vial should be dissolved in at least

10 ml and the 20 mg vial in at least 20 ml of the same solvents and administered by intravenous injection.

The dose should be adjusted according to the age and condition of the patient.

For administration to specific tissues, Mitomycin C Kyowa can be given also into the pleural and peritoneal cavities and, by the arterial route, directly into tumours.

Because of cumulative myelosuppression, patients should be fully re-evaluated after each course of Mitomycin C Kyowa and the dose reduced if the patient has experienced any toxic effects. Doses greater than 0.6 mg/kg have not been shown to be more effective and are more toxic than lower doses.

Treatment of superficial urinary bladder tumours: In the prevention of recurrent bladder tumours, the usual dose is the equivalent of 4–10 mg (0.06–0.15 mg/kg) potency of Mitomycin C Kyowa instilled into the bladder through a urethral catheter once or three times a week. In the treatment of bladder tumours, the usual dose is the equivalent of 10–40 mg (0.15–0.6 mg/kg) potency of Mitomycin C Kyowa instilled into the bladder either weekly or three times a week for a total of 20 doses. In either case, it should be dissolved in 20 ml–40 ml of water for injections before use. The dose should be adjusted in accordance with the age and condition of the patient.

Contra-indications, warnings, etc Mitomycin C Kyowa should be administered under the supervision of a physician experienced in cytotoxic cancer chemotherapy. Patients should be monitored closely during each course of treatment, paying particular attention to peripheral blood count including platelet count.

The principal toxicity of Mitomycin C Kyowa is bone marrow suppression, particularly thrombocytopenia and leucopenia. The nadir is usually around four weeks after treatment and toxicity is cumulative, with increasing risk after each course of treatment.

No repeat dosage should be given until leucocyte count has returned to $3.0 \times 10^9/l$ and platelet count to $90.0 \times 10^9/l$. If disease progression continues after two courses of treatment, the drug should be stopped since the chances of response are then minimal.

Severe renal toxicity has occasionally been reported after treatment and renal function should be monitored before starting treatment and again after each course.

Nausea and vomiting are sometimes experienced immediately after treatment but these are usually mild and of short duration. Local ulceration and cellulitis may be caused by tissue extravasation during intravenous injection and utmost care should be taken in administration. In the event of extravasation following an intravenous injection of Mitomycin C Kyowa, it is recommended that 5 ml of Sodium Bicarbonate 8.4% solution is immediately infiltrated into the area where extravasation has occurred followed by an injection of 4 mg Dexamethasone. In addition, a systemic injection of 200 mg Vitamin B6 may be of some value in promoting the regrowth of tissues that have been damaged.

Mitomycin C Kyowa should not normally be administered to patients who are pregnant or to mothers who are breast feeding. Teratological changes have been noted in animal studies. The effect of Mitomycin C Kyowa on fertility is unknown. Mitomycin C Kyowa is contraindicated in patients who have demonstrated a hypersensitive or idiosyncratic reaction to it in the past.

The person administering the injection of Mitomycin C Kyowa should not allow the solution to come into contact with his or her skin.

Treatment of skin or eye contact: Any Mitomycin C Kyowa substance or solution in contact with the skin should be washed several times with 8.4% sodium bicarbonate solution, followed by washing with soap and water. Use of handcreams or other emollient preparations is inappropriate as this may assist the penetration of any traces of Mitomycin C Kyowa into the epidermal tissue.

Contact with the eye. The eye should be rinsed several times with sodium bicarbonate eye lotion and the eye examined for several days after contact for evidence of corneal damage. If this occurs, appropriate treatment should be instituted.

Pharmaceutical precautions Unreconstituted Mitomycin C Kyowa remains stable for four years after manufacture when stored at room temperature. Reconstitution, as directed, should be accomplished using aseptic technique and the resulting solutions are best used immediately. If reconstituted Mitomycin C Kyowa must be stored prior to use, it should be protected from light and kept in a cool place – it should not be refrigerated. Solutions stored in this way should be discarded if unused after 12 hours.

When reconstituted solution is added to infusion fluids, especially where these contain dextrose, the resulting solution should be used immediately.

Legal category POM.

Package quantities 2 mg, 10 mg and 20 mg vials for intravenous injection.

Further information Mitomycin C Kyowa vials are available through hospital pharmacies for use in hospitals and hospital clinics and can be supplied to retail chemists for dispensing prescriptions for patients whose treatment has been initiated in hospital practice.

Product licence number 0156/5903.

PAMERGAN P100*

Presentation Pamergan P100 is a colourless solution for injection containing the following ingredients in each 2 ml ampoule:

Pethidine Hydrochloride BP	100 mg
Promethazine Hydrochloride BP	50 mg

Uses Promethazine hydrochloride is a powerful antihistamine agent possessing additional sedative, antiemetic and anticholinergic actions as well as a potentiating effect on central nervous system depressants.

Pethidine hydrochloride is a major analgesic which causes less respiratory depression than morphine.

Pamergan P100 is indicated for pre-anaesthetic medication, obstetrical analgesia and amnesia, and the management of severe pain.

Dosage and administration Pamergan P100 is usually injected intramuscularly; it may be given by the intravenous route after dilution to at least 10 ml with water for injections.

Pre-anaesthetic medication, obstetrical analgesia, severe pain: Administered by intramuscular injection.

Pre-anaesthetic medication: Adults: 2 ml (children: 8–12 years 0.75 ml; 12–16 years 1 ml). Administered 60–90 minutes before anaesthesia.

Obstetrical analgesia and amnesia: 1–2 ml when labour is well established, repeated at four-hourly intervals as required.

Severe pain: 1–2 ml every four to six hours in adults.

Contra-indications, warnings, etc The administration of Pamergan P100 solution to a patient who is or has recently been under treatment with a monoamine oxidase inhibitor may be followed by cerebral excitement, confusion and collapse, or by severe respiratory depression. It is important therefore that Pamergan P100 should not be given to patients receiving such treatment or within two weeks of its discontinuation.

Because of its pethidine content Pamergan P100 should not be given to patients with severe liver disease or for pain following cholecystectomy, biliary colic or increased intracranial pressure.

Because this preparation may cause or exacerbate respiratory depression, its use is contra-indicated in patients suffering from respiratory depression or obstructive airways disease.

Although no embryopathic effects have been reported with Pamergan P100 as with all drugs, it should only be used in pregnancy when the physician considers that the benefits outweigh the potential risks.

Precautions: This preparation may cause drowsiness: patients should not be allowed to drive or operate machinery until any such effects have worn off. Avoid the intake of alcohol during use. Administration during labour may cause some respiratory depression in the new born infant. In elderly patients, those with hypothyroidism or with chronic hepatic disease, a reduced dosage regime should be contemplated.

Warnings and adverse effects: Dryness of the mouth, blurring of vision, slight disorientation and dizziness occur in some patients and an occasional patient may develop a feeling of weakness or syncope accompanied by profuse perspiration.

Prolonged treatment with this preparation may give rise to tolerance and dependance to the pethidine component.

Overdosage: Accidental overdose may give rise to respiratory depression, hypotension, convulsions and circulatory collapse.

Treatment: Establish and maintain a patent airway, assisting respiration if necessary. If respiration is severely depressed give a small intravenous dose of naloxone (adults: 0.4 mg, children: 0.005–0.01 mg/kg, neonates: 0.01 mg/kg) repeated if necessary at intervals of 2–3 minutes. Hypotension may improve with improved oxygenation but may require treatment with an infusion of plasma or suitable electrolyte solution. Convulsions may be treated with a short acting muscle relaxant, intubation and controlled respiration.

Pharmaceutical precautions Protect from light. Pamergan P100 has a pH of 5.0–6.0 and is incompatible with alkaline preparations including thiopentone sodium injection.

Legal category CD (Sch 2) POM.

Package quantities Box of 10 × 2 ml ampoules.

Further information Nil.

Product licence number 0156/0020R.

SOLIWAX* EAR CAPSULES

Presentation Deep red, tube-shaped, soft gelatin capsules each containing docusate sodium 5% w/w in oil.

Uses Ear-wax solvent for removal of excessive or impacted cerumen or for cleaning the ear canal prior to examination or initiation of topical therapy in infections of the ear.

Dosage and administration The contents of a capsule should be squeezed into the ear canal after cutting off the tip of the capsule. The ear should then be loosely plugged with gauze or cotton wool and left for a time, depending on the amount and hardness of the wax. Where the deposit is light the ear may be cleansed after about half an hour, but where the wax is firmly impacted the solvent should be left in place overnight, followed by syringing if necessary.

Contra-indications, warnings, etc Contra-indicated in tympanic perforation.

Pharmaceutical precautions Store away from heat.

Legal category GSL.

Package quantities Containers of 10 capsules.

Further information Dioctyl Sodium Sulphosuccinate is a surface active agent which is able to penetrate and soften wax deposits in the ear. By wetting the surface of the organic matter it enables excess or impacted wax to be dislodged by simple manipulation or syringing.

Product licence number 0156/5902.

*Trade Mark

May & Baker Limited
Dagenham
Essex RM10 7XS

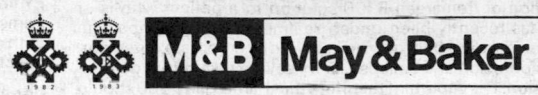

ANTHISAN*

Presentation Dark green, sugar-coated tablets containing 50 mg mepyramine maleate and marked 'Anthisan 50' in ivory print.
  Tablets contain tartrazine.

Uses Anthisan is a potent, rapidly acting antihistamine agent; it also possesses antipruritic properties. It is indicated in the treatment of allergic, anaphylactic and sensitisation reactions.

Dosage and administration *Orally – Adults:* 100 mg three times daily increased if necessary by steps of 50 or 100 mg daily to a maximum of 1 g daily.

Elderly: No specific dosage recommendations.

Children: up to 3 years, 12.5–25 mg three or four times daily. From 3 to 7 years, 25–50 mg three or four times daily. From 7 to 14 years, 25–75 mg three or four times daily.

Contra-indications, warnings, etc
Use in pregnancy: There is no evidence of the safety of the drug in human pregnancy but it has been widely used for many years without apparent ill consequence. Nevertheless Anthisan should not be used during pregnancy or lactation unless the physician considers it essential.

Precautions: Anthisan may cause drowsiness. Patients should not drive or operate machinery until the effect has been ascertained. Alcohol and CNS depressants should be avoided.

Side-effects: Drowsiness or fatigue may occur soon after the beginning of treatment but this tends to disappear after a few days. Gastric upset may be avoided by ensuring that Anthisan is taken with food or a well sweetened drink. Dizziness or dry mouth occurs infrequently. Asthmatic reactions and non-fatal blood dyscrasia have been reported.

Toxicity and treatment of overdosage: Fatal accidents have occurred in young children. Tablets should always be kept out of their reach.
  The chief symptom of overdosage is unconsciousness and there may be convulsions with unconsciousness in the intervening periods. The stomach should be washed out. Stimuli liable to provoke convulsions should be avoided, but if this complication should occur parenteral diazepam should be given; sedatives which are liable to increase respiratory depression should be avoided. Other measures such as artificial respiration and oxygen may also be required and an antibiotic can be given as a prophylactic against pneumonia.

Pharmaceutical precautions Protect from light.

Legal category P.

Package quantities Containers of 500 tablets.

Further information Nil.

Product licence number 0012/5099.

ASCABIOL*

Presentation Ascabiol is a mildly perfumed white emulsion containing 25% benzyl benzoate.

Uses Ascabiol is an efficient acaricide and is used in the treatment of scabies. It is also indicated in the treatment of pediculosis.

Dosage and administration *Scabies:* After a hot bath and drying, Ascabiol is applied to the whole body except the head and face. If the application is thorough, one treatment should suffice, but the possibility of failure is lessened if a second application is made within five days of the first.
  Alternatively, Ascabiol can be applied to the whole body, except the head and face, on three occasions at 12-hourly intervals. The patient has a hot bath 12 hours after the last application and changes to clean clothes and sheets.

Pediculosis: The affected region is coated with Ascabiol followed by a wash 24 hours later with soap and water. In severe cases this procedure may need to be repeated two or three times. An examination should always be made a week after the last treatment to confirm disinfestation.
  Ascabiol can be diluted with an equal quantity of water for older children and with three parts of water for babies.

Contra-indications, warnings, etc Ascabiol causes little skin irritation but may cause a slight transient burning sensation; it is also irritating to the eyes. The eyes should therefore be protected if it is applied to the scalp.
  If this preparation is accidentally taken by mouth, treatment should consist of gastric lavage or the administration of an emetic. An anticonvulsant should be given if necessary, otherwise treatment is symptomatic.

Pharmaceutical precautions Nil.

Legal category P.

Package quantities Bottle of 200 ml.

Further information Nil.

Product licence number 0012/5104.

AVOMINE*

Presentation Avomine is presented as white tablets, each containing 25 mg promethazine theoclate, indented 'Avomine' on one face and with a break line on the reverse.

Uses Long-acting anti-emetic, indicated for prevention and treatment of nausea and vomiting: including motion sickness, postoperative vomiting particularly following fenestration operation: and nausea and vomiting arising from other causes including drug-induced vomiting, and vomiting associated with gastro-enteritis. Vertigo due to Ménière's syndrome, labyrinthitis and other causes.

Kinetics: Promethazine is well absorbed after oral dosing and slowly excreted via urine and bile. It is distributed widely in the body. It enters the brain and crosses the placenta. Phenothiazines pass into the milk in low concentrations.

Dosage and administration *Motion sickness: Adults:* For prevention on long journeys: one 25 mg tablet each evening at bedtime, starting the day before setting out. The duration of action is such that a second dose in 24 hours is not often necessary.

For prevention of motion sickness on short journeys: one 25 mg tablet one or two hours before travelling or as soon after as possible.

Treatment of motion sickness: One 25 mg tablet as soon as possible and repeated the same evening followed by a third tablet on the following evening.

Nausea and vomiting due to other causes: Adults: One 25 mg tablet at night is often sufficient, but two or more of the 25 mg tablets, or more frequent administration twice or three times daily of one 25 mg tablet, may be necessary for some patients. It is not often necessary to give more than four of the 25 mg Avomine tablets in 24 hours.

Children: In the above indications children over 10 years of age may be given the lower adult doses described above. Children between 5 and 10 years may be given half the adult dose.

Elderly: No specific dosage recommendations.

Contra-indications, warnings, etc
Use in pregnancy: There is epidemiological evidence of the safety of promethazine in human pregnancy, animal studies have shown no hazard. Nevertheless it should not be used in pregnancy unless the physician considers it essential.

Ambulant patients receiving Avomine for the first time should not be in control of vehicles or machinery for the first few days until it is established that they are not hypersensitive to the central nervous effects of the drug and do not suffer from disorientation, confusion or dizziness.

Avomine will enhance the action of any sedative or hypnotic. Alcohol should be avoided during treatment.

In nausea and vomiting of unknown origin, it is essential to establish the diagnosis before giving an anti-emetic, to ensure that a serious underlying condition is not masked.

Side effects may be seen in a few patients: drowsiness, dizziness, disorientation. Photosensitive skin reactions have been reported; strong sunlight should be avoided during treatment.

Treatment of overdosage: Symptoms of severe overdosage are variable. They are characterised in children by various combinations of excitation, ataxia, inco-ordina-tion, athetosis and hallucinations, while adults may become drowsy and lapse into coma. Convulsions may occur in both adults and children; coma or excitement may precede their occurrence. Cardiorespiratory depression is uncommon.

If the patient is seen soon enough after ingestion, it should be possible to induce vomiting with ipecacuanha despite the anti-emetic effect of promethazine; alternatively, gastric lavage may be used.

Treatment is otherwise supportive with attention to maintenance of adequate respiratory and circulatory status. Convulsions should be treated with diazepam or other suitable anticonvulsant.

Pharmaceutical precautions Protect from light.

Legal category P.

Package quantities Containers of 250 × 25 mg tablets.

Further information Nil.

Product licence number 0012/5253.

CERVAGEM* ▼

Presentation Yellowish-white spindle shaped vaginal pessaries each containing 1.0 mg gemeprost.

Uses Softening and dilatation of the *cervix uteri* prior to trans-cervical intrauterine operative procedures in pregnant patients in the first trimester of gestation.

Dosage and administration Before administration, the pessary should be allowed to warm to room temperature away from direct heat and sunlight in the unopened foil sachet.

Adults: One pessary to be inserted into the posterior vaginal fornix 3 hours before surgery. Adequate dilatation and softening is generally maintained up to 12 hours after insertion. Beyond the recommended 3 hour interval the incidence of gastro-intestinal side-effects and uterine pain may increase.

Elderly: Not applicable.
Children: Not applicable.

Contra-indications, warnings, etc Gemeprost should not be administered to women with known hypersensitivity to prostaglandins.

Precautions: Gemeprost should be used with caution in patients with obstructive airways disease, those with cardiovascular insufficiency, elevated intraocular pressure, cervicitis or vaginitis.

Patients with the following diseases have not been studied: Ulcerative colitis, diabetes mellitus, sickle-cell anaemia, epilepsy, disorders of blood coagulation, cardiovascular or pulmonary disease. If it is necessary to postpone surgery much beyond the recommended 3 hour interval, patients should be kept under observation as there is a possibility that abortion may occur.

Adequate follow-up of patients having a pregnancy terminated is essential to ensure that the process has been completed as the effect of gemeprost on the foetus has not been established. Cervagem pessaries should not be used for the induction of labour or cervical softening at term as foetal effects have not been ascertained.

Side-effects: Vaginal bleeding and mild uterine pain, similar to menstrual pain, may occur in the interval between the administration of the pessary and surgery, especially if this interval is prolonged beyond the recommended 3 hours. Nausea, vomiting, loose stools or diarrhoea may occur but are rarely severe enough to require treatment. However, standard anti-emetic or anti-diarrhoeal agents may be administered if required. Other reported side-effects include: headache; muscle weakness; dizziness; flushing; chills; backache; dyspnoea; chest pain; palpitations and mild pyrexia. Anaphylactic reactions have not occurred with 'Cervagem' but such reactions have very rarely been noted with other prostaglandins.

Overdosage: The toxic dose of gemeprost in women has not been established. Cumulative dosage of 10 mg in 24 hours has been well tolerated. In animals the acute toxic effects are similar to those of Prostaglandin E_1; relaxation of smooth muscle, leading to hypotension; depression of the CNS. Clinically valuable signs of impending toxicity are likely to be sedation; tremor; convulsion; dyspnoea; abdominal pain and diarrhoea, which may be bloody; palpitations or bradycardia. Treatment should be symptomatic. A vaginal douche may be of value depending on the elapsed time since insertion of the pessary.

Pharmaceutical precautions Store below *minus* 10°C in the original pack. Temperature cycling should be avoided. Once the foil sachet has been opened, any pessary not used within 12 hours should be destroyed.

Legal category POM.

Package quantities Container of 5 unit dose foil sachets.

Further information Nil.

Product licence number 0012/0149.

CONRAY*

Presentation Ampoules or vials containing colourless sterile solutions of varying strengths of meglumine or sodium iothalamate.

Conray 280: Meglumine iothalamate injection 60% w/v containing 280 mg iodine in combined form per ml.

Conray 325: Sodium iothalamate injection 54% w/v containing 325 mg iodine in combined form per ml.

Conray 420: Sodium iothalamate injection 70% w/v containing 420 mg iodine in combined form per ml.

Uses X-ray contrast media are used for the opacification of the vascular and renal systems and female genital tract and do not normally possess any pharmacological action.

Kinetics: If renal function is not impaired Conray is rapidly excreted unchanged by glomerular filtration.

Dosage and administration See table on next page.
     There are no specific dosage recommendations for the elderly.

Contra-indications, warnings, etc *Pregnancy:* There is inadequate evidence as to the safety of Conray in human pregnancy. The pregnant female should not be submitted to X rays unless the radiologist considers it essential.
     Conray preparations must NEVER be injected into the subarachnoid space.
     For cerebral arteriography, Conray 280 should be used; Conray 325 and 420 should not be employed in this procedure and are not recommended in any peripheral arteriography.

Precautions: Following the use of any contrast medium of this type, there is the remote possibility of severe sensitivity reactions occurring. When they do, they tend to occur in the first few minutes following injection and the patient should be kept under observation during this period. It is essential to have immediately available emergency resuscitation equipment, including appropriate drugs, oxygen and means of administration.
     Subjects with a history of allergy or previous reactions to drugs or severe cardiovascular disease are more at risk than others.

Side-effects: Side-effects which may occur are nausea, vomiting, metallic taste, sensation of heat, weakness, headache, dizziness, thirst, coughing, sneezing, itching, urticaria, pallor, tachycardia and hypotension. Rarely: convulsions, circulatory failure and cardiac arrest. Pain may be felt at the site of injection.

Pharmaceutical precautions Protect from light.

Legal category POM.

Package quantities *Conray 280:* Box of 10 × 20 ml ampoules. Box of 10 × 50 ml bottles.
Conray 325: Box of 10 × 50 ml bottles.
Conray 420: Box of 10 × 20 ml ampoules. Box of 10 × 50 ml bottles.

Further information Nil.

Product licence numbers
Conray 280:   0012/5033
Conray 325:   0012/5034
Conray 420:   0012/5035

FLAGYL* & FLAGYL-S* SUSPENSION

Presentation Tablets containing 200 mg and 400 mg metronidazole. The 200 mg tablets are off white to cream, film coated, engraved 'Flagyl 200' around the outer margin. The 400 mg tablets are capsule shaped, off white to cream, film coated, engraved 'Flagyl 400' on one side.

Suspension: Buff-coloured, each 5 ml containing 320 mg metronidazole benzoate, equivalent to 200 mg metronidazole.
     Flagyl suspension contains 60% w/v sugars.

Suppositories containing 500 mg and 1.0 gram metronidazole.

Injection (for intravenous infusion) 0.5 per cent w/v in 100 ml bottles or 100 ml Viaflex containers or 20 ml ampoules.

Uses Flagyl is indicated in the prophylaxis and treatment of infections in which anaerobic bacteria have been identified or are suspected to be the cause.
     Flagyl is active against a wide range of pathogenic micro-organisms notably species of Bacteroides, Fusobacteria, Clostridia, Eubacteria, anaerobic cocci and Gardnerella vaginalis.
     It is also active against Trichomonas, Entamoeba histolytica, Giardia lamblia and Balantidium coli.
     It is indicated in:
     1. The prevention of postoperative infections due to anaerobic bacteria, particularly species of bacteroides and anaerobic streptococci.
     2. The treatment of septicaemia, bacteraemia, peritonitis, brain abscess, necrotising pneumonia, osteomyelitis, puerperal sepsis, pelvic abscess, pelvic cellulitis, and

Procedure	Conray 280	Conray 325	Conray 420
Intravenous urography	*Adults:* 40–80 ml. As for Conray 280. In the absence of preliminary dehydration 40–100 ml may be used. *Infants and children:* Under 12 kg: 2 ml/kg body weight. Over 12 kg: 1.5 ml/kg body weight (with a minimum of 24 ml). Over 10 years of age: Lower range of adult dosage.		40 ml is usually adequate but the schedule for Conray 280 can be used with safety.
Femoral and other peripheral arteriography.	15–20 ml injected into the femoral or iliac artery will provide excellent visualisation of the arterial tree of the leg. A similar or smaller dose is indicated for smaller arteries.	**Do not use**	**Do not use**
Cerebral angiography (carotid and vertebral)	Average adult dose is 6–10 ml for each injection. Exceptionally, up to 10 injections of 8 ml each have been made into the carotid artery.	**Do not use**	**Do not use**
Abdominal aortography (direct puncture or retrograde catheterisation)	*Adults:* 20–30 ml.	*Adults:* 20–30 ml.	*Adults:* 20–30 ml.
Thoracic aortography (including arch aortography)	Often adequate in children: 0.5–1 ml per kg body weight. May be used as a test dose in positioning catheter tip.	*Adults and children:* 0.5–1 ml per kg body weight. The usual volume employed in the adult is 20–40 ml.	
Intravenous aortography	—	—	*Adults and children:* 1 ml per kg body weight. In adults 80–100 ml or more per injection is often used. Frequently this amount is subdivided equally and given by rapid simultaneous bilateral injection.
Angiocardiography	May be used as test dose in positioning catheter tip. Volumes of up to 40 ml have been used for this purpose prior to the diagnostic dose of more concentrated medium.		*Adults and children over 14 years of age:* 20 to 50 ml per injection. *Small children and infants:* 0.5–1.0 ml per kg body weight with a minimum of 3 ml. Multiple injections may be required and the above doses may be repeated with confidence but 3 ml per kg body weight should not be exceeded.
Splenography, portal venography	*Adults;* 20–40 ml.	*Adults;* 20–40 ml.	*Adults:* 20–40 ml.
Femoral venography and/or inferior vena cavography	*Adults:* 20–60 ml.	*Adults:* 20–60 ml.	*Adults:* 20–60 ml.
Hysterosalpingography	About 10 ml are usually required, administered by slow injection into the uterine cervical canal via a syringe and suitable canula.	—	—

post-operative wound infections from which pathogenic anaerobes have been isolated.

3. Urogenital trichomoniasis in the female (trichomonal vaginitis) and in the male.

4. Non-specific vaginitis.

5. All forms of amoebiasis (intestinal and extra-intestinal disease and that of symptomless cyst passers)

6. Giardiasis.

7. Acute ulcerative gingivitis.

8. Anaerobically-infected leg ulcers and pressure sores.

9. Acute dental infections (e.g. acute pericoronitis and acute apical infections).

Kinetics: Metronidazole is rapidly and almost completely absorbed on administration of Flagyl Tablets; peak plasma concentrations occur after 20 min to 3 hours.

The bioavailability of metronidazole in Flagyl suppositories is 60–80%. Effective blood concentrations are achieved 5–12 hours after the first suppository and are maintained by the recommended 8 hourly regimen.

The elimination half-life of metronidazole is 7–8 hours.

Metronidazole can be used in chronic renal failure; it is rapidly removed from the plasma by dialysis.

Metronidazole is excreted in milk but the intake of a suckling infant of a mother receiving normal dosage would be considerably less than the therapeutic dosage for infants.

Dosage and administration *Flagyl injection* should be infused intravenously at an approximate rate of 5 ml/minute. Oral medication should be substituted as soon as feasible.

Flagyl suppositories are unsuitable for initiating treatment of serious conditions owing to slower absorption and lower plasma concentrations of metronidazole.

Flagyl tablets should be swallowed with water (Not CHEWED). It is recommended that the tablets be taken during or after a meal.

Flagyl suspension should be taken at least one hour before a meal.

Other antibiotics may be used concurrently; if the intravenous route is used, concomitant antibiotics should be administered separately and not mixed together.

Anaerobic infections: The duration of a course of Flagyl treatment is about 7 days but it will depend upon the seriousness of the patient's condition as assessed clinically and bacteriologically.

A. *Prophylaxis:* against anaerobic infection – chiefly in the context of abdominal (especially colorectal) and gynaecological surgery.

Intravenous: 500 mg shortly before operation, repeated 8 hourly, oral doses of 400 mg 8 hourly to be started as soon as feasible.

Children: 7.5 mg/kg (1.5 ml) 8 hourly.

Oral: 400 mg 8 hourly for 3–4 days followed by postoperative intravenous or rectal administration until patient is able to take tablets.

Shorter preoperative courses and higher oral doses (up to 1 g) have been used.

Children 7.5 mg/kg 8 hourly.

Rectal: 1 g 8 hourly.

Children: one half or a quarter suppository 8 hourly.

In Appendectomy prophylaxis may be started preoperatively with intravenous Flagyl. In general the duration of postoperative treatment will depend on the state of the appendix and/or degree of peritoneal soiling.

B. *Treatment of established anaerobic infection:*

Intravenous: to be used initially if patient's condition or symptoms preclude oral therapy: 500 mg 8 hourly.

Children: 7.5 mg/kg 8 hourly.

Oral: 800 mg followed by 400 mg 8 hourly.

Children: 7.5 mg/kg 8 hourly.

Rectal: 1 g 8 hourly. Substitute oral medication as early as possible. If rectal administration is prolonged beyond 3 days reduce dose to 1 g 12 hourly for remainder of course.

C. *Treatment of Protozoal and other infections:* See table.

Contra-indications, warnings, etc

Use in pregnancy: There is inadequate evidence of the safety of metronidazole in pregnancy. Flagyl should not therefore be given during pregnancy or during lactation unless the physician considers it essential; in these circumstances the short, high-dosage regimens are not recommended.

Contra-indication: known hypersensitivity to metronidazole.

Precautions: Regular clinical and laboratory monitoring are advised if administration of Flagyl for more than 10 days is considered to be necessary.

There is a possibility that after Trichomonas vaginalis has been eliminated a gonococcal infection might persist.

The elimination half-life of metronidazole remains unchanged in the presence of renal failure. The dosage of metronidazole therefore needs no reduction. Such patients however retain the metabolites of metronidazole. The clinical significance of this is not known at present. In patients undergoing haemodialysis metronidazole and metabolites are efficiently removed during an eight-hour period of dialysis. Metronidazole should therefore be re-administered immediately after haemodialysis.

No routine adjustment in the dosage of 'Flagyl' need be made in patients with renal failure undergoing intermittent peritoneal dialysis (IPD) or continuous ambulatory peritoneal dialysis (CAPD).

Patients should be advised not to take alcohol during metronidazole therapy because of the possibility of a disulfiram-like reaction.

Some potentiation of anticoagulant therapy has been reported when metronidazole has been used with the warfarin type oral anticoagulants. Dosage of the latter may require reducing. Prothrombin times should be monitored. There is no interaction with heparin.

Patients receiving phenobarbitone metabolise metronidazole at a much greater rate than normally, reducing the half life to approximately 3 hours.

Warnings and adverse effects: Serious adverse reactions occur very rarely with standard recommended regimens. Unpleasant taste in the mouth, furred tongue, nausea, vomiting gastro-intestinal disturbance, and urticaria and angioedema occur occasionally. Anaphylaxis may occur rarely.

Drowsiness, dizziness, headache, ataxia, skin rashes, pruritus, darkening of the urine (due to metronidazole metabolite) have been reported but very rarely.

During intensive and/or prolonged metronidazole therapy, a few instances of peripheral neuropathy or transient epileptiform seizures have been reported. In most cases neuropathy disappeared after treatment was stopped or when dosage was reduced. A moderate leucopenia has been reported in some patients but the

Dosage is given in terms of metronidazole or metronidazole equivalent

	Duration of dosage in days	Adults and children over 10 years‡	Children†		
			7 to 10 years	3 to 7 years	1 to 3 years
Urogenital trichomoniasis Where re-infection is likely, the consort should receive a similar course of treatment concurrently.	7	200 mg three times daily 400 mg twice daily	100 mg three times daily	100 mg twice daily	50 mg three times daily
	or 2	800 mg in the morning and 1,200 mg in the evening			
	or 1	2.0 g as a single dose			
Non-specific vaginitis	7	400 mg twice daily			
	1	2·0 g as a single dose			
Amoebiasis (a) Invasive intestinal disease in susceptible subjects	5	800 mg three times daily	400 mg three times daily	200 mg four times daily	200 mg three times daily
(b) Intestinal disease in less susceptible subjects and chronic amoebic hepatitis	5–10				
(c) Amoebic liver abscess also other forms of extra-intestinal amoebiasis	5	400 mg three times daily	200 mg three times daily	100 mg four times daily	100 mg three times daily
(d) Symptomless cyst passers	5–10	400–800 mg three times daily	200–400 mg three times daily	100–200 mg four times daily	100–200 mg three times daily
Giardiasis	3	2.0 g once daily	1.0 g once daily	600–800 mg once daily	500 mg once daily
Acute ulcerative gingivitis	3	200 mg three times daily	100 mg three times daily	100 mg twice daily	50 mg three times daily
Acute dental infections	3–7	200 mg three times daily			
Leg ulcers and pressure sores	7	400 mg three times daily			
Anaerobic infections (general)		See data sheet text			

† Children and babies weighing less than 10 kg should receive proportionately smaller dosages.
‡ *Elderly:* Flagyl is well tolerated by the elderly, but a pharmacokinetic study suggests cautious use of high dosage regimens in this age group.

white cell count has always returned to normal before or after treatment has been completed.

Treatment of overdosage: Uneventful recovery has followed attempts at suicide with quantities of 30 and 60 × 200 mg tablets.

There is no specific treatment for gross overdosage of Flagyl.

Pharmaceutical precautions Protect from light.

Legal category POM.

Package quantities Containers of 21 and 250 × 200 mg tablets. Calendar (blister) pack of 14 and container of 100 × 400 mg tablets.

Bottles of 50 and 100 ml suspension (metronidazole benzoate).

Containers of 10 × 500 mg and 10 × 1.0 gram suppositories.

Boxes of 10 × 100 ml bottles injection 0.5 per cent w/v.

Boxes of 20 × 100 ml injection 0.5 per cent w/v in VIAFLEX containers.

Carton of 10 × 20 ml ampoules 0.5 per cent w/v.

Further information Metronidazole has no useful direct activity against aerobic and facultatively anaerobic bacteria.

Flagyl injection does not contain a preservative; the 100 ml bottle is not, therefore, intended as a 'multi-dose'.

Dilution of Flagyl suspension, if necessary, should be carried out with syrup BP. The diluted suspension has a shelf life of 14 days.

In patients maintained on intravenous fluids, Flagyl injection may be diluted with appropriate volumes of normal saline, dextrose-saline, dextrose 5 per cent w/v or potassium chloride infusions (20 mmol and 40 mmol/ litre).

Aspartate amino transferase assays may give spuriously low values in patients taking metronidazole, depending on the method used.

Product licence numbers

Tablets 200 mg	0012/5256
Tablets 400 mg	0012/0084
Suppositories 500 mg	0012/0113
Suppositories 1.0 g	0012/0114
Injection 100 ml	0012/0107
Injection 20 ml	0012/0125
Suspension	0012/0131

FLAGYL COMPAK*

Presentation Flagyl Compak is a combined treatment pack containing: 21 × 200 mg Flagyl (metronidazole).

Tablets 14 × 100,000 units nystatin vaginal inserts, 1 vaginal insert applicator.

The 200 mg metronidazole tablets are off-white to cream, film coated, engraved 'Flagyl 200' around the outer margin.

The 100,000 units nystatin vaginal inserts are yellowish-cream, almond shaped, indented 'M&B' on one face.

Uses Flagyl is a potent trichomonacide. It is also active against other protozoa and anaerobic bacteria.

Nystatin is a fungistatic and fungicidal antibiotic which is active topically against Candida albicans.

Flagyl Compak is indicated in the treatment of vaginitis where a mixed trichomonal/candidal infection is diagnosed or suspected. Presenting symptoms may include vaginal discharge, pruritus vulvae and dyspareunia.

Kinetics: Metronidazole is rapidly and almost completely absorbed from the tablets leading to peak plasma concentrations after 20 min to 3 hours. Metronidazole is excreted in milk but the intake of a suckling infant of a mother receiving normal dosage would be considerably less than the therapeutic dosage for infants.

Nystatin is not absorbed through the skin or mucous membranes when applied topically.

Dosage and administration One Flagyl Tablet to be swallowed whole, with half a glassful of water during or after meals, three times daily for seven days.

Concurrently, one nystatin vaginal insert to be moistened and introduced high into the vagina night and morning for seven days. Some physicians may prefer to instruct patients to use one insert nightly, before retiring, for fourteen nights. Full patient instructions for use of the applicator are included in each Compak.

This product is not recommended for girls under 10 years of age.

Elderly: No specific dosage recommendations.

Where cross infection with Trichomonas vaginalis is confirmed or suspected the male consort should be treated concurrently with one Flagyl tablet by mouth three times daily for seven days.

Contra-indications, warnings, etc

Use in pregnancy: There is inadequate evidence of the safety of metronidazole in pregnancy.

Flagyl Compak should not therefore be given during pregnancy or during lactation unless the physician considers it essential.

Contra-indications: Known hypersensitivity to metronidazole.

Precautions: Regular clinical and laboratory monitoring are advised if administration of Flagyl for more than 10 days is considered to be necessary.

There is a possibility that after *Trichomonas vaginalis* has been eliminated a gonococcal infection might persist.

The elimination half-life of metronidazole remains unchanged in the presence of renal failure. The dosage of metronidazole therefore needs no reduction. Such patients however retain the metabolites of metronidazole. The clinical significance of this is not known at present.

Patients should be advised not to take alcohol during metronidazole therapy because of the possibility of a disulfiram-like reaction.

Some potentiation of anticoagulant therapy has been reported when metronidazole has been used with the warfarin type oral anticoagulants. Dosage of the latter may require reducing. Prothrombin times should be monitored. There is no interaction with heparin.

Patients receiving phenobarbitone metabolise metronidazole at a much greater rate than normally, reducing the half life to approximately 3 hours.

Warnings and adverse effects: Serious adverse reactions occur very rarely with standard recommended regimens. There have been reports of an unpleasant taste in the mouth, furred tongue, nausea, vomiting, gastro-intestinal disturbance, and of urticaria and angioedema. Anaphylaxis may occur rarely.

Drowsiness, dizziness, headache, ataxia, skin rashes, pruritus, inco-ordination of movements and darkening of the urine (due to metronidazole metabolite) have been reported but very rarely.

No adverse effects due to the use of nystatin vaginal inserts have been reported.

Pharmaceutical precautions Protect from light. Flagyl Compak should be stored in a cool place.

As nystatin loses potency slowly on storage, the vaginal inserts should be used within 18 months of the date of manufacture.

Legal category POM.

Package quantities Combined treatment pack containing 21 × 200 mg Flagyl Tablets, 14 × 100,000 units nystatin vaginal inserts, 1 vaginal insert applicator, full instructions for the patient.

Further information There is no evidence of resistant organisms developing to either Flagyl or nystatin.

Aspartate amino transferase assays may give spuriously low values in patients taking metronidazole, depending on the method used.

Product licence number 0012/5091.

FLAXEDIL*

Presentation Colourless injection solution containing gallamine triethiodide 4% w/v.

Uses Non-depolarising (competitive-blocking) muscle relaxant having a duration of action of 20–30 minutes. Flaxedil is used as a relaxant in surgery and to give suitable conditions for intubation. It is also given to potentiate the muscle-relaxant properties of halothane and to protect against the bradycardia it causes. Flaxedil is employed to aid the management of certain convulsive states and as a diagnostic agent for myasthenia gravis.

Dosage and administration Flaxedil is administered intravenously after the patient has been anaesthetised. Dosage must be adjusted to individual requirements, the nature of the general anaesthetic used, and the duration of the operation. Some anaesthetists recommend that a test dose of 20 mg should be given before anaesthesia is induced to exclude sensitivity.

As a guide the average adult requires 80–120 mg of Flaxedil for the provision of adequate muscular relaxation. Supplementary doses of 20–40 mg are given as required. Where no suitable vein is available, Flaxedil may be given intramuscularly with or without hyaluronidase.

Elderly: No specific dosage recommendations.

For children a dosage of 1.5 mg per kg should be given intravenously. In suspected myasthenia gravis a dosage of 0.025 mg per kg may be used as a diagnostic procedure.

Contra-indications, warnings, etc Flaxedil is contra-indicated in patients suffering from myasthenia gravis (except for diagnosis). Since gallamine is excreted by the kidneys extra care is necessary in its use in patients with renal dysfunction. In operative obstetrics, because gallamine passes rapidly through the placental barrier, it should be used with care until after delivery of the foetus. Flaxedil should only be used when facilities for securing an effective airway and providing controlled respiration with adequate oxygen are available. The action of muscle relaxants is enhanced by the antibiotics, amikacin, gentamicin, kanamycin, neomycin, streptomycin, polymixin, tobramycin and by potent anaesthetics such as halothane.

Muscular relaxation with Flaxedil is singularly free from side-effects, other than tachycardia which occurs in the majority of patients and which is associated with its vagolytic action. Ill effects of this have not been noted, but care is advised in its use in patients with heart conditions. Anaphylactic reactions have been reported occasionally.

Overdosage with Flaxedil is an unlikely event. If it is necessary to reverse the effects of Flaxedil rapidly, the antagonist neostigmine methylsulphate should be injected intravenously in a dosage of 1 mg initially followed by increments of 0.5 mg until the respiratory exchange is adequate. The use of neostigmine must always be preceded by the intravenous injection of atropine sulphate 0.5–1 mg. No patient who has received neostigmine should be left alone until all risk of excessive bradycardia and of recrudescence of muscular paralysis has passed.

Pharmaceutical precautions Protect from light.

Flaxedil is compatible with solutions of thiopentone sodium, but it is important to add the Flaxedil to the thiopentone solution, not vice versa. Flaxedil is incompatible with pethidine hydrochloride solutions.

Legal category POM.

Package quantities Boxes of 10 × 2 ml ampoules.

Further information Nil.

Product licence number 0012/5077.

GARDENAL SODIUM*

Presentation A clear, almost colourless injection solution containing 200 mg phenobarbitone sodium per ml in a propylene glycol/water mixture.

Uses Gardenal Sodium is a long-acting barbiturate with anticonvulsant properties. It may be used to control seizures in epilepsy and similar conditions.

Kinetics: Barbiturates are rapidly absorbed and widely distributed in the body. They diffuse across the placenta and appear in the milk. Phenobarbitone is excreted mainly unchanged in the urine. The plasma half life is shorter in children than adults but longer in neonates.

Dosage and administration May be injected undiluted by the subcutaneous or intramuscular route. Before intravenous administration Gardenal Sodium injection should be diluted to 10 times its own volume with Water for Injections immediately before use.

For the emergency control of convulsions:

Adults: 200 mg i.m. or s.c. repeated if necessary after 6 hours.

Elderly: No specific dosage recommendations, but see 'Precautions' below.

Children: 15 mg/kg i.m. is required as a loading dose to achieve adequate blood levels. This may be followed by 5 mg/kg daily by mouth (divided if appropriate).

In status epilepticus Gardenal Sodium is preferably given i.v. 400–800 mg in the adult, small doses being relatively ineffective.

Contra-indications, warnings, etc

Pregnancy and lactation: There is evidence of harmful effects in animals, therefore avoid its use during first trimester pregnancy unless there is no safer alternative. Hypo-prothrombinaemia and withdrawal symptoms have been seen in neonates whose mothers have been treated during late pregnancy. Barbiturates should be used with caution in the nursing mother.

Contra-indication: Acute intermittent porphyria is an absolute contra-indication.

Precautions: Gardenal Sodium should be used with care in infants, elderly or frail patients.

Dosage should be reduced in the presence of marked renal or hepatic failure.

Interactions: Gardenal Sodium should not be administered to patients known to have taken alcohol or other CNS depressants. In patients stabilized on phenytoin phenobarbitone may lead to lower serum concentrations of phenytoin. Sodium valproate could enhance the action of phenobarbitone. The following drugs may become less effective on administration of phenobarbitone: Warfarin, chloramphenicol, corticosteroids and oral contraceptives.

Warnings and adverse effects: Idiosyncratic reactions have occasionally occurred in the form of a hangover, followed by vertigo or gastro-intestinal upset or excitement or localised or diffuse pain. Hypersensitivity reactions appearing as localised swellings, particularly about the face have also been reported.

Toxicity and treatment of overdosage: Overdosage produces severe, persistent respiratory depression.

Treatment includes general measures for the support of the respiratory and cardiovascular systems.

Pharmaceutical precautions Protect from light.

Legal category POM.

Package quantities Box of 10 × 1 ml ampoules.

Further information Nil.

Product licence number 0012/5076.

HALOTHANE – M&B*

Presentation Halothane is an almost colourless liquid with a distinctive, pleasant odour.

Uses Halothane is a general anaesthetic used in inhalation anaesthesia. It is of particular value:

1. When cautery or diathermy is to be used.
2. In giving a pleasant and rapid induction particularly in children.
3. As it suppresses secretions from the salivary, bronchial and gastric glands.
4. In maintaining the required plane of anaesthesia which is easily reversed.
5. Since relaxation is adequate for most operations and respiration is readily controlled.
6. Since recovery is rapid and nausea and vomiting are rare.
7. As it is suitable for most types of surgery.
8. As it can be given with a very high percentage of oxygen when this is indicated.

Dosage and administration *The technique of halothane anaesthesia:*

1. *Pre-medication:* A small dose of pethidine with or without the addition of promethazine will produce satisfactory sedation in most patients and will reduce the tendency to tachypnoea. Atropine in an appropriate dose should be administered to all patients.

2. *Induction:* This is most conveniently carried out with a sleep dose of thiopentone sodium, to allow the application of a face mask. A gas flow of 8 litres/minute should be administered, of which at least 30% should be oxygen, and then the Halothane should slowly be introduced. Administration should start at 0.5% and be increased by a further 0.5% every few breaths until the inspired gases contain 3% Halothane. Intubation can be carried out after five minutes' inhalation of 3% Halothane in a carrier gas flow of 8 litres/minute or before exposure to Halothane if an intubating dose of suxamethonium is given. If intubation is performed before exposing the patient to Halothane, the introduction of Halothane must still be stepwise.

3. *Maintenance:* At a gas flow of 8 litres/minute, Halothane concentrations of between 0.5% and 1.5% are usually adequate. At a 2 litres/minute gas flow with the vaporiser out of circuit (VOC) a concentration of 2–2.5% fed into the absorber circuit will suffice. A low resistance vaporiser may be placed within the circle (VIC), but in this case controlled or assisted ventilation must not be used. A vaporiser for VIC use must not be capable of delivering a concentration greater than 3%.

4. *Recovery:* This is usually rapid and uneventful. If the Halothane is withdrawn as skin closure starts, reflexes will have returned by the time the dressings are in place.

Shivering is occasionally seen during recovery if there is a marked temperature differential between the theatre and the ward. This is readily controlled by the administration of a small dose of chlorpromazine, but supplementary oxygen may be required for a few minutes.

Methods of administration: Halothane is a potent anaesthetic and should, wherever possible, be administered via a specially calibrated and temperature-compensated vaporiser. A number of such vaporisers are now available.

Halothane can also be administered from the ordinary bottle vaporiser of a Boyle's machine, but the scale should be extended to allow fine adjustment in the concentration of Halothane delivered.

Open-drop anaesthesia with Halothane is not generally recommended; however, a few drops carefully applied to the mask may smooth the subsequent administration of ether.

Draw-over machines and inhalers can be satisfactorily used with Halothane, but if air is the carrier gas, supplementary oxygen or assisted respiration may be necessary to maintain full oxygenation.

Contra-indications, warnings, etc Whilst no absolute contra-indication to Halothane anaesthesia exists, particular care should be exercised in the following conditions:

1. In obstetrics – uterine relaxation and post-partum haemorrhage may result.
2. In neurosurgery – a rise in CSF pressure has been recorded, the effects of which may be mitigated by the use of moderate hyperventilation.
3. When Injection of Adrenaline is used concurrently – cardiac arrhythmias may occur.
4. In multiple anaesthesias and infectious hepatitis – the possibility that multiple exposure to Halothane and/or concomitant infectious hepatitis may cause liver failure. Unexplained pyrexia or jaundice occurring after an administration of Halothane should be regarded as a contra-indication to further Halothane anaesthesia until such time as the relationship between post-anaesthetic jaundice and Halothane has been elucidated. Multiple anaesthesias with any anaesthetic agent are more prone to be followed by hepatic damage than a single exposure. There is some evidence that a second exposure to Halothane within four weeks is undesirable and should be avoided.

The use of beta adrenergic blocking agents during Halothane anaesthesia is at the discretion of the anaesthetist.

Muscle relaxants: All commonly used muscle relaxants may be used in conjunction with Halothane, but, as Halothane potentiates the actions of gallamine and *d*-tubocurarine, the doses of these muscle relaxants must be reduced. The association of *d*-tubocurarine with Halothane may lead to a marked fall in blood pressure.

Ganglion blocking agents: Potentiation occurs between Halothane and the standard hypotensive agents such as pentolinium, pempidine and trimetaphan. These drugs must be used in reduced dosage when administered in conjunction with Halothane.

Vaporiser: Halothane must not be used in the EMO ether vaporiser as it attacks the metal; a vaporiser specially constructed for Halothane should be used.

Pharmaceutical precautions Store in a dark place below 25°C. Keep well closed. The vaporiser should be drained at regular intervals. Any discoloured Halothane should be discarded.

Legal category P.

Package quantities Bottle of 250 ml.

Further information Nil.

Product licence number 0012/0095.

HEXABRIX* ▼

Presentation

Hexabrix 320: Ampoules and bottles of a sterile solution of meglumine ioxaglate 39.30% w/v and sodium ioxaglate 19.65% w/v containing 320 mg iodine in combined form per ml.

Hexabrix 200: Bottles of a sterile solution of meglumine ioxaglate 24.56% w/v and sodium ioxaglate 12.28% w/v containing 200 mg iodine in combined form per ml.

Uses Low osmolar X-ray contrast medium for the opacification of the vascular system, urinary tract, joints and female genital tract, the indications for which are given in the table on the next page.

Kinetics: Hexabrix is rapidly eliminated by the kidneys with a half-life of about 90 minutes. 90% of the dose is eliminated in 24 hours. Some biliary excretion also occurs and opacification of the gall bladder may be observed 24 hours after administration. The compound is not metabolised.

Dosage and administration See accompanying table. For ease of injection it may be found helpful to warm Hexabrix to near body temperature.

Elderly: No specific dosage recommendations.

Contra-indications, warnings, etc Hexabrix must never be injected by the subarachnoid or epidural route. It is definitely contra-indicated for myelography.

Pregnancy: There is no evidence that this product is safe during pregnancy, nor is there evidence in animal work that it is free from hazard. The product should not be used during pregnancy unless benefit outweighs the risk and is considered essential by the physician. The ten day rule in women of childbearing age should be observed.

Precautions: Since the causes of severe reactions to iodinated water-soluble contrast media are unknown and preliminary testing is unreliable as an indication that a patient will react unfavourably, the only other safeguards are physical examination and a careful evaluation of the patient's history to screen out subjects known to suffer from allergy, asthma, or severe cardiovascular disease. The provision of facilities for resuscitation and the training of staff members in their prompt use is mandatory.

A positive history of allergy, asthma or of untoward reactions during previous similar investigations does not necessarily contra-indicate the use of the contrast agent, but it emphasises the need for extra caution, for a sensitivity-test dose before the definitive injection, possibly steroid cover, and for even greater than usual preparedness to deal promptly with any reaction that might occur.

Extra caution should be exercised in carrying out radiographic procedures with contrast media in patients with severe systemic disease, asthma, and in allergic subjects. In patients with advanced renal disease and inadequate renal function as reflected by a raised blood

urea, and in diabetics, the normally rapid excretion of the contrast medium may be markedly impaired. Even in patients with kidney disease substantial deterioration of renal function is minimised if the patient is well hydrated. Urine output must be carefully checked in these patients after the procedure.

Patients with hepatorenal insufficiency should not be examined unless the possibility of benefit clearly outweighs the additional risk. Re-examination should be delayed for five to seven days.

Special care should be exercised when Hexabrix is injected into the right heart or pulmonary artery in patients with pulmonary arterial hypertension. Right heart angiography is probably best avoided in patients with pulmonary arterial hypertension.

Special care should be exercised in patients being treated with a calcium ion antagonist (eg verapamil) and who are to undergo coronary angiography; in such circumstances, a few instances of serious arrhythmias have been reported.

Patients with MYELOMATOSIS, and to a lesser degree, DIABETES, show poor tolerance of all intravenous radio-diagnostic compounds, the use of which should be avoided unless the possibility of benefit clearly outweighs the risk. These patients must be particularly well hydrated should intravascular iodinated injections be necessary and urine output carefully monitored.

All organic iodine contrast media interfere with tests of thyroid function. If required, such diagnostic tests should be undertaken before procedures with Hexabrix or a few weeks after the procedures.

Sensitivity testing: Hypersensitivity to Hexabrix has been very rare but may be tested for by any of the standard techniques. It is doubtful, however, whether routine sensitivity testing is justified, providing careful enquiry has been made concerning a history of allergy or of untoward reactions on any previous occasion. A 'negative' sensitivity test-dose does not imply that the patient will tolerate a larger volume.

Resuscitation: It is essential to have at hand injections of adrenaline, a vasopressor, an anti-histaminic and hydrocortisone, together with appropriate sterile syringes, needles etc. Means for administering oxygen under positive pressure and maintaining an adequate air-way should always be available.

Because of the possibility, remote though it may be, of a delayed reaction to the contrast agent, the patient should never be left unsupervised for the thirty minutes immediately after the injection.

Warnings and adverse effects: In cerebral arteriography, the only frequent side-effect is facial heat, usually of mild degree. In femoral and iliac arteriography a warm feeling is usually experienced and very rarely slight pain may be felt but leg movement and/or vocal protests are unusual.

After the rapid injection of Hexabrix for angiocardiography or aortography, patients may experience a wave of mild warmth, associated with flushing passing over the body. Slight coughing may occur after right heart pulmonary artery injections. Other transient reactions reported rarely are nausea, vomiting, hypotension, headache and a metallic taste.

A few ventricular extrasystoles are common after any rapid intraventricular injection and the injection flow should not exceed 12 ml/sec in the adult ventricle. Ventricular fibrillation may occur very infrequently after intra-cardiac or intra-coronary injection and a DC defibrillator and other equipment necessary for defibrillation must always be available during these studies.

Procedure	Product	Dosage and administration
Femoral and other peripheral arteriographies	Hexabrix 320	15–20 ml injected into the femoral or iliac artery will provide excellent visualisation of the arterial tree of the leg. A similar or smaller dose is indicated for smaller arteries.
Cerebral angiography (carotid and vertebral)	Hexabrix 320	Average adult dose: 6–8 ml for each injection. Up to 10 injections each of 8 ml may be required.
Angio-cardiography	Hexabrix 320	Multiple small test injections may be used for positioning catheter tip. Adults and children over 14 years: 30–50 ml per injection. Children (14 years and under) and infants: 1–1.5 ml per kg bodyweight. Multiple injections may be required. Total dosage should not normally exceed 4 ml per kg bodyweight. In exceptional circumstances, this total dose may be exceeded according to the clinical condition.
Abdominal aortography (direct puncture or catheterisation)	Hexabrix 320	Adults: 20–30 ml. Up to 50 ml may be used particularly if films of the legs are also taken following the same injection.
Thoracic aortography (including arch aortography)	Hexabrix 320	Adults and children: 0.5–1 ml per kg bodyweight up to 40 ml per injection. This may be repeated if necessary. Total dosage should not normally exceed 4 ml per kg bodyweight.
Pulmonary angiography	Hexabrix 320	Adults: 20–40 ml. Children: 0.5–1 ml per kg bodyweight. Special care should be exercised in patients with pulmonary arterial hypertension.
Coronary arteriography	Hexabrix 320	Adults: 3–8 ml per injection, depending on size of artery. Several injections are usually given for complete demonstration, particularly in the left coronary artery.
Intravenous aortography	Hexabrix 320	Adults and children: 1–1.5 ml per kg bodyweight. In adults 100 ml is often used; frequently this amount is sub-divided equally and given by simultaneous rapid bilateral injection.
Femoral venography and/or inferior vena cavography	Hexabrix 320	Adults: 20–50 ml.
Leg phlebography	Hexabrix 200 Hexabrix 320	50–150 ml injected into a vein in the foot. 20–50 ml injected into a vein in the foot.
Intravenous urography	Hexabrix 320	Adults: 20–80 ml. 60–100 ml may be used provided that the patient is not dehydrated. Children: Under 12 kg–2 ml per kg bodyweight. Over 12 kg–1.5 ml per kg bodyweight (with a minimum of 24 ml). Over 10 years of age—lower range of adult dosage. Patients with severe renal disease or diabetes should be well hydrated. Particular care is necessary in these patients as temporary deterioration in renal function has been reported.
Splenography portal venography	Hexabrix 320	Adults: 20–40 ml by splenic puncture.
Knee arthrography (double contrast)	Hexabrix 320	By injection into the knee joint. Adults: 4.5 ml together with injections of air before and after the positive contrast medium.
Hysterosalpingography	Hexabrix 320	About 10 ml are usually required, administered by slow injection into the uterine cervical canal via a syringe and suitable cannula.

Following intracardiac, ascending aortic or coronary artery injection, the QRST complex of the ECG may be altered briefly. After prolonged cardiac catheterisation (with or without injection of a contrast medium), 5 to 10 per cent of patients may develop some degree of shivering or shock.

In intravenous urography, nausea, vomiting, dizziness and urticaria have been reported occasionally but have been of little consequence.

Toxicity and treatment of overdosage: In laboratory animals, the main signs of toxicity are convulsions, pulmonary congestion and oedema, respiratory depres-sion, prostration, darkening of the eyes and hypersaliva-tion; it is most unlikely that such toxic signs would occur in man, as it would be necessary to inject far greater doses than the maximum of those recommended. In man, overdosage as such should not arise but, since the causes of severe reactions to iodinated water-soluble contrast media are unknown, the information detailed under Precautions and resuscitation should be carefully studied.

Pharmaceutical precautions Protect from light.

Legal category POM.

Package quantities

Hexabrix 320: Box of 10 × 20 ml ampoules.
Box of 10 × 50 ml bottles.
Box of 10 × 100 ml bottles.

Hexabrix 200: Box of 10 × 50 ml bottles.

Further information Nil.

Product licence numbers
Hexabrix 320: 0012/0135
Hexabrix 200: 0012/0167

INTRAVAL* SODIUM

Presentation Vials or bottles of thiopentone sodium BP.

It is supplied in vials of 0.5 g and bottles of 2.5 g for extemporaneous preparation of 2.5% solutions, and in vials of 0.5 g and 1.0 g and bottles of 5 g for extemporaneous preparation of 5.0% solution. A sterile transfer device, with instructions for use, is supplied with each 2.5 g and 5 g bottle.

Uses Administered intravenously Intraval Sodium produces general anaesthesia of short duration; also used rectally.

Intraval Sodium is indicated for the induction of general anaesthesia; for general anaesthesia of short duration with or without the addition of a muscle relaxant; for the control of convulsive states. It is administered rectally for the induction of basal anaesthesia.

Other information: Although bound to plasma proteins it rapidly crosses the blood-brain barrier and reaches maximum concentration in the brain within 30 seconds of injection. Intraval Sodium is short-acting because the initial concentration in the brain is rapidly dispersed to other tissues. It is slowly metabolised by the liver. Only a small proportion of the active drug is excreted in the urine.

Dosage and administration Intraval Sodium is administered usually as a 2.5% solution, but a 5% solution is sometimes used. A 2.5% solution is advised for all elderly and bad-risk patients. The injection may be given through any superficial vein, but the most commonly used is the median cephalic at the elbow. Any other vein may be employed if the elbow site is inconvenient to the surgeon, so that the veins of the dorsum of the foot or back of the hand should be considered. Varicose veins should be avoided because of the sluggish state of blood flow in them.

Definite dosage cannot be stated for every case. The response of each patient must be observed and the dose regulated according to the onset of unconsciousness. Fractional administration is advised rather than the single-dose method, as this gives close control and greater flexibility of the anaesthetic and helps to prevent overdosage.

Most patients will require not more than 0.5 g otherwise recovery will be prolonged and possibly complicated. The patient should in all cases be premedicated with atropine and if necessary with an analgesic or tranquiliser, although the latter will increase materially the post-operative time. If chlorpromazine (Largactil) or promethazine (Phenergan) is used for premedication the amount of Intraval Sodium required for induction should be reduced.

Solutions are prepared by adding Water for Injections (BP). They must be used within 24 hours or discarded.

For induction: Inject 2–3 ml of the 5% or twice this volume of the 2.5% solution in 10–15 seconds, then pause for 30 seconds to 1 minute to observe the effect of the drug, depending on the state of the patient's circulation. Usually there is loss of consciousness and some relaxation. A further quantity of the solution may then be given if indicated, otherwise anaesthesia should be maintained by an appropriate inhalation agent.

For minor operations: Induction is as described above and additional quantities of the anaesthetic solution are given as required to maintain anaesthesia at a level adequate to obtund pain reflexes. The level of anaesthesia is best judged by the depth of respiration; surgical anaesthesia is usually present when respiration is depressed. It cannot be too strongly emphasised that the airway must be kept open with the patient breathing an adequate concentration of oxygen. In these circumstances the depressed respiration is not dangerous and the patient should remain a good colour with the skin warm, pink and dry.

Intravenous anaesthesia is not recommended for the maintenance of unconsciousness in lengthy procedures, so that for these, after induction, it should always be supplemented by the chosen inhalation agent.

Intraval Sodium may be employed rectally in the form of a solution for producing narcosis in 10–12 minutes. When given as a solution, it is usual to calculate dosage on the basis of 44 mg/kg body weight, which quantity is dissolved in 25 ml of water and instilled through a rectal catheter.

Children: Intraval Sodium is suitable for use in children as well as adults. The dosage is 2–7 mg/kg intravenously.

Contra-indications, warnings, etc

Use in pregnancy: There is epidemiological and clinical evidence of the safety of barbiturates in pregnancy including thiopenton. This drug readily crosses the placenta and appears in human milk. Dosage in the pregnant female should not exceed 250 mg.

Contra-indications: A history of acute intermittent porphyria is an absolute contra-indication to any barbiturate. Special care is required in patients with the following conditions: hypovolaemia; severe haemorrhage; burns; dehydration; severe anaemia; cardiovascular disease; status asthmaticus; severe liver disease; myasthenia gravis and muscular dystrophies; adrenocortical insufficiency even when controlled by cortisone; cachexia and severe toxaemia; raised intracranial pressure; raised blood urea; raised plasma potassium; metabolic disorders, e.g. thyrotoxicosis, myoedema, diabetes.

Precautions: Reduced doses are required in the elderly and in patients heavily pre-medicated with narcotics and other central depressants. On the other hand, those addicted to drugs are difficult subjects to anaesthetise with normal thiopentone dosage and it is advised that supplementary analgesic agents and relaxants be given as necessary.

The jaw drops rapidly after starting the injection and must be supported, since it is imperative to keep the airway open. The patient should always be in a recumbent position to avoid cerebral anaemia. If Intraval Sodium is used in dental work a mouth prop is inserted before injection is commenced. The throat must be properly packed to prevent access of blood, etc. to the larynx and the dose employed should not exceed 0.25 g otherwise recovery will be delayed. Facilities for intubation and administration of oxygen under positive pressure must always be available.

To prevent accidental intra-arterial injection the site of administration must be palpated carefully and after insertion of the needle a little blood should be drawn into the syringe to observe its colour. Intra-arterial injection produces severe arterial spasm with intense burning pain in the hand and fingers. The patient can sometimes warn the anaesthetist of this before losing consciousness. In the event of such accident, inject procaine hydrochloride directly into the artery and perform a stellate ganglion block. Early anticoagulant therapy is advisable.

Side-effects: Adverse effects: Coughing, sneezing or laryngeal spasm may occur during induction. Extravasation causes pain and possible tissue necrosis. Thrombophlebitis may result from the use of 5% solution. Skin rashes, fever, arthralgia and weakness are rare side-effects. Allergic reactions and hypersensitivity have been documented.

Toxicity and treatment of overdosage: Respiratory depression during thiopentone anaesthesia must be treated by artificial ventilation with oxygen, as also cardiac arrhythmia associated with anoxia or hypercardia. A fall in blood pressure is often noted initially, while overdose may lead to circulatory failure.

Apnoea or serious respiratory depression must be treated by controlled respiration with oxygen. Cardiovascular collapse requires immediate lowering of the head of the table; if the blood pressure fails to rise a pressor agent such as mephentermine or a plasma expander should be given. If the heart stops immediate massage should be given.

Pharmaceutical precautions Aqueous solutions of thiopentone sodium are strongly alkaline; a 2.5% solution has a pH about 10.5. The solution is incompatible with acids, acidic salts and oxidising agents. Solutions decompose on standing giving cloudiness, precipitation or crystallisation; any such solution must not be used.

Solutions should be freshly prepared and used within 24 hours or discarded.

Legal category POM.

Package quantities For the preparation of 2.5% solution: Vials of 0.5 g in boxes of 10 and 25. Multidose container of 2.5 g.

For the preparation of a 5% solution: Vials of 0.5 g and 1 g in boxes of 10 and 25. Multidose container of 5 g.

Further information Nil.

Product licence number 0012/5043.

LARGACTIL*

Presentation White sugar-coated tablets containing 10 mg, 25 mg, 50 mg and 100 mg chlorpromazine hydrochloride, printed in black 'Largactil' '10', '25', '50', and '100' respectively.

Pale straw coloured injection solution containing 2.5% w/v chlorpromazine hydrochloride in ampoules of 1 and 2 ml.

Syrup: A clear bright golden-brown syrupy liquid, each 5 ml containing 25 mg chlorpromazine hydrochloride and 68% w/v sugars.

Forte suspension coloured orange, each 5 ml containing 145 mg chlorpromazine embonate equivalent to 100 mg chlorpromazine hydrochloride.

Cream-coloured suppositories each containing 100 mg chlorpromazine base.

Uses Largactil is a phenothiazine neuroleptic. It is indicated in the following conditions:

– Schizophrenia and other psychoses (especially paranoid), mania and hypomania.
– In anxiety psychomotor agitation excitement, violent or dangerously impulsive behaviour. Largactil is used as an adjunct in the short term management of these conditions.
– Intractable hiccup.
– Nausea and vomiting of terminal illness (where other drugs have failed or are not available).
– Induction of hypothermia is facilitated by Largactil which prevents shivering causes vasodilatation.
– Childhood schizophrenia and autism.

Kinetics: Chlorpromazine is rapidly absorbed and widely distributed in the body. It is metabolised in the liver and excreted in the urine and bile. Whilst plasma concentration of chlorpromazine itself rapidly declines excretion of chlorpromazine metabolites is very slow. The drug is highly bound to plasma protein. It readily diffuses across the placenta. Small quantities have been detected in milk from treated women. Children require smaller dosages per kg than adults.

Dosage and administration See the general remarks below and Tables 1, 2 and 3. *Oral administration* should be used whenever possible. Patients unwilling to swallow tablets may be treated with suspension or syrup. Dosages should be low to begin with and gradually increased under close supervision until the optimum dosage for the individual is reached. Individuals vary considerably and the optimum dose may be affected by the formulation used.

Parenteral formulations may be used in emergencies. They may only be administered by *deep* intramuscular injection. Largactil is too irritant to give subcutaneously. Repeated injections should be avoided if possible.

Suppositories may be used if convenient. Each Largactil suppository contains 100 mg chlorpromazine base and has an effect approximately equivalent to 40 mg by mouth or 20 mg by injection.

Contra-indications, warnings, etc
Pregnancy: There is inadequate evidence of the safety of Largactil in human pregnancy but it has been widely used for many years without apparent ill consequence. There is evidence of harmful effects in animals. Like other drugs it should be avoided in pregnancy unless the physician considers it essential. It may occasionally prolong labour and at such a time should be withheld until the cervix is dilated 3–4 cm. Possible adverse effects on the foetus include lethargy or paradoxical hyperexcitability, tremor and low Apgar score. Largactil being excreted in milk, breastfeeding should be suspended during treatment.

Precautions: Largactil should be avoided in patients with liver or renal dysfunction, epilepsy, Parkinson's disease, hypothyroidism, cardiac failure, phaeochromocytoma, myasthenia gravis, prostate hypertrophy. It should be avoided in patients known to be hypersensitive to phenothiazines or with a history of narrow angle glaucoma. It should be used with caution in the elderly, particularly during very hot or very cold weather (risk of hyper-, hypothermia).

Patients should be warned about drowsiness during

Table 1: Dosage of chlorpromazine in schizophrenia, other psychoses, anxiety and agitation etc.

Route	Adult	Children under 1 year	Children 1–5 years	Children 6–12 years	Elderly or debilitated patients
Oral	Initially 25 mg t.d.s. or 75 mg at bedtime increasing by daily amounts of 25 mg to an effective maintenance dose. This is usually in the range 75 to 300 mg daily, but some patients may require up to 1 g daily.	Do not use unless need is life saving.	0.5 mg/kg bodyweight every 4–6 hours to a maximum recommended dose of 40 mg daily.	$\frac{1}{3}$ to $\frac{1}{2}$ the adult dose to a maximum recommended dose of 75 mg daily.	Start with $\frac{1}{3}$ to $\frac{1}{2}$ the usual adult dose with a more gradual increase in dosage.
i.m.	For acute relief of symptoms 25–50 mg every 6–8 hours.	As above.	0.5 mg/kg bodyweight every 6–8 hours. Dosage is not advised to exceed 40 mg daily.	0.5 mg/kg bodyweight every 6–8 hours. Dosage is not advised to exceed 75 mg daily.	Doses in the lower range for adults should be sufficient to control symptoms i.e. 25 mg 8 hourly.
Rectal	100 mg 6–8 hourly	—	—	—	—

Table 2: Hiccup. Induction of hypothermia

Indication	Route	Adult dose	Children under 1 year	Children 1–5 years	Children 6–12 years	Elderly or debilitated patients
Hiccups	Oral i.m.	25–50 mg t.d.s. or q.d.s. 25–50 mg and if this fails 25–50 mg in 500–1000 ml sodium chloride injection infused slowly.	No information available			
Induction of hypothermia to prevent shivering.	i.m.	25–50 mg every 6–8 hours.	Do not use.	Initial dose 0.5 mg to 1 mg/kg. Maintenance 0.5 mg/kg every 4–6 hours.	Initial dose 0.5 mg to 1 mg/kg. Maintenance 0.5 mg/kg every 4–6 hours.	No data available.

Table 3: Nausea and vomiting of terminal illness

Form	Adults	Children under 1 year	Children 1–5 years	Children 6–12 years	Elderly or debilitated patients
Oral	10–25 mg every 4–6 hours.	Do not use unless need is life saving.	0.5 mg/kg every 4–6 hours. Maximum daily dosage should not exceed 40 mg.	0.5 mg/kg every 4–6 hours. Maximum daily dosage should not exceed 75 mg.	Initially $\frac{1}{3}$ to $\frac{1}{2}$ the adult dose. The physician should then use his clinical judgment to obtain control.
Rectal	100 mg 6–8 hourly.	—	—	—	—
i.m.	25 mg initially then 25–50 mg every 3–4 hours until vomiting stops then drug to be taken orally.	Do not use unless need is life saving.	0.5 mg/kg 6–8 hourly. It is advised that maximum daily dosage should not exceed 40 mg.	0.5 mg/kg every 6–8 hours. It is advised that maximum daily dosage should not exceed 75 mg.	For oral use only.

the early days of treatment, and advised not to drive or operate machinery.

Postural hypotension with tachycardia as well as local pain or nodule formation may occur after i.m. administration. The patient should be kept supine and B.P. monitored when receiving parenteral chlorpromazine.

The elderly are particularly susceptible to postural hypotension.

Interactions of phenothiazine neuroleptics:

The CNS depressant actions of Largactil and other neuroleptic agents may be intensified (additively) by alcohol, barbiturates and other sedatives. Respiratory depression may occur.

The hypotensive effect of most antihypertensive drugs especially alpha adrenoceptor blocking agents may be exaggerated by Largactil.

The mild anticholinergic effect of Largactil may be enhanced by other anticholinergic drugs possibly leading to constipation, heat stroke, etc.

The action of some drugs may be opposed by Largactil; these include amphetamine, laevodopa clonidine, guanethidine, adrenaline.

Anticholinergic agents may reduce the antipsychotic effect of Largactil.

Some drugs interfere with absorption of neuroleptic agents: antacids, anti-Parkinson, lithium. Increases or decreases in the plasma concentrations of a number of drugs, e.g. propranolol, phenobarbitone have been observed but were not of clinical significance.

High doses of Largactil reduce the response to hypoglycaemic agents the dosage of which might have to be raised.

Documented adverse clinically significant interactions occur with alcohol, guanethidine and hypoglycaemic agents. Adrenaline must *not* be used in patients overdosed with Largactil. Other interactions are of a theoretical nature and not serious.

Minor side effects are nasal stuffiness, dry mouth, insomnia, agitation.

Adverse effects: Liver function: Jaundice, usually transient, occurs in a very small percentage of patients taking chlorpromazine. A premonitory sign may be a sudden onset of fever after one to three weeks of treatment followed by the development of jaundice. Chlorpromazine jaundice has the biochemical and other characteristics of obstructive jaundice and is associated with obstructions of the canaliculi by bile thrombi; the frequent presence of an accompanying eosinophilia indicates the allergic nature of this phenomenon. Treatment should be withheld on the development of jaundice.

Cardiorespiratory: Hypotension, usually postural, commonly occurs. Elderly or volume depleted subjects are particularly susceptible; it is more likely to occur after intramuscular administration.

Cardiac arrhythmias, including atrial arrhythmia, A-V block, ventricular tachycardia and fibrillation have been reported during neuroleptic therapy, possibly related to dosage. Pre-existing cardiac disease, old age, hypokalaemia and concurrent tricyclic antidepressants may predispose. ECG changes, usually benign, include widened QT interval, ST depression, U-waves and T-wave changes.

Respiratory depression is possible in susceptible patients.

Blood picture: A mild leukopaenia occurs in up to 30% of patients on prolonged high dosage. Agranulocytosis may occur rarely; it is not dose related. The occurrence of unexplained infections or fever requires immediate haematological investigation.

Extrapyramidal: Acute dystonias or dyskinesias, usually transitory are commoner in children and young adults, and usually occur within the first 4 days of treatment or after dosage increases.

Akathisia characteristically occurs after large initial doses.

Parkinsonism is commoner in adults and the elderly. It usually develops after weeks or months of treatment. One or more of the following may be seen: tremor, rigidity, akinesia or other features of Parkinsonism. Commonly just tremor.

Tardive dyskinesia: If this occurs it is usually, but not necessarily, after prolonged or high dosage. It can even occur after treatment has been stopped. Dosage should therefore be kept low whenever possible.

Skin and eyes: Contact skin sensitisation is a serious but rare complication in those frequently handling preparations of chlorpromazine; the greatest care must be taken to avoid contact of the drug with the skin. Skin rashes of various kinds may also be seen in patients treated with the drug. Patients on high dosage should be warned that they may develop photosensitivity in sunny weather and should avoid exposure to direct sunlight.

Occular changes and the development of a metallic greyish-mauve coloration of exposed skin have been noted in some individuals mainly females, who have received chloropromazine continuously for long periods (four to eight years).

Endocrine: Hyperprolactinaemia which may result in galactorrhoea, gynaecomastia, amenorrhoea; impotence.

Nouroleptic malignant syndrome (hyperthermia, rigidity autonomic dysfunction and altered consciousness) may occur with any neuroleptic.

Toxicity and treatment of overdosage: Symptoms of chlorpromazine overdosage include drowsiness or loss of consciousness, hypotension, tachycardia, E.C.G. changes, ventricular arrhythmias and hypothermia. Severe extra-pyramidal dyskinesias may occur.

If the patient is seen sufficiently soon (up to 6 hours) after ingestion of a toxic dose, gastric lavage may be attempted. Pharmacological induction of emesis is unlikely to be of any use. Activated charcoal should be given. There is no specific antidote. Treatment is supportive.

Generalised vasodilatation may result in circulatory collapse; raising the patient's legs may suffice, in severe cases, volume expansion by intravenous fluids may be needed; infusion fluids should be warmed before administration in order not to aggravate hypothermia.

Positive inotropic agents such as dopamine may be tried if fluid replacement is insufficient to correct the circulatory collapse. Peripheral vasoconstrictor agents are not generally recommended; avoid the use of adrenaline.

Ventricular or supraventricular tachy-arrhythmias usually respond to restoration of normal body temperature and correction of circulatory or metabolic disturbances. If persistent or life threatening, appropriate antiarrhythmic therapy may be considered. Avoid lignocaine and, as far as possible, long acting anti-arrhythmic drugs.

Pronounced central nervous system depression requires airway maintenance or, in extreme circumstances, assisted respiration. Severe dystonic reactions usually respond to procyclidine (5–10 mg) or orphenedrine (20–40 mg) administered intramuscularly or intravenously. Convulsions should be treated with intravenous diazepam.

Neuroleptic malignant syndrome should be treated with cooling. Dantrolene sodium may be tried.

Pharmaceutical precautions Protect from light. Largactil Injection Solutions, on exposure to light, rapidly develop a pink or yellow coloration; any such solution should be discarded. Largactil Injection Solutions have a pH of 5.0–6.5; they are incompatible with benzylpenicillin potassium, pentobarbitone sodium and phenobarbitone sodium. Largactil Forte Suspension and Syrup may be diluted, if required, with simple syrup (without preservatives).

Tablets should not be crushed and solutions should be handled with care because of the risk of contact dermatitis.

Legal category POM.

Package quantities *Tablets 10 mg and 25 mg:* Containers of 500; *50 mg and 100 mg:* Containers of 50 and 500.

Injection Solution 2.5%: Box of 10 × 1 ml ampoules.

Injection Solution 2.5%; Boxes of 10 × 2 ml ampoules.

Syrup: Bottles of 100 ml and 1 litre.

Forte Suspension: Bottle of 1 litre.

Suppositories: Boxes of 10.

Further information Nil.

Product licence numbers

Tablets 10 mg	0012/5108
Tablets 25 mg	0012/5109
Tablets 50 mg	0012/5110
Tablets 100 mg	0012/5111
Injection Solution 2.5%	0012/5308
Syrup	0012/5083
Forte Suspension	0012/5001
Suppositories	0012/5084

MYOCRISIN*

Presentation Ampoules containing injection solutions of varying strengths of sodium aurothiomalate. The solutions are pale yellow.

Uses Active Progressive Rheumatoid Arthritis (including Stills Disease).

Dosage and administration Myocrisin is administered by deep intramuscular injection, followed by gentle massage of the area.

Adults:

1. Remission Induction. Injections of 1 mg, 5 mg, and 10 mg at weekly intervals followed by 20–50 mg per week until remission occurs or a total of 1 gram has been given. Remission should occur around the 400–500 mg level.

2. Maintenance. 20–50 mg every 2–4 weeks should be administered according to response.

Elderly: No specific recommendations but elderly patients should be monitored with extra caution.

Children: (Stills Disease). The dosage is based on body weight. Therapy should be initiated with small weekly doses (1 mg/kg) up to a maximum weekly dose of:

Body weight under 20 kg	10 mg
Body weight 20–50 kg	20 mg
Body weight over 50 kg	30 mg

Treatment should be continued for six months. Response can be expected at the 300–500 mg level. If patients respond, maintenance therapy should be continued with the dosage administered over the previous 2–4 weeks for 1–5 years.

Contra-indications, warnings, etc Pregnancy, gross renal or hepatic disease, a history of blood dyscrasias, exfoliative dermatitis or systemic lupus erythematosus.

The absolute contra-indications should be positively excluded before considering gold therapy. Myocrisin should be administered with extra caution in the elderly and in patients with a history of urticaria, eczema or colitis. Extra caution should also be exercised if phenylbutazone or oxyphenbutazone are administered concurrently.

Before starting treatment and again before each injection, the urine should be tested for protein, the skin inspected for rash and a full blood count performed, including a numerical platelet count (not an estimate) and the readings plotted. Blood dyscrasias are most likely to occur when between 400 mg and 1 gram of gold have been given, or between the 10th and 20th week of treatment, but can also occur with as little as 40 mg or after only 2–4 weeks of therapy.

The presence of albuminuria, pruritus or rash, or an eosinophilia, are indications of developing toxicity; the Myocrisin should be withheld for one or two weeks until all signs have disappeared when the course may be restarted on a smaller dosage.

A complaint of sore throat, glossitis, buccal ulceration and/or easy bruising or bleeding, demands an immediate blood count, followed, if indicated by appropriate treatment for agranulocytosis and/or thrombocytopenia. Every patient treated with Myocrisin should be warned, both in writing and verbally, to report immediately the appearance of pruritus, metallic taste, sore throat or tongue, buccal ulceration or easy bruising, purpura, epistaxis, bleeding gums, menorrhagia or diarrhoea.

Hepatotoxicity with cholestatic jaundice is a rare complication which may occur early in the course of treatment; it subsides on withdrawing Myocrisin.

Diffuse unilateral or bilateral pulmonary fibrosis very rarely occurs. This progressive condition usually responds to drug withdrawal and steroid therapy – annual chest X-ray is recommended and attention should be paid to unexplained breathlessness and dry cough.

Side-effects may be largely avoided by the indicated careful titration of dosage. Minor reactions, usually manifest as skin rashes, are the most frequent and commonly benign, but as such reactions may be the forerunners of severe gold toxicity they must never be treated lightly. Significant skin complications are almost exclusively pruritic.

Treatment of overdosage: Minor side-effects resolve spontaneously on withdrawal of Myocrisin. Symptomatic treatment of pruritus with antihistamines may be helpful. Major skin lesions and serious blood dyscrasias demand hospital admission when dimercaprol or penicillamine may be used to enhance gold excretion. Fresh blood and/or platelet transfusions, corticosteroids and androgenic steroids may be required in the management of severe blood dyscrasias.

Pharmaceutical precautions Protect from light. Discoloured solutions should not be used.

Legal category POM.

Package quantities Boxes of 10 × 1 mg, 5 mg, 10 mg, 20 mg and 50 mg ampoules.

Further information Some rheumatologists provide their patients with a 'gold card' on which is recorded the amount of gold salt injected and results of laboratory tests, at the same time issuing a proforma for further treatment to the general practitioner responsible for the management of the patient. These are valuable aids in the early detection, and so reduce the incidence, of toxic reactions.

Product licence numbers

Injection 0.2%	0012/5116
Injection 1%	0012/5115
Injection 2%	0012/5114
Injection 4%	0012/5113
Injection 10%	0012/5006

NEULACTIL*

Presentation Tablets, uncoated, yellow, containing 2.5, 10 or 25 mg pericyazine, embossed 'Neulactil', 'Neulactil' 10 or 'Neulactil' 25 respectively on one face, with a break-line on the reverse. Neulactil tablets contain lactose.

Forte Syrup, clear orange brown syrupy liquid, each

5 ml containing 10 mg pericyazine. The content of sugars is about 68% w/v, and it contains 0.1% w/v of sodium sulphite and 0.1% w/v of sodium metabisulphite.

Uses Pericyazine is a neuroleptic with cardiovascular and antihistamine effects similar to those of chlorpromazine, but it has a stronger antiserotonin effect and a powerful central sedative effect.

Neulactil is indicated.

(a) In adults with schizophrenia or other psychoses, for the treatment of symptoms or prevention of relapse.

(b) In anxiety, psychomotor agitation, violent or dangerously impulsive behaviour. Neulactil is used as an adjunct to the short-term management of these conditions.

(c) In children with behaviour disorders or schizophrenia.

Kinetics: There is little information about plasma concentrations, distribution and excretion in humans. The rate of metabolism and excretion of phenothiazines decreases in old age.

Dosage and administration Dosage requirement varies with the individual and the severity of the condition being treated. Initial dosage should be low with progressive increases until the desired response is obtained, after which dosage should be adjusted to maintain control of symptoms.

Severe conditions Indication (a) or (c)	Mild or moderate conditions Indication (b)
Adults Initially 75 mg per day in divided doses. Dosage should be increased by 25 mg per day at weekly intervals until the optimum effect is achieved. Maintenance therapy would not normally be expected to exceed 300 mg per day.	Initially 15–30 mg daily, divided into two portions, with a larger dose being given in the evening.
Elderly Initially 15–30 mg per day in divided doses. If this is well tolerated the dosage may be increased if necessary for optimum control of behaviour.	5 to 10 mg per day is suggested as a starting dose. It may be divided so that a larger portion is given in the evening. Half or quarter the normal adult dose may be sufficient for maintenance therapy.
Children The initial daily dose should be calculated on bodyweight. A child weighing 10 kg should receive 0.5 milligram and this initial dose should be increased by 1 mg for each additional 5 kg of bodyweight up to a total daily dose of 10 mg daily. This dosage may be gradually increased until the desired effect is achieved but the daily maintenance dose should not exceed twice the initial amount. Neulactil is not recommended for use in children below 1 year of age.	Not recommended for children.

Contra-indications, warnings, etc

Pregnancy: There is inadequate evidence of the safety of Neulactil in human pregnancy but it has been widely used for many years without apparent ill consequence. There is evidence with some neuroleptics of harmful effects in animals. Like other drugs Neulactil should be avoided in pregnancy unless the physician considers it essential. It may occasionally prolong labour and at such a time should be withheld until the cervix is dilated 3–4 cm. Possible adverse effects on the foetus include lethargy or paradoxical hyperexcitability, tremor and low Apgar score. Phenothiazines may be excreted in milk therefore breastfeeding should be suspended during treatment.

Precautions: Neuroleptics should be avoided in patients with liver or renal dysfunction, epilepsy, Parkinson's disease, hypothyroidism, cardiac failure, phaeochromocytoma, myasthenia gravis, prostate hypertrophy. It should be avoided in patients known to be hypersensitive to phenothiazines or with a history of narrow angle glaucoma. It should be used with caution in the elderly, particularly during very hot or very cold weather (risk of hyper-, hypothermia).

Patients should be warned about drowsiness during the early days of treatment, and advised not to drive or operate machinery.

The elderly are particularly susceptible to postural hypotension.

Interactions of phenothiazine neuroleptics. The CNS depressant actions of neuroleptic agents may be intensified (additively) by alcohol, barbiturates and other sedatives. Respiratory depression may occur.

The hypotensive effect of most antihypertensive drugs especially alpha adrenoceptor blocking agents may be exaggerated by neuroleptics.

The mild anticholinergic effect of neuroleptics may be enhanced by other anticholinergic drugs possibly leading to constipation, heat stroke, etc.

The action of some drugs may be opposed by neuroleptics; these include amphetamine, laevodopa clonidine, guanethidine, adrenaline.

Anticholinergic agents may reduce the antipsychotic effect of neuroleptics.

Some drugs interfere with absorption of neuroleptic agents: antacids, anti-Parkinson, lithium. Increases or decreases in the plasma concentrations of a number of drugs, e.g. propranolol, phenobarbitone have been observed but were not of clinical significance.

High doses of neuroleptics may reduce the response to hypoglycaemic agents the dosage of which might have to be raised.

Adrenaline must *not* be used in patients overdosed with neuroleptics. Most of the above interactions are of a theoretical nature and not serious.

Minor side-effects are nasal stuffiness, dry mouth, insomnia, agitation.

Adverse effects: Liver function: Jaundice, occurs in a very small percentage of patients taking neuroleptics. A premonitory sign may be a sudden onset of fever after one to three weeks of treatment followed by the development of jaundice. Neuroleptic jaundice has the biochemical and other characteristics of obstructive jaundice and is associated with obstruction of the canaliculi by bile thrombi; the frequent presence of an accompanying eosinophilia indicates the allergic nature of this phenomenon. Treatment should be withheld on the development of jaundice.

Cardiorespiratory: Hypotension, usually postural, commonly occurs. Elderly or volume depleted subjects are particularly susceptible.

Cardiac arrhythmias, including atrial arrhythmia, A-V block, ventricular tachycardia and fibrillation have been reported during neuroleptic therapy, possibly related to dosage. Pre-existing cardiac disease, old age, hypokalaemia and concurrent tricyclic antidepressants may predispose. ECG changes, usually benign, include widened QT interval, ST depression, U-waves and T-wave changes.

Respiratory depression is possible in susceptible patients.

Blood picture: A mild leukopaenia occurs in up to 30% of patients on prolonged high dosage of neuroleptics. Agranulocytosis may occur rarely; it is not dose related. The occurrence of unexplained infections or fever requires immediate haematological investigation.

Extrapyramidal: Acute dystonias or dyskinesias, usually transitory are commoner in children and young adults, and usually occur within the first 4 days of treatment or after dosage increases.

Akathisia characteristically occurs after large initial doses.

Parkinsonism is commoner in adults and the elderly. It usually develops after weeks or months of treatment. One or more of the following may be seen: tremor, rigidity, akinesia or other features of Parkinsonism. Commonly just tremor.

Tardive dyskinesia: If this occurs it is usually, but not necessarily, after prolonged or high dosage. It can even occur after treatment has been stopped. Dosage should therefore be kept low whenever possible.

Skin and eyes: Contact skin sensitisation is a serious but rare complication in those frequently handling preparations of phenothiazines; the greatest care must be taken to avoid contact of the drug with the skin. Skin rashes of various kinds may also be seen in patients treated with the drug. Patients on high dosage should be warned that they may develop photosensitivity in sunny weather and should avoid exposure to direct sunlight.

Endocrine: hyperprolactinaemia which may result in galactorrhoea, gynaecomastia, amenorrhoea; impotence.

Neuroleptic malignant syndrome (hyperthermia, rigidity autonomic dysfunction and altered consciousness) may occur with any neuroleptic.

Toxicity and treatment of overdosage: Symptoms of neuroleptic overdosage include drowsiness or loss of consciousness, hypotension, tachycardia, E.C.G. changes, ventricular arrhythmias and hypothermia. Severe extra-pyramidal dyskinesias may occur.

If the patient is seen sufficiently soon (up to 6 hours) after ingestion of a toxic dose, gastric lavage may be attempted. Pharmacological induction of emesis is unlikely to be of any use. Activated charcoal should be given. There is no specific antidote. Treatment is supportive.

Generalised vasodilatation may result in circulatory collapse; raising the patient's legs may suffice, in severe cases, volume expansion by intravenous fluids may be needed; infusion fluids should be warmed before administration in order not to aggravate hypothermia.

Positive inotropic agents such as dopamine may be tried if fluid replacement is insufficient to correct the circulatory collapse. Peripheral vasoconstrictor agents are not generally recommended; avoid the use of adrenaline.

Ventricular or supraventricular tachy-arrhythmias usually respond to restoration of normal body temperature and correction of circulatory or metabolic disturbances. If persistent or life threatening, appropriate anti-arrhythmic therapy may be considered. Avoid lignocaine and, as far as possible, long acting anti-arrhythmic drugs.

Pronounced central nervous system depression requires airway maintenance or, in extreme circumstances, assisted respiration. Severe dystonic reactions usually respond to procyclidine (5–10 mg) or orphenedrine (20–40 mg) administered intramuscularly or intravenously. Convulsions should be treated with intravenous diazepam.

Neuroleptic malignant syndrome should be treated with cooling. Dantrolene sodium may be tried.

Pharmaceutical precautions Protect from light. Neulactil Forte Syrup can be diluted with Syrup BP without preservative. Such dilutions have a shelf-life of 14 days.

Legal category POM.

Package quantities Containers of 500 × 2.5 mg and 10 mg tablets and of 50 × 25 mg tablets.
Bottles of 1 litre Neulactil Forte Syrup.

Further information Nil.

Product licence numbers

Tablets 2.5 mg	0012/5276
Tablets 10 mg	0012/5277
Tablets 25 mg	0012/5278
Forte Syrup	0012/5016

NIVAQUINE*

Presentation White tablets, each containing 200 mg chloroquine sulphate (equivalent to 150 mg chloroquine base), embossed Nivaquine 200 on one face, with a break line on the reverse.

A red syrup, containing 68 mg chloroquine sulphate (equivalent to 50 mg chloroquine base), in each 5 ml.

Uses Nivaquine is a 4-aminoquinoline compound which has a high degree of activity against the asexual erythrocytic forms of all species of malaria parasites. It is indicated for the suppression and clinical cure of all forms of malaria and, in addition, produces radical cure of falciparum malaria.

Nivaquine also exerts a beneficial effect in certain collagen diseases and protects against the effects of solar radiation. It is employed in the treatment of rheumatoid arthritis, juvenile rheumatoid arthritis, discoid and systemic lupus erythematosus and skin conditions aggravated by sunlight.

Nivaquine is also active against *Entamoeba histolytica* and *Giardia lamblia* and when Flagyl (metronidazole) is not available it may be used in hepatic amoebiasis and giardiasis.

Dosage and administration

Elderly: No specific dosage recommendations.

Suppression of malaria: Adults: 2 × 200 mg tablets in a single dose, on the same day each week during exposure.

Children: 5 mg/kg (as chloroquine base) at weekly intervals.

This may be conveniently administered as Nivaquine syrup according to the following schedule:

1–2 years	1 × 5 ml spoonful
3–4 years	1½ × 5 ml spoonfuls
5–7 years	2 × 5 ml spoonfuls
8–10 years	3 × 5 ml spoonfuls
11–12 years	4 × 5 ml spoonfuls

It is advisable to start taking Nivaquine two weeks before entering an endemic area and to continue for six weeks after leaving.

Treatment of malaria: Adults and children over 10 years: for partially immune subjects a single dose of 4 × 200 mg tablets will provide a safe and effective course of treatment.

In non-immune subjects treatment should consist of 4 × 200 mg tablets in one dose, followed by 2 × 200 mg tablets after six hours and then 2 × 200 mg tablets daily for the next two days.

The above dosage is intended as a guide in the treatment of P. falciparum malaria; due to variation in strain sensitivity it may sometimes be necessary to increase the dosage up to 14 tablets (2,100 mg base) given over a period of five days.

Infants and children under 10 years: In partially immune subjects, the child should be given the number of 5 ml spoonfuls of Nivaquine Syrup equal to its age next birthday. The syrup or the equivalent dosage in tablets may be given as a single dose or divided into two with six hours between doses.

In non-immune subjects the dosage given above should be regarded as the first dose. This should be followed by a second dose, half the size of the first after six hours. This second dose should then be repeated once on each of the next two days.

In the above schemes tablets can be substituted for the syrup if desired (3 × 5 ml spoonfuls of Nivaquine Syrup are equivalent to 1 × 200 mg tablets).

Other indications *Adults: Rheumatoid arthritis:* 1 × 200 mg tablet daily. *Lupus erythematosus:* 1 × 200 mg tablet daily until maximum improvement is obtained, followed by a smaller maintenance dose. *Light sensitive skin eruptions:* 1 or 2 × 200 mg tablets daily during the period of maximum light exposure. *Children:* 3 mg/kg bodyweight daily.

Treatment should be discontinued if no improvement has occurred after six months.

Contra-indications, warnings, etc Nivaquine is generally contra-indicated in pregnancy. However, clinicians may decide to administer Nivaquine to pregnant women for the prevention or treatment of malaria. Ocular or inner ear damage may occur in infants born of mothers who receive high doses of chloroquine throughout pregnancy.

Caution is advised in cases of porphyria, hepatic or renal disease, severe gastro-intestinal, neurological and blood disorders and in patients receiving anticoagulant therapy.

Retinopathy: Irreversible retinal damage may occur with prolonged treatment. Ophthalmological examination should always be carried out before and regularly (3–6 monthly intervals) during treatment. Retinal damage is particularly likely to occur if treatment has been given for longer than one year, or if the total dosage has exceeded 1.6 g/kg bodyweight. These precautions also apply to patients receiving chloroquine continuously at weekly intervals as a prophylactic against malarial attack for more than three years.

Nivaquine has a temporary effect on visual accommodation and patients should be warned regarding driving or operating machinery. Bone marrow depression, including aplastic anaemia, occurs rarely. Full blood counts should therefore be carried out regularly during extended treatment.

The more common side-effects include gastro-intestinal disturbances, headache and skin eruptions. Depigmentation or loss of hair may also occur. Corneal opacities and visual disturbances may occur, apart from retinal damage. These usually disappear on cessation of treatment.

Treatment of overdosage: Prompt measures will be required to counteract the depressant effect of the drug on the respiratory and cardiovascular systems. Vomiting should be induced or gastric lavage carried out as soon as possible followed by appropriate resuscitative measures, such as tracheal intubation with artificial respiration and the administration of vasopressor agents or intravenous fluids. Intravenous $\frac{1}{6}$ molar sodium lactate solution has been used to counteract the quinidine-like action of chloroquine on the myocardium. The administration of enteric-coated ammonium chloride tablets 0.5 g every eight hours to promote excretion of the drug is also recommended.

Pharmaceutical precautions Nivaquine Syrup should be protected from light.

Legal category POM. When supplied for prevention of malaria in a container specifically labelled for that purpose P.

Package quantities Containers of 100 tablets and 60 ml bottle of syrup.

Further information Nil.

Product licence numbers
Tablets   0012/5260
Syrup   0012/5020

NOZINAN*

Presentation Colourless injection solution 2.5% methotrimeprazine hydrochloride in ampoules of 1 ml.

Uses Management of the terminally ill patient. Methotrimeprazine resembles chlorpromazine and promethazine in the pattern of its pharmacology. It possesses antiemetic, anti-histamine and anti-adrenaline activity and exhibits a strong sedative effect.

Nozinan potentiates the action of other central nervous system depressants but may be given in conjunction with appropriately modified doses of narcotic analgesics in the management of severe pain. Nozinan does not significantly depress respiration and is particularly useful where pulmonary reserve is low.

Nozinan is indicated in the management of terminal pain and accompanying restlessness or distress.

Kinetics: The substance is rapidly absorbed and slowly excreted with a half life of about 30 hours. It is excreted via the urine and faeces.

Dosage and administration Dosage varies with the condition and the individual response of the patient.

The usual dose for adults is 12.5–25 mg (0.5–1 ml) by the intramuscular, or after dilution immediately before use with an equal volume of normal saline, by the intravenous route: in cases of severe agitation up to 50 mg (2 ml) may be used, repeated every six to eight hours. Methotrimeprazine may induce postural hypotension requiring close observation of the patient.

Elderly: No specific dosage recommendations.

[Dosage may be changed to *oral* if more convenient, using 'Veractil' brand methotrimeprazine tablets 25 mg (May & Baker). See separate data sheet].

Contra-indications, warnings, etc Safety in pregnancy has not been established.

The hypotensive effects of Nozinan should be taken into account when it is administered to patients with cardiac disease and the elderly or debilitated. Patients receiving Nozinan should not drive or operate machinery.

Contra-indications: There are no absolute contra-indications to the use of Nozinan in terminal care.

Side-effects: Somnolence and asthenia are frequent side effects. Dry mouth is encountered occasionally. Hypotension may occur, especially in elderly patients. A raised ESR may occasionally be encountered. Agranulocytosis has been reported, as have photosensitivity and allergic skin reactions.

Parkinsonian-like reactions may occur in patients receiving prolonged high dosage. Jaundice is a rare side effect.

Overdosage: Treatments of overdosage should include countering acute hypotension by the adoption of either a supine or head-down position, and possibly the use of phenylephrine or noradrenaline by intravenous drip infusion: the acute symptomatic treatment of central nervous depression is not usually required. Haemodialysis is ineffective. Body temperature should be allowed to recover naturally unless it falls below about 29.4°C at which level cardiac arrhythmias may develop. A special watch should be kept for intestinal and urinary bladder distension.

Pharmaceutical precautions Protect from light. Nozinan Injection Solution, on exposure to light, rapidly develops a pink or yellow colouration and any such solution should be discarded. Nozinan Injection Solution is incompatible with alkaline solutions.

Legal category POM.

Package quantities Injection Solution 2.5% Box of 10 × 1 ml ampoules.

Further information Nil.

Product licence number Injection Solution 2.5% 0012/5007.

OCUSERT*

Presentation Ocusert Pilocarpine therapeutic systems are elliptically-shaped units designed to release pilocarpine continuously following placement into the upper or lower conjunctival sac. The systems consist of a core reservoir of pilocarpine surrounded by a membrane which controls the drug's diffusion from the system into the tear fluid. Two systems are available, Pilo-20 and Pilo-40, which release 20 and 40 mcg per hour, respectively, for one week. The Pilo-20 system is 5.7 × 13.4 mm across its axis, 0.3 mm thick, and contains 5 mg pilocarpine, the Pilo-40 system is 5.5 × 13 mm on its axis, 0.5 mm thick, and contains 11 mg pilocarpine. Except for the opaque white margin, the systems are clear.

Uses The Ocusert pilocarpine system is indicated for control of elevated intra-ocular pressure in glaucoma in pilocarpine-responsive patients.

Dosage and administration *Initiation of therapy:* The Ocusert Pilo-20 system will usually control a patient previously controlled by 1 per cent or 2 per cent pilocarpine eye drops; a patient who has used higher strengths of pilocarpine eye drops may require the Pilo-40. However, there is no direct correlation between the two strengths of Ocusert and the strength of pilocarpine eye drops necessary to achieve the required reduction of pressure. The Ocusert systems reduce the amount of pilocarpine necessary to achieve adequate reduction of intra-ocular pressure; therapy may be started therefore with the Ocusert Pilo-20 system irrespective of the strength of pilocarpine eye drops used previously by the patient. If the pressure is satisfactorily reduced with the Ocusert Pilo-20 system the patient should continue its use, replacing each unit every seven days; if greater reduction of intra-ocular pressure is required, the patient should be transferred to the Pilo-40 system. Depending on the patient's age, family history, and disease status, the ophthalmologist may elect to begin therapy with the Pilo-40 system.

Concomitant therapy: Where necessary, adrenaline or timolol eye drops or a diuretic of the carbonic anhydrase inhibitor type may be used concurrently with Ocusert systems. The release rate of pilocarpine from the Ocusert systems is not influenced by the beta adrenoceptor antagonist, by carbonic anhydrase inhibitors, adrenaline eye drops, fluorescein, or local anaesthetics, antibiotics or anti-inflammatory steroid eye drops.

Placement and removal of the Ocusert systems: Patient instructions for the placement of the Ocusert systems in the eye and their removal are included in each package. It is strongly recommended that the patient's ability to manage the placement and removal of the system be reviewed at the first patient visit after initiation of therapy.

Since pilocarpine-induced myopia from the Ocusert systems may occur during the first few hours of therapy, the patient should be advised to place the system into the conjunctival sac at bedtime. By morning the induced myopia is at a stable level.

Handling precautions: Patients should be instructed to wash their hands thoroughly with soap and water before touching or manipulating the Ocusert systems. If a displaced unit contacts unclean surfaces, rinsing with cool tap water before replacing is advisable. Biologically contaminated units should be discarded and replaced with fresh ones.

Retention in the eye: During the initial adaptation period, the Ocusert unit may slip out of the conjunctival sac on to the cheek. The patient is usually aware of such movement and can replace the unit without difficulty.

In those patients in whom retention of the Ocusert unit is a problem, placement in the upper conjunctival sac is often more acceptable. The Ocusert unit can be manipulated from the lower to the upper conjunctival sac by a gentle digital massage through the lid, a technique readily learned by the patient. For best retention, the unit should be moved before sleep to the upper conjunctival sac. Should the unit slip out of the conjunctival sac during sleep, its ocular hypotensive effect continues for a period of time comparable to that following instillation of eye drops. The patient should be instructed to check for the presence of the Ocusert unit before sleep and on rising.

Contra-indications, warnings, etc Ocusert systems are contra-indicated where pupillary constriction is undesirable, such as glaucomas associated with acute inflammatory disease of the anterior segment of the eye, and glaucomas occurring or persisting after extracapsular cataract extraction where posterior synechiae may occur.

Ocusert systems should not be used in patients with acute infectious conjunctivitis or keratitis except on specialist advice. Damaged or deformed systems should not be placed or retained in the eye. Systems believed to be associated with an unexpected increase in drug action should be removed and replaced with new systems.

The safety of Ocusert systems in patients with retinal detachment or with filtration blebs has not been established. Although eye drops have been used effectively in conjunction with the Ocusert systems, systemic reactions consistent with an increased rate of absorption from the eye of an autonomic drug, such as adrenaline, have been observed. In rare instances, reactions of this type can be severe. The conjunctival erythema and oedema associated with adrenaline eye drops are not substantially altered by concomitant use of an Ocusert system. The use of pilocarpine eye drops should be considered when intense miosis is desired in certain ocular conditions.

Ciliary spasm is encountered with pilocarpine usage but is not a contra-indication to continued therapy unless the induced myopia is debilitating to the patient. Irritation from pilocarpine has been frequently encountered and may require cessation of therapy depending on the judgement of the doctor. True allergic reactions are uncommon but require discontinuation of therapy if they occur.

Although withdrawal of the peripheral iris from the anterior chamber angle by miosis may reduce the tendency for narrow angle closure, miotics can occasionally precipitate angle closure by increasing the resistance to aqueous flow from posterior to anterior chamber. Miotic agents may also cause retinal detachment; thus, care should be exercised with all miotic therapy especially in young myopic patients.

Some patients may notice signs of conjuctival irritation, including mild erythema with or without a slight increase in mucous secretion when they first use Ocusert systems. These signs tend to lessen or disappear after the first week of therapy. In rare instances a sudden increase in pilocarpine effects has been reported.

Pharmaceutical precautions Store in a refrigerator at 2° to 8°C, i.e. not in the freezer compartment.

Legal category POM.

Package quantities Ocusert Pilo-20 or Ocusert Pilo-40 systems are available in containers of eight individual sterile systems.

Further information The decrease in intra-ocular pressure obtained with both the Pilo-20 and Pilo-40 systems is fully established within 1½ or 2 hours after placement in the conjunctival sac and is maintained for 24 hours a day for seven days. Intra-ocular pressure reduction with Ocusert systems for an entire week is achieved with either 3.4 mg or 6.7 mg pilocarpine (20 mcg or 40 mcg times 24 × 7, respectively), as compared with 28 mg of pilocarpine administered as a 2 per cent ophthalmic solution four times a day.

Ocusert systems may be used in association with contact lenses.

Product licence numbers
Pilo-20　0012/0118
Pilo-40　0012/0119

ORUDIS*

Presentation Capsules each containing 50 mg ketoprofen, bicoloured (opaque green/opaque purple) with each half printed 'Orudis 50' in white. Capsules each containing 100 mg ketoprofen (flesh opaque) printed 'Orudis 100' in black.

Suppositories each containing 100 mg ketoprofen.

Uses Orudis is a potent non-steroidal anti-inflammatory analgesic agent and a strong inhibitor of prostaglandin synthetase.

Orudis is recommended in the management of rheumatoid arthritis, osteoarthrosis, ankylosing spondylitis, acute articular and periarticular disorders (bursitis, capsulitis, synovitis, tendinitis), fibrositis, cervical spondylitis, low back pain (strain, lumbago, sciatica, fibrositis), painful musculo-skeletal conditions and dysmenorrhoea.

Orudis reduces joint pain and inflammation, and facilitates increase in mobility and functional independence. As with other non-steroidal anti-inflammatory agents, it does not cure the underlying disease.

Kinetics: Ketoprofen is completely absorbed from 'Orudis' capsules and maximum plasma concentration occurs after ½–1 hour. It declines thereafter with an elimination half-life of about 2–3 hours. There is no accumulation on continued daily dosing. Ketoprofen is rapidly absorbed from the suppository dosage form with maximum plasma concentration at 1–2 hours with an elimination half-life of 2–3 hours. Plasma levels obtained are comparable to those obtained from equal oral doses.

Dosage and administration Orudis is administered orally and/or rectally; to limit occurrence of gastrointestinal disturbance, capsules should always be taken with food (milk, meals).

Oral dosage is 50–100 mg twice daily, depending on patient weight and on severity of symptoms; medication should be taken early in the morning and late at night.

Rectal dosage is one suppository (100 mg) late at night supplemented as required with Orudis capsules during daytime.

If adverse effects (see below) develop on 100 mg orally twice daily, morning dosage, and if necessary night-time dosage also, should be reduced for several days to 50 mg night and morning, and then increased slowly, as tolerated; some patients are adequately controlled with oral night-time only treatment (100–200 mg).

Orudis suppositories are especially appropriate for controlling overnight symptoms (severity of night and morning pain; duration and severity of morning stiffness). Suppositories administered late at night provide more consistent effective control of overnight symptoms than oral medication.

Best results are obtained by titrating dosage to suit each patient; start with a low dosage in mild chronic disease and a high dosage in acute severe disease. Some patients derive greater benefit by treatment with capsules only; some with a combined capsule/suppository regimen; and others with a higher dosage at night-time than at early morning. Where patients require a maximum oral dosage initially, an attempt should be made to reduce this dosage for maintenance since lower dosage might be better tolerated for purposes of *long-term* treatment.

Elderly: Clinical and pharmacokinetic data have not yielded any evidence of an excess of adverse effects or cumulation in the elderly. There is therefore no need for dosage reduction in elderly patients unless they are frail, severely under weight.

Paediatric dosage not established.

Contra-indications, warnings, etc Active peptic ulceration; a history of recurrent peptic ulceration or chronic dyspepsia; severe renal dysfunction; disease in children (safety/dosage during long-term treatment has not been established).

Suppositories should not be used following recent proctitis or in association with haemorrhoids.

Ketoprofen should not be given to patients sensitive to aspirin or other non-steroidal anti-inflammatory agents known to inhibit prostaglandin synthetase. Severe bronchospasm might be precipitated in these subjects, and in patients suffering from, or with a history of, bronchial asthma or allergic disease.

Precautions *Pregnancy and lactation:* Embryopathic effects have not been recorded with this drug but it is recommended to avoid medication during pregnancy and lactation.

Plasma protein-binding drugs: Ketoprofen is highly protein-bound. Concomitant use of other protein-binding drugs, e.g. anticoagulants, sulphonamides, hydantoins, might necessitate modification of dosage in order to avoid increased levels of such drugs resulting from competition for plasma protein-binding sites.

Warning and adverse effects: Orudis capsules should always be prescribed 'To be taken with food' in case of gastrointestinal intolerance.

Care should be taken in patients with renal dysfunction.

Adverse effects, frequently transient, include indigestion, dyspepsia, flatulence, heartburn, abdominal discomfort, nausea and, very rarely, skin rashes. Bronchospasm might be precipitated in patients suffering from or with a history of bronchial asthma or allergy. Use of suppositories is sometimes associated with change in stool consistency, mostly of mild softening. In a study of 64 patients treated for up to six months with one suppository each night (supplemented during daytime with 'Orudis' capsules), local intolerance to suppositories sufficiently severe to discontinue treatment occurred in only four subjects.

Overdosage: Like other propionic acid derivatives, ketoprofen is of low toxicity in overdosage; symptoms after acute ketoprofen intoxication are largely limited to drowsiness, abdominal pain and vomiting, but adverse effects seen after overdosage with propionic acid derivatives such as hypotension, bronchospasm and gastrointestinal haemorrhage should be anticipated. Treatment is otherwise supportive and symptomatic.

Pharmaceutical precautions Store in a dry place, below 25°C.

Legal category POM.

Package quantities Orudis 50: Containers of 100 × 50 mg and 500 × 50 mg capsules.
Orudis 100: Containers of 100 × 100 mg capsules.
Blister pack of 7 × 100 mg suppositories.

Further information Nil.

Product licence numbers
50 mg capsules	0012/0122
100 mg capsules	0012/0133
100 mg suppositories	0012/0109

ORUVAIL* ▼

Presentation
Oruvail 100: Transparent pink capsules with opaque purple cap (each half printed 'Oruvail 100' in white), holding white pellets. Each capsule contains 100 mg ketoprofen in a pH sensitive controlled release delivery system.

Oruvail 200: Transparent pink capsules with opaque white cap (each half printed 'Oruvail' 200 in blue), holding white pellets. Each capsule contains 200 mg ketoprofen in a pH sensitive controlled release delivery system.

Uses Oruvail is a potent non-steroidal anti-inflammatory analgesic agent and a stong inhibitor of prostaglandin synthetase.

Oruvail is recommended in the management of rheumatoid arthritis, osteoarthritis, ankylosing spondylitis, acute articular and periarticular disorders (bursitis, capsulitis, synovitis, tendinitis), fibrositis, cervical spondylitis, low back pain (strain, lumbago, sciatica, fibrositis), painful musculo-skeletal conditions and dysmenorrhoea.

Oruvail reduces joint pain and inflammation, and facilitates increase in mobility and functional independence. As with other non-steroidal anti-inflammatory agents, it does not cure the underlying disease.

Kinetics: Ketoprofen is slowly but completely absorbed from Oruvail capsules. Maximum plasma concentration occurs after 6–8 hours. It declines thereafter with a half-life of about 8 hours. There is no accumulation on continued daily dosing.

Dosage and administration Oruvail is administered orally, usually with food.

Dosage is 100–200 mg once daily, depending on patient weight and on severity of symptoms.

Elderly: Clinical and pharmacokinetic data have not yielded any evidence of an excess of adverse effects or cumulation in the elderly. There is therefore no need for dosage reduction in elderly patients unless they are frail, severely under weight.

Paediatric dosage not established.

Contra-indications, warnings, etc Active peptic ulceration; a history of recurrent peptic ulceration or chronic dyspepsia. Severe renal dysfunction.

Ketoprofen should not be given to patients sensitive to aspirin or other non-steroidal anti-inflammatory agents known to inhibit prostaglandin synthetase. Severe bronchospasm might be precipitated in these patients and in those suffering from, or with a history of bronchial asthma or allergic disease.

Precautions: Pregnancy and lactation: embryopathic effects have not been recorded with this drug but it is recommended to avoid medication during pregnancy and lactation.

Plasma protein-binding drugs: Ketoprofen is highly protein-bound. Concomitant use of other protein-binding drugs, eg anticoagulants, sulphonamides, hydantoins, might necessitate modification of dosage in order to avoid increased levels of such drugs resulting from competition for plasma protein-binding sites.

Warning and adverse effects: Care should be taken in patients with renal dysfunction.

Oruvail capsules should always be prescribed to be taken with food in case of gastrointestinal intolerance.

Adverse effects, frequently transient, include, indigestion, dyspepsia, flatulence, heartburn, abdominal discomfort, nausea and, very rarely, skin rashes. Bronchospasm might be precipitated in patients suffering from or with a history of bronchial asthma or allergy.

Overdosage: Like other propionic acid derivatives, ketoprofen is of low toxicity in overdosage; symptoms after acute ketoprofen intoxication are largely limited to drowsiness, abdominal pain and vomiting, but adverse effects seen after overdosage with propionic acid derivatives such as hypotension, bronchospasm and gastrointestinal haemorrhage should be anticipated.

Owing to the slow release characteristics of Oruvail, it should be expected that ketoprofen will continue to be absorbed for up to 16 hours after ingestion.

Gastric lavage, aimed at recovering pellets that may still be in the stomach, should be performed if the patient is seen soon enough after ingestion. It should be possible to identify the pellets in the gastric contents. Treatment is otherwise supportive and symptomatic.

Administration of activated charcoal in an attempt to reduce absorption of slowly-released ketoprofen should be considered.

Pharmaceutical precautions Store in a dry place, below 25°C.

Legal category POM.

Package quantities
Oruvail 100: Containers of 100 capsules.
Oruvail 200: Calendar blister pack of 28 (2 × 14) capsules.

Further information Nil.

Product licence numbers
Oruvail 100: 0012/0143
Oruvail 200: 0012/0158

PHENERGAN*

Presentation *Tablets:* Blue, sugar-coated tablets containing 10 mg promethazine hydrochloride, marked M&B in reddish-brown print.

Blue, sugar-coated tablets containing 25 mg promethazine hydrochloride marked 'Phenergan 25' in reddish-brown print.

Phenergan 10 mg and 25 mg tablets contain lactose.

Elixir: A clear bright golden syrupy liquid containing 5 mg promethazine hydrochloride per 5 ml. The elixir contains 68% sugars, 0.1% sodium sulphite and 0.1% sodium metabisulphite.

Injection: A colourless injection solution containing 2.5% w/v promethazine hydrochloride.

Uses Potent long-acting antihistamine with additional, anti-emetic and sedative/calming effects. Indicated in symptomatic treatment of allergic conditions of the respiratory tract and skin: sensitisation reactions to drug or foreign proteins; anaphylactic reactions.

For sedation, hypnosis and insomnia.

For pre-medication for its sedative/calming effect, anti-emetic action and antisecretory effect.

In obstetrics.

As a paediatric sedative.

Kinetics: Promethazine is well absorbed after oral dosing and slowly excreted via urine and bile. It is distributed widely in the body. It enters the brain and crosses the placenta. Phenothiazines pass into the milk at low concentrations.

Dosage and administration *Adults: Oral administration:* Initial dose one 25 mg tablet at night – may be increased to two or three 25 mg tablets at night if necessary. In allergic conditions more frequent administration, twice or three times daily, may be necessary,

starting with one or two 10 mg tablets and increasing as required.

Parenteral administration: The usual adult dose is 25–50 mg by deep intramuscular injection or, in emergency, by slow intravenous injection after dilution of 2.5% solution to 10 times its volume with Water for Injections immediately before use. Maximum parenteral dose 100 mg.

Elderly: No specific dosage recommendations.

Children: They may be treated more conveniently by the elixir containing 5 mg per 5 ml.

As an antihistamine in allergy:
Infants from 6 months to 1 year   5–10 mg
Children of 1–5 years   5–15 mg
Children of 5–10 years   10–25 mg
  In cases where two doses in 24 hours are required the lower amount stated should be given.

As a hypnotic/sedative:
Infants from 6 months to 1 year   10 mg
Children of 1–5 years   15–20 mg
Children of 5–10 years   20–25 mg
  Given as a single night-time dose.

Parenteral: Half the oral dose, i.e. 6.25–12.5 mg for children from 5 to 10 years may be given by deep intramuscular injection.

Contra-indications, warnings, etc *Use in pregnancy:* There is epidemiological evidence for the safety of promethazine in pregnancy, and animal studies have shown no hazard, nevertheless it should not be used in pregnancy unless the physician considers it essential.

Ambulant patients receiving Phenergan for the first time should not be in control of vehicles or machinery for the first few days until it is established that they are not hypersensitive to the central nervous effects of the drug and do not suffer from disorientation, confusion or dizziness.

Phenergan will enhance the action of any sedative or hypnotic. Alcohol should be avoided during treatment.

Side-effects may be seen in a few patients: drowsiness, dizziness, disorientation. Photosensitive skin reactions have been reported; strong sunlight should be avoided during treatment.

Treatment of overdosage: Symptoms of severe overdosage are variable. They are characterised in children by various combinations of excitation, ataxia, inco-ordination, athetosis and hallucinations, while adults may become drowsy and lapse into coma. Convulsions may occur in both adults and children; coma or excitement may precede their occurrence. Cardiorespiratory depression is uncommon.

If the patient is seen soon enough after ingestion, it should be possible to induce vomiting with ipecacuanha despite the anti-emetic effect of promethazine; alternatively, gastric lavage may be used.

Treatment is otherwise supportive with attention to maintenance of adequate respiratory and circulatory status. Convulsions should be treated with diazepam or other suitable anticonvulsant.

Pharmaceutical precautions Protect from light. Solutions of Phenergan are incompatible with alkaline substances, which precipitate the insoluble promethazine base.

Legal category   Tablets, Elixir   P.
                       Injection Solution POM.

Package quantities Containers of 50 and 500 of both strength tablets.
Injection Solution 2.5%: Boxes of 10 × 1 ml and 10 × 2 ml ampoules.
Elixir: Bottles of 100 ml and 2 litres.

Further information Nil.

Product licence numbers
Tablets 10 mg   0012/5285
Tablets 25 mg   0012/5286
Elixir   0012/5025
Injection   0012/5054.

PHENERGAN* COMPOUND EXPECTORANT LINCTUS

Presentation Phenergan Compound Expectorant Linctus is presented as a straw-coloured linctus containing in each 5 ml:

Promethazine hydrochloride	5 mg
Ipecacuanha Liquid Extract BP	0.01 ml
Potassium guaiacolsulphonate	45.0 mg
Citric acid	65.0 mg

in a strawberry-flavoured vehicle containing 75% sugars.

Uses Cough linctus combining the antihistamine, anti-emetic, central sedative, local analgesic and anticholinergic actions of promethazine with the expectorant and mucolytic actions of ipecacuanha, potassium guaiacolsulphonate and citric acid.

Indicated for the symptomatic relief of nasal and bronchial congestion associated with coughs, colds and allied conditions of the respiratory tract.

Dosage and administration Phenergan Compound Expectorant Linctus should be administered two or three times daily in the following doses:

6 months to 5 years	2.5 ml
5–10 years	2.5–5 ml
Over 10 years	5–10 ml
Adults	5–10 ml

Elderly: No specific dosage recommendations.

Small infants should be treated under medical supervision only.

The linctus may be diluted with simple Syrup BP for the lower doses recommended above.

Contra-indications, warnings, etc
Use in pregnancy: There is epidemiological evidence for the safety of promethazine in human pregnancy and animal studies have shown no hazard. There is inadequate evidence of the safety of the other active ingredients but they have been in wide use for many years without ill-effect. Nevertheless Phenergan Compound Expectorant Linctus should not be used in pregnancy unless the physician considers it essential.

Apart from drowsiness, it is possible that a patient may prove hypersensitive to the central effects of promethazine and suffer from confusion or disorientation. It is therefore recommended that adults should not be in charge of vehicles or machinery during the first few days of taking the linctus, until it is established that their response has not been adversely affected. Avoid alcoholic drink.

It should be borne in mind that the promethazine in the linctus may tend to enhance the effects of any sedative, hypnotic or other central depressant drug given concurrently. Slight drowsiness may occur in some

patients and this can usually be avoided by reducing the dosage.

Overdosage: Symptoms of severe overdosage with promethazine are variable. They are characterised in children by various combinations of excitation, ataxia, inco-ordination, athetosis and hallucinations, while adults may become drowsy and lapse into coma. Convulsions may occur in both adults and children; coma or excitement may precede their occurrence. Cardiorespiratory depression is uncommon.

If the patient is seen soon enough after ingestion, it should be possible to induce vomiting with ipecacuanha despite the anti-emetic effect of promethazine; alternatively, gastric lavage may be used.

Treatment is otherwise supportive with attention to maintenance of adequate respiratory and circulatory status. Convulsions should be treated with diazepam or other suitable anticonvulsant.

Pharmaceutical precautions Protect from light.

Legal category P.

Package quantities Bottles of 100 ml.

Further information Nil.

Product licence number 0012/0093.

PHENERGAN* CREAM

Presentation Phenergan Cream is a white or off-white cream containing 2% w/w promethazine base and 0.15% w/w dibromopropamidine isethionate.

Uses Local antihistamine and local analgesic properties of promethazine are combined with the antibacterial action of dibromopropamidine. Indicated in early treatment of first and second degree burns and scalds in which it limits local reaction of erythema, blistering and oedema, relieves pain and prevents infection. For early application to insect bites and stings, particularly where there is a risk of secondary infection.

Dosage and administration In burns and scalds the cream is applied direct. Minor lesions on exposed parts may require no covering or only such as is necessary for their protection; for lesions on other parts of the body a gauze dressing and bandage may be indicated which should not be disturbed more often than necessary. Prolonged use of the cream for the treatment of burns or scalds is not indicated, since the antihistamine and local analgesic actions of promethazine are only effective and useful for the first few days; this applies also to insect bites and stings.

Contra-indications, warnings, etc Prolonged use and repeated applications may interfere with healing, and the period of applications should be restricted to three or four days.

Topical application of promethazine may occasionally give rise to a skin sensitisation reaction which may take the form of photosensitivity; exposure to bright sunlight should, therefore, be avoided.

Phenergan Cream is not suitable for application to eczematous skin, and should be applied sparingly and with caution where the skin is extensively broken or denuded.

It is possible that if very large areas of the skin are liberally covered with the cream, sufficient promethazine might be absorbed to cause drowsiness in an individual particularly sensitive to the central effects of the drug, but this is not likely to occur unless several grams of the cream have been used.

Phenergan Cream may stain clothing, bed linen, etc. and the stains may only become evident after laundering.

Pharmaceutical precautions Protect from light.

Legal category P.

Package quantities Tube of 25 g.

Further information Nil.

Product licence number 0012/5029.

PHENSEDYL* COUGH LINCTUS

Presentation Phensedyl Cough Linctus is presented as an orange-brown linctus, each 5 ml containing:

Promethazine hydrochloride	3.6 mg
Codeine phosphate	9.0 mg
Ephedrine hydrochloride	7.2 mg

The linctus contains 68% sugars.

Uses Combines central sedative, antihistamine, antiemetic, anticholinergic and local analgesic actions of promethazine hydrochloride with the antitussive action of codeine, and bronchodilator action of ephedrine, which also counteracts any excessive sedation.

Indicated for symptomatic relief of unproductive cough, including post-influenzal cough, cough due to pharyngitis and associated with bronchospasm, the spasms of whooping cough, cough due to smoking and other forms of irritation, cough which disturbs sleep.

Dosage and administration *Adults and children over 10 years:* 5–10 ml two to three times daily.

Elderly: No specific dosage recommendations.

Children of 5–10 years: 2.5–5 ml two or three times daily.

Children 2–5 years: 2.5 ml two or three times daily.

Contra-indications, warnings, etc
Use in pregnancy: There is epidemiological evidence of the safety of promethazine in human pregnancy, animal studies have shown no hazard. There is inadequate evidence of the safety of codeine and ephedrine but they have been in wide use for many years without ill-effect. Nevertheless Phensedyl should not be prescribed in pregnancy unless the physician considers it essential.

Because of ephedrine content do not use with monoamine oxidase inhibitors. Certain patients may be hypersensitive to the central effects of promethazine and suffer excessive drowsiness or disorientation or mental confusion. It is therefore recommended that those taking Phensedyl for the first time should not be in charge of vehicles or machinery for the first few days until it is established that their response has not been adversely affected. Avoid alcoholic drink. Promethazine may enhance the effects of sedatives, hypnotics or other central depressant drugs given concurrently. Phensedyl may cause slight drowsiness which is usually transitory.

In the event of overdosage, after inducing vomiting or washing out the stomach treatment is symptomatic.

Pharmaceutical precautions Protect from light.

Legal category CD (Sch 5), P.

Package quantities Bottles of 100 ml and 2 litres.

Further information Nil.

Product licence number 0012/5023.

PIPORTIL DEPOT* INJECTION ▼

Presentation Straw coloured viscous liquid containing pipothiazine palmitate 5.0% w/v (50 mg per ml) in sesame oil.

Uses Piportil Depot is a long-acting phenothiazine neuroleptic indicated for the maintenance treatment of schizophrenia and paranoid psychoses, and prevention of relapse, especially where compliance with oral medication is a problem.

Kinetics: There is little information about blood levels, distribution and excretion in humans. The rate of metabolism and excretion of phenothiazines decreases in old age.

Dosage and administration Patients should be stabilised on Piportil Depot under psychiatric supervision. Administration should be by deep intramuscular injection into the gluteal region.

Adults: Initially 25 mg (0.5 ml) should be given to assess the response of the patient to the drug. Further doses should be administered at appropriate intervals, increasing by increments of 25 or 50 mg until a satisfactory response is obtained. In clinical practice Piportil Depot has been shown to have a long duration of action, allowing intervals of 4 weeks between injections for maintenance therapy. Dosage should be adjusted under close supervision to suit each individual patient in order to obtain the best therapeutic response compatible with tolerance.

The duration of action depends on the dose administered, allowing dosage intervals to be varied to suit individual circumstances.

Most patients respond favourably to a dose of 50–100 mg (1–2 ml) every 4 weeks. The maximum recommended dose is 200 mg (4 ml) every four weeks.

Elderly: Neuroleptics should be used cautiously in the elderly; a reduced starting dose is recommended, i.e. 5–10 mg might be considered.

Children: Not recommended for use in children.

Contra-indications, warnings, etc Piportil Depot should not be administered to patients in comatose states or with marked cerebral atherosclerosis, phaeochromocytoma, renal or liver failure, severe cardiac insufficiency or hypersensitivity to other phenothiazine derivatives.

Precautions: Piportil Depot should be used with caution in patients suffering from or who have a history of, the following conditions: severe respiratory disease, epilepsy, alcohol withdrawal symptoms, brain damage, Parkinson's disease or marked extrapyramidal symptoms with previously used neuroleptics, personal or family history of narrow angle glaucoma, hypothyroidism, myaesthenia gravis, prostatic hypertrophy, thyrotoxicosis. Care is required in very hot or very cold weather particularly in elderly frail patients.

Pregnancy: There is inadequate evidence of safety of Piportil Depot in human pregnancy, although animal studies have shown no hazard. The drug should not be used during pregnancy or lactation unless the physician considers it essential.

Interactions of phenothiazine neuroleptics: The CNS depressant actions of neuroleptic agents may be intensified (additively) by alcohol, barbiturates and other sedatives. Respiratory depression may occur.

The hypotensive effect of most antihypertensive drugs

especially alpha adrenoceptor blocking agents may be exaggerated by neuroleptics.

The mild anticholinergic effect of neuroleptics may be enhanced by other anticholinergic drugs possibly leading to constipation, heat stroke, etc.

The action of some drugs may be opposed by phenothiazine neuroleptics; these include amphetamine, laevodopa clonidine, guanethidine, adrenaline.

Anticholinergic agents may reduce the antipsychotic effect of neuroleptics.

Some drugs interfere with absorption of neuroleptic agents: antacids, anti-Parkinson, lithium. Increases or decreases in the plasma concentrations of a number of drugs, e.g. propranolol, phenobarbitone have been observed but were not of clinical significance.

High doses of neuroleptics reduce the response to hypoglycaemic agents the dosage of which might have to be raised.

Adrenaline must *not* be used in patients overdosed with phenothiazine neuroleptics. Most of the above interactions are of a theoretical nature and not dangerous.

Adverse effects of neuroleptics: Minor side effects of neuroleptics are nasal stuffiness, dry mouth, insomnia, agitation and weight gain. Other possible adverse effects are listed below.

Liver function: jaundice, usually transient, occurs in a very small percentage of patients taking neuroleptics. A premonitory sign may be a sudden onset of fever after one to three weeks of treatment followed by the development of jaundice. Neuroleptic jaundice has the biochemical and other characteristics of obstructive jaundice and is associated with obstructions of the canaliculi by bile thrombi; the frequent presence of an accompanying eosinophilia indicates the allergic nature of this phenomenon. Treatment should be withheld on the development of jaundice.

Cardiorespiratory: Hypotension, usually postural, commonly occurs. Elderly or volume depleted subjects are particularly susceptible; it is more likely to occur after intramuscular administration.

Cardiac arrhythmias, including atrial arrhythmia, A-V block, ventricular tachycardia and fibrillation have been reported during neuroleptic therapy, possibly related to dosage. Pre-existing cardiac disease, old age, hypokalaemia and concurrent tricyclic antidepressants may predispose. ECG changes, usually benign, include widened QT interval, ST depression, U-waves and T-wave changes.

Respiratory depression is possible in susceptible patients.

Blood picture: A mild leukopaenia occurs in up to 30% of patients on prolonged high dosage of neuroleptics. Agranulocytosis may occur rarely; it is not dose related. The occurrence of unexplained infections or fever requires immediate haematological investigation.

Extrapyramidal: Acute dystonias or dyskinesias, usually transitory, are commoner in children and young adults, and usually occur within the first 4 days of treatment or after dosage increases.

Akathisia characteristically occurs after large initial doses.

Parkinsonism is commoner in adults and the elderly. It usually develops after weeks or months of treatment. One or more of the following may be seen: tremor, rigidity, akinesia or other features of Parkinsonism. Commonly just tremor.

Tardive dyskinesia: If this occurs it is usually, but not necessarily, after prolonged or high dosage. It can even

occur after treatment has been stopped. Dosage should therefore be kept low whenever possible.

Skin and eyes: Contact skin sensitisation is a serious but rare complication in those frequently handling preparations of phenothiazines; the greatest care must be taken to avoid contact of the drug with the skin. Skin rashes of various kinds may also be seen in patients treated with these drugs. Patients on high dosage should be warned that they may develop photosensitivity in sunny weather and should avoid exposure to direct sunlight.

Ocular changes and the development of a metallic greyish-mauve coloration of exposed skin have been noted in some individuals mainly females, who have received chlorpromazine continuously for long periods (four to eight years). Other neuroleptics have been implicated but less frequently.

Endocrine: hyperprolactinaemia which may result in galactorrhoea, gynaecomastia, amenorrhoea; impotence.

Neuroleptic malignant syndrome (hyperthermia, rigidity, autonomic dysfunction and altered consciousness) may occur with any neuroleptic.

Toxicity and treatment of neuroleptic overdosage: Symptoms of phenothiazine overdosage include drowsiness or loss of consciousness, hypotension, tachycardia, E.C.G. changes, ventricular arrhythmias and hypothermia. Severe extra-pyramidal dyskinesias may occur.

Generalised vasodilatation may result in circulatory collapse; raising the patient's legs may suffice, in severe cases, volume expansion by intravenous fluids may be needed; infusion fluids should be warmed before administration in order not to aggravate hypothermia.

Positive inotropic agents such as dopamine may be tried if fluid replacement is insufficient to correct the circulatory collapse. Peripheral vasoconstrictor agents are not generally recommended; avoid the use of adrenaline.

Ventricular or supraventricular tachy-arrhythmias usually respond to restoration of normal body temperature and correction of circulatory or metabolic disturbances. If they are persistent or life threatening, appropriate antiarrhythmic therapy may be considered. Avoid lignocaine and, as far as possible, long acting anti-arrhythmic drugs.

Pronounced central nervous system depression requires airway maintenance or, in extreme circumstances, assisted respiration. Severe dystonic reactions usually respond to procyclidine (5–10 mg) or orphenadrine (20–40 mg) administered intramuscularly or intravenously. Convulsions should be treated with intravenous diazepam.

Neuroleptic malignant syndrome should be treated with cooling. Dantrolene sodium may be tried.

Pharmaceutical precautions Piportil Depot should be protected from light. It can be stored at room temperature.

Legal category POM.

Package quantities Boxes of 10 × 1 ml (50 mg) and 10 × 2 ml (100 mg) ampoules.

Further information Nil.

Product licence number
Injection 5.0% w/v 0012/0117.

PRIMALAN*

Presentation White bi-convex tablets embossed Primalan on one side, unmarked on reverse. Each tablet contains 5 mg mequitazine.

Uses Antihistamine for the symptomatic treatment of allergic conditions such as hay fever, perennial rhinitis, urticaria, pruritus of allergic origin and allergic reactions associated with insect bites and stings.

Dosage and administration

Adults: One 5 mg tablet to be taken orally twice a day.

Elderly: There is no information on specific dosage recommendation in the elderly. Caution should therefore be exercised in this group of patients.

Children: At present Primalan is not recommended for children under the age of 12.

Contra-indications, warnings, etc Primalan should not be given to patients sensitive to phenothiazines or given concurrently with monoamine oxidase inhibitors. As with all antihistamines, it should be used with caution in epilepsy, prostatic hypertrophy, glaucoma and hepatic disease. Primalan should not be administered during pregnancy.

Although Primalan has been found to cause less drowsiness than other antihistamines of comparable efficacy, patients should be warned not to take charge of vehicles or machinery until it has been established that sedation has not occurred. Primalan may also potentiate the sedative effects of alcohol.

Side-effects: Primalan may potentiate sympathomimetic amines. Anticholinergic effects such as dryness of the mouth and disturbance of visual accommodation may occasionally occur, particularly in the early days of treatment.

Treatment of overdosage: Gastric lavage and supportive therapy. Avoid sedation with other phenothiazine derivatives.

Pharmaceutical precautions Store in a cool dry place and protect from light.

Legal category POM.

Package quantities Container of 100 tablets.

Further information Primalan has a prolonged action, allowing adequate control of symptoms with twice daily dosage.

Product licence numbers 0012/0161.

SECADREX ▼

Presentation Secadrex tablets are white, round, slightly biconvex, and film-coated, imprinted 'SECAD-REX' on one face; each contains the equivalent of 200 mg acebutolol (in the form of the hydrochloride) and 12.5 mg hydrochlorothiazide.

Uses Mild and moderate hypertension. Secadrex has been shown to be particularly suitable for elderly patients.

Dosage and administration One Secadrex tablet once daily, usually in the morning, is sufficient in most patients. If response is inadequate, dosage may be increased to two Secadrex tablets once daily. Two Secadrex tablets may be particularly suitable in moderately severe hypertension when satisfactory control of arterial blood pressure cannot be obtained with either a beta-blocker or a diuretic used alone.

Contra-indications, warnings, etc

(a) Cardiogenic shock is an absolute contra-indication to beta-blockade and caution is required in patients with blood pressures of the order of 100/60 or below.

(b) Heart block. Administration of any beta-adrenoceptor blocking agent is considered inadvisable (except perhaps in first degree block).

(c) Severe kidney and liver failure.

(d) Hypersensitivity to hydrochlorothiazide.

(e) Secadrex tablets should not be used with verapamil or within several days of verapamil therapy (and vice-versa).

(f) Insulin-dependent diabetes. Use in non-insulin dependent diabetics may be inadvisable since thiazide diuretics may cause further impairment of glucose tolerance.

(g) Gout or hyperuricaemia.

(h) *Pregnancy:* Secadrex should not be administered to female patients during the first trimester of pregnancy unless the physician considers it essential. Animal studies with acebutolol have shown no teratogenic hazard.

Thiazides are not generally recommended in the treatment of pregnancy hypertension; it may be preferable to use monotherapy with Sectral* or another suitable anti-hypertensive drug in pregnant patients.

Precautions: An increase in airways resistance may be provoked in asthmatic patients. Whilst the use of Secadrex tablets is not contra-indicated in patients with obstructive airways disease, care should be exercised when they are used in such subjects.

Caution should be exercised:

(a) If Secadrex tablets are administered in the presence of bradycardia (depending on the circumstances).

(b) If Secadrex tablets are to be prescribed with a catecholamine-depleting drug, such as reserpine.

(c) In the presence of signs of heart failure, since acebutolol has a slight but acceptable cardio-depressant action.

(d) In anaesthesia: some anaesthetists prefer to discontinue therapy 48 hours before anaesthesia, others do not consider this essential. Withdrawal should be made gradually. Thiazides may increase responsiveness to tubocurarine.

If Secadrex tablets and clonidine are given concurrently, the clonidine should not be discontinued until several days after the withdrawal of the beta-blocker (see also prescribing information on clonidine).

All patients receiving hydrochlorothiazide therapy (as in Secadrex tablets) should be monitored periodically for clinical signs of fluid or electrolyte imbalance, hypokalaemia, hyponatraemia and hypochloraemic alkalosis. Hypokalaemia can sensitise or exaggerate the response of the heart to the toxic effects of digitalis (eg increased ventricular irritability).

With the low dose of hydrochlorothiazide present in Secadrex tablets the possibility of significant imbalance becomes less likely.

Side effects: No serious side-effects have been reported with Secadrex treatment. The most common, ie those related to beta-blockade – hypotension, bradycardia, gastro-intestinal effects and depression have been met with infrequently, and usually do not require interruption or withdrawal of therapy.

There have been reports of skin rashes and/or dry eyes associated with the use of beta-adrenoceptor antagonists. The reported incidence is small and in most cases the symptoms have cleared when treatment was withdrawn. Discontinuation of the drug should be considered if any such reaction is not explicable. Cessation of treatment with a beta-blocker should be gradual.

Skin rashes and photosensitivity due to hydrochloro-thiazide have been reported as have blood dyscrasias including thrombocytopenia but these are rare.

Drug interactions: Tricyclic antidepressants and MAO inhibitors should not be used concurrently with Secadrex tablets. Lithium should generally not be given to patients receiving diuretics since the risk of lithium toxicity is very high in such patients.

Treatment of overdosage: In the rare event of excessive bradycardia or hypotension, 1 mg atropine sulphate administered intravenously should be given without delay. If this proves insufficient, it should be followed by a slow intravenous injection of isoprenaline (5 mcg per minute) with constant monitoring until a response occurs. In cases of severe poisoning with beta-adrenoceptor antagonists the injection of 10 mg glucagon intravenously has produced rapid improvement. If bradycardia becomes severe electrical pacing may be necessary.

Pharmaceutical precautions Store in a cool, dry place.

Legal category POM.

Package quantities Calendar (blister) pack of 28 (2 × 14) tablets.

Further information Secadrex is an effective anti-hypertensive agent, which combines Sectral, a cardio-selective beta-adrenoceptor antagonist with partial agonist activity and hydrochlorothiazide, an effective and acceptable diuretic/antihypertensive agent. The combination of these two medicaments in a single tablet may facilitate the management of hypertension and improve patient compliance.

Product licence number 0012/0137.

SECTRAL*

Presentation Sectral capsules each containing the equivalent of 100 mg acebutolol (in the form of the hydrochloride). The capsules are bi-coloured (opaque buff/opaque white) each half printed 'SECTRAL 100' in black.

Sectral 200 capsules each containing the equivalent of 200 mg acebutolol (in the form of the hydrochloride). The capsules are bi-coloured (opaque buff/opaque pink) each half printed 'SECTRAL 200' in black.

Sectral 400 tablets each containing the equivalent of 400 mg acebutolol (in the form of the hydrochloride). The tablets are off white, varnished.

Sectral injection – ampoules of 2 ml of an 0.5 per cent w/v injection of acebutolol (as hydrochloride), each ml containing the equivalent of 5 mg acebutolol.

Uses *Mode of action:* Sectral is a beta adrenoceptor antagonist which is cardioselective, ie acts preferentially on beta-I adrenergic receptors in the heart. Its principal effects are to reduce heart rate especially on exercise and to lower blood pressure in hypertensive subjects. Sectral and its equally active metabolite, diacetolol have anti-arrhythmic activity, the combined plasma half-life of the active drug and metabolite being 7–10 hours. Both have partial agonist activity (PAA) also known as intrinsic sympathomimetic activity (ISA). This property ensures that some degree of stimulation of beta receptors is

maintained. Under conditions of rest this tends to balance the negative chronotropic and negative inotropic effects. Sectral blocks the effects of excessive catecholamine stimulation resulting from stress.

Sectral is indicated in the following conditions:

1. The management of all grades of hypertension.
2. The management of angina pectoris.
3. The control of tachyarrhythmias.

Dosage and administration
There are no specific dosage recommendations for the elderly.

1. *Hypertension:* Initial dosage of 400 mg orally once daily at breakfast or 200 mg orally twice daily. If response is not adequate within two weeks, dosage may be increased up to 400 mg orally twice daily. If the hypertension is not adequately controlled consideration should be given to adding a second antihypertensive agent such as a compatible calcium antagonist or a small dose of a thiazide diuretic.

2. *Angina pectoris:* Initial dosage of 400 mg orally once daily at breakfast or 200 mg twice daily. In severe forms up to 300 mg three times daily may be required; up to 1,200 mg daily has been used.

3. *Cardiac arrhythmias*

(a) Intravenous administration in critical situations: Administer 20 mg (the contents of 2 ampoules) immediately over 3–5 minutes and monitor the patient's response for 5 to 10 minutes. If the desired effect is not observed, two further doses of 20 mg are to be injected at 10-minute intervals, or at shorter intervals if required by the urgency of the situation.

Depending on clinical response, doses up to 1 mg/kg may be used; in critical situations, this dose may be exceeded provided signs of excessive beta-blockage (bradycardia, hypotension) are not observed.

Effective beta blockade may be expected to last 3–4 hours after an initial effective intravenous dose. Depending on circumstances, further administration may be continued by intravenous infusion or oral administration. In the latter case, 200 mg of acebutolol may be administered orally shortly after achievement of the effective intravenous dose or concurrently with reduction of the intravenous infusion over a period of 60–90 minutes. Thereafter treatment may be continued with appropriate doses twice or thrice daily.

(b) Oral administration: Maximal anti-arrhythmic effect may not be achieved until up to 3 hours after oral administration.

The daily dose requirement for long term anti-arrhythmic activity should lie between 400 and 1200 mg daily. The dose can be gauged by response. Since the presence of more consistent beta-blockade may be necessary for the control of arrhythmias, better control may be achieved by divided doses rather than single daily doses.

Contra-indications, warnings, etc Cardiogenic shock is an absolute contra-indication and caution is required in patients with blood pressures of the order of 100/60 mm Hg or below. Sectral is also contra-indicated in patients with atrioventricular block, marked bradycardia and uncontrolled heart failure. Sectral should not be used with verapamil or within several days of verapamil therapy (and vice-versa).

Pregnancy: Sectral should not be administered to female patients during the 1st trimester of pregnancy unless the physician considers it essential. Animal studies have shown no teratogenic hazard. Beta blockers administered in late pregnancy may give rise to bradycardia of the foetus.

Renal impairment is not a contraindication to the use of Sectral which has both renal and non-renal excretory pathways. Some caution should be exercised when administering high doses to patients with severe renal failure as cumulation could possibly occur in these circumstances. Caution should be exercised in patients with obstructive airways disease and particularly if Sectral is to be administered intravenously in asthmatic subjects. Bronchospasm is usually at least partially reversible by the use of a suitable agonist.

In patients with labile and insulin-dependent diabetes the dosage of the hypoglycaemic agent may need to be reduced.

Cross reactions due to displacement of other drugs from plasma protein binding sites are unlikely due to the low degree of plasma protein binding exhibited by acebutolol and diacetolol. If a beta adrenoceptor antagonist is used concurrently with clonidine the latter should not be withdrawn until several days after the former is discontinued.

Sectral therapy should be brought to the attention of the anaesthetist prior to general anaesthesia. If treatment is continued, special care should be taken when using anaesthetic agents such as ether, cyclopropane and trichlorethylene.

Side-effects: Sectral possesses antihypertensive effects but these are unlikely to be noted in normotensive subjects. Those common to beta-blockade – bradycardia, gastrointestinal effects, cold extremities and lethargy have been met with infrequently. The low lipid solubility and lack of cumulation in CNS tissues of acebutolol and its active metabolite reduces the likelihood of sleep disturbances, depression or other central effects and such occurrences are rare.

There have been reports of skin rashes and/or dry eyes associated with the use of beta adrenoceptor blocking drugs. The reported incidence is small and in most cases the symptoms have cleared when treatment was withdrawn. Discontinuation of the drug should be considered if any such reaction is not otherwise explicable. Cessation of therapy with a beta blocker should be gradual.

Treatment of overdosage: In the rare event of excessive bradycardia or hypotension, 1 mg atropine sulphate administered intravenously should be given without delay. If this is insufficient it should be followed by a slow intravenous injection of isoprenaline (5 mcg per minute) with constant monitoring until a response occurs. In severe cases of self poisoning with circulatory collapse unresponsive to atropine and catecholamines the intravenous injection of glucagon 10–20 mg may produce a dramatic improvement. Cardiac pacing may be employed if bradycardia becomes severe.

Pharmaceutical precautions Sectral capsules should be stored in a dry place below 25°C.

Legal category POM.

Package quantities *Capsules 100 mg:* containers of 100 and 500.
Capsules 200 mg ('Sectral 200'): containers of 100.
Tablets 400 mg ('Sectral 400'): foil pack of 28 (2 × 14).
0.5% Injection Solution: Boxes of 10 × 2 ml ampoules.

Further information Sectral 400 tablets are available as a calendar pack containing 28 tablets for ease of use in once daily therapy for hypertension.

Product licence numbers

100 mg Capsules	0012/0100
200 mg Capsules ('Sectral 200')	0012/0101
400 mg Tablets ('Sectral 400')	0012/0124
Injection Solution	0012/0102

SONERYL*

Presentation Pink tablets each containing 100 mg butobarbitone, with the name 'Soneryl' indented on one face and a break line on the reverse.

Uses Soneryl is a barbiturate with a medium duration of action. It is a powerful hypnotic and is indicated for severe, intractable insomnia. Sleep is usually induced within 30–40 minutes and lasts for six to ten hours.

Dosage and administration One or two tablets at bedtime; may be increased to 3 or 4 in obstinate cases. These doses may be modified at the physician's discretion, but it is advisable not to exceed 6 tablets in 24 hours.

Elderly: Do not use.

Children: Do not use.

Contra-indications, warnings, etc
Contra-indications: Porphyria is an absolute contra-indication to the use of Soneryl. Patients with uncontrolled pain, or those with a history of alcohol or drug abuse should not be given Soneryl.

Soneryl should not be used in children, young adults, the elderly and the debilitated.

Pregnancy. Soneryl should not be administered during pregnancy or breast feeding.

Precautions: Reduced dosage should be used in patients with renal or hepatic failure.

Drug interactions: Barbiturates cause the induction of liver enzymes and this may affect the availability and blood concentrations of drugs given concurrently that are metabolised in the liver. These include the following: coumarin-type anticoagulants, synthetic steroids (including oral contraceptives), phenytoin, griseofulvin, rifampicin, phenothiazines such as chlorpromazine and tricyclic antidepressants.

Warnings and adverse effects: Drowsiness, sedation. Unsteadiness, vertigo and inco-ordination are common adverse effects.

Performance and alertness may be impaired during the first week of administration. Patients should be warned of the possible hazard when driving or operating machinery.

These effects may be potentiated by alcohol. Other adverse reactions may include a 'hangover' effect, paradoxical excitement, confusion, memory defects and skin rashes in patients who may be sensitive to this type of drug.

Treatment of overdosage: Soneryl overdosage should be treated by gastric lavage, artificial respiration with the administration of oxygen, maintenance of fluid balance and with an antibiotic to prevent pneumonia. Metaraminol may be used to treat hypotension, but if this is unsuccessful, blood volume expanders or intravenous hydrocortisone should be given.

Pharmaceutical precautions Nil.

Legal category CD (Sch 3), POM.

Package quantities Containers of 500 tablets.

Further information Barbiturates have a high addiction potential. Long-term use or use of high dosage for short periods may lead to tolerance and subsequently to physical and psychological dependence. Symptoms of dependence include confusion, defective judgement and loss of emotional control. Withdrawal symptoms occur after long-term normal use (and particularly after abuse) on rapid cessation of barbiturate treatment. Symptoms include nightmares, irritability and insomnia and in severe cases, tremors, delirium, convulsions and death. Withdrawal symptoms have been reported in neonates after barbiturate treatment during pregnancy and labour.

Product licence number 0012/5262.

STEMETIL*

Presentation Stemetil tablets are white, uncoated, indented on the face with name and strength; reverse is plain (break line for 25 mg tablet). They contain 5 mg or 25 mg prochlorperazine maleate.

Stemetil 1.25% Injection – colourless solution containing 12.5 mg prochlorperazine mesylate per ml in ampoules of 1 and 2 ml.

Stemetil Suppositories – cream-coloured suppositories containing base equivalents to 5 mg and 25 mg of maleate.

Stemetil Syrup: A dark straw-coloured syrupy liquid which contains 5 mg prochlorperazine mesylate in each 5 ml. The syrup contains 68% of sugars, 0.1% of sodium sulphite and 0.1% of sodium metabisulphite.

Uses Stemetil is a potent phenothiazine neuroleptic. It is used in vertigo due to Meniere's syndrome, labyrinthitis and other causes, and for nausea and vomiting from whatever cause. It may also be used for migraine, schizophrenia (particularly in the chronic stage), acute mania and as an adjunct to the short term management of anxiety.

There is little information about blood levels, distribution and excretion in humans. The rate of metabolism and elimination of antipsychotic drugs decreases in old age.

Dosage and administration

*Oral Administration
Adults*

Indication	Dosage
Prevention of nausea and vomiting.	5 to 10 mg b.d. or t.d.s.
Treatment of nausea and vomiting.	20 mg stat, followed if necessary by 10 mg two hours later.
Vertigo and Meniere's syndrome.	5 mg t.d.s. increasing if necessary to a total of 30 mg daily. After several weeks dosage may be reduced gradually to 5–10 mg daily.
Adjunct in the short-term management of anxiety.	15–20 mg daily in divided doses initially but this may be increased if necessary to a maximum of 40 mg daily in divided doses.

Schizophrenia and other psychotic disorders.	Usual effective daily oral dosage is in the order of 75–100 mg daily. Patients vary widely in response. The following schedule is suggested: Initially 12.5 mg twice daily for 7 days, the daily amount being subsequently increased by 12.5 mg at four to seven day intervals until a satisfactory response is obtained. After some weeks at the effective dosage, an attempt should be made to reduce this dosage. Total daily amounts as small as 50 mg or even 25 mg have sometimes been found to be effective.

*Intramuscular Administration
Adults*

Indication	Dosage
Treatment of nausea and vomiting.	12.5 mg by deep i.m. injection followed by oral medication six hours later, if necessary.
Schizophrenia and other psychotic disorders.	12.5 mg to 25 mg two or three times a day by deep i.m. injection until oral treatment becomes possible.

*Rectal Administration
Adults*

Indication	Dosage
Treatment of nausea and vomiting.	25 mg followed by oral medication 6 hours later if necessary.
Schizophrenia and psychotic disorders.	25 mg b.d. or t.d.s. until oral treatment possible.

Children's Dosage. Oral route only

Indication	Dosage
Prevention and treatment of nausea and vomiting	If it is considered unavoidable to use Stemetil for a child, the dosage is 0.25 mg/kg bodyweight two or three times a day. Stemetil is not recommended for children weighing less than 10 kg.

Intramuscular Stemetil should not be given to children.

Elderly: Stemetil should be used cautiously in this group in psychotic disorders. Elderly patients are susceptible to centrally-acting drugs hence lower initial dosage is recommended. Correct initial diagnosis of the disorder is important. Care should also be taken not to confuse adverse effects of Stemetil, e.g. orthostatic hypotension with effects due to the primary disorder.

Contra-indications, warnings, etc

Pregnancy: There is inadequate evidence of the safety of Stemetil in human pregnancy but it has been widely used for many years without apparent ill consequence. There is evidence of harmful effects in animals. Like other drugs it should be avoided in pregnancy unless the physician considers it essential. Neuroleptics may occasionally prolong labour and at such a time should be withheld until the cervix is dilated 3–4 cm. Possible adverse effects on the foetus include lethargy or paradoxical hyperexcitability, tremor and low Apgar score. Phenothiazines may be excreted in milk, breast-feeding should be suspended during treatment.

Precautions: Stemetil should be avoided in patients with liver or renal dysfunction, epilepsy, Parkinson's disease, hypothyroidism, phaeochromocytoma, myasthenia gravis, prostate hypertrophy. It should be avoided in patients known to be hypersensitive to phenothiazines or with a history of narrow angle glaucoma. It should be used with caution in the elderly, particularly during very hot or very cold weather (risk of hyper-, hypothermia).

Patients should be warned about drowsiness during the early days of treatment, and advised not to drive or operate machinery.

Postural hypotension with tachycardia as well as local pain or nodule formation may occur after i.m. administration.

The elderly are particularly susceptible to postural hypotension.

Children: Stemetil has been associated with dystonic reactions particularly after a cumulative dosage of 0.5 mg/kg. It should therefore be used cautiously in children.

Interactions of phenothiazine neuroleptics: The CNS depressant actions of neuroleptic agents may be intensified (additively) by alcohol, barbiturates and other sedatives. Respiratory depression may occur.

The hypotensive effect of most antihypertensive drugs especially alpha adrenoceptor blocking agents may be exaggerated by neuroleptics.

The mild anticholinergic effect of neuroleptics may be enhanced by other anticholinergic drugs possibly leading to constipation, heat stroke, etc.

The action of some drugs may be opposed by phenothiazine neuroleptics; these include amphetamine, laevodopa clonidine, guanethidine, adrenaline.

Anticholinergic agents may reduce the antipsychotic effect of neuroleptics.

Some drugs interfere with absorption of neuroleptic agents: antacids, anti-parkinson, lithium. Increases or decreases in the plasma concentrations of a number of drugs, e.g. propranolol, phenobarbitone have been observed but were not of clinical significance.

High doses of neuroleptics reduce the response to hypoglycaemic agents the dosage of which might have to be raised.

Adrenaline must *not* be used in patients overdosed with Stemetil. Most of the above interactions are of a theoretical nature and not dangerous.

Minor side effects of neuroleptics are nasal stuffiness, dry mouth, insomina, agitation.

Adverse effects of neuroleptics: Liver function: Jaundice, usually transient, occurs in a very small percentage of patients taking neuroleptics. A premonitory sign may be a sudden onset of fever after one to three weeks of treatment followed by the development of jaundice. Neuroleptic jaundice has the biochemical and other characteristics of obstructive jaundice and is associated with obstructions of the canaliculi by bile thrombi; the frequent presence of an accompanying eosinophilia indicates the allergic nature of this phenomenon. Treatment should be withheld on the development of jaundice.

Cardiorespiratory: Hypotension, usually postural, commonly occurs. Elderly or volume depleted subjects are particularly susceptible; it is more likely to occur after intramuscular administration.

Cardiac arrhythmias, including atrial arrhythmia, A-V block, ventricular tachycardia and fibrillation have been reported during neuroleptic therapy, possibly related to dosage. Pre-existing cardiac disease, old age, hypokalaemia and concurrent tricyclic antidepressants may predispose. ECG changes, usually benign, include widened QT interval, ST depression, U-waves and T-wave changes.

Respiratory depression is possible in susceptible patients.

Blood picture: A mild leukopaenia occurs in up to 30% of patients on prolonged high dosage. Agranulocytosis may occur rarely; it is not dose related. The occurrence of unexplained infections or fever requires immediate haematological investigation.

Extrapyramidal: Acute dystonias or dyskinesias, usually transitory are commoner in children and young adults, and usually occur within the first 4 days of treatment or after dosage increases.

Akathisia characteristically occurs after large initial doses.

Parkinsonism is commoner in adults and the elderly. It usually develops after weeks or months of treatment. One or more of the following may be seen: tremor, rigidity, akinesia or other features of Parkinsonism. Commonly just tremor.

Tardive dyskinesia: If this occurs it is usually, but not necessarily, after prolonged or high dosage. It can even occur after treatment has been stopped. Dosage should therefore be kept low whenever possible.

Skin and eyes: Contact skin sensitisation is a serious but rare complication in those frequently handling preparations of certain phenothiazines; the greatest care must be taken to avoid contact of the drug with the skin. Skin rashes of various kinds may also be seen in patients treated with the drug. Patients on high dosage should be warned that they may develop photosensitivity in sunny weather and should avoid exposure to direct sunlight.

Ocular changes and the development of a metallic greyish-mauve coloration of exposed skin have been noted in some individuals mainly females, who have received chlorpromazine continuously for long periods (four to eight years). This could possibly happen with Stemetil.

Endocrine: hyperprolactinaemia which may result in galactorrhoea, gynaecomastia, amenorrhoea; impotence.

Neuroleptic malignant syndrome (hyperthermia, rigidity, autonomic dysfunction and altered consciousness) may occur with any neuroleptic.

Toxicity and treatment of overdosage; Symptoms of phenothiazine overdosage include drowsiness or loss of consciousness, hypotension, tachycardia, E.C.G. changes, ventricular arrhythmias and hypothermia. Severe extra-pyramidal dyskinesias may occur.

If the patient is seen sufficiently soon (up to 6 hours) after ingestion of a toxic dose, gastric lavage may be attempted. Pharmacological induction of emesis is unlikely to be of any use. Activated charcoal should be given. There is no specific antidote. Treatment is supportive.

Generalised vasodilatation may result in circulatory collapse; raising the patient's legs may suffice, in severe cases, volume expansion by intravenous fluids may be needed; infusion fluids should be warmed before administration in order not to aggravate hypothermia.

Positive inotropic agents such as dopamine may be tried if fluid replacement is insufficient to correct the circulatory collapse. Peripheral vasoconstrictor agents are not generally recommended; avoid the use of adrenaline.

Ventricular or supraventricular tachy-arrhythmias usually respond to restoration of normal body temperature and correction of circulatory or metabolic disturbances. If persistent or life threatening, appropriate anti-arrhythmic therapy may be considered. Avoid lignocaine and, as far as possible, long acting anti-arrhythmic drugs.

Pronounced central nervous system depression requires airway maintenance or, in extreme circumstances, assisted respiration. Severe dystonic reactions usually respond to procyclidine (5–10 mg) or orphenadrine (20–40 mg) administered intramuscularly or intravenously. Convulsions should be treated with intravenous diazepam.

Neuroleptic malignant syndrome should be treated with cooling. Dantrolene sodium may be tried.

Pharmaceutical precautions Protect from light.

Legal category POM.

Package quantities Tablets 5 mg in containers of 25, 250 and 1,000.

Tablets 25 mg in containers of 50 and 500.

Injection solution of 1.25% in boxes of 10 × 1 ml and 2 ml ampoules.

Syrup presentation of 5 mg per 5 ml in bottles of 100 ml.

Suppositories of 5 mg and 25 mg in boxes of 10.

Further information Nil.

Product licence numbers

Tablets 5 mg	0012/5263
Tablets 25 mg	0012/5316
Injection	0012/5008
Suppositories 5 mg	0012/5117
Suppositories 25 mg	0012/5013
Syrup	0012/5022

STREPTOTRIAD*

Presentation Pink tablets, embossed 'Streptotriad' on one face with a break-line on the reverse. Each tablet contains:

Streptomycin (as sulphate)	65 mg
Sulphadiazine	100 mg
Sulphadimidine	100 mg
Sulphathiazole	100 mg

Uses Streptotriad is active against many strains of Shigella, the major causative organism of bacillary dysentery. Streptomycin is not absorbed and exerts its action locally in the gut, while the absorbed sulphonamides ensure activity within the wall of the gut. The combination of three different sulphonamides greatly reduces the risk of crystalluria.

Streptotriad is indicated in bacillary dysentery and for the treatment or prevention of non-specific diarrhoea, including 'traveller's diarrhoea'.

Dosage and administration *Treatment: Adults:* 2 tablets, three times a day.

Elderly: There are no specific dosage recommendations

for the elderly but for patients with renal or hepatic impairment see contra-indications below.

Children: 12 years or over, 1½ tablets, three times a day.
7–11 years, 1 tablet, three times a day.
3–6 years, ½ tablet, four times a day.
1–2 years, ¼ tablet, three times a day.

Treatment should be continued until the diarrhoea ceases; it is unlikely to be needed after the fourth day.

Prevention: For short-term prophylaxis in persons at risk: Adults: One or two tablets twice daily.

Children: Dosage should be about half that recommended for treatment.

Contra-indications, warnings, etc *Use in pregnancy:* There is inadequate evidence of safety of Streptotriad in human pregnancy. It is generally considered that sulphonamides given in late pregnancy may be a cause of kernicterus in the newborn. Streptotriad is therefore contra-indicated in the 3rd trimester of pregnancy.

Sulphonamides are excreted in the milk in small amounts. Streptotriad is therefore contra-indicated in nursing mothers.

Contra-indications: Sulphonamides are contra-indicated in hepatic and renal disease, acute porphyria, in patients known to be hypersensitive and in neonates and babies under 6 months old especially those with 6 GPD deficiency.

Precautions: An adequate fluid intake should be ensured, especially if the patient is dehydrated. Streptotriad should be given to infants under 6 months of age ONLY if truly indicated.

Interactions: Local anaesthetics which are hydrolyzed to PABA (procaine amylocaine etc) antagonise Sulphonamides and may lead to local abscess.

Sulphonamides potentiate thiopentone and the effect of Warfarin or tolbutamide could be enhanced.

Side-effects: These are unlikely with the recommended dosage, but in susceptible persons side-effects common to all sulphonamides could occur. These include nausea, vomiting, cyanosis, headache, depression, mental confusion and pyrexia. More rarely, rashes, blood dyscrasias and crystalluria and very rarely hepatitis and nephrosis. With oral streptomycin side-effects are very unlikely as the compound is not appreciably absorbed.

Treatment of overdosage: Gastric lavage should be carried out. Continuous forced fluids should be administered and the urine rendered alkaline to reduce the risk of crystalluria and increase the rate of excretion. Otherwise treatment is symptomatic.

Pharmaceutical precautions Store in a cool dark place. Care should be taken when dispensing Streptotriad as repeated handling of Streptomycin can result in skin sensitisation.

Legal category POM.

Package quantities Container of 50 tablets.

Further information Nil.

Product licence number 0012/5294.

SULPHADIAZINE INJECTION*

Presentation A colourless solution containing Sulphadiazine Sodium 27.2% w/v. Each 4 ml ampoule contains the equivalent of 1 g sulphadiazine.

Uses Sulphadiazine has a bacteriostatic action on a wide range of Gram-negative and Gram-positive micro-organisms including Neisseria meningitidis, pneumococci, B-haemolytic streptococci, Haemophilus influenzea, nocardia and other sulphonamide sensitive organisms.

Sulphadiazine injection is indicated for the treatment of severe meningitis.

Dosage and administration Sulphadiazine injection should preferably be administered intravenously. Because of the alkalinity of the solution, it should be diluted to a strength not exceeding 5% sulphadiazine with Water for Injections, or added to an appropriate volume of saline for infusion. The undiluted solution may be administered by deep intramuscular injection if the intravenous route is not available.

Adults: 2–3 g initially, followed by 1 g four times a day for the first two days of the infection. Subsequent treatment should be given by mouth, continuing for 2–3 days after clinical recovery.

Elderly: There are no specific dosage recommendations for the elderly but if renal or hepatic impairment exists the drug is contra-indicated.

Children: Over 2 months – 50 mg/kg initially followed by 25 mg/kg four times a day.

Sulphadiazine injection should be administered four times a day during the first two days of the infection after which the drug should be given orally.

Contra-indications, warnings, etc
Use in pregnancy and lactation: There is epidemiological evidence of the safety of sulphadiazine in human pregnancy, but the clinician should assess the risk benefit factors before administering sulphadiazine injection to pregnant women. It is generally considered that sulphonamides should not be given in late pregnancy because of the risk of kernicterus. However, recent work suggests that sulphadiazine does not cause kernicterus.

Sulphonamides are excreted in the milk in small amounts and should be used with caution in nursing mothers.

Contra-indications: In the presence of renal or hepatic disease, in acute porphyria and in patients known to be hypersensitive to sulphonamides.

In premature and newborn babies owing to the danger of kernicterus.

Sulphadiazine injection must never be given intrathecally or subcutaneously as its high alkalinity can cause necrosis.

Precautions: A high fluid intake (5–6 pints in 24 hours) should be maintained and urinary output should not be less than half that amount. In addition the urine should be rendered alkaline.

Side-effects: Those common to all sulphonamides could occur. Nausea, vomiting, cyanosis, headache, depression, mental confusion and pyrexia. More rarely rash, blood dyscrasias and crystalluria and very rarely hepatitis and nephrosis. Should crystalluria, followed by haematuria or oliguria occur, Sulphadiazine should be discontinued and large volumes of fluids administered, by intravenous infusion if necessary. Heat should be applied to the loins, and if the condition persists cystocopy and ureteric catheterisation followed by irrigation with warm sodium bicarbonate solution should be carried out. The catheters should be left in place for 24–28 hours or until urinary function is restored.

Treatment of overdosage: Continuous forced fluids may be necessary and the urine should be rendered alkaline. Otherwise treatment is symptomatic.

Pharmaceutical precautions Protect from light. Sulphadiazine injection is incompatible with acids, laevulose, iron salts and salts of heavy metals.

Store below 25°C but do not freeze.

Legal category POM.

Package quantities Box of 10 × 4 ml ampoules.

Further information Nil.

Product licence number 0012/5057.

SULPHATRIAD*

Presentation White tablets, with 'Sulphatriad 3' indented on one face and a break-line on the reverse. Each tablet contains 0.5 g sulphonamides, comprising:

Sulphadiazine	185 mg
Sulphamerazine	130 mg
Sulpathiazole	185 mg

Sulphatriad is bacteriostatic against a wide range of Gram-negative and Gram-positive micro-organisms. The use of three different derivatives to make up the total sulphonamide content reduces the risk of crystalluria. Sulphatriad is indicated in the treatment of acute infections with pneumococci, meningococci, B-haemolytic streptococci, *Escherichia coli, Haemophilus ducreyi* and other sulphonamide-sensitive organisms.

Kinetics: Sulphatriad is a combination of 3 sulphonamides having differing half lives: sulphathiazole 3–4 hr, sulphadiazine 10 hr, sulphamerazine 23–35 hr. All are readily absorbed after oral dosage and widely distributed.

Dosage and administration Sulphatriad is administered by mouth. If preferred, the tablets may be crushed and swallowed with water. The initial dose for treatment of adults is 2 g and this is followed by 1 g every four or six hours. Children are given half the adult dosage. For prophylaxis the dosage for adults is 0.5 g three times daily; for children of 6–12 years, 0.5 g twice daily; and for children of 1–5 years, 0.25 g three times daily.

Elderly: There are no specific dosage recommendations for the elderly but if renal or hepatic impairment exist the drug is contra-indicated.

Contra-indications, warnings, etc *Use in pregnancy and lactation:* There is epidemiological evidence of the safety of sulphonamides as a class in human pregnancy, but it is generally considered that sulphonamides given in late pregnancy may be a cause of kernicterus in the new born. Sulphonamides are excreted in the milk in small amounts and should be used with caution in nursing mothers.

Contra-indications: Sulphonamides are contra-indicated in hepatic and renal disease, acute porphyria, in patients known to be hypersensitive and in neonates and babies under 6 months especially those with G6PD deficiency.

Precautions: Because of the risk of crystalluria, although decreased in the case of sulphatriad, a high fluid intake should be maintained such as 5–6 pints in 24 hours. In addition the urine should be rendered alkaline.

Interactions: Local anaesthetics which are hydrolyzed to PABA (procaine, amylocaine, etc.) antagonize sulphonamides and may lead to a local abscess.

Sulphonamides potentiate thiopentone and the effect of Warfarin or tolbutamide could be enhanced.

Adverse effects: The side effects common to all sulphonamides could occur. These include nausea, vomiting, diarrhoea, cyanosis, headache, depression and mental confusion and pyrexia. More rarely hepatitis crystalluria and blood dyscrasias. Sulphatriad should be withdrawn if crystalluria, haematuria or oliguria occur. Copious amounts of fluid should be given by drip infusion. Heat should be applied to the loins, cystoscopy should be carried out. The ureters should be irrigated with warm 2·5% sodium bicarbonate solution.

Overdosage: In the event of overdosage an emetic should be given or the stomach should be washed out. Continuous forced fluids may be necessary and the urine should be made alkaline.

Pharmaceutical precautions Protect from light.

Legal category POM.

Package quantities Containers of 500.

Further information Nil.

Product licence numbers
Tablets   0012/5295

SURMONTIL*

Presentation Surmontil Tablets are compression-coated, white, each containing the equivalent of 10 mg or 25 mg trimipramine (as maleate). The face is indented with the name and strength; the reverse is plain. Surmontil Capsules (body white opaque with green cap, printed 'M & B SU50'), each contain the equivalent of 50 mg trimipramine (as maleate).

Uses Surmontil has a potent antidepressant action similar to that of other tricyclic antidepressants. It also possesses a pronounced sedative action. It is, therefore, indicated in the treatment of depressive illness, especially where sleep disturbance, anxiety or agitation is a presenting symptom. Sleep disturbance is controlled within 24 hours and true antidepressant action follows within 7–10 days.

Dosage and administration *Adults:* Mild/moderate depression in general practice. The recommended dosage is 50–75 mg orally given two hours before bedtime, the larger dose (75 mg) being preferable for those patients with more marked sleep disturbance. Treatment should be continued for at least three weeks.

Moderate/severe depression (patients under psychiatric supervision): Initial dosage – 75 mg orally per day. This is best given as a single dose late in the evening or as 25 mg midday and 50 mg late in the evening. Dosage should then be increased as necessary until the optimal therapeutic level is reached, usually 150–300 mg per day. Treatment at this dosage should be continued for four to six weeks, dosage then being reduced to a maintenance level, usually within the range of 75–150 mg per day, for two to three months.

Giving most of the total daily dosage at night induces a rapid return to normal sleep, reduces the need for night-time sedation and minimises daytime drowsiness.

Elderly: Initially 10–25 mg three times a day. The initial dose should be increased with caution under close supervision. Half the normal maintenance dose may be sufficient to produce a satisfactory clinical response.

Cyclothymic patients with recurrent depression may require maintenance therapy for up to one year or even longer.

Surmontil is not recommended for use in children.

Contra-indications, warnings, etc Recent myocardial infarction. Any degree of heart block or other cardiac arrhythmia. Mania, severe liver disease. During breast feeding.

The elderly are particularly liable to experience adverse reactions, especially agitation, confusion and postural hypotension (see Dosage).

Treatment should be avoided, if possible, in patients with narrow angle glaucoma, symptoms suggestive of prostatic hypertrophy and a history of epilepsy.

Patients posing a high suicidal risk require close initial supervision. The central nervous depressant action of alcohol is potentiated by Surmontil.

Anaesthetics given during tricyclic antidepressant therapy may increase the risk of arrhythmias and hypotension. If surgery is necessary, the anaesthetist should be made aware that a patient is being so treated.

Trimipramine should not be given concurrently with, or within 2 weeks of cessation of therapy with monoamine oxidase inhibitors. The anti-hypertensive effect of guanethidine, debrisoquine, bethanidine and possibly clonidine may be decreased by trimipramine.

It would be advisable to review all anti-hypertensive therapy during treatment with tricyclic anti-depressants. Trimipramine should not be given with sympathomimetic agents such as adrenaline, ephedrine, isoprenaline, noradrenaline, phenylephrine and phenylpropanolamine.

Barbiturates may increase the rate of metabolism of Surmontil.

Surmontil should be administered with care in patients receiving therapy for hyperthyroidism.

Use in pregnancy: Do not use during pregnancy, especially during the first and last trimester, unless there are compelling reasons. There is no evidence as to drug safety in human pregnancy nor is there evidence from animal work that it is free from hazard.

Patients should be monitored closely during the initial stages of treatment, as improvement may not occur during the first 2–4 weeks. Trimipramine may initially impair alertness. Patients should be warned of the possible hazard when driving or operating machinery. Cardiac arrhythmias and severe hypotension are likely to occur with high dosage or in deliberate overdosage. They may also occur in patients with pre-existing heart disease taking normal dosage. It may be advisable to monitor liver function in patients on long-term treatment with Surmontil.

Side-effects are similar to those of other tricyclic antidepressants; they are usually more evident during the first few days of treatment and are invariably controlled by modification of dosage. Drowsiness may occur, but this is minimised by giving the total daily dosage at night. Atropine-like side effects including dry mouth, disturbances of accommodation, tachycardia, constipation and hesitancy of micturition are common early in treatment, but usually lessen. Other adverse effects including sweating, postural hypotension, tremor and skin rashes. Interference with sexual function may occur.

Serious adverse effects are rare; the following have been reported: depression of the bone marrow including agranulocytosis, cholestatic jaundice, hypomania, convulsions and peripheral neuropathy. Psychotic manifestations, including mania and paranoid delusions, may be exacerbated during treatment with tricyclic anti-depressants. Withdrawal symptoms may occur on abrupt cessation of therapy and include insomnia, irritability and excessive perspiration. Adverse effects such as withdrawal symptoms, respiratory depression and agitation have been reported in neonates whose mothers had taken trimipramine during the last trimester of pregnancy.

Acute overdosage may be accompanied by hypotensive collapse, convulsions and coma. Provided coma is not present, gastric lavage should be carried out without delay even although some time may have passed since the drug was ingested. Patients in coma should have an endotracheal tube passed before gastric lavage is started. Absorption of trimipramine is slow but, as cardiac effects may appear soon after the drug is absorbed, a saline purge should be given. Electrocardiography monitoring is essential.

It is important to treat acidosis as soon as it appears with, for example, 20 ml per kg of M/6 sodium lactate injection by slow intravenous injection. Intubation is necessary and the patient should be ventilated before convulsions develop; convulsions should be treated with diazepam administered intravenously.

Ventricular tachycardia or fibrillation should be treated by electrical defibrillation; if supraventricular tachycardia develops, pyridostigmine bromide 1 mg (adults) intravenously or propranolol 1 mg (adults) intravenously should be administered at intervals as required.

Treatment should be continued for at least three days even if the patient appears to have recovered.

Pharmaceutical precautions Protect from light. Surmontil capsules should be stored in a dry place below 25°C.

Legal category POM.

Package quantities Tablets: Compression-coated – 10 mg in container of 50, and 25 mg in containers of 50 and 500. Capsules: 50 mg in containers of 50 and 500.

Further information Nil.

Product licence numbers
Tablets 10 mg   0012/5296
Tablets 25 mg   0012/5297
Capsules 50 mg   0012/5298

THALAZOLE*

Presentation White tablets each containing 0.5 g phthalylsulpathiazole. The tablets have the name 'Thalazole' embossed on one face and a break line on the reverse face.

Uses Thalazole is slowly hydrolyzed in the large intestine liberating sulpathiazole which has a bacteriostatic action on a variety of Gram positive and Gram negative organisms including Streptococci, Staphylococci, Nocardia, E. coli and Shigella.

It is used in the treatment or prevention of bacillary dysentery, and the eradication of the causative organism in convalescent and symptomless carriers. It is also indicated for reducing the bacterial count in the gut, both pre- and post-operatively in patients undergoing surgery of the intestinal tract. It can be used in association with specific treatment of intestinal amoebiasis when there is co-existing bacillary dysentery.

Kinetics: Only 5–10% of an oral dose is absorbed – some of it as sulpathiazole which is widely distributed in the body and rapidly excreted via the kidney.

Dosage and administration Thalazole is adminis-

tered by mouth. For treatment of acute bacillary dysentery the adult dose is 5 g or more daily in divided amounts: children are given half the adult dosage, and infants a quarter of the adult dosage. Thalazole should be continued until 24 hours after diarrhoea has ceased. Adequate fluid replacement is essential to combat dehydration. For prophylaxis, the dosage of Thalazole is 1 g twice daily for adults and children. For intestinal antisepsis in adults the dosage is 0.25 g per kg body weight initially, followed by 12 g daily in divided amounts given every three hours. Administration should start four days before the operation and continue for four days afterwards.

Elderly: No specific dosage recommendations.

Contra-indications, warnings, etc *Pregnancy and lactation:* There is epidemiological evidence of the safety of sulphonamides as a class in human pregnancy. Thalazole is sparingly absorbed and therefore the risk to foetus, neonate or suckling infant is minimal.

Contra-indication: Thalazole is contra-indicated in patients known to be hypersensitive to sulphonamides. In view of its limited absorption the risk of crystalluria is slight but patients should maintain an adequate fluid intake.

Adverse effects: Those common to the sulphonamides could occur, including nausea, vomiting, diarrhoea, rashes, headache, cyanosis, depression, mental confusion and pyrexia. More rarely hepatitis, crystalluria and blood dyscrasias.

Overdosage: In the event of overdosage gastric lavage should be carried out. Continuous forced fluids may be necessary and the urine should be rendered alkaline. Otherwise treatment is symptomatic.

Pharmaceutical precautions Protect from light.

Legal category POM.

Package quantities Tablets in container of 500.

Further information Nil.

Product licence number 0012/5266.

VALLERGAN*

Presentation *Tablets:* Dark blue, sugar-coated, imprinted M&B in ivory, each containing 10 mg trimeprazine tartrate. Vallergan tablets contain lactose.

Syrup: A clear bright straw-coloured syrupy liquid containing 7.5 mg trimeprazine tartrate in each 5 ml. It contains 68% w/v sugars.

Forte syrup: A clear colourless/pale yellow syrupy liquid containing 30 mg trimeprazine tartrate in each 5 ml, and 68% w/v of sugars.

Uses Vallergan has a central sedative effect comparable to that of chlorpromazine, but largely devoid of the latter's anti-adrenaline action. It has powerful anti-histamine and anti-emetic actions.

Vallergan is used in:
– Urticaria and pruritus.
– premedication for anaesthesia.
– short term sedation in children.

Dosage and administration *Urticaria and pruritus: Adults:* 10mg three or four times daily; up to 100 mg per day have been used in intractable cases.

Elderly: No specific dosage recommendations.

Children: 2.5–5 mg three or four times daily.

Pre-anaesthetic medication: Oral administration (children): The appropriate dosage of Vallergan Forte Syrup for this indication will depend to some extent on the preferences and objectives of the individual anaesthetist. In the age group 2–7 years, a dosage of 2 mg per kg body weight will give sedation, whilst 4 mg per kg body weight will usually induce sleep.

The drug is not recommended for infants.

Short-term sedation in children: Vallergan Forte Syrup may be given in divided dosage according to the following scheme:

– 3–6 years: 15–60 mg per day ($\frac{1}{2}$–2 × 5 ml spoonfuls).
– 7–12 years: 60–90 mg per day (2–3 × 5 ml spoonfuls).

Contra-indications, warnings, etc *Use in pregnancy and lactation:* There is no evidence of the safety of trimeprazine in human pregnancy, but it has been in wide use since 1957 without apparent ill consequence. The drug should not be used in pregnancy unless the physician considers it essential. Trimeprazine has been detected in human milk.

During the initiation of Vallergan therapy it is advisable that certain activities should be suspended for some days, e.g. the driving of vehicles or handling of power-operated tools, until it is evident that any undue drowsiness has either subsided or not appeared. Avoid alcoholic drink. Do not use in infants less than 6 months old.

Side-effects: The most frequent side-effect observed is drowsiness occurring in the early stages of treatment. Side-effects of rare occurrence are disturbing dreams, oral dryness, nasal stuffiness, headache, elation, depression, abdominal discomfort, galactorrhoea and skin rashes. Agranulocytosis is extremely rare. High dosage may give rise to parkinsonian-like effects and epileptiform convulsions. Malignant hyperpyrexia has been described.

Treatment of overdosage: Treatment of overdosage should include gastric lavage, countering of acute hypotension by the adoption of either a supine or head-down position, plasma expanders and possibly the use of phenylephrine or of noradrenaline by intravenous drip infusion; the active symptomatic treatment of central nervous depression as advocated for barbiturate poisoning, including parenteral penicillin and physiotherapy for the prevention of pneumonia. Haemodialysis is ineffective. Body temperature should be allowed to recover naturally unless it falls below about 30°C, at which level cardiac arrhythmias may become apparent. A special watch should be kept for intestinal and urinary bladder distension.

Pharmaceutical precautions Protect from light. Vallergan Syrup and Vallergan Forte Syrup may be diluted if required, using simple syrup.

Legal category POM.

Package quantities Tablets: Containers of 50 and 500.
Syrup: Bottles of 100 ml and 1 litre.
Forte syrup: Bottles of 100 ml and 1 litre.

Further information Nil.

Product licence numbers
Tablets   0012/5303
Syrup   0012/5019
Forte syrup 0012/5018.

VERACTIL*

Presentation White, varnished tablets containing 25 mg methotrimeprazine maleate indented 'Veractil', '25' on one face with break line on the reverse.

Uses Veractil is a neuroleptic with indications in psychiatry and general medicine, particularly in terminal illness. Clinically it is more sedative and more potent than chlorpromazine in the management of psychotic conditions and in the relief of chronic severe pain.

Psychiatry: As an alternative to Largactil in schizophrenia especially when it is desirable to reduce psychomotor activity.

General medicine: Alone, or together with appropriately modified doses of analgesics and narcotics, in the relief of severe pain and accompanying anxiety and distress.

Kinetics: Maximum serum concentrations are achieved in 1–3 hours; excretion is slow with a half life of 30 hours. It is excreted via the urine and faeces.

Dosage and administration Dosage varies with the condition under treatment and the individual response of the patient.

Adults: Ambulant patients: initially the total daily dose should not exceed 25–50 mg, usually divided into 3 doses; a larger portion of the dosage may be taken at bedtime to minimise diurnal sedation. The dosage is then gradually increased to the most effective level coupled with minimal side effects.

Bed patients: Initially the total daily dosage may be 100–200 mg, usually divided into 3 doses, gradually increased to 1 g daily if necessary. Attempts should be made when the patient is stable to reduce the dosage to an adequate maintenance level.

[Parenteral dosage may be preferred in patients suffering from severe pain. Methotrimeprazine 2·5% injection solution is available as 'NOZINAN' May & Baker (see 'NOZINAN' data sheet)].

Children: Children are very susceptible to the hypotensive and soporific effects of methotrimeprazine. It is advised that a total daily oral dosage of 40 mg should not be exceeded. The average effective daily intake for a 10-year-old is 15–20 mg.

Elderly patients: It is not advised to give methotrimeprazine to ambulant patients over 50 years of age unless the risk of a hypotensive reaction has been assessed.

Contra-indications, warnings, etc The safety of Veractil in pregnancy is not established.

The drug should be avoided or used with caution in patients with liver dysfunction or cardiac disease. Children and elderly patients are more susceptible to its postural hypotensive effect.

Patients having large initial doses should be kept in bed. It is advised that certain activities, e.g. the driving of vehicles or handling of power-operated tools, be suspended for a few days at the start of treatment until it is evident that drowsiness, disorientation, confusion or excessive hypotension have either subsided or not appeared.

Somnolence and asthenia are frequent, but subside as treatment progresses. Dry mouth is encountered infrequently. A raised ESR may occasionally be encountered; agranulocytosis is a rare complication.

Photosensitivity and allergic skin reactions have occasionally been reported. Parkinsonian-like reactions sometimes occur, but they are seldom noted except in patients receiving prolonged high dosage. Jaundice is a rare side-effect.

Overdosage: Treatment of overdosage should include gastric lavage; countering of acute hypotension by the adoption of either a supine or head-down position, plasma expanders and possibly the use of phenylephrine or noradrenaline by intravenous drip infusion; the active symptomatic treatment of central nervous depression is not usually required. Haemodialysis is ineffective. Body temperature should be allowed to recover naturally unless it falls below about 29.4°C, at which level cardiac arrhythmias may develop. A special watch should be kept for intestinal and urinary bladder distension.

Pharmaceutical precautions Protect from light.

Legal category POM.

Package quantities Tablets: containers of 500.

Further information Nil.

Product licence number 0012/5305.

Trade Mark

MCP Pharmaceuticals Limited
Simpson Parkway
Kirkton Campus
Livingston, West Lothian
EH54 7BH

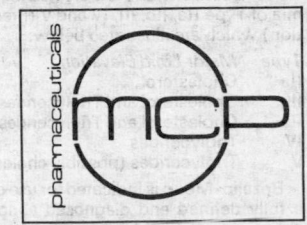

BEZALIP* ▼

Presentation Bezalip is available as white, film coated tablets each containing 200 mg bezafibrate. The tablets are marked BM on one face and G6 on the reverse.

Uses Bezalip is indicated for use in hyperlipidaemias of Type IIa, IIb, III, IV and V (Fredrickson Classification) which are illustrated below:

Type	Major Lipid Elevation
IIa	Cholesterol
IIb	Cholesterol and Triglycerides
III	Cholesterol and Triglycerides
IV	Triglycerides
V	Triglycerides (possibly cholesterol)

Bezalip is therefore indicated for use only in patients with a fully defined and diagnosed abnormality where diet alone is insufficient to correct the condition and in whom the long-term risks associated with the condition warrant treatment.

The rationale for the use of Bezalip to control abnormal elevations of serum lipids and lipoproteins is to reduce or prevent the long term adverse effects which have been shown by many major epidemiological studies to be positively and strongly correlated with such dyslipidaemias. The possible beneficial and adverse long-term consequences of some drugs used in the hyperlipidaemias are still the subject of scientific discussion, however, and there is currently no clinical evidence to demonstrate that Bezalip is effective in the prevention of heart disease.

Dosage and administration The recommended dosage of Bezalip is three tablets daily, equivalent to 600 mg bezafibrate. The tablets may be taken with or after food. Maintenance dosage may occasionally be reduced to two tablets daily, particularly in the treatment of hypertriglyceridaemia.

The initial response to therapy is normally rapidly apparent although a progressive response over a number of weeks may occur. The patient's response to Bezalip should be monitored at intervals. Treatment should be terminated if an adequate response has not been achieved within 4 to 6 months.

Contra-indications, warnings, etc Bezalip is contra-indicated in patients with severe liver dysfunction or primary biliary cirrhosis, and in those with severe renal disorders (serum creatinine values above 6 mg/100 ml). As bezafibrate is normally highly protein bound it should not be given to patients with the nephrotic syndrome. Although the drug substance has not been shown, in animal studies, to have any adverse effects on the foetus, it is recommended that Bezalip should not be administered either to pregnant women or to those who are breast-feeding. Bezalip is contra-indicated in patients hypersensitive to bezafibrate.

The chronic administration of the highest dose of bezafibrate to rats was associated with hepatic tumour formation in females. This dose was in the order of 30–40 times the human dose. No such adverse effect was apparent at reduced intake levels approximating more closely to the lipid-lowering dosage in humans.

Care is required in administering Bezalip to patients receiving anti-coagulant therapy. The dose of anti-coagulant should be reduced by 50 per cent initially and then titrated to the patient's needs. The dosage of Bezalip may need to be reduced in patients with mild to moderate renal dysfunction (contra-indicated in severe cases). At serum creatinine levels of 1.5 to 2.5 mg per 100 ml the dose of Bezalip should be reduced to two tablets daily, while one tablet daily is recommended when serum creatinine is in the range 2.6 to 6 mg per 100 ml.

Adverse effects in clinical use are rarely seen. Most commonly these effects are gastro-intestinal in nature, such as feelings of fullness of the stomach. This side effect is frequently transitory and does not normally require cessation of treatment. Other adverse effects may include a myositis-like syndrome and rarely disorders of potency and general hypersensitivity. The incidence of all these potential effects is low, and there is no evidence that administration is associated with an increased frequency of gallstones.

No serious clinical or biochemical effects are likely to occur in cases of acute overdosage and treatment in such cases, where necessary, should be symptomatic.

Pharmaceutical precautions Bezalip tablets require no special storage conditions. It is recommended, however, that they be stored in a cool, dry place in accordance with normal pharmaceutical practice.

Legal category POM.

Package quantities Packs of 100 and 500 tablets.

Further information The risks associated with hyperlipidaemia may be increased in a super-additive manner by the presence of other factors such as hypertension, obesity, smoking, genetic predisposition and diabetes. This increased risk of long term adverse effects should be taken into consideration when evaluating whether hyperlipidaemia in any particular patient warrants treatment with Bezalip.

Product licence number 0075/0036.

BEZALIP-MONO* ▼

Presentation Bezalip-Mono is a white, round, film-coated tablet with a white core and is imprinted BM/D9. Each tablet contains 400 mg bezafibrate.

Uses Bezalip-Mono is indicated for use in hyperlipidae-mia of Type IIa, IIb, III, IV and V (Fredrickson Classification) which are illustrated below:

Type	Major Lipid Elevation
IIa	Cholesterol
IIb	Cholesterol and Triglycerides
III	Cholesterol and Triglycerides
IV	Triglycerides
V	Triglycerides (possibly cholesterol)

Bezalip-Mono is indicated for use only in patients with a fully defined and diagnosed abnormality where diet alone is insufficient to correct the condition and in whom long-term risks associated with the condition warrant treatment.

The rationale for use of Bezalip-Mono to control abnormal elevations of serum lipids and lipoproteins is to reduce or prevent the long term adverse effects which have been shown by many major epidemiological studies to be positively and strongly correlated with such dyslipidaemias. The possible beneficial and adverse long term consequences of some drugs used in the hyperlipidaemias are still the subject of scientific discussion, however, and there is currently no clinical evidence to demonstrate that Bezalip-Mono is effective in the prevention of heart disease.

Dosage and administration The dosage of Bezalip-Mono is one tablet daily, equivalent to 400 mg bezafibrate. The tablets should be taken with or after the evening meal and should be swallowed whole without chewing.

The initial response to therapy is normally rapidly apparent although a progressive response over a number of weeks may occur. The patient's response should be monitored at intervals. Treatment should be terminated if an adequate response has not been achieved within 4 to 6 months.

Contra-indications, warnings, etc Bezalip-Mono is contra-indicated in patients with severe liver dysfunction and in those with severe renal disorders (serum creatinine values above 530 μ moles/l). As bezafibrate is normally highly protein-bound it should not be given to patients with the nephrotic syndrome. Although the drug substance has not been shown, in animal studies, to have any adverse effects on the foetus, it is recommended that Bezalip-Mono should not be administered either to pregnant women or to those who are breast-feeding. Bezalip-Mono is contra-indicated in patients hypersensitive to bezafibrate.

The chronic administration of the highest dose of bezafibrate to rats was associated with hepatic tumour formation in females. This dose was in the order of 30–40 times the human dose. No such adverse effect was apparent at reduced intake levels approximating more closely to the lipid-lowering dosage in humans.

Care is required in administering Bezalip-Mono to patients receiving anti-coagulant therapy. The dose of anti-coagulant should be reduced initially by 50 per cent and then titrated to the patient's needs. In patients with moderate renal impairment (serum creatinine 220 to 530 μ moles/l) Bezalip-Mono should not be employed. Such patients may be treated with conventional Bezalip tablets (200 mg bezafibrate) using a much reduced dosage.

Adverse effects in clinical use are rarely seen. Most commonly these effects are gastro-intestinal in nature, such as feelings of fullness of the stomach. This side effect is frequently transitory and does not normally require cessation of treatment. Other adverse effects may include a myositis-like syndrome and rarely disorders of potency and general hypersensitivity. The incidence of all these potential effects is low, and there is no evidence that administration is associated with an increased frequency of gallstones.

No serious clinical or biochemical effects are likely to occur in cases of acute overdosage and treatment in such cases, where necessary, should be symptomatic.

Pharmaceutical precautions Bezalip-Mono requires no special storage conditions. It is recommended, however, that the tablets be stored in a cool, dry place in accordance with normal pharmaceutical practice.

Legal category POM.

Package quantities Each pack contains 28 tablets.

Further information The risks associated with hyperlipidaemia may be increased in a super-additive manner by the presence of other factors such as hypertension, obesity, smoking, genetic predisposition and diabetes. This increased risk of long-term adverse effects should be taken into consideration when evaluating whether hyperlipidaemia in any patient warrants treatment with Bezalip-Mono.

Product licence number 0075/0051.

CANTIL*

Presentation Cantil is available as yellow, scored tablets each containing mepenzolate bromide 25 mg and as Cantil elixir, a clear, red, cherry-flavoured syrup containing in each 5 ml 12.5 mg of mepenzolate bromide.

Uses Cantil tablets and elixir contain mepenzolate bromide, a synthetic anticholinergic agent with a high degree of specificity for the smooth muscle of the lower gastro-intestinal tract.

Cantil is indicated for the relief of spasm or hyper-motility of the lower gastro-intestinal tract such as that associated with the irritable colon syndrome, mucous colitis, spastic colitis, spastic constipation, acute or chronic non-specific diarrhoeas, diverticulitis and ulcerative colitis.

Dosage and administration *Children, 6–12 years:* 5 ml of elixir three or four times daily by mouth.

Adults and older children: 1 or 2 tablets, or 10–20 mls of elixir, three or four times daily by mouth.

Contra-indications, warnings, etc Cantil is contra-indicated in glaucoma and should be used with caution in prostatic hypertrophy. Due to the specificity of action of mepenzolate bromide, typical anticholinergic effects occur only rarely with Cantil. Mild and transient blurring of vision occurs occasionally in patients with ulcerative colitis.

Treatment of overdosage is as for atropine and other anticholinergic drugs: empty the stomach by aspiration and lavage. Give a saline purgative to promote peristalsis (e.g. 30 g sodium sulphate in 250 ml warmed water). A short acting sedative or hypnotic (such as intravenous diazepam) may be given with caution if excitation occurs. Peripheral symptoms may be treated with i.m. or s.c. injection of neostigmine methylsulphate 5 mg at suitable intervals. Assisted respiration may be necessary. Fluids should be given freely and catheterisation may be required if urine is retained.

Pharmaceutical precautions The elixir is incompatible with alkaline solutions. Water is a suitable diluent if required.

Legal category POM.

Package quantities *Cantil Tablets:* Containers of 50 and 500.

Cantil Elixir: Bottles of 100 ml.

Further information Relief from the pain and discomfort of intestinal spasm usually occurs rapidly, typically within 10 to 20 minutes, and the action generally lasts for approximately four hours. Due to the relatively specific nature of the action of Cantil on the lower gastro-intestinal tract, particularly on the colon, Cantil has a low incidence of systemic anticholinergic effects.

Product licence numbers
Cantil Tablets 0075/5002
Cantil Elixir 0075/5003

CORO-NITRO* SPRAY ▼

Presentation A metered dose aerosol providing 0.4 mg glyceryl trinitrate per dose. Each aerosol contains 200 doses for buccal administration.

Uses Treatment and prophylaxis of angina pectoris.

Dosage and administration The normal dosage is one or two doses (0.4 to 0.8 mg glyceryl trinitrate) as required for relief of anginal pain or for short term prophylaxis before physical or emotional stress or other factors known to precipitate anginal attacks. Occasionally up to 3 doses (1.2 mg glyceryl trinitrate) may be needed at a single time in severe cases. In no circumstances should this be exceeded.

Coro-Nitro Spray is for buccal administration and patients must be warned not to inhale the spray. During use the aerosol should be held upright, close to the mouth. Pressure on the spray head will release a single dose of 0.4 mg glyceryl trinitrate. The spray should be directed into the mouth, preferably onto or under the tongue. Patients should be encouraged to practise using Coro-Nitro Spray, by test-firing into the air, when they first receive the product.

Coro-Nitro Spray is not recommended for children.

Contra-indications, warnings, etc Coro-Nitro Spray is contra-indicated in hypotensive disorders, including shock, in cases of significant cerebral trauma, and in patients hypersensitive to glyceryl trinitrate.

Use of Coro-Nitro Spray during pregnancy is not contra-indicated but is at the sole discretion of the prescribing doctor.

Adverse effects are similar to those normally seen with glyceryl trinitrate and may include headache, facial flushing, dizziness and nausea. Hypotensive effects may occur, especially when the patient has been consuming alcohol or is taking other hypotensive medication.

Excessive dosage may promote severe headache, facial flushing, hypotension and fainting and, rarely, cyanosis and methaemoglobinaemia. In some cases the effect of overdose will closely resemble shock. Recovery normally occurs spontaneously. The patient should lie in a supine position with the legs elevated to promote venous return. Symptomatic treatment may be needed if there is severe circulatory or respiratory collapse. Methaemoglobinaemia will respond to methylene blue infusion.

Note that if sprayed directly on to a naked flame the spray may briefly flare or sputter. Patients, especially those who smoke, should be warned not to use Coro-Nitro Spray near to a naked flame.

Pharmaceutical precautions Coro-Nitro Spray should not be stored in direct sunlight or near direct sources of heat. The aerosol container must not be punctured, broken or burnt, even if it appears to be empty.

Legal category P.

Package quantities Each Coro-Nitro Spray will deliver 200 metered doses of 0.4 mg glyceryl trinitrate.

Further information Coro-Nitro Spray is extremely stable and has a shelf life in excess of 3 years.

Coro-Nitro Spray may be employed together with other anti-anginal agents when necessary, including those used for long term prophylaxis such as isosorbide mononitrate and betablockers.

Product licence number 0075/0052.

GASTROCOTE*

Presentation Gastrocote is presented as white, uncoated tablets which are engraved on one side with the name Gastrocote. Each tablet contains:

Alginic Acid BPC	200 mg
Dried Aluminium Hydroxide Gel BP	80 mg
Magnesium Trisilicate BP	40 mg
Sodium Bicarbonate BP	70 mg

Uses Gastrocote acts to reduce the incidence of gastric reflux and thus of associated discomfort and pain. Gastrocote is indicated in heartburn, including heartburn of pregnancy, reflux oesophagitis, particularly where associated with hiatus hernia, and in all cases of epigastric distress associated with gastric reflux or regurgitation.

Dosage and administration *Adults and older children only:* 1 to 3 tablets to be chewed four times a day, that is, after main meals and at bedtime. Not to be given to children under 6 years.

Important: The tablets must be well chewed before swallowing.

Contra-indications, warnings, etc Care should be exercised in treating diabetic patients as the tablets each contain 1.03 g sucrose. Each tablet also contains 21 mg (0.91 mEq) of sodium which may be important for patients on a low sodium diet. There are no specific contra-indications to the use of Gastrocote and overdosage is virtually free of hazard although gastric bloating may occur.

Pharmaceutical precautions Gastrocote should be stored in a cool dry place.

Legal category P.

Package quantities Gastrocote tablets are supplied in containers of 100 tablets.

Further information When Gastrocote tablets are chewed sodium alginate is formed as a foam with the antacid constituents entrained. The foam coats the oesophagus with a demulcent, antacid layer when swallowed and then forms a viscous, colloidal foam gel floating on the stomach contents. This mild barrier physically impedes reflux. In the event of reflux being forced the demulcent alginate-antacid foam moves into the lower oesophagus before the stomach contents thus protecting the mucosa from further proteolytic attack and allowing healing to occur.

Product licence number 0075/0024

GLUCOTARD*

Presentation Each unit-dose sachet of Glucotard provides 5 grams of guar in the form of whitish-brown lemon flavoured mini-tablets.

Uses *Pharmacology:* Glucotard contains guar, an unabsorbable fibre of plant origin which, when taken with food, increases the consistency of the contents of the gastro-intestinal tract. Consequently, the absorption of dietary carbohydrate is retarded, although not diminished, thus preventing or reducing a post-prandial increase in blood glucose and facilitating an improved control of carbohydrate metabolism. Guar also interacts with the enterohepatic circulation of bile salts, promoting their increased excretion, and may influence intestinal transit time.

Indications for use: Glucotard is indicated for use in patients with diabetes mellitus to help to reduce post-prandial blood glucose concentrations, thus facilitating control and, where appropriate, allowing a reduction in the dosage of other anti-diabetic medication.

Dosage and administration *Dosage:* Diabetic patients whose metabolism is well controlled by diet, insulin or sulphonylurea drugs should take a single daily dose of Glucotard before breakfast to attenuate the hyperglycaemic response. For diabetic patients with excessive post-prandial blood glucose levels and/or with urinary excretion of glucose it is recommended that a dose of Glucotard should be taken 2 to 3 times daily before main meals. Concurrent anti-diabetic therapy with diet, insulin or sulphonylurea drugs normally should be continued unchanged.

Administration: Glucotard must be taken just before meals as, in order to be fully effective, it must mix with food in the stomach. Each individual dose of Glucotard should be taken in 3 to 4 portions, without chewing. Each portion should be placed dry onto the tongue and swallowed with several mouthfuls of water. At least a tumblerful (250 ml/8 fl oz) of water must be taken with each dose.

For those patients requiring more than a single dose of Glucotard each day it is recommended that the dosage should be increased gradually to reduce the possibility of gastro-intestinal disturbances which may follow a sudden increase in the fibre content of the diet.

Contra-indications, warnings, etc There are no specific contra-indications to the use of Glucotard. It is possible that Glucotard may alter the rate or extent of absorption of other drugs given orally at the same time. No clinically significant effects have been found with digoxin, paracetamol or bezafibrate. The bioavailability of sulphonylurea agents such as glibenclamide may be reduced although, due to the additive effects of Glucotard with these drugs, the control of carbohydrate metabolism is improved and no dosage adjustment is necessary. No information is available on the possibility of interaction with oral contraceptive medications. In the absence of such data it is recommended that patients using oral contraceptives either should not take Glucotard or they

should employ additional contraceptive precautions. There is no evidence that Glucotard reduces absorption of essential dietary components, such as vitamins, minerals and trace elements, and administration of such dietary supplements is unnecessary unless required for other reasons.

As Glucotard acts to improve the metabolic state in diabetic patients it is recommended that the blood and/or urine glucose concentrations should be monitored carefully, especially during the initial stages of therapy. Glucotard does not reduce the utilisation of carbohydrate in the diet and it should not be necessary to modify either diet or other anti-diabetic medication for most patients, although the possibility of such a need must be borne in mind.

The use of Glucotard in patients with oesophageal obstruction should be considered carefully as the mini-tablets may swell in-situ if oesophageal transit is delayed.

The adverse effects which may occur with use of Glucotard are those normally associated with bulking agents in the diet. They may include nausea, feelings of fullness and loss of appetite, flatulence, diarrhoea and related gastro-intestinal disturbances. These effects are generally transient and resolve within the first week of treatment. The incidence of such effects may be minimised by employing a gradual increase in the number of daily doses of Glucotard when treatment is started.

No information is available on the effects of overdosage. The effects anticipated include gastro-intestinal distension and an increase in the consistency of the gastro-intestinal contents. The patient should be given plenty of fluid to drink and otherwise treated symptomatically.

Pharmaceutical precautions Glucotard requires no special handling or storage conditions. As with all medicines it is recommended that it be stored in a cool, dry place in accordance with good pharmaceutical practice.

Legal category P.

Package quantities Glucotard is available in packs of 60 unit-dose sachets.

Further information Glucotard contains guar, a natural vegetable fibre derived from the seeds of the Cluster Bean (*Cyamopsis tetragonoloba, Leguminosae*).

Product licence number 0075/0054.

ISMO* 20 ▼

Presentation Ismo 20 tablets are white, circular, uncoated and are embossed on each side with a break line and the code BM/B3. Each tablet contains 20 mg isosorbide mononitrate.

Uses *Pharmacology:* Isosorbide mononitrate is an active metabolite of isosorbide dinitrate and exerts qualitatively similar effects. Unlike the dinitrate, however, isosorbide mononitrate demonstrates virtually complete systemic absorption after oral administration and is only slowly eliminated from the body. The therapeutic action of isosorbide mononitrate is thus predictable, reproducible and of long duration.

Indications: Ismo 20 tablets are indicated for use in prophylaxis and treatment of angina pectoris.

Dosage and administration A dosage of 40 to 60 mg isosorbide mononitrate daily (2 to 3 Ismo 20 tablets daily) provides control of angina pectoris in the majority of patients although the daily dosage may vary from 20 to 120 mg in appropriate cases. Ismo 20 tablets should be administered in divided doses using either a twice daily or three times daily dosage regime as appropriate. The tablets should be swallowed whole without chewing.

For patients who have not previously received prophylactic nitrate therapy it is recommended that the dosage should be 20 mg daily (half an Ismo 20 tablet twice daily) for the first two days and that it should be increased gradually until the desired therapeutic effect is achieved. Patients already accustomed to chronic nitrate therapy may normally be transferred directly to a therapeutic dose of Ismo 20. For patients previously treated with isosorbide dinitrate in conventional dose forms the dosage of Ismo 20 should be the same initially. Ismo 20 is effectively twice as potent as sustained release forms of isosorbide dinitrate and patients transferred from such treatment initially should receive Ismo 20 at half the previous dosage.

Contra-indications, warnings, etc Ismo 20 tablets are contra-indicated in patients with a known hypersensitivity to isosorbide mononitrate or isosorbide dinitrate. A number of nitrate-related adverse effects may occur during treatment, including headache and feelings of dizziness. The incidence of such effects is highest at the commencement of treatment and tends to decline with time. In sensitive patients postural hypotension may occur, especially after a high dose. Other reactions, similar to those associated with isosorbide dinitrate, may occur occasionally. In the event of overdosage the main sign is liable to be hypotension which should be treated by laying the patient in a supine position with the legs elevated to promote venous return.

Pharmaceutical precautions No special handling or storage precautions apply although it is recommended that Ismo 20 be stored in a cool, dry place in accordance with good pharmaceutical practice.

Legal category POM.

Package quantities Ismo 20 is available in packs of 60, 100 and 250 tablets.

Further information Ismo 20 provides long term nitrate prophylaxis for the treatment and control of angina pectoris in a form with complete biological availability due to the lack of any significant hepatic first-pass metabolism. This provides consistently uniform blood levels of drug substance and a more predictable clinical response. The onset of activity occurs within 20 minutes and is maintained for more than 8 hours.

Product licence number 0075/0044.

PALFIUM*

Presentation Palfium products contain Dextromoramide Tartrate BP, and the dose and strength are expressed as dextromoramide base. The presentations available cover the oral, parenteral and rectal routes of administration:

Palfium tablets, 5 mg: white, scored tablets for oral use (Dextromoramide Tablets BP, 5 mg).

Palfium tablets, 10 mg: peach, scored tablets for oral use (Dextromoramide Tablets BP, 10 mg).

Palfium injection, 5 mg and 10 mg per 1.0 ml of solution: a clear, colourless, aqueous solution for parenteral administration (Dextromoramide Tartrate Injection BP, 5 mg or 10 mg per 1 ml).

Palfium suppositories, 10 mg: light cream coloured suppositories for rectal administration.

Uses Palfium is a potent analgesic for relief of the severe pain of inoperable carcinoma and for the relief of other forms of severe and intractable pain.

Dosage and administration *Adult dosage: First dose:* Not more than 5 mg by mouth or by subcutaneous or intramuscular injection, or 10 mg rectally.

Subsequent doses: The size of subsequent doses depends upon the needs of the patient, that is, upon the severity of the pain. In cases of severe pain 10 mg Palfium may be required, repeated as necessary in order to maintain analgesia. The dose required may also be influenced by the patient's body weight. Regardless of body weight, however, not more than 20 mg should be given as a single dose and usually not more than 15 mg by injection. The dose frequency and the total daily dosage may vary significantly and should be titrated according to the needs of the individual patient.

In postoperative pain the initial dose of Palfium in the immediate postoperative period should be restricted, for example, to 2.5 mg, as the patient may still be under the influence of circulating anaesthetic agents and pre-medications. For subsequent postoperative care, 5 mg three or four times daily as required is usually sufficient.

Administration: Palfium is as effective orally as by injection. The oral route of administration thus is to be preferred. Palfium tablets should be given before food, if possible. Palfium is also fully effective rectally and a 10 mg dose may be administered by suppository, particularly at night. When oral administration is impracticable Palfium injection may be administered by the intramuscular or subcutaneous route. Administration by the intravenous route is not recommended in normal practice.

Child dosage: A paediatric dosage regime has not yet been established. Should the need arise to administer Palfium to a child, the initial dosage should be not more than 0.08 mg per Kg of body weight.

Contra-indications, warnings, etc Palfium is contra-indicated in patients with respiratory depression or obstructive airways disease, and in female patients during child-birth. It is also contra-indicated in patients receiving monoamine oxidase inhibitors and two to three weeks should be allowed to elapse before Palfium is administered to patients who have been treated with these agents.

The use of Palfium in pregnant patients is not recommended, although there is no evidence from animal studies to suggest that it is potentially harmful. In cases where the rate of metabolism of dextromoramide may be reduced, such as in the elderly and in patients with hypothyroidism or chronic hepatic insufficiency, it may be advisable to employ a reduced dosage regime.

Palfium may give rise to dizziness and sweating, especially in the ambulant patient. These effects may be minimised by advising the patient to rest, preferably supine, for a short period after administration of the first few doses. Nausea and vomiting may be troublesome but tend to occur only rarely. As with other potent analgesics tolerance and addiction may occur with continued use of Palfium. Concurrent administration of CNS depressants, including alcohol, must be carefully considered as such agents may enhance the central effects of Palfium and consequently the risk of respiratory depression.

Respiratory depression is unlikely to occur when Palfium is employed on its own in a normal therapeutic dosage. In the event of oral overdosage empty the stomach by aspiration and lavage using, for example, a 0.02% aqueous solution of potassium permanganate. If consciousness is impaired and respiration depressed suitable antagonists should be administered. Levallorphan tartrate 1.0 mg intravenously initially, followed by 1 or 2 doses of 0.5 mg may be used. Alternatively, nalorphine or naloxone may be administered using the appropriate dosage.

The circulation should be maintained with intravenous infusion of plasma or suitable electrolyte solutions and assisted respiration may be necessary until spontaneous breathing is restored.

Pharmaceutical precautions Palfium ampoules and tablets require no special precautions. As with all medicines, however, it is preferable that they be stored in a cool, dry place. Palfium suppositories must be stored in a cool location well away from radiators and other sources of heat.

Legal category CD (Sch 2) POM.

Package quantities Palfium tablets 5 mg and 10 mg, blister packs of 60.

Palfium injection, 5 mg and 10 mg per ml, packs of 10 1.1 ml ampoules.

Palfium suppositories, packs of 10.

Further information Palfium is as effective when given by mouth as when injected. The analgesic effect is rapid by all routes of administration (typically 20–30 minutes).

Palfium provides pain relief normally without clouding consciousness or mental activity, and does not cause constipation. It may be advantageous in some cases to provide simultaneous administration of a sedative, hypnotic or tranquilliser, such as chlorpromazine, with Palfium. A cautious approach should be made to establish the most satisfactory dosage regime. In most cases only half the normal dose of the ancillary drug will be required.

Product licence numbers

Palfium Tablets 5 mg	0075/5015R
Palfium Tablets 10 mg	0075/0035R
Palfium Injection 5 mg	0075/5012R
Palfium Injection 10 mg	0075/5013R
Palfium Suppositories	0075/5014R

PIPTALIN*

Presentation Piptalin elixir is an orange-flavoured and orange coloured suspension. Each 5 ml of elixir contains pipenzolate bromide 4 mg and simethicone (activated dimethicone) 40 mg.

Uses Piptalin is indicated for the alleviation of the discomfort and pain associated with spasm, hypermotility and gaseous distension in functional and organic digestive disorders, such as in infant colic, regurgitation and vomiting. Piptalin is also indicated for functional abdominal pain in the school child, and for flatulent dyspepsia, aerophagia, cardiospasm and pylorospasm.

Dosage and administration *Infants, up to 10 kg body weight:* 2.5 ml orally 15 minutes before each feed.

Young children, 10–20 kg body weight: 2.5 to 5.0 ml three or four times daily.

Older children, 20–40 kg body weight: 5 ml three or four times daily.

Adults: 10 ml three or four times daily.

Piptalin elixir should be taken approximately 15 minutes before meals. If necessary it may be diluted with water.

Contra-indications, warnings, etc Piptalin elixir is contra-indicated in bowel obstruction and in hypertrophic pyloric stenosis.

Typical anticholinergic side-effects due to pipenzolate bromide occur only rarely. In high doses Piptalin may cause constipation with tenesmus and, rarely, dermal flushing without fever. These effects usually disappear or diminish at lower dose levels.

Treatment of overdosage is as for other anticholinergic drugs. Empty the stomach by aspiration and lavage. Promote peristalsis with a saline purgative (30 g sodium sulphate in 250 ml warmed water is a suitable solution) and control excitation with a short acting sedative or hypnotic such as intravenous diazepam. Neostigmine methylsulphate may be injected i.m. or s.c. for control of peripheral symptoms. Assisted respiration may be necessary as may catheterisation if urine is retained. Fluids should be given freely.

Pharmaceutical precautions Piptalin elixir should be shaken thoroughly before use. It may be diluted with water or syrup and is incompatible with alkaline solutions.

Legal category POM.

Package quantities Piptalin elixir is available in bottles of 100 ml and 500 ml.

Further information Relief from discomfort and pain due to spasm and flatulence usually occurs within 10 to 20 minutes and the duration of antispasmodic action is normally approximately four hours.

Piptalin combines the antispasmodic activity of pipenzolate bromide with the deflatulant effects of simethicone. The former relieves spasm and reduces hypermotility and gastric secretion while simethicone assists in elimination of entrapped gas and in prevention of the formation of mucous-occluded gas pockets in the gastro-intestinal tract.

Product licence number 0075/5017.

SPIROCTAN*

Presentation Spiroctan products contain Spironolactone BP and are available as three dosage forms:

Spiroctan 25	light blue coated tablets marked BM B2 and containing 25 mg spironolactone BP.
Spiroctan 50	green coated tablets marked BM A8 and containing 50 mg spironolactone BP.
Spiroctan 100	light green hard gelatin capsules marked BM A7 and containing 100 mg spironolactone BP.

Uses *Pharmacology:* Spiroctan promotes diuresis by competitive inhibition of aldosterone, a sodium-retaining, potassium-excreting hormone. It acts on the distal portion of the renal tubule and may be used in conjunction with more proximally acting diuretics.

Indications for Use: Spiroctan is recommended for use

in the treatment of congestive heart failure, essential hypertension, idiopathic oedema, liver cirrhosis, ascites and nephrotic syndrome. For the prevention and treatment of peri-operative primary aldosteronism and also for the diagnosis and treatment of primary aldosteronism of different aetiology. Spiroctan is recommended for use in hypertension associated with diabetes particularly if the metabolic state deteriorates with other anti-hypertensive medication.

Dosage and administration *Adults:* Adequate maintenance dosage is usually between 50 and 200 mg daily, depending on the patients' response. This may be increased to 300 to 400 mg daily when necessary. An initial dosage of up to 600 mg daily may be employed in appropriate cases.

Children: The daily dosage for children is based on an intake of 1.5 to 3.0 mg per kg body weight, as shown in the following guidelines:

Age 1 to 3 years (up to approximately 15 kg): One tablet Spiroctan 25 every other day.

Age 4 to 7 years (up to approximately 23 kg): One tablet Spiroctan 25 each day.

Age 8 to 12 years (up to approximately 37 kg): One tablet Spiroctan 25 twice daily.

Spiroctan tablets and capsules should be taken with fluid. When the daily dosage does not exceed 200 mg it may normally be taken as a single dose. For children who cannot swallow solid dose forms the tablets may be crushed and taken with food or drink.

Contra-indications, warnings, etc Spiroctan is contra-indicated in cases of renal failure, acute renal insufficiency, where hyperkalaemia is present, and in patients hypersensitive to spironolactone.

Potassium supplements should not be administered with Spiroctan except initially in cases of hypokalaemia, and the use of Spiroctan with other potassium-sparing diuretics should be avoided.

The use of Spiroctan in women who are pregnant, who may become pregnant or who are breast-feeding is not recommended.

The action of other diuretics may be potentiated. The initial dose should be half that normally administered and the dosage should be adjusted to the patient's needs.

Although the dose of Spiroctan does not generally need to be reduced in hepatic dysfunction, such patients should be carefully monitored as hepatic coma may be precipitated in susceptible subjects.

Periodic estimation of serum electrolytes is recommended.

Adverse effects are infrequent and usually mild. They include drowsiness, mental confusion (especially in conjunction with alcohol) and gastro-intestinal effects. Drivers of vehicles or operators of dangerous machinery should be warned of the effects on alertness.

Gynaecomastia may occur rarely but is normally reversible on cessation of dosage. Very occasionally alterations in voice pitch occur and these may not be reversible. This risk should be carefully considered in patients for whom voice control is important, for example, in actors. Occasional reports of skin rashes, breast enlargement and nipple sensitivity have been made.

Carcinogenicity: Spironolactone has been shown to produce tumours in rats when administered at high doses over a long period of time. The significance of these findings with respect to clinical use is not certain. However, the long-term use of spironolactone in young

patients requires careful consideration of the benefits and the potential hazard involved.

Toxic effects in overdosage are due mainly to hyperkalaemia. Clinical symptoms include irregular pulse, lassitude, and muscular weakness and it may be difficult clinically to differentiate from hypokalaemia. Treatment is by cessation of therapy, administration of potassium-excreting diuretics, use of ion-exchange resins, etc.

Pharmaceutical precautions No special storage precautions are necessary. As with all medicines, however, it is recommended that Spiroctan be stored in a cool, dry place.

Legal category POM.

Package quantities
Spiroctan 25   Packs of 100 and 500 tablets.
Spiroctan 50   Packs of 100 tablets.
Spiroctan 100 Blister packs of 28 capsules.

Further information Spiroctan may be administered in combination with more proximally acting diuretics to increase diuresis and to prevent excessive potassium loss.

No metabolic changes occur with Spiroctan in incipient or overt diabetes.

In the treatment of essential hypertension and of oedema of varied aetiology the treatment should be continued for at least two weeks as an adequate response may not occur before this time.

Product licence numbers
Spiroctan 25   0075/0037
Spiroctan 50   0075/0038
Spiroctan 100 0075/0039

SPIROCTAN-M* INJECTION ▼

Presentation A clear, yellow, aqueous solution containing 200 mg potassium canrenoate in each 10 ml ampoule.

Pharmacology: Potassium canrenoate is converted in the body to canrenone, the major active metabolite of spironolactone. It is an aldosterone antagonist with clinical effects similar to those of spironolactone. As potassium canrenoate is administered intravenously, however, its clinical effects are more rapidly apparent. As with spironolactone, potassium canrenoate is capable of producing direct cardiac effects independent of its aldosterone antagonist actions. Potassium canrenoate thus demonstrates a clinically beneficial positive inotropic and anti-arrhythmic cardiac activity at the recommended dosage.

Indications: Spiroctan-M Injection is indicated for use in the treatment of oedema associated with cardiac dysfunction, particularly where cardiac arrhythmias and/or digitalis intolerance due to hypokalaemia occur. It is also indicated for use in the treatment of oedema associated with secondary aldosteronism in clinical cases such as ascites, oedema associated with liver dysfunction, oedema associated with the nephrotic syndrome and responsive oedema of different aetiology.

Spiroctan-M Injection is also indicated for the treatment of hypertension associated with an aldosterone excess.

Dosage and administration For use in adults only. The normal dose is up to 800 mg (up to 4 ampoules) daily by slow intravenous injection. This may be given in a single administration or in divided doses during the day.

In order to avoid irritation and pain at the site of infusion, Spiroctan-M Injection should be administered slowly, 2 to 3 minutes per ampoule, and preferably not into a thin vein.

An alternative method of administration is slow intravenous infusion following dilution with an appropriate vehicle.

In severe cases a potent diuretic may be administered together with Spiroctan-M Injection until satisfactory diuresis has been induced.

Contra-indications, warnings, etc *Contra-indications:* Spiroctan-M Injection is contra-indicated in patients with renal failure, hyperkalaemia or hyponatraemia and in those hypersensitive to potassium canrenoate. It should not normally be given together with potassium supplements.

Warnings and precautions: Spiroctan-M Injection is not recommended for administration to children, or to pregnant or breast-feeding women. The administration of undiluted Spiroctan-M Injection should occur slowly, 2 to 3 minutes per ampoule, to avoid local venous irritation. It is recommended that for patients on long term therapy the electrolyte balance should be monitored regularly. Normally, however, intravenous treatment is of short duration and therapy may be continued with spironolactone tablets or capsules given orally. As potassium canrenoate yields only one of several active metabolites of spironolactone its aldosterone antagonist potency relative to that of spironolactone in chronic dosage is approximately 0.7. This factor should be considered in transferring from intravenous potassium canrenoate to oral spironolactone tablets or capsules. Potassium canrenoate is metabolised to canrenone which is an active metabolite of spironolactone. Spironolactone has been shown to produce tumours in rats when administered in high doses over a long period of time. The significance of these findings with regard to clinical use is not certain. The long term use of potassium canrenoate in young patients requires careful consideration of the potential benefits and hazards involved.

Adverse effects: Some patients may experience irritation or pain at the site of injection, particularly if the injection is not administered slowly. A transient confusion syndrome has been observed during therapy with high doses (1,000 mg per day or more). This effect subsided when the dosage was reduced. Nausea and vomiting may also occur soon after a high dose and may be controlled by suitable anti-emetic medication.

It is theoretically possible that in chronic usage there may be anti-androgenic effects in females and gynaecomastia and sexual dysfunction in males. As Spiroctan-M Injection is not generally employed for chronic treatment no evidence of these effects has been reported.

Overdosage: The effects of acute overdosage may include nausea, vomiting, transient confusion and possibly hyperkalaemia. Treatment of overdose involves cessation of therapy, anti-emetic medication and the use of a potassium-eliminating drug if hyperkalaemia is present.

Pharmaceutical precautions Spiroctan-M Injection should be stored away from light.

For slow intravenous infusion Spiroctan-M Injection may be diluted with 250 ml of either dextrose solution 5% or sodium chloride solution 0.9%. No other drugs or nutrients may be added. Use the diluted preparation within 12 hours and check visually for the absence of precipitation before use.

Legal category POM.

Package quantities The ampoules are supplied in packs of 5.

Further information Potassium canrenoate is converted in the body to canrenone, which is the major active metabolite of spironolactone. The clinical effects of the two drugs are qualitatively similar although potassium canrenoate is more rapidly effective and is able to achieve higher blood levels of canrenone. Diuresis normally commences within the first 24 hours although latent periods of 10 days or more have been reported in very refractory cases. The direct cardiac actions of Spiroctan-M Injection occur soon after administration. After the acute phase of treatment dosage may be reduced and treatment may be continued with spironolactone tablets or capsules. Spiroctan-M Injection does not affect glucose metabolism, does not interfere with the treatment of diabetes, and does not promote hyperuricaemia.

Product licence number 0075/0040.

SUSTAMYCIN*

Presentation Sustamycin is presented as light blue/dark blue hard gelatin capsules. Each capsule contains 250 mg Tetracycline Hydrochloride BP in a sustained release formulation.

Uses Sustamycin is a sustained-action tetracycline formulation with an enhanced biological availability of tetracycline which allows for reduction of dose and of dose frequency. Sustamycin is indicated for the treatment of infections due to organisms susceptible to tetracycline including bronchitis, acute exacerbations of chronic bronchitis, acne and sexually transmitted diseases.

Dosage and administration *For adults and children over 12 years only:* Two capsules initially followed by 1 capsule every 12 hours. In more severe infections dosage may be increased at the discretion of the physician, for example, to 2 capsules twice daily. In acute cases treatment should be maintained for two to three days after the desired clinical response has been achieved. In the treatment of acne, therapy should continue for at least eight weeks although a lower dose, e.g. 1 capsule daily, may be used after the initial period.

Sustamycin should be taken preferably one hour before or two hours after main meals.

Contra-indications, warnings, etc Contra-indicated in patients with known hypersensitivity to tetracyclines.

Sustamycin should be used with caution in patients with renal or hepatic impairment.

If tetracycline is administered to young children (under eight years) or to pregnant women it is selectively taken up in developing bones and teeth and dental staining and enamel hypoplasia may occur. Sustamycin should not be used for such patients unless the potential benefits justify the risks.

The gastro-intestinal adverse effects common to the tetracyclines occur only rarely, due to the sustained release; skin photosensitivity reactions may be seen occasionally. Appropriate measures should be taken in the event of over-growth by a non-susceptible organism.

As with all tetracyclines, the concomitant intake of antacids, mineral supplements (calcium, magnesium and iron) and milk may diminish absorption from Sustamycin capsules.

Pharmaceutical precautions Store in well closed containers at a temperature below 30°C.

Legal category POM.

Package quantities Sustamycin is available in containers of 50 or 500 capsules.

Further information Sustamycin contains tetra-cycline hydrochloride in a sustained release form facilitating twice daily dosage which leads to increased patient compliance compared with the four times daily dosage regimen of conventional tetracycline. The formulation enables tetracycline to be absorbed throughout the gastro-intestinal tract, not just in the stomach. This enhanced absorption allows a reduction in total tetracycline dosage while maintaining full clinical efficacy.

Product licence number 0075/0017.

Trade Mark

Medo Pharmaceuticals Limited
East Street
Chesham
Bucks HP5 1DG

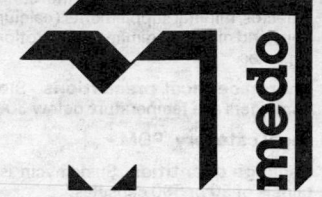

CELLUCON*

Presentation Chocolate coloured and flavoured uncoated tablet containing Methylcellulose BP 500 mg.

Uses To aid reduction of appetite, constipation, colitis, diverticulitis, irritable bowel syndrome and for the management of colostomies.

Dosage and administration
For appetite reduction, colitis, diverticulitis, constipation and irritable bowel syndrome:

Adults; 1 to 4 tablets to be chewed half an hour before meals followed by at least one glass of water or other liquid. In constipation, as normal function returns, the dose can be reduced.

Children: 1 to 2 tablets three to four times daily or as advised by the medical practitioner.

For Colostomies: The dose of Cellucon should be varied according to the fluid intake. An initial dose of three tablets two or three times a day should be tried and adjusted according to the patient's requirements. The tablets should be chewed or broken up and swallowed but the quantity of water should be reduced to a minimum, and no fluid should be taken for at least half an hour before and after the tablets. If the stools are too firm the dose of tablets should be decreased; if too loose the dose should be increased. If the bowels function at inconvenient times additional tablets can be taken to prevent unwanted evacuation.

Contra-indications, warnings, etc Cellucon should not be given if intestinal obstruction is suspected.

Pharmaceutical precautions Nil.

Legal category P.

Package quantities 100 and 250.

Further information Nil.

Product licence number 4147/5911.

DIOCTYL*

Presentation
Dioctyl Tablets: Yellow tablets containing docusate sodium 100 mg.

Dioctyl Paediatric Syrup: Pale yellow syrup containing docusate sodium 0.25% w/v (12.5 mg in 5 ml).

Dioctyl Syrup: Syrup containing docusate sodium 1% w/v (50 mg in 5 ml).

Uses Docusate sodium is an anionic wetting agent which acts as a faecal softener by allowing penetration of the accumulated, hard, dry faeces by water and fats.

Used for the prevention and treatment of chronic constipation.

Dosage and administration
For constipation

Adults: Up to 500 mg in divided doses daily. Treatment should be commenced with large doses which should be decreased as the condition of the patient improves.

Children: 12.5 to 25 mg three times daily.

Infants: 12.5 mg three times daily.

For barium meals: 400 mg to be taken with the meal.

Contra-indications, warnings, etc Anthraquinone derivatives should be taken in a reduced dose when administered with docusate sodium as it increases their absorption. Do not use when abdominal pain, nausea or vomiting is present. Do not take concurrently with mineral oil.

Pharmaceutical precautions In cold weather *Dioctyl Syrup* forms flaky crystals. These are readily re-dissolved by standing the container in water at 40°C or storage in a warm room for two or three days. Shaking also speeds redissolution.

Legal category P.

Package quantities *Dioctyl Tablets* 100 mg: 100; 250.
Dioctyl Paediatric Syrup 0.25% (12.5 mg in 5 ml): 125 ml; 1 litre.
Dioctyl Syrup (50 mg in 5 ml): 1 litre.

Further information Nil.

Product licence numbers
Dioctyl Tablets	4147/5910
Dioctyl Paediatric Syrup	4147/5908
Dioctyl Syrup	4147/5909

DIOCTYL* EAR DROPS

Presentation A clear liquid containing Docusate Sodium 5% w/w in Polyethylene Glycol in a 7 ml glass amber dropper bottle.

Uses For the softening of ear wax to facilitate its removal.

Dosage and administration Four drops should be instilled into the ear twice daily for 2–3 days. The head should be inclined to one side and the ear plugged with cotton wool soaked in Dioctyl Ear Drops if necessary. After 2–3 days the wax should be easy to remove with a cotton bud or a syringe. Patients prone to persistent problems with ear wax should use Dioctyl Ear Drops every two weeks.

Contra-indications, warnings, etc None.

Pharmaceutical precautions None.

Legal category GSL.

Package quantities Dioctyl Ear Drops are available in a 7 ml amber glass bottle with a removable glass dropper unit.

Further information Dioctyl Ear Drops are for use only in the ear. Docusate Sodium is the British Approved Name for Dioctyl Sodium Sulphosuccinate.

Product licence number 4147/0045.

HORMOFEMIN* CREAM

Presentation Smooth off-white cream containing Dienoestrol BP 0.025% w/w in a 40 g tube with a 4 g applicator.

Uses Senile vaginitis, atrophic vaginitis and pruritus vulvae when associated with the atrophic vaginal epithelium.

Dosage and administration Given for short term use only. The lowest dose that will control symptoms should be chosen and medication should be discontinued as promptly as possible.

Attempts to discontinue or taper medication should be made at three to six month intervals, following physical examination. The usual dosage range is a half to one applicator full per day for one or two weeks, then gradually reduced to one half initial dose for a similar period.

Treated patients with an intact uterus should be monitored closely for signs of endometrial cancer and appropriate diagnostic measures should be taken to rule out malignancy in the event of persistent or recurring abnormal vaginal bleeding. As a general rule it is advisable that patients receiving any form of oestrogen replacement therapy should have a complete physical examination at least once a year.

Contra-indications, warnings, etc Prolonged exposure to unopposed oestrogen may increase the risk of development of endometrial carcinoma, induction of other malignant neoplasms, and the risk of cancer of the breast. Long term continuous administration of natural and synthetic oestrogens in certain animal species increases the frequency of carcinomas of the breast, cervix, vagina and liver. There is now evidence that oestrogens increase the risk of carcinoma of the endometrium in humans.

At the present time there is no satisfactory evidence that oestrogens given to post-menopausal women increase the risk of cancer of the breast, although a recent long-term follow up of a single physician has raised the possibility. However, because of animal data there is a need for caution in prescribing oestrogens for women with a strong family history of breast cancer or who have breast nodules, fibrocystic disease or abnormal mammograms.

Pregnancy is an absolute contra-indication to the use of Dienoestrol cream since it may be harmful to the developing foetus.

Oestrogens should not be used in women with any of the other following conditions: known or suspected cancer of the breast, known or suspected oestrogen-dependent neoplasia, undiagnosed abnormal genital bleeding, active thrombophlebitis or thromboembolic disorders, a past history of thrombophlebitis, thrombosis, or thromboembolic disorders.

Thromboembolic disorders: While an increased rate of thromboembolic and thrombotic disease in post-menopausal users of oestrogens has not been found, this does not rule out the possibility that such an increase may be present or that subgroups of women who have underlying risk factors or who are receiving relatively large doses of oestrogens may have increased risk. Therefore oestrogens should not be used in persons with active thrombophlebitis or thromboembolic disorders, and they should not be used (except in treatment of malignancy) in persons with a history of such disorders. They should be used with caution in patients with cerebral vascular or coronary artery disease and only for those in whom oestrogens are clearly needed.

Gall bladder disease: A recent study has reported a two to three-fold increase in the risk of surgically confirmed gall bladder disease in women receiving post-menopausal oestrogens, similar to the two-fold increase previously noted in users of oral contraceptives.

Hepatic adenoma: Benign hepatic adenomas appear to be associated with the use of oral contraceptives. Although benign, and rare, these may rupture and may cause death through intra-abdominal haemorrhage. Such lesions have not yet been reported in association with other oestrogen or progestrogen preparations but should be considered in oestrogen users having abdominal pain and tenderness, abdominal mass, or hypovolemic shock.

Elevated blood pressure: It has been reported that this may occur with the use of oestrogens in the menopause and blood pressure should be monitored with oestrogen use, especially if high doses are used.

Precautions: A complete medical and family history should be taken prior to the initiation of any oestrogen therapy. The pretreatment and periodic physical examinations should include special reference to blood pressure, breasts, abdomen and pelvic organs, and should include a Papanicolaou smear.

A pathologist should be advised of oestrogen therapy when relevant specimens are submitted.

Certain patients may develop undesirable manifestations of excessive oestrogenic stimulations, such as abnormal or excessive uterine bleeding, mastodynia, etc. Pre-existing uterine fibroids may increase in size during oestrogen use.

Patients with a past history of jaundice during pregnancy have an increased risk of recurrence of jaundice while receiving oestrogen therapy. If jaundice develops in any patient receiving oestrogen, the medication should be discontinued while the cause is investigated.

Oestrogens may aggravate cases of porphyria.

Pharmaceutical precautions Store in a cool place.

Legal category POM.

Package quantities 40 g.

Further information Nil.

Product licence number 4147/5916.

MEDOCODENE*

Presentation Yellow scored uncoated tablets each containing Paracetamol PhEur 500 mg and Codeine Phosphate PhEur 8 mg

Uses The treatment of mild to moderate pain and as an antipyretic.

Dosage and administration
The tablets are for oral administration.

Adults: 1–2 tablets four times a day.

Children 6–12 years: ½–1 tablet 4 times a day.
Not suitable for children under 6 years of age, unless directed by a physician.
At least four hours should be allowed between doses. Not more than four doses in 24 hours.

Contra-indications, warnings, etc Codeine is a narcotic analgesic. Tolerance, psychological and physical dependence may occur. Constipation is common.

As Medocodene contains Paracetamol, an overdose can cause hepatic necrosis. Patients who have taken an overdose may appear well for several days, but they may then develop severe hepatic damage. Administration of Cysteamine, Methionine or Acetylcysteine within 12 hours of ingestion may prevent liver damage.

There is epidemiological evidence of the safety of Paracetamol in human pregnancy.

There is no, or inadequate, evidence of safety of Codeine in human pregnancy, but the drug has been widely used for many years without apparent ill consequence, and animal studies have not shown any hazard.

Pharmaceutical precautions Nil.

Legal category CD (Sch 5), P.

Package quantities Medocodene is available in 100, 250 and 1000 sizes.

Further information Nil.

Product licence number 4147/0034R.

PHOLCOMED* LINCTUS
PHOLCOMED*-D LINCTUS

Presentation A red, blackcurrant flavoured linctus containing:

Pholcodine BP	5 mg
Papaverine Hydrochloride BP	1.25 mg

Pholcomed-D linctus contains no sugar and has negligible calorific value.

Uses Pholcomed is used for the relief of irritating unproductive coughs. Pholcomed contains a combination of Pholcodine, a cough suppressant, and Papaverine acting on smooth muscle to relax the bronchi.
Pholcodine is less constipating than Codeine.

Dosage and administration *Adults:* Two to three 5 ml spoonfuls.

Children: Over 2 years: One 5 ml spoonful.

Infants: Half a 5 ml spoonful.
Three or four times daily after meals.

Contra-indications, warnings, etc Nil.

Pharmaceutical precautions Nil.

Legal category CD (Sch 5), P.

Package quantities Pholcomed: 125 ml. Pholcomed-D: 125 ml.

Further information Nil.

Product licence numbers

Pholcomed	4147/5901
Pholcomed-D	4147/5902

PHOLCOMED* FORTE LINCTUS
PHOLCOMED* FORTE DIABETIC LINCTUS

Presentation A red, blackcurrant flavoured linctus containing:

Pholcodine BP	19 mg
Papaverine Hydrochloride BP	5 mg

The diabetic linctus contains no sugar and has negligible calorific value.

Uses Pholcomed Forte is used for the relief of irritating unproductive coughs. Pholcomed contains a combination of Pholcodine, a cough suppressant, and Papaverine, acting on smooth muscle to relax the bronchi.
Pholcodine is less constipating than Codeine.

Dosage and administration *For adults only:* One 5 ml spoonful three times a day after meals.
Not suitable for children.

Contra-indications, warnings, etc Nil.

Pharmaceutical precautions Nil.

Legal category CD (Sch 5), P.

Package quantities
Pholcomed Forte: 125 ml and 2 litres.
Pholcomed Forte Diabetic: 125 ml.

Further information Nil.

Product licence numbers

Pholcomed Forte	4147/5903
Pholcomed Forte Diabetic	4147/5904

PHOLCOMED* PASTILLES

Presentation Blackcurrant flavoured, sugar coated disc shaped pastilles containing:

Pholcodine BP	4 mg
Papaverine Hydrochloride BP	1 mg

Uses Pholcomed Pastilles are used for the relief of irritating unproductive coughs. Pholcomed pastilles contain a combination of Pholcodine, a cough suppressant, and Papaverine, acting on smooth muscle to relax the bronchi.
Pholcodine is less constipating than Codeine.

Dosage and administration *Adults:* One to two pastilles hourly.

Children: One pastille hourly.
Maximum adult dose fifteen pastilles daily.
Maximum children's dose seven pastilles daily.

Contra-indications, warnings, etc Nil.

Pharmaceutical precautions Nil.

Legal category CD (Sch 5), P.

Package quantities 20 pastilles.

Further information Nil.

Product licence number 4147/5905.

PHOLCOMED* EXPECTORANT SYRUP

Presentation A red, cherry flavoured syrup containing:

Guaiphenesin BP	62.5 mg
Methylephedrine Hydrochloride	0.625 mg

Uses As an expectorant cough syrup with a broncho-dilator action.

Dosage and administration *Adults:* Two to four 5 ml spoonfuls.

Children: Half to one 5 ml spoonful.
Three times a day.

Contra-indications, warnings, etc The dose of Methylephedrine is very small, nevertheless, it should be used with caution in patients with heart disease, hyperthyroidism and closed angle glaucoma. It should not be given to patients treated with monoamine oxidase inhibitors.

Pharmaceutical precautions None.

Legal category P.

Package quantities 125 ml and 2 litres.

Further information Nil.

Product licence number 4147/5914.

*Trade Mark

E. Merck Limited
Four Marks
Alton
Hampshire GU34 5HG

MERCK

AMINOFUSIN* L600

Presentation A clear, sterile, pyrogen-free solution for intravenous feeding, containing pure L-amino acids which provide a high level of nitrogen in a low fluid volume.

Active ingredients:

L-*Amino acids*	g/litre
L-Isoleucine	1.55
L-Leucine	2.2
L-Lysine monohydrochloride	2.5
L-Methionine	2.1
L-Phenylalanine	2.2
L-Threonine	1.0
L-Tryptophan	0.45
L-Valine	1.5
L-Arginine (calc. as base)	4.0
L-Histidine (calc. as base)	1.0
L-Alanine	6.0
Glycine	10.0
L-Glutamic acid	9.0
L-Proline	7.0
Total	50.5

Carbohydrates	
Sorbitol	100.0

Vitamins	mg/litre
Ascorbic acid	400
Inositol	500
Nicotinamide	60
Pyridoxine HCl	40
Riboflavin 5'-phosphate-Na	2.5

Electrolytes	mmol/litre
Na^+	40
K^+	30
Mg^{++}	5
Acetate$^-$	10
Malate$^-$	15
(g/litre L-malic acid)	(2.01)
Cl$^-$	14
Total Nitrogen g/litre	7.6
kcal/litre approximately	600
pH	6.8

Osmolality approximately 1,300 mosm/kg

Uses For intravenous parenteral nutrition where the amino acids are in the optimum and balanced proportions together with a correctly balanced calorie supplement necessary to ensure maximum protein synthesis. Aminofusin is indicated whenever oral feeding is impossible or inadequate. Where extra calorie source is required Aminofusin L1000 is available containing 50 g of ethanol.

Dosage and administration The amount of Aminofusin to be administered daily is calculated according to individual patients' requirements of nitrogen, fluid, calories, etc. Adults should receive 0.8–1.6 g amino acids/kg body weight daily. Children, pregnant women and post-operative patients, 1.6–2.0 g amino acids/kg body weight daily. Newborn and premature infants 2.0–3.0 g amino acids/kg body weight daily.

Infusion rate 40–60 drops per minute (2–4 ml/kg/hr); it should not exceed 4 ml per kg/hour. Optimal utilisation is achieved when the daily dose is given in a continuous infusion over 24 hours. In patients who are unable to tolerate continuous infusions, two infusion periods of four or six hours each per day are recommended.

Contra-indications, warnings, etc Aminofusin L600 is contra-indicated in patients suffering shock, hyperkalaemia, severe disturbances of liver or kidney function and disturbance of amino acid metabolism; its effects should be carefully controlled when given to patients who tend towards elevated serum potassium or urea levels. Too rapid an infusion may result in renal losses, and nausea in sensitive patients.

A pre-existing deficiency of vitamins and, in particular, folic acid and Vitamin B_{12} may become clinically evident during intravenous nutrition with amino acids. Regular checks of the patients' Vitamin B_{12} status and folate demand are therefore recommended. Prophylactic administration of adequate vitamins should be given if required.

Overdosage: In the event of fluid or solute overload during parenteral therapy, re-evaluate the patient's condition and institute appropriate corrective treatment.

Pharmaceutical precautions Store between 15° and 25°C. The solution of Aminofusin should be clear at all times before infusion. Store away from light. If a precipitate or severe discoloration occurs, discard. Addition of drugs to the bottle of amino-acid solution or giving set should be avoided.

Legal category POM.

Package quantities 1,000 ml glass bottles. 6 bottles per case.

Further information Nil.

Product licence number 0493/0068.

AMINOFUSIN* L1000

Presentation A clear, sterile, pyrogen-free solution for intravenous feeding, containing pure L-amino acids which provide a high level of nitrogen in a low fluid volume, together with ethanol as a calorie supplement.

Active ingredients

L-*Amino acids*	g/litre
L-Isoleucine	1.55

L-Leucine		2.2
L-Lysine monohydrochloride		2.5
L-Methionine		2.1
L-Phenylalanine		2.2
L-Threonine		1.0
L-Tryptophan		0.45
L-Valine		1.5
L-Arginine (calc. as base)		4.0
L-Histidine (calc. as base)		1.0
L-Alanine		6.0
Glycine		10.0
L-Glutamic acid		9.0
L-Proline		7.0
	Total	50.5

Carbohydrates
Sorbitol	100
Ethanol	52.80

Vitamins	*mg/litre*
Ascorbic acid	400
Inositol	500
Nicotinamide	60
Pyridoxine HCl	40
Riboflavin 5'-phosphate-Na	2.5

Electrolytes	*mmol/litre*
Na^+	40
K^+	30
Mg^{++}	5
$Acetate^-$	10
$Malate^-$	15
(g/litre L-Malic acid)	(2.01)
Cl^-	14

Total Nitrogen g/litre	7.6
kcal/litre approximately	1000
pH	6.8

Osmolality approximately 2,700 mosm/kg

Uses For intravenous parenteral nutrition where the amino acids are in the optimum and balanced proportions together with a correctly balanced calorie supplement necessary to ensure maximum protein synthesis. Aminofusin is indicated whenever oral feeding is impossible or inadequate.

Dosage and administration
1. *Adults:* The amount of Aminofusin L1000 to be administered daily is calculated according to individual patients' requirements of nitrogen, fluid, calories, etc. Adults should receive 0.8–1.6 g amino acids/kg body weight daily.

2. *Children:* Not recommended.

Infusion rate 40–60 drops per minute (2–4 ml/kg/hr); it should not exceed 4 ml per kg per hour. Optimal utilisation is achieved when the daily dose is given in a continuous infusion over 24 hours. In patients who are unable to tolerate continuous infusions, two infusion periods of four or six hours each per day are recommended.

Contra-indications, warnings, etc Aminofusin L1000 is contra-indicated in patients suffering shock, hyperkalaemia, severe disturbances of liver or kidney function and disturbance of amino acid metabolism; its effects should be carefully controlled when given to patients who tend towards elevated serum potassium or urea levels. Too rapid an infusion may result in renal losses, and nausea in sensitive patients. This product contains alcohol, therefore its use is at the discretion of the attending physician.

A pre-existing deficiency of vitamins and, in particular, folic acid and Vitamin B_{12} may become clinically evident during intravenous nutrition with amino acids. Regular checks of the patients' Vitamin B_{12} status and folate demand are therefore recommended. Prophylactic administration of adequate vitamins should be given if required.

Overdosage: In the event of fluid or solute overload during parenteral therapy, re-evaluate the patient's condition and institute appropriate corrective treatment.

Pharmaceutical precautions Store between 15° and 25°C. The solution of Aminofusin should be clear at all times before infusion. Store away from light. If a precipitate or severe discoloration occurs, discard. Addition of drugs to the bottle of amino-acid solution or giving set should be avoided.

Legal category POM.

Package quantities 1,000 ml glass bottles. 6 bottles per case.

Further information Nil.

Product licence number 0493/0069.

AMINOFUSIN* L FORTE

Presentation A clear, sterile, pyrogen-free solution for intravenous feeding, containing pure L-amino acids which provide a high level of nitrogen in a low fluid volume. Aminofusin L Forte contains no calorie source, but is in the same proportion of L-amino acids but in twice the concentration with a total nitrogen content being 15.2 g/l instead of 7.6 g/l as in L1000.

Active ingredients

L-*Amino acids*		*g/litre*
L-Isoleucine		3.1
L-Leucine		4.4
L-Lysine monohydrochloride		5.0
L-Methionine		4.2
L-Phenylalanine		4.4
L-Threonine		2.0
L-Tryptophan		0.9
L-Valine		3.0
L-Arginine (calc. as base)		8.0
L-Histidine (calc. as base)		2.0
L-Alanine		12.0
Glycine		20.0
L-Glutamic acid		18.0
L-Proline		14.0
	Total	101.0

Vitamins	*mg/litre*
Inositol	500
Nicotinamide	60
Pyridoxine HCl	40
Riboflavin 5'-phosphate-Na	2.5

Electrolytes	*mmol/litre*
Na^+	40
K^+	30
Mg^{++}	5
$Acetate^-$	10
$Malate^-$	5
(g/litre L-malic acid)	(0.67)
Cl^-	27.5
Total Nitrogen g/litre	15.2

kcal/litre approximately   400
pH   5.3–5.5
Osmolality approximately 1050 mosm/kg.

Uses Aminofusin L Forte is indicated whenever oral feeding is impossible or inadequate, the Aminofusin L Forte solution can be used in special circumstances where there is a high N_2 requirement and in combination with other sources of energy such as hypertonic glucose or fat emulsion.

Dosage and administration
1. *Adults:* The amount of Aminofusin L Forte to be administered daily is calculated according to individual patient requirements of nitrogen, fluid, calories, etc. Adults should receive 0.8–1.6 g amino acids/kg body weight daily.
2. *Children:* Not recommended.

Infusion rate 35 drops per minute (1.5 ml/kg/hr); it should not exceed 1.5 ml per kg per hour. Optimal utilisation is achieved when the daily dose is given in a continuous infusion over 24 hours. In patients who are unable to tolerate continuous infusions, two infusion periods of four or six hours each per day are recommended.

Contra-indications, warnings, etc Aminofusin L Forte is contra-indicated in patients suffering shock, hyperkalaemia, severe disturbances of liver or kidney function and disturbance of amino acid metabolism; its effects should be carefully controlled when given to patients who tend towards elevated serum potassium or urea levels. Too rapid an infusion may result in renal losses, and nausea in sensitive patients.

A pre-existing deficiency of vitamins and, in particular, folic acid and Vitamin B_{12} may become clinically evident during intravenous nutrition with amino acids. Regular checks of the patients' Vitamin B_{12} status and folate demand are therefore recommended. Prophylactic administration of adequate vitamins should be given if required.

Overdosage: In the event of fluid or solute overload during parenteral therapy, re-evaluate the patient's condition and institute appropriate corrective treatment.

Pharmaceutical precautions Store between 15° and 25°C. The solution of Aminofusin L Forte should be clear at all times before infusion. Store away from light. If a precipitate or severe discoloration occurs, discard. Addition of drugs to the bottle of amino-acid solution or giving set should be avoided.

Legal category POM.

Package quantities 500 ml glass bottles, 10 bottles per case.

Further information Nil.

Product licence number 0493/0070.

BALNEUM*

Presentation A liquid preparation for external use. Each 100 ml contains 84.75 ml soya oil.

Uses Balneum has emollient properties and is recommended for the treatment of dry skin conditions including those associated with dermatitis and eczema.

Dosage and administration For full bath ($\sim$ 100 L)– 20 ml = 1 measure.

For bath for children ($\sim$ 25 L)–5 ml = ¼ measure.
For partial bath ($\sim$ 5L)–2.5 ml = ⅛ measure.
For particularly dry skin, 2–3 times the above quantities can be used.

Add Balneum to the bath water and mix well. The frequency and duration of bathing will depend on the type and severity of the condition. Generally 2–3 baths should be taken weekly. For babies and infants a daily bath is recommended.

Contra-indications, warnings, etc None.
No side-effects have been observed.

Pharmaceutical precautions None.

Legal category P.

Package quantities Bottles of 225 ml, 500 ml and 1000 ml.

Further information Balneum contains vegetable oil well tolerated by the skin. Since the product contains no wool alcohols or lanolin it can be safely used by patients sensitive to these materials. The bath can easily be cleaned after use.

Product licence number 0493/0064.

CISTOBIL*

Presentation Cistobil tablets are bi-convex tablets 13 mm in diameter and plain on both sides. Each tablet, white-cream in colour, contains 500 mg Iopanoic acid.

Uses Cistobil tablets are recommended as an oral contrast medium for cholecystography.

Dosage and administration *Adults:* The meal prior to ingestion of the tablets should be a normal meal containing some fat. 15–20 minutes later the standard adult dose of 6 tablets of Cistobil is taken one at a time during 5–10 minutes. The patient should have nothing to eat on the morning prior to the radiological examination which is usually carried out 10–14 hours after ingestion of the contrast medium. A double dose of Cistobil (12 tablets) may be prescribed in special cases, especially where the patient is heavy or obese. No more than 12 tablets should be given in 24 hours. The double dose should not be used in patients with renal insufficiency, this may include elderly patients.

Children: Not recommended.

Contra-indications, warnings, etc Like all iodinised media, Cistobil should be used with caution and is contra-indicated in diseases of the liver parenchyma, in renal insufficiency, iodine intolerance, thyrotoxicosis, in myocardial diseases, and in congestive heart failure.

X-ray examination of women should if possible be conducted during the pre-ovulation phase of the menstrual cycle and should be avoided during pregnancy; also since it has not been demonstrated that Cistobil is safe for use in pregnant women, it should be administered only if the procedure is considered essential by the physician.

Pharmaceutical precautions Nil.

Legal category P.

Package quantities Cartons of 30 tablets packed in unit doses, each unit dose consisting of 6 tablets.

Further information Nil.

Product licence number 0493/0072.

DIUREXAN*

Presentation Tablets each containing 20 mg Xipamide. The tablets are white, round, with bisecting score on one side and debossed A on the other, and have a diameter of 6 mm.

Uses Diurexan is a diuretic and antihypertensive agent having a gentle onset of action and gradual, prolonged effect. Whereas the main diuretic activity lasts for up to 12 hours, the antihypertensive effect is evident for 24 hours or more.

Hypertension: All grades of hypertension respond to treatment with Diurexan. It is an effective treatment on its own in mild to moderate hypertension, and may be used alone or combined with other antihypertensive agents in severe hypertension.

Oedema: Diurexan is indicated whenever diuretic therapy is required including congestive cardiac failure, hepatic oedema, renal oedema, peripheral oedema due to venous insufficiency and oedema of pregnancy in the second and third trimesters.

Dosage and administration For oral administration.

Hypertension: adults: The usual dose is 1 tablet (20 mg) daily, as a single early morning dose. In more severe grades of hypertension, 2 tablets daily, as a single early morning dose, may be required. When using Diurexan in combination with other antihypertensive therapy, the initial dose should not exceed 1 tablet daily.

Elderly: See precautions.

Children: No dose recommended.

Oedema: Adults: In the initial phase of treatment the usual dose is 2 tablets (40 mg) daily in a single early morning dose. Depending on the patient's response, the dose may be lowered to 1 tablet daily when sufficient control of oedema has been achieved. Higher doses, up to 4 tablets daily (80 mg), may be employed in resistant cases.

Elderly: See precautions.

Children: No dose recommended.

Contra-indications, warnings, etc

Contra-indications: Diurexan is contra-indicated in severe electrolyte deficiency, precomatose states associated with liver cirrhosis and severe renal insufficiency.

Side-effects and adverse reactions: Diurexan is generally well tolerated. Slight gastro-intestinal disturbances have been reported in a few cases as have episodes of mild dizziness.

Precautions: Like other diuretics, Diurexan may induce hypokalaemia in long-term therapy. Potassium supplements may be necessary particularly in the elderly where dietary potassium intake may be inadequate.

Animal experiments have indicated that Diurexan is devoid of teratogenic properties or effects on fertility and reproduction. Nevertheless, discretion is required before permitting therapy in pregnant patients. As with all drugs, treatment should be avoided in the first trimester of pregnancy.

Warnings: The dosage of other hypotensive drugs and cardiac glycosides may require adjustment when used in conjunction with Diurexan. In common with other diuretics, Diurexan may induce hyperuricaemia or changed glucose metabolism in patients predisposed to these conditions. Diabetic patients will probably require an adjustment of insulin dosage, or other hypoglycaemic agent therapy.

An increased risk of developing acute retention may arise in patients with prostatic hypertrophy.

Overdosage: General measures should be aimed at the maintenance of blood pressure, restoration of blood volume and correction of electrolyte imbalance.

Pharmaceutical precautions Store in a cool, dry place.

Legal category POM.

Package quantities Cartons of 140 tablets in blister packs of 14 tablets.

Further information Nil.

Product licence number 0493/0049.

ENDOBIL*

Presentation Endobil 100 ml bottle contains a 9.91% w/v concentration of the meglumine salt of iodoxamic acid for intravenous infusion, equivalent to an iodine content of 45 mg/ml.

Uses Intravenous cholecystography and cholangiography.

Dosage and administration *Endobil Infusion:* 100 ml.

Adults: The recommended duration of intravenous infusion is between fifteen and thirty minutes.

Patients undergoing cholegraphic procedures with Endobil should be adequately prepared with only a light meal on the night before examination and an enema. Endobil should be warmed to body temperature and administered intravenously with the patient lying down.

Elderly: Dosage as for adults.

Children: The use of Endobil in children is not recommended until further evidence has been accumulated and reviewed.

Contra-indications, warnings, etc

Contra-indications: Proven or suspected hypersensitivity to iodine-containing preparations.

Warnings, side-effects: Endobil should be used with caution in patients with severe functional impairment of the liver, kidneys or myocardium, severe hyperthyroidism and macroglobulinaemia (Waldenströms disease).

X-ray examination of women should if possible be conducted during the pre-ovulation phase of the menstrual cycle and should be avoided during pregnancy; also since it has not been demonstrated that Endobil is safe for use in pregnant women, it should be administered only if the procedure is considered essential by the physician.

Side-effects following the administration of Endobil are generally mild and relatively rare, the most common being facial flushing and nausea.

As with any contrast medium, injection solutions of adrenaline, a vasopressor, a corticosteroid and an antihistamine should be immediately available in case of hypersensitivity. To cover the remote possibility of delayed hypersensitivity the patient should be attended for 20 minutes following injection.

Pharmaceutical precautions Store away from light.

Legal category POM.

Package quantities *Endobil Infusion:* Box containing 10 × 100 ml bottles for intravenous infusion (4.5 g iodine).

Further information Nil.

Product licence number 0493/0074.

GAMANIL* ▼

Presentation Round, lacquered, brownish violet tablets with a spindle shaped scoring on one side, containing Lofepramine hydrochloride equivalent to 70 mg Lofepramine base.

Uses The treatment of symptoms of depressive illness.

Dosage and administration *Adults:* The usual dose is 140 mg to 210 mg per day in divided doses depending upon the severity of the condition. Higher doses can be given in severe cases.

Elderly: Elderly patients may respond to lower doses.

Children: Not recommended.

Contra-indications, warnings, etc The administration of Lofepramine in pregnancy and during breast feeding is not advised unless there are compelling medical reasons.

Lofepramine should be used with caution in patients with cardiovascular disease, severe liver or renal impairment, narrow angle glaucoma, symptoms suggestive of prostatic hypertrophy, or a history of epilepsy.

The elderly are particularly liable to experience adverse reactions to tricyclic antidepressants, especially agitation, confusion and, rarely, postural hypotension.

As with other antidepressants, ability to drive a car and operate machinery may be affected. Therefore caution should be exercised initially until the individual reaction to treatment is known.

As improvement may sometimes be delayed for two weeks, patients should be closely monitored during the initial treatment period.

Side-effects: Lofepramine has been shown to be well tolerated and side-effects when they occur tend to be mild and transient.

Reported side-effects have included dryness of mouth, constipation, disturbances of accommodation, tachycardia, hesitancy of micturition, dizziness, drowsiness, hypotension, sweating and tremor.

Rarely reported adverse effects include: allergic skin reactions, thrombocytopenia and transient increase in liver enzymes. Isolated cases of hypomania have occurred.

Comparative clinical trials have shown that Lofepramine is associated with a lower incidence of anticholinergic side-effects than amitriptyline or imipramine.

The following adverse effects have been encountered in patients under treatment with tricyclic antidepressants and should therefore be considered as theoretical hazards of Lofepramine even in the absence of substantiation: psychotic manifestations, including mania and paranoid delusions, may be exacerbated during treatment with tricyclic antidepressants; withdrawal symptoms may occur on abrupt cessation of therapy and include insomnia, irritability and excessive perspiration; adverse effects such as withdrawal symptoms, respiratory depression and agitation have been reported in neonates whose mothers have taken tricyclic antidepressants during the last trimester of pregnancy; interference with sexual function may occur.

Drug interactions: Lofepramine should not be administered concurrently with or within 2 weeks of cessation of therapy with monoamine oxidase inhibitors.

Lofepramine should not be given with sympathomimetic agents. Lofepramine may decrease the antihypertensive effect of adrenergic neurone blocking drugs; it is therefore advisable to review this form of antihypertensive therapy during treatment. Tricyclic antidepressants potentiate the central nervous depressant action of alcohol.

Anaesthetics given during tricyclic antidepressant therapy may increase the risk of arrhythmias and hypotension. If surgery is necessary, the anaesthetist should be informed that a patient is being so treated. Barbiturates may increase the rate of metabolism.

Overdosage: Treatment of overdosage is symptomatic and supportive. It should include immediate gastric lavage and routine close monitoring of cardiac function. Cardiac arrhythmias and severe hypotension are likely to occur with high dosage or in deliberate overdosage.

Reports of overdosage with Lofepramine, which include 23 patients who took quantities up to 5.6 g, have shown no serious sequelae directly attributable to the drug.

Pharmaceutical precautions The tablets should be stored at room temperature, in their original container, protected from light and moisture.

Legal category POM.

Package quantities Containers of 250 tablets 70 mg. Blister calendar packs of 4 × 14 tablets 70 mg.

Further information Nil.

Product licence number 0493/0060.

ILIADIN* MINI
ILIADIN* MINI PAEDIATRIC

Presentation A colourless, aqueous, buffered solution of Oxymetazoline hydrochloride 0.05% w/v in polythene unit-dose packs each containing 0.3 ml. Iliadin Mini Paediatric contains 0.025% w/v Oxymetazoline hydrochloride in 0.3 ml unit-dose packs.

Uses Iliadin has a vasoconstrictive and decongestive effect on the naso-pharyngeal mucosa which lasts for up to 12 hours.

Iliadin is indicated for the relief of nasal congestion associated with disorders of the upper respiratory tract including, infective and allergic rhinitis, sinusitis, nasopharyngitis and coryza.

Dosage and administration *Adults:* Instil half the contents of one mini unit into each nostril. Repeat every 8–12 hours as necessary.

N.B. The 0.05% solution is not recommended for children under the age of 6 years.

Infants and children: Instil half the contents of one mini unit of Iliadin Mini Paediatric into each nostril. Repeat every 8–12 hours as necessary, Iliadin Mini Paediatric can be used for infants whose nasal congestion interferes with feeding.

Contra-indications, warnings, etc Iliadin is contraindicated in patients with a known sensitivity to sympathomimetics; in patients who are receiving monoamine oxidase inhibitors, or within 14 days of stopping such treatment; and in acute coronary disease, cardiac asthma, hyperthyroidism or closed angle glaucoma. The excessive use of Iliadin may cause reactive hyperaemia.

Cases of rebound congestion and drug induced rhinitis following prolonged use of Iliadin are rare.

Iliadin should not be used during pregnancy unless considered essential by the physician.

Iliadin Paediatric: It is recommended that continuous therapy should not exceed 14 days and that it should be used with caution in infants under 12 weeks of age.

Pharmaceutical precautions Store at a temperature not exceeding 25°C.

Legal category P.

Package quantities Packs of 10 and 20 disposable mini units.

Further information Iliadin has been shown to provide more prolonged relief from nasal congestion than any other nasal decongestant. The unit-dose presentation is hygienic and eliminates the risk of cross infection.

Product licence numbers

Iliadin Mini	0493/0005
Iliadin Mini Paediatric	0493/0010

MERCK SKIN TESTING SOLUTIONS

Presentation Merck Skin Testing Solutions are aqueous allergen extracts containing 50% glycerin and preserved in 0.4% phenol with their strength expressed in PNU. There is a Merck Skin Testing Solution available for each extract in the Norisen range, and the following skin testing solutions are available:

POLLENS

Grasses: Grass Mix (Cocksfoot, Meadow Grass, Rye Grass, Tall Fescue, Timothy, Yorkshire Fog).

Barley, Maize, Oat (Cult.), Rye, Wheat.

Weeds: Weed Mix (Dandelion, Mugwort, Nettle, Pellitory, Plantain).

Dandelion, Mugwort, Nettle, Plantain, Pellitory.

Trees: Tree Mix (Early Blossoming) [Alder, Elm, Hazel, Poplar, Willow].

Tree Mix (Mid-Blossoming) [Beech, Birch, Oak, Plane].

Alder, Ash, Beech, Birch, Elder, Elm, False Acacia, Hazel, Oak, Plane, Poplar, Sycamore, Willow.

Flowers: Flower Mix (Aster, Chrysanthemum, Dahlia, Golden Rod, Marguerite [Daisy]).

Aster, Chrysanthemum, Dahlia, Golden Rod, Marguerite [Daisy].

OTHER ALLERGENS

Moulds: Fungi Mix I (Alternaria, Botrytis, Cladosporium, Curvularia, Fusarium, Helminthosporium).

Fungi Mix II (Aspergillus, Mucor, Pencillium, Pullularia, Rhizopus, Serpula).

Alternaria, Aspergillus, Botrytis, Candida, Chaetomium, Cladosporium, Curvularia, Fusarium, Helminthosporium, Mucor, Neurospora, Penicillium, Phoma, Pullularia, Rhizopus, Serpula (Dry Rot), Sporobolomyces, Trichophyton, Usitlago.

Epithelia: Feather Mix (Duck, Goose, Chicken).

Budgerigar, Cat, Cow, Dog, Goat, Golden Hamster, Guinea Pig, Horse, Pig, Rabbit, Sheep's Wool. (Extracts not available in Norisen range for Goat and Pig.)

Other inhalants: D. pteronyssinus (House Dust Mite). Hay Dust, House Dust, Rye Flour, Wheat Flour.

Stinging insects: Bee, Hornet, Wasp.

The following control solutions are available: Glycerosaline, histamine acid phosphate.

Form and appearance: The colour of an individual skin testing solution will depend on the source materials used, e.g. grass and weed extracts will be a pale green shade, house dust and house dust mite extracts will be a pale brown colour.

Uses Merck Skin Testing Solutions are used to confirm the provisional diagnosis of an allergic condition obtained from the detailed case history of the patient.

Dosage and administration Merck Skin Testing Solutions may be used for skin testing or nasal provocation testing. However, it is recommended that only an experienced allergist should attempt nasal provocation testing and that for the majority of cases, the modified prick test as described below will be satisfactory.

Modified prick test: The most suitable site for skin testing is on the flexor side of the fore-arm. The skin is first marked, using a ball point or felt tip pen, with those extracts to which the patient is suspected of being sensitive. The negative control is placed near the top of the arm, followed by the allergen extracts, usually with the house dust mite extract at the lower end, before the final positive control solution. The test sites should be approximately 4 cm apart. One small drop of the test solution is applied to the skin next to the mark for that allergen. A sterile lancet is then placed at an acute angle to the skin and a shallow lift is made. The lancet is raised for a second before the skin is released. This is repeated for each drop of solution, the lancet being wiped carefully on cotton wool before using each solution. Any excess solution remaining on the skin after the prick has been made is removed by placing a paper tissue over the arm for a moment or two.

The results are read after 15 to 20 minutes, when positive reactions will appear as weals and flares. Any weal or flare produced by the negative control must be subtracted from any reactions produced by the other allergens before they are assessed. Where both the weal and flare are only very small, i.e. the reaction is only mild, this is recorded as + against the particular allergen. Where there is a larger reaction, but not as large as the positive control, the reaction is recorded as ++ against the particular allergen. Where the reaction is similar to or greater than the positive control +++ should be recorded against the particular allergen.

Where a permanent record of the skin test reactions is required, the weals may be closely encircled by a ball point pen, and a piece of clear adhesive tape then applied to the arm, when an image of the reactions will be taken onto the tape. The tape may then be placed on the patient's record card.

Information on nasal provocation testing may be obtained from E. Merck Ltd.

Contra-indications, warnings, etc
Contra-indications: None known.

Precautions: Patients should be asked to discontinue any medication that they are receiving for their allergic condition prior to testing, as antihistamines and corticosteroids in high dosage may affect the results of the test. *Blood should not be drawn during testing.* Must not be used for intradermal testing. Adrenaline Injection BP should be available during testing. Particular care should be taken when testing with extracts of stinging insects, as patients may be exquisitely sensitive.

Overdosage: Not applicable.

Main side-effects/adverse reactions: Adverse reactions are extremely rare with the modified prick test, and would normally appear as large local reactions which will normally subside in three hours. In the event of persistent reactions, reference should be made to an experienced allergist. The patient may be assisted by the use of antihistamines.

In the unlikely event of a severe general reaction, a tourniquet should be applied to the upper arm proximal to the site of the skin test that has caused the reaction, and Adrenaline Injection BP should be injected around and beneath the site of the test. Adrenaline Injection BP may also be injected subcutaneously into the other arm if necessary.

Pharmaceutical precautions Merck Skin Testing Solutions should be stored between 2°C and 8°C. The solutions must not be allowed to freeze.

Legal category POM.

Package quantities Each solution is supplied in a 3 ml dropper bottle. Skin testing cases to hold up to 20 and 80 solutions are available.

Further information Nil.

Product licence number 0493/0038.

MICROK*

Presentation Hard gelatin capsules with opaque red cap and opaque white body each containing 600 mg potassium chloride equivalent to approximately 8 mmol of K+ in controlled release microcapsules (Microcaps).

Uses For the treatment and prevention of hypokalaemia which may be associated with the following:
Potassium deficiency states.
Long-term diuretic therapy.
Digitalis intoxication.
Primary or secondary aldosteronism.
Renal disease associated with increased potassium excretion, eg. nephrotic syndrome.
Liver cirrhosis.
Gastrointestinal disorders.
Hypochloraemic alkalosis.
Protracted treatment with corticosteroids, ACTH or carbenoxolone.
Cushings syndrome.
Initial treatment for megaloblastic anaemia.
Diabetic ketosis.

Dosage and administration *Adults:* The dosage of MicroK should be based on the condition and the degree of potassium depletion. Two to six capsules (16–48 mEqK+) daily are usually adequate. In severe potassium deficiency states, a higher dose of 3–4 capsules (24–32 mEqK+) every 6–8 hours may be required.

The capsules should be swallowed whole followed by a glass of water and should preferably be taken with or after meals.

Children: At the discretion of the physician.

Use in the elderly: It is not usually necessary to adjust

the dosage but concurrent renal insufficiency should be taken into account.

Contra-indications, warnings, etc
Contra-indications: Hyperkalaemia; gastro-intestinal tract ulceration; advanced renal failure; untreated Addison's disease; acute dehydration; obstruction of the digestive tract.

Precautions: Potassium chloride should be administered with caution to patients with renal or adrenal insufficiency. If severe vomiting or severe abdominal distress develops the preparation should be withdrawn at once. Monitoring of serum electrolytes is particularly necessary in patients with cardiac or renal disease. Potassium salts should not be administered with potassium-sparing diuretics.

In cases of metabolic acidosis, the hypokalaemia should be treated with an alkaline potassium salt.

Use in pregancy: Solid forms of oral potassium preparations should not be given to pregnant women except when considered essential.

Side-effects: In rare instances patients may experience abdominal discomfort or nausea.

Overdosage: Signs and symptoms include hypotension, cardiac arrhythmias, mental confusion, aesthenia and paraesthesia. Characteristic ECG changes are also seen (widening of the QRS complex and peaked T waves). Treatment: Gastric lavage, glucose and insulin infusions, forced diuresis and possibly peritoneal dialysis or haemodialysis. Mild hyperkalaemia can be treated with cation exchange resin. More severe forms may require intravenous infusion of sodium bicarbonate or intravenous injection of calcium chloride or calcium gluconate (10–20 ml of a 1% solution).

Pharmaceutical precautions The capsules should be stored in a cool, dry place protected from light.

Legal category P.

Package quantities Securitainers of 100 capsules.

Further information Each MicroK capsule contains microencapsulated potassium chloride; in this formulation each particle of powdered potassium chloride is coated with an inert membrane through which the active substance diffuses into the gastrointestinal tract by continuous dialysis over a period of 8 hours. This avoids dangerous blood potassium concentrations and keeps potassium concentrations uniformly low throughout the digestive tract thus ensuring gastrointestinal tolerance.

Product licence number 0493/0062.

MULTIBIONTA* for INFUSION

Presentation A 10 ml ampoule of an aqueous solution containing:

Vitamin A palmitate (corresponding to 10,000 Units of Vitamin A)	5.9 mg
Vitamin B₁ hydrochloride	50 mg
Vitamin B₂-5 phosphate sodium salt	10 mg
Nicotinamide	100 mg
Pantothenyl alcohol	25 mg
Vitamin B₆ hydrochloride	15 mg
Vitamin C	500 mg
Vitamin E acetate	5 mg

Uses Intravenous infusions of vitamins should only be considered when oral intake is impossible or inadequate.

Neonates and infants: Multibionta for infusion is indicated as part of a total parenteral feeding regimen in neonates and young children in the following conditions.

1. Neonatal surgery involving extensive resection or reimplantation.
2. Protracted diarrhoea unresponsive to dietary treatment.
3. Extreme prematurity.
4. Renal failure.

In older children and adults:

1. Obstructing lesions of the gastro-intestinal tract.
2. Massive bowel resection.
3. Extensive burns.
4. Major trauma and severe infections.
5. Acute states of inflammatory bowel disease.
6. Severe uncontrolled malabsorptive states with undernutrition.
7. Disorders of swallowing as might occur in poliomyelitis, tetanus or following severe trauma.
8. Prolonged coma.

Dosage and administration The exact requirements of intravenously administered vitamins (particularly in sick infants) are not known. For adults 10 ml of Multibionta in an average daily dose should be added to a full infusion bottle containing not less than 250 ml of the infusion. For neonates and small children 2 ml per litre of the infusion fluid is adequate; alternatively the dose can be calculated as 0.15 ml/kilogram/24 hours. However, if preferred, the adult dose may be used with complete safety.

There is no preparation which contains all the essential vitamins in recommended amounts. It is, therefore, suggested that the following are given during prolonged intravenous nutrition in the dosage indicated.

Folic acid   0.1–0.5 mg/day
Vitamin B$_{12}$ 100 mcg/month
Vitamin D   300 Units/day (administered IM as Calciferol. 1 ml contains 300,000 Units)
Vitamin K   3 mg twice weekly
Choline chloride   500 mg/day (normally present in adequate amounts as cholinephosphatides in fat emulsions)

Their compatibility with the carrier intravenous infusion should always be checked with the pharmacy before addition.

Additional information: The miscibility of 10 ml of Multibionta has been tested and it was found to be compatible with amino-acid solutions such as Aminofusin, carbohydrate solutions such as glucose at various concentrations, and fat solutions.

Although Multibionta is compatible with most commercially available infusion fluids like other additives it is best introduced into normal saline or dextrose-saline mixtures.

Contra-indications, warnings, etc Rarely, intravenous B$_1$ may act as an allergen.

In order to minimise possible loss of active substance in a mixture (masked incompatibility), it is recommended that solutions to which Multibionta is added should not be kept for longer than eight hours.

A mixture should be discarded if visible turbidity or crystallisation appear in the infusion solution.

Especial care should be taken to avoid exposure of a plastic bag or giving set to direct sunlight following addition of Multibionta infusion.

Pharmaceutical precautions Should be stored at a temperature not exceeding 20°C.

Legal category POM.

Package quantities 10 ml ampoules in packs of 3.

Further information Nil.

Product licence number 0493/0076.

NIOPAM* ▼

Presentation Ampoules or bottles containing sterile aqueous solutions of varying strengths of iopamidol.

Niopam 200: contains a 40.8% w/v concentration of the active constituent equivalent to 20% iodine or 200 mg Iodine/ml.

Niopam 300: contains a 61.2% w/v concentration of the active constituent equivalent to 30% iodine or 300 mg Iodine/ml.

Niopam 370: contains a 75.5% w/v concentration of the active constituent equivalent to 37% iodine or 370 mg Iodine/ml.

Uses X-ray contrast media for lumbar and thoraco-cervical myelography, cerebral angiography, peripheral arteriography and venography, angiocardiography, left ventriculography and coronary arteriography, aortography, selective visceral angiography, computer tomography enhancement, urography, arthrography.

Dosage and administration See table on next page.

Elderly: Dosage as for adults.

Contra-indications, warnings, etc

Contra-indications: Proven or suspected hypersensitivity to iodine containing preparations of this type.

Warnings: As with all other contrast media this product may provoke anaphylaxis or other manifestations of allergy with nausea, vomiting, dyspnoea, erythema, urticaria and hypotension. A positive history of allergy, asthma or untoward reaction during previous similar investigations indicates a need for extra caution; the benefit should clearly outweigh the risk in such patients. Appropriate resuscitative measures should be immediately available.

Care should be exercised in carrying out radiographic procedures with contrast media in patients with severe functional impairment of the liver or myocardium, severe systemic disease and in myelomatosis. In the latter condition patients should not be exposed to dehydration; similarly abnormalities of fluid or electrolyte balance should be corrected prior to use.

Care should also be exercised in patients with moderate to severe impairment of renal function (as reflected by a raised blood urea) or in diabetes. Substantial deterioration in renal function is minimised if the patient is well hydrated. Renal function parameters should be monitored after the procedure in these patients.

Patients with severe hepato-renal insufficiency should not be examined unless absolutely indicated. Re-examination should be delayed for 5–7 days.

Special care should be exercised when this product is injected into the right heart or pulmonary artery in patients with pulmonary hypertension. Right heart angiography should be carried out only when absolutely indicated.

NIOPAM – Recommended Dosage Schedule

Procedure	Niopam product and dosage	
Lumbar Myelography	Niopam 200 Niopam 300	Adults 5–15 ml Adults 5–10 ml
Thoraco-Cervical Myelography	Niopam 200 Niopam 300	Adults 5–15 ml Adults 5–10 ml
Cerebral Angiography	Niopam 300	Adults 5–10 ml* Children 5–7 ml**
Peripheral Arteriography	Niopam 300 Niopam 370	Adults 10–50 ml* Children **
Venography	Niopam 300	Adults 20–50 ml Children **
Angiocardiography & Left Ventriculography	Niopam 370	Adults 30–80 ml Children **
Coronary Arteriography	Niopam 370	Adults 4–8 ml per artery*
Aortography —retrograde	Niopam 370	Adults 30–80 ml
Selective Renal Arteriography	Niopam 370	Adults 5–10 ml Children **
Selective Visceral Angiography: Hepatic Coeliac Superior Mesenteric Inferior mesenteric	Niopam 370	Adults 30–70 ml 40–70 ml 25–70 ml 5–30 ml
Computer Tomography Enhancement	Niopam 200 Niopam 300	Adults *Brain Scanning* 50–100 ml *Whole Body Scanning* 40–100 ml
Intravenous Urography	Niopam 300 Niopam 370	Adults 40–80 ml In severe renal failure the usual high dose methods should be employed (up to 1.5 ml/kg) Children 1–2.5 ml/kg or**
Arthrography	Niopam 300	Adults 1–10 ml According to joint being examined.

* Repeat as necessary.
** According to body size and age.

During intracardiac and/or coronary arteriography, ventricular arrhythmias may infrequentlty occur.

In patients who are known epileptics or have a history of epilepsy, anticonvulsant therapy should be maintained before and following myelographic procedures. In some instances, anticonvulsant therapy may be increased for 48 hours before the examination.

Care should be taken in those patients receiving neuroleptic and antidepressant therapy who require myelographic investigations. If possible these drug types should be withdrawn for at least 48 hours before the myelographic examination.

Use of this product may interfere with tests for thyroid function.

Niopam should be used with caution in patients with hyperthyroidism. It is possible that hyperthyroidism may recur in patients previously treated for Graves' disease.

X-ray examination of women should if possibe be conducted during the pre-ovulation phase of the menstrual cycle and should be avioided during pregnancy; also since it has not been demonstrated that Niopam is safe for use in pregnant women, it should be administered only if the procedure is considered essential by the physician.

Side Effects: Side effects are infrequent and normally mild and may consist of headache, nausea, vomiting, heat sensation, dyspnoea and hypotension. Skin rashes may occur in some patients.

Following use in myelography, headaches, dizziness, nausea and vomiting may occasionally occur.

More severe reactions involving the cardiovascular system may call for emergency treatment; appropriate resuscitative measures should be immediately available.

No other drugs should be mixed with the contrast medium.

Pharmaceutical precautions Protect the solution from light.

Discard if solution is not clear of particulate matter.

Legal category POM.

Package quantities
Niopam 200: Box containing 5 × 10 ml ampoules
Box containing 5 × 20 ml ampoules
Niopam 300: Box containing 5 × 10 ml ampoules
Box containing 5 × 20 ml ampoules
Box containing 10 × 50 ml bottles
Box containing 10 × 100 ml bottles
Niopam 370: Box containing 5 × 10 ml ampoules
Box containing 5 × 20 ml ampoules
Box containing 10 × 50 ml bottles
Box containing 10 × 100 ml bottles
Box containing 10 × 200 ml bottles

Further information Niopam is one of the new generation of water soluble non-ionic contrast media. The development of this compound has led to considerable reduction in general toxicity particularly with regard to vascular endothelium and nervous tissues.

Product licence numbers
Niopam 200 0493/0065
Niopam 300 0493/0066
Niopam 370 0493/0067

NORISEN* ▼

Presentation Norisen is an aluminium adsorbed allergen extract for the specific hyposensitisation of patients sensitive to inhaled allergens or stinging insects. The extracts are suspended in normal saline containing 0.4% phenol as preservative, and their strength is expressed in protein nitrogen units (PNU).

Each treatment set is individually formulated and consists of 3 vials in graded strength as follows:

Vial 1 (Green Label) 100 PNU per ml
Vial 2 (Blue Label) 1,000 PNU per ml
Vial 3 (Red Label) 10,000 PNU per ml

Each maintenance set consists of one Vial 3 (Red Label).

The following allergen extracts are available:

POLLENS
Grasses: Grass Mix (Cocksfoot, Meadow Grass, Rye Grass, Tall Fescue, Timothy, Yorkshire Fog).
Barley, Maize, Oat (Cult.), Rye, Wheat.

Weeds: Weed Mix (Dandelion, Mugwort, Nettle, Pellitory, Plantain).
Dandelion, Mugwort, Nettle, Plantain, Pellitory.

Trees: Tree Mix (Early Blossoming) [Alder, Elm, Hazel, Poplar, Willow].
Tree Mix (Mid-Blossoming) [Beech, Birch, Oak, Plane].
Alder, Ash, Beech, Birch, Elder, Elm, False Acacia, Hazel, Oak, Plane, Poplar, Sycamore, Willow.

Flowers: Flower Mix (Aster, Chrysanthemum, Dahlia, Golden Rod, Marguerite [Daisy]).
Aster, Chrysanthemum, Dahlia, Golden Rod, Marguerite [Daisy].

OTHER ALLERGENS
Moulds: Fungi Mix I (Alternaria, Botrytis, Cladosporium, Curvularia, Fusarium, Helminthosporium).
Fungi Mix II (Aspergillus, Mucor, Pencillium, Pullularia, Rhizopus, Serpula).
Alternaria, Aspergillus, Botrytis, Candida, Chaetomium, Cladosporium, Curvularia, Fusarium, Helminthos-porium, Mucor, Neurospora, Penicillium, Pullularia, Phoma, Rhizopus, Serpula (Dry Rot), Sporobolomyces, Trichophyton, Ustilago.

Epithelia: Feather Mix (Duck, Goose, Chicken).
Budgerigar, Cat, Cow, Dog, Golden Hamster, Guinea Pig, Horse, Rabbit, Sheep's Wool.

Other inhalants: D. pteronyssinus (House Dust Mite), House Dust, Hay Dust, Rye Flour, Wheat Flour.

Stinging insects: Bee, Hornet, Wasp.
The extracts of stinging insects are available either individually or mixed with other stinging insect extracts, but may not be mixed with other allergen extracts.

The constituents of a course of treatment are determined by the allergist from the case history and the skin test reactions and indicated on the chart submitted with the order, and will be dependent upon the number of + signs against each allergen extract.

Where a patient is diagnosed as being extremely sensitive, a vial containing a special diluted extract of 10 PNU per ml can be supplied and should be administered before starting the treatment set.

Uses To hyposensitise those patients who have been shown to be sensitive to certain allergens as a result of case history and confirmation by skin testing.

Dosage and administration The dosage schedule, appropriate to the course of injections to be given, is enclosed with each treatment set. Detailed instructions on administration and the precautions that should be adopted are also supplied.

The injections must be given by the subcutaneous route only. As the allergens are slowly released from the aluminium depot, the interval between injections should be at least seven days and not more than two weeks. Before administration the vial must be shaken thoroughly so as to disperse the allergen suspension homogeneously. The course of hyposensitisation must commence with the lowest strength vial and the smallest injection from that vial.

For patients who are sensitive to seasonal allergens, the injections should be administered pre-seasonally and the course completed just before the particular allergens become airborne. For patients who are sensitive to perennial allergens the course of injections may be commenced at any time of the year.

Each course of treatment must be commenced using the initial three vial set, and one of the following dosage schedules should be followed, depending on the sensitivity of the patient. Where a patient suffers with severe symptoms, and has a large reaction to skin testing, it is advisable to start on the very sensitive dosage schedule while, in certain cases, e.g. for children under fourteen years of age and for extemely sensitive patients, the initial course should be preceded by a special dilution vial. Where the sensitivity of the patient is only considered to be average or mild, the mildly sensitive schedule set out on the next page may be used.

When a set contains *D.pteronyssinus*, the dose administered should not contain more than 1000 PNU *D.pteronyssinus* extract.

Where a patient on the very sensitive course has reached the third injection (0.25 ml) from the No. 3 vial without any adverse reaction, however small, then the two further injections from the No. 3 vial may be administered, providing, in the case of seasonal allergens, that there is sufficient time before the pollination season.

Vial	Very sensitive schedule (ml)	PNU	Mildly sensitive schedule (ml)	PNU
1	0.10	(10)	0.25	(25)
(Green Label)	0.20	(20)	0.50	(50)
100 PNU/ml	0.40	(40)		
	0.80	(80)		
2	0.15	(150)	0.10	(100)
(Blue Label)	0.30	(300)	0.30	(300)
1,000 PNU/ml	0.60	(600)	0.70	(700)
3	0.10	(1,000)	0.15	(1,500)
(Red Label)	0.15	(1,500)	0.25	(2,500)
10,000 PNU/ml	0.25	(2,500)	0.50	(5,000)
	(0.50)	(5,000)	1.00	(10,000)
	(1.00)	(10,000)		

Maintenance therapy for perennial allergens consists of repeating the top dose achieved on the above schedule at four to six week intervals for up to one year, commencing maintenance injections within six weeks of completing the course. Where seasonal allergens are involved it is recommended that hyposensitisation is carried out pre-seasonally for three successive years, using a three vial treatment set for each year. Where a patient has commenced on the very sensitive schedule, the mildly sensitive schedule should be administered on the second year and the mildly sensitive schedule repeated for the third year.

Where a slightly greater period than that recommended between injection occurs, the previous injection of the course should be repeated or in the case of maintenance injections, a reduced dose should first be given before continuing with the course. Where a considerable period has elapsed between injections, the initial treatment should be reduced further, or, in the case of a maintenance course, the initial treatment set should be repeated before attempting any further maintenance therapy.

A separate dosage schedule is provided with treatment sets containing extracts of stinging insects.

Contra-indications, warnings, etc

Contra-indications: Patients suffering from an acute infectious condition, or who are pregnant, particularly in the first trimester, should not be given a course of hyposensitisation. This also applies to patients during an acute attack of asthma, when 24 hours should be allowed to elapse before commencing the course of injections.

Precautions: Side-effects are relatively rare following the administration of hyposensitisation with Norisen extracts. It is recommended that patients should not eat a heavy meal immediately before the injections are given, and they should remain in the surgery for 20 minutes following the administration of each injection. It is recommended that they should not perform any physically strenuous work for several hours after an injection. Adrenaline Injection BP must be available whenever allergen extracts are administered.

Injections of Norisen must be administered only by the subcutaneous route and must not be injected into a blood vessel. The vial of extract must be shaken well before use, and care should be taken that the treatment is always commenced with the lowest strength vial and the smallest injection from that vial (see under Dosage and Administration). The interval beween injections must be at least one but not more than two weeks in the case of treatment sets, and maintenance set injections

should be given at intervals of not less than four weeks and not more than six weeks.

With seasonal allergens, the course of injections should be completed approximately three weeks before the pollens become airborne. In any event, pre-seasonal injections must be terminated before the pollination season commences.

Side-effects and adverse reactions: The occurrence of side-effects is rare, and any which occur normally take a mild course. Local swelling and pain which may appear several hours after the injection has been given can be blocked by oral or parenteral administration of anti-histamines.

If there are severe local reactions shortly after the injection, a tourniquet should be applied to the arm above the location of the injection and Adrenaline Injection BP should be injected subcutaneously in the vicinity of the injection site and, if necessary, adrenaline injection should be injected into the other arm as well. The tourniquet can then be released slowly and the patient kept under observation until the reaction has passed. For the next injection of the course, the same injection as caused the reaction may be repeated, or, if the reaction was very severe, the next lower dosage of the course should be repeated before proceeding with the increases in dosage.

A severe general reaction may require the subcutaneous injection of Adrenaline Injection BP which can be repeated if necessary. It may also be necessary to administer antihistamines and/or corticosteroids parenterally if so required.

Pharmaceutical precautions Norisen extracts should be stored between 2° and 8°C. The extracts must not be allowed to freeze.

Use aseptic precautions throughout. If the product is to be kept for more than 4 hours after withdrawing the first dose, the aseptic precautions taken must be sufficient to exclude the risk of microbial contamination.

Legal category POM.

Package quantities Each treatment set consists of three colour coded vials in graded strength numbered No. 1 (green label), No. 2 (blue label), No. 3 (red label). Each maintenance set consists of one No. 3 (red label) vial. All Norisen sets contain a supply of needle-attached syringes for each injection of the course, together with complete instructions on administration and a dosage schedule appropriate to the course of hyposensitisation to be administered.

Where a special dilution vial has been requested this is included in the treatment set and has an orange label.

Further information A Norisen set may be obtained by first completing a Norisen order form ensuring that those allergens that are to be included in the vaccine are clearly marked on the chart. The order form is then taken to a retail chemist or pharmacy together with the appropriate prescription, and the pharmacist then orders the set direct from E. Merck Ltd. All orders are acknowledged and delivery will normally take place within four weeks. Supplies of order forms and skin testing solutions may be obtained from E. Merck Ltd.

Product licence numbers 0493/0037

NORISEN* GRASS ▼

Presentation Norisen Grass is an aluminium adsorbed allergen extract of grass pollens (Cocksfoot, Meadow Grass, Rye Grass, Tall Fescue, Timothy and Yorkshire Fog) for the specific hyposensitisation of patients sensitive to grass pollens. The extract is suspended in normal saline containing 0.4% phenol as a preservative, and its strength is expressed in protein nitrogen units (PNU).

Each treatment set consists of three vials in graded strength as follows:

Vial 1 (Green Label)   100 PNU/ml
Vial 2 (Blue Label)   1,000 PNU/ml
Vial 3 (Red Label)   10,000 PNU/ml

Uses To hyposensitise those patients who are sensitive to grass pollen allergens and who suffer from hay fever.

Dosage and administration Two alternative dosage schedules are enclosed with each treatment set together with detailed instructions on administration and the precautions that should be adopted.

The injections must be given by the subcutaneous route only. As the allergens are slowly released from the aluminium depot, the interval between injections should be at least seven days and not more than two weeks. Before administration the vial must be shaken thoroughly so as to disperse the allergen suspension homogeneously. The course of hyposensitisation must commence with the lowest strength vial and the smallest injection from that vial.

The injections should be administered pre-seasonally and the course completed just before the grass pollens become airborne. This normally occurs at the end of May in the south of England, although the pollination may occur two weeks later in the north of England and Scotland.

The dosage schedule that should be followed will depend on the sensitivity of the patient. Where a patient suffers with severe symptoms, it is advisable to start on the very sensitive dosage schedule while, in certain cases, e.g. for children under fourteen years of age and for extremely sensitive patients, the initial course may be preceded by a special dilution vial, obtainable direct from E. Merck Ltd. Where the sensitivity of the patient is only considered to be average or mild, the mildly sensitive schedule set out below may be used.

Vial	Very sensitive schedule (ml)	PNU	Mildly sensitive schedule (ml)	PNU
1	0.10	(10)	0.25	(25)
(green label)	0.20	(20)	0.50	(50)
100 PNU/ml	0.40	(40)		
	0.80	(80)		
2	0.15	(150)	0.10	(100)
(blue label)	0.30	(300)	0.30	(300)
1,000 PNU/ml	0.60	(600)	0.70	(700)
3	0.10	(1,000)	0.15	(1,500)
(red label)	0.15	(1,500)	0.25	(2,500)
10,000 PNU/ml	0.25	(2,500)	0.50	(5,000)
	(0.50)	(5,000)	1.00	(10,000)
	(1.00)	(10,000)		

Where a patient on the very sensitive course has reached the third injection (0.25 ml) from the No. 3 vial without any adverse reaction, however small, then the two further injections from the No. 3 vial may be administered, providing that there is sufficient time before the pollination season.

It is recommended that hyposensitisation for grass pollen allergy is carried out pre-seasonally for three successive years, using a new Norisen Grass set for each year of treatment. Where a patient has commenced on the very sensitive schedule, the mildly sensitive schedule should be administered on the second year and the mildly sensitive schedule repeated for the third year.

Where a slightly greater period than that recommended between injections occurs, the previous injection of the course should be repeated. Where a considerable period has elapsed between injections, the next injection of the course should be reduced further.

Contra-indications, warnings, etc

Contra-indications: Patients suffering from an acute infectious condition, or who are pregnant, particularly in the first trimester, should not be given a course of hyposensitisation. This also applies to patients during an acute attack of asthma, when 24 hours should be allowed to elapse before commencing the course of injections.

Precautions: Side-effects are relatively rare following the administration of hyposensitisation with Norisen Grass extracts. It is recommended that patients should not eat a heavy meal immediately before the injections are given, and they should remain in the surgery for 20 minutes following the administration of each injection. It is recommended that they should not perform any physically strenuous work for several hours after an injection. Adrenaline Injection BP must be available whenever allergen extracts are administered.

Injections of Norisen Grass must be administered only by the subcutaneous route and must not be injected into a blood vessel. The vial of extract must be shaken well before use, and care should be taken that the treatment is always commenced with the lowest strength vial and the smallest injection from that vial (see under Dosage and Administration).

The interval between injections must be at least one but not more than two weeks, and the course of injections should be completed approximately three weeks before the grass pollens become airborne. In any event, injections of Norisen Grass must be terminated before the grass pollen season commences.

Side-effects and adverse reactions: The occurrence of side-effects is rare, and any which occur normally take a mild course. Local swelling and pain which may appear several hours after the injection has been given can be blocked by oral or parenteral administration of antihistamines.

If there are severe local reactions shortly after the injection, a tourniquet should be applied to the arm above the location of the injection and Adrenaline Injection BP should be injected subcutaneously in the vicinity of the injection site, and, if necessary, adrenaline solution should be injected into the other arm as well. The tourniquet can then be released slowly and the patient kept under observation until the reaction has passed. For the next injection of the course, the same injection as caused the reaction may be repeated, or, if the reaction was very severe, the next lower dosage of the course should be repeated before proceeding with the increases in dosage.

A severe general reaction may require the subcutaneous injection of Adrenaline Injection BP which can be repeated if necessary. It may also be necessary to administer antihistamines and/or corticosteroids parenterally if so required.

Pharmaceutical precautions Norisen Grass extracts should be stored between 2° and 8°C. The extracts must not be allowed to freeze.

Use aseptic precautions throughout. If the product is to be kept for more than 4 hours after withdrawing the first dose, the aseptic precautions taken must be sufficient to exclude the risk of microbial contamination.

Legal category POM.

Package quantities Each Norisen Grass set consists of three colour coded vials in graded strength numbered No. 1 (green label), No. 2 (blue label), No. 3 (red label). All Norisen sets contain sufficient needle-attached syringes for each injection of the course, together with complete instructions on administration and a dosage schedule (see under Dosage and Administration).

Further information Norisen Grass extracts are prepared by a process which avoids the use of pyridine, a solvent known to have a denaturing effect on allergen source materials. Thus the nature of the original allergic substance is preserved in the extract, and the risk of toxic effects is reduced. The allergens are slowly released from the site of the injection, and the dosage itself is completely flexible and may be modified for each individual patient.

Norisen Grass is immediately available from stock.

Where the patient is suspected of being allergic to allergens other than grass, the Merck range of skin testing solutions may be used to confirm the diagnosis and a specific Norisen treatment set prescribed.

Product licence number 0493/0048.

NUTRIZYM*

Presentation A white, oblong, double sugar-coated tablet. Each white, double-coated tablet contains:

Pancreatin BP	400 mg
Lipase	10,000 Units
Protease	560 Units
Amylase	10,000 Units
Ox bile	30 mg
Bromelains	50 mg

Uses Fibrocystic disease of the pancreas, chronic pancreatitis, steatorrhoea and other pancreatic deficiency states.

Dosage and administration *Adults:* 1–2 tablets during or after meals. In severe cases dosage may be increased. Up to six tablets after meals have been administered.

Children: 1–2 tablets to be taken with meals and further tablets may be taken according to the degree of pancreatic exocrine insufficiency.

Tablets should be swallowed whole with water.

Contra-indications, warnings, etc There are no known contra-indications or precautions.

Side-effects: Very rarely hypersensitivity reactions may occur.

Pharmaceutical precautions Store below 25° C in tightly closed containers.

Legal category P.

Package quantities Container of 100 tablets.

Further information Each Nutrizym Tablet has an enteric-coated pancreatin core and a shell of bromelains. The bromelain-proteolytic enzymes are active within the pH range of pH 3 and pH 8 (even pH 2 for short periods) and therefore act without loss of enzymatic effectiveness both in the stomach and small intestine.

Product licence number 3894/5900.

OPTIMAX*

Presentation Optimax Tablets: Yellow capsule shaped film coated tablets each containing 500 mg L-Tryptophan, 5 mg Pyridoxine Hydrochloride, 10 mg Ascorbic acid, bearing the name OPTIMAX on one side and a break line on the other.

Optimax tablets are available without vitamins; they are of similar appearance and are marked OPTIMAX WV.

Optimax Powder: A chocolate-flavoured powder for mixing into a drink with warm milk or water. Each 6 g of powder contains 1 g L-Tryptophan, 10 mg Pyridoxine hydrochloride, 20 mg Ascorbic acid.

Uses Optimax is indicated for the relief of symptoms of mild to moderate depressive illness. Long term efficacy and safety of L-Tryptophan have not been established; therefore, it is recommended that L-Tryptophan be used for short term therapy with a review at three monthly intervals. For the treatment of more severe depressive illness Optimax may be administered with other antidepressant drugs.

Dosage and administration
Adults: The usual dose is two tablets, three times daily or one sachet three times daily (equivalent to 3 g L-Tryptophan daily); for some patients up to 6 g L-Tryptophan may be required. There is no evidence to suggest that dosage in the elderly should be different.

Children: Not recommended.

When used in combination with other antidepressants it may be necessary to adjust the dosage of either component.

Contra-indications, warnings, etc
Contra-indications: No absolute contra-indications known.

Precautions and Drug Interactions: Where Optimax is combined with an MAO Inhibitor the side effects of the latter may be enhanced.

In patients taking Optimax in conjunction with phenothiazines or benzodiazepines there have been isolated reports of sexual disinhibition.

Pyridoxine should not be administered to patients undergoing treatment with L-Dopa.

L-Tryptophan is not advised, except for relatively short periods, in patients with active bladder disease or known bladder lesions.

Warnings and Adverse Effects: L-Tryptophan may produce drowsiness. Patients should be warned of the possible hazard when driving or operating machinery.

In some patients Optimax may cause a slight feeling of nausea which usually disappears within 2 or 3 days. Such nausea can be minimised by giving Optimax after food. Other adverse reactions include headache and lightheadedness.

Safety in pregnancy has not been established.

Overdosage: Drowsiness and vomiting may occur; supportive measures should be employed.

Pharmaceutical precautions Store in a cool dry place.

Legal category POM.

Package quantities *Optimax Tablets:* Securitainers of 100 and 500.

Optimax Powder: Cartons of 100 sachets.

Further information L-Tryptophan, one of the essential amino acids, is the major precursor of the brain amine 5-Hydroxytryptamine (5-HT). There is convincing evidence that levels of 5-HT are depleted in the CNS of depressed patients.

Abnormal tryptophan metabolism may occur in patients who are pyridoxine deficient. Such deficiency may occur in women taking oral contraceptives.

For some patients it may be beneficial to prescribe tablets for the morning and midday dose and powder for the night time dose.

Product licence numbers

Optimax Tablets	0493/5903R
Without vitamins	0493/5900R
Optimax Powder	0493/5902R

PENDRAMINE*

Presentation Tablets each containing 125 mg or 250 mg D-penicillamine base. The 125 mg tablets are white, elongated, film coated with bisecting score on one side, and have a length of 11 mm and a width of 5.5 mm. The 250 mg tablets are white, elongated, film coated with bisecting score on one side, debossed HB on the same side, and have a length of 16 mm and a width of 7 mm.

Uses Pendramine is indicated for the treatment of severe active rheumatoid arthritis, Wilson's disease, cystinuria and heavy metal poisoning, active chronic hepatitis, primary biliary cirrhosis.

Dosage and administration For oral administration:
(i) *Severe active rheumatoid arthritis: Adults:* A dose of 125–250 mg daily for the initial 4 week period, then increasing by similar amounts at intervals of not less than four weeks. The ultimate maintenance dose will depend on the response obtained in individual patients and is usually 500–750 mg in divided doses. Improvement may not occur for some months.

A few patients may require up to 2000 mg daily to obtain benefit.

The minimum maintenance dose to achieve suppression of symptoms should be used. Treatment should be discontinued if no benefit is obtained within 12 months.

When clinical assessment shows that suppression of disease activity has been achieved, the dose should be kept at this maintenance level for six months, thereafter reducing the daily dose by 250 mg at intervals of two or three months. Relapse may occur following withdrawal or when an inadequate dose level is reached, usually within three months, but most patients respond to further courses of Pendramine.

Children: 15–20 mg/kg/day is considered appropriate in the majority of cases. It is suggested that the initial dose is lower and increased at four weekly intervals over a period of three to six months.

(ii) *Wilson's Disease:*
D-penicillamine is a copper-chelating agent, and is most effectively used in conjunction with a low-copper diet (below 1 mg of copper per day).

Adults: 1500 to 2000 mg daily in divided doses, to be taken 30 minutes before food. The dose may be reduced to 750–1000 mg daily when disease control is achieved as evidenced by urinary copper excretion. (Twenty-four hour urine samples should be examined at 3-monthly intervals). A dose of 2000 mg daily should not be continued for more than one year.

Children: Up to 20 mg per kg body weight daily in divided doses before food. Maximum dose 500 mg/day.

(iii) *Cystinuria:* Prevention and treatment of cystine stones.

Treatment of stones: Adults: For the treatment of cystine stone, 750 mg daily in divided doses and especially at bedtime, increasing to 1500–2000 mg daily. The dose is adjusted to maintain urine levels of cystine below 100 mg per day. Maintain adequate fluid intake of 3 litres/day to provide a urine flow of 2 ml/min.

Children: Up to 30 mg per kg body weight daily in divided doses and especially at bedtime. The dose should be adjusted to maintain urine cystine levels below 100 mg/day.

Prophylaxis: Adults: (No history of stone formation but a cystine output in excess of 300 mg per day) 250–750 mg at night before retiring. The dose is adjusted to maintain overnight urine cystine levels below 100 mg/day.

Fluid intake should not be less than 3 litres/day.

Safety in pregnancy is not yet established but if treatment is unavoidable dosage should not exceed a maximum of 1000 mg/24 hours.

Children: Paediatric dosage not yet established.

(iv) *Heavy Metal Poisoning* (Lead): *Adults:* Daily oral dose of 1500–2000 mg in divided doses until urinary lead is stabilised at 0.5 mg/day.

Children: 20–25 mg per kg body weight daily in divided doses before food.

(v) *Active Chronic Hepatitis: Adults:* Pendramine is intended for the maintenance treatment of active chronic hepatitis. The diagnosis should be based on a history of at least three months duration with features of chronic aggressive hepatitis, with or without cirrhosis. Treatment with Pendramine should not be commenced until the disease process has been brought under control, initially by treatment with corticosteroids, e.g. 30 mg prednisone daily, some times with 75 mg azathioprine daily added to the regime. Disease control should be evidenced by biochemical analysis of liver function to include evaluation of serum bilirubin and transaminase activity.

Pendramine therapy should be commenced with 500 mg daily, in divided doses, increasing gradually over three months to the maintenance dose of 1250 mg daily. Concurrently, the dosage of corticosteroids should be reduced and phased out over a three-month period. Throughout therapy, liver function tests should be carried out at suitable intervals for assessment of the disease status.

Children: Not recommended.

(vi) *Primary Biliary Cirrhosis: Adults:* Diagnosis should be on the basis of mitochondrial antibody in the serum and a histological picture compatible with primary biliary cirrhosis. The presence of portal hypertension, manifested by splenomegaly, oesophageal varices, or both, is not a contraindication although patients with a history of bleeding from varices or of hepatic encephalopathy should be excluded.

Dosage should be started at 250 mg daily, increasing

weekly to the maintenance dose of 750–1000 mg daily, in divided doses.

Most patients with primary biliary cirrhosis have raised liver-copper concentrations, frequently above the level found in untreated Wilson's disease. Pendramine promotes a reduction in liver-copper, and a lowering of the maintenance dose is a reasonable step in patients whose liver-copper levels return to normal.

Children: Not recommended.

Contra-indications, warnings, etc
Contra-indications: Renal insufficiency. Lupus erythematosus. Hypersensitivity to D-penicillamine particularly if nephrotic syndrome or bone marrow depression has previously occurred.

Precautions: Known sensitivity to penicillamine. Throughout pregnancy.

Penicillamine should not be used in patients who are receiving concurrent gold therapy, antimalarial or cytotoxic drugs, oxyphenbutazone or phenylbutazone since these drugs have a propensity to cause similar serious haematologic and/or renal adverse reactions.

Establish the lowest effective dose of D-penicillamine by quantitative amino acid chromatography on urine. Urine protein estimations should be carried out initially weekly for the first three months of therapy and thereafter monthly. Renal function should be assessed monthly for 6 months and 3 monthly thereafter.

The observation of proteinuria necessitates repeated quantitative estimations. Heavy or steadily increasing proteinuria or significant haematuria necessitates withdrawal of Pendramine.

With the exception of Wilson's disease patients' (see later) platelet and white cell counts must be normal before commencing treatment. Because of the risk of blood dyscrasias and renal disturbances, full blood counts and urine examinations are essential during treatment. Weekly tests are recommended after each increase in dose as well as during the first eight weeks of therapy to monitor thrombocytopenia and neutropenia then monthly when dosage regimes have been stabilised.

Platelet counts below 120,000/cu.mm or leucocyte counts below 2,500/cu.mm necessitate withdrawal of D-penicillamine with resumption at a reduced dosage when counts return to normal. Recurrence of thrombocytopenia or leucopenia are an indication for cessation of treatment.

A low platelet or white cell count is not a contra-indication to commence treatment of Wilson's disease. Treatment should be discontinued however, if a low initial count falls further and/or excessive bruising or petechial haemorrhages occur.

Iron deficiency may occur in menstruating women. Should oral iron therapy be required it should not be given within 2 hours of taking penicillamine.

Allergic phenomena occurring early, unless severe, respond to cyproheptadine and temporary reductions of dose of D-penicillamine. Copper supplements may be necessary for alleviating taste impairment when treating conditions other than Wilson's disease.

Side Effects and Adverse Reactions: Both the frequency and severity of many side-effects and adverse reactions to D-penicillamine are found to be dose-related, hence the importance of initiating therapy at low doses and gradually increasing the quantity of drug given to the optimum level.

Nausea and vomiting may occur.

D-penicillamine may cause allergic reactions such as urticaria and erythema accompanied by hyperpyrexia. Transient rashes and fever may occur early in therapy; if persistent, temporary withdrawal of treatment with or without a short course of steroids may be necessary. Penicillamine may be reintroduced at a lower dosage. If steroids are given, penicillamine should be reintroduced before steroid withdrawal.

A later rash, which has been called both 'acquired epidermolysis bullosa' and 'penicillamine dermopathy' may occur, and also elastosis perforans serpiginosa – perhaps up to 2 years after treatment and may necessitate discontinuation of treatment.

Goodpastures syndrome, haemolytic anaemia and anorexia have been reported.

Other disorders of later onset and attributed to D-penicillamine are rheumatoid-like reactions, stomatitis and taste impairment. Reversible loss of taste occurs frequently. Reactions involving the appearance of thrombocytopenia, neutropenia or proteinuria may occur, particularly with higher dose levels. Less common are nephrotic syndrome and haematuria, purpura and increased skin friability due to increased collagen. Haematuria is rare, but if it occurs, treatment should be stopped immediately.

Serious complications include myasthenia gravis, pemphigus, nephrotic syndrome, Stevens-Johnson-like syndrome and lupus erythematosus. Deaths from agranulocytosis and aplastic anaemia have been recorded.

Pendramine should not be given concurrently with iron or other heavy metals with which it may form complexes.

Warnings: The safety of penicillamine in pregnancy has not been established. It has been shown to be teratogenic in rats when given in doses several times higher than those recommended for human use.

In the treatment of rheumatoid arthritis, response to Pendramine is often slow and the use of existing analgesics, anti-inflammatories or steroids should be continued and later gradually withdrawn, subject to patient improvement.

Treatment of Overdosage: Treatment of overdosage is symptomatic and withdrawal of the drug is necessary if serious side effects as mentioned above occur.

Pharmaceutical precautions Store in a dry place below 25°C. Keep containers tightly closed.

Legal category POM.

Package quantities
Tablets: 125 mg, plastic bottles of 100
Tablets: 250 mg, plastic bottles of 100

Further information Pendramine may be considered as an alternative to prednisone in the treatment of active chronic hepatitis when the latter drug causes complications such as diabetes, osteoporosis, etc. Occasionally, patients with rheumatoid arthritis who have responded to a particular dose begin to relapse. Most of these will respond to a dose increase which should be gradual.

Product licence numbers
Pendramine 125 mg 0493/0080
Pendramine 250 mg 0493/0081

PERIFUSIN*

Presentation A clear, slightly yellow, sterile, pyrogen-free solution for intravenous use through a peripheral vein, containing pure L-amino acids with added electrolytes.

Active Ingredients: g/litre
L-Glutamic acid	5.94
L-Alanine	3.96
L-Proline	4.62
Glycine	6.60
L-Arginine	2.64
L-Histidine	0.66
L-Valine	0.99
L-Tryptophan	0.33
L-Threonine	0.66
L-Phenylalanine	1.45
L-Methionine	1.39
L-Lysine HCl	1.65
L-Leucine	1.45
L-Isoleucine	1.06
Sodium hydroxide (100%)	1.60
Potassium hydroxide (100%)	1.68
Magnesium acetate $4H_2O$	1.07
L-malic acid	3.00

Electrolytes	*mmol/l*	*mg/l*
Na^+	40	920
K^+	30	1,171
Mg^{++}	5	121
Cl^-	9	320
Acetate$^-$	10.00	589
Malate$^-$	22.5	2,977
Total N g/litre	5.00	
Kcal/litre approximately	132	
pH	7.1	
Osmolality	376.5 mosm/kg	

Uses Perifusin which contains aminoacids in the optimum and balanced proportions with added electrolytes, is indicated for patients undergoing surgery and other cases of trauma in order to improve nitrogen balance and preserve muscle and visceral protein.

It improves patient tolerance to the catabolic phase of the post operative and post traumatic period and decreases susceptibility to complications.

Perifusin, being only slightly hypertonic, can be administered by intravenous infusion using a peripheral vein catheter.

Dosage and administration The amount of Perifusin to be administered daily is calculated according to individual patients' requirements of nitrogen, fluid, calories, etc. Adults should receive 0.8–1.6 g aminoacids/kg body weight daily. The average adult requirement is met by the infusion of 2–2½ litres of Perifusin per day. Children, pregnant women and post-operative patients, 1.6–2.0 g aminoacids/kg body weight daily. Newborn and premature infants, 2.0–3.0 g aminoacids/kg body weight daily.

Infusion rate 40–60 drops per minute (2–4 ml/kg/hr); it should not exceed 4 ml/kg/hr. Optimal utilisation is achieved when the daily dose is given in a continuous infusion over 24 hours. In patients who are unable to tolerate continuous infusions, two infusion periods of four or six hours each per day are recommended.

Contra-indications, warnings, etc Perifusin is contra-indicated in patients suffering shock, hyperkalaemia, severe infections (e.g. septicaemia), severe disturbances of liver or kidney function and disturbance of aminoacid metabolism: its effects should be carefully controlled when given to patients who tend towards elevated serum potassium or urea levels. Too rapid an infusion may result in renal losses, and nausea in sensitive patients.

Perifusin is not suitable for severely malnourished patients where total parenteral nutrition will be required. Shock should be treated before administration of Perifusin.

A pre-existing deficiency of vitamins and, in particular, folic acid and Vitamin B_{12} may become clinically evident during intravenous nutrition with aminoacids. Regular checks of the patients' Vitamin B_{12} status and folate demand are therefore recommended. Prophylactic administration of adequate vitamins should be given if required.

As with similar solutions which do not contain fat, the possible occurrence of hypophosphataemia should be monitored.

Pharmaceutical precautions Store between 15° and 25°C. The solution of Perifusin should be clear at all times before infusion. Store away from light. If a precipitate or severe discolouration occurs, discard. Addition of drugs to the bottle of amino acid solution or giving set should be avoided.

Legal category POM.

Package quantities 1 litre glass bottles, 6 bottles per case.

Further information Nil.

Product licence number 0493/0082.

SEPTOPAL* CHAINS

Presentation Methylmethacrylate-methylacrylate copolymer (PMMA) Beads (7 mm in diameter) each containing Gentamicin sulphate 7.5 mg (corresponding to 4.5 mg of Gentamicin base) and 20 mg of Zirconium dioxide as X-ray medium.

Chains consisting of 10 or 30 beads threaded on multiple-thread surgical wire.

Uses Gentamicin is a proven broad spectrum antibiotic active against both gram-positive and gram-negative organisms. Following insertion of the Chains, Gentamicin is released gradually from the PMMA beads over a prolonged period and the high bactericidal concentrations of the antibiotic reached at the site of infection enable the infection to be controlled, or provide protection against infection when used prophylactically.

Septopal Chains are indicated for short term and longer term administration in bone infection, e.g. chronic forms of osteomyelitis (post traumatic, haematogenous), infected pseudoarthroses, infected osteosyntheses.

Preventive treatment of potentially infected bone injuries.

Septopal Chains are also indicated for the prophylaxis and therapy of soft tissue infections (short term application only). Prophylactic indications include operative procedures on the small or large bowel and perineum, e.g. colonic resection, abdominoperineal resections and other procedures where the incidence of post operative wound infections may present a problem.

Therapeutic indications include post traumatic infections, peritonitis and abscesses of any origin.

Dosage and administration Septopal Chains have been sterilised in ethylene oxide. They are contained in a triple sachet. The two outer sachets are opened (aluminium covering followed by the non-sterile peel-off pack) and the chain in the inner, sterile sachet is then removed under aseptic conditions.

The cavity resulting after thorough surgical removal of the infected bone tissue sequestra is completely filled up with Septopal Chains; the number of Chains used will depend on the size of the cavity. Usually 1–3 Chains are inserted but up to 5 Chains have been used. Inserted Chains will be completely enclosed by primary wound closure.

It is recommended that the 10 bead chain is used for smaller cavities in bone and for smaller incision wounds and operations.

Septopal Chains may be used as follows:

1. *Bone Infections*
a) *Short Term Application:* For the implantation of Chains, it is recommended to take into account the direction in which the Chain will later be pulled out and to let the last bead project above the skin level in order that the Chain may be removed by careful, steady traction.

The Chains are in general removed 10–14 days following insertion and preferably not more than 10 days after the operation.

The less the Chains are fixed to connective tissue, the easier it is to remove them; this procedure is thus also less painful and more comfortable for the patient.

If the beads become fixed to connective tissue to an advanced extent, or if the traction of the beads is not adapted to the tissue conditions, one or several beads may rarely detach themselves from the multistranded wire or, in exceptional circumstances, the wire may break on the removal of the Chain. In such an event one should generally try to remove the single beads (together with the remaining wire). Should, however, extensive surgical procedures be necessary, the single beads may be left in the body, taking into consideration the comparative risk of reoperation.

b) *Longer Term Application:* If circumstances require it, the Chains may be implanted completely below the skin level, and removed by reoperation up to 3 months later. Control of local infection allows optimum conditions for subsequent surgical procedures, e.g. cancellous bone grafting.

2. *Soft Tissue Infections:* The application of chains is carried out as described under 1a above. In this indication, the chains are best removed by the sixth and the latest by the tenth day after the operation. In most cases it is advised that the chains are withdrawn gradually from about the second post insertion day.

Wherever possible, primary wound closure should be employed; this avoids excessive loss of secretion which would automatically reduce the Gentamicin concentration at the site of infection. An overflow drain can be employed only when considered necessary. Suction drainage is not employed but may be temporarily used in cases of obstructed wound secretion flow.

Contra-indications, warnings, etc There is no absolute contra-indication other than established intolerance of Gentamicin.

Since the beads are strung on surgical wire containing chrome and nickel, there is a potential for local sensitivity reactions to these metals.

Septopal can be used in all orthopaedic procedures where Gentamicin sensitive organisms are found to be present from routine bacteriological screening. Where resistant organisms are encountered to the standard 10 mcg disc test, a MIC determination is recommended.

In view of the high bactericidal Gentamicin concentration at the infection site, organisms found resistant to the standard 10 mcg sensitivity disc screen may in fact be sensitive and therefore results of such screening may not give a true reflection of clinical effectiveness.

In soft tissue, the chains should not be implanted intraperitoneally. If a wound is suspected of having an anaerobic infection or if anaerobic bacteria have been cultured, simultaneous systemic antibiotic treatment with appropriate antibiotics should be initiated.

Toxic effects due to the antibiotic are not anticipated since after use of Septopal Chains, barely detectable Gentamicin concentrations (no more than 0.5 mcg/ml) are found in serum for up to four days postoperatively following insertion of the Chains.

Pharmaceutical precautions Store at room temperature – do not freeze.

Septopal Chains should not be used beyond the expiry date (2 years).

Resterilisation of Septopal Chains should not be attempted under any circumstances.

Legal category POM.

Package quantities One Chain consisting of 10 or 30 beads threaded on surgical wire in a sterile inner sachet (peel-off pack).

Packs of 1 chain of 10 beads.
Packs of 1 Chain of 30 beads.
Packs of 5 Chains of 30 beads.

Further information Gentamicin is released in bactericidal concentrations at the site of infection, the flow of secretion during filling of the bone cavities is not inhibited and the biomechanics of the bone are not changed, granulation tissue grows into the hollow spaces between the beads during the healing process and only traces of the antibiotic are detectable in serum in spite of high local Gentamicin concentration. Local control of infection lessens the risk of secondary infection developing with subsequent bone grafting.

Product licence number 0493/0091.

TRIOSORBON*

Presentation A white soluble tasteless powder of high nutritional value which is readily absorbed and completely utilised. Triosorbon is packed in foil sachets containing 85 g of powder providing 400 kilocalories (1.67 MJ).

Triosorbon makes a palatable drink when mixed with water and it can be sprinkled over already prepared food.

The fat consists mainly of medium chain triglycerides.

The protein component is provided by a combination of whey protein, L-Cystine and Casein.

Carbohydrates are present in a well balanced mixture of mono, oligo and polysaccharides. The formulation is gluten free and virtually free of lactose.

Approximately 5 sachets of Triosorbon meet the adult daily nutritional requirements.

Composition: 100 g contains:

Protein	19 g
Nitrogen	3.05 g
Fat	19 g
Carbohydrates	56 g
Sodium 20 mmol	(0.46 g)
Potassium 20 mmol	(0.78 g)
Calcium 6 mmol	(0.24 g)
Magnesium 3.5 mmol	(0.085 g)
Phosphorus 9 mmol	(0.28 g)
Chloride 25 mmol	(0.9 g)

Additions of vitamins and other substances

Vitamin A	0.235 mg
Vitamin B_1	0.33 mg
Vitamin B_2	0.38 mg
Nicotinamide	4.24 mg
Vitamin B_6	0.52 mg
Vitamin B_{12}	0.71 mcg
Folic acid	94.1 mcg
Biotin	35.3 mcg
Pantothenic acid	1.29 mg
Vitamin C	21.2 mg
Vitamin D_3	2.36 mcg
Vitamin E	2.35 mg
Vitamin K_1	24.7 mcg
L-Cystine	300.0 mg
Ferrous sulphate, dried	13.25 mg
(Iron	4.24 mg)
Zinc Sulphate H_2O	9.7 mg
(Zinc	3.53 mg)
Copper Sulphate $5H_2O$	1.85 mg
(Copper	0.47 mg)
Manganese Sulphate H_2O	1.81 mg
(Manganese	0.59 mg)
Potassium Iodide	46.1 mcg
(Iodine	35.3 mcg)

Uses Triosorbon can be used as a complete diet or to supplement food intake, or as a tube feed (naso-gastric or via a jejunostomy) in diseases where normal ingestion is inadequate or impossible, e.g. short bowel syndrome, intractable malabsorption, pre-operative preparation of patients who are under-nourished, treatment for those with proven inflammatory bowel disease, treatment following total gastrectomy and dysphagia, bowel fistulae, anorexia nervosa. Not suitable as a sole source of nutrition for infants under one year or for children up to about five years.

Dosage and administration *Neonates and infants:* Up to one year 20 g of Triosorbon per kg body weight per day (1–2 sachets).

The calculated quantity is divided into 5–8 individual meals according to the age of the child.

Children and youths: They should receive 10–15 g Triosorbon per kg body weight per day (3–5 sachets).

Adults: Adults are given 7 g of Triosorbon per kg body weight per day (5 sachets).

Five sachets of Triosorbon meet the daily nutritional requirement approximately.

Dilution: One sachet of 85 g is mixed with 400 ml water.

Hints: It is recommended, particularly in bottle feeding and tube feeding, to follow the indicated dosage because of the hazards of hyperosmolar dehydration.

Triosorbon should not be cooked with meals but should be added to meals already prepared.

If indicated salt can be added.

Initially mix with a small amount of water into a smooth paste, then add the remainder of the water slowly.

Contra-indications, warnings, etc Not for intravenous use. Once Triosorbon has been mixed it should be used as soon as possible.

Pharmaceutical precautions Store in cool dry place.

Legal category No restrictions on sale or supply.

Package quantities Triosorbon is supplied in boxes containing 10 sachets of 85 g powder each.

Further information Borderline product.

Product licence number Not applicable.

TUTOPLAST* DURA

Presentation Tutoplast Dura is solvent dehydrated human dura mater in the form of absorbable collagen for homotransplantation. It is highly purified, free from antigens and enzymes, and sterilised by gamma irradiation.

Uses Tutoplast Dura may be used to effect a repair or closure in the following areas: Thoracic surgery, abdominal surgery, neurosurgery and urology.

Transplanted Tutoplast Dura provides the basis for the formation of endogenous connective tissue. Within a period of 3–4 months, about 85% of the transplant is absorbed and replaced by collagenous connective tissue. This endogenous tissue formation is contingent on the size of the transplant and the tissue reactivity in the surrounding transplant area.

Dosage and administration Tutoplast Dura, of suitable size for the area under transplantation, should be soaked in a sterile solution of 0.9% saline at room temperature for several minutes prior to use. This makes the Dura softer and easier to work with during surgery.

Contra-indications, warnings, etc
Contra-indication: Dura implantation is contra-indicated if local infection is present.

Pharmaceutical precautions Opened and unused material should be discarded.

Legal category POM.

Package quantities
1/1 calotte: pack containing 1 piece
1/2 calotte: pack containing 1 piece
4 × 5 cm: pack containing 2 pieces
1.5 × 3 cm: pack containing 5 pieces
2 × 10 cm: pack containing 2 pieces
4 × 10 cm: pack containing 1 piece
2 × 30 cm: pack containing 1 piece
Other sizes available on request from E Merck Ltd.

Further information Nil.

Product licence number 0493/0090.

UNGUENTUM MERCK*

Presentation Unguentum Merck is a stable emulsion system with a uniform distribution of fat and water (ambiphilic); thus it combines the properties of a) an oil in water emulsion (cream) and b) a water in oil emulsion (ointment), for use on dry or weeping conditions of the skin.

Composition:
Lipoid component: about 60%
Polyoxyethylene sorbitan fatty acid ester

Cetyl stearyl alcohol
Glycerin mono fatty acid ester
Propylene glycol
Paraffin hydrocarbons
Saturated neutral oil
Dispersed silicic acid
Sorbic acid
Water content: about 40%

Uses Unguentum Merck is to be used as a diluent for various topical corticosteroid formulations in those instances where a lower strength preparation is considered desirable by the physician and as a general base for extemporaneous dispensing.

Unguentum Merck has emollient properties and is recommended for the symptomatic treatment of dermatitis, nappy rash, ichthyosis, eczema, protection of raw and abraded skin areas, pruritus and related conditions where dry scaly skin is a problem, and as a pre-bathing emollient for dry/eczematous skin, to alleviate drying effects.

Dosage and administration *Administration:* A thin application of the cream should be gently massaged into the skin three times daily or at appropriate intervals.

When used as a protective cream Unguentum Merck should be applied sparingly to the affected areas of the skin before, or immediately after, exposure to a potentially harmful factor.

Contra-indications, warnings, etc Unguentum Merck should not be used for the treatment of patients sensitive to any of the ingredients.

Pharmaceutical precautions No special requirements.

Legal category P.

Package quantities Tubes of 50 g, 100 g. Jar of 900 g. 200 ml dispenser.

Further information Unguentum Merck contains no common allergens such as lanolin or parabens.

Product licence number 0493/0013.

UROMIRO* 300, 340, 380, 420
SODIUM UROMIRO* 300

Presentation Ampoules or bottles containing sterile aqueous solutions of varying strengths of meglumine and sodium iodamide.

Uromiro 300: Contains a 65% w/v concentration of the meglumine salt of iodamide equivalent to 30% iodine or 300 mg/ml.

Uromiro 340: Contains a concentration of 18.3% w/v meglumine iodamide and 43.4% w/v of sodium iodamide equivalent to 34% iodine or 340 mg/ml.

Uromiro 380: Contains a concentration of 70% w/v meglumine iodamide and 9.7% w/v sodium iodamide equivalent to 38% iodine or 380 mg/ml.

Uromiro 420: Contains a concentration of 40.8% w/v meglumine iodamide and 39.4% w/v sodium iodamide equivalent to 42% iodine or 420 mg/ml.

Sodium Uromiro 300: Contains a concentration of 52.66% w/v sodium iodamide equivalent to 30% iodine or 300 mg/ml.

Uses X-ray contrast media for the opacification of the vascular and renal systems, e.g. urography, cerebral angiography, peripheral arteriography, venography, op-

Intravenous Urography	Sodium Uromiro 300	Adults 40–80 ml	In severe renal failure the usual high dose methods of Urography should be applied (up to 1.5 ml/kg)
	Uromiro 300 Uromiro 340 Uromiro 380 Uromiro 420	Children 1 ml/kg	
Cerebral Angiography	Uromiro 300	Adults 8 ml Children 5–7 ml according to body size and age	
Angiocardiography	Uromiro 380 Uromiro 420	Adults 20–50 ml Children 1 ml/kg In both adults and children requiring frequent multiple injections, a total of 3–5 ml per kg should seldom be exceeded. Inject rapidly within 1–2 sec.	
Coronary Arteriography	Uromiro 380	Adults 5–8 ml per artery	
Peripheral Arteriography	Uromiro 300 Uromiro 340 Uromiro 380	Adults 20–30 ml Children according to body size and age	
Venography	Uromiro 300 Uromiro 340	Adults 20–30 ml Children according to body size and age	
Operative and T-tube Cholangiography	Uromiro 300	During the period of operation 10–15 ml of contrast medium are injected into the cystic duct or its stump by means of a fine needle. In the postoperative period this may be done through a T-tube left in situ at operation	
Aortography retrograde	Uromiro 380 Uromiro 420	Adults 20–40 ml Children according to body size and age	
Selective renal arteriography	Uromiro 380 Uromiro 420	Adults 8 ml Children according to body size and age	

erative and T-tube cholangiography, angiocardiography, coronary arteriography and aortography.

Dosage and administration See Table on previous page.

Elderly: Dosage as for adults.

Contra-indications, warnings, etc
Contra-indications: Proven or suspected hypersensitivity to iodine-containing preparations of this type.

Warnings, side-effects: Care should be exercised in patients with severe systemic disease, in hyperthyroidism, in allergic subjects and in myelomatosis; patients with this condition should not be exposed to dehydration.

X-ray examination of women should if possible be conducted during the pre-ovulation phase of the menstrual cycle and should be avoided during pregnancy; also since it has not been demonstrated that Uromiro is safe for use in pregnant women, it should be administered only if the procedure is considered essential by the physician.

Use of the product may give rise to side-effects including anaphylactoid or shock-like manifestations with nausea, vomiting, widespread reddening of the skin and heat sensation, headache, and sometimes coryza; oedema of the larynx, fever, sweating, asthenia, dizziness, pallor, dyspnoea, and moderate hypotension. Skin rashes of various description may occur in some patients.

More severe reactions involving the cardiovascular system may call for emergency treatment. Appropriate resuscitative measures should be immediately available. No other drugs should be mixed with the contrast medium.

Fluid intake should not be limited in neonates and small children.

Before using hypertonic contrast media any abnormalities of water and electrolyte balance should be corrected.

Pharmaceutical precautions Store away from light.

Legal category POM.

Package quantities
Uromiro 300:
Box containing 10 × 50 ml bottles.

Uromiro 340:
Box containing 5 × 20 ml ampoules.
Box containing 10 × 50 ml bottles.

Uromiro 380:
Box containing 10 × 50 ml bottles.

Uromiro 420:
Box containing 10 × 50 ml bottles.

Sodium Uromiro 300:
Box containing 10 × 50 ml bottles.

Further information Nil.

Product licence numbers
Uromiro 300   0493/0086
Uromiro 340   0493/0087
Uromiro 380   0493/0088
Uromiro 420   0493/0089
Sodium Uromiro 300   0493/0085

*Trade Mark

Merck Sharp & Dohme Limited
Hertford Road
Hoddesdon
Hertfordshire EN11 9BU

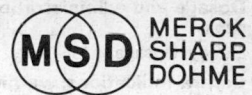

ALDOMET*

Presentation Yellow, film-coated tablets containing Methyldopa BP equivalent to the following amounts of anhydrous methyldopa: 125 mg (marked 'ALDOMET MSD 135'), 250 mg (marked 'ALDOMET MSD 401'), or 500 mg (marked 'ALDOMET MSD 516').

Fruit-flavoured, oral suspension containing 250 mg of methyldopa per 5 ml. The oral suspension contains sodium metabisulphite as preservative

Injection, ampoules containing, per millilitre, 50 mg Methyldopate Hydrochloride BP, as a colourless solution.

Uses Hypertension. Aldomet Injection is indicated for hypertension when parenteral medication is required. Treatment of acute hypertensive crises may be initiated with Aldomet Injection when an immediate effect is not necessary.

Dosage and administration *Oral therapy: Adults: Initial dosage:* Usually 250 mg two or three times a day, for two days.

Adjustment: Usually adjusted at intervals of not less than two days, until an adequate response is obtained. The maximum recommended daily dosage is 3 g.

Many patients experience sedation for two or three days when therapy with Aldomet is started or when the dose is increased. When increasing the dosage, therefore, it may be desirable to increase the evening dose first.

General considerations: Methyldopa is largely excreted by the kidney and patients with impaired renal function may respond to smaller doses.

Withdrawal of Aldomet is followed by return of hypertension, usually within 48 hours. This is not complicated generally by an overshoot of blood pressure.

Therapy with Aldomet may be initiated in most patients already on treatment with other antihypertensive agents by terminating these antihypertensive medications gradually if required (see manufacturer's recommendations on stopping these drugs). Following such previous antihypertensive therapy, Aldomet should be limited to an initial dose of not more than 500 mg daily and increased as required at intervals of not less than two days.

A thiazide may be added at any time during methyldopa therapy and is recommended if therapy has not been started with a thiazide or if effective control of blood pressure cannot be maintained on 2.0 g of methyldopa daily.

Aldomet may also be used concomitantly with Moduretic* (amiloride hydrochloride and hydrochlorothiazide, MSD) or beta-blocking agents, such as Blocadren* (timolol maleate MSD).

When methyldopa is given to patients on other antihypertensives the dose of these agents may need to be adjusted to effect a smooth transition.

Oral therapy: Children: Initial dosage is based on 10 mg/kg of body weight daily in 2–4 oral doses. The daily dosage then is increased or decreased until an adequate response is achieved. the maximum dosage is 65 mg/kg or 3.0 g daily, whichever is less.

Intravenous therapy: Aldomet Injection is for intravenous use only, it must not be given intramuscularly or subcutaneously. An effective dose will produce a fall in blood pressure that may begin in 4 to 6 hours and be maintained for 10 to 16 hours.

Usual adult dosage: 250–500 mg (5–10 ml) six-hourly. In severe cases, up to 1 g (20 ml) six-hourly may be needed, and this is the maximum recommended dosage. If there is renal impairment, lower dosages should suffice.

Children's dosage: The recommended intravenous dosage for children is 20–40 mg/kg of body weight in divided doses every six hours. The maximum dosage is 65 mg/kg or 3.0 g daily, whichever is less. If there is renal impairment, lower dosages should suffice.

The required dose should be added to 100 ml of 5% dextrose, and the resulting solution given by intravenous infusion over a period of 30–60 minutes. When practicable, oral therapy with Aldomet Tablets may be substituted, starting with the same dosage as that being used intravenously.

Use in the elderly: The initial dose in elderly patients should be kept as low as possible, not exceeding 250 mg daily; an appropriate starting dose in the elderly would be 125 mg b.d. increasing slowly as required, but not to exceed a maximum daily dosage of 2 g.

Contra-indications, warnings, etc

Contra-indications: Active hepatic disease, such as acute hepatitis and active cirrhosis; hypersensitivity (including hepatic disorders associated with previous methyldopa therapy), depression.

Precautions: Acquired haemolytic anaemia has occurred rarely. Should symptoms suggest anaemia, haemoglobin and/or haematocrit determinations should be made. If anaemia is confirmed, tests should be done for haemolysis. If haemolytic anaemia is present, Aldomet should be discontinued. Stopping therapy, with or without giving a corticosteroid, has usually brought prompt remission. Rarely, however, deaths have occurred.

Some patients on continued therapy with methyldopa develop a positive direct Coombs test. From the reports of different investigators, the incidence averages between 10% and 20%. A positive Coombs test rarely develops in the first six months of therapy, and if it has not developed within 12 months, it is unlikely to do so later on continuing therapy. Development is also dose-related, the lowest incidence occurring in patients receiving 1 g or less of methyldopa per day. The test becomes negative usually within weeks or months of stopping methyldopa.

Prior knowledge of a positive Coombs reaction will aid in evaluating a cross-match for transfusion. If a patient with a positive Coombs reaction shows an incompatible minor cross-match, an indirect Coombs test should be performed. If this is negative, transfusion with blood compatible in the major cross-match may be carried out. If positive, the advisability of transfusion should be determined by a haematologist.

Reversible leucopenia, with primary effect on granulocytes has been reported rarely. The granulocyte count returned to normal on discontinuing therapy. Reversible thrombocytopenia has occurred rarely.

Occasionally, fever has occurred within the first three weeks of therapy, sometimes associated with eosinophilia or abnormalities in liver function tests. Jaundice, with or without fever, also may occur. Its onset is usually within the first two or three months of therapy. In some patients the findings are consistent with those of cholestasis. Rare cases of fatal hepatic necrosis have been reported. Liver biopsy, performed in several patients with liver dysfunction, showed a microscopic focal necrosis compatible with drug hypersensitivity. Liver function tests and a total and differential white blood cell count are advisable at intervals during the first six weeks to twelve weeks of therapy, or whenever an unexplained fever occurs. Should fever, abnormality in liver function, or jaundice occur, therapy should be withdrawn. If related to methyldopa, the temperature and abnormalities in liver function will then return to normal. Methyldopa should not be used again in these patients. Methyldopa should be used with caution in patients with a history of previous liver disease or dysfunction.

When methyldopa is used with other antihypertensive drugs, potentiation of antihypertensive action may occur. The progress of patients should be carefully followed to detect side reactions or manifestations of drug idiosyncrasy.

A paradoxical pressor response has been reported with Aldomet Injection.

Patients may require reduced doses of anaesthetics when on methyldopa. If hypotension does occur during anaesthesia, it can usually be controlled by vasopressors. The adrenergic receptors remain sensitive during treatment with methyldopa.

Dialysis removes methyldopa; therefore, hypertension may recur after this procedure.

Rarely, involuntary choreo-athetotic movements have been observed during therapy with methyldopa in patients with severe bilateral cerebrovascular disease. Should these movements occur, therapy should be discontinued.

Interference with laboratory tests: Methyldopa may interfere with the measurement of urinary uric acid by the phosphotungstate method, serum creatinine by the alkaline picrate method, and AST (SGOT) by colorimetric method. Interference with spectrophotometric methods for AST (SGOT) analysis has not been reported.

As methyldopa fluoresces at the same wavelengths as catecholamines, spuriously high amounts of urinary catecholamines may be reported interfering with a diagnosis of phaeochromocytoma.

It is important to recognise this phenomenon before a patient with a possible phaeochromocytoma is subjected to surgery. Methyldopa does not interfere with measurement of VMA (vanillylmandelic acid) by those methods which convert VMA to vanillin. Methyldopa is not recommended for the treatment of patients with phaeochromocytoma.

Rarely, when urine is exposed to air after voiding, it may darken because of breakdown of methyldopa or its metabolites.

Pregnancy and nursing mothers: Aldomet has been used under close medical supervision for the treatment of hypertension during pregnancy. There was no clinical evidence that Aldomet caused fetal abnormalities or affected the neonate.

Methyldopa crosses the placental barrier and appears in cord blood and breast milk.

Although no obvious teratogenic effects have been reported, the possibility of fetal injury cannot be excluded and the use of the drug in women who are, or may become, pregnant or who are nursing their newborn infant requires that anticipated benefits be weighed against possible risks.

Side-effects: Sedation, usually transient, may occur during the initial period of therapy or whenever the dose is increased. Headache, asthenia or weakness may be noted as early and transient symptoms.

Significant side-effects due to Aldomet have been infrequent and this agent usually is well tolerated.

The following reactions have been reported:

Central nervous system: Sedation (usually transient, headache, asthenia or weakness), paraesthesiae, parkinsonism, Bell's palsy, involuntary choreoathetotic movements. Psychic disturbances including nightmares, impaired mental acuity and reversible mild psychoses or depression. Dizziness, light-headedness, and symptoms of cerebrovascular insufficiency (may be due to lowering of blood pressure).

Cardiovascular: Bradycardia, prolonged carotid sinus hypersensitivity, aggravation of angina pectoris. Orthostatic hypotension (decrease daily dosage). Oedema (and weight gain) usually relieved by use of a diuretic. (Discontinue methyldopa if oedema progresses or signs of heart failure appear.)

Gastro-intestinal: Nausea, vomiting, distension, constipation, flatus, diarrhoea, colitis, mild dryness of mouth, sore or 'black' tongue, pancreatitis, sialadenitis.

Haematological: Positive Coombs test, haemolytic anaemia, bone marrow depression, leucopenia, granulocytopenia, thrombocytopenia. Positive tests for antinuclear antibody, LE cells, and rheumatoid factor.

Allergic: Drug-related fever and abnormal liver function tests with jaundice and hepatocellular damage, lupus-like syndrome, myocarditis.

Dermatological: Rash as in eczema or lichenoid eruption, toxic epidermal necrolysis.

Other: Nasal stuffiness, rise in blood urea, breast enlargement, gynaecomastia, hyperprolactinaemia, amenorrhoea, lactation, impotence, decreased libido, mild arthralgia, myalgia.

Treatment of overdosage: If ingestion is recent, emesis may be induced or gastric lavage performed. There is no specific antidote. Methyldopa is dialysable. Treatment is symptomatic. Infusions may be helpful to promote urinary excretion. Special attention should be directed towards cardiac rate and output, blood volume, electrolyte balance, paralytic ileus, urinary function and cerebral activity. Administration of sympathomimetic agents may be indicated. When chronic overdosage is suspected,

Aldomet should be discontinued. Aldomet Suspension should not be diluted.

Pharmaceutical precautions Keep containers well closed and store the tablets and suspension below 25°C, protected from light. The injection should also be protected from freezing. Only 5% dextrose should be used as diluent for the injection.

Legal category POM.

Package quantities *Tablets 125 mg:* Bottles of 100. *Tablets 250 mg:* Bottles of 100 and 500. *Tablets 500 mg:* Bottles of 100 and 500. *Oral Suspension, 250 mg/5 ml:* Bottles of 200 ml. *Injection:* Ampoules of 5 ml.

Further information Aldomet reduces both supine and standing blood pressure. Symptomatic postural hypotension, exercise hypotension and diurnal blood pressure variations rarely occur. By adjustment of dosage, morning hypotension can be prevented without sacrificing control of afternoon blood pressure.

Methyldopa has no direct effect on cardiac function and usually does not reduce glomerular filtration rate, renal blood flow or filtration fraction. Cardiac output usually is maintained without cardiac acceleration. In some patients, the heart rate is slowed.

Because of its relative freedom from adverse effects on kidney function, methyldopa can be of benefit in the control of high blood pressure, even in the presence of renal impairment. It may help arrest or retard the progression of renal function impairment and damage due to sustained elevation of blood pressure.

Normal or elevated plasma renin activity may decrease in course of methyldopa therapy.

Product licence numbers

Tablets 125 mg	0025/0098
Tablets 250 mg	0025/0099
Tablets 500 mg	0025/0100
Oral Suspension 250 mg/5 ml	0025/0154
Injection	0025/5003

ARAMINE*

Presentation A clear, colourless solution containing, in each millilitre, Metaraminol Tartrate BP equivalent to 10 mg metaraminol. Aramine also contains methylparaben, propylparaben and sodium bisulphite as preservatives; with the solution made isotonic by the inclusion of sodium chloride.

Uses Sympathomimetic amine (vasopressor agent). For the treatment of acute hypotension due to loss of vasoconstrictor tone as may occur during spinal anaesthesia, and as an adjunct to accepted remedial procedures (e.g. tilting of patient and attention to fluid volumes). (See 'Precautions'.)

The pressor effect of a single dose of Aramine lasts from about twenty minutes up to one hour. Its onset is around one or two minutes after direct intravenous injection.

Dosage and administration Aramine Injection may be given intravenously either directly or by infusion. Because the maximum effect is not immediately apparent, allow at least ten minutes before increasing the dose. Since the vasopressor effect tapers off when therapy is stopped, be prepared to restart promptly if the blood pressure falls too rapidly. Patients with coexistent shock and acidosis may show poor response.

Direct intravenous injection is recommended only in grave emergencies. *Particular care should be taken to use the correct dose.*

Intravenous infusion (for adjunctive treatment of hypotension): 15–100 mg (1.5–10 ml) in 500 ml of Sodium Chloride Injection BP or 5% Dextrose Injection BP, adjusting the rate of infusion to maintain the blood pressure at the desired level. Higher concentrations of Aramine 150–500 mg per 500 ml of infusion fluid, have been used. If the patient needs additional saline or dextrose at a rate of flow that would provide an excessive dose of Aramine when used as recommended, the volume of infusion fluid should be increased accordingly. Aramine may also be added to *less* than 500 ml of infusion fluid if a smaller volume is desired.

Aramine is physically and chemically compatible with Injection Sodium Chloride BP, 5% Injection Dextrose BP, Ringer's Injection USP, Lactated Ringer's Injection USP, Dextran 70 Injection.

When Aramine is mixed with an infusion solution, sterile precautions should be observed. Mixtures should be used within 24 hours since infusion solutions do not contain preservatives.

Direct intravenous injection (to be employed only in grave emergencies, when immediate action is necessary to save life): 0.5–5 mg (0.05–0.5 ml), followed by an infusion of 15–100 mg (1.5–10 ml) in 500 ml of infusion liquid. *Particular care should be taken to use the correct dose when injecting undiluted Aramine.*

Use in the elderly: The dosage may not require modification for elderly patients; however geriatric patients may be more sensitive to sympathomimetic agents, therefore particular caution should be taken in this age group.

Contra-indications, warnings, etc
Contra-indications: Concurrent use with cyclopropane or halothane anaesthesia, unless clinical circumstances demand it. Hypersensitivity to any component of Aramine.

Precautions and side-effects: Caution should be exercised to avoid excessive blood pressure changes since response to treatment with Aramine is very variable and the ensuing control of the blood pressure may prove difficult.

In choosing the site for injection, it is important to avoid those areas generally recognised as being unsuitable for the use of any pressor agent and to discontinue the infusion immediately if infiltration or thrombosis occurs. Although the urgent nature of the patient's condition may force the choice of an unsuitable injection site, the preferred areas of injection should be used when possible. The larger veins of the antecubital fossa or thigh are preferred to the veins in the ankle or dorsum of the hand, particularly in patients with peripheral vascular disease, diabetes mellitus, Buerger's disease or conditions with coexistent hypercoagulability.

Monoamine oxidase inhibitors have been reported to potentiate the action of sympathomimetic amines. The pressor effect of Aramine is decreased but not reversed by alpha-adrenergic blocking agents.

Aramine should be used with caution in cases of heart disease, hypertension, thyroid disease or diabetes mellitus because of its vasoconstrictor action.

Sympathomimetic amines may provoke a relapse in patients with a history of malaria.

Sympathomimetic amines, including Aramine, may cause sinus or ventricular tachycardia, or other arrhythmias, especially in patients with myocardial infarction.

Abscess formation, tissue necrosis, and sloughing rarely may follow the use of Aramine.

Rapidly induced hypertensive responses have been reported to cause acute pulmonary oedema, cardiac arrhythmias and arrest. Aramine should be used with caution in patients with cirrhosis; electrolyte levels should be adequately restored if a diuresis ensues. A fatal ventricular arrhythmia was reported in a patient with Laënnec's cirrhosis while receiving metaraminol tartrate. In several instances, ventricular extrasystoles that appeared during infusion of Aramine promptly subsided when the rate of flow was reduced. Aramine should be used with caution in digitalised patients since the combination of digitalis and sympathomimetic amines is capable of causing ectopic arrhythmic activity.

With the prolonged action of Aramine, a cumulative effect is possible. An excessive vasopressor response may cause a prolonged elevation of blood pressure, even after discontinuation of therapy.

When vasopressor amines are used for long periods, the resulting vasoconstriction may prevent adequate expansion of circulating volume and may cause perpetuation of the shock state. There is evidence that plasma volume may be reduced in all types of shock, and that the measurement of central venous pressure is useful in assessing the adequacy of the circulating blood volume. Blood, or plasma-volume expanders, should therefore be employed when the principal reason for hypotension or shock is decreased circulating volume.

Treatment of overdosage: If the drug has been ingested, induce emesis or perform gastric lavage. If Aramine has been administered by subcutaneous or intramuscular injection, local ice packs may be applied to delay absorption. Intravenous infusion should be stopped immediately, but reinstated if hypotension occurs. If needed, an alpha-adrenergic blocking agent such as phenoxybenzamine may be used to reduce hypertension. Intravenous beta-adrenergic blocking agents may also be useful for reducing hypertension and may have a beneficial effect on cardiac arrhythmia, if present. Parenteral diazepam may be given for convulsions.

Pharmaceutical precautions Store below 25°C, protected from light and from freezing. Aramine is physically and chemically compatible with Injection Sodium Chloride BP, 5% Injection Dextrose BP, Ringer's Injection USP, Lactated Ringer's Injection USP, Dextran 70 Injection. The ampoule may be autoclaved.

Legal category POM.

Package quantities Ampoules of 1 ml.

Further information Aramine is a potent sympathomimetic amine which increases the force of myocardial contractions as well as having a peripheral vasoconstrictor action. It increases both systolic and diastolic blood pressures.

Renal, coronary, and cerebral blood flow are a function of perfusion pressure and regional resistance. In most instances of cardiogenic shock, the beneficial effect of sympathomimetic amines is attributable to their positive inotropic effect. In patients with insufficient or failing vasoconstriction, there is additional advantage to the peripheral action of Aramine, but in most patients with shock, vasoconstriction is adequate and any further increase is unnecessary. Therefore, blood flow to vital

organs may decrease with Aramine if the regional resistance increases excessively.

The pressor effect of Aramine is decreased but not reversed by alpha-adrenergic blocking agents. Primary or secondary fall in blood pressure and tachyphylactic response to repeated use are uncommon.

Product licence number 10 mg/ml injection 0025/5020.

BENEMID*

Presentation White, half-scored tablets, marked 'MSD 501', containing 500 mg Probenecid BP.

Uses Inhibits the reabsorption of urate ions in the renal tubules, thus increasing urinary excretion of uric acid and decreasing serum uric acid levels. This reduces the miscible urate pool, retards the deposition of urates, and promotes reabsorption of urate deposits. Also selectively inhibits the urinary excretion of β-lactam antibiotics (other than cephaloridine).

Gout and other forms of hyperuricaemia: Benemid is an effective uricosuric agent for the treatment of hyperuricaemia in gout and gouty arthritis. Time is required to achieve clinical results with Benemid despite its marked uricosuric activity. Although acute attacks may occur in the early stages of therapy, as therapy is continued, these attacks should become less frequent and less intense. With prolonged use, formation of new gouty tophi can be prevented; existing tophi decrease in size and may eventually disappear.

Benemid may also be given prophylactically to treat the asymptomatic hyperuricaemia that often occurs in 'gouty' families, in an attempt to forestall the development of acute gouty attacks and urate deposition in tissues.

Benemid may be used to control the hyperuricaemia induced or aggravated by diuretics employed in oedema and hypertension.

β-lactam antibiotic therapy: Benemid is indicated as an adjunctive therapy with β-lactam antibiotics (other than cephaloridine). It elevates and prolongs the plasma levels by whatever route the antibiotics are given. A twofold to fourfold increase in plasma concentration has been demonstrated for penicillin G, or V, the synthetic penicillins, ampicillin, methicillin, oxacillin, cloxacillin, and carbenicillin, and for the cephamycin, Mefoxin* (cefoxitin sodium, MSD), and the cephalosporins, cephalothin, cephalexin and cephaloglycin (but not cephaloridine).

Adjunctive therapy of this type is particularly useful when treating severe or resistant infections, such as gonorrhoea, subacute bacterial endocarditis, staphylococcal osteomyelitis, staphylococcal septicaemia, and meningitis due to Gram-positive organisms.

Dosage and administration *Uricosuric therapy: Usual adult dosage:* $\frac{1}{2}$ tablet (250 mg) twice a day for one week, followed thereafter by 1 tablet (500 mg) twice a day.

Some degree of renal impairment is common in patients with gout, therefore, a daily dosage of 2 tablets (1 g) may be adequate in many patients. If, however, symptoms of gouty arthritis remain uncontrolled or the 24-hour urate excretion is not above 700 mg, the daily dosage may be increased by 1 tablet (500 mg) every four weeks within tolerance [usually not more than 4 tablets (2 g) a day]. Benemid may not be effective in chronic renal insufficiency, particularly when the glomerular filtration rate is 30 ml/min or less.

Gastric intolerance may be indicative of overdosage, and may be corrected by reducing the dosage without losing the therapeutic response.

When acute attacks have been absent for at least six months and serum uric acid remains within normal limits, dosage may be reduced by 1 tablet (500 mg) a time over a period of months to the minimum effective dosage. The dosage should not be reduced to the point where serum uric acid levels tend to rise. Once a patient has been stabilised on Benemid, the usual restrictions on purine-producing foods may be somewhat relaxed.

β-lactam antibiotic therapy (general): Adults: 4 tablets (2 g) a day in divided doses. Elderly patients with suspected renal impairment should be given a smaller dosage, and Benemid should not be given concurrently with a β-lactam antibiotic in known cases of renal impairment.

Gonorrhoea: For uncomplicated gonorrhoea in men or women: a single dose of 2 tablets (1 g) with adequate doses of either oral ampicillin or intramuscular aqueous procaine penicillin or cefoxitin. If oral ampicillin is used, Benemid should be given simultaneously; if a parenteral antibiotic is administered, Benemid should be given at least 30 minutes beforehand.

Children over 2 years: 25 mg per kg body weight (or 0.7 g/m² body surface) initially, followed by 40 mg per kg (or 1.2 g/m²) a day in divided doses every six hours. For children weighing more than 50 kg, the adult dosage is recommended.

Use in the elderly: As with all drugs which are primarily renally excreted, care should be taken in the elderly whose renal function may be impaired.

Contra-indications, warnings, etc

Contra-indications: Known hypersensitivity to probenecid. History of blood dyscrasias. Uric acid kidney stones. Children under two years old. Therapy with Benemid should not be started until an acute gouty attack has subsided. Salicylates are contra-indicated in patients taking Benemid.

Precautions: Benemid should be used with caution in patients with a history of peptic ulcer. If hypersensitivity reactions appear during therapy, the drug should be withdrawn. If patients on Benemid need a mild analgesic, paracetamol is preferred.

Haematuria, renal colic, costovertebral pain and the formation of urate stones may be prevented by a liberal fluid intake and enough sodium bicarbonate (3–7.5 g daily) or potassium citrate (7.5 g daily) to keep the urine alkaline. When alkali is given, the acid-base balance of the patient should be carefully monitored.

Exacerbation of gout during therapy with Benemid may occur; if so, a full therapeutic dosage of colchicine, Indocid* (indomethacin) or other appropriate therapy should be given. A reducing substance may appear in the urine of patients receiving Benemid. This may give a false-positive Benedict's test, but the substance disappears when therapy is discontinued.

Drug interactions: The use of acetylsalicylic acid and pyrazinamide antagonises the uricosuric action of probenecid.

Probenecid produces an insignificant increase in free sulphonamide plasma concentrations but a significant increase in total sulphonamide plasma levels. Since probenecid decreases the renal excretion of conjugated sulphonamides, plasma concentrations of the latter should be determined from time to time when a sulphonamide and probenecid are given together for prolonged periods.

Probenecid may prolong or enhance the action of oral sulphonylureas and thereby increase the risk of hypoglycaemia.

When probenecid is given to patients receiving indomethacin, the plasma levels of indomethacin are likely to be increased. Therefore, a lower dosage of indomethacin may be required to produce a therapeutic effect, and increases in the dosage of indomethacin should be made cautiously and in small increments. Probenecid may increase plasma levels of rifampicin. The clinical significance of this is not known.

Benemid increases the plasma concentration of methotrexate. If Benemid is given with methotrexate, the dosage of methotrexate should be reduced and serum levels may need to be monitored.

In addition to its effects on the excretion of uric acid and the β-lactam antibiotics (other than cephaloridine). Benemid decreases the urinary excretion of ρ-aminosalicylic acid (PAS), ρ-aminohippuric acid (PAH), phenolsulphonylphthalein (PSP), pantothenic acid, 17-ketosteroids, sodium iodomethamate and related iodinated organic acids. Benemid decreases both hepatic and renal excretion of sulphabromophthalein (BSP). The renal tubular reabsorption of phosphorus is inhibited in hypoparathyroid but not in euparathyroid individuals.

Benemid does not affect the excretion of streptomycin, chloramphenicol, chlortetracycline, oxytetracycline, or neomycin. The effects on the excretion of cephaloridine are not clinically significant.

Use in pregnancy: Probenecid crosses the placental barrier and appears in cord blood. Its use in women of childbearing age requires that the anticipated benefit be weighed against possible hazards.

Side-effects: Headache, gastro-intestinal symptoms (e.g. anorexia, nausea, vomiting), frequency of micturition, hypersensitivity reactions (including anaphylaxis, dermatitis, pruritus, fever), sore gums, flushing, dizziness, anaemia and haemolytic anaemia (in some cases associated with genetic deficiency of glucose-6-phosphate dehydrogenase in red blood cells) have occurred. Rarely, the nephrotic syndrome, hepatic necrosis, and aplastic anaemia. In gouty patients, exacerbation of gout, and uric acid stones with or without haematuria, renal colic, or costovertebral pain, has been seen.

Treatment of overdosage: Emesis should be induced or gastric lavage performed. If signs of CNS excitation are present, a short-acting barbiturate should be given parenterally. Adrenaline should be give for anaphylactoid reactions. For less severe hypersensitivity reactions, antihistamines or corticosteroids may be given.

Pharmaceutical precautions Keep container tightly closed. Store in a cool place, protected from light.

Legal category POM.

Package quantities Bottles of 100.

Further information Benemid has been in use since 1952. It can generally be given indefinitely because of its low toxicity.

Product licence number 0025/5021.

BLOCADREN*

Presentation Blue, half-scored tablets, marked 'MSD 136' on one side with or without 'BLOCADREN' on the other, containing 10 mg Timolol Maleate BP.

Uses Beta-adrenergic-receptor blocking agent. For the treatment of essential hypertension and in angina pectoris due to ischaemic heart disease.

Blocadren is also indicated for the long-term prevention of myocardial infarction and cardiac death (including sudden death) in those who have survived the acute phase of a myocardial infarction.

Prophylactic management of common and classic migraine.

Dosage and administration

Hypertension: The initial dosage is 10 mg a day in a single or divided dosage. Depending on the response of the patient, increases in dosage can be made to a maximum of 60 mg daily. Daily dosages above 20 mg should be given on a divided dose schedule.

Use with Moduretic (amiloride hydrochloride and hydrochlorothiazide, MSD):* Studies have shown that Blocadren can be administered once daily when used concomitantly with Moduretic. The majority of patients will respond to a regimen of 10 or 20 mg of Blocadren once a day and 1 tablet of Moduretic.

Use with other antihypertensives: Blocadren may be used with thiazides, hydralazine, or methyldopa. Dosage adjustments are usually required.

For concomitant use with catecholamine-depleting drugs such as reserpine or guanethidine, see 'Precautions'.

Angina: Therapy should be initiated with 5 mg two or three times a day. Dosage increases may be necessary, depending on the symptomatic response, pulse rate, and blood pressure. The first increase should not exceed 10 mg a day in divided doses, and subsequent increases should not exceed 15 mg a day in divided doses. There should be an interval of at least three days between increases in dosage.

The usual dosage range is 15 to 45 mg a day. The majority of patients respond to a dosage in the range of 35 to 45 mg a day.

Preventive use in ischaemic heart disease: For long-term preventive use in patients who have survived the acute phase of myocardial infarction, the maintenance dose is 10 mg twice daily. Therapy should be initiated with 5 mg twice daily and the patient observed carefully. If no adverse reaction occurs, the dosage should then be increased after 2 days to 10 mg twice daily. In the studies evaluating Blocadren following myocardial infarction, treatment was begun 7 to 28 days after the acute phase.

Migraine: The recommended dosage in the prophylactic treatment of common and classic migraine is 10 to 20 mg administered once-a-day.

Use in the elderly: Initial dosage should be 5 mg b.d. Dosage may be increased cautiously depending on clinical response. *For the preventive use in ischaemic heart disease:* The dosage should be increased to 10 mg b.d. after the second day of treatment.

Contra-indications, warnings, etc

Contra-indications: Bronchospasm (including bronchial asthma) or severe chronic obstructive pulmonary disease; sinus bradycardia; second- and third-degree atrioventricular block; anaesthesia with agents that produce myocardial depression; congestive heart failure

(see 'Precautions'); right ventricular failure secondary to pulmonary hypertension; significant cardiomegaly; cardiogenic shock; hypersensitivity.

See also 'Use in pregnancy and nursing mothers', under 'Precautions'.

Precautions: Congestive heart failure: Blocadren may be given cautiously to patients with a history of cardiac failure who are well compensated, usually with digitalis or diuretics. Both digitalis and timolol maleate slow AV conduction. If cardiac failure persists, Blocadren should be withdrawn.

In patients without history of cardiac failure: At the first sign or symptom of cardiac failure, patients receiving Blocadren should be digitalised and/or given a diuretic, and the response closely observed. If cardiac failure still continues, Blocadren should be withdrawn.

Thyrotoxicosis: Patients suspected of developing thyrotoxicosis should be managed carefully to avoid abrupt withdrawal of Blocadren which might precipitate a thyroid storm.

Exacerbation of ischaemic heart disease following abrupt withdrawal: Hypersensitivity to catecholamines has been seen in patients withdrawn from beta-blocker therapy; exacerbation of angina and, in some cases, myocardial infarction has occurred after *abrupt* withdrawal of such therapy. When discontinuing chronically administered Blocadren, particularly in patients with ischaemic heart disease, the dosage should be gradually reduced over one to two weeks and the patient carefully monitored. If angina markedly worsens or acute coronary insufficiency develops, Blocadren should be reinstated promptly, at least temporarily, and other appropriate measures taken. Patients should be warned against interruption or discontinuation of Blocadren without advice. Because coronary artery disease is both common and may be unrecognised, it may be prudent not to discontinue Blocadren abruptly, even when only treating hypertension.

Major surgery: Because beta-adrenergic-receptor blockade impairs the heart's response to beta-adrenergic reflex stimuli, some patients on beta-adrenergic receptor blocking agents have shown protracted severe hypotension during anaesthesia. Difficulty in restarting and maintaining the heartbeat has also been reported.

Some authorities now recommend gradual withdrawal of beta-adrenergic receptor blocking agents from anginal patients before elective surgery. If necessary during surgery, the effects of Blocadren may be reversed by sufficient doses of such agonists as isoprenaline, dopamine, dobutamine or noradrenaline (see 'Overdosage').

Diabetes mellitus: Blocadren should be administered with caution to patients liable to spontaneous hypokalaemia, or to diabetic patients (especially those with labile diabetes) who are receiving insulin or oral hypoglycaemic agents. Beta-adrenergic receptor blocking agents may mask the premonitory signs and symptoms of acute hypoglycaemia.

Drug interactions: Close observation of the patient is recommended when Blocadren is administered to patients on catecholamine-depleting drugs such as reserpine, because of possible additive effects and the production of hypotension and/or marked bradycardia, which may produce vertigo, syncope, or postural hypotension.

Attenuation of the antihypertensive effect of beta-blockers by NSAIDs has been reported. Patients needing both agents should be monitored to confirm that the desired therapeutic effect has been obtained.

Oral calcium antagonists may be combined with Blocadren only when heart function is normal. When heart function is impaired, combination with dihydropyridine derivatives such as nifedipine may lead to hypotension; and combination with verapamil or diltiazem may cause AV conduction disturbances or left ventricular failure. Intravenous calcium antagonists and Blocadren should only be used together with caution.

Concomitant use of beta-blockers and digitalis with either diltiazem or verapamil may further prolong the AV conduction time.

Impaired hepatic or renal function: Since Blocadren is partially metabolised in the liver and excreted mainly by the kidney, dosage reduction may be necessary when hepatic and/or renal insufficiency is present.

In the presence of marked renal failure: Although the pharmacokinetics of Blocadren are not greatly altered by renal impairment, marked hypotensive responses have been seen in patients with marked renal impairment undergoing dialysis after 20 mg doses. Dosing in such patients should, therefore, be especially cautious.

Musculoskeletal: Timolol has been reported rarely to increase muscle weakness in some patients with myasthenic symptoms.

Cerebrovascular insufficiency: As an agent affecting both pulse and blood pressure, Blocadren should be used cautiously in patients with cerebrovascular insufficiency. Signs or symptoms suggesting reduced cerebral blood flow should prompt consideration of withdrawing therapy with Blocadren.

General: There have been reports of skin rashes and/or dry eyes associated with the use of beta-adrenoceptor-blocking drugs. The reported incidence is small and in most cases the symptoms have cleared when treatment was withdrawn. Discontinuation of the drug should be considered if any such reaction is not otherwise explicable. Cessation of therapy involving beta-blockade should be gradual.

Paediatric use: Safety and efficacy in children has not been established.

Use in pregnancy and nursing mothers: There are no adequate and well-controlled studies in pregnant women. Blocadren should only be used if the potential benefit justifies the risk to the fetus.

Because of the potential for serious adverse reactions in nursing babies, a decision to discontinue nursing, or Blocadren, should be made taking into account the importance of the drug to the mother.

Side-effects: Blocadren is usually well tolerated. Most adverse reactions are mild and transient. *General:* Asthenia, fatigue, headache, chest pain, extremity pain, decreased exercise tolerance, weight loss. *Cardiovascular:* Bradycardia, cardiac arrest, cerebral vascular accident, palpitation, arrhythmia, sino-atrial block, AV block (2nd or 3rd degree), syncope, hypotension, oedema, pulmonary oedema, cardiac failure, Raynaud's phenomenon, cold extremities, claudication, worsening of arterial insufficiency or angina pectoris, vasodilatation. *Digestive:* Dyspepsia, nausea, vomiting, diarrhoea, hepatomegaly. *Endocrine:* Hyperglycaemia, hypoglycaemia. *Integumentary:* Rash, pruritus, skin irritation, increased pigmentation, sweating, exfoliative dermatitis (one case). *Musculoskeletal:* Arthralgia. *Nervous system:* Dizziness, vertigo, paraesthesiae, local weakness.

Psychiatric: Nervousness, diminished concentration, hallucinations, nightmares, increased dreaming, insomnia, depression, somnolence, decreased libido. *Haematological:* Non-thrombocytopenic purpura. *Respiratory:* Dyspnoea, bronchial spasm, rales, cough. *Special senses:* Tinnitus, visual disturbances, diplopia, ptosis, eye irritation, dry eyes. *Urogenital:* Impotence, micturition difficulties *Clinical laboratory tests:* Changes in clinical laboratory tests are rare. Slight increases in blood urea, serum potassium and serum uric acid, and slight decreases in haemoglobin and haematocrit occurred, but were not progressive or associated with clinical manifestations.

Overdosage: No specific data are available. A study suggests that Blocadren does not readily dialyse.

The most common signs and symptoms to be expected following overdosage with a beta-adrenergic receptor blocking agent are symptomatic bradycardia, hypotension, bronchospasm, and acute cardiac failure. If overdosage occurs, the following measures are suggested. In all cases therapy with Blocadren should be stopped, and the patient closely observed.

1. Gastric lavage.
2. Symptomatic bradycardia: atropine sulphate, 0.25 to 2 mg intravenously, should be used to induce vagal blockade. If bradycardia persists, intravenous isoprenaline hydrochloride should be administered cautiously. In refractory cases, the use of a cardiac pacemaker may be considered.
3. Hypotension: a sympathomimetic pressor agent such as dopamine, dobutamine or noradrenaline should be used. In refractory cases, the use of glucagon has been reported to be useful.
4. Bronchospasm: isoprenaline hydrochloride should be used. Additional therapy with aminophylline may be considered.
5. Acute cardiac failure: conventional therapy with digitalis, diuretics, and oxygen should be instituted immediately. In refractory cases, the use of intravenous aminophylline is suggested. This may be followed, if necessary, by glucagon which has been reported useful.
6. Heart block: isoprenaline hydrochloride or a pacemaker should be used.

Pharmaceutical precautions Keep container well closed; store in a cool place, protected from light.

Legal category POM.

Package quantities Bottles of 100.

Further information Blocadren reduces blood pressure without acute hypotensive episodes in most patients with essential hypertension. The exact mechanism of action is still unknown. Blocadren does not usually affect normal blood pressure. Orally, Blocadren may lower intra-ocular pressure.

Blocadren effectively delays or prevents the development of anginal pain in most patients. It acts by modifying the cardiac response to stress or exercise. Blocadren antagonises the stimulation of the beta-adrenergic receptor sites caused by an excess of circulating catecholamines. In this way, Blocadren often increases the capacity for work and exercise in the patient with angina by reducing the incidence and severity of anginal attacks.

Product licence number 0025/0091.

CLINORIL*

Presentation Brilliant yellow, scored, hexagonal tablets, biconvex in shape, containing 200 mg and 100 mg Sulindac BP. The 200 mg tablets are marked 'MSD 942' and the 100 mg tablets are marked 'MSD 943'.

Uses Non-steroidal, analgesic/anti-inflammatory agent with antipyretic properties.

Indicated in osteoarthritis, rheumatoid arthritis, ankylosing spondylitis, acute gouty arthritis, peri-articular disorders such as bursitis, tendinitis, and tenosynovitis.

Dosage and administration The dosage should be taken twice a day and adjusted to the severity of the disease.

The usual dose is 400 mg a day. However, the dosage may be lowered depending on the response. Doses above 400 mg per day are not recommended.

In the treatment of acute gouty arthritis, therapy for seven days is usually adequate.

In peri-articular disorders, treatment should be limited to seven to ten days.

Clinoril should be adminstered with fluids or food.

Use in the elderly: The dosage does not require modification for the elderly patient.

Contra-indications, warnings, etc
Contra-indications: The use of Clinoril is contra-indicated in patients known to be allergic to the drug.

Clinoril should not be used in patients in whom acute asthmatic attacks, urticaria, or rhinitis have been precipitated by aspirin or other non-steroidal anti-inflammatory agents.

The drug should not be administered to patients with active gastro-intestinal bleeding.

The use of Clinoril should be avoided in patients with active peptic ulcer.

Since paediatric indications and dosage have not yet been established, Clinoril should not be given to children.

Clinoril should not be given to pregnant or lactating women, since safety for its use has not been established.

Precautions: Clinoril should be used with caution in patients having a history of gastro-intestinal haemorrhage or ulcers. In patients with renal functional impairment, since the major route of excretion of the drug is via the kidney, the dosage may need to be reduced. In a drug interaction study, an antacid (magnesium and aluminium hydroxides, in suspension, 30 ml) was administered with Clinoril with no significant difference in absorption.

While Clinoril has less effect on platelet function and bleeding time than aspirin, it is a moderate to weak inhibitor of platelet function and, therefore, patients who may be adversely affected by these actions should be carefully observed when Clinoril is administered.

A patient with signs and/or symptoms suggesting liver dysfunction, or in whom an abnormal liver function test has occurred, should be evaluated for evidence of a more severe hepatic reaction while on therapy. Significant elevations of AST(SGOT) and ALT(SGPT) (three times higher than normal) were seen in less than 1% of patients in controlled clinical trials.

Poor liver function may alter the blood levels of circulating metabolites of Clinoril. Patients with liver dysfunction on Clinoril should be monitored closely; daily dosage reduction may be required.

Cases of hepatitis, jaundice, or both, with or without fever, may occur within the first three months of therapy.

In some patients, the findings are consistent with those of cholestatic hepatitis.

Fever or other evidence of hypersensitivity including abnormalities in one or more liver function tests and skin reactions have occurred during therapy. Some fatalities have occurred.

Whenever a patient develops unexplained fever, rash or other dermatological reaction, or constitutional symptoms, Clinoril should be permanently stopped and liver function investigated. Fever and abnormal liver function are reversible.

Drug interactions: Dimethyl sulphoxide should not be used with Clinoril. Concomitant use has been reported to reduce plasma levels of the active metabolite of Clinoril, and also cause peripheral neuropathy.

Although sulindac and its sulphide metabolite are highly bound to protein, studies (in which Clinoril was given at a dose of 400 mg daily) have shown no clinically significant interaction with oral anticoagulants or oral hypoglycaemic agents. However, patients should be monitored carefully until it is certain that no change in their anticoagulant or hypoglycaemic dose is required.

Concomitant administration with aspirin in normal volunteers significantly depressed plasma levels of the active sulphide metabolite. Clinical study of the combination showed an increase in GI side effects with no improvement in the therapeutic response to Clinoril. The combination is not recommended.

Concomitant administration with diflunisal in normal volunteers reduced the plasma level of active sulphide metabolite by approximately one-third.

Probenecid given concomitantly with sulindac had only a slight effect on plasma sulphide levels, while plasma levels of sulindac and sulphone were increased. Sulindac was shown to produce a modest reduction in the uricosuric action of probenecid which probably is not usually significant.

Neither dextropropoxyphene hydrochloride nor paracetamol had any effect on the plasma levels of sulindac or its sulphide metabolite.

In contrast to most other non-steroidal anti-inflammatory drugs, Clinoril does not reduce the antihypertensive effect of a variety of agents used to treat mild-to-moderate hypertension. However, the blood pressure of patients taking Clinoril with antihypertensive agents should be closely monitored.

Side-effects: Clinoril is generally well tolerated. Those side-effects experienced are usually mild and may often respond to a reduction in dosage.

Gastro-intestinal: The most frequent types of side-effects occurring with Clinoril are gastro-intestinal; these include gastro-intestinal pain, dyspepsia, nausea with or without vomiting, diarrhoea, constipation, flatulence, anorexia, and gastro-intestinal cramps.

Dermatological: Rash, pruritus.

Central nervous system: Dizziness, headache, nervousness.

Special senses: Tinnitus.

Miscellaneous: Oedema.

The following side-effects were reported less frequently. The probability exists of a causal relationship between Clinoril and these side-effects:

Gastro-intestinal: Stomatitis, gastritis or gastro-enteritis. Peptic ulcer, as well as gastro-intestinal bleeding and perforations have been reported rarely. Fatalities have occurred. Liver function abnormalities, jaundice sometimes with fever, cholestasis, hepatitis, pancreatitis.

Dermatological: Sore or dry membranes, alopecia, photosensitivity. Erythema multiforme, toxic epidermal necrolysis, Stevens-Johnson syndrome, exfoliative dermatitis.

Cardiovascular: Congestive heart failure, especially in patients with marginal cardiac function, palpitation, hypertension.

Haematological: Thrombocytopenia, ecchymosis, purpura, leucopenia, agranulocytosis, neutropenia, bone marrow depression including aplastic anaemia, increased prothrombin time in patients on oral anticoagulants.

Genito-urinary: Urine discoloration, vaginal bleeding, haematuria, renal impairment, interstitial nephritis, nephrotic syndrome.

Nervous system: Vertigo, somnolence, insomnia, sweating, asthenia, paraesthesia, convulsions, syncope, depression, psychic disturbances including acute psychosis, aseptic meningitis.

Special senses: Blurred vision, decreased hearing, metallic or bitter taste.

Respiratory: Epistaxis.

Hypersensitivity reactions: Anaphylaxis and angioneurotic oedema. A potentially fatal hypersensitivity syndrome has been reported which may include constitutional symptoms (fever, rigors); dermatological findings such as rash or other cutaneous reactions listed above; involvement of major organs (changes in liver function tests, jaundice, pancreatitis, pneumonitis, leucopenia, eosinophilia, anaemia, renal impairment including renal failure); and less specific findings such as adenitis, arthralgia, fatigue, or chest pain.

Causal relationship unknown: Other reactions have been reported in clinical trials or since the drug was marketed, but occurred under circumstances where a causal relationship could not be established. However, in these rarely reported events, that possibility cannot be excluded. Therefore, these observations are listed to serve as alerting information to physicians.

Haematological: Haemolytic anaemia.

Nervous system: Neuritis.

Special senses: Transient visual disturbances.

Miscellaneous: Gynaecomastia.

Treatment of overdosage: Cases of overdosage have been reported and, rarely, fatalities have occurred. Stupor, coma, diminished urine output and hypotension have been seen. Isolated cases of patients receiving up to 900 mg a day have been reported, with no adverse effects.

In the event of acute overdosage, the stomach should be emptied by inducing vomiting or by gastric lavage, and the patient carefully observed and given symptomatic and supportive treatment.

Animal studies show that absorption is decreased by the prompt administration of activated charcoal and excretion is enhanced by alkalinisation of the urine.

Pharmaceutical precautions Keep container well closed; store in a cool place, protected from light.

Legal category POM.

Package quantities *200 mg:* Bottles of 100 and 500. *100 mg:* Bottles of 100.

Further information Clinoril usually provides symptomatic relief of inflammation, pain and tenderness and promotes early improvement in joint mobility. Clinoril has a prolonged duration of activity, which permits a twice-a-day dose schedule. Based on extensive studies, Clinoril has been shown to be suitable for the long-term relief of pain and inflammation.

Prostaglandin synthetase inhibition is hypothesised as the basis by which non-steroidal anti-inflammatory agents act. Following absorption, sulindac undergoes two major biotransformations: reversible reduction to the sulphide metabolite; and irreversible oxidation to the inactive sulphone metabolite. The sulphide metabolite is a potent inhibitor of prostaglandin synthesis and accounts for the activity of sulindac (Clinoril). Sulindac is thus a prodrug.

Product licence numbers
100 mg   0025/0121
200 mg   0025/0122

CODELSOL* INJECTION

Presentation A clear, colourless solution containing, per millilitre, Prednisolone Sodium Phosphate BP equivalent to 16 mg prednisolone (approximately 20 mg prednisolone phosphate).

Uses Corticosteroid.

For use in certain endocrine and non-endocrine disorders responsive to corticosteroid therapy.

Systemic administration: Recommended for systemic administration by intravenous or intramuscular injection when oral therapy is not feasible or desirable.

Endocrine disorders: Primary or secondary adrenocortical insufficiency (hydrocortisone or cortisone is the first choice; synthetic analogues may be used with mineralocorticoids where applicable, and in infancy mineralocorticoid supplementation is particularly important).

Non-endocrine disorders: Codelsol Injection may be used in the treatment of non-endocrine corticosteroid responsive conditions including:

Allergy and anaphylaxis: Angioneurotic oedema and anaphylaxis.

Gastro-intestinal disorders: Crohn's disease and ulcerative colitis.

Infections (with appropriate chemotherapy): Miliary tuberculosis and endotoxic shock.

Neurological disorders: Infantile spasms.

Respiratory: Bronchial asthma and aspiration pneumonitis.

Rheumatic disorders: Rheumatoid arthritis.

Skin disorders: Toxic epidermal necrolysis.

Local administration: Codelsol is suitable for intra-articular or soft-tissue injection as adjunctive therapy for short-term administration in:

Soft-tissue disorders such as carpal tunnel syndrome and tenosynovitis.

Intra-articular disorders such as rheumatoid arthritis and osteoarthrosis with an inflammatory component.

Codelsol may be injected intralesionally in selected skin disorders such as cystic acne vulgaris, localised lichen simplex, and keloids.

Dosage and administration The lowest possible dosage adequate to control the disease process should be used.

Dosage requirements are variable and must be determined individually on the basis of the disease and the response of the patient.

The usual initial daily dosage of Codelsol is 4–60 mg. In chronic use, the dosage should be restricted, where possible, to 7.5 mg daily. The daily parenteral dose of Codelsol is usually the same as the daily oral dose of prednisolone, and the usually recommended dosage interval is every four to eight hours. However, both the dose in the evening, which is useful in alleviating morning stiffness, and the divided dosage regimen are associated with greater suppression of the hypothalamo-pituitary-adrenal axis.

Intravenous and intramuscular injection: Codelsol Injection can be given directly from the vial, or added to sodium chloride injection or dextrose injection and given by intravenous drip. The slower rate of absorption by intramuscular administration should be recognised.

Because benzyl alcohol is associated with toxicity in premature infants, particular care should be taken to ensure that only preservative-free solutions are used to prepare mixtures for neonates, especially premature infants.

When Codelsol Injection is added to an infusion solution, the mixture must be used within 24 hours, since infusion solutions do not contain preservatives. The usual aseptic techniques governing injections should be observed.

Maintain or adjust the initial dosage until the patient's response is satisfactory. If satisfactory response does not occur after a reasonable time, discontinue Codelsol and transfer the patient to other therapy.

When symptoms have been controlled, the proper maintenance dose should be determined by decreasing dosage in small amounts to the lowest dose that maintains an adequate clinical response. If the drug is to be stopped after more than a few days, it should be withdrawn gradually.

Intra-articular, intralesional and soft-tissue injection: In general, intra-articular, intralesional, and soft-tissue injections are employed when only one or two joints or areas are affected.

Frequency of injection usually ranges from once every three to five days to once every two to three weeks, depending on the response. Frequent administration may result in tissue damage.

Use in children: Dosage should be limited to a single dose on alternate days to lessen retardation of growth and minimise suppression of hypothalamo-pituitary-adrenal axis.

Use in the elderly: Treatment of elderly patients, particularly if long term, should be planned bearing in mind the more serious consequences of the common side effects of corticosteroids in old age, especially osteoporosis, diabetes, hypertension, susceptibility to infection and thinning of the skin.

Contra-indications, warnings, etc

Contra-indications: Systemic fungal infection; hypersensitivity to any component.

Warnings: Frequent intra-articular injections over a prolonged period may lead to joint destruction with bone necrosis. Intra-articular injection of corticosteroids may produce systemic adverse reaction including adrenal suppression.

Precautions: Corticosteroids may exacerbate systemic fungal infections and should not be used unless they are needed to control drug reactions due to amphotericin.

Cases have been reported in which concomitant use of amphotericin and hydrocortisone was followed by cardiac enlargement and congestive heart failure.

Corticosteroids should be used cautiously in patients with ocular herpes simplex, because of possible corneal perforation.

The dosage of corticosteroid should be reduced gradually.

In patients on corticosteroid therapy subjected to unusual stress, dosage should be increased before, during and after the stressful situation.

Drug-induced secondary adrenocortical insufficiency may be minimised by gradual dosage reduction, but may persist for months after discontinuation of therapy. In any stressful situation during that period, therefore, corticosteroid therapy should be reinstated.

If the patient is receiving steroids already, the dosage may have to be increased. Since mineralocorticoid secretion may be impaired, salt and/or a mineralocorticoid should be administered concurrently.

Corticosteroids may mask some signs of infection, and new infections may appear during their use. There may be decreased resistance and inability to localise infection when corticosteroids are used.

A report shows that the use of corticosteroids in cerebral malaria is associated with a prolonged coma and an increased incidence of pneumonia and gastrointestinal bleeding.

Corticosteroids may activate latent amoebiasis. Therefore, it is recommended that latent or active amoebiasis be excluded before initiating corticosteroid therapy in any patient who has either spent time in the tropics, or has unexplained diarrhoea.

Prolonged use of corticosteroids may produce posterior subcapsular cataracts, and glaucoma with possible damage to the optic nerves, and may enhance the establishment of secondary ocular infections.

Average and large doses of hydrocortisone or cortisone can cause elevation of blood pressure, retention of salt and water, and increased excretion of potassium, but these effects are less likely to occur with synthetic derivatives, except when used in large doses. Dietary salt restriction and potassium supplementation may be necessary. All corticosteroids increase calcium excretion.

Administration of live virus vaccines is contraindicated in individuals receiving immunosuppressive doses of corticosteroids. If inactivated viral or bacterial vaccines are administered to individuals receiving immunosuppressive doses of corticosteroids, the expected serum antibody response may not be obtained. However, patients may be immunised if they are receiving corticosteroids as replacement therapy, e.g. for Addison's disease.

The use of Codelsol Injection in active tuberculosis should be restricted to those cases of fulminating or disseminated tuberculosis in which the corticosteroid is used for the management of the disease in conjunction with an appropriate antituberculosis regime. If corticosteroids are indicated in patients with latent tuberculosis or tuberculin reactivity, close observation is necessary as reactivation may occur. During prolonged corticosteroid therapy, these patients should receive prophylactic chemotherapy.

Because anaphylactoid reactions have occurred, rarely, in patients receiving parenteral corticosteroid therapy, appropriate precautions should be taken prior to administration, especially when the patient has a history of allergy to any drug.

Stopping corticosteroids after prolonged therapy may cause withdrawal symptoms, including fever, myalgia, arthralgia, and malaise. These reactions may occur in patients without evidence of adrenal insufficiency.

There is an enhanced effect of corticosteroids in patients with hypothyroidism and in those with cirrhosis.

Alterations in the patient's mental state may appear when corticosteroids are used, ranging from psychological dependence, euphoria, insomnia, mood swings, personality changes and severe depression, to frank psychotic manifestations.

Aspirin should be used cautiously in conjunction with corticosteroids in hypoprothrombinaemia.

Corticosteroids should be used with caution in renal insufficiency, congestive heart failure, hypertension, diabetes or in those with a family history of diabetes, epilepsy, osteoporosis, previous steroid myopathy, glaucoma (or previous history), myasthenia gravis, non-specific ulcerative colitis, diverticulitis, fresh intestinal anastomosis, active or latent peptic ulcer. Signs of peritoneal irritation following gastro-intestinal perforation in patients receiving large doses of corticosteroids may be minimal or absent. Fat embolism has been reported as a possible complication of hypercortisonism.

Corticosteroids may increase or decrease motility and number of spermatozoa.

As phenytoin, barbiturates, ephedrine, and rifampicin may enhance the metabolic clearance of corticosteroids, resulting in decreased blood levels and reduced physiological activity, the dosage of Codelsol may have to be adjusted.

The prothrombin time should be checked frequently in patients who are receiving corticosteroids and coumarin anticoagulants concurrently.

When corticosteroids are administered concomitantly with potassium-depleting diuretics, patients should be monitored closely for development of hypokalaemia.

Local steroid injection should be undertaken in an aseptic environment to reduce the particular risk of bacterial infection. Injection of a steroid into an infected site should be avoided. Appropriate examination of any joint fluid present is necessary to exclude a septic process.

A marked increase in pain accompanied by local swelling, further restriction of joint motion, fever, and malaise may be suggestive of septic arthritis. If this complication occurs and the diagnosis of sepsis is confirmed, appropriate antimicrobial therapy should be instituted.

Patients should understand the great importance of not over-using joints that are still diseased despite symptomatic improvement.

Corticosteroids should not be injected into unstable joints.

Frequent intra-articular injections have been reported to cause development of Charcot-like arthropathies.

The slower rate of absorption by intramuscular administration should be recognised.

Children: Corticosteroids cause growth retardation in infancy, childhood and adolescence. Treatment should be limited to the minimum dosage for the shortest possible time. In order to minimise suppression of the hypothalamo-pituitary-adrenal axis and growth retardation, treatment should be limited, where possible, to a single dose on alternate days.

Growth and development of infants and children on prolonged corticosteroid therapy should be carefully monitored.

Use in pregnancy and the nursing mother: There is inadequate evidence of safety in human pregnancy and there may be a very small risk of cleft palate and intra-uterine growth retardation in the fetus; there is evidence of harmful effects on pregnancy in animals.

Corticosteroids appear in breast milk and could suppress growth, interfere with endogenous corticosteroid production, or cause other unwanted effects. Mothers taking pharmacological doses of corticosteroids should be advised not to nurse.

Side-effects: Fluid and electrolyte disturbances: Sodium retention, fluid retention, congestive heart failure in susceptible patients, potassium loss, hypokalaemic alkalosis, hypertension, increased calcium excretion.

Musculoskeletal: Muscle weakness, steroid myopathy, loss of muscle mass, osteoporosis (especially in post-menopausal females), vertebral compression fractures, aseptic necrosis of femoral and humeral heads, pathological fracture of long bones, tendon rupture, and post-injection flare (following intra-articular use).

Gastro-intestinal: Peptic ulcer and possible subsequent perforation and haemorrhage, perforation of the small and large bowel particularly in patients with inflammatory bowel disease, pancreatitis, abdominal distension, ulcerative oesophagitis, dyspepsia, oesophageal candidiasis.

Dermatological: Impaired wound healing, thin fragile skin, petechiae, and ecchymoses, erythema, striae, telangiectasia, acne, increased sweating, suppression of skin tests, burning or tingling especially in the perineal area (after intravenous injection), other cutaneous reactions such as allergic dermatitis, urticaria, angioneurotic oedema, and hypo- or hyper-pigmentation.

Neurological: Convulsions, increased intracranial pressure with papilloedema (pseudotumour cerebri) usually after treatment, vertigo, headache, and rare instances of blindness associated with intra-lesional therapy around the face and head.

Endocrine: Menstrual irregularities, amenorrhoea, development of Cushingoid state, suppression of growth in children; secondary adrenocortical and pituitary unresponsiveness, particularly in times of stress, as in trauma, surgery or illness; decreased carbohydrate tolerance, manifestations of latent diabetes mellitus, increased requirements for insulin or oral hypoglycaemic agents in diabetes, hirsutism.

Ophthalmic: Posterior subcapsular cataracts, increased intra-ocular pressure, papilloedema, corneal or scleral thinning, exacerbation of ophthalmic viral disease, glaucoma, exophthalmos.

Metabolic: Negative nitrogen balance due to protein catabolism.

Other: Anaphylactoid or hypersensitivity reactions, leucocytosis, thrombo-embolism, weight gain, increased appetite, nausea, malaise, and sterile abscess.

Teratogenicity: See pregnancy warning under 'Use in pregnancy and the nursing mother'.

Treatment of overdosage: Codelsol Injection must be discontinued immediately. Anaphylactic and hypersensitivity reactions may be treated with adrenaline, positive-pressure artificial respiration, and aminophylline. The patient should be kept warm and quiet.

Pharmaceutical precautions Codelsol Injection is sensitive to heat and should not be autoclaved. Keep in a cool place, protected from light and freezing. Only sodium chloride injection or dextrose injection should be used as diluent. Any infusion mixture must be used within 24 hours.

Legal category POM.

Package quantities Vials of 2 ml.

Further information Nil.

Product licence number 0025/5041.

COGENTIN*

Presentation White, quarter-scored tablets, marked 'MSD 60', containing 2 mg Benztropine Mesylate BP.

An injection containing in each millilitre 1 mg Benztropine Mesylate BP, as a colourless solution.

Uses Anti-parkinsonian agent with powerful anticholinergic effects.

For symptomatic treatment of all types of 'classical' (arteriosclerotic, post-encephalitic, idiopathic) parkinsonism, and of extrapyramidal reactions induced by phenothiazines or reserpine.

Cogentin is particularly effective in the relief of rigidity and tremor. Among other symptoms which it can ameliorate are; sialorrhoea, drooling, mask-like facies, oculogyric crises, speech and writing difficulties, gait disturbances, dysphagia, and pain and insomnia due to muscle spasm and cramps.

Dosage and administration As Cogentin is cumulative in action, treatment should begin with a low dosage, which can be increased by amounts of 0.5 mg at intervals of five to six days, to the smallest dosage necessary for optimal relief without excessive side-effects. Maximum dosage, 6 mg a day.

Cogentin Injection may be used intramuscularly or intravenously in emergencies, or for patients unable to swallow tablets. (As there is no significant difference in time of onset of effect between intramuscular and intravenous administration, the intravenous route is not usually necessary.)

In emergencies, 1–2 ml (1–2 mg) of Cogentin Injection will normally provide quick relief. If signs of parkinsonism begin to return, the dose can be repeated.

'Classical' parkinsonism: Usual dosage: 1–2 mg a day, with a range of 0.5–6 mg a day, orally or parenterally. Dosage must be adjusted on an individual basis, taking into consideration the age and weight of the patient, and the type of parkinsonism. Older patients, thin patients and those with arteriosclerotic parkinsonism usually cannot tolerate large dosages. Most patients with post-encephalitic parkinsonism need and indeed tolerate fairly large dosages. Patients with a poor mental outlook may respond poorly. In arteriosclerotic and idiopathic parkinsonism, therapy may be initiated with a single daily dose of 0.5–1 mg at bedtime. This dosage will be adequate in some patients, whereas 4–6 mg a day may be required by others. In post-encephalitic parkinsonism, therapy may be initiated in most patients with 2 mg a day in one or more doses. In highly sensitive individuals, therapy may be initiated with 0.5 mg at bedtime, and increased as necessary.

Some patients obtain greatest relief by taking the entire dose at bedtime; others react more favourably to divided dosage, two to four times a day. One dose a day frequently is sufficient; divided doses may be unnecessary or even undesirable.

See also 'Further information'.

Drug-induced parkinsonism: Usual dosage range: 1–4 mg once or twice a day.

Acute dystonic reactions: 1–2 ml (1–2 mg) by intravenous injection followed usually by 1–2 mg orally twice a day.

Extrapyramidal reactions appearing soon after starting phenothiazine or reserpine therapy are likely to be temporary, and are usually controlled in one or two days by 1–2 mg of Cogentin orally two or three times a day. Cogentin should be withdrawn after one or two weeks to determine if it is still needed. It can be reinstated if necessary.

Certain extrapyramidal reactions which develop slowly (e.g. tardive dyskinesia) do not usually respond to Cogentin.

Use in the elderly: As with younger patients, dosage should be the smallest possible for optimum relief of symptoms. Initial dosage should be 0.5–1 mg preferably at night, increasing until optimum effect is seen. Older patients usually cannot tolerate large doses.

Contra-indications, warnings, etc

Contra-indications: Because of its atropine-like side-effects, Cogentin is contra-indicated in children under 3 years old and should be used with caution in older children.

Precautions: The safety of Cogentin for use during pregnancy has not been established.

Cogentin may impair the mental alertness and physical ability required for the performance of such hazardous tasks as driving a car or operating machinery.

Continued supervision of patients is recommended as Cogentin has a cumulative action. Patients with a tendency towards tachycardia and those with prostatic hypertrophy, should be closely observed.

Patients with mental disorders should be carefully supervised when Cogentin is used to control drug-induced extrapyramidal reactions, especially when therapy is started or the dosage of Cogentin is increased. Intensification of mental symptoms may occasionally occur. Cogentin should be temporarily withdrawn if the reactions are severe. (In such cases, increased dosage of the anti-parkinsonian agent could precipitate a toxic psychosis.)

Extra care should be taken when Cogentin is given concomitantly with phenothiazines or other drugs with anticholinergic or antihistaminic activity. Patients should be advised to report gastro-intestinal complaints promptly. Paralytic ileus, sometimes fatal, has occurred in patients taking anticholinergic-type anti-parkinsonian drugs, including Cogentin, in combination with phenothiazines and/or tricyclic antidepressants.

Tardive dyskinesia may appear in some patients on long-term therapy with phenothiazines or related agents, or after discontinuation of such therapy. Anti-parkinsonian agents do not usually alleviate symptoms of tardive dyskinesia, and in some cases may aggravate or unmask them. Cogentin is not recommended in tardive dyskinesia.

Cogentin has anticholinergic effects, and glaucoma is a possibility. Although Cogentin does not appear to have any adverse effect on simple glaucoma, its use is probably not advisable in narrow-angle glaucoma. It may cause anhidrosis; this should be borne in mind, particularly in hot weather, especially when given concomitantly with other atropine-like drugs to the chronically ill, alcoholics, or patients with a central nervous system disease. Cogentin should be used cautiously in patients with or prone to abnormalities of sweating. If there is evidence of anhidrosis, the possibility of hyperthermia should be considered. Dosage should be decreased as necessary to maintain body heat equilibrium by the action of perspiration. Severe anhidrosis and fatal hyperthermia have occurred.

Side-effects: Dry mouth, blurred vision, nervousness, nausea and (infrequently) vomiting; these may be controlled by dosage adjustment or temporary withdrawal. Constipation, numbness of the fingers, listlessness, depression, dysuria (rarely a problem). Mental confusion, excitement and visual hallucinations have been reported with high dosage or in particularly susceptible patients. Allergic reactions such as skin rash may require dosage reduction or withdrawal.

Treatment of overdosage: Physostigmine salicylate (1–2 mg, subcutaneously or intravenously) is reported to reverse symptoms of anticholinergic intoxication. A second injection may be given after two hours if needed. Otherwise, treatment is symptomatic and supportive.

Emesis should be induced or gastric lavage performed. A short-acting barbiturate may be used for CNS excitement, but with caution to avoid subsequent depression. Supportive care for CNS depression may be required (such convulsant stimulants as picrotoxin, leptazol or bemegride should be avoided). In severe respiratory depression, artificial respiration may be required. Also needed may be a local miotic for mydriasis and cycloplegia, ice bags or other cold applications and alcohol sponges for hyperpyrexia, a vasopressor and fluids for circulatory collapse, and a darkened room for photophobia.

Pharmaceutical precautions *Tablets:* Keep container tightly closed; store in a cool place, protected from light.

Injection: Store in a cool place, protected from light and freezing.

Legal category POM.

Package quantities *Tablets:* Bottles of 500. *Injection:* Ampoules of 2 ml.

Further information Cogentin may be used in combination with other agents employed in the treatment of parkinsonism; the dosage of such agents may be reduced or they may be gradually discontinued. Many patients obtain greatest relief with a combination of Cogentin and other agents.

Cogentin may be used concomitantly with levodopa, in which case the usual dosage of each may need to be reduced. However, if Cogentin is continued when Sinemet* (carbidopa and levodopa, MSD) is introduced the dosage of Cogentin may need to be adjusted.

Product licence numbers
Tablets   0025/5023
Injection   0025/5024

CONCORDIN*

Presentation Concordin-5, salmon-red, film-coated tablets, marked 'MSD 26', containing 5 mg Protriptyline Hydrochloride BP.

Concordin-10, white, film-coated tablets, marked 'MSD 47', containing 10 mg Protriptyline Hydrochloride BP.

Uses Symptoms of depressive illness.

It may be used successfully in depression that is a manifestation of psychosis or neurosis, whether endogenous or reactive. Endogenous depression is more likely to respond. Concordin is especially recommended in apathetic, withdrawn patients, because it promptly relieves anergia, and it lacks sedative activity.

The following 'target' symptoms of depression may be expected to respond well to Concordin: depressed mood; excessive crying; apathy; withdrawal; psychomotor retardation; loss of interest; fatigue; lassitude; feelings of guilt; anorexia; headache; functional somatic complaints (e.g. gastro-intestinal symptoms).

Dosage and administration Dosage should be adjusted for each patient, bearing in mind the cyclic nature and variable severity of depression, the danger of relapse, and the possibility of spontaneous remission.

Adults: Dosage range, 15–60 mg. Usual starting dosage, 30–40 mg a day, divided into 3 or 4 doses. Any increase in dosage should be made gradually, and added to the morning dose first. If insomnia is present, the last dose should be given no later than mid-afternoon. When a satisfactory response is noted, the dosage should be reduced to the smallest amount necessary to maintain relief. Maintenance therapy should be continued for at least three months after satisfactory improvement. If relapse occurs, Concordin may be reinstated.

If the dosage required for adequate antidepressant effect produces overstimulation, concurrent use of a tranquilliser will provide effective control. Overstimulation is unlikely if the dosage of Concordin is kept below 20 mg a day.

Therapy may be usefully initiated with a tranquilliser and preventive supervision in suicidal patients, because these patients usually have a high level of anxiety, and Concordin may relieve anergia before recovery from depression is complete.

Children: Concordin is not recommended for children under 16 years old.

Elderly patients: Initially 5 mg three times a day. These patients may not tolerate higher doses as well as other patients. If the elderly receive more than 20 mg a day, they should be observed for effects on the cardiovascular system.

Contra-indications, warnings, etc
Contra-indications: Concurrent use with a monoamine oxidase inhibitor. Hyperpyretic crises, severe convulsions, and deaths have occurred when tricyclic antidepressants and MAOIs have been given simultaneously (see also 'Precautions'); the acute recovery phase after recent myocardial infarction; known sensitivity to protriptyline. Any degree of heart block or other cardiac arrhythmias, mania, marked agitation, severe liver disease, during breast feeding. For 'Use in pregnancy', see 'Precautions'.

Precautions: A minimum of 14 days should elapse between discontinuing a monoamine oxidase inhibitor and introducing Concordin, which should then be started cautiously, with gradual increases in dosage until optimum response is achieved.

Protriptyline may block the antihypertensive effect of guanethidine, debrisoquine, bethanidine, and possibly clonidine or similar compounds. Review all antihypertensive therapy during treatment. It should be used with caution in patients with a history of epilepsy, impaired liver function, a tendency to urinary retention, prostatic hypertrophy, or increased intra-ocular pressure.

Concordin should be used cautiously in elderly patients and patients with cardiovascular disorders. Such patients should be closely observed because of the tendency of protriptyline to produce tachycardia, hypotension, arrhythmias, and prolongation of the conduction time. The elderly are particularly liable to experience agitation and confusion. Myocardial infarction and stroke have occurred with drugs of this class. On rare occasions, hyperthyroid patients or those receiving thyroid medication may develop arrhythmias when protriptyline is given.

Concordin may impair abilities needed for performing hazardous tasks, such as driving a vehicle or operating machinery.

Psychotic symptoms may be aggravated when Concordin is used in schizophrenic patients. Manic depressive patients may shift towards the manic phase. Paranoid delusions, with or without hostility, may be exaggerated. In any of these circumstances, it may be advisable to reduce the dosage, or to use a major tranquilliser concurrently. An antidepressant with a sedative component, such as amitriptyline hydrochloride may be given before bedtime to help relieve insomnia, and control lesser degrees of anxiety and agitation. There has been no evidence of potentiation when Concordin has been replaced immediately by Tryptizol* (see separate entry under Thomas Morson Pharmaceuticals), or vice versa.

Concordin may aggravate anxiety or agitation in overactive or agitated patients.

Protriptyline should not be given with sympathomimetic agents such as ephedrine, isoprenaline, noradrenaline, phenylephrine, and phenylpropanolamine. Protriptyline may enhance response to alcohol, barbiturates and other CNS depressants.

The possibility of suicide in depressed patients remains during treatment until significant remission has occurred: suicidal patients should not have access to large quantities of Concordin Tablets and should be carefully supervised.

Concurrent administration of Concordin may increase the hazards of electroconvulsive therapy. Such combined treatment should be limited to those for whom it is essential.

Anaesthetics given during tricyclic antidepressant therapy may increase the risk of arrhythmias and hypotension. If surgery is necessary, the anaesthetist should be informed that the patient is receiving protriptyline.

The natural course of depression often is of many months' duration. It is appropriate, therefore, to continue maintenance therapy for three months or longer to lessen the possibility of relapse.

Use during pregnancy: Avoid during pregnancy, especially during the first and last trimesters, unless there are compelling reasons.

There is no evidence as to drug safety in human pregnancy, nor is there evidence from animal work that it is free from hazard.

Warnings and adverse effects: Some of the adverse reactions below have not been specifically reported for Concordin, but are included because of the similar pharmacological properties of the tricyclic group of antidepressants. Concordin is more likely to aggravate anxiety and agitation and to produce such cardiovascular reactions as tachycardia and hypotension.

As improvement may not occur during the first two to four weeks of treatment, patients should be closely monitored during this period.

Cardiovascular: Hypotension, hypertension, tachycardia, palpitation, myocardial infarction, arrhythmias, heart block, stroke.

Psychiatric: Confusional states (especially in the elderly) with hallucinations, disorientation, delusions, anxiety, restlessness, agitation; insomnia, panic, and nightmares; hypomania; exacerbation of psychosis.

Neurological: Numbness, tingling, and paraesthesiae of extremities; incoordination, ataxia, tremors, peripheral neuropathy; extrapyramidal symptoms; seizures; alteration in EEG patterns, tinnitus.

Anticholinergic: Dry mouth and rarely associated sublingual adenitis; blurred vision, disturbance of accommodation, mydriasis; constipation, paralytic ileus; urinary retention, delayed micturition, dilatation of the urinary tract.

Allergic: Skin rash, petechiae, urticaria, itching, oedema (general, or of face and tongue), drug fever. Some rashes have been associated with photosensitisation. In view of this, patients should avoid excessive exposure to sunlight, including sunbathing.

Haematological: Bone-marrow depression; agranulocytosis; leucopenia; eosinophilia; purpura; thrombocytopenia.

Gastro-intestinal: Nausea and vomiting, anorexia, epigastric distress, diarrhoea, peculiar taste, stomatitis, abdominal cramps, black tongue.

Endocrine: Gynaecomastia in the male; breast enlargement and galactorrhoea in the female; increased or decreased libido, impotence; testicular swelling; elevation or depression of blood sugar levels.

Other: Jaundice (simulating obstructive); altered liver function; weight gain or loss; perspiration; flushing; urinary frequency, nocturia; drowsiness, dizziness, weakness, and fatigue; headache; parotid swelling; alopecia.

Withdrawal symptoms: Though not indicative of addiction, abrupt cessation of treatment after prolonged therapy may produce nausea, insomnia, irritability, excessive perspiration, headache, and malaise.

Withdrawal symptoms in neonates whose mothers received tricyclic antidepressants during the third trimester have also been reported.

Treatment of overdosage: Symptomatic and supportive; there is no specific antidote.

The stomach should be emptied as quickly as possible by emesis or gastric lavage. If the patient is stuporous but responds to some stimuli, only close observation and nursing care for a day or two may be needed. If the patient is comatose, supportive measures will be required. An open airway and an adequate fluid intake should be maintained, and body temperature regulated. Cardiac arrhythmias may be treated with neostigmine, pyridostigmine or propranolol. Close monitoring of cardiac function is advisable for not less than five days. Intravenous, physostigmine salicylate, 1 to 3 mg, has been reported to reverse the symptoms of amitriptyline poisoning in man. Animal studies have shown that physostigmine also reverses certain toxic effects of protriptyline. Because physostigmine is rapidly metabolised, the dosage should be repeated as required, particularly if life threatening signs such as arrhythmias, convulsions and deep coma recur or persist after the initial dose of physostigmine. If convulsions occur, they should be treated with anticonvulsants. Barbiturates should not be used. CNS depression may be treated with non-convulsant doses of CNS stimulants. Cardiac monitoring may be desirable, and use of digitalis should be considered if serious cardiovascular abnormalities occur. Standard measures may be used to manage shock and metabolic acidosis. Dialysis is not of value.

Treatment should be continued for at least 48 hours in patients who do not respond earlier. There have been instances where patients have been in coma for several days and have eventually recovered. Deaths by deliberate or accidental overdosage have occurred with this class of medicament. Since overdosage is often deliberate, patients may attempt suicide by other means during the recovery phase.

Pharmaceutical precautions Keep container well closed; store in a cool place, protected from light.

Legal category POM.

Package quantities *5 mg:* Bottles of 100.
10 mg: Bottles of 100.

Further information Concordin is a member of the tricyclic group of antidepressants. It is not a monoamine oxidase inhibitor, and dietary restrictions are not necessary. It has not produced addiction or habituation.

Concordin has a rapid onset of effect, which can be of particular importance where there is a risk of suicide. It is advisable, however, to administer a tranquilliser and to ensure preventative supervision when starting Concordin in suicidal patients since they usually have a high level of anxiety, and especially because Concordin may relieve the anergia before there is complete recovery from the depressed state.

When Concordin has to be used in conjunction with ECT, the total number of shock treatments required may be reduced.

Product licence numbers
5 mg   0025/5004
10 mg   0025/5005

CORTISONE ACETATE (MSD)

Presentation White tablets, marked 'MSD 126', containing 5 mg Cortisone Acetate BP.

White, half-scored tablets, marked 'MSD 219', containing 25 mg Cortisone Acetate BP.

Uses Corticosteroid.
For use in certain endocrine and non-endocrine disorders responsive to corticosteroid therapy.

Endocrine disorders: Primary, secondary and acute adrenocortical insufficiency.

Pre-operatively, and during serious trauma or illness in patients with known adrenal insufficiency or doubtful adrenocortical reserve.

Non-endocrine disorders: Cortisone may be used in the treatment of non-endocrine corticosteroid responsive conditions including:

Allergy and anaphylaxis: Angioneurotic oedema, anaphylaxis.

Arteritis collagenosis: Polymyalgia rheumatica, polyarteritis nodosa.

Blood disorders: Haemolytic anaemia, leukaemia, myeloma.

Cardiovascular disorders: Post-myocardial infarction syndrome.

Gastro-intestinal: Crohn's disease, ulcerative colitis.

Hypercalcaemia: Sarcoidosis.

Infections (with appropriate chemotherapy): Miliary tuberculosis.

Muscular disorders: Polymyositis.

Ocular disorders: Anterior and posterior uveitis, optic neuritis.

Renal disorders: Lupus nephritis.

Respiratory disease: Bronchial asthma, aspiration pneumonitis.

Rheumatic disorders: Rheumatoid arthritis.

Skin disorders: Pemphigus vulgaris.

Dosage and administration Dosage must be individualised on the basis of the disease and the response of the individual patient. The lowest possible dosage adequate to control the disease process should be used.

The initial dosage varies from 10 mg to 50 mg a day divided into 3 or 4 doses, the dosage depending on the disease being treated. In more severe diseases, doses higher than 50 mg may be required. The initial dose should be maintained or adjusted until the patient's response is satisfactory. Both the dose in the evening, which is useful in alleviating morning stiffness, and the divided dosage regimen are associated with greater suppression of the hypothalamo-pituitary-adrenal axis. If satisfactory clinical response does not occur after a reasonable period of time, discontinue Cortisone Acetate Tablets and transfer the patient to other therapy.

When symptoms have been controlled, the proper maintenance dosage should be determined by decreasing the dosage in small amounts to the lowest dose that maintains an adequate clinical response. Chronic dosage should preferably not exceed 30 mg Cortisone Acetate daily.

Patients should be monitored closely for signs that might require dosage adjustment, including changes in the clinical status resulting from remissions or exacerbations of the disease, individual drug responsiveness and the effect of stress (e.g. surgery, infection or trauma). During stress, it may be necessary to increase the dosage temporarily.

If the drug is to be stopped after more than a few days, treatment should be withdrawn gradually.

Specific dosage recommendations:
In chronic adrenocortical insufficiency: 10–25 mg a day or occasionally more, together with 4–6 g of sodium chloride or 1–3 mg of desoxycorticosterone acetate. When immediate support is mandatory, one of the soluble adrenocortical hormone preparations (e.g. Decadron* Injection, dexamethasone sodium phosphate, MSD), which may be effective within minutes after parenteral administration, can be life-saving.

In congenital adrenal hyperplasia: The usual daily dosage is 10–50 mg.

When an extremely rapid onset of action is desired, Decadron Injection may be administered intravenously for the first 2 or 3 doses.

Adrenaline is the drug of first choice in allergic reactions. Cortisone Acetate, MSD Tablets are useful either concurrently or as supplementary therapy.

Use in children: Dosage should be limited to a single dose on alternate days to lessen retardation of growth and minimise suppression of hypothalamo-pituitary-adrenal axis.

Use in the elderly: Treatment of elderly patients,

particularly if long term, should be planned bearing in mind the more serious consequences of the common side effects of corticosteroids in old age, especially osteoporosis, diabetes, hypertension, susceptibility to infection and thinning of the skin.

Contra-indications, warnings, etc

Contra-indications: Systemic fungal infections. Hypersensitivity to the drug.

Precautions: The dosage of corticosteroid should be reduced gradually.

Corticosteroids may exacerbate systemic fungal infections and should not be used unless they are needed to control drug reactions due to amphotericin.

Cases have been reported in which concomitant use of amphotericin and hydrocortisone was followed by cardiac enlargement and congestive heart failure.

A report shows that the use of corticosteroids in cerebral malaria is associated with a prolonged coma and an increased incidence of pneumonia and gastrointestinal bleeding.

Average and large doses of hydrocortisone or cortisone can cause elevation of blood pressure, salt and water retention, and increased excretion of potassium. These effects are less likely to occur with the synthetic derivatives except when used in large doses. Dietary salt restriction and potassium supplementation may be necessary. All corticosteroids increase calcium excretion.

In patients on corticosteroid therapy subjected to unusual stress, increased dosage of rapidly acting corticosteroids before, during and after the stressful situation is indicated.

Drug-induced secondary adrenocortical insufficiency may result from too rapid withdrawal of corticosteroids and may be minimised by gradual reduction of dosage. This type of relative insufficiency may persist for months after discontinuation of therapy; therefore, in any situation of stress occurring during that period, corticosteroid therapy should be reinstated. If the patient is receiving steroids already, the dosage may have to be increased. Since mineralocorticoid secretion may be impaired, salt and/or a mineralocorticoid should be administered concurrently.

Stopping corticosteroids after prolonged therapy may cause withdrawal symptoms including fever, myalgia, arthralgia, and malaise. This may occur in patients even without evidence of adrenal insufficiency.

Administration of live virus vaccines is contra-indicated in individuals receiving immunosuppressive doses of corticosteroids. If inactivated viral or bacterial vaccines are administered to individuals receiving immunosuppressive doses of corticosteroids, the expected serum antibody response may not be obtained. However, immunisation procedures may be undertaken in patients who are receiving corticosteroids as replacement therapy, e.g. for Addison's disease.

Aspirin should be used cautiously in conjunction with corticosteroids in hypoprothrombinaemia.

The use of Cortisone Acetate, MSD Tablets in active tuberculosis should be restricted to those cases of fulminating or disseminated tuberculosis in which the corticosteroid is used for the management of the disease in conjunction with an appropriate antituberculous regimen. If corticosteroids are indicated in patients with latent tuberculosis or tuberculin reactivity, close observation is necessary as reactivation of the disease may occur. During prolonged corticosteroid therapy, these patients should receive prophylactic chemotherapy.

Steroids should be used with caution in renal insufficiency, hypertension, diabetes or in those with a family history of diabetes, congestive heart failure, osteoporosis, previous steroid myopathy, glaucoma (or previous history), myasthenia gravis, non-specific ulcerative colitis, diverticulitis, fresh intestinal anastomoses, active or latent peptic ulcer. Signs of peritoneal irritation following gastro-intestinal perforation in patients receiving large doses of corticosteroids may be minimal or absent. Fat embolism has been reported as a possible complication of hypercortisonism.

Corticosteroids should be used cautiously in patients with ocular herpes simplex because of possible corneal perforation.

There is an enhanced effect of corticosteroids on patients with hypothyroidism and in those with cirrhosis.

Corticosteroids may mask some signs of infection, and new infections may appear during their use. There may be decreased resistance and inability to localise infection in patients on corticosteroids.

Corticosteroids may activate latent amoebiasis. Therefore, it is recommended that latent or active amoebiasis be excluded before initiating corticosteroid therapy in any patient who has either spent time in the tropics, or has unexplained diarrhoea.

Alterations in the patient's mental state may appear when corticosteroids are used, ranging from psychological dependence, euphoria, insomnia, mood swings, personality changes and severe depression, to frank psychotic manifestations.

Prolonged use of corticosteroids may produce posterior subcapsular cataracts, glaucoma with possible damage to the optic nerves, and may enhance the establishment of secondary ocular infections.

Steroids may increase or decrease motility and number of spermatozoa.

Phenytoin, barbiturates, ephedrine and rifampicin may enhance the metabolic clearance of corticosteroids, resulting in decreased blood levels and lessened physiological activity, thus requiring adjustment in corticosteroid dosage.

The prothrombin time should be checked frequently in patients who are receiving corticosteroids and coumarin anticoagulants concurrently.

When corticosteroids are administered concomitantly with potassium-depleting diuretics, patients should be monitored closely for development of hypokalaemia.

Children: Corticosteroids cause growth retardation in infancy, childhood and adolescence. Treatment should be limited to the minimum dosage for the shortest possible time. In order to minimise suppression of the hypothalamo-pituitary-adrenal axis and growth retardation, treatment should be limited, where possible, to a single dose on alternate days.

Growth and development of infants and children on prolonged corticosteroid therapy should be carefully monitored.

Use in pregnancy and the nursing mother: There is inadequate evidence of safety in human pregnancy and there may be a very small risk of cleft palate and intra-uterine growth retardation in the fetus; there is evidence of harmful effects on pregnancy in animals.

Corticosteroids appear in breast milk and could suppress growth, interfere with endogenous corticosteroid production, or cause other unwanted effects. Mothers taking pharmacological doses of corticosteroids should be advised not to nurse.

Side-effects: Fluid and electrolyte disturbances: Sodium

retention, fluid retention, congestive heart failure in susceptible patients, potassium loss, hypokalaemic alkalosis, hypertension, increased calcium excretion.

Musculoskeletal: Muscle weakness, steroid myopathy, loss of muscle mass, osteoporosis (especially in post-menopausal females), vertebral compression fractures, aseptic necrosis of femoral and humeral heads, pathological fracture of long bones, tendon rupture.

Gastro-intestinal: Peptic ulcer with possible perforation and haemorrhage, perforation of the small and large bowel particularly in patients with inflammatory bowel disease, pancreatitis, abdominal distension, ulcerative oesophagitis, dyspepsia, oesophageal candidiasis.

Dermatological: Impaired wound healing, thin fragile skin, petechiae and ecchymoses, erythema, striae, telangiectasia, acne, increased sweating, may suppress reactions to skin tests, other cutaneous reactions such as allergic dermatitis, urticaria, angioneurotic oedema.

Neurological: Convulsions, increased intracranial pressure with papilloedema (pseudotumour cerebri) usually after treatment, vertigo, headache.

Endocrine: Menstrual irregularities, amenorrhoea, development of Cushingoid state, suppression of growth in children, secondary adrenocortical and pituitary unresponsiveness (particularly in times of stress, as in trauma, surgery or illness), decreased carbohydrate tolerance, manifestations of latent diabetes mellitus, increased requirements for insulin or oral hypoglycaemic agents in diabetics.

Ophthalmic: Posterior subcapsular cataracts, increased intra-ocular pressure, papilloedema, corneal or scleral thinning, exacerbation of ophthalmic viral disease, glaucoma, exophthalmos.

Metabolic: Negative nitrogen balance due to protein catabolism.

Other: Hypersensitivity, leucocytosis, thrombo-embolism, weight gain, increased appetite, nausea, malaise.

Teratogenicity: See pregnancy warning under 'Use in pregnancy and the nursing mother'.

Treatment of overdosage: None indicated, unless patient has ingested a very large amount, and has one of the conditions which might predispose to adverse effects of adrenocortical steroids, in which case it is probably best to empty the stomach by inducing emesis or performing gastric lavage.

Pharmaceutical precautions Keep container well closed; store in a cool place, protected from light.

Legal category POM.

Package quantities *5 mg:* Bottles of 50.
25 mg: Bottles of 100.

Further information Nil.

Product licence numbers
5 mg   0025/5043
25 mg   0025/5044

COSMEGEN,* LYOVAC*

Presentation Yellow, lyophilised powder, in a vial containing 0.5 mg dactinomycin with 20 mg of mannitol.

Uses Cytotoxic, antineoplastic antibiotic with immuno-suppressant properties.

Mode of action: Cosmegen inhibits the proliferation of cells by forming a stable complex with DNA and interfering with DNA-dependent RNA synthesis.

Recommended only in the treatment, under appropriate supervision, of hospitalised patients with Wilms' tumour, rhabdomyosarcoma, and carcinoma of the testis or uterus. All other indications for dactinomycin are as yet experimental (e.g. Ewing's sarcoma, osteogenic sarcoma).

Wilms' tumour: The neoplasm responding most frequently to Cosmegen is Wilms' tumour. With low doses of both dactinomycin and radiotherapy, temporary objective improvement may be as good as, and may last longer than, that obtained with higher doses of each given alone.

Rhabdomyosarcoma: Temporary regression of the tumour and beneficial subjective results have occurred with dactinomycin in rhabdomyosarcoma, which, like most soft-tissue sarcomas, is comparatively radio-resistant.

Carcinoma of testis and uterus: The sequential use of dactinomycin and methotrexate, along with meticulous monitoring of human chorionic gonadotrophin levels until normal, has resulted in survival in the majority of women with metastatic choriocarcinoma.

Sequential therapy is used if there is:

1. Stability in gonadotrophin titres following two successive courses of an agent.
2. Rising gonadotrophin titres during treatment.
3. Severe toxicity preventing adequate therapy.

In patients with non-metastatic choriocarcinoma, dactinomycin or methotrexate or both, have been used successfully, with or without surgery.

Cosmegen has been beneficial as a single agent in the treatment of metastatic non-seminomatous testicular carcinoma.

Other neoplasms: Dactinomycin has been given intravenously or by regional perfusion, alone or with other antineoplastic compounds or with X-ray therapy, in the palliative treatment of Ewing's sarcoma and sarcoma botryoides. For non-metastatic Ewing's sarcoma, promising results were obtained when dactinomycin ($45 \, mcg/m^2$) and cyclophosphamide ($1,200 \, mg/m^2$) were given sequentially and with radiotherapy, over an eighteen-month period. Those with metastatic disease remain the subject of continued investigation with a more aggressive chemotherapeutic regimen employed initially.

Temporary objective improvement and relief of pain and discomfort have followed the use of dactinomycin, usually in conjunction with radiotherapy for sarcoma botryoides. This palliative effect ranges from transitory inhibition of tumour growth to a considerable but temporary regression in tumour size.

Cosmegen and radiation therapy: Much evidence suggests that Cosmegen potentiates the effects of X-ray therapy. The converse also appears likely; that Cosmegen may be more effective when radiation therapy is given concurrently.

With combined Cosmegen and radiation therapy, the normal skin, as well as the buccal and pharyngeal mucosa, shows early erythema. When given with dactinomycin, a smaller than usual X-ray dose causes erythema and vesiculation, which progresses more rapidly through the stages of tanning and desquamation. Healing may occur in four to six weeks rather than in two to three months. Erythema from previous X-ray therapy may be reactivated by the administration of Cosmegen alone, especially when the interval between the two forms of therapy is brief. This potentiation of radiation effects represents a special problem when the irradiation treatment area includes the mucous membrane. When irradiation is directed towards the nasopharynx, the combination may produce severe oropharyngeal mucositis.

Severe reactions may ensue if high doses of both Cosmegen and radiation therapy are used, or if the patient is particularly sensitive to such combined therapy.

Because of this potentiating effect, Cosmegen may be tried in radio-sensitive tumours not responding to doses of X-ray therapy that can be tolerated. Objective improvement in tumour size and activity may be observed when lower, better tolerated doses of both types of therapy are employed.

Isolation-perfusion technique: Cosmegen, alone or with other antineoplastic agents, has also been given by the isolation-perfusion technique, either as palliative treatment or as an adjunct to resection of a tumour. Some tumours that are considered resistant to chemotherapy and radiation therapy may respond when the drug is given by the perfusion technique. Neoplasms in which dactinomycin has been tried by this technique include various types of sarcoma, carcinoma and adenocarcinoma.

In some instances, tumours regressed, pain was relieved for variable periods, and surgery made possible. On other occasions, however, the outcome has been less favourable. Nevertheless, in selected cases, Cosmegen given by the perfusion technique may provide more effective palliation than when given systemically.

Dosage and administration Toxic reactions due to Cosmegen are frequent and may be severe, thus limiting the amount that may be given in many cases. However, the severity of toxicity varies markedly and is only partly dependent on the dosage used. Cosmegen must only be given in short courses.

The dosage of Cosmegen will vary with the tolerance of the patient, the size and location of the neoplasm, and the use of other forms of therapy. It may be necessary to reduce the usual dosage suggested below when other chemotherapy or X-ray therapy is used concurrently, or has been employed previously.

Intravenous use: Cosmegen is reconstituted by adding 1.1 ml of Water for Injections BP without preservative to the vial. For injection, 1.0 ml of the reconstituted solution, which will contain 0.5 mg of dactinomycin, is withdrawn into the syringe. Only Water for Injections BP (which does not contain preservatives) should be used. Other injection fluids may cause precipitation.

Cosmegen should be inspected for particulate matter and discoloration, whenever possible. The reconstituted solution is clear and gold-coloured.

When reconstituted, the solution of dactinomycin can be added to an infusion solution of 5% dextrose injection or sodium chloride injection, either directly or into the tubing of a running intravenous infusion.

Since dactinomycin is extremely corrosive to soft tissue, precautions for materials of this nature should be observed. To avoid extravasation, the calculated dose of Cosmegen should be given through the tubing of a running intravenous infusion, so that when administration is completed, the tubing can be flushed immediately to avoid damage to the vein. Partial removal of dactinomycin from intravenous solutions by cellulose ester membrane filters used in some intravenous in-line filters has been reported.

If Cosmegen is to be injected directly into the vein without the use of an infusion, the 'two-needle' technique should be used. The calculated dose should be reconstituted and withdrawn from the vial with one sterile needle; direct injection into the vein should then be performed with another sterile needle.

Any unused portion of the solution must be discarded.

Adults: Usually 0.5 mg (500 mcg) a day for a maximum of five days, given intravenously.

Children: 0.015 mg (15 mcg) per kg body weight a day for a maximum of five days, given intravenously. Alternatively, the dosage for children should not exceed 400–600 mcg/m² body surface intravenously for 5 days.

In both adults and children, a second course may be given, but not until at least three weeks have elapsed, and all evidence of toxicity has disappeared.

Isolation-perfusion technique: Administration by the isolation-perfusion technique offers certain advantages, provided leakage of the drug through the general circulation into other areas of the body is minimal. By this technique, dactinomycin is in continuous contact with the tumour for the duration of treatment. The dose may be increased well above that used by the systemic route, usually without adding to the danger of toxic effects. If the agent is confined to an isolated part, it should not interfere with the patient's defence mechanisms. Systemic absorption of toxic products from neoplastic tissue can be minimised by removing the perfusate when the procedure is finished.

The dosage schedules and the technique itself vary from one investigator to another; the published literature should, therefore, be consulted for details. In general, the following doses are suggested:

For a lower extremity or pelvis – 0.05 mg (50 mcg) per kg body weight.

For an upper extremity – 0.035 mg (35 mcg) per kg body weight.

It may be advisable to use lower doses in obese patients, or when previous chemotherapy or radiation therapy has been employed.

Use in the elderly: The general considerations already outlined also apply to elderly patients.

Contra-indications, warnings, etc

Contra-indications: If Cosmegen is given at or about the time of infection with chickenpox or herpes zoster, a severe generalised disease, which may be fatal, can occur.

Warning: Cosmegen should be administered only under the supervision of a physician who is experienced in the use of a cancer chemotherapeutic agent.

Precautions: Cosmegen, like all antineoplastic agents, is a toxic drug, and very careful and frequent observation of the patient for adverse reactions is necessary. These reactions may involve any tissue of the body. The possibility of an anaphylactoid reaction should be borne in mind.

Dactinomycin can affect male fertility adversely.

Use in children: As there is a greater frequency of toxic effects of dactinomycin in infants, Cosmegen should not normally be given to children less than 12 months old.

A variety of abnormalities of renal, hepatic and bone-marrow function have been reported in patients with neoplastic disease receiving dactinomycin. It is advisable to make frequent checks of renal, hepatic, and bone-marrow function.

An increased incidence of gastro-intestinal toxicity and bone-marrow depression has been reported when dactinomycin was given with X-ray therapy.

Particular caution is necessary when administering dactinomycin during the first two months after irradiation for the treatment of right-sided Wilms' tumour, since hepatomegaly and elevated AST (SGOT) levels have been seen.

Nausea and vomiting due to dactinomycin make it necessary to give Cosmegen intermittently. It is extremely important to observe the patient daily for toxic side-effects when combined therapy is employed, since a full course of therapy is occasionally not tolerated. If stomatitis, diarrhoea, or severe haemopoietic depression appear during therapy, these drugs should be discontinued until the patient has recovered.

Recent reports indicate an increased incidence of second primary tumours following treatment with radiation and anti-neoplastic agents, such as dactinomycin. Multi-modal therapy creates the need for careful, long-term observation of cancer survivors.

Drug/laboratory test interactions: It has been reported that dactinomycin may interfere with bioassay procedures for the determination of antibacterial drug levels.

Use in pregnancy and nursing mothers: This product has been shown to be teratogenic in animals and should not normally be given to pregnant women.

Dactinomycin should not be administered to mothers who are breast feeding.

Dactinomycin can affect male fertility adversely.

Side-effects: Toxic effects (except nausea and vomiting) do not usually become apparent until two to four days after a course of therapy is stopped, and may not reach a maximum before one to two weeks have elapsed. Deaths have been reported. However, side-effects are usually reversible on discontinuing therapy. They include the following:

General: Malaise, fatigue, lethargy, fever, myalgia, proctitis, hypocalcaemia.

Oral: Cheilitis, dysphagia, oesophagitis, ulcerative stomatitis, pharyngitis.

Gastro-intestinal: Anorexia, nausea, vomiting, abdominal pain, diarrhoea, gastro-intestinal ulceration. Nausea and vomiting, which occur early during the first few hours after administration, may be alleviated by giving anti-emetics.

Haematological: Anaemia (even to the point of aplastic anaemia, agranulocytosis, leucopenia, thrombocytopenia, pancytopenia, reticulocytopenia). Platelet and white blood cell counts should be done daily to detect severe haemopoietic depression. If either count shows a marked decrease, dactinomycin should be withheld to allow marrow recovery. This often takes up to three weeks.

Dermatological: Alopecia, skin eruptions, acne, flare-up of erythema or increased pigmentation of previously irradiated skin.

Soft tissues: Dactinomycin is extremely corrosive to soft tissues. If extravasation occurs during intravenous use, severe damage to soft tissues will occur. In at least one instance, this has led to contracture of the arms.

Side-effects relating especially to the isolation-perfusion technique: Complications of the perfusion technique are related mainly to the amount of drug that escapes into the systemic circulation and may consist of haemopoietic depression, increased susceptibility to infection, absorption of toxic products from massive destruction of neoplastic tissue, impaired wound healing, and superficial ulceration of the gastric mucosa. Other side-effects may include oedema of the extremity involved, damage

to the soft tissues of the perfused area, and potentially venous thrombosis.

Treatment of overdosage: There is no known antidote. Treatment is symptomatic after Cosmegen is discontinued.

Pharmaceutical precautions Store below 25°C protected from light. Avoid freezing.

It is recommended that Cosmegen is reconstituted only by trained personnel wearing protective gloves. A designated area should be set aside for this purpose and the work surface covered with disposable plastic-backed absorbent paper.

Luer-lock fittings on all syringes and sets are recommended, and use of large-bore needles or a venting needle will help to minimise back pressure and the possible formation of aerosols. Accidental splashing on to the skin or eye should be treated immediately with copious irrigation of isotonic saline. Pregnant staff should not handle Cosmegen.

Adequate care should be taken in the disposal of equipment after contact with Cosmegen.

Legal category POM.

Package quantities Vials containing 0.5 mg dactinomycin with 20 mg mannitol.

Further information Generally, the actinomycins inhibit Gram-positive and Gram-negative bacteria and some fungi. However, the toxic properties of the actinomycins (including dactinomycin) in relation to antibacterial activity preclude their use as antibiotics in the treatment of infectious diseases.

Because the actinomycins are cytotoxic, they have an antineoplastic effect which has been demonstrated in experimental animals with various types of tumour implant. This cytotoxic action is the basis for their use in the palliative treatment of certain types of cancer.

Dactinomycin is minimally metabolised. The terminal plasma half-life is approximately 36 hours. It tends to concentrate in nucleated cells and does not cross the blood-brain barrier.

Product licence number 0025/5075.

DARANIDE*

Presentation Yellow, half-scored tablets, marked 'MSD 49', containing 50 mg Dichlorphenamide BP.

Uses Carbonic anhydrase inhibitor.

For chronic simple (open-angle) glaucoma and secondary glaucoma. May be useful for pre-operative control of intra-ocular tension in acute angle-closure glaucoma.

Dosage and administration Although Daranide can be used alone, it is usually more effective when given concurrently with miotics.

Initial adult dosage: Usually 2–4 tablets followed by 2 tablets every 12 hours.

Maintenance dosage: ½–1 tablet one to three times a day.

Dosage must be carefully adjusted to the individual requirements of each patient. In acute angle-closure glaucoma, Daranide may be administered with miotics and osmotic agents. If this does not reduce the intra-ocular tension rapidly, surgery may be mandatory.

Use in the elderly: The dosage above also applies to the

elderly, but use with particular caution in this age group (see 'Precautions' and 'Side-effects').

Contra-indications, warnings, etc

Contra-indications: Hepatic insufficiency, renal failure, adrenocortical insufficiency, hyperchloraemic acidosis, depressed sodium or potassium levels or chronic non-congestive closed-angle glaucoma. Should not be used in patients with severe pulmonary obstruction who are unable to increase their alveolar ventilation, since acidosis may be increased. Hypersensitivity to dichlorphenamide.

See also 'Use in pregnancy' under 'Precautions'.

Precautions: Daranide increases potassium excretion, and hypokalaemia may develop under the following circumstances: when diuresis is brisk; in the presence of severe cirrhosis; during concomitant therapy with steroids or ACTH; interference with adequate oral electrolyte intake. Digitalised patients are particularly sensitive to the effects of potassium depletion. Hypokalaemia may be treated by administration of potassium chloride or giving foods with a high potassium content.

Like all carbonic anhydrase inhibitors, high doses of Daranide cause some decrease in renal blood flow and glomerular filtration rate.

Daranide should be used with caution in the presence of severe degrees of respiratory acidosis.

Carbonic anhydrase inhibitors may potentiate the effects of folic acid antagonists, hypoglycaemic agents, oral anticoagulants and local anaesthetics, and may increase the risk of salicylate toxicity in patients taking salicylates. Instances of severe osteomalacia have been reported in patients taking carbonic anhydrase inhibitors with anticonvulsants.

Use in pregnancy: Studies with dichlorphenamide in rats have demonstrated teratogenic effects (skeletal anomalies) at high dosages. There is no evidence of these effects in humans; however, dichlorphenamide is not recommended for use in women of child bearing age or in pregnant patients, especially during the first trimester. If pregnancy is present or suspected, the benefits of using Daranide should be weighed against possible hazards to the fetus.

Side-effects: The side-effects characteristic of carbonic anhydrase inhibitors may occur. These include: gastrointestinal disturbances (anorexia, nausea, and vomiting); loss of weight; constipation; urinary frequency; renal colic; renal calculi; skin eruptions; pruritus; leucopenia; agranulocytosis; thrombocytopenia; headache; weakness; nervousness; globus hystericus; sedation; lassitude; depression; confusion; disorientation; dizziness; ataxia; tremor; tinnitus; paraesthesiae of hands, feet and tongue.

Treatment of overdosage: Supportive; the stomach should be emptied by emesis or gastric lavage. Fluids and electrolytes should, if necessary, be replenished. The most likely electrolyte disturbance is a hyperchloraemic acidosis that may respond to bicarbonate administration.

Pharmaceutical precautions Keep container well closed; store in a cool place, protected from light.

Legal category POM.

Package quantities Bottles of 100.

Further information In glaucoma, Daranide has a rapid onset of action, lowering the pressure within an hour. It reaches maximal effect in two to four hours, and is effective for six to twelve hours.

Product licence number 0025/5025.

DECADRON* INJECTION

Presentation A clear, colourless solution containing, in each millilitre, Dexamethasone Sodium Phosphate BP equivalent to 4 mg dexamethasone phosphate or approximately 3.33 mg dexamethasone.

Uses Corticosteroid.

For use in certain endocrine and non-endocrine disorders responsive to corticosteroid therapy.

Systemic administration: Decadron Injection is recommended for systemic administration by intravenous or intramuscular injection when oral therapy is not feasible or desirable in the following conditions.

Endocrine disorders:

Primary or secondary adrenocortical insufficiency: (Hydrocortisone or cortisone is the first choice, but synthetic analogues may be used with mineralocorticoids where applicable and, in infancy, mineralocorticoid supplementation is particularly important.)

Non-endocrine disorders: Decadron Injection may be used in the treatment of non-endocrine corticosteroid responsive conditions including:

Allergy and anaphylaxis: Angioneurotic oedema and anaphylaxis.

Gastro-intestinal: Crohn's disease and ulcerative colitis.

Infection (with appropriate chemotherapy): Miliary tuberculosis and endotoxic shock.

Neurological disorders: Raised intracranial pressure secondary to cerebral tumours and infantile spasms.

Respiratory: Bronchial asthma and aspiration pneumonitis.

Skin disorders: Toxic epidermal necrolysis.

Shock: Adjunctive treatment where high pharmacological doses are needed. Treatment is an adjunct to, and not a substitute for specific and supportive measures the patient may require. Dexamethasone has been shown to be beneficial when used in the early treatment of shock, but it may not influence overall survival.

Local administration

Decadron Injection is suitable for intra-articular or soft-tissue injection as adjunctive therapy for short-term administration in:

Soft-tissue disorders such as carpal tunnel syndrome and tenosynovitis.

Intra-articular disorders such as rheumatoid arthritis and osteoarthritis with an inflammatory component.

Decadron Injection may be injected intralesionally in selected skin disorders such as cystic acne vulgaris, localised lichen simplex, and keloids.

Dosage and administration Decadron Injection can be given without mixing or dilution, but if preferred, can be added without loss of potency to sodium chloride injection or dextrose injection or compatible blood for transfusion, and given by intravenous drip. The infusion mixture must be used within 24 hours, and the usual aseptic techniques for injections should be observed.

Intravenous and intramuscular injection:

General considerations: Generally, initial and maintenance dosages must be determined individually according to the disease under treatment and to the response of the patient. The lowest possible dosage adequate to control the disease process should be used.

Usually the parenteral dosage ranges are one-third to one-half the oral dose, given every 12 hours.

The usual initial dosage is 0.5–20 mg (0.125–5 ml) a day. In situations of less severity, lower doses will generally suffice. However, in certain overwhelming, acute, life-threatening situations, administration in dosages exceeding the usual dosages may be justified. In these circumstances, the slower rate of absorption by intramuscular administration should be recognised.

The initial dosage should be maintained or adjusted until a satisfactory response is noted.

Both the dose in the evening, which is useful in alleviating morning stiffness, and the divided dosage regimen are associated with greater suppression of the hypothalamo-pituitary-adrenal axis. (If, after a reasonable time, there is a lack of satisfactory clinical response, Decadron Injection should be discontinued and the patient transferred to other appropriate therapy.) After a favourable response is noted, the proper maintenance dosage should be determined by decreasing the initial dosage by small amounts at appropriate intervals to the lowest dosage which will maintain an adequate clinical response. Chronic dosage should preferably not exceed 0.5 mg dexamethasone daily. Close monitoring is needed in regard to drug dosage.

If Decadron is to be stopped after it has been given for more than a few days, it should be withdrawn gradually rather than stopped abruptly.

Whenever possible, the intravenous route should be used for the initial dose and for as many subsequent doses as are given while the patient is in shock (because of the irregular rate of absorption of any medicament administered by any other route in such patients). When the blood pressure responds, use the intramuscular route until oral therapy can be substituted. For the comfort of the patient, not more than 2 ml should be injected intramuscularly at any one site.

In emergencies, the usual dose of Decadron Injection by intravenous or intramuscular injection is 1 ml–5 ml (4 mg–20 mg), depending on the severity of the condition (see also 'Shock'). This dose may be repeated until adequate response is discernible.

After initial improvement, single doses of 0.5 ml–1 ml (2 mg–4 mg) repeated as necessary, may be sufficient. The total daily dosage usually need not exceed 20 ml (80 mg), even in severe conditions.

When constant maximal effect is desired, dosage must be repeated at three-hour or four-hour intervals, or maintained by slow intravenous drip.

Intravenous and intramuscular injections are advised in acute illness. When the acute stage has passed, oral steroid therapy should be substituted as soon as feasible.

Shock (of haemorrhagic, traumatic, surgical or septic origin): Usually 2 to 6 mg/kg body weight as a single intravenous injection. This may be repeated in two to six hours if shock persists. Alternatively, this may be followed immediately by the same dose in an intravenous infusion. Therapy with Decadron Injection is an adjunct to, and not a replacement for conventional therapy.

Administration of these high doses should be continued only until the patient's condition has stabilised and usually no longer than 48–72 hours.

Cerebral oedema: Associated with primary or metastatic brain tumour, pre-operative preparation of patients with increased intracranial pressure secondary to brain tum-

our: initially 10 mg (2.5 ml) intravenously, followed by 4 mg (1 ml) intramuscularly every six hours until symptoms of cerebral oedema subside. Response is usually noted within 12–24 hours; dosage may be reduced after two to four days and gradually discontinued over five to seven days.

High doses of Decadron Injection are recommended for initiating short-term intensive therapy for acute life-threatening cerebral oedema. Following the high loading dose schedule of the first day of therapy, the dose is scaled down over the seven- to ten-day period of intensive therapy and subsequently reduced to zero over the next seven to ten days. When maintenance therapy is required, substitute oral Decadron as soon as possible. (See table below.)

Palliative management of recurrent or inoperable brain tumours: Maintenance therapy should be determined for each patient; 2 mg (0.5 ml) two or three times a day may be effective.

The smallest dosage necessary to control cerebral oedema should be used.

Suggested high dose schedule in cerebral oedema:

Adults:

Initial Dose	50 mg IV
1st day	8 mg IV every 2 hours
2nd day	8 mg IV every 2 hours
3rd day	8 mg IV every 2 hours
4th day	4 mg IV every 2 hours
5th–8th day	4 mg IV every 4 hours
Thereafter	decrease by daily reduction of 4 mg

Children (35 kg and over):

Initial Dose	25 mg IV
1st day	4 mg IV every 2 hours
2nd day	4 mg IV every 2 hours
3rd day	4 mg IV every 2 hours
4th day	4 mg IV every 4 hours
5th–8th day	4 mg IV every 6 hours
Thereafter	decrease by daily reduction of 2 mg

Children (below 35 kg):

Initial Dose	20 mg IV
1st day	4 mg IV every 3 hours
2nd day	4 mg IV every 3 hours
3rd day	4 mg IV every 3 hours
4th day	4 mg IV every 6 hours
5th–8th day	2 mg IV every 6 hours
Thereafter	decrease by daily reduction of 1 mg

Dual therapy: In acute self-limiting allergic disorders or acute exacerbations of chronic allergic disorders, the following schedule combining oral and parenteral therapy is suggested:

First day	Decadron Injection, 4 mg–8 mg (1 ml–2 ml) intramuscularly
Second day	Two 0.5 mg Decadron Tablets twice a day
Third day	Two 0.5 mg Decadron Tablets twice a day
Fourth day	One 0.5 mg Decadron Tablet twice a day
Fifth day	One 0.5 mg Decadron Tablet twice a day
Sixth day	One 0.5 mg Decadron Tablet
Seventh day	One 0.5 mg Decadron Tablet
Eighth day	Reassessment day

(For information on Decadron Tablets, see separate entry.)

Intrasynovial, intralesional, and soft-tissue injection: In general, these injections are employed when only one or two joints or areas are affected.

Some of the usual single doses are:

Site of injection	Amount of dexamethasone phosphate
Large joints (e.g. knee)	2–4 mg (0.5–1 ml)
Small joints (e.g. interphalangeal, temporomandibular)	0.8–1 mg (0.2–0.25 ml)
Bursae	2–3 mg (0.5–0.75 ml)
Tendon sheaths*	0.4–1 mg (0.1–0.25 ml)
Soft-tissue infiltration	2–6 mg (0.5–1.5 ml)
Ganglia	1–2 mg (0.25–0.5 ml)

* Injection should be made into the tendon sheath, and not directly into the tendon.

Frequency of injection: once every three to five days to once every two to three weeks, depending on response.

Use in children: Dosage should be limited to a single dose on alternate days to lessen retardation of growth and minimise suppression of the hypothalamo-pituitary-adrenal axis.

Use in the elderly: Treatment of elderly patients, particularly if long term, should be planned bearing in mind the more serious consequences of the common side effects of corticosteroids in old age, especially osteoporosis, diabetes, hypertension, susceptibility to infection and thinning of the skin.

Contra-indications, warnings, etc

Contra-indications: Systemic fungal infection; hypersensitivity to any component.

Warnings: Frequent intra-articular injections over a prolonged period may lead to joint destruction with bone necrosis. Intra-articular injection of corticosteroid may produce systemic adverse reactions including adrenal suppression.

Precautions: Corticosteroids may exacerbate systemic fungal infections and, therefore, should not be used in the presence of such infections unless they are needed to control drug reactions due to amphotericin. Moreover, there have been cases reported in which concomitant use of amphotericin and hydrocortisone was followed by cardiac enlargement and congestive failure.

The dosage of corticosteroid should be reduced gradually.

Average and large doses of hydrocortisone or cortisone can cause elevation of blood pressure, retention of salt and water, and increased excretion of potassium, but these effects are less likely to occur with synthetic derivatives, except when used in large doses. Dietary salt restriction and potassium supplementation may be necessary. All corticosteroids increase calcium excretion.

The slower rate of absorption by intramuscular administration should be recognised.

In patients on corticosteroid therapy subjected to unusual stress, dosage should be increased before, during and after the stressful situation. Drug-induced secondary adrenocortical insufficiency may be minimised by gradual dosage reduction, but may persist for months after discontinuation of therapy. In any stressful situation during that period, therefore, corticosteroid therapy should be reinstated. If the patient is already receiving corticosteroids, the dosage may have to be increased. Salt and/or a mineralocorticoid should be given concur-

rently, since mineralocorticoid secretion may be impaired.

Stopping corticosteroids after prolonged therapy may cause withdrawal symptoms including fever, myalgia, arthralgia, and malaise. This may occur in patients even without evidence of adrenal insufficiency.

Because anaphylactoid reactions have occurred, rarely, in patients receiving parenteral corticosteroid therapy, appropriate precautions should be taken prior to administration, especially when the patient has a history of allergy to any drug.

Administration of live virus vaccines is contra-indicated in individuals receiving immunosuppressive doses of corticosteroids. If inactivated viral or bacterial vaccines are administered to individuals receiving immunosuppressive doses of corticosteroids, the expected serum antibody response may not be obtained. However, immunisation procedures may be undertaken in patients who are receiving corticosteroids as replacement therapy, e.g. for Addison's Disease.

Aspirin should be used cautiously in conjunction with corticosteroids in hypoprothrombinaemia.

The use of Decadron Injection in active tuberculosis should be restricted to those cases of fulminating or disseminated tuberculosis in which the corticosteroid is used for the management of the disease in conjunction with an appropriate antituberculosis regimen. If the corticosteroids are indicated in patients with latent tuberculosis or tuberculin reactivity, close observation is necessary as reactivation may occur. During prolonged corticosteroid therapy, these patients should receive prophylactic chemotherapy.

Corticosteroids should be used with caution in renal insufficiency, hypertension, diabetes or in those with a family history of diabetes, congestive heart failure, osteoporosis, previous steroid myopathy, glaucoma (or previous history), myasthenia gravis, non-specific ulcerative colitis, diverticulitis, fresh intestinal anastomoses, active or latent peptic ulcer. Signs of peritoneal irritation following gastro-intestinal perforation in patients receiving large doses of corticosteroids may be minimal or absent. Fat embolism has been reported as a possible complication of hypercortisonism.

Corticosteroids should be used cautiously in patients with ocular herpes simplex because of possible corneal perforation.

There is an enhanced effect of corticosteroids in patients with hypothyroidism and in those with cirrhosis. Corticosteroids may increase or decrease motility and number of spermatozoa.

As phenytoin, barbiturates, ephedrine and rifampicin may enhance the metabolic clearance of corticosteroids, resulting in decreased blood levels and reduced physiological activity, the dosage may have to be adjusted. These interactions may interfere with dexamethasone suppression tests which should be interpreted with caution during administration of these drugs.

The prothrombin time should be checked frequently in patients who are receiving corticosteroids and coumarin anticoagulants at the same time.

When corticosteroids are administered concomitantly with potassium-depleting diuretics, patients should be observed closely for development of hypokalaemia.

Corticosteroids may mask some signs of infection, and new infections may appear during their use. There may be decreased resistance, and inability to localise infection.

A report shows that the use of corticosteroids in

cerebral malaria is associated with a prolonged coma and an increased incidence of pneumonia and gastro-intestinal bleeding.

Corticosteroids may activate latent amoebiasis. Therefore, it is recommended that latent or active amoebiasis be excluded before initiating corticosteroid therapy in any patient who has either spent time in the tropics, or has unexplained diarrhoea.

Alterations in the patient's mental state may appear when corticosteroids are used, ranging from psychological dependence, euphoria, insomnia, mood swings, personality changes and severe depression, to frank psychotic manifestations.

Prolonged use of corticosteroids may produce posterior subcapsular cataracts, glaucoma with possible damage to the optic nerves, and may enhance the establishment of secondary infections.

Local steroid injection should be undertaken in an aseptic environment to reduce the particular risk of bacterial infection. Injection of a steroid into an infected site should be avoided.

Appropriate examination of joint fluid is necessary to exclude a septic process.

A marked increase in pain accompanied by local swelling, further restriction of joint motion, fever, and malaise are suggestive of septic arthritis. If this complication occurs and the diagnosis of sepsis is confirmed, appropriate antimicrobial therapy should be instituted.

Patients should understand the great importance of not over-using joints that are still diseased despite symptomatic improvement.

Corticosteroids should not be injected into unstable joints.

Frequent intra-articular injections have been reported to cause development of Charcot-like arthropathies.

Children: Corticosteroids cause growth retardation in infancy, childhood and adolescence. Treatment should be limited to the minimum dosage for the shortest possible time. In order to minimise suppression of the hypothalamo-pituitary-adrenal axis and growth retardation, treatment should be limited, where possible, to a single dose on alternate days.

Growth and development of infants and children on prolonged corticosteroid therapy should be carefully monitored.

Use in pregnancy and the nursing mother: There is inadequate evidence of safety in human pregnancy and there may be a very small risk of cleft palate and intra-uterine growth retardation in the fetus; there is evidence of harmful effects on pregnancy in animals.

Corticosteroids appear in breast milk and could suppress growth, interfere with endogenous cortico-steroid production, or cause other unwanted effects. Mothers taking pharmacological doses of corticosteroids should be advised not to nurse.

Side-effects: Fluid and electrolyte disturbances: Sodium retention, fluid retention, congestive heart failure in susceptible patients, potassium loss, hypokalaemic alkalosis, hypertension, increased calcium excretion.

Musculoskeletal: Muscle weakness, steroid myopathy, loss of muscle mass, osteoporosis (especially in post-menopausal females), vertebral compression fractures, aseptic necrosis of femoral and humeral heads, pathological fracture of long bones, tendon rupture, and post-injection flare (following intra-articular use).

Gastro-intestinal: Peptic ulcer with possible perforation and haemorrhage, perforation of the small and large bowel, particularly in patients with inflammatory bowel disease, pancreatitis, abdominal distension, ulcerative oesophagitis, dyspepsia, oesophageal candidiasis.

Dermatological: Impaired wound healing, thin fragile skin, petechiae and ecchymoses, erythema, striae, telangiectasia, acne, increased sweating, possible suppression of skin tests, burning or tingling especially in the perineal area (after intravenous injection), other cutaneous reactions such as allergic dermatitis, urticaria, angioneurotic oedema, and hypo- or hyper-pigmentation.

Neurological: Convulsions, increased intracranial pressure with papilloedema (pseudotumour cerebri) usually after treatment, vertigo, headache, and rare instances of blindness associated with intra-lesional therapy around the face and head.

Endocrine: Menstrual irregularities, amenorrhoea, development of Cushingoid state, suppression of growth in children, secondary adrenocortical and pituitary unresponsiveness, particularly in times of stress, as in trauma, surgery or illness, decreased carbohydrate tolerance, manifestations of latent diabetes mellitus, increased requirements for insulin or oral hypoglycaemic agents in diabetes.

Ophthalmic: Posterior subcapsular cataracts, increased intra-ocular pressure, papilloedema, corneal or scleral thinning, exacerbation of ophthalmic viral disease, glaucoma, exophthalmos.

Metabolic: Negative nitrogen balance due to protein catabolism.

Other: Anaphylactoid or hypersensitivity reactions, leucocytosis, thrombo-embolism, weight gain, increased appetite, nausea, malaise, and sterile abscess.

Teratogenicity: See pregnancy warning under 'Use in pregnancy and the nursing mother'.

Treatment of overdosage: Anaphylactic and hypersensitivity reactions may be treated with adrenaline, positive-pressure artificial respiration and aminophylline. The patient should be kept warm and quiet.

Treatment is probably not indicated for reactions due to chronic poisoning unless the patient has a condition that would render him unusually susceptible to ill effects from corticosteroids. In this case, symptomatic treatment should be instituted as necessary.

Pharmaceutical precautions Decadron Injection is sensitive to heat and should not be autoclaved to sterilise the outside of the vial. Store below 25°C, protected from light and freezing. Only sodium chloride injection or dextrose injection should be used as diluent. Any infusion mixture must be used within 24 hours.

Legal category POM.

Package quantities Vials of 2 ml.

Further information Also available is Injection Decadron Shock-Pak containing, per millilitre, dexamethasone sodium phosphate equivalent to 20 mg dexamethasone, indicated exclusively for intravenous use as adjunctive therapy in severe shock. For information about this special high-dose form of Decadron Injection, see separate entry.

Decadron Injection is ready for immediate use. An adequate dose is contained in a small volume of vehicle, and small-bore needles can be used wherever appropriate.

Product licence number 0025/5045.

INJECTION DECADRON* SHOCK-PAK

Presentation An injection containing, per millilitre, dexamethasone sodium phosphate equivalent to 20 mg dexamethasone, as a colourless solution.

Uses Corticosteroid.

Only for the adjunctive treatment of shock where massive doses of corticosteroids are needed. It is an adjunct to, and not a substitute for, specific or supportive measures that the patient may require, e.g. restoration of circulating blood volume, correction of fluid and electrolyte balance, oxygen, surgical measures and antibiotics. Dexamethasone has been shown to be beneficial when used early in the treatment of septic shock, but it may not influence overall survival.

Dosage and administration Injection Decadron Shock-Pak is for administration by the intravenous route only.

Intravenous injection in shock: Injection Decadron Shock-Pak can be used without mixing or diluting. Injection should be made slowly.

The usual dosage by intravenous injection is 2–6 mg/kg body weight given as a single intravenous injection. This may be repeated in two to six hours, if shock persists. As an alternative, the initial intravenous injection may be followed immediately by an intravenous infusion containing the same dose. (Although Injection Decadron Shock-Pak was not primarily designed for intravenous infusion, it can be added to sodium chloride injection, or to dextrose injection, and administered by intravenous drip without loss of potency. When the Shock-Pak is added to an infusion solution, the mixture must be used within 24 hours as infusion solutions do not contain preservatives.)

These dosages are large in comparison with the usual recommended dosages of dexamethasone sodium phosphate. They are, however, for emergency use in acute conditions needing massive doses of corticosteroid, and reflect the tendency in current medical practice to use such high doses in the treatment of shock.

Therapy with Injection Decadron Shock-Pak is an adjunct to, and not a replacement for, conventional therapy. Administration of high doses of corticosteroids should be continued only until the patient's condition has stabilised, and usually no longer than 48–72 hours. Prolonged therapy at such high doses should be avoided to prevent possible complications, such as adrenal suppression or gastro-intestinal ulceration.

Use in the elderly: These dosage recommendations apply to all adults, including the elderly.

Contra-indications, warnings, etc
Contra-indications: Systemic fungal infections; hypersensitivity to any component.

Precautions: Injection Decadron Shock-Pak is for adjunctive use in the treatment of shock, and therapy must be accompanied by the usual standard measures employed in its management. In shock of septic origin, appropriate antibiotic therapy must be continued for as long as required.

The pronounced hormonal effects associated with prolonged corticosteroid therapy will probably not be seen when this injection is used for short-term adjunctive therapy in shock.

Use in pregnancy: There is inadequate evidence of safety in human pregnancy and there may be a very small risk of cleft palate and intra-uterine growth retardation in the fetus; there is evidence of harmful effects on pregnancy in animals.

Side-effects: Although adverse reactions associated with short-term corticosteroid therapy in high doses are uncommon, peptic ulceration may occur. However, for details of side-effects seen with prolonged dexamethasone therapy, please see previous entry on Decadron Injection. Some patients have reported transitory burning or tingling sensations, often in the perineal area, when intravenous injections of large doses of dexamethasone sodium phosphate were given. The usual aseptic techniques governing injections should be observed.

Treatment of overdosage: Anaphylactic and hypersensitivity reactions may be treated with adrenaline, positive-pressure artificial respiration and aminophylline. The patient should be kept warm and quiet.

Pharmaceutical precautions Injection Decadron Shock-Pak is sensitive to heat, and should not be autoclaved to sterilise the outside of the vial. It should be stored in a cool place and protected from freezing.

Only sodium chloride injection or dextrose injection should be used as diluents for infusion. Any infusion mixture must be used within 24 hours.

Legal category POM.

Package quantities Vials of 5 ml.

Further information Injection Decadron Shock-Pak is a special dosage form of dexamethasone sodium phosphate designed exclusively for intravenous use as adjunctive therapy in the treatment of severe shock. For other indications requiring an injectable steroid, Decadron Injection, a formulation containing, per millilitre, dexamethasone sodium phosphate equivalent to 4 mg dexamethasone phosphate (approximately 3.33 mg dexamethasone), is available.

Product licence number 0025/0077.

DECADRON* TABLETS

Presentation Yellow, half-scored tablets, marked 'MSD 41', containing 0.5 mg Dexamethasone BP.

Uses Corticosteroid.

For use in certain endocrine and non-endocrine disorders, in certain cases of cerebral oedema, and for diagnostic testing of adrenocortical hyperfunction.

Endocrine disorders: Primary or secondary adrenocortical insufficiency (the first choice is hydrocortisone or cortisone, but synthetic analogues may be used with mineralocorticoids where applicable; in infancy, mineralocorticoid supplementation is particularly important), congenital adrenal hyperplasia.

Non-endocrine disorders: Dexamethasone may be used in the treatment of non-endocrine corticosteroid responsive conditions including:

Allergy and anaphylaxis: Angioneurotic oedema, anaphylaxis.

Arteritis collagenosis: Polymyalgia rheumatica, polyarteritis nodosa.

Blood disorders: Haemolytic anaemia, leukaemia, myeloma.

Cardiovascular disorders: Post-myocardial infarction syndrome.

Gastro-intestinal: Crohn's disease, ulcerative colitis.

Hypercalcaemia: Sarcoidosis.

Infections (with appropriate chemotherapy): Miliary tuberculosis.

Muscular disorders: Polymyositis.

Neurological disorders: Raised intra-cranial pressure secondary to cerebral tumours.

Ocular disorders: Anterior and posterior uveitis, optic neuritis.

Renal disorders: Lupus nephritis.

Respiratory disease: Bronchial asthma, aspiration pneumonitis.

Rheumatic disorders: Rheumatoid arthritis.

Skin disorders: Pemphigus vulgaris.

Dosage and administration *General considerations:* Dosage must be individualised on the basis of the disease and the response of the patient. The lowest possible dosage adequate to control the disease process should be used.

The initial dosage varies from 0.5 mg to 9 mg a day depending on the disease being treated. In more severe diseases, doses higher than 9 mg may be required. The initial dosage should be maintained or adjusted until the patient's response is satisfactory. Both the dose in the evening, which is useful in alleviating morning stiffness, and the divided dosage regimen are associated with greater suppression of the hypothalamo-pituitary-adrenal axis. If satisfactory clinical response does not occur after a reasonable period of time, discontinue Decadron Tablets and transfer the patient to other therapy.

After a favourable initial response, the proper maintenance dosage should be determined by decreasing the initial dosage in small amounts to the lowest dosage that maintains an adequate clinical response. Chronic dosage should preferably not exceed 1.5 mg dexamethasone daily.

Patients should be monitored for signs that might require dosage adjustment, including changes in clinical status resulting from remissions or exacerbations of the disease, individual drug responsiveness, and the effect of stress (e.g. surgery, infection, trauma). During stress it may be necessary to increase dosage temporarily.

If the drug is to be stopped after more than a few days of treatment, it should be withdrawn gradually.

The following equivalents facilitate changing to Decadron from other glucocorticoids.

Milligram for milligram, dexamethasone is approximately equivalent to bethamethasone, 4 to 6 times more potent than methylprednisolone and triamcinolone, 6 to 8 times more potent than prednisone and prednisolone, 25 to 30 times more potent than hydrocortisone, and about 35 times more potent than cortisone.

In acute, self-limiting allergic disorders or acute exacerbations of chronic allergic disorders, the following dosage schedule combining parenteral and oral therapy is suggested.

First day	Decadron Injection, 4 mg or 8 mg (1 ml or 2 ml) intramuscularly
Second day	Two 0.5 mg Decadron Tablets twice a day
Third day	Two 0.5 mg Decadron Tablets twice a day
Fourth day	One 0.5 mg Decadron Tablet twice a day
Fifth day	One 0.5 mg Decadron Tablet twice a day
Sixth day	One 0.5 mg Decadron Tablet
Seventh day	One 0.5 mg Decadron Tablet
Eighth day	Reassessment day

This schedule is designed to ensure adequate therapy during acute episodes while minimising the risk of overdosage in chronic cases.

In cerebral oedema, Decadron Injection is generally administered initially in a dosage of 10 mg intravenously followed by 4 mg every six hours until the symptoms of cerebral oedema subside. Response is usually noted within 12 to 24 hours and dosage may be reduced after two to four days and gradually discontinued over a period of five to seven days.

For palliative management of patients with recurrent or inoperable brain tumours, maintenance therapy with either Decadron Injection or Tablets in a dosage of 2 mg two or three times daily may be effective.

Dexamethasone suppression tests:

1. *Tests for Cushing's syndrome:* Two milligrams of Decadron is given orally at 11 p.m., then blood is drawn for plasma cortisol determination at 8 a.m. the following morning.

For greater accuracy, 0.5 mg Decadron is given orally every 6 hours for 48 hours. Plasma cortisol is measured at 8 a.m. on the third morning. Twenty-four-hour urine collections are made for determination of 17-hydroxy-corticosteroid excretion.

2. *Test to distinguish Cushing's syndrome caused by pituitary ACTH excess from the syndrome induced by other causes:* Two milligrams of Decadron is given orally every 6 hours for 48 hours. Plasma cortisol is measured at 8 a.m. on the morning following the last dose. Twenty-four-hour urine collections are made for determination of 17-hydroxycorticosteroid excretion.

Use in children: Dosage should be limited to a single dose on alternate days to lessen retardation of growth and minimise suppression of hypothalamo-pituitary-adrenal axis.

Use in the elderly: Treatment of elderly patients, particularly if long term, should be planned bearing in mind the more serious consequences of the common side effects of corticosteroids in old age, especially osteoporosis, diabetes, hypertension, susceptibility to infection and thinning of the skin.

Contra-indications, warnings, etc
Contra-indications: Systemic fungal infections; hypersensitivity to the drug.

Precautions: The dosage of corticosteroid should be reduced gradually.

Corticosteroids may exacerbate systemic fungal infections and should not be used unless they are needed to control drug reactions due to amphotericin.

Cases have been reported in which concomitant use of amphotericin and hydrocortisone was followed by cardiac enlargement and heart failure.

A report shows that the use of corticosteroids in cerebral malaria is associated with a prolonged coma and an increased incidence of pneumonia and gastro-intestinal bleeding.

Average and large doses of hydrocortisone or cortisone can cause elevation of blood pressure, retention of salt and water, and increased excretion of potassium, but these effects are less likely to occur with synthetic derivatives, except when used in large doses. Dietary salt restriction and potassium supplementation may be necessary. All corticosteroids increase calcium excretion.

In patients on corticosteroid therapy subjected to unusual stress, dosage should be increased before, during and after the stressful situation. Drug-induced secondary adrenocortical insufficiency may result from too rapid withdrawal of corticosteroids and may be minimised by gradual dosage reduction, but may persist for months after discontinuation of therapy. In any stressful situation during that period, therefore, corticosteroid therapy should be reinstated. If the patient is already receiving corticosteroids, the dose may have to be increased. Salt and/or a mineralocorticoid should be given concurrently, since mineralocorticoid secretion may be impaired.

Stopping corticosteroids after prolonged therapy may cause withdrawal symptoms including fever, myalgia, arthralgia, and malaise. This may occur in patients even without evidence of adrenal insufficiency.

Administration of live virus vaccines is contraindicated in individuals receiving immunosuppressive doses of corticosteroids. If inactivated viral or bacterial vaccines are administered to individuals receiving immunosuppressive doses of corticosteroids, the expected serum antibody response may not be obtained. However, patients who are receiving corticosteroids as replacement therapy, e.g. for Addison's disease, may be immunised.

Aspirin should be used cautiously in conjunction with corticosteroids in hypoprothrombinaemia.

The use of Decadron Tablets in active tuberculosis should be restricted to those cases of fulminating or disseminated tuberculosis in which the corticosteroid is used for the management of the disease in conjunction with an appropriate antituberculous regimen. If corticosteroids are indicated in patients with latent tuberculosis or tuberculin reactivity, close observation of the disease is necessary as reactivation may occur. During prolonged corticosteroid therapy, these patients should receive prophylactic chemotherapy.

Corticosteroids should be used with caution in renal insufficiency, hypertension, diabetes or in those with a family history of diabetes, congestive heart failure, osteoporosis, previous steroid myopathy, glaucoma (or previous history), myasthenia gravis, non-specific ulcerative colitis, diverticulitis, fresh intestinal anastomosis, active or latent peptic ulcer. Signs of peritoneal irritation following gastro-intestinal perforation in patients receiving large doses of corticosteroids may be minimal or absent. Fat embolism has been reported as a possible complication of hypercortisonism.

Corticosteroids should be used cautiously in patients with ocular herpes simplex, because of possible corneal perforation.

There is an enhanced effect of corticosteroids in patients with hypothyroidism and in those with cirrhosis.

Corticosteroids may mask some signs of infection, and new infections may appear during their use. There may be decreased resistance and inability to localise infection in patients on corticosteroids.

Corticosteroids may activate latent amoebiasis. Therefore, it is recommended that latent or active amoebiasis be excluded before initiating corticosteroid therapy in any patient who has either spent time in the tropics, or has unexplained diarrhoea.

Alterations in the patient's mental state may appear when corticosteroids are used, ranging from psychological dependence, euphoria, insomnia, mood swings, personality changes and severe depression, to frank psychotic manifestations.

Prolonged use of corticosteroids may produce subcapsular cataracts, glaucoma with possible damage to the optic nerves, and may enhance the establishment of secondary infections.

Steroids may increase or decrease the motility and number of spermatozoa.

As phenytoin, barbiturates, ephedrine and rifampicin may enhance the metabolic clearance of corticosteroids, resulting in decreased blood levels and reduced physiological activity, the dosage of Decadron may have to be adjusted. These interactions may interfere with dexamethasone suppression tests which should be interpreted with caution during administration of these drugs.

The prothrombin time should be checked frequently in patients who are receiving corticosteroids and coumarin anticoagulants at the same time.

When corticosteroids are administered concomitantly with potassium-depleting diuretics, patients should be observed closely for development of hypokalaemia.

Children: Corticosteroids cause growth retardation in infancy, childhood and adolescence. Treatment should be limited to the minimum dosage for the shortest possible time. In order to minimise suppression of the hypothalamo-pituitary-adrenal axis and growth retardation, treatment should be limited, where possible, to a single dose on alternate days.

Growth and development of infants and children on prolonged corticosteroid therapy should be carefully monitored.

Use in pregnancy and the nursing mother: There is inadequate evidence of safety in human pregnancy and there may be a very small risk of cleft palate and intrauterine growth retardation in the fetus; there is evidence of harmful effects on pregnancy in animals.

Corticosteroids appear in breast milk and could suppress growth, interfere with endogenous corticosteroid production, or cause other unwanted effects. Mothers taking pharmacological doses of corticosteroids should be advised not to nurse.

Side-effects: Fluid and electrolyte disturbances: Sodium retention, fluid retention, congestive heart failure in susceptible patients, potassium loss, hypokalaemic alkalosis, hypertension, increased calcium excretion.

Musculoskeletal effects: Muscle weakness, steroid myopathy, loss of muscle mass, osteoporosis (especially in post-menopausal females), vertebral compression fractures, aseptic necrosis of femoral and humeral heads, pathological fracture of long bones, tendon rupture.

Gastro-intestinal: Peptic ulcer with possible perforation and haemorrhage, perforation of the small and large bowel particularly in patients with inflammatory bowel disease, pancreatitis, abdominal distension, ulcerative oesophagitis, dyspepsia, oesophageal candidiasis.

Dermatological: Impaired wound healing, thin fragile skin, petechiae and ecchymoses, erythema, striae, telangiectasia, acne, increased sweating, suppressed reaction to skin tests, other cutaneous reactions such as allergic dermatitis, urticaria, angioneurotic oedema.

Neurological: Convulsions, vertigo, headache. Increased intracranial pressure with papilloedema (pseudotumour cerebri) may occur usually after treatment.

Endocrine: Menstrual irregularities, amenorrhoea, development of Cushingoid state, suppression of growth in children, secondary adrenocortical and pituitary unresponsiveness (particularly in times of stress as in trauma, surgery or illness), decreased carbohydrate tolerance, manifestations of latent diabetes mellitus, increased need for insulin or oral hypoglycaemic agents in diabetics.

Ophthalmic: Posterior subcapsular cataracts, increased intra-ocular pressure, papilloedema, corneal or scleral thinning, exacerbation of ophthalmic viral disease, glaucoma, exophthalmos.

Metabolic: Negative nitrogen balance due to protein catabolism.

Other: Hypersensitivity, leucocytosis, thrombo-embolism, weight gain, increased appetite, nausea, malaise.

Teratogenicity: See pregnancy warning under 'Use in pregnancy and the nursing mother'.

Treatment of overdosage: Anaphylactic and hypersensitivity reactions may be treated with adrenaline, positive-pressure artificial respiration and aminophylline. The patient should be kept warm and quiet.

Treatment is probably not indicated for reactions due to chronic poisoning unless the patient has a condition that would render him unusually susceptible to ill effects from corticosteroids. In this case, the stomach should be emptied and symptomatic treatment should be instituted as necessary.

Pharmaceutical precautions Keep container well closed; store in a cool place, protected from light.

Legal category POM.

Package quantities *0.5 mg:* Bottles of 100.

Further information Decadron is a potent glucocorticoid with little mineralocorticoid activity. It has considerable anti-inflammatory properties, but its effect on electrolyte metabolism is slight, and thus, electrolyte imbalance is not normally a problem with Decadron. In low or average doses, Decadron does not usually cause elevation of blood pressure, salt and water retention, or excessive potassium excretion.

Product licence number
0.5 mg   0025/5046

DEMSER* ▼

Presentation Available as, two-tone blue, opaque capsules, marked 'MSD 690', and 'DEMSER', containing 250 mg metirosine.

Uses The treatment of phaeochromocytoma during: pre-operative preparation of patients for surgery; management of patients when surgery is contra-indicated; prolonged treatment of patients with malignant phaeochromocytoma.

Demser is not recommended for the control of essential hypertension.

Dosage and administration *Adults and children over 12 years of age:* Initially, 1 capsule (250 mg) four times a day. This may be increased by 1 or 2 capsules (250 or 500 mg) daily to a maximum of 4 g daily in divided doses. When used pre-operatively, the optimum dosage should be given for at least five to seven days before surgery.

The optimum dosage range is usually between 8 and 12 capsules (2 to 3 g) a day, titrated by monitoring clinical symptoms and catecholamine excretion. In patients who are hypertensive, dosage should be adjusted to lower blood pressure and control symptoms; in patients whose blood pressure is normal, adjust dosage until the urinary excretion of catecholamines and/or vanillylmandelic acid is reduced by 50% or more.

It is recommended that an alpha-adrenergic blocking agent such as phenoxybenzamine be added if control with Demser is not adequate.

The use of Demser in children under twelve years of age has been limited, and a dosage recommendation cannot be made.

Use in the elderly: These dosage recommendations apply to all adults, including the elderly.

Contra-indications, warnings, etc
Contra-indications: Hypersensitivity.

Warnings: When Demser is used pre-operatively, especially in combination with alpha-adrenoceptor blocking agents, blood volume must be maintained during and after surgery to avoid hypotension and decreased perfusion of vital organs. During surgery, life-threatening arrhythmias may occur requiring treatment with a beta-blocker or lignocaine. Blood pressure and ECG should be monitored continuously throughout surgery.

Demser does not eliminate the danger of arrhythmias or hypertensive crises occurring during manipulation of the tumour and additional alpha-blockade may be necessary.

Precautions: Crystalluria and urolithiasis have occurred in dogs; and crystalluria has been seen in a few patients. To minimise the risk, fluid intake should be sufficient to maintain a urine volume of 2,000 ml or more daily. Urine should be examined routinely, and if metirosine crystals (needles or rods) are seen, fluid intake should be increased. If crystalluria persists, the dosage of Demser should be reduced or discontinued.

Caution should be observed in administering Demser to patients receiving phenothiazines or haloperidol because the extrapyramidal effects of these drugs can be expected to be potentiated by inhibition of catecholamine synthesis; this has been documented to date only for haloperidol.

No evidence of adverse effects on hepatic, haematological or other functions (except for a few instances of increased AST) has been seen during clinical trials. However, total experience in man is limited to approximately 300 patients, and few patients have been studied long-term. Therefore, suitable laboratory tests should be carried out periodically in patients on prolonged therapy, particularly those with impaired hepatic or renal function.

Demser may cause spurious increases in urinary catecholamine measurements.

Nursing mothers: It is not known whether Demser is excreted in human milk. Mothers who need Demser should stop nursing.

Pregnancy: Complete reproduction studies have not been performed in animals to determine whether Demser affects fertility in males or females, has teratogenic potential, or has other adverse effects on the fetus. There are no well-controlled studies of Demser in pregnant women. The use of Demser in pregnant women should be avoided, if possible, but may be appropriate when anticipated benefits outweigh the potential risks.

Adverse reactions: The most common adverse reaction to Demser is moderate to severe sedation, which has been observed in almost all patients. It occurs at both low and high dosages. Sedative effects begin within the first 24 hours of therapy, are maximal after two to three days, and tend to wane during the next few days. Sedation usually is not obvious after one week unless the dosage is increased, but at dosages greater than 2,000 mg/day some degree of sedation or fatigue may persist.

When receiving Demser, patients should be warned about engaging in activities requiring mental alertness and motor co-ordination, such as driving a motor vehicle or operating machinery. Demser may have additive effects with alcohol and other CNS depressants, e.g. hypnotics, sedatives, tranquillisers, anti-anxiety agents.

In most patients who experience sedation, temporary changes in sleep pattern occur following withdrawal of the drug. Changes consist of insomnia that may last for two or three days and feelings of increased alertness and ambition. Even patients who do not experience sedation while on Demser may report symptoms of psychic stimulation when the drug is discontinued.

Extrapyramidal signs such as drooling, speech difficulty and tremor have been reported in approximately 10% of patients, occasionally with trismus and frank parkinsonism.

Anxiety, depression, hallucinations, disorientation and confusion have occurred but may disappear on reduction of the dosage.

Diarrhoea occurs in about 10% of patients, and may be severe. Infrequently, slight swelling of the breast, galactorrhoea, nasal stuffiness, decreased salivation, dry mouth, headache, nausea, vomiting, abdominal pain, and impotence or failure of ejaculation may occur. Crystalluria transient dysuria and haematuria have been seen in a few patients. Eosinophilia, increased AST levels, peripheral oedema, and hypersensitivity such as urticaria and pharyngeal oedema has been reported rarely.

Treatment of overdosage: There is no clinical experience with overdosage; consequently, the signs, symptoms and treatment have not been identified.

Pharmaceutical precautions Store in a cool place, protected from light.

Legal category POM.

Package quantities Bottles of 100.

Further information Nil.

Product licence number 0025/0132.

EDECRIN*

Presentation White, half-scored tablets, marked 'MSD 90', containing 50 mg Ethacrynic Acid BP.

Injection, vials containing sodium ethacrynate equivalent to 50 mg ethacrynic acid, as a dry, lyophilised powder.

Uses Diuretic.

For use in patients requiring an agent with greater diuretic potential than those commonly employed. For oedema of:

Congestive heart failure, including chronic congestive heart failure accompanying arteriosclerotic heart disease, rheumatic heart disease, hypertensive cardiovascular disease, pulmonary heart disease or congenital heart disease; *pulmonary oedema* (in emergency, Edecrin Injection is recommended); *renal oedema,* including that of the nephrotic syndrome and other renal diseases where a diuretic is indicated, even in many patients with marked impairment of renal function (Edecrin should be discontinued immediately, however, if there is further deterioration in renal function); *hepatic cirrhosis with ascites* (it is usually desirable to initiate therapy in hospital); *oedema due to other causes* including ascites due to malignancy, idiopathic oedema and lymphoedema. In children (over 2 years old) with oedema due

to the nephrotic syndrome or to congenital heart disease. (Edecrin Injection is not recommended for children.)

Edecrin Injection is useful in the treatment of acute pulmonary oedema and other conditions where urgent diuresis is required, or where patients are unable to swallow tablets.

Dosage and administration Dosage should be carefully regulated to prevent a more rapid or substantial diuresis than necessary. Response is usually closely related to the degree of oedema and to the dosage used; the presence and magnitude of aldosteronism largely determines the degree of potassium excretion. Excessive diuresis may be avoided if dosage increases are made by small amounts. Daily weighing of the patient under standard conditions and, where possible, serum electrolyte determinations will greatly contribute to the success of treatment.

Oral therapy: Usual initial adult dosage: 50 mg (1 tablet) a day given immediately after breakfast. When an urgent diuresis is essential, as in pulmonary oedema, an initial dosage substantially higher than 50 mg will be necessary. (In cases of emergency, Edecrin Injection is recommended.)

Adjustment: Increase, as necessary, by amounts of 25–50 mg ($\frac{1}{2}$–1 tablet) a day, to the lowest dosage which will produce a gradual weight loss (about $\frac{1}{2}$–1 kg a day).

Effective dosage range: Usually 50–150 mg (1–3 tablets) a day. Patients with severe refractory oedema may need a higher dosage. This should be achieved gradually, and in no case should exceed 400 mg (8 tablets) a day. When the total daily requirement is higher than 50 mg, it should be divided into 2 doses after meals.

Maintenance dosage: This should be adjusted to fit the changing needs of the patient. It is often less than the initial effective dosage. Treatment may be maintained by continuous or intermittent therapy. Intermittent therapy can usually be used without loss of therapeutic response. Edecrin may be administered on alternate days, or preferably for two- to three-day periods alternating with two or three days' rest, allowing more time for readjustment of any electrolyte imbalance.

Replacement of other diuretics: Transfer to Edecrin from other diuretic agents may be by simple substitution, as long as the recommended dosage schedule is followed.

Continuous or intermittent use of Edecrin may eliminate the need for injections or mercurials.

Children: Initially 25 mg ($\frac{1}{2}$ tablet) taken immediately after breakfast. If necessary, this should be carefully increased by 25 mg ($\frac{1}{2}$ tablet) a day until an effective dosage is achieved. A dosage for infants (under 2 years) has not been established.

Other considerations: The doses of Edecrin required to produce effective diuresis in renal oedema may be larger than those needed in congestive heart failure. Edecrin has additive effects when used with other diuretics. It may potentiate the effect of carbonic anhydrase inhibitors, increasing sodium and potassium excretion. If Edecrin is given to patients already receiving a carbonic anhydrase inhibitor, the initial dose and increments should be only 25 mg ($\frac{1}{2}$ tablet).

In severely oedematous patients. Edecrin may occasionally cause a massive diuresis with resultant imbalance. The dosage, therefore, must be carefully regulated.

Parenteral therapy: Usual adult intravenous dose: 50 mg, or 0.5–1 mg/kg of body weight. Some patients with renal oedema may require larger doses. Single intravenous doses of up to 100 mg have been used in critical situations.

To reconstitute the dry material, 50 ml of isotonic saline or 5% dextrose is added to the vial. (Some 5% dextrose injection solutions have a pH below 5. If such a preparation is used as diluent, the resulting solution may be cloudy or opalescent. The use of such a solution is not recommended.) The solution may be given slowly through the tubing of a running infusion, or by direct intravenous injection over several minutes. If repeated injections are necessary, the site of injections should be rotated to avoid possible thrombophlebitis. Edecrin Injection should not be given subcutaneously or intramuscularly because of local pain and irritation.

Edecrin Injection should not be mixed with whole blood or blood derivatives. If it is desired to administer it at the same time as a blood transfusion, it should be given independently.

Children: As paediatric experience with Edecrin Injection is limited, it is not recommended for children.

Use in the elderly: The general considerations on adjustment of dosage to meet individual needs apply equally to elderly patients (see 'Precautions').

Contra-indications, warnings, etc

Contra-indications: Anuria, infants (under 2 years). For 'Use in pregnancy and the nursing mother' see 'Precautions'. Hypersensitivity to any component of Edecrin.

Precautions: Edecrin should be given with caution to patients with advanced cirrhosis of the liver, particularly those with a history of episodes of electrolyte imbalance or hepatic encephalopathy. Edecrin may precipitate hepatic coma and death.

The effects of Edecrin on electrolytes are based on its renal pharmacology and are usually dose related. To minimise the possibility of profound electrolyte and water loss, therapy should be initiated with a low dosage and this carefully adjusted as necessary, intermittent dosage should be used where possible and the patient weighed regularly throughout treatment. If diuresis is excessive, Edecrin should be withdrawn until homeostasis is restored. When excessive electrolyte loss occurs, the imbalance should be corrected or the administration of Edecrin should be temporarily suspended.

Frequent serum electrolyte, alkali reserve and blood urea determinations should be made early in therapy, and periodically thereafter while active diuresis is taking place. Any electrolyte abnormality should be corrected or the drug temporarily withdrawn. If increasing electrolyte imbalance, azotaemia and/or oliguria occur during treatment of severe progressive renal disease, the diuretic should be discontinued.

Too vigorous a diuresis may induce an acute hypotensive episode. In elderly cardiac patients, severe diuresis may cause a rapid contraction of plasma volume and haemoconcentration which should be avoided to prevent the possible development of such thromboembolic episodes as cerebral thrombosis or pulmonary embolism.

Potassium supplements or a generous intake of potassium-rich foods is often advisable during treatment with Edecrin in patients receiving potassium-depleting steroids, and in patients receiving digitalis where hypokalaemia may precipitate digitalis toxicity. When metabolic alkalosis may be anticipated (e.g. in cirrhosis with ascites), a potassium-conserving agent or potassium chloride may mitigate or present hypokalaemia.

Weakness, muscle cramps, paraesthesiae, thirst, anorexia, and signs of hyponatraemia, hypokalaemia and/ or hypochloraemic alkalosis may follow vigorous or excessive diuresis or be accentuated by rigid salt restriction. Rarely, tetany has been reported following vigorous diuresis.

Note: Symptoms and signs which might indicate ulceration or obstruction of the small bowel in patients taking tablets or capsules containing potassium salts are indications for stopping treatment with such preparations immediately.

The chance of the chloruretic effect of Edecrin giving rise to bicarbonate retention and metabolic alkalosis may be corrected by giving chloride (ammonium or arginine chloride). Ammonium chloride should not be given to cirrhotic patients.

A reasonable salt intake will usually prevent hyponatraemia and hypochloraemia. However, cirrhotic patients usually require at least moderate salt restriction during diuretic therapy. Hypoproteinaemia may reduce the response to Edecrin and the use of salt-poor albumin considered.

A few patients on Edecrin have had a sudden onset of profuse, watery diarrhoea. If this occurs, and all other causative factors are ruled out, Edecrin should be discontinued and not readministered.

When Edecrin is given to patients receiving antihypertensive agents, the dosage of these agents may require adjustment; orthostatic hypotension may occur. The value and safety of Edecrin itself in the treatment of hypertension has not been established.

Edecrin has little or no effect on glomerular filtration rate or renal blood flow, except immediately after a pronounced reduction in plasma volume following rapid diuresis.

An increase in blood urea may occur. Although transient, it may usually be readily reversed by discontinuing Edecrin.

The concurrent use of such drugs as aminoglycosides with Edecrin should be avoided because of the risk of increasing their ototoxic potential.

Several drugs, including Edecrin, have been shown to displace warfarin from plasma protein. In patients receiving both types of drug, a reduction in the dosage of the anticoagulant may therefore be required.

Lithium should generally not be given to patients receiving diuretics, since the risk of lithium toxicity is very high in such patients.

Edecrin may increase the risk of gastric haemorrhage associated with corticosteroid treatment.

Use in pregnancy and the nursing mother: Edecrin is not recommended in pregnant patients. If administration in confirmed or suspected pregnancy is considered, the benefits should be weighed against possible hazards to the fetus. Safety and efficacy for use in toxaemia of pregnancy have not been established. Successive generation studies on laboratory animals have shown no foetal abnormalities. Edecrin is contra-indicated in nursing mothers. If its use is deemed essential, the patient should stop nursing.

Side-effects: Gastro-intestinal upsets include anorexia, malaise, abdominal discomfort or pain, dysphagia, nausea, vomiting and diarrhoea. They have occurred more frequently with large doses or after one to three months of continuous therapy. A few patients have had sudden onset of profuse, watery diarrhoea. Gastro-intestinal bleeding has occurred in some patients.

Reversible hyperuricaemia and decreased urinary urate excretion may occur. Acute gout may be precipitated. Acute symptomatic hypoglycaemia with convulsions occurred in two uraemic patients who received doses higher than those recommended.

Hyperglycaemia has occurred in a few patients, most of whom had decompensated cirrhosis of the liver. Rarely, acute pancreatitis has been reported in patients receiving diuretics, including Edecrin.

Jaundice, abnormal results of liver function tests, agranulocytosis, severe neutropenia and Henoch-Schönlein purpura (in rheumatic heart disease), have been reported rarely in seriously ill patients receiving several drugs including Edecrin. Thrombocytopenia has been reported rarely.

A number of possibly drug-related deaths have occurred in critically ill patients refractory to other diuretics. These have generally fallen into two categories: patients with severe myocardial disease who were receiving digitalis and presumably developed acute hypokalaemia with fatal arrhythmias; patients with severely decompensated hepatic cirrhosis with ascites, with or without accompanying encephalopathy, who were in electrolyte imbalance and died following intensification of the electrolyte deficit.

Skin rash, headache, fever, rigors, blurred vision, fatigue, apprehension and confusion have occurred infrequently. Rarely, haematuria has been reported. Deafness, tinnitus and vertigo with a sense of fullness in the ears, have occurred, most frequently in patients with severe impairment of renal function. These symptoms have been associated most often with intravenous administration and with doses in excess of those recommended. The deafness has usually been reversible and temporary (1–24 hours), but in some critically ill patients the hearing loss has been permanent. A number of these patients were also receiving drugs previously known to be ototoxic.

Edecrin Injection has occasionally caused local irritation and pain due to extravasation of injected fluid.

Treatment of overdosage: Symptomatic and supportive; no specific antidote. Dehydration, electrolyte imbalance, hepatic coma and hypotension should be corrected by standard methods. If respiration is impaired, oxygen or artificial respiration should be given.

Pharmaceutical precautions Keep tablet container well closed. Store tablets and injection in a cool place, protected from light. Injection: to reconstitute the lyophilised material, 50 ml of isotonic saline or 5% dextrose is added to the vial. (Some 5% dextrose injection solutions have a pH below 5. If such a preparation is used as diluent, the resulting solution may be cloudy. The use of such a solution is not recommended.) Any unused reconstituted solution should be discarded after 24 hours.

Legal category POM.

Package quantities *Tablets:* Bottles of 100. *Injection:* Vials containing sodium ethacrynate equivalent to 50 mg ethacrynic acid.

Further information Onset of action is usually apparent within 30 minutes of oral administration, peak effect is attained in about two hours, and diuresis lasts for six to eight hours. Onset of action is usually observed within five minutes after intravenous injection.

Product licence numbers
Tablets   0025/5006
Injection   0025/5007

HYDROCORTONE* TABLETS

Presentation White, quarter-scored tablets, marked 'MSD 619', containing 10 mg hydrocortisone. White, half-scored tablets, marked 'MSD 625', containing 20 mg hydrocortisone.

Uses Corticosteroid.
For use in certain endocrine and non-endocrine disorders responsive to corticosteroid therapy.

Endocrine disorders: Primary, secondary, or acute adrenocortical insufficiency.

Pre-operatively, and during serious trauma or illness in patients with known adrenal insufficiency or doubtful adrenocortical reserve.

Non-endocrine disorders: Hydrocortisone may be used in the treatment of non-endocrine corticosteroid responsive conditions including:

Allergy and anaphylaxis: Angioneurotic oedema, anaphylaxis.

Arteritis collagenosis: Polymyalgia rheumatica, polyarteritis nodosa.

Blood disorders: Haemolytic anaemia, leukaemia, myeloma.

Cardiovascular disorders: Post-myocardial infarction syndrome.

Gastro-intestinal: Crohn's disease, ulcerative colitis.

Hypercalcaemia: Sarcoidosis.

Infections (with appropriate chemotherapy): Miliary tuberculosis.

Muscular disorders: Polymyositis.

Ocular disorders: Anterior and posterior uveitis, optic neuritis.

Renal disorders: Lupus nephritis.

Respiratory disease: Bronchial asthma, aspiration pneumonitis.

Rheumatic disorders: Rheumatoid arthritis.

Skin disorders: Pemphigus vulgaris.

Dosage and administration Dosage must be individualised on the basis of the disease and the response of the individual patient. The lowest possible dosage adequate to control the disease process should be used.

The initial dosage varies from 10 mg to 40 mg a day divided into 3 or 4 doses. The dosage depends on the disease being treated. In more severe diseases, doses higher than 40 mg may be required. The initial dose should be maintained or adjusted until the patient's response is satisfactory. Both the dose in the evening, which is useful in alleviating morning stiffness, and the divided dosage regimen are associated with greater suppression of the hypothalamo-pituitary-adrenal axis. If satisfactory clinical response does not occur after a reasonable period of time, discontinue Hydrocortone Tablets and transfer the patient to other therapy.

When symptoms have been controlled, the proper maintenance dosage should be determined by decreasing the dosage in small amounts to the lowest dose that maintains an adequate clinical response. Chronic dosage should preferably not exceed 30 mg hydrocortisone daily.

Patients should be observed closely for signs that might require dosage adjustment, including changes in clinical status resulting from remissions or exacerbations of the disease, individual drug responsiveness, and the effect of stress (e.g. surgery, infection, trauma). During stress it may be necessary to increase the dosage temporarily.

If the drug is to be stopped after more than a few days of treatment, it should be withdrawn gradually.

When an extremely rapid onset of action is desired, Decadron Injection may be administered intravenously for the first 2 or 3 doses.

Adrenaline is the drug of first choice in severe allergic reactions. Hydrocortone Tablets are useful either concurrently or as supplementary therapy.

In chronic adrenocortical insufficiency, 10–20 mg a day, or occasionally more, together with 4–6 g of sodium chloride or 1–3 mg of desoxycorticosterone acetate. When immediate support is mandatory, one of the soluble adrenocortical hormone preparations (e.g. Decadron* Injection, dexamethasone sodium phosphate, MSD), which may be effective within minutes after parenteral administration, can be life-saving.

In congenital adrenal hyperplasia, the usual daily dosage is 10–30 mg.

Use in children: Dosage should be limited to a single dose on alternate days to lessen retardation of growth and minimise suppression of hypothalamo-pituitary-adrenal axis.

Use in the elderly: Treatment of elderly patients, particularly if long term, should be planned bearing in mind the more serious consequences of the common side effects of corticosteroids in old age, especially osteoporosis, diabetes, hypertension, susceptibility to infection and thinning of the skin.

Contra-indications, warnings, etc

Contra-indications: Systemic fungal infections. Hypersensitivity to the drug.

Precautions: The lowest possible dosage of corticosteroid should be used to control the condition under treatment, and when reduction in dosage is possible, the reduction should be gradual.

Average and large dosages of hydrocortisone or cortisone can cause elevation of blood pressure, salt and water retention, and increase excretion of potassium. These effects are less likely to occur with the synthetic derivatives except when used in large doses. Dietary salt restriction and potassium supplementation may be necessary. All corticosteroids increase calcium excretion.

In patients on corticosteroid therapy subjected to unusual stress, increased dosage of rapidly acting corticosteroids before, during and after the stressful situation is indicated.

Drug-induced secondary adrenocortical insufficiency may result from too rapid a withdrawal of corticosteroids and may be minimised by gradual reduction of dosage. This type of relative insufficiency may persist for months after discontinuation of therapy; therefore, in any situation of stress occurring during that period, corticosteroid therapy should be reinstated. If the patient is receiving steroids already, the dosage may have to be increased. Since mineralocorticoid secretion may be impaired, salt and/or a mineralocorticoid should be administered concurrently.

Stopping corticosteroids after prolonged therapy may cause withdrawal symptoms including fever, myalgia, arthralgia, and malaise. This may occur in patients even without evidence of adrenal insufficiency.

Administration of live virus vaccines is contra-indicated in individuals receiving immunosuppressive doses of corticosteroids. If inactivated viral or bacterial vaccines are administered to individuals receiving immunosuppressive doses of corticosteroids, the expected serum antibody response may not be obtained. However, immunisation procedures may be undertaken in patients who are receiving corticosteroids as replacement therapy, e.g. for Addison's disease.

Aspirin should be used cautiously in conjunction with corticosteroids in hypoprothrombinaemia.

The use of Hydrocortone Tablets in active tuberculosis should be restricted to those cases of fulminating or disseminated tuberculosis in which the corticosteroid is used for the management of the disease in conjunction with an appropriate antituberculous regimen. If corticosteroids are indicated in patients with latent tuberculosis or tuberculin reactivity, close observation is necessary as reactivation of the disease may occur. During prolonged corticosteroid therapy, these patients should receive prophylactic chemotherapy.

Corticosteroids should be used with caution in renal insufficiency, hypertension, diabetes or in those with a family history of diabetes, congestive heart failure, osteoporosis, previous steroid myopathy, glaucoma (or previous history), myasthenia gravis, non-specific ulcerative colitis, diverticulitis, fresh intestinal anastomoses, active or latent peptic ulcer. Signs of peritoneal irritation following gastro-intestinal perforation in patients receiving large doses of corticosteroids may be minimal or absent. Fat embolism has been reported as a possible complication of hypercortisonism.

Corticosteroids should be used cautiously in patients with ocular herpes simplex because of possible corneal perforation.

There is an enhanced effect of corticosteroids in patients with hypothyroidism and in those with cirrhosis.

Corticosteroids may mask some signs of infection, and new infections may appear during their use. There may be decreased resistance and inability to localise infection in patients on corticosteroids.

Corticosteroids may activate latent amoebiasis. Therefore, it is recommended that latent or active amoebiasis be excluded before initiating corticosteroid therapy in any patient who has either spent time in the tropics, or has unexplained diarrhoea.

Alterations in the patient's mental state may appear when corticosteroids are used, ranging from psychological dependence, euphoria, insomnia, mood swings, personality changes and severe depression, to frank psychotic manifestations.

Prolonged use of corticosteroids may produce posterior subcapsular cataracts, glaucoma with possible damage to the optic nerves, and may enhance the establishment of secondary ocular infections.

Growth and development of infants and children on prolonged corticosteroid therapy should be carefully monitored.

Corticosteroids may increase or decrease motility and number of spermatozoa.

Phenytoin, ephedrine, barbiturates and rifampicin may enhance the metabolic clearance of corticosteroids, resulting in decreased blood levels and lessened physiological activity, thus requiring adjustment in corticosteroid dosage.

The prothrombin time should be checked frequently in patients who are receiving corticosteroids and coumarin anticoagulants at the same time.

When corticosteroids are administered concomitantly with potassium-depleting diuretics, patients should be observed closely for development of hypokalaemia.

Children: Corticosteroids cause growth retardation in infancy, childhood and adolescence. Treatment should be limited to the minimum dosage for the shortest possible time. In order to minimise suppression of the hypothalamo-pituitary-adrenal axis and growth retardation, treatment should be limited, where possible, to a single dose on alternate days.

Growth and development of infants and children on prolonged corticosteroid therapy should be carefully monitored.

Use in pregnancy and the nursing mother: There is inadequate evidence of safety in human pregnancy and there may be a very small risk of cleft palate and intra-uterine growth retardation in the fetus; there is evidence of harmful effects on pregnancy in animals.

Corticosteroids appear in breast milk and could suppress growth, interfere with endogenous corticosteroid production, or cause other unwanted effects. Mothers taking pharmacological doses of corticosteroids should be advised not to nurse.

Side-effects: Fluid and electrolyte disturbances: Sodium retention, fluid retention, congestive heart failure in susceptible patients, potassium loss, hypokalaemic alkalosis, hypertension, increased calcium excretion.

Musculoskeletal effects: Muscle weakness, steroid myopathy, loss of muscle mass, osteoporosis (especially in post-menopausal females), vertebral compression fractures, aseptic necrosis of femoral and humeral heads, pathological fracture of long bones, tendon rupture.

Gastro-intestinal: Peptic ulcer with possible perforation and haemorrhage, perforation of the small and large bowel particularly in patients with inflammatory bowel disease, pancreatitis, abdominal distension, ulcerative oesophagitis, dyspepsia, oesophageal candidiasis.

Dermatological: Impaired wound healing, thin fragile skin, petechiae and ecchymoses, erythema, striae, telangiectasia, acne, increased sweating, may suppress reactions to skin tests, other cutaneous reactions such as allergic dermatitis, urticaria, angioneurotic oedema.

Neurological: Convulsions, increased intracranial pressure with papilloedema (pseudotumour cerebri) usually after treatment, vertigo, headache.

Endocrine: Menstrual irregularities, amenorrhoea, development of Cushingoid state, suppression of growth in children, secondary adrenocortical and pituitary unresponsiveness (particularly in times of stress, as in trauma, surgery, or illness), decreased carbohydrate tolerance, manifestations of latent diabetes mellitus, increased requirements for insulin or oral hypoglycaemic agents in diabetics.

Ophthalmic: Posterior subcapsular cataracts, increased intra-ocular pressure, papilloedema, corneal or scleral thinning, exacerbation of ophthalmic viral disease, glaucoma, exophthalmos.

Metabolic: Negative nitrogen balance due to protein catabolism.

Other: Hypersensitivity, leucocytosis, thrombo-embolism, weight gain, increased appetite, nausea, malaise.

Teratogenicity: See pregnancy warning under 'Use in pregnancy and the nursing mother'.

Treatment of overdosage: Anaphylactic and hypersensitivity reactions may be treated with adrenaline, positive-pressure artificial respiration and aminophylline. The patient should be kept warm and quiet.

Treatment is probably not indicated for reactions due to chronic poisoning unless the patient has a condition that would render him unusually susceptible to ill effects from corticosteroids. In this case, symptomatic treatment should be instituted as necessary.

Pharmaceutical precautions Keep container well closed, store in a cool place, protected from light.

Legal category POM.

Package quantities *10 mg:* Bottles of 100. *20 mg:* Bottles of 100.

Further information Nil.

Product licence numbers
10 mg 0025/5053
20 mg 0025/5054

HYDRODERM*

Presentation A white, translucent ointment containing, in each gram, 10 mg Hydrocortisone BP, 5 mg Neomycin Sulphate BP and 1,000 units Bacitracin Zinc BP, in an emollient base.

Uses Topical corticosteroid with topical antibiotics.

Hydroderm may be used for the short-term treatment of certain dermatological disorders responsive to low-potency topical corticosteroids where secondary infection by susceptible organisms is a significant factor, including exudative and secondary infected eczema and dermatitis, secondarily infected insect bite reactions, exudative flexural intertrigo, and acne vulgaris complicated by seborrhoeic eczema.

(Attention is drawn to the 'Contra-indications, warnings, etc' section.)

Dosage and administration A small amount of Hydroderm should be applied to the affected area two or three times a day. The area to be treated should be carefully cleansed before application, so that the possibility of introducing infection is minimised. Hydroderm should be applied gently to avoid damage to the skin.

Use in the elderly: These recommendations apply also to the elderly. (See 'Precautions'.)

Contra-indications, warnings, etc

Contra-indications: Tuberculosis of the skin, chickenpox, herpes simplex, vaccinia, or fungal infections; sensitivity to any of the components of Hydroderm. Hydroderm should not be used ophthalmically. Hydroderm is not for use in primary infections nor in eczema complicated by secondary beta-haemolytic streptococcal infection in which systemic antibiotics should be used.

Precautions: Hydroderm should be used with particular caution in patients with impaired renal or hepatic function. Hydroderm should always be applied sparingly and should never be applied to extensive, devitalised, infected or raw areas, and the period of treatment should not exceed 5 days if there is no clinical improvement. The use of occlusive dressings with Hydroderm is not recommended.

Extended recurrent application may increase the risk of contact sensitisation and should be avoided.

Hydroderm should be used with caution in elderly or

dehydrated patients and in patients being treated with drugs that are potentially nephrotic or ototoxic.

Elderly patients are more susceptible to nephrotoxic effects of aminoglycosides.

Topical corticosteroids may mask or enhance incipient infection. If any infection does not respond promptly, treatment with Hydroderm should be discontinued until the infection has been controlled by other means. If a new infection resistant to neomycin or bacitracin appears during therapy, it should be controlled by appropriate measures.

A few individuals may be sensitive to one or more components of Hydroderm, and therapy should always be stopped if this occurs.

Use in pregnancy and nursing mothers: Topical administration of corticosteroids to pregnant animals can cause abnormalities of fetal development. The relevance of this finding to human beings has not been established. There is risk of fetal ototoxicity if neomycin is used in pregnancy. Hydroderm is not recommended for use during pregnancy.

It is not known whether topical administration of corticosteroids could result in sufficient systemic absorption to produce detectable quantities in breast milk. Systemically-administered corticosteroids are secreted into breast milk in quantities not likely to have a deleterious effect on the infant. Nevertheless, caution should be exercised when topical corticosteroids are administered to a nursing mother.

Use in children: Paediatric patients may demonstrate greater susceptibility to topical corticosteroid induced hypothalamo-pituitary-adrenal axis suppression and Cushing's syndrome than mature patients because of a larger skin surface to body weight ratio.

Administration of topical corticosteroids to children should be limited to the least amount compatible with an effective therapeutic regimen. Chronic corticosteroid therapy may interfere with the growth and development of children.

Side-effects: The topical application of Hydroderm may be associated with both local and systemic side effects even when the treatment period is of short duration and occlusion dressings are omitted.

Local effects: Contact allergic dermatitis may occur and may be due to any of the three active constituents or to the vehicle.

Irritation of the skin, burning, itching, dryness, folliculitis, hypertrichosis, acneiform eruptions, hypopigmentation, maceration of the skin, perioral dermatitis, skin atrophy, striae, miliaria and tachyphylaxis may occur and are usually corticosteroid related.

Resistant strains of bacteria may develop when topical antibiotics are used and hypersensitivity reactions can occur.

Systemic effects: Topical use of hydrocortisone can suppress pituitary-adrenal function and produce a Cushingoid picture. Systemic side-effects are of particular importance in children in whom retardation of growth and pseudotumour cerebri have been reported. Although these side-effects are less likely to occur when a corticosteroid of low potency is employed (as in Hydroderm) over a short period of time, they should nevertheless be borne in mind.

Nephrotoxicity may be caused by the topical application of neomycin and less frequently of bacitracin.

Ototoxicity is a well known hazard of local treatment with neomycin.

The incidence of systemic side-effects accompanying the use of topical corticosteroid-antibiotic preparations rises if extensive or raw areas are treated, if treatment is prolonged and when occlusive dressings are used.

Treatment of overdosage: Not applicable.

Pharmaceutical precautions Store below 25°C.

Legal category POM.

Package quantities Tubes of 5 g.

Further information Hydroderm combines the anti-inflammatory, anti-allergic and antipruritic effects of a topical corticosteroid with the antibacterial action of two topically effective antibiotics.

Product licence number 0025/5055.

HYDROMET*

Presentation Salmon-pink, film-coated tablets, marked 'MSD 423', containing Methyldopa BP equivalent to 250 mg anhydrous methyldopa, and 15 mg Hydrochlorothiazide BP.

Uses Antihypertensive.

A highly effective combination of methyldopa and hydrochlorothiazide, two antihypertensive agents with complementary properties for the treatment of hypertension.

Dosage and administration *Initial dosage:* Usually 1 tablet twice a day for two days.

Adjustment: Upwards or downwards. Preferably at intervals of at least two days, until an adequate response is obtained.

The maximum recommended daily dosage of the components is 3 g of methyldopa and 200 mg hydrochlorothiazide.

Many patients experience sedation for two or three days when therapy with Hydromet is started or when the dose is increased. When increasing the dosage, therefore, it may be desirable to increase the evening dose first.

General considerations: Methyldopa is largely excreted by the kidney and patients with impaired kidney function may respond to smaller doses of Hydromet.

Withdrawal of Hydromet is followed by return of hypertension usually within 48 hours. This is not complicated by an overshoot of blood pressure.

Therapy with Hydromet may be initiated in most patients already on treatment with other antihypertensive agents by terminating these antihypertensive medications, gradually if required (see manufacturer's recommendations on stopping these drugs). Following such previous antihypertensive therapy, Hydromet should be limited to an initial dose of 1 tablet daily and increased as required at intervals of not less than two days.

When Hydromet is given to patients on other antihypertensives, the dose of these agents may need to be adjusted to effect a smooth transition.

Use in the elderly: The initial dose should not exceed 1 tablet daily. The dosage may be increased slowly as required by the initial response.

Contra-indications, warnings, etc

Contra-indications: Active liver disease (such as acute hepatitis and active cirrhosis); anuria; known sensitivity to methyldopa or hydrochlorothiazide, including hepatic disorders associated with previous methyldopa therapy. See 'Precautions' for use in pregnancy and the nursing mother.

Precautions: The precautions relating to the use of Hydromet are generally those of its components.

Methyldopa: Acquired haemolytic anaemia has occurred rarely. Should symptoms suggest anaemia, haemoglobin and/or haematocrit determinations should be made. If anaemia is confirmed, tests should be done for haemolysis. If haemolytic anaemia is present, Hydromet should be discontinued. Stopping therapy, with or without corticosteroids, has usually brought prompt remission. Rarely, however, deaths have occurred.

Some patients on continued therapy with methyldopa develop a positive direct Coombs test. From the reports of different investigators, the incidence averages between 10% and 20%. A positive Coombs reaction rarely develops in the first six months of therapy, and if it has not developed within 12 months, it is unlikely to do so later on continuing therapy. Development is also dose-related, the lowest incidence occurring in patients receiving 1 g or less of methyldopa per day. The test becomes negative usually within weeks to months after methyldopa is discontinued.

Prior knowledge of a positive Coombs reaction will aid in evaluation of cross-matching for transfusions. If a patient with a positive Coombs reaction shows an incompatible minor cross-match, an indirect Coombs test should be performed. If this is negative, transfusion with blood otherwise compatible in the major cross-match may be carried out. If positive, the advisability of transfusion should be determined by a haematologist.

Reversible leucopenia, with primary effect on granulocytes, has been reported rarely. The granulocyte count returned promptly to normal on discontinuing therapy. Reversible thrombocytopenia has occurred rarely.

Occasionally, fever has occurred within the first three weeks of therapy, sometimes associated with eosinophilia or abnormalities in liver function tests. Jaundice, with or without fever, also may occur. Its onset is usually within the first two or three months of therapy. In some patients the findings are consistent with those of cholestasis. Rare cases of fatal hepatic necrosis have been reported. Liver biopsy performed in several patients with liver dysfunction showed a microscopic focal necrosis compatible with drug hypersensitivity.

Liver function tests, and a total and differential white blood cell count, are advisable at intervals during the first six to twelve weeks of therapy, or whenever an unexplained fever occurs. Should fever, abnormality in liver function, or jaundice occur, therapy should be withdrawn. If related to methyldopa, the temperature and abnormalities in liver function have characteristically reverted to normal when methyldopa has been discontinued. Methyldopa should not be reinstated in these patients. Methyldopa should be used with caution in patients with a history of previous liver disease or dysfunction.

When methyldopa is used with other antihypertensive drugs, potentiation of antihypertensive action may occur. The progress of patients should be carefully followed to detect side reactions or unusual manifestations of drug idiosyncrasy.

Patients may require reduced doses of anaesthetics when on methyldopa. If hypotension does occur during anaesthesia, it can usually be controlled by vasopressors. The adrenergic receptors remain sensitive during treatment with methyldopa.

Dialysis removes methyldopa; therefore, hypertension may recur after this procedure.

Rarely, involuntary choreoathetotic movements have been observed during therapy with methyldopa in patients with severe bilateral cerebrovascular disease. Should these movements occur, therapy should be discontinued.

Interference with laboratory tests: Methyldopa may interfere with the measurement of urinary uric acid by the phosphotungstate method, serum creatinine by the alkaline picrate method, and AST (SGOT) by colorimetric method. Interference with spectrophotometric methods for AST analysis has not been reported.

As methyldopa fluoresces at the same wavelengths as catecholamines, spuriously high amounts of urinary catecholamines may be reported, giving rise to a false-positive diagnosis of phaeochromocytoma.

It is important to recognise this phenomenon before a patient with a possible phaeochromocytoma is subjected to surgery. Methyldopa does not interfere with measurement of VMA (vanillylmandelic acid) by those methods which convert VMA to vanillin. Methyldopa is not recommended for the treatment of patients with phaeochromocytoma.

Rarely, when urine is exposed to air after voiding, it may darken because of breakdown of methyldopa or its metabolites.

Hydrochlorothiazide: Azotaemia may be precipitated or increased by hydrochlorothiazide. Cumulative effects of hydrochlorothiazide may develop in patients with impaired renal function. If increasing azotaemia and oliguria occur during treatment of severe progressive renal disease, Hydromet should be discontinued.

Thiazides should be used with caution in patients with impaired hepatic function or progressive liver disease, since minor alterations of fluid and electrolyte balance or of serum ammonia may precipitate hepatic coma.

Sensitivity reactions may occur in patients with or without a history of allergy or bronchial asthma.

Hydrochlorothiazide adds to or potentiates the action of other antihypertensive agents. Potentiation occurs with ganglion or adrenergic blocking drugs.

The possibility of exacerbation or activation of systemic lupus erythematosus has been reported.

Patients should be carefully monitored for signs of fluid and electrolyte imbalance (hyponatraemia, hypomagnesaemia, hypochloraemic alkalosis and hypokalaemia). It is particularly important to make serum and urine electrolyte determinations if the patient is vomiting excessively or receiving parenteral fluids. Warning signs are dryness of the mouth, thirst, weakness, lethargy, drowsiness, restlessness, muscle pains or cramps, muscular fatigue, hypotension, oliguria, tachycardia and gastro-intestinal disturbance.

Hypokalaemia may develop, especially with brisk diuresis, when severe cirrhosis is present, or during concurrent steroid or ACTH administration. Interference with adequate electrolyte intake will contribute to hypokalaemia. Hypokalaemia can sensitise or exaggerate the response of the heart to the toxic effects of digitalis (e.g. increased ventricular irritability).

Hypokalaemia may be avoided or treated by giving potassium chloride or foods with a high potassium content. (Note that symptoms and signs which might indicate ulceration or obstruction of the small bowel in patients taking tablets or capsules containing potassium salts are indications for stopping treatment with such preparations immediately.)

Any chloride deficit is generally mild and does not usually require specific treatment except under unusual circumstances (as in liver or renal disease). Dilutional hyponatraemia may occur in oedematous patients in hot weather; except in rare instances when hyponatraemia is life-threatening, appropriate therapy is water restriction rather than administration of salt. In actual salt depletion, appropriate replacement is the therapy of choice.

Thiazides may increase responsiveness to tubocurarine. The antihypertensive effect of the thiazide may be enhanced in the post-sympathectomy patient. Hydrochlorothiazide may decrease arterial responsiveness to noradrenaline, but not enough to prevent noradrenaline being therapeutically useful. Orthostatic hypotension may occur, and may be potentiated by alcohol, barbiturates or narcotics.

Thiazides may decrease serum protein-bound iodine levels without signs of thyroid disturbance.

Calcium excretion is decreased by hydrochlorothiazide. Pathological changes in the parathyroid glands, with hypercalcaemia and hypophosphataemia, have been observed in a few patients on prolonged thiazide therapy.

The common complications of hyperparathyroidism such as renal lithiasis, bone reabsorption and peptic ulceration have not been seen. Thiazides should be discontinued before testing parathyroid function.

Hyperuricaemia may occur, or gout may be precipitated, in certain patients receiving thiazide therapy.

Insulin requirements in diabetic patients may be increased, decreased or unchanged. Latent diabetes mellitus may become manifest during thiazide administration.

Lithium should generally not be given to patients receiving diuretics, since the risk of lithium toxicity is very high in such patients.

Use of Hydromet in pregnancy and the nursing mother: Methyldopa has been used under close medical and obstetric supervision for the treatment of hypertension during pregnancy. There was no clinical evidence that methyldopa caused fetal abnormalities or affected the neonate. Methyldopa does cross the placental barrier and appears in cord blood and breast milk. Although no obvious teratogenic effects have been reported, the possibility of fetal injury cannot be excluded.

Thiazides also cross the placental barrier and appear in cord blood. Use of any drug in women who are or may become pregnant requires that anticipated benefits be weighed against possible risks. Hazards include foetal or neonatal jaundice, thrombocytopenia and possibly other adverse reactions which have occurred in the adult.

Thiazides also appear in breast milk. If use of Hydromet is deemed essential, the patient should stop nursing.

Side-effects: The side-effects of Hydromet are generally those of its components; combination of methyldopa and hydrochlorothiazide has not produced any additional side-effects.

Methyldopa: Significant side-effects due to methyldopa have been infrequent and this agent is usually well tolerated.

Sedation, usually transient, may occur initially or when the dosage is increased. Other early transient effects which may occur are headache, asthenia and weakness.

Central nervous system: Sedation (usually transient

headache, asthenia or weakness), paraesthesiae, parkinsonism, Bell's Palsy, involuntary choreoathetotic movements. Psychic disturbances including nightmares, impaired mental activity and reversible mild psychoses or depression. Dizziness, light-headedness, and symptoms of cerebrovascular insufficiency (may be due to lowering of blood pressure).

Cardiovascular: Bradycardia, prolonged carotid sinus hypersensitivity, aggravation of angina pectoris. Orthostatic hypotension (decrease daily dosage). Oedema (and weight gain) usually relieved by use of a diuretic. (Discontinue methyldopa if oedema progresses or signs of heart failure appear.)

Gastro-intestinal: Nausea, vomiting, distension, constipation, flatus, diarrhoea, colitis, mild dryness of the mouth, sore or 'black' tongue, pancreatitis, salivary gland inflammation.

Haematological: Positive Coombs test, haemolytic anaemia, bone-marrow depression, leucopenia, granulocytopenia, thrombocytopenia. Positive tests for antinuclear antibody, LE cells, and rheumatoid factor.

Allergic: Drug-related fever and abnormal liver function tests with jaundice and hepatocellular damage (see 'Precautions'), lupus-like syndrome, myocarditis.

Dermatological: Rash as in eczema or lichenoid eruption, toxic epidermal necrolysis.

Other: Nasal stuffiness, rise in blood urea, breast enlargement, gynaecomastia, hyperprolactinaemia, amenorrhoea, lactation, impotence, decreased libido, mild arthralgia, myalgia.

Hydrochlorothiazide: Gastro-intestinal system: Anorexia, gastric irritation, nausea, vomiting, cramps, diarrhoea, constipation, jaundice (intrahepatic cholestatic jaundice), pancreatitis, salivary gland inflammation.

Central nervous system: Dizziness, vertigo, paraesthesiae, headache, yellow vision.

Haematological: Leucopenia, agranulocytosis, thrombocytopenia, aplastic anaemia, haemolytic anaemia.

Cardiovascular: Orthostatic hypotension (may be aggravated by alcohol, barbiturates or narcotics).

Hypersensitivity: Purpura, photosensitivity, rash, urticaria, necrotising angiitis (vasculitis, cutaneous vasculitis), fever, respiratory distress including pneumonitis, anaphylactic reactions.

Other: Hyperglycaemia, glycosuria, hyperuricaemia, muscle spasm, weakness, restlessness, transient blurred vision.

Whenever side-effects are moderate to severe, dosage should be reduced or therapy withdrawn.

Treatment of overdosage: No specific antidote. If ingestion is recent, emesis may be induced or gastric lavage performed. When ingestion has been earlier, infusions may be helpful to promote urinary excretion. Otherwise, management is symptomatic treatment with special attention to cardiac rate and output, blood volume, electrolyte balance, dehydration, paralytic ileus, urinary function, hepatic coma and cerebral activity. Sympathomimetic agents may be indicated. Oxygen or artificial respiration may be required if breathing is impaired. If chronic overdosage is suspected, Hydromet should be discontinued.

Pharmaceutical precautions Keep container well closed; store in a cool place, protected from light.

Legal category POM.

Package quantities Bottles of 100 and 500.

Further information Hydromet reduces both supine and standing blood pressure. Symptomatic postural hypotension, exercise hypotension and diurnal blood pressure variations rarely occur. By adjustment of dosage, morning hypotension can be prevented without sacrificing control of afternoon blood pressure.

Product licence number 0025/5008.

HYDROSALURIC*

Presentation White, half-scored tablets, marked 'MSD 42', containing 25 mg Hydrochlorothiazide BP.

White, half-scored tablets, marked 'MSD 105', containing 50 mg Hydrochlorothiazide BP.

Uses Thiazide diuretic and hypertensive.

Oedema associated with congestive heart failure, hepatic cirrhosis, premenstrual tension and oedema due to various forms of renal dysfunction (i.e. the nephrotic syndrome, acute glomerulonephritis, chronic renal failure). Hypertension, either alone or as an adjunct to other antihypertensive drugs.

Dosage and administration Dosage should be determined on an individual basis, and the lowest dosage necessary to achieve the desired result should be used.

Adults – for oedema: Usually 50–100 mg once or twice a day. Many patients respond to intermittent therapy; for example, every other day, or three to five days a week. Intermittent therapy is less likely to produce excessive diuretic response with resulting undesirable electrolyte imbalance.

In oedema accompanying premenstrual tension: 25–50 mg once or twice a day, from the first morning of symptoms until the onset of the menses.

Adults – for control of hypertension: Usual starting dosage, 50 mg or 100 mg a day as a single or divided dose, increased or decreased according to response. Rarely some patients may require up to 200 mg daily in divided doses.

Thiazides may add to or potentiate the action of other antihypertensives. If HydroSaluric is used with other antihypertensive agents, it may be necessary to reduce the dosage of such agents so as to prevent an excessive drop in blood pressure.

Infants and children: Usually 2.5 mg per kg body weight a day, given in two doses. Infants under 6 months may need up to 3.5 mg per kg a day, in two doses. Infants up to 2 years of age may be given 12.5–37.5 mg of HydroSaluric a day in two doses. Children from 2 to 12 years of age may be given 37.5–100 mg a day in two doses. Dosage should be based on body weight.

Use in the elderly: Particular caution is needed in the elderly because of their susceptibility to electrolyte imbalance; the dosage should be carefully adjusted according to renal function and clinical response. If lower dosage is required, 25 mg tablets are available.

Contra-indications, warnings, etc
Contra-indications: Anuria, known hypersensitivity to hydrochlorothiazide or to other sulphonamide-derived drugs, severe renal or hepatic failure, Addison's disease, hypercalcaemia, concurrent lithium therapy. See also 'Use in pregnancy' and 'Use in nursing mothers', under 'Precautions'.

Warnings: Azotaemia may be precipitated or increased by HydroSaluric. Cumulative effects of hydrochlorothia-

zide may develop in patients with impaired renal function. If increasing azotaemia and oliguria occur during treatment of severe progressive renal disease, HydroSaluric should be discontinued.

Sensitivity reactions may occur in patients with or without a history of allergy or bronchial asthma.

HydroSaluric may add to or potentiate the action of other antihypertensive agents. Potentiation occurs with ganglionic- or adrenergic-blocking drugs.

The possibility of exacerbation or activation of systemic lupus erythematosus has been reported.

Hypokalaemia may develop, especially with brisk diuresis, when severe cirrhosis is present, or during concurrent steroid or ACTH administration, or after prolonged therapy. Interference with adequate electrolyte intake will contribute to hypokalaemia. Hypokalaemia can sensitise or exaggerate the response of the heart to the toxic effects of digitalis (e.g. increased ventricular irritability).

Hypokalaemia may be avoided or treated in the adult by concurrent use of amiloride hydrochloride (Midamor*), a potassium-conserving agent. It may also be avoided by giving potassium chloride or foods with a high potassium content.

Any chloride deficit is generally mild and does not usually require specific treatment except under unusual circumstances (as in liver or renal disease) when chloride replacement may be required in the treatment of metabolic alkalosis. Dilutional hyponatraemia may occur in oedematous patients in hot weather; appropriate therapy is water restriction rather than administration of salt except in rare instances when hyponatraemia is life-threatening. In actual salt depletion, appropriate replacement is the therapy of choice.

Thiazides may decrease serum protein-bound iodine levels without signs of thyroid disturbance.

Thiazides may decrease urinary calcium excretion, and may also cause intermittent and slight elevation of serum calcium in the absence of known disorders of calcium metabolism. Marked hypercalcaemia may be evidence of hidden hyperparathyroidism. Thiazides should be discontinued before carrying out tests for parathyroid function.

Hyperuricaemia may occur, or gout may be precipitated, in certain patients receiving thiazide therapy.

Drug interactions: Thiazides may increase responsiveness to tubocurarine. The antihypertensive effect of the thiazide may be enhanced in the post-sympathectomy patient.

Hydrochlorothiazide may decrease arterial responsiveness to noradrenaline, but not enough to prevent noradrenaline being therapeutically useful. Orthostatic hypotension may occur, and may be potentiated by alcohol, barbiturates or narcotics.

Insulin requirements in diabetic patients may be increased, decreased or unchanged. Latent diabetes mellitus may become manifest during thiazide administration.

Precautions: Thiazides should be used with caution in patients with impaired hepatic function or progressive liver disease, since minor alterations of fluid and electrolyte balance may precipitate hepatic coma.

Patients should be carefully monitored for signs of fluid and electrolyte imbalance (hyponatraemia, hypochloraemic alkalosis, hypomagnesaemia and hypokalaemia). It is particularly important to make serum and urine electrolyte determinations if the patient is vomiting excessively or receiving parenteral fluids. Warning signs or symptoms of fluid and electrolyte imbalance include dryness of the mouth, thirst, weakness, lethargy, drowsiness, restlessness, muscle pains or cramps, muscular fatigue, hypotension, oliguria, tachycardia and gastrointestinal disturbances.

Use in pregnancy: Thiazides appear in breast milk. If use of the drug is deemed essential, the patient should stop nursing. Thiazides cross the placental barrier and appear in cord blood. The use of HydroSaluric when pregnancy is present or suspected requires, therefore, that the benefits of the drug be weighed against possible hazards to the fetus. These hazards include fetal or neonatal jaundice, thrombocytopenia, and possibly other adverse reactions which have occurred in the adult. The routine use of diuretics in otherwise healthy pregnant women with or without mild oedema is not indicated because their use may be associated with hypovolaemia, increased blood viscosity and decreased placental perfusion.

Use in nursing mothers: Thiazides appear in breast milk. If use of the drug is deemed essential, the patient should stop nursing.

Side-effects: Gastro-intestinal system: Anorexia, gastric irritation, nausea, vomiting, cramps, diarrhoea, constipation, jaundice (intrahepatic cholestatic jaundice), pancreatitis, salivary gland inflammation.

Central nervous system: Dizziness, vertigo, paraesthesiae, headache, yellow vision.

Haematological: Leucopenia, agranulocytosis, thrombocytopenia, aplastic anaemia, haemolytic anaemia.

Cardiovascular: Orthostatic hypotension (may be aggravated by alcohol, barbiturates, or narcotics).

Hypersensitivity: Purpura, photosensitivity, rash, urticaria, necrotising angiitis (vasculitis, cutaneous vasculitis), fever, respiratory distress including pneumonitis, anaphylactic reactions.

Other: Hyperglycaemia, glycosuria, hyperuricaemia, muscle spasm, weakness, restlessness, transient blurred vision, impotence.

Whenever side-effects are moderate to severe, thiazide dosage should be reduced or therapy withdrawn.

Treatment of overdosage: Symptomatic and supportive; no specific antidote. If ingestion is recent the stomach should be emptied by emesis or gastric lavage. Dehydration, electrolyte imbalance, hepatic coma and hypotension should be corrected by standard methods. For impaired respiration, oxygen or artificial respiration should be given.

Pharmaceutical precautions Keep container tightly closed; store in a cool place, protected from light.

Legal category POM.

Package quantities *25 mg:* Bottles of 500. *50 mg:* Bottles of 500.

Further information Diuresis begins within two hours following administration, is at a peak after four hours and persists for six to twelve hours. No rigid dietary salt restriction required.

Product licence numbers
25 mg 0025/5009
50 mg 0025/5010

INNOVACE* ▼

Presentation Peach-coloured, triangular-shaped tablets, marked 'INNOVACE', containing 20 mg enalapril maleate, MSD.

Red, triangular-shaped tablets, marked 'INNOVACE', containing 10 mg enalapril maleate, MSD.

White, half-scored, triangular-shaped tablets, marked 'INNOVACE', containing 5 mg enalapril maleate, MSD.

Uses
Indications:
Hypertension: All grades of essential hypertension and renovascular hypertension where standard therapy is ineffective or inappropriate because of adverse effects.

Congestive heart failure: In congestive heart failure, Innovace should be used as an adjunctive therapy with digitalis and/or diuretics. Treatment with Innovace should always be initiated in hospital under close supervision.

Mode of action: Following oral administration, Innovace is rapidly absorbed and hydrolysed to enalaprilat, a highly specific, long-acting, non-sulphydryl angiotensin-converting enzyme inhibitor.

Innovace modulates a specific physiological mechanism, the renin-angiotensin-aldosterone system, which plays a major role in the regulation of blood pressure. Its onset of action begins smoothly and gradually within one hour and its effects continue usually for 24 hours after a single daily dose. Data indicate no loss of effect during long-term therapy. Rebound hypertension does not occur following abrupt cessation of therapy.

Congestive heart failure patients benefit particularly from reduction in pre-load and after-load of the heart, with an increase in cardiac output, without reflex tachycardia.

Dosage and administration The maximum daily dose is 40 mg.

The absorption of Innovace is not affected by food.

Essential and renovascular hypertension:
Treatment should be initiated with 5 mg once a day. Where concomitant therapy is a diuretic, the recommended initial dose of Innovace is 2.5 mg (see 'With concomitant diuretic therapy' section). The dose should be titrated to give optimum control of blood pressure. The usual maintenance dose is 10–20 mg given once daily. In severe hypertension, the dosage may be increased incrementally to a maximum of 40 mg once daily.

The dosage of other antihypertensive agents being used together with Innovace may need to be adjusted. Where Innovace replaces a beta-blocking drug in the therapeutic regime, the beta-blocking agent should not be discontinued abruptly; the dosage should be titrated down after commencing therapy with Innovace (see manufacturer's recommendations).

With concomitant diuretic therapy: The recommended initial dose of Innovace is 2.5 mg. Symptomatic hypotension can occur following the initial dose of Innovace; this is more likely when Innovace is added to previous diuretic therapy. Caution is recommended, therefore, since these patients may be volume or salt depleted. If possible, the diuretic therapy should be discontinued for 2–3 days prior to initiation of therapy with Innovace.

Innovace minimises the development of thiazide-induced hypokalaemia and hyperuricaemia.

Use in the elderly (over 65 years): The starting dose should be 2.5 mg. Innovace is effective in the treatment of hypertension in the elderly. Some elderly patients may be more responsive to Innovace than younger patients.

The dose should be titrated according to need for the control of blood pressure.

Congestive heart failure: Innovace can be used as adjunctive therapy with digitalis and/or diuretics in congestive heart failure. Therapy with Innovace should be initiated under close supervision in hospital, with a recommended starting dose of 2.5 mg. If possible, the dose of diuretic should be reduced before beginning treatment. Blood pressure and renal function should be monitored closely both before and during treatment with Innovace because severe hypotension and, more rarely, consequent renal failure have been reported (see 'Precautions').

In the absence of, or after effective management of, symptomatic hypotension following initiation of therapy with Innovace in congestive heart failure, the dose should be gradually increased, depending on the patient's response, to the usual maintenance dose (10–20 mg) given in a single or divided dose. This dose titration may be performed over a two- to four-week period, or more rapidly if indicated by the presence of residual signs and symptoms of heart failure.

The appearance of hypotension after the initial dose of Innovace does not preclude subsequent careful dose titration with the drug, following effective treatment of the hypotension.

Use in impaired renal function: (See 'Precautions') Innovace is excreted by the kidney. It should be used with caution in patients with renal impairment. The recommended starting dose is 2.5 mg. The dose should be titrated against the response, and should be kept as low as possible to maintain adequate control of blood pressure or heart failure.

Innovace is dialysable. Dialysis patients may be given the usual dose of Innovace on dialysis days. On the days when patients are not on dialysis the dosage should be tailored to the blood pressure response.

Contra-indications, warnings, etc

Contra-indications

Pregnancy: Innovace is contra-indicated in pregnancy because it has been shown to be fetotoxic in rabbits during middle and late pregnancy. If a woman who is receiving Innovace misses a menstrual period, she should be assessed for pregnancy by her doctor.

Hypersensitivity to enalapril.

Precautions

Pretreatment assessment of renal function: Evaluation of the patient should include assessment of renal function prior to initiation of therapy, and during treatment where appropriate.

Symptomatic hypotension has occurred after the initial dose of Innovace. It is more likely to occur in patients who have been volume-depleted by diuretic therapy, dietary salt restriction, dialysis, diarrhoea or vomiting.

In these patients, by discontinuing diuretic therapy or significantly reducing the diuretic dose for two to three days prior to initiating Innovace, the possibility of this occurrence is reduced. By initiating therapy with a small dose (2.5 mg Innovace) the duration of any hypotensive effect may be lessened.

Severe hypotension has been reported, mainly in patients with severe heart failure. Many of these patients were on high doses of loop diuretics, and some had hyponatraemia or functional renal impairment (see 'Dosage and administration'). If hypotension develops, the patient should be placed in a supine position. Volume repletion with oral fluids or intravenous normal saline may be required. Intravenous atropine may be necessary if there is associated bradycardia. Treatment with

Innovace may be restarted with careful dose titration following restoration of effective blood volume and pressure.

In some patients with congestive heart failure who have normal or low blood pressure, additional lowering of systemic blood pressure may occur with Innovace. If such hypotension becomes symptomatic, a reduction of dose or discontinuation of Innovace may become necessary.

The appearance of hypotension after the initial dose of Innovace does not preclude subsequent careful dose titration with the drug after effective management of the hypotension.

Impaired renal function: Innovace should be used with caution in patients with renal insufficiency as they may require reduced or less frequent doses (see 'Dosage'). Close monitoring of renal function during therapy should be performed as deemed appropriate in those with renal insufficiency. In the majority, renal function will not alter, or may improve.

Renal failure has been reported in association with Innovace and has been mainly in patients with severe congestive heart failure or underlying renal disease, including renal artery stenosis. If recognised promptly and treated appropriately, renal failure when associated with Innovace therapy is usually reversible.

Some hypertensive patients, with no apparent pre-existing renal disease have developed increases in blood urea and creatinine when Innovace has been given concurrently with a diuretic. Dosage reduction of Innovace and/or discontinuation of the diuretic may be required. This situation should raise the possibility of underlying renal artery stenosis (see 'Renovascular hypertension').

As with all antihypertensive agents, renal function should be assessed in patients with hypertension or congestive heart failure before initiating therapy.

Renovascular hypertension: Innovace can be used when surgery is not indicated, or prior to surgery. In some patients with bilateral renal artery stenosis or stenosis of the artery to a solitary kidney, increases of blood urea and creatinine, reversible upon discontinuation of therapy, have been seen. This is especially likely in patients treated with diuretics and/or those with renal insufficiency.

Surgery/anaesthesia: In patients undergoing major surgery or during anaesthesia with agents that produce hypotension, Innovace blocks angiotensin II formation secondary to compensatory renin release. This may lead to hypotension which can be corrected by volume expansion.

General: Where Innovace has been used as a single agent in hypertension, negro patients may show a reduced therapeutic response.

Innovace should not be used in patients with aortic stenosis or outflow obstruction.

Drug interactions: Combination with other antihypertensive agents such as beta-blockers, methyldopa, and diuretics may increase the antihypertensive efficacy. Ganglionic or adrenergic-blocking drugs should only be combined with Innovace under careful supervision. Concomitant propranolol may reduce the bioavailability of Innovace, but this does not appear to be of any clinical significance.

There is no experience in the use of Innovace with calcium antagonists.

Concomitant therapy with lithium may increase the serum lithium concentration.

Plasma potassium usually remains within normal limits. If Innovace is given with a diuretic, the likelihood of diuretic-induced hypokalaemia may be lessened. Innovace may elevate plasma potassium levels in patients with renal failure. Potassium supplements or potassium-sparing diuretics are not usually recommended, particularly in patients with impaired renal function, since they may lead to significant increases in plasma potassium.

If concomitant use of these agents is deemed appropriate, they should be used with caution and with frequent monitoring of plasma potassium.

Paediatric use: Innovace has not been studied in children.

Nursing mothers: Because it is not known whether Innovace is excreted in human milk, caution should be exercised if Innovace is given to nursing mothers.

Side-effects

Severe hypotension and renal failure have occurred in association with therapy with Innovace. These appear to occur in certain specific sub-groups (see 'Precautions').

Angioneurotic oedema has been reported with angiotensin-converting enzyme inhibitors, including Innovace. In such cases, Innovace should be discontinued immediately and the patient observed. Where swelling is confined to the face, lips and mouth the condition will usually resolve without further treatment, although antihistamines may be useful in relieving symptoms. These patients should be followed carefully until the swelling has resolved. However, where there is involvement of the tongue, glottis or larynx, likely to cause airways obstruction, subcutaneous adrenaline (0.5 ml 1:1000) should be administered promptly when indicated.

Other hypersensitivity reactions, including urticaria, have been reported.

Other adverse reactions: Dizziness and headaches are the more commonly reported side effects. Fatigue and asthenia were reported in 2–3% of patients. Other side-effects occurred in less than 2% of patients, and included nausea, diarrhoea, muscle cramps, rash, dysgeusia and cough.

Clinical laboratory test findings: Increases in blood urea and plasma creatinine, reversible on discontinuation of Innovace, are most likely in the presence of bilateral renal artery stenosis, especially in patients with renal insufficiency (see 'Precautions'). However, increases in blood urea and plasma creatinine may occur without evidence of pre-existing renal impairment, especially in patients taking diuretics. In this event undiagnosed renal artery stenosis should be suspected. Dosage reduction of Innovace and/or discontinuation of the diuretic should be considered.

Decreases in haemoglobin, haematocrit, platelets and white cell count, as well as elevation of liver enzymes, have been reported in a few patients, but a causal relationship to Innovace has not been established.

Overdosage: Available data are limited. The most likely manifestation of overdosage would be hypotension, which can be treated if necessary by intravenous infusion of normal saline solution. Innovace can be removed by haemodialysis.

Pharmaceutical precautions Store in a dry place below 25°C, protected from light.

Legal category POM.

Package quantities

Tablets 20 mg: Calendar packs of 28 tablets, bottles of 50 tablets

Tablets 10 mg: Calendar packs of 28 tablets, bottles of 50 tablets

Tablets 5 mg: Bottles of 50 tablets

Further information Nil.

Product licence numbers

5 mg tablet	0025/0194
10 mg tablet	0025/0195
20 mg tablet	0025/0196

MEFOXIN* INJECTION

Presentation In vials containing 1 g or 2 g of cefoxitin as the sodium salt. Each gram of cefoxitin contains approximately 2.3 mEq sodium.

Uses Mefoxin is indicated for the treatment of the following infections caused by sensitive bacteria: peritonitis and other intra-abdominal and intrapelvic infections; gonorrhoea; female genital tract infections; septicaemia; urinary tract infections; respiratory tract infections; bone and joint infections; and skin and soft-tissue infections.

Mefoxin is a broad-spectrum bactericidal antibiotic indicated for the treatment of infections caused by susceptible strains of Gram-positive and Gram-negative pathogens both aerobic and anaerobic.

Mefoxin has been clinically effective not only in infections due to antibiotic-sensitive organisms, but also in infections due to organisms resistant to one or more of the following antibacterial agents: penicillin, ampicillin, carbenicillin, tetracyclines, erythromycin, chloramphenicol, cephalosporins, kanamycin, gentamicin, tobramycin, and sulphamethoxazole-trimethoprim.

Many Gram-negative pathogens are resistant to penicillins and cephalosporins through the action of the beta-lactamases which are produced by these pathogens. Mefoxin is remarkably stable in the presence of these bacterial beta-lactamases, both penicillinases and cephalosporinases. Hence, the clinical efficacy of Mefoxin extends to many infections caused by such pathogens.

Mefoxin is indicated for the treatment of mixed infections caused by susceptible strains of aerobic and anaerobic bacteria. The majority of these mixed infections are associated with contamination from faecal flora originating from the vagina, skin, and mouth. In these mixed infections, *Bacteroides fragilis* is the most commonly encountered anaerobic pathogen and is usually susceptible to Mefoxin.

Mefoxin is also indicated for adjunctive therapy in the surgical treatment of infections, including abscesses, infection complicating hollow visceral perforations, cutaneous infections, and infections of serous surfaces, whether caused by aerobes, mixed aerobes and anaerobes, or anaerobes.

Clinical experience has demonstrated that Mefoxin can be administered to patients who are receiving carbenicillin, kanamycin, gentamicin, tobramycin, or amikacin.

Prevention: Mefoxin is indicated for the prevention of certain post-operative infections in patients undergoing contaminated or potentially contaminated surgical procedures or where the occurrence of post-operative infection could be serious.

Microbiology: Mefoxin is active in vitro *against:* Aerobic bacteria: *Gram-positive cocci* including: *Staphylococci:* (including coagulase-positive, coagulase-negative, and penicillinase-producing strains); Group A beta-haemolytic streptococci (*Streptococcus pyogenes*); Group B beta-haemolytic streptococci (*Streptococcus agalactiae*); *Streptococcus pneumoniae* (*Diplococcus pneumoniae*); other streptococci (except group D streptococci including enterococci, most strains of which are resistant, e.g. *Streptococcus faecalis*), *Gram-negative cocci* including: *Neisseria gonorrhoeae* (including penicillinase-producing strains); *Neisseria meningitidis. Gram-negative rods (facultative anaerobes)* including: *Escherichia coli; Klebsiella pneumoniae*; Klebsiella spp.; *Proteus mirabilis. Proteus* (indole-positive): *Proteus vulgaris; Proteus rettgeri; Proteus morganii; Haemophilus influenzae; Serratia marcescens*; Providencia spp.; Salmonella and Shigella spp.

Anaerobic bacteria: *Gram-positive cocci* including: Peptococcus spp.; Peptostreptococcus spp.; Microaerophilic streptococcus. *Gram-positive rods* including: *Clostridium perfringens*; Clostridium spp.; Eubacterium spp.; *Propionibacterium acnes. Gram-negative cocci* including: Veillonella spp. *Gram-negative rods* including: *Bacteroides fragilis; Bacteroides melaninogenicus*; Bacteroides spp. (including both penicillin-susceptible and penicillin-resistant strains); Fusobacterium spp.

Mefoxin is active against some strains of the following bacteria: *Acinetobacter calcoaceticus* var. *anitratum* (*Herellea vaginicola*); *Acinetobacter calcoaceticus* var. *Iwoffi* (*Mima polymorpha*); *Alcaligenes faecalis*; Citrobacter spp. and Flavo-bacterium spp.; Enterobacter spp.

Mefoxin is not active against Pseudomonas spp., most strains of enterococci, many strains of *Enterobacter cloacae*, methicillin-resistant staphylococci, and *Listeria monocytogenes.*

Human pharmacology: Mefoxin administered parenterally, produces high serum and urine concentrations. It is excreted virtually unchanged as active Mefoxin by the kidneys, and has a mean terminal serum half-life of approximately one hour. Mefoxin passes rapidly into body fluids such as pleural, bile, and ascitic fluids. Probenecid slows tubular excretion and increases and prolongs blood levels.

Intravenous: Peak serum concentration of Mefoxin following 1 g infused intravenously over three minutes was 125 mcg/ml, infused over 30 minutes was 72 mcg/ml, and infused over 120 minutes was 25 mcg/ml. Following 2 g infused intravenously over three minutes, peak serum concentration was 221 mcg/ml.

In a number of studies using 0.5 g, 1 g, or 2 g intravenous doses of Mefoxin mean total urinary recovery ranged from 77% to 99% of the cefoxitin dose.

Intramuscular: When Mefoxin was reconstituted for intramuscular injection with 0.5% or 1% lignocaine hydrochloride, the lignocaine had no effect on the absorption or elimination of Mefoxin.

Intramuscular injections of 1 g of Mefoxin in 0.5% lignocaine hydrochloride solution produced a peak serum concentration of 30 mcg/ml at 20 minutes. Approximately 85% of an intramuscular dose is excreted by the kidneys in the first six hours; this results in high urine levels (e.g. >3,000 mcg/ml between one and two hours after a 1 g dose).

Dosage and administration Mefoxin may be administered intravenously or intramuscularly. (See reconstitution directions for each route.) Dosage and route of administration should be determined by severity of

infection, susceptibility of the causative organisms, and condition of the patient.

Therapy may be started while awaiting the results of susceptibility testing.

Usual adult dosage			
Type of infection	Dose (g)	Frequency (hrs)	Total daily dosage
Uncomplicated	1	Every 8 (occasionally every 6)	3 g (4 g)
Moderately severe or severe	2	Every 8 (occasionally every 6)	6 g (8 g)
Infections generally needing antibiotics in higher dosage	3 (2)	Every 6 (every 4)	12 g

Maintenance dosage of Mefoxin in adults with reduced renal function			
Renal function	Creatinine clearance (ml/min)	Dose (g)	Frequency (hrs)
Mild impairment	50–30	1–2	Every 8–12
Moderate impairment	29–10	1–2	Every 12–24
Severe impairment	9–5	0.5–1	Every 12–24
Essentially no function	<5	0.5–1	Every 24–48

Adults Dosage: The usual dosage is 1 g or 2 g of Mefoxin every eight hours. (See 'Usual adult dosage' chart.)

In adults with renal insufficiency, an initial loading dose of 1 g to 2 g may be given. After a loading dose, the following recommendations for *maintenance dosage* may be used as a guide.

In the patients undergoing haemodialysis, the loading dose of 1–2 g should be given after each haemodialysis, and the maintenance dose should be given as indicated in the chart giving 'Maintenance dosage of Mefoxin in adults with reduced renal function'.

Neonates, infants and children:

Neonates
0–1 week of age   20–40 mg/kg every 12 hours
1–4 weeks of age   20–40 mg/kg every 8 hours
Infants   20–40 mg/kg every 6 hours or every 8 hours
Children   20–40 mg/kg every 6 hours or every 8 hours

In severe infections, the total daily dosage may be increased to 200 mg/kg, but not to exceed 12 g per day.

Mefoxin is not recommended for the therapy of meningitis. If meningitis is suspected an appropriate antibiotic should be used.

In children with renal insufficiency dosage frequency should be reduced as indicated for adults.

Uncomplicated urinary tract infections: In uncomplicated urinary tract infections due to susceptible organisms, 1 g intramuscularly twice a day has been shown to be effective.

Uncomplicated gonorrhoea: For single dose therapy of uncomplicated gonorrhoea, including that caused by penicillinase-producing strains, the recommended dose is 2 g of Mefoxin intramuscularly given with 1 g of probenecid by mouth (at the same time or up to one hour before).

Prophylactic administration for adults: 2 g intramuscularly or intravenously just prior to surgery (approximately $\frac{1}{2}$–1 hour before incision), then 2 g every 6 hours. Prophylactic therapy does not usually continue for more than 24 hours.

Prophylactic administration for neonates, infants and children: In infants and children, 30–40 mg/kg doses may be given at the same times as designated for adults. However, in neonates, 30–40 mg/kg doses may be given $\frac{1}{2}$ to 1 hour before initial incision and the second and third dose may be given every 8–12 hours.

Caesarean section: 2.0 g intravenously as soon as the umbilical cord is clamped; and 2.0 g intravenously or intramuscularly 4 and 8 hours after the initial dose. Subsequent doses may be given every six hours with usually no need to continue for more than 24 hours.

Intravenous administration: Reconstitute Mefoxin with Water for Injections BP: 1 g is soluble in 2 ml. Although Mefoxin is very soluble, for intravenous use it is preferable to add 10 ml of Water for Injections BP to the 1 g vial or to the 2 g vial. Shake to dissolve and then withdraw entire contents of vial into syringe.

Solutions of Mefoxin range from clear to light amber in colour. The pH of freshly reconstituted solutions usually ranges from 4.2 to 7.0.

For direct intravenous injection, Mefoxin may be slowly injected into the vein over a period of three to five minutes or may be given through the tubing when the patient is receiving parenteral solutions.

An intermittent intravenous infusion of Mefoxin may be employed when large amounts of fluid are to be given. However, during infusion of the solution containing Mefoxin, it may be advisable temporarily to discontinue administration of any other infusion solution at the same site (by using an appropriate IV infusion set).

A solution of Mefoxin may also be given by continuous intravenous infusion (see opposite for compatibility and stability).

Intramuscular administration ONLY: Reconstitute Mefoxin 1 g with 2 ml of Water for Injections BP, or 0.5% or 1% lignocaine hydrochloride (without adrenaline) solution. Mefoxin is given by deep injection into a large muscle mass. Avoid injection into a blood vessel.

Note: Some patients may be hypersensitive to lignocaine.

Preparation of solution: The following table is provided for convenience in reconstituting Mefoxin for both intravenous and intramuscular administration.

Strength	Amount of diluent to be added (ml*)	Approximate final volume (ml)	Approximate average concentration (mg/ml)
1 gram vial	2 (Intramuscular)	2.5	400
1 gram vial	10 (IV)	10.5	95
2 gram vial	10 or 20 (IV)	11 or 21	180 or 95

* Shake to dissolve and let stand until clear.

Compatibility and stability: A solution of Mefoxin in Water for Injections BP may be added to the following solutions: 0.9% Sodium Chloride Injection BP, 5% or 10% Dextrose Injection BP, Dextrose and Sodium Chloride Injection BP (5%/0.9%, 5%/0.45%, or 5%/

0.2%). Lactated Ringer's Injection USP, 5% Dextrose Injection in 0.02% sodium bicarbonate solution, 5% Dextrose in Lactated Ringer's Injection, 5% or 10% invert sugar in water, 10% invert sugar in saline solution, 4.2% Sodium Bicarbonate Injection BP, M/6 Sodium Lactate Injection BP, insulin (in normal saline or 10% invert sugar), heparin (100 units/ml and 0.1 units/ml), mannitol (2.5%, 5% and 10%).

Mefoxin has been shown to be chemically and visually compatible with aminoglycosides such as amikacin, gentamicin, kanamycin, and tobramycin mixed in 200 ml of 0.9% sodium chloride or 5% dextrose in water.

Use in the elderly: The dosage should be determined by the severity of the infection, the susceptibility of the causative organisms, the patient's clinical condition and renal function.

Contra-indications, warnings, etc

Contra-indications: Mefoxin is contra-indicated in persons who have shown hypersensitivity to cefoxitin. In the absence of clinical experience, Mefoxin should not be administered to patients who have shown hypersensitivity to cephalosporins.

Precautions: There is some clinical and laboratory evidence of partial cross-allergenicity between cephamycins and other beta-lactam antibiotics, penicillins, and cephalosporins. Severe reactions (including anaphylaxis) have been reported with most beta-lactam antibiotics.

Before therapy with Mefoxin, careful inquiry should be made concerning previous hypersensitivity reactions to beta-lactam antibiotics. Mefoxin should be given cautiously to penicillin-allergic patients.

Pseudomembranous colitis, reported with virtually all antibiotics, can range from mild to life threatening in severity. Antibiotics should be prescribed with caution in patients with a history of gastro-intestinal disease, particularly colitis. Treatment-related diarrhoea should always be considered as a pointer to this diagnosis. While studies indicate that a toxin of *Clostridium difficile* is one of the primary causes of antibiotic-related colitis, other causes should be considered.

Any patient who has demonstrated some form of allergy, particularly to drugs, should receive antibiotics cautiously. If an allergic reaction to Mefoxin occurs, the drug should be discontinued.

The total daily dosage should be reduced when Mefoxin is administered to patients with transient or persistent reduction of urinary output due to renal insufficiency because high and prolonged serum antibiotic concentrations can occur from usual doses.

Interference with laboratory tests: A false-positive reaction to glucose in the urine may occur with reducing substances but not with the use of specific glucose oxidase methods.

Using the Jaffe technique, falsely high creatinine values in serum may occur if Mefoxin serum concentrations exceed 100 mcg/ml. Serum samples from patients treated with Mefoxin should not be analysed for creatinine if withdrawn within two hours of drug administration.

Use in pregnancy: Use of the drug in women of childbearing potential requires that the anticipated benefits be weighed against possible hazards. Reproductive and teratogenic studies have been performed in mice and rats and have revealed no evidence of impaired fertility or harm to the fetus due to Mefoxin. There are no controlled studies with Mefoxin in pregnant women.

Nursing mothers: Mefoxin is excreted in human milk.

Side-effects: Mefoxin is generally well tolerated. Side-effects rarely require stopping treatment and usually have been mild and transient.

Local reactions: Thrombophlebitis has occurred with intravenous administration. Pain, induration and tenderness after intramuscular injections have been reported.

Allergic: Maculopapular rash, urticaria, pruritus, eosinophilia, fever and other allergic reactions have been noted rarely.

Gastro-intestinal: Symptoms of pseudomembraneous colitis can appear during or after antibiotic treatment. Nausea, vomiting, and diarrhoea have been reported rarely.

Blood: Transient leucopenia, neutropenia, haemolytic anaemia and thrombocytopenia has been reported. Some individuals particularly those with azotaemia, may develop positive direct Coombs tests during therapy with Mefoxin.

Liver function: Transient elevations in AST (SGOT), ALT (SGPT), serum LDH, and serum alkaline phosphatase have been reported rarely.

Kidney: Elevations in serum creatinine and/or blood urea levels have been observed. Acute renal failure has been reported rarely. The role of Mefoxin in changes in renal function tests is difficult to assess, since factors predisposing to pre-renal azotaemia or to impaired renal function usually have been present.

Treatment of overdosage: No information is available at present.

Pharmaceutical precautions Mefoxin, as reconstituted with Water for Injections BP, Water for Injections BP preserved with parabens or benzyl alcohol, 0.9% Sodium Chloride Injection BP, 5% Dextrose Injection BP, or 0.5% and 1.0% lignocaine hydrochloride (preserved in parabens), maintains satisfactory potency for 24 hours at room temperature, for one week under refrigeration (below 5°C) and for at least 30 weeks in the frozen state and will maintain potency after thawing for at least 24 hours at room temperature.

After reconstitution with Water for Injections BP and subsequent storage in disposable plastic syringes, Mefoxin is stable for 24 hours at room temperature and 48 hours under refrigeration.

When reconstituting Mefoxin for neonates, Water for Injections must be preservative free.

After the periods mentioned above, any unused solutions or frozen material should be discarded. Do not refreeze.

Note: Mefoxin in the dry state should be stored below 30°C. Avoid exposure to temperatures above 50°C. The dry material as well as solutions tend to darken, depending on storage conditions; product potency, however, is not adversely affected.

Legal category POM.

Package quantities Sterile Mefoxin is supplied in vials containing 1 g or 2 g of cefoxitin as the sodium salt.

Further information Nil.

Product licence numbers
1 g   0025/0130
2 g   0025/0131

MINTEZOL*

Presentation Orange-coloured chewable tablets, marked 'MSD 907', containing 500 mg Thiabendazole BP.

Uses Anthelmintic.

Mintezol is indicated as primary treatment against Strongyloidiasis; Cutaneous larva migrans (creeping eruption); Dracunculiasis (guinea worm); Visceral larva migrans.

Mintezol is indicated as secondary treatment against Enterobiasis (threadworm) when the infestation is mixed with a primary indication.

Mintezol can relieve the symptoms and fever of trichinosis during the invasion stage.

Mintezol is indicated only (a) when specific therapy is unavailable, (b) when other therapy cannot be used or (c) as additive therapy against *Necator americanus* and *Ancylostoma duodenale* (hookworm); *Trichuriasis* (whipworm); *Ascariasis* (large roundworm).

Dosage and administration Dosage depends on the body weight of the patient and is independent of the condition being treated. Usually, 2 doses are given each day. For patients weighing less than 60 kg (132 lb), each dose is based on 25 mg thiabendazole per kg body weight. For patients weighing 60 kg or more, each dose is 1.5 g thiabendazole. The maximum daily dosage for adults weighing 60 kg or more is 3 g.

Mintezol should be taken with meals and chewed before swallowing. Dietary restrictions, complementary medications and cleansing enemas are not necessary.

The table below relates dosage to body weight:

Patient's weight		Dose (twice daily)
kg	lb	Tablets (500 mg thiabendazole)
10	22	$\frac{1}{2}$
20	44	1
30	66	$1\frac{1}{2}$
40	88	2
50	110	$2\frac{1}{2}$
60 (or more)	132 (or more)	3

Duration of therapy does depend on the particular nematode infestation, and is as follows:

Strongyloidiasis, ascariasis, uncinariasis and trichuriasis: 2 doses a day for two successive days. Alternatively, a single dose of 50 mg/kg may be given, but a higher incidence of side-effects would be expected.

(Clinical experience with thiabendazole in the treatment of the conditions in the above paragraph in children weighing less than 15 kg has been limited.)

Cutaneous larva migrans: 2 doses a day for two successive days. If active lesions are still present two days after completion of this therapy, a second similar course is recommended.

Visceral larva migrans: 2 doses a day for 7 successive days. (Safety and efficacy data on this duration of treatment are limited.)

Trichinosis: 2 doses a day for two to four successive days, according to the response of the patient. The optimum dosage in trichinosis has not yet been established. (Clinical experience with thiabendazole in the treatment of this condition in children weighing less than 15 kg has been limited.)

Dracunculiasis: 50–100 mg/kg in two equally divided doses for one day. The lower dosage for patients with 1 or 2 visible worms; the higher dosage for patients with multiple infection (3 or more worms). In massive infections (10 worms or more), a second dose of 50 mg/kg can be given five to eight days after treatment, if required.

Further considerations: In certain patients, 2 doses a day may lead to a higher incidence of side-effects. In these circumstances, 25 mg per kg body weight may be given after the largest meal on the first day and repeated 24 hours later after a similar meal on the second day.

For mass treatment, a single dose of 50 mg/kg after the evening meal is highly effective and most convenient, though a higher incidence of side-effects may be expected.

Use in the elderly: Since CNS and hepatic side effects have been reported to occur and since excretion is primarily renal, use with caution in elderly patients who have renal, hepatic or CNS dysfunction. As with younger patients, the dosage should be calculated on the basis of body weight.

Contra-indications, warnings, etc

Contra-indication: A history of hypersensitivity to thiabendazole.

Precautions: If any hypersensitivity reactions occur, therapy should be discontinued immediately and not resumed. Erythema multiforme, including fatal cases of Stevens-Johnson syndrome, has been associated with thiabendazole therapy.

Mintezol may impair alertness in some patients, who should avoid driving, operating machinery, or other activities made hazardous by diminished alertness.

Mintezol is not suitable for the treatment of mixed infestations with ascaris because it may cause these worms to migrate.

Ideally, anaemic, dehydrated or malnourished patients should be given supportive therapy before starting treatment with Mintezol. Liver and renal function should be carefully monitored in patients with disorders of these organs.

Mintezol should not be used prophylactically.

Thiabendazole may compete with other drugs, such as theophylline, for sites of metabolism in the liver and thus elevate the serum levels of such drugs to potentially toxic levels. Therefore, when the concomitant use of thiabendazole and xanthine derivatives is anticipated, it may be necessary to monitor blood levels and/or reduce the dosage of such compounds. Such concomitant use should only be made under careful medical supervision.

Pregnancy and the nursing mother: Mintezol should not be used during pregnancy or lactation. Reports have suggested that thiabendazole is teratogenic in mice, although reproduction studies in generations of rabbits, rats, sheep, cattle and pigs have shown no fetal abnormalities attributable to the drug. Nevertheless, Mintezol should not be used in women of childbearing potential unless pregnancy has been excluded.

Side-effects: The most common are anorexia, nausea, vomiting and dizziness. Diarrhoea, epigastric distress, pruritus, weariness, giddiness, headache and drowsiness occur less often.

Rare side-effects are tinnitus, collapse, abnormal sensation in the eyes, blurring of vision, hyperirritability, numbness, hyperglycaemia, yellow vision, enuresis, hypotension, jaundice, transient leucopenia, perianal rash, crystalluria, haematuria, cholestasis and parenchymal liver damage, and a transitory rise in cephalin flocculation and SGOT. The appearance of live ascaris in the mouth and nose has been reported on rare occasions.

Hypersensitivity reactions include fever, facial flush, rigor, conjunctival injection, angioneurotic oedema, anaphylaxis, skin rashes, erythema multiforme including Stevens-Johnson syndrome, and lymphadenopathy.

Some patients excrete a metabolite which imparts a characteristic odour to their urine, similar to that which occurs after eating asparagus.

Treatment of overdosage: Symptomatic and supportive: there is no specific antidote. The stomach should be emptied by emesis or gastric lavage.

Pharmaceutical precautions Store in a dry place below 25°C.

Legal category P.

Package quantities *Tablets:* Packs of 6.

Further information Nil.

Product licence number 0025/5031.

MODURETIC*

Presentation Moduretic is available as peach-coloured, half-scored, diamond-shaped tablets, marked 'MSD 917', containing Amiloride Hydrochloride BP equivalent to 5 mg anhydrous amiloride hydrochloride and 50 mg Hydrochlorothiazide BP.

Moduretic is also available as an aniseed/peppermint-flavoured solution containing Amiloride Hydrochloride BP equivalent to 5 mg anhydrous amiloride hydrochloride and 50 mg Hydrochlorothiazide BP in each 5 ml.

Uses Potassium-conserving diuretic and antihypertensive.

For the treatment of patients with hypertension, congestive heart failure, or hepatic cirrhosis with ascites, in whom potassium depletion might be anticipated. The presence of amiloride hydrochloride minimises the likelihood of excessive potassium loss during vigorous diuresis for long-term therapy. The combination is thus particularly indicated in conditions where potassium balance is especially important, e.g. patients with congestive heart failure receiving digitalis.

In hypertension, Moduretic may be used alone or as an adjunct to other antihypertensive agents. In hepatic cirrhosis with ascites, Moduretic usually provides satisfactory diuresis with diminished potassium loss and less risk of metabolic alkalosis.

Dosage and administration The rate of loss of weight and the serum electrolyte levels should determine the dosage. The most satisfactory rate of weight loss after initiation of diuresis is about 0.5–1.0 kg/day.

Moduretic is not recommended for children (see 'Contra-indications').

Hypertension: Usually 1 or 2 Moduretic Tablets (or equivalent) once-a-day or in divided doses. Some patients may require only half a Moduretic Tablet a day. The dosage may be increased if necessary, but must not exceed the equivalent of 4 Moduretic Tablets a day.

Moduretic may be used alone or as an adjunct to other antihypertensive drugs, but since the antihypertensive effect of these agents may then be enhanced, their dosage may have to be reduced to avoid an excessive drop in blood pressure.

Studies have shown that therapy can be given on a

once-daily basis when Blocadren is given at the same time. The majority of patients will respond to a regimen of 10 or 20 mg of Blocadren once daily with the equivalent of 1 tablet of Moduretic.

Congestive heart failure: Initially the equivalent of 1 or 2 Moduretic Tablets a day, subsequently adjusted if required, but not exceeding 4 Moduretic Tablets (or equivalent) a day. Optimum dosage is determined by the diuretic response and the plasma potassium level. Once an initial diuresis has been achieved, reduction in dosage may be attempted for maintenance therapy. Maintenance therapy may be on an intermittent basis.

Hepatic cirrhosis with ascites: Initially the equivalent of 1 Moduretic Tablet a day, subsequently adjusted if required, but not exceeding 4 Moduretic Tablets (or equivalent) a day. A gradual weight reduction is especially desirable in cirrhotic patients, to reduce the likelihood of untoward reactions associated with diuretic therapy. Maintenance dosages may be lower than those required to initiate diuresis; dosage reduction should therefore be attempted when the patient's weight is stabilised.

Use in the elderly: Particular caution is needed in the elderly because of their susceptibility to electrolyte imbalance; the dosage should be carefully adjusted to renal function and clinical response.

Contra-indications, warnings, etc

Contra-indications: Hyperkalaemia (plasma potassium over 5.5 mmol/l); other potassium-conserving diuretics and potassium supplements (except in severe and/or refractory cases of hypokalaemia under careful monitoring); anuria; acute renal failure, severe progressive renal disease; severe hepatic failure; Addison's disease; hypercalcaemia, concurrent lithium therapy; diabetic nephropathy; patients with blood urea over 10 mmol/l or serum creatinine over 130 μmol/l, in whom serum electrolyte and blood urea levels cannot be monitored carefully and frequently; prior sensitivity to amiloride hydrochloride or hydrochlorothiazide. In renal impairment, use of potassium-conserving agent may result in rapid development of hyperkalaemia. Because the safety of amiloride hydrochloride for use in children has not been established, Moduretic is not recommended in children. For 'Use in pregnancy' and 'Use in nursing mothers', see 'Precautions'.

Precautions: Diabetes mellitus: Hyperkalaemia has commonly occurred in diabetic patients on amiloride hydrochloride, especially those with chronic renal disease or prerenal azotaemia. The status of renal function should therefore be determined before use in known or suspected diabetics.

The agents should be discontinued for at least 3 days before giving a glucose-tolerance test, as one patient with poorly controlled diabetes mellitus, who became severely hyperkalaemic while receiving amiloride hydrochloride, died following two repeated intravenous glucose-tolerance tests. The dosage of insulin or oral hypoglycaemic agents for diabetic patients may need to be changed. Diabetes mellitus which has been latent may become manifest during thiazide administration.

Metabolic or respiratory acidosis: Potassium-conserving therapy should be initiated only with caution in severely ill patients in whom metabolic or respiratory acidosis may occur, e.g. patients with cardiopulmonary disease or decompensated diabetes. Shifts in acid-base balance alter the balance of extracellular/intracellular potassium,

and the development of acidosis may be associated with rapid increases in plasma potassium.

Hyperkalaemia: This has been observed in patients receiving amiloride hydrochloride, either alone or with other diuretics, particularly in the aged, in diabetics, and in hospital patients with hepatic cirrhosis or congestive heart failure who had known renal involvement, were seriously ill, or were undergoing vigorous diuretic therapy. Such patients should be carefully observed for clinical, laboratory and ECG evidence of hyperkalaemia (not always associated with an abnormal ECG). Some deaths have been reported in this group of patients. Should hyperkalaemia develop, discontinue treatment immediately, and if necessary, take active measures to reduce the serum potassium to normal.

Electrolyte imbalance and blood urea increases: Hyponatraemia and hypochloraemia may occur. Hypochloraemic alkalosis may also occur, but its likelihood is reduced by the presence of amiloride in Moduretic.

Reversible increases in blood urea have been reported accompanying vigorous diuresis, especially in seriously ill patients, such as those with hepatic cirrhosis with ascites and metabolic alkalosis or those with resistant oedema; plasma electrolyte and blood urea levels should be carefully monitored in these patients.

Use with caution in patients with renal impairment. Special care should be taken to avoid cumulative or toxic effects due to a reduced excretion of its components. In addition, azotaemia may be precipitated or increased by hydrochlorothiazide. Renal function should be monitored. If increasing azotaemia and oliguria occur, treatment should be discontinued.

Effects in cirrhotic patients: Oral diuretic therapy is more frequently accompanied by adverse reactions in patients with hepatic cirrhosis and ascites because these patients are intolerant of acute shifts in electrolyte balance, and because they often have pre-existing hypokalaemia as a result of associated aldosteronism. Hepatic encephalopathy, manifested by tremors, confusion and coma, has been reported in patients on amiloride hydrochloride alone. Patients with liver disease on Moduretic should be observed for this complication. In cirrhotic patients receiving amiloride hydrochloride alone, a deepening of jaundice has occurred, but the relationship to amiloride is uncertain.

Metabolic and endocrine effects: Thiazides may decrease serum PBI levels without signs of thyroid disturbance.

Calcium excretion is decreased by thiazides. Pathological changes in the parathyroid glands accompanied by hypercalcaemia and hypophosphataemia have been seen in a few patients receiving prolonged thiazide therapy. However, the common complications of hyperparathyroidism have not been observed. Therapy should be discontinued before carrying out tests for parathyroid function.

Hyperuricaemia may occur, or gout may be precipitated or aggravated, in certain patients receiving thiazides.

Drug interactions: Hydrochlorothiazide potentiates the action of other antihypertensive drugs. Therefore the dosage of these agents, especially the adrenergic blockers, may need to be reduced when Moduretic is added to the regimen. NSAIDs may attenuate the antihypertensive effect of thiazide diuretics.

Thiazide-containing drugs may increase the responsiveness to tubocurarine. The antihypertensive effect of thiazides may be enhanced in the post-sympathectomy patient.

Hydrochlorothiazide may decrease arterial responsiveness to noradrenaline, but not enough to prevent noradrenaline being effective in therapeutic dosage.

Orthostatic hypotension may occur, and may be potentiated by alcohol, barbiturates, and narcotics.

Sensitivity reactions: Sensitivity reactions to thiazides may occur in patients with or without a history of allergy or bronchial asthma. The possibility that thiazides may activate or exacerbate systemic lupus erythematosus has been reported.

Use in pregnancy: As clinical experience is limited, Moduretic is not recommended for use during pregnancy. Since thiazides cross the placental barrier and appear in cord blood, use where pregnancy is present or suspected requires that the benefits of the drug be weighed against possible hazards to the fetus. These hazards include fetal or neonatal jaundice, thrombocytopenia, bone marrow depression, and possibly other side-effects that have occurred in the adult. The routine use of diuretics in otherwise healthy pregnant women with or without mild oedema is not indicated because they may be associated with hypovolaemia, increased blood viscosity and decreased placental perfusion.

Use in nursing mothers: Although it is not known whether amiloride hydrochloride is excreted in human milk, it is known that thiazides do appear in breast milk. If the drug is deemed essential, the patient should stop nursing.

Side-effects: The combination of amiloride and hydrochlorothiazide is usually well tolerated and significant side-effects are infrequent. No increase in the risk of adverse reactions has been seen over those of the individual components. The reported adverse reactions of the combination:

Body as a whole: Headache, weakness, fatigue, malaise, chest pain, and back pain.

Cardiovascular: Arrhythmias, tachycardia, digitalis toxicity, orthostatic hypotension, and angina pectoris.

Digestive: Anorexia, nausea, vomiting, diarrhoea, constipation, abdominal pain, GI bleeding, appetite changes, abdominal fullness, flatulence, thirst, and hiccups.

Metabolic: Elevated serum potassium levels (above 5.5 mmol/l), gout, and dehydration.

Integumentary: Rash, pruritus, and flushing.

Musculoskeletal: Leg ache, muscle cramps, and joint pain.

Nervous: Dizziness, vertigo, paraesthesiae, and stupor.

Psychiatric: Insomnia, nervousness, mental confusion, depression, and sleepiness.

Respiratory: Dyspnoea.

Special senses: Bad taste, visual disturbance, and nasal congestion.

Urogenital: Impotence, dysuria, nocturia, and incontinence.

The reported side-effects of amiloride:

Digestive: Abnormal liver function. Activation of probable pre-existing peptic ulcer.

Integumentary: Dry mouth.

Haematological: Aplastic anaemia, neutropenia.

Cardiovascular: One patient with partial heart block developed complete heart block.

The reported side-effects of hydrochlorothiazide:

Body as a whole: Anaphylactic reaction, fever.

Cardiovascular: Necrotising angiitis (vasculitis, cutaneous vasculitis).

Digestive: Jaundice (intrahepatic cholestatic jaundice), pancreatitis.

Endocrine/Metabolic: Glycosuria, hyperglycaemia, hyperuricaemia.

Integumentary: Photosensitivity, sialadenitis, urticaria.

Psychiatric: Restlessness.

Respiratory: Respiratory distress including pneumonitis.

Special senses: Transient blurred vision, xanthopsia.

Haematological: Agranulocytosis, aplastic anaemia, haemolytic anaemia, leucopenia, purpura, thrombocytopenia.

Overdosage: No specific data are available on overdosage with Moduretic. No specific antidote is available, and it is not known whether the drug is dialysable.

Treatment is symptomatic and supportive. Therapy should be discontinued and the patient watched closely. Emesis should be induced and/or gastric lavage performed. The most common signs and symptoms of overdosage with amiloride hydrochloride are dehydration and electrolyte imbalance. If hyperkalaemia occurs, active measures should be taken to reduce the plasma potassium levels.

Electrolyte depletion (hypokalaemia, hypochloraemia, hyponatraemia) and dehydration are the most common signs and symptoms of hydrochlorothiazide overdosage. Blood pressure should be monitored and corrected where necessary. If digitalis has been administered, hypokalaemia may accentuate cardiac arrhythmias.

Pharmaceutical precautions Keep container tightly closed; store in a cool place, protected from light.

Moduretic Solution should not be diluted.

Legal category POM.

Package quantities
Moduretic Tablets: Bottles of 100 and 500 tablets.
Moduretic Solution: Bottles of 200 ml solution.

Further information The combination of amiloride with hydrochlorothiazide causes less magnesium excretion than either the thiazides or the loop diuretics when used alone.

Onset of diuretic action begins within 2 to 4 hours after administration, and reaches a peak at about the fourth hour; there is detectable activity for about 24 hours.

Product licence numbers
Moduretic Tablets 0025/5016.
Moduretic Solution 0025/0165.

PERIACTIN*

Presentation White, half-scored tablets, marked 'MSD 62', containing Cyproheptadine Hydrochloride BP equivalent to 4 mg anhydrous cyproheptadine hydrochloride.

A yellow syrup containing, in each 5 ml, cyproheptadine hydrochloride equivalent to 2 mg anhydrous cyproheptadine hydrochloride.

Uses Periactin is a serotonin and histamine antagonist with anticholinergic and sedative properties.

In allergy and pruritus: Periactin has a wide range of anti-allergic and antipruritic activity, and can be used successfully in treatment of acute and chronic allergic and pruritic conditions, such as: dermatitis, including neurodermatitis and neurodermatitis circumscripta; eczema; eczematoid dermatitis; dermatographism; mild, local allergic reactions to insect bites; hay fever and other seasonal rhinitis; perennial allergic and vasomotor rhinitis; allergic conjunctivitis due to inhalant allergies and foods; urticaria; angioneurotic oedema; drug and serum reactions; anogenital pruritus; pruritus of chicken-pox.

Periactin is indicated as adjunctive therapy to adrenaline and other standard measures for the relief of anaphylactic reactions after the acute manifestations have been controlled.

In migraine headache: Periactin has been reported to have beneficial effects in a significant number of patients having vascular types of headache. Many patients who have responded inadequately to all other agents have reported amelioration of symptoms with Periactin. The characteristic headache and feeling of malaise may disappear within an hour or two of the first dose.

As an appetite stimulant: Periactin is recommended for those patients with decreased appetite where, in the opinion of the physician, stimulation of the appetite and consequent weight gain is desirable. Periactin is not a substitute for food: an adequate diet is essential for successful therapy. The physician should treat any underlying disease or condition which may be responsible for the weight loss.

Dosage and administration There is no recommended dosage for children under 2 years old. Periactin is not recommended for elderly debilitated patients.

In allergy and pruritus: Dosage must be determined on an individual basis. The effect of a single dose usually lasts for four to six hours. For continuous effective relief, the daily requirement should be given in divided doses, three or four times a day, or as often as necessary.

Adults: 4–20 mg a day, most patients requiring 12–16 mg a day.

Maximum: 32 mg a day.

Children aged 7–14 years: Usually 4 mg two or three times a day, according to the patient's weight and response. Any additional dosage should be given at bedtime. Maximum 16 mg a day.

Children aged 2–6 years: Initially 2 mg two or three times a day, adjusted according to the patient's weight and response. Any additional dosage should be given at bedtime. Maximum 12 mg a day.

In vascular headache and migraine: For both prophylactic and therapeutic use at an initial dose of 4 mg repeated if necessary after half an hour. Patients who respond usually obtain relief with 8 mg, and this dose should not be exceeded within a 4- to 6-hour period.

Maintenance: 4 mg every four to six hours.

As an appetite stimulant: Daily dosage may be given as a single dose once a day in the evening or alternatively in divided doses. Dosage should be individualised according to the needs and response of the patient.

Adults and adolescents: The usual dosage is 4 mg (1 tablet or two 5 ml spoonfuls) three times a day. Larger doses are neither required nor recommended for appetite stimulation.

Children aged 7–14 years: The dosage should not exceed 12 mg (3 tablets or six 5 ml spoonfuls) a day.

Children aged 2–6 years: The dosage should not exceed 8 mg (2 tablets or four 5 ml spoonfuls) a day.

The effect of Periactin on appetite and weight gain only occurs during the period of its administration. After therapy is stopped, there may be some weight loss, but usually not to pre-treatment levels.

Use in the elderly: Periactin should not be used in elderly, debilitated patients. Elderly patients are more likely to experience dizziness, sedation, and hypotension.

Contra-indications, warnings, etc
Contra-indications: Therapy of an acute asthmatic attack; newborn or premature infants; nursing mothers; known sensitivity to cyproheptadine hydrochloride or drugs with similar chemical structure; concurrent use with monoamine oxidase inhibitors; glaucoma; stenosing peptic ulcer; symptomatic prostatic hypertrophy; bladder neck obstruction; pyloroduodenal obstruction; elderly, debilitated patients; predisposition to urinary retention.

Precautions: Antihistamines should not be used to treat lower respiratory tract symptoms including those of acute asthma.

The safety and efficacy of Periactin is not established in children under 2 years old.

Antihistamines may diminish mental alertness; conversely, particularly in the young child, they may occasionally produce excitation.

Patients should be warned against engaging in activities requiring motor co-ordination and mental alertness such as driving a car or operating machinery.

Patients with severe appetite loss should be carefully assessed to exclude serious underlying pathology.

Rarely, prolonged therapy with antihistamines may cause blood dyscrasias.

Because Periactin has an atropine-like action, it should be used cautiously in patients with a history of bronchial asthma, increased intra-ocular pressure, hyperthyroidism, cardiovascular disease, or hypertension.

Drug interactions: MAO inhibitors prolong and intensify the anticholinergic effects of antihistamines.

Antihistamines may have additive effects with alcohol and other CNS depressants, e.g. hypnotics, sedatives, tranquillisers and anti-anxiety agents.

Pregnancy and nursing mothers: The use of any drug in pregnancy or in women of child-bearing age requires that the potential benefit of the drug should be weighed against possible hazards to the embryo or fetus. It is not known whether Periactin is excreted in human milk. Because many drugs are excreted in human milk, and because of the potential for serious adverse reactions in nursing infants from Periactin, a decision should be made whether to discontinue nursing or to discontinue the drug, taking into account the importance of the drug to the mother (see 'Contra-indications').

Side-effects: Side-effects reported with antihistamines are:

Central nervous system: Sedation, sleepiness (often transient), dizziness, disturbed co-ordination, confusion, restlessness, excitation, nervousness, tremor, irritability, insomnia, parasthesiae, neuritis, convulsions, euphoria, hallucinations, hysteria, faintness.

Integumentary: Allergic manifestations of rash and oedema, excessive perspiration, urticaria, photosensitivity.

Special senses: Acute labyrinthitis, blurred vision, diplopia, vertigo, tinnitus.

Cardiovascular: Hypotension, palpitation, tachycardia, extrasystoles, anaphylactic shock.

Haematological: Haemolytic anaemia, leucopenia, agranulocytosis, thrombocytopenia.

Digestive system: Dryness of mouth, epigastric distress, anorexia, nausea, vomiting, diarrhoea, constipation, jaundice.

Genito-urinary: Frequency and difficulty of micturition, urinary retention, early menses.

Respiratory: Dryness of the nose and throat, thickening of bronchial secretions, tightness of chest and wheezing, nasal stuffiness.

Miscellaneous: Fatigue, rigors, headache.

Overdosage: Antihistamine overdosage may vary from CNS depression or stimulation to convulsions and death, especially in infants and children. Atropine-like and GI symptoms may occur.

If vomiting has not occurred spontaneously, it should be induced in the conscious patient with syrup of ipecac. If the patient cannot vomit, gastric lavage with isotonic or half isotonic saline is indicated followed by activated charcoal.

Precautions against aspiration must be taken, especially in infants and children.

Life-threatening CNS signs and symptoms should be treated appropriately.

Saline cathartics usefully draw water into the bowel by osmosis to dilute bowel content rapidly.

Central stimulants must not be used, but vasopressors may be used to counteract hypotension.

Pharmaceutical precautions Periactin should be stored in a dry place below 25°C; the syrup should also be protected from freezing. Periactin Syrup may be diluted with Syrup BP; the mixture should be used within 14 days.

Legal category P.

Package quantities *Tablets:* Bottles of 100. *Syrup:* Bottles of 200 ml.

Further information Nil.

Product licence numbers
Tablets   0025/5017
Syrup   0025/5018

SALURIC*

Presentation White, half-scored tablets, marked 'MSD 432', containing 500 mg Chlorothiazide BP.

Uses Thiazide diuretic and antihypertensive.

Oedema associated with congestive heart failure, hepatic cirrhosis, premenstrual tension, and in oedema due to various forms of renal dysfunction (i.e. nephrotic syndrome, acute glomerulonephritis and chronic renal failure). Hypertension, either alone or as an adjunct to other antihypertensive drugs.

Dosage and administration *Adults – for oedema:* Usually 1 or 2 tablets (0.5–1.0 g) once or twice a day. Many patients respond to intermittent therapy: every other day, or three to five consecutive days a week. Intermittent therapy is less likely to produce excessive diuretic response with resulting electrolyte imbalance.

In oedema accompanying premenstrual tension: $\frac{1}{2}$–1 tablet once or twice a day, from the first morning of symptoms until the onset of the menses.

Adults – for control of hypertension: Initially, usually 0.5 g or 1.0 g a day as a single or divided dose, increased or decreased according to response. Some patients may need 4 tablets (2.0 g) a day (in divided doses).

Thiazides may add to or potentiate the action of other antihypertensives. If Saluric is added to therapy with other antihypertensive agents, dosage reduction of such agents may be necessary to prevent an excessive drop in blood pressure.

Infants and children: Usually 25 mg per kg body weight a day, given in 2 doses. Infants under 6 months may need up to 35 mg per kg a day, in 2 doses.

On this basis, infants up to 2 years of age may be given 125–375 mg of Saluric daily in 2 doses. Children from 2 to 12 years of age may be given 375 mg to 1.0 g daily in 2 doses. Dosage in both age groups should be based on body weight.

Use in the elderly: Particular caution is needed in the elderly because of their susceptibility to electrolyte imbalance; the dosage should be carefully adjusted according to renal function and clinical response.

Contra-indications, warnings, etc
Contra-indications: Anuria, known hypersensitivity to chlorothiazide or to other sulphonamide-derived drugs, severe renal or hepatic failure, Addison's disease, hypercalcaemia, concurrent lithium therapy. See 'Use in pregnancy' and 'Use in nursing mothers', under 'Precautions'.

Warnings: Azotaemia may be precipitated or increased by Saluric. Cumulative effects of chlorothiazide may develop in patients with impaired renal function. If increasing azotaemia and oliguria occur during treatment of severe progressive renal disease, Saluric should be discontinued.

Sensitivity reactions may occur in patients with or without a history of allergy or bronchial asthma.

Saluric may add to or potentiate the action of other antihypertensive agents. Potentiation occurs with ganglion- or adrenergic-blocking drugs.

The possibility of exacerbation or activation of systemic lupus erythematosus has been reported.

Hypokalaemia may develop, especially with brisk diuresis, when severe cirrhosis is present, during concurrent steroid or ACTH administration, or after prolonged therapy. Interference with adequate electrolyte intake will contribute to hypokalaemia. Hypokalaemia can sensitise or exaggerate the response of the heart to the toxic effects of digitalis (e.g. increased ventricular irritability).

Hypokalaemia may be avoided or treated in the adult by concurrent use of amiloride hydrochloride (Midamor*), a potassium-conserving agent. It may also be avoided by giving potassium chloride or foods with a high potassium content. (Note that symptoms and signs which might indicate ulceration or obstruction of the small bowel in patients taking tablets or capsules containing potassium salts are indications for stopping treatment with such preparations immediately.)

Any chloride deficit is generally mild and does not usually require specific treatment except under unusual circumstances (as in liver or renal disease) when chloride replacement may be required in the treatment of metabolic alkalosis. Dilutional hyponatraemia may occur in oedematous patients in hot weather; except in rare instances when hyponatraemia is life-threatening, appropriate therapy is water restriction rather than administration of salt. In actual salt depletion, appropriate replacement is the therapy of choice.

Thiazides may decrease serum protein-bound iodine levels without signs of thyroid disturbances.

Thiazides may decrease urinary calcium excretion, and may also cause intermittent and slight elevation of serum calcium in the absence of known disorders of calcium metabolism. Marked hypercalcaemia may be evidence of hidden hyperparathyroidism. Thiazides should be discontinued before carrying out tests for parathyroid function.

Hyperuricaemia may occur, or gout may be precipitated, in certain patients receiving thiazide therapy.

Drug interactions: Thiazides may increase responsiveness to tubocurarine. The antihypertensive effect of the thiazide may be enhanced in the post-sympathectomy patient.

Chlorothiazide may decrease arterial responsiveness to noradrenaline, but not enough to prevent noradrenaline being therapeutically useful. Orthostatic hypotension may occur, and may be potentiated by alcohol, barbiturates or narcotics.

Insulin requirements in diabetic patients may be increased, decreased or unchanged. Latent diabetes mellitus may become manifest during thiazide administration.

Precautions: Thiazides should be used with caution in patients with impaired hepatic function or progressive liver disease, since minor alterations of fluid and electrolyte balance may precipitate hepatic coma.

Patients should be carefully monitored for signs of fluid and electrolyte imbalance (hyponatraemia, hypomagnesaemia, hypochloraemic alkalosis and hypokalaemia). It is particularly important to make serum and urine electrolyte determinations when the patient is vomiting excessively or receiving parenteral fluids. Warning signs, irrespective of cause, are: dryness of mouth, thirst, weakness, lethargy, drowsiness, restlessness, muscle pains or cramps, muscular fatigue, hypotension, oliguria, tachycardia and gastro-intestinal disturbances.

Use in pregnancy: Thiazides appear in breast milk. If use of the drug is deemed essential the patient should stop nursing. Thiazides cross the placental barrier and appear in the cord blood. The use of Saluric when pregnancy is present or suspected, requires that the benefits of the drug be weighed against the possible hazards to the fetus. These hazards include fetal or neonatal jaundice, thrombocytopenia, and possibly other adverse reactions which have occurred in the adult. The routine use of diuretics in otherwise healthy, pregnant women with or without mild oedema is not indicated because their use may be associated with hypovolaemia, increased blood viscosity and decreased placental perfusion.

Use in nursing mothers: Thiazides appear in breast milk. If use of the drug is deemed essential, the patient should stop nursing.

Side-effects: Gastro-intestinal system: Anorexia, gastric irritation, nausea, vomiting, cramps, diarrhoea, constipation, jaundice (intrahepatic cholestatic jaundice), pancreatitis, salivary gland inflammation.

Central nervous system: Dizziness, vertigo, paraesthesiae, headache, yellow vision.

Haematological: Leucopenia, agranulocytosis, thrombocytopenia, aplastic anaemia, haemolytic anaemia.

Cardiovascular: Orthostatic hypotension (may be aggravated by alcohol, barbiturates, narcotics).

Hypersensitivity: Purpura, photosensitivity, rash, urticaria, necrotising angiitis (vasculitis, cutaneous vasculitis), fever, respiratory distress including pneumonitis, anaphylactic reactions.

Other: Hyperglycaemia, glycosuria, hyperuricaemia, muscle spasm, weakness, restlessness, transient blurred vision, impotence.

Whenever side-effects are moderate or severe, thiazide dosage should be reduced or therapy withdrawn.

Treatment of overdosage: Symptomatic and supportive; no specific antidote. If ingestion is recent the stomach should be emptied by emesis or gastric lavage. Dehydration, electrolyte imbalance, hepatic coma, and hypotension should be corrected by standard methods. For impaired respiration, oxygen or artificial respiration should be given.

Pharmaceutical precautions Keep container tightly closed; store in a cool place, protected from light.

Legal category POM.

Package quantities Bottles of 100.

Further information Diuresis usually begins within two hours, is at a peak after four hours and persists for six to twelve hours. No rigid dietary salt restriction required.

Product licence number 0025/5019.

SINEMET*

Presentation The standard strength is known as Sinemet-275 and is supplied as dapple-blue, half-scored, oval tablets, marked 'MSD 654', containing 25 mg Carbidopa BP (as carbidopa monohydrate) and 250 mg Levodopa BP.

Sinemet-Plus is available as yellow, half-scored, oval tablets, marked 'SINEMET PLUS', containing 25 mg carbidopa (as carbidopa monohydrate) and 100 mg levodopa.

Sinemet-110 is available as dapple-blue, half-scored, oval tablets, marked 'MSD 647', containing 10 mg Carbidopa BP (as carbidopa monohydrate) and 100 mg Levodopa BP.

Uses Antiparkinsonian agent.

For treatment of Parkinson's disease and syndrome. Sinemet is useful in relieving many of the symptoms of parkinsonism, particularly rigidity and bradykinesia. It is frequently helpful in the management of tremor, dysphagia, sialorrhoea, and postural instability associated with Parkinson's disease and syndrome.

When response to levodopa alone is irregular, and signs and symptoms of Parkinson's disease are not controlled evenly through the day, substitution of Sinemet usually reduces fluctuations in response. By reducing certain adverse reactions produced by levodopa alone, Sinemet permits more patients to obtain adequate relief of the symptoms of Parkinson's disease.

Sinemet may be given to patients with Parkinson's disease and syndrome who are taking vitamin preparations that contain pyridoxine.

Dosage and administration The optimum daily dosage of Sinemet must be determined by careful titration for each patient.

Sinemet Tablets are available as:

Sinemet-110 containing 10 mg carbidopa and 100 mg levodopa.

Sinemet-Plus containing 25 mg carbidopa and 100 mg levodopa.

Sinemet-275 containing 25 mg carbidopa and 250 mg levodopa.

General considerations: Studies show that the peripheral enzyme dopa decarboxylase is fully inhibited (saturated) by carbidopa at doses between 70 and 100 mg a day. The formulations of Sinemet are designed to provide a range of doses with sufficient carbidopa to inhibit peripheral dopa-decarboxylase and thus exert optimal therapy.

Patients who require less than 700 mg levodopa given as Sinemet-110 or Sinemet-275 will theoretically not receive sufficient carbidopa to saturate peripheral dopa decarboxylase. Sinemet-Plus may be helpful, especially for patients with nausea and vomiting.

Most patients can be maintained on divided doses of three to six tablets of Sinemet-275 a day. Tablets are scored for easy division should the frequency of daily dosage need to be increased. During the titration period, Sinemet-Plus may be more convenient.

Patients on Sinemet-Plus who need a higher dosage should be switched to Sinemet-275. Dosage with either form should not exceed eight tablets a day. If patients do show a need for higher doses, levodopa should be added.

Because both beneficial and adverse effects are seen more rapidly with Sinemet than with levodopa, patients should be carefully monitored during the dosage adjustment period. Involuntary movements, particularly blepharospasm, is a useful early sign of excess dosage in some patients.

Sinemet-110 can be used as an alternative to Sinemet-Plus.

Patients not receiving levodopa: Dosage may be initiated with one tablet of Sinemet-Plus three times a day, and adjusted as necessary by small increments to a maximum daily dosage of eight tablets. If patients need more levodopa, one tablet of Sinemet-275 should be substituted three or four times a day. If further titration is necessary, the dosage of Sinemet-275 may be increased gradually to a maximum of eight tablets a day.

Patients receiving levodopa: Discontinue levodopa at least twelve hours (24 hours for slow-release preparations) before starting therapy with Sinemet. The easiest way to do this is to give Sinemet as the first morning dose after a night without any levodopa. The dose of Sinemet should be approximately 20% of the previous daily dosage of levodopa.

The suggested starting dose for most patients is one tablet of Sinemet-275 three or four times a day.

Patients requiring less than 1,500 mg levodopa a day should be started on one tablet of Sinemet-Plus three or four times a day.

The dosage may then be adjusted gradually, but this should not exceed eight tablets a day.

Patients receiving levodopa with another decarboxylase inhibitor: When transferring a patient to Sinemet from levodopa combined with another decarboxylase inhibitor, its dosage should be discontinued at least twelve hours before Sinemet is started. Begin with a dosage of Sinemet that will provide the same amount of levodopa as contained in the other levodopa/decarboxylase inhibitor combination.

Patients receiving other antiparkinsonian agents: Current evidence indicates that other standard antiparkinsonian agents may be continued when Sinemet is introduced (as indicated above), though dosage may have to be adjusted.

Use in the elderly: There is wide experience in the use of this product in elderly patients. The recommendations set out above reflect the clinical data derived from this experience.

Contra-indications, warnings, etc

Contra-indications: Concurrent use with monoamine oxidase inhibitors (these must be discontinued at least two weeks before starting Sinemet), narrow-angle glaucoma; known hypersensitivity to this medication.

Because levodopa may activate a malignant melanoma, it should not be used in patients with suspicious undiagnosed skin lesions or a history of melanoma.

See also 'Pregnancy and lactation' under 'Precautions'.

Precautions: Sinemet may be given to patients already receiving levodopa alone; however, the levodopa must be discontinued at least 12 hours before Sinemet is started. Sinemet should be substituted at a dosage that will provide approximately 20% of the previous levodopa dosage (see 'Dosage and administration').

Sinemet is not recommended for the treatment of drug-induced extrapyramidal reactions. Sinemet should be administered cautiously to patients with severe cardiovascular or pulmonary disease, bronchial asthma, renal, hepatic or endocrine disease.

All patients should be monitored carefully for the development of mental changes, depression with suicidal tendencies, and other serious antisocial behaviour. Patients with current psychoses should be treated with caution. Patients with a history of severe involuntary movements or psychotic episodes when treated with levodopa alone should be observed carefully when Sinemet is substituted. These reactions are thought to be due to increased brain dopamine following administration of levodopa, and use of Sinemet may cause a recurrence. Concomitant administration of psychoactive drugs such as phenothiazines and butyrophenones should be carried out with caution, and the patient carefully observed for loss of antiparkinsonian effect. Patients with a history of convulsions should be treated with caution.

Phenytoin and papaverine have been reported to reverse the beneficial effects of levodopa.

Patients with chronic wide-angle glaucoma may be treated cautiously with Sinemet, provided the intra-ocular pressure is well controlled and the patient monitored carefully for changes in intra-ocular pressure during therapy.

Care should be exercised when Sinemet is administered to patients with a history of myocardial infarction who have atrial, nodal or ventricular arrhythmias. Cardiac function should be monitored with particular care in such patients during the period of initial dosage adjustment.

As symptoms of postural hypotension have occasionally been reported. Sinemet should be given with caution to patients receiving antihypertensive agents. Adjustment of the dosage of the antihypertensive agent may be required when Sinemet is started. (For patients on pargyline, see the contra-indication on monoamine oxidase inhibitors.)

As with levodopa, there is a possibility of upper gastrointestinal haemorrhage in patients with a history of peptic ulcer. If general anaesthesia is required, therapy with Sinemet may be continued as long as the patient is permitted to take fluids and medication by mouth. If therapy is interrupted temporarily, the usual daily dosage may be administered as soon as the patient is able to take oral medication.

Transient abnormalities in laboratory test results may occur, but have not been associated with clinical evidence of disease. These include elevated blood urea, AST (SGOT), ALT (SGPT), LDH, bilirubin, alkaline phosphatase, and protein-bound iodine levels.

Positive Coombs tests have been reported, both with Sinemet and levodopa alone, but haemolytic anaemia is extremely rare.

Usage in children: The safety of Sinemet in patients under 18 years of age has not been established.

Pregnancy and lactation: Although the effects of Sinemet on human pregnancy and lactation are unknown, both levodopa and combinations of carbidopa and levodopa have caused visceral and skeletal malformations in rabbits. Therefore, use of Sinemet in women of child-bearing potential requires that the anticipated benefits of the drug be weighed against possible hazards should pregnancy occur. Sinemet should not be given to nursing mothers.

Drug interactions: Clinical experience with concurrent administration of Sinemet and other standard antiparkinsonian drugs, e.g. benztropine mesylate, benzhexol hydrochloride, is limited. To date, however, there has been no indication of interactions that would preclude concurrent use. No adverse reactions have been reported that do not occur with the various agents alone.

Side-effects: Side-effects that occur frequently with Sinemet are those due to the central neuropharmacological activity of dopamine. These reactions can usually be diminished by dosage reduction. The most common are choreiform, dystonic and other involuntary movements. Muscle twitching and blepharospasm may be taken as early signs to consider dosage reduction.

Less common are mental changes, including paranoid ideation and psychotic episodes; depression, with or without development of suicidal tendencies; and dementia. Convulsions have occurred, but a causal relationship has not been established.

Less frequent side-effects are cardiac irregularities and/or palpitations, orthostatic hypotensive episodes, bradykinetic episodes (the 'on-off' phenomenon), anorexia, nausea, vomiting and dizziness.

Gastro-intestinal bleeding, development of duodenal ulcer, hypertension, phlebitis, leucopenia and agranulocytosis have occurred rarely.

Positive Coombs tests have been reported both with Sinemet and with levodopa alone, but haemolytic anaemia is extremely rare.

Other side-effects that have been reported include:

Psychiatric: Euphoria, lethargy, sedation, stimulation, fatigue and malaise, confusion, insomnia, nightmares, hallucinations and delusions, agitation and anxiety.

Neurological: Ataxia, faintness, headache, increased hand tremor, trismus, oculogyric crisis, weakness, numbness, bruxism.

Gastro-intestinal: Constipation, diarrhoea, epigastric and abdominal distress and pain, flatulence, hiccups, sialorrhoea, difficulty in swallowing, bitter taste, dry mouth, burning sensation of the tongue.

Dermatological: Sweating, oedema, hair loss, rash, unpleasant odour, dark sweat.

Respiratory: Hoarseness, bizarre breathing pattern.

Urogenital: Urinary retention, incontinence, haematuria, dark urine, priapism.

Special senses: Blurred vision, diplopia, dilated pupils, activation of latent Horner's syndrome.

Other: Hot flushes, weight gain or loss, flushing, abnormalities in laboratory tests (see 'Precautions').

Treatment of overdosage: General supportive measures should be employed, along with immediate gastric lavage. Intravenous fluids should be administered judiciously, and an adequate airway maintained. ECG monitoring should be instituted, and the patient carefully observed for the possible development of arrhythmias; if required, appropriate anti-arrhythmic therapy should be given.

The possibility that the patient may have taken other drugs as well as Sinemet should be taken into consideration. To date, no experience has been reported with dialysis, and hence its value in the treatment of overdosage is not known. Pyridoxine has no effect in reversing the effects of Sinemet.

Pharmaceutical precautions Keep container tightly closed; store in a cool place, protected from light.

Legal category POM.

Package quantities Bottles of 100.

Further information Levodopa relieves the symptoms of Parkinson's disease, presumably by being decarboxylated to dopamine in the brain. Carbidopa, which does not cross the blood-brain barrier, inhibits only the extracerebral decarboxylation of levodopa, making more levodopa available for transport to the brain and subsequent conversion to dopamine. This obviates the need for large doses of levodopa at frequent intervals. The lower dosage reduces or eliminates many adverse reactions, some of which are attributable to dopamine being formed in extracerebral tissues.

Product licence numbers

Sinemet-275	0025/0085
Sinemet-Plus	0025/0150
Sinemet-110	0025/0084

SODIUM PARA-AMINOHIPPURATE

Presentation A clear, colourless to slightly yellow solution for intravenous injection, containing in each 10 ml of sterile solution 2 g sodium para-aminohippurate. Inactive ingredient: Sodium Hydroxide BP.

Uses As a diagnostic agent for the estimation of effective renal plasma flow (RPF). In research procedures, for the measurement of the functional capacity of the renal tubular secretory mechanism (Tm_{PAH}).

Dosage and administration For intravenous use only.

For the measurement of RPF, the concentration of sodium para-aminohippurate in the plasma is maintained at 2 mg per 100 ml. As a research procedure for the measurement of Tm_{PAH}, the plasma level of sodium para-aminohippurate must be sufficient to saturate the capacity of the tubular secretory cells. Concentrations of from 40 to 60 mg per 100 ml are necessary.

Contra-indications, warnings, etc
Precautions: Intravenous solutions must be administered with caution in patients with low cardiac reserve, since a

rapid increase in plasma volume can precipitate congestive heart failure.

For measurement of RPF, small doses of sodium para-aminohippurate are used. However, in research procedures for Tm_{PAH} determinations high plasma levels are required to saturate the capacity of the tubular cells. During these procedures the intravenous administration of sodium para-aminohippurate solutions should be carried out slowly and with caution. The patient should be continuously observed for any adverse reactions.

Renal clearance measurement of sodium para-aminohippurate cannot be made with any significant accuracy in patients receiving sulphonamides, procaine or thiazolesulphone. These compounds interfere with chemical colour development essential to the analytical procedures.

Probenecid depresses tubular secretion of certain weak acids such as sodium para-aminohippurate. Therefore, patients receiving probenecid will have erroneously low RPF and Tm_{PAH} values. Clearance is also affected by penicillins and salicylates.

Side-effects: Vasomotor disturbances, flushing, tingling, nausea, vomiting, cramps. Patients may have a sensation of warmth or the desire to defaecate or urinate during or shortly after the administration of a primary dose.

Treatment of overdosage: Not applicable.

Pharmaceutical precautions No special requirements.

Legal category POM.

Package quantities Vials of 10 ml.

Further information Methods of calculating renal function are to be found in the package leaflet.

Product licence number 0025/5080.

TIMOPTOL* ▼

Presentation Clear, colourless to light yellow, sterile eye drops containing Timolol Maleate BP equivalent to 0.25% and 0.5% w/v solution of timolol. Each concentration is presented in:
Metered-dose Ocumeter* Dispensers containing 5 ml Ophthalmic Solution Timoptol with preservative.
Unit-dose dispensers containing 0.25 ml Ophthalmic Solution Timoptol without preservative.

Uses Timoptol Ophthalmic Solution is a beta-adrenergic receptor blocking agent used topically in the reduction of elevated intra-ocular pressure in various conditions including the following: patients with ocular hypertension; patients with chronic open-angle glaucoma including aphakic patients; some patients with secondary glaucoma.

Dosage and administration Recommended therapy is one drop 0.25% solution in the affected eye twice a day.

If clinical response is not adequate, dosage may be changed to one drop 0.5% solution in each affected eye twice a day. If needed, Timoptol may be used with miotics, adrenaline or systemically-administered carbonic anhydrase inhibitors.

Intra-ocular pressure should be reassessed approximately four weeks after starting treatment because response to Timoptol may take a few weeks to stabilise.

Provided that the intra-ocular pressure is maintained at satisfactory levels, many patients can then be placed on once-a-day therapy. Because of naturally occurring diurnal variations in intra-ocular pressure, satisfactory response is best determined by measuring the intra-ocular pressure at different times during the day.

Transfer from other agents: When only a single antiglaucoma agent is being used, continue the agent and add one drop of 0.25% Timoptol in each affected eye twice a day. On the following day, discontinue the previous agent completely, and continue with Timoptol. If a higher dosage of Timoptol is required, substitute one drop of 0.5% solution in each affected eye twice a day.

When several antiglaucoma agents are being used, the patient should be assessed individually. It may be possible to discontinue some or all the other agents; adjustments should be made to one agent at a time.

Clinical trials have shown the addition of Timoptol to be useful in patients who respond inadequately to maximum antiglaucoma drug therapy.

Timoptol Unit-dose: The Unit-dose Dispenser of Timoptol is free from preservative and should, therefore, be discarded after single use to one or both eyes. It may be used by patients who wear hydrophilic (soft) contact lenses, or who are sensitive to benzalkonium chloride.

Use in the elderly: There is wide experience with the usage of this product in elderly patients. The dosage recommendations above reflect the clinical data derived from this experience.

Contra-indications, warnings, etc
Contra-indications: Bronchial asthma, history of bronchial asthma, or severe chronic obstructive pulmonary disease; sinus bradycardia, second and third degree AV block, overt cardiac failure, cardiogenic shock; and hypersensitivity.

Precautions: Like other topically applied ophthalmic drugs, Timoptol may be absorbed systemically and adverse reactions seen with oral beta-blockers may occur.

Cardiac failure should be adequately controlled before beginning therapy with Timoptol. Patients with a history of severe cardiac disease should be watched for signs of cardiac failure and have their pulse rates checked.

Respiratory and cardiac reactions, including death due to bronchospasm in patients with asthma and, rarely, death associated with cardiac failure have been reported.

The effect on intra-ocular pressure or the known effects of systemic beta-blockade may be exaggerated when Timoptol is given to patients already receiving an oral beta-blocking agent. The response of these patients should be closely observed.

There have been reports of skin rashes and/or dry eyes associated with the use of beta-adrenergic receptor blocking drugs. The reported incidence is small and in most cases the symptoms have cleared when treatment was withdrawn. Discontinuation of the drug should be considered if any such reaction is not otherwise explicable. Cessation of therapy involving beta-blockade should be gradual.

The Ocumeter Dispenser of Timoptol contains benzalkonium chloride as a preservative and, therefore, should not be used in patients who continue to wear hydrophilic (soft) contact lenses.

The Unit-dose Dispenser of Timoptol is free from preservative and should, therefore, be discarded after single use to one or both eyes. It may be used in patients who wear hydrophilic (soft) contact lenses, or who are sensitive to benzalkonium chloride.

Drug interactions: Although Timoptol alone has little or

no effect on pupil size, mydriasis has occasionally been reported when Timoptol is given with adrenaline.

Timoptol may potentially add to the effects or oral calcium antagonists, rauwolfia alkaloids or beta-blockers to induce hypotension and/or marked bradycardia.

Nursing mothers: A decision for nursing mothers either to stop taking Timoptol or stop nursing should be based on the importance of the drug to the mother.

Use in pregnancy: Timoptol has not been studied in human pregnancy. The use of Timoptol requires that the anticipated benefit be weighed against possible hazards.

Use in children: Timoptol is not currently recommended for use in children.

Side-effects: Timoptol is usually well tolerated.

Special senses: Signs and symptoms of ocular irritation, including conjunctivitis, blepharitis, keratitis, and decreased corneal sensitivity. Visual disturbances, including refractive changes (due to withdrawal of miotic therapy in some cases), diplopia, and ptosis.

Cardiovascular: Bradycardia, arrhythmia, hypotension, syncope, heart block, cerebrovascular accident, cerebral ischaemia, congestive heart failure, palpitation, cardiac arrest.

Respiratory: Bronchospasm (predominantly in patients with pre-existing bronchospastic disease), respiratory failure, dyspnoea.

Body as a whole: Headache, asthenia, nausea, dizziness, depression.

Integumentary: Hypersensitivity reactions including localised and generalised rash and urticaria.

The adverse reactions seen with oral timolol maleate may occur with Timoptol.

Overdosage: No specific data are available.

The most common signs and symptoms to be expected following overdosage with a beta-blocker are symptomatic bradycardia, hypotension, bronchospasm, and acute cardiac failure. If overdosage occurs, the following measures are suggested.

1. Gastric lavage, if ingested.

2. Symptomatic bradycardia: Atropine sulphate, 0.25 to 2 mg intravenously, should be used to induce vagal blockade. If bradycardia persists, intravenous isoprenaline hydrochloride should be administered cautiously. In refractory cases, the use of a cardiac pacemaker may be considered.

3. Hypotension: A sympathomimetic pressor agent such as dopamine, dobutamine or noradrenaline should be used. In refractory cases, the use of glucagon has been reported to be useful.

4. Bronchospasm: Isoprenaline hydrochloride should be used. Additional therapy with aminophylline may be considered.

5. Acute cardiac failure: Conventional therapy with digitalis, diuretics, and oxygen should be instituted immediately. In refractory cases, the use of intravenous aminophylline is suggested. This may be followed, if necessary, by glucagon which has been reported useful.

6. Heart block (second or third degree): Isoprenaline hydrochloride or a pacemaker should be used.

Pharmaceutical precautions Timoptol is stable at room temperature. Protect from light.

Legal category POM.

Package quantities Both the 0.25% and 0.5% w/v solution are presented in:

Special metered-dose Ocumeter* Dispensers, each containing 5 ml.

Unit-dose Dispensers, available in cartons of 30 Unit doses.

Further information Unlike miotics, Timoptol reduces IOP with little or no effect on accommodation or pupil size. In patients with cataracts, the inability to see around lenticular opacities when the pupil is constricted is avoided. When changing patients from miotics to Timoptol a refraction might be necessary when these effects of the miotic have passed.

Diminished response after prolonged therapy with Timoptol has been reported in some patients.

Timoptol has been generally well tolerated in glaucoma patients wearing conventional hard contact lenses. Timoptol has not been studied in patients wearing lenses made with material other than polymethylmethacrylate (PMMA).

Product licence numbers

0.25%	Ophthalmic Solution	
	5 ml Ocumeter	0025/0134
	0.25 ml Unit-dose	0025/0210
0.5%	Ophthalmic Solution	
	5 ml Ocumeter	0025/0135
	0.25 ml Unit-dose	0025/0211

TYROZETS*

Presentation Pink, aniseed-flavoured lozenges, marked 'MSD' one side and Tyrozets the other, containing 1 mg tyrothricin and 5 mg Benzocaine BP.

Uses Antibiotic and local analgesic-anaesthetic.

For minor mouth and throat irritations; secondary irritation following tonsillectomy and other mouth and throat surgery.

Dosage and administration *Usual dosage:* 1 lozenge every three hours; maximum, 8 lozenges in 24 hours. If an adequate response is not evident within two days consider stopping Tyrozets.

To allow maximum contact with inflamed tissues, Tyrozets should not be chewed or swallowed whole, but allowed to dissolve slowly in the mouth.

Contra-indications, warnings, etc

Contra-indications: Hypersensitivity to tyrothricin or to benzocaine. If evidence of sensitivity occurs during therapy. Tyrozets should be discontinued.

Precautions: The use of antibiotics may cause overgrowth of non-susceptible organisms. If new infections due to bacteria or fungi appear during therapy, Tyrozets should be stopped and appropriate measures taken.

Topical use of Tyrozets as an aid to prevention of local infection in no way alters the need for adequate systemic therapy if an infection should develop.

Side-effects: Blackness or soreness of the tongue may occur, but usually disappears when therapy is stopped.

Treatment of overdosage: Symptomatic and supportive; emesis should be induced or gastric lavage performed.

Pharmaceutical precautions Store in a cool, dry place.

Legal category P.

Package quantities Twin vials of 12 lozenges.

Further information Since tyrothricin is used only locally and has a low index of sensitisation and toxicity, cross-sensitisation with antibiotics used systemically in more serious infections is unlikely.

Product licence number 0025/5072.

ZINAMIDE*

Presentation White, half-scored tablets, marked 'MSD 504', containing 500 mg Pyrazinamide BP.

Uses Antituberculous agent.

Zinamide is indicated in patients with active tuberculosis caused by *Mycobacterium tuberculosis*. Zinamide is not active against the atypical mycobacteria. Zinamide should only be given in combination with other antituberculous agents.

Dosage and administration *Usual adult dosage:* 20–35 mg/kg a day divided into three or four doses; the maximum daily dosage is 3 g regardless of body weight. Zinamide should be administered with at least one other effective antituberculous drug. The use of Zinamide in combination therapy does not modify the accepted dosages of other antituberculous agents.

Use in the elderly: The general considerations outlined above should also apply to elderly patients.

Contra-indications, warnings, etc
Contra-indications: Zinamide is contra-indicated in patients hypersensitive to it; in patients with hepatic disease; and in those with hyperuricaemia and/or gouty arthritis.

Safety for use in children has not been established (see also 'Precautions').

Zinamide is contra-indicated in nursing mothers. If its use is deemed essential, the patient should stop nursing.

Precautions: Zinamide should only be used when close daily observation of the patient is possible, and when laboratory facilities are available for performing frequent liver function tests and blood uric acid determinations. Pre-treatment examinations should include *in vitro* sensitivity tests of recent cultures of *M. tuberculosis* from the patient as measured against the usual antituberculous drugs.

Liver function tests, especially aspartate transferase (AST) and alanine transferase (ALT) determinations, should be carried out prior to therapy, and then every two to four weeks during therapy. Therapy with Zinamide should be withdrawn and not reinstated if signs of hepatocellular damage occur.

If hyperuricaemia accompanied by an acute gouty arthritis occurs, therapy should be discontinued and not reinstated. Close monitoring is advised to detect any increasing difficulty in the management of patients with a history of gout or diabetes mellitus.

Reduction in the size and/or frequency of dose is recommended for patients with renal insufficiency.

Children: The safety of Zinamide for use in children has not been established. Because of its potential toxicity, the use of Zinamide in children should be avoided unless it is considered crucial.

Pregnancy: There have been no adequate and well-controlled studies in pregnant women. Zinamide should only be used if the potential benefit justifies the risk to the foetus.

Side-effects: A hepatic reaction is the most common side-effect of Zinamide. This varies from a symptomless abnormality of hepatic cell function, detectable only by laboratory tests, through a mild syndrome of fever, anorexia, malaise, liver tenderness, hepatomegaly and splenomegaly, to more serious reactions such as clinical jaundice, and rare cases of progressive fulminating acute yellow atrophy and death.

Other side-effects – active gout, sideroblastic anaemia, arthralgias, anorexia, nausea and vomiting, dysuria, malaise, fever, urticaria, aggravation of peptic ulcer.

Overdosage: There has been no experience reported with pyrazinamide poisoning. Liver toxicity and hyperuricaemia may occur with overdosage.

The stomach should be emptied by gastric lavage if necessary.

There is no specific antidote. General supportive measures should be employed. Liver function should be monitored closely, and a high-carbohydrate, low-fat diet employed. Care should be taken to avoid exposure of the patient to other potential hepatotoxic agents, including alcohol. Benzodiazepines may be given if there is evidence of central nervous system stimulation. Probenecid may be given for hyperuricaemia.

Pharmaceutical precautions Keep container tightly closed; store in a cool place, protected from light.

Legal category POM.

Package quantities Bottles of 100. Pure pyrazinamide powder, for sensitivity tests, is available on request.

Further information Zinamide has been used with other agents, notably rifampicin, isoniazid or streptomycin. The use of such combinations has produced sputum conversion in a high proportion of patients able to continue therapy for at least six months.

Product licence number 0025/5038.

*Trade Mark

Merieux UK Ltd
Fulmer Hall
Hay Lane
Fulmer
Slough
Berkshire SL3 6HH

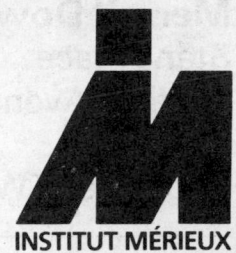

INSTITUT MÉRIEUX

MERIEUX TETAVAX* ▼
Adsorbed Tetanus Vaccine BP (Tet/Vac/Ads)

Presentation Merieux Tetavax is a sterile aqueous suspension of purified tetanus toxoid prepared by treating the toxin of *Clostridium tetani* with formaldehyde. The toxoid is adsorbed onto aluminium hydroxide and thiomersal is added as preservative.

Each 0.5 ml dose contains not less than 40 International Units (IU) of tetanus toxoid.

Uses Active immunisation against tetanus. Reinforcement of immunity to tetanus.

Dosage and administration By deep subcutaneous or intramuscular injection.

Primary immunisation: 3 injections each of 0.5 ml with an interval of 6–8 weeks between the first and second dose and 4–6 months between the second and third dose. Generally, the adsorbed combined vaccine (Diphtheria/Tetanus/Pertussis vaccine) is used for the primary immunisation of infants.

Reinforcing doses: In the United Kingdom, a reinforcing dose of 0.5 ml is recommended 5 years after the primary immunisation and subsequently at 5–15 year intervals.

In the event of injuries which may give rise to tetanus, the administration of a further single dose of 0.5 ml is recommended unless a booster dose is known to have been given in the preceding year.

A booster dose given any time after the primary immunisation schedule can be expected to provide reinforcement of immunity.

Adsorbed tetanus vaccine may be administered simultaneously with tetanus antitoxin or tetanus immunoglobulin but must be given at a separate site.

Shake well before use.

Contra-indications, warnings, etc
Contra-indication: Concurrent acute infectious disease except in the case of a tetanus prone wound.

Warnings: Not for intradermal use since it may give rise to a skin nodule at the injection site. At the time of injury likely to carry the risk of tetanus, a reinforcing dose is not usually necessary in patients who have received a booster within the preceding year and in such patients there is the risk of a hypersensitivity reaction.

Side effects: General reactions are uncommon but may include transient pyrexia, headache, malaise, local swelling, redness and tenderness (especially in adults), acute allergic reactions, pallor, dyspnoea, urticaria, angioneurotic oedema and acute anaphylactic reactions. A small painless nodule may form at the injection site especially if administered into the superficial layers of subcutaneous tissue.

Precautions: As for all injectable vaccines, in cases of emergency treatment of an allergic reaction, a sterile syringe and Adrenaline Injection BP or other means should be ready for use.

Pharmaceutical precautions Store at +2° to +8°C. Do not freeze.

Multidose containers which are partly used should be discarded at the end of the first day of use.

Legal category POM.

Package quantities Single dose pre-filled syringe; single dose ampoule (pack of 5) or 10 dose (5 ml) vial.

Further information All persons should be actively immunised against tetanus. Recovery from even severe tetanus may not lead to natural immunity. Adsorbed tetanus vaccine can be administered to persons of all ages.

Product licence numbers
Single dose   6745/0002
Multi dose   6745/0003

*Trade Mark

Merrell Dow Pharmaceuticals Limited
Stana Place
Fairfield Avenue
Staines
Middlesex TW18 4SX

Merrell Dow

CLOMID*

Presentation Pale yellow, round, flat, bevelled tablet. Upper surface bisected and the lower surface engraved 'M' within two circles. Each tablet contains 50 mg Clomiphene Citrate BP.

Uses Clomid (Clomiphene Citrate BP) is indicated for the treatment of ovulatory failure in women desiring pregnancy.

Clomid is indicated only for patients in whom ovulatory dysfunction is demonstrated, who meet the conditions described in this data sheet. Other causes of infertility must be excluded or adequately treated before giving Clomid.

Good levels of endogenous (as estimated from vaginal smears, endometrial biopsy, assay of urinary oestrogen, or endometrial bleeding in response to progesterone) provide a favourable prognosis for ovulatory response induced by Clomid. A low level of oestrogen, although clinically less favourable, does not preclude successful outcome of therapy.

Clomid therapy is ineffective in patients with primary pituitary or primary ovarian failure. Clomid therapy cannot be expected to substitute for specific treatment of other causes of ovulatory failure, such as thyroid or adrenal disorders. For hyperprolactinaemia there is other preferred specific treatment.

Clomid is not first line treatment for low weight related amenorrhoea, with infertility, and has no value if a high FSH blood level is observed following an early menopause.

Dosage and administration

General considerations: The work-up and treatment of candidates for Clomid therapy should be supervised by physicians experienced in management of gynaecological or endocrine disorders. Patients should be chosen for therapy with Clomid only after careful diagnostic evaluation. The plan of therapy should be outlined in advance. Other causes of infertility should be excluded or adequately treated before giving Clomid.

Many patients will respond to 50 mg daily for 5 days. In the determination of a recommended starting dose schedule, efficacy must be balanced against potential adverse effects. For example, the data available so far suggest that ovulation and pregnancy are slightly more attainable on 100 mg/day for 5 days than on 50 mg/day for 5 days. As the dosage is increased, however, ovarian hyperstimulation and other adverse effects may increase. Furthermore, although the data do not yet establish a relationship between dosage and multiple births, it would seem reasonable on pharmacological grounds that such a relationship does exist.

For these reasons it would seem prudent to begin the treatment of the usual patient with the lower dose, 50 mg daily for 5 days, and to increase the dose only in those patients who do not respond to the first course. Special care with lower dosage or duration of treatment for the first course is particularly recommended if unusual sensitivity to pituitary gonadotrophin is suspected, such as in patients with polycystic ovary syndrome.

Recommended dosage: The recommended dose for the first course of Clomid is 50 mg (1 tablet) daily for 5 days. Therapy may be started at any time in the patient who has had no recent uterine bleeding. If progestin-induced bleeding is planned, or if spontaneous uterine bleeding occurs before therapy, the regimen of 50 mg daily for 5 days should be started on or about the fifth day of the cycle. When ovulation occurs at this dosage, there is no advantage to increasing the dose in subsequent cycles of treatment.

If ovulation appears not to have occurred after the first course of therapy, a second course of 100 mg daily (two 50 mg tablets given as a single daily dose) for five days should be given. This course may be started as early as 30 days after the previous one. *Increase of the dosage or duration of therapy beyond 100 mg/day for 5 days should not be undertaken.*

The majority of patients who are going to respond will respond to the first course of therapy, and 3 courses should constitute an adequate therapeutic trial. If ovulatory menses have not yet occurred, the diagnosis should be re-evaluated. Treatment beyond this is not recommended in the patient who does not exhibit evidence of ovulation.

Pregnancy: The importance of properly timed coitus cannot be over-emphasised (i.e. at about the time of ovulation). For regularity of cyclic ovulatory response it is also important that each course of Clomid be started on or about the fifth cycle day, once ovulation has been established. As with other therapeutic modalities, Clomid therapy follows the rule of diminishing returns, such that likelihood of conception diminishes with each succeeding course of therapy. Before starting treatment, patients and their male partners should be advised of the possibility of multiple pregnancy and its potential hazards if conception occurs in relationship to Clomid therapy.

Long-term cyclic therapy: Not recommended.

Since the relative safety of long-term cyclic therapy has not yet been conclusively demonstrated, and since the majority of patients will ovulate following 3 courses, long-term cyclic therapy is not recommended.

Contra-indications, warnings, etc
Contra-indications

Use in pregnancy: Clomid is not indicated during pregnancy. Although there is no evidence that Clomid has a harmful effect on the human foetus, there is evidence that Clomid has a deleterious effect on rat and rabbit foetuses when given in high doses to the pregnant animal. To help avoid inadvertent Clomid administration during early pregnancy, the basal body temperature should be recorded throughout all treatment cycles and the patient should be carefully observed to determine whether ovulation occurs. If the basal temperature following Clomid is biphasic and is not followed by menses, the patient should be examined carefully and should have a pregnancy test.

Liver disease: Clomid therapy is contra-indicated in patients with liver disease or a history of liver dysfunction.

Abnormal uterine bleeding: Clomid is contra-indicated in patients with abnormal bleeding of undetermined origin.

Ovarian cyst: See 'Precautions'.

Precautions

Ovarian cyst: Pelvic examination is necessary prior to start of and before each subsequent course of Clomid treatment. Clomid should not be given in the presence of an ovarian cyst (including endometriosis involving the ovary), except polycystic ovary since further enlargement of the cyst may occur.

To minimise the hazard of the abnormal ovarian enlargement associated with Clomid therapy, the lowest dose consistent with expectation of good results should be used. The patient should be instructed to inform the physician of any abdominal or pelvic pain, discomfort or distension after taking Clomid. Maximal enlargement of the ovary may not occur until several days after discontinuation of the course of Clomid.

The patient who complains of abdominal or pelvic pain, discomfort, or distension after taking Clomid should be examined because of the possible presence of an ovarian cyst or other cause. If abnormal enlargement occurs, Clomid should not be given until the ovaries have returned to pre-treatment size. The ovarian enlargement and cyst formation associated with Clomid therapy usually regress spontaneously within a few days or weeks after discontinuing treatment. Most of these patients should be managed conservatively. The dosage and/or duration of the next dose should be reduced.

Multiple pregnancy: There is an increased chance of multiple pregnancy when conception occurs in relationship to Clomid therapy. During the clinical investigation studies, the incidence of multiple pregnancy was 7.9% (186 of 2369 Clomid associated pregnancies on which outcome was reported). Among these 2369 pregnancies, 2183 (92.1%) were single, 165 (6.9%) twin, 11 (0.5%) triplet, 7 (0.3%) quadruplet, and 3 (0.13%) quintuplet.

Pregnancy wastage and birth anomalies: The overall incidence of reported birth anomalies from pregnancies associated with maternal Clomid ingestion (before or after conception) during the investigational studies was within the range of that reported in published references for the general population. Among the birth anomalies spontaneously reported in the published literature as individual cases, the proportion of neural tube defects has been high among pregnancies associated with ovulation induced by Clomid, but this has not been supported by data from population-based studies.

The physician should explain so that the patient understands the assumed risk of any pregnancy whether the ovulation was induced with the aid of Clomid or occurred naturally.

The patient should be informed of the greater pregnancy risks associated with certain characteristics or conditions of any pregnant woman: e.g. age of female and male partner, history of spontaneous abortions, Rh genotype, abnormal menstrual history, infertility history (regardless of cause), organic heart disease, diabetes, exposure to infectious agents such as rubella, familial history of birth anomaly, and other risk factors that may be pertinent to the patient for whom Clomid is being considered. Based upon the evaluation of the patient, genetic counselling may be indicated.

Population-based reports have been published on possible elevation of risk of Down's Syndrome in ovulation induction cases and of increase in trisomy defects among spontaneously aborted foetuses from subfertile women receiving ovulation inducing drugs (no women with Clomid alone without additional inducing drug). However, as yet, the reported observations are too few to confirm or not confirm the presence of an increased risk that would justify amniocentesis, other than for the usual indications because of age and family history.

The experience from patients of all diagnoses during clinical investigation of Clomid shows a pregnancy wastage or foetal loss rate of 21.4% (abortion rate of 19.0% and other loss rate of 2.4%).

Clomid therapy after conception was reported for 158 of the 2369 delivered and reported pregnancies in the clinical investigations. Of these 158 pregnancies 8 infants (born of 7 pregnancies) were reported to have birth defects.

There was no difference in reported incidence of birth defects whether Clomid was given before the 19th day after conception or between the 20th and 35th day after conception. This incidence is within the anticipated range of general population.

Warnings

Visual symptoms: Patients should be advised that blurring or other visual symptoms may occasionally occur during or shortly after therapy with Clomid. Patients should be warned that visual symptoms may render such activities as driving a car or operating machinery more hazardous than usual, particularly under conditions of variable lighting. The significance of these visual symptoms is not understood. If the patient has any visual symptoms, treatment should be discontinued and ophthalmological evaluation performed.

Side-effects

Symptoms/signs/conditions: Adverse effects appeared to be dose related, occurring more frequently at higher dose and with the longer courses of treatment used in investigational studies. At recommended dosage, adverse effects are not prominent and infrequently interfere with treatment.

During investigational studies, the more common reported adverse effects included ovarian enlargement (13.6%), vasomotor flushes (10.4%), abdominal-pelvic discomfort (distension, bloating) (5.5%). The vasomotor symptoms resembling menopausal 'hot flushes' were rarely severe and disappeared promptly after treatment was discontinued. Abdominal symptoms were most often related to ovulatory (mittelschmerz) or premenstrual phenomena, or to ovarian enlargement.

Ovarian enlargement: At recommended dosage, abnormal ovarian enlargement is infrequent, although the usual cyclic variation in ovarian size may be exaggerated. Similarly, cyclic ovarian pain (mittelschmerz) may be accentuated. With higher or prolonged dosage, more frequent ovarian enlargement and cyst formation may occur, and the luteal phase of the cycle may be prolonged.

Rare instances of massive ovarian enlargement are recorded. Such an instance has been described in a patient with polycystic ovary syndrome whose Clomid therapy consisted of 100 mg daily for 14 days. Abnormal ovarian enlargement usually regresses spontaneously; most of the patients with this condition should be treated conservatively.

Eye/visual symptoms: Symptoms described usually as 'blurring' or spots or flashes (scintillating scotomata), increase in incidence with increasing total dose and usually disappear within periods ranging from a few days to a few weeks after Clomid is discontinued.

These symptoms appear to be due to intensification and prolongation of after-images. Symptoms often first appear or are accentuated with exposure to bright-lit environment. While measured visual acuity has not generally been affected, one investigational patient (not anovulatory) taking Clomid 200 mg daily developed visual blurring on the seventh day of treatment, which progressed to severe diminution of visual acuity by the tenth treatment day. No other abnormality was found and the visual acuity returned to normal on the third day after treatment was stopped.

Ophthalmologically definable scotomata and retinal cell function (electroretinographic) changes have been reported. A patient treated during clinical studies developed phosphenes and scotomata during prolonged Clomid administration, but they disappeared by the 32nd day after stopping therapy.

There are rare reports of cataracts. In a 34-year-old patient who had taken 3 courses of Clomid, slit-lamp microscopic examination showed a mild amount of posterior cortical subcapsular opacity in each eye. Ophthalmoscopic examination revealed normal findings. The diagnosis was reported as 'posterior cortical senile cataracts'. In another patient previously treated with Clomid posterior vitreous detachment was the reported diagnosis. Other conditions of which there were isolated reports include conditions such as: optic neuritis, retinal haemorrhage/thrombosis/vascular spasm, temporary loss of vision, and macular oedema.

Dermatoses: Dermatitis and rash were reported by investigational patients. Conditions such as rash and urticaria were the most common ones reported after prescription availability but also reported were conditions such as allergic reaction, erythema multiforme, ecchymosis and angioneurotic oedema. Hair thinning has been reported very rarely.

CNS symptoms: In investigational patients, CNS symptoms/signs/conditions of dizziness, light-headedness/ vertigo (0.9%), nervous tension/insomnia (0.8%), and fatigue/depression (0.7%) were reported. After prescription availability, there were isolated additional reports of these conditions and also of reports of other conditions such as syncope/fainting, cerebrovascular accident, cerebral thrombosis, psychotic reactions including paranoid psychosis, neurologic impairment, disorientation and speech disturbance.

Liver function: Bromsulphalein (BSP) retention of greater than 5% was reported in 32 of 141 patients in whom it was measured, including 5 of 43 patients who took approximately the dose of Clomid now recommended. Retention was usually minimal unless associated with prolonged continuous Clomid administration or with apparently unrelated liver disease. Other liver function tests were usually normal. In a later study in which patients were given 6 consecutive monthly courses of Clomid (50 or 100 mg daily for 3 days) or matching placebo, BSP tests were done on 94 patients. Values in excess of 5% retention were recorded in 11 patients, 6 of whom had taken drug and 5 placebo.

In a separate report, one patient taking 50 mg of Clomid daily developed jaundice on the 19th day of treatment; liver biopsy revealed bile stasis without evidence of hepatitis.

Overdosage: There is no experience of acute overdosage with Clomid.

Pharmaceutical precautions　Clomid tablets should be protected from light, moisture and excessive heat.

Legal category　POM.

Package quantities　Clomid is obtainable in packs of 30 and 100 tablets in blister packs.

Further information　Clomid is prescribable under the supervision of an appropriate specialist.

Pharmacological classification: Clomid is a triarylethylene compound (related to chlorotrianisene and tripáranol). It is a non-steroidal agent taken by mouth which stimulates ovulation in a high percentage of appropriately selected anovulatory women.

Actions: The ovulatory response to cyclic Clomid therapy appears to be mediated through increased output of pituitary gonadotrophins, which in turn stimulates the maturation and endocrine activity of the ovarian follicle and the subsequent development and function of the corpus luteum. The role of the pituitary is indicated by increased urinary excretion of gonadotrophins and the response of the ovary is manifested by increased urinary oestrogen excretion.

Clinical pharmacology: Clomid may induce ovulation in appropriately selected anovulatory women.

After Clomid is administered to appropriately selected anovulatory women, presumptive signs of ovulation may be observed. Criteria for ovulation include the observations such as a biphasic basal body temperature curve and the blood level of progesterone.

Orally administered 14C labelled clomiphene citrate was readily absorbed when administered to humans. Cumulative excretion of the 14C label by way of the urine and faeces averaged about 50% of the oral dose after 5 days in 6 subjects, with mean urinary excretion of 7.8% and mean faecal excretion of 42.4%. A mean rate of excretion of 0.73% per day of the 14C dose after 31 days to 35 days and 0.45% per day of the 14C dose after 42 days to 45 days was seen in faecal and urine samples collected from 6 subjects for 14 to 53 days after clomiphene citrate 14C administration. The remaining drug/metabolites may be slowly excreted from a sequestered enterohepatic recirculation pool.

Succcessful therapy, characterised by at least one pregnancy, occurred in 2012 of the 7578 investigational patients observed up to 1970 with ovulatory dysfunction (26.6%) who received Clomid. This group of 7578 patients included women who did not desire pregnancy at the time of treatment and additional patients who had impediments to achievement of pregnancy in addition to ovulatory dysfunction. In addition to the 2269 pregnancies in the 2012 patients, 366 pregnancies were reported during the investigational studies among 160 Clomid treated patients with diagnoses other than ovulatory dysfunction (normal ovulation and menstruation; poor luteal phase; infertility/sterility, cause undetermined; habitual abortion; and diagnosis not stated), to make a total of 2635 pregnancies in 2172 patients with all diagnoses. Outcome was reported on 2369 of the 2635 pregnancies.

Product licence number 4425/5900.

DESTOLIT* ▼

Presentation Plain white tablet containing 150 mg ursodeoxycholic acid on one side bisect line, marked Destolit on reverse.

Uses Destolit is indicated for the dissolution of radiolucent (i.e. non-radio opaque) cholesterol gallstones in patients with a functioning gallbladder.

Dosage and administration The daily dose for most patients is 3 or 4 tablets of 150 mg according to body weight. This dose should be divided into 2 administrations after meals, with one administration always to be taken after the evening meal.

A *daily dose* of about 8 to 10 mg/kg will produce cholesterol desaturation of bile in the majority of cases. The measurement of the lithogenic index on bile-rich duodenal drainage fluid after 4–6 weeks of therapy may be useful for determining the minimal effective dose. The lowest effective dose has been found to be 4 mg/kg.

The *duration of treatment* required to achieve gallstone dissolution will usually not be extended beyond 2 years and should be monitored by regular cholecystograms. Treatment should be continued for 3–4 months after the radiological disappearance of the gallstones.

Any temporary discontinuation of treatment, if prolonged for 3–4 weeks, will allow the bile to return to a state of supersaturation and will extend the total time required for litholysis. In some cases stones may recur after successful treatment.

Contra-indications, warnings, etc In common with all drugs, it is advised that ursodeoxycholic acid should not be given during the first trimester of pregnancy. (In the rabbit, embryotoxicity has been observed, but this has not been seen in the rat.) Treatment in women of child-bearing age should only be undertaken if measures to prevent pregnancy are used. Non-hormonal contraceptive measures are recommended. In cases of conception during treatment, therapy should be discontinued. Active gastric or duodenal ulcers are contra-indications, as are hepatic and intestinal conditions interfering with the enterohepatic circulation of bile acids (ileal resection and stoma, regional ileitis, extra and intra-hepatic cholestasis, severe, acute, and chronic liver diseases). A product of this class has been found to be carcinogenic in animals. The relevance of these findings to the clinical use of ursodeoxycholic acid has not been established.

Excessive dietary intake of calories and cholesterol should be avoided; a low cholesterol diet will probably improve the effectiveness of Destolit tablets. It is also recommended that drugs known to increase cholesterol elimination in bile, such as oestrogenic hormones, oral contraceptive agents and certain blood cholesterol lowering agents should also not be prescribed concomitantly.

Side-effects: Destolit is normally well tolerated. Diarrhoea has been found to occur only occasionally. No significant alterations have so far been observed in liver function.

Overdosage: It is unlikely that overdosage will cause serious adverse effects. Diarrhoea may occur and it is recommended that liver function tests be monitored. Ion-exchange resins may be useful to bind bile acids in the intestines.

Pharmaceutical precautions Destolit tablets have a shelf life of 3 years under normal room temperature storage conditions.

Legal category POM.

Package quantities Blister packs of 60 tablets.

Further information Nil.

Product licence number 4425/0045.

KOLANTICON* GEL

Presentation Kolanticon Gel is a white, viscous, peppermint-flavoured suspension, each 5 ml containing:

Dicyclomine Hydrochloride BP	2.5 mg
Dried Aluminium Hydroxide BP	200 mg
Light Magnesium Oxide BP	100 mg
Simethicone USP	20 mg

Uses Kolanticon is an antacid-antiflatulent-anti-spasmodic-demulcent indicated for the treatment and prophylaxis of symptoms of peptic ulcer and functional dyspepsia especially in patients in whom gastric distress results from hyperacidity, smooth muscle spasm and flatulence. Also indicated for symptomatic relief in oesophagitis, hiatus hernia, gastritis and iatrogenic gastritis.

Dosage and administration Two to four 5 ml spoonfuls every four hours as required.

Contra-indications, warnings, etc
Contra-indications: Known idiosyncrasy to any of the ingredients. Should not be used in patients with obstructive uropathy, obstructive disease of the gastro-intestinal tract, paralytic ileus and intestinal atony, severe ulcerative colitis, and myasthenia gravis.

Precautions: Magnesium salts in the presence of renal insufficiency may cause central nervous system depression. Aluminium hydroxide in the presence of low phosphorous diets may cause phosphorous deficiency. Aluminium hydroxide may reduce absorption of tetracyclines when given concomitantly. Products containing dicyclomine hydrochloride should be used with caution in any patient with or suspected of having glaucoma or prostatic hypertrophy. Use with care in patients with hiatus hernia associated with reflux oesophagitis because anticholinergic drugs may aggravate this condition.

Epidemiological studies in pregnant women with products containing dicyclomine hydrochloride (at doses up to 40 mg/day) have not shown that dicyclomine increases the risk of foetal abnormalities if administered during the first trimester of pregnancy. Reproduction studies have been performed in rats and rabbits at doses of up to 100 times the maximum recommended dose (based on 60 mg per day for an adult person) and have revealed no evidence of impaired fertility or harm to the foetus due to dicyclomine.

Since risk of teratogenicity cannot be excluded with absolute certainty for any product, the drug should be used during pregnancy only if clearly needed.

It is not known whether dicyclomine is secreted into human milk. Because many drugs are excreted in human milk, caution should be exercised when dicyclomine is administered to a nursing woman.

Side-effects: In particularly sensitive patients dicyclomine hydrochloride may cause atropine-like side-effects such as dry mouth, blurred vision, urinary retention or constipation.

Overdosage: Signs and symptoms of dicyclomine hydrochloride overdose include: headache, nausea and vomiting, blurred vision, dilated pupils, hot dry skin, dizziness, vertigo, dryness of mouth, difficulty in swallowing and CNS stimulation.

Treatment may include emetics, gastric lavage and symptomatic therapy if indicated.

Pharmaceutical precautions Store in a cool place. Shake well before use.

Legal category P.

Package quantities Amber glass bottles of 125 ml and 500 ml.

Further information Nil.

Product licence number 4425/0032.

KOLANTYL* GEL

Presentation Kolantyl Gel is a white viscous peppermint-flavoured suspension, each 5 ml containing:

Dicyclomine Hydrochloride BP	2.5 mg
Dried Aluminium Hydroxide BP	200 mg
Light Magnesium Oxide BP	100 mg

Uses Antacid and antispasmodic for the treatment of symptoms of peptic ulcer and for prophylaxis in the ulcer-prone patient: for the relief of symptoms of gastric hyperacidity with or without pylorospasm in conditions such as oesophagitis, hiatus hernia, and acute iatrogenic and chronic gastritis.

Dosage and administration Two to four 5 ml spoonfuls every four hours as required.

Contra-indications, warnings, etc Known idiosyncrasy to any of the ingredients. Should not be used in patients with obstructive uropathy, obstructive disease of the gastro-intestinal tract, paralytic ileus and intestinal atony, severe ulcerative colitis, and myasthenia gravis.

Precautions: Magnesium salts in the presence of renal insufficiency may cause central nervous system depression. Aluminium hydroxide in the presence of low phosphorous diets may cause phosphorous deficiency. Aluminium hydroxide may reduce absorption of tetracyclines when given concomitantly. Products containing dicyclomine hydrochloride should be used with caution in any patient with or suspected of having glaucoma or prostatic hypertrophy. Use with care in patients with hiatus hernia associated with reflux oesophagitis because anticholinergic drugs may aggravate this condition.

Epidemiological studies in pregnant women with products containing dicyclomine hydrochloride (at doses up to 40 mg/day) have not shown that dicyclomine increases the risk of foetal abnormalities if administered during the first trimester of pregnancy. Reproduction studies have been performed in rats and rabbits at doses of up to 100 times the maximum recommended dose (based on 60 mg per day for an adult person) and have revealed no evidence of impaired fertility or harm to the foetus due to dicyclomine.

Since risk of teratogenicity cannot be excluded with absolute certainty for any product, the drug should be used during pregnancy only if clearly needed.

It is not known whether dicyclomine is secreted into human milk. Because many drugs are excreted in human milk, caution should be exercised when dicyclomine is administered to a nursing woman.

Side-effects: Side-effects are uncommon. When they occur, they are usually related to the dicyclomine hydrochloride in the formula which, in a few susceptible individuals, may cause atropine-like side-effects. Such side-effects rarely necessitate a discontinuance of the drug.

Overdosage: Signs and symptoms of dicyclomine hydrochloride overdose include: headache, nausea and vomiting, blurred vision, dilated pupils, hot dry skin, dizziness, vertigo, dryness of mouth, difficulty in swallowing and CNS stimulation.

Treatment may include emetics, gastric lavage and symptomatic therapy if indicated.

Pharmaceutical precautions Store in a cool place. Shake well before use.

Legal category P.

Package quantities 500 ml.

Further information Nil.

Product licence number 4425/0034.

LURSELLE*

Presentation Lurselle is presented as plain white, non-coated tablets imprinted on one face with the name 'Lurselle' and a bisect line on the reverse face, each tablet containing 250 mg probucol [4-4' (iso-propylidenedithio) bis (2,6-di-t-butylphenol)].

Uses Lurselle is indicated as ancillary therapy to diet for the reduction of elevated serum cholesterol in patients with hypercholesterolaemia, or in patients with combined hypercholesterolaemia and hypertriglyceridaemia where levels of cholesterol are a cause of concern.

Dosage and administration The recommended dose for adults is two tablets of 250 mg twice a day with the morning and evening meals.

Paediatric dosage has not yet been established.

Contra-indications, warnings, etc Reproduction studies in animals have not demonstrated any impairment of fertility or any harm to the foetus or offspring due to Lurselle. As yet there are no adequate studies in pregnant women, and the use of Lurselle during pregnancy is therefore not recommended. If a patient wishes to become pregnant, it is recommended that the drug be withdrawn and birth control procedures should be continued for at least six months, due to the persistence of the drug in the fatty tissues of the body.

In animals it has been shown that some of the drug is excreted in the milk. It is recommended that nursing mothers should not be treated with Lurselle.

Before instituting therapy with Lurselle, an attempt should be made to control elevated serum cholesterol by appropriate dietary regimens, weight reduction, and the treatment of any underlying disorder which might be the cause of the hypercholesterolaemia. Serum cholesterol and triglyceride levels should be monitored during the first months of treatment with Lurselle and periodically thereafter.

A favourable trend in cholesterol reduction should be evident during the first two months of Lurselle administration. An assessment should be made by the sixth month whether adequate reduction is being attained. A discontinuation in Lurselle treatment is usually followed by a gradual return of cholesterol to pre-treatment values.

If a marked sustained rise in serum triglycerides occurs during Lurselle therapy, consideration should be given to improving dietary compliance, alcohol abstinence, further restriction of calories, or adjustment of carbohydrate intake. If hypertriglyceridaemia persists, Lurselle should be discontinued.

Overdosage: In cases of overdosage symptomatic treatment and supportive measures should be instituted according to the individual symptoms.

Side-effects: The side-effects associated with Lurselle are generally mild to moderate and of short duration. They include diarrhoea, which occurs in about 1 in 10 patients, flatulence, abdominal pain, nausea and vomiting. These reactions are usually transient and seldom require the drug to be discontinued.

During the clinical studies in which patients have been treated for as long as 9 years, Lurselle had to be discontinued in less than 3 percent of the patients because of adverse gastrointestinal reactions.

Angio-neurotic oedema has been observed very occasionally and a single hypersensitivity reaction with dizziness, palpitation and syncope has been reported.

Concomitant Therapy

The dosage of hypoglycaemic agents and oral anticoagulants need not usually be modified when given with Lurselle and these drugs do not alter the effect of Lurselle on serum cholesterol.

Administration of Lurselle with a second lipid lowering drug has been shown to produce further significant reductions in serum cholesterol. The most effective combinations were Lurselle with either ion exchange resins or nicotinic acid.

Pharmaceutical precautions Lurselle tablets should be stored in a well closed container, protected from light, heat and moisture.

Legal category POM.

Package quantities 120 tablets.

Further information Absorption of Lurselle from the gastrointestinal tract is limited; food intake improves absorption and consequently induces higher and less variable peak blood levels. Lurselle is eliminated slowly from the body; the major pathway of excretion is the biliary tract.

Studies in man on the mode of action of Lurselle are still underway but they have shown that Lurselle lowers serum cholesterol by increasing the excretion of bile acids and by inhibiting an early stage of cholesterol biosynthesis. In addition there may be a slight decrease in absorption of dietary cholesterol.

Studies with Lurselle have shown no evidence of biliary tract pathology or related gallstone formation.

Product licence number 4425/0043.

MERBENTYL* SYRUP

Presentation Merbentyl Syrup is colourless, and raspberry flavoured. Each 5 ml contains 10 mg Dicyclomine Hydrochloride BP.

Uses Merbentyl is a smooth muscle antispasmodic primarily indicated for the treatment of functional conditions involving smooth muscle spasm of the gastrointestinal tract. The commonest of these is irritable colon (mucous colitis, spastic colon).

Dosage and administration *Adults:* One to two 5 ml spoonfuls (10–20 mg) three times daily before or after meals.

Children (2–12 years): One 5 ml spoonful (10 mg) three times daily.

Children (6 months–2 years): 5–10 mg three or four times daily, 15 minutes before feeds. Do not exceed a daily dose of 40 mg. If it is necessary to dilute Merbentyl Syrup this may be done using Syrup BP or if diluted immediately prior to use with water.

Contra-indications, warnings, etc Known idiosyncrasy to Dicyclomine Hydrochloride BP. Infants under 6 months of age.

Precautions: Products containing dicyclomine hydrochloride should be used with caution in any patient with, or suspected of having, glaucoma or prostatic hypertrophy. Use with care in patients with hiatus hernia associated with reflux oesophagitis because anticholinergic drugs may aggravate the condition.

There are rare reports of infants, 3 months of age and under, administered dicyclomine hydrochloride syrup, who have evidenced respiratory symptoms (breathing difficulty, shortness of breath, breathlessness, respiratory collapse, apnoea), as well as seizures, syncope, asphyxia, pulse rate fluctuations, muscular hypotonia and coma. The above symptoms have occurred within minutes of ingestion and lasted 20–30 minutes. The symptoms were reported in association with dicyclomine hydrochloride syrup therapy but the cause and effect relationship has neither been disproved nor proved. The timing and nature of the reactions suggest that they were a consequence of local irritation and/or aspiration, rather than to a direct pharmacological effect. Although no causal relationship between these effects, observed in infants, and dicyclomine administration has been established, dicyclomine hydrochloride is contra-indicated in infants under 6 months of age. See 'Contra-indications' above.

Epidemiological studies in pregnant women with products containing dicyclomine hydrochloride (at doses up to 40 mg/day) have not shown that dicyclomine hydrochloride increases the risk of foetal abnormalities if administered during the first trimester of pregnancy. Reproduction studies have been performed in rats and rabbits at doses of up to 100 times the maximum recommended dose (based on 60 mg per day for an adult person) and have revealed no evidence of impaired fertility or harm to the foetus due to dicyclomine.

Since the risk of teratogenicity cannot be excluded with absolute certainty for any product, the drug should be used during pregnancy only if clearly needed.

It is not known whether dicyclomine is secreted in human milk. Because many drugs are excreted in human milk, caution should be exercised when dicyclomine is administered to a nursing woman.

Side-effects: Side-effects seldom occur with Merbentyl. However, in susceptible individuals, dry mouth, thirst and dizziness may occur. On rare occasions, fatigue, sedation, blurred vision, rash, constipation, anorexia, nausea and vomiting, headache, and dysuria have also been reported.

Overdosage: Symptoms of Merbentyl overdosage are

headache, dizziness, nausea, dry mouth, difficulty in swallowing, dilated pupils and hot dry skin. Treatment may include emetics, gastric lavage and symptomatic therapy if indicated.

Pharmaceutical precautions Should be stored and dispensed in amber glass bottles.

Legal category POM.
P – Preparations of Dicyclomine Hydrochloride for internal use with a maximum dose of 10 mg and a maximum daily dose of 60 mg.

Package quantities Amber glass bottles of 125 ml and 500 ml.

Further information Nil.

Product licence number 4425/0047.

MERBENTYL* TABLETS

Presentation Merbentyl Tablets are white, round, plain bi-convex tablets, stamped 'M' in two concentric circles, containing Dicyclomine Hydrochloride BP 10 mg.

Uses Merbentyl is a smooth muscle antispasmodic primarily indicated for the treatment of functional conditions involving smooth muscle spasm of the gastro-intestinal tract.

Dosage and administration *Adults:* 1–2 tablets (10–20 mg) three times daily before or after meals.
Children: (2–12 years): 1 tablet (10 mg) three times daily.

Contra-indications, warnings, etc Known idiosyncrasy to Dicyclomine Hydrochloride BP.
Precautions: Products containing dicyclomine hydrochloride should be used with caution in any patient with, or suspected of having glaucoma or prostatic hypertrophy. Use with care in patients with hiatus hernia associated with reflux oesophagitis because anticholinergic drugs may aggravate the condition.
Epidemiological studies in pregnant women with products containing dicyclomine hydrochloride (at doses up to 40 mg/day) have not shown that dicyclomine hydrochloride increases the risk of foetal abnormalities if administered during the first trimester of pregnancy. Reproduction studies have been performed in rats and rabbits at doses of up to 100 times the maximum recommended dose (based on 60 mg per day for an adult person) and have revealed no evidence of impaired fertility or harm to the foetus due to dicyclomine.
Since the risk of teratogenicity cannot be excluded with absolute certainty for any product, the drug should be used during pregnancy only if clearly needed.
It is not known whether dicyclomine is secreted in human milk. Because many drugs are excreted in human milk, caution should be exercised when dicyclomine is administered to a nursing woman.
Side-effects: Side-effects seldom occur with Merbentyl. However, in susceptible individuals, dry mouth, thirst and dizziness may occur. On rare occasions, fatigue, sedation, blurred vision, rash, constipation, anorexia, nausea and vomiting, headache and dysuria have also been reported.
Overdosage: Symptoms of Merbentyl overdosage are headache, dizziness, nausea, dry mouth, difficulty in swallowing, dilated pupils and hot dry skin. Treatment

may include emetics, gastric lavage and symptomatic therapy if indicated.

Pharmaceutical precautions None.

Legal category POM.
P – Preparations of Dicyclomine Hydrochloride for internal use with a maximum dose of 10 mg and a maximum daily dose of 60 mg.

Package quantities 100 tablets.

Further information Nil.

Product licence number 4425/0035.

MEROCAINE*

Presentation Merocaine lozenges are green, round, flat lozenges with 'M' indented on both sides. Each lemon/lime flavoured lozenge contains:
Cetylpyridinium Chloride BP 1.4 mg (1:1500)
Benzocaine Ph Eur 10 mg

Uses Merocaine lozenges provide rapid and profound local anaesthetic action and topical antibacterial effects for the temporary relief of pain and discomfort in sore throat and superficial mouth infections. Indicated for relief of minor throat irritations and, adjunctively, for symptomatic relief of pain and discomfort in more serious throat infections, such as tonsillitis and pharyngitis, and following dental procedures involving oral mucosa and gingival surfaces.

Dosage and administration Allow to dissolve slowly in the mouth. One lozenge every 2 hours as needed but not more than 8 lozenges in 24 hours. Not indicated for children under 12 years of age.

Contra-indications, warnings, etc
Contra-indications: Idiosyncrasy to any of the ingredients.
Side-effects: Allergic reactions and methaemoglobinaemia have been reported with benzocaine.
Overdosage: There is no experience of overdosage but normal procedures of gastric lavage and maintenance of respiration and circulation (using vasopressor drugs if necessary) should apply.

Pharmaceutical precautions None.

Legal category P.

Package quantities 3 strips of 8 lozenges per carton.

Further information Nil.

Product licence number 4425/0028.

MEROCETS* LOZENGES
MEROCET* SOLUTION

Presentation Merocets Lozenges are yellow, round, flat lozenges, peppermint flavoured, embossed with 'M' on each face within a raised edge. Each contains 1.4 mg Cetylpyridinium Chloride BP in a sugar base. Merocet Solution is a pale yellow cinnamon-peppermint flavoured solution containing 0.05% w/v Cetylpyridinium Chloride BP, Ethanol (96%) BP 14%, phosphate buffers and aromatics.

Uses Cetylpyridinium Chloride BP is a surface-active quaternary compound with bactericidal and antifungal properties. Merocets Lozenges and Merocet Solution are indicated for the symptomatic treatment of sore throat. They are also indicated for minor irritations of the mouth and throat and for use prophylactically in dentistry and after dental operations. The solution can also be used for daily oral hygiene.

Dosage and administration *Adults and children over three years:*
Lozenges: Allow to dissolve slowly in the mouth – 1 three-hourly or as often as required.

Adults and children over six years: Mouthwash/Gargle: The solution may be used full strength or diluted with an equal volume of water – warm if desired – every three hours, or as often as required.

Contra-indications, warnings, etc Known idiosyncrasy to cetylpyridinium chloride.

Precautions: None.

Side-effects: Infrequent and transient complaints of a burning sensation of the mouth.

Overdosage: There is no experience of overdosage.

Pharmaceutical precautions *Lozenges:* Store in a cool dry place.

Solution: Avoid storage at low temperatures.

Legal category GSL.

Package quantities *Merocets Lozenges:* 3 strips of 8 lozenges per carton.
Merocet Solution: White flint-glass bottles of 200 ml.

Further information Nil.

Product licence numbers
Merocets Lozenges 4425/5908
Merocet Solution 4425/0017

NETHAPRIN DOSPAN*

Presentation Nethaprin Dospan Tablets are white, round, flat, bevelled tablets, scored on one side and engraved 'N' on the other. Each tablet contains:

Nethamine* (etafedrine hydrochloride)	50 mg
Butaphyllamine* (bufylline)	180 mg
Decapryn* (Doxylamine Succinate USNF)	25 mg
Phenylephrine Hydrochloride BP	25 mg

Uses Nethaprin Dospan is a bronchodilator, antihistamine, mild sedative, decongestant indicated for bronchospasm (wheezing) associated with chronic bronchitis, bronchial asthma or emphysema. Also useful in allergic cough.

Dosage and administration *Adults and children over 12 years:* For relief of mild to moderate attacks and for 12-hour protection: one tablet every 12 hours as required.
Children 6–12 years: ½ tablet every 12 hours as required.
Not recommended for children under 6 years.

Contra-indications Do not administer concurrently with monoamine oxidase inhibitors (MAOI's). Hypersensitivity.

Precautions This preparation may cause drowsiness; patients should be advised not to drive or operate machinery if affected.
It is dangerous to exceed the stated dose.

Side-effects While significant sympathomimetic side-effects have not been reported, an occasional sensitive patient may experience side-effects characteristic of this class of medicine. Nausea or other gastro-intestinal upsets have been reported occasionally.

Overdosage Nethaprin Dospan is a sustained release formulation and releases active ingredients over 10–12 hours. Signs and symptoms of overdosage include salivation, diuresis, dryness of the mouth, excitement, hypertension, dilated pupils, convulsions, insomnia and tachycardia. Treatment may include emetics, gastric lavage, barbiturates, and the patient should be kept cool and quiet.

Pharmaceutical precautions Store in a cool dry place.

Legal category POM.

Package quantities Amber glass bottles of 50.

Further information Nil.

Product licence number 0027/5013.

NETHAPRIN* EXPECTORANT

Presentation Nethaprin Expectorant is an orange-red syrup, with a bitter-ginger flavour, each 5 ml containing:

Nethamine* (etafedrine hydrochloride)	20 mg
Butaphyllamine* (bufylline)	60 mg
Decapryn* (Doxylamine Succinate USNF)	6 mg
Glyceryl Guaiacolate (USNF 1970)	100 mg

Uses Nethaprin Expectorant is a bronchodilator, antihistamine, mild sedative, expectorant mixture indicated for the treatment of unproductive cough or excessive mucus production associated with bronchospasm (wheezing).

Dosage and administration *Adults and children over 12 years:* One to two 5 ml spoonfuls every three to four hours.
Children 6–12 years: One 5 ml spoonful every three to four hours.
Not recommended for children under 6 years.

Contra-indications Do not administer concurrently with monoamine oxidase inhibitors (MAOI's). Hypersensitivity.

Precautions This product may cause drowsiness: patients should be advised not to drive or operate machinery if affected.
It is dangerous to exceed the stated dose.

Side-effects While significant sympathomimetic side-effects have not been reported, an occasional sensitive patient may experience symptoms characteristic of this class of medicine. Nausea and other gastro-intestinal upsets have been reported occasionally.

Overdosage Signs and symptoms of overdosage include salivation, diuresis, dryness of the mouth, excitement, hypertension, dilated pupils, convulsions, insomnia and tachycardia. Treatment may include emetics gastric lavage, and barbiturates. The patient should be kept cool and quiet.

Pharmaceutical precautions Avoid extremes of temperature.

Legal category POM.

Package quantities Amber glass bottles of 500 ml.

Further information Nil.

Product licence number 0027/5014.

RIFADIN*

Presentation Rifadin capsules (blue and red) marked 'Lepetit', containing 150 mg Rifampicin BP.

Rifadin capsules (red) marked 'Lepetit', containing 300 mg Rifampicin BP.

Rifadin syrup (raspberry colour and flavour), containing 100 mg Rifampicin BP in each 5 ml.

Uses Rifadin, used in combination with other active antituberculosis drugs, is indicated in the treatment of all forms of tuberculosis, including fresh, advanced, chronic and drug-resistant cases. It is also effective against many atypical strains of Mycobacteria. Rifadin is active *in vitro* at low concentrations against Gram-positive organisms and at higher concentrations against Gram-negative organisms.

Dosage and administration The daily dose of Rifadin, calculated from the patient's body weight, should preferably be taken on an empty stomach or at least 30 minutes before a meal or 2 hours after a meal to ensure rapid and complete absorption. Rifadin should be given with other effective antituberculosis drugs to prevent the possible emergence of *rifampicin*-resistant strains of Mycobacteria.

Adults: The recommended single daily dose in tuberculosis is 8–12 mg/kg.

Usual daily dose:
　Patients weighing less than 50 kg – 450 mg.
　Patients weighing 50 kg or more – 600 mg.

Children: In children, oral doses of 10–20 mg/kg body weight daily are recommended, although a total daily dose should not usually exceed 600 mg.

Impaired liver function: A daily dose of 8 mg/kg should not be exceeded in patients with impaired liver function.

Use in the elderly: In elderly patients, the renal excretion of rifampicin is decreased proportionally with physiological decrease of renal function; due to compensatory increase of liver excretion, the serum terminal half-life is similar to that of younger patients. However, as increased blood levels have been noted in one study of rifampicin in elderly patients, caution should be exercised in using rifampicin in such patients, especially if there is evidence of liver function impairment.

Contra-indications, warnings, etc
Contra-indications: Rifadin is contra-indicated in the presence of jaundice, and in patients who are hypersensitive to the rifamycins.

Use in pregnancy and lactation: At very high doses in animals rifampicin has been shown to have teratogenic effects. There are no well controlled studies with rifampicin in pregnant women. Therefore, Rifadin should be used in pregnant women or in women of child bearing potential only if the potential benefit justifies the potential risk to the foetus. When Rifadin is administered during the last few weeks of pregnancy it may cause post-natal haemorrhages in the mother and infant for which treatment with Vitamin K 1 may be indicated.

Rifampicin is excreted in breast milk and infants should not be breast fed by a patient receiving rifampicin unless in the physician's judgement the potential benefit to the patient outweighs the potential risk to the infant.

Precautions: Patients with impaired liver function should only be given rifampicin in cases of necessity, and then with caution and under close medical supervision. In these patients, lower doses of rifampicin are recommended and careful monitoring of liver function, especially serum glutamic pyruvic transaminase (SGPT) and serum glutamic oxaloacetic transaminase (SGOT) should be carried out prior to therapy and then every two or four weeks during therapy. If signs of hepatocellular damage occur, rifampicin should be withdrawn. In patients with impaired liver function, elderly patients, malnourished patients, and possibly, children under two years of age, caution is particularly recommended when instituting therapeutic regimens in which isoniazid is to be used concurrently with rifampicin. It is rarely necessary, in the absence of clinical findings, to increase the frequency of performing routine liver function tests in patients with normal pretreatment liver function.

In some cases of hyperbilirubinaemia resulting from competition between rifampicin and bilirubin for excretory pathways of the liver at the cell level can occur in the early days of treatment. An isolated report showing a moderate rise in bilirubin and/or transaminase level is not in itself an indication for interrupting treatment; rather the decision should be made after repeating the tests, noting trends in the levels and considering them in conjunction with the patient's clinical condition.

Because of the possibility of immunological reaction (see Side-effects) occurring with intermittent therapy (less than 2 to 3 times per week) patients should be closely monitored. Patients should be cautioned against interruption of dosage regimens since these reactions may occur.

Drug/laboratory interactions: Rifampicin has been shown in animals and man to have liver enzyme inducing properties and may reduce the activity of anticoagulants, corticosteroids, cyclosporin, digitalis preparations, oral contraceptives, oral hypoglycaemic agents, dapsone, phenytoin, quinidine, narcotics and analgesics. It may be necessary to adjust the dosage of these drugs if they are given concurrently with Rifadin, particularly when it is initiated or withdrawn.

Patients on oral contraceptives should be advised to use alternative, non-hormonal methods of birth control during Rifadin therapy. Also diabetes may become more difficult to control.

If *p*-aminosalicylic acid and rifampicin are both included in the treatment regimen, they should be given not less than eight hours apart to ensure satisfactory blood levels.

Therapeutic levels of rifampicin have been shown to inhibit standard microbiological assays for serum folate and Vitamin B 12. Thus alternate assay methods should be considered. Transient elevation of BSP and serum bilirubin have been reported. Therefore, these tests should be performed before the morning dose of rifampicin.

Side-effects: Reactions occurring with either daily or intermittent dosage regimens include:

　Cutaneous reactions which are mild and self-limiting may occur and do not appear to be hypersensitivity reactions. Typically they consist of flushing and itching with or without a rash.

　Gastrointestinal reactions consist of anorexia, nausea, vomiting, abdominal discomfort, and diarrhoea. Pseudomembranous colitis has been reported with rifampicin therapy.

　Hepatitis can be caused by rifampicin and liver

function tests should be monitored. (See Warnings/Precautions).

Thrombocytopenia with or without purpura may occur, usually associated with intermittent therapy, but is reversible if drug is discontinued as soon as purpura occurs. Cerebral haemorrhage and fatalities have been reported when rifampicin administration has been continued or resumed after the appearance of purpura.

Eosinophilia, leukopenia, oedema, muscle weakness and myopathy have been reported to occur in a small percentage of patients treated with rifampicin.

Reactions usually occurring with intermittent dosage regimens and most probably of immunological origin include:

- 'Flu Syndrome' consisting of episodes of fever, chills, headache, dizziness, and bone pain appearing most commonly during the 3rd to the 6th month of therapy. The frequency of the syndrome varies but may occur in up to 50% of patients given once-weekly regimens with a dose of rifampicin of 25 mg/kg or more.
- Shortness of breath and wheezing.
- Decrease in blood pressure and shock.
- Acute haemolytic anaemia.
- Acute renal failure usually due to acute tubular necrosis or to acute interstitial nephritis.

If serious complications arise, e.g. renal failure, thrombocytopenia or haemolytic anaemia, rifampicin should be stopped and never restarted.

Occasional disturbances of the menstrual cycle have been reported in women receiving long term antituberculosis therapy with regimens containing rifampicin.

Rifampicin may produce a reddish discolouration of the urine, sputum and tears. The patient should be forewarned of this. Soft contact lenses may be permanently stained.

Overdosage: In cases of overdosage with Rifadin, gastric lavage should be performed as soon as possible. Intensive supportive measures should be instituted and individual symptoms treated as they arise.

Pharmaceutical precautions Rifadin capsules have a shelf life of four years when stored below 25°C. Rifadin syrup has a shelf life of three years. Rifadin syrup should not be diluted. It should be dispensed in clear or amber glass bottles.

Rifadin capsules should be protected from light and moisture.

Legal category POM.

Package quantities

Rifadin capsules 150 mg	Bottles of 100 capsules.
Rifadin capsules 300 mg	Bottles of 100 capsules.
Rifadin syrup 100 mg/5 ml	Bottles of 120 ml.

Further information An oral dose of 450–600 mg Rifadin produces therapeutically effective levels in the blood, with the peak concentrations being observed approximately 2 hours after administration. There is good distribution of rifampicin into body tissues and fluids including lung, bone, lymph nodes and inflammatory exudates. Rifampicin is excreted mainly in the bile and urine, and high concentrations are reached in both these fluids. No cross resistance has been shown between Rifadin and other antituberculosis drugs.

Product licence numbers

Rifadin capsules 150 mg	4425/5915
Rifadin capsules 300 mg	4425/5916
Rifadin syrup	4425/5917

RIFADIN* FOR INFUSION

Presentation

(i) 10 ml vial containing 300 mg Rifampicin BP (red lyophilised powder) with an accompanying 5 ml ampoule of clear colourless solvent solution (pyrogen free water plus polysorbate 81).

(ii) 20 ml vial containing 600 mg Rifampicin BP (red lyophilised powder) with an accompanying 10 ml ampoule of clear colourless solvent solution (pyrogen free water plus polysorbate 81).

Uses Rifadin For Infusion is indicated in patients with all forms of tuberculosis who are unable to tolerate oral therapy, e.g. post operative or comatose patients or patients in whom gastro-intestinal absorption is impaired. Rifadin is active *in vitro* at low concentrations against Gram-positive organisms and at higher concentrations against Gram-negative organisms.

Preparation of infusion: Rifadin For Infusion is prepared for use by aseptically adding the solvent to the vial of rifampicin powder and shaking vigorously and continuously for about 30 seconds. When the powder has completely dissolved, the solution should be immediately diluted in 500 ml (600 mg of rifampicin) or 250 ml (300 mg of rifampicin) of 5% glucose solution, or other suitable infusion fluid (see 'Pharmaceutical Precautions'). It is suggested that the infusion is administered over a period of 2–3 hours. The preparations should be used within 6 hours.

Dosage and administration Treatment with Rifadin For Infusion should include the concomitant use of other appropriate antibacterials to prevent the emergence of resistant strains of the causative organism.

Adults: In tuberculosis a single daily administration of 600 mg given in an intravenous infusion drip over 2 to 3 hours has been found to be effective and well tolerated for adult patients. Serum concentrations following this dosage regimen are similar to those obtained after 600 mg by mouth.

Children: Paediatric usage has not yet been established. However, the following regimen is suggested:

In tuberculosis: a single daily dose of up to 20 mg/kg bodyweight is recommended, although the total daily dose should not usually exceed 600 mg.

Impaired liver function: A daily dose of 8 mg/kg should not be exceeded in patients with impaired liver function.

Use in the elderly: In elderly patients, the renal excretion of rifampicin is decreased proportionally with physiological decrease of renal function; due to compensatory increase of liver excretion, the serum terminal half-life is similar to that of younger patients. However, as increased blood levels have been noted in one study of rifampicin in elderly patients, caution should be exercised in using rifampicin in such patients, especially if there is evidence of liver function impairment.

When patients are able to accept oral medication, they should be transferred to Rifadin Capsules or Syrup (for further information on these products see their separate data sheets).

Contra-indications, warnings, etc Rifadin For Infusion is contra-indicated in patients who are hypersensitive to rifamycins.

Although not recommended for use in patients with jaundice, the therapeutic benefit of Rifadin For Infusion should be weighed against the possible risks.

Use in pregnancy and lactation: At very high doses in

animals rifampicin has been shown to have teratogenic effects. There are no well controlled studies with rifampicin in pregnant women. Therefore, Rifadin For Infusion should be used in pregnant women or in women of child bearing potential only if the potential benefit justifies the potential risk to the foetus. When rifampicin is administered during the last few weeks of pregnancy it may cause post-natal haemorrhages in the mother and infant for which treatment with Vitamin K1 may be indicated.

Rifampicin is excreted in breast milk and infants should not be breast fed by a patient receiving rifampicin unless in the physician's judgement the potential benefit to the patient outweighs the potential risk to the infant.

Precautions: Patients with impaired liver function should only be given rifampicin in cases of necessity, and then with caution and under close medical supervision. In these patients, lower doses of rifampicin are recommended and careful monitoring of liver function, especially serum glutamic pyruvic transaminase (SGPT) and serum glutamic oxaloacetic transaminase (SGOT) should be carried out. If signs of hepatocellular damage occur, rifampicin should be withdrawn. In patients with impaired liver function, elderly patients, malnourished patients, and possibly, children under two years of age, caution is particularly recommended when instituting therapeutic regimens in which isoniazid is to be used concurrently with rifampicin.

It is rarely necessary, in the absence of clinical findings, to increase the frequency of performing routine liver function tests in patients with normal pretreatment liver function. In the presence of complete renal failure, rifampicin is excreted entirely in the bile: provided hepatic function is not impaired the dosage of rifampicin need not be adjusted.

In some cases hyperbilirubinaemia resulting from competition between rifampicin and bilirubin for excretory pathways of the liver at the cell level can occur in the early days of treatment. An isolated report showing a moderate rise in bilirubin and/or transaminase level is not in itself an indication for interrupting treatment; rather the decision should be made after repeating the tests, noting trends in the levels and considering them in conjunction with the patient's clinical condition.

Drug/laboratory interactions: Rifampicin has been shown in animals and man to have liver enzyme inducing properties and may reduce the activity of anticoagulants, corticosteroids, cyclosporin, digitalis preparations, oral contraceptives, oral hypoglycaemic agents, dapsone, phenytoin, quinidine, narcotics and analgesics. It may be necessary to adjust the dosage of these drugs if they are given concurrently with Rifadin, particularly when it is initiated or withdrawn.

Therapeutic levels of rifampicin have been shown to inhibit standard microbiological assays for serum folate and Vitamin B12. Thus alternate assay methods should be considered. Transient elevation of BSP and serum bilirubin have been reported. Therefore, these tests should be performed before the daily administration of Rifadin For Infusion.

Side-effects: Rifadin For Infusion is generally very well tolerated and accepted by patients, although hypersensitivity reactions have been described and occasionally patients have experienced fever, skin rashes and nausea/vomiting.

Occasional instances of phlebitis and pain at the infusion site have been reported.

Reactions occurring with either daily or intermittent dosage regimens include:

Cutaneous reactions which are mild and self-limiting may occur and do not appear to be hypersensitivity reactions. Typically they consist of flushing and itching with or without a rash.

Gastrointestinal reactions consist of anorexia, nausea, vomiting, abdominal discomfort, and diarrhoea. Pseudomembranous colitis has been reported with rifampicin therapy.

Hepatitis can be caused by rifampicin and liver function tests should be monitored. (See Warnings/Precautions).

Thrombocytopenia with or without purpura may occur, usually associated with intermittent therapy, but is reversible if drug is discontinued as soon as purpura occurs. Cerebral haemorrhage and fatalities have been reported when rifampicin administration has been continued or resumed after the appearance of purpura.

Eosinophilia, leukopenia, oedema, muscle weakness and myopathy have been reported to occur in a small percentage of patients treated with rifampicin.

Reactions usually occurring with intermittent dosage regimens and most probably of immunological origin include:
- 'Flu Syndrome' consisting of episodes of fever, chills, headache, dizziness, and bone pain appearing most commonly during the 3rd to the 6th month of therapy. The frequency of the syndrome varies but may occur in up to 50% of patients given once-weekly regimens with a dose of rifampicin of 25 mg/kg or more.
- Shortness of breath and wheezing.
- Decrease in blood pressure and shock.
- Acute haemolytic anaemia.
- Acute renal failure usually due to acute tubular necrosis or to acute interstitial nephritis.

If serious complications arise, e.g. renal failure, thrombocytopenia or haemolytic anaemia, rifampicin should be stopped and never restarted.

Occasional disturbances of the menstrual cycle have been reported in women receiving long term antituberculosis therapy with regimens containing rifampicin.

Rifampicin may produce a reddish discolouration of the urine, sputum and tears. The patient should be forewarned of this. Soft contact lenses may be permanently stained.

Pharmaceutical precautions Rifadin For Infusion should be freshly prepared. Unmixed rifampicin powder and the solvent both have a shelf life of 4 years when stored at room temperature.

Compatibilities: Rifadin For Infusion is compatible with the following infusion solutions for up to 6 hours: Mannitol 10% and 20%, Macrodex with Saline Solution, Macrodex with Glucose Solution, Rheomacrodex, Sodium Bicarbonate 1.4%, Laevulose 5% and 10%, Ringer Lactate, Ringer Acetate, Dextrose 5% and 10%, Saline Solution.

Incompatibilities: Rifadin For Infusion is incompatible with the following: Perfudex, Sodium Bicarbonate 5%, Sodium Lactate 0.167M, Ringer Acetate with Dextrose.

Legal category POM.

Package quantities *Rifadin For Infusion 300 mg.* Combined pack of: one vial containing 300 mg Rifampicin BP, *and* one ampoule containing 5 ml solvent.

Rifadin For Infusion 600 mg: Combined pack of: one

vial containing 600 mg Rifampicin BP, *and* one ampoule containing 10 ml solvent.

Further information Nil.

Product licence numbers
Rifadin For Infusion 300 mg   4425/0050
Rifadin For Infusion 600 mg   4425/0051

RIFATER* ▼

Presentation Smooth, round, shiny, pink-beige, sugar coated tablets containing Isoniazid BP 50 mg, Pyrazinamide BP 300 mg and Rifampicin BP 120 mg.

Uses Rifater is indicated in the treatment of pulmonary tuberculosis.

Dosage and administration Rifater is recommended in the initial intensive phase of the short-course treatment of pulmonary tuberculosis. During this phase, which lasts for 2 months, Rifater should be administered on a daily continuous basis. The concomitant administration of ethambutol or intramuscular streptomycin over the same period of time is advised.

Each Rifater tablet contains isoniazid (INH), pyrazinamide (Z) and rifampicin (RAMP) in such a ratio that the administration of 9–12 mg/kg RAMP, 4–5 mg/kg INH and 23–30 mg/kg Z can be achieved by giving 3 tablets daily to patients weighing less than 40 kg, 4 tablets to patients weighing 40–49 kg, 5 tablets to patients weighing 50–64 kg and 6 tablets to patients weighing 65 kg or more.

Once the initial intensive phase of treatment has been completed the treatment can be continued with the combination rifampicin-isoniazid (Rifinah*) always on a daily basis.

This regimen, if correctly applied, is 100% effective with very few, if any, relapses. The clinical evidence indicates that these occur generally in the first 6 months after stopping treatment with bacilli fully sensitive to the drugs employed, so that changes in the drugs to be utilised for further treatment are not required. The regimen has been found to be fully effective also in the presence of a bacillary population resistant to isoniazid, to streptomycin or to both drugs.

Children: The ratio of the three drugs in Rifater may not be appropriate in children (e.g. higher mg/kg doses of INH are usually given in children than in adults). Rifater can be used only in special cases, after careful consideration of the mg/kg dose of each component.

Use in the elderly: Caution should be exercised in such patients, in view of the possible decrease of the excretory function of the kidney and of the liver.

Contra-indications, warnings, etc
Contra-indications: Rifater is contra-indicated in patients who are hypersensitive to any one of the components of the combination. Rifater is contra-indicated in the presence of jaundice.

Use in pregnancy and lactation: At very high doses in animals rifampicin has been shown to have teratogenic effects. There are no well controlled studies with Rifater in pregnant women. Therefore, Rifater should be used in pregnant women or in women of child bearing potential only if the potential benefit justifies the potential risk to the foetus. When administered during the last few weeks of pregnancy, Rifater may cause post-natal haemorrhages in the mother and infant, for which treatment with Vitamin K1 may be indicated.

Rifampicin and isoniazid are excreted in breast milk and infants should not be breast fed by a patient receiving Rifater unless in the physician's judgement the potential benefit to the patient outweighs the potential risk to the infant.

Precautions: The precautions for the use of Rifater are the same as those considered when a triple individual administration of rifampicin, isoniazid and pyrazinamide is required. Each of these drugs has been associated with liver dysfunction. Patients with impaired liver function should only be given Rifater in cases of necessity and then with caution and under strict medical supervision. In these patients, careful monitoring of liver function, especially serum glutamic pyruvic transaminase (SGPT) and serum glutamic oxaloacetic transaminase (SGOT) should be carried out prior to therapy and then every two to four weeks during therapy. If signs of hepatocellular damage occur, Rifater should be withdrawn. Care should be exercised in the treatment of elderly or malnourished patients who may also require Vitamin B6 supplementation with the isoniazid therapy.

In some cases hyperbilirubinaemia resulting from competition between rifampicin and bilirubin for excretory pathways of the liver at the cell level can occur in the early days of treatment. An isolated report showing a moderate rise in bilirubin and/or transaminase level is not in itself an indication for interrupting treatment; rather, the decision should be made after repeating the tests, noting trends in the levels and considering them in conjunction with the patient's clinical condition.

Rifater should be used with caution in patients with a history of gout. If hyperuricaemia accompanied by an acute gouty arthritis occurs, the patient should be transferred to a regimen not containing pyrazinamide (e.g. Rifinah 150 or 300).

The possibility of pyrazinamide having an adverse effect on blood clotting time or vascular integrity should be borne in mind in patients with haemoptysis.

Because of the possibility of immunological reaction (see 'Adverse reactions') occurring with intermittent rifampicin therapy (less than 2 to 3 per week) patients should be closely monitored. Patients should be cautioned against interruption of dosage regimens since these reactions may occur.

Drug/laboratory interactions: Rifampicin has liver enzyme-inducing properties and may reduce the activity of a number of drugs including anticoagulants, corticosteroids, cyclosporin, digitalis preparations, quinidine, oral contraceptives, oral hypoglycaemic agents, dapsone, narcotics and analgesics. It may be necessary to adjust the dosage of these drugs if they are given concurrently with Rifater.

Patients using oral contraceptives should be advised to change to non-hormonal methods of birth control during Rifater therapy. Also diabetes may become more difficult to control.

If p-aminosalicylic acid and rifampicin are both included in the treatment regimen, they should be given not less than eight hours apart to ensure satisfactory blood levels.

Therapeutic levels of rifampicin have been shown to inhibit standard microbiological assays for serum folate and Vitamin B12. Thus alternate assay methods should be considered. Transient elevation of BSP and serum bilirubin have been reported. Therefore, these tests should be performed before the morning dose of rifampicin. Isoniazid may decrease the excretion of phenytoin or may enhance its effects. Appropriate adjustment of the anti-convulsant dose should be made.

Side-effects: Rifampicin: Reactions occurring with either daily or intermittent dosage regimens include:

Cutaneous reactions which are mild and self-limiting may occur and do not appear to be hypersensitivity reactions. Typically they consist of flushing and itching with or without a rash.

Gastrointestinal reactions consist of anorexia, nausea, vomiting, abdominal discomfort, and diarrhoea. Pseudomembranous colitis has been reported with rifampicin therapy.

Hepatitis can be caused by rifampicin and liver function tests should be monitored. (See Warnings/ Precautions).

Thrombocytopenia with or without purpura may occur, usually associated with intermittent therapy, but is reversible if drug is discontinued as soon as purpura occurs. Cerebral haemorrhage and fatalities have been reported when rifampicin administration has been continued or resumed after the appearance of purpura.

Eosinophilia, leukopenia, oedema, muscle weakness and myopathy have been reported to occur in a small percentage of patients treated with rifampicin.

Reactions usually occurring with intermittent dosage regimens and most probably of immunological origin include:

– 'Flu Syndrome' consisting of episodes of fever, chills, headache, dizziness, and bone pain appearing most commonly during the 3rd to the 6th month of therapy. The frequency of the syndrome varies but may occur in up to 50% of patients given once-weekly regimens with a dose of rifampicin of 25 mg/kg or more.
– Shortness of breath and wheezing.
– Decrease in blood pressure and shock.
– Acute haemolytic anaemia.
– Acute renal failure usually due to acute tubular necrosis or to acute interstitial nephritis.

If serious complications arise, e.g. renal failure, thrombocytopenia or haemolytic anaemia, Rifater should be stopped and never restarted.

Occasional disturbances of the menstrual cycle have been reported in women receiving long term antituberculosis therapy with regimens containing rifampicin.

Rifampicin may produce a reddish discolouration of the urine, sputum and tears. The patient should be forewarned of this. Soft contact lenses may be permanently stained.

Isoniazid: Severe and sometimes fatal hepatitis may occur with isoniazid therapy. Polyneuritis associated with isoniazid, presenting as paraesthesia, muscle weakness, loss of tendon reflexes, etc., is unlikely to occur with the recommended daily dose of Rifater. Various haematological disturbances have been identified during treatment with isoniazid, including eosinophilia, agranulocytosis, and anaemia. High doses of isoniazid can cause convulsions. The possibility that the frequency of seizures may be increased in patients with epilepsy should be borne in mind.

Pyrazinamide: Adverse reactions, other than hepatic reaction, which have been attributed to pyrazinamide are active gout (pyrazinamide has been reported to reduce urate excretion), sideroblastic anaemia, arthralgia, anorexia, nausea and vomiting, dysuria, malaise, fever, urticaria and aggravation of peptic ulcer. The hepatic reaction is the most common adverse reaction and varies from a symptomless abnormality of hepatic cell function

detected only through laboratory liver function tests, through a mild syndrome of fever, malaise and liver tenderness, to more serious reactions such as clinical jaundice and rare cases of acute yellow atrophy and death.

Overdosage: In cases of overdosage with Rifater, gastric lavage should be performed as soon as possible. Intensive supportive measures should be instituted and individual symptoms treated as they arise. Parenteral pyridoxine (Vitamin B6) should be given. Symptoms are more likely to be related to isoniazid, including coma, respiratory distress, hyperglycaemia and metabolic ketoacidosis.

Pharmaceutical precautions None.

Legal category POM.

Package quantities Blister strips of 20's in packs of 100's.

Further information Nil.

Product licence number 4425/0060.

RIFINAH*

Presentation *Rifinah 300:* orange, capsule-shaped tablets marked RH300 containing 300 mg Rifampicin BP and 150 mg Isoniazid BP.

Rifinah 150: cyclamen, round biconvex tablets marked RH150 containing 150 mg Rifampicin BP and 100 mg Isoniazid BP.

Uses Rifinah 300 and Rifinah 150 are indicated in the treatment of all forms of tuberculosis, including fresh, advanced and chronic cases.

Dosage and administration Another antituberculosis drug may be given concurrently with Rifinah until the susceptibility of the infecting organism to rifampicin and isoniazid has been confirmed.

Adults: Patients should be given the following single daily dose at least 30 minutes before a meal or 2 hours after a meal:

Rifinah 150: Patients weighing less than 50 kg – 3 tablets.

Rifinah 300: Patients weighing 50 kg or more – 2 tablets.

Use in the elderly: Caution should be exercised in such patients especially if there is evidence of liver impairment.

Contra-indications, warnings, etc

Contra-indications: Rifinah 300 and Rifinah 150 are contra-indicated in the presence of jaundice. Rifinah 300 and Rifinah 150 are contra-indicated in patients who are hypersensitive to rifamycins or isoniazid.

Use in pregnancy and lactation: Rifampicin has been shown to be teratogenic in rodents when given in large doses. There are no well controlled studies with Rifinah in pregnant women. Therefore, Rifinah should be used in pregnant women or in women of child bearing potential only if the potential benefit justifies the potential risk to the foetus.

When administered during the last few weeks of pregnancy, rifampicin can cause post-natal haemorrhages in the mother and infant, for which treatment with Vitamin K 1 may be indicated.

Rifampicin and isoniazid are excreted in breast milk and infants should not be breast fed by a patient receiving Rifinah unless in the physician's judgement the potential benefit to the patient outweighs the potential risk to the infant.

Precautions: Rifinah is a combination of 2 drugs, each of which has been associated with liver dysfunction.

Patients with impaired liver function should only be given Rifinah in cases of necessity, and then with caution and under close medical supervision. In these patients, careful monitoring of liver function, especially serum glutamic pyruvic transaminase (SGPT) and serum glutamic oxaloacetic transaminase (SGOT) should be carried out prior to therapy and then every two or four weeks during therapy. Similar care should be exercised in elderly patients, malnourished patients and children under two years of age. If signs of hepatocellular damage occur, Rifinah should be withdrawn. Care should be exercised in the treatment of elderly or malnourished patients who may also require Vitamin B_6 supplementation with the isoniazid therapy.

In some cases hyperbilirubinaemia resulting from competition between rifampicin and bilirubin for excretory pathways of the liver at the cell level can occur in the early days of treatment. An isolated report showing a moderate rise in bilirubin and/or transaminase level is not in itself an indication for interrupting treatment; rather the decision should be made after repeating the tests, noting trends in the levels and considering them in conjunction with the patient's clinical condition.

Because of the possibility of immunological reaction (see Side-effects) occurring with intermittent rifampicin therapy (less than 2 to 3 per week) patients should be closely monitored. Patients should be cautioned against interruption of dosage regimens since these reactions may occur.

Drug/laboratory interactions: Rifampicin has liver enzyme inducing properties and may reduce the activity of a number of drugs including anticoagulants, corticosteroids, cyclosporin, digitalis preparations, quinidine, oral contraceptives, oral hypoglycaemic agents, dapsone, narcotics and analgesics. It may be necessary to adjust the dosage of these drugs if they are given concurrently with Rifinah. Patients using oral contraceptives should be advised to change to non-hormonal methods of birth control during Rifinah therapy. Also, diabetes may become more difficult to control. When rifampicin is taken with para-aminosalicylic acid (P.A.S.), rifampicin levels in the serum may decrease. Therefore the drugs should be taken at least eight hours apart. Therapeutic levels of rifampicin have been shown to inhibit standard microbiological assays for serum folate and Vitamin B_{12}. Thus, alternate assay methods should be considered. Transient elevation of BSP and serum bilirubin have been reported. Therefore, these tests should be performed before the morning dose of rifampicin. Isoniazid may decrease the excretion of phenytoin or may enhance its effects. Appropriate adjustments of the anticonvulsant dose should be made.

Side-effects:

Rifampicin: Reactions to rifampicin occurring with either daily or intermittent dosage regimens include:

Cutaneous reactions which are mild and self-limiting may occur and do not appear to be hypersensitivity reactions. Typically they consist of flushing and itching with or without a rash. More serious hypersensitivity cutaneous reactions occur but are uncommon.

Gastrointestinal reactions consist of anorexia, nausea, vomiting, abdominal discomfort, and diarrhoea.

Pseudomembranous colitis has been reported with rifampicin therapy.

Hepatitis can be caused by rifampicin and liver function tests should be monitored. (See Warnings/Precautions).

Thrombocytopenia with or without purpura may occur, usually associated with intermittent therapy, but is reversible if drug is discontinued as soon as purpura occurs. Cerebral haemorrhage and fatalities have been reported when rifampicin administration has been continued or resumed after the appearance of purpura.

Eosinophilia, leukopenia, oedema, muscle weakness and myopathy have been reported to occur in a small percentage of patients treated with rifampicin.

Reactions usually occurring with intermittent dosage regimens and most probably of immunological origin include:

– 'Flu Syndrome' consisting of episodes of fever, chills, headache, dizziness, and bone pain appearing most commonly during the 3rd to the 6th month of therapy. The frequency of the syndrome varies but may occur in up to 50% of patients given once-weekly regimens with a dose of rifampicin of 25 mg/kg or more.

– Shortness of breath and wheezing.

– Decrease in blood pressure and shock.

– Acute haemolytic anaemia.

– Acute renal failure usually due to acute tubular necrosis or to acute interstitial nephritis.

If serious complications arise, e.g. renal failure, thrombocytopenia or haemolytic anaemia, rifampicin should be stopped and never restarted.

Occasional disturbances of the menstrual cycle have been reported in women receiving long term antituberculosis therapy with regimens containing rifampicin.

Rifampicin may produce a reddish discolouration of the urine, sputum and tears. The patient should be forewarned of this. Soft contact lenses may be permanently stained.

Isoniazid: Severe and sometimes fatal hepatitis may occur with isoniazid therapy. Polyneuritis associated with isoniazid, presenting as paraesthesia, muscle weakness, loss of tendon reflexes, etc., is unlikely to occur with the recommended daily dose of Rifinah. Various haematological disturbances have been identified during treatment with isoniazid, including eosinophilia, agranulocytosis, and anaemia. High doses of isoniazid can cause convulsions. The possibility that the frequency of seizures may be increased in patients with epilepsy should be borne in mind.

Overdosage: In cases of overdosage with Rifinah 300 or Rifinah 150, gastric lavage should be performed as soon as possible. Intensive supportive measures should be instituted and individual symptoms treated as they arise. Parenteral pyridoxine (Vitamin B_6) should be given. Symptoms are more likely to be related to isoniazid, including coma, respiratory distress, hyperglycaemia and metabolic ketoacidosis.

Pharmaceutical precautions Rifinah 300 and Rifinah 150 tablets have a shelf life of four years when stored below 25°C.

If it proves necessary to open a blister pack, Rifinah 300 and Rifinah 150 should be dispensed in amber glass or plastic containers. Protect from moisture.

Legal category POM.

Package quantities *Rifinah 300:* 4 weeks calendar packs – 56 tablets; bottles of 100 tablets.

Rifinah 150: 4 weeks calendar pack – 84 tablets; bottles of 100 tablets.

Further information The recommended daily dose of Rifinah 300 or Rifinah 150 produces therapeutically effective blood levels of rifampicin and isoniazid, two of the most powerful antituberculosis drugs. Serum concentrations and the biological half-life of the two component drugs do not differ significantly from values obtained when the drugs are given alone.

Product licence numbers
Rifinah 150   4425/0041
Rifinah 300   4425/0042

SYNDOL*

Presentation Syndol Tablets are yellow, round, flat-faced, bevelled-edge tablets. On one side there is an incised 'S' design and on the other a scored bisect line. Each tablet contains:

Paracetamol BP	450 mg
Codeine Phosphate BP	10 mg
Decapryn* (Doxylamine Succinate USNF)	5 mg
Caffeine BP	30 mg

Uses For the treatment of mild to moderate pain and as an antipyretic. Syndol is recommended for the symptomatic relief of headache, including muscle-contraction or tension headache, migraine, neuralgia, toothache, sore throat, dysmenorrhoea, muscular and rheumatic aches and pains, and for post-operative analgesia following surgical or dental procedures.

Dosage and administration *Adults and children over 12 years:* 1 or 2 tablets every four or six hours as needed for relief. Total dosage over a 24-hour period should not normally exceed 8 tablets.
Not recommended for children under 12 years.

Contra-indications, warnings, etc Idiosyncrasy to any of the ingredients.

Precautions: May cause drowsiness; if affected, patients should be advised not to drive or operate machinery.

Side-effects: Doxylamine succinate may cause drowsiness or dizziness in some patients. Mild constipation may occur associated with the codeine component of Syndol. Agranulocytosis is a very rare complication of treatment with paracetamol.

Overdosage: Treat symptomatically as for paracetamol and codeine.

Pharmaceutical precautions None.

Legal category CD (Sch 5), P.

Package quantities Blister strips of 10 in packs of 50 tablets and 20 tablets.

Further information Nil.

Product licence number 4425/0018.

TENUATE DOSPAN*

Presentation Tenuate Dospan Tablets are white, flat, bevelled, oblong tablets, scored on one side and stamped "Merrell" on the other side. Each contains Diethylpropion Hydrochloride BP 75 mg in a hydrophilic colloid gum designed to release the ingredient over a 10-hour period.

Uses An anoretic agent for short term use as an adjunct to the treatment of some patients with moderate or severe obesity when close support and supervision are also provided.

Dosage and administration *Adults:* One 75 mg tablet swallowed whole in mid-morning.
Not recommended for children or the elderly.
Current medical opinion supports intermittent use of an appetite suppressant. Courses of Tenuate Dospan may be given over periods of six to eight weeks with intervening periods of similar length without treatment and this may reduce the risk of dependence. The stated dose should not be exceeded. Efficacy in use for more than 3 to 6 months, and safety in long term use have not been established. Tenuate Dospan should be discontinued if weight loss does not occur or when patients stop losing weight.

Contra-indications, warnings, etc Tenuate Dospan should not be given concurrently with monoamine oxidase inhibitors (MAOI's) or other appetite suppressant drugs. It should not be given to patients hypersensitive to sympathomimetic agents, patients with uncontrolled thyrotoxicosis, emotionally unstable individuals or those with a history of psychiatric illness nor to patients known to be susceptible to drug or alcohol abuse. Although diethylpropion has less marked peripheral effects than the amphetamines, it should not be used in moderate/severe hypertension and severe cardivascular disease.

Use in pregnancy: Do not use during pregnancy.

Precautions and drug interactions: Tenuate Dospan should be used with caution when administered concurrently with antihypertensive medication, antidiabetic medication, psychotropic drugs (including sedatives) and sympathomimetic agents.

Warnings and adverse effects: Rarely severe enough to require discontinuation of therapy, side-effects associated with diethylpropion hydrochloride have been reported to occur in relatively low incidence. These have included dry mouth, restlessness, nervousness, euphoria, agitation, insomnia, palpitations, tachycardia, raised blood pressure, depression, psychosis, hallucinations, dependence, constipation and rashes. Gynaecomastia has been reported rarely. Infrequent occurrences of nausea and vomiting have been noted, but diarrhoea is exceedingly rare. Hypertensive crises may result from the administration during treatment with, or within 14 days of, monoamine oxidase inhibitors. Patients should be warned against driving or operating machinery until it is established that they are not over-stimulated or suffer from rebound sedation while taking, or after discontinuing, Tenuate Dospan. Alcoholic drink should be avoided.

Overdosage: Manifestations of acute overdosage include restlessness, tremor, hyper-reflexia, rapid respiration, confusion, assaultiveness, hallucinations, panic states. Fatigue and depression usually follow the central stimulation.
Cardiovascular effects include arrhythmias, hypertension or hypotension and circulatory collapse. Gastrointestinal symptoms include nausea, vomiting, diarrhoea and abdominal cramps. Overdose of pharmacologically similar compounds has resulted in fatal poisoning, usually terminating in convulsions and coma. Management of acute diethylpropion hydrochloride intoxication is largely symptomatic and includes lavage and sedation with a barbiturate. Experience with haemodialysis or peritoneal dialysis is inadequate to permit recommendation in this

regard. Intravenous phentolamine has been suggested on pharmacological grounds for possible acute, severe hypertension, if this complicates overdosage.

Pharmaceutical precautions Store in a cool dry place.

Legal category CD (Sch 3), POM.

Package quantities Tenuate Dospan tablets are in blister packs of 100.

Further information Prolonged use of diethylpropion may induce dependence with withdrawal syndrome on cessation of therapy. Hallucinations have occurred rarely following high doses of the drug. Several cases of toxic psychosis have been reported following the excessive use of the drug and a very small number have been reported in which the recommended dose appears not to have been exceeded. The psychosis was temporary and cleared up after the drug was discontinued.

Product licence number 4425/0015.

TRILUDAN* TABLETS AND SUSPENSION ▼

Presentation *Tablets:* White, round, flat faced, bevel edged tablets with 'M' in 2 concentric circles on one side and a scored bisect line with the code 084 on the other. Each tablet contains 60 mg terfenadine.

Suspension: A white oral suspension containing 30 mg terfenadine in 5 ml with a citrus-mint odour and taste.

Uses Triludan is an antihistamine which is indicated for the symptomatic relief of hay fever, allergic rhinitis and allergic skin conditions.

Dosage and administration
Adults and children over 12 years: One tablet twice daily or two 5 ml spoonfuls twice daily.

Children 6–12 years: Half a tablet twice daily or one 5 ml spoonful twice daily.

Contra-indications, warnings, etc Patients with known hypersensitivity to the drug.

Precautions: Although animal teratology studies have not indicated adverse effects, Triludan, like most medications, should not be used during pregnancy nor during lactation unless, in the opinion of the physician, the potential benefits outweigh any possible risk.

Side-effects: The following side-effects have been reported; their relationship to terfenadine has neither been proved nor disproved. These are: alopecia, anaphylaxis, angioedema, arrhythmias, bronchospasm, confusion, depression, dizziness, dry mouth, dyspnoea, fatigue, galactorrhoea, gastrointestinal distress, headache, insomnia, jaundice, liver dysfunction including transaminase elevations, menstrual disorders (including dysmenorrhoea), musculoskeletal pain, nightmares, oedema, palpitations, paraesthesia, photosensitivity reactions, skin rash, sweating, syncope, tremor, urinary frequency and visual disturbances. In objective tests Triludan has been shown to be free from central nervous system side effects. Reports of drowsiness are extremely rare.

Overdosage: One patient took 25 tablets (I.5G) and gastric lavage was performed one hour later with good recovery of tablets. There was a transient fall in blood pressure. Liver function tests initially and two days later were normal. No other problems were noted and there was no effect on consciousness.

Pharmaceutical precautions None.

Legal category P.

Package quantities Blister strips of 10 in cartons of 60 tablets. 125 ml amber bottle containing 120 ml suspension.

Further information Nil.

Product licence numbers
Tablets   4425/0024
Suspension   4425/0057

*Trade Mark

Thomas Morson Pharmaceuticals
Division of Merck Sharp & Dohme Limited
Hertford Road, Hoddesdon
Hertfordshire EN11 9BU

ATTENUVAX* ▼

Presentation Lyophilised powder for injection. When reconstituted, each dose of Attenuvax Injection contains not less than the equivalent of 1,000 $TCID_{50}$ (tissue culture infectious doses) of measles virus vaccine expressed in terms of the assigned titre of the FDA Reference Measles Virus. Attenuvax is a more attenuated line of measles virus derived from Enders' attenuated Edmonston strain.

Uses For general immunisation against measles.

Children: The Department of Health recommends that children 12 months of age or older be vaccinated against measles.

Attenuvax given immediately after exposure to natural measles may provide some protection. If, however, the vaccine is given a few days before exposure, substantial protection may be provided.

A single injection of Attenuvax has been shown to induce measles haemagglutination-inhibiting (HI) antibodies in more than 97% of vaccinees.

Dosage and administration After suitably cleansing the injection site, the total volume of reconstituted vaccine should be injected subcutaneously, preferably into the outer aspect of the arm. Attenuvax must not be given intravenously.

The dose of vaccine is the same for all patients.

Warning: A sterile syringe and Adrenaline Injection BP (1:1,000) should be ready for immediate use should an anaphylactoid reaction occur.

Reconstitution: To reconstitute the vaccine, all the diluent provided should be injected into a vial of lyophilised vaccine, and this agitated to ensure thorough mixing. All the reconstituted vaccine is then withdrawn into the syringe and injected subcutaneously.

Contra-indications, warnings, etc Children below the age of 12 months should not normally be given Attenuvax unless they are at special risk since the presence of maternal antibody may interfere with their ability to respond. Where immunisation below the age of 12 months is deemed necessary, a second dose should be given after the child has reached 15 months of age.

Any active or suspected infection is reason for delaying vaccination.

Patients with active untreated tuberculosis or malignant disease should not be vaccinated with Attenuvax.

Those with a family history of congenital or hereditary immunodeficiency should not be vaccinated until their immune competence is demonstrated.

Attenuvax should not be given to those with impaired immunoresponsiveness occurring naturally, or as a result of therapy. This contra-indication does not apply to patients receiving corticosteroids for replacement therapy, e.g. Addison's disease.

Attenuvax should not be used in patients with a history of anaphylactoid reaction to neomycin (each dose of reconstituted vaccine contains approximately 25 mcg of neomycin).

Hypersensitivity to eggs, chicken, or chicken feathers: Attenuvax is produced in cell cultures of chicken embryo. Patients with a history of anaphylactoid or other immediate reactions to eating eggs (e.g. hives, swelling of the mouth and throat, difficult breathing, hypotension and shock) should not be vaccinated. Evidence indicates, however, that those with other egg allergies are not at increased risk and there is no evidence to suggest that allergy to chicken or feathers increases the risk of reaction.

Pregnancy: Do not give Attenuvax to pregnant women, because the possible effects of the vaccine on fetal development or the mother's reproductive capacity are unknown at this time. It is recommended that pregnancy at the time of vaccination be ruled out, and that the possibility of pregnancy occurring in the three months following vaccination must be prevented by medically acceptable methods.

Warnings and adverse effects: Attenuvax is for subcutaneous injection only; *it must not be given intravenously.*

Children with a history of convulsions, or with parental history of epilepsy (non-traumatic) are considered to be at greater risk of convulsions.

In these cases, it is recognised that the simultaneous administration of normal immune globulint could be beneficial, although it should be recognised that the administration of immunoglobulin might increase the proportion of failures to immunise.

It may therefore be necessary to undertake a serological test to determine whether immunisation has been successful.

Attenuvax should not normally be given within three months of a transfusion with blood, or human plasma, or treatment with human immunoglobulin. If any of these substances have been used near to the time of vaccination, a test for the presence of measles antibody should be made at a later date.

---

† The dose of normal immune globulin used with Attenuvax should be between 0.4 and 0.8 units per kg bodyweight. It is important not to exceed this recommendation since excess immune globulin may completely inhibit the response to Attenuvax.

Typical dosage schedule

Bodyweight	5 kg	10 kg	15 kg	20 kg
Dose volume	0.25 ml	0.5 ml	0.75 ml	1.0 ml
Approximate strength	3 units	6 units	9 units	12 units

The dose of immune globulin should be given intramuscularly into the opposite limb.

There are no reports of transmission of live attenuated measles vaccine from vaccinees to susceptible contacts.

It has been reported that live attenuated measles virus vaccine may result in a temporary depression of tuberculin skin sensitivity. If a tuberculin test is to be done, it should be administered either before or with Attenuvax.

Children under treatment for tuberculosis have not experienced exacerbation of the disease when immunised with live measles virus vaccine, and no studies have been reported on the effect of measles virus vaccines on untreated tuberculous children.

Use with other vaccines: Routine administration of diphtheria, tetanus and pertussis vaccine and/or oral poliomyelitis vaccine with Attenuvax is not recommended because of insufficient data. However, if circumstances do dictate concurrent vaccination, separate syringes and separate sites for injection should be used.

Attenuvax should not be given less than one month before or after immunisation with other virus vaccines.

Nursing mothers: Because it is not known whether Attenuvax is secreted in human milk, caution should be exercised when considering the use of the vaccine in nursing mothers.

Because the vaccine is slightly acidic (pH 6.2–6.6), patients may complain of burning and/or stinging at the injection site for a short time.

Fever and rash may occur during the month after vaccination. Rarely, high fever or local reaction may occur. Children developing fever may, on rare occasions, exhibit febrile convulsions.

Thrombocytopenia and purpura have occurred rarely.

Forms of optic neuritis, including retrobulbar neuritis and papillitis, have been reported one to three weeks after inoculation with some live virus vaccines.

There have been isolated reports of both the Guillain-Barré syndrome being seen after vaccination and ocular palsies occurring 3–24 days after vaccination with a live attenuated measles virus vaccine, but no definite causal relationship between the vaccine and the disease syndromes has been established.

There have been reports of subacute sclerosing panencephalitis (SSPE) in children who did not have a history of natural measles but did receive measles vaccine. Some of these cases may have resulted from unrecognised measles in the first year of life or possibly from the measles vaccination. Based on estimated nationwide measles vaccine distribution in the USA, the association of SSPE cases to measles vaccination is about one case per million vaccine doses distributed. This is far less than the association with natural measles: 6–22 cases of SSPE per million cases of measles.

Local reactions characterised by marked swelling, redness and vesiculation at the injection site of attenuated live virus measles vaccines have occurred in children who have previously received killed measles vaccine. Rarely, there have been reports of more severe reactions, including prolonged high fevers, panniculitis, and extensive local reactions, which require hospitalisation.

Treatment of overdosage: Not applicable.

Pharmaceutical precautions During shipment, the vaccine should be maintained at a temperature below 10°C to insure that there is no loss of potency.

Prior to reconstitution, the vaccine should be shipped and stored between 2°–8°C. *Protect from light.*

A separate sterile disposable needle and syringe should be used for each vaccinee, free from preservatives, antiseptics, and detergents which may inactivate the vaccine.

Attenuvax contains no preservative; sorbitol and hydrolysed gelatin are added as stabilisers.

The vaccine should be reconstituted using only the diluent provided, and used immediately after reconstitution.

When reconstituted, the vaccine is yellow. It is acceptable for use only when clear and free from particulate matter.

Legal category POM.

Package quantities A single-dose vial of lyophilised vaccine with separate sterile diluent.

Further information Experience from more than 80 million doses of all live measles vaccines given in the USA through 1975 indicates that significant central nervous system reactions such as encephalitis and encephalopathy, occurring within 30 days after vaccination, have been temporally associated with measles vaccine approximately once for every million doses. In no case has it been shown that reactions were actually caused by vaccine. The risk of such serious neurological disorders following live measles virus vaccine administration remains far less than that for encephalitis and encephalopathy caused by natural measles (one per thousand reported cases).

A study suggests that the overall effect of measles vaccine has been to protect against SSPE by preventing measles with its inherent higher risk of SSPE.

The level of antibody response has been shown to persist for at least 13 years without substantial decline. If the present pattern continues, protection can be expected to be lifelong, but continued observation is necessary to demonstrate this point.

Product licence number 0025/0070.

DOLOBID*

Presentation Peach-coloured, capsule-shaped, film-coated tablets, marked 'DOLOBID', containing 250 mg Diflunisal BP; and orange-coloured, film-coated tablets, marked 'DOLOBID', containing 500 mg Diflunisal BP.

Uses Dolobid is indicated for the relief of pain.

Dolobid is also indicated in the relief of pain and inflammation associated with osteoarthritis and rheumatoid arthritis.

Dosage and administration The initial dosage is 500 mg given twice daily. For longer-term therapy, dosage can be adjusted to 250 mg or 500 mg given twice daily. Dosage should be adjusted to the nature and intensity of the pain being treated and should be given twice a day. Even if the initial dose is taken in the afternoon, a second dose should be taken at bedtime. Tablets should be swallowed whole, not crushed or chewed. The highest dose studied in patients was 1500 mg daily.

Use in the elderly: The dosage does not require modification for elderly patients.

Contra-indications, warnings, etc
Contra-indications: Hypersensitivity to the drug.

In patients who have previously experienced acute asthmatic attacks precipitated by aspirin or non-steroidal anti-inflammatory agents.

The drug should not be administered to patients with active gastro-intestinal bleeding.

The use of Dolobid should be avoided in patients with active peptic ulcer.

Dolobid should not be given to pregnant women, since the safety for this use has not been established. Nursing mothers should not take Dolobid, or should stop nursing.

Precautions: Although Dolobid has less effect on platelet function and bleeding time than aspirin, it does inhibit platelet function at higher doses; patients who may be adversely affected should be carefully observed.

Because of reports of adverse eye findings with agents of this class, eye complaints developing during treatment with Dolobid should be fully examined.

Dolobid should be used with caution in patients having a history of gastro-intestinal haemorrhage or ulcers. Fatalities have occurred, rarely.

Use with caution in patients receiving anticoagulant therapy since concomitant administration may prolong the prothrombin time.

The dosage of Dolobid may need to be reduced in patients with renal functional impairment since the major route of excretion is via the kidney. In patients with severe renal impairment, the drug should not be used.

No evidence of renal toxicity has been seen at therapeutic dose levels in man. In rats and dogs, high oral doses of diflunisal (50–200 mg/kg/day) as with aspirin, produced similar pathological changes (gastro-intestinal ulceration and renal papillary oedema). These dosages are approximately 3 to 12 times the maximum dosages recommended in man.

Laboratory tests: AST (SGOT) and ALT (SGPT) rose significantly by three times the upper limit of normal in less than 1% of patients in controlled clinical trials of non-steroidal anti-inflammatory drugs. A patient on Dolobid with signs or symptoms suggesting liver disease or in whom abnormal liver function tests have occurred should be evaluated for evidence of a more severe hepatic reaction. If liver tests persist or worsen, if signs or symptoms of liver disease develop or if systemic manifestations such as eosinophilia or rash occur, Dolobid should be discontinued.

Since paediatric indications and dosage have not yet been established, Dolobid should not be given to children.

Drug interactions: Indomethacin: The combined use of indomethacin and Dolobid has been associated with fatal gastro-intestinal haemorrhage. The combination should not be used. Co-administration of Dolobid with indomethacin increases the plasma level of indomethacin by about 30 to 35% with a concomitant decrease in renal clearance of indomethacin and its conjugate. *Aspirin:* Co-administration of aspirin causes approximately a 15% decrease in plasma levels of Dolobid. *Oral anticoagulant drugs:* The concomitant administration of Dolobid and warfarin or nicoumalone resulted in prolongation of prothrombin time in normal volunteers. This may occur because diflunisal competitively displaces coumarins from protein binding sites. Accordingly, prothrombin time should be monitored during and for several days after the concomitant drug administration of Dolobid and oral anticoagulants. Oral anticoagulants may require adjustment. *Tolbutamide:* No interaction has been seen between tolbutamide and Dolobid. *Hydrochlorothiazide:* Co-administration increases the plasma levels of hydrochlorothiazide by 25 to 35% with a concomitant decrease in renal clearance. This change is not clinically important. Dolobid counteracts the hyperuricaemic effect of hydrochlorothiazide. *Frusemide:* Co-administration did not affect the diuretic activity of frusemide in normal volunteers, but its hyperuricaemic activity was decreased by Dolobid. *Paracetamol:* Co-administration significantly increased the plasma levels of paracetamol by 50%, but the plasma levels of Dolobid were unaffected. *Antacids:* The clinical effect of occasional doses of antacid is insignificant, but this becomes significant when antacids are used continuously. Co-administration of aluminium hydroxide suspension significantly decreases the absorption of Dolobid by approximately 40%. *Other non-steroidal, anti-inflammatory agents:* No clinical data on the safety and efficacy of concomitant administration are available. No recommendations can be made. However, normal volunteers given sulindac and Dolobid showed significantly lower levels of the active sulphide metabolite of sulindac. Normal volunteers given naproxen and Dolobid showed no changes in plasma levels of either drug, but a significant decrease in urinary excretion of naproxen and its glucuronide metabolite.

Side effects: The side effects of Dolobid are related to the length of treatment: the incidence of reactions listed below were from 2 to 14 times less frequent in patients on short-term therapy.

3% to 9% incidence: Gastro-intestinal: Gastro-intestinal pain, dyspepsia, diarrhoea, nausea. *Dermatological:* Rash. *Miscellaneous:* Headache.

1% to 3% incidence: Gastro-intestinal: Vomiting, constipation, flatulence. *Psychiatric:* Somnolence, insomnia. *Central nervous system:* Dizziness. *Special senses:* Tinnitus. *Miscellaneous:* Fatigue/tiredness.

Less than 1% incidence: Gastro-intestinal: Peptic ulcer, gastro-intestinal perforation and bleeding, anorexia, eructation, cholestatic jaundice. *Dermatological:* Pruritus, sweating, dry mucous membranes, stomatitis, photosensitivity, erythema multiforme and Stevens-Johnson syndrome. *Haematological:* Thrombocytopenia. *Genito-urinary:* Dysuria, renal impairment including renal failure, interstitial nephritis. *Psychiatric:* Nervousness, depression. *Central nervous system:* Vertigo. *Hypersensitivity reactions:* Acute anaphylactic reaction with bronchospasm.

A potentially fatal hypersensitivity syndrome has been reported which may include constitutional symptoms (fever, rigors); dermatological findings listed above; involvement of major organs (changes in liver function, jaundice, leucopenia, thrombocytopenia, eosinophilia, renal impairment including renal failure); and less specific findings such as adenitis, arthralgia, arthritis, malaise, anorexia, and disorientation. *Miscellaneous:* Asthenia, and oedema.

Other reported reactions with an unknown causal relationship: Respiratory: Dyspnoea. *Cardiovascular:* Palpitation, syncope. *Special senses:* Transient visual disturbances. *Nervous system:* Paraesthesiae. *Musculoskeletal:* Muscle cramps. *Miscellaneous:* Chest pain.

Treatment of overdosage:

The initial plasma half-life following single oral doses of diflunisal seems to be dose dependent, ranging from approximately 7.5 hours for a 250 mg dose to 11 hours for a 500 mg dose.

Cases of overdosage have occurred and fatalities have been reported. The most common signs and symptoms observed with overdosage were drowsiness, vomiting, nausea, diarrhoea, hyperventilation, tachycardia, sweating, tinnitus, disorientation, stupor, and coma. Diminished urine output and cardiorespiratory arrest have also been reported. The lowest dose of Dolobid alone at which death was reported was 15 g; death has been reported from a mixed drug overdose that included 7.5 g Dolobid.

When an overdose is taken, the stomach should be emptied by inducing vomiting or gastric lavage, and the patient observed carefully and given symptomatic and supportive treatment.

To facilitate urinary elimination of the drug, attempt to maintain renal function. Because of the high degree of protein binding, haemodialysis is not recommended.

Pharmaceutical precautions Store in a cool place, protected from light.

Legal category POM.

Package quantities Dolobid 250 mg tablets are supplied in packs of 50, 100 and 1,000 tablets; the 500 mg tablets in packs of 100.

Further information Following a single therapeutic dose, significant relief of pain usually occurs within the first hour. Dolobid has a prolonged duration of action and can therefore be administered twice daily.

Dolobid has a dose-related effect on platelet function. In normal volunteers given Dolobid over eight days, 250 mg twice daily had no effect on platelet function and 500 mg twice daily affected platelet function only slightly. However, at 1,000 mg twice daily, which exceeds the maximum recommended dose, platelet function was inhibited. In contrast to aspirin, these effects were reversible.

Bleeding time was unaffected by 250 mg twice daily, slightly increased at 500 mg twice daily, and the greater increase at 1,000 mg twice daily was not statistically significant from placebo.

Faecal blood loss is significantly less following treatment with Dolobid (250 mg b.d.) than that associated with aspirin (600 mg q.i.d.).

Product licence numbers
250 mg tablet   0025/0128
500 mg tablet   0025/0146

H-B-VAX* ▼
Presentation
For recipients aged over 10 years: 1 ml single-dose vials of sterile suspension containing 20 mcg of hepatitis B surface antigen adsorbed on to alum.

For recipients aged under 10 years: 0.5 ml vial of sterile suspension containing 10 mcg of hepatitis B surface antigen adsorbed on to alum.

Uses H-B-Vax is indicated for immunisation against infection caused by hepatitis B virus, including all known subtypes. Vaccination is recommended for persons of all ages, especially those who are or will be at increased risk.

H-B-Vax will not prevent hepatitis caused by other organisms such as hepatitis A virus, non-A, non-B hepatitis viruses, or other viruses known to infect the liver.

The incidence of infection varies greatly in different parts of the world, and the vaccination strategy should be adjusted accordingly.

In areas of low prevalence, vaccination should be limited to those who are at increased risk of infection, such individuals would be found among:

Health-care personnel: Dentists: physicians and surgeons; nurses and hospital ancillary workers; dental hygienists; laboratory personnel handling blood products from known carriers; health-care students; especially those health-care personnel treating known carriers.

Patient and patient contacts: Patients in haemodialysis, haematology and oncology units; patients who need frequent and/or large-volume blood transfusions and clotting factor concentrates; residents and staff of mental institutions; intimate contacts of persons with persistent hepatitis B antigenaemia. Infants born to HBsAg positive mothers.

Plasma fractionation workers.

Persons at increased risk due to their sexual practices: Homosexually active males; prostitutes; persons who repeatedly contract sexually transmitted diseases.

Users of illicit injectable drugs.

Those living for prolonged periods in countries where hepatitis B is endemic.

Dosage and administration *H-B-Vax is for intramuscular use only; it must not be given intravenously, subcutaneously or intradermally.*

The deltoid muscle is the preferred site of injection in adults; the antero-lateral thigh is the preferred site in infants and children.

Shake well before use. After thorough agitation H-B-Vax is an opaque, white suspension.

The immunisation regimen consists of three doses of vaccine given intramuscularly.
1st dose: at elected date
2nd dose: 1 month later
3rd dose: 6 months after first dose, as a 'booster'

The volume of dose to be given on each occasion is:

Group	Initial	1 month	6 months
Children (birth to 10 years)	0.5 ml (10 mcg)	0.5 ml (10 mcg)	0.5 ml (10 mcg)
Infants born to HBsAg positive mothers	0.5 ml (at birth) plus immune globulin*	0.5 ml	0.5 ml
Adults and children over 10 years	1.0 ml (20 mcg)	1.0 ml (20 mcg)	1.0 ml (20 mcg)
Dialysis and immuno-compromised patients	2.0 ml† (40 mcg)	2.0 ml† (40 mcg)	2.0 ml† (40 mcg)

* Administer at a different site; advice on specific dosage to be obtained through the Public Health Laboratory Service. In clinical studies, the dosage range of HBIG used was 110–148 units.
† Two 1.0 ml doses given at different sites.

Contra-indications, warnings, etc
Contra-indications: Hypersensitivity to any component of the vaccine. Patients whose symptoms suggest hypersensitivity after an injection of H-B-Vax should not receive further injections.

Warnings: Patients with immunodeficiency or those receiving immunosuppressive therapy require larger vaccine doses and respond less well than healthy individuals.

Because of the prolonged incubation period of hepatitis B, infection may be present at the time of vaccination. H-B-Vax may be ineffective in such patients.

Although study is still needed to determine the

effectiveness of H-B-Vax after infection with hepatitis B, it has been shown that an injection of up to 5 ml of hepatitis B immunoglobulin does not interfere with the action of H-B-Vax injected at a different site.

Precautions: Adrenaline Injection BP (1:1000) should be available for immediate use should an anaphylactoid reaction occur.

Any serious active infection is reason for delaying vaccination unless, in the physician's opinion, this delay might entail even greater risk.

Caution should be exercised in administering H-B-Vax to individuals in whom a febrile or systemic reaction could pose a significant risk such as in patients with a severely compromised cardio-pulmonary status.

Nursing mothers: Although limited studies have shown no evidence that H-B-Vax is secreted in human milk, the physician should exercise caution before vaccinating nursing mothers with H-B-Vax.

Children: At the recommended doses, H-B-Vax has been shown to be well tolerated and highly immunogenic in newborns, infants, and children of all ages.

Antibodies acquired either from the mother or from hepatitis B immune globulin do not interfere with the active response to H-B-Vax.

Pregnancy: H-B-Vax is not recommended for pregnant women. Animal reproduction studies have not been conducted with the vaccine. It is also not known whether H-B-Vax can cause fetal harm when administered to pregnant women, or can affect reproductive capacity.

Adverse reactions: H-B-Vax is generally well tolerated.

In studies involving over 19,000 individuals, no serious adverse reactions were reported, and there was no tendency towards increased frequency or severity of complaints following successive doses of the vaccine.

In several other studies, it was found that both the incidence of adverse reactions and of elevations in ALT were not significantly different from those seen in placebo recipients.

Specific adverse reactions reported in a study of 1,255 healthy adults were:

Most commonly, injection site soreness including erythema, swelling, warmth and induration. Headache; upper respiratory tract reactions; GI complaints such as anorexia, nausea, vomiting, abdominal pain, and diarrhoea; fatigue/asthenia; fever ($\geq 100°F$), and myalgia.

Other less frequent adverse reactions classified by body system were:

Body as a whole: malaise, chills, sensation of warmth, irritability, diaphoresis. *Digestive:* abdominal cramps. *Haematological and lymphatic:* adenitis. *Musculoskeletal:* arthralgia. *Nervous system:* dizziness, disturbed sleep, paraesthesiae. *Integumentary:* nonspecific rash.

Other rare reactions include an immediate hypersensitivity reaction such as urticaria, angioneurotic oedema or pruritus; and a rare delayed reaction seen within days or weeks of vaccination as transient arthritis, fever, or such dermatological reactions as urticaria, erythema multiforme or ecchymosis.

No causal relationship has been established between H-B-Vax and the rare reports of paraesthesiae and acute radiculoneuropathy, including Guillain-Barré syndrome.

Treatment of overdosage: Not applicable.

Pharmaceutical precautions Store at 2°–8°C (35.6°–46.4°F). DO NOT FREEZE. The vaccine is used directly as supplied; no dilution or reconstitution is necessary. Thiomersal in 1:20,000 dilution is present in the vaccine as a preservative.

Legal category POM.

Package quantities One-ml vials of sterile suspension containing vaccine.

Further information The protective efficacy of H-B-Vax has been demonstrated in human populations. In a study involving individuals with a high risk of contracting hepatitis B virus infection, H-B-Vax has been shown to reduce the incidence of infection by over 90%. The vaccine protected against acute hepatitis B, asymptomatic infection, and chronic antigenaemia. There was evidence of immunity (protective antibody) in 78% of vaccinated subjects after administration of two doses of the three-dose vaccine regimen. However, the third dose was required to raise the proportion of seroconvertors to 92%, induce higher titres, and provide an extended period of protection.

Responsiveness is age dependent: children show a more vigorous response than adults.

The duration of protection and need for booster doses are not yet defined. Individuals who remain at high risk of exposure to hepatitis B virus may wish to determine periodically their anti-HBg level. If antibody levels fall below 10 i.u./l, administration of an additional dose of H-B-Vax should be considered.

Product licence number 0025/0164.

INDOCID*

Presentation Ivory, opaque capsules containing 25 mg or 50 mg Indomethacin BP, marked 'INDOCID 25' and 'INDOCID 50' respectively.

Opaque-ivory headed, transparent-blue based capsules carrying white and blue pellets containing 75 mg indomethacin in sustained-release form, marked 'INDOCID R 693'.

A fruit-flavoured suspension containing in each 5 ml, 25 mg indomethacin.

Polyethylene glycol suppositories containing 100 mg Indomethacin BP.

Uses Non-steroidal anti-inflammatory agent indicated for the active stages of rheumatoid arthritis; osteoarthritis; ankylosing spondylitis; degenerative joint disease of the hip; acute musculoskeletal disorders; low-back pain; and acute gout.

Also indicated in inflammation, pain and oedema following orthopaedic procedures; and the treatment of pain and associated symptoms of primary dysmenorrhoea.

Indocid Suppositories may be used where night pain and morning stiffness are prominent. One suppository at bedtime will frequently give relief from pain and stiffness for 13 to 16 hours after administration.

Indocid-R: Indocid-R may be substituted for all the indications of Indocid except acute gout, as clinical evidence is not currently available for this dosage form in this condition.

Dosage and administration The dosage of Indocid should be carefully adjusted to suit the needs of the individual patient.

Oral therapy: In order to reduce the possibility of gastrointestinal disturbances, *Indocid/Indocid-R Capsules and*

Suspension should always be taken with food, milk or an antacid. (Note, however, that Indocid Suspension should not be mixed with an antacid, but should be taken separately, because indomethacin is unstable in an alkaline medium.) Indocid Suspension should not be diluted.

In chronic conditions, starting therapy with a low dosage, increasing this gradually as necessary, and continuing a trial of therapy for an adequate period (in some cases, up to one month) will give the best results with a minimum of unwanted reactions.

The recommended oral dosage range is 50–200 mg daily. Paediatric dosage not established.

Dosage in dysmenorrhoea: Up to 75 mg a day, starting with onset of cramps or bleeding, and continuing for as long as the symptoms usually last.

Suppositories: Adults: 1 suppository to be inserted once or twice a day. One should be used at bedtime. If another is necessary, it should be used in the morning.

Dosage for Indocid-R: The sustained-release capsule may be given once or, where necessary, twice a day depending on patient needs and response.

Use in the elderly: Indocid should be used with particular care in older patients who are more prone to adverse reactions.

Contra-indications, warnings, etc

Contra-indications: Children (conditions for safe use not established); active peptic ulcer; a recurrent history of gastro-intestinal lesions; in patients who have nasal polyps associated with angioneurotic oedema, or who show sensitivity to indomethacin, aspirin, or other non-steroidal anti-inflammatory drugs. Indocid should not be used during pregnancy or lactation. Indocid is excreted in breast milk. Indocid Suppositories are contra-indicated in patients with a recent history of proctitis.

Precautions: Headache, sometimes accompanied by dizziness and lightheadedness, may occur, usually early in treatment. Starting therapy with a low dosage and increasing it gradually will minimise the incidence of headache. These symptoms frequently disappear on continuing therapy or reducing the dosage, but if headache persists despite dosage reduction, Indocid should be withdrawn. Patients should be warned that they may experience dizziness and, if they do, should not drive a car or undertake potentially dangerous activities needing alertness. Indocid should be used cautiously in patients with psychiatric disorders, epilepsy, or parkinsonism, as it may tend to aggravate these disorders.

Gastro-intestinal disturbances may be minimised by giving Indocid orally with food, milk or an antacid. They usually disappear on reducing the dosage; if not, the risks of continuing therapy should be weighed against the possible benefits.

Peptic ulcer has been reported in a small proportion of patients. Haemorrhage and perforation have occurred in a small proportion of patients, usually with a history of peptic ulcer or those receiving corticosteroids or salicylates concurrently. In some cases, however, there was no history of peptic ulcer, or of other agents being used. If gastro-intestinal bleeding does occur, Indocid should immediately be discontinued.

Tenesmus and irritation of the rectal mucosa (sigmoidoscopic examination of a number of patients showed no mucosal changes) have been reported with Indocid Suppositories.

Indocid may mask the signs and symptoms of infection. In patients with rheumatoid arthritis, eye changes may occur which may be related to the underlying disease or to the therapy. Therefore, in chronic rheumatoid disease, ophthalmological examinations are recommended.

Patients should be periodically observed to allow early detection of any unwanted effects on peripheral blood (anaemia), liver function or gastro-intestinal tract.

Indocid Suppositories should be used with caution in patients with a recent history of rectal bleeding.

Indocid can inhibit platelet aggregation. The effect usually disappears within 24 hours of discontinuing Indocid. Bleeding time is prolonged (but within normal range) in normal adults. Because this effect may be exaggerated in patients with underlying haemostatic defects, Indocid should be used cautiously in patients with coagulation defects.

Indocid should be used with caution in patients with impaired renal function. There have been reports of worsening renal impairment in such patients, some of whom developed hyperkalaemia. Similarly, there are reports of acute renal failure in patients with sodium retention associated with hepatic disease or congestive heart failure. Most of these renal abnormalities were reversible.

Laboratory tests: Borderline elevations of one or more liver tests may occur, and rarely, significant elevations of ALT (SGPT) or AST (SGOT) have been seen. If abnormal liver tests persist or worsen, if clinical signs and symptoms consistent with liver disease develop or if systemic manifestations such as rash or eosinophilia occur, Indocid should be stopped.

Drug interactions: Co-administration of aspirin may decrease blood levels of indomethacin. If Indocid is added to the treatment of patients receiving anticoagulant therapy, they should be observed closely for alterations of the prothrombin time.

Co-administration of diflunisal with Indocid increases the plasma level of indomethacin by about a third with a concomitant decrease in renal clearance. Fatal gastro-intestinal haemorrhage has occurred. The combination should not be used.

Co-administration of probenecid may increase plasma levels of indomethacin.

Because Indocid may reduce the antihypertensive effect of beta-blockers, patients receiving dual therapy should have the antihypertensive effect of their therapy reassessed.

If the patient is receiving corticosteroids concomitantly, a reduction in dosage of these may be possible, but should only be affected slowly under supervision.

Indocid is an inhibitor of prostaglandin synthesis and therefore the following drug interactions may occur:

Indocid may raise plasma lithium levels and reduce renal lithium clearance in subjects with steady state plasma lithium concentrations. At the onset of such combined therapy, plasma lithium concentration should be monitored more frequently.

Indocid may reduce the diuretic and antihypertensive effect of thiazides and frusemide in some patients. Indocid may cause blocking of the frusemide-induced increase in plasma renin activity.

Warnings and adverse reactions: CNS reactions – headache, dizziness, and lightheadedness. Mental confusion, anxiety, syncope, drowsiness, convulsions, coma, peripheral neuropathy, muscle weakness, involuntary muscle movements, insomnia, depression and other psychiatric disturbances such as depersonalisation may occur as transient reactions that often disappear with continued or reduced dosage. However, occasionally, severe reactions require stopping therapy.

Gastro-intestinal – the more frequent reactions are nausea, anorexia, vomiting, epigastric distress, abdominal pain, constipation, and diarrhoea. Others are ulceration (single or multiple) of oesophagus, stomach, duodenum or elsewhere in the small intestine, sometimes with haemorrhage and perforation (a few fatalities have been reported); gastro-intestinal bleeding without obvious ulcer formation; increased abdominal pain in patients with pre-existing ulcerative colitis. Rarely, intestinal ulceration followed by stenosis and obstruction has been reported. Reactions occurring infrequently are stomatitis; gastritis; bleeding from the sigmoid colon (occult or from a diverticulum); perforation of pre-existing sigmoid lesions such as diverticula and carcinomata; ulcerative colitis and regional ileitis (causal relationship not established). With suppositories, tenesmus and irritation of the rectal mucosa have occasionally been reported, but sigmoidoscopic examination in a number of cases has not revealed mucosal changes.

Hepatic – rarely, toxic hepatitis and jaundice (some fatalities reported).

Cardiovascular/renal – oedema, increased blood pressure, tachycardia, chest pain, arrhythmia, palpitation, congestive heart failure, blood urea elevation and haematuria (all infrequent).

Dermatological/hypersensitivity – pruritus, urticaria, angioneurotic oedema, angiitis, erythema nodosum, skin rash, exfoliative dermatitis, loss of hair, rapid fall in blood pressure resembling a shock-like state, and acute respiratory distress including sudden dyspnoea and asthma (all infrequent). Bronchospasm may be precipitated in patients suffering from or with a history of bronchial asthma or allergic disease.

Haematological – infrequently, blood dyscrasias may occur including leucopenia, petechiae or ecchymosis, purpura, aplastic and haemolytic anaemia, and particularly thrombocytopenia. Rarely, agranulocytosis and bone-marrow depression. Because some patients may develop anaemia secondary to obvious or occult gastrointestinal bleeding, appropriate blood determinations are recommended.

Ocular – infrequently, blurred vision, and orbital and periorbital pain. Corneal deposits and retinal disturbances including those of the macula reported in patients with rheumatoid arthritis on prolonged therapy, but similar changes seen in patients with rheumatoid arthritis who had not received Indocid.

Aural – infrequently, tinnitus (rarely, deafness).

Miscellaneous – vaginal bleeding, hyperglycaemia, glycosuria, epistaxis, ulcerative stomatitis.

The following adverse reactions have been associated with use of Indocid Suppositories: tenesmus; proctitis; rectal bleeding, burning, pain, discomfort, and itching.

Treatment of overdosage: If ingestion is recent, gastric lavage should be performed. Otherwise therapy is supportive; the progress of the patient should be followed for several days, as gastro-intestinal ulceration and haemorrhage are reported side-effects of indomethacin. Antacids may be helpful.

Pharmaceutical precautions Keep container well closed; store in a dry place below 25°C, protected from light. Indocid Suspension should also be protected from freezing.

Indocid/Indocid-R Capsules and Suspension should always be taken with food, milk or an antacid. (Note, however, that Indocid Suspension should not be mixed with an antacid but should be taken separately because indomethacin is unstable in an alkaline medium.) Indocid Suspension should not be diluted.

Legal category POM.

Package quantities *Capsules:* 25 mg, bottles of 100 and 500; 50 mg, bottles of 100; 75 mg, bottles of 100. *Suppositories:* Boxes of 10. *Suspension:* Bottles of 200 ml.

Further information Nil.

Product licence numbers

25 mg	0025/0111
50 mg	0025/0112
75 mg	0025/0125
Suppositories	0025/0062
Suspension	0025/0120

MERUVAX* II ▼

Presentation Lyophilised powder for injection. When reconstituted, Meruvax II Injection contains in each dose not less than the equivalent of 1,000 $TCID_{50}$ (tissue culture infective doses) of rubella virus vaccine expressed in terms of the assigned titre of the FDA (USA) Reference Rubella Virus. It is prepared from the Wistar Institute RA 27/3 strain of live attenuated rubella virus, adapted to and propagated in human diploid cell (WI-38) culture.

Uses Immunisation against rubella.
Children between 12 months of age and puberty: Meruvax II is indicated for immunisation against rubella in boys and girls from 12 months of age to puberty. No booster is needed. It is not recommended for infants less than a year old because they may retain maternal rubella-neutralising antibodies which may interfere with the immune response. Children in kindergarten and the first years at infants' school deserve priority for vaccination because they often are epidemiologically the major source of virus dissemination in the community. A history of rubella illness is usually not reliable enough to exclude children for immunisation.

Unimmunised children of susceptible pregnant women should receive live attenuated rubella vaccine. By this protection, children are less likely to acquire natural rubella and introduce the virus into the household.

Adolescent and adult males: Vaccination of adolescent or adult males may be useful in preventing or controlling outbreaks of rubella in circumscribed population groups.

Pregnant females: Pregnant females must NOT be given live attenuated rubella virus vaccine.

Animal reproduction studies have not been conducted with Meruvax II. It is also not known whether Meruvax II causes fetal harm in the pregnant woman or affects her reproductive capacity. There is evidence to suggest the transmission of rubella vaccine viruses to products of conception.

If a pregnant woman is inadvertently vaccinated or if she becomes pregnant within three months of vaccination, she should be counselled on the possible risks to the fetus. In a ten-year study involving 700 pregnant women who received rubella vaccination within three months of conception, none of their newborn infants had abnormalities compatible with congenital rubella syndrome.

Congenital malformations do occur in up to 7% of all live births. Their chance appearance after vaccination could lead to misinterpretation of the cause, particularly if the prior rubella-immune status of the vaccinee is unknown.

Non-pregnant adolescent and adult females: Immunisation of susceptible non-pregnant adolescent and adult females of child-bearing age with live attenuated rubella vaccine is indicated when:
(a) susceptibility to rubella has been established by the single radial haemolysis (radial diffusion) test;
(b) she agrees not to become pregnant for the next three months after vaccination and is informed of the reason for this precaution (this precaution also applies to women in the immediate post-partum period when it may be found most convenient to vaccinate – but see 'Nursing mothers');
(c) post-pubertal females are told of the frequent occurrence of self-limiting arthralgia and possible arthritis beginning two to four weeks after vaccination.

Vaccinating susceptible post-pubertal females confers individual protection against acquired rubella infection during pregnancy. This in turn prevents infection of the fetus and consequent congenital rubella injury.

Immunity is evidenced by a specific rubella antibody titre of 15 international units (1:16) or greater. Vaccination is then unnecessary.

Revaccination: Based on available evidence, there is no reason to revaccinate children who were vaccinated originally when 12 months of age or older; however, children vaccinated when younger than 12 months of age should be revaccinated. (Meruvax II is not recommended in infants less than 12 months of age.)

Use with other vaccines: Routine administration of diphtheria, tetanus and pertussis vaccine and/or oral poliomyelitis vaccine with Meruvax II is not recommended because of insufficient data. However, if circumstances do dictate concurrent vaccination, separate syringes and separate sites for injection should be used. Meruvax II should not be given less than one month before or after immunisation with other virus vaccines.

Dosage and administration The total volume reconstituted from the single-dose pack should be injected subcutaneously, preferably into the outer aspect of the upper arm, after suitably cleansing the immunisation site.

Meruvax II should not be injected intravenously, or administered intranasally.
Do not give immune serum globulin (ISG) with Meruvax II.

Reconstitution: To reconstitute the vaccine, all the diluent provided should be injected into a vial of lyophilised vaccine, and this agitated to ensure thorough mixing. All the reconstituted vaccine is then withdrawn into the syringe and injected subcutaneously.

Contra-indications, warnings, etc
Contra-indications: Do not give Meruvax II to pregnant females; the possible effects of the vaccine on fetal development or the mother's reproductive capacity are unknown at this time. When vaccination of post-pubertal females is undertaken, pregnancy must be avoided for three months following vaccination.

Anaphylactoid reaction to neomycin. (Each dose of reconstituted vaccine contains approximately 25 mcg of neomycin.)

Any febrile respiratory illness, or other active or suspected infection.

Active untreated tuberculosis.

Patients receiving immunosuppressive therapy. This contra-indication does not apply to patients who are receiving corticosteroids as replacement therapy, e.g. for Addison's disease.

Individuals with blood dyscrasias, leukaemia, lymphomas of any type, or other malignant neoplasms affecting the bone marrow or lymphatic systems.

Primary immunodeficiency states, including cellular immune deficiencies, hypogammaglobulinaemic and dysgammaglobulinaemic states.

Those with a family history of congenital or hereditary immunodeficiency, until their immune competence is demonstrated.

Precautions: Meruvax II is for subcutaneous administration; *it must not be given intravenously.*

Adrenaline should be available for immediate use should an anaphylactoid reaction occur.

Excretion of small amounts of live attenuated rubella virus from the nose and throat has occurred in the majority of susceptible individuals 7–28 days after vaccination. There is no definitive evidence to indicate that such virus is transmitted to susceptible persons who are in contact with vaccinated individuals. Consequently, transmission, while accepted as a theoretical possibility, has not been regarded as a significant risk. However, transmission of the vaccine virus via breast milk has been documented.

There is no evidence that live rubella virus vaccine given after exposure will prevent illness. There is, however, no contra-indication to vaccinating children already exposed to natural rubella.

Vaccination should be deferred for at least three months following blood or plasma transfusions or administration of human immune serum globulin. However, susceptible post-partum patients who received blood products may receive Meruvax II prior to discharge provided that a recent HI titre is drawn 6–8 weeks after vaccination to insure seroconversion. Similarly, although studies with other live rubella virus vaccines suggest that Meruvax II may be given in the immediate post-partum period to those non-immune women who have received anti-Rh_o (D) globulin (human) without interfering with vaccine effectiveness, a follow-up post-vaccination HI titre should also be determined.

It has been reported that live attenuated rubella vaccine may temporarily depress tuberculin skin sensitivity. If a tuberculin test is to be done, therefore, it should be administered before or simultaneously with Meruvax II.

Nursing mothers: Recent studies have shown that nursing mothers immunised with live attenuated measles vaccine may secrete and transmit the virus via breast milk. None of the nursed infants showed severe disease, although one did show mild clinical disease typical of acquired rubella. Caution should therefore be exercised when Meruvax II is administered to the nursing mother.

Adverse reactions: Because the vaccine is slightly acidic (pH 6.2–6.6), patients may complain of burning and/or stinging at the injection site for a short time.

Symptoms of the same kind as those seen following natural rubella may occur after vaccination. These include regional lymphadenopathy, urticaria, rash, malaise, sore throat, fever, headache, polyneuritis, and occasionally temporary arthralgia that is infrequently associated with signs of inflammation. Local pain, induration, wheal and flare, and erythema may occur at the injection site. Reactions are usually mild and transient.

Moderate fever (38.3° to 39.3°C/101° to 102.9°F) occurs occasionally, and high fever (above 39.4°C/103°F) occurs less commonly.

Reactions are usually mild and transient.

In children, joint reactions are rare and of brief duration if they do occur. In women, incidence rates for arthritis and arthralgia are generally higher than those seen in children (children: 0–3%; women: 12–20%) and the reactions tend to be more marked and of longer duration. Symptoms may persist for a matter of months or, on rare occasions, for years. In adolescent girls, the reactions appear to be intermediate in incidence between those seen in children and in adult women. Even in older women (35–45 years) these reactions are generally well tolerated and rarely interfere with normal activities.

Forms of optic neuritis, including retrobulbar neuritis and papillitis, have been reported one to three weeks after inoculation with some live virus vaccines.

Clinical experience with live virus rubella vaccines indicates that encephalitis and other nervous system reactions have occurred very rarely. A cause-and-effect relationship has not been established.

In view of the decreases in platelet counts that have been reported, thrombocytopenic purpura is a theoretical hazard.

Pharmaceutical precautions During shipment, to ensure that there is no loss of potency, the vaccine must be maintained at a temperature of 10°C (50°F) or less.

Before reconstitution, Meruvax II should be stored at 2° to 8°C (35.6° to 46.4°F), and *protected from light*.

A separate sterile disposable needle and syringe should be used for each vaccinee. Preservatives, antiseptics and detergents may inactivate the vaccine.

Meruvax II contains no preservative; sorbitol and hydrolysed gelatin are added as stabilisers.

Only the diluent supplied should be used for reconstitution. The vaccine should be used within one hour of reconstitution.

When reconstituted, the vaccine is yellow. It is acceptable for use only when clear and free from particulate matter.

Legal category POM.

Package quantities Single-dose vials of lyophilised vaccine with separate sterile diluent.

Further information A single injection of Meruvax II has been shown to induce rubella haemagglutination-inhibiting (HI) antibodies in over 97% of susceptible subjects.

Vaccine-induced antibody levels have been shown to persist for at least ten years without substantial decline. If the present pattern continues, it will provide a basis for the expectation that immunity following the vaccine will be permanent. However, continued surveillance will be required to demonstrate this point.

Product licence number 0025/0149.

MIDAMOR*

Presentation Yellow, diamond-shaped tablets, marked 'MSD 92', containing Amiloride Hydrochloride BP equivalent to 5 mg anhydrous amiloride hydrochloride.

Uses Potassium-conserving agent; diuretic.

Although Midamor has mild natriuretic, diuretic and antihypertensive activity when used alone which may be additive to the effects of thiazides and other saluretic-antihypertensive agents, its principal indication is as concurrent therapy with thiazides or more potent diuretics to conserve potassium during periods of vigorous diuresis and during long-term maintenance therapy.

In *congestive heart failure*, the positive effect of Midamor on potassium balance may be especially useful for patients also receiving digitalis, who are particularly sensitive to lowered potassium levels. In *hypertension*, it is used as an adjunct to therapy with thiazides and similar agents to prevent posassium depletion. When combined with hydrochlorothiazide, Midamor gives an additive antihypertensive action. In *hepatic cirrhosis with ascites*, Midamor usually provides adequate diuresis with diminished potassium loss and less risk of metabolic alkalosis, when used alone. It may be used with more potent diuretics when a greater diuresis is required.

Dosage and administration *Midamor alone:* The initial dosage should be 10 mg (as a single dose or 5 mg twice a day). This may be increased if necessary, but must not exceed 20 mg (4 tablets) a day. After diuresis has been achieved, the dosage may be reduced by 5 mg increments to the least amount required.

Midamor usually begins to act within two hours. Its effect upon electrolyte excretion reaches a peak between six and ten hours, and lasts about 24 hours. Most patients respond during the first day of treatment, but maximum therapeutic effect may not be seen for several days. As in all diuretic therapy, the rate of weight loss and the serum electrolyte levels should determine the dosage. The most satisfactory rate of weight loss is generally about 0.5–1.0 kg a day.

Midamor with other diuretic therapy: When Midamor is used with a diuretic which is given on an intermittent basis, it should be given at the same time as the diuretic.

Congestive heart failure: Initially, 5 or 10 mg (1 or 2 tablets) a day, together with the usual dosage of the diuretic concurrently employed. If diuresis is not achieved with minimal dosage of both agents, the dosage of both may be gradually increased, but that of Midamor should not exceed 20 mg (4 tablets) a day. Once diuresis has been achieved, reduction in dosage of both agents may be attempted for maintenance therapy. The dosage of both drugs is determined by the diuresis and the level of plasma potassium.

Hypertension: 5 or 10 mg (1 or 2 tablets) a day, together with the usual antihypertensive dosage of the thiazide concurrently employed. It is not usually necessary to exceed 10 mg of Midamor a day; in any event, not more than 20 mg (4 tablets) of Midamor a day should be given.

Hepatic cirrhosis with ascites: When used with another diuretic, treatment should be started with a small dose of Midamor, i.e. 5 mg (1 tablet), plus a low dosage of the other diuretic agent. If necessary, dosage of both agents may be increased gradually until there is effective diuresis.

The dosage of Midamor should not exceed 20 mg (4 tablets) a day. Maintenance doses may be lower than those required to initiate diuresis; reduction in the daily dosage should therefore be attempted when the patient's weight is stabilised. Gradual weight reduction in cirrhotic patients is especially desirable to reduce the likelihood of untoward reactions.

Use in the elderly: The elderly are more likely to experience hyperkalaemia since renal reserve may be reduced. The dosage should be carefully adjusted according to renal function, blood electrolytes and diuretic response.

Contra-indications, warnings, etc

Contra-indications: Hyperkalaemia (plasma potassium over 5.5 mmol/l); other potassium-conserving agents or potassium supplements; anuria, acute renal failure, severe progressive renal disease, diabetic nephropathy; patients with blood urea over 10 mmol/l, serum creatinine over 130 μmol/l, or with diabetes mellitus should not receive amiloride hydrochloride without careful frequent monitoring of serum electrolytes and blood urea levels; prior sensitivity to amiloride hydrochloride. In renal impairment, use of a potassium-conserving agent may result in rapid development of hyperkalaemia. Safety for use in children is not established. See also 'Use in pregnancy' under 'Precautions'.

Precautions – Diabetes mellitus: Hyperkalaemia has commonly occurred in diabetic patients, especially those with chronic renal disease or prerenal azotaemia. The status of renal function should therefore be determined before Midamor is given to known or suspected diabetic patients. Midamor should be discontinued for at least three days before a glucose-tolerance test, because one patient with poorly controlled diabetes mellitus, who became severely hyperkalaemic while receiving amiloride hydrochloride, died following two repeated intravenous glucose-tolerance tests.

Metabolic or respiratory acidosis: Potassium-conserving therapy should be initiated only with caution in severely ill patients in whom metabolic or respiratory acidosis may occur, e.g. patients with cardiopulmonary disease of decompensated diabetes. Shifts in acid-base balance alter the balance of extracellular-intracellular potassium, and the development of acidosis may be associated with rapid increases in plasma potassium.

Hyperkalaemia (plasma potassium levels over 5.5 mmol/litre): This has been observed in patients receiving amiloride hydrochloride, alone or with other diuretics, particularly in the aged, in diabetics, and in hospital patients with hepatic cirrhosis or cardiac oedema who had known renal involvement, were seriously ill, or were undergoing vigorous diuretic therapy. Such patients should be observed carefully for clinical, laboratory, and ECG evidence of hyperkalaemia (not always associated with an abnormal ECG).

Some deaths have been reported in this group of patients. If hyperkalaemia develops, Midamor should be discontinued immediately, and if necessary, active measures taken to reduce the plasma potassium to normal.

Electrolyte imbalance and blood urea increases: Hyponatraemia and hypochloraemia may occur when amiloride hydrochloride is used with other diuretics. Reversible increases in blood urea levels have been reported accompanying vigorous diuresis, especially when diuretics were used in seriously ill patients, such as those with hepatic cirrhosis with ascites and metabolic alkalosis, or those with resistant oedema. Careful monitoring of serum electrolytes and blood urea levels should therefore be carried out when Midamor is given with oral diuretics to such patients. Reports suggest that patients with pre-existing severe liver disease treated with diuretics, including amiloride hydrochloride, may experience hepatic encephalopathy, manifested by tremors, confusion and coma, and increased jaundice.

Drug interactions: Lithium should generally not be given

with diuretics because they reduce its renal clearance and add a high risk of lithium toxicity.

Effects in cirrhotic patients: Oral diuretic therapy is more frequently accompanied by adverse reactions in patients with hepatic cirrhosis and ascites, because these patients are intolerant of acute shifts in electrolyte balance, and because they often already have hypokalaemia as a result of associated aldosteronism.

Hepatic encephalopathy, manifested by tremors, confusion and coma, has been reported.

In cirrhotic patients, jaundice associated with the underlying disease process has deepened in a few instances, but the relationship to amiloride is uncertain.

Use in pregnancy and the nursing mother: Because clinical experience is limited. Midamor is not recommended for use during pregnancy. The potential benefits of the drug must be weighed against possible hazards to the fetus if it is administered to a woman of childbearing age.

It is not known whether Midamor is excreted in human milk. Because there is risk that it might take this route of excretion, and that it might then cause serious adverse reactions in the nursing infant, the mother should either stop nursing or stop taking the drug. The decision depends on the importance of the drug to the mother.

Side effects: Midamor is usually well tolerated and, except for hyperkalaemia, significant adverse effects are infrequent. Minor adverse reactions have been reported in about 20% of patients but their relationship to amiloride is uncertain. Nausea/anorexia, abdominal pain, flatulence, and mild skin rash are probably due to amiloride; but other effects are generally associated with diuresis or with the underlying disease being treated.

Body as a whole: Headache, weakness, fatigue, back pain, chest pain, neck/shoulder ache, pain in the extremities.

Cardiovascular: Angina pectoris, orthostatic hypotension, arrhythmias, palpitation, one patient with partial heart block developed complete heart block.

Digestive: Anorexia, nausea, vomiting, diarrhoea, constipation, abdominal pain, GI bleeding, jaundice, thirst, dyspepsia, heartburn, flatulence.

Metabolic: Elevated plasma potassium levels above 5.5 mmol/l.

Integumentary: Pruritus, rash, dryness of mouth, alopecia.

Musculoskeletal: Muscle cramps, joint pain.

Nervous: Dizziness, vertigo, paraesthesiae, tremors, encephalopathy.

Psychiatric: Nervousness, mental confusion, insomnia, decreased libido, depression, somnolence.

Respiratory: Cough, dyspnoea.

Special senses: Nasal congestion, visual disturbances, increased intra-ocular pressure, tinnitus.

Urogenital: Impotence, polyuria, dysuria, bladder spasms, frequency of micturition.

Reactions in which no causal relationship could be established were activation of probable pre-existing peptic ulcer, aplastic anaemia, neutropenia and abnormalities of liver function tests.

Overdosage: No data are available; and it is not known whether the drug is dialysable.

Therapy should be discontinued and the patient observed closely. No specific antidote is available. Emesis should be induced or gastric lavage performed. The most likely signs and symptoms are dehydration and electrolyte imbalance which should be treated by established methods. If hyperkalaemia occurs, active measures should be taken to reduce plasma potassium levels.

Pharmaceutical precautions Keep container well closed; store in a cool place, protected from light.

Legal category POM.

Package quantities Bottles of 100.

Further information Combined with hydrochlorothiazide, Midamor causes less magnesium excretion than either the thiazides or loop diuretics when used alone.

Product licence number 0025/5015.

MODUCREN* ▼

Presentation Blue, square, half-scored tablets, marked 'MODUCREN', containing 25 mg hydrochlorothiazide, 2.5 mg amiloride hydrochloride, and 10 mg timolol maleate.

Uses Mild to moderate hypertension.

Dosage and administration 1 to 2 tablets of Moducren once a day.

Use in the elderly: Moducren has been shown to be as well tolerated in the elderly as in younger patients. The recommended starting dose is 1 tablet daily.

Contra-indications, warnings, etc
Contra-indications: Patients with bronchial asthma or with a history of bronchial asthma, severe chronic obstructive pulmonary disease, sinus bradycardia, second- or third-degree AV block, overt cardiac failure, right ventricular failure secondary to pulmonary hypertension, significant cardiomegaly, and cardiogenic shock. Hyperkalaemia (plasma potassium over 5.5 mmol/l. Anuria, acute and chronic renal insufficiency, severe progressive renal disease and diabetic nephropathy. Patients with blood urea over 10 mmol/l or serum creatinine over 130 μmol/l or diabetes mellitus should not receive Moducren without careful and frequent serum urea and serum electrolyte monitoring.

Anaesthetic agents causing myocardial depression, hypersensitivity to any component of Moducren or to sulphonamide-derived drugs. Use of other potassium-conserving agents or potassium supplements except in severe and/or refractory cases of hypokalaemia when careful monitoring of the plasma potassium level is necessary.

See also *Children, Nursing mothers* and *Pregnancy* under *Precautions.*

Precautions: Congestive cardiac failure: Care should be exercised before and during treatment of patients with cardiomegaly or history of cardiac failure. *Cardiac arrhythmias:* Patients at risk of congestive heart failure should be carefully observed for bradycardia, AV block and respiratory distress. If congestive cardiac failure persists, Moducren should be withdrawn. Moducren should be withdrawn gradually in patients with angina pectoris because abrupt withdrawal of beta blockers has been associated with increase in pain, and reports of myocardial infarction, and ventricular arrhythmias. *Elective or emergency surgery:* Moducren should also be gradually withdrawn prior to elective surgery of anginal patients. Agonists such as isoprenaline or noradrenaline

may be used to counter the effects of beta-blockade in emergency surgery. *Renal and hepatic disease and electrolyte disturbances:* Moducren should be used with caution in patients with renal or hepatic disease and in those patients in whom fluid and electrolyte balance is critical. *Metabolic or respiratory acidosis:* Acid-base balance should be monitored frequently in severely ill patients at risk of respiratory or metabolic acidosis. *Electrolyte and fluid balance:* Plasma and urine electrolyte determinations should be made in patients vomiting excessively or receiving parenteral fluids. Dilutional hyponatraemia may occur in patients with oedema in hot weather which calls for appropriate therapy; hypochloraemia requires specific treatment only under exceptional circumstances. Hypokalaemia or hyperkalaemia may occur. If hyperkalaemia occurs, Moducren should be discontinued immediately. The degree of thiazide-induced hypomagnesaemia reduced. *Diabetes mellitus, hypoglycaemia:* Moducren should be given with caution to diabetic patients and to patients subject to spontaneous hypoglycaemia as the symptoms and signs of acute hypoglycaemia may be masked. Moducren should only be used in diabetic patients after determining the status of renal function. Moducren should be discontinued at least three days before glucose tolerance testing. Insulin requirements may need readjusting in patients taking Moducren. *Skin and sensitivity reactions:* There have been reports of skin rashes and/or dry eyes associated with the use of beta-adrenergic blocking drugs. The reported incidence is small and in most cases the symptoms have cleared when treatment was withdrawn. Discontinuation of the drug should be considered if any such reaction is not otherwise explicable. Withdrawal should be gradual. Sensitivity reactions to Moducren may occur with or without a history of allergy or bronchial asthma. Possible exacerbation or activation of systemic lupus erythematosus reactions have been reported with thiazide diuretics. *Metabolic and endocrine:* Beta-adrenergic blocking agents may mask the signs of hyperthyroidism. Hypercalcaemia and hypophosphataemia have been reported with thiazide diuretics. Moducren should be discontinued in patients prior to testing for parathyroid function. Hyperuricaemia or acute gout may be precipitated in some patients. *Musculoskeletal:* Beta-blockers have been reported to induce myasthenic symptoms such as diplopia, ptosis, and generalised weakness.

Drug interactions: Moducren may potentiate other antihypertensive agents, such as reserpine or guanethidine. Its effect may be enhanced in the post-sympathectomy patient. The antihypertensive effect of beta-blockers may be reduced by NSAIDS. Thiazides may increase the responsiveness to tubocurarine. Preparations containing lithium should not generally be given with diuretics because they reduce its renal clearance and add a high risk of lithium toxicity.

Oral calcium antagonists may be combined with Moducren only when heart function is normal. When heart function is impaired, combination with dihydropyridine derivatives such as nifedipine may lead to hypotension; and combination with verapamil or diltiazem may cause AV conduction disturbances or left ventricular failure.

Intravenous calcium antagonists and Moducren should only be used together with caution. Concomitant beta-blockers and digitalis with either diltiazem or verapamil may further prolong the AV conduction time.

Children: Because the safety and efficacy of Moducren

has not been established in children, it is not recommended for paediatric use.

Nursing mothers: Thiazides appear in breast milk, but it is not known whether timolol maleate or amiloride are also excreted. If the use of Moducren is deemed essential, the mother should stop nursing.

Pregnancy: Moducren is not recommended for use during pregnancy. The use of any drug in women of child-bearing age requires that the anticipated benefit be weighed against possible hazards, which include fetal or neonatal jaundice, thrombocytopenia, and possibly other adverse reactions which have occurred in the adult.

Side effects: Moducren is usually well tolerated with significant side effects only infrequently reported. Common effects experienced are dizziness, asthenia, fatigue, and bradycardia. Other side reactions reported are: *Body as a whole:* Headache; *Cardiovascular:* Tachycardia, cold extremities, hypotension, syncope, arrhythmia, angina pectoris; *Respiratory:* Dyspnoea, wheezing; *Digestive:* Nausea, dyspepsia, constipation, diarrhoea, vomiting, GI pain, anorexia, thirst, dry mouth, stomatitis; *Urogenital:* Impotence; *Nervous:* Vertigo, paraesthesiae, tremors; *Integumentary:* Sweating; *Musculoskeletal:* Muscle cramps; *Psychiatric:* Insomnia, nervousness, depression, somnolence, abnormal dreaming, sleep disturbance; *Special senses:* Visual disturbances.

The reported side effects of the individual components – see separate entries for Blocadren, HydroSaluric and Midamor – may be considered as potential adverse effects of Moducren.

Overdosage: No specific data are available regarding symptoms or the treatment of overdosage with Moducren. Little is known about the dialysability of its components: a study of patients with renal failure showed that timolol did not readily dialyse.

No antidote is available. Treatment is symptomatic and supportive.

Therapy with Moducren should be stopped and emesis and/or gastric lavage induced.

Hydrocholorothiazide and amiloride hydrochloride: The signs and symptoms most likely are dehydration and electrolyte imbalance. If hyperkalaemia occurs, active measures should be taken to reduce plasma potassium levels.

Timolol maleate: The most common signs and symptoms to be expected following overdosage with a beta-adrenergic receptor blocking agent are symptomatic bradycardia, hypotension, bronchospasm, and acute cardiac failure. If overdosage occurs, the following measures are suggested

1. *Gastric lavage*

2. *For symptomatic bradycardia:* Atropine sulphate 0.25 to 2 mg intravenously should be used to induce vagal blockade. If bradycardia persists, intravenous isoprenaline hydrochloride should be administered cautiously. In refractory cases, the use of a cardiac pacemaker may be considered.

3. *For hypotension:* A sympathomimetic pressor agent such as dopamine, dobutamine or noradrenaline should be used. In refractory cases, the use of glucagon has been reported to be useful.

4. *For bronchospasm:* Isoprenaline hydrochloride should be used. Additional therapy with aminophylline may be considered.

5. *For acute cardiac failure:* Conventional therapy with digitalis, diuretics, and oxygen should be instituted

immediately. In refractory cases, the use of intravenous aminophylline is suggested. This may be followed, if necessary, by glucagon which has been reported useful.

6. *For heart block:* Isoprenaline hydrochloride or a pacemaker should be used.

Pharmaceutical precautions Store in a dry place below 25°C, protected from light.

Legal category POM.

Package quantities Calendar packs of 28 tablets.

Further information Similar dosage schedules and similar bioavailability rationalise the combination of hydrochlorothiazide (a saluretic), timolol maleate (a beta-adrenergic receptor blocking agent), and amiloride hydrochloride (a potassium-conserving agent) for the treatment of hypertension.

Product licence number
Moducren Tablets   0025/0141.

MODURET 25*

Presentation Moduret 25 is available as off-white, diamond-shaped tablets, marked 'MSD 923', containing Amiloride Hydrochloride BP equivalent to 2.5 mg anhydrous amiloride hydrochloride and 25 mg Hydrochlorothiazide BP.

Uses Potassium-conserving diuretic and antihypertensive.

For the treatment of patients with congestive heart failure, hypertension, or hepatic cirrhosis with ascites, in whom potassium depletion might be anticipated. The presence of amiloride hydrochloride minimises the likelihood of potassium loss during diuresis for long-term maintenance therapy. The combination is thus indicated particularly in conditions where potassium balance is especially important, e.g. patients with congestive heart failure receiving digitalis.

In hypertension, Moduret 25 may be used alone or as an adjunct to other antihypertensive agents. In hepatic cirrhosis with ascites, Moduret 25 usually provides satisfactory diuresis with diminished potassium loss and less risk of metabolic alkalosis.

Dosage and administration The rate of loss of weight and the serum electrolyte levels should determine the dosage. The most satisfactory rate of weight loss after initiation of diuresis is about 0.5–1.0 kg/day.

Moduret 25 is not recommended for children (see 'Contra-indications').

Hypertension: Usually 2 or 4 Moduret 25 Tablets given once a day or in divided doses. Some patients may require only 1 Moduret 25 Tablet a day. The dosage may be increased if necessary, but must not exceed 8 Moduret 25 Tablets a day.

Moduret 25 may be used alone or as an adjunct to other antihypertensive drugs, but since the antihypertensive effect of these agents may be enhanced, their dosage may need to be reduced in order to reduce the risk of an excessive drop in pressure.

Studies have shown that therapy can be given on a once-daily basis when Blocadren* is given at the same time. The majority of patients will respond to a regimen of 10 or 20 mg Blocadren once daily with 2 tablets of Moduret 25.

Congestive heart failure: Initially 2 or 4 tablets of Moduret 25 a day, subsequently adjusted if required, but not exceeding 8 Moduret 25 Tablets a day. Optimal dosage is determined by the diuretic response and the plasma potassium level. Once an initial diuresis has been achieved, reduction in dosage may be attempted for maintenance therapy. Maintenance therapy may be on an intermittent basis.

Hepatic cirrhosis with ascites: Initiate therapy with a low dose. A single daily dose of 2 Moduret 25 Tablets may be increased gradually until there is an effective diuresis. Dosage should not exceed 8 Moduret 25 Tablets a day. A gradual weight reduction is especially desirable in cirrhotic patients to reduce the likelihood of untoward reactions associated with diuretic therapy. Maintenance dosages may be lower than those required to initiate diuresis; dosage reduction should therefore be attempted when the patient's weight is stabilised.

Use in the elderly: Particular caution is needed in the elderly because of their susceptibility to electrolyte imbalance; the dosage should be carefully adjusted to renal function and clinical response.

Contra-indications, warnings, etc

Contra-indications: Hyperkalaemia (plasma potassium over 5.5 mmol/l); other potassium-conserving diuretics. Potassium supplements or potassium-rich food (except in severe and/or refractory cases of hypokalaemia under careful monitoring); anuria; acute renal failure, severe progressive renal disease, severe hepatic failure, Addison's disease, hypercalcaemia, concurrent lithium therapy, diabetic nephropathy; patients with blood urea over 10 mmol/l, patients with diabetes mellitus, or those with serum creatinine over 130 μmol/l in whom serum electrolyte and blood urea levels cannot be monitored carefully and frequently; prior sensitivity to amiloride hydrochloride or hydrochlorothiazide. In renal impairment, use of a potassium-conserving agent may result in rapid development of hyperkalaemia. Because the safety of amiloride hydrochloride for use in children has not been established, Moduret 25 is not recommended for children. For 'Use in pregnancy' and 'Use in nursing mothers', see 'Precautions'.

Precautions
Diabetes mellitus: Hyperkalaemia has commonly occurred in diabetic patients on amiloride hydrochloride, especially those with chronic renal disease or prerenal azotaemia. The status of renal function should therefore be determined before use in known or suspected diabetics. The dosage of insulin or oral hypoglycaemic agents for diabetic patients may need to be changed. Diabetes mellitus which has been latent may become manifest during thiazide administration. The agents should be discontinued at least three days before giving a glucose tolerance test, as one patient with poorly controlled diabetes mellitus, who became severely hyperkalaemic while receiving amiloride hydrochloride, died following two repeated intravenous glucose-tolerance tests.

Metabolic or respiratory acidosis: Potassium-conserving therapy should be initiated only with caution in severely ill patients in whom metabolic or respiratory acidosis may occur, e.g. patients with cardiopulmonary disease or decompensated diabetes. Shifts in acid-base balance alter the balance of extracellular/intracellular potassium, and the development of acidosis may be associated with rapid increases in plasma potassium.

Hyperkalaemia: This has been observed in patients receiving amiloride hydrochloride, either alone or with other diuretics, particularly in the aged, in diabetics, and in hospital patients with hepatic cirrhosis or cardiac oedema who had known renal involvement, were seriously ill, or were undergoing vigorous diuretic therapy. Such patients should be carefully observed for clinical, laboratory, and ECG evidence of hyperkalaemia (not always associated with an abnormal ECG). Some deaths have been reported in this group of patients. Should hyperkalaemia develop, discontinue treatment immediately and, if necessary, take active measures to reduce the plasma potassium to normal.

Electrolyte imbalance and blood urea increase: Hyponatraemia and hypochloraemia may occur. Hypochloraemic alkalosis may also occur, but its likelihood is reduced by the presence of amiloride in Moduret 25.

Reversible increases in blood urea have been reported accompanying vigorous diuresis, especially in seriously ill patients, such as those with hepatic cirrhosis with ascites and metabolic alkalosis, or those with resistant oedema; plasma electrolyte and blood urea levels should be carefully monitored in these patients.

Use with caution in patients with renal impairment. Special care should be taken to avoid cumulative or toxic effects due to a reduced excretion of its components. In addition, azotaemia may be precipitated or increased by hydrochlorothiazide. Renal function should be monitored. If increasing azotaemia and oliguria occur, treatment should be discontinued.

Effects in cirrhotic patients: Oral diuretic therapy is more frequently accompanied by adverse reactions in patients with hepatic cirrhosis and ascites because these patients are intolerant to acute shifts in electrolyte balance, and because they often have pre-existing hypokalaemia as a result of associated aldosteronism. Hepatic encephalopathy, manifested by tremors, confusion and coma, has been reported in patients on amiloride hydrochloride alone. Patients with liver disease on Moduret 25 should be observed for this complication. In cirrhotic patients receiving amiloride hydrochloride alone, a deepening of jaundice has occurred, but the relationship of the drug is uncertain.

Metabolic and endocrine effects: Thiazides may decrease serum PBI levels without signs of thyroid disturbance.

Calcium excretion is decreased by thiazides. Pathological changes in the parathyroid glands accompanied by hypercalcaemia and hypophosphataemia have been seen in a few patients receiving prolonged thiazide therapy. However, the common complications of hyperparathyroidism have not been observed. Therapy should be discontinued before carrying out tests for parathyroid function.

Hyperuricaemia may occur, or gout may be precipitated or aggravated, in certain patients receiving thiazides.

Drug interactions: Hydrochlorothiazide potentiates the action of other antihypertensive drugs. Therefore, the dosage of these agents, especially the adrenergic-blockers, may need to be reduced when Moduret 25 is added to the regimen. NSAIDs may attenuate the antihypertensive effect of thiazide diuretics.

Thiazide-containing drugs may increase the responsiveness to tubocurarine. The antihypertensive effect of thiazides may be enhanced in the post-sympathectomy patient.

Hydrochlorothiazide may decrease arterial responsiveness to noradrenaline, but not enough to prevent noradrenaline being effective in therapeutic dosage.

Orthostatic hypotension may occur, and may be potentiated by alcohol, barbiturates, and narcotics.

Sensitivity reactions: Sensitivity reactions to thiazides may occur in patients with or without a history of allergy or bronchial asthma. The possibility that thiazides may activate or exacerbate systemic lupus erythematosus has been reported.

Use in pregnancy: As clinical experience is limited, Moduret 25 is not recommended for use during pregnancy. Since thiazides cross the placental barrier and appear in cord blood, use where pregnancy is present or suspected requires that the benefits of the drug be weighed against possible hazards to the fetus. These hazards include fetal or neonatal jaundice, thrombocytopenia, bone marrow depression, and possibly other side effects that have occurred in the adult. The routine use of diuretics in otherwise healthy pregnant women with or without mild oedema is not indicated because they may be associated with hypovolaemia, increased blood viscosity, and decreased placental perfusion.

Use in nursing mothers: Although it is not known whether amiloride hydrochloride is excreted in human milk, it is known that thiazides do appear in breast milk. If the use of the drug combination is deemed essential, the patient should stop nursing.

Side effects: The combination of amiloride and hydrochlorothiazide is usually well tolerated and significant clinical side effects are infrequent. No increase in the risk of adverse reactions has been seen over those of the individual components.

The reported adverse reactions of the combination:
Body as a whole: Headache, weakness, fatigue, malaise, chest pain, back pain.
Cardiovascular: Arrhythmias, tachycardia, digitalis toxicity, orthostatic hypotension, angina pectoris.
Digestive: Anorexia, nausea, vomiting, diarrhoea, constipation, abdominal pain, GI bleeding, appetite changes, abdominal fullness, flatulence, thirst, hiccups.
Metabolic: Elevated plasma potassium levels (above 5.5 mmol/l), gout, dehydration.
Integumentary: Rash, pruritus, flushing.
Musculoskeletal: Leg ache, muscle cramps, joint pain.
Nervous: Dizziness, vertigo, paraesthesiae, stupor.
Psychiatric: Insomnia, nervousness, mental confusion, depression, sleepiness.
Respiratory: Dyspnoea.
Special senses: Bad taste, visual disturbance, nasal congestion.
Urogenital: Impotence, dysuria, nocturia, incontinence.
The reported adverse reactions of amiloride:
Digestive: Abnormal liver function, activation of probable pre-existing peptic ulcer.
Integumentary: Dry mouth.
Haematological: Aplastic anaemia, neutropenia.
Cardiovascular: One patient with partial heart block developed complete heart block.
The reported adverse reactions of hydrochlorothiazide:
Body as a whole: Anaphylactic reaction, fever.
Cardiovascular: Necrotising angiitis (vasculitis, cutaneous vasculitis).
Digestive: Jaundice (intrahepatic cholestatic jaundice), pancreatitis.
Endocrine metabolic: Glycosuria, hyperglycaemia, hyperuricaemia.
Integumentary: Photosensitivity, sialadenitis, urticaria.
Psychiatric: Restlessness.
Respiratory: Respiratory distress, including pneumonitis.
Special senses: Transient blurred vision, xanthopsia.
Haematological: Agranulocytosis, aplastic anaemia,

haemolytic anaemia, leucopenia, purpura, thrombocytopenia.
Special senses: Transient blurred vision, xanthopsia.
Haematological: Agranulocytosis, aplastic anaemia, haemolytic anaemia, leucopenia, purpura, thrombocytopenia.

Overdosage: No specific data are available on overdosage. No specific antidote is available, and it is not known whether the drug is dialysable.

Treatment should be symptomatic and supportive. Therapy should be discontinued and the patient watched closely. Emesis should be induced and/or gastric lavage performed. The most common signs and symptoms of overdosage with amiloride hydrochloride are dehydration and electrolyte imbalance. Blood pressure should be monitored and corrected where necessary. If hyperkalaemia occurs, active measures should be taken to reduce the plasma potassium levels.

Electrolyte depletion (hypokalaemia, hypochloraemia, hyponatraemia) and dehydration are the most common signs and symptoms of hydrochlorothiazide overdosage. Blood pressure should be monitored and corrected where necessary. If digitalis has been administered, hypokalaemia may accentuate cardiac arrhythmias.

Pharmaceutical precautions Store in a dry place below 25°C, protected from light.

Legal category POM.

Package quantities Four calendar packs, each of 7 tablets.

Further information The combination of amiloride with hydrochlorothiazide has been shown to cause less magnesium excretion than either the thiazides or the loop diuretics when used alone.

Onset of diuretic action begins within 2 to 4 hours after administration, and reaches a peak at about the fourth hour; there is detectable activity for about 24 hours.

Product licence number 0025/0178.

MUMPSVAX*

Presentation Lyophilised powder which, when reconstituted, contains in each dose not less than 5,000 $TCID_{50}$ (tissue culture infectious doses) of mumps virus vaccine expressed in terms of the assigned titre of the FDA (USA) Reference Mumps Virus. It is prepared from the Jeryl Lynn (B Level) strain, named after the patient from whom the virus was initially recovered.

Uses Mumps virus vaccine.

Mumpsvax induces a modified, non-communicable mumps infection in susceptible persons. Clinical trials have shown Mumpsvax to be highly immunogenic and well tolerated. A single injection has been shown to induce antibody response in approximately 97% of susceptible children and 93% of susceptible adults.

The vaccine is indicated for immunisation against mumps in children over 12 months of age, or adults. It is not recommended for children younger than this because they may retain maternal mumps-neutralising antibodies which may interfere with the immune response.

Evidence indicates that the vaccine will not offer protection when given after exposure to natural mumps.

Revaccination: Based on available evidence, there is no need to revaccinate children who were originally vaccinated when 12 months or older. However, patients should be revaccinated if there is evidence that initial immunisation was ineffective.

Use with other vaccines: Routine administration of diphtheria, tetanus and pertussis vaccine and/or oral poliomyelitis vaccine with Mumpsvax is not recommended because of insufficient data. However, if circumstances do dictate concurrent vaccination, separate syringes and separate sites for injection should be used.

Mumpsvax should not be given less than one month before or after immunisation with other virus vaccines.

Dosage and administration After suitably cleansing the immunisation site, the total volume of reconstituted vaccine should be injected subcutaneously, preferably into the outer aspect of the upper arm. Mumpsvax must not be injected intravenously.

The dosage of vaccine is the same for all patients. *Do not give serum globulin (ISG) concurrently with Mumpsvax.*

To reconstitute the vaccine, all the diluent provided should be injected into the vial of lyophilised vaccine, and agitated to ensure thorough mixing. The entire contents of the vial should then be drawn back into the syringe.

Contra-indications, warnings, etc

Contra-indications: Do not give Mumpsvax to pregnant women, since the possible effects of the vaccine on fetal development are not known at this time. If vaccination of post-pubertal females is undertaken, pregnancy should be avoided for three months following vaccination (see 'Pregnancy').

Mumpsvax should not be given to children less than 1 year of age.

Anaphylactoid reaction to neomycin (each dose of reconstituted vaccine contains approximately 25 mcg of neomycin).

Patients with active untreated tuberculosis should not be given Mumpsvax.

Malignant disease. Those with impaired immune responsiveness, whether occurring naturally or as a result of treatment with steroids, radiotherapy, cytotoxic drugs or other therapy. This contra-indication does not apply to patients who are receiving corticosteroids as replacement therapy, e.g. for Addison's disease.

Any active or suspected infection is reason for delaying vaccination.

Those with a family history of congenital or hereditary immunodeficiency should not be vaccinated until their immune competence is demonstrated.

Hypersensitivity to eggs, chicken, or chicken feathers: Live mumps vaccine is produced in cell cultures of chick embryo.

Patients with a history of anaphylactoid or other immediate reactions to eating eggs (e.g. hives, swelling of the mouth and throat, difficult breathing, hypotension and shock) should not be vaccinated. Evidence indicates, however, that patients with egg allergies that are not anaphylactoid may be vaccinated in the usual way. There is also no evidence to suggest that allergy to chicken or feathers increases the risk of reaction.

Pregnancy: Animal reproduction studies have not been conducted with Mumpsvax. It is also not known whether Mumpsvax can damage the fetus or affect the mother's reproductive capacity.

Although mumps virus is capable of infecting the placenta and fetus, there is no good evidence that it causes congenital malformation in humans. Mumps vaccine virus has also been shown to affect the placenta, but the virus has not been isolated from fetal tissues taken from susceptible women who were vaccinated and underwent elective abortions.

Precautions. A sterile syringe and Adronaline Injection BP (1 : 1,000) should be ready for immediate use should an anaphylactoid reaction occur.

Vaccination should be deferred for at least three months following blood or plasma transfusions, or administration of human immune serum globulin. If any of these substances have been used near to the time of vaccination, a test for the presence of mumps antibody should be made at a later date.

It has been reported that live mumps virus vaccine may temporarily depress tuberculin skin sensitivity. Therefore, if a tuberculin test is to be done, it should be scheduled before or simultaneously with mumps vaccine.

As with any vaccine, Mumpsvax does not provide seroconversion in 100% of susceptible vaccinees.

Nursing mothers: Because it is not known whether Mumpsvax is secreted in human milk, caution should be exercised when considering the use of the vaccine in nursing mothers.

Adverse reactions: Because of the slight acidity of the vaccine (pH 6.2–6.6) patients may complain of burning and/or stinging at the injection site for a short time.

Mild fever occurs occasionally. Fever above 103°F (39.4°C) is uncommon.

Parotitis has been reported to occur in very low incidence, and orchitis rarely, in persons who were vaccinated. In most instances investigated, prior exposure to natural mumps was established. In other instances, whether or not this was due to vaccine, to prior natural mumps exposure or to other causes has not been established.

Reports of purpura and allergic reactions such as wheal and flare at the injection site, or urticaria have been extremely rare.

Forms of optic neuritis, including retrobulbar neuritis and papillitis, may infrequently follow viral infections and have been reported to occur one to three weeks following vaccination with some live virus vaccines.

Very rarely, encephalitis and other nervous system reactions have occurred in recipients of the vaccine. A cause-effect relationship has not been established.

Treatment of overdosage: Nil.

Pharmaceutical precautions During shipment, the vaccine should be maintained at a temperature below 10°C to insure that there is no loss of potency.

Prior to reconstitution, the vaccine should be stored between 2°C–8°C. *Protect from light.*

A separate sterile disposable needle and syringe should be used on each occasion, free from preservatives, antiseptics and detergents which may inactivate the vaccine.

The vaccine should be reconstituted using only the diluent provided, and used immediately after reconstitution.

When reconstituted, the vaccine is yellow. It is acceptable for use only when clear and free from particulate matter.

Legal category POM.

Package quantities One 0.5 ml single-dose vial of lyophilised vaccine with an ampoule containing diluent.

Further information Mumpsvax is grown in cell cultures of chick embryos free of avian leucosis and other adventitious agents.

Vaccine-induced antibody levels have persisted for at least 15 years without substantial decline. The pattern of antibody closely resembles that observed for natural mumps, although the antibody level is significantly lower than that following the natural infection. If this pattern continues, it will provide a basis for expectation that immunity following the vaccine will be permanent. However, continued observation will be required to demonstrate this point.

No reports have been received of transmission of mumps from vaccinees to susceptible contacts.

Product licence number 0025/0072.

TRYPTIZOL*

Presentation Tryptizol 75, clear orange, slow-release capsules, marked 'MSD 649', containing 75 mg amitriptyline hydrochloride as a pelleted formulation.

Blue, film-coated tablets, marked 'MSD 23', containing 10 mg Amitriptyline Hydrochloride BP; yellow, film-coated tablets, marked 'MSD 45', containing 25 mg; and brown, film-coated tablets, marked 'MSD 102', containing 50 mg.

Injection, a colourless solution containing per ml 10 mg amitriptyline hydrochloride.

Syrup, a pink suspension containing, in each 5 ml, Amitriptyline Embonate BP equivalent to 10 mg amitriptyline.

Uses Symptoms of depression (especially where sedation is required); also effective in nocturnal enuresis where organic pathology is excluded.

Dosage and administration *Depression.*

Oral therapy: Therapy should be started with a low dosage and increased gradually, according to the clinical response and any evidence of intolerance.

Adults – initial dosage: Usually 75 mg a day in divided doses (or a single dose at night). If necessary, this may be increased to a total of 150 mg a day, the additional doses being given in the late afternoon and/or at bedtime.

The sedative effect is usually rapidly apparent. The antidepressant activity may be seen within three or four days or may take up to 30 days to develop adequately.

Adults – maintenance dosage: usually 50–100 mg a day. For maintenance therapy, the total dosage may be given in a single dose preferably in the evening or at bedtime. When satisfactory improvement has been reached, dosage should be reduced to the lowest amount that will maintain relief of symptoms. Maintenance therapy should be continued for three months or longer to lessen the chances of relapse.

Parenteral therapy: Parenteral use of amitriptyline should be restricted to patients for whom oral therapy is inappropriate or difficult. Substitute oral therapy as soon as possible: 10–20 mg (1–2 ml) four times a day. The dosage should not exceed that for oral therapy and should always be given in divided doses, intramuscularly or intravenously.

Children: Due to lack of clinical experience, Tryptizol is not recommended for the treatment of *depression* in children under 16 years of age.

Enuresis: Children aged 6–10 years may receive 10–20 mg a day, while those aged 11–16 years may need 25–50 mg a day. The recommended dosage must not be exceeded, and therefore Tryptizol 75 is not suitable for the treatment of enuresis. Treatment should not exceed three months.

This medication should be kept out of the reach of children. Tryptizol Syrup can be diluted with Syrup BP.

Because of the wide variation in the absorption and distribution of tricyclic antidepressants in body fluids, dosage should be adjusted to clinical response and not based on plasma levels. However, plasma levels may be used as a guide to toxicity or to non-compliance.

Elderly patients: In general, lower dosages are recommended for these patients and an initial dosage of 10–25 mg t.d.s. is recommended, which should be increased slowly. A daily dosage of 50 mg may be satisfactory in elderly patients who may not tolerate higher dosages. The required dosage may be administered either as divided doses or as a single dose preferably in the evening or at bedtime.

Contra-indications, warnings, etc

Contra-indications: Co-administration with monoamine oxidase inhibitors; prior sensitisation to amitriptyline; during the recovery phase after myocardial infarction; arrhythmias, particularly heartblock of any degree; mania; severe liver disease; lactation; children under 6 years of age. See also 'Use in pregnancy and the nursing mother', under 'Precautions'.

Precautions: Tryptizol should be used with caution in patients with a history of epilepsy, in patients with impaired liver function and, because of its atropine-like action, in patients with a history of urinary retention, prostatic hypertrophy, narrow-angle glaucoma, or increased intra-ocular pressure. In patients with narrow-angle glaucoma, even average doses may precipitate an attack of glaucoma.

Patients with cardiovascular disorders, hyperthyroid patients, and those receiving thyroid medication or anticholinergic agents should be closely supervised and the dosage of all medications carefully adjusted.

Elderly patients are particularly liable to experience adverse reactions: especially agitation, confusion, and postural hypotension.

Tryptizol may impair alertness in some patients and activities made hazardous by diminished alertness (e.g. driving a car) should be avoided.

When Tryptizol is used for the depressive component of schizophrenia, psychotic symptoms may be aggravated. In manic-depressives, a shift towards the manic phase may occur; paranoid delusions, with or without associated hostility, may be aggravated. In such cases, a major tranquilliser should be given concurrently, or the dosage of Tryptizol reduced.

The risk of suicide remains during treatment of depressed patients and until significant remission occurs. Such patients require careful supervision.

Concurrent administration with ECT may increase the hazards of treatment, and should be limited to patients for whom it is deemed essential.

If possible, discontinue Tryptizol several days before surgery. But if emergency surgery is unavoidable, the anaesthetist should be informed that the patient is being treated with Tryptizol, because anaesthesia may increase the risk of hypotension and arrhythmias.

Behavioural changes have been observed in children receiving tricyclics for the treatment of enuresis.

Use in pregnancy: The safety of Tryptizol for use during pregnancy and lactation has not been established. Tryptizol is not recommended during pregnancy, especially during the first and third trimesters unless there are compelling reasons, and in these patients the benefits should be weighed against possible hazards to the fetus, child, or mother. Clinical experience of the use of Tryptizol in pregnancy has been limited. Animal studies have shown harmful effects at exceptionally high doses.

Drug interactions: The concurrent use of antidepressants having varying modes of action should be made only with due recognition of their possible potentiation and with a thorough knowledge of their respective pharmacologies. Monoamine oxidase inhibitors can potentiate the effects of tricyclic antidepressants such as Tryptizol, and hyperpyretic crises, severe convulsions, and fatalities have occurred. A minimum of 14 days should elapse between discontinuing an MAOI and starting Tryptizol, which should be introduced cautiously and dosage increased gradually.

Tryptizol may block the antihypertensive action of guanethidine, debrisoquine, bethanidine, and possibly clonidine. It would be advisable to review all antihypertensive therapy during treatment with tricyclic antidepressants.

Amitriptyline should not be given with sympathomimetic agents such as adrenaline, ephedrine, isoprenaline, noradrenaline, phenylephrine, and phenylpropanolamine.

Tryptizol may enhance the response to alcohol, barbiturates, and other CNS depressants. In turn, barbiturates may decrease, and methylphenidate may increase, the antidepressant action of amitriptyline. Delirium has been reported in patients taking amitriptyline with disulfiram.

Paralytic ileus may occur in patients taking tricyclic antidepressants in combination with drugs having an anticholinergic action.

Caution is advised if patients receive large doses of ethchlorvynol concurrently. Transient delirium has been reported in patients treated with 1 g ethchlorvynol and 75 mg to 150 mg of Tryptizol.

Warnings and adverse effects: In general, Tryptizol is well tolerated. The side effects given below are essentially a combined list of all those of the tricyclic group of antidepressants. Some of them have not been reported with Tryptizol, but are included because of the similar pharmacologies of the group members. As the antidepressant effects of Tryptizol may not become apparent for the first 2–4 weeks of therapy, patients should be closely monitored during this period.

Cardiovascular reactions: hypotension, postural hypotension, hypertension, tachycardia, palpitations, myocardial infarction, arrhythmias, heart block, stroke. Arrhythmias and severe hypotension are likely to occur with high dosage or overdosage.

CNS and neuromuscular: confusional states, disturbed concentration, disorientation, delusions, hallucinations, hypomania, excitement, anxiety, restlessness, insomnia, nightmares, numbness, tingling, and paraesthesiae of the extremities, peripheral neuropathy, incoordination, ataxia, tremors, convulsions, alteration of the EEG, extrapyramidal symptoms, tinnitus.

Anticholinergic: dry mouth, blurred vision, disturbance of accommodation, increased intra-ocular pressure, constipation, paralytic ileus, urinary retention, urinary tract dilatation.

Allergic: skin rash, urticaria, photosensitisation, oedema of face and tongue.

Haematological: bone-marrow depression including agranulocytosis, leucopenia, eosinophilia, purpura, thrombocytopenia.

Gastro-intestinal: nausea, epigastric distress, vomiting, anorexia, stomatitis, unpleasant taste, diarrhoea, parotid swelling, black tongue, rarely hepatitis (including altered liver function and jaundice).

Endocrine: testicular swelling, gynaecomastia; breast enlargement, galactorrhoea, increased or decreased libido, interference with sexual function, elevation or lowering of blood sugar levels, syndrome of inappropriate ADH (antidiuretic hormone) secretion.

Other reactions: dizziness, weakness, fatigue, headache, weight loss, increased perspiration, urinary frequency, mydriasis, alopecia, drowsiness, increased appetite and weight gain (may be a drug reaction or due to relief of the depression). Abrupt withdrawal after prolonged administration has caused nausea, headache and malaise. Reports have associated gradual withdrawal with transient symptoms including irritability, restlessness, as well as dream and sleep disturbances during the first two weeks of dosage reduction. These symptoms are not indicative of addiction.

Adverse reactions such as withdrawal symptoms, respiratory depression and agitation have been reported in neonates whose mothers had taken tricyclic antidepressants in the last trimester of pregnancy.

Mania or hypomania has been reported rarely within 2–7 days of stopping chronic therapy with tricyclic antidepressants.

Side effects in enuresis: Dosages used in enuresis are low compared with those used in depression, and side effects are therefore less frequent. The most common are drowsiness and anticholinergic effects. The only other side effects, reported infrequently at these dosages, have been mild sweating and itching.

The recommended dosage must not be exceeded.

Overdosage: High dosage may cause temporary confusion, disturbed concentration, or transient visual hallucinations. Overdosage may cause drowsiness; hypothermia; tachycardia and other arrhythmic abnormalities such as bundle branch block; ECG evidence of impaired conduction; congestive heart failure; dilated pupils; convulsions; severe hypotension; stupor, and coma. Other symptoms may be agitation, hyperactive reflexes, muscle rigidity, vomiting, hyperpyrexia, or any of those listed as adverse effects.

All persons suspected of having taken an overdosage should be admitted to hospital as soon as possible. Treatment is symptomatic and supportive. The stomach should be emptied as quickly as possible by emesis, followed by gastric lavage upon arrival at hospital. Following lavage, activated charcoal may be given during the first 24–48 hours at a dosage of 20–30 g every four to six hours. An ECG should be taken and close monitoring of cardiac function instituted if there is any sign of abnormality. An open airway and an adequate fluid intake should be maintained, and body temperature regulated.

Intravenous physostigmine salicylate, 1–3 mg, has been reported to reverse the symptoms of tricyclic antidepressant poisoning. Because physostigmine is rapidly metabolised, the dosage of physostigmine should be repeated as required, particularly if life-threatening signs such as arrhythmias, convulsions, and deep coma recur or persist after the initial dose of physostigmine. Because physostigmine itself may be toxic, it is not recommended for routine use.

Standard measures should be used to manage circulatory shock and metabolic acidosis. Cardiac arrhythmias may be treated with neostigmine, pyridostigmine or propanolol. Should cardiac failure occur, use of digitalis should be considered. Close monitoring of cardiac function for not less than five days is advisable.

If convulsions occur, they should be treated with paraldehyde, diazepam or an inhalation anaesthetic. Barbiturates should not be used because Tryptizol increases their CNS-depressant action.

Dialysis is of no value because of low plasma concentrations of amitriptyline. Since overdosage is often deliberate, patients may attempt suicide by other means during the recovery phase. Deaths by deliberate or accidental overdosage have occurred with this class of medicament.

Pharmaceutical precautions Keep containers well closed and store below 25°C, protected from light. The injection and the syrup should also be protected from freezing. Tryptizol Syrup may be diluted with Syrup BP; the mixture should be used within 14 days.

Legal category POM.

Package quantities *Capsules 75 mg:* Bottles of 100.
Tablets 10 mg: Bottles of 100 and 500.
Tablets 25 mg: Bottles of 100 and 500.
Tablets 50 mg: Bottles of 100.
Injection: Vials of 10 ml.
Syrup: Bottles of 200 ml and 1,000 ml.

Further information Tryptizol is a member of the tricyclic group of antidepressants. Its mode of action in man is not known, but it is not a monoamine oxidase inhibitor (special dietary restrictions are not necessary), and it does not act primarily by stimulating the CNS.

Product licence numbers

Capsules 75 mg	0025/0116
Tablets 10 mg	0025/0093
Tablets 25 mg	0025/0094
Tablets 50 mg	0025/0095
Injection	0025/5036
Syrup	0025/5037

*Trade Mark

Napp Laboratories Limited
Cambridge Science Park
Milton Road
Cambridge CB4 4GW

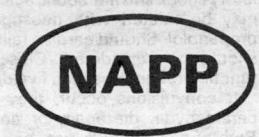

AUDAX* ANALGESIC EAR DROPS

Presentation Ear drops containing the Mundicylat* brand of choline salicylate 20% w/v.

Uses For relief of pain, particularly in acute otitis media. Also of use in acute and chronic painful otitis externa and painful chronic otitis media and otalgia generally.

Dosage and administration *Infants, children and adults:* With head tilted to one side the external auditory canal is filled with Audax ear drops. The ear should be plugged with cotton wool soaked with the ear drops or a wick may be inserted if preferred. Audax ear drops should be instilled four-hourly until permanent relief of symptoms is obtained. Cleansing of the ear where necessary facilitates therapy.

Contra-indications, warnings, etc Salicylate sensitivity.
    Where infection of the ear necessitates topical and/or systemic antibiotics, the Audax ear drops are designed as an adjuvant therapy.

Overdosage: In the event of deliberate or accidental oral ingestion of large volumes symptoms of salicylism may appear. For severe intoxication (plasma salicylate level in children above 300 mg/l) institute forced diuresis with i.v. infusions of saline and sodium bicarbonate or dextrose solution. Electrolyte levels should be monitored and corrected particularly if there is cardiac, renal or respiratory impairment.

Pharmaceutical precautions Store in a cool dry area protected from light.

Legal category P.

Package quantities Bottle containing 8 ml with dropper.

Further information The low surface tension of Audax ensures rapid penetration of the drops. The choline salicylate gives quick and prolonged analgesia. The pH of Audax ear drops is adjusted to approximate closely that normally found in the external auditory meatus.

Product licence number 0337/5004.

BETADINE* ANTISEPTIC SPRAY

Presentation Pressurised can containing a golden-brown solution of the Mundidone* brand of Povidone-Iodine USP 5% w/v.

Uses As a skin antiseptic for treatment or prevention of infection and to aid healing in ulcers, burns, minor injuries, incisions, etc.

Dosage and administration *Adults, children and infants:* Hold the Betadine antiseptic spray about 10 inches from the area to be treated; press valve firmly downwards to allow the spray to cover the desired area. Allow to dry.

Contra-indications, warnings, etc Do not spray into eyes. Avoid inhalation of spray. In rare instances of local irritation or sensitivity discontinue treatment. Administer with caution to patients with a history of hypersensitivity to iodine.

Treatment of overdosage: No cases of overdosage have been reported.

Pharmaceutical precautions Store in a cool dry place protected from light.

Legal category GSL.

Package quantities Antiseptic spray of 200 ml.

Further information Betadine antiseptic spray contains povidone-iodine, which retains the broad germicidal spectrum of iodine, but is non-stinging and non-irritating to sensitive denuded skin areas.
    Betadine antiseptic spray is rapidly microbicidal and quickly forms a protective film subjecting pathogens to the prompt and continued germicidal action of povidone-iodine.

Product licence number 0337/5022.

BETADINE* ANTISEPTIC PAINT

Presentation A golden brown, alcoholic solution containing the Mundidone* brand of Povidone-Iodine USP 10% w/v.

Uses As a general topical and quick drying antiseptic in the treatment and prevention of infection. It is ideal for Herpes simplex, Herpes zoster, grazes, abrasions, cuts and wounds, or any break in the skin which requires protection from infection.
    Betadine antiseptic paint is effective in the treatment of dermal infections caused by bacteria, fungi, yeasts, and viruses (e.g. Herpes virus Types I and II).

Dosage and administration Apply Betadine antiseptic paint undiluted, as necessary, to affected area and allow to dry. Use twice daily, and cover with a dressing if desired.
    Rinse the brush thoroughly after use.

Contra-indications, warnings, etc In rare instances of local irritation or sensitivity, discontinue treatment. Administer with caution to patients with a history of hypersensitivity to iodine.

Overdosage: No cases of overdosage have been reported.

Pharmaceutical precautions Store in a cool, dry place protected from light.

Legal category P.

Package quantities Glass bottles containing 8 ml with an applicator brush.

Further information Numerous studies have established the rapid microbicidal activity of the Mundidone* brand of Povidone-Iodine contained in Betadine antiseptic paint, both in vivo and in vitro, against Gram-negative and Gram-positive bacteria, fungi, viruses and yeasts. Betadine antiseptic paint is also sporicidal.

Betadine antiseptic paint is effective in the presence of serum, blood, purulent exudate and necrotic tissue.

The applicator brush provided with Betadine antiseptic paint is for ease of application to minor wounds and infections. Rapid, prolonged and complete antiseptic cover is afforded by the use of Betadine antiseptic paint when applied topically twice daily.

Product licence number 0337/0047.

STANDARDISED BETADINE* ANTISEPTIC SOLUTION
BETADINE* ALCOHOLIC SOLUTION
BETADINE* SURGICAL SCRUB

Presentation *Antiseptic Solution:* An aqueous solution containing the Mundidone* brand of Povidone-Iodine USP 10% w/v.

Alcoholic Solution: Contains the Mundidone* brand of Povidone-Iodine USP 10% w/v in an alcoholic solution.

Surgical Scrub: Contains the Mundidone* brand of Povidone-Iodine USP, 7.5% w/v with non-ionic surfactants.

All the preparations are golden-brown in colour.

Uses Degerming the skin pre-operatively and post-operatively for major and minor surgical procedures, and also in the case of the surgical scrub for pre-operative scrubbing and washing by surgeons and theatre staff.

Dosage and administration The antiseptic and alcoholic solutions should be applied full strength as often as needed. The surgical scrub should be used as a pre-operative antiseptic skin cleanser.

Contra-indications, warnings, etc A patch test should be performed in rare cases of iodine sensitivity. Administer with caution to patients with a history of hypersensitivity to iodine.

Overdosage: No cases of overdosage have been reported with Betadine preparations. In cases of deliberate or accidental ingestion of large quantities provide supportive and symptomatic treatment. Thyroid function may be monitored. In the case of alcoholic solution, treat as for ethyl alcohol.

Pharmaceutical precautions Store in a cool, dry place protected from light.

Legal category P.

Package quantities Containers of 500 ml and 5 litres.

Further information Numerous studies have established the rapid microbicidal activity of Povidone-Iodine contained in Betadine germicides, both in vitro and in vivo, against Gram-negative and Gram-positive bacteria,

fungi, protozoa, viruses and yeasts. Povidone-Iodine is also sporicidal.

The Standardised formulation of Betadine Antiseptic Solution gives a consistent level of active iodine between 2.5 and 3 ppm ensuring constant microbial activity at a pH compatible with that of human skin.

Betadine scrub and solutions have a rapid and prolonged germicidal action and with repeat usage a cumulative germicidal effect.

Betadine scrub and solutions are active in the presence of serum, blood, purulent exudate and necrotic tissue.

They can be used for the preparation of skin and mucous membranes and for burn and wound disinfection without the risk of systemic toxicity.

Povidone-Iodine as contained in Betadine germicides is not inactivated by soap.

Product licence numbers
Standardised Betadine antiseptic solution	0337/5901
Alcoholic solution	0337/5902
Surgical scrub	0337/5903

BETADINE* GARGLE AND MOUTHWASH

Presentation A pleasantly flavoured amber coloured solution containing the Mundidone* brand of Povidone-Iodine USP 1% w/v.

Uses For infected inflammatory conditions of the mouth and pharynx caused by bacterial or monilial infections, and in dental surgery.

Dosage and administration *Adults and children:* Use undiluted, or dilute with an equal volume of warm water. Gargle or rinse for at least 30 seconds. Repeat every two to four hours for as long as required.

Contra-indications, warnings, etc In rare instances of local irritation or sensitivity discontinue treatment.

Overdosage: No cases of overdosage have been reported.

Pharmaceutical precautions Store in a cool dry place protected from light.

Legal category P.

Package quantities Bottles containing 250 ml.

Further information Betadine gargle and mouthwash contains Povidone-Iodine, a complex of iodine which retains all the broad-spectrum germicidal activity of elemental iodine without its disadvantages.

The germicidal activity is maintained in the presence of blood, pus, serum and necrotic tissue.

Betadine gargle and mouthwash does not stain the skin, mucous membranes or teeth despite its powerful germicidal action.

Betadine gargle and mouthwash kills bacteria, viruses, fungi, spores and protozoa and rapidly reduces oral bacterial counts.

Product licence number 0337/0009.

BETADINE* OINTMENT

Presentation A golden-brown, water-soluble ointment containing the Mundidone* brand of Povidone-Iodine USP 10% w/w.

Uses For the treatment or prevention of infection in cuts and abrasions, minor surgical procedures and burns.

Treatment of mycotic and bacterial skin infections, decubitus and stasis ulcers and pyodermas.

Dosage and administration *Adults, children and infants:* The affected skin should be cleaned and dried. Apply Betadine ointment liberally. May be covered with a dressing or bandage. Betadine ointment may be used as often as is required. In the treatment of burns, every eight hours; in other treatments, apply once daily generally.

Contra-indications, warnings, etc In rare instance of local irritation or sensitivity, discontinue treatment. Administer with caution to patients with a history of hypersensitivity to iodine.

Overdosage: No cases of overdosage have been reported. In cases of deliberate or accidental ingestion of large quantities provide symptomatic and supportive treatment.

Pharmaceutical precautions Store in a cool, dry place.

Legal category GSL.

Package quantities Tubes of 80 g.

Further information Nil.

Product licence number 0337/5005.

BETADINE* SCALP AND SKIN CLEANSER

Presentation A golden-brown cleansing and sudsing surfactant solution containing the Mundidone* brand of Povidone-iodine USP 7.5% w/v.

Uses For seborrhoeic conditions of skin and scalp, acne vulgaris and other pyogenic skin conditions.

Dosage and administration *For hair and scalp:* Thoroughly wet the hair. Apply as a shampoo to the hair and scalp, rubbing well in. Allow to remain on the scalp for at least five minutes, rinse off with warm water. Reapply and work up into a rich lather before rinsing again.

For skin: Apply directly or with moistened sponge. Cleanse area thoroughly; repeat application and dry with clean or sterile towel or gauze.

Contra-indications, warnings, etc In rare instance of local irritation or sensitivity discontinue treatment.

Overdosage: No cases of overdosage have been reported. In cases of deliberate or accidental ingestion of large quantities provide symptomatic and supportive treatment.

Pharmaceutical precautions Store in a cool place protected from light.

Legal category GSL.

Package quantities Plastic bottle containing 250 ml.

Further information Betadine scalp and skin cleanser is neither a primary irritant nor a sensitiser.

It has a highly effective germicidal activity and is free from unpleasant odour.

Betadine scalp and skin cleanser is active in the presence of exfoliate debris and infected scalp lesions, and does not stain the skin.

Product licence number 0337/5023.

BETADINE* SHAMPOO

Presentation A golden-brown, cleansing and sudsing surfactant solution containing the Mundidone* brand of Povidone-Iodine USP 4% w/v and lanolin.

Uses Seborrhoeic conditions of the scalp associated with excessive dandruff, pruritus, scaling, exudation and erythema of the scalp. Pityriasis capitis. Infected lesions of the scalp – pyodermas (recurrent furunculosis, infective folliculitis and impetigo). Cradle-cap.

Dosage and administration *For adults, children and infants:*

1. Having first wetted the hair apply two or three capfuls of Betadine shampoo; use warm water to lather. Rinse.

2. Again apply two or three capfuls of Betadine shampoo and massage into the scalp with the tips of the fingers.

3. Work up to a golden lather using warm water.

4. Repeat treatment twice weekly until improvement is noted. Afterwards use Betadine shampoo once a week.

Contra-indications, warnings, etc In rare instance of local irritation or sensitivity, discontinue treatment.

Overdosage: No cases of overdosage have been reported. In cases of deliberate or accidental ingestion of large quantities provide symptomatic and supportive treatment.

Pharmaceutical precautions Store in a cool place protected from light.

Legal category GSL.

Package quantities Plastic bottle containing 250 ml.

Further information Betadine shampoo is neither a primary irritant nor a sensitiser.

It has a highly effective germicidal activity and is free from unpleasant odour.

Betadine shampoo is active in the presence of exfoliate debris and infected scalp lesions, and does not stain the skin.

Product licence number 0337/5033.

BETADINE* SKIN CLEANSER

Presentation A penetrating golden-brown, sudsing surfactant solution containing the Mundidone* brand of Povidone-Iodine USP 4% w/v.

Uses Acne vulgaris of the face and neck, and other pyogenic skin conditions. As an adjuvant to systemic antibiotic therapy in treating septic lesions. For disinfection of the skin (as a liquid soap).

Dosage and administration Apply directly or with moistened sponge to the affected areas, and work up a rich lather. Allow to remain on the skin for three to five minutes, then rinse off thoroughly with warm water and dry with clean or sterile towel or gauze. For pyodermas, repeat twice a day until improvement is noted, and then once a day.

Contra-indications, warnings, etc In rare instance of local irritation or sensitivity, discontinue treatment.

Overdosage: No cases of overdosage have been reported. In cases of deliberate or accidental ingestion of large quantities provide symptomatic and supportive treatment.

Pharmaceutical precautions Store in a cool place protected from light.

Legal category GSL.

Package quantities Plastic bottle containing 250 ml.

Further information Betadine skin cleanser is neither a primary irritant nor a sensitiser.

It has a highly effective germicidal activity and is free from unpleasant odour.

Betadine skin cleanser is active in the presence of exfoliate debris and infected skin lesions, and does not stain the skin.

Product licence number 0337/5034.

BETADINE* VAGINAL PESSARIES
BETADINE* VAGINAL GEL

Presentation Vaginal pessaries each containing the Mundidone* brand of Povidone-Iodine USP 200 mg in a water-soluble base.

Vaginal gel containing the Mundidone* brand of Povidine-Iodine USP 10% w/w.

Both preparations are golden-brown in colour.

Uses Vaginitis due to candidal, trichomonal, non-specific or mixed infections, and pre-operative preparation of the vagina.

Dosage and administration Use throughout the menstrual cycle for two to four weeks.

Pessaries: Insert one pessary with applicator night and morning. Each pessary should be wetted with water immediately prior to insertion, thus ensuring maximum dispersion of the active constituent and avoiding risk of local irritation.

Gel: Insert an applicator full of gel (5 g) every night. The regimen may be varied to combine the use of the two vaginal preparations or in combination with the Betadine* VC kit using one in the morning and one at night.

Contra-indications, warnings, etc If irritation, redness or swelling develop, discontinue use.

Patients with a history of iodine sensitivity should not use Betadine vaginal therapies without prior investigation.

These products are spermicidal and should not be used when conception is desired.

As with all drugs used in pregnancy, the therapeutic benefit to the patient must be balanced against possible effects on the foetus. Isolated reports have indicated that foetal absorption of iodine may occur following prolonged extensive intravaginal use of povidone-iodine in pregnancy, although the clinical significance of this remains to be established.

Overdosage: No cases of overdosage have been reported. In cases of deliberate or accidental ingestion of large quantities provide symptomatic and supportive treatment.

Pharmaceutical precautions Store in a cool dry place protected from light.

Legal category P.

Package quantities *Pessaries;* 28 with applicator.

Gel; 80 g with applicator.

Further information Betadine vaginal pessaries and vaginal gel are fungicidal, trichomonacidal and bacteri-

cidal to the pathogenic organisms which cause vaginitis. They retain their powerful germicidal effect in the presence of purulent exudate, blood, serum and necrotic tissue. The treatment does not cause stinging or staining in the vagina. The preparations are water soluble and the golden-brown colouration is easily removed by washing.

Product licence numbers
Pessaries   0337/5019
Gel   0337/5020

BETADINE* VC KIT

Presentation The Betadine VC kit consists of Betadine VC concentrate (containing the Mundidone* brand of Povidone-Iodine USP 10% w/v) 250 ml, with a plastic applicator bottle and vaginal applicator.

Uses As a vaginal cleanser in the treatment of vaginitis due to candidal, trichomonal, non-specific or mixed infections, and for pre-operative disinfection of the vagina.

Dosage and administration Once a day (preferably in the morning), for a fourteen-day period, including days of menstruation.

The Betadine VC concentrate should be diluted using the measuring cap on the concentrate bottle and used according to the patient instruction leaflet provided.

May be used in combination with Betadine vaginal pessaries or vaginal gel.

Contra-indications, warnings, etc As with other douches its use is not recommended in pregnancy.

If irritation, redness or swelling develop, discontinue use. Patients with a history of iodine sensitivity should not use Betadine VC kit without prior investigation.

This product is spermicidal and should not be used when conception is desired.

Overdosage: No cases of overdosage have been reported. In cases of accidental ingestion of large quantities provide symptomatic and supportive treatment.

Pharmaceutical precautions Store in a cool dry place protected from light.

Legal category P.

Package quantities Carton containing bottle of 250 ml Betadine VC concentrate, an empty applicator squeeze bottle and a plastic vaginal applicator, with patient instruction leaflet.

Further information Betadine VC kit (antiseptic vaginal cleansing kit) is fungicidal, trichomonacidal, bactericidal and virucidal. It retains its powerful germicidal effect in the presence of purulent exudate, blood, serum and necrotic tissue.

Product licence number 0337/5021.

BRADILAN* TABLETS

Presentation Enteric and white sugar coated tablets each containing tetranicotinoylfructose (nicofuranose) 250 mg.

Uses In peripheral vascular disease including primary and secondary Raynaud's disease, intermittent claudication, night cramps, perniosis and cerebrovascular disease.

In hyperlipidaemia, i.e. hypertriglyceridaemia, hypercholesterolaemia, and lipid abnormalities associated with atherosclerosis.

Dosage and administration Dosage needs to be adjusted to the individual. An average dose of 2 tablets three times a day is often sufficient, but doses of 3–4 tablets three times a day may be indicated in some patients. It is better to start therapy with 2 tablets three times a day and increase this dosage over a period of days until the effects of vasodilation are appreciated by the patient and noticed by the doctor. If minimal facial flushing is well tolerated by the patient the dosage should be maintained at this level. However, the beneficial effects of therapy are not lost by reducing the dosage slightly until flushing disappears.

Contra-indications, warnings, etc Adjust daily dosage to suit each patient individually to ambient temperature.

Patients entering an overheated room or going into a warm bed should not take Bradilan tablets immediately before doing so or they may experience increased vasodilator effects.

The vasodilator effect of Bradilan tablets is enhanced by alcoholic beverages, but their concomitant consumption is not contra-indicated.

Because of the special structure of Bradilan tablets they should not be chewed or broken, but swallowed whole.

Bradilan tablets should not be given in the 24 hours before a surgical operation.

Overdosage: In the event of accidental or deliberate overdosage, facial flushing, vasodilation and possibly hypotension, headache, gastric irritation, nausea, diarrhoea, hyperglycaemia and hyperthermia may occur. Gastric lavage should be performed and symptomatic treatment given in patients with diabetes, a history of gastro-intestinal ulceration and those susceptible to hyperthermia.

Pharmaceutical precautions Store in a well-closed container, in a cool dry place protected from light.

Legal category P.

Package quantities 50 and 250 tablets.

Further information With Bradilan tablet therapy a clinical response is observed within days.

Correct Bradilan tablet dosage and continued therapy do not result in continued facial flushing, headache, gastric irritation and nausea which are commonly associated with nicotinic acid and its salts. Because of its sustained therapeutic activity Bradilan tablets need be given only three to four times a day.

Product licence number 0337/5006.

BROVON* INHALANT SOLUTION

Presentation A solution for inhalation containing Atropine Methonitrate BP 0.14% w/v. Adrenaline (as hydrochloride) 0.50% w/v and Papaverine Hydrochloride BP 0.88% w/v.

Uses For relief and prevention of bronchospasm in asthma, chronic bronchitis and other respiratory diseases.

Dosage and administration Twice-daily and once-nightly use will prevent attacks. In acute episodes more frequent use may be necessary. No more than two puffs should be given within thirty minutes. In order to ensure that Brovon inhalant solution is atomised to form sufficiently small particles the Brovon Midget Inhaler must be used. By briskly pressing and releasing the rubber bulb a fine mist is produced which is inhaled through the mouth.

Contra-indications, warnings, etc Should not be prescribed with monoamine oxidase inhibitors or with sympathomimetic drugs.

Contra-indicated in patients with hypertension, thyrotoxicosis, acute coronary disease and cardiac asthma.

Overdosage: Administer alpha-adrenergic blocker by intravenous injection and a cardioselective beta blocker per os. Propranolol must not be given to asthmatics because of the risk of increasing bronchoconstriction.

Pharmaceutical precautions Store in cool dry place protected from light.

Legal category P.

Package quantities Bottles containing 20 ml and 50 ml.

Further information Nil.

Product licence number 0337/5009.

CARYLDERM* SHAMPOO

Presentation A pleasantly perfumed, clear yellow liquid shampoo containing carbaryl 1% w/v.

Uses For the treatment of head and pubic lice infestation.

Dosage and administration
The source of infestation should be sought and treated.

For head lice:
1. Wet the hair thoroughly with warm water and apply sufficient shampoo to work up a rich lather and ensure that no part of the scalp is left uncovered. Pay special attention to the back of the neck and area behind the ears. Take care to avoid the eyes.
2. Leave for at least five minutes.
3. Rinse thoroughly with clean, warm water and repeat procedure.
4. While the hair is still wet, comb with an ordinary comb. The fine-toothed Napp comb can then be used to remove the dead lice and eggs.
5. This treatment should be carried out a total of three times at three day intervals.

For pubic lice:
1. Wet area and apply shampoo directly to the pubic hair and the hair between the legs and around the anus.
2. Cover the skin and hair completely with the shampoo.
3. Work up a lather and leave for at least five minutes.
4. Rinse thoroughly.
5. Repeat procedure. The fine-toothed Napp comb can then be used to remove the dead lice and eggs.

Contra-indications, warnings, etc Children under the age of six months should be treated under medical supervision.

As with all shampoos, avoid contact with the eyes. When Carylderm Shampoo is used by a school nurse or other health officer in the mass treatment of large numbers of children, it is advisable that protective plastic or rubber gloves be worn.

Treatment of overdosage: In the event of deliberate or

accidental ingestion, empty stomach contents and keep patient warm. In the event of massive ingestion, atropine, in doses of 1 or 2 mg may be required to counteract cholinesterase inhibition.

Pharmaceutical precautions None.

Legal category P.

Package quantities Bottle of 100 ml.

Further information Carylderm Shampoo contains an insecticide of the carbamate group, which is rapidly lethal to both lice and their eggs.

Product licence number 0337/0044.

CARYLDERM* LOTION

Presentation A clear, colourless alcohol-based lotion containing carbaryl 0.5% w/v.

Uses For the treatment of head and pubic lice infestations.

Dosage and administration The source of infestation should be sought and treated.

For head lice:
1. Sprinkle the lotion on the hair and rub gently on to the head until the entire scalp is moistened. Pay special attention to the back of the neck and area behind the ears. Take care to avoid the eyes.
2. Allow to dry naturally – use NO heat.
3. As all lice and eggs will have been killed, the hair may be shampooed after 2 hours. If a residual effect is desired, however, it is recommended that shampooing be carried out after 12 hours.
4. While still wet, comb the hair with an ordinary comb. The fine-toothed Napp comb can then be used to remove the dead lice and eggs.

For pubic lice: Application and dosage etc. are as for the head. Apply the lotion to the pubic hair and the hair between the legs and around the anus. Allow to dry naturally using NO heat. Transient, mild stinging may be experienced due to the alcohol content.

Contra-indications, warnings, etc Contains flammable alcohol. Apply and dry with care. Avoid naked flames or lighted objects. Do not use artificial heat (e.g. electric dryers). Dry in a well-ventilated room. Do not cover the head before the lotion has dried completely.

Children under the age of six months should be treated under medical supervision.

When Carylderm Lotion is used by a school nurse or other health officer in the mass treatment of large numbers of children, it is advisable that protective plastic or rubber gloves be worn.

Treatment of overdosage: In the event of deliberate or accidental ingestion, as for ethyl alcohol, empty stomach contents and keep patient warm. In the event of massive ingestion, atropine, in doses of 1 or 2 mg may be required to counteract cholinesterase inhibition.

Pharmaceutical precautions Store in a cool place protected from light.

Legal category P.

Package quantities Sprinkler-top bottles of 55 ml and 110 ml.

Further information The volatile alcoholic base used in Carylderm Lotion evaporates quickly leaving a high concentration of Carbaryl on the hair. This is rapidly lethal to both lice and their eggs and may give several weeks' protection from reinfestation. For this protective effect to be optimal Carylderm Lotion should be left on the scalp for 12 hours before shampooing and no artificial heat used to dry the hair after shampooing.

Product licence number 0337/0038.

DIUMIDE*-K CONTINUS* TABLETS

Presentation White and orange film-coated bi-layered tablets. bi-convex in shape embossed DK on one side and (NAPP) on the other. Each tablet contains Frusemide BP 40 mg and Potassium Chloride 600 mg (8m Eq), the latter incorporated within the patented controlled release system.

Uses Diumide-K Continus tablets are indicated in patients requiring diuresis and concomitant potassium supplementation.

Indications include cardiac oedema, pulmonary oedema, hepatic oedema, renal oedema and peripheral oedema of various aetiologies.

Dosage and administration The usual adult dose is one tablet daily, normally in the morning. This may be adjusted depending on the condition.

N.B. Diumide-K Continus tablets should be swallowed whole with water preferably prior to or during a meal. The tablets should not be chewed so as not to destroy the controlled release system constituting the Potassium Chloride layer.

Diumide-K Continus tablets are not suitable for paediatric use.

Contra-indications, warnings, etc *Contra-indications;* Diumide-K Continus tablets are contra-indicated in hyperkalaemia, precomatose states associated with liver cirrhosis, Addison's disease and concomitant administration of potassium sparing diuretics.

Although the Continus controlled release system minimises the likelihood of oesophageal ulceration, all solid forms of potassium medication are contra-indicated in the presence of obstructions in the digestive tract (e.g. resulting from compression of the oesophagus due to dilation of the left atrium or from stenosis of the gut).

Warnings: Patients with prostatic hypertrophy or impairment of micturition have an increased risk of developing acute urinary retention.

Latent diabetes may become manifest or the insulin requirements of diabetic patients may increase.

Precautions; Care should be taken in patients being concurrently administered cardiac glycosides, hypotensive agents and cephaloridine. Care should also be exercised in patients with renal insufficiency where there is a risk of hyperkalaemia. Diumide-K Continus tablets should be administered with caution during the first trimester of pregnancy.

Side-effects: Frusemide is generally well tolerated and the patented Continus tablet ensures virtual absence of gastro-intestinal side-effects often associated with potassium administration.

In rare instance of allergic reaction treatment should be discontinued. Hyperuricaemia may occur with Frusemide therapy. Bone marrow depression has also been reported as a rare complication and therapy should be withdrawn.

Overdosage; Treatment of overdosage should be aimed

1016 NAPP LABORATORIES LIMITED

at fluid replacement and correction of the resulting electrolyte imbalance.

Pharmaceutical precautions Diumide-K Continus tablets should be stored in a cool dry place protected from light.

Legal category POM.

Package quantities Blister packs of 30 and containers of 250 and 1000 tablets.

Further information Frusemide produces a rapid and sustained diuresis which lasts for approximately four hours following administration. The potassium chloride content is released from the patented Continus tablet over a prolonged period ensuring maximum absorption, the avoidance of 'flushing out' of the potassium by the action of the diuretic, and virtual freedom from side-effects.

Product licence number 0337/0046.

ESODERM* LOTION

Presentation A clear colourless alcohol based lotion containing Lindane BP 1% w/v.

Uses Pesticide for the treatment of lice and scabies.

Dosage and administration
For scabies:
1. Use dampened cotton wool to apply to all parts of the body except face and scalp.
2. Rub well in and allow to dry naturally.
3. In severe cases repeat on two or three successive days.
4. Use clean underclothing and bed linen after final treatment, and bath.
For head lice:
1. Sprinkle the lotion onto dry hair. Rub gently into the scalp. Care should be taken to avoid contact with the eyes.
2. Repeat until hair is thoroughly moistened.
3. Allow to dry naturally – use no heat.
4. After 12 hours, shampoo the hair.
5. While the hair is still wet, comb with an ordinary comb. The fine-toothed Napp comb can now be used to remove all dead lice and eggs.
6. May be repeated after seven to nine days.

Contra-indications, warnings, etc Children under the age of six months should be treated under medical supervision.
When Esoderm lotion is used by a school nurse or other health officer in the mass treatment of large numbers of children, it is advisable that protective plastic or rubber gloves be worn.
Contains flammable alcohol. Apply and dry with care. Avoid naked flames (e.g. coal, gas or electric fire) or lighted objects (e.g. matches, cigarettes or lighters).
Do not use artificial heat (e.g. electric dryers).
Dry in a warm well-ventilated room.
For external use only.
Overdosage: As for ethyl alcohol, empty stomach contents and keep patient warm. In the event of massive ingestion diazepam or soluble barbiturates may be administered to control convulsions. Fat and oil should be avoided and adrenaline should not be given.

Pharmaceutical precautions Store in a cool place.

Legal category P.

Package quantities Sprinkler-top bottle of 55 ml.

Further information Lindane has a rapid action against *Sarcoptes Scabiei* and the alcoholic base aids penetration of burrows.

Product licence number 0199/5000.

ESODERM* SHAMPOO

Presentation Cream shampoo, cream in colour, containing: Lindane BP 1% w/w.

Uses Pesticide for the treatment of lice infestation.

Dosage and administration
1. Wet the hair thoroughly with warm water. Squeeze about two inches of cream shampoo into the hand and rub all over the hair, paying special attention to the roots and the scalp.
2. Apply sufficient shampoo to ensure that no part of the scalp or hair is left uncovered, and work up into a rich lather.
3. Leave for at least five minutes, rinse thoroughly with clean, warm water, and repeat procedure.
4. While the hair is still wet, comb with an ordinary comb. The fine-toothed Napp Comb can now be used to remove all dead lice and eggs.
5. Treatment may be repeated after seven to nine days.

Contra-indications, warnings, etc Children under the age of six months should be treated under medical supervision.
When Esoderm shampoo is used by a school nurse or other health officer in the mass treatment of large numbers of children, it is advisable that protective plastic or rubber gloves be worn.
For external use only.
Overdosage: Empty stomach contents and keep patient warm. In the event of massive ingestion diazepam or soluble barbiturates may be administered to control convulsions. Fat and oil should be avoided and adrenaline should not be given.

Pharmaceutical precautions None.

Legal category P.

Package quantities Tube of 40 g. Jar of 300 g.

Product licence number 0199/5001.

FERROCONTIN* CONTINUS* TABLETS

Presentation Red, film-coated, bi-convex tablets. Each tablet contains the equivalent of 100 mg Ferrous Iron in the form of Ferrous Glycine Sulphate within the patented controlled release system.

Uses Ferrocontin Continus tablets are indicated for the treatment and prophylaxis of iron deficiency anaemia.

Dosage and administration One tablet to be taken daily, or at the discretion of the physician. Ferrocontin Continus tablets should be swallowed whole and not chewed.

Contra-indications, warnings, etc None.
Overdosage: Symptoms of severe overdosage may include gastrointestinal irritation, haematemesis and diarrhoea. Inject Desferrioxamine 2 g intramuscularly.

Lavage stomach with 1% sodium bicarbonate. Administer 5 g Desferrioxamine per os. Maintain fluid and electrolyte balance. The physician should be aware that Ferrous Glycine Sulphate will be released into the blood stream for a period of hours from tablets in the intestine.

Pharmaceutical precautions Store in a cool dry place protected from light.

Legal category P.

Package quantities 30 and 250 tablets.

Further information The amino acid-iron chelate Ferrous Glycine Sulphate prevents oxidation to the ferric form in the gastro-intestinal tract, thus enhancing absorption. The use of the patented controlled release system optimises the bioavailability of ferrous iron and minimises the likelihood of side-effects.

Product licence number 0337/0041.

FERROCONTIN* FOLIC CONTINUS* TABLETS

Presentation Pale orange, film-coated bi-convex tablets. Each tablet contains the equivalent of 100 mg Ferrous Iron in the form of Ferrous Glycine Sulphate within the patented controlled release system and 0.5 mg Folic Acid BP.

Uses Ferrocontin Folic Continus tablets are indicated for the prophylaxis of iron and folic acid deficiencies during pregnancy.

Dosage and administration One tablet to be taken daily, or as directed by the physician. Ferrocontin Folic Continus tablets should be swallowed whole and not chewed.

Contra-indications, warnings, etc None.

Overdosage: Symptoms of severe overdosage may include gastrointestinal irritation, haematemesis, and diarrhoea. Inject Desferrioxamine 2 g intramuscularly. Lavage stomach with 1% sodium bicarbonate. Administer 5 g Desferrioxamine per os. Maintain fluid and electrolyte balance. The physician should be aware that Ferrous Glycine Sulphate will be released into the blood stream for a period of hours from tablets in the intestine.

Pharmaceutical precautions Store in a cool dry place protected from light.

Legal category POM.

Package quantities 30 and 250 tablets.

Further information The amino acid-iron chelate Ferrous Glycine Sulphate prevents oxidation to the ferric form in the gastro-intestinal tract, thus enhancing absorption. The use of the patented controlled release system optimises the bioavailability of ferrous iron and minimises the likelihood of side-effects. The folic acid content of 1 tablet is unlikely to mask the presence of pernicious anaemia.

Product licence number 0337/0042.

K-CONTIN* CONTINUS* TABLETS

Presentation A pale orange, film-coated, controlled release tablet containing Potassium Chloride BP 600 mg.

Uses For potassium therapy and supplementation in patients on diuretic therapy, geriatric patients, chronic diarrhoea, prolonged use of laxatives and megaloblastic anaemia.

Dosage and administration One K-Contin Continus tablet with each diuretic tablet is the average prescribed dose, but this should be adjusted to individual patient's requirements. The range of recommended dosage is 2–5 K-Contin Continus tablets daily (approximately 16–40 mEq K^+) or on alternate days if diuretic therapy has been so prescribed. The tablets should not be chewed but should be swallowed whole with water preferably prior to or during a meal.

Contra-indications, warnings, etc
Contra-indications: Although the Continus controlled release system minimises the likelihood of oesophageal ulceration, all solid forms of potassium medication are contra-indicated in the presence of obstructions in the digestive tract (e.g. resulting from compression of the oesophagus due to dilation of the left atrium or from stenosis of the gut).

Warnings: In patients with advanced renal failure, hyperkalaemia may develop if K-Contin Continus tablets are given injudiciously.

Signs or symptoms which may indicate ulceration or obstruction of the small bowel in patients taking tablets or capsules containing potassium salts are indications for stopping the treatment with potassium preparations.

Overdosage: Empty stomach contents. Treat mild to moderate hyperkalaemia with sodium polystyrene sulphate by mouth. Severe hyperkalaemia requires electrocardiogram monitoring and calcium gluconate i.v. injection (10 to 30 ml). The physician should be aware that potassium chloride will be released into the blood stream for a period of hours from tablets in the intestine.

Pharmaceutical precautions Store in a well-closed container, in a cool dry place protected from light.

Legal category P.

Package quantities Containers of 500 and 5,000 tablets.

Further information It is well recognised that potassium chloride is the correct salt for all patients who require potassium therapy. The K-Contin Continus tablet permits gradual release of the potassium chloride into the gut physiologically and continuously for 10–12 hours. The release mechanism is dependent on the physical structure of the K-Contin Continus tablet and does not depend on the pH of the gut.

Product licence number 0337/0025.

MORHULIN* OINTMENT

Presentation A white ointment containing Zinc oxide in a paraffin and lanolin base:

Cod liver oil BP	11.4% w/w
Zinc oxide BP	38.0% w/w

Uses For minor wounds, scalds, dermatitis, eczema, impetigo, boils, folliculitis, herpes etc.

Dosage and administration Spread thinly on gauze to cover affected area and about one inch of surrounding skin; on clean wounds dressing may remain for three days. If discharging wound, change dressing daily. For superficial wounds the ointment may be applied directly.

Contra-indications, warnings, etc None.

Pharmaceutical precautions None.

Legal category GSL.

Package quantities Tube of 50 g. Container of 350 g.

Further information Morhulin Ointment gives rapid relief of pain and irritation. It does not liquefy at body temperature and by preventing adhesion permits an easy and painless change of dressing.

Product licence number 0199/5012.

MST* CONTINUS* TABLETS

Presentation MST Continus tablets 10 mg are golden brown, film-coated and bi-convex. Each tablet contains 10 mg of Morphine Sulphate BP incorporated within the patented controlled release system. The tablets are marked (NAPP) on one side and $\frac{10}{mg}$ on the other side.

MST Continus tablets 30 mg are dark purple, film coated and bi-convex. Each tablet contains 30 mg of Morphine Sulphate BP incorporated within the patented controlled release system. The tablets are marked (NAPP) on one side and $\frac{30}{mg}$ on the other.

MST Continus tablets 60 mg are orange, film coated and bi-convex. Each tablet contains 60 mg of Morphine Sulphate B.P. incorporated within the patented controlled release system. The tablets are marked (NAPP) on one side and $\frac{60}{mg}$ on the other side.

MST Continus tablets 100 mg are grey, film coated and bi-convex. Each tablet contains 100 mg of Morphine Sulphate B.P. incorporated within the patented controlled release system. The tablets are marked (NAPP) on one side and $\frac{100}{mg}$ on the other side.

Uses MST Continus tablets are indicated for the prolonged relief of severe pain.

Dosage and administration MST Continus tablets must be swallowed whole and not chewed.

MST Continus tablets should be used twice daily, at 12 hourly intervals. The dosage is dependent upon the severity of the pain and the patient's previous history of analgesic requirements.

A patient presenting with severe pain should normally be started on a dosage of one or two MST Continus tablets 10 mg twice daily.

Increasing severity of pain or tolerance to morphine will require increased dosage of MST Continus tablets using 10 mg, 30 mg, 60 mg and 100 mg tablets alone or in combination to achieve the desired relief.

A patient transferred from other oral morphine preparations should normally receive the same total twenty-four hour morphine dosage divided between morning and evening administration.

Patients receiving MST Continus tablets in place of parenteral morphine should be given a sufficiently increased dosage to compensate for any reduction in analgesic effects associated with oral administration. Usually such increased requirement is of the order of 50% to 100%. In such patients individual dose adjustments are required.

Post-operative pain: MST Continus tablets are not recommended in the first 24 hours post-operatively; thereafter it is suggested that the following dosage schedule be observed at the physician's discretion:

(a) MST Continus tablets 20 mg 12 hourly to patients under 70 kilograms.

(b) MST Continus tablets 30 mg 12 hourly to patients over 70 kilograms.

Supplemental parenteral morphine may be given if required but with careful attention to the total dosage of morphine, and bearing in mind the prolonged effects of morphine in the MST Continus formulation.

As with all oral morphine preparations, MST Continus tablets should be used with caution post-operatively, and particularly in 'acute abdomen' and following abdominal surgery.

Contra-indications, warnings, etc Respiratory depression, obstructive airways disease, known morphine sensitivity, acute hepatic disease, concurrent administration of monoamine oxidase inhibitors or within two weeks of discontinuation of their use.

MST Continus tablets are not recommended for paediatric use or in pregnancy.

Pre-operative administration of MST Continus tablets is not recommended and is not an approved indication.

Precautions: As with all narcotics a reduction in dosage may be advisable in the elderly, in hypothyroidism, in renal and chronic hepatic disease.

Warnings and adverse effects: MST Continus tablets should not be used where there is a possibility of paralytic ileus occurring. Should paralytic ileus be suspected or occur during use, MST Continus tablets should be discontinued immediately. As with all morphine preparations, patients who are to undergo cordotomy or other pain relieving surgical procedures should not receive MST Continus tablets for 24 hours prior to surgery. If further treatment with MST Continus tablets is then indicated the dosage should be adjusted to the new post-operative requirement.

Tolerance and dependence may occur. When nausea and vomiting are troublesome, MST Continus tablets can be readily combined with phenothiazine antiemetics. It should be noted however, that morphine potentiates the effects of tranquillisers, anaesthetics, hypnotics and sedatives. As with all morphine preparations, constipation may occur, which may be treated with appropriate laxatives.

Overdosage: Signs of morphine toxicity and overdosage:

These are likely to consist of pin-point pupils, respiratory depression and hypotension. Circulatory failure and deepening coma may occur in more severe cases.

Treatment of morphine overdosage: Administer naloxone 0.4 mg intravenously. Repeat at 2–3 minute intervals as necessary, or by an infusion of 2 mg in 500 ml of normal saline or 5% dextrose (0.004 mg/ml).

The infusion should be run at a rate related to the previous bolus doses administered and should be in accordance with the patient's response. Empty the stomach. A 0.02% aqueous solution of potassium permanganate may be used for lavage. Assist respiration if necessary. Maintain fluid and electrolyte levels.

In the case of MST Continus tablets, the physician should be aware that tablets remaining in the intestine will continue to release morphine sulphate for a period of hours.

Pharmaceutical precautions MST Continus tablets should be stored in a cool, dry place protected from light.

Legal category CD (Sch 2) POM.

Package quantities Packs of 60 tablets.

Further information Morphine Sulphate BP is readily absorbed from the gastro-intestinal tract following oral administration. The patented controlled release system maintains plasma levels of morphine over a period of up to twelve hours and reduces the likelihood of morphine associated side-effects.

Product licence numbers
10 mg 0337/0055.
30 mg 0337/0059.
60 mg 0337/0087
100 mg 0337/0088

NITROCONTIN* CONTINUS* TABLETS

Presentation Nitrocontin Continus tablets 2.6 mg are flat, bevelled, pink, controlled release tablets containing Glyceryl Trinitrate BP 2.6 mg and embossed NC on one side and with the logo (NAPP) on the other.

Nitrocontin Continus tablets 6.4 mg are flat, bevelled, pink controlled release tablets containing Glyceryl Trinitrate BP 6.4 mg and embossed $\frac{NC}{64}$ on one side and with the logo (NAPP) on the other.

Uses For the prophylaxis and continued treatment of angina pectoris, whether or not associated with previous history of myocardial infarction. Nitrocontin Continus tablets are indicated in all cases in which sublingual nitroglycerin has provided temporary relief, whether these be cases of classical angina pectoris or the anginal pain subsequent to myocardial infarction.

Dosage and administration The tablets must be swallowed whole. Dosage should always be adjusted according to the response obtained by the individual patient and the severity of the anginal pain. Initially, the recommended dosage is one 2.6 mg tablet morning and evening.

If the symptoms have not been adequately controlled after a week on this regimen, the dosage should be increased to one 6.4 mg tablet morning and evening.

An increase in dosage to 6.4 mg three times daily may be found necessary in severe cases of angina pectoris which have not fully responded to the lesser recommended dosage.

Contra-indications, warnings, etc *Contra-indications:* As with all nitrites, cerebral haemorrhage and brain trauma, incipient glaucoma.

Side-effects: An infrequent side-effect of a transient nature which occurs with all nitrite administration is 'nitrite headache'. This disappears with continued treatment. Although patients develop tolerance to this symptom they do not develop tolerance to the drug. However, such side-effects are virtually absent or substantially diminished with Nitrocontin Continus tablet therapy due to the patented controlled release system.

Overdosage: Empty stomach contents. Administer oxygen if necessary. Treat methaemoglobinaemia with intravenous methylene blue. Keep unconscious patients horizontal and lower head. Physicians should be aware that tablets in the intestine will release Glyceryl Trinitrate for a period of hours.

Pharmaceutical precautions Store in a cool dry place protected from light.

Legal category P.

Package quantities *Tablets 2.6 mg:* 100 tablets.

Tablets 6.4 mg: 100 tablets.

Further information Glyceryl Trinitrate has a twofold action in relieving angina pectoris. It reduces cardiac work and dilates the coronary arteries. Thus, not only is the arterial oxygen requirement of the myocardium lessened, but the amount of oxygenated blood reaching the ischaemic heart is increased.

Nitrocontin Continus tablets provide adequate and continuous activity throughout the day and night on a simple b.d. dosage.

The need for sublingual glyceryl trinitrate is substantially reduced as the frequency and severity of anginal attacks are decreased.

Nitrocontin Continus tablets may be co-prescribed with β-blocking agents for enhanced prophylaxis from angina. Nitrocontin Continus tablets actively prevent anginal episodes and reduce heavy dependence on multiple doses of sublingual glyceryl trinitrate administration.

Product licence numbers
Tablets 2.6 mg   0337/5026
Tablets 6.4 mg   0337/5027

PHYLLOCONTIN* CONTINUS* TABLETS

Presentation Pale yellow, film-coated tablets with 'SA' on one side and (NAPP) on the other. Each tablet contains aminophylline 225 mg in the patented controlled release system.

Uses For the treatment and prophylaxis of bronchospasm associated with asthma, emphysema and chronic bronchitis. Phyllocontin Continus tablets are also indicated in the treatment of cardiac asthma and left ventricular or congestive cardiac failure.

Dosage and administration The usual daily dose is 2 tablets twice a day, taken morning and evening, following an initial week of therapy on 1 tablet twice daily.

Since patients vary in their response to xanthines, the dosage must be titrated individually, and may also need to be adjusted if concomitant medication is prescribed. If maximum response is not achieved, theophylline plasma levels should be measured. Smoking and consumption of alcohol may increase clearance of theophylline and therefore, the dosage requirement. While the usual dose is 2 tablets twice daily, factors such as viral infections, liver disease and heart failure, may reduce clearance of theophylline, and the dosage should be reduced if necessary. A reduction in dosage may be necessary in the elderly patient.

N.B. Tablets should be swallowed whole and not chewed.

Contra-indications, warnings, etc
Contra-indications: None.

Side-effects: The risk of side-effects usually associated with aminophylline and xanthine derivatives such as nausea, gastric irritation, headache and CNS stimulation are much diminished when Phyllocontin Continus tablets are given.

Overdosage: Empty stomach contents. Monitor electrocardiogram and maintain fluid balance. Oral activated charcoal has been found to reduce high theophylline blood levels. In severe poisoning employ charcoal-column haemoperfusion. Treat symptoms on appearance. The physician should be aware that tablets in the intestine will continue to release aminophylline for a period of hours.

Pharmaceutical precautions Store in a cool, dry place protected from light.

Legal category P.

Package quantities 60, 250 and 1000 tablets.

Further information Phyllocontin Continus tablets utilise the patented controlled release mechanism, in which aminophylline is released to give an effective therapeutic blood level, lasting up to 12 hours. This release mechanism therefore minimises the unpleasant side-effects usually associated with oral doses of aminophylline, e.g. nausea and gastric irritation.

Product licence number 0337/0026.

PHYLLOCONTIN* FORTE CONTINUS* TABLETS

Presentation Yellow, film coated capsule-shaped scored tablets with the logo (NAPP) and 350 embossed on one side and PHYLLOCONTIN FORTE on the other. Each tablet contains Aminophylline BP 350 mg in the patented controlled release system.

Uses For the treatment and prophylaxis of bronchospasm associated with asthma, emphysema and chronic bronchitis. Phyllocontin Forte Continus tablets are also indicated in the treatment of cardiac asthma and left ventricular or congestive cardiac failure.

Dosage and administration The usual daily dose is one or two tablets twice a day, taken morning and evening, following an initial week of therapy on 1 tablet twice daily.

Since patients vary in their response to xanthines, the dosage must be titrated individually and may also need to be adjusted if concomitant medication is prescribed.

If maximum response is not achieved, theophylline plasma levels should be measured. Smoking and consumption of alcohol may increase clearance of theophylline and therefore the dosage requirement. Factors such as viral infections, liver disease and heart failure, may reduce clearance of theophylline, and the dosage should be reduced if necessary. A reduction in dosage may be necessary in the elderly patient.

N.B. Tablets should not be chewed.

Contra-indications, warnings, etc
Contra-indications: None.

Side-effects: The risk of side-effects usually associated with aminophylline and xanthine derivatives such as nausea, gastric irritation, headache and CNS stimulation are much diminished when Phyllocontin Forte Continus tablets are given.

Overdosage: Empty stomach contents. Monitor electrocardiogram and maintain fluid balance. Oral activated medical charcoal has been found to reduce high theophylline blood levels. In severe poisoning employ charcoal-column haemoperfusion. Treat symptoms on appearance. The physician should be aware that tablets in the intestine will continue to release aminophylline for a period of hours.

Pharmaceutical precautions Store in a cool, dry place protected from light.

Legal category P.

Package quantities Containers of 60 tablets.

Further Information Phyllocontin Forte Continus tablets utilise the patented controlled release mechanism, in which aminophylline is released to give an effective therapeutic blood level lasting up to 12 hours. This release mechanism therefore minimises the unpleasant side-effects usually associated with oral doses of aminophylline, e.g. nausea and gastric irritation.

Product licence number 0337/0090

PHYLLOCONTIN* PAEDIATRIC CONTINUS* TABLETS

Presentation Pale orange bi-convex tablets with SA/2 on one side and (NAPP) on the other. Each tablet contains Aminophylline BP 100 mg in the patented controlled release system.

Uses For the treatment and prophylaxis of childhood bronchospasm associated with asthma, bronchitis and emphysema.

Dosage and administration The maintenance dose for children (expressed as mg aminophylline) is 12 mg/kg twice daily adjusted to the nearest 100 mg. It may be appropriate to give half the maintenance dose for the first week of therapy if the patient has not previously received xanthine preparations.

Some children with chronic asthma require and tolerate much higher doses (13–20 mg/kg twice daily). The dosage will therefore depend on the patient's clinical response and it is necessary to titrate the dosage to achieve optimal response. Viral infections and concomitant medication may reduce clearance of theophylline and the dosage should be reduced if necessary.

Lower dosages (based on usual adult dose) may be required by adolescents.

N.B. The tablets should be swallowed whole and not chewed.

Contra-indications, warnings, etc Should not be given concomitantly with ephedrine.

Side-effects: The risks of side-effects usually associated with aminophylline and xanthine derivatives such as nausea, gastric irritation, headache and CNS stimulation are much diminished when Phyllocontin Paediatric Continus tablets are given.

Overdosage: Empty stomach contents. Monitor electrocardiogram and maintain fluid balance. Oral activated medical charcoal has been found to reduce high theophylline blood levels. In severe poisoning employ charcoal-column haemoperfusion. Treat symptoms on appearance. The physician should be aware that tablets in the intestine will continue to release aminophylline for a period of hours.

Pharmaceutical precautions Store in a cool, dry place protected from light.

Legal category P.

Package quantities 50 and 250 tablets.

Product licence number 0337/0040.

PLESMET* SYRUP

Presentation Blackcurrant flavoured syrup containing the equivalent of 25 mg ferrous iron per 5 ml dose in the form of ferrous glycine sulphate.

Uses Treatment of iron deficiency anaemia.

Dosage and administration *Adults:* 5–10 ml three times a day.

Children: 2–5 ml two or three times per day according to age. Plesmet syrup may be diluted with Syrup Tolu BP to make up a 5 ml dose.

Contra-indications, warnings, etc None.

Overdosage: Symptoms of severe overdosage may include gastrointestinal irritation, haematemesis and diarrhoea. In the event of accidental or deliberate ingestion of large volumes, inject Desferrioxamine 2 g intramuscularly. Lavage stomach with 1% sodium bicarbonate. Administer 5 g Desferrioxamine per os. Maintain fluid and electrolyte balance.

Pharmaceutical precautions Store in a cool, dry place protected from light.

Legal category P.

Package quantities Bottles of 100 ml and 1 litre.

Further information Chelated iron is more readily absorbed and utilised than the more conventional forms of iron. Side effects are virtually absent.

Product licence number 0337/5904

PRESSURISED BROVON* INHALER

Presentation A green, transparent, shatterproof aerosol for inhalation containing Adrenaline 0.50% w/v (as hydrochloride) and Atropine Methonitrate BP 0.10% w/v in a freon-alcohol propellent solution.

Uses For the relief and prevention of bronchospasm in asthma, chronic bronchitis and other respiratory diseases.

Dosage and administration Having removed the dust cap, the unit is held upright, the mouthpiece inserted between the lips, and the patient breathes out. The adaptor is then depressed and at the same time patient inhales deeply. The breath is held for a moment, then the patient slowly exhales, releasing the adaptor at the same time. Each depression releases a consistently accurate measured dose of Pressurised Brovon inhalant containing adrenaline 0.25 mg and atropine 0.05 mg. Approximately 330 doses are obtained from each aerosol.

One 'puff' of Pressurised Brovon inhaler may be used four to six-hourly to prevent attacks. In an acute attack one or two puffs should suffice, repeated if necessary, not more often than every 30 minutes.

Contra-indications, warnings, etc Should not be prescribed with monoamine oxidase inhibitors or with sympathomimetic drugs.

Contra-indicated in patients with hypertension, thyrotoxicosis, acute coronary disease and cardiac asthma.

Overdosage may produce transitory tachycardia or dizziness. As with all atropine-containing preparations dryness of the mouth may occur.

It is highly inadvisable to exceed the recommended dose.

Overdosage: Administer alpha-adrenergic blocker by intravenous injection and a cardioselective beta-blocker per os. Propranolol must not be given to asthmatics because of the risk of increasing broncho-constriction.

Pharmaceutical precautions Store in a cool, dry area protected from light.

Legal category POM.

Package quantities Aerosol of 17 ml.

Further information The rapid sympathomimetic action of the adrenaline and the less rapid but more prolonged parasympatholytic action of the atropine methonitrate, are both complementary and mutually enhancing in relaxing bronchospasm.

Product licence number 0337/5011.

PRESSURISED ISO-BROVON* INHALER
PRESSURISED ISO-BROVON* PLUS INHALER

Presentation PIB Inhaler is a green, transparent, shatterproof aerosol for inhalation containing Isoprenaline Hydrochloride USP 0.35% w/v and Atropine Methonitrate BP 0.10% w/v in a freon/alcohol propellant solution.

The PIB Plus inhaler contains Isoprenaline Hydrochloride USP 1.00% w/v and Atropine Methonitrate BP 0.10% w/v in a freon/alcohol propellant solution.

Uses For the relief and prevention of bronchospasm in asthma, chronic bronchitis and other respiratory diseases.

Dosage and administration Having removed the dust cap the unit is held upright, the mouthpiece inserted between the lips and the patient breathes out. The adaptor is then depressed and at the same time the patient inhales deeply. The breath is held for a moment, then the patient slowly exhales, releasing the adaptor at the same time. Each depression releases a consistently accurate measured dose of PIB inhalant. Approximately 330 doses are obtained from each aerosol.

The PIB inhalers may be used four- to six-hourly to prevent attacks. In an acute attack one or two 'puffs' should suffice, repeated if necessary, not more often that every 30 minutes.

Contra-indications, warnings, etc Should not be prescribed with monoamine oxidase inhibitors or with sympathomimetic drugs.

Overdosage may produce transitory tachycardia or dizziness. As with all atropine-containing preparations dryness of the mouth may occur.

Contra-indicated in patients with hypertension, thyrotoxicosis, acute coronary disease and cardiac asthma.

It is highly inadvisable to exceed the recommended dose.

Overdosage: Administer alpha adrenergic blocker by intravenous injection and a cardioselective beta blocker per os. Propranolol must not be given to asthmatics because of the risk of increasing bronchoconstriction.

Pharmaceutical precautions Store in a cool dry place protected from light.

Legal category POM.

Package quantities Aerosol of 17 ml.

Further information Nil.

Product licence numbers
PIB   0337/5012
PIB Plus   0337/5010

PRIODERM* CREAM SHAMPOO

Presentation A light-orange pearlescent cream shampoo containing malathion 1.0% w/w.

Uses For the treatment of head and pubic lice infestation.

Dosage and administration The source of infestation should be sought and treated.

For head lice:
   1. Wet the hair thoroughly with warm water and apply sufficient shampoo to work up a rich lather and ensure that no part of the scalp is left uncovered. Pay special attention to the back of the neck and area behind the ears. Take care to avoid the eyes.
   2. Leave for at least five minutes.
   3. Rinse thoroughly with clean, warm water and repeat procedure.
   4. While the hair is still wet, comb with an ordinary comb. The fine-toothed Napp comb can then be used to remove the dead lice and eggs.
   5. This treatment should be carried out a total of three times at three day intervals.

For pubic lice:
   1. Wet area and apply shampoo directly to the pubic hair and the hair between the legs and around the anus.
   2. Cover the skin and hair completely with shampoo.
   3. Work up a lather and leave for at least five minutes.
   4. Rinse thoroughly.
   5. Repeat procedure. The fine-toothed Napp Comb can then be used to remove the dead lice and eggs.

Contra-indications, warnings, etc Children under the age of six months should be treated under medical supervision.

As with all shampoos, avoid contact with the eyes. When Prioderm Cream Shampoo is used by a school nurse or other health officer in the mass treatment of large numbers of children, it is advisable that protective plastic or rubber gloves be worn.

Treatment of overdosage: In the event of deliberate or accidental ingestion, empty stomach contents and keep patient warm. In the event of massive ingestion atropine and pralidoxime may be required to counteract cholinesterase inhibition.

Pharmaceutical precautions None.

Legal category P.

Package quantities Tube of 40 g.

Further information Prioderm Cream Shampoo contains the insecticide malathion which is rapidly lethal to both lice and their eggs.

Product licence number 0337/0036.

PRIODERM* LOTION

Presentation A clear, colourless, alcohol-based lotion containing malathion 0.5% w/v.

Uses For the treatment of head and pubic lice infestations and scabies.

Dosage and administration The source of infestation should be sought and treated.

For head lice:
   1. Sprinkle the lotion on the hair and rub gently on to the head until the entire scalp is moistened. Pay special attention to the back of the neck and area behind the ears. Take care to avoid the eyes.
   2. Allow the hair to dry naturally – use NO heat.
   3. As all lice and eggs will have been killed the hair may be shampooed after 2 hours. If a residual effect is desired, however, it is recommended that shampooing be carried out after 12 hours.
   4. While still wet, comb the hair with an ordinary comb. The fine-toothed Napp comb can then be used to remove the dead lice and eggs.

For pubic lice: Application and dosage, etc. are as for the head. Apply the lotion to the pubic hair and the hair between the legs and around the anus. Allow to dry naturally using NO heat. Transient, mild stinging may be experienced due to the alcohol content.

For scabies:
   1. Use cotton wool to apply lotion to all parts of the body except face and scalp.
   2. Rub in well and allow to dry naturally. Do not bathe until 12 hours after treatment.

Contra-indications, warnings, etc Contains flammable alcohol. Apply and dry with care. Avoid naked flames or lighted objects. Do not use artificial heat (e.g. electric dryers). Dry in a well-ventilated room. Do not cover the head before the lotion has dried completely.

Children under the age of six months should be treated under medical supervision.

When Prioderm Lotion is used by a school nurse or other health officer in the mass treatment of large numbers of children, it is advisable that protective plastic or rubber gloves be worn.

Treatment of overdosage: In the event of deliberate or accidental ingestion, as for ethyl alcohol, empty stomach contents and keep patient warm. In the event of massive ingestion atropine and pralidoxime may be required to counteract cholinsterase inhibition.

Pharmaceutical precautions Store in a cool place protected from light.

Legal category P.

Package quantities Sprinkler-top bottles of 55 ml and 110 ml.

Further information The volatile alcoholic base used in Prioderm Lotion evaporates quickly leaving a high concentration of Malathion on the hair. This is rapidly lethal to both lice and their eggs and may give several weeks' protection from reinfestation. For this protective effect to be optimal Prioderm Lotion should be left on the scalp for 12 hours before shampooing and no artificial heat used to dry the hair after shampooing.

Product licence number 0199/5002.

TRILISATE* TABLETS

Presentation Pale orange, capsule shaped, scored tablets containing 500 mg salicylate as Choline Magnesium Trisalicylate. The tablets embossed 'NAPP 500' on one side and 'TRILISATE' on the reverse.

Uses Trilisate tablets are indicated for relief of the signs and symptoms of rheumatoid arthritis, osteoarthritis and other arthroses.

Dosage and administration (a) One or two tablets twice a day for osteoarthritis and mild to moderate arthroses.

(b) Two or three tablets twice a day for rheumatoid arthritis and the more severe arthroses.

For maintenance therapy the total daily dosage may be given as a single daily dosage.

Contra-indications, warnings, etc *Contra-indications:* Hypersensitivity to aspirin. Active peptic ulceration. Haemophilia.

Precautions; Concurrent administration with other analgesics containing aspirin. As with other salicylates, Trilisate tablets should be used with caution in patients with chronic renal insufficiency, or with erosive gastritis or peptic ulcer.

Trilisate tablets should be used with caution in pregnancy.

Warnings and adverse effects: May induce gastrointestinal haemorrhage. Reports indicate that when salicylates are given with steroids, the butazones or alcohol, the risk of gastrointestinal ulceration is increased.

Trilisate tablets are not recommended for children under twelve years of age. As with all medicines, Trilisate tablets should be kept out of reach of children.

Overdosage: Empty stomach contents and lavage stomach with 5% sodium bicarbonate solution. Severe overdosage should be treated by diuresis induced by intravenous saline with sodium bicarbonate, or dextrose solution. Electrolyte levels and acid base balance should be monitored and corrected as necessary.

Pharmaceutical precautions Trilisate tablets should be stored in a cool, dry place, protected from light.

Legal category P.

Package quantities Containers of 60 tablets.

Further information When Trilisate tablets are administered, the salicylate is absorbed rapidly and reaches peak blood levels within two hours. At recommended doses, the therapeutic range of 5 to 30 mg/100 ml is achieved, and a steady state condition is normally reached after 4–5 doses.

Trilisate tablets do not cause any significant faecal blood loss nor do they affect platelet aggregation.

Trilisate tablets do not cause any observable stomach mucosal irritation as determined by endoscopic examination.

Product licence number 0337/0053.

UNIPHYLLIN* PAEDIATRIC CONTINUS* TABLETS

Presentation White, flat, bevelled-edged, scored tablets with the logo (NAPP) on one side. Each tablet contains Theophylline B.P. 200 mg in the patented controlled release system.

Uses For the treatment and prophylaxis of childhood bronchospasm associated with asthma, bronchitis and emphysema.

Dosage and administration The maintenance dose for children is a single daily dose of 18 mg/kg/day adjusted to the nearest 100 mg. It may be appropriate to give half the maintenance dose once daily for the first week of therapy if the patient has not previously received xanthine preparations.

Some children with chronic asthma require and tolerate much higher doses (20–35 mg/kg/day). The dosage will therefore depend on the patient's clinical response and it is necessary to titrate the dosage to achieve the optimum response. Viral infections may reduce clearance of theophylline and the dosage should be reduced if necessary.

Lower dosages (based on usual adult dose) may be required by adolescents.

N.B. Tablets should not be chewed.

Contra-indications, warnings, etc
Contra-indications: Should not be given concomitantly with ephedrine.

Side-effects: The risk of side-effects usually associated with theophylline and xanthine derivatives such as nausea, gastric irritation, headache and CNS stimulation are much diminished when Uniphyllin Paediatric Continus tablets are given.

Overdosage: Empty stomach contents. Monitor electrocardiogram and maintain fluid balance. Oral activated medical charcoal has been found to reduce high theophylline blood-levels. In severe poisoning employ charcoal-column haemoperfusion. Treat symptoms on appearance. The physician should be aware that tablets in the intestines will continue to release theophylline for a period of hours.

Pharmaceutical precautions Store in a cool, dry place protected from light.

Legal category P.

Package quantities Blister packs of 60.

Further information Uniphyllin Paediatric Continus tablets utilise the patented controlled release system from which theophylline is released to give an effective therapeutic blood level lasting up to 24 hours. This controlled release system also minimises the unpleasant side-effects usually associated with oral doses of theophylline, i.e. nausea and gastric irritation.

Product licence number 0337/0057.

UNIPHYLLIN CONTINUS* TABLETS

Presentation White, capsule-shaped, scored tablets with the logo (NAPP) and U400 embossed on one side and UNIPHYLLIN on the other. Each tablet contains Theophylline BP 400 mg in the patented controlled release system.

Uses For the treatment and prophylaxis of bronchospasm associated with asthma, emphysema and chronic bronchitis.

Uniphyllin Continus tablets are also indicated in the treatment of cardiac asthma and left ventricular and congestive cardiac failure.

Dosage and administration Patients 70 kg body weight or over: 800 mg to be taken as single daily dose following an initial week of therapy on 400 mg once daily.

Patients less than 70 kg body weight: 600 mg once daily following an initial week of therapy on 400 mg once daily.

Since patients vary in their response to xanthines, the dosage must be titrated individually and may also need to be adjusted if concomitant medication is prescribed. If maximum response is not achieved, theophylline plasma levels should be measured. Smoking and consumption of alcohol may increase clearance of theophylline and therefore, the dosage requirement. While the usual dose is 600–800 mg once daily, factors such as viral infections, liver disease, heart failure and cor pulmonale, may reduce clearance of theophylline and the dosage should be reduced if necessary. A reduction in dosage may be necessary in the elderly patient.

N.B. Tablets should not be chewed.

Contra-indications, warnings, etc
Contra-indications: None known.

Side-effects: The risk of side-effects usually associated with theophylline and xanthine derivatives such as nausea, gastric irritation, headache and CNS stimulation are significantly reduced when Uniphyllin Continus tablets are given.

Overdosage: Empty stomach contents. Monitor electrocardiogram and maintain fluid balance. In severe poisoning employ charcoal-column haemoperfusion. Treat symptoms on appearance. The physician should be aware that tablets in the intestine will release theophylline for a period of hours.

Pharmaceutical precautions Store in a cool, dry place protected from light.

Legal category P.

Package quantities Blister packs of 60 and containers of 250 and 1000 tablets.

Further information Uniphyllin Continus tablets utilise a patented controlled release system, from which the theophylline is released to give an effective therapeutic blood level lasting up to 24 hours. This controlled release system also minimises the unpleasant side-effects usually associated with oral doses of theophylline i.e. nausea and gastric irritation.

Product licence number 400 mg   0337/0074.

X-PREP* LIQUID
Presentation A chocolate-flavoured, brown liquid containing the Primolax* brand of purified, standardised extract of senna fruit equivalent to 72 mg total Sennosides in each 72 ml dose.

Uses A single-dose pre-radiographic purgative given the day prior to radiographic examination, particularly in gastro-intestinal and urological procedures.

Dosage and administration The following doses apply to all age groups:

Patients with bodyweight of 72 kgs or more – complete bottle, 72 ml (72 mg sennosides), should be taken between 2.00 and 4.00 pm on the day before the X-ray examination.

Patients with bodyweight of less than 72 kgs – dosage is 1 ml (1 mg sennosides) per kg bodyweight taken between 2.00 and 4.00 pm on the day before the X-ray examination.

In either case the dosage may be split into two equal volumes with one hour between each administration. Each administration should be followed by at least half a pint of water and the patient should drink a further half a pint of water every hour throughout the afternoon and evening.

Patients should be advised to expect a strong thorough bowel action to begin approximately six to eight hours later.

Contra-indications, warnings, etc
Contra-indications: The usual clinical contra-indications for purgatives apply to X-Prep Liquid. X-Prep Liquid should not be used in patients with bowel obstruction.

Warnings: Caution should be exercised in the elderly and in patients with inflammatory bowel disease or suspected diverticular disease.

As with all purgatives mild to severe griping and some nausea occasionally occur; however, these are generally less of a problem with X-Prep Liquid and are minimised by drinking at least the recommended volume of water.

A light, bland, fat-free meal should precede administration. No solid food should be taken after administration and nothing at all after 10.00 pm on the day before the X-ray examination.

In diabetic patients the doctor should be aware of the sugar content of X-Prep Liquid (47.52 g per 72 ml dose).

Overdosage: In the event of deliberate or accidental ingestion of large amounts where diarrhoea is severe, excessive loss of water and electrolytes may occur. Treatment is supportive with generous amounts of fluid. Electrolytes, especially potassium, should be monitored.

Pharmaceutical precautions Store in a cool, dry place protected from light.

Legal category P.

Package quantities Bottles containing 72 ml.

Further information Nil.

Product licence number 0337/5017.

*Trade Mark

Nicholas Laboratories Limited
PO Box 17
Slough
Berkshire SL1 4AU

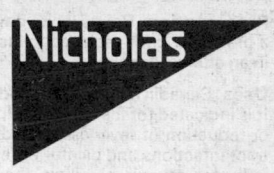

ALBUCID* EYE DROPS
ALBUCID* EYE OINTMENT

Presentation Albucid Eye Drops are sterile solutions containing 10% w/v, 20% w/v and 30% w/v Sulphacetamide Sodium PhEur. Sodium pentachlorophenate is included as a preservative.

Albucid Eye Ointments are sterile ointments containing 2½% w/w and 6% w/w Sulphacetamide Sodium PhEur in a greasy base and 10% w/w Sulphacetamide Sodium PhEur in a water-miscible base. Sodium Thiosulphate PhEur is included as a preservative.

Uses *Albucid Eye Drops:* Albucid Eye Drops 10%: Mild infections of the conjunctiva and eyelids. Industrial eye injuries. Prophylaxis against infection.

Albucid Eye Drops 20%: Conjunctivitis and ophthalmia neonatorum.

Albucid Eye Drops 30%: Severe conjunctivitis. Corneal ulceration including dendritic ulceration. Trachoma.

Albucid Eye Ointment: Albucid Eye Ointment 2½%: Mild infections of the conjunctiva and eyelids. Industrial eye injuries. Prophylaxis against infection.

Albucid Eye Ointment 6%: Conjunctivitis. Trachoma. Corneal ulceration including dendritic ulceration.

Albucid Eye Ointment 10%: Blepharitis and styes.

Dosage and administration *Albucid Eye Drops:* All ages: 2–4 drops two to six hourly.

Albucid Eye Ointment: All ages: 2½% and 6% at night. 10% apply to lids two to four times daily.

Contra-indications, warnings, etc
Contra-indicated: Known sensitivity to sulphonamides.

Side-effects: Some transient irritation may occur, especially with the higher concentrations.

Use in pregnancy: No special precautions required.

Overdosage: Not applicable.

Pharmaceutical precautions Store at room temperature. Do not freeze.

Legal Category POM.

Package quantities Albucid Eye Drops (all strengths): Opaque white polythene bottles with coloured caps, containing 10 ml sterile solution. Colour coding of caps: 10% drops – green; 20% drops – brown; 30% drops – red.

Albucid Eye Ointment (all strengths): Tube containing 4 g sterile ointment.

Product licence numbers

Albucid Eye Drops	10%	0188/5912
	20%	0188/5911
	30%	0188/5910
Albucid Eye Ointment	2½%	0188/5915
	6%	0188/5914
	10%	0188/5916

ASMAPAX*

Presentation Buff-coloured circular, bevelled-edge tablets impressed with 'ASMAPAX' and 'N' on one side and a break-line on the other. Each tablet contains:

Ephedrine resinate (equivalent to Ephedrine Hydrochloride PhEur 50 mg)	123 mg
Theophylline Hydrate PhEur	65 mg

Uses Prolonged action bronchodilator.
Relief of bronchospasm in chronic bronchitis, asthma and similar disorders.

Dosage and administration *Adults:* 1–2 tablets two or three times a day.

Children 5–12 years: ½ tablet two or three times a day, or as directed.

Use in the elderly: No special dosage regimen required but care should be taken to observe contra-indications below.

Contra-indications, warnings, etc A known sensitivity to ephedrine is the only absolute contra-indication, but Asmapax should be used with caution in patients with cardiac conditions, hypertension, hyperthyroidism, impaired liver function or prostatic enlargement. Like all sympathomimetic amines, ephedrine should not be used in conjunction with monoamine oxidase inhibitors.

Use in pregnancy: The use of this product should be avoided in pregnancy.

Theophylline and ephedrine are excreted in breast milk and therefore breast-feeding should be avoided.

Overdosage: Gastric lavage should be undertaken if vomiting has not occurred; followed by symptomatic supportive treatment, including correction of electrolyte disturbance, and mild sedation.

Pharmaceutical precautions Store at room temperature.

Legal category POM.

Package quantities Containers of 30 and 250 tablets.

Further information Ephedrine may increase blood glucose levels.

Product licence number 0188/5920.

CLARADIN*

Presentation Round white bevelled edge tablets with a breakline. Each tablet contains Aspirin PhEur 300 mg in an effervescent base.

Uses Claradin has analgesic and anti-pyretic properties. It is indicated for the relief of mild to moderate pain and/or reduction of fever associated with upper respiratory tract infections and painful or febrile disorders, such as influenza, pyrexia, neuralgia, rheumatic pain, dysmenorrhoea, and migraine pain.

Claradin also has anti-inflammatory properties, and is indicated in rheumatoid arthritis, osteoarthrosis and acute and chronic rheumatic conditions.

Dosage and administration Claradin Tablets should be dissolved in water before administration.

As an analgesic and antipyretic.

Adults: 2–3 tablets every four hours. Do not exceed 13 tablets in 24 hours unless so directed.

Children: 4–6 years: Half a tablet every four hours. Do not exceed 3 tablets in 24 hours.

7–12 years: 1 tablet every four hours. Do not exceed 6 tablets in 24 hours.

As an anti-inflammatory.

Usual dose, Adults: 300–1200 mg (1–4 tablets) up to 4 g daily in divided doses. In acute rheumatic conditions up to 8 g daily (26 tablets) in divided doses.

Children (up to age 12): Up to 80 mg/kg/day, in divided doses.

Elderly persons: No special dosage regimen required, but exercise caution when renal function is impaired.

Contra-indications, warnings, etc
Contra-indications: Claradin, as other aspirin products, is contra-indicated in patients with active peptic ulceration, haemophilia, or who have hypersensitivity to aspirin. Breast-feeding is contra-indicated at high doses, because of the theoretical risk of affecting clotting mechanisms.

Precautions and warnings: Aspirin may precipitate bronchospasm, and induce asthmatic attacks in susceptible subjects; it may induce gastro-intestinal haemorrhage, occasionally major.

Drug interactions: Aspirin may enhance the effects of anti-coagulants, and may inhibit the action of uricosuric agents.

Use in pregnancy: There is clinical and epidemiological evidence of safety of aspirin in pregnancy, but it may prolong labour and contribute to maternal and neo-natal bleeding, and so is best avoided at term.

Overdosage: Gastric lavage, forced alkaline diuresis and supportive therapy may be employed. Restoration of acid-base balance may be necessary.

Pharmaceutical precautions Store at room temperature, in a dry place.

Legal category P.

Package quantities Claradin tablets are packed in moisture-proof aluminium foil, in cartons of 100 tablets.

Further information In high dosage, aspirin has a uricosuric effect, and may reduce plasma bicarbonate, and prolong prothrombin time. Claradin is formulated to achieve rapid absorption of aspirin, and high plasma levels of acetylsalicylic acid. This is of value in ensuring rapid onset of analgesia, particularly when there is gastro-intestinal stasis, as in migraine.

Claradin is well tolerated, on account of its administration in buffered solution.

Claradin has a sodium content of 7.1 mmol per tablet.

Product licence number 0188/0010.

CORTUCID* EYE CREAM

Presentation Cortucid is a bland, sterile fluid cream containing Sulphacetamide Sodium PhEur 10.0% w/w, and Hydrocortisone Acetate PhEur 0.5% w/w in a water miscible cream base. Sodium Thiosulphate PhEur is included as a preservative.

Uses Cortucid gives prompt relief of inflammatory conditions of the eye, whilst protecting the eye against the increased hazard of infection resulting from the use of a corticosteroid.

Cortucid is for the treatment of inflammatory eye conditions of either bacterial or allergic origin.

Dosage and administration For all ages: It is suggested that the cream should be dropped into the eye every three to six hours until the condition improves (about two days). Thereafter the number of applications per day may be reduced, but treatment should be continued for at least two days after the condition has subsided.

Contra-indications, warnings, etc Cortucid should not be used in patients with ocular tuberculosis, herpes simplex ophthalmicus, corneal ulceration, trachoma or glaucoma.

Cortucid is also contra-indicated in patients exhibiting true sensitivity to one of the ingredients.

Use in pregnancy: Topical administration of any corticosteroid to pregnant animals can cause abnormalities of foetal development. The relevance of this finding in human beings has not been established. However, topical steroids should not be used extensively in pregnancy i.e. in large amounts or for prolonged periods.

Precautions: Long term continuous topical therapy should be avoided. In infants, adrenal suppression can occur even without occlusion.

Overdosage: Not applicable.

Pharmaceutical precautions Store in a cool, dry place.

Legal category POM.

Package quantities Cortucid is packed in tubes containing 3 g.

Further information Inflammation of the eye, if allowed to persist, may result in the formation of vision-impairing scar tissue. Cortucid is formulated with hydrocortisone to safely suppress the inflammation and with sodium sulphacetamide, a suitable bacteriostat for local application in the eye.

Product licence number 0188/5923.

GENTICIN* CREAM
GENTICIN* OINTMENT

Presentation Genticin Cream is a white, smooth cream which contains Gentamicin Sulphate PhEur ≡ 0.3% w/w gentamicin base in a water-miscible base. Methylhydroxybenzoate PhEur and Butylhydroxybenzoate PhEur are included as preservatives.

Genticin Ointment is a colourless, opaque ointment which contains Gentamicin Sulphate PhEur ≡ 0.3% w/w gentamicin base in a greasy base. Methylhydroxybenzoate PhEur and Propylhydroxybenzoate PhEur are included as preservatives.

Uses The unique broad spectrum of activity of Genticin Cream and Ointment makes them ideally suitable for the topical treatment of all bacterial skin conditions.

Genticin Cream and Ointment are indicated particularly in infected wounds, impetigo, varicose ulcers, Decubitus ulcers, Sycosis barbae, folliculitis and burns.

Dosage and administration For all ages: Genticin Cream and Ointment are intended for topical use only and should be applied three to four times daily to the infected area, covering with a gauze dressing if necessary. Cream preparations are recommended for moist lesions and ointment for dry conditions.

Contra-indications, warnings, etc There are no specific contra-indications except in cases of true sensitivity to one of the ingredients.

Precautions: If irritation, sensitization or super-infection develop, treatment with Genticin should be discontinued and appropriate therapy instituted.

Overdosage: Not applicable.

Use in pregnancy: No additional precautions required.

Pharmaceutical precautions Store at room temperature. Do not freeze.

In order to preserve the therapeutic activity of these products they should not be diluted.

Legal category POM.

Package quantities Genticin Cream and Ointment are available in 15 g and 100 g tubes.

Further information The wide range and degree of antibacterial activity of Genticin coupled with freedom from troublesome side effects make it particularly suitable for bacterial skin conditions, where the pathogens involved or their sensitivity to antibiotics are unknown.

Product licence numbers
Genticin Cream   0188/5926
Genticin Ointment   0188/5927

GENTICIN* EYE/EAR DROPS

Presentation Gentamicin Sulphate PhEur ≡ 0.3% w/v gentamicin base in a sterile, aqueous, isotonic solution in a 10 ml dropper bottle. Benzalkonium Chloride BP and Borax PhEur are included as preservatives.

Uses Genticin (gentamicin) is a proven bactericidal antibiotic active against an extremely broad spectrum of Gram-positive and Gram-negative bacteria. Genticin Eye/Ear Drops are therefore particularly useful in all external bacterial infections of the eye, where the bacterial organisms are often very varied.

In particular Genticin Eye/Ear Drops are indicated in conjunctivitis, blepharitis, styes, corneal ulcers, and prophylaxis in trauma.

Genticin Eye/Ear Drops have also been used extensively in infected ear conditions.

Dosage and administration For all ages:
Eyes: 1–3 drops instilled in affected eye three to four times a day or as required.

Ears: The area should be cleaned and 2–4 drops instilled three to four times a day and at night. In middle ear infections the cavity may be filled with drops.

Contra-indications, warnings, etc There are no specific contra-indications except true sensitivity to one of the ingredients.

Precautions: If irritation, sensitization or super-infection develop, treatment with Genticin shoud be discontinued and appropriate therapy instituted.

Use in pregnancy: No additional precautions required.

Pharmaceutical precautions Store at room temperature. Do not freeze.

Legal category POM.

Package quantities Genticin Eye/Ear Drops are available in 10 ml opaque, white, polythene dropper bottles with white plastic caps.

Further information Gentisone HC Ear Drops are also available where a mild steroid (hydrocortisone acetate 1.0% w/v) is required in addition to Genticin (gentamicin sulphate 0.3% w/v) to treat infections complicated by an inflammatory condition such as often occurs in the outer ear.

Product licence number 0188/5924.

GENTICIN* EYE OINTMENT ▼

Presentation Genticin Eye Ointment is a sterile, colourless, opaque ointment which contains Gentamicin Sulphate PhEur ≡ 0.3% w/w gentamicin base in a greasy base.

Methylhydroxybenzoate PhEur and Propylhydroxybenzoate PhEur are included as preservatives.

Uses Genticin (gentamicin) is a proven bactericidal antibiotic active against an extremely broad spectrum of Gram-positive and Gram-negative bacteria. Genticin Eye Ointment is therefore particularly useful in all external bacterial infections of the eye, where the bacterial organisms are often very varied.

In particular Genticin Eye Ointment is indicated in conjunctivitis, blepharitis, styes, corneal ulcers, and prophylaxis in trauma.

Dosage and administration For all ages: Genticin Eye Ointment should be applied three to four times daily to the infected area.

Contra-indications, warnings, etc There are no specific contra-indications except in cases of true sensitivity to one of the ingredients.

Precautions: If irritation, sensitization or super-infection develop, treatment with Genticin should be discontinued and appropriate therapy instituted.

Overdosage: Not applicable.

Pharmaceutical precautions Store at room temperature.

Legal category POM.

Package quantities Genticin Eye Ointment is available in 3g tubes.

Further information The wide range and degree of

antibacterial activity of Genticin coupled with freedom from troublesome side effects make it particularly suitable for bacterial eye conditions where the pathogens involved or their sensitivity to antibiotics are unknown.

Product licence number 0188/0057.

GENTICIN* HC CREAM
GENTICIN* HC OINTMENT

Presentation Genticin HC Cream is a smooth, white cream which contains Hydrocortisone Acetate PhEur 1.0% w/w, and Gentamicin Sulphate PhEur ≡ 0.3% w/w gentamicin base in a water-miscible base. Methylhydroxybenzoate PhEur and Butylhydroxybenzoate PhEur are included as preservatives.

Genticin HC Ointment is a colourless, opaque ointment which contains Hydrocortisone Acetate PhEur 1.0% w/w and Gentamicin Sulphate PhEur ≡ 0.3% w/w gentamicin base in a greasy base. Methylhydroxybenzoate PhEur and Propylhydroxybenzoate PhEur are included as preservatives.

Uses Genticin has been combined with 1.0% w/w hydrocortisone for the treatment of those inflammatory skin conditions where secondary bacterial infections may be involved.

Genticin HC Cream and Ointment are indicated particularly in infective eczemas (infantile, atopic, allergic, seborrhoeic, etc), infective contact dermatitis, infected pemphigus, otitis externa, and infected pruritus.

Dosage and administration For all ages: Genticin HC Cream and Ointment are intended for topical use only and should be applied three to four times daily to the infected area, covering with a gauze dressing if necessary. Cream preparations are recommended for moist lesions and ointment for dry conditions.

Contra-indications, warnings, etc There are no specific contra-indications except in cases of true sensitivity to one of the ingredients.

Use in pregnancy: Topical administration of any corticosteroid to pregnant animals can cause abnormalities of foetal development. The relevance of this finding to human beings has not been established. However, topical steroids should not be used extensively in pregnancy i.e. in large amounts or for prolonged periods.

Precautions: If irritation, sensitization or super-infection develop, treatment with Genticin should be discontinued and appropriate therapy instituted.

Long term continuous topical therapy should be avoided. In infants, adrenal suppression can occur even without occlusion.

Steroids may delay the healing of leg ulcers or pressure sores.

Overdosage: Not applicable.

Pharmaceutical precautions Store at room temperature. Do not freeze.

In order to preserve the therapeutic activity of these products they should not be diluted.

Legal category POM.

Package quantities Genticin HC Cream and Ointment are available in tubes of 15 g.

Further information The wide range and degree of antibacterial activity of Genticin coupled with freedom from troublesome side-effects make it particularly suit-

able for bacterial skin conditions, where the pathogens involved or their sensitivity to antibiotics are unknown.

Product licence numbers
Genticin HC Cream   0188/5922
Genticin HC Ointment   0188/5928

GENTICIN* INJECTABLE
GENTICIN* PAEDIATRIC INJECTION

Presentation *Genticin Injectable:* Each 2 ml multidose vial and snap-off ampoule contains a 2 ml solution of Gentamicin Sulphate PhEur ≡ 80 mg gentamicin base. Methylhydroxybenzoate PhEur and Propylhydroxybenzoate PhEur are included as preservatives.

Genticin Paediatric Injection: Each 2 ml multidose vial contains a 2 ml solution of Gentamicin Sulphate PhEur ≡ 20 mg gentamicin base. Methylhydroxybenzoate PhEur and Propylhydroxybenzoate PhEur are included as preservatives.

Uses Genticin (gentamicin) is a proven bactericidal antibiotic active against an extremely broad spectrum of Gram-positive and Gram-negative pathogens including *E. coli,* Klebsiella, Proteus, *Pseudomonas aeruginosa* and penicillin-resistant strains of *Staph. aureus.*

Indications for the use of Genticin are bacteraemia, septicaemia, urinary-tract infections, severe chest infections, severe neonatal infections and other systemic infections due to susceptible bacteria.

Dosage and administration Genticin is normally administered intramuscularly, but may be given intravenously if required.

If intravenous administration is necessary the normal intramuscular dose should be given as a bolus injection into the tubing of the giving set or directly into the venous system over a period of two to three minutes. Genticin should not be given as a slow infusion or mixed with other drugs before use (see below for incompatibilities).

With either intramuscular or intravenous administration the following dosage applies for normal renal function:

Adults: 60 kg and over: 80 mg eight-hourly.
Less than 60 kg: 60 mg eight-hourly.

The following table applies in cases of impaired renal function.

Blood urea (mg/100 ml)	Creatinine clearance (GFR) (ml/min)	Dose and frequency of administration
<40	>70	80 mg† 8-hourly
40–100	30–70	80 mg† 12-hourly
100–200	10–30	80 mg† daily
>200	5–10	80 mg† every 48 hours
Twice-weekly intermittent haemodialysis	<5	80 mg† after dialysis

† 60 mg if body weight <60 kg.

Urinary-tract infections: As above.

Alternatively, if renal function is not impaired, 160 mg once daily may be used.

In life-threatening infections the frequency of dosage may need to be increased to six-hourly and the quantity of each dose may also be increased at the discretion of the clinician up to a total dosage of 5 mg/kg in 24 hours. In such cases it is advisable to monitor gentamicin serum levels.

Elderly persons: Adjust dosage according to weight and renal function. Periodic serum monitoring is desirable.

Children: Genticin Paediatric Injection is one quarter the strength of Genticin Injectable (see above).

In children and in neonates, it can be expected that serum levels will be lower than those found in adults at equivalent dosage per body weight.

The recommended paediatric dosage is therefore as follows:

Up to 12 years: 6.0 mg/kg in 24 hours in 3 equally divided doses (i.e. 2.0 mg/kg eight-hourly).

In infants up to two weeks this dosage should be given in 2 equally divided doses (i.e. 3.0 mg/kg 12-hourly). Serum levels should preferably be monitored daily.

In neonates, infants and children, subsequent dosage will often need to be increased to achieve therapeutic serum levels. Peak levels should be measured about one hour after intramuscular or intravenous injection and should reach 4 mcg/ml, but not exceed 10 mcg/ml.

Contra-indications, warnings, etc There are no absolute contra-indications other than sensitivity to one of the ingredients.

Since those toxic symptoms that can be elicited are usually reversible, and since the conditions predisposing towards excess serum levels are well defined, it is considered that gentamicin is a relatively safe antibiotic for systemic therapy. As with all aminoglycosides, at critical levels gentamicin exhibits toxicity. With gentamicin the vestibular mechanism may be affected when serum levels of 10 mcg/ml or when a trough level of 2 mcg/ml are exceeded. This is usually reversible if observed promptly and the dose adjusted. In the patient with normal renal function it is virtually impossible to achieve these levels at standard dosage. Where renal function is impaired through disease or old age the frequency, but not the amount, of each dose should be reduced according to the degree of impairment. Gentamicin is excreted by simple glomerular filtration, and dosage frequency may be predicted by assessing creatinine clearance rates or blood urea and reducing the frequency accordingly. The table detailed in *Dosage and administration* may be useful when treating adults.

It is also advisable to check serum levels to confirm that peak (one hour) levels do not exceed 10 mcg/ml and that trough levels (before next injection) do not exceed 2 mcg/ml.

Use in pregnancy: Although there is no animal evidence of teratogenicity, gentamicin crosses the placenta and there is a risk of ototoxicity in the foetus and gentamicin should only be used where the seriousness of the mother's condition justifies the risk.

Pharmaceutical precautions Genticin is a remarkably stable antibiotic and does not require to be kept under refrigerated conditions. In general we would not advise mixing Genticin injectables with any other drug prior to administration.

In particular the following are incompatible in mixed solution with Genticin injectables: penicillins, cephalosporins, Erythromycin, Lipiphysan, heparins, †sodium bicarbonate.

†Carbon dioxide may be liberated on addition of the two solutions. Normally this will dissolve in the solution, but under some circumstances small bubbles may form.

Dilution in the body will obviate the danger of physical and chemical incompatibility and enable Genticin injectables to be given concurrently with the drugs listed above either as a bolus injection into the drip tubing, with adequate flushing, or at separate sites. However, in the case of carbenicillin and gentamicin they should only be given at separate sites.

There is evidence that any potential nephrotoxicity of cephalosporins may be increased in the presence of gentamicin and we would recommend monitoring of kidney function if this combination is used. (For further information on mixed antibiotic therapy see section on 'Further information'.)

Neuromuscular blockade and respiratory paralysis have occasionally been reported from administration of aminoglycosides to patients who have received curare-type muscle relaxants during anaesthesia.

Legal category POM.

Package quantities *Genticin Injectable:* Ampoules and vials are packed in boxes of 5 and 25.

Genticin Paedriatric Injection: Vials are packed in boxes of 5.

Further information Genticin has been shown to have a uniquely broad spectrum of activity and its use is recommended in bacterial infection where urgent, effective and, often, blind chemotherapy is called for. For combined antibiotic therapy with Genticin Injectable and Genticin Paediatric Injection the following rules of thumb may apply:

1. Genticin Injectable (or Genticin Paediatric Injection) act synergistically with penicillins and this combination is particularly useful against enterococci.

2. Genticin Injectable (or Genticin Paediatric Injection) and bacteriostatic antibiotics may give an antagonistic interaction (e.g. as with chloramphenicol). In the specific case of clindamycin and lincomycin the disadvantage of antagonism may be outweighed by the addition of activity against anaerobic organisms.

Product licence numbers
Genticin Injectable   0188/5905
Genticin Paediatric Injection   0188/5909

GENTICIN* INTRATHECAL

Presentation Genticin Intrathecal 2 ml snap-off ampoule. Each 1 ml contains Gentamicin Sulphate PhEur ≡ 1.0 mg gentamicin base (1,000 units) and Sodium Chloride PhEur (8.5 mg) to render the solution isotonic.

Uses Genticin (gentamicin) is a proven bactericidal antibiotic active against an extremely broad spectrum of Gram-positive and Gram-negative pathogens, including *E. coli, H. influenzae,* Proteus, Pseudomonas, *Neisseria meningitidis* and staphylococci which are the pathogens often associated with infection of the CSF.

Genticin Intrathecal is recommended for bacterial meningitis and ventriculitis.

Although gentamicin crosses the blood-brain barrier it has been shown, as with other antibiotics, that parenteral therapy should be supported with intrathecal or intraventricular administration.

Dosage and administration The recommended daily dose is 1 mg gentamicin base intrathecally or intraventricularly plus 2.4 mg/kg/day intramuscularly in three equally divided doses at eight-hourly intervals in adult patients.

In children the supportive dosage is: Up to 12 years: 6 0 mg/kg in 24 hours in three equally divided doses (i.e. 2.0 mg/kg eight hourly).

In infants up to two weeks this dosage should be given in two equally divided doses (i.e. 3.0 mg/kg 12 hourly).

Elderly persons: No special dosage regimen required.

The intraventricular/intrathecal dose may need to be increased at the discretion of the Clinician to obtain adequate CSF levels which can be controlled by assay, particularly if a severe degree of hydrocephalus is present. Treatment should continue until the CSF is shown to be bacteriologically clear.

Contra-indications, warnings, etc There are no absolute contra-indications, except true sensitivity to gentamicin.

The precautions specified for Genticin Injectable for concomitant intramuscular and intravenous treatment should be observed.

Use in pregnancy: Although there is no animal evidence of teratogenicity, gentamicin crosses the placenta and there is a risk of ototoxicity in the foetus and gentamicin should only be used where the seriousness of the mother's condition justifies the risk.

Pharmaceutical precautions Genticin is a remarkably stable antibiotic and does not require to be kept under refrigerated conditions. In general we would not advise mixing Genticin Intrathecal with any other antibiotic prior to administration.

Legal category POM.

Package quantities Genticin Intrathecal ampoules are made available in boxes of 5.

Further information Nil.

Product licence number 0188/0004.

GENTICIN* PURE POWDER

Approved name: Gentamicin Sulphate

Presentation Available as a 1 g non-sterile hygroscopic powder in a securitainer pack. The weight of powder will vary according to potency but will be approximately 1.8 g Gentamicin Sulphate PhEur ≡ 1 g gentamicin base (1 million units). Also available as a 0.5 g sterile vial, each vial containing 0.9 g Gentamicin Sulphate PhEur ≡ 0.5 g gentamicin base (500,000 units) sterilised by irradiation.

Uses Genticin Pure Powder is supplied for the preparation of preservative-free solutions of gentamicin for intrathecal and intraventricular administration in meningitis and ventriculitis and other indications where a preservative free solution, or different concentrations are required.

Dosage and administration The recommended daily dose is 1 mg gentamicin base intrathecally or intraventricularly plus 2.4 mg/kg/day intramuscularly in three equally divided doses at eight hourly intervals in adult patients.

In children the supportive dosage is: Up to 12 years: 6.0 mg/kg in 24 hours in three equally divided doses (i.e. 2.0 mg/kg eight hourly). In infants up to two weeks this doage should be given in two equally divided doses (i.e. 3.0 mg/kg 12 hourly).

Elderly persons: No special dosage regimen required.

The intraventricular/inthrathecal dose may need to be increased at the discretion of the Clinician to obtain adequate CSF levels which can be controlled by assay, particularly if a severe degree of hydrocephalus is present. Treatment should continue until the CSF is shown to be bacteriologically clear.

Contra-indications, warnings, etc There are no absolute contra-indications, except true sensitivity to gentamicin.

Where renal function is impaired the frequency of dosage by the systemic route should be reduced to avoid serum levels in excess of 10 mcg/ml as a peak (one hour) level and 2 mcg/ml as a trough. In the patient with normal renal function it is virtually impossible to achieve these levels with the standard dosage, but with gentamicin the vestibular mechanism may be affected when these levels are exceeded. This is usually reversible if observed in time and the dose adjusted.

Use in pregnancy: Although there is no animal evidence of teratogenicity, gentamicin crosses the placenta and there is a risk of ototoxicity in the foetus and Gentamicin should only be used where the seriousness of the mother's condition justifies the risk.

Pharmaceutical precautions Genticin Pure Powder should be stored at room temperature and has a shelf-life of three years in unopened vials.

Care should be taken after the container has been opened to replace the stopper immediately.

Genticin Pure Powder may be dissolved in water or in normal saline for injection purposes in order to obtain a preservative-free solution. This should be sterilised before use, preferably by membrane filtration.

Legal category POM.

Package quantities Genticin Pure Powder is available in airtight, moisture-proof containers containing 1 g of gentamicin base and in a glass vial containing 0.5 g sterile gentamicin base.

Further information The package leaflet contained in every pack gives a suggested method for the preparation of intrathecal injection based on 1 mg of gentamicin base per 1 ml.

Product licence number 0188/5906.

GENTISONE* HC EAR DROPS

Presentation Gentamicin Sulphate PhEur ≡ 0.3% w/v gentamicin base plus Hydrocortisone Acetate PhEur 1.0% w/v in a sterile aqueous suspension in a 10 ml polythene dropper bottle. Borax PhEur and Benzalkonium Chloride BP are included as preservatives.

Uses Genticin (gentamicin) is a proven bactericidal antibiotic active against an extremely broad spectrum of Gram-positive and Gram-negative bacteria. Gentisone HC Ear Drops are therefore particularly useful in combating bacterial infections of the ear where the offending organisms are often varied and difficult to identify.

Gentisone HC Ear Drops are indicated in otitis externa, chronic suppurative otitis media, prophylaxis in trauma and pre- and post-operatively in surgery to the ear including infected mastoidectomy cavities.

Dosage and administration For all ages: The area should be cleaned and 2–4 drops instilled three to four times a day and at night. In middle ear infections the cavity may be filled with drops.

Contra-indications, warnings, etc
There are no specific contra-indications except in cases of true sensitivity to one of the ingredients.

Use in pregnancy: Topical administration of any corticosteroid to pregnant animals can cause abnormalities of foetal development. The relevance of this finding in human beings has not been established, however, topical steroids should not be used extensively in pregnancy i.e. in large amounts or for prolonged periods.

Precautions: If irritation, sensitization or super-infection develop, treatment with Genticin should be discontinued and appropriate therapy instituted.

Long term continuous topical therapy should be avoided. In infants, adrenal suppression can occur even without occlusion.

Overdosage: Not applicable.

Pharmaceutical precautions Store at room temperature. Do not freeze.

Legal category POM.

Package quantities Gentisone HC Ear Drops are available in 10 ml opaque white polythene dropper bottles with orange plastic caps.

Further information Genticin Eye/Ear Drops are also available where a plain antibiotic solution is required for topical application, for example, in the treatment of simple infections of the eye and ear.

Product licence number 0188/5925.

HALIN* ▼

Presentation White, bi-convex, sugar coated repeat action tablets. Each tablet contains: Dexbrompheniramine Maleate USP 6 mg and Pseudoephedrine Sulphate USP 120 mg. These ingredients are equally distributed between the tablet core and the coating.

Uses Decongestant and antihistamine. For relief of symptoms of upper respiratory mucosal congestion associated with the common cold, seasonal and perennial nasal allergies, acute rhinitis, rhinosinusitis, influenza, eustachian catarrh and obstruction.

Dosage and administration *Adults and children over 12 years of age:* One tablet every 12 hours in the morning and at bedtime.

Children under 12 years: Not recommended.

Elderly persons: No special dosage regimen required, but care should be taken to observe the contra-indications and precautions below.

Contra-indications, warnings, etc
Contra-indications: Hypertension and severe coronary artery disease. Patients under treatment with monoamine oxidase inhibiting drugs and for two weeks after stopping these drugs.

Use in pregnancy: Halin should not be given to pregnant women or to nursing mothers.

Precautions and warning: May cause drowsiness and this effect would be enhanced by alcohol or other CNS depressants such as hypnotics, sedatives and tranquillisers.

This product may occasionally act as a cerebral stimulant in adults, giving rise to insomnia, nervousness, hyperpyrexia, tremors and epileptiform convulsions.

Caution in patients with prostatic hypertrophy, hyperthyroidism, glaucoma, severe hepatic and renal disease.

Overdosage: Gastric lavage and symptomatic supportive treatment.

Pharmaceutical precautions Store at room temperature.

Legal category POM.

Package quantities Box of 100 tablets (strips of 10 tablets).

Further information Halin tablets combine in repeat action form the antihistamine actions of dexbrompheniramine maleate with the vasoconstrictor properties of pseudoephedrine.

Product licence number 0188/0061.

HAMARIN* 100 TABLETS ▼
HAMARIN* 300 TABLETS ▼

Presentation Hamarin 100 – White biconvex tablets, engraved on one side with a break-line and 'Hamarin' and '100', and with a triangle logo on the other side. Each tablet contains Allopurinol BP 100 mg.

Hamarin 300 – White biconvex tablets, engraved on one side with a break-line and 'Hamarin' and '300', and with a triangle logo on the other side. Each tablet contains Allopurinol BP 300 mg.

Uses Gout: Primary hyperuricaemia.
Secondary hyperuricaemia: Prophylaxis of uric acid and calcium oxalate stones.

Dosage and administration *Adults:* The initial dose should be in the range 100–300 mg per day, as a single daily dose. The dose should be adjusted by monitoring serum uric acid levels at appropriate intervals, until the desired effect is achieved, which may take one to three weeks.

The maintenance dose is normally 200–600 mg per day. It is rarely found necessary to exceed 900 mg per day. Doses in excess of 300 mg should be administered in divided doses.

Children: Dosage should be in the range 10–20 mg/kg/ day. Use in children is indicated largely in leukaemia and other malignant conditions, and enzyme disorders such as Lesch-Nyhan syndrome.

Elderly persons: Use of allopurinol in elderly persons should take full cognizance of the increased risk of renal or hepatic impairment in such patients, and the dose reduced accordingly.

Contra-indications, warnings, etc
Contra-indications: Acute gout. Known intolerance of allopurinol.

Precautions: Treatment with allopurinol should not be started during an acute attack of gout. Prophylactic therapy with allopurinol may be started when the acute attack has completely subsided; anti-inflammatory agents should be given concurrently.

Dosage should be reduced in patients with renal or hepatic disorders.

Fluid intake should ensure adequate urinary output.

Use with caution in pregnancy.

Use in pregnancy and lactation: There is no evidence that allopurinol taken orally in humans caused foetal abnormalities. However, allopurinol should be used with caution in pregnancy. Allopurinol has been associated with foetal abnormalities in mice after intraperitoneal administration, but oral administration in animals has shown no such effects.

There is no data on the excretion of allopurinol and metabolites in breast milk.

Drug interactions: When administered concurrently with allopurinol the dose of 6-mercaptopurine and azathioprine should be reduced to one quarter of the usual dose. The activity of these drugs is prolonged by inhibition of xanthine oxidase.

The possibility of interaction with anti-coagulants whose activity may be enhanced should be borne in mind when allopurinol is concurrently administered. Prothrombin times should be checked.

There may be an increased risk of prolonged hypoglycaemic activity when allopurinol is administered with chlorpropamide, in patients with impaired renal function.

Allopurinol may interact with uricosuric agents.

Adverse effects: Adverse effects are usually rare and mainly of a minor nature. They are more common in patients with renal impairment.

An acute attack of gouty arthritis may be precipitated during the early stages of treatment with allopurinol. (See initiation of therapy).

Skin reactions: Skin reactions are the most common adverse effect, and may occur at any time during treatment. They may be pruritic, maculopapular, sometimes scaly or purpuric and, rarely, exfoliative.

Allopurinol should be withdrawn immediately should such reactions occur.

After recovery from mild skin reactions, allopurinol may be re-introduced at low dose (e.g. 50 mg/day); this may be gradually increased.

If the rash recurs, allopurinol should be withdrawn immediately and permanently.

General hypersensitivity: Skin reactions may rarely be associated with exfoliation, fever, lymphadenopathy, arthralgia and eosinophilia.

In such cases, allopurinol should be withdrawn immediately and permanently.

Corticosteroids may be beneficial in treating such reactions, which occur usually in patients with pre-existing hepatic or renal disorders.

Gastro-intestinal disorders: Nausea and vomiting can be avoided by taking allopurinol after meals.

Blood and lymphatic system: Transient reduction in the numbers of blood cells and platelets have been occasionally reported, usually in association with hepatic and/or renal disorder. The clinical significance has yet to be demonstrated.

Miscellaneous: In conditions which give rise to an increased miscible urate pool (e.g. malignant disease and its treatment, Lesch-Nyhan syndrome), allopurinol rarely leads to tissue deposition of xanthine. High fluid intake and alkalinisation should ensure adequate urinary output. Xanthine crystals seen in muscle tissue of patients receiving allopurinol appear to have no clinical significance.

The following have been reported, but do not have a clear cause and effect relationship with administration of allopurinol: nausea, vomiting, abdominal pain, diarrhoea, alopecia, headache, drowsiness, general malaise, granulomatous hepatitis, hepatic necrosis, cataracts, visual disorders, macular changes, impotence, diabetes, furunculosis, hypertension, haematuria, oedema.

Initiation of therapy: In common with uricosuric agents, allopurinol may precipitate an acute attack of gouty arthritis during the early stages of treatment. It is therefore advisable to give concurrently a suitable anti-inflammatory agent, or colchicine, for at least one month.

Use with uricosuric agents: Allopurinol may be given concurrently with uricosuric agents; this may be useful in patients with large tophaceous deposits. The possibility of interactions between allopurinol and uricosuric agents, perhaps necessitating dosage adjustment of one or both drugs, should be borne in mind.

When changing from uricosuric therapy to allopurinol, one to three weeks overlap of treatments is advisable, to ensure continuous hypouricaemic effect.

Use with cytotoxic drugs: When used to prevent uric acid nephropathy in neoplastic conditions, allopurinol treatment should be started before cytotoxic therapy.

When allopurinol is administered concurrently with 6-mercaptopurine or azathioprine, only one quarter of the usual dose of cytotoxic agent should be given. There is no unequivocal evidence that allopurinol potentiates the action of other cytotoxic drugs.

Dosage in impaired renal function, and renal dialysis: Allopurinol and its metabolites are excreted via the kidney. Impairment of kidney function may lead to retention of the drug and its metabolites, with consequent prolongation of action. The amount and frequency of dosage may need to be reduced, as indicated by monitoring serum uric acid levels.

Allopurinol and metabolites are removed by dialysis. The table below gives recommended doses for adults.

Creatinine clearance	Dose
> 20 ml/minute	Standard dose
10–20 ml/minute	100–200 mg/day
< 10 ml/minute	100 mg/day, or at longer intervals.
Renal dialysis	300–400 mg after each dialysis (none in the interim).

Interference with tests: Allopurinol has been reported to interfere with liver function tests.

Toxicity and treatment of overdosage: The most likely effect of overdosage is gastro-intestinal disturbance.

Massive absorption of allopurinol may lead to marked xanthine oxidase inhibition. This should have no untoward effect, unless 6-mercaptopurine and/or azathioprine is being taken concurrently, when the activity of these drugs may be increased.

Adequate hydration to maintain diuresis facilitates excretion of allopurinol and its metabolites.

Dialysis may rarely be needed if clinically appropriate.

Pharmaceutical precautions Store in a cool dry place.

Legal category POM.

Package quantities Hamarin 100: Containers of 100 tablets.
Hamarin 300: Containers of 30 tablets.

Further information Hamarin may also be used in the treatment of hyperuricaemia that may be associated with neoplastic disease or its treatment, enzyme disorders, especially the Lesch-Nyhan syndrome, diuretic therapy and psoriasis.

Product licence numbers Hamarin 100: 0188/0068.
Hamarin 300: 0188/0069.

METRAMID* TABLETS ▼

Presentation White, round, flat, bevelled edged tablets, engraved on one side with 'Metramid', and with a break-line and two triangular logos on the other side.

Each tablet contains Metoclopramide Hydrochloride BP equivalent to 10 mg of the anhydrous substance.

Uses 1. *Digestive disorders:* Metramid restores normal co-ordination and tone to the upper gastro-intestinal tract, and relieves symptoms of heartburn, dyspepsia, flatulence, associated with reflux oesophagitis, hiatus, hernia, gastritis, duodenitis, peptic ulcer, regurgitation of bile.

2. *Nausea and vomiting:* Metramid is used as an anti-emetic for the treatment of nausea and vomiting associated with gastro-intestinal disorders such as peptic ulcer, gastritis and the results of gastrectomy, and induced by drugs such as digitalis, cytotoxics and antibacterial agents.

3. *Migraine:* Metramid relieves symptoms of nausea and vomiting and overcomes gastric stasis associated with migraine. The absorption of analgesics in migraine patients may be enhanced by concomitant administration of Metramid.

Dosage and administration The total daily dose should not exceed 0.5 mg/kg body weight, and should be administered in divided doses. This precaution is especially necessary in young adults.

1. *Adults:* One tablet (10 mg) three times daily.

2. *Young Adults (15–20 years):* Metramid tablets should only be used in cases of severe intractable vomiting such as may be associated with radiotherapy and intolerance to cytotoxic drugs; in gastric radiology and duodenal intubation. The dose should not exceed 0.5 mg/kg body weight per day unless directed by the physician.

3. *Children:* Metramid tablets are not recommended for children under 15 years.

4. *Elderly persons:* Clearance of metoclopramide is reduced in patients with renal impairment. Use of Metramid in elderly persons should take full cognizance of the increased risk of renal impairment in such patients, and the dose reduced accordingly.

5. *Use in pregnancy and lactation:* Although no teratogenic effects have been shown in tests in several mammalian species, use of metoclopramide is not advised during pregnancy.

Metoclopramide may raise serum prolactin levels, with consequent increase in milk volume. The drug is excreted in breast milk.

Contra-indications, warnings, etc

Precautions: Care should be taken to ensure that maximum dosage recommendations are not exceeded, as this increases the likelihood of dystonic reactions.

If vomiting persists despite treatment with metoclopramide, the possibility of any underlying disorder, e.g. cerebral irritation should be investigated.

Metoclopramide should not be administered within three to four days after gastro-intestinal surgery, as vigorous muscle contractions may impair healing.

Metoclopramide should not be used in patients with breast cancer, which may be prolactin-dependent.

Drug interactions: Concomitant administration of metoclopramide and phenothiazines should be undertaken with caution, as both drugs may give rise to extrapyramidal symptoms.

The action of metoclopramide is antagonised by atropine and other anticholinergic drugs.

Metoclopramide may affect the absorption of other concomitantly administered drugs.

Adverse effects: Metoclopramide may produce extrapyramidal reactions, usually dystonic in type. These are more common at doses in excess of 0.5 mg/kg body weight per day, in children and young adults under 20 years, particularly young women, and in patients with low body weight or renal impairment.

The acute dyskinesias include trismus, torticollis, facial spasms and oculogyric crisis. There may be generalised increase in muscle tone.

Most such reactions occur within 36 hours of starting drug treatment, and disappear within 24 hours of withdrawal of the drug.

Should treatment of extrapyramidal reactions be required, an anti-Parkinsonian drug or benzodiazepine may be used.

Other side-effects are generally minor or transient in nature, and include dizziness, faintness, bowel disturbances and drowsiness. Metoclopramide may be associated with hyperprolactinaemia and galactorrhoea.

Interference with tests: Metoclopramide has not been reported to interfere with biochemical tests.

Toxicity and treatment of overdosage: Extrapyramidal reactions are more likely to occur with overdosage. Gastric lavage and intensive supportive therapy should be initiated. Dystonic symptoms should be treated with anticholinergic agents.

Pharmaceutical precautions Store in a cool, dark place.

Legal category POM.

Package quantities Container of 100 tablets.

Further information Nil.

Product licence number 0188/0070.

MICROPAQUE* D.C.

Presentation A low viscosity white suspension with a bland taste containing 100% w/v of Barium Sulphate PhEur.

Uses Radiological investigations of the gastro-intestinal tract. Micropaque D.C. is particularly suited to the Double Contrast Technique.

Dosage and administration The volume of Micropaque D.C. used will depend on the patient, the procedure and technique involved. The following dosages represent a basic guide to the quantities suitable for routine examinations:

Barium swallow.	40–60 ml undiluted
Double contrast stomach and duodenum examination	100–150 ml undiluted
Follow through small bowel examination	150–250 ml undiluted
Barium enema	250–500 ml diluted with 500–1000 ml water.

Elderly persons: No special dosage regimen is required,

but care should be taken to observe contra-indications and warnings below.

Contra-indications, warnings, etc Perforation of any region of the gastro-intestinal tract. Intestinal obstruction. Pyloric stenosis might be considered as a contra-indication to the use of barium sulphate. Administration of a barium enema should proceed with particular care in patients with existing intestinal disease, in children, the elderly or the debilitated.

In choosing the route of administration, the possibility of actual or incipient bowel obstruction should be borne in mind.

Overdosage: Not applicable.

Use in pregnancy: Micropaque is not absorbed.

Pharmaceutical precautions Shake well before use. Store at room temperature. Do not freeze. A light brown supernatant layer may appear and is quite normal. It will disappear when the bottle is shaken.

Legal category P.

Package quantities 300 ml plastic bottle containing 250 ml suspension and 50 ml 'shake space'. 15 bottles in each pack.

Further information Micropaque D.C., having a high density combined with a low viscosity, has been formulated to demonstrate particularly fine definition in conjunction with a suitable effervescent distending agent such as Nicholas CO_2 Granules for Double Contrast Technique in the gastro-intestinal tract.

Product licence number 0188/0013.

MICROPAQUE* HD ▼

Presentation A fine white powder with a bland taste of vanilla containing 96% w/w Barium Sulphate PhEur.

Uses Double contrast radiological investigations of the gastrointestinal tract.

Dosage and administration Micropaque HD Powder must be reconstituted before use by adding water.

A table of dilutions is provided to enable the user to select the concentration most suited to their technique.

% w/v Barium sulphate	Water (mls)	Final volume (mls)
200	83	150
210	76	143
220	69	136
230	63	130
240	58	125

As a guide, findings indicate that a concentration of around 220% w/v will give optimum results.

Optimum dispersion is obtained by shaking for approximately one minute.

Although the volume of suspension used will depend on the patient, the procedure and technique involved, the following dosages of Micropaque HD represent a basic guide to the quantities suitable for routine examinations of the upper gastrointestinal tract.

Barium swallow   40–60 ml
Double contrast stomach and duodenum
examination   100–150 ml

Follow-through examination of the small
bowel   150–250 ml

Elderly persons: No special dosage regimen is required, but care should be taken to observe the contra-indications and warnings below.

Contra-indications, warnings, etc Perforation of any region of the gastrointestinal tract and intestinal obstruction. Pyloric stenosis might be considered as a contra-indication to the use of barium sulphate. Administration of a barium enema should proceed with particular care in patients with existing intestinal disease, in children, the elderly or the debilitated. In choosing the route of administration, the possibility of actual or incipient bowel obstruction should be borne in mind.

Overdosage: Not applicable.

Use in pregnancy: Micropaque is not absorbed.

Pharmaceutical precautions Store at room temperature in a dry place. Micropaque HD should be used as soon as possible after reconstitution and in any event within two hours of adding water.

Legal category P.

Package quantities 500 ml polypropylene beaker containing 312 g barium sulphate (96% w/w). 20 beakers in each pack.

Further information Micropaque HD produces a high density, low viscosity suspension on reconstitution that is especially designed for double contrast examinations of the upper gastrointestinal tract. It should be used in conjunction with a compatible gas producing agent such as Nicholas CO_2 Granules.

Product licence number 0188/0055.

MICROPAQUE* STANDARD

Presentation A creamy-white suspension with a bland characteristic taste of butterscotch/vanilla, containing 100% w/v Barium Sulphate PhEur.

Uses Radiological investigations of the gastro-intestinal tract.

Dosage and administration *Adults: Oesophagus:* Use undiluted Micropaque Standard orally as required. For prolonged adhesion use Microtrast Oesophageal Paste.

Stomach and duodenum: To demonstrate the mucosal pattern use up to 50 ml of undiluted Micropaque Standard orally, follow this with a further 100 ml of Micropaque Standard diluted with 100 ml of water for demonstration of stomach distension and emptying function. If this biphased technique is not used, 150 ml of Micropaque Standard diluted with 50 ml of water may be given.

Small intestine: Use 100 ml of Micropaque Standard diluted with 150 ml of water or follow through from stomach examination.

Colon: For examination by barium enema using the filled colon technique, use 1 volume of Micropaque Standard to 2 volumes of water made up to the required quantity. For double contrast studies use 1–2 volumes of Micropaque Standard to 1 volume of water. 400 ml total volume is usually sufficient. An important pre-requisite is a thorough cleansing preparation of the colon and an examination time of preferably not greater than 15 minutes.

Children: No children's dosage is recommended as such investigations in children are rare and specialised. The dosage will therefore be tailored by the radiologist to suit the special requirements in each case.

Elderly persons: No special dosage regimen required, but care should be taken to observe the contra-indications and warnings below.

Contra-indications, warnings, etc Perforation of any region of the gastro-intestinal tract. Intestinal obstruction. Pyloric stenosis might be considered as a contra-indication to the use of barium sulphate preparations. Administration of a barium enema should proceed with particular care in patients with existing intestinal disease, in children, the elderly or the debilitated. In choosing the route of administration, the possibility of actual or incipient bowel obstruction should be borne in mind.

Overdosage: Not applicable.

Use in pregnancy: Micropaque is not absorbed.

Pharmaceutical precautions Shake before use.
Store at room temperature. Do not freeze. A light brown supernatant layer may appear and is quite normal. It will disappear when the bottle is shaken.

Legal category P.

Package quantities Plastic bottles containing 250 ml and 2 litres.

Further information Nil.

Product licence number 0188/5903

MICROPAQUE* POWDER

Presentation A cream-coloured, free-flowing fine powder, which, when reconstituted with water, has a pleasant bland characteristic butterscotch/vanilla flavour. The powder contains 92% w/w Barium Sulphate PhEur.

Uses Radiological investigations of the gastro-intestinal tract.

Dosage and administration *Standard mix. Method of preparation:*
1. Measurement by volume. To 8 volumes of powder add 7 volumes of water, e.g. to 800 ml of powder add 700 ml of water to make 1 litre of liquid dispersion.
2. Measurement by weight. Add to 1 kg of powder sufficient water to make up to 1 litre of liquid dispersion.
Water should always be added to the powder with slow stirring.

Adults: Oesophagus: Use undiluted Micropaque standard mix orally as required. For prolonged adhesion use Microtrast Oesophageal Paste.

Stomach and duodenum: To demonstrate the mucosal pattern use up to 50 ml of undiluted Micropaque standard mix orally. Follow this with a further 100 ml of Micropaque standard mix diluted with 100 ml of water for demonstration of stomach distension and emptying function. If this biphased technique is not used, 150 ml of Micropaque Standard diluted with 50 ml of water may be given.

Small intestine: Use 100 ml of Micropaque standard mix diluted with 150 ml of water or follow through from stomach examination.

Colon: For examination by barium enema using the filled colon technique use 1 volume of Micropaque standard mix to 2 volumes of water made up to the required quantity. For double contrast studies use 1–2 volumes of Micropaque standard mix to 1 volume of water. 400 ml total volume is usually sufficient. An important prerequisite is a thorough cleansing of the colon and an examination time of preferably not greater than 15 minutes.

Children: No children's dosage is recommended as such investigations in children are rare and specialised. The dosage will therefore be tailored by the radiologist to suit the special requirements in each case.

Elderly persons: No special dosage regimen required but care should be taken to observe the contra-indications and warnings below.

Contra-indications, warnings, etc Perforation of any region of the gastro-intestinal tract. Intestinal obstruction. Pyloric stenosis might be considered as a contra-indication to the use of barium sulphate preparations. Administration of a barium enema should proceed with particular care in patients with existing intestinal disease, in children, the elderly or the debilitated. In choosing the route of administration, the possibility of actual or incipient bowel obstruction should be borne in mind.

Overdosage: Not applicable.

Use in pregnancy: Micropaque is not absorbed.

Pharmaceutical precautions Store at room temperature in a dry place.

Legal category P.

Package quantities 3.5 kg in a plastic container.

Further information Nil.

Product licence number 0188/5904.

MICROTRAST*

Presentation An off-white, viscous paste with a faint odour of vanilla and a bland, pleasant and characteristic faintly butterscotch/vanilla flavour. Contains 70% w/w Barium Sulphate PhEur.

Uses Radiographic study of the mucosal outline and pattern of the entire oesophagus, swallowing mechanism, oesophageal peristalsis, heart size and configuration.

Dosage and administration *Adults:* A large teaspoonful (10 g) to a tablespoonful (45 g) as required, orally.

Children: No children's dosage recommended as such investigations in children are rare and specialised. The dosage will therefore be tailored by the radiologist to suit the special requirements in each case.

Elderly persons: No special dosage regimen required, but care should be taken to observe the contra-indications and warnings below.

Contra-indications, warnings, etc Perforation of any region of the gastro-intestinal tract. Pyloric stenosis might be considered as a contra-indication to the use of barium sulphate preparations. Administration of a barium enema should proceed with particular care in patients with existing intestinal disease, in children, the elderly or the debilitated. In choosing the route of administration, the possibility of actual or incipient bowel obstruction should be borne in mind.

Overdosage: Not applicable.

Use in pregnancy: Micropaque is not absorbed.

Pharmaceutical precautions Store at room temperature. Do not freeze.

Legal category P.

Package quantities 800 g in a plastic tube.

Further information Nil.

Product licence number 0188/5902.

NEO-MERCAZOLE* TABLETS

Presentation Circular, shallow-convex, pink, compression-coated tablets containing a white core. Impressed with a tear-drop symbol enclosing the letters 'BS' on one side and a break-line on the other. Each tablet contains 5 mg Carbimazole BP.

Uses Anti-thyroid agent. Neo-Mercazole is indicated in all conditions where reduction of thyroid synthesis is required.

    1. Thyrotoxicosis (as the sole treatment).
    2. Preparation prior to thyroidectomy (selected patients).
    3. In combination with radioactive iodine ablative therapy.

Dosage and administration *Adults:* The usual initial total daily dose is 30 mg, but this may be increased to 40–60 mg daily in divided doses, in severe cases. Once control is achieved, dosage is gradually reduced to the lowest maintenance level, compatible with adequate control.

Children: The usual daily dosage is 15 mg or as directed by the physician.

Elderly persons: No special dosage regimen is required, but care should be taken to observe the contra-indications and warnings below.

Contra-indications, warnings, etc If reactions to Neo-Mercazole are to be encountered, they normally occur within the first eight weeks of starting treatment. The most common minor side-effects are nausea, headache, arthralgia, mild gastric distress and skin rashes. Occasional hair loss has been reported. These side-effects are usually self-limiting and may not require withdrawal of the drug.

    Bone-marrow depression has been reported, but this serious side-effect is rare and does not appear to be time or dose related. Routine blood tests are not necessary and, because of the nature of the disorder, are impractical, but it is imperative that patients be warned about the onset of sore throats or other manifestations which might suggest the early development of bone-marrow depression. It is important that the drug is stopped and the physician concerned contacted immediately. There is some evidence that early withdrawal of the drug will lead to complete recovery.

Use in pregnancy: Carbimazole is known to cross the placenta but provided that the mother's dose is within the standard range and that her thyroid state is monitored there is no evidence of neonatal thyroid abnormalities.

    The dose of Neo-Mercazole must be regulated by the patient's clinical condition. It is most important to appreciate that the basic metabolic rate is raised during pregnancy (the rise averages 25% above normal and occurs mainly in the second half of pregnancy) and that the dosage must be adjusted accordingly.

    The smallest dose compatible with rendering the patient symptom-free should be employed and during the last three months should, if possible, not exceed 15 mg daily.

    If the patient's condition is satisfactory, Neo-Mercazole should be discontinued three to four weeks before delivery. Neo-Mercazole is secreted in breast milk, and if treatment is continued during lactation, the patient should not be allowed to breast feed her baby.

Pharmaceutical precautions Store at room temperature.

Legal category POM.

Package quantities Containers of 100 and 500 tablets.

Further information Nil.

Product licence number 0188/5907.

NEUTRADONNA* POWDER

Presentation White/off white powder. Each level 5 ml spoonful of powder contains aluminium sodium silicate 1.27 g and belladonna alkaloids 0.096 mg (calculated as hyoscyamine).

Uses Neutradonna is recommended for use in gastro-intestinal disorders, including peptic ulcer, hiatus hernia, and other hyperacidic dyspepsias.

Dosage and administration *Adults:* 1–2 level 5 ml spoonfuls up to four times a day after meals, and at bedtime. The powder should be taken stirred into a little milk or water.

Children: Not recommended for children under 12 years.

Elderly persons: No special dosage regimen required, but care should be taken to observe the contra-indications below, which may be particularly applicable to elderly persons.

Contra-indications, warnings, etc
Contra-indications: Neutradonna is contra-indicated in glaucoma, and in patients with renal failure, or who are severly debilitated. Belladonna alkaloids are excreted in breast milk, and neonates may be particularly susceptible to their effects. Breast-feeding is therefore a contra-indication to the use of this product.

Warnings: Neutradonna should be used with caution in patients with enlarged prostate, or with known sensitivity to belladonna. Side-effects include constipation, dryness of the mouth, and blurred vision.

Drug interactions: As with other antacids, Neutradonna may inhibit the absorption of other drugs, e.g. tetracyclines, digoxin and vitamins. This may be avoided if such drugs are not administered within two hours of taking Neutradonna.

    Anticholinergic effects of other drugs may be potentiated.

Use in Pregnancy: Use in pregnancy is not recommended.

Overdosage: Effects of overdosage include blurred vision, photophobia, ataxia, mental confusion, tachycardia, hypertension, cardiac arrhythmia, dryness of the mouth, urinary urgency and possible retention, and hyperpyrexia. Treatment is by gastric lavage, and intensive symptomatic and supportive treatment.

Pharmaceutical precautions Store at room temperature in a dry place.

Legal category P.

Package quantities Container of 100 g powder.

Further information Aluminium sodium silicate has a rapid and prolonged antacid action, and belladonna relaxes spasm of the gastrointestinal tract, and also reduces acid secretion by the stomach.

Neutradonna Powder contains 6.1 mmol sodium per level 5 ml spoonful (1.27 g).

Product licence number 0188/5908.

NEUTRADONNA* TABLETS

Presentation White, circular, flat-faced, bevelled-edge tablets. One face is plain and the other is impressed with a break-line and bears two tear-drop symbols enclosing the letters 'BS'. Each tablet contains aluminium sodium silicate 650 mg and belladonna alkaloids 0.048 mg (calculated as hyoscyamine).

Uses Neutradonna is recommended for use in gastrointestinal disorders, including peptic ulcer, hiatus hernia, and other hyperacidic dyspepsias.

Dosage and administration *Adults:* 2–3 tablets up to four times a day after meals. The last dose each day should be taken at bedtime. The tablet should be chewed before swallowing.

Children: Not recommended for children under 12 years.

Elderly persons: No special dosage regimen required, but care should be taken to observe the contra-indications below, which may be particularly applicable to elderly persons.

Contra-indications, warnings, etc
Contra-indications: Neutradonna is contra-indicated in glaucoma, and in patients with renal failure, or who are severely debilitated. Belladonna alkaloids are excreted in breast milk, and neonates may be particularly susceptible to their effects. Breast-feeding is therefore a contra-indication to the use of this product.

Warnings: Neutradonna should be used with caution in patients with enlarged prostate, or with known sensitivity to belladonna. Side-effects include constipation, dryness of the mouth and blurred vision.

Drug interactions: As with other antacids, Neutradonna may inhibit the absorption of other drugs, e.g. tetracyclines, digoxin and vitamins. This may be avoided if such drugs are not administered within two hours of taking Neutradonna. Anticholinergic effects of other drugs may be potentiated.

Use in pregnancy: Use in pregnancy is not recommended.

Overdosage: Effects of overdosage include blurred vision, photophobia, ataxia, mental confusion, tachycardia, hypertension, cardiac arrhythmia, dryness of the mouth, urinary urgency and possible retention, and hyperpyrexia. Treatment is by gastric lavage, and intensive symptomatic and supportive treatment.

Pharmaceutical precautions Store at room temperature.

Legal category P.

Package quantities Box of 120 tablets (10 cartons of 12).

Further information Aluminium sodium silicate has a rapid and prolonged antacid action, and belladonna relaxes spasm of the gastrointestinal tract, and also reduces acid secretion by the stomach. Neutradonna Tablets have a sodium content of 1.9 mmol per tablet.

Product licence number 0188/5913.

NICHOLAS CO$_2$ GRANULES ▼

Presentation Sachet containing:

Betaine hydrochloride	1830.0 mg
Sodium Bicarbonate PhEur	1000.0 mg
Dimethicone BPC	75.0 mg

Uses Gas producing agent for double contrast radiography of the gastro-intestinal tract.

Each sachet generates approximately 267 ml CO_2.

Dosage and administration 1–2 sachets as required per examination. Each sachet should be administered with a little water or barium suspension at the beginning of the examination.

The films should be taken as rapidly as possible after coating of the stomach wall with barium suspension, and the patient should be instructed to suppress eructation for as long as possible.

Elderly persons: No special dosage regimen required.

Contra-indications, warnings, etc There are no specific contra-indications.

Use in pregnancy: No special precautions.

Overdosage: not applicable.

Pharmaceutical precautions Store in a cool, dry place.

Legal category P.

Package quantities Supplied in boxes of 10 sachets.

Further information Nicholas CO_2 Granules contain a defoaming agent which reduces excessive bubbling during formulation of gas and enhances the visualisation of mucosal detail.

Product licence number 0188/0007.

PALAPRIN FORTE*

Presentation Pale orange, oval tablets, with 'PALAPRIN FORTE' impressed on one face. The other face has a break-line and bears two tear-drop symbols enclosing the letters 'BS'. Each tablet contains Aloxiprin BP 600 mg, equivalent to aspirin 500 mg.

Uses As an analgesic/anti-inflammatory agent in rheumatoid arthritis, osteo-arthritis, various forms of spondylitis and other 'rheumatic' conditions where high dosage salicylate therapy is indicated.

Dosage and administration *Adults:* Usual dose 300–1200 mg, up to four times a day (max 4.8 g per day). In acute rheumatic conditions, up to 9.6 g per day, in divided doses.

In order to ensure the maintenance of plasma salicylate

levels adequate for anti-inflammatory, as well as analgesic effect, dosage may be calculated on a body-weight basis, at the rate of one tablet (600 mg) per 6 kg body weight per day, in divided doses.

Dosage should be carefully controlled, and in conditions where high dosage therapy is used, e.g. Still's disease, plasma salicylate levels should be monitored.

The tablets should preferably be dispersed in water before administration, but can be chewed, sucked or swallowed whole with a draught of water.

Children up to age 12: In acute rheumatic conditions, dosage is calculated on a body weight basis, at the rate of 100 mg/kg per day, in divided doses.

Elderly persons: No special dosage regimen required but exercise caution where renal function is impaired.

Contra-indications, warnings, etc

Contra-indications: Palaprin Forte, as other aspirin products, is contra-indicated in patients with active peptic ulceration, haemophilia, or who have hypersensitivity to aspirin. Breast-feeding is contra-indicated at high doses, because of the theoretical risk of affecting clotting mechanisms.

Precautions and warnings: Aspirin may precipitate bronchospasm, and induce asthmatic attacks in susceptible subjects; it may induce gastro-intestinal haemorrhage, occasionally major. May cause constipation and tinnitus at high doses. Should tinnitus occur, dosage should be reduced.

Drug interactions: Aspirin may enhance the effects of anti-coagulants, and may inhibit the action of uricosuric agents.

Use in pregnancy: There is clinical and epidemiological evidence of safety of aspirin in pregnancy, but it may prolong labour and contribute to maternal and neo-natal bleeding, and so is best avoided at term.

Overdosage: Gastric lavage, forced alkaline diuresis and supportive therapy may be employed. Restoration of acid-base balance may be necessary.

Pharmaceutical precautions Store at room temperature.

Legal category P.

Package quantities Containers of 250 tablets.

Further information In high dosage aspirin has a uricosuric effect, and may reduce plasma bicarbonate, and prolong prothrombin time.

Aloxiprin releases salicylate largely in the small intestine, thereby reducing the likelihood of salicylate induced dyspepsia.

Product licence number 0188/5011.

POLYCROL* GEL

Presentation A white peppermint-flavoured suspension containing in each 5 ml:

Activated methylpolysiloxane   25 mg
Magnesium Hydroxide PhEur   100 mg
Aluminium hydroxide gel   4.75 ml

Uses Disorders of the upper gastrointestinal tract, including dyspepsia, peptic ulcer, duodenitis, gastritis, flatulent dyspepsia, aerophagy, oesophagitis and hiatus hernia. Polycrol Gel rapidly relieves acid pain, disperses gastric foam and assists eructation of gas and air.

Dosage and administration *Adults:* One or two 5 ml spoonfuls of gel between meals and at bedtime.

Children: Under 5 years: Half 5 ml spoonful with food, up to 6 doses per day.

5–12 years: One 5 ml spoonful with food, up to 6 doses per day.

Elderly persons: No special dosage regimen required but care should be taken to observe the contra-indications below which may be particularly applicable to elderly persons.

Contra-indications, warnings, etc

Contra-indications: Polycrol Gel should not be administered to patients with renal failure, or who are severely debilitated.

Warnings: Polycrol Gel may rarely give rise to nausea.

Drug interactions: As with other antacids, Polycrol Gel may inhibit the absorption of other drugs, e.g. tetracyclines, digoxin and vitamins. This may be avoided if such drugs are not administered within two hours of taking Polycrol.

Use in pregnancy: There is no evidence to contra-indicate the use of Polycrol Gel in pregnancy.

Overdosage: Not applicable.

Pharmaceutical precautions Store at room temperature.

Legal category P.

Package quantities Plastic bottle containing 300 ml.

Further information Polycrol contains a balanced mixture of antacids (aluminium and magnesium hydroxides) together with a deflatulent (methylpolysiloxane).

The antacids are balanced to reduce the risk of any bowel reaction and with Polycrol Gel neither constipation nor diarrhoea should occur.

Polycrol Gel contains 0.075 mmol sodium per 5 ml.

Product licence number 0188/5930.

POLYCROL* TABLETS

Presentation Circular, flat bevelled-edge tablet consisting of two layers, green and white. The green face is impressed with the letter 'N'. Each tablet contains:

Activated methylpolysiloxane   25 mg
Aluminium hydroxide/magnesium   275 mg
   carbonate co-dried gel
Magnesium Hydroxide PhEur   100 mg

Uses Disorders of the upper gastrointestinal tract including dyspepsia, peptic ulcer, duodenitis, gastritis, flatulent dyspepsia, aerophagy, oesophagitis and hiatus hernia. Polycrol Tablets rapidly relieve acid pain, disperse gastric foam and assist eructation of gas and air.

Dosage and administration *Adults:* 1 or 2 tablets to be chewed between meals and at bedtime.

Children: Under 5 years: Half a tablet to be chewed two or three times a day.

5–12 years: 1 tablet to be chewed two to three times a day.

Elderly persons: No special dosage regimen required, but care should be taken to observe the contra-indications below, which may be particularly applicable to elderly persons.

Contra-indications, warnings, etc

Contra-indications: Polycrol Tablets should not be administered to patients with renal failure, or who are severely debilitated.

Warnings: Polycrol Tablets may rarely give rise to nausea.

Drug interactions: As with other antacids, Polycrol Tablets may inhibit the absorption of other drugs, e.g. tetracyclines, digoxin and vitamins. This may be avoided if such drugs are not administered within two hours of taking Polycrol.

Use in pregnancy: There is no evidence to contra-indicate the use of Polycrol Tablets in pregnancy.

Overdosage: Not applicable.

Pharmaceutical precautions Store at room temperature.

Legal category P.

Package quantities Box of 200 tablets (10 cartons of 20 tablets).

Further information Polycrol Tablets contain a balanced mixture of antacids (aluminium and magnesium hydroxides) together with a deflatulent (methylpolysiloxane).

The antacids are balanced to reduce the risk of any bowel reaction and with Polycrol Tablets neither constipation nor diarrhoea should occur.

Product licence number 0188/5919.

POLYCROL* FORTE GEL

Presentation A white, viscous, peppermint-flavoured gel containing in 5 ml:

Activated methylpolysiloxane	125 mg
Magnesium Hydroxide PhEur	100 mg
Aluminium hydroxide gel	4.75 ml

Uses In antacid/deflatulent therapy in conditions such as dyspepsia of functional or organic origin, heartburn, hiatus hernia, flatulence and abdominal distension, oesophagitis, gastritis, symptomatic treatment of peptic ulcer and other conditions where flatulence and hyperacidity may be present.

Polycrol Forte Gel rapidly relieves acid pain, disperses gastric foam and assists eructation of gas and air.

Dosage and administration *Adults:* One to two 5 ml spoonfuls of gel between meals and at bedtime.

Children: Under 5 years: Half 5 ml spoonful with food up to 6 doses per day.

5–12 years: One 5 ml spoonful with food up to 6 doses per day.

Elderly persons: No special dosage regimen required, but care should be taken to observe the contra-indications below, which may be particularly applicable to elderly persons.

Contra-indications, warnings, etc

Contra-indications: Polycrol Forte Gel should not be administered to patients with renal failure, or who are severely debilitated.

Warnings: Polycrol Forte Gel may rarely give rise to nausea.

Drug interactions: As with other antacids, Polycrol Forte Gel may inhibit the absorption of other drugs, e.g. tetracyclines, digoxin and vitamins. This may be avoided if such drugs are not administered within two hours of taking Polycrol.

Use in pregnancy: There is no evidence to contra-indicate the use of Polycrol Forte Gel in pregnancy.

Overdosage: Not applicable.

Pharmaceutical precautions Store at room temperature.

Legal category P.

Package quantities Plastic bottle containing 300 ml.

Further information Polycrol Forte Gel contains a balanced mixture of antacids (aluminium and magnesium hydroxides) together with a deflatulent (methylpolysiloxane).

The antacids are balanced to reduce the risk of any bowel reaction and with Polycrol Forte Gel, neither constipation nor diarrhoea should occur.

Polycrol Forte Gel contains 0.075 mmol sodium per 5 ml.

Product licence number 0188/5929.

POLYCROL* FORTE TABLETS

Presentation White, circular, flat-faced tablets. One face is plain and the other is impressed with a triangle and the words 'POLYCROL FORTE' round the periphery. Each tablet contains:

Activated methylpolysiloxane	250 mg
Aluminium hydroxide/magnesium carbonate co-dried gel	275 mg
Magnesium Hydroxide PhEur	100 mg

Uses In antacid/deflatulent therapy in conditions such as dyspepsia of functional or organic origin, heartburn, hiatus hernia, flatulence and abdominal distension, oesophagitis, gastritis, symptomatic treatment of peptic ulcer and other conditions where flatulence and hyperacidity may be present.

Polycrol Forte Tablets rapidly relieve acid pain, disperse gastric foam and assist eructation of gas and air.

Dosage and administration *Adults:* One or two tablets to be chewed between meals and at bedtime.

Children: Not recommended for children under 12 years.

Elderly persons: No special dosage regimen required, but care should be taken to observe the contra-indications below, which may be particularly applicable to elderly persons.

Contra-indications, warnings, etc

Contra-indications: Polycrol Forte Tablets should not be administered to patients with renal failure, or who are severely debilitated.

Warnings: Polycrol Forte Tablets may rarely give rise to nausea.

Drug interactions: As with other antacids, Polycrol Forte Tablets may inhibit the absorption of other drugs, e.g. tetracyclines, digoxin and vitamins. This may be avoided if such drugs are not administered within two hours of taking Polycrol.

Use in pregnancy: There is no evidence to contra-indicate the use of Polycrol Forte Tablets in pregnancy.

Overdosage: Not applicable.

Pharmaceutical precautions Store at room temperature, in a dry place.

Legal category P.

Package quantities Box of 120 tablets.

Further information Polycrol Forte Tablets contain a balanced mixture of antacids (aluminium and magnesium hydroxides) together with a deflatulent (methylpolysiloxane).

The antacids are balanced to reduce the risk of any bowel reaction and with Polycrol Forte Tablets, neither constipation nor diarrhoea should occur.

Product licence number 0188/5918.

VASCARDIN*

Presentation Vascardin 10 mg tablets are circular, white, flat-faced, bevelled edge tablets with a break-line on one side and '10' within a triangle impressed on the reverse. Each tablet contains Diluted Isosorbide Dinitrate BP $\equiv$ 10 mg isosorbide dinitrate.

Vascardin 30 mg tablets are circular, white, flat-faced, bevelled edge tablets with a break-line on one side and '30' within a triangle impressed on the reverse. Each tablet contains Diluted Isosorbide Dinitrate BP $\equiv$ 30 mg isosorbide dinitrate.

Uses Angina pectoris – reduction of frequency and severity of attacks. Reduction of cardiac workload and oxygen consumption. Used alone or in combination with β-blockade in certain patients.

Congestive cardiac failure as adjunctive therapy.

Dosage and administration For adults only.

Angina: Treatment: As directed, $\frac{1}{2}$–1 10 mg tablet sublingually at the onset, or for prevention of acute anginal attacks.

Prophylaxis: 30–120 mg orally in divided doses daily, or as required. Dosage should be increased gradually to minimise the possibility of nitrate headache and achieve tolerance. If the headache does occur it can be relieved by simple analgesics.

Congestive cardiac failure: 10–30 mg orally four times daily, according to patient requirements. The dose should be increased gradually to an optimum, using continuous haemodynamic monitoring to determine the level. Vascardin should be used as adjunctive therapy to other standard drugs (cardiac glycosides and diuretics) in cases of severe congestive cardiac failure.

Elderly persons: No special dosage regimen required.

Contra-indications, warnings, etc *Contra-indications:* Use with caution in patients with glaucoma. If used concurrently with anticoagulant therapy, aspirin or other salicylates should not be taken. This product may antagonise the effects of noradrenaline, histamine and acetylcholine. Pulmonary capillary pressure should not usually be allowed to fall below 15 mm Hg, or the systolic blood pressure below the physiological range in normal and hypertensive patients. There should be no fall at all in patients with hypotension in the range of 90–110 mm Hg of systolic pressure. In certain sensitive patients, vasodilators including Vascardin, may cause excessive hypotension leading to increased ischaemia, extension of myocardial damage and progressive congestive heart failure. This product should not be used in patients with severe anaemia, head trauma or cerebral haemorrhage, nor in patients with known sensitivity to nitrates. Obstructive and restrictive cardiac conditions such as valvular stenosis and pericarditis are contraindications.

Use in pregnancy: Vascardin should not be used during pregnancy unless considered essential by the physician.

There is no evidence that isosorbide dinitrate is excreted in breast milk however treatment of nursing mothers must be at the discretion of the physician.

Side-effects: During the first few days treatment, some patients may experience nitrate headache (see under Dosage and Administration). Hypotension may occur if the dose is increased too rapidly.

Overdosage: Although isosorbide dinitrate is quickly absorbed, gastric lavage is advised. The main effect of overdosage is hypotension, which should be treated by raising the patient's legs.

Pharmaceutical precautions Store at room temperature.

Legal category P.

Package quantities Vascardin 10 mg, containers of 250 tablets. Vascardin 30 mg, containers of 100 tablets.

Further information Nil.

Product licence numbers 0188/5931 and 0188/0065.

*Trade Mark

Nordisk-UK
Highview House
Tattenham Crescent
Epsom Downs
Epsom
Surrey KT18 5QJ

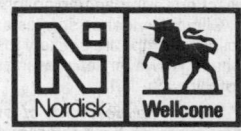

HUMAN VELOSULIN* ▼
HUMAN INSULATARD* ▼
HUMAN MIXTARD* 30/70 ▼
HUMAN INITARD* 50/50 ▼

Presentation Human Velosulin (Neutral Insulin Injection) is a neutral solution of highly purified human insulin (emp).

Human Insulatard (Isophane Insulin Injection [NPH]) is a neutral suspension of highly purified microcrystalline human insulin (emp).

Human Mixtard 30/70 is a neutral suspension of highly purified human insulin (emp) comprising 30% Neutral Insulin in solution and 70% Isophane Insulin in microcrystalline form.

Human Initard 50/50 is a neutral suspension of highly purified human insulin (emp) comprising 50% Neutral Insulin in solution and 50% Isophane Insulin in microcrystalline form.

All the above insulins are available in 100 iu/ml strength. The vials are fitted with orange-coloured disposable plastic caps as a security safeguard. No attempt should be made to refit the caps after removal. Additionally, to aid identification, Human Velosulin has one, Human Insulatard two, Human Mixtard 30/70 three and Human Initard 50/50 four raised tactile marks on the aluminium closure ring.

Uses The treatment of insulin-requiring diabetic patients. Human Velosulin has a rapid onset and a short duration of action making it particularly suitable for the treatment of diabetic coma and pre-coma.

Dosage and administration The dosage of insulin is determined by the physician according to the needs of the patient. Human Velosulin, Human Insulatard, Human Mixtard 30/70 and Human Initard 50/50 may be mixed in all proportions without changing the characteristic effect of any of the types of insulin.

Human Velosulin may be given by subcutaneous, intramuscular or intravenous injection or infusion. It has an onset of action of approximately 30 minutes after subcutaneous injection with duration of about 8 hours, the maximum effect being 1 to 3 hours after injection.

Human Insulatard, Human Mixtard 30/70 and Human Initard 50/50 should be well mixed by gently inverting the vial several times before being given either once or twice daily by subcutaneous or intramuscular injection. Human Insulatard, Human Mixtard 30/70 and Human Initard 50/50 should not be given intravenously.

Human Insulatard has an onset of action of approximately 1½ hours after subcutaneous injection with an overall duration of action which may extend to 24 hours, the maximum effect occurring 4 to 12 hours after injection.

Human Mixtard 30/70 and Human Initard 50/50 each have a duration of action of some ½ to 24 hours after subcutaneous injection, the maximum effect occurring 4 to 8 hours after injection. Human Initard 50/50 has a stronger initial effect than Human Mixtard 30/70.

Onset of action is more rapid and overall duration of action shorter following intramuscular injection than with the subcutaneous route assuming adequate vascular perfusion.

Use in pregancy and lactation: It is essential to maintain continuous good control of the insulin-requiring diabetic patient throughout pregnancy. In the insulin-treated (gestational or insulin-dependent) pregnant diabetic patient, the insulin requirements fall during the first trimester and increase during the second and third trimesters.

Use in the elderly: Clearance rates may be reduced in the elderly due to falling renal function. Insulin may therefore have a more prolonged action. Dose requirements should be regularly reviewed.

Contra-indications, warnings, etc
Contra-indications: Insulin is contra-indicated in hypoglycaemia.

Precautions: Variations in lifestyle and other factors, eg, infection and pregnancy, can affect insulin requirements.

Patients previously treated with insulin of beef or mixed beef/pork origin may require a dosage adjustment on transfer to highly purified human insulin (emp).

Hypoglycaemia can be enhanced by drugs including the following: aspirin; sulphonylureas and agents affecting them; certain steroids.

Hyperglycaemia can be enhanced by drugs including the following: triiodothyronine; thyroxine; various natural and synthetic steroids, including some oral contraceptives; diuretics, including thiazides; cyclophosphamide.

Certain β-blockers, especially propranolol, may affect insulin requirements and mask the signs of hypoglycaemia mediated by the sympathetic nervous system.

Monoamine oxidase inhibitors (MAOI) may potentiate the action of insulin.

Side-and adverse effects: The most important side-effect is hypoglycaemia. Reduction of hyperglycaemia in newly diagnosed diabetics may alter visual refraction.

Insulin, and protamine, like any other injected proteins, are potentially immunogenic. This may or may not have clinical implications. Local reactions at the injection site may include transient erythema, induration, urticaria and oedema. The incidence is minimal with highly purified human insulin (emp). These usually resolve with continuing usage of insulin. True generalised hypersensitivity reactions approaching anaphylaxis are very rare.

Clinical evidence suggests that highly purified human insulins (emp) are unlikely to cause localised lipodystrophies, However, at present, this possibility cannot be totally excluded.

Toxicity and treatment of overdosage: The symptoms and signs of hypoglycaemia depend on the patient's clinical state and on the rate and extent of the fall in blood glucose levels.

If possible, glucose, sucrose, or rapidly absorbable carbohydrate should be taken by mouth. Failing this, hypoglycaemia should be reversed as rapidly as possible by intravenous injection of glucose 50% solution. Alternative emergency treatments include the subcutaneous injection of up to 1 ml of adrenaline solution 1:1000 or the subcutaneous, intramuscular or intravenous injection of lyophilised glucagon 0.5-1.0 mg (1 unit = 1.0 mg). Both adrenaline and glucagon injections mobilise hepatic glycogen, but the effect is short lived and must be supplemented by freely available carbohydrate as soon as possible.

Pharmaceutical precautions Nordisk Wellcome highly purified human insulins (emp) should be stored between 2 and 8°C, protected from sunlight. Insulin which has been frozen should not be used.

Legal category P.

Package quantities 10 ml glass vials.

Further information Mixing of these highly purified human insulins (emp) with preparations of other species is not recommended.

Product licence numbers

Nordisk-UK Ltd		The Wellcome Foundation Ltd
Human Velosulin	3132/0031	0003/0211
Human Insulatard	3132/0034	0003/0212
Human Mixtard 30/70	3132/0037	0003/0213
Human Initard 50/50	3132/0040	0003/0214

VELOSULIN*
INSULATARD*
MIXTARD* 30/70
INITARD* 50/50

Presentation Velosulin (Neutral Insulin Injection BP) is a neutral solution of highly purified pork insulin.

Insulatard (Isophane Insulin Injection BP [NPH]) is a neutral suspension of highly purified microcrystalline pork insulin.

Mixtard 30/70 is a neutral suspension of highly purified pork insulin comprising 30% Neutral Insulin in solution and 70% Isophane Insulin in microcrystalline form.

Initard 50/50 is a neutral suspension of highly purified pork insulin comprising 50% Neutral Insulin in solution and 50% Isophane Insulin in microcrystalline form.

All the above insulins are available in 100 iu/ml strength. The vials are fitted with orange coloured disposable plastic caps as a security safeguard. No attempt should be made to refit the caps after removal. Additionally, to aid identification, Velosulin has one,

Insulatard two, Mixtard 30/70 three and Initard 50/50 four raised tactile marks on the aluminium closure ring.

Uses The treatment of insulin-requiring diabetic patients. Velosulin has a rapid onset and a short duration of action making it particularly suitable for the treatment of diabetic coma and pre-coma.

Dosage and administration The dosage of insulin is determined by the physician according to the needs of the patient. Velosulin, Insulatard, Mixtard 30/70 and Initard 50/50 may be mixed in all proportions without changing the characteristic effect of any of the types of insulin.

Velosulin may be given by subcutaneous, intramuscular or intravenous injection or infusion. It has an onset of action of approximately 30 minutes after subcutaneous injection with duration of about 8 hours, the maximum effect being 1 to 3 hours after injection.

Insulatard, Mixtard 30/70 and Initard 50/50 should be well mixed by gently inverting the vial several times before being given either once or twice daily by subcutaneous or intramuscular injection. Insulatard, Mixtard 30/70 and Initard 50/50 should not be given intravenously.

Insulatard has an onset of action of approximately $1\frac{1}{2}$ hours after subcutaneous injection with an overall duration of action which may extend to 24 hours, the maximum effect occurring 4 to 12 hours after injection.

Mixtard 30/70 and Initard 50/50 each have a duration of action of some $\frac{1}{2}$ to 24 hours after subcutaneous injection, the maximum effect occurring 4 to 8 hours after injection. Initard 50/50 has a stronger initial effect than Mixtard 30/70.

Onset of action is more rapid and overall duration of action shorter following intramuscular injection than with the subcutaneous route assuming adequate vascular perfusion.

Use in pregnancy and lactation: It is essential to maintain continuous good control of the insulin-requiring diabetic patient throughout pregnancy. In the insulin-treated (gestational or insulin-dependent) pregnant diabetic patient, the insulin requirements fall during the first trimester and increase during the second and third trimesters.

Use in the elderly: Clearance rates may be reduced in the elderly due to falling renal function. Insulin may therefore have a more prolonged action. Dose requirements should be regularly reviewed.

Contra-indications, warnings, etc
Contra-indications: Insulin is contra-indicated in hypoglycaemia.

Precautions: Variations in lifestyle and other factors, eg. infection and pregnancy, can affect insulin requirements.

Patients previously treated with insulin of beef or mixed beef/pork origin may require a dosage adjustment on transfer to highly purified pork insulin.

Hypoglycaemia can be enhanced by drugs including the following: aspirin; sulphonylureas and agents affecting them; certain steroids.

Hyperglycaemia can be enhanced by drugs including the following: triiodothyronine; thyroxine; various natural and synthetic steroids, including some oral contraceptives; diuretics, including thiazides; cyclophosphamide.

Certain β-blockers, especially propranolol, may affect insulin requirements and mask the signs of hypoglycaemia mediated by the sympathetic nervous system.

Monoamine oxidase inhibitors (MAOI) may potentiate the action of insulin.

Side- and adverse effects: The most important side-effect is hypoglycaemia. Reduction of hyperglycaemia in newly diagnosed diabetics may alter visual refraction.

Insulin, and protamine, like any other injected proteins, are potentially immunogenic. This may or may not have clinical implications. Local reactions at the injection site may include transient erythema, induration, urticaria and oedema. The incidence is minimal with highly purified pork insulin. These usually resolve with continuing usage of insulin. True generalised hypersensitivity reactions approaching anaphylaxis are very rare.

Clinical evidence suggests that highly purified pork insulins are unlikely to cause localised lipodystrophies. However, at present, this possibility cannot be totally excluded.

Toxicity and treatment of overdosage: The symptoms and signs of hypoglycaemia depend on the patient's clinical state and on the rate and extent of the fall in blood glucose levels.

If possible, glucose, sucrose, or rapidly absorbable carbohydrate should be taken by mouth. Failing this, hypoglycaemia should be reversed as rapidly as possible by intravenous injection of glucose 50% solution. Alternative emergency treatments include the subcutaneous injection of up to 1 ml of adrenaline solution 1:1000 or the subcutaneous, intramuscular or intravenous injection of lyophilised glucagon 0.5–1.0 mg (1 unit = 1.0 mg). Both adrenaline and glucagon injections mobilise hepatic glycogen, but the effect is short lived and must be supplemented by freely available carbohydrate as soon as possible.

Pharmaceutical precautions Nordisk Wellcome highly purified pork insulins should be stored between 2 and 8°C, protected from sunlight. Insulin which has been frozen should not be used.

Legal category P.

Package quantities 10 ml glass vials.

Further information Mixing of these highly purified pork insulins with preparations of other species is not recommended.

Product licence numbers

Nordisk-UK Ltd		The Wellcome Foundation Ltd
Velosulin	3132/0019	0003/0188
Insulatard	3132/0018	0003/0191
Mixtard 30/70	3132/0021	0003/0194
Initard 50/50	3132/0020	0003/0197

VELOSULIN* CARTRIDGE ▼
Neutral Insulin Injection BP, highly purified pork

Presentation Velosulin Cartridge is a neutral solution of highly purified pork insulin available in 5.7 ml glass cartridge vials containing 100 iu/ml for use only in the Nordisk Infuser.

Uses The treatment of insulin-requiring diabetic patients. To be used only with the Nordisk Infuser.

Dosage and administration Velosulin Cartridge is intended to be administered as subcutaneous infusion using the Nordisk Infuser System.

Basal rate and prandial doses are to be determined by the physician.

Velosulin Cartridge should only be used with the infusion set supplied with the Nordisk Infuser. No attempt should be made to refill the cartridges. When empty, they should be discarded and a fresh cartridge inserted. In order to minimise the risk of infusion site irritation or infection, it is recommended that the infusion set is changed every 2–3 days. The infusion site should be cleansed thoroughly and the needle taped securely in place. The infusion site should be changed according to a suitable routine and should be cleansed regularly. The procedure (given in the User's Manual) should be followed when the cartridge or infusion set is changed. The maximum in-use life of Velosulin Cartridge used in the Nordisk Infuser is 14 days.

Velosulin Cartridge is stable at normal Infuser operating temperatures (30–37°C if worn under outdoor clothing), although care must be taken to avoid extremes of temperature, eg. when sunbathing, winter sports, etc.

Use in pregnancy and lactation: It is essential to maintain continuous good control of the insulin-requiring diabetic patient throughout pregnancy. In the insulin-treated (gestational or insulin-dependent) pregnant diabetic patient, the insulin requirements fall in the first trimester and increase during the second and third trimesters.

Use in the elderly: No specific studies regarding continuous subcutaneous insulin infusion (CSII) in the elderly have yet been conducted. Clearance rates may be reduced in the elderly due to falling renal function. Insulin may therefore have a more prolonged action. Dose requirements should be regularly reviewed.

Contra-indications, warnings, etc
Contra-indications: Insulin is contra-indicated in hypoglycaemia.

Precautions: Variations in lifestyle and other factors, eg. infection and pregnancy, can affect insulin requirements.

Patients previously treated by subcutaneous insulin injection may require a dosage adjustment when transferred to subcutaneous infusion.

Hypoglycaemia can be enhanced by drugs including the following: aspirin; sulphonylureas, and agents affecting them; certain steroids.

Hyperglycaemia can be enhanced by drugs including the following: triiodothyronine; thyroxine; various natural and synthetic steroids, including some oral contraceptives; diuretics, including thiazides; cyclophosphamide.

Certain β-blockers, especially propranolol, may affect insulin requirements and mask the signs of hypoglycaemia mediated by the sympathetic nervous system.

Monoamine oxidase inhibitors (MAOI) may potentiate the action of insulin.

Side- and adverse effects: The most important side-effect is hypoglycaemia. Reduction of hyperglycaemia in newly diagnosed diabetics may alter visual refraction.

Insulin, like many other injected substances, is potentially immunogenic. This may or may not have clinical implications. Local reactions at the infusion site may include transient erythema, induration, urticaria and oedema. The incidence is minimal with highly purified pork insulin. These usually resolve with continuing usage of insulin. True generalised hypersensitivity reactions approaching anaphylaxis are very rare.

Clinical evidence suggests that highly purified pork insulins are unlikely to cause localised lipodystrophies. However, at present, this possibility cannot be totally excluded.

Toxicity and treatment of overdosage: The symptoms and signs of hypoglycaemia depend on the patient's clinical state and on the rate and extent of the fall in blood glucose levels.

Infusion with Velosulin Cartridge should be reduced or suspended until normal blood glucose levels are restored.

If possible, glucose, sucrose, or rapidly absorbable carbohydrate should be taken by mouth. Failing this, hypoglycaemia should be reversed as rapidly as possible by intravenous injection of glucose 50% solution. Alternative emergency treatments include the subcutaneous injection of up to 1 ml of adrenaline solution 1:1000 or the subcutaneous, intramuscular or intravenous injection of lyophilised glucagon 0.5–1.0 mg (1 unit = 1.0 mg). Both adrenaline and glucagon injections mobilise hepatic glycogen, but the effect is short lived and must be supplemented by freely available carbohydrate as soon as possible.

Pharmaceutical precautions Velosulin Cartridge should be stored between 2 and 8°C, protected from sunlight. Insulin which has been frozen should not be used. Velosulin Cartridge insulin which appears turbid (cloudy) should not be used.

Legal category P.

Package quantities 1 × 5.7 ml glass cartridge vials.

Further information Nil.

Product licence numbers
Nordisk-UK Ltd   *The Wellcome Foundation Ltd*
3132/0043   0003/0208

*Trade Mark

Norgine Limited
116–120 London Road
Headington
Oxford OX3 9BA

ALCOS ANAL*

Presentation A white ointment containing:

Sodium oleate	10%
Hydroxypolyethoxydodecane	2%
Chlorothymol	0.1%

White suppositories, each containing:

Sodium oleate	200 mg
Hydroxypolyethoxydodecane	20 mg
Chlorothymol	0.7 mg

Uses Haemorrhoids and pruritus ani.

Dosage and administration Ointment for rectal and topical administration; suppositories for rectal administration.

Adults (including the elderly) and children: For internal haemorrhoids, one application of ointment or one suppository should be introduced into the anus at night, in the morning, and after defaecation.

For external haemorrhoids and pruritus ani, the ointment should be applied to the affected area at night, in the morning, and after defaecation.

Contra-indications, warnings, etc
Contra-indications: None known.

Precautions: None known.

Use in pregnancy: No teratogenic effects have been reported, but caution should be exercised during the first trimester of pregnancy.

Side-effects: Rarely, initial application may produce a burning sensation.

Pharmaceutical precautions Store in a cool, dry place.

Legal category P.

Package quantities Ointment: Tubes of 20 g with applicator.
Suppositories: Box of 10 suppositories.

Further information Nil.

Product licence numbers
Ointment	0322/0032.
Suppositories	0322/0033.

CAMCOLIT*

Presentation *Camcolit 250:* White film coated tablets with 'Camcolit' engraved on one side and a break line on the reverse, each containing 250 mg Lithium Carbonate BP (equivalent to 6.8 millimoles).

Camcolit 400: White film coated tablets, with 'Camcolit S' engraved on one side and a break line on the reverse, each containing 400 mg Lithium Carbonate BP (equivalent to 10.8 millimoles).

Uses Treatment and prophylaxis of mania, manic-depressive illness and recurrent depression.

Dosage and administration Tablets for oral administration. Camcolit 400 may be given in divided or single daily doses, whereas Camcolit 250 should be given in divided dosage.

Acute mania: Treatment of mania should be initiated in hospital where regular monitoring of serum lithium levels can be conducted.

The dosage of Camcolit should be adjusted to produce a serum lithium level between 0.6 and 1.2 mmol/l 12 hours after the last dose. The required serum lithium level may be achieved in one of two ways but, whichever is adopted, regular estimations must be carried out to ensure maintenance of levels within the therapeutic range. For consistent results it is essential that the blood samples for serum lithium estimations are taken 12 hours after the last dose of lithium.

1. 1,500–2,000 mg of lithium carbonate are administered daily for the first five or seven days. A blood sample for serum lithium estimation is taken 12 hours after the last dose on the fifth or seventh day, and the dosage of Camcolit is adjusted to keep the serum lithium level within the therapeutic range.

Subsequently, regular serum lithium estimations must be carried out and, where necessary, the dosage of Camcolit adjusted accordingly.

The precise initial dose of lithium should be decided in the light of the age and weight of the patient; young patients often require a dose higher than average and older patients a lower dose.

2. A lithium clearance test is carried out and the initial dosage calculated from the results. Even when the initial dosage is calculated in this way, it is still desirable that serum lithium levels should be determined at weekly intervals during the first three weeks of treatment, and any necessary adjustments to dosage made as a result of the levels actually obtained.

Most of the above applies in the treatment of hypomania as well as mania, but the patient (if not too ill) can be started on treatment as an outpatient provided that facilities for periodic serum lithium monitoring are available.

Prophylaxis of recurrent affective disorders (including unipolar mania, unipolar depressions and bipolar manic-depressive illness): A dosage of 500–1,200 mg of lithium carbonate can be administered daily for the first seven days. A blood sample for serum lithium estimation is then taken 12 hours after the last dose, and the dosage of Camcolit is adjusted to keep the plasma lithium level within the effective range. Clinical improvement is usually associated with serum concentrations of 0.5 mmol/l or above. Toxic symptoms are usually associated with concentrations exceeding 1.5 mmol/l.

Use in elderly: Usually 500–1,000 mg/day.

Toxic symptoms are likely with serum concentrations above 1.0 mmol/l.

Use in children: Not recommended.

Measurement of serum lithium concentrations: Lithium therapy should not be initiated unless adequate facilities for routine monitoring of serum concentrations are available. On initiation of therapy serum concentrations should be measured weekly until stabilisation is achieved, then weekly for one month and at monthly intervals thereafter. Additional measurements should be made if signs of lithium toxicity occur (see below), on dosage alteration, development of significant intercurrent disease, signs of manic or depressive relapse and if significant change in sodium or fluid intake occurs.

As bioavailability varies from product to product a change of product should be regarded as initiation of new treatment. Blood levels should therefore be monitored weekly until re-stabilisation is achieved. More frequent monitoring is required if patients are receiving diuretics.

Contra-indications, warnings, etc The first consideration in lithium therapy is the selection of proper candidates. The second is the physical state of the patient, which must be adequate to handle the lithium ion when it is introduced into the body.

Contra-indications: Patients with renal disease, cardiovascular disease, Addison's disease or those breast feeding.

Precautions: Pre-treatment and periodic routine clinical monitoring is essential. This should include assessment of renal function, urine analysis, assessment of thyroid function and cardiac function, especially in patients with cardiovascular disease.

Patients should be euthyroid before the initiation of lithium therapy.

Clear instructions regarding the symptoms of impending toxicity should be given by the doctor to all patients receiving long-term lithium therapy (see Warnings and Adverse Effects). Patients should also be warned to report if polyuria or polydipsia develop. Episodes of nausea and vomiting or other conditions leading to salt/water depletion (including severe dieting) should also be reported. Patients should be advised to maintain their usual salt and fluid intake.

Elderly patients are particularly liable to lithium toxicity. Lower doses of lithium may be needed during diuretic therapy as lithium clearance is reduced.

Raised plasma levels of ADH may occur during treatment.

Symptoms of nephrogenic diabetes are particularly prevalent in patients receiving concurrent treatment with tri/tetracyclic antidepressants.

Serum lithium concentrations may increase during concomitant therapy with indomethacin or tetracycline.

Warnings: Long-term treatment with lithium may result in permanent changes in the kidney and impairment of renal function. High serum concentrations of lithium, including episodes of acute lithium toxicity may enhance these changes. The minimum clinically effective dose of lithium should always be used. Patients should be maintained on lithium after 3–5 years only if, on assessment, benefit persists.

Renal function should be routinely monitored in patients with polyuria and polydipsia.

Use in pregnancy: There is epidemiological evidence that the drug may be harmful in human pregnancy. Should the use of lithium be unavoidable, close monitoring of serum concentrations should be made throughout the pregnancy and during parturition.

Side-effects: Side effects are usually related to serum lithium concentrations and are infrequent at levels below 1.0 mmol/l.

Mild gastro-intestinal effects, nausea, vertigo, muscle weakness and a dazed feeling may occur, but frequently disappear after stabilisation. Fine hand tremore, polyuria and mild thirst may persist. Some studies suggest that the tremor can be controlled by relatively small doses of propranolol.

Long term treatment with lithium is frequently associated with disturbances of thyroid function including goitre and hypothyroidism. These can be controlled by administration of small doses of thyroxine (0.05–0.2 mg daily) concomitantly with lithium. Thyrotoxicosis has also been reported.

Mild cognitive impairment may occur during long term use.

Hypercalcaemia, hypermagnesaemia, hyperparathyroidism and an increase in antinuclear antibodies have also been reported.

Exacerbation of psoriasis may occur.

Signs of impending toxicity: Appearance or aggravation of gastro-intestinal symptoms, muscle weakness, lack of co-ordination, drowsiness or lethargy may be early signs of intoxication. With increasing toxicity there is ataxia, giddiness, tinnitus, blurred vision, coarse tremor, muscle twitching and a large output of dilute urine. At blood levels above 2–3 mmol/l, there is increasing disorientation, seizures, coma and death.

Pharmaceutical precautions Store in a cool, dry place.

Legal category POM.

Package quantities *Camcolit 250:* Packs of 100 and 1,000 tablets.
Camcolit 400: Packs of 100 and 500 tablets.

Further information The authors of a comparison between Camcolit and two types of 'slow release' or 'controlled-release' lithium concluded that there was no significant difference in humans in the rate of absorption or excretion of the different products.

A second study demonstrated that patients who had been receiving their daily dose of lithium carbonate in the form of another 'controlled-release' preparation could be changed to the same daily dose of lithium carbonate in the form of Camcolit 400 without significant change in plasma lithium levels or clinical conditions.

Product licence numbers
Camcolit 250 0322/5900
Camcolit 400 0322/0015

CYCLOBRAL*

Presentation Pink/brown hard gelatin capsules imprinted CYCLOBRAL. Each capsule contains 400 mg cyclandelate.

Uses As an adjunct to the management of elderly patients with arterio-sclerotic dementia, and for peripheral vascular disorders such as intermittent claudication, Raynaud's syndrome, night cramps, acrocyanosis, cold extremities, chilblains and 'restless legs'.

Dosage and administration Capsules for oral administration.

Adults (including the elderly): 1 capsule three or four times daily.

Children: Not recommended.

Contra-indications, warnings, etc
Contra-indications: Acute phase of cerebrovascular accidents or recent myocardial infarction. Actual or incipient peripheral gangrene or frostbite.

Precautions: Glaucoma.

Use in pregnancy: No teratogenic effects have been reported, but caution should be exercised during the first trimester of pregnancy.

Side-effects: Nausea, gastro-intestinal distress or flushing may occasionally occur.

Overdosage: Gastric lavage, followed, if necessary, by administration of vasopressors.

Pharmaceutical precautions Store in a cool, dry place.

Legal category P.

Package quantities Packs of 250 capsules.

Further information Cyclandelate has a low order of toxicity and for maximum therapeutic effect it is recommended that four capsules daily should be given.

Product licence number 0322/0036.

FYBRANTA*

Presentation Mottled, light brown tablets containing bran 2 g.

Uses The treatment of all colonic and other gastro-enterological diseases where administration of bran is indicated, including the treatment of constipation, symptomatic relief in diverticular disease and the 'irritable bowel' syndrome. Treatment of conditions requiring a high-fibre regimen.

Dosage and administration *Adults (including the elderly):* Usually 1–3 tablets three or four times daily, preferably with meals.

At the discretion of the physician, larger quantities may be prescribed in individual cases.

Children: A lower dose, at the discretion of the physician.

Fybranta tablets should be chewed, part of a tablet at a time if necessary, and swallowed with a drink.

No attempt should be made to swallow the tablets whole.

Contra-indications, warnings, etc
Contra-indications: Intestinal obstruction, gluten enteropathies.

Precautions: None known.

Use in pregnancy: There is no evidence to suggest that Fybranta should not be taken during pregnancy.

Side-effects: None reported.

Pharmaceutical precautions Store in a cool, dry place.

Legal category GSL.

Package quantities Packs of 100 tablets.

Further information Fybranta tablets contain calcium phosphate which ensures neutralisation of the phytic

acid in bran, which may otherwise interfere with calcium absorption.

Product licence number 0322/0016.

GUARINA*

Presentation A fine off-white dispersible granulate in unit dose sachets. Each sachet contains 5 g of guar gum (USNF).

Uses As an adjunct in the treatment of diabetes mellitus.

Dosage and administration
Dosage: Adults: initially, one sachet daily, increasing if necessary to a maximum of three sachets daily from the third week of therapy. It is important that all doses should be taken before meals.

Children: No specific recommendations can be made for children.

To be taken immediately before meals. The contents of one sachet should be added to 150 ml ($\frac{1}{4}$ pint) of a cold drink, stirred briskly and taken straight away. Cold sugar-free still drinks or fruit juice may be used, instead of water. If a sugar sweetened drink is used, its sugar content should be taken into account.

Contra-indications, warnings, etc
Contra-indications: 1. Oesophageal disease or dysfunction. 2. Intestinal obstruction.

Precautions: Careful monitoring is required during the initial stages of treatment, to minimise the dangers of hypoglycaemia.

Side-effects: Flatulence, some alteration in bowel habit or nausea may occur in a few patients, but these effects are usually transient.

Pharmaceutical precautions Store in a cool, dry place, below 25°C.

Legal category P.

Package quantities Cartons of 60 sachets.

Further information Guar is used to slow the rate of glucose absorption, thereby reducing the post-prandial peak in the blood-glucose level. This may allow a reduction in dosage of insulin or oral hypoglycaemic agents.

Product licence number 0322/0053.

KAMILLOSAN* OINTMENT

Presentation Light brown ointment containing:

Chamomile extract	10.0%
Oil of chamomile	0.5%

in a base containing lanolin.

Uses Prophylaxis and treatment of sore and cracked nipples in nursing mothers, nappy rash, nappy chafe and chapped hands.

Dosage and administration Ointment for topical application.

Sore and cracked nipples: Apply after breastfeeding.

Nappy rash: Apply at every nappy change.

Other conditions: Apply twice daily as necessary.

Contra-indications, warnings, etc
Contra-indications: None known.

Precautions: None known.

Use in pregnancy: There is no evidence to suggest that Kamillosan should not be used during pregnancy.

Side-effects: None reported.

Pharmaceutical precautions Store in a cool, dry place.

Legal category GSL.

Package quantities Tubes of 20 g and 5 g.

Further information Nil.

Product licence number 0322/5914.

MURIPSIN*

Presentation Orange, film-coated tablets, each containing:

Glutamic Acid Hydrochloride USNF X111	500 mg
Pepsin BPC 1959	35 mg

Uses The symptomatic treatment of gastric hydrochloric acid deficiency.

Dosage and administration Tablets for oral administration. *Adults (including the elderly):* 1 or 2 tablets with each meal.

Children: No specific dosage can be recommended.

Contra-indications, warnings, etc
Contra-indications: None known.

Precautions: None known.

Use in pregnancy: No teratogenic effects have been reported, but caution should be exercised during the first trimester of pregnancy.

Side-effects: None reported.

Pharmaceutical precautions Store in a cool, dry place.

Legal category GSL.

Package quantities Packs of 50 tablets.

Further information Each Muripsin tablet is approximately equivalent to the oral administration of 1 ml Dilute Hydrochloric Acid BP.

Product licence number 0322/5005.

NORMACOL*

Presentation White, coated granules containing Sterculia BP 62%.

Uses Treatment of constipation, particularly simple or idiopathic constipation, and constipation arising in pregnancy.

Management of colostomies and ileostomies.

The 'high residue diet' management of diverticular disease of the colon and other conditions requiring a high fibre regime.

The initiation and maintenance of bowel action after rectal and anal surgery.

Administration after ingestion of sharp foreign bodies to provide a coating and reduce the possibility of intestinal damage during transit.

Dosage and administration Granules for oral administration.

Adults: (including the elderly): 1 or 2 sachets or 1–2 heaped 5 ml spoonfuls, once or twice daily after meals.

Children (6–12 years): One half of the above amount.

The granules should be placed dry on the tongue and, without chewing or crushing, swallowed immediately with plenty of liquid (water or a cool drink).

Contra-indications, warnings, etc
Contra-indications: Intestinal obstruction, faecal impaction, and total atony of the colon.

Precautions: Not to be taken immediately before retiring, especially in the elderly. Adequate fluid intake should be maintained. Caution should be exercised in cases of ulcerative colitis.

Use in pregnancy: Normacol is indicated for use in pregnancy.

Side-effects: Abdominal distension. Intestinal obstruction is possible if the product is taken in overdosage or if it is not adequately washed down with fluid.

Pharmaceutical precautions Store in a cool, dry place.

Legal category GSL.

Package quantities Packs of 60 sachets (2 × 30), each sachet containing 7 g of granules, or packs of 500 g.

Further information Each 7 g sachet of granules contains 1.72 g of available carbohydrate, equivalent to 6.75 kcal.

Product licence number 0322/5010.

NORMACOL* ANTISPASMODIC

Presentation Orange, coated granules containing:

Sterculia BP	62% ·
Alverine Citrate USNF X111	0.5%

Uses Treatment of spastic and hypertonic constipation and the 'irritable bowel' syndrome.

Dosage and administration Granules for oral administration. *Adults (including the elderly):* 1–2 heaped 5 ml spoonfuls once or twice daily after meals.

Children (6–12 years): One half the above amount.

The granules should be placed dry on the tongue and, without chewing or crushing, swallowed immediately with plenty of water.

Contra-indications, warnings, etc
Contra-indications: Intestinal obstruction, faecal impaction, and total atony of the colon.

Precautions: Not to be taken immediately before retiring, especially in the elderly. Adequate fluid intake should be maintained.

Use in pregnancy: No teratogenic effects have been reported but caution should be exercised during the first trimester of pregnancy.

Side-effects: Abdominal distension. Intestinal obstruction is possible if the product is taken in overdosage or is not adequately washed down with fluid.

Pharmaceutical precautions Store in a cool, dry place.

Legal category P.

Package quantities Packs of 500 g.

Further information Nil.

Product licence number 0322/5009.

NORMACOL* STANDARD

Presentation Brown, coated granules containing:

Sterculia BP 62%
Frangula BPC 1949 8%

Uses Treatment of constipation, particularly hypotonic or slow transit constipation resistant to bulk alone.

The initiation and maintenance of bowel action after rectal surgery and after haemorrhoidectomy.

Dosage and administration Granules for oral administration.

Adults (including the elderly): 1–2 heaped 5 ml spoonfuls once or twice daily after meals.

Children (6–12 years): One half the above amount.

The granules should be placed dry on the tongue and, without chewing or crushing, swallowed immediately with plenty of water.

Contra-indications, warnings, etc

Contra-indications: Intestinal obstruction, faecal impaction, and total atony of the colon.

Precautions: Not to be taken immediately before retiring, especially in the elderly. Adequate fluid intake should be maintained. Caution should be exercised in cases of ulcerative colitis.

Use in pregnancy: No teratogenic effects have been reported, but caution should be exercised during the first trimester of pregnancy.

Use during lactation: There is no evidence to suggest that Normacol Standard is unsuitable for use during lactation, though Normacol is available without frangula, if preferred.

Side-effects: Abdominal distension. Intestinal obstruction is possible if the product is taken in overdosage or is not adequately washed down with fluid.

Pharmaceutical precautions Store in a cool, dry place.

Legal category GSL.

Package quantities Packs of 200 g and 500 g.

Further information Nil.

Product licence number 0322/5011.

NORMACOL* STANDARD SUGAR FREE FORMULA

Presentation Brown, sugarless, coated granules containing:

Sterculia BP 62%
Frangula BPC 1949 8%

Uses Treatment of constipation, particularly hypotonic or slow transit constipation resistant to bulk alone.

The initiation and maintenance of bowel action after rectal surgery and after haemorrhoidectomy.

This formulation is particularly useful where patients must, or wish to, restrict carbohydrate intake.

Dosage and administration Granules for oral administration.

Adults (including the elderly): 1–2 heaped 5 ml spoonfuls once or twice daily after meals.

Children (6–12 years): One half the above amount.

The granules should be placed dry on the tongue and, without chewing or crushing, swallowed immediately with plenty of water.

Contra-indications, warnings, etc

Contra-indications: Intestinal obstruction, faecal impaction, and total atony of the colon.

Precautions: Not to be taken immediately before retiring, especially in the elderly. Adequate fluid intake should be maintained. Caution should be exercised in cases of ulcerative colitis.

Use in pregnancy: No teratogenic effects have been reported, but caution should be exercised during the first trimester of pregnancy.

Use during lactation: There is no evidence to suggest that Normacol Standard Sugar Free Formula is unsuitable for use during lactation, though Normacol is available without frangula, if preferred.

Side-effects: Abdominal distension. Intestinal obstruction is possible if the product is taken in overdosage or is not adequately washed down with fluid.

Pharmaceutical precautions Store in a cool, dry place.

Legal category GSL.

Package quantities Packs of 500 g.

Further information Nil.

Product licence number 0322/5017.

POSALFILIN*

Presentation Dark brown ointment containing:

Podophyllum Resin BP 20%
Salicylic Acid BP 25%

Uses Treatment of plantar warts.

Dosage and administration Ointment for topical administration. *Adults (including the elderly) and children:*

1. Place a felt corn ring around the wart, if necessary adjusting the size of the hole by snipping, allowing the wart to protrude through the hole.
2. Apply the ointment (using a minimum amount) to exposed wart only. Cover with a piece of plaster.
3. The dressing may be renewed two or three times weekly. When wart appears soft and spongy leave exposed to the air for a day or two when it will usually drop off. If not, repeat the above procedure.
4. Wash hands thoroughly after applying the ointment, and if a waterproof plaster is used normal washing will not effect the efficacy of the treatment.

Contra-indications, warnings, etc
Contra-indications: Pregnancy.

Precautions: The patient should be warned that Posalfilin Ointment is caustic to healthy skin.

Use in pregnancy: Contra-indicated.

Side-effects: Inflammation of the surrounding skin may occur, in which case treatment should be suspended.

Pharmaceutical precautions Store in a cool, dry place.

Legal category P.

Package quantities Tubes of 10 g.

Further information Nil.

Product licence number 0322/5901.

PREFIL*

Presentation Brown, coated granules containing Sterculia BP 55%.

Uses Treatment of obesity, in conjunction with a calorie-controlled diet.

Dosage and administration Granules for oral administration. *Adults (including the elderly):* Two rounded 5 ml spoonfuls, ½ to 1 hour before each meal. The granules should be placed dry on the tongue, in small quantities if necessary, and without chewing or crushing, swallowed with ½ pint of low-calorie drink.

Children: At the discretion of the physician, when a reduced dosage may be given.

Contra-indications, warnings, etc
Contra-indications: Intestinal obstruction.

Precautions: None known.

Use in pregnancy: There is no evidence to suggest that Prefil should not be used during pregnancy.

Side-effects: Some patients who have become accustomed to an unusually low residue diet may experience slight abdominal discomfort from the increase in bulk which follows the administration of full doses of Prefil. These patients may be advised to take a smaller dose initially, increasing to the full dose over a period of one week. In these circumstances, the full clinical effect may not be experienced until the end of the first week.

Pharmaceutical precautions Store in a cool, dry place.

Legal category GSL.

Package quantities Packs of 200 g and 500 g.

Further information Available carbohydrate content approx. 1.6 g per spoonful (as sucrose) equivalent to 6 Cals.

Product licence number 0322/0035.

PYRALVEX*

Presentation Brown liquid containing:

Extract of Anthraquinone glycosides	5%
Salicylic Acid BP	1%

Uses Treatment of inflammatory conditions of the oral mucosa.

Dosage and administration *Adults (including the elderly) and children:* To be applied to the inflamed oral mucosa (after removing any dentures worn) three or four times daily using the brush provided.

Contra-indications, warnings, etc
Contra-indications: None known.

Precautions: None known.

Use in pregnancy: There is no evidence to suggest that Pyralvex should not be used during pregnancy.

Side-effects: Transient stinging may occur immediately after application.

Pharmaceutical precautions Store in a cool, dry place.

Legal category P.

Package quantities 10 ml bottle with brush.

Further information Nil.

Product licence number 0322/5013.

SOMNITE*

Presentation *Tablets:* Round, white, uncoated, flat, bevel-edged tablets of 12 mm diameter with a single break line on one side and sailing boat design on the other. Each tablet contains Nitrazepam BP 5 mg.

Suspension: An off-white, translucent, thixotropic suspension with a cherry flavour. Each 5 ml spoonful contains Nitrazepam BP 2.5 mg.

Uses Short term treatment of insomnia where daytime sedation is acceptable.

Dosage and administration Tablets and suspension for oral administration. *Adults:* 5 mg (one tablet or two 5 ml spoonfuls suspension) before retiring. This dose may, if necessary, be increased to 10 mg.

Elderly patients: 2.5 mg before retiring. This dose may, if necessary, be increased to 5 mg.

Children: Not recommended.

Contra-indications, warnings, etc
Contra-indications: Known sensitivity to benzodiazepines. Acute pulmonary insufficiency.

Precautions: Chronic pulmonary insufficiency. In chronic renal or hepatic disease. In labour. High single doses or repeated low doses have been reported to produce hypotonia, poor sucking and hypothermia in the neonate and irregularities in the foetal heart. Avoid if possible in lactation. The concurrent use of other CNS depressant drugs should be avoided.

Use in pregnancy: There is no evidence as to drug safety in human pregnancy nor is there evidence from animal work that it is free from hazard. Do not use during pregnancy, especially during the first and last trimesters, unless there are compelling reasons.

Side-effects: Common adverse effects include drowsiness, sedation, blurring of vision, unsteadiness and ataxia. These effects occur following single as well as repeated dosage and may persist well into the following day. Performance at skilled tasks and alertness may be impaired. Patients should be warned of this hazard and advised not to drive or operate machinery during treatment. These effects are potentiated by alcohol. The elderly are particularly liable to experience these symptoms together with confusion especially if organic brain symptoms are present. See also Dependence Potential and Withdrawal Symptoms below.

Abnormal psychological reactions to benzodiazepines have been reported. Rare behavioural adverse effects include paradoxical aggressive outbursts, excitement, confusion, and the uncovering of depression with suicidal tendencies.

Other rare adverse effects including hypotension, gastro-intestinal and visual disturbances, skin rashes urinary retention, headache, vertigo, changes in libido; blood dyscrasias and jaundice have also been reported.

Dependence potential and withdrawal symptoms: In general the dependence potential of benzodiazepines is low but this increases when high dosages are attained, especially when given over long periods. This is particularly so in patients with a history of alcoholism, drug abuse or in patients with marked personality disorders. Regular monitoring of treatment in such patients is essential and routine repeat prescriptions should be avoided.

Treatment in all patients should be withdrawn gradually as symptoms such as depression, nervousness, rebound insomnia, irritability, sweating and diarrhoea have been reported following abrupt cessation of treatment in patients receiving even normal therapeutic doses for short periods of time.

Abrupt withdrawal following excessive dosage may produce confusion, toxic psychosis, convulsions or a condition resembling delirium tremens.

Overdosage: The primary symptoms of overdosage are drowsiness, dizziness, ataxia and slurred speech. Treatment is symptomatic but gastric lavage may be useful if performed soon after ingestion.

Pharmaceutical precautions Somnite tablets should be stored in a cool, dry place and protected from light and moisture. Somnite suspension should be stored in a cool place, protected from light.

Somnite Suspension may be diluted to a maximum of 1 in 5 with Syrup BP (preserved). The shelf life of the diluted suspension is not more than 14 days.

Legal category CD (Sch 4) POM.

Package quantities Somnite tablets 5 mg: Packs of 100 and 500.
Somnite suspension: 2.5 mg/5 ml: Bottles of 150 ml

Further information Somnite is a long acting benzodiazepine. Repeated dosage will lead to accumulation of whole drug and metabolites. The elderly and patients with impaired renal and/or hepatic function will be particularly susceptible to the adverse effects listed above. Treatment should be kept to a minimum and given only under close medical supervision.

Little is known regarding efficacy or safety of benzodiazepines in long-term use. It is advisable to review treatment regularly and to discontinue use as soon as possible.

Somnite does not induce microsomal enzymes as may occur with barbiturates and may be given together with commonly used cardiovascular drugs, anticoagulants, antihypertensives, stimulants, spasmolytics, antidepressants and chemotherapeutic agents.

Product licence numbers
Tablets   0322/0034.
Suspension   0322/0039

SPASMONAL*

Presentation Blue/grey, opaque, hard gelatin capsules, marked '78' on one half and with a sailing boat design on the other. Each capsule contains 60 mg Alverine Citrate USNF XIII.

Uses Selective smooth muscle spasmolytic.

Dosage and administration Capsules for oral administration. *Adults (including the elderly):* 1 or 2 capsules one to three times daily.

Children: No specific dosage can be recommended.

Contra-indications, warnings, etc
Contra-indications: None known.

Precautions: None known.

Use in pregnancy: No teratogenic effects have been reported, but caution should be exercised during the first trimester of pregnancy.

Side-effects: None reported at normal therapeutic doses.

Pharmaceutical precautions Store in a cool, dry place.

Legal category P.

Package quantities Containers of 100 capsules.

Further information Alverine citrate is a synthetic, non-narcotic, non-habit-forming spasmolytic of a low order of toxicity in comparison with other anti-spasmodics. It is related to (but more than twice as active as) papaverine, and has a specific effect on the smooth muscle of the intestine and uterus, but not on those of the respiratory or cardiovascular system.

Product licence number 0322/5014.

TAMPOVAGAN* STILBOESTROL AND LACTIC ACID

Presentation Off-white, hard, vaginal pessaries, each containing:
Stilboestrol BP 0.5 mg in a base including Lactic Acid BP 5%.

Uses Treatment of atrophic vaginitis, senile vaginitis and menopausal vaginitis.

Dosage and administration *Adults (including the elderly):* Two pessaries to be inserted high into the vagina at night.
Children: Not recommended.

Contra-indications, warnings, etc
Contra-indications: Pregnancy, suspected pregnancy or women who might become pregnant. Not for use in children.

Precautions: None known.

Use in pregnancy: Contra-indicated.

Side-effects: None reported.

Pharmaceutical precautions Store in a cool, dry place.

Legal category POM.

Package quantities Cartons of 10 pessaries.

Further information Nil.

Product licence number 0322/5910.

WAXSOL*

Presentation Colourless liquid containing:
Docusate sodium 0.5% in a water-miscible base.

Uses Cerumenolytic.

Dosage and administration For aural use only.
Adults (including the elderly) and children: The patient

should be directed to fill the ear with Waxsol on not more than two consecutive nights, before attending for syringing.

Contra indications, warnings, etc

Contra-indications: Perforation of the ear drum; inflammation of the ear.

Precautions: If pain or inflammation is experienced, treatment should be discontinued.

Use in pregnancy: There is no evidence to suggest that Waxsol should not be used during pregnancy.

Side-effects: Rarely, transient stinging or irritation may occur.

Pharmaceutical precautions Store in a cool place.

Legal category GSL.

Package quantities 10 ml bottle with dropper.

Further information Waxsol, because of its low surface tension and its water-miscibility, rapidly penetrates the dry matrix of the ceruminous mass, reducing the solid material to a semi-solid debris which can be syringed away readily or, in less severe and in chronic cases, is ejected by normal physiological processes.

Product licence number 0322/5016.

*Trade Mark

Norwich Eaton Limited
Hedley House
St Nicholas Avenue, Gosforth
Newcastle Upon Tyne NE3 1LR

Norwich Eaton

ALPHADERM*

Presentation Alphaderm contains hydrocortisone 1% w/w and urea 10% w/w in a specially formulated base which assists the percutaneous transportation of the active ingredients to the site of action. The base is self-occlusive and fulfils the functions of both an ointment and a cream. Alphaderm does not contain lanolin, parabens or any preservative.

Uses Alphaderm is indicated for the treatment of all ichthyotic, eczematous or dry inflammatory states of skin not due to pathogenic organisms, including atopic, infantile and hyperkeratotic eczema; intertrigo; neurodermatitis and all lichenoid conditions; contact dermatitis; photosensitivity reactions and prurigo.

Dosage and administration Alphaderm is applied topically. Wash affected areas well, dry and apply directly to the lesions twice daily. Occlusive dressings may be used but are usually unnecessary because of the self-occlusive nature of the special base.

Contra-indications, warnings, etc Alphaderm is contra-indicated in bacterial, viral and fungal diseases of the skin.
Precautions: In pregnant animals, administration of corticosteroids can cause abnormalities of foetal development. The relevance of this finding in human beings has not been established. However, topical steroids should not be used extensively in pregnancy, i.e. in large amounts or for long periods. In infants, long-term continuous topical therapy should be avoided; adrenal suppression can occur even without occlusion.
In some instances Alphaderm may cause irritation when applied to sensitive skin.

Pharmaceutical precautions Store at a temperature not exceeding 25°C.

Legal category POM.

Package quantities Alphaderm is available in tubes of 30 g and 100 g.

Further information Optimum rehydration of dry skin is achieved without the use of occlusive dressings.

Product licence number 0364/0019.

AQUADRATE*

Presentation Aquadrate contains urea 10% w/w in a specially formulated base. It has keratolytic action and helps to hydrate the skin. The base is self-occlusive and it fulfils the functions of both an ointment and a cream. Aquadrate does not contain lanolin, parabens or any preservative.

Uses Aquadrate is indicated in atopic eczema, ichthyosis, xeroderma, hyperkeratosis and other chronic dry skin conditions.

Dosage and administration Aquadrate is applied topically. Wash affected areas well, rinse off all traces of soap, dry, and apply sparingly twice daily. Occlusive dressings may be used but are usually unnecessary because of the self-occlusive nature of the base.

Contra-indications, warnings, etc In some instances, Aquadrate may cause irritation when applied to sensitive skin.

Pharmaceutical precautions Store at a temperature not exceeding 30°C.

Legal category P.

Package quantities Aquadrate is available in tubes of 30 g and 100 g.

Further information Nil.

Product licence number 0364/0018.

CHLORASEPTIC* LIQUID

Presentation Chloraseptic liquid consists of a dark green, aqueous solution containing phenol BP and sodium phenolate (total phenol 1.4%), menthol, thymol and glycerin.

Uses Chloraseptic liquid is recommended for the relief of the pain associated with sore throat (pharyngitis), tonsillitis and superficial mucosal lesions as well as aphthous ulcers, Vincent's ulcers, moniliasis, and denture ulcers. Chloraseptic will also relieve post-operative pain following dental surgery. Chloraseptic will also control halitosis associated with minor mouth and throat infections.

Dosage and administration *Spray:* For sore throat – use full strength – Adults should spray throat five times at first; children from 6–12 years, three times. Repeat every two hours if necessary.

Gargle: As a gargle for sore throat – use full strength or dilute with equal parts of water. Rinse thoroughly, then expel remainder.

Mouthwash: For mouth and gum irritations – use full strength. Rinse for 15 seconds, then expel remainder. As a deodorising mouthwash – use full strength or dilute with equal parts of water. Rinse thoroughly, then expel remainder.

Contra-indications, warnings, etc Not to be given to children under six years unless directed by physician. Consult physician if sore throat is severe or lasts more than two days, or is accompanied by high fever, headache, nausea or vomiting.

Pharmaceutical precautions Nil.

Legal category P.

Package quantities 115 ml with spray attachment and 150 ml bottle.

Further information Nil.

Product licence number 0364/0023.

DANTRIUM*

Presentation Dantrium capsules are available in two strengths, containing either 25 mg or 100 mg dantrolene sodium per capsule.

Dantrium is presented in orange/light brown capsules. The 25 mg capsule carries the monogram Dantrium 25 mg on the cap and 0149, 0030 and a single coding bar on the body. The 100 mg capsule carries the monogram Dantrium 100 mg on the cap and 0149, 0033 and triple coding bars on the body.

Uses Dantrium produces relaxation of contracted skeletal muscle by affecting the contractile response at a site beyond the myoneural junction. Dantrium produces a dissociation of excitation-contraction coupling, probably by interfering with the release of Ca^{++} from the sarcoplasmic reticulum. The effect is seen in both fast and slow fibres but is more pronounced in the former.

Dantrium is indicated for the treatment of chronic, severe spasticity in adults resulting from such disorders as stroke, multiple sclerosis, spinal cord injury and cerebral palsy. It is useful in these conditions whenever spasticity is so severe that increased muscular resistance to stretch, clonus or exaggerated reflex posturing interfere with the activities of daily living such as exercise, posture, equilibrium, walking, transfer manoeuvres or the use of braces.

Occasionally, only a subtle but perceptible improvement in spasticity may occur with Dantrium therapy. In such instances information regarding improvement should be sought from the patient and those who are in constant daily contact and attendance on him. Brief withdrawal of Dantrium for a period of two to four days will frequently demonstrate exacerbation of the spasticity and may help to reinforce a previously indefinable clinical impression.

Dosage and administration Before commencing Dantrium therapy, it is important to set an attainable therapeutic goal for the individual patient. Such a goal would be a reduction in spasticity which allows the patient or his attendants to carry out a function which could not previously be performed or one that he or his attendants consider important.

The need for patience and attention to the individual patient's needs in titrating Dantrium dosage is of paramount importance.

Dosage should be increased until the maximum benefit compatible with the patient's neurological deficit is achieved.

The lowest dose compatible with optimal response is recommended. Dosage in excess of 400 mg/day is not recommended.

A recommended dosage increment scale is shown below:

Week	Recommended dosage
First	One 25 mg capsule daily
Second	One 25 mg capsule twice daily
Third	Two 25 mg capsules twice daily
Fourth	Two 25 mg capsules three times daily
Fifth	Three 25 mg capsules three times daily
Sixth	Three 25 mg capsules four times daily
Seventh	One 100 mg capsule four times daily

Most patients will achieve their therapeutic goal at a titrated dose of 75 mg three times daily.

If no observable benefit is derived from the administration of Dantrium after a total of 45 days, therapy should be discontinued.

Many patients experience side effects such as weakness and fatigue during the first four weeks of therapy whilst the patient adjusts to the changes in muscle tone induced by the drug. They are usually transient and mild in nature. Patients should be warned of them and encouraged to persevere with treatment. Should it be necessary the dosage of Dantrium may be reduced and then gradually increased according to the patient's tolerance. It may be possible to reduce the duration of each dosage stage to four days, depending on the patient's reaction to the drug.

Contra-indications, warnings, etc
Contra-indications: Dantrium is contra-indicated where spasticity is utilised to sustain upright posture and balance in locomotion or whenever spasticity is utilised to obtain or maintain increased function.

Dantrium is contra-indicated in patients with evidence of hepatic dysfunction. Isolated cases of jaundice in patients receiving Dantrium have been reported.

Dantrium should not be administered to children.

Warnings: Usage in pregnancy: Although teratological studies in animals have proved satisfactory, the safety of Dantrium in pregnancy has not been established. In such patients, the potential benefits must be weighed against the possible hazards.

Precautions: Dantrium has a potentially hepatotoxic action. Before beginning Dantrium therapy, liver function tests should be performed in all patients (serum AST (SGOT) or serum ALT (SGPT), alkaline phosphatase, total bilirubin, LDH, or their equivalents) to establish a base-line, and to rule out pre-existing liver disease. These tests should be repeated upon hospital discharge or at six weeks after starting therapy; further tests may be carried out at the physician's discretion. Generally, if these studies reveal abnormal values, therapy should not be commenced or should be discontinued when other causes for these abnormalities cannot be found. Some patients have reverted to normal laboratory values during continuation of therapy, whilst others have not.

The use of Dantrium with other potentially hepatotoxic drugs should be avoided.

Dantrium should be used with caution in patients with impaired pulmonary function, particularly those with obstructive pulmonary disease, and in patients with severely impaired cardiac function due to myocardial disease.

Patients should be advised not to drive a motor vehicle or to undertake potentially dangerous work until Dantrium therapy has been stabilised.

Although the primary pharmacological effect of Dantrium is exerted directly on skeletal muscle, caution should be exercised in the concomitant administration of tranquillising agents.

Action in event of overdosage: For acute overdosage, general supportive measures should be employed along with immediate gastric lavage.

Fluids should be administered in large quantities to avert the theoretical possibility of crystalluria.

Side-effects and adverse reactions: The most frequently occurring side-effects of Dantrium have been drowsiness, dizziness, weakness, general malaise, fatigue and diarrhoea. These effects are generally transient, occur early in treatment, and can often be obviated by careful determination and regulation of the dosage. An acne-like rash has been reported on rare occasions.

Pharmaceutical precautions Dantrium capsules should be stored at room temperature.

Legal category POM.

Package quantities Dantrium capsules 25 mg and Dantrium capsules 100 mg are supplied in containers of 100 capsules.

Further information The duration and intensity of skeletal muscle relaxation in patients on Dantrium is related to the dosage and blood levels. The mean biological half-life of Dantrium is about nine hours after a 100 mg dose.

Studies specifically designed to determine compatibility with diazepam and phenobarbitone revealed that neither of these drugs appears to affect Dantrium metabolism.

Product licence numbers
Dantrium capsules 25 mg   0364/0015
Dantrium capsules 100 mg   0364/0016

DANTRIUM* INTRAVENOUS

Presentation Dantrium Intravenous is available as a sterile, lyophilized orange powder which is a mixture of 20 mg dantrolene sodium, 3000 mg mannitol and sufficient sodium hydroxide to yield a pH of approximately 9.5 when reconstituted with 60 ml of water for injection PhEur.

Uses Dantrium Intravenous is indicated for the treatment of malignant hyperthermia. It is for intravenous use only.

In isolated muscle preparations, dantrolene sodium uncouples the excitation and contraction of skeletal muscle, probably by interfering with the release of calcium from the sarcoplasmic reticulum.

In the malignant hyperthermia syndrome, evidence points to an intrinsic abnormality of muscle tissue. It has been postulated that 'triggering agents' (i.c. skeletal muscle relaxants and inhalation anaesthetics) induce a sudden rise in myoplasmic calcium, either by preventing the sarcoplasmic reticulum from accumulating calcium adequately, or by accelerating its release. This rise in myoplasmic calcium activates the acute catabolic processes involved in the malignant hyperthermia crisis.

Dantrolene sodium may prevent the increases in myoplasmic calcium and the acute catabolism within the muscle cell by interfering with the release of calcium from the sarcoplasmic reticulum to the myoplasm. Thus the physiological, metabolic and biochemical changes associated with the crisis may be reversed or attenuated.

Dosage and administration As soon as the malignant hyperthermia syndrome is recognised all anaesthetic agents should be discontinued. An initial Dantrium intravenous dose of 1 mg/kg should be given rapidly into the vein. It must not be mixed with other intravenous infusions. If the physiological and metabolic abnormalities persist or reappear, this dose may be repeated up to a cumulative dose of 10 mg/kg. Clinical experience to date has shown that the average dose of Dantrium Intravenous required to reverse the manifestations of malignant hyperthermia has been 2.5 mg/kg. If a relapse or recurrence occurs, Dantrium Intravenous should be readministered at the last effective dose.

Contra-indications, warnings, etc
Precautions: 1. In some subjects as much as 10 mg/kg of Dantrium Intravenous has been needed to reverse the crisis. In a 70 kg man this dose would require approximately 36 vials. Such a volume has been administered in approximately one and a half hours.

2. Because of the high pH of the intravenous formulation of Dantrium, care must be taken to prevent extravasation of the intravenous solution into the surrounding tissues.

3. *Pregnancy:* The safety of Dantrium Intravenous in pregnant women has not been established; it should be given only when the potential benefits have been weighed against the possible risk to mother and child.

4. *Drug interactions:* The combination of therapeutic doses of intravenous dantrolene sodium and verapamil in halothane/alpha-chloralose anaesthetized swine has resulted in ventricular fibrillation and cardiovascular collapse in association with marked hyperkalaemia. It is recommended that the combination of intravenous dantrolene sodium and calcium channel blockers, such as verapamil, not be used during the reversal of a malignant hyperthermia crisis until the relevance of these findings to humans is established.

Warnings: The use of Dantrium Intravenous in the management of malignant hyperthermia is not a substitute for previously known supportive measures. It will be necessary to discontinue the suspect triggering agents, attend to increased oxygen requirements and manage the metabolic acidosis. When necessary institute cooling, attend to urinary output and monitor for electrolyte imbalance.

Side-effects and adverse reactions: No side-effects have been attributed to Dantrium Intravenous in patients treated with short-term therapy for malignant hyperthermia. The nature of the emergency and the complexity of concomitant therapy will make it extremely difficult to isolate cause and effect relationships for any of the drugs used. Hepatotoxic reactions have been noted in a small number of subjects given long term oral dantrolene therapy.

Pharmaceutical precautions Each vial of Dantrium Intravenous should be reconstituted by adding 60 ml of water for injection PhEur, and shaking until the solution is clear. The contents of the vial must be protected from direct light and used within six hours of reconstitution. Protect the reconstituted solutions from temperatures above 30°C and below 15°C.

Unreconstituted product should be protected from light and stored below 30°C.

Legal category POM.

Package quantities Dantrium Intravenous is available

in packs of twelve vials each containing 20 mg dantrolene sodium.

Further information Nil.

Product licence number 0364/0030.

DIDRONEL* TABLETS ▼

Presentation White, rectangular tablets, marked with 'P&G' on one face and '402' on the other. Each tablet contains Etidronate Disodium USP 200 mg.

Uses

Indications:

(a) Paget's disease of bone: Didronel is indicated for the treatment of Paget's disease of bone (osteitis deformans). Effectiveness has been demonstrated primarily in patients with polyostotic Paget's disease with symptoms of pain and with clinically significant elevations of urinary hydroxyproline and serum alkaline phosphatase. In other circumstances in which there is extensive involvement of the skull or the spine with the prospect of irreversible neurological damage, or when a weight-bearing bone may be involved, the use of Didronel may be considered.

(b) Heterotopic ossification: Didronel is also indicated for the prevention and treatment of heterotopic ossification following hip replacement or due to spinal injury.

Dosage and administration 5 mg/kg/day to 20 mg/kg/day as detailed below.

(a) Paget's disease:

Adults: The recommended initial dose of Didronel for most patients is 5 mg/kg body weight/day, for a period not exceeding six months. Doses above 10 mg/kg should be reserved for use when there is an overriding requirement for suppression of increased bone turnover associated with Paget's disease or when the patient requires more prompt reduction of elevated cardiac output. Treatment with doses above 10 mg/kg/day should be approached cautiously and should not exceed three months duration. Doses in excess of 20/mg/kg/day are not recommended.

Retreatment should be undertaken only after a drug-free period of at least three months and after it is evident that reactivation of the disease has occurred and biochemical indices of the disease have become substantially re-elevated or approach pre-treatment values (approximately twice the upper limit of normal or 75% of pre-treatment value). In no case should duration of retreatment exceed the maximum duration of the initial treatment. Premature retreatment should be avoided. In clinical trials the biochemical improvements obtained during drug therapy have generally persisted for a period of three months to, in some cases, up to two years after drug withdrawal.

Children: Disorders of bone in children, referred to as juvenile Paget's disease, have been reported rarely. The relationship to adult Paget's disease has not been established. Didronel has not been studied in children for Paget's disease.

(b) Heterotopic ossification:

Hip replacement: For the prevention and treatment of heterotopic ossification following hip replacement, the recommended adult dose is 20 mg/kg/day for one month pre-operatively followed by 20 mg/kg/day for three months post-operatively. The total treatment period is four months. There is no evidence that Didronel therapy will affect mature heterotopic bone.

Spinal cord injury: In heterotopic ossification due to spinal cord injury the recommended adult dose of Didronel is 20 mg/kg/day for two weeks followed by 10 mg/kg/day for ten weeks. The total treatment period is twelve weeks. This recommended dosage should be instituted as soon as is medically feasible following the injury, preferably prior to any radiographic evidence of heterotopic ossification.

Directions for use: Didronel should be administered as a single, oral dose, two hours before a meal. It may be given with fruit juice or water. Food in the stomach or upper portions of the small intestine, particularly materials with a high calcium content such as milk, may reduce absorption. Therefore, eating should be avoided for two hours before and after drug administration.

Daily dosage guide

Body weight		Required daily regimen of 200 mg tablets		
Kilograms	Stones	5 mg/kg*	10 mg/kg*	20 mg/kg†
50	8	1	3	5
60	9.5	2	3	6
70	11	2	4	7
80	12.5	2	4	8
90	14	2	5	9

* Course of therapy – 6 months
† Course of therapy – 3 months

Contra-indications, warnings, etc At present, clinical trials have demonstrated no absolute contra-indications to Didronel.

Precautions:

1. *General:* Didronel retards mineralisation of osteoid laid down during the bone accretion process. This effect is dose and time dependent. There may be an overlap of beneficial and mineralisation inhibition effects in some patients at higher doses. Extended periods of medication should be approached cautiously. When administered at doses of 20 mg/kg/day Didronel suppresses bone turnover and essentially stops mineralisation of new bone in Pagetic lesions and, to a lesser extent, in the uninvolved skeleton. Mineralisation of Pagetic lesions has been demonstrated to occur normally after discontinuation of the drug.

At lower doses (5 mg/kg/day), mineralisation inhibition is uncommon and when it occurs it is focal in nature. This does not usually present a clinical problem. However, should a patient present with significant osteolysis in a weight-bearing bone, special efforts should be taken to prevent the possibility of a combination of mineralisation inhibition and a failure of the drug to inhibit resorption leading to an adverse effect on bone.

It is recommended that serum phosphate and serum alkaline phosphatase levels and if possible urinary hydroxyproline levels, be measured before commencing therapy. The serum phosphate level should be repeated at one month and if it has risen more than 0.5 mg/dl (0.16 SI) above the upper limit of normal the patient may be receiving more drug than required and the mineralisation of new osteoid may be impaired. In these cases, where 200 mg per day (a single tablet) may be excessive, the tablet may be split or doses may be administered less frequently.

The serum alkaline phosphatase and/or urinary hydroxyproline levels should be repeated at three months. If the elevated pre-treatment level has not been reduced by 25%, the patient may be relatively resistant to therapy. If the serum phosphate level is normal at three months, consideration should be given to increasing the dose. If the patient has increased serum phosphate levels, consideration should be given to discontinuing the drug and substituting alternative therapy.

Patients with Paget's disease of bone should maintain an adequate nutritional status, and particularly, an adequate intake of calcium and vitamin D. Patients with restricted vitamin D and calcium intake may be particularly sensitive to drugs that affect calcium homeostasis and should be closely monitored during Didronel therapy.

In the treatment of heterotopic ossification following hip replacement no problems relating to loosening of prosthetic devices have been encountered. The incidence of migration of the trochanter has not been observed to be increased with Didronel therapy.

Didronel is not metabolised but excreted unchanged via the kidney; therefore, treatment of patients with impaired renal function should be approached very cautiously, if at all.

Didronel therapy has been withheld from patients with enterocolitis because increased frequency of bowel movements and diarrhoea are seen in some patients when Didronel is administered at a dose of 20 mg/kg/day and may be increased occasionally at lower doses.

2. *Pregnancy:* Reproduction studies have been performed in rats and rabbits. In some of these studies there was a decrease in the number of live born foetuses. There were no teratogenic effects. Because Didronel does not cross the placental barrier in these species, the decrease in number of live foetuses may have been due to a metabolic effect of Didronel in the mother. There is no experience in pregnant women given Didronel. Didronel should be used only when clearly needed in women who are or may become pregnant.

3. *Nursing mothers:* It is not known whether this drug is secreted in human milk. As a general rule, breast feeding should not be undertaken while a patient is on a drug since many drugs are secreted in human milk.

Warnings: The physician should adhere to the recommended dose regimen in order to avoid overtreatment of Didronel. The response to therapy may be of slow onset and may continue even for months after treatment when the drug has been discontinued. Dosage should not be increased prematurely nor should treatment be resumed before there is clear evidence of reactivation of the disease process. Retreatment should not be initiated until the patient has had at least a three-month drug-free interval.

Increased or recurrent bone pain at existing Pagetic sites and/or the appearance of pain at sites previously asymptomatic has been reported. At the recommended dose (5 mg/kg/day) 1 out of 10 patients reported the phenomena; at higher doses the figure rose to 2 out of 10. In placebo-treated patients, the occurrence was 1 out of 15. In Didronel treated patients, the pain resolved while therapy was continued in some patients but persisted for several months in others.

Fractures are recognised as a common feature in patients with Paget's disease. There has been no evidence of increased risk at the recommended dose of 5 mg/kg/day for six months. The risk of fracture may be increased when Didronel is taken at a dose level of 20 mg/kg/day in excess of three months. This risk may be greater in patients with extensive and severe disease, a history of multiple fractures, and/or rapidly advancing osteolytic lesions. It is recommended that the drug be discontinued when fractures occur and that the therapy not be reinstated until fracture healing is complete.

The incidence of osteogenic sarcoma is known to be increased in Paget's disease. Pagetic lesions, with or without therapy, may appear by X-ray to progress markedly, possibly with some loss of definition of periosteal margins. Such lesions should be evaluated carefully to differentiate these from osteogenic sarcoma.

Concomitant fractures are common in patients with spinal cord injury. In controlled studies, no problems of fracture healing or stabilisation of the spine were encountered. In cases with multiple long bone fractures, it may be advisable to delay therapy for a short time until callus formation is evidenced.

Side-effects: Gastro-intestinal complaints such as diarrhoea and nausea are increased in some patients when Didronel is administered at doses greater than 5 mg/kg/day. The incidence is about 1 out of 15 in both placebo-treated patients and in patients on Didronel, 5 mg/kg/day. The incidence rises to approximately 2 out of 10 patients with Didronel at the dose of 20 mg/kg/day.

Overdosage: While there is no experience with acute overdosage, it is theoretically possible that enough Didronel could be taken to result in hypocalcaemia. Treatment should be by cessation of therapy, correction of hypocalcaemia with intravenous calcium gluconate and maintenance of an adequate nutritional status, artificially supplemented if necessary.

Pharmaceutical precautions Normal pharmaceutical storage and handling are indicated.

Legal category POM.

Package quantities 60 × 200 mg tablets.

Further information Didronel is also known as EHDP (the disodium salt of ethane-1-hydroxy-1, 1-diphosphonate).

Product licence number 0166/0101.

Product licence holder: Brocades Great Britain Ltd, West Byfleet, Surrey.

FURACIN*

Presentation Furacin Soluble Ointment is a yellow ointment containing 0.2% Nitrofurazone BP in a water-soluble polyethylene glycol base.

Furacin Solution (Sterile) is a yellow liquid containing 0.2% Nitrofurazone BP in a water-miscible vehicle.

Uses Furacin is a broad-spectrum topical antibacterial effective in the presence of blood, pus and serum.

Furacin is indicated in bacterial skin infections including pyodermas, infected dermatoses and infections of wounds, burns and ulcers. Furacin is also of value in the treatment of skin-graft donor sites. Furacin Solution (Sterile) may be used as a bladder irrigant or instillate (diluted 1 in 6 with sterile water for injection).

Dosage and administration Furacin Soluble Ointment: Furacin Soluble Ointment is administered topically. Apply directly to the wound with sterile tongue-depressor or other spatula. Alternatively, melt the ointment in a beaker at a little above body temperature and pour gently on to the wound.

The ointment may also be applied on a gauze dressing. Bandages may be prevented from absorbing Furacin Soluble Ointment by covering the Furacin impregnated gauze with an impermeable layer, such as jaconet or gauze saturated with petroleum jelly. If bandages stick, remove them by saturating with sterile saline. Dressings may be left undisturbed on burns, cuts and wounds for 7–10 days

Furacin Solution (Sterilo): Furacin Solution (Sterile) may be administered either topically or as a bladder instillate.

Furacin may be used for children at the doctor's discretion.

Contra-indications, warnings, etc Furacin is contra-indicated in patients with known sensitivity to nitrofurazone.

It is not recommended to continue using Furacin when the infection is cleared.

Furacin Solution and Furacin Ointment should be used with caution in patients with known or suspected renal impairment. The polyethylene glycols in the base can be absorbed through denuded skin and may not be excreted normally by the compromised kidney. This may lead to symptoms of progressive renal impairment.

Side-effects and adverse reactions: Sensitisation to Furacin has been reported. Should this occur, treatment should be discontinued. Since the drug is not used systemically, sensitisation does not carry the implications for the patient that sensitisation to systemic therapy with antibiotics or sulphonamides may.

Pharmaceutical precautions Furacin Soluble Ointment is supplied in aluminium collapsible tubes. The ointment should be stored in light-proof containers and contact with metals other than stainless steel or aluminium should be avoided. There are no other special storage requirements.

Furacin Solution is supplied as a sterile product in 50 ml amber bottles. The product should be protected from light by storing in a dark place. Once opened Furacin Solution (Sterile) should be used immediately. Any unused solution must be discarded.

Legal category POM.

Package quantities Furacin Soluble Ointment is available in tubes of 25 g. Furacin Solution (Sterile) is available in bottles of 50 ml.

Further information Nil.

Product licence numbers
Furacin Soluble Ointment 0364/0013
Furacin Solution (Sterile) 0364/0012

FURADANTIN*

Presentation Furadantin Tablets are yellow in colour and have a pentagonal shape. Each tablet has a break line on one face and the tablet strength is shown on the opposite face. Furadantin Tablets are available in two strengths, containing 100 mg or 50 mg Nitrofurantoin PhEur.

Furadantin Suspension is a yellow suspension containing 25 mg Nitrofurantoin PhEur per 5 ml.

Uses Furadantin is a broad-spectrum antibacterial agent, active against the majority of urinary pathogens. It is bactericidal in renal tissue and throughout the urinary tract. After oral administration the nitrofurantoin is rapidly excreted in the urine, up to 45% being unchanged.

Therapeutic: Cystitis, pyelitis, pyelonephritis; also postoperative infections of the genito-urinary tract, particu-

larly after the passage of instruments and after prostatectomy.

Prophylactic and suppressive: As cover for catheterisation or instrumentation of the urinary tract. To prevent reinfection in susceptible individuals.

Dosage and administration Furadantin is administered orally. The dose should be taken with each meal and at bedtime, with food or milk.

In the event of severe nausea the dose may be reduced, but not below the adult equivalent of 200 mg in 24 hours. Should it persist the drug should be withdrawn.

Therapeutic – Adults: Tablets 50–100 mg four times daily – the lower dosage level is recommended for uncomplicated urinary tract infections.

Suspension: Four 5 ml spoonfuls four times a day.

Therapeutic – Children: Furadantin Suspension or Furadantin Tablets 50 mg may be used. Dosage recommendations for children are given in the table below.

Body weight	Average age for weight	Dose to be taken four times daily	
kg		Suspension	50 mg Tablets
5–13	3–30 months	2.5 ml	$\frac{1}{4}$
13–23	2$\frac{1}{2}$–6 years	5 ml	$\frac{1}{2}$
23–36	6–11 years	10 ml	1
36–50	11–14 years	15 ml	1$\frac{1}{2}$

Treatment at this dose level for more than 14 days is seldom necessary.

Prophylactic and suppressive: When such therapy is desirable one quarter to one half of the therapeutic dose is suggested.

Elderly patients: The therapeutic dose may be reduced to 50 mg four times a day. Significant impairment of renal function is a contra-indication to the use of Furadantin (see below).

Contra-indications, warnings, etc Infants under one month should not be given Furadantin.

Furadantin is contra-indicated in patients suffering from anuria, oliguria or significant impairment of renal function. Treatment of this type carries an increased risk of toxicity because of impaired excretion of the drug.

A small number of negroes and some people from the Eastern Mediterranean area suffer from a deficiency of glucose-6-phosphate dehydrogenase in their blood cells. In such people, nitrofurantoin in common with many other therapeutic agents may cause haemolysis. This enzyme deficiency is extremely rare in Caucasians. Any sign of haemolysis is an indication to discontinue the drug. Haemolysis ceases when the drug is withdrawn.

Precautions: Furadantin should only be used in pregnancy if considered essential by the physician. Foetal studies in animals with nitrofurantoin do not suggest that it causes any increase in the incidence of congenital abnormalities. This is confirmed by over 30 years of clinical usage. However, it is recognised that caution should be observed when prescribing for the pregnant patient.

Action in event of overdosage: Excessive intake would probably cause vomiting. In case vomiting does not occur soon after an excessive dose, induction of emesis or stomach wash-out is recommended. A high fluid intake should be maintained to promote urinary excretion of the drug.

Antidote: There is no known specific antidote to nitrofurantoin.

Side-effects: Nausea or vomiting may occur, but this can be minimised or eliminated by taking the drug with food or milk, or adjustment of dosage.

Adverse reactions: Peripheral neuropathy has been reported after treatment with Furadantin. Predisposing conditions include renal impairment, anaemia, diabetes, electrolyte imbalance, vitamin B deficiency and debilitating disease. Should numbness or tingling occur in any part of the body, treatment should be discontinued.

Drug rashes, pyrexia and hepatitis associated with nitrofurantoin therapy have been reported. The hepatitis is of an allergic type and may be associated with antinuclear factor and lymphocyte sensitisation.

A respiratory syndrome with bronchospasm and/or dyspnoea, cough and sometimes chest pain has been reported. These symptoms have occasionally been associated with transitory pulmonary infiltration or pleural effusion.

These adverse reactions to nitrofurantoin therapy are rare.

Pharmaceutical precautions Furadantin Tablets are supplied in polypropylene containers with polythene pilfer-proof caps. The tablets should be stored in light-proof and preferably moisture-proof containers. There are no other special storage requirements.

Furadantin Suspension is supplied in amber bottles and should be protected from light as exposure will cause darkening of the active principle. Because of this, amber bottles should be used in dispensing. The glass should preferably be neutral since discoloration will occur on contact with alkaline materials.

It is not recommended to dilute Furadantin Suspension.

Legal category POM.

Package quantities Furadantin Tablets 100 mg and 50 mg are supplied in packs of 100 and 1,000. Furadantin Suspension is supplied in bottles of 300 ml.

Further information Furadantin is not a sulphonamide; there is no need to increase fluid intake or give alkalis; forcing fluids beyond normal merely dilutes the antibacterial concentration in the urine.

The urine of patients receiving Furadantin may be coloured a dark yellow or brown. This results from the presence of metabolites and is quite harmless. Furadantin can interfere with certain laboratory tests. False positive or spuriously high readings may be produced with urine glucose tests utilising the copper sulphate reduction method, e.g. Benedict's reagent, Clinitest (Ames).

Product licence numbers

Furadantin Tablets 50 mg	0364/0008
Furadantin Tablets 100 mg	0364/0009
Furadantin Suspension	0364/0010

MACRODANTIN*

Presentation Macrodantin is presented in hard gelatin capsules, and is available in two strengths, containing 100 mg and 50 mg Nitrofurantoin PhEur macrocrystals.

The 100 mg capsule has an opaque yellow body and cap, and bears the monogram 'Macrodantin 100'.

The 50 mg capsule has an opaque yellow cap, an opaque white body and bears the monogram 'Macrodantin 50'.

Uses Macrodantin is a broad-spectrum antibacterial agent, active against the majority of urinary pathogens. It is bactericidal in renal tissue and throughout the urinary tract.

The nitrofurantoin macrocrystals of Macrodantin are specially formulated. The controlled crystal size is designed to control the speed of absorption and thus reduce the incidence of nausea. Clinical and animal studies indicate that Macrodantin therapy decreases the likelihood of nausea in patients who might experience these symptoms on nitrofurantoin therapy. This special reformulation of nitrofurantoin has not caused any decrease in its bioavailability.

Therapeutic: Cystitis, pyelitis, pyelonephritis; also post-operative infections of the genito-urinary tract, particularly after the passage of instruments and after prostatectomy.

Prophylactic and suppressive: As cover for catheterisation or instrumentation of the urinary tract. To prevent reinfection in susceptible individuals.

Dosage and administration Macrodantin is administered orally. The dose should be taken with each meal and at bedtime, with food or milk.

In the event of severe nausea the dose may be reduced, but not below the adult equivalent of 200 mg in 24 hours. Should it persist the drug should be withdrawn.

Therapeutic – Adults: Capsules: 50–100 mg four times daily – the lower dosage level is recommended for uncomplicated urinary tract infections.

Children: For children, Macrodantin 50 mg capsules may be used. Dosage recommendations for children are given in the table below. Treatment at this dose level for more than 14 days is seldom necessary.

| Body weight | Average age | Dosage, 50 mg |
| kg | for weight | capsules |
	(years)	
13–23	2½–6	1 capsule twice a day
23–36	6–11	1 capsule four times a day
36–50	11–14	2 capsules three times a day

Prophylactic and suppressive: When such therapy is desirable one quarter to one half of the therapeutic dose is suggested.

Elderly patients: The therapeutic dose may be reduced to 50 mg four times a day. Significant impairment of renal function is a contra-indication to the use of Macrodantin (see below).

Contra-indications, warnings, etc Infants under one month should not be given Macrodantin.

Macrodantin is contra-indicated in patients suffering from anuria, oliguria or significant impairment of renal function. Treatment of this type carries an increased risk of toxicity because of impaired excretion of the drug.

A small number of negroes and some people from the Eastern Mediterranean area suffer from a deficiency of glucose-6-phosphate dehydrogenase in their blood cells. In such people, nitrofurantoin in common with many other therapeutic agents may cause haemolysis. This enzyme deficiency is extremely rare in Caucasians.

Any sign of haemolysis is an indication to discontinue the drug. Haemolysis ceases when the drug is withdrawn.

Precautions: Macrodantin should only be used in pregnancy if considered essential by the physician. Foetal studies with the active ingredient nitrofurantoin, do not suggest that Macrodantin causes any increase in the incidence of congenital abnormalities. This is confirmed by over 30 years of clinical use of nitrofurantoin. However it is recognised that caution should always be observed when prescribing for the pregnant patient.

Action in event of overdosage: Excessive intake would probably cause vomiting. In case vomiting does not occur soon after an excessive dose, induction of emesis or stomach wash-out is recommended. A high fluid intake should be maintained to promote urinary excretion of the drug.

Antidote: There is no known specific antidote to nitrofurantoin.

Side-effects: Nausea or vomiting may occur, but this can be minimised or eliminated by taking the drug with food or milk, or adjustment of dosage.

Adverse reactions: Peripheral neuropathy has been reported after treatment with nitrofurantoin. Predisposing conditions include renal impairment, anaemia, diabetes, electrolyte imbalance, vitamin B deficiency and debilitating disease. Should numbness or tingling occur in any part of the body, treatment should be discontinued.

Drug rashes, pyrexia and hepatitis associated with nitrofurantoin therapy have been reported. The hepatitis is of an allergic type and may be associated with antinuclear factor and lymphocyte sensitisation.

A respiratory syndrome with bronchospasm and/or dyspnoea, cough and sometimes chest pain has been reported. These symptoms have occasionally been associated with transitory pulmonary infiltration or pleural effusion.

These adverse reactions to nitrofurantoin therapy are rare.

Pharmaceutical precautions Macrodantin Capsules are supplied in polypropylene containers with polythene pilfer-proof caps. The capsules should be stored in light-proof and preferably moisture-proof containers. There are no other special storage requirements.

Legal category POM.

Package quantities Macrodantin Capsules 100 mg and 50 mg are supplied in containers of 100.

Further information Macrodantin is not a sulphonamide: there is no need to increase fluid intake or give alkalis; forcing fluids beyond normal merely dilutes the antibacterial concentration in the urine.

The urine of patients receiving Macrodantin may be coloured a dark yellow or brown. This results from the presence of metabolites and is quite harmless. Macrodantin can interfere with certain laboratory tests. False positive or spuriously high readings may be produced with urine glucose tests utilising the copper sulphate reduction method, e.g. Benedict's reagent, Clinitest (Ames).

Product licence numbers
Macrodantin Capsules 50 mg   0364/0005
Macrodantin Capsules 100 mg   0364/0006

PSORADRATE CREAM*

Presentation Psoradrate cream is a smooth textured, unperfumed, bland, yellow cream containing 0.1% w/w Dithranol BP; 0.2% w/w Dithranol BP or 0.4% w/w Dithranol BP in a specially formulated powder-in-cream base which includes stabilised, hypermolar urea to assist percutaneous transportation of the active ingredient. Psoradrate cream does not contain lanolin, parabens or preservatives.

Uses Psoradrate cream is indicated for the treatment of subacute and chronic psoriasis. In addition, Psoradrate 0.1% is indicated for the treatment of psoriasis of the scalp.

Dosage and administration Wash affected areas well, dry thoroughly and apply directly to the lesions twice daily. If so directed by the physician, Psoradrate may be applied once a day using short contact therapy techniques (remove with soap and water). An application time of two hours has been shown to produce optimum improvement although shorter contact times do give satisfactory results. Treatment should be continued until the raised lesions have disappeared and the skin is smooth. Occlusive dressings should not be used because they may increase the incidence of staining and stinging on normal skin. For use on the scalp, shampoo and dry hair, then rub Psoradrate 0.1% into the lesions, preferably at night. Remove the next morning with shampoo.

Contra-indications, warnings, etc Psoradrate cream is contra-indicated in pustular psoriasis.

The active ingredient of Psoradrate cream, dithranol, may cause a tingling or stinging sensation when applied to skin or lesions. It is irritant to the eyes and mucosa. If eye contact occurs wash out immediately with a neutral solution. If mucosal contact occurs wash out with plenty of water. Exercise care when applying to the face and intertrigenous areas. Skin staining may occur and clothing may occasionally be discoloured. For external use only.

Before using creams containing high concentrations of dithranol it is advisable to establish the patient's tolerance. In cases in which tolerance has not been established, treatment of psoriatic lesions should be commenced with a low concentration of dithranol, namely Psoradrate 0.1%. If the patient's skin can tolerate Psoradrate 0.1% cream, but the lesions appear resistant, then treatment should be changed to increased strength Psoradrate creams to aid the clearance of the lesions. If, however, the patient is known to have a high tolerance to dithranol then therapy can be commenced using Psoradrate 0.2% cream, or Psoradrate 0.4% cream.

Pharmaceutical precautions Store in a cool place.

Legal category P.

Package quantities Psoradrate 0.1% and 0.2% are available in tubes of 30 g and 100 g. Psoradrate 0.4% is available in 100 g tubes.

Further information Use of a descaling agent such as salicylic acid is not necessary with Psoradrate creams. The creams are absorbed into the skin and the inconvenience of removing the applications is avoided. Relapse rate with dithranol therapy has been reported as being less than that seen with steroids. Stains on clothes can be removed with a solvent such as trichloroethylene.

Product licence numbers
Psoradrate Cream 0.1%   0364/0027
Psoradrate Cream 0.2%   0364/0031
Psoradrate Cream 0.4%   0364/0037

TOPICYCLINE* ▼

Presentation Topicycline is presented in two separate bottles as a yellow powder and a solvent which must be combined prior to use.

The powder contains 154 mg of Tetracycline Hydrochloride PhEur as the active ingredient, as well as 230 mg 4-epitetracycline hydrochloride and 70 mg sodium bisulphite.

The solvent contains 1.25 mg per ml of n-decyl methyl sulphoxide (DecMSO) and citric acid in a 40% ethanol solution.

Once reconstituted, Topicycline contains 2.2 mg per ml of tetracycline hydrochloride. The n-decyl methyl sulphoxide enhances penetration of tetracycline into the skin.

Uses Topicycline is indicated in the treatment of acne vulgaris.

Dosage and administration Topicycline is first prepared according to the manufacturer's instructions.

Topicycline is applied topically, twice daily. It should be applied generously, to the entire affected area, not just to individual lesions, until the skin is thoroughly wet.

The average amount of Topicycline delivered to the skin by application to the face and neck twice a day is approximately 1.3 ml/day. This quantity of the medication contains approximately 2.9 mg of tetracycline hydrochloride. Twice-daily use of Topicycline on other acne-involved areas, in addition to the face and neck, has resulted in an average application of about 2.2 ml/day, or 4.8 mg of tetracycline hydrochloride.

Contra-indications, warnings, etc Topicycline is contra-indicated in patients who have shown hypersensitivity to any of its ingredients or to any of the other tetracyclines.

Topicycline is for external use only, and care should be taken to keep it out of the eyes, nose and mouth.

Because the serum level of tetracycline resulting from the use of Topicycline (less than 0.1 mcg/mg) is less than 7% of that associated with a therapeutic dose of 500 mg/day of tetracycline administered orally, liver damage from the use of Topicycline is highly unlikely, even in patients with renal impairment. Nevertheless, the warnings associated with the use of tetracycline orally should be considered before prescribing Topicycline for patients with renal impairment.

Reproduction studies in rats and rabbits have revealed no evidence of impaired fertility or harm to the foetus from Topicycline. There are no data, however, on the use of this product in pregnant women.

It is not known whether tetracycline or any other component of Topicycline administered in this topical form, is secreted in human milk. Because many drugs are secreted in human milk, caution should be exercised if Topicycline is administered to nursing mothers.

Safety and effectiveness in children below the age of eleven have not been established.

Side-effects: Some patients may experience a stinging or burning sensation upon application of Topicycline. The sensation normally lasts no more than a few minutes, and does not occur at every application. There has been

no indication that patients experience sufficient discomfort to reduce the frequency of use or to discontinue use of the product.

Pharmaceutical precautions Unreconstituted product should be stored at a temperature not exceeding 25°C.

Reconstituted Topicycline should be used within 8 weeks of reconstitution, and should be stored at room temperature or below.

Any unused material should be discarded.

Legal category POM.

Package quantities Topicycline is supplied in a single carton containing one plastic bottle of powder (454 mg) and one of liquid (70 ml); these two phases must be combined prior to use. At the time of dispensing, the liquid is poured into the powder-containing bottle and the powder contents are dissolved by shaking the bottle. An applicator and overcap are supplied. Reconstituted Topicycline contains 154 mg of tetracycline hydrochloride, 70 ml of medication is dispensed.

Further information Reconstituted Topicycline provides about an eight-week supply for treating the face and neck, or about a four week supply for treating the face, neck and additional acne-involved areas.

Product licence number 0522/0010.

Product licence holder: Proctor & Gamble Ltd., Newcastle upon Tyne.

VIVONEX* STANDARD

Presentation Vivonex Standard is an off-white, unflavoured water-soluble powder. The contents of one packet supply 300 kilocalories (1.256 MJ) and the following:

	Grams	% by weight
Available nitrogen in the form of pure amino acids (amino acid content 6.18 g)	0.98	1.22
Fat as highly purified safflower oil (80% as triglyceride of linoleic acid)	0.435	0.54
Carbohydrate as glucose solids	69.0	86.3

Caloric contribution:

Amino acids	*8.2%*
Fat	*1.3%*
Carbohydrate	*90.5%*

Six packets of Vivonex Standard supply 5.88 g of available nitrogen, 2.61 g fat, 414 g carbohydrate and the vitamins, amino acids and minerals shown in the following table.

Vitamins	Per 80 g packet	In six 80 g packets
Vitamin A (Retinol) IU	833.33	5,000
Vitamin D$_3$ (Cholecalciferol) IU	66.67	400
Vitamin E IU	5	30
Vitamin C (Ascorbic acid) mg	10	60
Folic Acid mg	0.07	0.4
Vitamin B$_1$ (Thiamine) mg	0.25	1.5
Vitamin B$_2$ (Riboflavine) mg	0.28	1.7
Nicotinamide mg	3.33	20
Vitamin B$_6$ mg	0.33	2
Vitamin B$_{12}$ mcg	1	6
Biotin mg	0.05	0.3
Pantothenic Acid mg	1.67	10
Vitamin K mcg	11.17	67
Choline mg	12.28	73.7

Amino acids

Essential amino acids	% total amino acids	g/6 packets
L-Isoleucine	4.55	1.69
L-Leucine	7.20	2.67
L-Lysine	5.41	2.00
L-Methionine	4.66	1.73
L-Phenylalanine	5.18	1.93
L-Threonine	4.55	1.69
L-Tryptophan	1.41	0.52
L-Valine	5.02	1.86
Total	37.98	14.09

Non-essential amino acids	% total amino acids	g/6 packets
L-Alanine	4.85	1.80
L-Arginine	8.87	3.29
L-Aspartic acid	10.35	3.84
L-Glutamine	17.07	6.33
Glycine	7.91	2.93
L-Histidine	2.21	0.82
L-Proline	6.48	2.41
L-Serine	3.34	1.24
L-Tyrosine	0.94	0.35
Total	62.02	23.01

Electrolytes

Cations	In normal dilution 80 g in 300 ml m-equiv/100 ml	In powder form mg/80 g packet	mg/6 packets
Sodium	3.74	258	1,548
Potassium	2.99	351.5	2,109
Calcium	2.77	166.7	1,000
Magnesium	1.83	66.67	400
Manganese	0.00567	0.468	2.81
Iron	0.0358	3	18
Copper	0.0035	0.333	2
Zinc	0.0255	2.5	15

Anions	m-equiv/100 ml	mg/80 g packet	mg/6 packets
Chloride	5.185	551.6	3,310
Phosphate (as P)	5.40	166.6	1,000
Acetate	0.029	5.202	31.2
Iodide	0.000066	0.025	0.150
Gluconate	1.69	991.8	5,950
Sorbate	0.447	149	894

Six packets also contain 0.25 mcg Cobalt as Vitamin B$_{12}$.

Uses Vivonex Standard provides total enteral nutrition which requires minimal digestion and produces no exogenous residue.

It is indicated in the treatment of bowel fistulae, bowel obstruction, Crohn's disease, ulcerative colitis and other disorders of the digestive organs or of the alimentary tract where elemental nutrition with low fat and minimal residue is considered of value.

Vivonex Standard can be used to ensure a clear operative field for bowel surgery or diagnostic procedures. Use of Vivonex Standard pre-operatively can help to ensure that the negative nitrogen balance, often seen post-operatively in undernourished patients, is minimised or avoided.

Post-operatively Vivonex Standard provides a balanced, low residue, low fat, milk free nutritional regimen to maintain a positive nitrogen balance during the catabolic phase, and to simplify nursing during the recovery period. Vivonex Standard may also be used as an alternative to parenteral feeding and as supplementary feeding when a high energy intake is required.

Dosage and administration *Dosage – Adults:* Six packets (1,800 kilocalories) a day, which may be increased if thought necessary to meet the nutritional demands of some patients.

Children: Vivonex Standard may be given to children. However, when used for children under 10 years it may be necessary to adjust the quantity of Vivonex Standard consumed daily to meet the projected nutritional requirements for the patient involved.

Vivonex Standard may be used as a nutritional source in both infants and children. Vivonex Standard contains no cystine, a semi-essential amino acid in the newborn. The amount of Vivonex Standard required to maintain weight and nitrogen balance will vary with each individual.

As the recommended daily intake varies with the age of the infant or child, daily administration of a mineral and vitamin supplement may be necessary to meet individual needs, particularly when Vivonex Standard is used as the sole source of nutrition for more than a few days.

If Vivonex Standard, in standard dilution, is administered as the sole source of nutrition, additional fluid will be required to avoid dehydration.

Administration: Vivonex Standard may be administered orally, as a drink or frozen, or by nasogastric or enteric tube.

Contra-indications, warnings, etc
Contra-indications: There are no contra-indications.

Warnings: Vivonex Standard must not be administered parenterally.

Precautions: Because of the high caloric contribution from carbohydrates some depleted individuals may manifest elevated blood sugar levels requiring insulin for regulation. Vivonex Standard should be used with care in diabetics.

The electrolyte content of Vivonex Standard is based on requirements of normal individuals and may be excessive for patients with electrolyte imbalance.

Use during pregnancy or lactation may require supplementary vitamins and minerals.

Use for children under 10 years may require adjustment of the daily consumption to meet the projected nutritional requirements for the patient involved.

Most patients should be started slowly on Vivonex Standard. Begin the first day with Vivonex Standard at half strength and on the second day the patient may be tried with the standard dilution. Each 300 ml feed must be sipped slowly over at least a one hour period for best results.

Action in event of overdosage: Overdosage is unlikely to occur and would result in vomiting and/or diarrhoea. Should overdosage occur, stop feeding Vivonex Standard and give water to avoid dehydration.

Pharmaceutical precautions *Storage:* When packaged in cartons or in packets, Vivonex Standard should be stored in a cool, dry place.

In normal dilution Vivonex Standard is a perishable liquid. A full day's supply may be prepared at one time and stored in the refrigerator for up to 24 hours. Shake the liquid briefly before serving. Never leave at room temperature for more than a few hours.

Diluents: In no circumstances should Vivonex Standard be mixed with less than 250 ml of water per 80 g packet.

Legal category POM.

Package quantities Vivonex Standard is supplied in cartons of six packets, each packet containing 80 g soluble powder.

Further information Vivonex Standard is a complete, elemental, minimal residue nutrition requiring little digestion. It is absorbed in the upper small intestine, leaving the lower bowel at rest. Vivonex Standard leaves no exogenous residue. On a Vivonex Standard-only regimen faecal volume and frequency are much reduced, and a bowel action every five to seven days is to be expected.

In severe catabolic states the Vivonex Standard formulation may fail to achieve positive nitrogen balance. In such circumstances Vivonex HN is recommended.

Adult patients receiving Vivonex Standard do not normally require any additional supplements.

Vivonex Standard is available solely as an unflavoured powder. To ensure patient acceptance when feeding Vivonex orally, the drink should be served flavoured and chilled. Vivonex Flavour sachets are available in Orange, Strawberry, Beef Broth and Tomato flavours. Beef Broth and Tomato flavours may be blended with warm water. Alternatively, Vivonex may be flavoured using commercially available carbonated or still soft drinks.

Where accurate nutritional control is required, allowance must be made for any added calorie or mineral content, and for indigestible matter.

Vivonex Standard may be administered as a slow continuous naso-enteric infusion via any suitable naso-enteric feeding system.

For details of prescribing under the ACBS ruling see the current edition of MIMS.

Product licence number 0364/0014.

VIVONEX* HN

Presentation Vivonex HN is an off-white, unflavoured water-soluble powder. The contents of one packet supply 300 kilocalories (1.256 MJ) and the following:

	Grams	% by weight
Available nitrogen in the form of pure amino acids (amino acid content 13.31 g)	2	2.5
Fat as highly purified safflower oil (80% as triglyceride of linoleic acid)	0.261	0.326
Carbohydrate as glucose solids	63.3	79.1

Caloric contribution.

Amino acids	17.7%
Fat	0.78%
Carbohydrate	81.5%

Ten packets of Vivonex HN supply 20 g of available nitrogen, 2.61 g fat, 633 g carbohydrate and the vitamins, amino acids and minerals shown in the following table.

Vitamins	Per 80 g packet	In ten 80 g packets
Vitamin A (Retinol) IU	500	5,000
Vitamin D_3 (Cholecalciferol) IU	40	400
Vitamin E IU	3	30
Vitamin C (Ascorbic acid) mg	6	60
Folic Acid mg	0.04	0.4
Vitamin B_1 (Thiamine) mg	0.15	1.5
Vitamin B_2 (Riboflavine) mg	0.17	1.7
Nicotinamide mg	2	20
Vitamin B_6 mg	0.2	2
Vitamin B_{12} mcg	0.6	6
Biotin mg	0.03	0.3
Pantothenic Acid mg	1	10
Vitamin K mcg	6.7	67
Choline mg	7.37	73.7

Amino acids

Essential amino acids	% total amino acids	g/10 packets
L-Isoleucine	4.15	5.53
L-Leucine	6.57	8.75
L-Lysine	4.94	6.58
L-Methionine	4.58	6.10
L-Phenylalanine	7.10	9.45
L-Threonine	4.16	5.53
L-Tryptophan	1.28	1.71
L-Valine	4.58	6.10
Total	37.36	49.75

Non-essential amino acids	% total amino acids	g/10 packets
L-Alanine	5.18	6.90
L-Arginine	4.07	5.41
L-Aspartic Acid	11.06	14.72
L-Glutamine	18.22	24.25
Glycine	9.84	13.09
L-Histidine	2.36	3.14
L-Proline	6.92	9.21
L-Serine	4.15	5.52
L-Tyrosine	0.84	1.12
Total	62.64	83.36

Electrolytes

Cations	In normal dilution 80 g in 300 ml m-equiv/100 ml	In powder form mg/80 g packet	mg/10 packets
Sodium	3.35	231.3	2,313
Potassium	1.79	210.5	2,105
Calcium	1.66	100.0	1,000
Magnesium	1.097	40.0	400
Manganese	0.00341	0.281	2.81
Iron	0.02148	1.8	18
Copper	0.002098	0.2	2
Zinc	0.0153	1.5	15

Anions	m-equiv/100 ml	mg/80 g packet	mg/10 packets
Chloride	5.24	557.3	5,573
Phosphate (as P)	3.16	100	1,000
Acetate	0.018	3.131	31.3
Iodide	0.000039	0.015	0.15
Gluconate	0.967	565.7	5,657
Sorbate	0.268	89.2	892

Ten packets also contain 0.25 mcg Cobalt as Vitamin B_{12}.

Uses Vivonex HN provides total enteral nutrition for patients who have increased calorie and nitrogen requirements. Vivonex HN requires minimal digestion and produces no exogenous residue.

Use of Vivonex HN prior to major surgery can help to avoid or minimise negative nitrogen balance.

The high nutritional value and minimal residue properties of Vivonex HN make it useful in the management of malabsorption states, short bowel syndrome, bowel fistulae, bowel obstruction, Crohn's disease, ulcerative colitis and as a treatment following total gastrectomy; or for other conditions of the digestive organs or of the alimentary tract where elemental nutrition with low fat, minimal residue and a high nutritional contribution is considered of value.

Post-operatively Vivonex HN provides a balanced, low residue, low fat, milk free nutritional regimen to maintain a positive nitrogen balance during the catabolic phase and to simplify nursing during the recovery period.

Vivonex HN, which may be given orally or by continuous nasoenteric infusion may be used as an alternative to parenteral feeding and/or as supplementary feeding when a high intake is required.

Dosage and administration *Dosage – Adults:* Ten packets (3,000 kilocalories) a day, which may be increased if thought necessary to meet the nutritional demands of some patients.

Children: Vivonex HN may be given to children. However, when used for children under 10 years it may be necessary to adjust the quantity of Vivonex HN consumed daily to meet the projected nutritional requirements for the patient involved.

Vivonex HN may be used as a nutritional source in both infants and children. Vivonex HN contains no cystine, a semi-essential amino acid in the newborn. The amount of Vivonex HN required to maintain weight and nitrogen balance will vary with each individual.

As the recommended daily intake varies with the age of the infant or child, daily administration of a mineral and vitamin supplement may be necessary to meet individual needs, particularly when Vivonex HN is used as the sole source of nutrition for more than a few days.

If Vivonex HN, in standard dilution, is administered as the sole source of nutrition, additional fluid will be required to avoid dehydration.

Administration: Vivonex HN may be administered orally, as a drink or frozen, or by nasogastric or enteric tube.

Contra-indications, warnings, etc
Contra-indications: There are no contra-indications.

Warnings: Vivonex HN must not be administered parenterally.

Precautions: Because of the high caloric contribution from carbohydrates some depleted individuals may manifest elevated blood sugar levels requiring insulin for regulation. Vivonex HN should be used with care in diabetics.

The electrolyte content of Vivonex HN is based on requirements of normal individuals and may be excessive for patients with electrolyte imbalance.

Use during pregnancy or lactation may require supplementary vitamins and minerals.

Use for children under 10 years may require adjustment of the daily consumption to meet the projected nutritional requirements for the patient involved.

Most patients should be started slowly on Vivonex HN. Details of a suggested regimen for initiating tube feeding are given on the package insert inside each carton of Vivonex HN.

For oral feeding a similar regimen should be adopted to allow the body to adjust to liquid nutrition. It is essential that each 300 ml feed be sipped slowly over a period of at least an hour.

Action in event of overdosage: Overdosage is unlikely to occur and would result in vomiting and/or diarrhoea. Should overdosage occur, stop feeding Vivonex HN and give water to avoid dehydration.

Pharmaceutical precautions *Storage:* When packaged in cartons or in packets, Vivonex HN should be stored in a cool, dry place.

In normal dilution, Vivonex HN is a perishable liquid. A full day's supply may be prepared at one time and stored in the refrigerator for up to 24 hours. Shake the liquid briefly before serving. Never leave at room temperature for more than a few hours.

Diluents: In no circumstances should Vivonex HN be mixed with less than 250 ml of water per 80 g packet.

Legal category POM.

Package quantities Vivonex HN is supplied in cartons

of 10 packets, each packet containing 80 g soluble powder.

Further information Vivonex HN is a complete, elemental, minimal residue, nutrition requiring little digestion. It is absorbed in the upper small intestine, leaving the lower bowel at rest. Vivonex HN leaves no exogenous residue. On a Vivonex HN only regimen faecal volume and frequency are much reduced, and a bowel action every five to seven days is to be expected.

When severe catabolic states do not exist the Vivonex Standard formulation may be the preparation of choice.

Adult patients receiving Vivonex HN do not normally require any additional supplements.

Vivonex HN is available solely as an unflavoured powder. To ensure patient acceptance when feeding Vivonex HN orally, the drink should be served flavoured and chilled. Vivonex Flavour sachets are available in

Orange, Strawberry, Beef Broth and Tomato flavours. Beef Broth and Tomato flavours may be blended with warm water. Alternatively, Vivonex HN may be flavoured using commercially available carbonated or still soft drinks.

Where accurate nutritional control is required, allowance must be made for any added calorie or mineral content, and for indigestible matter.

Vivonex HN may be administered as a slow continuous nasoenteric infusion via any suitable naso-enteric feeding system.

For details of prescribing under ACBS ruling see the current edition of MIMS.

Product licence number 0364/0017.

Trade Mark

Novo Laboratories Ltd
Ringway House
Bell Road Daneshill East
Basingstoke, Hants, RG24 0QN

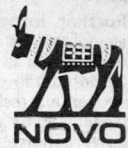

HUMAN ACTRAPID* PENFILL*

Presentation Human Actrapid Penfill (Neutral Insulin Injection) is a clear, neutral solution of monocomponent Human insulin (emp), 100 iu/ml contained in a 1.5 ml cartridge.

Uses The treatment of insulin requiring diabetics.

Dosage and administration The dosage is determined by the physician according to the needs of the patient.

Human Actrapid Penfill is intended for use in the NovoPen* injection device. NovoPen is a mechanical device the size and shape of a large fountain pen, for accurately delivering the required insulin dose. It is designed to be carried in the pocket or handbag of the diabetic.

Instructions for the use of Human Actrapid Penfill in NovoPen are included with the device and must be carefully followed.

Injections using the Human Actrapid Penfill – NovoPen – needle assembly may be given subcutaneously or intramuscularly.

Human Actrapid Penfill has a duration of action of some ½ to 8 hours and its maximum effect is exerted between 2½ and 5 hours, following subcutaneous injection.

Human Actrapid Penfill may be used in regimens utilising this insulin alone, usually as three or more injections daily, or in regimens where an intermediate or long acting insulin injected with a conventional syringe, is given in addition.

Human Actrapid Penfill must not be used or refilled with conventional syringes.

A spare syringe and vial of insulin corresponding to the Penfill preparation should always be kept, in case the pen or cartridges get lost or damaged.

Use in pregnancy: It is essential to maintain continuous good control of the insulin requiring diabetic patient throughout pregnancy. In the insulin treated (gestational or insulin dependent) pregnant diabetic patient the insulin requirements usually fall in the first trimester and increase during the second and third trimester.

Use in the elderly: There are no precautions concerning the use of insulin which are specific to the elderly diabetic. However, injection procedures may be difficult for the infirm or the confused patient, and the simplest regimen consistent with keeping the patient symptom-free should be considered.

Contra-indications, warnings, etc
Contra-indications: Insulin is contra-indicated in hypoglycaemia.

Precautions: Owing to its strong early effect, the injection of Human Actrapid Penfill should be followed by a meal within approximately 30 minutes of administration.

When patients are transferred from other insulins to Human Monocomponent insulin, the change should be made according to the following general guidelines:

For patients currently controlled on Human Monocomponent, porcine monocomponent or other highly purified human or porcine insulin preparations, no dosage change is anticipated other than the routine adjustments made in order to maintain stable diabetic control.

Patients currently stabilised on mixed species or bovine insulin may require a dosage adjustment dependent upon dosage, purity, species and formulation of the insulin preparation(s) currently administered. Variations in glycaemic control may occur and adjustments in therapy should be made under the guidance of a physician.

Insulin resistant patients receiving over 100 units daily should be referred to hospital for transfer.

The addition of corticosteroids, oral contraceptives or initiation of thyroid hormone replacement therapy may lead to an increase in insulin requirements. The addition of a beta-adrenergic blocking agent or a monoamine oxidase inhibitor (MAOI), may also necessitate an adjustment of insulin dosage.

Warnings: Lipodystrophy, insulin resistance and hypersensitivity reactions have been associated with insulin therapy, but the incidence and severity of these unwanted effects is minimal with the Human Monocomponent insulins.

Severe local or generalised allergic reactions require immediate treatment and, in some cases, desensitisation may be necessary.

Toxicity and treatment of overdosage: In the event of an overdose, glucose should be given orally if the patient is conscious. Where the patient is unconscious, an intramuscular, subcutaneous or intravenous injection of glucagon should be given and oral carbohydrate administered when the patient responds. Alternatively, intravenous glucose may be administered; it must be given if there is no response to glucagon.

Pharmaceutical precautions Human Actrapid Penfill cartridges not in use should be stored between 2° and 8°C, and should not be allowed to freeze.

When in use or carried as a spare, Human Actrapid Penfill may be kept at ambient temperature (e.g. in the pocket or handbag) for up to one month, but should not be exposed to excessive heat or sunlight. Penfill cartridges in use must not be stored in a refrigerator.

Human Actrapid Penfill has a shelf life of 2 years from the date of manufacture.

Legal category P

Package quantities Pack of 5 × 1.5 ml cartridges, 100 iu/ml.

Further information Sole distributor: Farillon Ltd, Bryant Avenue, Romford, Essex RM3 0PJ. Tel: Ingrebourne 71136.

Product licence number 4668/0009.

HUMAN ACTRAPID* ▼
HUMAN MONOTARD* ▼
HUMAN PROTAPHANE* ▼
HUMAN ACTRAPHANE*
HUMAN ULTRATARD*

Presentation Human Actrapid (Neutral Insulin Injection) is a clear neutral solution of monocomponent human insulin (emp).

Human Monotard (Insulin Zinc Suspension) is a neutral suspension of amorphous (30%) and crystalline (70%) monocomponent human insulin (emp).

Human Protaphane (Isophane Insulin Injection) is a neutral suspension of monocomponent human isophane insulin (emp).

Human Actraphane (Neutral 30 iu/Isophane 70 iu Insulin Injection) is a neutral suspension of human insulin (emp), consisting of soluble human monocomponent insulin and isophane human monocomponent insulin in the ratio 3:7.

Human Ultratard (Insulin Zinc Suspension Crystalline) is a neutral suspension of crystalline monocomponent human insulin (emp).

When shaken the suspensions appear white and cloudy.

The Human Monocomponent insulin preparations are available in a strength of 100 iu/ml.

Uses The treatment of insulin-requiring diabetic patients.

Dosage and administration *Adults and children:* The dosage of insulin is determined by the physician according to the needs of the patient.

Human Actrapid may be given by injection subcutaneously, intramuscularly or intravenously. It has a duration of action of some $\frac{1}{2}$ to 8 hours and its maximum effect is exerted between $2\frac{1}{2}$ and 5 hours after injection.

Human Monotard, Human Protaphane, Human Actraphane and Human Ultratard may be given by subcutaneous or intramuscular injection. The vial should be gently shaken before use to ensure that the insulin is uniformly distributed throughout the liquid. The dose should then be immediately drawn into the syringe and injected.

Human Monotard and Human Protaphane may be given once, or more commonly, twice a day.

Human Monotard has a duration of action of some $2\frac{1}{2}$ to 22 hours and its maximum effect is exerted between 7 and 15 hours after injection.

Human Protaphane has a duration of action of some $1\frac{1}{2}$ to 24 hours and its maximum effect is exerted between 4 and 12 hours after injection.

Human Actraphane may be given once or more commonly, twice daily especially when a strong initial effect is desired. It has a duration of action of some $\frac{1}{2}$ to 24 hours and its maximum effect is exerted between 2 and about 12 hours after injection.

Human Ultratard is usually given as a once daily injection but may also be given twice daily if required. It may be used as a once daily injection (if necessary with the addition of short acting insulin) in maturity onset diabetes when diet or oral hypoglycaemic drugs fail to produce good control.

The approximate duration of action of Human Ultratard is some 4 to 28 hours and its maximum effect is exerted between 8 and 24 hours after injection.

Human insulin suspensions may be mixed in the syringe with Human Actrapid to intensify the initial effect. When mixing with insulin zinc suspension the injection should be given immediately after mixing. When longer acting insulins are mixed with short acting soluble insulins, the short acting insulin should be drawn into the syringe first.

100 iu/ml insulin must only be used with syringes specifically designed for this strength of insulin.

Infusion pumps: Peristaltic pumps (roller pumps) are not suitable for use with Human Actrapid due to the risk of precipitation.

Human insulin suspensions must not be used in insulin infusion pumps.

Use in pregnancy: It is essential to maintain continuous good control of the insulin requiring diabetic patient throughout pregnancy. In the insulin-treated (gestational or insulin dependent) pregnant diabetic patient the insulin requirements usually fall in the first trimester and increase during the second and third trimester.

Use in the elderly: There are no precautions concerning the use of insulin which are specific to the elderly diabetic. However the injection procedure may be difficult for the infirm, the poorly sighted, or the confused patient, and the simplest regimen consistent with keeping the patient symptom-free should be considered.

Contra-indications, warnings, etc
Contra-indications: Insulin is contra-indicated in hypoglycaemia.

Precautions: Owing to their strong early effect injections of Human Actrapid or Human Actraphane should be followed by a meal within 30 minutes of administration.

On transfer from porcine monocomponent or other highly purified porcine insulin preparation to Human Monocomponent insulin preparations, or on transfer from one Human Monocomponent insulin, or other highly purified human insulin preparation, to another Human Monocomponent insulin preparation, no change in dosage is anticipated other than the routine adjustments made in order to maintain stable diabetic control.

Patients currently stabilised on mixed species or bovine insulin may require a dosage adjustment dependent upon the dosage, purity, species and formulation of the insulin(s) currently administered. Variations in glycaemic control may occur and adjustments in therapy should be made under the guidance of a physician.

In particular, on transfer of patients stabilised on mixed species or bovine insulins to Human Ultratard there is a small risk of hypoglycaemia since patients may require a smaller dosage. The decrease in insulin requirements may occur immediately or gradually over a period of weeks or months and varies from patient to patient. Some patients may experience a more pronounced onset of action with Human Ultratard compared with Ultratard MC.

Insulin resistant patients receiving over 100 units daily should be referred to hospital for transfer.

The addition of corticosteroids, oral contraceptives or thyroid hormone replacement therapy may lead to an increase in insulin requirements. The addition of a beta-adrenergic blocking agent or a monoamine oxidase inhibitor (MAOI) may also necessitate an adjustment of insulin dosage.

Side-effects: Lipodystrophy, insulin resistance and hypersensitivity reactions have been associated with insulin therapy, but the incidence and severity of these unwanted effects is minimal with the Human Monocomponent insulins. Severe local or generalised allergic reactions require immediate treatment and, in some cases, desensitisation may be necessary.

Overdosage: In the event of an overdose, glucose should be given orally if the patient is conscious. Where the patient is unconscious, an intramuscular, subcutaneous or intravenous injection of glucagon should be given and oral carbohydrate administered when the patient responds. Alternatively, intravenous glucose may be administered; it must be given if there is no response to glucagon.

Pharmaceutical precautions The mixing of phosphate containing insulin preparations with insulin zinc suspensions should be avoided.

The Human Monocomponent insulin preparations should be stored between 2°C and 8°C. They should not be exposed to excessive heat or sunlight, neither should they be frozen. The vial in use may be kept at room temperature (max. 25°C) for one month.

Legal category P.

Package quantities 10 ml glass vials.

Further information Sole distributor: Farillon Limited, Bryant Avenue, Romford, Essex, RM3 0PJ. Tel: Ingrebourne 71136.

Product licence numbers

Human Actrapid	100 iu/ml	4668/0003
Human Monotard	100 iu/ml	4668/0006
Human Protaphane	100 iu/ml	4668/0007
Human Actraphane	100 iu/ml	4668/0010
Human Ultratard	100 iu/ml	4668/0008

**ACTRAPID* MC
SEMITARD* MC
RAPITARD* MC
MONOTARD* MC
LENTARD* MC**

Presentation Actrapid MC (Neutral Insulin Injection BP) is a neutral solution of porcine MC insulin.

Semitard MC (Insulin Zinc Suspension Amorphous BP) is a neutral suspension of amorphous porcine MC insulin.

Rapitard MC (Biphasic Insulin Injection BP) is a neutral suspension comprising porcine MC insulin (25%) in solution and crystalline bovine MC insulin (75%).

Monotard MC (Insulin Zinc Suspension BP) is a neutral suspension of amorphous (30%) and crystalline (70%) porcine MC insulin.

Lentard MC (Insulin Zinc Suspension BP) is a neutral suspension of amorphous porcine MC insulin (30%) and crystalline bovine MC insulin (70%).

When shaken the suspensions appear white and cloudy.

The MC insulin preparations are available in a strength of 100 iu/ml.

Uses The treatment of insulin requiring diabetic patients.

Dosage and administration *Adults and children:* The dosage of insulin is determined by the physician according to the needs of the patient.

Actrapid MC may be given by injection subcutaneously, intra-muscularly or intravenously. It has a duration of action of some $\frac{1}{2}$ to 8 hours and its maximum effect is exerted between $2\frac{1}{2}$ and 5 hours after subcutaneous injection.

Suspensions may be given by subcutaneous or intramuscular injection. The vial should be gently shaken before use to ensure that the insulin is uniformly distributed throughout the liquid. The dose should then be immediately drawn into the syringe and injected.

Semitard MC is usually given twice daily. It has a duration of action of some $1\frac{1}{2}$ to 16 hours and its maximum effect is exerted between 5 and 10 hours after injection.

Rapitard MC has a duration of action of some $\frac{1}{2}$ to 22 hours and its maximum effect is exerted between 4 and 12 hours after injection. Rapitard MC may be used once or twice daily.

Monotard MC is given once or more commonly twice a day. It has a duration of action of some $2\frac{1}{2}$ to 22 hours and its maximum effect is exerted between 7 and 15 hours after injection.

Lentard MC has a duration of action of some $2\frac{1}{2}$ to 24 hours and its maximum effect is exerted between 7 and 15 hours after injection. It may be given once or twice daily.

The MC insulin suspensions may be mixed in the syringe with Actrapid MC to intensify the initial effect. The insulin mixture should be injected immediately. When longer acting insulins are mixed with short acting soluble insulins, the short acting insulin should be drawn into the syringe first.

100 iu/ml insulin must only be used with syringes specifically designed for this strength of insulin.

Infusion pumps: Peristaltic pumps are not suitable for use with Actrapid MC due to the risk of precipitation. Insulin suspensions must not be used in insulin infusion pumps.

Use in pregnancy: It is essential to maintain continuous good control of the insulin requiring diabetic patient throughout pregnancy. In the insulin treated (gestational or insulin dependent) pregnant diabetic patient the insulin requirements usually fall in the first trimester and increase during the second and third trimester.

Use in the elderly: There are no precautions concerning the use of insulin which are specific to the elderly diabetic. However the injection procedure may be difficult for the infirm, the poorly sighted, or the confused patient, and the simplest regimen consistent with keeping the patient symptom-free should be considered.

Contra-indications, warnings, etc
Contra-indications: Insulin is contra-indicated in hypoglycaemia.

Precautions: Owing to their strong early effect injections of Actrapid MC or Rapitard MC should be followed by a meal within 30 minutes of administration.

Patients transferred from conventional (predominantly bovine) insulins may require a smaller dosage. The dosage reduction may occur immediately after transfer or gradually over a period of weeks or months. In order to reduce the risk of hypoglycaemia, the patient and the physician should be aware of the possibility that the insulin requirement may be reduced.

If the daily insulin dosage is below 40 iu the risk is considered minimal. However, when higher dosages are required, stricter supervision of the patient is necessary and possibly a 20% reduction should be made initially on transfer to the porcine MC insulins. Insulin resistant patients receiving over 100 units daily should be referred to hospital for transfer.

The addition of corticosteroids, oral contraceptives or thyroid hormone replacement therapy may lead to an increase in insulin requirements. The addition of a beta-adrenergic blocking agent or a monoamine oxidase inhibitor (MAOI), may also necessitate an adjustment of insulin dosage.

Side-effects: Lipodystrophy, insulin resistance and hypersensitivity reactions have been associated with insulin therapy, but the incidence and severity of these unwanted effects is minimal with the MC insulins.

Severe local or generalised allergic reactions require immediate treatment and, in some cases, desensitisation may be necessary.

Overdosage: In the event of an overdose, glucose should be given orally if the patient is conscious. Where the patient is unconscious, an intramuscular, subcutaneous or intravenous injection of glucagon should be given and oral carbohydrate administered when the patient responds. Alternatively, intravenous glucose may be administered; it must be given if there is no response to glucagon.

Pharmaceutical precautions The mixing of phosphate containing insulin preparations with insulin zinc suspensions should be avoided.

The MC insulin preparations should be stored between 2°C and 8°C. They should not be exposed to excessive heat or sunlight, neither should they be frozen. The vial in use may be kept at room temperature (max. 25°C) for one month.

Legal category P.

Package quantities 10 ml glass vials.

Further information Sole distributor: Farillon Limited, Bryant Avenue, Romford, Essex, RM3 0PJ. Tel: Ingrebourne 71136.

Product licence numbers

Actrapid MC	100 iu/ml	0542/0026
Semitard MC	100 iu/ml	0542/0027
Rapitard MC	100 iu/ml	0542/0029
Monotard MC	100 iu/ml	0542/0028
Lentard MC	100 iu/ml	0542/0030

GLUCAGON NOVO

Presentation Glucagon Novo is available as the hydrochloride in lyophilised freeze-dried form with accompanying diluent in two pack sizes:

1 mg – a vial containing glucagon hydrochloride 1 mg (1 i.u.) and lactose 107 mg; a vial containing 1.1 ml Water for Injections, and a sterile plastic disposable syringe.

10 mg – a vial containing glucagon hydrochloride 10 mg (10 i.u.) and lactose 140 mg, and a vial containing 10 ml of diluent (comprising glycerol 200 mg, methyl hydroxybenzoate 10 mg and propyl hydroxy-benzoate 1.5 mg as added preservatives, Water for Injections to 10 ml).

Uses

Indications: Treatment of severe hypoglycaemic reactions which may occur in the management of diabetic patients receiving insulin or oral hypoglycaemic agents.

Termination of insulin coma during insulin shock therapy in psychiatric patients.

As an adjunct for examinations of the gastro-intestinal tract by radiography or endoscopy.

Actions: Glucagon is a hyperglycaemic agent that mobilises hepatic glycogen which is released into the blood as glucose.

Independent of its hyperglycaemic effect glucagon also has an inhibitory action on the motility of the gastro-intestinal tract.

Dosage and administration *Adults and children:*

1. Treatment of severe hypoglycaemic reactions. Dissolve the lyophilised glucagon in the accompanying diluent. Give 0.5 to 1 mg (0.5 to 1 i.u.) of Glucagon Novo by subcutaneous, intramuscular or intravenous injection. If the patient does not awaken within 10 minutes, intravenous glucose must be given. When the patient responds, administer oral carbohydrate to restore the liver glycogen and prevent secondary hypoglycaemia.

2. Termination of insulin shock therapy. Dissolve the lyophilised glucagon in the accompanying diluent. 1–2 mg (1–2 iu) of Glucagon Novo is administered by subcutaneous, intramuscular or intravenous injection. If the patient does not awaken within 10 minutes, intravenous glucose must be given. When the patient responds, administer oral carbohydrate to restore the liver glycogen and prevent secondary hypoglycaemia.

In very deep states of coma, intravenous glucose may be given concurrently with Glucagon Novo.

3. Radiography and endoscopy of the gastro-intestinal tract. Doses range from 0.2–2 mg depending on the diagnostic technique used and the route of administration. The usual diagnostic dose for relaxation of the stomach, duodenal bulb, duodenum and small bowel is 0.2–0.5 mg given intravenously or 1 mg given intramuscularly; the usual dose to relax the colon is 0.5–0.75 mg intravenously or 1–2 mg intramuscularly.

Onset of action after an intravenous injection of 0.2–0.5 mg occurs within one minute and the duration of the effect is between 5 and 20 minutes depending on the organ under examination. The onset of action after an intramuscular injection of 1–2 mg occurs after 4–14 minutes and lasts approximately 10–40 minutes depending on the organ.

Contra-indications, warnings, etc *Contra-indications:* Glucagon Novo is contra-indicated in phaeochromocytoma, insulinoma and glucagonoma.

The presence of fibril formation or solid particles in the solution is a contra-indication to its use at any time.

Warnings: Glucagon reacts antagonistically towards insulin.

Precautions: Caution must be observed if Glucagon Novo is used in diabetic patients as an adjunct in radiography or endoscopy of the gastro-intestinal tract. Since glucagon is a protein, there is a theoretical possibility of hypersensitivity.

Side-effects: Nausea and vomiting may occur occasionally especially with doses above 1 mg, or if the injection is given too fast. No evidence of toxicity has been reported.

Pharmaceutical precautions Glucagon as the dry substance should be stored below 25°C.

1 mg pack: The solution should be prepared immediately prior to use.

10 mg pack: The solution should be prepared immediately prior to use but can be stored at 4°C for up to one week. Do not use solution unless clear.

Legal category POM.

Package quantities A single dose pack consisting of a vial containing 1 mg glucagon hydrochloride, a vial containing 1.1 ml Water for Injection, and a sterile plastic disposable syringe. A multiple dose pack consisting of a vial containing 10 mg glucagon hydrochloric and a vial containing 10 ml diluent.

Further information *Sole distributors:* Farillon Limited, Bryant Avenue, Romford, Essex. RM3 0PJ. Tel: Ingrebourne 71136.

Product licence numbers
1 mg   0542/0016
10 mg   0542/0017

TRISEQUENS*

Presentation Trisequens is supplied in a calendar dial-pack of 28 sequential tablets:

12 blue biconvex tablets marked NOVO 270 on one side, blank on the other side, each containing 2 mg oestradiol and 1 mg oestriol.

10 white biconvex tablets marked NOVO 271 on one side, blank on the other side, each containing 2 mg oestradiol, 1 mg oestriol and 1 mg Norethisterone Acetate BP.

6 red biconvex tablets marked NOVO 272 on one side, blank on the other side, each containing 1 mg oestradiol, and 0.5 mg oestriol.

Uses Trisequens is indicated for the treatment of symptoms due to oestrogenic deficiency.

The oestrogen components of Trisequens counteract falling oestrogen levels during the menopause, whilst the progestogen component counteracts hyper-stimulation of the endometrium. A regular shedding of the endometrium is normally induced by Trisequens during the red tablet phase or at the end of the white tablet phase.

Dosage and administration Trisequens is administered orally without chewing, one tablet daily without interruption, starting with the blue tablets. In menstruating women the first tablet should be taken on the fifth day of menstrual bleeding. If menstruation has stopped altogether or is infrequent and sporadic (2–4 monthly intervals) the first tablet can be taken at any time. Treatment may be stopped at approximately 6–12 monthly intervals to establish whether continued therapy for relief of menopausal symptoms is still required.

Not intended for children or males.

Contra-indications, warnings, etc

Contra-indications: Known or suspected mammary or genital carcinoma. Known or suspected oestrogen-dependent tumours. Thrombophlebitis, thromboembolic disorders or patients with a past history of these conditions.

Undiagnosed irregular vaginal bleeding. Acute or chronic liver disease or history of liver disease where the liver function tests have failed to return to normal. Jaundice or history of jaundice in pregnancy. Rotor syndrome or Dubin-Johnson syndrome. Haemoglobinopathies or sickle-cell anaemia. Porphyria. Hyperlipoproteinaemia, especially in the presence of other risk factors which may indicate a predisposition to cardiovascular or cerebrovascular disorders. Patients with existing cerebrovascular or cardiovascular disease. A history during pregnancy of severe pruritus, herpes gestationis, or a deterioration of otosclerosis. Pregnancy or suspected pregnancy.

Precautions and warnings: Before initiation of therapy with Trisequens it is advisable to undertake a thorough examination to exclude any possibility of genital or mammary tumours. Women receiving long-term therapy with Trisequens should be given a similar examination every 6 months. Special attention should be paid to body weight, blood pressure, heart, breasts, pelvic organs, legs and skin.

The indications for immediate withdrawal of therapy are as follows: thrombophlebitis; thromboembolic disorders; the appearance of jaundice; the occurrence of migraine-like headaches; sudden visual disturbances or a significant increase in blood pressure.

It is also advisable to withdraw treatment 6 weeks before elective surgery and during prolonged periods of immobilisation.

Patients with epilepsy, migraine, diabetes, asthma, or cardiac dysfunction should be carefully controlled as oestrogens may worsen these conditions.

Trisequens may potentiate the side-effects of phenothiazines. Drugs such as barbiturates, phenytoin, and rifampicin, which induce the activity of hepatic microsomal drug-metabolizing enzymes, may decrease the effectiveness of Trisequens. Mineral oil may decrease the intestinal absorption of Trisequens.

Trisequens has no contraceptive effect.

Pre-existing uterine fibromyomata may increase in size under the influence of oestrogens and if this is observed administration of the preparation should be discontinued.

Side-effects: During the first few months of treatment, tension in the breasts, spotting or break-through bleeding can occur. These side effects are usually of a temporary character and normally disappear after continued treatment. Other side effects such as headache, oedema or nausea seldom occur.

Pharmaceutical precautions Protect from light.

Legal category POM.

Package quantities Trisequens is supplied in a calendar dial-pack of 28 tablets.

Further information *Sole distributor:* Farillon Ltd, Bryant Avenue, Romford, Essex RM3 0PJ. Tel: Ingrebourne 71136.

Product licence number 0542/0020

*Trade Mark

Organon Laboratories Limited
Cambridge Science Park
Milton Road
Cambridge CB4 4FL

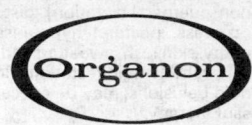

BOLVIDON*

Presentation White, film-coated, bi-convex tablets 6 mm in diameter, coded CT4 on one side and 'Organon' on the reverse side, each containing *10 mg* Mianserin Hydrochloride BP.

White, film-coated, bi-convex tablets 7 mm in diameter, coded CT6 on one side and 'Organon' on the reverse side, each containing *20 mg* Mianserin Hydrochloride BP.

White, film-coated, bi-convex tablets 8 mm in diameter, coded CT7 on one side and 'Organon' on the reverse side, each containing *30 mg* Mianserin Hydrochloride BP.

Uses Symptoms of depressive illness.

Dosage and administration The tablets should be swallowed whole without chewing.

Adults: Bolvidon can be taken either in divided doses or as a single dose at night. Treatment should usually commence with 30 mg or 40 mg per day for the first few days. The effective daily dosage usually lies between 30 mg and 90 mg. Divided daily doses up to 200 mg are well tolerated.

It is often advantageous to maintain antidepressant treatment for several months after initial clinical improvement has occurred.

Elderly: Not more than 30 mg a day initially. The dose should be slowly increased under close supervision. A lower than the normal maintenance dose may be sufficient to produce a satisfactory clinical response.

Children: Not recommended.

Contra-indications, warnings, etc
Contra-indications: Mania. Severe liver disease. During breast feeding. Breast feeding should be discontinued if treatment with Bolvidon is considered essential.

Do not use during pregnancy unless there are compelling reasons. There is no evidence of safety in human pregnancy. Animal studies have not shown hazard.

Precautions and warnings: Care should always be taken in patients with recent myocardial infarction or heart block. Serious cardiotoxic effects appear to be rare at therapeutic dosage, even in patients with pre-existing cardiac disease, recent myocardial infarction or cardiac insufficiency.

The elderly are less liable to experience adverse reactions such as agitation, confusion and postural hypotension with Bolvidon than with tricyclics or bridged tricyclics, but all anti-depressant therapy should be used with caution in this group of patients.

Patients posing a high suicidal risk require close initial supervision.

Avoid if possible in patients with epilepsy. When treating patients with diabetes, hepatic or renal insufficiency, normal precautions should be exercised and the dosages of any concurrent therapy kept under review. Patients with narrow angle glaucoma or symptoms suggestive of prostatic hypertrophy should also be monitored even though anticholinergic side-effects are not anticipated with Bolvidon therapy.

There are indications that Bolvidon, like other antidepressants, may precipitate hypomania in susceptible subjects with bipolar affective illness. In such a case treatment with Bolvidon should be withdrawn.

Bolvidon may potentiate the central nervous depressant action of alcohol.

If surgery is necessary during Bolvidon therapy the anaesthetist should be informed of the treatment being given.

Drug interactions: Bolvidon should not be given concurrently with, or within two weeks of cessation of therapy with monoamine oxidase inhibitors.

Phenytoin plasma levels should be monitored in patients treated concurrently with Bolvidon.

Interactions with sympathomimetic agents have not been reported, and are unlikely.

Clinical experience has shown that Bolvidon does not interact with the anti-hypertensives bethanidine, clonidine, hydralazine, guanethidine or propranolol (either alone or in combination with hydralazine). Nevertheless, the monitoring of blood pressure is recommended for those patients receiving concurrent antihypertensive therapy.

Concurrent anticoagulant therapy of the coumarin type (e.g. warfarin) is also permissible, but close additional monitoring procedures should be carried out.

Warnings and adverse effects: As an improvement may not occur during the first 2–4 weeks of treatment, patients should be closely monitored during this period.

It is advisable to maintain treatment with Bolvidon for several months after initial clinical improvement.

The most commonly occurring side effect is drowsiness, particularly during the first few days of treatment. Patients should be warned of the possible hazard in driving or operating machinery. Any drowsiness may be potentiated by alcohol.

Serious adverse effects are uncommon. A small number of cases of bone marrow depression, usually presenting as an agranulocytosis or granulocytopenia, and generally reversible on stopping of treatment, have been reported. If a patient develops symptoms of infection e.g. fever, sore throat, stomatitis or other inflammatory conditions during treatment with Bolvidon, treatment should be stopped and a full blood count obtained. This adverse reaction has been observed in all age groups but appears to be more common in the elderly.

Jaundice, usually mild, hypomania and convulsions have also been reported at therapeutic dosage and under such circumstances treatment should be withdrawn.

Additional adverse effects that may occur include breast disorders (gynaecomastia, nipple tenderness and non-puerperal lactation), disturbances of liver function, dizziness, postural hypotension, oedema, polyarthropathy, skin rash, sweating and tremor.

Psychotic manifestations, including mania and paranoid delusions, may be exacerbated during antidepressant therapy.

The following adverse effects although not reported with Bolvidon can occur with tricyclics and bridged tricyclics: interference with sexual function; withdrawal symptoms in adults; withdrawal symptoms (e.g. neuromuscular irritability) in neonates whose mothers received tricyclic or bridged tricyclic antidepressants during pregnancy.

Overdosage: There is no specific antidote. Treatment is by gastric lavage with appropriate supportive therapy. Symptoms of overdosage are normally confined to prolonged sedation.

Cardiac arrhythmias, convulsions, severe hypotension and respiratory depression are unlikely to occur.

Pharmaceutical precautions Protect from light.

Legal category POM.

Package quantities

Bolvidon tablets 10 mg are supplied in push-through PVC/foil blister strips of 30 tablets. Packed in cartons containing three strips (90 tablets).

Bolvidon tablets 20 mg are supplied in push-through PVC/foil blister strips of 21 tablets. Packed in cartons containing three strips (63 tablets).

Bolvidon tablets 30 mg are supplied in push-through PVC/foil blister strips of 14 tablets. Packed in cartons containing three strips (42 tablets).

All strengths also available in Securitainers of 100 and 500 tablets.

Further information Bolvidon is a tetracyclic antidepressant which is structurally distinct from classical tricyclics and from bridged tricyclics; this difference is reflected in its pharmacology.

Bolvidon produces fewer and milder side effects than the tricyclics and bridged tricyclics especially in terms of anticholinergic effects and effects on the cardiovascular system. Bolvidon does not cause the severe complications in overdosage associated with tricyclics and bridged tricyclics, e.g. severe cardiac arrhythmias, respiratory depression, convulsions and coma.

Elderly: Pharmacokinetic studies of Bolvidon in the elderly patient suggest a longer half-life and slower metabolic clearance. This information implies that a single night-time dose of Bolvidon should be preferable to divided doses in the elderly patient; in addition, a lower than the normal maintenance dose may be sufficient to produce a satisfactory clinical response.

Product licence numbers
10 mg tablets – 0065/0031R
20 mg tablets – 0065/0057R
30 mg tablets – 0065/0061R

COTAZYM*

Presentation Dark green gelatine capsules, containing pancreatic enzymes in powder form.

Each capsule contains not less than 14,000 BP-U lipase, not less than 10,000 BP-U amylase, and not less than 500 BP-U protease.

Uses As an adjunct in the treatment of pancreatic exocrine deficiency.

Dosage and administration The usual dose is 6 capsules daily in divided doses. The capsules should be opened and the contents sprinkled on to the food.

Contra-indications, warnings, etc
Contra-indications: Patients with a known allergy to the active ingredients (porcine protein).

Precautions and warnings: Buccal and perianal irritation may occur, and rarely inflammation, when large doses are used.

This product contains lactose and this should be taken into account when treating patients with lactose intolerance.

Use during pregnancy: There is no evidence of safety in use during pregnancy and animal reproduction-toxicological studies are lacking. Therefore, during pregnancy the benefits of the use of Cotazym capsules should be weighed against the possible hazards to the foetus.

Adverse reactions: As with any pancreatic extract, Cotazym capsules may have adverse effects in high dosages. These may include hyperuricosuria or hyperuricaemia (due to the purine content of the product), and buccal or perianal irritation, rarely amounting to frank inflammation.

Pharmaceutical precautions Store in a cool, dry place between 2 and 15°C and protect the capsules from light.

Legal category P.

Package quantities Securitainer of 100 capsules.

Further information Nil.

Product licence number 0065/5054.

DECA-DURABOLIN*

Presentation Deca Durabolin is a clear, sterile, oily, solution for injection containing nandrolone decanoate, 25 mg or 50 mg per ml.

Uses Deca Durabolin is a protein-anabolic preparation with a duration of action up to three weeks after injection.

Dosage and administration
Indications: Adults: During chronic debilitating diseases; during prolonged glucocorticosteroid therapy; during radiotherapy; after major surgery and trauma – 25–50 mg every three weeks.

Higher and more frequent dosages may be indicated for adults in the following conditions: For the symptomatic treatment of osteoporosis – 50 mg every 2–3 weeks; for the palliative treatment of selected cases of disseminated mammary carcinoma in women – 50 mg every 2–3 weeks.

Children:
more than 30 kg: 15 mg　　　every 3 weeks
　　　20–30 kg: 7.5–10.0 mg every 3 weeks
　　　10–20 kg: 5.0–7.5 mg　every 3 weeks
less than 10kg: 5.0 mg　　　every 3 weeks

N.B.: For an optimal therapeutic effect it is necessary to administer adequate amounts of vitamins, minerals and proteins in a calorie-rich diet.

Deca Durabolin should be administered by deep intramuscular injection.

Contra-indications, warnings, etc
Contra-indications: Pregnancy. Known or suspected carcinoma of prostate or mammary carcinoma in the male.

Precautions and warnings: If signs of virilisation develop, discontinuation of the treatment should be considered.

Patients, especially the elderly, with the following conditions should be monitored: Latent or overt cardiac failure, renal dysfunction, hypertension, epilepsy or migraine (or a history of these conditions), since anabolic steroids may occasionally induce sodium and water retention;

Diabetes, or latent diabetes, since anabolic steroids may improve the glucose tolerance and decrease the need for insulin or other antidiabetic drugs;

Incomplete statural growth, since anabolic steroids in high dosages may accelerate epiphyseal closure;

Skeletal metastases, since anabolic steroids may induce hypercalcaemia and hypercalciuria in these patients;

Liver dysfunction.

Adverse reactions: Deca-Durabolin at the *recommended* dosages is unlikely to produce virilising effects.

High dosages, prolonged treatment and/or too frequent administration may cause:

Virilisation which appears in sensitive women as hoarseness, acne, hirsutism and increase of libido; in prepubertal boys as an increased frequency of erections and phallic enlargement, and in girls as an increase of pubic hair and clitoral hypertrophy. Hoarseness may be the first symptom of vocal change which may end in long-lasting, sometimes irreversible deepening of the voice;

Amenorrhoea and inhibition of spermatogenesis;

Premature epiphyseal closure;

Sodium and water retention.

Interactions: It is advisable to check the prothrombin time regularly when Deca Durabolin is used in conjunction with an oral anticoagulant.

Concurrent administration of liver enzyme inducing drugs such as rifampicin, barbiturates, carbamazepine, dichloralphenazone, phenylbutazone, phenytoin or primidone may decrease the effect of Deca Durabolin.

Pharmaceutical precautions Protect from light. Store at room temperature (15° to 25°C).

After storage at lower temperatures precipitation of the arachis oil vehicle may occur. By heating the ampoules at 100°C for a few minutes or at 40°C for one hour the solution becomes clear. The precipitation and rewarming does not affect the activity of the injection.

Legal category POM.

Package quantities
25 mg per ml: 1 ml ampoules in boxes of 3 and 1 ml Orgaject Disposable Syringes singly.
50 mg per ml: 1 ml ampoules in boxes of 3 and 1 ml Orgaject Disposable Syringes singly.

Further information Nil.

Product licence numbers
25 mg/ml   0065/5005
50 mg/ml   0065/5063.

DECA-DURABOLIN* 100
Presentation Deca Durabolin 100 is a clear, sterile, oily, solution for injection containing nandrolone decanoate, 100 mg per ml.

Uses Deca Durabolin 100 is a higher dosage form of nandrolone decanoate intended for adjuvant therapy in the treatment of certain blood disorders.

Indicated in such conditions as: Anaemia of chronic renal failure (including patients on haemodialysis); aplastic anaemia; anaemia due to cytotoxic disease.

The aetiology of anaemia may be complex and concurrent use of other drugs e.g. Folic Acid, Iron, Vitamin B12 etc. should be employed when the haematological picture indicates their usage.

Treatment with Deca-Durabolin 100 is not a substitute for other therapeutic measures.

The onset of a therapeutic effect may vary widely among patients. If no satisfactory response occurs after 3–6 months of treatment, administration should be discontinued.

After a satisfactory improvement or a normalisation of the red blood picture has been obtained, treatment should be withdrawn gradually on the basis of regular monitoring of the haematological parameters.

Should a relapse occur at any time whilst the dose is being reduced or after stopping the treatment, re-institution of therapy should be considered.

Dosage and administration Deca Durabolin 100 should be administered by deep intramuscular injection.

Adults: Anaemia of chronic renal failure (including patients on haemodialysis) – males 200 mg weekly; females 100 mg weekly.

Aplastic anaemia – 50–150 mg weekly.

Anaemia due to cytotoxic therapy – 200 mg weekly, starting 2 weeks prior to the course of cytotoxic therapy. This treatment should be continued throughout cytotoxic therapy and thereafter during the recovery period until the blood count has returned to normal.

Children: A dosage scheme for children cannot be given because of insufficient clinical experience.

Contra-indications, warnings, etc
Contra-indications: Pregnancy.

Known or suspected carcinoma of prostate and mammary carcinoma in the male.

Precautions and warnings: The recommended doses should not be exceeded.

If signs of virilisation develop, discontinuation of the treatment should be considered.

Deca-Durabolin 100 injection should not be used in conjunction with heparin.

Patients, especially the elderly, with the following conditions should be monitored: Latent or overt cardiac failure, renal dysfunction, hypertension, epilepsy or migraine (or a history of these conditions), since anabolic steroids may occasionally induce sodium and water retention;

Diabetes, or latent diabetes, since anabolic steroids may improve the glucose tolerance and decrease the need for insulin or other antidiabetic drugs;

Incomplete statural growth, since anabolic steroids in high dosages may accelerate epiphyseal closure;

Skeletal metastases, since anabolic steroids may induce hypercalcaemia and hypercalciuria in these patients;

Liver dysfunction.

Adverse reactions: The high dosages which are required to obtain a therapeutic effect in the indications mentioned may cause: Virilisation which appears in sensitive women as hoarseness, acne, hirsutism and increase of libido; in prepubertal boys as an increased frequency of erections and phallic enlargement, and in girls as an increase of pubic hair and clitoral hypertrophy. Hoarseness may be the first symptom of vocal change which may end in long-lasting, sometimes irreversible deepening of the voice;

Amenorrhoea and inhibition of spermatogenesis;

Premature epiphyseal closure;

Sodium and water retention.

Occasionally, abnormal values in some liver function tests. These changes appear to be reversible after completion of the treatment course.

Interactions: Although only one possible case of interaction with an oral anticoagulant has been observed, it is advisable to check the prothrombin time regularly when Deca Durabolin 100 is used in conjunction with such an agent.

Concurrent administration of liver enzyme inducing drugs such as rifampicin, barbiturates, carbamazepine, dichloralphenazone, phenylbutazone, phenytoin or primidone may decrease the effect of Deca Durabolin 100.

Pharmaceutical precautions Protect from light. Store at room temperature (15° to 25°C).

After storage at lower temperatures precipitation of the arachis oil vehicle may occur. By heating the ampoules at 100°C for a few minutes or at 40°C for one hour the solution becomes clear. The precipitation and rewarming does not affect the activity of the injection.

Legal category POM.

Package quantities 100 mg per ml: 1 ml ampoules in boxes of 3.

Further information Deca Durabolin 100 stimulates erythropoiesis in anaemia whether this is due to hypoplasia of the stem cells in the bone marrow or to a decreased production of erythropoietin. This action may be useful as an adjunct to chemotherapy or radiotherapy in malignant disease. There are indications that leucopoiesis and thrombopoieses are also favourably stimulated.

Product licence number 0065/0036.

DURABOLIN*

Presentation Durabolin is a clear, sterile, oily, solution for injection containing nandrolone phenylpropionate, 25 mg or 50 mg per ml.

Uses Durabolin is a protein-anabolic preparation with a duration of action of one week after injection.

Dosage and administration
Indications: Adults: During chronic debilitating diseases; during prolonged glucocorticoid therapy; during radiotherapy; after major surgery and trauma – 25–50 mg weekly.

Higher and more frequent dosages may be indicated for adults in the following conditions: For the symptomatic treatment of osteoporosis – 50 mg weekly; for the palliative treatment of selected cases of disseminated mammary carcinoma in women – 50 mg weekly.

Children:

more than 30 kg: 15 mg	weekly	
20– 30 kg: 7.5–10.0 mg	weekly	
10– 20 kg: 5.0–7.5 mg	weekly	
less than 10 kg: 5.0 mg	weekly	

N.B.: For an optimal therapeutic effect it is necessary to administer adequate amounts of vitamins, minerals and proteins in a calorie-rich diet.

Durabolin should be administered by deep intramuscular injection.

Contra-indications, warnings, etc
Contra-indications: Pregnancy. Known or suspected carcinoma of prostate or mammary carcinoma in the male.

Precautions and warnings: If signs of virilisation develop, discontinuation of the treatment should be considered.

Patients, especially the elderly, with the following conditions should be monitored: Latent or overt cardiac failure, renal dysfunction, hypertension, epilepsy or migraine (or a history of these conditions), since anabolic steroids may occasionally induce sodium and water retention.

Diabetes, or latent diabetes, since anabolic steroids may improve the glucose tolerance and decrease the need for insulin or other antidiabetic drugs;

Incomplete statural growth, since anabolic steroids in high dosages may accelerate epiphyseal closure.

Skeletal metastases, since anabolic steroids may induce hypercalcaemia and hypercalciuria in these patients.

Liver dysfunction.

Adverse reactions: Durabolin at the *recommended* dosages is unlikely to produce virilising effects.

High dosages, prolonged treatment and/or too frequent administration may cause: Virilisation which appears in sensitive women as hoarseness, acne, hirsutism and increase of libido; in prepubertal boys as an increased frequency of erections and phallic enlargement, and in girls as an increase of pubic hair and clitoral hypertrophy. Hoarseness may be the first symptom of vocal change which may end in long-lasting, sometimes irreversible deepening of the voice;

Amenorrhoea and inhibition of spermatogenesis;

Premature epiphyseal closure;

Sodium and water retention.

Interactions: It is advisable to check the prothrombin time regularly when Durabolin is used in conjunction with an oral anticoagulant.

Concurrent administration of liver enzyme inducing drugs such as rifampicin, barbiturates, carbamazepine, dichloralphenazone, phenylbutazone, phenytoin or primidone may decrease the effect of Durabolin.

Pharmaceutical precautions Protect from light. Store at room temperature (15° to 25°C). After storage at lower temperatures precipitation of the arachis oil vehicle may occur. By heating the ampoules at 100°C for a few minutes or at 40°C for one hour the solution becomes clear. The precipitation and rewarming does not affect the activity of the injection.

Legal category POM.

Package quantities
25 mg per ml: 1 ml ampoules in boxes of 3 and 1 ml Orgaject Disposable Syringes singly.
50 mg per ml: 1 ml Orgaject Disposable Syringes singly.

Further information Nil.

Product licence numbers
25 mg/ml: 1 ml ampoules and
    1 ml Orgajects   0065/5007
50 mg/ml: 1 ml Orgajects   0065/5091

GESTANIN*

Presentation Round, flat, white tablets, diameter 6.5 mm, code-marked 'GK4' on one side, with 'Organon' and a star on the reverse side. Each tablet contains 5 mg of allylestrenol.

Uses Gestanin is an orally active gestagen. Allylestrenol has a pronounced pregnancy maintaining action in castrated animals without producing hormonal side effects.

Indications: Threatened abortion and habitual abortion.

Dosage and administration

In threatened abortion: 1 tablet three times daily for 5–7 days. If necessary, the treatment period may be extended. After disappearance of the symptoms the dosage should be gradually reduced unless symptoms return.

In habitual abortion: 1–2 tablets daily as soon as pregnancy has been diagnosed. The administration should be continued until at least one month after the end of the critical period.

    Gestanin tablets are for oral administration.

Contra-indications, warnings, etc

Contra-indications: Patients with a history of, or existent thromboembolic disorders, or with mammary or genital carcinoma.

    Patients with impaired liver function, or with active liver disease.

    Patients with undiagnosed, irregular vaginal bleeding.

Precautions and warnings: A decreased glucose tolerance may occur in diabetic patients on this treatment and their control must be carefully supervised.

    Patients receiving treatment with a progestogen should be kept under regular surveillance, and should have a thorough physical examination regularly.

Side-effects: Gastrointestinal complaints (nausea, vomiting) have been occasionally reported.

Overdosage: There is no specific antidote. Patients should be given appropriate supportive therapy using standard resuscitative measures as required.

Pharmaceutical precautions Protect from light.

Legal category POM.

Package quantities Bottles of 100 tablets.

Further information Administration of Gestanin, in combination with bedrest, can remove or prevent the threat of abortion in early pregnancy. Gestanin is generally well tolerated. Serious adverse reactions have been reported neither in the mother nor in the offspring.

Product licence number 0065/5030.

MARVELON* ▼

Presentation White, round, biconvex tablets, diameter 6 mm, coded TR5 on one side and ORGANON* on the reverse side.

    Each tablet contains 150 micrograms of desogestrel and 30 micrograms ethinyloestradiol.

Uses Oral contraception.

Dosage and administration The tablets are to be taken orally, without chewing, at the same time each day, e.g. at the time of the evening meal.

First course: One tablet daily for 21 days, starting on the first day of the menstrual cycle, with a tablet which is marked with the appropriate day of the week. If menstruation has already progressed beyond day 1, the course should then be started on day 5. For a day 5 start, an additional method of non-hormonal contraception should be used for the first fourteen days.

Subsequent courses: Each subsequent course is started after seven tablet-free days. Provided the last pack is taken correctly, the patient is protected from pregnancy during the tablet-free days as well. Subsequent packs should be taken in exactly the same way as the first pack.

Post-partum use: After delivery, oral contraception should start on the first day of the first spontaneous menstruation or 4–6 weeks after delivery. Since the first post-partum ovulation may precede the first bleeding, additional non-hormonal precautions should be taken for the first 14 days of tablet-taking. In general, Marvelon appears to have no adverse effect on lactation and the excretion of desogestrel in the milk is negligible. However, suppression of lactation may occur when administration is started immediately post-partum.

After a miscarriage or abortion: Marvelon should be taken immediately. The patient is then fully protected against pregnancy and no additional precautions are required.

Changing from a 21 or 22 day pill: All tablets in the old pack should be finished. The first Marvelon tablet is taken on the *first day* of the withdrawal bleed, provided that this bleeding starts within seven days of taking the last tablet. In the absence of bleeding within 7 days of taking the previous tablet, pregnancy should first be excluded. Additional precautions are not required.

Changing from a combined every day pill (28 day tablets) to Marvelon: Withdrawal bleeding should begin while the patient is still taking the inactive tablets. Marvelon should be started on the first day of this period. Remaining tablets from the every day pack should be discarded. Additional precautions are not required.

Changing from a progestogen-only pill (POP or Mini Pill) to Marvelon: The first Marvelon tablet should be taken on the first day of the period, even if the patient has already taken a mini pill on that day. All the remaining progestogen-only pills in the mini pill pack should be discarded. Additional contraceptive precautions are not required.

    If the patient is breast feeding and taking a progestogen-only (mini) pill, then she may not have a period. The first Marvelon tablet should be taken on the day *after* stopping the mini pill. All remaining tablets in the mini pill packet must be discarded. Additional contraceptive precautions must be taken for the first fourteen days.

Contra-indications, warnings, etc

Contra-indications: Pregnancy or suspected pregnancy.

    Cardiovascular or cerebrovascular disorders, or a history of these conditions e.g. thrombophlebitis, phlebothrombosis, pulmonary embolism, arterial thrombosis, stroke or myocardial infarction.

    Hyperlipoproteinaemia, especially in the presence of other risk factors which may indicate a predisposition to cardiovascular or cerebrovascular disorders.

    Moderate to severe hypertension.

Acute or chronic liver disease or a history of liver disease where the liver function tests have failed to return to normal, e.g., jaundice or history of jaundice in pregnancy, Rotor syndrome or Dubin-Johnson syndrome.

N.B. The use of oral contraceptives is not contraindicated in patients with a history of hepatitis whose liver functions are normal. However, treatment should be stopped if liver function tests become abnormal or cholestatic jaundice appears.

Known or suspected oestrogen-dependent tumours, e.g. mammary, genital carcinoma.

Endometrial hyperplasia.

Undiagnosed irregular vaginal bleeding.

Haemoglobinopathies e.g. sickle cell anaemia.

Porphyria.

A history during pregnancy, or previous oestrogen/progestogen use, of severe pruritus, herpes gestationis or a deterioration of otosclerosis.

Precautions and warnings: Physical examination should precede the prescribing of any oral contraceptive and should be repeated regularly, generally once every six months. Special attention should be paid to duration of the cycle, body weight, blood pressure, heart, breasts, pelvic organs, legs and skin.

A cervical smear should be taken at regular intervals.

Pregnancy must be excluded before treatment is started. Whenever there is a reason to suspect pregnancy during treatment, this must be investigated by the physician. If pregnancy is confirmed, tablet-taking must be stopped immediately.

Patients with the following conditions should be monitored very closely:

Diabetes, since glucose tolerance may deteriorate during oral contraceptive use.

Mild hypertension. Some women experience an increase in blood pressure during pregnancy and/or during oral contraceptive use. In these women, the blood pressure should be checked regularly. In cases where moderate to severe hypertension develops, the pill should be stopped.

Sickle cell trait, since in special conditions, e.g. during infections or anoxia, oestrogens may induce thrombo-embolic processes.

Migraine, epilepsy, asthma, myocardial or renal disease, or a history of these conditions, or a disease exacerbated by pregnancy, since fluid retention has been observed during continued use of oral contraceptives and may exacerbate these conditions.

Oestrogen-sensitive gynaecological disorders, e.g. uterine fibromyomata which may increase in size, and endometriosis which may be aggravated by oestrogen treatment.

Forgotten tablets: If the patient forgets to take a tablet, she should take it as soon as she remembers, continuing with the rest of the pack as usual. Provided she is not more than 12 hours late in taking her tablet, Marvelon will still give contraceptive protection during this cycle.

However, if any one tablet is forgotten for more than 12 hours, then two tablets should be taken the next day (the forgotten tablet plus the usual one) at the normal time. The rest of the pack should be taken as usual. In these circumstances, another method of non-hormonal contraception, such as the sheath, should be used either until the next period or for the next fourteen days, whichever is the longer.

Vomiting or diarrhoea: If the patient has severe vomiting or diarrhoea, a tablet may not be absorbed properly. This may reduce contraceptive reliability. The patient should continue taking her tablets as normal. Additional non-hormonal contraceptive precautions are required until the end of the current cycle.

Bleeding whilst taking Marvelon: If the patient experiences any bleeding between periods, she should *not* stop taking Marvelon. The bleeding usually ceases in a day or two. It does not necessarily mean that contraceptive protection is lost. Some women may experience a reduced amount and/or duration of blood-loss during the withdrawal bleed.

Absence of withdrawal bleeding: Occasionally the withdrawal bleeding may fail to occur at all. Provided all tablets have been taken correctly and there is no obvious reason why reliability should be reduced e.g. drug interaction or recent episode of vomiting or diarrhoea, then pregnancy is unlikely and there is no reason to discontinue Marvelon. However, if the withdrawal bleeding had previously been regular and suddenly fails to occur, pregnancy must then be excluded. If there are any reasons to suspect pregnancy, then successive pregnancy tests may need to be performed at intervals of one week. Whilst awaiting the outcome of these tests, the patient should stop tablet-intake and use another method of non-hormonal contraception.

Caution should be observed when prescribing oral contraceptives to young women whose cycles are not yet stabilised.

Cardiovascular system: The risk of arterial thrombosis associated with combined oral contraceptives increases with age and this risk is aggravated by cigarette smoking. The use of combined oral contraceptives by women in the older age group, especially those who are cigarette smokers, should therefore be discouraged and alternative methods advised.

Since oral contraceptives may increase the risk of thrombosis they should be discontinued where possible approximately six weeks prior to elective surgery and not recommended until the patient has recovered and is mobile.

If any signs of thrombo-embolic processes occur, tablet intake must be discontinued immediately.

In the presence of severe varicose veins the benefits of oestrogen therapy must be weighed against the possible risks.

Hepato-biliary system: There are reports indicating an association between the use of oestrogen-containing preparations and the occurrence of cholelithiasis; however contradictory findings have been reported.

Hepatic cell adenomas have been reported in women on oral contraceptive preparations. The adenoma may present itself as an abdominal mass or with the signs and symptoms of an acute abdomen. A bleeding hepatic cell adenoma, although rare, should be considered if the patient has abdominal pain or evidence of intra-abdominal bleeding.

Central nervous system: The combined oral contraceptive pill can produce headache, migraine and mood changes. In some women, frank depression may occur. In a number of these women there may be a disturbance of tryptophan metabolism and in such cases the administration of vitamin B6 might be of therapeutic value.

Skin: Chloasma is occasionally seen during the use of oral contraceptives, especially in women with a history of chloasma gravidarum. Women with a tendency to chloasma should avoid exposure to the sun whilst taking this preparation.

Effect on laboratory tests

Thyroid function tests: The radio-iodine uptake shows that thyroid function is unchanged. There is a rise in serum protein-bound iodine, similar to that in pregnancy and during the administration of oestrogens. This is due to the increased capacity of the plasma proteins for binding thyroid hormones, rather than to any change in glandular function. In women taking oral contraceptives, the content of protein-bound iodine in the blood serum should, therefore, not be used for the evaluation of thyroid function.

ACTH function test: Oral contraceptives have no significant influence on adrenocortical function. The ACTH function test for the adrenal cortex remains unchanged. The reduction in corticosteroid excretion and the elevation of plasma corticosteroids are due to an increased cortisol-binding capacity of the plasma proteins.

Effect on erythrocyte sedimentation rate (ESR): Oral contraceptives may accelerate erythrocyte sedimentation in the absence of any disease. This effect is due to a change in the proportion of the plasma protein fractions.

Oral contraceptive preparations may also influence the results of other laboratory tests. Increases in plasma copper, iron and alkaline phosphatase have also been recorded.

Side-effects and adverse reactions: The following side effects and adverse reactions have been associated with either oestrogen or progestogen therapy:

Genito-urinary tract: Intermenstrual bleeding, post-pill amenorrhoea, changes in cervical secretion, increase in size of uterine leiomyomata, aggravation of endometriosis, certain vaginal infections e.g. candidiasis.

Breast: Tenderness, pain, enlargement, secretion.

Gastro-intestinal tract: Nausea, vomiting, cholelithiasis, cholestatic jaundice.

Cardiovascular system: Rise of blood pressure, phlebitis, thrombosis.

Skin: Chloasma, erythema nodosum, rash, recurrence of herpes gestationis.

Eyes: Discomfort of the cornea if contact lenses are used.

CNS: Headache, migraine, mood changes.

Metabolic: Sodium and water retention, reduced glucose tolerance, changes in body weight.

Interactions: Irregular cycles and reduced reliability of oral contraceptives may occur when these preparations are used concomitantly with liver enzyme inducing drugs such as rifampicin, barbiturates, carbamazepine, dichloralphenazone, phenylbutazone, phenytoin, primidone, or with certain antibiotics (e.g. ampicillin or tetracycline). If no withdrawal bleeding occurs, then possible drug interactions should be considered where applicable. Pregnancy is possible and must be excluded. In such patients, the pill should be stopped immediately until pregnancy has been excluded or confirmed. During this time other forms of non-hormonal contraception should be used.

Interactions have also been reported between oral contraceptives and tricyclic antidepressants, anticoagulants and corticosteroids. Steroids affect drug metabolism and the therapeutic or toxic effects of other drugs may be modified.

The response to metyrapone is less pronounced in women receiving oral contraceptives and is similar to the response during pregnancy. This should be borne in mind if a metyrapone test is required for any reason.

Overdosage: There have been no reports of serious ill-effects from overdosage. In general, it is therefore unnecessary to treat overdosage. However, if overdosage is discovered within two or three hours and is substantial, then gastric lavage can be safely used.

There are no specific antidotes and further treatment should be symptomatic.

Pharmaceutical precautions Store in a cool, dry place and protect from light.

Legal category POM.

Package quantities Pack of 21 tablets (one month's supply).

Further information Nil.

Product licence number 0065/0071.

MINILYN*

Presentation White, round, biconvex tablets, diameter 6 mm, coded with a circle on one side and Organon* on the reverse side. Each tablet contains 2.5 mg Lynoestrenol BP and 50 micrograms of Ethinyloestradiol BP.

Uses Oral contraception.

Dosage and administration The tablets are to be taken orally, without chewing, at the same time each day, e.g. at the time of the evening meal.

First course: One tablet daily for 22 days, starting on the first day of the menstrual cycle, with a tablet which is marked with the appropriate day of the week. If menstruation has already progressed beyond day 1, the course should then be started on day 5. For a day 5 start, an additional method of non-hormonal contraception should be used for the first fourteen days.

Subsequent courses: Each subsequent course is started after six tablet-free days. Provided the last pack is taken correctly, the patient is protected from pregnancy during the tablet-free days as well. Subsequent packs should be taken in exactly the same way as the first pack.

Post-partum use: After delivery, oral contraception should start on the first day of the first spontaneous menstruation or 4–6 weeks after delivery. Since the first post-partum ovulation may precede the first bleeding, additional non-hormonal precautions should be taken for the first 14 days of tablet-taking. In general, Minilyn appears to have no adverse effect on lactation and the excretion of the active substances in the milk is negligible. However, suppression of lactation may occur when administration is started immediately post-partum.

After a miscarriage or abortion: Minilyn should be taken immediately. The patient is then fully protected against pregnancy and no additional precautions are required.

Changing from a 21-day pill: All tablets in the old pack should be finished. The first Minilyn tablet is taken on the *first day* of the withdrawal bleed, provided that this bleeding starts within six days of taking the last tablet. In the absence of bleeding within six days of taking the previous tablet, pregnancy should first be excluded. Additional precautions are not required.

Changing from a combined every day pill (28 day tablets) to Minilyn: Withdrawal bleeding should begin while the patient is still taking the inactive tablets. Minilyn should be started on the first day of this period. Remaining tablets from the every day pack should be discarded. Additional precautions are not required.

Changing from a progestogen-only pill (POP or Mini

Pill) to Minilyn: The first Minilyn tablet should be taken on the first day of the period, even if the patient has already taken a mini pill on that day. All the remaining progestogen-only pills in the mini pill pack should be discarded. Additional contraceptive precautions are not required.

If the patient is breast feeding and taking a progestogen-only (mini) pill, then she may not have a period. The first Minilyn tablet should be taken on the day *after* stopping the mini pill. All remaining tablets in the mini pill packet must be discarded. Additional contraceptive precautions must be taken for the first fourteen days.

Contra-indications, warnings, etc

Contra-indications: Pregnancy or suspected pregnancy.

Cardiovascular or cerebrovascular disorders, or a history of these conditions e.g. thrombophlebitis, phlebo-thrombosis, pulmonary embolism, arterial thrombosis, stroke or myocardial infarction.

Hyperlipoproteinaemia, especially in the presence of other risk factors which may indicate a predisposition to cardiovascular or cerebrovascular disorders.

Moderate to severe hypertension.

Acute or chronic liver disease or a history of liver disease where the liver function tests have failed to return to normal, e.g., jaundice or history of jaundice in pregnancy, Rotor syndrome or Dubin-Johnson syndrome.

N.B. The use of oral contraceptives is not contraindicated in patients with a history of hepatitis whose liver functions are normal. However, treatment should be stopped if liver function tests become abnormal or cholestatic jaundice appears.

Known or suspected oestrogen-dependent tumours, e.g. mammary, genital carcinoma.

Endometrial hyperplasia.

Undiagnosed irregular vaginal bleeding.

Haemoglobinopathies e.g. sickle cell anaemia.

Porphyria.

A history during pregnancy or previous oestrogen/ progestogen use of severe pruritus, herpes gestationis or a deterioration of otosclerosis.

Precautions and warnings: Physical examination should precede the prescribing of any oral contraceptive and should be repeated regularly, generally once every six months. Special attention should be paid to duration of the cycle, body weight, blood pressure, heart, breasts, pelvic organs, legs and skin.

A cervical smear should be taken at regular intervals.

Pregnancy must be excluded before treatment is started. Whenever there is a reason to suspect pregnancy during treatment, this must be investigated by the physician. If pregnancy is confirmed, tablet taking must be stopped immediately.

Patients with the following conditions should be monitored very closely:

Diabetes, since glucose tolerance may deteriorate during oral contraceptive use.

Mild hypertension. Some women experience an increase in blood pressure during pregnancy and/or during oral contraceptive use. In these women, the blood pressure should be checked regularly. In cases where moderate to severe hypertension develops, the pill should be stopped.

Sickle cell trait, since in special conditions, e.g. during infections or anoxia, oestrogens may induce thrombo-embolic processes.

Migraine, epilepsy, asthma, myocardial or renal dis-

ease, or a history of these conditions, or a disease exacerbated by pregnancy, since fluid retention has been observed during continued use of oral contraceptives and may exacerbate these conditions.

Oestrogen-sensitive gynaecological disorders, e.g. uterine fibromyomata which may increase in size, and endometriosis which may be aggravated by oestrogen treatment

Forgotten tablets: If the patient forgets to take a tablet, she should take it as soon as she remembers, continuing with the rest of the pack as usual. Provided she is not more than 12 hours late in taking her tablet, Minilyn will still give contraceptive protection during this cycle.

However, if any one tablet is forgotten for more than 12 hours, then two tablets should be taken the next day (the forgotten tablet plus the usual one) at the normal time. The rest of the pack should be taken as usual. In these circumstances, another method of non-hormonal contraception, such as the sheath, should be used either until the next period or for the next fourteen days, whichever is the longer.

Vomiting or diarrhoea: If the patient has severe vomiting or diarrhoea, a tablet may not be absorbed properly. This may reduce contraceptive reliability. The patient should continue taking her tablets as normal. Additional non-hormonal contraceptive precautions are required until the end of the current cycle.

Bleeding whilst taking Minilyn: If the patient experiences any bleeding between periods, she should *not* stop taking Minilyn. The bleeding usually ceases in a day or two. It does not necessarily mean that contraceptive protection is lost. Some women may experience a reduced amount and/or duration of blood-loss during the withdrawal bleed.

Absence of withdrawal bleeding: Occasionally the withdrawal bleeding may fail to occur at all. Provided all tablets have been taken correctly and there is no obvious reason why reliability should be reduced e.g. drug interaction or recent episode of vomiting or diarrhoea, then pregnancy is unlikely and there is no reason to discontinue Minilyn. However, if the withdrawal bleeding had previously been regular and suddenly fails to occur, pregnancy must then be excluded. If there are any reasons to suspect pregnancy, then successive pregnancy tests may need to be performed at intervals of one week. Whilst awaiting the outcome of these tests, the patient should stop tablet-intake and use another method of non-hormonal contraception.

Caution should be observed when prescribing oral contraceptives to young women whose cycles are not yet stabilised.

Cardiovascular system: The risk of arterial thrombosis associated with combined oral contraceptives increases with age and this risk is aggravated by cigarette smoking. The use of combined oral contraceptives by women in the older age group, especially those who are cigarette smokers, should therefore be discouraged and alternative methods advised.

Since oral contraceptives may increase the risk of thrombosis they should be discontinued where possible approximately six weeks prior to elective surgery and not recommended until the patient has recovered and is mobile.

If any signs of thrombo-embolic processes occur, tablet intake must be discontinued immediately.

In the presence of severe varicose veins the benefits

of oestrogen therapy must be weighed against the possible risks.

Hepato-biliary system: There are reports indicating an association between the use of oestrogen-containing preparations and the occurrence of cholelithiasis; however contradictory findings have been reported.

Hepatic cell adenomas have been reported in women on oral contraceptive preparations. The adenoma may present itself as an abdominal mass or with the signs and symptoms of an acute abdomen. A bleeding hepatic cell adenoma, although rare, should be considered if the patient has abdominal pain or evidence of intra-abdominal bleeding.

Central nervous system: The combined oral contraceptive pill can produce headache, migraine and mood changes. In some women, frank depression may occur. In a number of these women there may be a disturbance of tryptophan metabolism and in such cases the administration of vitamin B6 might be of therapeutic value.

Skin: Chloasma is occasionally seen during the use of oral contraceptives, especially in women with a history of chloasma gravidarum. Women with a tendencey to chloasma should avoid exposure to the sun whilst taking this preparation.

Effect on laboratory tests

Thyroid function tests: The radio-iodine uptake shows that thyroid function is unchanged. There is a rise in serum protein-bound iodine, similar to that in pregnancy and during the administration of oestrogens. This is due to the increased capacity of the plasma proteins for binding thyroid hormones, rather than to any change in glandular function. In women taking oral contraceptives, the content of protein-bound iodine in the blood serum should, therefore, not be used for the evaluation of thyroid function.

ACTH function test: Oral contraceptives have no significant influence on adrenocortical function. The ACTH function test for the adrenal cortex remains unchanged. The reduction in corticosteroid excretion and the elevation of plasma corticosteroids are due to an increased cortisol-binding capacity of the plasma proteins.

Effect on erythrocyte sedimentation rate (ESR): Oral contraceptives may accelerate erythrocyte sedimentaion in the absence of any disease. This effect is due to a change in the proportion of the plasma protein fractions.

Oral contraceptive preparations may also influence the results of other laboratory tests. Increases in plasma copper, iron and alkaline phosphatase have also been recorded.

Side-effects and adverse reactions: The following side-effects and adverse reactions have been associated with either oestrogen or progestogen therapy:

Genito-urinary tract: Intermenstrual bleeding, post-pill amenorrhoea, changes in cervical secretion, increase in size of uterine leiomyomata, aggravation of endometriosis, certain vaginal infections e.g. candidiasis.

Breast: Tenderness, pain, enlargement, secretion.

Gastro-intestinal tract: Nausea, vomiting, cholelithiasis, cholestatic jaundice.

Cardiovascular system: Rise of blood pressure, phlebitis, thrombosis.

Skin: Chloasma, erythema nodosum, recurrence of herpes gestationis.

Eyes: Discomfort of the cornea if contact lenses are used.

CNS: Headache, migraine, mood changes.

Metabolic: Sodium and water retention, reduced glucose tolerance, changes in body weight.

Interactions: Irregular cycles and reduced reliability of oral contraceptives may occur when these preparations are used concomitantly with liver enzyme inducing drugs such as rifampicin, barbiturates, carbamazepine, dichloralphenazone, phenylbutazone, phenytoin, primidone, or with certain antibiotics (e.g. ampicillin or tetracyline). If no withdrawal bleeding occurs, then possible drug interactions should be considered where applicable. Pregnancy is possible and must be excluded. In such patients, the pill should be stopped immediately until pregnancy has been excluded or confirmed. During this time other forms of non-hormonal contraception should be used.

Interactions have also been reported between oral contraceptives and tricyclic antidepressants, anticoagulants and corticosteroids. Steroids affect drug metabolism and the therapeutic or toxic effects of other drugs may be modified.

The response to metyrapone is less pronounced in women receiving oral contraceptives and is similar to the response during pregnancy. This should be borne in mind if a metyrapone test is required for any reason.

Overdosage: There have been no reports of serious ill-effects from overdosage. In general, it is therefore unnecessary to treat overdosage. However, if overdosage is discovered within two or three hours and is substantial, then gastric lavage can be safely used.

There are no specific antidotes and further treatment should be symptomatic.

Pharmaceutical precautions Store in a cool, dry place and protect from light.

Legal category POM.

Package quantities Pack of 22 tablets (one month's supply).

Further information Nil.

Product licence number 0065/5041.

MIXOGEN* TABLETS

Presentation Round, white tablets, diameter 8 mm, code-marked SZ7 on one side, and Organon* on the reverse side.

Each tablet contains 4.4 micrograms Ethinyloestradiol BP and 3.6 mg Methyltestosterone BP.

Uses A combination of oestrogen and androgen which provides treatment for climacteric symptoms in women.

Dosage and administration 1–2 tablets daily. In women with an intact uterus, oestrogens should be administered cyclically (e.g., 3 weeks on, one week off).

N.B. Dosage may be adjusted according to the requirements of the individual patient.

Contra-indications, warnings, etc

Contra-indications: Pregnancy or suspected pregnancy.

Cardiovascular or cerebrovascular disorders, e.g. thrombophlebitis, thrombo-embolic processes or a history of these conditions.

Moderate to severe hypertension.

Acute or chronic liver disease or history of liver disease where the liver function tests have failed to return to normal. Jaundice or history of jaundice in pregnancy. Rotor syndrome or Dubin-Johnson syndrome. *N.B.* The use of oestrogen/androgen-containing preparations is not contra-indicated in patients with a history of hepatitis whose liver functions are normal.

Known or suspected oestrogen-dependent tumours, e.g. mammary, genital carcinoma.

Endometrial hyperplasia.

Undiagnosed vaginal bleeding.

Haemoglobinopathies e.g. sickle cell anaemia.

Porphyria.

Hyperlipoproteinaemia, especially in the presence of other risk factors which may indicate a predisposition to cardiovascular or cerbrovascular disorders.

A history during pregnancy, or previous oestrogen use, of severe pruritus, herpes gestationis or a deterioration of otosclerosis.

Precautions and warnings: Pregnancy must be excluded before treatment is started. Whenever there is a reason to suspect pregnancy during treatment, this possibility must be investigated by the physician. If pregnancy has been confirmed, tablet-intake must be discontinued immediately.

Physical examination should precede the prescribing of any oestrogen/androgen preparation and should be repeated regularly. Special attention should be paid to duration of the cycle, body weight, blood pressure, heart, breasts, pelvic organs, legs and skin.

Prolonged exposure to unopposed oestrogens may increase the risk of the development of endometrial carcinoma. Therefore, a cervical smear should be taken at regular intervals.

Oestrogen-containing preparations may increase the risk of thrombosis and this should be taken into account when surgery is to be performed in patients using these preparations. Where possible oestrogen-containing preparations should be discontinued approximately six weeks prior to elective surgery or during enforced bedrest and not recommended until the patient has recovered and is mobile.

If any signs of thrombo-embolic processes occur, tablet-intake must be discontinued immediately.

In the presence of severe varicose veins the benefits of oestrogen therapy must be weighed against the possible risks.

There are reports indicating an association between the use of oestrogen-containing preparations and the occurrence of cholelithiasis; however contradictory findings have been reported.

Tumours of the liver have been reported occasionally in patients subjected to prolonged treatment with C-17-alpha-alkylated androgenic-anabolic steroids. The possibility that these compounds may induce or enhance the development of hepatic tumours cannot at present be excluded, and this should be considered when the use of this product is proposed, especially in young people who are not suffering from life-threatening disorders.

Treatment should be discontinued if liver function tests become abnormal or cholestatic jaundice appears.

Pain in the breasts or excessive production of cervical mucus may be indicative of too high a dosage.

The use of oestrogen/androgen-containing preparations may influence the results of certain laboratory tests (e.g. thyroid function tests).

Patients, especially the elderly, with the following conditions should be monitored:

Myocardial, renal or hepatic disease, epilepsy, migraine, or asthma (or a history of these conditions) or a disease exacerbated by pregnancy, since sodium and water retention have been observed during continued use of oestrogen/androgen preparations and this may exacerbate the above conditions.

Diabetes, since oestrogen/androgens may influence glucose tolerance and change the need for insulin or other antidiabetic drugs.

Sickle cell trait, since in special conditions, e.g. during infections or anoxia, oestrogens may induce thrombo-embolic processes.

Oestrogen-sensitive gynaecological disorders, e.g. uterine fibromyomata which may increase in size, and endometriosis which may be aggravated by oestrogen treatment.

A history of hypertension; if hypertension develops, treatment should be discontinued.

Adverse reactions: The following adverse reactions have been associated with oestrogen or androgen therapy or a combination of the two:

Genito-urinary tract: Intermenstrual bleeding, endometrial proliferation, excessive production of cervical mucus, increase in size of uterine fibromyomata, aggravation of endometriosis, enlarged clitoris.

Breast: Tenderness, pain, enlargement, secretion.

Gastro-intestinal tract: Nausea, vomiting, cholelithiasis, cholestatic jaundice.

Cardiovascular system: Thrombosis, rise of blood pressure.

Skin: Erythema nodosum, rash, oily skin, acne, hirsutism.

Eyes: Discomfort of the cornea if contact lenses are used.

CNS: Headache, migraine, mood changes.

Metabolic: Sodium and water retention, reduced glucose tolerance and change in body weight.

Other: Hoarseness or deepening of the voice.

Interactions: Concurrent administration of liver enzyme inducing drugs such as rifampicin, barbiturates, carbamazepine, dichloralphenazone, phenylbutazone, phenytoin or primidone may decrease the effect of Mixogen tablets.

Overdosage: There is no specific antidote. Patients should be given appropriate supportive therapy using standard resuscitative measures as required.

Pharmaceutical precautions Protect from light.

Legal category POM.

Package quantities Bottles of 100 tablets.

Further information Combined administration of oestrogens and androgens may offer special advantages in the treatment of conditions of oestrogen deficiency. In the female, androgens are thought to oppose the action of oestrogens on the genital organs by competing for oestrogen-binding receptors.

In addition, the androgenic hormone contributes to the overall efficacy of the product by improving the sense of well-being and exerting a favourable influence on libido.

Product licence number 0065/5042.

MULTILOAD CU250* ▼

Presentation The Multiload Cu250 is an intrauterine device made of polyethylene, 3.6 cm in length, with 27 cm of copper wire 0.3 mm diameter wrapped around the stem, giving a total surface area of 250 mm² of copper. The flexible side arms ensure that the Multiload Cu250 remains in position as high as is possible against the fundus without the uterine cavity being stretched in any way. The device is preloaded in its inserter and a monofilament nylon thread is attached to the stem.

Uses Intrauterine contraception.

Method of insertion Although IUD's may be inserted at any time during the menstrual cycle, insertion during or shortly after the menstrual period reduces the possibility of an existing undiagnosed pregnancy. In the case of nulliparous women it may be of advantage to have it fitted during menstruation.

Multiload Cu250 may be inserted immediately (no later than 15 minutes) post-abortion or post-placenta. If the device is not inserted immediately post-abortion or post-placenta, insertion should be delayed until at least 6 weeks after delivery or abortion (delayed post-partum insertion).

The Multiload Cu250 is suitable for both multiparous and nulliparous patients (however, see following procedure for inserting the Multiload Cu250). Pain during and after insertion is more likely to occur in nulliparous than in multiparous women. An expeller is not necessary.

It is imperative that a sterile no-touch technique is employed throughout the insertion procedure.

It is recommended that the Multiload Cu250 be replaced every three years.

Recommended insertion procedure
Preparation

1. Perform a careful bimanual examination to determine the version, flexion axis and other aspects of the uterus.
2. Insert a bivalve speculum to expose the cervix. Cleanse the cervix and vaginal walls with sterile cotton wool dipped in antiseptic solution. Wipe all secretion away from the external os.
3. Grasp the anterior lip of the cervix with a single-tooth tenaculum, taking a good bite through the cervical lip so that *steady downward traction to straighten the uterine axis* can be maintained without risk of cervical laceration.
   Reflex contraction, which causes cramp of the uterus when the tenaculum is applied, can be prevented by injection of a local anaesthetic into the anterior lip or a paracervical block.
4. Carefully sound the uterus to determine its depth and to confirm the direction of its axis. If the sound meets more than normal resistance at the internal os, it may be advisable to gently dilate the cervical canal to 4–5 mm, using sterile, tapered rather than cylindrical dilators. In the absence of other instruments for measurement of the internal dimensions of the uterine cavity, the sound may be used to obtain an idea of its configuration.

Inserting the Multiload Cu250

1. Lay the Multiload pack on a flat surface. Strip the wrapping from the Multiload by lifting the transparent front sheet of the pack from the distal end.
2. The vertical stem of the Multiload is already preloaded in the introducer tube. The side arms do not require loading into the tube. They are sufficiently flexible to adapt to the shape of the cervical canal.
3. Pick up the introducer tube (with pre-loaded IUD) grasping the tube at the indentation near its distal end and move the cervical stop to the numbered mark corresponding to the sounded length in cm.
4. Lift the introducer tube (with pre-loaded IUD) from

its tray. The distal end of the introducer tube may be held without risk of contaminating the device. Hold the introducer tube and pre-loaded IUD upwards, so that the IUD does not fall from the tube.

5. Carefully insert the Multiload into the uterus until it touches the fundus and the cervical stop rests against the external os while *maintaining steady downward traction with the tenaculum to straighten the uterine axis.* No attempt should be made to force insertion.
6. When the Multiload touches the fundus, it is released into the uterine cavity by simply withdrawing the introducer tube. During this procedure continue to apply downward traction with the tenaculum. No push-rod is required to insert the Multiload. Check the cervical canal with the sound to ensure that the tail of the Multiload is entirely within the uterine cavity. Trim the threads of the Multiload to 2 to 3 cm measured from the external os.

Immediate post-placental insertion

1. Insert a bivalve speculum to expose the cervix after delivery of the placenta and membranes (no later than 15 minutes). Cleanse the cervix and vaginal walls with sterile cotton wool dipped in antiseptic solution.
2. Grasp both the anterior and the posterior lips with one or two ring forceps and draw the cervix down for close inspection.
3. Take the introducer tube (with pre-loaded IUD) and insert the Multiload along the palmar aspect of two fingers into the uterine cavity until it touches the fundus. Check the position of the Multiload with the flat hand on the abdominal wall covering the fundal region.
4. When the Multiload touches the fundus, it is released into the uterine cavity by very gentle withdrawal of the inserter tube. Take care not to pull on the threads which are left uncut until the first follow-up visit.

Removal procedure

Prepare the vulva, insert the speculum, cleanse the cervix and *straighten the uterine axis* with the tenaculum as for insertion.

Use a forceps to grasp both threads of the Multiload as near to their exit from the external os as possible. Steady traction should easily withdraw the Multiload from the uterus.

Contra-indications, warnings, etc
Contra-indications

Absolute: Pregnancy or suspected pregnancy, history of ectopic pregnancy.

Congenital or acquired abnormalities of the uterine cavity or cervical canal

Pelvic inflammatory disease either pre-existing or in a patient with a history of such conditions including: cervicitis, acute or sub-acute salpingitis, and endometritis or infected abortion in the past three months.

Suspected or proven carcinoma of the cervix or endometrium, including unresolved abnormal cervical smear or cervical dysplasia.

Dysfunctional uterine bleeding.

Use with organic mercurial pessaries.

Wilson's Disease or hypersensitivity to copper.

Relative: Uterine polyps or fibroids.

Disturbance of the blood clotting mechanism.

Severe anaemia.

Previous Caesarean section, uterine incision or perforation.

Patients receiving anticoagulants, steroids or non-steroidal anti-inflammatory drugs.

Use during breast feeding:
The Multiload Cu250 may be used during breast feeding.

Precautions and warnings: Every potential IUD user should be fully informed of the risks and benefits of IUDs and how these may affect them.

The patient should always be given a copy of the leaflet contained in the pack which explains the importance of seeking medical advice in the very unlikely event of pregnancy or if complications occur.

The patient should be advised to contact her doctor immediately if she misses a menstrual period or has any other reason to think she may be pregnant or if any signs or symptoms of a genito-urinary infection appear.

As with all IUDs, the patient must be left in no doubt about the very slight chance of pregnancy.

Prior to insertion of an IUD a thorough history and physical examination, including a pelvic examination and Papanicolaou smear, should be performed. After insertion the patient should be taught to examine herself to confirm the presence of the thread.

The patient should be re-examined within three months after insertion or within a month after immediate post-placental insertion and thereafter at regular intervals. If the retrieval thread is not visible at the cervix on follow-up examination, it may have been drawn up into the uterus or cervical canal and may reappear during the next menstrual period. If it cannot be found, it may have broken off, or the device may have perforated or been expelled. Ultrasound or X-ray may be used to locate the device. If partial expulsion occurs, removal is indicated and another Multiload may be inserted.

Intrauterine devices should be used with caution in women with anaemia.

Medical diathermy (shortwave and microwave) of the abdominal and sacral areas should be applied with caution as it may induce heat injuries because of the presence of metallic copper on the IUD.

If pelvic infection occurs which is unresponsive to treatment, the Multiload Cu250 should be removed. An increased incidence of pelvic inflammatory disease and menorrhagia associated with the use of IUDs has been reported. Pelvic infection may result in future infertility.

Use of an IUD in women with valvular or congenital heart disease represents a potential source of septic emboli. Appropriate antibiotic cover should be given three days prior to, and for at least ten days after insertion, in patients with a past history of rheumatic fever and certain known or suspected cardiac abnormalities, in order to preclude the possibility of precipitating subacute bacterial endocarditis.

Pain during and after insertion is more likely to occur in nulliparous than in multiparous women.

After insertion some women are troubled by uterine cramp. Syncope, bradycardia and other neuro-vascular episodes may occur during or immediately after insertion or removal of IUDs. Intermittent bleeding, prolongation of menstruation and an increase in menstrual blood loss are to be expected, especially during the first two or three cycles.

The possibility of a seizure being precipitated in a patient suffering from epilepsy during, or shortly after, the insertion of an IUD, should be borne in mind.

Uterine or cervical perforation, embedment and allergic reactions have also been reported.

Pregnancy: If pregnancy occurs with a Multiload Cu250 in situ and the thread is visible, then as with all IUDs the device should be removed. If the thread is not visible or device removal would be difficult, the patient should be investigated by a specialist. Patients who are pregnant with an IUD in situ should be closely observed and told to report immediately all abnormal symptoms such as 'flu-like' symptoms, fever, cramping pain, bleeding or excesive discharge, as the onset of septicaemia associated with septic abortion may be insidious with general symptoms rather than initial signs of spontaneous abortion. It has been demonstrated that the presence of an IUD in a pregnant uterus increases the risk of abortion and sepsis.

The long-term effects of intrauterine copper on the foetus are unknown.

The risk of ectopic pregnancy is reported to be greater in women who conceive with an IUD in situ than in those without an IUD. Therefore, if a patient becomes pregnant with a Multiload Cu250 in situ, she should be carefully evaluated for possible ectopic pregnancy.

Reasons for removal: Pregnancy (see above).

Pelvic inflammatory disease (see Precautions and Warnings).

Excessive and persistent bleeding or cramping.

Perforation of the uterus or uterine wall. This is extremely rare with Multiload Cu250 but if it should happen, the IUD should be removed.

Partial downward displacement of the device into the cervical canal.

Translocation of stemmed IUDs may occur after immediate post-placental insertion. If translocation occurs, the IUD should be removed.

Pharmaceutical precautions The Multiload Cu250 is supplied sterile in a peel-open pouch, which should not be opened until required for insertion. Aseptic precautions should be carried out when handling the device. Care should be taken to ensure that the sterile packages are not damaged; they should be stored in cool dry conditions.

Legal category POM.

Package quantities 1 outer package containing 10 Multiload Cu250.

10 inner packs each containing 1 Multiload Cu250 ready for immediate use and fitted with a disposable inserter.

Further information The Multiload Cu250 can be regarded as a third generation IUD. As a result of its special shape the Multiload Cu250 represents a breakaway from the principle that IUDs must be firmly embedded into the uterine cavity in order to prevent expulsion.

Contractions of the uterus are cushioned by the wide upper end of the Multiload Cu250, resulting in flexure of the side arms which are designed to prevent expulsion.

In addition, with 250 mm² of copper wound around the vertical stem a very low pregnancy rate is obtained without using a maximum surface area.

The ability to become pregnant is normally restored a short time after removal of the Multiload Cu250.

The amount of copper eluted from copper IUDs is well below the daily dietary intake of copper. No changes in blood levels of copper have been detected.

There is a tendency for small quantities of calcium to form a sediment on the surface of all IUDs.

Product licence number 0065/0062.

MULTILOAD CU250* SHORT ▼

Presentation The Multiload Cu250 SHORT is an intrauterine device made of polyethylene, 2.5 cm in length with 21 cm of copper wire 0.4 mm diameter wrapped around the stem, giving a total surface area of 250 mm^2 of copper. The flexible side arms ensure that the Multiload Cu250 SHORT remains in position as high as is possible against the fundus without the uterine cavity being stretched in any way. The device is preloaded in its inserter and a monofilament nylon thread is attached to the stem.

Uses Intrauterine contraception.

Method of insertion Although IUDs may be inserted at any time during the menstrual cycle, insertion during or shortly after the menstrual period reduces the possibility of an existing undiagnosed pregnancy. In the case of nulliparous women it may be of advantage to have it fitted during menstruation.

Multiload Cu250 SHORT may be inserted immediately (no later than 15 minutes) post-abortion or post-placenta. If the device is not inserted immediately post-abortion or post-placenta, insertion should be delayed until at least 6 weeks after delivery or abortion (delayed post-partum insertion).

The Multiload Cu250 SHORT is suitable for both multiparous and nulliparous patients having a uterine sound length between 5 cm and 7 cm (however, see following procedure for inserting the Multiload Cu250 SHORT). Pain during and after insertion is more likely to occur in nulliparous than in multiparous women. An expeller is not necessary.

It is imperative that a sterile no-touch technique is employed throughout the insertion procedure.

It is recommended that the Multiload Cu250 SHORT be replaced every three years.

Recommended insertion procedure
Preparation
1. Perform a careful bimanual examination to determine the version, flexion axis and other aspects of the uterus.
2. Insert a bivalve speculum to expose the cervix. Cleanse the cervix and vaginal walls with sterile cotton wool dipped in antiseptic solution. Wipe all secretion away from the external os.
3. Grasp the anterior lip of the cervix with a single-tooth tenaculum, taking a good bite through the cervical lip so that *steady downward traction to straighten the uterine axis* can be maintained without risk of cervical laceration.

Reflex contraction, which causes cramp of the uterus when the tenaculum is applied, can be prevented by injection of a local anaesthetic into the anterior lip or a paracervical block.
4. Carefully sound the uterus to determine its depth and to confirm the direction of its axis. If the sound meets more than normal resistance at the internal os, it may be advisable to gently dilate the cervical canal to 4–5 mm, using sterile, tapered rather than cylindrical dilators. In the absence of other instruments for measurement of the internal dimensions of the uterine cavity, the sound may be used to obtain an idea of its configuration.

Inserting the Multiload Cu250 SHORT
1. Lay the Multiload Cu250 SHORT pack on a flat surface. Strip the wrapping from the Multiload Cu250 SHORT by lifting the transparent front sheet of the pack from the distal end.
2. The vertical stem of the Multiload Cu250 SHORT is already preloaded in the introducer tube. The side arms

do not require loading into the tube. They are sufficiently flexible to adapt to the shape of the cervical canal.
3. Pick up the introducer tube (with pre-loaded IUD) grasping the tube at the indentation near its distal end and move the cervical stop to the numbered mark corresponding to the sounded length in cm.
4. Lift the introducer tube (with pre-loaded IUD) from its tray. The distal end of the introducer tube may be held without risk of contaminating the device. Hold the introducer tube and pre-loaded IUD upwards, so that the IUD does not fall from the tube.
5. Carefully insert the Multiload Cu250 SHORT into the uterus until it touches the fundus and the cervical stop rests against the external os while *maintaining steady downward traction with the tenaculum to straighten the uterine axis.* No attempt should be made to force insertion.
6. When the Multiload Cu250 SHORT touches the fundus, it is released into the uterine cavity by simply withdrawing the introducer tube. During this procedure continue to apply downward traction with the tenaculum. No push-rod is required to insert the Multiload Cu250 SHORT. Check the cervical canal with the sound to ensure that the tail of the Multiload Cu250 SHORT is entirely within the uterine cavity. Trim the threads of the Multiload Cu250 SHORT to 2 to 3 cm measured from the external os.

Immediate post-placental insertion
1. Insert a bivalve speculum to expose the cervix after delivery of the placenta and membranes (no later than 15 minutes). Cleanse the cervix and vaginal walls with sterile cotton wool dipped in antiseptic solution.
2. Grasp both the anterior and the posterior lips with one or two ring forceps and draw the cervix down for close inspection.
3. Take the introducer tube (with pre-loaded IUD) and insert the Multiload Cu250 SHORT along the palmar aspect of two fingers into the uterine cavity until it touches the fundus. Check the position of the Multiload Cu250 SHORT with the flat hand on the abdominal wall covering the fundal region.
4. When the Multiload Cu250 SHORT touches the fundus, it is released into the uterine cavity by very gentle withdrawal of the inserter tube. Take care not to pull on the threads which are left uncut until the first follow-up visit.

Removal procedure
Prepare the vulva, insert the speculum, cleanse the cervix and *straighten the uterine axis* with the tenaculum as for insertion.

Use a forceps to grasp both threads of the Multiload Cu250 SHORT as near to their exit from the external os as possible. Steady traction should easily withdraw the Multiload Cu250 SHORT from the uterus.

Contra-indications, warnings, etc
Contra-indications
Absolute: Pregnancy or suspected pregnancy, history of ectopic pregnancy.

Congenital or acquired abnormalities of the uterine cavity or cervical canal

Pelvic inflammatory disease either pre-existing or in a patient with a history of such conditions including: cervicitis, acute or sub-acute salpingitis, and endometritis or infected abortion in the past three months.

Suspected or proven carcinoma of the cervix or endometrium, including unresolved abnormal cervical smear or cervical dysplasia.

Dysfunctional uterine bleeding.

Use with organic mercurial pessaries.

Wilson's Disease or hypersensitivity to copper.

Relative: Uterine polyps or fibroids.

Disturbance of the blood clotting mechanism.

Severe anaemia.

Previous Caesarean section, uterine incision or perforation.

Patients receiving anticoagulants, steroids or nonsteroidal anti-inflammatory drugs.

Use during breast feeding:

The Multiload Cu250 SHORT may be used during breast feeding.

Precautions and warnings: Every potential IUD user should be fully informed of the risks and benefits of IUDs and how these may affect them.

The patient should always be given a copy of the leaflet contained in the pack which explains the importance of seeking medical advice in the very unlikely event of pregnancy or if complications occur.

The patient should be advised to contact her doctor immediately if she misses a menstrual period or has any other reason to think she may be pregnant or if any signs or symptoms of a genito-urinary infection appear.

As with all IUDs, the patient must be left in no doubt about the very slight chance of pregnancy.

Prior to insertion of an IUD a thorough history and physical examination, including a pelvic examination and Papanicolaou smear, should be performed. After insertion the patient should be taught to examine herself to confirm the presence of the thread.

The patient should be re-examined within three months after insertion or within a month after immediate post-placental insertion and thereafter at regular intervals. If the retrieval thread is not visible at the cervix on follow-up examination, it may have been drawn up into the uterus or cervical canal and may reappear during the next menstrual period. If it cannot be found, it may have broken off, or the device may have perforated or been expelled. Ultrasound or X-ray may be used to locate the device. If partial expulsion occurs, removal is indicated and another Multiload may be inserted.

Intrauterine devices should be used with caution in women with anaemia.

Medical diathermy (shortwave or microwave) of the abdominal and sacral areas should be applied with caution as it may induce heat injuries because of the presence of metallic copper on the IUD.

If pelvic infection occurs which is unresponsive to treatment, the Multiload CU250 SHORT should be removed. An increased incidence of pelvic inflammatory disease and menorrhagia associated with the use of IUDs has been reported. Pelvic infection may result in future infertility.

Use of an IUD in women with valvular or congenital heart disease represents a potential source of septic emboli. Appropriate antibiotic cover should be given three days prior to, and for at least ten days after insertion, in patients with a past history of rheumatic fever and certain known or suspected cardiac abnormalities, in order to preclude the possibility of precipitating subacute bacterial endocarditis.

Pain during and after insertion is more likely to occur in nulliparous than in multiparous women.

After insertion some women are troubled by uterine cramp. Syncope, bradycardia and other neuro-vascular episodes may occur during or immediately after insertion or removal of IUDs. Intermittent bleeding, prolongation of menstruation and an increase in menstrual blood loss are to be expected, especially during the first two or three cycles.

The possibility of a seizure being precipitated in a patient suffering from epilepsy during, or shortly after, the insertion of an IUD, should be borne in mind.

Uterine or cervical perforation, embedment and allergic reactions have also been reported.

Pregnancy: If pregnancy occurs with a Multiload Cu250 SHORT in situ and the thread is visible, then as with all IUDs the device should be removed. If the thread is not visible or device removal would be difficult, the patient should be investigated by a specialist. Patients who are pregnant with an IUD in situ should be closely observed and told to report immediately all abnormal symptoms such as 'flu-like' symptoms, fever, cramping pain, bleeding or excessive discharge, as the onset of septicaemia associated with septic abortion may be insidious with general symptoms rather than initial signs of spontaneous abortion. It has been demonstrated that the presence of an IUD in a pregnant uterus increases the risk of abortion and sepsis.

The long-term effects of intrauterine copper on the foetus are unknown.

The risk of ectopic pregnancy is reported to be greater in women who conceive with an IUD in situ than in those without an IUD. Therefore, if a patient becomes pregnant with a Multiload Cu250 SHORT in situ, she should be carefully evaluated for possible ectopic pregnancy.

Reasons for removal: Pregnancy (see above).

Pelvic inflammatory disease (see Precautions and Warnings).

Excessive and persistent bleeding or cramping.

Perforation of the uterus or uterine wall. This is extremely rare with Multiload Cu250 SHORT but, if it should happen, the IUD should be removed.

Partial downward displacement of the device into the cervical canal.

Translocation of stemmed IUDs may occur after immediate post-placental insertion. If translocation occurs, the IUD should be removed.

Pharmaceutical precautions The Multiload Cu250 SHORT is supplied sterile in a peel-open pouch, which should not be opened until required for insertion. Aseptic precautions should be carried out when handling the device. Care should be taken to ensure that the sterile packages are not damaged; they should be stored in cool dry conditions.

Legal category POM.

Package quantities 1 outer package containing 10 Multiload Cu250 SHORT.

10 inner packs each containing 1 Multiload Cu250 SHORT ready for immediate use and fitted with a disposable inserter.

Further information The Multiload Cu250 SHORT can be regarded as a third generation IUD. As a result of its special shape the Multiload Cu250 SHORT represents a breakaway from the principle that IUDs must be firmly embedded into the uterine cavity in order to prevent expulsion.

Contractions of the uterus are cushioned by the wide upper end of the Multiload Cu250 SHORT, resulting in flexure of the side arms which are designed to prevent expulsion.

In addition, with 250 mm^2 of copper wound around

the vertical stem a very low pregnancy rate is obtained without using a maximum surface area.

The ability to become pregnant is normally restored a short time after removal of the Multiload Cu250 SHORT.

The amount of copper eluted from copper IUDs is well below the daily dietary intake of copper. No changes in blood levels of copper have been detected.

There is a tendency for small quantities of calcium to form a sediment on the surface of all IUDs.

Product licence number 0065/0075.

OESTRADIOL IMPLANTS (Organon)

Presentation Pellets of fused, crystalline oestradiol for implantation. Each pellet contains either 25 mg, 50 mg, or 100 mg of Oestradiol.

The 25 mg weight has a diameter of 2.2 mm and the 50 mg and 100 mg weights have a diameter of 4.5 mm.

Uses Indicated in females for long-term treatment requiring oestrogen replacement e.g. climacteric symptoms.

Dosage and administration 25–100 mg.

Frequency of replacement depends on the duration of activity of the implants administered and the severity of the symptoms. Patients require a further implant when symptoms return, usually every 4 to 8 months.

Oestradiol Implants should be inserted subcutaneously (either by means of a trocar and cannula or by open surgery), into an area where there is comparatively little movement, such as the lower abdominal wall or the buttock. Insertion is made under local anaesthesia and the wound closed either with an adhesive dressing or a fine suture.

Precautions should be taken to avoid the formation of a haematoma at the site by inserting the implant into the subcutaneous fatty layer of the abdominal wall.

Full aseptic 'no-touch' technique should be adopted.

Because of the sustained absorption, the endometrium is liable to progressive hypertrophy. For this reason, where the uterus is intact, a cyclically administered oral progestogen for 7 to 13 days in each calendar month is necessary to prevent endometrial hyperplasia.

Contra-indications, warnings, etc

Contra-indications: Pregnancy or suspected pregnancy.

Cardiovascular or cerebrovascular disorders, e.g. thrombophlebitis, thrombo-embolic processes or a history of these conditions.

Moderate to severe hypertension.

Acute or chronic liver disease or history of liver disease where the liver function tests have failed to return to normal. Jaundice or history of jaundice in pregnancy. Rotor syndrome or Dubin-Johnson syndrome. *N.B.* The use of oestrogens is not contra-indicated in patients with a history of hepatitis whose liver functions are normal.

Known or suspected oestrogen-dependent tumours, e.g. mammary, genital carcinoma.

Endometrial hyperplasia.

Undiagnosed vaginal bleeding.

Haemoglobinopathies e.g. sickle cell anaemia.

Porphyria.

Hyperlipoproteinaemia, especially in the presence of other risk factors which may indicate a predisposition to cardiovascular or cerebrovascular disorders.

A history during pregnancy or previous oestrogen use of severe pruritus, herpes gestationis or a deterioration of otosclerosis.

Precautions and warnings: Pregnancy must be excluded before treatment is started. Whenever there is a reason to suspect pregnancy during treatment, this possibility must be investigated by the physician. If pregnancy has been confirmed, the implant must be removed immediately.

Physical examination should precede the prescribing of any oestrogen and should be repeated regularly. Special attention should be paid to duration of the cycle, body weight, blood pressure, heart, breasts, pelvic organs, legs and skin.

Prolonged exposure to unopposed oestrogens may increase the risk of the development of endometrial carcinoma. Therefore a cervical smear should be taken at regular intervals.

Oestrogen preparations may increase the risk of thrombosis and this should be taken into account when surgery is to be performed. Where possible, oestrogen preparations should be discontinued approximately six weeks prior to elective surgery or during enforced bedrest and not recommenced until the patient has recovered and is mobile.

If any signs of thrombo-embolic processes occur, the implant must be removed immediately.

In the presence of severe varicose veins the benefits of oestrogen therapy must be weighed against the possible risks.

There are reports indicating an association between the use of oestrogen-containing preparations and the occurrence of cholelithiasis; however contradictory findings have been reported.

Treatment should be discontinued if liver function tests become abnormal or cholestatic jaundice appears.

Pain in the breasts or excessive production of cervical mucus may be indicative of too high a dosage.

The use of oestrogen preparations may influence the results of certain laboratory tests (e.g. thyroid function tests).

Patients, especially the elderly, with the following conditions should be monitored:

Myocardial, renal or hepatic disease, epilepsy migraine, or asthma (or a history of these conditions), or a disease exacerbated by pregnancy, since sodium and water retention have been observed during continued use of oestrogen/androgen preparations and this may exacerbate the above conditions.

Diabetes, since oestrogens may influence the glucose tolerance and change the need for insulin or other antidiabetic drugs.

Sickle cell trait, since in special conditions, e.g. during infections or anoxia, oestrogen-containing preparations may induce thrombo-embolic processes.

Oestrogen-sensitive gynaecological disorders, e.g. uterine fibromyomata which may increase in size and endometriosis which may be aggravated by oestrogen treatment.

A history of hypertension; if hypertension develops the implant should be removed.

Incomplete statural growth, since oestrogens in high dosages may accelerate epiphyseal closure.

Hypernephroma, bronchial carcinoma and skeletal metastases, since these conditions may produce hypercalcaemia or hypercalciuria which may in turn be exacerbated by oestrogen therapy. If hypercalcaemia or hypercalciuria develops the implant should be removed.

Adverse reactions: The following adverse reactions have been associated with oestrogen therapy:

Genito-urinary tract: Intermenstrual bleeding, endometrial proliferation, excessive production of cervical mucus, increase in size of uterine fibromyomata, aggravation of endometriosis.

Breast: Tenderness, pain, enlargement, secretion.

Gastro-intestinal tract: Nausea, vomiting, cholelithiasis, cholestatic jaundice.

Cardiovascular system: Thrombosis, rise of blood pressure.

Skin: Erythema nodosum, rash.

Eyes: Discomfort of the cornea if contact lenses are used.

CNS: Headache, migraine, mood changes.

Metabolic: Sodium and water retention, reduced glucose tolerance, premature epiphyseal closure, and change in body weight.

When high dosages and prolonged treatment are necessary, e.g. in the management of mammary and prostatic carcinoma, psychotic disturbances may occur. Additionally, gynaecomastia, reduced libido, impotence and disturbances of spermatogenesis may occur in male patients.

Interactions: Concurrent administration of liver enzyme inducing drugs such as rifampicin, barbiturates, carbamazepine, dichloralphenazone, phenylbutazone, phenytoin or primidone may decrease the effect of Oestradiol Implants.

Pharmaceutical precautions Protect from light.

Legal category POM.

Package quantities Each sterile implant is supplied singly, in a sealed glass tube, available in the following weights: 25 mg, 50 mg, and 100 mg.

Further information Implantation of fused implants of oestradiol provides a slow release of the hormone. A 2.2 mm diameter trocar and cannular should be used to introduce the 25 mg Oestradiol Implant and a 4.5 mm trocar and cannula should be used to introduce either a 50 mg or 100 mg Oestradiol Implant. On each occasion before reuse it is important to sterilise the trocar and cannula set by washing and subsequent heat sterilisation. This may be carried out by boiling in water for 30 minutes or through the use of an autoclave.

Product licence numbers   25 mg   0065/5074
                              50 mg   0065/5075
                             100 mg   0065/5076

ORABOLIN*

Presentation Round, flat, white tablets, diameter 9 mm, code-marked 'SB3' on one side, with 'Organon' and a star on the reverse side. Each tablet contains 2 mg Ethyloestrenol BP.

Uses Orabolin is an orally active protein-anabolic preparation.

Indications: During chronic debilitating diseases, particularly in elderly patients; after major surgery; cases of anorexia, weight loss and poor general condition such as cachexia, in which causal treatment or dietary measures alone proved unsatisfactory.

Dosage and administration
Adults: 1–2 tablets daily. N.B. For an optimal therapeutic effect, it is necessary to administer adequate amounts of vitamins, minerals and protein in a calorie-rich diet.

The duration of treatment will depend on the response.

If after 4 weeks no beneficial effect is observed, treatment should be discontinued.

Contra-indications, warnings, etc
Contra-indications: Pregnancy.
   Known or suspected prostatic or mammary carcinoma in the male.
   Abnormal liver function.

Precautions and warnings: The recommended dosages should not be exceeded.

If signs of virilization develop, treatment should be discontinued.

Caution should be exercised in young women whose cycles are not yet stabilised.

Treatment should be discontinued if liver function tests become abnormal or cholestatic jaundice appears.

Tumours of the liver have been reported occasionally in patients subjected to prolonged treatment with C-17 alpha-alkylated androgenic-anabolic steroids. The possibility that these compounds may induce or enhance the development of hepatic tumours cannot at present be excluded and this should be considered when the use of this product is proposed especially in young people who are not suffering from life-threatening disorders.

Patients, especially the elderly, with the following conditions should be monitored: Latent or overt cardiac failure, renal dysfunction, hypertension, epilepsy or migraine (or a history of these conditions), since anabolic steroids may occasionally induce sodium and water retention; this precaution particularly applies to the elderly patient.

Diabetes, or latent diabetes, since anabolic steroids may improve the glucose tolerance and decrease the need for insulin or other antidiabetic drugs.

Incomplete statural growth, since anabolic steroids in high dosages may accelerate epiphyseal closure.

Hypernephroma, bronchial carcinoma, and skeletal metastases, since these conditions may produce hypercalcaemia or hypercalciuria which may in turn be exacerbated by androgen therapy. If hypercalcaemia or hypercalciuria develops treatment should be discontinued.

Adverse reactions: Orabolin at the recommended dosages is unlikely to cause virilising effects.

High dosages and/or prolonged treatment may cause: Virilisation, which appears in sensitive women as hoarseness, acne, hirsutism and increase of libido; in prepubertal boys as an increased frequency of erections and phallic enlargement, and in girls as an increase of pubic hair and clitoral hypertrophy. Hoarseness may be the first symptom of vocal change which may end in a long-lasting, sometimes irreversible deepening of the voice.

Amenorrhoea and inhibition of spermatogenesis.

Premature epiphyseal closure.

Sodium and water retention.

Nausea.

Occasionally, abnormal values in some liver function tests. These changes appear to be reversible after discontinuation of the treatment.

Interactions: C-17 alpha-alkylated anabolic steroids have been reported to potentiate the action of oral anticoagulants. This interaction has not been reported with Orabolin. However, this should be borne in mind when Orabolin is administered concomitantly with oral anticoagulants, in which case reduction of the anticoagulant dosage may be necessary.

Pharmaceutical precautions Protect from light.

Legal category POM.

Package quantities Bottles of 100 tablets.

Further information Metabolic studies have shown positive effects on protein metabolism, a nitrogen saving and anticatabolic action. Orabolin can be used as an adjuvant in the treatment of conditions characterised by a negative nitrogen balance.

Product licence number 0065/5043.

ORADEXON-ORGANON* INJECTION

Presentation A clear aqueous solution for injection, available as 1 ml ampoules containing dexamethasone sodium phosphate 5 mg per ml, and as 2 ml vials containing the equivalent of 4 mg dexamethasone per ml. (5 mg/ml dexamethasone sodium phosphate is approximately equivalent to 4 mg/ml dexamethasone).

Uses Oradexon-Organon can be used for all forms of general and local glucocorticoid injection therapy and all acute conditions in which intravenous glucocorticoids may be life-saving.

Dosage and administration
N.B. All dosages are expressed as mg dexamethasone sodium phosphate.

In general, glucocorticoid dosage depends on the severity of the condition and response of the patient. Under certain circumstances, for instance in stress, extra dosage adjustments may be necessary. If no favourable response is noted within a couple of days, glucocorticoid therapy should be discontinued.

Adults: Once the disease is under control the dosage should be reduced or tapered off to the lowest suitable level under continuous monitoring and observation of the patient. This should be done by giving one early morning dose, daily (or preferably every other morning), of an oral glucocorticoid with a shorter biological half-life than dexamethasone e.g. prednisolone.

For acute life-threatening situations (e.g. anaphylaxis, acute severe asthma) substantially higher dosages may be needed. Cerebral oedema (adults): initial dose 10–20 mg IV followed by 6 mg IV or IM every 6 hours, until a satisfactory result has been obtained. In brain surgery these dosages may be necessary until several days after the operation. Thereafter, the dosage has to be tapered off gradually. Increase of intracranial pressure associated with brain tumours can be counteracted by continuous treatment.

For local treatment, the following dosages can be recommended:
Intra-articularly: 2–4 mg large joints, 0.8–1 mg small joints;
Intrabursally: 2–4 mg; in tendon sheaths: 0.4–1 mg. The frequency of these injections may vary from every 3–5 days to every 2–3 weeks.

For rectal drip in cases of ulcerative colitis: 5 mg diluted in 120 ml saline.

Suggested doses for children: Dosage requirements are variable and may have to be changed according to individual needs. Usually 0.25 mg/kg to 0.50 mg/kg of body weight daily.

Administration: Oradexon-Organon may be administered intravenously, subcutaneously, intramuscularly, by local injection or as a rectal drip. For administration by intravenous infusion: see section on compatibility with infusion fluids. With intravenous administration high plasma levels can be obtained rapidly.

Rapid intravenous injection of massive doses of glucocorticoids may sometimes cause cardiovascular collapse; the injection should therefore be given slowly over a period of several minutes.

Intra-articular injections should be given under strictly aseptic conditions.

Discontinuation of prolonged therapy should be carried out by gradual reduction of dosage and under strict medical supervision, since withdrawal may result in acute exacerbation of the disease, acute adrenocortical insufficiency and polyarteritis.

Use with infusion fluids: Oradexon-Oraganon has been shown to retain its potency for at least 24 hours at room temperature, and in daylight conditions, when diluted with one of the following infusion fluids:
Sodium chloride 0.9%
Anhydrous glucose 5%
Invert sugar 10%
Sorbitol 5%
Ringer's solution
Hartmann's solution (Ringer-lactate)
Rheomacrodex
Haemaccel

Using these infusion fluids, Oradexon-Organon can also be injected directly into the infusion line without causing precipitation of the ingredients. Direct injection into the infusion line is also possible with the following infusion fluids:
Mannitol 10%
Vamin N

Contra-indications, warnings, etc
Contra-indications: No contraindications exist when glucocorticoids, in a large single dose, are used in conditions where life is endangered.

Systemic glucocorticoids are generally contraindicated in patients with Cushing's Syndrome, gastrointestinal ulcers, glaucoma, hypersensitivity to glucocorticoids, systemic fungal infections or certain viral infections, e.g. varicella and herpes genitalis and ocular herpes infections, active tuberculosis and acute psychosis.

Local injection of a glucocorticoid is contraindicated in bacteraemia, and systemic fungal infections, unstable joints, hypersensitivity to glucocorticoids, and infections at the injection site e.g. septic arthritis resulting from gonorrhoea or tuberculosis.

Precautions and warnings: Patients, especially the elderly, with the following conditions should be monitored: Latent or overt cardiac failure, renal dysfunction, hypertension, epilepsy or migraine, since glucocorticoids may induce fluid retention.

Osteoporosis, since glucocorticoids have a negative effect on the calcium balance.

A history of psychotic illness.

Latent tuberculosis, since glucocorticoids may induce reactivation.

Certain parasitic infestations, in particular amoebiasis.

Incomplete statural growth, since glucocorticoids on prolonged administration may accelerate epiphyseal closure.

Glucocorticoid therapy is non-specific, suppresses the symptoms and signs of disease and decreases the resistance to infections. Appropriate antimicrobial therapy should accompany glucocorticoid therapy when necessary, e.g. in tuberculosis, and viral and fungal infections of the eye.

If a live vaccine is to be administered it should be borne in mind that glucocorticoids exert an immunosuppressive effect.

Patients on long-term glucocorticoid therapy should be regularly examined for increased intra-ocular pressure and posterior subcapsular cataracts.

Patients on long-term glucocorticoid therapy should be regularly examined with respect to their glucose metabolism.

Before, during and after stressful situations, dosage may need to be increased in patients currently on glucocorticoids or resumed in patients who have undergone prolonged glucocorticoid treatment in the previous year.

Local injection of a glucocorticoid may produce systemic effects.

After parenteral administration of glucocorticoids serious anaphylactoid reactions, such as glottis oedema, urticaria, and bronchospasm, have occasionally occurred, particularly in patients with a history of allergy. If such an anaphylactoid reaction occurs, the following measures are recommended: immediate slow intravenous injection of 0.1–0.5 ml of adrenaline (solution of 1:1000, 0.1–0.5 mg adrenaline dependent on body weight), intravenous administration of aminophylline and artificial respiration if necessary.

Cases of ruptured tendon have been reported following the injection of glucocorticoids directly into a tendon. In the treatment of conditions such as tendinitis or tenosynovitis care should be taken to inject into the space between the tendon sheath and the tendon.

Use during pregnancy and breast feeding: During pregnancy, the benefits of the use of glucocorticoids should be weighed against the possible hazards to the mother or foetus. Infants whose mothers received substantial doses of glucocorticoids during pregnancy should be carefully observed for signs of adrenal insufficiency.

Glucocorticoids appear in breast milk in very small quantities. Mothers taking high doses of glucocorticoids should be advised not to breast-feed.

Adverse reactions: Adverse reactions associated with prolonged systemic glucocorticoid therapy are unlikely when high doses are administered over a short period of time. Nevertheless, gastric and duodenal ulceration, with possible perforation and haemorrhage, may occasionally occur.

The following adverse reactions have been associated with prolonged systemic glucocorticoid therapy:

Endocrine and metabolic disturbances: Cushing-like syndrome, hirsutism, menstrual irregularities, premature epiphyseal closure, secondary adrenocortical and pituitary unresponsiveness, decreased glucose tolerance, negative nitrogen and calcium balance.

Fluid and electrolyte disturbances: Sodium and water retention, abdominal distension, hypertension, potassium loss, hypokalaemic alkalosis.

Muscular-skeletal effects: Myopathy, osteoporosis, aseptic necrosis of femoral and humeral heads.

Gastro-intestinal effects: Gastric and duodenal ulceration, perforation and haemorrhage.

Dermatologic effects: Impaired wound healing, skin atrophy, striae, petechiae and ecchymoses, bruising, facial erythema, increased sweating, acne.

C.N.S. effects: Psychic disturbances ranging from euphoria to frank psychotic manifestations, convulsions, in children pseudotumour cerebri (benign intracranial hypertension) with vomiting and papilloedema.

Ophthalmic effects: Glaucoma, increased intraocular pressure, posterior subcapsular cataracts.

Immunosuppressive effects: Diminished lymphoid tissue and immune response, increased susceptibility to infections, decreased responsiveness to vaccination and skin tests, diminished inflammatory response.

Hypersensitivity reactions may occasionally occur.

A transient burning or tingling sensation, mainly in the perineal area, following intravenous injection of large doses of corticosteroid phosphates.

Local adverse reactions include post-injection flare, and a painless destruction of the joint reminiscent of Charcot's arthropathy, especially with repeated intra-articular injections.

Interactions: Patients concomitantly using glucocorticoids and the following drugs should be monitored: Diuretics and/or cardiac glycosides, since potassium loss may be enhanced. This is a particular risk in patients using cardiac glycosides, since hypokalaemia increases the toxicity of these drugs.

Antidiabetics, since glucocorticoids may impair glucose tolerance, thereby increasing the need for antidiabetic drugs.

Non-steroidal, anti-inflammatory drugs, since the incidence and/or severity of gastro-intestinal ulceration may increase.

Oral anticoagulants, since glucocorticoids increase blood coagulability and therefore alter the need for these drugs.

Glucocorticoids may be less effective when used concomitantly with liver enzyme-inducing drugs, such as rifampicin, ephedrine, barbiturates, phenytoin, primidone and phenylbutazone.

If patients undergoing long-term therapy with glucocorticoids are concomitantly given salicylates, any reduction in glucocorticoid dosage should be made with caution, since salicylate intoxication has been reported in such cases. Additionally, there may be interaction with salicylates in patients with hypoprothrombinaemia.

Pharmaceutical precautions Protect from light.

Legal category POM.

Package quantities Single 2 ml vials containing the equivalent of 8 mg Dexamethasone BP (4 mg/ml).

Boxes of 25 × 1 ml ampoules. Each ampoule containing 5 mg/ml Dexamethasone Sodium Phosphate BP.

Further information After administration of Oradexon-Organon, dexamethasone sodium phosphate is rapidly converted into dexamethasone. This is a synthetic glucocorticoid whose anti-inflammatory potency is 7 times greater than prednisolone and 30 times that of the natural glucocorticoid, hydrocortisone. Like other glucocorticoids, dexamethasone also has anti-allergic, antipyretic and immunosuppressive properties. Dexamethasone has practically no sodium and water-retaining properties and is, therefore, particularly suitable for use in patients with cardiac failure or hypertension.

Because of its long biological half-life (36–54 hours), dexamethasone is especially suitable in conditions where continuous glucocorticoid action is desired.

Product licence number 0065/5013.

ORADEXON-ORGANON* TABLETS

Presentation Round, flat white tablets in two strengths; 0.5 mg Dexamethasone BP – code marked 'XC4' with 'Organon' and a star on the reverse side; 2.0 mg Dexamethasone BP – code marked 'XC8' with 'Organon' and a star on the reverse side.

Uses Indicated in a wide variety of disorders amenable to glucocorticoid therapy, as well as an adjunct in the control of cerebral oedema.

Dosage and administration In general, glucocorticoid dosage depends on the severity of the condition and response of the patient. Under certain circumstances, for instance in stress, extra dosage adjustments may be necessary. If no favourable response is noted within a couple of days, glucocorticoid therapy should be discontinued.

Adults: Once the disease is under control the dosage should be reduced or tapered off to the lowest suitable level under continuous monitoring and observation of the patient. This should be done by giving one early morning dose, daily (or preferably every other morning), of an oral glucocorticoid with a shorter biological half-life than dexamethasone e.g. prednisolone.

For a short dexamethasone suppression test, 1 mg dexamethasone is given at 11 p.m. and plasma cortisol measured the next morning. Patients who do not show a decrease in cortisol can be exposed to a longer test: 0.5 mg dexamethasone is given at 6 hourly intervals for 48 hours followed by 2 mg every 6 hours for a further 48 hours. 24 hour-urine collections are made before, during and at the end of the test for determination of 17-hydroxycorticosteroids.

Discontinuation of prolonged therapy should be carried out by gradual reduction of dosage and under strict medical supervision, since withdrawal may result in acute exacerbation of the disease and acute adrenocortical insufficiency and polyarteritis.

Children: 0.01–0.04 mg/kg of body weight daily.

Dosage of glucocorticoids should be adjusted on the basis of the individual patient's response.

Contra-indications, warnings, etc

Contra-indications: No contraindications exist when glucocorticoids, in a large single dose, are used in conditions where life is endangered.

Glucocorticoids are generally contraindicated in patients with Cushing's Syndrome, gastro-intestinal ulcers, glaucoma, hypersensitivity to glucocorticoids, systemic fungal infections or certain viral infections, e.g. varicella and herpes genitalis and ocular herpes infections, active tuberculosis and acute psychosis.

Precautions and warnings:

Patients, especially the elderly, with the following conditions should be monitored: Latent or overt cardiac failure, renal dysfunction, hypertension, epilepsy or migraine, since glucocorticoids may induce fluid retention.

Osteoporosis, since glucocorticoids have a negative effect on the calcium balance.

A history of psychotic illness.

Latent tuberculosis, since glucocorticoids may induce reactivation.

Certain parasitic infestations, in particular amoebiasis.

Incomplete statural growth, since glucocorticoids on prolonged administration may accelerate epiphyseal closure.

Glucocorticoid therapy is non-specific, suppresses the symptoms and signs of disease and decreases the resistance to infections. Appropriate antimicrobial therapy should accompany glucocorticoid therapy when necessary, e.g. in tuberculosis, and viral and fungal infections of the eye.

If a live vaccine is to be administered it should be borne in mind that glucocorticoids exert an immunosuppresive effect.

Patients on long-term glucocorticoid therapy should be regularly examined for increased intra-ocular pressure and posterior subcapsular cataracts.

Patients on long-term glucocorticoid therapy should be regularly examined with respect to their glucose metabolism.

Before, during and after stressful situations, dosage may need to be increased in patients currently on glucocorticoids or resumed in patients who have undergone prolonged glucocorticoid treatment in the previous year.

Use during pregnancy and breast feeding: During pregnancy, the benefits of the use of glucocorticoids should be weighed against the possible hazards to the mother or foetus. Infants whose mothers received substantial doses of glucocorticoids during pregnancy should be carefully observed for signs of adrenal insufficiency.

Glucocorticoids appear in breast milk in very small quantities. Mothers taking high doses of glucocorticoids should be advised not to breast-feed.

Adverse reactions: Adverse reactions associated with prolonged systemic glucocorticoid therapy, are unlikely when high doses are administered over a short period of time. Nevertheless, gastric and duodenal ulceration, with possible perforation and haemorrhage, may occasionally occur.

The following adverse reactions have been associated with prolonged systemic glucocorticoid therapy:

Endocrine and metabolic disturbances: Cushing-like syndrome, hirsutism, menstrual irregularities, premature epiphyseal closure, secondary adrenocortical and pituitary unresponsiveness, decreased glucose tolerance, negative nitrogen and calcium balance.

Fluid and electrolyte disturbances: Sodium and water retention, abdominal distension, hypertension, potassium loss, hypokalaemic alkalosis.

Muscular-skeletal effects: Myopathy, osteoporosis, aseptic necrosis of femoral and humeral heads.

Gastro-intestinal effects: gastric and duodenal ulceration, perforation and haemorrhage.

Dermatologic effects: Impaired wound healing, skin atrophy, striae, petechiae and ecchymoses, bruising, facial erythema, increased sweating, acne.

C.N.S. effects: Psychic disturbances ranging from euphoria to frank psychotic manifestations, convulsions, in children pseudotumour cerebri (benign intracranial hypertension) with vomiting and papilloedema.

Ophthalmic effects: Glaucoma, increased intraocular pressure, posterior subcapsular cataracts.

Immunosuppressive effects: Increased susceptibility to infections, decreased responsiveness to vaccination and skin tests, diminished inflammatory response.

Hypersensitivity reactions may occasionally occur.

Interactions:

Patients treated concomitantly with glucocorticoids and one of the following drugs should be monitored: Diuretics and/or cardiac glycosides, since potassium loss may be enhanced. This is a particular risk in patients using cardiac glycosides, since hypokalaemia increases the toxicity of these drugs.

Antidiabetics, since glucocorticoids may impair glucose tolerance, thereby increasing the need for antidiabetic drugs.

Non-steroidal anti-inflammatory drugs since the incidence and/or severity of gastro-intestinal ulceration may increase.

Oral anticoagulants, since glucocorticoids may alter the need for these drugs.

Glucocorticoids may be less effective when used concomitantly with liver enzyme-inducing drugs, such as rifampicin, ephedrine, barbiturates, phenytoin, primidone and phenylbutazone.

If patients undergoing long-term therapy with glucocorticoids are concomitantly given salicylates, any reduction in glucocorticoid dosage should be made with caution, since salicylate intoxication has been reported in such cases. Additionally, there may be interaction with salicylates in patients with hypoprothrombinaemia.

Antacids, especially those containing magnesium trisilicate, have been reported to impair the gastro-intestinal absorption of glucocorticoids. Therefore doses of one agent should be spaced as far as possible from the other.

Pharmaceutical precautions Protect from light.

Legal category POM.

Package quantities Oradexon-Organon 0.5 mg tablets: bottles of 500
Oradexon-Organon 2.0 mg tablets: bottles of 100 and 500.

Further information Dexamethasone is a synthetic glucocorticoid whose anti-inflammatory potency is 7 times greater than prednisolone. Like other glucocorticoids, dexamethasone also has anti-allergic, antipyretic and immunosuppressive properties.

Dexamethasone has practically no water and salt-retaining properties and is, therefore, particularly suitable for use in patients with cardiac failure or hypertension. Because of its long biological half-life (36–54 hours), dexamethasone is especially suitable in conditions when continuous glucocorticoid action is desired.

Product licence numbers 0.5 mg 0065/5044
2.0 mg 0065/5045.

OVESTIN* CREAM

Presentation An intravaginal cream containing oestriol 0.1% w/w.

Uses Vulvo-vaginal complaints due to oestrogen deficiency associated with the climacteric and the post-menopause or after oophorectomy: Atrophic vaginitis; kraurosis vulvae; pruritus vulvae; dyspareunia due to an atrophic vaginal mucosa; as pre-surgery therapy for vaginal operations and during subsequent convalescence.

Dosage and administration Ovestin Cream should be given at the lowest dose to control the symptoms and for as short a time as is found necessary.

Ovestin Cream is administered intravaginally by means of a calibrated applicator.

One applicator-dose (applicator filled to the red mark) is 0.5 g Ovestin Cream containing 0.5 mg oestriol.

Usual dose for vulvo-vaginal complaints associated with the menopause: One application per day for 2 to 3 weeks.

As maintenance dosage, one application twice a week is recommended.

Medication should be discontinued every 2 to 3 months for a period of 4 weeks to assess the necessity for further treatment.

Pre-surgery therapy (one application per day) should begin 2 weeks before the operation. Following surgery a period of at least 2 weeks should be allowed before resuming therapy.

The following 'Instructions for use' should be given to the patient and are included in the package interior leaflet:

Instructions for use
Apply the cream before retiring.
Remove the cap from the tube.
Withdraw the plunger to the red mark and screw the nozzle end of the applicator on to the tube.
Squeeze the tube to force sufficient cream into the applicator to fill it to the red mark.
Unscrew the applicator from the tube and replace the cap on the tube.
To apply cream, lie down, insert the end of the applicator deeply into the vagina and slowly push the plunger all the way in.
After use, pull the plunger out of the barrel and wash both in warm, soapy water. Rinse well afterwards. Do not use detergent.
DO NOT PUT THE APPLICATOR IN HOT OR BOILING WATER.

Contra-indications: Pregnancy or suspected pregnancy and during lactation.

Thrombophlebitis, thrombo-embolic processes, or a history of these conditions.

Known or suspected oestrogen-dependent tumours, e.g. mammary, genital carcinoma.

Undiagnosed vaginal bleeding.

Acute or chronic liver disease or history of liver disease where the liver function tests have failed to return to normal. Jaundice or history of jaundice in pregnancy. Rotor syndrome or Dubin-Johnson syndrome.

Porphyria.

Cerebrovascular or cardiovascular disease.

Hyperlipoproteinaemia, especially in the presence of other risk factors which may indicate a predisposition to cerebrovascular or cardiovascular disorders.

A history during pregnancy or previous oestrogen use of severe pruritus, herpes gestationis or a deterioration of otosclerosis.

Precautions and warnings: In the event of persistent or recurring vaginal bleeding, appropriate diagnostic measures should be taken to rule out malignancy. In case of vaginal infections these should be treated before therapy with Ovestin Cream is started.

As with any preparation that is to be applied to mucosal surfaces, Ovestin Cream may cause local irritation or itching at the beginning of treatment. During the first weeks of therapy, occasional mastodynia may occur. In general, these complaints are transient in nature.

Prolonged exposure to unopposed oestrogens may increase the risk of the development of endometrial carcinoma.

Pain in the breasts or excessive production of cervical mucus may be indicative of too high a dosage.

During prolonged treatment with oestrogens, periodic medical examinations are advisable.

A cervical smear should be taken at regular intervals.

Oestrogen preparations may increase the risk of thrombosis and this should be taken into account when surgery is to be performed in patients using these preparations. Where possible, oestrogens should be discontinued approximately six weeks prior to elective surgery and not recommended until the patient has recovered and is mobile.

Patients, especially the elderly, with the following conditions should be monitored: Latent or overt cardiac failure; renal or hepatic dysfunction; hypertension; epilepsy or migraine or a history of these conditions; a history of thromboembolic disorders (since oestrogens may cause sodium and water retention and exacerbate the above conditions); endometriosis; fibrocystic mastopathy; diabetes mellitus.

Pharmaceutical precautions The preparation should be stored at room temperature (15–25°C).

Legal category POM.

Package quantities Tube (+applicator) containing 15 g cream.

Further information In conditions of oestrogen deficiency, atrophic changes occur in the vagina and vulva. The signs and symptoms associated with these changes in the vaginal and vulval epithelia may be alleviated by the topical application of oestriol.

During the use of Ovestin Cream systemic resorption of oestriol may occur to some degree.

Product licence number 0065/0074.

OVESTIN* TABLETS

Presentation Round, flat, white tablets, diameter 8 mm, code-marked 'DG4' on one side, with 'Organon' and a star on the reverse side.

Each tablet contains 250 micrograms of Oestriol.

Uses For the treatment of vaginal and cervical disorders and symptoms of oestrogen deficiency associated with the climacteric.

Dosage and administration 1 or 2 tablets daily. The tablets should be taken orally without being chewed. It is important that the total daily dose is taken at one time.

Contra-indications, warnings, etc
Contra-indications: Pregnancy or suspected pregnancy and during lactation.

Thrombophlebitis, thrombo-embolic processes, or a history of these conditions.

Known or suspected oestrogen-dependent tumours, e.g. mammary, genital carcinoma.

Undiagnosed vaginal bleeding.

Acute or chronic liver disease or history of liver disease where the liver function tests have failed to return to normal. Jaundice or history of jaundice in pregnancy. Rotor syndrome or Dubin-Johnson syndrome.

Porphyria.

Cerebrovascular or cardiovascular disease.

Hyperlipoproteinaemia, especially in the presence of other risk factors which may indicate a predisposition to cerebrovascular or cardiovascular disorders.

A history during pregnancy or previous oestrogen use of severe pruritus, herpes gestationis or a deterioration of otosclerosis.

Precautions and warnings: Prolonged exposure to unopposed oestrogens may increase the risk of the development of endometrial carcinoma.

Pain in the breasts or excessive production of cervical mucus may be indicative of too high a dosage.

During prolonged treatment with oestrogens, periodic medical examinations are advisable.

A cervical smear should be taken at regular intervals.

With vaginal infections, a concomitant specific treatment is recommended.

Oestrogen preparations may increase the risk of thrombosis and this should be taken into account when surgery is to be performed in patients using these preparations. Where possible, oestrogens should be discontinued approximately six weeks prior to elective surgery and not recommended until the patient has recovered and is mobile.

Patients, especially the elderly, with the following conditions should be monitored: Latent or overt cardiac failure; renal or hepatic dysfunction; hypertension; epilepsy or migraine or a history of these conditions; a history of thromboembolic disorders (since oestrogens may cause sodium and water retention and exacerbate the above conditions); endometriosis; fibrocystic mastopathy; diabetes mellitus.

Adverse reactions: Adverse reactions are rare and only appear if the dosage is too high or treatment is prolonged. These include nausea and vomiting, headache, sodium and water retention, tenderness, pain, and increase in size of the breasts, menstrual disturbances, uterine bleeding (during or on withdrawal of therapy), excessive production of cervical mucus, and psychotic disturbances.

Symptoms such as sudden severe headaches, pains in the chest, visual disturbances, or swelling of the arms or legs require immediate medical examination.

Interactions: Concurrent administration of liver enzyme inducing drugs such as rifampicin, barbiturates, carbamazepine, dichloralphenazone, phenylbutazone, phenytoin or primidone may decrease the effect of Ovestin Tablets.

Overdosage: There is no specific antidote. Patients should be given appropriate supportive therapy using standard resuscitative measures as required.

Pharmaceutical precautions Protect from light.

Legal category POM.

Package quantities Bottles of 100 tablets.

Further information Oestriol is a naturally-occurring oestrogen with a selective action on the cervix and vagina; unlike most other oestrogens, oestriol in therapeutic doses, has relatively little proliferative effect on the endometrium, so that uterine bleedings only rarely occur.

Product licence number 0065/5049.

RESTANDOL* ▼

Presentation Soft, oval, reddish-brown gelatin capsules each containing 40 mg of testosterone undecanoate in oleic acid. Code marked D_3V and ORG.

Uses Restandol is an orally active testosterone preparation.

Indications:

Testosterone replacement therapy in male hypogonadal disorders, for example: After castration; eunuchoidism;

hypopituitarism; endocrine impotence; male climacteric symptoms like decreased libido and decreased mental and physical activity; certain types of infertility due to disorders of spermatogenesis.

Testosterone therapy may also be indicated in osteoporosis due to androgenic deficiency.

Dosage and administration

Adults: The initial dosage required will usually be 120–160 mg daily for 2–3 weeks. Subsequent dosage (40–120 mg daily) should be based on the clinical effect obtained during the first weeks of therapy.

Elderly: It should be noted that smaller and less frequent doses may achieve the same response.

The capsules should be taken after meals, if necessary with a little water, and be swallowed whole without chewing. It is preferable that half of the daily dose be taken in the morning and the other half in the evening. If an uneven number of capsules is taken daily, the greater part should be taken in the morning.

Contra-indications, warnings, etc

Contra-indications: Known or suspected prostatic or mammary carcinoma; hypercalcaemia, hypercalcaemia, nephrotic syndrome, ischaemic heart disease or untreated congestive heart failure.

Precautions and warnings:
Patients, especially the elderly, with the following conditions should be monitored: Latent or overt cardiac failure, renal or hepatic dysfunction, hypertension, epilepsy or migraine (or a history of these conditions), since androgens may occasionally induce sodium and water retention.

Mammary carcinoma, hypernephroma, bronchial carcinoma, and skeletal metastases, since these conditions may produce hypercalcaemia or hypercalciuria which may in turn be exacerbated by androgen therapy. If hypercalcaemia or hypercalciuria develops treatment should be discontinued.

A decrease in protein-bound iodine (PBI) may occur, but this has no clinical significance.

Androgens should be used cautiously in prepubertal boys to avoid premature epiphyseal closure or precocious sexual development.

Androgen therapy should only be used in male hypogonadism in which testosterone levels have been demonstrated to be low.

In treating males, stimulation to the point of increasing nervous, mental and physical activities beyond the patient's cardiovascular capacity should be avoided.

Tumours and other histological abnormalities and disturbances of liver function have been reported in patients subjected to prolonged treatment with some testosterone derivatives. Most of these compounds were 17-alpha alkyl derivatives but a smaller number of cases has occurred with certain 17-beta esters of testosterone. The possibility that such changes result from the use of Restandol has not been excluded.

Adverse reactions: Restandol, like any other androgen therapy, may give rise to the following adverse reactions:

Priapism and other signs of excessive sexual stimulation.

Precocious sexual development, an increased frequency of erections, phallic enlargement and premature epiphyseal closure in pre-pubertal males.

Sodium and water retention.

Oligospermia and a decreased ejaculatory volume.

Treatment should be interrupted until these symptoms have disappeared after which it should be continued at a lower dosage.

Hoarseness of the voice may be the first symptom of vocal change which may lead to irreversible lowering of the voice. If signs of virilisation, particularly lowering of the voice, develop, treatment should be discontinued.

Interactions: Concurrent administration of liver enzyme inducing drugs such as rifampicin, barbiturates, carbamazepine, dichloralphenazone, phenylbutazone, phenytoin or primidone may decrease the effect of Restandol.

Overdosage: Treatment of overdosage is by gastric lavage with appropriate supportive therapy. Standard resuscitative measures should be given as required.

Pharmaceutical precautions Store in a cool (6–15°C) dry place. Protect from light.

Legal category POM.

Package quantities 60 capsules.

Further information Restandol is an orally effective testosterone preparation. The therapeutic substance is tesosterone undecanoate, a fatty acid ester of the natural androgen testosterone. Testosterone is inactive on oral administration because it is prematurely inactivated by the liver. Testosterone undecanoate is able to by-pass the liver via the lymphatic system and is therefore orally active.

Product licence number 0065/0059.

SUSTANON* 100

Presentation Sustanon 100 is a clear, sterile, oily solution containing in each millilitre 20 mg Testosterone Propionate BP, 40 mg Testosterone Phenylpropionate BP and 40 mg Testostrone Isocaproate BP.

Uses Sustanon 100 is an androgenic preparation for intramuscular administration containing three different esters of the natural hormone testosterone.

Indications: Testosterone replacement therapy in male hypogonadal disorders, for example: After castration; eunuchoidism; hypopituitarism; endocrine impotence; male climacteric symptoms like decreased libido and decreased mental and physical activity; certain types of infertility due to disorders of spermatogenesis.

Testosterone therapy may also be indicated in osteoporosis due to androgen deficiency.

Dosage and administration In general, dosage should be adjusted to the individual response of the patient.

Usually, one injection of 1 ml per two weeks will be adequate.

Sustanon 100 should be administered by deep intramuscular injection.

Contra-indications, warnings, etc

Contra-indications: Hypercalciuria, hypercalcaemia, nephrotic syndrome, ischaemic heart disease or untreated congestive heart failure; known or suspected prostatic or mammary carcinoma.

Precautions and warnings:
Patients, especially the elderly, with the following conditions should be monitored: Latent or overt cardiac failure, renal or hepatic dysfunction, hypertension, epilepsy or migraine (or a history of these conditions), since

androgens may occasionally induce fluid and sodium retention.

Hypernephroma, bronchial carcinoma, and skeletal metastases, since these conditions may produce hypercalcaemia or hypercalciuria which may in turn be exacerbated by androgen therapy. If hypercalcaemia or hypercalciuria develops treatment should be discontinued.

A decrease in protein-bound iodine (PBI) may occur, but this has no clinical significance.

Androgens should be used cautiously in prepubertal boys to avoid premature epiphyseal closure or precocious sexual development.

Androgen therapy should only be used in male hypogonadism in which testosterone levels have been demonstrated to be low.

In treating males, stimulation to the point of increasing nervous, mental and physical activities beyond the patient's cardiovascular capacity should be avoided.

Adverse reactions:
Sustanon 100 like any other androgen therapy, may give rise to the following adverse reactions: Priapism and other signs of excessive sexual stimulation.

Precocious sexual development, an increased frequency of erections, phallic enlargement and premature epipyseal closure in pre-pubertal males.

Sodium and water retention.

Oligospermia and a decreased ejaculatory volume.

Treatment should be interrupted until these symptoms have disappeared, after which it should be continued at a lower dosage.

Hoarseness of the voice may be the first symptom of vocal change which may lead to irreversible lowering of the voice. If signs of virilisation, particularly lowering of the voice, develop, treatment should be discontinued.

Interactions: Concurrent administration of liver enzyme inducing drugs such as rifampicin, barbiturates, carbamazepine, dichloralphenazone, phenylbutazone, phenytoin or primidone may decrease the effect of Sustanon 100.

Pharmaceutical precautions Protect from light.
Store at room temperature (15 to 25°C).

After storage at lower temperatures precipitation of the arachis oil vehicle may occur. By heating the ampoules at 100°C for a few minutes or at 40°C for one hour, the solution will become clear. The precipitation and rewarming does not affect the activity of the injection.

Legal category POM.

Package quantities 1 ml ampoules in boxes of 3.

Further information Testosterone propionate has a rapid onset and short duration of action. Testosterone phenylpropionate and isocaproate have an intermediate onset and long duration of action. By combining these testosterone esters the action of Sustanon 100 starts shortly after injection and is maintained for about two weeks.

Product licence number 0065/5019.

SUSTANON* 250

Presentation Sustanon 250 is a clear, sterile, oily solution containing in each millilitre 30 mg Testosterone Propionate BP, 60 mg Testosterone Phenylpropionate BP, 60 mg Testosterone Isocaproate BP, and 100 mg Testosterone Decanoate BP.

Uses Sustanon 250 is an androgen preparation for intramuscular administration containing four different esters of the natural hormone testosterone.

Indications: Testosterone replacement therapy in male hypogonadal disorders, for example: after castration; eunuchoidism; hypopituitarism; endocrine impotence; male climacteric symptoms like decreased libido and decreased mental and physical activity; certain types of infertility due to disorders of spermatogenesis.

Testosterone therapy may also be indicated in osteoporosis due to androgen deficiency.

Dosage and administration In general, dosage should be adjusted to the individual response of the patient.

Usually, one injection of 1 ml per three weeks will be adequate.

Sustanon 250 should be administered by deep intramuscular injection.

Contra-indications, warnings, etc

Contra-indications: Known or suspected prostatic or mammary carcinoma; hypercalciuria, hypercalcaemia, nephrotic syndrome, ischaemic heart disease or untreated congestive heart failure.

Precautions and warnings: Patients, especially the elderly, with the following conditions should be monitored: Latent or overt cardiac failure, renal or hepatic dysfunction, hypertension, epilepsy or migraine (or a history of these conditions), since androgens may occasionally induce fluid and sodium retention.

Hypernephroma, bronchial carcinoma, and skeletal metastases, since these conditions may produce hypercalcaemia or hypercalciuria which may in turn be exacerbated by androgen therapy. If hypercalcaemia or hypercalciuria develops treatment should be discontinued.

A decrease in protein-bound iodine (PBI) may occur, but this has no clinical significance.

Androgens should be used cautiously in prepubertal boys to avoid premature epiphyseal closure or precocious sexual development.

Androgen therapy should only be used in male hypogonadism in which testosterone levels have been demonstrated to be low.

In treating males, stimulation to the point of increasing nervous, mental and physical activities beyond the patient's cardiovascular capacity should be avoided.

Adverse reactions: Sustanon 250 like any other androgen therapy, may give rise to the following adverse reactions: Priapism and other signs of excessive sexual stimulation.

Precocious sexual development, an increased frequency of erections, phallic enlargement and premature epiphyseal closure in pre-pubertal males.

Sodium and water retention.

Oligospermia and a decreased ejaculatory volume.

Treatment should be interrupted until these symptoms have disappeared, after which it should be continued at a lower dosage.

Hoarseness of the voice may be the first symptom of vocal change which may lead to irreversible lowering of the voice. If signs of virilisation, particularly lowering of the voice, develop, treatment should be discontinued.

Interactions: Concurrent administration of liver enzyme inducing drugs such as rifampicin, barbiturates, carbamazepine, dichloralphenazone, phenylbutazone, phenytoin or primidone may decrease the effect of Sustanon 250.

Pharmaceutical precautions Protect from light. Store at room temperature (15 to 25°C).

After storage at lower temperatures precipitation of the arachis oil vehicle may occur. By heating the ampoules at 100°C for a few minutes or at 40°C for one hour, the solution will become clear. The precipitation and rewarming does not affect the activity of the injection.

Legal category POM.

Package quantities 1 ml ampoules in boxes of 3.

Further information Testosterone propionate has a rapid onset and short duration of action. Testosterone phenylpropionate and isocaproate have an intermediate onset and long duration of action. Testosterone decanoate has a slow onset and long duration of action. By combining these testosterone esters the action of Sustanon 250 starts shortly after injection and is maintained for about three weeks.

Product licence number 0065/5086.

TESTORAL SUBLINGS*

Presentation Round, bi-convex, white to creamy white tablets, diameter 8 mm, code-marked with a 'T' surrounded by 'Subling' on one side, with 'Organon' and a star on the reverse side. Each tablet contains 10 mg Testosterone BP.

Uses Androgen replacement therapy.

Indications: Testosterone replacement therapy in male hypogonadal disorders, for example: After castration; eunuchoidism; hypopituitarism; endocrine impotence; male climacteric symptoms like decreased libido and decreased mental and physical activity; certain types of infertility due to disorders of spermatogenesis.

Testosterone therapy may also be indicated in osteoporosis due to androgenic deficiency.

Dosage and administration
Adults: The usual initial dosage is 10 to 30 mg daily with a subsequent maintenance dose of 10 mg daily.

Elderly: It should be noted that smaller and less frequent doses may achieve the same response.

Testoral subling tablets should not be swallowed whole but allowed to dissolve under the tongue or between cheek and gum.

Contra-indications, warnings, etc
Contra-indications: Known or suspected prostatic or mammary carcinoma.

Hypercalciuria, hypercalcaemia, nephrotic syndrome, ischaemic heart disease or untreated congestive heart failure.

Precautions and warnings: Patients, especially the elderly, with the following conditions should be monitored: Latent or overt cardiac failure, renal or hepatic dysfunction, hypertension, epilepsy or migraine (or a history of these conditions), since androgens may occasionally induce sodium and water retention.

Hypernephroma, bronchial carcinoma, and skeletal metastases, since these conditions may produce hypercalcaemia or hypercalciuria which may in turn be exacerbated by androgen therapy. If hypercalcaemia or

hypercalciuria develops treatment should be discontinued.

A decrease in protein-bound iodine (PBI) may occur, but this has no clinical significance.

Androgens should be used cautiously in prepubertal boys to avoid premature epiphyseal closure or precocious sexual development.

Androgen therapy should only be used in male hypogonadism in which testosterone levels have been demonstrated to be low.

In treating males, stimulation to the point of increasing nervous, mental and physical activities beyond the patient's cardiovascular capacity should be avoided.

Adverse reactions: Testoral Sublings, like any other androgen therapy, may give rise to the following adverse reactions: Priapism and other signs of excessive sexual stimulation.

Precocious sexual development, an increased frequency of erections, phallic enlargement and premature epiphyseal closure in pre-pubertal males.

Sodium and water retention.

Oligospermia and a decreased ejaculatory volume.

Treatment should be interrupted until these symptoms have disappeared, after which it should be continued at a lower dosage.

Hoarseness of the voice may be the first symptom of vocal change which may lead to irreversible lowering of the voice. If signs of virilisation, particularly lowering of the voice, develop, treatment should be discontinued.

Interactions: Concurrent administration of liver enzyme inducing drugs such as rifampicin, barbiturates, carbamazepine, dichloralphenazone, phenylbutazone, phenytoin or primidone may decrease the effect of Testoral Sublings.

Overdosage: There is no specific antidote. Patients should be given appropriate supportive therapy using standard resuscitative measures as required.

Pharmaceutical precautions Protect from light.

Legal category POM.

Package quantities Bottles of 100 tablets.

Further information The male hormone testosterone, although inactivated when swallowed, can be absorbed through the buccal mucosa. Testoral Sublings provide testosterone in smooth, textured tablets, specially prepared for sublingual absorption.

Product licence number 0065/5051.

TESTOSTERONE IMPLANTS (Organon)

Presentation Pellets of fused, crystalline testosterone for implantation. Each pellet contains 100 or 200 mg of Testosterone BP and has a diameter of 4.5 mm.

Uses Testosterone replacement therapy in male hypogonadal disorders, for example: After castration; eunuchoidism; hypopituitarism; endocrine impotence; male climacteric symptoms like decreased libido and decreased mental and physical activity; certain types of infertility due to disorders of spermatogenesis.

Testosterone implantation is also used in certain inoperable mammary carcinomas in the female.

Dosage and administration
Adults: Male: 100–600 mg depending on individual requirements.

Female: Mammary carcinoma 500–1500 mg.

Published data and clinical experience suggest that a dosage of 600 mg usually maintains plasma testosterone levels within the normal physiological range for 4–5 months.

Implants are inserted, either by means of a trocar and cannula or by open surgery, into an area where there is comparatively little movement, such as the lower abdominal wall or the buttock. Insertion is made under local anaesthesia and the wound is closed either with an adhesive dressing or a fine suture.

Whichever method is used for the insertion of implants, the following principles apply: Full aseptic 'no touch' technique should be adopted.

Precautions should be taken to avoid the formation of haematoma at the site.

The rate of absorption of the active ingredient depends on the surface area of the implant. Thus the daily rate of absorption can be increased by supplying the total dose in a number of separate implants each sited on a separate track.

Contra-indications, warnings, etc

Contra-indications: Androgens are contra-indicated in pregnancy, and in cases of mammary or prostatic carcinoma in males.

Hypercalciuria, hypercalcaemia, nephrotic syndrome, ischaemic heart disease or untreated congestive heart failure.

Precautions and warnings: Patients, especially the elderly, with the following conditions should be monitored: Latent or overt cardiac failure, renal or hepatic dysfunction, hypertension, epilepsy, migraine or asthma (or a history of these conditions), since androgens may occasionally induce sodium and water retention.

Mammary carcinoma, hypernephroma, bronchial carcinoma, and skeletal metastases, since these conditions may produce hypercalcaemia or hypercalciuria which may in turn be exacerbated by androgen therapy. If hypercalcaemia or hypercalciuria develops treatment should be discontinued.

A decrease in protein-bound iodine (PBI) may occur, but this has no clinical significance.

Androgens should be used cautiously in prepubertal boys to avoid premature epiphyseal closure or precocious sexual development.

Androgen therapy should only be used in male hypogonadism in which testosterone levels have been demonstrated to be low.

In treating males, stimulation to the point of increasing nervous, mental and physical activities beyond the patient's cardiovascular capacity should be avoided.

Adverse reactions: Testosterone Implants, like any other androgen therapy, may give rise to the following adverse reactions:

Priapism and other signs of excessive sexual stimulation.

Precocious sexual development, an increased frequency of erections, phallic enlargement and premature epiphyseal closure in pre-pubertal males.

Sodium and water retention.

Oligospermia and a decreased ejaculatory volume.

Hoarseness of the voice may be the first symptom of vocal change which may lead to irreversible lowering of the voice. If signs of virilisation, particularly lowering of the voice develop, treatment should be discontinued.

Interactions: Concurrent administration of liver enzyme inducing drugs such as rifampicin, barbiturates, carba-mazepine, dichloralphenazone, phenylbutazone, phenytoin or primidone may decrease the effect of Testosterone Implants.

Pharmaceutical precautions Protect from light.

Legal category POM.

Package quantities Each sterile implant is supplied singly, in a sealed glass tube. Available in 100 mg and 200 mg weights.

Further information Implantation of fused implants of testosterone provides slow release of the hormone. A 4.5 mm trocar and cannula should be used for insertion.

On each occasion before reuse it is important to sterilise the trocar and cannula set by washing and subsequent heat sterilisation. This may be carried out by boiling in water for 30 minutes or through the use of an autoclave.

Product licence numbers 100 mg   0065/5083
200 mg   0065/5084.

TETRABID-ORGANON*

Presentation Hard gelatin capsules (purple cap/yellow body). Each capsule contains 250 mg Tetracycline Hydrochloride PhEur.

Uses The treatment of all infections caused by organisms sensitive to tetracycline, bronchitis, and for the treatment and prophylaxis of acute exacerbations of chronic bronchitis. Tetrabid-Organon is also indicated in the treatment of acne vulgaris.

Dosage and administration *Adults and children over 12 years:* Two capsules initially, followed by one capsule every 12 hours. For more severe infections, dosage may be increased at the discretion of the physician. Treatment should continue for at least two or three days after achievement of the desired clinical response.

In treatment of acne vulgaris: one capsule daily for at least three months.

Capsules should preferably by taken one hour before, or two hours after meals.

Contra-indications, warnings, etc

Contra-indications: Patients with chronic renal failure, a history of tetracycline sensitivity, pregnancy or suspected pregnancy (unless specifically indicated by bacterial sensitivity tests and where the risk involved is justified) and during lactation.

Tetracycline should not be administered to children under seven years of age.

Precautions and warnings: Tetracycline should be administered with caution in patients with renal or hepatic impairment or those receiving potentially hepatotoxic drugs, this may be of particular relevance to the elderly group of patients in whom such impairment is relatively more common; a reduction of the dosage or a longer time interval between doses is indicated.

Broad-spectrum antibiotic therapy may result in overgrowth of non-susceptible organisms. If such superinfection should occur, resulting in the development of oral thrush, pruritus ani or gastrointestinal side-effects, the antibiotic therapy should be discontinued and appropriate measures taken.

In long-term therapy laboratory monitoring of certain functions (including haemopoietic, renal and hepatic studies) should be performed.

Adverse reactions: Skin photosensitivity reactions are occasionally observed in patients on tetracycline therapy. Treatment should be discontinued at the first evidence of skin erythema.

Tetracycline is selectively taken up in developing bones and teeth of foetus and children, causing dental staining and enamel hypoplasia.

Nausea, vomiting and diarrhoea may occasionally occur.

It is advisable to avoid administering tetracycline in conjunction with penicillin since bacteriostatic drugs may interfere with the bactericidal action of penicillin.

Interactions: Antacids, iron, calcium, magnesium and zinc salts have been reported to impair the intestinal absorption of tetracycline. Therefore doses of one agent should be spaced as far as possible from the other.

Concurrent use of milk products interferes with absorption of tetracyclines to a variable degree, and should be avoided.

In general, the physician should be aware that interactions may occur when tetracycline is administered concomitantly with various drugs, e.g. the reliability of oral contraceptives may be reduced. The concurrent use of the anaesthetic methoxyflurane in patients receiving tetracycline therapy increases the risk of kidney failure. In addition, tetracycline has been reported to interfere with some diagnostic tests.

Tetracycline has been shown to depress plasma prothrombin activity, therefore patients who are on anticoagulant therapy may require a reduction of their anticoagulant dosage.

Overdosage: In cases of overdosage, allergic reactions such as drug fever, anaphylactic shock and rashes may occur. If anaphylactic reactions occur the following measures may be advisable: immediate intravenous injection of adrenaline (0.1–0.5 mg dependent on body weight), intermittent positive-pressure ventilation and administration of aminophylline if necessary.

Pharmaceutical precautions Store at a temperature below 30°C and in dry conditions.

Legal category POM.

Package quantities Securitainer of 100 or 500 capsules.

Further information Tetrabid-Organon is a sustained-action tetracycline formulation which requires only half the daily dose and half the frequency of administration of conventional tetracycline.

Twice-daily Tetrabid-Organon provides tetracycline therapy with a reduced incidence of side-effects. The formulation allows sustained release of tetracycline throughout the gastro-intestinal tract and fumaric acid (33 mg) provides a localised low pH environment at the point of release which favours increased absorption.

Product licence number 0065/0028.

*Trade Mark

Organon Teknika Ltd
Science Park
Milton Road
Cambridge

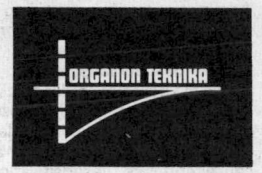

NORCURON* ▼

Presentation Vial containing 10 mg vecuronium bromide in a buffered freeze-dried form, with a 5 ml ampoule of Water for Injections as solvent.

Uses Norcuron is a neuromuscular blocking agent of the non-depolarising type with a short to medium duration of action. It is used as an adjuvant in surgical anaesthesia to obtain relaxation of the skeletal muscles in a wide range of surgical procedures. Norcuron has no ganglion blocking properties, lacks vagolytic action and histamine release is not expected to occur.

Norcuron has no cumulative effects. Several maintenance doses can therefore be given in succession. These properties make Norcuron highly suitable for short as well as for long-lasting operations. The relatively low renal elimination and the transient liver storage of Norcuron suggest that biliary excretion is the major excretion route. The elimination half-life ranges from 30–70 minutes. Norcuron is well tolerated by the patient.

Dosage and administration Norcuron is administered intravenously.

The following may be used as a general guide to dosage: For intubation and subsequent surgical procedures.

Initial dose: 0.08–0.10 mg/kg (good to excellent intubation conditions within 90–120 seconds).

Incremental doses: 0.03–0.05 mg/kg.
Skeletal muscle relaxation lasts for 20–30 minutes.
Not for use in neonates or children, since dosage regimens have not been established.

In obese patients a reduction of the dose is recommended.

When calculating the dose of neuromuscular blocking agents the following factors must be taken into account: the anaesthetic technique used, potential interactions with the drugs used during and before anaesthesia, and the condition of the individual patient.

In general it is not recommended that Norcuron should be mixed with other agents in the same syringe or with solutions for intravenous infusion, except for the following intravenous infusion fluids which have been shown to be compatible with Norcuron: 0.9% Sodium Chloride solution; 5.0% Glucose solution; Ringer's solution; Ringer-glucose solution.

When administered by intravenous infusion the Norcuron freeze-dried substance should first be dissolved in the 5 ml of solvent (Water for Injections) provided and the resultant solution added to the infusion fluid. The diluted solution will remain stable for 24 hours at room temperature and in daylight. In practice the infusion containing Norcuron will only be used as long as muscle relaxation is required, at maximum for a few hours. Afterwards the solution should be discarded.

Contra-indications, warnings, etc

Contra-indications: There are no known contra-indications for the use of Norcuron.

Use in pregnancy: Since there is no experience with the use of Norcuron in pregnant women, it cannot be recommended during pregnancy.

Clinical studies show that Norcuron can be used in childbirth by Caesarian section without effect on the newly born child.

Precautions and warnings: Generally speaking it is advisable to monitor the degree of neuromuscular block. Before the administration of Norcuron conditions such as electrolyte disturbance, altered pH and dehydration should if possible be corrected. Care should be exercised if there is a danger of regurgitation when intubating the patient.

In patients with renal insufficiency a slight prolongation of the neuromuscular blockade can be expected after the use of Norcuron.

Extreme caution should be exercised, and very small doses used, in patients with myasthenia gravis or myasthenic syndrome, unless it is intended to administer prolonged post-operative respiratory assistance. In case of myopathy (such as dystrophia myotonica), neuromuscular disease, severe obesity, electrolyte disturbances (e.g. excessive potassium loss), altered pH and after poliomyelitis or dehydration, Norcuron should be dosed carefully as unwanted effects may occur.

Patients with liver disease or liver insufficiency do not usually require a reduction of the initial dose. In some patients the required dose may even be higher.

In operations requiring hypothermia the neuromuscular blockade of non-depolarising drugs is decreased and increases when re-warming the patient.

Norcuron should be administered only by anaesthetists familiar with its use, and only when facilities for controlled ventilation, insufflation with oxygen and endotracheal intubation are available for immediate use.

Since Norcuron in clinically effective doses affects the respiratory muscles, as well as other skeletal muscles, respiration must be assisted in all patients. It is essential to ensure that the patient is breathing spontaneously, deeply and regularly before leaving the theatre after anaesthesia. The neuromuscular blockade achieved with Norcuron can be reversed with a cholinesterase inhibiting agent (e.g. neostigmine) in an adequate dose, together with atropine as an anticholinergic agent.

Interactions: Prior to surgery and during anaesthesia a number of medicines are commonly administered to the patient. This creates the possibility of interaction.

In addition, the condition of the patient may influence the neuromuscular blocking (n.m.b.) activity of Norcuron.

The following medicines and conditions of the patient

may interact with the n.m.b. activity of Norcuron: Administration of depolarising drugs (e.g. suxamethonium chloride) following a non-depolarising drug (e.g. Norcuron) is dangerous.

The non-depolarising drug increases resistance towards the neuromuscular blocking effect of the depolarising drug. Therefore high doses of a depolarising drug are necessary before muscular relaxation can be obtained. These high doses of a depolarising drug may cause endplate desensitisation and prolonged postoperative apnoea.

Unlike a non-depolarising block, a depolarising block cannot be overcome by an anticholinesterase agent and may even be worsened.

Recent evidence suggests that alkylating drugs (nitrogen mustards) should be considered a possible hazard when given to patients during anaesthesia involving the use of muscle relaxants.

Anaesthetics: The following anaesthetics may influence the neuromuscular blocking activity of Norcuron: Increased effect: Halothene, ether, enflurane, isoflurane (Forane), methoxyflurane, cyclopropane, thiopentone, methohexitone, ketamine, fentanyl, gammahydroxybutyrate, etomidate, propanidid.

The following drugs may influence the magnitude and/or duration of action of non-depolarising neuromuscular blocking agents:
Increased effect: other non-depolarising muscle relaxants, prior administration of suxamethonium, aminoglycoside and polypeptide antibiotics, diuretics, beta-adrenergic blocking agents, thiamine, M.A.O. inhibiting agents, quinidine, protamine, alpha-adrenergic blocking agents, imidazole, metronidazole and calcium antagonists e.g. Verapamil.
Decreased effect: neostigmine, edrophonium, corticosteroids, noradrenaline, azathioprine, theophylline, potassium chloride, sodium chloride and calcium chloride.
Variable effect: depolarising muscle relaxants given after the administration of Norcuron may produce potentiation or attenuation of the neuromuscular blocking effect.

Condition of the patient: The following conditions may influence the neuromuscular blocking activity of Norcuron:
Increased effect: Hypokalaemia (e.g. after severe vomiting, diarrhoea, digitalisation and diuretic therapy), hypermagnesaemia, hypocalcaemia (after massive transfusion), hypoproteinaemia, dehydration, acidosis, hypercapnoea, cachexia, myasthenia gravis, myasthenic syndrome, profound anaesthesia.
Decreased effect: Hypothermia, superficial anaesthesia.

Disturbances in renal function and hypocalcaemia are factors favouring the development of a syndrome resembling that of myasthenia gravis following administration of antibiotics. A disturbed plasma protein pattern requires prudence.

Like pancuronium bromide, d-tubocurarine or other non-depolarising neuromuscular blocking agents, Norcuron may cause a reduction in the partial thromboplastin time and the prothrombin time.

With respect to the frequently reported interactions involving other non-depolarising neuromuscular blocking agents the anaesthetist should be aware of the possibility that similar interactions may occur with Norcuron.

Side-effects: So far during extensive clinical testing no side-effects have been reported with Norcuron.

Overdosage: The spontaneous reversal of the neuromuscular blockade caused by Norcuron is rapid. However, when needed, standard reversal agents, e.g. neostigmine or pyridostigmine, will readily antagonise its neuromuscular effects.

Pharmaceutical precautions Norcuron can be kept for three years, provided it is stored in the dark at a temperature below 25°C.

Legal category POM.

Package quantities 20 vials each containing 10 mg vecuronium bromide.

20 ampoules each containing 5 ml solvent (Water for Injections PhEur.)

Further information Norcuron is an amino-steroidal derivative which is a highly active non-depolarising neuromuscular blocking agent. The drug is highly selective in its action at the neuromuscular junction and therefore much larger doses would be required to produce ganglion block, vagal block, histamine release and noradrenaline uptake block. Overall a highly significant lack of cardiovascular side-effects has been observed even with doses much higher than those producing neuromuscular block.

Norcuron offers a shorter time to intubation, a shorter duration of action and a consistently more rapid rate of recovery in comparison to standard non-depolarisers. Further, its lack of cumulative effect, particularly in renal failure patients, offers a distinct advantage over the present armamentarium of both non-depolarising and depolarising drugs. Norcuron induced block is readily reversed by standard agents and the predictability of duration of action relative to dose employed, in addition to rapid rate of recovery, promise that an antagonist will on occasion be unnecessary at the end of surgery.

Extensive clinical studies show Norcuron to cause little or no change in cardiovascular parameters and that it is even less active than pancuronium in causing histamine release. Hence Norcuron should be most useful where little change in cardiovascular or pulmonary systems is desirable. This stability, in conjunction with the predictability of its action, allows Norcuron to be used safely and reliably over prolonged periods by infusion where this is desirable as well as in short surgical procedures where a fast time to intubation and short duration of action are required of a non-depolarising neuromuscular blocking agent.

Product licence number 3524/0013.

PAVULON*

Presentation Pancuronium bromide BP 2 ml ampoules. A clear, aqueous solution. Active ingredient: Each 2 ml ampoule contains pancuronium bromide BP 4 mg. Other ingredients: sodium chloride BP 16 mg, acetate buffers to pH 4, 1% benzyl alcohol.

Uses Pavulon is a neuromuscular blocking agent of the non-depolarising type with a medium duration of action. It is used as an adjuvant in surgical anaesthesia to obtain relaxation of the skeletal muscles in a wide range of surgical procedures.

Pavulon is also used for neuromuscular blockade during intensive care therapy for a variety of pathologies, including intractable status asthmaticus and tetanus. Pavulon is the relaxant of choice when other muscle relaxants might be inappropriate, e.g. shock, allergy, renal and hepatic insufficiency.

Dosage and administration Pavulon is administered intravenously. When calculating dosages of neuromuscular blocking agents the following factors must be taken into account: the anaesthetic technique used, the anticipated duration of the operation, potential interactions with the drugs used during (and before) anaesthesia, and the condition of the individual patient. The following may be used as a general guide to dosage:

Adult surgery: Initial dose: 0.05–0.08 mg/kg (intubation accomplished within 150–120 seconds) or 0.08–0.1 mg/kg (intubation accomplished within 120–090 seconds). Incremental doses: 0.01–0.02 mg/kg.

Child surgery: Initial dose: 0.06–0.1 mg/kg. Incremental doses: 0.01–0.02 mg/kg.

Neonatal surgery: 0.03–0.04 mg/kg intravenously. Incremental doses: As neonates are sensitive this dose should be adjusted according to the initial response but generally incremental doses lie in the range 0.01–0.02 mg/kg body weight.

Following the administration of suxamethonium the dosage of Pavulon may be considerably reduced.

Adults: Initial dose: 0.02–0.06 mg/kg. Incremental doses: 0.01–0.02 mg/kg.

Children: Initial dose: 0.02–0.06 mg/kg. Incremental doses: 0.01–0.02 mg/kg.

If the recommended doses of Pavulon are exceeded this will increase the risk of prolonged neuromuscular block, difficulties with the reversal, and marked side effects. In heavy or obese patients calculation of the dosage of Pavulon on the basis of mg/kg leads to overdosing.

Pavulon is longer-acting in the intensive-care patient, and an intravenous dose of 0.06 mg/kg every one to one and a half hours, or even less frequently, is usually adequate. It can also be given by intramuscular injection in a dose of 0.03–0.06 mg/kg every one to two hours. Onset of effect by this route is about 10 minutes.

The duration of action depends upon the clinical condition of the patient and the dose administered, but in normal subjects receiving preoperative muscle relaxant doses the duration of action is usually 40–45 minutes.

In the control of tetanus, duration of Pavulon relaxation probably depends on the severity of the spasm: duration of effect can therefore be variable.

Pavulon should not be mixed with other agents in the same syringe, or with solutions for intravenous infusion, as a change in pH may induce precipitation.

Contra-indications, warnings, etc
Contra-indications: Patients with a known hypersensitivity to Pavulon injection.

Concurrent use of a depolarising neuromuscular blocking drug e.g. suxamethonium.

Precautions and warnings: Generally speaking it is advisable to monitor the degree of neuromuscular block. Before the administration of Pavulon conditions such as electrolyte disturbance, altered pH and dehydration should if possible be corrected. Care should be exercised if there is a danger of regurgitation when intubating the patient.

Pavulon should be used with particular care in neonates, in ill or cachectic patients, in the presence of liver disease or obstructive jaundice (resistant to effects of drug) in states with altered plasma protein levels or when there is diminished renal blood flow or renal disease.

Care should be taken in patients with renal insufficiency since Pavulon is partially excreted, unchanged, in the urine.

Pavulon should be used cautiously in patients with a tendency to hypertension, as in adrenogenital syndrome, phaeochromocytoma or hypertension caused by renal disease.

Extreme caution should be exercised, and very small doses used, in patients with myasthenia gravis or myasthenic syndrome, unless it is intended to administer prolonged post-operative respiratory assistance. In case of myopathy (such as dystrophia myotonica), severe obesity, electrolyte disturbances (e.g. excessive potassium loss), altered pH and after poliomyelitis or dehydration, Pavulon should be dosed carefully as unwanted effects may occur.

In the presence of liver disease the usual dose should be administered, but in certain cases a higher dose may be required, since, in some patients, there is increased resistance to the action of non-depolarising neuromuscular blocking agents.

In operations requiring hypothermia the neuromuscular blockade of non-depolarising drugs is decreased and increases when re-warming the patient. Hypothermia in neonates, therefore, requires a reduced dosage of Pavulon.

Care should be exercised during pregnancy, particularly during the first 12 weeks. Since the consequences of the use of neuromuscular blocking agents on the developing foetus are extremely difficult to assess, one should carefully consider the advantages and the risks.

Pavulon should be administered only by anaesthetists familiar with its use, and only when facilities for controlled ventilation, insufflation with oxygen and endotracheal intubation are available for immediate use.

Since Pavulon in clinically effective doses affects the respiratory muscles, as well as other skeletal muscles, respiration must be assisted in all patients. It is essential to ensure that the patient is breathing spontaneously, deeply and regularly before leaving the theatre after anaesthesia. The neuromuscular blockade achieved with Pavulon can be reversed with a cholinesterase inhibiting agent (e.g. neostigmine) in an adequate dose, together with atropine as an anticholinergic agent.

Pavulon should be used with extreme caution in patients with acid base disturbances, (particularly metabolic acidosis), or electrolyte imbalance. Hypokalaemia or hypocalcaemia may cause an increased effect.

Pavulon may cause a rise in blood pressure and this should be borne in mind when used concurrently with other agents, e.g. halothane, ketamine.

Special care should be exercised if given to the same patient more than once in 24 hours, as a cumulative effect may develop.

Patients with carcinomatosis, especially when associated with bronchial carcinoma, may exhibit a marked sensitivity to this agent, and the neuromuscular block produced may respond poorly to neostigmine.

Allergic reactions including bronchospasm and hypotension occur rarely with Pavulon.

Interactions: Prior to surgery and during anaesthesia a number of medicines are commonly administered to the patient. This creates the possibility of interaction. In addition, the condition of the patient may influence the neuromuscular blocking (n.m.b.) activity of Pavulon.

The following medicines and conditions of the patient may interact with the n.m.b. activity of Pavulon:

Administration of depolarising drugs (e.g. suxamethonium chloride) following a non-depolarising drug (e.g. Pavulon) is not advisable.

The non-depolarising drug increases resistance towards the neuromuscular blocking effect of the depolarising drug. Therefore high doses of a depolarising drug are necessary before muscular relaxation can be obtained. These high doses of a depolarising drug may cause endplate desensitisation and prolonged postoperative apnoea.

Unlike a non-depolarising block, a depolarising block cannot be overcome by an anticholinesterase agent and may even be worsened.

Recent evidence suggests that alkylating drugs (nitrogen mustards) should be considered a possible hazard when given to patients during anaesthesia involving the use of muscle relaxants.

There is a selective interaction between Pavulon and nitroglycerin in that the latter affects the process of recovery from neuromuscular blockade. When nitroglycerin infusion precedes Pavulon injection prolongation of the blockade will occur.

Care should be taken with anaesthesia involving the use of halothane and Pavulon in patients receiving chronic tricyclic antidepressant therapy, as this predisposes to the development of cardiac arrhythmias.

Anaesthetics: The following anaesthetics may influence the neuromuscular blocking activity of Pavulon:

Increased effect: halothane, ether, enflurane, isoflurane (Forane), methoxyflurane, cyclopropane, thiopentone, methohexitone.

Decreased effect: neurolept analgesia (NLA), propanidid.

Influence on the cardiovascular system: Pavulon does not intensify the hypotension induced by halothane; in addition the cardiac depression is partly restored. The excessive bradycardia induced by neurolept analgesia and some of the cholinergic effects of morphine derivatives are counteracted by Pavulon.

The following drugs may influence the duration of action of Pavulon and the intensity of the neuromuscular block:

Increased effect: other muscle relaxants (e.g. d-tubocurarine), antibiotics of the polypeptide and aminoglycoside groups (e.g. neomycin, streptomycin, kanamycin), diazepam, propranolol, thiamine (high dose), M.A.O. inhibiting agents, quinidine, magnesium sulphate, protamine, nitroglycerin.

Decreased effect: neostigmine, edrophonium, corticosteroids (high dose), adrenaline, potassium chloride, sodium chloride, calcium chloride, heparin (temporary decrease), azathioprine, theophylline.

Condition of the patient: The following conditions may influence the neuromuscular blocking activity of Pavulon:

Increased effect: Hypokalaemia (e.g. after severe vomiting, diarrhoea, digitalisation), hypermagnesaemia, hypocalcaemia (after massive transfusion), hypoproteinaemia, dehydration, acidosis, hypercapnoea, cachexia, myasthenia gravis, myasthenic syndrome, renal and liver failure, profound anaesthesia.

Decreased effect: Hypothermia, hyperdiuresis, superficial anaesthesia.

Disturbances in renal function and hypocalcaemia are factors favouring the development of a syndrome resembling that of myasthenia gravis following administration of antibiotics. A disturbed plasma protein pattern requires prudence. Pavulon (like d-tubocurarine) causes a reduction in the partial thromboplastin time and the prothrombin time.

With respect to the frequently reported interactions involving other non-depolarising neuromuscular blocking agents the anaesthetist should be aware of the possibility that similar interactions may occur with Pavulon.

Side-effects: After Pavulon a slight to moderate rise in arterial pressure may occur. Increased pulse rate and cardiac output are frequently reported, showing Pavulon to have weak vagolytic activity. In general this is considered to be a favourable effect. Pavulon decreases intra-ocular pressure and induces miosis, both effects being favourable in ophthalmic surgery. A few cases of localised reactions at the site of injection have been reported.

Overdosage: In the event of an overdosage the patient should continue to be ventilated, and at the same time receive a cholinesterase inhibiting agent (e.g. pyridostigmine, neostigmine) in an adequate dose, as an antidote.

Pharmaceutical precautions In the pharmacy, Pavulon should be stored at 2–8°C and protected from light, when it will retain its stability for two years. Pavulon is stable for six weeks at 25°C.

Opened ampoules of Pavulon should be discarded if the contents are not used within a few hours.

Legal category POM.

Package quantities Boxes of 25 ampoules 2 ml.

Further information The active substance of Pavulon is pancuronium bromide, an amino steroid which effectively blocks transmission of motor nerve impulses to the striated muscle receptors. Endplate depolarisation does not occur. Pancuronium bromide has no hormonal activity. An initial dose of Pavulon of 0.08 mg/kg IV has a mean onset of action of 45 seconds, a maximum effect after 90–120 seconds, and a mean duration of action of 60 minutes (these data are approximations since, as is well-known, all muscle relaxants display dose-response variability). The potency ratio of Pavulon/d-tubocurarine is approximately 6–7 : 1.

Pavulon is accepted as one of the standard preparations in anaesthesia, and is widely used in all fields of surgery. It has a smooth onset of action, extremely low toxicity and the virtual absence of such side-effects as histamine release, and although rare instances of bronchospasm have been reported Pavulon has, in general, a lack of associated bronchospasm. There is lack of ganglion blockade and thus no hypotensive effect, unlike some other muscle relaxants.

Pavulon is of considerable value when used in conjunction with halothane, since it helps to counteract the cardiovascular depression normally induced by halothane. Pavulon is particularly suitable for use in poor risk patients and in intensive-care units. Pavulon is used widely with good results in Caesarean section.

Product licence number 0065/5014.

*Trade Mark

Ortho-Cilag Pharmaceutical Limited

PO Box 79, Saunderton
High Wycombe
Buckinghamshire HP 14 4HJ.

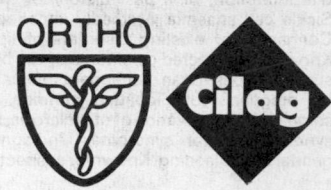

ACI-JEL* THERAPEUTIC VAGINAL JELLY

Presentation Acetic acid 0.92% w/w in a buffered (pH 4). gel base.

Uses In any case where the restoration and maintenance of vaginal acidity is desirable, as in the treatment of non-specific vaginal infection and in the milder forms of simple cervicitis. Aci-Jel Therapeutic Vaginal Jelly is also useful as an adjunct to systemic therapy in trichomoniasis, and prophylactically after courses of other, more specific therapy.

Dosage and administration One applicatorful intra-vaginally in the morning and upon retiring. The frequency of the application and duration of treatment depend upon the type of case and the degree of progress.

Contra-indications, warnings, etc
Contra-indications: None known.

Warnings: Rarely, local irritation and inflamation have been reported.

Precautions: Use during pregnancy: In view of the nature of the active ingredients Aci-Jel can be used with caution during pregnancy.

Overdosage: Aci-Jel Therapeutic Vaginal Jelly is intended for intravaginal use. If accidental ingestion of large quantities of the product occurs, an appropriate method of gastric emptying may be used if considered desirable.

Pharmaceutical precautions Store at room temperature.

Legal category GSL.

Package quantities Tube containing 85 g. with the ORTHO* Plastic Vaginal Applicator.

Further information Nil.

Product licence number 0076/5015.

BINOVUM*

Presentation ¼-inch diameter, circular tablets with flat faces and bevelled edges. The 7 white tablets are engraved C over 535 on both faces and contain 0.5 mg Norethisterone PhEur and 35 mcg Ethinyloestradiol BP. The 14 peach tablets are engraved C over 135 on both faces and contain 1.0 mg Norethisterone PhEur and 35 mcg Ethinyloestradiol BP.

Uses Contraception and the recognised indications for such oestrogen/progestogen combinations.

Action: Through the mechanism of gonadotrophin suppression by the oestrogenic and progestational actions of the ingredients. Although the primary mechanism of action is inhibition of ovulation, alterations to the cervical mucus and to the endometrium may also contribute to the efficacy of the product.

Dosage and administration The basic dosage regimen is a 28 day cycle, of 1 tablet daily for 21 days, followed by 7 tablet-free days. A white tablet is taken every day for 7 days, then a peach coloured tablet is taken every day for 14 days. For initial therapy, the first white tablet is taken on the first day of bleeding of the menstrual cycle. If BiNovum* Tablets are first taken later than the first day of bleeding of the first menstrual cycle of medication, contraceptive reliance should be not placed on this product until after the first 14 consecutive days of administration.

Subsequent cycles: Each subsequent course is started after 7 tablet-free days have followed the preceding course.

Changing from another combined oral contraceptive: The first white tablet should be taken on the first day of the withdrawal bleed after the completion of the previous course of tablets.

Changing from a progestogen-only contraceptive: The first white tablet should be taken on the first day of bleeding that occurs either during the last course of tablets or following completion of the tablet course.

Post-partum use: After pregnancy, oral contraception may be initiated immediately post-partum in the non-nursing patient or as soon as spontaneous menstruation has been resumed. Another method of contraception should be used in the interval between delivery and the first course of tablets, unless it is started within seven days of delivery. After a miscarriage or first-trimester abortion, oral contraception may be started immediately.

If the patient forgets more than one tablet, she should recommence the course as soon as she remembers, taking the appropriate tablet for that day and omitting any tablets delayed more than 12 hours. She should then use an additional method of contraception until the next withdrawal bleed. To obtain maximum contraceptive effectiveness, all contraceptive tablets should be taken exactly as directed and at approximately the same time each day.

If the patient has vomiting or diarrhoea, absorption of the hormones will be impaired, making it advisable to use an additional reliable method of contraception until her next menstrual period. Should a bleeding fail to occur at the usual time, the possibility of pregnancy should be excluded before starting the next pack.

Contra-indications, warnings, etc
Contraindications: Existing thrombophlebitis, throm-

boembolic disorders, cerebrovascular disease, myocardial infarction, or a past history of these conditions. Sickle-cell anaemia. Markedly impaired liver function. Congenital or existing disorders of lipid metabolism. Known or suspected carcinoma of the breast. Known or suspected oestrogen-dependent neoplasia. History during pregnancy of idiopathic jaundice, severe pruritus, shingles or deterioration of otosclerosis. Dubin-Johnson syndrome. Rotor syndrome. Undiagnosed abnormal genital tract bleeding. Known or suspected pregnancy.

Warnings: An increased risk of thrombophlebitis, cerebrovascular disorders, myocardial infarction and pulmonary embolism associated with the use of oral contraceptives has been reported in several retrospective case control studies. The increased risk has been estimated in these studies to be approximately 4 to 11 times higher (for cerebral haemorrhage two times higher) for users when compared to non users. This reported risk according to two of the studies is not related to duration of use nor does it persist after discontinuance according to one of the studies. An interim report of a large scale continuing prospective study has tended to confirm these retrospective studies for thrombophlebitis and possible cerebrovascular disorders. This study also reported that the risk of superficial and deep vein thrombosis was lower in women using preparations containing 50 mcg of oestrogen or less. There may not be full recovery from such disorders and it should be realised that in a few cases they are fatal.

Because of a possible increased risk of post surgical thromboembolic complications in oral contraceptive users, therapy should be discontinued at least six weeks prior to elective surgery. Caution should be exercised in administering oestrogen/progestogen combinations to women with a history of hypertension. An increased risk of surgically confirmed gall bladder disease associated with the use of oral contraceptives has been reported in a retrospective case control study.

Liver tumours, occasionally fatal, have been reported in women using oral contraceptives. These tumours may present as an abdominal mass, intra-abdominal bleeding and/or with signs and symptoms of acute abdomen. These have been reported in short term as well as long term users of oral contraceptives.

A small fraction of the active ingredients in oral contraceptives has been identified in the milk of mothers receiving these drugs. The effects, if any, on the breast-fed child have not been determined. If possible the use of oral contraceptives should be deferred until the infant is weaned.

When women have taken hormones during pregnancy there have been some reports of the possibility of adverse effects on the developing child. A direct relationship between such effects and oral contraceptives has not been confirmed, but as with any other drug, avoidance of continuing oral contraception in early pregnancy is desirable. Therefore pregnancy should be ruled out before initiating or continuing the administration of oral contraceptives to patients who have missed one menstrual period.

Certain factors may entail some risk of thrombosis, e.g. smoking, obesity, varicose veins, cardiovascular diseases, diabetes, and migraine. The suitability of a combined oral contraceptive should be judged according to the severity of such conditions in the individual case, and should be discussed with the patient before she decides to take it. The risk of arterial thrombosis associated with combined oral contraceptives increases with age and this risk is aggravated by cigarette smoking. The use of combined oral contraceptives in women in the older age group, especially those who are cigarette smokers, should therefore be discouraged and alternative methods advised.

Reduced efficacy and increased incidence of breakthrough bleeding have been associated with concomitant use of oral contraceptives and rifampicin. A similar association has been suggested with oral contraceptives and barbiturates, phenytoin sodium, ampicillin, tetracycline and griseofulvin.

Reasons for stopping oral contraceptives immediately: Early manifestations of thrombotic or thromboembolic disorders, thrombophlebitis, cerebrovascular disorders (including haemorrhage), myocardial infarction, pulmonary embolism or retinal thrombosis. Hypertension. Gradual or sudden, partial or complete loss of vision. Proptosis or diplopia. Onset or aggravation of migraine or development of headaches of a new pattern which are recurrent, persistent or severe. Papilloedema or any evidence of retinal vascular lesions. During periods of immobility (e.g. after accidents). Pregnancy. Manifestations of liver tumours.

Precautions: Examination of the pelvic organs, breasts and blood pressure should precede the prescribing of any oral contraceptive, and should be repeated regularly.

The following are some of the conditions reported to be influenced by oral contraceptive therapy, and where the physician will have to exercise medical judgement to commence, continue or discontinue therapy as appropriate.

(a) Pre-existing uterine fibromyomata may increase in size.
(b) A decrease in glucose tolerance in a significant number of women.
(c) An increase in blood pressure in a small but significant number of women.
(d) Cholestatic jaundice. Patients with a history of cholestatic jaundice of pregnancy are more likely to develop cholestatic jaundice during oral contraceptive therapy.
(e) Amenorrhoea during and after oral contraceptive therapy. Women with a past history of oligomenorrhoea or secondary amenorrhoea or women with irregular cycles are more likely to remain anovulatory or to become amenorrhoeic post oral contraceptive therapy.
(f) Depression.
(g) Fluid retention. Conditions which might be influenced by this factor include epilepsy, migraine, asthma, cardiac or renal dysfunction.
(h) Varicose veins.
(i) Multiple sclerosis.
(j) Porphyria.
(k) Tetany.
(l) Wearing of contact lenses.
or any condition that is prone to worsen during pregnancy.

The following laboratory determinations may be altered in patients using oral contraceptives:

Hepatic: Increased BSP retention and other tests.
Coagulation: Increased prothrombin, Factors VII, VIII, IX and X, decreased antithrombin III, increased platelet aggregability.
Endocrine: Increased PBI and butanol extractable protein bound iodine and decreased T_3 uptake, increased glucose blood levels.

Other: Increased phospholipids and tri-glycerides, decreased serum folate values and disturbance in tryptophan metabolism, decreased pregnanediol excretion, reduced response to metyrapone test.

These tests usually return to pre-therapy values after discontinuing oral contraceptive use. However, the physician should be aware that these altered determinations may mask an underlying disease.

Side effects: Those most commonly reported in early cycles of oral contraceptive therapy include breakthrough bleeding, spotting, nausea, vomiting and other gastrointestinal disturbances. These frequently decrease with continued use. Other common side-effects include: change in menstrual flow, change in weight, oedema, chloasma (which may persist post therapy), amenorrhoea, breast changes (tenderness, enlargement and secretion).

In addition to the conditions and disorders discussed above, the following have been reported as adverse reactions in patients using combined oral contraceptives:

Neuro-ocular lesions	Haemorrhagic eruptions
Rash	Cystitis-like syndrome
Cervical erosion and secretions	Headache
	Nervousness
Suppression of lactation	Fatigue
Pre-menstrual like syndrome	Hirsutism
	Loss of scalp hair
Changes in libido	Erythema multiforme
Leg cramp	Erythema nodosum
Relative pyridoxine deficiency	Itching
	Vaginal candidiasis
	Porphyria

Overdosage: Serious ill effects have not been reported following acute ingestion of large doses of oral contraceptives by young children. Overdosage may cause nausea, and withdrawal bleeding may occur in females. An appropriate method of gastric emptying may be used if considered desirable.

Pharmaceutical precautions Protect from light.

Legal category POM.

Package quantities Carton containing 3 pushpaks each of 21 tablets – sufficient for 3 cycles.

Further information Nil.

Product licence number 0076/0090.

DELFEN* CONTRACEPTIVE CREAM

Presentation Delfen Contraceptive Cream contains nonoxynol-9 5.0% w/w in a white, oil and water emulsion at pH 4.5.

Uses Delfen Contraceptive Cream is a spermicidal cream for the control of conception. A higher degree of protection against pregnancy will be afforded by using another method of contraception in addition to a spermicidal contraceptive.

Dosage and administration One applicatorful (5 cc) intravaginally prior to coitus. A fresh application must be made if intercourse is repeated or delayed by more than one hour. If a douche is desired, it should be deferred for at least six hours after intercourse.

Contra-indications, warnings, etc Hypersensitivity to the product.
Warnings: Where avoidance of pregnancy is essential

the choice of contraceptive should be made in consultation with a doctor or a family planning clinic.
Side-effects: Irritation of the vagina or penis has been reported. In such cases the medication should be discontinued.
Overdosage: Delfen Contraceptive Cream is intended for intravaginal use only, and if taken orally by mistake is likely to taste unpleasant. If excess quantities are swallowed this may give rise to gastric irritation as the product contains a surfactant, and general supportive therapy should be carried out if necessary.

Pharmaceutical precautions None known.

Legal category GSL.

Package quantities Tube containing 70 g.

ORTHO* Plastic Vaginal Applicator available separately.

Further information Nil.

Product licence number 0076/5004.

DELFEN* CONTRACEPTIVE FOAM

Presentation Delfen Contraceptive Foam is a white, non-staining aerosol foam which contains nonoxynol-9 12.5% w/w and buffered to normal vaginal pH of 4.5.

Uses Delfen Contraceptive Foam is a spermicidal foam for the control of conception. It provides rapid dispersion and extensive, uniform coverage of the cervix. A higher degree of protection against pregnancy will be afforded by using another method of contraception in addition to a spermicidal contraceptive. It is suitable for use with an occlusive device.

Dosage and administration One applicatorful intravaginally prior to coitus. A fresh application must be made if intercourse is repeated or delayed by more than one hour. If a douche is desired, it should be deferred for at least six hours after intercourse.

Contra-indications, warnings, etc Hypersensitivity to the product.
Warnings: Where avoidance of pregnancy is essential, the choice of contraceptive should be made in consultation with a doctor or a family planning clinic.
Side-effects: Irritation of the vagina or penis has been reported. In such cases the medication should be discontinued.
Overdosage: Delfen Contraceptive Foam is intended for intravaginal use only, and if taken orally by mistake is likely to taste unpleasant. If excess quantities are swallowed this may give rise to gastric irritation as the product contains a surfactant, and general supportive therapy should be carried out if necessary.

Pharmaceutical precautions Contents are under pressure. Do not burn or puncture container. Store at room temperature, not over 49°C (120°F).

Legal category GSL.

Package quantities 20 g aerosol container with or without the DELFEN* Contraceptive Foam Applicator.

Further information Nil.

Product licence number 0076/5003.

DERMONISTAT* CREAM

Presentation A smooth, white non-staining cream containing miconazole nitrate 2% w/w.

Uses A potent antimycotic cream for the treatment of fungal infections of the skin, hair and nails.

Dosage and administration May be applied topically to both adults and children.

Fungal infections of the skin: The cream should be applied to the lesions twice daily and continued for 10 days after the lesions have disappeared.

Fungal infections of the nail: The cream should be applied thinly to the infected nail once daily and the nail covered with a non-perforated plastic bandage. Nails should be clipped short at regular intervals and treatment continued until the growth of the new nail is established and a definite cure can be observed.

Contra-indications, warnings, etc Hypersensitivity to the product.

Side-effects: Isolated cases of sensitisation and irritation have been reported. If this occurs administration of the product should be discontinued.

Precautions: Dermonistat Cream is only absorbed in small amounts following application to the skin. Hence no special precautions are necessary in elderly patients. In view of the low level of absorption and the lack of teratogenic effects in animals, Dermonistat can be used with caution during pregnancy.

Overdosage: Dermonistat Cream is intended for topical use. If accidental ingestion of large quantities of the product occurs, an appropriate method of gastric emptying may be used if considered desirable.

Pharmaceutical precautions None known.

Legal category P.

Package quantities 30 g tubes. A patient-instruction leaflet is enclosed in each package.

Further information Nil.

Product licence number 0076/0041.

GYNOL* II CONTRACEPTIVE JELLY

Presentation Gynol II Contraceptive Jelly is a clear, unscented, unflavoured water-dispersible spermicidal jelly which contains nonoxynol-9 2% w/w buffered to normal vaginal pH.

Uses Gynol II Contraceptive Jelly is a spermicidal jelly for use in conjunction with an occlusive vaginal diaphragm, whenever the control of conception is desirable.

A higher degree of protection against pregnancy will be afforded by using another method of contraception in addition to a spermicidal contraceptive.

Dosage and administration The jelly should be spread over the surface of the diaphragm which will be in contact with the cervix and on the rim. The diaphragm must be allowed to remain in situ for at least six to eight hours after coitus. A fresh application of jelly or other spermicides, e.g. Orthoforms* Contraceptive Pessaries, must be made prior to any subsequent act of coitus within this period of time, without removing the diaphragm. (A vaginal applicator should be used for inserting more cream or jelly.)

Contra-indications, warnings, etc
Contra-indications: Hypersensitivity to the product.

Warnings: Where avoidance of pregnancy is essential, the choice of contraceptive should be made in consultation with a doctor or family planning clinic.

Occasional irritation of the vagina or penis has been reported. In such cases the medication should be discontinued.

The diaphragm should not remain in position for longer than 24 hours.

Overdosage: Gynol II Contraceptive Jelly is intended for intravaginal use only. If excess quantities are taken orally by mistake this may give rise to gastric irritation as the product contains a surfactant, and general supportive therapy should be carried out if necessary.

Pharmaceutical precautions None known.

Legal category GSL.

Package quantities Tube containing 81 g. Ortho* Vaginal Applicator available separately.

Further information Nil.

Product licence number 0076/0127.

GYNO-PEVARYL* 1 VAGINAL PESSARY

Presentation A white egg shaped pessary containing 150 mg of econazole nitrate and melting at 37°C.

Uses Vaginitis due to candida albicans and other yeasts.

Dosage and administration The pessary should be inserted as high as possible into the vagina in the evening prior to retiring.

Contra-indications, warnings, etc
Contra-indications: None known.

Side-effects: None known.

Overdose: Not applicable.

Precautions: Hypersensitivity has rarely been recorded.

Gyno-Pevaryl 1 Vaginal Pessary is effective in the treatment of vaginal candidiasis associated with pregnancy. However, as with any new product, caution should be exercised when prescribing during the first trimester of pregnancy.

Pharmaceutical precautions Store in a cool place.

Legal category POM.

Package quantities Each pack contains one pessary and a patient instruction leaflet.

Further information Anogenital hygiene is important to help prevent re-infection.

Product licence number 0076/0097.

GYNO-PEVARYL*150 VAGINAL PESSARIES
GYNO-PEVARYL*150 VAGINAL PESSARIES AND CREAM COMBIPACK

Presentation *Pessaries:* White egg-shaped pessaries each containing 150 mg econazole nitrate and melting at 37°C.

Combipack: A combination pack comprising 3 Gyno-Pevaryl vaginal pessaries (each containing 150 mg econazole nitrate) plus a 15 g tube of Gyno-Pevaryl cream (containing 1% econazole nitrate).

Uses *Pessaries:* Vaginitis due to *Candida albicans* and other yeasts.

Combipack: Pessaries for vaginitis; cream for associated vulvitis and to treat the sexual partner to help prevent re-infection.

Dosage and administration *Pessaries:* One pessary should be inserted high into the vagina each evening for three consecutive days.

Combipack: Pessaries as above. The cream should be applied to the vulva and perianal region and/or to the sexual partner's penis, including under the foreskin.

Contra-indications, warnings, etc
Contra-indications: None known.

Side-effects: Rarely, transient local mild irritation may occur immediately after application.

Precautions: Hypersensitivity has rarely been recorded, if it should occur, administration should be discontinued. Gyno-Pevaryl Pessaries and Cream are only absorbed in small amounts following topical application. Hence no special precautions are necessary in elderly patients.

Gyno-Pevaryl 150 Vaginal Pessaries are effective in the treatment of vaginal candidiasis associated with pregnancy, but as with any product, caution should be exercised when prescribing during the first trimester.

Overdosage: Gyno-Pevaryl Vaginal Pessaries and Cream are intended for intravaginal use. If accidental ingestion of large quantities of the product occurs, an appropriate method of gastric emptying may be used if considered desirable.

Pharmaceutical precautions Store in a cool place.

Legal category POM.

Package quantities *Pessaries:* Each pack contains 3 pessaries and a patient instruction leaflet. The pessaries are individually sealed in a white plastic strip marked Gyno-Pevaryl 150 at regular intervals.

Combipack: Each pack contains 3 pessaries, a 15 g tube of cream and a patient instruction leaflet.

Further information Anogenital hygiene is important to help prevent re-infection.

Product licence numbers
Pessaries   0076/0058
Combipack   0076/0058 and 0076/0060

LIPPES LOOP* INTRAUTERINE CONTRACEPTIVE DEVICE

Presentation The Lippes Loop is manufactured from polyethylene in the shape of a double 'S'. Four different sizes are available to allow for the variability in the size of the uterus (see below). A fine double thread 'tail' made of polyethylene suture material (monofilament) is attached to the lower end to facilitate removal. In addition, palpation of the tail in the vagina by the patient, or visualization by the physician, can assist in determining whether or not an undetected expulsion has occurred. The Lippes Loop comes prepacked and sterilized with an introducer and insertion tube in a sealed envelope. The insertion tube is equipped with a flange which is used to determine the depth to which the tube should be inserted through the cervical canal and into the uterine cavity. The four available sizes are as follows:

Loop A – 22.5 mm. Blue thread. For nulliparous patients.

Loop B – 27.5 mm WITH REDUCED RADII. Black thread. Suggested for patients who have experienced premature pregnancy losses, and multiparous patients whose uteri measure less than 6 cm.

Loop C – 30 mm WITH REDUCED RADII. Yellow thread. Suggested for use in patients with one or more children.

Loop D – 30 mm. White thread. Suggested for use in multiparous patients where the risk of expulsion is thought to be greater than usual.

Uses Contraception.

Dosage and administration The Lippes Loop is inserted by a doctor into the patient's uterus. The insertion technique is described on the leaflet provided with each device.

Contra-indications, warnings, etc Contraindications: IUCD's should not be inserted when the following conditions exist:

1. Pregnancy or suspicion of pregnancy.
2. Abnormalities of the uterus resulting in distortion of the uterine cavity.
3. Pelvic inflammatory disease or a history of repeated pelvic inflammatory disease.
4. Postpartum endometritis or infected abortion in the past three months.
5. Known or suspected uterine or cervical malignancy including unresolved abnormal cervical smear.
6. Genital bleeding of unknown aetiology.
7. Cervicitis, until infection is controlled.
8. Large or multiple fibroids.
9. Menorrhagia and/or intermenstrual bleeding.
10. Severe dysmenorrhoea.

Warnings:

1. Pregnancy:
(a) Long-term effects: Long-term effects on the offspring, when pregnancy occurs with the Lippes Loop *in situ*, are unknown.
(b) Septic abortion: Reports have indicated an increased incidence of septic abortion associated in some instances with septicaemia, septic shock, and, rarely, death in patients becoming pregnant with an IUCD *in situ*. Most of these reports have been associated with the mid-trimester of pregnancy. In some cases the initial symptoms have been insidious and not easily recognised. If pregnancy should occur with an IUCD *in situ*, it is recommended that the IUCD be removed if the thread is visible. If the thread is not visible or device removal proves to be or would be difficult, the IUCD may be left *in situ* until the pregnancy goes to term or until a decision is made to terminate the pregnancy.
(c) Continuation of pregnancy: If the patient chooses to continue the pregnancy with the IUCD *in situ* there is an increased risk of spontaneous abortion and of sepsis, including, rarely, death. If the pregnancy is continued the patient should be closely observed and advised to report immediately all abnormal symptoms, such as flu-like syndrome, fever, abnormal cramping and pain, bleeding or vaginal discharge. The onset of septicaemia may be insidious with general symptoms rather than initial signs of spontaneous abortion.

2. Ectopic Pregnancy:

(a) A pregnancy that occurs with an IUCD *in situ* is more likely to be ectopic than a pregnancy occurring without an IUCD *in situ*. Accordingly, patients who become pregnant whilst using the IUCD require careful evaluation for the possibility of an ectopic pregnancy.

(b) Special attention as to whether an ectopic pregnancy has occurred is required for patients with delayed menses, slight metrorrhagia, and/or unilateral pelvic pain and for patients who wish to terminate the pregnancy with the device *in situ*.

3. Pelvic Infection: An increased risk of pelvic infection has been reported with the IUCD in situ. This, at times, may result in the development of bilateral or unilateral tubo-ovarian abscesses or general peritonitis which may lead to infertility if left untreated. Appropriate aerobic and anaerobic bacteriological studies are indicated at the time of initiation of antibiotic therapy. Removal of the IUCD is advised with reassessment of continuing treatment, based upon these bacteriological and sensitivity tests.

4. Embedding: Partial penetration or embedding of the IUCD in the endometrium may cause subsequent removal to be a difficult procedure.

5. Perforation: Partial or total perforation of the uterine wall or cervix may occur with the use of IUCD's. The possibility of perforation must be kept in mind during insertion and at the time of any subsequent examination. If perforation occurs, the IUCD should be removed. Adhesions, foreign body reactions, and intestinal obstruction may result if an IUCD is left in the peritoneal cavity. It is possible for the IUCD to penetrate the uterine wall at any time following insertion.

Precautions: Prior to insertion of an IUCD, a thorough history and physical examination, including a pelvic examination and Papanicolaou smear, should be performed.

Insertion of an IUCD into a uterine cavity measuring less than 6.5 cm may increase the incidence of expulsion, bleeding, pain and perforation.

The patient should be re-examined within 3 months after insertion and thereafter at yearly intervals to ensure the device is still *in situ*. The patient should be advised to contact her doctor immediately if she misses a menstrual period or has any other reason to think she may be pregnant.

IUCD's should be used with caution in patients:

a) With anaemia.

b) Receiving anticoagulant therapy or having any disorder of coagulation.

c) Receiving steroid therapy (possible masking of pelvic inflammatory disease should be borne in mind).

d) With known or suspected rheumatic or congenital heart disease. The need for appropriate antibiotic cover during insertion of the device should be carefully considered.

e) With a history of a previous uterine incision or perforation of the uterus.

f) With a history of previous ectopic pregnancy.

Syncope, bradycardia or other neuro-vascular episodes may occur during insertion or removal of IUCD's, especially in patients susceptible to these conditions. The possibility of a seizure being precipitated in a patient suffering from epilepsy, at or shortly after the insertion of an IUCD, should also be borne in mind.

No method of contraception can be described as absolutely effective. In some cases it may be appropriate to recommend the use of an additional reliable method of contraception at mid-cycle.

Time of insertion: The Lippes Loop should be inserted preferably during or immediately after a normal menstrual period. Lippes Loop normally is not inserted until 6 weeks or more after delivery or an abortion.

To remove: To remove the Lippes Loop, pull gently on the exposed tail.

Spontaneous expulsion: Expulsion of the Lippes Loop occurs in some patients spontaneously. This expulsion occurs most frequently during the first or second cycle of use, usually at the time of the menstrual period. Expulsion can, however, occur at any time, even several months after insertion.

Confirmation of the expulsion of the device is necessary prior to inserting a second device. Pregnancy must be ruled out before any method of locating the device is undertaken.

Adverse reactions:

1. *Effect on menstrual patterns:* Post-insertion: Almost all patients will experience varying amounts of vaginal bleeding after insertion of the Lippes Loop. In approximately 25% of patients, post-insertion bleeding should cease in a few days.

Intermenstrual Bleeding: Spotting or light bleeding may occur intermenstrually in approximately 25% of patients in the first cycle following insertion. A few patients may experience mid-cycle spotting for several consecutive cycles.

Menstrual Periods: Variation in the first menstrual period following insertion is frequent. This occurs most often as spotting or a brown discharge for 2 days before the period. The first menstrual flow will be longer and slightly heavier than usual, and occasionally the bleeding may be extremely heavy. If this bleeding persists, consideration may be given to removal of the device. A few patients may have heavier than normal bleeding during the second postinsertion menstrual period. The bleeding pattern usually returns to normal by the third cycle. Pelvic pathology should be considered if heavy bleeding occurs beyond this point.

2. *Cramps:* Insertion of the Lippes Loop in multiparous patients usually causes no pain. Slight cramps lasting a few minutes are reported by about 10% of patients in this group and rarely require analgesic therapy.

In contrast, most nulliparous patients complain of moderate to severe cramps which may last for several days following insertion. Analgesics are often required for relief of discomfort in this group: occasionally, removal of the device may be necessary.

3. *Syncope:* Syncope may occur immediately following insertion, particularly in nulliparous patients: it is uncommon in the multiparous patient. A few minutes in a horizontal position may be needed for stabilisation in some patients.

4. *Pelvic inflammatory disease:* Recent studies have indicated that there may be an increased incidence of pelvic inflammatory disease amongst patients fitted with any intrauterine contraceptive device.

Handling precautions If the seal of the sterile envelope is broken, the device inside should not be used.

Legal category POM. Also available through family planning clinics.

Package Quantities Each sterile Lippes Loop is

supplied in a sealed envelope. A 'Direction for the Patient' leaflet is also supplied.

Further information Nil.

Product licence numbers
Size A 0076/0077
Size B 0076/0078
Size C 0076/0079
Size D 0076/0080

MASSE* BREAST CREAM

Presentation A white oil in water cream containing glycerin, lanolin, arachis oil, sorbitan monostearate, glyceryl monostearate, cetyl alcohol, stearic acid, polysorbate 60, propyl p-hydroxybenzoate, methyl-p-hydroxybenzoate, sodium benzoate, purified water.

Uses For pre-natal and post-natal nipple care. Use prenatally for preparing the nipples for breast feeding including the massage of flat and inverted nipples. Use post-natally for routine application to the nipples of lactating women.

Dosage and administration *Pre-natal nipple care:* Masse Breast Cream is applied once or twice daily during the last two or three months of pregnancy. A 1" ribbon of cream is massaged gently into the nipples and the surrounding pigmented area with the fingertips until the cream is absorbed. The massage should be with gentle outward motion from the areola to the apex of the nipple.

Post-natal nipple care: Masse Breast Cream is massaged gently around the nipple and areola after the breast has been cleansed after each nursing.

Contra-indications, warnings, etc Acute mastitis or breast abscess. Lanolin sensitivity.

Hypersensitivity to the product: In cases of excess soreness or irritation consult your physician.

Local irritation has been reported in rare cases.

Overdosage: Masse Breast Cream is intended for topical use. If accidental ingestion of large quantities of the product occurs, an appropriate method of gastric emptying may be used if considered desirable.

Pharmaceutical precautions None known.

Legal category GSL.

Package 28 g tubes. A patient instruction leaflet is enclosed in each package.

Further information Nil.

Product licence number 0076/5009.

MICRONOR* ORAL CONTRACEPTIVE TABLETS

Presentation White, $\frac{1}{4}$ inch diameter, circular tablets with flat faces and bevelled edges, bearing on each face the engraving C over 035. Micronor Oral Contraceptive Tablets each contain 0.35 mg Norethisterone PhEur.

Uses Contraception.

Action: Micronor has a progestational effect on the endometrium and on the cervical mucus. The exact mechanism of how it prevents conception has not been confirmed.

Dosage and administration Micronor is administered orally on a continuous daily dosage regimen starting on the first day of menstruation. One tablet is taken at the same time each day, every day of the year, whether menstruation occurs or not. When starting Micronor therapy the patient should be instructed to use an additional reliable non-hormonal method of contraception during the first 14 days of the first cycle.

The non-nursing patient may be prescribed Micronor in the post partum period whether or not menstruation has resumed provided the possibility of pregnancy has been excluded.

The possibility of ovulation and conception prior to initiation of medication should be considered.

Strict adherence to the dosage regimen is important. If the patient should fail to take 1 tablet at the usual time protection is reduced. She should take the missed tablet as soon as she remembers and take the next tablet on the day it is due. When a tablet is missed an additional reliable means of contraception should be used in addition to taking Micronor until her next period occurs.

If the patient does not have a period within 45 days of her last period, pregnancy should be excluded.

If the patient has vomiting or diarrhoea, absorption of the hormone will be impaired, making it advisable to use an additional reliable method of contraception until the next menstrual period.

Contra-indications, warnings, etc Any of the following conditions should be regarded as contra-indications for the use of Micronor. Existing thrombophlebitis, thromboembolic disorders, cerebral vascular disease, myocardial infarction, or a past history of these conditions. Markedly impaired liver function. Known or suspected hormone dependent neoplasia. Known or suspected carcinoma of the breast. Undiagnosed abnormal genital tract bleeding. Known or suspected pregnancy.

Warnings: Because of a possible increased risk of post surgery thromboembolic complications in oral contraceptive users, therapy should be discontinued six weeks prior to elective surgery.

Masculinisation of the female foetus has occurred when progestogens have been used in pregnant women, although this has been observed at doses much higher than that contained in Micronor. Pregnancy should be ruled out before continuing administration of Micronor to patients who have gone 45 days without a menstrual period.

A small fraction of the active ingredients in oral contraceptives has been identified in the milk of mothers receiving these drugs. The effects, if any, on the breast-fed child have not been determined. If possible the use of oral contraceptives should be deferred until the infant is weaned.

Reduced efficacy and increased incidence of breakthrough bleeding have been associated with concomitant use of oral contraceptives and rifampicin. A similar association has been suggested with oral contraceptives and barbiturates, phenytoin sodium, ampicillin, tetracycline and griseofulvin.

Reasons for stopping oral contraceptives immediately: Early manifestations of thrombotic or thromboembolic disorders, thrombophlebitis, cerebrovascular disorders (including haemorrhage), myocardial infarction, pulmonary embolism. Gradual or sudden, partial or complete loss of vision. Proptosis or diplopia. Onset or aggravation of migraine or development of headaches of a new pattern which are recurrent, persistent or severe. Papilloedema or any evidence of retinal vascular lesions. During periods of immobility (e.g. after accidents). Pregnancy. Manifestations of liver tumours.

Precautions: Examination of the pelvic organs, breasts and blood pressure should precede the prescribing of any oral contraceptive, and should be repeated regularly. The following are some of the medical conditions reported to be influenced by the combined pill, and may be affected by Micronor. The physician will have to exercise medical judgement to commence, continue or discontinue therapy as appropriate.

a) Pre-existing uterine fibromyomata may increase in size.

b) A decrease in glucose tolerance in a significant number of women.

c) An increase in blood pressure in a small but significant number of women.

d) Cholestatic jaundice. Patients with a history of cholestatic jaundice of pregnancy are more likely to develop cholestatic jaundice during oral contraceptive therapy.

e) Amenorrhoea during and after oral contraceptive therapy. Women with a past history of oligomenorrhoea or secondary amenorrhoea or women with irregular cycles may be more likely to remain anovulatory or to become amenorrhoeic post oral contraceptive therapy.

f) Depression.

g) Fluid retention. Conditions which might be influenced by this factor include epilepsy, migraine, asthma, cardiac or renal dysfunction.

h) Varicose veins.

i) Multiple sclerosis.

j) Porphyria.

k) Tetany.

l) Wearing of contact lenses.

or any condition that is prone to worsen during pregnancy.

The following laboratory determinations may be altered in patients using oral contraceptives.

Hepatic: Increased BSP retention and other tests.

Coagulation: Increased prothrombin, Factors VII, VIII, IX and X, decreased antithrombin III, increased platelet aggregability.

Endocrine: Increased PBI and butanol extractable protein bound iodine and decreased T^3 uptake, increased glucose blood levels.

Other: Increased phospholipids and tri-glycerides, decreased serum folate values and disturbance in tryptophan metabolism, decreased pregnanediol excretion, reduced response to metyrapone test.

These tests usually return to pre-therapy values after discontinuing oral contraceptive use. However, the physician should be aware that these altered determinations may mask an underlying disease.

Side-effects: Micronor has been found to be a well tolerated drug. Side-effects are usually self-limiting and of relatively short duration. Amongst the symptoms reported are headaches, nausea, vomiting, breast changes, change in weight, chloasma, break-through bleeding and spotting. Particularly in the early cycles of therapy the menstrual pattern becomes irregular, some cycles being short and others long. It is important that patients should be advised that whilst on Micronor therapy they will experience that variation in cycle length.

Overdosage: Serious ill effects have not been reported following acute ingestion of large doses of oral contraceptives by young children. Overdosage may cause nausea, and withdrawal bleeding may occur in females. An appropriate method of gastric emptying may be used if considered desirable.

Pharmaceutical precautions Protect from light.

Legal category POM.

Package quantities Carton containing 3 pushpaks each of 28 tablets – sufficient for 3 cycles.

Further information Nil.

Product licence number 0076/0017.

MONISTAT* CREAM
MONISTAT* PESSARIES

Presentation *Cream:* A white, water-miscible cream containing miconazole nitrate 2% w/w.

Pessaries: White egg-shaped pessaries each containing 100 mg miconazole nitrate and melting at 37°C.

Uses A potent antimycotic agent for the local treatment and rapid symptomatic relief of vulvovaginal moniliasis and balanitis.

Dosage and administration *Cream:* One applicatorful (approx. 5 g) intravaginally, with additional cream smeared onto other affected areas, once daily, preferably at night, for 14 days.

Pessaries: One pessary should be inserted high into the vagina at night for the same period.

Patients should be instructed not to discontinue treatment upon relief of symptoms, but to complete the prescribed course. The simultaneous treatment of the partner with Monistat Cream is advisable.

Contra-indications, warnings, etc Hypersensitivity to the product.

Side-effects: Isolated cases of vulvo-vaginal burning, itching and irritation have been reported after using the product. If this occurs administration of the product should be discontinued.

Precautions: Monistat Cream and Pessaries are only absorbed in small amounts following topical application. Hence no special precautions are necessary in elderly patients. In view of the low level of absorption and lack of teratogenic effects in animals, the products can be used with caution during pregnancy.

Overdosage: Monistat Cream and Pessaries are intended for intravaginal use. If accidental ingestion of large quantities of the product occurs, an appropriate method of gastric emptying may be used if considered desirable.

Pharmaceutical precautions Cream – none known. Pessaries – store in a cool place.

Legal category POM.

Package quantities *Cream:* 78 g tube with ORTHO* Plastic Vaginal applicator.

Pessaries: Each pessary is completely sealed in PVC strips with seven pessaries to a strip. Each carton contains two strips of seven pessaries.

Both packs contain full patient instructions.

Further information Monistat Cream or Pessaries are particularly useful in the treatment of those patients with predisposing conditions for monilial vulvovaginitis –

pregnancy, diabetes and those taking oral contraceptives or broad-spectrum antibiotics.

Product licence numbers
Cream   0076/0040
Pessaries   0076/0048

NEOCON* 1/35

Presentation Peach coloured ¼ inch diameter, circular tablets with flat faces and bevelled edges, bearing the engraving C over 135 on each face. Each tablet contains 1 mg Norethisterone PhEur and 35 mcg Ethinyloestradiol BP.

Uses Contraception and the recognised indications for such oestrogen/progestogen combinations.

Action: Through the mechanism of gonadotrophin suppression by the oestrogenic and progestational actions of the ingredients. Although the primary mechanism of action is inhibition of ovulation, alteration to the cervical mucus and to the endometrium may also contribute to the efficacy of the product.

Dosage and administration The basic dosage regimen is a 28-day cycle of 1 tablet daily for 21 days followed by seven tablet-free days. For initial therapy the first tablet is taken on the fifth day of the menstrual cycle, counting the first day of bleeding as Day 1. Each subsequent course is started after seven tablet-free days have followed the preceding course. To obtain maximal contraceptive effectiveness, all contraceptive tablets should be taken exactly as directed and at approximately the same time each day. Contraception can be initiated immediately post partum in the non-nursing patient. The possibility of ovulation and conception prior to initiation of medication should be considered.

The patient should be advised that during the first 14 days of the first course an additional reliable non-hormonal form of contraception should be used. If the patient misses more than 1 tablet, she should begin taking tablets again as soon as remembered and an additional reliable method of contraception used until the next withdrawal bleed. If the patient has vomiting or diarrhoea, absorption of the hormones will be impaired, making it advisable to use an additional reliable method of contraception until her next menstrual period. Should a bleeding fail to occur at the usual time, the possibility of pregnancy should be excluded before starting the next pack.

Contra-indications, warnings, etc Existing thrombophlebitis, thromboembolic disorders, cerebral vascular disease, myocardial infarction, or a past history of these conditions. Sickle-cell anaemia. Markedly impaired liver function. Congenital or existing disorders of lipid metabolism. Known or suspected carcinoma of the breast. Known or suspected oestrogen-dependent neoplasia. History during pregnancy of idiopathic jaundice, severe pruritus, shingles or deterioration of otosclerosis. Dubin-Johnson syndrome. Rotor Syndrome. Undiagnosed abnormal genital tract bleeding. Known or suspected pregnancy.

Warnings: An increased risk of thrombophlebitis, cerebrovascular disorders, myocardial infarction and pulmonary embolism associated with the use of oral contraceptives has been reported in several retrospective case control studies. The increased risk has been estimated in these studies to be approximately 4 to 11 times higher (for cerebral haemorrhage two times higher) for users when compared to non users. This reported risk according to two of the studies is not related to duration of use nor does it persist after discontinuance according to one of the studies. An interim report of a large scale continuing prospective study has tended to confirm these retrospective studies for thrombophlebitis and possible cerebrovascular disorders. This study also reported that the risk of superficial and deep vein thrombosis was lower in women using preparations containing 50 mcg of oestrogen or less. There may not be full recovery from such disorders and it should be realised that in a few cases they are fatal.

Because of a possible increased risk of post surgery thromboembolic complications in oral contraceptive users, therapy should be discontinued at least six weeks prior to elective surgery. Caution should be exercised in administering oestrogen/progestogen combinations to women with a history of hypertension. An increased risk of surgically confirmed gall bladder disease associated with the use of oral contraceptives has been reported in a retrospective case control study.

Liver tumours, occasionally fatal, have been reported in women using oral contraceptives. These tumours may present as an abdominal mass, intra-abdominal bleeding and/or with signs and symptoms of acute abdomen. These have been reported in short-term as well as long-term users of oral contraceptives.

A small fraction of the active ingredients in oral contraceptives has been identified in the milk of mothers receiving these drugs. The effects, if any, on the breast-fed child have not been determined. If possible the use of oral contraceptives should be deferred until the infant is weaned.

When women have taken hormones during pregnancy there have been some reports of the possibility of adverse effects on the developing child. A direct relationship between such effects and oral contraceptives has not been confirmed, but as with any other drug, avoidance of continuing oral contraception in early pregnancy is desirable. Therefore pregnancy should be ruled out before initiating or continuing the administration of oral contraceptives to patients who have missed one menstrual period.

Certain factors may entail some risk of thrombosis, eg smoking, obesity, varicose veins, caridovascular diseases, diabetes, and migraine. The suitability of a combined oral contraceptive should be judged according to the severity of such conditions in the individual case, and should be discussed with the patient before she decides to take it. The risk of arterial thrombosis associated with combined oral contraceptives increases with age and this risk is aggravated by cigarette smoking. The use of combined oral contraceptives in women in the older age group, especially those who are cigarette smokers, should therefore be discouraged and alternative methods advised.

Reduced efficacy and increased incidence of breakthrough bleeding have been associated with concomitant use of oral contraceptives and rifampicin. A similar association has been suggested with oral contraceptives and barbiturates, phenytoin sodium, ampicillin, tetracycline and griseofulvin.

Reasons for stopping oral contraception immediately: Early manifestation of thrombotic or thromboembolic disorders, thrombophlebitis, cerebrovascular disorders (including haemorrhage), myocardial infarction, pulmonary embolism or retinal thrombosis. Hypertension.

Gradual or sudden, partial or complete loss of vision. Proptosis or diplopia. Onset or aggravation of migraine or development of headaches of a new pattern which are recurrent, persistent or severe. Papilloedema or any evidence of retinal vascular lesions. During periods of immobility (eg. after accidents). Pregnancy. Manifestations of liver tumours.

Precautions: Examination of the pelvic organs, breasts and blood pressure should precede the prescribing of any oral contraceptive, and should be repeated regularly. The following are some of the conditions reported to be influenced by oral contraceptive therapy, and where the physician will have to exercise medical judgement to commence, continue or discontinue therapy as appropriate.

a) Pre-existing uterine fibromyomata may increase in size.
b) A decrease in glucose tolerance in a significant number of women.
c) An increase in blood pressure in a small but significant number of women.
d) Cholestatic jaundice. Patients with a history of cholestatic jaundice of pregnancy are more likely to develop cholestatic jaundice during oral contraceptive therapy.
e) Amenorrhoea during and after oral contraceptive therapy. Women with a past history of oligomenorrhoea or secondary amenorrhoea or women with irregular cycles may be more likely to remain anovulatory or to become amenorrhoeic post oral contraceptive therapy.
f) Depression.
g) Fluid retention. Conditions which might be influenced by this factor including epilepsy, migraine, asthma, cardiac or renal dysfunction.
h) Varicose veins.
i) Multiple sclerosis.
j) Porphyria.
k) Tetany.
l) Wearing of contact lenses
or any condition that is prone to worsen during pregnancy.

The following laboratory determinations may be altered in patients using oral contraceptives:

Hepatic: Increased BSP retention and other tests.
Coagulation: Increased prothrombin, Factors VII, VIII, IX and X; decreased antithrombin III; increased platelet aggregability.
Endocrine: Increased PBI and butanol extractable protein bound iodine and decreased T3 uptake, increased glucose blood levels.
Other: Increased phospholipids and tri-glycerides, decreased serum folate values and disturbance in tryptophan metabolism. Decreased pregnanediol excretion, reduced response to metyrapone test.

These tests usually return to pre-therapy values after discontinuing oral contraceptive use. However, the physician should be aware that these altered determinations may mask an underlying disease.

Side-effects: Side-effects most commonly reported in early cycles of oral contraceptive therapy include breakthrough bleeding, spotting, nausea, vomiting and other gastrointestinal disturbances. These frequently decrease with continued use. Other common side-effects include: change in menstrual flow, change in weight, oedema, chloasma (which may persist post

therapy), amenorrhoea, breast changes (tenderness, enlargement and secretion).

In addition to the conditions and disorders discussed above, the following have been reported as adverse reactions in patients using combined oral contraceptives:

Neuro-ocular lesions	Haemorrhagic eruptions
Rash	Cystitis-like syndrome
Cervical erosion and secretions	Headache
	Nervousness
Suppression of lactation	Fatigue
Pre-menstrual like syndrome	Hirsutism
	Loss of scalp hair
Changes in libido	Erythema multiforme
Leg cramp	Erythema nodosum
Relative pyridoxine deficiency	Itching
	Vaginal candidiasis
	Porphyria

Overdosage: Serious ill effects have not been reported following acute ingestion of large doses of oral contraceptives by young children. Overdosage may cause nausea, and withdrawal bleeding may occur in females. An appropriate method of gastric emptying may be used if considered desirable.

Pharmaceutical precautions Protect from light.

Legal category POM.

Package quantities Carton containing 3 pushpaks each of 21 tablets – sufficient for 3 cycles.

Further information Nil.

Product licence number 0074/0054.

ORTHO-CREME* CONTRACEPTIVE CREAM

Presentation Ortho-Creme Contraceptive Cream is a white spermicidal cream which contains nonoxynol-9 2.0% w/w, buffered to normal vaginal pH.

Uses Ortho-Creme Contraceptive Cream is a spermicidal cream for the control of conception. A higher degree of protection against pregnancy will be afforded by using another method of contraception in addition to a spermicidal contraceptive.

Dosage and administration The cream should be spread over the surface of the diaphragm which will be in contact with the cervix, and on the rim. The diaphragm, and spermicide must be allowed to remain undisturbed for at least six to eight hours after coitus. A fresh application of cream or other spermicides, e.g. Orthoforms Contraceptive Pessaries, must be made prior to any subsequent act of coitus within this period of time, without removing the diaphragm. (A vaginal applicator should be used for inserting more cream or jelly.)

Douching is not recommended; but if it is desired it should be deferred for at least six hours after intercourse.

Contra-indications, warnings, etc Hypersensitivity to the product.

Warning: Where avoidance of pregnancy is essential, the choice of contraceptive should be made in consultation with a doctor or a family planning clinic.

Occasional irritation of the vagina or penis has been reported. In such cases the medication should be discontinued.

The diaphragm should not remain in position for longer than 24 hours.

Overdosage: Ortho-Creme Contraceptive Cream is ir

tended for intravaginal use only, and if taken orally by mistake is likely to taste unpleasant. If excess quantities are swallowed, this may give rise to gastric irritation as the product contains a surfactant, and general supportive therapy should be carried out if necessary.

Pharmaceutical precautions None known.

Legal category GSL.

Package quantities Tubes containing 70 g.
ORTHO* Plastic Vaginal Applicator available separately.

Further information Nil.

Product licence number 0076/5008.

ORTHO* DIENOESTROL CREAM

Presentation A white non-staining cream containing 0.01% w/w dienoestrol.

Uses For intravaginal use only. Indicated in the treatment of atrophic vaginitis and kraurosis vulvae in post menopausal women, and for the treatment of pruritis vulvae and dyspareunia when associated with the atrophic vaginal epithelium.

Dosage and administration Given for short term use only. The lowest dose that will control symptoms should be chosen and medication should be discontinued as promptly as possible.

Attempts to discontinue or taper medication should be made at three to six month intervals, following physical examination. The usual dosage range is one or two applicatorfuls per day for one or two weeks, then gradually reduced to one half initial dosage for a similar period. A maintenance dose of one applicatorful, one to three times a week, may be used after restoration of the vaginal mucosa has been achieved. Treated patients with an intact uterus should be monitored closely for signs of endometrial cancer and appropriate diagnostic measures should be taken to rule out malignancy in the event of persistent or recurring abnormal vaginal bleeding. As a general rule it is advisable that patients receiving any form of oestrogen replacement therapy should have a complete physical examination at least once a year.

Contra-indications, warnings, etc Prolonged exposure to unopposed oestrogen may increase the risk of development of endometrial carcinoma, induction of other malignant neoplasms, and the risk of cancer of the breast: long term continuous administration of natural and synthetic oestrogens in certain animal species increases the frequency of carcinomas of the breast, cervix, vagina and liver. There is now evidence that oestrogens increase the risk of carcinoma of the endometrium in humans.

At the present time there is no satisfactory evidence that oestrogens given to post-menopausal women increase the risk of cancer of the breast, although a recent long-term follow up of a single physician has raised this possibility. However, because of animal data there is a need for caution in prescribing oestrogens for women with a strong family history of breast cancer or who have breast nodules, fibrocystic disease, or abnormal mammograms.

Pregnancy is an absolute contra-indication to the use of Dienoestrol cream since it may be harmful to the developing foetus.

Oestrogens should not be used in women with any of the other following conditions: known or suspected cancer of the breast, known or suspected oestrogen-dependent neoplasia, undiagnosed abnormal genital bleeding, active thrombophlebitis or thromboembolic disorders, a past history of thrombophlebitis, thrombosis, or thromboembolic disorders.

Thromboembolic disorders: While an increased rate of thromboembolic and thrombotic disease in postmenopausal users of oestrogens has not been found, this does not rule out the possibility that such an increase may be present or that subgroups of women who have underlying risk factors or who are receiving relatively large doses of oestrogens may have increased risk. Therefore oestrogens should not be used in persons with active thrombophlebitis or thromboembolic disorders, and they should not be used (except in treatment of malignancy) in persons with a history of such disorders. They should be used with cau ion in patients with cerebral vascular or coronary artery disease and only for those in whom oestrogens are clearly needed.

Gall bladder disease: A recent study has reported a two to three-fold increase in the risk of surgically confirmed gall bladder disease in women receiving post-menopausal oestrogens, similar to the two-fold increase previously noted in users of oral contraceptives.

Hepatic adenoma: Benign hepatic adenomas appear to be associated with the use of oral contraceptives. Although benign, and rare, these may rupture and may cause death through intra-abdominal haemorrhage. Such lesions have not yet been reported in association with other oestrogen or progestogen preparations but should be considered in oestrogen users having abdominal pain and tenderness, abdominal mass, or hypo-volemic shock.

Elevated blood pressure: It has been reported that this may occur with the use of oestrogens in the menopause and blood pressure should be monitored with oestrogen use, especially if high doses are used.

Precautions: A complete medical and family history should be taken prior to the initiation of any oestrogen therapy. The pretreatment and periodic physical examinations should include special reference to blood pressure, breasts, abdomen, and pelvic organs, and should include a Papanicolaou smear.

A pathologist should be advised of oestrogen therapy when relevant specimens are submitted. Certain endocrine and liver function tests may be affected by oestrogen containing products. These are:

Increased B.S.P. retention
Increased prothrombin and factors VII, VIII, IX, and X; decreased antithrombin 3, increased norepinephrine-induced platelet aggregability
Impaired glucose tolerance.
Increased thyroid binding globulin (TBG) leading to increased circulating total thyroid hormone, as measured by PBI, T4 by column or T4 by RIA. Free T3 resin uptake is decreased, reflecting the elevated TRG; free T4 is unaltered
Decreased pregnanediol excretion
Reduced response to metyrapone
Reduced serum folate concentration
Increased serum triglyceride and phospholipid concentration

Certain patients may develop undesirable manifestations of excessive oestrogenic stimulations, such as abnormal or excessive uterine bleeding, mastodynia, etc.

Pre-existing uterine fibroids may increase in size during oestrogen use.

Patients with a past history of jaundice during pregnancy have an increased risk of recurrence of jaundice while receiving oestrogen therapy. If jaundice develops in any patient receiving oestrogen, the medication should be discontinued while the cause is investigated.

Oestrogens may aggravate cases of porphyria.

Oestrogens may cause fluid retention. Conditions possibly affected by this factor such as epilepsy, migraine and cardiac or renal dysfunction require careful monitoring.

Oestrogens should be used with caution in patients with:

Metabolic bone diseases that are associated with hypercalcaemia
Impaired liver function
A history of mental depression
Diabetes

Oestrogens should be used judiciously in patients in whom bone growth is not complete.

Ortho Dienoestrol is generally well tolerated. There have been occasional reports of burning, itching and irritation. The doctor should also be aware of those adverse reactions reported to occur with systemic administration of oestrogens.

Overdosage: Ortho Dienoestrol Cream is intended for intravaginal use. If accidental ingestion of large quantities of the product occurs, an appropriate method of gastric emptying may be used if considered desirable. Overdosage may cause nausea, and in females withdrawal bleeding may occur.

Pharmaceutical precautions Store at room temperature.

Legal category POM.

Package quantities Tubes of 78 g with the ORTHO* Plastic Vaginal Applicator.

Further information Nil.

Product licence number 0076/5010.

ORTHOFORMS* CONTRACEPTIVE PESSARIES

Presentation White, opaque pessaries. Each pessary contains nonoxynol-9 5% w/w.

Uses Whenever the control of conception is desired. Placed in the vagina, the pessary melts and rapidly forms a smooth emollient cream which spreads, mixing intimately with secretions and seminal fluid. Orthoforms Contraceptive Pessaries melt rapidly between 34°C and 37°C – the normal vaginal temperature range.

Orthoforms Contraceptive Pessaries are intended to add reliability to the use of other methods, such as the diaphragm, the sheath, the cervical cap, the IUCD, or when intercourse is repeated without removing the appliance.

A higher degree of protection against pregnancy will be afforded by using another method of contraception in addition to a spermicidal contraceptive.

Dosage and administration The Orthoforms Contraceptive Pessary should be inserted as high as possible into the vagina approximately 5 minutes before intercourse to permit the pessary to melt. It retains its spermicidal activity for approximately 1 hour. Any subsequent acts of intercourse should not be undertaken before the insertion of an additional pessary.

Contra-indications, warnings, etc Hypersensitivity to the product.

Side-effects: Irritation of the vagina or penis has been reported. In such cases the medication should be discontinued.

Warnings: Where avoidance of pregnancy is essential the choice of contraceptive should be made in consultation with a doctor or a family planning clinic.

Overdosage: Orthoforms Contraceptive Pessaries are intended for intravaginal use only, and if taken orally by mistake are likely to taste unpleasant. If excess quantities are swallowed this may give rise to gastric irritation as the product contains a surfactant, and general supportive therapy should be carried out if necessary.

Pharmaceutical precautions Orthoforms Contraceptive Pessaries should be stored in a cool place.

Legal category GSL.

Package quantities Pack of 15 pessaries.

Further information Nil.

Product licence number 0076/5006.

ORTHO* GYNE-T* INTRAUTERINE COPPER CONTRACEPTIVE DEVICE

Presentation Each device consists of a polyethylene 'T' shaped support with 120 mg pure copper wire (providing a surface area of 200 sq. mm) wound around the vertical section of the 'T'.

The support is impregnated with a radiopaque substance and has a polyethylene suture attached to the base of the 'T'.

Uses Contraception.

Dosage and administration Ortho Gyne-T Intrauterine Copper Contraceptive Device may be used in any woman of child-bearing age including nulligravidous patients.

One device is inserted by its introducer into the uterus. The device should be removed after three years of use. If continued contraception is required a new device should be inserted. The device should be placed as high as possible within the uterine cavity and the patient should check periodically, particularly after menstruation, to ensure that the threads still protrude from the cervix. She should return to her doctor if she becomes aware that the device has been expelled. When the threads cannot be felt by the patient and cannot be seen by her doctor further investigation is necessary.

Contra-indications, warnings, etc
Contra-indications: The use of the device is contraindicated in the following conditions:

1. Pregnancy or suspicion of pregnancy.
2. Abnormalities of the uterus resulting in distortion of the uterine cavity.
3. Pelvic inflammatory disease or a history of repeated pelvic inflammatory disease.
4. Post-partum endometritis or infected abortion in the past three months.
5. Known or suspected uterine or cervical malignancy including unresolved abnormal cervical smear.
6. Uterine bleeding of unknown aetiology.

7. Cervicitis until infection is controlled.
8. Known allergy to copper.

Warnings: The expulsion, perforation and removal rates may be increased when insertions are made before normal uterine involution occurs post partum.

The device should be removed for the following reasons:

1. Excessive and persistent bleeding or cramping.
2. Perforation of the uterus and location of the device outside the uterine cavity. In this case hospital investigation and surgical removal will be required.
3. Partial downward displacement of the device within the cervical canal.

Pregnancy: If a patient is found to be pregnant with an Ortho Gyne-T *in situ* and the thread is visible it is recommended that in the absence of reasons to the contrary the device be removed as soon as possible. As with other intrauterine devices the possibility exists that should a second trimester abortion occur sepsis may supervene, and hence the desirability of removing the device as early as possible. If the thread is not visible then it is recommended that the device is left *in situ* until the pregnancy goes to term or a decision is made to terminate the pregnancy.

Ectopic pregnancy: A pregnancy that occurs with an IUCD in place is more likely to be ectopic than a pregnancy that occurs without an IUCD in place. Accordingly patients who become pregnant while using an IUCD should be carefully evaluated for the possibility of ectopic pregnancy.

Pelvic infection: An increased risk of pelvic infection has been reported in women with IUCD's *in situ.*

Precautions: Prior to insertion of an IUCD a thorough history and physical examination, including a pelvic examination and Papanicolaou smear, should be performed. Insertion of an IUCD into a uterine cavity measuring less than 6.5 cm by sounding may increase the incidence of expulsion, bleeding, pain and perforation. The patient should be re-examined within three months after insertion and thereafter at yearly intervals to ensure the device is still in place. The patient should be advised to contact her doctor immediately if she misses a menstrual period or has any other reason to think she may be pregnant.

IUCDs should be used with caution in patients with anaemia, menorrhagia or hypermenorrhoea or in patients receiving anticoagulants or having any disorder of coagulation.

Syncope, bradycardia or other neuro-vascular episodes may occur during insertion or removal of IUCDs especially in patients susceptible to these conditions. Patients with known or suspected cardiac abnormalities should receive appropriate antibiotic cover during insertion of the device. No method of contraception is 100% effective. In some cases it may be appropriate to recommend the use of an additional reliable method of contraception at mid-cycle.

Overdosage: Not applicable.

Pharmaceutical precautions If the seal of the sterile pack is broken the device inside should not be used.

Legal category POM. Also available through family planning clinics.

Package quantities Each sterile Ortho Gyne-T Intrauterine Copper Contraceptive Device unit is supplied in a sealed transparent envelope together with a sterile disposable GYNEPROBE* intrauterine sound for measuring the depth of the uterus. Full fitting instructions and advice for the patient are supplied with each device.

Further information Nil.

Product licence number 0076/0046.

ORTHO-GYNOL* CONTRACEPTIVE JELLY

Presentation Ortho-Gynol Contraceptive Jelly is a water-dispersible spermicidal jelly having a pH of 4.5, which contains p-diisobutylphenoxypolyethoxyethanol 1.0% w/w.

Uses Ortho-Gynol Contraceptive Jelly is a spermicidal jelly for use in conjunction with an occlusive vaginal diaphragm, whenever the control of conception is desirable.

A higher degree of protection against pregnancy will be afforded by using another method of contraception in addition to a spermicidal contraceptive.

Dosage and administration The jelly should be spread over the surface of the diaphragm which will be in contact with the cervix and on the rim. The diaphragm and spermicide must be allowed to remain undisturbed for at least six to eight hours after coitus. A fresh application of jelly or other spermicides, e.g. Orthoforms Contraceptive Pessaries, must be made prior to any subsequent act of coitus within this period of time, without removing the diaphragm. (A vaginal applicator should be used for inserting more cream or jelly.)

Douching is not recommended; but if desired it should be deferred for at least six hours after intercourse.

Contra-indications, warnings, etc Hypersensitivity to the product.

Warning: Where avoidance of pregnancy is essential, the choice of contraceptive should be made in consultation with a doctor or family planning clinic.

Occasional irritation of the vagina or penis has been reported. In such cases the medication should be discontinued.

The diaphragm should not remain in position for longer than 24 hours.

Overdosage: Ortho-Gynol Contraceptive Jelly is intended for intravaginal use only, and if taken orally by mistake is likely to taste unpleasant. If excess quantities are swallowed this may give rise to gastric irritation as the product contains a surfactant, and general supportive therapy should be carried out if necessary.

Pharmaceutical precautions None known.

Legal category GSL.

Package quantities Tube containing 81 g.
ORTHO* Plastic Vaginal Applicator available separately.

Further information Nil.

Product licence number 0076/5007.

ORTHO-NOVIN* 1/50 ORAL CONTRACEPTIVE TABLETS

Presentation White $\frac{1}{4}$ inch diameter, circular tablets with flat faces and bevelled edges, bearing on each face the engraving C over 150. Each tablet contains 1 mg Norethisterone PhEur and 50 mcg Mestranol BP.

Uses Contraception and the recognised indications for such oestrogen/progestogen combinations.

Action: Through the mechanism of gonadotrophin suppression by the oestrogenic and progestational actions of the ingredients. Although the primary mechanism of action is inhibition of ovulation, alterations to the cervical mucus and to the endometrium may also contribute to the efficacy of the product.

Dosage and administration The basic dosage regimen is a 28-day cycle of 1 tablet daily for 21 days followed by seven tablet-free days. For initial therapy the first tablet is taken on the fifth day of the menstrual cycle, counting the first day of bleeding as Day 1. Each subsequent course is started after seven tablet-free days have followed the preceding course. To obtain maximal contraceptive effectiveness all contraceptive tablets should be taken exactly as directed and at approximately the same time each day. Contraception can be initiated immediately post partum in the non-nursing patient. The possibility of ovulation and conception prior to the initiation of medication should be considered. The patient should be advised that during the first 14 days of the first course an additional reliable non-hormonal form of contraception should be used. If the patient misses more than one tablet she should begin taking tablets again as soon as remembered and an additional reliable method of contraception used until the next withdrawal bleed.

If the patient has vomiting or diarrhoea, absorption of the hormones will be impaired, making it advisable to use an additional reliable method of contraception until her next menstrual period. Should a bleeding fail to occur at the usual time, the possibility of pregnancy should be excluded before starting the next pack.

Contra-indications, warnings, etc

Contra-indications: Existing thrombophlebitis, thromboembolic disorders, cerebral vascular disease, myocardial infarction, or a past history of these conditions. Sickle-cell anaemia. Markedly impaired liver function. Congenital or existing disorders of lipid metabolism. Known or suspected carcinoma of the breast. Known or suspected oestrogen-dependent neoplasia. History during pregnancy of idiopathic jaundice, severe pruritus, shingles or deterioration of otosclerosis. Dubin-Johnson syndrome. Rotor syndrome. Undiagnosed abnormal genital tract bleeding. Known or suspected pregnancy.

Warnings: An increased risk of thrombophlebitis, cerebrovascular disorders, myocardial infarction and pulmonary embolism associated with the use of oral contraceptives has been reported in several retrospective case control studies. The increased risk has been estimated in these studies to be approximately 4 to 11 times higher (for cerebral haemorrhage two times higher) for users when compared to non users. This reported risk according to two of the studies is not related to duration of use nor does it persist after discontinuance according to one of the studies. An interim report of a large scale continuing prospective study has tended to confirm these retrospective studies for thrombophlebitis and possible cerebrovascular disorders. This study also reported that the risk of superficial and deep vein thrombosis was lower in women using preparations containing 50 mcg of oestrogen or less. There may not be full recovery from such disorders and it should be realised that in a few cases they are fatal.

Because of a possible increased risk of post surgery thromboembolic complications in oral contraceptive users, therapy should be discontinued at least six weeks prior to elective surgery. Caution should be exercised in administering oestrogen/progestogen combinations to women with a history of hypertension. An increased risk of surgically confirmed gall bladder disease associated with the use of oral contraceptives has been reported in a retrospective case control study.

Liver tumours, occasionally fatal, have been reported in women using oral contraceptives. These tumours may present as an abdominal mass, intra-abdominal bleeding and/or with signs and symptoms of acute abdomen. These have been reported in short term as well as long term users of oral contraceptives.

A small fraction of the active ingredients in oral contraceptives has been identified in the milk of mothers receiving these drugs. The effects, if any, on the breast-fed child have not been determined. If possible the use of oral contraceptives should be deferred until the infant is weaned.

When women have taken hormones during pregnancy there have been some reports of the possibility of adverse effects on the developing child. A direct relationship between such effects and oral contraceptives has not been confirmed, but as with any other drug, avoidance of continuing oral contraception in early pregnancy is desirable. Therefore pregnancy should be ruled out before initiating or continuing the administration of oral contraceptives to patients who have missed one menstrual period.

Certain factors may entail some risk of thrombosis, e.g. smoking, obesity, varicose veins, cardiovascular diseases, diabetes, and migraine. The suitability of a combined oral contraceptive should be judged according to the severity of such conditions in the individual case, and should be discussed with the patient before she decides to take it. The risk of arterial thrombosis associated with combined oral contraceptives increases with age and this risk is aggravated by cigarette smoking. The use of combined oral contraceptives in women in the older age group, especially those who are cigarette smokers, should therefore be discouraged and alternative methods advised.

Reduced efficacy and increased incidence of breakthrough bleeding have been associated with concomitant use of oral contraceptives and rifampicin. A similar association has been suggested with oral contraceptives and barbiturates, phenytoin sodium, ampicillin, tetracycline and griseofulvin.

Reasons for stopping oral contraceptives immediately: Early manifestations of thrombotic or thromboembolic disorders, thrombophlebitis, cerebrovascular disorders (including haemorrhage), myocardial infarction, pulmonary embolism or retinal thrombosis. Hypertension. Gradual or sudden, partial or complete loss of vision. Proptosis or diplopia. Onset or aggravation of migraine or development of headaches of a new pattern which are recurrent, persistent or severe. Papilloedema or any evidence of retinal vascular lesions. During periods of immobility (e.g. after accidents). Pregnancy. Manifestations of liver tumours.

Precautions: Examination of the pelvic organs, breasts and blood pressure should precede the prescribing of any oral contraceptive, and should be repeated regularly. The following are some of the medical conditions reported to be influenced by oral contraceptive therapy, and where the physician will have to exercise medical judgement to commence, continue or discontinue therapy as appropriate:

1. Pre-existing uterine fibromyomata may increase in size.

2. A decrease in glucose tolerance in a significant number of women.

3. An increase in blood pressure in a small but significant number of women.

4. Cholestatic jaundice. Patients with a history of cholestatic jaundice of pregnancy are more likely to develop cholestatic jaundice during oral contraceptive therapy.

5. Amenorrhoea during and after oral contraceptive therapy. Women with a past history of oligomenorrhoea or secondary amenorrhoea or women with irregular cycles may be more likely to remain anovulatory or to become amenorrhoeic post oral contraceptive therapy.

6. Depression.

7. Fluid retention. Conditions which might be influenced by this factor include epilepsy, migraine, asthma, cardiac or renal dysfunction.

8. Varicose veins.

9. Multiple sclerosis.

10. Porphyria.

11. Tetany.

12. Wearing of contact lenses

or any condition that is prone to worsen during pregnancy.

The following laboratory determinations may be altered in patients using oral contraceptives:

Hepatic: Increased BSP retention and other tests.

Coagulation: Increased prothrombin, Factors VII, VIII, IX and X; decreased antithrombin III; increased platelet aggregability.

Endocrine: Increased PBI and butanol extractable protein bound iodine and decreased T^3 uptake; increased glucose blood levels.

Other: Increased phospholipids and tri-glycerides, decreased serum folate values and disturbance in tryptophan metabolism. Decreased pregnanediol excretion, reduced response to metyrapone test.

These tests usually return to pre-therapy values after discontinuing oral contraceptive use. However, the physician should be aware that these altered determinations may mask an underlying disease.

Side-effects: Side-effects most commonly reported in early cycles of oral contraceptive therapy include breakthrough bleeding, spotting, nausea, vomiting and other gastro-intestinal disturbances. These frequently decrease with continued use. Other common side-effects include: change in menstrual flow, change in weight, oedema, chloasma (which may persist post therapy), amenorrhoea, breast changes (tenderness, enlargement and secretion).

In addition to the conditions and disorders discussed above, the following have been reported as adverse reactions in patients using combined oral contraceptives:

Neuro-ocular lesions
Rash
Cervical erosion and secretions
Suppression of lactation
Pre-menstrual-like syndrome
Changes in libido
Leg cramp
Relative pyridoxine deficiency
Haemorrhagic eruptions
Cystitis like syndrome
Headache
Nervousness
Fatigue
Hirsutism
Loss of scalp hair
Erythema multiforme
Erythema nodosum
Itching
Vaginal candidiasis
Porphyria

Overdosage: Serious ill effects have not been reported following acute ingestion of large doses of oral contraceptives by young children. Overdosage may cause nausea, and withdrawal bleeding may occur in females. An appropriate method of gastric emptying may be used if considered desirable.

Pharmaceutical precautions Protect from light.

Legal category POM.

Package quantities Carton containing 3 pushpaks each of 21 tablets – sufficient for 3 cycles.

Further information Nil.

Product licence number 0076/5000.

OVYSMEN* 0.5/35 ORAL CONTRACEPTIVE TABLETS

Presentation White $\frac{1}{4}$ inch diameter, circular tablets with flat faces and bevelled edges, bearing the engraving C over 535 on each face. Each tablet contains 0.5 mg Norethisterone PhEur and 35 mcg Ethinyloestradiol BP.

Uses Contraception and the recognised indications for such oestrogen/progestogen combinations.

Action: Through the mechanism of gonadotrophin suppression by the oestrogenic and progestational actions of the ingredients. Although the primary mechanism of action is inhibition of ovulation, alterations to the cervical mucus and to the endometrium may also contribute to the efficacy of the product.

Dosage and administration The basic dosage regimen is a 28-day cycle of 1 tablet daily for 21 days followed by seven tablet-free days. For initial therapy the first tablet is taken on the fifth day of the menstrual cycle, counting the first day of bleeding as Day 1. Each subsequent course is started after seven tablet-free days have followed the preceding course. To obtain maximal contraceptive effectiveness, all contraceptive tablets should be taken exactly as directed and at approximately the same time each day. Contraception can be initiated immediately post partum in the non-nursing patient. The possibility of ovulation and conception prior to initiation of medication should be considered. The patient should be advised that during the first 14 days of the first course an additional reliable non-hormonal form of contraception should be used. If the patient misses more than 1 tablet, she should begin taking tablets again as soon as remembered and an additional reliable method of contraception used until the next withdrawal bleed.

If the patient has vomiting or diarrhoea, absorption of the hormones will be impaired, making it advisable to use an additional reliable method of contraception until her next menstrual period. Should a bleeding fail to occur at the usual time, the possibility of pregnancy should be excluded before starting the next pack.

Contra-indications, warnings, etc
Contra-indications: Existing thrombophlebitis, throm-

boembolic disorders, cerebral vascular disease, myocardial infarction, or a past history of these conditions. Sickle-cell anaemia. Markedly impaired liver function. Congenital or existing disorders of lipid metabolism. Known or suspected carcinoma of the breast. Known or suspected oestrogen-dependent neoplasia. History during pregnancy of idiopathic jaundice, severe pruritus, shingles or deterioration of otosclerosis. Dubin-Johnson syndrome. Rotor syndrome. Undiagnosed abnormal genital tract bleeding. Known or suspected pregnancy.

Warnings: An increased risk of thrombophlebitis, cerebrovascular disorders, myocardial infarction and pulmonary embolism associated with the use of oral contraceptives has been reported in several retrospective case control studies. The increased risk has been estimated in these studies to be approximately 4 to 11 times higher (for cerebral haemorrhage two times higher) for users when compared to non users. This reported risk according to two of the studies is not related to duration of use nor does it persist after discontinuance according to one of the studies. An interim report of a large scale continuing prospective study has tended to confirm these retrospective studies for thrombophlebitis and possible cerebrovascular disorders. This study also reported that the risk of superficial and deep vein thrombosis was lower in women using preparations containing 50 mcg of oestrogen or less. There may not be full recovery from such disorders and it should be realised that in a few cases they are fatal.

Because of a possible increased risk of post surgery thromboembolic complications in oral contraceptive users, therapy should be discontinued at least six weeks prior to elective surgery. Caution should be exercised in administering oestrogen/progestogen combinations to women with a history of hypertension. An increased risk of surgically confirmed gall bladder disease associated with the use of oral contraceptives has been reported in a retrospective case control study.

Liver tumours, occasionally fatal, have been reported in women using oral contraceptives. These tumours may present as an abdominal mass, intra-abdominal bleeding and/or with signs and symptoms of acute abdomen. These have been reported in short-term as well as long-term users of oral contraceptives.

A small fraction of the active ingredients in oral contraceptives has been identified in the milk of mothers receiving these drugs. The effects, if any, on the breast-fed child have not been determined. If possible the use of oral contraceptives should be deferred until the infant is weaned.

When women have taken hormones during pregnancy there have been some reports of the possibility of adverse effects on the developing child. A direct relationship between such effects and oral contraceptives has not been confirmed, but as with any other drug, avoidance of continuing oral contraception in early pregnancy is desirable. Therefore pregnancy should be ruled out before initiating or continuing the administration of oral contraceptives to patients who have missed one menstrual period.

Certain factors may entail some risk of thrombosis, e.g. smoking, obesity, varicose veins, cardiovascular diseases, diabetes, and migraine. The suitability of a combined oral contraceptive should be judged according to the severity of such conditions in the individual case, and should be discussed with the patient before she decides to take it. The risk of arterial thrombosis associated with combined oral contraceptives increases with age and this risk is aggravated by cigarette smoking. The use of combined oral contraceptives in women in the older age group, especially those who are cigarette smokers, should therefore be discouraged and alternative methods advised.

Reduced efficacy and increased incidence of breakthrough bleeding have been associated with concomitant use of oral contraceptives and rifampicin. A similar association has been suggested with oral contraceptives and barbiturates, phenytoin sodium, ampicillin, tetracycline and griseofulvin.

Reasons for stopping oral contraceptives immediately: Early manifestations of thrombotic or thromboembolic disorders, thrombophlebitis, cerebrovascular disorders (including haemorrhage), myocardial infarction, pulmonary embolism or retinal thrombosis. Hypertension. Gradual or sudden, partial or complete loss of vision. Proptosis or diplopia. Onset or aggravation of migraine or development of headaches of a new pattern which are recurrent, persistent or severe. Papilloedema or any evidence of retinal vascular lesions. During periods of immobility (e.g. after accidents). Pregnancy. Manifestations of liver tumours.

Precautions: Examination of the pelvic organs, breasts and blood pressure should precede the prescribing of any oral contraceptive, and should be repeated regularly. The following are some of the conditions reported to be influenced by oral contraceptive therapy, and where the physician will have to exercise medical judgement to commence, continue or discontinue therapy as appropriate.

a) Pre-existing uterine fibromyomata may increase in size.

b) A decrease in glucose tolerance in a significant number of women.

c) An increase in blood pressure in a small but significant number of women.

d) Cholestatic jaundice. Patients with a history of cholestatic jaundice of pregnancy are more likely to develop cholestatic jaundice during oral contraceptive therapy.

e) Amenorrhoea during and after oral contraceptive therapy. Women with a past history of oligomenorrhoea or secondary amenorrhoea or women with irregular cycles may be more likely to remain anovulatory or to become amenorrhoeic post oral contraceptive therapy.

f) Depression.

g) Fluid retention. Conditions which might be influenced by this factor including epilepsy, migraine, asthma, cardiac or renal dysfunction.

h) Varicose veins.

i) Multiple sclerosis.

j) Porphyria.

k) Tetany.

l) Wearing of contact lenses.

or any condition that is prone to worsen during pregnancy.

The following laboratory determinations may be altered in patients using oral contraceptives:

Hepatic: Increased BSP retention and other tests.

Coagulation: Increased prothrombin, Factors VII, VIII, IX and X; decreased antithrombin III; increased platelet aggregability.

Endocrine: Increased PBI and butanol extractable protein bound iodine and decreased T^3 uptake, increased glucose blood levels.

Other: Increased phospholipids and tri-glycerides, decreased serum folate values and disturbance in tryptophan metabolism. Decreased pregnanediol excretion, reduced response to metyrapone test.

These tests usually return to pre-therapy values after discontinuing oral contraceptive use. However, the physician should be aware that these altered determinations may mask an underlying disease.

Side-effects: Side-effects most commonly reported in early cycles of oral contraceptive therapy include breakthrough b.,eding, spotting, nausea, vomiting and other gastro-intestinal disturbances. These frequently decrease with continued use. Other common side-effects include: change in menstrual flow, change in weight, oedema, chloasma (which may persist post therapy), amenorrhoea, breast changes (tenderness, enlargement and secretion).

In addition to the conditions and disorders discussed above, the following have been reported as adverse reactions in patients using combined oral contraceptives:

Neuro-ocular lesions
Rash
Cervical erosion and secretions
Suppression of lactation
Pre-menstrual like syndrome
Changes in libido
Leg cramp
Relative pyridoxine deficiency
Haemorrhagic eruptions
Cystitis-like syndrome
Headache
Nervousness
Fatigue
Hirsutism
Loss of scalp hair
Erythema multiforme
Erythema nodosum
Itching
Vaginal candidiasis
Porphyria

Overdosage: Serious ill effects have not been reported following acute ingestion of large doses of oral contraceptives by young children. Overdosage may cause nausea, and withdrawal bleeding may occur in females. An appropriate method of gastric emptying may be used if considered desirable.

Pharmaceutical precautions Protect from light.

Legal category POM.

Package quantities Carton containing 3 pushpaks each of 21 tablets – sufficient for 3 cycles

Further information Nil.

Product licence number 0076/0047.

PANCREASE* CAPSULES

Presentation Hard, white, gelatin capsules printed 0095 on the body, containing enteric coated beads of porcine Pancreatin BP equivalent to Pancrelipase USP. Each capsule has a protease activity of not less than 330 BP Units, an amylase activity of not less than 2,900 BP Units and lipase activity of not less than 5,000 BP Units.

Uses Exocrine pancreatic enzyme deficiency as in cystic fibrosis, chronic pancreatitis, post-pancreatectomy, post-gastrointestinal bypass surgery (e.g. Billroth

II gastroenterostomy), ductal obstruction from neoplasm (e.g. of the pancreas or common bile duct).

The enzymes catalyse the hydrolysis of fats into glycerol and fatty acids, protein into proteoses and derived substances and starch into dextrins and sugars.

Dosage and administration For adults and children 1 or 2 capsules during each meal and one capsule with snacks. Occasionally a third capsule with meals may be required depending upon individual requirements. Where swallowing of capsules is difficult, they may be opened and the beads taken with liquids or soft foods which do not require chewing. To protect the enteric coating the beads should not be crushed or chewed.

Contra-indications, warnings, etc Hypersensitivity to pork protein. The safety of Pancrease during pregnancy has not yet been established. Such use is not recommended.

The most frequently reported adverse reactions to Pancrease Capsules are gastrointestinal in nature. Less frequently allergic-type reactions have also been observed.

Extremely high doses of exogenous pancreatic enzymes have been associated with hyperuricosuria and hyperuricaemia.

Contact of the beads with food having a pH higher than 5.5 can dissolve the protective enteric shell.

Pharmaceutical precautions Keep bottle tightly closed. Store at room temperature in a dry place. Do not refrigerate.

Legal category P.

Package quantities Containers of 100 capsules.

Further information The enteric coated Pancrease beads resist gastric inactivation and deliver predictable, high levels of biologically active enzymes into the duodenum.

Product licence number 0076/0129.

PEVARYL* CREAM
PEVARYL* LOTION
PEVARYL* SPRAY POWDER

Presentation *Cream:* A white cream containing 1% econazole nitrate.

Lotion: A white water-miscible lotion containing 1% econazole nitrate.

Spray Powder: A white powder containing 1% econazole nitrate, emitted as a spray by means of an aerosol container.

Uses Econazole nitrate is a broad-spectrum antifungal agent.

Cream: All fungal skin infections due to dermatophytes (e.g., Trichophyton species), yeasts (e.g., Candida species), moulds and other fungi. These include ringworm (tinea) infections, athlete's foot, paronychia, pityriasis versicolor, erythrasma and vulvitis, balanitis and napkin rash due to Candida.

Lotion: As Pevaryl Cream, but particularly suitable for hairy and moist areas and for fungal otitis externa.

Spray Powder: As Pevaryl Cream, but particularly suitable in intertriginous areas. Also for the protection of areas at risk and as yet unaffected by such infections.

Dosage and administration *Cream:* Apply to the affected area 2-3 times daily and rub in gently.

In nail infections, apply once daily and cover with an occlusive dressing.

Lotion. As for Pevaryl* Cream.

Spray Powder: Apply to the affected area twice daily until the lesions have healed.

In order to prevent relapse, treatment should be continued for 2 weeks after clinical cure.

Contra-indications, warnings, etc *Contra-indications:* None known.

Side effects: Rarely, transient local mild irritation may occur immediately after application.

Precautions: Cream and Lotion: Hypersensitivity has rarely been recorded, if it should occur, administration of the product should be discontinued.

Spray Powder: As for Pevaryl Cream and Pevaryl Lotion. The spray should be kept away from the eyes and mucous membranes.

Pevaryl Cream, Lotion and Spray Powder are only absorbed in small amounts following application to the skin. Hence no special precautions are necessary in elderly patients. In view of the low level of absorption and the lack of teratogenic effects in animals, the products can be used with caution during pregnancy.

Overdosage: Pevaryl Cream, Lotion and Spray Powder are intended for topical use. If accidental ingestion of large quantities of the product occurs, an appropriate method of gastric emptying may be used if considered desirable.

Pharmaceutical precautions
Cream and Lotion: None.

Spray Powder: Shake well before use. Contents are under pressure. Store in a cool place away from heat and sunlight; do not burn or puncture, even when empty.

Legal category
Cream: P.
Lotion: P.
Spray Powder: P.

Package quantities *Cream:* Each tube contains 30 g.
Lotion: Each bottle contains 30 ml.
Spray Powder: 200 g aerosol can contains 20 g econazole nitrate powder 1%.

Further information The infected area should be kept clean and dry during treatment.

Pevaryl Spray Powder is suitable for use in conjunction with Pevaryl Cream or Pevaryl Lotion. It is also useful for the treatment of clothing such as shoes and socks in cases of tinea pedis.

Cream: 0076/0059
Lotion: 0076/0066
Spray powder   0076/0063

RETIN-A* ACNE TREATMENT

Presentation Retin-A* Acne Treatment is available as either a clear yellow solution of 0.025% w/w tretinoin supplied in amber bottles or in tubes of tretinoin gel 0.025% w/w or tretinoin cream 0.05% w/w.

Uses For topical application in the treatment of acne vulgaris in which comedones, papules and pustules predominate.

Retin-A Lotion is best suited for large areas such as the back.

Retin-A Gel is best suited for severe acne, for initial therapy and for oily and dark skin.

Retin-A Cream is best suited for use on dry and fair skin.

Dosage and administration Retin-A Acne treatment should be applied once or twice daily to the area of skin where acne lesions occur. Only apply sufficient to cover the affected area lightly, using a gauze swab, cotton wool or the tips of clean fingers. Avoid over-saturation to the extent that excess medication could run into eyes, angles of the nose or other areas where treatment is not intended.

Initial application may cause transitory stinging and a feeling of warmth. The correct frequency of administration should produce no more than an erythema similar to that of mild sunburn. In patients with sensitive skin, application once daily may be sufficient. In patients with normal skin, increasing the frequency of application to twice daily is usually necessary.

If Retin-A is applied excessively, no more rapid or better results will be obtained and marked redness, peeling or discomfort may occur. Should this occur accidentally or through over-enthusiastic use, application should be discontinued for a few days.

Patience is needed in this treatment, since therapeutic effects will not usually be observed until after 6-8 weeks of treatment. During the early weeks of treatment, an apparent exacerbation of inflammatory lesions may occur. This is due to the action of the medication on deep, previously unseen comedones and papules. Once the acne lesions have responded satisfactorily, it should be possible to maintain the improvement with less frequent applications.

Cosmetics may be used, but the areas to be treated should be thoroughly washed beforehand. Astringent toiletries should be avoided.

Contra-indications, warnings, etc Use of the product should be discontinued if hypersensitivity to any of the ingredients should occur. Retin-A Acne Treatment should be kept away from the eye and eyelids, the mouth and other mucous membranes. Care should also be taken not to let the medication accumulate in folds of the skin and the angles of the nose. Retin-A should not be applied to eczematous skin, nor to cuts and abrasions.

Caution should be exercised when Retin-A is used concomitantly with other skin medications, particularly those containing peeling agents such as sulphur, resorcinol, benzoylperoxide or salicyclic acid. It is also advisable to 'rest' a patients skin until the effects of peeling agents subside before use of Retin-A is begun.

Recent studies in mice treated with the active ingredient (tretinoin) of Retin-A and exposed to artificial sunlight suggest that tretinoin may speed up the appearance of sunlight induced skin tumours. Laboratory mice treated with tretinoin but not exposed to sunlight did not develop skin tumours. The significance of these studies as related to human beings is unknown. However it is important to avoid or minimise exposure of Retin-A treated areas to sunlight or sunlamps during the course of treatment. Patients with sunburn should be advised not to use the product until fully recovered because of heightened susceptibility to sunlight as a result of the use of tretinoin. Weather extremes such as wind or cold, also may be irritating to patients under treatment with tretinoin.

Retin-A should not be used in patients with a personal or family history of cutaneous epithelioma.

Side effects: The application of excessive amounts of Retin-A to the skin may cause severe erythema, irritation and discomfort. Should this occur, the frequency of application should be reduced or the use of Retin-A discontinued temporarily. Temporary hypo or hyperpigmentation has been reported in a few individuals treated with Retin-A. All side effects so far reported have been reversible upon discontinuation of Retin-A therapy.

This drug should only be used during pregnancy if clearly needed, since there are no adequately controlled human studies.

Overdosage: Retin-A is intended for topical use only. Excessive use is dealt with under side effects. Taken orally by mischance Retin-A is liable to taste unpleasant. Unless the amount is small an appropriate method of gastric emptying should be used as soon as possible.

Pharmaceutical precautions Store in a cool place. The 80 ml bottle of lotion should be protected from light and any remaining medicine discarded on completion of treatment.

Legal category POM.

Package quantities *Lotion:* Amber glass bottle containing 80 ml.

Gel and Cream: Tubes containing 60 g.

Further information Nil.

Product licence numbers
Lotion 0076/0037
Gel 0076/0050
Cream 0076/0056

SULTRIN* TRIPLE SULFA CREAM

Presentation A white, non-staining cream containing Sulphathiazole 3.42% w/w, Sulphacetamide 2.86% w/w and Sulphabenzamide 3.70% w/w.

Uses For the treatment of infections caused by *Haemophilus Vaginalis* and non-specific bacterial vaginitis and cervicitis. It may also be used in the prevention of bacterial complications following cervical and vaginal surgery and vulvectomy and as an anti-infective in the post-partum state.

Dosage and administration One applicatorful intravaginally twice daily for 10 days. The dosage may then be reduced to once a day if necessary.

Contra-indications, warnings, etc Sulphonamide sensitivity and kidney disease.

The effects of Sultrin on the outcome of pregnancy are not known. Therefore caution should be exercised when using the product during pregnancy.

The safety and effectiveness for use in children have not been established.

The most frequent adverse reaction to Sultrin is localised irritation and/or allergy.

Precautions: Since the primary route of excretion of Sultrin cream is renal, caution should be used in prescribing the product to elderly patients who potentially may have impaired renal function.

Overdosage: Sultrin Triple Sulfa Cream is intended for intravaginal use. If accidental ingestion of large quantities of the product occurs, an appropriate method of gastric emptying may be used if considered desirable. Elimination of sulphonamides in the urine may be assisted by giving alkalis such as sodium bicarbonate and increasing fluid intake.

Pharmaceutical precautions Store at room temperature, avoid excessive heat.

Legal category POM.

Package quantities Tube containing 78 g with or without the ORTHO* Plastic Vaginal Applicator.

Further information The three sulphonamides exert optimal bacteriostatic action at different specific pH levels. The point of optimal activity for each drug is:

Sulphathiazole pH 7.0
Sulphacetamide pH 5.2
Sulphabenzamide pH 4.6

Product licence number 0076/5012.

SULTRIN* VAGINAL TABLETS

Presentation Sultrin Vaginal Tablets are white, non-staining, water-dispersible, lozenge-shaped tablets engraved on one side with the Ortho shield design and on the reverse with C. Each tablet contains:

Sulphathiazole 172.5 mg
Sulphacetamide 143.75 mg
Sulphabenzamide 184.0 mg

in a rapidly disintegrating base.

Uses For the treatment of infections caused by *Haemophilus Vaginalis* and non-specific bacterial vaginitis and cervicitis. It may also be used in the prevention of bacterial complications following cervical and vaginal surgery and vulvectomy and as an anti-infective in the post-partum state.

Dosage and administration One tablet placed high in the vagina twice daily for 10 days. Repeat if necessary.

Contra-indications, warnings, etc Sulphonamide sensitivity; renal disease.

The effects of Sultrin on the outcome of pregnancy are not known. Therefore caution should be exercised when using the product during pregnancy.

The safety and effectiveness for use in children have not been established.

The most frequent adverse reaction to Sultrin is localised irritation and/or allergy.

Precaution: Since the primary route of excretion of Sultrin Tablets is renal, caution should be used in prescribing the product to elderly patients who potentially may have impaired renal function.

Overdosage: Sultrin Vaginal Tablets are intended for intravaginal use. If accidental ingestion of large quantities of the product occurs, an appropriate method of gastric emptying may be used if considered desirable. Elimination of sulphonamides in the urine may be assisted by giving alkalis such as sodium bicarbonate and increasing fluid intake.

Pharmaceutical precautions None known.

Legal category POM.

Package quantities Packages of 20 foil-wrapped tablets with vaginal applicator.

Further information The three sulphonamides exert

optimal bacteriostatic action at different specific pH levels. The point of optimal activity for each drug is:

Sulphathiazole   pH 7.0
Sulphacetamide   pH 5.2
Sulphabenzamide   pH 4.6

Product licence number 0076/5013.

SUPROL* CAPSULES ▼

Presentation Size 1 – hard gelatin capsules with an ivory body and a green cap. Each capsule contains 200 mg of suprofen, a substituted aryl-acetic acid.

Uses Suprol is indicated for the treatment of mild to moderate pain associated with the following conditions.
Musculo-skeletal pain.
Post partum episiotomy pain.
Post operative pain following general surgery.
Post operative dental pain.
Pain in osteoarthritis or rheumatoid arthritis.
Dysmenorrhoea.

Dosage and administration The recommended oral dose of Suprol is 200 mg three or four times a day.

Contra-indications, warnings, etc Suprol should not be used in patients in whom salicylates or other non-steroidal anti-infammatory drugs induce bronchospasm, rhinitis, urticaria, or other sensitivity reactions.

Patients presenting with an allergic reaction to Suprol should be evaluated as to the severity of the reaction and treated appropriately with conventional therapy. This may include the use of adrenaline, antihistamines, pressors, fluids, and/or steroids.

Peptic ulceration and gastrointestinal bleeding have rarely been reported in patients receiving Suprol capsules. The drug should be given under close supervision to patients with a history of gastrointestinal ulcers and should not be administered to patients with diagnosed gastrointestinal ulcers.

Suprol has been shown to inhibit platelet aggregation and template bleeding time *in vivo*, but the effect begins to normalise within 4 hours and approaches normal within 24 hours after the last dose of Suprol. The *in vitro* binding of warfarin, diphenylhydantoin and tolbutamide to human plasma proteins is unaffected by suprofen. However, as with aspirin, patients with coagulation disorders and those stabilised on warfarin should be closely monitored when Suprol is administered.
As with other non-steroidal anti-inflammatory drugs, elevation of BUN has been reported in clinical studies with Suprol. Since suprofen is predominantly eliminated from the body by urinary excretion via glomerular filtration it should be used with caution in patients with impaired renal function, such as the elderly, and those on long-term therapy should be monitored and may require lower doses. Rarely, elevations of liver enzymes have been reported.

Mild peripheral oedema has been observed in some patients receiving long-term therapy. Therefore, Suprol should be used with caution in patients with fluid retention, heart failure or hypertension.

No teratogenic effects have been found in animals, but as in the case of all new drugs, caution should be exercised in prescribing Suprol to pregnant women. Safety for use during pregnancy has not been established. Small quantities of Suprol are excreted in human milk. Hence, caution should be exercised in prescribing the drug for nursing mothers.

The safety and effectiveness of Suprol has not been established in children.

Side-effects: Most adverse reactions reported are related to the gastrointestinal tract and include nausea, dyspepsia, gastrointestinal distress and diarrhoea. Other reactions reported less frequently, include headache, dizziness, sedation, fluid retention and rash.

Overdosage: Insufficient experience with acute overdosage precludes characterisation of sequelae and assessment of antidotal efficacy at this time. It is reasonable to assume however, that the standard practices of gastric evacuation, activated charcoal administration and general supportive therapy would apply.

Pharmaceutical precautions Protect from light.

Legal category POM.

Package quantities Containers of 100 capsules.

Further information Suprol produces significant analgesia within $\frac{1}{2}$ hour and maximum analgesia within 1–2 hours following oral administration. The duration of analgesia is generally 4–6 hours.

Suprol is a non narcotic analgesic and in clinical studies no patient tolerance has been observed.

The presence of food and, to a lesser extent, milk, in the gastrointestinal tract appears to diminish the rate of absorption of Suprol and lower the peak plasma levels of the drug. However, the extent of absorption was only slightly reduced by food and unaffected by milk.

Concomitant administration of Suprol with antacids did not reduce the bioavailability of the drug.

Product licence number 0076/0083.

TOLECTIN* TABLETS ▼
TOLECTIN* DS CAPSULES

Presentation *Tablets:* White, flat, circular tablet (12 mm diameter) with bevelled edges. The word TOLECTIN is engraved on one side with a score line on the reverse. For oral administration.

Tolectin (tolmetin sodium) 200 mg tablets each contain 246 mg of tolmetin sodium dihydrate, which is equivalent to 200 mg tolmetin. Each tablet contains 18 mg (0.784 m Eq) of sodium.

Capsules: A size 'O' hard gelatin capsule with an ivory opaque body and a light blue opaque cap containing a yellow powder. For oral administration.

Tolectin (tolmetin sodium) 400 mg capsules each contain 490 mg of tolmetin sodium dihydrate, which is equivalent to 400 mg of tolmetin. Each capsule contains 36 mg (1.568 m Eq) of sodium.

Uses Tolectin is a non-steroidal anti-inflammatory agent with analgesic and antipyretic properties. It is indicated for:

rheumatoid arthritis
juvenile rheumatoid arthritis (Still's Disease)
osteoarthritis
ankylosing spondylitis
peri-articular disorders such as fibrositis and bursitis

Dosage and administration The initial adult dosage is 400 mg three times daily. This may be adjusted within the range 600–1800 mg daily in 2, 3 or 4 divided doses depending on patient response and the severity of the disease.

In juvenile rheumatoid arthritis the dosage is 20–25

mg/kg/day in 3–4 divided doses. The maximum dose is 30 mg/kg/day or 1800 mg/day whatever the body weight. Half a tablet (100 mg) is a suitable unit for most children's doses.

Contra-indications, warnings, etc *Contra-indications:* active peptic ulcer; previous sensitivity to Tolectin, aspirin, or other non-steroidal anti-inflammatory agents, which have induced symptoms of asthma, rhinitis or urticaria.

Warnings: Tolectin should be used with caution in patients with a history of upper gastrointestinal tract disease. Tolectin prolongs bleeding time and patients who may be adversely affected should be carefully monitored during Tolectin therapy.

No teratogenic effects have been found in animals, but, as in the case of all new drugs, caution should be exercised in the prescribing of Tolectin to pregnant women. Safety for use during pregnancy or lactation has not been established.

Renal papillary necrosis has occurred in animals after long term administration although there has been no evidence of renal toxicity in clinical trials. However, since Tolectin is eliminated primarily by the kidneys, caution should be observed and patients with impaired renal function, such as the elderly, should be closely monitored and may require lower doses.

In patients with rheumatoid arthritis who have received certain anti-rheumatic drugs, eye changes have been observed. During clinical studies of up to 2 years with Tolectin no such changes have occurred.

Side effects: epigastric discomfort, headache (rare), water and sodium retention, skin rash. Gastro-intestinal disturbance may occur but blood loss due to Tolectin is rare.

Small and transient decreases in haemoglobin and haematocrit not associated with gastrointestinal bleeding have occurred. A few cases of granulocytopenia have been observed.

Management of overdosage: In the event of overdosage, the stomach should be emptied by inducing vomiting or by gastric lavage followed by the administration of activated charcoal. Studies in rats indicate that the urinary excretion of the drug is enhanced when the urine is made alkaline with sodium bicarbonate.

Pharmaceutical precautions *Tablets and Capsules:* Extremes of temperature and humidity should be avoided.

Legal category POM.

Package quantities Containers of 100 tablets or 100 capsules.

Further information In clinical trials Tolectin has shown no interaction with concomitantly administered drugs, such as gold, corticosteroids and paracetamol.

Preliminary studies indicate that Tolectin does not interact with anti-coagulant drugs.

In adult diabetic patients under treatment with either sulphonylureas or insulin no changes have been observed in the clinical effects of either Tolectin or the hypoglycaemic agents.

The metabolites of tolmetin in urine have been found to give positive tests for proteinuria using tests which rely on acid precipitation as their endpoint. No interference is seen in the tests for proteinuria using dye-impregnated commercially available reagent strips.

Product licence numbers
Tablets: 0076/0021
Capsules: 0076/0075

TRINOVUM*

Presentation $\frac{1}{4}$ inch diameter, circular tablets with flat faces and bevelled edges engraved on each face as follows: the seven white tablets each contain 0.5 mg Norethisterone PhEur and 35 mcg Ethinyloestradiol BP and are engraved C535; the seven light peach coloured tablets each contain 0.75 mg Norethisterone PhEur and 35 mcg Ethinyloestradiol BP and are engraved C735; the seven peach coloured tablets each contain 1.0 mg Norethisterone PhEur and 35 mcg Ethinyloestradiol BP and are engraved C135.

Uses Contraception and the recognised indications for such oestrogen/progestogen combinations.

Action: Through the mechanism of gonadotrophin suppression by the oestrogenic and progestational actions of the ingredients. Although the primary mechanism of action is inhibition of ovulation, alterations to the cervical mucus and to the endometrium may also contribute to the efficacy of the product.

Dosage and administration The basic dosage regimen is a 28-day cycle of one tablet daily for 21 days followed by seven tablet-free days. A white tablet is taken on every day for 7 days, a light peach coloured tablet is taken every day for 7 days, followed by a peach coloured tablet every day for 7 days. For initial therapy, the first white tablet is taken on the first day of bleeding of the menstrual cycle. If Trinovum* tablets are first taken later than the first day of bleeding of the first menstrual cycle of medication, contraceptive reliance should be not placed on the product until after the first 14 consecutive days of administration.

Subsequent cycles: Each subsequent course is started after 7 tablet-free days have followed the preceding course.

Changing from another combined oral contraceptive: The first white tablet should be taken on the first day of the withdrawal bleed after the completion of the previous course of tablets.

Changing from a progestogen-only contraceptive: The first white tablet should be taken on the first day of bleeding that occurs either during the last course of tablets or following completion of the tablet course.

Post-partum use: After pregnancy, oral contraception may be initiated immediately post-partum in the non-nursing patient or as soon as spontaneous menstruation has been resumed. Another method of contraception should be used in the interval between delivery and the first course of tablets, unless it is started within seven days of delivery. After a miscarriage or first-trimester abortion, oral contraception may be started immediately.

If the patient forgets more than one tablet, she should recommence the course as soon as she remembers, taking the appropriate tablet for that day and omitting any tablets delayed more than 12 hours. She should then use an additional method of contraception until the next withdrawal bleed.

If a patient has vomiting or diarrhoea, absorption of the hormones will be impaired, making it advisable to use an additional method of contraception until her next menstrual period. Should a bleeding fail to occur at the usual time, the possibility of pregnancy should be excluded before starting the next pack.

Contra-indications, warnings, etc

Contra-indications: Existing thrombophlebitis, thromboembolic disorders, cerebral vascular disease, myocardial infarction, or a past history of these conditions. Sickle-cell anaemia. Markedly impaired liver function. Congenital or existing disorders of lipid metabolism. Known or suspected carcinoma of the breast. Known or suspected oestrogen-dependent neoplasia. History during pregnancy of idiopathic jaundice, severe pruritus, shingles or deterioration of otosclerosis. Dubin-Johnson syndrome. Rotor syndrome. Undiagnosed abnormal genital tract bleeding. Known or suspected pregnancy.

Warnings: An increased risk of thrombophlebitis, cerebrovascular disorders, myocardial infarction and pulmonary embolism associated with the use of oral contraceptives has been reported in several retrospective case control studies. The increased risk has been estimated in these studies to be approximately 4 to 11 times higher (for cerebral haemorrhage two times higher) for users when compared to non users. This reported risk according to two of the studies is not related to duration of use nor does it persist after discontinuance according to one of the studies. An interim report of a large scale continuing prospective study has tended to confirm these retrospective studies for thrombophlebitis and possible cerebrovascular disorders. This study also reported that the risk of superficial and deep vein thrombosis was lower in women using preparations containing 50 mcg of oestrogen or less. There may not be full recovery from such disorders and it should be realised that in a few cases they are fatal.

Because of a possible increased risk of post surgery thromboembolic complications in oral contraceptive users, therapy should be discontinued at least six weeks prior to elective surgery. Caution should be exercised in administering oestrogen/progestogen combinations to women with a history of hypertension. An increased risk of surgically confirmed gall bladder disease associated with the use of oral contraceptives has been reported in a retrospective case control study.

Liver tumours, occasionally fatal, have been reported in women using oral contraceptives. These tumours may present as an abdominal mass, intra-abdominal bleeding and/or with signs and symptoms of acute abdomen. These have been reported in short term as well as long term users of oral contraceptives.

A small fraction of the active ingredients in oral contraceptives has been identified in the milk of mothers receiving these drugs. The effects, if any, on the breast-fed child have not been determined. If possible the use of oral contraceptives should be deferred until the infant is weaned.

When women have taken hormones during pregnancy there have been some reports of the possibility of adverse effects on the developing child. A direct relationship between such effects and oral contraceptives has not been confirmed, but as with any other drug, avoidance of continuing oral contraception in early pregnancy is desirable. Therefore pregnancy should be ruled out before initiating or continuing the administration of oral contraceptives to patients who have missed one menstrual period.

Certain factors may entail some risk of thrombosis e.g. smoking, obesity, varicose veins, cardiovascular diseases, diabetes, and migraine. The suitability of a combined oral contraceptive should be judged according to the severity of such conditions in the individual case, and should be discussed with the patient before she decides to take it. The risk of arterial thrombosis associated with combined oral contraceptives increases with age and this risk is aggravated by cigarette smoking. The use of combined oral contraceptives in women in the older age group, especially those who are cigarette smokers, should therefore be discouraged and alternative methods advised.

Reduced efficacy and increased incidence of breakthrough bleeding have been associated with concomitant use of oral contraceptives and rifampicin. A similar association has been suggested with oral contraceptives and barbiturates, phenytoin sodium, ampicillin, tetracycline and griseofulvin.

Reasons for stopping oral contraceptives immediately: Early manifestations of thrombotic or thromboembolic disorders, thrombophlebitis, cerebrovascular disorders (including haemorrhage), myocardial infarction, pulmonary embolism or retinal thrombosis. Hypertension. Gradual or sudden, partial or complete loss of vision. Proptosis or diplopia. Onset or aggravation of migraine or development of headaches of a new pattern which are recurrent, persistent or severe. Papilloedema or any evidence of retinal vascular lesions. During periods of immobility (e.g. after accidents). Pregnancy. Manifestations of liver tumours.

Precautions: Examination of the pelvic organs, breasts and blood pressure should precede the prescribing of any oral contraceptive, and should be repeated regularly.

The following are some of the conditions reported to be influenced by oral contraceptive therapy, and where the physician will have to exercise medical judgement to commence, continue or discontinue therapy as appropriate.

a) Pre-existing uterine fibromyomata may increase in size.
b) A decrease in glucose tolerance in a significant number of women.
c) An increase in blood pressure in a small but significant number of women.
d) Cholestatic jaundice. Patients with a history of cholestatic jaundice of pregnancy are more likely to develop cholestatic jaundice during oral contraceptive therapy.
e) Amenorrhoea during and after oral contraceptive therapy. Women with a past history of oligomenorrhoea or secondary amenorrhoea or women with irregular cycles may be more likely to remain anovulatory or to become amenorrhoeic post oral contraceptive therapy.
f) Depression.
g) Fluid retention. Conditions which might be influenced by this factor include epilepsy, migraine, asthma, cardiac or renal dysfunction.
h) Varicose veins.
i) Multiple sclerosis.
j) Porphyria.
k) Tetany.
l) Wearing of contact lenses.
or any condition that is prone to worsen during pregnancy.

The following laboratory determinations may be altered in patients using oral contraceptives:

Hepatic: Increased BSP retention and other tests.
Coagulation: Increased prothrombin, Factors VII, VIII, IX

and X: decreased antithrombin III, increased platelet aggregability.

Endocrine: Increased PBI and butanol extractable protein bound iodine and decreased T3 uptake, increased glucose blood levels.

Other: Increased phospholipids and tri-glycerides, decreased serum folate values and disturbance in tryptophan metabolism, decreased pregnanediol excretion, reduced response to metyrapone test.

These tests usually return to pre-therapy values after discontinuing oral contraceptive use. However, the physician should be aware that these altered determinations may mask an underlying disease.

Side-effects: Most commonly reported in early cycles of oral contraceptive therapy include breakthrough bleeding, spotting, nausea, vomiting and other gastrointestinal disturbances. These frequently decrease with continued use. Other common side-effects include: change in menstrual flow, change in weight, oedema, chloasma (which may persist post therapy), amenorrhoea, breast changes (tenderness, enlargement and secretion).

In addition to the conditions and disorders discussed above, the following have been reported as adverse reactions in patients using combined oral contraceptives:

Neuro-ocular lesions	Haemorrhagic eruptions
Rash	Cystitis-like syndrome

Cervical erosion and secretions	Headache
Suppression of lactation	Nervousness
Pre-menstrual like syndrome	Fatigue
	Hirsutism
Changes in libido	Loss of scalp hair
Leg cramp	Erythema multiforme
Relative pyridoxine deficiency	Erythema nodosum
	Itching
	Vaginal candidiasis
	Porphyria

Overdosage: Serious ill effects have not been reported following acute ingestion of large doses of oral contraceptives by young children. Overdosage may cause nausea, and withdrawal bleeding may occur in females. An appropriate method of gastric emptying may be used if considered desirable.

Pharmaceutical precautions Protect from light.

Legal category POM.

Package quantities Carton containing 3 pushpaks each of 21 tablets – sufficient for 3 cycles.

Further information Nil.

Product licence number 0076/0095.

*Trade Mark

Paines & Byrne Limited
Pabyrn Laboratories
Greenford
Middlesex UB6 7HG

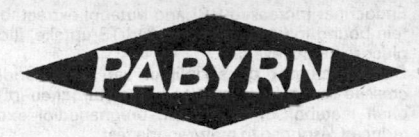

BENZTRONE*

Presentation Ampoules of a sterile, straw coloured solution of Oestradiol Benzoate BP in Ethyl Oleate BP for injection.

Uses Benztrone may be used for oestrogen replacement therapy associated with the menopause, primary amenorrhoea and female hypogonadism.

Dosage and administration Benztrone is given by intramuscular injection.

Oestrogen replacement therapy: 1–5 mg injection given every 14 days or more frequently if indicated.

Contra-indications, warnings, etc Oestrogen-dependent carcinoma. Prolonged exposure to unopposed oestrogens may increase the risk of development of endometrial carcinoma. History of thrombo-embolism, hepatic impairment. Caution is advised in pregnancy, breast-feeding, diabetes, epilepsy, cardiac or renal disease.

Pharmaceutical precautions Protect from light. On storage, solid matter may separate and this should be redissolved by warming before use.

Legal category POM.

Package quantities
1 mg in 1 ml ampoules – box of 10.
5 mg in 1 ml ampoules – box of 10.

Further information Nil.

Product licence numbers
1 mg   0051/5022
5 mg   0051/5024

CE-COBALIN*

Presentation Ce-Cobalin is a raspberry-flavoured syrup. Each 5 ml contains 30 mcg Vitamin B_{12} and 10 mg Vitamin C.

Uses Ce-Cobalin provides Vitamin B_{12} and vitamin C supplementation in deficiency states such as self-imposed dietary restrictions as in strict vegetarianism.

Dosage and administration Ce-Cobalin is taken orally and provides an adequate supplement to the diet at the following dosages:

Children: One 5 ml spoonful 3 times daily.

Adults: One or two 5 ml spoonsful 3 times daily.

Contra-indications, warnings, etc No known contra-indications. Ce-Cobalin is not intended for use in the treatment of pernicious anaemia.

Pharmaceutical precautions Store in a cool place.

Legal category P.

Package quantities 100 ml.

Further information Only about 2 mcg of vitamin B_{12} can be absorbed through the ileum from a single oral dose, so it should be given daily.

Initial treatment of clinical deficiency should be by injection of hydroxocobalamin (Cobalin-H).

Product licence number 0051/5019.

COBALIN-H*

Presentation 1 ml ampoules containing a sterile, clear, red solution providing 1000 mcg hydroxocobalamin per millilitre for injection. Cobalin-H complies with the specification for Hydroxocobalamin Injection BP.

Uses Addisonian pernicious anaemia. Prophylaxis and treatment of other macrocytic anaemias due to B_{12} deficiency. Tobacco amblyopia and Leber's atrophy.

Dosage and administration The following dosages are suitable for children and adults. Addisonian pernicious anaemia and other macrocytic anaemias *without* neurological involvement: *Initially* – 250 mcg to 1000 mcg intramuscularly on alternate days for one or two weeks then 250 mcg weekly until blood count is normal. *Maintenance* – 1000 mcg every two or three months.

Addisonian pernicious anaemia and other macrocytic anaemias *with* neurological involvement: *Initially* – 1000 mcg on alternate days as long as improvement continues. *Maintenance* – 1000 mcg every two months.

Prophylaxis of macrocytic anaemias associated with Vitamin B_{12} deficiency resulting from gastrectomy, ileal resection, certain malabsorption states and vegetarianism: 1000 mcg every two or three months.

Tobacco amblyopia and Leber's optic atrophy: *Initially* – 1000 mcg daily by intramuscular injection for two weeks then twice weekly as long as improvement is maintained. *Maintenance* – 1000 mcg every three months or as required.

Contra-indications, warnings, etc
Contra-indications: Sensitivity to hydroxocobalamin.

Precautions: Should not be given before a megaloblastic marrow has been demonstrated.

Pharmaceutical precautions Store in a cool place protected from light.

Legal category POM.

Package quantities Box of 10 ampoules.

Further information Hydroxocabalamin injection has

completely replaced Cyanocobalamin injection and is now the form of Vitamin B_{12} therapy of choice.

Product licence number 0051/5041.

DALIVIT*

Presentation *Capsules:* Oval red, soft gelatine capsules containing oily yellow suspension.

Drops: Deep yellow liquid with a characteristic taste and odour in a 15 ml amber glass bottle with integral dropper.

Syrup: Pale yellow liquid with a characteristic taste and odour

Formula		Capsules	Drops	Syrup
Vitamin A		7,500 Units	5,000 Units	5,000 Units
Vitamin D		1,000 Units	400 Units	1,000 Units
Thiamine	Hydrochloride BP	–	1 mg	2.5 mg
Thiamine	Mononitrate USP	3 mg	–	–
Riboflavin BP		3 mg	0.4 mg	1 mg
Pyridoxine	Hydrochloride BP	1 mg	0.5 mg	1 mg
Ascorbic Acid BP		75 mg	50 mg	25 mg
Nicotinamide BP		25 mg	5 mg	10 mg
Calcium pantothenate		5 mg	–	5 mg
		in each capsule	in each 0.6 ml	in each 5 ml

Actions and uses *Drops:* These are intended principally for administration to infants and very young children for the prevention and treatment of vitamin deficiency states and for the maintenance of normal health and growth in early childhood.

Capsules and syrup: For the prevention and treatment of vitamin deficiency in older children and adults. Indicated particularly in febrile and infective conditions or to provide essential vitamins for patients on restrictive diets.

Dosage and administration *Adults:* 1 Dalivit Capsule or 5 ml Dalivit Syrup daily.

Infants: Drops.
Up to 12 months: 0.3 ml daily (7 drops).
Over 12 months: 0.6 ml daily (14 drops).

In conditions of impaired absorption or frank vitamin deficiency, these doses may be increased at the discretion of the physician.

Contra-indications, warnings, etc Hypersensitivity to any of the active ingredients is a contra-indication. Excessive doses of vitamins A and D can lead to hypervitaminosis. When multivitamin preparations are prescribed allowance must be made for vitamins from other sources. This is particularly important during the first trimester of pregnancy when large doses of Vitamin A may be teratogenic.

Pharmaceutical precautions *Capsules:* Store in a cool dry place.

Drops: Store in a cool place protected from light.

Syrup: Store in a cool place protected from light.

Legal category Capsules and Syrup P.
Drops GSL.

Package quantities *Capsules:* 100, 500.
Drops: 15 ml.
Syrup: 100 ml.

Further information Dalivit Drops are prescribable under the NHS.

Product licence numbers
Capsules 0051/5018
Drops 0051/5016
Syrup 0051/5017

DI-SIPIDIN*

Presentation Transparent, hard gelatine insufflation capsules containing pituitary posterior lobe, standardised in terms of antidiuretic activity. Each capsule contains pituitary posterior lobe powder mixed with lactose to provide 30 antidiuretic units.

Uses The antidiuretic effect of posterior pituitary is well known and the intranasal route is an acceptable alternative to the injections of the hormone. Indicated for the treatment of diabetes insipidus.

Dosage and administration Di-Sipidin is administered by high nasal insufflation using the Pabyrn insufflator. Diabetes insipidus: 2–3 capsules daily. Children: 1–2 capsules daily. Administered in divided doses throughout the day by means of the special insufflator.

Contra-indications, warnings, etc Contra-indicated in hypertension. Allergic rhinitis, asthma and alveolitis have occasionally been reported following the use of pituitary posterior lobe insufflation. Chronic rhinitis or other nasal obstruction may impair or prevent absorption; the nasal passage should be completely cleared before insufflation of the powder.

Legal category POM.

Package quantities 25 or 100 capsules. Outfit comprising 25 capsules and insufflator. Pabyrn insufflator available separately.

Further information Nil.

Product licence number 0051/5143.

FOLICIN*

Presentation White sugar-coated tablets each containing: Dried Ferrous Sulphate 200 mg (Approx. 60 mg of iron), Copper Sulphate BPC 2.5 mg, Manganese Sulphate BPC 2.5 mg, Folic Acid BP 2.5 mg.

Uses For the prophylaxis and treatment of pregnancy anaemia.

Dosage and administration 1–2 tablets daily throughout the ante-natal period.

This product is not suitable for administration to children.

Contra-indications, warnings, etc Diagnosis of pernicious anaemia should be excluded before folic acid therapy is instituted. Folicin may cause gastro-intestinal discomfort, diarrhoea or vomiting in some patients. Constipation may follow long term use.

Overdosage with iron: Induce emesis and follow by gastric lavage with sodium bicarbonate 1% solution. Dissolve 2 g of desferrioxamine in Water for Injections and inject intramuscularly. Also give orally or by stomach tube 5 g of desferrioxamine dissolved in 50 ml of water.

Pharmaceutical precautions Store in a cool dry place.

Legal category POM.

Package quantities 100 and 500.

Further information Folicin is prescribable under the NHS.

Product licence number 0051/5030.

GESTONE*

Presentation Ampoules of a sterile straw coloured solution of Progesterone BP 10, 25 or 50 mg per ml in ethyl oleate for injection.

Uses Treatment of premenstrual syndrome. Also indicated for habitual and threatened abortion and dysfunctional uterine bleeding.

Dosage and administration
1. *Premenstrual syndrome:* Nulliparous women; 50 mg. Parous women; 100 mg IM daily, starting at signs of ovulation (day 12–14) continuing until the onset of menstruation. After initial treatment, dosage may be varied to that which gives full symptomatic control. Higher doses are normally required by women of high parity, a history of pre-eclampsia or postnatal depression and of slim build.

2. *Habitual abortion:* 10–20 mg twice weekly for first four months of pregnancy. Start as soon after conception as possible.

3. *Threatened abortion:* 25–50 mg daily for four days. Continuing at 10–25 mg twice weekly until fourth month of pregnancy.

4. *Dysfunctional uterine bleeding:* 5–10 mg daily 5–10 days before anticipated onset of menstruation.

Contra-indications, warnings, etc
Contra-indications: Undiagnosed vaginal bleeding, missed or incomplete abortion, history of thromboembolism, mammary carcinoma.

Pharmaceutical precautions Store in a cool place protected from light. On storage solid matter may separate and this should be re-dissolved by warming before use.

Legal category POM.

Package quantities Ampoules containing: 10 mg in 1 ml; 25 mg in 1 ml; 50 mg in 1 ml; 100 mg in 2 ml; in boxes of 10.

Further information Gestone should be injected deep into the buttock, rather than the thigh or deltoid using a 1.5 inch (3.8 cm) needle. This site has ample fat cells where a depot of progesterone can be formed for slow release.

Product licence numbers
10 mg   0051/5035
25 mg   0051/5036
50 mg   0051/5037
100 mg   0051/5038

GONADOTRAPHON FSH*

Presentation Gonadotraphon FSH is presented in ampoules containing a white, sterile, freeze-dried plug of 1000 Units Serum Gonadotrophin BP (Pregnant Mares' Serum) in a lactose base, for injection. A 2 ml ampoule of solvent for reconstitution is provided with each ampoule of freeze-dried material.

Uses In the male: Sterility due to defective spermatogenesis. In the female: Secondary amenorrhoea, anovulatory sterility.

Dosage and administration By deep intramuscular injection, preferably into the gluteal muscle.

Sterility due to defective spermatogenesis: 1500 Units twice weekly for 6 weeks followed by 500 Units once a week for 4 weeks.

Secondary amenorrhoea: 3000 Units daily for 5 days, followed by 3 injections of 1500 Units Gonadotraphon LH (chorionic gonadotrophin) on alternate days. May be repeated at monthly intervals or varied according to patient's response.

Anovulatory sterility: Treatment to start on fifth day of the cycle with, 500 Units daily for 10 days. Followed by 5000 Units Gonadotraphon LH daily for 10 days.

Contra-indications, warnings, etc
Contra-indications: Pregnancy, ovarian cysts, adrenal or thyroid disorders, intracranial lesions.

Warnings: Exclude endocrine disorders before treatment. A routine scratch test should be performed on patients prone to allergy. Intravenous injection is not recommended as it is liable to cause allergic reaction.

Treatment with FSH and HCG preparations should be carefully managed and monitored in order to avoid overstimulation of the ovary.

If pregnancy follows treatment with FSH and HCG preparations the possibility of multiple births is greater than usual.

Pharmaceutical precautions Aqueous solutions of gonadotrophic hormones are unstable but the freeze-dried powder will remain stable if stored at a temperature not exceeding 20°C.

Legal category POM.

Package quantities Twin ampoules of powder and solvent.

Further information Solvent contains 0.5% Phenol BP in Water for Injections BP. This has been found to reduce the pain of injections.

Product licence number 0051/5077.

GONADOTRAPHON LH*

Presentation Gonadotraphon LH is presented in ampoules containing a white, sterile, freeze-dried plug of 500, 1000, or 5000 Units of Chorionic Gonadotrophin BP (HCG) in a lactose base, for injection. All strengths are supplied with 2 ml ampoules of solvent for reconstitution of the powder.

Uses In the male: Delayed puberty, undescended testes, oligospermia or aspermia with inactive testes.

In the female: Induction of ovulation, recurrent abortion, menorrhagia due to persistent follicular phase, secondary amenorrhoea.

Dosage and administration Gonadotraphon LH is given by intramuscular injection.

In the male:
Delayed puberty: 500 Units twice weekly for four to six weeks.

Undescended testes: Optimum age range is 7–10 years but treat before puberty. 500 Units 3 times weekly for 6–10 weeks. In males over 17 years of age 1000 Units twice weekly. Treatment should be continued for one or two months after testicular descent.

Oligospermia or aspermia with inactive testes: 500 Units 2 or 3 times weekly for 16 weeks.

In the female:
Induction of ovulation: Gonadotraphon FSH (Serum Gonadotrophin) 500 Units intramuscularly daily from the 5th to the 14th day of the cycle followed by Gonadotraphon LH 5000 Units daily from the 15th to the 24th day of the cycle. If there is no response to the first course of injections, after one month a further course should be given with doubled dosage.

Recurrent abortion: 1000 Units to 2000 Units twice weekly from the earliest evidence of pregnancy to the 14th week of gestation.

Menorrhagia due to persistent follicular phase: 1000 Units twice weekly for the last two weeks of cycle.

Secondary amenorrhoea: 3000 Units Gonadotraphon FSH intramuscularly daily for 5 days, followed by 3 injections of 1500 Units Gonadotraphon LH on alternate days. This treatment should be repeated for 2 or 3 cycles; menstruation will normally occur 8 to 10 days after the last injection in each course of treatment.

Contra-indications, warnings, etc Caution should be exercised in patients with cardiac or renal impairment, asthma, epilepsy, migraine and patients predisposed to allergies.

Evidence of sexual precocity is an indication for withdrawal of treatment. However, in those cases where continuation of therapy is necessary, treatment may be resumed on a reduced dosage regime.

Administration of high dosages may occasionally lead to development of oedema in males, dosage should be considerably reduced in such cases.

Treatment with FSH and HCG preparations should be carefully managed and monitored in order to avoid overstimulation of the ovary.

If pregnancy follows treatment with FSH and HCG preparations the possibility of multiple births is greater than usual.

Pharmaceutical precautions In the dry state, in sealed ampoules, Gonadotraphon LH will remain stable if protected from light and stored at a temperature not exceeding 20°C. Solutions are unstable and should be freshly prepared.

Legal category POM.

Package quantities Twin ampoules: 500 Units – Boxes of 5 or 50; 1000 Units – Boxes of 5 or 50; 5000 Units – Box of 1 or 5.

Further information The solvent contains 0.5% Phenol BP in Water for Injections BP. This has been found to reduce the pain of injections.

Product licence numbers
500 Units   0051/5026
1000 Units 0051/5027
5000 Units 0051/5028

HEPARIN INJECTION BP (PABYRN)

Presentation A sterile, pyrogen-free, clear, colourless solution for injection of Heparin Sodium BP (Mucous)

in concentrations of 1,000, 5,000, 10,000 or 25,000 Units per ml.

Actions and uses Heparin has an anticoagulant action and its principal use is in the prophylaxis and treatment of thrombo-embolic disorders. It is of particular value in the treatment of deep vein thrombosis following major surgery and is used routinely in extra corporeal circulation procedures involving heart-lung and renal dialysis machines.

Dosage and administration An initial intravenous injection of 12,500 Units followed by 7,500–10,000 Units at four hourly intervals as required. May also be administered by continuous infusion via Dextrose/Saline solutions. The aim of treatment is to extend clotting time to about 15 minutes, which is two to three times the normal rate. In the prophylaxis and treatment of post-operative deep vein thrombosis, a subcutaneous dose of 5,000 Units two hours pre-operatively followed by 5,000 Units every 8–12 hours for 7–10 days.

Contra-indications, warnings, etc Heparin is contra-indicated in haemophilia, purpura and other haemorrhagic states. Also in bacterial endocarditis, gastric and duodenal ulcers, threatened abortion and advanced renal or hepatic disease. Idiosyncracies to Heparin treatment have been seen and dosage may need to be individually adjusted and monitored.

Haemorrhage due to overdosage can often be controlled by discontinuing Heparin therapy. Severe bleeding may be reduced by administering 1 mg of protamine sulphate for each 100 Units of Heparin to be neutralised. Hypersensitivity reactions are rare.

Pharmaceutical precautions Heparin injections should be stored in a cool place protected from light and should not be used after expiry date indicated. As Heparin loses potency in solutions with a pH less than 6 (e.g. Dextrose 5%) it should only be added to such solutions immediately prior to infusion. Heparin is incompatible in aqueous solutions with certain substances including antibiotics, antihistamines, phenothiazines, narcotic analgesics, hydrocortisone and hyaluronidase.

Legal category POM.

Package quantities Preservative-free ampoules containing 1,000 U in 1 ml, 5,000 U in 1 ml in packs of 50. 10,000 U in 1 ml, 25,000 U in 1 ml, 5,000 U in 5 ml, 25,000 U in 5 ml and 5,000 U in 0.2 ml in packs of 10 and 5 ml vials with preservative in strengths of 1,000 U/ml, 5,000 U/ml and 25,000 U/ml in packs of 10.

Further information Nil.

Product licence numbers
5 ml vials and 1 ml ampoules
  1,000 Units/ml   0051/5069
  5,000 Units/ml   0051/5070
10,000 Units/ml   0051/0020
25,000 Units/ml   0051/5071

0.2 ml ampoules
  5,000 Units/0.2 ml   0051/5071

5 ml ampoules
  5,000 Units/5 ml   0051/5044
25,000 Units/5 ml   0051/5144

HEPARINISED SALINE

Presentation A sterile, pyrogen-free, clear, colourless solution of Heparin Sodium BP (mucous) 10 Units per ml in Sodium Chloride Injection BP, contained in 5 ml ampoules. (50 Units per ampoule).

Uses Heparin has an anticoagulant action. The principal use of Heparinised Saline is for flushing intravascular catheters and indwelling cannulae, attendant llnes and heparin locks. This maintains patency by preventing the clotting of blood within an in-situ needle or catheter device, without alteration of systemic clotting factors.

Dosage and administration Use one 5 ml ampoule (50 Units) to flush every four hours or as required.

Contra-indications, warnings, etc Established heparin hypersensitivity. Heparinised Saline is not intended for therapeutic use and the low levels of heparin reaching the blood should not have any systemic effect.

Pharmaceutical precautions Heparinised Saline may not be compatible with some other drug solutions.

Legal category POM.

Package quantities Boxes of 10 × 5 ml ampoules.

Further information Nil.

Product licence number 0051/0019.

KETOVITE*

Presentation *Ketovite Tablets:* Yellow tablets each containing:

Thiamine hydrochloride	1.0 mg
Riboflavine	1.0 mg
Pyridoxine hydrochloride	0.33 mg
Nicotinamide	3.3 mg
Calcium pantothenate	1.16 mg
Ascorbic Acid	16.6 mg
α-Tocopheryl Acetate	5.0 mg
Inositol	50.0 mg
Biotin	0.17 mg
Folic Acid	0.25 mg
Acetomenapthone	0.5 mg

Ketovite Liquid: Pale straw coloured liquid for oral administration containing in each 5 ml:

Vitamin A	2,500 Units
Vitamin D	400 Units
Choline Chloride	150 mg
Cyanocobalamin	12.5 mcg

Uses The artificial nature of many therapeutic diets means that certain essential vitamins are not available from food and must, therefore, be provided in alternative form. It is for this purpose that Ketovite is used. Ketovite Tablets when used in conjunction with Ketovite Liquid will provide a complete vitamin supplementation in conditions such as phenylketonuria, disaccharide intolerance, galactosaemia and other disorders of carbohydrate or amino-acid metabolism. Ketovite is also of value in other restricted diets, such as those in renal conditions, malabsorption states and allergic conditions.

Ketovite tablets and Ketovite liquid do not contain sucrose, lactose, glucose, starch, fructose, sodium, or artificial colouring material.

Note: Ketovite Tablets and Ketovite Liquid are not interchangeable. For complete vitamin supplementation, both products should be administered.

Dosage and administration As a complete vitamin supplement for infants, young children or adults on restricted or synthetic diets: 1 Ketovite Tablet three times a day plus 5 ml Ketovite Liquid daily.

Contra-indications, warnings, etc Hypersensitivity to any of the vitamins present.

Pharmaceutical precautions Tablets: Store in a cool dry place. Liquid: Store at 5°C to 15°C.

Legal category
Tablets: POM.
Liquid: P.

Package quantities
Tablets 100 and 500.
Liquid 100 ml.

Further information Ketovite is prescribable under the NHS.

Product licence numbers
Tablets 0051/5079.
Liquid 0051/5080.

PABRINEX*

Presentation Pairs of amber ampoules of Vitamins B and C Injection BPC for intravenous and intramuscular injection:
I/V High Potency – 5 ml No. 1 + 5 ml No. 2 Printed Blue
I/M High Potency – 5 ml No. 1 + 2 ml No. 2 Printed Red
I/M Maintenance – 2 ml No. 1 + 2 ml No. 2 Printed Pink
Active ingredients: See table overleaf.

Uses Rapid therapy of severe depletion or malabsorption of the water soluble vitamins B and C, particularly in alcoholism, after acute infections, post-operatively and in psychiatric states.

Also used to maintain levels of Vitamins B and C in patients on chronic intermittent haemodialysis.

Dosage and administration
Intravenous: The contents of each pair of ampoules (total 10 ml) are drawn up into a syringe to mix them just before use, then injected slowly into a vein. For drip injection dilute with normal saline. *Not for intramuscular use.*

Intramuscular: The contents of each pair of ampoules (total: 7 ml – High Potency, 4 ml – Maintenance) are drawn up into a syringe to mix them just before use, then injected slowly high into the gluteal muscles, 5 cm below the iliac crest. *Not for intravenous use.*

Adult dose: Pabrinex is indicated for rapid therapy of severe vitamin depletion or malabsorption reported to occur in the following conditions:

Coma or delirium from alcohol, narcotics or barbiturates; collapse following continuous narcosis: The contents of 2–3 pairs of ampoules Intravenous High Potency (Blue No 1 and No 2) injected at intervals of 8 hours or at the discretion of the physician.

Psychosis following narcosis or ECT; toxicity from acute infections: The contents of one pair of ampoules Intravenous High Potency (Blue No 1 and No 2) or Intramuscular High Potency (Red No 1 and No 2) twice daily for up to 7 days.

Psychiatric states due to continued ill-health, old age, post operative debility and chronic infections; stress conditions: The contents of one pair of ampoules Intramuscular Maintenance (Pink No 1 and No 2) twice daily until maximum improvement is observed and maintained.

	Intravenous		Intramuscular			
	High potency		High potency		Maintenance	
Colour code	Blue label		Red label		Pink label	
Composition	No 1	No 2	No 1	No 2	No 1	No 2
Thiamine Hydrochloride BP (Vitamin B$_1$)	250 mg		250 mg		100 mg	
Riboflavine (as Phosphate Sodium BP) (Vitamin B$_2$)	4 mg		4 mg		4 mg	
Pyridoxine Hydrochloride BP (Vitamin B$_6$)	50 mg		50 mg		50 mg	
Nicotinamide BP		160 mg		160 mg		160 mg
Ascorbic Acid BP (as Sodium Ascorbate) (Vitamin C)		500 mg		500 mg		500 mg
Anhydrous Dextrose BP		1 g†				
Benzyl Alcohol BP			140 mg*		80 mg*	
Volume per Ampoule	5 ml	5 ml	5 ml	2 ml	2 ml	2 ml
Dose Volume	10 ml		7 ml		4 ml	

(* provides 2% w/v in mixed ampoules)
(† provides 10% w/v in mixed ampoules)

Haemodialysis: The contents of one pair of ampoules Intravenous High Potency (Blue No 1 and No 2) every two weeks diluted with saline and given at the end of the dialysis.

Children's dose: Pabrinex is rarely indicated for administration to children, but suitable doses are:

Under 6 years	$\frac{1}{4}$ adult dose
6–10 years	$\frac{1}{3}$ adult dose
10–14 years	$\frac{1}{2}$–$\frac{2}{3}$ adult dose
14 years and over	adult dose

Contra-indications, warnings, etc Sensitivity to any of the vitamins present, though this is rarely encountered. Occasionally hypotension or mild paraesthesia may result from continued high doses of Thiamine (Vitamin B$_1$).

Pharmaceutical precautions Store in a cool place and protect from light.

Legal category POM.

Package quantities Packs of 5 pairs and 10 pairs of ampoules.

Further information Nil.

Product licence numbers
I/V High Potency	0051/5008
I/M High Potency	0051/5005
I/M Maintenance	0051/5006

PANCREX*

Presentation

Pancrex V Forte Tablets (Pancreatin Tablets BP). White sugar and enteric coated tablets each containing not less than the following BP units of activity: Free protease 330, lipase 5,600, amylase 5,000.

Pancrex V Tablets (Pancreatin Tablets BP). White sugar and enteric coated tablets each containing not less than the following BP units of activity: Free protease 110, lipase 1,900, amylase 1,700.

Pancrex V Capsules: Ivory coloured opaque hard gelatine capsules imprinted 'Pancrex V' and company logo, containing Pancreatin BP and providing not less than the following BP units of activity per capsule: Free protease 430, lipase 8,000, amylase 9,000.

Capsules provide a simple and convenient method of dose measurement of the powder for administration to younger children requiring a low dose.

Pancrex V Capsules '125': Clear hard gelatine capsules containing Pancreatin BP and providing not less than the following BP units of activity: Free protease 160, lipase 2,950, amylase 3,300.

These low dose capsules may be used when small amounts of Pancrex are required, for example for neonates.

Pancrex Granules (Pancreatin Granules BP). Enteric coated granules containing not less than the following BP units of activity in each gram: Free protease 300, lipase 5,000, amylase, 4,000.

Pancrex V Powder (Pancreatin BP). A white or buff coloured powder having not less than the following BP units of activity in each gram: Free protease 1,400, lipase 25,000, amylase 30,000.

Uses To compensate for reduced intestinal enzyme activity in pancreatic deficiency states.

Indications: Fibrocystic disease of the pancreas (cystic fibrosis), chronic pancreatitis and pancreatic steatorrhoea following pancreatectomy. May also be indicated following gastrectomy as an aid to digestion.

Dosage and administration It is generally accepted that dosage may vary considerably according to the needs of the individual patient, but the following dosage scale provides a suitable basis for adjustment. Variations in response may be due to enteric coating.

Pancrex V Forte Tablets: 6–10 tablets four times daily half an hour before meals swallowed whole.

Pancrex V Tablets: 5–15 tablets four times daily half an hour before meals swallowed whole.

Pancrex V Capsules: Infants – The contents of 1–2 capsules mixed with feeds. Older children and adults – 2–6 capsules four times daily with meals swallowed whole, or the contents mixed with a drink or fruit purée.

The capsules may provide a suitable alternative to the enteric coated presentations in cases where the pH of the duodenum is not sufficiently alkaline to dissolve the enteric coat.

Pancrex V Capsules '125': Neonates – The contents of 1–2 capsules with feeds.

Pancrex Granules: 5–10 g swallowed dry or mixed with a little water or milk, four times daily before meals.

Pancrex V Powder: 0.5–2 g swallowed dry or mixed with a little water or milk four times daily with meals.

In the case of newborn infants, a dose of from 0.25–0.5 g of Pancrex V may be indicated.

Contra-indications, warnings, etc It is possible that some irritation of the skin of the mouth may occur if tablets are chewed or preparations retained in the mouth. Irritation of the anus may also occur. A barrier cream may prevent this local irritation. Allergic/asthmatic reactions have occasionally occurred on handling the powder.

Rare cases of hyperuricosuria and hyperuricaemia have been reported when extremely high doses of Pancreatin have been taken.

If Pancrex V is mixed with liquids or feeds, the resulting mixture should not be allowed to stand for more than one hour prior to use.

Safety in pregnancy has not been established. However no teratogenic effects have been observed in clinical cases.

Pharmaceutical precautions The preparations should be stored in a well-closed container in a cool place and used before the expiry date indicated on the label.

Legal category GSL.

Package quantities

Pancrex V Forte Tablets	100 and 500
Pancrex V Tablets	100 and 500
Pancrex V Capsules	100 and 500
Pancrex V Capsules '125'	500
Pancrex Granules	100 g and 500 g
Pancrex V Powder	100 g and 250 g

Further information Some of the activity of Pancrex V Powder and the powder from Pancrex V Capsules is destroyed by the acidity of the stomach. Dosage recommendations reflect this. However, cimetidine given 30–45 minutes before meals has been found to potentiate the action of the enzyme by reducing gastric acid secretion.

The following gives the approximate equivalence of the different dosage forms to 1 gram of Pancrex V Powder:

3 Capsules
9 '125' Capsules
5 Forte Tablets
15 Tablets
5 grams of Granules

Palatability of capsule contents, powder and granules may be improved by mixing with fruit juice or puree.

Pancrex is prepared from Pancreatin of porcine origin.

Product licence numbers

Pancrex V Forte Tablets	0051/5000
Pancrex V Tablets	0051/5002
Pancrex V Capsules	0051/5043
Pancrex V Capsules '125'	0051/5104
Pancrex Granules	0051/5003
Pancrex V Powder	0051/5004

VIRORMONE*

Presentation
Virormone Injection: Ampoules of 25, 50 and 100 mg of Testosterone Propionate BP in ethyl oleate for intramuscular injection.

Virormone Oral: White tablets of Methyltestosterone BP: 5 mg, 10 mg and 25 mg for oral or sublingual use.

Uses Testosterone is the androgenic hormone of male testis. It is used as replacement therapy in castrated adults and in those who are hypogonadal due to either pituitary or testicular disease.

May also be used for control of carcinoma of the breast in post-menopausal women.

Dosage and administration
In the male: Hypogonadism (adults), delayed puberty, cryptorchidism.

In the female: Carcinoma of the breast.

	Virormone (By IM injection)	Virormone oral (swallowed or sublingually)
Hypogonadism	50 mg 2–3 times weekly	50 mg daily
Delayed puberty cryptorchidism	50 mg weekly	10–20 mg daily
Carcinoma of the breast	100 mg 2–3 times weekly	50–100 mg daily

Contra-indications, warnings, etc
Cautions: Do not use before puberty in males, unless for treatment of delayed puberty. In any case caution is advised since the fusion of the epiphyses is hastened and may lead to short stature.

Use with care in patients with cardiac, renal or hepatic impairment, circulatory failure, hypertension or epilepsy. A reduced dosage may be advisable in elderly male patients since hyperstimulation can occur.

Virilism may occur in female patients on high doses.

Contra-indications: Breast cancer in men, prostatic carcinoma, pregnancy, breast feeding and nephrosis.

Warning: Tumours of the liver have been reported occasionally in patients subjected to prolonged treatment with androgenic-anabolic steroids. The possibility that these compounds may induce or enhance the development of hepatic tumours cannot at present be excluded and this should be considered when the use of this product is proposed, especially in young people who are not suffering with life threatening disorders.

Pharmaceutical precautions Protect from light.

Legal category POM.

Package quantities Virormone: 25 or 50 mg in 1 ml ampoules; 100 mg in 2 ml ampoules. Boxes of 10. Virormone Oral: Tablets of 5, 10, or 25 mg – packs of 100.

Further information Virormone and Virormone Oral are potent anabolic steroids. Replacement therapy is usually instituted with Virormone injection and Virormone Oral tablets are used for maintenance therapy. The

effects of Virormone Oral are increased about two-fold when used sublingually.

Product licence numbers

Virormone

25 mg/1 ml	0051/5057
50 mg/1 ml	0051/5058
100 mg/2 ml	0051/5059

Virormone Oral

5 mg	0051/5060
10 mg	0051/5061
25 mg	0051/5062

*Trade Mark

Parke-Davis Research Laboratories
Mitchell House
Southampton Road
Eastleigh
Hampshire SO5 5RY

PARKE-DAVIS
RESEARCH LABORATORIES

ABIDEC*

Presentation Oral drops: a clear yellow liquid, with a characteristic odour and taste.
Capsules: bright yellow oval gelatin capsule containing an oily yellow brown suspension.

Composition	Drops Each 0.6 ml contains	Capsules
Vitamin A PhEur	4000 units	4000 units
Vitamin B₁ (thiamine hydrochloride PhEur)	1 mg	1 mg
Vitamin B₂ (riboflavine Ph Eur)	0.4 mg	1 mg
Vitamin B₆ (pyridoxine hydrochloride PhEur)	0.5 mg	0.5 mg
Vitamin C (ascorbic acid PhEur)	50 mg	25 mg
Vitamin D₂ (calciferol Ph Eur)	400 units	400 units
Nicotinamide PhEur	5 mg	10 mg

Uses
Drops: The prevention and treatment of vitamin deficiencies and for the maintenance of normal growth and health during the early years of infancy and childhood; multivitamin supplement.

Capsules; The prevention of vitamin deficiencies, particularly when depletion is suspected; pregnancy and lactation; convalescence following debilitating illness; restricted diets.

Dosage and administration Oral.
Infants and children
0–6 years: 0.3 ml daily.
7 years and over:
Drops: 0.6 ml daily.
Capsules: One capsule daily.

Adults
Capsules: One capsule daily.
Drops: 0.6 ml daily.

Elderly (over 65 years): As for adults.

Contra-indications, warnings, etc Hypersensitivity to any of the active constituents. Excessive dosage of vitamin A and D can lead to hypervitaminosis. When prescribing *Abidec*, as with other multivitamin preparations, allowance should be made for vitamins obtained from other sources.
Treatment of overdosage: Not applicable.

Pharmaceutical precautions
Oral drops: Product has an expiry date of 2 years. Store below 25°C.

Capsules: Product has an expiry date of 3 years.

Legal category GSL.

Package quantities *Oral drops:* 50 ml pack (2 × 25 ml + 2 droppers graduated at 0.3 ml and 0.6 ml)
Capsules: Containers of 250.

Further information Nil.

Product licence numbers
Oral drops   0018/5021
Capsules   0018/5020

AGAROL*
Presentation A stable, white emulsion containing the following active constituents per 5 ml:

Phenolphthalein BP	66 mg
Liquid paraffin BP	1.6 ml
Agar	10 mg

Uses Agarol provides balanced cathartic and laxative properties. For the treatment of constipation. Agarol may be especially required when straining at stool is a hazard e.g. in patients with hernia, cardiac or hypertensive conditions, during convalescence after surgery, pre and post operatively in the surgical treatment of haemorrhoids and other allied ano-rectal conditions, obstetric patients and patients confined to bed.

Dosage and administration Oral
Adults: One to three 5 ml spoonfuls to be taken at bedtime. If necessary the dose may be repeated 2 hours after breakfast.

Elderly (over 65 years): As for adults. Long term overindulgence in laxatives has been reported. This is of particular importance in the elderly where a degree of dehydration may already exist.

Children (5–12 years) One 5 ml spoonful to be taken at bedtime or 2 hours after breakfast. Agarol may be mixed with water, milk or fruit juices.

Contra-indications, warnings, etc
Contra-indications: Sensitivity to phenolphthalein.

Warnings: None applicable.

Precautions: Agarol should not be taken within 2 hours of a meal since there is a theoretical risk that the liquid paraffin content could interfere with absorption of fat soluble vitamins.

Side-effects: Rarely, sensitivity to phenolphthalein.

Overdosage: Overdosage may cause excessive purgation and may produce skin eruptions or rash in sensitive persons. Gastric lavage is unnecessary, but fluid (and electrolyte) replacement may be required. Skin rash should be treated symptomatically.

Pharmaceutical precautions Protect from excessive heat (greater than 30°C).

Legal category P.

Package quantities Bottles containing 200 ml, 500 ml.

Further information Nil.

Product licence number 0019/5000.

ALOPHEN*

Presentation Brown film-coated pills.

Composition: Each pill contains:

Aloin BPC 1973	15 mg
Belladonna dry extract BP	5 mg
Prepared Ipecacuanha PhEur	4 mg
Phenolphthalein BP	30 mg

Uses Alophen Pill is for the relief of constipation due to torpidity of the lower bowel. It acts promptly, evacuation normally occurring within 8–10 hours.

Dosage and administration Oral.
Adults: 1 to 3 pills at bedtime.

Elderly (over 65 years): As for adults. Long term overindulgence in laxatives has been reported. This is of particular importance in the elderly where a degree of dehydration may already exist.

Children: Not recommended.

Contra-indications, warnings, etc Should not be used without the advice of a physician when nausea, vomiting or abdominal pain are present. Should not be given to patients with inflammatory bowel diseases or with glaucoma. Use with caution in patients with prostatic enlargement.
  Prolonged continuous use is not recommended.

Treatment of overdosage: Treatment should be supportive together with fluid replacement.

Pharmaceutical precautions Store below 30°C.

Legal category P.

Package quantities Packs of 50.

Further information Nil.

Product licence number 0018/0062.

AMSIDINE* CONCENTRATE FOR INFUSION ▼

Presentation Amsidine is formulated as two sterile liquids that are combined prior to use: *Drug ampoule* – a 2 ml clear, neutral glass printed ampoule containing a clear bright orange/red coloured solution; *Diluent vial* – a 20 ml amber glass vial containing a clear colourless solution.
  Each 2 ml ampoule contains 1.5 ml of amsacrine solution in anhydrous N,N-dimethylacetamide in a strength of 50 mg amsacrine per ml. That is, each ampoule contains 75 mg amsacrine. Each 20 ml amber vial contains 13.5 ml of 0.0353M L-lactic acid. Exactly 1.5 ml of the solution from the ampoule is removed by the aid of a graduated glass syringe and immediately added to the vial with L-lactic acid and the contents are mixed thoroughly by shaking. The resulting red solution contains 5 mg/ml Amsidine.

Uses
Action: Amsidine is a sterile antitumour chemotherapeutic agent for intravenous infusion. Although not completely clarified, the mode of action of amsacrine is related to its property of binding the DNA through intercalation and external (electrostatic) forces. Amsacrine inhibits the synthesis of DNA while the RNA may not be directly affected. An additional mode of action, involving modification of cell membrane function, has been suggested.

Indications: Amsidine is indicated for the induction and maintenance of remission in acute leukaemia of adults. It is effective in patients refractory to the anthracycline antibiotics used singly or in combination with other chemotherapeutic agents, and in patients who were formerly treated with maximum cumulative doses of these antibiotics.

Dosage and administration Amsidine must be diluted in 500 ml 5% Dextrose Injection BP and infused over 60 to 90 minutes because phlebitis or pain at the injection site may occur at doses greater than $70 mg/m^2$. (*Note: do not use other diluents. Amsidine is incompatible with saline.*) Care must be taken that no extravasation occurs which might produce severe irritation or necrosis. Caution in the handling and preparation of the solution should be exercised, and the use of polyethylene gloves is recommended. If the solution of Amsidine contacts the skin or mucosae, immediately wash thoroughly with soap and water. (See enclosure leaflet.)

Adults
Induction of remission phase: The usual dosage of Amsidine in the induction phase is $90 mg/m^2$ every day for five consecutive days (total dose $450 mg/m^2$ per course of treatment). If bone marrow biopsy performed on day six displays over 50% cellularity and the blasts count is over 30%, the treatment may be extended for an additional three days, bringing the total dose per course of treatment to $720 mg/m^2$.
  More than one course of treatment may be required to achieve induction. Depending on the effectiveness of the first course in producing myelosuppression, the subsequent courses are given at two-week (if not effective) to four-week (if effective) intervals. In cases where a hypocellular marrow has not been achieved after the first course of treatment, the daily dose of Amsidine may be escalated to $120 mg/m^2$ per day for the subsequent courses, provided that this is not contraindicated for reasons of non-myelosuppressive toxicity.
  For patients with impaired liver function or impaired renal function, the dose of Amsidine should be decreased by 20–30% (to $60–75 mg/m^2$ per day).

Maintenance phase: The maintenance dose is about one third the induction dose, given either as a single IV infusion or divided in three daily doses, e.g. $150 mg/m^2$ given once every 3–4 weeks or $50 mg/m^2$ per day for three consecutive days, repeated every 3–4 weeks. Each maintenance course should bring down the granulocyte count to $1,000–1,500/mm^3$ and the platelet count to $50,000–100,000/mm^3$. If this is not accomplished the maintenance dose may be escalated by 20% every second course. The granulocyte and platelet counts should be allowed to recover between the courses to over $1,500/mm^3$ and $100,000/mm^3$ respectively; otherwise the subsequent course should be delayed.

Children under 12 years: None.

Contra-indications, warnings, etc

Contra-indications: Treatment with Amsidine should not be started in patients who have pre-existing marked bone marrow suppression induced by other chemotherapeutic agents or radiotherapy.

Precautions: Patients should be hospitalised during the induction phase of treatment for close observation and extensive laboratory monitoring. Amsidine should be used only by physicians experienced in cancer chemotherapy. The drug may cause severe myelosuppression, and complete blood counts must be performed frequently. Leucocyte, red cell and platelet transfusions should be available.

With recommended dose schedules, leucopenia is usually transient, reaching its nadir at 10–13 days after treatment, with recovery usually following by the 17th to 25th day. White blood cell counts of 1,000/mm³ or lower are to be expected during treatment with appropriate doses of Amsidine. Doses higher than recommended may produce more severe or more prolonged marrow suppression. The potential for cardiotoxicity may be increased particularly by hypokalaemia, also concurrent use of diuretics, aminoglycosides or other nephrotoxic drugs and previous exposure to other anthracycline therapy. Periodic monitoring of bone marrow, cardiac, liver, kidney and CNS functions should be carried out in patients receiving Amsidine and particularly in those with pre-existing disorders of these systems. In the case of an exceedingly large fall in white cell count and excessive depression of bone marrow, suspension of treatment or reduction of dosage may be necessary.

Studies have demonstrated a mutagenic potential. No carcinogenic studies have been carried out. As with other antineoplastic agents there is a possibility that prolonged use may lead to a carcinogenic effect. This should be borne in mind when undertaking long-term treatment.

Use in pregnancy: Animal studies have indicated that amsacrine has foetotoxic and teratogenic properties. In addition there may be an effect on fertility. There is no information on use in human pregnancy, therefore, the benefit/risk considerations should be carefully weighed when administering Amsidine.

Adverse reactions
Haematopoietic system: The dose-limiting toxicity associated with Amsidine is myelosuppression and pancytopenia, requiring supportive treatment with white and red blood cells and platelets. Major complications during therapy were infections and haemorrhages treated respectively, with antibiotics and platelet transfusions.

Gastro-intestinal: Nausea with or without vomiting occurred frequently, but these symptoms were usually mild to moderate. Mucositis (stomatitis and oesophagitis) was almost as frequent and ranged in severity from mild to life-threatening; its frequency and severity were not strictly dose-related.

Central nervous system: A few cases of grand mal seizures in acute leukaemia patients have occurred during treatment with Amsidine. These patients were suffering, however, from a number of conditions related to far-advanced disease and were heavily pretreated; and it is unclear whether the seizures were attributable to Amsidine. The seizures generally were responsive to standard treatment, such as phenytoin.

Hepatic: Liver function tests showed occasional transient elevations of serum bilirubin and alkaline phosphatase, sometimes accompanied by jaundice, which required lowering the dose of Amsidine.

Renal: Occasional occurrence of haematuria, anuria, and rarely acute renal failure have been reported.

Cardiac: Cardiotoxicity occurred in several patients. It ranged from grand mal seizures followed by ventricular tachycardia to congestive heart failure or cardiac arrest.

Cutaneous: Local tissue irritation, necrosis and phlebitis have been reported. This problem is related to the concentration of drug infused per unit time; it is ameliorated by diluting the drug in a large volume of 5% Dextrose Injection BP and infusing over a longer period of time (1 to 2 hours).

Alopecia occurred in about 1 in 7 patients, sometimes precipitously. Since most patients were previously treated with other chemotherapeutic agents and/or radiation, it is not clear whether this was a cumulative effect of all treatments.

Treatment of overdosage: Treatment of overdosage should be supportive and the blood picture should be closely monitored with appropriate blood transfusions being given if necessary.

Pharmaceutical precautions Caution in handling and preparation of solution should be exercised, and the use of polyethylene gloves is recommended (see enclosure leaflet). If the solution of Amsidine contacts the skin or mucosae, immediately wash thoroughly with soap and water.

Amsidine must be diluted in 500 ml 5% Dextrose Injection BP and infused over 60 to 90 minutes. (*Note: do not use other diluents. Amsidine is incompatible with saline*).

The solution when diluted for infusion is stable for eight hours at room temperature. It should be protected from exposure to sunlight, and any unused solution should be discarded (see enclosure leaflet). *Glass syringes must be used. Amsidine in solution reacts with plastic syringes.*

Legal category POM.

Package quantities Each carton contains six 2 ml ampoules containing amsacrine solution and six 20 ml vials of diluent.

Further information Nil.

Product licence number 0018/0124.

ANUGESIC*-HC CREAM

Presentation Buff-coloured cream with the characteristic odour of Balsam Peru. Each 100 g of cream contains:

Pramoxine Hydrochloride USP	1.00 g
Hydrocortisone Acetate PhEur	0.50 g
Benzyl Benzoate BP	1.20 g
Bismuth Oxide	0.875 g
Balsam Peru BPC 1973	1.85 g
Zinc Oxide PhEur	12.35 g
Resorcinol BP	0.875 g

Uses Anugesic-HC Cream provides antiseptic, astringent, emollient and decongestant properties. In addition the anti-inflammatory action of hydrocortisone helps to reduce swelling and hyperaemia. Pramoxine is a rapidly acting local anaesthetic. The cream may be used to provide lubrication for suppositories.

Anugesic-HC Cream is indicated for the comprehensive symptomatic treatment of severe and acute discomfort or pain associated with internal and external haemorrhoids, proctitis, cryptitis, anal fissures, pruritus ani and perianal sinuses. It is also indicated postoperatively in ano-rectal surgical procedures.

Dosage and administration Topical.
Adults: Apply cream to the affected area at night, in the morning and after each evacuation.
Not to be taken orally.
Thoroughly cleanse the affected area, dry and apply cream by gently smoothing onto the affected area. For internal conditions use rectal nozzle provided and clean it after each use.

Elderly (over 65 years): As for adults.

Children: Not recommended.

Contra-indications, warnings, etc
Contra-indications: Tubercular, fungal and most viral lesions including herpes simplex, vaccinia and varicella. History of sensitivity to any of the constituents.

Warnings: As with all products containing topical steroids the possibility of systemic absorption should be borne in mind. Prolonged or excessive use may produce systemic corticosteroid effects. During the first trimester of pregnancy long-term therapy with topical corticosteroids should be avoided.

Precautions: Following symptomatic relief definite diagnosis should be established.

Side-effects: Rarely, sensitivity reactions.
Patients may occasionally experience transient burning on application, especially if the anoderm is not intact.

Overdosage: If swallowed, main toxic ingredient is resorcinol, which may cause shock, collapse, rash, convulsion and coma, but only if more than about 100 g Anugesic-HC Cream is swallowed.
Fever, nausea, vomiting, stomach cramps and diarrhoea may develop 3–12 hours after ingestion.
Pramoxine is relatively non-toxic and less sensitising than other local anaesthetics.
Hydrocortisone normally does not produce toxic effects in an acute single overdose.
Treatment of a large acute overdosage should include gastric lavage, purgation with magnesium sulphate and complete bed rest. If necessary, give oxygen, and general supportive measures. Methaemoglobinaemia should be treated by intravenous methylene blue.

Pharmaceutical precautions Store at a temperature not exceeding 25°C.

Legal category POM.

Package quantity Tubes containing 15 g.

Further information Anugesic-HC Cream is prepared in a water-miscible base which provides intimate contact with the area to be treated without having to cross an anhydrous barrier. A cream is also more convenient to use being aesthetically more acceptable than ointments.

Product licence number 0019/5005.

ANUGESIC*-HC SUPPOSITORIES

Presentation Buff-coloured suppositories. Each 2.8 g suppository contains:

Pramoxine Hydrochloride USP	27 mg
Hydrocortisone Acetate PhEur	5 mg
Benzyl Benzoate BP	33 mg
Bismuth Oxide	24 mg
Bismuth Subgallate BP	59 mg
Balsam Peru BPC 1973	49 mg
Zinc Oxide PhEur	296 mg

Uses Anugesic-HC Suppositories provide antiseptic, astringent, emollient and decongestant properties. In addition the anti-inflammatory action of hydrocortisone helps to reduce swelling and hyperaemia. Pramoxine is a rapidly acting local anaesthetic.
Anugesic-HC Suppositories are indicated for the comprehensive symptomatic treatment of severe and acute discomfort or pain associated with internal haemorrhoids, proctitis, cryptitis, anal fissures, pruritus ani and perianal sinuses. Also indicated post-operatively in ano-rectal surgical procedures.

Dosage and administration *Adults:* Remove plastic cover and insert one suppository into the anus at night, in the morning and after each evacuation.
Not to be taken orally.

Elderly (over 65 years): As for adults.

Children: Not recommended.

Contra-indications, warnings, etc
Contra-indications: Tubercular, fungal and most viral lesions including herpes simplex, vaccinia and varicella. History of sensitivity to any of the constituents.

Warnings: As with all products containing topical steroids the possibility of systemic absorption should be borne in mind. Prolonged or excessive use may produce systemic corticosteroid effects. During the first trimester of pregnancy long-term therapy with topical corticosteroids should be avoided.

Precautions: Following symptomatic relief definite diagnosis should be established.

Side-effects: Rarely, sensitivity reactions.
Patients may occasionally experience transient burning on application, especially if the anoderm is not intact.

Overdosage: If swallowed, fever, nausea, vomiting, stomach cramps and diarrhoea may develop 3–12 hours after ingestion.
Pramoxine is relatively non-toxic and less sensitising than other local anaesthetics.
Hydrocortisone normally does not produce toxic effects in an acute single overdose.
Treatment of a large acute overdosage should include gastric lavage, purgation with magnesium sulphate and complete bed rest. If necessary, give oxygen, and general supportive measures. Methaemoglobinaemia should be treated by intravenous methylene blue.

Pharmaceutical precautions Store in a dry place, at a temperature not exceeding 25°C.

Legal category POM.

Package quantity Box of 12 suppositories.

Further information Nil.

Product licence number 0019/5006.

ANUSOL* CREAM & OINTMENT

Presentation *Anusol Cream:* A buff-coloured cream having the characteristic odour of Balsam Peru. Each 100 g of cream contains:

Bismuth Oxide	2.14 g
Balsam Peru BPC 1973	1.80 g
Zinc Oxide PhEur	10.75 g.

Anusol Ointment: A light buff coloured ointment having the characteristic odour of Balsam Peru. Each 100 g of ointment contains:

Bismuth Subgallate BP	2.25 g
Bismuth Oxide	0.875 g
Balsam Peru BPC 1973	1.875 g
Zinc Oxide PhEur	10.75 g.

Uses Anusol Cream and Anusol Ointment provide antiseptic, astringent and emollient properties which help to relieve discomfort associated with minor ano-rectal conditions. Anusol Cream also provides lubricating properties for use with suppositories. Indicated for the symptomatic relief of uncomplicated internal and external haemorrhoids, pruritus ani, proctitis and fissures. Also indicated post-operatively in ano-rectal surgical procedures and after incision of thrombosed or sclerosed ano-rectal veins.

Dosage and administration Topical

Adults: Apply to the affected area at night, in the morning and after each evacuation until the condition is controlled. Thoroughly cleanse the affected area, dry and apply cream or ointment. Anusol Ointment should be applied on a gauze dressing. Anusol Cream is prepared in a vanishing cream base and may be gently smoothed onto the affected area without the need to apply a gauze dressing. For internal conditions use rectal nozzle provided, and clean it after each use.

Not to be taken orally.

Elderly (over 65 years): As for adults.

Children: Not recommended.

Contra-indications, warnings, etc

Contra-indications: History of sensitivity to any of the constituents.

Warnings: None applicable.

Precautions: None applicable.

Side-effects: Rarely, sensitivity reactions. Patients may occasionally experience transient burning on application, especially if the anoderm is not intact.

Overdosage: Treatment of a large acute overdose should include gastric lavage, purgation with magnesium sulphate and complete bed rest. If necessary, apply oxygen, and give general supportive measures.

Pharmaceutical precautions Store at a temperature not exceeding 25°C.

Legal category GSL.

Package quantities Anusol Cream: Tubes containing 23 g., Anusol Ointment: Tubes containing 25 g.

Further information The formula of Anusol Cream is similar to that of Anusol Ointment. The advantage of the cream preparation is that the water-miscible base gives intimate contact with the area to be treated and the medicaments do not have to cross an anhydrous barrier. A cream is also more convenient to use, being aesthetically more acceptable than ointments.

Product licence numbers

Anusol Cream	0019/0040.
Anusol Ointment	0019/5002.

ANUSOL* SUPPOSITORIES

Presentation White suppositories. Each 2.8 g suppository contains:

Bismuth Subgallate BP	59 mg
Bismuth Oxide	24 mg
Balsam Peru BPC 1973	49 mg
Zinc Oxide PhEur	296 mg

Uses Anusol Suppositories provide antiseptic astringent and emollient properties which help to relieve discomforts associated with minor ano-rectal conditions.

Indicated for the symptomatic relief of uncomplicated internal haemorrhoids and proctitis. Also indicated post-operatively in ano-rectal surgical procedures and after incision of thrombosed or sclerosed ano-rectal veins.

Dosage and administration *Adults:* Remove wrapper and insert one suppository into the anus at night, in the morning and after each evacuation.

Not to be taken orally.

Elderly (over 65 years): As for adults.

Children: Not recommended.

Contra-indications, warnings, etc

Contra-indications: History of sensitivity to any of the constituents.

Warnings: None applicable.

Precautions: None applicable.

Side-effects: Rarely, sensitivity reactions. Patients may occasionally experience transient burning on application, especially if the anoderm is not intact.

Overdosage: Treatment of a large acute overdose should include gastric lavage, purgation with magnesium sulphate and complete bed rest. If necessary, give oxygen and general supportive measures.

Pharmaceutical precautions Store at a temperature not exceeding 25°C.

Legal category GSL.

Package quantities Box of 12 or 24 suppositories.

Further information Nil.

Product licence number 0019/5001.

ANUSOL*-HC OINTMENT

Presentation A buff-coloured ointment having a characteristic odour of Balsam Peru. Each 100 g of ointment contains:

Hydrocortisone Acetate PhEur	0.25 g
Benzyl Benzoate BP	1.25 g
Bismuth Subgallate BP	2.25 g
Bismuth Oxide	0.875 g
Balsam Peru BPC 1973	1.875 g
Zinc Oxide PhEur	10.75 g
Resorcinol BP	0.875 g

Uses Anusol-HC Ointment provides antiseptic, astringent, emollient and decongestant properties which help to relieve discomforts associated with minor ano-rectal conditions. In addition the anti-inflammatory action of hydrocortisone helps reduce swelling and hyperaemia.

Indicated for the symptomatic relief of external and internal haemorrhoids, proctitis, cryptitis, anal fissures, pruritus ani and perianal sinuses. Also indicated post-operatively in ano-rectal surgical procedures.

Dosage and administration Topical
Adults: Apply ointment to the affected area at night, in the morning and after each evacuation.

Thoroughly cleanse the affected area, dry and apply ointment on a gauze dressing. For internal conditions use rectal nozzle provided and clean it after each use.

Not to be taken orally.

Elderly (over 65 years): As for adults.

Children: Not recommended.

Contra-indications, warnings, etc
Contra-indications: Tubercular, fungal and most viral lesions including herpes simplex, vaccinia and varicella. History of sensitivity to any of the constituents.

Warnings: As with all products containing topical steroids the possibility of systemic absorption should be borne in mind. Prolonged or excessive use may produce systemic corticosteroid effects. During the first trimester of pregnancy long-term therapy with topical corticosteroids should be avoided.

Precautions: Following symptomatic relief definite diagnosis should be established.

Side-effects: Rarely, sensitivity reactions.

Patients may occasionally experience transient burning on application, especially if the anoderm is not intact.

Overdosage: If swallowed, main toxic ingredient is resorcinol, which may cause shock, collapse, rash, convulsion and coma, but only if more than about 100 g Anusol-HC Ointment is swallowed.

Fever, nausea, vomiting, stomach cramps and diarrhoea may develop 3–12 hours after ingestion.

Hydrocortisone normally does not produce toxic effects in an acute single overdose.

Treatment of a large acute overdose should include gastric lavage, purgation with magnesium sulphate and complete bed rest. If necessary, give oxygen, and general supportive measures. Methaemoglobinaemia should be treated by intravenous methylene blue.

Pharmaceutical precautions Store at a temperature not exceeding 25°C.

Legal category POM.

Package quantities Tubes containing 15 g.

Further information Nil

Product licence number 0019/5004.

ANUSOL*-HC SUPPOSITORIES

Presentation Olive green suppositories. Each 2.8 g suppository contains:

Hydrocortisone Acetate PhEur	10 mg
Benzyl Benzoate BP	33 mg
Bismuth Subgallate BP	59 mg
Bismuth Oxide	24 mg
Balsam Peru BPC 1973	49 mg
Zinc Oxide PhEur	296 mg
Resorcinol BP	24 mg

Uses Anusol-HC Suppositories provide antiseptic, astringent, emollient and decongestant properties which help to relieve discomforts associated with minor ano-

rectal conditions. In addition the anti-inflammatory action of hydrocortisone helps reduce swelling and hyperaemia.

Anusol-HC Suppositories are indicated for the symptomatic relief of internal haemorrhoids, proctitis, cryptitis, anal fissures, pruritus ani and perianal sinuses. Also indicated post-operatively in ano-rectal surgical procedures.

Dosage and administration *Adults:* Remove wrapper and insert one suppository into the anus at night, in the morning and after each evacuation.

Not to be taken orally.

Elderly (over 65 years): As for adults.

Children: Not recommended.

Contra-indications, warnings, etc
Contra-indications: Tubercular, fungal and most viral lesions including herpes simplex, vaccinia and varicella. History of sensitivity to any of the constituents.

Warnings: As with all products containing topical steroids the possibility of systemic absorption should be borne in mind. Prolonged or excessive use may produce systemic corticosteroid effects. During the first trimester of pregnancy long-term therapy with topical corticosteroids should be avoided.

Precautions: Following symptomatic relief definite diagnosis should be established.

Side-effects: Rarely, sensitivity reactions.

Patients may occasionally experience transient burning on application, especially if the anoderm is not intact.

Overdosage: If swallowed, main toxic ingredient is resorcinol, which may cause shock, collapse, rash, convulsion and coma, but only if more than about 40 suppositories are ingested.

Fever, nausea, vomiting, stomach cramps and diarrhoea may develop 3–12 hours after ingestion.

Hydrocortisone normally does not produce toxic effects in an acute single overdose.

Treatment of a large acute overdose should include gastric lavage, purgation with magnesium sulphate and complete bed rest. If necessary, give oxygen, and general supportive measures. Methaemoglobinaemia should be treated by intravenous methylene blue.

Pharmaceutical precautions Store at a temperature not exceeding 25°C.

Legal category POM.

Package quantities Box of 12 suppositories.

Further information Nil.

Product licence number 0019/5003.

BENADRYL*

Presentation 25 mg capsule – pink/pink gelatin capsule imprinted PARKE-DAVIS, PD 25.

Composition: Each capsule contains:
Diphenhydramine Hydrochloride PhEur 25 mg.

Action: Benadryl (diphenhydramine hydrochloride PhEur Parke-Davis), is a potent antihistamine agent, which possesses anticholinergic (antispasmodic), antitussive, antiemetic, antipruritic and sedative effects.

Uses Indicated in the treatment of hay fever, urticaria, vasomotor rhinitis, angioneurotic oedema, drug sensitisation, bee and jelly fish stings and serum and penicillin reactions. Good responses have been observed in contact dermatitis, erythema multiforme, atopic eczema and other allergic dermatoses, characterised by tissue oedema, erythema and pruritus. Successful results have also been reported in food sensitivity, migraine, Meniere's disease, dermographism and in some cases of bronchial asthma. Clinical experience has indicated that, as an antispasmodic, it is useful in controlling symptoms of spastic colitis, nocturnal cramps and dysmenorrhoea. It has also proved beneficial in Parkinsonism and it has been reported as the drug of choice in drug-induced extrapyramidal reactions.

Dosage and administration Oral.

Adults: Most allergic conditions are controlled by one 25 mg capsule taken three times a day supplemented by a 50 mg dose at bedtime to allay symptoms throughout the night. In severe, acute or chronic states intensive dosage may be necessary. In no instance should the daily dosage exceed 400 mg. When partial or complete relief is obtained 50 to 100 mg daily will often be sufficient to prevent recurrence of symptoms.

Elderly (over 65 years): As for adults.

Children: No dose recommended.

Contra-indications, warnings, etc May cause drowsiness. If affected the patient should not drive or operate machinery. Avoid alcoholic drink.

Other side-effects reported include dryness of mouth, dizziness and nausea.

Contra-indicated in patients with known hypersensitivity to the active constituent.

As with other medicines care should be taken in administration during pregnancy.

Treatment of overdosage: Gastric lavage in the conscious patient and intensive supportive therapy where necessary, as with cases of overdosage of antihistamine drugs.

Pharmaceutical precautions Store in a dry place at a temperature not exceeding 30°C.

Legal category P.

Package quantities 25 mg capsules available in packs of 50.

Further information Nil.

Product licence number 0018/5006.

CENTRAX* ▼

Presentation Blue, slightly mottled, circular, biconvex tablets, having a single breakline on one face marked W and 10. Each tablet contains 10 mg prazepam.

Uses Centrax is indicated for the symptomatic relief of anxiety-tension states associated with stressful circumstances, organic or psychosomatic illness.

Dosage and administration Oral

Adults: The usual dosage is 30 mg daily in single or divided doses. The dose should be adjusted within the range 10 mg to 60 mg daily in accordance with response of the patient.

Elderly (over 65 years): Half the normal adult dose may be sufficient for a therapeutic response in the elderly. As with other benzodiazepines the elderly are particularly liable to experience the symptoms listed in the Warnings and adverse effects section together with confusion, especially if organic brain symptoms are present. There-

fore in elderly or debilitated patients, the initial dose should be small, and increments should be made gradually, in accordance with the response of the patient, to preclude ataxia or excessive sedation.

Children: None.

Contra-indications, warnings, etc

Contra-indications: Known sensitivity to benzodiazepines, acute pulmonary insufficiency.

Use in pregnancy: There is no evidence as to drug safety in human pregnancy, nor is there evidence from animal work that it is free from hazard. Do not use during pregnancy, especially during the first and last trimesters, unless there are compelling reasons.

Precautions: Chronic pulmonary insufficiency, and in renal or hepatic disease.

In labour: High single doses or repeated low doses have been reported to produce hypotonia, poor sucking and hypothermia in the neonate, and irregularities in the fetal heart. In view of their molecular size, prazepam and its metabolites are probably excreted in human milk, therefore Centrax should not be given to nursing mothers.

Caution must be exercised in patients with glaucoma or myasthenia gravis because of possible deleterious effects attributed to the benzodiazepines in such patients.

Warnings and adverse effects: As with other benzodiazepines drowsiness, sedation, blurring of vision, unsteadiness and ataxia have been reported. The effects occur following single as well as repeated dosage and may persist well into the following day. Performance at skilled tasks and alertness may be impaired. Patients should be warned of this hazard and advised not to drive or operate machinery during treatment. The effects are potentiated by alcohol, phenothiazines, narcotics, barbiturates, other CNS depressant drugs, MAO inhibitors, and other anti-depressants. The elderly are particularly liable to experience these symptoms together with confusion especially if organic brain symptoms are present. Therefore in elderly or debilitated patients, the initial dose should be small, and increments should be made gradually, in accordance with the response of the patient, to preclude ataxia or excessive sedation. See also Dependence potential and withdrawal symptoms below. Abnormal psychological reactions to benzodiazepines have been reported. Rare behavioural adverse effects include paradoxical aggressive outbursts, excitement, confusion, and the uncovering of depression with suicidal tendencies. Other rare adverse effects include slight decreases in blood pressure, gastro-intestinal and visual disturbances, skin rashes, urinary retention, headache, vertigo, change in libido, blood dyscrasias and jaundice.

Dependence potential and withdrawal symptoms: In general, the dependence potential of benzodiazepines is low but this increases when high doses are attained, especially when given over long periods. This is particularly so in patients with a history of alcoholism or drug abuse, or in patients with marked personality disorders. Regular monitoring of treatment in such patients is essential and routine repeat prescriptions should be avoided. Treatment in all patients should be withdrawn gradually as symptoms such as depression, nervousness, rebound insomnia, irritability, sweating, and diarrhoea have been reported following abrupt cessation of treatment in patients receiving even normal therapeutic doses for short periods of time. Abrupt withdrawal following excessive dosage may produce confusion, toxic psychosis, convulsions, or a condition resembling delirium tremens.

Treatment of overdosage: Clinical features of benzodiazepine overdosage include impaired level of consciousness, dizziness, ataxia, slurred speech and respiratory depression. Gastric lavage or emesis is rarely necessary, and the mainstay of management is general supportive therapy.

Pharmaceutical precautions Store in a dark, dry place at a temperature not exceeding 25°C.

Legal category CD (Sch 4), POM.

Package quantities Packs of 100 tablets.

Further information This is a long acting benzodiazepine. Repeated dosage will lead to accumulation of drug metabolites. The elderly and patients with impaired renal and/or hepatic function will be particularly susceptible to adverse effects listed above. Treatment should be kept to a minimum and given only under close medical supervision. Little is known regarding efficacy or safety of benzodiazepines in long term use. It is advisable to review treatment regularly, and to discontinue use as soon as possible.

Product licence number 0019/0054

CHLOROMYCETIN* CAPSULES 250 mg and PALMITATE SUSPENSION

Presentation
Chloromycetin Capsules 250 mg: Hard gelatin capsule with white opaque body/light grey opaque cap imprinted 'PARKE-DAVIS'.

Chloromycetin Palmitate Suspension: A white suspension with no bitter taste.

Composition: Each capsule contains:
Chloramphenicol PhEur 250 mg.
Each 5 ml suspension contains:
Chloramphenicol palmitate BP equivalent to Chloramphenicol PhEur 125 mg.

Action: Chloramphenicol palmitate which contains the effective polymorph is hydrolysed to the free antibiotic before absorption. Resulting blood concentrations are similar to those produced by the administration of other oral forms of chloramphenicol.

Chloramphenicol exerts mainly a bacteriostatic effect on a wide range of gram-negative and gram-positive bacteria, and is particularly active against Salmonella typhi and Haemophilus influenzae. The mode of action is through interference with or inhibition of protein synthesis in intact cells. Development of resistance to chloramphenicol, both experimentally and in man, appears to be low in contrast to other antibiotics.

Chloramphenicol administered orally is absorbed rapidly from the gastro-intestinal tract producing detectable concentrations in the blood within one half hour after administration. Average peak serum levels of free chloramphenicol after the first dose generally occur within one or two hours.

The principal route of excretion of chloramphenicol is through the kidneys, total urinary excretion ranging from 68 to over 90 per cent. Small amounts of active drug are found in the bile and faeces. Chloramphenicol diffuses rapidly throughout tissues and body fluids. Chloramphenicol enters cerebrospinal fluid even in the absence of meningeal inflammation. Measurable levels are also detectable in pleural and ascitic fluids, saliva and milk. It diffuses readily into the aqueous, vitreous humours of the eye. Transport across the placental barrier occurs with somewhat lower concentration in cord blood than in maternal blood.

Uses Chloramphenicol is a potent therapeutic agent and should not be used for trivial infections. It should be administered according to the instructions of a medical practitioner. It is recommended that chloramphenicol should be reserved for use in typhoid fever, H. influenzae meningitis, serious chest infections and situations where clinical assessment usually supplemented by laboratory studies indicates that no other antibiotic would suffice.

Dosage and administration
Adults and children over 2 weeks old: The conventional dosage of chloramphenicol of 50 mg/kg of bodyweight per day in divided doses at six-hour intervals is recommended for the average patient. In exceptional cases, such as with patients having infections due to moderately resistant organisms or suffering from infections such as septicaemia or meningitis, dosage schedules up to 100 mg/kg/day may be prescribed. However, these higher doses should be decreased as soon as clinically indicated. To prevent relapses, treatment should be continued after the temperature has returned to normal for 4 days in rickettsial diseases and for 8–10 days in typhoid fever.

In instances of impaired hepatic or renal function, the ability to metabolise or excrete chloramphenicol may be reduced and the medical practitioner should adjust the dose accordingly.

Elderly (over 65 years): As for adults.

Chloramphenicol has been used successfully at normal dosage in elderly patients. The pattern and incidence of adverse effects does not appear to differ from younger adults. Chloramphenicol is mainly conjugated in the liver to form an inactive glucoronide. Mildly decreased renal function in the elderly will not therefore significantly affect levels of chloramphenicol.

Premature and newborn infants and children with immature metabolic processes: (see gray syndrome under Adverse reactions).

A total of 25 mg/kg/day divided into four doses at six-hour intervals usually produces and maintains a concentration of chloramphenicol in blood and tissues adequate to control most infections in premature and new born infants and children with immature metabolic processes. After the first two weeks of life, full term infants ordinarily may receive up to a total of 50 mg/kg/day equally divided into four doses at six-hour intervals. Precise control of serum chloramphenicol levels should be achieved through analytical methods, wherever this is feasible.

Contra-indications, warnings, etc Chloramphenicol is contra-indicated in individuals with a history of previous hypersensitivity and/or toxic reaction to the drug.

Blood dyscrasias including aplastic anaemia may be associated with the administration of chloramphenicol. If facilities are available, it is well to determine the routine blood profile before therapy, and blood studies should be repeated at appropriate intervals especially during prolonged or intermittent therapy. The intervals at which such studies should be performed depends on the circumstances of each individual case. Consideration should be given to discontinuing the drug if evidence of depression of any of the blood elements appears attributable to chloramphenicol, weighing these effects against the seriousness and course of the disease under treatment. Repeated courses of chloramphenicol and concurrent therapy with other drugs known to cause bone marrow depression or even aplastic anaemia should be avoided. Chloramphenicol should be administered according to the direction of a medical practitioner, and it should not be used for the treatment of trivial infections. Excessive blood levels, as with other antibiotics may result from administration of the recommended dose to patients with impaired liver or kidney function, including those due to immature metabolic processes in the premature and full-term infant. Chloramphenicol should not be administered intravenously during labour. The medical practitioner should also remember that chloramphenicol is excreted in the milk of the lactating mother. Therefore mothers taking this drug should not breast-feed their infants.

Chloramphenicol should not be used during pregnancy unless considered essential by the physician.

As with other antibiotics, the use of chloramphenicol may result in an overgrowth of non-susceptible organisms including fungi.

Chloramphenicol is not alone in the phenomenon of drug interaction and when patients are concurrently receiving anti-coagulants or anti-convulsants, dosage adjustment of these agents may be necessary. The half-life of chloramphenicol is considerably prolonged in patients receiving paracetamol (acetaminophen). Concurrent administration of these drugs should be avoided.

Adverse reactions: Haematological reactions: Blood dyscrasias including aplastic anaemia have been attributed to the administration of chloramphenicol. Two types of bone marrow depression have been observed. One type may occur during therapy, is reversible on cessation of treatment and is dose related. The second type which may occur weeks to months after therapy is rare; it may be genetically related, and is not dose related. In more than half the cases, it is irreversible. It may lead to aplastic anaemia which may be fatal. The reported incidence of aplastic anaemia varies throughout the world.

Hypoplastic anaemia, thrombocytopenia and agranulocytosis have also been described following administration of chloramphenicol.

Gastro-intestinal reactions: Nausea, vomiting, glossitis and stomatitis, diarrhoea and enterocolitis may occur; incidence is low.

Neurological reactions: Optic and peripheral neuritis have been reported usually following long-term dosage.

Hypersensitivity reactions: Sensitivity reactions are sometimes encountered.

Gray syndrome: Toxic reactions including fatalities have occurred in the premature and newborn infant; the signs and symptoms associated with these reactions are known as the 'gray syndrome'. Single reports have appeared in an infant as old as three months, and in an infant born of a mother receiving chloramphenicol intravenously during labour. The following points summarise the studies of the 'gray syndrome'.

1. In most instances therapy has been instituted within the first 48 hours of life.
2. Symptoms first appeared after 3 to 4 days of continued treatment with conventional adult dosage of chloramphenicol not tolerated by and incorrect for this age group.
3. The symptoms appeared in the following order.
 (a) Abdominal distension with or without vomiting.
 (b) Progressive pallid cyanosis.

(c) Vasomotor collapse, frequently accompanied by irregular respiration.
 (d) Death within a few hours of onset of symptoms.
4. Progression of symptoms from onset to exitus was accelerated with higher dosage schedules.
5. In some cases upon early recognition of the associated symptomatology, termination of therapy frequently reversed the process with complete recovery.

Treatment of overdosage: If more than 120 ml suspension or 12 capsules are swallowed, the stomach should be emptied and any symptoms treated accordingly.

Pharmaceutical precautions Store at a temperature not exceeding 30°C; protect from light.

Chloromycetin Palmitate Suspension: Suitable diluent Syrup BP. When diluted use within 14 days of preparation.

Legal category POM.

Package quantities Chloromycetin Capsules 250 mg: Available in packs of 100 capsules.

Chloromycetin Palmitate Suspension: Available in packs of 100 ml.

Further information Nil.

Product licence numbers

Chloromycetin Capsules 250 mg	0018/5097
Chloromycetin Palmitate Suspension	0018/5076.

CHLOROMYCETIN* EAR DROPS

Presentation Pale yellow viscous ear drops.

Composition: Each ml contains: Chloramphenicol PhEur 100 mg in Propylene Glycol PhEur.

Action: Chloramphenicol is a broad spectrum antibiotic. It is primarily bacteriostatic and acts by inhibition of protein synthesis by interfering with the transfer of activated amino-acids from soluble RNA to ribosomes. Resistance to chloramphenicol is slow to develop; moderate in degree and not necessarily permanent.

Uses Treatment of ear infections including chronic otorrhoea, suppurative otitis media and infections of fenestration and mastoid operation cavities.

Dosage and administration
Topical: Adults: Apply the solution on a piece of wick and leave in the site for up to 48 hours, or instil as drops two or three times daily.

Elderly (over 65 years): As for adults.

Children and infants: All age groups – as for adults.

Contra-indications, warnings, etc Hypersensitivity to chloramphenicol.

Aplastic anaemia has been reported following topical use of chloramphenicol. Whilst the hazard is a rare one, it should be borne in mind when assessing the benefits expected from the use of this compound.

Treatment of overdosage: None.

Pharmaceutical precautions To be protected from light. Store below 25°C.

Legal category POM.

Package quantities Bottles of 5 ml.

Further information Nil.

Product licence number 0018/5048.

CHLOROMYCETIN*
HYDROCORTISONE OPHTHALMIC
OINTMENT

Presentation Chloromycetin Hydrocortisone Ophthalmic Ointment 1%.
White translucent sterile ointment.

Composition
Chloromycetin Hydrocortisone Ophthalmic Ointment 1% contains:
Chloramphenicol PhEur   1%
Hydrocortisone Acetate PhEur   0.5%

Action: Chloromycetin (chloramphenicol PhEur) has a wide range of antibacterial activity and is effective against virtually all bacterial pathogens known to cause diseases of the eye. It penetrates the non-inflamed eye better than any other antibiotic regardless of the mode of administration and resistance is slow to develop, moderate in degree and not necessarily permanent.

Indications Ocular inflammation due to allergy when this is coexistent with a bacterial infection sensitive to chloramphenicol.

Dosage and administration Topical to the eye.
Adults: The frequency of administration of the ointment depends on the type and severity of the disease and varies from every hour to once or twice a day. Treatment should not be stopped abruptly.
Elderly (over 65 years): As for adults.
Children and infants: All age groups: as for adults.

Contra-indications, warnings, etc Chloromycetin Hydrocortisone Ophthalmic Ointment should not be administered to patients hypersensitive to chloramphenicol. The prolonged use of antibiotics may occasionally result in overgrowth of non-susceptible organisms including fungi. If any new infection appears during treatment the antibiotic should be discontinued and appropriate measures taken. Chloramphenicol should be reserved for use only in infections for which it is specifically indicated. Aplastic anaemia has been reported following topical use of chloramphenicol. Whilst the hazard is a rare one, it should be borne in mind when assessing the benefits expected from the use of this compound.

In treating bacterial diseases of the eye it is considered that the use of steroids is dangerous unless the organism is already under antibiotic control, for although the external appearance improves, the progress of the disease may be concealed.

Pharmaceutical precautions Store at a temperature not exceeding 30°C.

Legal category POM.

Package quantities Available in 4 g Tube.

Further information Nil.

Product licence number 0018/5050R.

CHLOROMYCETIN* OPHTHALMIC
PREPARATIONS

Presentation Eye drops, eye ointment.

Composition: Chloromycetin Redidrops* (Ophthalmic) 0.5% (Chloramphenicol Eye Drops BP):

Chloromycetin Redidrops conform to the requirements of the BP 1980 for chloramphenicol eye drops containing 0.5% w/v Chloramphenicol PhEur in a sterile solution of purified water containing suitable buffering agents and 0.002% w/v phenyl mercuric acetate as a preservative.

Chloromycetin Ophthalmic Ointment (Chloramphenicol Eye Ointment BP) contains 1% chloramphenicol Ph Eur in a petrolatum base.

Action Chloromycetin (Chloramphenicol Ph Eur) has a wide range of antibacterial activity and is effective against virtually all bacterial pathogens known to cause diseases of the eye. It penetrates the non-inflamed eye better than any other antibiotic regardless of the mode of administration, and resistance to it is slow to develop, moderate in degree and not necessarily permanent. Clinical studies have shown that preparations of Chloromycetin for local treatment of ocular conditions are well tolerated.

Indications Treatment of bacterial conjunctivitis caused by the organisms *Escherichia coli, Haemophilus influenzae, Staphylococcus aureus, Streptococcus haemolyticus,* Morax-Axenfeld and others.

Dosage and administration The recommended dosage for adults, children and infants of all age groups is 2 drops, or a small amount of ointment to be applied to the affected eye every three hours or more frequently if required: treatment should be continued for at least 48 hours after the eye appears normal.

Elderly (over 65 years): As for adults.
Chloromycetin has been used successfully at normal dosage in elderly patients. The pattern and incidence of adverse effects does not appear to differ from younger adults.

Contra-indications, warnings, etc Chloromycetin Ophthalmic Preparations should not be administered to patients hypersensitive to chloramphenicol.

In severe infections the topical use of chloramphenicol should be supplemented by appropriate systemic treatment. The prolonged use of antibiotics may occasionally result in overgrowth of non-susceptible organisms, including fungi. If any new infection appears during treatment the antibiotic should be discontinued and appropriate measures taken. Chloramphenicol should be reserved for use only in infections for which it is specifically indicated.

Aplastic anaemia has been reported following topical use of chloramphenicol. Whilst the hazard is a rare one, it should be borne in mind when assessing the benefits expected from the use of this compound.

Treatment of overdosage: Not applicable.

Pharmaceutical precautions *Chloromycetin Redidrops:* Store between 2 and 8°C. Protect from light. Contents must be used within four weeks of being dispensed.

Chloromycetin Ophthalmic Ointment 1%: Store at a temperature not exceeding 30°C. Use within one month of opening.

Legal category POM.

Package quantities *Chloromycetin Redidrops:* 5 ml and 10 ml in polythene dropper bottle.
Chloromycetin Ophthalmic Ointment 1%: Tube of 4 g.

Further information Nil

Product licence numbers
Chloromycetin Redidrops   0018/0065R
Chloromycetin Ophthalmic Ointment 1% 0018/5074R

CHLOROMYCETIN* SUCCINATE

Presentation A plug of freeze-dried sterile powder which when reconstituted with Water for Injection makes a clear solution for injection.

Composition: Each 1.2 g vial contains: Chloramphenicol Sodium Succinate BP equivalent to Chloramphenicol PhEur 1.2 g.

Each 300 mg vial contains: Chloramphenicol Sodium Succinate BP equivalent to Chloramphenicol PhEur 300 mg.

Action: Chloramphenicol sodium succinate when administered intravenously is hydrolysed to the free antibiotic within the body. Part of the parenterally administered chloramphenicol sodium succinate is excreted by the kidneys prior to hydrolysis and although serum levels of free chloramphenicol are lower than when a comparable dose of chloramphenicol is given orally, they are clinically effective.

Chloramphenicol exerts mainly a bacteriostatic effect on a wide range of gram-negative and gram-positive bacteria and is also active against rickettsial organisms and the lymphogranuloma-psittacosis group. It is particularly active against *Salmonella typhi* and *Haemophilus influenzae*. The mode of action is through interference with or inhibition of protein synthesis in intact cells. Development of resistance to chloramphenicol both experimentally and in man, appears to be low in contrast to other antibiotics. The principal route of excretion of chloramphenicol is through the kidneys, total urinary excretion ranging from 68 to over 90 per cent. Small amounts of active drug are found in the bile and faeces. Chloramphenicol diffuses rapidly throughout the tissues and body fluids. Chloramphenicol enters cerebrospinal fluid even in the absence of meningeal inflammation. Measurable levels are also detectable in pleural and ascitic fluids, saliva, and in milk. It diffuses readily into the aqueous and vitreous humours of the eye. Transport across the placental barrier occurs with somewhat lower concentration in cord blood than in maternal blood.

Uses Chloramphenicol is a potent therapeutic agent and should not be used for trivial infections. It should be administered according to the instructions of a medical practitioner. It is recommended that chloramphenicol should be reserved for use in typhoid fever, H. influenzae meningitis, serious chest infections and situations where clinical assessment usually supplemented by laboratory studies indicates that no other antibiotic would suffice.

Dosage and administration

Adults and children over 2 weeks old: The conventional dosage of chloramphenicol of 50 mg/kg of bodyweight per day in divided doses at six-hour intervals is recommended for the average patient. In exceptional cases, such as with patients having infections due to moderately resistant organisms or suffering from infections such as septicaemia or meningitis, dosage schedules up to 100 mg/kg/day may be prescribed. However, these high dosages should be decreased as soon as clinically indicated. To prevent relapses treatment should be continued after the temperature has returned to normal for 4 days in rickettsial diseases and for 8–10 days in typhoid fever. Chloramphenicol in the form of chloramphenicol succinate should be administered intravenously in seriously ill patients or under conditions in which the patient is not able to take the drug by mouth. In such instances, it is highly desirable that the physician change over to orally administered chloramphenicol as soon as is practicable. In instances of impaired hepatic or renal function, the ability to metabolise or excrete chloramphenicol may be reduced and the medical practitioner should adjust the dose accordingly.

Elderly (over 65 years): As for adults.

Chloramphenicol has been used successfully at normal dosage in elderly patients. The pattern and incidence of adverse effects does not appear to differ from younger adults.

Premature and newborn infants and children with immature metabolic processes: (see Gray syndrome under Adverse reactions).

25 mg/kg/day divided into four doses at six-hour intervals usually produces and maintains a concentration of chloramphenicol in blood and tissues adequate to control most infections in premature and newborn infants and children with immature metabolic processes. After the first two weeks of life, full term infants ordinarily may receive up to a total of 50 mg/kg/day equally divided into four doses at six hour intervals. Precise control of serum chloramphenicol levels should be achieved through analytical methods, wherever this is feasible.

For administration to young children, infants, and neonates in particular, the Chloromycetin Succinate 300 mg vial is recommended for preparation of the solution. The Chloromycetin Succinate 1.2 g vial is more suitable for preparation of the solution for older children and adults. See above for actual dosage to be given.

Method of preparation.

Chloromycetin 300 mg vial: Prepare a solution of 25 mg/ml (2.5%) by the addition of 11.75 ml of aqueous diluent. This solution should be injected intravenously over at least a one minute period, the amount administered depending on the bodyweight of the patient.

Chloromycetin 1.2 g vial: Prepare a solution of 100 mg/ml (10%) by the addition of 11 ml of aqueous diluent. This solution should be injected intravenously over at least a one minute period, the amount administered depending on the bodyweight of the patient.

Further information is contained in the package insert, which should be consulted before preparation and administration.

Contra-indications, warnings, etc Chloramphenicol succinate is contra-indicated in persons with a history of previous hypersensitivity and/or toxic reaction to the drug.

Blood dyscrasias including aplastic anaemia may be associated with the administration of chloramphenicol succinate. If facilities are available, it is well to determine the routine blood profile before therapy, and blood studies should be repeated at appropriate intervals especially during prolonged or intermittent therapy.

The intervals at which such studies should be performed depends on the circumstances of each individual case. Consideration should be given to discontinuing the drug if evidence of depression of any of the blood elements appear attributable to chloramphenicol, weighing these effects against the seriousness and course of the disease under treatment. Repeated courses of chloramphenicol succinate and concurrent therapy with other drugs known to cause bone marrow depression or even aplastic anaemia should be avoided. Chloramphenicol succinate should be administered according to the direction of a medical practitioner, and it should not be used for the treatment of trivial infections. Excessive blood levels, as with other antibiotics, may result from administration of the recommended dose to patients with impaired liver or kidney function, including those due to immature metabolic processes in the premature and full-term infant. Chloramphenicol succinate should not be administered intravenously during labour. The medical practitioner should also remember that chloramphenicol is excreted in the milk of the lactating mother. Therefore mothers taking this drug should not breast-feed their infants. Chloramphenicol should not be used during pregnancy unless considered essential by the physician.

As with other antibiotics, the use of chloramphenicol succinate may result in an overgrowth of non-susceptible organisms including fungi.

Chloramphenicol succinate is not alone in the phenomenon of drug interaction and when patients are concurrently receiving anti-coagulants or anti-convulsants, dosage adjustment of these agents may be necessary. The half-life of chloramphenicol is considerably prolonged in patients receiving paracetamol (acetaminophen). Concurrent administration of these drugs should be avoided.

Adverse reactions:
Haematological reactions: Blood dyscrasias including aplastic anaemia have been attributed to the administration of chloramphenicol. Two types of bone marrow depression have been observed. One type may occur during therapy, is reversible on cessation of treatment, and is dose related.

The second type which may occur weeks to months after therapy is rare; it may be genetically related and is not dose related. In more than half of the cases, it is irreversible. It may lead to aplastic anaemia which may be fatal. The reported incidence of aplastic anaemia varies throughout the world.

Hypoplastic anaemia, thrombocytopenia and agranulocytosis have also been described following the administration of chloramphenicol.

Gastro-intestinal reactions: Nausea, vomiting, glossitis and stomatitis, diarrhoea and enterocolitis may occur; incidence is low.

Neurological reactions: Optic and peripheral neuritis have been reported usually following long-term dosage.

Hypersensitivity reactions: Sensitivity reactions are sometimes encountered.

Gray syndrome: Toxic reactions including fatalities have occurred in the premature and newborn infant; the signs and symptoms associated with these reactions are known as the 'gray syndrome'. Single reports have appeared in an infant as old as three months, and in an infant born of a mother receiving chloramphenicol intravenously during labour. The following points summarise the studies of the 'gray syndrome'.

1. In most instances therapy has been instituted within the first 48 hours of life.

2. Symptoms first appeared after 3 to 4 days of continued treatment with conventional adult dosage of chloramphenicol not tolerated by and incorrect for this age group.

3. The symptoms appeared in the following order.
   (a) Abdominal distension with or without vomiting.
   (b) Progressive pallid cyanosis.
   (c) Vasomotor collapse, frequently accompanied by irregular respiration.
   (d) Death within a few hours of onset of symptoms.

4. Progression of symptoms from onset to exitus was accelerated with higher dosage schedules.

5. In some cases upon early recognition of the

associated symptomatology, termination of therapy frequently reversed the process with complete recovery.

Treatment of overdose: There is no known antidote. General supportive therapy to prevent cardiovascular collapse.

Pharmaceutical precautions Protect from light.
Store at a temperature not exceeding 30°C.

To reduce the risk of microbial and particulate contamination the reconstituted solution should be used on one occasion only, immediately after preparation.

Legal category POM.

Further information 300 mg vial: prepare a solution of 25 mg/ml (2.5%) by the addition of 11.75 ml of aqueous diluent. This solution should be injected intravenously over at least a one minute period, the amount administered depending on the bodyweight of the patient. 1.2 g vial: prepare a solution of 100 mg/ml (10%) by the addition of 11 ml of aqueous diluent. This solution should be injected intravenously over at least a one minute period, the amount administered depending on the bodyweight of the patient.

Further information is contained in the package insert, which should be consulted before preparation and administration.

Chloramphenicol sodium succinate is generally compatible with infusion fluids when the pH range is 5.5 to 7.0. For further information contact the manufacturer.

Package quantities Vials of 1.2 mg and 300 mg.

Product licence numbers
Chloromycetin Succinate 1.2 g   0018/5078
Chloromycetin Succinate 300 mg   0018/5077

CHOLEDYL*

Presentation Coated pink, bi-convex tablets with a debossed 'Choledyl 100' on one side, containing 100 mg Choline Theophyllinate BP.

Coated yellow, bi-convex tablets with a debossed 'Choledyl 200' on one side, containing 200 mg Choline Theophyllinate BP.

An amber-coloured, chocolate-flavoured, clear syrup. Each 5 ml spoonful contains Choline Theophyllinate BP 62.5 mg.

Uses For the relief and prophylaxis of bronchospasm in chronic bronchitis and asthma.

Dosage and administration *Tablets:* Oral administration.

Adults: 400–1,600 mg daily in divided doses. The usual adult dose is 100–400 mg four times daily.

Elderly (over 65 years): As for adults. Theophylline clearance tends to decrease slightly with age and elderly patients will, therefore, tend to have higher serum theophylline levels. They should, therefore, be monitored closely for signs of toxicity during dosage adjustment.

Children (over 6 years): 3–4 × 100 mg tablets daily in divided doses. The 200 mg tablet should not be administered to children.

Syrup: Oral administration.

Children: (3-6 years): One to two 5 ml spoonfuls three times daily.

Contra-indications, warnings, etc
Contra-indications: Use in patients with a known

hypersensitivity to the xanthine group of drugs. An initial dose of 5 mg/kg may be increased slowly over three-day periods until an optimum clinical response is achieved. The peak serum theophylline level should not reach values greater than 20 mcg/ml. Use in children at more than six-hourly intervals.

Precautions and warnings: Caution should be exercised in its use in patients with cardiac disease. Care should be taken in its use in patients suffering from insomnia and in its concomitant use with β-adrenergic agonists, glucagon and the other xanthine drugs as these will potentiate the effect of theophylline. The incidence of toxic effects may be enhanced by the concomitant use of ephedrine. There is no evidence of safety of this drug in human pregnancy but it has been in wide use for many years without apparent ill consequences; animal studies have shown no hazard. Choledyl syrup contains invert sugar syrup (3.7 ml/5 ml) and due care should be taken where it is prescribed for patients with diabetes mellitus.

Side-effects: Gastro-intestinal upsets, palpitations and CNS stimulation may occur occasionally.

Overdosage: Characterised by nausea, vomiting, gastro-intestinal irritation, unusual thirst, CNS stimulation including convulsions in severe cases, tachycardia, arrhythmias, fall in BP and collapse.

Treatment: Gastric lavage. For fall in blood pressure, nurse in head-down position and treat with fluid replacement if necessary. Use general supportive measures and treat symptoms accordingly. Diazepam i.v. may be given to control convulsions. Charcoal haemoperfusion can be considered in severely intoxicated patients.

Pharmaceutical precautions Choledyl Syrup should be stored in a dry place at a temperature not exceeding 25°C, and protected from light.

Legal category P.

Package quantities *Tablets 100 mg:* Bottles containing 100 and 500 tablets.
Tablets 200 mg: Bottles containing 100 and 500 tablets.
Choledyl Syrup: Bottles containing 200 ml and 1 litre.

Further information Nil.

Product licence numbers
Tablets 100 mg   0019/0049
Tablets 200 mg   0019/0050
Syrup   0019/0048

COSYLAN*

Presentation An amber coloured peach flavoured syrup.

Composition: Each 5 ml contains: Dextromethorphan Hydrobromide PhEur 13.5 mg.

Action: Clinical trials in patients with acute and chronic cough have demonstrated dextromethorphan to have a significant cough suppressant action.

Uses For the treatment of a persistent dry irritating cough.

Dosage and administration
Oral: Adults; 5 ml three or four times daily.

Elderly (over 65 years): As for adults.

Children:
6 to 12 years: 2.5 ml three or four times daily.
1 to 5 years: 1.25 ml three or four times daily.

Contra-indications, warnings, etc Known hypersensitivity to the active constituent. Use with caution in patients with hepatic dysfunction.

Dextromethorphan hydrobromide occasionally causes drowsiness, dizziness and gastro-intestinal upsets.

Treatment of overdosage: Gastric lavage and general supportive measures should be used.

Pharmaceutical precautions Store below 30°C in a dry place.

Suitable diluent: Syrup BP. Use within 14 days of preparation.

Legal category P.

Package quantities Available in packs of 125 ml.

Further information Nil.

Product licence number 0018/0103.

EPANUTIN* CAPSULES AND SUSPENSION

Presentation Epanutin Capsules (Phenytoin Capsules BP) contain 25 mg, 50 mg or 100 mg Phenytoin Sodium Ph Eur.

Epanutin Suspension (Phenytoin Mixture BPC 1973) contains 30 mg Phenytoin BPC 1973 in 5 ml.

Epanutin Capsules 25 mg: A white powder in a No. 4 hard gelatin capsule with a white opaque body and a purple opaque cap radially imprinted Epanutin 25.

Epanutin Capsules 50 mg: A white powder in a No. 4 hard gelatin capsule with white opaque body and a pale pink opaque cap radially imprinted Epanutin 50.

Epanutin Capsules 100 mg: A white powder in a No. 3 hard gelatin capsule with a white opaque body and orange cap radially imprinted Epanutin 100.

Epanutin Suspension: Cherry-red suspension.

Action Anticonvulsant which appears to stabilise rather than raise the seizure threshold and prevent spread of seizure activity rather than abolish the primary focus of seizure discharge.

Indications Control of grand mal epilepsy, temporal lobe seizures and certain other convulsive states. Epanutin has also been employed in the treatment of migraine, trigeminal neuralgia and certain psychoses.

Dosage and administration *Epanutin Capsules:* Oral.

Adults: 100 mg two to four times daily before meals, with a maximum total of 600 mg a day.

Elderly (over 65 years): As with adults the dosage of Epanutin should be titrated carefully to the patient's individual requirements using the same guidelines.

Elderly patients as a group tend to receive multiple drug therapies and the possibility of increased risk of drug interactions should be borne in mind.

Infants and children up to 3 years: The initial dose is up to 50 mg two or three times daily.

Children 4-6 years: The dosage may be increased above the infant dose.

Children 7-12 years: As for adults.

Each dose of Epanutin should be followed by at least ½ tumblerful of water. In cases showing a tendency to nausea and a feeling of fullness of the stomach, the dose may be given with or following meals.

Epanutin Suspension: Oral.

Adults: 15 ml three times daily. Subsequent dosage should be adjusted according to the therapeutic response.

Elderly (over 65 years): As with adults the dosage of Epanutin should be titrated carefully to the patient's individual requirements using the same guidelines.

Elderly patients as a group tend to receive multiple drug therapies and the possibility of increased risk of drug interactions should be borne in mind.

Children under 6 years: 5 ml twice daily increasing to 5 ml three or four times daily.

Children 6 years and over: As for adults.

These dosages are a guide only and the generally accepted principles of anticonvulsant treatment should be carried out, i.e. Epanutin Capsules or Suspension should be introduced in small dosage with gradual increments until control is achieved (or therapeutic blood levels reached, if facilities for estimation of these exist) or until toxic effects appear. If toxic effects do appear, the dose should be decreased, and if control is not achieved, the drug should be withdrawn gradually and an alternative anticonvulsant substituted. Maintenance of treatment should be the lowest dose of anticonvulsant consistent with control of seizures.

Contra-indications, warnings, etc Hypersensitivity to hydantoins.

There is some evidence that phenytoin may produce congenital abnormalities in the offspring of a small number of epileptic patients, therefore it should not be used as the first drug in pregnancy, especially early pregnancy, unless in the judgement of the physician the potential benefits outweigh the risk. Small quantities of phenytoin are excreted in breast milk.

If the patient has been receiving other anticonvulsants, such as phenobarbitone, the sudden withdrawal of the drugs may precipitate a series of attacks before Epanutin has been given in sufficient amounts to exercise control. This may be avoided by gradually replacing with Epanutin the anticonvulsant previously used.

During initial treatment, minor side-effects may include gastric distress, nausea, transient nervousness, weight loss, sleeplessness and a feeling of unsteadiness. Side-effects usually subside with continued use. Allergic phenomena such as polyarthropathy, fever, skin eruptions and hepatitis may occur. Eruptions usually subside upon discontinuance of therapy. Lupus erythematosus and erythema multiforme have occurred. Though mild and rarely an indication for stopping dosage, gingival hypertrophy, hirsutism and excessive motor activity are occasionally encountered in the younger age groups. Haematological disorders including megaloblastic anaemia, leucopenia, agranulocytosis, thrombocytopenia, pancytopenia and aplastic anaemia have been reported. The occasional occurrence of lymphadenopathy indicates the need to differentiate such a condition from other lymph-gland pathology. Nystagmus in combination with diplopia and ataxia indicates that dosage should be reduced.

Phenytoin should be used with caution in the presence of liver dysfunction.

Certain drugs have been shown to elevate phenytoin plasma levels including antituberculous agents, dicoumarol anticoagulants, sulthiame, pheneturide, disulfiram, chloramphenicol, halothane, thyroid preparations and viloxazine. The levels of phenytoin are decreased by carbamazepine. The effect of phenytoin may be diminished by alcohol and altered by phenobarbitone. Phenytoin induced enzyme induction can enhance the metabolism of oral contraceptives and therefore may lead to a diminished contraceptive effect. Phenytoin may affect blood calcium and blood sugar metabolism and dexamethasone and metyrapone tests.

Treatment of overdosage: The mean lethal dose for adults is estimated to be 2 to 5 g. The cardinal initial symptoms are nystagmus, ataxia and dysarthria. The patient then becomes comatose, the pupils are unresponsive and hypotension occurs followed by respiratory depression and apnoea. Treatment is non-specific since there is no known antidote. First, the stomach should be emptied. If the gag reflex is absent, the airway should be supported. Oxygen, vasopressors and assisted ventilation may be necessary for central nervous system respiratory and cardiovascular depression. Total exchange transfusion has been utilised in the treatment of severe intoxication in children.

Pharmaceutical precautions *Capsules:* Store at a temperature not exceeding 30°C.

Epanutin Suspension: Store at a temperature not exceeding 25°C. Suitable diluent – Syrup BP. When diluted use within 14 days of preparation.

Legal category POM.

Package quantities Epanutin Capsules 100 mg are available in containers of 500 and 1,000.

Epanutin Capsules 50 mg and 25 mg are available in containers of 500.

Epanutin Suspension (30 mg per 5 ml) is available in bottles of 500 ml.

Further information Conventional doses of phenytoin will produce a therapeutically desirable serum level (between 10 and 20 micrograms/ml) only in a proportion of patients under treatment. Levels below 10 micrograms/ml may result in ineffective treatment, whilst it has been reported that with levels above 20 to 25 micrograms/ml toxic effects begin to appear.

The 25 mg Epanutin Capsule has been introduced because incremental doses of the drug should become progressively smaller as the serum concentration increases, since there is no linear relationship between dose and serum level – for example, an incremental dose of 50 mg may be enough to increase a serum level in a particular patient from 10 micrograms/ml to a toxic level.

Product licence numbers

Epanutin Capsules 25 mg	0018/0112
Epanutin Capsules 50 mg	0018/5079
Epanutin Capsules 100 mg	0018/5080
Epanutin Suspension	0018/5106

EPANUTIN* INFATABS*

Presentation Yellow, triangular, flat, chewable tablets with breaking line on one side and with a spearmint flavour. Each Infatab contains 50 mg Phenytoin BPC 1973.

Action Anticonvulsant which appears to stabilise rather than raise the seizure threshold and prevent spread of seizure activity rather than abolish the primary focus of seizure discharge.

Indications Control of grand mal epilepsy, temporal lobe seizures and certain other convulsant states.

Dosage and administration Oral – to be chewed.

Initially: Under 1 year: ½ tablet twice daily.

1-6 years: ½ tablet two to four times daily.

7-12 years: 1 tablet two to four times daily.

Adults: 2 tablets two to four times daily.

Elderly (over 65 years): As with adults the dosage of Epanutin should be titrated carefully to the patient's individual requirements using the same guidelines.

Elderly patients as a group tend to receive multiple drug therapies and the possibility of increased risk of drug interactions should be borne in mind.

These dosages are a guide only and the generally accepted principles of anticonvulsant treatment should be carried out, i.e. Epanutin Infatabs should be introduced in small dosage with gradual increments until control is achieved (or therapeutic blood levels reached, if facilities for estimation of these exist) or until toxic effects appear. If toxic effects do appear, the dose should be decreased, and if control is not achieved, the drug should be withdrawn gradually and an alternative anticonvulsant substituted. Maintenance of treatment should be the lowest dose of anticonvulsant consistent with control of seizures.

Equal doses of Epanutin Infatabs and Capsules may not give rise to equivalent blood levels.

Contra-indications, warnings, etc Hypersensitivity to hydantoins.

There is some evidence that phenytoin may produce congenital abnormalities in the offspring of a small number of epileptic patients, therefore it should not be used as first drug during pregnancy, especially in early pregnancy, unless in the judgement of the physician, the potential benefits outweigh the risks. Small quantities of phenytoin are excreted in breast milk.

If the patient has been receiving other anticonvulsants, the sudden withdrawal of the drugs may precipitate a series of seizures before Epanutin Infatabs have been given in sufficient amounts to exercise control. This may be avoided by gradually replacing the anticonvulsant previously used with Epanutin Infatabs. During initial treatment, minor side-effects may include gastric distress, nausea, transient nervousness, weight loss, sleeplessness and a feeling of unsteadiness. Side-effects usually subside with continued use. Allergic phenomena such as polyarthropathy, fever, skin eruptions and hepatitis may occur. Eruptions usually subside upon discontinuance of therapy. Lupus erythematosus and erythema multiforme have occurred. Though mild and rarely an indication for stopping dosage, gingival hypertrophy, hirsutism and excessive motor activity are occasionally encountered in the younger age groups. Haematological disorders including megaloblastic anaemia, leucopenia, agranulocytosis, thrombocytopenia, pancytopenia and aplastic anaemia have been reported. The occasional occurrence of lymphadenopathy indicates the need to differentiate such a condition from other lymph-gland pathology. Nystagmus in combination with diplopia and ataxia indicates that dosage should be reduced.

Phenytoin should be used with caution in the presence of liver dysfunction.

Certain drugs have been shown to elevate phenytoin plasma levels including anti-tuberculous agents, dicoumarol anticoagulants, sulthiame, pheneturide, disulfiram, chloramphenicol, halothane, thyroid preparations and viloxazine. The levels of phenytoin are decreased by carbamazepine. The effect of phenytoin may be diminished by alcohol and altered by phenobarbitone. Phenytoin induced enzyme induction can enhance the metabolism of oral contraceptives and therefore may lead to a diminished contraceptive effect. Phenytoin may affect blood calcium and blood sugar metabolism and dexamethasone and metyrapone tests.

Treatment of overdosage: The mean lethal dose for adults is estimated to be 2 to 5 g. The cardinal initial symptoms are nystagmus, ataxia and dysarthria. The patient then becomes comatose, the pupils are unresponsive and hypotension occurs followed by respiratory depression and apnoea. Treatment is non-specific since there is no known antidote. First, the stomach should be emptied. If the gag reflex is absent, the airway should be supported. Oxygen, vasopressors and assisted ventilation may be necessary for central nervous system, respiratory and cardiovascular depression. Total exchange transfusion has been utilised in the treatment of severe intoxication in children.

Pharmaceutical precautions Store at a temperature not exceeding 30°C.

Legal category POM.

Package quantities Packs of 100 tablets

Further information Nil.

Product licence number 0018/0069.

EPANUTIN* READY MIXED PARENTERAL

Presentation Epanutin Ready Mixed Parenteral (Phenytoin Injection BP) contains 250 mg Phenytoin Sodium Ph Eur in each 5 ml ampoule.

Action Anticonvulsant which appears to stabilise rather than raise the seizure threshold and prevent spread of seizure activity rather than abolish the primary focus of seizure discharge.

Indications Epanutin Ready Mixed Parenteral is indicated for the control of status epilepticus and other persistent convulsive disorders; for the prophylactic control of seizures in neurosurgery. It is of use in the treatment of certain cardiac arrhythmias, especially when these are digitalis induced.

Dosage and administration *Use in status epilepticus: Adults:* By slow intravenous injection, at a rate not exceeding 50 mg per minute, 150–250 mg, followed if necessary, after 30 minutes, by 100–150 mg. Where it is impossible to immobilise an extremity, or veins are inaccessible, the intramuscular route may be used initially. Great care should be taken to avoid the risk of breaking the injection needle.

Elderly (over 65 years): As for adults. However, complications may occur more readily in elderly patients.

Children: Dosage is usually determined according to weight, in proportion to the dosage for a 150 lb (70 kg) adult.

Use in neurosurgery: 2–4 ml (100–200 mg) intramuscularly three to four times daily during the period encompassing surgery and the post-operative phase.

Use in cardiac arrhythmias: 3.5–5 mg per kg of body weight intravenously initially, repeated once if necessary. The solution should be injected slowly intravenously and at a uniform rate which should not exceed 1 ml (50 mg) per minute.

Contra-indications, warnings, etc Hypersensitivity

to hydantoins. Heart block. Intra-arterial administration must be avoided in view of the high pH of the preparation.

Fatalities due to cardiac arrest, ventricular fibrillation, tonic seizures and respiratory arrest have been reported following intravenous administration of phenytoin in cases with cardiac arrhythmias. Alterations of cardiac and respiratory function can be produced by too rapid administration of the drug intravenously. Complications may occur more readily in elderly and gravely ill patients. In all cases optimal dosage of Epanutin Ready Mixed Parenteral must be determined by trial. Dosage in excess of the minimum required to prevent convulsions is not recommended. Subcutaneous or perivascular injection should be avoided because of the highly alkaline nature of the solution, which may cause local tissue damage. Solutions of Epanutin Ready Mixed Parenteral should not be added to intravenous solutions because of the precipitation of the free acid.

There is some evidence that phenytoin may produce congenital abnormalities in the offspring of a small number of epileptic patients, therefore it should not be used as first drug during pregnancy, especially early pregnancy, unless in the judgement of the physician the potential benefits outweigh the risks. Small quantities of phenytoin are excreted in breast milk.

Caution: The use of Epanutin by the intravenous route should be considered an emergency procedure. Continuous electrocardiographic monitoring is recommended. As with the administration of any potent cardiac antiarrhythmic drug, cardiac resuscitative equipment should be available.

Treatment of overdosage: The mean lethal dose in adults is estimated to be 2–5 g. The cardinal initial symptoms are nystagmus, ataxia and dysarthria. The patient then becomes comatose, pupils unresponsive and hypotension occurs followed by respiratory depression and apnoea. Treatment is non-specific since there is no known antidote. If the gag reflex is absent, the airway should be supported. Oxygen, vasopressors and assisted ventilation may be necessary for central nervous system, respiratory and cardiovascular depression. Total exchange transfusion has been utilised in the treatment of severe intoxication in children.

Pharmaceutical precautions Store at a temperature not exceeding 25°C. Protect from light. The product should not be used if a precipitate or haziness develops in the solution in the ampoule. Epanutin Ready Mixed Parenteral should not be added to intravenous infusion fluids because of precipitation of the acid.

Legal category POM.

Package quantities 10 × 5 ml ampoules.

Further information Nil.

Product licence number 0018/0070.

ERYMAX* ▼

Presentation Capsules containing 250 mg Erythromycin PhEur; orange and white enteric coated pellets in a size 0 capsule with an opaque orange cap and a colourless body.

Uses Erythromycin is an antibiotic effective in the treatment of bacterial disease caused by susceptible organisms.

Examples of its use are in the treatment of upper and lower respiratory tract infections of mild to moderate severity; skin and soft tissue infections including pustular acne. Erythromycin is usually active against the following organisms *in vitro* and in clinical infection: *Streptococcus pyogenes;* Alpha haemolytic streptococci; *Staphylococcus aureus; Streptococcus pneumoniae; Mycoplasma pneumoniae; Treponema pallidum; Corynebacterium diphtheriae; Corynebacterium minutissimum; Entamoeba histolytica; Listeria monocytogenes; Neisseria gonorrhoeae; Bordetella pertussis; Legionella pneumophila.*

Dosage and administration Oral.

Adults: 250 mg every six hours – before or with meals. 500 mg every twelve hours may be given if desired; b.i.d. dosage should not be used if dosage exceeds one gram.

Elderly (over 65 years): As for adults.

Children: 30–50 mg/kg/day in divided doses given every six hours or twice daily. For the treatment of more severe infections, this dose may be doubled; elevated doses should be given every six hours. The drug should be given before or with meals. This product may be given to children of any age group who can swallow the intact capsules.

Streptococcal infections

For active infection – a full therapeutic dose is given for at least ten days.

For continuous prophylaxis against recurrences of streptococcal infections in patients with evidence of rheumatic fever heart disease, the dose is 250 mg b.i.d.

For the prevention of bacterial endocarditis in patients with valvular disease scheduled for dental or surgical procedures of the upper respiratory tract, adult dose is 1.0 gram (children 20 mg/kg) 2 hours before surgery. Following surgery, 500 mg for adults (children 10 mg/kg) orally every six hours for 8 doses.

Primary syphilis: 30–40 grams given in divided doses over a period of 10–15 days.

Intestinal amoebiasis: 250 mg four times daily for 10 to 14 days for adults: 30 to 50 mg/kg/day in divided doses for 10 to 14 days for children.

Legionnaires' disease: 1–4 g daily until clinical signs and symptoms indicate a clinical cure. Treatment may be prolonged.

Pertussis: 30–50 mg/kg/day given in divided doses for 5–14 days, depending upon eradication of a positive culture.

Use in pregnancy: Like all drugs, erythromycin should be used in pregnancy only when clearly indicated.

Nursing mothers: Erythromycin is excreted in human milk.

Contra-indications, warnings, etc

Contra-indications: Erymax is contra-indicated in patients with known hypersensitivity to erythromycin.

Precautions: In patients with impaired hepatic function, liver function should be monitored, since a few reports of hepatic dysfunction have been received in patients taking erythromycin as the estolate, base or stearate.

Prolonged use of erythromycin has caused overgrowth of nonsusceptible bacteria or fungi; this is a rare occurrence.

In a few patients receiving high doses of theophylline, concomitant use of erythromycin has caused increase of serum theophylline levels and signs of toxicity.

Serious allergic reaction, including anaphylaxis, has been reported.

Side effects: Rarely, hypersensitivity and superinfections. Nausea and abdominal discomfort can occur at elevated doses; diarrhoea and vomiting are less common.

Overdosage: Nausea, vomiting and diarrhoea have been reported.

Treatment: Gastric lavage and general supportive therapy.

Pharmaceutical precautions Store below 25°C. Protect from moisture and light.

Legal category POM.

Package quantities Securitainers containing 100 capsules.

Further information Nil.

Product licence number 0018/0133.

ESTROVIS*

Presentation Pink-coloured, bi-convex tablets having one side debossed with 'W' monogram, the other side debossed 'Estrovis 4'. Each tablet contains Quinestrol 4.0 mg.

Uses Quinestrol is a synthetic oestrogen which is stored to a considerable extent in body fat.

Estrovis is indicated both for the inhibition of lactation and the suppression of established lactation.

Dosage and administration *Adults:* Oral administration.

Inhibition: 1 tablet given within six hours of delivery. Symptoms of lactation may occasionally develop on the fourth to sixth day and should be treated expectantly. Only if these symptoms persist and prove troublesome should a second tablet of Estrovis be necessary.

Suppression: 1 tablet to be given immediately the decision to suppress lactation has been made, followed by a second tablet 48 hours later. In many cases one tablet only will suffice to suppress an already failing lactation.

When 2 tablets are given it is advisable to inform the patient that she may experience a heavier than normal period when her menses resume.

Contra-indications, warnings, etc

Contra-indications: Use in patients with a history of, or existent thromboembolic disorders, or with breast or genital cancer (known or suspected to be oestrogen dependent). Use in patients with existing thrombophlebitis or cerebrovascular disease or cardiovascular disease. Use in patients with undiagnosed, irregular vaginal bleeding. Use in pregnancy or suspected pregnancy and in patients with impaired liver function or with active liver disease.

Warnings and precautions: Use in patients suffering from epilepsy, or a history of migraine, asthma or cardiac dysfunction, may result in exacerbation of these disorders because of fluid retention. A decreased glucose tolerance may occur in diabetic patients on this treatment and their control must be carefully supervised. It is important that oestrogens or oestrogen/progestogen combinations should be used at the lowest possible dosage and for the shortest time period compatible with the requisite response.

Side-effects: Clinical studies have indicated an extremely low incidence of side-effects due to Estrovis: very rarely, nausea and vomiting have been reported.

Overdosage: Acute overdosage is seldom attended by any symptoms though there may be nausea and vomiting. Treatment is rarely required except symptomatically.

Pharmaceutical precautions Store in a cool dry place, not exceeding 25°C.

Legal category POM.

Package quantities Estrovis Tablets are supplied in packs of 2 or 20 designed so that the tablets may be dispensed one or two at a time.

Further information Nil.

Product licence number 0019/5009.

GELUSIL* SUSPENSION

Presentation A viscous white suspension, each 5 ml containing:

Magnesium Trisilicate Ph Eur	620 mg
Dried Aluminium Hydroxide Gel BP	310 mg

Uses Gelusil Suspension is a liquid antacid indicated for the relief of hyperacidity, indigestion and heartburn when occurring alone or in association with peptic ulcer.

Dosage and administration Oral

Adults: One to four 5 ml spoonfuls of the liquid to be administered with water after meals or whenever symptoms arise.

Elderly (over 65 years): As for adults. No clinical or pharmacokinetic data specific to this age group is available. However, at normal dosage no problems have been reported.

Children (6–12 years): Half the adult dose.

Contra-indications, warnings, etc

Contra-indications: None known.

Warnings: None applicable.

Precautions: Prolonged or intensive therapy in patients with severe renal insufficiency may lead to hypermagnesaemia.

Antacids are known to interfere with the absorption of certain drugs including cimetidine, mexiletine, chlorpromazine, diflunisal, ketaconazole, penicillamine, pivampicillin and the tetracyclines.

Side-effects: None is observed at the therapeutic dosage.

Overdosage: Symptoms are unlikely and treatment is rarely required.

Pharmaceutical precautions Store at a temperature not exceeding 25°C.

Legal category GSL.

Package quantities Plastic bottle containing 500 ml.

Further information Nil.

Product licence number 0019/5012.

GELUSIL* TABLETS

Presentation A white bevel-edge tablet marked GELUSIL on one side containing:

Magnesium Trisilicate Ph Eur	500 mg
Dried Aluminium Hydroxide Gel BP	250 mg

Uses Gelusil is an antacid indicated for the relief of gastric hyperacidity, indigestion and heartburn when occurring alone or in association with peptic ulcer.

Dosage and administration Oral.

Adults: One or two tablets to be chewed or sucked after meals or whenever symptoms arise.

Elderly (over 65 years): As for adults. No clinical or pharmacokinetic data specific to this age group is available. However, at normal dosage no problems have been reported.

Children (6–12 years): Half the adult dose or as directed by the physician.

Contra-indications, warnings, etc
Contra-indications: None known.

Warnings: None applicable.

Precautions: Prolonged or intensive therapy in patients with severe renal insufficiency may lead to hypermagnesaemia.

Antacids are known to interfere with the absorption of certain drugs including cimetidine, mexiletine, chlorpromazine, diflunisal, ketaconazole, penicillamine, pivampicillin and the tetracyclines.

Gelusil tablets contain 561 mg sugar per tablet and due care should be taken when they are prescribed for patients with diabetes mellitus.

Side-effects: None is observed at the therapeutic dosage.

Overdosage: Symptoms are unlikely and treatment is rarely required.

Pharmaceutical precautions No special precautions.

Legal category GSL.

Package quantities Gelusil Tablets are packed in bottles containing 250 and 500 tablets and in foil-wrapped tubes of 20 and 50.

Further information Nil.

Product licence number 0019/5011R.

KETALAR*

Presentation Parenteral general anaesthetic.

Ketalar: (ketamine hydrochloride) dl 2-(o-chlorophenyl)-2-(methylamino) cyclohexanone hydrochloride, is a white crystalline solid, soluble in water to 20% clear and colourless solution.

The base component is 86.7% of the salt. It is supplied as a slightly acid (pH 3.5–5.5) solution for intravenous or intramuscular injection in concentrations containing the equivalent of either 10, 50 or 100 mg ketamine base per ml. The latter two concentrations contain 1:10,000 Phemeride* (benzethonium chloride) as a preservative. The 10 mg per ml solution has been made isotonic with sodium chloride.

Uses Ketalar *is recommended:*

1. As the sole anaesthetic agent for diagnostic and surgical procedures. Although best suited for short procedures, Ketalar can be used, with additional doses, for longer procedures. If skeletal muscle relaxation is desired, a muscle relaxant should be used and respiration should be supported.

2. For the induction of anaesthesia prior to the administration of other general anaesthetic agents.

3. To supplement other anaesthetic agents.

Specific areas of application or types of procedures:

1. When the intramuscular route of administration is preferred.

2. Debridement, painful dressings, and skin grafting in burned patients, as well as other superficial surgical procedures.

3. Neurodiagnostic procedures such as pneumoencephalograms, ventriculograms, myelograms, and lumbar punctures.

4. Diagnostic and operative procedures of the eye, ear, nose, and mouth, including dental extractions.

Note: Eye movements may persist during ophthalmological procedures.

5. Anaesthesia in poor-risk patients with depression of vital functions or where depression of vital functions must be avoided, if at all possible.

6. Orthopaedic procedures such as closed reductions, manipulations, femoral pinning, amputations, and biopsies.

7. Sigmoidoscopy and minor surgery of the anus and rectum, circumcision and pilonidal sinus.

8. Cardiac catheterization procedures.

9. Caesarian section; as an induction agent in the absence of elevated blood pressure.

10. Anaesthesia in the asthmatic patient, either to minimise the risks of an attack of bronchospasm developing, or in the presence of bronchospasm where anaesthesia cannot be delayed.

Dosage and administration

Adults, elderly (over 65 years) and children: For surgery in elderly patients ketamine has been shown to be suitable either alone or supplemented with other anaesthetic agents.

Preoperative preparations:

1. Ketalar has been safely used alone when the stomach was not empty.

However, since the need for supplemental agents and muscle relaxants cannot be predicted, when preparing for elective surgery it is advisable that nothing be given by mouth for at least six hours prior to anaesthesia.

2. Atropine, scopolamine, or another drying agent should be given at an appropriate interval prior to induction.

3. The use of droperidol (0.1 mg/kg IM) as premedication has been effective in reducing the incidence of emergence reactions.

Onset and duration: As with other general anaesthetic agents, the individual response to Ketalar is somewhat varied depending on the dose, route of administration, age of patient, and concomitant use of other agents, so that dosage recommendation cannot be absolutely fixed. The dose should be titrated against the patient's requirements.

Because of rapid induction following intravenous injection, the patient should be in a supported position during administration. An intravenous dose of 2 mg/kg (1 mg/lb) of body-weight usually produces surgical anaesthesia within 30 seconds after injection and the anaesthetic effect usually lasts 5 to 10 minutes. An intramuscular dose of 10 mg/kg (5 mg/lb) of body-weight usually produces surgical anaesthesia within 3 to 4 minutes following injection and the anaesthetic effect usually lasts 12 to 25 minutes. Return to consciousness is gradual.

A. Ketalar as the sole anaesthetic agent:

Induction:

Intravenous route: The initial dose of Ketalar administered intravenously may range from 1 mg/kg to 4.5 mg/kg

(0.5 to 2 mg/lb). † The average amount required to produce 5 to 10 minutes of surgical anaesthesia has been 2.0 mg/kg (1 mg/lb.) It is recommended that intravenous administration be accomplished slowly (over a period of 60 seconds). More rapid administration may result in respiratory depression.

Intramuscular route: The initial dose of Ketalar administered intramuscularly may range from 6.5 to 13 mg/kg (3 to 6 mg/lb.) † A low initial intramuscular dose of 4 mg/kg (2 mg/lb) has been used in diagnostic manoeuvres and procedures not involving intensely painful stimuli. A dose of 10 mg/kg (5 mg/lb) will usually produce 12 to 25 minutes of surgical anaesthesia.

Maintenance of anaesthesia: Lightening of anaesthesia may be indicated by nystagmus, movements in response to stimulation, and vocalization. Anaesthesia is maintained by the administration of additional doses of Ketalar by either the intravenous or intramuscular route.

Each additional dose is from ½ to the full induction dose recommended above for the route selected for maintenance, regardless of the route used for induction.

The larger the total amount of Ketalar administered, the longer will be the time to complete recovery.

Purposeless and tonic-clonic movements of extremities may occur during the course of anaesthesia. These movements do not imply a light plane and are not indicative of the need for additional doses of the anaesthetic.

B. Ketalar as induction agent prior to the use of other general anaesthetics: Induction is accomplished by a full intravenous or intramuscular dose of Ketalar as defined above. If Ketalar has been administered intravenously and the principal anaesthetic is slow-acting, a second dose of Ketalar may be required 5 to 8 minutes following the initial dose. If Ketalar has been administered intramuscularly and the principal anaesthestic is rapid-acting, administration of the principal anaesthetic may be delayed up to 15 minutes following the injection of Ketalar.

C. Ketalar as supplement to anaesthetic agents: Ketalar is clinically compatible with the commonly used general and local anaesthetic agents when an adequate respiratory exchange is maintained. The dose of Ketalar for use in conjunction with other anaesthetic agents is usually in the same range as the dosage stated above; however, the use of another anaesthetic agent may allow a reduction in the dose of Ketalar.

Management of patients in recovery: Following the procedure the patient should be observed but left undisturbed. This does not preclude the monitoring of vital signs. If, during the recovery, the patient shows any indication of emergence delirium, consideration may be given to the use of one of the following agents: diazepam (5 to 10 mg IV in an adult) or droperidol (2.5 to 7.5 mg IV or IM). A hypnotic dose of a thiobarbiturate (50 to 100 mg IV) may be used to terminate severe emergence reactions. If any one of these agents is employed, the patient may experience a longer recovery period.

Contra-indications, warnings, etc

Contra-indications: Ketalar is contra-indicated in persons in whom an elevation of blood pressure would constitute a serious hazard (see Adverse Reactions section). Ketalar should not be used in patients with eclampsia or pre-eclampsia.

† *In terms of ketamine base.*

Precautions:

1. To be used only in hospitals by or under the supervision of experienced medically qualified anaesthetists except under emergency conditions.

2. As with any general anaesthetic agent, resuscitative equipment should be available and ready for use.

3. Barbiturates and Ketalar, being chemically incompatible because of precipitate formation, should not be injected from the same syringe.

4. Prolonged recovery time may occur if barbiturates and/or narcotics are used concurrently with Ketalar.

5. Emergence delirium phenomena may occur during the recovery period.

The incidence of these reactions may be reduced if verbal and tactile stimulation of the patient is minimised during the recovery period. This does not preclude the monitoring of vital signs.

6. Because pharyngeal and laryngeal reflexes usually remain active, mechanical stimulation of the pharynx should be avoided unless muscle relaxants, with proper attention to respiration, are used.

7. Although aspiration of contrast medium has been reported during Ketalar anaesthesia under experimental conditions (Taylor, P. A., and Towey, R. M., *Brit. med. J.* 1971, **2**: 688) in clinical practice aspiration is seldom a problem.

8. Cardiac function should be continually monitored during the procedure in patients found to have hypertension or cardiac decompensation.

9. Since an increase in cerebrospinal fluid pressure has been reported during Ketalar anaesthesia, Ketalar should be used with special caution in patients with preanaesthetic elevated cerebrospinal fluid pressure.

10. Respiratory depression may occur with overdosage of Ketalar, in which case supportive ventilation should be employed. Mechanical support of respiration is preferred to the administration of analeptics.

11. The intravenous dose should be administered over a period of 60 seconds. More rapid administration may result in transient respiratory depression or apnoea.

12. In surgical procedures involving visceral pain pathways, Ketalar should be supplemented with an agent which obtunds visceral pain.

13. Use with caution in the chronic alcoholic and the acutely alcohol-intoxicated patient.

14. When Ketalar is used on an outpatient basis, the patient should not be released until recovery from anaesthesia is complete and then should be accompanied by a responsible adult.

Adverse reactions:

Cardiovascular: Temporary elevation of blood pressure and pulse rate is frequently observed following administration of ketamine hydrochloride. However, hypotension and bradycardia have been reported. Arrhythmia has also occurred. The medium peak rise of blood pressure has ranged from 20 to 25 per cent of preanaesthetic values. Depending on the condition of the patient, this elevation of blood pressure may be considered an adverse reaction or a beneficial effect.

Respiratory: Depression of respiration or apnoea may occur following too rapid intravenous administration or high doses of ketamine hydrochloride. Laryngospasm and other forms of airway obstruction have occurred during ketamine hydrochloride anaesthesia.

Ocular: Diplopia and nystagmus may occur following ketamine hydrochloride administration. A slight elevation in intraocular pressure may also occur.

Psychological: During recovery from anaesthesia the patient may experience emergence delirium, characterised by vivid dreams (pleasant or unpleasant), with or without psychomotor activity, manifested by confusion and irrational behaviour. The fact that these reactions are observed less often in the young (15 years of age or less) makes Ketalar especially useful in paediatric anaesthesia. These reactions are also less frequent in the elderly (over 65 years of age) patient. The incidence of emergence reactions is reduced as experience with the drug is gained. No residual psychological effects are known to have resulted from the use of Ketalar.

Neurological: In some patients, enhanced skeletal muscle tone may be manifested by tonic and clonic movements sometimes resembling seizures. These movements do not imply a light plane of anaesthesia and are not indicative of a need for additional doses of the anaesthetic.

Gastro-intestinal: Anorexia, nausea, and vomiting have been observed, however, these are minimal and are not usually severe. The great majority of patients are able to take liquids by mouth shortly after regaining consciousness.

Other: Local pain and exanthema at the injection site have infrequently been reported. Transient erythema and/or morbilliform rash have also been reported. Increased salivation leading to respiratory difficulties may occur unless an antisialogogue is used.

Symptoms and treatment of overdosage: Respiratory depression can result from an overdosage of ketamine hydrochloride. Supportive ventilation should be employed. Mechanical support of respiration that will maintain adequate blood oxygen saturation and carbon dioxide elimination is preferred to administration of analeptics.

Ketalar has a wide margin of safety; several instances of unintentional administration of overdoses of Ketalar (up to 10 times that usually required) have been followed by prolonged but complete recovery.

Pharmaceutical precautions Barbiturates and Ketalar, being chemically incompatible because of precipitation formation, should not be injected from the same syringe. Protect from light. Store at a temperature not exceeding 30°C.

Legal category POM.
Ketamine hydrochloride is to be used only in hospitals by or under the supervision of experienced medically qualified anaesthetists.

Package quantities Vials of 20 ml containing 10 mg ketamine base per ml.
Vials of 10 ml containing 50 mg ketamine base per ml.
Vials of 5 ml containing 100 mg ketamine base per ml.

Further information Nil.

Product licence numbers
Ketalar 10 mg per ml   0018/5117
Ketalar 50 mg per ml   0018/5118
Ketalar 100 mg per ml   0018/0015

LENTIZOL*

Presentation Capsules containing 50 mg Amitriptyline Hydrochloride BP – white pellets in a size 2 capsule with a pink body and a red cap radially marked 'LENTIZOL 50'.

Capsules containing 25 mg Amitriptyline Hydrochloride BP – white pellets in a size 3 all-pink capsule radially marked 'LENTIZOL 25'.

The pellets are prepared in a special sustained-release presentation which allows the active constituent to be released over a period of up to 12 hours.

Uses Symptoms of depressive illness especially where sedation is required.

Dosage and administration Oral administration:
Adults and adolescents over 16 years old: Initially 50-100 mg as a single dose at night, increasing to 200 mg/day according to clinical response. Maintenance dose 50-100 mg at night.

Elderly (over 65 years): 25-75 mg a day initially. The initial dose should be increased with caution under close supervision. Half the normal maintenance dose may be sufficient to produce a satisfactory clinical response.

The elderly are particularly liable to experience adverse reactions especially agitation, confusion and postural hypotension.

Children (under 16 years): Not recommended.

Use in pregnancy: Do not use during pregnancy, especially during the first and last trimesters, unless there are compelling reasons. There is no, or inadequate, evidence of safety of the drug in human pregnancy; although it has been in wide use for many years without apparent ill-consequence. There is evidence of harmful effects in pregnancy in animals, when given in exceptionally high doses.

Contra-indications, warnings, etc
Contra-indications: Recent cardiac infarction and patients with any degree of heart block or disorders of cardiac rhythm, and those suffering from coronary artery insufficiency. Patients with mania, severe liver disease, or known hypersensitivity to dibenzazepines. Lentizol should not be given to mothers during breast feeding.

Precautions: Unless essential it is inadvisable to combine Lentizol with ECT.

Avoid if possible in patients with narrow angle glaucoma, symptoms suggestive of prostatic hypertrophy and a history of epilepsy. Lentizol should be used with caution in hyperthyroid patients.

Patients posing a high suicidal risk require close initial supervision.

Tricyclic anti-depressants potentiate the central nervous depressant action of alcohol.

Anaesthetics given during tri/tetracyclic anti-depressant therapy may increase the risk of arrhythmias and hypotension. If surgery is necessary, the anaesthetist should be informed that a patient is being so treated.

Drug interactions: Lentizol should not be administered concurrently or within 14 days of termination of treatment with MAO inhibitors. It should not be given with directly acting sympathomimetic agents such as adrenaline, ephedrine, isoprenaline, noradrenaline, phenylephrine, and phenylpropanolamine, and should be used with caution when administered concurrently with anticholinergic drugs.

Lentizol may counteract the effect of adrenergic neurone blocking agents, and possibly clonidine, and therefore it would be advisable to review all antihypertensive therapy during treatment.

The action of Lentizol may be decreased by barbiturates, and potentiated by methyl phenidate.

Warnings: As improvement may not occur during the

first 2 4 weeks of treatment, patients should be closely monitored during this period.

Amitriptyline may initially impair alertness. Patients should be warned of the possible hazard when driving or operating machinery.

Cardiac arrhythmias and severe hypotension are likely to occur with high dosage or in deliberate overdosage. They may also occur in patients with pre-existing heart disease taking normal dosage.

Adverse effects: The following adverse effects, although not necessarily all reported with amitriptyline, have occurred with other tricyclic anti-depressants.

Amitriptyline may produce excessive perspiration and has some anticholinergic activity which may cause dryness of mouth, blurred vision, constipation, tachycardia and urinary retention. These symptoms are common but usually lessen on continuing therapy.

Other common adverse effects include postural hypotension, tremor and skin rashes. Interference with sexual function, nausea, anorexia and dizziness may also occur. Drowsiness may occur in some patients but this can usually be controlled by reducing the dose. If necessary the dose may subsequently be gradually increased.

Serious adverse effects are rare; those reported include:

depression of the bone marrow, including agranulocytosis, cholestatic jaundice, hypomania, convulsions and peripheral neuropathy, paralytic ileus.

Psychotic manifestations, including mania and paranoid delusions, may be exacerbated during treatment with tricyclic anti-depressants.

Withdrawal symptoms may occur on abrupt cessation of therapy and include insomnia, irritability and excessive perspiration.

Adverse effects such as withdrawal symptoms, respiratory depression and agitation have been reported in neonates whose mothers had taken amitriptyline during the last trimester of pregnancy.

Overdosage: Amitriptyline exerts an anticholinergic effect as well as antihistamine and adrenaline blocking actions. Large doses produce convulsions, coma, apnoea and cardiac irregularities, with intestinal stasis.

Treatment: Gastric lavage and emesis if appropriate. Vital signs should be continuously monitored and patients should be treated in ICUs wherever possible. General supportive measures with careful attention to electrolyte balance. Cardiac irregularities may need controlling with antiarrhythmic drugs and physostigmine salicylate is also indicated. Forced diuresis and haemodialysis have no place in treatment.

Pharmaceutical precautions Store in a dry place at a temperature not exceeding 25°C.

Legal category POM.

Package quantities *50 mg:* Bottles containing 50 and 250 capsules.
25 mg: Bottles containing 50 and 250 capsules.

Further information Nil.

Product licence numbers
50 mg   0019/5046
25 mg   0019/5045

LOESTRIN*

Presentation Loestrin 20: A pale blue-grey film-coated tablet. Each tablet contains Norethisterone Acetate BP 1 mg and Ethinyloestradiol PhEur 0.02 mg. Loestrin 30: A green film-coated tablet. Each tablet contains Norethisterone acetate BP 1.5 mg and Ethinyloestradiol PhEur 0.03 mg.

Action Loestrin achieves contraceptive effect primarily by inhibition of ovulation through gonadotrophin suppression. It is possible that other sites of action such as changes in cervical mucus and in the endometrium may contribute to the efficacy of combined oral contraceptives.

Indications Control of conception.

Dosage and administration *Oral:* One Loestrin 20 tablet or one Loestrin 30 tablet should be taken daily for three weeks, starting on the fifth day of menstrual bleeding, and then an interval of one week allowed before commencing the second course of tablets. In the first cycle only, it is advisable to use another method of contraception for the first 14 days in addition to taking the tablets. Second and subsequent courses should be taken for three weeks with one week without tablets between courses. Thus each new course of tablets is always started on the same day of the week. It is important that the tablets are taken as directed. Tablets should be taken without regard to menstrual bleeding except in the initial cycle.

If a tablet is not taken at the usual time, it must be taken within the next 12 hours. If the delay exceeds 12 hours the course should be continued by taking the tablets in the pack at their proper times and leaving the missed tablet(s). Additional contraceptive methods should be used until the next withdrawal bleed.

Vomiting and/or diarrhoea may reduce the effectiveness of the pill. If this occurs extra contraceptive measures should be taken for the rest of the cycle.

It has been suggested that certain drugs may produce increased metabolism of oral contraceptive steroids. Patients receiving additional drugs, including phenobarbitone, phenytoin and some antibiotics, might be advised to use non-hormonal additional methods of contraception for the rest of the cycle.

Post-partum: Oral contraception is usually started as soon as spontaneous menstruation has resumed after childbirth. However, oral contraception can be started within 7–12 days of a vaginal delivery, provided that the patient is ambulant and there are no puerperal complications. If medication is started within 12 days of delivery, additional contraceptive precautions are unnecessary. After a first trimester abortion, oral contraceptives can normally be started immediately.

Children: None.

Contra-indications, warnings, etc
Contra-indications: Thromboembolic disorders, or a past history of these conditions; sickle cell anaemia; known or suspected disorders of lipid metabolism; markedly impaired liver function; known or suspected carcinoma of the breast; known or suspected oestrogen dependent neoplasms; undiagnosed abnormal vaginal bleeding. Loestrin should not be given during pregnancy, or to patients with a history of severe pruritus during pregnancy or of herpes of pregnancy. Loestrin should not be given to patients with a history of otosclerosis, idiopathic

jaundice; Dubin-Johnson or Rotor syndromes or any significant liver disease.

Warnings: The use of oral contraceptives has been shown to be associated with an increased risk of thromboembolic disorders. The physician should be alert to the earliest manifestations of these disorders, (thrombophlebitis, cerebrovascular disorders, pulmonary embolism, and retinal thrombosis). Should any of these occur or be suspected, Loestrin should be discontinued immediately.

Certain factors may predispose to the development of thrombosis, e.g. smoking, obesity, age, the presence of varicose veins, cardiovascular disease, diabetes and migraine. The suitability of combined oral contraceptives for patients with any of these conditions should be discussed with the patient before a final decision is taken.

The risk of arterial thrombosis associated with combined oral contraceptives increases with age, and the risk is aggravated by cigarette smoking. The use of combined oral contraceptives by women in the older age group, especially those who are cigarette smokers, should therefore be discouraged, and alternative methods advised.

Very rarely, hepatic tumours have been reported in users of combined oral contraceptives, generally for a protracted period of time. A hepatic tumour should be considered in the differential diagnosis when upper abdominal pain, enlarged liver or signs of intra-abdominal haemorrhage occur.

Medication should be discontinued pending examination if there is a sudden onset of proptosis, diplopia or migraine.

Patients with a history of depression should be carefully observed and the drug discontinued if the depression recurs to a serious degree.

Since the safety of Loestrin in pregnancy has not been demonstrated, it is recommended that for any patient who has missed a period, the absence of pregnancy should be established before continuing the contraceptive regimen.

Combined oral contraceptives should be stopped at least six weeks before elective surgery and during immobilisation, e.g. after accidents etc.

Loestrin should be discontinued if the patient becomes jaundiced or has a significant rise in blood pressure.

Precautions: The pre-treatment and periodic physical examination should include special reference to breast and pelvic organs, including Papanicolaou smear since oestrogens have been known to produce tumours, some of them malignant in five species of subprimate animals.

Oestrogen-progestogen preparations should be used with caution in patients with a history of hypertension. Some women experience an increase in blood pressure following administration of contraceptive steroids. Pregnancy should be excluded before starting treatment.

Because these agents may cause some degree of fluid retention, patients with conditions which might be influenced by this such as epilepsy, migraine, asthma and cardiac or renal dysfunction, should be carefully observed.

A decrease in glucose tolerance has been observed in a significant percentage of patients on oral contraceptives. The mechanism of this decrease is obscure. For this reason, diabetic patients should be carefully observed while receiving Loestrin.

Under the influence of oestrogen-progestogen prep-

arations, pre-existing uterine fibroleiomyatoma may increase in size.

The following conditions also require careful consideration: multiple sclerosis, porphyria, tetany, disturbed liver function, gallstones, cardiovascular disease, renal disease, chloasma, the wearing of contact lenses or any disease that is prone to worsen during pregnancy. The deterioration or first appearance of any of these conditions may indicate that the oral contraceptive should be stopped.

Loestrin may mask the onset of the climacteric.

The following laboratory results may be altered by the use of oral contraceptives: hepatic function (increased sulphobromophthalein retention and other tests); thyroid function (thyroid-binding globulin, T3, T4 serum levels); haematological tests (increase in prothrombin factors VII, VIII, IX, and X; decreased antithrombin; increased adrenalin-induced platelet aggregation); measurement of pregnanediol excretion (reduced). Therefore, if such tests are abnormal in a patient taking Loestrin, it is recommended that they be repeated after Loestrin has been withdrawn for two months.

The pathologist should be advised of the administration of Loestrin when relevant specimens are submitted.

Any possible influence of prolonged administration of Loestrin on pituitary, ovarian, adrenal, hepatic and uterine functions is unknown at present.

A small fraction of the hormonal agents in oral contraceptives have been identified in the milk of mothers receiving these drugs. The long range effect to the nursing infant is at present unknown.

Adverse effects: The following adverse effects which have been reported in patients receiving oral contraceptives are believed to be drug-related.

Nausea, vomiting, gastro-intestinal symptoms (such as abdominal cramps and bloating), breakthrough bleeding, spotting, change in menstrual flow, amenorrhoea during and after treatment, oedema, chloasma or melasma, breast changes (tenderness, enlargement and secretion), change in weight, cervical erosion and changes in cervical secretion, suppression of lactation when given immediately post-partum, cholestatic jaundice, migraine, rash (allergic), rise in blood pressure, depression, and thromboembolic disorders.

Although the following adverse effects have been reported in women taking oral contraceptives, an association has been neither confirmed nor refuted: prolonged amenorrhoea after discontinuing oral contraceptives, pre-menstrual like syndrome, headache, nervousness, dizziness, fatigue, cataract, backache, hirsutism, loss of scalp hair, erythema multiforme, erythema nodosum, haemorrhagic eruption and itching.

In most women the menstrual flow is reduced and occasionally may be missed altogether. This reduced flow is not normally indicative of pregnancy, particularly if the tablets have been taken correctly, but pregnancy should be ruled out before a new course of tablets is started.

Breakthrough bleeding happens more often in the first two or three cycles after starting the tablets. The patient should continue taking the tablets according to the schedule if breakthrough bleeding occurs. Probably it will amount to no more than spotting and will not last more than a day or two. If breakthrough bleeding is experienced after the third cycle, the patient should consult her physician.

Treatment of overdosage: The usual effects in children

are nausea, and drowsiness. Slight vaginal bleeding occasionally occurs in girls. In view of the low toxicity following overdosage with oral contraceptives, it is suggested that treatment should be conservative.

Pharmaceutical precautions Store below 30°C in a dry place.

Legal category POM.

Package quantities Available in packs of 21 tablets.

Further information Nil.

Product licence numbers
Loestrin 20: 0018/0086
Loestrin 30: 0018/0087

MUCOLEX* ▼

Presentation *Mucolex Syrup:* Clear reddish syrup with a raspberry-menthol flavour containing carbocisteine 250 mg/5ml.
Mucolex Tablets: Round, convex orange tablet, each tablet containing 375 mg carbocisteine.

Uses Mucolytic agent for use in disorders of the respiratory tract in which an increase in the amount or viscosity of mucus is a prominent feature.

Dosage and administration Oral administration.
Mucolex Syrup: Adults: Three 5 ml spoonfuls three times a day initially; after a satisfactory response, this may be reduced to two 5 ml spoonfuls three times daily.
Elderly (over 65 years): As for adults. No clinical or pharmacokinetic data specific to this age group is available. However, at normal dosage no problems have been reported.
Children: (6–12 years): One 5 ml spoonful three times a day.
(2–5 years): 5–10 ml daily in divided doses.
Not recommended for children under 2 years.

Mucolex Tablets: Adults: Two tablets three times daily initially, after a satisfactory response, this may be reduced to one tablet four times daily.
Elderly (over 65 years): As for adults. No clinical or pharmacokinetic data specific to this age group is available. However, at normal dosage no problems have been reported.
Children: Not recommended.

Contra-indications, warnings, etc Carbocisteine is contra-indicated in cases of peptic ulcer, and is not recommended during the first trimester of pregnancy. Side-effects of carbocisteine are rare. The most common are gastro-intestinal disorders and nausea which usually subside with the lowering of dosage or discontinuation of treatment.
Treatment of overdosage: Gastric lavage and supportive therapy.

Pharmaceutical precautions Protect from light. Recommended diluent: Syrup BP. When diluted use within 14 days of preparation.

Legal category POM.

Package quantities
Mucolex Syrup is contained in 250 ml glass bottles.
Mucolex Tablets are available in containers of 100.

Further information Nil.

Product licence numbers
Mucolex Syrup   0019/0066
Mucolex Tablets 0019/0069

NARDIL*

Presentation Orange, film-coated tablets each containing 15 mg phenelzine (as the sulphate BP).

Uses Phenelzine is a monoamine oxidase inhibitor. Nardil is indicated as follows:
Symptoms of depressive illness, especially where phobic symptoms are present or where treatment with other anti-depressants has failed.

Dosage and administration Oral.
Adults: One 15 mg tablet three times a day. A response is usually seen within the first week. If no response is evident after two weeks, the dosage may be increased to a maximum of one 15 mg tablet four times a day. Doses of up to two 15 mg tablets three times a day may be used in hospitals. The effectiveness of the drug may not become apparent in less than four weeks' therapy. After a satisfactory response has been achieved, the dosage may be reduced very gradually to a suitable maintenance level. This may be as low as one 15 mg tablet every other day.
Elderly (over 65 years): As for adults.
Postural hypotension may be an unwanted effect of MAOIs in the elderly. Elderly patients as a group tend to receive multiple drug therapies and the possibility of increased risk of drug interactions should be borne in mind. Nardil should only be used with great caution in elderly patients. Despite these problems, MAOIs (including Nardil) have been found to be useful in the treatment of depression in the elderly.
Children: Nardil is not indicated for children.

Contra-indications, warnings, etc
Contra-indications: Nardil should not be given where there is any history of hepatic damage or insufficiency. Toxic hepatitis due to Nardil, as well as other monoamine oxidase inhibitors, has been reported. Incidence is low, occurring no more than once in every 37,500 courses of treatment with Nardil. Contra-indicated in cerebrovascular disease. In general tricyclic anti-depressants, e.g. clomipramine, imipramine, desipramine, butriptyline, nortriptyline, protriptyline, should not be given with, or within 14 days of treatment with MAOI therapy, although it is recognised that there is some division of consultant opinion on this matter.
Nardil tablets contain gluten and are therefore contra-indicated in coeliac disease or gluten enteropathy.

Use in pregnancy: Do not use during pregnancy, especially during the first and last trimesters, unless there are compelling reasons. There is no evidence as to drug safety in human pregnancy nor is there evidence from animal work that it is free from hazard.

Precautions: Nardil may potentiate the action of pethidine, morphine, adrenaline, amphetamines and other sympathomimetic amines such as fenfluramine, ephedrine, phenylpropanolamine, dopamine and levodopa. Many patients on Nardil react quite normally to therapeutic doses of pethidine or morphine. However, if it is necessary to administer either of these drugs to a patient on Nardil, a trial dose of one-tenth to one-fifth of the normal dose should be given initially. If this is without adverse effect the dosage may be built up to the normal over a further period of two to three hours. Nardil may also potentiate the effects of anti-hypertensives, hypo-glycaemic agents, sympathomimetics, anti-parkinson drugs, local anaesthetics and CNS depressants including barbiturates.

Nardil should be withdrawn two weeks before elective surgery/dentistry.

Patients under treatment with Nardil should avoid cheese, cooked or plain, and foods containing a high proportion of degraded protein – Oxo, Bovril, Marmite, etc – during treatment, and up to 14 days after ceasing treatment. Flavoured textured vegetable protein, hung game, pickled herrings or broad bean pods may also present a hazard. Patients should severely restrict their alcohol intake and heavy red wines, particularly Chianti, should be avoided completely. Patients should be warned against self-medication, particularly cold cures. Where a reaction between Nardil and certain foodstuffs occurs the intensity of the reaction is usually related to the tyramine content of the food. The reaction is now well recognised and serious hypertensive episodes are ex-tremely rare. Should such a reaction occur, the hyperten-sion should promptly be controlled by slow administration of phentolamine 5–10 mg i.v., repeated if necessary. Care should be taken in administering Nardil with trimipramine or amitriptyline.

Nardil should only be used with great caution in elderly or agitated patients, or those who have cardiovascular disease, epilepsy, blood dyscrasias, phaeochromocy-toma or patients with liver toxicity, or diabetes; patients taking diuretics. Nardil may also potentiate the effects of alcohol.

Warnings and adverse effects: Minor side-effects are: dizziness, drowsiness, weakness and fatigue, oedema and gastro-intestinal disturbances (nausea, vomiting, dryness of the mouth, constipation), insomnia, blurred vision, adverse effects on driving ability and postural hypotension. Less common side-effects are: headache, nervousness, euphoria, paraesthesia, sweating, in-creased appetite and weight, rash, difficulty in micturi-tion, muscle tremor, peripheral neuritis, behavioural changes, arrhythmias, convulsions, impotence and de-layed ejaculation, purpura and blood dyscrasias.

Overdosage: Large doses may produce hypomania, euphoria, followed by coma with hypotension, or acute hypertension with sometimes sub-arachnoid haemor-rhage. In a few cases, extra-pyramidal symptoms have been recorded.

Treatment: Gastric lavage (tablets dissolve slowly in stomach). Absolute bed rest: raise feet in hypotension. Vasopressors are best avoided. Hypertension should be urgently controlled with phentolamine i.v. Avoid hyp-notics, such as morphine, pethidine, barbiturates. Use phenothiazine derivates (chlorpromazine) to control restlessness and intravenous therapy to maintain fluid and electrolyte balance. In deep coma and severe hypotension hydrocortisone by injection may be tried. There is no specific antidote for Nardil.

Pharmaceutical precautions Store in a dry place at a temperature not exceeding 25°C.

Legal category POM.

Package quantity Bottles of 100 tablets.

Further information Nil.

Product licence number 0019/5018R.

OPILON* AMPOULES

Presentation Ampoules containing a sterile, colourless aqueous solution, free from turbidity and foreign parti-cles. Each 1 ml Opilon Ampoule contains:

Thymoxamine hydrochloride BP (Moxisylyte Hydro-chloride INN) equivalent to thymoxamine base 5.00 mg.

Each 2 ml Opilon Forte Ampoule contains:

Thymoxamine hydrochloride BP (Moxisylyte Hydro-chloride INN) equivalent to thymoxamine base 30.00 mg.

Uses All conditions characterised by peripheral ischae-mia responsive to alpha adrenergic blockade.

Intravenously, as a continuous drip, to relieve vaso-spasm and pain during surgery for acute and chronic arterial disease.

Intra-arterially, to counteract vasospasm in recon-structive surgery and before withdrawal of a needle or catheter.

As an intra-arterial perfusion for treatment of rest pain and incipient gangrene.

Dosage and administration *Adults:* Parenteral ad-ministration.

1. As a single dose of 0.1 mg/kg body weight i.v. This dose may be given four times a day.

2. As a single dose of 0.1 mg/kg body weight i.v. which may be followed by oral therapy.

3. As a continuous i.v. drip using 30 mg in 500 ml normal saline every six hours.

4. As an intra-arterial perfusion for treatment of rest pain and incipient gangrene. It is not recommended that this technique be carried out prior to consultation with the Product Licence Holder.

5. As a single dose of 5 mg into the distal end of an artery following arterial surgery or before withdrawal of a cardiac catheter.

Elderly (over 65 years): As for adults. No clinical or pharmacokinetic data specific to this age group is available. However, at normal dosage no problems have been reported.

Children: No dose recommended.

Contra-indications, warnings, etc

Contra-indications: Hypersensitivity to any of the ingre-dients.

Warnings: The alpha adrenergic blocking action of Opilon may potentiate the effect of a number of drugs used in the management of hypertension. In practice, with the recommended dosage of Opilon, difficulties have not been reported.

Precautions: Opilon should be used with caution in diabetes as, theoretically, insulin requirements may be reduced. Tricyclic antidepressants may increase any hypotensive effect produced by α-blockade. Opilon should also be used with caution in patients with anginal symptoms and in subjects who have had a recent coronary infarction.

The safety of Opilon for use during pregnancy and lactation has not been established.

Side-effects: Occasionally mild nausea, diarrhoea, ver-tigo, headache, and facial flushing may be encountered. These are, however, rare and transient.

Overdosage: In excessive overdosage, a fall in blood pressure is the main symptom. Nurse in head-down position and give an i.v. infusion of noradrenaline until the blood pressure has been restored to normal.

Pharmaceutical precautions Store at a temperature of 2 to 8°C. Do not freeze. Protect from light.

Legal category POM.

Package quantities Opilon and Opilon Forte Ampoules are supplied in boxes of 10.

Further information Nil.

Product licence numbers
Opilon Ampoules　　　0019/5019
Opilon Forte Ampoules　　0019/5020

OPILON* TABLETS

Presentation Pale yellow, bi-convex tablets approximately 11 mm in diameter debossed 'Opilon' on one side and a bisecting score on the other. Each tablet contains:

Thymoxamine hydrochloride BP
(Moxisylyte Hydrochloride INN)
equivalent to thymoxamine base　　40.00 mg

Uses Thymoxamine is an alpha adrenergic blocking agent. Opilon is indicated in all conditions characterised by peripheral ischaemia responsive to alpha adrenergic blockade, in particular those due to vasospasm such as Raynaud's phenomenon, chilblains, acrocyanosis, erythrocyanosis, excessively cold hands and feet and labyrinthine ischaemia (Ménière's syndrome).

Dosage and administration Oral.
Adults: One tablet to be swallowed four times a day. For those conditions affected by climatic environment 1 tablet should be administered every three hours during the 12-hour period when symptoms are most likely to occur.
Elderly (over 65 years): As for adults. No clinical or pharmacokinetic data specific to this age group is available. However, at normal dosage no problems have been reported.
Children: Opilon is not indicated for use in children.

Contra-indications, warnings, etc
Contra-indications: Hypersensitivity to any of the ingredients.
Warnings: The alpha adrenergic blocking action of Opilon may potentiate the effect of a number of drugs used in the management of hypertension. In practice, with the recommended dosage of Opilon, difficulties have not been reported.
Precautions: Opilon should be used with caution in diabetes as, theoretically, insulin requirements may be reduced. Tricyclic antidepressants may increase any hypotensive effect produced by α-blockade. Opilon should also be used with caution in patients with anginal symptoms and in subjects who have had a recent coronary infarction.
　The safety of Opilon for use during pregnancy and lactation has not been established.
Side-effects: Occasionally mild nausea, diarrhoea, vertigo, headache and facial flushing may be encountered. These are, however, rare and transient.
Overdosage: In excessive overdosage, a fall in blood pressure is the main symptom. Nurse in head-down position and give an i.v. infusion of noradrenaline until the blood pressure has been restored to normal.

Pharmaceutical precautions Store in a cool dry place at a temperature not exceeding 25°C.

Legal category POM.

Package quantities Bottles containing 50 and 250 tablets.

Further information Nil.

Product licence number 0019/5021.

ORALDENE*

Presentation A clear, red-coloured solution containing hexetidine 0.10%.

Uses Oraldene is an anti-infective agent indicated for mouth infections such as gingivitis, chronic periodontitis, stomatitis. Also of value in aphthous ulcers, dental ulcers, halitosis, pre- and post-dental surgery and oral thrush and in geriatric nursing. It is also of value as an adjuvant to systemic therapy in tonsillitis and pharyngitis.

Dosage and administration *Adults, elderly (over 65 years) and children:* Rinse the mouth or gargle with at least 15 ml of Oraldene two to three times a day. Oraldene should not be diluted.

Contra-indications, warnings, etc
Contra-indications: None known.
Warning: Oraldene is not to be taken internally.
Precautions: None applicable.
Side-effects: Very rarely, mild local irritation of the buccal tissues.
Overdosage: Hexetidine is a bactericide and fungicide. It is non-toxic in the strength used in this preparation. Acute intoxication with alcohol contained in the vehicle is unlikely even with massive doses.
Treatment: Treatment is rarely necessary.

Pharmaceutical precautions Store away from direct light at a temperature not exceeding 25°C.

Legal category GSL.

Package quantities Oraldene is supplied in clear glass bottles containing 100 ml and 200 ml.

Further information Nil.

Product licence number 0019/5022.

PENTOVIS*

Presentation Green opaque soft gelatin capsules, each containing 0.25 mg quinestradol in solution in sesame oil.

Uses Quinestradol exerts an oestrogenic effect on the lower segment of the genital tract (below the level of the external os). Pentovis is indicated in atrophic vaginitis, Kraurosis vulvae and other vulval and vaginal conditions arising in post-menopausal oestrogen deficiency states. Peri- and post-menopausal urinary incontinence. Pre- and post-operative gynaecology.

Dosage and administration Oral.
Adults: Atrophic vaginitis: 2 capsules twice daily for 2 to 3 weeks depending on the severity of the condition.
　The course may be repeated if adequate clinical response is not obtained.
　Patients awaiting plastic repair operation: 2 capsules daily for 10 to 14 days prior to operation.
　Post operatively: 2 capsules daily for 7 to 10 days as required.

Urinary incontinence: 4 to 8 capsules daily for approximately 4 weeks.

The duration of treatment should not exceed 6 months.

Elderly (over 65 years): As for adults.

Children: Pentovis is not indicated for children.

Contra-indications, warnings, etc
Contra-indications: Use in patients with a history of, or existent thrombo-embolic disorder or with breast or genital cancer (known or suspected to be oestrogen-dependent). Use in patients with impaired liver function, or with active liver disease. Use in patients with undiagnosed, irregular vaginal bleeding. Use in pregnancy or suspected pregnancy. Prolonged exposure to unopposed oestrogen may increase the risk of the development of endometrial carcinoma. Pentovis is not recommended in pre-pubertal patients.

Warnings and precautions: The use of this product in patients suffering from epilepsy, or history of migraine, asthma, or cardiac dysfunction may result in exacerbation of these disorders, because of fluid retention. A decreased glucose tolerance may occur in diabetic patients on this treatment, and their control must be carefully supervised. However, experience to date suggests a minimal problem in this regard.

The patients on such treatments should be kept under regular surveillance in view of the possibility of development of such conditions as thromboembolism, coronary insufficiency, hepatic tumours. These hazards are particularly significant in patients over the age of 35 years.

It is important that oestrogens should be used at the lowest possible dosage and for the shortest time compatible with the requisite response.

Side-effects: The side-effects commonly associated with other oestrogen fractions have not been experienced with Pentovis.

Overdosage: Acute overdose is attended only by nausea and vomiting. Treatment is rarely necessary except symptomatically.

Pharmaceutical precautions Store in a dry place, at a temperature not exceeding 25°C.

Legal category POM.

Package quantities Bottles of 30 and 250 soft gelatin capsules.

Further information Nil.

Product licence number 0019/5023.

PERITRATE*
Presentation Light green biconvex tablets containing pentaerythritol tetranitrate 10.0 mg.

Uses For prophylaxis in angina pectoris and coronary insufficiency generally and for management of post-coronary conditions.

Dosage and administration Oral.
Adults: The basic prophylactic dose is two tablets (20 mg) four times a day before meals but an additional tablet taken half-an-hour before exertion gives protection for stair climbing, walking and the daily rush to and from work.

Up to ten extra Peritrate tablets may be safely taken in 24 hours.

Elderly (over 65 years): As for adults. No clinical or pharmacokinetic data specific to this age group is available. However, at normal dosage no problems have been reported.

Children: No dose recommended.

Contra-indications, warnings, etc
Contra-indications: Sensitivity to nitrates or nitrites.

Warnings: Peritrate can act as a physiological antagonist to adrenaline, noradrenaline, acetylcholine and histamine.

Use in pregnancy: Due to the nature of the indications for Peritrate experience in pregnancy is limited. Safety in pregnancy has not been established.

Precautions: Peritrate should not be used immediately following coronary thrombosis and it should be used with caution in patients with glaucoma. Tolerance may develop.

Side-effects: Rash, headache, gastro-intestinal distress, cutaneous vasodilation and flushing, transient dizziness, and postural hypotension.

Overdosage: Peritrate is a vasodilator; possible toxic effects are headache, flushing of face, palpitations, weakness, nausea, syncope and methaemoglobinaemia.

Treatment: Bed rest with the head lowered. Give oxygen and maintain respiration. Avoid adrenaline. Methylene blue 1 or 2 mg/kg body weight may be given i.v. for methaemoglobinaemia.

Pharmaceutical precautions Store in a dry place at a temperature not exceeding 25°C. Protect from light.

Legal category P.

Package quantities Peritrate tablets are supplied in glass bottles containing 50 and 500 tablets.

Further information Nil.

Product licence number 0019/5024.

PHOLCOLIX*
Presentation An orange coloured and flavoured syrup.

Composition: Each 5 ml contains:

Paracetamol PhEur	150.00 mg
Pholcodine PhEur	5.00 mg
Phenylpropanolamine Hydrochloride BP	12.50 mg

Action: Pholcolix combines the cough suppressant action of pholcodine with the analgesic and antipyretic properties of paracetamol and the decongestant action of phenylpropanolamine.

Uses Treatment of cough associated with symptoms of the common cold.

Dosage and administration Oral.
Adults: Two 5 ml spoonfuls four times a day.

Elderly (over 65 years): As for adults.

Children: 6–12 years: One 5 ml spoonful four times a day.

2–5 years: 2.5 ml four times a day.
The product may be diluted with Syrup BP.

Contra-indications, warnings, etc Pholcolix should not be administered to persons whose sensitivity to small doses of sympathomimetic agents is manifested by sleeplessness, dizziness, light-headedness, weakness, tremors or cardiac arrhythmias.

Pholcolix is contra-indicated in hyperthyroidism, hypertension, cardiac dysfunction, diabetes mellitus and liver disorders.

Pholcolix is not to be taken during pregnancy.

Precautions: Pholcolix should not be administered to patients during, or for two weeks after, treatment with monoamine oxidase (MAO) inhibitors.

Overdosage: Drowsiness, palpitations, weakness and incoordination; delayed acute liver failure.

Treatment: Gastric lavage. If possible determine plasma paracetamol levels. Within 10 hours of ingestion give methionine orally or cysteamine i.v. Otherwise general supportive treatment should be carried out.

Pharmaceutical precautions Store at a temperature not exceeding 25°C.

Legal category CD (Sch 5), P.

Package quantities Bottles containing 1 litre.

Further information Nil.

Product licence number 0018/0123.

PITRESSIN*

Presentation A clear, sterile, colourless solution for injection.

Composition: Each ml contains: Argipressin 20 international units.

Action: Pitressin has a direct antidiuretic action on the kidney. It also constricts peripheral vessels and causes contraction of the smooth muscle of the intestine, gall bladder and urinary bladder.

Uses For use in diabetes insipidus and control of bleeding from oesophageal varices.

Dosage and administration
Adults
Diabetes insipidus: 0.25 ml to 1 ml (5 to 20 units) by subcutaneous or intramuscular injection every four hours.

Oesophageal varices: For the initial control of variceal bleeding Pitressin should be given intravenously. Pitressin, 20 units diluted in 100 ml Dextrose 5% w/v may be infused over a 15 minute period (Shields R, Brit J Hosp Med, p. 126, February 1977).

Elderly (over 65 years): As for adults. No clinical or pharmacokinetic data specific to this age group is available. However, at normal dosage no problems have been reported.

Children and infants: No dose recommended.

Contra-indications, warnings, etc Anaphylaxis or hypersensitivity to the drug or its components.

Warnings: This drug should not be used in patients with vascular disease, especially disease of the coronary arteries, except with extreme caution. In such patients, even small doses may precipitate anginal pain, and with larger doses, the possibility of myocardial infarction should be considered.

Pitressin may produce water intoxication. The early signs of drowsiness, listlessness, and headaches should be recognized to prevent terminal coma and convulsions.

Precautions: Pitressin should be used cautiously in the presence of epilepsy, migraine, asthma, heart failure, or any state in which a rapid addition to extracellular water may produce hazard for an already overburdened system.

Chronic nephritis with nitrogen retention contraindicates the use of Pitressin until reasonable nitrogen blood levels have been attained.

Adverse effects: Local or systemic allergic reactions may occur in hypersensitive individuals. The following side-effects have been reported following the administration of Pitressin: tremor, sweating, vertigo, circumoral pallor, 'pounding' in head, abdominal cramps, passage of gas, nausea, vomiting, urticaria, bronchial constriction. Anaphylaxis (cardiac arrest and/or shock) has been observed shortly after injection of Pitressin.

Treatment of overdosage: If water intoxication occurs, no fluids should be given. In severe cases, small amounts of hypertonic saline may be administered. Urea and mannitol infusions may be helpful in cases of cerebral oedema. If a patient should experience anginal pain after administration of Pitressin, amyl nitrate by inhalation, or glyceryl trinitrate sublingually, may be given.

Pharmaceutical precautions Store between 2°C and 8°C. Do not freeze.

Legal category POM.

Package quantities Available in packs of 10 × 1 ml ampoules.

Further information Nil.

Product licence number 0018/5056.

PONSTAN* Capsules
(Mefenamic Acid Capsules BP)

PONSTAN* Paediatric Suspension
(Mefenamic Acid Suspension 50 mg/5 ml)

Presentation *Capsules:* An off-white powder in a No. 1 hard gelatin capsule with an ivory opaque body and aqua-blue opaque cap, radially printed PONSTAN 250. Each capsule contains Mefenamic Acid BP 250 mg.

Paediatric Suspension: An off-white suspension, with a typical aroma and taste. Each 5 ml suspension contains Mefenamic Acid BP 50 mg.

Action Mefenamic acid is a non-steroidal anti-inflammatory agent with analgesic properties and a demonstrable antipyretic effect. It has also been shown to inhibit prostaglandin activity.

Indications 1. As an anti-inflammatory analgesic for the symptomatic relief of rheumatoid arthritis (including Still's Disease), osteoarthritis, and pain including muscular, traumatic and dental pain, headaches of most aetiology, post-operative and post-partum pain; pyrexia in children.

2. Primary dysmenorrhoea.

3. Menorrhagia due to dysfunctional causes and presence of an IUD when other pelvic pathology has been ruled out.

Dosage and administration Oral.
Adults: 2 capsules (500 mg) three times daily.

In menorrhagia to be administered on the first day of excessive bleeding and continued according to the judgement of the physician.

In dysmenorrhoea to be administered at the onset of menstrual pain and continued according to the judgement of the physician.

Elderly (over 65 years): As for adults. Whilst no pharmacokinetic or clinical studies specific to the elderly have been undertaken with Ponstan, it has been used at normal dosage in trials which included many elderly patients.

Ponstan should be used with caution in elderly patients suffering from dehydration and renal disease.

Non oliguric renal failure and proctocolitis have been reported mainly in elderly patients who have not discontinued Ponstan after the development of diarrhoea.

Children: It is recommended that children under 12 years of age should be given Ponstan Paediatric Suspension (50 mg/5 ml) in the following dosage regime.
Infants over 6 months – 25 mg/kg of body weight daily in divided doses, or
6 months–1 year – one 5 ml spoonful.
2 years–4 years – two 5 ml spoonfuls.
5 years–8 years – three 5 ml spoonfuls.
9 years–12 years – four 5 ml spoonfuls.
Dose may be repeated as necessary, up to three times daily.

Apart from the treatment of Still's Disease, therapy should not be continued for longer than seven days in children.

Contra-indications, warnings, etc Mefenamic acid is contra-indicated in inflammatory bowel disease and in patients suffering from peptic and/or intestinal ulceration, and in patients with renal or hepatic impairment.

Precautions: Safety in pregnancy has not been established. In patients suffering from dehydration and renal disease, particularly the elderly. Concurrent therapy with other plasma protein binding drugs may necessitate a modification in dosage. In the case of anticoagulants the dose of the anticoagulant may need to be reduced.

In dysmenorrhoea and menorrhagia lack of response should alert the physician to investigate other causes.

Warnings and adverse effects: Diarrhoea occasionally occurs following the use of mefenamic acid. Although this may occur soon after starting treatment, it may also occur after several months of continuous use. The diarrhoea has been investigated in some patients who have continued this drug in spite of its continued presence. These patients were found to have associated proctocolitis.

If diarrhoea does develop, the drug should be withdrawn immediately and this patient should not receive mefenamic acid again.

Skin rashes have been observed following the administration of mefenamic acid and occurrence of a rash is a definite indication to withdraw medication.

As with other prostaglandin inhibitors allergic glomerulonephritis has occurred occasionally: non-oliguric renal failure has been reported on a few occasions in elderly patients with dehydration usually from diarrhoea. It has been suggested that the recovery is more rapid and complete than with other forms of analgesic induced renal impairment.

Rarely, thrombocytopenia has been reported with mefenamic acid.

In some cases reversible haemolytic anaemia has occurred. Temporary lowering of the white blood cell count, which may have been due to mefenamic acid, has been reported. Blood studies should therefore be carried out during long-term administration.

Bronchospasm may be precipitated in patients suffering from, or with a previous history of, bronchial asthma or allergic disease. Patients on prolonged therapy should also be kept under surveillance with particular attention to liver dysfunction. Should this appear it is an indication to discontinue therapy.

Drowsiness and dizziness have rarely been reported.

Note: A positive reaction in certain tests for bile in the urine of patients receiving mefenamic acid has been demonstrated to be due to the presence of the drug and its metabolites and not to the presence of bile.

Treatment of overdosage: Gastric lavage in the conscious patient and intensive supportive therapy where necessary. Activated charcoal has been shown to be a powerful adsorbent for mefenamic acid and its metabolites. Studies in experimental animals and humans showed that a 5 to 1 ratio of charcoal to mefenamic acid resulted in considerable suppression of absorption of the drug.

Pharmaceutical precautions Store at a temperature not exceeding 30°C. Recommended diluent for Suspension – Syrup BP. When diluted use within 14 days of preparation.

Legal category POM.

Package quantities *Capsules:* Available in packs of 100 and 500.

Suspension: Available in packs of 125 ml.

Further information Nil.

Product licence numbers
Ponstan Capsules	0018/0094R
Ponstan Paediatric Suspension	0018/5025R

PONSTAN* DISPERSIBLE TABLETS

Presentation A blue, flat, bevel-edged tablet with 'Ponstan D' debossed on one side. Each tablet contains mefenamic acid BP 250 mg.

Uses
Action: Mefenamic acid is a non-steroidal anti-inflammatory agent with analgesic properties, and a demonstrable antipyretic effect. It has also been shown to inhibit prostaglandin activity.

Indications:
1. As an anti-inflammatory analgesic for the symptomatic relief of rheumatoid arthritis (including Still's Disease), osteoarthritis and pain, including muscular, traumatic and dental pain, headaches of most aetiology, post-operative and post-partum pain; pyrexia in children.
2. Primary dysmenorrhoea.
3. Menorrhagia due to dysfunctional causes and presence of an IUD when other pelvic pathology has been ruled out.

Dosage and administration Oral.

Adults: 2 tablets (500 mg) dissolved in half a tumbler of water three times daily. In menorrhagia, to be administered on the first day of excessive bleeding and continued according to the judgement of the physician. In dysmenorrhoea to be administered at the onset of menstrual pain and continued according to the judgement of the physician.

Elderly (over 65 years): As for adults.
Whilst no pharmacokinetic or clinical studies specific to the elderly have been undertaken with Ponstan, it has been used at normal dosage in trials which included many elderly patients.

Ponstan should be used with caution in elderly patients suffering from dehydration and renal disease.

Non oliguric renal failure and proctocolitis have been reported mainly in elderly patients who have not discontinued Ponstan after the development of diarrhoea.

Children: It is recommended that children under 12 years of age should be given Ponstan Paediatric Suspension.

Contra-indications, warnings, etc

Contra-indications: Mefenamic acid is contra-indicated in inflammatory bowel disease and in patients suffering from peptic and/or intestinal ulceration, and in patients with renal or hepatic impairment.

Precautions: Safety in pregnancy has not been established.

In patients suffering from dehydration and renal disease, particularly the elderly.

Concurrent therapy with other plasma protein binding drugs may necessitate a modification in dosage. In the case of anticoagulants the dose of the anticoagulant may need to be reduced.

In dysmenorrhoea and menorrhagia lack of response should alert the physician to investigate other causes.

Warnings and adverse effects: Diarrhoea occasionally occurs following the use of mefenamic acid. Although this may occur soon after starting treatment, it may also occur after several months of continuous use. The diarrhoea has been investigated in some patients who have continued this drug in spite of its continued presence; these patients were found to have associated proctocolitis.

If diarrhoea does develop, the drug should be withdrawn immediately and this patient should not receive mefenamic acid again.

Skin rashes have been observed following the administration of mefenamic acid and the occurrence of a rash is a definite indication to withdraw medication.

As with other prostaglandin inhibitors allergic glomerulonephritis has occurred occasionally: non-oliguric renal failure has been reported on a few occasions in elderly patients with dehydration usually from diarrhoea. It has been suggested that the recovery is more rapid and complete than with other forms of analgesic induced renal impairment. Rarely, thrombocytopenia has been reported with mefenamic acid. In some cases reversible haemolytic anaemia has occurred. Temporary lowering of white blood cell count, which may have been due to mefenamic acid, has been reported. Blood studies should therefore be carried out during long term administration.

Bronchospasm may be precipitated in patients suffering from, or with a previous history of, bronchial asthma or allergic disease. Patients on prolonged therapy should also be kept under surveillance with particular attention to liver dysfunction. Should this appear it is an indication to discontinue therapy.

Drowsiness and dizziness have rarely been reported.

Note: A positive reaction in certain tests for bile in the urine of patients receiving mefenamic acid has been demonstrated to be due to the presence of the drug and its metabolites and not to the presence of bile.

Treatment of overdosage: Gastric lavage in the conscious patient and intensive supportive therapy where necessary. Activated charcoal has been shown to be a powerful adsorbent for mefenamic acid and its metabolites. Studies in experimental animals and humans showed that a 5 to 1 ratio of charcoal to mefenamic acid resulted in considerable suppression of absorption of the drug.

Pharmaceutical precautions Store in a dry place at a temperature not exceeding 25°C.

Legal category POM.

Package quantities Available in packs of 100.

Further information Nil.

Product licence number 0018/0129.

PONSTAN FORTE*

Presentation Yellow film-coated ovoid tablet inscribed PONSTAN FORTE on one side.

Composition: Each tablet contains Mefenamic Acid BP 500 mg.

Action Mefenamic acid is a non-steroidal anti-inflammatory agent with analgesic properties and a demonstrable antipyretic effect. It has also been shown to inhibit prostaglandin activity.

Indications

1. As an anti-inflammatory analgesic for the symptomatic relief of rheumatoid arthritis (including Still's Disease) osteoarthritis, and pain including muscular, traumatic and dental pain, headaches of most aetiology, post-operative and post-partum pain.

2. Primary dysmenorrhoea.

3. Menorrhagia due to dysfunctional causes and presence of an IUD when other pelvic pathology has been ruled out.

Dosage and administration Oral.

Adults: 1 tablet (500 mg) three times daily.

In menorrhagia to be administered on the first day of excessive bleeding and continued according to the judgement of the physician. In dysmenorrhoea to be administered at the onset of menstrual pain and continued according to the judgement of the physician.

Elderly (over 65 years): As for adults. Whilst no pharmacokinetic or clinical studies specific to the elderly have been undertaken with Ponstan, it has been used at normal dosage in trials which included many elderly patients.

Ponstan should be used with caution in elderly patients suffering from dehydration and renal disease.

Non oliguric renal failure and proctocolitis have been reported mainly in elderly patients who have not discontinued Ponstan after the development of diarrhoea.

Children: It is recommended that children under 12 years of age should be given Ponstan Paediatric Suspension (see Ponstan data sheet).

Contra-indications, warnings, etc Mefenamic acid is contra-indicated in inflammatory bowel disease and in patients suffering from peptic and/or intestinal ulceration, and in patients with renal or hepatic impairment.

Precautions: Safety in pregnancy has not been established. In patients suffering from dehydration and renal disease, particularly the elderly. Concurrent therapy with other plasma protein binding drugs may necessitate a modification in dosage. In the case of anticoagulants the dose of the anticoagulant may need to be reduced. In dysmenorrhoea and menorrhagia, lack of response should alert the physician to investigate other causes.

Warnings and adverse effects: Diarrhoea occasionally occurs following the use of mefenamic acid. Although this may occur soon after starting treatment, it may also occur after several months of continuous use. The diarrhoea has been investigated in some patients who have continued this drug in spite of its continued presence. These patients were found to have associated proctocolitis.

If diarrhoea does develop, the drug should be withdrawn immediately and this patient should not receive mefenamic acid again.

Skin rashes have been observed following the administration of mefenamic acid and the occurrence of a rash is a definite indication to withdraw medication.

As with other prostaglandin inhibitors allergic glomerulonephritis has occurred occasionally: non-oliguric renal failure has been reported on a few occasions in elderly patients with dehydration usually from diarrhoea. It has been suggested that the recovery is more rapid and complete than with other forms of analgesic induced renal impairment.

Rarely, thrombocytopenia has been reported with mefenamic acid.

In some cases reversible haemolytic anaemia has occurred. Temporary lowering of the white blood cell count, which may have been due to mefenamic acid, has been reported. Blood studies should therefore be carried out during long-term administration.

Bronchospasm may be precipitated in patients suffering from, or with a previous history of, bronchial asthma or allergic disease.

Patients on prolonged therapy should also be kept under surveillance with particular attention to liver dysfunction. Should this appear it is an indication to discontinue therapy.

Drowsiness and dizziness have rarely been reported.

Note: A positive reaction in certain tests for bile in the urine of patients receiving mefenamic acid has been demonstrated to be due to the presence of the drug and its metabolites and not to the presence of bile.

Treatment of overdosage: Gastric lavage in the conscious patient and intensive supportive therapy where necessary. Activated charcoal has been shown to be a powerful adsorbent for mefenamic acid and its metabolites. Studies in experimental animals and humans showed that a 5 to 1 ratio of charcoal to mefenamic acid resulted in considerable suppression of absorption of the drug.

Pharmaceutical precautions Store at a temperature not exceeding 30°C.

Legal category POM.

Package quantities Available in packs of 100.

Further information Nil.

Product licence number 0018/0095R.

RINUREL* LINCTUS

Presentation Yellow-coloured linctus. Each 5 ml contains:

Paracetamol Ph Eur	150.00 mg
Phenylpropanolamine hydrochloride BP	12.50 mg
Phenyltoloxamine citrate	11.00 mg
Pholcodine Ph Eur	5.00 mg

Uses Rinurel Linctus provides analgesic, antipyretic, decongestant, antihistamine and antitussive properties.

Rinurel Linctus is indicated for symptomatic relief of unproductive cough, headache, sinus and facial pain, nasal and sinus congestion often associated with acute and chronic sinusitis, allergic and vasomotor rhinitis and upper and lower respiratory tract infections including influenza and the common cold.

Dosage and administration Oral.

Adults: Two 5 ml spoonfuls to be taken orally four times daily.

Elderly (over 65 years): As for adults.

Children (6–12 years): One 5 ml spoonful to be taken orally four times daily.

(2–5 years): 2.5 ml to be taken orally four times daily.

Contra-indications, warnings, etc

Contra-indications: Contra-indicated in persons whose sensitivity to small doses of sympathomimetic agents is manifested by sleeplessness, dizziness, light-headedness, weakness, tremors or cardiac arrhythmias.

Warnings: If drowsiness occurs, patients should not drive or operate machinery.

Alcohol or barbiturates should not be taken concomitantly.

Not to be taken during pregnancy.

Precautions: Caution should be exercised in patients with hyperthyroidism, hypertension, cardiac dysfunction, diabetes mellitus and liver disorders. Rinurel Linctus should not be used during treatment with MAO inhibitors or for two weeks after completion of therapy.

Side-effects: Drowsiness, dryness of mouth and mild stimulation have been occasionally reported.

Overdosage: Drowsiness, palpitations, weakness and inco-ordination. Later delayed acute liver failure.

Treatment: Gastric lavage. If possible check plasma paracetamol level. Within 10 hours of ingestion give methionine orally or cysteamine i.v. Otherwise take generally supportive measures.

Pharmaceutical precautions Store at a temperature not exceeding 25°C.

Legal category CD (Sch 5), P.

Package quantities Bottles containing 200 ml.

Further information Rinurel Linctus may be diluted with Syrup BP when prescribing for young children.

Product licence number 0019/5031.

RINUREL* TABLETS

Presentation Pink tablets, scored once. Each tablet contains:

Paracetamol Ph Eur	300.0 mg
Phenylpropanolamine Hydrochloride BP	25.0 mg
Phenyltoloxamine citrate	22.0 mg

Uses Rinurel Tablets provide analgesic, antipyretic, decongestant and antihistamine properties.

Rinurel Tablets are indicated for the symptomatic relief of headache, sinus and facial pain, nasal and sinus congestion often associated with acute and chronic sinusitis, allergic and vasomotor rhinitis, influenza and the common cold.

Dosage and administration Oral.

Adults: 1 tablet every four hours. Do not exceed 6 tablets in 24 hours.

Elderly (over 65 years): As for adults.

Children under 12 years: Not recommended.

Contra-indications, warnings, etc

Contra-indications: Contra-indicated in persons whose sensitivity to small doses of sympathomimetic agents is manifested by sleeplessness, dizziness, light-headedness, weakness, tremors or cardiac arrhythmias.

Warnings: If drowsiness occurs, patients should not drive or operate machinery.

Alcohol or barbiturates should not be taken concomitantly.

Not to be taken during pregnancy.

Precautions: Caution should be exercised in patients with hyperthyroidism, hypertension, cardiac dysfunction, diabetes mellitus and liver disorders. Rinurel should not be used during treatment with MAO inhibitors or for two weeks after completion of therapy.

Side-effects: Drowsiness, dryness of mouth and mild stimulation have been occasionally reported.

Overdosage: Drowsiness, palpitations, weakness and inco-ordination. Later delayed acute liver failure.

Treatment: Gastric lavage. If possible check plasma paracetamol level. Within 10 hours of ingestion give methionine orally or cysteamine i.v. Otherwise take generally supportive measures.

Pharmaceutical precautions Store in a dry place at a temperature not exceeding 30°C.

Legal category P.

Package quantity Bottles containing 250 tablets.

Further information Nil.

Product licence number 0019/5029.

SYTRON*

Presentation A clear red mixture with a cherry taste.

Composition: Each 5 ml contains:
Sodium Ironedetate   190 mg
(Equivalent to 27.5 mg of Iron)

Action: Sodium ironedetate is not an iron salt as it contains iron in an un-ionised form. In this compound the iron is 'insulated' or 'sequestered' with the sodium salt of ethylenediamine tetra-acetic acid to form a chelate. This accounts for the fact that Sytron is not astringent and does not discolour teeth. Studies using radio-active tracers, have shown that iron chelate is split within the gastro-intestinal tract, releasing elemental iron which is absorbed and rendered available for haemoglobin regeneration.

Uses Iron deficiency anaemia, in paediatrics, in anaemias complicating rheumatoid arthritis. It is especially suitable in pregnancy when other forms of oral iron are not well tolerated.

Dosage and administration *Oral: Adults:* 5 ml increasing gradually to 10 ml three times daily.

Elderly (over 65 years): As for adults.

Children: (including premature infants) up to 1 year: 2.5 ml twice daily; somewhat smaller doses should be used initially. 1 to 5 years: 2.5 ml three times daily. 6 to 12 years: 5 ml three times daily.

Contra-indications, warnings, etc Patients have occasionally complained of nausea or mild diarrhoea in the early stages of treatment. In such cases it has been found that if treatment is withdrawn for a short time,

these symptoms quickly disappear and subsequently the patient will tolerate further doses, which should be on a somewhat reduced scale. Normal individuals have taken Sytron in twice the recommended dosage and some of these have experienced mild diarrhoea. This should be taken into account if dosage is increased much higher than the recommended scale.

Treatment of overdosage: Probably not required but if indicated, treatment should be according to any symptoms that may arise.

Pharmaceutical precautions Store below 30°C. Recommended diluent: Water. When diluted use within 14 days of preparation.

Legal category P.

Package quantities Containers of 500 ml and 2.25 litre.

Further information Nil.

Product licence number 0018/5029.

TEDRAL* ELIXIR

Presentation Clear, yellow liquid each 5 ml of which contains:
Theophylline PhEur   30.00 mg
Ephedrine Hydrochloride PhEur   6.00 mg

Uses Tedral elixir is for symptomatic relief of bronchospasm in bronchial asthma, chronic bronchitis and hay fever.

Dosage and administration Oral.
Adults: Four 5 ml spoonfuls every four hours.

Elderly (over 65 years): As for adults. Theophylline clearance tends to decrease slightly with age and elderly patients will, therefore, tend to have higher serum theophylline levels. They should, therefore, be monitored closely for signs of toxicity during dosage adjustment.

Children: (6–12 years): Two 5 ml spoonfuls every four hours.

Children (2–5 years): One 5 ml spoonful every four hours. The medication should preferably be taken after meals.

Contra-indications, warnings, etc

Contra-indications: Sensitivity to any of the ingredients.

Precautions and warnings: Tedral elixir should not be administered to patients who are receiving MAO inhibitors or have received these within the previous 14 days. It should not normally be administered during pregnancy and lactation. Tedral elixir should be used with caution in patients who are suffering from cardiovascular disorders, severe hypertension, hyperthyroidism, prostatic hypertrophy or glaucoma.

Side-effects: Difficulty in micturition, mild epigastric distress, palpitations, tremulousness, insomnia and C.N.S. stimulation have been reported.

Overdosage: Irritation of alimentary tract. Nausea, vomiting and giddiness.

Treatment: Gastric lavage. Use general supportive measures.

Pharmaceutical precautions Protect from light. Store at a temperature not exceeding 25°C.

Legal category POM.

Package quantities Tedral elixir is available in bottles containing 200 ml.

Further information Nil.

Product licence number 0019/0073.

TEDRAL* TABLETS

Presentation Each white, bi-convex tablet inscribed TEDRAL on one side contains:

Theophylline Ph Eur	120 mg
Ephedrine Hydrochloride Ph Eur	24 mg

Uses Tedral is for symptomatic relief of chronic asthma in adults.

Dosage and administration Oral.

Adults: 1 tablet every four hours.

Elderly (over 65 years): As for adults. Theophylline clearance tends to decrease slightly with age and elderly patients will, therefore, tend to have higher serum theophylline levels. They should, therefore, be monitored closely for signs of toxicity during dosage adjustment.

Children: Not recommended.

Contra-indications, warnings, etc

Contra-indications: Sensitivity to any of the ingredients.

Precautions and warnings: Tedral should not be administered to patients who are being treated with MAO inhibitors, or have received them within the preceding 14 days. It should be used with caution in patients who are suffering from cardiovascular disorders, severe hypertension, hyperthyroidism, prostatic hypertrophy or glaucoma.

Theophylline clearance may be decreased in critically ill patients with severe obstructive pulmonary disease and/or cor pulmonale; acute pulmonary oedema; congestive heart failure; hepatic cirrhosis and pneumonia with fever.

Theophylline clearance may be increased in heavy smokers.

Theophylline clearance may be decreased by concurrent administration of cimetidine, corticosteroids, erythromycin influenza vaccine and oral contraceptives.

Theophylline clearance may be increased by concurrent administration of barbiturates, carbamazepine, phenytoin, rifampicin and sulphinpyrazone.

The anti-hypertensive effect of guanethidine and related drugs may be decreased by the concurrent administration of ephedrine.

Pregnancy and lactation: There is some evidence linking in utero exposure to sympathomimetics (including ephedrine) to minor malformations, therefore the use of Tedral is not advised during pregnancy.

Theophylline is excreted in breast milk, therefore the use of Tedral is not advised during lactation.

Side-effects: Difficulty in micturition, mild epigastric distress, palpitations, tremulousness, insomnia and CNS stimulation have been reported.

Overdosage: Irritation of alimentary tract. Nausea, vomiting and giddiness.

Treatment: Gastric lavage. Use general supportive measures.

Pharmaceutical precautions Store in a dry place at a temperature not exceeding 30°C.

Legal category POM.

Package quantities Tedral Tablets are packed in brown glass bottles containing 50 and 500 tablets.

Further information Nil.

Product licence number 0019/5036R.

VIRA-A*

Presentation An ophthalmic ointment.

Composition: Vira-A (Vidarabine) Ophthalmic Ointment contains: Vidarabine (9-β-D-arabinofuranosyladenine) 3% in a sterile, inert, petrolatum base.

Action Vira-A is a purine nucleoside which possesses antiviral activity. Vira-A possesses virostatic activity against the DNA family of viruses including herpes simplex (types I and II), varicella, vaccinia, and cytomegalovirus in both tissue culture and experimental animal infections.

Vira-A is rapidly metabolised to arabinosyl-hypoxanthine (Ara-Hx), the principal metabolite. Ara-Hx also possesses antiviral activity but it is significantly less than that of the parent compound. Following topical ocular administration in humans, trace amounts of both Vira-A and Ara-Hx can be detected in the aqueous humour only if the cornea is severely defective. If the cornea is intact, only trace amounts of Ara-Hx can be recovered from the aqueous humour.

Systemic absorption of Vira-A should not occur following ocular administration and swallowing tears from the lacrimal duct. In laboratory animals, Vira-A is rapidly deaminated in the gastro-intestinal tract to Ara-Hx. Vira-A interferes with corneal wound healing less than other forms of antiviral ocular chemotherapy such as idoxuridine.

Indications Vira-A Ophthalmic Ointment is indicated for the treatment of herpes keratoconjunctivitis manifested by dendritic keratitis or geographic corneal ulcers. The drug is effective against both fresh corneal lesions and those which have not responded to idoxuridine. Vira-A is also indicated in patients who have developed toxic or allergic reactions to idoxuridine. The diagnosis is established by finding the typical dendritic or geographic lesions on slit-lamp examination. Generally, an average of seven days' continuous therapy is required to achieve corneal re-epithelisation of previously untreated lesions. Approximately 90% of treated eyes will re-epithelise by the end of three weeks' therapy. Lesions which have not healed previously on idoxuridine require an average of 11 days to re-epithelise. Approximately 75% of patients with idoxuridine-refractory lesions will heal by the end of four weeks of therapy with Vira-A. Continuation of therapy for an additional seven days after corneal re-epithelisation is recommended to prevent relapses of the infection.

Vira-A is less effective against stromal keratitis and uveitis as compared to epithelial disease secondary to the herpes virus.

Vira-A is not effective against RNA-virus and adenoviral ocular infections. It is also not effective against bacterial infections of the cornea or non-viral ulcers such as trophic or disciform keratitis.

Dosage and administration Topical. The proper dose is to extrude one half inch of the ointment into the conjunctival sac five times daily until corneal re-epithelisation has occurred. Treatment may then be continued at a reduced frequency, such as twice daily, for an additional seven days.

Contra-indications, warnings, etc Vira-A Ophthalmic Ointment is contra-indicated in patients who develop intolerance to it. The possibility of development of viral resistance to vidarabine cannot be ruled out. If there is no response after seven days' treatment, other forms of therapy should be considered.

Precautions: The diagnosis of herpes keratoconjunctivitis should be established clinically prior to prescribing Vira-A.

Patients should be forewarned that Vira-A, like any ophthalmic ointment, may produce a temporary visual haze.

Usage in pregnancy: Vira-A parenterally is teratogenic in rats and mice. Topically, 10% Vira-A ointment applied to 10% of the body surface of rabbits during organogenesis induced foetal abnormalities. When 10% Vira-A ointment was applied to 2% to 3% of the body surface of rabbits, no foetal abnormalities were found. This dose greatly exceeds the total recommended human dose. Since a risk of producing foetal damage is present if Vira-A is administered to pregnant women, it should be used in women who are or may become pregnant only when it is clearly needed and the anticipated benefit to the patient outweighs this potential risk to the foetus.

It is not known whether Vira-A is secreted in human milk. As a general rule, nursing should not be undertaken while a patient is under treatment since many drugs are excreted in human milk.

Side-effects: Lacrimation, foreign body sensation, conjunctival injection, burning, irritation, superficial punctate keratitis, pain, photophobia, punctal occlusion, and sensitivity have been reported. The following have also been reported but appear disease-related: uveitis, stromal oedema, secondary glaucoma, trophic defects, corneal vascularisation, and hyphaemia.

Treatment of overdosage: Acute massive overdosage by oral ingestion of the ophthalmic ointment has not occurred. However, the rapid deamination to arabinosyl-hypoxanthine should preclude any serious consequences. The oral LD_{50} for pure Vira-A is greater than 5,020 mg/kg in mice and rats. Thus, no untoward effects should result from ingestion of the entire contents of a tube (105 mg).

Ocular overdosage is unlikely because any excess is quickly expelled from the conjunctival sac. Too frequent administration should be avoided.

Pharmaceutical precautions Store between 2°–8°C.

Legal category POM.

Package quantities Available in tubes of 3.5 g.

Further information Nil.

Product licence number 0018/0072.

VIRA-A* PARENTERAL

Presentation A suspension which, when diluted with a recommended fluid, forms a solution for intravenous administration.

Composition: Each ml of suspension contains 200 mg of vidarabine monohydrate equivalent to 187.4 mg of vidarabine (ara-A, adenine arabinoside). Each millilitre contains Phemeride* (benzethonium chloride), not more than 0.1 mg, as a preservative; disodium hydrogen

phosphate, 0.957 mg, and sodium dihydrogen phosphate, 4.138 mg, as buffering agents. Hydrochloric acid may have been added to adjust pH.

Uses *Action:* Vira-A is a purine nucleoside obtained from fermentation cultures of *Streptomyces antibioticus.* Vira-A possesses *in vitro* and *in vivo* antiviral activity against herpes simplex types 1 and 2, varicella-zoster, and vaccinia viruses.

The antiviral mechanism of action has not yet been established. Vira-A appears to interfere with the early steps of viral DNA synthesis. Vira-A is rapidly deaminated to arabinosylhypoxanthine (Ara-Hx), the principal metabolite. Ara-Hx also possesses *in vitro* antiviral activity but this activity is significantly less than Vira-A.

Following IV administration, Vira-A is rapidly distributed into tissues and metabolised into Ara-Hx, resulting in low plasma levels of the parent compound. The Ara-Hx plasma levels reflect the rate of infusion, showing no accumulation with time. The mean half-life is 3.3 hours. Excretion is principally via the kidneys. Urinary excretion is constant over 24 hours. Forty-one to 53% of the daily dosage is recovered in the urine as Ara-Hx.

Indications and Usage: Varicella-zoster (herpes-zoster) infection: Vira-A is indicated in the treatment of varicella-zoster infections in the immunosuppressed patient, either localised or disseminated, and chickenpox in the immunosuppressed or immunocompromised patient. These infections are diagnosed by the typical clinical appearance. To be effective, therapy with Vira-A should be initiated within six days of the onset of the disease, when new lesions are forming. The recommended dosage is 10 mg/kg/day intravenously for at least five days. Vira-A does not inhibit the rate of lesion crusting and scabbing.

Vira-A should only be administered to patients with serious varicella-zoster infections where the benefits clearly outweigh the risks.

Vira-A is not effective against RNA viral or adenoviral infections. It is also not effective against bacterial or fungal infections. There is no clinical data to indicate efficacy against cytomegalovirus, vaccinia, or variola infections.

Dosage and administration Important – the contents of the vial must be diluted prior to administration.

Method of Preparation: Each vial contains 200 mg of Vira-A per ml of suspension. The solubility of Vira-A in intravenous infusion fluids is limited. Each one mg of Vira-A requires 2.22 ml of intravenous infusion fluid for complete solubilisation. Therefore, each one litre of intravenous infusion fluid will solubilise a maximum of 450 mg of Vira-A.

The following intravenous infusion fluids have been evaluated as being compatible with Vira-A Parenteral: 5% Dextrose Injection, 5% Dextrose and 0.33% Sodium Chloride Injection, 5% Dextrose and 0.45% Sodium Chloride Injection, 5% Dextrose and 0.9% Sodium Chloride Injection, Lactated Ringers Injection.

Vira-A has been shown to be pharmaceutically compatible with ampicillin, gentamicin and chloramphenicol.

Prepare the Vira-A solution for intravenous administration by aseptically transferring the proper dose of Vira-A into an appropriate intravenous infusion fluid. Shake the Vira-A vial well to obtain a homogeneous suspension before measuring and transferring. The intravenous infusion fluid used to prepare the Vira-A solution may be prewarmed to 35° to 40°C to facilitate dissolution of the drug following its transference. Depending on the dose to be given, more than one litre of intravenous infusion fluid may be required. Thoroughly agitate the prepared mixture until *completely* clear. Complete dissolution of the drug, as indicated by a completely clear solution, is ascertained by careful visual inspection. Final filtration with an in-line membrane filter (0.45 μ or smaller) is recommended.

Once in solution, the drug has been found to be chemically stable at room temperature (below 30°C) for at least two weeks. However, as with all intravenous mixtures dilution should be made just prior to administration. Subsequent agitation, shaking, or inversion of the bottle is unnecessary once the drug is completely in solution.

Dosage: Chickenpox and localised or disseminated varicella-zoster – 10 mg/kg/day for at least five days.

Elderly (over 65 years): As above. Although no pharmacokinetic studies specific to the elderly have been undertaken, Vira-A parenteral has been used successfully at normal dosage in elderly patients.

Administration: Using aseptic technique, slowly infuse the total daily dose by intravenous infusion (prepared as discussed above) at a constant rate over a 12- to 24-hour period.

Rapid or bolus injections must be avoided.

Contra-indications, warnings, etc Vira-A is contra-indicated in patients who develop intolerance to it.

Vira-A must not be administered by the intramuscular or subcutaneous route due to the low solubility and poor absorption.

Precautions: Patients with impaired kidney function, such as following renal transplant, may have a slower rate of renal excretion of Ara-Hx. Therefore, the dosage of Vira-A may need to be adjusted according to the severity of impairment.

The volume of intravenous fluids necessary requires special care when administering Vira-A to patients susceptible to fluid overloading or cerebral oedema. Examples are patients with CNS infections and impaired renal function.

A platelet count and complete blood count are recommended during Vira-A administration since haemoglobin, haematocrit, white blood cells, and platelets may be depressed during therapy.

Because Vira-A is virostatic, some degree of immunocompetence must be present in order to achieve clinical response.

Usage in Pregnancy: Vira-A given parenterally is teratogenic in rats and rabbits.

Dosages of 5 mg/kg or higher given intramuscularly to pregnant rabbits during organogenesis induced foetal abnormalities. Dosages of 3 mg/kg or less did not induce teratogenic changes in pregnant rabbits. Vira-A doses ranging from 30 to 250 mg/kg were given intramuscularly to pregnant rats during organogenesis; signs of maternal toxicity were induced at dosages of 100 mg/kg or higher and frank foetal abnormalities were found at dosages of 150 to 250 mg/kg.

A safe dose for the human embryo or foetus has not been established. Consequently, Vira-A should be used in pregnant patients only for life-threatening illnesses where the possible benefits to be derived outweigh the potential risks involved.

It is not known whether Vira-A is excreted in human milk. As a general rule, nursing should not be undertaken while a patient is under treatment because many drugs are excreted in human milk. If Vira-A is present in breast milk, it is unlikely that nursing infants would absorb appreciable amounts of drug because Vira-A is rapidly deaminated in the gastrointestinal tract.

Side-Effects: The principal side effects involve the gastrointestinal tract: anorexia, nausea, vomiting, and diarrhoea. In controlled and uncontrolled studies, the incidence of anorexia, nausea, vomiting, and/or diarrhoea was 14% in a dosage range of 10 to 15 mg/kg/day. These reactions are mild to moderate and seldom require termination of Vira-A.

CNS disturbances have been occasionally reported at therapeutic dosages. These are: tremor (1.8%), dizziness, hallucinations, confusion, psychosis, and ataxia.

Haematological clinical laboratory changes noted in controlled and uncontrolled studies were, a decrease in haemoglobin or haematocrit (16.5%), white blood cell count (6.8%), and platelet count (6.9%). SGOT elevations were observed in 6.6%. Other changes occasionally observed were decreases in reticulocyte count and elevated bilirubin.

Other symptoms reported were: weight loss, malaise, pruritus, rash, haematemesis, and pain at injection site.

Treatment of overdosage: Acute massive overdosage of the intravenous form has not been reported. Acute water overloading would pose a greater threat to the patient than Vira-A, due to its low solubility. Dosages of Vira-A two to three times the antiviral dosages can produce haematopoietic depression, principally thrombocytopenia. If a massive overdose of the intravenous form occurs, haematological, liver, and renal functions should be observed.

Acute massive oral ingestion should not be toxic because drug absorption from the gastrointestinal tract is minimal. The oral LD_{50} for Vira-A is greater than 5,020 mg/kg in mice and rats.

Pharmaceutical precautions Store below 30°C. Protect from freezing. Shake well before diluting.

Legal category POM.

Package quantities Vials of 5 ml containing 200 mg/ml vidarabine monohydrate in the form of a sterile suspension. 10 × 5 ml vials per pack.

Further information Nil.

Product licence number 0018/0073.

VI-SIBLIN*

Presentation Brown Granules. Ispaghula Husks BP (obtained from *Plantago ovata*) 66.0%.

Action Plantago absorbs and retains 30 times its own volume of water and is therefore used as a bulk laxative.

Indications For the treatment of chronic constipation.

Dosage and administration Oral.

Adults: Two 5 ml spoonfuls with a glassful of water one or more times daily.

Elderly (over 65 years): As for adults.

Children: None.

Contra-indications, warnings, etc Should not be used in patients with intestinal obstruction. Intestinal obstruction has been reported after the administration of bulk-forming agents. Patients who have difficulty swallowing should be warned not to take these preparations dry, and generous quantities of water should accompany the administration.

Treatment of overdosage: None.

Pharmaceutical precautions Store below 30°C.

Legal category GSL.

Package quantities Available in packs containing 250 g.

Further information Nil.

Product licence number 0018/5063.

ZARONTIN*

Presentation Zarontin Syrup (Ethosuximide Elixir BP) is a clear red, raspberry-flavoured syrup. Each 5 ml contains Ethosuximide BP 250 mg.

Zarontin Capsules (Ethosuximide Capsules BP) are orange, 8 minim, oblong soft gelatin capsules containing a clear liquid and printed 'P-D' in ivory ink. Each capsule contains Ethosuximide BP 250 mg.

Action Ethosuximide suppresses the paroxysmal spike and wave pattern common to petit mal seizures. The frequency of epileptiform attacks is reduced, apparently by depression of the motor cortex and elevation of the threshold of the central nervous system to convulsive stimuli. Compared with other succinimide anticonvulsants, ethosuximide is more specific for pure petit mal.

Indications Primarily useful in petit mal epilepsy. When grand mal and other forms of epilepsy co-exist with petit mal, Zarontin may be administered in combination with other anticonvulsants such as phenobarbitone, Epanutin* (Phenytoin Sodium Ph Eur) and primidone.

Dosage and administration Oral.
Adults and children over 6 years: initially 2 capsules or two 5 ml spoonfuls daily and adjusted thereafter to the patient's needs; daily dosage should be increased by small increments, for example, by 1 capsule or 5 ml every four to seven days, until control is achieved with minimal side-effects; although 4–6 capsules or 20–30 ml daily in divided doses often produce control of seizures, 7–8 capsules or 35–40 ml daily is not an unusual requirement.

Children and infants under 6 years: The initial dose is 5 ml daily which is adjusted by small increments until control is achieved with minimal side-effects.

Contra-indications, warnings, etc Hypersensitivity to succinimides.

There is some evidence that the succinimides may produce congenital abnormalities in the offspring of a small number of epileptic patients, and therefore they should only be used in pregnancy if in the judgement of the physician the potential benefits outweigh the risk. Ethosuximide may be excreted in breast milk. Zarontin should be used with caution in patients with impaired hepatic or renal function.

Mild side-effects, which are usually transient, may occur initially. These include apathy, drowsiness, depression, mild euphoria, headache, ataxia, dizziness, anorexia, gastric upset, nausea and vomiting. Psychotic states thought to be induced or exacerbated by anticonvulsant therapy have been reported. Skin rashes have been seen in a few patients. Systemic lupus erythematosus has occasionally been associated with the use of ethosuximide. Haematological reactions to ethosuximide appear to be uncommon. Cases of leucopenia, agranulocytosis and aplastic anaemia have been reported. The extent to which ethosuximide is implicated in these reactions is yet to be determined. Monocytosis, leucocytosis and transitory mild eosinophilia have also been noted. In most cases of leucopenia, the blood picture has been restored to normal on reduction of the dosage or discontinuation of the drug. Where leucopenia has occurred with other drugs, the polymorph count has in some cases increased steadily after starting treatment with ethosuximide and discontinuing previous medication. If the patient has been receiving other anticonvulsants the sudden withdrawal of the drugs may precipitate a series of attacks before Zarontin has been given in sufficient amounts to exercise control. This may be avoided by gradually replacing with Zarontin the anticonvulsant previously used.

Treatment of overdosage: If less than 2 g have been taken, fluids should be given by mouth. If a larger dose has been taken the stomach should be emptied, respiration maintained and any other symptoms treated accordingly.

Pharmaceutical precautions *Capsules:* Store at a temperature not exceeding 30°C.

Syrup: Store at a temperature not exceeding 25°C.
Recommended diluent – Syrup BP. When diluted use within 14 days of preparation.

Legal category POM.

Package quantities *Capsules 250 mg:* 50 and 500. *Syrup:* 250 ml.

Further information Nil.

Product licence numbers
Zarontin Syrup   0018/5040
Zarontin Capsules   0018/0078

Trade Mark

Pfizer Limited
Sandwich
Kent CT13 9NJ

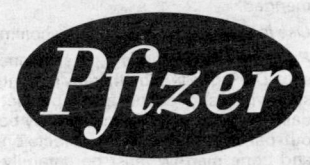

ALEXAN* INJECTABLE SOLUTION ▼

Presentation Alexan (cytarabine) is available as an isotonic solution in ampoules ready for injection. Ampoules contain either 2 ml or 5 ml of a solution of 20 mg/ml cytarabine.

Uses Alexan is a cytostatic agent for induction of clinical remission and/or maintenance therapy in patients with:
Acute myeloid leukaemia
Acute non-lymphoblastic leukaemias
Acute lymphoblastic leukaemias
Blast crises of chronic myeloid leukaemia
Diffuse histiocytic lymphomas (non Hodgkin's lymphomas of high malignancy)

Dosage and administration Alexan is administered by continuous intravenous infusion, intravenous injection, intrathecal injection, intramuscular or subcutaneous injection. Due to the short half-life of cytarabine, use of a rapid i.v. injection will result, in most patients, in a plasma concentration below the minimal therapeutic level in less than one hour. If it is desirable to give a rapid i.v. injection then it is necessary to divide the daily recommended dosage into two or more administrations at equal time intervals.

To prepare an infusion solution, Alexan can be added to sodium chloride intravenous infusion or dextrose intravenous infusion.

Continuous infusions have ranged from 8–12 hours to 120–168 hours. In comparision with single i.v. injections, continuous infusions of the same dosage show more pronounced side effects on the gastro-intestinal tract. Intrathecal, lumbar or intraventricular administration of Alexan can be carried out with the original solution. It is recommended that 5–8 ml of cerebrospinal fluid (CSF) be drawn up, mixed with the injection solution in the syringe and slowly re-injected. Systemic toxicity is not to be expected using this route of administration.

Intramuscular and subcutaneous injections are usually only used in maintenance therapy. Intracutaneous injections should be avoided due to the risk of oedema.

Effective cytotoxic plasma levels may be expected to lie in the range 0.01–0.15 mcg/ml.

The dosage required should be as exact as possible for each individual and is best calculated according to body surface area. Unless otherwise indicated in special combinations, Alexan should be used in the following doses:

Remission Induction Therapy:

Acute leukaemias: 100–200 mg/m²/day or 3–6 mg/kg/day
Current medical practice recommends 100 mg/m² twice daily when rapid intravenous injection is used. However, when continuous infusion is employed 100 mg/m²/day is recommended as a starting dose. The duration will depend on clinical and morphological (bone marrow) findings.

Either Treat the patient for up to seven days and allow 7–14 days treatment free to allow the bone marrow to recover before applying consolidation cycles (often of reduced duration of treatment) until remission or toxicity occurs.

Or Continue to treat the patient until the appearance of bone marrow hypoplasia which may be considered a tolerance limit. Before repeating the therapy cycle (often of reduced duration) there should be a treatment free period of at least 14 days, or until the bone marrow has recovered. For remission induction therapy patients should be supervised in a centre with laboratory and supportive resources sufficient to monitor drug tolerance and protect and maintain a patient compromised by drug toxicity.

Remission Maintenance: Leukaemias: 75–100 mg/m²/day or 1.5–3 mg/kg/day for five consecutive days once a month or one day each week. CNS leukaemias: 10–30 mg/m² three times weekly intrathecally. Lymphomas: these conditions are normally treated with a suitable combination of agents.

Contra-indications, warnings, etc

Contra-indications: Patients who already have bone marrow suppression should be excluded from treatment with Alexan unless the clinician considers that the benefit of such treatment outweighs its risk for the individual patient. Hypersensitivity to cytarabine.

Warnings: Hyperuricaemic prophylaxis is an absolute requirement, particularly in patients with high blast counts with acute monoblastic leukaemia or with large tumour masses. The clinician should monitor the patient's blood uric acid level and be prepared to use such supportive and pharmacological measures as might be necessary to control this. Because of the possible teratogenic effect of cytarabine on male and female germ cells adequate conception control should be established during, and for a sufficient period after, treatment.

To minimise the risks associated with remission induction therapy (granulocytopenia and associated infection, haemorrhage secondary to thrombocytopenia) Alexan should only be used in centres where adequate supportive therapy is available. Cytarabine has also been reported to cause chromosome breaks in human leucocytes in vitro. It inhibits DNA synthesis in mammalian cell cultures. These factors should be considered in long term administration.

Use in pregnancy: Alexan is known to be teratogenic in some animal species and should be used in women who are or who may become pregnant only after due consideration of the benefit/risk potential.

The use of Alexan in nursing mothers is not recommended.

Use in the elderly: No special recommendations.

Precautions: Alexan is a potent bone marrow suppressant. During induction therapy patients should be closely supervised and leucocyte and platelet counts performed daily. Remission maintenance may be carried out under out-patient conditions but effects on the blood picture and bone marrow must be carefully monitored. If the platelet count falls below 50,000/mm^3 or the leucocyte count falls below 1,000/mm^3 suspension or modification of therapy should be considered. The blood count may continue to fall following discontinuation of Alexan. Treatment may be recommenced if indicated, when bone marrow recovery is confirmed by bone marrow biopsy.

Haemopoietic, renal and hepatic function should be regularly monitored.

Side-effects: With high dosage continuous infusion (more than 200 mg/m^2/day) over 5–7 days the gastro-intestinal complications are more pronounced and can exceptionally lead to paralytic ileus. Rash, thrombophlebitis and bleeding are among the most frequent side-effects.

The following may also occur during treatment with Alexan: bone marrow suppression (such as thrombocytopenia, leucopenia, anaemia), megaloblastosis, immunosuppression, nausea, vomiting, diarrhoea, oral inflammation or ulceration, fever, pneumonia, anorexia, hepatic dysfunction.

Pharmaceutical precautions Store below 15°C.

The increasing use of cytotoxic drugs and the potential hazards associated with them, require special precautions to be taken in their handling, preparation and administration. These recommendations provide a basis for the safe handling of Alexan.

1. All staff working with Alexan should receive special training.

2. Dilution of Alexan should be performed in a designated aseptic area which gives maximum protection to the surrounding environment.

3. Adequate protective clothing including gloves and safety spectacles should be worn.

Should spillage on the skin occur, the affected area should be washed with copious quantities of water.

Should spillage into the eye occur, immediately cleanse thoroughly using copious quantities of sodium chloride eye wash. (If sodium chloride eye wash is not available water can be used as an alternative.) Should eye irritation continue medical help should be sought.

4. Alexan should not be handled by pregnant staff.

5. Adequate care and precautions should be taken in the disposal of items used to dilute Alexan.

Disposal procedure
Unopened ampoules: Place in a suitable container† and incinerate at 300°C.

Diluted solution: Inactivate with hydrochloric acid adjusting to pH2. Absorb diluted liquid on to paper, ash or sawdust. Place in a high risk waste disposal bag† and incinerate at 300°C.

Disposal of swabs, etc: Swabs, etc, should be placed in a high risk waste disposal bag† and incinerated at 300°C.

Accidental spillage: Should spillage on the floor or breakage of an ampoule occur, suitable protective clothing should be donned including PVC gloves. With rubber gloves as over protection, the area should be cleaned with absorbent paper and the floor wiped with cloths soaked in hydrochloric acid solution at pH2, then the floor should be washed with copious quantities of water. The absorbent paper, cloths, gloves and other materials used in the management of the spillage should be placed in a high risk waste disposal bag† and incinerated at 300°C. Care should be taken in disposing of broken glass from ampoules, which should go into a closed container† for incineration.

Legal category POM.

Package quantities Alexan is a solution (20 mg/ml) ready prepared for use.
It is packed as:
2 ml ampoule (40 mg cytarabine) in packs of 10.
5 ml ampoule (100 mg cytarabine) in packs of 10.

Further information There is extensive literature available on the effectiveness of cytarabine both alone and in combination with other agents in the treatment of conditions for which it is indicated.

Product licence number 0057/0190.

† The containers and bags should be those specified in the 'Safe disposal of clinical waste'. Health & Safety Advisory Committee, HMSO, 1982.

ATARAX*

Presentation Atarax (hydroxyzine hydrochloride) is available as:
10 mg sugar-coated tablets, coloured orange and coded on one side with 'Pfizer'.
25 mg sugar-coated tablets, coloured green and coded on one side with 'Pfizer'. Syrup 10 mg/5 ml clear, flavoured with sugar, peppermint and spearmint.

Uses *Actions:* Atarax is unrelated chemically to phenothiazine, reserpine, and meprobamate. Atarax has demonstrated its clinical effectiveness in the management of neuroses and emotional disturbances manifested by anxiety, tension, agitation, apprehension or confusion.

Atarax has been shown clinically to be a rapid-acting true ataractic with a wide margin of safety. It induces a calming effect in anxious, tense, psychoneurotic adults and also in anxious, hyperkinetic children without impairing mental alertness. It is not a cortical depressant, but its action may be due to a suppression of activity in certain key regions of the subcortical area of the central nervous system.

Primary skeletal muscle relaxation has been demonstrated experimentally. Secondary skeletal muscle relaxation due to ataraxia should be regarded as additive to this primary effect.

Atarax has been shown experimentally to have antispasmodic properties, apparently mediated through interference with the mechanism that responds to spasmogenic agents such as serotonin, acetylcholine, and histamine. Antihistamine effects have been demonstrated experimentally and confirmed clinically.

An anti-emetic effect, both by the apomorphine test and the veriloid test, has been demonstrated.

Atarax is rapidly absorbed in the gastro-intestinal tract and effects are usually noted within 15 to 30 minutes after oral administration.

Pharmacological and clinical studies indicate that Atarax in therapeutic dosage does not increase gastric secretion or acidity and in most cases provides mild antisecretory benefits.

Indications: The total management of anxiety, tension, and psychomotor agitation in conditions of emotional stress, requires in most instances a combined approach of psychotherapy and chemotherapy. Atarax has been found to be particularly useful for this latter phase of therapy in its ability to render the disturbed patient more amenable to psychotherapy in long term treatment of the psychoneurotic and psychotic, although it should not be used as the sole treatment of psychosis or of clearly demonstrated cases of depression.

Atarax is also useful in alleviating the manifestations of anxiety and tension as in the preparation for dental procedures and in acute emotional problems. It has also been recommended for the management of anxiety associated with organic disturbances and as adjunctive therapy in alcoholism and allergic conditions with strong emotional overlay, such as asthma.

It is useful in the management of pruritus due to allergic conditions such as chronic urticaria and atopic and contact dermatoses, and in histamine-mediated pruritus.

Atarax benefits the cardiac patient by its ability to allay the associated anxiety and apprehension attendant to certain types of heart disease. Atarax is not known to interfere with the action of digitalis in any way and may be used concurrently with this agent.

Dosage and administration For symptomatic relief of anxiety and tension associated with psychoneurosis and as an adjunct in organic disease states in which anxiety is manifested: in adults, 50–100 mg four times daily; children under 6 years, 50 mg daily in divided doses and over 6 years, 50–100 mg daily in divided doses.

For use in the management of pruritus due to allergic conditions such as chronic urticaria and atopic and contact dermatoses, and in histamine-mediated pruritus: in adults, 25 mg three or four times daily; children under 6 years, 50 mg daily in divided doses and over 6 years, 50–100 mg daily in divided doses.

As a sedative when used as a premedication and following general anaesthesia: 50–100 mg in adults, and 0.6 mg/kg in children.

As with all medications, the dosage should be adjusted according to the patient's response to therapy.

Use in the elderly: Atarax may be used in elderly patients with no special precautions other than the care always necessary in this age group. The lowest effective maintenance dose and careful observation for side effects are important.

Contra-indications, warnings, etc
Contra-indications: Atarax is contra-indicated in patients who have shown a previous hypersensitivity to it.

Warnings: It is not known whether Atarax is excreted in human milk. Since many drugs are so excreted, Atarax should not be given to nursing mothers.

Use in pregnancy: Atarax, when administered to the pregnant mouse, rat and rabbit, induced foetal abnormalities in the rat at doses substantially above the human therapeutic range. Clinical data in human beings are inadequate to establish safety in early pregnancy. Until such data are available, Atarax is contra-indicated in early pregnancy.

Side-effects: Therapeutic doses of Atarax seldom produce impairment of mental alertness. However, drowsiness may occur; if so, it is usually transitory and may disappear in a few days of continued therapy or upon reduction of the dose. Dryness of the mouth may be encountered at higher doses. Extensive clinical use has substantiated the absence of toxic effects on the liver or bone marrow when administered in the recommended doses for over four years of uninterrupted therapy. The absence of side-effects has been further demonstrated in experimental studies in which excessively high doses were administered.

Involuntary motor activity, including rare instances of tremor and convulsions, have been reported, usually with doses considerably higher than those recommended. Continuous therapy with over 1 g/day has been employed in some patients without these effects having been encountered.

Overdosage: The most common manifestation of Atarax overdosage is hypersedation. As in the management of overdosage with any drug, it should be borne in mind that multiple agents may have been taken.

If vomiting has not occurred spontaneously, it should be induced. Immediate gastric lavage is also recommended. General supportive care, including frequent monitoring of the vital signs and close observation of the patient, is indicated. Hypotension, though unlikely, may be controlled with intravenous fluids and noradrenaline, or metaraminol. Do not use adrenaline as Atarax counteracts its pressor action. Caffeine and Sodium Benzoate Injection may be used to counteract central nervous system depressant effects.

There is no specific antidote. It is doubtful that haemodialysis would be of any value in the treatment of overdosage with Atarax. However, if other agents such as barbiturates have been ingested concomitantly, haemodialysis may be indicated. There is no practical method to quantitate Atarax in body fluids or tissue after its ingestion or administration.

Pharmaceutical precautions Store below 25°C.

Legal category POM.

Package quantities
Tablets 10 mg: Packs of 100
Tablets 25 mg: Packs of 100
Syrup: Bottle of 150 ml.

Further information 10 mg tablets contain the azo-dye, sunset yellow (E110). 25 mg tablets contain the azo-dye, tartrazine (E102) and lissamine green (E142).

Product licence numbers
Tablets 10 mg   0057/5003
Tablets 25 mg   0057/5004
Syrup   0057/5005.

COMBANTRIN* ▼

Presentation Combantrin is available as orange tablets containing 125 mg pyrantel as pyrantel pamoate.

Uses *Actions:* Combantrin is an anthelmintic agent highly effective against infections due to pinworm (*Enterobius vermicularis*), roundworm (*Ascaris lumbricoides*), hookworm (*Ancylostoma duodenale* and *Necator americanus*), and *Trichostrongylus colubriformis* and *orientalis.* Combantrin has some activity against whipworm (*Trichuris trichiura*).

Combantrin exercises a neuromuscular blocking effect on susceptible helminths. By virtue of its action, Combantrin immobilises ascarides and brings about their expulsion without producing excitation, or stimulating migration of the affected worms. Within the intestinal tract Combantrin is effective against mature and immature forms of susceptible helminths. The normal migratory stages of worms are unaffected. Combantrin is poorly absorbed from the gastro-intestinal tract. More than 50% is oxcreted unchanged in the faeces following oral administration; less than 7% is found in the urine unchanged and in the form of metabolites.

Indications: Combantrin is specifically indicated for the treatment of infection with any of the following gastro-intestinal parasites when these are present either alone or as a mixed infection.

1. *Enterobius vermicularis* (threadworm, pinworm)
2. *Ascaris lumbricoides* (roundworm)
3. *Ancylostoma duodenale* (hookworm)
4. *Necator americanus* (hookworm)
5. *Trichostrongylus colubriformis* and *orientalis.*

Combantrin should be used for the treatment of infection with one or more of these parasites in both adults and children. It is well tolerated and will not stain the oral mucosa upon ingestion or the clothing by faecal contamination. The presence of an infection with any of the five parasites in one member of a family or group of persons in close proximity may indicate unidentified infection in other members. In these circumstances, Combantrin administration to all the family or group members is recommended. (Rigorous cleaning of living quarters and clothing to destroy helminthic ova will help prevent reinfection.)

Dosage and administration The recommended dose of Combantrin for the treatment of infections with *Enterobius vermicularis, Ascaris lumbricoides, Ancylostoma duodenale, Necator americanus, Trichostrongylus colubriformis* and *orientalis* is 10 mg/kg of patient body weight, administered orally as a single dose. A simplified dosage schedule, based on the above and on estimated weights at various ages follows:

Age of patient	Weight	Tablets of 125 mg
6 months to 2 years	less than 12 kg	1
2 to 6 years	12 to 22 kg	2
6 to 12 years	22 to 41 kg	4
over 12 years	41 to 75 kg	6
	Adults over 75 kg	8

For more severe infections of *Necator americanus*, the recommended dosage is 20 mg/kg bodyweight administered as a single dose on each of two consecutive days, or 10 mg/kg bodyweight administered as a single dose on each of three consecutive days.

Infection due to *Ascaris lumbricoides* alone can be successfully treated with a dose of 5 mg/kg bodyweight administered as a single dose.

A simplified dosage schedule for ascariasis based on the above and on estimated weights at various ages follows:

Age of patient	Weight	Tablets of 125 mg
6 months to 2 years	less than 12 kg	$\frac{1}{2}$
2 to 6 years	12 to 22 kg	1
6 to 12 years	22 to 41 kg	2
over 12 years	41 to 75 kg	3
	adults over 75 kg	4

In mass treatment programmes directed against *Ascaris lumbricoides* infestation alone, a single dose of 2.5 mg/kg bodyweight can be used. A simplified dosage schedule based on the preceding and on estimated weight at various ages follows:

Age of patient	Weight	Tablets of 125 mg
6 months to 2 years	less than 12 kg	$\frac{1}{4}$
2 to 6 years	12 to 22 kg	$\frac{1}{2}$
6 to 12 years	22 to 41 kg	1
over 12 years	41 to 75 kg	$1\frac{1}{2}$
	adults over 75 kg	2

Contra-indications, warnings, etc

Use in pregnancy: Although animal reproductive studies have not demonstrated any teratogenic effects, Combantrin has not been studied in the pregnant patient. Accordingly, it should not be used during pregnancy unless in the judgement of the physician it is essential for the welfare of the patient.

Use in the elderly: No additional precautions.

Precautions: Combantrin should be used with caution in patients with pre-existing hepatic dysfunction, as minor transient elevations of the SGOT have occurred in a small percentage of patients.

Side-effects: Clinical experience has shown Combantrin to be extremely well tolerated. Side-effects, if encountered, usually relate to the gastro-intestinal tract – anorexia, abdominal cramps, nausea, vomiting and diarrhoea. Other side effects that may occur are: headache, dizziness, drowsiness, insomnia and rash.

Pharmaceutical precautions Store below 25°C.

Legal category POM.

Package quantities Pack of 6 tablets.

Further information Nil.

Product licence number 0057/0057.

DELTACORTRIL* ENTERIC

Presentation Deltacortril Enteric tablets 2.5 mg uniformly brown in colour and coded 'Pfizer'.

Deltacortril Enteric tablets 5 mg uniformly red in colour and coded 'Pfizer'.

Deltacortril is the synthetic crystalline steroid prednisolone.

Uses *Actions:* Naturally occurring glucocorticoids (hydrocortisone and cortisone), which also have salt-retaining properties, are used as replacement therapy in adrenocortical deficiency states. Their synthetic analogues are primarily used for their potent anti-inflammatory effects in disorders of many organ systems.

Deltacortril Enteric is one of the highly potent glucocorticoid steroids having anti-inflammatory, hormonal, and metabolic effects similar to those of cortisone and hydrocortisone.

Glucocorticoids cause profound and varied metabolic effects. In addition, they modify the body's immune responses to diverse stimuli.

Indications: Endocrine disorders: Primary or secondary adrenocortical insufficiency (hydrocortisone or cortisone is the first choice; synthetic analogues may be used in conjunction with mineralocorticoids where applicable;

in infancy mineralocorticoid supplementation is of particular importance).

Congenital adrenal hyperplasia.
Non-suppurative thyroiditis.
Hypercalcaemia associated with cancer.

Rheumatic disorders: As adjunctive therapy for short term administration (during an acute episode or exacerbation) in:

Psoriatic arthritis.
Rheumatoid arthritis including juvenile rheumatoid arthritis (selected cases may require low-dose maintenance therapy).
Ankylosing spondylitis.
Acute and subacute bursitis.
Acute nonspecific tenosynovitis.
Acute gouty arthritis.
Post traumatic oesteoarthritis.
Synovitis of osteoarthritis.
Epicondylitis.

Collagen diseases: During an exacerbation or as maintenance therapy in selected cases of:

Systematic lupus erythematosus.
Systematic dermatomyositis (polymyositis).
Acute rheumatic carditis.

Dermatological diseases: Pemphigus.
Bullous dermatitis herpetiformis.
Exfoliative dermatitis.
Mycosis fungoides.
Severe seborrhoeic dermatitis.

Allergic states: Control of severe or incapacitating allergic conditions intractable to adequate trials of conventional treatment.

Seasonal or perennial allergic rhinitis.
Bronchial asthma.
Contact dermatitis.
Atopic dermatitis.
Serum sickness.
Drug hypersensitivity reactions.

Ophthalmic diseases: Severe acute and chronic allergic and inflammatory processes involving the eye and its adnexa such as:

Allergic conjunctivitis.
Keratitis.
Allergic corneal marginal ulcers.
Herpes zoster ophthalmicus.
Iritis and iridocyclitis.
Chorioretinitis.
Anterior segment inflammation.
Diffuse posterior uveitis and choroiditis.
Optic neuritis.
Sympathetic ophthalmia.

Respiratory diseases: Symptomatic sarcoidosis.
Loeffler's syndrome not manageable by other means.
Berylliosis.
Fulminating or disseminated pulmonary tuberculosis when used concurrently with appropriate antituberculous chemotherapy.
Aspiration pneumonitis.

Haematological disorders: idiopathic thrombocytopenic purpura in adults.

Secondary thrombocytopenia in adults.
Acquired (autoimmune) haemolytic anaemia.
Erythroblastopenia (red blood cell anaemia).
Congenital (erythroid) hypoplastic anaemia.

Neoplastic diseases: For management of:
Leukaemias and lymphomas in adults.

Acute leukaemia of childhood.

Oedematous states: To induce a diuresis or remission of proteinuria in the idiopathic nephrotic syndrome, without ureaemia, or that due to lupus erythematosus.

Gastro-intestinal diseases: To assist the patient during a critical period of disease in:

Ulcerative colitis.
Regional enteritis.

Miscellaneous: Tuberculous meningitis with subarachnoid block or impending block when used concurrently with appropriate antituberculous chemotherapy.

Trichinosis with neurological or myocardial involvement.

Dosage and administration The initial dosage of Deltacortril Enteric may vary from 5 mg to 60 mg/day depending on the specific disease entity being treated. In situations of less severity lower doses will generally suffice, while in selected patients higher initial doses may be required. The initial dosage should be maintained or adjusted until a satisfactory response is noted. If after a reasonable period of time there is a lack of satisfactory clinical response, Deltacortril Enteric should be discontinued and the patient transferred to other appropriate therapy. It should be emphasised that dosage requirements are variable and must be individualised on the basis of the disease under treatment and the response of the patient. After a favourable response is noted, the proper maintenance dosage should be determined by decreasing the initial drug dosage in small amounts at appropriate time intervals until the lowest dosage which will maintain an adequate clinical response is reached. It should be kept in mind that constant monitoring is needed in regard to drug dosage. Included in the situations which may make dosage adjustments necessary are changes in clinical status secondary to remissions or exacerbations in the disease process, the patient's individual drug responsiveness, and the effect of patient exposure to stressful situations not directly related to the disease entity under treatment; in this latter situation it may be necessary to increase the dosage of Deltacortril Enteric for a period of time consistent with the patient's condition. If after long-term therapy the drug is to be stopped, it is recommended that it be withdrawn gradually rather than abruptly.

Contra-indications, warnings, etc
Contra-indications: Systemic fungal infections.

Warnings: Deltacortril Enteric should be used with caution in the presence of a diminished cardiac reserve or congestive heart failure, diabetes mellitus, infectious diseases, chronic renal failure, uraemia and in elderly persons.

Patients on corticosteroid therapy subjected to unusual stress require increased dosage before, during and after the stressful situation.

Corticosteroids may mask some signs of infection, and new infections may appear during their use. There may be decreased resistance and inability to localise infection when corticosteroids are used.

Prolonged use of corticosteroids may produce posterior subcapsular cataracts, glaucoma with possible damage to the optic nerves, and may enhance the establishment of secondary ocular infections due to fungi or viruses.

Average and large doses of hydrocortisone or cortisone can cause elevation of blood pressure, salt and water retention, and increased excretion of potassium. These effects are less likely to occur with the synthetic derivatives except when used in large doses. Dietary salt restrictions and potassium supplementation may be necessary. All corticosteroids increase calcium excretion.

Immunisation procedures should not be undertaken in patients who are on corticosteroids, especially on high dose, because of possible hazards of neurological complications and a lack of antibody response.

The use of Deltacortril Enteric in active tuberculosis should be restricted to those cases of fulminating or disseminated tuberculosis in which the corticosteroid is used for the management of the disease in conjunction with an appropriate antituberculous regimen.

If corticosteroids are indicated in patients with latent tuberculosis or tuberculin reactivity, close observation is necessary as reactivation of the disease may occur. During prolonged corticosteroid therapy, these patients should receive chemoprophylaxis.

Use in pregnancy: There is inadequate evidence of safety in human pregnancy and there may be a very small risk of cleft palate and intra-uterine growth retardation in the foetus; there is evidence of harmful effects on pregnancy in animals. The use of these drugs in pregnancy, nursing mothers or women of childbearing potential requires that the possible benefits of the drug be weighed against the potential hazards to the mother and foetus. Infants born of mothers who have received substantial doses of corticosteroids during pregnancy should be carefully observed for signs of hypoadrenalism.

Use in the elderly: Elderly patients are particularly liable to adverse metabolic effects and care is necessary to use the lowest possible maintenance dose whenever corticosteroid therapy is prolonged. The more serious consequence of the common side effects of corticosteroids in old age, especially osteoporosis, diabetes, hypertension, susceptibility to infection and thinning of the skin should be borne in mind.

Use in children: Corticosteroids cause growth retardation in infancy, childhood and adolescence. Treatment should be limited to the minimum dosage for the shortest possible time. In order to minimise suppression of the hypothalamo-pituitary adrenal axis and growth retardation, treatment should be administered where possible as a single dose on alternate days.

Precautions: Drug-induced secondary adrenocortical insufficiency may be minimised by gradual reduction of dosage. This type of relative insufficiency may persist for months after discontinuation of therapy; therefore, in any situation of stress occurring during that period, hormone therapy should be reinstituted. Since mineralocorticoid secretion may be impaired, salt and/or a mineralocorticoid should be administered concurrently.

There is an enhanced effect of corticosteroids on patients with hypothyroidism and in those with cirrhosis.

Corticosteroids should be used cautiously in patients with ocular herpes simplex because of possible perforation.

The lowest possible dose of corticosteroid should be used to control the condition under treatment, and when reduction in dosage is possible, the reduction should be gradual.

Psychic derangements may appear when corticosteroids are used, ranging from euphoria, insomnia, mood swings, personality changes and severe depression, to frank psychic manifestation. Also, existing emotional instability of psychotic tendencies may be aggravated by corticosteroids.

Aspirin should be used cautiously in conjunction with corticosteroids in hypoprothrombinaemia.

Steroids should be used with caution in nonspecific ulcerative colitis, if there is a probability of impending perforation, abscess or other pyogenic infection, diverticulitis, fresh intestinal anastomoses; active or latent peptic ulcer, renal insufficiency; hypertension, osteoporosis; and myasthenia gravis.

Side-effects:
Fluid and electrolyte disturbances:
  Sodium retention.
  Fluid retention.
  Congestive heart failure in susceptible patients.
  Potassium loss.
  Hypokalaemic alkalosis.
  Hypertension.
Musculoskeletal:
  Muscle weakness.
  Steroid myopathy.
  Loss of muscle mass.
  Osteoporosis.
  Vertebral compression fractures.
  Aseptic necrosis of femoral and humeral heads.
  Pathological fracture of long bones.
Gastro-intestinal:
  Peptic ulcer with possible perforation and haemorrhage.
  Pancreatitis.
  Abdominal distension.
  Ulcerative oesophagitis.
Dermatological:
  Mild hirsutism.
  Impaired wound healing.
  Thin fragile skin.
  Petechiae and ecchymoses.
  Facial erythema.
  Increased sweating.
  May suppress reactions to skin tests.
Neurological:
  Convulsions.
  Increased intracranial pressure with papilloedema (pseudo-tumour cerebri) usually after treatment.
  Vertigo.
  Headache.
Endocrine:
  Menstrual irregularities.
  Development of Cushingoid state.
  Suppression of growth in children.
  Secondary adrenocortical and pituitary unresponsiveness, particularly in times of stress, as in trauma, surgery or illness.
  Decreased carbohydrate tolerance.
  Manifestations of latent diabetes mellitus.
  Increased requirements for insulin or oral hypoglycaemic agents in diabetics.
Ophthalmic:
  Posterior subcapsular cataracts.
  Increased intraocular pressure.
  Glaucoma.
  Exophthalmos.
Metabolic:
  Negative nitrogen balance due to protein catabolism.

Overdosage: Treat symptomatically with attention to serum electrolytes.

Pharmaceutical precautions Store below 25°C.

Legal category POM.

Package quantities *Deltacortril Enteric Tablets 2.5 mg and 5 mg:* Packs of 100 and 500.

Further information The 5 mg tablets contain an azo dye, (E124).

Product licence numbers
2.5 mg tablets   0057/5012
5 mg tablets   0057/0128.

DIABINESE*

Presentation Diabinese (chlorpropamide) is available as a white scored tablet in two different strengths:

Diabinese 100 mg tablet coded DIA/100 on one side and 'Pfizer' on the other.

Diabinese 250 mg tablet coded DIA/250 on one side and 'Pfizer' on the other.

Diabinese is classified as an arylsulphonylurea.

Uses *Actions:* Diabinese brand of chlorpropamide is an oral hypoglycaemic agent. The precise mechanism of action is not completely understood but is believed to be that of stimulation of synthesis and release of endogenous insulin. Extrapancreatic effects may play a part in the mechanism of action of oral sulphonylureas.

Diabinese is a potent, active, oral hypoglycaemic agent indicated for the treatment of selected diabetic patients. It is generally used alone to control the mild to moderately severe maturity-onset, stable diabetic (Type II diabetic). While Diabinese is a sulphonamide derivative, it is devoid of antibacterial activity.

Diabinese is rapidly absorbed from the gastrointestinal tract. Within one hour after a single oral dose, it is readily detectable in the blood, and reaches a maximum within two to four hours. It is metabolised and excreted in the urine as unchanged drug and as hydroxylated or hydrolyzed metabolites. The biological half-life of chlorpropamide averages about 36 hours. Within 96 hours, 80 to 90% of a single oral dose is excreted in the urine. However, long-term administration of therapeutic doses does not result in undue accumulation in the blood, since absorption and excretion rates become stabilized in about 5 to 7 days after the initiation of therapy.

Diabinese exerts a hypoglycaemic effect in normal humans within one hour, becoming maximal at 3 to 6 hours and persisting for at least 24 hours. The potency of Diabinese is approximately six times that of tolbutamide. Some experimental results suggest that its increased effectiveness may be the result of slower excretion and absence of significant deactivation.

There is now evidence that improvement in pancreatic beta cell function, with consequent improvement in glucose tolerance, may occur with prolonged administration of Diabinese. Accordingly, in individuals with asymptomatic diabetes mellitus, principally manifested by an abnormal glucose tolerance, continuous use of Diabinese may result in 'normalization' of their tolerance to glucose.

Diabinese does not interfere with the usual tests to detect albumin in the urine.

Some patients fail to respond initially, or gradually lose their responsiveness to sulphonylurea drugs, including Diabinese. Alternatively, Diabinese, may be effective in some patients who have not responded or have ceased to respond to other sulphonylureas.

Indications: Diabinese is indicated as an adjunct to diet to lower the blood glucose in patients with non-insulin-dependent diabetes mellitus (NIDDM/Type II), whose hyperglycaemia cannot be controlled by diet alone.

In initiating treatment for non-insulin-dependent diabetes, diet should be emphasized as the primary form of treatment. Caloric restriction and weight loss are essential in the obese diabetic patient. Proper dietary management alone may be effective in controlling the blood glucose and symptoms of hyperglycaemia. The importance of regular physical activity should also be stressed, and cardiovascular risk factors (such as smoking, obesity and hypertension) should be identified and corrective measures taken where possible.

Use of Diabinese must be viewed by both the physician and patients as a treatment in addition to diet, and not as a substitute for diet or as a convenient mechanism for avoiding dietary restraint. Furthermore, loss of blood glucose control on diet alone may be transient, thus requiring only short-term administration of Diabinese.

During maintenance programmes, Diabinese should be discontinued if satisfactory lowering of blood glucose is no longer achieved. Judgments should be based on regular clinical and laboratory evaluations.

In considering the use of Diabinese in asymptomatic patients, it should be recognized that controlling the blood glucose in non-insulin-dependent diabetes has not been definitely established to be effective in preventing the long-term cardiovascular or neurological complications of diabetes.

It may also prove effective in controlling certain patients who have shown an inadequate response or true primary or secondary failure to other sulphonylurea agents. In patients requiring high doses or frequent administration of another oral agent, control may be facilitated through its use.

Patient selection: The most likely patient for therapy is one in whom diabetes is of the NIDDM type, stable, and not controllable by dietary regulation alone. A past history of diabetic coma does not necessarily preclude successful therapeutic control with Diabinese. A trial period may be indicated in certain patients who might be expected to respond to this type of medication, but who failed in initial trials with, or after having been on other oral sulphonylurea agents, or in patients whose diabetic control on such agents has not been satisfactory. Diabinese may prove effective and provide improved control of the diabetes. The final evaluation of response in patients who qualify as candidates for Diabinese is a therapeutic trial for a period of at least seven days. During the trial period, the absence of ketonuria together with a satisfactory control, indicates that the patient is responsive and amenable to control with the drug. However, the development of ketonuria within 24 hours after withdrawal of insulin usually will be indicative of a poor response. The patient is considered nonresponsive if he fails to achieve satisfactory lowering of blood sugar levels or fails to obtain objective or subjective clinical improvement and if he develops ketonuria or glycosuria. Insulin is indicated for the therapy of such patients.

Concurrent Diabinese – biguanide therapy: The concurrent use of Diabinese with a biguanide is indicated in the treatment of uncomplicated diabetes mellitus of the stable, nonketotic, NIDDM type which cannot be controlled by diet alone, by diet and insulin, or by diet and sulphonylurea agents. The appropriate biguanide data sheet should be consulted for complete details of patient selection, indications, warnings and dose.

Diabinese in diabetes insipidus: Limited studies to date have shown that Diabinese is also useful in the treatment of idiopathic diabetes insipidus. In using Diabinese for this purpose, the physician must remain constantly aware of the possible occurrence of hypoglycaemic reactions in such individuals, particularly when unrelated illness, or other causes, reduce food intake. When Diabinese must be temporarily discontinued, in such cases, therapy with antidiuretic hormone should be substituted.

In the treatment of diabetes insipidus, daily dosage has been in the range of 100–500 mg daily for older children and adults. Because of the risk of hypoglycaemia that can develop in these individuals, it is desirable to start therapy at the lower range, gradually adjusting the dose as indicated. Patients and particularly the parents of children who are patients, should be warned of the possibility and treatment of hypoglycaemic reactions, especially during intercurrent infections or other periods of impaired food intake. In such circumstances, Diabinese therapy should be promptly discontinued and the patient's physician contacted.

When physicians are considering Diabinese for the treatment of diabetes insipidus, it is essential that they read this product document completely and particularly those paragraphs relating to Precautions and Side-effects.

Dosage and administration There is no fixed dosage regimen for the management of diabetes mellitus with Diabinese or other hypoglycaemic agents. In addition to the usual monitoring of urinary glucose, the patient's blood glucose must also be monitored periodically to determine the minimum effective dose for the patient; to detect primary failure, i.e. inadequate lowering of blood glucose at the maximum recommended dose of medication; and to detect secondary failure, i.e. loss of an adequate blood glucose lowering response after an initial period of effectiveness. Glycosylated haemoglobin levels may also be of value in monitoring the patient's response to therapy.

Short-term administration of Diabinese may be sufficient during periods of transient loss of control in patients usually controlled well on diet.

The total daily dosage is generally taken at a single time each morning with breakfast. Occasionally cases of gastrointestinal intolerance may be relieved by dividing the daily dosage. A loading or primary dose is not necessary and should not be used.

Initial therapy: The mild to moderately severe, middle-aged, stable diabetic patient should be started on 250 mg daily.

Use in the elderly: Because the elderly diabetic patient appears to be more sensitive to the hypoglycaemic effect of sulphonylurea drugs, older patients should be started on smaller mounts of Diabinese, in the range of 100 to 125 mg daily.

No transition period is necessary when transferring patients from other oral hypoglycaemic agents to Diabinese. The other agent may be discontinued abruptly and Diabinese started at once. In prescribing Diabinese, due consideration must be given to its greater potency.

The large majority of mild to moderately severe, middle-aged, stable diabetic patients receiving insulin can be placed directly on the oral drug and their insulin abruptly discontinued. For patients requiring more than 40 units of insulin daily, therapy with Diabinese may be initiated with a 50 per cent reduction in insulin for the first few days, with subsequent further reductions dependent upon the response.

During the insulin withdrawal period, patients should

test their urine for sugar and ketone bodies at least three times daily and report the results frequently to their physician. If they are abnormal, the physician should be notified immediately. In some cases it may be advisable to consider hospitalisation during the transition period.

Five to seven days after the initial therapy, the blood level of chlorpropamide reaches a plateau. Dosage may subsequently be adjusted upward or downward by increments of not more than 50 to 125 mg at intervals of three to five days to obtain optimal control. More frequent adjustments are usually undesirable.

Maintenance therapy: Most moderately severe, middle-aged stable diabetic patients are controlled by approximately 250 mg daily. Many investigators have found that some milder diabetics do well on daily doses of 100–125 mg or less. Many of the more severe diabetics may require 500 mg daily for adequate control. Patients who do not respond completely to 500 mg daily will usually not respond to higher doses. Maintenance doses above 500 mg daily should be avoided.

In elderly patients, debilitated or malnourished patients, and patients with impaired renal or hepatic function, the initial and maintenance dosing should be conservative to avoid hypoglycaemic reactions (see Precautions section).

Diabinese/Metformin dosage: The dosage of Diabinese should be maintained at or increased to 500 mg. If control is still inadequate, metformin may be added at a dosage of 0.5 gram twice daily, increasing by 0.5 to 1.0 gram every one to two weeks to a maximum of 3 grams daily.

If adequate control is obtained without side-effects, reduction in dosage of both Diabinese and metformin should be undertaken slowly (reducing the dosage of one drug at a time) in an attempt to maintain control with the least possible medication.

Contra-indications, warnings, etc
Contra-indications: Hypersensitivity to Diabinese; juvenile or growth-onset diabetes mellitus; severe or unstable 'brittle' diabetes; diabetes complicated by ketosis and acidosis, diabetic coma, major surgery, severe infection, or severe trauma; patients with serious impairment of hepatic, renal or thyroid function.

Precautions
General: Hypoglycaemic: All sulphonylurea drugs are capable of producing severe hypoglycaemia. Proper patient selection, dosage and instructions are important to avoid hypoglycaemic episodes. Renal or hepatic insufficiency may cause elevated blood levels of Diabinese and the latter may also diminish gluconeogenic capacity, both of which increase the risk of serious hypoglycaemic reactions. Elderly, debilitated or malnourished patients, and those with adrenal or pituitary insufficiency are particularly susceptible to the hypoglycaemic action of glucose-lowering drugs. Hypoglycaemia may be difficult to recognise in the elderly, and in people who are takeing beta-adrenergic blocking drugs. Hypoglycaemia is more likely to occur when caloric intake is deficient, after severe or prolonged exercise, when alcohol is ingested, or when more than one glucose-lowering drug is used.

Because of the long half-life of Diabinese, patients who become hypoglycaemic during therapy require careful supervision of the dose and frequent meals for at least 3 to 5 days. Hospitalisation and intravenous glucose may be necessary.

Loss of control of blood glucose: When a patient

stabilised on any diabetic regimen is exposed to stress such as fever, trauma, infection, or surgery, a loss of control may occur. At such times, it may be necessary to discontinue Diabinese and administer insulin.

The effectiveness of any oral hypoglycaemic drug, like Diabinese, in lowering blood glucose to a desired level, decreases in many patients over a period of time. This may be due to progression of the severity of the diabetes or to diminished responsiveness to the drug. This phenomenon is known as secondary failure, to distinguish it from primary failure in which the drug is ineffective in an individual patient when first given.

Information for patients: Patients should be informed of the potential risks and advantages of Diabinese and of alternative modes of therapy. They should also be informed about the importance of adherence to dietary instructions, of a regular exercise programme, and of regular testing of urine and/or blood glucose.

The risks of hypoglycaemia, its symptoms and treatment, and conditions that predispose to its development should be explained to patients and responsible family members. Primary and secondary failure should also be explained.

Patients should be instructed to contact their physician promptly if they experience symptoms of hypoglycaemia or other adverse reactions.

Laboratory tests: Blood and urine glucose should be monitored periodically. Measurement of glycosylated haemoglobin may be useful.

Drug interactions: The hypoglycaemic action of sulphonylurea may be potentiated by certain drugs including nonsteroidal anti-inflammatory agents and other drugs that are highly protein bound, salicylates, sulphonamides, chloramphenicol, probenecid, coumarins, monoamine oxidase inhibitors and beta-adrenergic blocking agents. When such drugs are administered to a patient receiving Diabinese, the patient should be observed closely for hypoglycaemia. When such drugs are withdrawn from a patient receiving Diabinese, the patient should be observed closely for loss of control.

A disulfiram-like reaction may be produced by the ingestion of alcohol.

Certain drugs tend to produce hyperglycaemia and may lead to loss of control. These drugs include the thiazides and other diuretics, corticosteroids, phenothiazines, thyroid products, oestrogens, oral contraceptives, phenytoin, nicotinic acid, sympathomimetics, calcium channel blocking drugs and isoniazid. When such drugs are administered to or withdrawn from a patient receiving Diabinese, the patient should be closely observed for loss of control. Diabetic control may be altered in patients also treated with cyclophosphamide.

Use in pregnancy: Diabinese is contra-indicated during pregnancy. Serious consideration should be given to the potential hazard of using Diabinese in women of childbearing age who may become pregnant.

Nursing mothers; Diabinese is excreted in breast milk and it is not recommended that a woman breast feed while taking this medication.

Use in children: Safety and effectiveness in children have not been established.

Side-effects: The majority of side-effects have been dose-related, transient, and have responded to dose reduction or withdrawal of the medication. However, clinical experience thus far has shown that, as with other sulphonylureas, some side-effects associated with hypersensitivity may be severe and deaths have been reported in some instances.

Hypoglycaemia: See 'Precautions' and 'Overdosage' sections.

Gastrointestinal reactions: Cholestatic jaundice may occur rarely; Diabinese should be discontinued if this occurs. Gastrointestinal disturbances are the most common reactions; nausea has been reported in less than 5% of patients and diarrhoea, vomiting, anorexia, and hunger in less than 2%. Other gastrointestinal disturbances have occurred in less than 1% of patients. They tend to be dose related and may disappear when dosage is reduced.

Dermatological reactions: Pruritis has been reported in less than 3% of patients. Other allergic skin reactions, e.g., urticaria and maculopapular eruptions have been reported in approximately 1% or less of patients. These may be transient and may disappear despite continued use of Diabinese; if skin reactions persist the drug should be discontinued.

Porphyria cutanea tarda and photosensitivity reactions have been reported with sulphonylureas.

Skin eruptions progressing to erythema multiforme and exfoliative dermatitis have also been reported.

Haematological reactions: Leucopenia, agranulocytosis, thrombocytopenia, haemolytic anaemia, aplastic anaemia, and pancytopenia have been reported with sulphonylureas.

Metabolic reactions: Hepatic porphyria and disulfiram-like reactions have rarely been reported with Diabinese. See 'Drug interactions' section.

Endocrine reactions: On rare occasions, Diabinese has caused a reaction identical to the syndrome of inappropriate antidiuretic hormone (ADH) secretion. The features of this syndrome result from excessive water retention and include hyponatraemia, low serum osmolality, and high urine osmolality.

Overdosage: Overdosage of sulphonylureas including Diabinese can produce hypoglycaemia. Mild hypoglycaemic symptoms without loss of consciousness or neurological findings should be treated aggressively with oral glucose and adjustments in drug dosage and/or meal patterns. Close monitoring should continue until the physician is assured that the patient is out of danger. Severe hypoglycaemic reactions with coma, seizure, or other neurological impairment occur infrequently, but constitute medical emergencies requiring immediate hospitalisation. If hypoglycaemic coma is diagnosed or suspected, the patient should be given a rapid intravenous injection of concentrated (50%) glucose solution. This should be followed by a continuous infusion of a more dilute (10%) glucose solution at a rate that will maintain the blood glucose at a level above 5.6 mmol/l (100 mg/dl). Patients should be closely monitored for a minimum of 24 to 48 hours since hypoglycaemia may recur after apparent clinical recovery.

Pharmaceutical precautions Store below 25°C.

Legal category POM.

Package quantities Diabinese 100 mg and 250 mg tablets are packed into blister strips of twenty tablets each. These are available in packs of 100 tablets.

Further information Nil.

Product licence numbers
100 mg Tablets   0057/5015
250 mg Tablets   0057/5016

EXIREL* METERED INHALER ▼

Presentation Exirel is presented as a metered dose inhaler, delivering 0.2 mg pirbuterol as the acetate per actuation. Each canister is capable of delivering at least 200 individual doses. Pirbuterol acetate is a white crystalline powder which is very soluble in water.

Uses *Actions:* Exirel is a beta-adrenergic receptor agonist, which has been shown *in vitro* and in *in vivo* animal studies to exert a more selective action on $beta_2$-adrenergic receptors located in the lung than on $beta_1$-receptors in the heart muscle. No data exist to confirm this in man.

Indications: Exirel inhaler is indicated for the treatment or prophylaxis of bronchial asthma and the reversible bronchospasm which may be associated with bronchitis and emphysema.

Dosage and administration The dose of Exirel for adults and children over 12 years is 1 or 2 inhalations (0.2 mg or 0.4 mg). For maintenance or prophylactic therapy the recommended dosage is 2 inhalations (0.4 mg) three or four times daily which can be increased, but the total should not exceed 12 inhalations (2.4 mg) daily. With repetitive dosing, inhalation should usually not be repeated more often than every four hours. To use the Exirel inhaler, patients should actuate the valve shortly after the beginning of a slow inhalation which should be followed by at least 10 second breath holding.

Contra-indications, warnings, etc

Contra-indications: Exirel inhaler is contra-indicated in patients known to be sensitive to sympathomimetic agents, and in patients who are receiving non-selective beta-adrenergic blocking agents.

Warnings: If the recommended dose of Exirel inhaler fails to maintain effective relief, patients should be advised to seek immediate medical attention.

Excessive use of sympathomimetic inhalants has been associated with an increased incidence of adverse reactions including life-threatening dysrhythmias.

Use in pregnancy: Animal tests show no teratogenic effects, but the safety of Exirel inhaler during pregnancy or lactation has not yet been established. The expected therapeutic effects of the drug should be weighed against the possible hazard to the mother or child in these situations.

Use in children: Exirel inhaler is not presently recommended for children below the age of 12 due to lack of clinical data in this age group. For children between the ages of 6 and 12 years the use of Exirel Syrup is recommended.

Use in the elderly: No additional recommendations are made for elderly patients. Use of the lowest dose giving adequate clinical efficacy is advised.

Precautions: As with other sympathomimetic agents, Exirel inhaler should be used with caution in patients with thyrotoxicosis.

Side-effects: Side-effects such as tremors, headache, nervousness, insomnia, palpitations have been reported infrequently and are similar to those reactions recorded with other $beta_2$-adrenergic agonists.

Overdosage: In the event of overdosage with Exirel inhaler, supportive and symptomatic treatment is indicated. Cardioselective beta-blocking drugs may be useful but should be used with caution in patients with a history of bronchospasm.

Pharmaceutical precautions The Exirel inhaler should be stored below 30°C. It must not be exposed to heat or punctured.

Legal category POM.

Package quantities Each canister of Exirel inhaler contains sufficient material to give at least 200 metered doses of pirbuterol as pirbuterol acetate.

Further information Following administration of Exirel inhaler a clinically significant improvement in pulmonary function is usually observed within 5–10 minutes with maximum effect within 15–30 minutes. The duration of action of Exirel is at least five hours. The efficacy of Exirel is not diminished on chronic administration.

In man plasma levels of drug following inhaler administration were undetectable. However urine contained approximately 15% of the dose as unchanged drug and approximately 36% as the sulphate conjugate after oral dosing.

Product licence number Exirel inhaler 0057/0184.

EXIREL* CAPSULES AND SYRUP ▼

Presentation Exirel is available as capsules containing 10 mg or 15 mg or as a syrup containing 7.5 mg/5 ml of pirbuterol as the hydrochloride.

The 10 mg capsule has a turquoise body and an olive cap printed 'Exirel 10' and 'Pfizer'. The 15 mg capsule has a turquoise body and a beige cap printed 'Exirel 15' and 'Pfizer'. The syrup is a clear, colourless to pale yellow, cherry burgundy flavoured, liquid.

Pirbuterol hydrochloride is a white crystalline powder which is very soluble in water.

Uses *Actions:* Exirel is a beta-adrenergic receptor agonist, which has been shown *in vitro* and in *in vivo* animal studies to exert a more selective action on $beta_2$-adrenergic receptors located in the lung than on $beta_1$ receptors in the heart muscle. No data exist to confirm this in man.

Indications: Exirel capsules and syrup are indicated for the treatment and prophylaxis of bronchial asthma and the reversible bronchospasm which may be associated with bronchitis and emphysema.

Dosage and administration For adults, and children 12 years and above, the effective dosage of Exirel capsules or syrup is 10 mg or 15 mg administered three or four times daily.

For children between the age of 6 and 12 years, the dose is 7.5 mg (5 ml syrup) four times daily.

The maximum total daily recommended dose is 60 mg for adults and 30 mg for children 6–12 years of age.

Contra-indications, warnings, etc

Contra-indications: Exirel capsules and syrup are contra-indicated in patients known to be sensitive to sympathomimetic agents, and in patients who are receiving non-selective beta-adrenergic blocking agents.

Warnings: If the recommended dose of Exirel capsules or syrup fails to maintain effective relief, patients should be advised to seek immediate medical attention.

Use in pregnancy: Animal tests show no teratogenic effects, but the safety of Exirel capsules and syrup for use during pregnancy or lactation has not yet been established. The expected therapeutic effects of the drug should be weighed against the possible hazard to the mother or child in these situations.

Use in young children: The efficacy and safety of oral dosage forms of Exirel has not yet been established in children below the age of 6 years.

Use in the elderly: No additional recommendations are made for elderly patients. Use of the lowest dose giving adequate clinical efficacy is advised.

Precautions: As with other sympathomimetic agents, Exirel capsules and syrup should be used with caution in patients with thyrotoxicosis, coronary artery disease or cardiac dysrhythmias.

Side-effects: Side-effects such as tremors, headache, nervousness, insomnia, palpitations have been reported infrequently and are similar to those reactions recorded with other beta$_2$-adrenergic agonists.

Overdosage: In the event of overdosage with Exirel, supportive and symptomatic treatment is indicated. Cardioselective beta-blocking drugs may be useful but should be used with caution in patients with a history of bronchospasm.

Pharmaceutical precautions Exirel capsules should be stored below 30°C. Exirel syrup should be stored below 25°C.

Legal category POM.

Package quantities Exirel capsules, 10 mg or 15 mg are supplied in packs of 100.

Exirel syrup is supplied in bottles containing 150 ml. (7.5 mg/5 ml).

Further information Following administration of Exirel capsules or syrup a clinically significant improvement in pulmonary function is usually observed within one hour with maximum effect within 1–2 hours. Following oral administration the duration of action of Exirel is six hours or more. The efficacy of Exirel is not diminished on chronic administration.

In man maximum levels of drug appear in plasma 1–3 hours after oral dosing. The half life is approximately two hours. The drug is extensively metabolised with the sulphate conjugate being the chief urinary excretion product.

Product licence numbers
Exirel Capsules 10 mg 0057/0229
Exirel Capsules 15 mg 0057/0230
Exirel Syrup 0057/0208.

FASIGYN*

Presentation Fasigyn (tinidazole) is available as 500 mg film coated white tablets or as an intravenous formulation presented in bottles of 400 ml (800 mg) and 800 ml (1600 mg) tinidazole.

Uses *Actions:* Fasigyn is rapidly and completely absorbed after oral therapy. Peak serum levels usually occur within two hours after administration and decline slowly, with an elimination half-life of 12 to 14 hours.

In healthy volunteers, peak plasma concentrations at 2 hours after a single oral 2 g dose vary between 40–51 mcg/ml. At 24 hours the values are between 11–19 mcg/ml. Detectable levels of approximately 1 mcg/ml are still observed up to 72 hours.

In healthy volunteers, Fasigyn 1600 mg given as a single intravenous infusion over 10–15 minutes gives peak plasma concentrations of 32 mcg/ml declining to

8.6 mcg/ml at 24 hours, 2.1 mcg/ml at 48 hours and 0.5 mcg/ml at 72 hours.

In healthy volunteers, Fasigyn 800 mg given as a single intravenous infusion over 10–15 minutes gives peak plasma concentrations of between 14–21 mcg/ml. At 24 hours post-infusion the values are between 4–5 mcg/ml, justifying once daily dosage administration.

Studies with labelled Fasigyn in humans show that Fasigyn is excreted mainly in the urine and to a lesser extent in faeces in a proportion of 5 to 1 measured as radioactivity excreted after 5 days. The urinary recovery of unchanged Fasigyn is around 25% of administered drug while metabolites account for approximately 12%.

In patients with moderate to severe renal impairment the pharmacokinetic characteristics are not markedly changed in comparison with those in normal volunteers. Thus modification of the dosage in patients with impaired renal function is not necessary.

The plasma protein binding is approximately 12%.

Following dosing with Fasigyn the compound is well distributed into body tissues in clinically effective concentrations and effectively passes the blood brain barrier.

Fasigyn is active against both protozoa and obligate anaerobic bacteria. The activity against protozoa involves *Trichomonas vaginalis, Entamoeba histolytica* and *Giardia lamblia.*

The mode of action of Fasigyn against anaerobic bacteria and protozoa involves penetration of the drug into the cell of the micro-organism and subsequent damage of DNA strands or inhibition of their synthesis.

Fasigyn is active against *Gardnerella vaginalis* and most anaerobic bacteria including *Bacteroides fragilis, Bacteroides melaninogenicus, Bacteroides* spp., *Clostridium* spp., *Eubacterium* spp., *Fusobacterium* spp., *Peptococcus* spp., *Peptostreptococcus* spp., and *Veillonella* spp.

Indications: 1. *Prophylaxis:* The prevention of post-operative infections caused by anaerobic bacteria, especially those associated with colonic, gastro-intestinal and gynaecological surgery.

2. *Treatment of anaerobic infections such as:*
Intraperitoneal infections: peritonitis, abscess.
Gynaecological infections: endometritis, endomyometritis, tubo-ovarian abscess.
Bacterial septicaemia.
Post-operative wound infections.
Skin and soft tissue infections.
Upper and lower respiratory tract infections: pneumonia, empyema, lung abscess.
3. Non-specific vaginitis.
4. Acute ulcerative gingivitis.
5. Urogenital trichomoniasis in both male and female patients.
6. Giardiasis.
7. Intestinal amoebiasis.
8. Amoebic involvement of the liver.

Intravenous Fasigyn is indicated in the prophylaxis or treatment of anaerobic infections and in those conditions where oral treatment is impractical or impossible.

Dosage and administration

1. *Prevention of post-operative infections: Adult: Oral:* A single oral dose of 2 g approximately 12 hours before surgery.

Intravenous: A total dose of 1600 mg given either as a single pre-operative infusion or in two divided doses: the first dose just prior to surgery, the second peri-operatively or post-operatively no later than 12 hours after completion of surgical intervention.

Children less than 12 years: Data are not available to allow dosage recommendations for children below the age of 12 years in the prevention of post-operative infections.

2. *Treatment of anaerobic infections: Adults: Oral:* An initial dose of 2 g the first day followed by 1 g daily given as a single dose or as 500 mg twice daily.

Intravenous: An initial dose of 800 mg intravenously followed by 800 mg/day, given as a single daily dose or in 2 divided doses until oral therapy is feasible.

Intravenous therapy should be discontinued when feasible and oral therapy continued in a daily dosage of 1 g given as a single dose or as 500 mg twice daily.

Treatment for 5 to 6 days will generally be adequate but clinical judgement must determine the duration of therapy, particularly when eradication of infection from certain sites may be difficult.

Regular clinical and laboratory observation is advised if it is considered necessary to continue therapy for more than 7 days.

Children less than 12 years: Data are not available to allow dosage recommendations for children below the age of 12 years in the treatment of anaerobic infections.

3. *Non-specific vaginitis: Adults:* Non-specific vaginitis is treated with a single oral dose of 2 g. Higher cure rates have been achieved with 2 g single daily doses on two consecutive days (total dosage 4 g).

4. *Acute ulcerative gingivitis: Adults:* A single oral dose of 2 g.

5. *Urogenital trichomoniasis:* When infection with *Trichomonas vaginalis* is confirmed, simultaneous treatment of the consort is recommended.

Adult preferred regimen: A single dose of 2 g.

Children: A single dose of 50 to 75 mg/kg of body weight. It may be necessary to repeat this dose once in some cases.

6. *Giardiasis: Adults:* A single dose of 2 g orally.

Children: A single dose of 50 to 75 mg/kg of body weight. It may be necessary to repeat this dose once in some cases.

7. *Intestinal amoebiasis: Adults:* A single daily dose of 2 g orally for two or three days.

Children: A single daily dose of 50 to 60 mg/kg of body weight on each of three successive days.

8. *Amoebic involvement of the liver: Adults:* Total dosage varies from 4.5 to 12g, depending on the virulence of the *Entamoeba histolytica.*

Treatment should be initiated with 1.5 to 2 g orally as a single daily dose for 3 days. In the occasional instance where a three-day course is ineffective, treatment may be continued for up to a total of five days.

Children: A single daily dose of 50 to 60 mg/kg of body weight on each of five successive days.

In amoebic involvement of the liver, the aspiration of pus may be required in addition to therapy with Fasigyn.

Oral administration: It is recommended that oral Fasigyn be taken during or after a meal.

Intravenous administration: Intravenous Fasigyn should be given as an infusion of 400 mg (200 ml) over 20 minutes or 800 mg (400 ml) over 40 minutes.

Infusion with other intravenous solutions: Intravenous Fasigyn may be co-administered with the following frequently used intravenous solutions: 5% Dextrose in Water, 20% Dextrose in Water, isotonic saline, potassium chloride (20 mEq and 40 mEq).

Contra-indications, warnings, etc

Contra-indications: As with other drugs of similar structure, Fasigyn is contra-indicated in patients having, or with a history of blood dyscrasia although no persistent haematological abnormalities have been noted in clinical or animal studies.

Fasigyn should be avoided in patients with organic neurological disorders.

Fasigyn should not be administered to patients with known hypersensitivity to the drug.

Use in pregnancy: Fasigyn crosses the placental barrier and is present in the breast milk when administered to nursing mothers. Since the effects of compounds of this class on foetal development and in the newborn are not definitely known, Fasigyn is contra-indicated during the first trimester of pregnancy and in nursing mothers during the neo-natal period. While there is no evidence that Fasigyn is harmful during the later stages of pregnancy, its use during the last two trimesters of pregnancy requires that the potential benefits be weighed against possible hazards to mother and foetus.

Use in the elderly: There are no special recommendations for this age group.

Precautions: Although believed not to occur with Fasigyn, related compounds when taken together with alcoholic beverages have caused abdominal cramps, flushing, and vomiting.

Drugs of similar chemical structure have also produced various neurological disturbances such as dizziness, vertigo, inco-ordination, and ataxia. If, during therapy with Fasigyn, abnormal neurological signs develop, therapy should be discontinued.

Side-effects: Reported side-effects have generally been infrequent, mild and self-limiting. Side-effects from the gastro-intestinal tract include nausea, vomiting, anorexia, diarrhoea and metallic taste.

Hypersensitivity reactions, occasionally severe, may occur in rare cases in the form of skin rash, pruritus, urticaria and angioneurotic oedema.

As with related compounds, Fasigyn may produce transient leucopenia. Other rarely reported side-effects are headache, tiredness, furry tongue and dark urine.

With the intravenous dosage form, thrombophlebitis has occasionally been observed at the infusion site.

Overdosage: There is no specific treatment for gross overdosage of Fasigyn, but early gastric lavage is recommended following overdosage by mouth.

Pharmaceutical precautions Tablets – Store below 25°C in a dry place, away from light.
Intravenous – Store below 25°C, away from light.
Discard any unused solution following withdrawal of dose.

Legal category POM.

Package quantities 20 × 500 mg tablets. Bottles of 400 ml or 800 ml intravenous infusion (2 mg/ml).

Further information Each 100 ml Fasigyn intravenous infusion includes 5.5 g dextrose monohydrate PhEur.

Product licence numbers
500 mg tablet   0057/0150
Intravenous   0057/0189.

FELDENE*
FELDENE* 20

Presentation Feldene is available as maroon and blue capsules, coded 'Pfizer' and 'FEL 10' containing 10 mg piroxicam and maroon capsules coded 'Pfizer' and 'FEL 20' containing 20 mg piroxicam.

Feldene suppositories (white to off-white) containing 20 mg piroxicam.

Feldene dispersible tablets are available in two strengths: 10 mg – white to off-white flat round tablets coded 'FEL' and '10' on one side, with an incised line between, and 'Pfizer' on the other. 20 mg – white to off-white capsular tablets coded 'FEL20' on one side and lettered 'PFIZER' on the other. The dispersible tablet should be dropped into a small amount of water and stirred.

Uses Feldene is a non-steroidal anti-inflammatory agent indicated for a variety of conditions requiring anti-inflammatory and/or analgesic activity, such as rheumatoid arthritis, oesteoarthritis (arthrosis, degenerative joint disease) ankylosing spondylitis, acute musculoskeletal disorders and acute gout.

Dosage and administration
Rheumatoid arthritis, osteoarthritis, ankylosing spondylitis: The recommended starting dose is 20 mg given as a single daily dose. The majority of patients will be maintained on 20 mg daily. A relatively small group of patients may be maintained on as little as 10 mg daily. Some patients may require up to 30 mg daily given in single or divided doses. Long-term administration of doses 30 mg or higher carries an increased risk of gastro-intestinal side-effects.

Acute gout: Therapy should be initiated by a single dose of 40 mg followed on the next four to six days with 40 mg daily, given in a single or divided daily dosage. Feldene is not indicated for the long-term management of gout.

Acute musculoskeletal disorders: Therapy should be initiated with 40 mg daily for the first two days, given in single or divided doses. For the remainder of the seven to fourteen day treatment period, the dose should be reduced to 20 mg daily.

Feldene dispersible tablets can be swallowed whole with a fluid, or may be dispersed in a minimum of 50 ml of water and then swallowed.

Combined administration: The total daily dosage of Feldene administered as capsules, dispersible tablets and suppositories should not exceed the maximal recommended daily dosage as indicated above.

Use in the elderly: Elderly, frail or debilitated patients may tolerate side-effects less well and such patients should be carefully supervised.

As with other NSAID's, caution should be used in the treatment of elderly patients who are more likely to be suffering from impaired renal, hepatic or cardiac function.

Rectal: For each indication, the dosage of Feldene suppositories, when used alone, is identical with the dosage of Feldene capsules. Feldene suppositories offer an alternative route of administration for those physicians who may wish to prescribe them in certain patients, or for those patients who prefer them.

Contra-indications, warnings, etc
Contra-indications:
  1. Active peptic ulceration or a history of recurrent ulceration.
  2. Feldene should not be used in those patients who have previously shown a hypersensitivity to the drug. The potential exists for cross sensitivity to aspirin and other non-steroidal anti-inflammatory drugs.
  3. Feldene should not be given to patients in whom aspirin and other non-steroidal anti-inflammatory drugs induce the symptoms of asthma, rhinitis, angioedema or urticaria.
  4. Feldene suppositories should not be used in patients with any inflammatory lesions of the rectum or anus, or in patients with a recent history of rectal or anal bleeding.

Warnings
Use in pregnancy: Although no teratogenic effects were seen in animal testing, the safety of Feldene during pregnancy or during lactation has not yet been established. Feldene inhibits prostaglandin synthesis and release through a reversible inhibition of the cyclo-oxygenase enzyme. This effect, as with other non-steroidal anti-inflammatory drugs has been associated with an increased incidence of dystocia and delayed parturition in pregnant animals when drug administration was continued into late pregnancy. Non-steroidal anti-inflammatory drugs are also known to induce closure of the ductus arteriosus in infants. A preliminary study indicates that piroxicam is found in maternal milk in a concentration of approximately 1% of that reached in plasma. Feldene is not recommended for use in nursing mothers as clinical safety has not been established.

Use in children: Dosage recommendations and indications for use in children have not been established.

Precautions: Peptic ulceration and gastro-intestinal bleeding, in rare cases fatal, have been reported with Feldene.

Drug administration should be closely supervised in patients with a history of upper gastro-intestinal disease. Feldene should be withdrawn if peptic ulceration or gastro-intestinal bleeding occurs.

Feldene suppositories should be given with caution to patients with any rectal or anal pathology.

In rare cases, non-steroidal anti-inflammatory drugs may cause interstitial nephritis, glomerulitis, papillary necrosis and the nephrotic syndrome. Such agents inhibit the synthesis of renal prostaglandin which plays a supportive role in the maintenance of renal perfusion in patients whose renal blood flow and blood volume are decreased. In these patients, administration of a non-steroidal anti-inflammatory drug may precipitate overt renal decompensation which is typically followed by recovery to pretreatment state upon its discontinuation of non-steroidal anti-inflammatory therapy. Patients at greatest risk of such a reaction are those with congestive heart failure, liver cirrhosis, nephrotic syndrome and overt renal disease. Because of the extensive renal excretion of piroxicam and its biotransformation products (less than 5% of the daily dose excreted unchanged, see Further Information), lower doses of Feldene should be anticipated in patients with impaired renal function and they should be carefully monitored.

Non-steroidal anti-inflammatory drugs may cause sodium, potassium and fluid retention, and may interfere with the natriuretic action of diuretic agents. These properties should be kept in mind when treating patients with compromised cardiac function or hypertension since they may be responsible for a worsening of those conditions.

As with other non steroidal anti-inflammatory drugs, bleeding has been reported rarely when Feldene has been administered to patients on coumarin-type anticoagulants. Patients should be monitored closely if Feldene and oral anticoagulants are administered together.

Feldene, like other non-steroidal anti-inflammatory drugs, decreases platelet aggregation and prolongs bleeding time. This effect should be kept in mind when bleeding times are determined.

As with other non-steroidal anti-inflammatory drugs, the use of Feldene in conjunction with aspirin or the concomitant use of two non-steroidal anti-inflammatory drugs is not recommended because data are inadequate to demonstrate that the combination produces greater improvement than that achieved with the drug alone and the potential for adverse reactions is increased.

Because of reports of adverse eye findings with non-steroidal anti-inflammatory drugs, it is recommended that patients who develop visual complaints during treatment with Feldene have ophthalmic evaluation.

Feldene is highly protein-bound, and therefore might be expected to displace other protein-bound drugs. The physician should closely monitor patients for change in dosage requirements when administering Feldene to patients on highly protein-bound drugs. Non-steroidal anti-inflammatory drugs, including Feldene, have been reported to increase steady state plasma lithium levels. It is recommended that these levels are monitored when initiating, adjusting and discontinuing Feldene.

Studies in man have shown that the concomitant administration of Feldene and aspirin resulted in a reduction of plasma levels of piroxicam to about 80% of the normal values. Concomitant administration of antacids had no effect on piroxicam plasma levels. Neither did concurrent therapy with Feldene and digoxin affect the plasma levels of either drug.

Side-effects: Gastro-intestinal symptoms are the most commonly encountered side-effects but in most instances do not interfere with the course of therapy. These side-effects include stomatitis, anorexia, epigastric distress, nausea, constipation, abdominal discomfort, flatulence, diarrhoea, abdominal pain and indigestion. Objective evaluations of gastric mucosal appearances and intestinal blood loss show that 20 mg/day of Feldene administered either in single or divided daily doses is significantly less irritating to the gastro-intestinal tract than aspirin.

Long-term administration of doses of 30 mg or higher carries an increased risk of gastro-intestinal side-effects.

As with other non-steroidal anti-inflammatory drugs, oedema, mainly ankle oedema, has been reported in a small percentage of patients and the possibility of precipitating congestive cardiac failure in elderly patients or those with compromised cardiac function should therefore be borne in mind. CNS effects, such as dizziness, headache, somnolence, insomnia, depression, nervousness, hallucinations, mood alterations, dream abnormalities, mental confusion, paraesthesias and vertigo have been reported rarely. Swollen eyes, blurred vision and eye irritations have been reported. Routine ophthalmoscopy and slit-lamp examination have revealed no evidence of ocular changes. Malaise and tinnitus may occur.

Dermal hypersensitivity reactions, usually in the form of rash and pruritus have been reported. Onycholysis and alopecia have rarely been reported. Photo-allergic reactions have infrequently been associated with therapy. As with other non-steroidal anti-inflammatory drugs, toxic epidermal necrolysis (Lyell's disease) and Stevens-Johnson syndrome may develop in rare cases. Vesiculo bullous reactions have been reported rarely.

Ano-rectal reactions to suppositories have presented as local pain, burning, pruritus, tenesmus. Rare instances of rectal bleeding have occurred.

Reversible elevations of BUN and creatinine have been reported (see Precautions).

Decreases in haemoglobin and haematocrit, unassociated with obvious gastro-intestinal bleeding, have occurred. Anaemia has been reported. Thrombocytopenia and non-thrombocytopenic purpura (Henoch-Schoenlein), leucopenia and eosinophilia have been reported. Rare cases of aplastic anaemia are also reported. Epistaxis has rarely been reported. Changes in different liver function parameters have been observed. As with most other non-steroidal anti-inflammatory drugs, some patients may develop increased serum transaminase levels during treatment with Feldene.

Palpitations and dyspnoea have been reported rarely. Anecdotal cases of positive ANA have been reported rarely in patients receiving Feldene.

Metabolic abnormalities such as hypoglycaemia, hyperglycaemia, weight increase or decrease have been reported rarely.

Overdosage: In the event of overdosage with Feldene, supportive and symptomatic therapy is indicated. Preliminary studies indicate that administration of activated charcoal may result in reduced re-absorption of piroxicam thus reducing the total amount of active drug available.

Pharmaceutical precautions Capsules and Dispersible Tablets: Store below 30°C. Suppositories: Store below 25°C. Do not refrigerate.

Legal category POM.

Package quantities
Feldene Capsules 10 mg: Pack of 60
Feldene 20 Capsules 20 mg: Pack of 30
Feldene Suppositories 20 mg: Pack of 10
Feldene Dispersible Tablets 10 mg: Pack of 60
Feldene Dispersible Tablets 20 mg: Pack of 30.

Further information Feldene is smoothly absorbed following oral or rectal administration. The extent and rate of absorption are not influenced by administration in the fasting state. The plasma half-life is approximately 50 hours in man and stable plasma concentrations are maintained throughout the day on once-daily dosage. Continuous treatment with 20 mg/day for periods of 1 year produces similar blood levels to those seen once steady state first is achieved.

Feldene is extensively metabolised and less than 5% of the daily dose is excreted unchanged in urine and faeces. One important metabolic pathway is hydroxylation of the pyridyl ring of the Feldene side chain, followed by conjugation with glucuronic acid and urinary elimination.

Product licence numbers

Feldene Capsules 10 mg	0057/0145
Feldene 20 Capsules 20 mg	0057/0146
Feldene Suppositories 20 mg	0057/0219
Feldene Dispersible Tablets 10 mg	0057/0240
Feldene Dispersible Tablets 20 mg	0057/0242.

GLIBENESE*

Presentation Glibenese (glipizide) is available as white oblong tablets marked GBS/5 on the scored side and 'Pfizer' on the other. Each tablet contains 5 mg glipizide.

Uses *Actions:* Glibenese is an orally active sulphony- lurea which effectively reduces blood glucose to the normal range in properly selected patients with non- insulin-dependent diabetes mellitus (NIDDM). It elimi- nates or diminishes glycosuria and ameliorates symptoms such as polyuria, polydipsia and pruritus.

The primary mode of action of Glibenese in experimen- tal animals is the stimulation of insulin secretion from the beta-cells of pancreatic islet tissue. In man, stimulation of insulin secretion by Glibenese in response to a meal is undoubtedly of major importance. Fasting insulin levels are not elevated even on long-term Glibenese adminis- tration, but the post-prandial insulin response continues to be enhanced after at least 6 months of treatment. The insulinotropic response to a meal occurs within 30 minutes after an oral dose of Glibenese in diabetic patients, but elevated insulin levels do not persist beyond the time of the meal challenge. There is also increasing evidence that extrapancreatic effects involving potentia- tion of insulin action form a significant component of the activity of Glibenese.

Blood sugar control persists for up to 24 hours after a single dose of Glibenese even though plasma levels have declined to a small fraction of peak levels by that time. Once-daily administration of doses up to 15 mg has been shown to be safe and effective maintenance therapy in selected patients.

Some patients fail to respond initially, or gradually lose their responsiveness to sulphonylurea drugs, including Glibenese. Alternatively, Glibenese, may be effective in some patients who have not responded or have ceased to respond to other sulphonylureas.

Gastrointestinal absorption of Glibenese in man is uniform, rapid and essentially complete. Peak plasma concentrations occur 1–3 hours after a single oral dose. The half-life of elimination ranges from 2–4 hours in normal subjects, whether given intravenously or orally. The metabolic and excretory patterns are similar with the two routes of administration, indicating that first-pass metabolism is not significant. Glibenese does not accu- mulate in plasma on repeated oral administration. Total absorption and disposition of an oral dose was unaffected by food in normal volunteers, but absorption was delayed by about 40 minutes. Thus, Glibenese was more effective when administered about 30 minutes before, rather than with a test meal in diabetic patients. Protein binding was studied in serum from volunteers who received either oral or intravenous Glibenese and found to be 98–99% one hour after either route of administration. The apparent volume of distribution of Glibenese after intravenous administration was 11 litres, indicative of localisation within the extracellular fluid compartment.

The metabolism of Glibenese is extensive and occurs mainly in the liver. The primary metabolites are inactive hydroxylation products and polar conjugates and are excreted mainly in the urine. Less than 10% unchanged Glibenese is found in the urine.

In a placebo-controlled, crossover study in normal volunteers, Glibenese showed no anti-diuretic activity, and, in fact, led to a slight increase in free water clearance.

Indications: Glibenese is indicated as an adjunct to diet to lower the blood glucose in patients with non-insulin- dependent diabetes mellitus (type II, NIDDM), formerly known as maturity onset of diabetes, whose hypergly- caemia cannot be controlled by diet alone.

In initiating treatment for non-insulin dependent diabetes, diet should be emphasised as the primary form of treatment. Caloric restriction and weight loss are essential in the obese diabetic patient. Proper dietary management alone may be effective in controlling the blood glucose and symptoms of hyperglycaemia. The importance of regular physical activity should also be stressed, cardiovascular risk factors should be identified and corrective measures taken where possible.

Use of Glibenese must be viewed by both the physician and patient as a treatment in addition to diet, and not as a substitute for diet or as a convenient mechanism for avoiding dietary restraint. Furthermore, loss of blood glucose control on diet alone also may be transient, thus requiring only short-term administration of Glibenese.

During maintenance programmes, Glibenese should be discontinued if satisfactory lowering of blood glucose is no longer achieved. Judgments should be based on regular clinical and laboratory evaluation.

In considering the use of Glibenese in asymptomatic patients, it should be recognised that controlling the blood glucose in non-insulin-dependent diabetes, has not been definitely established to be effective in pre- venting the long-term cardiovascular or neurological complications of diabetes.

Patient selection: The most likely patient for therapy is one in whom diabetes is of the NIDDM type, stable, and not controlled by dietary regulation alone. A past history of diabetic coma does not necessarily preclude success- ful therapeutic control with Glibenese. A trial period may be indicated on certain patients who might be expected to respond to this type of medication, but who failed in initial trials with, or after having been on other oral sulphonylurea agents, or in patients whose diabetic control on such agents has not been satisfactory. Glibenese may prove effective and provide improved control of the diabetes. The final evaluation of response in patients who qualify as candidates for Glibenese is a therapeutic trial for a period of at least seven days. During the trial period, the absence of ketonuria together with a satisfactory control, indicates that the patient is respon- sive and amenable to control with the drug. However, the development of ketonuria within 24 hours after withdrawal of insulin usually will be indicative of a poor response. The patient is considered unresponsive if he fails to achieve satisfactory lowering of blood sugar levels or fails to obtain objective or subjective clinical improvement and if he develops ketonuria or glycosuria. Insulin is indicated for the therapy of such patients.

Dosage and administration There is no fixed dosage regimen for the management of diabetes mellitus with Glibenese or any other hypoglycaemic agent. In addition to the usual monitoring of urinary glucose, the patient's blood glucose must also be monitored periodically to determine the minimum effective dose for the patient, to detect primary failure: i.e. inadequate lowering of blood glucose at the maximum recommended dose of medica- tion, and to detect secondary failure, i.e. loss of adequate blood-glucose-lowering response after an initial period of effectiveness. Glycosylated haemoglobin levels may also be of value in monitoring the patient's response to therapy.

Short term administration of Glibenese may be suffi- cient during period of transient loss of control in patients usually controlled well on diet.

In general, Glibenese should be given approximately 30 minutes before a meal to achieve the greatest reduction in post-prandial hyperglycaemia.

Initial dose: The recommended starting dose is 5 mg, given before breakfast or the midday meal. Mild diabetics, elderly patients or those with liver disease may be started on 2.5 mg

Titration: Dosage adjustments should ordinarily be in increments of 2.5 to 5 mg, as determined by blood glucose response. At least several days should elapse between titration steps. The maximum recommended single dose is 15 mg. Doses above 15 mg should ordinarily be divided.

Maintenance: Some patients may be effectively controlled on a once-a-day regimen. Total daily dosage above 15 mg should ordinarily be divided. Total daily dosage above 30 mg has been given safely on a twice daily basis to long term patients. Patients can usually be stabilised on a dosage ranging from 2.5 to 30 mg daily. The maximum recommended daily dosage is 40 mg.

Use in the elderly: Because the elderly patient appears to be more sensitive to the hypoglycaemic effect of sulphonylurea drugs, older patients should be started on 2.5 mg daily.

In elderly patients, debilitated or malnourished patients, and patients with an impaired renal or hepatic function, the initial and maintenance dosing should be conservative to avoid hypoglycaemic reactions (see Precautions section).

Patients receiving insulin: As with other sulphonylurea class hypoglycaemics, many stable non-insulin-dependent diabetic patients receiving insulin may be safely placed on Glibenese. When transferring patients from insulin to Glibenese, the following general guidelines should be considered.

For patients whose daily insulin requirement is 20 units or less, insulin may be discontinued and Glibenese therapy begun at usual dosages. Several days should elapse between Glibenese titration steps.

For patients whose daily insulin requirement is greater than 20 units, the insulin dose should be reduced by 50% and Glibenese therapy initiated at usual dosages. Subsequent reductions in insulin dosage should depend on individual patient response. Several days should elapse between Glibenese steps.

During the insulin withdrawal period, the patient should test urine samples for sugar and ketone bodies at least three times daily. Patients should be instructed to contact the prescriber immediately if these tests are abnormal. In some cases, especially when the patient has been receiving greater than 40 units of insulin daily, it may be advisable to consider hospitalisation during the transition period.

Patients receiving other oral hypoglycaemic agents: As with other sulphonylurea class hypoglycaemics, no transition period is necessary when transferring patients to Glibenese. Patients should be observed carefully (1–2 weeks) for hypoglycaemia when being transferred from longer half-life sulphonylureas (e.g. chlorpropamide) to Glibenese due to potential overlapping of drug effect.

Concurrent biguanide therapy: As with other sulphonylureas, a proportion of patients who do not achieve optimal control with Glibenese alone, or who experience secondary failure, may be expected to have their control improved or restored by the addition of a biguanide.

For such patients, it is suggested that the dosage of Glibenese should be maintained and the biguanide chosen should be added using low doses initially and increasing the dosage of the biguanide progressively

until adequate control is achieved or restored. Should gastrointestinal side-effects appear, an attempt should be made to reduce the dosage of the biguanide.

Contra-indications, warnings, etc
Contra-indications: Glibenese is contra-indicated in the following conditions:
1. Patients who are hypersensitive to Glibenese.
2. Juvenile-onset diabetes.
3. Severe or unstable 'brittle' diabetes.
4. Diabetes complicated by ketosis and acidosis, major surgery, severe sepsis or severe trauma.
5. Severe renal, hepatic or thyroid impairment, coexistent renal and hepatic disease.

Precautions
General: Hypoglycaemia: All sulphonylurea drugs are capable of producing severe hypoglycaemia. Proper patient selection, dosage, and instructions are important to avoid hypoglycaemic episodes. Renal or hepatic insufficiency may cause elevated blood levels of Glibenese and the latter may also diminish gluconeogenic capacity, both of which increase the risk of serious hypoglycaemic reactions. Elderly, debilitated or malnourished patients, and those with adrenal or pituitary insufficiency are particularly susceptible to the hypoglycaemic action of glucose-lowering drugs. Hypoglycaemia may be difficult to recognise in the elderly, and in people who are taking beta-adrenergic blocking drugs. Hypoglycaemia is more likely to occur when caloric intake is deficient, after severe or prolonged exercise, when alcohol is ingested, or when more than one glucose-lowering drug is used.

Loss of control of blood glucose: When a patient stabilised on any diabetic regimen is exposed to stress such as fever, trauma, infection, or surgery, a loss of control may occur. At such times, it may be necessary to discontinue Glibenese and administer insulin.

The effectiveness of any oral hypoglycaemic drug, including Glibenese, in lowering blood glucose to a desired level decreases in many patients over a period of time, which may be due to progression of the severity of the diabetes or to diminished responsiveness to the drug. This phenomenon is known as secondary failure, to distinguish it from primary failure in which the drug is ineffective in an individual patient when first given.

Information for patients: Patients should be informed of the potential risks and advantages of Glibenese and of alternative modes of therapy. They should also be informed about the importance of adherence to dietary instructions, of a regular exercise programme, and of regular testing of urine and/or blood glucose.

The risk of hypoglycaemia, its symptoms and treatment, and conditions that predispose to its development should be explained to patients and responsible family members. Primary and secondary failure should also be explained.

Laboratory tests: Blood and urine glucose should be monitored periodically. Measurement of glycosylated haemoglobin may be useful.

Drug interaction: The hypoglycaemic action of sulphonylurea may be potentiated by certain drugs including nonsteroidal anti-inflammatory agents and other drugs that are highly protein bound, salicylates, sulphonamides, chloramphenicol, probenecid, coumarins, monoamine oxidase inhibitors and beta-adrenergic blocking agents. When such drugs are administered to a patient receiving Glibenese, the patient should be observed closely for hypoglycaemia. When such drugs are withdrawn from a patient receiving Glibenese, the patient should be observed closely for loss of control.

Certain drugs tend to produce hyperglycaemia and may lead to loss of control. These drugs include the thiazides and other diuretics, corticosteroids, phenothiazines, thyroid products, oestrogens, oral contraceptives, phenytoin, nicotinic acid, sympathomimetics, calcium channel blocking drugs and isoniazid. When such drugs are administered to or withdrawn from a patient receiving Glibenese, the patient should be closely observed for loss of control. Diabetic control may be altered in patients also treated with cyclophosphamide.

In the mouse, Glibenese pre-treatment did not cause an accumulation of acetaldehyde after ethanol administration. Clinical experience has confirmed the virtual absence of an alcohol interaction in man.

Use in pregnancy: Glibenese is contra-indicated during pregnancy. Serious consideration should be given to the potential hazard of using Glibenese in women of childbearing age who may become pregnant.

Nursing mothers: Although it is not known whether Glibenese is excreted in human milk, some sulphonylurea drugs are known to be so. It is therefore not recommended that a woman breast feed while taking this medication.

Use in children: Safety and effectiveness in children have not been established.

Side-effects: The majority of side-effects have been dose related, transient, and have responded to dose reduction or withdrawal of the medication. However, clinical experience thus far has shown that, as with other sulphonylureas some side-effects associated with hypersensitivity may be severe and deaths have been reported in some instances.

Hypoglycaemia: See 'Precautions' and 'Overdosage' sections.

Gastrointestinal: Gastrointestinal complaints include nausea, diarrhoea, constipation and gastralgia. They appear to be dose related and usually disappear on division or reduction of dosage.

Dermatological: Allergic skin reactions including erythema, morbilliform or maculopapular reactions, urticaria, pruritis and eczema have been reported. They frequently disappear with continued therapy. However, if they persist, the drug should be discontinued.

Miscellaneous: Dizziness, drowsiness and headache have each been reported in patients treated with Glibenese. They are usually transient and seldom require discontinuance of therapy.

Laboratory tests: The pattern of laboratory test abnormalities observed with Glibenese is similar to that for other sulphonylureas. Occasional mild to moderate elevations of SGOT, LDH, alkaline phosphatase, BUN and creatinine were noted. One case of jaundice was reported. The relationship of these abnormalities to Glibenese is uncertain, and they have rarely been associated with clinical symptoms.

Overdosage: There is no well documented experience with Glibenese overdosage. The acute oral toxicity was extremely low in all species tested (LD_{50} greater than 4g/kg).

Overdosage of sulphonylureas including Glibenese can produce hypoglycaemia. Mild hypoglycaemic symptoms without loss of consciousness or neurological findings should be treated aggressively with oral glucose and adjustments in drug dosage and/or meal patterns.

Close monitoring should continue until the physician is assured that the patient is out of danger. Severe hypoglycaemic reactions with coma, seizure, or other neurological impairment occur infrequently, but constitute medical emergencies requiring immediate hospitalisation. If hypoglycaemic coma is diagnosed or suspected, the patient should be given a rapid intravenous injection of concentrated (50%) glucose solution. This should be followed by continuous infusion of a more dilute (10%) glucose solution at a rate that will maintain the blood glucose at a level above 5.6 mmol/l (100 mg/dl). Patients should be closely monitored for a minimum of 24 to 48 hours since hypoglycaemia may recur after apparent clinical recovery. Clearance of Glibenese from plasma would be prolonged in persons with liver disease. Because of the extensive protein binding of Glibenese, dialysis is unlikely to be of benefit.

Pharmaceutical precautions Store below 25°C.

Legal category POM.

Package quantities Glibenese tablets 5 mg are packed into blister strips of ten tablets each. Available in cartons of 60 tablets.

Further information Nil.

Product licence number 0057/0113.

HYPOVASE*

Presentation Hypovase is available in tablets containing prazosin hydrochloride as follows:

0.5 mg white tablets, unscored: marked 'Pfizer' on one side.

1 mg scored orange tablets: marked HYP/1 on one side.

2 mg scored white tablets: marked HYP/2 on one side and 'Pfizer' on the other.

5 mg scored white tablets: marked HYP/5 on one side and 'Pfizer' on the other.

Uses *Actions:* Hypovase causes a decrease in total peripheral vascular resistance, but the exact mechanism of action is unknown. Animal studies suggest that the vasodilator effect of Hypovase is related to blockade of postsynaptic alpha-1-adrenoceptors. The results of forearm plethysmographic studies in humans demonstrate that the peripheral vasodilatation is a balanced effect on both resistance vessels (arterioles) and capacitance vessels (veins). Unlike non-selective alpha-adrenergic blocking agents, the antihypertensive action of Hypovase is usually not accompanied by reflex tachycardia.

Clinical studies have shown that Hypovase therapy is not associated with adverse changes in the serum lipid profile.

Studies indicate that chronic therapy with Hypovase has little effect on plasma renin activity.

Haemodynamic studies have been carried out in hypertensive patients following single dose administration and during the course of long term maintenance therapy. The results confirm that the usual therapeutic effect is a fall in blood pressure unaccompanied by a clinically significant change in cardiac output, heart rate, renal blood flow, or glomerular filtration rate.

Clinically, the antihypertensive effect is believed to be a direct result of peripheral vasodilatation. In man, blood pressure is lowered in both the supine and standing positions. This effect is more pronounced on the diastolic blood pressure. Tolerance has not been observed in long-term clinical use. Rebound elevation of blood pressure does not occur following abrupt cessation of Hypovase therapy.

Haemodynamic studies carried out in patients with congestive cardiac failure (left ventricular failure) following initial oral therapy and during the course of longer term maintenance therapy, both at rest and on exercise indicate that the therapeutic effect in these patients is due to a reduction in left ventricular filling pressure, reduction in cardiac impedence and an augmentation of cardiac output. These effects are associated with a balanced vasodilator effect on both arterioles and veins. The use of Hypovase in congestive heart failure does not provoke a reflex tachycardia and blood pressure reduction is minimal in normotensive patients.

Raynaud's phenomenon and Raynaud's disease have been successfully treated with Hypovase. The vasodilator action of the drug increases blood flow to affected parts to reduce severity of the signs, symptoms, frequency and duration of attacks.

Following oral administration in normal volunteers and hypertensive patients, plasma concentrations reach a peak in one to two hours, with a plasma half-life of two to three hours. Pharmacokinetic data in a limited number of patients with congestive heart failure, most of whom showed evidence of hepatic congestion, indicates that peak plasma concentrations are reached in 2.5 hours and plasma half-life is approximately 7 hours. Hypovase is highly bound to plasma protein. Animal studies indicate that Hypovase is extensively metabolised, primarily by demethylation and conjugation, and excreted mainly via bile and faeces. Similar metabolism and excretion has been documented in human studies.

Hypovase has been administered without any adverse drug interaction in clinical experience to date with the following;

(1) cardiac glycosides – digitalis and digoxin;

(2) hypoglycaemic agents – insulin, chlorpropamide, phenformin, tolazamide and tolbutamide;

(3) tranquillisers and sedatives – chlordiazepoxide, diazepam and phenobarbitone;

(4) agents for treatment of gout – allopurinol, colchicine and probenecid;

(5) anti-arrhythmic agents – procainamide and quinidine;

(6) analgesic, antipyretic, and anti-inflammatory agents – dextropropoxyphene, aspirin, indomethacin and phenylbutazone;

Uses *Indications:* Hypertension: Hypovase is indicated in the treatment of all grades of essential (primary) hypertension and of all grades of secondary hypertension of varied aetiology. It can be used as the initial and sole agent or it may be employed in a treatment regimen in conjunction with diuretic and/or other antihypertensive drugs as needed for proper patient response.

Renal blood flow and glomerular filtration rate are not impaired by long term oral administration and thus Hypovase can be used with safety in hypertensive patients with impaired renal function.

Congestive cardiac failure: Hypovase is indicated in the treatment of congestive cardiac failure. Hypovase may be added to the therapeutic regimen in those patients who have not shown a satisfactory response or who have become refractory to conventional therapy with diuretics, and/or cardiac glycosides.

Raynaud's phenomenon and Raynaud's disease: Hypovase is indicated in the treatment of Raynaud's phenomenon and Raynaud's disease.

Dosage and administration *Hypertension:* The dosage range is from 0.5–20 mg daily and treatment is best initiated at a low starting dose. It is recommended that the starting dose of 0.5 mg be given with food preferably with the evening meal, at least two or three hours before retiring.

The b.d. starter pack is available for the convenience of prescribers to initiate treatment up to 2 mg twice daily.

Specific recommendations: The following are given as guides to administration.

Patients receiving no antihypertensive therapy: It is recommended that therapy be initiated at 0.5 mg twice or three times daily for three to seven days, with the starting dose administered in the evening. Unless poor acceptance suggests the patient is unusually sensitive, this dose should be increased to 1 mg twice or three times daily for a further three to seven days. Thereafter, if necessary, the daily dose should be increased gradually as determined by the patients response to the blood pressure lowering effect. A significant number (of the order of 60–70%) of patients are likely to be maintained on a dosage regimen of Hypovase alone of up to 15 mg daily in divided doses. Maximum recommended daily dosage: 20 mg in divided doses.

Patients receiving diuretic therapy with inadequate control of blood pressure: The diuretic should be reduced to a maintenance dose level for the particular agent and Hypovase initiated with 0.5 mg at bedtime then continuing with 0.5 mg twice or three times daily. After the initial period of observation, the dosage of Hypovase should be gradually increased as determined by the patient's response.

Patients receiving other antihypertensive agents but with inadequate control: As some additive effect is anticipated, the other agent dosage level (e.g., beta-adrenergic blocking agents, methyldopa, reserpine, clonidine† etc.) should be reduced and Hypovase initiated at 0.5 mg at bedtime then continuing with 0.5 mg twice or three times daily. Subsequent dosage increase, should be made depending upon the patient's response.

There is evidence that adding Hypovase to beta-adrenergic blocking agent therapy may bring about a substantial reduction in blood pressure. Therefore, the low initial dosage regimen is recommended.

Use in the elderly: Since the elderly may be more susceptible to hypotension, therapy should be initiated with the lowest possible dose.

Patients with moderate to severe grades of renal impairment: Evidence to date shows that Hypovase does not further compromise renal function when used in patients with renal impairment. As some patients in this category have responded to small doses of Hypovase, it is recommended that therapy be initiated at 0.5 mg daily and that dosage increases be instituted cautiously.

Congestive cardiac failure (left ventricular failure): The recommended starting dose is 0.5 mg two, three or four times daily. Dosage should be titrated according to the patients's clinical response, based on careful monitoring of cardiopulmonary signs and symptoms, and when

† The manufacturer's instructions should be followed to avoid possible rebound hypertension with clonidine dose reduction.

indicated, haemodynamic studies. Dosage may be adjusted as often as every two to three days in patients under close medical supervision. In severely ill, decompensated patients, rapid dosage titration over one to two days may be indicated and is best done when haemodynamic monitoring is available. In clinical studies, the therapeutic dosages ranged from 4 mg to 20 mg daily in divided doses. Adjustment of dosage may be required in the course of Hypovase therapy in some patients to maintain optimal clinical improvement.

Suggested starting dosage: 0.5 mg two, three or four times daily, increasing to 4 mg in divided doses.

Usual daily maintenance dosage: 4 mg to 20 mg in divided doses.

Raynaud's phenomenon and Raynaud's disease: The recommended starting dosage is 0.5 mg twice daily given for a period of three to seven days and should be adjusted according to the patient's clinical response. Usual maintenance dosage 1 mg or 2 mg twice daily.

Contra-indications, warnings, etc
Contra-indications: Sensitivity to Hypovase.

Warnings – Use in pregnancy or lactation: Although no teratogenic effects were seen in animal testing, the safety of Hypovase during pregnancy has not yet been established. Accordingly, under these circumstances, it should be used only when in the opinion of the physician, potential benefit outweighs potential risk. Hypovase has been shown to be excreted in small amounts in human milk. Caution should be exercised when Hypovase is administered to nursing mothers.

Use in children: Hypovase is not recommended for the treatment of children under the age of 12 years since safe conditions for its use have not been established.

In patients with congestive cardiac failure: Hypovase is not recommended in the treatment of congestive cardiac failure due to mechanical obstruction such as aortic valve stenosis, mitral valve stenosis, pulmonary embolism and restrictive pericardial disease. Adequate data are not yet available to establish efficacy in patients with left ventricular failure due to recent myocardial infarction.

Precautions
In patients with hypertension: A very small percentage of patients may respond in an abrupt and exaggerated manner to the initial dose of Hypovase. Postural hypotension evidenced by dizziness and weakness, or rarely loss of consciousness, has been reported, particularly with the commencement of therapy, but this effect is readily avoided by initiating treatment with a low dose of Hypovase and with small increases in dosage during the first one to two weeks of therapy. The effect when observed, is not related to the severity of hypertension, is self-limiting and in most patients does not recur after the initial period of therapy or during subsequent dose titration steps.

When instituting therapy with any effective antihypertensive agent, the patient should be advised how to avoid symptoms resulting from postural hypotension and what measures to take should they develop. The patient should be cautioned to avoid situations where injury could result should dizziness or weakness occur during the initiation of Hypovase therapy. (e.g. driving or operating machinery).

In patients with congestive cardiac failure: When Hypovase is initially administered to patients with congestive cardiac failure who have undergone vigorous

diuretic or other vasodilator treatment, particularly in higher than the recommended starting dose, the resultant decrease in left ventricular filling pressure may be associated with a significant fall in cardiac output and systemic blood pressure. In such patients, observance of the recommended starting dose of Hypovase followed by gradual titration is particularly important. (See 'Dosage and administration').

Infrequently, the clinical efficacy of Hypovase in patients with congestive cardiac failure has been reported to diminish after several months of treatment. In these patients there is usually evidence of weight gain or peripheral oedema indicating fluid retention. Since spontaneous deterioration may occur in such severely ill patients a causal relationship to prazosin therapy has not been established. Thus, as with all patients with congestive cardiac failure, careful adjustment of diuretic dosage according to the patient's clinical condition is required to prevent excessive fluid retention and consequent relief of symptoms. In those patients without evidence of fluid retention, when clinical improvement has diminished, an increase in the dosage of Hypovase will usually restore clinical efficacy.

Raynaud's phenomenon and Raynaud's disease: Because Hypovase decreases peripheral vascular resistance, careful monitoring of blood pressure during initial administration and titration of Hypovase is suggested. Close observation is especially recommended for patients already taking medications that are known to lower blood pressure.

Drug/laboratory test interactions: False positive results may occur in screening tests for phaeochromocytoma (urinary vanillylmandelic acid (VMA) and methoxyhydroxyphenyl glycol (MHPG) metabolites of noradrenaline) in patients who are being treated with Hypovase.

Side-effects – In patients with hypertension: The most common side-effects associated with Hypovase therapy are: dizziness, headache, drowsiness, lack of energy, weakness, nausea, and palpitations. In most instances side-effects will disappear with continued therapy or may be tolerated with no decrease in dosage of the drug.

In addition, the following reactions have been associated with Hypovase therapy: vomiting, diarrhoea, constipation, abdominal discomfort and/or pain, liver function abnormalities, pancreatitis, oedema, dyspnoea, faintness, transient temporary loss of consciousness, tachycardia, nervousness, vertigo, hallucinations, depression, paraesthesia, rash, pruritus, alopecia, urinary frequency, impotence, incontinence, priapism, blurred vision, reddened sclera, epistaxis, tinnitus, dry mouth, nasal congestion, diaphoresis and sweating.

Some of these side-effects have occurred rarely, and in many instances the exact causal relationships have not been established.

In patients with congestive cardiac failure (left ventricular failure): The following side-effects have been observed in patients being managed for congestive cardiac failure with Hypovase when used in conjunction with cardiac glycosides and diuretics: Drowsiness, dizziness, postural hypotension, blurred vision, oedema, dry mouth, palpitations, nausea, diarrhoea, impotence, headache, and nasal congestion. In most instances these occurrences have been mild to moderate in severity and have resolved with continued therapy or have been tolerated with no decrease in drug dosage.

Raynaud's phenomenon and Raynaud's disease: The

most common, although infrequently reported side-effect, was mild dizziness.

Overdosage: Accidential ingestion of at least 50 mg of Hypovase in a two year old child resulted in profound drowsiness and depressed reflexes. No decrease in blood pressure was noted. Recovery was uneventful. Should overdosage lead to hypotension, support of the cardio vascular system is of first importance. Restoration of blood pressure and normalisation of heart rate may be accomplished by keeping the patient in the supine position. If this measure is inadequate, shock should first be treated with volume expanders. If necessary vaso-pressors including angiotensin should then be used. Renal function should be monitored and supported as needed. Laboratory data indicate Hypovase is not dialysable because it is protein bound.

Pharmaceutical precautions Store below 30°C.

Legal category POM

Package quantities b.d. starter pack, for the conven-ience of patients initiating Hypovase therapy, containing 8 × 0.5 mg Hypovase tablets and 32 × 1 mg Hypovase tablets (See 'Further information').

Hypovase 0.5 mg:	packs of 100
Hypovase 1 mg:	packs of 100
Hypovase 2 mg:	packs of 100
Hypovase 5 mg:	packs of 100

Further information The two week b.d. starter pack has the following instructions to the patient: 'Step 1 (0.5 mg tablets) – 4 days, first dose in the evening.

Step 2 (1 mg tablets) – 4 days, first dose in the evening.

Step 3 (2 × 1 mg tablets) – 6 days, first dose in the evening.

Your doctor will wish you to follow further dosage instructions beyond Step 3 and you should follow these instructions or see your doctor before the end of Step 3.'

The tablets (0.5 and 1 mg) are carefully packed in sequence, in blister strips to ensure correct usage.

The 1 mg tablets contain FD & C Yellow No 6 Dye, E110

Product licence numbers

0.5 mg tablet	0057/0149
1 mg tablet	0057/0106
2 mg tablet	0057/0107
5 mg tablet	0057/0108

MITHRACIN*

Presentation Mithracin (mithramycin) is available in vials as a freeze-dried preparation for intravenous administration. Each vial contains 2500 mcg of mithra-mycin with 100 mg of mannitol and sufficient disodium phosphate to adjust to pH 7.

Mithramycin is a yellow crystalline compound which is produced by a micro-organism, *Streptomyces plicatus*. It has an empirical formula of $C_{52}H_{76}O_{24}$.

Uses *Actions:* Although the exact mechanism by which Mithracin causes tumour inhibition is not yet known, studies have indicated that this compound forms a complex with deoxyribonucleic acid (DNA) and inhibits cellular ribonucleic acid (RNA) and enzymic RNA synthesis. The binding of Mithracin to DNA in the presence of Mg^{++} (or other divalent cations) is respons-ible for the inhibition of DNA-directed RNA synthesis.

This action presumably accounts for the biological properties of Mithracin.

Mithracin shows potent cytotoxicity against malignant cells of human origin (Hela cells) growing in tissue culture. Mithracin is lethal to Hela cells in 48 hours at concentrations as low as 0.5 mcg/ml of tissue culture medium. Mithracin has shown significant antitumour activity against experimental leukaemia in mice when administered intraperitoneally.

In mice the average intravenous LD_{50} of Mithracin is 2,000 mcg/kg of body weight. When administered orally, it is not toxic to mice even at doses of 100 times greater than the intravenous LD_{50}. In rats the average intra-venous LD_{50} of Mithracin is 1,700 mcg/kg of body weight. It is not toxic to rats when administered orally at doses 17 times greater than the intravenous LD_{50}. In dogs and monkeys Mithracin is essentially nontoxic when administered intravenously for 24 days at daily doses as high as 50 and 24 mcg/kg of body weight, respectively.

However, at higher doses of 100 mcg/kg/day intra-venously it is lethal to dogs and monkeys. Signs of toxicity in dogs and monkeys included anorexia, vomit-ing, listlessness, melaena, anaemia, lymphopenia, ele-vated alkaline phosphatase, serum glutamic oxalo-acetic transaminase, serum glutamic pyruvic transaminase values, hypochloraemia, and azotaemia. Dogs also showed marked thrombocytopenia, hyponatraemia, hy-pokalaemia, hypocalcaemia, and decreased prothrombin consumption. Necropsy findings consisted of necrosis of lymphoid tissue and multiple generalised haemor-rhages. Mithracin was only mildly irritating when injected intramuscularly in rabbits and subcutaneously in guinea pigs. Histological evidence of inhibition of spermatoge-nesis was observed in a substantial number of male rats receiving doses of 0.6 mg/kg/day and above. This preclinical finding of selective drug effect constituted the scientific rationale for clinical trials in testicular tumours.

Indications: Mithracin is a potent antineoplastic agent which has been shown to be useful in the treatment of carefully selected hospitalised patients with malignant tumours of the testis in whom successful treatment by surgery and/or radiation is impossible.

Also, on the basis of limited clinical experience to date, it may be considered in the treatment of certain symptomatic patients with hypercalcaemia and hyper-calciuria associated with a variety of neoplasms.

The use of Mithracin in other types of neoplastic disease is not recommended at the present time.

Dosage and administration (please see *Warnings* section). The daily dose of Mithracin is based on the patient's body weight. If a patient has abnormal fluid retention such as oedema, hydrothorax, or ascites, the patient's ideal weight rather than actual body weight should be used to calculate the dose.

Treatment of testicular tumours: In the treatment of patients with testicular tumours the recommended daily dose of Mithracin is 25 to 30 mcg/kg of body weight. Therapy should be continued for a period of eight to ten days unless significant side-effects or toxicity occur during therapy. A course of therapy consisting of more than ten daily doses is not recommended.

Individual daily doses should not exceed 30 mcg/kg of body weight.

In those patients with responsive tumours, some degree of tumour regression is usually evident within three or four weeks following the initial course of therapy. If tumour masses remain unchanged following an initial course of therapy, additional courses of therapy at monthly intervals are warranted.

When a significant tumour regression is obtained, it is suggested that additional courses of therapy be given at monthly intervals until a complete regression of tumour masses is achieved or until definite tumour progression or new tumour masses occur in spite of continued courses of therapy.

Treatment of hypercalcaemia and hypercalciuria: Reversal of hypercalcaemia and hypercalciuria can usually be achieved with Mithracin at doses considerably lower than those recommended for use in the treatment of testicular tumours.

In hypercalcaemia and hypercalciuria associated with advanced malignancy the recommended course of treatment with Mithracin is 25 mcg/kg body weight/day for three to four days.

If the desired degree of reversal of hypercalciuria is not achieved with the initial course of therapy, additional courses of therapy may then be administered at intervals of one week or more to achieve the desired result or to maintain serum calcium and urinary calcium excretion at normal levels. It may be possible to maintain normal calcium balance with single weekly doses or with a schedule of 2 or 3 doses each week.

Note: Because of the drug's toxicity and the limited clinical experience to date in these indications, the following recommendations should be kept in mind by the physician.

1. Consider cases of hypercalcaemia and hypercalciuria not responsive to conventional treatment.

2. Apply same contra-indications and precautionary measures as in antitumour treatment.

3. Renal function should be carefully monitored before, during and after treatment.

4. Benefits of use during pregnancy or in women of child-bearing age should be weighed against potential toxicity to embryo or foetus.

Clinical report: Treatment of patients with inoperable testicular tumours: In a combined series of 305 patients with inoperable testicular tumours treated with Mithracin, 33 patients (10.8%) showed a complete disappearance of tumour masses and an additional 80 patients (26.2%) responded with significant, partial regression of tumour masses. The longest duration of a continuing complete response is now over 8.5 years. The therapeutic responses in this series of patients have been summarised by type of testicular tumour in the table below.

Results in 305 Testicular Tumour cases by tumour type:

Type of testicular tumour	Total	Complete response	Partial response	No response
Embryonal cell	173	26	42	105
Teratoma	5	0	1	4
Teratocarcinoma	23	0	5	18
Seminoma	18	0	7	11
Choriocarcinoma	13	1	6	6
Mixed tumour	73	6	19	48
Totals	305	33	80	192

Mithracin may be useful in the treatment of patients with testicular tumours which are resistant to other chemotherapeutic agents. Prior radiation therapy or prior chemotherapy did not alter the response rate with Mithracin. This suggests that there is no significant cross-resistance between Mithracin and other chemotherapeutic agents.

Treatment of patients with hypercalcaemia and hypercalciuria: A limited number of patients with hypercalcaemia (range: 12.0 to 25.8 mg%) and patients with hypercalciuria (range: 215 to 492 mg/day) associated with malignant disease, were treated with Mithracin. Hypercalcaemia and hypercalciuria were promptly reversed in all patients. In some patients, the primary malignancy was of nontesticular origin.

Administration: Mithracin should be administered intravenously only. The appropriate daily dose of Mithracin should be diluted in one litre of 5% dextrose in water and administered by slow intravenous infusion over a period of 4 to 6 hours. Rapid direct intravenous injection of Mithracin should be avoided as it may be associated with a higher incidence and greater severity of gastrointestinal side-effects. Extravasation of solutions of Mithracin may cause local irritation and cellulitis. Should thrombophlebitis or perivascular cellulitis occur, the infusion should be terminated and reinstituted at another site. The application of moderate heat to the site of extravasation may help to disperse the compound and minimise discomfort and local tissue irritation. The use of anti-emetic compounds prior to and during treatment with Mithracin may be helpful in relieving nausea and vomiting.

To reconstitute, add aseptically 4.9 ml of Sterile Water for Injection to the contents of the vial and shake to dissolve. Each ml of the resulting solution will then contain 500 mcg of Mithracin. After removal of the appropriate dose, the remaining unused solution must be discarded. Fresh solution must be prepared in the above manner each day of therapy.

Contra-indications, warnings, etc

Contra-indications: Mithracin is contra-indicated in patients with thrombocytopenia, thrombocytopathy, coagulation disorder or an increased susceptibility to bleeding due to other causes. Mithracin should not be administered to any patient with impairment of bone marrow function.

Mithracin should not be used in the treatment of patients who are not hospitalised and who cannot be observed carefully and frequently during and after therapy, or whenever appropriate laboratory facilities are unavailable.

Warnings: The information contained in this Data Sheet should be thoroughly reviewed before administering the preparation: In the treatment of each patient, the physician must weigh carefully the possibility of achieving therapeutic benefit versus the risk of toxicity which may occur with Mithracin therapy.

It is recommended that Mithracin be administered only to hospitalised patients by or under the supervision of a qualified physician who is experienced in the use of cancer chemotherapeutic agents, because of the possibility of severe reactions. Facilities for the determination of necessary laboratory studies must be available.

Severe thrombocytopenia, a haemorrhagic tendency and even death, may result from the use of Mithracin. Although severe toxicity is more apt to occur in patients who have far-advanced disease or are otherwise considered poor risks for therapy, serious toxicity may also occasionally occur even in patients who are in relatively good condition.

Use in pregnancy: Mithracin should not normally be

administered to patients who are pregnant or to mothers who are breast feeding.

Precautions: Mithracin should be administered only to patients who are hospitalised and who can be observed frequently and carefully during and after therapy.

Electrolyte imbalance, especially hypocalcaemia, hypokalaemia, and hypophosphataemia, should be corrected with appropriate electrolyte therapy prior to treatment with Mithracin.

Mithracin should be used with extreme caution in patients with significant impairment of renal or hepatic function.

In the treatment of each patient, the physician must weigh carefully the possibility of achieving therapeutic benefit versus the risk of toxicity which may occur with Mithracin therapy.

The following laboratory studies should be obtained frequently during therapy and for several days following the last dose: platelet count, prothrombin time, bleeding time. The occurrence of thrombocytopenia or a significant prolongation of prothrombin time or bleeding time is an indication for the termination of therapy.

Side-effects: The most important form of toxicity associated with the use of Mithracin consists of a bleeding syndrome which usually begins with an episode of epistaxis. This bleeding tendency may only consist of a single or several episodes of epistaxis and progress no further. However, in some cases, this haemorrhagic syndrome can start with an episode of haematemesis which may progress to more widespread haemorrhage in the gastro-intestinal tract or to a more generalised bleeding tendency. This haemorrhagic diathesis is most likely due to abnormalities in multiple clotting factors.

A detailed analysis of the clinical data in 1,160 patients treated with Mithracin indicates that the haemorrhagic syndrome is dose-related. With doses of 30 mcg/kg/day or less for 10 or fewer doses, the incidence of bleeding episodes has been 5.4%, with an associated drug-related mortality rate of 1.6%. With doses greater than 30 mcg/kg/day and/or for more than 10 doses, a significantly larger number of bleeding episodes occurred (11.9%) and the associated drug-related mortality rate was also significantly higher (5.7%).

The most common side-effects reported with the use of Mithracin consist of gastro-intestinal symptoms: anorexia, nausea, vomiting, diarrhoea, and stomatitis. Other less frequently reported side-effects include fever, drowsiness, weakness, lethargy, malaise, headache, depression, phlebitis, facial flushing, and skin rash.

The following laboratory abnormalities have been reported during therapy with Mithracin and in most instances were reversible following cessation of treatment.

Haematological abnormalities: Depression of platelet count, white blood cell count, haemoglobin and prothrombin content; elevation of clotting time and bleeding time; abnormal clot retraction.

Thrombocytopenia may be rapid in onset and may occur at any time during the therapy or within several days following the last dose. With the occurrence of severe thrombocytopenia, the infusion of platelet concentrates or platelet-rich plasma may be helpful in elevating the platelet count.

The occurrence of leucopenia with the use of Mithracin is relatively uncommon, occurring only in approximately 6% of patients.

It has been uncommon for abnormalities in clotting time or clot retraction to be demonstrated prior to the onset of an overt bleeding episode noted in some patients treated with Mithracin. Nevertheless, the performance of these tests periodically is recommended because in a few instances an abnormality in one of these studies may have served as a warning to terminate therapy because of impending serious toxicity.

Abnormal liver function tests: Increased levels of serum glutamic oxalacetic transaminase, serum glutamic pyruvic transaminase, lactic dehydrogenase, alkaline phosphatase, serum bilirubin, ornithine carbamyl transferase, isocitric dehydrogenase, and increased retention of bromsulphalein.

Abnormal renal function: Increased blood urea nitrogen and serum creatinine; proteinuria.

Abnormalities in electrolyte concentrations: Depression of serum calcium, phosphorus and potassium.

Pharmaceutical precautions Store at 2°C to 8°C.

The increasing use of cytotoxic drugs and the potential hazards associated with them, requires special precautions to be taken in their handling, preparation and administration. These recommendations provide a basis for the safe handling of Mithracin.

1. All staff working with Mithracin should receive special training.

2. Reconstitution of Mithracin should be performed in a designated aseptic area which gives maximum protection to the surrounding environment.

3. Adequate protective clothing including gloves and safety spectacles should be worn.

Should spillage on the skin occur, the affected area should be washed with copious quantities of water.

Should spillage into the eye occur, immediately cleanse thoroughly using copious quantities of sodium chloride eye wash. (If sodium chloride eye wash is not available water can be used as an alternative). Should eye irritation continue medical help should be sought.

4. Mithracin should not be handled by pregnant staff.

5. Adequate care and precautions should be taken in the disposal of items used to reconstitute Mithracin.

Disposal procedure
Unopened vials: Place in a suitable closed container† and incinerate at 300°C.

Reconstituted solution: Dilute small volumes with larger volumes of 100% w/v trisodium phosphate solution. Absorb diluted liquid on to paper, ash or sawdust. Place in high risk waste disposal bag† and incinerate at 300°C.

Disposal of swabs, etc: Swabs etc. should be placed in a high risk waste disposal bag† and incinerated at 300°C.

Accidental spillage: Should spillage on the floor or breakage of a vial of reconstituted solution occur, suitable protective clothing should be donned including PVC gloves. With rubber gloves as over protection, the area should be cleaned with absorbent paper and the floor wiped with cloths soaked in 10% trisodium phosphate solution or 0.1N sodium hydroxide solution, then washed with copious quantities of water. The absorbent paper, cloths, gloves and other materials used in the management of the spillage should be placed in a high risk waste disposal bag† and incinerated at 300°C.

If Mithracin is still as the freeze dried powder, damp down quickly to avoid dispersion and proceed as above.

Care should be taken in disposing of broken glass from

† The containers and bags should be those specified in 'safe disposal of clinical waste'. Health and Safety Advisory Committee, HMSO, 1982.

vials, which should go into a closed container† for incineration.

Legal category POM.

Package quantities Vial containing 2500 mcg.

Further information Nil.

Product licence number 0057/5022.

NEPHRIL*

Presentation Nephril is available as white scored tablets coded NEP/1 on one side and 'Pfizer' on the other, each containing 1 mg polythiazide.

Uses *Actions:* The mechanism of action results in an interference with the renal tubular mechanism of electrolyte reabsorption. At maximal therapeutic dosage, all thiazides are approximately equal in their diuretic potency. The mechanism whereby thiazides function in the control of hypertension is unknown.

Indications: Nephril is an orally effective, non-mercurial diuretic, saluretic and antihypertensive agent. Nephril is indicated as adjunctive therapy in oedema associated with congestive cardiac failure, hepatic cirrhosis and corticosteroid and oestrogen therapy.

Nephril has also been found useful in oedema due to various forms of renal dysfunction, such as nephrotic syndrome, acute glomerulonephritis and chronic renal failure.

Nephril is indicated in the management of hypertension either as the sole therapeutic agent or to enhance the effectiveness of other antihypertensive drugs in the more severe forms of hypertension.

Dosage and administration The usual dosage of Nephril for diuretic therapy is 1 to 4 mg daily. For antihypertensive therapy the usual maintenance dose is between 2 and 4 mg daily although some patients may be optimally controlled on doses of 0.5 mg or 1 mg daily. However, few patients will require doses as high as 4 mg daily and at such a dose level serum electrolytes should be monitored frequently. Dosage should be individualised according to response and should be titrated to gain the maximum therapeutic effect with the minimum dose required to maintain that therapeutic response.

Contra-indications, warnings, etc
Contra-indications: Anuria. Hypersensitivity to polythiazide or other sulphonamide derived drugs.

Warnings: Thiazides should be used with caution in severe renal disease. In patients with renal disease, thiazides may precipitate azotaemia. Cumulative effects of the drug may develop in patients with impaired renal function. If progressive renal impairment becomes evident, as indicated by a rising nonprotein nitrogen or blood urea nitrogen, a careful reappraisal of therapy is necessary with consideration given to withholding or discontinuing diuretic therapy. Thiazides should be used with caution in patients with impaired hepatic function or progressive liver disease, since minor alterations of fluid and electrolyte balance may precipitate hepatic coma.

Thiazides may add to or potentiate the action of other antihypertensive drugs. Potentiation occurs with ganglionic or peripheral adrenergic blocking drugs.

Sensitivity reactions may occur in patients with a history of allergy or bronchial asthma. The possibility of exacerbation or activation of systemic lupus erythematosus has been reported.

Use in pregnancy: The routine use of diuretics in healthy pregnant women is inappropriate and may expose mother and foetus to unnecessary hazard. Diuretics do not prevent development of toxaemia of pregnancy and there is no satisfactory evidence that they are useful in the treatment of established toxaemia.

Oedema during pregnancy may arise from pathological causes or from physiological and mechanical consequences of pregnancy. Physiological hypervolaemia during pregnancy may be associated with generalised oedema including dependent oedema. This oedema is properly treated by recumbency and support hose. Thiazides may be indicated in pregnancy when oedema is due to pathological causes other than toxaemia. Rarely short courses of thiazides are indicated where physiological oedema is unrelieved by rest and where the oedema causes extreme discomfort.

Thiazides cross the placental barrier and appear in cord blood. The use of thiazides in pregnant women requires that the anticipated benefit be weighed against possible hazards to the foetus. These hazards include foetal or neonatal jaundice, thrombocytopenia and possibly other side-effects which have occurred in the adult.

Use in nursing mothers: Thiazides appear in breast milk. If use of Nephril is deemed essential, breast feeding should be discontinued.

Use in children: Nephril is not recommended for use in children.

Use in the elderly: Elderly patients are especially liable to the adverse effects of diuretics. It is important that the lowest clinically effective dose is used.

Precautions: All patients receiving thiazide therapy should have periodic determinations of serum electrolytes at appropriate intervals to detect possible electrolyte imbalance. Such patients should also be observed for clinical signs of fluid or electrolyte imbalance; namely hyponatraemia, hypochloraemic alkalosis and hypokalaemia. Serum and urine electrolyte determinations are particularly important when the patient is vomiting or receiving parenteral fluids. Warning signs of possible electrolyte imbalance, irrespective of cause, are: dryness of mouth, thirst, weakness, lethargy, drowsiness, restlessness, muscle pains or cramps, muscular fatigue, hypotension, oliguria, tachycardia and gastro-intestinal disturbances such as nausea and vomiting.

Hypokalaemia may develop with thiazides as with any other potent diuretic, especially with brisk diuresis, when severe cirrhosis is present, or during concomitant use of corticosteroids or ACTH.

Interference with adequate oral electrolyte intake will also contribute to hypokalaemia. Hypokalaemia may exaggerate metabolic effects of digitalis therapy especially with reference to myocardial activity.

Any chloride deficit is generally mild and usually does not require specific treatment except under extraordinary circumstances (as in liver disease or renal disease). Dilutional hyponatraemia may occur in oedematous patients in hot weather; appropriate therapy is water restriction, rather than administration of salt except in rare instances, when the hyponatraemia is life threatening. In actual salt depletion, appropriate replacement is the therapy of choice. Hyperuricaemia may occur or frank gout may be precipitated in certain patients receiving thiazide therapy.

Insulin requirements in diabetic patients may be increased, decreased or unchanged. Latent diabetes mellitus may become manifest during thiazide administration.

Thiazide drugs may increase the responsiveness to tubocurarine.

The antihypertensive effects of thiazides may be enhanced in the post-sympathectomy patient. Thiazides may decrease arterial responsiveness to noradrenaline. This diminution is not sufficient to preclude effectiveness of the pressor agent for therapeutic use.

If progressive renal impairment becomes evident, as indicated by a rising non-protein nitrogen or blood urea nitrogen a careful reappraisal of therapy is necessary with consideration given to withholding or discontinuing diuretic therapy.

Thiazides may decrease serum protein-bound iodine levels without signs of thyroid disturbance.

Side-effects:

Gastro-intestinal – anorexia, gastric irritation, nausea, vomiting, cramping, diarrhoea, constipation, jaundice (intrahepatic cholestatic jaundice), pancreatitis.

Central nervous system – dizziness, vertigo, paraesthesia, headache, xanthopsia.

Haematological – leucopenia, agranulocytosis, thrombocytopenia, aplastic anaemia.

Dermatological – purpura, photosensitivity, rash, urticaria, necrotising angiitis (vasculitis) (cutaneous vasculitis).

Cardiovascular – orthostatic hypotension may occur and be aggravated by alcohol, barbiturates or narcotics.

Other – hyperglycaemia, glycosuria, hyperuricaemia, muscle spasm, weakness, restlessness.

Whenever adverse reactions are moderate or severe, thiazide dosage should be reduced or therapy withdrawn.

Overdosage: Gastric lavage and supportive therapy. Treatment of acute renal failure if present. Potassium supplements.

Pharmaceutical precautions Store below 25°C.

Legal category POM.

Package quantities Tablets 1 mg packs of 100 and 500.

Further information Nil.

Product licence number 0057/5024.

SINEQUAN*

Presentation Sinequan (doxepin hydrochloride) is available in capsules of four strengths. All capsules bear the name 'Pfizer'.

The four sizes of capsules are distinguished by their colour and coding as follows:

Sinequan 10 mg capsule coded 'SQN 10' (opaque orange).

Sinequan 25 mg capsule coded 'SQN 25' (opaque blue cap/opaque orange body).

Sinequan 50 mg capsule coded 'SQN 50' (opaque blue).

Sinequan 75 mg capsule coded 'SQN 75' (opaque blue cap/opaque rich yellow body).

Sinequan is a tricyclic antidepressant.

Uses *Actions:* The mechanism of action of Sinequan is not definitely known. It is not a central nervous stimulant nor a monoamine oxidase inhibitor. The current hypothesis is that the clinical effects are due, at least in part, to influences on the adrenergic activity at the synapses so that deactivation of noradrenaline by reuptake into the nerve terminals is prevented. In animal studies anticholinergic, antiserotonin and antihistamine effects on smooth muscle have been demonstrated. At higher than usual clinical doses, adrenaline response was potentiated in animals. This effect was not demonstrated in humans.

Indications: Symptoms of depressive illness, especially where sedation is required.

Sinequan may be used with benefit where symptoms are of short or long duration prior to treatment and in patients with a wide range of intensity of illness.

As with other psychotherapeutic agents, the degree of response varies with each patient. In patients exhibiting a beneficial response, this may be seen within a few days of commencing therapy, while others may not respond for two weeks or longer.

Due to its excellent toleration, Sinequan is particularly useful in ambulatory patients seen in general practice as well as in the treatment of hospitalised patients.

Use in children: The use of Sinequan in children under 12 years is not recommended, because safe conditions for its use have not been established.

Dosage and administration The optimum oral dose depends on the severity of the condition and the individual patient's response. The dose varies from 30–300 mg daily, and is usually administered in three divided doses daily.

For the majority of patients with moderate or severe symptoms, it is recommended that treatment commences with an initial dose of 75 mg daily. Many of these patients will respond satisfactorily at this dose level. For patients who do not, the dosage may be adjusted according to individual response. In more severely ill patients, it may be necessary to administer a dose of up to 300 mg a day to obtain a clinical response.

As an alternative regimen, the total daily dosage, up to 100 mg may be given as a single dose without loss of effectiveness. This dose may be given at bedtime.

In patients where insomnia is a troublesome symptom, it is recommended that the total daily dose be divided so that a higher proportion is given for the evening dose; similarly, if drowsiness is experienced as a side effect of treatment. Sinequan may be administered by this regimen, or the dosage may be reduced.

It is often possible, having once obtained a satisfactory therapeutic response, to reduce the dose for maintenance therapy.

The optimal antidepressant effect may not be evident for two to three weeks.

Use in the elderly: In general, lower dosages are recommended. Where the presenting symptoms are mild in nature, it is advisable to initiate treatment at a dose of 10–50 mg daily. A satisfactory clinical response is obtained in many of these patients at a daily dose of 30–50 mg. The dosage may be adjusted according to the individual response.

Contra-indications, warnings, etc
Contra-indications: Hypersensitivity, mania, severe liver disease, lactation, glaucoma, tendency to urinary retention.

Precautions: The once-a-day dosage regimen of Sinequan in patients with intercurrent illness or patients taking other medications should be carefully adjusted. This is especially important in patients receiving other medications with anticholinergic effects.

The use of Sinequan on a once-a-day dosage regimen in geriatric patients should be adjusted carefully on the basis of the patient's condition. The elderly are particularly liable to experience toxic effects, especially agitation, confusion and postural hypotension. The initial dose should be increased with caution under close supervision. Half the normal maintenance dose may be sufficient to produce a satisfactory clinical response.

Use with caution in patients who have experienced a recent myocardial infarction.

Combined use with other antidepressants, alcohol or antianxiety agents should be undertaken with due recognition of the possibility of potentiation. It is known, for example, that monoamine oxidase inhibitors may potentiate other drug effects, therefore Sinequan should not be given concurrently, or within two weeks of cessation of therapy, with monoamine oxidase inhibitors.

Anaesthetics given during tricyclic or tetracyclic antidepressant therapy may increase the risk of arrhythmias and hypotension. If surgery is necessary, the anaesthetist should be informed that a patient is being so treated.

Use with caution in patients with a history of epilepsy.

Sinequan may decrease the antihypertensive effect of agents such as debrisoquine, bethanidine, guanethidine and possibly clonidine. It usually requires daily doses of Sinequan in excess of 150 mg before any effect on the action of guanethidine is seen. It would be advisable to review all antihypertensive therapy during treatment with tricyclic antidepressants.

Sinequan should not be given with sympathomimetic agents, such as ephedrine, isoprenaline, noradrenaline, phenylephrine and phenylpropanolamine.

Barbiturates may increase the rate of metabolism of Sinequan.

The dose of thyroid hormone medication may need reducing if Sinequan is being given concurrently.

Since drowsiness may occur with the use of Sinequan, patients should be warned of the possibility and cautioned against driving a car or operating machinery while taking this drug.

Since suicide is an inherent risk in any depressed patient until significant improvement has occurred, patients should be closely supervised during early therapy.

Use in pregnancy: There is inadequate evidence of safety in human pregnancy but the drug has been widely used for many years without apparent ill consequences and animal studies have not shown any hazard.

Side-effects: Note: Some of the side-effects noted below have not been specifically reported with Sinequan. However, due to the close pharmacological similarities amongst the tricyclics, the reactions should be considered when prescribing Sinequan.

Anticholinergic effects: Dry mouth, blurred vision, constipation and urinary retention have been reported. If they do not subside with continued therapy, or if they become severe, it may be necessary to reduce the dosage.

Central nervous system effects: Drowsiness is the most commonly noticed side-effect. This tends to disappear as therapy is continued. Other infrequently reported CNS side-effects are confusion, disorientation, hallucinations,

paraesthesiae, ataxia and extrapyramidal symptoms, tremor and convulsions.

Psychotic manifestations, including mania and paranoid delusions may be exacerbated during treatment with tricyclic antidepressants.

Cardiovascular: Although Sinequan carries less risk than other tricyclic antidepressants, caution should be observed in the treatment of patients with heart block or cardiac arrhythmias. Cardiovascular effects including hypotension and tachycardia have been reported occasionally.

Allergic: Skin rash, facial oedema, photosensitisation and pruritus have occasionally occurred.

Haematological: Eosinophilia has been reported in a few patients. There have been occasional reports of bone marrow depression manifesting as agranulocytosis, leucopenia, thrombocytopenia and purpura.

Gastro-intestinal: Nausea, vomiting, indigestion, taste disturbances, diarrhoea and anorexia have been reported. (See Anticholinergic effects).

Endocrine: Raised or lowered libido, testicular swelling, gynaecomastia, enlargement of breasts and galactorrhoea in the female, raising or lowering of blood sugar levels and inappropriate antidiuretic hormone secretion have been reported following the administration of tricyclics.

Other: Dizziness, tinnitus, weight gain, sweating, chills, fatigue, weakness, flushing, jaundice and alopecia have been occasionally observed as adverse effects.

Withdrawal: Withdrawal symptoms may occur on abrupt cessation of tricyclic antidepressant therapy and include insomnia, irritability, and excessive perspiration. Withdrawal symptoms in neonates whose mothers received tricyclic antidepressants during the third trimester have also been reported and include respiratory depression, convulsions and 'jitteriness' (hyper-reflexia).

Overdosage:

A. *Signs and Symptoms:*

1. Mild: Drowsiness, stupor, blurred vision, excessive dryness of mouth.

2. Severe: Respiratory depression, hypotension, coma, convulsions, cardiac arrhythmias and tachycardias.

Also: urinary retention (bladder atony), decreased gastro-intestinal motility (paralytic ileus), hyperthermia (or hypothermia), hypertension, dilated pupils, hyperactive reflexes.

B. *Management and Treatment:*

1. Mild: Observation and supportive therapy is all that is usually necessary.

2. Severe: Medical management of severe Sinequan overdosage consists of aggressive supportive therapy. If the patient is conscious, gastric lavage, with appropriate precautions to prevent pulmonary aspiration, should be performed even though Sinequan is rapidly absorbed. The use of activated charcoal has been recommended, as has been continuous gastric lavage with saline for 24 hours or more. An adequate airway should be established in comatose patients and assisted ventilation used if necessary. ECG monitoring may be required for several days, since relapse after apparent recovery has been reported. Arrhythmias should be treated with the appropriate anti-arrhythmic agent. It has been reported that many of the cardiovascular and CNS symptoms of tricyclic antidepressant poisoning in adults may be reversed by the slow intravenous administration of 1 mg

to 3 mg of physostigmine salicylate. Because physostigmine is rapidly metabolised, the dosage should be repeated as required. Convulsions may respond to standard anticonvulsant therapy. However, barbiturates may potentiate any respiratory depression. Dialysis and forced diuresis generally are not of value in the management of overdosage due to high tissue and protein binding of Sinequan.

Pharmaceutical precautions Store below 25°C.

Legal category POM.

Package quantities
Capsules 10 mg: Packs of 100 and 500.
Capsules 25 mg: Packs of 100 and 500.
Capsules 50 mg: Pack of 100.
Capsules 75 mg: Pack of 60.

Further information Nil.

Product licence numbers
10 mg capsules   0057/5032R
25 mg capsules   0057/5033R
50 mg capsules   0057/5034R
75 mg capsules   0057/0133

TERRAMYCIN*

Presentation Terramycin (oxytetracycline) is available as:

Tablets 250 mg: Each sugar-coated yellow tablet contains 250 mg oxytetracycline as the dihydrate and coded 'Pfizer'.

Capsules 250 mg: Hard gelatin capsules, opaque yellow cap and body printed TER250 and 'Pfizer', each containing 250 mg oxytetracycline as the hydrochloride.

Uses *Actions:* Terramycin is a product of the metabolism of Streptomyces rimosus and is one of the family of tetracycline antibiotics.

Terramycin is primarily bacteriostatic and is thought to exert its antimicrobial effect by the inhibition of protein synthesis. Terramycin is active against a wide range of Gram-negative and Gram-positive organisms.

The drugs in the tetracycline class have closely similar antimicrobial spectra and cross-resistance among them is common.

Tetracyclines are readily absorbed and are bound to plasma proteins in varying degrees. They are concentrated by the liver in the bile and excreted in the urine and faeces in high concentrations and in a biologically active form.

Terramycin diffuses readily through the placenta into the foetal circulation, into the pleural fluid and, under some circumstances, into the cerebrospinal fluid.

Indications: Terramycin is a broad-spectrum antibiotic.

Terramycin is indicated in infections caused by the following micro-organisms:

Rickettsiae (Rocky Mountain spotted fever, typhus fever and the typhus group, Q fever, rickettsialpox and tick fevers).
Mycoplasma pneumoniae (PPLO, Eaton Agent).
Agents of psittacosis and ornithosis.
Agents of lymphogranuloma venereum and granuloma inguinale.
The spirochaetal agent of relapsing fever (Borrelia recurrentis).

The following Gram-negative micro-organisms:
Haemophilus ducreyi (chancroid).
Pasteurella pestis and *Pasteurella tularensis.*
Bartonella bacilliformis.
Bacteroides species.
Vibrio comma and *Vibrio fetus.*
Brucella species (in conjunction with streptomycin).

Because many strains of the following groups of micro-organisms have been shown to be resistant to tetracyclines, culture and susceptibility testing are recommended.

Terramycin is indicated for treatment of infections caused by the following Gram-negative micro-organisms, when bacteriological testing indicates appropriate susceptibility to the drug:

Escherichia coli.
Enterobacter aerogenes.
Shigella species.
Mima species and *Herellea* species.
Haemophilus influenzae (respiratory infections).
Klebsiella species (respiratory and urinary infections).

Terramycin is indicated for treatment of infections caused by the following Gram-positive micro-organisms when bacteriological testing indicates appropriate susceptibility to the drug:

Streptococcus species.
Diplococcus pneumoniae.
Staphylococcus aureus. (Skin and soft tissue infections).

When penicillin is contra-indicated, tetracyclines are alternative drugs in the treatment of infections due to:

Neisseria gonorrhoeae.
Treponema pallidum and *Treponema pertenue* (syphilis and yaws).
Listeria monocytogenes.
Clostridium species.
Bacillus anthracis.
Fusiformis fusiformis (Vincent's infection).
Actinomyces species.

In acute intestinal amoebiasis, the tetracyclines may be a useful adjunct to amoebicides. In severe acne, the tetracyclines may be useful adjunctive therapy.

Tetracyclines are indicated in the treatment of trachoma, although the infectious agent is not always eliminated, as judged by immunofluorescence.

Inclusion conjunctivitis may be treated with oral tetracyclines or with a combination of oral and topical agents.

Dosage and administration Oral administration:

Adults: The suggested minimum adult dosage for Terramycin is 1 g daily in divided doses given as 250 mg four times daily. Higher doses, such as 500 mg four times daily, may be required for severe infections or for those infections which do not respond to the smaller dose.

Children: Usual daily dose 25–50 mg/kg (10–20 mg/lb) of body weight divided in four equal doses.

Elderly: Terramycin may be given at the usual adult dosage. The possibility of sub-clinical renal insufficiency should be kept in mind, as it may lead to drug accumulation.

Therapy should be continued for at least 24–48 hours after symptoms and fever have subsided.

Antacids containing aluminium, calcium or magnesium impair absorption and should not be given to patients taking oral tetracyclines.

Food and some dairy products also interfere with

absorption. Oral forms of tetracyclines should be given one hour before or two hours after meals.

In patients with renal impairment: Total dosage should be decreased by reduction of recommended individual doses and/or by extending time intervals between doses.

In the treatment of streptococcal infections, a therapeutic dose of Terramycin should be administered for at least ten days.

For treatment of brucellosis, 500 mg Terramycin four times daily accompanied by streptomycin.

Gonococcal infections: Male and female, 1.5 g initially followed by 0.5 g four times daily for a total of 9 g.

For treatment of syphilis, a total of 30–40 g in equally divided doses over a period of ten to fifteen days should be given. Close follow-up, including laboratory tests, is recommended.

Administration of adequate amounts of fluid with capsule and tablet forms is recommended to reduce the risk of oesophageal irritation and ulceration. (see *Side-effects*.)

Contra-indications, warnings, etc

Contra-indications: Terramycin is contra-indicated in persons who have shown hypersensitivity to any of the tetracyclines.

Warnings: The use of drugs of the tetracycline class during tooth development (last half of pregnancy, infancy and childhood to the age of 8 years) may cause permanent discoloration of the teeth (yellow-grey-brown). This side-effect is more common during long term use of the drugs but has been observed following repeated short-term courses. Enamel hypoplasia has also been reported. Tetracycline drugs, therefore, should not be used in this age group unless other drugs are not likely to be effective or are contra-indicated.

If renal impairment exists, even usual oral or parenteral doses may lead to excessive systemic accumulation of the drug and possible liver toxicity. Under such circumstances, lower than usual total doses are indicated and, if therapy is prolonged, serum level determinations of the drug may be advisable.

The antianabolic action of the tetracyclines may cause an increase in BUN. While this in not a problem in those with normal renal function, in patients with significantly impaired renal function, higher serum levels of tetracycline may lead to azotaemia, hyperphosphataemia and acidosis.

Photosensitivity manifested by an exaggerated sunburn reaction has been observed in some individuals taking tetracyclines.

As with other antibiotic preparations, Terramycin may result in overgrowth of nonsusceptible organisms, including fungi. If superinfection occurs, the antibiotic should be discontinued and appropriate therapy instituted.

In venereal diseases when coexistent syphilis is suspected a dark field examination should be performed before treatment is started and the blood serology repeated monthly for at least four months.

Because tetracyclines have been shown to depress plasma prothrombin activity, patients who are on anticoagulant therapy may require downward adjustment of their anticoagulant dosage.

In long-term therapy, periodic laboratory evaluation of organ systems, including heamatopoietic, renal and hepatic studies should be performed.

All infections due to Group A beta-haemolytic streptococci should be treated for at least ten days.

Since bacteriostatic drugs may interfere with the bactericidal action of penicillin, it is advisable to avoid giving tetracyclines in conjunction with penicillin.

Use in pregnancy: Results of animal studies indicate that tetracyclines cross the placenta, are found in foetal tissues and can have toxic effects on the developing foetus (often related to retardation of skeletal development). Evidence of embryotoxicity has also been noted in animals treated early in pregnancy.

Use in newborns, infants and children: All tetracyclines form a stable calcium complex in any bone forming tissue. A decrease in the fibula growth rate has been observed in prematures given oral tetracycline in doses of 25 mg/kg every six hours. This reaction was shown to be reversible when the drug was discontinued.

Tetracyclines are present in the milk of lactating women who are taking a drug in this class.

Use in the elderly: Evidence is not available to suggest an increased incidence of adverse reactions in this age group. However, the possibility of sub-clinical renal insufficiency should be considered, as it may lead to drug accumulation.

Side-effects: Gastro-intestinal: Anorexia, nausea, vomiting, diarrhoea, glossitis, dysphagia, enterocolitis and inflammatory lesions (with monilial overgrowth) in the anogenital region. These side-effects have been caused by both the oral and parenteral administration of tetracyclines. Rare instances of oesophagitis and oesophageal ulcerations have been reported in patients receiving capsule and tablet forms of drugs in the tetracycline class. Most of these patients took medications immediately before going to bed.

Skin: Maculopapular and erythematous rashes. Exfoliative dermatitis has been reported but is uncommon. Photosensitivity.

Renal toxicity: Rise in BUN has been reported and is apparently dose related.
(See *Warnings.*)

Hypersensitivity reactions: Urticaria, angioneurotic oedema, anaphylaxis, anaphylactoid purpura, pericarditis and exacerbation of systemic lupus erythematosus.

Blood: Haemolytic anaemia, thrombocytopenia, neutropenia and eosinophilia have been reported.

Other: Bulging fontanelles have been reported in young infants following full therapeutic dosage. This sign disappeared rapidly when the drug was discontinued.

When given over prolonged periods, tetracyclines have been reported to produce brown-black microscopic discoloration of thyroid glands. No abnormalities of thyroid function studies are known to occur.

Pharmaceutical precautions Store below 25°C. Protect from light.

Legal category POM.

Package quantities *Tablets 250 mg:* Packs of 100 and 1,000.
Capsules 250 mg: Pack of 100.

Further information Nil.

Product licence numbers
Tablets 250 mg	0057/5080
Capsules 250 mg	0057/5036

TERRA-CORTRIL* EAR SUSPENSION

Presentation Terra-Cortril Ear Suspension contains 15 mg of Hydrocortisone Acetate PhEur, 5 mg of Oxytetracycline as the Hydrochloride PhEur and 10,000 units of Polymyxin B Sulphate PhEur in each millilitre of a controlled-viscosity, gel-like base.

Uses *Actions:* This single preparation provides a potent anti-inflammatory, anti-allergic hormone which controls excessive tissue reaction to infections, allergens and trauma, and effective antibiotic activity to curtail the growth of the causative and secondary infecting organism(s).

The broad antimicrobial spectrum of oxytetracycline commends its use in the treatment of infections due to staphylococci, streptococci, pneumococci, H. influenzae (Koch-Weeks bacillus), the diplo-bacillus of Morax-Axenfeld, Friedlander's bacillus, E. coli. and A. aerogenes. The effectiveness of oxytetracycline against both Gram-positive and Gram-negative organisms is enhanced by the particular potency of polymyxin B against infections caused by Pseudomonas pyocyanea, (B. pyocyaneus), where polymyxin B is the antibiotic of choice.

Indications: Terra-Cortril Ear Suspension is recommended for the topical treatment of ear conditions in which hydrocortisone is indicated and where there is the possibility of the presence of infection by organisms sensitive to the tetracyclines or polymyxin B.

Terra-Cortril Ear Suspension is recommended for infections of the external ear canal due to organisms sensitive to the tetracyclines, particularly those of mixed bacterial origin and where the aetiology remains obscure and which are accompanied by inflammatory reactions for which hydrocortisone is indicated. The suspension is also recommended in the treatment of impetigo, diffuse otitis externa and for localised lesions which have become super infected.

In addition, Terra-Cortril Ear Suspension may be used in allergic external otitis of mixed origin, atopic external otitis, excessive inflammatory reactions, pruritus and chronic eczema of the external ear canal.

If the infection is found to be deep-seated or spreading, the topical effect of the suspension should be reinforced by the systemic administration of Terramycin.

Dosage and administration For the treatment of affections of the external ear canal it is recommended that 2 to 4 drops be instilled three times daily, or as prescribed by the physician. The patient should be instructed to avoid contamination of the nozzle with exudate from the infected site.

Contra-indications, warnings, etc
Contra-indications: Terra-Cortril is contra-indicated in the presence of fungal infections. Acute purulent infections may be masked or enhanced by the presence of the steroid.

The use of topical hydrocortisone preparations is contra-indicated in tuberculous lesions of the skin, herpes simplex, vaccinia and varicella.

Hypersensitivity to any of the components of the preparation.

Warnings: Specific antimicrobial therapy by the systemic route is indicated for treatment of deep infections of the ear.

Precautions: Allergic reactions to oxytetracycline may occur occasionally, but are rare. If such reactions occur, the use of Terra-Cortril Ear Suspension should be discontinued.

The use of oxytetracycline and other antibiotics may result in an overgrowth of resistant organisms – particularly monilia and staphylococci. Constant observation of the patient for this possibility is required. If new infections due to non-susceptible bacteria or fungi appear during therapy, appropriate measures should be taken.

Topical administration of corticosteroids to pregnant animals can cause abnormalities of foetal development. The relevance of this to human beings has not been established. Topical steroids should not be used extensively in the first trimester of pregnancy, i.e. in large amounts or for prolonged periods. However, the unproven theoretical teratogenic hazard must be placed in perspective against the need for corticosteroids to maintain the health of the patient.

Caution should be exercised in the use of topical steroids in the treatment of infantile eczema because of the risk of suppression of adrenal function following absorption. To date this effect has not been reported with Terra-Cortril Ear Suspension.

Use in the elderly: No special precautions.

Pharmaceutical precautions Store below 25°C.

Legal category POM.

Package quantities Tube 5 ml.

Further information The tube has a specially designed narrow nozzle.

Product licence number 0057/5073.

TERRA-CORTRIL* SPRAY

Presentation Terra-Cortril Spray contains oxytetracycline hydrochloride PhEur and hydrocortisone PhEur in finely divided form as a pressure packed presentation for topical application when both anti-inflammatory and anti-infective action is required. Terra-Cortril Spray is available as an aerosol in:

42 g (30 ml) container (50 mg hydrocortisone PhEur and 150 mg oxytetracycline as the hydrochloride PhEur).
84 g (60 ml) container (100 mg hydrocortisone PhEur and 300 mg oxytetracycline as the hydrochloride PhEur).

Uses *Actions:* Terra-Cortril Spray contains both the anti-infective activity of Terramycin and the anti-inflammatory activity of hydrocortisone.

Terramycin is a potent broad-spectrum antibiotic which is useful topically for prevention or treatment of superficial cutaneous infections due to a variety of pyogenic bacteria, both Gram-positive and Gram-negative.

Hydrocortisone is primarily effective because of its anti-inflammatory, anti-pruritic, and vasoconstrictive actions.

In the treatment of superficial infections of skin amenable to Terramycin therapy, the anti-inflammatory action of the hydrocortisone in this preparation will afford prompt symptomatic relief while the Terramycin is acting against the causative organisms.

Where topical therapy with hydrocortisone is of value, the added presence of Terramycin will serve to prevent or eradicate secondary bacterial complications. Since varying degrees of bacterial infection frequently complicate those skin conditions for which hydrocortisone topical therapy is indicated, this combined preparation may offer therapeutic advantages over the use of hydrocortisone alone.

Terra-Cortril Spray is thus useful in the treatment of

skin conditions in which antibacterial and anti-inflammatory effects are desired.

In the allergic dermatoses, the inciting allergens in the food or environment should be determined and eliminated. Patch tests, intradermal tests or other suitable procedures should be employed to determine the allergens. In patients with widespread dermatitis, oral steroid therapy may be advisable.

Supplementary therapy with oral Terramycin is advisable in the treatment of severe infections or those which may become systemic.

Indications: Cutaneous infections: Including superficial pyogenic infections, pyoderma, pustular dermatitis, and infections associated with minor burns or wounds (under close supervision).

Atopic dermatitis: Including allergic eczema, both disseminated and circumscribed neurodermatitis, pruritus with lichenification, eczematoid dermatitis, food eczema and infantile eczema.

Contact dermatitis: Due to plants, drugs, cosmetics, clothing material, and miscellaneous substances.

Nonspecific pruritus: Of the anus, vulva or scrotum.

Dosage and administration After thorough cleansing of the affected skin area, a small amount of the spray should be applied, covering the whole surface and keeping the container at a proper distance (approximately 20–25 cm). Applications should be made two to four times daily. When actual infection is present, the spray may be applied and then covered with a sterile gauze in order to keep the affected area protected. Care should be taken not to discontinue therapy too soon after the initial response has been obtained.

Supplementary therapy with oral Terramycin is advisable in the treatment of severe infections or those which may become systemic.

Terra-Cortril Spray can be used in infants, children and adults.

Contra-indications, warnings, etc
Contra-indications: Hypersensitivity to any of the components of the preparation.

Acute herpes simplex, vaccinia and varicella.
Tuberculosis of the skin.
Fungal diseases of the skin.

Warnings: When used on the face, the eyes should be closed and protected. Inhalation of the spray should be avoided.

Precautions: If irritation develops, the product should be discontinued and appropriate therapy instituted.

The use of Terramycin and other antibiotics may result in an overgrowth of resistant organisms – particularly monilia and staphylococci. Constant observation of the patient for this possibility is essential.

If new infections due to nonsusceptible bacteria or fungi appear during therapy, appropriate measures should be taken.

If a favourable response does not occur promptly, the corticosteroid should be discontinued until the infection has been adequately controlled.

If extensive areas are treated or if the occlusive technique is used there will be increased systemic absorption of the corticosteroid and suitable precautions should be taken, particularly in children and infants.

Although topical steroids have not been reported to have an adverse effect on human pregnancy, the safety of their use in pregnant women has not been absolutely established. In laboratory animals, increases in incidence of foetal abnormalities have been associated with exposure of gestating females to topical corticosteroids, in some cases at rather low dosage levels. Therefore, drugs of this class should not be used extensively on pregnant patients, in large amounts, or for prolonged periods of time.

Terra-Cortril Spray is not for ophthalmic use.

Use in the elderly: No special precautions.

Side-effects: Hydrocortisone and Terramycin are well tolerated by the epithelial tissues and may be used topically with minimal untoward effects. Allergic reactions may occur occasionally, but are rare.

The following local side-effects have been reported with topical corticosteroids, especially under occlusive dressings: burning, itching, irritation, dryness, folliculitis, hypertrichosis, acneiform eruptions, hypopigmentation, perioral dermatitis, allergic contact dermatitis, maceration of the skin, secondary infection, skin atrophy, striae, and miliaria.

The use of Terra-Cortril Spray should be discontinued if such reactions occur.

Pharmaceutical precautions Store below 25°C.

Legal category POM.

Package quantities 42 g (30 ml) aerosol
84 g (60 ml) aerosol

Further information Nil.

Product licence number 0057/5074.

TERRA-CORTRIL* TOPICAL OINTMENT

Presentation Terra-Cortril Topical Ointment contains 30 mg oxytetracycline as the hydrochloride PhEur and 10 mg hydrocortisone PhEur in each gram of petroleum base.

Uses *Actions:* Terra-Cortril Topical Ointment contains both the anti-infective activity of Terramycin and the anti-inflammatory activity of hydrocortisone.

Terramycin is a potent broad-spectrum antibiotic which is useful topically for prevention of treatment of superficial cutaneous infections due to a variety of pyogenic bacteria, both Gram-positive and Gram-negative.

Hydrocortisone is primarily effective because of its anti-inflammatory, anti-pruritic, and vasoconstrictive actions.

In the treatment of superficial infections of the skin amenable to Terramycin therapy, the anti-inflammatory action of the hydrocortisone in this ointment will afford prompt symptomatic relief while the Terramycin is acting against the causative organisms.

Where topical therapy with hydrocortisone is of value, the added presence of Terramycin will serve to prevent or eradicate secondary bacterial complications. Since varying degrees of bacterial infection frequently complicate those skin conditions for which hydrocortisone topical therapy is indicated, this combined preparation may offer therapeutic advantages over the use of hydrocortisone alone.

Terra-Cortril Topical Ointment is thus useful in the treatment of skin conditions in which antibacterial and anti-inflammatory effects are desired.

In the allergic dermatoses, the inciting allergens in the food or environment should be determined and eliminated. Patch tests, intradermal tests or other suitable procedures should be employed to determine the allergens. In patients with widespread dermatitis, oral therapy with hydrocortisone may be advisable.

Supplementary therapy with oral Terramycin is advisable in the treatment of severe infections or those which may become systemic.

Indications: Cutaneous infections: Including superficial pyogenic infections, pyoderma, pustular dermatitis, and infections associated with minor burns or wounds (under close supervision).

Atopic dermatitis: Including allergic eczema, both disseminated and circumscribed neurodermatitis, pruritus with lichenification, eczematoid dermatitis, food eczema, and infantile eczema.

Contact dermatitis: Due to plants, drugs, cosmetics, clothing material, and miscellaneous substances.

Nonspecific pruritus: Of the anus, vulva, or scrotum.

Dosage and administration After thorough cleansing of the affected skin areas, a small amount of the ointment should be applied gently. Applications should be made two to four times daily. When actual infection is present, the ointment may be applied on sterile gauze and, by this means, kept in contiguous contact with the affected area. Care should be taken not to discontinue therapy too soon after the initial response has been obtained.

Contra-indications, warnings, etc
Contra-indications: Hypersensitivity to any of the components of the preparation.
    Acute herpes simplex, vaccinia and varicella.
    Tuberculosis of the skin.
    Fungal diseases of the skin.

Precautions: If irritation develops, the product should be discontinued and appropriate therapy instituted.

The use of Terramycin and other antibiotics may result in an overgrowth of resistant organisms – particularly *Candida* and staphylococci. Constant observation of the patient for this possibility is essential. If new infections due to nonsusceptible bacteria or fungi appear during therapy, appropriate measures should be taken.

If a favourable response does not occur promptly, the corticosteroid should be discontinued until the infection has been adequately controlled.

If extensive areas are treated or if the occlusive technique is used, there will be increased systemic absorption of the corticosteroid and suitable precautions should be taken, particularly in children and infants.

Although topical steroids have not been reported to have an adverse effect on human pregnancy, the safety of their use in pregnant women has not been absolutely established. In laboratory animals, increases in incidence of foetal abnormalities have been associated with exposure of gestating females to topical corticosteroids, in some cases at rather low dosage levels. Therefore, drugs of this class should not be used extensively on pregnant patients, in large amounts or for prolonged periods of time.

Terra-Cortril Ointment is not recommended for ophthalmic use.

Use in the elderly: No special precautions.

Side-effects: Hydrocortisone and Terramycin are well tolerated by the epithelial tissues and may be used topically with minimal untoward effects. Allergic reactions may occur occasionally, but are rare.

The following local side-effects have been reported with topical corticosteroids, especially under occlusive dressings: burning, itching, irritation, dryness, folliculitis, hypertrichosis, acneiform eruptions, hypopigmentation, perioral dermatitis, allergic contact dermatitis, maceration of the skin, secondary infection, skin atrophy, striae, miliaria.

The use of Terra-Cortril Topical Ointment should be discontinued if such reactions occur.

Pharmaceutical precautions Store below 25°C.

Legal category POM.

Package quantities 15 g tube
                        30 g tube

Further information Nil.

Product licence number 0057/5076.

TERRA-CORTRIL* NYSTATIN CREAM

Presentation Terra-Cortril Nystatin Cream is an homogeneous yellow cream containing 30 mg oxytetracycline as calcium di-oxytetracycline USP, 10 mg hydrocortisone PhEur and 100,000 units nystatin BP in each gram of perfumed cream.

Uses *Actions:* Terra-Cortril Nystatin Cream is ideal for use in conditions where topical, nonsystemic action is desired. The Terramycin present will prevent or overcome superficial infections caused by organisms susceptible to it. Concomitantly, the concentration of hydrocortisone supplied is ample for inflammatory reactions resulting from allergy, infection or trauma. Nystatin is an antifungal antibiotic which is both fungistatic and fungicidal *in vitro* against a wide variety of yeasts and yeast-like fungi. It is effective for the treatment of cutaneous infections caused by *Candida albicans* and other Candida as well as other yeasts.

Thus this product provides the combined broadspectrum activity of Terramycin against the primarily causative or secondarily infecting organisms, and the effectiveness of hydrocortisone, an anti-allergic, anti-inflammatory hormone, which controls excessive tissue reaction to infections, allergens, and trauma along with nystatin which prevents or eradicates secondary fungal infections.

Indications: The use of Terra-Cortril Nystatin Cream is indicated in the treatment of steroid-responsive dermatoses. The added presence of Terramycin and nystatin will serve to prevent or eradicate secondary bacterial and fungal complications. Since varying degrees of bacterial and/or fungal infection frequently complicate those skin conditions for which hydrocortisone topical therapy is indicated, this combined preparation may offer therapeutic advantages over the use of hydrocortisone alone.

Among these conditions are: Atopic dermatitis: including allergic eczema, both disseminated and circumscribed neurodermatitis, pruritus with lichenification, eczematoid dermatitis, food eczema, and infantile eczema.

Cutaneous infections: including superficial pyogenic infections, pyoderma, pustular dermatitis, and infections associated with minor burns or wounds.

Contact dermatitis: due to plants, drugs, cosmetics, clothing material and miscellaneous substances.

Non-specific pruritus: of the anus, vulva or scrotum.

Dosage and administration After thorough cleansing of the affected skin areas, a small amount of the cream should be applied gently. Applications should be made two to four times daily. When actual infection is present, the cream may be applied on sterile gauze and, by this means, kept in contiguous contact with the affected area. Care should be taken not to discontinue therapy too soon after the initial response has been obtained.

Supplementary therapy with oral Terramycin is advisable in the treatment of severe infections or those which may become systemic.

Terra-Cortril Nystatin Cream can be used in infants, children and adults.

Contra-indications, warnings, etc
Contra-indications: 1. Acute herpes simplex, vaccinia and varicella.

2. Tuberculosis of the skin.

3. Hypersensitivity to any of the components of the cream.

4. Acute purulent infections.

Precautions: The use of Terramycin and other antibiotics may result in an overgrowth of resistant organisms. Observation of the patient for this possibility is required.

If irritation develops, the product should be discontinued and appropriate therapy instituted.

If a favourable response does not occur promptly, the corticosteroid should be discontinued until the infection has been adequately controlled.

If extensive areas are treated or if the occlusive technique is used there will be increased systemic absorption of the corticosteroid and suitable precautions should be taken, particularly in children and infants.

Although topical steroids have not been reported to have an adverse effect on human pregnancy, the safety of their use in pregnant women has not been absolutely established. In laboratory animals, increase in incidence of foetal abnormalities have been associated with exposure of gestating females to topical corticosteroids, in some cases at rather low dosage levels. Therefore, drugs of this class should not be used extensively on pregnant patients, in large amounts, or for prolonged periods of time.

Terra-Cortril Nystatin Cream is not for opthalmic use.

Use in the elderly: No special precautions.

Side-effects: Hydrocortisone and Terramycin are well tolerated by the epithelial tissues and may be used topically with minimal untoward effects. Allergic reactions may occur occasionally, but are rare.

The following local side-effects have been reported with topical corticosteroids, especially under occlusive dressings: burning, itching, irritation, dryness, folliculitis, hypertrichosis, acneiform eruptions, hypopigmentation, perioral dermatitis, allergic contact dermatitis, maceration of the skin, secondary infection, skin atrophy, striae, miliaria.

The use of Terra-Cortril Nystatin Cream should be discontinued if such reactions occur.

Pharmaceutical precautions Store below 25°C.

Legal category POM.

Package quantities 30 g tube.

Further information Nil.

Product licence number 0057/0099.

VIBRAMYCIN*

Presentation Vibramycin is available as: green capsules containing 100 mg doxycycline as the hydrochloride, coded 'Pfizer' and 'VBM 100'.

Vibramycin 50, green and cream capsules containing 50 mg doxycycline as the hydrochloride, coded 'Pfizer' and 'VBM 50'.

Vibramycin D (dispersible) tablets, off white-buff tablets coded D9 on the one side and 'Pfizer' on the other, each containing 100 mg doxycycline as the monohydrate.

Syrup: 30 ml (5 ml containing the equivalent of 50 mg doxycycline as the calcium chelate), coloured red and fruit flavoured.

Vibramycin is a broad-spectrum antibiotic synthetically derived from oxytetracycline. The chemical designation of this light yellow crystalline powder is alpha-6-deoxy-5-oxytetracycline.

Vibramycin has a high degree of lipid solubility and a low affinity for calcium. It is highly stable in normal human serum. Vibramycin will not degrade into an epianhydro form.

Uses *Actions:* Vibramycin is primarily bacteriostatic and is believed to exert its antimicrobial effect by the inhibition of protein synthesis. Vibramycin is active against a wide range of Gram-positive and Gram-negative bacteria and certain other micro-organisms.

Tetracyclines are readily absorbed and are bound to plasma proteins in varying degrees. They are concentrated by the liver in the bile and excreted in the urine and faeces at high concentrations and in a biologically active form. Vibramycin is virtually completely absorbed after oral administration. Studies reported to date indicate that the absorption of Vibramycin, unlike certain other tetracyclines, is not notably influenced by the ingestion of food or milk.

Following a 200 mg dose, normal adult volunteers averaged peak serum levels of 2.6 mcg/ml of Vibramycin at 2 hours decreasing to 1.45 mcg/ml at 24 hours. Studies have shown no significant difference in serum half-life of Vibramycin (range 18 to 22 hours) in individuals with normal and severely impaired renal function.

Haemodialysis does not alter the serum half-life of Vibramycin.

Indications: Vibramycin has been found clinically effective in the treatment of a variety of infections caused by susceptible strains of Gram-positive and Gram-negative bacteria and certain other micro-organisms.

Pneumonia: Single and multiple pneumonia and bronchopneumonia due to susceptible strains of pneumococci and other *Streptococcus* species, *Staphylococcus* species, *H. influenzae, Klebsiella pneumoniae,* and *Mycoplasma pneumoniae.*

Other respiratory tract infections: Pharyngitis, tonsillitis, otitis media, bronchitis and sinusitis caused by susceptible strains of beta-haemolytic streptococci, *Staphylococcus* species, pneumococci and *H. Influenzae.*

Genito-urinary tract infections: Pyelonephritis, cystitis, urethritis, caused by susceptible strains of the *Klebsiella-Enterobacter* group, *Escherichia coli, Staphylococcus* species, *Neisseria gonorrhoeae,* and *Chlamydia trachomatis.* Acute gonococcal anterior urethritis in the adult male has been effectively treated with a single large dose of Vibramycin. The highest cure rates were achieved with more extended therapy.

Soft tissue infections: Impetigo, furunculosis, cellulitis, abscess, infected traumatic and postoperative wounds and paronychia caused by susceptible strains of *Staphylococcus aureus, Staphylococcus albus, Streptococcus* species, *E. coli,* and susceptible strains of the *Klebsiella-*

Enterobacter group. In the treatment of soft tissue infections, indicated surgical procedures should be carried out in conjunction with Vibramycin treatment.

Dermatological infections: Acne vulgaris and acne conglobata.

Since Vibramycin is a member of the tetracycline series of antibiotics, it may be expected to be useful in the treatment of infections which respond to other tetracyclines, such as:

Ophthalmic infections: Due to susceptible strains of gonococci, staphylococci, and *H. Influenzae*. Vibramycin is indicated in the treatment of trachoma, although the infectious agent is not always eliminated, as judged by immunofluorescence. Inclusion conjunctivitis may be treated with oral Vibramycin alone or in combination with topical agents.

Gastro-intestinal infections: Due to susceptible strains of such organisms as *Entamoeba histolytica*, enteropathogenic *E. coli*, *Shigella* species, and *Salmonella* species.

Miscellaneous: Psittacosis. Prostatis and trigonitis due to *Proteus* species. Other infections due to susceptible strains of *Bacteroides* species, *Yersinia* species, *Brucella* species (in combination with streptomycin), *Listeria* species, *Rickettsia* species and *Bordetella pertussis*, *Bacillus anthracis*, *Clostridium welchii*, *Neisseria meningitis*, spirochaetes, (*Treponema* species), *Calymmatobacterium granulomatis*.

In acute intestinal amoebiasis Vibramycin may be a useful adjunct to amoebicides.

Dosage and administration The usual dose of Vibramycin for the treatment of acute infections in adults is 200 mg on the first day of treatment (administered as a single dose or divided into two equal doses with a 12 hour interval), followed by a maintenance dose of 100 mg/day. In the management of more severe infections (particularly chronic infections of the urinary tract), 200 mg daily should be given throughout the treatment period. Vibramycin-D tablets are administered by drinking a suspension of the tablet in half a cup of water.

The recommended dosage schedule for children weighing 50 kg or less is 4 mg/kg of body weight on the first day of treatment (given as a single dose or divided into two equal doses with a 12 hour interval), followed by 2 mg/kg of body weight on subsequent days. For more severe infections up to 4 mg/kg of body weight may be used daily. For children over 50 kg the usual adult dose should be used. (See *Warnings* section about use in children).

Administration of adequate amounts of fluid along with capsule forms of drugs in the tetracycline class is recommended to reduce the risk of oesophageal irritation and ulceration.

If gastric irritation occurs, it is recommended that Vibramycin be given with food or milk. Studies indicate that the absorption of Vibramycin is not markedly influenced by simultaneous ingestion of food or milk.

Exceeding the recommended dosage may result in an increased incidence of side-effects. Therapy should be continued at least 24 to 48 hours after symptoms and fever have subsided. When used in streptococcal infections, therapy should be continued for ten days to prevent the development of rheumatic fever or glomerulonephritis.

Acne vulgaris: In the treatment of acne vulgaris the recommended dose is 50 mg daily with food. Duration

of treatment will vary from 6 to 12 weeks or longer dependent upon the response.

Acute gonococcal anterior urethritis in males: A single dose of 300 mg or 100 mg twice daily for two to four days. The dose should be administered with food, including milk or carbonated beverage, as required.

Acute gonococcal infections in the adult female: Doses of 100 mg twice daily until cure is effected.

Uncomplicated urethral, endocervical, or rectal infection in adults caused by *Chlamydia trachomatis:* 100 mg, by mouth, twice daily for at least seven days.

Primary and secondary syphilis: 300 mg daily in divided doses for at least ten days. Louse-borne typhus has been successfully treated with a single oral dose of 100 to 200 mg according to severity.

Concomitant therapy: antacids containing aluminium, calcium or magnesium impair absorption and should not be given to patients taking Vibramycin.

Studies to date have indicated that administration of Vibramycin at the usual recommended doses does not lead to excessive accumulation of the antibiotic in patients with renal impairment.

Use in the elderly: Vibramycin may be prescribed in the usual dose with no special precautions. No dosage adjustment is necessary in the presence of renal impairment.

Contra-indications, warnings, etc
Contra-indications: Vibramycin is contra-indicated in persons who have shown hypersensitivity to any of the tetracyclines.

Warnings: The use of drugs of the tetracycline class during tooth development (last half of pregnancy, infancy and childhood to the age of 8 years) may cause permanent discoloration of the teeth (yellow-grey-brown). This adverse reaction is more common during long term use of the drugs but has been observed following repeated short term courses. Enamel hypoplasia has also been reported.

Vibramycin, therefore, should not be used in these groups of patients unless other drugs are not available, are not likely to be effective or are contra-indicated.

Photosensitivity manifested by an exaggerated sunburn reaction has been observed in some individuals taking tetracyclines. Patients likely to be exposed to direct sunlight or ultraviolet light should be advised that this reaction can occur with tetracycline drugs and treatment should be discontinued at the first evidence of skin erythema.

The antianabolic action of the tetracyclines may cause an increase in BUN. Studies to date indicate that this does not occur with the use of Vibramycin in patients with impaired renal function.

Use in pregnancy: (See *Warnings* section about use during tooth development.)

Vibramycin has not been studied in pregnant patients. It should not be used in pregnant women unless, in the judgement of the physician, it is essential for the welfare of the patient.

Results of animal studies indicate that tetracyclines cross the placenta, are found in foetal tissues and can have toxic effects on the developing foetus (often related to retardation of skeletal development). Evidence of embryotoxicity has also been noted in animals treated early in pregnancy.

Use in children: (See *Warnings* section about use during tooth development). As with other tetracyclines, Vibramycin forms a stable calcium complex in any bone-forming tissue. A decrease in the fibula growth rate has been observed in prematures given oral tetracycline in doses of 25mg/kg every 6 hours. This reaction was shown to be reversible when the drug was discontinued.

Tetracyclines are present in the milk of lactating women who are taking a drug of this class and should therefore be avoided in nursing mothers.

Precautions: The use of antibiotics may occasionally result in over-growth of nonsusceptible organisms. Constant observation of the patient is essential. If a resistant organism appears, the antibiotic should be discontinued and appropriate therapy instituted.

When treating venereal disease when co-existent syphilis is suspected, proper diagnostic procedures, including dark-field examinations, should be utilized. In all such cases monthly serological tests should be made for at least four months.

Infections due to group A beta-haemolytic streptococci should be treated for at least ten days.

In long term therapy because the tetracyclines have been shown to depress plasma prothrombin activity, patients who are on anticoagulant therapy may require downward adjustment of their anticoagulant dosage.

Since bacteriostatic drugs may interfere with the bactericidal action of penicillin, it is advisable to avoid giving Vibramycin in conjunction with penicillin.

Side-effects: Due to virtually complete absorption of Vibramycin gastro-intestinal side-effects are infrequent. The following side-effects have been observed in patients receiving tetracyclines.

Gastro-intestinal: anorexia, nausea, vomiting, diarrhoea, glossitis, dysphagia, enterocolitis, and inflammatory lesions (with monilial overgrowth) in the anogenital region. These reactions have been caused by both the oral and parenteral administration of tetracyclines. Rare instances of oesophagitis and oesophageal ulcerations have been reported in patients receiving capsule and tablet forms of drugs in the tetracycline class. Most of these patients took medications immediately before going to bed.

Skin: Maculopapular and erythematous rashes. Exfoliative dermatitis has been reported but is uncommon. Photosensitivity is discussed in the *Warnings* section.

Hypersensitivity reactions: Urticaria, angioneurotic oedema, anaphylaxis, anaphylactoid purpura, pericarditis, and exacerbation of systemic lupus erythematosus.

Bulging fontanelles in infants and benign intracranial hypertension in adults has been reported in individuals receiving full therapeutic dosages. These conditions disappeared rapidly when the drug was discontinued.

Blood: haemolytic anaemia, thrombocytopenia, neutropenia and eosinophilia have been reported with tetracyclines.

When given over prolonged periods, tetracyclines have been reported to produce brown-black microscopic discoloration of thyroid tissue. No abnormalities of thyroid function are known to occur.

Overdose and toxic effects: Acute overdosage with antibiotics is rare. Toxic effects are usually due to hypersensitivity reactions and should be treated as such.

Pharmaceutical precautions *Storage:* Capsules and syrup: Store below 25°C. Dispersible tablets: Store below 25°C. Protect from light.

When Vibramycin Syrup is dispensed to meet prescriptions for 2.5 ml (25 mg) doses, the product should be diluted with an equal amount of simple syrup. This ensures that each 25 mg dose is taken in the minimum statutory volume of 5 ml. When thus dispensed the syrup should be used within fourteen days.

Legal category POM.

Package quantities 50 mg capsules in calendar packs of 28. 100 mg capsules in blister packs of 10 and 50. Syrup 30 ml bottle (50mg/5 ml). Dispersible tablets 100 mg in blister packs of 10.

Further information Nil.

Product licence numbers

Capsules 50 mg	0057/0238
Capsules 100 mg	0057/5059
Syrup	0057/5060
Dispersible tablets	0057/0188

*Trade Mark

Pharmaceutical Manufacturing Company
Home Park Estate
Kings Langley, Herts WD4 8DH

XYLOTOX* 2% E.80

Presentation Sterile clear aqueous solution: ligno-caine hydrochloride 20 mg/ml, Adrenaline BP 1:80,000.

Uses Local anaesthetic solution with vasoconstrictor for dental infiltration anaesthesia where a vasoconstrictor is indicated. For all dental nerve-block techniques.

Dosage and administration *Infiltration:* 1 ml. *Nerve block:* 1.5 to 2 ml. *Extensive surgery:* 3 to 10 ml. Adult maximum dose 500 mg.

In children the maximum dose is considerably less and should be calculated in relation to the body weight.

Contra-indications, warnings, etc Patients with thyrotoxicosis and cardiac disease, particularly with arrhythmia or hypertension. Known hypersensitivity to local anaesthetics of the amide type.

Adverse reactions: The type of toxic reaction is unpredictable and depends on dosage, route of administration and state of patient, the reactions are primarily of two types, typified by stimulation and depression of the cerebral cortex and medulla respectively. Slow onset – stimulation leading to nervousness, dizziness, blurred vision, nausea, tremor convulsions and respiratory arrest. Rapid onset – depression leading primarily to respiratory arrest, cardiovascular collapse and cardiac arrest. Symptoms occur rapidly and with little warning.

Precautions: Adequate resuscitation equipment must be available whenever local or general anaesthesia is administered. Though clinical tolerance is remarkably good, overdosage or accidental intravenous injection may give rise to toxic reactions. These are best avoided by aspiration before making an injection in order to avoid accidental intravascular injection.

Care should be observed in patients taking tricyclic anti-depressants.

Pharmaceutical precautions Store in a cool place.

Legal category POM.

Package quantities Glass cartridges of 2.2 ml and 1.8 ml in boxes of 100.

Further information Nil.

Product licence number 0017/0141.

*Trade Mark

Pharmacia Ltd
Pharmacia House
Midsummer Boulevard
Milton Keynes MK9 3HP

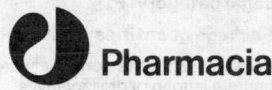

CALMURID*

Presentation A white shiny cream containing Carbamide (urea) BP 10% and lactic acid 5% in a stabilising emulsified base.

Uses For correction of hyperkeratosis and dryness in ichthyosis and allied conditions characterised by dry, rough, scaly skin.

Dosage and administration A thick layer of Calmurid is applied twice daily after washing the affected area. The cream is left on the skin for three to five minutes and then lightly rubbed in. Excess cream can be wiped off with a tissue. Frequency of application can be reduced as patient progresses. In hyperkeratosis of the feet apply Calmurid as above after soaking the feet in warm water for 15 minutes and drying with a rough towel.

Elderly: No special instructions.

Contra-indications, warnings, etc *Adverse effects:* Calmurid is acidic and can cause smarting when applied to raw areas, fissures or mucous membranes. Where this is a barrier to therapy, use of Calmurid diluted 50% with Aqueous Cream BP for one week should result in freedom from smarting on application of Calmurid.

Pharmaceutical precautions Store in a cool place but do not freeze. Do not put in alloy containers.

Legal category GSL.

Package quantities Tubes of 50 g, 100 g and 300 g.

Further information Calmurid, besides being keratolytic, replaces the small water-binding molecules of which dry skin may be deficient. It does not contain lanolin, steroids or preservatives.

Product licence number 0009/5009.

CALMURID* HC

Presentation A white shiny cream containing:

Carbamide (urea) BP	10%
Hydrocortisone	1%
Lactic acid	5%

in a stabilising emulsified base.

Uses Atopic eczema; Besnier's prurigo; acute and chronic allergic eczema; neurodermatitis and other hyperkeratotic skin conditions with accompanying inflammation.

Dosage and administration Apply the cream twice daily after washing and drying the lesion.

Elderly: No special instructions.

Contra-indications, warnings, etc *Adverse effects:* Because Calmurid HC is acidic it may cause smarting if applied to raw or fissured areas. Moist lesions should be encouraged to dry before beginning therapy.

Where smarting is a barrier to therapy, use of a mixture of Calmurid HC with an equal amount of Aqueous Cream BP for a week should result in freedom from smarting when undiluted Calmurid HC is applied.

In pregnant animals, administration of corticosteroids can cause abnormalities of foetal development. The relevance of this finding to human beings has not been established. However, topical steroids should not be used extensively in pregnancy, i.e. in large amounts or for long periods.

In infants, long-term continuous topical therapy should be avoided. Adrenal suppression can occur even without occlusion.

Contra-indications: Do not use in tubercular, viral or syphilitic skin infections. Antimycotic treatment should complement Calmurid HC in dermal fungal infections.

Pharmaceutical precautions Keep in a cool place but do not freeze. Do not pack in alloy containers.

Legal category POM.

Package quantities Tubes of 30 g and 100 g.

Further information Calmurid HC has keratolytic, antipruritic, anti-inflammatory and re-hydrating effects on the skin. It does not contain lanolin or preservatives.

Product licence number 0009/5003.

CALMURID* SOLUTION

Presentation Solution containing 20% urea, 5% lactic acid in a stabilising aqueous vehicle.

Uses For the treatment of dry scalp conditions – seborrhoea, seborrhoeic eczema, atopic eczema, ichthyosis. As part of the treatment of psoriasis of the scalp.

Dosage and administration Apply the solution to the scalp twice a day.

Wash the hair every other day with a mild shampoo during the course of treatment.

Elderly and children: No special instructions.

Contra-indications, warnings, etc Calmurid Solution can cause smarting temporarily when applied to raw or fissured areas.

Over-use may cause matting of the hair. The dried lotion will readily dissolve off the hair.

A feeling of scalp dryness has occasionally been noted early in treatment, but it generally soon passes off. A persistent feeling of scalp dryness may be due to too frequent use or the use of a harsh shampoo when the hair is washed.

Pharmaceutical precautions Store in a cool place but do not freeze.

Legal category P.

Package quantities Plastic bottle of 125 ml.

Further information Calmurid Solution does not contain lanolin or preservatives.

Product licence number 0009/0017.

DEBRISAN*

Presentation Sterile, straw-coloured spherical beads of dextranomer of 0.1–0.3 mm diameter, packed in plastic castors or single-use sachets.

Uses A dressing for moist wounds and indolent ulcers, whether clean or infected and small area burns.

Dosage and administration A 3 mm layer of Debrisan should be sprinkled onto the wound and kept in place by a pad of lint or a perforated plastic sheet. Debrisan is hydrophilic and the tissue exudate is drawn up into the layer. The Debrisan should be renewed before saturation occurs. Depending on the rate of exudation this may be necessary from one to five times a day. Once or twice daily is usually adequate. When Debrisan is changed the old material is readily rinsed off with water or saline and new material may then be sprinkled onto the wound.

Shallow wounds, or those in awkward positions, may be dressed more easily by using Debrisan Paste, or by mixing four parts of Debrisan with one part of sterile glycerol to form a stiff paste. This should be spread into the wound with a spatula to a depth of 3 mm or more. Dressing continues as above. The paste should be prepared freshly at each application. Once wound is clean and poorly secreting, change therapy to an antiseptic dressing, e.g. chlorhexidine tulle, or a sterile pad.

Full instructions for use are enclosed with each pack. Treated in this manner the wound will remain soft and pliable during healing.

Elderly: No special instructions.

Contra-indications, warnings, etc
1. Do not leave Debrisan for more than 24 hours on wounds with a very low exudation rate as it may dry and form a crust which may be difficult to wash off.
2. Occlusive dressings may lead to maceration of skin round the wound under treatment.
3. When deep infected wounds are treated, care must be taken to wash Debrisan from the depths of the wound.
4. No side-effects have been reported.

Warning: Debrisan spillage can render surfaces very slippery. Clear spillages promptly.

Precautions:
1. Not to be used on dry wounds.
2. When exudate has been markedly removed by Debrisan alternative treatment should be substituted.
3. In order to avoid cross-infection it is recommended that the contents of a castor be confined to the treatment of a single patient for one day.

Pharmaceutical precautions Keep in a dry place in well-closed containers.

Package quantities Castors of 60 g.
Sachets of 4 g in boxes of ten sachets.

Legal category POM.

Further information Each gram of Debrisan absorbs 4 grams of exudate. Capillary action carries debris and bacteria away from the wound surface. Local oedema is reduced so that the wound may look larger initially. Debrisan is non sensitising and controls malodour.

Product licence number 0009/0021.

DEBRISAN* ABSORBENT PAD ▼

Presentation Foil sachet containing sterile off-white paste in textile bag. Paste consists of Dextranomer 90%, polyethylene glycol and water 10%.

Uses For topical application to exudating wounds, whether clean or infected, such as surgical wounds, post traumatic wounds, pressure sores and leg ulcers.

Dosage and administration Frequency of change of the pad will be dictated by the rate of exudation of the wound. This may vary from twice daily to every two days. The textile has little tendency to adhere to the wound, but when it does sterile saline should readily loosen it. No special regimes of age groups.

Contra-indications, warnings, etc
Precautions: Use with caution near the eyes.

Warnings: Transient pain may occur in the wound area. This can often be avoided by wetting the wound before pad application.

Pharmaceutical precautions None.

Legal category POM.

Package quantities Box containing 7 × 3 g pads.

Further information Nil.

Product licence number 0009/0048.

DEBRISAN* PASTE ▼

Presentation Foil-plastic laminate pouches containing 10 g of a sterile soft, white, granular paste consisting of: Dextranomer 6.4 g, polyethylene glycol 600 and water to 10 g.

Uses Treatment of exudative and infected wounds such as surgical or post-traumatic wounds, decubital ulcers and leg ulcers. As the paste is adherent it may be preferred to Debrisan beads on shallow wounds, or those where retention of the beads is a problem.

Dosage and administration After cleaning the wound with sterile water or saline the Paste is applied firmly with a spatula to a depth of not less than 3 mm. The wound is covered and the Paste changed at intervals governed by the exudation rate of the wound, the Paste being renewed before it is entirely discoloured and saturated with secretion and debris. Debrisan Paste should be changed from twice daily to every two days according to the rate of exudation. Stop Debrisan Paste once the wound is granulating and free of exudate, changing to sterile or antiseptic dressings.

Elderly: No special instructions.

Contra-indications, warnings, etc Use with caution: When applied near the eyes; in deep fistulae etc. with a narrow opening where paste removal might be difficult.
Occasionally pain may be experienced in the wound

after application. This can be avoided by wetting the wound before applying the Paste.

Pharmaceutical precautions Stored at room temperature the shelf life is 3 years.

Legal category POM.

Package quantities 6 × 10 g; 4 × 10 g.

Product licence number 0009/0044.

HEALONID* ▼

Presentation Disposable single-use syringes containing Healonid of the following composition per ml:

Sodium hyaluronate	10 mg
Sodium chloride	8.5 mg
Disodium hydrogen phosphate dihydrate	0.28 mg
Sodium dihydrogen phosphate hydrate	0.04 mg
Water for injections	to 1 ml

The syringe membrane must be perforated before use, (see directions for use).

Uses Sodium hyaluronate is a visco-elastic polymer normally found in the aqueous and vitreous humour. Healonid, which contains sodium hyaluronate is a highly viscous clear solution at rest, yet it will readily flow through a fine cannula or needle under pressure. Introduction of Healonid into the anterior or posterior chamber keeps tissues separated during the operative procedure and protects them from trauma from other tissues or instruments. The anterior chamber depth is maintained, vitreous bulge can be reduced, and the loss of irreplaceable endothelial cells which inevitably accompanies surgery can be greatly reduced.

Indications: Surgical procedures on the eye, including intraocular lens insertion, intra and extra capsular lens extraction, glaucoma surgery, corneal graft, surgery for accidental trauma, retinal detachment and vitreal replacement procedures.

Dosage and administration The syringe is assembled and made ready for use according to the instruction sheet with each syringe.

It is recommended that Healonid be removed from the refrigerator to attain room temperature 30–60 mins before use.

Cataract surgery: A sufficient volume of Healonid is gently introduced into the anterior chamber at an early stage in the operation prior to lens extraction to protect the tissues from trauma.

Intraocular lens insertion: Healonid is introduced into the anterior chamber before lens extraction and is also used to coat the lens and instruments prior to introduction into the eye. Further Healonid may be injected to replace losses.

Glaucoma filtration surgery: Prior to trabeculectomy Healonid is injected slowly through a corneal paracentesis to maintain the anterior chamber volume. Injection may be continued to allow Healonid to flow through the sutured outer scleral flap to the conjunctival filtration site.

Corneal transplant surgery: After removal of the corneal button the anterior chamber is filled with Healonid. The donor graft is then placed on the bed of Healonid and sutured into place. Healonid may be put into the anterior chamber of the donor eye to protect the corneal endothelium.

Trauma: In various kinds of perforating trauma Healonid can be instilled to refill the anterior chamber, prevent prolapse of the iris and formation of synechiae. Blood contaminated Healonid should be replaced with new Healonid before closure.

Precautions: The anterior chamber should not be overfilled with Healonid, except in glaucoma surgery. At close of surgery some of the Healonid should be removed by irrigation or aspiration. Intraocular pressure should be monitored during the post operative period and any excessive rises treated with appropriate therapy.

Elderly: No special instructions.

Contra-indications, warnings, etc There are no known contra-indications to Healonid. Because the drug is extracted from avian tissues, despite rigorous purification procedures minute amounts of protein are present, and thus the remote possibility of idiosyncratic reactions remains.

Adverse reactions: The drug is very well tolerated and the only untoward effect reported has been a transient rise in intraocular pressure in a few cases.

Pharmaceutical precautions Healonid has a shelf life of 3 years when stored at 2–8°C protected from light and freezing. These conditions should be adhered to routinely. However, Healonid may be stored at room temperature for up to 4 weeks by the user.

Legal category POM.

Package quantities Disposable syringes containing 0.4 ml, 0.75 ml and 2.0 ml.

Further information Healonid does not interfere with the healing process. Its use may reduce incidence of synechiae and adhesions. Evidence from animal experiments indicates that Healonid is no longer present in the anterior chamber six days after introduction.

Product licence number 0009/0045.

HYSKON*

Presentation A sterile viscous aqueous solution of dextran 70 (M_w 70,000) and dextrose.
100 ml solution contains:

Dextran 70 (M_w 70,000) Pharmacia	32 g
Dextrose	10 g
Water for injections	to 100 ml

Viscosity at 20°C 220 cSt (255 cP).

Uses Hyskon is indicated for use with the hysteroscope. It is used both as a rinsing fluid and for dilatation of the uterus.

Dosage and administration *Dosage:* 50–100 ml for one examination. The amount of Hyskon required per patient depends on a number of factors, such as the type and length of the diagnostic procedure, whether or not manipulation or surgery is performed. Most often, however, the amount of Hyskon instilled into the uterus will be between 50 and 100 millilitres.

Administration: Hyskon should be introduced into the uterine cavity through the cannula of a hysteroscope under low pressure (approximately 100 mmHg) until the uterus is sufficiently distended to permit adequate visualisation. During the hysteroscopic examination, Hyskon should be infused at a rate that keeps the cavity suitably distended. To avoid injection of the fluid into the tissues of the uterus and parametria and to avoid having unnecessary amounts of the fluid pass into peritoneal cavity, pressures greater than 150 mmHg should be used with great care. Small amounts of fluid may occasionally escape into the peritoneal cavity.

Elderly: No special instructions.

Contra-indications, warnings, etc (1) Hyskon should not be used in patients known to be hypersensitive to dextran. Other contra-indications are those relative to the hysteroscopic procedure itself, such as pregnancy and upper genital tract infection.

(2) No other local or systemic reactions have been reported.

Pharmaceutical precautions (1) Use only if solution is clear.

(2) Store at an even temperature, preferably not exceeding 30°C.

Legal category POM.

Package quantities Carton containing 6 × 100 ml bottles.

Further information Hyskon has excellent optical properties.

The viscosity of Hyskon is adjusted to achieve optimum dilatation without too rapid escape of solution from the uterus. Its viscosity also prevents admixture with mucus and blood which would otherwise reduce visibility.

Product licence number 0009/0018.

MACRODEX* IN DEXTROSE

Presentation Macrodex in Dextrose contains:

Dextran of weight average molecular weight

70,000	30 g
Dextrose	25 g
Water for Injections	to 500 ml

Colourless, clear, slightly viscous solution. Bottle has a yellow seal.

Uses
1. As a plasma volume expander.
2. The prevention of thrombo-embolic episodes.
3. As a low sodium content alternative to Macrodex in Normal Saline.

Dosage and administration Dose may be adjusted to the needs and progress of the case.

Hypovolaemic shock: Give 500–1,000 ml i.v. as initial dose, the rate dependent on the patient's needs. Thereafter give equal volumes of Macrodex and blood. Haematocrit should be kept above 25%. Total Macrodex dose should not exceed 2,500 ml.

Shock prophylaxis at surgery: 500–1,000 ml is run in during operation, the rate being governed by pulse, skin colour, BP, etc.

Burns: Use to correct haemoconcentration. In general 3–5 litres can be given daily for 48 hours.

Prophylaxis of post-operative thrombosis: Slowly infuse 500 ml during or at the end of surgery over four to six hours, followed by a further 500 ml over four to six hours next day. In high-risk cases (hip fractures, history of thrombosis, etc) continue the treatment on alternate days for up to two weeks.

Elderly: Care not to overload.

Contra-indications, warnings, etc *Precautions:*

Give with caution to patients vulnerable to vascular overloading (congestive heart failure, renal disease, etc).

Adverse reactions: Very rarely spontaneous hypersensitivity – urticaria, rigors and flushing, occasionally with asthma and hypotension. Usually occurs in cases not under stress and appears within a few minutes of starting the infusion. *Action:* Stop the infusion and give symptomatic anti-allergic therapy.

Pharmaceutical precautions Store at steady room temperature. Poor storage can produce dextran flakes, which can be re-dissolved by autoclaving.

Legal category POM.

Package quantities Infusion bottles of 500 ml.

Further information Macrodex infusions have not been reported to produce difficulties with blood cross matching when given in volumes up to 1500 mls.

Product licence number 0009/5001.

MACRODEX* IN NORMAL SALINE

Presentation Macrodex in Normal Saline contains:

Dextran of weight average molecular weight

70,000	30 g
Sodium Chloride	4.5 g
Water for Injections	to 500 ml

Colourless, clear, slightly viscous solution. Bottle has a green seal.

Uses
1. As a plasma volume expander.
2. The prevention of thrombo-embolic episodes.
3. In certain cases of renal or cardiac disease Macrodex in 5% Dextrose may be preferred for its low sodium content.

Dosage and administration Dose may be adjusted to the needs and progress of the case.

Hypovolaemic shock: Give 500–1,000 ml i.v. as initial dose, the rate dependent on the patient's needs. Thereafter give equal volumes of Macrodex and blood. Haematocrit should be kept above 25%. Total Macrodex dose should not exceed 2,500 ml.

Shock prophylaxis at surgery: 500–1,000 ml is run in during operation, the rate being governed by pulse, skin colour, BP, etc.

Burns: Use to correct haemoconcentration in general 3 litres can be given daily for 48 hours.

Prophylaxis of post-operative thrombosis: Slowly infuse 500 ml during or at the end of surgery over four to six hours, followed by a further 500 ml over four to six hours, next day. In high-risk cases (hip fractures, history of thrombosis, etc) continue the treatment on alternate days for up to two weeks.

Elderly: Care not to overload.

Contra-indications, warnings, etc Give with caution to patients vulnerable to vascular overloading (congestive heart failure, renal disease, etc). Where a sodium load is undesirable, use Macrodex in 5% Dextrose.

Adverse reactions: Very rarely spontaneous hypersensitivity – urticaria, rigors and flushing, occasionally with asthma and hypotension. Usually occurs in cases not under stress and appears within a few minutes of starting the infusion. *Action:* Stop the infusion and give sympto-matic anti-allergic therapy.

Pharmaceutical precautions Store at steady room temperature. Poor storage can produce dextran flakes, which can be re-dissolved by autoclaving.

Legal category POM.

Package quantities Infusion bottles of 500 ml.

Further information Macrodex infusions have not been reported to produce difficulties with blood cross matching when given in volumes up to 1500 mls.

Product licence number 0009/5000.

RELAXIT*

Presentation A sterile viscous solution contained in a 5 ml applicator pack.

Relaxit contains:

Sodium citrate (dihydrate)	450 mg
Sodium lauryl sulphate	75 mg
Sorbic acid	5 mg
Glycerol and Sorbitol Solution to	5 ml

Uses Relaxit is a micro-enema for the relief of constipation.

Dosage and administration *Adults and children over the age of three:* The nozzle of the micro-enema is inserted fully into the rectum and the contents squeezed out.

Children under the age of three: Insert only half the length of the nozzle then squeeze the contents out.

Elderly: As adults.

Contra-indications, warnings, etc None.

Pharmaceutical precautions Store in a cool place. Shelf life two years.

Legal category P.

Package quantities Boxes of 4 or 100.

Further information Relaxit liberates bound water in the faecal mass, thus producing a soft motion which may be easily evacuated. Defaecation usually occurs within 15 minutes.

Product licence number 0009/0019.

RHEOMACRODEX* IN DEXTROSE

Presentation Rheomacrodex 10% in 5% Dextrose contains:

Dextran 40	50 g
Dextrose	25 g
Water for Injections to	500 ml

It complies with the monograph for Dextran 40 Injection BP. The solution is clear and slightly viscous. The infusion bottle has a red seal.

Uses
1. As a plasma volume expander.
2. To counteract diminution of the blood flow in the circulatory system.
3. The prevention and management of thrombotic episodes.
4. As a low sodium content alternative to Rheoma-crodex in Normal Saline.

Dosage and administration Adjust dosage to needs and progress of the case.

1. *Adults*

Reduced capillary circulation in shock, etc: 500–1,000 ml i.v. over 30–60 minutes, with further 500 ml later same day. Thence 500 ml/day for up to five days.

Impaired arterial or venous circulation: Initially 500–1,000 ml i.v. over four to six hours. Give 500 ml next day, then alternate days for up to two weeks.

Prophylaxis of post-operative thrombosis: Infuse 500 ml i.v. during or at the end of surgery followed by 500 ml given over four to six hours next day. In high-risk cases (hip fractures, history of thrombosis etc) continue the infusions, giving 500 ml over four to six hours alternate days for up to two weeks.

Vascular and plastic surgery: 500 ml i.v. immediately before surgery over 30–60 minutes with another 500 ml given during the operation. A further 500 ml over four to six hours is given post-operatively and on alternate days for up to two weeks.

Open cardiovascular surgery: 10–20 ml per kg body weight is added to perfusion fluid. Concentration of dextran should never exceed 3%.

2. *Children*

Infants: 5 ml/kg body weight.

Children: 10 ml/kg body weight.

3. *Elderly:* Dosage as adults, but with extra care regarding dehydration overloading and renal function.

Contra-indications, warnings, etc
Contra-indications: Severe bleeding tendency, e.g. thrombocytopenia. Severe congestive cardiac failure. Established renal failure with anuria.

Precautions:
1. Correct existing dehydration in patients before giving Rheomacrodex. Give adequate fluids during therapy (keep urine flow above 250 ml/6 hours, Urine SG below 1,065).
2. Extra care with patients vulnerable to vascular overloading (congestive heart failure, renal failure).
3. If Rheomacrodex is given with heparin, reduce heparin dose by 35–70% because of synergism.

Adverse reactions:
1. Very rarely spontaneous hypersensitivity as urti-caria, rigors and flushing, occasionally with asthma and hypotension. Usually occurs in cases not under stress and appears within a few minutes of starting the infusion. *Action:* Stop the infusion and give symptomatic therapy.
2. Capillary oozing of wound surfaces due to improved perfusion pressure and capillary flow.

Pharmaceutical precautions Store at steady room temperature. Poor storage can produce dextran flakes. These re-dissolve on autoclaving.

Legal category POM.

Package quantities Infusion bottles of 500 ml.

Further information Rheomacrodex infusions have not been reported to produce difficulties with blood cross matching when given in volumes up to 1500 mls.

Product licence number 0009/5005.

RHEOMACRODEX* IN NORMAL SALINE

Presentation   Rheomacrodex 10% in Normal Saline contains:

Dextran 40	50 g
Sodium Chloride	4.5 g
Water for Injections to	500 ml

It complies with the monograph for Dextran 40 Injection BP. The solution is clear and slightly viscous. The infusion bottle has a blue seal.

Uses

1. As a plasma volume expander.
2. To counteract diminution of blood flow in the circulatory system.
3. The prevention and management of thrombotic episodes.

In certain cases of renal or cardiac disease where an additional sodium load is undesirable Rheomacrodex 10% in 5% Dextrose may be preferred.

Dosage and administration   Adjust dosage to needs and progress of the case.

1. *Adults*

Reduced capillary circulation in shock, etc: 500–1,000 ml i.v. over 30–60 minutes, with further 500 ml later same day. Thence 500 ml/day for up to five days.

Impaired arterial or venous circulation: Initially 500–1,000 ml i.v. over four to six hours. Give 500 ml next day, then alternate days for up to two weeks.

Prophylaxis of post-operative thrombosis: Infuse 500 ml i.v. during or at the end of surgery followed by 500 ml given over four to six hours next day. In high risk cases (hip fractures, history of thrombosis, etc) continue the infusions, giving 500 ml over four to six hours alternate days for up to two weeks.

Vascular and plastic surgery: 500 ml i.v. immediately before surgery over 30–60 minutes with another 500 ml given during the operation. A further 500 ml over four to six hours is given post-operatively and on alternate days for up to two weeks.

Open cardiovascular surgery: 10–20 ml per kg body weight is added to perfusion fluid. Concentration of dextran should never exceed 3%.

2. *Children*

Infants: 5 ml/kg body weight.

Children: 10/kg body weight.

3. *Elderly:* Dosage as adults but with extra care regarding dehydration, overloading and renal function.

Contra-indications, warnings, etc

Contra-indications: Severe bleeding tendency, e.g. thrombocytopenia. Severe congestive cardiac failure. Established renal failure with anuria.

Precautions:

1. Correct existing dehydration in patients before giving Rheomacrodex. Give adequate fluids during therapy (keep urine flow above 250 ml/6 hours, Urine SG below 1,065).
2. Extra care with patients vulnerable to vascular overloading (congestive heart failure, renal failure). Rheomacrodex in 5% Dextrose may be preferred in these cases.
3. If Rheomacrodex is given with heparin, reduce heparin dose by 35–70% because of synergism.

Adverse reactions:

1. Very rarely spontaneous hypersensitivity as urticaria, rigors and flushing, occasionally with asthma and hypotension. Usually occurs in cases not under stress and appears within a few minutes of starting the infusion. *Action:* Stop the infusion and give symptomatic anti-allergic therapy.
2. Capillary oozing of wound surfaces due to improved perfusion pressure and capillary flow.

Pharmaceutical precautions   Store at steady room temperature. Poor storage can produce dextran flakes. These re-dissolve on autoclaving.

Legal category   POM.

Package quantities   Infusion bottle of 500 ml.

Further information   Rheomacrodex infusions have not been reported to produce difficulties with blood cross matching when given in volumes up to 1500 mls.

Product licence number   0009/5004.

SALAZOPYRIN* TABLETS, ENEMAS AND SUPPOSITORIES

Presentation

Tablets: Yellow, 13.5 mm diameter tablets, tasteless, scored deeply on one side, with a Pharmacia logo on the other side, containing sulphasalazine (USP) 0.5 g.

Enema: Soft plastic disposable enema bottles containing sulphasalazine 3 g, vehicle to 100 mls.

Suppositories: Yellow, odourless, torpedo-shaped containing sulphasalazine 0.5 g.

Uses   Treatment of ulcerative colitis and Crohn's disease.

Dosage and administration

Adults and elderly: The dose is adjusted according to the severity of the disease and the patient's tolerance to the drug, as detailed below.

1. Tablets: Induction and maintenance of remission of ulcerative colitis; treatment of active Crohn's disease.

Severe attack: Salazopyrin 2–4 tablets four times a day may be given in conjunction with steroids as part of an intensive management regime. Rapid passage of the tablets may reduce effect of the drug. Night-time interval between doses should not exceed eight hours.

Mild-moderate attack: 2–4 tablets four times a day may be given in conjunction with steroids.

Maintenance therapy: With induction of remission reduce the dose gradually to 4 tablets per day. This dosage should be continued indefinitely, since discontinuance even several years after an acute attack is associated with a four fold increase in risk of relapse.

2. Enemas: Treatment of ulcerative colitis and Crohn's colitis.

One enema should be given daily, preferably at bedtime.

3. Suppositories: Treatment of ulcerative colitis and Crohn's colitis affecting the rectum.

Two suppositories to be inserted in the morning and two at bedtime after defaecation. After three weeks it may be possible to gradually reduce the dosage as the patient improves.

Adjunct to oral therapy: In severe generalised disease affecting the rectum or rectosigmoid, and in cases slow to respond to oral therapy, one or two suppositories may be given morning and evening in addition.

Children
1. Tablets: The dose is reduced in proportion to body weight.

    Severe: 40–60 mg/kg per day
    Mild–moderate: 40–60 mg/kg per day
    Maintenance: 20–30 mg/kg per day

2. Enema: The enema presentation contains an adult dose and is not recommended for children.
3. Suppositories: Reduce the adult dosage on the basis of body weight.

Contra-indications, warnings, etc
Contra-indications:
(a) History of sensitivity to sulphonamides or salicylates.
(b) Infants under 2 years of age.
(c) In the case of the Enema, subjects sensitive to methyl or propyl parabens.

Precautions: Haematological and hepatic side effects may occur. Differential white cell, red cell and platelet counts should be performed initially and at monthly intervals for the first three months of treatment. Liver function tests should be carried out at monthly intervals for the first three months of treatment.

Patients with allergy, or renal or hepatic disease should be treated with caution. Patients with glucose-6-phosphate dehydrogenase deficiency should be closely observed for signs of haemolytic anaemia (Heinz body anaemia).

The uptake of digoxin and folate may be reduced. An acute attack may be precipitated in patients with porphyria.

Adverse effects: Since sulphasalazine is metabolised to sulphapyridine and 5-amino salicylic acid, side effects of sulphonamides or salicylates may occur. Patients with slow acetylator status are more likely to experience adverse effects due to sulphapyridine. The most commonly encountered reactions are nausea, headache, rash, loss of appetite and raised temperature.

The following adverse reactions have been reported:

Haematological: Heinz body anaemia, methaemoglobulinaemia, hypoprothrombinaemia, haemolytic anaemia, leucopenia, agranulocytosis, aplastic anaemia, megaloblastic anaemia, thrombocytopenia.

Hypersensitivity reactions: Generalised skin eruptions, Stevens–Johnson syndrome, exfoliative dermatitis, epidermal necrolysis, pruritis, urticaria, photosensitisation, anaphylaxis, serum sickness, drug fever, periorbital oedema, conjunctival and scleral injection, arthralgia, allergic myocarditis, polyarteritis nodosa, LE-phenomenon and lung complications with dyspnoea, fever, cough, eosinophilia, fibrosing alveolitis.

Gastro-intestinal reactions: Stomatitis, parotitis, pancreatitis, hepatitis.

CNS reactions: Vertigo, tinnitus, peripheral neuropathy, ataxia, convulsions, insomnia, mental depression and hallucinations.

Fertility: Oligospermia, reversible on discontinuance of drug.

Renal reactions: Crystalluria, haematuria, proteinuria and nephrotic syndrome.

Overdosage: There is no specific antidote to Salazopyrin.

Pregnancy and lactation: Long term clinical usage and experimental studies have failed to reveal any teratogenic or icteric hazards. The amounts of drug present in the milk should not present a risk to a healthy infant.

Pharmaceutical precautions
Store suppositories in a cool place.

Legal category POM.

Package quantities
Tablets: Bottles of 100 and 500.
Suppositories: Boxes of 10 and 50.
Enemas: Boxes of 7 × 100 mls.

Further information
The drug may colour the urine orange-yellow.

When gastro-intestinal intolerance to Salazopyrin tablets occurs, Salazopyrin EN-tabs may be used instead. These film-coated enteric tablets are subject to a separate Data Sheet.

Product licence numbers
Tablets: 0009/5006R
Suppositories: 0009/5008R
Enemas: 0009/0023

SALAZOPYRIN* EN-TABS

Presentation
Yellow elliptical convex film coated enteric tablets, containing 0.5 g of sulphasalazine. One side of the tablet has Pharmacia logo on it.

Uses
1. The treatment of Rheumatoid Arthritis which has failed to respond to non-steroidal anti-inflammatory drugs (NSAIDs).
2. Induction and maintenance of remission of Ulcerative Colitis.
3. The treatment of active Crohn's disease.

Dosage and administration
Rheumatoid arthritis
Adults including the elderly: Commence treatment with 0.5 g daily (one tablet) for one week, thereafter increasing the dose by one tablet each week, to a maximum of 3 g/day (six tablets) as in the following table.

	1st Week	2nd Week	3rd Week	4th Week
Morning —		1 tablet	1 tablet	2 tablets
Evening	1 tablet	1 tablet	2 tablets	2 tablets†

† etc to 3 g/day maximum.

Should a patient experience nausea, the dose should be reduced to a previously tolerated dose for one week and then increased. EN-tabs should not be broken or crushed. Alternatively, the total daily dose may be divided and taken three times or four times daily.

In rheumatoid arthritis Salazopyrin EN-tabs have a 'disease-modifying' action: clinical and haematological response is often seen after one month but may be delayed for up to 12 weeks following the commencement of treatment.

Salazopyrin EN-tabs do not possess analgesic activity, therefore NSAIDs or analgesic treatment should not be reduced or stopped abruptly until clinical response has been achieved.

Patients have been maintained on Salazopyrin EN-tabs for several years.

No recommendations are made for the treatment of children with rheumatoid arthritis.

Ulcerative colitis
Adults:
Severe: 2–4 tablets four times a day given in conjunction with steroids as part of an intensive management

regime. The night-time interval between doses should not exceed eight hours. In severe disease rapid passage of the tablets may reduce the effect of the drug.

Mild–moderate: 2–4 tablets four times a day given in conjunction with steroids.

Maintenance: With induction of remission reduce the dose gradually to four tablets per day in divided doses. This dosage should be continued indefinitely, since discontinuance even several years after an acute attack has been shown to be associated with a four fold increase in the risk of relapse.

Salazopyrin EN-tabs should not be broken or crushed.

Children: The dose is reduced in proportion to body weight.

Severe:	40–60 mg/kg per day
Mild–Moderate:	40–60 mg/kg per day
Maintenance:	20–30 mg/kg per day

Crohn's Disease

In active Crohn's disease, Salazopyrin EN-tabs should be administered as for severe ulcerative colitis.

Contra-indications, warnings, etc
Contra-indications:
(a) History of sensitivity to sulphonamides or salicylates.
(b) Infants under 2 years of age.

Precautions: Haematological and hepatic side effects may occur. Differential white cell, red cell and platelet counts should be performed initially and at monthly intervals for the first three months of treatment. Liver function tests should be carried out at monthly intervals for the first three months of treatment.

Patients with allergy, or renal or hepatic disease should be treated with caution. Patients with glucose-6-phosphate dehydrogenase deficiency should be closely observed for signs of haemolytic anaemia (Heinz body anaemia).

The uptake of digoxin and folate may be reduced. An acute attack may be precipitated in patients with porphyria.

Adverse effects: Since sulphasalazine is metabolised to sulphapyridine and 5-amino salicylic acid, effects of sulphonamides or salicylates may occur. Patients with slow acetylator status are more likely to experience adverse effects due to sulphapyridine. The most commonly encountered reactions are nausea, headache, rash, loss of appetite and raised temperature.

The following adverse reactions have been reported:

Haematological: Heinz body anaemia, methaemoglobulinaemia, hypoprothrombinaemia, haemolytic anaemia, leucopenia, agranulocytosis, aplastic anaemia, megaloblastic anaemia, thrombocytopenia.

Hypersensitivity reactions: Generalised skin eruptions, Stevens–Johnson syndrome, exfoliative dermatitis, epidermal necrolysis, pruritis, urticaria, photosensitisation, anaphylaxis, serum sickness, drug fever, periorbital oedema, conjunctival and scleral injection, arthralgia, allergic myocarditis, polyarteritis nodosa, LE-phenomenon and lung complications with dyspnoea, fever, cough, eosinophilia, fibrosing alveolitis.

Gastro-intestinal reactions: Stomatitis, parotitis, pancreatitis, hepatitis.

CNS reactions: Vertigo, tinnitus, peripheral neuropathy, ataxia, convulsions, insomnia, mental depression and hallucinations.

Fertility: Oligospermia, reversible on discontinuance of drug.

Renal reactions: Crystalluria, haematuria, proteinuria and nephrotic syndrome.

Overdosage: There is no specific antidote to Salazopyrin EN-tabs.

Pregnancy and lactation: Long term clinical usage and experimental studies have failed to reveal any teratogenic or icteric hazards. The amounts of drug present in the milk should not present a risk to a healthy infant.

Legal category POM.

Package quantities EN-tabs: Containers of 100 (special easily-opened pack for the disabled) and 500.

Further information The drug may colour the urine orange-yellow.

Product licence number 0009/5007R.

SENTIAL* ▼

Presentation Cream containing 4% urea, 4% sodium chloride, 0.5% hydrocortisone in a stabilising emulsified base.

Uses Atopic eczema and other dry eczemas of various genesis.

Dosage and administration Apply a thin layer twice daily to the affected areas.

Elderly and children: No special instructions.

Contra-indications, warnings, etc
Adverse effects: Sential may cause a smarting sensation of short duration when applied to the skin.

Contra-indications: Not to be used in the presence of skin infections unless effective specific therapy for the infection is being given.
Not to be used as a wound treatment.
Avoid contact with the eyes.

Pharmaceutical precautions Store in a cool place but do not freeze.

Legal category POM.

Package quantities Tubes of 30 g and 100 g.

Further information Nil.

Product licence number 0009/0051.

SPRILON*

Presentation A 200 g aerosol spray contains: Dimethicone 1.2 g (Dimethicone 350 BPC 73% Dimethicone 200 BPC 27%). Zinc Oxide BP 14.4 g. Base to 60 g (wool fat, wool alcohols, cetyl alcohol, dextran, liquid paraffin, white soft paraffin and water). Propellants to 200 g (Dichlorofluoromethane BPC and Trichlorofluoromethane BPC.)

Uses For prophylaxis and treatment of pressure sores, skin maceration due to faeces or urine, or around fistulae and ileostomies. Protection and treatment of fissures, leg ulcers, moist eczemas. Protection of skin beneath plaster casts.

Dosage and administration Shake can well. Spray surface at right angles from distance of eight inches. Two to three seconds should be sufficient for an area the size of the buttocks.

Elderly: No special instructions.

Contra-indications, warnings, etc *Precautions:*
Protect the eyes. Keep out of the reach of children. Do
not use on cases allergic to wool fat.

Warning: Do not puncture, incinerate or heat can over
50°C even when empty.

Pharmaceutical precautions Nil.

Legal category GSL.

Package quantities 200 g.

Further information The spray rapidly forms a white,
durable, flexible film which while protecting the skin and
assisting healing also allows normal transepidermal water
loss.

Product licence number 0009/5002.

*Trade Mark

Pharmacia Diagnostics
A Division of Pharmacia Limited
Pharmacia House
Midsummer Boulevard
Milton Keynes MK9 3HP

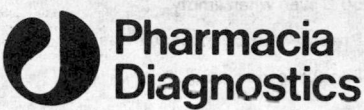

Pharmacia Diagnostics

PHARMALGEN* BEE VENOM (*Apis Mellifera*)

Presentation Venom, freeze dried with mannitol and Albumin Human (formerly called Normal Serum Albumin, 'NSA').

Initial Treatment Sets: Four vials, colour coded and labelled as below, together with vials of diluent. Upon dilution a range of concentrations is produced suited to initial treatment and intradermal testing.

GREEN	1	To give 0.1 mcg venom/ml when reconstituted
YELLOW	2	To give 1 mcg venom/ml when reconstituted
RED	3	To give 10 mcg venom/ml when reconstituted
BROWN	4	To give 100 mcg venom/ml when reconstituted

Maintenance Sets: These consist of four silver capped vials each containing 100 mcg/ml of venom when reconstituted with the diluent supplied.

Diluent Vials: Contain 4.5 ml of Albumin Human Diluent (Albumin Human 0.3 mg, sodium chloride 9 mg, phenol 3 mg, water for injections to 1 ml). Available, separate from the above sets in boxes of 10.

Uses Diagnosis and treatment of allergy to bee stings.

Dosage and administration See package insert.

Contra-indications, warnings, etc
Contra-indications: Other serious immunological illness, infections and pregnancy. Pregnancy is not an absolute contra-indication but the risk to the foetus of an anaphylactic reaction must be considered.

Precautions:
1. Read instructions carefully before use.
2. Use as directed by a specialist.
3. Follow sterile procedure for injections. Use a disposable tuberculin syringe for subcutaneous injections.
4. Avoid intravascular injection: check by aspiration of the syringe.
5. Observe the patient for an hour after each injection, and have the means of treatment of possible anaphylactic reactions, (e.g. adrenaline) immediately available.

Pharmaceutical precautions Store refrigerated, at 2–8°C.
Shelf life is 3 years in freeze-dried condition for venoms, and 3 years for diluent whilst sealed.
After reconstitution: see package insert.
Precaution: The container permits the withdrawal of

successive doses provided that adequate aseptic precautions are taken to ensure the maintenance of sterility of the product over the intended period of use.

Note: Do not re-freeze reconstituted venom.

Legal category POM.

Package quantities
See Presentation above.

Further information Patients desensitized with Pharmalgen will require monthly injections to maintain their protection. Regular investigations of venom specific IgE and IgG levels will indicate changes in their immunity, but at present treatment is recommended to continue for 3 years.

Product licence number Bee Venom, with diluent 0009/0024.

PHARMALGEN* WASP VENOM (*Vespula spp*)

Presentation Venom, freeze dried with mannitol and Albumin Human (formerly called Normal Serum Albumin, 'NSA').

Initial Treatment Sets: Four vials, colour coded and labelled as below, together with vials of diluent. Upon dilution a range of concentrations is produced suited to initial treatment and intradermal testing.

GREEN	1	To give 0.1 mcg venom/ml when reconstituted
YELLOW	2	To give 1 mcg venom/ml when reconstituted
RED	3	To give 10 mcg venom/ml when reconstituted
BROWN	4	To give 100 mcg venom/ml when reconstituted

Maintenance Sets: These consist of four silver capped vials each containing 100 mcg/ml of venom when reconstituted with the diluent supplied.

Diluent Vials: Contain 4.5 ml of Albumin Human Diluent (Albumin Human 0.3 mg, sodium chloride 9 mg, phenol 3 mg, water for injections to 1 ml). Available, separate from the above sets in boxes of 10.

Uses Diagnosis and treatment of allergy to wasp stings.

Dosage and administration See package insert.

Contra-indications, warnings, etc
Contra-indications: Other serious immunological illness, infections and pregnancy. Pregnancy is not an absolute

contra-indication but the risk to the foetus of an anaphylactic reaction must be considered.

Precautions:
1. Read instructions carefully before use.
2. Use as directed by a specialist.
3. Follow sterile procedure for injections. Use a disposable tuberculin syringe for subcutaneous injections.
4. Avoid intravascular injection: check by aspiration of the syringe.
5. Observe the patient for an hour after each injection, and have the means of treatment of possible anaphylactic reactions, (e.g. adrenaline) immediately available.

Pharmaceutical precautions Store refrigerated, at 2–8°C.

Shelf life is 3 years in freeze-dried condition for venoms. and 3 years for diluent whilst sealed.

After reconstitution: see package insert.

Precautions: The container permits the withdrawal of successive doses provided that adequate aseptic precautions are taken to ensure the maintenance of sterility of the product over the intended period of use.

Note: Do not re-freeze reconstituted venom.

Legal category POM.

Package quantities
See Presentation above.

Further information Patients desensitized with Pharmalgen will require monthly injections to maintain their protection. Regular investigations of venom specific IgE and IgG levels will indicate changes in their immunity, but at present treatment is recommended to continue for 3 years.

Product licence number Wasp Venom, with diluent 0009/0025.

SPECTRALGEN* POLLENS (SINGLE SPECIES) ▼

Presentation *Availability:* Spectralgen Pollens are available for the diagnosis and treatment of allergy to grass pollens (Rye grass, Timothy, Rye (cultivated) and Velvet grass/Yorkshire Fog) and tree pollens (Grey Alder, Common Silver Birch, Hazel).

Mixtures of the four grass pollens or the three tree pollens are also available (see following Data Sheets).

Initial treatment sets: Each pack contains four vials of freeze dried allergen and four vials of diluent.

There is a ten-fold increase in potency from one vial to the next, a colour coding of the vial caps aiding identification. When the vials are each reconstituted with 4.5 ml of diluent they have the following composition per ml, ignoring the diluent solutes.

		Capped vial	No.
Glycine	0.24 mg/ml		
Purified Pollen	100 BU*/ml	Green	1
Allergens	1,000 BU/ml	Yellow	2
	10,000 BU/ml	Red	3
	100,000 BU/ml	Brown	4

Maintenance treatment sets: Single vials of 10,000 BU/ml or 100,000 BU/ml are supplied with a vial of either NSA or Depot Diluent, as a kit for maintenance injections.

Each pack may be ordered with either Albumin (human) diluent or Depot diluent, according to intended procedure.

(1) Albumin (human) – suitable for diagnosis and all forms of therapy.

Each ml contains:

Normal Serum Albumin (Human)	0.3 mg
Sodium Chloride	9 mg
Phenol	4 mg

(2) Depot Diluent – suitable for conventional desensitization and maintenance. Each ml contains:

Sodium Chloride	9 mg
Phenol	5 mg
Aluminium Hydroxide corresponding to Aluminium Oxide	1.3 mg
Water for injections to	1 ml

Uses Diagnosis and treatment of allergy to grass or tree pollen.

Dosage and administration An initial treatment course can usually be completed in 3–12 weeks. For full details see package insert which gives conventional and semi-rush dosage schedules.

Contra-indications, warnings, etc
Contra-indications: Other serious immunological illness, infections and pregnancy. Pregnancy is not an absolute contra-indication but the risk to the foetus of an anaphylactic reaction must be considered.

Precautions: (1) read the instructions carefully before use.

(2) Follow sterile procedure for injections. Use a disposable tuberculin syringe for subcutaneous injections.

(3) Do not inject into a blood vessel or muscle.

(4) Observe the patient for at least half an hour after each injection and have the means of treatment of possible anaphylactic reactions (e.g. adrenalin), immediately available.

(5) If drugs which modify the allergic response such as antihistamines or bronchodilators, have been given within the previous twenty-four hours the patient's tolerance of an allergen injection may be increased. A consistent policy with respect to concurrent medications should be followed.

(6) Other vaccines should not be given within seven days before or after an allergen injection.

(7) Use on the advice or guidance of a specialist.

(8) In order to avoid possible contamination it is advised that solutions, once made up, should be discarded after four hours. However, the containers do permit the withdrawal of successive doses provided that aseptic precautions are taken to maintain the sterility of the product over the intended period of use.

Pharmaceutical precautions: *Shelf-life:* The shelf-life of freeze dried Spectralgen pollen when protected from light, is three years at 2–8°C. The shelf-life of albumin and Depot diluent, sealed and protected from light, is three years at 2–8°C.

Spectralgen pollen preparations in solution (reconstituted) should be kept at 2–8°C and not frozen. At concentrations of 100 BU/ml and above, allergens in solution have a shelf-life of at least twelve weeks at 2–8°C.

Contents of vials should not be mixed with other preparations and materials should not be transferred to other vials, as stability would be adversely affected. Only Sprectralgen diluents are suitable for reconstituting the freeze dried material.

Legal category POM.

Package quantities *Initial treatment set;* Each pack consists of four 5 ml colour coded allergen vials together with four 5 ml vials of the diluent requested (specify NSA or Depot diluent).

Maintenance treatment set: Each pack consists of one colour coded allergen vial (No. 3, 10,000 BU/ml or No. 4, 100,000 BU/ml as specified) with one vial of either NSA or Depot diluent.

Further information For *in vivo* testing and initial semi-rush or rush treatment dilution with albumin diluent is recommended. For maintenance treatment, the Depot diluent alternative may be used. See package insert for details. Treatment with Spectralgen is recommended only after a full specific allergy diagnosis has shown that the patient is allergic to the particular allergens, and that the condition is mediated by IgE, which can be verified by measuring specific IgE with Phadebas RAST. Additional vials of albumin diluent are routinely available.

Note: 1,000 biological units (BUs) are equivalent to one Histamine Equivalent Prick, 1 HEP i.e. in a panel of known sensitive patients 1,000 BUs or one HEP will give the same skin test reaction as a skin prick test with 0.1% Histamine chloride solution. This procedure is used to establish the allergenic potency of the reference material for each species, but for batch to batch quality control an inhibition RAST method is used.

Product licence numbers

Trees

t2	*Alnus incana*	0009/0034 (in NSA)
	(Grey Alder)	0009/0035 (in Depot)
t3	*Betula verrucosa*	0009/0036 (in NSA)
	(Common Silver Birch)	0009/0037 (in Depot)
t4	*Corylus avellana*	0009/0038 (in NSA)
	(Hazel)	0009/0039 (in Depot)

Grasses

g5	*Lolium perenne*	0009/0026 (in NSA)
	(Rye grass)	0009/0027 (in Depot)
g6	*Phleum pratense*	0009/0028 (in NSA)
	(Timothy grass)	0009/0029 (in Depot)
g12	*Secale cereale*	0009/0030 (in NSA)
	(Rye – cultivated)	0009/0031 (in Depot)
g13	*Holcus lanatus*	0009/0032 (in NSA)
	(Velvet grass/ Yorkshire Fog)	0009/0033 (in Depot)

SPECTRALGEN POLLENS (4 GRASS MIX) ▼

Presentation *Availability:* Spectralgen mixed grass pollens are available for the treatment of multiple allergy to grass pollen. The mixture contains purified pollen from allergens of four members of the Gramineae – Rye grass (*Lolium perenne*), Timothy grass (*Phleum pratense*), Cultivated Rye (*Secale cereale*), and Velvet grass/ Yorkshire Fog (*Holcus lanatus*). Closely related grasses have allergens in common with those named above so the mixture induces tolerance to related species and these four species will cover all the important grasses found in Britain.

Diagnosis of allergy to specify species may be made by Phadebas RAST if the condition is IgE mediated or by

in vivo testing with Spectralgen pollens individual species. The mixture may be used where no single species features dominantly in the diagnosis.

Initial treatment sets: Each pack contains four vials of freeze dried allergen and four vials of diluent.

There is a ten-fold increase in potency from one vial to the next, a colour coding of the vial caps aiding identification. When the vials are each reconstituted with 4.5 ml of diluent they have the following composition per ml, ignoring the diluent solutes.

		Capped vial	No.
Glycine	0.24 mg/ml		
Purified Pollen	100 BU*/ml	Green	1
Allergens	1,000 BU/ml	Yellow	2
	10,000 BU/ml	Red	3
	100,000 BU/ml	Brown	4

Maintenance treatment sets: Single vials of 10,000 BU/ml or 100,000 BU/ml are supplied with a vial of either albumin or Depot Diluent, as a kit for maintenance injections.

Each pack may be ordered with either albumin diluent or Depot diluent, according to intended procedure.

(1) Albumin (human) Diluent – suitable for diagnosis and all forms of therapy.
Each ml contains:

Normal Serum Albumin (Human)	0.3 mg
Sodium Chloride	9 mg
Phenol	4 mg
Water for injections to	1 ml

(2) Depot Diluent – suitable for conventional desensitization and maintenance. Each ml contains:

Sodium Chloride	9 mg
Phenol	5 mg
Aluminium Hydroxide corresponding to Aluminium Oxide	1.3 mg
Water for injections to	1 ml

Uses Treatment of allergy to grass pollen.

Dosage and administration An initial treatment course can usually be completed in 3–12 weeks. For full details see package insert which gives conventional and semi-rush dosage schedules.

Contra-indications, warnings, etc
Contra-indications: Other serious immunological illness, infections and pregnancy. Pregnancy is not an absolute contra-indication but the risk to the foetus of an anaphylactic reaction must be considered.

Precautions: (1) Read instructions carefully before use.
(2) Follow sterile procedure for injections. Use a disposable tuberculin syringe for subcutaneous injections.
(3) Do not inject into a blood vessel or muscle.
(4) Observe the patient for at least half an hour after each injection and have the means of treatment of possible anaphylactic reactions (e.g. adrenalin), immediately available.
(5) If drugs which modify the allergic response such as antihistamines or bronchodilators, have been given within the previous twenty-four hours the patient's tolerance of an allergen injection may be increased. A

consistent policy with respect to concurrent medications should be followed.

(6) Other vaccines should not be given within seven days before or after an allergen injection.

(7) Use on the advice or guidance of a specialist.

(8) In order to avoid possible contamination it is advised that solutions, once made up, should be discarded after four hours. However, the containers do permit the withdrawal of successive doses provided that aseptic precautions are taken to maintain the sterility of the product over the intended period of use.

Pharmaceutical precautions

Shelf-life: The shelf-life of freeze dried Spectralgen pollen when protected from light, is three years at 2–8°C. The shelf-life of albumin and Depot diluent, sealed and protected from light, is three years at 2–8°C.

Spectralgen pollen preparations in solution (reconstituted) should be kept at 2–8°C and not frozen. At concentrations of 100 BU/ml and above, allergens in solution have a shelf-life of twenty-four weeks in albumin diluent, and twelve weeks in Depot diluent, at 2–8°C.

Contents of vials should not be mixed with other preparations and materials should not be transferred to other vials, as stability would be adversely affected. Only Spectralgen diluents are suitable for reconstituting the freeze dried material.

Legal category POM.

Package quantities

Initial treatment set: Each pack consists of four 5 ml colour coded allergen vials together with four 5 ml vials of the diluent requested (specify NSA or Depot diluent).

Maintenance treatment set: Each pack consists of one colour coded allergen vial (No. 3, 10,000 BU/ml or No. 4, 100,000 BU/ml as specified) with one vial of either NSA or Depot diluent.

Further information For *in vivo* testing and initial semi-rush or rush-treatment dilution with albumin diluent is recommended. For maintenance treatment, the Depot diluent alternative may be used. See package insert for details. Treatment with Spectralgen is recommended only after a full specific allergy diagnosis has shown that the patient is allergic to the particular allergens, and that the condition is mediated by IgE, which can be verified by measuring specific IgE with Phadebas RAST. Additional vials of albumin diluent are routinely available.

*Note: 1,000 biological units (BUs) are equivalent to one Histamine Equivalent Prick, (1 HEP) i.e. in a panel of known sensitive patients 1,000 BUs or one HEP will give the same skin test reaction as a skin prick test with 0.1% Histamine chloride solution. This procedure is used to establish the allergenic potency of the reference material for each species, but for batch to batch quality control, an inhibition RAST method is used.

Product licence numbers

| gm4 | Spectralgen Pollen | 0009/0040 (in NSA) |
| | (4 Grass Mix) | 0009/0041 (in Depot) |

SPECTRALGEN* POLLENS (3 TREE MIX) ▼

Presentation *Availability:* Spectralgen mixed tree pollens are available for the treatment of multiple allergy to tree pollens. The mixture contains purified allergens from pollen of Grey Alder (*Alnus incana*), Common Silver Birch (*Betula verrucosa*), and Hazel (*Corylus avellana*). Closely related trees have allergens in common

with those named above, so the mixture induces tolerance to related species.

Diagnosis of allergy to specific species may be made if the condition is IgE mediated by the Phadebas RAST test for those species or by *in vivo* testing with individual species. The mixture may be used where no single species features dominantly in the diagnosis.

Initial treatment sets: Each pack contains four vials of freeze dried allergen and four vials of diluent.

There is a ten-fold increase in potency from one vial to the next, a colour coding of the vial caps aiding identification. When the vials are each reconstituted with 4.5 ml of diluent they have the following composition per ml, ignoring the diluent solutes.

		Capped vial	No.
Glycine	0.24 mg/ml		
Purified Pollen	100 BU*/ml	Green	1
Allergens	1,000 BU/ml	Yellow	2
	10,000 BU/ml	Red	3
	100,000 BU/ml	Brown	4

Maintenance treatment sets: Single vials of 10,000 BU/ml and 100,000 BU/ml are supplied with a vial of either albumin (human) or Depot Diluent, as a kit for maintenance injections.

Each pack may be ordered with either NSA diluent or Depot diluent, according to intended procedure.

(1) Albumin (human) Diluent – suitable for diagnosis and all forms of therapy.
Each ml contains:

Normal Serum Albumin (Human)	0.3 mg
Sodium Chloride	9 mg
Phenol	4 mg
Water for injections to	1 ml

(2) Depot Diluent – suitable for conventional desensitization and maintenance.
Each ml contains:

Sodium Chloride	9 mg
Phenol	5 mg
Aluminium Hydroxide corresponding to Aluminium Oxide	1.3 mg
Water for injections to	1 ml

Uses Treatment of allergy to tree pollen.

Dosage and administration An initial treatment course can usually be completed in 3–12 weeks. For full details see package insert which gives conventional and semi-rush dosage schedules.

Contra-indications, warnings, etc

Contra-indications: Other serious immunological illness, infections and pregnancy. Pregnancy is not an absolute contra-indication but the risk to the foetus of an anaphylactic reaction must be considered.

Precautions: (1) Read instructions carefully before use.

(2) Follow sterile procedure for injections. Use a disposable tuberculin syringe for subcutaneous injections.

(3) Do not inject into a blood vessel or muscle.

(4) Observe the patient for at least half an hour after each injection and have the means of treatment of

possible anaphylactic reactions (e.g. adrenalin), immediately available.

(5) If drugs which modify the allergic response such as antihistamines or bronchodilators, have been given within the previous twenty-four hours the patient's tolerance of an allergen injection may be increased. A consistent policy with respect to concurrent medications should be followed.

(6) Other vaccines should not be given within seven days before or after an allergen injection.

(7) Use on the advice or guidance of a specialist.

(8) In order to avoid possible contamination it is advised that solutions once made up, should be discarded after four hours. However, the containers do permit the withdrawal of successive doses provided that aseptic precautions are taken to maintain the sterility of the product over the intended period of use.

Pharmaceutical precautions

Shelf-life: The shelf-life of freeze dried Spectralgen pollen when protected from light, is three years at 2–8°C. The shelf-life of albumin and Depot diluent, sealed and protected from light, is three years at 2–8°C.

Spectralgen pollen preparations in solution (reconstituted) should be kept at 2–8°C and not frozen. At concentrations of 100 BU/ml and above, allergens in solution have a shelf-life of twenty-four weeks in albumin diluent, and twelve weeks in Depot diluent, at 2–8°C.

Contents of vials should not be mixed with other preparations and materials should not be transferred to other vials, as stability would be adversely affected. Only Spectralgen diluents are suitable for reconstituting the freeze dried material.

Legal category POM.

Package quantities *Initial treatment set:* Each pack consists of four 5 ml colour coded allergen vials together with four 5 ml vials of the diluent requested (specify NSA or Depot diluent).

Maintenance treatment set: Each pack consists of one colour coded allergen vial (No. 3, 10,000 BU/ml or No. 4, 100,000 BU/ml as specified) with one vial of either NSA or Depot diluent.

Further information For *in vivo* testing and initial semi-rush or rush treatment dilution with albumin diluent is recommended. For maintenance treatment, the Depot diluent alternative may be used. See package insert for details. Treatment with Spectralgen is recommended only after a full specific allergy diagnosis has shown that the patient is allergic to the particular allergens, and that the condition is mediated by IgE, which can be verified by measuring specific IgE with Phadebas RAST. Additional vials of albumin diluent are routinely available.

*Note: 100 biological units (BUs) are equivalent to one Histamine Equivalent Prick (1 HEP), i.e. in a panel of known sensitive patients 1,000 BUs or one HEP will give the same skin test reaction as a skin prick test with 0.1% Histamine chloride solution. This procedure is used to establish the allergenic potency of the reference material for each species, but for batch to batch quality control, an inhibition RAST method is used.

Product licence numbers

tm1	Spectralgen Pollen	0009/0042 (in NSA)
	(3 Tree Mix)	0009/0043 (in Depot)

*Trade Mark

Pharmax Limited
Bourne Road
Bexley
Kent DA5 1NX

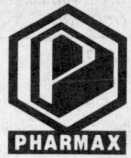

COLOMYCIN* INJECTION

Presentation Colomycin Injection is Colistin Sulphomethate Injection BP presented as a neutral glass vial containing a creamy-white crystalline powder (before reconstitution). Available as:
1. Colistin Sulphomethate Sodium BP 500,000 units
2. Colistin Sulphomethate Sodium BP 1,000,000 units.

Uses Colomycin Injection is used in the treatment of systemic infections caused by sensitive Gram-negative organisms, e.g. in urinary tract infection, respiratory infection, meningitis, septicaemia, osteomyelitis.

Dosage and administration Colomycin Injection is usually administered intramuscularly or intravenously, but when indicated can be introduced via other routes such as intrathecally, subconjunctivally, by aerosol inhalation and by local instillation.

Normal recommendations for systemic treatment are:

Children (up to 60 kg): 50,000 units/kg body weight in 24 hours, divided into three eight-hourly doses.

Adults (over 60 kg): 6,000,000 units in 24 hours (i.e. 2 × 1,000,000 unit vials every eight hours).

Infusion therapy: Daily dosage as above. Infusion, should preferably be completed within six hours.

Aerosol therapy: Daily dosage as above, concomitant with parenteral administration. For the aerosol, colistin is dissolved in water or saline for use in a suitable nebuliser attached to an air/oxygen supply.

Bladder irrigation: 1,000,000 units are dissolved in 50 ml water or saline and instilled during catheterisation. In the presence of infection, administration is carried out twice daily.

The above are expressed as average doses. Should clinical or bacteriological response be slow, dosage may be increased as indicated by the patient's condition. Minimum of five days treatment is recommended.

Where there is moderate or severe renal impairment, excretion of the antibiotic is delayed. Therefore, size of dose and dosage interval should be adjusted in relation to renal function. The table overleaf is a guide to dosage modifications in order to prevent accumulation of Colomycin. It is stressed that adjustments may still have to be made on evaluation of the individual patient.

Blood level estimations are recommended. 10–15 mcg/ml should be adequate.

Contra-indications, warnings, etc Colomycin Injection is contra-indicated in patients with known sensitivity to colistin. With appropriate dosage modifications, Colomycin need not be withheld in cases of renal impairment. Curariform muscle relaxants should be used with extreme caution in patients receiving Colomycin Injection.

Adverse reactions may include transient sensory disturbances such as perioral paraesthesia and vertigo. Therapy need not be discontinued and reduction of dosage may alleviate symptoms. Adverse effects on renal function have been reported but this generally returns to normal following discontinuation of therapy. Permanent nerve damage, such as deafness or vestibular damage, has not been reported. Local irritation at the site of injection is minimal.

Overdosage can result in renal insufficiency, muscle weakness and apnoea. There is no specific antidote; management is supportive treatment plus attempts to increase the rate of elimination of colistin, e.g. mannitol diuresis, prolonged haemodialysis, or peritoneal dialysis.

Pharmaceutical precautions Vials should be stored in a cool dry place protected from light. Solutions of Colomycin for parenteral administration should preferably be freshly prepared. Compatible infusion solutions are Normal Saline; 5% dextrose; 5% fructose; Ringer's solution; 10% Dextran 40 in Normal Saline. Infusions should be completed within six hours.

Mixed infusions or injections involving Colomycin should be avoided.

Colomycin Injection is compatible with the preservative phenylmercuric nitrate, and with the mucolytic agents acetylcysteine and superinone.

Legal category POM.

Package quantities Boxes of 10 × 500,000 unit vials and 10 × 1,000,000 unit vials.

Further information Colistin is a polypeptide antibiotic which possesses bactericidal activity against most Gram-negative organisms. Clinically it is of particular value in serious infections caused by pathogens such as *Pseudomonas aeruginosa, Escherichia coli,* Klebsiella spp. It cannot be recommended for Proteus spp.

Susceptible organisms do not readily develop or acquire resistance, and R factor mediated resistance has not been encountered.

(1 mg Colistin Sulphomethate Sodium is approx 12,500 units.)

Product licence numbers
500,000 units 0108/5005
1,000,000 units 0108/5006.

COLOMYCIN* TABLETS
COLOMYCIN* SYRUP
COLOMYCIN* STERILE POWDER

Presentation *Colomycin Tablets (Colistin Tablets BP):* 1,500,000 unit tablet; white tablet with P in hexagon on one face and two crossed score-marks on

Creatinine clearance (ml/min)	B.U.N. (mg/100 ml)	(mmol/l)	Adult dosage	Childrens' dosage
20–72	>60	>10	1½–2 million units every 8 hr	12,500–16,000 units/kg every 8 hr
10–20	>100	>16.5	1½ million units every 12–18 hr	12,500 units/kg every 12–18 hr
<10	>200	>33	1 million units every 18–24 hr	8,000 units/kg every 18–24 hr

reverse, containing Colistin Sulphate BP 1,500,000 units.

Syrup: Pale pink powder for reconstitution, containing Colistin Sulphate BP 4,000,000 units per bottle (i.e. 250,000 units/5 ml, when dispensed).

Sterile powder: White crystalline powder in neutral glass vial, containing Colistin Sulphate BP 1 g.

Uses The treatment of gastro-intestinal infections caused by sensitive Gram-negative organisms. Also bowel preparation. In addition, the sterile powder can be used for topical infections. Colistin Sulphate is not absorbed from the gastro-intestinal tract, and must *not therefore be used for systemic infections.*

Dosage and administration *Oral therapy (tablets, syrup or solution): Children up to 15 kg:* 250,000–500,000 units (i.e. 5–10 ml syrup) every eight hours.

Children of 15–30 kg: 750,000–1,500,000 units every eight hours.

Adults, and children over 30 kg: 1,500,000–3,000,000 units every eight hours.

Minimum of five days treatment is recommended. Should clinical or bacteriological response be slow, dosage may be increased.

Bowel preparation: A 24-hour course of Colistin Sulphate at the normal dosage above. Treatment should preferably finish 12 hours before surgery.

Topically: Usually applied at a 1% concentration as a solution, powder or ointment, according to the nature of the infection.

COLOMYCIN STERILE POWDER MUST NOT BE USED FOR PREPARATION OF INJECTABLE SOLUTIONS.

Contra-indications, warnings, etc There are no absolute contra-indications to oral therapy, and side-effects are rare. The syrup base contains sucrose. In cases of intolerance a solution of Colomycin Sterile Powder can be used.

Topical therapy is well tolerated; transient irritation at the site of application has been reported infrequently. Allergic sensitisation has not occurred.

Pharmaceutical precautions Colomycin preparations should be stored in a cool dry place, protected from light.

After reconstitution with water, Colomycin Syrup is stable for two weeks at room temperature.

Suitable ointment bases for colistin with stability of one month at room temperature include Simple Cream BP; Simple Cream plus hydrous lanolin (90:10); Hydrous Ointment BP; Macrogol Ointment BPC.

For a topical powder, Colomycin can be dispensed with lactose or Biosorb.

Eye and ear drops can be made in water or saline, 0.002% phenylmercuric nitrate is a suitable preservative.

Topical solutions of Colistin can be stored for one month at room temperature.

Legal category POM.

Package quantities *1,500,000 units Tablet:* Securitainers of 50 tablets.

Syrup: Bottle for reconstitution to 80 ml.

Sterile Powder: Vials of 1 g.

Further information 1 mg Colistin Sulphate is approx. 19,500 units.

Product licence numbers
1,500,000 units Tablet   0108/5008
Syrup   0108/5009
1 g Sterile Powder   0108/5010

FLETCHERS'* ARACHIS OIL RETENTION ENEMA

Presentation Ready-to-use, self-contained single-dose, disposable enema containing Arachis Oil BP 130 ml.

Uses To soften impacted faeces.

Dosage and administration *Adults:* 1 enema as required.

Children: In proportion, according to age.

The enema should be warmed before use.

Contra-indications, warnings, etc Nil.

Pharmaceutical precautions Store at room temperature.

Legal category P.

Package quantities Box of 10 × enemas.

Further information Nil.

Product licence number 0108/5016.

FLETCHERS' ENEMETTE*

Presentation Ready-to-use, self-contained single-dose, disposable microenema of 5 ml liquid containing: Dioctyl Sodium Sulphosuccinate BPC 90 mg (Docusate Sodium INN).

Uses Routine treatment of constipation. Pre- and post-operative cleansing of the bowel, in obstetrics and prior to proctoscopy, sigmoidoscopy or X-ray examination.

Dosage and administration *Adults:* 1 enema as required. *Children:* Under 3 years, not recommended. Over 3 years as for adults.

Contra-indications, warnings, etc Nil.

Pharmaceutical precautions Protect from heat.

Legal category P.

Package quantities Box of 25 microenemas.

Further information The formulation of dioctyl sodium sulphosuccinate, a faecal softening agent, in glycerol (which when administered rectally promotes peristalsis and evacuation of the lower bowel) and polyethylene glycol, provides an easy-to-use, efficacious, low-volume enema.

Product licence number 0108/0078.

FLETCHERS'* PHOSPHATE ENEMA

Presentation Fletchers' Phosphate Enema is Phosphate Enema BPC, Formula B, in a ready-to-use, self-contained, disposable, single-dose enema of 128 ml aqueous solution containing:

Sodium Acid Phosphate BP	12.80 g
Sodium Phosphate PhEur	10.24 g

Available with standard or long rectal tube.

Uses Routine treatment of constipation. Pre- and post-operative cleansing of the bowel, in obstetrics and prior to proctoscopy, sigmoidoscopy or X-ray examination.

Dosage and administration *Adults:* 1 enema, as required.

Children: In proportion, according to age.

The enema may be administered at room temperature, or warmed in warm water before use. The long-tube variety will provide better operating distance for staff and easier control for self-administration.

Contra-indications, warnings, etc Contra-indicated in patients with inflammatory or ulcerative conditions of the large bowel, in those with increased colonic absorptive capacity e.g. Hirschsprung's disease, and in those with acute gastrointestinal conditions.

Prolonged use may lead to irritation of the anal canal. This product should be used with caution in patients requiring a reduced sodium intake and electrolyte balance should be maintained during extended use.

Pharmaceutical precautions Store in a cool place.

Legal category P.

Package quantities *Standard:* Box of 10 enemas; also box of 50 enemas.

Long Tube; Box of 10 enemas; also box of 50 enemas.

Further information Nil.

Product licence number 0108/5015.

LASMA*

Presentation White capsule shaped tablets, imprinted 'PHARMAX' on one side and single scored on the reverse. Lasma is a sustained release tablet containing Theophylline PhEur 300 mg.

Uses Lasma tablets are indicated for the treatment and prophylaxis of bronchospasm associated with asthma, emphysema and bronchitis.

Dosage and administration Lasma may be administered as a single daily dose or in divided doses.

Divided dosage schedule: One tablet every 12 hours, preferably after food. The given dose may be increased, if necessary, by half-tablet increments.

Single daily dosage schedule: In appropriate cases, 24-hour maintenance therapy may be achieved by administration of a single dose. Therapy should commence with 2 tablets (600 mg) daily, preferably after food. In patients of 70 kg body weight or over, dosage should be increased after 1 week to 3 tablets (900 mg) daily.

Lasma tablets should be swallowed and not chewed.

Contra-indications, warnings, etc
Contra-indications: There are no absolute contra-indications to theophylline.

Precautions: Care should be exercised in the treatment of patients with cardiac arrhythmias, peptic ulcers or severe hypertension. Cardiac failure or hepatic dysfunction decreases theophylline clearance and patients with such conditions should be carefully monitored. Lasma should not be used concurrently with other preparations containing xanthine derivatives.

Side-effects: Side-effects (particularly tremor) are rare at plasma theophylline concentrations of less than 20 mcg/ml but may include gastro-intestinal disturbances, headache, CNS stimulation and tremor.

Overdosage: Symptoms may include nausea, vomiting, gastro-intestinal irritation, cramps, convulsions, tachycardia and hypotension.

The stomach contents should be emptied and supportive measures employed to maintain circulation, respiration and fluid and electrolyte balance. Electrocardiographic monitoring should be carried out and in severe poisoning charcoal haemoperfusion should be used.

Pregnancy: Safety in human pregnancy has not been established. Theophylline crosses the placental barrier and is secreted in breast milk.

Pharmaceutical precautions None.

Legal category P.

Package quantities Bottles of 100 tablets.

Further information Lasma is a sustained release formulation of theophylline designed to facilitate the control of plasma theophylline levels within the optimum range. This reduced diurnal variation in plasma levels provides for:

(i) Reduced risk of rapid and excessive absorption of theophylline and hence improved safety.

(ii) Maintenance of the desired plasma levels, so providing continuous protection.

(iii) Improved convenience of dosing for the patient.

Product licence number 0108/0075.

MEGACLOR* CAPSULES

Presentation Red, oblong, soft gelatin capsules containing Clomocycline Sodium 170 mg.

Uses Megaclor is a methylol derivative of chlortetracycline used in the treatment of infections caused by tetracycline-sensitive organisms, including infections associated with the genito-urinary tract, respiratory tract, ENT and soft tissue. It may also be used for specific infections such as brucellosis, and for long-term therapy in acne.

Dosage and administration *Adults:* 1 or 2 capsules three or four times daily. Suggested dosage for acne in adults is: 4 capsules daily for one week, 2 capsules daily for one week then 1 capsule daily for seven weeks, or maintenance as required.

Contra-indications, warnings, etc Tetracyclines are contra-indicated in severe renal or hepatic failure, or where there is a history of hypersensitivity to tetracyclines. Tetracycline may cause a yellow or brown discoloration of teeth in children or the developing foetus. For this reason it should be avoided during pregnancy, and in children where ever possible. Absorption of Megaclor may be impaired by concomitant administration of calcium, magnesium, iron or aluminium salts (e.g. in antacids). Gastro-intestinal side-effects may occur, but are infrequent and seldom troublesome. Photosensitive reactions are uncommon. In the event of overdosage, employ gastric lavage and supportive therapy; there is no specific antidote.

Pharmaceutical precautions Store in a cool dry place and protect from light. Dispense in an airtight container.

Legal category POM.

Package quantities Securitainers of 100 capsules.

Further information Megaclor is highly soluble and is rapidly and almost competely absorbed from the small intestine.

Product licence number 0108/5020.

MUCOGEL* SUSPENSION

Presentation A white mint flavoured suspension. Each 5 ml contains:

Aluminium Hydroxide equivalent to dried gel BP	
	220 mg
Magnesium Hydroxide BP	195 mg

Uses Antacid therapy in gastric and duodenal ulcer, gastritis, heartburn, gastric hyperacidity. Treatment of indigestion.

Dosage and administration Usual adult doses are: 10–20 ml three times daily preferably between meals and at bedtime, or as required.

Contra-indications, warnings, etc
Contra-indications: Mucogel Suspension should not be used in patients who are severely debilitated or suffering from kidney failure. Antacids inhibit the absorption of tetracyclines and vitamins and should not be taken concomitantly.

Adverse effects: Gastrointestinal side-effects are uncommon. This formulation minimises the problems of diarrhoea and constipation.

Use in pregnancy and lactation: Unnecessary drug therapy should be avoided in the first trimester of pregnancy.

Overdosage: Serious symptoms are unlikely to follow overdosage.

Pharmaceutical precautions Mucogel suspension may be stored at room temperature. Do not freeze.

Legal category GSL.

Package quantities Bottles of 300 and 500 ml.

Further information Mucogel is a pleasant-tasting, well tolerated antacid containing balanced quantities of aluminium and magnesium.

Product licence number 0108/0074.

PREDENEMA*

Presentation Ready-to-use, self-contained, single-dose, disposable enema of 100 ml buffered aqueous solution containing Prednisolone Metasulphobenzoate Sodium, equivalent to Prednisolone 20 mg.

Uses Local treatment of ulcerative colitis.

Dosage and administration *Adults only:* 1 enema nightly for two to four weeks, extending the course when a good response is being obtained. The long tube presentation facilitates self-administration.

The enema may be administered at room temperature or warmed in warm water before use.

Contra-indications, warnings, etc Administration of prednisolone via this route for this indication is seldom associated with adverse effects. It is contra-indicated in local conditions where it might mask infection or impair healing, such as peritonitis, sinusitis, fistulae, intestinal obstruction, perforation of the bowel.

Precautions: Symptoms of adrenal insufficiency have not been reported, but prolonged therapy should be carefully monitored.

Topical administration of corticosteroids to pregnant animals can cause abnormalities of foetal development. The relevance of this finding to human beings has not been established. However, topical steroids should not be used extensively in pregnancy, (i.e. in large amounts or for prolonged periods.)

Pharmaceutical precautions Store in a cool place, protected from light.

Legal category POM.

Package quantities Long tube box of 7 enemas
Standard tube box of 10 enemas.

Further information Nil

Product licence number 0108/5018.

SAVENTRINE* TABLETS

Presentation White sustained release tablet with grey/brown surface speckling and 'P' in hexagon embossed on one face. Each tablet contains Isoprenaline Hydrochloride BP 30 mg.

Uses Beta-adrenergic stimulant for use in chronic atrioventricular block and Stokes-Adams attacks, heart block induced at cardiac surgery, carotid sinus, syncope; bradycardia.

Dosage and administration Dosage must be tailored to the requirements of the individual patient. Treatment is best initiated under observation in hospital with facilities available for monitoring ECG and for cardiac resuscitation.

ECG should be monitored during intravenous infusion of isoprenaline (5 mg in 500 ml of 5% dextrose solution at 10–30 drops per minute) or a 20 mg sublingual tablet. Following a favourable increase in ventricular rate without appearance or increase in the ventricular ectopic beats, oral Saventrine therapy can be started.

The usual initial dosage is 1 tablet (30 mg) eight-hourly and this can be increased quite rapidly if required. Daily dosage may range from 90 mg in some patients to 840 mg in others, with frequency of administration varying from eight-hourly to two-hourly. Optimum dosage is that which satisfactorily controls the heart rate with minimum side-effects.

Tablets must be swallowed whole, they are not for sublingual administration.

Children: Monitor and proceed as for adults.

Contra-indications, warnings, etc Saventrine is contra-indicated in acute coronary disease and in patients prone to episodes of ventricular fibrillation or tachycardia secondary to their slow rate.

Side-effects may include palpitations, tremor, tachycardia, precordial pain. Sweats, facial flushing, headache and diarrhoea have also been reported. Incidence of side-effects with this presentation is less than with sublingual isoprenaline, and side-effects usually respond to dosage adjustment.

In the event of overdosage, toxic effects may be diminished by a beta-adrenergic blocking drug.

Pharmaceutical precautions Store at room temperature.

Legal category POM.

Package quantities Securitainers of 30 and 250 tablets.

Further information Saventrine contains granules of Isoprenaline Hydrochloride coated with varying numbers of layers of ethylcellulose. Following ingestion there is sustained release of active ingredient over several hours unimpeded by changes of pH, digestive enzymes or intestinal motility.

Isoprenaline is a potent sympathomimetic amine acting almost exclusively via beta-adrenergic receptors, and exerts positive chronotropic and inotropic effects on the heart. An intravenous preparation of Isoprenaline Hydrochloride (Saventrine i.v.) is also available for monitoring purposes.

Product licence number 0108/5028.

SAVENTRINE* i.v.

Presentation Glass ampoules containing a stabilised solution of Isoprenaline Hydrochloride BP for injection. Each ampoule contains 2 ml of 1 mg/ml solution.

Uses Beta-adrenergic stimulant for use in:
1. Monitoring of patients with heart block to determine their suitability for treatment on a long-term basis with Saventrine sustained action oral tablets.
2. Cardiogenic or endotoxic shock states.
3. Acute Stokes-Adams attacks and other cardiac emergencies.
4. Certain other slow heart states, e.g. severe bradycardia precipitated by beta-adrenergic antagonists.
5. Evaluation of congenital heart defects.

Dosage and administration The usual route is by intravenous infusion, in 5% dextrose solution or Water for Injections. Widely varying doses have been used with success.
1. Monitoring heart block: 5–40 mcg/min.

2. Shock states: 0.5–10 mcg/min.
3. Acute Stokes-Adams attack: 4–8 mcg/min or alternatively, intracardiac injection of 0.1 mg in 10 ml water.
4. Slow heart states: 1–4 mcg/min.
5. Congenital cardiac defects: 1.5–4 mcg/min.

Children: Adjust above dosage in proportion to weight.

Contra-indications, warnings, etc Isoprenaline may precipitate ventricular extrasystoles and arrhythmias, especially in patients who may be hypersensitive to the drug. In such cases the infusion rate should be reduced or possibly discontinued.

Side-effects may include palpitations, tremor, precordial pain, sweats, facial flushing, headache.

In the event of overdosage, a beta-adrenergic blocking drug may diminish toxic effects.

Pharmaceutical precautions Store in a cool place protected from light.

Legal category POM.

Package quantities Carton of 6 ampoules.

Further information Isoprenaline Hydrochloride is a sympathomimetic amine with potent activity at beta-adrenergic receptors. See also Saventrine tablets.

Product licence number 0108/5030.

SUSCARD* BUCCAL TABLETS ▼

Presentation White biconvex tablets, marked with 'P' inside a hexagon on one face; dosage strength on other face. Suscard is a sustained release presentation of glyceryl trinitrate in four strengths, 1 mg, 2 mg, 3 mg and 5 mg, for buccal administration (see below).

Uses The management and treatment of angina pectoris; congestive cardiac failure.

Administration The Suscard tablet is placed high up between the upper lip and the gum to either side of the front teeth.

The diagrams below show the correct placement of the tablet.

The onset of action of Suscard tablets is extremely rapid, and the tablets may be substituted for sublingual glyceryl trinitrate tablets in the treatment of acute angina pectoris. The duration of action of the Suscard tablet, once in place, as shown above, correlates with the dissolution time of the tablet. This is normally 3–5 hours. However, the first few doses may dissolve more rapidly until the patient is used to the presence of the tablet.

During the dissolution period the tablet will soften and adhere to the gum; in practice the presence of the tablet is not noticeable to the patient after a short time.

Patients should be instructed as to the correct placement of the tablet and should note the following points:

(a) The tablet should not be moved about the mouth with the tongue, as this will cause it to dissolve more rapidly.
(b) A slight stinging sensation (as for sublingual glyceryl trinitrate) may be felt for a few minutes after placement of the tablet.
(c) If a tablet is **accidentally** swallowed it may be replaced by a further tablet.

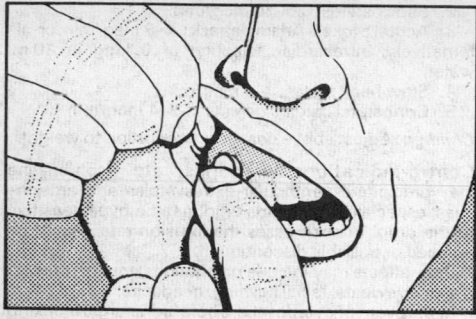

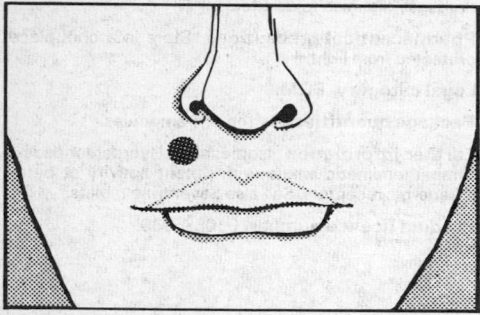

THE TABLETS SHOULD *NOT* BE PLACED UNDER THE TONGUE, CHEWED OR INTENTIONALLY SWALLOWED.

(d) In patients who wear dentures, the tablet may be placed in any comfortable position between the lip and the gum.

(e) The patient may alternate the placement of successive tablets on the right and left sides of the front teeth.

Suscard tablets do not interfere with the ingestion of food or liquids.

Dosage *Angina:* administration of Suscard tablets should start with the 1 mg strength. If angina occurs while the tablet is in place, the dosage strength used should be increased to 2 mg and then to the 3 mg where necessary. The 5 mg dosage strength should be reserved for patients with severe angina pectoris refractory to treatment with the lower dosage strengths.

Suggested dosage frequency in angina:

(a) For patients suffering only occasional angina pectoris – The tablets may be administered on a p.r.n. basis, to relieve the acute attack.

(b) For patients suffering angina pectoris in response to known stimuli – The tablet may be administered a few minutes prior to encountering the angina-precipitating stimulus.

(c) For patients in whom chronic therapy is indicated – The tablet should be administered on a thrice daily basis or as dictated by the dissolution rate of the tablet in an individual patient. If angina occurs during the period between the disappearance of one tablet and the time the next tablet is due to be put in place, dosage frequency should be increased.

Note that if an acute attack of angina pectoris is suffered while a tablet is in place, an additional tablet may be positioned on the opposite side of the mouth.

Congestive cardiac failure: Dosage should commence with the 5 mg strength, administered three times daily. In moderately severe or severe cases, particularly where patients have not responded to standard therapy (digitalis/diuretics), the dosage may need to be increased to 10 mg (2 × 5 mg tablets) t.i.d. over a period of three or four days. In such instances one tablet should be placed between the upper lip and the gum, on each side of the front teeth.

Contra-indications, warnings, etc Contra-indications are as for glyceryl trinitrate. Suscard tablets should not be used in patients with marked anaemia, head trauma, cerebral haemorrhage or closed angle glaucoma.

Side-effects are predominantly headache and facial flushing. In the unlikely event of severe side-effects, the tablet may simply be removed from the mouth.

Toxic effects of glyceryl trinitrate include vomiting, restlessness, cyanosis, methaemoglobinaemia and syncope. Overdosage (i.e. if large numbers of tablets have been swallowed) should be treated with gastric aspiration and lavage, plus attention to respiratory and circulatory symptoms.

Pharmaceutical precautions Can be stored at room temperature. Dispense in glass.

Legal category P.

Package quantities 1, 2, and 3 mg-bottles of 100 tablets, 5 mg-bottles of 60 tablets.

Further information Nil.

Product licence numbers
1 mg   0108/0067
2 mg   0108/0069
3 mg   0108/0073
5 mg   0108/0071.

SUSTAC*

Presentation Pink tablets with surface speckling and 'P' in hexagon embossed on one face. Sustac is a sustained release presentation of glyceryl trinitrate in three strengths; 2.6 mg, 6.4 mg and 10.0 mg.

Uses Prophylactic therapy of angina pectoris.

Dosage and administration Sustac tablets must be swallowed whole. They are not for sublingual administration. Dosage should be tailored to the requirements of the individual patient, but is usually 1 or 2 tablets of the 2.6 mg or 6.4 mg strength taken two or three times daily, or 1 tablet of the 10 mg strength two or three times daily.

Suggested initial doses: Mild angina: One 2.6 mg tablet three times daily.

Moderate angina: One 6.4 mg tablet two or three times daily.

Severe angina: One or two 6.4 mg tablets three times daily, or one 10 mg tablet three times daily.

Contra-indications, warnings, etc
Contra-indications are as for glyceryl trinitrate. Sustac should not be used in patients with marked anaemia, head trauma, cerebral haemorrhage, incipient glaucoma.

Side-effects include facial flushing and headache. Toxic effects of glyceryl trinitrate include vomiting, restlessness, cyanosis, methaemoglobinaemia and syncope.

Overdosage should be treated with gastric aspiration and lavage, plus attention to respiratory and circulatory defects.

Pharmaceutical precautions Can be stored at room temperature.

Legal category P.

Package quantities 2.6 mg and 6.4 mg: Securitainers of 250 tablets. 10 mg: Bottles of 100 tablets.

Further information Sustac tablets contain granules of glyceryl trinitrate coated with varying numbers of layers of ethycellulose. Following ingestion there is sustained release of active ingredient over several hours, unimpeded by changes of pH, digestive enzymes or intestinal motility.

Sustac can be used in combination with reduced beta-blockade dosage to give a patient full anti-anginal support, and at the same time reduce the likelihood of beta-blockade side-effects.

Product licence numbers
2.6 mg   0108/5031
6.4 mg   0108/5032
 10 mg   0108/0064

*Trade Mark

Quinoderm Limited
Manchester Road
Oldham OL8 4PB

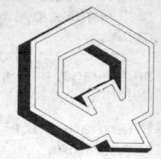

CEANEL* CONCENTRATE

Presentation *Appearance:* Ceanel Concentrate is a clear, viscous amber-coloured liquid.

Active ingredients:

Phenylethyl Alcohol BPC	7.5%
Cetrimide BP	10%
Undecenoic Acid BP	1%

Uses *Main pharmacological action:* Cetrimide is particularly active against Gram-positive organisms. This feature combined with the bactericidal action of phenylethyl alcohol and the fungicidal properties of undecenoic acid makes Ceanel Concentrate particularly effective in the treatment of dermatological conditions. Ceanel Concentrate is effective in removing debris and scale in seborrhoea capitis, and psoriasis of the scalp.

Indications: Psoriasis of the scalp, seborrhoeic dermatitis, dandruff, psoriasis of the trunk and limbs.

Dosage and administration *Adults and children:* *Scalp conditions:* Wet the scalp and hair with warm water. Protect the eyes with a towel to avoid discomfort. Apply $\frac{1}{2}$–1 teaspoonful of Ceanel to the wetted scalp. Then apply a small amount of water and work up into a lather. Rinse and repeat. Finally rinse the hair and scalp *thoroughly*. Use three times in the first week and twice weekly thereafter.

Other areas of the body: Wet the area to be treated with warm water; apply sufficient Ceanel Concentrate by gentle massage to cover the wetted area. Allow to remain in contact for two minutes. Remove the Ceanel by thorough rinsing with warm water. Use as required.

Contra-indications, warnings, etc *Precaution:* The eyes should be protected during treatment. A simple way to do this is with a towel.

Overdosage: Ceanel Concentrate is for external use only. If Ceanel Concentrate is accidentally taken by mouth treat as for cetrimide poisoning.

For external use only. Keep out of the reach of children.

Pharmaceutical precautions *Storage:* No special precaution required.

Diluents: Ceanel Concentrate is easily removed by warm water.

Legal category P.

Package quantities Available in packs of 50 ml, 150 ml and 500 ml.

Further information In clinical trials Ceanel Concentrate was used on 31 patients suffering from psoriasis, seborrhoeic eczema, atopic eczema or infected eczema of the scalp. A complete clearing of scaling was obtained in 24 of the 25 patients with psoriasis, and in all six patients with eczema.

Greasiness of the scalp was eliminated in 20 of the 21 patients with psoriasis who showed this feature.

Product licence number 0291/5002.

ECZEDERM* CREAM

Presentation *Appearance:* Eczederm is a pink-coloured cream.

Active ingredients:

Calamine BP	20.88%
Arachis Oil BP	12.5%

Uses *Pharmacological actions:* The soothing and healing properties of Calamine have been combined with the bland cooling effect from the special emollient base. This has produced a unique blend of useful therapeutic properties.

Indications: Mild dermatoses including both wet and dry eczema especially where steroid containing preparations should be avoided.

Dosage and administration *Adults and children:* Spread thinly over the affected area up to three times a day. The use of occlusive dressings may be considered in dry scaly dermatoses.

Contra-indications, warnings, etc Eczederm cream is for topical use only. There are no known contra-indications except true hypersensitivity to one of the ingredients. Ingestion should be avoided.

Pharmaceutical precautions *Storage:* Eczederm should be stored in a cool place and extremes of temperature avoided.

Diluents etc: Eczederm is not suitable for dilution or reformulation.

Legal category P.

Package quantities Eczederm is supplied in tubes of 25 g and 50 g. Also available in plastic containers of 500 g.

Further information This preparation does not contain parabens type compounds or lanolin. It is of special use where steroid containing preparations are contra-indicated.

Product licence number 0291/0003.

ECZEDERM* CREAM WITH HYDROCORTISONE 0.5%

Presentation *Appearance.* Eczederm Cream with Hydrocortisone 0.5% is a pink-coloured cooling cream.

Active ingredients:

Calamine BP	20.88%
Starch (Maize) BP	2.09%
Hydrocortisone BP	0.5%

Uses *Main pharmacological action:* The combination of the properties of hydrocortisone, with the mild astringent properties of calamine in a bland cooling-cream base results in a preparation which can have anti-inflammatory soothing and emollient properties.

Indications: Dry scaly eczematous dermatoses and wet exudative eczematous dermatoses.

Dosage and administration *Adults and children:* Spread thinly over the affected area up to three times daily in both forms of eczema.

Contra-indications, warnings, etc *Warning:* In pregnant animals, administration of corticosteroids can cause abnormalities of foetal development. The relevance of this finding to human beings has not been established. However, topical steroids should not be used extensively in pregnancy, i.e. in large amounts or for long periods.

In infants, long-term continuous topical therapy should be avoided. Adrenal suppression can occur even without occlusion.

This preparation is for external use only.

Keep out of the reach of children.

Pharmaceutical precautions *Storage:* Eczederm Cream with Hydrocortisone 0.5% should be stored in a cool place, avoiding extremes in temperature.

Legal category POM.

Package quantities Eczederm Cream with Hydrocortisone 0.5% is available in tubes of 25 g.

Further information This preparation does not contain any parabens type compounds or lanolin.

Product licence number 0291/5004.

GELCOTAR*

Presentation *Active ingredients:* Strong Coal Tar Solution BPC 5% (w/w).

Tar BP (Pine tar) 5% (w/w).

Appearance: Gelcotar is a light-brown thixotropic gel which spreads easily and cleanly on the skin. It is non-sticky, non-greasy and being water-miscible is easily removed and does not permanently stain the skin.

Uses *Main pharmacological action:* The combination of two different tars in Gelcotar provides a preparation with antipruritic, keratolytic and antiseptic properties. The combination also provides the usual therapeutic activity of tars.

The base has been developed with the objective of providing a cosmetically acceptable thixotropic formulation at the same time as retaining the efficacy of crude tar.

Indications: Treatment of psoriasis.

Treatment of dermatitis in the chronic phase.

Dosage and administration *Adults and children:* By gentle massage over all the affected area twice daily.

Contra-indications, warnings, etc

Contra-indications: Known sensitivity or intolerance to any of the ingredients.

Precautions: For external use only.

Keep away from the eyes and other mucosal surfaces.

Overdosage: Not applicable.

Main side-effects/adverse reactions: None reported.

Pharmaceutical precautions *Storage:* Store in a cool place.

Legal category P.

Package quantities 50 g and 500 g.

Further information If sensitivity occurs or infection appears discontinue use and institute appropriate therapy.

Gelcotar is water-miscible and does not permanently stain the skin.

Product licence number 0291/0011.

HIOXYL* CREAM

Presentation A smooth, white, non-greasy cream with virtually no odour, containing stabilised Hydrogen Peroxide 1.5%.

Uses The antiseptic effect of Hydrogen Peroxide is a result of its ready release of oxygen when applied to tissues. The effect only lasts as long as oxygen is being released, and for solutions of Hydrogen Peroxide, this is only of short duration.

Hioxyl Cream is a unique formulation in which Hydrogen Peroxide has been stabilised in a soothing, easy to apply, cream to give prolonged antiseptic action.

Indications: The treatment of leg ulcers, pressure sores, minor wounds and infections.

Dosage and administration Hioxyl Cream is applied freely using a piece of lint or gauze. If necessary it may be covered with a dressing. The application can be repeated as required.

Contra-indications, warnings, etc There are no known contra-indications or warnings to the use of Hioxyl Cream.

Pharmaceutical precautions Store in a cool place.

Legal category P.

Package quantities Tubes of 25 g and 100 g.

Further information Care should be taken to avoid usage with other topical medicaments due to possible chemical interaction negating the active principle.

Product licence number 0291/0008.

QUINOCORT* CREAM

Presentation

Active ingredients:

Potassium Hydroxyquinoline Sulphate BPC	0.5%
Hydrocortisone BP	1.0%

Appearance: The active ingredients are formulated in a vanishing cream base and the preparation is faintly yellow in appearance.

Uses *Main pharmacological action:* Hydrocortisone provides anti-inflammatory action yet is the least potent topical corticosteroid available. Potassium hydroxyquinoline sulphate provides broad spectrum antibacterial and anticandidal activity. The combination facilitates treatment of steroid responsive dermatoses where complication by infection with bacteria or yeast is evident, suspected, or a possibility.

Indications: The treatment of infected eczema, intertrigo and other steroid responsive dermatoses where anti-infective cover is appropriate.

Dosage and administration *Adults and children:* By gentle massage over all the affected area two to three times daily.

Contra-indications, warnings, etc
Precautions: Caution should be exercised when using this preparation in infants.

Avoid contact with eyes and other mucosal surfaces.

Warning: In pregnant animals administration of corticosteroids can cause abnormalities of foetal development. The relevance of this finding in human beings has not been established. However topical steroids should not be used extensively in pregnancy i.e. in large amounts or for long periods.

In infants long term continuous topical therapy should be avoided. Adrenal suppression can occur even without occlusion.

Contra-indications: Known sensitivity or intolerance to any of the ingredients.

Pharmaceutical precautions *Storage:* Store in a cool place avoiding extremes of temperature.

Legal category POM.

Package quantities Tubes of 30 g.

Further information Nil.

Product licence number 0291/0014.

QUINODERM* CREAM

Presentation *Appearance:* Quinoderm Cream is a creamy white astringent vanishing cream.

Active ingredients:

Benzoyl Peroxide	10%
Potassium Hydroxyquinoline Sulphate BPC	0.5%

Uses *Main pharmacological action:* The combination of the mild keratolytic properties of benzoyl peroxide and the antibacterial, antifungal and deodorant properties of potassium hydroxyquinoline sulphate in a specially formulated bland water-miscible base makes this preparation valuable in the treatment of pustular affections of the skin, particularly when associated with staphylococcal infection.

Indications: Acne vulgaris, acne rosacea, acneform eruptions, acne varioliformis, impetigo, sycosis barbae, folliculitis.

Dosage and administration *Adults and children:* By gentle massage over all the affected area, two or three times daily.

Contra-indications, warnings, etc Quinoderm Cream is used topically.

Precaution: In a few isolated cases overreaction to Quinoderm Cream may occur. To minimise this possibility, select a small area of skin behind the ear, apply the cream and leave for 12 hours. If severe irritation or pronounced redness occurs do not proceed.

For external use only. Keep out of the reach of children.

Pharmaceutical precautions *Storage:* Quinoderm Cream should be stored in a cool place, avoiding extremes of temperature.

Diluents, etc: Quinoderm Cream can be easily removed by warm water and soap.

Legal category P.

Package quantities Quinoderm Cream is supplied in tubes of 25 g and 50 g.

Further information In clinical trials in acne vulgaris 81 patients out of 106 showed a good or very good response to Quinoderm Cream. In acne rosacea 7 out of 11 patients showed a good or very good response to this preparation.

Product licence number 0291/5000.

QUINODERM* CREAM 5

Presentation *Appearance:* Quinoderm Cream 5 is a creamy white astringent vanishing cream.

Active ingredients:

Benzoyl Peroxide	5.0%
Potassium Hydroxyquinoline Sulphate BPC	0.5%

Uses *Main pharmacological action:* The combination of the mild keratolytic properties of benzoyl peroxide and the antibacterial, antifungal and deodorant properties of potassium hydroxyquinoline sulphate in a specially formulated bland water-miscible base make this preparation valuable in the treatment of pustular affections of the skin particularly when associated with staphylococcal infection.

Indications: Acne vulgaris, acneform eruptions, folliculitis.

Dosage and administration *Adults and children:* By gentle massage over all the affected area, two or three times daily.

Contra-indications, warnings, etc Quinoderm Cream 5 is contra-indicated in acne rosacea. Patients with known sensitivity to either of the active ingredients should not use Quinoderm Cream 5. Quinoderm Cream 5 is used topically.

Precaution: In a few isolated cases overreaction to Quinoderm Cream 5 may occur. To minimise this possibility, select a small area of skin behind the ear, apply the cream and leave for 12 hours. If severe irritation or pronounced redness occurs do not proceed.

All medicines should be kept out of the reach of children.

Pharmaceutical precautions *Storage:* Quinoderm Cream 5 should be stored in a cool place, avoiding extremes of temperature.

Diluents, etc: Quinoderm Cream 5 can be easily removed by warm water and soap.

Excipients, incompatibles: Not applicable.

Legal category P.

Package quantities Quinoderm Cream 5 is supplied in tubes of 50 g.

Further information Contact with mouth and eyes should be avoided. Care should be taken to avoid contact with dyed fabrics as this preparation may adversely affect dye fastness.

Product licence number 0291/0012.

QUINODERM* CREAM WITH HYDROCORTISONE 1%

Presentation *Appearance:* Quinoderm Cream with Hydrocortisone 1% is a creamy white astringent vanishing cream.

Active ingredients:

Benzoyl Peroxide	10%
Potassium Hydroxyquinoline Sulphate BPC	0.5%
Hydrocortisone BP	1%

Uses *Main pharmacological action:* The combination of the anti-inflammatory properties of hydrocortisone, the keratolytic action of benzoyl peroxide and the antibacterial, antifungal and deodorant properties of potassium hydroxyquinoline sulphate in an astringent cream base makes this preparation valuable in the treatment of pustular affections of the skin, particularly when associated with staphylococcal infection.

Indications: Severe acne vulgaris, acne rosacea, acneform eruptions, acne varioliformis, impetigo, sycosis barbae, folliculitis and perifolliculitis.

Dosage and administration *Adults and Children:* Spread thinly over the affected area and then gently massage until no trace of the cream can be seen on the skin surface. Apply two or three times daily. It is important that the whole of the area be treated, not just individual spots or blemishes.

Contra-indications, warnings, etc
Contra-indications: None.

Warning: In pregnant animals, administration of corticosteroids can cause abnormalities of foetal development. The relevance of this finding to human beings has not been established. However, topical steroids should not be used extensively in pregnancy, i.e. in large amounts or for long periods.

In infants, long-term continuous topical therapy should be avoided. Adrenal suppression can occur even without occlusion.

This preparation is for external use only.

Keep out of the reach of children.

Pharmaceutical precautions *Storage:* Quinoderm Cream with Hydrocortisone 1% should be stored in a cool place, avoiding extremes of temperature.

Diluents: The cream is easily removed by warm water and soap.

Legal category POM.

Package quantities Quinoderm Cream with Hydrocortisone is available in tubes of 30 g.

Further information In clinical trials in acne vulgaris 41 patients out of 46 showed a good or very good response to Quinoderm Cream with hydrocortisone 1% and in acne rosacea 21 patients out of 21 showed a good or very good response to this preparation.

Product licence number 0291/5001.

QUINODERM LOTIO-GEL*

Presentation Quinoderm Lotio-Gel contains colloidal Benzoyl Peroxide 10% and Potassium Hydroxyquinoline Sulphate BPC 0.5% in a homogeneous astringent gel formulated to give the colour and consistency of a creamy white lotion.

Uses Quinoderm Lotio-Gel is indicated in the treatment of acne.

The main pharmacological action of benzoyl peroxide is considered to be keratolytic and comedolytic. Potassium hydroxyquinoline sulphate has broad spectrum antibacterial activity. This combination is formulated in a specifically researched and developed base and is designed to aid the resolution of the polymorphic lesions of acne.

The base has been developed with the objective of providing a stable pharmaceutical form which maximises the advantages of a gel and lotion in a system which does not employ organic solvents and therefore has a correspondingly lower irritancy, toxicity and abuse potential.

Dosage and administration The preparation should be applied by gentle massage over all the affected area, one to three times daily.

Contra-indications, warnings, etc Patients with known sensitivity to either of the active constituents should not use Quinoderm Lotio-Gel.

In a few isolated cases overreaction to Quinoderm Lotio-Gel may occur. To minimise this possibility, select a small area of skin behind the ear, apply the Lotio-Gel and leave for 12 hours. If severe irritation or pronounced redness occurs, do not proceed.

All medicines should be kept out of the reach of children.

Contact with mouth and eyes should be avoided.

Care should be taken to avoid contact with dyed fabrics as this preparation may adversely affect dye fastness.

Pharmaceutical precautions Quinoderm Lotio-Gel should be stored in a cool place avoiding extremes of temperature.

Legal category P.

Package quantities Quinoderm Lotio-Gel is available in plastic bottles of 30 ml.

Further information Patients may vary in their response to benzoyl peroxide preparations. The stability of benzoyl peroxide in Quinoderm Lotio-Gel is enhanced to minimise any variation in response which may be attributable to variations in the concentration of this active constituent.

Product licence number 0291/0007.

QUINODERM* LOTIO-GEL 5%

Presentation Quinoderm Lotio-Gel 5% contains colloidal Benzoyl Peroxide 5% and Potassium Hydroxyquinoline Sulphate BPC 0.5% in a homogeneous astringent gel formulated to give the colour and consistency of a creamy white lotion.

Uses Quinoderm Lotio-Gel 5% is indicated in the treatment of acne.

The main pharmacological action of benzoyl peroxide is considered to be keratolytic and comedolytic. Potassium hydroxyquinoline sulphate has broad spectrum antibacterial activity. This combination is formulated in a specifically researched and developed base and is designed to aid the resolution of the polymorphic lesions of acne.

The base has been developed with the objective of providing a stable pharmaceutical form which maximises the advantages of a gel and lotion in a system which does not employ organic solvents and therefore has a correspondingly lower irritancy, toxicity and abuse potential.

Dosage and administration The preparation should be applied by gentle massage over all the affected area, one to three times daily.

Contra-indications, warnings, etc Patients with known sensitivity to either of the active constituents should not use Quinoderm Lotio-Gel 5%.

In a few isolated cases overreaction to Quinoderm Lotio-Gel 5% may occur. To minimise this possibility, select a small area of skin behind the ear, apply the Lotio-Gel and leave for twelve hours. If severe irritation or pronounced redness occurs, do not proceed.

All medicines should be kept out of the reach of children.

Contact with mouth and eyes should be avoided.

Care should be taken to avoid contact with dyed fabrics as this preparation may adversely affect dye fastness.

Pharmaceutical precautions Quinoderm Lotio-Gel 5% should be stored in a cool place avoiding extremes of temperature.

Legal category P.

Package quantities Quinoderm Lotio-Gel 5% is available in plastic bottles of 30 ml.

Further information Patients may vary in their response to benzoyl peroxide preparations. The stability of benzoyl peroxide in Quinoderm Lotio-Gel 5% is enhanced to minimise any variation in response which may be attributable to variations in the concentration of this active constituent.

Product licence number 0291/0009.

QUINOPED* CREAM

Presentation *Appearance:* Quinoped Cream is a cream-coloured astringent cream.

Active ingredients:
Benzoyl Peroxide 5%
Potassium Hydroxyquinoline Sulphate BPC   0.5%

Uses *Main pharmacological action:* Benzoyl peroxide functions as a keratolytic and facilitates the removal of macerated tissue and associated debris. Potassium hydroxyquinoline sulphate has antifungal and deodorant properties.

Indications: Athlete's foot (tinea pedis) and related fungal infections.

Dosage and administration *Adults and children:* Spread thinly over all the affected area and gently massage until no trace of the cream can be seen on the skin surface. Apply morning and night.

Contra-indications, warnings, etc For external use only. Keep out of the reach of children.

Pharmaceutical precautions *Storage:* Quinoped Cream should be stored in a cool place, avoiding extremes of temperature.

Diluents: The cream is easily removed with warm water and soap.

Legal category P.

Package quantities Quinoped Cream is available in tubes of 25 g.

Further information Quinoped Cream is a balanced formulation to counteract the effect of *T. rubrum, T. interdigitale* and *E. floccosum.*

Product licence number 0291/0002.

*Trade Mark

Reckitt & Colman Pharmaceutical Division
Dansom Lane
Hull HU8 7DS

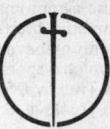

Associated companies:
Lloyd-Hamol Ltd
Westminster Laboratories Ltd

CODIS*
(Co-codaprin dispersible)

Presentation White tablets engraved on one side with the code U4 the other side being plain. Each tablet contains Aspirin BP 400 mg and codeine phosphate PhEur 8 mg (co-codaprin) and when dissolved in water provides a palatable solution of calcium acetylsalicylate and codeine phosphate.

Uses As an analgesic and antipyretic for the relief of mild to moderate pain, including headaches, migraine, neuralgia, toothache, period pains, aches and pains and the symptoms of colds, influenza and feverish conditions. The symptomatic relief of sprains, strains, rheumatic pain, sciatica, lumbago, fibrositis, muscular aches and pains, joint swelling and stiffness.

Dosage and administration
Adults: 1–2 tablets, dissolved in water; the dose may be repeated after four hours; maximum 8 tablets daily, in divided doses. Codis is not recommended for children under 12 years of age.
There is no indication that dosage need be modified for the elderly.

Contra-indications, warnings, etc The unwanted effects of Codis are those normally associated with soluble aspirin and codeine. It should not be given to patients known to be allergic to aspirin, or suffering from active peptic ulceration or haemophilia.
There is clinical and epidemiological evidence for the safety of aspirin in human pregnancy, but it may prolong labour and contribute to maternal and neonatal bleeding, and is therefore best avoided in the last trimester of pregnancy. Aspirin may precipitate bronchospasm, and induce attacks of asthma in susceptible subjects; it may also induce gastro-intestinal haemorrhage, occasionally major. Aspirin may enhance the effects of anticoagulants and inhibit the effects of uricosurics.
For *overdosage*, water or milk, given immediately, may delay absorption. The usual procedures for aspirin overdosage should be followed, including general supportive measures and gastric lavage if necessary. For respiratory depression caused by the codeine, nalorphine or naloxone should be given by injection. It is advisable for the patient to be sent to hospital for appropriate biochemical assessment and treatment.

Pharmaceutical precautions Keep in a cool, dry place.

Legal category CD (Sch 5), P.

Package quantities Cartons of 500 tablets in foil.

Further information Because the aspirin and codeine phosphate are taken in solution, effective blood levels and relief of pain may be achieved more rapidly than with ordinary aspirin or codeine tablets. The superiority of soluble aspirin over ordinary aspirin in the rapid achievement of high levels of acetylsalicyclic acid in blood have been demonstrated.
Codis has no known effects on diagnostic laboratory tests.

Product licence number 0044/5003R.
Product licence held by Reckitt & Colman Pharmaceutical Division.

COLVEN*

Presentation Colven is presented as grapefruit flavoured granules of yellowish-brown colour contained in a sachet.
Active ingredients: Each sachet contains Ispaghula Husk BP 3.5 g and mebeverine hydrochloride 135 mg.

Uses Colven is indicated for the treatment of conditions where abdominal pain and bowel dysfunction occur, such as irritable bowel syndrome, or where these symptoms occur in patients with gastrointestinal diseases such as colitis, Crohn's disease, ulcerative colitis or gastritis.

Dosage and administration
Adults, children over 12: One sachet morning and evening, half an hour before meals. An additional sachet may be taken before the midday meal if symptoms are not controlled at this time.
The contents of one sachet of Colven should be stirred into a glass of cold water and taken immediately.

Contra-indications, warnings, etc Colven is contra-indicated in cases of intestinal obstruction and colonic atony such as senile megacolon. As this product contains 6.1 mmol of sodium per sachet, its use is contra-indicated where strict control of salt intake is required, for example, in severe renal and cardiovascular conditions. The product is not at present recommended for children under 12 and, in common with most drugs, care should be taken in prescribing during pregnancy.
In the event of overdosage, conservative measures should be taken. The patient may notice abdominal discomfort and flatulence and attention should be paid to maintaining an adequate fluid intake, particularly if the granules have been taken without water, contrary to the administration instructions.

Pharmaceutical precautions Store in a cool dry place.

Legal category POM.

Package quantities Carton of 60 (6 × 10) sachets.

Further information Studies by Ritchie and Truelove

(1979, 1980) have demonstrated that a combination of ispaghula and mebeverine gave better overall relief of the symptoms of irritable bowel syndrome when compared to bran or another antispasmodic agent. Ispaghula with meboverine is presented as effervescent granules which disperse readily in water. References: Ritchie, J.A. & Truelove, S.C. (1979) Br.Med.J., 1, 376. Ritchie, J.A. & Truelove, S.C. (1980) Br.Med.J., 281, 1317.

Product licence number 0044/0075.

DISPROL* PAEDIATRIC

Presentation A sugar-free suspension of Paracetamol PhEur in a pale yellow banana-flavoured liquid. Each 5 ml dose contains 120 mg of paracetamol.

Uses For the treatment of mild to moderate pain, including headache, migraine, neuralgia, toothache, pain in teething, sore throat, aches and pains. Symptomatic relief of rheumatic aches and pains. Symptomatic relief of influenza, feverishness, feverish colds.

Dosage and administration
Children 3–12 months: Half to one 5 ml spoonful every four hours.

1 year to under 6 years: One to two 5 ml spoonfuls every four hours.

6 years to 12 years: Two to four 5 ml spoonfuls every four hours.
Dosage for children under 3 months is at physician's discretion.
Not more than 4 doses should be administered in any 24-hour period.

Contra-indications, warnings, etc Hypersensitivity to paracetamol.
Precautions: Use with caution in patients with hepatic or renal dysfunction or diabetes.
Drug interactions: Drugs which induce hepatic microsmal enzymes such as alcohol, barbiturates and tricyclic antidepressants may increase the hepatotoxicity of paracetamol particularly after overdosage.
Side-effects: Side-effects from paracetamol administered in normal doses are rare and there is epidemiological evidence of the safety of paracetamol in human pregnancy.
There have been isolated reports of agranulocytosis, methaemoglobinaemia and thrombocytopenic purpura, and after overdosage or prolonged administration isolated cases of chronic hepatic necrosis, acute pancreatitis and nephrotoxicity.
Treatment of overdosage: Overdosage should be treated promptly by gastric lavage followed by I.V. N-acetylcysteine or oral methionine since liver damage following overdosage does not become apparent for 1 to 6 days after ingestion. Initial mild symptoms consist of nausea, vomiting and pallor. Measurements of the blood paracetamol level and the time elapsed since ingestion is important in order to determine whether further therapy with N-acetylcysteine is necessary.

Pharmaceutical precautions Store below 25°C and protect from light, avoid freezing.

Legal category P.

Package quantities 500 ml bottles.

Further information Disprol Paediatric contains no

sugar. The sweetening agent is Lycasin which is non-cariogenic. Each 5 mls of suspension can provide up to 12 Kcal and this should be taken into account when treating diabetic children.

Product licence number 0044/0085.

FYBOGEL*
FYBOGEL* ORANGE

Presentation Fybogel: Flaky granules of a pale buff colour.
Fybogel Orange: Flaky granules of a pale orange colour with an orange flavouring.
One sachet of granules contains Ispaghula Husk BP 3.5 g.

Uses Fybogel is recommended for the treatment of patients requiring a high-fibre regimen.

Dosage and administration Adults: children over 12: One sachet morning and evening.
Children under 12: $\frac{1}{2}$–1 level 5 ml spoonful depending on age and size morning and evening.
Fybogel should be stirred into water and taken as soon as possible, preferably after meals.
There is no indication that dosage need be modified for the elderly.

Contra-indications, warnings, etc Fybogel is contra-indicated in cases of intestinal obstruction and colonic atony such as senile megacolon.
In the event of overdosage conservative measures should be taken. The patient may notice abdominal discomfort and flatulence, and attention should be paid to maintaining an adequate fluid intake particularly if the granules have been taken without water contrary to the administration instructions.

Pharmaceutical precautions Nil.

Legal category GSL.

Package quantities Carton of 60 (6 × 10) sachets.

Further information Daily Fybogel therapy provides a high-fibre regimen. Ispaghula husk is capable of retaining 40 times its weight of water, promoting easy evacuation and avoiding episodes of straining. Fybogel effervescent granules disperse readily to form a palatable drink in water. The unflavoured form of Fybogel may be mixed with fruit squash to vary the flavour. Each sachet of Fybogel contains 6.0 mmol sodium. Each sachet of Fybogel Orange contains 6.1 mmol sodium.
Fybogel has no known effects on diagnostic laboratory tests.

Product licence numbers
Fybogel   0044/0041
Fybogel Orange   0044/0068.
Product licence held by Reckitt & Colman Pharmaceutical Division.

LIQUID GAVISCON*

Presentation A pink suspension with a flavour of fennel (similar to aniseed).
10 ml of Liquid Gaviscon contains sodium alginate 500 mg, Sodium Bicarbonate PhEur 267 mg, calcium carbonate 160 mg.

Uses Gaviscon alleviates the painful conditions resulting from the reflux of gastric acid and bile into the oesophagus by suppressing the reflux itself. It is indicated in heartburn, including heartburn of pregnancy, dyspepsia associated with gastric reflux, hiatus hernia, reflux oesophagitis, regurgitation and all cases of epigastric and retrosternal distress where the underlying cause is gastric reflux.

Dosage and administration *Adults, children over 12:* 10–20 ml after meals and at bedtime.

Children under 12: 5–10 ml after meals and at bedtime. Infants not recommended. See Infant Gaviscon. If desired, the standard dose of Liquid Gaviscon may be taken diluted with not more than an equal quantity of water, well stirred.

There is no indication that dosage need be modified for the elderly.

Contra-indications, warnings, etc There are no specific contra-indications.

As Gaviscon's mode of action is physical, overdosage presents virtually no hazard. The only likely consequence is abdominal distension, which is best treated conservatively.

Pharmaceutical precautions Store below 30°C; avoid freezing.

Legal category GSL.

Package quantities Amber bottles of 500 ml.

Further information On ingestion Gaviscon reacts with gastric acid to produce in the stomach a floating viscous gel of near neutral pH which effectively impedes reflux. In severe cases the gel itself may be refluxed into the oesophagus, where it protects the inflamed mucosa, thus allowing healing to take place and preventing further inflammation.

The sodium content of a dose of 10 ml liquid is 141 mg (6.2 mmol). This may be of importance when a highly restricted salt diet is required as in some renal and cardiovascular conditions.

Liquid Gaviscon has no known effects on diagnostic laboratory tests.

Product licence number 0044/0058.
Product licence held by Reckitt & Colman Pharmaceutical Division.

GAVISCON* TABLETS

Presentation White, mint-flavoured tablet engraved on both sides with the word 'Gaviscon' and a sword symbol. Each tablet contains Alginic Acid BPC 500 mg, Magnesium Trisilicate PhEur 25 mg, Dried Aluminium Hydroxide Gel BP 100 mg, Sodium Bicarbonate PhEur 170 mg in a peppermint flavoured base.

Uses Gaviscon alleviates the painful conditions resulting from the reflux of gastric acid and bile into the oesophagus by suppressing the reflux itself. It is indicated in heartburn, including heartburn of pregnancy, dyspepsia associated with gastric reflux, hiatus hernia, reflux oesophagitis, regurgitation and all cases of epigastric and retrosternal distress where the underlying cause is gastric reflux.

Dosage and administration *Adults, children over 12:* 1 or 2 tablets after meals and at bedtime.

Children under 12: 1 tablet after meals and at bedtime. Infants not recommended. See Infant Gaviscon.

Tablets should be thoroughly chewed. It is recommended they be broken in half and chewed a little at a time. This may be followed by a drink of water.

There is no indication that dosage need be modified for the elderly.

Contra-indications, warnings, etc There are no specific contra-indications.

As Gaviscon's mode of action is physical, overdosage presents virtually no hazard. The only likely consequence is abdominal distension which is best treated conservatively.

Pharmaceutical precautions Nil.

Legal category GSL.

Package quantities Carton containing 3 tubes of 20 tablets.

Further information On ingestion, Gaviscon reacts with gastric acid to produce in the stomach a floating viscous gel of near neutral pH which effectively impedes reflux. In severe cases the gel itself may be refluxed into the oesophagus, where it protects the inflamed mucosa, thus allowing healing to take place and preventing further inflammation.

Care should be taken when treating diabetic patients, owing to the sugar content of the tablets. The sodium content of a tablet is 47 mg (2.25 mmol).

Gaviscon Tablets have no known effects on diagnostic laboratory tests.

Product licence number 0044/0021.
Product licence held by Reckitt & Colman Pharmaceutical Division.

GAVISCON* GRANULES

Presentation Brown, chocolate-flavoured granules. One sachet of granules contains Alginic Acid BPC 481 mg, Sodium Alginate 521 mg, Magnesium Trisilicate PhEur 52 mg, Dried Aluminium Hydroxide Gel BP 208 mg, Sodium Bicarbonate PhEur 177 mg in an inert base including Sucrose PhEur 2.083 g.

Uses Gaviscon alleviates the painful conditions resulting from the reflux of gastric acid and bile into the oesophagus by forming an alginate raft which floats on top of the stomach contents and physically impedes reflux. It is indicated in heartburn, including heartburn of pregnancy, dyspepsia associated with gastric reflux, hiatus hernia, reflux oesophagitis, regurgitation, and all cases of epigastric and retrosternal distress where the underlying cause is gastric reflux.

Dosage and administration *Adults, children over 12:* 1 sachet after meals and at bedtime.

Children under 12: ½ sachet (1 level 5 ml spoonful granules) after meals and at bedtime. Infants: Not recommended. See Infant Gaviscon.

Granules should be thoroughly chewed and may be followed by a drink of water.

There is no indication that dosage need be modified for the elderly.

Contra-indications, warnings, etc There are no specific contra-indications. As Gaviscon's mode of action is physical, overdosage presents virtually no hazard. The only likely consequence is abdominal distension which is best treated conservatively.

Pharmaceutical precautions Nil.

Legal category GSL.

Package quantities Cartons of 10 sachets.

Further information On ingestion, Gaviscon reacts with gastric acid to produce in the stomach a floating viscous gel of near neutral pH which effectively impedes reflux. In severe cases the gel itself may be refluxed into the oesophagus, where it protects the inflamed mucosa, thus allowing healing to take place and preventing further inflammation.

Care should be taken when treating diabetic patients owing to the sugar content of the granules. The sodium content of a sachet is 118 mg (5.2 mmol).

Gaviscon Granules have no known effects on diagnostic laboratory tests.

Product licence number 0044/5008.
Product licence held by Reckitt & Colman Pharmaceutical Division.

INFANT GAVISCON*

Presentation Infant Gaviscon is a fine white powder, packed in a sachet and sterilised. Each sachet contains Alginic Acid BPC 924 mg, Magnesium Trisilicate PhEur 50 mg, Dried Aluminium Hydroxide Gel BP 200 mg and Sodium Bicarbonate PhEur 340 mg, in a base containing colloidal silica (Aerosil) and Mannitol BP.

Uses Infant Gaviscon helps to prevent gastric regurgitation in infants, where competence of the cardiac sphincter has not been fully established.

Its indications are gastric regurgitation, gastro-oesophageal reflux and reflux associated with hiatus hernia in infants and young children.

Dosage and administration *Young children:* The contents of 1 sachet mixed with half a tumbler of water after each meal.

Infants up to 2 months: Not more than $\frac{1}{2}$ sachet mixed with made up feed immediately before use.

Infants over 2 months: $\frac{1}{2}$–1 sachet mixed with the made-up feed immediately before use.

Breast fed infants: Mix powder with 10–20 ml of boiled, cooled water and give after feeding using a spoon or feeding bottle. Any unused powder should be discarded.

Contra-indications, warnings, etc Not to be used in premature infants, or in situations where excessive water-loss is likely, e.g. fever or high room-temperature. Care should be taken when treating infants with gastroenteritis or known or suspected renal disease or impairment, as the sodium content (93 mg, or 4 mmol per sachet) may add to the risk of hypernatraemia.

As Infant Gaviscon's mode of action is physical there are virtually no systemic unwanted effects resulting from overdosage. Overdosage may lead to gastric distension, which is best treated conservatively. Gross overdosage has been reported as causing an intragastric mass.

Pharmaceutical precautions Nil.

Legal category GSL.

Package quantities Carton of 10 sachets.

Further information Infant Gaviscon thickens a water or milk feed, and in the stomach reacts with acid gastric contents to form a viscous gel which suppresses gastro-oesophageal reflux.

Infant Gaviscon has no known effects on diagnostic laboratory tests.

Product licence number 0044/5007.
Product licence held by Reckitt & Colman Pharmaceutical Division.

PRIPSEN*

Presentation Pripsen is a cream-coloured powder presented in a dual sachet pack. The powder forms a fine red suspension in milk or water.

Each individual sachet contains 4 g Piperazine Phosphate BP and standardised senna equivalent to 15.3 mg total sennosides calculated as sennoside B.

Uses Pripsen is a potent anthelmintic recommended for the eradication of threadworm and roundworm.

Dosage and administration
Adults and children over 6: 1 sachet. Repeat after 14 days.

Children aged 1–6 years: $\frac{2}{3}$ sachet (2 level 5 ml spoonsful). Repeat after 14 days.

Infants – 3 months to 1 year: $\frac{1}{3}$ sachet (1 level 5 ml spoonful). Repeat after 14 days.

Pripsen should be stirred into a small glass of milk or water and drunk immediately.

When treating roundworms, additional single prophylactic doses at monthly intervals may be necessary to eliminate the risk of reinfestation.

There is no indication that dosage need be modified for the elderly.

Contra-indications, warnings, etc Pripsen should not be used in patients with severe bilateral renal dysfunction or epilepsy.

As doses are normally separated by at least 14 days the rare neurotoxic side-effects of piperazine (transient visual disturbance and vertigo), which are due to cumulative blood-levels, are unlikely to occur.

Although Pripsen has not been associated with any reports of teratogenicity, in common with most drugs, its use in the first trimester of pregnancy is not advised.

Overdose: Effects of overdosage will most likely be due to the piperazine content. Treatment by gastric lavage and supportive measures is indicated.

Pharmaceutical precautions Any unused powder should be discarded.

Legal category P.

Package quantities Carton of 12 dual-sachets.

Further information Pripsen has an effective cure rate of virtually 100%, the piperazine paralysing the worms which are then evacuated before recovery by the efficient laxative action of standardised senna. Threadworms may be still in the larval stage when Pripsen is first administered so the follow-up dose should be taken after 14 days to eliminate this reinfestation.

Pripsen is ideal for mass administration where cross-infestation is likely.

Pripsen has no known effects on diagnostic laboratory tests.

Product licence number 0063/5004.
Product licence held by Westminster Laboratories Ltd.

SENOKOT*

Presentation *Tablets:* Small brown tablets engraved on one side only with the word Senokot and a sword symbol. One tablet contains standardised senna equivalent to 7.5 mg total sennosides calculated as sennoside B.

Granules: Brown chocolate-flavoured granules. One 5 ml level spoonful (2.73 g) contains standardised senna equivalent to 15 mg total sennosides calculated as sennoside B.

Syrup: Brown, fruit-flavoured syrup. One 5 ml spoonful contains standardised senna extract equivalent to 7.5 mg total sennosides calculated as sennoside B.

Uses In the management of constipation, including: Simple constipation, whether self-induced or environmental, e.g. neglect of the call to stool or poor sanitary conditions.

Constipation in old age, especially where maintenance treatment is required.

Constipation in pregnancy and the puerperium.
Idiopathic slow-transit constipation.
Constipation in the irritable bowel syndrome.
Conservative treatment of haemorrhoids.
Avoidance of straining after surgery and in cerebral and cardiovascular disease.

Dosage and administration The correct dose of Senokot is the smallest required to produce a comfortable soft-formed motion. It varies between individuals, but is generally found within the following ranges:

Adults: 2 to 4 tablets, or 1 to 2 level 5 ml spoonfuls of granules or 2 to 4 × 5 ml spoonfuls of syrup.

Children over 6 years: Half the adult dosages.

Children 2–6 years: Senokot syrup ½ to one 5 ml spoonful for preference.

New users should start with the lowest doses and, if necessary increase it by half the initial dose each day until a comfortable formed motion is produced. If no bowel action has occurred after three days' progressively increased dosage a further medical examination should be considered.

Senokot is best taken as a single dose, at bedtime by adults and in the morning by children. The tablets can be taken with a drink, the granules can be stirred into hot milk, sprinkled on food, or eaten as they are.

There is no indication that dosage need be modified for the elderly.

Contra-indications, warnings, etc Senokot like all laxatives, should not be given when any undiagnosed acute or persistent abdominal symptoms are present. Temporary mild griping may occur during adjustment of dosage. In case of gross accidental overdosage, where diarrhoea is severe, conservative measures are usually sufficient: generous amounts of fluid especially fruit drinks should be given.

Pharmaceutical precautions The tablets and granules should be kept in closed airtight containers, and the syrup in amber bottles as supplied. Store in a cool place.

Legal category P.

Package quantities *Tablets:* Pack of 1,000.
Granules: Tins of 500 g.
Syrup: Bottles of 500 ml.

Further information The physiological action of the natural anthrone glycosides in Senokot is virtually colon-specific. The active glycosides are protected by a natural sugar moiety which safeguards their transport to the large bowel, where bacterial action breaks the sugar–anthrone bond and releases the active fraction. Peristalsis is then stimulated via the submucosal and myenteric nerve plexuses.

Being colon-specific, Senokot does not affect the vital nutritional functions of the upper gastro-intestinal tract.

Diabetic patients should use the tablets as these have a low sugar content.

Clinical studies have shown that breast fed infants of mothers taking Senokot did not show any side effects to the drug.

Senokot has no known effects on diagnostic laboratory tests.

Product licence numbers
Tablets   0063/5000
Granules   0063/5002
Syrup   0063/5003

Product licences held by Westminster Laboratories Ltd.

SOLPRIN*

Presentation White tablets engraved on both sides with a sword symbol. Each tablet contains Aspirin PhEur 300 mg, and when dissolved in water provides a palatable solution of calcium acetylsalicylate.

Uses As an analgesic, antipyretic and anti-inflammatory, for the relief of pain in headache, toothache, neuralgia, sciatica and period pains, and the reduction of inflammation in rheumatism and associated conditions.

Dosage and administration *Adults:* 1–3 tablets dissolved in water. The dose may be repeated after four hours; maximum 12 tablets daily in divided doses (in acute rheumatic conditions up to 24 tablets daily in divided doses).

Children 6–12 years: 1 tablet dissolved in water, repeated after four hours if necessary; maximum 80 mg/kg body weight daily in divided doses.

There is no indication that dosage need be modified for the elderly.

Contra-indications, warnings, etc Unwanted effects are those of soluble aspirin. Solprin should not be given to patients suffering from active peptic ulceration or haemophilia or known to be allergic to aspirin.

There is clinical and epidemiological evidence of the safety of aspirin in pregnancy, but it may prolong labour and contribute to maternal and neonatal bleeding and is best avoided in the last trimester of pregnancy.

Aspirin may precipitate bronchospasm, and induce attacks of asthma in susceptible subjects; it may also induce gastro-intestinal haemorrhage, occasionally major.

Aspirin may enhance the effects of anticoagulants and inhibit the action of uricosurics.

For overdosage, the usual procedures for aspirin overdosage should be followed, including general supportive measures and gastric lavage if necessary.

Pharmaceutical precautions Nil.

Legal category GSL.

Package quantities 500 tablets in foil.

Further information Solprin is aspirin in a soluble form. Because the aspirin is taken in solution, effective blood levels and the relief of pain and inflammation may be achieved more rapidly than with ordinary aspirin; further, it is less likely to cause gastric upsets.

Solprin has no known effects on diagnostic laboratory tests.

Product licence number 0044/5000.
Product licence held by Reckitt & Colman Pharmaceutical Division.

TEMGESIC* INJECTION

Presentation Temgesic Injection is a colourless liquid containing 0.3 mg/ml buprenorphine, as the hydrochloride, in a 5% dextrose solution, adjusted to pH range 3.5–5.5. Clear glass snap-ampoules of 1 ml (0.3 mg) or 2 ml (0.6 mg).

Uses As a strong analgesic for the relief of moderate to severe pain.

Dosage and administration *Adults:* The recommended dosage is 1 to 2 ml (0.3–0.6 mg buprenorphine), by IM or slow IV injection, every six to eight hours or as required. Temgesic is not at present recommended for children under 12 years. There is no evidence that dosage need be modified for the elderly.

Contra-indications, warnings, etc There are no absolute contra-indications. Because Temgesic can show antagonist properties, it may precipitate mild withdrawal symptoms in narcotic addicts or in patients who have been maintained on high doses of morphine.

Temgesic may cause some drowsiness; this could be potentiated by other centrally-acting agents, including alcohol, tranquillisers, sedatives and hypnotics. Ambulant patients should be warned not to drive or operate machinery if affected.

As with other strong centrally acting analgesics care should be taken when treating patients with impaired respiratory function. However, Temgesic rarely causes significant respiratory depression. Although volunteer studies have indicated that opiate antagonists may not fully reverse the effects of Temgesic, clinical experience has shown that naloxone may be of benefit in reversing a reduced respiratory rate. Respiratory stimulants such as doxapram are also effective.

Since buprenorphine is metabolised in the liver, the intensity and duration of its action may be enhanced in patients with impaired liver function. Temgesic should be used with caution in patients who are receiving monoamine oxidase inhibitors.

Until further information is available Temgesic is not recommended for use during pregnancy. Although buprenorphine is excreted in breast milk, the drug concentrations are very low and unlikely to be of clinical significance to the baby. There is indirect evidence in animal studies to suggest that Temgesic may cause a reduction in milk flow during lactation. Although this occurred only at doses well in excess of the human dose, it should be borne in mind when treating lactating women.

Overdosage: Temgesic has a wide safety margin, and in clinical practice doses well in excess of those recommended have been used without untoward effect. Supportive measures should be instituted and, if appropriate, naloxone or respiratory stimulants can be used.

The expected symptoms of overdosage would be drowsiness, nausea and vomiting; marked miosis may occur.

Side-effects: Drowsiness, or sleep from which the patient can easily be aroused, may occur particularly in the postoperative period. In common with other strong analgesics, nausea, vomiting, dizziness and sweating have been reported which may be more frequent in ambulant patients. Should nausea and vomiting occur, concurrent administration of an anti-emetic is advised. The psychotomimetic effects sometimes observed with other antagonist-analgesics are only rarely encountered with Temgesic.

Pharmaceutical procautions Temgesic Injection, though stable, should be kept cool and protected from light. It may be diluted with 5% Injection Dextrose BP or Injection Sodium Chloride BP.

Legal category POM.

Package quantities Pack of 5 ampoules (1 ml or 2 ml).

Further information There is evidence to indicate that therapeutic doses of buprenorphine do not reduce the analgesic efficacy of standard doses of an opiate agonist, and that when buprenorphine is employed within the normal therapeutic range, standard doses of narcotic agonist may be administered before the effects of the former have ended without compromising analgesia.

Clinical experience to date suggests that Temgesic may be usefully employed both as premedication and an analgesic supplement to balanced anaesthesia.

Human and animal studies indicate that buprenorphine has a substantially lower dependence profile than pure agonist analgesics.

Temgesic Injection contains 50 mg dextrose per ml, but no sodium, potassium or preservative.

Temgesic has no known effects on diagnostic laboratory tests.

Product licence numbers
Temgesic Injection 1 ml   0044/0056
Temgesic Injection 2 ml   0044/0057

TEMGESIC* SUBLINGUAL

Presentation Temgesic Sublingual is a white, biconvex tablet engraved on one side with a sword-symbol, containing 0.2 mg buprenorphine, as the hydrochloride.

Uses As a strong analgesic for the relief of moderate to severe pain.

Dosage and administration 1–2 tablets (0.2–0.4 mg buprenorphine) to be dissolved under the tongue, every 6–8 hours or as required.

The recommended starting dose for moderate to severe pain of the type typically presenting in general practice is 1–2 tablets 8 hourly.

The tablet should not be chewed or swallowed as this will reduce efficacy.

Temgesic Sublingual is not at present recommended for children under 12 years. There is no evidence that dosage need be modified for the elderly.

Contra-indications, warnings, etc There are no absolute contra-indications. Because Temgesic has antagonistic properties, it may precipitate mild withdrawal symptoms in narcotic addicts or in patients who have been maintained on high doses of morphine.

Temgesic may cause some drowsiness; this could be potentiated by other centrally-acting agents, including alcohol, tranquillisers, sedatives and hypnotics. Ambulant patients should be warned not to drive or operate machinery if affected.

As with other strong centrally acting analgesics care should be taken when treating patients with impaired respiratory function. However, Temgesic rarely causes significant respiratory depression. Although volunteer studies have indicated that opiate antagonists may not fully reverse the effects of Temgesic, clinical experience has shown that naloxone may be of benefit in reversing a reduced respiratory rate. Respiratory stimulants such as doxapram are also effective.

Since buprenorphine is metabolised in the liver, the intensity and duration of its action may be affected in patients with impaired liver function. Temgesic should be used with caution in patients who are receiving monoamine oxidase inhibitors.

Until further information is available Temgesic is not recommended for use during pregnancy. Although buprenorphine is excreted in breast milk, the drug concentrations are very low and unlikely to be of clinical significance to the baby. There is indirect evidence in animal studies to suggest that Temgesic may cause a reduction in milk flow during lactation. Although this occurred only at doses well in excess of the human dose, it should be borne in mind when treating lactating women.

Overdosage: Temgesic Sublingual has a wide safety margin and in clinical practice doses of buprenorphine well in excess of those recommended have been used without untoward effect.

Overdosage by the sublingual route is unlikely. The expected symptoms would be drowsiness, nausea and vomiting; marked miosis may occur.

If tablets are swallowed overdosage is less likely because the absorbed active ingredient is rapidly metabolised in the gut wall and by the liver. Gastric lavage should be carried out and supportive measures instituted. If appropriate, naloxone or respiratory stimulants can be used.

Side-effects: No serious toxic reactions have been observed where Temgesic Sublingual has been given in normal therapeutic doses.

In common with other strong analgesics, nausea, vomiting, dizziness, sweating and drowsiness have been reported and may be more frequent in ambulant patients.

Should nausea and vomiting occur, concurrent administration of an anti-emetic is advised.

The psychotomimetic effects sometimes observed with other antagonist-analgesics are only rarely encountered with Temgesic Sublingual.

Pharmaceutical precautions Store in a cool place.

Legal category POM.

Package quantities Carton of 50 tablets, blister-packs of 10 tablets each.

Further information There is evidence to indicate that therapeutic doses of buprenorphine do not reduce the analgesic efficacy of standard doses of an opiate agonist, and that when buprenorphine is employed within the normal therapeutic range, standard doses of narcotic agonist may be administered before the effects of the former have ended without compromising analgesia.

Temgesic Sublingual has been formulated to allow the active ingredient to be absorbed through the buccal mucosa within minutes.

Human and animal studies indicate that buprenorphine has a substantially lower dependence profile than full agonist analgesics.

Temgesic has no known affects on diagnostic laboratory tests.

Product licence number 0044/0063.

TIMODINE*

Presentation Pale yellow cream containing (w/w):

Nystatin BP	100,000 i.u./g
Hydrocortisone BP	0.5%
Benzalkonium Chloride Solution BP	0.2%
Dimethicone 350 BP	10.0%

Uses For the treatment of dermatoses, including intertrigo, eczema, seborrhoeic dermatitis, "housewife's eczema" and pruritus ani and vulvae, in which *Candida albicans* is a factor. For the treatment of severe napkin rash involving *Candida albicans*.

Dosage and administration

Dermatoses: Sufficient Timodine should be applied to cover the lesion in a thin layer. It should then be massaged into the skin until the cream disappears. The treatment should be repeated three times a day until the lesion has healed.

There is no indication that dosage need be modified for the elderly.

Napkin Rash: After removal of the soiled napkin, the affected area should be cleaned and dried and a thin layer of Timodine applied. The treatment should be repeated after every napkin change until the lesion has healed.

Contra-indications, warnings, etc

Contra-indications: Sensitivity to benzalkonium chloride or nystatin.

Precaution: Keep away from the eyes.

Topical administration of corticosteroids to pregnant animals can cause abnormalities of foetal development. The relevance of this finding to human beings has not been established; however, topical steroids should not be used extensively in pregnancy, i.e. in large amounts or for prolonged periods.

Side-effects: None have been reported.

Pharmaceutical precautions Store in a cool place.

Legal category POM.

Package quantities Tubes of 30 g.

Further information Timodine is particularly indicated in the treatment of dermatoses occurring in sites, such as the skin folds, in which the special environmental conditions present predispose to maceration and chafing, leading to secondary infection with *Candida albicans* and bacteria, and causing additional inflammation and persistent pruritus.

Timodine has no known effects on diagnostic laboratory tests.

Product licence number 1839/0001.
Product licence held by Lloyd-Hamol Ltd.

TIMOPED* CREAM

Presentation A white cream containing Tolnaftate BP 1.0%; Triclosan 0.25%.

Uses For the topical treatment of athletes foot (tinea pedis) and other cutaneous mycotic infections due to *Trichophyton*, *Epidermophyton*, and *Microsporum* spp.

Dosage and administration Timoped Cream should be massaged into the affected area and allowed to dry to a white powder. Two applications per day are recommended. Symptomatic relief is usually rapid, with lesions generally clearing within two to three weeks.

There is no indication that dosage need be modified for the elderly.

Contra-indications, warnings, etc There are no known contra-indications to the use of Timoped Cream, however, treatment should be discontinued if dermatitis, irritation or pruritus develops.

Pharmaceutical precautions Store in a cool place.

Legal category GSL.

Package quantities Tubes of 30 g.

Further information Tolnaftate is a potent fungicidal agent that is effective in the treatment of superficial cutaneous fungal infections. Timoped Cream also contains drying agents which help treatment of conditions involving macerated skin.

Timoped has no known effects on diagnostic laboratory tests.

Product licence number 0044/0077.

TRANSVASIN*

Presentation Creamy-white, water-miscible cream containing (w/w):

Ethyl nicotinate	2.0%
Hexyl nicotinate	2.0%
Tetrahydrofurfuryl salicylate	14·0%
Benzocaine PhEur	2.0%

Uses For the relief of rheumatic and muscular pain and the treatment of sprains and strains.

Dosage and administration *Directions for use:* Massage gently into the affected area until the cream is entirely absorbed.

Transvasin should be applied at least twice daily until the pain abates.

There is no indication that dosage need be modified for the elderly.

Contra-indications, warnings, etc
Contra-indications: Sensitivity to salicylates, nicotinates or benzocaine.

Pharmaceutical precautions Keep in a cool place.

Legal category P.

Package quantities Tubes of 30 g.

Further information Transvasin is a rubefacient, and within a few minutes of application a sensation of warmth is felt, followed by a reddening of the skin. This erythema does not indicate intolerance.

Transvasin has no known effects on diagnostic laboratory tests.

Product licence number 1839/5001.
Product licence held by Lloyd-Hamol Ltd.

*Trade Mark

Riker Laboratories
Morley Street
Loughborough
Leics LE 11 1EP

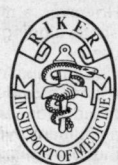

ACUPAN*

Presentation *Acupan Tablets:* White, film-coated, circular, biconvex tablets, 7 mm in diameter, marked APN on one side. Each tablet contains nefopam hydrochloride 30 mg.

Acupan Injection: Each 2 ml ampoule contains 1 ml of a solution of nefopam hydrochloride 20 mg/ml.

Uses Acupan is indicated for the relief of acute and chronic pain, including: post-operative pain; dental pain; musculo-skeletal pain; acute traumatic pain and cancer pain.

Acupan is a potent and rapidly-acting analgesic. It is totally distinct from other centrally-acting analgesics such as morphine, codeine, pentazocine and propoxyphene.

Unlike the narcotic agents, Acupan has been shown not to cause respiratory depression. There is no evidence from pre-clinical research of habituation occurring with Acupan.

Dosage and administration *Adults: Acupan Tablets:* Dosage may range from 1 to 3 tablets three times daily depending on response. The recommended starting dosage is 2 tablets three times daily.

Acupan Injection: 20 mg (1 ml) intramuscularly repeated if necessary every six hours (see instructions for administration). Onset of effect after intramuscular injection is within 15–20 minutes and peak effect is reached at one to one-and-a-half hours after administration.

Treatment started with Acupan injection may be continued with Acupan Tablets. 60 mg Acupan (2 tablets) is approximately bioequivalent to 20 mg (1 ampoule) given by injection.

Instructions for administration of Acupan Injection: Acupan Injection should always be given with the patient lying down and after injection the patient should remain lying down for 15–20 minutes. The patient should then get up slowly.

Elderly: Elderly patients may require reduced dosage due to slower metabolism. Suggested starting dose 1 tablet 3 times a day.

Children: Since Acupan has not been evaluated in children no dosage recommendation can be given for patients under 12 years.

Contra-indications, warnings, etc *Side-effects:* Nausea, nervousness, dry mouth and lightheadedness may occur. Less frequently, vomiting, blurred vision, drowsiness, sweating, insomnia, headache and tachycardia have been reported.

Caution: The side-effects of Acupan may be additive to those of other agents with anticholinergic or sympathomimetic activity. It should not be used in the treatment of myocardial infarction since there is no clinical experience in this indication. Hepatic and renal insufficiency may interfere with the metabolism and excretion of nefopam. Caution should be exercised when nefopam is administered concurrently with tricyclic antidepressants.

Use in pregnancy: There has been little human usage but there has been no adverse animal evidence.

Contra-indications: Acupan is contra-indicated in patients with a history of convulsive disorders and should not be given to patients taking mono-amine-oxidase (MAO) inhibitors.

Overdosage: A few cases of overdosage with Acupan have been reported and successfully treated. Diazepam should be given, preferably by mouth, to prevent the onset of CNS excitement. Other treatment should consist of general supportive measures.

In dogs given abnormally high doses of paracetamol, correspondingly excessive doses of nefopam potentiated the known hepatotoxicity of paracetamol. These studies indicated that repeated oral doses of 236 mg/kg/day of paracetamol with 24 mg/kg/day of nefopam showed potentiation of paracetamol hepatotoxicity. These doses are about six to eight times higher than the average human doses. Lower doses equivalent to three to four times the human dose produced no evidence of hepatotoxicity potentiation.

Pharmaceutical precautions Store in a cool, dry place.

Package quantities *Acupan Tablets;* Packs of 40 and 100 tablets.
Acupan Injection; Boxes containing 5 × 2 ml ampoules filled with 1 ml of solution.

Legal category POM.

Further information Nil.

Product licence numbers
Acupan Tablets   0068/0061
Acupan Injection   0068/0069

ALU-CAP*

Presentation Opaque green/red hard gelatin capsule, size 0, marked 'RIKER'. Each capsule contains 475 mg Dried Aluminium Hydroxide Gel BP as a white powder.

Uses Alu-Cap is recommended for use as a phosphate-binding agent in the management of renal failure. It may also be used as an antacid.

In the gut, aluminium hydroxide adsorbs phosphate ions. This reduces absorption of phosphate into the body, and thereby reduces serum phosphate levels. In patients with renal failure, the problem of high serum phosphate levels may be partially solved by a diet low in phosphorus. However, a more liberal diet is feasible when a phosphate-binding agent, such as aluminium hydroxide, is used.

Aluminium hydroxide gel is a slow-acting antacid. It is used to provide symptomatic relief in gastric hyperacidity. In addition, the antipeptic and demulcent activity of aluminium hydroxide helps to protect inflamed gastric mucosa against further irritation by gastric secretions.

Dosage and administration *For phosphate-binding: Adults and children:* The dosage must be selected in accordance with individual patient requirements, and may range from 4 to 20 capsules of Alu-Cap daily (approximately 2–10 g dried aluminium hydroxide gel), taken with meals.

As an antacid: Adults: One Alu-Cap four times daily and on retiring. Alu-Cap is not suitable for antacid therapy in children.

Elderly: No special dosage recommendations are made for elderly patients.

Contra-indications, warnings, etc
Side-effects: Aluminium hydroxide is astringent and may cause constipation.

Precautions: Serum phosphate levels should be monitored in all patients receiving phosphate binders, to prevent the development of a phosphate depletion syndrome.

Aluminium hydroxide may form complexes with certain antibiotics (tetracyclines); concomitant administration may result in reduced absorption of the antibiotic.

Pregnancy: There is no evidence of safety of the drug in human pregnancy but it has been in wide use for many years without apparent ill consequence – animal studies having shown no hazard.

Contra-indications: Patients with hypophosphataemia.

Overdosage: Symptoms and treatment: A single massive dose of aluminium hydroxide is unlikely to have harmful sequelae, as aluminium is not absorbed systemically to any great extent. Gastric lavage should be administered, followed by a mild aperient if required.

Pharmaceutical precautions Store in a cool, dry place.

Legal category P.

Package quantities Bottles of 100 capsules.

Further information Nil.

Product licence number 0068/0052.

CALCISORB*

Presentation Creamy-white to beige fibrous powder. The active ingredient is the sodium salt of the phosphate ester of cellulose. Each dose of 5 g is supplied in sachet form and contains approximately 4.7 g of the active ingredient and 0.3 g of moisture.

Uses Sodium cellulose phosphate is an ion-exchange compound with a particular affinity for divalent cations. The product binds calcium ions in the lumen of the stomach and intestine and thus prevents hyperabsorption of dietary calcium. Calcium bound by cellulose phosphate is no longer available for absorption and is therefore excreted in the faeces.

Each 5 g dose will bind approximately 350 mg of calcium.

Calcisorb is used to diminish calcium absorption from the diet: 1) in the treatment of hypercalciuria and recurrent formation of renal stones: 2) in osteopetrosis; 3) as a basis of a test for calcium absorption.

Other possible uses are: 1) treatment of idiopathic hypercalcaemia of infancy; 2) treatment of hypercalcaemic sarcoidosis; 3) treatment of vitamin D intoxication.

Dosage and administration
Adults: 15 g daily, divided as three 5 g doses with meals.

Children: 10 g daily, divided as three doses with meals.

The required dose should be dispersed in water and taken orally. Alternatively the powder may be sprinkled onto food.

Elderly: No special dosage recommendations are made for elderly patients.

Contra-indications, warnings, etc
Contra-indications: Renal failure. Congestive heart failure and other conditions in which a low sodium intake is essential.

Side-effects: Side-effects are rare. Isolated cases of diarrhoea have been reported. One patient with mild renal disease developed a moderate magnesium deficiency. This was readily corrected by halving the dose.

No signs of calcium deficiency have been reported during the continuous use of cellulose phosphate for up to 11 years. This theoretical hazard is particularly relevant to pregnancy, but in view of the absence of data on the effect of cellulose phosphate on calcium levels in pregnant women it is recommended that treatment is discontinued during pregnancy and lactation. Likewise growing children should be prescribed Calcisorb only at the discretion of a senior physician and under his direct supervision.

Pharmaceutical precautions Since cellulose phosphate is an ester, some hydrolysis occurs on storage, the rate increasing with temperature. Calcisorb should therefore be kept in a refrigerator for long-term storage.

For short-term storage by the patient, i.e. of the order of one month, refrigeration is unnecessary. The product is supplied with a minimum expiry date of two years from manufacture.

Legal category P.

Package quantities Supplied in packs of 100 sachets.

Further information Calcisorb should be used in conjunction with a low calcium diet in which dairy products in particular are severely restricted.

During treatment with Calcisorb restriction of oxalate-rich foods, such as spinach, rhubarb, peanuts, beetroot and chocolate, may be beneficial. An oral magnesium supplement of 58–87 mg elemental magnesium, twice daily, in patients receiving 10 and 15 g sodium cellulose phosphate daily, respectively, is also recommended.

Product licence number 0068/5900

DIFFLAM* CREAM

Presentation Difflam is a white, pleasant-smelling cream, containing benzydamine hydrochloride 3% w/w.

Uses Difflam cream is a topical analgesic and anti-inflammatory treatment for the relief of symptoms associated with painful inflammatory conditions of the musculo-skeletal system, including:

Acute inflammatory disorders such as myalgia and bursitis.

Traumatic conditions such as sprains, strains, contusions and the after-effects of fractures.

Difflam cream is well absorbed through the skin. It concentrates in inflamed tissue where it has been shown to have anti-inflammatory and local anaesthetic actions.

Dosage and administration Difflam cream should be massaged lightly into the affected area three times daily and at the discretion of the doctor, up to six times daily in more severe conditions.

Elderly: No special dosage recommendations are made for elderly patients.

Contra-indications, warnings, etc *Side-effects:* Benzydamine is very well tolerated; the only adverse effect that occurred in clinical studies was a local skin reaction which varied from erythema to a papular eruption; the incidence was low (less than two per cent of patients) and the skin returned to normal on stopping treatment.

Use in pregnancy: There is inadequate evidence of safety of the drug in human pregnancy but it has been in wide use for many years without apparent ill consequence, animal studies having shown no hazard.

Caution: To avoid possible irritation, Difflam cream should be kept away from eyes and mucosal surfaces.

Overdosage: Difflam is unlikely to cause adverse systemic effects, even if accidental ingestion should occur. No special measures are required.

Pharmaceutical precautions Avoid extremes of temperature. Store in a cool dry place.

Legal category P.

Package quantities Tubes containing 30 g and 80 g.

Further information Nil.

Product licence number 0068/0088.

DIFFLAM* ORAL RINSE

Presentation Difflam Oral Rinse is a pleasant tasting, clear, green solution, containing benzydamine hydrochloride 0.15% w/v.

Uses Difflam Oral Rinse is a locally acting analgesic and anti-inflammatory treatment for the relief of painful inflammatory conditions of the mouth and throat including:

Traumatic conditions: Pharyngitis following tonsillectomy or the use of a naso-gastric tube.

Inflammatory conditions: Pharyngitis, aphthous ulcers and oral ulceration due to radiation therapy.

Dentistry: For use prophylactically and after dental operations.

Benzydamine is absorbed into inflamed tissue. It is a unique preparation which concentrates in inflamed tissue, where it exerts an anti-inflammatory and analgesic action by stabilising the cellular membrane and inhibiting prostaglandin synthesis.

Dosage and administration Rinse or gargle with 15 ml (approximately 1 tablespoonful) every $1\frac{1}{2}$ to 3 hours as required for pain relief. Not suitable for children aged 12 years or under. The solution should be expelled

from the mouth after use. Difflam Oral Rinse should generally be used undiluted, but if 'stinging' occurs the rinse may be diluted with water. Uninterrupted treatment should not exceed seven days, unless under medical supervision.

Elderly: No special dosage recommendations are made for elderly patients.

Contra-indications, warnings, etc *Side-effects:* Benzydamine is well tolerated; side-effects are minor. Occasionally, oral tissue numbness or 'stinging' sensations may occur.

Overdosage: Difflam is unlikely to cause adverse systemic effects, even if accidental ingestion should occur. No special measures are required.

Use in pregnancy: There is inadequate evidence of safety of the drug in human pregnancy, but it has been in wide use for many years without apparent ill consequence, animal studies having shown no hazard.

Pharmaceutical precautions Do not leave the uncartonned bottle in direct sunlight.

Legal category P.

Package quantities Bottle containing 200 ml

Further information Nil.

Product licence number 0068/0096.

DIFFLAM* SPRAY

Presentation Difflam Spray is a metered-dose pump spray which delivers a pleasant tasting, clear, green solution, containing benzydamine hydrochloride 0.15% w/v, 150 µl per puff.

Uses Difflam Spray is a locally acting analgesic and anti-inflammatory treatment for the throat and mouth.

It is especially useful for the relief of pain in traumatic conditions such as following tonsillectomy or the use of a naso-gastric tube; dental surgery.

Benzydamine is absorbed into inflamed tissue. It is a unique preparation which concentrates in inflamed tissue, where it exerts an anti-inflammatory and analgesic action by stabilising the cellular membrane and inhibiting prostaglandin synthesis.

Dosage and administration

Adults and elderly: 4 to 8 puffs, $1\frac{1}{2}$ to 3 hourly.

Children (6 to 12): 4 puffs, $1\frac{1}{2}$ to 3 hourly.

Children under 6: 1 Puff to be administered per 4 kg body weight, up to a maximum of 4 puffs, $1\frac{1}{2}$–3 hourly.

The spray should be directed on to the affected area.

Contra-indications, warnings, etc

Side-effects: Benzydamine is well tolerated; side-effects are minor. Occasionally, oral tissue numbness or 'stinging' sensations may occur. The stinging has been reported to disappear upon continuation of the treatment, however, if it persists, it is recommended that treatment be discontinued.

Overdosage: Difflam is unlikely to cause adverse systemic effects, even if accidental ingestion should occur. No special measures are required.

Use in pregnancy: There is inadequate evidence of safety of the drug in human pregnancy, but it has been in wide use for many years without apparent ill consequence, animal studies having shown no hazard.

Pharmaceutical precautions After use the nozzle should be wiped with a tissue to prevent blockage.

It is important that the unit be used and stored upright.

Legal category P.

Package quantities Bottle containing 30 ml.

Further information Nil.

Product licence number 0068/0112.

DISALCID*

Presentation Grey and orange hard gelatin capsule, size 0, marked DS on one half and RIKER on the other.

Each 'Disalcid' capsule contains Salsalate BP 500 mg.

Uses Disalcid is indicated in the treatment of chronic inflammatory conditions of joints, tendons, muscles and connective tissue – for example, osteoarthritis, rheumatoid arthritis, tendinitis, bursitis, fibrositis and polymyalgia.

Salsalate is an ester which after absorption is slowly hydrolysed to two molecules of free salicylic acid. Its insolubility in gastric juice renders it very unlikely to cause the gastric irritation, erosion and haemorrhage associated with acetylsalicylic acid. Moreover, its prolonged biological half-life is a real therapeutic advantage at night and in the relief of morning stiffness.

Dosage and administration *Adults:* 4 capsules daily in divided doses. Where a greater anti-inflammatory effect is required dosage may be increased to 2 capsules three or four times daily.

The last dose should be taken at bedtime. Disalcid should be taken immediately before or with food.

Children: Disalcid has not yet been evaluated in children. No dosage recommendation can therefore be made for children under the age of 12.

Elderly: Use with caution in elderly patients at a reduced dosage.

Contra-indications, warnings, etc
Side-effects: Allergic reactions may occur rarely with salsalate, as with other salicylates. If tinnitus and deafness occur they are usually signs of overdosage and are reversible by reducing dosage.

Caution: Although Disalcid is relatively free from the risk of gastric erosion usually associated with anti-inflammatory agents, caution should be observed in patients with active peptic ulcer.

Disalcid should be used with caution in patients with renal impairment.

Disalcid may enhance the activity of anticoagulants and hypoglycaemic agents.

Pregnancy: There is no evidence of safety of the drug in human pregnancy; it has been in wide use for many years without apparent ill consequence; there is evidence of harmful effects of salicylates in pregnancy in animals. It is recommended that Disalcid Capsules should not be taken by breast feeding mothers.

Contra-indications: Disalcid is contra-indicated in patients with known hypersensitivity to salicylic acid or its derivatives.

Overdosage: Symptoms: Overdosage with Disalcid produces the usual symptoms of salicylism: tinnitus and deafness, vertigo, headache, sweating, hyperventilation and confusion are likely to occur.

Treatment: The stomach should be emptied by lavage with sodium bicarbonate or water.

Patients suffering from severe intoxication should in addition have forced alkaline diuresis by intravenous infusions of sodium bicarbonate solution. Haemodialysis or peritioneal dialysis may be needed in extreme cases, especially in the presence of cardiac or renal impairment.

Pharmaceutical precautions Disalcid should be stored in a cool, dry place. The container should be kept tightly closed.

Legal category POM.

Package quantities *Disalcid Capsules:* Bottles of 100.

Further information Nil.

Product licence number 0068/0089.

DORBANEX*
DORBANEX* FORTE

Presentation Dorbanex is available in three forms – as capsules and two strengths of liquid.

Each yellow size 1 capsule, marked 'RIKER' contains: Poloxamer 188 200 mg and Danthron BP 25 mg (Codanthramer).

Dorbanex Liquid is peach flavoured and orange coloured. Each 5 ml spoonful contains: Poloxamer 188 200 mg and Danthron BP 25 mg (Co-danthramer).

Dorbanex Forte is peach flavoured and orange coloured. Each 5ml spoonful contains: Poloxamer 188 1,000 mg and Danthron BP 75 mg.

Uses Dorbanex is indicated whenever a laxative needs to be prescribed for acute or chronic constipation. It is particularly useful in: painful defaecation associated with anal fissures, ulcers and haemorrhoids; restoring normal bowel habit in children and the elderly; post-operative patients and those confined to bed; preparation of patients for surgery and radiography; the prevention of faecal impaction; drug-induced constipation.

Dorbanex Forte is indicated for the patient with chronic, intractable constipation, or who may have become resistant to laxative treatment at normal dosage.

Poloxamer increases the penetration of water into faecal material, thus preventing the faecal mass from drying and hardening excessively. Faecal softening plus the surface activity of poloxamer has a useful lubricant effect on the gut content.

Poloxamer is not absorbed from the gut and does not directly stimulate peristalsis. It is excreted almost completely in the faeces.

Danthron is an anthraquinone compound. It acts on the nerve endings of the myenteric plexus to stimulate the muscle of the large intestine. Onset of effect is between six and twelve hours after administration.

Dosage and administration *Dorbanex Capsules: Adults:* One or two capsules.

Children: One capsule.

Before or after surgery or before radiography: 2 to 4 capsules.

Dorbanex Liquid: Adults: One or two 5 ml spoonfuls.

Children: A half to one 5 ml spoonful, as required.

Before or after surgery or before radiography: Two to four 5 ml spoonfuls.

Dorbanex Forte: Adults: One 5 ml spoonful, or as directed by the physician.

Dorbanex Forte is not recommended for children under 12 years.

Treatment should be taken at bedtime.

Elderly: No special dosage recommendations are made for elderly patients.

Contra-indications, warnings, etc

Side-effects: Danthron may cause temporary harmless pink or red colouring of the urine and perianal skin and, in prolonged use or high dosage, of the mucosa of the large intestine.

Caution: Dorbanex may cause staining of the buttocks in incontinent patients and in babies or children wearing napkins. This may proceed to superficial sloughing of the skin. For this reason Dorbanex is not recommended for the treatment of infants and children in napkins, and should be used with caution in all incontinent patients.

Pregnancy: There is inadequate evidence of safety of the drug in human pregnancy but it has been in wide use for many years without apparent ill consequence, animal studies having shown no hazard.

Contra-indications: In common with other gastro-intestinal evacuants, Dorbanex should not be given when acute, painful conditions of the abdomen are present, or the cause of constipation is suspected to be intestinal obstruction.

Overdosage: Patients should be given plenty of fluids. An anticholinergic preparation such as atropine methonitrate would help to offset the excessive intestinal motility.

Pharmaceutical precautions Store in a cool, dry place.

Diluents: Tragacanth Mucilage BP or Syrup BP should be used as diluents if required.

Attention is drawn to the fact that it is not possible to dilute Dorbanex Forte to fulfil prescriptions for Dorbanex because of the different ratio of the ingredients.

Legal category
Capsules P.
Liquid P.
Forte P.

Package quantities *Dorbanex Capsules:* Packs of 30 and 500.

Dorbanex Liquid: Bottles of 100 ml, 250 ml and 1,000 ml.

Dorbanex Forte: Bottles of 250 ml and 1,000 ml.

Further information Dorbanex capsules contain 65 mg lactose and 50 mg starch per capsule and so may be used for the treatment of constipation in patients with diabetes mellitus.

Product licence numbers
Dorbanex Capsules   0068/5067
Dorbanex Liquid   0068/5033
Dorbanex Forte   0068/5007

DUO-AUTOHALER*
MEDIHALER-DUO*

Presentation

Duo-Autohaler is a breath-actuated, pressurised aerosol for inhalation therapy. The vial contains a creamy-white suspension of Isoprenaline Hydrochloride BP 8 mg/ml

and phenylephrine bitartrate 12 mg/ml in aerosol propellent and delivers 400 measured doses, each containing 160 mcg Isoprenaline Hydrochloride BP and 240 mcg phenylephrine bitartrate.

Medihaler-duo is a pressurised aerosol for inhalation therapy. The vial contains a creamy-white suspension of Isoprenaline Hydrochloride BP 8 mg/ml and phenylephrine bitartrate 12 mg/ml in aerosol propellent and delivers 400 measured doses each containing 160 mcg Isoprenaline Hydrochloride BP and 240 mcg phenylephrine bitartrate.

Uses

Duo-Autohaler/Medihaler-duo is a potent bronchodilator and is indicated for the immediate and prolonged relief of bronchospasm in bronchial asthma and chronic bronchitis.

Isoprenaline is a directly acting sympathomimetic amine which activates both β_1 and β_2 adrenergic receptors. It has virtually no affinity for α-receptors. As a result it is a bronchodilator which also produces vasodilatation in all blood vessels, including those of the pulmonary system. Pulse rate and cardiac output are increased, the degree of cardiac stimulation being proportional to the blood level. Isoprenaline is quickly eliminated from the blood and therefore has no cumulative effect. It inhibits histamine release in the lungs and has a beneficial effect on cilia and mucus flow.

By inhalation, isoprenaline has a rapid onset of bronchodilatation. Cardiac stimulation does not usually occur and the maximum possible bronchodilatation is produced at doses below those which result in significant tachycardia. Appreciable cardiac stimulation occurs only at the upper end of the therapeutic dose range.

Phenylephrine acts primarily on α-receptors. It complements and modifies the action of isoprenaline in several respects. It augments bronchodilatation. It delays the absorption of isoprenaline from the lungs and helps to prolong the bronchodilator activity. Phenylephrine also tends to offset the cardiovascular effects of isoprenaline.

Paradoxically, the improved ventilation produced by bronchodilators is often accompanied by impairment of oxygenation of venous blood as it passes through the lungs, with consequent falls in arterial oxygen levels. This results from the non-selective relaxation of smooth muscle both of bronchioles and the pulmonary blood vessels. Phenylephrine opposes this effect and *Duo-Autohaler/Medihaler-duo* is thus less likely to cause falls in the arterial oxygen tension than isoprenaline alone.

Dosage and administration Each puff from *Duo Autohaler/Medihaler duo* delivers a measured dose of 160 mcg isoprenaline hydrochloride and 240 mcg phenylephrine bitartrate.

One, two or at most three puffs should be sufficient to provide relief in most cases. It should not be necessary for the patient to take further treatment for at least 30 minutes, or more than eight treatments in any 24 hour period.

Children: Duo-Autohaler/Medihaler-duo should be administered to children only under the supervision of a responsible adult.

Elderly: No special dosage recommendations are made for elderly patients.

Contra-indications, warnings, etc
Side-effects: Overdosage may cause dry mouth, palpitations or nervousness.

Contra-indications: *Duo-Autohaler/Medihaler-duo* should be used with caution in the presence of cardiac disease, hypertension or hyperthyroidism.

Pregnancy: There is clinical and epidemiological evidence of safety of the drug in human pregnancy.

Overdosage: Acute poisoning in non-asthmatics: No cases have been reported. In the absence of details of such practical experience, the following guidance is based on theoretical considerations.

Symptoms: The toxic effects of isoprenaline (namely those of tachycardia, palpitations, peripheral vasodilatation and fall in blood pressure) are likely to be counterbalanced by the vasoconstrictor action of phenylephrine. Treatment: General symptomatic therapy.

Chronic poisoning in asthmatics: No cases have been reported. Excessive use of *Duo-Autohaler/Medihaler-duo* during an attack of asthma indicates lack of response. This is a grave sign suggestive of status asthmaticus. It is recommended that 100 mg hydrocortisone be given immediately by intravenous injection, and the patient admitted to hospital without delay. Beta-blocking drugs should not be used.

Pharmaceutical precautions *Duo-Autohaler/Medihaler-duo* should be stored in a cool place, protected from frost and sunlight. The shelf-life of *Duo-Autohaler/Medihaler-duo* is three years.

The *Duo-Autohaler/Medihaler-duo* vial is pressurised and therefore no attempt should be made to puncture it or to dispose of it by burning.

Legal category POM.

Package quantities *Duo-Autohaler* is supplied as complete units for which replacement cartridges are available. Each vial delivers 400 doses.

Medihaler-duo: Standard pack (complete unit) vial containing 400 doses.

Further information Nil.

Product licence numbers
Duo-Autohaler   0068/5012
Medihaler-duo   0068/5070

DUROMINE*

Presentation *Duromine* is available in two strengths. Each capsule contains phentermine 15 mg or 30 mg as an ion-exchange resin complex.

Duromine 15 mg: Opaque green/grey size number three capsules printed *Duromine* 15.

Duromine 30 mg: Opaque maroon/grey size number three capsules printed *Duromine* 30.

Uses *Duromine* is an appetite-depressant for short-term use as an adjunct to the treatment of some patients with moderate to severe obesity, for whom close control and supervision should be provided.

After ingestion, the active constituent phentermine is gradually released from the ion-exchange resin complex over a period of 10–14 hours.

The prolonged release of phentermine gives sustained plasma levels devoid of absorption peaks, thus minimising the risk of adverse CNS reactions.

Dosage and administration *Adults:* One 15 mg or 30 mg capsule daily at breakfast time. *Duromine* is not recommended for the elderly or children.

Intermittent dosage: Treatment for 4 to 8 weeks followed by a similar period without medication may be as effective as continuous treatment, and reduces the risk of dependence.

Efficacy in use for more than 3–6 months and safety in long-term use has not been established and may carry an increased risk of dependence.

The stated dose should not be exceeded.

Treatment should be discontinued if weight loss does not occur or ceases.

Contra-indications, warnings, etc
Contra-indications: *Duromine* is contra-indicated in patients under treatment with monoamine-oxidase (MAO) inhibitors, and should not be given within 2 weeks of stopping such treatment. It is also contra-indicated in thyrotoxicosis, severe hypertension, and in patients sensitive to sympathomimetic agents.

Duromine should not be given to patients with a history of psychiatric illness, emotionally unstable or vulnerable personalities, or those with previous drug or alcohol abuse. It should not be used concurrently with other appetite depressant drugs or by women during lactation.

Use in pregnancy: Do not use in pregnancy. There is inadequate evidence of safety in human pregnancy, and there is no information from animal studies.

Caution: *Duromine* should be used with caution in patients under treatment with antihypertensive agents, since it may cause some loss of blood pressure control, and in patients receiving psychotropic drugs, including sedatives and sympathomimetic agents.

Side-effects: Patients have been withdrawn from trials due to the following adverse reactions: insomnia, CNS stimulation, vomiting, dry mouth, facial oedema, rash and headache. Other side-effects which were well tolerated included constipation, urinary frequency, nausea, dizziness, nervousness and depression.

Palpitations, tachycardia, high blood pressure, psychosis and hallucinations may also occur.

Patients may be at risk whilst driving or operating machinery, and there may be an interaction with alcohol. There is also a possibility of dependence.

Overdosage
Symptoms: Initially irritability, agitation, disorientation and tremor may occur, followed by cardiac arrhythmias, convulsions, hallucinations and coma.

Treatment: The stomach should be emptied by emesis or stomach tube and washed out with water if the preparation has been ingested within the last three or four hours. Diazepam, preferably by mouth (cautiously by intravenous injection) should be used to control marked excitement and convulsions. Provided renal function is adequate, elimination of phentermine may be assisted by acidification of the urine by agents such as lysine hydrochloride or arginine hydrochloride.

Pharmaceutical precautions Store in a cool, dry place.

Legal category CD (Sch 3), POM.

Package quantities
Duromine 15 mg: Bottles of 30 capsules.
Duromine 30 mg: Bottles of 30 capsules.

Further information There is a possibility that amphetamine-type dependence may occur and *Duromine* may be socially abused for euphoriant effect.

Product licence numbers
Duromine 15 mg: 0068/5055R
Duromine 30 mg: 0068/5056R

DUROPHET*

Presentation 7.5 mg strength: Opaque white/white size 3 capsules printed RIKER. Each capsule contains amphetamine 3.75 mg, dexamphetamine 3.75 mg as ion-exchange resin complexes.

12.5 mg strength: Opaque white/charcoal grey size 3 capsules printed RIKER. Each capsule contains amphetamine 6.25 mg, dexamphetamine 6.25 mg as ion-exchange resin complexes.

20 mg strength: Opaque charcoal grey/charcoal grey size 3 capsules printed RIKER. Each capsule contains amphetamine 10 mg, dexamphetamine 10 mg as ion-exchange resin complexes.

Uses 'Durophet' is indicated in narcolepsy.

Durophet contains equal parts of amphetamine and dexamphetamine as ion-exchange resin complexes from which they are slowly released. The extended absorption reduces the chance of side-effects and simplifies dosage.

Dosage and administration *Adults:* A starting dose of 7.5 mg or 12.5 mg, gradually increasing if necessary, up to a maximum of 60 mg a day. The total daily dose should be taken first thing in the morning.

Children: Not recommended.

Elderly: Unless absolutely necessary, the use of Durophet is best avoided in elderly patients.

In those patients receiving a high dose, treatment should be stopped gradually to prevent withdrawal symptoms, notably depression.

Contra-indications, warnings, etc *Side-effects:* Dryness of the mouth, hyperactivity and other signs of mild central nervous stimulation may occur in some patients. Drug dependence may occur as tolerance develops, but this is unlikely.

Cautions: Durophet should be used with caution in severe hypertension, anorexia, hyperthyroidism, impaired kidney function and in patients hypersensitive to sympathomimetic agents. It should be used with care in patients of unstable personality and those with a history of drug abuse.

Contra-indications: Durophet is contra-indicated in patients under treatment with monoamine oxidase (MAO) inhibitors or within 14 days of such treatment. It should not be given to patients with thyrotoxicosis, cardiovascular disease, anxiety, hyperexcitability or restlessness.

Overdosage: Symptoms: These would be, initially, insomnia and irritability, but larger doses may give rise to fatigue, mental depression, an increase in blood pressure, fever, cardiovascular reactions, respiratory failure and cyanosis, disorientation, hallucinations, convulsions and coma.

Treatment: The stomach should be emptied by emesis or stomach tube and washed out with water if the preparation has been ingested within the last three or four hours.

If respiration is irregular or cyanosis is present, artificial respiration or oxygen should be given. The patient should be kept quiet and warm. For marked excitement, chlorpromazine 1 to 1.5 mg per kg body weight may be given intramuscularly or intravenously. Alternatively, a short-acting barbiturate, such as quinalbarbitone sodium or cyclobarbitone should be given by mouth, or if necessary, thiopentone sodium should be administered by intravenous injection. Providing renal function is adequate, elimination of the amphetamine may be assisted by acidification of the urine with ammonium chloride in conjunction with an adequate fluid intake.

Use in pregnancy: There is epidemiological evidence that the drug may be harmful in human pregnancy and animal studies have also shown hazard.

Pharmaceutical precautions Store in a cool, dry place.

Legal category CD (Sch 2), POM.

Package quantities
Capsules	7.5 mg	Bottles of 30
Capsules	12.5 mg	Bottles of 30
Capsules	20 mg	Bottles of 30

Further information Nil.

Product licence numbers
Capsules	7.5 mg	0068/5064
Capsules	12.5 mg	0068/5065
Capsules	20 mg	0068/5066

HIPREX*

Presentation White to creamy-white, oblong tablet with breakline, marked HX on one side. Each Hiprex tablet contains methenamine hippurate 1 g.

Uses
Hiprex is indicated in the prophylaxis and treatment of urinary tract infections:

1. As maintenance therapy after successful initial treatment of acute infections with antibiotics.

2. As long-term therapy in the prevention of recurrent cystitis.

3. To suppress urinary infection in patients with indwelling catheters and to reduce the incidence of catheter blockage.

4. To provide prophylaxis against the introduction of infection into the urinary tract during instrumental procedures.

5. Asymptomatic bacteriuria.

Methenamine hippurate is readily absorbed from the gastro-intestinal tract and excreted via the kidney.

With Hiprex, as with other specific urinary antibacterial agents of this type, antibacterial activity is confined to the urinary tract. The chemical structure of methenamine hippurate is such that a two-fold antibacterial action is obtained:

1. The slow release of the bactericidal formaldehyde, from the methenamine part, in the urine; acid pH is necessary for this reaction to occur. It is obtained and maintained there by the presence of hippuric acid.

2. The bacteriostatic effect of hippuric acid itself on urinary tract pathogens.

Hiprex has a wide antibacterial spectrum covering both gram-positive and gram-negative organisms. It is active against the bacteria which most commonly cause urinary tract infection – *Escherichia coli, Aerobacter aerogenes,* Pseudomonas and some strains of Proteus. Urinary antibacterial activity can be shown within 30 minutes of administration.

Hiprex is particularly useful for long-term treatment because neither tolerance to its effect nor bacterial resistance occurs. The incidence of side-effects is extremely low.

Dosage and administration *Adults:* 1 g twice daily.

In patients with catheters the dosage may be increased to 1 g three times daily.

Elderly: Hiprex is well tolerated at standard dosages in elderly patients.

Children: 6–12 years: 500 mg twice daily.

The tablets may be halved, or they can be crushed and taken with a drink of milk or fruit juice if the patient prefers.

Contra-indications, warnings, etc *Side-effects:* Occasionally rashes, gastric irritation or irritation of the bladder may occur.

All side-effects are reversible on withdrawal of the drug.

Contra-indications: Severe dehydration, metabolic acidosis, or severe renal failure (serum creatinine > 5 mg%). Hiprex may be used where mild to moderate renal insufficiency is present.

Hiprex should not be administered concurrently with sulphonamides because of the possibility of crystalluria, or with alkalising agents, such as mixture of potassium citrate.

Use in pregnancy: There is inadequate evidence of safety of the drug in human pregnancy but it has been in wide use for many years without apparent ill consequence, animal studies having shown no hazard.

Methenamine is excreted in breast milk but the quantities will be insignificant to the infant.

Overdosage: Vomiting and haematuria may occur. Bladder symptoms can be treated by the consumption of copious quantities of water and 2–3 teaspoonfuls of bicarbonate of soda.

Pharmaceutical precautions The container should be kept tightly closed.

Legal category P.

Package quantities Bottles of 100 tablets.

Further information Nil.

Product licence number 0068/5003

INTRALGIN*

Presentation Intralgin contains Benzocaine BP 2 per cent w/w and salicylamide 5 per cent w/w in an alcoholic vehicle. Intralgin is a clear, pleasant-smelling preparation – non-greasy and non-staining.

Uses Intralgin is indicated for the relief of muscle pain from strains, sprains and injuries, and pain associated with fibrositis, lumbago and non-articular rheumatism.

Intralgin combines two ingredients to relieve muscular aches and pains by absorption through the skin into the muscle.

Benzocaine is a widely used, well-tolerated local anaesthetic, acting rapidly on nerve endings. The action of the analgesic, salicylamide, is similar to that of salicylates.

The use of isopropyl alcohol as a vehicle for the medicaments contributes significantly to the action of Intralgin. Isopropyl alcohol because of its penetrative properties facilitates the percutaneous absorption of benzocaine and salicylamide so that they reach underlying tissue to relieve pain rapidly. Vigorous massage is

not needed with Intralgin, unlike traditional rubs which rely for effect on erythema or counter-irritation.

Dosage and administration Intralgin Gel should be applied liberally and rubbed gently into the skin until penetration is complete. Vigorous massage is unnecessary.

Elderly: No special dosage recommendations are made for elderly patients.

For more rapid absorption the painful area should be warmed before applying Intralgin.

Contra-indications, warnings, etc
Side-effects: Local sensitivity reactions to the benzocaine constituent have occasionally been reported.

Caution: If irritation or itching occurs due to hypersensitivity, Intralgin should be discontinued and a soothing cream applied.

Pregnancy: There is inadequate evidence of safety of Intralgin in human pregnancy but it has been in wide use for many years without apparent ill consequence.

Excretion in breast milk, if any, is expected to be too low to affect the infant.

Overdosage: Not applicable.

Pharmaceutical precautions The tube should be kept tightly closed and kept away from direct heat.

Legal category P.

Package quantities Tubes of 50 g.

Further information Nil.

Product licence number 0068/5076.

ISO-AUTOHALER*
MEDIHALER-ISO*
MEDIHALER-ISO* FORTE

Presentation *Iso-Autohaler, Medihaler-iso* and *Medihaler-iso Forte* are pressurised aerosols for inhalation therapy.

Iso-Autohaler is a breath-actuated, pressurised aerosol for inhalation therapy. The vial contains a creamy white suspension of Isoprenaline Sulphate BP 4 mg/ml in aerosol propellent, and delivers 400 measured doses, each containing 80 mcg Isoprenaline Sulphate BP.

The *Medihaler-iso* vial contains a creamy-white suspension of Isoprenaline Sulphate BP 4 mg/ml in aerosol propellent, and delivers 400 measured doses, each containing 80 mcg Isoprenaline Sulphate BP.

The *Medihaler-iso Forte* vial contains a creamy-white suspension of Isoprenaline Sulphate BP 20 mg/ml in aerosol propellent, and delivers 400 measured doses, each containing 400 mcg Isoprenaline Sulphate BP.

Uses *Iso-Autohaler/Medihaler-iso* and *Medihaler-iso Forte* are potent bronchodilators, and are indicated for the relief of bronchospasm in bronchial asthma and chronic bronchitis.

Isoprenaline is a directly acting sympathomimetic amine which activates both β_1 and β_2 adrenergic receptors. It has virtually no affinity for α-receptors. As a result it is a bronchodilator which also produces vasodilatation in all blood vessels, including those of the pulmonary system. Pulse rate and cardiac output are increased, the degree of cardiac stimulation being proportional to the blood level. Isoprenaline is quickly eliminated from the blood and therefore has no cumulative effect. It inhibits histamine release in the lungs and has a beneficial effect on cilia and mucus flow.

By inhalation, isoprenaline has a rapid onset of bronchodilatation. Cardiac stimulation does not usually occur and the maximum possible bronchodilatation is produced at doses below those which result in significant tachycardia. Appreciable cardiac stimulation occurs only at the upper end of the therapeutic dose range.

Dosage and administration Each puff from *Iso-Autohaler/Medihaler-iso* delivers a measured dose of 80 mcg isoprenaline sulphate and from *Medihaler-iso Forte*, 400 mcg isoprenaline sulphate. One, two or at the most three puffs should be sufficient to provide relief in most cases. It should not be necessary for the patient to take further treatment for at least 30 minutes, or more than eight treatments in any 24-hour period.

Children: Iso-Autohaler/Medihaler-iso should be administered to children only under the supervision of a responsible adult. *Medihaler-iso Forte* is not recommended for children.

Elderly: No special dosage recommendations are made for elderly patients.

Contra-indications, warnings, etc
Side-effects: Overdosage may cause dry mouth, palpitations or nervousness.

Contra-indications: Iso-Autohaler/Medihaler-iso and *Medihaler-iso Forte* should be used with caution in the presence of cardiac disease, hypertension or hyperthyroidism.

Pregnancy: There is clinical and epidemiological evidence of safety of the drug in human pregnancy.

Overdosage: Acute poisoning in non-asthmatics: No cases have been reported. In the absence of details of such practical experience, the following guidance is based on theoretical considerations.

Symptoms of acute isoprenaline poisoning are likely to be mainly cardiovascular effects, e.g. tachycardia, palpitations, peripheral vasodilatation and fall in blood pressure.

Treatment: General symptomatic therapy.

Chronic poisoning in asthmatics: Some cases have been reported, but no details of treatment have been given, other than withdrawal of the aerosol.

Excessive use of during an attack of asthma indicates lack of response. This is a grave sign suggestive of status asthmaticus. It is recommended that 100 mg hydrocortisone be given immediately by intravenous injection, and the patient admitted to hospital without delay. Beta-blocking drugs should not be used.

Pharmaceutical precautions Iso-Autohaler/Medihaler-iso and Medihaler-iso Forte should be stored in a cool place, protected from frost and sunlight. The shelf-life of *Iso-Autohaler, Medihaler-iso* and *Medihaler-iso Forte* is three years.

As the *Autohaler/Medihaler* vial is pressurised, no attempt should be made to puncture it or to dispose of it by burning.

Legal category POM.

Package quantities *Iso-Autohaler* is supplied as complete units for which replacement cartridges are available. Each vial delivers 400 doses.

Medihaler-iso, Medihaler-iso Forte: Standard pack (complete unit) vial containing 400 doses.

Further information Nil.

Product licence numbers
Iso-Autohaler 0068/5017
Medihaler-iso 0068/5082
Medihaler-iso Forte 0068/5072

LERGOBAN*

Presentation Creamy-white, circular, bi-convex tablets, 0.25 inch (6.4 mm) in diameter. The markings are 'LB' on one side and 'RIKER' on the other. Each Lergoban Tablet contains Diphenylpyraline Hydrochloride BP 5 mg.

Uses Lergoban is indicated in: allergic rhinitis, allergic conjunctivitis, angioneurotic oedema, hay fever, urticaria, allergic skin conditions and irritation.

Diphenylpyraline is an antihistamine with the general properties of antihistamine compounds, but with a low incidence of side-effects. In Lergoban its therapeutic usefulness is greatly increased by the long-acting presentation. Lergoban Tablets consist of a porous plastic matrix in which the diphenylpyraline is dispersed. In the gastro-intestinal tract, the active ingredient is gradually leached from the pores of the matrix and absorbed systemically. The release rate is not affected by changes in pH, digestive enzymes, viscosity, surface tension or electrolyte concentration. The small plastic skeleton is insoluble and is excreted unchanged in the faeces.

The duration of effect from each dose of Lergoban is about 10 hours, so that only two doses every 24 hours are required.

Dosage and administration *Adults:* One or two 5 mg tablets every 12 hours, or as directed by the physician.

Children: Older children may be given one 5 mg tablet every 12 hours.

Lergoban is not recommended for children under 10 years.

Elderly: Elderly patients may require a reduced dosage due to slower metabolism.

Contra-indications, warnings, etc
Side-effects: Although side-effects are less likely with this sustained release tablet, slight drowsiness and dizziness, flushing, headache, anorexia and dryness of the mouth may occur.

Pregnancy: There is inadequate evidence of safety of Lergoban in human pregnancy but it has been in wide use for many years without apparent ill consequence, animal studies having shown no hazard.

Contra-indications: None.

Caution: Doses greater than those recommended may cause sedation and drowsiness. Patients undergoing treatment with an antihistamine should be warned of this possibility if they are in control of vehicles or machinery, where loss of attention may lead to accidents.

In some patients, the action of antihistamines may be potentiated by alcohol or other CNS depressants.

Overdosage: In adults, overdosage of antihistamines usually causes sedation, varying from drowsiness to deep sleep. Conversely in children, antihistamines often act as cerebral stimulants and may cause convulsions and hyperpyrexia. Stimulation may also occur in some adults.

Treatment: If the drug has recently been taken, the stomach should be emptied by gastric lavage, using a tube greater than 7 mm in diameter. Excitement may be controlled with diazepam given by mouth; the ECG should be monitored.

Pharmaceutical precautions Store in a cool, dry place.

Legal category P.

Package quantities Bottles of 50 and 200 tablets.

Further information Nil.

Product licence number 0068/5002.

MEDIHALER-EPI*

Presentation Medihaler-epi is a pressurised aerosol for inhalation therapy. The vial contains a creamy-white suspension of Adrenaline Acid Tartrate BP 14 mg/ml in aerosol propellent, and delivers 400 measured doses, each containing 280 mcg Adrenaline Acid Tartrate BP.

Uses Medihaler-epi is a potent bronchodilator, and is indicated for the relief of bronchospasm in bronchial asthma, chronic bronchitis and drug sensitivity reactions.

Adrenaline is a sympathomimetic amine which activates both α- and β-adrenergic receptors. As a result, it causes vasoconstriction, bronchodilatation, relieves mucosal congestion and is a cardiac stimulant.

By inhalation adrenaline relaxes bronchial smooth muscle and constricts bronchial mucosal vessels, relieving congestion and oedema. However, tolerance to adrenaline can develop after repeated use and the action of adrenaline in reducing bronchial secretion may make mucus more viscid.

Dosage and administration Each puff from Medihaler-epi delivers a measured dose of 280 mcg adrenaline acid tartrate. One, two or at the most three puffs should be sufficient to provide relief in most cases. It should not be necessary for the patient to take further treatment for at least 30 minutes or more than eight treatments in any 24-hour period.

Correct technique is essential if the patient is to obtain full benefit from each treatment. Probably the most reliable way of ensuring this is for the doctor to show the patient how to use Medihaler-epi by personal demonstration, using a Demonstration Unit containing no active medicament. These units are available on request.

Children: Medihaler-epi should be administered to children only under the supervision of a responsible adult.

Elderly: No special dosage recommendations are made for elderly patients.

Instructions for use: With the adapter dust cap removed, Medihaler-epi should be shaken to disperse the particles of medicament in the propellent.

The mouthpiece should then be placed well into the mouth and the lips closed firmly around it. (When the adapter is held at the correct angle, the spray will go right to the back of the throat and down into the lungs.) The patient should now breathe out fully through the adapter.

As soon as the patient starts to breathe in, the vial should be pressed firmly down into the adapter. This releases a dose.

The adapter should now be taken from the mouth and the inspired breath held for as long as possible to avoid exhaling particles of medicament.

Before taking a further inhalation, the patient should wait at least one minute to allow the full effect of the puff to become apparent.

Contra-indications, warnings, etc

Side-effects: Overdosage may cause dry mouth, palpitations or nervousness.

Contra-indications: Medihaler-epi should be used with caution in the presence of cardiac disease, hypertension or hyperthyroidism.

Prolonged use of adrenaline may lead to the development of tolerance (adrenaline 'fastness'). When this occurs, isoprenaline is a most effective alternative.

Pregnancy: There is clinical and epidemiological evidence of safety of the drug in human pregnancy.

Overdosage: Acute poisoning in non-asthmatics: No cases have been reported. The following guidance is based on acute adrenaline poisoning following parenteral administration.

Symptoms: Restlessness, palpitations, rapid pulse, tremor, weakness, dizziness, headache, coldness of extremities; elevated blood pressure, tachycardia; the symptoms are rapid in onset and of short duration.

Treatment: It is essential to administer immediately intravenous injections of quick-acting sympatholytics, e.g. phentolamine or piperoxan.

Chronic poisoning in asthmatics: Some cases have been reported, but no details of treatment have been given, other than withdrawal of the aerosol.

Excessive use of Medihaler-epi during an attack of asthma indicates lack of response. This is a grave sign suggestive of status asthmaticus. It is recommended that 100 mg hydrocortisone be given immediately by intravenous injection, and the patient admitted to hospital without delay. Beta-blocking drugs should not be used.

Pharmaceutical precautions Medihaler-epi should be stored in a cool place, protected from frost and sunlight. The shelf-life of Medihaler-epi is three years.

As the Medihaler vial is pressurised, no attempt should be made to puncture it or to dispose of it by burning.

Legal category POM.

Package quantities Standard pack (complete unit): vial contains 400 doses.

Further information Nil.

Product licence number 0068/5060.

MEDIHALER* ERGOTAMINE

Presentation Creamy-white suspension in pressurised container. Medihaler Ergotamine contains a suspension of Ergotamine Tartrate BP 9 mg/ml in aerosol propellent, and delivers to the patient 75 measured doses, each containing 360 mcg ergotamine tartrate.

Uses Medihaler Ergotamine is indicated for rapid relief in migraine, recurrent vascular headache, histaminic cephalalgia, occipital neuralgia.

Micronised ergotamine tartrate taken by inhalation is rapidly absorbed from the highly vascular epithelium of the respiratory tract into the systemic circulation. Two factors make this route of administration particularly effective: speed of absorption and lack of interference with the drug's action by either the digestive tract or the liver. Another advantage is that the dose is retained in spite of vomiting.

One or two inhalations from Medihaler Ergotamine

can abort the migraine attack before cephalic vasodilatation becomes fixed and before oedema of the vascular wall and perivascular tissues has developed. In the majority of patients, full therapeutic effect is achieved within 15 minutes.

Dosage and administration
Adults and children aged 10 or over: One inhalation should be taken at the first sign of attack and should be repeated if necessary after five minutes.

Caution: No more than 6 inhalations should be taken in any 24-hour period. Maximum dosage in one week should not exceed 15 inhalations.

Elderly: No special dosage recommendations are made for elderly patients.

Children: Medihaler Ergotamine is not recommended for children younger than 10 years of age.

To obtain full benefit from treatment, the patient should follow these simple steps:
Remove the dust-cap and shake the unit.
Place the mouthpiece well into the mouth with lips closed firmly around it.
Breathe out fully.
Start to breathe in and then press the vial firmly down into the adapter with the forefinger. This operates Medihaler Ergotamine and the dose is released.
Release pressure on the vial. Remove the unit from the mouth and hold the breath as long as possible before breathing out.
After use, replace the dust cap.

Contra-indications, warnings, etc
Side-effects: Ergotamine tartrate may cause nausea and vomiting in some patients. As these symptoms can occur in migraine attacks, it may be difficult to determine whether the illness or the medication is responsible.

Muscular pain may occasionally be experienced. This can be controlled by reduction of dosage.

Contra-indications: Septic conditions, coronary disease, peripheral vascular disease, renal or hepatic dysfunction, hypertension or pregnancy.

Overdosage: Symptoms: Acute poisoning is rare. Symptoms are nausea, vomiting, diarrhoea, thirst, coldness of the skin, pruritus, rapid and weak pulse, numbness and tingling of the extremities, confusion and unconsciousness.

Treatment: Treatment of poisoning is symptomatic. Vasodilators such as choline esters, nitrites or papaverine may be used, together with mechanical procedures to restore the circulation. Nausea and vomiting may be relieved by atropine.

Pharmaceutical precautions
Medihaler Ergotamine has a shelf-life of 2 years and should be stored at 5°C until dispensed.

Once dispensed the shelf life is 6 months.

As the Medihaler Ergotamine vial is pressurised no attempt should be made to puncture it or to dispose of it by burning.

Legal category POM.

Package quantities
Standard pack (complete unit): pressurised vial containing 75 doses.

Further information Nil.

Product licence number 0068/5014

NORFLEX*

Presentation *Injection:* Each 2 ml ampoule contains Orphenadrine Citrate BP 30 mg/ml.

Tablets: White, circular, bi-convex tablets, 8.7 mm diameter, marked NX on one side and 'RIKER' on the reverse. Each tablet contains Orphenadrine Citrate BP 100 mg in a slow-release base.

Uses Norflex is indicated for the relief of acute skeletal muscle spasm associated with muscle injury, sprains and strains, prolapsed intervertebral disc, 'whiplash' injuries, fractures before and after reduction and immobilisation, acute torticollis and hiccough.

Orphenadrine acts centrally by blocking reticular facilitation, i.e. it blocks preferentially those pathways whose hyperactivity leads to an exaggeration of motor function such as spasticity, rigidity or muscle spasm.

Norflex is a potent skeletal muscle relaxant which provides relief of acute muscle spasm and associated pain. It relaxes only muscle in spasm without impairment of normal muscle tone or voluntary movement. Action is rapid in onset, particularly in the case of Norflex Injection, and relatively prolonged. The effect of orphenadrine on skeletal muscle spasm has been demonstrated objectively by means of electromyography.

Dosage and administration *Parenteral:* 60 mg (one 2 ml ampoule) administered intramuscularly or intravenously. Further 60 mg doses may be given at 12-hour intervals, if required.

Note: An intravenous injection should be administered over a period of about five minutes.

Oral: 2 tablets daily, 1 in the morning and 1 in the evening. This may be increased to 3 tablets daily if required.

The cautions and contra-indications apply particularly to elderly patients.

Norflex is not recommended for children under 12 years.

Contra-indications, warnings, etc
Side-effects: Dry mouth, nausea, blurring of vision, dizziness and restlessness may occur in some patients susceptible to the parasympatholytic action of orphenadrine. These symptoms rapidly disappear following reduction of dosage or cessation of treatment. Some patients may experience a transient feeling of lightheadedness or dizziness following an injection of Norflex.

Caution: Norflex should be used with caution in patients with tachycardia.

Pregnancy: There is inadequate evidence of safety of the drug in human pregnancy but it has been in wide use for many years without apparent ill consequence, animal studies having shown no hazard.

Orphenadrine is probably excreted into breast milk, but the quantity is unlikely to be significant at therapeutic doses.

Contra-indications: Contra-indications to Norflex result from the parasympatholytic action of orphenadrine. Norflex should not be given to patients with glaucoma, urinary retention (e.g. due to prostatic hypertrophy or obstruction of the bladder neck) and myasthenia gravis.

Overdosage: Symptoms of orphenadrine citrate overdosage: Excitement, confusion and delirium leading to coma, convulsions, tachycardia. Dilated pupils and urinary retention may occur.

Treatment: Gastric lavage should be carried out immediately regardless of the estimated ingested dose. Convulsions and delirium respond to relatively large doses of diazepam, preferably by mouth. Adequate hydration of the patient is important.

Pharmaceutical precautions Store in a cool, dry place.

Legal category POM.

Package quantities *Ampoules (30 mg/ml):* 3 × 2 ml. *Tablets:* Packs of 100.

Further information Nil.

Product licence numbers
Norflex Tablets   0068/5008
Norflex Injection   0068/5078

NORGESIC*

Presentation A white circular, compressed tablet 12.7 mm diameter. Markings are 'N/G' on one side and 'RIKER' on the other. Each tablet contains Orphenadrine Citrate BP 35 mg and Paracetamol BP 450 mg.

Uses Norgesic is indicated for the relief of painful skeletal muscle spasm associated with chronic low back pain, sprains and strains, prolapsed intervertebral disc, muscle injury, non-articular rheumatism (fibrositis, myositis and myalgia), 'whiplash' injuries, acute torticollis, tension headache, dysmenorrhoea, other acute or chronic painful muscular conditions.

Orphenadrine acts centrally by blocking reticular facilitation, i.e. it blocks preferentially those pathways whose hyperactivity leads to an exaggeration of motor function such as spasticity, rigidity or muscle spasm. Orphenadrine relaxes only muscle in spasm without impairment of normal muscle tone or voluntary movement. Action is rapid in onset and relatively prolonged. The effect of orphenadrine on skeletal muscle spasm has been demonstrated objectively by means of electromyography.

Paracetamol is a well-tolerated analgesic and antipyretic. Its analgesic action is rapid in onset (within 30 minutes) and lasts for three to four hours. It has been found to be particularly effective for the relief of pain in muscles and joints.

Paracetamol does not produce gastric upset or bleeding. Hepatic and renal necrosis have been associated with the ingestion of paracetamol in amounts greatly in excess of normal therapeutic dosage.

Dosage and administration *Adults:* Two tablets three times a day.

Norgesic is not recommended for children under 12 years old.

Elderly: Elderly patients may require a reduced dose due to slower metabolism.

Contra-indications, warnings, etc
Side-effects: Dry mouth, nausea, blurring of vision, dizziness and restlessness may occur in some patients susceptible to the parasympatholytic action of orphenadrine. These symptoms disappear rapidly following reduction of dosage or withdrawal of treatment.

Contra-indications: Contra-indications to Norgesic result from the parasympatholytic action of orphenadrine. Norgesic should not be given to patients with glaucoma, urinary retention (e.g. due to prostatic hypertrophy or

obstruction of the bladder neck) or myasthenia gravis. It should be used with caution in patients with tachycardia.

There is inadequate evidence of safety of the drug in human pregnancy but it has been in wide use for many years without apparent ill consequence, animal studies having shown no hazard.

Orphenadrine and paracetamol are excreted into breast milk but the quantities are unlikely to be significant at therapeutic doses.

Overdosage: Symptoms of orphenadrine citrate overdosage are excitement, confusion, and delirium leading to coma. Convulsions, tachycardia, dilated pupils and urinary retention may occur.

Paracetamol overdosage may cause acute liver damage but symptoms may not appear for up to several days after ingestion.

Treatment: Gastric lavage should be carried out immediately, regardless of the estimated ingested dose. Convulsions and delirium respond to relatively large doses of diazepam, preferably by mouth. Adequate hydration of the patient is important. It is recommended that the patient be referred to a hospital where early and regular monitoring of plasma paracetamol levels can be carried out. If instituted sufficiently early, treatment with N-acetylcysteine, l-methionine or l-cysteamine will minimise liver damage.

Pharmaceutical precautions Store in a cool, dry place.

Legal category POM.

Package quantities Packs of 100 and 500.

Further information Nil.

Product licence number 0068/5059.

NUELIN*

Presentation White, circular, biconvex tablet with breakline, 9 mm in diameter, marked NL/125 on one side and 'RIKER' on the other.

Each Nuelin tablet contains Theophylline BP 125 mg in microcrystalline form.

Uses Nuelin is indicated for the relief of bronchospasm.

Theophylline is well established in the treatment of bronchospasm. In Nuelin, the theophylline is present as microfine particles to give a very high rate of dissolution which results in rapid and predictable absorption.

Dosage and administration *Adults:* One tablet three or four times daily, preferably after food; this can be increased to two tablets three or four times daily depending on response.

Elderly: Elderly patients may require lower doses due to reduced theophylline clearance.

Children: 7–12 years (20–35 kg): Half or 1 tablet three or four times daily, preferably after food.

The difficulty of dividing the tablet accurately makes Nuelin unsuitable for use in children under the age of seven.

Nuelin tablets are soluble in water.

Contra-indications, warnings, etc
Side-effects: Nausea or other gastric distress may occur rarely. Palpitations and insomnia have been reported occasionally.

Pregnancy: There is inadequate evidence of safety of the

drug in human pregnancy but it has been in wide use for many years without apparent ill consequence; there is evidence of harmful effects in pregnancy in animals.

Theophylline is excreted in breast milk and has been shown to cause irritability in infants. It is therefore recommended that the mother nurse her infant just prior to taking her next dose, when plasma theophylline levels are expected to be low.

Contra-indications: There are no known contra-indications to theophylline therapy.

Precaution: Cimetidine and erythromycin delay the elimination of theophylline. A reduction of the theophylline dosage is recommended.

Overdosage: Symptoms: Characterised by nausea, vomiting and gastro-intestinal irritation. Tachycardia and hypotension may also occur.

Treatment: Gastric lavage and general supportive measures are recommended.

Pharmaceutical precautions Store in a cool, dry place.

Legal category P.

Package quantities Packs of 100 tablets.

Further information Nil.

Product licence number 0068/0064.

NUELIN* LIQUID

Presentation Clear, light brown, pleasantly flavoured liquid. Each 5 ml dose of Nuelin Liquid contains the equivalent of 60 mg Theophylline Hydrate BP as the sodium glycinate salt.

Uses Nuelin Liquid is indicated for the relief of bronchospasm. Nuelin in tablet form (microcrystalline theophylline 125 mg) is established as a highly effective bronchodilator. Nuelin Liquid is designed to offer comparable relief of bronchospasm with the same low incidence of side-effects, for patients who prefer a liquid presentation. Each 10 ml of Nuelin Liquid approximates to one 125 mg Nuelin tablet.

Dosage and administration *Adults:* 10–20 ml (two to four 5 ml spoonfuls) three or four times daily, preferably after food.

Children: 7–12 years: One-and-a-half or two 5 ml spoonfuls three or four times daily, preferably after food.

2–6 years: One or one-and-a-half 5 ml spoonfuls three or four times daily, preferably after food.

Under 2 years: It is recommended that dosage is calculated at 5 mg/kg theophylline hydrate per dose (0.4 ml/kg Nuelin Liquid) and given three or four times daily, preferably after food. Nuelin Liquid may be diluted with Syrup BP if required.

Elderly: Elderly patients may require lower doses due to reduced theophylline clearance.

Contra-indications, warnings, etc

Contra-indications: There are no known contra-indications to theophylline therapy.

Pregnancy: There is inadequate evidence of safety of the drug in human pregnancy; it has been in wide use for many years without apparent ill consequence; there is evidence of harmful effects in pregnancy in animals.

Theophylline is excreted in breast milk and has been shown to cause irritability in infants.

Side-effects: Nausea or other gastric distress may occur rarely. Palpitations and insomnia have been reported occasionally.

Precaution: Cimetidine and erythromycin delay the elimination of theophylline. A reduction of the theophylline dosage is recommended.

Overdosage: Symptoms: Nausea, vomiting and gastrointestinal irritation.

Treatment: Gastric lavage and general supportive measures are recommended.

Pharmaceutical precautions Store in a cool, dry place.

Legal category P.

Package quantities Bottles of 500 ml.

Further information Each 5 ml spoonful of Nuelin Liquid contains 0.38 mEq sodium (8.7 mg Na).

Product licence number 0068/0084.

NUELIN* SA

Presentation *Nuelin SA:* White, biconvex, round tablets, 9 mm in diameter and marked NLS 175 on one side and RIKER on the other.

Each Nuelin SA tablet contains 175 mg anhydrous theophylline in a slow release formulation which gives a particularly smooth release of medicament over a prolonged period.

Nuelin SA-250: White, biconvex, round tablets with breakline, 11 mm in diameter and marked NLS 250 on one side and RIKER on the other. Each Nuelin SA-250 tablet contains 250 mg anhydrous theophylline in a slow release formulation.

Uses Nuelin SA and Nuelin SA-250 tablets are indicated for the treatment and prophylaxis of bronchospasm.

Because effective plasma levels are maintained for up to twelve hours from a single dose, less frequent dosing is required than with conventional theophylline preparations.

Dosage and administration *Nuelin SA: Adults:* One tablet twice daily, preferably after food, increasing to two tablets twice daily if necessary.

Children: 6 to 12 years: one tablet twice daily, preferably after food.

Nuelin SA-250: Adults: One tablet twice daily, preferably after food, increasing to two tablets twice daily if necessary.

Children: 6 to 12 years: Half or one tablet twice daily, preferably after food.

Nuelin SA and Nuelin SA-250 tablets are not recommended for children under six years.

Nuelin SA tablets should be swallowed whole and not crushed or chewed.

Nuelin SA-250 tablets are scored and may be halved but should not be crushed or chewed.

Elderly: Elderly patients may require lower dosage due to reduced theophylline clearance.

Contra-indications, warnings, etc

Side-effects: The side-effects commonly associated with

xanthine derivatives such as nausea, gastric irritation, palpitations and insomnia are much diminished when a sustained action preparation such as Nuelin SA is used.

Caution: In the case of an acute asthmatic attack in a patient receiving a sustained action theophylline preparation, great caution must be taken when administering intravenous aminophylline. Half the recommended loading dose of aminophylline (generally 6 mg/kg) should be given i.e. 3 mg/kg, cautiously.

Cimetidine and erythromycin delay the elimination of theophylline. A reduction of the theophylline dosage is recommended.

Pregnancy: There is inadequate evidence of safety of the drug in human pregnancy; it has been in wide use for many years without apparent ill consequence; there is evidence of harmful effects in pregnancy in animals.

Theophylline is excreted in breast milk and has been shown to cause irritability in infants. As it is recommended that the mother nurse her infant just prior to taking her next dose when theophylline plasma levels are expected to be low, a non-sustained release form such as Nuelin is preferable for nursing mothers.

Contra-indications: There are no known contra-indications to theophylline therapy.

Overdosage: Symptoms: Nausea, vomiting and gastric irritation. Tachycardia and hypotension may also occur.

Treatment: Gastric lavage and general supportive measures are recommended.

Pharmaceutical precautions Store in a cool, dry place.

Legal category P.

Package quantities *Nuelin SA:* Packs of 100 and 500.
Nuelin SA-250: Packs of 100 tablets.

Further information Nil.

Product licence numbers
Nuelin SA   0068/0092
Nuelin SA-250   0068/0093

NUMOTAC*

Presentation White to creamy-white, circular biconvex tablets 7.14 mm diameter, marked 'NT' on one side and 'RIKER' on the other. Each tablet contains Isoetharine Hydrochloride USP 10 mg in a porous plastic matrix.

Uses Numotac is indicated for the relief of bronchospasm in chronic bronchitis, bronchial asthma and pulmonary emphysema.

Isoetharine is a sympathomimetic amine with a marked bronchodilator action. It is rapidly absorbed from the gastro-intestinal tract and has a relatively fast onset of action.

A notable feature of isoetharine is that at normal dosage levels it acts selectively on the β_2-receptors of bronchial muscle and has little effect on the β_1 cardiac receptors. Cardiac side-effects are therefore reduced to negligible levels, and occur only at higher doses or in hypersensitive patients.

Numotac contains isoetharine hydrochloride embedded in a porous plastic matrix. By this means, the release of isoetharine is controlled, giving Numotac a duration of action of between four and six hours. This formulation reduces the possibility of side-effects associated with uneven blood levels.

Dosage and administration *Adults:* One or two tablets three or four times daily.

For patients who have not previously been prescribed oral bronchodilator therapy or who are known to be sensitive to the action of sympathomimetic amines, treatment should be started on the lower dosages (3 or 4 tablets daily). Dosage may then be adjusted upwards, if necessary, to achieve optimum response.

Clinical and pharmacological studies have shown that 'Numotac' acts for between four and six hours. In susceptible patients administration at shorter intervals may give rise to side-effects. When this occurs dosage should be adjusted accordingly.

Children: The 10 mg tablet should not be broken, and this dose is not recommended for children aged 12 years or under.

Elderly: Elderly patients may require a reduced dosage due to slower metabolism.

Contra-indications, warnings, etc
Side-effects: With higher doses, or in persons sensitive to sympathomimetic amines, tachycardia, palpitations, tremor or vertigo may occur.

Cautions and contra-indications: Numotac should be used with caution in the presence of cardiac disease, or hypertension. The use of Numotac is contra-indicated in thyrotoxicosis.

There is no evidence as to the drug safety in human pregnancy nor is there evidence from animal work that it is free from hazard.

Overdosage: Symptoms: The blood pressure may fall and cause dizziness and fainting. Other symptoms may include headache, nervousness, tremor and weakness.

Treatment: General symptomatic treatment. If the drug has recently been taken, the stomach should be emptied by gastric lavage, using a tube greater than 8 mm in diameter.

Pharmaceutical precautions Store in a cool, dry place.

Legal category POM.

Package quantities Bottles of 100 and 500 tablets.

Further information Nil.

Product licence number 0068/5054.

PEPTARD*

Presentation Creamy-white, circular, biconvex tablet, 7 mm in diameter. The markings are 'RIKER' on one side, and letters 'PTD' on the other. Each Peptard tablet contains L-Hyoscyamine Sulphate BP 200 mcg.

Uses Peptard is indicated for the treatment of peptic ulcer, irritable colon, hyperhidrosis and conditions in which the oral administration of an antispasmodic/antisecretory agent is beneficial.

Naturally occurring atropine consists of a racemic mixture of hyoscyamine isomers of which the l-isomer has the greater physiological activity. With l-hyoscyamine it is possible to adjust the dose more readily to obtain a selective action on the gastro-intestinal tract with fewer anticholinergic side-effects than with atropine.

l-Hyoscyamine reduces the volume of gastric secretion

and total acid output. Secretion during both psychic and gastric phases is reduced, but not abolished. A decrease in pepsin output contributes to the overall effects.

In Peptard, the slow release of l-hyoscyamine sulphate from the plastic matrix provides more even blood levels and response.

Dosage and administration *Adults:* In general, two or three tablets (400–600 mcg) twice daily.

Children: Older children (over 10 years) one or two tablets twice daily.

Elderly: No special dosage recommendations are made for elderly patients.

Individual cases may be increased, for example, with peptic ulcer therapy, up to 3 mg a day in three divided doses.

The tablets should be swallowed whole.

Contra-indications, warnings, etc
Side-effects: At the optimum effective dose, the only side-effects that have occurred are dry mouth, slight visual disturbance and occasional hesitancy of micturition.

Pregnancy: There is no evidence as to the drug safety in human pregnancy nor is there evidence from animal work that it is free from hazard.

Contra-indications: Peptard should not be given to patients with, or suspected of suffering from glaucoma or with obstruction of the neck of the urinary bladder, pyloric stenosis or myasthenia gravis.

Overdosage – Symptoms: The main symptoms of toxicity are dryness of mucous membranes and intense thirst, dilation of pupils and blurred vision, a hot, dry skin, with or without a rash, hyperpyrexia, tachycardia, palpitations and elevated blood pressure, urinary urgency and hesitation; and restlessness, excitement and confusion.

Treatment: If the drug has recently been taken, the stomach should be emptied by gastric lavage, using a tube greater than 7 mm in internal diameter. Symptomatic treatment should be given.

Pharmaceutical precautions The tablets should be stored at room temperature.

The shelf-life of Peptard is two years.

Legal category POM.

Package quantities Bottles of 100 tablets.

Further information Nil.

Product licence number 0068/0054.

PHOLTEX*

Presentation Each 5 ml dose contains Pholcodine BP 15 mg and phenyltoloxamine 10 mg in a pleasantly flavoured, orange-coloured, thixotropic vehicle.

Uses For antitussive action.

Pholtex is well accepted by children and is valuable in the treatment of whooping cough and the cough associated with measles.

Pholtex contains the cough depressant pholcodine, the action of which is potentiated and reinforced by the antihistamine phenyltoloxamine.

Phenyltoloxamine complements the action of pholcodine not only because it potentiates the activity of the cough depressant but also because of its antihistaminic

and antispasmodic actions which help to relieve associated symptoms.

Dosage and administration *Adults:* One 5 ml dose two or three times daily.

Elderly: Elderly patients may require a reduced dosage due to slower metabolism.

Children: Half to full adult dosage, according to age.

Pholtex contains no sugar and is therefore suitable for cough treatment in diabetic patients.

Contra-indications, warnings, etc
Side-effects: In common with all preparations which contain antihistamines, Pholtex may cause drowsiness, although this is very unlikely to occur in the recommended dosage.

Pregnancy: There is no evidence as to the drug safety in human pregnancy nor is there evidence from animal work that it is free from hazard.

Contra-indications: None.

Overdosage: The symptoms of antihistamine overdosage would probably predominate. These include nausea and vomiting, diarrhoea, colic and epigastric pain. Overdosage may cause sedation, but large doses could cause convulsions and hyperpyrexia, particularly in children.

Treatment: The stomach should be emptied by aspiration and lavage. The respiration may require assistance. The patient, particularly if a child, should be kept quiet.

Pharmaceutical precautions Store in a cool, dry place.

Diluents: Tragacanth Mucilage BP or Syrup BP should be used as diluents if required.

Legal category CD (Sch 5), P.

Package quantities Bottles of 100 ml and 1,000 ml.

Further information Nil.

Product licence number 0068/5030.

PULMADIL* INHALER
PULMADIL* AUTO

Presentation Pulmadil Inhaler is a pressurised aerosol for bronchodilator inhalation therapy. The vial contains a suspension of rimiterol hydrobromide 10 mg/ml in aerosol propellent and delivers to the patient 300 measured doses each containing 200 mcg rimiterol hydrobromide.

Pulmadil Auto is a breath-actuated, pressurised aerosol for bronchodilator inhalation therapy. The vial contains a suspension of rimiterol hydrobromide 10 mg/ml in aerosol propellent and delivers to the patient 300 measured doses each containing 200 mcg rimiterol hydrobromide.

Uses Pulmadil is indicated for the relief of bronchospasm in bronchial asthma and chronic bronchitis.

Rimiterol hydrobromide is a sympathomimetic agent which has a rapid and highly selective action on β_2-adrenergic receptors in bronchial muscle. At therapeutic dose levels it has virtually no effect on β_1-adrenergic receptors. Cardiac stimulation is therefore reduced to negligible levels and occurs only at high doses or in hypersensitive patients. The plasma half life of rimiterol in man is less than five minutes.

Dosage and administration One to three puffs should provide relief in most cases. This treatment dose should not be repeated in less than thirty minutes. No more than eight treatments should be taken in any 24-hour period.

Children: Pulmadil Inhaler and Pulmadil Auto should be administered to children only under the supervision of a responsible adult.

Elderly: No special dosage recommendations are made for elderly patients.

Instructions for use: Pulmadil Inhaler: With the dust cap removed, Pulmadil Inhaler should be shaken to disperse the particles of medicament in the propellent.

The mouthpiece should then be placed well into the mouth and the lips closed firmly around it. The patient should now breathe out fully through the adapter.

As soon as the patient starts to breathe in, the vial should be pressed firmly down into the adapter. This releases a dose. The adapter should now be taken from the mouth and the breath held for as long as possible to avoid exhalation of particles of medicament.

Before taking a further inhalation, the patient should wait at least one minute to allow the full effect of the first to become apparent.

Pulmadil Auto: To obtain full benefit from Pulmadil Auto the patient should follow these simple steps:

1. Shake the unit with the mouthpiece cover closed. Then open the mouthpiece cover downwards.
2. Breathe out as much as possible, then close the lips tightly round the mouthpiece. Keep the teeth apart and the tongue flat (to allow the flow of medicament into the lungs).
3. Suck in air through the mouthpiece as rapidly and deeply as possible. When the unit operates a click will be heard. *Continue to breathe in after the click* until the lungs are full. Hold the breath for a few seconds. Then take the inhaler away from the mouth and breathe out slowly through pursed lips. If no click is heard, repeat step 3, making sure that the lips are well sealed round the mouthpiece.
4. *The unit must be reset before another dose can be taken,* by closing the mouthpiece cover upwards. It is important to keep the cover closed when it is not in use.

Contra-indications, warnings, etc *Side-effects:* No side-effects of any significance have been reported.

Pregnancy: There is inadequate evidence of safety of the drug in human pregnancy but it has been in wide use for many years without apparent ill consequence, animal studies having shown no hazard.

It is very unlikely that sufficient drug will be excreted in the breast milk to affect the infant.

Contra-indications: There are no known contra-indications, but 'Pulmadil' should be administered with care to patients with thyrotoxicosis.

Overdosage: As rimiterol is rapidly eliminated from the blood it carries little risk of accumulation even if used excessively. No cases of overdosage have been reported and the following guidance is based on theoretical considerations.

Symptoms: The blood pressure may fall and cause dizziness and fainting. Anxiety, tremor and tachycardia may be present.

Treatment: General symptomatic therapy.

Excessive use in asthmatics: Excessive use of any bronchodilator aerosol can indicate lack of response. This is a grave sign suggestive of status asthmaticus. It is recommended that 100 mg of hydrocortisone be given intravenously immediately and the patient admitted to hospital without delay.

Pharmaceutical precautions Pulmadil Inhaler and Pulmadil Auto should be stored in a cool place, protected from frost and direct sunlight.

As the Pulmadil vial is pressurised, no attempt should be made to puncture or dispose of it by burning.

The shelf-life of both Pulmadil preparations is three years.

Legal category POM.

Package quantities Pulmadil Inhaler is supplied as a complete standard pack, comprising a vial delivering 300 doses and an adapter.

Pulmadil Auto is supplied as a complete unit for which replacement cartridges are available. Each cartridge delivers 300 doses.

Further information Nil.

Product licence number 0068/0030.

RAUWILOID*

Presentation Dark cream circular, bi-convex tablets, diameter 8 mm, marked 'RD' on one side and 'RIKER' on the other. Each tablet contains 2 mg alseroxylon fraction (selected alkaloid hydrochlorides) of *Rauwolfia serpentina.*

Uses Rauwiloid is indicated for the treatment of mild to moderate hypertension.

When a more pronounced fall in blood pressure is needed, Rauwiloid can be combined with other antihypertensive agents, such as the thiazide diuretics. Rauwiloid reduces blood pressure by interfering with transmission at sympathetic nerve endings, and depleting the myocardium of its catecholamines (chiefly noradrenaline).

The antihypertensive activity of Rauwiloid is complemented by mild bradycardic and tranquillising effects.

Rauwiloid causes a slow but prolonged release of serotonin and catecholamines from stores in various parts of the body. This release leads eventually to the depletion of noradrenaline at the post-ganglionic nerve endings of the sympathetic nervous system, in the blood-vessel walls, and in other organs such as the heart and spleen. Depletion of noradrenaline results in a generalised reduction of sympathetic transmission. Since the sympathetic system is the pathway for vasoconstrictor impulses, vasomotor tone is reduced. This reduction is particularly noticeable in vascular areas such as the skin and splanchnic circulation, and the resulting peripheral vasodilatation produces a lowering of blood pressure.

Dosage and administration Initially, two tablets (4 mg) daily. This may be taken as a single dose at night or in divided doses. When the blood pressure is stable at the lower level a maintenance dose of one tablet daily may be sufficient.

Onset of antihypertensive effect is graded and may not be apparent for four weeks or more after the start of treatment.

Elderly: The cautions and contra-indications apply particularly to elderly patients.

Contra-indications, warnings, etc
Side-effects: Nasal stuffiness, drowsiness and a slight looseness of the bowel (although diarrhoea is rare) may

occur. There might also be a slight increase in appetite and an increase in weight. As with other Rauwolfia preparations, the possibility of mental depression must be considered. However, serious mental depression has not been reported as a result of Rauwiloid therapy.

Pregnancy: There is no evidence as to the drug safety in human pregnancy nor is there evidence from animal work that it is free from hazard.

Contra-indications: There are no absolute contra-indications to the use of Rauwiloid. It should, however, be administered with caution to patients who have a history of depression or peptic ulcer.

Overdosage: Symptoms: Mild overdosage can produce nasal congestion, gastro-intestinal upsets such as vomiting and diarrhoea, drowsiness, apathy, fatigue, headache, vertigo, hallucinations.

Higher doses may cause flushing, insomnia, vasodilatation, bradycardia, severe depression, sodium retention, oedema, peptic ulceration.

After a single massive dose most of the above effects are not encountered. Instead, the patient becomes sleepy and eventually comatose. Coma may last for several days.

Treatment: In the acutely poisoned patient, who is not in a coma, an emetic should be administered, or gastric lavage performed, even several hours after ingestion of the alkaloid. A saline cathartic should be left in the stomach. Nasal congestion, excessive salivation, gastro-intestinal upsets and other parasympathetic side-effects may also be controlled by small doses of atropine.

Epigastric pain and peptic ulcer may be treated with local antacid therapy.

Unless the blood pressure becomes very low, vasopressor drugs which may prove inactive (e.g. ephedrine) or which may lead to exaggerated cardiovascular response (e.g. adrenaline or noradrenaline) should be avoided. Blankets and external application of mild heat should be used to maintain normal body temperature.

Pharmaceutical precautions Store in a cool, dry place.

Legal category POM.

Package quantities Bottles of 200 tablets.

Further information Nil.

Product licence number 0068/5010.

RIKOSPRAY* BALSAM

Presentation Brown solution in a pressurised aerosol canister. Pressurised canister contains:

Dissolved solids of Benzoin BP (equivalent to Sumatra Benzoin BP 12.5% w/w)	9% w/w
Prepared Storax BP	2.5% w/w
Solvent and aerosol propellent to	100% w/w

Uses Rikospray Balsam is indicated in all conditions where tincture of benzoin is, or would be, applied topically, e.g. under adhesive plaster dressings; in colostomy and ileostomy hygiene; in the prevention of bedsores and the treatment of pressure points and other ischaemic areas; in the treatment of cracked nipples and skin fissures.

Rikospray Balsam delivers benzoin and storax to the skin in a thin transparent film which is protective and non-irritant.

Benzoin and storax are naturally occurring balsamic oleoresins containing mixtures of resins and benzoic and cinnamic acids. The natural resins provide protection against the physical and chemical irritation of adhesive plaster; against skin maceration in ileostomy and colostomy; and against irritation leading to the breakdown of underlying tissues in bedsores and other dry ischaemic areas.

The benzoic and cinnamic acid compounds are mild antiseptics and can reduce the destructive effect of bacteria on debilitated tissue.

Administration *Directions for use:* Shake the canister. The affected part should be sprayed sparingly, keeping the nozzle about 15 to 20 cm from the skin. To obtain an adequate and evenly distributed film, the canister should be kept moving during application.

Contra-indications, warnings, etc
Side-effects: None reported.

Contra-indications: Rikospray Balsam should not be applied over areas of obvious infection. It is not intended for use by inhalation.

Overdosage: Not applicable.

Pharmaceutical precautions As the Rikospray Balsam canister is pressurised, it should not be punctured, incinerated or exposed to heat, including the sun, even when empty.

Rikospray Balsam is inflammable and should not be used near a fire or flame.

To clear a blocked valve, invert can and spray in this position for 2–3 seconds.

Legal category GSL.

Package quantities Canisters of 150 g.

Further information Nil.

Product licence number 0068/5028.

RIKOSPRAY* SILICONE

Presentation White suspension in a pressurised aerosol container. The application of Rikospray Silicone delivered to the skin contains:

Aluminium dihydroxyallantoinate	0.5% w/w
Cetylpyridinium Chloride BP	0.02% w/w
Dimethicone 1,000 BP to	100%

Uses Rikospray Silicone is indicated in: the prevention and treatment of bedsores, particularly in incontinent patients; the prevention and treatment of napkin rash; colostomy hygiene.

Rikospray Silicone delivers a spray which coats the skin with a film of virtually 100% silicone. The silicone compounds are well known for their water-repellent and protective properties. The protective film is instantly impervious to water, urine or faeces.

Aluminium dihydroxyallantoinate is an amphoteric substance which is insoluble in water and alcohol. It combines the astringent and bacteriostatic activity of aluminium with the healing properties of allantoin, and is also a mild antiperspirant. No irritant or sensitising properties have been reported from its use.

Cetylpyridinium chloride possesses bactericidal properties.

Administration *Directions for use:* Before applying Rikospray Silicone, the affected area should be washed thoroughly and the skin dried carefully.

The canister should be shaken before use, and then held about 15 to 20 cm from the skin. Rikospray Silicone should be applied sparingly to cover the entire area. This should be done twice daily for at least one week, then application once daily will often be sufficient.

Contra-indications, warnings, etc
Side-effects: None reported.

Contra-indications: None.

Overdosage: Not applicable.

Pharmaceutical precautions The shelf life of Rikospray Silicone is five years.

As the Rikospray Silicone canister is pressurised, it should not be punctured, incinerated or exposed to heat, including the sun, even when empty.

Legal category GSL.

Package quantities Canisters of 200 g.

Further information As Silicone can make some surfaces slippery, care should be taken to avoid the spray coming into contact with the floor.

Product licence number 0068/5080.

SALBULIN* INHALER

Presentation *Salbulin* Inhaler is a pressurised aerosol for bronchodilator inhalation therapy. It delivers to the patient 200 measured doses each containing 100 mcg Salbutamol BP.

Uses *Salbulin* Inhaler is indicated for the treatment and prophylaxis of bronchial asthma and for the treatment of reversible airways obstruction associated with bronchitis and emphysema. It is also suitable for routine maintenance therapy in chronic asthma and chronic bronchitis, because of its prolonged action. *Salbulin* Inhaler may be used to relieve attacks of acute dyspnoea and may also be taken prophylactically before exertion or to prevent exercise-induced asthma. It is suitable for treating bronchospasm in patients with co-existing heart disease or hypertension, including those taking beta-blocking drugs, because of its selective action on the bronchial receptors and lack of effects on the cardiovascular system. Salbutamol is a sympathomimetic agent which has a highly selective action on beta-adrenergic receptors in bronchial muscle. At therapeutic levels it has little activity on cardiac receptors.

Dosage and administration
Adults: For the relief of acute bronchospasm and for managing intermittent episodes of asthma: one or two inhalations as a single dose; for chronic maintenance or prophylactic therapy: two inhalations, three or four times daily; for prevention of exercise-induced bronchospasm: two inhalations before exertion.

Children: For the relief of acute bronchospasm, management of episodic asthma or before exercise: one inhalation; for routine maintenance or prophylaxis: one inhalation three or four times a day, increasing if necessary to two inhalations three or four times daily.

Elderly: The dosage is the same as for other adults.

Contra-indications, warnings, etc
Contra-indications: There are no contra-indications to *Salbulin* Inhaler therapy.

Precautions: Administer cautiously to patients with thyrotoxicosis. The patient should be advised to seek medical advice if the treatment ceases to be effective.

Side-effects: None reported.

Overdosage: Treatment: A cardioselective beta-blocking agent should be administered, but these should be used with caution in patients with a history of bronchospasm.

Use in pregnancy: The use of inhaled salbutamol during the first trimester of pregnancy is not recommended unless the clinical need outweighs the risk.

Pharmaceutical precautions *Salbulin* Inhaler should be stored in a cool place, protected from frost and direct sunlight. As the vial is pressurised, no attempt should be made to puncture or dispose of it by burning.

Legal category POM.

Package quantities Each canister provides 200 inhalations.

Further information *Salbulin* Inhaler is not contra-indicated in patients under treatment with MAOIs (monoamine oxidase inhibitors). It does not cause difficulty in micturition as salbutamol does not stimulate alpha-adrenoceptors.

Product licence number 68/0108.

SALBULIN* TABLETS
SALBULIN* SYRUP

Presentation *Salbulin* Tablets 2 mg: White, circular, flat tablets, 6.5 mm in diameter and marked SBT 2 on one side and 'RIKER' on the other. Each tablet contains Salbutamol Sulphate BP equivalent to Salbutamol BP 2 mg.

Salbulin Tablets 4 mg: White, circular, flat tablets, 8.5 mm in diameter and marked SBT 4 on one side and 'RIKER' on the other. Each tablet contains Salbutamol Sulphate BP equivalent to Salbutamol BP 4 mg.

Salbulin Syrup: Colourless, fruit-flavoured liquid. Each 5 ml contains Salbutamol Sulphate BP equivalent to Salbutamol BP 2 mg.

Uses *Salbulin* tablets and *Salbulin* syrup are indicated for the relief of bronchospasm in chronic bronchitis, bronchial asthma and pulmonary emphysema.

Salbulin syrup is designed for patients, particularly children and the elderly, who prefer a liquid presentation.

Salbutamol is a sympathomimetic agent which has a highly selective action on beta-adrenergic receptors in bronchial muscle. At therapeutic dose levels it has little activity on cardiac receptors.

Dosage and administration
Adults: 2–4 mg three or four times daily. This may be increased if necessary to 8 mg three or four times daily.

Elderly: Initially 2 mg three or four times a day. The dose may be increased, if necessary, to 4 mg three or four times daily.

Children: 2–6 years – 1–2 mg, (half to one tablet or 2.5–5 ml liquid) three or four times daily.

6–12 years – 2 mg (one tablet or 5 ml liquid) three or four times daily.

Over 12 years – 2–4 mg (one 2 mg tablet or one 4 mg tablet) three or four times daily.

Contra-indications, warnings, etc
Contra-indications: Concurrent administration of beta-blocking drugs, such as propranolol.

Precautions: Salbutamol should be administered cautiously to patients with thyrotoxicosis.

Side-effects: As with all beta-adrenergic stimulants, skeletal muscle tremor occurs in some patients.

Overdosage: Symptoms: Peripheral vasodilatation and a compensatory small increase in heart rate; occasionally headaches.

Treatment: Preferably a cardioselective beta-blocking agent but beta-blocking drugs should be used with caution in patients with a history of bronchospasm.

Use in pregnancy: The use of oral salbutamol during the first trimester of pregnancy is not recommended, unless the clinical need outweighs the risk.

Pharmaceutical precautions *Salbulin* tablets and syrup should be stored in a cool dry place. *Salbulin* syrup may be diluted with Purified Water BP and this mixture, if protected from light, will keep for 28 days at room temperature.

Legal category POM.

Package quantities
Salbulin tablets 2 mg: Bottles of 100 and 500 tablets
Salbulin tablets 4 mg: Bottles of 100 and 500 tablets
Salbulin syrup: Bottles of 150 ml and 2000 ml

Further information *Salbulin* tablets and *Salbulin* syrup are not contra-indicated in patients under treatment with MAOIs (monoamine oxidase inhibitors). They do not cause difficulty in micturition as salbutamol does not stimulate alpha-adrenoceptors.

Salbulin syrup is sugar free.

Product licence numbers
Salbulin tablets 2 mg 0068/0106
Salbulin tablets 4 mg 0068/0107
Salbulin syrup 0068/0109

TAMBOCOR* ▼

Presentation *Tambocor tablets:* White, circular, biconvex tablets, 8.5 mm in diameter marked RIKER on one side and TR 100 with a break-line on the other. Each tablet contains flecainide acetate 100 mg.

Tambocor injection: Each ampoule contains 15 ml of a solution of flecainide acetate 10 mg/ml, for intravenous use only.

Uses Tambocor is a Class I anti-arrhythmic (local anaesthetic) agent for the treatment of the conditions listed below when these are resistant to other therapy or when other treatment is unsatisfactory. It is recommended that treatment with Tambocor should be initiated in hospitals.

Tambocor slows conduction through the heart, having its greatest effect on His bundle conduction. It also acts selectively to increase anterograde and particularly retrograde accessory pathway refractoriness. Its actions may be reflected in the ECG by prolongation of the PR interval and widening of the QRS complex. The effect on the JT interval is insignificant.

Indications: Tablets: Tambocor tablets are indicated for:

a) Chronic prophylaxis of ventricular tachyarrhythmias, unifocal and multi-focal ventricular extrasystoles;

b) AV nodal reciprocating tachycardia; Wolff-Parkinson-White Syndrome and similar conditions with accessory pathway and anterograde or retrograde conduction.

Tambocor tablets can be used for the maintenance of normal rhythm following conversion by other means.

Injection: Tambocor injection is indicated when rapid control or short term prophylaxis of the following arrhythmias is the main clinical requirement:

a) Ventricular tachycardia, ventricular extrasystoles;

b) AV nodal reciprocating tachycardia; Wolff-Parkinson-White Syndrome and similar conditions with accessory pathway and anterograde or retrograde conduction.

Dosage and administration *Tablets: Adults:* The recommended dosage is one to two tablets twice daily (200 to 400 mg). The maximum daily dose is 400 mg. This is normally reserved for patients of large build or where rapid control of the arrhythmia is required. After 3–5 days it is recommended that the dosage be progressively adjusted to the lowest level which maintains control of the arrhythmia. It may be possible to reduce dosage during long-term treatment.

Children: Tambocor is not recommended in children under 12, as there is no evidence of its use in this age group.

Elderly patients: The rate of flecainide elimination from plasma may be reduced in elderly people. An initial dose of one tablet twice daily will usually be adequate, and it may well be possible to reduce this dose for maintenance therapy after one week.

Injection:
a) *Bolus injection:* Tambocor can be given in an emergency or for rapid effect by a slow injection of 2 mg/kg over not less than ten minutes. If preferred the dose may be diluted with 5% dextrose and given as a mini-infusion.
It is recommended that Tambocor should be administered more slowly to patients in sustained ventricular tachycardia with careful monitoring of the electrocardiogram. Similar caution should apply to patients with a history of cardiac failure, who may become decompensated during the administration. For such patients it is recommended that the initial dose is given over 30 minutes.
The maximum recommended bolus dose is 150 mg.

b) *Intravenous infusion:* When prolonged parenteral administration is required, it is recommended that therapy is initiated by slow injection over 30 minutes as above and continued by intravenous infusion at the following rates:
First hour: 1.5 mg/kg per hour. *Second and later hours:* 0.25 mg/kg per hour.
Transfer to oral dosage is accomplished by administering 1 × 100 mg tablet of Tambocor and then withdrawing the infusion over four hours by hourly decrements of 20% of the maintenance rate. An oral dose of 1–2 × 100 mg Tambocor tablets is given 12 hours after the first oral dose. Oral maintenance is then continued as indicated in the oral dosage instructions.

Dosage in impaired renal function: A reduced maintenance dosage in cases of moderate or greater degree of renal insufficiency is recommended.

Use in Pregnancy and Lactation: There is no evidence as to drug safety in human pregnancy.

In New Zealand White rabbits high doses of flecainide caused some foetal abnormalities, but these effects were not seen in Dutch Belted rabbits or rats. The relevance of these findings to humans has not been established.

The possibility of flecainide being excreted in milk should be considered.

Contra-indications, warnings, etc

Contra-indications: Tambocor is contra-indicated by the oral and intravenous route:

i) In cardiac failure;

ii) Unless pacing rescue is available Tambocor should not be given to patients with sinus node dysfunction, atrial conduction defects, second degree or greater atrio-ventricular block, bundle branch block or distal block.

Precautions: Electrolyte disturbances should be corrected before using Tambocor.

Tambocor is known to increase endocardial pacing thresholds – ie. to decrease endocardial pacing sensitivity. This effect is reversible and is more marked on the acute pacing threshold than on the chronic.

Tambocor should thus be used with caution in all patients with permanent pacemakers or temporary pacing electrodes, and should not be administered to patients with existing poor thresholds or non-programmable pacemakers unless suitable pacing rescue is available.

Generally, a doubling of either pulse width or current is sufficient to regain capture, but it may be difficult to obtain ventricular thresholds less than 1 Volt at initial implantation in the presence of Tambocor.

The minor negative inotropic effect of flecainide may assume importance in patients predisposed to cardiac failure. Difficulty has been experienced in defibrillating some patients. Most of the cases reported had pre-existing heart disease with cardiac enlargement, a history of myocardial infarction, arterio-sclerotic heart disease and cardiac failure.

Use of flecainide with other Class I antiarrhythmics is not recommended. Treatment with Tambocor is compatible with use of β-blockers and oral anticoagulants. Flecainide can cause the plasma digoxin level to rise by about 15%, which is unlikely to be of clinical significance for patients with plasma levels in the therapeutic range. It is recommended that the digoxin plasma level in digitalised patients should be measured not less than six hours after any digoxin dose, before or after administration of flecainide.

A few cases of elevated liver enzymes and jaundice have been reported which were possibly related to treatment with 'Tambocor'.

Side-effects: Most commonly giddiness, dizziness and lightheadedness. Visual disturbances, such as double vision and blurring of vision, may occur. More rarely nausea and vomiting have been reported. These effects are usually transient and disappear upon continuing or reducing the dosage.

Pro-arrhythmic effects have been reported in a small number of patients.

Overdosage: No specific antidote is known. There is no known way of rapidly removing flecainide from the system, but forced acid diuresis may be helpful. Neither dialysis nor haemoperfusion are helpful and injections of anticholinergics are not recommended. Treatment may include therapy with an inotropic agent, intravenous calcium, giving circulatory assistance (e.g. balloon pumping) mechanically assisting respiration, or temporarily inserting a transvenous pacemaker if there are severe conduction disturbances or the patient's left ventricular function is otherwise compromised.

Pharmaceutical precautions

Storage: Shelf-life tablets – 2 years
injection – 3 years

Tambocor tablets should be stored in a cool, dry place. Tambocor injection should be protected from light.

Dilution: When necessary Tambocor injection should be diluted with, or injected into, sterile solutions of 5% dextrose. If chloride containing solutions, such as sodium chloride or Ringer's lactate are used, the injection should be added to a volume of not less than 500 ml, otherwise a precipitate will form.

Legal category POM.

Package quantities *Tablets* – packs of 100 tablets.
Injection – 5 × 15 ml ampoules.

Further information Nil.

Product licence numbers
Tablets 0068/0102
Injection 0068/0101

THEODROX*

Presentation White to creamy-white, circular, bi-convex tablets, 12.0 mm diameter, marked TX on one side and 'RIKER' on the other. Each tablet contains Dried Aluminium Hydroxide Gel BP 260 mg and Aminophylline BP 195 mg.

Uses Theodrox is indicated in the prophylaxis of bronchospasm in asthma and chronic bronchitis.

Aminophylline is a combination of theophylline and ethylenediamine. It has properties very similar to those of theophylline but is more soluble. It relaxes involuntary muscle and relieves bronchial spasm. In common with other xanthine compounds, aminophylline has a diuretic action.

Administered orally, aminophylline can cause gastric irritation. However, in Theodrox this possibility is reduced by the simultaneous administration of aluminium hydroxide gel, which counteracts gastric acidity and retards the breakdown of aminophylline to theophylline in the stomach. By this means, larger doses of aminophylline can be given with less risk of side-effects such as nausea and vomiting.

Dosage and administration *Adults:* 1 tablet three times daily and one at night.

Theodrox is not recommended for children.

Elderly: Elderly patients may require a reduced dosage due to slower drug clearance.

Contra-indications, warnings, etc

Side-effects: Occasionally, nausea or vomiting may occur in some patients.

Caution: Theodrox should be administered with caution to patients with peptic ulcer.

Pregnancy: There is inadequate evidence of safety of the drug in human pregnancy but it has been in wide use for many years without apparent ill consequence; There is evidence of harmful effects in pregnancy in animals.

Theophylline is excreted in breast milk and has been shown to cause irritability in infants.

Overdosage: Symptoms: Nausea and vomiting.

Treatment: If necessary the stomach should be emptied by aspiration and lavage.

Pharmaceutical precautions Store in a cool, dry place.

Legal category P.

Package quantities Bottles of 100 tablets.

Further information Nil.

Product licence number 0068/5011.

TITRALAC*

Presentation White, circular, bi-convex tablets, 11.2 mm in diameter, marked 'TC' on one side and 'Riker' on the other. Each tablet contains Calcium Carbonate BP 420 mg and Glycine BP 180 mg.

Uses Titralac is indicated as a calcium supplement or phosphate binding agent in the management of renal failure.

Dosage and administration As calcium supplement: According to the requirements of the patient. Each Titralac tablet contains 4.2 mmol (168 mg) calcium.

As phosphate binding agent: According to the requirements of the patient. Each Titralac tablet binds, in vitro, about 340 mg phosphate.

These dosage instructions apply to adults, elderly and children.

Titralac tablets may be chewed, allowed to dissolve in the mouth or swallowed whole as desired.

Contra-indications, warnings, etc
Side-effects: None reported.

Precautions: Serum phosphate levels should be monitored in all patients receiving phosphate binders, to prevent the development of a phosphate depletion syndrome.

In long-term treatment, serum and urinary calcium levels should be monitored to prevent hypercalcaemia occurring.

Pregnancy: There is clinical and epidemiological evidence of safety of Titralac in human pregnancy.

Contra-indications: Patients with hypophosphataemia, hypercalcaemia or hypercalciuria.

Overdosage: Not applicable.

Pharmaceutical precautions Store in a cool, dry place.

Legal category GSL.

Package quantities Bottles of 100 and 500 tablets.

Further information Nil.

Product licence number 0068/5004.

TRIBIOTIC* SPRAY

Presentation Pressurised aerosol canister contains creamy-white suspension of:

Neomycin Sulphate BP	500,000 units
Bacitracin Zinc BP	10,000 units
Polymyxin B Sulphate BP	150,000 units
Aerosol propellent to	110 g

The contents of the canister are sterile.

Uses Tribiotic Spray is indicated for the prevention and control of bacterial infection in surgery, at any stage of surgical procedures.

Because neomycin is well absorbed from broken or inflamed skin, the spray should not be used on large denuded areas, including those due to burns, sunburn, chronic ulcers and chronic inflammatory dermatoses.

Also, it is not indicated for pruritis and minor skin disorders.

The combination of neomycin, bacitracin and polymyxin B in Tribiotic Spray provides an almost complete spectrum of activity against the common pathogenic organisms likely to occur in wounds and infected skin conditions. It provides a quick non-touch application; the antibiotic powders are micronised during manufacture to produce a fine dry spray which is evenly distributed over the skin.

Neomycin is a broad-spectrum antibiotic, primarily bactericidal rather than bacteriostatic. It is not inactivated by pus, exudates, gastro-intestinal secretions, bacterial growth products or enzymes. Hypersensitivity reactions are uncommon.

Bacitracin is effective against most Gram-positive organisms. However, it is not destroyed by Gram-negative bacteria and can be of value in the control of mixed infections.

Polymyxin B is selectively bactericidal to Gram-negative bacteria (particularly *Pseudomonas aeruginosa, Escherichia coli, Aerobacter aerogenes, Haemophilus influenzae,* Friedlander's bacillus and the dysentery group) but exerts no action on *Proteus*. Topical applications of polymyxin B have been found effective in the prophylaxis and treatment of infection in granulating surfaces.

Dosage and administration *Directions for use:* The canister should be shaken before and between applications, and held 15 to 25 cm from the skin.

The spray should be applied sparingly to cover the affected area and should be kept clear of the eyes.

Important: During use, the canister should not be inverted or inclined at an angle greater than 45°.

Application of Tribiotic Spray should be limited in adults to a maximum of one canister per day for no more than seven days. Patients with renal impairment are particularly vulnerable to neomycin ototoxicity and the dose should be appropriately reduced.

Dosage should not exceed 15 mg neomycin/kg body weight/day in children. Each 1 second spray contains approximately 15 mg neomycin.

Greater caution should be exercised when treating infants.

Occasionally, blockage may occur from agglomeration of the powder in the outlet of the actuating button. This can easily be cleared with a sterile hypodermic needle (No. 15–17).

Elderly: Use with caution in the elderly as they are more susceptible to ototoxicity, particularly if renal insufficiency is present.

Use in pregnancy: Due to lack of sufficient information, the product should not be administered during the first trimester of pregnancy or during lactation unless the clinical need outweighs the possible risk.

Contra-indications, warnings, etc
Contra-indications: Because of the risk of systemic absorption Triobiotic Spray is not recommended for the treatment of burns. The only other contra-indication is allergic sensitivity to one or more of the constituents.

Precautions: The quantity of neomycin absorbed after topical administration is usually small. However, if high doses are applied, sufficient absorption can occur to cause permanent loss of hearing; the maximum recommended dose should not therefore be exceeded. Nephrotoxicity, resulting in ototoxicity may also occur. Care should be taken in patients with a hearing loss.

The concurrent use with other aminoglycoside antibiotics is not recommended and caution should be exercised in case of cross hypersensitivity to other aminoglycoside antibiotics.

The possibility of resistant organisms should be considered.

Neomycin has inherent neuromuscular blocking activity and may potentiate the action of similar agents, causing respiratory depression.

Overdosage: Overdosage only occurs with chronic use rather than acute.

Pharmaceutical precautions
Storage: Store in a cool place. The shelf-life of Tribiotic Spray is three years.
Container: As the Tribiotic Spray canister is pressurised, it should not be punctured, incinerated or exposed to heat, including the sun, even when empty.

Legal category POM.

Package quantities Canister of 110 g.

Further information Nil.

Product licence number 0068/5075.

VIDENE* POWDER

Presentation Videne Powder is a cream coloured powder containing red/brown particles, presented in a translucent polythene squeeze bottle. Contains Povidone-Iodine USP 5% w/w.

Uses Videne powder is a wide spectrum antiseptic for topical use. It presents all the bactericidal, fungicidal and virucidal properties of iodine, normally without the risk of skin sensitisation encountered with elemental iodine.

Videne powder is indicated for topical application to superficial wounds and minor burns, in the treatment and prevention of infection.

Dosage and administration Apply a light dusting of powder to the affected area. When dry this forms a protective antiseptic layer over the area treated.

There are no special dosage recommendations for children or elderly patients.

Contra-indications, warnings, etc
Precautions: Care must be taken when used on known iodine sensitive subjects, although they do not normally react to povidone iodine.

Excess powder can be washed off readily with warm water.
Contra-indications: Not to be administered internally.
Pregnancy: Videne powder is not recommended for use during pregnancy because of the possibility of absorption through broken skin and subsequent interference with tests of thyroid function.
Overdosage:
Symptoms: Symptoms of overdosage include metabolic acidosis, hypernatraemia and renal impairment.
Treatment: In cases where Videne powder has been taken orally, gastric lavage with dilute starch mucilage or a 1% solution of sodium thiosulphate should be admin-

istered. The electrolyte balance must be corrected and any lost fluids replaced.

Pharmaceutical precautions Videne powder should be stored away from heat, and direct sunlight. It should be used directly from the container. Videne powder is sterile until open.

Legal category GSL.

Package quantities Videne powder is supplied as 15 g polythene squeeze bottles.

Further information Nil.

Product licence number 0068/0116.

VIDENE* SOLUTION

Presentation Videne Solution is a red-brown liquid with a slight tendency to froth. It is an aqueous solution of 10% w/w Povidone-Iodine USP.

Uses Videne Solution is a broad-spectrum antiseptic for topical use. It presents all the bactericidal, fungicidal, and virucidal properties of iodine without the risk of skin sensitisation encountered with elemental iodine.

Videne Solution may be used wherever an effective antiseptic is required for the skin, e.g. in casualty work or for pre-operative skin preparation. It will give a colour delineation to the skin which effectively indicates which areas of the skin remain antiseptic.

Dosage and administration Videne Solution is applied undiluted to the skin in the area to be disinfected and painted on with a gauze swab. It can then be allowed to dry to form a protective antiseptic film or it may be removed with sterile gauze swabs.

Videne Solution may also be applied on impregnated gauze swabs which are then held onto the skin with tapes.

There are no special dosage recommendations for children or elderly patients.

Contra-indications, warnings, etc
Contra-indications: Videne Solution must never be administered orally.
Precautions: Care should be taken with known iodine-sensitive subjects, although these do not normally react to povidone iodine.
Side-effects: In very rare instances Videne Solution may produce skin reactions in iodine-sensitive subjects. These reactions subside when treatment is stopped.
Overdosage: Gastric lavage with dilute starch mucilage or a 1% solution of sodium thiosulphate should be carried out in cases of oral administration. The electrolyte balance should be corrected and lost fluids restored.

Pharmaceutical precautions Videne Solution must be stored away from heat and must not be exposed to direct sunlight. it must not be stored in plastic containers not approved by the manufacturer. Glass vessels are suitable for storing the product. It should be used undiluted.

Legal category P.

Package quantities Videne Solution is supplied in 500 ml bottles and 5 litre polythene containers.

Further information Nil.

Product licence number 0068/0114.

VIDENE* SURGICAL SCRUB

Presentation Videne Surgical Scrub is a red-brown liquid with a pronounced tendency to froth. It is a preparation of 7.5% w/w Povidone-Iodine USP in a detergent base.

Uses Videne Surgical Scrub is a broad-spectrum antiseptic for topical use. It presents all the bactericidal, fungicidal and virucidal properties of iodine without the risk of skin sensitisation encountered with elemental iodine.

Videne Surgical Scrub may be used for pre-operative hand disinfection by the surgical team, or for disinfecting the site of incision prior to elective surgery.

Dosage and administration *(a) Pre-operative hand disinfection:* After first wetting the hands and arms with water, approximately 3.5 ml of Videne Surgical Scrub is applied and rubbed thoroughly onto these areas. A brush may be used to scrub the nails. A little water is added to develop a lather and finally this is rinsed off with running water. Various dispensers which are designed to deliver 3.5 ml of the Surgical Scrub are available from the manufacturers.

(b) Skin disinfection prior to surgery: The site of incision should be washed with Videne Surgical Scrub two or three times a day for at least two days prior to the operation. Immediately before surgery the skin should be moistened with water, Videne Surgical Scrub applied and rubbed thoroughly into the area for several minutes. A sterile gauze swab is used to develop a lather, which is finally rinsed off with sterile water.

Only water should be used to dilute Videne Surgical Scrub.

There are no special dosage recommendations for children or elderly patients.

Contra-indications, warnings, etc
Contra-indications: Videne Surgical Scrub must never be administered orally.

Precautions: Care must be taken when Videne Surgical Scrub is used on known iodine-sensitive subjects, although these do not normally react to povidone iodine.

Side-effects: In very rare instances Videne Surgical Scrub may produce skin reactions in iodine-sensitive subjects. These reactions subside when treatment is stopped.

Overdosage: Gastric lavage with dilute starch mucilage or a 1% solution of sodium thiosulphate should be carried out in cases of oral administration. The electrolyte balance should be corrected and lost fluids restored.

Pharmaceutical precautions Videne Surgical Scrub must be stored away from heat, with exposure to direct sunlight minimised. It must not be stored in plastic containers not approved by the manufacturer, although glass vessels are suitable. Only water should be used as a diluent.

Legal category P.

Package quantities Videne Surgical Scrub is available in 500 ml bottles for use with a wall dispenser, and in 5 litre non-returnable polythene containers.

Further information Nil.

Product licence number 0068/0113.

VIDENE* TINCTURE

Presentation Videne Tincture is a red-brown liquid with an odour of methylated spirits. It is a preparation of 10% w/w Povidone-Iodine USP in a solution of methylated spirits.

Uses Videne Tincture is a broad-spectrum antiseptic for topical application. It presents all the bactericidal, fungicidal and virucidal properties of iodine without the risk of skin sensitisation encountered with elemental iodine.

Videne Tincture is indicated for quick drying pre-operative skin disinfection, particularly in orthopaedic surgery. Being coloured, it gives a useful delineation of the prepared area.

Dosage and administration Videne Tincture is applied undiluted to the area to be incised and thoroughly painted on using a gauze swab. The solution may be allowed to dry to form a protective film or may be removed, using a sterile gauze swab.

There are no special dosage recommendations for children or elderly patients.

Contra-indications, warnings, etc
Contra-indications: Videne Tincture must never be administered orally.

Precautions: Care must be exercised when it is used on known iodine-sensitive subjects, although these do not normally react to povidone iodine. Videne Tincture must not be used on broken skin because of the intense stinging produced by the alcohol present.

Side-effects: In very rare instances Videne Tincture may produce skin reactions in iodine-sensitive subjects. These reactions subside on cessation of treatment.

Overdosage: In cases where Videne Tincture has been taken orally, gastric lavage with dilute starch mucilage or a 1% solution of sodium thiosulphate should be administered. The electrolyte balance should be corrected and any lost fluids replaced.

Pharmaceutical precautions Videne Tincture must be stored away from heat and flames. Exposure to direct sunlight should be minimised. It is recommended that Videne Tincture should be used undiluted. It must not be stored in plastic containers not recommended by the manufacturer, although glass vessels are suitable for storage.

Legal category P.

Package quantities Videne Tincture is available in 500 ml bottles and 5 litre polythene containers.

Further information Videne Tincture must not be used near a naked flame as the solution is flammable. Stains on linen or clothing due to Videne Tincture may easily be removed by washing in water.

Product licence number 0068/0115.

*Trade Mark

A. H. Robins Company Limited
Langhurst
Horsham
West Sussex RH13 5QP

A·H·ROBINS

ALLBEE* WITH C

Presentation *Allbee with C:* Yellow and green, size 1 capsule monogrammed AHR in black. Each capsule contains:

Thiamine Mononitrate USP	15.0 mg
Riboflavine PhEur	10.0 mg
Pyridoxine Hydrochloride PhEur	5.0 mg
Nicotinamide PhEur	50.0 mg
Calcium Pantothenate PhEur	10.0 mg
Ascorbic Acid PhEur	300.0 mg

Uses Vitamin B and C deficiencies.

Dosage and administration *Oral:*

Adults: 1 to 3 capsules daily.

Older patients: Normal adult dosage is recommended since experience has not indicated that this dosage is inappropriate for older patients.

Children: 6–12 years: 1 capsule daily.

Under 6 years: Not recommended.

Contra-indications, warnings, etc

Contra-indications: Known hypersensitivity to the active constituents. Ascorbic acid in doses greater than one gram daily should not be taken during pregnancy since the effects of large doses on the foetus is unknown. Ascorbic acid supplements should not be given to patients with hyperoxaluria.

Precautions and warnings: When Allbee with C is co-prescribed with levodopa, care should be exercised as the pyridoxine may antagonise the therapy. Yellow colouration of urine is normal on recommended dosage. Large doses of ascorbic acid may cause diarrhoea. Ascorbic acid has caused haemolytic anaemia in certain individuals with a deficiency of glucose 6-phosphate dehydrogenase. Increased intake of ascorbic acid over a prolonged period may result in an increase in renal clearance of ascorbic acid and deficiency may result if it is withdrawn rapidly.

Pharmaceutical precautions Nil.

Legal category GSL.

Package quantities
Allbee with C: Bottles of 30 capsules.

Further information Nil.

Product licence number 0100/5001

DIMOTANE* L.A.
DIMOTANE* TABLETS
DIMOTANE* ELIXIR

Presentation *Dimotane L.A.:* Sugar-coated, peach-coloured tablet monogrammed AHR in black. Each tablet contains Brompheniramine Maleate USP 12.0 mg (one-third of active ingredient in coating for immediate release: two-thirds of active ingredient in delayed-release core).

Dimotane Tablets: Scored, peach-coloured compressed tablet stamped AHR. Each tablet contains Brompheniramine Maleate USP 4.0 mg.

Dimotane Elixir: Cola-flavoured, pale yellow-green-coloured liquid. Each 5 ml contains Brompheniramine Maleate USP 2.0 mg.

Uses Antihistaminic in the treatment of allergic conditions and reactions such as hay fever and urticaria.

Dosage and administration *Oral:* Dimotane LA:

Adults: 1 to 2 tablets night and morning.

Older patients: Normal adult dosage is recommended since experience has not indicated that this dosage is inappropriate for older patients.

Children: 6–12 years: 1 tablet at night on retiring, a further tablet may be taken in the morning if necessary.

Dimotane tablets:

Adults: 1 to 2 tablets three or four times daily.

Older patients: Normal adult dosage is recommended since experience has not indicated that this dosage is inappropriate for older patients.

Children: 6–12 years: ½ to 1 tablet three or four times daily.

Dimotane Elixir:

Adults: 10 to 20 ml three or four times daily.

Older patients: Normal adult dosage is recommended since experience has not indicated that this dosage is inappropriate for older patients.

Children: 6–12 years: 5 to 10 ml three or four times daily.
 3–6 years: 5 ml three or four times daily.
 Under 3 years: 0.4–1 mg/kg per 24 hours in four divided doses or at the discretion of the physician.

Contra-indications, warnings, etc

Contra-indications: Hypersensitivity to the active ingredient. Coma or pre-coma states. Known brain damage or epilepsy.

Precautions and warnings: Drowsiness may occur. Patients receiving Dimotane should not drive nor operate machinery unless it has been shown that their physical and mental capacity remains unaffected. May potentiate the effects of CNS depressants including alcohol. In common with many other antihistamines, brompheniramine has an atropine-like action and should therefore be used with caution in patients with bronchial asthma, especially children. The effects of anti-cholinergic drugs may be potentiated. May act as a cerebral stimulant in children and occasionally in adults. If this occurs, it is possible that insomnia, nervousness, hyperpyrexia and tremors may occur and, very rarely, epileptiform convulsions. Therefore children taking Dimotane should not be left unattended for long periods. This product should not be used during pregnancy unless considered essential by the physician.

Treatment of overdosage: Gastric lavage together with appropriate supportive therapy dependent upon individual response to the preparation.

Pharmaceutical precautions Discolouration of tablets may occur when exposed to prolonged strong sunlight.

Legal category P.

Package quantities
Dimotane LA: Bottles of 100 and 500 tablets
Dimotane: Bottles of 100 tablets
Dimotane Elixir: Bottles of 500 ml

Further information
Dimotane Elixir contains Ethanol (96%) BP 3.2% v/v.
Dimotane Tablets, Dimotane LA and Dimotane Elixir are tartrazine free. These products contain the following quantities of sucrose:

Dimotane LA: 132 mg per tablet

Dimotane Tablets: No sucrose

Dimotane Elixir: 2050 mg per 5 ml.

Product licence numbers
Dimotane Tablets   0100/5004
Dimotane Elixir   0100/5005
Dimotane LA   0100/5006

DIMOTANE* EXPECTORANT

Presentation Raspberry-flavoured, pale pink-coloured liquid. Each 5 ml contains:

Guaiphenesin BP	100.0 mg
Phenylephrine Hydrochloride BP	5.0 mg
Phenylpropanolamine Hydrochloride BP	5.0 mg
Brompheniramine Maleate USP	2.0 mg

Uses Treatment of cough to facilitate expectoration. Dimotane Expectorant has been formulated to combine the expectorant properties of guaiphenesin together with decongestants, and an antihistamine.

Dosage and administration *Oral:*

Adults: 5 to 10 ml three or four times daily.

Older patients: Normal adult dosage is recommended since experience has not indicated that this dosage is inappropriate for older patients.

Children: 6–12 years: 5 ml three or four times daily
  3–6 years: 2.5 to 5 ml three or four times daily
  Under 3 years: At the discretion of the physician. Suggested dosage 1.0 to 2.5 ml three or four times daily.

Contra-indications, warnings, etc
Contra-indications: Hypersensitivity to the active ingredients. Coma or pre-coma states. Known brain damage or epilepsy. Use in patients with acute ischaemic heart disease, thyrotoxicosis, glaucoma, or urinary retention. Patients currently receiving, or who have within two weeks received, monoamine oxidase inhibitors or tricyclic antidepressants. Patients receiving other sympathomimetic drugs.

Precautions and warnings: Drowsiness may occur. Patients receiving Dimotane Expectorant should not drive nor operate machinery unless it has been shown that their physical and mental capability remains unaffected. May potentiate the effects of CNS depressants including alcohol. In common with many other antihistamines, brompheniramine has an atropine-like action and should therefore be used with caution in patients with bronchial asthma, especially children. The effects of anticholinergic drugs may be potentiated. May act as a cerebral stimulant in children and occasionally in adults. If this occurs it is possible that insomnia, nervousness, hyperpyrexia or tremor may occur and, very rarely, epileptiform convulsions. Therefore children taking Dimotane Expectorant should not be left unattended for long periods. Should be used with caution in patients receiving digitalis, adrenergic blockers or anti-hypertensive agents. This product should not be used during pregnancy unless considered essential by the physician.

Treatment of overdosage: Gastric lavage together with appropriate supportive therapy dependent upon individual response to the various constituents of the preparation.

Pharmaceutical precautions Avoid prolonged storage at low temperatures.

Legal category P.

Package quantities Bottles of 100 ml and 200 ml.

Further information Recommended diluent: Syrup BP.
  Dimotane Expectorant contains: Ethanol (96%) BP 3.6% v/v.
  This product contains 2500 mg sucrose per 5 ml.

Product licence number 0100/5007.

DIMOTANE* WITH CODEINE
DIMOTANE* WITH CODEINE PAEDIATRIC

Presentation *Dimotane with Codeine:* Clear, dark pink coloured liquid with an odour of raspberry. Each 5 ml contains:

Brompheniramine Maleate USP	2.0 mg
Pseudoephedrine Hydrochloride BP	30.0 mg
Codeine Phosphate PhEur	10.0 mg

Dimotane with Codeine Paediatric: Clear, dark pink coloured liquid with an odour of raspberry. Each 5 ml contains:

Brompheniramine Maleate USP	2.0 mg
Pseudoephedrine Hydrochloride BP	15.0 mg
Codeine Phosphate PhEur	3.0 mg

Uses Cough suppressant and nasal decongestant in coughs associated with colds and other similar conditions of the upper respiratory tract.

Dosage and administration Oral.
Dimotane with Codeine:

Adults: 10 ml three times daily

Older patients: Normal adult dosage is recommended since experience has not indicated that this dosage is inappropriate for older patients.

Children: 6–12 years: 7.5 ml three times daily.
  Under 6 years: At the discretion of the physician. Dimotane with Codeine Paediatric is recommended.

Dimotane with Codeine Paediatric:
Children: 6–12 years: 15 ml three times daily
  3–6 years: 10 ml three times daily
  2–3 years: 5 ml three times daily

Under 2 years: Not to be used.

Contra-indications, warnings, etc

Contra-indications: Hypersensitivity to the active ingredients. Coma or pre-coma states. Known brain damage or epilepsy. Use in patients with acute ischaemic heart disease, thyrotoxicosis, glaucoma, or urinary retention. Patients currently receiving, or who have within two weeks received, monoamine oxidase inhibitors or tricyclic antidepressants. Patients receiving other sympathomimetic drugs.

Precautions and warnings: Codeine is a narcotic analgesic. Drowsiness may occur. Patients receiving this product should not drive nor operate machinery unless it has been shown that their physical and mental capability remains unaffected. May potentiate the effects of CNS depressants including alcohol. In common with many other antihistamines, brompheniramine has an atropine-like action and should therefore be used with caution in patients with bronchial asthma, especially children. Tolerance, psychological and physical dependence and constipation may occur. The effects of anticholinergic drugs may be potentiated. May act as a cerebral stimulant in children and occasionally in adults. If this occurs it is possible that insomnia, nervousness, hyperpyrexia or tremor may occur and very rarely epileptiform convulsions. Therefore children taking this product should not be left unattended for long periods. Should be used with caution in patients receiving digitalis, adrenergic blockers, anti-hypertensive agents or non-steroidal anti-inflammatory drugs. This product should not be used during pregnancy unless considered essential by the physician.

Treatment of overdosage: Gastric lavage together with appropriate supportive therapy dependent upon individual response to the various constituents of the preparation.

Pharmaceutical precautions   Nil.

Legal category   CD (Sch 5), P.

Package quantities   Bottles of 100 ml and 200 ml.

Further information   Recommended diluent: 70% glycerol v/v.

These products contain Ethanol (96%) BP 2.5% v/v.

These products are sugar-free. The sweetener in these products will not cause dental caries.

Product licence numbers

Dimotane with Codeine	0100/0080
Dimotane with Codeine Paediatric	0100/0084

DOPRAM* INFUSION
DOPRAM* INJECTION

Presentation

Dopram infusion: Clear colourless solution. Each 500 ml flexible plastic bag contains Doxapram Hydrochloride BP 2 mg per ml in 5% Glucose Intravenous Infusion BP.

Dopram injection: Clear colourless solution. Each 5 ml ampoule contains Doxapram Hydrochloride BP 20 mg per ml.

Uses   Respiratory stimulant.

The principal pharmacological action of Dopram is an increase in minute volume produced primarily by an increase in tidal volume and to a lesser extent by changes in respiratory rate. Neuropharmacological studies have shown that the primary sites of action of Dopram are the peripheral chemoreceptors. It is considered that this site of action of Dopram is responsible for its relative specificity of action; it is only following large doses of doxapram hydrochloride that non-specific central nervous system stimulation occurs.

Dopram is specifically indicated in the following situations:

Acute respiratory failure (Dopram Infusion): To stimulate respiration in patients whose blood gas status or clinical condition suggests that severe carbon dioxide retention would occur during controlled oxygen therapy.

To stimulate respiration in patients showing a progressive increase in PCO_2 with mental status changes during or after controlled oxygen therapy.

Following anaesthesia:

1. To stimulate ventilation in the postoperative period as an aid to the reduction of postoperative pulmonary complications. (Dopram Infusion or Dopram Injection.)

2. To permit the use of effective doses of narcotic analgesics without associated problems of respiratory depression. (Dopram Infusion or Dopram Injection.)

3. To increase the rate of recovery from inhalational anaesthesia and also over-sedation due to intravenous diazepam, when this would be beneficial. (Dopram Injection.)

Dosage and administration   For intravenous use only.

Adults:

Acute respiratory failure: Dopram Infusion 1.5 mg per minute to 4.0 mg per minute dependent upon the condition and response of the patient. Whenever possible the condition of the patient should be monitored by frequent measurement of blood gas tensions.

Following anaesthesia: Dopram Injection 1.0 to 1.5 mg/kg body weight which may be repeated at one hour intervals. Alternatively, Dopram Infusion may be given at a rate of 2 to 3 mg per minute. Appropriate adjustments to the administration rate should be made according to the response of the patient.

Older patients: Normal adult dosage is recommended since experience has not indicated that this dosage is inappropriate for older patients.

Children: The use of Dopram in children is not recommended.

Contra-indications, warnings, etc

Contra-indications: Severe hypertension, status asthmaticus, coronary artery disease, thyrotoxicosis, epilepsy, physical obstruction of the respiratory tract.

Precautions and warnings: Dopram should be administered concurrently with oxygen to patients with severe irreversible airways obstruction or severely decreased lung compliance, due to the increased work of breathing in these patients. Clinical data suggest that there may be interaction between doxapram and aminophylline which is manifested by agitation and increased skeletal muscle activity. Care should thus be taken when these two drugs are used concomitantly. Dopram should also be administered with great care to patients being treated concurrently with monoamineoxidase inhibitors. Animal studies have shown that the action of doxapram, in common with a large number of drugs, is potentiated after pretreatment with a monoamineoxidase inhibitor. Dopram potentiates the effects of sympathomimetic agents. In patients presenting with bronchoconstriction, Dopram should always be used in conjunction with bronchodilator drugs in order to reduce the amount of respiratory effort.

Although there is no recognised hazard, this product is not recommended for use in pregnancy unless there are compelling clinical reasons to do so.

On recommended dosage a moderate increase in blood pressure and a slight increase in heart rate have been reported. This should be borne in mind when Dopram is considered for use in those patients with hypertension or with impaired cardiac functional reserves. Dizziness and perineal warmth have also been reported. Other side effects have been reported in the post anaesthetic period but these are also commonly observed during recovery from anaesthesia, and include muscle fasciculation, hyperactivity, sweating, confusion, hallucinations, cough, dyspnoea, laryngospasm, bronchospasm, sinus tachycardia, bradycardia, extrasystoles, nausea and/or vomiting and salivation.

Treatment of overdosage: Gross overdosage may result in hypertension, tachycardia, and increased skeletal muscle activity. The hypertension should be treated with appropriate supportive therapy and the increase in skeletal muscle activity controlled with intravenous barbiturates.

Pharmaceutical precautions Dopram is incompatible with alkaline solutions such as aminophylline, frusemide and thiopentone sodium. Store at room temperature. Do not refrigerate Dopram Injection.

Legal category POM.

Package quantities Dopram infusion: Packs of 5 flexible plastic bags each containing 500 ml.
Dopram injection: Packs of 5 ampoules each containing 5 ml.

Further information It has been shown that, when used in the postoperative situation, Dopram does not affect the quality of analgesia produced by narcotics such as morphine or pethidine.

Product licence numbers
Dopram Infusion   0100/5019
Dopram Injection   0100/5018

MALINAL* TABLETS
MALINAL* SUSPENSION

Presentation *Malinal tablets:* White, biconvex, bevel-edged, round, peppermint flavoured, chewable tablets, scored and stamped AHR, containing Almasilate 500 mg.

Malinal suspension: White, peppermint flavoured suspension containing in each 5 ml, Almasilate 500 mg.

Uses Antacid for the relief of symptoms due to hyperacidity including acid reflux and gastritis.

Dosage and administration
Malinal tablets: Oral
Adults: Chew two tablets at mealtimes and at bedtime, or when symptoms occur.
Older patients: Normal adult dosage is recommended since experience has not indicated that this dosage is inappropriate for older patients.

Malinal suspension: Oral
Adults: 10 ml at mealtimes and at bedtime or when symptoms occur.
Older patients: Normal adult dosage is recommended

since experience has not indicated that this dosage is inappropriate for older patients.

Contra-indications, warnings, etc
Contra-indications: There are no known contra-indications to Malinal, but it is probably wise to avoid taking preparations containing antacids in the first trimester of pregnancy.

Precautions and warnings: In common with some other antacids Almasilate may lead to a phosphate depletion syndrome, particularly in patients on a low phosphate diet, e.g. malnutrition. Almasilate may form complexes with certain drugs e.g. tetracyclines, digoxin and vitamins, resulting in decreased absorption. This should be borne in mind when concomitant administration is considered.

Magnesium salts may cause central nervous depression in the presence of renal insufficiency.

Treatment of overdosage: Treatment of overdosage is not necessary.

Pharmaceutical precautions Nil.

Legal category P.

Package quantities
Malinal Tablets: Packs containing 36 tablets
Malinal Suspension: Bottles of 200 ml.

Further information 500 mg of Almasilate contains 2.63 mEq (32 mg) magnesium. Each tablet or 5 ml of suspension contains approximately 0.5 mmol of Sodium.
Malinal Tablets contain 250 mg sucrose per tablet.

Product licence numbers
Malinal Tablets: 0100/0068
Malinal Suspension: 0100/0065

RHEUMOX* 600
RHEUMOX* CAPSULES

Presentation *Rheumox 600 Tablets:* Pale orange, film-coated, capsule shaped tablets both sides scored with a breakline and one side printed RHEUMOX 600, containing Azapropazone Dihydrate 600 mg.

Rheumox Capsules: Two-tone orange size 1 capsule, monogrammed AHR Rheumox containing Azapropazone Dihydrate 300 mg.

Uses Rheumox is a non-steroidal anti-inflammatory analgesic agent indicated in the treatment of rheumatoid arthritis, ankylosing spondylitis, osteoarthrosis and painful musculoskeletal conditions. Rheumox is also indicated in attacks of acute gouty arthritis and in the long term prophylaxis of gout and the control of hyperuricaemia.

Dosage and administration Rheumatoid arthritis, ankylosing spondylitis, osteoarthrosis and painful musculoskeletal conditions.
Rheumox is recommended for adults only.
Rheumox 600 Tablets: Oral – One 600 mg tablet night and morning.
Rheumox Capsules: Oral – One 300 mg capsule four times daily or two 300 mg capsules night and morning.

Older patients: Azapropazone is principally excreted unchanged by the kidney. In patients over 65 whose renal function may be reduced, it is therefore suggested that the dose be 300 mg in the morning and 600 mg to be taken last thing at night. In patients much older than this, a suitable regimen is 600 mg at night or 300 mg twice daily. This dosage can be subsequently adjusted since some elderly patients have excellent renal function.

Acute gout: 2,400 mg in divided doses during the first 24 hours followed by 1,800 mg per day until the attack is resolving after which 1,200 mg per day is used until symptoms have disappeared. In treating acute gout it is good practice to ensure that the patient increases his fluid intake.

Chronic gout: Azapropazone reduces serum urate levels by enhancing urate excretion. The usual dosage for this purpose is 600 mg night and morning (either Rheumox 600 or Rheumox Capsules may be used). In patients over 65 the dosage should be as described above.

Contra-indications, warnings, etc
Contra-indications: Rheumox increases the plasma concentration of phenytoin and should not be given to patients taking this drug.

Rheumox potentiates the action of warfarin in many patients and should not be used with this or other oral anticoagulants. If it is essential that Rheumox be given to a patient already taking an oral anticoagulant, this should not be done until the dose of the anticoagulant has been reduced to a very low level. Rheumox can then be introduced and the dose of the anticoagulant increased until the required effect is produced. Prothrombin determinations should be carried out daily throughout this procedure. Rheumox is not recommended in the presence of a peptic ulcer or where there is a history of blood dyscrasia. Patients on long term treatment should be regularly reviewed.

Precautions and warnings: Patients with a history of peptic ulcer have been treated safely with Rheumox but in this situation constant supervision is recommended as in some, ulceration may recur. Azapropazone may interfere with the blood sugar lowering effect of oral hypoglycaemic agents. Concurrent use of these drugs is not recommended. Data at present available does not indicate that interaction occurs with sulphonamides but adjustments of the dosage of these drugs may be necessary in some instances.

Specific renal function tests in man and long term administration to animals have not revealed any adverse effects of Rheumox on the kidney but since its clearance is predominantly renal it is not recommended for use in patients with overt renal dysfunction. Animal reproduction studies did not result in foetal abnormalities but safety in human pregnancy cannot be assumed and its use should be avoided in pregnancy whenever possible.

Skin rashes occur occasionally and a proportion of these are photo-allergic reactions. Fluid retention and gastro-intestinal upsets also occur occasionally. Gastro-intestinal bleeding has been reported as has angioneurotic oedema. Very rarely, fibrosing alveolitis and Coombs positive haemolytic anaemia have been reported in association with Rheumox therapy. Should either occur, therapy should be discontinued.

Treatment of overdosage: If overdosage should occur, two specific courses of action are suggested on theoretical grounds. Firstly, since Rheumox is poorly soluble in gastric juice, stomach lavage should recover any gastric residue of the drug, provided of course that it is done early enough.

Secondly, since Rheumox is predominantly excreted by the kidney, forced alkaline diuresis is theoretically indicated.

Pharmaceutical precautions Protect from light.

Legal category POM.

Package quantities *Rheumox 600 Tablets:* Bottles of 100 and 500 tablets.
Rheumox Capsules: Bottles of 100 and 500 capsules.

Further information Nil.

Product licence numbers
Rheumox 600 Tablets: 0100/0059
Rheumox Capsules: 0100/0037

ROBAXIN*-750

Presentation Scored white compressed capsule-shaped tablet embossed AHR containing: Methocarbamol USP   750 mg.

Uses As a short-term adjunct to the symptomatic treatment of acute musculoskeletal disorders associated with painful muscle spasms.

Dosage and administration *Oral: Adults:* The usual dose is 2 tablets qid (6.0 g) but therapeutic response has been achieved with doses as low as 1 tablet three times daily.

Older patients: Half the maximum adult daily dose, or less, may be sufficient to produce a therapeutic response in the elderly.

Children: Not recommended.

Contra-indications, warnings, etc
Contra-indications: Hypersensitivity to methocarbamol. Coma or pre-coma states. Known brain damage or epilepsy. Myasthenia gravis.

Use in pregnancy: There is no evidence of safety in human pregnancy, nor is there evidence from animal work that it is free from hazard. Do not use during pregnancy, especially the first trimester, or lactation, unless there are compelling reasons to do so.

Precautions and warnings: This product may cause drowsiness and patients receiving it should not drive nor operate machinery unless their physical and mental capability remain unaffected – especially if other medication capable of causing drowsiness is also being taken.

This product may potentiate the effects of other central nervous system depressants and stimulants including alcohol, barbiturates, anaesthetics and appetite suppressants. The effects of anti-cholinergics e.g. atropine and some psychotropic drugs may be potentiated by methocarbamol. Little is known about the possibility of interactions with other drugs.

Robaxin may give rise to manifestations of allergy including skin rash, urticaria and angioneurotic oedema. This product may very rarely give rise to restlessness, anxiety, vertigo, tremor, confusion and convulsions. Light-headedness and dizziness have been reported. Nausea and vomiting have also been reported during use of Robaxin. Robaxin should be used with caution in patients with renal and hepatic insufficiency.

Treatment of overdosage: Gastric lavage with appropriate supportive therapy for 24 hours as methocarbamol is excreted within that time.

Pharmaceutical precautions Nil.

Legal category POM.

Package quantities Bottles of 100 tablets.

Further information Nil.

Product licence number 0100/5026.

ROBAXIN* INJECTABLE

Presentation 10 ml sterile ampoules each containing:
Methocarbamol USP 1.0 g
Vehicle 50% aqueous polyethylene glycol 300.

Uses In the treatment of acute painful muscle spasm, due to musculoskeletal disorders or trauma.

Dosage and administration For intravenous use only.

Adults: 10–30 ml dependent on the severity of the condition and therapeutic response. Should not exceed 30 ml per day. Not to be administered for more than three consecutive days.

Older patients: Half the maximum adult dose or less may be sufficient for a therapeutic response in the elderly.

Children: Not recommended.

Rate of administration: Administer by slow intravenous injection or infusion directly into the vein at a maximum rate of 3 ml per minute.

Diluent: May be added to an intravenous drip of sterile isotonic saline, or sterile 5% dextrose. 10 ml of Robaxin Injectable should not be diluted to more than 250 ml.

Contra-indications, warnings, etc
Contra-indications: Hypersensitivity to methocarbamol or sulphite. Coma or pre-coma states. Known brain damage or epilepsy. Myasthenia gravis.

Use in pregnancy: There is no evidence of safety in human pregnancy, nor is there any evidence from animal work that it is free from hazard. Do not use during pregnancy, especially the first trimester, or lactation, unless there are compelling reasons to do so.

Precautions and warnings: This product may cause drowsiness and patients receiving it should not drive nor operate machinery unless their physical and mental capabilities remain unaffected – especially if other medication capable of causing drowsiness is also being taken. This product may potentiate the effects of other central nervous system depressants and stimulants including alcohol, barbiturates, anaesthetics and appetite suppressants. The effects of anti-cholinergics, e.g. atropine, and some psychotropic drugs, may be potentiated by methocarbamol. Little is known about the possibility of interactions with other drugs.

Robaxin may give rise to manifestations of allergy including skin rash, urticaria and angioneurotic oedema. This product may very rarely give rise to restlessness, anxiety, vertigo, tremor, confusion and convulsions. Lightheadedness and dizziness have been reported. Nausea and vomiting have also been reported during use of Robaxin.

Robaxin Injectable should be used with extreme caution in patients with impaired renal function as the solvent used may cause raised urea levels and acidosis. Robaxin should be used with caution in patients with hepatic insufficiency.

Treatment of overdosage: Appropriate supportive therapy for 24 hours as methocarbamol is excreted within that time.

Pharmaceutical precautions Nil.

Legal category POM.

Package quantities Boxes containing 5 ampoules.

Further information Nil.

Product licence number 0100/5027.

ROBAXISAL* FORTE

Presentation A two-layer, pink and white compressed tablet scored and stamped AHR, containing:
Methocarbamol USP 400 mg
Acetylsalicylic Acid PhEur 325 mg

Uses In the short term management of pain and skeletal muscle spasm associated with musculoskeletal disorders such as lumbago, fibrositis, sprains, strains etc.

Dosage and administration *Oral:*
Adults: 2 tablets four times daily.

Older patients: Half the adult dose may be sufficient to produce a therapeutic response.

Children: Not recommended.

Contra-indications, warnings, etc
Contra-indications: Hypersensitivity to methocarbamol or aspirin. Coma or pre-coma states. Known brain damage or epilepsy. Myasthenia gravis. Active peptic ulceration and haemophilia.

Use in pregnancy: There is no evidence of safety in human pregnancy, nor is there evidence from animal work that it is free from hazard. Do not use during pregnancy especially the first trimester, or lactation, unless there are compelling reasons to do so.

Robaxisal Forte contains aspirin and is therefore best avoided at term because of possible effect on platelet function in the newborn. It may enhance the effects of anticoagulants.

Precautions and warnings: This product may cause drowsiness and patients receiving it should not drive nor operate machinery unless their physical and mental capability remain unaffected – especially if other medication capable of causing drowsiness is also being taken. This product may potentiate the effects of other central nervous system depressants and stimulants including alcohol, barbiturates, anaesthetics and appetite suppressants. The effects of anti-cholinergics, e.g. atropine and some psychotropic drugs, may be potentiated by methocarbamol. Little is known about the possibility of interaction with other drugs.

Robaxisal Forte should be used with caution in patients with renal and hepatic insufficiency.

Robaxisal Forte contains aspirin and therefore may give rise to gastrointestinal bleeding, and may precipitate bronchospasm especially in asthmatic patients. Patients currently on anti-coagulant therapy should have blood coagulation parameters regularly monitored.

Robaxisal Forte may give rise to manifestations of allergy including skin rash, urticaria and angioneurotic oedema. This product may very rarely give rise to restlessness, anxiety, vertigo, tremor, confusion and convulsions. Nausea and vomiting have been reported.

Treatment of overdosage: Supportive therapy for 24 hours, as methocarbamol is excreted within that time. If salicylate intoxication occurs, especially in children, the hyperpnoea may be controlled with sodium bicarbonate. Judicious use of 5% CO_2 with 95% O_2 may be of benefit. Abnormal electrolyte patterns should be corrected with appropriate fluid therapy.

Pharmaceutical precautions Nil.

Legal category POM.

Package quantities Bottles of 100 tablets.

Further information Nil.

Product licence number 0100/5028.

ROBINUL*

Presentation Round, pink, compressed tablet one side monogrammed $\frac{AHR}{2}$, the other side scored with a break line.

Each tablet contains Glycopyrrolate USP 2.0 mg

Uses Treatment of gastro-intestinal hypermotility and adjunctive therapy in the treatment of peptic ulcer.

Dosage and administration *Oral.*

Adults: ½–2 tablets two or three times daily.

Older patients: Normal adult dosage is recommended since experience has not indicated that this dosage is inappropriate for older patients.

Contra-indications, warnings, etc

Contra-indications: Glaucoma and pyloric obstruction.

Precautions and warnings: Because of the increase in heart rate produced by the administration of anticholinergics, use with caution in patients with coronary artery disease, congestive heart failure, cardiac arrhythmias, hypertension or thyrotoxicosis. This product should be used very cautiously in pyrexial patients due to inhibition of sweating. Due to the anticholinergic side effects of glycopyrrolate, care is required in treating patients with known or suspected prostatic disease. Anticholinergic effects such as blurred vision, dry mouth, tachycardia, drowsiness and mild abdominal discomfort may occur. Glycopyrrolate may cause drowsiness. Patients should therefore not drive nor operate machinery unless it has been shown not to affect their physical or mental ability.

Glycopyrrolate should not be used during pregnancy as safety in this condition has not been established. Reproduction studies in rats and rabbits revealed no teratogenic effects from glycopyrrolate. However, diminished rates of conception and of survival at weaning were observed in rats, in a dose related manner. Studies in dogs suggest that this may be due to diminished seminal secretion which is evident at high doses of glycopyrrolate. The significance of this for man is not clear.

Treatment of overdosage: Gastric lavage or induced emesis is advised. Catheterisation may be necessary.

Pharmaceutical precautions Nil.

Legal category POM.

Package quantities Bottles of 100 tablets.

Further information Nil.

Product licence number 0100/5029.

ROBINUL* INJECTION ▼

Presentation 3 ml and 1 ml ampoule (snap-open ampoule) of isotonic aqueous solution containing in each 1 ml:
Glycopyrrolate USP 0.2 mg

Uses *Properties:* Robinul (glycopyrrolate) is a quaternary ammonium anticholinergic agent. The quaternary ammonium moiety renders Robinul highly ionised at physiological pH and it thus penetrates the blood brain and placental barriers poorly. The effect of Robinul on secretory organs is particularly marked and prolonged and good control of salivary and pharyngeal secretions can be obtained with doses which do not produce marked changes in heart rate. Gastric secretions are, similarly, reduced by Robinul.

Indications: 1. To protect against the peripheral muscarinic actions of anticholinesterases such as neostigmine and pyridostigmine, used to reverse neuromuscular blockade produced by nondepolarising muscle relaxants.

2. As a preoperative antimuscarinic agent to reduce salivary, tracheobronchial and pharyngeal secretions, and to reduce the acidity of the gastric contents.

3. As a preoperative or intra-operative antimuscarinic to attenuate or prevent intraoperative bradycardia associated with the use of suxamethonium or due to cardiac vagal reflexes.

Dosage and administration *Premedication – Adults:* 0.2 mg to 0.4 mg intravenously or intramuscularly before the induction of anaesthesia. Alternatively, a dose of 0.004 to 0.005 mg/kg up to a maximum of 0.4 mg may be used. Larger doses may result in profound and prolonged antisialogogue effect which may be unpleasant for the patient.

Older patients: Normal adult dosage is recommended since experience has not indicated that this dosage is inappropriate for older patients.

Children: 0.004 to 0.008 mg/kg up to a maximum of 0.2 mg intravenously or intramuscularly before the induction of anaesthesia. Larger doses may result in profound and prolonged antisialogogue effect which may be unpleasant for the patient.

Intraoperative use – Adults: In those situations where intraoperative use is indicated, a single dose of 0.2 to 0.4 mg (or 0.004 to 0.005 mg/kg up to a maximum of 0.4 mg) by intravenous injection should be used. This dose may be repeated if necessary.

Older patients: Normal adult dosage is recommended since experience has not indicated that this dosage is inappropriate for older patients.

Children: In those situations where intraoperative use is indicated, a single dose of 0.004 to 0.008 mg/kg or up to a maximum of 0.2 mg by intravenous injection should be used. This dose may be repeated if necessary.

Reversal – Adults: 0.2 mg intravenously per 1 mg neostigmine or the equivalent dose of pyridostigmine. Alternatively, a dose of 0.01–0.015 mg/kg intravenously with 0.05 mg/kg neostigmine or equivalent dose of pyridostigmine. Robinul may be administered simultaneously from the same syringe with the anticholinesterase; greater cardiovascular stability results from this method of administration.

Older patients: Normal adult dosage is recommended since experience has not indicated that this dosage is inappropriate for older patients.

Children: 0.01mg/kg intravenously with 0.05 mg/kg neostigmine or the equivalent dose of pyridostigmine. Robinul may be administered simultaneously from the same syringe with the anticholinesterase; greater cardiovascular stability results from this method of administration.

Contra-indications, warnings, etc

Contra-indications: Apart from established hypersensitivity to glycopyrrolate, there are no absolute contraindications to Robinul.

Precautions and warnings: Reproduction studies in rats and rabbits revealed no teratogenic effects from glycopyrrolate. Safety in human pregnancy and lactation has not been established. However, diminished rates of conception and of survival at weaning were observed in rats, in a dose-related manner. Studies in dogs suggest that this may be due to diminished seminal secretion which is evident at high doses of glycopyrrolate. The significance of this for man is not clear.

Because of the increase in heart rate produced by the administration of anticholinergics, use with caution in patients with coronary artery disease; congestive heart failure; cardiac arrhythmias; hypertension; thyrotoxicosis. This product should be used very cautiously in pyrexial patients due to inhibition of sweating.

Large doses of quaternary ammonium anticholinergic compounds have been shown to block end plate nicotinic receptors. This should be considered before using glycopyrrolate in patients with myasthenia gravis.

It is known that the administration of anticholinergic agents during inhalation anaesthesia can result in ventricular arrhythmias.

Side-effects: Robinul may produce the following effects which are extensions of its fundamental pharmacological actions, dry mouth, difficulty in micturition, disturbances in visual accommodation, tachycardia, palpitation, inhibition of sweating.

Treatment of overdosage: Since glycopyrrolate is a quarternary ammonium agent symptoms of overdosage are peripheral rather than central in nature. To combat peripheral anticholinergic effects a quaternary ammonium anticholinesterase such as neostigmine methyl sulphate may be given in a dose of 1.0 mg for each 1.0 mg of glycopyrrolate known to have been administered by the parenteral route.

Pharmaceutical precautions

Robinul Injection has been shown to be physically compatible with the following agents commonly used in anaesthetic practice: Butorphanol, Lorazepam, Droperidol and Fentanyl Citrate, Levorphanol Tartrate, Pethidine Hydrochloride, Morphine Sulphate, Neostigmine, Promethazine and Pyridostigmine.

Robinul Injection has been shown to be physically incompatible with the following agents commonly used in anaesthetic practice:

Diazepam, Dimenhydrinate, Methohexitone Sodium, Pentazocine, Pentobarbitone Sodium, Thiopentone Sodium.

Robinul Injection should be stored at ambient temperature.

Legal category POM.

Package quantities
Packs of 10 ampoules each containing 1 ml or 3 ml.

Further information
Robinul Injection has been used successfully as an adjunct to reversal by neostigmine when atropine has been used as the preoperative anticholinergic.

The use of Robinul Injection as a preoperative anticholinergic is associated with less effect on the cardiovascular system, compared to atropine.

The use of Robinul Injection as an adjunct to reversal by neostigmine of non depolarising muscle relaxants is associated with less initial tachycardia and better protection against the cholinergic effects of neostigmine compared to reversal with a mixture of neostigmine and atropine.

Product licence number 0100/0054.

ROBINUL* POWDER

Presentation A white, crystalline powder, Glycopyrrolate USP

Uses Iontophoretic treatment of the plantar and palmar skin for idiopathic hyperhidrosis.

Dosage and administration A 0.05% solution in distilled water of Glycopyrrolate USP is applied to palmar or plantar skin. When treating the foot or hand sufficient solution to cover the palm or sole is placed in a non-metallic container and the anode, of sheet metal larger in area than the part being treated, is placed in the solution. The sole or palm is separated from the anode by 5 mm of plastic foam or a layer of lint or sponge sheet.

In all cases an electrical circuit is completed by placing another limb in lukewarm tap water containing the cathode, similarly shielded from direct contact with the skin.

Recommended average conditions are 90 volts DC at 10–20 mA for adults (including older patients) and 2–10 mA for children, for 12 minutes at each site, depending on the patient's skin tolerance, body weight and size. Only one site should be treated at a time, and only two sites in any one day. Treatments should not be repeated within seven days, but may be repeated later varying the precise conditions according to the recurrence and severity of hyperhidrosis. See also Warnings section below.

Contra-indications, warnings, etc

Contra-indications: Glaucoma. Do not use during pregnancy.

Precautions and warnings: Glycopyrrolate may cause tachycardia. Since this drug may cause drowsiness, patients receiving glycopyrrolate should not drive nor operate machinery immediately after treatment unless it has been shown not to affect their physical or mental ability. It should be used with great caution in patients with cardiovascular disease, thyrotoxicosis and obstructive disorders of the lower urinary tract. Patients with mycotic or other skin infection should not be treated.

Dryness of mouth, blurred vision and mild abdominal discomfort may occur. Exercise care in patients with prostatic hypertrophy. Due to the effect of anti-cholinergics on mucous secretions, it is advisable not to treat people with chronic bronchitis. Occasionally difficulty in eating may occur and micturition may be temporarily affected for some hours after treatment. A mild tingling feeling may occur in the immersed areas during treatment and any recent cuts or cracks in the skin may smart when the current is increased at the start of iontophoresis. The latter can be avoided by covering the lesion with a thin smear of petroleum jelly. Avoid over-exertion especially in hot weather, until any side effects have disappeared.

The product should only be used by specialist units experienced in iontophoretic technique.

The electrodes and treated skin areas *must* be placed in non-metallic containers and separated carefully by layers of, for example, sponge or lint. Direct contact between electrodes and skin must be avoided otherwise burns may result.

The current must be very slowly increased from zero mA and decreased to zero mA at the beginning and end of the treatment period respectively to avoid any Faradic discharge between the electrode and skin on removal of the patient's limb from the container of solution. Instruct patient that contact must not be broken during treatment.

Do not use during pregnancy as safety in this condition has not been established. Reproduction studies in rats and rabbits revealed no teratogenic effects from glycopyrrolate. However, diminished rates of conception and of survival at weaning were observed in rats, in a dose related manner. Studies in dogs suggest that this may be due to diminished seminal secretion which is evident at high doses of glycopyrrolate. The significance of this for man is not clear.

Pharmaceutical precautions Robinul Powder is supplied in amber-glass bottles containing 5 grams. The powder is slightly hygroscopic and the container should not be left open. For use by iontophoresis the powder should be dissolved in freshly distilled or deionised water to the recommended concentration.

Prior to use a stock solution (e.g. 0.1% or 0.5% w/v) may be made up with freshly boiled and cooled distilled or deionised water. This stock solution should be stored in a refrigerator to minimise possible microbial growth and should be kept in thoroughly clean amber-glass, capped containers. Glycopyrrolate does hydrolyse very slowly at pH 7 and room temperature and it is recommended that stock solutions be kept for no more than 14 days. Do not keep solutions once used for iontophoretic treatment. The solution must not be alkaline, otherwise the glycopyrrolate will hydrolyse more rapidly.

Legal category POM.

Package quantities Supplied in amber-glass bottles containing 5 grams Glycopyrrolate USP.

Further information Further recommendations concerning treatment are given in the package insert.

Product licence number 0100/0052.

*Trade Mark

Roche Products Limited
PO Box 8
Welwyn Garden City
Hertfordshire AL7 3AY

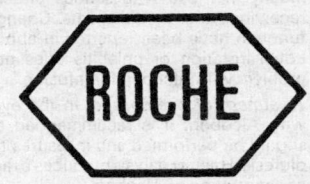

ALCOBON*

Presentation Round, white tablets with 'ROCHE' imprinted on one face and a single break bar on the other, containing 500 mg flucytosine.

Infusion bottles containing 2.5 g flucytosine in 250 ml aqueous saline solution. The solution is colourless to slightly yellow.

Uses *Properties:* Alcobon is a fluorinated pyrimidine effective in the treatment of certain systemic fungal infections. In fungi sensitive to the preparation it acts as a competitive inhibitor of uracil metabolism. In man it is excreted largely unchanged almost entirely in the urine. Flucytosine can be removed by haemodialysis.

Indications: Alcobon is indicated for the treatment of systemic infections with *Cryptococcus neoformans, Candida albicans* and certain other *Candida* species, *Torulopsis glabrata, Hansenula* and fungi which cause chromomycosis; *Phialophora verrucosa, Phialophora pedrosoi* and *Cladosporium carrionii.*

Alcobon for Infusion is indicated only when the patient is unable to accept oral Alcobon.

Dosage and administration For severe infections the total daily oral dose in adults and children is 200 mg/kg body weight divided into 4 doses. In patients harbouring extremely sensitive organisms a total daily dose of 100–150 mg/kg body weight may be sufficient.

Alcobon for Infusion should be administered using a giving set incorporating a 15 micron filter. It may be administered directly into a vein, through a central venous catheter, or by intraperitoneal infusion. The recommended dosage is the same as for oral Alcobon, the total daily dose being divided over the 24 hours. Adequate effects can, however, often be obtained with a lower dose of Alcobon when the intravenous route is used.

It is suggested that the duration of the infusion should be of the order of 20 to 40 minutes provided this is balanced with the fluid requirements of the patient. As a rule, treatment with Alcobon for Infusion should rarely be required for periods of more than one week. The patient should be started on oral therapy with Alcobon tablets as soon as this becomes practicable.

Since Alcobon is excreted primarily by the kidneys, patients with renal impairment should be given smaller doses. The following is suggested as a guide for dosage in patients with severe infection associated with renal impairment:

In patients with creatinine clearance
<40 to >20 ml/min: 50 mg/kg every 12 hours.
<20 to >10 ml/min: 50 mg/kg every 24 hours.
< 10 ml/min: an initial single dose of 50 mg/kg; subsequent doses should be calculated according to the results of regular monitoring of the serum concentration of the drug, which should not be allowed to exceed 80 mcg/ml. Blood levels of 25–50 mcg/ml are normally effective.

The duration of treatment should be determined on an individual basis. The outcome of therapy will be affected by variations in the sensitivity of the infecting organism, its accessibility and its susceptibility to Alcobon, as well as by differences in the response of individual patients. In cases of cryptococcal meningitis, treatment should last for at least four months.

Elderly: Although no specific studies have been performed to establish the use of Alcobon in the elderly, documented use indicates that dosage requirements and side-effect profile are similar to those of younger patients. Particular attention should be paid to renal function in this group.

Alcobon tablets are for oral administration.

Alcobon for Infusion is for intravenous or intraperitoneal administration.

Alcobon for Infusion may be given concurrently with other infusions of normal saline, dextrose or dextrose/saline. No other agent should be added to or mixed with Alcobon for Infusion.

Contra-indications, warnings, etc

Use in pregnancy: Teratogenic effects have been seen in rats, in which species flucytosine is metabolised to fluorouracil. The metabolism may differ in man; nevertheless, the use of Alcobon in pregnancy and in women of childbearing age requires that the potential benefits of therapy be weighed against its possible hazards.

Precautions: Blood levels should be closely monitored in patients with renal insufficiency. If, for any reason, repeated measurements of the blood levels cannot be performed in cases of severe renal failure, Alcobon should not be given.

Because the levels of the drug in blood samples taken during or immediately after administration of Alcobon for Infusion are not a reliable guide to subsequent levels, it is advisable to remove blood for monitoring of blood levels of Alcobon shortly before starting the next infusion.

Special care should be taken in patients with blood dyscrasias and those in whom the bone marrow may be depressed because of disease or treatment. Regular blood counts and tests of liver function should be performed in all patients.

In calculating the fluid and electrolyte intake of patients with impaired renal function, cardiac failure or electrolyte imbalance, due allowance should be made for the volume and chloride content (138 millimole/litre) of Alcobon for Infusion.

Side-effects: At the recommended doses, Alcobon is well tolerated. Nausea, vomiting, diarrhoea and skin rashes have occurred but are usually of a transient nature. Thrombocytopenia and leucopenia have been reported, mostly in those with serious underlying disease and receiving other medicaments. Changes in tests of liver function have been reported in about 10% of patients. Local irritation or phlebitis does not appear to be a problem with Alcobon for Infusion.

Treatment of overdosage: In the event of overdosage with Alcobon, it is recommended that gastric lavage should be performed and measures taken to encourage diuresis. Haemodialysis produces a rapid fall in the serum concentration of Alcobon.

Pharmaceutical precautions *Storage:* Alcobon tablets should be stored in a well-closed container, protected against moisture.

Alcobon for Infusion should be stored between 15 and 23°C. If stored below 15°C, precipitation of Alcobon substance may occur, which should be redissolved by heating to 80°C for not more than 30 minutes. Prolonged storage above 23°C could lead to the decomposition of Alcobon resulting in the formation of 5-fluorouracil.

Additives: Alcobon for Infusion may be given concurrently with other infusions of normal saline, dextrose or dextrose/saline. No other agent should be added to or mixed with Alcobon for Infusion.

Legal category POM.

Package quantities Alcobon tablets are available in packings of 100.

Alcobon for Infusion 2.5 g in 250 ml in packings of 5.

Further information *Availability:* Alcobon tablets and Alcobon for Infusion are available to hospitals only.

Sensitivity testing: It is recommended that cultures for sensitivity testing be taken before treatment and repeated at regular intervals during therapy. However, it is not necessary to delay treatment until results of these tests are known. To determine sensitivities, the methods of Shadomy (*Appl. Microbiol,* 1969, **17**, 871) and Scholer (*Mykosen,* 1970, **13**, 179) are recommended.

For sensitivity testing it is essential that culture media are free of antagonists to flucytosine.

Product licence numbers
Tablets   0031/0069
Infusion   0031/0094

ALLOFERIN*

Presentation Ampoules containing 10 mg alcuronium chloride in 2 ml. The ampoule solution is almost colourless to pale yellow.

Uses *Properties:* Alloferin is a medium-acting neuromuscular blocking agent. It is a derivative of toxiferine, an alkaloid of calabash curare producing muscle relaxation of the non-depolarizing type.

Indications: Muscle relaxation: Alloferin is used for surgical and anaesthetic procedures in which a muscle relaxant is required.

Dosage and administration Response to Alloferin, as to other non-depolarizing relaxants, is subject to individual variation; underlying disease conditions or concurrently administered agents may significantly alter dosage requirements (see Precautions). The following doses are intended as a guide.

Adults: An initial dose of 0.20 to 0.25 mg/kg body-weight intravenously is usually adequate to achieve 95 per cent neuromuscular block. If endotracheal intubation

is to be performed after administration of Alloferin, adequate laryngeal relaxation may be expected after a pause of 90–120 seconds. Profound muscle relaxation will continue for approximately 20–30 minutes when non-potentiating anaesthetic agents are employed. With an initial dose of 0.3 mg/kg body-weight, which may be used when intubating before longer procedures, muscle relaxation is obtained for approximately 40 minutes.

Incremental doses of one-sixth to one-quarter of the initial dose should provide relaxation for additional periods of similar duration to the first.

The following table is given as a more detailed guide to doses for a 70 kg patient

Anaesthetic	Intubation with Alloferin (mg)	Intubation with suxamethonium		
		Abdominal (mg)	Pelvic floor (mg)	Upper abdomen and thorax (mg)
N$_2$O/O$_2$	14–17.5	9	7	11
Halothane 1.5 to 2 vol. %	8.5–11	6	4.5	6.5

Elderly: No specific data are available on the use of Alloferin in the elderly; however, there is no indication from the published literature that the problems encountered in the elderly need be any greater than with the younger adult.

Children: There is insufficient information to recommend a dosage for Alloferin in neonates (up to 28 days of age). Older infants and children should be given 0.125 to 0.20 mg/kg body-weight.

Alloferin ampoules are for intravenous injection.

Alloferin ampoule solution may be diluted with Water for Injection immediately before use.

Maintenance of stability cannot be guaranteed when Alloferin ampoule solution is diluted.

Contra-indications, warnings, etc

Contra-indications: Alloferin is contra-indicated in patients with a history of hypersensitivity to the agent. Use of muscle relaxants is preferably avoided in patients with myasthenia gravis or myasthenic (Eaton-Lambert) syndrome.

Use in pregnancy: No information is available on the effects of Alloferin on the developing foetus and its use in pregnancy should therefore be avoided. Studies indicate that Alloferin does not cross the placenta in amounts that would affect the foetus at or near term.

Precautions: Like other neuromuscular blocking agents, Alloferin should only be administered in the presence of an experienced anaesthetist. The patient's ventilation should be controlled.

Alloferin is mainly excreted in the urine and may therefore accumulate in patients with renal impairment when repeated doses are given. Dosage should be reduced accordingly.

Alloferin is partly bound to serum albumin. Dosage requirements may therefore be altered in patients with hepatic or other disease in which serum protein levels are disturbed.

Increased sensitivity to non-depolarizing drugs may be seen in most neuromuscular diseases, especially amyotrophic lateral sclerosis, poliomyelitis, Duchenne muscular dystrophy and multiple neurofibromatosis.

Sensitivity to non-depolarizing relaxants may be increased by the following drugs: Antibiotics of the polymyxin and aminoglycoside groups (streptomycin, neomycin, kanamycin, gentamicin, amikacin, tobramycin), lincomycin; volatile anaesthetics (ether, halothane, methoxyflurane, cyclopropane, isoflurane, enflurane); drugs with local anaesthetic properties (including quinidine, beta-blocking drugs, phenytoin, penicillamine); ganglion-blocking agents (e.g. trimetaphan), diazepam.

In high concentrations, Mg may increase, whilst K, Na and Ca decrease non-depolarizing neuromuscular block. The action of Alloferin is reportedly not significantly altered by changes in blood pH within the physiological range. Where marked electrolyte or acid-base disturbances are present these should be corrected, if possible, before Alloferin is administered. Care should be taken with dosage especially in acidosis.

During hypothermia non-depolarizing neuromuscular blockade may be decreased. However, care is required during subsequent re-warming to ensure that increased effect does not lead to recurrence of paralysis.

Side-effects: At doses producing adequate neuromuscular block Alloferin does not have marked ganglion-blocking, histamine-releasing or vagolytic actions. Nevertheless, its administration is usually followed by a transient (2–5 minute) lowering of blood pressure due to a fall in peripheral vascular resistance. Less regularly, there may be a moderate increase in heart rate; cardiac output is not significantly altered. Intraocular pressure remains stable.

A few cases of anaphylactoid reaction have been recorded following administration of Alloferin, in most cases in patients who have had previous anaesthesia or a history of allergy.

Effects of overdosage and their treatment: Prolonged respiratory and muscular paralysis are symptoms of overdosage. Artificial ventilation must be continued, and the patient kept under observation until neuromuscular function is restored and there is no risk of recurrence of paralysis.

Prostigmin (neostigmine methylsulphate), given in a dose of 1 to 5 mg (0.05–0.07 mg/kg in children) with atropine 0.4 to 1.25 mg (0.02–0.03 mg/kg in children) by intravenous injection, is routinely used to speed reversal of the neuromuscular block.

Pharmaceutical precautions *Storage:* The recommended maximum storage temperature for Alloferin ampoules is 25°C; the ampoules should be protected from light.

Alloferin should not be administered in the same syringe as thiopentone.

Legal category POM.

Package quantities Alloferin ampoules in packings of 10.

Further information Nil.

Product licence number 0031/5000.

ARFONAD*

Presentation Ampoules containing 250 mg trimetaphan camsylate in 5 ml. The ampoule solution is colourless.

Uses *Properties:* Arfonad is a ganglion-blocking agent which also has a direct dilator effect on peripheral vessels. It has a rapid, short and readily reversible action,

which permits minute-to-minute control of the blood pressure.

Indications: Arfonad is used to induce controlled hypotension during certain surgical procedures. These may include: neurosurgery; vascular surgery; prostatectomy; chest surgery; thyroidectomy; bone and joint surgery.

Dosage and administration *Adults and children:*
(a) Dilution to 250 ml with normal saline or dextrose-saline gives a 0.1% solution (1 mg per ml) which is the strength usually used for an intravenous drip. The Arfonad drip is started at an average of 60 drops (approximately 3 to 4 mg) per minute and, having ascertained the patient's response, the rate of administration is then adjusted to maintain the desired level of hypotension. Since there is marked variation in individual response, continuous blood pressure monitoring is essential to maintain proper control.

(b) If a weaker solution is preferred, a 0.05% solution can be prepared by diluting the 5% ampoule solution to 500 ml.

(c) It may be necessary to use a more concentrated solution in operations in which intravenous fluid should be restricted. For such patients a solution containing 0.25% Arfonad should be prepared by diluting the original 5% solution to 100 ml with normal saline or dextrose-saline. The rate at which the drip is given should be correspondingly reduced.

(d) The undiluted solution has also been used by intermittent intravenous injection.

As with other hypotensive drugs. Arfonad should be stopped before wound closure to allow the blood pressure to rise.

Elderly: No specific data are available on the use of Arfonad in the elderly.

Whilst there is no indication that this is accompanied by particular problems, it is known that the elderly may be more sensitive to hypotensive drugs.

Arfonad ampoules are for administration by intravenous drip and intermittent intravenous injection.

Arfonad ampoule solution may be diluted with Water for Injection, normal saline or dextrose-saline immediately before use.

Contra-indications, warnings, etc
Contra-indications: Arfonad should not be used for hypotensive surgery in patients with severe arteriosclerosis, severe cardiac disease, or pyloric stenosis.

Use in pregnancy: Use of Arfonad in pregnancy should be avoided due to the risk of producing paralytic ileus or meconium ileus in the newborn.

Precautions: Extreme caution should be exercised when using Arfonad in patients with degenerative diseases of the central nervous system, Addison's disease and diabetes mellitus.

Arfonad should be used with particular caution in patients with coronary artery disease, prostatic hypertrophy or glaucoma (cf. pupillary dilatation effect).

Owing to its histamine-releasing effects, Arfonad should be used with caution in subjects with a history of allergy. Caution is also required in the elderly, in patients with cerebral or coronary vascular insufficiency, and in patients with hepatic or renal insufficiency. Care should also be taken in patients receiving neuromuscular blocking agents (especially suxamethonium), myocardial depressants or systemic corticosteroids.

Since the effect of Arfonad is neutralised by vasopressor drugs such as adrenaline, noradrenaline and ephedrine, local adrenaline infiltration at the site of incision is contra-indicated.

Side-effects: Ganglionic blockade due to Arfonad may reduce gastro-intestinal motility and bladder function and affect visual accommodation. Constipation, mydriasis, increased intra-ocular pressure, decreased oral and nasal secretion, respiratory arrest (on rapid infusion of greater than 5 mg/minute), hypoglycaemia and hypokalaemia may also rarely occur.

Treatment of overdosage: The major effect will be a marked fall in blood pressure below the desired level of hypotension. Tachycardia and respiratory depression may result, particularly if Arfonad is used concomitantly with a muscle relaxant. Vasopressor agents such as phenylephrine, ephedrine or noradrenaline are antidotes and may be used to effect a rapid return to normotensive level.

Pharmaceutical precautions *Storage:* The recommended maximum storage temperature is 6°C; avoid freezing.

Additives: It is inadvisable to use the Arfonad drip as a vehicle for administering other drugs. Arfonad is known to be incompatible with thiopentone, gallamine triethiodide, strongly alkaline solutions, iodides and bromides.

Legal category POM.

Package quantities Arfonad ampoules in packings of 10.

Further information Nil.

Product licence number 0031/5001.

BACTRIM* ROCHE

Approved name: Co-trimoxazole.

Presentation Bactrim dispersible tablets: round, pale yellow tablets with 'ROCHE' in a hexagon imprinted on one face, a single break bar on the other, containing 80 mg trimethoprim and 400 mg sulphamethoxazole.

Bactrim Drapsules*; capsuliform, orange, film-coated tablets with 'ROCHE' imprinted on one side, containing 80 mg trimethoprim and 400 mg sulphamethoxazole.

Bactrim Double Strength tablets: oval, biconvex, white tablets with $\frac{ROCHE}{800+160}$ imprinted on one face, a single break bar on the other, containing 160 mg trimethoprim and 800 mg sulphamethoxazole.

Bactrim Paediatric tablets; round, white tablets with 'ROCHE' imprinted on one face, containing 20 mg trimethoprim and 100 mg sulphamethoxazole.

Bactrim suspension (adult); pale yellow, aniseed-flavoured suspension containing 80 mg trimethoprim and 400 mg sulphamethoxazole in 5 ml.

Bactrim paediatric syrup; sugar-free, pale creamy yellow, banana-flavoured suspension containing 40 mg trimethoprim and 200 mg sulphamethoxazole in 5 ml.

Uses *Properties:* Bactrim is bactericidal *in vitro* to a wide range of Gram-positive and Gram-negative organisms, including *Streptococcus, Staphylococcus, Pneumococcus, Neisseria, Escherichia coli, Klebsiella, Proteus* spp., *Haemophilus, Salmonella, Shigella, Vibrio cholerae, Brucella, Pneumocystis carinii, Nocardia* and *Bordetella.* A particularly high degree of activity is exhibited against *Haemophilus influenzae, E. coli* and *Proteus* spp., making

Bactrim particularly suitable for the treatment of chronic bronchitis and urinary tract infections.

Bactrim exerts its bactericidal action by the sequential blockade of two bacterial enzyme systems in the same metabolic pathway. The synergy thus produced accounts for the high degree of bactericidal activity.

Indications: Respiratory infections, including acute and chronic bronchitis (treatment and prophylaxis), also bronchiectasis, lung abscess, lobar and broncho-pneumonia, *Pneumocystis carinii* pneumonitis, sinusitis and otitis media. Urinary tract infections, including urethritis, cystitis, pyelitis, pyelonephritis and prostatitis. Gastro-intestinal tract infections caused by *Salmonella typhi* and *paratyphi*, including the chronic carrier state; bacillary dysentery and cholera (as an adjuvant to fluid and electrolyte replacement). Skin infections, including pyoderma, abscesses and wound infections. Septicaemias. Gonorrhoea. Other infections caused by a wide range of pathogenic bacteria, including acute and chronic osteomyelitis, acute brucellosis, nocardiosis and actinomycetoma, and in South American blastomycosis.

Dosage and administration *Adults and children over 12 years: Bactrim tablets (adult) and Double Strength tablets.* Usual dosage 2 tablets (adult) or 1 Double Strength tablet twice daily. Minimum dosage and dosage for long-term treatment (more than 14 days), 1 tablet (adult) or $\frac{1}{2}$ Double Strength tablet twice daily. For severe infections and septicaemias, 3 tablets (adult) or $1\frac{1}{2}$ Double Strength tablets twice daily. For uncomplicated gonorrhoea, 4 doses of 4 tablets (adult) or 2 Double Strength tablets at 12-hourly intervals over two days may be given. Alternatively 2 doses of 5 tablets (adult) or $2\frac{1}{2}$ Double Strength tablets at an interval of up to 12 hours but not less than eight hours. (The same number of Drapsules* instead of tablets (adult) may be given.) Bactrim Adult suspension 5 ml = 1 tablet (adult) or Drapsule.*

Bactrim tablets (adult) may be dispersed in water or swallowed whole.

Elderly: Clinical and pharmacokinetic studies in elderly patients have shown no need to alter dosage recommendations from those for younger adults.

Children under 12 years: Bactrim tablets (adult).
  6–12 years: 1 tablet twice daily.

Bactrim paediatric tablets:
  2–5 years: 2 paediatric tablets twice daily.
  6–12 years: 4 paediatric tablets twice daily.

Bactrim paediatric syrup
  6 weeks to 5 months: 2.5 ml twice daily.
  6 months to 5 years: 5 ml twice daily.
  6–12 years: 10 ml twice daily.

In children, this corresponds to an approximate dose of 6 mg trimethoprim/kg body weight/day plus 30 mg sulphamethoxazole/kg body weight/day, divided into 2 equal doses.

The dosage required for the treatment of *Pneumocystis carinii* pneumonitis is generally higher than that recommended for other conditions. In children a dosage of 20 mg trimethoprim/kg body weight/day, plus 100 mg sulphamethoxazole/kg body weight/day, given in equally divided doses every six hours for 14 days is suggested. For this reason, treatment should be undertaken only if facilities for regular monitoring of blood levels of the sulphamethoxazole component are available.

Duration of therapy: In acute infections Bactrim should

be given for at least five days or until the patient has been symptom-free for two days. Treatment for prostatitis and acute brucellosis should be maintained for a period of at least four weeks, whilst nocardiosis, actinomycetoma and South American blastomycosis require long-term therapy.

All dosage forms are for oral administration.

Bactrim adult suspension may be diluted with Syrup BP. Maintenance of stability cannot be guaranteed when Bactrim adult suspension is diluted. Dilution of Bactrim paediatric syrup is not recommended.

Contra-indications, warnings, etc

Contra-indications: Bactrim is contra-indicated in patients showing marked liver parenchymal damage or blood dyscrasias, and in severe renal insufficiency where repeated measurements of the plasma concentration cannot be performed. Bactrim should not be given to patients with a history of sensitivity to sulphonamides or trimethoprim. Treatment must be immediately discontinued on the appearance of a skin rash.

Bactrim should not be given to premature babies nor during the first few weeks of life.

Use in pregnancy: The drug should not be given during pregnancy. The usual caution in prescribing any drug for women of childbearing age should also be exercised with Bactrim. Both trimethoprim and sulphamethoxazole are excreted in breast milk. This does not contra-indicate the use of Bactrim in lactating mothers but due account should be taken of the age of the infant being breast-fed.

Precautions: An adequate urinary output should be maintained. In cases with renal impairment a reduced or more widely spaced dosage is indicated to avoid accumulation of the drug. In such patients, measurement of the plasma concentration of the drug is advisable. Regular blood counts are necessary whenever long-term therapy is used.

In the elderly regular monthly blood counts are particularly advisable if Bactrim is to be given for a prolonged period (i.e. exceeding three months), since it has been suggested that elderly patients are more susceptible to blood dyscrasias.

Special caution should be exercised in treating patients with conditions predisposing to folate deficiency and in patients who are also receiving other preparations containing folate inhibitors (e.g. antimalarial drugs containing pyrimethamine; methotrexate) or anticonvulsant drugs.

Care should be taken when giving Bactrim to patients receiving sulphonylurea hypoglycaemic agents or coumarin anticoagulants as the action of these drugs may be increased.

Side-effects: At the recommended dosage Bactrim is well tolerated. Nausea, vomiting, glossitis and skin rashes, including, rarely, erythema multiforme (Stevens-Johnson syndrome) and toxic epidermal necrolysis (Lyell syndrome), can occur.

As Bactrim contains a sulphonamide, the possibility of blood dyscrasias like those associated with sulphonamides should be borne in mind. The changes reported with Bactrim mainly consist of thrombocytopenia, purpura, leucopenia, neutropenia and, very rarely, agranulocytosis. They have usually proved to be reversible on withdrawal of the drug. Elderly patients are more susceptible to these blood changes. During long-term therapy, isolated cases of megaloblastic changes in the bone marrow have been reported; these are reversible by folinic acid therapy.

Effects of overdosage and their treatment: Symptoms of overdosage may include vomiting, mental and visual disturbances, petechiae, purpura and jaundice. Haematuria, crystalluria and anuria may occur in severe cases.

Treatment is symptomatic and may include gastric lavage and forced diuresis. Alkalinisation of the urine may aid the elimination of the sulphamethoxazole component of Bactrim.

Hypersensitivity reactions may require treatment with steroids. Calcium folinate, 3 to 6 mg intramuscularly for five to seven days, may be given to counteract the effects of trimethoprim on haemopoiesis.

Pharmaceutical precautions *Storage:* The recommended maximum storage temperature for Bactrim adult suspension and paediatric syrup is 30°C. No special precautions are required for other oral presentations of Bactrim.

Legal category POM.

Package quantities Bactrim tablets (adult) in packings of 100 and 500.
Bactrim Drapsules in packings of 100 and 500.
Bactrim Double Strength tablets in packings of 50.
Bactrim paediatric tablets in packings of 100.
Bactrim adult suspension in bottles of 100 ml.
Bactrim paediatric syrup in bottles of 100 ml.

Further information Bactrim IM Injection and, to hospitals only, Bactrim for Infusion are also available for patients in whom parenteral administration is indicated. See separate data sheets.

Product licence numbers

Tablets (adult)	0031/0075
Drapsules	0031/5044
Double Strength tablets	0031/0110
Paediatric tablets	0031/5045
Paediatric syrup	0031/5046
Adult suspension	0031/5047

BACTRIM* ROCHE IM INJECTION

Approved name: Co-trimoxazole

Presentation Each 3 ml ampoule contains 160 mg trimethoprim and 800 mg sulphamethoxazole in a vehicle containing 52% glycofurol. The pH of the solution, which is faintly yellow, is approximately 9–10.

Uses *Properties:* Bactrim is bactericidal *in vitro* to a wide range of Gram-positive and Gram-negative organisms, including *Streptococcus, Staphylococcus, Pneumococcus, Neisseria, Escherichia coli, Klebsiella, Proteus* spp., *Haemophilus, Salmonella, Shigella, Vibrio cholerae, Brucella, Pneumocystis carinii, Nocardia* and *Bordetella*. A particularly high degree of activity is exhibited against *Haemophilus influenzae, E. coli* and *Proteus* spp., making Bactrim particularly suitable for the treatment of chronic bronchitis and urinary tract infections.

Bactrim exerts its bactericidal action by the sequential blockade of two bacterial enzyme systems in the same metabolic pathway. The synergy thus produced accounts for the high degree of bactericidal activity.

Indications: Clinical experience with oral Bactrim indicates its therapeutic value in the following conditions:
Respiratory tract infections.
Renal and urinary tract infections.
Genital tract infections.
Gastro-intestinal tract infections caused by *Salmonella*

typhi and *paratyphi*; bacillary dysentery and cholera (as an adjuvant to fluid and electrolyte replacement).

Skin and wound infections.

Septicaemias, osteomyelitis, acute brucellosis, nocardiosis and other infections caused by sensitive organisms.

Bactrim IM Injection is for use when intramuscular administration is preferable to oral therapy.

Dosage and administration Bactrim IM Injection is suitable only for intramuscular administration as described below. It is *not* suitable for any other route or method of administration.

Adults and children over 12 years: One 3 ml ampoule twice daily.

Maximum dosage (for severe infections): One and a half ampoules (4.5 ml) twice daily or one 3 ml ampoule three times daily.

Elderly: Clinical and pharmacokinetic studies in elderly patients have shown no need to alter dosage recommendations from those for younger adults.

Children 6–12 years: The recommended dosage is approximately 6 mg trimethoprim/kg body weight/day plus 30 mg sulphamethoxazole/kg body weight/day divided into two equal doses. As a guide, half an ampoule (1.5 ml) twice daily may be used. The dosage required for the treatment of *Pneumocystis carinii* pneumonitis is generally higher than that recommended for other conditions.

Bactrim IM Injection should not be given to children under the age of six years because of their small muscle mass.

Duration of treatment: it is recommended that Bactrim IM Injection should not be administered in the standard dosage (as indicated above) for more than five successive days, or in the maximum dosage for more than three successive days.

Mode of administration of Bactrim IM: Bactrim IM Injection should be given by deep intramuscular injection into the upper and outer quadrant of the buttock. Successive injections should be given alternately on opposite sides.

Any unused ampoule solution should be discarded.

The ampoule solution of Bactrim IM Injection should not be diluted.

Contra-indications, warnings, etc

Contra-indications: Bactrim is contra-indicated in patients showing marked liver parenchymal damage or blood dyscrasias and in severe renal insufficiency where repeated measurements of the plasma concentration cannot be performed. Bactrim should not be given to patients with a history of sensitivity to sulphonamides or trimethoprim. Treatment must be immediately discontinued on the appearance of a skin rash.

Bactrim should not be given to premature babies nor during the first few weeks of life.

Use in pregnancy: The drug should not be given during pregnancy. The usual caution in prescribing any drug for women of childbearing age should also be exercised with Bactrim. Both trimethoprim and sulphamethoxazole are excreted in breast milk. This does not contra-indicate the use of Bactrim in lactating mothers but due account should be taken of the age of the infant being breast-fed.

Precautions: An adequate urinary output should be maintained. In cases with renal impairment a reduced or more widely spaced dosage is indicated to avoid accumulation of the drug. In such patients, measurement of the plasma concentration of the drug is advisable.

Regular blood counts are necessary whenever long-term therapy is used.

Special caution should be exercised in treating patients with conditions predisposing to folate deficiency and in patients who are also receiving other preparations containing folate inhibitors, e.g. anti-malarial drugs containing pyrimethamine, methotrexate or anticonvulsant drugs.

Care should be taken when giving Bactrim to patients receiving sulphonylurea hypoglycaemic agents or coumarin anticoagulants as the action of these drugs may be increased.

Side-effects: At the recommended dosage. Bactrim is well tolerated. Nausea, vomiting, glossitis and skin rashes, including, rarely, erythema multiforme (Stevens-Johnson syndrome) and toxic epidermal necrolysis (Lyell syndrome), can occur.

As Bactrim contains a sulphonamide, the possibility of blood dyscrasias like those associated with sulphonamides should be borne in mind. The changes reported with Bactrim mainly consist of thrombocytopenia, purpura, leucopenia, neutropenia and, very rarely, agranulocytosis. They have usually proved to be reversible on withdrawal of the drug. Elderly patients are more susceptible to these blood changes. During long-term therapy, isolated cases of megaloblastic changes in the bone marrow have been reported: these are reversible by folinic acid therapy.

Local reactions to Bactrim IM Injection do not appear to be a clinical problem and mainly consist of mild to moderate pain at the injection site; induration is uncommon.

Effects of overdosage and their treatment: Symptoms of overdosage may include vomiting, mental and visual disturbances, petechiae, purpura and jaundice. Haematuria, crystalluria and anuria may occur in severe cases.

Treatment is symptomatic and may include gastric lavage and forced diuresis. Alkalinisation of the urine may aid the elimination of the sulphamethoxazole component of Bactrim.

Hypersensitivity reactions may require treatment with steroids. Calcium folinate, 3–6 mg intramuscularly for five to seven days, may be given to counteract the effects of trimethoprim on haemopoiesis.

Pharmaceutical precautions *Storage:* Bactrim IM Injection should be protected from light. The recommended maximum storage temperature is 30°C.

Additives: The ampoule solution of Bactrim IM Injection should not be diluted.

Legal category POM.

Package quantities Bactrim IM Injection, ampoules containing 160 mg trimethoprim and 800 mg sulphamethoxazole, in packings of 10.

Further information *Availability:* Bactrim is also available as dispersible tablets, Drapsules*, Double Strength tablets, paediatric tablets, adult suspension, paediatric syrup and, to hospitals only, as Bactrim Roche for Infusion. See separate data sheets.

Product licence number 0031/0118.

BACTRIM* ROCHE FOR INFUSION

Approved name: Co-trimoxazole

Presentation Each 5 ml ampoule contains 80 mg trimethoprim and 400 mg sulphamethoxazole in a vehicle containing 40% propylene glycol. The solution, which is almost colourless to very pale yellow, has a pH of approximately 10.5.

Uses *Properties:* Bactrim is bactericidal *in vitro* to a wide range of Gram-positive and Gram-negative organisms, including *Streptococcus, Staphylococcus, Pneumococcus, Neisseria, Escherichia coli, Klebsiella, Proteus* spp., *Haemophilus, Salmonella, Shigella, Vibrio cholerae, Brucella, Pneumocystis carinii, Nocardia* and *Bordetella*. A particularly high degree of activity is exhibited against *Haemophilus influenzae, E. coli* and *Proteus* spp. making Bactrim particularly suitable for the treatment of chronic bronchitis and urinary tract infections.

Bactrim exerts its bactericidal action by the sequential blockade of two bacterial enzyme systems in the same metabolic pathway. The synergy thus produced accounts for the high degree of bactericidal activity.

Indications: Clinical experience with oral Bactrim indicates its therapeutic value in the following conditions. Respiratory tract infections. Renal and urinary tract infections. Genital tract infections. Gastro-intestinal tract infections caused by *Salmonella typhi* and *paratyphi;* bacillary dysentery and cholera (as an adjuvant to fluid and electrolyte replacement). Skin and wound infections. Septicaemias, osteomyelitis, acute brucellosis, nocardiosis and other infections caused by sensitive organisms.

Parenteral administration of Bactrim for Infusion is indicated where oral dosage is not possible, for example: Pre- and post-operative infections and severe trauma. Other clinical situations where the patient is unable to take or tolerate oral therapy.

Dosage and administration (ONLY to be given when DILUTED in an intravenous infusion – see below.)

Adults and children over 12 years: 10 ml twice daily.
Maximum dosage (for severe cases): 15 ml twice daily.

Elderly: Clinical and pharmacokinetic studies in elderly patients have shown no need to alter dosage recommendations from those for younger adults.

Children up to 12 years: The recommended dosage is approximately 6 mg trimethoprim/kg body weight/day, plus 30 mg sulphamethoxazole/kg body weight/day, divided into 2 equal doses. As a guide, the following dosage regimes may be used:

6 weeks to 5 months: 1.25 ml twice daily.
6 months to 5 years: 2.5 ml twice daily.
6–12 years: 5 ml twice daily.

The dosage required for the treatment of *Pneumocystis carinii* pneumonitis is generally higher than that recommended for other conditions. A dosage of 20 mg trimethoprim/kg body weight/day plus 100 mg sulphamethoxazole/kg body weight/day, given in equally divided doses every six hours is suggested. For this reason, treatment should be undertaken only if facilities for monitoring of blood levels of the sulphamethoxazole component are available.

Duration of treatment: It is intended that Bactrim for Infusion should be used only during such a period as the patient is unable to accept oral therapy with Bactrim. In general, administration is unlikely to be required for more than a few days. At present it is recommended that the maximum dose (as indicated above) should not be administered for more than three successive days.

Mode of administration of Bactrim for Infusion: Bactrim for Infusion is suitable only for use as described below

after addition to intravenous infusions. It is NOT suitable for any other route or method of administration.

Bactrim for Infusion must ONLY be given by the intravenous route and MUST BE DILUTED according to the schedule given below.

Bactrim for Infusion should only be mixed with one of the following infusion solutions: Dextrose Injection BP 5% and 10%. Laevulose Injection BP 5%. Compound Sodium Lactate Injection BP (Hartmann's Solution). Compound Sodium Chloride Injection BPC 1959 (Ringer's Solution). Sodium Chloride Injection BP. Sodium Chloride and Dextrose Injection BP (0.45% sodium chloride and 2.5% dextrose). Dextran 40 Injection BP. Dextran 70 Injection BP. No other agent should be added to or mixed with the infusion.

Dilution should be carried out as follows: One ampoule Bactrim for Infusion (5 ml) to 125 ml infusion solution.

Two ampoules Bactrim for Infusion (10 ml) to 250 ml infusion solution.

Three ampoules Bactrim for Infusion (15 ml) to 500 ml infusion solution.

Dilution should be carried out **immediately** before use. After addition of Bactrim for Infusion to the infusion solution, the mixture should be well shaken in order to ensure thorough mixing. Should visible turbidity or crystallisation appear in the solution at any time before or during the infusion, the mixture should be discarded.

It is suggested that the duration of the infusion should be of the order of $1\frac{1}{2}$ hours, but this should be balanced against the fluid requirements of the patient.

Contra-indications, warnings, etc
Contra-indications: Bactrim is contra-indicated in patients showing marked liver parenchymal damage or blood dyscrasias and in severe renal insufficiency where repeated measurements of the plasma concentration cannot be performed. Bactrim should not be given to patients with history of sensitivity to sulphonamides or trimethoprim. Treatment must be immediately discontinued on the appearance of a skin rash.

Bactrim should not be given to premature babies nor during the first few weeks of life.

Use in pregnancy: The drug should not be given during pregnancy. The usual caution in prescribing any drug for women of childbearing age should also be exercised with Bactrim. Both trimethoprim and sulphamethoxazole are excreted in breast milk. This does not contra-indicate the use of Bactrim in lactating mothers but due account should be taken of the age of the infant being breast-fed.

Precautions: An adequate urinary output should be maintained. In cases with renal impairment a reduced or more widely spaced dosage is indicated to avoid accumulation of the drug. In such patients, measurement of the plasma concentration of the drug is advisable. Special caution should be exercised in treating patients with conditions predisposing to folate deficiency and in patients who are also receiving other preparations containing folate inhibitors (e.g. antimalarial drugs containing pyrimethamine; methotrexate) or anticonvulsant drugs.

Care should be taken when giving Bactrim to patients receiving strongly serum-protein-bound drugs such as oral hypoglycaemic agents or coumarin anticoagulants as the action of these drugs may be increased.

Side-effects: At the recommended dosage, Bactrim is well tolerated. Nausea, vomiting, glossitis and skin rashes, including, rarely, erythema multiforme (Stevens-

Johnson syndrome) and toxic epidermal necrolysis (Lyell syndrome), can occur.

As Bactrim contains a sulphonamide, the possibility of blood dyscrasias like those associated with sulphonamides should be borne in mind. The changes reported with Bactrim mainly consist of thrombocytopenia, purpura, leucopenia, neutropenia and, very rarely, agranulocytosis. They have usually proved to be reversible on withdrawal of the drug. Elderly patients are more susceptible to these blood changes. During long-term therapy, isolated cases of megaloblastic changes in the bone marrow have been reported, these are reversible by folinic acid therapy.

Bactrim for Infusion has occasionally given rise to local side-effects in the form of pain and phlebitis.

Effects of overdosage and their treatment: Symptoms of overdosage may include vomiting, mental and visual disturbances, petechiae, purpura and jaundice. Haematuria, crystalluria and anuria may occur in severe cases.

Treatment is symptomatic and may include forced diuresis. Alkalinisation of the urine may aid the elimination of the sulphamethoxazole component of Bactrim for Infusion.

Hypersensitivity reactions may require treatment with steroids. Calcium folinate, 3–6 mg intramuscularly for five to seven days, may be given to counteract the effects of trimethoprim on haemopoiesis.

Pharmaceutical precautions *Storage:* Bactrim for Infusion should be protected from light.

Legal category POM.

Package quantities Bactrim for Infusion, ampoules containing 80 mg trimethoprim and 400 mg sulphamethoxazole in 5 ml, in packings of 10.

Further information *Availability:* Bactrim for Infusion is available to hospitals only.

Bactrim is also available as dispersible tablets (adult), Drapsules*, Double Strength tablets, paediatric tablets, adult suspension and paediatric syrup and as Bactrim Roche IM Injection. See separate data sheets.

Product licence number 0031/0070.

BECOSYM*

Presentation Becosym tablets: round, dark brown, film-coated tablets with BECOSYM imprinted on one face. They are known as Vitamin B Tablets, Compound, Strong BPC.

Becosym Forte tablets: round, dark brown, film-coated tablets with BECOSYM FORTE imprinted on one face.

Becosym syrup: dark red-orange, fruit-flavoured syrup.

The vitamin content of these preparations is shown below.

	Each tablet (mg)	Each Forte tablet (mg)	Syrup 5 ml (mg)
Thiamine hydrochloride	5	15	5
Riboflavine	2	15	2
Nicotinamide	20	50	20
Pyridoxine hydrochloride	2	10	2

Uses *Properties:* The vitamin B-complex comprises a group of water-soluble factors more or less closely associated in their natural occurrence. It is known that nearly every vitamin of the B-complex forms part of a co-enzyme essential for the metabolism of protein, carbohydrate or fatty acid.

Manifestations of deficiency of the B-vitamins include glossitis, stomatitis, cheilosis, the heart manifestations of beriberi, the skin manifestations of pellagra, corneal vascularisation and polyneuritis.

Indications: Becosym has been found of value in: clinical and subclinical vitamin deficiency states; supplementation of diet in old age and as an aid to recovery from illness and surgery; adjunct to treatment with broad-spectrum antibiotics.

Dosage and administration

Becosym and Becosym Forte tablets and Becosym syrup are for oral administration.

Becosym syrup may be diluted with Syrup BP. Maintenance of stability cannot be guaranteed when Becosym syrup is diluted.

	Prophylactic	Therapeutic
Adults	1–3 tablets or 5–15 ml syrup daily	2 or 3 Forte tablets daily
Children	5 to 15 ml syrup daily	1–3 tablets daily
Infants	5 ml syrup daily	

Elderly: Although no specific studies have been performed to establish the use of Becosym in the elderly, it has been used extensively and the dosage requirements appear to be similar to those of younger adults.

Contra-indications, warnings, etc

Use in pregnancy: Becosym and other vitamin B preparations have been widely used during pregnancy without apparent ill consequence; animal studies have shown no hazard.

Pharmaceutical precautions *Storage:* The recommended maximum storage temperature for Becosym, Becosym Forte tablets and Becosym syrup is 25°C. Becosym syrup should be protected from light.

Legal category Tablets GSL
Forte tablets GSL
Syrup GSL

Package quantities Becosym tablets in packings of 100 and 500.

Becosym Forte tablets in packings of 25, 100 and 250. Becosym syrup in packings of 100 ml.

Further information Nil.

Product licence numbers
Tablets 0031/5005
Forte tablets 0031/5006
Syrup 0031/5007

BENERVA*

Presentation Round, white tablets with 'BENERVA' imprinted on one face, '3' in the centre of the other, containing 3 mg thiamine hydrochloride.

Round, white tablets with 'BENERVA 10' imprinted on one face, containing 10 mg thiamine hydrochloride.

Round, white tablets with 'BENERVA 25' imprinted on one face, containing 25 mg thiamine hydrochloride.

Round, white tablets with 'BENERVA 50' imprinted on one face, containing 50 mg thiamine hydrochloride.

Round, white tablets with 'BENERVA 100' imprinted on one face, containing 100 mg thiamine hydrochloride.

Round, white tablets with 'ROCHE' imprinted on one face, containing 300 mg thiamine hydrochloride.

Ampoules containing 25 mg thiamine hydrochloride in 1 ml. The ampoule solution is almost colourless to faintly yellow.

Ampoules containing 100 mg thiamine hydrochloride in 1 ml. The ampoule solution is almost colourless to faintly yellow.

Uses *Properties:* Vitamin B_1, in the form of thiamine pyrophosphate (co-carboxylase), is involved in several key steps of carbohydrate metabolism. It is a coenzyme for the oxidative decarboxylation of pyruvate to acetyl-coenzyme A (an intermediate in the biosynthesis of fatty acids, steroids and the neurotransmitter acetylcholine) and of 2-oxo-glutarate to succinyl-coenzyme A (in the citric acid cycle), and is a coenzyme for transketolase in the pentose phosphate pathway. Thiamine is particularly important for nerve-cell function. Chronic deficiency of the vitamin is accompanied by polyneuritis and brady-cardia, whilst marked deficiency is characterized by muscle weakness, paraesthesiae and paralysis ('dry' beriberi), and by dilatation of the right heart, often with oedema ('wet' beriberi); Wernicke's encephalopathy may occur in severe cases.

Indications: Benerva is specific in the treatment of the various manifestations of thiamine deficiency such as the classic severe form (beri-beri) and also conditions such as Wernicke's encephalopathy. Supplementary Benerva may be indicated prophylactically in conditions where there is low dietary intake or impaired gastro-intestinal absorption of thiamine (e.g. alcoholism) or where requirements are increased (pregnancy, carbo-hydrate-rich diet).

Dosage and administration *Adults:*

Prophylaxis	3–10 mg daily.
Mild chronic deficiency	10–25 mg daily.
Severe deficiency	200–300 mg daily.

Elderly: Although no specific studies have been per-formed to establish the use of Benerva in the elderly, it has been used extensively and the dosage requirements and side-effects appear to be similar to those of younger adults.

Children: If, on the recommendation of a physician, a children's dosage is required, then it is suggested that 5 to 20 mg daily may be given. If a parenteral dose is required, 2.5 to 100 mg daily, depending on body-weight, may be given.

Benerva tablets are for oral administration.

Benerva ampoules are for intramuscular or intravenous injection.

Benerva ampoule solution may be diluted with Water for Injection.

Maintenance of stability cannot be guaranteed when Benerva ampoule solution is diluted.

Contra-indications, warnings, etc *Contra-indica-tions:* Known hypersensitivity to thiamine (vitamin B_1).

Use in pregnancy: There is no evidence as to the safety of Benerva in human pregnancy, nor is there evidence from animal work that it is free from hazard.

Precautions: Although Benerva is very well tolerated, it is now recognised that an anaphylactic reaction may sometimes occur after an injection of vitamin B_1, probably due to sensitisation to the vitamin. A patient may tolerate one or more courses of injection without trouble but then experience a reaction to a later injection. Mild allergic phenomena, such as sneezing or mild asthma, are warning signs that further injection may give rise to anaphylactic shock. To avoid this possibility it is advisable to start a second course of injections with a dose considerably lower than that previously used. Because of the above, injections of B_1 should not be given intravenously, except in the case of comatose patients who are often given large doses of vitamins by intravenous drip.

Pharmaceutical precautions *Storage:* Recom-mended maximum storage temperature 30°C. Benerva tablets and ampoules should be protected from light.

Legal category Tablets GSL.
Ampoules POM.

Package quantities Benerva tablets 3 mg in packings of 100.

Benerva tablets 10 mg in packings of 100.
Benerva tablets 25 mg in packings of 100.
Benerva tablets 50 mg in packings of 100.
Benerva tablets 100 mg in packings of 100.
Benerva tablets 300 mg in packings of 100.
Benerva ampoules 25 mg in 1 ml in packings of 10.
Benerva ampoules 100 mg in 1 ml in packings of 10.

Further information Nil.

Product licence numbers

Tablets 3 mg	0031/5050
Tablets 10 mg	0031/5051
Tablets 25 mg	0031/5052
Tablets 50 mg	0031/5053
Tablets 100 mg	0031/5054
Tablets 300 mg	0031/5055
Ampoules 25 mg	0031/5056
Ampoules 100 mg	0031/5057

BENERVA* COMPOUND

Presentation Round, yellow tablets with 'ROCHE' imprinted on one face, containing 1 mg thiamine hydrochloride, 1 mg riboflavine and 15 mg nicotinamide. They are known as Vitamin B Tablets Compound BPC.

Uses *Properties:* Benerva Compound tablets contain the three principal members of the vitamin B-complex.

The vitamin B-complex comprises a group of water-soluble factors more or less closely associated in their natural occurrence. It is known that nearly every vitamin of the B-complex forms part of a co-enzyme essential for the metabolism of protein, carbohydrate or fatty acid.

Indications: Treatment of minor degrees of vitamin B-complex deficiency.

Dosage and administration

	Prophylactic	Therapeutic
Adults	1–2 tablets daily	1–3 tablets three times daily
Children:		
Over 12 years	1½–2 tablets daily	1½–2 tablets three times daily
Under 12 years	½–1 tablet daily	½–1 tablet three times daily

Benerva Compound tablets are for oral administration.

Elderly: Although no specific studies have been performed to establish the use of Benerva Compound in the elderly, it has been used extensively and dosage requirements appear to be similar to those of younger adults.

Contra-indications, warnings, etc
Use in pregnancy: Benerva Compound and other vitamin B complex preparations have been widely used during pregnancy without apparent ill consequence; animal studies have shown no hazard.

Pharmaceutical precautions *Storage:* Recommended maximum storage temperature 25°C. Benerva Compound tablets should be protected from light.

Legal category GSL.

Package quantities Benerva Compound tablets in packings of 200.

Further information Nil.

Product licence number 0031/5009.

DALMANE*

Presentation Capsules with opaque grey cap and opaque yellow body with 'ROCHE 15' printed in red on both cap and body, containing 16.4 mg flurazepam monohydrochloride (equivalent to 15 mg flurazepam). Capsules with black cap and opaque grey body with 'ROCHE 30' printed in red on both cap and body, containing 32.8 mg flurazepam monohydrochloride (equivalent to 30 mg flurazepam).

Uses *Properties:* Dalmane is a benzodiazepine drug with hypnotic properties.

Indications: The short-term treatment of insomnia. Dalmane is helpful in overcoming difficulties in getting to sleep and also in the problem of frequent nocturnal awakenings. Its properties make it particularly indicated where the total duration of sleep is less than adequate.

Dosage and administration *Adults:* The dosage of Dalmane should be determined on an individual basis taking into account the severity of the insomnia and the patient's response to treatment. Dosage is important in determining the duration of effect and the occurrence of residual effects. For most patients the optimum dose is 15 mg – this will ensure a full night's sleep with minimal residual effects on wakening. Patients with severe insomnia may require 30 mg but residual effects on awakening, associated with an anxiolytic effect, are more frequent at this dose. The following doses are indicated as a guide:

Mild to moderate insomnia	15 mg
Severe insomnia	30 mg.

Elderly or debilitated patients: The initial dose should not exceed 15 mg.

Dalmane is not for paediatric use.

Dalmane capsules are for oral administration.

Contra-indications, warnings, etc *Contra-indications:* Patients with known sensitivity to benzodiazepines; acute pulmonary insufficiency; respiratory depression.

Use in pregnancy: There is no evidence as to drug safety in human pregnancy, nor is there evidence from animal work that it is free from hazard. Do not use during pregnancy, especially during the first and last trimesters, unless there are compelling reasons.

The administration of high doses or prolonged administration of low doses of benzodiazepines in the last trimester of pregnancy has been reported to produce irregularities in the foetal heart, and hypotonia, poor sucking and hypothermia in the neonate.

No data regarding the passage of flurazepam in breast milk are available. However, in common with other benzodiazepines, its passage into breast milk might be expected. If possible, the use of Dalmane during lactation should be avoided.

Precautions: In patients with chronic pulmonary insufficiency, and in patients with chronic renal or hepatic disease, dosage may need to be reduced.

Patients should be advised that, like all medicaments of this type, Dalmane may modify patients' performance at skilled tasks (driving, operating machinery, etc.) to a varying degree depending upon dosage, administration and individual susceptibility. Patients should further be advised that alcohol may intensify any impairment, and should, therefore be avoided during treatment. If the patient awakens for short intervals during the period of drug activity (as indeed during non-drug induced sleep) ability to recall these events may be impaired.

Excessive or prolonged use of benzodiazepines may occasionally result in the development of some psychological dependence, with withdrawal symptoms on sudden discontinuation of the drug. This is particularly so in patients with a history of alcoholism or drug abuse or in patients with marked personality disorders. Regular monitoring in such patients is essential, routine repeat prescriptions should be avoided and treatment should be withdrawn gradually. Symptoms such as depression, nervousness, rebound insomnia, irritability, sweating, and diarrhoea have been reported following abrupt cessation of treatment in patients receiving even normal therapeutic doses for short periods of time.

In rare instances, withdrawal following excessive dosages may produce confusional states, psychotic manifestations and convulsions.

Abnormal psychological reactions to benzodiazepines have been reported. Rare behavioural effects include paradoxical aggressive outbursts, excitement, confusion and the uncovering of depression with suicidal tendencies.

If Dalmane is combined with centrally-acting drugs such as neuroleptics, tranquillisers, antidepressants, hypnotics, analgesics and anaesthetics, the sedative effects are likely to be intensified. The elderly require special supervision.

When Dalmane is used in conjunction with antiepileptic drugs, side-effects and toxicity may be more evident, particularly with hydantoins or barbiturates or combinations including them. This requires extra care in adjusting dosage in the initial stages of treatment.

Side-effects and adverse reactions: Common adverse effects include drowsiness, sedation, unsteadiness and ataxia; these are dose-related and may persist into the following day, even after a single dose. The elderly are particularly sensitive to the effects of central depressant drugs and may experience confusion, especially if organic brain changes are present; therefore dosage in these patients should not exceed 15 mg.

Other adverse effects are rare and include headache, vertigo, hypotension, gastro-intestinal upsets, skin rashes, visual disturbances, changes in libido, and urinary retention. Isolated cases of blood dyscrasias and jaundice have also been reported

Occasionally patients treated with Dalmane experience a bitter after-taste.

Treatment of overdosage: When taken alone in overdosage, Dalmane presents few problems in management. Signs may include drowsiness, ataxia and dysarthria, with coma in severe cases. Treatment is symptomatic. Gastric lavage is useful only if performed soon after ingestion. There is no specific antidote to Dalmane.

When taken with centrally-acting drugs, especially alcohol, the effects of overdosage are likely to be more severe and, in the absence of supportive measures, may prove fatal.

Pharmaceutical precautions *Storage:* Dalmane capsules in blister packings should be stored in a dry place.

Legal category CD (Sch. 4), POM.

Package quantities Dalmane capsules 15 mg and 30 mg in blister packs of 30.

Further information The pharmacokinetic properties of Dalmane make it particularly indicated for patients whose total duration of sleep is less than adequate. The dosage of the drug is important in balancing the duration of effect with the occurrence of residual effects. On repeated dosing there is accumulation of an active metabolite, desalkylflurazepam, with steady state levels being reached within two to three weeks. Psychomotor studies have demonstrated, however, that a dose of 15 mg given for seven consecutive nights did not significantly affect performance on the morning after final administration. However, impairment of performance was recorded on the morning after final administration of 30 mg for seven consecutive nights. This dose is associated with daytime anxiolytic effects.

The elderly, and patients with impaired renal and/or hepatic function, will be particularly susceptible to the adverse effects listed above. It is advisable to review treatment regularly and to discontinue use as soon as possible.

Treatment should be kept to minimum and given only under close medical supervision. Little is known regarding the efficacy or safety of benzodiazepines in long-term use.

Product licence numbers
Capsules 15 mg   0031/0065
Capsules 30 mg   0031/0066

DECLINAX*

Presentation Round, white tablets with 'ROCHE 10' imprinted on one face and a single break bar on the other, containing 12.8 mg debrisoquine sulphate (equivalent to 10 mg base).

Round, pale blue tablets with 'ROCHE 20' imprinted on one face and two break bars on the other, containing 25.6 mg debrisoquine sulphate (equivalent to 20 mg base).

Uses *Properties:* Declinax lowers blood pressure markedly and promptly in the hypertensive patient. It does this by blocking the transmission of sympathetic nerve impulses at the nerve terminals, thereby decreasing peripheral vascular resistance. Reduction in post-ganglionic sympathetic transmission is achieved by interfering with the physiological release of noradrenaline, without depleting major catecholamine stores in cardio-vascular tissues and without impairing the cardiac contractile mechanism. The action, as with other alpha-adrenergic agents, is most marked in the standing position. Declinax normally acts within 4–10 hours and its effects usually last for 9–24 hours, although an occasional patient may show a longer response. There is no accumulation on maintenance dosage.

Indications: Declinax is indicated for the treatment of all grades of hypertension. It can be given either alone or together with other antihypertensive drugs or diuretics.

Dosage and administration *Adults: Mild to moderate hypertension:* 10 mg once or twice daily. This dose can be increased by 10 mg at three-day intervals. The total dose usually falls within the range 20–60 mg daily.

Severe hypertension: 20 mg once or twice daily. This dose can be increased, depending on response, by 10–20 mg every three or four days provided a close check is kept on the blood pressure. The total dose usually falls within the range 40–120 mg, but in cases of very severe hypertension 300 mg or more daily may be given.

Should postural hypotension occur with a dosage that controls the blood pressure, the total daily dose should be adjusted to give a small dose in the morning, a relatively large dose at midday and a moderate evening dose.

Elderly: There is inadequate evidence of the safety of Declinax in the elderly, although it has been in wide use for many years without apparent ill consequence specifically relating to elderly populations. However, as with other potent hypotensive agents, including alpha-adrenergic blockers, the possibility of postural hypotension occurring should be borne in mind.

Children: No dosage recommendations are made for the administration of Declinax to children.

Declinax tablets are for oral administration.

Contra-indications, warnings, etc
Contra-indications: Declinax should not be given to patients with a phaeochromocytoma or with a recent history of cerebral or myocardial infarction. It is contra-indicated in patients who have shown hypersensitivity to the drug.

Use in pregnancy: There is inadequate evidence of safety of Declinax in human pregnancy but it has been in wide use for many years without apparent ill consequence, animal studies having shown no hazard.

Precautions: Declinax should be used with caution in patients with renal insufficiency; smaller or more widely spread doses may be appropriate.

Declinax may give rise to exertional and postural hypotension (see *Side-effects*). Caution should therefore be exercised in patients with coronary or cerebral insufficiency.

The possibility of an enhanced hypotensive effect should be borne in mind when any drug with a tendency to lower blood pressure is given concomitantly with Declinax.

As with other potent hypotensive agents, including alpha-adrenergic blockers, the possibility of postural hypotension occurring in the elderly should be borne in mind.

Patients on antihypertensive drugs often have a lower blood pressure in warm weather, therefore in hot climates their dose of Declinax may need to be reduced. Evidence from both animal experiments and clinical observation suggests that the hypotensive action of adrenergic neurone-blocking drugs such as Declinax may be inhibited by simultaneous treatment with tricyclic anti-depressants. Extra care should be taken when prescribing antihypertensive drugs in patients being treated with levodopa. Patients taking Declinax are sensitive to sympathomimetic drugs.

If anaesthesia for surgery or dentistry is necessary, the anaesthetist should be informed that the patient is being treated with Declinax.

Abrupt cessation of Declinax should be avoided as this may lead to rebound hypertension.

Side-effects: Declinax is well tolerated. Overdosage causes postural hypotension, most noticeable in the early morning or with long standing and associated with weakness, giddiness and fatigue. The patient should be warned of the possibility of these symptoms occurring. This can be minimised by reducing the dose. Other side-effects include malaise, nausea, headache, sweating, failure of ejaculation in the male, and sometimes frequency of micturition and nocturia. Diarrhoea, common with some other antihypertensive agents, is seen only very rarely. Aggravation of angina pectoris has been reported in a few cases.

Effects of overdosage and their treatment: Excessive fall in blood pressure will be shown by orthostatic collapse. This will usually respond rapidly to placing the patient in a recumbent position. Patients receiving Declinax are particularly sensitive to the effects of catecholamines. Sympathomimetic agents should therefore be administered only with great caution.

Pharmaceutical precautions *Storage:* Declinax tablets should be stored in well-closed containers.

Legal category POM.

Package quantities Declinax tablets 10 mg in packings of 100 and 500.
Declinax tablets 20 mg in packings of 100 and 500.

Further information The metabolism of debrisoquine is subject to genetic polymorphism such that non-metabolisers may show a marked response (e.g. orthostatic hypotension) to doses that have little or no effect in metabolisers.

New patients should be carefully monitored during the initial treatment to determine possible non-metabolisers (approximately 8% of Caucasian populations).

Product licence numbers
Tablets 10 mg   0031/5059
Tablets 20 mg   0031/5060

DROMORAN* ROCHE

Presentation Round, white tablets with 'ROCHE' imprinted on one face, two concentric circles on the other, containing 1.5 mg levorphanol tartrate. Ampoules containing 2 mg levorphanol tartrate in 1 ml. The ampoule solution is colourless to pale yellow.

Uses *Properties:* Dromoran Roche is a more potent and longer-acting analgesic than morphine. The analgesic effect begins within 10–30 minutes after administration and may continue for as long as eight hours. Dromoran Roche is effective by mouth. Only in acute pain, when it is desirable to obtain rapid relief, is it necessary to give the drug by injection.

Indications: Relief of severe pain; pre-operative medication; supplement to nitrous oxide/oxygen anaesthesia.

Dosage and administration *Adults: Oral:* Single dose of 1.5–4.5 mg once or twice daily.

Adults: Injection: When immediate relief of very severe pain is required, the following doses may be given by injection.

Subcutaneous or intramuscular injection: The usual single dose is 2–4 mg.

Intravenous injection: 1–2 mg.
Thereafter maintenance doses by mouth can be given as above.

Premedication: Single dose of 1–2 mg by injection one hour before operation.

Supplement to nitrous oxide/oxygen anaesthesia: Total dose usually 1.5–2 mg given in divided doses of 0.25–0.5 mg.

Elderly: Elderly patients are more sensitive to the actions of narcotic analgesics; the initial dose of Dromoran should be at the lower end of the ranges recommended for adults.

Children: Paediatric dose not established.

Dromoran Roche tablets are for oral administration.
Dromoran Roche ampoules are for intramuscular, intravenous or subcutaneous injection.
Dromoran Roche ampoule solution may be diluted with Water for Injection.
Maintenance of stability cannot be guaranteed when Dromoran Roche ampoule solution is diluted.

Contra-indications, warnings, etc
Contra-indications: Dromoran Roche should not be given to comatose patients or to patients with respiratory depression or obstructive airways disease. It should not be administered to patients who are receiving mono-amine oxidase inhibitors or within two weeks of their withdrawal.

Dromoran Roche should not be given to patients with a history of hypersensitivity or idiosyncratic response to the drug.

Use in pregnancy: There is little reported human usage of Dromoran Roche in pregnancy. Although no adverse effects have been found in animals, the established medical principle of prescribing medicaments in early pregnancy only when absolutely indicated should be observed.

Dromoran Roche crosses the placenta and may also be secreted in breast milk. This should be borne in mind when considering its use in patients during pregnancy or breast feeding. Administration in labour may cause respiratory depression in the newborn infant.

Precautions: Dromoran Roche should only be given with caution, and in reduced dosage, to neonates and premature infants, elderly and debilitated patients, and in patients with head injuries, severe hepatic or renal impairment, biliary tract disorders, hypothyroidism, adrenocortical insufficiency, shock, prostatic hypertrophy, and supraventricular tachycardia.

Caution is also required in patients exhibiting acute alcoholism, raised intracranial pressure or convulsive disorders. Dromoran Roche depresses respiratory function and should be administered with particular care in patients with respiratory insufficiency.

The effects of Dromoran Roche may be potentiated by concurrent administration of other central nervous system depressants, including anaesthetic agents. Concomitant administration of Dromoran Roche with phenothiazines may induce severe hypotension. Patients should be instructed to avoid alcohol while under treatment, since the individual response cannot be foreseen.

Dromoran Roche may modify patients' reactions (driving ability, operation of machinery, etc.) to a varying extent, depending on dosage, administration and individual susceptibility.

Repeated administration of Dromoran Roche may induce tolerance to the drug, with a tendency to increasing dosage requirements to obtain the desired effect, or to physical and psychological dependence of the morphine type, with the development of withdrawal symptoms after abrupt cessation of therapy. Cross-tolerance between narcotic analgesics can occur.

Side-effects: Dromoran Roche is usually well tolerated. Neither circulatory disturbances nor effects on the blood-picture are likely. Appetite, gastro-intestinal and renal functions are less likely to be affected by Dromoran Roche than by morphine; however, nausea, vomiting, constipation and confusion may be troublesome. The drug has a less pronounced hypnotic effect than morphine, and is, therefore, useful for the relief of pain during the day.

Effects of overdosage and their treatment: In overdosage pin-point pupils, tremors and convulsions, depressed respiration and impaired level of consciousness or coma may occur. In severe poisoning there may be dilatation of pupils, shock, severe respiratory depression and pulmonary oedema.

Gastric aspiration and lavage should be performed soon after ingestion and intensive supportive therapy carried out. Naloxone is the preferred antidote.

Pharmaceutical precautions *Storage:* The recommended maximum storage temperature for Dromoran Roche ampoules is 25°C; the ampoules should be protected from light.

Dromoran Roche tablets in blister packs should be stored in a dry place.

Legal category CD (Sch. 2), POM.

Package quantities Dromoran Roche tablets in 5 packs of 10 in a labelled carton or 10 packs of 50 in unlabelled shrinkwrap.

Dromoran Roche ampoules in packings of 10.

Further information Nil.

Product licence numbers
Tablets   0031/5061R
Ampoules   0031/5062R

EFUDIX* ▼

Presentation White, opaque cream containing 5% w/w fluorouracil.

Uses *Properties:* Efudix is a topical cytostatic preparation which exerts a beneficial therapeutic effect on neoplastic and pre-neoplastic skin lesions without damaging normal skin. The pattern of response follows this sequence: erythema, vesication, erosion, ulceration, necrosis and epithelisation.

Indications: Efudix is used for the topical treatment of superficial pre-malignant and malignant skin lesions; keratoses, including senile, actinic and arsenical forms; keratoacanthoma; Bowen's disease; superficial basal-cell carcinoma.

Deep, penetrating or nodular basal cell and squamous cell carcinomas do not usually respond to Efudix therapy. It should be used only as a palliative therapy in such cases where no other form of treatment is possible.

Dosage and administration *Pre-malignant conditions:* The cream should be applied thinly to the affected area once or twice daily: an occlusive dressing is not essential.

Malignant conditions: The cream should be applied once or twice daily under an occlusive dressing where this is practicable.

The cream should not harm healthy skin. Treatment should be continued until there is a marked inflammatory response from the treated area, preferably with some erosion in the case of pre-malignant conditions. Severe discomfort may be alleviated by the use of topical steroid cream. The usual duration of treatment for an initial course of therapy is three to four weeks, but this may be prolonged. Lesions on the face usually respond more quickly than those on the trunk or lower limbs whilst lesions on the hands and forearms respond more slowly. Healing may not be complete until one or two months after therapy is stopped.

Elderly: Many of the conditions for which Efudix is indicated are common in the elderly. No special precautions are necessary.

Children: In view of the lack of clinical data available, Efudix is not recommended for use in children.

Efudix cream is for topical application.
Efudix cream should not be diluted.

Contra-indications, warnings, etc
Contra-indications: Efudix is contra-indicated in patients with known sensitivity to Efudix or parabens.

Use in pregnancy: Fluorouracil has been shown to be teratogenic. Efudix should not normally be administered to patients who are pregnant. It should also be regarded as contra-indicated in mothers who are breast-feeding.

Precautions: Efudix is for topical use only and care should be taken to avoid contact with mucous membranes or the eyes. The hands should be washed carefully after applying the cream.

The total area of skin being treated with Efudix at any one time should not exceed 500 cm^2 (approx 23×23 cm). Larger areas should be treated a section at a time.

Side-effects: Efudix is well tolerated and systemic toxicity is negligible. Transient erythema may occur in healthy skin surrounding the area being treated. Pre-existing subclinical lesions may become apparent. Exposure to sunlight may increase the intensity of the reaction.

Effects of overdosage and their treatment: If Efudix is accidentally ingested, signs of fluorouracil overdosage may include nausea, vomiting and diarrhoea. Stomatitis and blood dyscrasias may occur in severe cases. Appropriate measures should be taken for the prevention of systemic infection and daily white cell counts should be performed.

Pharmaceutical precautions *Storage:* The recommended maximum storage temperature for Efudix cream is 30°C.

Legal category POM.

Package quantities Efudix cream in tubes of 20 g.

Further information Efudix should be used only under specialist medical supervision.

Availability: Efudix cream is available through hospital

pharmacies for use in hospitals and hospital clinics and can be supplied to retail pharmacies for dispensing prescriptions for patients whose treatment has been initiated in hospital practice.

Product licence number   0031/0027

EPHYNAL*

Presentation   Round, white tablets with 'EPHYNAL' imprinted on one face, the other being plain, containing 3 mg tocopheryl acetate.

Round, white tablets with 'EPHYNAL' imprinted on one face and 'TEN' on the other, containing 10 mg tocopheryl acetate.

Round, white tablets with 'EPHYNAL 50' imprinted on one face with a single break bar on the other, containing 50 mg tocopheryl acetate.

Round, white to pale cream tablets with 'EPHYNAL 200' imprinted on one face and a single break bar on the other, containing 200 mg tocopheryl acetate.

Uses   *Properties:* Ephynal is a synthetic vitamin E preparation. The exact role of vitamin E in the animal organism has not yet been established. Vitamin E is known to exert an important physiological function as an anti-oxidant for fats, with a sparing action on vitamin A, carotenoids and on unsaturated fatty acids. Other work has demonstrated that vitamin E is connected with the maintenance of certain factors essential for the normal metabolic cycle.

Vitamin E deficiency produces a wide variety of manifestations in many organs and tissues of the body of most animal species that have been studied.

Indications: Ephynal is indicated in high dosage for the treatment of intermittent claudication of moderate severity.

There is occasionally evidence of tocopheryl deficiency resulting in clinical signs in the following disorders: malabsorption syndromes, e.g. fibrocystic disease of the pancreas; sprue; premature infants on unsupplemented artificial feeds.

Dosage and administration   *Adults:* The recommended daily intake as a vitamin is from 3 to 15 mg but more may be required when large amounts of unsaturated fats are contained in the diet.

For treatment of intermittent claudication doses of 400–600 mg a day should be administered for three months or more.

Elderly: There is epidemiological evidence for the safety of vitamin E supplementation in the elderly. There have been no adverse effects reported in elderly patients treated with high doses of vitamin E for intermittent claudication.

Children (infants): 1–10 mg/kg body weight daily.

Ephynal tablets are for oral administration.

Contra-indications, warnings, etc   Known hypersensitivity to vitamin E.

Warnings: Diarrhoea and abdominal pain may occur with large doses of vitamin E (i.e. greater than 1 gram daily).

Vitamin E has been reported to increase the risk of thrombosis in patients who have any predisposition thereto, or who are taking oestrogens; these findings have not been confirmed.

Use in pregnancy: There is no evidence of the safety of high dosages (above the normal recommended daily

dosage) of vitamin E in pregnancy nor is there evidence from animal work that it is free from hazard.

Pharmaceutical precautions   *Storage:* Ephynal tablets should be stored in well-closed containers.

Legal category   GSL.

Package quantities   Ephynal tablets 3 mg in packings of 100.

Ephynal tablets 10 mg in packings of 100.
Ephynal tablets 50 mg in packings of 100.
Ephynal tablets 200 mg in packings of 50.

Further information   Nil.

Product licence numbers

Tablets 3 mg	0031/5012
Tablets 10 mg	0031/5013
Tablets 50 mg	0031/5014
Tablets 200 mg	0031/5015

FANSIDAR*   ▼

Presentation   Round, white tablets with ROCHE and a hexagon imprinted on one face and two break bars on the other, containing 500 mg sulfadoxine and 25 mg pyrimethamine.

Uses   *Properties:* The mode of action of Fansidar is based on the reciprocal potentiation of its two components. Fansidar blocks the action of two enzymes which catalyse consecutive stages in the biosynthesis of folinic acid in malaria parasites. Larger doses of the components of Fansidar are necessary if they are given independently and the effect obtained is inferior to that of the combination.

Fansidar is effective against plasmodial strains which are resistant to chloroquine and/or pyrimethamine and other antifolate preparations.

With Fansidar, the danger of emergence of resistance is reduced. However, in certain malarious areas, particularly South-East Asia and South America, strains of *Plasmodium falciparum* may be encountered which have developed resistance to Fansidar. Fansidar affects all developmental stages of the parasites. It has a prolonged action, yet effective plasma concentrations are rapidly attained after a single dose. Trophozoites and schizonts quickly disappear from the blood. Pre-erythrocytic stages are also affected and the gametocytes, although increased in number, are rendered much less infective for the vector. A protective effect persists for up to two to four weeks depending on the dose given and the immune state of the subject.

Indications: Treatment and prophylaxis of *Plasmodium falciparum* malaria.

Treatment of malaria: Fansidar is indicated for the treatment of *Plasmodium falciparum* malaria when the infection is contracted in an area of chloroquine resistance.

Prophylaxis of malaria: Malaria prophylaxis with Fansidar is indicated for travellers to areas where chloroquine-resistant *Plasmodium falciparum* malaria is endemic. Whenever malaria prophylaxis is prescribed, the malaria situation and in particular, resistance trends at the traveller's destination and any stop-over point must be considered. At present, there is no antimalarial agent which provides absolute protection against malaria, but conscientiously performed drug prophylaxis can usually prevent serious progression of the disease.

Dosage and administration

Curative treatment of malaria: The appropriate amount of the drug is given in one single dose. This dose should not be repeated for at least seven days.

Adults		2 to 3 tablets
(higher dose for persons over 60 kg)		

Children	10–14 years	(31–45 kg)	2 tablets
	7–9 years	(21–30 kg)	1½ tablets
	4–6 years	(11–20 kg)	1 tablet
	under 4 years	(5–10 kg)	½ tablet

In very severe cases, quinine may be added, preferably parenterally. An adequate supply of fluids and electrolytes should be maintained.

Prophylactic management: The following dose of Fansidar should be taken every seven days:

Adults		1 tablet

Children	9–14 years	(30–45 kg)	¾ tablet
	4–8 years	(11–29 kg)	½ tablet
	under 4 years	(5–10 kg)	¼ tablet

Regular dosage is important for continuous protection to be maintained.

Routine measures to protect against mosquito bites should not be omitted.

Fansidar prophylaxis should be started about one week before entering the endemic area in order to assess tolerance; this will enable an alternative drug to be selected in the infrequent case where Fansidar is poorly tolerated.

IMPORTANT: Fansidar prophylaxis should be continued for four to six weeks after returning to a non-malarious area to ensure elimination of possible falciparum infections (malignant malaria). However, as with other prophylactic drugs, infections of benign malaria (vivax and malariae infections) may give rise to clinical attacks up to several months after return, despite regular prophylaxis.

Travellers should be instructed to report to a doctor any fever that occurs during or after their stay in a malarious area.

Use in the elderly: Although no specific studies have been performed to establish the use of Fansidar in the elderly, it has been used extensively and the dosage requirements and side-effects appear to be similar to those of younger adults.

Fansidar tablets are for oral administration.

Contra-indications, warnings, etc

Contra-indications: Patients with known sulphonamide hypersensitivity.

Prophylactic (repeated) use of Fansidar is contra-indicated in patients with severe renal insufficiency, marked liver parenchymal damage or blood dyscrasias.

Treatment must be immediately discontinued upon the appearance of any mucocutaneous signs or symptoms such as pruritus, erythema, rash, orogenital lesions or pharyngitis and a medical practitioner consulted.

Like all other preparations containing sulphonamides, Fansidar is contra-indicated in premature babies and during the first few weeks of life.

Use in pregnancy: Foetal damage has been observed in the rat when any drug containing a folate inhibitor, including Fansidar, is administered in early gestation.

The damage is caused by the folic acid antagonist, pyrimethamine, a component of Fansidar; the damage can be prevented by the concomitant administration of folinic acid.

However, no such adverse effects attributed to Fansidar have been reported during human clinical use and the preparation is, therefore, not contra-indicated during pregnancy. The usual medical practice of avoiding the use of Fansidar during early pregnancy should be followed unless considered essential by a medical practitioner. Pregnant women should be made aware of the particular risks of contracting malaria during pregnancy, and should be advised not to undertake unnecessary journeys to endemic areas. A folate supplement should be given to pregnant women receiving Fansidar.

Both pyrimethamine and sulfadoxine are excreted in maternal breast milk. Nursing mothers should not take Fansidar.

Precautions: Excessive exposure to the sun should be avoided.

Regular blood counts are recommended during long-term prophylactic use (over three months) of Fansidar.

Drug interactions: Concurrent administration of other preparations containing folate antagonists (e.g. co-trimoxazole, methotrexate, anticonvulsants) can result in increased impairment of folic acid metabolism which leads to haematological side-effects. Such concomitant therapy should be avoided if possible.

Side-effects: Fansidar is usually well tolerated at the recommended dosage.

As with other drugs containing sulphonamides and/or pyrimethamine, the following side-effects and hypersensitivity reactions may occur:

Skin reactions: Drug rash, pruritus and slight hair loss have been observed. These reactions are usually mild and disappear spontaneously upon withdrawal of the drug. In very rare instances, particularly in hypersensitive patients, cases of erythema multiforme, Stevens–Johnson syndrome and Lyell's syndrome have occurred, some of which have been fatal.

Gastro-intestinal reactions: Feeling of fullness, nausea, rarely vomiting, stomatitis. There have been isolated reports of hepatitis occurring conjointly with administration of Fansidar.

Haematological changes: In rare cases, leucopenia (usually asymptomatic), thrombocytopenia and megaloblastic anaemia have been observed. In extremely rare cases, they take the form of agranulocytosis or purpura. As a rule, all these changes disappear after withdrawal of the drug.

Other side-effects: Fatigue, headache, fever and polyneuritis may occasionally occur.

Adverse reactions occurring after the administration of the sulfadoxine component of Fansidar are not normally more prolonged than those occurring after shorter-acting sulphonamides despite the continued presence of the drug in the body.

Treatment of overdosage: Possible symptoms of overdosage include anorexia, nausea, vomiting, signs of excitation, and possibly convulsions and haematological changes (megaloblastic anaemia, leucopenia, thrombocytopenia).

Treatment is symptomatic and may include forced diuresis. Vigorous gastric lavage should be carried out as early as possible after ingestion. Alkalinization of the urine may aid elimination of the sulfadoxine component of Fansidar. Possible convulsions due to the pyrimethamine components of Fansidar should be watched for and may require anticonvulsant therapy.

Hypersensitivity reactions may require treatment with steroids. Calcium folinate may be given to counteract the effects of pyrimethamine on haemopoiesis.

Pharmaceutical precautions *Storage:* No special precautions are required.

Legal category POM.

Package quantities Fansidar tablets are available in foil strips in packs of 12 and 150.

Further information
Pharmacokinetics
Absorption: After administration of 1 tablet, peak plasma levels for pyrimethamine (0.21 mg per litre) and for sulfadoxine (63.2 mg per litre) are reached after about four hours (means obtained from 14 test subjects).

Elimination: A relatively long elimination half-life is characteristic of both components. The mean values are 96 hours for pyrimethamine and 184 hours for sulfadoxine. Both pyrimethamine and sulfadoxine are eliminated mainly via the kidneys.

Accumulation: Patients taking 1 tablet a week (recommended adult dose for malaria prophylaxis) can be expected to have mean steady state plasma concentrations of 0.15 mg per litre for pyrimethamine (after about four weeks) and 98.4 mg per litre for sulfadoxine (after about seven weeks).

Protein binding: The following values were determined for binding to plasma protein: pyrimethamine 84.9% and sulfadoxine 91.4%.

Product licence number 0031/5097

FLUORO-URACIL ROCHE

Presentation Ampoules containing 250 mg fluorouracil in the form of the sodium salt in 10 ml Water for Injection BP. The ampoule solution is colourless to slightly yellow.

Capsules with powder blue opaque cap and medium orange opaque body with ROCHE printed in black along both cap and body, containing 250 mg fluorouracil.

Uses *Properties:* Fluoro-uracil Roche, a cytostatic agent, is a fluorinated pyrimidine belonging to the category of antimetabolites. It inhibits cell division by interfering with the synthesis of deoxyribonucleic acid (DNA) and to a lesser extent of ribonucleic acid (RNA).

Indications: The palliative treatment of carcinoma.

Dosage and administration Various techniques are employed when using Fluoro-uracil Roche in the treatment of carcinoma. The following examples are given for guidance.

Adults: By the intravenous route: Fluoro-uracil Roche may be administered by intravenous infusion or by intravenous injection. Dosages are generally based on the patient's body weight. If the patient is obese or there has been a spurious gain due to oedema, ascites or other forms of fluid retention, the patient's ideal weight should be used in calculating the dosage. The initial doses given below should be reduced by one-third to a half if the following conditions are present; poor nutritional state; after major surgery (within the previous 30 days); inadequate bone-marrow function (anaemia, leucopenia with white cell count less than 3,500 per mm^3, throm-

bocytopenia with platelet count less than 100,000 per mm^3); impaired hepatic or renal function.

Initial treatment: This may be in the form of an infusion or injection, the former usually being preferred because of lesser toxicity.

Infusion: A daily dose of 15 mg/kg but not more than 1 g per infusion is diluted in 500 ml dextrose 5% solution or 500 ml 0.9% sodium chloride solution and given by intravenous infusion at the rate of 40 drops per minute over four hours. Alternatively, the daily dose may be infused over 30–60 minutes, or given as a continuous infusion over 24 hours. This daily dose is given on successive days until toxicity occurs or until 12–15 g have been given. This sequence of injections constitutes a 'course' of therapy. Some patients have received up to 30 g at a maximum rate of 1 g daily. The daily dose should never exceed 1 g. An interval of four to six weeks should be allowed between any two 'courses' of Fluorouracil Roche.

Injection: A dose of 12 mg/kg i.v. daily on three consecutive days. If there are no signs of toxicity the patient receives 6 mg/kg i.v. on the fifth, seventh and ninth days. If toxicity occurs the signs should be allowed to regress before further doses are administered.

Maintenance therapy consists of 5–15 mg/kg i.v. once weekly.

A more recent alternative method is to give 15 mg/kg i.v. once a week throughout the course of treatment. This obviates the need for an initial period of daily administration.

Regional perfusion intra-arterially: Continuous infusion of Fluoro-uracil Roche into an artery supplying a localised growth has been shown to produce a better result in some tumours than would have been expected from systemic administration by the intravenous route, together with a decrease in toxicity. The usual dose is 5–7.5 mg/kg daily.

In combination with radiotherapy: Irradiation combined with Fluoro-uracil Roche has been found to be useful in the treatment of certain types of metastatic lesions in the lungs and for relief of pain caused by recurrent, inoperable growth. The standard dose of Fluoro-uracil Roche is used.

By the oral route: Fluoro-uracil Roche may be administered orally using either the capsule or the ampoule solution.

Oral administration is not recommended when Fluorouracil Roche is being used initially as the sole agent in palliative treatment of carcinoma. Oral administration may be useful in: palliative therapy employing a combination of drugs; long-term maintenance or post-operative prophylactic therapy in weekly doses; and where therapy with Fluoro-uracil Roche is indicated, but it is impracticable to administer the drug parenterally.

The usual dosage for maintenance treatment is 15 mg/kg once weekly. For palliative therapy a more rapid onset of therapeutic effect may be obtained by giving a daily dose of 15 mg/kg on six successive days. This is followed by maintenance therapy of 15 mg/kg once weekly. The daily dose should not exceed 1 g.

The capsules should be taken with water after a meal.

The solution may be mixed with fruit juice or other similar beverages immediately before oral ingestion to mask its rather bitter taste. Multi-dose preparations must not be made up.

Elderly: Fluoro-uracil Roche should be used in the elderly with similar consideration as in younger adults, notwithstanding that incidence of concomitant medical illness is higher in the former group.

Children: No dosage recommendations are made for the administration of Fluoro-uracil Roche to children.

Fluoro-uracil Roche ampoules are for intra-arterial, intravenous or oral administration.

Fluoro-uracil Roche capsules are for oral administration.

Contra-indications, warnings, etc

Contra-indications: Fluoro-uracil Roche should not be used in the management of non-malignant disease.

Use in pregnancy: Fluoro-uracil Roche has been shown to be teratogenic. It therefore should not normally be administered to patients who are pregnant. Fluoro-uracil Roche should also be regarded as contra-indicated in mothers who are breast-feeding.

Precautions: It is recommended that Fluoro-uracil Roche be given only by or under the supervision of a physician who is experienced in cancer chemotherapy and who is well versed in the use of potent antimetabolites. Because of the possibility of severe toxic reactions, all patients should be admitted to hospital for initial treatment. Fluoro-uracil Roche should be used with great care in debilitated patients.

The margin between the effective and toxic doses of Fluoro-uracil Roche is narrow and a therapeutic response is unlikely without some evidence of toxicity. Even with meticulous selection of patients and careful adjustment of dosage, there may be severe haematological toxicity and gastro-intestinal haemorrhage. Severe toxicity is more likely in poor-risk patients.

Treatment should be discontinued promptly whenever one of the following signs of toxicity appears: Leucopenia (WBC under 3,500 per mm³). Thrombocytopenia (platelets under 100,000 per mm³). Stomatitis (the first small ulceration at the inner margin of the lips is a signal for stopping treatment). Severe diarrhoea (frequent bowel movements and watery stools). Gastro-intestinal ulceration and bleeding. Haemorrhage at any site.

Isolated cases of angina, ECG abnormalities and rarely myocardial infarction have been reported following Fluoro-uracil administration. Caution should therefore be exercised in treating patients who experience chest pain during courses of therapy, or patients with a history of heart disease.

The carcinogenic potential of Fluoro-uracil Roche has not been evaluated but, as with all cystostatic drugs, this possibility should be borne in mind when designing long-term management of patients.

Side-effects: During treatment, diarrhoea, nausea and vomiting commonly occur, but may be controlled by the use of appropriate drugs.

Leucopenia usually follows an adequate course of treatment with Fluoro-uracil Roche. The lowest white cell count commonly occurs between the seventh and fourteenth days after the first dose, but it may be delayed for as long as the twentieth day. By the thirtieth day, the count has usually returned to the normal range. Because of the importance of leucopenia, the white cell count should be checked frequently throughout the course. If it falls, it is advisable to obtain differential counts. If the total is less than 2,000 per mm³, and especially if there is granulocytopenia, it is recommended that the patient be placed in protective isolation in the hospital and treated with appropriate measures for the prevention of systemic infection.

Alopecia and dermatitis may occur in a substantial proportion of cases. Female patients particularly should be warned as to the possibility of alopecia. Since the alopecia seems to be reversible, special measures do not seem to be indicated.

Effects of overdosage and their treatment: Signs and symptoms are qualitatively similar to the side-effects, and similar measures should be taken to treat them.

Pharmaceutical precautions *Storage:* Fluoro-uracil Roche ampoule solution should be stored between 10°C and 30°C and should be protected from light.

Fluorouracil Roche capsules in blister packings should be stored in a dry place; the recommended maximum storage temperature is 25°C.

Additives: Fluoro-uracil Roche ampoule solution may be diluted with Dextrose Injection, Sodium Chloride Injection or Water for Injection BP immediately before parenteral use.

Fluoro-uracil Roche ampoule solution may be diluted with fruit juice or other similar beverages immediately before use to facilitate ingestion by the oral route. Fluoro-uracil Roche ampoule solution must not be made up into multi-dose preparations.

Legal category POM.

Package quantities Fluoro-uracil Roche ampoules in packings of 10.

Fluoro-uracil Roche capsules in blister packings of 50.

Further information *Availability:* Fluoro-uracil Roche ampoules are available through hospital pharmacies for use in hospitals and hospital clinics and can be supplied to retail chemists for dispensing prescriptions for patients whose treatment has been initiated in hospital practice.

Product licence numbers
Ampoules   0031/5079
Capsules   0031/0139

GANTRISIN*

Presentation Round, white tablets with 'Gantrisin' imprinted on one face, containing 500 mg sulphafurazole.

White, fruit-flavoured syrup containing 591.5 mg N'-acetylsulphafurazole (equivalent to 500 mg sulphafurazole) in 5 ml.

Uses *Properties:* Gantrisin is a sulphonamide which is characterised by high therapeutic activity, ready solubility and low toxicity. High concentrations are obtained in the blood and urine. Its relatively high solubility, even in slightly acid media, reduces the likelihood of crystalluria and renal complications to a minimum. It is effective against sulphonamide-sensitive organisms.

Indications: Infections of the respiratory tract and ear, infections of the urinary tract, bacillary dysentery; skin and soft tissue infections, prophylactic treatment of secondary infections.

Dosage and administration

	Tablets		Syrup in ml	
	Initial	Mainten-ance 4–6 hourly	Initial	Mainten-ance 4–6 hourly
Adults and older children	4	2	20	10
Children 9–14 years	3	1½	15	7.5
5–8 years	2	1	10	5
2–4 years	1	½	5	2.5
Infants			2.5	1.25

For severe infections twice these doses are given.

Elderly: Gantrisin is not precluded from use in the elderly. However, such patients should be treated with caution and the dosage adjusted or the drug withdrawn should an adverse reaction occur.

Gantrisin tablets and syrup are for oral administration. Gantrisin syrup may be diluted with Syrup BP. Maintenance of stability cannot be guaranteed when Gantrisin syrup is diluted.

Contra-indications, warnings, etc

Contra-indications: Like all other sulphonamides, Gantrisin is contra-indicated in premature and newborn infants during the first month of life. Because of immaturity of liver enzyme systems, such infants may have difficulty in conjugating sulphonamides normally.

Gantrisin should not be given to patients with a history of sulphonamide sensitivity or patients suffering from porphyria or jaundice.

Use in pregnancy: The use of Gantrisin in late pregnancy should be avoided because of the possible risk of kernicterus in the neonate. Gantrisin has been in wide use in human pregnancy for many years without apparent ill consequence. There is evidence of harmful effects in pregnancy in animals, when given in high doses. Sulphonamides are excreted in breast milk. This does not contra-indicate the use of Gantrisin in lactating mothers but due account should be taken of the age of the infant being breast-fed.

Precautions: An adequate urinary output should be maintained. Gantrisin, like other sulphonamides, should only be used with caution in patients with renal or hepatic dysfunction or in the presence of blood dyscrasias.

Haemolytic anaemia may occur with sulphonamide therapy in individuals with glucose-6-phosphate dehydrogenase deficiency or other conditions predisposing to haemoglobin disorders. The use of sulphonamides in patients receiving concomitant therapy with folic acid antagonists or oral hypoglycaemic agents may increase the effects of these agents.

Side-effects: Clinical experience has shown Gantrisin to be exceptionally free from serious side-effects, although, occasionally, patients may experience the reactions common to sulphonamides, including nausea, vomiting, glossitis and skin rashes. Leucopenia may rarely occur over long periods of treatment, hence regular blood counts are recommended during long-term treatment.

Effects of overdosage and their treatment: Symptoms of overdosage may include vomiting, mental and visual disturbances, petechiae, purpura and jaundice. In acute cases, haematuria, crystalluria and anuria may occur.

Treatment is symptomatic; gastric lavage may be useful. An adequate fluid intake should be maintained and the urine made alkaline. Hypersensitivity reactions may require treatment with steroids.

Pharmaceutical precautions *Storage:* All Gantrisin preparations should be protected from light. Gantrisin tablets should be stored in well-closed containers. The recommended maximum storage temperature of Gantrisin syrup is 25°C; the syrup should be stored in glass containers.

Legal category POM.

Package quantities Gantrisin tablets in packings of 100.

Gantrisin syrup in packings of 100 ml.

Further information Nil.

Product licence numbers
Tablets　　0031/5019
Syrup　　　0031/5020

GLUTRIL*

Presentation Round, white tablets with 'ROCHE' imprinted on one face and a single break bar on the other, containing 25 mg glibornuride.

Uses *Properties:* Glutril is an effective and long-acting hypoglycaemic agent. In common with other substances of the sulphonylurea group, the action of Glutril is attributed to the release of endogenous insulin from the beta cells of the pancreatic islets of Langerhans. There is evidence that Glutril also exhibits extra-pancreatic activity.

Indications: The treatment of maturity-onset diabetes mellitus which is not adequately controlled by dietary measures alone and does not require insulin. Glutril is particularly suitable for the treatment of elderly maturity-onset diabetics.

Dosage and administration *Adults:* The dosage of Glutril varies from individual to individual and only a guide can be given.

Patients not previously treated with hypoglycaemic agents: Treatment should begin with ½ tablet (12.5 mg) Glutril daily taken with breakfast. This dosage may be increased to 1 tablet (25 mg) or 2 tablets (50 mg) daily if necessary. Some patients may require a higher dose to control hyperglycaemia and they may be given 2½ (62.5 mg) or 3 tablets (75 mg) daily.

Where higher doses are required, the total daily dose should be divided. Two tablets should be administered in the morning and the remainder of the dose in the evening.

It is recommended that the dose of Glutril should not exceed 75 mg daily.

Oral hypoglycaemic agents of the biguanide type may be added to the Glutril regimen in instances where a dose of 75 mg daily is reached without satisfactory control of hyperglycaemia.

Patients previously treated with oral hypoglycaemic agents: Patients may be transferred from other oral hypoglycaemic agents to Glutril, the dosage of the latter being based on the amount of the previous therapy required to control hyperglycaemia. The following equivalents may be used as a basis:

Glutril 25 mg is equivalent to 1,000 mg tolbutamide, 250 mg chlorpropamide or 5 mg glibenclamide.

Patients previously treated with insulin: Some patients previously treated with low doses of insulin (less than 40 units daily) may be suitable for transfer to Glutril therapy.

Children: No dosage recommendations are made for the administration of Glutril to children.

Elderly: There are no specific dosage recommendations for elderly patients. Glutril is particularly suitable for the treatment of maturity-onset diabetes.

Glutril tablets are for oral administration.

Contra-indications, warnings, etc

Contra-indications: Glutril is contra-indicated in the presence of ketoacidosis and severe renal, hepatic, adrenal and thyroid dysfunction. It should not be used in patients with known intolerance to sulphonylurea derivatives. Juvenile diabetes should not be treated with Glutril.

Use in pregnancy: Glutril is not indicated for use in pregnancy.

Precautions: The action of oral hypoglycaemic agents including Glutril may be influenced by other therapeutic agents. Sulphonamides, salicylates, phenylbutazone, coumarin derivatives, adrenergic beta-receptor blocking drugs, monoamine oxidase inhibitors, cyclophosphamide, chloramphenicol, and tuberculostatics may enhance the effects of Glutril whilst thiazide diuretics, frusemide, ethacrynic acid, diazoxide, oral contraceptives containing oestrogens and corticosteroids may diminish its effects. Alcohol and tetracycline derivatives may also alter the action of Glutril.

In patients suffering from intercurrent infections or trauma, the dosage of Glutril may need to be adjusted. If such complications are severe, diabetic control may be lost and this will necessitate the withdrawal of Glutril and the maintenance of diabetic control with insulin. Glutril should be reintroduced when the patient has recovered from the infection or trauma.

If the patient requires an anaesthetic, it is recommended that the last dose the patient would normally receive prior to the procedure be omitted and oral glucose be given as soon as the patient recovers. If major surgery is undertaken, control should be maintained with insulin and/or intravenous glucose.

Side-effects: Glutril is well tolerated and, despite its potency, hypoglycaemic reactions are rare. Skin reactions and gastro-intestinal disturbances, such as nausea and vomiting, have been observed, but they occur in only a small proportion of patients. Transient depression of the platelet count has been observed.

Effects of overdosage and their treatment: If a hypoglycaemic reaction should occur, it may be rapidly controlled by the ingestion of appropriate carbohydrates. In the event of severe hypoglycaemia occurring, intravenous glucose or intramuscular glucagon should be given. Gastric lavage may be useful if performed soon after ingestion.

Pharmaceutical precautions *Storage:* Glutril tablets should be stored in their original packing. The recommended maximum storage temperature for Glutril tablets is 30°C.

Legal category POM.

Package quantities Glutril tablets in blister packs of 100, each pack containing 10 strips each of 10 tablets.

Further information Glutril is rapidly and almost completely absorbed, with peak blood levels being attained two to four hours after administration. The plasma half-life is in the region of eight hours. Glutril is extensively metabolised following oral administration, six metabolites having been identified. The metabolites are either inactive or possess hypoglycaemic properties which are considerably less than those of the parent compound.

Product licence number 0031/0059

HYPNOVEL* AMPOULES 10 mg/2 ml ▼

Presentation Colourless glass ampoules containing 10 mg of midazolam base as the hydrochloride in 2 ml aqueous solution. The ampoule solution is colourless.

Uses *Properties:* Midazolam is a potent imidazobenzodiazepine, forming water-soluble salts which are stable and well tolerated by injection. Midazolam possesses the typical pharmacological properties of the benzodiazepines, namely hypnotic, anxiolytic, muscle-relaxant and anticonvulsant activity. In clinical use the induction of sleep is the main action.

At sedative and anaesthetic doses, given intravenously, the action is rapid in onset and of short duration; anterograde amnesia frequently accompanies the period of peak sedation.

When given by intramuscular injection, Hypnovel is very rapidly absorbed and has a bioavailability of greater than 90%. The onset of action is relatively rapid and may be accompanied by anterograde amnesia. On intramuscular injection, Hypnovel is well tolerated locally.

The mean elimination half-life of midazolam is about 2 hours.

Indications: As intravenous sedative cover before and during minor medical, dental and surgical procedures such as gastroscopy, endoscopy, cystoscopy, bronchoscopy and cardiac catheterization.

As an intramuscular premedication for patients with physical status ASA I-IV who are to undergo surgical procedures.

As an alternative intravenous agent for the induction of anaesthesia in high risk and elderly patients, especially where cardiovascular stability is of particular importance. Induction is more reliable when heavy opiate premedication has been administered or when Hypnovel is given with a narcotic analgesic such as fentanyl.

Dosage and administration *Intravenous sedation:* One or more intravenous administrations over a single operating session.

Adults: Usual dosage range: 2.5 mg to 7.5 mg total dose (equivalent to around 0.07 mg/kg body-weight).

The dose should be titrated against the response of the patient. At the desired sedative end-point the patient will be drowsy, speech will be slurred but response to command will be maintained.

As a guide, it is recommended that 0.75 ml of Hypnovel 10 mg/2 ml solution (equivalent to 3.75 mg midazolam) be administered intravenously over 30 seconds. If, after 2 minutes, sedation is not adequate, incremental doses of 0.1 to 0.2 ml of Hypnovel solution (0.5 to 1 mg midazolam) should be given. The initial dose should be reduced in patients of low body-weight.

Elderly: The elderly are more sensitive to the effects of benzodiazepines and in these patients the lower dose of 2.5 mg may be adequate.

Children: Hypnovel has not been evaluated for use as an intravenous sedative in children.

Intramuscular premedication: Adults: A single intramuscular injection of 0.07–0.1 mg/kg body-weight, administered 30–60 minutes pre-operatively, has been shown to be adequate in most cases. The usual dose is about 5 mg.

Atropine or hyoscine hydrobromide may be given concomitantly, bearing in mind that hyoscine hydrobromide will enhance and prolong the sedative and amnesic effects of Hypnovel.

Hypnovel can be combined with atropine or hyoscine hydrobromide in the same syringe to be given as a single intramuscular injection.

Elderly: The elderly are more sensitive to the effects of benzodiazepines and in these patients the lower dose of 2.5 mg may be adequate.

Children: Hypnovel has not been evaluated for use as an intramuscular premedicant in children.

Intravenous induction of anaesthesia: One or more bolus intravenous injections over a single anaesthetic session.

Adults: The dose should be titrated against the individual response of the patient. Hypnovel should be given by slow intravenous injection until there is a loss of eyelid reflex, response to commands and voluntary movements.

In anticipating the required dose of Hypnovel, both the premedication already given and the age of the patient are important. Young, fit unpremedicated patients may require at least 0.3 mg/kg body-weight, whereas patients premedicated with an opiate usually require only 0.2 mg/kg body-weight.

Elderly: The elderly are more sensitive to the effects of benzodiazepines. Induction may be adequate with 0.1 mg/kg body-weight in premedicated patients and 0.2 mg/kg body-weight in unpremedicated patients.

Children over 7 years: Hypnovel has been shown to be an effective agent for induction of anaesthesia in children over 7 years of age, at a dose of 0.15 mg/kg body-weight.

Mode of administration: For the administration of Hypnovel the patient should be placed in a supine position and remain there throughout the procedure. A second person should always be present and facilities for resuscitation should always be available. It is recommended that patients should remain under medical supervision until at least 1 hour has elapsed from the time of injection. They should always be accompanied home by a responsible adult.

Patients who have received Hypnovel alone for IV sedation prior to minor procedures should be warned not to drive or operate machinery for 8 hours. Where Hypnovel is used concurrently with other central nervous system depressants (e.g. potent analgesics) recovery may be prolonged. Patients should therefore be assessed carefully before being allowed to go home or resume normal activities.

When Hypnovel is given with potent analgesics, the latter should be administered first and the sedative effects of Hypnovel can then be safely titrated on top of any sedation caused by the analgesic.

Contra-indications, warnings, etc

Contra-indications: Benzodiazepine sensitivity; acute pulmonary insufficiency; respiratory depression.

Use in pregnancy: Animal experiments have not indicated any teratogenic risk with Hypnovel but evaluation in human pregnancy has not been undertaken.

The administration of high single doses of benzodiazepines in the last trimester of pregnancy has been reported to produce irregularities in the foetal heart, and hypotonia, poor sucking and hypothermia in the neonate. Hypnovel ampoule solution should not be used during the last trimester.

Hypnovel may pass into breast milk and caution should be exercised with its use in lactating mothers.

Precautions: When Hypnovel is given along with centrally-acting drugs, such as potent analgesics, the sedative effect may be intensified and the possibility of severe respiratory or cardiovascular depression should be considered.

Patients should be instructed to avoid alcohol before and for at least 8 hours after administration of Hypnovel since the individual response cannot be foreseen.

Hypnovel should be given with caution to patients with impairment of renal or hepatic function, to elderly or debilitated patients, and to patients with myasthenia gravis.

Side-effects: Hypnovel is well tolerated and changes in arterial blood pressure, heart rate and respiration are usually slight. However, the rapid injection of a high dose can induce soft-tissue airway obstruction or apnoea of short duration.

Other side-effects reported include headache, dizziness and hiccoughs. Local effects on veins are infrequent. However, pain on injection and thrombophlebitis may occur.

Treatment of overdosage: Hypnovel has a wide safety margin. Overdosage may produce airway obstruction, apnoea, hypotension and coma in severe cases. There is no specific antidote to Hypnovel and treatment is supportive.

Pharmaceutical precautions *Storage:* The recommended maximum storage temperature for Hypnovel ampoules is 30°C.

Additives: Hypnovel ampoule solution is stable, both physically and chemically, for up to 1 hour at room temperature when mixed in the same syringe with Atropine Sulphate Injection 500 mcg/ml, or Hyoscine Hydrobromide Injection 0.4 mg/ml. Admixtures with other injections in the same syringe have not been tested and are therefore not recommended.

There is no evidence of the adsorption of midazolam into the plastic of infusion apparatus or syringes.

Legal category POM.

Package quantities Hypnovel ampoules in packings of 10.

Further information The 'second peak' effect, which is known to occur following intravenous diazepam, has not been observed with Hypnovel.

The metabolites of Hypnovel do not contribute significantly to the clinical effects of the drug.

Although admixture with large-volume parenteral fluids is not recommended for use in the indications described above, Hypnovel ampoule solution is stable both physically and chemically, for up to 24 hours at room temperature when mixed with 500 ml infusion fluids containing Dextrose 4% with Sodium Chloride 0.18%, Dextrose 5% or Sodium Chloride 0.9%.

Admixture with Hartmann's solution is not recommended, as the potency of midazolam decreases.

Hypnovel ampoules 10 mg/5 ml are also available, and are recommended especially for intravenous administration of the drug where careful titration is required (see separate literature).

Product licence number 0031/0126

HYPNOVEL* AMPOULES 10 mg/5 ml ▼

Presentation Colourless glass ampoules containing 10 mg of midazolam base as the hydrochloride in 5 ml aqueous solution. The ampoule solution is colourless.

Uses

Properties: Midazolam is a potent imidazobenzodiazepine, forming water-soluble salts which are stable and well tolerated by injection. Midazolam possesses the typical pharmacological properties of the benzodiazepines, namely hypnotic, anxiolytic, muscle-relaxant and anticonvulsant activity. In clinical use the induction of sleep is the main action.

At sedative and anaesthetic doses, given intravenously, the action is rapid in onset and of short duration; anterograde amnesia frequently accompanies the period of peak sedation.

The mean elimination half-life of midazolam is about 2 hours.

Indications: As intravenous sedative cover before and during minor medical, dental and surgical procedures such as gastroscopy, endoscopy, cystoscopy, bronchoscopy and cardiac catheterisation.

As an alternative intravenous agent for the induction of anaesthesia in high risk and elderly patients, especially where cardiovascular stability is of particular importance. Induction is more reliable when heavy opiate premedication has been administered or when Hypnovel is given with a narcotic analgesic such as fentanyl.

Dosage and administration

Intravenous sedation: One or more intravenous administrations over a single operating session.

Adults: Usual dosage range: 2.5 mg to 7.5 mg total dose (equivalent to around 0.07 mg/kg body-weight).

The dose should be titrated against the response of the patient. At the desired sedative end-point the patient will be drowsy, speech will be slurred but response to command will be maintained.

As a guide, it is recommended that 1.75 ml of Hypnovel 10 mg/5 ml solution (equivalent to 3.5 mg midazolam) be administered intravenously over 30 seconds. If, after 2 minutes, sedation is not adequate, incremental doses of 0.25 to 0.5 ml of Hypnovel 10 mg/5 ml solution (0.5 to 1 mg midazolam) should be given. The initial dose should be reduced in patients of low body-weight.

Elderly: The elderly are more sensitive to the effects of benzodiazepines and in these patients the lower dose of 2.5 mg (1.25 ml of Hypnovel 10 mg/5 ml solution) may be adequate.

Children: Hypnovel has not been evaluated for use as an intravenous sedative in children.

Intravenous induction of anaesthesia: One or more bolus intravenous injections over a single anaesthetic session.

Adults: The dose should be titrated against the individual response of the patient. Hypnovel should be given by slow intravenous injection until there is a loss of eyelid reflex, response to commands and voluntary movements.

In anticipating the required dose of Hypnovel, both the premedication already given and the age of the patient are important. Young, fit unpremedicated patients may require at least 0.3 mg/kg body-weight, whereas patients premedicated with an opiate usually require only 0.2 mg/kg body-weight.

Elderly: The elderly are more sensitive to the effects of benzodiazepines. Induction may be adequate with 0.1 mg/kg body-weight in premedicated patients and 0.2 mg/kg body-weight in unpremedicated patients.

Children over 7 years: Hypnovel has been shown to be an effective agent for induction of anaesthesia in children over 7 years of age, at a dose of 0.15 mg/kg body-weight.

Mode of administration: For the administration of Hypnovel the patient should be placed in a supine position and remain there throughout the procedure. A second person should always be present and facilities for resuscitation should always be available. It is recommended that patients should remain under medical supervision until at least 1 hour has elapsed from the time of injection. They should always be accompanied home by a responsible adult.

Patients who have received Hypnovel alone for IV sedation prior to minor procedures should be warned not to drive or operate machinery for 8 hours. Where Hypnovel is used concurrently with other central nervous system depressants (e.g. potent analgesics) recovery may be prolonged. Patients should therefore be assessed carefully before being allowed to go home or resume normal activities.

When Hypnovel is given with potent analgesics, the latter should be administered first and the sedative effects of Hypnovel can then be safely titrated on top of any sedation caused by the analgesic.

Contra-indications, warnings, etc

Contra-indications: Benzodiazepine sensitivity; acute pulmonary insufficiency; respiratory depression.

Use in pregnancy: Animal experiments have not indicated any teratogenic risk with Hypnovel but evaluation in human pregnancy has not been undertaken.

The administration of high single doses of benzodiazepines in the last trimester of pregnancy has been reported to produce irregularities in the foetal heart, and hypotonia, poor sucking and hypothermia in the neonate. Hypnovel ampoule solution should not be used during the last trimester.

Hypnovel may pass into breast milk and caution should be exercised with its use in lactating mothers.

Precautions: When Hypnovel is given along with centrally-acting drugs, such as potent analgesics, the sedative effect may be intensified and the possibility of severe respiratory or cardiovascular depression should be considered.

Patients should be instructed to avoid alcohol before and for at least 8 hours after administration of Hypnovel since the individual response cannot be foreseen.

Hypnovel should be given with caution to patients with impairment of renal or hepatic function, to elderly or debilitated patients, and to patients with myasthenia gravis.

Side-effects: Hypnovel is well tolerated and changes in arterial blood pressure, heart rate and respiration are usually slight. However, the rapid injection of a high dose can induce soft-tissue airway obstruction or apnoea of short duration.

Other side-effects reported include headache, dizziness and hiccoughs. Local effects on veins are infrequent. However, pain on injection and thrombophlebitis may occur.

Treatment of overdosage: Hypnovel has a wide safety margin. Overdosage may produce airway obstruction, apnoea, hypotension and coma in severe cases. There is no specific antidote to Hypnovel and treatment is supportive.

Pharmaceutical precautions *Storage:* The recommended maximum storage temperature for Hypnovel ampoules is 30°C. *Additives:* Admixtures of Hypnovel 10 mg/5 ml solution with other injections have not been tested and are therefore not recommended.

There is no evidence of the adsorption of midazolam onto the plastic of infusion apparatus or syringes.

Legal category POM.

Package quantities Hypnovel ampoules 10 mg/5 ml in packings of 10.

Further information The second peak effect, which is known to occur following intravenous diazepam, has not been observed with Hypnovel.

The metabolites of Hypnovel do not contribute significantly to the clinical effects of the drug.

Although admixture with large-volume parenteral fluids is not recommended for use in the indications described above, Hypnovel ampoule solution is stable, both physically and chemically, for up to 24 hours at room temperature when mixed with 500 ml infusion fluids containing Dextrose 4% with Sodium Chloride 0.18%, Dextrose 5% or Sodium Chloride 0.9%.

Admixture with Hartmann's solution is not recommended, as the potency of midazolam decreases.

Hypnovel ampoules 10 mg/2 ml are also available, and are recommended especially for use as an intramuscular premedication (see separate literature).

Product licence number 0031/0189.

KONAKION*

Presentation White, sugar-coated tablets with 'ROCHE' printed in black across one face, containing 10 mg phytomenadione.

Ampoules containing 1 mg phytomenadione in 0.5 ml.
Ampoules containing 10 mg phytomenadione in 1 ml.

The ampoule solution, which is clear to opalescent greenish-yellow in colour, contains a polyethoxylated castor oil as a non-ionic surfactant.

Uses *Properties:* Konakion is a synthetic preparation of vitamin K_1. The presence of vitamin K (i.e. vitamin K_1 itself or substances with vitamin K activity) is essential for the formation within the body of prothrombin, factor VII, factor IX and factor X. Lack of vitamin K leads to increased tendency to haemorrhage. When an antidote to an anticoagulant is necessary it is essential to use vitamin K_1 itself, as vitamin K analogues are much less effective.

Indications: Konakion is indicated in the treatment of haemorrhage or threatened haemorrhage associated with a low blood level of prothrombin or factor VII. The main indications are: An antidote to anticoagulant drugs of the dicoumarol type. Prevention and treatment of neonatal haemorrhage.

Dosage and administration *Adults: As an antidote to anticoagulant drugs*

For potentially fatal and severe haemorrhage: Konakion therapy should be accompanied by a more immediate effective treatment such as transfusions of whole blood or blood clotting factors. The anticoagulant should be withdrawn and an intravenous injection of Konakion given slowly in a dose of 10–20 mg (1 or 2 ampoules). The prothrombin level should be estimated three hours later, and if the response has been inadequate, the dose should be repeated. Not more than 40 mg of Konakion should be given intravenously in 24 hours.

Less severe haemorrhage: Konakion is given orally in doses of 10–20 mg (1–2 tablets). The prothrombin level is estimated 8–12 hours later and if the response has been inadequate, the dose should be repeated. Intramuscular injections of Konakion may also be given in doses of 10–20 mg (1 or 2 ampoules), repeated if necessary.

Lowering of prothrombin to dangerous level but no haemorrhage: A dose of 5–10 mg Konakion orally may be given to bring the prothrombin level back to within safe limits. In such instances it is not usually necessary to discontinue the anticoagulant.

Adults: Other indications: Doses of 10–20 mg as required.

Children: If, on the recommendation of a physician, a children's dosage is required, then it is suggested that 5–10 mg be given.

Elderly: Elderly patients tend to be more sensitive to reversal of anticoagulation with Konakion; dosage in this group should be at the lower end of the ranges recommended for adults.

Treatment of newborn infants: Prophylactic: 1 mg by intramuscular injection.

Therapeutic: 1 mg by intramuscular injection, repeated at eight-hourly intervals if necessary.

Konakion tablets are for oral administration and should be chewed or allowed to dissolve slowly in the mouth.

Konakion ampoules are for intramuscular or intravenous injection.

Konakion ampoule solution should not be diluted.

Contra-indications, warnings, etc
Contra-indications: Use in patients with a known hypersensitivity to any of the constituents (see *Precautions*).

Use in pregnancy: There is no specific evidence regarding the safety of Konakion in early pregnancy, but as with most drugs, the administration during pregnancy should only occur if the benefits outweigh the risks.

Precautions: Konakion ampoules contain a polyethoxylated castor oil as a non-ionic surfactant. In animal studies, polyethoxylated castor oil can produce severe anaphylactoid reactions associated with histamine release. There is strong circumstantial evidence that similar reactions occurring in patients may have been caused by polyethoxylated castor oil. Polyethoxylated castor oil, when given to patients over a period of several days, can also produce abnormal lipoprotein electrophoretic patterns, alterations in blood viscosity and erythrocyte aggregation.

In potentially fatal and severe haemorrhages due to overdosage of coumarin anticoagulants, intravenous injections of Konakion must be administered slowly and not more than 40 mg should be given during a period of 24 hours. Konakion therapy should be accompanied by a more immediate effective treatment such as transfusions of whole blood or blood clotting factors. When patients with prosthetic heart valves are given transfusions for the treatment of severe or potentially fatal haemorrhages, fresh frozen plasma should be used.

Side-effects: The too rapid intravenous administration of vitamin K_1 has caused reactions, including flushing of the face, sweating, a sense of chest constriction, cyanosis and peripheral vascular collapse.

Repeated intramuscular injection of vitamin K_1 preparations, usually over prolonged periods in patients with hepatic disease, may give rise to local cutaneous and subcutaneous changes.

Pharmaceutical precautions *Storage:* Konakion ampoule solution should be protected from light; it should not be allowed to freeze. The recommended maximum storage temperature for Konakion ampoules is 30°C.

Konakion tablets should be stored in well-closed containers, protected from light and in a cool place.

Legal category POM.

Package quantities Konakion tablets in packings of 25.

Konakion ampoules 1 mg in 0.5 ml and 10 mg in 1 ml in packings of 10.

Further information Large doses of Konakion should be avoided if it is intended to continue with anticoagulant therapy. If haemorrhage is severe, a transfusion of fresh whole blood may be necessary whilst awaiting the effect of the vitamin K_1. Vitamin K_1 is not an antidote to heparin.

Product licence numbers

Tablets	0031/5022R
Ampoules 1 mg	0031/5023R
Ampoules 10 mg	0031/5077R

LARODOPA*

Presentation Round, white tablets with 'ROCHE' in a hexagon imprinted on one face and two break bars on the other, containing 500 mg levodopa.

Uses *Properties:* Larodopa is an anti-Parkinsonian agent. Levodopa is the metabolic precursor of dopamine. The latter is severely depleted in the striatum, pallidum and substantia nigra of Parkinsonian patients and it is considered that administration of Larodopa raises the level of available dopamine in these centres.

Treatment with Larodopa gives worthwhile sustained relief in about two-thirds of these patients. Akinesia usually responds first, then rigidity and then tremor. Amelioration may be seen in other symptoms, including oculogyric crises. It may take six months or more before maximal improvement is achieved.

Indications: Parkinsonism – idiopathic, post-encephalitic. Previous neurosurgery is not a contra-indication to Larodopa.

Dosage and administration Dosage and administration are variable and no more than a guide can be given.

Adults: Hospitalised patients: Initially 0.25–1 g daily in up to five divided doses immediately after food. Dosage should be increased by 0.5–1 g every three to four days until adequate improvement results or intolerable side-effects appear. If severe side-effects appear, the dosage should be gradually decreased to the maximum tolerated. Patients in whom intolerance prevents the achievement of an effective drug level will usually benefit from a

change of treatment to Madopar* (levodopa combined with a peripheral decarboxylase inhibitor).

General practice patients and out-patients: Initially 0.125 g twice daily immediately after food. After one week, the dose may be increased to 0.125 g four or five times daily. Thereafter dosage should be increased at weekly intervals by 0.375 g daily, the total daily dose being given in four or five divided doses. The response of individual patients varies and some patients may tolerate a more rapid rate of increase, e.g. by 0.25–0.5 g daily at intervals of three to four days.

Improvement is usually seen in two to three weeks with the normal dosage range being 2.5–8g daily, but further improvement may occur up to six months or even longer.

When the optimum daily dosage for any particular patient has been reached, it may need to be redistributed throughout the day to meet fluctuations in the individual's requirements. Most patients find a four or five times daily dosage scheme satisfactory; some obtain a smoother effect with two-hourly administration; others, who develop akinetic crises at particular times of the day, learn by experience the daily dosage scheme most suited to their needs.

After a period at the maximum tolerated dosage level, side-effects may slowly develop, usually in the form of involuntary movements. These generally regress without loss of therapeutic effect if the dosage is slightly reduced.

Anticholinergic drugs should be continued during Larodopa therapy. As treatment with Larodopa proceeds and the therapeutic effect is found, the dosage of the anticholinergic drugs may need to be changed. Bromocriptine may be given with Larodopa.

Elderly: Elderly patients with Parkinson's disease have been treated with levodopa. However, levodopa tolerance is less in the elderly and produces more severe hypotensive side effects in older patients with Parkinson's disease, especially those with a history of myocardial infarction.

Children: No dosage recommendations are made for the administration of Larodopa to children.

Larodopa tablets are for oral administration.

Contra-indications, warnings, etc

Contra-indications: Larodopa is contra-indicated in narrow-angle glaucoma (it may be used in wide-angle glaucoma provided that the intra-ocular pressure remains under control); severe psychoneuroses or psychoses.

It should not be given in conjunction with monoamine oxidase inhibitors or within two weeks of their withdrawal.

Suspicion has arisen that levodopa may activate a malignant melanoma. Therefore Larodopa should not be used in persons who have a history of, or who may be suffering from, a malignant melanoma.

Use in pregnancy: There is inadequate evidence of safety of the drug in human pregnancy; it has been in wide use for many years without apparent ill consequence; there is evidence of harmful effects in pregnancy in animals.

Precautions: Pyridoxine (vitamin B_6) which is often included in multivitamin preparations is known to block the effects of levodopa.

Drugs which interfere with central amine mechanisms, such as rauwolfia alkaloids (reserpine), phenothiazines, thioxanthenes, butyrophenones and amphetamines, should be avoided where possible. If, however, their administration is considered essential, extreme care should be exercised and a close watch kept for any signs of potentiation, antagonism or other interactions and for any unusual side-effects.

In the event of general anaesthesia being required. Larodopa therapy may be continued as long as the patient is able to take fluids and medication by mouth. If therapy is temporarily interrupted, the usual daily dosage may be administered as soon as the patient is able to take oral medication. Whenever therapy has been interrupted for longer periods, dosage should again be adjusted gradually; however, in many cases the patient can rapidly be returned to his previous therapeutic dosage.

When other drugs must be given in conjunction with Larodopa, the patient should be carefully observed for unusual side-effects or potentiating effects.

Care should be taken when using Larodopa in the following circumstances: in endocrine, renal, hepatic, pulmonary or cardiovascular disease; particularly where there is a history of myocardial infarction and in patients with peptic ulcer; where sympathomimetic drugs may be required, e.g. bronchial asthma; where antihypertensive drugs are being used. Periodic evaluation of hepatic, haemopoietic, renal and cardiovascular functions is advised.

Patients who improve on Larodopa therapy should be advised to resume normal activities gradually as rapid mobilisation may increase the risk of injury.

Animal experiments in different species have shown no evidence of deleterious effects of Larodopa on the physiology of reproduction or embryonic development. However, the established medical principle of prescribing medicaments in early pregnancy only when absolutely indicated should be observed.

Side-effects: Tolerance to Larodopa varies widely between patients and is often related to the rate of dosage increase. Post-encephalitic Parkinsonian patients tolerate the drug less well. Side-effects, usually dose-related, occur at some time in most patients. During the initiation of therapy nausea and vomiting, anorexia, weakness and hypotension, which is usually postural (but a labile hypertension may rarely be seen), are most frequent. Nausea and vomiting may be minimised by administering Larodopa immediately after food, an anti-emetic, e.g. cyclizine hydrochloride 50 mg three times daily, may also be helpful.

Psychiatric disturbances are common in Parkinsonian patients including those being treated with levodopa. They include mild elation, anxiety, agitation, insomnia, depression and dementia.

Anxiety and insomnia may be treated with a benzodiazepine drug, e.g. Valium and Mogadon respectively. Depression may be treated with tricyclic anti-depressants and ECT may be administered if appropriate. Monoamine oxidase inhibitors must not be used.

Involuntary movements, commonly in the form of oral dyskinesias, often accompanied by 'paddling' foot movements, or of the choreoathetoid type, are common, particularly on long-term administration. They are usually dose-dependent and may disappear or become tolerable after dose reduction. With long-term administration, fluctuations in the therapeutic response may be encountered. They include 'freezing' episodes ('on-off') effect and end-of-dose deterioration. Patients may be helped by dosage reduction or by giving smaller and more frequent doses.

Transient rises in SGOT, SGPT and alkaline phosphatase values have been noted; serum uric acid and blood urea nitrogen levels are occasionally increased. On some occasions the urine passed during Larodopa treatment may be altered in colour; usually red-tinged, this will turn dark on standing. These changes are due to metabolites and are no cause for concern. In rare instances, headache and peripheral neuropathy have been reported.

Effects of overdosage and their treatment: Symptoms of overdosage are qualitatively similar to the side-effects but may be of greater magnitude.

Treatment should include gastric lavage, general supportive measures, intravenous fluids and the maintenance of an adequate airway. Electrocardiographic monitoring should be instituted and the patient carefully observed for the possible development of arrhythmias. If necessary, anti-arrhythmic therapy should be given and other symptoms treated as they arise.

Pharmaceutical precautions *Storage:* Larodopa tablets should be stored in well-closed containers, protected from light.

Legal category POM.

Package quantities Larodopa tablets in packings of 200.

Further information Nil.

Product licence number 0031/5063.

LEXOTAN* ▼

Presentation Lilac, hexagonal biconvex tablets having L1.5 imprinted on one face and a single break bar on the other, containing 1.5 mg bromazepam.

Pink, hexagonal biconvex tablets having L3 imprinted on one face and a single break bar on the other, containing 3 mg bromazepam.

Uses *Properties:* Lexotan is a pyridylbenzodiazepine compound with anxiolytic properties.

Indications: Lexotan is indicated for the short-term treatment of anxiety and associated symptoms such as tension and agitation.

Dosage and administration *Adults:* The optimum dosage and frequency of administration of Lexotan should be based on the individual patient, the severity of symptoms and previous psychotropic drug history.

The usual dosage in general practice is from 3 mg to 18 mg daily in divided doses.

In exceptional circumstances, in hospitalised patients, up to the maximum daily dosage of 60 mg, in divided doses, may be given.

Elderly: Elderly patients are more sensitive to the actions of Lexotan; doses should not exceed half those normally recommended.

Children: Lexotan is not for paediatric use.

Lexotan tablets are for oral administration.

Contra-indications, warnings, etc
Contra-indications: Patients with known sensitivity to benzodiazepines; acute pulmonary insufficiency; respiratory depression.

Use in pregnancy: The use of Lexotan during pregnancy should be avoided.

The administration of high doses or prolonged administration of low doses of benzodiazepines in the last trimester of pregnancy or during labour has been reported to produce irregularities in the foetal heart, and hypotonia, poor sucking and hypothermia in the neonate.

Benzodiazepines have been detected in breast milk. If

possible, the use of Lexotan should be avoided during lactation.

Precautions: In patients with chronic pulmonary insufficiency, and in patients with chronic renal or hepatic disease, dosage may need to be reduced.

If Lexotan is combined with centrally-acting drugs such as neuroleptics, tranquillisers, antidepressants, hypnotics, analgesics and anaesthetics, the sedative effects may be intensified.

Patients should be advised that, like all medicaments of this type, Lexotan may modify patients' performance at skilled tasks (driving, operating machinery, etc.) to a varying degree depending upon dosage and individual susceptibility. Patients should further be advised that alcohol may intensify any impairment and should therefore be avoided during treatment.

The dependence potential of the benzodiazepines is low but this increases when high doses are used, especially when given over long periods. This is particularly so in patients with a history of alcoholism or drug abuse or in patients with marked personality disorders. Regular monitoring in such patients is essential, routine repeat prescriptions should be avoided and treatment should be withdrawn gradually. Symptoms such as depression, nervousness, rebound insomnia, irritability, sweating and diarrhoea have been reported following abrupt cessation of treatment with normal therapeutic doses. In rare instances, withdrawal following excessive dosages may produce confusional states, psychotic manifestations and convulsions.

Abnormal psychological reactions to benzodiazepines have been reported. Rare behavioural effects include paradoxical aggressive outbursts, excitement, confusion, and the uncovering of depression with suicidal tendencies.

Side-effects: Common adverse effects include drowsiness, sedation, unsteadiness and ataxia; these are dose-related and may persist into the following day, even after a single dose. Drowsiness may be a particular problem when Lexotan is used in higher dosage in some patients, especially if they are unused to this form of therapy. The elderly are particularly sensitive to the effects of central depressant drugs and may experience confusion, especially if organic brain changes are present; the dosage of Lexotan should not exceed one-half that recommended for other adults.

Other adverse effects are rare and include headache, vertigo, hypotension, gastro-intestinal upsets, skin rashes, visual disturbances, changes in libido, and urinary retention. Isolated cases of blood dyscrasias and jaundice have also been reported.

Treatment of overdosage: When taken alone in overdosage Lexotan presents few problems in management. Signs may include drowsiness, ataxia and dysarthria, with coma in severe cases. Treatment is symptomatic. Gastric lavage is useful only if performed soon after ingestion. There is no specific antidote to Lexotan.

When taken with centrally acting drugs, especially alcohol, the effects of overdosage are likely to be more severe and, in the absence of supportive measures, may prove fatal.

Pharmaceutical precautions *Storage:* Lexotan tablets should be stored in well-closed containers in a dry place, protected from light.

Legal category CD (Sch. 4), POM.

Package quantities Lexotan tablets 1.5 mg in original blister packings of 20.
Lexotan tablets 3 mg in blister packings of 100.

Further information Lexotan is rapidly absorbed from the gastro-intestinal tract. The mean half-life for elimination of Lexotan in man is about 16 hours. Metabolites of Lexotan do not contribute significantly to the effects of the drug.

Product licence numbers
Tablets 1.5 mg   0031/0127
Tablets 3 mg   0031/0128.

LIBRAXIN*

Presentation   Round, yellow-green, film-coated tablets with 'LIBRAXIN' imprinted on one face, containing 5 mg chlordiazepoxide and 2.5 mg clidinium bromide.

Uses *Properties:* Libraxin combines the anti-anxiety properties of Librium* and the antispasmodic and antisecretory properties of clidinium bromide. Accepted concepts of gastro-intestinal physiology and physiopathology recognise two important components in gastro-intestinal dysfunction: the emotional factor and the somatic factor. Librium is an effective and well-tolerated drug for the treatment of patients in whom anxiety and tension are contributory or causative factors in a psychosomatic illness. Clidinium bromide is a synthetic anticholinergic agent which has been shown in experimental and clinical studies to have a pronounced antispasmodic and antisecretory effect on the gastro-intestinal tract. Its anticholinergic action appears to be approximately equal to that of atropine but its side-effects are milder and less frequent.

Indications: For the control of hypersecretion, hypermotility and emotional factors associated with gastro-intestinal disorders, such as nervous dyspepsia, peptic ulcer, cardiospasm, pylorospasm, irritable bowel syndrome.

Dosage and administration *Adults:* 1 or 2 tablets three or four times daily – before meals and at bedtime. In the majority of patients, 1 tablet three times daily gives excellent results.

Elderly: In elderly patients it is recommended that the initial dose be 1 tablet twice daily.

Children: No dosage recommendations are made for the administration of Libraxin to children.

Libraxin tablets are for oral administration.

Contra-indications, warnings, etc
Contra-indications: Patients with known sensitivity to benzodiazepines; acute pulmonary insufficiency; respiratory depression.

Because of its anticholinergic effects, Libraxin should not be given to patients suffering from glaucoma or prostatic enlargement.

Use in pregnancy: The use of Libraxin during pregnancy should be avoided.

The administration of high doses or prolonged administration of low doses of benzodiazepines in the last trimester of pregnancy or during labour has been reported to produce irregularities in the foetal heart and hypotonia, poor sucking and hypothermia in the neonate.

Benzodiazepines have been detected in breast milk. If possible, the use of Libraxin should be avoided during lactation.

Precautions: In patients with chronic pulmonary insufficiency, and in patients with chronic renal or hepatic disease, dosage may need to be reduced.

Patients should be advised that, like all medicaments of this type, I ibraxin may modify patients' performance at skilled tasks (driving, operating machinery, etc.) to a varying degree depending on dosage, administration and individual susceptibility. Patients should further be advised that alcohol may intensify any impairment and should therefore be avoided during treatment.

If Libraxin is combined with centrally-acting drugs such as neuroleptics, tranquillizers, anaesthetics, monoamine oxidase inhibitors and antidepressants, the sedative effect may be intensified.

The dependence potential of the benzodiazepines is low but this increases when high doses are used, especially when given over long periods. This is particularly so in patients with a history of alcoholism or drug abuse or in patients with marked personality disorders. Regular monitoring in such patients is essential, routine repeat prescriptions should be avoided and treatment should be withdrawn gradually. Symptoms such as depression, nervousness, rebound insomnia, irritability, sweating, and diarrhoea have been reported following abrupt cessation of treatment in patients receiving even normal therapeutic doses for short periods of time.

In rare instances, withdrawal following excessive dosages may produce confusional states, psychotic manifestations and convulsions.

Abnormal psychological reactions to benzodiazepines have been reported. Rare behavioural effects include paradoxical aggressive outbursts, excitement, confusion, and the uncovering of depression with suicidal tendencies.

Side-effects: Libraxin is very well tolerated. Minor side-effects are infrequent and are controlled by reduction of dosage. They include drowsiness, muscle weakness, dryness of the mouth, blurring of vision, constipation and hesitancy of micturition.

Elderly and debilitated patients are particularly sensitive to the effects of central depressant drugs and may experience confusion especially if organic brain changes are present; the dosage of Libraxin should not exceed one-half that recommended for other adults.

Isolated cases of blood dyscrasias and jaundice with benzodiazepines have also been reported.

Treatment of overdosage: Primary signs and symptoms of overdosage may include drowsiness, confusion, dry mouth, urinary retention, dilated pupils and coma.

Gastric lavage should be performed within a few hours of ingestion, and symptoms treated as they arise.

Pilocarpine is an antidote to clidinium overdosage. Noradrenaline may be given to correct hypotension, if it develops, and diazepam or pentobarbitone sodium for severe excitement states.

Pharmaceutical precautions *Storage:* Libraxin tablets should be stored in well-closed containers. The recommended maximum storage temperature for Libraxin tablets is 30°C.

Legal category CD (Sch. 4), POM.

Package quantities Libraxin tablets in packings of 100 and 500.

Further information Nil.

Product licence number 0031/5024.

LIBRIUM*

Presentation Capsules with opaque green cap and opaque yellow body with $\frac{LIB}{5}$ printed in red-brown along both cap and body, containing 5 mg chlordiazepoxide hydrochloride.

Capsules with black cap and opaque green body with $\frac{LIB}{10}$ printed in red-brown along both cap and body, containing 10 mg chlordiazepoxide hydrochloride.

Round, yellowish-green, film-coated tablets with $\frac{LIB}{5}$ imprinted around the periphery, containing 5 mg chlordiazepoxide.

Round, light bluish-green, film-coated tablets with $\frac{LIB}{10}$ imprinted around the periphery, containing 10 mg chlordiazepoxide.

Round, dark bluish-green, film-coated tablets with $\frac{LIB}{25}$ imprinted around the periphery, containing 25 mg chlordiazepoxide.

Ampoules containing 100 mg chlordiazepoxide (in the form of 112 mg chlordiazepoxide hydrochloride) accompanied by ampoules of 2 ml of solvent.

Uses *Properties:* Librium has anxiolytic and central muscle-relaxant properties. It has little autonomic activity.

Indications: Capsules and tablets:
Short-term treatment of the symptoms of anxiety.
Psychosomatic disorders; anxiety complicating organic illness; anxiety accompanying psychoses.
Short-term treatment of insomnia associated with anxiety where daytime anxiolytic effects are desirable.
Muscle spasm of varied aetiology.
Symptomatic relief of acute alcohol withdrawal.

Ampoules:
Symptomatic relief of alcohol withdrawal where oral administration is not possible.
Relief of acute anxiety where oral administration is not possible.

Dosage and administration *Capsules and tablets: Adults:* Mild to moderate anxiety states: up to 30 mg daily in divided doses.
Severe anxiety states: 40 to 100 mg daily in divided doses.
Insomnia associated with anxiety: 10 to 30 mg before retiring.
Symptomatic relief of acute alcohol withdrawal: 25 to 100 mg repeated if necessary in 2 to 4 hours.
Muscle spasm of varied aetiology: 10 to 30 mg daily in divided doses.

Elderly and debilitated patients: Doses should not exceed half those normally recommended.

Librium capsules and tablets are for oral administration.

Ampoules – Adults: Symptomatic relief of acute alcohol withdrawal: 50 to 100 mg by intramuscular injection, repeated if necessary in 2 to 4 hours.

Relief of acute anxiety: 50 to 100 mg by intramuscular injection followed by 25 to 100 mg 3 or 4 times daily if necessary.

Elderly and debilitated patients: Doses should not exceed half those normally recommended.

Intramuscular injection: Add 2 ml of the special solvent to the contents of one 5 ml dry-filled amber ampoule of Librium hydrochloride sterile powder. Avoid excessive pressure in injecting the solvent into the ampoule containing the Librium as this may cause bubbles to form on the surface of the solution. Agitate gently until completely dissolved. The solution should be prepared immediately before administration and should be colourless to pale yellow when reconstituted. Administer slowly by deep intramuscular injection.

Caution: Librium preparations made with the special solvent should not be given intravenously.

Do not use the solvent if opalescent or hazy.

Librium ampoule solution made with the special solvent should not be diluted.

Contra-indications, warnings, etc

Contra-indications: Patients with known sensitivity to benzodiazepines; acute pulmonary insufficiency; respiratory depression.

Use in pregnancy: There is no evidence as to drug safety in human pregnancy, nor is there evidence from animal work that it is free from hazard. Do not use during pregnancy, especially during the first and last trimesters, unless there are compelling reasons.

The administration of high doses or prolonged administration of low doses of benzodiazepines in the last trimester of pregnancy has been reported to produce irregularities in the foetal heart, and hypotonia, poor sucking and hypothermia in the neonate.

Chlordiazepoxide may appear in breast milk. If possible, the use of Librium should be avoided during lactation.

Precautions: In patients with chronic pulmonary insufficiency, and in patients with chronic renal or hepatic disease, dosage may need to be reduced.

Patients should be advised that, like all medicaments of this type, Librium may modify patients' performance at skilled tasks (driving, operating machinery, etc.) to a varying degree depending upon dosage, administration and individual susceptibility. Patients should further be advised that alcohol may intensify any impairment and should therefore be avoided during treatment.

The dependence potential of the benzodiazepines is low but this increases when high doses are used, especially when given over long periods. This is particularly so in patients with a history of alcoholism or drug abuse or in patients with marked personality disorders. Regular monitoring in such patients is essential, routine repeat prescriptions should be avoided and treatment should be withdrawn gradually. Symptoms such as depression, nervousness, rebound insomnia, irritability, sweating, and diarrhoea have been reported following abrupt cessation of treatment in patients receiving even normal therapeutic doses for short periods of time.

In rare instances, withdrawal following excessive dosages may produce confusional states, psychotic manifestations and convulsions.

Abnormal psychological reactions to benzodiazepines have been reported. Rare behavioural effects include paradoxical aggressive outbursts, excitement, confusion, and the uncovering of depression with suicidal tendencies.

If Librium is combined with centrally-acting drugs such as neuroleptics, tranquillizers, antidepressants, hypnotics, analgesics and anaesthetics, the sedative effects are likely to be intensified. The elderly require special supervision.

When Librium is used in conjunction with anti-epileptic drugs, side-effects and toxicity may be more evident, particularly with hydantoins or barbiturates or combinations including them. This requires extra care in adjusting dosage in the initial stages of treatment.

Side-effects and Adverse Reactions: Common adverse effects include drowsiness, sedation, unsteadiness and ataxia; these are dose-related and may persist into the following day even after a single dose. The elderly are particularly sensitive to the effects of central depressant drugs and may experience confusion, especially if organic brain changes are present; the dosage of Librium should not exceed one-half that recommended for other adults.

Other adverse effects are rare and include headache, vertigo, hypotension, gastrointestinal upsets, skin rashes, visual disturbances, changes in libido, and urinary retention. Isolated cases of blood dyscrasias and jaundice have also been reported.

Treatment of overdosage: When taken alone in overdosage Librium presents few problems in management. Signs may include drowsiness, ataxia and dysarthria, with coma in severe cases. Treatment is symptomatic. Gastric lavage is useful only if performed soon after ingestion. There is no specific antidote to Librium.

When taken with centrally-acting drugs, especially alcohol, the effects of overdosage are likely to be more severe and, in the absence of supportive measures, may prove fatal.

Pharmaceutical precautions *Storage:* The recommended maximum storage temperature of Librium capsules and tablets is 25°C.

Librium capsules and tablets should be stored in well-closed containers and protected from light.

Librium ampoules should be kept in a refrigerator; the recommended maximum storage temperature is 6°C.

Legal category CD (Sch. 4), POM.

Package quantities Librium capsules 5 mg and 10 mg and Librium tablets 5 mg, 10 mg and 25 mg in packings of 100 and 500.

Librium ampoules 100 mg accompanied by ampoules with 2 ml solvent, in boxes of 10.

Further information Librium is well absorbed, with peak blood levels being achieved one or two hours after administration. The drug has a half-life of 6–30 hours. Steady-state levels are usually reached within three days.

Chlordiazepoxide is metabolised to desmethylchlordiazepoxide. Demoxepam and desmethyldiazepam are also found in the plasma of patients on continuous treatment. The active metabolite desmethylchlordiazepoxide has an accumulation half-life of 10–18 hours; that of demoxepam has been recorded as 21–78 hours.

Steady-state levels of these active metabolites are reached after 10–15 days, with metabolite concentrations which are similar to those of the parent drug.

No clear correlation has been demonstrated between the blood levels of Librium and its clinical effects.

The elderly and patients with impaired renal and/or hepatic function will be particularly susceptible to the adverse effects listed above. It is advisable to review treatment regularly and to discontinue use as soon as possible.

Treatment should be kept to a minimum and given only under close medical supervision. Little is known regarding the efficacy of benzodiazepines in long-term use.

Product licence numbers

Capsules 5 mg	0031/5025R
Capsules 10 mg	0031/5026R
Tablets 5 mg	0031/5027R
Tablets 10 mg	0031/5028R
Tablets 25 mg	0031/5029R
Dry ampoules 100 mg	0031/5078R
Solvent ampoules	0031/5030R

LIMBITROL*

Presentation Limbitrol 5 capsules with opaque green cap and opaque pink body marked 'LOL 5', containing 5 mg chlordiazepoxide and 14.15 mg amitriptyline hydrochloride (equivalent to 12.5 mg amitriptyline base).

Limbitrol 10 capsules with opaque, dark green cap and opaque pink body marked 'LOL 10', containing 10 mg chlordiazepoxide and 28.3 mg amitriptyline hydrochloride (equivalent to 25 mg amitriptyline base).

Uses *Properties:* Limbitrol combines the anxiolytic effect of chlordiazepoxide with the antidepressant action of amitriptyline.

Indications: The treatment of the symptoms of depressive illness with associated anxiety.

Dosage and administration *Adults:* It is recommended that patients should be started on one capsule Limbitrol 5 three times daily. If the response is inadequate the dose should be increased to one capsule Limbitrol 10 three times daily.

In more severe cases it may be necessary to initiate treatment with one capsule Limbitrol 10 three times daily. If necessary, dosage may be increased to two or three capsules three times daily.

Elderly patients: Limbitrol is not for geriatric use.

Children: Limbitrol is not for paediatric use.

Limbitrol capsules are for oral administration.

Contra-indications, warnings, etc

Contra-indications: Patients with known sensitivity to benzodiazepines; acute pulmonary insufficiency.

Recent myocardial infarction; heart block of any degree; cardiac arrhythmias. Patients with mania, whose condition may be exacerbated by tricyclic antidepressants.

Because of its anticholinergic effects, Limbitrol should not be given to patients suffering from narrow-angle glaucoma or symptoms suggestive of prostatic hypertrophy. Limbitrol should not be taken with monoamine oxidase inhibitors. A minimum of 14 days should elapse between discontinuation of an MAOI and starting Limbitrol, which should be introduced cautiously and dosage increased gradually.

Use in pregnancy: The use of Limbitrol during pregnancy, especially in the first trimester, should be avoided.

The administration of high doses or prolonged administration of low doses of benzodiazepines in the last trimester of pregnancy and during labour has been reported to produce irregularities in the foetal heart, and hypotonia, poor sucking and hypothermia in the neonate.

Tricyclic antidepressants, when administered during the last trimester of pregnancy, have also been associated with adverse effects such as withdrawal symptoms, respiratory depression and agitation in the foetus.

Chlordiazepoxide and amitriptyline may appear in breast milk. Limbitrol should therefore be avoided during lactation.

Precautions: In patients with chronic pulmonary insufficiency, and patients with chronic renal or hepatic disease, dosage may need to be modified.

Limbitrol should be used with caution in patients with hyperthyroidism or cardiovascular disorders.

Limbitrol should be avoided in patients with a history of epilepsy.

If Limbitrol is combined with centrally-acting drugs such as neuroleptics, tranquillizers, antidepressants, hypnotics, analgesics and anaesthetics, the sodative effects may be intensified.

Patients should be advised that, like all medicaments of this type, Limbitrol may modify patients' performance at skilled tasks (driving, operating machinery, etc.) to a varying degree depending on dosage, administration and individual susceptibility. Patients should further be advised that alcohol may intensify any impairment and should therefore be avoided during treatment.

Anaesthesia given during tricyclic antidepressant therapy may increase the risk of arrhythmias and hypotension. If anaesthesia is necessary, the anaesthetist should be informed that the patient is being treated with Limbitrol.

Amitriptyline may decrease the antihypertensive effect of adrenergic neurone-blocking drugs such as guanethidine, bethanidine or debrisoquine (Declinax*), and possibly also clonidine. It is advisable to review all antihypertensive therapy during treatment with Limbitrol.

Limbitrol should not be given with sympathomimetic agents such as adrenaline, ephedrine, isoprenaline, noradrenaline, phenylephrine and phenylpropanolamine.

Barbiturates may decrease and methylphenidate may increase the antidepressant action of amitriptyline.

The possibility of suicide in depressed patients should be borne in mind, and patients should be carefully supervised, especially during the early stages of treatment.

The dependence potential of the benzodiazepines is low, but this increases when high doses are used, especially when given over long periods. This is particularly so in patients with marked personality disorders. Regular monitoring in such patients is essential, routine repeat prescriptions should be avoided and treatment should be withdrawn gradually. Symptoms such as depression, nervousness, rebound insomnia, irritability, sweating, and diarrhoea have been reported following abrupt cessation of treatment in patients receiving even normal therapeutic doses for short periods of time.

In rare instances, withdrawal following excessive dosages may produce confusional states, psychotic manifestations and convulsions.

Abnormal psychological reactions to benzodiazepines have been reported. Rare behavioural effects include paradoxical aggressive outbursts, excitement, confusion, and the uncovering of depression with suicidal tendencies.

The efficacy and safety of Limbitrol in elderly patients has not been demonstrated.

The fixed dosage of chlordiazepoxide and amitriptyline provided in Limbitrol may not be appropriate for some patients, for whom the alternative of prescribing the two active ingredients separately in the necessary amounts should be considered.

Side-effects: The most common side-effects are drowsiness, dry mouth and dizziness during the first few days of treatment, and anticholinergic effects such as constipation, disturbances of accommodation, tachycardia and hesitancy of micturition, which also usually lessen or disappear with time.

Other adverse effects are rare and include headache, hypotension, gastro-intestinal upsets, skin rashes, tremor, interference with sexual function, and urinary retention. Isolated cases of blood dyscrasias, jaundice, hypomania, convulsions, and peripheral neuropathy have also been reported.

Cardiac arrhythmias and severe hypotension are likely to occur with high dosage and in deliberate overdosage of amitriptyline. They may also occur with normal dosage in patients with pre-existing heart disease.

Psychotic manifestations, including mania and paranoid delusions, may be exacerbated during treatment with tricyclic antidepressants.

Treatment of overdosage: Deaths by deliberate or accidental overdosage of amitriptyline have occurred. Symptoms of amitriptyline overdosage may include drowsiness, stupor and coma; tachycardia and other cardiac arrhythmias including ventricular fibrillation; severe hypotension and congestive cardiac failure; agitation, hyper-reflexia and convulsions; hyperpyrexia, dilated pupils and paralytic ileus.

Symptoms of chlordiazepoxide overdosage may include drowsiness, ataxia and dysarthria, with coma in severe cases.

Treatment is symptomatic and supportive. Gastric lavage should be performed as quickly as possible and followed by the use of activated charcoal. Maintain an open airway and adequate fluid intake. Continuous ECG monitoring is essential; serious cardiac arrhythmias may be treated with neostigmine (Prostigmin*), pyridostigmine (Mestinon*) or propranolol. Intravenous fluids may be required to maintain the blood pressure. Body temperature should be regulated. Intravenous diazepam (Valium Roche*) is recommended for the control of convulsions.

There is no specific antidote to amitriptyline and chlordiazepoxide overdosage but the intravenous administration of physostigmine (1 to 3 mg) has been reported to reverse the symptoms. This dose should be repeated as indicated.

When taken with centrally-depressant drugs, especially alcohol, the effects of overdosage are likely to be more severe.

Pharmaceutical precautions *Storage:* Recommended maximum storage temperature 30°C.

Legal category CD (Sch. 4), POM.

Package quantities Limbitrol 5 capsules in packings of 100 and 500.
Limbitrol 10 capsules in packings of 100 and 500.

Further information Nil.

Product licence numbers
Limbitrol 5 Capsules   0031/5066R
Limbitrol 10 Capsules   0031/5067R

MADOPAR*

Presentation Madopar 62.5 capsules with blue cap and grey body with 'ROCHE' printed in black on both cap and body, containing 50 mg levodopa and 14.25 mg benserazide hydrochloride (equivalent to 12.5 mg of the base).

Madopar 125 capsules with blue cap and pink body with 'ROCHE' printed in black on both cap and body, containing 100 mg levodopa and 28.5 mg benserazide hydrochloride (equivalent to 25 mg of the base).

Madopar 250 capsules with blue cap and caramel body with 'ROCHE' printed in black on both cap and body, containing 200 mg levodopa and 57 mg benserazide hydrochloride (equivalent to 50 mg of the base).

Uses *Properties:* Madopar is an anti-Parkinsonian agent. Levodopa is the metabolic precursor of dopamine. The latter is severely depleted in the striatum, pallidum and substantia nigra of Parkinsonian patients and it is considered that administration of levodopa raises the level of available dopamine in these centres. However, conversion of levodopa into dopamine by the enzyme dopa decarboxylase also takes place in extracerebral tissues. As a consequence the full therapeutic effect may not be obtained and side-effects occur.

Administration of a peripheral decarboxylase inhibitor, which blocks the extracerebral decarboxylation of levodopa, in conjunction with levodopa has significant advantages: these include reduced gastro-intestinal side-effects, a more rapid response at the initiation of therapy and a simpler dosage regimen.

Madopar is a combination of levodopa and benserazide in the ratio of 4:1 which in clinical trials has been shown to be the most satisfactory. Like every replacement therapy, treatment with Madopar will be a permanent one.

Indications: Parkinsonism – idiopathic, post-encephalitic. Previous neurosurgery is not a contra-indication to Madopar.

Dosage and administration Dosage and administration are variable and no more than a guide can be given.

Patients not previously treated with levodopa: The initial recommended dose is 1 capsule of Madopar 125 twice daily. This dose may be increased by 1 capsule per day every third or fourth day until a full therapeutic effect is obtained, or side-effects supervene. Individual patient response varies, and some patients may only tolerate a slower rate of increase, e.g. 1 capsule of Madopar 125 at weekly intervals.

The effective dose usually lies within the range of 4–8 capsules of Madopar 125 (2–4 capsules of Madopar 250) daily in divided doses, most patients requiring no more than 6 capsules of Madopar 125 daily.

Madopar 62.5 capsules may be used to facilitate adjustment of dosage to the needs of the individual patient. Patients who experience fluctuations in response may be helped by dividing the dosage into smaller, more frequent doses with the aid of Madopar 62.5 capsules.

Optimal improvement is usually seen in one to three weeks, but the full therapeutic effect of Madopar may not be apparent for some time. It is advisable, therefore, to allow several weeks to elapse before contemplating dosage increments above the average dose range. If satisfactory improvement is still not achieved, the dose of Madopar may be increased, but with caution. It is rarely necessary to give more than 10 capsules of Madopar 125 (5 capsules of Madopar 250) per day.

Treatment should be continued for at least six months before failure is concluded from the absence of a clinical response.

Madopar 250 capsules are only for maintenance therapy once the optimal dosage has been determined using Madopar 125 capsules.

Patients previously treated with levodopa: The following procedure is recommended:

Levodopa alone should be discontinued and Madopar started on the following day. The patient should be initiated on a total of one less Madopar 125 capsule daily than the total number of 500 mg levodopa tablets or capsules previously taken (for example, if the patient had previously taken 2 g levodopa daily, then he should start on 3 capsules Madopar 125 daily on the following day).

Observe the patient for one week and then, if necessary, increase the dosage in the manner described for new patients.

Patients previously treated with other levodopa/ decarboxylase inhibitor combinations: Previous therapy should be withdrawn for 12 hours. Madopar therapy should then be started with 1 capsule of Madopar 125 twice daily. This dose may then be increased in the manner described for patients not previously treated with levodopa.

Other anti-Parkinsonian drugs may be given with Madopar. Existing treatment with other anti-Parkinsonian drugs, e.g. anticholinergics or amantadine, should be continued during initiation of Madopar treatment. However, as treatment with Madopar proceeds and the therapeutic effect becomes apparent, the dosage of the other drugs may need to be reduced or the drugs gradually withdrawn.

Elderly: Although there may be an age-related decrease in tolerance to levodopa in the elderly, Madopar appears to be well-tolerated and side-effects are generally not troublesome. In some elderly patients it may suffice to initiate treatment with 1 capsule of Madopar 62.5 once or twice daily, increasing by 1 capsule every third or fourth day.

Children: Not to be given to patients under 25 years of age; therefore, no dosage recommendations are made for the administration of Madopar to children.

Madopar capsules are for oral administration.

Madopar capsules must always be swallowed whole. They should be taken with, or immediately after, meals.

Contra-indications, warnings, etc

Contra-indications: Madopar is contra-indicated in narrow-angle glaucoma (it may be used in wide angle glaucoma provided that the intra-ocular pressure remains under control); severe psychoneuroses or psychoses.

It should not be given in conjunction with monoamine oxidase inhibitors, or within two weeks of their withdrawal.

It should not be given to patients under 25 years of age.

Suspicion has arisen that levodopa may activate a malignant melanoma. Therefore Madopar should not be used in persons who have a history of, or who may be suffering from, a malignant melanoma.

Use in pregnancy: Madopar should not be given to pregnant women. Should a woman become pregnant, she should immediately discontinue therapy. Patients taking Madopar should not breast-feed their infants.

Precautions: When other drugs must be given in conjunction with Madopar, the patient should be carefully observed for unusual side-effects or potentiating effects.

Drugs which interfere with central amine mechanisms, such as rauwolfia (reserpine), tetrabenazine (Nitoman), metoclopramide, phenothiazines, thioxanthenes, butyrophenones and amphetamines, should be avoided where possible. If, however, their administration is considered essential, extreme care should be exercised and a close watch kept for any signs of potentiation, antagonism or other interactions and for any unusual side-effects.

In the event of general anaesthesia being required,

Madopar therapy may be continued as long as the patient is able to take fluids and medication by mouth. If therapy is temporarily interrupted, the usual daily dosage may be administered as soon as the patient is able to take oral medication. Whenever therapy has been interrupted for longer periods, dosage should again be adjusted gradually; however, in many cases the patient can rapidly be returned to his previous therapeutic dosage.

Pyridoxine (vitamin B_6) may be given with Madopar, but not with levodopa alone.

Care should be taken when using Madopar in the following circumstances: in endocrine, renal, pulmonary or cardiovascular disease; particularly where there is a history of myocardial infarction or arrhythmia, hepatic disorder or peptic ulcer; where sympathomimetic drugs may be required, e.g. bronchial asthma; where antihypertensive drugs are being used.

Periodic evaluation of hepatic, haemopoietic, renal and cardiovascular functions is advised.

Patients who improve on Madopar therapy should be advised to resume normal activities gradually as rapid mobilisation may increase the risk of injury.

Side-effects: Tolerance to Madopar varies widely between patients and is often related to the rate of dosage increases. Side-effects such as nausea and vomiting, which are frequently observed during the initial stages of levodopa therapy, are much less common in patients treated with Madopar. Also, cardiovascular disturbances such as arrhythmias and orthostatic hypotension may occur, but are less frequent than in patients treated with levodopa alone.

Psychiatric disturbances are common in Parkinsonian patients including those being treated with levodopa. They include mild elation, anxiety, agitation, insomnia, depression, aggression, hallucination and delusions.

Anxiety and insomnia may be treated with a benzodiazepine drug, e.g. diazepam (Valium Roche) and nitrazepam (Mogadon) respectively. Depression may be treated with tricyclic anti-depressants and ECT may be administered if appropriate. Monoamine oxidase inhibitors must not be used.

Involuntary movements, commonly in the form of oral dyskinesias, often accompanied by 'paddling' foot movements, or of the choreoathetoid type, are common, particularly on long-term administration. They are usually dose-dependent and may disappear or become tolerable after dose reduction.

With long-term administration, fluctuations in the therapeutic response may be encountered. They include 'freezing' episodes, end-of-dose deterioration and the so-called 'on-off' effect. Patients may be helped by dosage reduction or by giving smaller and more frequent doses.

Transient rises in SGOT, SGPT and alkaline phosphatase values have been noted; serum uric acid and blood urea nitrogen levels are occasionally increased.

Effects of overdosage and their treatment: Symptoms of overdosage are qualitatively similar to the side effects but may be of greater magnitude.

Treatment should include gastric lavage, general supportive measures, intravenous fluids and the maintenance of an adequate airway. Electrocardiographic monitoring should be instituted and the patient carefully observed for the possible development of arrhythmias. If necessary, anti-arrhythmic therapy should be given and other symptoms treated as they arise.

Pharmaceutical precautions *Storage;* Madopar capsules should be protected from moisture. The recommended maximum storage temperature is 25°C.

Legal category POM.

Package quantities Madopar 62.5 capsules containing 50 mg levodopa and 12.5 mg benserazide in bottles of 100.

Madopar 125 capsules containing 100 mg levodopa and 25 mg benserazide in bottles of 100.

Madopar 250 capsules containing 200 mg levodopa and 50 mg benserazide in bottles of 100.

Further information Nil.

Product licence numbers
Madopar 62.5 Capsules 0031/0125
Madopar 125 Capsules 0031/0073
Madopar 250 Capsules 0031/0074

MADRIBON*

Presentation Round, white tablets with 'ROCHE' imprinted on one face with two break bars on the other, containing 500 mg sulphadimethoxine.

Uses *Properties:* Madribon is a long-acting sulphonamide. Therapeutic blood levels are maintained for at least 24 hours after each dose; consequently, a single daily dose is sufficient.

Madribon differs from most sulphonamides in that only small amounts are conjugated in the form of the acetyl derivative, whereas the greater part is conjugated as glucuronide, and excreted in the urine as such. This glucuronide, unlike the acetyl derivatives of most sulphonamides, is highly soluble and, as a result, the risk of renal complications with Madribon is minimal.

Indications: Madribon is indicated in all infections due to organisms which are sulphonamide-sensitive. Trials have shown Madribon to be effective in the treatment of: bronchitis; ear, nose and throat infections; pneumonia; infections of the urinary tract; bacillary dysentery; skin and soft tissue infections; prophylactic treatment of secondary infections.

Dosage and administration

	Tablets	
	Initial	Maintenance 24-hourly
Adults and older children	4	2
Children		
9–14 years	3	1½
5–8 years	2	1
2–4 years	1	½

For mild infections half the above doses are given. For long-term prophylaxis half the maintenance dose is given daily.

Elderly: There is no evidence to indicate that the pharmacokinetics of Madribon differs in the elderly as compared with younger patients. Madribon has been used extensively in elderly patients, with no apparent ill effect.

Madribon tablets are for oral administration.

Contra-indications, warnings, etc
Contra-indications: Like all other sulphonamides, Madribon is contra-indicated in premature and new-born

infants during the first weeks of life. Madribon should not be given to patients suffering from porphyria or jaundice.

Madribon should not be given to patients with a history of sulphonamide sensitivity. As with many other compounds, rare, but sometimes serious, allergo-toxic skin conditions have been reported in connection with long-acting sulphonamides. Although no direct evidence exists to associate Madribon as the causative agent of such conditions, if a rash occurs during therapy, treatment should be immediately discontinued.

Use in pregnancy: Madribon has been in wide use in human pregnancy for many years, without apparent ill consequence. There is evidence of harmful effects in pregnancy in animals when given in high doses. It should not be given to pregnant women in the week before term. Sulphonamides are excreted in breast milk. This does not contra-indicate the use of Madribon in lactating mothers but due account should be taken of the age of the infant being breast-fed.

Precautions: An adequate urinary output should be maintained. Madribon, like other sulphonamides, should only be used with caution in patients with renal or hepatic dysfunction or in the presence of blood dyscrasias. Haemolytic anaemia may occur with sulphonamide therapy in individuals with glucose-6-phosphate dehydrogenase deficiency or other conditions predisposing to haemoglobin disorders. The use of sulphonamides in patients receiving concomitant therapy with folic acid antagonists or oral hypoglycaemic agents may increase the effects of these agents.

Side-effects: Clinical experience has shown Madribon to be exceptionally free from serious side-effects although, occasionally, patients may experience the reactions common to sulphonamides, including nausea, vomiting, glossitis and skin rashes. Leucopenia may rarely occur over long periods of treatment, hence regular blood counts are recommended during long-term treatment.

Effects of overdosage and their treatment: Symptoms of overdosage may include vomiting, mental and visual disturbances, petechiae, purpura and jaundice. In severe cases, haematuria, crystalluria and anuria may occur, but this is less likely with Madribon than with other sulphonamides since it is excreted mainly as a soluble glucuronide.

Treatment is symptomatic; gastric lavage may be useful. An adequate fluid intake should be maintained and the urine made alkaline. Hypersensitivity reactions may require treatment with steroids.

Pharmaceutical precautions *Storage:* Madribon tablets should be stored in well-closed containers, protected from light.

Legal category POM.

Package quantities Madribon tablets in packings of 50.

Further information Nil.

Product licence number 0031/5032.

MARPLAN*

Presentation Round, dull pink tablets with ROCHE imprinted across one face and a single break bar on the other, containing 10 mg isocarboxazid.

Uses *Properties:* Marplan is a monoamine oxidase inhibitor, effective in small doses. Its antidepressant action is thought to be related to its effect on physiological amines such as serotonin and noradrenaline, and this effect is cumulative and persistent.

Indications Treatment of the symptoms of depressive illness.

Dosage and administration *Adults:* A daily dose of 30 mg, in single or divided doses, should be given until improvement is obtained. The maximal effect is only observed after a period varying from 1–4 weeks. If no improvement has been seen by 4 weeks, doses up to 60 mg may be tried, according to the patient's tolerance, for no longer than 4–6 weeks, provided the patient is closely monitored because of the increased risk of adverse reactions occurring. Once the optimal effect is achieved, the dose should be reduced to the lowest possible amount sufficient to maintain the improvement. Clinical experience has shown this to be usually 10–20 mg daily but up to 40 mg daily may be required in some cases.

Elderly: The elderly are more likely to experience adverse reactions such as agitation, confusion and postural hypotension. Half the normal maintenance dose may be sufficient to produce a satisfactory clinical response.

Children: Marplan is not indicated for paediatric use.
Marplan tablets are for oral administration.

Contra-indications, warnings, etc
Contra-indications: Marplan is contra-indicated in patients with any impairment of hepatic function, cerebrovascular disorders or severe cardiovascular disease, and in those with actual or suspected phaeochromocytoma.

Use in pregnancy: Do not use in pregnancy, especially during the first and last trimesters, unless there are compelling reasons. There is no evidence as to drug safety in human pregnancy, nor is there evidence from animal work that it is free from hazard. In addition, the effect of psychotropic drugs on the fine brain structure of the foetus is unknown. Since there is no information on the secretion of the drug into breast milk, Marplan is contra-indicated during lactation.

Warnings: Like other monoamine oxidase inhibitors, Marplan potentiates the action of a number of drugs and foods. Patients being treated with a monoamine oxidase inhibitor should not receive indirectly-acting sympathomimetic agents, such as amphetamines, metaraminol, fenfluramine or similar anorectic agents, ephedrine or phenylpropanolamine (contained in many proprietary 'cold-cure' medications), dopamine or levodopa.

Patients should also be warned to avoid foodstuffs and beverages with a high tyramine content: mature cheeses (including processed cheeses), hydrolysed yeast or meat extracts, heavy red wines such as Chianti, and other foods which are not fresh and are fermented, pickled, 'hung', 'matured' or otherwise subject to protein degradation before consumption. Broad bean pods (which contain levodopa) and banana skins may also present a hazard.

In extreme cases interactions may result in severe hypertensive episodes. Marplan should therefore be discontinued immediately upon the occurrence of palpitations or frequent headaches.

Pethidine should not be given to patients receiving monoamine oxidase inhibitors as serious, potentially fatal reactions, including central excitation, muscle rigidity, hyperpyrexia, circulatory collapse, respiratory depression and coma, can result. Such reactions are less likely with morphine, but experience of the interaction of Marplan with narcotic analgesics other than pethidine is limited and extreme caution is therefore necessary when administering morphine to patients undergoing therapy with Marplan.

Marplan should not be administered together with, or immediately following, other monoamine oxidase inhibitors or most tricyclic antidepressants (clomipramine, desipramine, imipramine, butriptyline, nortriptyline or protriptyline). Although there is no proof that combined therapy will be effective, refractory cases of depression may be treated with Marplan in combination with amitriptyline or trimipramine, provided appropriate care is taken. Hypotensive and other adverse reactions are likely to be increased.

An interval of 1–2 weeks should be allowed after treatment with Marplan before the administration of antidepressants with a different mode of action or any other drug which may interact. On the other hand, Marplan may be given immediately following treatment with antidepressants having a different mode of action.

Marplan should be discontinued for at least 2 weeks prior to elective surgery requiring general anaesthesia. The anaesthetist should be warned that a patient is being treated with Marplan, in the event of emergency surgery being necessary.

Precautions: Concurrent administration of Marplan with other central nervous system depressants (especially barbiturates and phenothiazines), stimulants, local anaesthetics, ganglion-blocking agents and other hypotensives (including methyldopa and reserpine), diuretics, vasopressors, anticholinergic drugs and hypoglycaemic agents may lead to potentiation of their effects. This should be borne in mind if dentistry, surgery or a change in treatment of a patient becomes necessary during treatment with Marplan.

All patients taking Marplan should be warned against self-medication with proprietary 'cold-cure' preparations and nasal decongestants and advised of the dietary restrictions listed under 'Warnings'.

With Marplan, as with other drugs acting on the central nervous system, patients should be instructed to avoid alcohol while under treatment, since the individual response cannot be foreseen. Like all medicaments of this type, Marplan may modify patients' reactions (driving ability, operation of machinery, etc.) to a varying extent, depending on dosage and individual susceptibility.

Some monoamine oxidase inhibitors have occasionally caused hepatic complications and jaundice in patients, therefore regular monitoring of liver function should be carried out during Marplan therapy. If there is any evidence of a hepatotoxic reaction, the drug should be withdrawn immediately.

The drug should be used cautiously in patients with impaired renal function, to prevent accumulation taking place, and also in the elderly or debilitated and those with cardiovascular disease, diabetes or blood dyscrasias.

In restless or agitated patients, Marplan may precipitate states of excessive excitement. Marplan appears to have varying effects in epileptic patients; while some have a decrease in frequency of seizures, others have more seizures.

Side-effects: In general, Marplan is well tolerated by the majority of patients. Side-effects, if they occur, are those common to the group of monoamine oxidase inhibitors. The most frequently reported have been orthostatic hypotension, associated in some patients with disturbances in cardiac rhythm, peripheral oedema, complaints of dizziness, dryness of the mouth, nausea and vomiting, constipation, blurred vision, insomnia, drowsiness, weakness and fatigue. These side-effects can usually be controlled by dosage reduction.

There have been infrequent reports of mild headaches, sweating, paraesthesia, peripheral neuritis, hyperreflexia, agitation, overactivity, muscle tremor, confusion and other behavioural changes, difficulty in micturition, impairment of erection and ejaculation, and skin rashes. Although rare, blood dyscrasias (purpura, granulocytopenia) have been reported. Response to Marplan may be accompanied by increased appetite and weight gain.

Treatment of overdosage: The primary symptoms of overdosage include dizziness, ataxia and irritability. In acute cases, hypotension or hypertension, tachycardia, pyrexia, psychotic manifestations, convulsions, respiratory depression and coma may occur and continue for 8–14 days before recovery.

Gastric lavage should be performed soon after ingestion and intensive supportive therapy carried out.

Sympathomimetic agents should not be given to treat hypotension but plasma expanders may be used in severe cases. Hypertensive crises may be treated by pentolinium or phentolamine, severe shock with hydrocortisone. Diazepam may be used to control convulsions or severe excitement. Dialysis is of value in eliminating the drug in severe cases.

Pharmaceutical precautions *Storage:* Marplan tablets should be stored in well-closed containers. The recommended maximum storage temperature is 25°C.

Legal category POM.

Package quantities Marplan tablets in packings of 50.

Further information Nil.

Product licence number 0031/5080R.

MARSILID*

Presentation Round, white tablets with 'm' imprinted on one face and a single break bar on the other, containing 39.1 mg iproniazid phosphate (equivalent to 25 mg iproniazid).

Round, white tablets with 'm' imprinted on one face and a double break bar on the other, containing 78.2 mg iproniazid phosphate (equivalent to 50 mg iproniazid).

Uses *Properties:* Marsilid is a potent monoamine inhibitor. Its antidepressant action is thought to be related to its effects on physiological amines such as serotonin and noradrenaline, and this effect is cumulative and persistent.

Indications: Treatment of the symptoms of severe depressive illness.

Dosage and administration *Adults:* A single daily dose of 100 to 150 mg should be given, normally in the morning, until improvement is observed. Thereafter the dose may be reduced gradually until the patient is taking a maintenance dose as small as 25 or 50 mg daily.

Elderly: The elderly are more likely to experience adverse reactions such as agitation, confusion and postural hypotension. Half the normal maintenance dose may be sufficient to produce a satisfactory clinical response.

Children: Marsilid is not indicated for paediatric use. Marsilid tablets are for oral administration.

Contra-indications, warnings, etc
Contra-indications: Marsilid is contra-indicated in patients with any impairment of hepatic function, cerebrovascular disorders or severe cardiovascular disease, and in those with actual or suspected phaeochromocytoma.

Use in pregnancy: Do not use in pregnancy, especially during the first and last trimesters, unless there are compelling reasons. There is no evidence as to drug safety in human pregnancy, nor is there evidence from animal work that it is free from hazard. In addition the effect of psychotropic drugs on the fine brain structure of the foetus is unknown. Since there is no information on the secretion of the drug into breast milk, Marsilid is contra-indicated during lactation.

Warnings: Like other monoamine oxidase inhibitors, Marsilid potentiates the action of a number of drugs and foods. Patients being treated with a monoamine oxidase inhibitor should not receive indirectly-acting sympathomimetic agents, such as amphetamines, metaraminol, fenfluramine or similar anorectic agents, ephedrine or phenylpropanolamine (contained in many proprietary 'cold-cure' medications), dopamine or levodopa. Patients should also be warned to avoid foodstuffs and beverages with a high tyramine content: matured cheeses (including processed cheeses), hydrolysed yeast or meat extracts, heavy red wines such as Chianti, and other foods which are not fresh and are fermented, pickled, 'hung', 'matured' or otherwise subject to protein degradation before consumption. Broad bean pods (which contain levodopa) and banana skins may also present a hazard.

In extreme cases interactions may result in severe hypertensive episodes. Marsilid should therefore be discontinued immediately upon the occurrence of palpitations or frequent headaches.

Circulatory collapse, respiratory depression, central excitement and coma have been reported from the combination of monoamine oxidase inhibitors and pethidine. If a narcotic analgesic is required in a patient receiving Marsilid a drug other than pethidine should be used, initially in a small dose which should be increased cautiously.

Marsilid should not be administered together with, or immediately following, other monoamine oxidase inhibitors or tricyclic antidepressants. An interval of two weeks should be allowed after treatment with Marsilid before the administration of another antidepressant or any other drug which may interact.

Marsilid should be discontinued for at least two weeks prior to elective surgery requiring general anaesthesia. The anaesthetist should be warned that a patient is being treated with Marsilid, in the event of emergency surgery being necessary.

Precautions: The use of Marsilid should be restricted to patients who have failed to respond to other forms of treatment and, in the first instance, should be initiated in hospital.

Concurrent administration of Marsilid with other central nervous system depressants (especially barbiturates and phenothiazines), stimulants, local anaesthetics, ganglion-blocking agents and other hypotensives (including methyldopa and reserpine), diuretics, vasopressors, anticholinergic drugs and hypoglycaemic agents lead to potentiation of their effects. This should be borne in mind if dentistry, surgery or a change in treatment of a patient becomes necessary during treatment with Marsilid.

All patients taking Marsilid should be warned against self-medication with proprietary 'cold-cure' preparations (including nasal decongestants) and advised of the dietary restrictions listed under *Warnings*.

With Marsilid, as with other drugs acting on the central nervous system, patients should be instructed to avoid alcohol while under treatment, since the individual response cannot be foreseen. Like all medicaments of this type, Marsilid may modify patients' reactions (driving ability, operation of machinery, etc) to a varying extent, depending on dosage and individual susceptibility.

Hepatic complications and jaundice are known to have occurred during treatment with Marsilid, therefore regular monitoring of liver function should be carried out in patients who receive the drug. If there is any evidence of a hepatotoxic reaction, Marsilid should be withdrawn immediately.

The drug should be used cautiously in patients with impaired renal function, to prevent accumulation taking place, and also in the elderly or debilitated and those with cardiovascular disease, diabetes or blood dyscrasias.

In restless or agitated patients, Marsilid may precipitate states of excessive excitement. Higher doses of Marsilid may precipitate epileptiform fits, especially in patients with a history of epilepsy.

Side-effects: Side-effects caused by Marsilid are those common to the group of monoamine oxidase inhibitors. The most frequently reported have been orthostatic hypotension, associated in some patients with disturbances in cardiac rhythm, peripheral oedema, complaints of dizziness, dryness of the mouth, nausea and vomiting, constipation, difficulty in micturition, impairment of erection and ejaculation, blurred vision, insomnia, drowsiness, headaches, weakness and fatigue. These side-effects can usually be controlled by dosage reduction. There have been less frequent reports of sweating, paraesthesiae, hyperreflexia, agitation, overactivity, muscle tremor, confusion and other behavioural changes, and skin rashes. Peripheral neuritis has sometimes been observed and can be prevented by giving pyridoxine (vitamin B_6) to patients on high doses of Marsilid. Response to Marsilid may be accompanied by increased appetite and weight gain.

Treatment of overdosage: The primary symptoms of overdosage include dizziness, ataxia and irritability. In acute cases, hypotension or hypertension, tachycardia, pyrexia, psychotic manifestations, convulsions, respiratory depression and coma may occur and continue for eight to fourteen days before recovery.

Gastric lavage should be performed soon after ingestion and intensive supportive therapy carried out.

Sympathomimetic agents should not be given to treat hypotension but plasma expanders may be used in severe cases. Hypertensive crises may be treated by pentolinium or phentolamine, severe shock with hydrocortisone. Diazepam may be given to control convulsions or severe excitement. Dialysis is of value in eliminating the drug in severe cases.

Pharmaceutical precautions *Storage:* Marsilid tablets should be stored in well-closed containers. The recommended maximum storage temperature is 30°C.

Legal category POM.

Package quantities Marsilid tablets 25 mg in packings of 50.

Marsilid tablets 50 mg in packings of 100.

Further information Nil.

Product licence numbers
Tablets 25 mg   0031/5068R
Tablets 50 mg   0031/5069R

MESTINON*

Presentation Round, white tablets with 'ROCHE' imprinted across one face with two break bars on the other, containing 60 mg pyridostigmine bromide.

Ampoules containing 1 mg pyridostigmine bromide in 1 ml. The ampoule solution is colourless to faintly yellow.

Uses *Properties:* Mestinon is an antagonist to cholinesterase, the enzyme which normally destroys acetylcholine. The action of Mestinon can briefly be described, therefore, as the potentiation of naturally occurring acetylcholine. Mestinon has a more prolonged action than Prostigmin* (neostigmine), although it is somewhat slower to take effect; because it has a weaker 'muscarinic' action than Prostigmin, it is usually much better tolerated by myasthenic patients in whom the longer action is also an advantage.

Indications: Myasthenia gravis; paralytic ileus; postoperative urinary retention.

Dosage and administration Mestinon has a gradual onset of effect (generally 30–60 minutes), whether given orally or parenterally. To facilitate change of treatment from one route of administration to another, the following doses are approximately equivalent in effect: 2 mg intramuscularly, subcutaneously or intravenously = 60 mg orally.

Administration of Mestinon by the intravenous route, if required, should be by very slow injection. When Mestinon is given by injection a syringe of atropine sulphate should always be available to counteract severe cholinergic reactions, should they occur.

Myasthenia gravis: Adults: Doses of 30 to 120 mg by mouth or 1–4 mg by intramuscular or subcutaneous injection are given at intervals throughout the day when maximum strength is needed (for example, on rising and before mealtimes).

The usual duration of action of a dose is three to four hours in the daytime but a longer effect (six hours) is often obtained with a dose taken on retiring for bed.

The total daily dose is usually in the range of 5–20 tablets (or 10–40 mg by injection) but doses higher than these may be needed by some patients.

Newborn infants: Neostigmine has generally been preferred in the treatment of neonatal myasthenia. However, Mestinon can be given, particularly if neostigmine proves unsuitable on account of pronounced cholinergic effects. The dosage requirements of Mestinon range from 0.2 to 0.4 mg (0.05–0.15 mg/kg bodyweight) by intramuscular injection or 5–10 mg orally every four hours, given 30–60 minutes before feeding.

Treatment is not usually required beyond eight weeks of age except in the rare conditions of congenital and familial infantile myasthenia.

Older children: Children under 6 years old should receive an initial dose of half a tablet (30 mg) of Mestinon; children 6–12 years old should receive one tablet (60 mg). Dosage should be increased gradually, in increments of 15–30 mg daily, until maximum improvement is obtained. Total daily requirements are usually in the range of 30–360 mg by mouth (1–12 mg by injection).

The requirement for Mestinon is usually markedly decreased after thymectomy or when additional therapy (steroids, immunosuppressant drugs) is given.

When relatively large doses of Mestinon are taken by myasthenic patients it may be necessary to give atropine or other anticholinergic drugs to counteract the muscarinic effects. It should be noted that the slower gastrointestinal motility caused by these drugs may affect the absorption of oral Mestinon.

In all patients the possibility of 'cholinergic crisis', due to overdosage of Mestinon, and its differentiation from 'myasthenic crisis', due to increased severity of the disease, must be borne in mind. Both types of crisis are manifested by increased muscle weakness, but whereas myasthenic crisis may require more intensive anticholinesterase treatment, cholinergic crisis calls for immediate discontinuation of this treatment and institution of appropriate supportive measures, including respiratory assistance.

Other indications: Adults: The usual dose is 1 to 4 tablets by mouth or 1–5 mg by intramuscular or subcutaneous injection.

Children: 15–60 mg by mouth or 0.25–1 mg by injection. The frequency of these doses may be varied according to the needs of the patient.

Elderly: There are no specific dosage recommendations for Mestinon in elderly patients.

Mestinon tablets are for oral administration, Mestinon ampoules for intramuscular, intravenous or subcutaneous injection.

Mestinon ampoule solution may be diluted with Water for Injection. However, maintenance of stability cannot be guaranteed when Mestinon preparations are diluted.

Contra-indications, warnings, etc

Contra-indications: Mestinon should not be given to patients with mechanical gastro-intestinal or urinary obstruction.

Mestinon is contra-indicated in patients with known hypersensitivity to the drug and to bromides.

Mestinon should not be used in conjunction with depolarizing muscle relaxants such as suxamethonium as neuromuscular blockade may be potentiated and prolonged apnoea may result.

Use in pregnancy: The safety of Mestinon during pregnancy or lactation has not been established. Although the possible hazards to mother and child must be weighed against the potential benefits in every case, experience with Mestinon in pregnant patients with myasthenia gravis has revealed no untoward effect of the drug on the course of pregnancy.

As the severity of myasthenia gravis often fluctuates considerably, particular care is required to avoid cholinergic crises, due to overdosage of the drug, but otherwise management is no different from that in non-pregnant patients.

Observations indicate that only negligible amounts of Mestinon are excreted in breast milk; nevertheless, due regard should be paid to possible effects on the breast-feeding infant.

Precautions: Extreme caution is required when administering Mestinon to patients with bronchial asthma.

Care should also be taken in patients with bradycardia, recent coronary occlusion, hypotension, vagotonia, epilepsy or Parkinsonism.

Bradycardia may occur, to a possibly dangerous level,

on intravenous injection of Mestinon unless atropine is given simultaneously.

There is no evidence to suggest that Mestinon has any special effects in the elderly. However, elderly patients may be more susceptible to dysrhythmias than the younger adult.

Mestinon should not be given during cyclopropane or halothane anaesthesia; however, it may be used after withdrawal of these agents.

Side-effects: These may include nausea and vomiting, increased salivation, diarrhoea and abdominal cramps.

Treatment of overdosage: Signs of overdosage due to muscarinic effects may include abdominal cramps, increased peristalsis, diarrhoea, nausea and vomiting, increased bronchial secretions, salivation, diaphoresis and miosis. Nicotinic effects consist of muscular cramps, fasciculations and general weakness. Bradycardia and hypotension may also occur.

Artificial respiration should be instituted if respiratory depression is severe. Atropine sulphate 1 to 2 mg intravenously is an antidote to the muscarinic effects.

Pharmaceutical precautions *Storage:* Recommended maximum storage temperature for ampoules and tablets is 25°C. Mestinon tablets and ampoule solution should be protected from light. Mestinon tablets should be protected from moisture.

Legal category POM.

Package quantities Mestinon tablets in packings of 200.
Mestinon ampoules in packings of 10.

Further information Nil.

Product licence numbers
Tablets   0031/5036
Ampoules   0031/5037

MOGADON*

Presentation Round, white tablets with ROCHE and two semi-circles imprinted on one face with a single break bar on the other, containing 5 mg nitrazepam.

Capsules with black cap and translucent purple body with ROCHE printed in red-brown along both cap and body, containing 5mg nitrazepam.

Uses *Properties:* Mogadon is a benzodiazepine compound with sedative properties.

Indications: Short-term treatment of insomnia where daytime sedation is acceptable.

Dosage and administration *Adults:* 5 mg before retiring. This dose may, if necessary, be increased to 10 mg.

Elderly and debilitated patients: Doses should not exceed half those normally recommended.

Mogadon 5 mg tablets and 5 mg capsules are not for paediatric use.

Mogadon tablets and capsules are for oral administration.

Contra-indications, warnings, etc

Contra-indications: Patients with known sensitivity to benzodiazepines; acute pulmonary insufficiency; respiratory depression.

Use in pregnancy: There is no evidence as to drug safety

in human pregnancy, nor is there evidence from animal work that it is free from hazard. Do not use during pregnancy, especially during the first and last trimesters, unless there are compelling reasons.

The administration of high doses or prolonged administration of low doses of benzodiazepines in the last trimester of pregnancy has been reported to produce irregularities in the foetal heart, and hypotonia, poor sucking and hypothermia in the neonate.

Nitrazepam has been detected in breast milk. If possible, the use of Mogadon should be avoided during lactation.

Precautions: In patients with chronic pulmonary insufficiency, and in patients with chronic renal or hepatic disease, dosage may need to be reduced.

Patients should be advised that, like all medicaments of this type, Mogadon may modify patients' performance at skilled tasks (driving, operating machinery, etc.) to a varying degree depending upon dosage and individual susceptibility. Patients should further be advised that alcohol may intensify any impairment, and should, therefore, be avoided during treatment. If the patient awakens for short intervals during the period of drug activity (as indeed during non-drug induced sleep) ability to recall these events may be impaired.

Excessive or prolonged use of benzodiazepines may occasionally result in the development of some psychological dependence, with withdrawal symptoms on sudden discontinuation of the drug. This is particularly so in patients with a history of alcoholism or drug abuse or in patients with marked personality disorders. Regular monitoring in such patients is essential; routine repeat prescriptions should be avoided and treatment should be withdrawn gradually. Symptoms such as depression, nervousness, rebound insomnia, irritability, sweating, and diarrhoea have been reported following abrupt cessation of treatment in patients receiving even normal therapeutic doses for short periods of time.

In rare instances, withdrawal following excessive dosages may produce confusional states, psychotic manifestations and convulsions.

Abnormal psychological reactions to benzodiazepines have been reported. Rare behavioural effects include paradoxical aggressive outbursts, excitement, confusion and the uncovering of depression with suicidal tendencies.

If Mogadon is combined with centrally-acting drugs such as neuroleptics, tranquillisers, antidepressants, hypnotics, analgesics and anaesthetics, the sedative effects are likely to be intensified. The elderly require special supervision.

When Mogadon is used in conjunction with anti-epileptic drugs, side-effects and toxicity may be more evident, particularly with hydantoins or barbiturates or combinations including them. This requires extra care in adjusting dosage in the initial stages of treatment.

Side-effects and adverse reactions: Common adverse effects include drowsiness, sedation, unsteadiness and ataxia; these are dose-related and may persist into the following day, even after a single dose. The elderly are particularly sensitive to the effects of central depressant drugs and may experience confusion, especially if organic brain changes are present; the dosage of Mogadon should not exceed one-half that normally recommended for other adults.

Other adverse effects are rare and include headache, vertigo, hypotension, gastro-intestinal upsets, skin rashes, visual disturbances, changes in libido, and urinary retention. Isolated cases of blood dyscrasias and jaundice have also been reported.

Treatment of overdosage: When taken alone in overdosage Mogadon presents few problems in management. Signs may include drowsiness, ataxia and dysarthria, with coma in severe cases. Treatment is symptomatic. Gastric lavage is useful only if performed soon after ingestion. There is no specific antidote to Mogadon.

When taken with centrally-acting drugs, especially alcohol, the effects of overdosage are likely to be more severe and, in the absence of supportive measures, may prove fatal.

Pharmaceutical precautions *Storage:* Recommended maximum storage temperature for Mogadon tablets is 25°C and for Mogadon capsules is 30°C.

Mogadon tablets and capsules should be protected from light.

Legal category CD (Sch. 4), POM.

Package quantities Mogadon tablets 5 mg and capsules 5 mg in packings of 100 and 500.

Further information Mogadon is well absorbed with peak blood levels being achieved within two hours after administration.

The half-life of nitrazepam is on average 24 hours. Steady-state levels are achieved within five days. Nitrazepam undergoes biotransformation to a number of metabolites none of which possesses significant clinical activity.

No clear correlation has been demonstrated between the blood levels of Mogadon and its clinical effects.

The elderly, and patients with impaired renal and/or hepatic function, will be particularly susceptible to the adverse effects listed above. It is advisable to review treatment regularly and to discontinue use as soon as possible.

Treatment should be kept to a minimum and given only under close medical supervision. Little is known regarding the efficacy or safety of benzodiazepines in long-term use.

Product licence numbers

Tablets	0031/0062R
Capsules	0031/0083R

NATULAN*

Presentation Capsules with opaque ivory cap and body with 'ROCHE' printed in red-brown along both cap and body, containing 58.3 mg procarbazine hydrochloride (equivalent to 50 mg of procarbazine).

Uses *Properties:* Natulan, a methylhydrazine derivative, is a cytostatic agent. It is effective in patients who have become resistant to radiation therapy and other cytostatic agents.

Indications: The main indication is Hodgkin's disease (lymphadenoma).

Natulan may also be useful in other advanced lymphomata and a variety of solid tumours which have proved resistant to other forms of therapy.

Dosage and administration *In combination chemotherapeutic regimens:* Natulan is usually administered concomitantly with other appropriate cytostatic drugs in repeated four- to six-weekly cycles. In most such combination chemotherapy regimens currently in use (e.g. the so-called MOPP schedule with mustine, vincristine and prednisone) Natulan is given daily on the first 10–14 days of each cycle in a dosage of 100 mg per sq. metre of body surface (to nearest 50 mg).

As sole therapeutic agent: Adults: Treatment should begin with small doses which are increased gradually up to a maximum daily dose of 250 or 300 mg divided as evenly as possible throughout the day.

Initial dosage scheme

1st day	50 mg	4th day	200 mg
2nd day	100 mg	5th day	250 mg
3rd day	150 mg	6th day et seq.	250–300 mg

Further procedure: Treatment should be continued with 250 or 300 mg daily until the greatest possible remission has been obtained, after which a maintenance dose is given.

Maintenance dose: 50–150 mg daily. Treatment should be continued until a total dose of at least 6 g has been given. Otherwise, a negative result is not significant.

Elderly: Natulan should be used with caution in the elderly. Patients in this group should be observed very closely for signs of early failure or intolerance of treatment.

Children: If, on the recommendation of a physician, a children's dosage is required, 50 mg daily should be given for the first week. Daily dosage should then be maintained at 100 mg per sq metre of body surface (to nearest 50 mg) until leucopenia or thrombocytopenia occurs or maximum response is obtained.

Natulan capsules are for oral administration.

Contra-indications, warnings, etc

Contra-indications: Pre-existing severe leucopenia or thrombocytopenia from any cause; severe hepatic or renal damage.

Natulan should not be used in the management of non-malignant disease.

Use in pregnancy: Natulan is teratogenic in animals. Therefore it should not be administered to patients who are pregnant unless considered absolutely essential by the physician. Its use should be avoided in breastfeeding mothers.

Precautions: Natulan should be given only under the supervision of a physician who is experienced in cancer chemotherapy and having facilities for regular monitoring of clinical and haematological effects during and after administration.

Introduction of therapy should only be effected under hospital conditions.

Caution is advisable in patients with hepatic or renal dysfunction, cardiovascular or cerebrovascular disease, phaeochromocytoma, or epilepsy.

Regular blood counts are of great importance and if during the initial treatment the total white cell count falls to 3,000 per mm^3 or the platelet count to 80,000 per mm^3, treatment should be suspended temporarily until the leucocyte and/or platelet levels recover, when therapy with the maintenance dose may be resumed.

Treatment should be interrupted on the appearance of allergic skin reactions.

Natulan is a weak MAO inhibitor and therefore interactions with certain foodstuffs and drugs, although very rare, must be borne in mind. Thus, owing to possible potentiation of the effect of barbiturates, narcotic analgesics (especially pethidine), drugs with anticholinergic effects (including phenothiazine derivatives and tricyclic antidepressants), other central nervous system depressants (including anaesthetic agents) and anti-

hypertensive agents, these drugs should be given concurrently with caution and in low doses. Intolerance to alcohol (disulfiram-like reaction) may occur.

Natulan has been shown to be carcinogenic in animals. The possibility of a similar effect should be borne in mind when planning long-term management of patients.

Side-effects: Loss of appetite and nausea occur in most cases, sometimes with vomiting. These symptoms are usually confined to the first few days of treatment and then tend to disappear.

Natulan causes leucopenia and thrombocytopenia. These haematological changes are almost always reversible and seldom require complete cessation of therapy.

Effects of overdosage and their treatment: Signs of overdosage include severe nausea and vomiting, dizziness, hallucinations, depression and convulsions; hypotension or tachycardia may occur.

Gastric lavage and general supportive treatment should be performed, with prophylactic treatment against possible infection, and frequent blood counts.

Pharmaceutical precautions *Storage:* Recommended maximum storage temperature 25°C. Natulan capsules in blister packings should be stored in a dry place.

Legal category POM.

Package quantities Natulan capsules in blister packings of 50.

Further information Nil.

Product licence number 0031/5038

NIPRIDE*

Presentation Ampoules containing the equivalent of 50 mg sodium nitroprusside for reconstitution with 5% Dextrose Injection BP.

Uses *Properties:* Nipride is a potent, rapidly-acting peripheral vasodilator. Vasodilatation is achieved by a direct and balanced action on both arterial and venous blood vessels. The action is directly on vascular musculature and is achieved independently of the autonomic nervous system. The resultant circulatory effects depend on the initial haemodynamic status of the patient. Thus in hypertensive and normotensive patients without heart failure a fall in systemic blood pressure is produced with little or no effect on cardiac output. In patients with heart failure, reduction of resistance to left ventricular outflow ('afterload') and lowering of raised ventricular pressure ('preload') regularly lead to increased cardiac output, usually without significant hypotension.

Duration of effect is brief due to rapid conversion to cyanide and then thiocyanate. This permits minute-by-minute control of the haemodynamic effects.

Indications: Nipride is indicated for the immediate reduction of blood pressure of patients in hypertensive crises. Oral antihypertensive therapy should be started whilst the blood pressure is being controlled with Nipride.

Nipride may be used for surgical procedures where a hypotensive technique is appropriate.

Nipride may also be used to improve cardiac function in acute myocardial infarction, aortic or mitral valve disease, cardiomyopathy and other associated causes of acute or chronic heart failure. This includes its intraoperative or post-operative administration in patients undergoing surgery. Haemodynamic improvement is generally associated with an improvement in clinical symptoms of cardiac failure.

Dosage and administration Nipride is to be given as an intravenous infusion only. It is not recommended for administration by any other route or method. The infusion rate has to be determined for each individual patient by continuous monitoring of blood pressure. The maximum doses listed below should not be exceeded. Nipride should preferably be administered using a micro-drip regulator, infusion pump or any similar device which allows precise control of the flow rate. To prevent or reduce a marked compensatory reaction – which occurs particularly in younger patients – associated with a sharp rise in plasma catecholamine and renin levels, with tachycardia and corresponding tachyphylaxis of the effect of Nipride, the dose should be *increased slowly* until the desired effect occurs. The infusion *should not be terminated abruptly*, but rather over a period of 10–30 minutes, in order to prevent an excessive rise in blood pressure (rebound effect).

The dose required to achieve a given reduction in blood pressure decreases with increasing age of the patient.

If therapy is required for several days blood and plasma cyanide levels should be monitored regularly to ensure that concentrations of 100 mcg/100 ml (38 micromole/l) and 8 mcg/100 ml (3 micromole/l), respectively, are not exceeded. If an infusion is administered for more than three days, serum thiocyanate concentration should also be monitored and should not exceed 6 mg/100 ml (1 millimole/l).

Adults: Hypertensive crises: In patients who are not receiving antihypertensive drugs, treatment with Nipride should be instituted with a dose of 0.3 to 1.0 mcg/kg body-weight/minute.

As soon as a response is obtained the dosage should be adjusted to individual requirements; this will normally be within the range of 0.5 to 6 mcg/kg/minute (average: 3 mcg/kg/minute). Usually, an average of 200 mcg/minute (range of 20 to 400 mcg/minute) is sufficient to maintain the blood pressure at a level 30 to 40 per cent lower than the pre-treatment diastolic blood pressure. The rate of administration should be adjusted to maintain the desired antihypertensive effect, as determined by frequent blood pressure measurements.

In order to avoid excessive levels of cyanide, an end-product of Nipride metabolism, and to lessen the possibility of a precipitous fall in blood pressure, the maximum recommended dose during short-term use (several hours) is 8 mcg/kg/minute. If a marked reduction of blood pressure is not obtained within 10 minutes with the maximum dosage, administration of Nipride should be stopped.

Patients who are being treated with antihypertensive drugs are more sensitive to the effects of Nipride and therefore require smaller doses. Nipride is pharmacologically compatible with other drugs commonly used to treat hypertension. The hypotensive effect of Nipride is augmented by ganglion-blocking agents.

Nipride infusion may be continued until the patient can be safely treated with oral antihypertensive agents alone.

Adults: Hypotensive procedures
When Nipride is used for the induction of deliberate hypotension during anaesthesia, lower doses than the above should be employed. The intrinsic hypotensive action of many anaesthetic agents (e.g. halothane) must be borne in mind.

It is suggested that the maximum dose should not exceed 1.5 mcg/kg/minute. The usual practices and precautions for hypotensive techniques should be observed.

Adults: Cardiac failure
Nipride should ideally only be used when facilities for intensive monitoring of the patient are available.

The Nipride infusion should be started at a rate of 10 to 15 mcg/minute and the dosage raised in increments of 10 to 15 mcg/minute every five to ten minutes until an initial response is observed. Thereafter the dosage should be adjusted until the optimal therapeutic effect is achieved. Larger initial increments may be tolerated by hypertensive patients. The therapeutic dosage is usually in the range of 10 to 200 mcg/minute.

It is suggested that dosage should not exceed 400 mcg/minute (6 mcg/kg body-weight/minute); if no significant improvement is achieved with this rate of administration, Nipride infusion should be stopped.

If signs of hypotension or hypoperfusion occur during administration of Nipride, the infusion rate should be reduced or treatment discontinued. Changes in mental status, neurological signs, oliguria, further chest pain or arrhythmias, nausea and vomiting are indications for such dosage adjustment.

Nipride infusion may be given in conjunction with diuretics, inotropic agents or other measures conventionally used in the management of cardiac failure.

Nipride should be continued until the patient can be stabilised on appropriate oral therapy. Normally this should not be for longer than 72 hours.

Elderly: Nipride should be used with caution in the elderly. Treatment should begin with low doses since they may be more sensitive to the hypotensive effects of Nipride.

Children: No dosage recommendations are made for the administration of Nipride to children.

Preparation of Nipride infusion: The infusion solution must be prepared according to the schedule given below.

The contents of a Nipride ampoule should be dissolved in the 2 ml Dextrose Injection BP provided. No other diluent may be used. The resulting solution should be diluted in 250 ml to 1,000 ml of 5% Dextrose Injection and the infusion bottle promptly wrapped in the aluminium foil provided or other opaque materials to protect it from light. A self-adhesive label is provided for attaching to the container of the diluted infusion. Both the initial solution and the infusion solution should be prepared immediately before use and any unused portion discarded. The freshly-prepared solution for infusion has a faint orange-brownish tint. If it is highly coloured, it should not be used.

Once prepared, the solution should not be stored or administered for a period longer than four hours. No preparation other than 5% Dextrose Injection should be added to the Nipride ampoule or mixed with the Nipride infusion solution.

Contra-indications, warnings, etc
Contra-indications: Nipride should not be used in the treatment of compensatory hypertension, e.g. that associated with conditions such as coarctation of the aorta or arteriovenous shunt.

Cyanide and thiocyanate may interfere with the metabolism of cyanocobalamin (vitamin B_{12}). Nipride is therefore contra-indicated in patients who are deficient in this vitamin, have impaired liver function or suffer from Leber's optic atrophy.

Use in pregnancy: The safety of Nipride in pregnant women has not been established.

Precautions: In patients with known disturbance of cerebral blood flow, Nipride should be used to lower blood pressure only with extreme caution. Thiocyanate inhibits both the uptake and binding of iodine. Caution should therefore be exercised in treating patients with hypothyroidism or severe renal impairment.

Blood pressure should be monitored frequently during Nipride administration since the hypotensive effect is rapid. When the rate of infusion is slowed or administration is stopped, the blood pressure usually begins to rise immediately and returns to pre-treatment levels within one to ten minutes.

If higher infusion rates of Nipride are required to control the blood pressure, especially during hypotensive procedures, there is a possibility that a metabolic acidosis may occur.

Side-effects: Nausea, retching, diaphoresis, apprehension, headache, restlessness, muscle-twitching, retrosternal discomfort, palpitations, dizziness and abdominal pain have been noted with a too-rapid reduction in blood pressure. The symptoms rapidly disappear with slowing of the rate of infusion of Nipride or temporary withdrawal of the drug. When administration is continued at a slower rate of infusion symptoms do not usually recur.

Cyanide inhibits cellular oxidative metabolism. Excessive concentrations of cyanide (plasma levels greater than 8 mcg/100 ml), which may occur when levels of available endogenous thiosulphate are depleted, would be manifested by tachycardia, sweating, hyperventilation, cardiac arrhythmias and profound metabolic acidosis. Unexplained cyanosis whilst receiving Nipride may be due to methaemoglobinaemia.

Effects of overdosage and their treatment: Overdosage will be manifest by a marked fall in blood pressure below the desired level. The duration of action of Nipride is very short, the hypotensive effects ceasing almost immediately upon discontinuation of the infusion. Pre-treatment blood pressure levels are usually regained within one to ten minutes. Discontinuation of administration or a reduction in the rate of administration are usually sufficient measures for managing overdosage of Nipride.

If cyanide intoxication is diagnosed the following measures should be taken *immediately*:
1. Discontinue the infusion of Nipride.
2. Administer as a cyanide antidote either
   A. Sodium thiosulphate, 12.5 g in 25 ml or 50 ml of 5% Dextrose Injection, infused intravenously over 10 minutes. This dose may be repeated if necessary. (The value of prior administration of sodium nitrite or amyl nitrite has been questioned as this carries the risk that excessive methaemoglobin formation may adversely affect the already critically low oxygen utilisation of a cyanide-poisoned patient.)
   or
   B. Dicobalt edetate, 300 mg in 20 ml, injected intravenously over about one minute, followed by 50 ml of 50% Dextrose Injection. These doses may be repeated immediately if the response is inadequate, and a third dose given after five minutes if necessary.
3. Institute ancillary treatment (oxygen, resuscitation) to support respiration. Haemodialysis enhances removal of thiocyanate and may thereby assist recovery from cyanide poisoning.

Hydroxocobalamin has been suggested as an alternative antidote but is impractical in the acute treatment of cyanide poisoning because of the large dosage requirements. However, hydroxocobalamin 1.5 mg/kg body-weight or sodium thiosulphate 75 mg/kg body-weight have been used prophylactically to reduce plasma cyanide concentration in patients receiving close to the recommended maximum doses of Nipride.

Pharmaceutical precautions Nipride ampoules and infusion solution should be protected from light. When the infusion solution is prepared the container should be wrapped in aluminium foil or other opaque material. Solutions of Nipride should not be stored for more than four hours or administered over a period longer than four hours.

In aqueous solution Nipride yields the nitroprusside ion which reacts with minute quantities of a wide variety of inorganic or organic substances to form reaction products which are frequently highly coloured. If coloration is observed, the solution should be discarded.

No preparation other than 5% Dextrose Injection should be added to the Nipride ampoule or mixed with the Nipride infusion solution.

Storage: Nipride ampoules and infusion should be protected from light.

Legal category POM.

Package quantities Nipride ampoules 50 mg accompanied by ampoules of 2 ml 5% Dextrose Injection BP in packings of 5.

Further information At therapeutic doses, nitroprusside is completely metabolised in contact with erythrocytes within a few minutes, with the formation of cyanomethaemoglobin, and cyanide.

Cyanide is mostly retained within the erythrocytes ('bound' cyanide), without significantly affecting the function of the latter, and released only slowly into the plasma ('free' cyanide). In the liver, 'free' cyanide is transformed into relatively non-toxic thiocyanate in the presence of thiosulphate and rhodanase, a high-capacity enzyme. The toxicity of Nipride that has been observed in cases of overdosage and/or absence of endogenous thiosulphate is due almost entirely to the presence of excessive concentrations (> 8 mcg per 100 ml) of 'free' cyanide in the plasma. As a result of its physicochemical similarity to the iodide ion, thiocyanate is subjected to repeated enterohepatic recirculation prior to being eliminated via the kidneys. In patients with normally functioning kidneys, the biological half-life of thiocyanate is several days, but in renal insufficiency the half-life may be considerably longer. When Nipride is administered in high doses for more than three days, potentially toxic levels of thiocyanate (> 6 mg per 100 ml) may therefore accumulate.

Availability: Nipride is available to hospitals only.

Product licence number 0031/0102.

NITOMAN*

Presentation Round, pale yellowish-buff tablets with 'Roche' imprinted across one face and a single break bar on the other, containing 25 mg tetrabenazine.

Uses *Properties:* The central effects of Nitoman closely resemble those of reserpine, but it differs from the latter in having less peripheral activity and being much shorter-acting.

It is known from animal experiments that Nitoman intervenes in the metabolism of biogenic amines, such as serotonin and noradrenaline, and that this activity is mainly limited to the brain. It is thought that the effect of Nitoman on brain amines explains its clinical effects in man.

Indications: Movement disorders associated with organic central nervous system conditions, e.g. Huntington's chorea, hemiballismus and senile chorea.

Dosage and administration *Adults:* Dosage and administration are variable and only a guide is given. An initial starting dose of 25 mg three times a day is recommended. This can be increased by 25 mg a day every three or four days until 200 mg a day is being given or the limit of tolerance, as dictated by unwanted effects, is reached, whichever is the lower dose. If there is no improvement at the maximum dose in seven days, it is unlikely that the compound will be of benefit to the patient, either by increasing the dose or by extending the duration of treatment.

Elderly: No specific studies have been performed in the elderly, but Nitoman has been administered to elderly patients in standard dosage without apparent ill effect.

Children: No specific dosage recommendations are made for the administration of Nitoman to children although it has been used without ill effect.

Nitoman tablets are for oral administration.

Contra-indications, warnings, etc
Contra-indications: Nitoman blocks the action of reserpine.

Use in pregnancy: There is inadequate evidence of safety of the drug in human pregnancy and no evidence from animal work, but it has been in wide use for many years without apparent ill consequence. Nitoman should be avoided in breast-feeding mothers.

Precautions: Levodopa should be administered with caution in the presence of Nitoman.

Patients should be advised that Nitoman may cause drowsiness and therefore may modify their performance at skilled tasks (driving ability, operation of machinery, etc.) to a varying degree, depending on dose and individual susceptibility.

Side-effects: Side-effects are usually mild with little hypotensive action and few digestive disorders. The main unwanted effect reported to date has been drowsiness, which occurs with higher doses. If depression occurs, it can be controlled by reducing the dose or by giving antidepressant drugs such as the monoamine oxidase inhibitors. However, Nitoman should not be given immediately after a course of any of the monoamine oxidase inhibitors as such treatment may lead to a state of restlessness, disorientation and confusion. In man, a Parkinsonian-like syndrome has been reported on rare occasions, usually in doses above 200 mg per day, but this disappears on reducing the dose.

Effects of overdosage and their treatment: Signs and symptoms of overdosage may include drowsiness, sweating, hypotension and hypothermia. Treatment is symptomatic.

Pharmaceutical precautions *Storage:* Nitoman tablets should be stored in well-closed containers.

Legal category POM.

Package quantities Nitoman tablets in packings of 500.

Further information Nil.

Product licence number 0031/5073.

NOBRIUM

Presentation Capsules with yellow opaque cap and orange opaque body with 'ROCHE 5' printed in red along both cap and body, containing 5 mg medazepam.

Capsules with black cap and coral opaque body with 'ROCHE 10' printed in red along both cap and body, containing 10 mg medazepam.

Uses *Properties:* Nobrium has anxiolytic properties. It has little autonomic activity.

Indications: Short-term treatment of the symptoms of anxiety.

Dosage and administration *Adults:*

Mild anxiety states: 15 to 30 mg daily in divided doses.

Severe anxiety states: 20 to 40 mg daily in divided doses.

Elderly and debilitated patients: Doses should not exceed half those normally recommended.

Nobrium is not for paediatric use.
Nobrium capsules are for oral administration.

Contra-indications, warnings, etc
Contra-indications: Patients with known sensitivity to benzodiazepines; acute pulmonary insufficiency; respiratory depression.

Use in pregnancy: There is no evidence as to drug safety in human pregnancy, nor is there evidence from animal work that it is free from hazard. Do not use during pregnancy, especially during the first and last trimesters, unless there are compelling reasons.

The administration of high doses or prolonged administration of low doses of benzodiazepines in the last trimester of pregnancy or during labour has been reported to produce irregularities in the foetal heart, and hypotonia, poor sucking and hypothermia in the neonate.

Medazepam and its metabolites may appear in breast milk. If possible, the use of Nobrium should be avoided during lactation.

Precautions: In patients with chronic pulmonary insufficiency, and in patients with chronic renal or hepatic disease, dosage may need to be reduced.

Patients should be advised that, like all medicaments of this type, Nobrium may modify patients' performance at skilled tasks (driving, operating machinery, etc.) to a varying degree depending upon dosage, administration and individual susceptibility. Patients should further be advised that alcohol may intensify any impairment, and should, therefore, be avoided during treatment.

The dependence potential of the benzodiazepines is low but this increases when high doses are used, especially when given over long periods. This is particularly so in patients with a history of alcoholism or drug abuse or in patients with marked personality disorders. Regular monitoring in such patients is essential, routine repeat prescriptions should be avoided and treatment should be withdrawn gradually. Symptoms such as depression, nervousness, rebound insomnia, irritability, sweating, and diarrhoea have been reported following abrupt cessation of treatment in patients receiving even normal therapeutic doses for short periods of time.

In rare instances, withdrawal following excessive dosages may produce confusional states, psychotic manifestations and convulsions.

Abnormal psychological reactions to benzodiazepines have been reported. Rare behavioural effects include paradoxical aggressive outbursts, excitement, confusion, and the uncovering of depression with suicidal tendencies.

If Nobrium is combined with centrally-acting drugs such as neuroleptics, antidepressants, hypnotics, analgesics and anaesthetics, the sedative effects are likely to be intensified. The elderly require special supervision.

When Nobrium is used in conjunction with anti-epileptic drugs, side-effects and toxicity may be more evident, particularly with hydantoins or barbiturates or combinations including them. This requires extra care in adjusting dosage in the initial stages of treatment.

Side-effects and adverse reactions: Common adverse effects include drowsiness, sedation, unsteadiness and ataxia; these are dose-related and may persist into the following day, even after a single dose. The elderly are particularly sensitive to the effects of central depressant drugs and may experience confusion, especially if organic brain changes are present; the dosage of Nobrium should not exceed one-half that recommended for other adults.

Other adverse effects are rare and include headache, vertigo, hypotension, gastro-intestinal upsets, skin rashes, visual disturbances, changes in libido, and urinary retention. Isolated cases of blood dyscrasias and jaundice have also been reported.

Treatment of overdosage: When taken alone in overdosage Nobrium presents few problems in management. Signs may include drowsiness, ataxia and dysarthria, with coma in severe cases. Treatment is symptomatic. Gastric lavage is useful only if performed soon after ingestion. There is no specific antidote to Nobrium.

When taken with centrally-acting drugs, especially alcohol, the effects of overdosage are likely to be more severe and, in the absence of supportive measures, may prove fatal.

Pharmaceutical precautions *Storage:* No special precautions are required.

Legal category CD (Sch. 4), POM.

Package quantities Nobrium capsules 5 mg, 10 mg in packings of 100 and 500.

Further information Nobrium is rapidly absorbed, and peak blood levels are reached within two hours of dosing. The drug itself has a short half-life and is metabolised to normedazepam and diazepam, then to N-desmethyldiazepam. These active metabolites have longer half-lives and accumulate during repeated administration.

The active metabolite, N-desmethyldiazepam, accumulates to reach concentrations five to ten times those of the parent compound. Ten to fifteen days continuous administration are thought to produce steady state plasma levels, although a longer period may be required in some individuals, particularly the elderly.

No clear correlation has been demonstrated between the blood levels of Nobrium and its clinical effects.

The elderly, and patients with impaired renal and/or hepatic function, will be particularly susceptible to the adverse effects listed above. It is advisable to review treatment regularly and to discontinue use as soon as possible.

Treatment should be kept to a minimum and given only under close medical supervision. Little is known regarding the efficacy or safety of benzodiazepines in long-term use.

Product licence numbers
Capsules 5 mg   0031/5039R
Capsules 10 mg   0031/5040R

NOLUDAR*

Presentation Round, white tablets with 'Noludar' imprinted across one face with two break bars on the other, containing 200 mg methyprylone.

Uses *Properties:* Noludar has sedative properties.

Indications: The short-term treatment of intractable insomnia.

Dosage and administration *Adults:* 200–400 mg to be taken 15 minutes before bedtime.

Elderly and debilitated patients: Doses should not exceed half those normally recommended.

Noludar tablets are not for paediatric or adolescent use.

Noludar tablets are for oral administration.

Contra-indications, warnings, etc *Contra-indications:* Patients with a history of alcohol or drug abuse, those suffering from acute intermittent porphyria, or sleep apnoea are not suitable candidates for Noludar treatment. Noludar should not be used for the treatment of uncontrolled pain.

Use in pregnancy: There is no evidence of safety in human pregnancy, nor is there evidence from animal work that it is free from hazard. Noludar should not, therefore, be given to pregnant or lactating females.

Precautions: Caution should be exercised when treating patients with hepatic or renal insufficiency.

As with other drugs acting on the central nervous system, patients should be instructed to avoid alcohol whilst receiving Noludar, since the individual response cannot be foreseen.

Like all medicaments of this type, Noludar may modify patients' reactions (driving ability, operation of machinery, etc.) to a varying extent depending on dosage and individual susceptibility. The concurrent use of other CNS depressant drugs should also be avoided.

There is insufficient evidence on the interaction of methyprylone with oral contraceptives and anticoagulants, therefore caution should be exercised during concomitant therapy.

Warnings: Although the potential for induction of liver enzymes exists in animals treated with high doses of methyprylone, the relevance to man has not been documented.

Noludar has a high addiction potential of the barbiturate-alcohol type. Long-term use or use of high doses for short periods may lead to tolerance and subsequently to physical and psychological dependence. Symptoms of dependence include confusion, defective judgement and loss of emotional control.

Withdrawal symptoms consisting of nightmares and insomnia have been reported following short-term use in normal dosage. Such symptoms are likely to be more common and severe after longer-term use or after abrupt cessation of higher doses. In severe cases delirium tremens or convulsions may be observed.

Side-effects: Common adverse effects include headache, dizziness, drowsiness and vertigo. Other adverse effects include nausea, ataxia, incoordination, paradoxical excitement, vomiting, diarrhoea, pruritus, skin rashes, hypotension, confusion and memory impairment.

Treatment of overdosage: In all cases of overdosage with Noludar, especially when other agents have been ingested simultaneously, the potential for serious, possibly fatal toxicity should be recognised. Close monitoring and active management of the patient are therefore appropriate.

Signs and symptoms of overdosage may include drowsiness, pyrexia, hypotension, respiratory depression and slight bradycardia. Later, hyperactivity, coma and convulsions may occur.

Gastric lavage should be performed, with general supportive therapy, including oxygen and airway maintenance and intravenous fluids. Plasma expanders should be given to correct hypotension; dialysis may be of use.

Pharmaceutical precautions *Storage:* Noludar tablets should be protected from moisture and light.

Legal category CD (Sch 3), POM.

Package quantities Noludar tablets in packings of 100.

Further information Nil.

Product licence number 0031/5041R.

OMNOPON*

Presentation Round, white to buff tablets marked 'ROCHE' on one side, containing 10 mg papaveretum.

Ampoules containing 20 mg papaveretum in 1 ml. The ampoule solution is colourless to pale brown. Hydroxybenzoates are included in the formulation as preservatives.

Uses *Properties:* Omnopon, a potent analgesic, contains both the phenanthrene and isoquinoline groups of opium alkaloids. The former includes codeine and morphine which exert a marked narcotic action on the central nervous system. The second group is represented by papaverine, which acts mainly at the periphery as an antispasmodic, and noscapine.

Indications: Pre-operative medication; relief of postoperative pain; relief of severe chronic pain, particularly that of inoperable carcinoma, relief of pain in coronary thrombosis.

Dosage and administration *Adults:* Single dose of 10 to 20 mg by mouth or by injection, usually not to be repeated more often than 4 hourly.

Elderly and debilitated patients: Elderly patients are more sensitive to the actions of narcotic analgesics: the initial dose of Omnopon should not exceed 10 mg.

Children 1 to 12 years: Usual dosage 0.2–0.3 mg papaveretum/kg body-weight, as a maximum single dose.
　　Example.

Age	1 year	12 years
Weight on 50th centile (approx.)	10 kg	40 kg
Dose of papaveretum required (0.2–0.3 mg/kg)	2–3 mg	8–12 mg
Quantity of Omnopon 20 mg/ml solution required	0.10–0.15 ml	0.4–0.6 ml

The use of a small graduated syringe is recommended for the accurate administration of dosages given to children. In the absence of graduated syringes, Omnopon ampoule solution should be diluted with Water for Injections before measuring the dose.

Omnopon tablets are for oral administration. They are not recommended for use in children under 12 years of age.

Omnopon ampoules are for intramuscular, intravenous or subcutaneous injection. They are not recommended for use in babies under one year of age.

Omnopon ampoule solution contains hydroxybenzoates as preservatives and therefore should not be given by the intrathecal route.

Maintenance of stability cannot be guaranteed when Omnopon ampoule solution is diluted.

Contra-indications, warnings, etc

Contra-indications: Omnopon should not be given to comatose patients or patients with respiratory depression or obstructive airways disease. It should not be administered to patients who are receiving monoamine oxidase inhibitors or within two weeks of their withdrawal.

Omnopon should not be given to patients with a history of hypersensitivity or idiosyncratic response to opium alkaloids.

Use in pregnancy: There is inadequate evidence of safety of Omnopon in human pregnancy, but the drug has been widely used for many years without apparent ill-consequence, and animal studies have not shown any hazard. Nevertheless, the established medical principle of prescribing medicaments in early pregnancy only when absolutely indicated should be observed.

Omnopon crosses the placenta and is also secreted in breast milk. This should be borne in mind when considering its use in patients during pregnancy or breast feeding. Administration in labour may cause respiratory depression in the newborn infant.

Precautions: Omnopon should only be given with caution, and in reduced dosage, to neonates and premature infants, elderly and debilitated patients, and in patients with head injuries, severe hepatic or renal impairment, biliary tract disorders, hypothyroidism, adrenocortical insufficiency, shock, prostatic hypertrophy, and supraventricular tachycardia.

Caution is also required in patients exhibiting acute alcoholism, raised intracranial pressure or convulsive disorders. Omnopon depresses respiratory function and should be administered with particular care in patients with respiratory insufficiency.

The effects of Omnopon may be potentiated by concurrent administration of other central nervous system depressants, including anaesthetic agents. Concomitant administration of Omnopon with phenothiazines may induce severe hypotension. Patients should be instructed to avoid alcohol while under treatment, since the individual response cannot be foreseen.

Omnopon may modify patients' reactions (driving ability, operation of machinery, etc.) to a varying extent, depending on dosage, administration and individual susceptibility.

Repeated administration of Omnopon may induce tolerance to the drug, with a tendency to increasing dosage requirements to obtain the desired effect, or to physical and psychological dependence of the morphine type, with the development of withdrawal symptoms after abrupt cessation of therapy. Cross-tolerance between narcotic analgesics can occur.

Side-effects: Nausea and vomiting may be troublesome. Constipation and confusion may occur.

Treatment of overdosage: Signs of overdosage are similar to those with morphine: they include pin-point pupils, depressed respiration and coma. In severe poisoning there may be dilatation of the pupils, shock, severe respiratory depression and pulmonary oedema.

Gastric lavage should be performed soon after ingestion and intensive supportive therapy carried out. Naloxone is the preferred antidote.

Pharmaceutical precautions *Storage:* Omnopon ampoules should be protected from light. Omnopon tablets in blister packs should be stored in a dry place and protected from light. The recommended maximum storage temperature for Omnopon ampoules is 25°C and for Omnopon tablets is 30°C.

Legal category CD (Sch. 2), POM.

Package quantities Omnopon tablets in cartons of 500, each carton containing 10 packs of 50 tablets in blister strips of 10 tablets.

Omnopon ampoules in packings of 10.

Further information Omnopon is also available as Paediatric ampoules (10 mg/ml) to facilitate parenteral administration to young children (see separate prescribing information).

Product licence numbers
Ampoules 20 mg   0031/5100R
Tablets 10 mg   0031/5098R

OMNOPON* PAEDIATRIC AMPOULES

Presentation Ampoules containing 10 mg papaveretum in 1 ml. The ampoule solution is colourless to pale brown. Hydroxybenzoates are included in the formulation as preservatives.

Uses *Properties:* Omnopon, a potent analgesic, contains both the phenanthrene and isoquinoline groups of opium alkaloids. The former includes codeine and morphine, which exert a marked narcotic action on the central nervous system. The second group is represented by papaverine, which acts mainly at the periphery as an antispasmodic, and noscapine.

Indications: Pre-operative medication; relief of post-operative pain; relief of severe chronic pain, particularly that of inoperable carcinoma; relief of pain in coronary thrombosis.

Dosage and administration *Adults:* Single dose of 10 to 20 mg by injection, usually not to be repeated more often than four hourly.

Elderly: Elderly patients are more sensitive to the actions of narcotic analgesics: the initial dose should not exceed 10 mg.

Children 1–12 years: Usual dosage: 0.2–0.3 mg/kg body-weight, as a maximum single dose.

Example

Age	Weight on 50th centile (approx.)	Dose of papaveretum (0.2–0.3 mg/kg) required	Quantity of Omnopon 10 mg/ml solution required
1 year	10 kg	2–3 mg	0.2–0.3 ml
12 years	40 kg	8–12 mg	0.8–1.2 ml

Children 1–12 months: Usual dosage: 0.15–0.2 mg/kg body-weight, as a maximum single dose.

Example

Age	Weight on 50th centile (approx.)	Dose of papaveretum (0.15–0.2 mg/kg) required	Quantity of Omnopon 10 mg/ml solution required
3 months	5 kg	0.75–1 mg	0.075–0.1 ml
12 months	10 kg	1.5–2 mg	0.15–0.2 ml

Neonates aged up to 1 month
Usual dosage: 0.15 mg/kg body-weight, as a maximum single dose.

Age	Weight on 50th centile (approx.)	Dose of papaveretum (0.15 mg/kg) required	Quantity of Omnopon 10 mg/ml solution required
Newborn	3.5 kg	0.525 mg	0.0525 ml
1 month	4.0 kg	0.6 mg	0.06 ml

Omnopon Paediatric ampoules 10 mg/ml are for intramuscular, intravenous or subcutaneous injection and are recommended for use in babies under one year of age.

Omnopon Paediatric ampoule solution 10 mg/ml contains hydroxybenzoates as preservatives and therefore should not be given by the intrathecal route.

The use of a small graduated syringe is recommended for the accurate administration of dosages given to children. In the absence of graduated syringes, Omnopon Paediatric ampoule solution should be diluted with Water for Injections before measuring the dose.

Maintenance of stability cannot be guaranteed when Omnopon Paediatric ampoule solution is diluted.

Contra-indications, warnings, etc
Contra-indications: Omnopon should not be given to comatose patients or to patients with respiratory depression or obstructive airways disease. It should not be administered to patients who are receiving monoamine oxidase inhibitors or within two weeks of their withdrawal.

Omnopon should not be given to patients with a history of hypersensitivity or idiosyncratic response to opium alkaloids.

Use in pregnancy: There is inadequate evidence of safety of Omnopon in human pregnancy, but the drug has been widely used for many years without apparent ill-consequence, and animal studies have not shown any hazard. Nevertheless, the established medical principle of prescribing medicaments in early pregnancy only when absolutely indicated should be observed.

Omnopon crosses the placenta and is also excreted in breast milk. This should be borne in mind when considering its use in patients during pregnancy or breast feeding. Administration in labour may cause respiratory depression in the newborn infant.

Precautions: Omnopon should only be given with caution, and in reduced dosage, to neonates and premature infants, elderly and debilitated patients, and in patients with head injuries, severe hepatic or renal impairment, biliary tract disorders, hypothyroidism, adrenocortical insufficiency, shock, prostatic hypertrophy, and supraventricular tachycardia.

Caution is also required in patients exhibiting acute alcoholism, raised intracranial pressure or convulsive disorders. Omnopon depresses respiratory function and should be administered with particular care in patients with respiratory insufficiency.

The effects of Omnopon may be potentiated by concurrent administration of other central nervous system depressants, including anaesthetic agents. Concomitant administration of Omnopon with phenothiazines may induce severe hypotension.

Patients should be instructed to avoid alcohol while under treatment, since the individual response cannot be foreseen.

Omnopon may modify patients' reactions (driving ability, operation of machinery, etc.) to a varying extent, depending on dosage, administration and individual susceptibility.

Repeated administration of Omnopon may induce tolerance to the drug, with a tendency to increasing dosage requirements to obtain the desired effect, or to physical and psychological dependence of the morphine type, with the development of withdrawal symptoms after abrupt cessation of therapy. Cross-tolerance between narcotic analgesics can occur.

Side-effects: Nausea and vomiting may be troublesome. Constipation and confusion may occur.

Treatment of overdosage: Signs of overdosage are similar to those with morphine; they include pin-point pupils, depressed respiration and coma. In severe poisoning there may be dilatation of the pupils, shock, severe respiratory depression and pulmonary oedema.

Gastric lavage should be performed soon after ingestion and intensive supportive therapy carried out. Naloxone is the preferred antidote.

Pharmaceutical precautions *Storage:* Omnopon Paediatric ampoules 10 mg/ml should be protected from light; the recommended maximum storage temperature is 25°C.

Legal category CD (Sch. 2), POM.

Package quantities Omnopon Paediatric ampoules 10 mg/ml in packings of 10.

Further information Omnopon is also available as ampoules 20 mg/ml and 10 mg tablets (see separate data sheet).

Product licence number 0031/0156.

OMNOPON*-SCOPOLAMINE

Presentation Ampoules containing 20 mg of papaveretum and 0.4 mg of hyoscine (scopolamine) hydrobromide in 1 ml. The ampoule solution is almost colourless to pale yellow. Hydroxybenzoates are included in the formulation as preservatives.

Uses *Properties:* Omnopon-scopolamine combines the properties of the opium alkaloids with those of scopolamine. Thus it is an analgesic and sedative and has a marked inhibitory effect on the secretions.

Indication: Pre-anaesthetic medication.

Dosage and administration *Adults:* Usually ½ to one ampoule injected ¾–1 hour before anaesthesia.

Elderly: No specific studies have been performed in the elderly but this group is more sensitive to the actions of narcotic analgesics and hyoscine: the dose of Omnoponscopolamine should not exceed ½ ampoule.

Children 1–12 years: Usual dosage: 0.2–0.3 mg/kg body-weight, as a maximum single dose.
Example:

Age	1 year	12 years
Weight 50th centile (approx.)	10 kg	40 kg
Dose of papaveretum required (0.2–0.3 mg/ kg)	2–3 mg	8–12 mg
Quantity of Omnoponscopolamine required	0.10–0.15 ml	0.4–0.6 ml

The use of a small graduated syringe is recommended for the accurate administration of dosages given to children. In the absence of graduated syringes, Omnopon-scopolamine ampoule solution should be diluted with Water for Injections before measuring the dose.

Omnopon-scopolamine ampoules are for intramuscular or subcutaneous injection and are not recommended for use in babies under one year of age.

Omnopon-scopolamine ampoule solution contains hydroxybenzoates as preservatives and therefore should not be given by the intrathecal route.

Maintenance of stability cannot be guaranteed when Omnopon-scopolamine ampoule solution is diluted.

Contra-indications, warnings, etc
Contra-indications: Omnopon-scopolamine should not be given to comatose patients or to patients with respiratory depression or obstructive airways disease. It should not be administered to patients who are receiving monoamine oxidase inhibitors or within two weeks of their withdrawal.

Omnopon-scopolamine should not be given to patients with a history of hypersensitivity or idiosyncratic response to opium alkaloids.

Use in pregnancy: There is inadequate evidence of safety of Omnopon-scopolamine in human pregnancy, but the drug has been widely used for many years without apparent ill-consequence, and animal studies have not shown any hazard. Nevertheless, the established medical principle of prescribing medicaments in early pregnancy only when absolutely indicated should be observed.

Omnopon-scopolamine crosses the placenta and is also secreted in breast milk. This should be borne in mind when considering its use in patients during pregnancy or breast feeding. Administration in labour may cause respiratory depression in the newborn infant.

Precautions: Omnopon-scopolamine should only be given with caution, and in reduced dosage, to neonates and premature infants, elderly and debilitated patients, and in patients with head injuries, severe hepatic or renal impairment, biliary tract disorders, hypothyroidism, adrenocortical insufficiency, shock, prostatic hypertrophy, and supraventricular tachycardia.

Caution is also required in patients exhibiting acute alcoholism, raised intracranial pressure or convulsive disorders. Omnopon-scopolamine depresses respiratory function and should be administered with particular care in patients with respiratory insufficiency.

The effects of Omnopon-scopolamine may be potentiated by concurrent administration of other central nervous system depressants, including anaesthetic agents. Concomitant administration of Omnopon-scopolamine with phenothiazines may induce severe hypotension. Patients should be instructed to avoid alcohol while under treatment, since the individual response cannot be foreseen.

Omnopon-scopolamine may modify patients' reactions (driving ability, operation of machinery, etc.) to a varying extent, depending on dosage, administration and individual susceptibility.

Repeated administration of Omnopon-scopolamine may induce tolerance to the drug, with a tendency to increasing dosage requirements to obtain the desired effect, or to physical and psychological dependence of the morphine type, with the development of withdrawal symptoms after abrupt cessation of therapy. Cross-tolerance between narcotic analgesics can occur.

Side-effects: Nausea and vomiting may be troublesome. Constipation and confusion may also occur. Dryness of the mouth usually occurs.

Treatment of overdosage: Signs of overdosage are similar to those seen with morphine. Pin-point pupils, depressed respiration and impaired level of consciousness or coma may occur. In severe poisoning there may be dilatation of the pupils, shock, severe respiratory depression and pulmonary oedema.

Intensive supportive therapy should be carried out. Naloxone is the preferred antidote. If excitement due to scopolamine occurs, Valium Roche (diazepam) or short-acting barbiturates may be helpful.

Pharmaceutical precautions *Storage:* Omnopon-scopolamine ampoules should be protected from light. The recommended maximum storage temperature is 25°C.

Legal category CD (Sch. 2), POM.

Package quantities Omnopon-scopolamine ampoules in packings of 10.

Further information Nil.

Product licence number 0031/5096R.

PETHIDINE ROCHE

Presentation Round, white tablets with 'ROCHE' imprinted on one face, containing 25 mg pethidine hydrochloride.

Round white tablets with 'ROCHE' imprinted on one face, containing 50 mg pethidine hydrochloride.

Ampoules containing 50 mg pethidine hydrochloride in 1 ml. The ampoule solution is colourless to pale yellow.

Ampoules containing 100 mg pethidine hydrochloride in 2 ml. The ampoule solution is colourless to pale yellow.

Uses *Properties:* Pethidine Roche combines analgesic and antispasmodic properties; it is relatively short-acting and has little soporific effect. These properties make Pethidine Roche particularly useful for pain relief in labour and as an adjunct to nitrous oxide-oxygen anaesthesia.

Indications: Obstetric analgesia; moderate to severe pain; premedication and analgesia during anaesthesia.

Dosage and administration *Adults:* The normal single dose, usually not to be repeated more often than four-hourly, is as follows:

Oral: 50–150 mg.

Intramuscular or subcutaneous injection: 25–100 mg.

Intravenous injection: 25–50 mg.

Elderly and debilitated patients: Initial doses should not exceed 50 mg orally or 25 mg by injection as elderly and debilitated patients are likely to be particularly sensitive to the central depressant effects of the drug.

Children: Single dose of 0.5–2 mg/kg body weight orally or intramuscularly. This dose may be repeated if clinically necessary but it should not be repeated more often than four-hourly.

The use of a small graduated syringe is recommended for the accurate administration of dosages given to children. In the absence of graduated syringes, Pethidine Roche ampoule solution should be diluted with Water for Injections before measuring the dose.

Pethidine Roche tablets are for oral administration. Pethidine Roche ampoules are for intramuscular, intravenous or subcutaneous injection.

Pethidine Roche ampoule solution may be diluted with Water for Injection. Such dilution is recommended for accurate titration of children's doses.

Maintenance of stability cannot be guaranteed when Pethidine Roche ampoule solution is diluted.

Contra-indications, warnings, etc

Contra-indications: Pethidine should not be given to comatose patients or to patients with respiratory depression or obstructive airways disease. It should not be administered to patients who are receiving monoamine oxidase inhibitors or within two weeks of their withdrawal.

Pethidine Roche should not be given to patients with a history of hypersensitivity or idiosyncratic response to the drug.

Use in pregnancy: There is inadequate evidence of safety of pethidine in human pregnancy, but the drug has been widely used for many years without apparent ill-consequence, and animal studies have not shown any hazard. Nevertheless, the established medical principle of prescribing medicaments in early pregnancy only when absolutely indicated should be observed.

Pethidine crosses the placenta and is also secreted in breast milk. This should be borne in mind when considering its use in patients during pregnancy or breast feeding. Administration in labour may cause respiratory depression in the newborn infant.

Precautions: Pethidine should only be given with caution, and in reduced dosage, to neonates and premature infants, elderly and debilitated patients, and in patients with head injuries, severe hepatic or renal impairment, biliary tract disorders, hypothyroidism, adrenocortical insufficiency, shock, prostatic hypertrophy, and supraventricular tachycardia.

Caution is also required in patients exhibiting acute alcoholism, raised intracranial pressure or convulsive disorders. Pethidine depresses respiratory function and should be administered with particular care in patients with respiratory insufficiency.

The effects of pethidine may be potentiated by concurrent administration of other central nervous system depressants, including anaesthetic agents. Concomitant administration of pethidine with phenothiazines may induce severe hypotension. Patients should be instructed to avoid alcohol while under treatment, since the individual response cannot be foreseen.

Pethidine may modify patients' reactions (driving ability, operation of machinery, etc.) to a varying extent, depending on dosage, administration and individual susceptibility.

Repeated administration of pethidine may induce tolerance to the drug, with a tendency to increasing dosage requirements to obtain the desired effect, or to physical and psychological dependence of the morphine type, with the development of withdrawal symptoms after abrupt cessation of therapy. Cross-tolerance between narcotic analgesics can occur.

Side-effects: Pethidine may cause mild euphoria, dizziness, nausea and vomiting, hypotension and respiratory depression.

Treatment of overdosage: In acute overdosage, signs and symptoms may include incoordination, tremors and convulsions followed by respiratory depression and coma.

Gastric lavage should be performed soon after ingestion, and intensive supportive therapy carried out. Naloxone is the preferred antidote. The urinary excretion can be increased by rendering the urine acid by the administration of ammonium chloride.

Pharmaceutical precautions *Storage:* Pethidine Roche tablets in blister packs should be stored in a dry place protected from moisture.

The recommended maximum storage temperature for Pethidine Roche ampoules is 30°C.

Legal category CD (Sch. 2), POM.

Package quantities Pethidine Roche tablets 25 mg and 50 mg shrink wrapped in packs of 500 containing cartons of 50 tablets in blister strips of 10 tablets.

Pethidine Roche ampoules containing 50 mg in 1 ml in packings of 10.

Pethidine Roche ampoules containing 100 mg in 2 ml packings of 10.

Further information Nil.

Product licence numbers

Tablets 25 mg	0031/5102R
Tablets 50 mg	0031/5103R
Ampoules 50 mg	0031/5105R
Ampoules 100 mg	0031/5106R

PROSTIGMIN*

Presentation Round, white tablets with 'PROSTIGMIN' imprinted on one face with a single break bar on the other, containing 15 mg neostigmine bromide.

Ampoules containing 0.5 mg neostigmine methylsulphate in 1 ml. The ampoule solution is almost colourless to pale yellow.

Ampoules containing 2.5 mg neostigmine methylsulphate in 1 ml. The ampoule solution is almost colourless to pale yellow.

Uses *Properties:* Prostigmin is an antagonist to cholinesterase, the enzyme which normally destroys acetylcholine. The action of Prostigmin can briefly be described, therefore, as the potentiation of naturally occurring acetylcholine.

Indications: Myasthenia gravis; antagonist to non-depolarising neuromuscular blockade; paralytic ileus; post-operative urinary retention; paroxysmal supraventricular tachycardia.

Dosage and administration Prostigmin has a slower onset of effect when given orally than when given parenterally, but the duration of action is longer and the intensity of action more uniform.

To facilitate change of treatment from one route of administration to another, the following doses are approximately equivalent in effect:

0.5 mg intravenously = 1–1.5 mg intramuscularly or subcutaneously = 15 mg orally.

Administration of Prostigmin by the intravenous route, if required, should be by very slow injection. When Prostigmin is given by injection a syringe of atropine sulphate should always be available to counteract severe cholinergic reactions, should they occur.

Myasthenia gravis

Adults: Doses of 15 to 30 mg by mouth or 1–2.5 mg by intramuscular or subcutaneous injection are given at intervals throughout the day when maximum strength is needed (for example, on rising and before mealtimes). The usual duration of action of a dose is two to four hours.

The total daily dose is usually in the range of 5–20 tablets (or 5–20 mg by injection) but doses higher than these may be needed by some patients.

Newborn infants: An initial dose of Prostigmin 0.1 mg should be given intramuscularly (or 1–2 mg orally if preferred). Thereafter dosage must be titrated individually but is usually 0.05–0.25 mg by injection or 1–5 mg orally every four hours, given half an hour before feeding.

Treatment is not usually required beyond eight weeks of age except in the rare conditions of congenital and familial infantile myasthenia.

Older children: Children under 6 years old should receive an initial dose of half a tablet (7.5 mg) of Prostigmin; children 6–12 years old should receive one tablet (15 mg). Alternatively, 0.2–0.5 mg may be given by injection as required. Dosage requirements should be adjusted according to the response but are usually in the range of 15–90 mg orally per day.

The requirement for Prostigmin is usually markedly decreased after thymectomy, or when additional therapy (steroids, immunosuppressant drugs) is given.

When relatively large doses of Prostigmin are taken by myasthenic patients, it may be necessary to give atropine or other anticholinergic drugs to counteract the muscarinic effects. It should be noted that the slower gastrointestinal motility caused by these drugs may affect the absorption of oral Prostigmin.

In all patients the possibility of 'cholinergic crisis', due to overdosage of Prostigmin, and its differentiation from 'myasthenic crisis', due to increased severity of the disease, must be borne in mind. Both types of crisis are manifested by increased muscle weakness, but whereas myasthenic crisis may require more intensive anticholinesterase treatment, cholinergic crisis calls for immediate discontinuation of this treatment and institution of appropriate supportive measures, including respiratory assistance.

Antagonist to non-depolarising neuromuscular blockade

Generally, reversal of neuromuscular block with Prostigmin should not be attempted until there is evidence of spontaneous recovery from paralysis. It is recommended that the patient be well ventilated and a patent airway maintained until complete recovery of normal respiration is assured.

Adults and children: A single dose of Prostigmin 0.05–0.07 mg/kg body-weight and atropine 0.02–0.03 mg/kg body-weight, by slow intravenous injection over one minute, is usually adequate for complete reversal of non-depolarising muscle relaxants within 5–15 minutes. The maximum recommended dose of Prostigmin in adults is 5 mg and in children 2.5 mg. The two drugs are often given simultaneously, but in patients who show brady-cardia the pulse rate should be increased to about 80/minute with atropine before administering Prostigmin.

The speed of recovery from neuromuscular blockade is primarily determined by the intensity of the block at the time of antagonism but it is also subject to other factors, including the presence of drugs (e.g. anaesthetic agents, antibiotics, antiarrhythmic drugs) and physiological changes (electrolyte and acid-base imbalance, renal impairment). These factors may prevent successful reversal with Prostigmin or lead to re-curarisation after apparently successful reversal. Therefore it is imperative that patients should not be left unattended until these possibilities have been excluded.

Other indications
Adults: The usual dose is 1 to 2 tablets orally or 0.5 to 2.5 mg by subcutaneous or intramuscular injection.
Children: 2.5–15 mg orally or 0.125–1 mg by injection. The frequency of these doses may be varied according to the needs of the patient.

Elderly: There are no specific dosage recommendations for Prostigmin in elderly patients.

Prostigmin tablets for oral administration, Prostigmin ampoules for intramuscular, intravenous or subcutaneous injection.

Prostigmin ampoule solution may be diluted with Water for Injection. However maintenance of stability cannot be guaranteed when Prostigmin preparations are diluted.

Contra-indications, warnings, etc
Contra-indications: Prostigmin should not be given to patients with mechanical gastro-intestinal or urinary obstruction.

Prostigmin is contra-indicated in patients with known hypersensitivity to the drug and, in the case of Prostigmin tablets, to bromides.

Prostigmin should not be used in conjunction with depolarising muscle relaxants such as suxamethonium as neuromuscular blockade may be potentiated and prolonged apnoea may result.

Use in pregnancy: The safety of Prostigmin during pregnancy or lactation has not been established. Although the possible hazards to mother and child must therefore be weighed against the potential benefits in every case, experience with Prostigmin in pregnant patients with myasthenia gravis has revealed no untoward effect of the drug on the course of pregnancy.

As the severity of myasthenia gravis often fluctuates considerably, particular care is required to avoid cholinergic crisis, due to overdosage of the drug, but otherwise management is no different from that in non-pregnant patients.

Observations indicate that only negligible amounts of Prostigmin are excreted in breast milk; nevertheless due regard should be paid to possible effects on the breast-feeding infant.

Precautions: Extreme caution is required when administering Prostigmin to patients with bronchial asthma.

Care should also be taken in patients with bradycardia, recent coronary occlusion, hypotension, vagotonia, epilepsy or Parkinsonism.

Bradycardia may occur, to a possibly dangerous level, on intravenous injection of Prostigmin unless atropine is given simultaneously.

There is no evidence to suggest that Prostigmin has any special effects in the elderly. However, elderly patients may be more susceptible to dysrhythmias than the younger adult.

Prostigmin should not be given during cyclopropane or halothane anaesthesia; however, it may be used after withdrawal of these agents.

Side-effects: These may include nausea and vomiting, increased salivation, diarrhoea and abdominal cramps.

Treatment of overdosage: Signs of overdosage due to muscarinic effects may include abdominal cramps, increased peristalsis, diarrhoea, nausea and vomiting, increased bronchial secretions, salivation, diaphoresis and miosis. Nicotinic effects consist of muscular cramps, fasciculations and general weakness. Bradycardia and hypotension may also occur.

Artificial respiration should be instituted if respiratory depression is severe. Atropine sulphate 1–2 mg intravenously is an antidote to the muscarinic effects.

Pharmaceutical precautions *Storage:* The recommended maximum storage temperature for Prostigmin ampoules 2.5 mg is 25°C. All Prostigmin preparations should be protected from light.

Legal category
Tablets   POM
Ampoules   POM

Package quantities Prostigmin tablets in packings of 100.
Prostigmin ampoules 0.5 mg in 1 ml in packings of 10.
Prostigmin ampoules 2.5 mg in 1 ml in packings of 10.

Further information Nil.

Product licence numbers
Ampoules 0.5 mg   0031/5084
Ampoules 2.5 mg   0031/5085
Tablets   0031/5086

RIMIFON*
Presentation Ampoules containing 50 mg isoniazid in 2 ml. The ampoule solution is almost colourless.

Uses *Properties:* Rimifon is a highly active tuberculostatic drug. It has a high rate of diffusion so that the tuberculostatic action affects intracellular as well as extracellular bacilli.

Indications: All forms of pulmonary and extra-pulmonary tuberculosis.

Dosage and administration Rimifon ampoules are for intramuscular, intravenous, intrathecal or intrapleural injection.

Adults and children: The usual intramuscular or intravenous dose for adults is 200 to 300 mg as a single daily dose, for children 100 to 300 mg daily (10–20 mg/kg), but doses much larger than these are sometimes given, especially in conditions such as tuberculous meningitis.

Neonates: The recommended intravenous or intramuscular dose for neonates is 3–5 mg/kg with a maximum of 10 mg/kg daily. Isoniazid may be present in the milk of lactating mothers (see Use in Pregnancy).

Elderly: No dosage reduction is necessary in the elderly.

Intrapleural use: 50–250 mg may be instilled intrapleurally after aspiration of pus, the dosage of oral isoniazid on that day being correspondingly reduced. The ampoule solution is also used for the local treatment of tuberculous ulcers, for irrigation of fistulae, etc.

Intrathecal use: It should be noted that CSF concentrations of isoniazid are approximately 90% of plasma concentrations. Where intrathecal use is required 25–50 mg daily has been given to adults and 10–20 mg daily for children, according to age.

It is usual to give Rimifon together with other antituberculous therapy, as determined by current practice and/or sensitivity testing.

It is recommended that pyridoxine 10–50 mg daily be given during Rimifon therapy to minimise adverse reactions, especially in malnourished patients and those predisposed to neuropathy (e.g. diabetics and alcoholics).

Use in renal and hepatic impairment: No dosage reduction of Rimifon is necessary when given to patients with mild renal failure. Patients with severe renal failure (glomerular filtration rate of less than 10 ml/minute) and slow acetylator status might require a dose reduction of about 100 mg to maintain trough plasma levels less than 1 mcg/ml.

The possible risks of administration of Rimifon to patients with pre-existing non-tuberculous hepatic disease should be balanced against the benefits expected from treating tuberculosis.

Rimifon ampoule solution may be diluted with Water for Injection.

Maintenance of stability cannot be guaranteed when Rimifon ampoule solution is diluted.

Contra-indications, warnings, etc
Contra-indications: Rimifon should not be given to patients with a history of sensitivity to isoniazid.

Use in pregnancy: While Rimifon is generally regarded to be safe in pregnancy, there is a possibility of an increased risk of foetal malformations occurring when isoniazid is given in early pregnancy. If pregnancy cannot be excluded possible risks should be balanced against therapeutic benefits.

Isoniazid is excreted in breast milk at concentrations equivalent to those found in maternal plasma, 6–12 mcg/ml. This could result in an infant ingesting up to 2 mg/kg/day.

Precautions: For use in renal and hepatic impairment see *Dosage and administration.*

Isoniazid may inhibit the metabolism of phenytoin, primidone and carbamazepine. Plasma levels of these drugs should be monitored if concurrent therapy with Rimifon is necessary.

Side-effects: Rimifon is generally well tolerated. Side-effects have been reported mainly in association with high doses or in slow acetylators who develop higher blood levels of the drug. Fever, peripheral neuropathy (preventable with pyridoxine), allergic skin conditions and, rarely, lupoid syndrome, pellagra, purpura and haematological reactions have occurred during isoniazid therapy. Convulsions and psychotic reactions have also occurred, especially in patients with a previous history of these conditions. These manifestations usually subside rapidly when the drug is withdrawn.

Hepatitis may develop after 4–8 weeks treatment. Monthly review is suggested to detect and limit the severity of this side-effect by stopping treatment if plasma transaminases exceed three times the upper limit of normal. There is no evidence that this side-effect is related to acetylator status.

Care should be taken when prescribing isoniazid for patients with pre-existing hepatitis (see *Dosage and administration*).

Treatment of overdosage: In severe poisoning the main risk is of epileptiform convulsions. In addition any of the side-effects listed above may occur together with metabolic acidosis and hyperglycaemia. Treatment should be directed to the control of convulsions; large doses of pyridoxine may limit the occurrence of other adverse effects. Metabolic acidosis may require sodium bicarbonate infusion. The drug is removed by dialysis.

Pharmaceutical precautions *Storage:* The recommended maximum storage temperature for Rimifon ampoules is 25°C; the ampoules should be protected from light.

Legal category POM.

Package quantities Rimifon ampoules in packings of 10.

Further information Nil.

Product licence number 0031/5109.

RIVOTRIL*
Presentation Round, dull pinkish-buff tablets with 'RIV 0.5' imprinted on one face and two break bars on the other, containing 0.5 mg clonazepam.

Round, white tablets with 'RIV 2' imprinted on one face and two break bars on the other, containing 2 mg clonazepam.

Ampoules containing 1 mg clonazepam in 1 ml solvent, each accompanied by an ampoule containing 1 ml Water for Injection USP as a diluent. The ampoule solution is colourless.

Uses *Properties:* Rivotril is a benzodiazepine derivative exhibiting marked anticonvulsant properties. These have been demonstrated in the many tests in animals which are employed to establish the anti-epileptic properties of a drug. Animal experiments and electroencephalographic studies in man have shown that Rivotril prevents generalisation of convulsive activity and raises the seizure threshold. In many cases, abnormal electroencephalograms become normal. Rivotril improves both focal seizures and primarily generalised attacks. Administered intravenously, Rivotril quickly controls status epilepticus.

Indications: All clinical forms of epileptic disease and seizures in infants, children or adults, especially: typical or atypical petit mal; generalised primary or secondary tonic-clonic seizures including grand mal; status epilepticus in all clinical forms; focal seizures with elementary or complex symptomatology, various forms of myoclonus and associated abnormal movements.

Dosage and administration *Tablets:* Treatment should be started with low doses. These should not exceed 1 mg/day for adults, 0.5 mg/day for children and 0.25 mg/day for infants and small children. If desired, the total dose may be given at night for the first four days of treatment. The dose may be increased progressively until the maintenance dose suited to the individual patient has been found.

The dosage of Rivotril must be adjusted to the needs of each individual and depends on the age of the patient and the individual response to therapy. The maintenance dosage must be determined according to clinical response and tolerance.

The normal daily dosage for various age groups falls in the following ranges:

Adults	4–8 mg
School children (5–12 years)	3–6 mg
Small children (1–5 years)	1–3 mg
Infants (0–1 year)	0.5–1 mg

Elderly: The elderly are particularly sensitive to the effects of central depressant drugs and may experience confusion. It is recommended that the initial dosage of Rivotril should not exceed 0.5 mg/day.

These are total daily dosages which should be divided into three or four doses taken at intervals throughout the day. If necessary, larger doses may be given at the discretion of the physician. The maintenance dose should be attained after two to four weeks of treatment.

In some forms of childhood epilepsy, certain patients may cease to be adequately controlled by Rivotril. Control may be re-established by increasing the dose, or interrupting treatment with Rivotril for two to three weeks. During the interruption in therapy careful observation and other drugs may be needed.

Simultaneous administration of more than one anti-epileptic drug is a common practice in the treatment of epilepsy and may be undertaken with Rivotril. The dosage of each drug may be required to be adjusted to obtain the optimum effect. If status epilepticus occurs in a patient receiving oral Rivotril, intravenous Rivotril may still control the status.

Rivotril tablets are for oral administration.

Ampoules: for the treatment of status epilepticus the dose and rate of administration is governed by the response of the patient. As a guide, we suggest:

Adults: 1 mg (1 ampoule of active substance mixed with 1 ampoule of diluent) by slow intravenous injection.

Infants and children: 0.5 mg (equivalent to ½ ampoule of active substance mixed with ½ ampoule of diluent) by slow intravenous injection.

This dose should be repeated if needed. It may be given by slow intravenous infusion if preferred.

Intravenous injection of Rivotril should be into a large vein of the antecubital fossa. The injection should be given slowly – in adults, 1 mg over approximately 30 seconds. This will greatly diminish the rare possibility of hypotension or apnoea occurring. Nevertheless, facilities for resuscitation should always be available.

The contents of the diluent ampoule which contains 1 ml of Water for Injection USP, *must* be added to the contents of the other ampoule, which contains 1 mg clonazepam in 1 ml, *immediately* before injection.

Rivotril ampoule solution may be diluted when given in intravenous infusions of saline or dextrose, such as are customary in the treatment of status epilepticus. Thus, up to 3 mg (3 ampoules) in 250 ml of the following solutions is permissible: Sodium Chloride Injection BP. Dextrose Injection BP 5% and 10%. Sodium Chloride and Dextrose Injection BP (0.45% sodium chloride and 2.5% dextrose). This infusion dilution should be made up freshly and used within 12 hours.

Rivotril ampoules are for intravenous administration. Maintenance of stability cannot be guaranteed when Rivotril ampoule solution is diluted.

Contra-indications, warnings, etc

Contra-indications: Patients with known sensitivity to benzodiazepines; acute pulmonary insufficiency; respiratory depression.

Use in pregnancy: The use of Rivotril during pregnancy or lactation should be avoided.

The administration of high doses or prolonged administration of low doses of benzodiazepines in the last trimester of pregnancy or during labour has been reported to produce irregularities in the foetal heart, and hypotonia, poor sucking and hypothermia in the neonate.

Precautions: Rivotril should be used with caution in patients with chronic pulmonary insufficiency, or with impairment of renal or hepatic function, and in debilitated patients. In these cases dosage may need to be reduced.

Since alcohol can provoke epileptic seizures, irrespective of therapy, patients should be advised not to drink alcohol while under treatment. In combination with Rivotril, alcohol may modify the effects of the drug, compromise the success of therapy or give rise to unpredictable side-effects.

As a general rule, epileptic patients are not allowed to drive. Even when adequately controlled on Rivotril, it should be remembered that any increase in dosage or alteration in timings of dosage may modify patients' reactions, depending on individual susceptibility. If a patient is allowed to operate machinery, he should also be warned of these possible effects.

When Rivotril is used in conjunction with other anti-epileptic drugs, side-effects and toxicity may be more evident, particularly with hydantoins or phenobarbitone and combinations including them. This requires extra care in adjusting dosage in the initial stages of treatment.

As with all other anti-epileptic drugs, treatment with Rivotril must not be abruptly interrupted but must be withdrawn by gradually reducing the dose. This precaution must also be taken when withdrawing another drug while the patient is still receiving Rivotril therapy.

Side-effects: The side-effects observed consist of fatigue, somnolence, occasional muscular hypotonia and co-ordination disturbances. Such effects are usually transitory and disappear spontaneously as treatment continues or with dosage reduction. They tend to occur early in treatment and can be greatly reduced, if not avoided, by commencing with low dosages followed by progressive increases.

In infants and small children, and particularly those with a degree of mental impairment, Rivotril may give rise to salivary or bronchial hypersecretion with drooling. Supervision of the airway may be required.

As with other benzodiazepines, isolated cases of blood dyscrasias and abnormal liver function tests have been reported.

Rivotril generally has a beneficial effect on behaviour disturbances in epileptic patients. In certain cases, paradoxical effects such as aggressiveness, irritability, agitation, psychotic disorders and activation of new types of seizures may be precipitated. If these occur, the addition to the regimen of another suitable drug may be necessary.

Although Rivotril has been given uneventfully to patients with porphyria, rarely it may induce convulsions in these patients.

Treatment of overdosage: As with other benzodiazepine drugs, overdosage should not present undue problems of management or threat to life. Patients have recovered from overdoses in excess of 60 mg without special treatment. Severe somnolence with muscle hypotonia will be present. Treatment is symptomatic and may include the need to maintain an airway. Gastric lavage may be useful if performed soon after ingestion.

Pharmaceutical precautions *Storage:* Rivotril tablets should be stored in well-closed containers, in a cool place. Rivotril tablets and ampoules should be protected from light.

Legal category CD (Sch. 4), POM.

Package quantities Rivotril tablets 0.5 mg in packings of 100 and 500.

Rivotril tablets 2 mg in packings of 100 and 500.

Rivotril ampoules 1 mg in packings of 10, accompanied by 1 ml ampoules Water for Injection USP as diluent.

Further information Nil.

Product licence numbers
Tablets 0.5 mg   0031/0076
Tablets 2 mg   0031/0077
Ampoules 1 mg   0031/0078

ROACCUTANE* ▼

Presentation Oval, soft-gelatine capsules (spherical diameter approximately 5.8 mm), one-half pale red-violet and the other half white, marked 'R5', containing 5 mg isotretinoin.

Oval, soft-gelatine capsules (spherical diameter approximately 8.2 mm), one-half pale red-violet and the other half white, marked 'R20', containing 20 mg isotretinoin.

Uses *Properties:* Isotretinoin is a stereoisomer of tretinoin (all-*trans*-retinoic acid), an established preparation for topical treatment of acne vulgaris. Taken orally, Roaccutane has marked therapeutic efficacy in severe forms of acne, which are difficult to control with other means. The exact mechanism of action of Roaccutane is not known but clinical improvement is associated with a dose-related suppression of the size and activity of sebaceous glands.

Indications: Roaccutane is indicated for the treatment of cystic and conglobate acne and severe acne which has failed to respond to an adequate course of a systemic antimicrobial agent.

Dosage and administration The therapeutic response to Roaccutane is dose-related and varies between patients. This necessitates individual adjustment of dosage according to the response of the condition and the patient's tolerance of the drug. In most cases complete or near-complete remission of acne is achieved with a 12- to 16-week course of treatment. It is recommended that repeat courses of treatment should not normally be given.

The daily dosage, to the nearest number of whole capsules, should be taken with food either as a single dose or in two divided doses during the day, whichever is more convenient.

Adults: Initial dosage: All patients initially should receive Roaccutane 0.5 mg/kg body-weight daily for a period of 4 weeks, when their responsiveness to the drug will usually be apparent. Acute exacerbation of acne is occasionally seen during the initial period but this subsides, usually within 7–10 days, with continued treatment.

Subsequent dosage: Patients who show early improvement should continue to receive the initial dosage of 0.5 mg/kg body-weight daily for the remainder of the course.

In patients who show little or no initial improvement, and who are tolerating the drug well, dosage should be increased up to 1 mg/kg body-weight daily for the remainder of the course.

In patients who show intolerance to the initial dosage, treatment should be continued with a reduced dosage of 0.1 to 0.2 mg/kg body-weight daily.

Repeated courses of therapy are not normally indicated.

With effective treatment, complete clearing of acne is usually achieved and prolonged remission ensues. However, patients whose acne is not completely cleared at the end of treatment can be expected to show continuing improvement for up to several months thereafter. Only if a definite relapse is seen in the post-treatment period should a repeated course be considered.

Concomitant therapy: As a rule, other drugs conventionally used for the treatment of acne, including antibiotics, keratolytics and exfoliants, are not indicated but non-irritant topical preparations may be applied if required.

Patients should be instructed to avoid taking preparations containing high doses of vitamin A, i.e. more than the recommended dietary allowance of 4,000–5,000 iu per day.

Children: Roaccutane is not indicated for the treatment of prepubertal acne.

Roaccutane capsules are for oral administration.

Contra-indications, warnings, etc

Contra-indications: Roaccutane is contra-indicated in hepatic and renal impairment. It should not be given to breast-feeding mothers.

Roaccutane is teratogenic; major foetal abnormalities have been reported in humans. It is therefore contra-indicated in pregnancy. In any woman of childbearing potential the risk of its use must be weighed against the expected therapeutic benefit under all circumstances, taking into account the precautions specified below.

Precautions: For all women of childbearing potential the following precautions must be strictly observed.

1. Pregnancy should be excluded before instituting therapy with Roaccutane.

2. Any woman of childbearing potential who is receiving Roaccutane must practise effective contraception during the treatment period and for at least 4 weeks following its cessation.

3. Contraceptive measures must also be taken in the case of repeated courses of treatment.

4. Any pregnancy occurring during treatment with Roaccutane, or immediately following its completion, carries a risk of foetal malformation. This would raise the question of the termination of pregnancy for medical reasons. Therefore, before instituting Roaccutane therapy in a woman of childbearing potential the treating physician must explain clearly and in detail what precautions must be taken. This should include the risks involved and the possible consequences of a pregnancy occurring during Roaccutane treatment or in the first 4 weeks following its completion.

In view of the importance of the foregoing precautions, Roaccutane Patient Information Cards are available to doctors and it is strongly recommended that these be given to all patients.

Liver function and blood lipids (fasting value) should be measured in all patients at the start of treatment, after the first month of administration and thereafter as appropriate before discontinuation of Roaccutane.

At the completion of a lifespan study in rats there was an increased incidence of phaeochromocytoma in animals given isotretinoin at dosages of 32 and 8 mg/kg/day, but not 2 mg/kg/day. Since rats are particularly prone to develop this tumour type, the significance of this finding for use of Roaccutane in man is uncertain;

nevertheless, repeated courses of treatment are not normally recommended.

Patients should not donate blood either during or for at least one month following discontinuation of therapy with Roaccutane. Theoretically there would be a small risk to a woman in the first trimester of pregnancy who received blood donated by a patient on Roaccutane therapy.

Side-effects: Most of the clinical side-effects of Roaccutane are dose-related and are usually well-tolerated at the recommended dosages. The side-effects may recede during continued treatment and in all cases have proved reversible with reduction of dosage or discontinuation of therapy.

The skin and mucous membranes are most commonly affected. Dryness of the skin may be associated with scaling, thinning, erythema (especially of the face) and pruritus. An increase in epidermal fragility has been reported, and frictional trauma may lead to epidermal blistering. Dryness of the nasal mucosa may be associated with mild epistaxis. Dryness of the conjunctivae has been reported and may lead to mild to moderate conjunctivitis which may be alleviated by use of topical antibiotics. Corneal opacities have been reported in a few patients but spontaneous resolution has usually occurred on discontinuation of Roaccutane.

Hair thinning may occur but is uncommon at dosages below 1 mg/kg/day and is reversible following discontinuation of Roaccutane. Nevertheless, patients should be warned that this is a possibility during treatment.

Non-specific symptoms such as nausea, malaise, drowsiness and sweating have been reported infrequently. Benign intracranial hypertension has been reported, particularly in association with concomitant antibiotic therapy.

Myalgia and arthralgia may occur and may be associated with reduced tolerance to vigorous exercise. Isolated instances of raised serum CPK values have been reported in patients receiving Roaccutane, particularly those undertaking vigorous physical activity. In these cases the clinical significance is unknown.

A rise in serum levels of liver enzymes may occur. In a few cases significant increases have occurred, necessitating dosage reduction or discontinuation of Roaccutane.

Elevation of serum triglycerides above the normal range has been observed, especially where predisposing factors such as a family history of lipid disorders, obesity, alcohol abuse, diabetes mellitus or smoking are present. The changes are dose-related and may be controlled by dietary means (including restriction of alcohol intake) and/or by reduction of dosage of Roaccutane.

Rare instances have been reported of elevated blood glucose levels in diabetic patients receiving Roaccutane, therefore, careful monitoring of glucose levels during treatment is advised.

Isotretinoin has been shown to affect diaphyseal and spongy bone adversely in animals at high doses in excess of those recommended for use in man.

Bone changes, including early epiphyseal closure, have occurred in man after several years' administration of Roaccutane in very high doses for disorders of keratinization. Prospective X-ray examination of some patients treated for severe cystic acne with Roaccutane revealed evidence of skeletal hyperostosis without clinical symptoms.

Treatment of overdosage: Isotretinoin is a derivative of vitamin A and overdosage should be expected to induce symptoms of hypervitaminosis A.

Manifestations of acute vitamin A toxicity include severe headache, nausea or vomiting, drowsiness, irritability, and pruritus. Signs and symptoms of accidental or deliberate overdosage with Roaccutane would probably be similar. They would be expected to be reversible and to subside without need for treatment. Because of the variable absorption of the drug, gastric lavage may be worthwhile in the first few hours after ingestion.

Pharmaceutical precautions *Storage:* Roaccutane capsules should be stored in a well-closed container and protected from light; the recommended maximum storage temperature is 30°C.

Legal category POM.

Package quantities Roaccutane capsules 5 mg in packings of 100.

Roaccutane capsules 20 mg in packings of 100.

Further information *Availability:* Roaccutane capsules are available through hospital pharmacies for use in hospitals and hospital clinics and it is recommended that Roaccutane should be given only by, or under supervision of, a dermatological specialist.

Product licence numbers
Capsules 5 mg   0031/0158
Capsules 20 mg   0031/0160

RO-A-VIT*

Presentation Round, cream, sugar-coated tablets with 'ROCHE' printed in red on one face, containing 50,000 i.u. retinol (vitamin A) as the acetate (15 mg retinol equivalent).

Ampoules containing 300,000 i.u. retinol as the palmitate (90 mg retinol equivalent) in 1 ml oily solution.

Uses *Properties:* Ro-A-Vit is a synthetic vitamin A preparation. Vitamin A may be considered to act chiefly as a regulator of the growth and activity of epithelial tissues. It plays an essential role in the visual cycle through its participation in the synthesis of visual purple by the retina.

The cardinal signs and symptoms of vitamin A deficiency are those affecting the eyes, such as xerosis, swelling and destruction of the cornea and night-blindness. Changes in the skin and changes in the mucous membranes of the respiratory, digestive and urinary tracts have been reported.

Indications: Prevention and treatment of vitamin A deficiencies.

Ro-A-Vit ampoules are indicated when oral therapy is inappropriate (e.g. in malabsorption syndrome).

Dosage and administration *Tablets – Adults:* 1–6 tablets daily (50,000–300,000 i.u.).

Children: If, on the recommendation of a physician, a children's dosage is required, then it is suggested that up to 50,000 i.u. daily be given according to age.

Ampoules: Adults and children: A maintenance dosage of ½–1 ampoule by deep intramuscular injection once monthly is usually sufficient but in acute deficiency states the same dosage may be given once weekly. When prolonged therapy with high, weekly dosages of vitamin A is required it is suggested that Ro-A-Vit ampoules be given in courses of no longer than six weeks separated by treatment-free intervals of two weeks so that the patient can be observed for signs of possible hypervitaminosis A.

Elderly: No specific studies of vitamin A have been performed in elderly patients but Ro-A-Vit has been widely used for many years without apparent ill consequence.

Ro-A-Vit tablets are for oral administration.

Ro-A-Vit ampoule solution is only suitable for deep intramuscular injection.

Contra-indications, warnings, etc
Contra-indication: Hypersensitivity to vitamin A.

Use in pregnancy: High doses of vitamin A can be teratogenic. Ro-A-Vit is therefore contra-indicated during pregnancy.

Effects of overdosage and their treatment: Massive doses of vitamin A are required to produce toxicity and therefore it is extremely unlikely that even exceptionally large single doses would cause hypervitaminosis A except possibly in children. Manifestations of acute overdosage in children include severe headache, nausea or vomiting, drowsiness, irritability and pruritus. In chronic overdosage in children the following have been noted after periods of $2\frac{1}{2}$–15 months: hydrocephaly, alopecia, painful swellings over the long bones, with bone and joint pains, hyperosteosis, and deep, hard, tender swellings in the extremities. Adults are likely to complain of bone and joint pains. The vitamin should be discontinued. Symptoms of acute overdosage subside within 72 hours and of chronic overdosage over a period of several months, without further treatment.

Pharmaceutical precautions
Storage: Ro-A-Vit tablets should be stored in well-closed containers. The recommended maximum storage temperature for Ro-A-Vit tablets is 25°C.

Ro-A-Vit ampoules should be protected from light. Recommended maximum storage temperature 25°C.

Legal category
POM.

Package quantities
Ro-A-Vit Tablets in packings of 100.

Ro-A-Vit ampoules in packings of 10.

Further information
Nil.

Product licence numbers
Tablets   0031/5111
Ampoules 0031/0124

ROCALTROL*

Presentation Soft gelatine capsules, one length red opaque and the other white opaque, containing 0.25 microgram calcitriol. Soft gelatine capsules, both lengths brown red opaque, containing 0.5 microgram calcitriol.

Uses *Properties:* Calcitriol has the greatest biological activity of the known vitamin D metabolites and is normally formed in the kidneys from its immediate precursor, 25-hydroxycholecalciferol. In physiological amounts it augments the intestinal absorption of calcium and phosphate and plays a significant part in the regulation of bone mineralisation. The defective production of calcitriol in chronic renal failure contributes to the abnormalities of mineral metabolism found in that disorder.

Rocaltrol is a synthetic preparation of calcitriol. Oral administration of Rocaltrol to patients with chronic renal failure compensates for impaired endogenous production of calcitriol which is decreased when the glomerular filtration rate falls below 30 ml/min. Consequently, intestinal malabsorption of calcium and phosphate and the resulting hypocalcaemia are improved, thereby reversing the signs and symptoms of bone disease.

The onset and reversal of the effects of Rocaltrol are more rapid than those of other compounds with vitamin D activity and adjustment of the dose can be achieved sooner and more precisely. The effects of inadvertent overdosage can also be reversed more readily.

Indications: Rocaltrol is indicated for the correction of the abnormalities of calcium and phosphate metabolism in patients with renal osteodystrophy.

Dosage and administration The dose of Rocaltrol should be carefully adjusted for each patient according to the biological response so as to avoid hypercalcaemia. The effectiveness of treatment depends in part on an adequate daily intake of calcium, which should be augmented by dietary changes or supplements if necessary. The capsules should be swallowed with a little water.

Adults: It is suggested that treatment should be started with two to four 0.5 mcg capsules of Rocaltrol daily and serum calcium levels monitored at weekly intervals. The daily dose may be increased by increments of 0.25–0.5 mcg to a total of 2 or 3 mcg daily according to the biological response. When dose requirements are stable serum calcium levels may be monitored at intervals of two to four weeks.

When there is biochemical or radiographic evidence of bone healing the requirements for Rocaltrol generally decrease. The dose should then be adjusted to avoid hypercalcaemia.

Higher doses of Rocaltrol may be required when barbiturates or anticonvulsants are given concurrently but this should rarely exceed 5 mcg daily. Reduction of dose is necessary if such drugs are withdrawn.

Elderly: Clinical experience with Rocaltrol in elderly patients indicates that the dosage recommended for use in younger adults may be given without apparent ill consequence.

Children: Dosage in children has not been established.

Rocaltrol capsules are for oral administration only.

Contra-indications, warnings, etc
Contra-indications: Rocaltrol should not be given to patients with hypercalcaemia or evidence of metastatic calcification.

Use in pregnancy: The safety of Rocaltrol during pregnancy has not been established and it should be given only when the potential benefit has been weighed against the possible hazard. The usual caution in prescribing any drug for women of child-bearing age should be observed.

Precautions: All other vitamin D compounds and their derivatives, including proprietary compounds or foodstuffs which may be 'fortified' with vitamin D, should be withheld during treatment with Rocaltrol.

Treatment does not obviate the need to control plasma phosphate with phosphate binding agents. Since Rocaltrol affects phosphate transport in the gut and bone, the dose of phosphate binding agent may need to be modified.

Side-effects: Hypercalcaemia and hypercalciuria are the major side-effects of Rocaltrol and indicate excessive dosage. The clinical features of hypercalcaemia include anorexia, nausea, vomiting, headache, weakness, apathy and somnolence. More severe manifestations may include thirst, dehydration, polyuria, nocturia, abdominal pain, paralytic ileus and cardiac arrhythmias. Rarely, overt psychosis and metastatic calcification may occur. The relatively short biological half-life of Rocaltrol permits rapid elimination of the compound when treatment is stopped and hypercalcaemia will recede within two to seven days. The rate of reversal of biological effects is more rapid than when other vitamin D derivatives are used.

Mild, non-progressive and reversible elevations in levels of liver enzymes (SGOT, SGPT) have been noted in a few patients treated with Rocaltrol, but no pathological changes in the liver have been reported.

Effects of overdosage and their treatment: In acute overdose gastric lavage should be considered as soon after ingestion as possible provided that the drug was taken within the previous six to eight hours.

Should hypercalcaemia occur, Rocaltrol should be discontinued until plasma calcium levels have returned to normal. A low-calcium diet will speed this reversal. Rocaltrol can then be restarted at a lower dose or given in the same dose but at less frequent intervals than previously. Severe hypercalcaemia may be treated by ensuring adequate hydration, inducing a diuresis where practicable and by general supportive measures. Calcitonin may increase the rate of fall of serum calcium when bone resorption is increased.

In patients treated by intermittent haemodialysis, a low concentration of calcium in the dialysate may also be used.

Pharmaceutical precautions *Storage:* Rocaltrol capsules should be protected from heat.

Legal category POM.

Package quantities Capsules 0.25 mcg in packings of 100.
Capsules 0.5 mcg in packings of 100.

Further information Nil.

Product licence numbers
Capsules 0.25 mcg   0031/0122
Capsules 0.5 mcg   0031/0123

ROHYPNOL* ▼

Presentation A purple film-coated, bi-convex diamond-shaped tablet with a single break bar on one side and 'ROHYPNOL' on the other side, containing 1 mg flunitrazepam.

Uses *Properties:* Rohypnol is a benzodiazepine compound with hypnotic properties.

Indications: The short-term treatment of sleep disturbances, particularly in patients who have difficulty in falling asleep.

The induction of sleep at unusual times on a short-term or irregular basis.

Dosage and administration *Adults:* 0.5–1 mg before retiring.

Adults with severe sleep disturbances: 1–2 mg.

Elderly or debilitated patients: It is recommended that the initial dose to be taken before retiring should not exceed 0.5 mg; tolerability at this dosage level is excellent. In exceptional cases, where the hypnotic effect

is less than adequate but tolerability is satisfactory, the dose may be increased to 1 mg.
Rohypnol tablets are not for paediatric use.
Rohypnol tablets are for oral administration.

Contra-indications, warnings, etc

Contra-indications: Patients with known sensitivity to benzodiazepines; acute pulmonary insufficiency; respiratory depression.

Use in pregnancy: The use of Rohypnol during pregnancy should be avoided.

The administration of high doses or prolonged administration of low doses of benzodiazepines in the last trimester of pregnancy or during labour has been reported to produce irregularities in the foetal heart, and hypotonia, poor sucking and hypothermia in the neonate.

Rohypnol has been detected in breast milk. If possible, the use of Rohypnol should be avoided during lactation.

Precautions: In patients with chronic pulmonary insufficiency, and in patients with chronic renal or hepatic disease, dosage may need to be reduced.

If Rohypnol is combined with centrally-acting drugs such as neuroleptics, tranquillizers, antidepressants, hypnotics, analgesics and anaesthetics, the sedative effects may be intensified.

Patients should be advised that, like all medicaments of this type, Rohypnol may modify patients' performance at skilled tasks (driving, operating machinery, etc.) to a varying degree depending upon dosage and individual susceptibility. Patients should further be advised that alcohol may intensify any impairment and should, therefore, be avoided during treatment.

The dependence potential of the benzodiazepines is low but this increases when high doses are used, especially when given over long periods. This is particularly so in patients with a history of alcoholism or drug abuse or in patients with marked personality disorders. Regular monitoring in such patients is essential; routine repeat prescriptions should be avoided and treatment should be withdrawn gradually. Symptoms such as depression, nervousness, rebound insomnia, irritability, sweating, and diarrhoea have been reported following abrupt cessation of treatment with normal therapeutic doses.

In rare instances, withdrawal following excessive dosages may produce confusional states, psychotic manifestations and convulsions.

Abnormal psychological reactions to benzodiazepines have been reported. Rare behavioural effects include paradoxical aggressive outbursts, excitement, confusion and the uncovering of depression with suicidal tendencies.

Side-effects: Adverse effects include drowsiness, unsteadiness and ataxia; these are dose-related and are likely to be uncommon with the recommended dosage. The elderly are particularly sensitive to the effects of central depressant drugs and may experience confusion. If organic brain changes are present, the dosage of Rohypnol should not exceed 0.5 mg in these patients.

Other adverse effects are less common and include headache, vertigo, hypotension, gastro-intestinal upsets, skin rashes, visual disturbances, changes in libido, and urinary retention. Isolated cases of blood dyscrasias and jaundice have also been reported.

Treatment of overdosage: When taken alone in overdosage Rohypnol presents few problems in management. Signs may include drowsiness, ataxia, and dysarthria, with coma in severe cases. Treatment is symptomatic.

Gastric lavage is useful only if performed soon after ingestion. There is no specific antidote to Rohypnol.

When taken with centrally-acting drugs, especially alcohol, the effects of overdosage are likely to be more severe and, in the absence of supportive measures, may prove fatal.

Pharmaceutical precautions *Storage:* Rohypnol tablets should be stored in a dry place and protected from light.

Legal category CD (Sch. 4), POM.

Package quantities Rohypnol tablets 1 mg are blister-packed in packings of 100.

Further information The distribution half-life of flunitrazepam is about three hours; the elimination half-life is, on average, 22 hours.

The onset of effect is rapid and the duration of effect is dose-dependent.

Treatment should be kept to a minimum and given only under close medical supervision. Little is known regarding the efficacy or safety of benzodiazepines in long-term use.

Product licence number 0031/0104.

RONICOL*

Presentation Round, white tablets with *'RONICOL'* imprinted across one face with a single break bar on the other, containing 59.4 mg nicotinyl alcohol tartrate (equivalent to 25 mg nicotinyl alcohol).

Uses *Properties:* Ronicol is the alcohol corresponding to nicotinic acid and has similar vasodilator properties. Its action is more sustained than that of nicotinic acid because, in addition to the vasodilator effect of the alcohol itself, partial metabolism of the alcohol results in the gradual release of nicotinic acid. Ronicol exerts a direct vasodilator action on the walls of small arteries and arterioles; there is a slight transient tendency towards a fall in blood pressure and slowing of the pulse.

Indications: Circulatory disorders, including peripheral vascular disease, vascular spasm (e.g. Raynaud's disease and acrocyanosis). Ménière's syndrome, chilblains, eye conditions due to deficient retinal circulation.

Dosage and administration *Adults:* 1–2 tablets four times daily.

Elderly: No specific precautions are required for the use of Ronicol in elderly patients.

Children: No dosage recommendations are made for the administration of Ronicol to children.

Ronicol tablets are for oral administration.

Contra-indications, warnings, etc
Use in pregnancy: There is no evidence of the safety of Ronicol in human pregnancy but it has been in wide use for many years without apparent ill consequence, animal studies having showed no hazard.

Precautions: Care should be taken in the long-term administration of high doses of Ronicol in patients with pre-diabetic or diabetic metabolic disorders.

Side-effects: Ronicol is very well tolerated and may be given over long periods without toxic effects. Mild, transient flushing of the face and a feeling of warmth in the region of the head may be experienced when the patient is taking an optimal dose.

Effects of overdosage and their treatment: In overdosage, gastric irritation, diarrhoea, flushing and general vasodilatation and possibly hypotension may occur.

Gastric lavage should be performed and symptoms treated as they arise.

Pharmaceutical precautions *Storage:* Ronicol should be stored in well-closed containers.

Legal category P.

Package quantities Ronicol tablets in packings of 100.

Further information Nil.

Product licence number 0031/5113.

RONICOL* TIMESPAN*

Presentation Brown-red, sugar-coated tablets with 'ROCHE' printed in black across one face containing 357 mg nicotinyl alcohol tartrate (equivalent to 150 mg nicotinyl alcohol).

Uses *Properties:* Ronical Timespan tablets are slow-release tablets, the active principle being Ronicol, which is the alcohol corresponding to nicotinic acid and has similar vasodilator properties. In addition to the vasodilator effect of the alcohol itself, partial metabolism of the alcohol results in the gradual release of nicotinic acid. The compound exerts a direct vasodilator action on the walls of small arteries and arterioles which is maintained for 12 hours. There is a slight transient tendency towards a fall in blood pressure and slowing of the pulse.

Indications: Circulatory disorders, including peripheral vascular disease, vascular spasm (e.g. Raynaud's disease and acrocyanosis). Ménière's syndrome, chilblains, eye conditions due to deficient retinal circulation.

Dosage and administration *Adults:* 1 or 2 tablets night and morning, depending on the severity of the condition. They should be swallowed whole.

Elderly: No specific precautions are required for the use of Ronicol Timespan in elderly patients.

Children: No dosage recommendations are made for the administration of Ronicol Timespan to children.

Ronicol Timespan tablets are for oral administration.

Contra-indications, warnings, etc
Use in pregnancy: There is no evidence of the safety of Ronicol Timespan in human pregnancy but it has been in wide use for many years without apparent ill consequence, animal studies having shown no hazard.

Precautions: Care should be taken in the long-term administration of high doses of Ronicol in patients with pre-diabetic or diabetic metabolic disorders.

Side-effects: Ronicol Timespan is very well tolerated and may be given over long periods without toxic effects. Mild, transient flushing of the face and a feeling of warmth in the region of the head may be experienced when the patient is taking an optimal dose.

Effects of overdosage and their treatment: In overdosage, gastric irritation, diarrhoea, flushing and general vasodilatation and possibly hypotension may occur.

Gastric lavage should be performed and symptoms treated as they arise.

Pharmaceutical precautions *Storage:* Ronicol Timespan should be stored in well-closed containers.

Legal category P.

Package quantities Ronicol Timespan tablets in packings of 100.

Further information Nil.

Product licence number 0031/5114.

SYNKAVIT*
Alternative name: Menadiol sodium diphosphate.

Presentation Round, white tablets with 'SYNKAVIT' imprinted on one face with a single break bar across the other, containing 12.63 mg of the tetra-sodium salt of 2-methyl-1,4-naphthahydroquinone diphosphate (equivalent to 10 mg of the free ester).

Ampoules containing 12.63 mg of the tetra-sodium salt of 2-methyl-1,4-naphthahydroquinone diphosphate (equivalent to 10 mg of the free ester) in 1 ml. The ampoule solution is colourless to pale yellow.

Uses *Properties:* Synkavit is a water-soluble vitamin K analogue. The presence of vitamin K is essential for the formation within the body of prothrombin, factor VII, factor IX and factor X. Lack of vitamin K leads to increased tendency to haemorrhage.

Indications: Synkavit is indicated in the treatment of haemorrhage or threatened haemorrhage associated with a low blood level of prothrombin or factor VII.

The main indications include: obstructive jaundice (before and after surgery); haemorrhage after dental extractions; prevention of neonatal haemorrhage.

Dosage and administration *Adults:* Usual therapeutic dose – 10–40 mg daily.

Elderly: Recommendations for the elderly do not differ from those for younger adults.

Children: If, on the recommendation of a physician, a children's dosage is required, it is suggested that 5–20 mg daily be given.

For haemorrhagic disease of the newborn: Administered prophylactically to the mother: 10 mg by mouth daily for three to four days before labour, or 5 mg by injection during labour.

In the peri-natal period do not use Synkavit as vitamin K_1 (Konakion*) is the drug of choice (see separate data sheet).

Administered to the infant: Do not use Synkavit as vitamin K_1 (Konakion*) is the drug of choice (see separate data sheet). Also refer to Contra-indications and warnings.

Synkavit tablets are for oral administration.

Synkavit ampoules are for intramuscular, intravenous or subcutaneous injection.

Synkavit ampoule solution may be diluted with Water for Injection.

Maintenance of stability cannot be guaranteed when Synkavit ampoule solution is diluted.

Contra-indications, warnings, etc
Contra-indications: The administration of Synkavit to neonates or to mothers in the peri-natal period is contra-indicated in the treatment of haemorrhagic disease of the newborn as vitamin K_1 (Konakion*) is the drug of choice.

Use in pregnancy: There is no specific evidence regarding the safety of Synkavit in pregnancy but, as with most drugs, the administration during pregnancy should only occur if the benefits outweigh the risks.

Precautions: Caution should be exercised in administering Synkavit and other vitamin K analogues to newborn (especially premature) infants.

Moderate doses of Synkavit have produced haemolytic anaemia, hyperbilirubinaemia and kernicterus, especially in premature infants even when administered prior to delivery. In the perinatal period, vitamin K_1 (Konakion) is the drug of choice. Synkavit may induce haemolysis (especially in the newborn infant) in the presence of erythrocyte glucose-6-phosphate dehydrogenase deficiency or low concentrations of alpha-tocopherol in the blood.

Pharmaceutical precautions *Storage:* Recommended maximum storage temperature for Synkavit tablets is 30°C, for Synkavit ampoules 10 mg 25°C. All Synkavit preparations should be protected from light.

Legal category Tablets P
Ampoules POM.

Package quantities Synkavit tablets in packings of 100.
Synkavit ampoules 10 mg in 1 ml in packings of 10.

Further information In almost all circumstances Synkavit is as effective as the natural vitamin (vitamin K_1). For severe cases of drug-induced hypoprothrombinaemia or bleeding produced in association with coumarin or indanedione anticoagulants or salicylates, Konakion (vitamin K_1) should be used.

Product licence numbers
Tablets   0031/5115
Ampoules 10 mg   0031/5116

TARACTAN*
Presentation Round, pink, sugar-coated tablets with 'ROCHE' printed in red across one face, containing 15 mg chlorprothixene.

Round, dark red-brown, sugar-coated tablets with 'ROCHE' printed in white across one face, containing 50 mg chlorprothixene.

Uses *Properties:* Taractan is a major tranquillising drug of the thioxanthene group. It has sedative and anti-adrenergic properties, similar to those of chlorpromazine, but it has greater anticholinergic and some antihistamine activity.

Indications: In schizophrenia, other psychoses and psychoneuroses for the management of severe anxiety, tension, agitation, hallucinations, delusions and associated disturbances.

Dosage and administration Dosage should be individually adjusted according to the severity of the condition. In general, small doses should be used initially and increased to the optimal effective level according to the clinical response. Unwanted lethargy and drowsiness are usually controlled by dosage reduction.

Adults: Ambulatory treatment of agitation and anxiety, tension, excitation or irritability: initially 15 mg three times daily. Dosages exceeding 100 mg daily are rarely required.

Severe psychosis: initially 15–50 mg three or four times daily, to be increased as needed at intervals of 2–3 days. Dosages exceeding 600 mg daily are rarely required.

Elderly and debilitated patients: In general, lower doses should be given, especially in patients with cerebral arteriosclerosis. Initially, dosage should not exceed 15 mg three times daily and subsequent increases should be gradual.

Children: Not recommended.

Taractan tablets are for oral administration.

Contra-indications, warnings, etc

Contra-indications: Circulatory collapse; comatose states; known hypersensitivity to the drug or other similar drugs (e.g. chlorpromazine).

Use of Taractan should be avoided in patients with severe renal, hepatic or cardiovascular disease or in marked cerebral arteriosclerosis.

Use in pregnancy and lactation: There is insufficient evidence of safety in human pregnancy, nor is there evidence from animal studies that it is free from hazard. Do not use in pregnancy.

Chlorprothixene is found in breast milk. Do not use during lactation.

Precautions: Because of its structural similarity to the phenothiazines, the precautions appropriate to pheno-thiazine therapy should also be exercised with Taractan.

In patients suspected to be suffering from cardiac insufficiency, with disturbances of heart rhythm or conduction, in chronic pulmonary insufficiency, in Par-kinsonism and in patients with a history of epilepsy, care is required, especially in the elderly (including confu-sional states).

The elderly are specially prone to experience adverse effects such as sedation, hypotension, confusion and temperature changes.

Care is required in patients with narrow-angle glau-coma, prostatic hypertrophy, myasthenia gravis, hypo-thyroidism, phaeochromocytoma and during very hot weather ('heat stroke' is a possible side-effect).

When necessary, Taractan may be used concomitantly with anticonvulsant drugs but it should be borne in mind that Taractan may lower the convulsive threshold and, therefore, dosage of the anticonvulsant may need to be adjusted.

Caution is required when administering other central nervous system depressants, including anaesthetics, analgesics, hypnotics, tricyclic antidepressants and monoamine oxidase inhibitors as their sedative and cardiovascular effects may be intensified by Taractan. The anticholinergic effects of atropine and other drugs may also be increased and undesirable anticholinergic effects can be enhanced by anti-Parkinsonism drugs.

Patients should be instructed to avoid alcohol while under treatment with Taractan since the individual response cannot be foreseen. Patients should further be advised that, like all medicaments of this type, Taractan may modify performance at skilled tasks (driving, oper-ating machinery, etc.) to a varying degree, depending on dosage and individual susceptibility.

Chlorprothixene antagonises the action of adrenaline and other sympathomimetic agents and reverses the blood-pressure-lowering effects of clonidine and adre-nergic blocking agents such as guanethidine. It may impair the metabolism of tricyclic antidepressants, the anti-Parkinsonian effect of levodopa and the effects of anticonvulsants.

In high acute doses, Taractan, like other neuroleptics, may interfere with insulin secretion and thereby affect the control of diabetes.

The possibility of increased anticoagulant effect due to inhibition of hepatic metabolism, as reported with phenothiazines, should be borne in mind.

Antacids can impair absorption; tea and coffee may prevent absorption by causing insoluble precipitates.

Taractan may enhance the cardiac depressant effect of quinidine, the absorption of corticosteroids and digoxin, the effect of diazoxide and of neuromuscular blocking agents. Interactions with propranolol have been reported.

The possibility of interaction with lithium should be borne in mind.

In patients who require prolonged therapy with Taractan, the possibility of liver damage, pigmentary retinopathy, lenticular or corneal opacities, and the development of irreversible dyskinesias should be kept in mind, although these adverse effects appear to be less frequent with Taractan than with phenothiazine com-pounds. Regular and careful monitoring of the blood picture, hepatic function and ECG is advisable, particu-larly if these may be affected by other concurrently administered drugs.

Withdrawal: Taractan is not known to produce physical dependence, but gastritis, nausea and vomiting, dizziness and tremulousness have been reported following abrupt withdrawal of high-dose therapy.

Side-effects: Drowsiness is the most common side-effect, particularly during the first or second week, after which it generally recedes. If troublesome, dosage should be lowered. Anticholinergic effects, including dry mouth, nasal congestion, constipation, urinary retention and mydriasis, may be experienced.

Postural hypotension, leading to faintness or dizziness and tachycardia, may occur, especially when dosage is suddenly increased. On rare occasions (e.g. in heat stroke) the hypotensive effect may produce a shock-like condition.

Obstructive jaundice, usually occurring between the second and fourth weeks of treatment and regarded as a sensitivity reaction, has been associated with Taractan. This has usually been reversible but chronic jaundice has been reported.

Blood dyscrasias may occur, most often in the form of leucopenia but including rare cases of agranulocytosis, eosinophilia, thrombocytopenic purpura, and pancyto-penia. The appearance of signs of bone-marrow depres-sion requires immediate cessation of treatment.

Extrapyramidal reactions in the form of acute dystonias, Parkinsonism rigidity, tremor or akinesia, akathisia and oculogyric crises may occur. These tend to be dosage-related and subside within 24–48 hours of discontinuing the drug or reducing dosage.

Anti-Parkinsonian agents should not be prescribed routinely because of the possible risks of aggravating anticholinergic side-effects of chlorprothixene, of pre-cipitating toxic confusional states and tardive dyskinesia or of impairing its therapeutic efficacy. They should only be given as required.

As with all neuroleptic drugs, persistent or tardive dyskinesias may appear during long-term therapy or after drug withdrawal. Tardive dyskinesia is a syndrome of irregularly repetitive involuntary movements affecting the oro-facial muscles and sometimes the limbs and trunk. Although more commonly associated with high-potency neuroleptic drugs given in relatively large doses for prolonged periods, it has also been reported with short-term neuroleptic therapy at low dosages. The potential irreversibility and seriousness as well as unpre-dictability of the syndrome require especially careful assessment of risk versus benefit and the lowest possible dosage and duration of treatment consistent with therapeutic efficacy.

Other side-effects reported include convulsions (particularly in patients with a history of epilepsy or EEG abnormalities) and slight peripheral oedema. Chlorprothixene can cause increased susceptibility to sunburn and patients should be warned to avoid excessive exposure. Skin rashes (urticaria, photosensitivity) have been reported. Amenorrhoea, lactation and other signs of endocrine disturbance are seen only infrequently at high dosages.

Chlorprothixene, even in low dosage in susceptible (especially non-psychotic) individuals, may cause unpleasant subjective feelings of being mentally dulled or slowed down, nausea, dizziness, headache or paradoxical effects of excitement, agitation or insomnia.

ECG changes, with prolongation of the QT interval and T-wave changes, have been reported in patients treated with moderate to high doses; they are reversible on reducing the dose.

Sexual function, including erection and ejaculation, may be impaired by chlorprothixene. Moderate weight gain (1–2 kg) is commonly seen; in the occasional cases where the gain is excessive, this may be prevented by reducing the dose.

Chlorprothixene may impair the control of body temperature and cases of hyperthermia have occurred rarely. The possible development of hypothermia, particularly in the elderly, should be borne in mind.

Treatment of overdosage: The primary symptoms of overdosage are drowsiness, moderate to severe hypotension with shock, general weakness, cyanosis, pyrexia, contracted pupils, tachycardia (which may occur after a delay of several hours), respiratory depression and coma. Convulsions and hyperactivity may occur later during the recovery period. Acute renal failure has been reported. There is no specific antidote to Taractan.

Early gastric lavage should be performed. If hypotension occurs, the patient should be placed in a head-down position and oxygen and intravenous fluids administered. If an adequate blood pressure is still not obtained, noradrenaline or metaraminol may be given, but not adrenaline. Respiration should be maintained by artificial methods. Intravenous diazepam (Valium Roche) or short-acting barbiturates may be used to control convulsions. Continuous cardiac monitoring is essential for at least 48 hours; in some cases a longer period may be necessary.

Pharmaceutical precautions *Storage:* Taractan tablets should be stored in well-closed containers.

Legal category POM.

Package quantities Taractan tablets 15 mg in packings of 50.
Taractan tablets 50 mg in packings of 50.

Further information Nil.

Product licence numbers
Tablets 15 mg   0031/5118R
Tablets 50 mg   0031/5129R

TEMETEX*

Presentation White cream containing 0.1% w/w diflucortolone valerate in an oil-in-water emulsion.

White to yellowish-white fatty ointment containing 0.1% w/w diflucortolone valerate in an anhydrous base.

White to yellowish-white ointment containing 0.1% w/w diflucortolone valerate in a water-in-oil emulsion.

Uses *Properties:* Diflucortolone valerate, the active ingredient of Temetex preparations, is a highly effective topical corticosteroid with rapid onset of action, marked anti-inflammatory action and good cutaneous tolerance. In addition to inhibiting inflammation in inflammatory and allergic skin diseases, it ameliorates the subjective complaints such as itching, burning and pain.

Three different presentations are available, each designed to suit a particular condition of the patient's skin, thereby aiding the achievement of the optimal clinical response.

Indications: Temetex preparations are indicated for the treatment of non-infected eczemas, dermatitis, psoriasis and other corticosteroid-responsive dermatoses.

Dosage and administration *Adults and children:* Initially, the Temetex preparation best suited to the particular skin condition (see below) should be applied as a thin film two or three times daily according to the severity of the condition. Once clinical improvement has been obtained, maintenance treatment with one application daily should be sufficient.

Temetex cream is suitable for weeping skin lesions and moist skin regions (anus, flexures) which require a base with a high water-content. It allows secretions to drain and ensures rapid drying of the skin.

Temetex fatty ointment is designed for use in chronic and very dry or scaly conditions. The anhydrous, greasy base retains moisture thereby softening the thickened horny layer of the skin, and so improving the penetration of the active substance. As the fatty ointment has an occlusive effect, this largely dispenses with the need for occlusive dressings.

Temetex ointment has the broadest range of applications, being suitable for conditions which are neither weeping nor very dry. The base, which has a balanced fat and water content, greases the skin lightly without having an occlusive effect.

In refractory cases either Temetex ointment or Temetex fatty ointment may be applied under an occlusive dressing large enough to cover completely the affected area of skin and affixed to healthy skin. The dressing should not be left on for more than two days but it may be replaced intermittently, if necessary. However, if the lesion becomes infected during treatment the use of occlusive dressings should be suspended until the infection has been controlled.

Elderly: No special precautions are required for the use of Temetex preparations in the elderly.

Temetex preparations are for external application only.

Contra-indications, warnings, etc
Contra-indications: Temetex should not be applied in the presence of syphilitic, tuberculous or viral (chickenpox, vaccinia) infections that involve the skin. It is not suitable for the treatment of ophthalmic conditions.

Temetex fatty ointment should not be applied to weeping lesions.

Use in pregnancy: In pregnant animals, topical application of corticosteroids can cause abnormalities of foetal development. The relevance of these findings to human beings has not been established and there is inadequate evidence of safety of the drug in pregnancy, even though it has been in wide use for many years without apparent ill effect.

Nevertheless, topical steroids should not be used extensively (i.e. in large amounts or for prolonged periods) during the first trimester of pregnancy.

Precautions: With Temetex, as with all topical corticosteroid preparations, long-term continuous therapy in infants should be avoided as adrenal suppression can occur, even without the use of occlusive dressings. Babies and infants up to four years of age should not therefore be treated for a period of more than three weeks, especially in areas covered by napkins, which may act as an occlusive dressing.

Care should be taken to avoid contact with the eyes. The hands should be washed carefully after applying Temetex.

Infections in the treated area require additional specific antimicrobial therapy. This treatment can often be topical, but for severe bacterial infections systemic therapy may be necessary. If fungal infections are present a topically active antimycotic agent should be applied.

Side-effects: Temetex is well tolerated locally. Very occasionally a mild burning, itching or irritation may occur at the site of application.

As with all topical corticosteroids, there is a risk of skin atrophy, telangiectasia, striae and acneiform eruptions following extensive use of Temetex, particularly with the fatty ointment or where occlusive dressings are applied. The face is more susceptible to such atrophic changes than other areas of the body. The application of unusually large amounts of Temetex preparations may result in the absorption of systemically active amounts of corticosteroid.

In the event of any untoward reaction, treatment should be discontinued.

Treatment of overdosage: It is anticipated that ingestion of Temetex preparations is unlikely to present any problems of management. No specific recommendations for treatment are made.

Pharmaceutical precautions *Storage:* Recommended maximum storage temperature 30°C.

Legal category POM.

Package quantities Temetex cream, fatty ointment and ointment in tubes of 30 g.

Further information Nil.

Product licence numbers
Cream   0031/0080
Fatty ointment   0031/0082
Ointment   0031/0081

TENSILON*

Presentation Ampoules containing 10 mg edrophonium chloride in 1 ml. The ampoule solution is almost colourless.

Uses *Properties:* Tensilon is an antagonist to cholinesterase, the enzyme which normally destroys acetylcholine. The action of Tensilon can briefly be described, therefore, as the potentiation of naturally occurring acetylcholine. It differs from Prostigmin* (neostigmine) and Mestinon* (pyridostigmine) in the rapidity and brevity of its action.

Indications: Myasthenia gravis, as a diagnostic test; to distinguish between overdosage and underdosage of cholinergic drugs in myasthenic patients; diagnosis of suspected 'dual block'; antagonist to non-depolarising neuromuscular blockade; treatment of paroxysmal supraventricular tachycardia.

Dosage and administration *Adults – Test for myasthenia gravis:* A syringe is filled with the contents of 1 ampoule Tensilon (10 mg) and 2 mg is given intravenously, the needle and syringe being left *in situ.* If no response occurs within 30 seconds, the remaining 8 mg is injected. In adults with unsuitable veins, 10 mg is given by intramuscular injection.

To differentiate between 'myasthenic' and 'cholinergic' crises: In a myasthenic patient who is suffering from marked muscle weakness, in spite of taking large doses of Mestinon or Prostigmin, a test dose of 2 mg Tensilon is given intravenously one hour after the last dose of the cholinergic compound. If therapy has been inadequate, there is a rapid, transient increase of muscle strength; if the patient has been overtreated, Tensilon causes a transient increase of muscle weakness.

Diagnosis of suspected 'dual block': Tensilon 10 mg intravenously. If the block is due to depolarisation, it is briefly potentiated, whereas in a 'dual block', it is reversed.

Children: Diagnostic tests: A total dose of 0.1 mg/kg body-weight may be given intravenously. One fifth of this dose should be injected initially; if no response occurs, the remainder of the dose is administered 30 seconds later.

Antagonist to non-depolarising neuromuscular blockade: Generally, reversal of neuromuscular block with Tensilon should not be attempted until there is evidence of spontaneous recovery from paralysis. It is recommended that the patient be well ventilated and a patent airway maintained until complete recovery of normal respiration is assured.

Adults and children: Tensilon 0.5–0.7 mg/kg body-weight and atropine 0.007 mg/kg body-weight, by slow intravenous injection over several minutes, is usually adequate for reversal of non-depolarising muscle relaxants within 5–15 minutes. The two drugs are usually given simultaneously, but in patients who show bradycardia the pulse rate should be increased to about 80/minute with atropine before administering Tensilon.

The speed of recovery from neuromuscular blockade is primarily determined by the intensity of the block at the time of antagonism but it is also subject to other factors, including the presence of drugs (e.g. anaesthetic agents, antibiotics, antiarrhythmic drugs) and physiological changes (electrolyte and acid-base imbalance, renal impairment). These factors may prevent successful reversal with Tensilon or lead to recurarisation after apparently successful reversal. Therefore it is imperative that patients should not be left unattended until these possibilities have been excluded.

Treatment of paroxysmal supraventricular tachycardia: Tensilon 10 to 20 mg intravenously, combined with carotid sinus pressure if necessary.

Elderly: There are no specific dosage recommendations for Tensilon in elderly patients.

Tensilon ampoules are for intramuscular or intravenous injection.

Tensilon ampoules may be diluted with Water for Injections. However, maintenance of stability cannot be guaranteed when Tensilon ampoule solution is diluted.

Contra-indications, warnings, etc

Contra-indications: Tensilon should not be given to patients with mechanical intestinal or urinary obstruction.

Tensilon is contra-indicated in patients with known hypersensitivity to the drug.

With doses above 10 mg, especially the higher dosage employed to antagonise neuromuscular blockade, Tensilon should not be used in conjunction with depolarising muscle relaxants such as suxamethonium as neuromuscular blockade may be potentiated and prolonged apnoea may result.

Use in pregnancy: The safety of Tensilon during pregnancy or lactation has not been established. Although the possible hazards to mother and child must be weighed against the potential benefits in every case, experience with Tensilon in pregnant patients with myasthenia gravis has revealed no untoward effect of the drug on the course of pregnancy.

There is no information on the excretion of Tensilon into breast milk. Although only negligible amounts would be expected to be present, due regard should be paid to possible effects on the breast-feeding infant.

Precautions: Extreme caution is required when administering Tensilon to patients with bronchial asthma.

Care should also be taken in patients with bradycardia, recent coronary occlusion, vagotonia, hypotension, epilepsy or Parkinsonism.

In diagnostic uses of Tensilon, a syringe containing 1 mg of atropine should be kept at hand to counteract severe cholinergic reactions, should they occur.

When Tensilon is used as an antagonist to neuromuscular blockade bradycardia may occur, to a possibly dangerous level, unless atropine is given simultaneously. In this indication, Tensilon should not be given during cyclopropane or halothane anaesthesia; however, it may be used after withdrawal of these agents.

There is no evidence to suggest that Tensilon has any special effects in the elderly. However, elderly patients may be more susceptible to dysrhythmias than younger adults.

Side-effects: These may include nausea and vomiting, increased salivation, diarrhoea and abdominal cramps.

Effects of overdosage and their treatment: Tensilon overdosage may give rise to bradycardia, arrhythmias, hypotension and bronchiolar spasm. Perspiration, gastro-intestinal hypermotility and visual disturbances may also occur.

Atropine sulphate 1–2 mg intravenously is an antidote to the muscarinic effects.

Pharmaceutical precautions *Storage:* Tensilon ampoule solution should be protected from light.

Legal category POM.

Package quantities Tensilon ampoules in packings of 10.

Further information Nil.

Product licence number 0031/5095.

TIGASON* ▼

Presentation Capsules with buff-yellow cap and buff-yellow body with ROCHE printed in black on both cap and body, containing 10 mg etretinate.

Capsules with orange-yellow cap and buff-yellow body with ROCHE printed in black on both cap and body, containing 25 mg etretinate.

Uses *Properties:* Retinol (vitamin A) is known to be essential for normal epithelial growth and differentiation, though the mode of this effect is not yet established.

Both retinol and retinoic acid are capable of reversing hyperkeratotic and metaplastic skin changes. However, these effects are generally only obtained at dosages associated with considerable local or systemic toxicity.

Tigason, a synthetic aromatic derivative of retinoic acid, has a more favourable therapeutic ratio, with a greater and more specific inhibitory effect on psoriasis and disorders of epithelial keratinization. The usual therapeutic response to Tigason consists of desquamation (with or without erythema) followed by more normal re-epithelization.

Indications: Severe extensive psoriasis which is resistant to other forms of therapy.

Palmo-plantar pustular psoriasis.

Congenital ichthyosis.

Darier's disease (keratosis follicularis).

Dosage and administration There is a wide variation in the absorption and rate of metabolism of Tigason. This necessitates individual adjustment of dosage. For this reason the following dosage recommendations can serve only as a guide.

Adults: Other dermatological therapy, particularly with keratolytics, should normally be stopped before administration of Tigason, though use of topical corticosteroids or bland emollient ointment may be continued if indicated.

Tigason should be started at a dose of 0.75–1 mg/kg body-weight per day (in most cases 50–75 mg daily), taken in divided doses, for two to four weeks. By this time involved areas of skin will usually show a marked response and/or side-effects should be apparent. If no therapeutic effect is seen by four weeks, and in the absence of toxicity, daily dosage may then be increased in increments of 10 mg at weekly intervals until a response is observed or a total daily dose of 1.5 mg/kg body-weight is reached.

Once a response has been observed, the dosage of Tigason should be reduced to 0.5 mg/kg body-weight per day, taken in divided doses, for a further six to eight weeks, when the maximum therapeutic effect should usually have been obtained.

When maximum clearing of lesions has occurred, especially in patients with psoriasis and Darier's disease, treatment with Tigason should normally be discontinued for an interval in order to assess whether a worthwhile period of remission ensues. Subsequent exacerbations may then be treated intermittently as necessary. However, in some patients, especially those with congenital ichthyosis, the period of remission may be brief and continued maintenance therapy, at the lowest dose which will prevent recurrences (usually 0.25–0.5 mg/kg body-weight per day), may be appropriate.

Elderly: Dosage is the same as for younger adults.

Children: Dosage should be carried out as outlined above for adults. Clinical experience indicates that Tigason is generally better tolerated by children.

Tigason capsules are for oral administration.

Contra-indications, warnings, etc Tigason is contra-indicated in patients with hepatic or renal impairment. It should not be given to breast-feeding mothers.

Use in pregnancy: Tigason is teratogenic. Therefore, in

any woman of childbearing potential, the risk must be weighed against the expected therapeutic benefit under all circumstances, taking into account the precautions specified below.

Precautions: For all women of childbearing potential the following precautions must be strictly observed.

1. Pregnancy must be excluded before instituting therapy with Tigason.

2. Any woman of childbearing potential who is receiving Tigason must practise effective contraception for at least one month before treatment, during the treatment period and for at least 12 months following its cessation.

3. The same contraceptive measures must also be taken in the case of repeated treatment for recurrences of the disease.

4. Any pregnancy occurring during treatment with Tigason, or in the 12 months following its completion, carries a high risk of foetal malformation. This would raise the question of the termination of pregnancy for medical reasons. Therefore, before instituting Tigason the treating physician must explain clearly and in detail what precautions must be taken. This should include the risks involved and the possible consequences of pregnancy occurring during Tigason treatment or in the 12 months following its completion.

In view of the importance of the above precautions, Tigason Patient Information Cards are available to doctors and it is strongly recommended that these be given to all patients.

Liver function and blood lipids (fasting value) should be measured at the start of treatment, after the first month of administration and at three-monthly intervals thereafter.

Patients should be warned of the possibility of alopecia occurring (see 'Side-effects').

Patients should also be instructed to avoid taking preparations containing high doses of Vitamin A, i.e. more than the recommended dietary allowance of 4,000–5,000 iu per day.

Patients should not donate blood either during or for at least one year following discontinuation of therapy with Tigason. Theoretically there would be a small risk to a woman in the first trimester of pregnancy who received blood donated by a patient on Tigason therapy.

Side-effects: Most of the clinical side-effects of Tigason are dose-related and are usually well-tolerated at the recommended dosages. However, the toxic dose of Tigason is close to the therapeutic dose and most patients experience some side-effects during the initial period whilst dosage is being adjusted. They are reversible with reduction of dosage or discontinuation of therapy.

The skin and mucous membranes are most commonly affected. Dryness of the mucous membranes, sometimes with erosion, involving the lips, mouth, conjunctivae and nasal mucosa are seen. Dryness of the skin may be associated with scaling, thinning, erythema (especially of the face) and pruritus. Palmar and plantar exfoliation, epistaxis and epidermal fragility have been reported, as well as paronychia. Dryness of the conjunctivae may lead to mild-to-moderate conjunctivitis alleviated by the use of topical antibiotics.

Hair thinning and frank alopecia may occur, usually noted four to eight weeks after starting therapy, and is reversible following discontinuation of Tigason. Patients should be warned that this is a possibility during treatment.

Non-specific symptoms such as nausea, malaise,

drowsiness and sweating have been reported infrequently. Myalgia and arthralgia may occur and be associated with reduced tolerance to exercise.

Benign intracranial hypertension has been reported.

A rise in serum levels of liver enzymes may occur. When significant, dosage reduction or discontinuation of therapy may be necessary.

Elevation of serum triglycerides above the normal range has been observed, especially where predisposing factors such as a family history of lipid disorders, obesity, alcohol abuse, diabetes mellitus or smoking are present. The changes are dose-related and may be controlled by dietary means (including restriction of alcohol intake) and/or by reduction of dosage of Tigason.

Extraosseous calcification has been reported following long-term administration of etretinate.

Treatment of overdosage: Manifestations of acute vitamin A toxicity include severe headache, nausea or vomiting, drowsiness, irritability and pruritus. Signs and symptoms of accidental or deliberate overdosage with Tigason would probably be similar. They would be expected to be reversible and to subside without need for treatment.

Because of the variable absorption of the drug, gastric lavage may be worthwhile within the first few hours after ingestion.

Pharmaceutical precautions *Storage:* Tigason capsules should be stored in a well-closed container and protected from light. The recommended maximum storage temperature is 30°C.

Legal category POM.

Package quantities Tigason capsules 10 mg in packings of 100.
Tigason capsules 25 mg in packings of 100.

Further information *Availability:* Tigason capsules are available only through hospital pharmacies for use in hospitals and hospital clinics.

It is recommended that Tigason be given only by, or under supervision of, a dermatological specialist.

Product licence numbers
Capsules 10 mg   0031/0134
Capsules 25 mg   0031/0135

TRH-ROCHE
Approved name: Protirelin.

Presentation Plain glass ampoules containing 0.2 mg TRH-Roche (thyrotrophin-releasing hormone) in 2 ml. The ampoule solution is almost colourless to faintly yellow.

Round, white tablets with 'ROCHE' imprinted on one face and a single break bar on the other and imprinted (TRH/TRH) containing 40 mg TRH-Roche (thyrotrophin releasing hormone).

Uses *Properties:* TRH-Roche stimulates the secretion of thyroid-stimulating hormone (TSH). Intravenous injection results in a prompt rise in serum TSH levels in normal subjects, peak levels being observed about 20 minutes after administration. There is a concomitant rise in serum levels of prolactin. TRH-Roche is also active orally, the maximum TSH response being apparent some two to four hours after ingestion. The maximum responses of protein-bound iodine (PBI), tri-iodothyronine (T_3) and thyroxine (T_4) occur up to five hours after the administration of a single oral dose.

Indications: The administration of TRH-Roche provides a means of assessing thyroid function and the reserve of TSH in the pituitary gland and is recommended as a test procedure where such assessment is indicated. It is particularly useful as a diagnostic test for: mild hyperthyroidism; ophthalmic Graves' disease; mild or preclinical hypothyroidism; hypopituitarism; hypothalamic disease. It may also be used in place of the T_3 suppression test.

Dosage and administration *Intravenous injection:* Tests employing intravenous TRH-Roche are based on the serum TSH response to a standard dose. They provide a means of both quantitative and qualitative assessment of thyroid function. It is essential for each laboratory to establish its own normal range of values for serum TSH before attempting quantitative assessment of TRH-Roche responses by this means.

Intravenous TRH-Roche test:
1. Blood sample taken for control TSH assay.
2. TRH-Roche 0.2 mg given as a single bolus injection.
3. Blood sample taken 20 minutes after injection for peak TSH assay.
4. If necessary, a further blood sample may be taken 60 minutes after injection to detect a delayed TSH response.

The ampoule solution should not be diluted.

Oral TRH-Roche test: Responses to oral TRH-Roche have not been defined within precise limits and they therefore provide a means of qualitative rather than quantitative assessment.

1. Blood sample taken either immediately before TRH-Roche administration or, if more convenient, on the previous day for control TSH assay and/or PBI, T_3 or T_4 estimations.
2. TRH-Roche 40 mg (1 tablet) administered with half a glass of water to the patient fasted overnight.
3. Patient to fast for one hour after taking the tablet.
4. Blood sample taken four to five hours after dosing for repeat estimations of TSH and/or PBI, T_3 or T_4.

TRH-Roche tablets are for oral administration.

Elderly: Although no specific studies have been performed to establish the use of TRH-Roche in the elderly, its use has been well documented. Dosage requirements and the side-effect profile are similar to those of younger adults.

Children: The procedure for administering TRH-Roche to children are identical with those outlined above. An intravenous dose of 1 mcg/kg body-weight may be used.

Interpretation of results: Interpretation of the responses to TRH-Roche is based on the increase in TSH and/or PBI, T_3 or T_4 levels from the basal values. In normal subjects, there is a prompt rise in serum levels of TSH. The changes observed in various conditions are briefly outlined below:

1. Hyperthyroidism – no rise in serum TSH or thyroid hormone levels.
2. Ophthalmic Graves' disease – often no rise in serum TSH or thyroid hormone levels.
3. Primary hypothyroidism – exaggerated and prolonged rise in serum TSH but no change in thyroid hormone levels.
4. Hypopituitarism – absent or impaired TSH or thyroid hormone response implies diminished TSH reserve.

5. Hypothalamic disease – a rise in serum TSH or thyroid hormone levels can occur in the presence of hypothyroidism; delayed responses are common.

The TRH-Roche test provides, in most instances, information similar to that obtained from a T_3 suppression test in that an absent or impaired response usually correlates with an absent or impaired response to T_3 suppression.

The response to TRH-Roche may be modified in subjects taking T_3, T_4, antithyroid drugs, corticosteroids, oestrogens, levodopa, phenothiazines, metoclopramide, bromocriptine, salicylates or theophylline.

Contra-indications, warnings, etc
Use in pregnancy: There is some clinical evidence of safety in human pregnancy, animal studies having shown no hazard. Nevertheless, the established medical principle of not administering drugs during early pregnancy should be observed.

Precautions: There are no absolute contra-indications to TRH-Roche. In view of the postulated effect of bolus injections of TRH-Roche on smooth muscle, administration orally would seem more appropriate in patients with bronchial asthma or other types of obstructive airways disease. Caution should also be observed in patients with myocardial ischaemia. TRH-Roche administration is not normally associated with a fall in blood sugar, but caution is recommended when giving the drug orally to patients with severe hypopituitary disease in the fasting state because of the possibility of hypoglycaemia.

Side-effects: TRH-Roche is well tolerated. No impairment of hepatic, renal or haematological function has been reported. Following rapid intravenous injection, side-effects of a mild and transient nature may be experienced. They comprise nausea, a desire to micturate, a feeling of flushing, slight dizziness and a peculiar taste, and have been attributed to a local action of the bolus of TRH-Roche on the plain muscle of the gastrointestinal and genito-urinary tracts. Side-effects after oral administration are very rare, nausea being the only one so far observed. No reactions of an allergic nature have been noted with TRH-Roche.

Effects of overdosage: No symptoms of overdosage have been noted in patients receiving up to 1 mg intravenously.

Pharmaceutical precautions *Storage:* The recommended maximum storage temperature for TRH-Roche ampoules is 30°C. No special precautions are required for the tablets.

Legal category POM.

Package quantities TRH-Roche ampoules containing 0.2 mg TRH-Roche in 2 ml in packings of 10. TRH-Roche 40 mg tablets in packings of 10.

Further information *Availability:* TRH-Roche is available to hospitals only.

Product licence numbers
Ampoules 0031/0064
Tablets 0031/0063

VALIUM* ROCHE TABLETS, CAPSULES, SYRUP AND SUPPOSITORIES
Presentation Round, white tablets with ROCHE 2

imprinted on one face and a single break bar on the other, containing 2 mg diazepam.

Round, pale yellow tablets with ROCHE 5 imprinted on one face and a single break bar on the other, containing 5 mg diazepam.

Round, blue tablets with ROCHE 10 imprinted on one face and a single break bar on the other, containing 10 mg diazepam.

Capsules with opaque blue cap and opaque white body with ROCHE 2 printed in red-brown along both cap and body, containing 2 mg diazepam.

Capsules with opaque blue cap and opaque yellow body with ROCHE 5 printed in red-brown along both cap and body, containing 5 mg diazepam.

Pink, raspberry-flavoured syrup containing 2 mg diazepam in 5 ml.

Suppositories containing 5 mg diazepam.
Suppositories containing 10 mg diazepam.

Uses *Properties:* Valium Roche has anxiolytic, anticonvulsant and central muscle-relaxant properties. It has little autonomic activity.

Indications: Adults: Short-term treatment of symptoms of anxiety.

Anxiety associated with, or precipitating, psychosomatic illness; anxiety complicating organic illness.

Treatment of anxiety accompanying psychoses.

Short-term treatment of conditions where anxiety may be a precipitating or aggravating factor, e.g. tension headaches or migraine attacks.

Short-term treatment of insomnia associated with anxiety where daytime anxiolytic effects are desirable.

Symptomatic treatment of acute alcohol withdrawal.

Muscle spasm. As an adjunct to the control of muscle spasm in tetanus.

May be useful in the management of cerebral spasticity in selected cases.

As an adjunct to the management of some types of epilepsy, e.g. myoclonus.

Premedication.

Children: Night terrors and somnambulism.

May be useful in controlling tension and irritability in cerebral spasticity in selected cases.

As an adjunct to the control of muscle spasm in tetanus.

Premedication.

Dosage and administration

Anxiety states: Adults: Mild anxiety states – 2 mg three times daily.

Severe anxiety states – 15 to 30 mg daily in divided doses.

Symptomatic relief of acute alcohol withdrawal – 5 to 20 mg, repeated if necessary in 2 to 4 hours.

Insomnia associated with anxiety – 5 to 15 mg before retiring.

Night terrors and somnambulism: Children: 1 to 5 mg at bedtime.

Conditions associated with muscle spasm: Adults: Muscle spasm – 2 to 15 mg daily in divided doses.

Management of cerebral spasticity in selected cases – 2 to 60 mg daily in divided doses.

Adjunct to control of muscle spasm in tetanus – 3 to 10 mg/kg body-weight daily by nasoduodenal tube. The selected dose should relate to the severity of the case

and in extremely severe cases higher doses have been used. Intravenous Valium Roche is recommended initially (see separate data sheet).

Children: Control of tension and irritability in cerebral spasticity in selected cases – 2 to 40 mg daily in divided doses.

As an adjunct to the control of muscle spasm in tetanus – As for adults.

Adjunct to the management of some types of epilepsy: Premedication: 2 to 60 mg daily in divided doses.

Adults: 5 to 20 mg.

Children: 2 to 10 mg.

Elderly or debilitated patients: Doses should not exceed half those normally recommended.

Valium Roche capsules, tablets and syrup are for oral administration.

Valium Roche suppositories are for rectal administration.

Valium Roche syrup may be diluted with Sorbitol Solution BPC or Syrup BP.

Contra-indications, warnings, etc

Contra-indications: Patients with known sensitivity to benzodiazepines; acute pulmonary insufficiency; respiratory depression.

Use in pregnancy: There is no evidence as to drug safety in human pregnancy, nor is there evidence from animal work that it is free from hazard. Do not use during pregnancy, especially during the first and last trimesters, unless there are compelling reasons.

The administration of high doses or prolonged administration of low doses of benzodiazepines in the last trimester of pregnancy or during labour has been reported to produce irregularities in the foetal heart, and hypotonia, poor sucking and hypothermia in the neonate.

Diazepam has been detected in breast milk. If possible, the use of Valium Roche should be avoided during lactation.

Precautions: In patients with chronic pulmonary insufficiency, and in patients with chronic renal or hepatic disease, dosage may need to be reduced.

Patients should be advised that, like all medicaments of this type, Valium Roche may modify patients' performance at skilled tasks (driving, operating machinery, etc.) to a varying degree depending on dosage, administration and individual susceptibility. Patients should further be advised that alcohol may intensify any impairment and should, therefore, be avoided during treatment.

The dependence potential of the benzodiazepines is low but this increases when high doses are used, especially so when given over long periods. This is particularly so in patients with a history of alcoholism or drug abuse or in patients with marked personality disorders. Regular monitoring in such patients is essential, routine repeat prescriptions should be avoided and treatment should be withdrawn gradually. Symptoms such as depression, nervousness, rebound insomnia, irritability, sweating, and diarrhoea have been reported following abrupt cessation of treatment in patients receiving even normal therapeutic doses for short periods of time.

In rare instances, withdrawal following excessive dosages may produce confusional states, psychotic manifestations and convulsions.

Abnormal psychological reactions to benzodiazepines have been reported. Rare behavioural effects include paradoxical aggressive outbursts, excitement, confusion, and the uncovering of depression with suicidal tendencies.

If Valium Roche is given concomitantly with centrally-acting drugs such as neuroleptics, antidepressants, hypnotics, analgesics and anaesthetics, the sedative effects are likely to be intensified. The elderly require special supervision.

Pharmacokinetic studies on potential interactions between Valium Roche and anti-epileptic drugs have produced conflicting results. Both depression and elevation of drug levels, as well as no change, have been reported. When Valium Roche is used in conjunction with anti-epileptic drugs, side-effects and toxicity may be more evident, particularly with hydantoins or barbiturates or combinations including them. This requires extra care in adjusting dosage in the initial stages of treatment.

Side-effects and adverse reactions: Common adverse effects include drowsiness, sedation, unsteadiness and ataxia. These effects occur following single as well as repeated dosage, and may persist into the following day. The elderly are particularly sensitive to the effects of central depressant drugs and may experience confusion, especially if organic brain changes are present; the dosage of Valium Roche should not exceed one-half that recommended for other adults.

Other adverse effects are rare and include headache, vertigo, hypotension, gastrointestinal upsets, skin rashes, visual disturbances, changes in libido, and urinary retention. Isolated cases of blood dyscrasias and jaundice have also been reported.

Treatment of overdosage: When taken alone in overdosage Valium Roche presents few problems in management. Signs may include drowsiness, ataxia and dysarthria, with coma in severe cases. Treatment is symptomatic. Gastric lavage is useful only if performed soon after ingestion. There is no specific antidote to Valium Roche.

When taken with centrally-acting drugs, especially alcohol, the effects of overdosage are likely to be more severe and, in the absence of supportive measures, may prove fatal.

Pharmaceutical precautions *Storage:* The recommended maximum storage temperature for Valium Roche syrup and suppositories is 30°C.

All Valium Roche presentations should be protected from light.

Additives and pharmaceutical precautions: Valium Roche syrup may be diluted with Sorbitol Solution BPC or Syrup BP.

Maintenance of stability cannot be guaranteed if this advice is not followed.

Legal category CD (Sch. 4), POM.

Package quantities Valium 2 Roche tablets 2 mg, Valium 5 Roche tablets 5 mg, Valium 10 Roche tablets 10 mg, capsules 2 mg and capsules 5 mg in packings of 100 and 500.

Valium Roche syrup in packings of 100 ml.

Valium Roche suppositories 5 mg and 10 mg in packings of 5.

Further information Valium Roche is well absorbed, with peak blood levels being achieved one to two hours after administration, producing a rapid onset of clinical effects.

Diazepam is a long-acting benzodiazepine. It is metabolised to the active metabolites, N-desmethyldi-

azepam and oxazepam. Excretion is via the kidney in the form of conjugated oxazepam and temazepam. The half-life of diazepam varies from 20 to 50 hours whilst that of desmethyldiazepam ranges up to 100 hours.

Repeated doses will lead to accumulation of whole drug and metabolites. The latter may take two weeks to reach steady state and can reach higher concentrations than the parent compound.

No clear correlation has been demonstrated between the blood levels of Valium Roche and its clinical effects.

The elderly, and patients with impaired renal and/or hepatic function, will be particularly susceptible to the adverse effects listed above. It is advisable to review treatment regularly and to discontinue use as soon as possible.

Treatment should be kept to a minimum and given only under close medical supervision. Little is known regarding the efficacy or safety of benzodiazepines in long-term use.

Valium Roche is also available as 10 mg and 20 mg ampoules (see separate data sheet).

Product licence numbers

Tablets 2 mg	0031/5121R
Tablets 5 mg	0031/5122R
Tablets 10 mg	0031/5123R
Capsules 2 mg	0031/5124R
Capsules 5 mg	0031/5125R
Syrup	0031/5126R
Suppositories 5 mg	0031/0119
Suppositories 10 mg	0031/0120

VALIUM* ROCHE AMPOULES

Presentation Ampoules containing 10 mg diazepam in 2 ml.

Ampoules containing 20 mg diazepam in 4 ml.

The ampoule solution is almost colourless to greenish-yellow.

Uses *Properties:* Valium Roche has anxiolytic, anticonvulsant and central muscle-relaxant properties. It has little autonomic activity.

Indications: Severe acute anxiety or agitation; delirium tremens.

Acute muscle spasm; tetanus.

Acute convulsions including status epilepticus, those due to poisoning, and febrile convulsions.

Pre-operative medication or premedication for a wide variety of procedures, e.g. in dentistry, surgery, radiology, endoscopy, cardiac catheterisation, cardioversion.

Dosage and administration *Adults:* Severe acute anxiety or agitation – 10 mg by IV or IM injection which may be repeated after an interval of not less than 4 hours.

Delirium tremens – 10 to 20 mg IV or IM. Higher doses may be needed, depending on severity of symptoms.

Acute muscle spasm – 10 mg by IV or IM injection which may be repeated after an interval of not less than 4 hours.

Tetanus – Initially an IV dose of 0.1 to 0.3 mg/kg body-weight, repeated at intervals of 1 to 4 hours. Continuous IV infusion of 3 to 10 mg/kg body-weight per 24 hours can also be used. Alternatively, the same dose of oral Valium Roche may be administered by nasoduodenal tube. The selected dose should relate to the severity of the case and in extremely severe cases higher doses have been used.

Status epilepticus, convulsions due to poisoning – 10

to 20 mg IV or IM, repeated if necessary 30–60 minutes later. If indicated, this may be followed by a slow intravenous infusion (maximum dose: 3 mg/kg body-weight over 24 hours).

Pre-operative medication or premedication – 0.2 mg/kg body-weight. The usual adult dose is 10 to 20 mg but higher doses may be necessary according to the clinical response.

Elderly or debilitated patients: Doses should not exceed half those normally recommended.

Children:

Status epilepticus, convulsions due to poisoning, febrile convulsions – 0.2 to 0.3 mg/kg body-weight IV (or IM) or 1 mg per year of life.

Tetanus – As for adults.

Pre-operative medication or premedication – 0.2 mg/kg body-weight.

In order to reduce the likelihood of untoward effects during intravenous sedation the injection should be given slowly (0.5 ml of the solution per half-minute) until the patient becomes drowsy, the eyelids droop and the speech becomes slurred but the patient is still able to respond to requests.

It is strongly recommended that intravenous injections of Valium Roche should be given into a large vein of the antecubital fossa, the patient having been placed in a supine position and kept there throughout the procedure.

If these conditions are adhered to for administration of Valium Roche intravenously the possibility of hypotension or apnoea occurring will be greatly diminished.

Except in emergencies, a second person should always be present during intravenous use and facilities for resuscitation should always be available. It is recommended that patients should remain under medical supervision until at least one hour has elapsed from the time of injection. They should always be accompanied home by a responsible adult, with a warning not to drive or to operate machinery for 24 hours.

Valium Roche ampoule solution should not normally be diluted. An exception to this is when given slowly in large intravenous infusions of normal saline or dextrose, such as are given in the treatment of tetanus and status epilepticus. Not more than 40 mg (8 ml ampoule solution) should be added to 500 ml of infusion solution. The solution should be freshly made up and used within six hours.

Valium Roche ampoule solution should not be mixed with other drugs in the same infusion solution or in the same syringe.

Maintenance of stability cannot be guaranteed if this advice is not followed.

Valium Roche ampoules are for intravenous or intramuscular administration.

Contra-indications, warnings, etc

Contra-indications: Patients with known sensitivity to benzodiazepines; acute pulmonary insufficiency; respiratory depression.

Use in pregnancy: There is no evidence as to drug safety in human pregnancy, nor is there evidence from animal work that it is free from hazard. Do not use during pregnancy, especially during the first and last trimesters, unless there are compelling reasons.

The administration of high doses or prolonged administration of low doses of benzodiazepines in the last trimester of pregnancy or during labour has been reported to produce irregularities in the foetal heart, and hypotonia, poor sucking and hypothermia in the neonate.

Diazepam has been detected in breast milk. If possible the use of Valium Roche should be avoided during lactation.

Precautions: Parenteral Valium Roche should not normally be used in patients with organic brain changes (particularly arteriosclerosis) or with chronic pulmonary insufficiency. However, in emergency or when such patients are treated in hospital, Valium Roche may be given parenterally in reduced dosage. For IV administration, the injection should be given slowly.

In patients with chronic pulmonary insufficiency, and in patients with chronic renal or hepatic disease, dosage may need to be reduced.

Patients should be advised that, like all medicaments of this type, Valium Roche may modify patients' performance at skilled tasks (driving, operating machinery, etc.) to a varying degree depending upon dosage, administration and individual susceptibility. Patients should further be advised that alcohol may intensify any impairment and should, therefore, be avoided during treatment.

Abnormal psychological reactions to benzodiazepines have been reported. Rare behavioural effects include paradoxical aggressive outbursts, excitement, confusion, and the uncovering of depression with suicidal tendencies.

If Valium Roche is combined with centrally-acting drugs such as neuroleptics, antidepressants, hypnotics, analgesics and anaesthetics, the sedative effects are likely to be intensified. Furthermore, if such centrally depressant drugs are given parenterally in conjunction with intravenous Valium Roche, severe respiratory and cardiovascular depression may occur. The elderly require special supervision.

When intravenous Valium Roche is to be administered concurrently with a narcotic analgesic agent, e.g. in dentistry, it is recommended that Valium Roche be given after the analgesic and that the dose be carefully titrated to meet the patient's needs.

Pharmacokinetic studies on potential interactions between Valium Roche and anti-epileptic drugs have produced conflicting results. Both depression and elevation of drug levels, as well as no change, have been reported. When Valium Roche is used in conjunction with anti-epileptic drugs, side-effects and toxicity may be more evident, particularly with hydantoins or barbiturates or combinations including them. This requires extra care in adjusting dosage in the initial stages of treatment.

Side-effects and adverse reactions: Intravenous injection may be associated with local reactions, and thrombophlebitis and venous thrombosis may occur. In order to minimise the likelihood of these effects, intravenous injections of Valium Roche should be given into a large vein of the antecubital fossa.

Apnoea or hypotension may rarely occur following intravenous injection. The incidence may be minimised by not exceeding the recommended rate of administration. Patients should always be managed in the supine position and kept there throughout the procedure.

Other adverse effects include drowsiness, sedation, unsteadiness and ataxia; these are dose-related and may persist into the following day. The elderly are particularly sensitive to the effects of centrally depressant drugs and may experience confusion, especially if organic brain symptoms are present. The dosage of Valium Roche in these patients should not exceed one-half that recommended for other adults.

Rare adverse effects include headache, vertigo, hypotension, gastrointestinal upsets, skin rashes, visual disturbances, changes in libido, and urinary retention. Isolated cases of blood dyscrasias and jaundice have also been reported.

Treatment of overdosage: Treatment is symptomatic. There is no specific antidote to Valium Roche.

Pharmaceutical precautions *Storage:* The recommended maximum storage temperature for Valium Roche ampoules is 30°C. They should be protected from light.

Dilution, additives and pharmaceutical precautions: Valium Roche ampoule solution should not normally be diluted. An exception to this is when given slowly in large intravenous infusions of normal saline or dextrose such as are given in the treatment of tetanus and status epilepticus. Not more than 40 mg (8 ml ampoule solution) should be added to 500 ml of infusion solution. The solution should be freshly made up and used within six hours.

Over 50% of diazepam in solution may be adsorbed onto the walls of plastic containers of infusion solution; these should not therefore be used for diazepam solutions. Adsorption onto plastic drip tubing causes an initial significant reduction of delivered diazepam concentration which then gradually rises over the next few hours. The drip rate should frequently be titrated against the patient's condition.

Bolus injection allows a more accurate and rapid titration of dosage than slow intravenous infusion. It is therefore to be preferred for the management of acute problems.

Valium Roche ampoule solution should not be mixed with other drugs in the same infusion solution or in the same syringe.

Maintenance of stability cannot be guaranteed if this advice is not followed.

Legal category CD (Sch. 4), POM.

Package quantities Valium Roche ampoules 10 mg in 2 ml and 20 mg in 4 ml, in packings of 10.

Further information Diazepam is a long-acting benzodiazepine. It is metabolised to the active metabolites, N-desmethyldiazepam and oxazepam. Excretion is via the kidney in the form of conjugated oxazepam and temazepam. The half-life of diazepam varies from 20 to 50 hours whilst that of desmethyldiazepam ranges up to 100 hours.

Repeated doses will lead to accumulation of whole drug and metabolites. The latter may take two weeks to reach steady state and can reach higher concentrations than the parent compound.

Intramuscular injection of Valium Roche can lead to a rise in serum creatine phosphokinase activity, with a maximum level occurring between 12 and 24 hours after the injection. This fact should be taken into account in the differential diagnosis of myocardial infarction.

The absorption from intramuscular injection of Valium Roche may be variable, particularly from the gluteal muscles. This route of administration should only be used when oral or intravenous dosing is not possible or advisable.

The elderly, and patients with impaired renal and/or hepatic function, will be particularly susceptible to the adverse effects listed above. It is advisable to review treatment regularly and to discontinue use as soon as possible.

Treatment should be kept to a minimum and given only under close medical supervision. Little is known regarding the efficacy or safety of benzodiazepines in long-term use.

Availability: Valium Roche is also available as 2 mg, 5 mg and 10 mg tablets, 2 mg and 5 mg capsules, syrup (2 mg/5 ml) and as 5 mg and 10 mg suppositories. See separate data sheet.

Product licence numbers
Ampoules 10 mg 0031/0068R
Ampoules 20 mg 0031/5128R

VALRELEASE* ▼

Presentation Capsules with opaque blue cap and opaque light blue body with ROCHE printed in red along both cap and body, containing 10 mg diazepam in a controlled-release form.

Uses *Properties:* Valrelease has the characteristics of the benzodiazepine tranquillizers. The active ingredient, diazepam, is released in a controlled manner thus avoiding the peaks and troughs in plasma levels which are encountered with conventional three-times daily administration.

Indications: Treatment of the symptoms of anxiety – this includes both psychic and somatic manifestations.

Dosage and administration *Adults:* One capsule daily to be taken usually early in the evening.

Elderly: No dosage recommendations are made for elderly patients.

Children: No dosage recommendations are made for children.

Valrelease capsules are for oral administration.
Valrelease capsules should be taken with water.

Contra-indications, warnings, etc *Contra-indications:* Patients with known sensitivity to benzodiazepines; acute pulmonary insufficiency; respiratory depression.

Use in pregnancy: The use of diazepam during pregnancy should be avoided unless there are compelling reasons for administration.

Diazepam crosses the placenta and the administration of high doses or prolonged administration of low doses in the last trimester of pregnancy or labour has been reported to produce irregularities in the foetal heart, and hypotonia, poor sucking and hypothermia in the neonate.

Diazepam has been detected in breast milk. If possible, the use of Valrelease should be avoided during lactation.

Precautions: In patients with chronic pulmonary insufficiency, and in patients with chronic renal or hepatic disease, dosage may need to be modified.

If diazepam is combined with centrally-acting drugs such as neuroleptics, tranquillizers, antidepressants, hypnotics, analgesics and anaesthetics, the sedative effects may be intensified.

Patients should be advised that, like all medicaments of this type, diazepam may modify patients' performance at skilled tasks (driving, operating machinery, etc.) to a varying degree depending upon dosage, administration and individual susceptibility. Patients should further be advised that alcohol may intensify any impairment, and should therefore be avoided during treatment.

The dependence potential of the benzodiazepines is low but this increases when high doses are used, especially when given over long periods. This is particularly so in patients with a history of alcoholism or drug abuse or in patients with marked personality disorders. Regular monitoring in such patients is essential and routine repeat prescriptions should be avoided. Treatment should be withdrawn gradually. Symptoms such as depression, nervousness, rebound insomnia, irritability, sweating, and diarrhoea have been reported following abrupt cessation of treatment with normal therapeutic doses.

In rare instances, withdrawal following excessive dosages may produce confusional states, psychotic manifestations and convulsions.

Abnormal psychological reactions to benzodiazepines have been reported. Rare behavioural effects include paradoxical aggressive outbursts, excitement, confusion, and the uncovering of depression with suicidal tendencies.

Side-effects: Common adverse effects include drowsiness, sedation, unsteadiness and ataxia; these are dose-related and may persist into the following day even after a single dose.

Other adverse effects are rare and include headache, vertigo, hypotension, gastro-intestinal upsets, skin rashes, visual disturbances, changes in libido, and urinary retention. Isolated cases of blood dyscrasias and jaundice have also been reported.

Treatment of overdosage: When taken in overdosage, diazepam presents few problems in management. Signs may include drowsiness, ataxia and dysarthria, with coma in severe cases. Treatment is symptomatic. Gastric lavage is useful only if performed soon after ingestion. There is no specific antidote to diazepam.

When taken with centrally-acting drugs, especially alcohol, the effects of overdosage are likely to be more severe and, in the absence of supportive measures, may prove fatal.

Pharmaceutical precautions *Storage:* Valrelease capsules should be protected from light and stored in a dry place. Recommended maximum storage temperature is 30°C.

Legal category CD (Sch. 4), POM.

Package quantities Valrelease capsules 10 mg in packings of 50.

Further information Nil.

Product licence number 0031/0140

*Trade Mark

Rorer Pharmaceuticals
Stepfield, Witham
Essex CM8 3AG

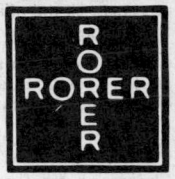

AGIOLAX*

Presentation Brown, sugar-coated granules, each 100 grams of which contains: Seeds of Plantago Ovata 54.2 g, Senna Pods 12.4 g.

Uses For the relief of constipation.
It is particularly suitable for bowel regulation in bedridden patients and pregnant women. It is also useful in facilitating pain-free evacuation in patients with haemorrhoids.

Dosage and administration Agiolax should be placed dry on the tongue and, without chewing or crushing, swallowed with a glass of water or warm drink.
Adults and children over 12 years: One or two level 5 ml spoonfuls after supper and, if necessary, before breakfast. In obstinate cases two level 5 ml spoonfuls every six hours for 1 to 3 days.
Children (5 to 12 years): Half the adult dosage.

Contra-indications, warnings, etc Should not be used in cases of intestinal obstruction.
Treatment of overdosage: Excessive use of purgatives may produce excessive loss of water and electrolytic loss. Treat symptomatically with careful attention to body electrolytes, particularly potassium.

Pharmaceutical precautions No special storage precautions required.

Legal category P.

Package quantities Containers of 100 grams and 250 grams.

Further information Special note for diabetics: Each level 5 ml spoonful contains approximately 4 g of Agiolax equivalent to 0.7 g of sucrose.

Product licence number 4638/0001.

ANANASE* FORTE

Presentation Orange yellow, enteric-coated tablets each containing Bromelain Concentrate equivalent to 100,000 Rorer Units of activity.

Uses Ananase Forte is a proteolytic enzyme for use in the treatment of inflammatory oedema associated with:
Soft tissue trauma – contusions, lacerations, sprains, strains, haematomas, dislocations, fractures, burns.
Post-operative tissue reactions – as in general orthopaedic, ocular, oral and gynaecological surgery.
Skin conditions – cellulitis, furunculosis.
Ulceration – varicose, decubitus, diabetic.

Dosage and administration Usual adult dose is 1 tablet four times daily, taken orally.

Children's dosage is at the discretion of the physician.

Contra-indications, warnings, etc Contra-indicated in patients with known sensitivity to the drug or to pineapple or its products.
Ananase Forte should be used with caution in patients with abnormalities of the blood-clotting mechanism, such as haemophilia, or with severe hepatic or renal disease.
Patients on anticoagulant therapy should be observed carefully because of possible potentiation of the anticoagulant effect.
Side-effects are seldom observed. Sensitivity manifested by skin rash has occurred. There has been no report of anaphylactic reaction. Cases of metrorrhagia and menorrhagia may possibly be related to the drug. Nausea, vomiting or diarrhoea are rare. In the event of any adverse reaction, the drug should be discontinued.
Use in pregnancy: The product should not be used during pregnancy or lactation unless the physician considers it essential.
Treatment of overdosage: Symptomatic treatment observing closely blood clotting factors.

Pharmaceutical precautions Can be stored at room temperature.

Legal category P.

Package quantities Securitainers of 25 and 250 tablets.

Further information Ananase Forte is intended to supplement and augment standard therapeutic procedures for reduction of inflammation and oedema, to ease pain, speed healing and accelerate tissue repair. It contains a concentrate of proteolytic enzymes derived from the pineapple plant. While the mode of action of proteolytic enzymes has not been finally established, it is probable that depolymerisation of fibrin and permeability modifications of venules and lymphatics underlie the action.

Product licence number 0050/5005.

AURALTONE*

Presentation A clear, colourless or very pale yellow liquid, odourless and very hygroscopic. It contains:
Phenazone BPC 5.0% w/v
Benzocaine BP 1.0% w/v

Uses For the treatment of acute otitis media, inflammatory conditions of the tympanic membrane and generally for the relief of ear-ache.

Dosage and administration For external use.
It is administered to the ear with the dropper provided.

In the absence of specific instructions from the physician fill the affected ear with Auraltone and plug the ear lightly with dry cotton wool.

Contra-indications, warnings, etc *Phenazone toxic effects:* Phenazone is liable to give rise to skin eruptions and in susceptible individuals even small doses may have this effect.

Warning: Keep out of the reach of children.

Pharmaceutical precautions Keep in a cool, dry place, tightly capped. Do not warm or use with wet dressings.

Legal category P.

Package quantities 15 ml in a bottle fitted with a dropper cap.

Further information Nil.

Product licence number 0208/5000.

COPHOLCO*

Presentation A dark brown syrupy linctus, odour and taste of aniseed. Each 5 ml contains the following active ingredients:

Pholcodine BP	5.63 mg
Terpin Hydrate BPC (1968)	2.82 mg
Menthol BP	1.41 mg
Cineole BPC	0.0026 ml

Uses For the relief of cough in laryngitis, tracheitis and for all unproductive and 'ticklish' coughs.

Dosage and administration For oral administration.

Children over 5 years: Half to one 5 ml spoonful without water four or five times daily.

Adults: Two 5 ml spoonfuls without water four or five times daily.

Contra-indications, warnings, etc *Pholcodine toxic effects:* Nausea and drowsiness occasionally occur.

Terpin hydrate toxic effects: Epigastric pain may follow the administration of terpin hydrate on an empty stomach.

Warning: Keep out of the reach of children.

Use in pregnancy: The safety of Copholco in pregnancy has not been established and its use in pregnant women should be avoided unless considered necessary.

Treatment of overdosage: Gastric lavage within two hours. Afterwards symptomatic treatment as required.

Pharmaceutical precautions Nil.

Legal category CD (Sch 5), P.

Package quantities Glass bottle containing 100 ml.

Further information Nil.

Product licence number 0208/5002.

COPHOLCOIDS*

Presentation Blackish, hard, sugar coated pastilles. Odour and taste of aniseed. Each pastille contains:

Pholcodine BP	4.0 mg
Terpin Hydrate BPC (1968)	16.0 mg
Menthol BP	2.0 mg
Cineole BPC	0.004 ml

Uses Copholcoids are for the relief of cough in laryngitis, tracheitis and all unproductive and 'ticklish' coughs.

Dosage and administration For oral administration.

Children over 5 years: Suck 1 pastille three times daily at four hourly intervals.

Adults: Suck 1 or 2 pastilles three or four times daily according to the severity of the condition.

Contra-indications, warnings, etc *Pholcodine toxic effects:* Nausea and drowsiness occasionally occur.

Terpin hydrate toxic effects: Epigastric pain may follow the administration of terpin hydrate on an empty stomach.

Warning: Keep out of the reach of children.

Use in pregnancy: The safety of Copholcoids in pregnancy has not been established, and its use in pregnant women should be avoided unless considered necessary.

Treatment of overdosage: Gastric lavage within two hours. Afterwards symptomatic treatment as required.

Pharmaceutical precautions Store in a cool, dry place.

Legal category CD (Sch 5), P.

Package quantities Cartons containing 50 g.

Further information Nil.

Product licence number 0208/5003.

EMETROL* SOLUTION

Presentation A yellow solution with odour and taste of peppermint. Each 5 ml contains:

Laevulose (fructose)	1.87 g
Dextrose (glucose)	1.87 g
Phosphoric Acid BP	21.5 mg

Uses Functional nausea or vomiting, morning sickness, regurgitation in infants, motion sickness.

Dosage and administration For oral administration.
1. *Functional nausea/vomiting: Adults:* 15 to 30 ml (three to six 5 ml spoonfuls) repeated at 15 minute intervals until distress ceases.
   Infants & children: 5 to 10 ml (one to two 5 ml spoonfuls) in the same manner.
2. *Morning sickness:* 15 to 30 ml on arising, repeated three hourly or when nausea threatens.
3. *Regurgitation:* 5 to 10 ml ten to fifteen minutes before each feed. In refractory cases 10 to 15 ml thirty minutes before feeding.
4. *Motion sickness: Adults:* 15 to 30 ml before starting trip repeated at convenient intervals if required.
   Children: 5 to 10 ml before starting trip repeated at convenient intervals if required.

Contra-indications, warnings, etc This product contains sugar and should not be taken by diabetics except under the advice and supervision of a physician.

This product contains fructose and should not be taken by persons with hereditary fructose intolerance (HFI).

Caution: Emetrol should not be taken for more than one hour (5 doses) without consulting the physician.

Do not dilute Emetrol or drink fluids of any kind immediately before or at least 15 minutes after taking a dose.

Pharmaceutical precautions Store at room temperature.

Legal category P.

Package quantities Glass bottles containing 100 ml and 500 ml.

Further information Emetrol contains balanced amounts of laevulose (fructose) and dextrose (glucose) with orthophosphoric acid, stabilised at an optimum pH. The mode of action is based on the local reduction of smooth muscle tone, thus providing rapid, effective relief.

Emetrol should not be diluted as dilution alters the stabilised pH necessary for optimal effect.

Product licence number 0050/5001.

FRUSENE* ▼

Presentation Pale yellowish, scored tablets 9 mm diameter. Each tablet containing 40 mg frusemide (furosemide rINN) and 50 mg triamterene.

Uses
Indications: Cardiac or hepatic oedema.

Properties: Frusene contains frusemide and triamterene, thus minimising the possible hypokalaemia produced by frusemide and the hyperkalaemia produced by triamterene. It has been demonstrated that when Frusene is used no decrease in serum potassium level is observed whilst the diuretic response is similar to an equivalent dose of frusemide.

Frusene does not raise the creatinine level in patients with normal renal function. If the patient has an elevated creatinine level at initiation of therapy the use of Frusene may further raise it.

The fact that Frusene prevents hypokalaemia is of importance when treating out-patients with severe cardiac insufficiency or other patients needing potent diuretic therapy. In geriatric patients who are especially sensitive to the development of hypokalaemia the use of Frusene should be considered even when diuretics are only needed every other day. In hypertensive patients the use of Frusene may be more advisable than frusemide by itself.

Potassium replacement during Frusene treatment should only be considered in special cases and is not normally required.

Dosage and administration The dosage will depend on individual requirements.

The usual adult dose is 1 tablet 1–2 times daily.

Contra-indications, warnings, etc
Contra-indications: Frusene is contra-indicated in severe renal or hepatic failure, elevated serum potassium level.

Precautions: Frusene should be used with caution during the first trimester of pregnancy.

Side effects: As Frusene is a combination of frusemide and triamterene side effects due to either component are possible. Reported side effects are as follows:

Triamterene: nausea, diarrhoea, fatigue, headache, dry mouth or rash have been reported. If renal function is impaired triamterene has been reported to cause elevation of BUN and the uric acid level. Some leukopenia cases have been reported due to triamterene.

Frusemide: Frusemide is generally well tolerated. Side effects of a minor nature such as nausea, malaise or gastric upset may occur but are not usually severe enough to cause withdrawal of treatment. The incidence of allergic reactions such as skin rashes is very low but when these occur treatment should be withdrawn. In common with other sulphonamide-based diuretics hyperuricaemia may occur and in rare cases, clinical gout may be precipitated. Bone marrow depression has been reported as a rare complication and necessitates withdrawal of treatment.

Frusene: The use of a combination of frusemide and triamterene minimises the possible hypokalaemia caused by frusemide.

Pharmaceutical precautions Frusene should be stored in a dry place protected from light.

Legal category POM.

Package quantities Frusene is available in containers of 100 tablets and 1000 tablets.

Further information Nil.

Product licence number 0339/0018.

MAALOX* SUSPENSION AND TABLETS

Presentation White peppermint-flavoured suspension. Each 5 ml contains:

Dried Aluminium Hydroxide Gel BP	220 mg
Magnesium Hydroxide BPC	195 mg

White peppermint-flavoured tablet containing:

Dried Aluminium Hydroxide Gel BP	400 mg
Magnesium Hydroxide BPC	400 mg

Uses Antacid therapy in gastric and duodenal ulcer, gastritis, heartburn and gastric hyperacidity.

Dosage and administration Maalox is administered orally and can be taken with milk or water if required.

Usual adult doses are: 10–20 ml taken 20 minutes to one hour after meals and at bedtime, or as required. One or two tablets well chewed, 20 minutes to one hour after meals and at bedtime, or as required.

Contra-indications, warnings, etc Maalox should not be used in patients who are severely debilitated or suffering from kidney failure.

Maalox will inhibit absorption of tetracyclines and vitamins if taken concurrently. Gastro-intestinal side-effects are uncommon.

Treatment of overdosage: Serious symptoms are unlikely following overdosage.

Pharmaceutical precautions The suspension must be kept from freezing and the bottle kept tightly closed.

Legal category GSL

Package quantities Suspension: Plastic bottle containing 500 ml. Carton containing 20 sachets of 10 ml.
Tablets: Carton containing 50 strip-packed tablets.

Further information Maalox is a highly palatable balanced combination of two reliable antacids and has minimal gastro-intestinal side-effects. It is therefore especially suitable when prolonged therapy is necessary.

Product licence numbers
Suspension 0050/5002
Tablets 0050/5003

MAALOX* PLUS SUSPENSION AND TABLETS

Presentation White lemon/cream flavoured suspension. Each 5 ml contains the equivalent of:

Dried Aluminium Hydroxide Gel BP	220 mg
Magnesium Hydroxide BPC	195 mg
Simethicone	25 mg

Yellow/white tablet marked Maalox Plus on one face and Rorer on the other face. Each tablet contains:

Dried Aluminium Hydroxide Gel BP	200 mg
Magnesium Hydroxide BPC	200 mg
Simethicone	25 mg

Uses As an antacid/antiflatulent for relief of hyperacidity and/or flatulence associated with all gastric disorders of a functional or organic nature.

Dosage and administration Maalox Plus suspension and tablets are for oral administration and can be taken with milk or water if required.

Adult doses: 10–20 ml four times a day, taken twenty minutes to one hour after meals and at bedtime, or as required.

Two to four tablets well chewed, four times a day, taken twenty minutes to one hour after meals and at bedtime, or as required.

Contra-indications, warnings, etc Maalox Plus should not be used in patients who are severely debilitated or suffering from kidney failure.

Maalox Plus will inhibit absorption of tetracyclines and vitamins if taken concurrently.

Gastro-intestinal side-effects are uncommon.

Treatment of overdosage: Serious symptoms are unlikely following overdosage.

Pharmaceutical precautions The suspension must be kept from freezing and the bottle kept tightly closed.

Legal category GSL.

Package quantities *Suspension:* Plastic bottle containing 180 ml. Carton containing 6 sachets of 10 ml. *Tablets:* Carton containing 10 strip-packed tablets.

Further information Maalox Plus is a highly palatable, balanced combination of two reliable antacids together with a potent antiflatulent. The antacids are balanced such that gastro-intestinal side-effects (constipation and diarrhoea) are minimal. It is therefore especially suitable when prolonged therapy is necessary. The simethicone disperses gastric foam and assists eructation of gases. It accelerates the penetration of antacids throughout the gastric contents and provides mucosal protection from the effects of excess acid.

Product licence numbers
Suspension   3384/0002
Tablets   3384/0001

NEURODYNE* CAPSULES

Presentation No. 0 white hard gelatin capsules, marked 'NEURODYNE' containing a white odourless powder. Each capsule contains:

| Paracetamol BP | 500 mg |
| Codeine Phosphate BP | 8 mg |

Uses For the treatment of mild to moderate pain, and symptomatic relief of muscular and rheumatic aches and pains, period pains and influenza.

Dosage and administration For oral administration.

For adults only: 1 or 2 capsules to be taken every four hours or as directed by the physician. Maximum daily dose up to 8 capsules (in divided doses).

Contra-indications, warnings, etc An overdose of paracetamol can cause hepatic necrosis. Codeine is a narcotic analgesic. Tolerance psychological and physical dependance may occur.

Constipation is common.

Use in pregnancy: There is epidemiological evidence of safety of paracetamol and inadequate evidence of safety of codeine in human pregnancy.

Codeine has been used for many years without apparent ill consequences, and animal studies have not shown any hazard.

Warning: Keep out of the reach of children.

Treatment of overdosage: Gastric lavage and saline purgative. Assist respiration if necessary. Observe closely for signs of paracetamol liver toxicity.

Pharmaceutical precautions Keep in a tightly closed container and store in a cool, dry place.

Legal category CD (Sch 5), P.

Package quantities Containers of 100 and 250 capsules.

Further information Nil.

Product licence number 0208/5004R.

PHYTOCIL* CREAM

Presentation A white, semi-translucent, homogeneous cream with the odour of menthol. It contains:

1-Phenoxypropan-2-ol	2.0% w/w
Salicylic Acid BP	1.5% w/w
2-p-Chlorophenoxyethanol	1.0% w/w
Menthol BP	1.0% w/w

Uses For the treatment of tinea pedis, tinea cruris, tinea circinata and other fungal infections of the skin.

Dosage and administration For external use only.

Apply sufficient to treat the affected area of the skin twice or three times a day.

Contra-indications, warnings, etc No side-effects reported.

Warning: Keep out of the reach of children.

Pharmaceutical precautions Store in a cool, dry place.

Legal category P.

Package quantities Tubes containing 25 g.

Further information Nil.

Product licence number 0208/5005.

PHYTOCIL* POWDER

Presentation A fine uniform white powder with a sweetish odour, characteristic of the phenoxetols. It contains:

Zinc Undecenoate BP	5.8% w/w
1-Phenoxy-propan-2-ol	2.0% w/w
2-p-Chlorophenoxyethanol	1.0% w/w

Uses For the treatment of tinea pedis, tinea cruris, tinea circinata and other fungal infections of the skin.

Dosage and administration For external use only.
Apply to the affected areas of the skin twice daily and also dust into hosiery and shoes.

Contra-indications, warnings, etc No side-effects reported.

Warning: Keep out of the reach of children.

Pharmaceutical precautions Store in dry place.

Legal category P.

Package quantities Powder tins containing 50 g.

Further information Nil.

Product licence number 0208/5006.

SECADERM* SALVE

Presentation A green, translucent ointment with the odour of phenol, terebene and melaleuca oil. It contains:

Resin BP	26.0% w/w
Turpentine Oil BP	6.00% w/w
Melaleuca Oil BPC (1949)	5.60% w/w
Terebene	5.25% w/w
Phenol BP	2.40% w/w

Uses Indicated in the relief and treatment of boils, abscesses, whitlow, bunions and chilblains.

Dosage and administration For external use only.
Apply once or twice daily to the affected parts and cover with a light dressing of gauze.

Contra-indications, warnings, etc No side-effects reported.

Warning: Keep out of the reach of children.

Pharmaceutical precautions Store in a cool place.

Legal category GSL.

Package quantities Tubes containing 15 g.

Further information Nil.

Product licence number 0208/5007.

*Trade Mark

Roussel Laboratories Limited
Broadwater Park
North Orbital Road
Uxbridge
Middlesex UB9 5HP

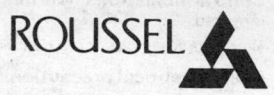

ROUSSEL

ACTINAC*

Presentation Actinac is presented as a pale yellow dry powder, together with a solvent for the preparation of a lotion. Each gram of powder contains:

Chloramphenicol BP	40 mg
Hydrocortisone Acetate BP	40 mg
Butoxyethyl nicotinate	24 mg
Allantoin	24 mg
Precipitated Sulphur BP	320 mg

The solvent is Purified Water BP, containing an approved lavender perfume and bacteriostat.

Uses Actinac is for use in the topical treatment of acne vulgaris and other acneiform conditions. It is formulated to control local infection and suppress inflammation with its consequent scarring effects.

Dosage and administration The lotion should be prepared according to the manufacturer's literature and applied with cotton wool or lint night and morning for the first four days and only at night thereafter. In order to prevent recurrence, treatment should be continued for three nights after the lesions have disappeared.

Contra-indications, warnings, etc Actinac is contra-indicated in patients who have a known hypersensitivity to any of the ingredients.

Avoid Actinac coming into contact with the eyes and mouth.

Early in the course of treatment, erythema may occur at the site of application and the patient may experience a sensation of warmth due to the vasodilator action of the nicotinate. In the unlikely event of a severe reaction, the patient is instructed to consult the doctor before further use of Actinac.

In pregnant animals, administration of corticosteroids can cause abnormalities of foetal development. The relevance of this finding to human beings has not been established. However, topical steroids should not be used extensively in pregnancy, i.e. in large amounts or for long periods. It is advisable to remove jewellery before applying the lotion.

Pharmaceutical precautions Store cool. The lotion when constituted will remain active for 21 days. Any lotion remaining after this time must be discarded and a fresh supply of lotion prepared.

Legal category POM.

Package quantities Each pack of Actinac contains two bottles of powder (each 5 g), two bottles of solvent (each 16 ml) and an instruction leaflet for the patient.

Further information Nil.

Product licence number 0109/0037.

ALTACAPS* ▼

Presentation Available as capsules containing a suspension of hydrotalcite and activated dimethicone. Each capsule contains 500 mg of hydrotalcite and 125 mg of activated dimethicone in a lemon and mint flavoured, yellow-beige, suspension. The capsule shell consists of soft gelatin flavoured with lemon and lime and coloured yellow.

Uses Altacaps have antacid, mucosal protective and anti-flatulent properties. As an antacid, hydrotalcite buffers in the optimal range of pH 3 to 5 for over 2 hours.

Altacaps are indicated for and provide symptomatic relief in the following conditions: Gastritis; peptic ulceration; hyperacidity; dyspepsia; flatulence and abdominal distension; heartburn, especially when associated with oesophagitis or hiatus hernia, and heartburn in pregnancy.

Dosage and administration
Adults: Two capsules between meals and at bedtime or as directed by the physician.

The capsules should be sucked or chewed to release the liquid content. The remaining capsule shell should then be chewed and swallowed or may be discarded.

Not recommended for children.

Contra-indications, warnings, etc There are no known contra-indications to Altacaps, but it is wise to avoid any drug, including antacids, during the first trimester of pregnancy. As with other compounds containing aluminium or magnesium, Altacaps may reduce intestinal absorption of tetracycline.

Altacaps contain the same active ingredients as Altacite Plus for which side-effects are generally uncommon although some reports of diarrhoea and vomiting have been received.

Pharmaceutical precautions Store in a cool, dry place. Protect from light.

Legal category P.

Package quantities Carton containing 50 capsules in 5 blister strips of 10.

Further information Although not an essential part of treatment, chewing of the citrus flavoured capsule shell will stimulate saliva flow and so help to dissolve the gelatin and wash down the antacid suspension. Alternatively, the shell can be discarded once the liquid has been expelled.

The sodium content of Altacaps is low (0.036 mmol per capsule).

Product licence number 0109/0125.

HYDROTALCITE (formerly Altacite*)

Presentation Hydrotalcite is available as white, buttermint-flavoured tablets marked 'altacite' and 'ROUSSEL', and as an aqueous suspension, slightly off-white, viscous and flavoured with peppermint.

Each tablet and each 5 ml of suspension contains 500 mg of hydrotalcite.

Uses Antacid, buffering in the optimum range of pH 3–5 for over two hours.

Hydrotalcite is indicated for symptomatic relief in the following conditions: peptic ulceration; dyspepsia; hyperacidity; gastritis; heartburn, especially when associated with reflux oesophagitis or hiatus hernia, and heartburn in pregnancy.

Dosage and administration *Adults:* 2 tablets or 10 ml of suspension between meals and at bedtime or as directed by a physician.

Elderly: No specific recommendations in the elderly.

Children (6–12 years): Half the adult dose.

The tablets should be chewed or crushed before swallowing.

Contra-indications, warnings, etc There are no contra-indications to Hydrotalcite but it is wise to avoid any drug, including antacids, during the first trimester of pregnancy. As with other compounds containing aluminium or magnesium, Hydrotalcite may reduce intestinal absorption of tetracycline. Side-effects are uncommon. Diarrhoea and vomiting have been reported but have ceased on withdrawal of therapy.

Pharmaceutical precautions No special storage requirements.

Legal category P.

Package quantities *Hydrotalcite Tablets:* Carton of 12 blister strips each containing 10 tablets.

Hydrotalcite Suspension: Polypropylene bottle containing 500 ml.

Further information There is no evidence of absorption of Hydrotalcite in man. Investigations in healthy human volunteers have shown no elevation of serum aluminium or magnesium levels on administering Hydrotalcite at therapeutic dosage for a continuous period of 28 days.

The sodium content of Hydrotalcite is 0.22 mmol per tablet or 5 ml of suspension.

Product licence numbers

Hydrotalcite Tablets	0109/0040
Hydrotalcite Suspension	0109/0041

ALTACITE PLUS*

Presentation *Suspension:* Viscous, slightly off-white aqueous suspension, flavoured with spearmint. Each 5 ml of suspension contains 500 mg of hydrotalcite and 125 mg of activated dimethicone.

Uses Altacite Plus has antacid, mucosal protective and anti-flatulent properties. As an antacid, Altacite Plus buffers in the optimal range of pH 3–5 for over two hours.

It is indicated for symptomatic relief in the following conditions: dyspepsia; flatulence and abdominal distension; hyperacidity; gastritis; peptic ulceration; heartburn, especially when associated with oesophagitis or hiatus hernia; and heartburn in pregnancy.

Dosage and administration *Adults:* 10 ml suspension between meals and at bedtime or as directed by the physician.

Elderly: No specific recommendations in the elderly.

Children (8–12 years): Half the adult dose.

Contra-indications, warnings, etc There are no known contra-indications to Altacite Plus, but it is wise to avoid any drug, including antacids, during the first trimester of pregnancy. As with other compounds containing aluminium or magnesium, Altacite Plus may reduce intestinal absorption of tetracycline. Side-effects are uncommon. Diarrhoea and vomiting have been reported but have ceased on withdrawal of therapy.

Pharmaceutical precautions No special storage requirements.

Legal category P.

Package quantities *Altacite Plus Suspension:* Polypropylene bottle containing 500 ml.

Further information There is no evidence of absorption of hydrotalcite in man. Investigations in healthy human volunteers have shown no elevation of serum aluminium or magnesium levels on administration of hydrotalcite at therapeutic dosage for a continuous period of 28 days.

The sodium content of Altacite Plus suspension is 0.078 mmol/5 ml.

Product licence number

Altacite Plus Suspension	0109/0062

CIDOMYCIN*
GENTAMICIN INJECTION BP
GENTAMICIN INTRATHECAL INJECTION
GENTAMICIN SULPHATE BP

Presentation Cidomycin for parenteral use is available as:

Cidomycin Injectable in 2 ml vials or ampoules each containing the equivalent of 80 mg gentamicin base as sulphate.

Cidomycin Injectable 160 mg in 2 ml ampoules each containing the equivalent of 160 mg gentamicin base as sulphate.

Cidomycin Injectable Paediatric in 2 ml vials each containing the equivalent of 20 mg gentamicin base as sulphate.

Cidomycin Intrathecal Injectable in 1 ml ampoules each containing 5 mg gentamicin base as sulphate.

Cidomycin Sterile Powder is whitish in colour and is available in packs of 1 g (base activity).

Uses Gentamicin is an aminoglycoside antibiotic with broad-spectrum bactericidal activity. It is usually active against most strains of the following organisms: *Escherichia coli, Klebsiella spp., Proteus spp.* (indole positive and indole negative), *Pseudomonas aeruginosa,* staphylococci, *Enterobacter spp., Citrobacter spp* and *Providencia spp.*

Gentamicin injection and gentamicin paediatric injection are indicated in urinary-tract infections, chest infections, bacteraemia, septicaemia, severe neonatal infections, infections following burns, infected traumatic or surgical wounds and other systemic infections due to sensitive organisms.

Gentamicin intrathecal injection is indicated as a supplement to systemic therapy in bacterial meningitis, ventriculitis and other bacterial infections of the central nervous system.

Gentamicin sterile powder prepared as a sterile injection may be used for serious intra-ocular infections and prophylactically prior to intra-ocular surgery.

Dosage and administration *Gentamicin injection: Adults: Serious infections:* If renal function is not impaired, 5 mg/kg daily in divided doses at six- or eight-hourly intervals. The total daily dose may be subsequently increased or decreased as clinically indicated.

Systemic infections: 80 mg eight-hourly for 7–10 days is usually an effective dose. If body weight is less than 60 kg, 60 mg eight hourly should be used.

Urinary-tract infections: As 'systemic infections'. Or, if renal function is not impaired, 160 mg once daily may be used.

Children: Up to 2 weeks of age: 3 mg/kg 12-hourly. *2 weeks to 12 years:* 2 mg/kg eight-hourly.

The elderly: There is some evidence that elderly patients may be more susceptible to aminoglycoside toxicity whether secondary to previous eighth nerve impairment or borderline renal dysfunction. Accordingly, therapy should be closely monitored by frequent determination of gentamicin serum levels, assessment of renal function and signs of ototoxicity.

Renal impairment: Gentamicin is excreted by simple glomerular filtration and therefore reduced dosage is necessary where renal function is impaired. Nomograms are available for the calculation of dose, which depends on the patient's age, weight and renal function. The following table may be useful when treating adults.

Blood urea		Creatinine clearance (GFR) (ml/min)	Dose and frequency of administration
(mg/100 ml)	(mmol/l)		
<40	6–7	>70	80 mg* 8-hourly
40–100	6–17	30–70	80 mg* 12-hourly
100–200	17–34	10–30	80 mg* daily
>200	>34	5–10	80 mg* every 48 hours
Twice-weekly intermittent haemodialysis		<5	80 mg* after dialysis

*60 mg if body weight <60 kg. Frequency of dosage in hours may also be approximated as serum creatinine (mg%) × eight or in SI units, as serum creatinine (μmol/l) divided by 11. If these dosage guides are used peak serum levels must be measured. Peak levels of gentamicin occur approximately one hour after intramuscular injection and 15 minutes after bolus intravenous injection. Trough levels are measured just prior to the next injection. Assay of peak serum levels gives confirmation of adequacy of dosage and also serves to detect levels above 10 mg/l, at which the possibility of ototoxicity should be considered.

The recommended dose and precautions for intramuscular and intravenous administration are identical. Gentamicin when given intravenously should be injected directly into a vein or into the drip set tubing over no less than three minutes. If administered by infusion, this should be over no longer than 20 minutes and in no greater volume of fluid than 100 ml.

Gentamicin intrathecal injection: Bacterial meningitis and ventriculitis: the starting dose of gentamicin intrathecal injection for both children and adults is 1 mg daily, intrathecally or intraventricularly, together with 1 mg/kg every eight hours intramuscularly. The MIC of the infecting organism in the CSF should be assessed and, if necessary, the intrathecal/intraventricular dose increased to 5 mg daily, whilst keeping the intramuscular dose at 1 mg/kg eight-hourly. Treatment should be continued for at least seven days but longer if necessary. Periodic serum and CSF gentamicin assays should be carried out to ensure that adequate antibiotic levels are maintained and that serum and CSF levels do not exceed 10 mg/l.

Gentamicin sterile powder: Serious bacterial intra-ocular infections and prophylaxis prior to surgery: gentamicin sulphate equivalent to 20–40 mg base should be injected subconjunctivally once or twice daily until infection subsides. This may require continuation of therapy for two or more days. In the majority of cases concomitant intramuscular therapy is not required. This dosage regimen is suitable for children and adults.

Contra-indications, warnings, etc
Contra-indications: Hypersensitivity; myasthenia gravis. Pregnancy and lactation: There are no proven cases of intrauterine damage caused by gentamicin. However, in common with most drugs known to cross the placenta, usage in pregnancy should only be considered in life-threatening situations where the expected benefits outweigh possible risks. In the absence of gastro-intestinal inflammation, the amount of gentamicin ingested from the milk is unlikely to result in significant blood levels in breast-fed infants.

Warnings: Ototoxicity has been recorded following the use of gentamicin. Groups at special risk include patients with impaired renal function and possibly the elderly. Consequently, renal, auditory and vestibular functions should be monitored in these patients and serum levels determined so as to avoid peak concentrations above 10 mg/l and troughs above 2 mg/l. As there is some evidence that risk of both ototoxicity and nephrotoxicity is related to the level of total exposure, duration of therapy should be the shortest possible compatible with clinical recovery. In some patients with impaired renal function there has been a transient rise in blood-urea-nitrogen which has usually reverted to normal during or following cessation of therapy. It is important to adjust the frequency of dosage according to the degree of renal function (see table).

Interaction with other substances: Concurrent administration of gentamicin and other potentially ototoxic or nephrotoxic drugs should be avoided. Potent diuretics such as ethacrynic acid and frusemide are believed to enhance the risk of ototoxicity whilst amphotericin B, cis-platinum and cyclosporin are potential enhancers of nephrotoxicity. Any potential nephrotoxicity of cephalosporins, and in particular cephaloridine, may also be increased in the presence of gentamicin. Consequently, if this combination is used monitoring of kidney function is advised.

Neuromuscular blockade and respiratory paralysis have been reported from administration of aminoglycosides to patients who have received curare-type muscle relaxants during anaesthesia.

Overdosage: Haemodialysis and peritoneal dialysis will aid removal from blood but the former is probably more efficient. Calcium salts given intravenously have been used to counter the neuromuscular blockade caused by gentamicin.

Pharmaceutical precautions Gentamicin is a remarkably stable antibiotic and does not require refrigeration. Avoid freezing.

In general gentamicin injection should not be mixed. In particular the following are incompatible in mixed solution with gentamicin injection: penicillins, cephalosporins, erythromycin, Lipiphysan, heparins, sodium bicarbonate.† Dilution in the body will obviate the danger of physical and chemical incompatibility and enable gentamicin to be given concurrently with the drugs listed above either as a bolus injection into the drip tubing, with adequate flushing, or at separate sites. In the case of carbenicillin, administration should only be at a separate site.

Legal category POM.

Package quantities *Cidomycin Injectable:* Packs of 25 × 2 ml vials or ampoules.
Cidomycin Injectable 160 mg/2 ml: Pack of 1 × 2 ml ampoule.
Cidomycin Injectable Paediatric: Packs of 5 × 2 ml vials.
Cidomycin Intrathecal Injectable: Packs of 5 × 1 ml ampoules.
Cidomycin Sterile Powder: Bottles containing 1 g.

Further information Nil.

† Carbon dioxide may be liberated on addition of the two solutions. Normally this will dissolve in the solution but under some circumstances small bubbles may form.

Product licence numbers

Cidomycin Injectable	0109/5065
Cidomycin Injectable 160 mg/2 ml	0109/0066
Cidomycin Injectable Paediatric	0109/5066
Cidomycin Intrathecal Injectable	0109/0057
Cidomycin Sterile Powder	0109/5067

CIDOMYCIN* (TOPICAL)

Presentation Available as a white cream which contains gentamicin sulphate in a water-miscible base and as a translucent ointment in a petroleum base. Each gram of ointment or cream contains gentamicin sulphate equivalent to 3 mg gentamicin base.

Uses Cidomycin is a wide-spectrum antibiotic and the ointment and cream are recommended for the treatment of primary and secondary skin infections due to susceptible bacteria.
Primary infections: Impetigo contagiosa, superficial folliculitis, ecthyma, furunculosis, sycosis barbae and pyoderma gangrenosum.
Secondary infections: Infected, contact, seborrhoeic, and eczematoid dermatitis, pustular acne, infected burns and wounds, ulcers and paronychia.

Dosage and administration A small amount of ointment or cream should be applied to the lesions three or four times daily or as prescribed. If necessary this may be covered with a dressing.

Contra-indications, warnings, etc Cidomycin is contra-indicated when there is a known hypersensitivity to any ingredient of the preparation.
Precautions: If irritation, sensitisation or super-infection develop, treatment with Cidomycin should be discontinued and appropriate therapy instituted.
Overdosage: Haemodialysis or peritoneal dialysis will aid the removal of gentamicin from the blood.

Pharmaceutical precautions Store cool. In order to preserve their antibacterial activity Cidomycin Cream and Ointment should not be diluted by the addition of excipient.

Legal category POM.

Package quantities *Cidomycin cream:* Tubes of 15 g and 30 g.
Cidomycin ointment: Tubes of 15 g and 30 g.

Further information Nil.

Product licence numbers

Cidomycin Cream	0109/5063
Cidomycin Ointment	0109/5064

CLAFORAN* ▼

Presentation Claforan is available in vials containing 500 mg, 1 g or 2 g of cefotaxime as cefotaxime sodium.

Claforan is a white to slightly creamy powder which, when dissolved in Water for Injections BP forms a straw coloured solution suitable for intravenous or intramuscular administration. Variations in the intensity of colour of the freshly prepared solution do not indicate change in potency or safety.

Uses
Properties: Claforan is a broad spectrum bactericidal cephalosporin antibiotic. Claforan is exceptionally active

in vitro against Gram-negative organisms sensitive or resistant to first or second generation cephalosporins. It is similar to other cephalosporins in activity against Gram-positive bacteria.

Indications: Claforan is indicated in the treatment of the following infections either before the infecting organism has been identified or when caused by bacteria of established sensitivity.

Septicaemia

Respiratory tract infections: acute and chronic bronchitis, bacterial pneumonia, infected bronchiectasis, lung abscess and post-operative chest infections.

Urinary tract infections: acute and chronic pyelonephritis, cystitis and asymptomatic bacteriuria.

Soft tissue infections: cellulitis, peritonitis and wound infections.

Bone and joint infections: osteomyelitis, septic arthritis.

Obstetric and gynaecological infections: pelvic inflammatory disease.

Gonorrhoea: particularly if penicillin-resistant.

Other bacterial infections: meningitis and other sensitive infections suitable for parenteral antibiotic therapy.

The administration of Claforan prophylactically may reduce the incidence of certain post-operative infections in patients undergoing surgical procedures that are classified as contaminated or potentially contaminated or in clean operations where infection would have serious effects.

Protection is best ensured by achieving adequate local tissue concentrations at the time contamination is likely to occur. Claforan should therefore be administered immediately prior to surgery and if necessary continued in the immediate post-operative period. Administration should usually be stopped within 24 hours since continuing use of any antibiotic in the majority of surgical procedures does not reduce the incidence of subsequent infections.

Bacteriology: The following organisms have shown in vitro sensitivity to Claforan.

Gram-positive: Staphylococci, including coagulase-positive, coagulase-negative and penicillinase-producing strains. Beta-haemolytic and other streptococci such as *Streptococcus mitis* (*viridans*). Many strains of enterococci, e.g. *Streptococcus faecalis*, are relatively resistant. *Streptococcus* (*Diplococcus*) *pneumoniae*. *Clostridium spp.*

Gram-negative:
Escherichia coli
Haemophilus influenzae including ampicillin-resistant strains
Klebsiella spp.
Proteus spp. both indole-positive and indole-negative
Enterobacter spp.
Neisseria spp. including β-lactamase producing strains of *N. gonorrhoeae*
Salmonella spp. including *Salm. typhi*
Shigella spp.
Providencia spp.
Serratia spp.
Citrobacter spp.

Claforan has frequently exhibited useful in vitro activity against *Pseudomonas* and *Bacteroides* species although some strains of *Bacteroides fragilis* are resistant.

There is in vitro evidence of synergy between Claforan and aminoglycoside antibiotics such as gentamicin against some species of Gram-negative bacteria including some strains of *Pseudomonas*. No in vitro antagonism has been noted. In severe infections caused by *Pseudomonas spp.* the concurrent use of an aminoglycoside antibiotic may be indicated.

Dosage and administration Claforan may be administered intravenously or intramuscularly. Dosage, route and frequency of administration should be determined by severity of infection, sensitivity of causative organisms and condition of the patient. Therapy may be started before the result of sensitivity tests are known.

Adults: The usual dose in adults is 2 to 6 g daily, depending upon the severity of the infection. However, dosage may be varied according to the severity of the infection, sensitivity of causative organisms and condition of the patient. For infections caused by sensitive *Pseudomonas spp.* daily doses of more than 6 g are usually required.

Guidelines for dosage: Mild to moderate or uncomplicated infections such as U.T.I. 1 g every 12 hours. Moderate to serious infections 1 g every 8 hours. Life threatening infections 2 g every 8 hours.

In exceptional circumstances of life threatening infections caused by an organism less sensitive to cefotaxime, e.g. pseudomonas, up to 12 g per day (in divided dosages) may occasionally be of advantage.

Gonorrhoea 1 g single dose.

Children: The usual dosage is 100–150 mg/kg/day in 2 to 4 divided doses. In very severe infections up to 200 mg/kg/day, in divided doses, may be required.

Neonates: The recommended dosage is 50 mg/kg/day in 2 to 4 divided doses. In severe infections, 150–200 mg/kg/day, in divided doses, have been given.

Dosage in renal impairment: Because of extra-renal elimination, it is only necessary to reduce the dosage of Claforan in severe renal failure (GFR <5 ml/min). After an initial loading dose of 1 g, the daily dose should be halved without change in the frequency of dosing, e.g. 1 g 12 hourly becomes 0.5 g 12 hourly, 1 g 8 hourly becomes 0.5 g 8 hourly, 2 g 8 hourly becomes 1 g 8 hourly, etc. As in all other patients, dosage may require further adjustment according to the course of the infection and the general condition of the patient.

Intravenous and intramuscular administration: Dissolve Claforan in Water for Injections BP as shown. Shake well until dissolved and then withdraw the entire contents of the vial into the syringe and use immediately.

Vial size	Volume of Water for Injections to be added
500 mg	2 ml
1 g	4 ml
2 g	10 ml

Intravenous infusion: Claforan may be administerd by intravenous infusion. 1–2 g are dissolved in 40–100 ml of Water for Injections BP or in the infusion fluids listed under 'Pharmaceutical precautions'. The prepared infusion should be administered over 20–60 minutes.

Elderly: No specific recommendations for the elderly.

Contra-indications, warnings, etc
Contra-indications: Known allergy to cephalosporins.

Precautions: Cephalosporin antibiotics may usually be given safely to patients who are hypersensitive to penicillins, although cross reactions have been reported. Special care is indicated in patients who have had an anaphylactic response to penicillin.

Patients with severe renal dysfunction – see 'Dosage and administration'.

Cephalosporin antibiotics at high dosage should be given with caution to patients receiving aminoglycoside antibiotics or potent diuretics such as frusemide as these combinations are thought to have an adverse effect on renal function. However, at the recommended doses, enhancement of nephrotoxicity is unlikely to be a problem with Claforan.

As with all cephalosporins, pseudomembranous colitis may rarely occur during treatment. If this occurs, the drug should be stopped and specific treatment instituted.

Interference with laboratory tests: A false-positive reaction to glucose may occur with reducing substances but not with the use of specific glucose oxidase methods.

Pregnancy: Although studies in animals have not shown an adverse effect on the developing foetus, the safety of Claforan in human pregnancy has not been established. Consequently, Claforan should not be administered during pregnancy especially during the first trimester, without carefully weighing the expected benefits against the possible risks.

Lactation: Claforan is excreted in the milk.

Side effects: Adverse reactions to Claforan have occurred relatively infrequently and have generally been mild and transient. Effects reported include diarrhoea, candidiasis, rashes, fever, eosinophilia, leukopenia and transient rises in liver transaminase and alkaline phosphatase.

Transient pain may be experienced at the site of injection. This is more likely to occur with higher doses. Occasionally, phlebitis has been reported in patients receiving intravenous Claforan. However, this has rarely been a cause for discontinuation of treatment.

Overdosage: Serum levels of Claforan may be reduced by peritoneal dialysis or haemodialysis.

Pharmaceutical precautions The dry powder in vials should be stored away from heat and protected from light. Whilst it is preferable to use only freshly prepared solutions for both intravenous and intramuscular injection, Claforan is compatible with several commonly used intravenous infusion fluids and will retain satisfactory potency for up to 24 hours refrigerated in the following:

   Water for Injections BP
   Sodium Chloride Injection BP
   5% Dextrose Injection BP
   Dextrose and Sodium Chloride Injection BP
   Compound Sodium Lactate Injection BP (Ringer-Lactate Injection).

After 24 hours any unused solution should be discarded.

Claforan is also compatible with 1% lignocaine. Freshly prepared solutions should be used.

Some increase in colour of prepared solutions may occur on storage. However, provided the recommended storage conditions are observed, this does not indicate change in potency or safety.

Legal category POM.

Package quantities Individually packed vials containing 500 mg or 1 g cefotaxime as cefotaxime sodium (for use by intramuscular or intravenous injection) in packs of 10.

Individually packed vials containing 2 g cefotaxime as cefotaxime sodium (for intravenous use only) in packs of 10.

Further information Each gram of Claforan contains approximately 48 mg (2.09 mmol) of sodium. Claforan has been used with other beta-lactam antibiotics such as carbenicillin in the treatment of neutropenic patients. Claforan may also be administered separately with metronidazole in the treatment of mixed infections caused by anaerobic and aerobic organisms.

Claforan usually passes the blood-brain barrier in levels above the MIC of common sensitive pathogens when the meninges are inflamed.

The laboratory abbreviation for cefotaxime is CTX.

Product licence number 0109/0074

EUGLUCON*

Presentation Euglucon is available as:

1. White, circular, biconvex tablets, 6 mm in diameter, marked EU on one side and 2.5 on the reverse. Each tablet contains 2.5 mg Glibenclamide BP.

2. White, oblong 10 mm × 5 mm tablets containing 5 mg Glibenclamide BP. Each side has a breakline and is inscribed BM/EU, such that when a tablet is broken into half, one side is marked BM, and the other EU.

Uses Euglucon is an oral hypoglycaemic agent of the sulphonylurea type.

Euglucon is indicated for the treatment of maturity-onset diabetes which is not adequately controlled by dietary measures alone.

Dosage and administration Euglucon should be taken with or immediately after food. The total daily dosage is preferably given as a single dose at breakfast or with the first main meal, but due consideration should be given to the patient's meal habits and daily activity when apportioning dosage.

1. *New Diabetics*: In maturity-onset diabetes of mild to moderate severity, treatment should be started with 5 mg daily or 2.5 mg in debilitated or elderly patients. If this dosage is not sufficient for proper control it should be increased by 2.5 mg at intervals of one week, or as directed by the clinician. The total daily dose of Euglucon rarely exceeds 15 mg. Increasing dosage beyond this level is unlikely to produce further response.

2. *Transfer from other sulphonylureas:* Transfer to Euglucon can usually be carried out without any break in therapy.

Euglucon treatment should be started with 5 mg daily and, if necessary, adjusted in steps of 2.5 or 5 mg. A dose of 5 mg Euglucon is approximately equivalent to 1000 mg tolbutamide, 250 mg chlorpropamide, 25 mg glibornuride or 5 mg glipizide.

3. *Changeover from biguanides:* Euglucon treatment should be started with 2.5 mg of Euglucon and the biguanide withdrawn. Dosage should then be adjusted by increments of 2.5 mg to achieve control.

Combination with biguanides: If adequate control is not possible with diet and 15 mg of Euglucon, control can often be re-established by a combination of Euglucon and a biguanide derivative.

4. *Euglucon and insulin:* While it is appreciated that most patients who are on insulin therapy will continue to need it, there may be a few patients, particularly those on low daily dosages, who will remain stabilised if transferred to Euglucon.

No dosage recommendations can be made for the administration of Euglucon to children.

Contra-indications, warnings, etc Euglucon is contra-indicated in:

1. The treatment of juvenile or unstable diabetes.

2. Patients who have had serious metabolic decompensation with ketosis and, in particular, diabetic pre coma and coma.

3. Serious impairment of renal, hepatic, thyroid or adrenocortical function.

4. Pregnancy. After delivery, Euglucon therapy can be started or resumed.

5. Hypersensitivity to glibenclamide.

Precautions: The hypoglycaemic action of oral antidiabetic agents including Euglucon may be enhanced by sulphonamides, salicylates, phenylbutazone, coumarin derivatives, beta-blocking agents, monoamine-oxidase inhibitors, cyclophosphamide, benzafibrate, clofibrate, fenfluamine, tetracyclines, sulphinpyrazone and chloramphenicol. Conversely, thiazide diuretics, frusemide, ethacrynic acid, oral contraceptives containing oestrogens/gestagens, thyroid hormones and corticosteroids may diminish hypoglycaemic activity. Hypoglycaemic activity may also be affected by tuberculostatics.

In patients suffering from intercurrent infections or trauma, the dosage of Euglucon may need to be increased. If such complications are severe, diabetic control may be lost necessitating withdrawal of Euglucon and maintenance of diabetic control with insulin. Euglucon should be re-introduced when the patient has recovered from the infection or trauma.

Pregnancy: There is no information on the use of Euglucon in human pregnancy but it has been in wide, general use for many years without apparent ill consequence. Animal studies have shown no hazard.

Nursing mothers: It has not been established whether glibencamide is secreted in human milk. Other sulphonylureas have been found in milk. There is no evidence that glibenclamide differs from the group in this respect.

Side-effects: Euglucon is well tolerated and side-effects serious enough to necessitate withdrawal are uncommon. Gastro-intestinal symptoms (nausea, anorexia and diarrhoea) are uncommon and allergic skin reactions are seldom encountered.

Reversible leucopenia and thrombocytopenia have been reported but are rare. Transient changes in liver enzyme concentrations and liver function tests during treatment with glibenclamide have been reported, but these are not known to be directly attributable to the product. As with other agents, hypoglycaemia can occur with Euglucon, but is not usually prolonged and responds to appropriate therapeutic measures.

Effects of overdosage and their treatment: If a hypoglycaemic reaction should occur, the conscious patient may be treated with dextrose or 3–4 lumps of table sugar with water. This may be repeated, if necessary, in 15 minutes.

If the patient is comatose, sucrose or dextrose may be given by stomach tube or dextrose given intravenously. Glucagon may be administered in a dose of 1 mg subcutaneously or intramuscularly to produce consciousness.

Pharmaceutical precautions No special storage requirements.

Legal category POM.

Package quantities 5 mg tablets: Blister packs of 100. 2.5 mg tablets: Blister packs of 100.

Further information Absorption studies in healthy human volunteers using labelled glibenclamide formulated as Euglucon tablets showed a mean absorption of $84 \pm 9\%$.

Excretion was approximately 50% in the urine and 50% in the faeces. Absorbed glibenclamide was completely metabolised and the three isolated metabolites in the concentrations found had no significant hypoglycaemic activity.

Product licence numbers

Euglucon 2.5 mg Tablets   0109/0073
Euglucon 5 mg Tablets   0109/5023

LANITOP*

Presentation Lanitop tablets contain 0.1 mg medigoxin. The tablets are round (6 mm diameter), yellow and with a score line. They are engraved one side with LAN on the left side and TOP on the right side of the breakline.

Uses Lanitop is indicated in all cases in which digitalis therapy is required, e.g. congestive heart failure and certain cardiac arrhythmias, especially atrial fibrillation.

Dosage and administration Dosage is dependent upon the glycoside requirement of the heart in individual patients. It has been shown that 95% of patients may be treated successfully, using the following schedule.

1. *Adults and children over 14:*
Digitalisation: 2 tablets twice daily for three to five days.
Maintenance: 1 tablet two or three times daily.

In emergencies a more rapid digitalisation may be achieved by giving: 2 tablets three times daily for two to four days.

2. *Elderly:* It is recommended that digitalis therapy in elderly patients be carried out gradually, and with smaller doses, except in an emergency.

3. *Infants and children under 14 years:* Digitalisation may be effected by using 0.01 mg/kg repeated six-hourly until therapeutic result is obtained, 2–4 doses usually being sufficient. Maintenance is usually achieved with 0.01 mg/kg daily, which should be adjusted as necessary.

Contra-indications, warnings, etc All cardiac glycosides are contra-indicated in digitalis intoxication, hypercalcaemia and before electro-cardioversion. Special care should be taken if the patient is already receiving or has recently been receiving a cardiac glycoside. In addition, glycoside therapy may be contra-indicated or may require additional therapeutic measures in manifest hypokalaemia, disorders of atrio-ventricular conduction and in pathological bradycardia, depending on its severity.

Parenteral administration of calcium, particularly simultaneously, should be avoided during any glycoside therapy.

The effects of digitalis therapy may be potentiated by quinidine and lithium. Some antacid constituents affect the bioavailability of digitalis if taken simultaneously.

As with all digitalis therapy, gastric disturbance, arrhythmias and visual disturbances may occur, particularly in those patients who are hypersensitive to glycosides or who have an electrolyte imbalance such as that caused by diuretic therapy.

A reduced glycoside requirement may be expected in the elderly and when there is renal insufficiency. The recommended doses may produce evidence of toxicity in patients with acute myocardial infarction, severe pulmonary disease, advanced heart failure, and in premature infants.

Teratogenic studies have been conducted in animals without adverse effects. However, the likely benefit from the administration of Lanitop should be weighed against possible adverse effects during the first trimester of pregnancy.

Treatment of overdosage: Gastric lavage should be given and the ECG monitored. Potassium should be administered for hypokalaemia; glucose and insulin for hyperkalaemia; atropine for bradycardia; antiarrhythmic agents as appropriate for tachycardia and arrhythmia.

Pharmaceutical precautions Store in a cool dry place. Protect from light.

Legal category POM.

Package quantities *Lanitop Tablets:* Bottles of 100.

Further information Absorption of Lanitop is rapid (5–20 minutes) and virtually complete. Its duration of action is similar to that of digoxin. These characteristics fulfil the pharmacokinetic requirements of an ideal cardiac glycoside.

The stated dosages are less than those normally used when digoxin is administered. Under steady state conditions 0.3 mg Lanitop daily is therapeutically equivalent to 0.5 mg of digoxin daily.

Product licence number
Lanitop Tablets   0109/0053

LOPRAZOLAM* TABLETS 1 mg ▼

Presentation Loprazolam tablets 1 mg. Yellow, circular tablets, 7 mm in diameter, marked Dormonoct 1 on one face with breakline on reverse. Each tablet contains loprazolam mesylate equivalent to 1 mg loprazolam.

Uses Loprazolam is indicated for the short-term treatment of insomnia including difficulty in falling asleep and/or frequent nocturnal awakenings.

Dosage and administration
Adults: The recommended dose is 1 mg at bedtime. This may be increased to 1.5 mg or 2 mg if necessary.

Elderly: Dosage in the elderly should be limited to 1 mg at bedtime.

Frail, debilitated or aged patients: A starting dose of a half tablet may be appropriate. Dosage should not exceed 1 mg.

Children: There is insufficient evidence to recommend the use of Loprazolam in children.

Contra-indications, warnings, etc
Contra-indications: Sensitivity to benzodiazepines, acute pulmonary insufficiency, myasthenia gravis.

Pregnancy and lactation: The use of loprazolam during pregnancy should be avoided. The possibility of loprazolam being excreted in the milk should also be considered in nursing mothers.

Precautions: As with all CNS-active drugs, patients should be warned of the possible hazard of driving or operating machinery, and that loprazolam may be potentiated by alcohol or other drugs acting on the CNS.

Loprazolam should be used with caution in chronic pulmonary insufficiency, cerebrovascular disease and chronic renal or hepatic impairment.

In general, the dependence potential of benzodiazepines is low but this increases when high doses are attained, especially when given over long periods, and particularly in patients with a history of alcoholism or drug abuse. Regular monitoring of treatment of such patients is desirable and withdrawal of treatment should be gradual.

Side-effects: In general, loprazolam is very well tolerated. However, the common side effects of benzodiazepines, including headaches, nausea, drowsiness, blurring of vision, dizziness and ataxia may occur on the following day, particularly in unusually sensitive patients or when dosage has been excessive.

Rare behavioural adverse effects of benzodiazepines include paradoxical aggressive outbursts, excitement, confusion, and the uncovering of depression with suicidal tendencies. Even more rare side effects reported with some benzodiazepines have been hypotension, gastrointestinal and visual disturbances, skin rashes, urinary retention, changes in libido, blood dyscrasias and jaundice.

Overdosage: As with other benzodiazepines, overdosage does not usually present a threat to life. Treatment is symptomatic and gastric lavage may be of use if performed shortly after ingestion.

Pharmaceutical precautions Store in a dry place, protected from light.

Legal category CD (Sch 4) POM.

Package quantities Loprazolam Tablets 1 mg are blister packed in strips of 10 and presented in cartons of 30.

Further information Loprazolam is an intermediate acting benzodiazepine. There are no long-lived sedative metabolites. Therefore there is a reduced likelihood of the occurrence of daytime drowsiness or impairment in the performance of skilled tasks, associated with the long acting products. Equally, there is less likelihood of rebound insomnia, which may occur with the ultra-short acting benzodiazepines.

Loprazolam was previously known as Dormonoct.*

Product licence number 0109/0080.

MOLIPAXIN*

Presentation Molipaxin (trazodone hydrochloride) is available as: Molipaxin 50 mg Size No. 3 opaque violet/green capsules printed R365B and **⋏**. Each capsule contains 50 mg trazodone hydrochloride.

Molipaxin 100 mg. Size No. 2, opaque violet/fawn capsules printed R365C and **⋏**. Each capsule contains 100 mg trazodone hydrochloride.

Molipaxin 150 mg, salmon-pink, film coated, round biconvex tablets, approximately 11 mm in diameter with a white core. The tablet is embossed with 'Molipaxin' and '150' on one face and a breakline on the other face.

Molipaxin Liquid for oral use is a clear colourless solution with an orange odour and taste. Each 5 ml contains 50 mg trazodone hydrochloride.

Uses *Properties:* Molipaxin is a potent antidepressant. It also has anxiety reducing activity. Molipaxin is a triazolopyridine derivative chemically unrelated to known tricyclic, tetracyclic and other antidepressant agents. It has negligible effect on noradrenaline reuptake mechanisms. Whilst the mode of action of

Molipaxin is not known precisely, its antidepressant activity may concern noradrenergic potentiation by mechanisms other than uptake blockade. A central anti-serotonin effect may account for the drug's anxiety reducing properties.

Indications: Relief of symptoms in all types of depression including depression accompanied by anxiety. Symptoms of depression likely to respond in the first week of treatment include depressed mood, insomnia, anxiety, somatic symptoms and hypochondriasis.

Dosage and administration The starting dose of Molipaxin is initially 150 mg in single or divided doses after food (50 mg twice daily in the elderly or frail). This should be increased to 200 or 300 mg per day according to severity at the second consultation, but not before 7 days of treatment. The usual maintenance dose in patients with moderate-to-severe depression is 300 mg per day. In cases of mild depression, as seen in general practice, the usual maintenance dose is 200 mg per day. Maximum dosage in very severe depression is 600 mg per day in divided doses. To utilise Molipaxin's sedative properties, most of the daily maintenance dose may be given at night, avoiding single doses above 100 mg in the elderly and frail.

In conformity with current psychiatric opinion, it is suggested that Molipaxin be continued for several months after remission. Cessation of Molipaxin treatment should be gradual.

Children: There are insufficient data to recommend the use of Molipaxin in children.

Contra-indications, warnings, etc
Contra-indications: None.

Precautions: As with all other drugs acting on the central nervous system, patients should be warned against the risks of handling machinery and driving.

Although no untoward effects have been reported, Molipaxin may enhance the effects of muscle relaxants and volatile anaesthetics. Similar considerations apply to combined administration with sedative and antidepressant drugs, including alcohol. Molipaxin has been well tolerated in depressed schizophrenic patients receiving standard phenothiazine therapy and also in depressed parkinsonian patients receiving therapy with levodopa.

Interactions between Molipaxin and monoamine oxidase inhibitors have not been reported. However, on grounds of clinical caution, Molipaxin is not recommended for concurrent administration with monoamine oxidase inhibitors or within two weeks of terminating treatment with these compounds.

Since Molipaxin is only a very weak inhibitor of noradrenaline re-uptake and does not modify the blood pressure response to tyramine, interference with the hypotensive action of guanethidine-like compounds is unlikely. However, studies in laboratory animals suggest that Molipaxin may inhibit most of the acute actions of clonidine. In the case of other types of antihypertensive drug, although no clinical interactions have been reported, the possibility of potentiation should be considered.

Current clinical experience suggests that Molipaxin does not cause seizures. Nevertheless, care should be exercised when administering Molipaxin to patients suffering from epilepsy, avoiding in particular, abrupt increases or decreases in dosage.

Molipaxin should be administered with care in patients with severe hepatic or renal disease.

Pregnancy and lactation: Although studies in animals have not shown any direct teratogenic effect, the safety of Molipaxin in human pregnancy has not been established. On basic principles, therefore, its use during the first trimester should be avoided. The possibility of Molipaxin being excreted in the milk should also be considered in nursing mothers.

Side-effects: Molipaxin is a sedative antidepressant and drowsiness, sometimes experienced during the first days of treatment, usually disappears on continued therapy.

The incidence of anticholinergic-like symptoms is not different from placebo.

No major side effects have been reported even in patients treated continuously for periods in excess of one year. The following symptoms, most of which are commonly reported in cases of untreated depression, have also been recorded in small numbers of patients receiving Molipaxin therapy: dizziness, headache, nausea and vomiting, weakness, decreased alertness, weight loss, tremor, dry mouth, bradycardia, tachycardia, postural hypotension, oedema, constipation, diarrhoea, blurred vision, restlessness, confusional states, insomnia and skin rash.

As with other drugs with alpha-adrenolytic activity, Molipaxin has been associated with priapism. At the date of issue, there has been only one report in the UK. However, reports from the United States suggest an association between trazodone and priapism which has on occasion required surgical intervention or led to permanent sexual dysfunction. Patients developing this suspected adverse reaction should cease Molipaxin therapy immediately.

Overdosage: There is no specific antidote to Molipaxin. The stomach should be emptied as quickly as possible. Treatment should be symptomatic and supportive in the case of hypotension and excessive sedation.

Pharmaceutical precautions *Molipaxin Capsules:* No special storage conditions are required.
Molipaxin Tablets: Store in a dry place.
Molipaxin Liquid: Protect from light and store at room temperature. N.B. Molipaxin Liquid is primarily intended for in-patient use. If dispensed for out-patient use a standard childproof cap should be fitted.

Legal category POM.

Package quantities *Molipaxin Capsules:* Molipaxin 50 mg and 100 mg capsules presented in blister strips of 20 each in pack sizes of 100.

Molipaxin Tablets: Molipaxin 150 mg in blister strips of 30 tablets.

Molipaxin Liquid: Bottle of 150 ml oral liquid.

Further information In contrast to the tricyclic antidepressants, Molipaxin is devoid of anticholinergic activity. Consequently, troublesome side effects such as dry mouth, blurred vision and urinary hesitancy have occurred no more frequently than in patients receiving placebo therapy. This may be of importance when treating depressed patients who are at risk from conditions such as glaucoma, urinary retention and prostatic hypertrophy.

Studies in animals have shown that Molipaxin is less cardiotoxic than the tricyclic antidepressants and clinical studies suggest that the drug may be less likely to cause cardiac arrhythmias in man.

Molipaxin has had no effect on arterial blood pCO_2 or

pO_2 levels in patients with severe respiratory insufficiency due to chronic bronchial or pulmonary disease.

Product licence numbers

Molipaxin Capsules 50 mg	0109/0045
Molipaxin Capsules 100 mg	0109/0046
Molipaxin Tablets 150 mg	0109/0133
Molipaxin Liquid 50 mg/5 ml	0109/0117

PROCTOFIBE*

Presentation Proctofibe is available as beige biconvex film-coated tablets, 12 mm in diameter, each containing 375 mg of a fibrous extract of grain and 94 mg of a fibrous extract of citrus.

Uses Colonic and gastro-intestinal disorders where a high-fibre regimen is indicated including uncomplicated diverticular disease, irritable colon, simple constipation, haemhorrhoidal disorders, anal fissure, pregnancy, myocardial infarction and other conditions where straining at stool should be avoided.

Dosage and administration *Adults:* 4–12 tablets daily in divided doses, or as directed by the physician.

Elderly: No specific recommendations in the elderly.

Children: Over three years of age, as adults.

The tablets should be swallowed with ample water. (Alternatively, they may be crushed and dispersed in water.)

Contra-indications, warnings, etc Intestinal obstruction, gluten enteropathies, coeliac disease. As with other fibre presentations, transient bloating and flatulence may occasionally be reported in the first two weeks of treatment.

Pharmaceutical precautions Store in a cool, dry place.

Legal category P.

Package quantities Bottles of 125 tablets.

Further information Nil.

Product licence number 0109/0081.

PROCTOSEDYL*

Presentation Proctosedyl is available as smooth, off-white suppositories and as an odourless, yellowish-white, translucent, greasy ointment. Each suppository or gram of ointment contains the following active ingredients:

Cinchocaine Hydrochloride BP	5 mg
Hydrocortisone BP	5 mg
Framycetin Sulphate BP (Soframycin)	10 mg
Aesculin	10 mg

Uses The local anaesthetic cinchocaine relieves pain and relaxes sphincteric spasm. Pruritus and inflammation are relieved by hydrocortisone, which also decreases serous discharge, while Soframycin controls local infection (a cause of inflammation and irritation).

Proctosedyl is thus used for the following: internal and external haemorrhoids; prophylaxis between attacks to prevent recurrences; haemorrhoidal complications-anal pruritus, perianal eczema, proctitis, fissure; pre-operative and post-operative treatment of haemorrhoidectomy patients; post-partum haemorrhoidal conditions.

Dosage and administration A suppository is inserted morning and evening, and after each stool.

Apply the ointment in small quantity with the finger, on the painful or pruritic area, morning and evening and after each stool. For deep application attach cannula to tube, insert to full extent and squeeze tube gently from lower end whilst withdrawing.

The ointment may be used separately or concurrently with the suppositories.

Contra-indications, warnings, etc Known hypersensitivity to any of the ingredients.

In pregnant animals, administration of corticosteroids can cause abnormalities of foetal development. The relevance of this finding to human beings has not been established. However, topical steroids should not be used extensively in pregnancy, i.e. in large amounts or for long periods.

As with all preparations containing topical corticosteroids, the possibility of systemic absorption should be considered. In particular, long-term continuous therapy should be avoided in infants. Adrenal suppression can occur even without occlusion.

Pharmaceutical precautions Store cool.

Legal category POM.

Package quantities *Proctosedyl Suppositories:* Packs of 12.
Proctosedyl Ointment: Tubes of 30 g (with cannula).

Further information Nil.

Product licence numbers

Proctosedyl ointment	0109/5038
Proctosedyl Suppositories	0109/5039

RYTHMODAN* CAPSULES
RYTHMODAN* RETARD TABLETS ▼
RYTHMODAN INJECTION

Presentation
Oral.

Rythmodan Capsules: Capsules with opaque green cap and opaque beige body with 'RY' and 'RL' printed in black, containing 100 mg of disopyramide base.

Capsules with opaque white cap and body with 'RY' and '150' printed in black, containing 150 mg disopyramide base.

Rythmodan Retard Tablets: White, circular biconvex tablets, 12 mm in diameter, film-coated with a break line. Tablets are marked 'RY' and 'R' on one side and ⚗ on the reverse. Each tablet contains disopyramide phosphate equivalent to 250 mg disopyramide base in a sustained release formulation.

Intravenous Injection.

Rythmodan Injection: Ampoules for intravenous use only. 5 ml ampoules containing disopyramide phosphate equivalent to 50 mg disopyramide base in solution.

Uses *Properties:* Rythmodan is able to prevent and control a wide variety of cardiac arrhythmias, probably by slowing conduction in the His-Purkinje system and by increasing the effective refractory period of the atria and ventricles.

Indications: Oral Rythmodan is indicated in:

1. Maintenance of normal rhythm following conversion by Rythmodan Injection, other parenteral drugs or electroconversion.

2. Prevention of arrhythmias after myocardial infarction.

3. Treatment of persistent ventricular and atrial extrasystoles, paroxysmal supraventricular tachycardia, Wolff-Parkinson-White syndrome.

4. Suppression of arrhythmias during surgical procedures.

5. Control of arrhythmias following the use of digitalis or similar glycosides.

Rythmodan Injection is intended for intravenous use only and is indicated in the following conditions:

1. Conversion of ventricular and supraventricular arrhythmias after myocardial infarction, including those not responding to lignocaine or other i.v. treatment.

2. Control of ventricular and atrial extrasystoles, supraventricular tachycardia, and Wolff-Parkinson-White syndrome.

3. Control of arrhythmias following digitalis or similar glycosides when Rythmodan cannot be administered orally.

Dosage and administration
Oral

Rythmodan Capsules: The recommended daily dosage in adults is 300–800 mg in divided doses adjusted according to the response of the patient.

Rythmodan Retard Tablets: The recommended dose for stabilised patients or those receiving Rythmodan for the first time is 1 to $1\frac{1}{2}$ tablets (250–375 mg) twice daily. Patients being transferred from intravenous therapy with Rythmodan should be stabilised on standard Rythmodan capsules for the first 24 hours (see below). Tablets should be swallowed and not crushed or chewed.

Intravenous Injection

Rythmodan Injection: The recommended dosage can be given by two different regimes.

1. An initial direct intravenous injection of 2 mg/kg (but not exceeding 150 mg (15 ml) irrespective of body weight) should be given SLOWLY OVER NOT LESS THAN FIVE MINUTES, i.e. the rate of injection must not exceed 30 mg (3 ml) per minute in order to reduce or avoid unwanted haemodynamic effects. If conversion occurs during this time the injection should be stopped. If the arrhythmia is to respond to Rythmodan it will usually do so within 10–15 minutes after completion of the injection.

Transfer to oral maintenance therapy is accomplished by giving 200 mg orally, immediately on cessation of intravenous administration, followed by 200 mg every 8 hours for 24 hours. Most patients may be maintained subsequently on a daily dosage of 500–750 mg of Rythmodan, preferably administered as 1 to $1\frac{1}{2}$ Rythmodan Retard tablets (250–375 mg) twice daily. Where the need for lower dosage outweighs the convenience of twice daily administration, appropriate doses of conventional capsules (100 or 150 mg) may be administered.

If conversion is achieved by intravenous Rythmodan but the arrhythmia subsequently recurs, a further slow direct intravenous injection over not less than five minutes may be administered cautiously and preferably under ECG control. The total administration by the intravenous route should not exceed 4 mg/kg (maximum 300 mg) in the first hour, nor should the combined administration by the intravenous and oral routes exceed 800 mg in 24 hours.

2. An initial direct intravenous injection as above, i.e. over not less than five minutes, maintained by intravenous infusion by drip of 20–30 mg/hour (or 0.4 mg/kg/hour) up to a maximum of 800 mg daily. This regime should be employed if the patient is unable to take oral medication or in particularly serious arrhythmias being treated in *coronary care units.*

Heart failure: In determining the intervals between administration of Rythmodan capsules it should be borne in mind that whilst the elimination half-life in normal volunteers is approximately seven hours, in patients with heart failure, half-life values of 12 hours or more have been recorded.

Impaired renal function (Disease state or the elderly): Standard capsules should be used in patients in renal failure. A reduced dosage, preferably accompanied by assay of disopyramide plasma levels in cases of severe renal failure (creatinine clearance <8 ml/min) is recommended. The following table may be helpful as a guide.

Creatinine clearance (ml/min)	Dosage 100 or 150 mg capsules
Normal	Normal dosage
20–60	100 mg 8-hourly or 150 mg 12-hourly
8–20	100 mg 12-hourly
<8	150 mg daily

Children: There are insufficient data to recommend the use of Rythmodan in children.

Contra-indications, warnings, etc
Contra-indications: Disopyramide is contra-indicated in second or third degree heart block and sinus node disease if no pacemaker is present, cardiogenic shock and severe uncompensated heart failure and hypersensitivity to disopyramide.

Warnings and precautions: There have been reports of ventricular tachycardia or ventricular fibrillation or Torsade de Pointes in patients receiving disopyramide. These have been usually, but not always, associated with significant widening of the QRS complex or prolonged QT interval. If these ECG changes or arrhythmias develop the drug should be discontinued.

Disopyramide should be used only with caution in patients with atrial flutter or atrial tachycardia with block as conversion of a partial AV block to a 1:1 response may occur. Accordingly, the need for prior digitalisation should be considered.

Owing to its negative inotropic effect, disopyramide should be used with caution in patients suffering from significant cardiac failure. Such patients should be fully digitalised or controlled with other therapy before initiating treatment with disopyramide.

The occurrence of hypotension following disopyramide administration, which has been observed especially in patients with cardiomyopathy or inadequately compensated congestive heart failure, requires prompt discontinuation of the drug. Any resumption of therapy should be at a lower dose with close patient monitoring.

The use of disopyramide in combination with other negative inotropic drugs such as beta adrenoceptor antagonists is not recommended especially in intravenous therapy.

In view of the serious nature of many of the conditions being treated it is suggested that *Rythmodan Injection should only be used when facilities exist for cardiac monitoring or defibrillation, should the need arise.*

Disopyramide should be used with caution in patients receiving concurrent therapy with diuretics likely to give rise to hypokalaemia since this may reduce patient response to disopyramide.

Disopyramide should be used with caution in the treatment of digitalis intoxication.

Care should be taken when prescribing disopyramide for patients with bundle branch block as the effect of disopyramide in this condition is unpredictable. If first degree heart block develops in a patient receiving disopyramide, dosage should be reduced and may require discontinuation if the block persists.

Since disopyramide is eliminated predominantly by glomerular filtration the dose administered to patients with significant renal impairment may require adjustment. Patients with renal impairment should not be treated with sustained release disopyramide.

Hepatic impairment causes an increase in the plasma half-life of Rythmodan and a reduced dosage may be required.

Due to its anticholinergic properties, patients with glaucoma, a tendency to urinary retention, or any patient receiving a drug with anticholinergic activity may be unsuitable for Rythmodan therapy.

Pregnancy: Although Rythmodan has undergone animal tests for teratogenicity without evidence of any effect on the developing foetus, the benefits of using Rythmodan in the first trimester of pregnancy should be weighed against possible risks.

Lactation: Studies have shown that Rythmodan is excreted in breast milk. Therefore, if the drug is considered essential, an alternative method of infant feeding should be used.

Side effects: Rythmodan is usually well tolerated. Most common side effects (dry mouth, blurred vision, urinary hesitancy) are attributable to the drug's mild anticholinergic action. Exceptionally this may be marked. Gastrointestinal irritation may also occur. Very rarely, disopyramide therapy has been associated with acute psychosis, cholestatic jaundice and hypoglycaemia. Side effects usually disappear rapidly with reduction of dosage or cessation of therapy. Profuse sweating may indicate too rapid intravenous injection.

Overdosage: Animal studies indicate that overdosage may lead to cardiac arrest or atrio-ventricular block or to disorders of ventricular excitability leading to terminal ventricular fibrillation. Intracardiac conduction defects and ventricular hyperexcitability may be controlled by general intensive supportive therapy.

Infusion studies in dogs and man have shown the effectiveness of isoprenaline in restoring any marked fall in blood pressure.

Pharmaceutical precautions Store in a cool place. Rythmodan Injection is physically compatible with the following: Sodium Chloride Injection BP, Dextrose Injection BP, Compound Sodium Chloride Injection BPC, Compound Sodium Lactate Injection BP.

Legal category POM.

Package quantities

Rythmodan Capsules 100 mg	Packs of 100
Rythmodan Capsules 150 mg	Packs of 100
Rythmodan Retard 250 mg	Packs of 100
Rythmodan Injection 50 mg/5 ml	Packs of 5 ampoules

Further information Nil.

Product licence numbers

Rythmodan Capsules 100 mg	0109/0022
Rythmodan Capsules 150 mg	0109/0075
Rythmodan Retard Tablets▼ 250 mg	0109/0094
Rythmodan Injection	0109/0060

SOFRADEX*

Presentation Sofradex is available as a sterile, yellow-white, translucent ear/eye ointment and as sterile, clear colourless ear/eye drops.

Each gram of ointment contains Framycetin Sulphate BP (Soframycin) 5 mg, gramicidin 0.05 mg and Dexamethasone BP 0.5 mg.

Each millilitre of drops contains Framycetin Sulphate BP (Soframycin) 5 mg, gramicidin 0.05 mg and dexamethasone sodium metasulphobenzoate 0.5 mg.

Uses Sofradex is used in the ear and eye to counter irritation, inflammation and infection. It is especially effective in those conditions with an associated seborrhoeic background.

The ear: Otitis externa (acute and chronic).

The eye: Eyelid: blepharitis and infected eczema.
Conjunctiva: allergic, infective (non-purulent) and rosacea conjunctivitis.
Cornea: rosacea keratitis.
Sclera: scleritis and episcleritis.
Anterior segment: iridocyclitis.

Dosage and administration *Sofradex Drops: In the ear:* 2 or 3 drops should be instilled into the ear three or four times daily; alternatively, a gauze wick kept saturated with the drops should be inserted into the external auditory meatus.

In the eye: For rapid effect, 1 or 2 drops every one or two hours should be instilled in acute conditions (generally for two, or three days), reducing to 1 or 2 drops three or four times daily.

Sofradex Ointment: In the ear: Sofradex should be applied twice or thrice daily, and especially at bedtime, to the meatus, concha or over the pinna and to adjacent skin areas if extension to these parts has occurred.

In the eye: 2 or 3 applications of the ointment daily, or at bedtime if drops have been used during the day.

Contra-indications, warnings, etc Sofradex is contra-indicated in: herpes simplex infections and other virus diseases of the cornea and conjunctiva; tuberculosis of the eye; fungal diseases of the eye; trachoma.

Purulent infections of the eye could be masked and indeed enhanced by the presence of the steroid, particularly when the infecting organism is not sensitive to the antibiotics contained in Sofradex.

Hypersensitivity to any of the active ingredients.

Preparations containing framycetin should not be used for treating otitis externa when the ear drum is perforated, because of the risk of ototoxicity.

Side effects:
1. Raised intra-ocular pressure may result from extended use of topical steroid therapy in some individuals.
2. In conditions causing thinning of the cornea, any topical steroid may cause perforation.
3. Cataract has been reported to have occurred after unduly prolonged treatment of eye conditions with topical corticosteroids.

Note:
In pregnant animals, administration of corticosteroids

can cause abnormalities of foetal development. The relevance of this finding to human beings has not been established. However, topical corticosteroids should not be used extensively in pregnancy, i.e. in large amounts or for long periods.

Although it is unlikely that infants will be treated long-term with Sofradex, it must be remembered that if steroids are applied to the skin of infants for continued periods of time, there is a risk of adrenal suppression occurring, even without occlusion.

Pharmaceutical precautions Store cool.

Legal category POM.

Package quantities *Sofradex Ear/Eye Drops:* Bottles of 8 ml.
Sofradex Ear/Eye Ointment: Tubes of 5 g (fitted with ophthalmic nozzle).

Further information Nil.

Product licence numbers
Sofradex Ear/Eye Drops   0109/0030
Sofradex Ear/Eye Ointment   0109/0031

SOFRAMYCIN* STERILE EYE DROPS/OINTMENT

Presentation Soframycin is available as a sterile eye ointment and as colourless, sterile eye drops.

Each gram of ointment contains Framycetin Sulphate BP (Soframycin) 5 mg in a sterile, non-irritating greasy base.

Each millilitre of drops contains Framycetin Sulphate BP (Soframycin) 5 mg in a sterile, buffered, isotonic, aqueous solution.

Uses Soframycin is used for the treatment of bacterial infections of the eye, notably conjunctivitis and blepharitis, for styes, corneal abrasions and burns, and prophylactically following the removal of foreign bodies. It is also indicated for corneal ulcers (alone or as a complement to the use of Soframycin by subconjunctival injection).

Dosage and administration *Soframycin Drops:* For rapid effect, preferably during the daytime, 1 or 2 drops every one or two hours should be instilled in acute conditions (generally for two or three days), reducing to 1 or 2 drops three or four times daily.
Soframycin Ointment: For continued effect, 2 or 3 applications of the ointment daily, or at bedtime if drops have been used during the day.

Contra-indications, warnings, etc Soframycin is contra-indicated when there is a known hypersensitivity to any ingredient of the preparation.

Pharmaceutical precautions Store cool.

Legal category POM.

Package quantities *Soframycin Eye Drops:* 8 ml in ophthalmic dispenser.
Soframycin Eye Ointment: Tubes of 5 g (fitted with ophthalmic nozzle).

Further information Nil.

Product licence numbers
Soframycin Eye Drops   0109/5040
Soframycin Eye Ointment   0109/5041

SOFRA-TULLE*

Presentation Sofra-Tulle is a sterile, lightweight, lano-paraffin gauze dressing impregnated with Framycetin Sulphate BP 1% (Soframycin).

Uses Sofra-Tulle has a wide range of antibacterial activity and is an ideal dressing for immediate use in a variety of infected lesions.

Thermal: Burns, scalds.

Traumatic: Lacerations, abrasions, bites, puncture wounds, crush injuries.

Ulcerative: Varicose, diabetic, decubitus and tropical ulcers.

Elective: Skin grafts (donor and receptor sites), avulsion of finger and/or toe nails, circumcision, suture lines.

Miscellaneous: Secondarily infected skin conditions (e.g. eczema, dermatitis, herpes zoster), colostomies, ileostomies, tracheostomies, incised abscesses, incised perionychia.

Dosage and administration If necessary, the lesion should first be cleansed, then a single layer of Sofra-Tulle applied and covered with a suitable dressing. When dressing ulcers, the tulle should be shaped to fit the ulcer crater. If the lesion exudes profusely it is advisable to change the dressings at least once a day.

Contra-indications, warnings, etc Sofra-Tulle is contra-indicated where there is known allergy to lanolin or to Soframycin, or where organisms are known to be resistant to the latter.

Precautions: Cross-sensitisation to Soframycin may occur in patients known to be allergic to Streptomyces-derived antibiotics (neomycin, paramomycin, kanamycin).

In most cases, absorption of the antibiotic is negligible. However, where large body areas are involved, e.g. 30% or more body burn, the possibility of ototoxicity being produced by prolonged applications should be borne in mind.

Pharmaceutical precautions Store cool.

Legal category POM.

Package quantities Cartons of 10 and 50 units; each unit pack contains one sterile antibiotic gauze dressing 10 cm × 10 cm placed between two layers of parchment. Also available as a continuous gauze strip 30 cm × 10 cm packed in cartons of 10 units.

Further information Nil.

Product licence number 0109/5047

SURGAM* ▼

Presentation White, convex tablets, 11 mm in diameter, marked SURGAM 300 on one side and ⚚ on the reverse. Each tablet contains 300 mg tiaprofenic acid.

White, convex tablets, 10 mm in diameter, marked SURGAM 200 on one side and ⚚ on the reverse. Each tablet contains 200 mg tiaprofenic acid.

Uses *Properties:* Surgam is a non-steroidal anti-inflammatory agent with marked analgesic properties.

Indications: Rheumatoid arthritis, osteoarthritis; low back pain; musculo-skeletal disorders such as fibrositis, capsulitis, epicondylitis and other soft-tissue inflammatory conditions; sprains and strains, post-operative inflammation and pain, and other soft-tissue injuries.

Dosage and administration *Adults:* 600 mg daily in divided doses.

300 mg twice daily.
Alternatively 200 mg three times daily.

Elderly: Current research suggests that it is not necessary to modify the dosage of Surgam in the elderly or in cases of mild to moderate renal impairment. In severe renal impairment, it is suggested that the dosage should be reduced to 200 mg twice daily.

Children: There are insufficient data to recommend use of Surgam in children.

Contra-indications, warnings, etc

Contra-indications: Active peptic ulceration, hypersensitivity to the drug.

Precautions: Surgam should be used with care in patients with a history of peptic ulceration, severe renal or hepatic insufficiency, asthma or previous sensitivity to aspirin or other non-steroidal anti-inflammatory agents. Non-steroidal anti-inflammatory drugs may cause some sodium and fluid retention. This should be borne in mind in patients with incipient or actual congestive heart failure. Since Surgam is highly protein-bound, it may be necessary to modify the dosage of other highly protein-bound drugs, e.g. anticoagulants, sulphonamides, hypoglycaemic agents, phenytoin and certain potent diuretics when these are administered concurrently.

Pregnancy: Although animal studies have not revealed evidence of teratogenicity, safety in human pregnancy and lactation cannot be assumed and, in common with other non-steroidal anti-inflammatory agents, administration during the first trimester should be avoided.

Lactation: There are no data on the passage of Surgam into the breast milk.

Side effects: Surgam is generally well tolerated. However, there have been occasional reports of gastro-intestinal upset, headache, drowsiness and skin rash.

Treatment of overdosage: In the event of overdosage with Surgam, supportive and symptomatic therapy is indicated.

Pharmaceutical precautions Store in a cool place and protect from light.

Legal category POM.

Package quantities 300 mg tablets in bottles of 60.
200 mg tablets in bottles of 100.

Further information Nil.

Product licence numbers
Surgam 300 mg   0109/0109
Surgam 200 mg   0109/0108

*Trade Mark

Rybar Laboratories Limited
Amersham
Buckinghamshire HP6 5BX

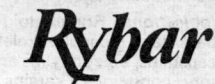

C.A.M.*
BRONCHODILATOR SYRUP

Presentation Rybar C.A.M. is a pale-green coloured liquid. Each 5 ml contains:

Butethamate citrate INN	4 mg
Ephedrine Hydrochloride BP	4 mg

Uses C.A.M. is indicated in the symptomatic treatment of bronchospasm in children and adults with asthma or bronchitis. C.A.M.'s antitussive action may also be useful in children with unproductive cough.

Dosage and administration *Age 1½–2 years:* half a 5 ml spoonful three times daily.

Age 2–4 years: One 5 ml spoonful three times daily.

Age over 4 years: Two 5 ml spoonsful three times daily.

Adults: Four 5 ml spoonsful, 3–4 times daily.

Contra-indications, warnings, etc C.A.M. is contra-indicated in children and adults with severe heart disease, hypertension, thyrotoxicosis and in patients recently or currently taking monoamine oxidase inhibitors.

Overdosage: Patients who have taken an overdosage of C.A.M. should have gastric lavage performed within four hours of the overdosage occurring. If overdosage is extreme, or there is delay in removing the drug from the stomach, symptomatic treatment of cardiac or respiratory embarrassment should be considered.

Side-effects: The synergistic action of butethamate citrate with ephedrine hydrochloride allows the dose of ephedrine to be kept low. This means that normal sympathomimetic side-effects, such as nausea, restlessness and sweating, due to overdosage of ephedrine are virtually absent.

Pharmaceutical precautions C.A.M. should not be exposed to bright sunlight, as this may cause the chemical degradation of ephedrine hydrochloride.

Legal category P.

Package quantities C.A.M. is available in bottles of 150 ml and 1 litre.

Further information Does not contain tartrazine.

Product licence number 0237/5014.

FOLEX*-350 TABLETS

Presentation Each pink, sugar-coated Folex-350 Tablet contains:

Ferrous Fumarate BP	308 mg (equivalent to 100 mg ferrous iron)
Folic Acid BP	350 mcg

Each pink tablet is overprinted with the word 'Folex-350'.

Uses The prevention and treatment of iron deficiency anaemia of pregnancy; the prevention of megaloblastic anaemia of pregnancy; nutritional anaemia.

Dosage and administration One tablet a day. In pregnancy it is recommended that Folex-350 should be started at the first ante-natal consultation and continued until 3 months after delivery.

Contra-indications, warnings, etc Folex-350 is contra-indicated in megaloblastic anaemia due to vitamin B_{12} deficiency.

Overdosage: Patients who have taken an overdosage of Folex-350 should have gastric lavage performed, if possible within four hours of the overdosage occurring. In addition, patients should have such symptomatic treatment as appears necessary. In order to eliminate excess free iron, a chelating agent such as desferrioxamine may be administered.

Side-effects: Side-effects of iron and folic acid preparations which have been reported include nausea, vomiting, gastro-intestinal symptoms, constipation and diarrhoea.

Pharmaceutical precautions No special precautions are required.

Legal category P.

Package quantities Folex-350 is supplied in containers of 30 (child-resistant), 100, 1000 and 5000 tablets.

Further information The high incidence of iron and folate deficiencies in pregnant women may result in possible obstetrical abnormalities. It is now considered advisable to administer daily iron and folic acid routinely, in one tablet, throughout pregnancy.

Product licence number 0237/5008.

GUAREM* GRANULES ▼

Presentation Sachets, each containing guar gum granules 5 gramms. The fine pale cream granules, which are tasteless, are readily water-miscible, for the preparation of palatable fluid drinks.

Uses For use in diabetes to help control post-prandial glucose levels, thereby facilitating control, and where appropriate, allowing reduction of insulin or oral hypoglycaemic dosage levels.

Action: Guar gum which is derived from natural sources is a high molecular weight polysaccharide, galactomannan. In solution it slows the rate of absorption of other carbohydrates leading to a reduction in post-prandial hyperglycaemia and insulin secretion. Guar gum is not absorbed and remains chemically unchanged until it reaches the colon where it is broken down before excretion. Reduction in plasma cholesterol (LDL) levels have also been reported.

Dosage and administration

Adults: One 5 g sachet to be taken three times daily with each main meal. The contents of a sachet may be stirred into a fruit flavoured drink (tumblerful) and swallowed promptly before each main meal. Alternatively, it may be sprinkled evenly over a meal on the plate or stirred into suitable foods (e.g. tomato juice, yoghurt, muesli, etc), in which case the food must be accompanied by a drink of 200 ml (orange, tea, etc).

Children (12 and over): As for adults.

Children (under 12): Not recommended at present.

Contra-indications, warnings, etc

To avoid any risk of oesophageal obstruction or rupture, this product should not be given to patients with a history of oesophageal disease or difficulty in swallowing.

Guarem should not be ingested as dry granules.

During initial therapy, blood glucose levels should be carefully monitored and concurrent treatment adjusted where necessary, to minimise the possibility of hypoglycaemia.

Side effects: Gastro-intestinal symptoms (flatulence, diarrhoea) are quite common at the commencement of treatment. These can be reduced or avoided by initiating treatment gradually in accordance with pack instructions.

Pharmaceutical precautions Guarem should be stored in a dry place.

Legal category P.

Package quantities Cartons of 50 and 100 sachets.

Further information Each sachet is individually printed with simple and clear administration instructions.

Product licence number 0237/0023.

RBC*CREAM

Presentation Slightly pink cream, in internally lacquered aluminium tubes, containing (W/W):

Antazoline Hydrochloride BP	1.8%
Calamine BP	8.0%
Camphor BP	0.1%
Cetrimide BP	0.5%

Uses For the immediate relief of sunburn, insect stings and bites, nettle rash, hives and itching due to minor skin irritation. Also for itching e.g. as accompanying chicken pox and herpes zoster.

Dosage and administration Cleanse affected area and apply every 3 hours, as necessary.

Contra-indications, warnings, etc None.

Side effects: In rare cases of sensitivity, application should be discontinued.

Pharmaceutical precautions Store below 25°C.

Legal category P.

Package quantities 25 g.

Further information Nil.

Product licence number 0150/5002.

RYBARVIN* INHALANT

Presentation Rybarvin Inhalant is a colourless liquid which contains:

Atropine Methonitrate BP	0.1% w/v
Papaverine Hydrochloride BP	0.08% w/v
Adrenaline BP	0.4% w/v
Benzocaine BP	0.08% w/v
Saline base to 100%	

Uses Rybarvin is indicated for the symptomatic relief of asthma.

Dosage and administration *Adults:* Rybarvin should be inhaled deeply, using a Rybar Inhaler for one to two minutes three times daily. Further inhalations may be taken at other times to relieve acute asthmatic attack.

Children: The length of inhalation should be reduced to a half to one minute. Inhalations should be taken twice daily in the morning and evening.

In conditions in which there is inflammation of the bronchial mucous membrane the full effect of Rybarvin may not be obtained, owing to poor absorption of the active ingredients.

Contra-indications, warnings, etc Rybarvin Inhalant is contra-indicated in patients with heart conditions or hypertension.

Pharmaceutical precautions The activity of Rybarvin Inhalant is destroyed by the action of light and metal. It is very important that the specially designed Rybar Inhaler is used by patients using Rybarvin.

Legal category P.

Package quantities Rybarvin is available in 30 ml bottles.

Further information Rybarvin has not been shown to be habit-forming.

The Rybar Inhaler is made of glass and fitted with a rubber bulb so that no metal parts come into contact with Rybarvin Inhalant.

The Rybar Inhaler provides a very fine mist of droplets which enables rapid absorption of the active ingredients from the lungs. Full instructions for the patient are given with each inhaler.

Product licence number 0237/5016.

*Trade Mark

Sandoz Pharmaceuticals
A division of Sandoz Products Limited
Sandoz House
98 The Centre
Feltham, Middlesex TW13 4EP

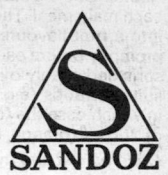

BRINALDIX* K

Presentation Flat, round, white, effervescent tablets with a rough surface, of 22 mm diameter, 4.0 to 4.4 mm thick and 2.4 g weight. Each effervescent tablet contains 20 mg clopamide, 600 mg Potassium Chloride PhEur and 400 mg Potassium Bicarbonate BPC and provides 470 mg potassium (12 mmol: 12 mEq K^+), 286 mg chloride (8 mmol: 8 mEq Cl^-) and 800 mg anhydrous citric acid (787.5 mg citrate ion).

Uses
Principal actions: Brinaldix K effervescent tablets provide a combined diuretic/potassium preparation.

The onset of diuresis is generally within two hours of administration; the maximum diuretic effect is attained in the first three to six hours and the major diuresis is over within 12 to 24 hours. The urinary excretion of sodium and chloride ions remains in the ratio of approximately 1:1 throughout the dosage range, thus minimising the risk of disturbance to acid/base balance. The sodium/potassium excretion ratio of clopamide is high.

Each effervescent tablet provides 12 mmol K^+ and 8 mmol Cl^- thus reducing the risk of hypokalaemic, hypochloraemic alkalosis.

Indications: Hypertension and oedema of cardiac, renal or hepatic origin.

Dosage and administration
Hypertension: One to two effervescent tablets daily dissolved in 60 ml ($\frac{1}{3}$ to $\frac{1}{2}$ a tumblerful) of water in the morning.

Oedema – initial treatment: Two to three effervescent tablets daily dissolved in 60 ml ($\frac{1}{3}$ to $\frac{1}{2}$ a tumblerful) of water in the morning.

Oedema–maintenance: One to three effervescent tablets dissolved in 60 ml ($\frac{1}{3}$ to $\frac{1}{2}$ a tumblerful) of water in the morning either on consecutive days or intermittently according to the patient's condition or response.

Children: Brinaldix K is not recommended for children.

Use in the elderly: No evidence exists that the dosage or tolerance of Brinaldix K is directly affected by advanced age; however, elderly patients should be carefully supervised as factors sometimes associated with ageing, such as poor diet, impaired renal function or susceptibility to electrolyte imbalance, may indirectly affect dosage or tolerance of the drug.

Contra-indications, warnings, etc
Contra-indications: Acute glomerulonephritis, severe impairment of renal or hepatic function, hypersensitivity to the drug and sulphonamides, Addison's disease, hypercalcaemia or concurrent lithium therapy.

Precautions: Brinaldix K should be used with care in patients receiving concomitant antihypertensive therapy, non-steroidal anti-inflammatory drugs and corticosteroids.

Although Brinaldix K has been formulated to minimise the occurrence of hypokalaemia, the latter may develop in certain patients. Hypokalaemia may result in increased sensitivity to cardiac glycosides and possible cardiac arrhythmias. It is recommended that patients be monitored for renal function and for early signs of fluid and electrolyte imbalance. Potassium supplements may be required.

In common with other thiazide diuretics, Brinaldix K may precipitate or aggravate diabetes and gout.

Pregnancy/breast feeding: Diuretics are best avoided for the management of oedema of pregnancy or hypertension in pregnancy as their use may be associated with hypovolaemia, increased blood viscosity and reduced placental perfusion.

There is inadequate evidence of thiazide safety in human pregnancy and some workers have described foetal bone marrow depression and thrombocytopenia. Foetal and neonatal jaundice have also been reported.

Lactation warning: As thiazide diuretics pass into breast milk Brinaldix K should be avoided in mothers who wish to breast feed.

Overdosage: Symptoms of overdosage may include thirst, nausea, vomiting, polyuria, hypokalaemia, drowsiness, confusion, hypotension and convulsions. Treatment should be directed to the removal of ingested material by induced emesis or gastric lavage as appropriate. Blood pressure, fluid and electrolyte balance should be monitored and correction made, if required. However deliberate overdosage is unlikely with effervescent preparations.

Side-effects: Brinaldix K is well tolerated and side-effects are rare. In a small number of patients nausea and headache have been reported, and skin rash has occurred. Impotence, blood dyscrasias and pancreatitis have been reported with thiazide diuretics.

Pharmaceutical precautions Brinaldix K Tablets are hygroscopic and should be dispensed in their original containers which carry a note to the patient requesting that the containers be kept tightly closed in a cool dry place.

Legal category POM.

Package quantities Containers of 100 effervescent tablets (5 tubes of 20).

Further information Brinaldix K Tablets each contain

501.5 mg sucrose. Approximate calorific value – 4 kcals per tablet.

Product licence number 0101/5022R.

CAFERGOT*

Presentation *Tablets:* Very pale pink, round, coated tablets, 9.5–10 mm diameter, 5.4–5.6 mm thick, weighing 370 mg. Branded CAFERGOT on one face. Each tablet contains 1 mg Ergotamine Tartrate PhEur and 100 mg Caffeine PhEur.

Suppositories: Off-white suppositories weighing 1.98 g. Each suppository contains 2 mg Ergotamine Tartrate PhEur and 100 mg Caffeine PhEur.

Uses *Principal action:* Cafergot contains a combination of ergotamine and caffeine specially developed for the treatment of the acute migraine attack. Ergotamine aborts attacks of migraine and related vascular headaches by a direct vasoconstrictor effect on distended extracranial arteries. Concomitant administration of caffeine enhances the absorption of ergotamine.

Cafergot suppositories are specially valuable for patients who have nausea and vomiting early in the attack and cannot retain or absorb anything taken by mouth. To be fully effective the tablets must be taken, or the suppositories used, as early as possible in the attack.

Indications: Migraine. Migraine variants.

Dosage and administration *Tablets:* Two tablets should be taken at the first warning of an attack. This dose is normally sufficient, but if relief is not obtained within half an hour a further tablet should be taken, repeated if necessary at half-hourly intervals up to a maximum of 6 tablets. Subsequently, the total dose found effective in a previous attack should be taken immediately prodromal symptoms are experienced. Maximum dosage is 6 tablets per day and 10 in any one week.

Suppositories: One suppository should be administered at the first warning of an attack. This dose is normally sufficient, but if relief is not obtained additional doses may be taken up to a maximum of 3 suppositories. Subsequently, the total dose found effective in a previous attack should be administered immediately prodromal symptoms are experienced. Maximum dosage is 3 suppositories per day and 5 in any one week.

Use in the elderly: No evidence exists that elderly patients require different dosages or show different side effects from younger patients.

Contra-indications, warnings, etc *Contra-indications:* Pregnancy, peripheral vascular disorders, coronary disease, impaired hepatic or renal function, sepsis, obliterative vascular disease, severe hypertension, breast feeding.

Precautions: Concomitant use of erythromycin and ergotamine should be avoided.

Overdosage: Treatment should be directed to the elimination of ingested material by aspiration and gastric lavage.

Arterial spasm may be corrected by the administration of a vasodilator. General supportive measures should be applied with particular reference to the respiratory and cardiovascular systems.

Side-effects: Nausea, vomiting and occasionally weakness in the legs and muscle pain may occur; numbness and tingling of the extremities can be indicative of peripheral vascular disturbance and treatment must be stopped immediately if signs of circulatory impairment appear. Failure to observe this precaution can lead to the development of ergotism.

Pharmaceutical precautions Keep suppositories in a cool place.

Legal category POM.

Package quantities *Tablets:* Cartons of 100
Suppositories: Boxes of 6 and 30

Further information Nil.

Product licence numbers
Tablets: 0101/5023
Suppositories: 0101/5001

CEDILANID*

Presentation White, uncoated tablets weighing 85 mg. Flat and of 6 mm diameter with a bevelled edge, coded GO and scored on one side with SANDOZ engraved on the other. Each tablet contains 250 mcg lanatoside C.

Uses *Principal action:* In common with all cardio-active glycosides of digitalis, Cedilanid improves cardiac function in the failing heart by increasing the force of myocardial contraction and by correcting disturbances of heart rhythm by a direct effect on the excitatory mechanism and the conduction system probably mediated by ion transport mechanisms.

Indications: Acute heart failure. Routine digitalisation and maintenance of the patient in congestive heart failure.

Dosage and administration Dosage should be reduced in the presence of chronic cor pulmonale, coronary insufficiency, electrolyte disturbances and renal or hepatic insufficiency.

Adults
Digitalisation: 1.5–2 mg (6 to 8 tablets) daily over a 3–5 day period.

Maintenance: 250 mcg–1.5 mg (1 to 6 tablets) per day as indicated by the patient's requirements.

Children: 10–30 mcg/kg body weight/day in 3 divided doses.

Use in the elderly: Elderly patients may be unusually sensitive to digitalis preparations. Special care is indicated when increasing the dosage and a low initial dose should be used. This sensitivity may be due to a direct effect of ageing but changes in renal function with age may also contribute.

Contra-indications, warnings, etc
Contra-indications: Complete AV block and 2nd degree AV block (especially 2 : 1), excessive sinus bradycardia (particularly when associated with Stokes-Adams seizures).

Precautions: Digitalised patients should not be given calcium by parenteral injection. The dose of Cedilanid administered should be adjusted to compensate for any other digitalis preparations administered in the recent past. High dose oral calcium supplements, psychotropic drugs (including lithium) and sympathomimetics should be given with caution to digitalised patients. Potassium depletion sensitises the heart to cardiac glycosides.

Overdosage: Fatalities from ingestion of massive oral doses of Cedilanid are rare because vomiting usually occurs. Common symptoms of overdosage include anorexia, nausea, vomiting, headache, visual disturbances and disorientation. Slow or irregular pulse, fall of blood pressure and a wide range of cardiac arrythmias and conduction defects have been reported as a result of digitalis toxicity. Death is usually due to ventricular fibrillation and is sometimes preceded by delirium and convulsions. Chronic poisoning by cumulation produces gradual onset of these symptoms.

Treatment: Activated charcoal may reduce absorption. Emesis or gastric lavage within eight hours, to empty the stomach. Check and carefully monitor serum potassium. Correct hypo- or hyperkalaemia. Treat arrhythmias. Atropine 0.3–0.6 mg will reverse profound bradycardia. A cardiac pacemaker may be required.

In severe cases treatment with digitalis antibodies may be considered.

Side-effects: Toxic effects occur if the dose of Cedilanid has not been carefully tailored to the specific requirements and tolerance of each individual patient.

The most frequent side-effects noted are: *CNS and gastro-intestinal disturbances:* anorexia, nausea, vomiting; in rare instances (especially in elderly arteriosclerotics), confusion, disorientation, aphasia and visual disturbances including chromatopsia.

Cardiac: Disturbances of heart rate, conduction and rhythm (bigeminy), lowering of the S-T segment with preterminal T-wave inversion.

Allergic skin reactions: Pruritus, urticaria, macular rashes occur very occasionally.

Pharmaceutical precautions Protect from light.

Legal category POM.

Package quantities Containers of 100 and 500 tablets.

Further information Nil.

Product licence number 0101/5025.

DESERIL*

Presentation Canary-yellow, coated, round, biconvex tablets weighing 100 mg, 6 mm diameter, 3.4 to 3.9 mm thick, branded DSL one side. Each tablet contains 1.33 mg Methysergide Maleate BP (equivalent to 1 mg methysergide base).

Uses *Principal action:* Deseril is a potent serotonin antagonist. In addition to inhibiting the pain-facilitating and permeability-increasing actions of serotonin, Deseril can potentiate the effects of vasoconstrictor stimuli.

Indications: Prophylactic treatment of migraine, cluster headache and other vascular headaches in patients who, despite other attempts at control, experience headaches of such severity or regularity that their social or economic life is seriously disrupted. (Note: Deseril is not recommended for treatment of the acute attack.)

Control of profuse diarrhoea associated with carcinoid disease.

Dosage and administration *Prophylactic treatment of headache:* 1 or 2 tablets two or three times a day, with meals.

Treatment should start with one tablet at bedtime and dosage should then be increased gradually over about two weeks until effective levels are reached. The minimum effective dose should be used – often that which will prevent 75% of attacks rather than all headaches.

From the outset, patients should understand that regular clinical supervision and periodic withdrawal of treatment are essential so that adverse effects can be recognised and minimised.

Carcinoid syndrome: High doses are usually necessary. In most reported cases dosage ranged between 12 and 20 tablets daily.

Children: Deseril is not recommended for the treatment of children.

Use in the elderly: No evidence exists that elderly patients require different dosages or show different side effects from younger patients.

Contra-indications, warnings, etc *Contra-indications:* Pregnancy, lactation, peripheral vascular disorders, progressive arteriosclerosis, severe hypertension, coronary heart disease, valvular heart disease, phlebitis or cellulitis of the lower extremities, pulmonary disease, collagen disease, impaired kidney or liver function, diseases of the urinary tract, cachectic or septic conditions.

Warnings: Continuous Deseril administration should not exceed six months without a drug-free interval of at least one month for reassessment; dosage should be reduced gradually over two or three weeks to avoid rebound headaches. In patients undergoing treatment with Deseril the dose of ergotamine required to control acute attacks may have to be reduced.

Precautions: Regular clinical supervision of patients treated with Deseril is essential. Particular attention should be paid to complaints of urinary dysfunction, pain in the loin, flank or chest, and pain, coldness or numbness in the limbs. Patients should be regularly examined for the presence of cardiac murmurs, vascular bruits, pleural or pericardial friction rubs and abdominal or flank masses or tenderness. Treatment with Deseril should be stopped should any of these symptoms or signs occur.

Caution is also advised during drug administration to patients with a past history of peptic ulceration.

In carcinoid syndrome the risk of adverse reactions due to the higher dosage must be weighed against the therapeutic benefit.

Overdosage: Treatment should be directed to elimination of the ingested material by aspiration and gastric lavage. General supportive measures should be applied. The patient should be carefully observed for peripheral vasospasm which may be treated by warmth, care being taken to protect ischaemic limbs. If there is evidence of impending tissue damage vasodilators may be used.

Side-effects:

General: The most commonly reported side-effects are nausea, heartburn, abdominal discomfort, vomiting, dizziness, lassitude and drowsiness. These side-effects can often be minimised by taking Deseril with food. Tissue oedema, insomnia, leg cramps and weight gain have occurred, and skin eruptions or loss of scalp hair have occasionally been reported. Mental and behavioural disturbances have occurred in isolated instances.

Inflammatory fibrosis: Retroperitoneal fibrosis: Continuous long-term Deseril administration has been associated with the development of retroperitoneal fibrosis. This is very rare when continuous treatment has not exceeded 6 months. Retroperitoneal fibrosis usually presents with symptoms of urinary tract obstruction such as persistent loin or flank pain, oliguria, dysuria, increased blood nitrogen and vascular insufficiency of the lower limbs. Deseril must be withdrawn if retroperitoneal fibrosis develops; drug withdrawal is often associated with clinical improvement over a few days to several weeks.

Fibrosis in other areas: Fibrotic processes involving lungs, pleura, heart valves and major vessels have been reported in a small number of patients. Presenting symptoms include chest pain, dyspnoea or pleural friction rub and pleural effusion. Cardiac murmurs or vascular bruits have also been reported. Appearance of these symptoms demands immediate withdrawal of Deseril. These fibrotic manifestations are often reversible although less readily so than retroperitoneal fibrosis.

Vascular: Vascular reactions, including arterial spasm, have been seen in some patients. The following have all been described: arterial spasm in a limb causing coldness, numbness, pain or intermittent claudication; renal artery spasm giving rise to transitory hypertension; mesenteric artery spasm causing abdominal pain; retinal artery spasm causing reversible loss of vision; coronary artery spasm causing angina and questionably resulting in myocardial infarction. Arterial spasm is rapidly reversible following drug withdrawal.

Pharmaceutical precautions Nil.

Legal category POM.

Package quantities Blister pack of 50 tablets.

Further information Nil.

Product licence number 0101/5026.

DIHYDERGOT*

Presentation *Tablets:* Off-white, uncoated, round tablets weighing 100 mg, 6 mm diameter, 2.6 to 2.8 mm thick, flat with bevelled edge. Single break line coded OL on one side, branded 'SANDOZ' the other. Each tablet contains 1 mg dihydroergotamine mesylate (equivalent to 860 mcg dihydroergotamine base).

Ampoules: Clear, colourless solution. Each 1 ml contains 1 mg dihydroergotamine mesylate.

Uses The hydrogenation of ergotamine to dihydroergotamine reduces the uterotonic effect and the pressor effect is modified. Dihydergot contracts hypotonic vessels by stimulation of the alpha-adrenoceptors. It also possesses alpha-adrenergic blocking properties (i.e. it is a partial agonist). Its tonic effect on capacitance vessels is more pronounced than its effect on resistance vessels. This activity results in increased venous tone and prevents excessive venous pooling.

During prolonged oral administration, Dihydergot induces a stabilization of the tone of extracranial vessels and therefore is of value for the prophylactic treatment of the migraine attack. It may be used orally or by injection as an alternative to ergotamine for the symptomatic relief of the migraine attack.

Dihydergot injection is effective in the prophylactic treatment of postoperative deep vein thrombosis. This activity is considerably enhanced by administration in combination with a low-dose heparin regimen. In this way impaired venous return and activation of clotting factors, two conditions contributing to the development of postoperative thrombosis, can be controlled.

Indications: Prophylactic treatment of migraine. May also be used for the symptomatic treatment of the migraine attack.

Prophylactic treatment of postoperative deep vein thrombosis using Dihydergot Injection in conjunction with a low dose heparin regimen.

Dosage and administration *Prevention of migraine:* 1–2 tablets three times daily reduce the frequency and severity of attacks in most patients.

Treatment of migraine: 2–3 tablets repeated half-hourly if necessary, up to a total of 10 tablets per day.

Intramuscular or subcutaneous injection of 1–2 mg (1–2 ml) given as soon as the prodromal symptoms appear usually aborts the attack within half an hour. If the attack is not relieved by this time a further dose may be given.

Prevention of postoperative deep vein thrombosis Injection only: Individual injections of Dihydergot 500 mcg (0.5 ml) with heparin 5000 iu given subcutaneously every 8–12 hours. Treatment is started 1–2 hours before surgery and continued not less than 6 hours postoperatively. Subsequent doses are given 8–12 hourly for at least 7–10 days depending on the risk of thrombosis.

Use in the elderly: No evidence exists that elderly patients require different dosages or show different side effects from younger patients.

Contra-indications, warnings, etc *Contra-indications:* Parenteral administration of Dihydergot is contra-indicated in patients suffering from uncontrolled cardiac failure, coronary artery disease (see also precautions), inadequately controlled hypertension and in pregnancy.

Precautions: A small number of patients with coronary insufficiency have been treated with twice daily injections of Dihydergot 500 mcg intramuscularly under resting conditions and only in severe coronary disability were anginal attacks precipitated. However, due to the possibility of increased cardiac filling pressure, great care should be exercised in treating such patients, and the dose of 500 mcg (0.5 ml) should not be exceeded.

Intra-arterial injection of Dihydergot must be avoided. Should this occur by accident an alpha-blocker should be administered. Caution is indicated where Dihydergot is being given on a long-term basis to patients with severe renal disease unless they are receiving dialysis and for patients with severe liver disease. In such cases the dosage should be reduced.

Concomitant use of the antibiotic triacetyloleandomycin, which is not available in the UK, or erythromycin and Dihydergot by mouth should be avoided.

When using heparin in combination with Dihydergot Injection the general contra-indications and precautions implicit with the use of heparin should be observed. Mean plasma heparin levels have been reported to be higher in patients receiving Dihydergot concurrently.

In rare cases vascular spasms may occur during parenteral Dihydergot therapy, in particular in the lower extremities. Caution is advised in the use of Dihydergot/heparin treatment in patients with multiple injuries and severe soft tissue damage, in paraplegia, shock and sepsis. If signs and symptoms of impaired vascular perfusion develop, treatment should be withdrawn and therapy with a peripheral vasodilator such as sodium-nitroprusside, hydralazine or glyceryl trinitrate should be initiated.

The tendency to haemorrhage and total intra-operative and postoperative blood loss in patients on Dihydergot/

heparin treatment has been found to be similar to that encountered with low-dose heparin therapy.

Subcutaneous administration may give rise to local discomfort at the injection site.

Overdosage: Symptoms might include nausea, vomiting, abdominal pain; numbness, tingling, pain and cyanosis of the extremities with absent or diminished peripheral pulses; respiratory depression; hypertension and/or hypotension; convulsions, confusion, delirium, coma. Treatment should be directed to elimination of unabsorbed drug by emesis or gastric lavage and to general supportive measures with particular reference to the cardiovascular and respiratory systems.

Side-effects: Nausea and vomiting may occasionally occur. Following parenteral treatment, in rare cases vascular spasms may occur; numbness and tingling of the fingers and toes as well as precordial pain have been reported in a few cases. With oral use, however, such effects are extremely rare.

Pharmaceutical precautions Protect from light.

Once Ampoule is opened the contents should be used immediately. Dihydergot and heparin injections should be administered individually.

Legal category POM.

Package quantities *Tablets:* Containers of 50. *Ampoules:* Boxes of 5 × 1 ml.

Further information Snap ampoule: no file required.

Product licence numbers
Tablets   0101/5027
Ampoules   0101/5007

HYDERGINE*

Presentation *1·5 mg Tablets:* Hydergine 1.5 mg is available as white, flat, bevel-edged tablets, scored on one side with HYDERGINE 1.5 engraved on the other, and of 240 mg weight, 9 mm diameter and 2.9 mm thickness. Each tablet contains 1.5 mg Co-dergocrine Mesylate BP.

4·5 mg Tablets: Hydergine 4.5 mg is available as white, round, biconvex tablets coded HYDERGINE in circular form on one side with 4.5 engraved on the other, and of 240 mg weight and 9 mm diameter. Each tablet contains 4.5 mg Co-dergocrine Mesylate BP.

Uses *Indications:* As an adjunct in the management of elderly patients with mild to moderate dementia.

Dosage and administration 1.5 mg three times a day or a once daily dosage of 4.5 mg.

Hydergine should be taken before meals.

The effect of Hydergine is not immediate: alleviation of symptoms is usually gradual and may not be apparent for two to three weeks. Continuing improvement may be expected for at least three months.

Contra-indications, warnings, etc *Contra-indications:* Known hypersensitivity to the drug.

Precautions: Caution should be exercised in the administration of Hydergine to patients with severe bradycardia.

Overdosage: Supportive measures are all that are likely to be needed.

Side-effects: Side-effects are infrequent following administration of Hydergine and even relatively large doses are well tolerated. Minor side-effects including gastro-

intestinal disturbances, flushes, rashes, nasal stuffiness, abdominal cramps, headaches, dizziness and postural hypotension in hypertensive patients have on occasion been reported.

Pharmaceutical precautions Protect from light.

Legal category POM.

Package quantities *1.5 mg Tablets:* containers of 100.
4.5 mg Tablets: calendar pack of 28.

Further information Double-blind studies have shown that improvement occurs with all the symptoms listed in the Sandoz Clinical Assessment-Geriatric (SCAG) scale except for hostility; significant improvement can be expected for nine of the symptoms, namely confusion, impairment of recent memory, disorientation, anxiety, depression, emotional lability, irritability, unsociability and the overall impression of the patient.

Product licence numbers
1.5 mg Tablets   0101/0042R
4.5 mg Tablets   0101/0117

LACTULOSE SOLUTION BP

Presentation Lactulose Solution BP is available as a clear, almost colourless to pale yellow syrup. Each 5 ml spoonful contains 3.35 g lactulose and 1.34 g of other sugars (lactose, galactose, tagatose and other ketosugars).

Uses *Principal action:* Lactulose prevents the formation of hard stools and encourages normal bowel movement. Unlike traditional laxative preparations which act either on the innervation or musculature of the intestine or by bulk stimulus, lactulose provides a natural substrate for the saccharolytic bacterial flora in the colon.

Lactulose is a disaccharide which is not hydrolysed in the small intestine. Therefore it cannot be absorbed and is transported to the colon with water to retain the osmotic balance. In the colon, several species of bacteria can hydrolyse lactulose to the monosaccharides galactose and fructose.

By encouraging this normal metabolic activity of the bacteria, the osmotic pressure of the colonic contents is doubled and more water is drawn into the bowel.

Further metabolism of the monosaccharides leads to the production of acetic and lactic acids and the subsequent lowering of colonic pH. This acidification of the colonic contents is considered to be the main reason for the effectiveness of lactulose solution. In chronic portal-systemic encephalopathy it may be associated with the decrease in the relative concentration of free ammonia, the major agent involved in the cerebral disturbance.

Indications: Chronic constipation. Chronic portal-systemic encephalopathy.

Dosage and administration
Chronic constipation: Because lactulose acts naturally to encourage the normal activity of the bowel, it may be two or three days before the full benefit of the treatment is obtained. It is important, therefore, to follow the dosage regimen set out below.

Adults:
Initially: Three to six 5 ml spoonfuls for the first two to three days of treatment. (Nine spoonfuls may be given in obstinate cases).

Maintenance: Two to three 5 ml spoonfuls daily or according to the needs of the patient.

Children:

Initially: Two to five 5 ml spoonfuls for the first two or three days of treatment.

Maintenance: One to three 5 ml spoonfuls daily or according to the needs of the patient.

Chronic portal-systemic encephalopathy: Six to ten 5 ml spoonfuls three times daily according to the requirements of the patient, for adequate acidification of the colonic contents.

Use in the elderly: No evidence exists that elderly patients require different dosages or show different side-effects from younger patients.

Contra-indications, warnings, etc

Contra indications: In common with other preparations used for the treatment of constipation, lactulose solution should not be used in patients with gastrointestinal obstruction. Lactulose solution should not be given to patients with galactosaemia or lactose intolerance.

Precautions: Lactulose solution should be used with caution during the first trimester of pregnancy.

Overdosage: No cases of intoxication due to deliberate or accidental overdosage with lactulose solution have been reported to the Company.

Side-effects: Side-effects rarely occur after the administration of lactulose solution. Mild transient effects such as abdominal distension or cramps and flatulence, which subside after the initial stages of treatment, have occasionally been reported.

High doses may provoke nausea in some patients. This can be minimised by administration with water, fruit juice, or with meals.

Pharmaceutical precautions Lactulose solution should be stored in a cool place.

Dilution of the solution is not recommended.

Legal category P.

Package quantities Bottles of 200 ml, 300 ml and 1 litre.

Further information Approximate calorific value – 19 kcals per 5 ml spoonful.

Product licence number 0101/0076

MELLERIL*

Presentation

Suspension: An opaque, creamy/white, semi-viscous fluid, available in two strengths: 25 mg in 5 ml (0.5%): Each 5 ml spoonful contains 25 mg thioridazine base equivalent to 27.5 mg of thioridazine hydrochloride.

100 mg in 5 ml (2%): Each 5 ml spoonful contains 100 mg thioridazine base equivalent to 110 mg of thioridazine hydrochloride.

Syrup: A clear, orange liquid. Each 5 ml spoonful contains 25 mg thioridazine base equivalent to 27.5 mg of thioridazine hydrochloride.

Tablets: White, film coated tablets with a bevel edge, available in four strengths:

10 mg Thioridazine Tablets BP are 6.0 mm in diameter, approximately 2.7 mm thick and weigh 92 mg. They are embossed MEL on one side and 10 on the other.

25 mg Thioridazine Tablets BP are 7.0 mm in diameter, approximately 2.7 mm thick and weigh 143 mg. They are embossed MEL on one side and 25 on the other.

50 mg Thioridazine Tablets BP are 9 mm in diameter, approximately 4.0 mm thick and weigh 287 mg. They are embossed MEL on one side and 50 on the other.

100 mg Thioridazine Tablets BP are 10 mm in diameter, approximately 4.2 mm thick and weigh 359 mg. They are embossed MEL on one side and 100 on the other.

Uses *Principal action:* Melleril is a phenothiazine antipsychotic.

Although the basic pharmacological actions of Melleril are similar to those of phenothiazines generally, the antipsychotic activity is its principal action, and other effects such as antiemetic and antihistaminic activities are minimal. It has a wide therapeutic margin and is well tolerated in the recommended dosage range.

Indications

Adults: Schizophrenia: treatment of symptoms and prevention of relapse. Mania and hypomania.

As an adjunct to the short-term management of anxiety, moderate to severe psychomotor agitation, excitement, violent or dangerously impulsive behaviour.

Agitation and restlessness in the elderly.

Children: Behaviour disorders and epilepsy – only where there are severe mental or behavioural problems such as senseless hyperactivity, aggressiveness, temper tantrums, self-injury or mutilation, or agitation.

Dosage and administration

	Daily dose range in terms of the hydrochloride (Tablets)†
Adults	
Schizophrenia, mania, hypomania. For acute schizophrenia, an initial loading dose of 200 mg may be given. In hospitalised, resistant patients under specialist supervision, up to 800 mg daily may be administered *for not more than 4 weeks.*	150–600 mg
Moderate to severe: psychomotor agitation, excitement, violent or dangerously impulsive behaviour.	75–200 mg
Anxiety, agitation and restlessness in the elderly.	30–100 mg

There may be great variability in individual response and dosage requirements. In underweight patients, or in those suffering from kidney or liver disease, lower initial doses and more gradual increases are indicated.

Use in the Elderly

In elderly patients lower initial doses and more gradual increases are indicated.

	Daily dose range in terms of the hydrochloride (Tablets)†
Children	
Under 5 years of age	1 mg/kg bodyweight

† Liquid formulations of Melleril contain thioridazine base. To convert from hydrochloride to base, multiply by 0.91. As might be expected the in-vitro dissolution profiles of the suspension and tablets differ; bioequivalence of the liquid and solid dose formulations should not, therefore, be assumed.

5 years and over	Usually 75–150 mg/day. In severe cases up to 300 mg/day may be used.

Contra-indications, warnings, etc

Contra-indications: Comatose states, severe depression of the CNS or a history of blood dyscrasia.

Use in pregnancy: Do not use during pregnancy unless there are compelling reasons. There is inadequate evidence for safety of the drug in human pregnancy, and there is some evidence of harmful effect in a few, but not all, animal studies. The newborn of mothers treated with Melleril in late pregnancy may show signs of intoxication such as excessive sleepiness, tremor and hyperactivity.

Do not use during lactation. If the use of Melleril is considered essential, breast feeding should be discontinued.

Precautions: Melleril should be used with caution in patients with cardiac arrhythmias, cardiac disease, severe respiratory disease, renal failure, Parkinson's disease, a personal or family history of narrow angle glaucoma, in prostatic hypertrophy, myasthenia gravis, epilepsy, phaeochromocytoma and in patients who have shown hypersensitivity to other phenothiazines. In patients with liver disease, regular monitoring of liver function is essential. Phenothiazines should be administered with caution to patients who participate in activities requiring complete mental alertness. Regular blood counts should be carried out during the first three to four months of treatment or if any clinical signs of blood dyscrasias appear. Phenothiazines generally may affect temperature regulation and decrease serum thyroxine concentrations, although this is very unlikely with Melleril.

Acute withdrawal symptoms including nausea, vomiting and insomnia have rarely been described after abrupt cessation of high dose Melleril. Gradual withdrawal is advisable. Drug withdrawal in children may lead to rapid clinical relapse and neurological symptoms, although this is less common with Melleril than with other antipsychotics.

Melleril may enhance the central nervous system depression produced by other CNS depressant drugs including alcohol, hypnotics, sedatives or narcotic analgesics. In common with other phenothiazines, Melleril antagonises the action of adrenaline and other sympathomimetic agents, and may reverse the blood pressure lowering effects of adrenergic-blocking agents such as guanethidine and clonidine. Phenylpropanolamine has been reported to interact with phenothiazines and cause ventricular arrhythmias. It may affect the metabolism of tricyclic antidepressants, phenytoin and other anticonvulsants. It may also impair the antiparkinsonian effects of levodopa; it may possibly affect the control of diabetes or the action of anticoagulants. It may enhance the cardiac depressant effects of quinidine. Antacids should not be used within two hours of taking phenothiazines. Undesirable anticholinergic effects can be enhanced by anticholinergic drugs. Neurotoxicity resulting from combination with lithium has been reported rarely.

Side-effects and warnings: Common side-effects, particularly with higher dosage and at the start of treatment, include drowsiness, sedation, dry mouth and nasal stuffiness. Dose-related postural hypotension may occur, particularly in the elderly. Other dose-related anticholinergic-type side-effects include blurring of vision, tachycardia, constipation and urinary hesitancy or retention.

Even in low dosage, in susceptible (especially non-psychotic) individuals, Melleril may cause feelings of being mentally dulled or slowed down, nausea, dizziness, headache, or paradoxical effects of excitement, agitation or insomnia. Confusional states or epileptic fits can occur.

At higher dose levels, as with other phenothiazines, ECG changes such as prolongation of the Q-T interval, flattening of the T-wave and the appearance of U-waves have been reported. These changes are more likely to occur in the presence of a low potassium blood level. Like all phenothiazines, Melleril may induce arrhythmias.

Pigmentary retinopathy has been observed in a small number of patients receiving long-term therapy with daily doses above the recommended maximum of 600 mg and has been seen rarely in patients taking less. It is characterised by decreased visual acuity, chromatopsia (usually brown-tinted vision) and impairment of dark adaptation; progressive loss of vision may occur. Fundoscopic examination discloses deposits of pigment. The patient should be told of the importance of reporting any change in vision. If prolonged high-dose treatment is envisaged full ophthalmic examinations should be carried out at appropriate intervals.

The possibility of pigmentary retinopathy, together with the possibility of cardiotoxic reactions, emphasises the need not to increase doses beyond the recommended maximum daily dose of 600 mg. Extra-pyramidal reactions may occur but are uncommon within the recommended dosage range; antiparkinsonian agents are therefore rarely required and should be prescribed with caution. Whenever an antipsychotic agent is used, the possible risk of development of tardive dyskinesia should be considered, and the patients monitored for early signs. With Melleril the risk is less than with other phenothiazines, and tardive dyskinesia tends to be seen particularly with prolonged treatment at high doses. The potential seriousness and unpredictability of tardive dyskinesia and the fact that it has occasionally been reported to occur when neuroleptic antipsychotic drugs have been prescribed for relatively short periods in low dosage means that the prescribing of such agents requires especially careful assessment of risks versus benefit. Tardive dyskinesia can be precipitated or aggravated by antiparkinsonian drugs. Short lived dyskinesias may occur after abrupt drug withdrawal.

Antipsychotic drugs such as Melleril may cause hyperprolactinaemia resulting in galactorrhoea and oligo- and amenorrhoea. Sexual function, including erection and ejaculation may be impaired. Weight gain is occasionally seen with Melleril and oedema has been reported. These effects may be prevented by reduction in dosage.

Blood dyscrasias have been reported: transient leucopenia can occur and agranulocytosis has been reported very rarely, most commonly in the first three months of treatment, but occasionally later. Blood counts should be performed if a patient develops signs of persistent infection.

Melleril very rarely may cause a photosensitivity reaction. The critical dose for this to occur is 400 to 600 mg daily. Other rare side-effects include skin rashes, altered seizure control, jaundice, hepatitis and liver dysfunction.

Long-term usage at doses above the recommended maximum can very rarely cause increased melanin pigmentation of the skin, which may be irreversible. Although not reported with Melleril, phenothiazines have been reported to cause raised serum cholesterol, rarely hyperglycaemia, faecal impaction, severe paralytic ileus or megacolon.

Overdosage: Acute overdosage of Melleril usually gives rise to coma with shallow breathing, hypotension and absence of reflexes. Motor restlessness, hyperflexia, cardiac arrhythmias and epileptiform convulsions may occur. Treatment should be directed to the elimination of the ingested material by emesis and gastric lavage. General supportive measures should be applied with particular reference to the cardiovascular and respiratory systems.

Acute hypotension should be treated with plasma expanders. If treatment with a vasopressor (*not* adrenaline) proves necessary (as it might in resistant cases) careful monitoring of the patient, particularly of cardiac function, is indicated. Attention should be paid to symptoms of metabolic acidosis and delayed cardiac effects.

Pharmaceutical precautions Melleril Suspension should not be diluted with any of the usual diluents, but the two strengths may be admixed to give a dosage range of between 25 mg and 100 mg per 5 ml spoonful. If an electric stirrer is used, care should be taken to avoid the incorporation of air.

Melleril Syrup and Suspension should be protected from light.

Legal category POM.

Package quantities Melleril Suspension 25 mg in 5 ml and 100 mg in 5 ml: Bottles of 1 litre.
Melleril Syrup: Bottles of 100 ml, 500 ml and 1 litre.
Melleril Tablets
10 mg: Containers of 100 tablets.
25 mg, 50 mg and 100 mg: Containers of 100, 1,000 and 5,000 tablets.

Further information Melleril tablets were formerly sugar coated.

Both strengths of Melleril Suspension contain 3.16 g of sucrose per 5 ml spoonful. Approximate calorific value – 13 kcals per 5 ml.

Melleril Syrup contains 2.25 g of sucrose per 5 ml spoonful. Approximate calorific value – 15 kcals per 5 ml.

Product licence numbers
Suspension 25 mg/5 ml   0101/0052R
Suspension 100 mg/5 ml   0101/0053R
Syrup   0101/5034R
Tablets 10 mg   0101/5033R
Tablets 25 mg   0101/5053R
Tablets 50 mg   0101/5054R
Tablets 100 mg   0101/5055R

PARLODEL*

Presentation
1 mg tablets: White, flat, bevel-edged tablets, 8 mm in diameter scored on one side with 'PARLODEL' impressed circumferentially and a '1' centrally on the other side. Each tablet nominally weighs 180 mg and contains 1.147 mg of bromocriptine mesylate equivalent to 1 mg bromocriptine base.

2.5 mg tablets: White, round, flat, bevel-edged tablets, 7 mm in diameter, 2.7 to 2.9 mm thick, scored on one side with 'PARLODEL 2.5' impressed circumferentially on the other side, weight 140 mg. Each tablet contains 2.87 mg bromocriptine mesylate equivalent to 2.5 mg bromocriptine base.

5 mg capsules: Opaque, hard gelatin capsules, size 3, upper part powder blue, lower part white, printed PS in red. Each capsule contains 5.735 mg bromocriptine mesylate equivalent to 5 mg bromocriptine base.

10 mg capsules: Opaque, white, hard gelatin capsules, size 1, each containing 11.47 mg bromocriptine mesylate equivalent to 10 mg bromocriptine base.

Uses *Principal action:* Parlodel is a dopaminergic-receptor stimulant or dopamine agonist. This pharmacological action is manifest in normal individuals and those with hyperprolactinaemic states by an inhibition of the secretion of prolactin by the pituitary; in many acromegalic patients a lowering of elevated circulating growth hormone levels results.

In patients with prolactin secreting adenomas there is radiological evidence to indicate tumour regression in some cases. Improvement in visual field defects and in general anterior pituitary function may also occur.

Because of its dopaminergic activity Parlodel is also effective in idiopathic Parkinson's disease, which is characterised by a specific nigro-striatal dopamine deficiency.

Indications: The inhibition or suppression of puerperal lactation.

The treatment of hyperprolactinaemia in men and women with hypogonadism and/or galactorrhoea.

The treatment of hyperprolactinaemic infertility.

Parlodel has been used successfully in the treatment of a number of infertile women who do not have demonstrable hyperprolactinaemia.

In a number of specialized units, patients who have been shown to have prolactin secreting adenomas have been treated successfully with Parlodel.

In particular Parlodel can be considered as a first choice of treatment in patients with macroadenomas and as an alternative to the surgical procedure, transsphenoidal hypophysectomy, in patients with microadenomas.

The treatment of cyclical benign breast disease/cyclical pronounced mastalgia.

Cyclical menstrual disorders have also responded to Parlodel, particularly breast symptomatology, but, in the premenstrual syndrome, there is also some evidence that other symptoms, such as headache, mood changes and bloatedness, may be alleviated.

Parlodel has been used in a number of specialised units, as an adjunct to surgery and/or radiotherapy, to reduce circulating growth hormone levels in the management of acromegalic patients.

In the treatment of idiopathic Parkinson's disease, Parlodel has been used both alone and in combination with levodopa in the management of previously untreated patients and those disabled by 'on-off' phenomena. Parlodel has been used with occasional benefit in patients who do not respond to, or are unable to tolerate, levodopa and those whose response to levodopa is declining.

Dosage and administration Parlodel should always be taken during a meal.

A number of disparate conditions are amenable to treatment with Parlodel, and for this reason, the recommended dosage regimens are variable. In most indications, irrespective of the final dosage, the optimum response with the minimum of side effects is best achieved by gradual introduction of Parlodel. The following scheme is suggested:

Initially 1 mg to 1.25 mg at bedtime, increasing after 2 to 3 days to 2 mg to 2.5 mg at bedtime. Dosage may then be increased by 1 mg to 2.5 mg at 2 to 3 day intervals, until a dosage of 2.5 mg twice daily is achieved. Further dosage increments, if necessary, should be added in a similar manner.

Prevention of lactation: 2.5 mg on the day of delivery, followed by 2.5 mg twice daily for 14 days. Gradual introduction of Parlodel is not necessary in this indication.

Suppression of lactation: 2.5 mg on the first day, increasing after 2 to 3 days to 2.5 mg twice daily for 14 days. Gradual introduction of Parlodel is not necessary in this indication.

Hypogonadism/galactorrhoea syndromes/infertility: Introduce Parlodel gradually according to the suggested scheme.

Most patients with hyperprolactinaemia have responded to 7.5 mg daily, in divided doses, but doses of up to 30 mg daily have been used. In infertile patients without demonstrably elevated serum prolactin levels, the usual dosage is 2.5 mg twice daily.

Prolactinomas: Introduce Parlodel gradually according to the suggested scheme. Dosage may then be increased by 2.5 mg daily at 2 to 3 day intervals as follows: 2.5 mg eight-hourly, 2.5 mg six-hourly, 5 mg six-hourly. Patients have responded to doses of up to 30 mg daily.

Cyclic benign breast disease/cyclical pronounced mastalgia/cyclical menstrual disorders: Introduce Parlodel gradually, according to the suggested scheme, until the recommended dosage of 2.5 mg twice daily is reached.

Acromegaly: Introduce Parlodel gradually, according to the suggested scheme. Dosage may then be increased by 2.5 mg daily at 2 to 3 day intervals as follows: 2.5 mg eight-hourly, 2.5 mg six-hourly, 5 mg six-hourly. Patients have responded to doses of between 20 mg and 60 mg daily.

Parkinson's disease: Introduce Parlodel gradually, as follows: Week 1: 1 mg to 1.25 mg at bed time. Week 2: 2 mg to 2.5 mg at bed time. Week 3: 2.5 mg twice daily. Thereafter, take three times a day increasing by 2.5 mg every 3 to 14 days depending on the patient's response. Continue until the optimum dose is reached. This will usually be between 10 and 80 mg daily. In patients already receiving levodopa the dosage of this drug may be gradually decreased, while the dosage of Parlodel is increased until the optimum balance is determined.

Use in the elderly: There is no clinical evidence that Parlodel poses a special risk to the elderly.

Contra-indications, warnings, etc

Contra-indications: No absolute contra-indications to treatment with Parlodel are known. For procedure during pregnancy see 'Precautions' and 'Further information'.

Precautions: Hyperprolactinaemia may be idiopathic, drug-induced, or due to hypothalamic or pituitary disease. The possibility that hyperprolactinaemic patients may have a pituitary tumour should be recognised and complete investigation at specialized units to identify such patients is advisable. Parlodel will effectively lower prolactin levels in patients with pituitary tumours but does not obviate the necessity for radiotherapy or surgical intervention where appropriate in acromegaly. Rare reports have been made of rapid expansion of preexisting pituitary tumours during pregnancy and this may also occur in patients who have been able to conceive as a result of Parlodel therapy. As a precautionary measure, in cases of established pregnancy, visual fields should be monitored to detect untoward effects of

pituitary enlargement so that Parlodel may be reintroduced or other appropriate treatment instituted.

If pregnancy occurs it is advisable to withdraw Parlodel after the first missed menstrual period for most patients. However, with increasing evidence of lack of teratogenic and embryopathic effect in the human subject, consideration should be given to maintaining treatment in those cases where there is evidence of a large tumour or of expansion.

Treatment of women suffering from hyperprolactinaemic amenorrhoea with Parlodel results in ovulation. Patients in whom pregnancy is undesirable, or unwanted, should be advised to take contraceptive measures other than an oral contraceptive. When women of childbearing age are treated with Parlodel for conditions not associated with hyperprolactinaemia the lowest effective dose should be used. This is in order to avoid suppression of prolactin to below normal levels, with consequent impairment of luteal function.

Gynaecological assessment, preferably including cervical and endometrial cytology, is recommended for women receiving Parlodel for extensive periods. Six-monthly assessment is suggested for post-menopausal women and annual assessment for women with regular menstruation.

Hypotensive reactions may be disturbing in some patients during the first few days of treatment and particular care should be exercised when driving vehicles or operating machinery.

Tolerance to Parlodel may be reduced by alcohol.

In acromegalic patients, whilst Parlodel may effectively lower growth hormone levels, treatment to limit expansion of the tumour is also indicated. Acromegalic patients should be carefully assessed for peptic ulceration prior to treatment with Parlodel and advised to report gastro-intestinal side-effects promptly, as gastro-intestinal bleeding has been reported, though the connection with treatment is not proven.

Caution is required where Parlodel is being given in high doses to patients with a history of psychotic disorders or severe cardiovascular disease.

Among Parkinsonian patients on long-term, high-dose Parlodel treatment, pleural effusions have been observed in some cases. While a causal relationship between Parlodel and these findings is uncertain, patients presenting with unexplained pleuro-pulmonary signs or symptoms should be examined thoroughly and discontinuation of Parlodel therapy should be contemplated.

Overdosage: Overdosage with Parlodel is likely to result in vomiting and other symptoms which could be due to over-stimulation of dopaminergic receptors and might include confusion, hallucinations and hypotension. General supportive measures should be undertaken to remove any unabsorbed material and maintain blood pressure if necessary.

Side-effects: Nausea is the most commonly occurring side-effect. Postural hypotension, dizziness, headache, vomiting, and mild constipation have also occasionally been reported. The occurrence of side-effects is minimised by taking Parlodel during a meal and by gradual introduction of the dose. If side-effects do occur, a reduction of dosage, followed in a few days by a more gradual increase, will ameliorate the symptoms.

In acromegalic and Parkinsonian patients receiving high doses of Parlodel, digital vasospasm induced by cold has occasionally occurred. Drowsiness, and less frequently, confusion, psychomotor excitation, hallucinations, dyskinesia, dry mouth and leg cramps have been reported during high-dose treatment of Parkinson's disease with Parlodel. All these side-effects are dose-dependent and can usually be controlled by a reduction in dosage and a more gradual implementation of dosage increments.

Pharmaceutical precautions Protect tablets and capsules from heat and damp.

Legal category POM.

Package quantities 1 mg Tablets: Containers of 100. 2.5 mg Tablets: Containers of 30, 100 and 500. 5 mg Capsules: Containers of 100. 10 mg Capsules: Containers of 100.

Further information Based on the outcome of over 1400 completed pregnancies in mothers who were given Parlodel at some stage in the early weeks of pregnancy, it may be concluded that the use of Parlodel to restore fertility is not associated with an increased risk of abortion, premature delivery, multiple pregnancy or occurrence of malformation in infants.

Product licence numbers
1 mg Tablets	0101/0176
2.5 mg Tablets	0101/0061
5 mg Capsules	0101/0131
10 mg Capsules	0101/0108

PHOSPHATE-SANDOZ*

Presentation Flat, round, white, effervescent tablets with a rough surface, weight 3.7 g, 25.4 mm diameter and 4.4 to 4.9 mm thick. Citrus flavoured. Each effervescent tablet contains 1.936 g Anhydrous Sodium Acid Phosphate BP, 350 mg Sodium Bicarbonate PhEur and 315 mg Potassium Bicarbonate BPC. This provides the equivalent of 500 mg elemental phosphorus (16.1 mmol phosphate), 468.8 mg sodium (20.4 mmol: 20.4 mEq Na^+), 123 mg potassium (3.1 mmol: 3.1 mEq K^+), also 800 mg anhydrous citric acid (787.4 mg citrate ion).

Uses *Principal action:* Oral administration of inorganic phosphates produces a fall in serum calcium in patients with hypercalcaemia. The main effect of oral phosphate in hypercalcaemia is to bind calcium in the gut thus reducing absorption.

High-dose phosphate supplement.

Indications: Hypercalcaemia associated with such conditions as hyperparathyroidism, multiple myelomatosis and malignancy. Hypophosphataemia associated with vitamin D resistant rickets and vitamin D resistant hypophosphataemic osteomalacia.

Dosage and administration Phosphate-Sandoz Effervescent Tablets should be dissolved in $\frac{1}{3}$ to $\frac{1}{2}$ a tumblerful of water.

Dosage should be adjusted to suit the requirements of individual patients. Excessive dosage has been reported to produce hypocalcaemia in isolated cases. Particular care should therefore be taken to ensure appropriate dosage in the elderly.

Adults
Hypercalcaemia: Up to 6 tablets daily (adjustment being made according to requirements).

Vitamin D resistant hypophosphataemic osteomalacia: 4 to 6 tablets daily.

Children under 5 years
Hypercalcaemia: Up to 3 tablets daily (adjustment being made according to requirements).

Vitamin D resistant rickets: 2 to 3 tablets daily.

Contra-indications, warnings, etc
Precautions: In cases of impaired renal function associated with hypercalcaemia and in cases where restricted sodium intake is required, e.g. congestive cardiac failure, hypertension or pre-eclamptic toxaemia, the sodium (20.4 mmol per tablet) and potassium (3.1 mmol per tablet) content of Phosphate-Sandoz should be taken into consideration. In cases of hypercalcaemia associated with impaired renal function and hyperphosphataemia, the main effect of oral phosphate is to bind calcium in the gut and thus reduce calcium absorption. The effect of oral phosphate on serum phosphate is likely to be minimal, but close monitoring of serum levels is recommended.

Concurrent administration of antacids, containing agents such as aluminium hydroxide, may result in displacement of calcium from binding to oral phosphate, thus reducing efficacy.

Soft-tissue calcification and nephrocalcinosis have been reported in isolated cases following intravenous therapy with phosphate. This is thought to be a function of dosage and rapidity of phosphate administration. While such effects appear less likely to occur following treatment with oral phosphates, careful surveillance of patients is recommended, especially if on long-term therapy.

Use in pregnancy: The safety of Phosphate-Sandoz in human pregnancy has not been formally studied, but the drug has been widely used for many years without ill-consequence.

Side-effects: Apart from gastro-intestinal upsets, nausea and diarrhoea, very few side-effects have been reported.

Overdosage: Excessive dosage has been reported to produce hypocalcaemia in isolated cases. This has proved reversible when dosage has been adjusted.

Pharmaceutical precautions Protect from heat and moisture. Since Phosphate-Sandoz Tablets are hygroscopic they should be dispensed in their original containers.

Legal category GSL.

Package quantities Boxes of 100 (5 tubes of 20 effervescent tablets).

Further information Phosphate-Sandoz Tablets each contain 136 mg sucrose. Approximate calorific value – 3 kcals per tablet.

Product licence number 0101/5038R

SANDIMMUN* ▼

Presentation *Oral solution:* Clear, yellow, oily solution containing 100 mg cyclosporin per ml. *Concentrate for intravenous infusion:* Each ml of concentrate contains 50 mg cyclosporin in a clear, brown-yellow, oily solution containing 650 mg polyethoxylated castor oil and 33% ethanol by volume. Sandimmun concentrate is available in 1 ml (50 mg) and 5 ml (250 mg) ampoules.

Uses *Principal action:* Cyclosporin is a cyclic polypeptide consisting of 11 amino acids. It is a potent immunosuppressive agent which prolongs survival of allogeneic transplants involving skin, heart, kidney, pancreas, bone marrow, cornea, small intestine and lung in animals. Successful solid organ and bone marrow allogeneic transplants have been performed in man using cyclosporin to prevent and treat rejection and graft-versus-host disease.

Studies in animals suggest that cyclosporin inhibits the development of cell-mediated reactions. It appears to block the resting lymphocytes in the G_0 or early G_1 phase of the cell cycle, and also inhibits lymphokine production and release, including interleukin 2 (T cell growth factor, TCGF). The available evidence suggests that cyclosporin acts specifically and reversibly on lymphocytes. It does not depress haemopoiesis and has no effect on the function of phagocytic cells.

Indications

Organ transplantation: Prevention of graft rejection following kidney, liver, pancreas, heart or heart-lung transplantation.

Treatment of transplant rejection in patients previously receiving other immunosuppressive agents.

Bone marrow transplantation: Prevention of graft rejection following bone marrow transplantation and prophylaxis of graft-versus-host disease.

Treatment of established graft-versus-host disease.

Dosage and administration

Organ transplantation: Initially, a single dose of Sandimmun Oral Solution, 14 to 17.5 mg/kg body weight, should be given 4 to 12 hours before transplantation. As a general rule, treatment with Sandimmun Oral Solution should continue at a dosage of 14 to 17.5 mg/kg/day for one to two weeks post-operatively. Dosage should then be reduced by about 2 mg/kg/day at monthly intervals until a maintenance dose of 6 to 8 mg/kg/day is reached. Dosage may be gradually adjusted until trough *blood* cyclosporin levels, determined by radioimmunoassay, are within the desired range of about 250 to 1000 ng/ml (equivalent to *serum/plasma* levels of 50 to 200 ng/ml). Following this procedure will minimise the risk of overdosage. (See also Precautions.) When Sandimmun is given with corticosteroids, some patients will require doses lower than 5 mg/kg/day as early as one month post-transplant.

The total daily dosage of Sandimmun Oral Solution may be given as a single dose or in two divided doses. If the taste needs to be masked the solution may be diluted with milk, chocolate drink or fruit juice immediately before being taken.

The Concentrate for intravenous infusion may be used during episodes of gastrointestinal disturbance when absorption of the Oral Solution might be impaired. It can also be used to initiate Sandimmun therapy but it is recommended that patients be transferred to the Oral Solution as soon as possible after surgery. Sandimmun Concentrate should be diluted 1:20 to 1:100 with normal saline or 5% dextrose before use. The recommended dosage is one-third of the previously administered oral dose (3 to 5 mg/kg/day if initiating therapy), given by slow intravenous infusion over 2 to 6 hours.

Bone marrow transplantation/Prevention of graft-versus-host disease (GVHD): Sandimmun Concentrate for intravenous infusion is usually preferred for initiation of therapy, although the Oral Solution may be used. The recommended dosage by the intravenous route is 3 to 5 mg/kg/day, starting on the day before transplantation and continuing during the immediate post-transplant period of up to two weeks until oral maintenance therapy begins. The Concentrate should be diluted 1:20 to 1:100 with normal saline or 5% dextrose before use and should

be given by slow intravenous infusion over about 2 to 6 hours.

Treatment with Sandimmun should continue using the Oral Solution at a dosage of 12.5 mg/kg/day for at least three and preferably six months before tailing off to zero, although dosages of up to 25 mg/kg/day have been used. In some cases it may not be possible to withdraw Sandimmun therapy until a year after bone marrow transplantation. If GVHD develops after Sandimmun is withdrawn it should respond to reinstitution of therapy. Low doses should be used for mild, chronic GVHD.

The total daily dosage of Sandimmun Oral Solution may be given as a single dose or in two divided doses. If the taste needs to be masked the Solution may be diluted with milk, chocolate drink or fruit juice immediately before being taken.

If Sandimmun Oral Solution is used to initiate therapy, the recommended dosage is 12.5 to 25 mg/kg/day for about 5 days.

Sandimmun Concentrate for intravenous infusion may be used for maintenance therapy during episodes of gastrointestinal disturbance where absorption of the Oral Solution might be impaired or where a patient is unable to tolerate the oral preparation. One third of the previously administered oral dose should be given.

Use in the elderly: The indications for Sandimmun make it unlikely that it will be used in elderly patients. Experience in the elderly is, therefore, limited but no particular problems have been reported following the use of the drug at the recommended dose.

Note: Experience with Sandimmun in young children is still limited. Children from three months of age have received the drug at the recommended dosage with no particular problems although at dosages at the upper end of the recommended range, and above, children seem to be more susceptible to fluid retention, convulsions and hypertension. This responds to dosage reduction.

Contra-indications, warnings, etc

Contra-indications: Known hypersensitivity to cyclosporin. Sandimmun concentrate for intravenous infusion should not be used in patients known to be hypersensitive to polyethoxylated castor oils.

Precautions: The concentrate for intravenous infusion contains polyethoxylated castor oil, which has been reported to cause anaphylactoid reactions. Sandimmun should not be administered with other immunosuppressive agents except corticosteroids. Oversuppression can lead to increased susceptibility to infection and the possible development of lymphoma.

Sandimmun may affect liver and kidney function (*see Side-effects*). Close monitoring of serum creatinine, urea, bilirubin and liver enzymes is required and dosage adjustments may be necessary. Steady-state trough *blood* levels of cyclosporin (i.e. those before the next dose) of about 250 to 1000 ng/ml (equivalent to *serum/plasma* levels of 50 to 200 ng/ml) have been recommended, using the radioimmunoassay method to determine cyclosporin levels.

A machine perfusion time of more than 24 hours and a reanastomosis time of more than 45 minutes can have a significant effect on renal graft function in Sandimmun treated patients. Both factors appear to enhance the nephrotoxic effect of Sandimmun.

Care should be taken using Sandimmun with systemic antibiotics or compounds which are known to have nephrotoxic effects, e.g. aminoglycosides, amphotericin B. The trimethoprim component of co-trimoxazole, given together with Sandimmun may cause a reversible deterioration in renal function.

Ketoconazole, an antifungal agent, has been reported to increase the plasma concentration of cyclosporin. Phenytoin, rifampicin and isoniazid have been reported to decrease serum and blood cyclosporin levels. Intravenous (but not oral) administration of sulphadimidine and trimethoprim has also resulted in a marked reduction of serum cyclosporin levels. Concomitant administration of such drugs with Sandimmun should therefore be avoided. Where combined administration is unavoidable, careful monitoring of cyclosporin blood levels and adjustment of Sandimmun dosage are essential.

Animal studies indicate that cyclosporin is not teratogenic. However, its safety in pregnant and nursing women has not been established. Cyclosporin passes into the breast milk and mothers receiving treatment with Sandimmun should not, therefore, breast feed their infants.

Side-effects: Side-effects are usually mild to moderate and usually respond to dosage reduction.

The most frequently observed side-effects in organ transplant patients are hypertrichosis, tremor, impaired renal function, hepatic dysfunction, gingival hypertrophy and gastrointestinal disturbances (anorexia, nausea, vomiting). Hyperkalaemia can occur during Sandimmun therapy. It can be treated successfully and has also disappeared spontaneously.

Hypertension has been observed in most heart transplant patients treated with Sandimmun. In renal transplant recipients there is very little difference in the incidence of hypertension between Sandimmun treated and conventionally treated patients.

The most frequently observed side-effects in bone marrow transplant patients are tremor, gastrointestinal disturbances (anorexia, nausea and vomiting), impaired renal function and hypertrichosis. Facial oedema has also been observed. Infrequently, a combination of hypertension, fluid retention and convulsions has occurred, mainly in children.

A dose-dependent and reversible increase in serum creatinine and urea is the most frequent and potentially the most serious complication of Sandimmun therapy. In about one-quarter of patients, reversible impairment of renal function has been observed; this is generally responsive to dosage reduction. Sandimmun may also cause increases in serum bilirubin and liver enzymes and these changes also appear to be dose dependent and reversible.

A subjective burning sensation may occur in the hands and feet usually in the first week of oral administration.

Overdosage: Little experience is available with overdosage. Symptomatic treatment and general supportive measures should be followed in all cases of overdosage. Forced emesis could be of value within the first few hours after intake. Signs of nephrotoxicity might occur which would be expected to resolve following drug withdrawal. Sandimmun is not dialysable to any great extent nor is it well cleared by charcoal haemoperfusion. Hypertension and convulsions have been reported in some patients receiving Sandimmun therapy at dosages above the recommended range and in others with high trough blood levels of cyclosporin. This might, therefore, be expected as a feature of overdosage.

Pharmaceutical precautions The polyethoxylated castor oil contained in the concentrate for intravenous infusion can cause phthalate stripping from PVC.

Once an ampoule is opened the contents should be used immediately. The oral solution should be used within 2 months of opening the bottle.

Refrigeration of the oral solution is not recommended as this may result in precipitation.

Legal category POM.

Package quantities Oral Solution: Bottles of 50 ml Concentrate for infusion: Boxes of 10 × 5 ml ampoules. Boxes of 10 × 1 ml ampoules

Further information Sandimmun therapy requires careful monitoring and follow up and the drug should only be used in units with experience of immunosuppressive therapy and organ and bone marrow transplantation where adequate equipment, laboratory and supportive medical resources are available.

A radioimmunoassay kit is available for determining blood cyclosporin levels.

The Sandimmun Oral Solution pack contains a patient leaflet, copies of which are available on request.

Product licence numbers
Oral Solution   0101/0124
Concentrate for infusion   0101/0153

SANDOCAL*
CALCIUM-SANDOZ*

Presentation *Sandocal:* Orange, slightly speckled, flat-faced, round, effervescent tablets with a rough surface, weighing 6.3 g, 33 mm diameter and 5.6 mm thick. Orange-flavoured. Each effervescent tablet contains 3.08 g calcium lactate gluconate, equivalent to 4.5 g calcium gluconate and provides 400 mg calcium (10 mmol: 20 mEq Ca^{++}), 137 mg sodium (6 mmol: 6 mEq Na^+), 176 mg potassium (4.5 mmol: 4.5 mEq K^+) and 1.1 g anhydrous citric acid (1.08 g citrate ion).

Calcium-Sandoz Syrup: Colourless to pale straw coloured, fruit-flavoured syrup. Each 15 ml contains 3.27 g calcium glubionate and 2.17 g calcium lactobionate. Three 5 ml spoonfuls provide 325 mg calcium (8.1 mmol: 16.2 mEq Ca^{++}).

Calcium-Sandoz Ampoules 10%: Clear, colourless solution. Each 10 ml contains 1.375 g calcium glubionate, equivalent to 10% calcium gluconate (93 mg calcium–2.32 mmol: 4.64 mEq Ca^{++}).

Uses *Principal action:* Calcium in convenient dosage forms to correct deficiency states.

Indications: High-dose oral calcium in the form of Sandocal Effervescent Tablets and Calcium-Sandoz Syrup is indicated in the treatment of pregnancy cramps and neonatal tetany, and as a therapeutic supplement in osteoporosis, post-gastrectomy malabsorption, osteomalacia, rickets, pregnancy and lactation.

Parenteral administration is indicated when the pharmacological action of a high calcium ion concentration is required.

Dosage and administration *Oral:* See table.

Indication	Daily dosage Effervescent Tablets (The tablets must be dissolved in ⅓–½ tumblerful of water)	Syrup (ml)
Osteoporosis Post-gastrectomy malabsorption Osteomalacia and rickets Lactation	3–5 tablets	60–100
Pregnancy supplement Pregnancy cramps	1–3 tablets	20–60
Neonatal tetany		5 ml four-hourly, mixed with milk feed

Parenteral: 5–10 ml of Calcium-Sandoz 10% i.v. or i.m. daily or every other day.

Children require about half the adult dosage.

Intramuscular injections should be given deep in the gluteus medius muscle using a long needle; this route is not recommended for children.

Intravenous injections should be given very slowly (three minutes for 10 ml).

Calcium-Sandoz should not be injected subcutaneously.

Use in the elderly: No evidence exists that dosage or tolerance of Sandocal or Calcium-Sandoz is directly affected by advanced age; however, elderly patients should be supervised as factors sometimes associated with ageing, such as poor diet or impaired renal function, may indirectly affect dosage or tolerance (see also Precautions).

Contra-indications, warnings, etc

Contra-indications: Severe hypercalcaemia and hypercalciuria (e.g. in hyperparathyroidism, vitamin D overdosage, decalcifying tumours such as plasmocytoma and skeletal metastases, in severe renal failure and in osteoporosis due to immobilisation). Parenteral calcium therapy is strictly contra-indicated in patients receiving cardiac glycosides.

Precautions: Consideration should be given to the sodium and potassium content of Sandocal Effervescent Tablets (see under 'Presentation') before administration to patients suffering from conditions associated with significant electrolyte imbalance, impaired renal function or where limitation in sodium intake is indicated e.g. in the treatment of congestive cardiac failure, hypertension, pre-eclamptic toxaemia, etc. In these cases Calcium-Sandoz Syrup, which contains neither sodium nor potassium, may be substituted for the tablet. Careful monitoring of blood levels and urinary calcium excretion is especially necessary when high-dose parenteral calcium therapy is administered, particularly in children and elderly patients. Treatment should be suspended immediately if blood calcium exceeds 105–110 mg/l or if the 24 hour urinary calcium excretion exceeds 5 mg/kg when it is also necessary to be alert to the possibility of cardiac dysrhythmias.

Overdosage: No cases of intoxication with calcium due to deliberate or accidental overdosage have been reported to the Company. Deliberate overdose is unlikely with effervescent preparations.

Side-effects: Diarrhoea has occurred in a very small number of patients receiving Sandocal. If intravenous injection is administered too rapidly, nausea, vomiting, hot flushes, sweating, hypotension and even vasomotor collapse may ensue.

Pharmaceutical precautions Sandocal Tablets must be stored in a cool dry place. They are hygroscopic and should be dispensed in their original containers.

Calcium-Sandoz Syrup may be diluted with Syrup BP; the diluted syrup should be used within 14 days.

Legal category   Sandocal   P.
                   Calcium-Sandoz Syrup   P.
                   Calcium-Sandoz Injection   POM.

Package quantities *Sandocal Effervescent Tablets:* Boxes of 100 (5 tubes of 20). *Calcium-Sandoz Syrup:* Bottles of 500 ml. *Calcium-Sandoz Ampoules:* Boxes 5 × 10 ml.

Further information Sandocal Tablets contain 935.5 mg sucrose per tablet. Approximate calorific value 18 kcals per tablet.

Calcium-Sandoz Syrup contains 1.512 g sucrose per 5 ml (4.536 g sucrose per 15 ml dose). Approximate calorific value – 13 kcals per 5 ml (39 kcals per 15 ml dose).

Product licence numbers

Effervescent Tablets	0101/5043
Syrup	0101/5024
Ampoules	0101/5003

SANDOGLOBULIN

Presentation Freeze-dried substance for preparation of an intravenous solution of human normal immunoglobulin. Sodium chloride 0.9% w/v (normal saline) for reconstitution.

Sandoglobulin is a polyvalent antibody preparation containing, in concentrated form, all the antibodies normally occurring in the donor pool. The distribution of IgG subclasses in the preparation corresponds closely to that found in normal plasma.

Sandoglobulin is available in two pack sizes, one containing 3 g protein, 5 g sucrose as stabiliser and a 100 ml bottle of normal saline; the other containing 6 g protein, 10 g sucrose and a 200 ml bottle of normal saline. It does not contain any preservative.

Uses *Principal actions:* Sandoglobulin contains intact immunoglobulin which possesses unchanged Fab and Fc functional activity. The anticomplementary activity of the preparation is only detectable at very low levels, but in the presence of an appropriate antigen it activates complement by the classical pathway.

The exact mechanism of action in idiopathic thrombocytopenic purpura remains to be elucidated. Changes have been shown to occur in the function of Fc receptors in mononuclear phagocytes, leading to a decreased binding affinity and prolonged clearance rates within the reticulo-endothelial system. It would appear that Sandoglobulin may block platelet removal by temporary competitive inhibition.

Indications: Replacement therapy for congenital agammaglobulinaemia and hypogammaglobulinaemia in patients who are unable to tolerate intramuscular injections.

Treatment of idiopathic thrombocytopenic purpura.

Dosage and administration

Dosage: Replacement therapy for congenital agamma-globulinaemia and hypogammaglobulinaemia: 0.1 to 0.3 g/kg body weight every 2 to 4 weeks according to severity of clinical signs and symptoms.

Idiopathic thrombocytopenic purpura: 0.4 g/kg body weight/day on 5 successive days. Maintenance doses of 0.4 g/kg body weight may be given as required in order to maintain platelet count.

Reconstitution: Prepare the solution immediately before use. Dissolve the contents of the bottle in sodium chloride injection 0.9% w/v (normal saline) as follows:
3 g in 100 ml to produce a 3% solution.
6 g in 200 ml to produce a 3% solution.
3 g in 50 ml to produce a 6% solution.
6 g in 100 ml to produce a 6% solution.

After disinfecting the stoppers, use the transfer needle provided to connect the bottles of normal saline and Sandoglobulin. Invert the connected bottles to allow the saline to flow into the Sandoglobulin bottle. Discard the empty saline bottle and transfer needle. Turn the Sandoglobulin bottle to wet any undissolved substance. Avoid frothing and *do not shake the solution.* Sandoglobulin usually dissolves in a few minutes, but in exceptional cases may take up to 20 minutes.

Administration: Sandoglobulin is for intravenous use. Infuse only clear solutions at close to body temperature. The first infusion of Sandoglobulin should be of a 3% solution, infused at a rate not exceeding 10 to 20 drops per minute. This is because the first infusion of immunoglobulin, particularly in previously untreated agammaglobulinaemic patients, may lead to inflammatory side-effects as a result of the reaction between the antibodies administered and the free antigen in the blood and tissues of the recipient. After 15 minutes the rate of infusion may be increased to 20 to 30 drops per minute and, after 30 minutes, it may be further increased to 40 to 50 drops per minute. Subsequent infusions may be administered at a rate of 40 to 50 drops per minute. For repeated administration of high doses a 6% solution may be used. In this case the initial rate of infusion should again be 20 to 30 drops per minute, increasing after 15 minutes to a maximum of 50 drops per minute. Antihistamines may be administered to prevent inflammatory reactions in agammaglobulinaemic patients being treated for the first time.

Note: 20 drops = approximately 1 ml.

Contra-indications, warnings, etc

Contra-indications: Rarely, anaphylactoid reactions may occur in sensitised patients with a selective IgA deficiency who possess antibodies to IgA. In such cases the administration of immunoglobulin or of other blood products containing IgA is contraindicated.

Side-effects: If the correct dosage and administration routine is followed (Dosage and Administration) severe adverse reactions rarely occur. Nevertheless, the patient should be closely monitored for signs of anaphylactoid reactions such as a sensation of pressure in the chest, hypotension and cyanosis. In such cases the infusion should be stopped until the symptoms have passed.

Delayed inflammatory reactions including headache, nausea, mild pyrexia, shivering and tachycardia are more likely to occur in agammaglobulinaemic and hypogammaglobulinaemic patients who have never received immunoglobulin substitution therapy before or who have not received therapy within the previous 8 weeks. These

reactions usually occur 30 to 60 minutes after the start of the infusion and disappear after it has been completed.

Overdosage: An overdosage of Sandoglobulin has never been reported, but is unlikely to leave harmful effects either on blood circulation or on other body functions. The only consequence of an abnormally increased level of IgG is the accelerated catabolic rate of this protein.

Pharmaceutical precautions Sandoglobulin should be protected from light and stored below 25°C.

Once the freeze-dried substance has been reconstituted it should be used without delay.

Do not shake the Sandoglobulin solution.

Any solution remaining after infusion must be discarded. Open bottles must not be used again because of the danger of bacterial contamination.

Infuse only clear solutions at close to body temperature.

Sodium chloride 0.9% w/v (normal saline) should be used to reconstitute Sandoglobulin. No other compatibilities have yet been evaluated so due consideration should be given to the advisability of adding other intravenous fluids or medications to Sandoglobulin.

Legal category POM.

Package quantities 3 g pack including 100 ml normal saline, transfer needle and giving set. 6 g pack including 200 ml normal saline, transfer needle and giving set.

Further information Sandoglobulin is prepared by cold alcohol fractionation of pooled plasma from blood donors and contains at least 96% IgG.

Individual donor units of plasma are screened for hepatitis B surface antigen which, combined with careful plasma selection, minimises the risk of hepatitis transmission. To date, no new antigenic properties have been shown to be acquired during fractionation and sensitisation has not been recognised as a clinical problem even after repeated administration. At least 90% of the immunoglobulin is intact monomeric and dimeric (7S) IgG; the remainder consists of a small amount of polymeric IgG and traces of IgA, IgM and immunoglobulin fragments.

Product licence numbers
3 g pack   0101/0182
6 g pack   0101/0186

SANDO-K*

Presentation Flat, round, white, effervescent tablets with a slightly rough surface, weighing 2.4 g and of 22 mm diameter and 4.25 mm thickness. Salty taste. Each tablet contains 600 mg Potassium Chloride PhEur, 400 mg Potassium Bicarbonate BPC and 800 mg of anhydrous citric acid. This provides the equivalent of 470 mg potassium (12 mmol: 12 mEq K$^+$) and 285 mg chloride (8 mmol: 8 mEq Cl$^-$); also 2.2 mg sodium content.

Uses *Principal action:* Sando-K Effervescent Tablets provide a high-dose, palatable potassium supplement in solution.

Enteric-coated and matrix-type solid-dose forms of potassium have been incriminated in the development of small-bowel ulceration, obstruction, perforation, stenosis and haemorrhage, probably produced by a high local potassium concentration. Sando-K Effervescent Tablets when dissolved in water prevent such local concentration, thus minimising gastro-intestinal irritation. Sando-K Effervescent Tablets contain 8 mmol of chloride ion, now believed to be of significance in limiting hypokalaemic, hypochloraemic alkalosis.

Indications: Prevention and treatment of hypokalaemic states such as those associated with: administration of diuretics of the sulphamoyl group (includes thiazides, etc.); ulcerative colitis; renal tubular acidosis; Cushing's syndrome.

Dosage and administration Sando-K Effervescent Tablets must be dissolved in $\frac{1}{3}-\frac{1}{2}$ a tumblerful of water and may be taken with food if preferred.

Dosage will depend upon the clinical conditions and diet of the patient and will vary widely, but 2–4 tablets daily (24 to 48 mmol K+) are likely to provide an adequate prophylactic or therapeutic dose in most patients. Large doses may be indicated in more severe hypokalaemic conditions when the dose should be regulated by the patient's response as determined by serum electrolyte levels.

Use in the elderly: No evidence exists that elderly patients require different dosages or show different side-effects from younger patients. However, elderly patients should be carefully supervised as factors sometimes associated with ageing, such as poor diet or impaired renal function, may indirectly affect the dosage or tolerance.

Contra-indications, warnings, etc
Contra-indications and precautions: Care should be taken to avoid dosage in excess of requirements for patients with impaired renal function.

Side-effects: Side-effects are rare with Sando-K. If there are any signs of gastric irritancy, Sando-K, in common with all other potassium salts, should be given with or after food.

Overdosage: Hyperkalaemia. Deliberate overdosage is unlikely with effervescent preparations. Poisoning is usually minimal below 6.5 mmol: mEq/l, moderate between 6.5 and 8 mmol: mEq/l and severe above that level. The absolute toxicity is governed by both pH and associated sodium levels. Hyperkalaemic symptoms, and particularly the ECG effects, may be transiently controlled by calcium gluconate, administration of glucose or glucose and insulin, sodium bicarbonate or hypertonic sodium infusions, cation exchange resins or by haemodialysis and peritoneal dialysis. Caution should be exercised in patients who are digitalised and who may experience acute digitalis intoxication in the course of potassium removal.

Pharmaceutical precautions Store in a cool dry place. Sando-K Effervescent Tablets are hygroscopic and should be dispensed in their original containers.

Legal category P.

Package quantities Boxes of 100 (5 × 20 effervescent tablets).

Further information Sando-K Tablets each contain 522.1 mg sucrose. Approximate calorific value – 4 kcals per tablet.

Product licence number 0101/5044.

SANOMIGRAN*
Presentation
0.5 mg Tablets: Ivory/yellow, coated, bi-convex tablets of 5.5 to 5.6 mm diameter, weighing 90 mg. Printed SMG on one face. Each tablet contains 725 mcg pizotifen hydrogen malate (equivalent to 500 mcg pizotifen base).

1.5 mg Tablets: Ivory/yellow, coated, bi-convex tablets of 9.0 mm diameter, weighing 280 mg. Printed SMG 1.5 on one face. Each tablet contains 2.175 mg pizotifen hydrogen malate (equivalent to 1.5 mg pizotifen base).

Elixir 0.25 mg in 5 ml: Clear, colourless, fruit flavoured elixir. Each 5 ml spoonful contains 365 mcg pizotifen hydrogen malate (equivalent to 250 mcg pizotifen base).

Uses *Principal action:* Pharmacodynamic studies demonstrate that Sanomigran has a broad antagonistic activity against biogenic amines. Tests show powerful antiserotin and antitryptaminic properties, marked antihistaminic effects, some antagonistic activity against kinins, a weak anticholinergic effect and useful sedative and antidepressant properties.

Sanomigran also possesses appetite-stimulating properties.

The prophylactic effect of Sanomigran in migraine is associated with its ability to modify the humoral mechanisms of headache. It inhibits the permeability-increasing effect of serotonin and histamine on the affected cranial vessels, thereby checking the transudation of plasmakinin so that the pain threshold of the receptors is maintained at 'normal' levels. In the sequence of events leading to the migraine attack, depletion of plasma serotonin contributes to loss of tone in the extracranial vessels. Sanomigran inhibits serotonin re-uptake by the platelets, thus maintaining plasma serotonin and preventing the loss of tome and passive distension of the extracranial arteries.

Indications: Prophylactic treatment of recurrent vascular headaches, including classical migraine, common migraine and cluster headache (periodic migrainous neuralgia).

Dosage and administration
Adults: Usually 1.5 mg daily. This may be taken as a single dose at night or in three divided doses, using 1.5 mg tablets, 0.5 mg tablets or elixir as appropriate. Dosage should be adjusted to individual patients' requirements up to a maximum of 6 mg daily. Up to 3 mg may be given as a single daily dose.

Children: Up to 1.5 mg daily, usually as a divided dose although up to 1 mg has been given as a single daily dose at night. Tablets or elixir may be used.

Use in the elderly: No evidence exists that elderly patients require different dosages or show different side-effects from younger patients.

Contra-indications, warnings, etc
Contra-indications: There are no known contra-indications to treatment with Sanomigran.

Precautions: Patients should be cautioned about the possibility of drowsiness and informed of its significance in the driving of vehicles and the operation of machinery. The central effects of sedatives, hypnotics, antihistamines (including certain common cold preparations) and alcohol may be enhanced by Sanomigran.

Although the anticholinergic activity of Sanomigran is relatively weak, caution is required in the presence of closed angle glaucoma and in patients with a predisposition to urinary retention. Dosage adjustment may be necessary in patients with kidney insufficiency.

Clinical data with Sanomigran in pregnancy are very limited. Although there is no evidence that Sanomigran has a teratogenic effect, like other drugs it should only be administered during pregnancy under compelling circumstances.

Although the concentrations of Sanomigran measured in the milk of treated mothers are not likely to affect the infant, its use in nursing mothers is not recommended.

Overdosage: Symptoms of overdosage may include drowsiness, dizziness, hypotension, dryness of the mouth, confusion, excitatory states (in children), ataxia, nausea, vomiting, dyspnoea, cyanosis, tachycardia, convulsions (particularly in children), coma and respiratory paralysis. Treatment should be directed to the elimination of the drug by gastric lavage and diuresis. Severe hypotension must be corrected (*cave:* adrenaline may produce paradoxical effects). Convulsions may be treated with short-acting barbiturates or benzodiazepines. General surveillance measures are indicated.

Side-effects: The most commonly occurring side-effects are drowsiness, a gain in weight and/or an increased appetite. Other side-effects such as dizziness and nausea have been reported infrequently.

Pharmaceutical precautions Protect tablets from direct light.

Legal category POM.

Package quantities 0.5 mg tablets: Containers of 100.
1.5 mg tablets: Calendar packs of 28.
Elixir: Bottles of 300 ml.

Further information Sanomigran elixir does not contain sucrose.

Product licence numbers
0.5 mg tablets 0101/0036
1.5 mg tablets 0101/0129
Elixir 0101/0163

SYNTOCINON* NASAL SPRAY

Presentation Syntocinon Spray is available as a solution containing 40 Units of synthetic oxytocin in 1 ml for intranasal administration.

Uses *Principal action:* Syntocinon is synthetic oxytocin, identical to the polypeptide hormone released by the posterior lobe of the pituitary gland.

Oxytocin has a physiological function in the neurohumoral reflex which makes milk available to the suckling infant. Stimulation of the nipple by suckling causes nervous impulses to pass by an unknown pathway to the hypothalamus and thence to the posterior lobe of the pituitary which releases oxytocin into the bloodstream. The hormone is carried by the blood to the breast, where it causes contraction of the myoepithelial cells surrounding the alveoli and small ductules forcing their milk content into the larger ducts converging on the nipple. This reflex is known as the milk let-down or milk ejection reflex and may be inhibited in conditions of stress. It is possible to counteract the inhibitory processes by administering oxytocin. By allowing a free flow of milk, breast feeding is facilitated and the possibility of damage to the nipple is reduced as is milk engorgement and breast abscess formation. There is evidence to suggest that when the milk let-down reflex is established by the routine administration of oxytocin there is an increase in milk production.

Syntocinon is administered intranasally in the form of a fine spray from which oxytocin is sufficiently well absorbed from the nasal mucosa to elicit the milk let-down response.

Indications: To facilitate the establishment of breast feeding by eliciting the milk let-down reflex and allowing a free flow of milk. Thereby a) permitting a satisfactory feed; b) reducing damage to the nipples; c) preventing or relieving milk engorgement of the breasts; d) preventing breast abscess formation.

Dosage and administration The patient should be advised to hold the spray upright, insert the nozzle into the nostril and give the container one firm squeeze (approximately 2 Units) into one or both nostrils as directed by the doctor.

The spray should be used two to five minutes before the baby is put to the breast.

Contra-indications, warnings, etc
Contra-indications: Pregnancy, hypersensitivity.

Overdosage: It is considered that intoxication resulting from injudicious usage is unlikely to occur with oxytocin administered by this route as it is rapidly inactivated by proteolytic enzymes in the alimentary tract.

Pharmaceutical precautions Store at temperature below 5°C, but do NOT freeze. Use within one month of opening.

Legal category POM.

Package quantities Spray bottles of 5 ml.

Further information Nil.

Product licence number 0101/5011.

SYNTOCINON* PARENTERAL SOLUTION

Presentation Syntocinon is available as Oxytocin Injection BP containing 2 units in 2 ml, 5 units in 1 ml, 10 units in 1 ml or 50 units in 5 ml.

Uses *Principal action:* Syntocinon is synthetic oxytocin which is identical to the polypeptide hormone released by the posterior lobe of the pituitary gland. Unlike oxytocin from natural sources, Syntocinon is completely free from vasopressin and extraneous animal protein.

At normal therapeutic doses, Syntocinon selectively stimulates the contraction of uterine smooth muscle.

Indications: Syntocinon Parenteral Solution may be used for: Induction of labour; stimulation of labour in hypotonic uterine inertia; management of missed and incomplete abortion; postpartum haemorrhage in the occasional patient who does not respond to ergometrine.

Dosage and administration By intravenous drip infusion: 1 Unit of oxytocin in 1 litre 5% dextrose solution delivers approximately 1 mUnit/min when infused at a rate of 15 drops per minute.

For induction or stimulation of labour:
1. Physiological oxytocin infusion. The range of dosage is between 2 mUnits and 5 mUnit/min.
2. Pharmacological oxytocin infusion. Initially $1\frac{1}{2}$–3 mUnit/min adjusted gradually until contractions occur every two to five minutes; rate of infusion not exceeding 12 mUnit/min.
3. Oxytocin titration: Initially 1 mUnit/min, then double the rate of flow every 10 minutes until contractions commence. Thereafter double the rate of flow every 20 minutes until contractions lasting 40–50 seconds occur

at intervals of two to three minutes. Doses of oxytocin up to 128 mUnit/min have been used.

Missed abortion: 10 to 20 Units per 500 ml of 5% dextrose solution increasing by 10 to 20 Units per 500 ml every hour to a maximum of 100 Units per 500 ml if necessary. The rate of infusion recommended is 10 to 30 drops per minute.

Contra-indications, warnings, etc

Contra-indications: The use of Syntocinon is contra-indicated in hypertonic uterine inertia, mechanical obstruction to delivery, failed trial labour, severe toxaemia, predisposition to amniotic fluid embolism, foetal distress and placenta praevia.

Precautions: Considerable caution should be exercised in abnormal presentation, multiple pregnancy, excessive parity and previous caesarian section. High doses of oxytocin should only be used in fully equipped centres where patients can be kept under constant observation. In patients with cardiovascular disorders the infusion volume should be low.

Overdosage: The fatal dose of Syntocinon has not been established. Syntocinon is subject to inactivation by proteolytic enzymes of the alimentary tract. Hence it is not absorbed from the intestine and is not likely to have toxic effects when ingested.

Where high doses of Syntocinon are given with large volumes of electrolyte-free fluid, the following symptoms of water intoxication may occur:

1. Headache, anorexia, nausea, vomiting and abdominal pain.
2. Lethargy, drowsiness, unconsciousness and grand-mal type seizures.
3. Low blood electrolyte concentration.

Treatment: All fluid intake should be restricted. Diuresis should be promoted as soon as possible and the electrolyte imbalance should be corrected. Convulsions may be controlled by judicious use of diazepam. In the case of coma, a free airway should be maintained with other routine measures normally employed in the nursing of the unconscious patient.

Side-effects: As there is a wide variation in uterine sensitivity, uterine spasm may be caused in some instances by what are normally considered to be low doses.

Very high doses may cause violent uterine contractions leading to uterine rupture, tissue damage and asphyxia of the foetus.

Pharmaceutical precautions Protect from light. Store between 4° and 22°C.

Syntocinon should not be infused via the same apparatus as blood or plasma, because the peptide linkages are rapidly inactivated by oxytocinase. Syntocinon is incompatible with solutions containing sodium metabisulphite as a stabiliser.

Syntocinon is compatible with the following infusion fluids, but due attention should be paid to the advisability of using electrolyte fluids in individual patients. Dextrose 5%, Sodium/potassium chloride (103 mmol Na$^+$ and 51 mmol K$^+$), Laevulose 20%, Macrodex 6%, Sodium bicarbonate 1.39%, Sodium chloride 0.9%, Sodium lactate 1.72%, Rheomacrodex 10%, Ringer's solution.

Legal category POM.

Package quantities
50 Units/5 ml: Boxes of 5.
10 Units/1 ml: Boxes of 10.
5 Units/1 ml: Boxes of 10.
2 Units/2 ml: Boxes of 10.

Further information Nil.

Product licence numbers
50 Units/5 ml   0101/0071
10 Units/1 ml   0101/0070
5 Units/1 ml   0101/0069
2 Units/2 ml   0101/0068

SYNTOMETRINE*

Presentation Syntometrine is available as a parenteral solution containing Ergometrine Maleate PhEur 500 mcg and 5 Units of oxytocin in 1 ml.

Uses *Principal action:* Designed for intramuscular injection, Syntometrine combines the known sustained oxytocic action of ergometrine with the more rapid action of oxytocin on the uterus. The latent period following an intramuscular injection of Syntometrine is considerably shorter than with any other ergot preparation.

Indications: Syntometrine is indicated in the active management of the third stage of labour or, routinely following the birth of the placenta, to prevent or treat postpartum haemorrhage.

Dosage and administration Intramuscular injection of 1 ml. May also be administered by intravenous injection in a dose of $\frac{1}{2}$ to 1 ml.

Contra-indications, warnings, etc

Contra-indications: Severe disorders of liver or kidney function.

Precautions: When the intravenous route is employed, care should be exercised in patients of doubtful cardiac status.

Caution should be exercised in the presence of hypertension, sepsis, obliterative vascular disorders and liver or kidney failure.

Side-effects: Occasional reports of nausea, vomiting and abdominal pain.

Overdosage: No case of maternal intoxication with Syntometrine has been reported to the Company. Inadvertent administration to the newborn infant has proved fatal. In reported accidental neonatal overdosage cases, respiratory and cardiovascular support have been required.

Pharmaceutical precautions Protect from light. Store between 4° and 22°C.

Legal category POM.

Package quantities Boxes of 10 × 1 ml.

Further information Snap ampoules: no file required.

Product licence number 0101/5046.

SYNTOPRESSIN* NASAL SPRAY

Presentation Syntopressin is available as a solution containing lypressin 50 Units per ml for use as a nasal spray.

Uses *Principal action:* Syntopressin is synthetic 8-lysine-vasopressin (lypressin). It is completely free of oxytocin and extraneous animal protein. Syntopressin has a direct antidiuretic action. It is used for the control of polyuria in diabetes insipidus.

Indications: Diabetes insipidus, spontaneous or induced.

Dosage and administration One or two applications of the spray (2.5 to 5.0 Units) to one or both nostrils, repeated three to seven times a day according to the response of the patient.

The patient should be advised to hold the bottle upright and to spray the inside of one or both nostrils by squeezing the bottle firmly then removing from the nostril to release the pressure. This should be repeated one or more times at intervals as required to produce the desired dose.

Use in the elderly: No evidence exists that elderly patients require different doses, or show different side-effects from younger people.

Contra-indications, warnings, etc Coronary heart disease, anaesthesia with halothane or cyclopropane.

Precautions: As with other forms of vasopressin, caution is advised in the administration of this drug to patients suffering from advanced arteriosclerosis, peripheral vascular disease, hypertension, epilepsy and during pregnancy, particularly toxaemic.

Overdosage: No cases of overdosage have been reported to the Company.

Side-effects: Nausea, abdominal pain or urge to defaecate may follow injudicious use. On rare occasions nasal congestion with ulceration of the nasal mucosa has been reported.

Pharmaceutical precautions Store in a cool place, but do NOT freeze.

Legal category POM.

Package quantities Spray bottles of 5 ml.

Further information Nil.

Product licence number 0101/5047.

TAVEGIL*

Presentation

Tablets: White, uncoated, round tablets, 7 mm in diameter, with bevelled edges, branded TAVEGIL on one side with a single break line on the other. Each tablet contains 1.34 mg clemastine hydrogen fumarate (equivalent to 1 mg clemastine base).

Elixir: A clear, colourless liquid with an odour of peaches. Each 5 ml spoonful contains 670 mcg (0.67 mg) clemastine hydrogen fumarate (equivalent to 500 mcg (0.5 mg) clemastine base).

Uses *Principal action:* Tavegil is a potent, specific antihistamine which is innately long-acting.

Indications: Allergic rhinitis, including hay fever and perennial rhinitis, vasomotor rhinitis. Allergic dermatoses, including pruritus, atopic eczema and contact dermatitis. Urticaria. Angioneurotic oedema. Drug allergy.

Dosage and administration *Tablets: Adults:* 1 tablet night and morning. In individual cases the dose may be increased to 6 tablets daily if necessary.

Children up to 12 years: ½ to 1 tablet night and morning according to age.

Elixir: Adults: Two 5 ml spoonfuls night and morning. In individual cases the dose may be increased to 12 spoonfuls daily if necessary.

Children up to 12 years: One or two 5 ml spoonfuls night and morning according to age.

Use in the elderly: No evidence exists that elderly patients require different dosages or show different side-effects from younger patients.

Contra-indications, warnings, etc *Precautions:* Patients should be warned not to take charge of vehicles or machinery until the effect of Tavegil treatment on the individual is known. Tavegil may potentiate the effects of sedatives and alcohol and patients should be advised to avoid alcoholic drinks.

Tavegil should not be given during pregnancy and breast feeding unless it is strictly indicated.

Overdosage: May give rise to confusion, nausea and vomiting. Treatment should be directed to the removal of ingested material by induced emesis or gastric lavage as appropriate. Routine supportive measures are indicated to combat respiratory depression and hypotension.

Side-effects: Of the side-effects associated with anti-histamine drugs, excessive sedation is the most common and troublesome. With Tavegil at normal dosage, drowsiness is infrequent and when it occurs it is usually mild and transient. Very occasional miscellaneous side-effects such as weakness, dizziness, fatigue, dry mouth, palpitations, gastro-intestinal disturbance, heartburn and skin rash have occurred. In general, these adverse effects can be controlled by a diminution of dosage.

Pharmaceutical precautions Protect tablets from light. Tavegil Elixir may be diluted with Syrup BP or Sorbitol Syrup (70%). The diluted elixir should be used within 14 days.

Legal category P.

Package quantities *Tavegil Tablets:* Containers of 50 and 500.

Tavegil Elixir: Bottles of 150 ml.

Further information Tavegil Elixir is sucrose free and is suitable for diabetic patients. It has an approximate calorific value of 11 kcals per 5 ml spoonful.

Product licence numbers
Tavegil Tablets   0101/0033
Tavegil Elixir   0101/0058

TERONAC*

Presentation White, flat, bevel-edged tablets of 7 mm diameter, each weighing 220 mg. Breakline on one side with TERONAC imprinted on the other side. Each tablet contains 2 mg mazindol base.

Uses *Principal action:* Teronac is an appetite suppressant with potent anorexic activity.

It is unrelated to amphetamine and is not metabolised to an amphetamine derivative.

Indications: An aid to the establishment of a diet in the treatment of obesity, accompanied by close support and supervision.

Teronac may be used in patients with stable heart disease, and in diabetic patients (see Precautions).

Dosage and administration *Adults:* 1 tablet after breakfast or as directed by the physician.

Use in the elderly: Not recommended.

Children: Not recommended.

A continuous treatment period of not more than three months is recommended as an aid to the establishment of a controlled diet. The recommended dosage should not be exceeded in an attempt to increase the effect. Administration should not continue if weight loss does not occur within one month of starting treatment, or if weight loss ceases.

Contra-indications, warnings, etc

Contra-indications: Teronac should not be used in patients with peptic ulcer or glaucoma, severe renal, hepatic or cardiac insufficiency, cardiac arrhythmias and severe hypertension or in patients who are breast feeding. Teronac is contra-indicated in patients with a history of psychiatric illness, emotional instability, or those who are liable to drug or alcohol abuse.

Teronac does not inhibit monoamine oxidase (MAO) but potentiates the pressor effects of catecholamines. It can therefore be anticipated that Teronac will interact with the following: MAO inhibitors and antihypertensive agents of the adrenergic neurone blocking type, e.g. guanethidine and debrisoquine.

These medicinal agents should not be taken until one month has elapsed from the cessation of treatment with Teronac.

Use in Pregnancy: Teronac should not be used during pregnancy. There is no evidence as to the safety of the drug in human pregnancy, nor is there evidence from animal work that it is free from hazard.

Precautions: Teronac should be used with caution in patients with prostatic hypertrophy, coronary heart disease, severely agitated states, and in patients taking thyroid medication, psychostimulants or antihypertensive agents. Patients should be cautioned against taking cough and cold remedies containing sympathomimetic decongestants during treatment with Teronac and for one month after ceasing treatment, without first seeking the doctor's advice. This caution is also applicable to patients undergoing local anaesthesia for dental procedures with products containing adrenaline or other sympathomimetic haemostatics.

Diabetic patients' response to insulin and oral antidiabetic agents may be affected by Teronac and dietary control, and the metabolic status of such patients should therefore be monitored and the dosage of insulin or oral antidiabetic agents adjusted if necessary.

Patients driving vehicles or operating machinery should be alerted to the possibility of impaired reactions and be advised to avoid alcohol.

Overdosage: Treatment should be directed to the removal of ingested material by induced emesis and gastric lavage as appropriate. Hyperactivity and anxiety are major factors of overdosage, excess CNS stimulation should be controlled if necessary with chlorpromazine. There is no reported use of forced acid diuresis, but it may be of theoretical value.

Side-effects: The most commonly occurring side-effects include constipation, sweating, dry-mouth and insomnia. Less frequently nervousness, headache, syncope, dizziness, chills, skin rashes, reversible disturbances of micturition and sexual function may also occur. Mild tachycardia has occasionally been reported at higher dosage levels. On rare occasions, euphoria and hallucinations have been reported in the first few days of therapy.

Pharmaceutical precautions Store in a dry place at a temperature not exceeding 21°C.

Legal category CD (Sch 3), POM.

Package quantities Containers of 30 tablets.

Further information Dependence and abuse for stimulant effect have rarely been reported. Weight loss is steady and consistent during treatment with Teronac.

Product licence number 0101/0079R.

TORECAN*

Presentation *Tablets:* White, bi-convex, sugar-coated tablets of 7 mm diameter, weighing 180 mg and printed 'SANDOZ' on one face. Each tablet contains thiethylperazine maleate equivalent to 6.33 mg base (10 mg salt).

Ampoules: Clear, colourless-to-yellow-tinged parenteral solution. Each 1 ml ampoule contains thiethylperazine malate equivalent to 6.5 mg base (10.86 mg salt).

Suppositories: White to pale-yellow suppositories weighing 1.93 g. Each suppository contains thiethylperazine maleate equivalent to 6.5 mg base (10.28 mg salt).

Uses *Principal action:* Torecan is an anti-emetic and antinauseant. It controls vomiting, nausea and vertigo.

Torecan is a phenothiazine derivative which, unlike many other compounds in this group, exhibits specific anti-emetic and antivertiginous properties with little or no tranquillising, sedative or other effects.

The present concept of the vomiting mechanism is that emesis may be induced by direct action on the vomiting centre in the medulla or by lowering its threshold to stimulation. Excitation of the vomiting centre may result from direct visceral impulses or be secondary to stimulation of the chemoreceptor trigger zone. Pharmacological studies have shown that Torecan in similar doses will control vomiting induced by stimulation of both the chemoreceptor trigger zone and the vomiting centre. This suggests that Torecan may possess a more effective action than other anti-emetic agents.

Indications: Torecan is indicated for the relief of vertigo and the control of nausea and vomiting associated with various causes, notably:

1. Labyrinthine disturbances – Ménière's disease, labyrinthitis, surgery, motion sickness, cerebral irritation and damage or disease of the inner ear.

2. Miscellaneous conditions–uraemia, drug idiosyncrasy, hepatic disorders, biliary diseases, migraine, alcoholism and malignant disease.

3. Gastro-intestinal disturbances – gastroenteritis.

4. Radiotherapy and treatment with cytostatic agents.

5. Post-operative nausea, vomiting and vertigo.

Dosage and administration

Adults: Tablets: 1 tablet two or three times daily.

Ampoules: 1 ml by intramuscular injection. Effective in 30 to 60 minutes.

Suppositories: 1 suppository night and morning.

Children: Not recommended for children under 15 years.

Use in the elderly: See *Precautions.*

Contra-indications, warnings, etc

Contra-indications: Severely depressed or comatose states. Hypersensitivity to phenothiazines.

Precautions: No case of bone marrow depression or renal toxicity has been reported. As with many synthetic drugs, the physician should nevertheless be alert to this possibility in susceptible individuals. On a very few occasions, jaundice has occurred following administration of Torecan, but a drug-effect relationship has not been established. Like most phenothiazines, Torecan may occasionally provoke extrapyramidal side-effects; females under 30 and particularly children appear more susceptible. Consequently, Torecan is not recommended for children under 15 years. These symptoms respond to withdrawal of the drug, or to treatment with sedatives and anti-parkinsonian agents.

In elderly patients on long-term Torecan therapy tardive dyskinesia has been observed rarely. As a rule patients over 60 years of age should not be treated for more than 2 months and should be carefully monitored for the occurrence of untoward neurological symptoms.

Torecan may impair reaction time and can potentiate the effects of sedatives and alcohol. Torecan should be given in pregnancy and during breast feeding only if strictly indicated.

Side-effects: Drowsiness, dryness of the mouth and occasional postural hypotension may occur, particularly if the maximum recommended dosage of 30 mg daily is exceeded.

Extra-pyramidal side effects – see 'Precautions'.

Overdosage: The symptoms of Torecan overdosage are similar to those of other phenothiazines with the exception that there is less CNS depression with Torecan. There is no specific antidote for acute phenothiazine poisoning therefore treatment is directed at minimising the amount of the drug absorbed, eliminating the absorbed drug from the body and combating the toxic effects of the overdose by gastric lavage, maintenance of adequate pulmonary ventilation and general supportive measures. Emetics are obviously of less value. If emetics are given and do not work, then do not exceed the normal dose.

Peritoneal dialysis and haemodialysis are ineffective in treatment of phenothiazine poisoning.

Symptoms of hypotension should be corrected. Severe extrapyramidal reactions usually respond to intravenous administration of anti-parkinsonian agents, e.g. Benztropine 2 mg i.v. or i.m. Prophylactic antibiotic therapy is generally favoured. Hypothermia; body temperature should be allowed to recover naturally unless it falls below 30°C.

Pharmaceutical precautions Suppositories should be stored in a cool place.

Ampoules should be protected from light.

Legal category POM.

Package quantities *Tablets:* Containers of 50. *Ampoules:* Boxes of 5 × 1 ml. *Suppositories:* Boxes of 6.

Further information Nil.

Product licence numbers

Tablets	0101/5048
Ampoules	0101/5012
Suppositories	0101/5013

TREMONIL*

Presentation White, uncoated, bi-convex tablets of 8 mm diameter, each weighing 155 mg. Break line on one side, with TREMONIL imprinted on the other side. Each tablet contains 5 mg methixene hydrochloride.

Uses *Principal actions:* Tremonil is a parasympatholytic agent and has spasmolytic and antihistaminic properties.

Indications: Tremonil is indicated in the treatment of Parkinsonism. It is more effective in controlling the tremors than in reducing the rigidity of this syndrome.

Tremonil is also indicated in the treatment of senile tremor.

Dosage and administration *Adults:* Treatment should be started with single doses of 2.5 mg ($\frac{1}{2}$ tablet), three times daily. The dose may then be slowly and gradually raised by small increments until the most effective dose is reached. The optimum effective dosage lies between 15 mg and 60 mg daily in divided dosage, depending upon the severity of symptoms initially and their response to treatment.

Use in the elderly: In elderly patients, the optimum maintenance dosage is often lower than that required by younger subjects with comparable disease, e.g. 15 to 30 mg daily.

Children: There are no dosage recommendations for children.

Contra-indications, warnings, etc

Contra-indications: Prostatic hypertrophy and other conditions causing urinary retention, narrow angle glaucoma, cardiac arrhythmias, intestinal hypotonia, myasthenia gravis, acute intoxication with alcohol, hypnotics, analgesics or psychotropics.

Precautions: Autonomic disturbances occasionally occur during the initial stages of treatment and due caution should be observed in patients who have to drive or perform tasks requiring precision. If these do not disappear spontaneously as treatment proceeds, the dose should be lowered until the highest well-tolerated dose is reached. Treatment should be continued at this level for several days and then gradually increased.

Special care is needed in the adjustment of the daily dosage in patients with marked autonomic lability.

When changing treatment from another anti-Parkinson drug, the small starting dose of Tremonil should be substituted for a part of the dosage of the drug already in use. As the dose of Tremonil is increased, that of the drug for which it is being substituted should be reduced accordingly.

When adding Tremonil to another anticholinergic drug, it is advisable to reduce slightly the dose of the latter for a few days. In this way the occurrence of undesirable side-effects due to the sudden increase in the total dosage of parasympatholytic agents may be avoided. When Tremonil is administered concurrently with phenothiazine tranquillisers to control extrapyramidal side-effects, the average total daily dose of Tremonil is around 15 mg.

Tremonil should be given in the early stages of pregnancy and during breast feeding only if strictly indicated.

Side-effects: Tremonil is generally well tolerated but signs of autonomic imbalance, e.g. dryness of mucous membranes, transient visual disturbances, tachycardia, flushing and dizziness, may occur in some patients during the early stages of treatment. These symptoms tend to disappear spontaneously during treatment, but a temporary reduction in dosage may be required. See recommendations under 'Dosage'.

Nausea, sensations of abdominal pressure, weakness and fatigue may occur half to one hour after a single dose of 10 to 15 mg.

Constipation and urinary retention have been noted.

Mental confusion may result from the use of synthetic anti-Parkinson drugs, especially when given in high dosage, or to elderly patients, and the possibility of this side-effect should be borne in mind, especially when several drugs are given concurrently.

If signs of mental confusion are observed the drug should be discontinued immediately.

Overdosage: Toxic effects are anticholinergic in nature.

Treatment should consist of gastric lavage, routine supportive measures and giving fluids freely. Atropine antagonists such as neostigmine methylsulphate may relieve the peripheral symptoms.

Although physostigmine (1 to 4 mg i.v.) will antagonise the central effects, it is rarely indicated.

Pharmaceutical precautions Nil.

Legal category POM.

Package quantities Containers of 50 tablets.

Further information Nil.

Product licence number 0101/5904.

VISKALDIX*

Presentation White, uncoated, round, flat, bevel edged tablets of 7 mm diameter and weighing 120 mg. The tablets are marked VISKALDIX on one side with a single break line on the other. Each tablet contains 10 mg pindolol and 5 mg clopamide.

Uses *Principal action:* Viskaldix is a combination of the beta-adrenoceptor blocking agent pindolol and the diuretic clopamide; each component lowers blood pressure through a different mechanism of action. Clinical studies have shown that the combination is an effective and well-tolerated antihypertensive agent, that both components contribute to this effect, and that the combination is more effective than pindolol alone.

Pindolol is a specific beta-adrenoceptor blocking agent with some intrinsic sympathomimetic activity which minimises myocardial depression and other undesirable effects of beta-blockade, including bradycardia and bronchoconstriction. Clopamide, in the dosage present in Viskaldix, contributes to a lowering of blood pressure without marked diuresis. The hypotensive effect of the combination is often seen after five to seven days but the maximum effect may not be achieved for two to three weeks.

Indication: Mild to moderate hypertension.

Dosage and administration 1 tablet daily in the morning. If blood pressure is not satisfactorily lowered after two to three weeks, two tablets may be taken as a single dose in the morning. A maximum dose of three tablets daily may be taken if necessary.

Use in the elderly: No evidence exists that the dosage or tolerability of Viskaldix is directly affected by advanced age: however, because of the diuretic component, elderly patients should be carefully supervised as factors sometimes associated with aging, such as poor diet or impaired renal function, may indirectly affect the dosage or tolerability.

Contra-indications, warnings, etc

Contra-indications: Cardiac failure unless satisfactorily controlled by digitalis (see also precautions). Atrioventricular block, pronounced bradycardia, obstructive pulmonary disease, cor pulmonale, severe renal or hepatic failure, metabolic acidosis, prolonged fasting, hypokalaemia, pregnancy.

Viskaldix should not be taken in conjunction with agents which inhibit calcium transport, e.g. verapamil, during concomitant administration of lithium, or by patients with known hypersensitivity to sulphonamides.

Precautions: Patients with a poor cardiac reserve should be stabilised with digitalis before treatment with Viskaldix to prevent impairment of myocardial contractility. Viskaldix should be used with caution in patients with a history of bronchial asthma or recent myocardial infarction and also in patients with spontaneous hypoglycaemia and diabetics under treatment with insulin or oral hypoglycaemic agents. Viskaldix should be administered during breast feeding only in compelling circumstances.

During treatment with Viskaldix, patients should not undergo anaesthesia with agents causing myocardial depression (e.g. halothane, cyclopropane, trichlorethylene, ether, chloroform). Viskaldix should be gradually withdrawn before elective surgery. In emergency surgery or cases where withdrawal of Viskaldix would cause deterioration in cardiac condition, atropine sulphate 1 to 2 mg intravenously should be given to prevent severe bradycardia.

If a beta-blocker is indicated in a patient with a phaeochromocytoma it must always be given in conjunction with an alpha-blocker. Pre-existing peripheral vascular disorders may be aggravated by beta-blockers.

In severe renal failure a further impairment of renal function following beta-blockade has been reported in a few cases. Potassium levels should be checked in patients with kidney or liver failure, and urate levels in patients suffering from gout.

There have been reports of skin rashes and/or dry eyes associated with the use of beta-adrenoreceptor blocking drugs. The reported incidence is small and in most cases the symptoms have cleared when treatment was withdrawn. Discontinuance of the drug should be considered if any such reaction is not otherwise explicable. Cessation of therapy with a beta-blocker should be gradual.

Overdosage: Overdosage may cause alterations in heart rate, nausea, vomiting, orthostatic disturbances, collapse, hypokalaemia and its accompanying disorders.

Treat by elimination of any unabsorbed drug and general supportive measures. Plasma electrolytes should be closely monitored. Marked bradycardia, as a result of overdosage or idiosyncrasy, should be treated with atropine sulphate 1 to 2 mg intravenously. If necessary isoprenaline hydrochloride can be administered by slow intravenous injection, under constant supervision, beginning with 25 mcg (5 mcg/min) until the desired effect is achieved. A cardiac pacemaker may be required. Intravenous glucagon (5 to 10 mg) has been reported to overcome some of the features of serious overdosage with beta-blockers and may be useful.

Side-effects: Few serious side-effects have been reported. Depression, diarrhoea, insomnia, headaches, sleep disturbance, epigastric pain, fatigue, dizziness, hypotension have occurred but are usually transient and disappear if dosage is reduced.

Pharmaceutical precautions Nil.

Legal category POM.

Package quantities Calendar pack of 28.

Product licence number 0101/0113.

VISKEN*

Presentation *5 mg Tablets:* Visken 5 mg is available as white, round, flat, bevel-edged tablets of 7 mm diameter, and weighing 120 mg. The tablets are marked VISKEN 5 on one side with a single break line on the reverse. Each tablet contains 5 mg of pindolol base.

15 mg Tablets: Visken 15 mg is available as white, round, flat, bevel-edged tablets of 9 mm diameter and weighing 200 mg. Branded SANDOZ on one side, and coded JU with a single break line on the reverse. Each tablet contains 15 mg of pindolol base.

Uses *Principal action:* Visken is a specific beta-adrenoceptor blocking agent with low cardiodepressant activity at therapeutic dose. Its beta-blocking activity prevents excessive sympathetic drive to the heart, resulting in a fall in heart rate, and a decrease in cardiac work and myocardial oxygen consumption. Visken possesses some intrinsic sympathomimetic activity even at low dosage which may prevent reduction of resting sympathetic tone to an undesirably low level and minimise myocardial depression.

Indications: Hypertension: For reduction of blood pressure in essential hypertension. Onset of action of Visken is usually rapid, most patients showing a response within the first one to two weeks of treatment. However, maximum response may take several weeks to develop.

Angina pectoris: Prophylactic treatment with Visken reduces the frequency and severity of anginal attacks and increases work capacity.

Dosage and administration *Hypertension:* Initially one 15 mg tablet daily, with breakfast or 5 mg two or three times daily. Most patients respond to a once-daily dose of from 15 mg to 30 mg.

If necessary, dosage may be increased at weekly intervals up to a maximum of 45 mg daily in single or divided doses. Patients not responding after three to four weeks at this dosage level rarely benefit from further elevations in dosage. Addition of Visken to existing diuretic therapy increases the hypotensive effect and combination with other anti-hypertensives enables reduction in dosage of these agents.

Angina pectoris: Usually half to one 5 mg tablet up to three times a day according to response.

Use in the elderly: No evidence exists that elderly patients require different dosages or show different side-effects from younger patients.

Contra-indications, warnings, etc
Contra-indications: Cardiac failure unless satisfactorily controlled by digitalis (see also 'Precautions'). Atrioventricular block, pronounced bradycardia, obstructive pulmonary disease, cor pulmonale, metabolic acidosis, prolonged fasting, severe renal failure, pregnancy.

Visken should not be taken in conjunction with agents which inhibit calcium transport, e.g. verapamil.

Precautions: Patients with a poor cardiac reserve should be stabilised with digitalis before treatment with Visken to prevent impairment of myocardial contractility.

As with all beta-blockers, Visken should be used with caution in patients with a history of bronchial asthma or recent myocardial infarction and in the treatment of patients with spontaneous hypoglycaemia or diabetics under treatment with insulin or oral hypoglycaemic agents. Visken should be administered during breast feeding only in compelling circumstances.

During treatment with Visken patients should not undergo anaesthesia with agents causing myocardial depression (e.g. halothane, cyclopropane, trichlorethylene, ether, chloroform). Visken should be gradually withdrawn before elective surgery. In emergency surgery or cases where withdrawal of Visken would cause deterioration in cardiac condition, atropine sulphate 1 to 2 mg intravenously should be given to prevent severe bradycardia.

If a beta-blocker is indicated in a patient with a phaeochromocytoma it must always be given in conjunction with an alpha-blocker. Pre-existing peripheral vascular disorders may be aggravated by beta-blockers.

In severe renal failure a further impairment of renal function following beta blockade has been reported in a few cases.

There have been reports of skin rashes and/or dry eyes associated with the use of beta-adrenoreceptor blocking drugs. The reported incidence is small and in most cases the symptoms have cleared when treatment was withdrawn. Discontinuance of the drug should be considered if any such reaction is not otherwise explicable. Cessation of therapy with a beta-blocker should be gradual.

Overdosage: Treat by elimination of any unabsorbed drug and general supportive measures. Marked bradycardia as a result of overdosage or idiosyncrasy should be treated with atropine sulphate 1 to 2 mg intravenously. If necessary, isoprenaline hydrochloride can be administered by a slow intravenous injection, under constant supervision, beginning with 25 mcg (5 mcg/min) until the desired effect is achieved. A cardiac pacemaker may be required; i.v. glucagon (5 to 10 mg) has been reported to overcome some of the features of serious overdosage and may be useful.

Side-effects: Few serious side-effects have been reported. Depression, diarrhoea, insomnia, headaches, sleep disturbance, epigastric pain, fatigue, dizziness, hypotension have occurred but are usually transient and disappear if dosage is reduced. Allergic skin reactions have occasionally been reported.

Pharmaceutical precautions Nil.

Legal category POM.

Package quantities *5 mg tablets:* Containers of 100. *15 mg tablets:* Containers of 30.

Further information Nil.

Product licence numbers
Tablets 5 mg   0101/0065
Tablets 15 mg   0101/0110

ZADITEN*

Presentation *1 mg capsules:* White, opaque, oblong, gelatin capsules, size 4, weighing 182 mg. Each capsule contains 1.38 mg ketotifen hydrogen fumarate (equivalent to 1 mg ketotifen base). Coded CS.

1 mg tablets: Off-white, uncoated, round, flat, bevel-edged tablets weighing 190 mg, 7 mm diameter. Single breakline one side and marked ZADITEN 1 on the other. Each tablet contains 1.38 mg ketotifen hydrogen fumarate (equivalent to 1 mg ketotifen base).

Elixir: Clear, colourless, strawberry flavoured elixir. Each 5 ml spoonful contains 1.38 mg ketotifen hydrogen fumarate (equivalent to 1 mg ketotifen base).

Uses *Principal action:* Zaditen possesses marked anti-anaphylactic properties and is effective in preventing asthmatic attacks.

Laboratory experiments indicate that this anti-anaphylactic activity may be due in the main to the inhibition of release of myotonic mediators from tissue mast cells and basophils, in particular SRS (slow reacting substance) and histamine, to the inhibition of SRS-induced bronchospasms in vivo and to calcium antagonistic properties. In addition, Zaditen exerts a sustained inhibitory effect on histamine reactions which can be clearly dissociated from its anti-anaphylactic properties.

Experimental investigations in asthmatic subjects have shown that Zaditen is as effective orally as a selective mast cell stabiliser administered by inhalation: antihistamines are ineffective in these tests.

The effectiveness of Zaditen in the prevention of bronchial asthma has been studied in long term clinical trials. Asthma attacks were reduced in number, severity and duration and in some cases the patients were completely freed from attacks. Progressive reduction of corticosteroids and/or bronchodilators was also possible.

The prophylactic activity of Zaditen may take several weeks to become fully established.

Zaditen will not abort established attacks of asthma.

Indications: Prophylactic treatment of bronchial asthma. Symptomatic treatment of allergic conditions including rhinitis and conjunctivitis.

Dosage and administration *Adults:* 1 mg twice daily with food. If necessary the dose may be increased to 2 mg twice daily.

Children from two years: 1 mg twice daily with food. Patients known to be easily sedated should begin treatment with 0.5 to 1 mg at night for the first few days.

Use in the elderly: No evidence exists that elderly patients require different dosages or show different side effects from younger patients.

Contra-indications, warnings, etc
Contra-indications: A reversible fall in the thrombocyte count in patients receiving Zaditen concomitantly with oral antidiabetic agents has been observed in a few cases. This combination of drugs should therefore be avoided until this phenomenon has been satisfactorily explained.

Although there is no evidence of any teratogenic effect, recommendations for Zaditen in pregnancy or when breast feeding cannot be given.

Precautions: Post-marketing surveillance has shown exacerbation of asthma in approximately 2 per 1000 patients. Since some of these asthmatic attacks might

have been related to stopping existing treatment, it is important to continue such treatment for a minimum of two weeks after starting Zaditen. This applies especially to systemic corticosteroids and ACTH because of the possible existence of adrenocortical insufficiency in steroid-dependent patients; in such cases recovery of a normal pituitary-adrenal response to stress may take up to one year.

If intercurrent infection occurs Zaditen treatment must be supplemented by specific antimicrobial therapy.

During the first days of treatment with Zaditen reactions may be impaired. Patients should be warned not to take charge of vehicles or machinery until the effect of Zaditen treatment on the individual is known. Patients should be advised to avoid alcoholic drinks.

Zaditen may potentiate the effects of sedatives, hypnotics, antihistamines and alcohol.

Overdosage: The reported features of overdosage include confusion, drowsiness, nystagmus, headache and disorientation. One patient became unconscious and one developed convulsions. Bradycardia and respiratory depression should be watched for. Elimination of the drug with gastric lavage or emesis is recommended. Otherwise general supportive treatment is all that is required.

Side-effects: Drowsiness and, in isolated cases, dry mouth and slight dizziness may occur at the beginning of treatment, but usually disappear spontaneously after a few days.

Pharmaceutical precautions Protect from heat and moisture. Zaditen Elixir may be diluted with Syrup BP containing parahydroxybenzoate preservatives. Diluted elixir should be used within 14 days of preparation.

Legal category POM.

Package quantities *1 mg capsules:* Containers of 60 capsules.
1 mg tablets: Containers of 60 tablets.
Elixir 1 mg/5 ml: Bottles of 150 ml.

Further information Zaditen Elixir contains 1.5 g sucrose per 5 ml dose. Approximate calorific value 14 kcals per 5 ml dose.

Product licence numbers
1 mg capsules   0101/0105
1 mg tablets   0101/0125
Elixir 1 mg/5 ml   0101/0137

*Trade Mark

Schering Pharmaceuticals

Division of Schering Health Care Limited

The Brow, Burgess Hill
West Sussex RH15 9NE

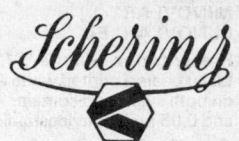

ANDROCUR*

Presentation Each round, white, 9 mm tablet is impressed on one side with 'BV' in a regular hexagon, and is scored on the other. It contains 50 mg cyproterone acetate.

Uses Control of libido in severe hypersexuality and/or sexual deviation in the adult male.

Dosage and administration The daily dose should be divided and taken after the morning and evening meals. The usual dose is 1 tablet twice daily.

Contra-indications, warnings, etc *Contra-indications:* Liver diseases. Malignant tumours (other than prostatic cancer for which cyproterone acetate is indicated. See data sheet for Cyprostat*) and wasting diseases (because of transient catabolic action). A history of thrombosis or embolism. Severe chronic depression. Androcur should not be given to youths under 18 or those whose bone maturation and testicular maturation are incomplete.

Warnings/side-effects: Liver, Cyproterone acetate has been found to cause liver abnormalities in animals, including the development of tumours. Liver function tests should be performed regularly during treatment.

Inhibition of spermatogenesis. The sperm count and the volume of ejaculate are reduced. Infertility is usual, and there may be azoospermia after eight weeks. There is usually slight atrophy of the seminiferous tubules. Follow-up examinations have shown these changes to be reversible, spermatogenesis usually reverting to its previous state about three to five months after stopping Androcur, or, in some users, up to 20 months. That spermatogenesis can recover even after very long treatment is not yet known. There is evidence that abnormal sperms which might give rise to malformed embryos are produced during treatment with Androcur.

Tiredness. Fatigue and lassitude are common in the first few weeks but become much less from the third month.

Gynaecomastia. About one patient in five develops transient or perhaps in some cases permanent enlargement of the mammary glands. In rare cases galactorrhoea and tender benign nodules have been reported. Symptoms mostly subside after discontinuation of treatment or reduction of dosage.

Bodyweight. During long-term treatment, changes in body weight have been reported, chiefly weight gains.

Other changes that have been reported include reduction of sebum production and consequently improvement of existing acne vulgaris, transient patchy loss and reduced growth of body hair, increased growth of scalp hair, lightening of hair colour and female type of pubic hair growth.

Rarely cases of osteoporosis have been reported.

Precautions and special information: Adrenocortical function: During treatment, adrenocortical function should be supervised, since suppression has been observed.

Diabetes: Androcur can influence carbohydrate metabolism. Parameters of carbohydrate metabolism should be examined carefully in all diabetics before and regularly during treatment.

Chronic alcoholism: Alcohol appears to reduce the effect of Androcur, which is of no value in chronic alcoholics.

Haemoglobin: Hypochromic anaemia has been found rarely during long-term treatment, and blood counts before and at regular intervals during treatment are advisable.

Nitrogen balance: A negative nitrogen balance is usual at the start of treatment, but does not persist.

Spermatogenesis: A spermatogram should be recorded before starting treatment in patients of procreative age, as a guard against attribution of pre-existing infertility to Androcur at a later stage.

It should be noted that the decline in spermatogenesis is slow, and Androcur should, therefore, not be regarded as a male contraceptive.

Medico-legal considerations: Doctors are advised to ensure that the fully informed consent of the patient to Androcur treatment is obtained and can be verified.

Road safety: The marked lassitude and asthenia that may be experienced, particularly during the first few weeks of treatment, necessitate especial care while driving.

Overdosage: There have been no reports of ill-effects from overdosage, which it is, therefore, generally unnecessary to treat. If overdosage is discovered within two or three hours and is so large that treatment seems desirable, gastric lavage can safely be used. There are no specific antidotes, and further treatment should be symptomatic.

Pharmaceutical precautions Store in cool, dry conditions away from strong sunlight: shelf-life five years.

Legal category POM.

Package quantities Bottles of 50 tablets.

Further information Cyproterone acetate acts as an antiandrogen by blocking androgen receptors. It also has progestogenic activity which exerts a negative feedback effect on the hypothalamic receptors, so leading to a reduction in gonadotrophin release, and hence to diminished production of testicular androgens.

Product licence number 0053/0023.

ANOVLAR* 21
GYNOVLAR* 21
MINOVLAR*
MINOVLAR* ED

Presentation *Anovlar 21:* Each green, sugar-coated tablet bears a printed white A in a white regular hexagon on both sides, and contains 4 mg norethisterone acetate and 0.05 mg ethinyloestradiol.

Gynovlar 21: Each pink, sugar-coated tablet bears a printed black A in a black regular hexagon on both sides and contains 3 mg norethisterone acetate and 0.05 mg ethinyloestradiol.

Minovlar: Each ochre, sugar-coated tablet bears a printed black A in a black regular hexagon on both sides, and contains 1 mg norethisterone acetate and 0.05 mg ethinyloestradiol.

Minovlar ED: 21 Minovlar tablets plus 7 inactive bridging tablets.

Uses Oral contraception and the recognised gynaecological indications for such oestrogen-progestogen combinations. The mode of action includes the inhibition of ovulation by suppression of the mid-cycle surge of luteinising hormone, the inspissation of cervical mucus so as to constitute a barrier to sperm, and the rendering of the endometrium unreceptive to implantation.

Dosage and administration *Anovlar 21, Gynovlar 21 and Minovlar.*

First treatment cycle: 1 tablet daily for 21 days, starting on the fifth day of the menstrual cycle (the first day of menstruation counting as day 1). In the first cycle only, an additional form of contraception (except the rhythm, temperature or cervical-mucus methods) must be used for the first 14 days of tablet-taking.

Subsequent cycles: Each subsequent course is started after seven tablet-free days have followed the preceding course.

Minovlar ED: First treatment cycle: 1 tablet daily for 28 days, starting in the red sector on the the first day of bleeding, the starting tablet being the one marked with the appropriate day of the week.

Subsequent cycles: Each subsequent course is started in the red sector on the day after the previous one has been finished. Pack, therefore, follows pack without interval. In the first cycle only, an additional form of contraception (except the rhythm, temperature or cervical-mucus methods) must be used for the first 14 days of tablet-taking.

Changing from high-dosed to low-dosed preparations: Additional (non-hormonal) precautions, other than the rhythm, temperature or cervical-mucus methods, should also be used for the first 14 days when changing product.

Post-partum and post-abortum use: After pregnancy oral contraception is usually started as soon as spontaneous menstruation has been resumed. However, oral contraception can be started within 7–12 days of a vaginal delivery, provided that the patient is fully ambulant and there are no puerperal complications. Starting within 12 days of delivery obviates additional contraceptive precautions. After a first-trimester abortion, oral contraception may be started immediately.

Special circumstances requiring additional contraception: Incorrect administration: If a tablet is delayed, it should be taken as soon as possible, and if it is taken within 12 hours of the correct time additional contraception is not needed. Further tablets should then be taken at the usual time. However, if the delay exceeds 12 hours, ovulation may occur. In those circumstances, any tablet or tablets delayed more than 12 hours should be omitted, the remaining tablets should be taken on the correct days at the usual time, and extra precautions (except the rhythm, temperature and cervical-mucus methods) should be used until the next withdrawal bleed.

Gastro-intestinal upset: Vomiting or diarrhoea may reduce the effectiveness of the tablets by preventing them from being fully absorbed. Therefore, it is advisable that an additional method of contraception be used throughout the remainder of the course concerned. Mild laxatives do not impair contraceptive action.

Interaction with other drugs: Some drugs accelerate the metabolism of oral contraceptives taken concurrently. Drugs suspected of having the capacity to reduce the efficacy of oral contraceptives include barbiturates, phenytoin, phenylbutazone, rifampicin, ampicillin and other antibiotics. It is, therefore, advisable to use non-hormonal methods of contraception (except the rhythm, temperature or cervical-mucus methods) in addition to the oral contraceptive as long as an extremely high degree of protection must be provided during treatment with such drugs.

Contra-indications, warnings, etc
Contra-indications: Pregnancy. Thrombotic disorders and a history of these conditions, sickle-cell anaemia, disorders of lipid metabolism and other conditions in which, in individual cases, there is known or suspected to be a much increased risk of thrombosis. Acute or severe chronic liver diseases. Dubin-Johnson syndrome. Rotor syndrome. History, during pregnancy, of idiopathic jaundice or severe pruritus. History of herpes gestationis. Mammary or endometrial carcinoma, or a history of these conditions. Abnormal vaginal bleeding of unknown cause. Deterioration of otosclerosis during pregnancy.

Warnings: There is a general opinion, based on statistical evidence, that users of combined oral contraceptives experience, more often than non-users, venous thromboembolism, arterial thrombosis, including cerebral and myocardial infarction, and subarachnoid haemorrhage. Full recovery from such disorders does not always occur, and it should be realised that in a few cases they are fatal. How often these disorders occur in users of the modern low-dose pills is not known, but there are reasons for suggesting that they may occur less often than with older pills.

Certain factors may entail some risk of thrombosis, e.g. smoking, obesity, varicose veins, cardiovascular diseases, diabetes and migraine. The suitability of a combined oral contraceptive should be judged according to the severity of such conditions in the individual case, and should be discussed with the patient before she decides to take it. The risk of arterial thrombosis associated with oral contraceptives increases with age, and this risk is aggravated by cigarette-smoking. The use of combined oral contraceptives by women in the older age-group, especially those who are cigarette-smokers should therefore be discouraged, and alternative methods advised.

The possibility cannot be ruled out that certain chronic diseases may occasionally deteriorate during the use of combined oral contraceptives (see 'Precautions'). Hepatic tumours have been reported very rarely in women taking combined oral contraceptives, generally for a protracted period of time. A hepatic tumour should be considered in the differential diagnosis when upper abdominal pain, enlarged liver or signs of intra-abdominal haemorrhage occur.

Reasons for stopping oral contraception immediately: Occurrence of migraine in patients who have never previously suffered from it. Exacerbation of pre-existing migraine. Any unusually frequent or unusually severe headaches. Any kind of acute disturbance of vision. Suspicion of thrombosis or infarction. Six weeks before elective operations and during immobilisation, e.g. after accidents, etc. Significant rise in blood-pressure. Jaundice. Clear exacerbation of conditions known to be capable of deteriorating during oral contraception or pregnancy. Pregnancy is a reason for stopping immediately because it has been suggested by some investigations that oral contraceptives taken in early pregnancy may slightly increase the risk of foetal malformations. Other investigations have failed to support these findings. The possibility therefore cannot be excluded, but it is certain that if a risk exists at all, it is very small.

Precautions: Examination of the pelvic organs, breasts and blood-pressure should precede the prescribing of any combined oral contraceptive, and should be repeated regularly. Before starting treatment, pregnancy must be excluded.

The following conditions require careful consideration: a history of severe depressive states, varicose veins, diabetes, hypertension, epilepsy, otosclerosis, multiple sclerosis, porphyria, tetany, disturbed liver function, gallstones, cardiovascular diseases, renal diseases, chloasma, uterine fibroids, asthma, the wearing of contact lenses, or any disease that is prone to worsen during pregnancy. The first appearance or deterioration of any of these conditions may indicate that the oral contraceptive should be stopped.

The risk of the deterioration of chloasma, which is often not fully reversible, is reduced by the avoidance of excessive exposure to sunlight.

Side-effects: Occasional side-effects may include nausea, vomiting, headaches, breast tension, changed body weight or libido, depressive moods and chloasma.

Menstrual changes:

1. *Reduction of menstrual flow:* This is not abnormal and it is to be expected in some patients. Indeed, it may be beneficial where heavy periods were previously experienced.

2. *Missed menstruation:* Occasionally, withdrawal bleeding may not occur at all. If the tablets have been taken correctly, pregnancy is very unlikely, but should be ruled out before a new course of tablets is started.

Intermenstrual bleeding: Very light 'spotting' or heavier 'breakthrough bleeding' may occur during tablet-taking, especially in the first few cycles. It appears to be generally of no significance, except where it indicates errors of tablet-taking, or where the possibility of interaction with other drugs exists (q.v.). However, if irregular bleeding is persistent, an organic cause should be considered.

Effect on adrenal and thyroid glands: Oral contraceptives have no significant influence on adrenocortical function. The ACTH function test for the adrenal cortex remains unchanged. The reduction in corticosteroid excretion and the elevation of plasma corticosteroids are due to an increased cortisol-binding capacity of the plasma proteins.

The response to metyrapone is less pronounced than in untreated women and is thus similar to that during pregnancy.

The radio-iodine uptake shows that thyroid function is unchanged. There is a rise in serum protein-bound iodine, similar to that in pregnancy and during the administration of oestrogens. This is due to the increased capacity of the plasma proteins for binding thyroid hormones, rather than to any change in glandular function. In women taking oral contraceptives, the content of protein-bound iodine in blood serum should, therefore, not be used for evaluation of thyroid function.

Effect on blood chemistry: Oral contraceptives may accelerate erythrocyte sedimentation in the absence of any disease. This effect is due to a change in the proportion of the plasma protein fractions. Increases in plasma copper, iron and alkaline phosphatase have also been recorded.

Overdosage: There have been no reports of serious ill-effects from overdosage, even when a considerable number of tablets have been taken by a small child. In general, it is, therefore, unnecessary to treat overdosage. However, if overdosage is discovered within two or three hours and is so large that treatment seems desirable, gastric lavage can be safely used.

There are no specific antidotes and further treatment should be symptomatic.

Pharmaceutical precautions Store in cool, dry conditions: shelf-life five years.

Legal category POM.

Package quantities All Schering combined oral contraceptives are available in packs containing one month's supply.

Further information Nil.

Product licence numbers
Anovlar 21   0053/5019
Gynovlar 21   0053/5000
Minovlar   0053/5010
Minovlar ED   0053/5016

BILIGRAM*

Presentation *Biligram* is a 35% w/v aqueous solution of ioglycamide (meglumine ioglycamate), with an iodine content of 176 mg/ml.

Biligram for infusion is a 17% aqueous solution of ioglycamide (meglumine ioglycamate), with an iodine content of 85 mg/ml.

Uses Cholegraphy, infusion cholegraphy.

Intravenous cholegraphy should be performed as the first examination only when there is strong evidence of disease involving the biliary tract. In all other cases for diagnosis—especially in obscure upper abdominal complaints—oral cholegraphy (Biloptin, Solu-Biloptin) is to be preferred.

Dosage and administration The infusion should always be started at a low rate and then increased to the final higher rate after three to five minutes. This technique reduces heterotopic excretion and improves the tolerance.

Dosage

1. *Adults: Injection* 30 ml Biligram ensures optimum contrast for normal to overweight adults. Injection time not less than 5 minutes.

Infusion: One 100 ml bottle. Infusion time not less than 30 min.

2. *Children aged 12 years and over:*

Injection: 0.4 ml/kg body weight. Injection time not less than 10 minutes.

Infusion: 0.8–1.0 ml/kg body weight. Infusion time one drop every two seconds.

3. *Children aged under 12 years:*

Injection: (under 1 yr) 0.8 ml/kg body weight. (1–6 years) 0.6 ml/kg body weight. (6–11 yrs) 0.45 ml/kg body weight. Injection time: not less than 10 minutes.

Contra-indications, warnings, etc

Contra-indications: Severe cardiovascular insufficiency, particularly right ventricular failure. Proven or suspected hypersensitivity to iodine-containing contrast media. Manifest thyrotoxicosis. Severe functional disturbance of the liver or kidneys. Monoclonal IgM gammopathy e.g. macroglobulinaemia (Waldenström's disease).

Warnings/side-effects: In patients with multiple myeloma, other severe diseases, poor general health or thyroid hyperfunction, the need for examination merits particularly careful consideration. This applies to patients with a history of allergy (e.g. bronchial asthma, endogenous eczema), since experience has shown that they may exhibit hypersensitivity to drugs. Pre-testing does not give a reliable warning of allergic reactions to iodine-containing contrast media. Some radiologists give an antihistamine or a corticoid prophylactically to patients with a history of allergy. Because of the possibility of precipitation, contrast medium and prophylactic agents must not be administered mixed together.

Since radiation should, if possible, be avoided during pregnancy, and moreover it has not yet been demonstrated whether it is safe to use Biligram in pregnant patients, Biligram should be administered during pregnancy only if the doctor regards the examination as essential.

Thyroid hyperfunction can increase for some time after the administration of biliary contrast media.

If iodine isotopes are to be administered for diagnosing thyroid disease, it should be borne in mind that the capacity of the thyroid tissue to take up iodine will be reduced for eight to ten weeks or more by iodinated biliary contrast media.

Some investigators have reported temporary and reversible changes in liver-function tests after Biligram. These changes are not thought to reflect liver damage.

The opinion has been expressed that intravenous cholegraphy should not be performed immediately after negative oral cholegraphy. A large number of radiologists do not share this view – provided that the patient is adequately hydrated and renal function is not impaired.

The patient should be recumbent during the administration of Biligram. Thereafter, the patient must be kept under close observation for at least 15 minutes, since about 90% of all severe incidents occur within that time, and must not be left unsupervised until the end of the examination. If the administration does not take place on the X-ray table, any patient with a labile circulation should be brought to the X-ray machine sitting or lying down. Inadvertent paravenous administration of Biligram can cause pain, but experience has shown that it is very rarely followed by serious tissue reactions. A local anaesthetic helps to relieve the pain. With more extensive paravenous infiltration, it is recommended that a hyaluronidase preparation be injected into the affected area to hasten absorption.

The greater the rate of administration of Biligram, the higher the incidence of common side-effects, such as an unpleasant taste, nausea, vomiting or a sensation of heat. These side-effects are rare if the recommended rate of administration is adhered to. Too rapid an administration may put the patient's life at risk – particularly if he has cardiovascular damage, whether manifest or not, or if his general condition is poor. Each bottle of Biligram for infusion should be used for one investigation only, and any remaining medium should be discarded.

Particular caution should be exercised in allergic patients who have previously tolerated injectable iodine-containing contrast media without any complication, since they may have become sensitised to these substances. As with any contrast medium, the possibility of hypersensitivity must always be considered. If marked side-effects or suspected allergic reactions occur during infusion or injection and persist or even worsen when the administration is interrupted, it is probable that the patient has such a hypersensitivity. Therefore, the investigation must be abandoned. The needle or cannula should be left in the vein for some time in order to maintain access for intravenous therapy. Even relatively minor symptoms, such as itching of the skin, sneezing, violent yawns, tickling in the throat, hoarseness or attacks of coughing may be early signs of a severe reaction and, therefore, merit careful attention.

Very rarely, severe or even life-threatening incidents, such as severe hypotension and collapse, circulatory failure, ventricular fibrillation, cardiac arrest, pulmonary oedema, anaphylactic shock or other allergic manifestations, convulsions or other cerebral symptoms may occur.

At present there is no clinical test that is suitable for predicting an incident. It must be emphasised that every use of a contrast medium therefore entails a certain risk and requires appropriate precautions. Ready availability of all drugs and equipment for emergency treatment and familiarity with the various procedures are prerequisites for the effective management of contrast-medium incidents.

Some guidance in the treatment of such incidents is contained in the leaflet supplied with the pack.

Pharmaceutical precautions Storage: Protect from light and heat. Shelf-life five years.

Legal category POM.

Package quantities
Biligram	Packs of 5 × 30 ml ampoules
Biligram for infusion	Packs of 5 × 100 ml vials

Further information Nil.

Product licence numbers
Biligram	0053/0054
Biligram for infusion	0053/0055

BILISCOPIN* ▼

Presentation Ampoules or bottles containing sterile solutions of meglumine iotroxate.

	Volume ml	Iodine mg/ml	Iodine Total, g	Osmoles/l at 37°C
Biliscopin:	30	180	5.4	0.46
Biliscopin for infusion:	100	50	5.0	0.28

Uses Cholegraphy, infusion cholegraphy.

Intravenous cholegraphy should be performed as the first examination only when there is strong evidence of disease involving the biliary tract. In all other cases for diagnosis – especially in obscure upper abdominal complaints – oral cholegraphy (Biloptin, Solu-Biloptin) is to be preferred.

Dosage and administration
1. Adults: Injection: 30 ml Biliscopin provides good contrast in most normal or overweight adults. In underweight patients, 20 ml is generally sufficient.

Injection time: not less than 5 minutes.

Infusion: one 100 ml bottle of Biliscopin for infusion in not less than 15 minutes.

The infusion should always be started at a low rate and then increased to the final higher rate after three to five minutes. This technique reduces heterotopic excretion and improves tolerance.

2. Children: Because of insufficient experience in the use of Biliscopin in children, optimal paediatric dosages have not been established.

Contra-indications, warnings, etc
Contra-indications: Severe cardiovascular insufficiency, particularly right ventricular failure. Proven or suspected hypersensitivity to iodine-containing contrast media. Manifest thyrotoxicosis. Severe functional disturbance of the liver or kidneys. Monoclonal IgM gammopathy e.g. macroglobulinaemia (Waldenström's disease).

Warnings/side-effects: In patients with multiple myeloma, other severe diseases, poor general health or thyroid hyperfunction, the need for examination merits particularly careful consideration. This applies to patients with a history of allergy (e.g. bronchial asthma, endogenous eczema), since experience has shown that they may exhibit hypersensitivity to drugs. Pre-testing does not give a reliable warning of allergic reactions to iodine-containing contrast media. Some radiologists give an antihistamine or a corticoid prophylactically to patients with a history of allergy. Because of the possibility of precipitation, contrast medium and prophylactic agents must not be administered mixed together. Since radiation should, if possible, be avoided during pregnancy, and moreover it has not yet been demonstrated whether it is safe to use Biliscopin in pregnant patients, Biliscopin should be administered during pregnancy only if the doctor regards the examination as essential.

Thyroid hyperfunction can increase for some time after the administration of biliary contrast media.

If iodine isotopes are to be administered for diagnosing thyroid disease, it should be borne in mind that the capacity of the thyroid tissue to take up iodine will be reduced for eight to ten weeks or more by iodinated biliary contrast media.

Some investigators have reported temporary and reversible changes in liver-function tests after Biliscopin. These changes are not thought to reflect liver damage.

The opinion has been expressed that intravenous cholegraphy should not be performed immediately after negative oral cholegraphy. A large number of radiologists do not share this view – provided that the patient is adequately hydrated and renal function is not impaired.

The patient should be recumbent during the administration of Biliscopin. Thereafter, he must be kept under close observation for at least 15 minutes, since about 90% of all severe incidents occur within that time, and must not be left unsupervised until the end of the examination. If the administration does not take place on the X-ray table, any patient with a labile circulation should be brought to the X-ray machine sitting or lying down. Inadvertent paravenous administration of Biliscopin can cause pain, but experience has shown that it is very rarely followed by serious tissue reactions. A local anaesthetic helps to relieve the pain. With more extensive paravenous infiltration, it is recommended that a hyaluronidase preparation be injected into the affected area to hasten absorption.

The greater the rate of administration of Biliscopin, the higher the incidence of common side-effects, such as an unpleasant taste, nausea, vomiting or a sensation of heat. These side-effects are rare if the recommended rate of administration is adhered to. Too rapid an administration may put the patient's life at risk – particularly if he has cardiovascular damage, whether manifest or not, or if his general condition is poor. Each bottle of Biliscopin for infusion should be used for one investigation only, and any remaining medium should be discarded.

Particular caution should be exercised in allergic patients who have previously tolerated injectable iodine-containing contrast media without any complication, since they may have become sensitised to these substances. As with any contrast medium, the possibility of hypersensitivity must always be considered. If marked side-effects or suspected allergic reactions occur during infusion or injection and persist or even worsen when the administration is interrupted, it is probable that the patient has such a hypersensitivity. Therefore, the investigation must be abandoned. The needle or cannula should be left in the vein for some time in order to maintain access for intravenous therapy. Even relatively minor symptoms, such as itching of the skin, sneezing, violent yawns, tickling in the throat, hoarseness or attacks of coughing may be early signs of a severe reaction and, therefore, merit careful attention.

Very rarely, severe or even life-threatening incidents, such as severe hypotension and collapse, circulatory failure, ventricular fibrillation, cardiac arrest, pulmonary oedema, anaphylactic shock or other allergic manifestations, convulsions or other cerebral symptoms may occur.

At present there is no clinical test that is suitable for predicting an incident. It must be emphasised that every use of a contrast medium therefore entails a certain risk and requires appropriate precautions. Ready availability of all drugs and equipment for emergency treatment and familiarity with the various procedures are prerequisites for the effective management of contrast-medium incidents.

Some guidance in the treatment of such incidents is contained in the leaflet supplied with the pack.

Pharmaceutical precautions
Storage: Protect from light and heat.
Shelf-life: Five years.

Legal category POM.

Package quantities *Biliscopin:* Packs of 10 × 30 ml ampoules. *Biliscopin for infusion:* Packs of 10 × 100 ml infusion bottles.

Further information Nil.

Product licence numbers
Biliscopin   0053/0109
Biliscopin for infusion   0053/0110

BILOPTIN* AND SOLU-BILOPTIN*

Presentation *Biloptin:* Capsules of sodium iopodate.
6 Biloptin capsules, containing a total 1.84 g iodine in 3 g of sodium iopodate.

Solu-Biloptin: Sachets, each containing 1.85 g iodine in 3 g of calcium iopodate.

Uses Oral contrast media for cholecystography and cholangiography.

Dosage and administration See table below.

Routine cholecystography

Solu-Biloptin	Biloptin

Both media should be taken after the last meal on the evening before the examination.
Adults

The contents of 1 sachet.	6 capsules

Children:

Under 4 yrs or under 20 kg body weight 0.30 g of powder/kg body weight.	Solu-Biloptin is recommended.
Over 4 yrs or over 20 kg body weight 0.15 g of powder/kg body weight.	

Neonates and infants:
Biligram is recommended, but a trial by the oral route may be undertaken using 0.45 g of Solu-Biloptin powder/kg body weight.

The results are improved if an enema is given on the preceding evening and another immediately before the examination.

Other examination techniques in adults only

Biloptin	Solu-Biloptin
Rapid cholecystography 6 capsules or double dose of 12 capsules.	The contents of 1 sachet or double dose of 2 sachets.
Cholangiography 12 capsules	The contents of 2 sachets.
Fractionated oral cholecystography 6 capsules 10–12 hrs before the examination and another 6 capsules 3 hrs before the examination.	The contents of 1 sachet 10–12 hrs before the examination and another 1 sachet 3 hrs before the examination.

Contra-indications, warnings, etc
Contra-indications: Proven or suspected hypersensitivity to iodine-containing contrast media. Thyrotoxicosis. Severe impairment of hepatic or renal function.

Warnings/side-effects: Biloptin and Solu-Biloptin are well tolerated and side-effects, even of a trivial nature, are extraordinarily rare. Sensitive patients may occasionally complain of mild sensations of pressure in the stomach or nausea. Attacks of diarrhoea and vomiting are exceptional. Very few cases of urticaria have been observed.

If iodine isotopes are to be administered for diagnosing thyroid disease, it should be borne in mind that the capacity of the thyroid tissue to take up iodine will be reduced for 8–10 weeks or more by iodinated biliary X-ray contrast media.

Apart from the fact that X-ray examinations should, if possible, be avoided during pregnancy, it must be pointed out that it has not yet been proved beyond question that Biloptin may be used without hesitation in pregnant patients. Therefore, such an examination with a contrast medium during pregnancy should be carried out only if considered absolutely necessary by the physician.

Pharmaceutical precautions Store in cool, dry conditions. Shelf-life five years.

Legal category P.

Package quantities
Biloptin capsules. 0.5 g 20 × 6
Solu-Biloptin sachets. 3 g × 20

Further information Nil.

Product licence numbers
Biloptin   0053/5048
Solu-Biloptin   0053/5049

BRONCHODIL AEROSOL ▼
BRONCHODIL RESPIRATOR SOLUTION
BRONCHODIL TABLETS
BRONCHODIL ELIXIR

Presentation Aerosol dispenser with metered-dose unit, containing 20 ml suspension. Each metered dose provides 0.5 mg reproterol hydrochloride.

An aqueous colourless respirator solution of reproterol hydrochloride, in a concentration of 10 mg/ml.

White, half-scored, oval, film-coated tablets, each containing 20 mg reproterol hydrochloride.

A red, fruit-flavoured elixir, each 5 ml of which contains 10 mg reproterol hydrochloride. The elixir contains no sugar.

Uses Bronchodil, a selective β_2-adrenergic stimulant with very little action on cardiac receptors, is indicated for the treatment of conditions involving reversible airways obstruction, such as bronchial asthma, including that of an allergic origin, acute and chronic bronchitis and emphysema.

It is effective in the prophylaxis of acute attacks of bronchospasm.

Because of its selective action on the bronchi, Bronchodil may be used in the treatment of bronchospasm in patients with co-existing heart disease or hypertension.

Bronchodil elixir is especially useful as oral therapy for children and those adults who prefer a liquid medicine, and for diabetics, as it contains no sugar.

Bronchodil respirator solution is indicated in the treatment of status asthmaticus or other forms of bronchospasm e.g. acute exacerbations of chronic bronchitis or severe bronchial asthma.

Dosage and administration *Inhalation: Aerosol:*

Adults: For acute attacks of bronchospasm, the usual dose is 1 or 2 inhalations, repeated every 3–6 hours as required.

For chronic reversible obstruction of the airways, and the prophylaxis of recurrent attacks of acute bronchospasm, the usual dose is 2 inhalations three times a day.

Children: 6–12 years: No more than 1 inhalation every

3–6 hours for acute attacks, or three times a day for prophylaxis.

Inhalation: Respirator Solution:
Bronchodil Respirator Solution is designed to be given by intermittent positive-pressure ventilation in oxygen-enriched air or by a suitable nebulizer.

The recommended dose is 10 mg–20 mg (1–2 mls) which should be diluted in 3 ml sterile, normal saline. This dose should be given over a 10 min. period.

Whilst the dose should not normally be altered, the dilution and duration of administration may be adjusted to suit the particular nebulizer in use.

At present there are no clinical trial data relating to use in children of Bronchodil Respirator Solution. However, experience with Bronchodil tablets, elixir and aerosol indicates that the Respirator Solution can be used for children by reduction of the adult dose in proportion to the child's weight, according to established principles of dosage in children.

Oral: Tablets
Adults: The usual adult dose is one tablet three times daily. If side-effects occur, the dosage should be reduced to half a tablet three times daily.

Children: 6–12 years: Usually half a tablet three times daily.
Over 12 years, usually half to one tablet 3 times daily, according to bodyweight.

Oral: Elixir
Adults: The usual adult dosage is 10 ml orally three times daily. If side-effects occur, the dosage should be reduced to 5 ml three times daily.

Children: 6–12 years: 5 ml orally three times daily.

Over 12 years: 5–10 ml orally three times daily, according to bodyweight.

Contra-indications, warnings, etc
Contra-indications: There are no known contra-indications.

Side-effects: Bronchodil is generally well tolerated but, as with other β-adrenergic stimulants, digital tremor, palpitations, slight tachycardia and restlessness may occasionally occur.

Precautions: Care should be taken with patients suffering from myocardial infarction, thyrotoxicosis or phaeochromocytoma. Bronchodil should be used with caution in patients already receiving sympathomimetic agents. Bronchodil should not be prescribed with β-blocking drugs. Although no teratogenic effects have been observed in animal experiments, caution is recommended during the first trimester of pregnancy.

Exceeding the stated dose does not produce an enhanced therapeutic effect, and should be avoided.

Overdosage: Reversal of the therapeutic action on the bronchi is never required, since excessive bronchodilatation cannot result from overdosage. General blockade of the β-adrenergic stimulus is therefore never appropriate, and if a β-blocker is used, it should be of the cardioselective type. Such a drug is the recommended antidote. However, β-blockade is not mandatory unless there is severe tachycardia or cardiac arrhythmia threatens, and β-blockers should be used with caution in patients with existing or potential cardiac failure, which may be precipitated by the negative inotropic effect of β-blockade on the myocardium. Muscle tremor and restlessness can be treated with benzodiazepines, which are particularly useful in children.

Pharmaceutical precautions Store in a cool, dry place.

Shelf-lives: tablets 5 years, respirator solution 4 years, aerosol and elixir 3 years.
The elixir should be protected from light.
The aerosol canister should be kept away from heat, and must not be punctured or incinerated, even when empty.
Solutions in nebulizers should be replaced daily.

Legal category POM.

Package quantities Each aerosol canister provides 400 metered doses.
The tablets are supplied as blister packs of 100.
The elixir is supplied in amber bottles of 100 ml.
Amber bottles containing 50 ml respirator solution.

Further information The elixir may be diluted with purified water BP. The resulting mixture should be protected from light, and will then keep for 14 days.

Product licence numbers

Aerosol	0053/0130
Tablets	0053/0131
Elixir	0053/0139
Respirator solution	0053/0137.

CONTROVLAR*

Presentation Each pink, sugar-coated tablet bears a printed black A in a black regular hexagon on both sides and contains 3 mg norethisterone acetate and 0.05 mg ethinyloestradiol.

Uses Controvlar inhibits ovulation, which is of value in the treatment of dysmenorrhoea, since anovulatory cycles are almost always painless. Mittelschmerz is also prevented by the suppression of ovulation. Controvlar prevents the oestrogenic overstimulation that is responsible for menorrhagia, metropathia haemorrhagica and the symptoms of endometriosis. It imposes a regular cycle of bleeding and is, therefore, suitable for the treatment of menstrual irregularities, i.e. polymenorrhoea and oligomenorrhoea.

Dosage and administration *First treatment cycle:* One tablet daily for 21 days, starting on the fifth day of the menstrual cycle (the first day of menstruation counting as day 1).

Subsequent cycles: Each subsequent course is started after seven tablet-free days have followed the preceding course, irrespective of the menstrual pattern, with the proviso that, if no bleeding occurs at all, pregnancy should be excluded before treatment is resumed.

Contra-indications, warnings, etc
Contra-indications: Pregnancy. Thrombotic disorders and a history of these conditions, sickle-cell anaemia, disorders of lipid metabolism and other conditions in which, in individual cases, there is known or suspected to be a much increased risk of thrombosis. Acute or severe chronic liver disease. Dubin-Johnson syndrome. Rotor syndrome. History, during pregnancy of idiopathic jaundice or severe pruritus. History of herpes gestationis. Mammary or endometrial carcinoma, or a history of these conditions. Deterioration of otosclerosis during pregnancy.

Warnings: There is a general opinion, based on statistical evidence, that users of this type of oestrogen-progestogen combination experience, more often than non-users, venous thromboembolism, arterial thrombosis, including cerebral and myocardial infarction, and subarachnoid haemorrhage. Full recovery from such disorders does not always occur, and it should be realised that in a few cases they are fatal.

Certain conditions may entail some risk of thrombosis, e.g. smoking, obesity, varicose veins, cardiovascular diseases, diabetes and migraine. The advisability of prescribing Controvlar should be judged according to the severity of such conditions in the individual case and should be discussed with the patient.

The possibility cannot be ruled out that certain chronic diseases may occasionally deteriorate during the use of Controvlar (see 'Precautions').

Hepatic tumours have been reported very rarely in women taking oestrogen-progestogen combinations of this type, generally for a protracted period of time. A hepatic tumour should be considered in the differential diagnosis when upper abdominal pain, enlarged liver or signs of intra-abdominal haemorrhage occur.

Reasons for stopping Controvlar immediately: Occurrence of migraine in patients who have never previously suffered from it. Exacerbation of pre-existing migraine. Any unusually frequent or unusually severe headaches. Any kind of acute disturbance of vision. Suspicion of thrombosis or infarction. Six weeks before elective operations and during immobilisation, e.g. after accidents, etc. Significant rise in blood pressure. Jaundice. Clear exacerbation of conditions known to be capable of deteriorating during oral contraception or pregnancy. Pregnancy is a reason for stopping Controvlar immediately because it has been suggested by some investigations that oestrogen-progestogen combinations taken in early pregnancy may slightly increase the risk of foetal malformations. Other investigations have failed to support these findings. The possibility therefore cannot be excluded, but it is certain that, if a risk exists at all, it is very small.

Precautions: Examination of the pelvic organs, breasts and blood-pressure should precede the prescribing of Controvlar, and should be repeated regularly. Before starting treatment, pregnancy must be excluded.

The following conditions require careful consideration: a history of severe depressive states, varicose veins, diabetes, hypertension, epilepsy, otosclerosis, multiple sclerosis, porphyria, tetany, disturbed liver function, gallstones, cardiovascular diseases, renal diseases, chloasma, uterine fibroids, asthma, the wearing of contact lenses, or any disease that is prone to worsen during pregnancy. The first appearance or deterioration of any of these conditions may indicate that Controvlar should be stopped. The risk of the deterioration of chloasma, which is often not fully reversible, is reduced by the avoidance of excessive exposure to sunlight.

Side-effects: Occasional side-effects may include: nausea, vomiting, headaches, breast tension, changed body weight or libido, depressive moods and chloasma.

Effect on adrenal and thyroid glands: Controvlar has no significant influence on adrenocortical function. The ACTH function test for the adrenal cortex remains unchanged. The reduction in corticosteroid excretion and the elevation of plasma corticosteroids are due to an increased cortisol-binding capacity of the plasma proteins.

The response to metyrapone is less pronounced than in untreated women and is thus similar to that during pregnancy.

The radio-iodine uptake shows that thyroid function is unchanged. There is a rise in serum protein-bound iodine, similar to that in pregnancy and during the administration of oestrogens. This is due to the increased capacity of the plasma proteins for binding thyroid hormones, rather than to any change in glandular function. In women taking Controvlar, the content of protein-bound iodine in blood serum should, therefore, not be used for the evaluation of thyroid function.

Effect on blood chemistry: Controvlar may accelerate erythrocyte sedimentation in the absence of any disease. This effect is due to a change in the proportion of the plasma protein fractions. Increases in plasma copper, iron and alkaline phosphatase have also been recorded.

Overdosage: There have been no reports of serious ill-effects from overdosage, even when a considerable number of tablets have been taken by a small child. In general, it is, therefore, unnecessary to treat overdosage. However, if overdosage is discovered within two or three hours and is so large that treatment seems desirable, gastric lavage can be safely used. There are no specific antidotes and further treatment should be symptomatic.

Pharmaceutical precautions Store in cool, dry conditions; shelf-life five years.

Legal category POM.

Package quantities 21 tablets.

Further information Nil.

Product licence number 0053/5014.

CYCLO-PROGYNOVA* 1 mg
CYCLO-PROGYNOVA* 2 mg

Presentation *Cyclo-Progynova 1 mg:* The circular memo-pack holds 11 beige tablets, each containing 1 mg oestradiol valerate, and 10 light-brown tablets, each containing 1 mg oestradiol valerate and 0.25 mg levonorgestrel. All tablets have a lustrous, sugar coating, and bear a black B in a black regular hexagon printed on both sides.

Cyclo-Progynova 2 mg: The circular memo-pack holds 11 white tablets, each containing 2 mg oestradiol valerate, and 10 pale brown tablets, each containing 2 mg oestradiol valerate and 0.5 mg norgestrel. All tablets have a lustrous, sugar coating and bear a red B in a red regular hexagon printed on both sides.

Uses The treatment of the climacteric syndrome. The prophylaxis and treatment of the postmenopausal sequelae of oestrogen withdrawal, e.g. osteoporosis and senile vaginitis.

Cyclo-Progynova 1 mg and Cyclo-Progynova 2 mg are designed to provide hormone replacement therapy during and after the climacteric. The addition of a progestogen in the second half of each course helps to provide good control of the irregular cycles that are characteristic of the premenopausal phase and opposes the production of endometrial hyperplasia. Whilst natural hormone production is little affected, Cyclo-Progynova 1 mg and Cyclo-Progynova 2 mg abolish or improve the characteristic symptoms of the climacteric such as hot flushes, sweating attacks and sleep disorders.

Cyclo-Progynova 1 mg and Cyclo-Progynova 2 mg do not consistently inhibit ovulation and are therefore unsuitable for contraception.

Dosage and administration If the patient is still

menstruating freely, treatment should begin on the 5th day of menstruation. Patients whose periods are very infrequent or who are postmenopausal may start at any time, provided pregnancy has been excluded (see Precautions and special information).

Initial treatment should be with Cyclo-Progynova 1 mg. One beige tablet is taken daily for 11 days, followed by one light-brown tablet daily for 10 days. An interval of seven days follows, during which bleeding will normally occur. Cyclo-Progynova 2 mg should be substituted if the control of climacteric symptoms or dysfunctional bleeding is not fully achieved at the lower dosage. One white tablet is taken daily for 11 days, followed by one pale brown tablet for 10 days. An interval of seven days again follows, during which bleeding is to be expected.

When symptoms have been controlled, Cyclo-Progynova 1 mg will usually suffice for maintenance, but it should be borne in mind that the appropriate dosage will be determined by the rate of metabolism of Cyclo-Progynova, rather than by the initial severity of the symptoms.

Contra-indications, warnings, etc

Contra-indications: Pregnancy, (see Precautions and special information) severe disturbances of liver function, jaundice or general pruritus during a previous pregnancy, Dubin-Johnson syndrome, Rotor syndrome, existing or previous thromboembolic processes, sickle-cell anaemia, suspected or existing hormone-dependent disorders or tumours of the uterus and breast, congenital disturbances of lipid metabolism, a history of herpes gestationis, otosclerosis with deterioration in previous pregnancies.

Warnings/side-effects: Hormonal contraception should be stopped when Cyclo-Progynova is started and the patient should be advised to take non-hormonal contraceptive precautions. The following symptoms have been reported during treatment: anxiety, increased appetite, bloating, breast symptoms, cardiac symptoms, depression, dizziness, dyspepsia, leg pains and swelling, altered libido, nausea, rashes, vomiting and altered weight.

Some women are predisposed to cholestasis during steroid therapy.

Diseases that are known to be subject to deterioration during pregnancy (e.g. multiple sclerosis, epilepsy, diabetes, hypertension, porphyria, tetany and otosclerosis) should be carefully observed during treatment.

Precautions and special information: Before starting treatment, pregnancy must be excluded. If withdrawal bleeding fails to occur at about 28-day intervals, treatment should be stopped until pregnancy has been ruled out.

Treatment should be stopped at once if migrainous or frequent and unusually severe headaches occur for the first time, or if there are other symptoms that are possible prodromata of vascular occlusion.

Treatment should also be stopped if trauma, illness or impending surgery is considered to entail a risk of thrombosis.

Treatment should be stopped at once if jaundice or pregnancy occurs, or if there is a significant rise in blood-pressure.

In patients with mild chronic liver disease, liver function should be checked every 8–12 weeks.

Examination of the pelvic organs, endometrium, breasts and blood-pressure is advised before and periodically during treatment with Cyclo-Progynova.

Irregular bleeding during tablet-taking should be investigated.

Prolonged exposure to unopposed oestrogens may increase the risk of development of endometrial carcinoma. The general consensus of opinion is that the addition of 10 days progestogen towards the end of the cycle, as in Cyclo-Progynova, diminishes the possibility of such a risk, and some investigators consider that it might be protective.

Overdosage: There have been no reports of ill-effects from overdosage which it is, therefore, generally unnecessary to treat. If overdosage is discovered within two or three hours and is so large that treatment seems desirable, gastric lavage can safely be used. There are no specific antidotes, and further treatment should be symptomatic.

Pharmaceutical precautions Store in cool, dry conditions. Shelf-life five years.

Legal category POM.

Package quantities Each outer carton contains a memo-pack containing 21 tablets.

Further information Nil.

Product licence numbers
Cyclo-Progynova 1 mg   0053/0108
Cyclo-Progynova 2 mg   0053/0053

CYPROSTAT*

Presentation Each round white, 9 mm tablet is impressed on one side with 'BV' in a regular hexagon, and is scored on the other. It contains 50 mg cyproterone acetate.

Uses Palliative treatment of prostatic carcinoma.

Cyprostat may be used alone or in conjunction with surgery. (See Further Information.)

Dosage and administration The usual daily dose is 300 mg (6 tablets) orally, divided into 2–3 doses and taken after meals. Cyprostat therapy should not be discontinued when remission or improvement occurs. The dose may be reduced if side-effects are troublesome, but should be kept within the range of 200–300 mg daily.

Contra-indications, warnings, etc
Contra-indications: None.

Warnings, Side-effects: Liver: Cyproterone acetate has been found to cause liver abnormalities in animals, including the development of tumours. Liver function tests are sometimes altered during treatment with Cyprostat and should therefore be performed regularly.

Inhibition of spermatogenesis: The sperm count and the volume of ejaculate are reduced. Infertility is usual, and there may be azoospermia after 8 weeks. There is usually slight atrophy of seminiferous tubules. Follow-up examinations have shown these changes to be reversible, spermatogenesis usually reverting to its previous state about 3–5 months after stopping Cyprostat, or in some users, up to 20 months. That spermatogenesis can recover even after very long treatment is not yet known. There is evidence that abnormal sperms which might give rise to malformed embryos are produced during treatment with Cyprostat.

Thromboembolism: Patients with a history of thrombosis may be at risk of recurrence of the disease during Cyprostat therapy.

Chronic depression: It has been found that some patients

with severe chronic depression deteriorate whilst taking Cyprostat therapy.

Tiredness: Fatigue and lassitude are common in the first few weeks of therapy but usually become much less from the third month. The marked lassitude and asthenia necessitate especial care when driving or operating machinery.

Gynaecomastia: Transient, and perhaps in some cases permanent, enlargement of the mammary glands has been reported. In rare cases, galactorrhoea and tender benign nodules have been reported. Symptoms generally subside after discontinuation of treatment or on reduction of dosage, but this should be weighed against the risk to the tumour of using inadequate doses.

Body weight: During long-term treatment, changes in body weight have been reported. Both increases and decreases have been seen.

Other changes that have been reported include reduction of sebum production leading to dryness of the skin, and transient patchy loss of body hair.

Adrenocortical function: During treatment adrenocortical function should be supervised, since suppression has been observed in children taking cyproterone acetate.

Diabetes: Cyprostat can influence carbohydrate metabolism. Parameters of carbohydrate metabolism should be examined carefully in all diabetics before and regularly during treatment.

Chronic alcoholism: The chronic abuse of alcohol appears to reduce the effect of cyproterone acetate in male hypersexuality, but the relevance of this to the treatment of prostatic carcinoma is not known.

Haemoglobin: Hypochromic anaemia has been found rarely during long-term treatment, and blood-counts before and at regular intervals during treatment are advisable.

Nitrogen balance: A negative balance is usual at the start of treatment, but does not persist.

Overdosage: There have been no reports of ill-effects of overdosage, which it is, therefore, generally unnecessary to treat. If overdosage is discovered within two or three hours and is so large that treatment seems desirable, gastric lavage can safely be used. There are no specific antidotes, and further treatment should be symptomatic.

Pharmaceutical precautions Store in cool, dry conditions away from strong sunlight. *Shelf-life:* five years.

Package quantities: Containers of 200 tablets.

Legal category: POM.

Further information: Prostatic carcinoma and its metastases are in general androgen-dependent. Cyprostat exerts a direct antiandrogenic action on the tumour and its metastases, and in addition it exerts a negative feedback effect on the hypothalamic receptors, so leading to a reduction in gonadotrophin release, and hence to diminished production of testicular androgens.

Product licence number 0053/0133.

DEPOSTAT*

Presentation Gestronol hexanoate in oily solution for intramuscular administration. Ampoules containing 200 mg in 2 ml.

Uses Endometrial carcinoma. Benign prostatic hyper-

plasia. Depostat is a depot progestogen, in a concentrated injectable non-aqueous solution, and is 25 times more potent than its parent substance progesterone. In the female, the action of Depostat is concentrated on the endometrium. This action is direct and does not involve suppression via the pituitary. Except in some highly anaplastic tumours, Depostat has a strong antimitotic effect, with regression or arrest of primary endometrial carcinoma and of soft-tissue metastases.

In the male, Depostat has been shown to reduce prostatic weight significantly. It may effect an objective improvement in peak urine flow rates and residual urine and in subjective symptoms such as nocturia.

Dosage and administration Endometrial carcinoma, before hysterectomy and for advanced disease. A well-tolerated adjunct to other therapy. To inhibit metastatic spread before and after operation, 200–400 mg intramuscularly every 5–7 days, starting immediately following diagnosis and continuing for a minimum of 12 weeks.

For treating existing metastases: 200–400 mg intramuscularly every 5–7 days. If the metastases are hormone-responsive, improvement will be observed within 8-12 weeks of therapy. Treatment should then be continued as long as it appears beneficial.

Benign prostatic hyperplasia where a) the patient is an operation risk; b) symptoms are mild; c) there is a waiting list for operation: standard dosage is 200 mg weekly by intramuscular injection, but in view of Depostat's good tolerance, this dosage can confidently be increased. In trials, 300 mg and 400 mg weekly have been used. The full benefit of treatment is unlikely to be established in a shorter period than three months, and trial results suggest that improvement can continue during substantially longer periods.

Contra-indications, warnings, etc
Contra-indications: Pregnancy, History of herpes gestationis.

Warning/side-effects: Rarely, local reactions may occur at the site of injection. Exacerbation of bronchial asthma, epilepsy and migraine may sometimes occur.

Side-effects are infrequent. In males, a reversible depression of libido and mammary discomfort have been reported by a few patients. Spermatogenesis is temporarily inhibited. In rare cases coughing, dyspnoea and circulatory irregularities may develop during or immediately after the injection.

Tolerance: In patients with chronic liver damage it is advisable to check liver function at intervals during long-term treatment or repeated courses of Depostat. Transient moderate rises in bromsulphthalein retention and serum transaminases have occasionally been observed but have always proved harmless.

Pharmaceutical precautions Store in cool dry conditions away from strong sunlight: shelf-life five years.

Legal category POM.

Package quantities 5 ampoules of 2 ml.

Further information Nil.

Product licence number 0053/0018.

DIANE ▼

Presentation Each pink, sugar-coated tablet, bearing a printed 'c' in a regular hexagon on both sides, contains

2 mg of the anti-androgen cyproterone acetate and 0.05 mg of the oestrogen ethinyloestradiol.

Uses *In women only:* (a) Severe acne, refractory to prolonged oral antibiotic therapy and (b) Idiopathic hirsutism of mild to moderate degree.

Diane blocks androgen-receptors. It also reduces androgen synthesis both by a negative feedback effect on the hypothalamo-pituitary-ovarian systems and by the inhibition of androgen-synthesising enzymes.

Although Diane also acts as an oral contraceptive, it is not recommended in women solely for contraception, but should be reserved for those women requiring treatment for the androgen-dependent skin conditions described.

Complete remission of acne is to be expected in nearly all cases, often within a few months, but in particularly severe cases treatment for longer may be necessary before the full benefit is seen. It is recommended that treatment be withdrawn when the acne or hirsutism has completely resolved. Repeat courses of Diane may be given if the condition recurs.

Dosage and administration *First treatment course:* 1 tablet daily for 21 days, starting on the 5th day of the menstrual cycle (the first day of mestruation counting as Day 1).

Subsequent courses: Each subsequent course is started after 7 tablet-free days have followed the preceding course.

When the contraceptive action of Diane is also to be employed, it is essential that the above instructions be rigidly adhered to. Other contraceptive precautions (excluding oral contraceptives and other hormonal methods and the rhythm, temperature or cervical-mucus methods) should be taken during the first 14 days of tablet-taking. Should bleeding fail to occur at the usual time, the possibility of pregnancy **must** be excluded before the next pack is started. In addition, the following circumstances in which the contraceptive action of Diane may be diminished should be noted:

Special circumstances requiring additional contraception – incorrect administration: If a tablet is delayed, it should be taken as soon as possible, and if it is taken within 12 hours of the correct time additional contraception is not needed. Further tablets should then be taken at the usual time. However, if the delay exceeds 12 hours, ovulation may occur. In those circumstances, any tablet or tablets delayed more than 12 hours should be omitted, the remaining tablets should be taken on the correct days at the usual time, and extra precautions (except the rhythm, temperature or cervical-mucus methods) should be used until the next withdrawal bleed.

Gastro-intestinal upset: Vomiting or diarrhoea may reduce the contraceptive effectiveness of the tablets by preventing them from being fully absorbed. Therefore, it is advisable that an additional method of contraception be used throughout the remainder of the course concerned. Mild laxatives do not impair contraceptive action.

Interaction with other drugs: Some drugs taken concurrently accelerate the metabolism of Diane. Drugs suspected of having the capacity to reduce the contraceptive efficacy of Diane include barbiturates, phenytoin, phenylbutazone, rifampicin, ampicillin and other antibiotics. The possibility cannot be ruled out that oral tetracyclines, if used in conjunction with Diane may have such an effect, although it has not been shown. When drugs of these classes are being taken, it is, therefore, advisable to use additional methods of contraception (excluding oral contraceptives and other hormonal methods) since an extremely high degree of protection must be provided when Diane is being taken.

Contra-indications, warnings, etc
Contra-indications: Pregnancy (see second paragraph of 'Warnings'). Lactation. Thrombotic disorders and a history of these conditions, sickle-cell anaemia, disorders of lipid metabolism and other conditions in which, in individual cases, there is known or suspected to be a much increased risk of thrombosis. Acute or severe chronic liver diseases. Dubin–Johnson syndrome. Rotor syndrome. History, during pregnancy, of idiopathic jaundice or severe pruritus. History of herpes gestationis. Mammary or endometrial carcinoma, or a history of these conditions. Abnormal vaginal bleeding of unknown cause. Deterioration of otosclerosis during pregnancy.

Warnings: Like many other steroids, Diane, when given in very high doses and for the majority of the animal's life-span, has been found to cause an increase in the incidence of tumours, including carcinoma, in the liver of rats. The relevance of this finding to humans is unknown. Diane has been shown to have good liver tolerance in women given prolonged treatment.

Animal studies have revealed that feminisation of male foetuses may occur if cyproterone acetate is administered during the phase of embryogenesis at which differentiation of the external genitalia occurs. Although the results of these tests are not necessarily relevant to man, the possibility must be considered that administration of Diane to women after the 45th day of pregnancy could cause feminisation of male foetuses. It follows from this that pregnancy is an absolute contra-indication for treatment with Diane, and must be excluded before such treatment is begun.

Although its strong anti-androgenic effect is distinctive, Diane has many properties in common with combined oral contraceptives, which must not be taken during treatment with Diane. There is a general opinion, based on statistical evidence, that users of combined oral contraceptives experience, more often than non-users, venous thromboembolism, arterial thrombosis, including cerebral and myocardial infarction, and subarachnoid haemorrhage. Full recovery from such disorders does not always occur, and it should be realised that in a few cases they are fatal.

Certain factors may entail some risk of thrombosis, e.g. smoking, obesity, varicose veins, cardiovascular diseases, diabetes and migraine. The risk of arterial thrombosis associated with combined oral contraceptives increases with age, and this risk is aggravated by cigarette-smoking. The suitability of Diane should be judged according to the severity of such conditions in the individual case, and should be discussed with the patient before she decides to take it.

The possibility cannot be ruled out that certain chronic diseases may occasionally deteriorate during the use of Diane (see 'Precautions').

Reasons for stopping medication immediately: Occurrence of migraine in patients who have never previously suffered from it. Exacerbation of pre-existing migraine. Any unusually frequent or unusually severe headaches. Any kind of acute disturbances of vision. Suspicion of thrombosis or infarction. Jaundice. Six weeks before elective operations and during immobilisation, e.g. after accidents, etc. Significant rise in blood pressure. Clear exacerbation of conditions known to be capable of deteriorating during oral contraception or pregnancy. Pregnancy is a reason for stopping immediately, not only because of the possible specific risk to a male foetus referred to above, but also because it has been suggested by some investigations that oral contraceptives taken in early pregnancy may slightly increase the risk of foetal malformations in general. Other investigations have failed to support these findings. The possibility therefore cannot be excluded, but it is certain that, if a risk of general malformations exists at all, it is very small.

Precautions: Examination of the pelvic organs, breasts and blood-pressure should precede the prescribing of Diane, and should be repeated regularly.

The following conditions require careful observation during medication: a history of severe depressive states, varicose veins, diabetes, hypertension, epilepsy, otosclerosis, multiple sclerosis, porphyria, tetany, disturbed liver function, gall-stones, cardiovascular diseases, renal diseases, chloasma, uterine fibroids, asthma, the wearing of contact lenses or any disease that is prone to worsen during pregnancy. The deterioration or first appearance of any of these conditions may indicate that Diane should be stopped.

It should be borne in mind that the use of ultraviolet lamps for the treatment of acne, or prolonged exposure to sunlight, increases the risk of the deterioration of chloasma.

Side-effects: Occasional side-effects may include: nausea, vomiting, headaches, breast tension, changed body weight or libido, depressive moods and chloasma.

Menstrual changes: 1. Reduction of flow. This is not abnormal and it is to be expected in some patients.

2. Missed menstruation. If withdrawal bleeding does not occur, pregnancy must be excluded by a pregnancy test after a suitable interval before a new course of tablets is started.

Intermenstrual bleeding: Very light 'spotting' or heavier 'breakthrough bleeding' may occur during tablet-taking, especially in the first few cycles. It appears to be generally of no significance, except where it indicates errors of tablet-taking, or where the possibility of interaction with other drugs exist (*q.v.*). However, if irregular bleeding is persistent, an organic cause should be considered.

Effect on thyroid glands: The radio-iodine uptake shows that thyroid function is unchanged. There is a rise in serum protein-bound iodine, similar to that in pregnancy and during the administration of oestrogens. This is due to the increased capacity of the plasma proteins for binding thyroid hormones, rather than to any change in glandular function. In women taking Diane, the content of protein-bound iodine in blood serum should, therefore, not be used for the evaluation of thyroid function.

Effect on blood chemistry: Diane may accelerate erythrocyte sedimentation in the absence of any disease. This effect is due to change in the proportion of the plasma protein fractions. Increases in plasma copper, iron and alkaline phosphates have also been recorded.

Overdose: There have been no reports concerning overdosage, but, on general principles from a knowledge of the pharmacological actions of the constituents of Diane, it would seem unnecessary to treat. However, if overdose is discovered within two or three hours and is so large that treatment seems desirable, gastric lavage can be safely used. There are no specific antidotes and further treatment should be symptomatic.

Pharmaceutical precautions Storage: cool, dry conditions. Shelf-life: five years.

Legal category POM.

Package quantities Outer carton contains three memo-packs; each containing 21 tablets.

Further information Nil.

Product licence number 0053/0116.

EUGYNON* 30
EUGYNON* 50
MICROGYNON* 30

Presentation *Eugynon 30:* Each white, sugar-coated tablet bears a printed black C in a regular hexagon on both sides and contains 0.25 mg levonorgestrel and 0.03 mg ethinyloestradiol.

Eugynon 50: Each white, sugar-coated tablet contains 0.25 mg levonorgestrel in 0.5 mg norgestrel, and 0.05 mg ethinyloestradiol.

Microgynon 30: Each beige, sugar-coated tablet bears a black A in a black hexagon printed on both sides and contains 0.15 mg levonorgestrel and 0.03 mg ethinyloestradiol.

Uses Oral contraception and the recognised gynaecological indications for such oestrogen-progestogen combinations. The mode of action includes the inhibition of ovulation by suppression of the mid-cycle surge of luteinising hormone, the inspissation of cervical mucus so as to constitute a barrier to sperm, and the rendering of the endometrium unreceptive to implantation.

Dosage and administration *First treatment cycle:* 1 tablet daily for 21 days, starting on the fifth day of the menstrual cycle (the first day of menstruation counting as day 1). In the first cycle only, an additional form of contraception (except the rhythm, temperature or cervical-mucus methods) must be used for the first 14 days of tablet-taking.

Subsequent cycles: Each subsequent course is started after seven tablet-free days have followed the preceding course.

Changing from high-dosed to low-dosed preparations: Additional (non-hormonal) precautions, other than the rhythm, temperature or cervical-mucus methods, should also be used for the first 14 days when changing products.

Post-partum and post-abortum use: After pregnancy oral contraception is usually started as soon as spontaneous menstruation has been resumed. However, oral contraception can be started within 7–12 days of a vaginal delivery, provided that the patient is fully ambulant and there are no puerperal complications. Starting within 12 days of delivery obviates additional contraceptive precautions. After a first-trimester abortion, oral contraception may be started immediately.

Special circumstances requiring additional contraception: Incorrect administration: If a tablet is delayed, it should be taken as soon as possible, and if it is taken within 12 hours of the correct time additional contraception is not needed. Further tablets should then be taken at the usual time. However, if the delay exceeds 12 hours, ovulation may occur. In those circumstances, any tablet or tablets delayed more than 12 hours should be omitted, the remaining tablets should be taken on the correct days at the usual time, and extra precautions (except the rhythm, temperature and cervical-mucus methods) should be used until the next withdrawal bleed.

Gastro-intestinal upset: Vomiting or diarrhoea may reduce the effectiveness of the tablets by preventing them from being fully absorbed. Therefore, it is advisable that an additional method of contraception be used throughout the remainder of the course concerned. Mild laxatives do not impair contraceptive action.

Interaction with other drugs: Some drugs accelerate the metabolism of oral contraceptives taken concurrently. Drugs suspected of having the capacity to reduce the efficacy of oral contraceptives include barbiturates, phenytoin, phenylbutazone, rifampicin, ampicillin and other antibiotics. It is, therefore, advisable to use non-hormonal methods of contraception (except the rhythm, temperature or cervical-mucus methods) in addition to the oral contraceptive as long as an extremely high degree of protection must be provided during treatment with such drugs.

Contra-indications, warnings, etc
Contra-indications: Pregnancy. Thrombotic disorders and a history of these conditions, sickle-cell anaemia, disorders of lipid metabolism and other conditions in which, in individual cases, there is known or suspected to be a much increased risk of thrombosis. Acute or severe chronic liver diseases. Dubin-Johnson syndrome. Rotor syndrome. History, during pregnancy, of idiopathic jaundice or severe pruritus. History of herpes gestationis. Mammary or endometrial carcinoma, or a history of these conditions. Abnormal vaginal bleeding of unknown cause. Deterioration of otosclerosis during pregnancy.

Warnings: There is a general opinion, based on statistical evidence, that users of combined oral contraceptives experience, more often than non-users, venous thromboembolism, arterial thrombosis, including cerebral and myocardial infarction, and subarachnoid haemorrhage. Full recovery from such disorders does not always occur, and it should be realised that in a few cases they are fatal. How often these disorders occur in users of the modern low-dose pills is not known, but there are reasons for suggesting that they may occur less often than with older pills.

Certain factors may entail some risk of thrombosis, e.g. smoking, obesity, varicose veins, cardiovascular diseases, diabetes and migraine. The suitability of a combined oral contraceptive should be judged according to the severity of such conditions in the individual case, and should be discussed with the patient before she decides to take it. The risk of arterial thrombosis associated with oral contraceptives increases with age, and this risk is aggravated by cigarette-smoking. The use of combined oral contraceptives by women in the older age-group, especially those who are cigarette-smokers should therefore be discouraged, and alternative methods advised.

The possibility cannot be ruled out that certain chronic diseases may occasionally deteriorate during the use of combined oral contraceptives (see 'Precautions'). Hepatic tumours have been reported very rarely in women taking combined oral contraceptives, generally for a protracted period of time. A hepatic tumour should be considered in the differential diagnosis when upper abdominal pain, enlarged liver or signs of intra-abdominal haemorrhage occur.

Reasons for stopping oral contraception immediately: Occurrence of migraine in patients who have never previously suffered from it. Exacerbation of pre-existing migraine. Any unusually frequent or unusually severe headaches. Any kind of acute disturbance of vision. Suspicion of thrombosis or infarction. Six weeks before elective operations and during immobilisation, e.g. after accidents, etc. Significant rise in blood-pressure. Jaundice. Clear exacerbation of conditions known to be capable of deteriorating during oral contraception or pregnancy. Pregnancy is a reason for stopping immediately because it has been suggested by some investigations that oral contraceptives taken in early pregnancy may slightly increase the risk of foetal malformations. Other investigations have failed to support these findings. The possibility therefore cannot be excluded, but it is certain that if a risk exists at all, it is very small.

Precautions: Examination of the pelvic organs, breasts and blood-pressure should precede the prescribing of any combined oral contraceptive, and should be repeated regularly. Before starting treatment, pregnancy must be excluded.

The following conditions require careful consideration: a history of severe depressive states, varicose veins, diabetes, hypertension, epilepsy, otosclerosis, multiple sclerosis, porphyria, tetany, disturbed liver function, gallstones, cardiovascular diseases, renal diseases, chloasma, uterine fibroids, asthma, the wearing of contact lenses, or any disease that is prone to worsen during pregnancy. The first appearance or deterioration of any of these conditions may indicate that the oral contraceptive should be stopped.

The risk of the deterioration of chloasma, which is often not fully reversible, is reduced by the avoidance of excessive exposure to sunlight.

Side-effects: Occasional side-effects may include nausea, vomiting, headaches, breast tension, changed body weight or libido, depressive moods and chloasma.

Menstrual changes:

1. *Reduction of menstrual flow:* This is not abnormal and it is to be expected in some patients. Indeed, it may be beneficial where heavy periods were previously experienced.

2. *Missed menstruation:* Occasionally, withdrawal bleeding may not occur at all. If the tablets have been taken correctly, pregnancy is very unlikely, but should be ruled out before a new course of tablets is started.

Intermenstrual bleeding: Very light 'spotting' or heavier 'breakthrough bleeding' may occur during tablet-taking, especially in the first few cycles. It appears to be generally of no significance, except where it indicates errors of tablet-taking, or where the possibility of interaction with other drugs exists (q.v.). However, if irregular bleeding is persistent, an organic cause should be considered.

Effect on adrenal and thyroid glands: Oral contraceptives have no significant influence on adrenocortical function. The ACTH function test for the adrenal cortex remains unchanged. The reduction in corticosteroid excretion and the elevation of plasma corticosteroids are due to an increased cortisol-binding capacity of the plasma proteins.

The response to metyrapone is less pronounced than in untreated women and is thus similar to that during pregnancy.

The radio-iodine uptake shows that thyroid function is unchanged. There is a rise in serum protein-bound iodine, similar to that in pregnancy and during the administration of oestrogens. This is due to the increased capacity of the plasma proteins for binding thyroid hormones, rather than to any change in glandular function. In women taking oral contraceptives, the content of protein-bound iodine in blood serum should, therefore, not be used for evaluation of thyroid function.

Effect on blood chemistry: Oral contraceptives may accelerate erythrocyte sedimentation in the absence of any disease. This effect is due to a change in the proportion of the plasma protein fractions. Increases in plasma copper, iron and alkaline phosphatase have also been recorded.

Overdosage: There have been no reports of serious ill-effects from overdosage, even when a considerable number of tablets have been taken by a small child. In general, it is, therefore, unnecessary to treat overdosage. However, if overdosage is discovered within two or three hours and is so large that treatment seems desirable, gastric lavage can be safely used.

There are no specific antidotes and further treatment should be symptomatic.

Pharmaceutical precautions Store in cool, dry conditions.

Shelf-life:
Eugynon 30 and Microgynon 30 – 5 years.
Eugynon 50 – 7 years.

Legal category POM.

Package quantities All Schering combined oral contraceptives are available in packs containing one month's supply.

Further information Nil.

Product licence numbers
Eugynon 30   0053/0049
Eugynon 50   0053/0061
Microgynon 30   0053/0064

GASTROGRAFIN*

Presentation Gastrografin contains 10% sodium diatrizoate and 66% meglumine diatrizoate in aqueous solution, with added flavouring and wetting agents. The iodine content is 370 mg/ml.

Uses Gastrografin is designed for investigation of the gastro-intestinal tract. It can be used either orally or as an enema. Follow-through examinations with barium can often be improved by combining it with Gastrografin. Gastrografin is of considerable value in the following instances.

1. Suspected partial or complete stenosis.
2. Acute haemorrhage.
3. Threatening perforation (peptic ulcer, diverti-culum).
4. Megacolon.
5. Foreign bodies or tumours.
6. Gastro-colic fistula.
7. Before endoscopy.

Gastrografin is also recommended for the treatment of uncomplicated meconium ileus.

Dosage and administration *Oral – Adults and children of 10 years of age or over:* 60 ml Gastrografin are sufficient for the visualisation of the stomach. Up to 100 ml may be needed for a follow-through examination of the gastro-intestinal tract.

For computerised tomography 1 to 1.5 litres of a 3% solution of Gastrografin in water (30 ml/litre).

For elderly or cachetic patients: Dilution with an equal volume of water is recommended.

Children up to 10 years of age: 15–30 ml are usually sufficient. This dose may be diluted with twice its volume of water.

For infants and young children: It is recommended that the contrast medium be diluted with three times its volume of water.

Rectal – Adults: The contrast medium should be diluted with three to four times its volume of water. Not more than 500 ml of Gastrografin solution should normally be required.

Children: The contrast medium should be diluted with four to five times its volume of water; up to five years of age the weaker dilution should be used.

Gastrografin and Barium Sulphate: Oral and rectal administration.

Adults: 30 ml Gastrografin plus the usual dose of barium should be adequate.

Children: 10 ml Gastrografin may be added to the barium.

For children up to five years of age: from 2–5 ml Gastrografin to 100 ml barium may be preferable. Further dilution which does not affect the contrast may be used if necessary in cases of pylorospasm or pyloric stenosis.

For the early diagnosis of a perforation or anastomosis in the oesophagus or gastro-intestinal tract, the patient should drink 100 ml Gastrografin. After 30–60 minutes (later, if the defect is suspected of being in the distal gut), a urine specimen should be taken and 5 ml mixed with 5 drops of concentrated hydrochloric acid. The contrast medium which has undergone renal excretion will appear within two hours as a typical crystal formation in the precipitate.

Technique for the treatment of uncomplicated meconium ileus: Gastrografin can be given by enema to infants for non-operative treatment of uncomplicated meconium ileus, i.e. in the absence of volvulus, gangrene, perforation, peritonitis or atresia, all of which require immediate operation.

A large syringe and soft rubber catheter, No. 8 French, are recommended. The buttocks can be taped tightly together to minimise leakage but a Foley catheter should not be used. The procedure must be carried out slowly and only under fluoroscopic control. Injection should stop as soon as Gastrografin is seen to enter the ileum. Owing to its high osmolality, Gastrografin may cause the loss of a large amount of fluid into the intestines. An intravenous drip must therefore be set up before the enema is given and plasma should be infused as required. If the Gastrografin is not expelled during the first hour after removal of the rectal catheter, an X-ray should be taken to ensure that over-distension of the bowel as a result of the high osmolarity of Gastrografin has not occurred.

Contra-indications, warnings, etc
Contra-indications: Hypersensitivity to iodine-containing contrast media.

Warnings/side-effects: In dehydrated patients, especially in severely dehydrated infants and young children, the need for examination merits particularly careful consideration. Disturbances in water or electrolyte balance must first be corrected.

Because of its high osmotic pressure and minima

absorption, Gastrografin should not be administered to infants in higher doses than those recommended above.

Caution should be observed in patients with thyroid disease. Aspiration of Gastrografin into the lungs may cause pulmonary oedema. Caution is needed with oesophagotracheal fistulae to avoid passage of the medium into the lungs. Systemic effects are rare, since Gastrografin is only minimally absorbed from the alimentary tract.

Owing to its hypertonicity, Gastrografin may occasionally cause diarrhoea.

Existing enteritis or colitis may be temporarily exacerbated.

Pharmaceutical precautions *Storage:* Protect from light and heat. Shelf-life five years.

Legal category P.

Package quantities Bottles 5 × 100 ml.

Further information Nil.

Product licence number 0053/5023.

GONDAFON*

Presentation Each white, half-scored, torpedo-shaped tablet contains 500 mg of glymidine (the sodium salt of 2-benzene-sulphonamido-5-methoxyethoxy-pyrimidine).

Uses Non-insulin-dependent mellitus (type II) not adequately controlled by diet alone.

Dosage and administration Generally, initial dosage of 2–3 tablets daily with breakfast, or rarely 2 with breakfast and 1 in the late afternoon. After stabilisation, 1 or 2 tablets with breakfast often suffices.

The maximum permissible dosage of 4 tablets daily should be taken as 3 tablets with breakfast and 1 in the late afternoon.

Contra-indications, warnings, etc

Contra-indications: Pregnancy: diabetic coma and pre-coma; acetonuria, all forms of metabolic decompensation during infection, operations and severe stress conditions. Severe hepatic and renal disease.

As with all benzenesulphonamides, treatment should be stopped immediately if allergies or blood dyscrasias occur. Similarly, any patient likely to undergo a major operation should probably be transferred temporarily to insulin therapy.

Although Gondafon has a short biological half-life, care should be taken to avoid insidious hypoglycaemia in the elderly patient. This can be mistaken for a stroke.

There is no known cross-allergy between Gondafon and other sulphonylureas or sulphonamides. However, caution is recommended in giving Gondafon to a person with a history of allergy to either of these classes of compound.

Gondafon reduces the tolerance of ethyl alcohol.

Hypoglycaemia: Mild symptoms of hypoglycaemia should be treated with a sandwich. Severe hypoglycaemia in the conscious patient should be treated with 5 tablespoonfuls of sugar in a cup of tea or water or by 1 mg of glucagon intramuscularly and should be followed by a sandwich after symptoms have improved. Hypoglycaemic coma should be treated by 1 mg of glucagon intramuscularly or subcutaneously and 50–100 ml of 40% glucose or 50% dextrose solution intravenously.

After recovery, the patient should be watched for three days, and should be questioned so that the circumstances in which the hypoglycaemic attack occurred can be identified and its recurrence prevented.

Warnings: side-effects: Adverse reactions occur infrequently with Gondafon, but the commonest appear to be skin eruptions and gastro-intestinal disorders. Very rarely, leucopenia and purpura have been reported.

Pharmaceutical precautions Store in cool, dry conditions: shelf-life five years.

Legal category POM.

Package quantities Packs of 100 tablets.

Further information Nil.

Product licence number 0053/5004.

LOGYNON* (21-day)

Presentation The memo-pack holds six light-brown tablets containing 30 mcg ethinyloestradiol and 50 mcg levonorgestrel, five white tablets containing 40 mcg ethinyloestradiol and 75 mcg levonorgestrel and ten ochre tablets containing 30 mcg ethinyloestradiol and 125 mcg levonorgestrel.

All tablets have a lustrous, sugar coating. The light-brown tablets bear a black C in a regular hexagon on both sides. The white and the ochre tablets bear a black B in a regular hexagon on both sides.

Uses Oral contraception and the recognised gynaecological indications for such oestrogen-progestogen combinations. The mode of action includes the inhibition of ovulation by suppression of the mid-cycle surge of luteinising hormone, the inspissation of cervical mucus so as to constitute a barrier to sperm, and the rendering of the endometrium unreceptive to implantation.

Dosage and administration *First treatment cycle:* 1 tablet daily for 21 days, starting with the tablet marked number 1, on the first day of the menstrual cycle.

Subsequent cycles: Each subsequent course is started when seven tablet-free days have followed the preceding course.

Changing from another combined oral contraceptive: The first tablet of Logynon should be taken on the first day of the withdrawal bleed which follows the previous oral contraceptive course. Alternatively where it is desirable to retain the previous routine of tablet-taking, Logynon may be started on the same day that the previous combined oral contraceptive would have been resumed, provided the patient has had a withdrawal bleed. In this case, however, additional (non-hormonal) contraceptive precautions, other than the rhythm, temperature or cervical-mucus methods, should also be used for the first 14 days.

Post-partum and post-abortum use: After pregnancy oral contraception is usually started as soon as spontaneous menstruation has been resumed. However, oral contraception can be started within 7–12 days of a vaginal delivery, provided that the patient is fully ambulant and there are no puerperal complications. Starting within 12 days of delivery obviates additional contraceptive precautions. After a first-trimester abortion, oral contraception may be started immediately.

Special circumstances requiring additional contraception: Incorrect administration: If a tablet is delayed, it should be taken as soon as possible, and if it is taken within 12 hours of the correct time additional contraception is not needed. Further tablets should then be taken at the usual time. However, if the delay exceeds 12 hours, ovulation may occur. In those circumstances, any tablet or tablets delayed more than 12 hours should be omitted, the remaining tablets should be taken on the correct days at the usual time, and extra precautions (except the rhythm, temperature or cervical-mucus methods) should be used until the next withdrawal bleed.

Gastro-intestinal upset: Vomiting or diarrhoea may reduce the effectiveness of the tablets by preventing them from being fully absorbed. Therefore, it is advisable that an additional method of contraception be used throughout the remainder of the course concerned. Mild laxatives do not impair contraceptive action.

Interaction with other drugs: Some drugs accelerate the metabolism of oral contraceptives taken concurrently. Drugs suspected of having the capacity to reduce the efficacy of oral contraceptives include barbiturates, phenytoin, phenylbutazone, rifampicin, ampicillin and other antibiotics. It is, therefore, advisable to use non-hormonal methods of contraception (except the rhythm, temperature or cervical-mucus methods) in addition to the oral contraceptive as long as an extremely high degree of protection must be provided during treatment with such drugs.

Contra-indications, warnings, etc

Contra-indications: Pregnancy. Thrombotic disorders and a history of these conditions, sickle-cell anaemia, disorders of lipid metabolism and other conditions in which, in individual cases, there is known or suspected to be a much increased risk of thrombosis. Acute or severe chronic liver diseases. Dubin-Johnson syndrome. Rotor syndrome. History, during pregnancy, of idiopathic jaundice or severe pruritus. History of herpes gestationis. Mammary or endometrial carcinoma, or a history of these conditions. Abnormal vaginal bleeding of unknown cause. Deterioration of otosclerosis during pregnancy.

Warnings: There is a general opinion, based on statistical evidence, that users of combined oral contraceptives experience, more often than non-users, venous thromboembolism, arterial thrombosis, including cerebral and myocardial infarction, and subarachnoid haemorrhage. Full recovery from such disorders does not always occur, and it should be realised that in a few cases they are fatal. How often these disorders occur in users of the modern low-dose pills is not known, but there are reasons for suggesting that they may occur less often than with older pills.

Certain factors may entail some risk of thrombosis, e.g. smoking, obesity, varicose veins, cardiovascular diseases, diabetes and migraine. The suitability of a combined oral contraceptive should be judged according to the severity of such conditions in the individual case, and should be discussed with the patient before she decides to take it. The risk of arterial thrombosis associated with oral contraceptives increases with age, and this risk is aggravated by cigarette-smoking. The use of combined oral contraceptives by women in the older age-group, especially those who are cigarette-smokers should therefore be discouraged, and alternative methods advised.

The possibility cannot be ruled out that certain chronic diseases may occasionally deteriorate during the use of combined oral contraceptives (see 'Precautions'). Hepatic tumours have been reported very rarely in women

taking combined oral contraceptives, generally for a protracted period of time. A hepatic tumour should be considered in the differential diagnosis when upper abdominal pain, enlarged liver or signs of intra-abdominal haemorrhage occur.

Reasons for stopping oral contraception immediately: Occurrence of migraine in patients who have never previously suffered from it. Exacerbation of pre-existing migraine. Any unusually frequent or unusually severe headaches. Any kind of acute disturbance of vision. Suspicion of thrombosis or infarction. Six weeks before elective operations and during immobilisation, e.g. after accidents, etc. Significant rise in blood-pressure. Jaundice. Clear exacerbation of conditions known to be capable of deteriorating during oral contraception or pregnancy. Pregnancy is a reason for stopping immediately because it has been suggested by some investigations that oral contraceptives taken in early pregnancy may slightly increase the risk of foetal malformations. Other investigations have failed to support these findings. The possibility therefore cannot be excluded, but it is certain that if a risk exists at all, it is very small.

Precautions: Examination of the pelvic organs, breasts and blood-pressure should precede the prescribing of any combined oral contraceptive, and should be repeated regularly. Before starting treatment, pregnancy must be excluded.

The following conditions require careful consideration: a history of severe depressive states, varicose veins, diabetes, hypertension, epilepsy, otosclerosis, multiple sclerosis, porphyria, tetany, disturbed liver function, gallstones, cardiovascular diseases, renal diseases, chloasma, uterine fibroids, asthma, the wearing of contact lenses, or any disease that is prone to worsen during pregnancy. The first appearance or deterioration of any of these conditions may indicate that the oral contraceptive should be stopped.

The risk of the deterioration of chloasma, which is often not fully reversible, is reduced by the avoidance of excessive exposure to sunlight.

Side-effects: Occasional side-effects may include nausea, vomiting, headaches, breast tension, changed body weight or libido, depressive moods and chloasma.

Menstrual changes:

1. *Reduction of menstrual flow:* This is not abnormal and it is to be expected in some patients. Indeed, it may be beneficial where heavy periods were previously experienced.

2. *Missed menstruation:* Occasionally, withdrawal bleeding may not occur at all. If the tablets have been taken correctly, pregnancy is very unlikely, but should be ruled out before a new course of tablets is started.

Intermenstrual bleeding: Very light 'spotting' or heavier 'breakthrough bleeding' may occur during tablet-taking, especially in the first few cycles. It appears to be generally of no significance, except where it indicates errors of tablet-taking, or where the possibility of interaction with other drugs exists (q.v.). However, if irregular bleeding is persistent, an organic cause should be considered.

Effect on adrenal and thyroid glands: Oral contraceptives have no significant influence on adrenocortical function. The ACTH function test for the adrenal cortex remains unchanged. The reduction in corticosteroid excretion and the elevation of plasma corticosteroids are due to an increased cortisol-binding capacity of the plasma proteins.

The response to metyrapone is less pronounced than in untreated women and is thus similar to that during pregnancy.

The radio-iodine uptake shows that thyroid function is unchanged. There is a rise in serum protein-bound iodine, similar to that in pregnancy and during the administration of oestrogens. This is due to the increased capacity of the plasma proteins for binding thyroid hormones, rather than to any change in glandular function. In women taking oral contraceptives, the content of protein-bound iodine in blood serum should, therefore, not be used for evaluation of thyroid function.

Effect on blood chemistry: Oral contraceptives may accelerate erythrocyte sedimentation in the absence of any disease. This effect is due to a change in the proportion of the plasma protein fractions. Increases in plasma copper, iron and alkaline phosphatase have also been recorded.

Overdosage: There have been no reports of serious ill-effects from overdosage, even when a considerable number of tablets have been taken by a small child. In general, it is, therefore, unnecessary to treat overdosage. However, if overdosage is discovered within two or three hours and is so large that treatment seems desirable, gastric lavage can be safely used.

There are no specific antidotes and further treatment should be symptomatic.

Pharmaceutical precautions Store in cool, dry conditions: shelf-life five years.

Legal category POM.

Package quantities All Schering combined oral contraceptives are available in packs containing one month's supply.

Further information Nil.

Product licence number 0053/0085.

LOGYNON* ED

Presentation The memo-pack holds six light-brown tablets containing 30 mcg ethinyloestradiol and 50 mcg levonorgestrel, five white tablets containing 40 mcg ethinyloestradiol and 75 mcg levonorgestrel, ten ochre tablets containing 30 mcg ethinyloestradiol and 125 mcg levonorgestrel and seven white placebo tablets.

All tablets have a lustrous, sugar coating. The light-brown tablets bear a black C in a regular hexagon printed on both sides. The white active tablets and the ochre tablets bear a black B in a regular hexagon on both sides. The white placebo tablets are larger and bear a black O in a regular hexagon.

Uses Oral contraception and the recognised gynaecological indications for such oestrogen-progestogen combinations. The mode of action includes the inhibition of ovulation by suppression of the mid-cycle surge of luteinising hormone, the inspissation of cervical mucus so as to constitute a barrier to sperm, and the rendering of the endometrium unreceptive to implantation.

Dosage and administration *First treatment cycle:* 1 tablet daily for 28 days, starting in the red sector on the first day of bleeding, the initial tablet being the one marked with the appropriate day of the week. In the first cycle only, an additional form of contraception (except the rhythm, temperature or cervical-mucus methods) must be used for the first 14 days of tablet-taking.

Subsequent cycles. Each subsequent course is started in the red sector on the day after the previous one has been finished. Pack, therefore, follows pack without interval.

Changing from high-dosed to low-dosed preparations: Additional (non-hormonal) precautions, other than the rhythm, temperature or cervical-mucus methods, should also be used for the first 14 days when changing products.

Post-partum and post-abortum use: After pregnancy oral contraception is usually started as soon as spontaneous menstruation has been resumed. However, oral contraception can be started within 7–12 days of a vaginal delivery, provided that the patient is fully ambulant and there are no puerperal complications. Starting within 12 days of delivery obviates additional contraceptive precautions. After a first-trimester abortion, oral contraception may be started immediately.

Special circumstances requiring additional contraception: Incorrect administration: If a tablet is delayed, it should be taken as soon as possible, and if it is taken within 12 hours of the correct time additional contraception is not needed. Further tablets should then be taken at the usual time. However, if the delay exceeds 12 hours, ovulation may occur. In those circumstances, any tablet or tablets delayed more than 12 hours should be omitted, the remaining tablets should be taken on the correct days at the usual time, and extra precautions (except the rhythm, temperature or cervical-mucus methods) should be used until the next withdrawal bleed.

Gastro-intestinal upset: Vomiting or diarrhoea may reduce the effectiveness of the tablets by preventing them from being fully absorbed. Therefore, it is advisable that an additional method of contraception be used throughout the remainder of the course concerned. Mild laxatives do not impair contraceptive action.

Interaction with other drugs: Some drugs accelerate the metabolism of oral contraceptives taken concurrently. Drugs suspected of having the capacity to reduce the efficacy of oral contraceptives include barbiturates, phenytoin, phenylbutazone, rifampicin, ampicillin and other antibiotics. It is, therefore, advisable to use non-hormonal methods of contraception (except the rhythm, temperature or cervical-mucus methods) in addition to the oral contraceptive as long as an extremely high degree of protection must be provided during treatment with such drugs.

Contra-indications, warnings, etc

Contra-indications: Pregnancy. Thrombotic disorders and a history of these conditions, sickle-cell anaemia, disorders of lipid metabolism and other conditions in which, in individual cases, there is known or suspected to be a much increased risk of thrombosis. Acute or severe chronic liver diseases. Dubin-Johnson syndrome. Rotor syndrome. History, during pregnancy, of idiopathic jaundice or severe pruritus. History of herpes gestationis. Mammary or endometrial carcinoma, or a history of these conditions. Abnormal vaginal bleeding of unknown cause. Deterioration of otosclerosis during pregnancy.

Warnings: There is a general opinion, based on statistical evidence, that users of combined oral contraceptives experience, more often than non-users, venous thromboembolism, arterial thrombosis, including cerebral and myocardial infarction, and subarachnoid haemorrhage. Full recovery from such disorders does not always occur, and it should be realised that in a few cases they are fatal. How often these disorders occur in users of the modern low-dose pills is not known, but there are reasons for suggesting that they may occur less often than with older pills.

Certain factors may entail some risk of thrombosis, e.g. smoking, obesity, varicose veins, cardiovascular diseases, diabetes and migraine. The suitability of a combined oral contraceptive should be judged according to the severity of such conditions in the individual case, and should be discussed with the patient before she decides to take it. The risk of arterial thrombosis associated with oral contraceptives increases with age, and this risk is aggravated by cigarette-smoking. The use of combined oral contraceptives by women in the older age-group, especially those who are cigarette-smokers should therefore be discouraged, and alternative methods advised.

The possibility cannot be ruled out that certain chronic diseases may occasionally deteriorate during the use of combined oral contraceptives (see 'Precautions'). Hepatic tumours have been reported very rarely in women taking combined oral contraceptives, generally for a protracted period of time. A hepatic tumour should be considered in the differential diagnosis when upper abdominal pain, enlarged liver or signs of intra-abdominal haemorrhage occur.

Reasons for stopping oral contraception immediately: Occurrence of migraine in patients who have never previously suffered from it. Exacerbation of pre-existing migraine. Any unusually frequent or unusually severe headaches. Any kind of acute disturbance of vision. Suspicion of thrombosis or infarction. Six weeks before elective operations and during immobilisation, e.g. after accidents, etc. Significant rise in blood-pressure. Jaundice. Clear exacerbation of conditions known to be capable of deteriorating during oral contraception or pregnancy. Pregnancy is a reason for stopping immediately because it has been suggested by some investigations that oral contraceptives taken in early pregnancy may slightly increase the risk of foetal malformations. Other investigations have failed to support these findings. The possibility therefore cannot be excluded, but it is certain that if a risk exists at all, it is very small.

Precautions: Examination of the pelvic organs, breasts and blood-pressure should precede the prescribing of any combined oral contraceptive, and should be repeated regularly. Before starting treatment, pregnancy must be excluded.

The following conditions require careful consideration: a history of severe depressive states, varicose veins, diabetes, hypertension, epilepsy, otosclerosis, multiple sclerosis, porphyria, tetany, disturbed liver function, gallstones, cardiovascular diseases, renal diseases, chloasma, uterine fibroids, asthma, the wearing of contact lenses, or any disease that is prone to worsen during pregnancy. The first appearance or deterioration of any of these conditions may indicate that the oral contraceptive should be stopped.

The risk of the deterioration of chloasma, which is often not fully reversible, is reduced by the avoidance of excessive exposure to sunlight.

Side-effects: Occasional side-effects may include nausea, vomiting, headaches, breast tension, changed body weight or libido, depressive moods and chloasma.

Menstrual changes:

1. *Reduction of menstrual flow:* This is not abnormal and it is to be expected in some patients. Indeed, it may be beneficial where heavy periods were previously experienced.

2. *Missed menstruation:* Occasionally, withdrawal bleeding may not occur at all. If the tablets have been taken correctly, pregnancy is very unlikely, but should be ruled out before a new course of tablets is started.

Intermenstrual bleeding: Very light 'spotting' or heavier 'breakthrough bleeding' may occur during tablet-taking, especially in the first few cycles. It appears to be generally of no significance, except where it indicates errors of tablet-taking, or where the possibility of interaction with other drugs exists (q.v.). However, if irregular bleeding is persistent, an organic cause should be considered.

Effect on adrenal and thyroid glands: Oral contraceptives have no significant influence on adrenocortical function. The ACTH function test for the adrenal cortex remains unchanged. The reduction in corticosteroid excretion and the elevation of plasma corticosteroids are due to an increased cortisol-binding capacity of the plasma proteins.

The response to metyrapone is less pronounced than in untreated women and is thus similar to that during pregnancy.

The radio-iodine uptake shows that thyroid function is unchanged. There is a rise in serum protein-bound iodine, similar to that in pregnancy and during the administration of oestrogens. This is due to the increased capacity of the plasma proteins for binding thyroid hormones, rather than to any change in glandular function. In women taking oral contraceptives, the content of protein-bound iodine in blood serum should, therefore, not be used for evaluation of thyroid function.

Effect on blood chemistry: Oral contraceptives may accelerate erythrocyte sedimentation in the absence of any disease. This effect is due to a change in the proportion of the plasma protein fractions. Increases in plasma copper, iron and alkaline phosphatase have also been recorded.

Overdosage: There have been no reports of serious ill-effects from overdosage, even when a considerable number of tablets have been taken by a small child. In general, it is, therefore, unnecessary to treat overdosage. However, if overdosage is discovered within two or three hours and is so large that treatment seems desirable, gastric lavage can be safely used.

There are no specific antidotes and further treatment should be symptomatic.

Pharmaceutical precautions Store in cool, dry conditions: shelf-life five years.

Legal category POM.

Package quantities All Schering combined oral contraceptives are available in packs containing one month's supply.

Further information Nil.

Product licence number 0053/0115.

NEOGEST*

Presentation Each round, dark brown, sugar-coated tablet bears a printed white D in a white regular hexagon on both sides and contains 37.5 mcg levonorgestrel contained in 75 mcg norgestrel.

Uses Oral contraception.

Mode of action: The contraceptive action of Neogest may be explained as follows.

It changes the cervical mucus so that a barrier is formed against the migration of sperm into the uterine cavity. Nidation is impeded because of changes in the structure of the endometrium. As a rule there is no inhibition of ovulation. Evidence suggests that a reduction in corpus-luteum function may also contribute to the contraceptive action.

Dosage and administration The first tablet is taken on the first day of menstrual bleeding at a time chosen by the patient. All subsequent tablets must then be taken at this time. The contraceptive effect is likely to be reduced if a tablet is delayed more than three hours. The tablets are taken daily and pack follows pack without interruption for as long as protection against conception is required. The contraceptive action begins after 14 tablets have been taken.

When starting oral contraception with Neogest, additional precautions other than the rhythm or temperature or combined-pill methods must be used for the first 14 days of tablet-taking.

Use after delivery or abortion: Although after delivery or abortion it is customary to start oral contraception at the end of the first biphasic menstrual cycle, Neogest may be started as early as the 7th day post partum.

Use during breast feeding: There is no evidence that Neogest diminishes the yield of breast milk. Radioactivity can be found in the milk after the administration of labelled levonorgestrel. However, it is not known whether the metabolites which appear in minute amounts in the milk and do not accumulate in the infant's tissues are biologically active.

Contra-indications, warnings, etc

Contra-indications: History during pregnancy of idiopathic jaundice or severe pruritus. Dubin-Johnson and Rotor syndromes, acute and severe chronic liver diseases. Pregnancy. History of herpes gestationis. Although no association between progestogen-only oral contraceptives and thromboembolic disorders has been shown, it is at present required that a history of such disorders be described as a contra-indication to Neogest, as it is to oestrogen-containing oral contraceptives.

Warnings/side-effects: Clinical investigations indicate that, in general, Neogest is very well tolerated. Symptoms reported in isolated cases include nausea, vomiting, dizziness, headaches, migraine, depressive moods, disturbances of appetite, allergic reactions. Amenorrhoea and changes in the pattern of the menstrual cycle have also been observed (For details see 'Menstrual pattern'.)

Circumstances requiring additional contraceptive precautions, other than the temperature, rhythm and cervical-mucus methods.

1. If a tablet is taken more than three hours late (i.e. if it is more than 27 hours since the last tablet was taken), protection against conception may be impaired. From the time of such an error, extra nonhormonal methods must be employed until 14 consecutive tablets have been taken in the correct manner.

2. When changing over to Neogest from other hormonal contraceptives, additional contraceptive measures must be employed until 14 consecutive tablets have been taken regularly.

3. Vomiting or diarrhoea may reduce the effectiveness of the tablets by preventing them from being fully absorbed. If vomiting occurs shortly after a tablet has been taken, the contraceptive protection may be maintained if a second tablet is taken within three hours of the normal time, provided that vomiting does not recur. It is advisable to take the last tablet of the pack for this purpose, so as to avoid confusion.

In the case of repeated vomiting, or continued diarrhoea, additional contraceptive measures should be employed until 14 days after the symptoms have subsided.

4. Interaction with other drugs. Some drugs accelerate the metabolism of oral contraceptives taken concurrently. Drugs suspected of having the capacity to reduce the efficacy of oral contraceptives include barbiturates, phenylbutazone, phenytoin, rifampicin, ampicillin and other antibiotics. It is, therefore, advisable to use nonhormonal methods of contraception (except the rhythm, temperature or cervical-mucus methods) during treatment with such drugs.

Menstrual pattern: A usual feature of all progestogen-only oral contraceptives is that they produce an initial irregularity of the bleeding pattern, but such irregularity tends to decrease with time.

The patient should be informed before starting Neogest that her menstrual pattern is likely to alter.

Procedure in the case of cycle disturbances: Irregular bleeding is from a medical point of view no reason for discontinuing therapy, as long as organic causes and pregnancy can be ruled out.

If amenorrhoea lasts longer than three months, or occurs repeatedly, administration of Neogest should be suspended until regular cyclical bleeding has been re-established.

No attempt must be made to control irregular cycles by the additional administration of oestrogens since they would reverse the effect of Neogest on the cervical mucus, thus seriously reducing the contraceptive efficacy.

Reasons for stopping oral contraception immediately: First signs of thrombophlebitis or thromboembolism. Jaundice. Pregnancy.

Overdosage: There have been no reports of serious ill-effects from overdosage even when a considerable number of tablets have been taken by a small child. In general, it is, therefore, unnecessary to treat overdosage. However, if overdosage is discovered within two or three hours and is so large that treatment seems desirable, gastric lavage can be safely used. There are no specific antidotes and further treatment should be symptomatic.

Pharmaceutical precautions Store in cool, dry conditions.

Shelf-life: Seven years.

Legal category POM.

Package quantities Memo-pack containing 35 tablets.

Further information Nil.

Product licence number 0053/0062.

NERICUR* GEL 5
NERICUR* GEL 10

Presentation Nericur Gel is an aqueous gel containing either 5% or 10% benzoyl peroxide.

Uses All stages of acne vulgaris. Benzoyl peroxide has a strong antibacterial action against Propionibacterium acnes. It also has keratolytic and sebostatic actions, which cause some dryness and desquamation.

Dosage and administration Treatment should be initiated with Nericur Gel 5%. Once daily, the affected areas should be washed with soap and water and then dried, before Nericur Gel is applied. For stubborn cases treatment may be continued with Nericur Gel 10%, provided that Nericur Gel 5% has been well tolerated. For particularly sensitive skin, Nericur Gel 5% should be applied every other day.

For optimal effect, Nericur Gel should be applied in the evening, sufficient time being allowed for it to dry before the patient goes to bed, in order to avoid any bleaching of bed-linen.

Contra-indications, warnings, etc
Contra-indications: Known hypersensitivity to benzoyl peroxide.

Precautions: For external use only. Avoid contact with eyes and mucosae. If the skin is exposed to strong or prolonged sunlight, Nericur Gel should be applied at longer intervals, and a highly-protective sun-screening agent should be used. Nericur Gel should only be applied to dry skin, to avoid unnecessary irritation.

Side-effects: As with all keratolytic substances, itching, reddening, burning and a feeling of skin tension may occur. This may be relieved by the use of a moisturising cream or by temporary interruption of use.

In rare cases, a contact dermititis may occur, in which event treatment should be stopped immediately.

Pharmaceutical precautions Store in a cool place. Shelf-life 2 years from date of manufacture.

Legal category P.

Package quantities Tubes containing 30 g.

Further information Nil.

Product licence numbers
Nericur 5   0053/0168
Nericur 10   0053/0169.

NERISONE* CREAM, OILY CREAM AND OINTMENT

Presentation *Cream* (oil-in-water emulsion), *oily cream* (water-in-oil emulsion) and *ointment* (anhydrous base): 1 g of each Nerisone presentation contains 1 mg (0.1%) diflucortolone valerate.

Uses Corticoid-responsive dermatoses in the absence of infection.

Dosage and administration Initially 2-3 applications daily, according to the severity of the condition. For maintenance, one application daily.

Nerisone is available in three bases. The base chosen for an individual case should depend on the physical characteristics of the lesion. For example, in very dry and chronic skin conditions, the occlusive effect of the Nerisone ointment base aids the healing process.

Contra-indications, warnings, etc
Contra-indications: Rosacea and peri-oral dermatitis. Viral infections. Bacterial or fungal infections of the skin in the absence of appropriate anti-infective therapy. Nerisone is not suitable for the treatment of ophthalmic conditions.

Warnings/side-effects: In infants, long-term continuous therapy with topical corticosteroids should be avoided. Adrenal suppression can occur, even without occlusion. Topical administration of corticosteroids to pregnant animals can cause abnormalities of foetal development. The relevance of this finding to human beings has not been established. However, topical steroids should not be used extensively during the first trimester of pregnancy, i.e. in large amounts or for prolonged periods.

In common with all other topical corticoids, side-effects may occur when Nerisone is applied to large areas of the body (10% or more) and for long periods of time (more than four weeks), especially if the ointment or an occlusive dressing is being used. These may be local signs such as atrophy of the skin, telangiectasia, striae and acneform changes; or systemic corticoid effects caused by absorption. Therefore, caution should be exercised when using occlusive dressings, as there is a possibility that natural steroid production may be depressed.

Babies and children up to the age of 4 years should not be treated with Nerisone for longer than three weeks – particularly on skin areas covered by napkins.

Nerisone may be applied under an occlusive dressing. However, each dressing should not be left on for more than 24 hours. Although occlusive dressings may be used repeatedly, it should be noted that systemic corticoid absorption is likely to be increased with a consequent increased risk of adrenal suppression. Should secondary infection occur during treatment, the use of occlusive dressings should be postponed until the infection has been controlled.

Pharmaceutical precautions Store in cool, dry conditions.

Shelf-life: Five years.

Legal category POM.

Package quantities 30 g tubes.

Further information Nil.

Product licence numbers
Nerisone Cream   0053/0075
Nerisone Oily Cream   0053/0073
Nerisone Ointment   0053/0074

NERISONE* FORTE OILY CREAM AND OINTMENT

Presentation *Oily cream* (water-in-oil emulsion) and *ointment* (anhydrous base). 1 gram of each Nerisone Forte presentation contains 3 mg (0.3%) diflucortolone valerate.

Uses Initial and intermittent treatment of severe and recalcitrant corticoid-responsive dermatoses in the absence of infection. These include psoriasis, neurodermatitis (endogenous eczema, atopic eczema), lichen planus, discoid lupus erythematosus and severe chronic eczema.

Dosage and administration Initially, two or three thin applications daily, according to the severity of the condition. Once the clinical picture has improved, the patient should be changed from Nerisone Forte to Nerisone, for maintenance therapy.

Nerisone Forte is available in two bases.

Nerisone Forte Oily Cream: This is an emulsion of water in oil. Because it is an emulsion, it allows heat and exudate to pass freely through, while the oil component protects against undesirable drying out of the skin.

Nerisone Forte Ointment: This has an anhydrous fatty base, which is particularly indicated in chronic and dry skin conditions. The softening and occlusive properties of this base often aid the healing process.

Contra-indications, warnings, etc
Contra-indications: Rosacea, acne and peri-oral dermatitis. Viral infections. Bacterial or fungal infections of the skin in the absence of appropriate anti-infective therapy. Nerisone is not suitable for the treatment of ophthalmic conditions.

Warnings/side-effects: In infants, long-term continuous therapy with topical corticosteroids should be avoided. Adrenal suppression can occur, even without occlusion. Topical administration of corticosteroids to pregnant animals can cause abnormalities of foetal development. The relevance of these findings to human beings has not been established. However, topical steroids should not be used extensively during the first trimester of pregnancy, i.e. in large amounts or for prolonged periods.

Only in rare cases, and preferably under the guidance of a dermatologist, should Nerisone Forte be considered for use on the face, or in babies and children up to the age of four, and then only briefly for the initial control of *very severe* lesions.

In view of the high efficacy and potency of Nerisone Forte, no more than 60 g a week should be applied, and it is suggested that treatment for one or two weeks should generally be sufficient to obtain control of even the most refractory lesion, after which a change to Nerisone can usually be made if maintenance therapy is necessary.

Since prolonged therapy with potent topical corticosteroids may cause local atrophic changes such as striae, thinning and telangiectasia, particularly in skin folds and where occlusive dressings are used, it is recommended that the progress of patients under treatment for more than one week with Nerisone Forte be reviewed weekly, and that repeat prescriptions be written only when the prescribing physician has again seen the patient.

Since absorption is increased with the use of occlusive dressings, these should not be left on for more than 24 hours. If secondary infection occurs during treatment, the use of occlusive dressings should be stopped until the infection has been eliminated, and appropriate treatment of the infection should be instituted if it persists.

Pharmaceutical precautions Store in cool, dry conditions.

Shelf-life: Five years.

Legal category POM.

Package quantities 15 g tubes.

Further information Nerisone Forte preparations contain neither parabens nor lanolin.

Product licence numbers
Nerisone Forte Oily Cream 0053/0099
Nerisone Forte Ointment 0053/0100

NOCTAMID* ▼
Presentation Round, white, scored tablets. Those marked CG in a regular hexagon contain 0.5 mg lorme-

tazepam. Those marked CF in a regular hexagon contain 1.0 mg lormetazepam.

Uses Noctamid is indicated for the short-term treatment of insomnia, including difficulty in falling asleep and/or frequent nocturnal awakenings.

Dosage and administration
Adults: Normally 1.0 mg orally before retiring. In elderly patients 0.5 mg is recommended. Tablets may be swallowed or taken sublingually. Subsequently, the initial dosage may be doubled in individual cases if this proves necessary.

Children: Noctamid has not been evaluated for the treatment of children.

Contra-indications, warnings, etc
Contra-indications: Known sensitivity to benzodiazepines. Myasthenia gravis.

Precautions and warnings: Noctamid and other centrally-acting drugs such as phenothiazines enhance each other's actions, and hence careful monitoring of dosage is advised during co-prescription.

The effects of Noctamid are potentiated by alcohol.

Metabolic interactions between Noctamid and other drugs have not been studied and a close watch should be kept for possible interactions.

Prolonged use of benzodiazepines, especially in high dosage, may occasionally result in the development of some psychological dependence, with withdrawal symptoms on sudden discontinuation. Treatment in these cases should be withdrawn gradually. Careful usage seldom results in the development of dependence.

Patients taking Noctamid should be warned about the possible hazard from dizziness or drowsiness when driving or operating machinery. Elderly patients are particularly susceptible to these effects, and to confusion, as are those with organic brain disease.

The use of Noctamid during pregnancy is not recommended, both in accordance with the general principle that drugs should not be administered to pregnant women unless essential, and because the possibility of a harmful effect on the human foetus cannot be totally ruled out, although extensive animal tests have shown no teratogenic actions.

Side-effects: In general, Noctamid is very well tolerated. However the common side-effects of benzodiazepines, including headaches, nausea, drowsiness, blurring of vision, dizziness and ataxia may occur on the following day, particularly in unusually sensitive patients or when dosage has been excessive.

Rare behavioural adverse effects of benzodiazepines include paradoxical aggressive outbursts, excitement, confusion, and the uncovering of depression with suicidal tendencies. Even more rare side-effects reported with some benzodiazepines have been hypotension, gastrointestinal and visual disturbances, skin rashes, urinary retention, changes in libido, blood dyscrasias, and jaundice, but they have not been reported with Noctamid.

Overdosage: As with other benzodiazepines, overdosages should not present a threat to life. General supportive measures should be used. Treatment is symptomatic, and gastric lavage may be of use if performed shortly after ingestion. If the patient is conscious, an emetic such as ipecacuanha may be given. The patient is likely to sleep, and a clear airway should be maintained.

Pharmaceutical precautions Store in a cool, dry place.

Shelf-life: five years.

Legal category CD (Sch 4), POM.

Package quantities 1 mg-30 tablets and 100 tablets (blister packs), 0.5 mg-30 tablets and 100 tablets (blister packs).

Further information Lormetazepam is rapidly absorbed from the gastrointestinal tract and is conjugated in a simple one-step process to a pharmacologically inactive glucuronide.

There are no major metabolites.

Product licence numbers
0.5 mg tablets   0053/0117
1 mg tablets   0053/0118

NORGESTON*

Presentation Each round, white, sugar-coated tablet bears a printed black E in a black regular hexagon on both sides and contains 30 mcg levonorgestrel.

Uses Oral contraception.

Mode of action: The contraceptive action of Norgeston may be explained as follows:

It changes the cervical mucus so that a barrier is formed against the migration of sperm into the uterine cavity. Nidation is impeded because of changes in the structure of the endometrium. As a rule there is no inhibition of ovulation. Evidence suggests that a reduction in corpus-luteum function may also contribute to the contraceptive action.

Dosage and administration The first tablet is taken on the first day of menstrual bleeding at a time chosen by the patient. All subsequent tablets must then be taken at this time. The contraceptive effect is likely to be reduced if a tablet is delayed more than three hours. The tablets are taken daily and pack follows pack without interruption for as long as protection against conception is required. The contraceptive action begins after 14 tablets have been taken.

When starting oral contraception with Norgeston, additional precautions other than the rhythm or temperature methods must be used for the first 14 days of tablet-taking.

Use after delivery or abortion: Although after delivery or abortion it is customary to start oral contraception at the end of the first biphasic menstrual cycle, Norgeston may be started as early as the seventh day post-partum.

Use during breast feeding: There is no evidence that Norgeston diminishes the yield of breast milk. Radioactivity can be found in the milk after the administration of labelled levonorgestrel. However, it is not known whether the metabolites which appear in minute amounts in the milk, and do not accumulate in the infant's tissues, are biologically active.

Contra-indications, warnings, etc
Contra-indications: History, during pregnancy, of idiopathic jaundice or severe pruritus; Dubin-Johnson and Rotor syndromes; acute and severe chronic liver diseases; pregnancy. History of herpes gestationis. Although no association between progestogen-only oral contraceptives and thromboembolic disorders has been shown, it is at present required that a history of such

disorders be described as a contra-indication to Norgeston, as it is to oestrogen-containing oral contraceptives.

Warnings/side-effects: Clinical investigations indicate that, in general, Norgeston is very well tolerated. Symptoms reported in isolated cases include nausea, vomiting, dizziness, headaches, migraine, depressive moods, disturbances of appetite, allergic reactions. Amenorrhoea and changes in the pattern of the menstrual cycle have been observed. (For details, see 'Menstrual pattern'.)

Circumstances requiring additional contraceptive precautions, other than the temperature, rhythm and cervical-mucus methods.

1. If a tablet is taken more than three hours late (i.e. if it is more than 27 hours since the last tablet was taken), protection against conception may be impaired. From the time of such as error, extra non-hormonal methods must be employed until 14 consecutive tablets have been taken in the correct manner.

2. When changing over to Norgeston from other hormonal contraceptives, additional contraceptive measures must be employed until 14 consecutive tablets have been taken regularly.

3. Vomiting or diarrhoea may reduce the effectiveness of the tablets by preventing them from being fully absorbed. If vomiting occurs shortly after a tablet has been taken, the contraceptive protection may be maintained if a second tablet is taken within three hours of the normal time, provided that vomiting does not recur. It is advisable to take the last tablet of the pack for this purpose, so as to avoid confusion.

In the case of repeated vomiting, or continued diarrhoea, additional contraceptive measures should be employed for a further 14 days after the symptoms have subsided.

4. Interaction with other drugs. Some drugs accelerate the metabolism of oral contraceptives taken concurrently. Drugs suspected of having the capacity to reduce the efficacy of oral contraceptives include barbiturates, phenylbutazone, phenytoin, rifampicin, ampicillin and other antibiotics. It is, therefore, advisable to use non-hormonal methods of contraception (except the rhythm, temperature or cervical-mucus methods) during treatment with such drugs.

Menstrual pattern: A usual feature of all progestogen-only oral contraceptives is that they produce an initial irregularity of the bleeding pattern, but such irregularity tends to decrease with time.

The patient should be informed before starting Norgeston that her menstrual pattern is likely to alter.

Procedure in the case of cycle disturbances: Irregular bleeding is, from a medical point of view, no reason for discontinuing therapy, as long as organic causes and pregnancy can be ruled out.

If amenorrhoea lasts longer than three months, or occurs repeatedly, administration of Norgeston should be suspended until regular cyclical bleeding has been re-established.

No attempt must be made to control irregular cycles by the additional administration of oestrogens, since they would reverse the effect of Norgeston on the cervical mucus, thus seriously reducing the contraceptive efficacy.

Reasons for stopping oral contraception immediately: First signs of thrombophlebitis or thromboembolism. Jaundice. Pregnancy.

Overdosage: There have been no reports of serious ill-effects from overdosage, even when a considerable number of tablets have been taken by a small child. In general, it is, therefore, unnecessary to treat overdosage. However, if overdosage is discovered within two or three hours and is so large that treatment seems desirable, gastric lavage can be safely used. There are no specific antidotes and further treatment should be symptomatic.

Pharmaceutical precautions Store in cool, dry conditions.

Shelf-life: Five years.

Legal category POM.

Package quantities Memo-pack containing 35 tablets.

Further information Nil.

Product licence number 0053/0068.

NORISTERAT* ▼

Presentation Norethisterone oenanthate in oily solution for intramuscular administration. Ampoules contain 200 mg in 1 ml.

Uses Noristerat is a depot contraceptive. It is intended for short-term use when a high level of efficacy independent of possible errors by the patient is required. It has been licensed for short-term use for wives of men undergoing vasectomy, until the vasectomy is effective, and women immunised against rubella, to prevent pregnancy during the period of activity of the virus.

Use after delivery or abortion: Noristerat can generally be used immediately after delivery or abortion (but see following 'Use during lactation').

Use during lactation: Noristerat has not been reported to inhibit milk production, which is an advantage when the mother wishes to breast-feed. However, traces of the hormone appear in the milk, and although considered harmless to a healthy neonate might theoretically, like other steroids, impair the degradation of bilirubin, especially during the first week of life. If the mother has received Noristerat, breast-feeding should therefore be withheld from neonates with severe or persistent jaundice requiring medical treatment.

Dosage and administration 200 mg Noristerat intramuscularly provides contraception for eight weeks. The first injection should be given within the first five days of a menstrual cycle (the first day of menstruation counting as day 1), unless it is given so soon after delivery or abortion that no possibility of pregnancy exists. The injection may be repeated once, after eight weeks. Noristerat must always be injected deep into the gluteal muscles, care being taken that no liquid runs back from the injection site, which could result in loss of efficacy. The viscosity of the liquid at low temperatures is high, necessitating considerable pressure of injection. Therefore it is suggested that the ampoule be immersed in warm water before injection. A needle of at least medium bore should be used, and care taken to ensure that the needle is securely attached to the syringe.

Contra-indications, warnings, etc
Interaction with other drugs: Some drugs may accelerate the metabolism of Noristerat. Drugs suspected of having this capacity, which may reduce the efficacy of the preparation, include barbiturates, phenytoin and rifampicin.

Contra-indications: Acute and severe chronic liver disease. History, during pregnancy, of idiopathic jaundice or general pruritus, or of herpes gestationis. Dubin-Johnson and Rotor syndromes. Pregnancy.

Warnings: Although there have so far been no observations of thromboembolic disease during the use of Noristerat, as a precaution it is recommended that this preparation should not be used where there is a history of thromboembolic processes.

Side-effects: Subjective symptoms reported consist mainly of bloating, breast discomfort, headaches, dizziness and transient nausea. Marked increases of weight are rare.

Menstrual pattern: The patient should be informed before starting Noristerat that her menstrual pattern is likely to alter.

Menstrual changes: These, in the form of spotting, breakthrough bleeding and delayed menstruation are relatively frequent, and generally do not require treatment. With persistent bleeding, however, it may be expedient to administer progestogen/oestrogen tablets, e.g. combined oral contraceptives, for 10 days to create a withdrawal bleed 1–4 days later.

Amenorrhoea: If, when the second injection is due, bleeding has not occurred in the preceding eight weeks, the second injection should not be given until pregnancy has been ruled out.

Precautions: Women with a history of severe depressive states, disturbed liver function or any disease that is prone to worsen during pregnancy should be carefully observed during medication.

Effect on blood chemistry: No influence of Noristerat on basal plasma cortisol, the ACTH test or the metyrapone test has been observed. In the acute dexamethasone suppression test, however, a higher plasma cortisol value than expected was found in four out of 10 women, although there were no clinical indications of disturbed adrenocortical function. A shortening of the recalcification time and of the thromboplastin time (Quick's test) were observed in studies of the blood coagulation system.

Pharmaceutical precautions Store away from strong sunlight. Shelf life 5 years.

Legal category POM.

Package quantities Single packs of 1 ampoule.

Further information Nil.

Product licence number 0053/0095.

NOVA-T* ▼

Presentation Nova-T is an intra-uterine contraceptive device (IUCD) in the form of a T, made of polyethylene impregnated with barium sulphate to make the device radio-opaque. Around the stem is wrapped a wire of surface area about 200 square mm, the outer layer consisting of 103–143 mg of copper, and the core of 11–29 mg of silver. The silver core, which is resistant to corrosion, is designed to prevent fracture of the wire when the copper is substantially corroded, and to enable the device to be retained for up to five years.

Uses Intra-uterine contraception.

Administration After a pelvic examination to exclude contra-indications, and to determine the size and position of the uterus, the presterilised device is inserted into the uterus by means of the inserter, and according to the instructions provided, using non-touch technique.

Contra-indications, warnings, etc

Contra-indications: Pregnancy. Known or suspected malignant tumours in the genital tract. Large or multiple fibroids. Uterine polyps. Hypoplasia (external os to fundus, less than 6.5 cm), malformation, or extreme malposition of the uterus. Severe dysmenorrhoea. Genital infections. Postpartum endometritis or infected abortion in the last three months. Endometriosis. Active pelvic inflammatory disease. History of repeated pelvic inflammatory disease. Genital bleeding of unknown origin. Menorrhagia and/or intermenstrual bleeding. Coagulation deficiencies. Wilson's disease. Allergy to copper.

Warnings: Medical diathermy must not be applied to the user's abdomen or sacral region, since heating of the copper may cause injury.

Perforation of the uterus may occur during insertion or subsequently, and demands early removal of the device, the copper of which may cause peritoneal adhesions.

IUCD's may, in general, predispose to uterine infections. The use of IUCD's may rarely jeopardise subsequent fertility. IUCD's should be used with caution in patients with anaemia and those receiving anticoagulants, in whom additional menstrual bleeding may be of clinical consequence. Caution is necessary in patients receiving steroid therapy, which may mask pelvic inflammatory disease.

Pregnancy: The user must be instructed to inform her doctor at once if she suspects herself to be pregnant.

If a pregnancy should occur, the possibility that it is ectopic should be carefully considered, since intrauterine contraceptive devices provide less protection against ectopic than against intra-uterine pregnancies, and a pregnancy occurring with an IUCD in situ is therefore more likely to be ectopic than a pregnancy occurring without an IUCD in situ.

The device should be removed by traction on the threads, since, although this procedure may itself entail some risk of increasing abortion, retention of the device in the uterus may increase the risk of sepsis and spontaneous abortion at a later stage. Moreover, the long-term effects of the intra-uterine copper on the foetus are not fully known. If the device cannot be removed, termination of the pregnancy should be considered.

If, after the discussion of the above recommendation, the patient insists on continuing a pregnancy with the device still present, she should be closely observed and told to report all abnormal symptoms such as flu-like symptoms, fever, cramping pain, vaginal bleeding or discharge, since the onset of septicaemia associated with septic abortion may be insidious, with initial general symptoms rather than localising symptoms and signs of spontaneous abortion.

Precautions: Appropriate precautions, including administration of antibiotics, should be considered when inserting an IUCD in patients with known or suspected rheumatic or congenital heart disease. Caution is advised in patients with a history of previous uterine incision or perforation of the uterus or previous ectopic pregnancy. The possibility of a seizure's being precipitated in an epileptic patient at or shortly after the insertion of an IUCD should be borne in mind.

Side-effects: Insertion and removal may be associated with some pain and bleeding, and rarely a vasovagal attack. Otherwise pain, especially cramps, in the lower abdomen or sacral area, is most common in the first few days after insertion. Menses are often somewhat heavier than before, especially in patients who are taking anticoagulants, but intermenstrual bleeding or spotting is usually transient. Dysmenorrhoea may occur. Rashes, disappearing on removal of the device, and probably due to allergy to copper, have been reported.

Medical indications for removal of the device: Persistent pain or heavy bleeding. Differential diagnosis of persistent irregular uterine bleeding. Signs and symptoms of uterine infections or other pelvic inflammatory disease. Pregnancy. Displacement of the device. Development of allergy to copper.

Pharmaceutical precautions Nova-T is supplied in a sterile pack, which should not be opened until just before insertion of the device, which must be handled with aseptic precautions. If the seal of the sterile envelope is broken, the device inside should not be used.

Shelf-life 5 years.

Legal category POM.

Package quantities 1 IUCD per envelope.

Further information Nil.

Product licence number 0053/0128.

PRIMOLUT N*

Presentation Each white, uncoated tablet is impressed with 'AN' in a regular hexagon on one side and contains 5 mg norethisterone BP.

Uses Metropathia haemorrhagica. Premenstrual syndrome. Postponement of menstruation. Endometriosis. Menorrhagia. Dysmenorrhoea.

A total dose of about 100–150 mg Primolut N (10–15 mg on each of 10 consecutive days) will produce complete secretory transformation of an endometrium which has been pretreated with oestrogens.

A particular advantage is that the menstruation-like withdrawal bleeding occurs consistently two to three days after stopping Primolut N.

During treatment with Primolut N the basal body temperature rises, as it does under the influence of endogenous progesterone in the second half of the menstrual cycle.

Dosage and administration The use of Primolut N is restricted to patients in whom there is no possibility of early pregnancy in the cycle concerned.

Metropathia haemorrhagica (dysfunctional uterine bleeding): 1 tablet 3 times daily for 10 days. Bleeding is arrested usually within 1–3 days. A withdrawal bleeding resembling normal menstruation occurs within 2–4 days after discontinuing treatment.

Prophylaxis against recurrence of dysfunctional bleeding: If there are no signs of resumption of normal ovarian function (no rise in the second half of the cycle of the morning temperature, which should be measured daily) recurrence must be anticipated. Cyclical bleeding can be established with 1 tablet twice daily from the 19th to the 26th day of the cycle.

Premenstrual syndrome (including premenstrual mastalgia): Premenstrual symptoms such as headache, migraine, breast discomfort, water retention, tachycardia and psychic disturbances may be relieved by the administration of 2–3 tablets daily from the 19th to the 26th day of the cycle. Treatment should be repeated for several cycles. When treatment is stopped, the patient may remain symptom-free for a number of months.

Postponement of menstruation: In cases of too frequent menstrual bleeding, and in special circumstances (e.g. operations, travel, sports) the postponement of menstruation is possible, 1 tablet Primolut N three times daily, starting 3 days before the expected onset of menstruation. A normal period should occur 2–3 days after the patient has stopped taking tablets.

Dysmenorrhoea: Functional or primary dysmenorrhoea is almost invariably relieved by the suppression of ovulation. 1 tablet three times daily for 20 days, starting on the fifth day of the cycle (the first day of menstruation counting as day 1). Treatment should be maintained for three to four cycles followed by treatment-free cycles. A further course of therapy may be employed if symptoms return.

Endometriosis (pseudo-pregnancy therapy): Longterm treatment is commenced on the 5th day of the cycle with 2 tablets Primolut N daily for the first few weeks. In the event of spotting, the dosage is increased to 4 and, if necessary, 5 tablets daily.

After bleeding has ceased, the initial dose is usually sufficient. Duration of treatment: 4–6 months continuously, or longer if necessary.

Menorrhagia (hypermenorrhoea): 1 tablet 2–3 times a day from the 19th to the 26th day of the cycle (counting the first day of menstruation as day 1).

Note: If menstrual bleeding should fail to follow a course of Primolut N, the possibility of pregnancy must be ruled out before a further course is given.

Contra-indications, warnings, etc
Contra-indications: Pregnancy. Severe disturbance of liver function. Dubin-Johnson and Rotor syndromes. History during pregnancy of idiopathic jaundice, severe pruritus or herpes gestationis.

Warnings/side-effects: Rarely occur in doses of 15 mg daily. Amongst those recorded are slight nausea, exacerbation of epilepsy and migraine. With extremely high dosage there may be cholestatic liver changes.

Overdosage: There have been no reports of ill-effects from overdosage and treatment is generally unnecessary. If overdosage is discovered within two or three hours and is so large that treatment seems desirable, gastric lavage can safely be used.

There are no special antidotes, and further treatment should be symptomatic.

Pharmaceutical precautions Store in cool dry conditions: shelf-life five years.

Legal category POM.

Package quantities Bottles of 100 tablets. Containers of 500 tablets.

Further information Nil.

Product licence number 0053/5033.

PRIMOTESTON* DEPOT 250 mg

Presentation Primoteston Depot 250 mg contains testosterone oenanthate 250 mg per ml in clear non-aqueous solution for intramuscular injection.

Uses Mammary carcinoma in the female. Androgen deficiency in the male.

Primoteston Depot is a depot androgen for use when male sex hormones are indicated. Testosterone oenanthate has not only a sustained androgenic effect but also a very powerful one, since testosterone in this depot form is particularly well utilised by the body.

Dosage and administration *In the female. Advanced mammary carcinoma:* In advanced mammary carcinoma with metastases or recurrences, high-dosage therapy causes objective remission in some cases and frequently subjective improvement. In responsive cases, pain is diminished and the general condition considerably improved. Bone metastases are often affected favourably. In order to sustain a remission for as long as possible, it is sometimes necessary after a time to shorten the interval between injections. If hypercalcaemia occurs, treatment must be discontinued. In women over 60 years of age, treatment with oestrogens is often more effective.

Dosage: 250 mg Primoteston Depot intramuscularly every two weeks.

In the male: Hypogonadism: To stimulate development of underdeveloped androgen-dependent organs and for initial treatment of deficiency symptoms, 250 mg Primoteston Depot intramuscularly every two to three weeks.

For maintenance treatment: 250 mg Primoteston Depot intramuscularly every three to six weeks, according to individual requirement.

Contra-indications, warnings, etc
Contra-indications: Prostatic carcinoma and pregnancy.

Warnings/side-effects: With high dosage and prolonged testosterone therapy, an increased tendency to fluid retention and oedema is seen occasionally. In patients with a tendency to oedema, therefore, caution is indicated unless the oedema is due to lack of protein, when the protein-anabolic effect of Primoteston Depot is beneficial.

With prolonged use and high dosage of androgens in women, symptoms of virilisation must be expected. Regular examination of the prostate is advisable for men receiving androgen therapy.

Pharmaceutical precautions Store in cool, dry conditions away from strong sunlight: shelf-life five years.

Legal category POM.

Package quantities Ampoules of 250 mg, 3 × 1 ml.

Further information Nil.

Product licence number 0053/5037.

PROGYNOVA* 1 mg
PROGYNOVA* 2 mg

Presentation *Progynova 1 mg:* Each beige, sugar-coated tablet bears a printed black B in a black regular hexagon and contains 1 mg of oestradiol valerate.

Progynova 2 mg: Each pale blue, sugar-coated tablet bears a printed red B in a red regular hexagon and contains 2 mg of oestradiol valerate.

Uses The treatment of climacteric symptoms in the short term in postmenopausal women (i.e. who have had no uterine bleeding for at least 12 months).

Dosage and administration One tablet of Progynova 1 mg daily for 21 days, followed by an interval of at least seven days before the next course. If the response is inadequate, Progynova 2 mg may be substituted, but the lowest dose compatible with the control of symptoms should always be used, and an attempt should he made to revert to Progynova 1 mg after symptoms have been satisfactorily controlled. However, it should be realised that the appropriate dosage will be determined by the individual patient's rate of metabolism of Progynova, rather than by the initial severity of the symptoms.

Alternatively, if the response to Progynova 1 mg is inadequate, Cyclo-Progynova can be substituted, and in general when high-dose oestrogen therapy is required, oestrogen-progestogen combinations are recommended.

Bleeding: If possible, a dosage should be found that will abolish climacteric symptoms without inducing endometrial bleeding. Non-recurrent bleeding of short duration in the tablet-free intervals is usually due to oestrogen withdrawal. Any recurrent bleeding occurring during tablet-taking should be investigated to exclude endometrial hyperplasia or carcinoma. If recurrent bleeding is found to be non-pathological, then Cyclo-Progynova, which produces controlled shedding of the endometrium, should be substituted. (For further information, see the data sheet for Cyclo-Progynova.)

The treatment of recurrences: If, after completion of short-term treatment and the withdrawal of Progynova, climacteric symptoms should recur, further treatment should be with Cyclo-Progynova (except in hysterectomised patients, who may take Progynova without any limit on the duration of treatment, and without intervals).

Contra-indications, warnings, etc
Contra-indications: Pregnancy. Severe disturbances of liver function, jaundice or general pruritus during a previous pregnancy, Dubin-Johnson syndrome, Rotor syndrome, existing or previous thromboembolic processes, sickle-cell anaemia, suspected or existing hormone-dependent disorders or tumours of the uterus or breast, congenital disturbances of lipid metabolism, otosclerosis with deterioration in previous pregnancies.

Warnings/side-effects: Prolonged exposure to unopposed oestrogens may increase the risk of the development of endometrial carcinoma. The following have been reported during treatment: dyspepsia, flatulence, nausea, vomiting, abdominal pain and bloating, weight-gain, breast tension and pain, palpitations, cardiac symptoms, increased libido, headaches, dizziness, vertigo, epistaxis, biliary stasis, hypertension, urticaria and other rashes, thrombophlebitis, uterine bleeding, mucous vaginal discharge, general pruritus.

Diseases that are known to be subject to deterioration during pregnancy (e.g. multiple sclerosis, epilepsy, diabetes, hypertension, porphyria, tetany and otosclerosis) should be carefully observed during treatment.

Precautions and special information: Treatment should be stopped at once if migrainous or frequent and unusually severe headaches occur for the first time, or if there are any other symptoms that are possible prodromata of vascular occlusion.

Treatment should also be stopped if trauma, illness or impending surgery is considered to entail a risk of thrombosis.

Treatment should be stopped at once if jaundice occurs, or if there is a significant rise in blood-pressure.

In patients with mild chronic liver disease, liver function should be checked every 8–12 weeks.

Women with a family history of endometrial carcinoma should be carefully observed.

Examination of the pelvic organs, endometrium, breasts and blood-pressure is advised before and periodically during treatment with Progynova.

Overdosage: There have been no reports of ill-effects from overdosage, which it is, therefore, generally unnecessary to treat. If overdosage is discovered within two or three hours and is so large that treatment seems desirable, gastric lavage can safely be used. There are no specific antidotes, and further treatment should be symptomatic.

Pharmaceutical precautions Store in cool, dry conditions:

Shelf-life:
Progynova 1 mg 5 years.
Progynova 2 mg 7 years.

Legal category POM.

Package quantities Memo-packs of 21 tablets.

Further information Nil.

Product licence numbers
Progynova 1 mg 0053/0057
Progynova 2 mg 0053/0058

PROLUTON* DEPOT
(formerly PRIMOLUT DEPOT)

Presentation Hydroxyprogesterone hexanoate BP 250 mg and 500 mg in ampoules for intramuscular injection.

Uses Habitual abortion, when associated with proven progesterone-deficiency.

Dosage and administration 250–500 mg Proluton Depot at weekly intervals during the first half of pregnancy.

Contra-indications, warnings, etc
Contra-indications: A history of herpes gestationis.

Warnings: Many medicinal products, including female sex hormones, have been suspected of being capable of affecting the normal development of a child in the early stages of pregnancy. Many researchers consider that in relation to sex hormones such a suspicion is ill founded but one has to accept that for no medicinal product can a teratogenic activity be excluded with absolute certainty. Therefore, the general principle is now widely accepted that inessential use of drugs during pregnancy should be avoided. Following this general principle, Proluton Depot should be used to maintain pregnancy only if it is strictly indicated, i.e. if there is an urgent desire to have a child, especially if luteal insufficiency is present.

Since Proluton Depot may prevent spontaneous evacuation of a dead foetus (missed abortion) the progress of the pregnancy should be regularly monitored by appropriate means, including immunological tests.

Side-effects: Very rarely, local reactions may occur at the site of injection.

Pharmaceutical precautions Store in cool, dry conditions away from strong sunlight. Shelf-life five years.

Legal category POM.

Package quantities *250 mg:* Packs of 3 and 20 ampoules 1 ml.

500 mg: Packs of 3 and 20 ampoules 2 ml.

Further information Nil.

Product licence numbers
Proluton Depot 250 mg   0053/5031
Proluton Depot 500 mg   0053/5032

PRO-VIRON*

Presentation Each white tablet has AX in a regular hexagon impressed on one side and is scored on the reverse. It contains 25 mg mesterolone.

Uses Androgen deficiency. Male infertility.

Pro-viron is an orally active androgen with properties quite distinct from those of older products. It offers unusual therapeutic possibilities because it can be given in high dosage over long periods. The presence of a methyl group at C-1 confers special properties on this steroid which, unlike testosterone and all its derivatives that are used for androgen therapy, is not metabolised to oestrogen.

This difference almost certainly accounts for the observation that in its usual therapeutic dosage in normal men, Pro-viron does not significantly depress the release of gonadotrophins from the pituitary. Hence (1) spermatogenesis is unimpaired. (2) unlike other androgens, which suppress and therefore replace endogenous androgens, Pro-viron supplements endogenous androgens.

Furthermore, in contrast to other orally active androgens, liver tolerance is excellent (a fact probably related to the absence of 17-alkyl substitution of the steroid nucleus).

Dosage and administration *Androgen deficiency:* Initially: 1 tablet three to four times daily, i.e. 75–100 mg daily for several months, followed by maintenance therapy of 2–3 tablets (50–75 mg) daily.

Male infertility: 100 mg daily for several months.

Contra-indications, warnings, etc
Contra-indications: In common with other androgens, Pro-viron is contra-indicated in the presence of prostatic carcinoma, since androgens can stimulate the growth of an existing carcinoma.

Warnings/side-effects: Reported side-effects have been rare, transient and minor. Regular examination of the prostate during treatment is advised, in order to exclude prostatic carcinoma.

Overdosage: There have been no reports of ill-effects from overdosage and treatment is generally unnecessary. If overdosage is discovered within two or three hours and is so large that treatment seems desirable, gastric lavage can safely be used.

There are no special antidotes and further treatment should be symptomatic.

Pharmaceutical precautions Store in cool, dry conditions, away from strong sunlight. Shelf-life five years.

Legal category POM.

Package quantities Bottles of 50 tablets.

Further information Nil.

Product licence number 0053/0030.

SCHERING PC4* ▼

Presentation Four white, sugar-coated tablets, each containing 0.25 mg levonorgestrel (in 0.5 mg dl-norgestrel) and 0.05 mg ethinyloestradiol.

Uses Post-coital contraception within 72 hours of unprotected coitus as an occasional emergency measure. Schering PC4 is primarily aimed to prevent implantation of the fertilised ovum in the endometrium.

Dosage and administration The first two tablets should be taken as soon as possible after coitus (up to a maximum of 72 hours afterwards) and the remaining two tablets twelve hours after the first two.

Contra-indications, warnings, etc
Contra-indications: Therapy should not be administered to a patient whose menstrual bleeding is overdue. Treatment is inappropriate also for a patient who has had unprotected intercourse more than 72 hours previously in the current menstrual cycle.

Other contra-indications: Thrombotic disorders and a history of these conditions, sickle-cell anaemia, disorders of lipid metabolism and other conditions in which, in individual cases, there is known or suspected to be a much increased risk of thrombosis. Acute or severe chronic liver diseases. Dubin-Johnson syndrome. Rotor syndrome. History, during pregnancy, of idiopathic jaundice or severe pruritus. History of herpes gestationis. Mammary or endometrial carcinoma, or a history of these conditions. Abnormal vaginal bleeding of unknown cause. Deterioration of otosclerosis during pregnancy.

Warnings: Schering PC4 does not appear to be as effective as some regularly-used methods of contraception and is suitable only as an occasional emergency measure. Schering PC4 is not effective if started later than 72 hours after coitus and should not be so used.

Patients who become pregnant despite post-coital contraception should be carefully evaluated for possible ectopic pregnancy. Since Schering PC4 appears to affect only endometrial implantation, tubal pregnancy may occur at the expected rate, and it is thus possible that there will be a relative increase in ectopic pregnancy in patients who become pregnant despite the use of Schering PC4 therapy.

The safety of use during lactation has not been established.

The effect of Schering PC4 on the conceptus in the event of failure to prevent conception is not definitely known. Some investigators have suggested that sex hormones taken in the first trimester of pregnancy may slightly increase the risk of foetal malformations, but numerous other investigators have failed to support these findings. The consensus of opinion amongst teratologists is that even known teratogens will not produce malformations before organogenesis starts, which is much later than the 72 hours after fertilisation to which the use of Schering PC4 is restricted.

Malabsorption: Vomiting, severe diarrhoea or other causes of malabsorption might impair the efficacy of Schering PC4.

Drug interactions: The efficacy of Schering PC4 might be impaired by interaction with concurrently-used drugs including barbiturates, phenylbutazone, phenytoin, rifampicin, ampicillin and other antibiotics.

Precautions: Examination of the pelvic organs, breasts and blood pressure should normally precede the prescribing of any combined oral contraceptive. The following conditions require careful consideration: a history of severe depressive states, diabetes, hypertension, epilepsy, porphyria, tetany, disturbed liver function, gallstones, cardiovascular diseases, renal diseases.

The importance of follow-up and the possibility of an early or late onset of the next period should be explained to the patient. The practice of abstinence or careful use of a barrier method until the onset of the next period should also be advised. Follow-up should be carried out 3 weeks after administration of therapy to assess the effectiveness of the method, to discuss future management if a period has not occurred, and to counsel the patient about future contraception.

Side-effects: Nausea and vomiting are common side-effects, and the latter may reduce the efficacy of therapy if it occurs within about 2 hours after the ingestion of either dose of tablets, in which event consideration should be given to the taking of more pills.

The concomitant administration of an anti-emetic has been favoured by some practitioners.

The pattern of menstrual bleeding is often temporarily disturbed. Breast discomfort and headaches also may occur.

Overdosage: There have been no reports of serious ill-effects from overdosage.

Pharmaceutical precautions Store in cool, dry conditions: shelf-life five years.

Legal category POM.

Package quantities Single pack of four tablets.

Further information Nil.

Product licence number 0053/0162.

SCHERIPROCT* OINTMENT AND SUPPOSITORIES

Presentation Each white suppository contains:

Prednisolone hexanoate	1.3 mg
Dibucaine hydrochloride	1.0 mg
Clemizole undecylate	5.0 mg

A white ointment containing in 1 g:

Prednisolone hexanoate	1.9 mg
Dibucaine hydrochloride	5.0
Clemizole undecylate	10.0 mg

Uses Haemorrhoids, fissures, proctitis, pruritus ani and vulvae, and other inflammatory and allergic processes in the anal region.

Dosage and administration *Suppositories:* 1 Scheriproct Suppository to be inserted daily. In severe cases 1 suppository two to three times daily at the beginning of treatment. After complete disappearance of symptoms it is advisable to insert 1 suppository every second day for one further week. The suppositories should be inserted after defaecation.

Ointment: Apply in a thin layer twice daily. In order to obtain a more rapid improvement, Scheriproct Ointment may be applied three to four times on the first day. To avoid relapses, Scheriproct Ointment should be applied once a day for a few days after complete disappearance of the symptoms. The nozzle provided facilitates intra-rectal application.

Contra-indications, warnings, etc
Contra-indications: Viral infections. Bacterial or fungal infections of the skin in the absence of appropriate anti-infective therapy.

Warnings/side-effects: In infants, long-term continuous therapy with topical corticosteroids should be avoided. Adrenal suppression can occur, even without occlusion. Topical administration of corticosteroids to pregnant animals can cause abnormalities of foetal development. The relevance of these findings to human beings has not been established. However, topical steroids should not be used extensively during the first trimester of pregnancy, i.e. in large amounts or for prolonged periods. As with all topical steroids, there is a risk of developing skin atrophy following extensive therapy. The application of unusually large quantities of topical corticoids may result in the absorption of systemically active amounts of corticoid. Infections or secondarily infected dermatoses definitely require additional therapy with antibiotics or chemotherapeutic agents. This treatment can often be topical, but for heavy infections systemic antibacterial therapy may be necessary. If fungal infections are present, a topically active antimycotic should be applied.

Pharmaceutical precautions In order to restore the consistency of suppositories which have become soft owing to warm temperature, they should be put into cold water before the covering is removed.

Store in cool, dry conditions: shelf-life five years.

Legal category POM.

Package quantities *Suppositories:* Packs of 12.
Ointment: Tubes of 30 g.

Further information Nil.

Product licence numbers

Scheriproct Suppositories	0053/5001
Scheriproct Ointment	0053/5002

SH420*

Presentation Each uncoated, white tablet has AR in a regular hexagon impressed on one side, with quarter-scoring on the reverse. It contains 10 mg norethisterone acetate.

Uses Inoperable mammary carcinoma. As an adjunct to surgery and/or radiotherapy.

Note: Hormone therapy can never replace surgery or radiotherapy.

SH420 is a potent progestogen with a clinical efficacy which appears to be at least comparable to that of androgens and oestrogens in the treatment of inoperable mammary carcinoma. It does not, however, have the disadvantage of virilisation as with androgens and is unlikely to cause uterine bleeding as is the case with oestrogens. It may be used in the treatment of both pre- and post-menopausal women.

Although the mode of action of the various classes of hormone in inhibiting the growth of mammary carcinoma is not well understood, the very important role of the pituitary seems to be generally agreed on, as is shown by the response to pituitary ablation and hence to pituitary suppression by hormonal means.

SH420 is a powerful inhibitor of the pituitary. The effect of the progestogen may not depend wholly, however, on pituitary inhibition and it may be that an anti-oestrogenic effect as well as a direct effect on the tumour plays a part. Clinically SH420 has yielded subjective improvement (relief of pain and improvement in the general condition) and objective improvement (regression of tumour and/or bone and soft-tissue metastases).

Dosage and administration The recommended initial dosage of SH420 is 1 tablet three times a day (30 mg norethisterone acetate daily). If, after 6 weeks, no response is apparent, this can be increased to 2 tablets three times daily (60 mg daily).

Any remission obtainable should be apparent by the end of two months. If regression or arrest of tumour growth is obtained, treatment should be maintained as long as it continues to appear beneficial. If after about 9 weeks no response is apparent, none is to be expected and some other form of therapy should be tried.

Contra-indications, warnings, etc

Contra-indications:
Pregnancy. History of herpes gestationis.

Warnings/side-effects: The great advantage of SH420 over oestrogens and androgens is the almost complete freedom from side-effects.

Side-effects such as nausea, uterine bleeding and reversible cholestatic liver changes have occasionally been observed.

Overdosage: There have been no reports of ill-effects from overdosage and treatment is generally unnecessary. If overdosage is discovered within two or three hours and is so large that treatment seems desirable, gastric lavage can safely be used.

There are no special antidotes and further treatment should be symptomatic.

Pharmaceutical precautions Store in cool, dry conditions, away from strong sunlight. Shelf-life five years.

Legal category POM.

Package quantities Bottles of 100 tablets.

Further information Nil.

Product licence number 0053/5012.

TRAVOGYN ▼

Presentation (a) *Vaginal tablets:* White, almond-shaped vaginal tablets, impressed with CT in a regular hexagon on one side, and containing 300 mg isoconazole nitrate.

(b) *Cream:* A white cream containing 1% isoconazole nitrate.

Uses Travogyn exhibits a broad spectrum of activity against fungal pathogens, including yeasts and yeast-like fungi (particularly those belonging to Candida spp. and Torulopsis glabrata), and against dermatophytes and hyphomycetes. Travogyn also has bactericidal activity against some gram-positive bacteria, including staphylococci, streptococci and micrococci, which may cause secondary infection of inflammatory skin lesions.

(a) *Vaginal tablets:* Travogyn vaginal tablets may be used for vaginal mycoses, particularly those due to Candida, or for mixed infections with fungi and gram-positive bacteria.

(b) *Cream:* Travogyn cream should be used, in conjunction with Travogyn vaginal tablets, to treat vulval or perianal spread of susceptible vaginal infections. It may be used to treat balanitis of possible candidal

origin and its prophylactic use in the partners of infected women is advisable.

Travogyn cream may be used alone for perineal or intertriginous infections of probable fungal origin that do not appear to be secondary to vaginal mycoses.

N.B. Travogyn formulations should not be the treatment of first choice for pure trichomonal infections.

Dosage and administration (a) *Vaginal tablets:* Two 300 mg vaginal tablets should be inserted together deep into the vagina. Only one application is required and may be done by the doctor at the time of consultation, or by the patient, preferably at night.
(b) *Cream:* Where treatment of the external genital or peri-anal regions, or simultaneous treatment of the partner, is required, Travogyn cream should be applied twice daily until symptoms have disappeared.

Contra-indications, warnings, etc There are no known contra-indications.

Occasionally during the first 12 to 24 hours, symptoms of intolerance such as burning or itching of the vagina and vulva, may occur. Although in order to avoid any possibility of adverse effects on the foetus, the general principle is now widely accepted that the administration of drugs to women during pregnancy should, as far as possible, be avoided, nothing that is known about the effect of isoconazole nitrate, either from animal experiments, or from clinical experience, suggests that Travogyn therapy should not be used during pregnancy.

Pharmaceutical precautions Store in a cool place.

Shelf-life: Five years.
The cream should be used within 28 days of opening.

Legal category POM.

Package quantities Two vaginal tablets in foil-backed blister packs.
Tubes of 20 g cream.

Further information Nil.

Product licence numbers
Vaginal tablets: 0053/0124
Cream: 0053/0122

ULTRABASE*

Presentation Ultrabase is a white oil-in-water cream for topical application.

Components: Polyoxyl 40 stearate, white soft paraffin, liquid paraffin, stearyl alcohol, carbopol 934, sodium hydroxide, methylhydroxybenzoate (methyl-paraben), propylhydroxybenzoate (propyl-paraben), disodium-edetate, demineralised water, crematest perfume oil.

Uses Ultrabase is intended for general use as an emollient and as a diluent for dermatological preparations and a vehicle for other medicaments. Additionally, it may be alternated with topical corticosteroids when the latter are being gradually withdrawn, and may be continued alone after complete withdrawal of the topical corticosteroid.

Dosage and administration The cream should be smoothed into the skin as often as required.

Contra-indications, warnings, etc There are no specific contra-indications to the use of Ultrabase, other than known allergy to any of the components.

Side-effects: No side-effects have been reported.

Pharmaceutical precautions Store in cool, dry conditions, away from strong sunlight: shelf-life five years.

Legal category GSL.

Package quantities Tubes containing 50 g. Jars containing 500 g.

Further information Ultrabase is suitable as a diluent for Schering's corticoid cream preparations and as a vehicle for coal tar solutions, urea, resorcinol, zinc oxide and precipitated sulphur.

Product licence number 0053/0063.

ULTRADIL* OINTMENT PLAIN AND CREAM PLAIN
ULTRALANUM* OINTMENT PLAIN AND CREAM PLAIN

Presentation White creams (oil-in-water emulsions) and ointments (water-in-oil emulsions) with the following ingredients.

Ultradil Ointment plain and Cream plain: 0.1% fluocortolone pivalate BP and 0.1% fluocortolone hexanoate BP.

Ultralanum Ointment plain: 0.25% fluocortolone and 0.25% fluocortolone hexanoate BP.

Ultralanum Cream plain: 0.25% fluocortolone pivalate BP and 0.25% fluocortolone hexanoate BP.

Ultradil plain and Ultralanum plain are dilute and full-strength preparations respectively of the corticoid, fluocortolone, and its esters.

Uses *Ultradil Cream and Ointment plain:* Most eczemas, dermatoses and other corticoid-responsive skin conditions in the absence of infection. Ultradil is particularly indicated when the patient is young, the skin area large or the treatment schedule prolonged.

Ultralanum Cream and Ointment plain: More severe corticoid-responsive skin conditions in the absence of infection.

Dosage and administration *Ultradil plain: (ointment and cream):* The usual initial dosage is 1 application three times a day, reducing to 1 application twice daily.
For maintenance one application daily.

Ultralanum plain: (ointment and cream): Initially 2–3 applications daily, according to severity of condition. For maintenance one application daily.

Contra-indications, warnings, etc
Contra-indications: Rosacea and peri-oral dermatitis. Viral infections. Bacterial or fungal infections of the skin in the absence of appropriate anti-infective therapy. Not suitable for the treatment of ophthalmic conditions.

Warnings/side-effects: In infants long-term continuous therapy with topical corticosteroids should be avoided. Adrenal suppression can occur even without occlusion. Topical administration of corticosteroids to pregnant animals can cause abnormalities of foetal development. The relevance of these findings to human beings has not been established. However, topical steroids should not be used extensively during the first trimester of pregnancy, i.e. in large amounts or for prolonged periods. As with all topical steroids, there is a risk of skin atrophy following extensive therapy. The application of unusually large quantities of topical corticoids may result in the absorption of systemically active amounts of corticoid.

Infections or secondarily infected dermatoses definitely require additional therapy with antibiotics or chemotherapeutic agents. This treatment can often be topical, but for heavy infections systemic antibacterial therapy may be necessary. If fungal infections are present, a topically active antimycotic should be applied.

Pharmaceutical precautions Store in cool, dry conditions: shelf-life five years.

Legal category POM.

Package quantities *Ultradil Ointment plain:* Tubes of 50 g and 100 g.
Ultradil Cream plain: Tubes of 50 g and 100 g.
Ultralanum Ointment plain: Tubes of 30 g and 50 g.
Ultralanum Cream plain: Tubes of 30 g and 50 g.

Further information Nil.

Product licence numbers
Ultradil Ointment plain	0053/5015
Ultradil Cream plain	0053/5017
Ultralanum Cream plain	0053/5011
Ultralanum Ointment plain	0053/5005

ULTRAPROCT* OINTMENT
ULTRAPROCT* SUPPOSITORIES

Presentation Each white suppository contains:
Fluocortolone pivalate BP	0.61 mg
Fluocortolone hexanoate BP	0.63 mg
Dibucaine hydrochloride	1.00 mg
Clemizole undecylate	5.00 mg

A white ointment containing in 1 g:
Fluocortolone pivalate BP	0.92 mg
Fluocortolone hexanoate BP	0.95 mg
Dibucaine hydrochloride	5.00 mg
Clemizole undecylate	10.00 mg

Uses Haemorrhoids, fissures, proctitis, pruritus ani and vulvae, and other inflammatory and allergic processes in the anal region.

Dosage and administration *Suppositories:* 1 Ultraproct Suppository to be inserted daily. In severe cases 1 suppository two to three times daily at the beginning of treatment. After complete disappearance of symptoms, it is advisable to insert one suppository every second day for one further week. The suppositories should be inserted after defaecation.

Ointment: Apply in a thin layer twice daily. In order to obtain a more rapid improvement, Ultraproct Ointment may be applied three or four times on the first day. To avoid relapses, Ultraproct Ointment should be applied once a day for a few days after complete disappearance of the symptoms. The nozzle provided facilitates intra-rectal application.

Contra-indications, warnings, etc
Contra-indications: Viral infections. Bacterial or fungal infections of the skin in the absence of appropriate anti-infective therapy.

Warnings/side-effects: In infants, long-term continuous therapy with topical corticosteroids should be avoided. Adrenal suppression can occur even without occlusion. Topical administration of corticosteroids to pregnant animals can cause abnormalities of foetal development. The relevance of these findings to human beings has not been established. However topical steroids should not be used extensively during the first trimester of pregnancy i.e. in large amounts or for prolonged periods. As with all topical steroids, there is a risk of skin atrophy following extensive therapy. The application of unusually large quantities of topical corticoids may result in the absorption of systemically active amounts of corticoid. Infections or secondarily-infected dermatoses definitely require additional therapy with antibiotics or chemotherapeutic agents. This treatment can often be topical but for heavy infections systemic antibacterial therapy may be necessary. If fungal infections are present, a topically active antimycotic should be applied.

Pharmaceutical precautions In order to restore the consistency of suppositories which have become soft owing to warm temperature, they should be put into cold water before the covering is removed.

Store in cool dry conditions: shelf-life five years.

Legal category POM.

Package quantities *Suppositories:* Packs of 12.

Ointment: Tubes of 10 g and 30 g.

Further information Nil.

Product licence numbers
Ultraproct Suppositories   0053/5009
Ultraproct Ointment   0053/5008

UROGRAFIN*

Presentation Ampoules, vials or bottles containing colourless sterile solutions of varying strengths of meglumine diatrizoate and meglumine/sodium diatrizoates.

Urografin 150: An intravenous injection of meglumine diatrizoate 26.1% w/v and sodium diatrizoate 3.9% w/v, containing 146 mg iodine per ml.

Urografin 290: An intravascular injection of meglumine diatrizoate 52.1% w/v and sodium diatrizoate 7.9% w/v, containing 292 mg iodine per ml.

Urografin 310M: An intravascular injection of meglumine diatrizoate 65% w/v, containing 306 mg iodine per ml.

Urografin 325: An intravenous injection of meglumine diatrizoate 18% w/v and sodium diatrizoate 40% w/v, containing 325 mg iodine per ml.

Urografin 370: An intravascular injection of meglumine diatrizoate 66% w/v and sodium diatrizoate 10% w/v, containing 370 mg iodine per ml.

Uses X-ray contrast media for the delineation of the vascular and renal systems.

Dosage and administration See table on following pages.

Contra-indications, warnings, etc
Contra-indications: Proven or suspected hypersensitivity to iodine-containing contrast media, manifest thyrotoxicosis and decompensated cardiac insufficiency.

Hysterosalpingography must not be carried out during pregnancy or in patients with acute inflammatory conditions in the pelvic cavity.

Warnings/side-effects: For patients with severe impairment of hepatic or renal function, cardiac or circulatory insufficiency, cerebral arteriosclerosis, cerebral spasmodic conditions, epilepsy, juvenile-onset diabetes, long-standing diabetes, pulmonary emphysema, poor general health, hyperthyroidism or multiple myeloma the need for examination with X-ray contrast media merits careful consideration.

This also applies to patients with a history of allergy, e.g. bronchial asthma, since experience shows that they may exhibit hypersensitivity to drugs. Because of possible precipitation, X-ray contrast media and prophylactic agents must not be injected as mixed solutions.

Particular caution should be exercised in allergic persons who have previously tolerated an injectable iodine-containing contrast medium without any complication because they may have become sensitized to these substances in the meantime.

The patient should be recumbent during the administration of Urografin. Thereafter, the patient must be kept under close observation for at least 15 minutes, since about 90% of all severe incidents occur within that time. If the administration does not take place on the X-ray table, any patient with a labile circulation should be brought to the X-ray machine sitting or lying down.

In patients with multiple myeloma, juvenile-onset diabetes, long-standing diabetes, polyuria, oliguria or gout, and in infants, young children and marasmic patients the fluid supply should not be restricted. Existing disturbances of the balance of water and electrolytes must be corrected before the administration of a hypertonic contrast-medium solution.

Premedication with an alpha-blocker is recommended in patients with phaeochromocytoma.

X-ray examinations should if possible be avoided during pregnancy. It has not yet been proved beyond question that Urografin may be used without hesitation in pregnant patients. Therefore an examination with a contrast medium during pregnancy should be carried out only if considered absolutely necessary by the physician.

If iodine isotopes are to be administered for diagnosing thyroid disease, it should be borne in mind that after the administration of iodised contrast media which are excreted via the kidneys, the capacity of the thyroid tissue to take up iodine will be reduced for a few days, and sometimes up to 6 weeks.

Mild subjective symptoms, such as a feeling of heat and nausea, occur very seldom and disappear rapidly when the injection is slowed down or briefly interrupted. Transient pain may occur, in particular during the examination of peripheral vascular regions. Extravasations give rise to serious tissue reactions only in very rare cases.

If marked side-effects or suspected allergic reactions occur during injection and do not disappear, or even get worse, when the injection is briefly interrupted, it is probable that the patient has such a hypersensitivity and the investigation must be abandoned. Even relatively minor symptoms such as itching of the skin, sneezing, violent yawns, tickling in the throat, hoarseness or attacks of coughing may be early signs of a severe reaction and, therefore, merit careful attention.

Very rarely, severe or even life-threatening side-effects such as severe hypotension and collapse, circulatory failure, ventricular fibrillation, cardiac arrest, pulmonary oedema, anaphylactic shock or other allergic manifestations, convulsions, or other cerebral symptoms may occur.

Ready availability of all drugs and equipment for emergency treatment and familiarity with the respective procedures are prerequisites for the effective management of contrast-medium incidents. Some guidance in the treatment of such incidents is contained in the leaflet supplied with the pack.

Pharmaceutical precautions *Storage:* Protect from light and heat. Shelf-life five years.

Legal category POM.

Package quantities
Urografin 150: Packs of 10 × 10 ml ampoules and 10 × 20 ml ampoules.
Urografin 150 for Infusion: Packs of 1 × 250 ml bottles and 1 × 500 ml bottles.
Urografin 290: Packs of 10 × 20 ml ampoules and 10 × 50 ml vials.
Urografin 310M: Packs of 10 × 20 ml ampoules and 10 × 50 ml vials.

Urografin 325: Packs of 10 × 20 ml ampoules and 10 × 50 ml vials.

Urografin 370: Packs of 10 × 20 ml ampoules and 10 × 50 ml vials. In addition packs of 1 × 100 ml vials and 1 × 200 ml vials.

Further information Nil.

Product licence numbers
Urografin 150	0053/5041
Urografin 150 for infusion	0053/5007
Urografin 290	0053/5043
Urografin 310M	0053/5018
Urografin 325	0053/5006
Urografin 370	0053/5044

UROGRAFIN MEDIA – DOSAGE AND ADMINISTRATION

1. Adults only

The table on this and the next page shows the medium/media Schering suggest for each investigation. Alternative medium/media (shown by asterisk) may be used in the same dose. Schering media may be used at the discretion of the radiologist for other established permutations of medium and examination which, for the sake of simplicity, have been omitted from the table.

Examination	150	290	310M	325	370
Intravenous urography		Up to 70 ml	Up to 70 ml	Up to 70 ml	Up to 70 ml
High-dose urography		100 ml	100 ml	100 ml	
Drip-infusion urography	2–4 ml/kg body wt up to 250 ml				
Retrograde urography	5–10 ml				
Cystography	Up to 500 ml				
Angiocardiography			*		30–50 ml
Right-heart catheterisation			*		40–80 ml
Left-heart catheterisation			*		40–60 ml
Pulmonary angiography			*		30–40 ml
Coronary arteriography			DO NOT USE		4–8 ml per artery[a] *
Renal arteriography		*	5–8 ml		
Coeliac-axis arteriography		*	35–50 ml		
Superior mesenteric arteriography		*	20–30 ml		
Inferior mesenteric arteriography		*	15–20 ml		
Peripheral arteriography (leg)		*	15–25 ml		
Peripheral arteriography (arm)					
Subclavian			20 ml		
Axillary			15 ml		
Brachial			10 ml		
Hepatic arteriography		*	25 ml		
Thoracic aortography		*			30–60 ml
Percutaneous retrograde abdominal aortography		*	25–30 ml. No more than 2 inj.		
Pelvic aortography		*			20–25 ml
Lower limb aortography		*	35–50 ml		
Translumbar abdominal aortography		*			20–30 ml *
Placentography			25 ml		
Carotid angiography (internal)			8–10 ml		
Carotid angiography (external)			6–8 ml. Not more than 3 inj. per artery		
Vertebral angiography			6 ml. Not more than 2 inj. per vessel		

Table continued on next page

Urografin Media – Dosage and administration. Table continued from previous page.

Examination	150	290	310M	325	370
Pelvic venography		*	25–30 ml	*	
Venacavography					
Inferior			30–50 ml	*	
Superior			25–35 ml	*	
Renal venography		*	10–15 ml		
Peripheral venography					
Leg			30–50 ml		
Arm			20–30 ml per injection		
Splenoportography			40–50 ml		40–50 ml
Splenoportography – indirect		*	30–50 ml Higher doses required to demonstrate splenic and portal veins		
Hysterosalpingography				*	4–7 ml
Arthrography		*		1–10 ml	
Percutaneous cholangiography		20–30 ml			

[a] 100 ml and 200 ml vials are available for coronary arteriography
(Other indications include selective visceral angiography, limb venography, jugular venography, vesiculography, sialography, sinusography, amniography, lymphangiography, intramuscular urography, operative cholangiography, fistulography, oesophageal and anal atresia.)
Urografin media are not suitable for myelography

2. Children and neonates

Intravenous urography: The fact that urograms of infants and young children generally show a lower contrast density than those of adults is explained by the physiologically less effective function of the immature nephron. Relatively high doses of media are therefore indicated.

Drip-infusion urography: Dosage of Urografin 150 should not exceed 4 ml/kg body weight.

Angiocardiography: In neonates up to 5 kg body weight, 8 ml of Urografin 310M or Urografin 370. Infants over 5 kg body weight, 1 ml/kg body weight up to 25 ml per injection.

	Urografin 310M/290		Urografin 325/370
Up to 1 year	8–12 ml	Up to 1 year	7–10 ml
1–2 years	12–15 ml	1–2 years	10–12 ml
2–6 years	15–20 ml	2–6 years	12–15 ml
6–10 years	20–25 ml	6–12 years	15–20 ml
10–15 years	25–30 ml	over 12 years	adult dose

Right and left-heart catheterisation: 1–1.2 ml/kg body weight of Urografin 310M or Urografin 370, with a maximum of 15 ml per injection for the right heart and 25 ml per injection for the left heart.

Pulmonary angiography: 0.5–0.6 ml/kg body weight up to 8 ml Urografin 310M or Urografin 370 per injection.

*Trade Mark

Schwarz Pharmaceuticals Ltd
Schwarz House
East Street
Chesham
Bucks HP5 1DG

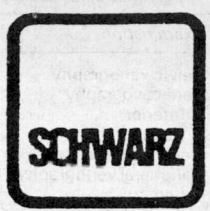

DEPONIT 5 ▼

Presentation Deponit is a transdermal drug delivery system in the form of a self-adhesive, skin-coloured patch. The adhesive film of Deponit has a surface area of 16 cm² and contains 16 mg of glyceryl trinitrate. Each patch is designed to release glyceryl trinitrate at an average rate of 5 mg per 24 hours.

Uses Deponit is indicated for the prophylaxis of angina pectoris either alone, or in combination with other antianginal therapy. The glyceryl trinitrate is formulated in the adhesive layer in the form of dissolved and adsorbed molecules. By simple diffusion across the skin, the active constituent is thus released at a rate of 5 mg per 24 hours.

Glyceryl trinitrate reduces the tone of vascular smooth muscle. This action is more marked on the venous capacitance vessels than the arterial vessels. There is a reduction in venous return to the heart and a lowering of elevated filling pressure. This lowering of filling pressure reduces the left ventricular end diastolic volume and preload. The net effect is a reduction in myocardial oxygen consumption.

Systemic vascular resistance, pulmonary vascular resistance and arterial pressure are also reduced and there is a net reduction in afterload.

Glyceryl trinitrate improves the myocardial oxygen supply by redistributing the blood flow along collateral channels and from the epicardial to the endocardial regions.

Dosage and administration

Adults: One patch to be applied to the lateral chest wall daily.

Children: The safety and efficacy of Deponit in children has yet to be established.

Each patch is packaged in individually sealed sachets and should only be removed prior to administration. There is a convenient break in the covering foil which can be easily peeled off by the patient. The exposed patch may then be applied to the lateral chest wall and should be removed after no longer than 24 hours.

Subsequent applications should always be made to a new area of skin and several days should be allowed to elapse before applying a fresh patch to the same area.

Safety, efficacy and tolerability beyond 28 days therapy have yet to be established.

Use in the elderly: No specific information on use in the elderly is available, but there is no evidence to suggest that an alteration in dose is required.

Contra-indications, warnings, etc

Contra-indications: Deponit should not be given to patients who are sensitive to nitrates or with increased intracranial pressure. Marked anaemia, acute circulatory failure (shock) or severe hypotension are other contra-indications to Deponit.

Side-effects: Headaches may develop initially, but these will usually disappear after a few days. There is also the possibility of reflex tachycardia. Postural hypotension, syncope or dizziness occur rarely, and these effects may be potentiated by alcohol. Nausea may also occur infrequently.

Allergic reactions may occur in sensitive patients.

When the patch is removed, there may be a slight reddening of the skin which will usually subside in a few hours.

Precautions: Deponit should not be used during pregnancy or lactation unless considered absolutely essential by the physician.

Deponit is not suitable for acute anginal attacks. If these occur during therapy then additional medication should be considered. Deponit dilates peripheral blood vessels and may increase the antihypertensive properties of vasodilators, calcium antagonists, tricyclic antidepressants and alcohol.

In patients with a recent history of myocardial infarction or acute heart failure, Deponit should be used with caution. As with all anti-anginal nitrate preparations, withdrawal of treatment should be gradual (over 4–6 weeks) by replacement with decreasing doses of long-acting oral nitrates. This product should be used with extreme caution in patients pre-disposed to closed angle glaucoma.

Deponit should be removed prior to electrical defibrillation to prevent the possibility of 'arcing' across the patch.

Pharmaceutical precautions Store below 25°C.

Legal category P.

Package quantities Deponit 5 is packaged in cartons of 30 patches.

Further information Deponit consists of an adhesive layer containing glyceryl trinitrate which is approximately 300 μ thick. This adhesive layer is covered by two aluminium foils which are impermeable to the active constituent thus ensuring no loss of glyceryl trinitrate during the shelf life of the product.

When applied to the skin, Deponit adheres to the whole area of application without risk of becoming detached even during activities like swimming and bathing.

Glyceryl trinitrate is also known as nitroglycerin, trinitrin or trinitroglycerin.

Product licence number 4438/0014.

ELANTAN* 20 ▼

Presentation White tablets with break score, containing 20 mg Isosorbide mononitrate. Each tablet is marked with the code E20.

Use Prophylaxis of angina pectoris.

Dosage and administration Long term treatment, one tablet to be taken two or three times a day after meals taken unchewed with a little fluid. The dosage may be increased to two tablets three times a day.

Contra-indications, warnings, etc Elantan should not be used in cases of acute circulatory failure (shock, vascular collapse), very low blood pressure or low filling pressure. The drug should not be used during the first three months of pregnancy. Symptoms of circulatory collapse may arise after the first dose in patients with labile circulation and nitrate headache may also occur. Both symptoms can be largely avoided if the treatment is started with half a tablet of Elantan morning and evening.

Reaction capacity may be reduced if alcohol is consumed during treatment.

Pharmaceutical precautions None.

Legal category POM.

Package quantities Elantan 20 is blister-packed in cartons of 50 and 100 tablets and in a hospital-only dispensing pack of 500 tablets.

Further information Isosorbide mononitrate is the British approved name for isosorbide 5-mononitrate.

Elantan lacks any significant first pass metabolism providing consistently uniform plasma levels of Isosorbide mononitrate, thereby laying the foundation for improved clinical response.

Product licence number 4438/0005.

ELANTAN 40*

Presentation White uncoated tablets with break score, containing 40 mg Isosorbide mononitrate. Each tablet is marked with the code E40.

Use Prophylaxis of angina pectoris.

Dosage and administration Long-term treatment: 1 tablet twice a day after meals taken unchewed with a little fluid.

Contra-indications, warnings, etc Elantan should not be used in cases of acute circulatory failure (shock, vascular collapse), very low blood pressure or low filling pressure. The drug should not be used during the first three months of pregnancy. Symptoms of circulatory collapse may arise after the first dose in patients with labile circulation and nitrate headache may also occur. Both symptoms can be largely avoided if the treatment is started with a lower dose of Elantan initially. Reaction capacity may be reduced if alcohol is consumed during treatment.

Pharmaceutical precautions None.

Legal category POM.

Package quantities Elantan 40 is blister-packed in cartons of 50 tablets.

Further information Isosorbide mononitrate is the British Approved Name for Isosorbide 5-mononitrate.

Elantan lacks any significant first pass metabolism providing consistently uniform plasma levels of Isosorbide mononitrate, thereby laying the foundation for improved clinical response.

Product licence number 4438/0008.

ISOKET* I.V.

Presentation Isoket i.v. is a solution of isosorbide dinitrate 1 mg/ml in sterile isotonic saline. It is supplied in 10 ml ampoules, 50 ml bottles and 100 ml bottles. The solution contains no alcohol.

Uses Isoket is indicated in the treatment of unresponsive left ventricular failure secondary to acute myocardial infarction, unresponsive left ventricular failure of various aetiology and severe or unstable angina pectoris. Isosorbide dinitrate is a vasodilator, reducing the afterload and especially the preload of the heart. It influences the oxygen supply to ischaemic myocardium by causing the redistribution of blood flow along the collateral channels and from epicardial to endocardial regions. It also reduces oxygen demand by increasing venous capacitance, causing pooling of blood in peripheral veins thereby reducing ventricular volume and heart wall distension.

Dosage and administration

Dosage: The dose employed must be adjusted according to the patient's response. In general, a dose of between 2 and 7 mg per hour is suitable, although doses as high as 10 mg per hour may be necessary.

Children: The safety and efficacy of Isoket has not yet been established in children.

Administration: Isoket is a concentrated solution and should never be injected directly in the form of a bolus. Isoket can be administered as an intravenous admixture with a suitable vehicle such as Sodium Chloride Injection BP or Dextrose Injection BP. Prepared Isoket admixtures are always given by intravenous infusion or with the aid of a syringe pump incorporating a glass or rigid plastic syringe. During administration, there should be close monitoring of the patient's blood pressure and pulse. Admixtures are prepared by exchanging the required volume of Isoket with an equal volume of the infusion vehicle. For example, if a dose of 6 mg per hour is required, 50 ml of Isoket (equivalent to 5×10 ml ampoules or 1×50 ml bottle) should be added to 450 ml of the infusion vehicle to give a final volume of 500 ml. This admixture now contains 1 mg in 10 ml and the required dosage can be obtained by giving 60 ml per hour which is equivalent to a drip rate of 60 paediatric microdrops per minute or 20 standard drops per minute. This drip rate provides enough solution for an infusion time of 8 hours and 20 minutes. When it is necessary to further reduce the fluid intake, a more concentrated solution may be obtained by using a 100 ml bottle (100 mg) of Isoket made up to 500 ml with a suitable infusion vehicle. This admixture now contains 200 mcg/ml (2 mg in 10 ml). With a concentration of 200 mcg/ml, the patient requiring 6 mg Isoket per hour would need a drip rate of 30 paediatric microdrops per minute (which is the same as 30 ml per hour) *or* 10 standard drops per minute. The Admixture should be made up under aseptic conditions.

Contra-indications, warnings, etc

Contra-indications: Isoket should not be used in the treatment of cardiogenic shock unless some means of maintaining an adequate diastolic aortic pressure are undertaken. Isoket is contra-indicated in circulatory collapse, severe hypotension or low filling pressure.

Precautions: Close attention to pulse and blood pressure is necessary during the administration of Isoket infusions.

Adverse effects: Whilst sharp falls in systemic arterial pressure can give rise to symptoms of cerebral flow deficiency and decreased coronary perfusion, clinical experience with Isoket has shown that this is not normally a problem. This is consistent with the known vasodilatory effects of Isosorbide dinitrate which occur predominantly on the venous rather than the arterial side of the circulation. In common with other nitrates, headaches and nausea may occur during administration.

Pharmaceutical precautions *Compatibility:* Isoket contains isosorbide dinitrate in isotonic saline and is compatible with commonly employed infusion solutions. No incompatibilities have so far been demonstrated. Isoket is compatible with glass infusion bottles and infusion packs made of polyethylene, e.g. Polyfusor* (Boots). Isoket may also be infused slowly using a syringe pump with a glass or plastic syringe (Gillette Sabre* syringe, B.D. Plastipak* syringe or Monoject* disposable syringe. Sherwood Medical Ltd.) Isoket is incompatible with infusion bags and administration sets made from PVC and a loss of activity of up to 40% is possible on prolonged contact, e.g. 8 hours. Loss after 1 hour is approximately 30%. The use of PVC containers should therefore be avoided, e.g. Viaflex* (Travenol) or Steriflex* (Boots). A high pressure polyethylene tubing known to be compatible with Isoket i.v. is available from Vygon U.K. Limited under the name of Lectrocath.*

Legal category POM.

Package quantities 10 ml ampoules: Each pack contains ten ampoules of Isoket i.v. (10 mg/10 ml).
50 ml bottles: Each pack contains one bottle of Isoket i.v. (50 mg/50 ml).
100 ml bottles: Each pack contains one bottle of Isoket i.v. (100mg/100 ml).

Further information Nil.

Product licence number 4438/0001.

ISOKET* RETARD 20

Presentation Circular yellow tablets, scored on one side, and containing 20 mg Isosorbide dinitrate in a sustained release formulation.

Uses For the prevention of anginal attacks.

Dosage and administration The tablets are for oral administration. The deep score-line permits easy division of the tablets when low dosages are prescribed.

The usual dose for long-term treatment is one tablet every 12 hours; the tablets should be swallowed without chewing. Up to four tablets daily may be taken if necessary.

Contra-indications, warnings, etc

Contra-indications: A history of sensitivity to the drug. Very low blood pressure.

Warnings: Headaches may develop in sensitive persons, and these may be minimized by commencing with low, gradually increasing doses. Cutaneous vasodilatation, postural hypotension and dry rashes may occasionally occur.

Precautions: Alcohol intake may enhance the effect of the drug and induce hypotension. The product should not be used during pregnancy or lactation except under the direction of a doctor.

Pharmaceutical precautions None.

Legal category P.

Package quantities The tablets are supplied in blister-packs of 50 tablets.

Further information The special sustained release formulation of Isoket Retard tablets permits onset of action within 20 minutes and a duration of up to 12 hours.

Product licence number 4438/0004

NITROCINE*

Presentation Nitrocine is presented as ampoules containing 10 mg nitroglycerin in 10 ml isotonic sterile solution or as glass bottles containing 50 mg nitroglycerin in 50 ml isotonic sterile solution. Nitrocine does not contain alcohol or potassium.

Uses Nitroglycerin reduces the tone of vascular smooth muscle. This action is more marked on the venous capacitance vessels than the arterial vessels. There is a reduction in venous return to the heart and a lowering of elevated filling pressure. This lowering of filling pressure reduces the left ventricular end diastolic volume and preload. The net effect is a lowering of myocardial oxygen consumption.

Systemic vascular resistance, pulmonary vascular resistance and arterial pressure are also reduced by nitroglycerin and there is a net reduction in afterload.

Nitroglycerin reduces the work load on the heart by reducing the preload and the afterload.

Nitroglycerin improves the myocardial oxygen supply by redistributing blood flow along collateral channels and from epicardial to endocardial regions.

Surgery: Nitrocine may be used for the rapid control of hypertension during cardiac surgery.

Nitrocine may be used to reduce blood pressures and maintain controlled hypotension during surgical procedures.

Nitrocine may also be used to control myocardial ischaemia during and after cardiovascular surgery.

Unresponsive congestive heart failure: Nitrocine may be used to treat unresponsive congestive heart failure secondary to acute myocardial infarction.

Unstable angina: Nitrocine may be used to treat unstable angina which is refractory to treatment with beta blockers and sublingual nitrates.

Dosage and administration Nitrocine solution is a concentrate which should be diluted prior to intravenous administration. The product is normally administered intravenously as an admixture using a suitable vehicle such as Sodium Chloride Injection BP or Dextrose Injection BP.

Admixtures are prepared by exchanging the required volume of Nitrocine with an equal volume of infusion vehicle. For example to obtain an admixture of nitrogly-cerin at a concentration 100 mcg/ml 50 ml Nitrocine solution (containing 50 mg nitroglycerin) is added to 450 ml of the infusion vehicle to give a final volume of 500 ml. If a dosage of 100 mcg/min is required, this can be obtained by giving 60 ml of the admixture per hour. This is equivalent to a drip rate of 60 paediatric microdrops per minute or 20 standard drops per minute. At this drip rate, the admixture provides enough solution for an infusion time of 8 hours 20 minutes. For full details it is advisable to consult the dosage chart on the package insert.

Nitrocine may be given by intravenous infusion or with the aid of syringe pump. During Nitrocine administration there should be close haemodynamic monitoring of the patient.

The dose of Nitrocine should be adjusted to meet the individual needs of the patient and the responses of the monitored haemodynamic parameters.

The recommended dosage range is 10–200 mcg/min but up to 400 mcg/min may be necessary during some surgical procedures.

Surgery: A starting dose of 25 mcg/min is recommended for the control of hypertension, or to produce hypoten-sion during surgery. This may be increased by increments of 25 mcg/min at 5 minute intervals until the blood pressure is stabilized. Doses between 10–200 mcg are usually sufficient during surgery although doses of up to 400 mcg/min have been required in some cases.

The treatment of perioperative myocardial ischaemia may be started with a dose of 15–20 mcg/min, with subsequent increments of 10–15 mcg/min until the required effect is obtained.

Unresponsive congestive heart failure: The recom-mended starting dose is 20–25 mcg/min. This may be decreased to 10 mcg/min or increased in steps of 20–25 mcg/min every 15–30 minutes until the desired effect is obtained.

Unstable angina: An initial dose of 10 mcg/min is recommended with increments being made at approxi-mately 30 minute intervals according to the needs of the patient.

Children: The safety and efficacy of Nitrocine has not yet been established in children.

Contra-indications, warnings, etc

Contra-indications: Nitrocine should not be used in the following cases:

Known hypersensitivity to nitrates.

Marked anaemia, severe cerebral haemorrhage, un-corrected hypovolaemia or severe hypotension.

Patients predisposed to closed angle glaucoma.

Nitrocine should not be used during pregnancy or lactation except under the direction of a doctor.

Precautions: Close attention to pulse and blood pressure is necessary during the administration of Nitrocine infusions.

Nitrocine should be used with caution in patients suffering from hypothyroidism, severe liver or renal disease, hypothermia and malnutrition.

Adverse effects: In common with other nitrates, head-aches and nausea may occur during administration. Other possible adverse reactions include hypotension, tachycardia, retching, diaphoresis, apprehension, rest-lessness, muscle twitching, retrosternal discomfort, pal-pitations, dizziness and abdominal pain. Paradoxical bradycardia has also been observed. Mild overdose usually results in hypotension and tachycardia. This may be reversed by elevating the legs and decreasing or terminating the infusion. In the event of severe overdose, intravenous administration of methoxamine or phenyle-phrine is recommended.

Pharmaceutical precautions Admixtures are stable for approximately 24 hours at room temperature in the recommended containers. Open ampoules or bottles should be used immediately and any unused drug discarded. Nitrocine contains nitroglycerin and no drug incompatibilities have been reported so far.

Compatibility: Nitrocine is compatible with glass infusion bottles and with rigid infusion packs made of polyethyl-ene, e.g. Polyfusor (Boots). Nitrocine may also be infused slowly using a syringe pump with a glass or plastic syringe (Gillette Sabre syringe, B.D. Plastipak syringe or Monoject disposable syringe, Sherwood Medical Ltd.)

Nitrocine is incompatible with PVC and severe losses of nitroglycerin (over 40%) may occur if this material is used. Contact with PVC bags such as Viaflex (Travenol) or Steriflex (Boots) should be avoided. A high pressure tubing known to be compatible with nitroglycerin is Lectrocath tubing from Vygon U.K. Limited.

Legal category POM.

Package quantities

Ampoules: Each pack contains 10 × 10 ml ampoules of Nitrocine.

Bottles: Each contains 50 ml of Nitrocine.

Further information Nitrocine contains no alcohol or potassium since these substances have been reported to be deleterious to patients with coronary heart disease. The effects reported after infusion of small quantities of alcohol include diminished left ventricular function, shown by a decrease in stroke volume and a rise in end diastolic pressure, with associated deterioration in the electrocardiograph.

The effects of alcohol are known to persist beyond 5 hours.

The effects reported after administration of parenteral preparations containing potassium include exacerbation of myocardial ischaemia and near fatal ventricular fibrillation.

Nitroglycerin is also known as glyceryl trinitrate, trinitroglycerin or trinitrin.

Product licence number 4438/0006.

*Trade Mark

Searle Pharmaceuticals
Division of G. D. Searle & Company Limited
PO Box 53
Lane End Road
High Wycombe
Bucks HP12 4HL

SEARLE

ALDACTONE* 100 mg
ALDACTONE* 50 mg
ALDACTONE* 25 mg

Presentation *Aldactone 100 mg:* Buff, film-coated tablets engraved SEARLE 134 on one side, containing Spironolactone BP 100 mg.

Aldactone 50 mg: Off-white, film-coated tablets engraved SEARLE 916 on one side, containing Spironolactone BP 50 mg.

Aldactone 25 mg: Buff, film-coated tablets engraved SEARLE 39 on one side, containing Spironolactone BP 25 mg.

Uses Congestive heart failure; Hepatic cirrhosis with ascites and oedema; Malignant ascites; Nephrotic syndrome; Idiopathic oedema including premenstrual oedema; Diagnosis and treatment of primary aldosteronism; Essential hypertension.

Dosage and administration Food has been reported to increase the bioavailability of Aldactone. It is recommended that tablets are taken with meals.

Adults: Congestive heart failure: Usual dose – 100 mg/day. In difficult or severe cases the dosage may be gradually increased up to 400mg/day. When oedema is controlled, the usual maintenance level is 75–200 mg/day.

Hepatic cirrhosis with ascites and oedema: If urinary Na+ /K+ ratio is greater than 1.0, 100 mg per day. If the ratio is less than 1.0, 200–400 mg/day. Maintenance dosage should be individually determined.

Malignant ascites: Initial dose usually 100–200 mg/day. In severe cases the dosage may be gradually increased up to 400 mg/day. When oedema is controlled, maintenance dosage should be individually determined.

Nephrotic syndrome: Usual dose – 100–200 mg/day. Spironolactone has not been shown to be anti-inflammatory, nor to affect the basic pathological process. Its use is only advised if glucocorticoids by themselves are insufficiently effective.

Idiopathic oedema including premenstrual oedema: Usual dose – 100 mg/day.

Diagnosis and treatment of primary aldosteronism: Aldactone may be employed as an initial diagnostic measure to provide presumptive evidence of primary hyperaldosteronism while patients are on normal diets.

Long test: Aldactone is administered at a daily dosage of 400 mg for three to four weeks. Correction of hypoka-

laemia and of hypertension provides presumptive evidence for the diagnosis of primary hyperaldosteronism.

Short test: Aldactone is administered at a daily dosage of 400 mg for four days. If serum potassium increases during Aldactone administration but drops when Aldactone is discontinued, a presumptive diagnosis of primary hyperaldosteronism should be considered.

After the diagnosis of hyperaldosteronism has been established by more definitive testing procedures, Aldactone may be administered in doses of 100 mg to 400 mg daily in preparation for surgery. For patients who are considered unsuitable for surgery, Aldactone may be employed for long-term maintenance therapy at the lowest effective dosage determined for the individual patient.

Essential hypertension: Usual dose – 50–100 mg per day, which for difficult or severe cases may be gradually increased at two weekly intervals up to 200 mg/day.

Treatment should be continued for two weeks or longer since an adequate response may not occur before this time. Dosage should subsequently be adjusted according to the response of the patient.

Elderly: It is recommended that treatment is started with the lowest dose and titrated upwards as required to achieve maximum benefit. Care should be taken in severe hepatic and renal impairment which may alter drug metabolism and excretion.

Children: Initial daily dosage should provide 3 mg of spironolactone per kilogram body weight, given in divided doses. Dosage should be adjusted on the basis of response and tolerance. If necessary a suspension may be prepared by crushing Aldactone tablets. A suitable suspending vehicle is methylcellulose mixture '450' (900 mg/10 ml) [Cologel*] 20% v/v, purified water to 100%. Such a suspension is chemically stable for one month when refrigerated.

Contra-indications, warnings, etc
Contra-indications: Aldactone is contra-indicated in patients with anuria, acute renal insufficiency, rapidly deteriorating or severe impairment of renal function, hyperkalaemia, Addison's disease and in patients who are hypersensitive to spironolactone.

Aldactone should not be administered concurrently with other potassium-conserving diuretics and potassium supplements should not be given routinely with Aldactone as hyperkalaemia may be induced.

Warnings: Carcinogenicity: Spironolactone has been shown to produce tumours in rats when administered at high doses over a long period of time. The significance of these findings with respect to clinical use is not certain. However, the long-term use of spironolactone in young patients requires careful consideration of the benefits and the potential hazard involved.

Precautions: Fluid and electrolyte balance: Fluid and electrolyte status should be regularly monitored, particularly in the elderly and in those with significant renal impairment.

Hyperkalaemia may occur in patients with impaired renal function or excessive potassium intake and can cause cardiac irregularities which may be fatal. Should hyperkalaemia develop Aldactone should be discontinued, and if necessary, active measures taken to reduce the serum potassium to normal.

Hyponatraemia may be induced, especially when Aldactone is administered in combination with other diuretics.

Reversible hyperchloraemic metabolic acidosis usually in association with hyperkalaemia has been reported to occur in some patients with decompensated hepatic cirrhosis, even in the presence of normal renal function.

Urea: Reversible increases in blood urea have been reported in association with Aldactone therapy, particularly in the presence of impaired renal function.

Drug interactions: Potentiation of the effect of other antihypertensive drugs occurs and their dosage may need to be reduced when Aldactone is added to the treatment regime, and then adjusted as necessary.

As carbenoxolone may cause sodium retention and thus decrease the effectiveness of Aldactone, concurrent use should be avoided.

Spironolactone reduces vascular responsiveness to noradrenaline. Caution should be exercised in the management of patients subjected to regional or general anaesthesia while they are being treated with Aldactone.

Pregnancy: Spironolactone or its metabolites may cross the placental barrier. The use of Aldactone in pregnant women requires that the anticipated benefit be weighed against the possible hazards to the mother and foetus.

Nursing mothers: Canrenone, a metabolite of spironolactone, appears in breast milk. If use of Aldactone is considered essential, an alternative method of infant feeding should be instituted.

Adverse effects: Gynaecomastia may develop in association with the use of spironolactone. Development appears to be related to both dosage level and duration of therapy and is normally reversible when spironolactone is discontinued. In rare instances some breast enlargement may persist. Other adverse reactions reported in association with spironolactone include: gastrointestinal intolerance, drowsiness, lethargy, headache, mental confusion, ataxia, drug fever, skin rashes, menstrual irregularities, impotence and mild androgenic effects.

Overdosage: Acute overdosage may be manifested by drowsiness, mental confusion, nausea, vomiting, dizziness or diarrhoea. Hyponatraemia or hyperkalaemia may be induced but these effects are unlikely to be associated with acute overdosage. Symptoms of hyperkalaemia may manifest as paraesthesia, weakness, flaccid paralysis or muscle spasm and may be difficult to distinguish clinically from hypokalaemia. Electrocardiographic changes are the earliest specific signs of potassium disturbances. No specific antidote has been identified. Improvement may be expected after withdrawal of the drug. General supportive measures including replacement of fluids and electrolytes may be indicated. For hyperkalaemia, reduce potassium intake, administer potassium-excreting diuretics, intravenous glucose with regular insulin, or oral ion-exchange resins.

Pharmaceutical precautions Store below 30°C (86°F).

Legal category POM.

Package quantities *Aldactone 100 mg:* Calendar pack of 28 tablets and bottles containing 100 and 500 tablets.

Aldactone 50 mg: Bottles containing 100 tablets.

Aldactone 25 mg: Bottles containing 100 and 500 tablets.

Further information Aldactone as a competitive aldosterone antagonist increases sodium excretion whilst reducing potassium loss at the distal renal tubule. It has a gradual and prolonged action, maximum response being usually attained after 2–3 days' treatment.

Combination of Aldactone with a conventional, more proximally acting diuretic usually enhances diuresis without excessive potassium loss.

Product licence numbers
Aldactone 100 mg   0020/0048
Aldactone 50 mg   0020/0088
Aldactone 25 mg   0020/5000

REHIDRAT*

Presentation Foil/laminate sachet containing 14 g of lemon and lime flavoured greyish-white granular powder with green particles. Each sachet contains:

Sodium Chloride PhEur	0.44 g
Potassium Chloride PhEur	0.38 g
Sodium Bicarbonate PhEur	0.42 g
Citric Acid PhEur	0.44 g
Glucose	4.09 g
Sucrose PhEur	8.07 g
Fructose	0.07 g
Plus flavourings	

Uses Oral electrolyte mixture for prevention and correction of mild and moderate dehydration. In the management of diarrhoea in infants, children and adults.

Maintenance and replacement of fluid and electrolytes following corrective parenteral therapy for dehydration. As a supplement to corrective parenteral therapy for dehydration.

Dosage and administration
General advice: The contents of one 14 g sachet should be dissolved in 250 ml (approximately half a pint) of drinking water. For infants the water should be freshly boiled AND COOLED. The solution should be freshly made immediately prior to use. Any unused solution remaining an hour after reconstitution should be discarded unless stored in a refrigerator where it may be kept and used for up to 24 hours. Advise patients that the solution should not be boiled after reconstitution, and that it should always be used at the recommended dilution.

The degree of dehydration should be assessed. Patients with mild or moderate dehydration may appear almost normal, they may be thirsty and may have normal or slightly diminished skin elasticity or, in children, slightly sunken fontanelle. Urine flow may be reduced. Patients with signs of severe dehydration who are usually too weak to drink will initially require parenteral therapy. Oral therapy should only be instituted when shock is corrected.

The volume of reconstituted Rehidrat required will depend on the weight of the patient.

General guidelines for oral therapy

1. Rehydration: Replacement of fluid and electrolyte losses. Mild or moderate dehydration – 50–120 ml per kilogram body weight orally, usually given in divided doses over 4 to 6 hours. Adults may need up to 1000 ml per hour. A continuous nasogastric infusion may be used if necessary.

2. Maintenance: Mild to moderate diarrhoea – 100–200 ml per kilogram body weight orally over a period of 24 hours in divided doses. Continuing diarrhoea – 15 ml per kilogram body weight orally every hour. Observe carefully to confirm adequate maintenance of hydration.

Where nausea or vomiting is present Rehidrat should be administered in small frequent doses, in sips. If vomiting persists appropriate intravenous therapy should be instituted. The patient instruction leaflet included in each carton advises patients to consult their doctor if there is no improvement in 24–48 hours.

Elderly: Administer Rehidrat in amounts appropriate to correct dehydration. Also see Precautions.

Infants and children: For bottle fed infants advise mothers to make the feed up for a 24 hour period and to store the reconstituted solution in the refrigerator.

Diarrhoea can have serious consequences in children under 3 years old. For this age group, the patient instruction leaflet included in each carton advises that management should be on medical advice. Breast feeding should continue and Rehidrat should be given after feeds. In other infants and children administration of Rehidrat should begin with discontinuation of cow's milk and solids for 24 hours. Regrading of feeds is advisable and should be adjusted to meet individual needs. Cow's milk should gradually be introduced over a period of about five days as treatment with Rehidrat continues.

A suggested regimen for regrading of feeds in infants is given below. Regrading may be carried out more quickly for older children.

Day	Volume of Rehidrat solution (ml)	Volume of milk (ml)	Total volume in 24 hours (ml)
1	150 × wt*	0	150 × wt
2	120 × wt	30 × wt	150 × wt
3	90 × wt	60 × wt	150 × wt
4	60 × wt	90 × wt	150 × wt
5	30 × wt	120 × wt	150 × wt
6	0	150 × wt	150 × wt

† Weight in kilograms

Solids are usually reintroduced when the infant is receiving full strength milk but introduction may be sooner to suit individual needs.

Simplified oral dosage guidelines: For mild diarrhoea a simplified dosage scheme may be suggested. Young children may be given Rehidrat solution in quantities usual for their normal feeds, in conjunction with an appropriate graduated feeding regimen.

Older children and adults may be allowed to drink Rehidrat solution to satisfy their thirst.

Contra-indications, warnings, etc Rehidrat is con-tra-indicated in patients with renal impairment manifesting as oliguria or anuria, intestinal obstruction, paralytic ileus, intractable vomiting and in patients with severe dehydration which requires parenteral fluid therapy. Rehidrat should not be mixed or given with electrolyte-containing solutions. Salt or sugar should not be added to Rehidrat.

Precautions: When Rehidrat is used as a supplement to parenteral fluid therapy, care must be taken not to exceed the total water and electrolyte requirements.

The sugar content of Rehidrat should be considered when treating diabetics.

Administration of oral sugar-electrolyte solutions to patients with sugar malabsorption may worsen diarrhoea.

Adverse effects: Incorrect dilution could result in abnor-malities of carbohydrate and electrolyte balance.

Overdosage: Toxicity resulting from overdosage of oral electrolyte solutions is rare. In the event of overdosage hypernatraemia or hyperkalaemia could occur.

Pharmaceutical precautions Store below 30°C (86°F).

Legal category P.

Package quantities Boxes of 24 sachets with instructions for use.

Further information The reconstituted Rehidrat and water solution has the following composition:

	mmol/l
Sodium	50
Potassium	20
Chloride	50
Bicarbonate	20
Citrate	9
Glucose	91
Sucrose	94
Fructose	2
Total osmolarity	336

Product licence number 0020/0093.

SERENACE* AMPOULES
SERENACE* TABLETS
SERENACE* LIQUID
SERENACE* CAPSULES

Presentation *Serenace 5 mg and 20 mg Ampoules:* Clear glass ampoules containing Haloperidol BP 5 mg in 1 ml aqueous solution.

Clear glass ampoules containing Haloperidol BP 20 mg in 2 ml aqueous solution.

Serenace 1.5 mg; 5 mg; 10 mg and 20 mg Tablets: White, biconvex, scored tablets engraved 'SEARLE 41' on one side, containing Haloperidol BP 1.5 mg.

Bright pink, biconvex, scored tablets engraved 'SEARLE 12' on one side, containing Haloperidol BP 5 mg.

Pale pink, biconvex, scored tablets engraved 'SEARLE 919' on one side, containing Haloperidol BP 10 mg.

Dark pink, biconvex, scored tablets engraved 'SEARLE 920' on one side, containing Haloperidol BP 20 mg.

Serenace Liquid: Clear, odourless, colourless liquid containing Haloperidol BP 2 mg per ml.

Serenace Capsules: Two-tone green capsules printed 'SEARLE' on both halves, containing Haloperidol 500 mcg (0.5 mg).

Uses Psychotic disorders – schizophrenia, mania and hypomania, especially paranoid psychoses. Mental or behavioural problems such as aggression, hyperactivity and self-mutilation in the mentally retarded. Moderate to severe psychomotor agitation, excitement, violent or dangerously impulsive behaviour. Gilles de la Tourette syndrome and severe tics. Childhood behaviour disorders, especially when associated with hyperactivity and aggression. Restlessness and agitation in the elderly. Adjunct to short-term management of anxiety.

Dosage and administration There is considerable variation from patient to patient in the response to treatment and the dosage required. As with all antipsychotics, dosage should be individualised according to the needs and response of each patient.

To determine the initial dosage, consideration should be given to the patient's age, severity of symptoms and previous response to other antipsychotic therapy. Oral dosage may be given in single or divided doses. Administration twice daily is sufficient in most cases.

Adults: Psychotic disorders; mental or behavioural problems; moderate to severe psychomotor agitation or impulsive behaviour.

Initial treatment: Parenteral administration; For rapid emergency treatment 5 or 10 mg or, infrequently, up to 30 mg by intramuscular injection may be required. Depending on the response of the patient, subsequent doses may be given as frequently as every 30 to 60 minutes, although 6–12 hourly intervals may be satisfactory. There is a wide variation among individual patients, so that cumulative dosage is not predictable in advance. Some patients may have an optimal early response after as little as 10 mg, whereas others may require up to 40 or 50 mg. Higher doses are not usually necessary.

Serenace injection may also be administered intravenously.

Oral administration: Initial dosage may range from as little as 1.5 mg daily to 20 mg daily, dependent on the characteristics, severity of symptoms and response of each individual patient. It may be necessary to increase the dosage gradually to obtain maximum control of symptoms. Severely disturbed or resistant patients may require up to 100 mg daily or, infrequently, up to 200 mg daily.

Maintenance treatment: Once a satisfactory therapeutic response has been achieved, dosage should be reduced gradually to the lowest effective maintenance level which is often as low as 3 to 10 mg daily, dependent on the characteristics and response of each individual patient.

Gilles de la Tourette Syndrome: Initial dosage is usually 2 mg daily. During the acute phase of treatment, dosage can be increased gradually to obtain maximum control of symptoms and may range between 6 and 50 mg or, exceptionally, up to 180 mg daily.

Once a satisfactory therapeutic response has been achieved dosage should be reduced gradually to the lowest effective maintenance level which for most patients is 4 mg daily.

Elderly: Half the recommended adult starting dose may be sufficient for therapeutic response in the elderly. The maximum and maintenance dose will generally be lower for debilitated or geriatric patients who may be more sensitive to Serenace.

Anxiety: 500 mcg (0.5 mg) (one capsule) twice daily.

Children: Oral administration: 25 to 50 mcg (0.025 to

0.05 mg) per kg body weight per day to a maximum of 10 mg, although adolescents may require up to 30 mg or, exceptionally, up to 60 mg daily.

Parenteral administration: Not recommended.

Contra-indications, warnings, etc
Contra-indications: Comatose states, patients with Parkinson's disease or a sensitivity to haloperidol and use during lactation.

Precautions: Liver disease, renal failure, phaeochromocytoma, conditions predisposing to epilepsy (e.g. alcohol withdrawal or brain damage). May be given to epileptics, but usual anticonvulsant therapy should be continued.

Use cautiously in thyrotoxic patients and those with arteriosclerosis who may have occult or manifest lesions of the basal ganglia. Such patients may be more prone to develop extrapyramidal symptoms.

Administer with care to patients with severe cardiovascular disorders, because of the possibility of transient hypotension. Should hypotension occur and a vasopressor be required, adrenaline should not be used since haloperidol may block its vasopressor activity and paradoxical further lowering of the blood pressure may occur.

Drug interactions: Serenace may potentiate the central nervous system depression produced by other CNS-depressant drugs including alcohol, hypnotics, sedatives or strong analgesics.

Enhanced CNS effects (sedation, mental disturbances) have been reported with the combined use of methyldopa and haloperidol.

Severe neuromuscular symptoms with impairment of consciousness and fever have been reported with combined use of lithium and haloperidol. A causal relationship has not been established, however, patients receiving such combined therapy should be carefully observed for early evidence of neurological toxicity and treatment should be discontinued if such signs appear.

Serenace may antagonise the action of adrenaline and other sympathomimetic agents.

Pregnancy: The safety of Serenace in pregnancy has not been established.

Reproduction studies in rodents have shown an increased incidence of resorption, reduced fertility and pup mortality. No specific teratogenic effect has been reported in rats, rabbits or dogs but cleft palate and open eye syndrome have been observed in mice.

No well controlled studies of haloperidol use in pregnant women have been conducted. Two cases of foetal limb malformation have been reported following maternal use of haloperidol combined with other drugs during the first trimester. No causal relationship has been established. Use of haloperidol during pregnancy requires that the anticipated benefit be weighed against the possible hazards to mother and foetus.

Lactation: Haloperidol has been detected in breast milk. If use of haloperidol is considered essential, breast feeding should be discontinued.

Warnings and adverse effects: Haloperidol may impair alertness, especially at the start of treatment. These effects may be potentiated by alcohol. Patients should be warned of the risks of sedation and advised not to drive or operate machinery during treatment, until their susceptibility is known.

Extrapyramidal symptoms such as Parkinson-like symptoms, akinesia, akathisia, dyskinesia, dystonia may develop during haloperidol treatment. Very rarely dystonia has been reported to produce laryngeal/pharyngeal spasm associated with gagging, cyanosis, respiratory distress and asphyxia. Such symptoms may be promptly controlled by parenteral administration of a short-acting barbiturate, an antihistamine or an antiparkinsonian drug. The occurrence and severity of most extrapyramidal symptoms are generally, but not always, dose related. Extrapyramidal reactions have on occasions been reported during treatment at relatively low dose levels in both children and adults. Administration of anti-Parkinsonian drugs may be required for control of such reactions.

In common with other antipsychotics haloperidol has been associated with persistent tardive dyskinesia. Tardive dyskinesia may develop in some patients on long term therapy or may develop after drug therapy has been discontinued. The risk is reported to be greater in elderly patients on high dose therapy. Characteristic symptoms are rhythmical involuntary movements of the tongue, face, mouth or jaw sometimes accompanied by involuntary movements of the extremities. They may persist for many months or even years and, while they gradually disappear in some patients, they appear to be permanent in others. Gradual reduction of dosage to reveal persisting dyskinesia has been suggested, so that treatment may be stopped if necessary. Anti-Parkinsonian agents have proved of little value in this syndrome.

In schizophrenia, the response to antipsychotic drug treatment may be delayed. If drugs are withdrawn, recurrence of symptoms may not become apparent for several weeks or months.

Some degree of sedation may occur, particularly with higher doses and at the start of treatment. The elderly appear more susceptible. At low doses in susceptible (especially non-psychotic) individuals, haloperidol may cause unpleasant subjective feelings of being mentally dulled or slowed down, dizziness, headaches or paradoxical effects of excitement, agitation or insomnia.

Other adverse effects reported include gastrointestinal symptoms, nausea, loss of appetite, dyspepsia, autonomic effects such as blurring of vision and, infrequently, tachycardia. Dose-related hypotension is uncommon, but can occur, particularly in the elderly or after parenteral administration.

Impairment of sexual function, including erection and ejaculation; oedema; blood dyscrasias, including agranulocytosis and transient leucopenia; skin reactions including exfoliative dermatitis, erythema multiforme and photosensitisation and jaundice, are rarely reported. Transient abnormalities of liver function tests may occur in the absence of jaundice.

Impairment of body temperature could occur at high doses. In common with other antipsychotics, hormonal effects include hyperprolactinaemia which could cause galactorrhoea, gynaecomastia and oligo- or amenorrhoea. Abrupt discontinuation of high doses of antipsychotics has very rarely resulted in acute withdrawal symptoms, including nausea, vomiting and insomnia. Gradual withdrawal is advisable.

Rare cases of sudden and unexplained death have been reported in psychiatric patients receiving treatment with antipsychotics including haloperidol. The nature of the evidence makes it impossible to determine the contributory role, if any, of the drug.

In common with other antipsychotics, haloperidol has been associated with rare cases of neuroleptic malignant syndrome, an idiosyncratic response characterised by hyperthermia, muscle rigidity, autonomic instability, altered consciousness and coma. Signs of autonomic dysfunction such as tachycardia, labile arterial pressure, and sweating may precede the onset of hyperthermia, acting as early warning signs. Recovery usually occurs within five to seven days of antipsychotic withdrawal. Affected patients should be carefully monitored.

Overdosage: Intensification of the known pharmacological and adverse effects may occur. The most prominent would be severe extrapyramidal symptoms, hypotension or sedation. The patient may appear comatose with respiratory depression and hypotension which could be severe enough to produce a shock-like state. Extrapyramidal reactions may include muscular weakness or rigidity and a generalised or localised tremor. With accidental overdosage hypothermia, bradycardia, sinus arrhythmia and hypertension have been reported in young children.

No specific antidote has been identified.

In the event of overdosage the stomach should be emptied by aspiration and lavage. Emetics should not be used. Establishment of a patent airway and artificial ventilation may be needed. Hypotension may be counteracted by placing the patient in the head-down position and by use of a plasma expander and careful use of a vasopressor agent such as noradrenaline. Adrenaline should not be used. Severe extrapyramidal reactions should be treated with parenteral antihistamines or antiparkinsonian drugs. The relatively long plasma elimination half-life of haloperidol should be considered. (See Further Information).

Pharmaceutical precautions Store below 30°C (86°F). Serenace Ampoules should be protected from light.

Serenace Liquid can be diluted to meet individual patient requirements. The diluted solution should be stored in amber glass, screw-cap bottles at 4°C. If a concentration of 0.1 mg haloperidol per 5 ml diluted solution or less is required, Syrup B.P. is the recommended diluent. If a concentration greater than 0.1 mg haloperidol per 5 ml diluted solution is required, Syrup B.P. or distilled water are the recommended diluents. When following these recommendations the diluted solution has been found to be chemically stable for at least 8 weeks. However, it is advised that it be used as soon as possible. It may be considered advisable to restore the concentration of preservatives to original levels of 0.5 mg/ml and 0.05 mg/ml methyl- and propyl-hydroxybenzoate respectively.

Legal category POM.

Package quantities
5 mg Ampoules: Boxes of 6.
20 mg Ampoules: Boxes of 10.
1.5 mg Tablets: Bottles of 50, 250 and 1000.
5 mg Tablets: Bottles of 50, 250 and 1000.
10 mg Tablets: Bottles of 50, 250 and 1000.
20 mg Tablets: Bottles of 50 and 250.
2mg/ml Liquid: Bottles of 100 ml and 500 ml.
500 mcg Capsules: Bottles of 50, 250 and 1000.

Further information Haloperidol is a butyrophenone. Its pharmacological profile of activity includes a pronounced capacity to induce extrapyramidal reactions and a low incidence of autonomic side-effects, such as hypotension.

The pharmacokinetics of haloperidol have been studied in healthy volunteers and patients. In volunteers, following a single intravenous or oral dose, serum elimination half-life ranged from 10 to 19 hours and 12 to 38 hours respectively. Similar elimination half-lives were observed in patients after administration of a single oral or intramuscular dose of the drug or after withdrawal of the drug from patients who were in a steady-state. Steady-state serum levels were usually achieved within 6 days on a fixed oral dosage.

Product licence numbers

5 mg Ampoules	0020/5036
20 mg Ampoules	0020/0078
1.5 mg Tablets	0020/5033
5 mg Tablets	0020/5034
10 mg Tablets	0020/0076
20 mg Tablets	0020/0079
2 mg/ml Liquid	0020/5035
500 mcg Capsules	0020/5038

SPIROPROP* ▾

Presentation Pink, film-coated tablets engraved 'SEARLE 997' on one side. Each tablet contains 80 mg Propranolol Hydrochloride BP and 50 mg Spironolactone BP.

Uses *Actions:* Spironolactone, as a competitive aldosterone antagonist, is a potassium-sparing diuretic with sustained antihypertensive activity.

Propranolol is a non-selective beta-adrenergic receptor blocking drug with antihypertensive properties. It exerts a competitive and reversible blockade of the beta-adrenergic receptors, thereby protecting the cardiovascular system against excessive or inappropriate sympathetic activity.

The combination of spironolactone and propranolol in a single tablet has a number of advantages:

1. Spironolactone and propranolol have different modes of antihypertensive activity, but their therapeutic actions are complementary.

2. Clinical evaluation has demonstrated that spironolactone and propranolol have a synergistic action in the treatment of mild to moderate hypertension.

3. Once daily dosage aids patient compliance.

4. Plasma concentrations of both potassium and magnesium are well maintained.

Indications: Mild to moderate hypertension.

Dosage and administration Food has been reported to increase the bioavailability of both propranolol and spironolactone. It is recommended that tablets are taken with meals.

Adults: The usual dosage is one tablet daily. The single daily dose may be increased to two tablets if response is not adequate after 4 weeks.

Elderly: It is recommended that treatment is started with the lowest dose and titrated upwards as required to achieve maximum benefit. Care should be taken in severe hepatic and renal impairment which may alter drug metabolism and excretion.

Children: Not recommended.

Contra-indications, warnings, etc
Contra-indications: Spiroprop is contra-indicated in patients with second or third degree heart block, sinus bradycardia, cardiogenic shock, right ventricular failure secondary to pulmonary hypertension, bronchial asthma and a previous history of bronchospasm, acute renal insufficiency, rapid deteriorating or severe impairment of renal function, anuria, hyperkalaemia, Addison's disease, sensitivity to propranolol or spironolactone and should

not be used after prolonged fasting. Spiroprop should not be given with calcium channel blockers of the verapamil type and neither drug should be administered within several days of discontinuing the other.

Spiroprop should not be administered concurrently with other potassium-conserving diuretics and potassium supplements should not be given routinely with Spiroprop as hyperkalaemia may be induced.

Warnings: Carcinogenicity: Spironolactone has been shown to produce tumours in rats when administered at high doses over a long period of time. The significance of these findings with respect to clinical use is not certain. However, the long term use of spironolactone in young patients requires careful consideration of the benefits and the potential hazard involved.

Precautions: Use with care in patients whose cardiac reserve is poor. Inhibition of sympathetic stimulation with beta-blockade has the potential of further depressing myocardial contractility and precipitating heart failure. Cardiac failure should be considered a contraindication to beta-blockade, unless or until signs of failure are controlled by digitalis or diuretics. The action of digitalis, which tends to augment contractility, may be reduced by beta-blockers because they reduce contractility. The effects of beta-blockers and digitalis are additive in depressing AV conduction. Exercise caution during combined use of these drugs.

In patients with ischaemic heart disease treatment with beta-blockers should be discontinued gradually. This may be achieved by treating with progressively smaller doses of propranolol alone.

Propranolol may mask signs of hyperthyroidism. Sudden withdrawal may result in exacerbation of symptoms of hyperthyroidism, including thyroid storm. Propranolol does not interfere with thyroid function tests.

In common with other beta-blockers, propranolol may mask signs of acute hypoglycaemia. This is especially important in patients with labile diabetes. Hypoglycaemic attacks may be accompanied by a precipitous elevation of blood pressure.

Fluid and electrolyte status should be regularly monitored to detect possible hyperkalaemia, hyponatraemia and elevated urea, particularly in the elderly and in those with significant renal impairment.

Drug interactions: Spiroprop should not be given with calcium channel blockers of the verapamil type, or with other potassium-sparing agents. Potassium supplements should not be given routinely with Spiroprop as hyperkalaemia may be induced. Exercise caution during combined use of Spiroprop and digitalis (see Precautions).

As with all beta-blockers great caution should be observed if Spiroprop is administered prior to or during anaesthesia. Spironolactone reduces vascular responsiveness to noradrenaline. Caution should be exercised in the management of patients subjected to regional or general anaesthesia. Consider withdrawal before surgery except for cases of phaeochromocytoma when used together with an alpha-adrenergic blocker.

Patients receiving catecholamine-depleting drugs, such as reserpine, in combination with Spiroprop should be carefully observed, since an excessive reduction in sympathetic drive to the heart might occur. Care should be taken when administering Spiroprop during and within 2 weeks of administration of adrenergic augmenting psychotropic drugs such as monoamine oxidase inhibitors.

As carbenoxolone may cause sodium retention and

thus decrease the effectiveness of spironolactone, concurrent use should be avoided.

Pregnancy: Although there is no evidence of teratogenicity in rats and rabbits, both constituents cross the placental barrier. Use of Spiroprop during pregnancy requires that the anticipated benefit be weighed against the possible hazards to mother and foetus.

Nursing mothers: A metabolite of spironolactone, canrenone, and propranolol have been detected in breast milk. If use of Spiroprop is considered essential, an alternative method of infant feeding should be instituted.

Adverse reactions: Spiroprop is usually well tolerated. There is no evidence to suggest that Spiroprop produces adverse reactions that do not occur with spironolactone or propranolol alone.

Side-effects of spironolactone are infrequent and usually reversible upon discontinuing the drug. These include drowsiness, lethargy, mental confusion, ataxia, drug fever, impotence, mild androgenic effects, menstrual irregularities, headache, gastrointestinal disturbances and skin rashes.

Gynaecomastia may develop in association with the use of spironolactone. The development of gynaecomastia appears to be related to both dosage level and duration of therapy and is normally reversible when spironolactone is discontinued. In rare instances some breast enlargement may persist.

Side-effects of propranolol are generally mild and include nausea, fatigue, diarrhoea, dizziness, lassitude, insomnia, cold extremities, and paraesthesia. These are usually transient and resolve when the drug is withdrawn. Bronchospasm may occur particularly in susceptible individuals. There are also reports that beta-blockers can produce depression, disturbances of vision, hallucinations, skin rashes and/or dry eyes. If any such reaction occurs that is otherwise inexplicable, withdrawal of the drug should be considered.

If intolerance to the drug occurs, manifested as bradycardia (heart rate below 55 per minute), hypotension, congestive cardiac failure or heart block, the drug should be withdrawn and, if necessary, treatment for overdose instituted (see below).

Overdosage: Treat fluid depletion and electrolyte imbalances if present. For hyperkalaemia reduce potassium intake, administer potassium-excreting diuretics, intravenous glucose with regular insulin or oral ion-exchange resins.

Excessive bradycardia can usually be corrected with atropine. If there is no response to vagal blockade, isoprenaline or orciprenaline may be administered with caution.

Cardiac failure should be managed with digitalisation and diuretics. Do not administer potassium-retaining diuretics.

Hypotension may be managed with vasopressors such as noradrenaline or dopamine.

Bronchospasm may be treated with isoprenaline or aminophylline.

Pharmaceutical precautions Store below 30°C (86°F).

Legal category POM.

Package quantities Calendar pack of 28 tablets.

Further information Spiroprop is designed to aid drug compliance by providing a simple convenient and acceptable presentation of the most widely prescribed beta-adrenergic receptor blocking drug, propranolol hydrochloride, with the potassium sparing diuretic, spironolactone, for the treatment of mild to moderate hypertension. A synergistic effect of the two active ingredients in lowering blood pressure has been demonstrated in a clinical evaluation.

Product licence number 0020/0104.

*Trade Mark

Serono Laboratories (UK) Ltd
2 Tewin Court
Welwyn Garden City
Hertfordshire AL7 1AU

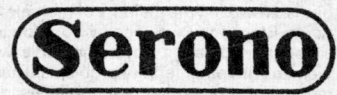

ARES-SERONO GROUP

METRODIN*

Presentation Metrodin ampoules contain urofollitrophin in a freeze-dried, sterile powder form. Urofollitrophin is the Approved Name given to a preparation of menopausal gonadotrophin extracted from human urine but possessing no luteinising hormone (LH) activity.

Each Metrodin ampoule contains:
Human follicle stimulating hormone (FSH)   75 IU
Lactose   10 mg

Each Metrodin ampoule is accompanied by a solvent ampoule containing:
Sodium Chloride Injection BP   1 ml

Uses Metrodin, followed by chorionic gonadotrophin (hCG, Profasi*), is indicated for the induction of ovulation in patients with amenorrhoea or other anovulatory states associated with elevated LH:FSH ratios. These high ratios usually occur in a form of polycystic ovary syndrome. Where endogenous LH levels are raised the administration of exogenous LH in the follicular phase is unwarranted. Metrodin therefore offers a more physiological approach to gonadotrophin therapy in these patients.

Dosage and administration Metrodin is given by intramuscular injection only. The injection should be reconstituted with the solvent provided immediately before use. Up to 5 ampoules of Metrodin may be dissolved in 1 ml solvent.

The object of Metrodin therapy is to develop a single mature Graafian follicle over several days of treatment and then to give Profasi to release the ovum. Follicular development is judged by the concentration of oestrogen, measured in blood or urine. Ultrasound measurement of follicular growth is a possible alternative to biochemical monitoring. Clinical assessment of the response to Metrodin, including pelvic examination and cervical mucus studies, should also be performed. Metrodin administration should continue until adequate follicular development is achieved. Although the patient produces LH, a positive feedback defect may interfere with the normal endogenous LH surge needed to induce ovulation. Follicular rupture should therefore be achieved by the intramuscular administration of Profasi, which mimics the mid-cycle LH surge.

If the patient wishes to conceive, she is recommended to have coitus on the day when Profasi is given and on the following day.

Metrodin may be given as a course of daily or alternate day injections. The recommended starting dose of Metrodin is 2 ampoules (150 IU FSH) for daily injections or 5 ampoules (375 IU FSH) if injections are to be given on alternate days. Treatment with Metrodin should continue until an adequate, but not excessive, response is achieved, as indicated by oestrogen measurements and/or ultrasonography. The dosage of Metrodin may be increased stepwise at approximately weekly intervals, depending on biochemical, ultrasound and clinical responses.

When an optimal response is obtained, a single intramuscular injection of 10,000 IU Profasi should be administered 24–48 hours after the last dose of Metrodin.

If a patient fails to respond satisfactorily after 3 weeks of Metrodin treatment, that cycle should be abandoned. The patient should be reassessed if she fails to conceive after 6 ovulatory cycles.

The dose of Metrodin required to evoke the desired response is critical and varies both from patient to patient and in the same patient at different times. Monitoring of Metrodin therapy by hormonal assay or by ultrasound measurement of follicle size is therefore essential.

Oestrogen values of less than 180 nmol/24 h (50 ug/24 h) for total urinary oestrogens or 1100 pmol/l (300 pg/ml) for plasma oestradiol-17β may indicate inadequate follicular development. Conversely, if the levels are higher than either 514 nmol/24 h (140 ug/24 h) for total urinary oestrogens or 3000 pmol/l (800 pg/ml) for plasma oestradiol-17β, there is an increased risk of ovarian hyperstimulation and Profasi should be withheld. A very steep rise in oestrogens may also indicate an increased risk of hyperstimulation.

When monitoring Metrodin therapy by ultrasound, a follicular diameter of 16–25 mm should indicate the presence of a mature follicle and therefore the optimal time for the administration of Profasi. If the follicular diameter is less than 16 mm, further Metrodin injections may be required. However, if the follicle diameter exceeds 25 mm there is an increased risk of hyperstimulation and so Profasi should not be given in that cycle. Profasi should also be withheld when several mature follicles are visualised, in view of the risk of multiple ovulation.

Further details concerning Metrodin dosage and monitoring are available on request.

Contra-indications, warnings, etc Metrodin may cause local reactions at the injection site.

Metrodin therapy is precluded when a satisfactory outcome cannot be expected, e.g. with ovarian dysgenesis, absent uterus, premature menopause or tubal occlusion. Appropriate treatment should first be given for any other endocrine disorder such as hypothyroidism, adrenocortical deficiency, hyperprolactinaemia or pituitary tumour. Other possible causes of infertility in either partner should be excluded before commencing Metrodin therapy.

Although the absence of LH reduces the risk of severe hyperstimulation, the possibility of hyperstimulation should be considered and careful monitoring performed. Excessive oestrogen responses to Metrodin do not generally give rise to significant side-effects unless Profasi is given to induce ovulation. Profasi administration should therefore be withheld if hormone assays or ultrasound measurement detect an excessive response.

Gonadotrophin therapy increases the risk of multiple births. However, the majority of multiple conceptions are twins. Pregnancy wastage by abortion is higher than in a normal population but comparable with the rates in women with other fertility problems. There have been no reports of congenital abnormalities associated with Metrodin therapy.

Pharmaceutical precautions Metrodin should be stored below 25°C and protected from light.

Legal category POM.

Package quantities Boxes containing 3 ampoules Metrodin plus 3 ampoules solvent.

Further information One IU of human urinary FSH is defined as the activity contained in 0.11388 mg of the 1st International Standard.

Product licence number 3400/0012.

PERGONAL*

Presentation Pergonal ampoules contain human menopausal gonadotrophin (HMG) in a freeze-dried, sterile powder form (Approved Name: Menotrophin BP).

Each Pergonal ampoule contains:
Human follicle stimulating hormone (FSH)	75 IU
Human luteinising hormone (LH)	75 IU
Lactose	10 mg

Each Pergonal ampoule is accompanied by a solvent ampoule containing: Sodium Chloride Injection BP — 1 ml

Uses
Women: Pergonal and subsequently chorionic gonadotrophin (hCG, Profasi) are indicated for the induction of ovulation in the amenorrhoeic patient or anovulatory woman with regular or irregular cycles.

Men: Pergonal with concomitant Profasi therapy is indicated for the stimulation of spermatogenesis in men who have primary or secondary hypogonadotrophic hypogonadism.

Dosage and administration Pergonal is given by intramuscular injection only. The injection should be reconstituted with the solvent provided immediately prior to use. Up to 5 ampoules of Pergonal may be dissolved in 1 ml solvent.

Women: The object is to develop a single mature Graafian follicle with individually tailored doses of Pergonal over several days and then give Profasi to release the ovum. Follicular development is judged by the concentration of oestrogen, measured in blood or urine. Clinical assessment of the response including pelvic examination and cervical mucus studies should also be performed. Pergonal administration should continue until an adequate oestrogen level is achieved.

If the oestrogen values are less than either 180 nmol/24 h (50 mcg/24 h) for total urinary oestrogens or 1100 pmol/l (300 pg/ml) for plasma oestradiol-17 β, follicular development may be inadequate. Conversely, if the levels are higher than either 514 nmol/24 h (140 mcg/24 h) for total urinary oestrogens or 3000 pmol/l (800 pg/ml) for plasma oestradiol-17 β, there is an increased risk of ovarian hyperstimulation and

Profasi should be withheld. The optimal time for Profasi administration is the day of the urinary oestrogen peak or the day after the plasma oestradiol-17 β peak.

In the anovulatory patient the stimulated follicles will not liberate ova spontaneously. Follicular rupture has to be achieved by injecting Profasi, which simulates the normal surge of LH at ovulation.

If the patient wishes to conceive, she is recommended to have coitus on the day when Profasi is given and on the following day.

The dose of Pergonal required to evoke the desired response is critical and varies both from patient to patient and in the same patient at different times. Monitoring by hormone assay is therefore essential.

Two Pergonal dosage schedules are commonly employed:

Schedule 1: Alternate day therapy
Three equal doses of Pergonal are given on alternate days. In a menstruating woman the initial injection of Pergonal should be given on day 7, 8 or 9 of the cycle. A single dose of 10,000 IU Profasi is given one week after the first injection of Pergonal, provided the clinical and biochemical responses are adequate and not excessive.

Schedule 2: Daily therapy
Daily injections of Pergonal are given until an adequate response is achieved. This is judged on the basis of daily oestrogen determinations. In the absence of a response the dose of Pergonal may be increased or the course abandoned. A single injection of 10,000 IU Profasi is administered 24–48 hours after the last dose of Pergonal.

Further details concerning Pergonal dosage and monitoring are available on request.

Men: Treatment should begin with Profasi 2000 IU 2–3 times a week to produce evidence of adequate masculinisation.

If the only response to Profasi is androgenic in nature, Pergonal (1 ampoule 3 times a week) and Profasi 2000 IU (twice a week) should be given for a minimum period of four months.

If the patient has not responded with evidence of increased spermatogenesis at the end of four months, therapy may be continued with Pergonal (1 or 2 ampoules 3 times a week) and Profasi 2000 IU (twice a week).

Pergonal should only be used by clinicians who are thoroughly familiar with infertility problems.

Contra-indications, warnings, etc Pergonal may occasionally cause local reactions at the injection site. Fever and joint pains have been reported rarely.

Women: Pergonal therapy is precluded when an effective response cannot be obtained, e.g. with ovarian dysgenesis, absent uterus, premature menopause or tubal occlusion. Appropriate treatment should first be given for hypothyroidism, adrenocortical deficiency, hyperprolactinaemia or pituitary tumour. An acceptable semen analysis should be available before Pergonal treatment.

Adherence to the recommended Pergonal dosage and monitoring schedules will minimise the possibility of ovarian hyperstimulation. Excessive oestrogenic responses to Pergonal do not generally give rise to significant side effects unless Profasi is given to induce ovulation. Hormone assays will detect an excessive oestrogen response to Pergonal and Profasi administration should be withheld.

The incidence of multiple births following Pergonal/Profasi therapy has been variously reported between

10% and 40%. However, the majority of multiple conceptions are twins.

Pregnancy wastage by abortion is higher than in a normal population but comparable with the rates in women with other fertility problems. The risks of congenital abnormalities are not increased by Pergonal.

Men: Elevated endogenous FSH levels are indicative of primary testicular failure. Such patients are usually unresponsive to Pergonal/Profasi therapy.

No adverse reactions have been reported in men.

Pharmaceutical precautions Pergonal should be stored below 25°C.

Legal category POM.

Package quantities Boxes containing 10 ampoules Pergonal plus 10 ampoules solvent.

Further information One IU of human urinary FSH and one IU of human urinary LH are defined as the activities contained in 0.11388 mg and 0.13369 mg of the 1st International Standard, respectively.

Product licence number 3400/0007.

PROFASI*

Presentation Ampoules of Profasi (Chorionic Gonadotrophin Injection BP) contain chorionic gonadotrophin (hCG) in freeze-dried, sterile powder form. Four strengths are available (500, 1000, 2000 and 5000 IU). Each ampoule is accompanied by a solvent ampoule containing Sodium Chloride Injection BP.

Uses Chorionic gonadotrophin (hCG) is a hormonal substance obtained from human pregnancy urine. Its action is predominantly luteinising.

Profasi is used in the treatment of anovulatory infertility, where its administration would form part of a recognised treatment regimen involving the prior stimulation of follicular maturation and endometrial proliferation, e.g. with Pergonal (Menotrophin Injection BP).

In the male, Profasi stimulates the interstitial cells of the testes and consequently the secretion of androgens and the development of secondary sexual characteristics. With concomitant Pergonal therapy, Profasi stimulates the induction and maintenance of spermatogenesis. Profasi is also indicated in the treatment of hypogonadotrophic hypogonadism and of cryptorchidism.

Dosage and administration Profasi is given by intramuscular injection only.

Anovulatory Infertility: Profasi 10,000 IU in mid-cycle, following treatment with Pergonal according to a recognised scheme.

Details of Pergonal dosage and monitoring are available on request.

Hypogonadotrophic hypogonadism: Profasi 2000 IU twice weekly with concomitant Pergonal (1 ampoule three times a week), if necessary, for a minimum period of four months.

Cryptorchidism: Profasi 500 to 1000 IU on alternate days for several weeks.

Contra-indications, warnings, etc Stimulation of ovulation with Pergonal may lead to superovulation and the hyperstimulation syndrome. Oestrogen assays will detect an excessive response so that Profasi may be withheld in that particular treatment cycle.

In the male, high dosage of Profasi may lead to oedema and in such cases dosage should be considerably reduced.

If signs of sexual precocity are observed, treatment should be stopped. If continued therapy is considered necessary, a reduced dosage regimen should be instituted.

Pharmaceutical precautions Profasi should be stored below 25°C and protected from light. Solutions of Profasi should be used immediately after preparation.

Legal category POM.

Package quantities Ampoules of Profasi 500, Profasi 1000, and Profasi 2000 are packed in boxes of two. Ampoules of Profasi 5000 are packed singly and in boxes of 10.

For all strengths, each ampoule is accompanied by an ampoule of Sodium Chloride Injection BP as solvent.

Further information One IU of chorionic gonadotrophin is defined as the activity contained in 0.001279 mg of the 2nd International Standard Preparation.

Product licence numbers
Profasi 500 IU 3400/0003
Profasi 1000 IU 3400/0004
Profasi 2000 IU 3400/0005
Profasi 5000 IU 3400/0006

SEROPHENE*

Presentation White, round, flat, bevelled tablet, single scored on one side, each containing 50 mg Clomiphene Citrate B.P.

Uses Serophene is indicated for the treatment of anovulation and infertility due to impaired hypothalamic pituitary function.

The best response to Serophene is generally obtained in women with evidence of follicular function and endogenous oestrogen production. These patients lack adequate, cyclic stimulation of pituitary gonadotrophic function. Serophene may also be of benefit in patients with limited oestrogen production.

Dosage and administration The recommended dose for the first treatment course of Serophene is 50 mg (one Serophene tablet) daily for five consecutive days starting within the first five days of spontaneous or induced menstrual bleeding. The commencement date of Serophene therapy is arbitrary in women who have not experienced recent uterine bleeding.

Reponse to Serophene, suggestive of ovulation, is indicated by a biphasic basal body temperature, a mid-cycle rise in LH output, an increase in serum progesterone during the presumptive mid-luteal phase or by menstrual bleeding in an amenorrhoeic patient. If ovulation occurs, but pregnancy does not result, the same dose of Serophene should be repeated in the next treatment course. If presumptive evidence of ovulation is not followed by menstrual bleeding, the possibility of pregnancy should be considered and excluded before Serophene treatment is restarted.

In the absence of ovulation, the daily dose of Serophene may be increased by increments of 50 mg (one Serophene tablet) each successive month to a maximum of 200 mg (four Serophene tablets) given as a single daily dose for five days. This dose level of Serophene should not be exceeded. If ovulation does not occur, a single intramuscular injection of up to

10,000 IU chorionic gonadotrophin (hCG, Profasi) may be given 7 to 10 days after the last Serophene tablet, in order to reinforce the LH surge.

If the patient wishes to conceive, coitus particularly around the expected time of ovulation is advised. A maximum of six apparently ovulatory treatment courses with the lowest effective dose of Serophene is suggested. If at this stage pregnancy has not occurred, then patients should be reinvestigated and sequential Pergonal (Menotrophin BP)/Profasi therapy may be considered.

Contra-indications, warnings, etc Serophene should not be administered to patients with active liver disease or with hereditary defect in bilirubin metabolism.

Serophene therapy is precluded when an effective response cannot be obtained, e.g. ovarian dysgenesis or premature menopause. Appropriate treatment should first be given for hypothyroidism, adrenocortical deficiency, hyperprolactinaemia or pituitary tumour. Other possible causes of infertility in either partner should first be excluded.

Patients with very low baseline levels of endogenous gonadotrophins and oestrogens are usually less responsive to Serophene treatment, and consideration should be given to gonadotrophin (Pergonal/Profasi) therapy.

Patients receiving Serophene should be instructed to report any abdominal discomfort immediately and a pelvic examination should be performed to determine whether ovarian enlargement has occurred or not. While the incidence of clinically significant hyperstimulation is low with the recommended Serophene dosage scheme, the presence of excessive ovarian enlargement may require the dosage scheme to be modified. Rare occurrences of lutein cyst rupture with intraperitoneal haemorrhage have been reported. Vasomotor symptoms resembling 'hot flushes' may occur with Serophene.

Other side effects of Serophene are generally mild, not dose related and readily reversible on drug withdrawal. These include vomiting, breast discomfort, skin reactions (dermatitis or urticaria), dizziness and hair loss. Serophene should be withdrawn if visual disturbances occur, e.g. blurring, spots or flashes (in rare cases scotomata).

The multiple pregnancy rate is approximately 8%, twins representing 90% of this figure.

Although a higher abortion rate than in a normal population has been reported, this is comparable with that in women with other fertility problems. There is no evidence that this is drug related.

Care should be taken to avoid administration of Serophene if pregnancy is suspected. Although Serophene has been shown to be embryotoxic in animals at high doses, there is no evidence to suggest that it increases the incidence of congenital malformations in humans at therapeutic levels. The incidence of congenital malformations following Serophene treatment is similar to that observed in women with other fertility problems.

There is evidence that some women ovulate spontaneously for some cycles after cessation of Serophene treatment. There is no experience of acute poisoning with Serophene.

Pharmaceutical precautions Serophene should be stored below 25°C and protected from light and moisture.

Legal category POM.

Package quantities Serophene is blister packed in boxes of 10, 30 and 100 tablets.

Further information The mode of action of Serophene at the recommended dose appears to be through

competition for available oestrogen receptor sites in the hypothalamus. Oestrogen is thus displaced from sites which were responsible for the suppression of gonadotrophin-releasing hormone; pituitary secretion of FSH and LH follows which initiates the normal menstrual cycle.

Product licence number 3400/0009.

UKIDAN*

Presentation Ukidan 5000 and Ukidan 25,000 are available in single vials containing urokinase as a sterile, white, freeze-dried powder. Vials of 5000 and 25,000 International Units (IU) of urokinase.

Uses Ukidan is a protein substance isolated from human male urine. Ukidan brings about the dissolution of blood clots by provoking the activation of plasminogen; the latter is the inactive precursor of plasmin, the proteolytic enzyme responsible for the breakdown of fibrin into small peptide molecules which are dispersible through the blood stream. Being of human origin, Ukidan is non-antigenic in man and is free from inherent toxicity.

Ukidan 5000 and Ukidan 25,000 are indicated as thrombolytic agents in localised conditions such as a non-resolving vitreous haemorrhage and hyphaema. They are also used for the removal of clots in other 'closed' situations such as arterio-venous haemodialysis shunts and intravenous cannulae.

Dosage and administration

Vitreous haemorrhage: The following general technique is used: After pre-operative acetazolamide treatment, an incision is made through the conjunctiva 6 mm from the supratemporal limbus. A similar 2 mm incision is made through the sclera into the suprachoroidal space and a mattress suture is placed across the edges of the wound. Ukidan 25,000 IU is drawn up in 0.3 ml Water for Injections using a fine bore retro-ocular needle and a rotating technique for insertion. The drug is injected 10 mm into the centre of the vitreous. The mattress suture is tightened and the needle is withdrawn rapidly to prevent loss of vitreous or Ukidan. Finally, the wound is sealed with cryopexy.

Improvement in visual acuity occurs during a three month post-operative period though good results in the first week are quite common. Recurrent haemorrhages may be treated by second and subsequent injections.

Hyphaema: When saline irrigation is unsuccessful in removing the blood clot, Ukidan may be considered for the management of hyphaema, particularly when the clot completely fills the anterior chamber and there is an accompanying rise in intra-ocular pressure. The following general technique is used: an incision of about 3 mm is made inside the temporal limbus of the cornea. 5000 IU Ukidan is dissolved in Sodium Chloride Injection (2 ml) and drawn up into the syringe fitted with a suitable irrigator. The tip of the irrigator is introduced through the incision so as to be over the iris rather than the pupillary space (thus avoiding risk of damage to the lens), with the aperture directed towards the corneal endothelium or parallel to the plane of the iris. The solution is injected and withdrawn repeatedly with minimal pressure. Clot disintegration commonly begins within five minutes, facilitating injection of the solution. If residual clot remains a small quantity of the solution (e.g. 0.3 ml) may be left in the anterior chamber for 24–48 hours.

Clotted A.V. shunts: Generally, 5000–25,000 IU Ukidan

in 2–3 ml Sodium Chloride Injection is instilled into the affected limb of the shunt which is then clamped off for 2–4 hours. This may be repeated if necessary. For the venous side an infusion of 5000 IU in 200 ml, run in over 30 minutes, has been used but this may be less satisfactory than the use of more concentrated solutions.

Contra-indications, warnings, etc Ukidan is generally contra-indicated in vitreous haemorrhage complicated by severe retinal disturbances (e.g. retinal detachment, tumour or diabetic proliferative retinopathy). Normal intraocular pressure and normal gonioscopy should be evident. Mild, transient, sterile hypopyon, anterior uveitis and glaucoma have been observed post-operatively.

Local use of Ukidan 5000 or Ukidan 25,000 does not require haematological monitoring.

Pharmaceutical precautions Ukidan should be stored at 0–6°C.

Legal category POM.

Package quantities Ukidan injections are packed as single vials.

Further information The activity of Ukidan is expressed in International Units (IU). One IU is approximately equivalent to one CTA unit, and to about 0.7 Ploug units.

Product licence number 3400/0001.

*Trade Mark

Servier Laboratories Limited
Fulmer Hall
Windmill Road
Fulmer, Slough SL3 6HH

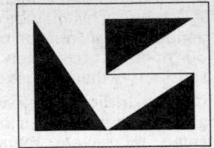

DIAMICRON*

Presentation *Diamicron tablets:* White, circular tablets with a cross scoring on one side each containing 80 mg gliclazide. Gliclazide is 1-(3-azabicyclo (3,3,0) oct-3-yl)-3-(p-tolylsulphonyl) urea.

Pharmacology Gliclazide is a hypoglycaemic sulphonylurea differing from other related compounds by the addition of an azabicyclo octane ring. The drug is well absorbed and its half-life in man is approximately 10–12 hours. Gliclazide is metabolised in the liver; less than 5% of the dose is excreted unchanged in the urine.

In man, apart from having similar hypoglycaemic effect to the other sulphonylureas, gliclazide has been shown to reduce platelet adhesiveness and aggregation and increase fibrinolytic activity. These factors are thought to be implicated in the pathogenesis of long term complications of diabetes mellitus.

Uses For the treatment of maturity onset diabetes in patients who cannot be controlled on diet alone.

Dosage and administration *Adults:* The total daily dose may vary from 40 to 320 mg taken orally. The dose should be adjusted according to the individual patient's response commencing with 40–80 mg daily ($\frac{1}{2}$–1 tablet) and increasing until adequate control is achieved. Higher doses should be divided according to the main meals of the day.

In obese patients or those not showing adequate response to Diamicron alone, a biguanide may be added.

Elderly: Plasma clearance of gliclazide is not altered in the elderly and steady state plasma levels can therefore be expected to be similar to those in adults under 65 years. Clinical experience in the elderly to date shows that Diamicron is effective and well tolerated. Care should be exercised, however, when prescribing sulphonylureas in the elderly due to a possible age-related increased tendency for hypoglycaemia.

Children: Diamicron, as with other sulphonylureas, is not indicated for the treatment of juvenile onset diabetes mellitus.

Contra-indications, warnings, etc
Contra-Indications: Diamicron should not be used in:
1. Juvenile onset diabetes.
2. Diabetes complicated by ketosis and acidosis.
3. Pregnancy.
4. Diabetics undergoing surgery, after severe trauma or during infections.
5. Patients known to have hypersensitivity to other sulphonylureas and related drugs.

Precautions: Diamicron is generally well tolerated but nausea, headache, rashes and gastro-intestinal disturbances have been reported. Care should be exercised in patients with hepatic and/or renal impairment and a small starting dose should be used with careful patient monitoring. As with other sulphonylureas, hypoglycaemia will occur if the patients' dietary intake is reduced or if they are receiving a larger dose of Diamicron than required.

Care should be taken when giving Diamicron with drugs which are known to alter the diabetic state or potentiate the drug's action, such as sulphonamides, salicylates, phenylbutazone, β-blocking agents, MAOI's, thiazide diuretics and steroid hormones.

Overdosage: The symptom to be expected of overdose would be hypoglycaemia. The treatment is gastric lavage and correction of the hypoglycaemia by appropriate means with continued monitoring of the patient's blood sugar until the effect of the drug has ceased.

Pharmaceutical precautions Nil.

Legal category POM.

Package quantities Cartons of 60 tablets (containing three push-through blister strips of 20 tablets).

Further information Nil.

Product licence number 0093/0024.

IMOTEST*-TUBERCULIN ▼
Merieux Tuberculin Test Ring (Purified Tuberculin)

Presentation Each Imotest unit consists of a plastic ring with a 9 mm square setting on which is mounted a platform with nine points arranged in three rows of three. A plastic tube fitted over the platform is filled with protein purified tuberculin (PPD) (0.05 ml) prior to being heat sealed. The entire unit has been sterilised. The reactivity of Imotest is comparable to the intermediate strength Mantoux test (5TU PPD). The ring is designed to fit onto the thumb of the administrator.

Uses Imotest-Tuberculin is an intradermal test for the detection of tuberculin sensitivity and is used for screening for tuberculosis.

Dosage and administration *Adults and children:* Tuberculin testing may be done during the first year of life. The frequency of repeated testing may be increased in groups where there is a higher risk of tuberculosis. The recommended site for accurate tuberculin testing is the volar surface of the mid-forearm. The skin should be cleaned with alcohol, ether or acetone and allowed to dry.

Method of application: Place the ring on the thumb so the points protrude from the pulp surface. Carefully remove the tube surrounding the points by a slight twist which breaks the seal. Squeeze the tuberculin from the plastic tube onto the Imotest points until they are covered. Grasp the patient's arm firmly with the free hand stretching the skin of the forearm tightly. Press the loaded points firmly into the cleansed site.

Sufficient pressure should be exerted to produce nine visible puncture sites and an imprint of the square base. Do not wipe the puncture site and allow 3 or 4 minutes exposure before the patient dresses.

Reading the reaction: The test should be read at 48 to 72 hours after administration. Slight local erythema may be observed but the sole criterion for a positive reaction is a palpable induration. It is important to measure exactly the broadest transverse diameter of the induration by examining under adequate light. This procedure is facilitated by using the millimeter callipers which may be obtained from Servier Laboratories on application. Identification of the application site is usually easy because of the distinct imprint of the points.

Positive reaction: The presence of a palpable induration of transverse diameter measuring 3 mm and more constitutes a positive reaction.

Negative reaction: If the diameter of induration measures less than 1 mm the reaction is considered negative.

Doubtful reaction: Induration diameters between 1 mm and 3 mm are considered doubtful reactions.

Contra-indications, warnings, etc
Contra-indication: Erythema nodosum.

Precautions: In the case of severe positive reactions, investigations for pathological causes should be carried out.

Tuberculin testing should be carried out with caution in persons with active tuberculosis. However, activation of quiescent lesions is not to be expected.

Reactivity to the test may be suppressed in patients who are receiving corticosteroids or immunosuppressive agents, or those who have recently been vaccinated with live virus vaccine such as measles.

Do not apply Imotest on areas of acne, hairy areas and areas without adequate subcutaneous tissue.

Discard the Imotest ring and the tube containing tuberculin after use. Do not re-use.

Side effects: Vesiculation, ulceration, or necrosis may occur at the test site in highly sensitive persons. Pain, pruritus and discomfort at the test site may be relieved by cold packs or by a topical corticosteroid preparation.

Pharmaceutical precautions Imotest should be stored at room temperature in the original pack.

Legal category POM.

Package quantities Box of 10 tests.

Further information Nil.

Product licence number 0093/0041.

LOCABIOTAL*

Presentation 10 ml of 0.25% solution of fusafungine in a pressurised aerosol container designed to give approximately 200 metered doses. Each metered dose contains approximately 125 mcg fusafungine. Two attachments, one for nasal use, one for oral use, are supplied.

Fusafungine is an antibiotic produced by *Fusarium lateritium* strain 437.

Uses A topical antibiotic with anti-inflammatory prop-

erties for the treatment of infections and inflammatory conditions of the upper respiratory tract.

Dosage and administration *Administration:* By inhalation using the appropriate attachment.

Dosage: Adults: Nasal – 3 metered doses in each nostril five times a day.

Oral – 5 metered doses five times a day.

Children	Nasal – in each nostril five times a day	Oral – three times a day
3–5 years	1 metered dose	2 metered doses
6–12 years	2 metered doses	3 metered doses
12 years	3 metered doses	4 metered doses

Contra-indications, warnings, etc
Contra-indication: Sensitivity to fusafungine or excipients.

Warnings: Avoid directing the spray into the eyes, as aerosol sprays can cause irritation.

Side-effects: Some patients may experience a transient stinging sensation.

Pharmaceutical precautions *Storage:* Store at room temperature.

Note. Do not throw full or empty aerosol containers into a fire or subject them to excessive heat.

Legal category POM.

Package quantities Unit pack of one 10 ml aerosol container with one oral and one nasal attachment.

Further information An insert leaflet for patients is included in each pack.

Product licence number 0093/5003.

MFV-JECT* ▼

Presentation MFV-JECT is available in mono-dose pre-filled syringes and multidose vials. MFV-JECT is Inactivated Influenza Vaccine (Split Virion) BP, purified by zonal ultra-centrifugation and extraction with ether. The strains of influenza virus contained in the vaccine are those currently recommended each year by the World Health Organisation. Each dose also contains not more than 0.05 mg of thiomersal as preservative.

Uses Prophylaxis against influenza.

Dosage and administration By subcutaneous or intramuscular injection.

Adults and children over 13 years: Single dose; 0.5 ml.

Children under 13 years: Not recommended.

The vaccine should be allowed to reach room temperature before use.

Contra-indications, warnings, etc
Contra-indications: Persons known to have sensitivity to egg protein.

Side-effects: The incidence of side-effects with the vaccine is minimal due to the purification method; however, a transient erythema, tenderness or pain at the site of injection or mild fever may appear within the first 48 hours.

Precautions: The vaccine should be used with caution in patients with a history of allergy.

Overdosage: Not applicable.

Pharmaceutical precautions Protect from light and store at 4°C. Do not freeze.

Legal category POM.

Package quantities Monodose in prefilled syringe (0.5 ml), unit dose pack; 10 dose (5 ml) vial; 50 dose (25 ml) vial.

Further information The vaccine has been widely used in the elderly.

Product licence number 0093/0033.

MERIEUX HUMAN ALBUMIN 20%

Presentation Merieux Human Albumin 20% is a sterile aqueous solution of human serum albumin of placental origin. It is presented as a solution for intravenous injection or infusion. The solution varies in colour from yellow to orange, contains acetyltryptophanate and sodium caprylate as stabilisers and has a pH of 6.7–7.3. It contains 20% protein of which at least 96% is albumin. No preservatives are added.

Uses Treatment of acute hypoalbuminaemia in shock from loss of plasma, following acute trauma, surgery, septicaemia, haemorrhage or in the acute phase following severe and extensive burns or acute nephrosis. Albumin increases intravascular volume and maintains oncotic pressure thereby counteracting hypovolemia. Albumin may also be used for treating neonatal hyperbilirubinaemia.

Dosage and administration *Route of administration:* By slow intravenous injection or infusion. The rate of infusion should be adjusted to the clinical situation and the desired therapeutic results.

Shock: Adults 125–250 ml
        Children 1–2 ml/kg bodyweight

Burns: Adults   First hour 125–250 ml
                First day a further 125–250 ml
                Subsequent therapy 125–250 ml/day
        Children First hour 2–4 ml/kg
                Subsequent therapy 1–2 ml/kg/day

Immediate therapy should be instituted during the first 24 hours based on the severity of the patient's condition. Continuation therapy beyond 24 hours may be necessary in order to replace the losses due to the continuing increased protein catabolism and and increased albumin leakage. The albumin is infused either together with or alternating with isotonic glucose solution in a proportion of 1 volume of albumin solution to 3 volumes of glucose solution.

Neonatal hyperbilirubinaemia: 10–15 ml (1 g/kg) associated with exchange transfusions.

Acute nephrosis: Adults 125–250 ml/day
                 Children 2–5 ml/kg/day

Contra-indications, warnings, etc Circulatory overload and severe changes in systemic circulation should be avoided.

Central venous pressure should be monitored in case of risk of circulatory overload.

In the case of associated dehydration, albumin treatment should be associated or alternated with adequate rehydration treatment.

Side-effects: As with all blood products, rare cases of febrile reactions may occur, especially in cases of known sensitisation to blood or its derivatives. These reactions are generally brief and without recurrence.

Pharmaceutical precautions Merieux Human Albu-

min 20% should be stored protected from light at a temperature between +2° and +8°C. The shelf-life is 5 years.

The solution must not be used if it is cloudy or has a deposit. Once the cap has been pierced by a needle, the contents must be used immediately.

Legal category POM.

Package quantities Merieux Human Albumin 20% is supplied in rubber capped bottles of 10 ml, 50 ml and 100 ml.

Further information Nil.

Product licence number 0093/0044.

MERIEUX* INACTIVATED RABIES VACCINE (MIRV)

Presentation Human Diploid Cell Rabies Vaccine.

The vaccine is a lyophilised, stabilised suspension of inactivated Wistar rabies virus strain PM/WI 38 1503-3M, cultured on human diploid cells and inactivated by beta-propiolactone. The dry vaccine is coloured off-white but after reconstitution with the diluent supplied it turns a pinkish colour due to the presence of phenol red.

The potency of the reconstituted vaccine is not less than $2.5 \times$ the International Standard per dose (1 ml).

Uses 1. Prophylactic immunisation against rabies.

2. Treatment of patients following suspected rabies contact.

Dosage and administration The dose of reconstituted vaccine in all cases is 1 ml given by deep subcutaneous injection.

Reconstitution: Inject diluent from syringe into vaccine vial, shake to ensure complete reconstitution and withdraw contents back into syringe.

1. Prophylaxis: 1 ml of reconstituted vaccine followed by a second dose (1 ml) after a one month interval. A booster dose should be given a further 6–12 months later. To maintain high antibody titres, a further booster should be given every three years if risk of infection continues.

2. Treatment: The first injection should be given as soon as possible after the suspected contact (day 0) and followed by five further doses on days 3, 7, 14, 30 and 90. The treatment schedule may be stopped if the animal concerned is found conclusively to be free of rabies.

Contra-indications, warnings, etc There are no absolute contra-indications to inactivated rabies vaccine cultured on human diploid cells. Redness, swelling or tenderness at the site of injection may occur during the first 48 hours. A mild fever has been reported in about 1% of cases during the first 24 hours. In subjects with a history of allergy there may be an increased risk of side-effects and this possibility should be taken into account.

Pharmaceutical precautions Store at 4°C, do not freeze. Use immediately after reconstituting the vaccine.

Legal category POM.

Package quantities A vial of lyophilised vaccine containing one dose together with a disposable syringe containing 1 ml of diluent. The diluent is sterile water for injection without preservatives.

Further information Nil.

Product licence number 0093/0028.

MERIEUX* ORAL POLIOMYELITIS VACCINE
Poliomyelitis Vaccine (Oral) ▼

Presentation The product is available in single dose ampoules and multi-dose vials. The vaccine is a sterile aqueous suspension of suitable live attenuated strains of poliomyelitis virus types 1, 2 and 3 grown in monkey kidney cell cultures. The virus strains are those chosen by Sabin for their antigenic potency and safety.

Each dose contains:

Poliomyelitis virus type 1 $\geqslant 3 \times 10^5$ TCID$_{50}$
Poliomyelitis virus type 2 $\geqslant 1 \times 10^5$ TCID$_{50}$
Poliomyelitis virus type 3 $\geqslant 3 \times 10^5$ TCID$_{50}$

and magnesium chloride and human serum albumin as stabilisers. The vaccine may appear pink due to the presence of phenol red and may contain traces of neomycin.

Uses Prophylaxis against poliomyelitis.

Dosage and administration By oral administration only. The contents of a single dose ampoule (0.5 ml) or two drops (0.1 ml) of vaccine from a multi-dose vial can be conveniently administered on a lump of sugar or directly into the mouth.

Primary Immunisation – Adults and children: 3 doses at intervals of not less than 4 weeks.

In the United Kingdom, oral polio vaccine is normally given to infants at the same time as routine vaccination against diphtheria, tetanus and pertussis.

Reinforcing doses – Adults: Reinforcing doses may be given to adults if they are likely to be exposed to special risk of contracting the disease.

Children: 1 dose upon school entry and again at 15–19 years of age or upon leaving school.

Contra-indications, warnings, etc

Contra-indications: Acute febrile illness or any suspected infection, malignant disease, impaired immune responsiveness e.g. steroid treatment, radiotherapy. The vaccine should not be administered to pregnant women, unless they are known to be at definite risk from poliomyelitis.

Precautions: The efficacy of the vaccine may be impaired if given when the subject has diarrhoea or gastrointestinal dysfunction. The vaccine should not generally be administered within 3–4 weeks of another live vaccine.

Warnings: The vaccine may contain trace amounts of neomycin. Administration of vaccine to subjects known to be hypersensitive to this antibiotic should be avoided.

The vaccine may contain minute traces of penicillin carried over from the original Sabin strains but this does not normally contra-indicate use except in extreme cases of hypersensitivity.

Other unvaccinated members of the household, including adults, are advised to have a vaccination at the same time as the vaccinee.

Overdosage: Not applicable.

Pharmaceutical precautions If stored at −20°C, the vaccine can be expected to retain its potency up to the expiry date indicated on the pack. After thawing, store at +4°C for no longer than 6 months. Do not re-freeze. Once opened, any unused vaccine must be discarded after 4 hours.

Legal category POM.

Package quantities Single-dose snap-open ampoules (0.5 ml), unit dose pack; 10 dose (1 ml) vial.
Box of 10 droppers for use with multi-dose vials.

Further information Nil.

Product licence number 0093/0042.

NATRILIX* ▼

Presentation Pink biconvex sugar-coated tablets each containing 2.5 mg indapamide hemihydrate.

Uses For the treatment of hypertension.
Natrilix may be used as sole therapy or combined with other antihypertensive agents.

Dosage and administration *Adults:* The dosage is 1 tablet, containing 2.5 mg indapamide hemihydrate, daily to be taken in the morning. The action of Natrilix is progressive and the reduction in blood pressure may continue and not reach a maximum until several months after the start of therapy. A larger dose than 2.5 mg Natrilix daily is not recommended as there is no appreciable additional antihypertensive effect but a diuretic effect may become apparent. If a single daily tablet of Natrilix does not achieve a sufficient reduction in blood pressure, another antihypertensive agent may be added; those which have been used in combination with Natrilix include beta-blockers, methyldopa, clonidine and other adrenergic blocking agents. The co-administration of Natrilix with diuretics which may cause hypokalaemia is not recommended.

There is no evidence of rebound hypertension on withdrawal of Natrilix.

Elderly: There are no significant changes in the pharmacokinetics of indapamide in the elderly. Numerous clinical studies have shown that it can be used without problems and indeed has a particular benefit on systolic blood pressure in the elderly.

Children: There is no experience of the use of this drug in children.

Contra-indications, warnings, etc There are no absolute contra-indications to the use of Natrilix but caution should be exercised when prescribing it in cases of severe renal or hepatic impairment.

As with all new drugs, the administration of Natrilix should be avoided during pregnancy although no teratological effects have been seen in animals.

In a very small number of predisposed patients, hypokalaemia has been observed and awareness of this possibility should be borne in mind when prescribing Natrilix.

At doses higher than that recommended, Natrilix has a diuretic effect, therefore it is not recommended to prescribe it with a diuretic agent which may cause hypokalaemia. Also, slight weight loss has been reported in some patients taking Natrilix. Reported side-effects have included nausea and headache, but they are generally uncommon and mild in nature. Serum urate levels may rise slightly but there is no evidence that glucose tolerance is adversely affected.

Overdosage: Symptoms of overdosage would be those associated with a diuretic effect: electrolyte disturbances, hypotension and muscular weakness. Treatment would be symptomatic, directed at correcting the electrolyte abnormalities and gastric lavage or emesis should be considered.

Pharmaceutical precautions Nil.

Legal category POM.

Package quantities Cartons of 30 tablets (containing two push-through blister strips of 15 tablets) and cartons of 60 tablets (containing three push-through blister strips of 20 tablets).

Further information No interactions have been reported between Natrilix and oral hypoglycaemic agents, anticoagulants, uricosurics and anti-inflammatory agents.

Product licence number 0093/0022.

PONDERAX PACAPS*
PONDERAX* 20 mg

Presentation
Ponderax Pacaps: Prolonged action formulation in hard gelatine capsule with clear body and opaque blue cap, printed in black with PxPA 60 containing small white pellets. Each prolonged action capsule contains 60 mg fenfluramine hydrochloride BP.

Ponderax 20 mg: Pale blue, sugar-coated tablet, containing 20 mg fenfluramine hydrochloride BP.

Uses As an adjunct to the dietary treatment of moderate to severe obesity including obesity associated with maturity-onset diabetes.

Patients should be given close support and supervision.

Dosage and administration
Adults
Ponderax 20 mg: Initially 20 mg twice a day increasing after the first week in gradual steps to 40 mg, 60 mg or 80 mg twice a day as required. It has been shown that effective weight loss is related to achieving adequate blood levels of fenfluramine.

Ponderax Pacaps: Initially one 60 mg capsule daily. The dosage may be increased if necessary after the first few weeks to 2 capsules once daily. The capsules need only be taken once daily because of the slow release of the active constituent.

If weight loss does not occur at the maximum therapeutic dose, treatment should be gradually withdrawn. If weight loss ceases, treatment may be continued where there is evidence that the lower body weight is maintained but treatment beyond a total of 6 months is not recommended.

Treatment with Ponderax tablets or Ponderax Pacaps should not be stopped suddenly. Stepwise reduction of dosage over one or more weeks is recommended to avoid the possibility of precipitating depression which occasionally has been severe.

Do not exceed the maximum stated dose.

If possible, the tablets or capsules should be taken half an hour before food.

Elderly: Care should be taken when prescribing for patients over 65 years of age because drowsiness is more likely to occur.

Children: Not recommended.

Contra-indications, warnings, etc
Contra-indications: Ponderax should not be used in patients with a history of depressive illness and concurrent treatment with antidepressants. It should not be used concurrently with neuroleptic or antidepressant therapy especially MAOI's. There should be an interval of three weeks between stopping MAOI's and starting Ponderax.

Ponderax should not be used in patients with a known history of drug or alcohol abuse.

It is recommended that Ponderax is not given concomitantly with other appetite suppressants. There should be an interval of two weeks between stopping any other appetite suppressant and starting Ponderax to allow for any possible withdrawal symptoms to subside.

Ponderax should not be used in epilepsy, although exacerbation of this condition has only been reported very infrequently.

Precautions and warnings: Ponderax may potentiate the action of anti-hypertensive, anti-diabetic and sedative drugs. The dosage of these drugs should be reassessed when Ponderax is prescribed.

Ponderax may cause drowsiness. It may affect the ability to drive or operate machinery and increase the effects of alcohol.

Dependence has been rarely reported and has occurred very seldom in subjects without a history of drug abuse. Although fenfluramine is chemically related to amphetamine, the introduction of a CF_3 group into the molecule alters the pharmacological characteristics of the compound which is evident from its lack of central nervous system stimulation and its low risk of abuse or dependence.

Care should be exercised in patients with a history of psychiatric illness and in those in whom there is underlying emotional instability.

Following sudden withdrawal of Ponderax, severe depression has occasionally been reported. This risk may be avoided by a gradual reduction of dosage.

Medicines should not be used in pregnancy, especially the first trimester, unless the benefits outweigh any possible risk. Although no harmful effects on the foetus have been demonstrated, it is not recommended that Ponderax be administered during pregnancy. Fenfluramine may be excreted in breast milk and administration during lactation is not recommended.

Side-effects: The most common side-effects are diarrhoea, drowsiness, dizziness and lethargy. Dry mouth, urinary frequency, nausea, vomiting, nervousness, irritability and headache have also been reported.

Depression may occur after abrupt withdrawal and most commonly about 4 days after cessation of treatment, although it has also been reported during therapy.

Infrequent occurrences of insomnia, bad dreams, visual disorder, hypotension, impotence and loss of libido have been reported.

Rashes, reversible pulmonary hypertension, purpura and blood dyscrasias have been rarely reported.

Side-effects may be reduced by using a gradual build-up of dosage; in other patients the effects are often transient and a temporary reduction of dosage will usually eliminate them. Side-effects seldom necessitate any interruption of therapy.

Overdosage: The following symptoms have been reported: Dilated pupils, tachycardia, facial flushing, hypertension, agitation, fine tremor; these can progress to vomiting, convulsions, unconsciousness, hyperpyrexia, depression of respiration, cardiac arrhythmias, ventricular fibrillation and death may occur following very high overdosage.

Action to be taken in the event of an overdose:

Continuously monitor ECG; (ii) use diazepam to control convulsions; (iii) reduce hyperthermia; (iv) use anti-arrhythmic drugs (e.g. beta-blockers) to control cardiac tachyarrhythmias.

Pharmaceutical precautions Ponderax Pacaps should be stored in a cool, dry place.

Legal category POM.

Package quantities Ponderax Pacaps: Push-through blister strips of ten capsules. Carton of 60 capsules (six strips). Ponderax 20 mg: Push-through blister strips of 20 tablets. Carton of 100 tablets (five strips).

Further information Ponderax is not a controlled drug under the Misuse of Drugs Act 1971 and the Misuse of Drugs Regulation 1973.

The 29th session of the U.N. Commission on Narcotic Drugs endorsed the WHO recommendation that 'fenfluramine does not have amphetamine-like abuse potential nor is there evidence of significant public health or social problems arising from its use'.

Product licence numbers

Pacaps	0093/0013R
20 mg tablets	0093/5004R

Trade Mark

Smith & Nephew Pharmaceuticals Ltd

Bampton Road,
Harold Hill,
Romford,
Essex RM3 8SL

Smith+Nephew

CLINITAR* CREAM

Presentation Greenish-brown oil in water cream containing 1% w/w Stantar*.

Uses For the treatment of sub-acute and chronic psoriasis and eczema.

Dosage and administration *All age groups:* Apply to the affected areas once or twice daily.

Contra-indications, warnings, etc The use of Clinitar cream is not recommended in generalised pustular psoriasis, infections of the skin, or for patients allergic to coal tar. Coal tar can sensitise the skin to UV light, leading to sunburn. Clinitar cream should therefore be used cautiously in the sun. Before any irradiation treatment, Clinitar cream should be removed completely.

Pharmaceutical precautions None.

Legal category P.

Package quantities 60 g tube.

Further information Clinitar cream contains Stantar, which is an extract of coal tar standardized to have a photosensitising activity corresponding to that of crude coal tar. By using Stantar instead of crude coal tar a product is obtained which is easy to apply, has no unpleasant smell, and is cosmetically inconspicuous.

Product licence number 0033/0110.

CLINITAR* GEL

Presentation A clear brown gel with a slightly greenish fluorescence, containing 2.5% w/w Stantar*.

Uses For the treatment of psoriasis of the scalp and of the body. Other dermatoses responding to tar treatment, such as seborrhoeic dermatitis and chronic eczema.

Dosage and administration Apply to the affected areas once or twice daily.

Contra-indications, warnings, etc The use of Clinitar Gel is not recommended in generalised pustular psoriasis, infections of the skin, or for patients allergic to coal tar. Coal tar can sensitise the skin to U.V. light, leading to sunburn. Clinitar Gel should therefore be used cautiously in the sun. Before any irradiation treatment, Clinitar Gel should be removed completely. During summer, it is advisable to apply Clinitar Gel only once a day at bedtime followed by a bath the next morning.

Simultaneous treatments with a coal tar product and drugs which may provoke photosensitivity may create a potential risk for the patient to acquire unintended sunburn on exposure to the sun or sunlight from an artificial source.

Pharmaceutical precautions None.

Legal category P.

Package quantities 40 g tube.

Further information Clinitar Gel contains Stantar, which is an extract of coal tar standardized to have a photosensitising activity corresponding to that of crude coal tar. By using Stantar instead of crude coal tar a product is obtained which is easy to apply, has no unpleasant smell, and is cosmetically inconspicuous.

Product licence number 0033/0115.

CLINITAR* SHAMPOO

Presentation A clear, brown shampoo with a slightly greenish fluorescence, containing 2% w/w Stantar*.

Uses For the treatment of pityriasis simplex capitis (dandruff), seborrhoeic dermatitis of the scalp, and psoriasis of the scalp.

Dosage and administration *All age groups:* Moisten the hair and rub a little shampoo into the hair and scalp. Rinse and repeat the treatment, this time producing a heavy lather. Leave the lather in the hair for 5 minutes after the second treatment and then rinse carefully. Use 1–3 times a week.

Contra-indications, warnings, etc The use of Clinitar shampoo is not recommended for patients allergic to coal tar.

Avoid getting shampoo into the eyes.

Pharmaceutical precautions None. Store at room temperature.

Legal category P.

Package quantities 60 g tube.

Further information Clinitar shampoo contains Stantar, which is an extract of coal tar standardized to have a photosensitising activity corresponding to that of crude coal tar. By using Stantar instead of crude coal tar a product is obtained which is easier to rub in and wash out, and has a pleasant smell.

Product licence number 0033/0109.

CUPLEX*

Presentation A clear, brownish-yellow viscous gel containing Salicylic Acid PhEur 11% w/w, Lactic Acid PhEur 4% w/w and copper (II) acetate (corresponding to 1.1 mg of copper per 100 g) in a collodion base.

Uses Topical treatment of common, juvenile, plantar and mosaic warts: corns and callouses.

Dosage and administration *All age groups:*
1. Every night soak the wart in hot water for 5 minutes.
2. Dry thoroughly.
3. Apply one or two drops of Cuplex to the wart and allow to spread.
4. In the morning, remove elastic film and re-apply.
5. Twice or three times per week, rub away the wart surface carefully (excessive rubbing will cause stinging when Cuplex is applied) with an emery board or pumice stone, then apply Cuplex.

Contra-indications, warnings, etc Do not apply to facial or anogenital warts. Avoid contact with the eyes. Only apply to the affected area. Keep away from naked flames.

Pharmaceutical precautions Store in a cool place. Highly inflammable.

Legal category P.

Package quantities 5 g tubes.

Further information Warts are contagious and any person suffering from warts should always use their own towel.

Most warts will disappear after 6 to 12 weeks of treatment with Cuplex, providing instructions are carefully and consistently followed.

Product licence number 0033/0100.

EPPY*

Presentation L-adrenaline base 1% in an isotonic buffered ophthalmic solution, containing phenylmercuric acetate 0.002% w/v as the preservative.

Uses For the treatment of primary open angle and secondary glaucoma. It may be used in conjunction with miotic or carbonic anhydrase inhibitor therapy.

Dosage and administration *Adults (including the elderly):* One drop instilled into the eye once or twice a day.
Children: At the discretion of the physician.

When used with pilocarpine or other miotics, Eppy should be instilled 5 to 10 minutes afterwards.

Contra-indications, warnings, etc Eppy should not be used in the case of a narrow angle between the iris and cornea as pupillary dilation may precipitate angle closure. Occasionally patients may complain of orbital discomfort or red eye. Rarely headache, irritation and local skin reactions may occur. As with other adrenaline preparations, melanosis may occasionally occur, but this has no pathological significance. Systemic effects are rare but can include tachycardia, extrasystoles and elevation of blood pressure. Although only one case of a possible systemic reaction has been reported, caution is recommended in patients with thyrotoxicosis, hypertension, or cardiovascular problems including tachycardia.

Pharmaceutical precautions Eppy should not be diluted or dispensed from any container other than the original bottle. It should be stored, in its carton, in a cool place away from strong light. Eppy should not be used if the solution has become dark amber. Eppy should be discarded one month after opening.

Eppy is fully potent for two years unopened.

Legal category P.

Package quantities Eppy is supplied as a sterile ophthalmic solution in a 7.5 ml bottle, with a separate sterile dropper.

Further information An air-excluding filling process and strict control of sterilisation ensure the long shelf-life of Eppy.

In common with other sympathomimetic agents Eppy does not affect accommodation.

Product licence number 0033/5022.

FLAMAZINE*

Presentation A white hydrophilic cream containing silver sulphadiazine 1% w/w. The cream is a semi-solid oil in water emulsion. The silver sulphadiazine is in a fine micronised form.

Uses Topical broad spectrum antibacterial. Flamazine is indicated in the treatment of infected leg ulcers and pressure sores, burns and skin graft donor sites, cuts, wounds and other skin conditions where infection may prevent healing.

It is particularly effective against gram-negative organisms such as *Pseudomonas aeruginosa.*

Dosage and administration Flamazine should be applied by means of a sterile spatula or a hand covered with a sterile glove in a layer approximately 3–5 mm thick.

In leg ulcers Flamazine should be applied followed by an absorbent gauze dressing and a support bandage, e.g. 10 cm Elastocrepe. Care should be taken not to spread Flamazine on to non-ulcerated skin, and it should not be used on very wet ulcers. The dressing should be changed at least three times a week and desloughing and cleansing carried out at the same time.

In the treatment of burns Flamazine should be applied every 24 hours.

Contra-indications, warnings, etc Teratology tests have been carried out in rabbits (Dutch-belted strain) and no evidence of teratogenicity has been found. Nevertheless the use of this drug during pregnancy must be at the clinician's discretion. Further, because sulphonamide therapy is known to increase the incidence of kernicterus, silver sulphadiazine cream should be used with caution in pregnancy at term, in premature infants or in newborn infants during the first months of life.

Although reports of leucopenia following the use of Flamazine in the treatment of burns have been published, these reports do not appear to have been fully substantiated. However, in view of the reports it is as well to be aware of the possibility of low white blood cell counts occurring.

Sensitivity has been shown to occur but the incidence is lower than with other sulphonamides.

Flamazine should be used with caution if hepatic and/or renal function become impaired.

Pharmaceutical precautions The container should be stored in a cool place away from light. One container of Flamazine should be reserved for one patient; any remaining cream should be discarded after the completion of treatment.

Legal category POM.

Package quantities The preparation is obtainable in jars containing 250 g or 500 g and also tubes of 50 g.

Further information As well as its prophylactic effect, Flamazine may also exert a therapeutic action in wounds which are already infected. Flamazine is painless on application, does not cause electrolyte disturbance, is easy to apply and remove and does not stain.

Product licence number 0033/0056.

FLUORETS*

Presentation Sterile, individually wrapped paper strips each impregnated with approximately 1 mg Fluorescein Sodium BP.

Uses Fluorescein does not stain a normal cornea but conjunctival abrasions are stained yellow or orange, corneal abrasions or ulcers are stained a bright green and foreign bodies are surrounded by a green ring.

Fluorescein can be used in diagnostic examinations including Goldmann tonometry and the fitting of hard contact lenses.

Dosage and administration Pull tabs apart at right-hand end of envelope and withdraw Fluoret. Moisten tip with tear fluid from lower fornix, sterile water or sterile ophthalmic solution. Then gently stroke the Fluoret across the conjunctiva. For the best result the patient should blink several times.

Contra-indications, warnings, etc The applicator should be used once and then discarded. Care should be taken to handle the strip by the non-impregnated end only.

Pharmaceutical precautions No special precautions.

Legal category P.

Package quantities Gravity-delivered cartons of 100 individually wrapped Fluorets.

Further information Nil.

Product licence number 0033/5095.

GANDA*

Presentation Ganda is a clear, viscous, colourless to almost colourless liquid, available in four strengths.

Ganda 1+0.2 (Guanethidine Monosulfate PhEur 1% w/v+Adrenaline BP 0.2% w/v)

Ganda 3+0.5 (Guanethidine Monosulfate PhEur 3% w/v+Adrenaline BP 0.5% w/v)

Ganda 5+0.5 (Guanethidine Monosulfate PhEur 5% w/v+Adrenaline BP 0.5% w/v)

Ganda 5+1 (Guanethidine Monosulfate PhEur 5% w/v+Adrenaline BP 1% w/v)

in a buffered solution containing benzalkonium chloride 0.01% w/v as the preservative. It is supplied in a plastic dropper bottle packed in a nitrogen-filled pouch.

Uses For the treatment of primary open angle or secondary glaucoma. It may be used in conjunction with miotics or carbonic anhydrase inhibitor therapy.

Dosage and administration *Adult (including the elderly):* One drop to be instilled into the eye once or twice daily or at the discretion of the physician.

Children: At the discretion of the physician.

When used in conjunction with miotics, Ganda should follow the miotic after an interval of 5–10 minutes.

Contra-indications, warnings, etc Ganda should not be used in the case of a narrow angle between the iris and cornea as pupillary dilation may precipitate angle closure.

Occasionally a patient may complain of orbital discomfort or red eye. Rarely, headache, irritation and local skin reactions may occur. As with other adrenaline preparations, melanosis may occasionally occur, but this has no pathological significance. Systemic effects are rare but can include tachycardia, extrasystoles, and elevation of blood pressure. Although no reports of such reactions to Ganda have been received, caution is recommended in patients with thyrotoxicosis, hypertension or cardiovascular problems including tachycardia.

One clinical investigator has reported that in two cases out of 21, a paradoxical increase of I.O.P. occurred for which no explanation was offered.

Some degree of ptosis may represent an adverse effect in glaucoma, but will usually respond to a reduction in dosage or in the frequency of administration.

At prolonged high dosage a tendency to superficial punctate keratitis has been reported, responding either to a reduction in dosage or termination of treatment.

Pharmaceutical precautions Ganda is supplied in a plastic dropper bottle in a nitrogen-filled pouch, inside a carton. It should be stored in its carton in a cool place away from strong light. The carton only should be removed before supplying to the patient. Ganda should not be diluted, nor should it be dispensed from any container other than the original bottle. Ganda should not be used if the solution has become dark amber. The contents of the bottle should be discarded one month after removal from the pouch. Ganda is fully potent for two years providing the pouch remains unopened.

Legal category POM.

Package quantities Ganda is supplied as a sterile ophthalmic solution in a 7.5 ml plastic dropper bottle. Each bottle is enclosed in a nitrogen-filled, double-sealed, nylon/aluminium foil pouch inside a carton.

Further information The use of the nitrogen-filled overwrap ensures the long shelf-life of Ganda.

Ganda is a unique combination of Adrenaline BP and Guanethidine Monosulfate PhEur in a plastic dropper bottle which has been specially designed for patient convenience. Its special formulation gives improved stability, and includes a viscoliser to enhance comfort and effectiveness.

In common with other sympathomimetic agents Ganda does not affect accommodation.

Product licence numbers

Ganda 1+0.2	0033/0075
Ganda 3+0.5	0033/0071
Ganda 5+0.5	0033/0070
Ganda 5+1	0033/0069

MINIMS* AMETHOCAINE HYDROCHLORIDE

Presentation Single-use, clear, colourless, sterile eye drops. Two strengths are available: Amethocaine (Tetracaine) Hydrochloride PhEur 0.5% and 1% w/v solutions.

Uses As a topical anaesthetic.

Dosage and administration One drop as required.

Contra-indications, warnings, etc Amethocaine may give rise to dermatitis in hypersensitive patients. Amethocaine is hydrolysed in the body to p-amino-benzoic acid and should not therefore be used in patients being treated with sulfonamides. On instillation an initial burning sensation may be complained of but this passes off in less than half a minute. The anaesthetised eye should be protected from dust and bacterial contamination. The cornea may be damaged by prolonged application of anaesthetic eye drops.

Each Minims unit should be discarded after a single use.

Pharmaceutical precautions Minims should be stored in a cool place, and should not be exposed to strong light.

Legal category POM.

Package quantities Cartons of 20 units, each containing approximately 0.5 ml.

Further information Nil.

Product licence numbers
Amethocaine Hydrochloride 0.5%   0033/5000
Amethocaine Hydrochloride 1%   0033/5001

MINIMS* ATROPINE SULFATE

Presentation Single-use, clear, colourless, sterile eye drops, available as a 1% w/v solution of Atropine Sulfate PhEur.

Uses As a mydriatic and cycloplegic.

Dosage and administration One drop as required.

Contra-indications, warnings, etc The protracted mydriasis which is difficult to reverse, may be a disadvantage. All mydriatics and cycloplegics are contra-indicated in eyes where the filtration angle is narrow, as an acute attack of angle closure glaucoma may be precipitated. If in doubt it is recommended that homatropine is used, since its action can be reversed by eserine (physostigmine).

Each Minims unit should be discarded after a single use.

Pharmaceutical precautions Minims should be stored in a cool place, and should not be exposed to strong light.

Legal category POM.

Package quantities Cartons of 20 units, each unit containing approximately 0.5 ml.

Further information Dilation of the pupil occurs within half an hour after application.

Product licence number 0033/5002.

MINIMS* BENOXINATE (OXYBUPROCAINE) HYDROCHLORIDE

Presentation Single-use, clear, colourless, sterile eye drops, available as a 0.4% w/v solution of Benoxinate (Oxybuprocaine) Hydrochloride USP.

Uses As a topical anaesthetic.

Dosage and administration One drop of benoxinate 0.4% is sufficient when dropped into the conjunctival sac to anaesthetise the surface of the eye to allow tonometry after one minute. A further drop after 90 seconds provides adequate anaesthesia for the fitting of contact lenses.

Three drops at 90 second intervals provides sufficient anaesthesia after five minutes for a foreign body to be removed from the corneal epithelium, or for incision of a Meibomian cyst through the conjunctiva.

Corneal sensitivity is normal again after about one hour.

Contra-indications, warnings, etc The anaesthetised eye should be protected from dust and bacterial contamination. The cornea may be damaged by prolonged application of anaesthetic eye drops.

Each Minims unit should be discarded after a single use.

Pharmaceutical precautions Minims should be stored in a cool place, and should not be exposed to strong light.

Legal category POM.

Package quantities Cartons of 20 units, each unit containing approximately 0.5 ml.

Further information When applied to the conjunctiva benoxinate is less irritant than amethocaine in normal concentrations.

Product licence number 0033/5004.

MINIMS* CASTOR OIL

Presentation Single-use, clear, almost colourless or slightly yellow, viscous sterile eye drops.

Uses As a lubricant and emollient.

Dosage and administration One or two drops as required.

Contra-indications, warnings, etc Each Minims unit should be discarded after a single use.

Pharmaceutical precautions Minims should be stored in a cool place and should not be exposed to strong light.

Legal category P.

Package quantities Cartons of 20 units, each unit containing approximately 0.5 ml.

Further information Nil.

Product licence number 0033/5018.

MINIMS* CHLORAMPHENICOL

Presentation Single-use, clear, colourless, sterile eye drops, available as a 0.5% w/v solution of Chloramphenicol PhEur containing buffering agents.

Uses As a topical antibacterial. Chloramphenicol is a broad spectrum antibiotic with bacteriostatic activity and is effective against a wide range of Gram-negative and Gram-positive organisms.

Dosage and administration *Adult:* One or more drops as required.

Children: One drop as required.

Contra-indications, warnings, etc Treatment with chloramphenicol should be discontinued immediately on the appearance of toxic symptoms or allergic skin rashes. Aplastic anaemia has been reported following topical use of chloramphenicol. Whilst the hazard is a rare one, it should be borne in mind when assessing the benefits expected from use of this compound.

Each Minims unit should be discarded after a single use.

Pharmaceutical precautions Chloramphenicol Minims should be stored between 2°C and 8°C. Do not freeze. Discard one month after removal from refrigerated storage.

Legal category POM.

Package quantities Cartons of 20 units, each unit containing approximately 0.5 ml.

Further information Nil.

Product licence number 0033/0055.

MINIMS* CYCLOPENTOLATE HYDROCHLORIDE

Presentation Single-use, clear, colourless, sterile eye drops. Two strengths are available: Cyclopentolate Hydrochloride BP 0.5% and 1% w/v solutions.

Uses As a mydriatic and cycloplegic.

Dosage and administration *Adult:* One or two drops as required. Maximum effect is induced 30–60 minutes after instillation. In iritis or iridocyclitis 1 or 2 drops of a 0.5% w/v solution are instilled every six to eight hours. One or two drops of a 0.5% w/v solution are also used for breaking down adhesions of the iris to the lens. For refraction the instillation of 1 drop of a 0.5% w/v solution repeated after five minutes is usually sufficient. Deeply pigmented eyes may require a 1% w/v solution.

Children: At the discretion of the physician.

Contra-indications, warnings, etc Recovery of accommodation occurs within 24 hours.

All mydriatics and cycloplegics are contra-indicated in eyes where the filtration angle is narrow, as an acute attack of angle closure glaucoma may be precipitated.

Each Minims unit should be discarded after a single use.

Pharmaceutical precautions Minims should be stored in a cool place, and should not be exposed to strong light.

Legal category POM.

Package quantities Cartons of 20 units, each unit containing approximately 0.5 ml.

Further information Nil.

Product licence numbers
Cyclopentolate Hydrochloride 0.5%   0033/5005
Cyclopentolate Hydrochloride 1%   0033/5006

MINIMS* FLUORESCEIN SODIUM

Presentation Single-use, clear, orange-red, sterile eye drops. Two strengths are available: Fluorescein Sodium BP 1% and 2% w/v solutions.

Uses Fluorescein does not stain a normal cornea but conjunctival abrasions are stained yellow or orange, corneal abrasions or ulcers are stained a bright green and foreign bodies are surrounded by a green ring.

Fluorescein can be used in diagnostic examinations including Goldmann tonometry and the fitting of hard contact lenses.

Dosage and administration Sufficient solution should be applied to stain the damaged areas. Excess may be washed away with sterile saline solution.

Contra-indications, warnings, etc Special care should be taken to avoid microbial contamination.

Each Minims unit should be discarded after a single use.

Pharmaceutical precautions Minims should be stored in a cool place, and should not be exposed to strong light.

Legal category P.

Package quantities Cartons of 20 units, each unit containing approximately 0.5 ml.

Further information *Pseudomonas aeruginosa* grows well in fluorescein solutions, therefore a single use preparation is to be preferred.

Product licence numbers
Fluorescein Sodium 1%   0033/0079
Fluorescein Sodium 2%   0033/5008

MINIMS* GENTAMICIN SULFATE

Presentation Single-use, clear, colourless sterile eye drops containing Gentamicin Sulfate BP equivalent to 0.3% w/v gentamicin base, and additional ingredients.

Uses As a broad-spectrum bactericidal antibiotic, for the treatment of infections of the eye caused by both Gram-positive and Gram-negative organisms, including *Pseudomonas aeruginosa*.

Dosage and administration One drop as required.

Contra-indications, warnings, etc Gentamicin should not be used in patients with hypersensitivity to gentamicin and/or other aminoglycosides. Each Minims unit should be discarded after a single use.

Pharmaceutical precautions Minims should be stored in a cool place, and should not be exposed to strong light. Do not freeze.

Legal category POM.

Package quantities Cartons of 20 units, each unit containing approximately 0.5 ml.

Further information Nil.

Product licence number 0033/0094.

MINIMS* HOMATROPINE HYDROBROMIDE

Presentation Single-use, clear, colourless, sterile eye drops, available as a 2% w/v solution of Homatropine Hydrobromide PhEur.

Uses As a mydriatic and cycloplegic.

Dosage and administration One drop as required.

Contra-indications, warnings, etc All mydriatics and cycloplegics are contra-indicated in eyes where the filtration angle is narrow, as an acute attack of angle closure glaucoma may be precipitated.

Each Minims unit should be discarded after a single use.

Minims Homatropine should not be used in patients allergic to atropine.

Pharmaceutical precautions Minims should be stored in a cool place, and should not be exposed to strong light.

Legal category POM.

Package quantities Cartons of 20 units, each unit containing approximately 0.5 ml.

Further information Homatropine hydrobromide has properties similar to those of atropine and is often used in preference to the latter because its action is more rapid in onset and it has a less prolonged mydriatic action.

Product licence number 0033/5010.

MINIMS* LIGNOCAINE AND FLUORESCEIN

Presentation Single-use, clear, yellow, sterile eye drops containing Lignocaine (Lidocaine) Hydrochloride PhEur 4.0% w/v, Fluorescein Sodium BP 0.25% w/v and stabilising agents.

Uses As a diagnostic stain and topical anaesthetic combined. Minims Lignocaine and Fluorescein units are used in the measurement of intra-ocular pressure by Goldman tonometry.

Dosage and administration *Adult:* One or more drops as required.

Children: At the discretion of the physician.

Contra-indications, warnings, etc Known hypersensitivity to Lignocaine and other local anaesthetics.

Special care should be taken to protect the anaesthetised eye from foreign body contamination, particularly in elderly patients in whom the duration of anaesthesia may exceed 30 minutes. The cornea may be damaged by prolonged application of anaesthetic eye drops.

Each Minims unit should be discarded after a single use.

Pharmaceutical precautions Minims should be stored in a cool place and should not be exposed to strong light.

Legal category POM.

Package quantities Cartons of 20 units, each unit containing approximately 0.5 ml.

Further information Nil.

Product licence number 0033/0073.

MINIMS* NEOMYCIN SULFATE

Presentation Single-use, clear, colourless, sterile eye drops, available as a 0.5% w/v solution of Neomycin Sulfate PhEur containing stabilising agents.

Uses As a topical antibacterial preparation. Neomycin sulfate has a broad spectrum of antibiotic activity, being effective against most strains of staphylococci and some strains of *Proteus vulgaris* and *Pseudomonas aeruginosa*. It has no action against fungi and viruses.

Dosage and administration One or more drops as required.

Contra-indications, warnings, etc It should not be used in patients with known hypersensitivity to neomycin and/or other aminoglycosides. Caution is necessary if it is applied to patients with eczema.

Each Minims unit should be discarded after a single use.

Pharmaceutical precautions Minims should be stored in a cool place, and should not be exposed to strong light.

Legal category POM.

Package quantities Cartons of 20 units, each unit containing approximately 0.5 ml.

Further information Nil.

Product licence number 0033/5012.

MINIMS* PHENYLEPHRINE HYDROCHLORIDE

Presentation Single-use, clear, colourless, sterile eye drops, available as a 10% w/v solution of Phenylephrine (Metaoxedrine) Hydrochloride BP containing stabilising agents.

Uses As a mydriatic agent.

Dosage and administration *Adult:* One drop as required.

Children: The use of Minims phenylephrine in infants is not recommended.

Contra-indications, warnings, etc All mydriatics and cycloplegics are contra-indicated in eyes where the filtration angle is narrow, as an acute attack of angle closure glaucoma may be precipitated.

Phenylephrine should not be used in patients with thyrotoxicosis, hypertension, or cardiovascular problems including tachycardia, and patients on β blockers.

Each Minims unit should be discarded after a single use.

Pharmaceutical precautions Minims should be stored in a cool place, and should not be exposed to strong light.

Legal category P.

Package quantities Cartons of 20 units, each unit containing approximately 0.5 ml.

Further information Nil.

Product licence number 0033/5021.

MINIMS* PILOCARPINE NITRATE

Presentation Single-use, clear, colourless, sterile eye drops. Three strengths are available: Pilocarpine Nitrate PhEur 1%, 2%, and 4% w/v solutions.

Uses As a miotic for reversing the action of the weaker mydriatics and in emergency treatment of glaucoma.

Dosage and administration To induce miosis one or two drops should be used. In cases of emergency treatment of acute narrow angle glaucoma, one drop should be used every five minutes until miosis is achieved.

Contra-indications, warnings, etc Pilocarpine induces spasm of the ciliary muscle which may last up to two hours.

Each Minims unit should be discarded after a single use.

Pharmaceutical precautions Minims should be stored in a cool place, and should not be exposed to strong light.

Legal category POM.

Package quantities Cartons of 20 units, each unit containing approximately 0.5 ml.

Further information Nil.

Product licence numbers
Pilocarpine Nitrate 1%　0033/5013
Pilocarpine Nitrate 2%　0033/5014
Pilocarpine Nitrate 4%　0033/5016

MINIMS* PREDNISOLONE SODIUM PHOSPHATE

Presentation Single-use, clear, colourless, sterile eye drops, available as a 0.5% w/v solution of Prednisolone Sodium Phosphate BP containing additional ingredients.

Uses Non-infected inflammatory conditions of the eye.

Dosage and administration
Adult: One or two drops as required.
Children: At the discretion of the physician.

Contra-indications, warnings, etc Use is contra-indicated in viral, fungal, tuberculous and other bacterial infections. Prolonged application to the eye of preparations containing corticosteroids has caused increased intra-ocular pressure and therefore the drops should not be used in patients with glaucoma. Topical administration of corticosteroids to pregnant animals can cause abnormalities of foetal development and although the relevance of this finding to human beings has not been established, the use of Minims Prednisolone during pregnancy should be avoided.

In children, long-term continuous topical corticosteroid therapy should be avoided due to possible adrenal suppression.

Each Minims unit should be discarded after a single use.

Pharmaceutical precautions Minims should be stored in a cool place, and should not be exposed to strong light.

Legal category POM.

Package quantities Cartons of 20 units, each unit containing approximately 0.5 ml.

Further information Nil.

Product licence number 0033/0091.

MINIMS* ROSE BENGAL

Presentation Single-use, clear, dark-red, sterile eye drops, available as a 1% w/v solution of rose bengal.

Uses As a diagnostic stain. Rose bengal solution stains degenerated conjunctival and corneal epithelial cells. It is particularly useful in demonstrating these changes in Sjogren's syndrome, where lack of tears has caused damage. Pressure marks from contact lenses are shown

by rose bengal indicating that alteration of the lens may be necessary.

Dosage and administration One or two drops as required.

Contra-indications, warnings, etc Can produce severe stinging in dry eyes where it should be used with care.

Each Minims unit should be discarded after a single use.

Pharmaceutical precautions Minims should be stored in a cool place, and should not be exposed to strong light.

Legal category P.

Package quantities Cartons of 20 units, each unit containing approximately 0.5 ml.

Further information Nil.

Product licence number 0033/0048.

MINIMS* SODIUM CHLORIDE

Presentation Single-use, clear, colourless, sterile eye drops, available as a 0.9% w/v solution of Sodium Chloride PhEur.

Uses As an irrigating solution.

Dosage and administration Adequate solution should be used to irrigate the eye.

Contra-indications, warnings, etc Each Minims unit should be discarded after a single use.

Pharmaceutical precautions Minims should be stored in a cool place, and should not be exposed to strong light.

Legal category P.

Package quantities Cartons of 20 units, each unit containing approximately 0.5 ml.

Further information Nil.

Product licence number 0033/5017.

MINIMS* SULFACETAMIDE SODIUM

Presentation Single-use, clear, colourless or slightly yellow, sterile eye drops, available as a 10% w/v solution of Sulfacetamide Sodium PhEur containing stabilising agents.

Uses For the treatment of conjunctivitis. Sulfacetamide sodium is active against both Gram-positive and Gram-negative organisms.

Dosage and administration *Adult:* One drop as required.
Children: At the discretion of the physician.

Contra-indications, warnings, etc Local application to the eye may cause burning or stinging, but this is rarely severe enough to necessitate discontinuation of treatment. Sulfacetamide sodium should not be used in persons who have shown hypersensitivity to sulfonamides.

Each Minims unit should be discarded after a single use.

Pharmaceutical precautions Minims should be stored in a cool place, and should not be exposed to strong light.

Legal category POM.

Package quantities Cartons of 20 units, each unit containing approximately 0.5 ml.

Further information Nil.

Product licence number 0033/5019.

MINIMS* THYMOXAMINE HYDROCHLORIDE

Presentation Single-use, clear, colourless, sterile eye drops, available as a 0.5% w/v solution of Thymoxamine Hydrochloride BP.

Uses Reversal of the mydriasis caused by phenylephrine and other sympathomimetics.

Dosage and administration One drop as required.

Contra-indications, warnings, etc Upon instillation an initial transient burning sensation may be experienced. Minimal conjunctival hyperaemia generally occurs but this passes after a few hours. A transient ptosis may occasionally occur. Each Minims unit should be discarded after a single use.

Pharmaceutical precautions Thymoxamine Minims should be stored between 2°C and 8°C. Do not freeze. Do not expose to strong light. Discard one month after removal from refrigerated storage.

Legal category POM.

Package quantities Cartons of 20 units, each unit containing approximately 0.5 ml.

Further information Clinical studies with thymoxamine have shown that it produces miosis without causing a significant change in the depth of the anterior chamber or altering facility of outflow. Unlike parasympathomimetic miotics thymoxamine does not cause spasm of the ciliary muscle.

Product licence number 0033/0101.

MINIMS* TROPICAMIDE

Presentation Single-use, clear, colourless, sterile eye drops. Two strengths are available: Tropicamide BP 0.5% and 1% w/v solutions.

Uses As a mydriatic and cycloplegic.

Dosage and administration *Adult:* 2 drops at five minute intervals, with a further 1 or 2 drops after 30 minutes if required.

Children: At the discretion of the physician.

Contra-indications, warnings, etc All mydriatics and cycloplegics are contra-indicated in eyes where the filtration angle is narrow, as an acute attack of angle closure glaucoma may be precipitated.

Each Minims unit should be discarded after a single use.

Pharmaceutical precautions Minims units should be stored in a cool place and should not be exposed to strong light.

Legal category POM.

Package quantities Cartons of 20 units, each unit containing approximately 0.5 ml.

Further information The 0.5% solution in particular may be expected to cause little or no cycloplegia.

Product licence numbers
Tropicamide 0.5%　0033/0077
Tropicamide 1.0%　0033/0078

NARPHEN*

Presentation Narphen is available as white, biconvex compressed tablets embossed SNP/2 on one side and scored on the reverse. Each tablet contains 5 mg Phenazocine Hydrobromide BP (1973).

Uses Narphen is a powerful analgesic for the relief of severe pain. Pain relief usually occurs within 20 minutes and lasts for five to six hours. Narphen is indicated for acute and chronic pain, including pre- and postoperative pain and for obstetric analgesia. Narphen is particularly suitable for the treatment of intractable pain such as that of carcinoma as it produces minimal sedation.

In treating biliary or pancreatic pain constriction of the Sphincter of Oddi is undesirable and the low spasmogenic activity of Narphen may be advantageous.

Dosage and administration *Adults (including the elderly):* One tablet every four to six hours sublingually or orally; up to 20 mg may be administered in a single dose if necessary.

Children: Paediatric dosage not established.

Contra-indications, warnings, etc Narphen is contra-indicated in coma, convulsive disorders, delirium tremens, myxoedema, alcoholism, respiratory depression and obstructive airways disease. Narphen should not be given concurrently with monoamine oxidase inhibitors, nor within two weeks of discontinuation of treatment with them.

It is wise to reduce dosage in the elderly, and in hypothyroidism or chronic hepatic disease. Administration in labour may cause respiratory depression in the new-born infant.

Care is required in the presence of renal insufficiency or concurrent administration of other narcotic analgesics, sedatives/hypnotics or anaesthetics.

At the commencement of dosage some patients may experience a feeling of light-headedness or dizziness which soon passes.

Nausea and vomiting may be troublesome although emetic symptoms and constipation are less than with other narcotic analgesics. If nausea and vomiting occur anti-emetics such as those of the phenothiazine type may be effective.

Pruritus and occasionally dryness of the mouth and sweating have occurred. Hypotension is rare. As with other narcotics respiratory depression, tolerance and dependence may occur.

Although there is insufficient evidence of the safety of this drug in human pregnancy, animal studies have not shown any hazard. Nevertheless the use of phenazocine during pregnancy is not recommended.

Treatment of overdosage: Naloxone may be used as an antidote to overdosage or to antagonise any respiratory depression that may occur.

Pharmaceutical precautions Protect from light.

Legal category CD (Sch 2) POM.

Package quantities Tablets of 5 mg in securitainers of 25 and 100.

Further information Nil.

Product licence number 0033/5047R.

SIMPLENE*

Presentation Simplene is a clear, viscous, colourless to almost colourless liquid, containing Adrenaline BP in a buffered solution preserved with benzalkonium chloride 0.01% w/v. It is supplied in a plastic dropper bottle packed in a nitrogen-filled pouch and is available in two strengths.
Simplene 0.5% (Adrenaline BP 0.5% w/v)
Simplene 1%   (Adrenaline BP 1% w/v)

Uses For the treatment of primary open angle or secondary glaucoma. It may be used in conjunction with miotics or carbonic anhydrase inhibitor therapy.

Dosage and administration *Adults (including the elderly):* One drop to be instilled into the eye once or twice daily.
Children: At the discretion of the physician.
When used with pilocarpine or other miotics, Simplene should be instilled 5 to 10 minutes afterwards.

Contra-indications, warnings, etc Simplene should not be used in the case of a narrow angle between the iris and cornea as pupillary dilation may precipitate angle closure. Occasionally patients may complain of orbital discomfort or red eye. Rarely, headache, irritation and local skin reactions occur. As with other adrenaline preparations, melanosis may occasionally occur, but this has no pathological significance. Systemic effects are rare but include tachycardia, extrasystoles, and elevation of blood pressure. Although no reports of such reactions to Simplene have been received, caution is recommended in patients with thyrotoxicosis, hypertension or cardiovascular problems including tachycardia.

Pharmaceutical precautions Simplene is supplied in a plastic dropper bottle in a nitrogen-filled pouch, inside a carton. It should be stored in its carton in a cool place away from strong light. The carton only should be removed before supplying to the patient. Simplene should not be diluted, nor should it be dispensed from any container other than the original bottle. Simplene should not be used if the solution has become dark amber. The contents of the bottle should be discarded one month after removal from the pouch. Simplene is fully potent for 2 years providing the pouch remains unopened.

Legal category POM.

Package quantities Simplene is supplied as a sterile ophthalmic solution in a 7.5 ml plastic dropper bottle. Each bottle is enclosed in a nitrogen-filled, double-sealed, nylon/aluminium foil pouch, inside a carton.

Further information The use of the nitrogen-filled overwrap ensures the long shelf-life of Simplene.
Simplene is a unique presentation of adrenaline in a plastic dropper bottle, which has been specially designed for patient convenience. Its special formulation gives improved stability, and includes a visco liser to enhance comfort and effectiveness.
In common with other sympathomimetic agents Simplene does not affect accommodation.

Product licence numbers
Simplene 1.0%   0033/0057
Simplene 0.5%   0033/0072

SNO* PHENICOL

Presentation Multi-dose, colourless to pale straw coloured eye drops containing Chloramphenicol PhEur 0.5% w/v supplied in a plastic dropper bottle. This solution contains chlorhexidine acetate 0.01% w/v as the preservative.

Uses As a topical antibacterial. Chloramphenicol is a broad spectrum antibiotic with bacteriostatic activity and is effective against a wide range of Gram-negative and Gram-positive organisms.

Dosage and administration *Adults (including the elderly):* One or more drops as required.
Children: One drop as required.

Contra-indications, warnings, etc This product is not intended as a long term treatment for dry eye syndromes.
Treatment with chloramphenicol should be discontinued immediately on the appearance of toxic symptoms or allergic skin rashes. Aplastic anaemia has been reported following topical use of chloramphenicol. Whilst the hazard is a rare one, it should be borne in mind when assessing the benefits expected from the use of this compound.

Pharmaceutical precautions Sno phenicol should not be diluted or dispensed from any container other than the original bottle and should be stored at 2°C–8°C. Do not freeze.
Sno phenicol is fully potent for two years unopened.
Sno phenicol, like other eye drops, should be discarded one month after opening.

Legal category POM.

Package quantities Sno phenicol is supplied as a sterile ophthalmic solution in a 10 ml plastic dropper bottle.

Further information The solution is formulated with a viscoliser for patient comfort.

Product licence number 0033/0076.

SNO* PILO

Presentation Multi-dose, clear, colourless to pale yellow, eye drops supplied in a plastic dropper bottle. Three strengths are available: 1.0%, 2.0% and 4.0% w/v Pilocarpine Hydrochloride BP preserved with 0.01% benzalkonium chloride.

Uses For the treatment of glaucoma.

Dosage and administration *Adults (including the elderly):* One or two drops four times a day or as required.
Children: At the discretion of the physician.

Contra-indications, warnings, etc Sno pilo is contra-indicated where pupillary constriction is undesirable e.g. in cases of acute iritis.
Ciliary spasm with a temporary reduction of visual acuity occurs. Sensitivity is only rarely observed but if reaction occurs the use of the drops should be discontinued.

Sno pilo should not be used in patients fitted with soft contact lenses.

Pharmaceutical precautions Sno pilo should not be diluted or dispensed from any container other than the original bottle and should be stored in a cool place. Sno pilo is fully potent for three years unopened. Sno pilo, like other eye drops, should be discarded one month after opening.

Legal category POM.

Package quantities Sno pilo is supplied as a sterile ophthalmic solution in a 10 ml plastic dropper bottle.

Further information The solution is formulated with a viscoliser for patient comfort.

Product licence numbers
Sno pilo 1.0% w/v   0033/0065
Sno pilo 2.0% w/v   0033/0066
Sno pilo 4.0% w/v   0033/0068

SNO* TEARS

Presentation Sno tears is a clear, colourless slightly viscous solution in a plastic dropper bottle. It contains polyvinyl alcohol 1.4% w/v together with benzalkonium chloride 0.004% w/v and disodium edetate 0.02% w/v as an antibacterial system.

Uses As an artificial tear and lubricant in cases of tear deficiency.

Dosage and administration One or more drops as required.

Contra-indications, warnings, etc Sno tears should not be used in patients fitted with soft contact lenses.

Pharmaceutical precautions Sno tears should not be diluted or dispensed from any container other than the original bottle and should be stored in a cool place.
Sno tears is fully potent for three years unopened, but as with other eye drops, it should be discarded one month after opening.

Legal category P.

Package quantities Sno tears is supplied as a sterile ophthalmic solution in a 10 ml plastic dropper bottle.

Further information Nil.

Product licence number 0033/0097.

WELLDORM*

Presentation An elongated, oval, film-coated tablet. The coated tablet has a uniform smooth, film coat, of bluish-purple colour. Each tablet contains 650 mg of Dichloralphenazone BP. The tablets are packed in blister strips.

Uses For the treatment of insomnia in all age groups; and for administration in the early stages of labour.

Dosage and administration *Adult dose:* The hypnotic dose is two or three tablets to be taken with a drink 20 minutes before bedtime.
Elderly dose: One to three tablets as above.
Paediatric dose: For children under the age of 12 Welldorm Elixir would provide an adequate dose range.

Contra-indications, warnings, etc Acute intermittent porphyria. An acute attack may be precipitated.
There have been occasional reports of skin rashes, nausea, vomiting, headache, hangover, anaphylaxis and occasional sensitivity reactions. Blood dyscrasias are extremely rare. Welldorm has been extensively used for over 25 years, during which time only one case of thrombocytopenia attributable to the drug has been reported.
A study has shown that withdrawal or omission of Welldorm therapy in patients receiving anticoagulant therapy with coumarin derivatives, e.g. warfarin, can lead to marked lengthening of the prothrombin time.
Although there is insufficient evidence of the safety of this drug in human pregnancy, animal studies have not shown any hazard. Nevertheless the use of dichloralphenazone during pregnancy is not recommended except in the early stages of labour.
Treatment of overdosage: Gastric lavage and supportive therapy. In severe cases haemoperfusion should be used.

Pharmaceutical precautions The tablets should be stored in a cool dry place.

Legal category POM.

Package quantities The tablets are packed in blister strips of 15, two strips (30 tablets) per carton.

Further information Welldorm is a chloral hydrate derivative which induces a near natural sleep and does not interfere with the paradoxical/orthodox (REM/Non-REM) ratio.

Product licence number 0033/0032.

WELLDORM* ELIXIR

Presentation Welldorm Elixir is a clear, red syrup, with a pleasant passion-fruit flavour. Welldorm Elixir contains 225 mg Dichloralphenazone BP in each 5 ml dose.

Uses Welldorm Elixir is for the treatment of insomnia in all age groups and for sedation in children.

Dosage and administration *Adult dose (including the elderly):* 15–45 ml as an hypnotic dose.
Children: Hypnotic:
   Up to 1 year: 2.5–5 ml
   1–5 years: 5–10 ml
   6–12 years: 10–20 ml
Sedative: Sedative doses are half the above hypnotic dose (Syrup BP should be used as a diluent).

Contra-indications, warnings, etc Acute intermittent porphyria. An acute attack may be precipitated.
There have been occasional reports of skin rashes, nausea, vomiting, headache, hangover and occasional sensitivity reactions. Blood dyscrasias are extremely rare. Welldorm has been extensively used for over 25 years, during which time only one case of thrombocytopenia attributable to the drug has been reported.
A study has shown that withdrawal or omission of Welldorm therapy in patients receiving anticoagulant therapy with coumarin derivatives, e.g. warfarin, can lead to marked lengthening of the prothrombin time.
Although there is insufficient evidence of the safety of this drug in human pregnancy, animal studies have not shown any hazard. Nevertheless the use of dichloralphenazone during pregnancy is not recommended.

Treatment of overdosage: Gastric lavage and supportive therapy. In severe cases haemoperfusion should be used.

Pharmaceutical precautions Syrup BP should be used as a diluent. Welldorm Elixir should be stored in a well-stoppered bottle away from direct sunlight.

Legal category POM.

Package quantities Welldorm Elixir is supplied in bottles containing 150 ml and 500 ml.

Further information Welldorm Elixir is a chloral hydrate derivative which induces a near natural sleep and does not interfere with the paradoxical/orthodox (REM/Non-REM) ratio.

Product licence number 0033/5025.

*Trade Mark

Smith Kline & French Laboratories Limited
Mundells
Welwyn Garden City
Hertfordshire AL7 1EY

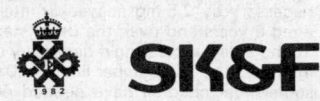

CENDEVAX*
Rubella vaccine, live BP
(Cendehill* strain)

Presentation Cendevax rubella vaccine is a live attenuated vaccine prepared in rabbit kidney cells. It is available in glass vials containing a pink freeze-dried pellet; a clear, colourless, sterile diluent is provided in a separate ampoule (monodose) or vial (10-dose). Each 0.5 ml of reconstituted vaccine contains not less than 1,000 $TCID_{50}$ of live attenuated Cendehill strain of rubella virus, together with not more than 25 μg (17 i.u.) neomycin sulphate.

Uses Routine immunisation of pre-pubertal girls against rubella. Also indicated in seronegative women of child-bearing age *who are not pregnant* and in whom the possibility of pregnancy can be excluded for at least three months following vaccination, including post-partum mothers, and for immunisation of children and adults to prevent transmission of rubella to the at-risk pregnant woman.

Dosage and administration *Adults and children:* 0.5 ml of the reconstituted vaccine administered by the subcutaneous route only.

The vaccine should be reconstituted using only the sterile diluent supplied with each dose. With multi-dose vials, the whole of the sterile diluent (7 ml) should be transferred into the vial containing the vaccine, keeping the latter upright. It should then be shaken to ensure complete solution. The syringe should be dry sterilised; the vaccine is readily inactivated by alcohol and other chemical disinfectants and antiseptics, and care is needed to avoid contact with these substances when sterilising syringes and skin before vaccination.

Contra-indications, warnings, etc
Contra-indications: **Never give to pregnant women, or to women of child-bearing age not fully aware of the need to avoid pregnancy for three months after vaccination,** since the vaccine virus may have an effect on the foetus.

Do not use in the presence of acute febrile illness, or in states of altered immunity including those which may accompany conditions such as leukaemia, lymphoma or generalised malignancy, or treatment with corticosteroids, cytotoxic drugs or irradiation. Do not give to those known to be hypersensitive to rabbit protein or fur or neomycin. Facilities should be available to treat rare cases of anaphylaxis should they occur.

Cautions: While there is no evidence to indicate that the vaccine virus is transmissible to susceptible contacts, the theoretical possibility remains.

The possibility of interference from passive antibodies following administration of gamma globulin or anti-D immunoglobulin or blood transfusion should be borne in mind. Serum antibodies may be checked after three months.

It is not usually recommended that live vaccines be given within three weeks of each other.

Adverse reactions: Mild rash, slight temperature elevation and slight enlargement of the posterior cervical glands have been reported. Arthralgia, and less commonly arthritis, have occurred even more rarely and almost exclusively in adult women. These reactions have been mild and transient. Rare cases of myeloradiculoneuritis have been reported with rubella vaccines.

Overdosage: Not a problem.

Pharmaceutical precautions Protect from light. Reconstitute only with the diluent supplied. The colour of reconstituted vaccine may vary from light orange to light red. Although the vaccine should be used promptly after reconstitution, it may when necessary be kept at a temperature between 2°C and 8°C for not longer than one hour before being used. Cendevax rubella vaccine should be stored between 2°C and 8°C and should not be frozen (lower temperatures will not harm the vaccine but may damage the diluent ampoule or vial).

Legal category POM.

Package quantities Monodose vials and 10-dose vials, each with a separate ampoule or vial containing 0.5 ml or 7 ml sterile diluent respectively.

Further information Because of possible interference from persisting maternal antibodies, there is little value in giving the vaccine to infants under one year of age.

While there is no evidence that vaccination during the incubation period of natural rubella will prevent the disease, there is no contra-indication to the use of the vaccine in these circumstances.

Product licence number 0002/5004.

DEXEDRINE* TABLETS

Presentation Half-scored, yellow tablets, marked SK&F, each containing 5 mg dexamphetamine sulphate.

Uses Dexedrine is a sympathomimetic amine with central stimulant and anorectic activity.

It is indicated in narcolepsy. It is also indicated for children with refractory hyperkinetic states under the supervision of a physician specialising in child psychiatry.

Dosage and administration *Adults:* In narcolepsy, the usual starting dosage is 10 mg Dexedrine a day, given in divided doses. Dosage may be increased if necessary by 10 mg a day at weekly intervals to a suggested maximum of 60 mg a day.

Elderly: Start with 5 mg a day, and increase by increments of 5 mg at weekly intervals.

Children: In hyperkinetic states, the usual starting dosage for children aged 3–5 years is 2.5 mg a day, increased if necessary by 2.5 mg at weekly intervals; for children aged 6 years and over, the usual starting dosage is 5–10 mg a day, increasing if necessary by 5 mg at weekly intervals. The usual upper limit is 20 mg a day, though some older children have needed 40 mg or more for optimal response.

Contra-indications, warnings, etc

Contra-indications: Do not use in patients known to be intolerant of sympathomimetic amines, during, or for 14 days after, treatment with an MAO inhibitor, in those with a history of drug abuse, with symptomatic cardiovascular disease and/or moderate or severe hypertensive disease, or in those suffering from hyperthyroidism or hyperexcitability.

Cautions: Use with caution in patients on guanethidine, since the action of this drug may be antagonised by Dexedrine; and in patients with glaucoma.

Height and weight should be carefully monitored in children as growth retardation may occur.

In common with other drugs acting on the CNS, Dexedrine may affect ability to drive or operate machinery.

Use in pregnancy: Dexamphetamine has been thought to produce embryotoxic effects in rodents, and retrospective evidence of uncertain significance in man has suggested a similar possibility. Dexedrine should therefore be avoided in pregnancy, especially during the first trimester.

Adverse reactions: Insomnia (especially with dosage later in the day), restlessness, irritability, euphoria, tremor, dizziness, headache and other symptoms of overstimulation have been reported. Also dry mouth, unwanted anorexia and other gastro-intestinal symptoms, sweating, and cardiovascular effects such as tachycardia, palpitation and minor increases in blood pressure.

Drug dependence, with consumption of increasing doses to levels many times those recommended, may occur as tolerance develops. At such levels, a psychosis, which may be clinically indistinguishable from schizophrenia, can occur. Treatment should be stopped gradually since abrupt cessation may produce extreme fatigue and mental depression.

Overdosage: Symptoms of overdosage include excitement, hallucinations, convulsions leading to coma; tachycardia and cardiac arrhythmias; and respiratory depression. Treatment consists of the induction of vomiting and/or gastric lavage, together with supportive and symptomatic measures. Excessive stimulation or convulsions may be treated with diazepam. Excretion of dexamphetamine may be increased by forced acid diuresis.

Pharmaceutical precautions No special storage precautions are required.

Legal category CD (Sch 2), POM.

Package quantities Containers of 100 tablets.

Further information Nil.

Product licence number 0002/5008R.

DIBENYLINE* CAPSULES

Presentation Opaque white capsules with clear ruby-red caps, double-marked SKF, each containing 10 mg phenoxybenzamine hydrochloride as a white powder.

Uses Dibenyline is a non-competitive long-acting α-adrenergic receptor antagonist.

It is indicated in the short-term management of severe hypertensive episodes associated with phaeochromocytoma. Dibenyline should only be used after careful consideration of the likely benefit of treatment compared with the mutagenic and carcinogenic risk (see *Cautions* below).

Dosage and administration *Adults:* The usual starting dose is 10 mg daily. This may be increased by 10 mg daily until control of hypertensive episodes is achieved, or postural hypotension occurs. Usually the dosage required is 1 to 2 mg/kg body weight daily in two doses. Concomitant β-adrenergic blockade may be necessary to control tachycardia and arrhythmias notably when tumours are secreting an appreciable amount of adrenaline as well as noradrenaline.

Elderly: Use with caution: 10 mg a day should be sufficient (see *Contra-indications* and *Cautions* below).

Children: There is little experience in children, but doses of 1 to 2 mg/kg daily have been used successfully.

Contra-indications, warnings, etc

Contra-indications: Do not use in patients who have had a cerebrovascular accident; or in the recovery period (usually 3 to 4 weeks) after acute myocardial infarction.

Cautions: Use with great caution in patients in whom a fall in blood pressure and/or tachycardia may be undesirable, such as the elderly or those with severe heart disease, congestive heart failure, cerebrovascular disease or renal damage. The mode of action should be borne in mind if used concurrently with α-sympathomimetics or myocardial depressants.

Phenoxybenzamine is carcinogenic in the rat and has shown mutagenic activity in the bacterial Ames test and the mouse lymphoma assay. It should, therefore, be used only after very careful consideration of the risks, in patients in whom alternative treatment is inappropriate.

Use in pregnancy: There is little evidence as to the safety of Dibenyline in pregnancy and it should not be used in pregnancy unless essential.

Adverse reactions: Side-effects are generally mild and transient, but may include postural hypotension with dizziness and compensatory tachycardia, nasal congestion, inhibition of ejaculation, miosis and lassitude. Gastro-intestinal upset has also been reported.

Overdosage: The main effect of overdosage is profound hypotension, which may last several hours, tachycardia and collapse. Treatment consists of the induction of vomiting and/or gastric lavage together with appropriate symptomatic and supportive measures. Treat hypotension with plasma expanders and the 'head down' position. Noradrenaline is of little value when α-adrenergic receptors are blocked. Adrenaline should not be used since stimulation of β-adrenergic receptors will further decrease blood pressure.

Pharmaceutical precautions Store in a dry place at a temperature not exceeding 30°C.

Legal category POM.

Package quantities Containers of 100 capsules.

Further information Treatment should be started as soon as possible after diagnosis, and time allowed for stabilisation of the condition before invasive investigations or operations are carried out. Operative cover with intravenous phenoxybenzamine may be given. In a few inoperable cases long-term treatment with Dibenyline has been used.

Product licence number 0002/5009.

DYAZIDE* TABLETS

Presentation Peach-coloured, half-scored, circular tablets bearing the mark SKF E93, each containing 50 mg triamterene and 25 mg hydrochlorothiazide.

Uses Dyazide is a potassium-conserving diuretic preparation with antihypertensive activity.

It is recommended for the treatment of mild to moderate hypertension, alone or in combination with other antihypertensive drugs. It is also indicated in the control of oedema in cardiac failure, cirrhosis of the liver or the nephrotic syndrome, and in drug-induced and premenstrual oedema.

Dosage and administration *Adults only: In hypertension:* Initially 1 tablet a day after the morning meal, thereafter adjusted to the patient's needs. If Dyazide is added to already established therapy with another antihypertensive drug, the dosage of the latter should be reduced, and later adjusted if necessary. If another antihypertensive drug is added to Dyazide therapy, the dosage of the latter will not normally be reduced.

In oedema: The usual starting dosage is 1 Dyazide tablet twice a day after meals. The optimal dosage may be 3 tablets a day, 2 after breakfast and 1 after lunch. Maintenance dosage: Once a diuresis has been established, dosage should be reduced. Usually 1 tablet a day, or two tablets on alternate days, will suffice.

A dosage of 4 tablets a day should not be exceeded; at this level adverse reactions such as raised blood urea are more likely.

Elderly: Dosage as above. Dyazide has been widely used and is usually well tolerated in patients over the age of 60 years. The normally occurring reduction in glomerular filtration with age should be borne in mind.

Contra-indications, warnings, etc
Contra-indications: Do not give Dyazide to patients with hyperkalaemia, progressive renal failure, or known hypersensitivity to either constituent of the product. Potassium supplements, or other potassium-conserving drugs, including ACE inhibitors, should not be given routinely with Dyazide.

Cautions: Use Dyazide with caution in patients with hepatic or renal insufficiency; in those predisposed to gout since both components can elevate uric acid levels; and in diabetic patients since thiazide diuretics can provoke hyperglycaemia and glycosuria.

It is advisable to monitor blood urea and serum potassium levels periodically. This is important in the elderly, those with renal impairment and those receiving concomitant treatment with indomethacin (see *Adverse reactions*).

Thiazides reduce excretion of lithium and may thus precipitate intoxication.

Use in pregnancy and lactation: Dyazide has been in clinical use for a number of years, and there is no experimental or clinical evidence to suggest associated foetal abnormalities. Nevertheless, thiazides have been shown to pass through the placenta and also into breast milk. In rare instances, thrombocytopenia, pancreatitis or hypoglycaemia have been reported in newborn infants of mothers treated with thiazides. The use of Dyazide in pregnant or nursing mothers should therefore be avoided unless essential.

Adverse reactions: Nausea, vomiting, diarrhoea, muscle cramps, weakness, dizziness, headache, dry mouth and rash have been reported. Photosensitivity is rare.

Minor serum electrolyte changes have been observed infrequently, and marked fluctuations in serum potassium levels are uncommon. Metabolic acidosis occasionally occurs. Electrolyte imbalance may also indicate excessive dosage or be secondary to the condition under treatment.

In common with most diuretics, Dyazide may reduce glomerular filtration rate and cause a temporary increase in blood urea levels; again this may also indicate excessive dosage or be secondary to the condition under treatment.

Renal failure, reversible on stopping treatment, has been reported very rarely and has been due to acute interstitial nephritis or an interaction between triamterene and indomethacin.

Rare cases of thrombocytopenic purpura and megaloblastic anaemia have been reported with triamterene; thiazides alone have caused jaundice, acute pancreatitis and, rarely, blood dyscrasias including agranulocytosis, thrombocytopenia and leucopenia.

Overdosage: Symptoms of electrolyte imbalance, hypotension, gastro-intestinal disturbance and muscular weakness may occur. Treatment consists of the induction of vomiting and/or gastric lavage, correction of fluid depletion and electrolyte imbalance, and symptomatic and supportive therapy. If hypotension persists after adequate fluid replacement, dopamine may be used.

Pharmaceutical precautions No special storage precautions are required.

Legal category POM.

Package quantities Containers of 100 and 500 tablets.

Further information Triamterene may cause a blue fluorescence of the urine under certain light conditions.

Long-term use has confirmed that little change occurs in serum potassium and sodium levels in most patients.

Product licence number 0002/0050.

DYTAC* CAPSULES

Presentation Opaque, maroon-coloured capsules, double-marked SKF, each containing 50 mg triamterene as a yellow, granular powder.

Uses Triamterene is a potassium-conserving diuretic, thought to act by directly inhibiting the exchange of sodium for potassium and hydrogen in the distal renal tubule.

Dytac is recommended for the control of oedema in cardiac failure, cirrhosis of the liver or the nephrotic syndrome, and in drug-induced and premenstrual oedema. When Dytac is used as an adjuvant to potassium-depleting diuretics, such loss may be inhibited and diuresis enhanced.

Dosage and administration *Adults only:* When given

alone, the usual dosage range is from 3 to a maximum of 5 Dytac capsules a day. The optimal daily dosage is 4 capsules, given in divided doses after breakfast and lunch. After the first week, treatment should preferably be given on alternate days to ensure satisfactory maintenance diuresis without an increase in blood urea levels. When given with another diuretic, lower dosages of both should be used initially.

Elderly: Dosage as above. The normally occurring reduction in glomerular filtration with age should be borne in mind.

Contra-indications, warnings, etc
Contra-indications: Do not give Dytac to patients with hyperkalaemia, progressive renal failure, or known hypersensitivity to the drug. Potassium supplements, or other potassium-conserving drugs, including ACE inhibitors, should not be given routinely with Dytac.

Cautions: Use Dytac with caution in patients with hepatic or renal insufficiency; in those predisposed to gout since Dytac has been shown in rare instances to elevate uric acid levels; and with hypotensive agents since an additive effect may result.

It is advisable to monitor blood urea and serum potassium levels periodically. This is important in the elderly, those with renal impairment and those receiving concomitant treatment with indomethacin (see *Adverse reactions*).

Use in pregnancy: Dytac has been available since 1962, and there is no experimental or clinical evidence to suggest any associated hazard to the foetus. Nevertheless, drugs should be avoided in pregnancy unless essential, especially during the first trimester.

Adverse reactions: Nausea, vomiting, diarrhoea, weakness, headache, dry mouth, minor decreases in blood pressure, and rash have been reported. Photosensitivity is very rare.

Hyperkalaemia and/or hyponatraemia have been observed in some patients, and hypokalaemia has been described rarely in cirrhotic patients. Metabolic acidosis occasionally occurs. Electrolyte imbalance may also indicate excessive dosage or be secondary to the condition under treatment.

In common with most diuretics, Dytac may reduce glomerular filtration rate and cause a temporary increase in blood urea levels; again this may also indicate excessive dosage or be secondary to the condition under treatment.

Renal failure, reversible on stopping treatment, has been reported very rarely and has been due to acute interstitial nephritis or an interaction between triamterene and indomethacin.

Rare cases of thrombocytopenic purpura and megaloblastic anaemia have been reported.

Overdosage: Symptoms of electrolyte imbalance, especially hyperkalaemia are likely. Gastro-intestinal disturbances, muscular weakness and possibly hypotension may occur. Treatment consists of the induction of vomiting and/or gastric lavage, correction of electrolyte imbalance and fluid depletion, and symptomatic and supportive measures.

Pharmaceutical precautions Store in a dry place.

Legal category POM.

Package quantities Containers of 30 and 250 capsules.

Further information Triamterene may cause a blue fluorescence of the urine under certain light conditions.

Product licence number 0002/5014.

DYTIDE* CAPSULES
Presentation Clear, colourless capsules with opaque, maroon caps, double-marked SKF, each containing 50 mg triamterene and 25 mg benzthiazide as a yellow, granular powder.

Uses Dytide is a potassium-conserving diuretic preparation for the control of oedema in cardiac failure, cirrhosis of the liver or the nephrotic syndrome, and in drug-induced and premenstrual oedema.

Dosage and administration *Adults only:* The optimal dosage is 3 Dytide capsules a day, 2 being taken after breakfast and 1 after lunch. After the first week, treatment should preferably be given on alternate days, to ensure satisfactory maintenance diuresis without an increase in blood urea levels. Maintenance dosage may be reduced to 1 or 2 capsules every other day, taken after breakfast or after breakfast and lunch.

Elderly: Dosage as above. The normally occurring reduction in glomerular filtration with age should be borne in mind.

Contra-indications, warnings, etc
Contra-indications: Do not give Dytide to patients with hyperkalaemia, progressive renal failure, or known hypersensitivity to either constituent of the product. Potassium supplements, or other potassium-conserving drugs, including ACE inhibitors, should not be given routinely with Dytide.

Cautions: Use Dytide with caution in patients with hepatic or renal insufficiency; in those predisposed to gout since both components can elevate uric acid levels; with hypotensive agents, since an additive effect may result; and in diabetic patients since thiazides can provoke hyperglycaemia and glycosuria.

It is advisable to monitor blood urea and serum potassium levels periodically. This is important in the elderly, those with renal impairment and those receiving concomitant treatment with indomethacin (see *Adverse reactions*).

Thiazides reduce excretion of lithium and may thus precipitate intoxication.

Use in pregnancy and lactation: Dytide has been available since 1963, and there is no experimental or clinical evidence to suggest associated foetal abnormalities. Nevertheless, thiazides have been shown to pass through the placenta and also into breast milk. In rare instances, thrombocytopenia, pancreatitis or hypoglycaemia have been reported in newborn infants of mothers treated with thiazides. The use of Dytide in pregnant or nursing mothers should therefore be avoided unless essential.

Adverse reactions: Nausea, vomiting, diarrhoea, muscle cramps, weakness, dizziness, headache, dry mouth, decreases in blood pressure, and rash have been reported. Photosensitivity is rare.

Minor serum electrolyte changes have been observed infrequently, and marked fluctuations in serum potassium levels are uncommon. Metabolic acidosis occasionally occurs. Electrolyte imbalance may also indicate excessive dosage or be secondary to the condition under treatment.

In common with most diuretics, Dytide may reduce glomerular filtration rate and cause a temporary increase in blood urea levels; again this may also indicate excessive dosage or be secondary to the condition under treatment.

Renal failure, reversible on stopping treatment, has been reported very rarely and has been due to acute interstitial nephritis or an interaction between triamterene and indomethacin.

Rare cases of thrombocytopenic purpura and megaloblastic anaemia have been reported with triamterene; thiazides alone have caused jaundice, acute pancreatitis and, rarely, blood dyscrasias including agranulocytosis, thrombocytopenia and leucopenia.

Overdosage: Symptoms of electrolyte imbalance, hypotension, gastro-intestinal disturbance and muscular weakness may occur. Treatment consists of the induction of vomiting and/or gastric lavage, correction of fluid depletion and electrolyte imbalance and symptomatic and supportive therapy. If hypotension persists after adequate fluid replacement, dopamine may be used.

Pharmaceutical precautions Store in a dry place.

Legal category POM.

Package quantities Containers of 30 and 250 capsules.

Further information Triamterene may cause a blue fluorescence of the urine under certain light conditions.

Product licence number 0002/5015.

ERVEVAX* ▼
Rubella vaccine, live BP
(RA27/3 strain)

Presentation Ervevax rubella vaccine is a live attenuated vaccine prepared in human diploid cells. It is presented as a pink pellet in a glass vial; clear, colourless sterile diluent is provided in a separate container. Each 0.5 ml dose of the reconstituted vaccine contains not less than 1,000 $TCID_{50}$ of the RA27/3 live attenuated strain of rubella virus with not more than 25 µg (17 i.u.) neomycin sulphate.

Uses Routine immunisation of pre-pubertal girls against rubella. Also indicated in seronegative women of child-bearing age *who are not pregnant* and in whom the possibility of pregnancy can be excluded for at least three months following vaccination, including post-partum mothers, and for immunisation of children and adults to prevent transmission of rubella to the at-risk pregnant woman.

Dosage and administration
Adults and children: 0.5 ml of the reconstituted vaccine administered by the subcutaneous route only.

The vaccine should be reconstituted using only the sterile diluent supplied. The whole of the sterile diluent should be transferred into the vial containing the vaccine, keeping the latter upright. The vaccine pellet should be completely dissolved by shaking. The syringe should be dry sterilised; the vaccine is readily inactivated by alcohol and other chemical disinfectants and antiseptics, and care is needed to avoid contact with these substances when sterilising skin before vaccination.

Contra-indications, warnings, etc
Contra-indications: **Never give to pregnant women, or to women of child-bearing age not fully aware of the need to avoid pregnancy for three months after vaccination,** since theoretically the vaccine virus could have an effect on the foetus.

Do not use in the presence of acute febrile illness, or in states of altered immunity including those which may accompany conditions such as leukaemia, lymphoma or generalised malignancy or treatment with corticosteroids, cytotoxic drugs or irradiation. Do not give to those with known systemic hypersensitivity to this vaccine or to neomycin. Although anaphylactic reactions are rare, facilities for management should always be available.

Cautions: Transmission of vaccine virus to susceptible contacts, while accepted as a theoretical possibility, has not been regarded as a significant risk.

The possibility of interference from passive antibodies following administration of gamma globulin or anti-D immunoglobulin or blood transfusion should be borne in mind. Serum antibodies may be checked three months after injection.

It is not usually recommended that live vaccines be given within three weeks of each other. Ervevax can however be given at the same time as oral polio vaccine.

Adverse reactions: Mild rash, temperature elevation and slight enlargement of the posterior cervical glands, transient arthralgia and arthritis with or without joint effusion, and extremely rarely transient polyneuropathy have been reported. Such effects are more common and tend to be more marked in adults than in children. Symptoms, when they do occur, usually begin 1 to 3 weeks following vaccination and are normally transient.

Overdosage: Not a problem.

Pharmaceutical precautions Protect from light. The vaccine should be stored between 2°C and 8°C (lower temperatures will not harm the vaccine, but may damage the diluent container). At room temperature (20–25°C) the unreconstituted vaccine is stable for up to 10 weeks.

Reconstitute only with the diluent supplied. The reconstituted vaccine should be used immediately, and certainly within one hour. The reconstituted vaccine may vary in colour from light orange to light red.

Legal category POM.

Package quantities Monodose vials, each with a separate ampoule of sterile diluent, or 10-dose vials, each with a separate vial of sterile diluent.

Further information Latest data indicate that satisfactory antibody titres have persisted for up to 16 years so far.

Because of possible interference from persisting maternal antibodies, there is little value in giving the vaccine to infants under one year of age.

Product licence number 0002/0125.

ESKAMEL* CREAM

Presentation A smooth, brown, non-greasy cream, which dries rapidly to a flesh colour when applied to the skin. It contains 2% w/w resorcinol and 8% w/w precipitated sulphur.

Uses Eskamel has mild antiseptic, keratolytic and exfoliative properties, and is indicated in the treatment of acne.

Dosage and administration *Adults and children:* Wash the affected areas with soap and water, and dry carefully. Apply Eskamel thinly to the skin with the fingers but do not rub in. Once a day is usually enough, but if the patient has a very oily skin, the cream may be applied more often. Eskamel may be used under make-up to mask the spots and lesions of acne.

Contra-indications, warnings, etc
Contra-indications: Do not use in patients who are sensitive to sulphur or resorcinol, or in the presence of acute local infection.

Cautions: Use with care on acutely inflamed areas or near the eyes and mouth.

Adverse reactions: Moderate erythema and scaling are the expected effects of Eskamel. If these are excessive or if inflammation occurs, stop treatment until the reaction has subsided, and then apply Eskamel less often.

Overdosage: If ingestion occurs, mild gastro-intestinal disturbance might occur. Treatment consists of rinsing out the mouth together with symptomatic measures if required.

Pharmaceutical precautions Store at a temperature not exceeding 30°C. Keep in the original specially lined tubes to prevent evaporation.

Legal category P.

Package quantities Tubes containing 25 g.

Further information Nil.

Product licence number 0002/5000.

ESKORNADE* SPANSULE* CAPSULES
ESKORNADE* SYRUP

Presentation Clear, colourless capsules, grey-capped and filled with a mixture of red, grey and white pellets. Each Spansule sustained-release capsule contains 50 mg phenylpropanolamine hydrochloride and 5 mg diphenylpyraline hydrochloride. Two-thirds of the phenylpropanolamine and diphenylpyraline is formulated for sustained release over a period of six to eight hours.

A pale green syrup, greengage-flavoured, each 5 ml dose containing 12.5 mg phenylpropanolamine hydrochloride and 1.5 mg diphenylpyraline hydrochloride.

Uses Eskornade is a combination of an oral nasal decongestant and an antihistamine (H_1-receptor antagonist).

It is indicated in the relief of congestion and hypersecretion in the nasal cavity and paranasal sinuses, associated with the common cold, allergic rhinitis, acute and chronic rhinitis, sinusitis and influenza.

Dosage and administration The stated dose should not be exceeded. *Adults:* One Eskornade Spansule capsule every 12 hours or two 5 ml doses of Eskornade syrup up to four times a day.

Elderly: Use with great caution (see *Contra-indications* and *Cautions* below).

Eskornade Spansule capsules are not recommended in children under 12 years, and Eskornade syrup is not recommended in children under 2 years.

Children aged 2 to 5 years: One 2.5 ml dose of Eskornade syrup up to four times a day.

Children aged 6 to 12 years: One 5 ml dose up to four times a day.

Contra-indications, warnings, etc
Contra-indications: Do not use in patients with hypertensive disease, including those treated with antihypertensive drugs, whose action may be impaired by phenylpropanolamine, severe heart disease, or hyperthyroidism; or hypersensitivity to either of the ingredients; or during, or for 14 days after, treatment with an MAO inhibitor.

Cautions: Patients who drive or operate machinery should be warned of the possibility of drowsiness. Alcoholic drinks should be avoided. Administer with caution to patients with organic heart disease or angina of effort or with prostatic hypertrophy or glaucoma. Potentiation may occur if this product is used with other CNS depressants.

Use in pregnancy: Eskornade has been available since 1960, and there is no experimental or clinical evidence to suggest any associated hazard to the foetus. Nevertheless, drugs should be avoided in pregnancy unless essential, especially during the first trimester.

Adverse reactions: Blurred vision, dry mouth, urinary hesitancy or retention, palpitations, drowsiness or insomnia, and dizziness may occur.

Overdosage: Signs and symptoms may be related to any of the product's constituents and may include nausea and vomiting, irritability, convulsions, fever, tachycardia, arrhythmias or increased blood pressure. Absorption of phenylpropanolamine and diphenylpyraline from the sustained-release Spansule capsule is likely to be prolonged, and this should be borne in mind. Treatment consists of gastric lavage, together with appropriate supportive and symptomatic measures. Central excitation or convulsions may require treatment with diazepam. Excretion of phenylpropanolamine may be increased by forced acid diuresis.

Pharmaceutical precautions Store Spansule capsules in a dry place at a temperature not exceeding 30°C. If the syrup is refrigerated or stored below about 15°C, cloudiness may occur. However, this readily disappears if the product is stored at normal room temperature. Dilute only with Syrup BP; a 50/50 dilution is stable for one month at temperatures of up to 30°C.

Legal category P.

Package quantities Blister packs of 30 and containers of 250 Spansule capsules. Bottles containing 150 ml syrup.

Further information Nil.

Product licence numbers
Eskornade Spansule capsules   0002/5019
Eskornade syrup   0002/5020

EXPANSYL* SPANSULE* CAPSULES

Presentation Clear, colourless capsules, black-capped and filled with a mixture of blue, lime-green, and white pellets. Each Spansule sustained-release capsule contains 50 mg ephedrine sulphate, 2 mg trifluoperazine present as the hydrochloride and 5 mg diphenylpyraline hydrochloride. Two-thirds of the dose of ephedrine and diphenylpyraline is formulated for sustained release over a period of six to eight hours.

Uses Expansyl combines the properties of an adrenergic bronchodilator, a phenothiazine tranquilliser and an antihistamine (H_1-receptor antagonist) for the relief of episodes of bronchospasm in chronic bronchitis and mild bronchial asthma.

Dosage and administration *Adults only:* 1 Expansyl Spansule capsule night and morning, increasing if necessary to a maximum of 3 capsules a day.

Elderly: Use with great caution (see *Contra-indications* and *Cautions* below).

Contra-indications, warnings, etc
Contra-indications: Do not use in patients with hypertensive disease, severe heart disease, hyperthyroidism or hypersensitivity to any of the ingredients; during, or for 14 days after, treatment with an MAO inhibitor; or in patients with existing blood dyscrasias or known liver damage.

Cautions: Patients who drive or operate machinery should be warned of the possibility of drowsiness. Alcoholic drinks should be avoided. Use with caution in patients with organic heart disease or angina of effort, or with prostatic hypertrophy. Potentiation may occur if this product is used with other CNS depressants.

Nausea and vomiting as a sign of organic disease may be masked by the anti-emetic action of trifluoperazine.

Use in pregnancy: Expansyl has been available since 1961, and there is no experimental or clinical evidence to suggest any associated hazard to the foetus. Nevertheless drugs should be avoided in pregnancy unless essential, especially during the first trimester.

Adverse reactions: Drowsiness, dizziness, restlessness, insomnia, dry mouth, blurred vision, palpitation, and difficulty in micturition may occur.

Extrapyramidal symptoms due to trifluoperazine are very unlikely at the recommended dosage. Extremely rarely, long-term therapy with trifluoperazine in low dosage has been associated with tardive dyskinesia, which can be long-lasting or even irreversible.

Overdosage: Signs and symptoms may be related to any of the product's constituents, but those of ephedrine would usually predominate. They may include nausea and vomiting, irritability, convulsions, fever, tachycardia, arrhythmias, extrapyramidal symptoms and hypotension. Absorption of ephedrine and diphenylpyraline from the sustained-release Spansule capsule is likely to be prolonged and this should be borne in mind. Treatment consists of gastric lavage, together with appropriate supportive and symptomatic measures. Do not induce vomiting. Extrapyramidal symptoms may be treated with an anticholinergic antiparkinsonism drug. Treat hypotension with fluid replacement; if severe or persistent, noradrenaline may be considered. Adrenaline is contra-indicated. Excretion of ephedrine may be increased by forced acid diuresis.

Pharmaceutical precautions Store in a dry place at a temperature not exceeding 30°C and protect from light.

Legal category POM.

Package quantities Containers of 30 and 250 Spansule capsules.

Further information Nil.

Product licence number 0002/5021.

FEFOL* SPANSULE* CAPSULES

Presentation Clear, colourless capsules, transparent green-capped and filled with a mixture of coral-red, pale yellow, and white pellets. Each Spansule sustained-release capsule contains 150 mg dried ferrous sulphate and 500 mcg folic acid. Four-fifths of the iron is specially formulated for sustained release over a period of several hours.

Uses Fefol is a haematinic preparation for prophylaxis of iron and folic-acid deficiency during pregnancy.

Dosage and administration *Adults only:* 1 Fefol Spansule capsule a day throughout pregnancy. Some pregnant patients may need a higher prophylactic dose of iron because of dietary or other factors.

Contra-indications, warnings, etc
Cautions: The folic acid content of one capsule a day is unlikely to mask pernicious anaemia should this condition be present; pregnancy during pernicious anaemia is very rare.

Iron chelates with tetracyclines, and absorption of both agents may be impaired.

Adverse reactions: Nausea and other gastro-intestinal symptoms sometimes encountered during iron therapy are unlikely to occur with Fefol Spansule capsules.

Overdosage: Symptoms of overdosage with iron salts include epigastric pain, nausea and vomiting, haematemesis and circulatory collapse. In severe cases, encephalopathy, acute hepatic necrosis and acute renal failure may develop after a latent period. The sustained-release Spansule capsule presentation of ferrous sulphate may delay excessive absorption of iron and allow more time for the initiation of appropriate counter-measures. Treatment consists of gastric lavage followed by the introduction of 5 g desferrioxamine into the stomach. Serum iron levels should be monitored and in severe cases intravenous desferrioxamine should be given together with supportive and symptomatic measures as required.

Pharmaceutical precautions Store in a dry place at a temperature not exceeding 30°C.

Legal category POM.

Package quantities Pack containing 2 or 144 blister strips each of 14 Spansule capsules. Containers of 250 and 5,000 Spansule capsules.

Further information Fefol Spansule capsules are formulated to release most of the iron in the upper small intestine where absorption is greatest, and not in the stomach where gastric irritation may be caused.

Product licence number 0002/5022.

FEFOL Z* SPANSULE* CAPSULES

Presentation Clear, colourless capsules, transparent dark blue-capped and filled with a mixture of coral-red, pale yellow and white pellets. Each Spansule sustained-release capsule contains 150 mg dried ferrous sulphate (47 mg elemental iron), 61.8 mg zinc sulphate monohydrate (22.5 mg elemental zinc) and 500 mcg folic acid. Four-fifths of the iron is specially formulated for sustained release over several hours. The zinc sulphate is formulated for release over one to two hours.

Uses Fefol Z is an oral iron, zinc and folic acid preparation for the prophylaxis of iron and folic acid deficiency during pregnancy for use when inadequate diet calls for supplementary zinc and when the need for such therapy has been determined by a physician.

Dosage and administration

Adults only: 1 Fofol Z Spansule Capsule a day throughout pregnancy. Some pregnant patients may need a higher prophylactic dose of iron because of dietary or other factors.

Contra-indications, warnings, etc

Cautions: The folic acid content of one capsule a day is unlikely to mask pernicious anaemia should this condition be present; pregnancy during pernicious anaemia is very rare.

Iron and zinc chelate with tetracyclines and absorption of all three agents may be impaired.

The absorption of zinc may be reduced in the presence of iron.

In patients with renal failure, a risk of zinc accumulation could exist.

Adverse reactions: Mild gastro-intestinal upset is occasionally produced by both ferrous sulphate and zinc sulphate but the sustained-release presentation is designed to minimise this effect.

Overdosage: The features of iron overdosage are likely to predominate. Symptoms include epigastric pain, nausea and vomiting, haematemesis and circulatory collapse. In severe cases, encephalopathy, acute hepatic necrosis and acute renal failure may develop after a latent period. Treatment consists of gastric lavage except where signs of the corrosive effect of zinc are present (see below) followed by the introduction of 5 g desferrioxamine into the stomach. Serum iron levels should be monitored and in severe cases intravenous desferrioxamine should be given.

Zinc sulphate in gross overdosage is corrosive. Symptoms are those of gastro-intestinal irritation, leading in severe cases to haemorrhage, corrosion of the mucosa and possible later stricture formation. Gastric lavage or emesis should be avoided. Demulcents such as milk should be given. Chelating agents such as dimercaprol, penicillamine or edetic acid have been recommended.

Symptomatic and supportive therapy should be given. Absorption of both iron and zinc may be slowed by the sustained-release presentation.

Pharmaceutical precautions Store in a dry place at a temperature not exceeding 30°C.

Legal category POM.

Package quantities Containers of 30 Spansule capsules.

Further information Nil.

Product licence number 0002/0100.

FEFOL-VIT* SPANSULE* CAPSULES

Presentation Clear, colourless capsules, opaque white-capped and filled with a mixture of coral-red, orange-yellow, pale yellow, and white pellets. Each Spansule sustained-release capsule contains 150 mg dried ferrous sulphate, 500 mcg folic acid, 2 mg thiamine mononitrate, 2 mg riboflavine, 1 mg pyridoxine hydrochloride, 10 mg nicotinamide and 50 mg ascorbic acid. Four-fifths of the iron is specially formulated for sustained release over a period of several hours.

Uses Fefol-Vit is a haematinic with added vitamins, for prophylaxis of iron and folic-acid deficiency during pregnancy, particularly when inadequate diet calls for supplementary vitamins B and C.

Dosage and administration *Adults only:* 1 Fefol-Vit Spansule capsule a day throughout pregnancy. Some pregnant patients may need a higher prophylactic dose of iron because of dietary or other factors.

Contra-indications, warnings, etc

Cautions: The folic acid content of one capsule a day is unlikely to mask pernicious anaemia should this condition be present; pregnancy during pernicious anaemia is very rare.

Iron chelates with tetracyclines, and absorption of both agents may be impaired.

Adverse reactions: Nausea and other gastro-intestinal symptoms sometimes encountered during iron therapy are unlikely to occur with Fefol-Vit Spansule capsules.

Overdosage: Symptoms of overdosage with iron salts include epigastric pain, nausea and vomiting, haematemesis and circulatory collapse. In severe cases, encephalopathy, acute hepatic necrosis and acute renal failure may develop after a latent period. The sustained-release Spansule capsule presentation of ferrous sulphate may delay excessive absorption of iron and allow more time for the initiation of appropriate counter-measures. Treatment consists of gastric lavage followed by the introduction of 5 g desferrioxamine into the stomach. Serum iron levels should be monitored and in severe cases intravenous desferrioxamine should be given together with supportive and symptomatic measures as required.

Pharmaceutical precautions Store in a dry place at a temperature not exceeding 30°C.

Legal category POM.

Package quantities Containers of 30, 250 and 4,000 Spansule capsules.

Further information Fefol-Vit Spansule capsules are formulated to release most of the iron in the upper small intestine where absorption is greatest, and not in the stomach where gastric irritation may be caused.

Product licence number 0002/0049.

FENBID* SPANSULE* CAPSULES

Presentation Opaque maroon capsules, opaque pink-capped, containing off-white pellets. Each capsule contains 300 mg ibuprofen in a sustained release formulation which provides a prolonged therapeutic effect.

Uses Ibuprofen is a non-steroidal anti-inflammatory agent with analgesic and antipyretic properties. Fenbid is indicated for the treatment of rheumatoid arthritis, osteoarthritis, ankylosing spondylitis and other sero-negative (non-rheumatoid) arthropathies. It is also indicated in acute periarticular disorders such as bursitis, capsulitis of the shoulder, tendinitis, tenosynovitis and for the relief of mild to moderate pain in sprains, strains, low back pain, dysmenorrhoea, dental and post-operative pain.

Dosage and administration

Adults and children over 12 years: Usual starting dose is two capsules (600 mg) twice daily, taken night and morning. This may be increased to three capsules

(900 mg) twice daily until the acute phase is controlled. Maintenance dose: One or two capsules twice daily.

Elderly: Dosage as above.

Patients should be instructed not to chew or suck the capsules as this destroys the sustained release properties. Providing this is ensured, the contents of a capsule may be sprinkled onto a spoonful of soft food, yoghurt, or similar substance, for patients who experience difficulty in swallowing the capsules.

The evening dose of Fenbid Spansule capsules will maintain a prolonged therapeutic effect throughout the night and help to prevent morning stiffness.

Contra-indications, warnings, etc
Contra-indication: Active peptic ulceration.

Cautions: Fenbid may be used, with caution, in patients with gastro-intestinal disease, but may be tolerated by patients with intolerance to other anti-rheumatic drugs. The possibility of cross-sensitivity with aspirin and other non-steroidal anti-inflammatory agents should be borne in mind.

Bronchospasm may be precipitated in patients suffering from, or with a history of, bronchial asthma or allergic disease.

If given to patients receiving anticoagulant therapy, prothrombin time should be monitored daily for the first few days of combined treatment.

Use in pregnancy and lactation: As with other non-steroidal anti-inflammatory agents, Fenbid Spansule capsules should be avoided during pregnancy and lactation unless essential. Traces of ibuprofen have been detected in breast milk, but no adverse effects have been reported.

Adverse reactions: Generally well-tolerated with a low incidence of side-effects. Adverse effects may include gastro-intestinal upsets, rashes, headache, nervousness, tinnitus and oedema. Gastro-intestinal haemorrhage may rarely occur. Blurred vision, toxic amblyopia, thrombocytopenia and oliguric renal failure have been reported during ibuprofen treatment, but were resolved on cessation of treatment.

Overdosage: The following signs and symptoms have been reported: headache, vomiting, drowsiness, loss of consciousness and hypotension. Symptomatic treatment is recommended, directed at maintaining normal blood pressure and correcting any electrolyte imbalance, particularly potassium. In children, emesis, and in adults, gastric lavage, may need to be considered, but only after careful assessment of the patient's condition, in particular the level of consciousness.

Pharmaceutical precautions Store in a dry place at a temperature not exceeding 30°C and protect from light.

Legal category POM.

Package quantities Containers of 120 Spansule capsules.

Further information Nil.

Product licence number 0002/0111.

FEOSPAN* SPANSULE* CAPSULES

Presentation Clear, colourless capsules, ruby-red-capped and filled with a mixture of green and coral-red pellets. Each Spansule sustained-release capsule contains 150 mg dried ferrous sulphate. Four-fifths of the iron is specially formulated for sustained release over a period of several hours.

Uses Feospan is a haematinic for the prevention and treatment of iron deficiency.

Dosage and administration *Adults:* 1 Feospan Spansule capsule a day. In more severe cases, 2 capsules a day may be required.

Elderly: Dosage as above.

Children aged over 1 year: 1 capsule a day. The capsule may be opened and the pellets mixed with soft, cool food, but they must not be chewed.

Contra-indications, warnings, etc
Caution: Iron chelates with tetracyclines, and absorption of both agents may be impaired.

Adverse reactions: Nausea and other gastro-intestinal symptoms sometimes encountered during iron therapy are unlikely to occur with Feospan Spansule capsules.

Overdosage: Symptoms of overdosage with iron salts include epigastric pain, nausea and vomiting, haematemesis and circulatory collapse. In severe cases, encephalopathy, acute hepatic necrosis and acute renal failure may develop after a latent period. The sustained-release Spansule capsule presentation of ferrous sulphate may delay excessive absorption of iron and allow more time for the initiation of appropriate counter-measures. Treatment consists of gastric lavage followed by the introduction of 5 g desferrioxamine into the stomach. Serum iron levels should be monitored and in severe cases intravenous desferrioxamine should be given together with supportive and symptomatic measures as required.

Pharmaceutical precautions Store in a dry place at a temperature not exceeding 30°C.

Legal category P.

Package quantities Containers of 30, 250 and 5,000 Spansule capsules.

Further information Feospan Spansule capsules are formulated to release most of the iron in the upper small intestine where absorption is greatest, and not in the stomach where gastric irritation may be caused.

Product licence number 0002/5023.

FEOSPAN Z* SPANSULE* CAPSULES

Presentation Clear, colourless capsules, transparent pink-capped and filled with a mixture of coral-red, green and white pellets. Each Spansule sustained-release capsule contains 150 mg dried ferrous sulphate (47 mg elemental iron) and 61.8 mg zinc sulphate monohydrate (22.5 mg elemental zinc). Four-fifths of the iron is specially formulated for sustained release over several hours. The zinc sulphate is formulated for release over one to two hours.

Uses Feospan Z is an oral iron and zinc preparation for the prevention of iron deficiency for use when inadequate diet calls for supplementary zinc and when the need for such therapy has been determined by a physician.

Dosage and administration
Adults: 1 Feospan Z Spansule capsule a day. In more severe cases, 2 capsules a day may be required.

Elderly: Dosage as above.

Children aged over 1 year: 1 capsule a day. The capsule

may be opened and the pellets mixed with soft cool food, but they must not be chewed.

Contra-indications, warnings, etc

Cautions: Iron and zinc chelate with tetracyclines, and absorption of all three agents may be impaired.

The absorption of zinc may be reduced in the presence of iron.

In patients with renal failure, a risk of zinc accumulation could exist.

Adverse reactions: Mild gastro-intestinal upset is occasionally produced by both ferrous sulphate and zinc sulphate but the sustained-release presentation is designed to minimise this effect.

Overdosage: The features of iron overdosage are likely to predominate. Symptoms include epigastric pain, nausea and vomiting, haematemesis and circulatory collapse. In severe cases, encephalopathy, acute hepatic necrosis and acute renal failure may develop after a latent period. Treatment consists of gastric lavage except where signs of the corrosive effect of zinc are present (see below) followed by the introduction of 5 g desferrioxamine into the stomach. Serum iron levels should be monitored and in severe cases intravenous desferrioxamine should be given.

Zinc sulphate in gross overdosage is corrosive. Symptoms are those of gastro-intestinal irritation, leading in severe cases to haemorrhage, corrosion of the mucosa and possible later stricture formation. Gastric lavage or emesis should be avoided. Demulcents such as milk should be given. Chelating agents such as dimercaprol, penicillamine or edetic acid have been recommended.

Symptomatic and supportive therapy should be given. Absorption of both iron and zinc may be slowed by the sustained-release presentation.

Pharmaceutical precautions Store in a dry place at a temperature not exceeding 30°C.

Legal category P.

Package quantities Containers of 30 Spansule capsules.

Further information Nil.

Product licence number 0002/0099.

FESOVIT* SPANSULE* CAPSULES

Presentation Clear, colourless capsules, opaque yellow-capped and filled with a mixture of coral-red, orange-yellow, and white pellets. Each Spansule sustained-release capsule contains 150 mg dried ferrous sulphate, 2 mg thiamine mononitrate, 2 mg riboflavine, 1 mg pyridoxine hydrochloride, 10 mg nicotinamide and 50 mg ascorbic acid. Four-fifths of the iron is specially formulated for sustained release over a period of several hours.

Uses Fesovit is a haematinic with added vitamins, for the prevention and treatment of iron deficiency, particularly in the elderly patient where inadequate diet calls for supplementary vitamins B and C.

Dosage and administration *Adults:* 1 Fesovit Spansule capsule a day. In more severe cases, 2 capsules a day may be required.

Elderly: Dosage as above.

Children aged over 1 year: 1 Fesovit Spansule capsule a

day. The capsule may be opened and the pellets mixed with soft, cool food, but they must not be chewed.

Contra-indications, warnings, etc

Caution: Iron chelates with tetracyclines, and absorption of both agents may be impaired.

Adverse reactions: Nausea and other gastro-intestinal symptoms sometimes encountered during iron therapy are unlikely to occur with Fesovit Spansule capsules.

Overdosage: Symptoms of overdosage with iron salts include epigastric pain, nausea and vomiting, haematemesis and circulatory collapse. In severe cases, encephalopathy, acute hepatic necrosis and acute renal failure may develop after a latent period. The sustained-release Spansule capsule presentation of ferrous sulphate may delay excessive absorption of iron and allow more time for the initiation of appropriate counter-measures. Treatment consists of gastric lavage followed by the introduction of 5 g desferrioxamine into the stomach. Serum iron levels should be monitored and in severe cases intravenous desferrioxamine should be given together with supportive and symptomatic measures as required.

Pharmaceutical precautions Store in a dry place at a temperature not exceeding 30°C and protect from light.

Legal category P.

Package quantities Blister packs of 30 and containers of 250 and 5,000 Spansule capsules.

Further information Fesovit Spansule capsules are formulated to release most of the iron in the upper small intestine where absorption is greatest, and not in the stomach where gastric irritation may be caused.

Product licence number 0002/0029.

FESOVIT Z* SPANSULE* CAPSULES

Presentation Clear, colourless capsules, transparent orange-capped and filled with a mixture of coral-red, orange-yellow and white pellets. Each Spansule sustained-release capsule contains 150 mg dried ferrous sulphate (47 mg elemental iron), 61.8 mg zinc sulphate monohydrate (22.5 mg elemental zinc), 2 mg thiamine mononitrate, 2 mg riboflavine, 1 mg pyridoxine hydrochloride, 10 mg nicotinamide, and 50 mg ascorbic acid. Four-fifths of the iron is specially formulated for sustained release over several hours. The zinc sulphate is formulated for release over one to two hours.

Uses Fesovit Z is an oral iron and zinc preparation, with added vitamins, for the prevention of iron deficiency for use when inadequate diet calls for supplementary zinc and vitamins B and C and when the need for such therapy has been determined by a physician.

Dosage and administration

Adults: 1 Fesovit Z Spansule capsule a day. In more severe cases, 2 capsules a day may be required.

Elderly: Dosage as above.

Children aged over 1 year: 1 capsule a day. The capsule may be opened and the pellets mixed with soft, cool food, but they must not be chewed.

Contra-indications, warnings, etc

Cautions: Iron and zinc chelate with tetracyclines and absorption of all three agents may be impaired.

The absorption of zinc may be reduced in the presence of iron.

In patients with renal failure, a risk of zinc accumulation could exist.

Adverse reactions: Mild gastro-intestinal upset is occasionally produced by both ferrous sulphate and zinc sulphate but the sustained-release presentation is designed to minimise this effect.

Overdosage: The features of iron overdosage are likely to predominate. Symptoms include epigastric pain, nausea and vomiting, haematemesis and circulatory collapse. In severe cases, encephalopathy, acute hepatic necrosis and acute renal failure may develop after a latent period. Treatment consists of gastric lavage except where signs of the corrosive effect of zinc are present (see below) followed by the introduction of 5 g desferrioxamine into the stomach. Serum iron levels should be monitored and in severe cases intravenous desferrioxamine should be given.

Zinc sulphate in gross overdosage is corrosive. Symptoms are those of gastro-intestinal irritation, leading in severe cases to haemorrhage, corrosion of the mucosa and possible later stricture formation. Gastric lavage or emesis should be avoided. Demulcents such as milk should be given. Chelating agents such as dimercaprol, penicillamine or edetic acid have been recommended.

Symptomatic and supportive therapy should be given. Absorption of both iron and zinc may be slowed by the sustained-release presentation.

Pharmaceutical precautions Store in a dry place at a temperature not exceeding 30°C.

Legal category P.

Package quantities Containers of 30 Spansule capsules.

Further information Nil.

Product licence number 0002/0101.

HISTRYL* SPANSULE* CAPSULES
HISTRYL* PAEDIATRIC SPANSULE* CAPSULES

Presentation Clear, colourless capsules, opaque pink-capped and filled with a mixture of white and two shades of pink pellets in two strengths. Each Spansule sustained-release capsule, size No. 2, contains 5 mg diphenylpyraline hydrochloride, and each paediatric Spansule capsule, size No. 4, contains 2.5 mg diphenylpyraline hydrochloride. Two-thirds of the dose of diphenylpyraline is specially formulated for sustained release over a period of six to eight hours.

Uses Histryl is an antihistamine (H_1-receptor antagonist) for relief of allergic and vasomotor rhinitis, urticaria, angioneurotic oedema, allergic eczema, insect bites and stings, food and drug allergy, and the urticarial and oedematous lesions of serum sickness.

Dosage and administration *Adults:* 1 or 2 Histryl Spansule capsules (5 mg) night and morning. The higher dosages should be reserved for more severe conditions.

Elderly: Start with the lower dosage.

Children aged 7 years and over: 1 Histryl paediatric spansule capsule (2.5 mg) twice a day.

Contra-indications, warnings, etc

Contra-indications: Do not use in patients hypersensitive to the active ingredient.

Cautions: Patients who drive or operate machinery should be warned of the possibility of drowsiness. Alcoholic drinks should be avoided. Potentiation may occur if this product is used with other CNS depressants.

Use in pregnancy: Histryl has been available since 1957, and there is no experimental or clinical evidence to suggest any associated hazard to the foetus. Nevertheless, drugs should be avoided in pregnancy unless essential, especially during the first trimester.

Adverse reactions: Drowsiness, dryness of the mucous membranes, dizziness and blurred vision may occasionally occur.

Overdosage: Symptoms of overdosage may include nausea and vomiting, and effects of CNS excitation and/or depression including coma. Absorption of diphenylpyraline from the sustained-release Spansule capsule is likely to be prolonged and this should be borne in mind. Treatment consists of the induction of vomiting and/or gastric lavage together with symptomatic and supportive measures.

Pharmaceutical precautions Store in a dry place at a temperature not exceeding 25°C.

Legal category P.

Package quantities Both strengths in containers of 30 and 250 Spansule capsules.

Further information Nil.

Product licence numbers
Histryl Spansule capsules	0002/5031
Histryl paediatric Spansule capsules	0002/5032

LISKONUM* TABLETS

Presentation White, oblong, film-coated tablets, with convex faces and a breakline on both sides, each containing 450 mg lithium carbonate (12.2 mmol Li^+) in controlled-release form.

Uses Liskonum is a controlled-release tablet, designed to reduce fluctuations in serum lithium levels and the likelihood of adverse reactions.

It is indicated for the treatment of acute episodes of mania or hypomania and for the prophylaxis of recurrent manic-depressive illness.

Dosage and administration *Adults only:* Liskonum should be given twice a day.

Treatment of acute mania or hypomania: Patients should be started on one or one and a half tablets twice a day. Dosage should then be adjusted to achieve a serum lithium level of 0.8 to a maximum of 1.5 mmol/l. Serum concentration of lithium should be measured after four to seven days' treatment and then at least once a week until dosage has remained constant for 4 weeks. When the acute symptoms have been controlled, recommendations for prophylaxis should be followed.

Prophylaxis: The usual starting dosage is one tablet twice a day. Dosage should then be adjusted until a serum level of 0.5 to 1.0 mmol/l is maintained. Serum concentration of lithium should be measured after four to seven days' treatment and then every week until dosage has remained constant for four weeks. Frequency of monitoring may then be gradually decreased to a minimum of once every two months but should be increased following any situation where changes in lithium levels are possible (see *Cautions*).

Blood samples for measurement of serum lithium concentration should be taken just before a dose is due and not less than 12 hours after the previous dose.

Levels of more than 2 mmol/l *must* be avoided.

Tablets may be halved but should not be chewed or broken up.

Elderly: Use with caution. Start with half a tablet twice a day and adjust serum levels to the lower end of the above ranges (see also *Cautions*).

The full prophylactic effect of lithium may not be evident for 6 to 12 months, and treatment should be continued through any recurrence of the illness.

Contra-indications, warnings, etc

Contra-indications: Do not use in patients with impaired renal function, cardiac disease, or untreated hypothyroidism. Lithium should not be given to patients with low body sodium levels, including, for example, dehydrated patients, those on low sodium diets, or those with Addison's disease.

Cautions: Vomiting, diarrhoea, intercurrent infection, fluid deprivation and drugs likely to upset electrolyte balance, such as diuretics, may all reduce lithium excretion and thereby precipitate intoxication; reduction of dosage may be required. In elderly patients, lithium excretion may also be reduced. Diuretics should only be used with caution during treatment; thiazides show a paradoxical diuretic effect resulting in possible water retention and lithium intoxication. Lithium retention may also follow combined use with indomethacin and other prostaglandin-synthetase-inhibiting drugs. The possibility of hypothyroidism and of renal dysfunction arising during prolonged treatment should be borne in mind and periodic assessments made.

There have been reports of interaction between lithium and some neuroleptics, particularly haloperidol at higher dosages, also between lithium and methyldopa or phenytoin.

Patients should be warned of the symptoms of impending intoxication (see below), of the urgency of immediate action should these symptoms appear, and also of the need to maintain a constant and adequate salt and water intake.

Use in pregnancy and lactation: Lithium crosses the placental barrier. In animal studies, lithium has been reported to interfere with fertility, gestation and foetal development. There is epidemiological evidence that the drug may be harmful in human pregnancy. Lithium therapy should not be used during pregnancy, especially during the first trimester, unless the benefits are considered to outweigh the risks. If given, however, serum levels should be measured frequently because of the changes in renal function associated with pregnancy and parturition.

Since lithium is secreted in breast milk, bottle feeding is advisable.

Adverse reactions: At therapeutic serum levels, mild nausea and diarrhoea, fine tremor of the hands, muscle weakness, vertigo, giddiness, weight gain, oedema, and a dazed feeling may occur. Hypothyroidism has been reported. Rarely hyperthyroidism may occur and mild hyperparathyroidism has been reported. Mild polyuria and polydipsia are not infrequent and, occasionally, nephrogenic diabetes insipidus may be present. Histological renal changes, with interstitial fibrosis, have been

observed in some patients on long-term treatment; while there may be an association with impaired reabsorption, a relationship between these changes and a reduction in glomerular filtration rate or development of renal insufficiency has not been established.

Skin reactions including acne or acneiform eruptions, papular skin disorders, rashes, and exacerbation of psoriasis have been reported.

Intoxication: Vomiting, diarrhoea, drowsiness, lack of co-ordination and/or a coarse tremor of the extremities and lower jaw may occur, especially with serum levels above the therapeutic range. Ataxia, giddiness, blurred vision, dysarthria, tinnitus, muscle hyperirritability, choreoathetoid movements and toxic psychosis have also been described.

If any of the above symptoms appear, treatment should be stopped immediately and arrangements made for serum lithium measurement.

Overdosage: Symptoms are similar to those listed above under *Intoxication* but more marked, particularly those of central nervous system origin. In severe cases, seizures, coma and death may ensue.

Treatment consists of the induction of vomiting and/or gastric lavage together with supportive and symptomatic measures. Particular attention should be paid to maintenance of fluid and electrolyte balance and of adequate renal function. Where convulsions are present, diazepam may be used. Forced alkaline diuresis, peritoneal dialysis or haemodialysis may help eliminate the lithium ion. The latter method is preferable, particularly where serum lithium exceeds 4 mmol/l.

Pharmaceutical precautions   Store in a dry place.

Legal category   POM.

Package quantities   Boxes containing 60 tablets in blister packs. Securitainers containing 1,000 tablets.

Further information   Nil.

Product licence number   0002/0083.

MICRALAX* MICRO-ENEMA

Presentation   A disposable plastic tube with a 2-inch pliable plastic nozzle, which contains 5 ml of a colourless viscous liquid incorporating 450 mg sodium citrate, 45 mg sodium alkylsulphoacetate and 5 mg sorbic acid, together with glycerin, sorbitol and purified water.

Uses   Micralax combines the action of sodium citrate, a 'peptizing' agent which can displace bound water present in the faeces; sorbitol, which enhances this action; and sodium alkylsulphoacetate, a wetting agent.

Micralax is indicated whenever an enema is necessary to relieve constipation: in dyschezia, especially in bedridden patients; in geriatrics, paediatrics and obstetrics; and in preparation for X-ray examination, proctoscopy and sigmoidoscopy.

Dosage and administration   *Adults and children aged 3 years and over:* Administer the contents of one micro-enema rectally, inserting the full length of the nozzle.

No lubricant is needed as a drop of the mixture is sufficient.

Contra-indications, warnings, etc

Contra-indication: Do not use in patients with inflammatory bowel disease.

Adverse reactions: No side-effects have been reported Excessive use may cause diarrhoea and fluid loss, which should be treated symptomatically.

Pharmaceutical precautions Store in a cool place.

Legal category P.

Package quantities Packs of 12 and 100.

Further information Nil.

Product licence number 0002/5037.

OCTOVIT* TABLETS

Presentation Maroon, oblong, film-coated tablets, engraved SK&F on one side, each containing: 2500 i.u. vitamin A present as the acetate, 1 mg thiamine present as the mononitrate, 1.5 mg riboflavine, 20 mg nicotinamide, 2 mg pyridoxine present as the hydrochloride, 2 mcg cyanocobalamin, 30 mg ascorbic acid, 100 i.u. cholecalciferol, 10 mg tocopherol present as the acetate, 100 mg calcium present as the hydrogen-phosphate dihydrate, 10 mg iron present as dried ferrous sulphate, 10 mg magnesium present as the hydroxide, and 5 mg zinc present as the sulphate monohydrate.

Uses Octovit is a multivitamin/mineral product indicated where supplementation with the vitamins and minerals specified above may be of benefit and for those at risk of developing a deficiency state.

Dosage and administration *Adults and children over 12 years:* One tablet a day or as prescribed by the physician.

Contra-indications, warnings, etc Iron and zinc chelate with tetracyclines and absorption of all three agents may be impaired.

Overdosage: Overdosage is unlikely to occur. However, prolonged administration of extremely large doses of vitamin A and cholecalciferol may result in hypervitaminosis. Early symptoms include irritability, nausea and vomiting, loss of appetite, headache, and dry and pruritic skin.

Pharmaceutical precautions Store in a dry place at a temperature not exceeding 25°C and protect from light.

Legal category P.

Package quantities Tablets in blister packs of 14 and 70.

Further information Nil.

Product licence number 0002/0113.

PARNATE* TABLETS

Presentation Geranium-red, sugar-coated tablets, marked SKF, each containing 10 mg tranylcypromine present as the sulphate.

Uses Parnate is a non-hydrazine monoamine oxidase inhibitor for the treatment of symptoms of depressive illness especially where phobic symptoms are present or where treatment with other types of antidepressant has failed. It is not recommended for mild depressive states resulting from temporary situational difficulties.

Dosage and administration *Adults only:* Initially, one tablet morning and afternoon. If the response is not adequate after the first week, add a further tablet at midday, and continue for at least a week. A dosage of 3 tablets a day should only be exceeded with caution. When a satisfactory response has been obtained, dosage

may be reduced to a maintenance level, often of 1 tablet a day.

When given with a tranquilliser, the dosage of Parnate is not affected. When given concurrently with electroconvulsive therapy, the usual dosage is 1 tablet twice a day during the series and 1 tablet a day afterwards as maintenance therapy.

Elderly: Use with great caution (see *Contra-indications* and *Cautions* below).

Contra-indications, warnings, etc
Contra-indications: Do not give Parnate less than a week after stopping treatment with any other antidepressant drug including other MAO inhibitors, because of persisting effects, then give half the usual dosage for the first week. Similarly, after stopping Parnate, allow at least two weeks to elapse before starting treatment with any drug that may interact.

Do not give Parnate with indirectly-acting sympathomimetic amines such as amphetamine, fenfluramine or similar anti-obesity agents, ephedrine or phenylpropanolamine (certain 'cold-cures' may contain such agents), or with levodopa or dopamine, as severe hypertensive reactions may result; with pethidine and closely related narcotic analgesics as potentiation may occur; or with other MAO inhibitors, as symptoms of overdosage are possible.

Reports of hyperactivity, hypertonicity, hyperpyrexia, coma and death have been associated with the use of Parnate in combination with tricyclic antidepressants; tetracyclic antidepressants should also be avoided. The use of clomipramine in patients already on Parnate may be particularly hazardous.

Do not use Parnate in patients with actual or suspected cerebrovascular disease or severe cardiovascular disease; in those with actual or suspected phaeochromocytoma, or with hyperthyroidism; or in those with known liver damage or blood dyscrasias.

Dietary precautions: High levels of tyramine in certain foods have been the cause of severe hypertensive reactions in patients on MAO inhibitor therapy (see *Adverse reactions*). Accordingly, patients must be warned to avoid the following: matured cheeses, hydrolysed protein extracts such as Marmite or Bovril, alcoholic drinks, particularly red wines such as Chianti, non-alcoholic beer and lager, and protein foods that are not fresh or whose preparation involved hydrolysis, fermentation, pickling, or 'hanging'; also broad-bean pods, which contain levodopa, and banana skins.

Cautions: Caution should be exercised when giving Parnate with the following: guanethidine, as its action may be antagonised; reserpine, as hyperactivity may occur; methyldopa, as central excitation may result; other hypotensive agents because of possible additive effects; oral hypoglycaemic agents or insulin, as their action may be potentiated; anticholinergic antiparkinsonism drugs, as potentiation has been reported; narcotic analgesics, except pethidine which is contra-indicated (see above), because of possible potentiation; and carbamazepine, which has similarities with tricyclic antidepressants. Although the effects of barbiturates may be enhanced, and this possibility should be borne in mind, they have frequently been given with Parnate, particularly at night. Metrizamide should be avoided in patients on MAO inhibitors since they may lower the seizure threshold.

Patients should be specifically asked if they are taking

any other medication because of the possibility of drug interactions.

Use Parnate with great caution in elderly patients; in those with cardiovascular disease in whom physical activity should be regulated, as the drug may suppress anginal pain; and in epileptic patients, as tranylcypromine has a variable effect on the convulsive threshold in animals. Parnate may aggravate some co-existing symptoms in depression such as anxiety and agitation. Parnate should preferably be withdrawn at least two weeks before elective surgery because of possible drug interaction.

Caution should be exercised in prescribing Parnate for patients with a previous history of dependence on drugs or alcohol.

In common with other drugs acting on the CNS, Parnate may affect ability to drive or operate machinery.

Use in pregnancy and lactation: Do not use in pregnancy, especially during the first and last trimesters, unless there are compelling reasons. There is no evidence as to drug safety in human pregnancy nor is there evidence from animal work that it is free from hazard. Tranylcypromine passes into the milk of lactating dogs.

Adverse reactions: Severe hypertensive reactions may occur, notably in association with foods containing tyramine (see *Dietary precautions*). Such reactions may be presaged by palpitations and unusually frequent headaches; patients should be warned to discontinue the drug if such symptoms occur. As well as a rapid rise in blood pressure, severe occipital headache, which may radiate frontally, is virtually always present, and pain and stiffness in the neck are usual; other features include multiple extrasystoles, often with bradycardia though sometimes with tachycardia, other arrhythmias, substernal pain, nausea and vomiting, sweating, pallor, sometimes followed by flushing, mydriasis and photophobia. Rarely, hypotension may dominate the clinical picture. ECG changes may be seen. The symptoms can mimic subarachnoid haemorrhage or may actually be associated with intracranial bleeding. Exceptionally, hemiparesis, hemiplegia or death has resulted.

Severe hypertensive reactions should be treated at once by reducing the blood pressure; slow intravenous injection of 5 mg phentolamine mesylate should be effective. Injectable or oral chlorpromazine is suitable for milder reactions. Acute symptoms generally subside within 24 hours.

Insomnia is the most frequent side-effect; it may usually be overcome by giving the last dose of the day not later than 3 pm, by reducing dosage, or by prescribing a mild hypnotic.

Mild headache, drowsiness, weakness, dizziness, palpitation, transient restlessness, dry mouth, blurred vision, nausea, oedema, weight gain, increased appetite and rash have been reported. Overstimulation, including anxiety and agitation, developing rarely into hypomania, has also been observed; the dosage should be reduced. Hypotension, which may be postural, may occur; it is usually temporary, but if it persists the drug should be stopped. Peripheral neuritis and difficulty in micturition have occurred rarely.

Dependence on Parnate, with tolerance to high doses, has been reported rarely, and can occur in patients without a past history of drug dependence. This should be distinguished from the return of features of the original illness on cessation of treatment.

Liver dysfunction has occurred very rarely, and isolated instances of purpura and blood dyscrasias have been reported.

Overdosage: Signs and symptoms are usually of the type already described as adverse reactions, but may be more intense, may include hyperpyrexia, tremor and convulsions, and may follow a latent period. Treatment consists of the induction of vomiting and/or gastric lavage together with supportive and symptomatic measures. External cooling is recommended for hyperpyrexia. Treat hypotension with fluid replacement; if severe or persistent, noradrenaline may be considered. Hypertension, if it occurs, may be relieved by slow intravenous injection of phentolamine mesylate. Pancuronium with mechanical ventilation may help reverse muscle spasm and pyrexia. Beta-adrenergic receptor blockade has been used successfully.

Pharmaceutical precautions Store in a dry place.

Legal category POM.

Package quantities Containers of 50 and 500 tablets.

Further information It is generally considered that no particular hazard is attached to the use of local anaesthetics containing small amounts of adrenaline in patients receiving Parnate unless cardiovascular disease is present.

Product licence number 0002/5040R.

PARSTELIN* TABLETS

Presentation Leaf-green, sugar-coated tablets, marked SKF, each containing 10 mg tranylcypromine present as the sulphate and 1 mg trifluoperazine present as the hydrochloride.

Uses Parstelin is a combination of a non-hydrazine monoamine oxidase inhibitor and a phenothiazine tranquilliser, for the treatment of symptoms of depressive illness complicated by anxiety, especially where phobic symptoms are present or where treatment with other types of antidepressant has failed. It is not recommended for mild depressive states resulting from temporary situational difficulties.

Dosage and administration *Adults only:* Initially, 1 tablet morning and afternoon. If the response is not adequate after the first week, add a further tablet at midday, and continue for at least a week. A dosage of 3 tablets a day should only be exceeded with caution. When a satisfactory response has been obtained, dosage may be reduced to a maintenance level, often of 1 tablet a day.

Elderly: Use with great caution (see *Contra-indications* and *Cautions* below).

Contra-indications, warnings, etc
Contra-indications: Do not give Parstelin less than a week after stopping treatment with any other antidepressant drug including other MAO inhibitors, because of persisting effects, then give half the usual dosage for the first week. Similarly, after stopping Parstelin, allow at least two weeks to elapse before starting treatment with any drug that may interact.

Do not give Parstelin with indirectly-acting sympathomimetic amines such as amphetamine, fenfluramine, or similar anti-obesity agents, ephedrine or phenylpropanolamine (certain 'cold-cures' may contain such agents) or with levodopa or dopamine, as severe hypertensiv reactions may result; with pethidine and closely related narcotic analgesics, as potentiation may occur; or with other MAO inhibitors, as symptoms of overdosage are possible.

Reports of hyperactivity, hypertonicity, hyperpyrexia, coma and death have been associated with the use of tranylcypromine in combination with tricyclic antidepressants; tetracyclic antidepressants should also be avoided. The use of clomipramine in patients already on Parstelin may be particularly hazardous.

Do not use Parstelin in patients with actual or suspected cerebrovascular disease or severe cardiovascular disease; in those with actual or suspected phaeochromocytoma, or with hyperthyroidism; in those with existing blood dyscrasias or known liver damage; or in those hypersensitive to the ingredients.

Dietary precautions: High levels of tyramine in certain foods have been the cause of severe hypertensive reactions in patients on MAO inhibitor therapy (see *Adverse reactions*). Accordingly, patients must be warned to avoid the following: matured cheese, hydrolysed protein extracts such as Marmite or Bovril, alcoholic drinks, particularly red wines such as Chianti, non-alcoholic beer and lager, and protein foods that are not fresh or whose preparation involved hydrolysis, fermentation, pickling, or 'hanging'; also broad-bean pods, which contain levodopa, and banana skins.

Cautions: Caution should be exercised when giving Parstelin with the following: guanethidine, as its action may be antagonised; reserpine, as hyperactivity may occur; methyldopa, as central excitation may result; other hypotensive agents because of possible additive effects; oral hypoglycaemic agents or insulin, as their action may be potentiated; anticholinergic antiparkinsonism drugs, as potentiation has been reported; narcotic analgesics, except pethidine which is contra-indicated (see above), because of possible potentiation; and carbamazepine, which has similarities with tricyclic antidepressants. Although the effects of barbiturates may be enhanced, and this possibility should be borne in mind, they have frequently been given with Parstelin, particularly at night. Metrizamide should be avoided in patients on MAO inhibitors since they may lower the seizure threshold. Potentiation may occur if trifluoperazine is used with other CNS depressants.

Patients should be specifically asked if they are taking any other medication because of the possibility of drug interactions.

Use Parstelin with great caution in elderly patients; in those with cardiovascular disease in whom physical activity should be regulated, as tranylcypromine may suppress anginal pain; and in epileptic patients as tranylcypromine has a variable effect on the convulsive threshold in animals. Tranylcypromine may aggravate some co-existing symptoms in depression such as anxiety and agitation. Parstelin should preferably be withdrawn at least two weeks before elective surgery because of possible drug interaction.

Nausea and vomiting as a sign of organic disease may be masked by the anti-emetic action of trifluoperazine.

Caution should be exercised in prescribing Parstelin for patients with a previous history of dependence on drugs or alcohol.

In common with other drugs acting on the CNS, Parstelin may affect ability to drive or operate machinery.

Use in pregnancy and lactation: Do not use in pregnancy, especially during the first and last trimesters, unless there are compelling reasons. There is no evidence as to drug safety in human pregnancy nor is there evidence from animal work that it is free from hazard. Both tranylcypromine and trifluoperazine pass into the milk of lactating dogs.

Adverse reactions: Severe hypertensive reactions may occur, notably in association with foods containing tyramine (see *Dietary precautions*). Such reactions may be presaged by palpitations and unusually frequent headaches; patients should be warned to discontinue the drug if such symptoms occur. As well as a rapid rise in blood pressure, severe occipital headache, which may radiate frontally, is virtually always present, and pain and stiffness in the neck are usual; other features include multiple extrasystoles, often with bradycardia though sometimes with tachycardia, other arrhythmias, substernal pain, nausea and vomiting, sweating, pallor, sometimes followed by flushing, mydriasis and photophobia. Rarely, hypotension may dominate the clinical picture. ECG changes may be seen. The symptoms can mimic subarachnoid haemorrhage or may actually be associated with intracranial bleeding. Exceptionally, hemiparesis, hemiplegia or death has resulted.

Severe hypertensive reactions should be treated at once by reducing the blood pressure; slow intravenous injection of 5 mg phentolamine mesylate should be effective. Injectable or oral chlorpromazine is suitable for milder reactions. Acute symptoms generally subside within 24 hours.

Insomnia is the most frequent side-effect; it may usually be overcome by giving the last dose of the day not later than 3 pm, by reducing dosage, or by prescribing a mild hypnotic.

Mild headache, drowsiness, weakness, dizziness, palpitation, transient restlessness, dry mouth, blurred vision, nausea, oedema, weight gain, increased appetite and rash have been reported. Overstimulation, including anxiety and agitation, developing rarely into hypomania, has also been observed; the dosage should be reduced. Hypotension, which may be postural, may occur; it is usually temporary, but if it persists the drug should be stopped. Peripheral neuritis and difficulty in micturition have occurred rarely.

Dependence on tranylcypromine, with tolerance to high doses, has been reported rarely, and can occur in patients without a past history of drug dependence. This should be distinguished from the return of features of the original illness on cessation of treatment.

Extrapyramidal symptoms due to the trifluoperazine component are very unlikely at the recommended dosage. Extremely rarely, long-term therapy with trifluoperazine in low dosage has been associated with tardive dyskinesia, which can be long-lasting or even irreversible.

Liver dysfunction has occurred very rarely, and isolated instances of purpura and blood dyscrasias have been reported.

Overdosage: Signs and symptoms are usually of the type already described as adverse reactions to tranylcypromine, but may be more intense, may include hyperpyrexia, tremor and convulsions, and may follow a latent period. In the unlikely event of symptoms from the trifluoperazine component, these are extrapyramidal in type. Treatment consists of gastric lavage together with supportive and symptomatic measures. Do not induce vomiting. External cooling is recommended for hyperpyrexia. Treat hypotension with fluid replacement; if severe or persistent, noradrenaline may be considered; adrenaline is contraindicated. Hypertension, if it occurs, may be relieved by slow intravenous injection of phentolamine mesylate.

Pancuronium with mechanical ventilation may help reverse muscle spasm and pyrexia. Beta-adrenergic receptor blockade has been used successfully.

Pharmaceutical precautions Store in a dry place at a temperaturo not exceeding 30°C and protect from light.

Legal category POM.

Package quantities Containers of 50 and 500 tablets.

Further information It is generally considered that no particular hazard is attached to the use of local anaesthetics containing small amounts of adrenaline in patients receiving tranylcypromine unless cardiovascular disease is present.

Parstelin should normally only be used on the recommendation of a specialist in psychiatry.

Product licence number 0002/5041R.

PHENOBARBITONE SPANSULE* CAPSULES

Presentation Clear, colourless capsules, blue-capped and filled with a mixture of dark blue, pale blue, and white pellets, in two strengths. Each Spansule sustained-release capsule, size No. 3, contains 60 mg, and each size No. 2 capsule, 100 mg phenobarbitone. Two-thirds of the dose is formulated for sustained release over a period of six to eight hours.

Uses Phenobarbitone Spansule capsules are anticonvulsant and are indicated in the treatment of epilepsy.

Dosage and administration *Adults:* Dosage depends on the need of the individual patient, and may vary from one 60 mg capsule a day in the morning or at night, to three 100 mg capsules a day.

Elderly: Lower dosages are likely to be required (see *Cautions*).

Children aged 6 years and over: As in adults, the dosage requirement may vary, the highest usual dosage being two 60 mg capsules a day. The capsules may be opened and the pellets mixed with soft, cool food, but they must not be chewed.

Contra-indications, warnings, etc
Contra-indications: Do not use in patients with porphyria, severe liver damage, or known hypersensitivity to barbiturates.

Cautions: Patients who drive or operate machinery should be warned of the possibility of drowsiness. Potentiation is likely if phenobarbitone is used with other CNS depressants. Patients should also be warned that alcohol may potentiate the effects of phenobarbitone. The drug should be used with care in the elderly, and in those with kidney or liver damage.

Because phenobarbitone can induce liver microsomal enzymes, the rate of metabolism of certain drugs can be increased. Those drugs whose expected effect may be reduced in this way include coumarin-type anticoagulants and some steroid hormones.

Prolonged use may lead to dependence of the barbiturate-alcohol type, and particular care should be taken in treating patients with a history of dependence on drugs or alcohol.

Use in pregnancy and lactation: It has been suggested that certain anticonvulsants, possibly including phenobarbitone, may produce embryotoxic effects in man. Although this drug has been available for very many years, it should be avoided in pregnancy unless essential, especially during the first trimester.

Barbiturates can pass into breast milk and should, unless essential, be avoided by nursing mothers.

Adverse reactions: Drowsiness, which may be marked, and allergic reactions including skin reactions, may occur. Paradoxically in children irritability may be observed.

Overdosage: Absorption of phenobarbitone from the sustained-release Spansule capsule is likely to be prolonged, and this should be borne in mind. Treatment consists of the induction of vomiting and/or gastric lavage, together with intensive supportive and symptomatic measures. In severe poisoning, forced alkaline diuresis, haemodialysis or charcoal haemoperfusion may help to eliminate the drug.

Pharmaceutical precautions Store in a dry place at a temperature not exceeding 30°C.

Legal category CD (Sch 3), POM.

Package quantities Both strengths in containers of 30 and 250 Spansule capsules.

Further information Nil.

Product licence numbers
Phenobarbitone Spansule capsules 60 mg
0002/5043
Phenobarbitone Spansule capsules 100 mg
0002/5042

POLIOMYELITIS VACCINE, LIVE (ORAL) BP (Sabin strains)

Presentation Poliomyelitis Vaccine, Live (Oral) BP, as supplied by Smith Kline & French, is a light orange to pink liquid stabilised with molar magnesium chloride. Each dose (3 drops) provides at least $10^6 TCID_{50}$ type 1 (LS-c,2ab), $10^5 TCID_{50}$ type 2 (P712, Ch, 2ab) and $10^{5.5} TCID_{50}$ type 3 (Leon 12a$_1$b) live attenuated strains of poliomyelitis virus grown in monkey kidney cell cultures, and contains not more than 7 μg (5 i.u.) neomycin sulphate.

Uses Active immunisation against poliomyelitis.

Dosage and administration *Adults and children: For oral use only:* NOT FOR INJECTION. Three drops of the vaccine constitute one dose which may be given with syrup or on a lump of sugar to mask the bitter salty taste of the magnesium chloride.

For a complete schedule, three doses of the vaccine should be given at intervals of at least four weeks (see also *Further information*).

Other unvaccinated members of the same household (including adults) should be advised vaccination at the same time as the vaccinee.

Contra-indications, warnings, etc
Contra-indications: The vaccine should not be used in the presence of acute febrile illness or intercurrent infection, diarrhoea, vomiting or other gastro-intestinal disturbance, neither should it be given in the presence of impaired immune response including leukaemia, lymphoma, generalised malignancy or treatment with corticosteroids, cytotoxic drugs or irradiation. Do not give to those known to be hypersensitive to neomycin (see also *Cautions*).

Cautions: The vaccine may contain trace amounts of

penicillin and streptomycin which should not contra-indicate its use except in those with a history of severe anaphylaxis due to either antibiotic.

It is not normally recommended that live vaccines are given within three weeks of each other.

Use in pregnancy: Pregnant women should not be given oral poliomyelitis vaccine unless they are at definite risk from poliomyelitis.

Adverse reactions: Paralysis temporally associated with vaccination has been reported very rarely in recipients or contacts.

Overdosage: Not applicable.

Pharmaceutical precautions Protect from light and store between 2°C and 6°C. Under these conditions there is no significant loss of virus titre for 12 months.

When tubes of vaccine have been opened there is a risk of contamination with bacteria and moulds which may result in a reduction of vaccine potency. It is good practice, therefore, to discard vaccine remaining in opened tubes at the end of the vaccinating session. Any unopened vaccine should be returned to storage between 2°C and 6°C as soon as possible. Potency is maintained for two weeks at room temperature (20°C to 25°C).

Legal category POM.

Package quantities Plastic dropper tube containing 10 doses.

Further information Current policy recommends that the first dose of oral poliomyelitis vaccine should be given at three months of age. The first and second doses should be separated by six to eight weeks and the second and third doses by four to six months. For convenience the vaccine may be given at the same time as the three-dose basic course of diphtheria/tetanus/pertussis vaccine.

It is currently recommended that a reinforcing dose of poliomyelitis vaccine should be given at school entry and at 15 to 19 years of age. Adults need not be offered a reinforcing dose unless they are at special risk.

Product licence number 0002/0076.

PRAGMATAR* OINTMENT

Presentation A pale, buff-coloured, oil-in-water cream containing 4% w/w cetyl alcohol-coal tar distillate, 3% w/w precipitated sulphur, and 3% w/w salicylic acid.

Uses Pragmatar has mild antipruritic, antiseptic, and keratolytic properties. It is indicated in the treatment of dandruff, other seborrhoeic conditions, and common scaly skin disorders.

Dosage and administration *Adults and children:* For mild dandruff, apply the ointment once a week when the hair is washed. For more severe cases, treat the entire scalp daily at bedtime, applying lightly but thoroughly with the fingertips. The ointment can be washed out the next morning or left as a pleasant hair dressing. For other indicated subacute or chronic skin disorders, apply daily in small quantities to affected areas only.

For use in infants, the ointment may be diluted by mixing with a few drops of water in the palm of the hand.

Contra-indications, warnings, etc
Contra-indications: Do not use in patients who are sensitive to sulphur, or in the presence of acute local infection.

Caution: Use with care near the eyes, mucous membranes or on acutely inflamed areas. If any ointment should accidentally enter the eye, flush with normal saline solution.

Adverse reactions: No side-effects are to be expected if the ointment is used according to directions. Excessive use, however, may cause erythema and irritation.

Overdosage: If ingestion occurs, gastro-intestinal disturbances may follow. Treatment consists of rinsing out the mouth together with symptomatic measures if necessary. Even with massive ingestion, salicylate poisoning seems unlikely.

Pharmaceutical precautions Store in a cool place.

Legal category P.

Package quantities Tubes containing 25 g.

Further information Nil.

Product licence number 0002/5044.

REDEPTIN* INJECTION

Presentation Each ampoule or vial of Redeptin contains an opalescent white aqueous suspension containing 2 mg fluspirilene in each 1 ml.

Uses Fluspirilene is a major tranquilliser of the diphenylbutylpiperidine group. It is slowly absorbed after intramuscular injection. Detectable blood levels are reached within four hours of injection, and the antipsychotic action usually lasts for about a week, with a range of 5 to 15 days.

Redeptin is recommended for the symptomatic treatment of schizophrenia, and has proved especially useful for maintenance therapy. It is of particular value in patients who are unreliable in taking oral medication.

Dosage and administration *Adults only:* The recommended starting dose is 2 mg a week by deep intramuscular injection; this may be increased by 2 mg a week according to response. Do not massage the injection site. The maintenance dosage for most patients is from 2 to 8 mg a week, but some may require up to 12 mg a week. Dosage should not exceed 20 mg a week. Gradual withdrawal from high dosage treatment is advisable.

Elderly: A quarter to half the usual starting dosage may be sufficient. See also *Cautions.*

Because individual response and dosage requirements can vary considerably, treatment should be started and dosage increased under close supervision.

As with all major tranquillisers clinical improvement may not be evident for several weeks after starting treatment, and there may also be delay before recurrence of symptoms after stopping treatment.

Administration: Before administration the container should be shaken well. The 6 ml vial should be used on one occasion only.

Contra-indications, warnings, etc

Contra-indications: Do not use in patients who have suffered uncontrollable adverse effects during previous treatment with diphenylbutylpiperidine derivatives or in those hypersensitive to such compounds.

Do not use in pregnancy; especially during the first and last trimesters, unless there are compelling reasons. There is no evidence of safety in human pregnancy, and there is some evidence of harmful effects in animal studies. Fluspirilene may be excreted into breast milk. Since the effect of even small quantities of fluspirilene on the infant brain is not established, nursing mothers should be advised to stop breast feeding.

Cautions: Patients who drive or operate machinery should be warned of the possibility of drowsiness.

Potentiation may occur if antipsychotic drugs are combined with CNS depressants such as alcohol, hypnotics and strong analgesics.

Elderly patients may be particularly sensitive, especially as regards extrapyramidal effects.

Care should be exercised in patients with known liver damage, and, because Redeptin contains povidone, in those with kidney damage.

In patients with Parkinson's disease, symptoms may be worsened, and the effects of levodopa reversed. Since fluspirilene may lower the convulsive threshold, patients with epilepsy or conditons pre-disposing to epilepsy, such as alcohol or brain damage, should be treated with caution, and metrizamide avoided; the effect of anticonvulsants may be impaired.

Although no neurotoxic interactions with lithium have been reported, this possibility should be borne in mind.

Nausea and vomiting as a sign of organic disease may be masked by the anti-emetic action of fluspirilene.

The possibilities of interaction with anticoagulants and of effects on control of diabetes have been raised with antipsychotic drugs but there have been no reports to date of such effects with fluspirilene.

Adverse reactions: The majority of side-effects occur during the first two days after injection. Extrapyramidal reactions are common in moderate to high dosage, and include, especially dyskinesia and akathisia but also tremor, salivation, acute dystonias and oculogyric crises. They may occur within 6 to 12 hours after injection and usually disappear within 48 hours; they can normally be controlled by reduction of dosage or, when necessary, by the use of anticholinergic antiparkinsonism drugs.

Tardive dyskinesia may occur during or after long-term treatment with antipsychotic drugs. Symptoms (persistent dyskinesia of facial muscles, sometimes with involuntary movements of the extremities) may persist for prolonged periods, in some cases being irreversible. Elderly patients and those with organic brain damage are at particular risk. Periodic gradual reduction of dosage to reveal persisting dyskinesia has been suggested so that treatment may be stopped if necessary. Anticholinergic antiparkinsonism drugs may aggravate the condition. Since the occurrence of tardive dyskinesia may be related to length of treatment and dosage, Redeptin should be given for as short a time and at as low a dose as possible.

Subcutaneous nodules at the site of injection have been reported, usually in patients on high doses for long periods. These nodules tend to disappear when treatment is stopped. They may be minimised by using as many different injection sites as possible. Other reactions reported include fatigue and drowsiness, which may be dose-related and be particularly marked at the start of treatment, upper gastro-intestinal symptoms such as

nausea and vomiting, insomnia, restlessness, excitement, anxiety, headache and sweating. There have also been occasional reports of autonomic symptoms such as blurred vision, hypotension and dizziness, rash, weight gain, and EEG and ECG changes. Increased prolactin levels, with galactorrhoea, gynaecomastia or amenorrhoea have been reported. In some patients side-effects may become progressively more marked over a period of weeks or months; these signs of accumulation can be eliminated by omitting one injection every four or five weeks.

Jaundice has been rarely reported during treatment with Redeptin; transient abnormalities of liver function tests have also occurred.

Overdosage: In the unlikely event of accidental overdosage, signs and symptoms are likely to be predominantly extrapyramidal, possibly with some excitation. Treatment would consist of supportive and symptomatic measures. Extrapyramidal symptoms should be treated with an anticholinergic antiparkinsonism drug. The long-acting properties of the presentation should be borne in mind.

Pharmaceutical precautions　Redeptin ampoules and vials should be stored upright at room temperature and protected from light.

Legal category　POM.

Package quantities　Redeptin ampoules, each containing either 2 mg fluspirilene in 1 ml or 6 mg fluspirilene in 3 ml, are available in boxes of 10. Redeptin vials, each containing 12 mg fluspirilene in 6 ml, are available in packs of 5.

Further information　Maximal plasma levels of fluspirilene are found 4 to 8 hours after administration; it has a very prolonged excretion half-life of approximately 3 weeks.

Product licence number　0002/0056R.

RIMEVAX*
Measles vaccine, live BP
(Schwarz strain)

Presentation　Rimevax measles vaccine, prepared in chicken embryo fibroblasts, is presented as a pink freeze-dried pellet in a glass vial with a separate ampoule of clear, colourless, sterile diluent. Each 0.5 ml dose of reconstituted vaccine contains not less than 1,000 $TCID_{50}$ of the highly attenuated live Schwarz strain measles virus and not more than 25 µg (17 i.u.) of neomycin sulphate.

Uses　Rimevax is indicated for active immunisation against measles (rubeola).

If given to contacts within three days of exposure to measles, the full clinical disease may be suppressed.

Dosage and administration　*Adults and children:* 0.5 ml of the reconstituted vaccine subcutaneously or intramuscularly. The vaccine should be reconstituted using the sterile diluent provided.

The vaccine is quickly inactivated by ether, alcohol and detergents and care should be taken to avoid contact with these substances when cleaning skin prior to vaccination. Syringes need to be dry sterilised.

Contra-indications, warnings, etc
Contra-indications: Do not use Rimevax in the presence of acute illness, whether active or expected, following exposure to infection other than measles. This applies

particularly to active tuberculosis and respiratory tract infection. It is also contra-indicated in states of altered immunity including those which may accompany conditions such as leukaemia, lymphoma, generalised malignancy or treatment with corticosteroids, cytotoxic drugs or irradiation.

Rimevax may contain traces of chick embryo protein, but this does not normally contra-indicate its use except in cases of severe hypersensitivity to eggs (past anaphylactoid reactions to egg ingestion). Rimevax should not be given to those known to be hypersensitive to neomycin. A solution of 1:1000 adrenaline should be available for injection in rare cases of anaphylactic reaction.

Do not use during pregnancy.

Cautions: Measles vaccine should only be given to children with a history of convulsions with the simultaneous administration of human normal immunoglobulin [recommended dosage 1.3 mg protein/kg (0.6 mg protein/lb) body weight]. In such children or those with a family history of convulsions, consideration should be given to delaying immunisation until after the second birthday.

Because of the possibility of interference from passive antibodies, measles vaccine should not normally be given to infants below the age of one year, or to subjects who have received blood or human plasma transfusions or human immunoglobulin within the previous three months. If the vaccine is given in these circumstances, serum antibodies should be checked at a later date.

Tuberculin testing should be delayed for about eight weeks after measles vaccination since false-negative results may be obtained during this period.

It is not usually recommended that live vaccines be given within three weeks of each other.

Adverse reactions: These are usually mild and are more likely around the eighth day after vaccination. They may include rash, malaise, cough, pharyngitis, coryza, pyrexia and headache. In a very few subjects convulsions may accompany the fever. Immediate allergic-type reactions have been reported rarely. Very rarely encephalitis has been reported in association with measles vaccination.

Pharmaceutical precautions Protect from light. Rimevax measles vaccine should be stored between 2°C and 8°C and should not be frozen (lower temperatures will not harm the vaccine but may damage the diluent ampoule). At room temperature (20°–25°C) Rimevax is stable for up to four weeks.

The vaccine should be reconstituted using the sterile diluent provided. The colour of reconstituted vaccine may vary from light orange to light red. Once reconstituted Rimevax should be used immediately and certainly within one hour.

Legal category POM.

Package quantities Single-dose vials, each with a separate ampoule containing sterile diluent, singly and in packs of 50.

Further information Current policy recommends routine vaccination against measles for children between 1 and 2 years of age. Rimevax may also be used for older children and adults known to be susceptible to measles.

The following groups of children at special risk may in particular benefit from vaccination: children from the age of one year upwards in residential care; those entering nursery school or other establishments accepting children for day care; those with chronic conditions affecting physical development such as cystic fibrosis or congenital heart disease; and those with a history of convulsions provided the appropriate cautions (see *Cautions* above) are observed.

Maximum periods of stability of freeze-dried Rimevax:

2°–8°C	2 years
20°–25°C	4 weeks
37°C	14 days
41°C	7 days

It is recommended that the vaccine is stored at 2°–8°C (see **Pharmaceutical precautions**).

Product licence number 0002/0088.

STELABID* TABLETS

Presentation Dull yellow, sugar-coated tablets, marked SKF in grey, each containing 5 mg isopropamide present as the iodide and 1 mg trifluoperazine present as the hydrochloride.

Uses Stelabid is a combination of two long-acting compounds, an anticholinergic agent and a phenothiazine tranquilliser. It is indicated in the short term symptomatic treatment of peptic ulcer, and other gastrointestinal disorders in which hypersecretion and/or painful spasms are a problem as, for example, in irritable or spastic colon and functional diarrhoea. Stelabid is especially indicated when such conditions are complicated by emotional factors such as tension and anxiety.

Dosage and administration *Adults only:* 2 or 3 tablets a day, according to the severity of the condition. The dosage should be divided and taken in the morning and at bedtime. At the higher dosage, and particularly in patients troubled by night pain, 2 tablets may be taken at bedtime.

Elderly: Use with great caution (see *Contra-indications* and *Cautions* below).

Contra-indications, warnings, etc

Contra-indications: Do not use in patients with glaucoma, intestinal obstruction of organic origin or intestinal atony, reflux oesophagitis, prostatic hypertrophy or incipient urinary retention from any cause, or ulcerative colitis; in those sensitive to iodine; or in patients with existing blood dyscrasias or known liver damage.

Cautions: Care should be exercised when treating elderly patients or those with cardiovascular disease.

Patients who drive or operate machinery should be warned of the possibility of drowsiness.

Potentiation may occur if this product is used with other drugs with anticholinergic properties or with central nervous system depressants.

The iodine present may interfere with some tests of thyroid function.

Nausea and vomiting as a sign of organic disease may be masked by the anti-emetic action of trifluoperazine.

Use in pregnancy: Combinations of isopropamide and trifluoperazine have been available since 1960, and there is no experimental or clinical evidence to suggest any associated hazard to the foetus. Nevertheless, drugs should be avoided in pregnancy unless essential, especially during the first trimester.

Adverse reactions: Blurred vision, mydriasis, dry mouth, restlessness, insomnia, urinary hesitancy or retention, constipation, tachycardia, palpitations, and drowsiness may occur.

Extrapyramidal symptoms due to the trifluoperazine component are very unlikely at the recommended dosage. Extremely rarely, long-term therapy with trifluoperazine in low dosage has been associated with tardive dyskinesia, which can be long-lasting or even irreversible.

Overdosage: Signs and symptoms may be those of either isopropamide or trifluoperazine, or both, and may include extrapyramidal symptoms, CNS depression and hypotension. Treatment consists of gastric lavage, together with symptomatic and supportive measures. Do not induce vomiting. Central excitation may require a sedative such as diazepam. Neostigmine, 0.25 mg subcutaneously in an adult, may reverse the peripheral effects of anticholinergic poisoning. Treat hypotension with fluid replacement; if severe or persistent, noradrenaline may be considered. Adrenaline is contra-indicated.

Pharmaceutical precautions Store in a dry place and protect from light.

Legal category POM.

Package quantities Containers of 100 and 500 tablets.

Further information Nil.

Product licence number 0002/5073.

STELAZINE* TABLETS
STELAZINE* SPANSULE* CAPSULES
STELAZINE* SYRUP
STELAZINE* CONCENTRATE
STELAZINE* INJECTION

Presentation Blue, sugar-coated tablets, marked SKF, containing either 1 mg or 5 mg trifluoperazine present as the hydrochloride.

Clear, colourless capsules, opaque yellow-capped and filled with a mixture of dark and light blue and white pellets. Each Spansule capsule, size No. 4, contains 2 mg, size No. 2, 10 mg, and size No. 1, 15 mg trifluoperazine present as the hydrochloride. Two-thirds of the dose of trifluoperazine is formulated for release over a period of six to eight hours.

A clear, pale yellow, peach-flavoured syrup, each 5 ml dose containing 1 mg trifluoperazine present as the hydrochloride.

A clear, pale yellow, peach-flavoured concentrate with a bitter numbing after-taste. Before dilution, each 1 ml of concentrate contains 10 mg trifluoperazine present as the hydrochloride.

Ampoules containing 1 mg trifluoperazine present as the hydrochloride in 1 ml.

Uses Stelazine is a piperazine phenothiazine tranquilliser with potent antipsychotic, anxiolytic, and antiemetic activity, and a pharmacological profile of moderate sedative and hypotensive properties, and fairly pronounced tendency to cause extrapyramidal reactions.

Low dosage: Stelazine is indicated as an adjunct in the short term management of anxiety states, depressive symptoms secondary to anxiety, and agitation. It is also indicated in the symptomatic treatment of nausea and vomiting.

High dosage: Stelazine is indicated for the treatment of symptoms and prevention of relapse in schizophrenia and in other psychoses, especially of the paranoid type, but not in depressive psychoses. It may also be used as an adjunct in the short term management of severe psychomotor agitation and of dangerously impulsive behaviour in, for example, mental subnormality.

Dosage and administration *Adults: Low dosage:* 2–4 mg a day as tablets or syrup, given in divided doses, or one or two 2 mg Spansule capsules a day, according to the severity of the patient's condition. If necessary, dosage may be increased to 6 mg a day, but above this level extrapyramidal symptoms are more likely to occur in some patients.

High dosage: The recommended starting dose for physically fit adults is 5 mg twice a day (or one 10 mg Spansule capsule a day); after a week this may be increased to 15 mg a day (which may be given as one 15 mg Spansule capsule). If necessary, further increases of 5 mg may be made at three-day intervals, but not more often. When satisfactory control has been achieved, dosage should be reduced gradually until an effective maintenance level has been established. Stelazine Spansule capsules are particularly useful for such maintenance therapy.

As with all major tranquillisers clinical improvement may not be evident for several weeks after starting treatment, and there may also be delay before recurrence of symptoms after stopping treatment. Gradual withdrawal from high dosage treatment is advisable.

Intramuscular use: For a more rapid and intense effect or when oral administration presents difficulties, Stelazine may be given by deep intramuscular injection; the recommended dosage is 1–3 mg a day, given in divided doses. Higher dosages may sometimes be necessary up to a suggested maximum of 6 mg a day. Oral therapy should be substituted as soon as possible.

Elderly: Reduce starting dose in elderly or frail patients by at least half.

Children: Low dosage: For children aged 3–5 years, up to 1 mg a day as the syrup, given in divided doses. For children aged 6–12 years, the dosage may be increased to a maximum of 4 mg a day.

High dosage: For children aged under 12 years, the initial oral dosage should not exceed 5 mg a day, given in divided doses. Any subsequent increase should be made with caution, at intervals of not less than three days, and taking into account age, body weight and severity of symptoms.

Intramuscular use: There has been little experience in the use of intramuscular Stelazine in children. If required, a starting dose of 1 mg per 20 kg (44 lb) body weight a day, given in divided doses, is suggested.

Use of liquid presentations: Dilute Stelazine Concentrate before use with either purified water containing 0.1% benzoic acid or Syrup BP containing 0.05% w/v parahydroxybenzoic acid esters. Dilution at the rate of 1 in 10 volumes gives a concentration of 5 mg trifluoperazine in each 5 ml dose. Stelazine Syrup may be diluted with Syrup BP, with or without 0.05% parahydroxybenzoic acid esters.

Both Stelazine Syrup and Concentrate may be administered with a drink of demineralised water, orange juice or Syrup BP.

Contra-indications, warnings, etc

Contra-indications: Do not use Stelazine in comatose patients, or in those with existing blood dyscrasias or known liver damage, or in those hypersensitive to the active ingredient or related compounds.

Cautions: Care should be taken when treating elderly

patients, and initial dosage should be reduced. Such patients can be especially sensitive, particularly to extrapyramidal and hypotensive effects. Patients with cardiovascular disease including arrhythmias should also be treated with caution. Because Stelazine may increase activity, care should be taken in patients with angina pectoris.

In patients with Parkinson's disease, symptoms may be worsened, and the effects of levodopa reversed. Since phenothiazines may lower the convulsive threshold, patients with epilepsy should be treated with caution, and metrizamide avoided. Although Stelazine has minimal anticholinergic activity, this should be borne in mind when treating patients with narrow angle glaucoma, myasthenia gravis and prostatic hypertrophy.

Nausea and vomiting as a sign of organic disease may be masked by the anti-emetic action of Stelazine.

Potentiation may occur if antipsychotic drugs are combined with CNS depressants such as alcohol, hypnotics and strong analgesics. Phenothiazines may antagonise the action of guanethidine.

Patients who drive or operate machinery should be warned of the possibility of drowsiness.

Use in pregnancy and lactation: Stelazine has been available since 1958, and there is no experimental or clinical evidence (including follow-up surveys in over 800 women who had taken low-dosage Stelazine during pregnancy) to suggest any associated hazard to the foetus. Nevertheless, drug treatment should be avoided in pregnancy unless essential, especially during the first trimester. Trifluoperazine passes into the milk of lactating dogs.

Adverse reactions: Lassitude, drowsiness, dizziness, transient restlessness, insomnia, dry mouth, blurred vision, muscular weakness, anorexia, mild postural hypotension, skin reactions including photosensitivity reactions, weight gain, oedema and confusion may occasionally occur. Tachycardia, constipation, urinary hesitancy and retention, and hyperpyrexia have been reported very rarely. Adverse reactions tend to be dose related and to disappear. Hyperprolactinaemia may occur at higher dosages with associated effects such as galactorrhoea or amenorrhoea. Phenothiazines can produce ECG changes with prolongation of the QT interval and T-wave changes; serious arrhythmias have been reported. Such effects are rare with Stelazine. In some patients, especially non-psychotic patients, Stelazine even at low dosage may cause unpleasant symptoms of being dulled or paradoxically of being agitated.

Extrapyramidal symptoms are rare at daily dosages of 6 mg or less; they are considerably more common at higher dosage levels. These symptoms include parkinsonism; akathisia, with motor restlessness and difficulty in sitting still; and acute dystonia or dyskinesia, which may occur early in treatment and may present with torticollis, facial grimacing, trismus, tongue protrusion and abnormal eye movements including oculogyric crises. Such reactions may often be controlled by reducing the dosage or by stopping medication. In more severe dystonic reactions, an anticholinergic antiparkinsonism drug should be given.

Tardive dyskinesia of the facial muscles, sometimes with involuntary movements of the extremities, has occurred in some patients on long-term high dosage and, more rarely, low-dosage phenothiazine therapy, including Stelazine. Symptoms may appear for the first time either during or after a course of treatment; they may become worse when treatment is stopped. The symptoms may persist for many months or even years, and while they gradually disappear in some patients, they appear to be permanent in others. Patients have most commonly been elderly, with organic brain damage. Particular caution should be observed in treating such patients. Periodic gradual reduction of dosage to reveal persisting dyskinesia has been suggested, so that treatment may be stopped if necessary. Anticholinergic antiparkinsonism agents may aggravate the condition. Since the occurrence of tardive dyskinesia may be related to length of treatment and dosage, Stelazine should be given for as short a time and at as low a dosage as possible.

Mild cholestatic jaundice, and blood dyscrasias such as agranulocytosis, pancytopenia, leucopenia and thrombocytopenia have been reported very rarely. Signs of persistent infection should be investigated.

Very rare cases of skin pigmentation and lenticular opacities have been reported with Stelazine.

Overdosage: Signs and symptoms will be predominantly extrapyramidal; hypotension may occur. Absorption of trifluoperazine from the Spansule capsule is likely to be prolonged, and this should be borne in mind. Treatment consists of gastric lavage together with supportive and symptomatic measures. Do not induce vomiting. Extrapyramidal symptoms may be treated with an anticholinergic antiparkinsonism drug. Treat hypotension with fluid replacement; if severe or persistent, noradrenaline may be considered. Adrenaline is contra-indicated.

Pharmaceutical precautions Store tablets in a dry place and protect from light. Store Spansule capsules in a dry place at a temperature not exceeding 30°C and protect from light. Protect syrup from light. If it is necessary to dilute the syrup, use Syrup BP either without preservatives or containing 0.05% w/v parahydroxybenzoic acid esters; the diluted syrup is stable for 14 days. Store concentrate at a temperature not exceeding 30°C and protect from light. The concentrate must be diluted before use, if possible with Syrup BP containing 0.05% w/v parahydroxybenzoic acid esters; alternatively it may be diluted with purified water containing 0.1% w/v benzoic acid. The diluted concentrate when stored at a temperature not exceeding 30°C and protected from light is stable for up to 3 months. Cloudiness of syrup and concentrate may result if diluents containing sodium salts of parahydroxybenzoic acid esters are used. Protect ampoules from light.

Legal category POM.

Package quantities Tablets, 1 mg, in containers of 100 and 1,000. Tablets, 5 mg, in containers of 100, 1,000 and 5,000.

Spansule capsules, 2 mg, in containers of 30, 250 and 5,000. Spansule capsules, 10 mg and 15 mg, in containers of 100 and 5,000.

Syrup, in bottles containing 200 ml.

Concentrate, in bottles containing 100 ml and one litre.

Ampoules, each containing 1 ml, in boxes of 10.

Further information Nil.

Product licence numbers

Stelazine tablets, 1 mg	0002/5081R
Stelazine tablets, 5 mg	0002/5082R
Stelazine Spansule capsules, 2 mg	0002/5077R
Stelazine Spansule capsules, 10 mg	0002/5078R
Stelazine Spansule capsules, 15 mg	0002/5079R
Stelazine syrup	0002/5080R

| Stelazine concentrate | 0002/5076R |
| Stelazine injection | 0002/5075R |

TAGAMET* TABLETS
TAGAMET* SYRUP
TAGAMET* INJECTION
TAGAMET* INFUSION

Presentation Pale green, oval, film-coated tablots, engraved SK&F T800 on one side, containing 800 mg cimetidine.

Pale green, oblong, film-coated tablets, engraved TAGAMET on one side and SK&F 400 on reverse, containing 400 mg cimetidine.

Pale green, circular, film-coated tablets, engraved TAGAMET on one side and SK&F 200 on reverse, containing 200 mg cimetidine.

A clear, orange-coloured, peach-flavoured syrup, each 5 ml dose containing 200 mg cimetidine.

Ampoules containing 200 mg cimetidine in 2 ml solution.

Infusion bags (flexible plastic containers) containing 400 mg cimetidine in 100 ml 0.9% w/v sodium chloride.

Uses Tagamet is a histamine H_2-receptor antagonist which rapidly inhibits both basal and stimulated gastric secretion of acid and reduces pepsin output.

Tagamet is indicated in the treatment of duodenal and benign gastric ulceration, recurrent and stomal ulceration, oesophageal reflux disease and other conditions where reduction of gastric acid by Tagamet has been shown to be beneficial: persistent dyspeptic symptoms with or without ulceration, particularly meal-related upper abdominal pain; the prophylaxis of gastro-intestinal haemorrhage from stress ulceration in seriously ill patients; before general anaesthesia in patients thought to be at risk of acid aspiration (Mendelson's) syndrome, particularly obstetric patients during labour; and to reduce malabsorption and fluid loss in the short bowel syndrome. Tagamet is also recommended in the management of the Zollinger-Ellison syndrome.

Dosage and administration Tagamet is usually given orally, but parenteral or nasogastric dosing may be substituted for all or part of the recommended oral dose in cases where oral dosing is impracticable or considered inappropriate.

The total daily dose by any route should not normally exceed 2.4 g. Dosage should be reduced in patients with impaired renal function (see *Cautions*).

Adults: Oral: The usual dosage is 400 mg twice a day with breakfast and at bedtime. For patients with duodenal or benign gastric ulceration, a single daily dose of 800 mg at bedtime is recommended. Other effective regimens are 200 mg three times a day with meals and 400 mg at bedtime (1.0 g/day) and, if inadequate, 400 mg four times a day (1.6 g/day) also with meals and at bedtime.

Symptomatic relief is usually rapid. Treatment should be given initially for at least four weeks (six weeks in benign gastric ulcer). Most ulcers will have healed by that stage, but those which have not will usually do so after a further course of treatment.

Treatment may be continued for longer periods in those patients who may benefit from reduction of gastric secretion and the dosage may be reduced as appropriate to 400 mg at bedtime or 400 mg in the morning and at bedtime.

In patients with benign peptic ulcer disease, relapse may be prevented by continued treatment, usually with 400 mg at bedtime; 400 mg in the morning and at bedtime has also been used.

In oesophageal reflux disease, 400 mg four times a day, with meals and at bedtime, for four to eight weeks is recommended to heal oesophagitis and relieve associated symptoms.

In patients with very high gastric acid secretion (e.g. Zollinger-Ellison syndrome) it may be necessary to increase the dose to 400 mg four times a day, or in occasional cases further.

Antacids can be made available to all patients until symptoms disappear.

In the prophylaxis of haemorrhage from stress ulceration in seriously ill patients, doses of 200–400 mg can be given every four to six hours by oral, nasogastric or parenteral routes. By direct intravenous injection a dose of 200 mg should not be exceeded: see below.

In patients thought to be at risk of acid aspiration syndrome an oral dose of 400 mg can be given 90–120 minutes before induction of general anaesthesia or, in obstetric practice, at the start of labour. While such a risk persists, a dose of up to 400 mg may be repeated (parenterally if appropriate) at four-hourly intervals as required up to the usual daily maximum of 2.4 g. Tagamet syrup should not be used. The usual precautions to avoid acid aspiration should be taken.

In the short bowel syndrome, e.g. following substantial resection for Crohn's disease, the usual dosage range (see above) can be used according to individual response.

Parenteral: Tagamet may be given intravenously or intramuscularly.

The usual dosage for intravenous administration is 200–400 mg which may be repeated four- to six-hourly.

For direct intravenous injection, 200 mg should be given **slowly** over at least 2 minutes, and may be repeated four- to six-hourly. If there is cardiovascular impairment, or if a larger dose is needed, the dose should be diluted and given over at least 10 minutes. In such cases infusion is preferable.

For intermittent intravenous infusion, the contents of one Tagamet Infusion bag (containing cimetidine 400 mg in 100 ml 0.9% w/v sodium chloride) should be infused over 30 minutes to 1 hour, and may be repeated every four to six hours.

If continuous intravenous infusion is required, Tagamet may be given at an average rate of 50 to 100 mg/hour over 24 hours.

The dose by intramuscular injection is normally 200 mg which may be repeated at four- to six-hourly intervals.

Elderly: The normal adult dosage may be used unless renal function is markedly impaired (see *Cautions* and *Adverse reactions*).

Children: Experience in children is less than that in adults. In children more than one year old, Tagamet 25–30 mg/kg body weight per day in divided doses may be administered by either the oral or parenteral route.

The use of Tagamet in infants under one year old is not fully evaluated; 20 mg/kg body weight per day in divided doses has been used.

Contra-indications, warnings, etc
No known contra-indications.

Cautions: Dosage should be reduced in patients with impaired renal function according to creatinine clearance. The following dosages are suggested: creatinine clearance of 0 to 15 ml per minute, 200 mg twice a day; 15 to 30 ml per minute, 200 mg three times a day; 30 to

50 ml per minute, 200 mg four times a day; over 50 ml per minute, normal dosage. Cimetidine is removed by haemodialysis, but not to any significant extent by peritoneal dialysis.

Tagamet can prolong the elimination of drugs metabolised by oxidation in the liver. Although pharmacological interactions with a number of drugs, e.g. diazepam, propranolol, have been demonstrated, only those with oral anticoagulants, phenytoin and theophylline appear, to date, to be of clinical significance. Close monitoring of patients on Tagamet receiving oral anticoagulants or phenytoin is recommended and a reduction in the dosage of these drugs may be necessary.

Clinical trials of over five years' continuous treatment and more than nine years' widespread use have not revealed unexpected adverse reactions related to long-term therapy. The safety of prolonged use is not, however, fully established and care should be taken to observe periodically patients given prolonged treatment.

Tagamet treatment can relieve the symptoms and allow superficial healing of gastric cancer. The potential delay in diagnosis should particularly be borne in mind in patients of middle age and over with new or recently changed dyspeptic symptoms.

In patients on drug treatment or with illnesses that could cause falls in blood cell count, the possibility that H_2-receptor antagonism could potentiate this effect should be borne in mind.

Use in pregnancy and lactation: Although tests in animals have not revealed any hazards from the administration of Tagamet during pregnancy or lactation, both these and studies in women have shown that it does cross the placental barrier and is excreted in milk. As with most drugs, the use of Tagamet should be avoided during pregnancy and lactation unless essential.

Adverse reactions: More than 35 million patients have been treated with Tagamet worldwide and adverse reactions have been infrequent. Diarrhoea, dizziness or rash, usually mild and transient, and tiredness have been reported. Gynaecomastia has been reported and is almost always reversible on discontinuing treatment. Biochemical or biopsy evidence of reversible liver damage has been reported occasionally. Reversible confusional states have occurred, usually in elderly or already very ill patients, e.g. those with renal failure. There have been very rare reports of interstitial nephritis, acute pancreatitis, thrombocytopenia, headache, myalgia and arthralgia, all reversible on withdrawal of treatment. Alopecia has been reported but no causal relationship has been established. Reversible impotence has also been very rarely reported but no causal relationship has been established at usual therapeutic doses. Isolated increases of plasma creatinine have been of no clinical significance.

Overdosage: Acute overdosage of up to 20 grams has been reported several times with no significant ill effects. Induction of vomiting and/or gastric lavage may be employed together with symptomatic and supportive therapy.

Pharmaceutical precautions Store syrup below 25°C, and ampoules below 30° C, protected from light.

Store infusion bags below 25°C, and protect from light except during use.

Legal category POM.

Package quantities Tablets, 800 mg, in calendar packs of 30 and blister packs of 150. Tablets, 400 mg, in calendar packs of 60, ward packs of 50 and in containers of 2,500. Tablets, 200 mg in blister packs of 120 and containers of 500 and 5,000. Syrup in bottles containing 500 ml. Ampoules in boxes of 20. Infusion bags in boxes of 20.

Further information Tagamet has been shown to be compatible with electrolyte and dextrose solutions commonly used for intravenous infusion.

Product licence numbers

Tagamet tablets 800 mg	0002/0128
Tagamet tablets 400 mg	0002/0092
Tagamet tablets 200 mg	0002/0063
Tagamet syrup	0002/0073
Tagamet injection	0002/0059
Tagamet infusion	0002/0112

VERTIGON* SPANSULE* CAPSULES

Presentation Clear, colourless capsules, opaque purple-capped and filled with a mixture of yellow-green and white pellets, in two strengths. Each Spansule sustained-release capsule, size No. 4, contains 10 mg, and each capsule, size No. 3, 15 mg prochlorperazine present as the maleate. Two-thirds of the dose is specially formulated for sustained release over a period of six to eight hours.

Uses Vertigon is a potent phenothiazine tranquilliser, anti-emetic, and vestibular sedative.

Vertigon Spansule capsules are indicated in the short term symptomatic treatment of vertigo due to Menière's disease, labyrinthitis or other causes; nausea and vomiting associated with vertigo or other causes; and minor mental and emotional disturbances.

Dosage and administration *Adults and children aged 12 years and over:* Usually one 15 mg Vertigon Spansule capsule once or twice a day. In less severe cases one 10 mg capsule once or twice a day may be adequate. When satisfactory control has been achieved, a daily maintenance dosage of one 10 mg or 15 mg capsule may be given.

Elderly: Start with 10 mg once a day (see *Cautions*).

Contra-indications, warnings, etc

Contra-indications: Vertigon is contra-indicated in patients with existing blood dyscrasias, known liver damage or those hypersensitive to the active ingredient.

Cautions: Caution should be exercised when treating elderly patients or those with cardiovascular disease because of the possibility of hypotension.

Nausea and vomiting as a sign of organic disease may be masked by the anti-emetic action of Vertigon.

Potentiation may occur if this product is used with other CNS depressants.

Patients who drive or operate machinery should be warned of the possibility of drowsiness.

Use in pregnancy and lactation: Prochlorperazine has been available for many years, and there is no experimental or clinical evidence to suggest any associated hazard to the foetus. Nevertheless, drugs should be avoided in pregnancy unless essential, especially during the first trimester. Prochlorperazine passes into the milk of lactating dogs.

Adverse reactions: Drowsiness, dizziness, skin reactions, dry mouth and, rarely, hypotension may occur; effects such as amenorrhoea are extremely unusual at this dosage level.

Extrapyramidal reactions are very unlikely at the

recommended dosage, but at the higher dosage levels used in psychiatry they are considerably more common. If prolonged, such dosage with phenothiazines may be associated with skin pigmentation, and lenticular opacities. Tardive dyskinesia has occurred in some patients on long-term high-dosage and, more rarely, low-dosage phenothiazine therapy; this may be long-lasting or even irreversible.

Rare cases of toxic hepatitis of a cholestatic type, and leucopenia and agranulocytosis have been reported with prochlorperazine.

Overdosage: Signs and symptoms will be predominantly extrapyramidal; hypotension may occur. Absorption of prochlorperazine from the sustained-release Spansule capsule is likely to be prolonged, and this should be borne in mind. Treatment consists of gastric lavage together with appropriate supportive and symptomatic measures. Do not induce vomiting. Extrapyramidal symptoms may be treated with an anticholinergic antiparkinsonism drug. Treat hypotension with fluid replacement; if severe or persistent, noradrenaline may be considered. Adrenaline is contra-indicated.

Pharmaceutical precautions Store in a dry place at a temperature not exceeding 30°C and protect from light.

Legal category POM.

Package quantities Both strengths in containers of 100 Spansule capsules.

Further information Nil.

Product licence numbers
Vertigon Spansule capsules, 10 mg   0002/0036
Vertigon Spansule capsules, 15 mg   0002/0037

Z SPAN* SPANSULE* CAPSULES

Presentation Clear, colourless capsules, opaque light blue-capped and filled with a mixture of white and grey pellets. Each Spansule sustained-release capsule contains 61.8 mg zinc sulphate monohydrate (22.5 mg elemental zinc) formulated for release over one to two hours.

Uses Z Span is an oral zinc preparation for use when inadequate diet calls for supplementary zinc and when the need for such therapy has been determined by a physician, and for the treatment of zinc deficiency which has been demonstrated.

Dosage and administration *Adults and children over 1 year:* As a dietary supplement, 1 Z Span Spansule capsule a day. For the treatment of frank zinc deficiency, 1 capsule three times a day, to be adjusted thereafter according to response. The capsule may be opened and the pellets mixed with soft, cool food, but they must not be chewed.

Elderly: Dosage as above.

Contra-indications, warnings, etc
Cautions: Zinc chelates with tetracyclines and absorption of both agents may be impaired.

Excessive zinc intake over long periods may affect absorption of other metals such as iron or copper, but no clinically significant effect is expected at the dose of one capsule a day.

In patients with renal failure, a risk of accumulation could exist.

Adverse reactions: Mild gastro-intestinal upset is occasionally produced by zinc sulphate but the sustained-release presentation is designed to minimise this effect.

Overdosage: A single dose in excess of 10 capsules may be emetic. A fatal dose of zinc sulphate is unlikely to be less than 10 g (equivalent to more than 150 capsules). Zinc sulphate in gross overdosage is corrosive. Symptoms are those of gastro-intestinal irritation, leading in severe cases to haemorrhage, corrosion of the mucosa and possible later stricture formation. Gastric lavage or emesis should be avoided. Demulcents such as milk should be given. Chelating agents such as dimercaprol, penicillamine or edetic acid have been recommended.

Symptomatic and supportive therapy should be given. Absorption of zinc may be slowed by the sustained-release presentation.

Pharmaceutical precautions Store in a dry place at a temperature not exceeding 30°C.

Legal category P.

Package quantities Containers of 30 Spansule capsules.

Further information Nil.

Product licence number 0002/0098.

*Trade Mark

E. R. Squibb & Sons Limited
Squibb House
Staines Rd
Hounslow TW3 3JA

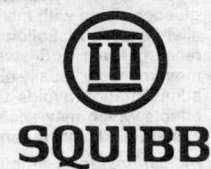

SQUIBB

ADCORTYL* CREAM, OINTMENT AND ADCORTYL* IN ORABASE*

Presentation *Cream:* White cream containing triamcinolone acetonide 0.1% in an aqueous vanishing cream base.

Ointment: White, nearly translucent, containing triamcinolone acetonide 0.1% in Plastibase.*

Adcortyl in Orabase: White to light tan crystalline paste containing triamcinolone acetonide 0.1% in Orabase (gelatin, pectin and sodium carboxymethylcellulose in Plastibase*).

Uses *Actions:* Triamcinolone acetonide is a potent fluorinated corticosteroid with rapid anti-inflammatory, antipruritic and anti-allergic actions.

Indications: Adcortyl Cream and Ointment are recommended in steroid-responsive conditions which may include: atopic eczema, contact eczema, follicular eczema, infantile eczema, otitis externa, anogenital eczema (pruritus ani et vulvae), nummular eczema, seborrhoeic or flexural eczema, neurodermatitis, psoriasis, sunburn, insect bites.

Adcortyl in Orabase is indicated for aphthous ulcers, ulcerative stomatitis, denture stomatitis, desquamative gingivitis, erosive lichen planus and lesions of traumatic origin.

Dosage and administration *Adults and children:*
Cream: To be applied to moist, weeping lesions two to four times daily.

Ointment: To be applied to dry, scaly lesions two to four times daily.

Adcortyl in Orabase: To be applied to the lesion two to four times daily. Apply to the affected area; do not rub in.

Elderly: Natural thinning of the skin occurs in the elderly; hence corticosteroids should be used sparingly and for short periods of time.

Contra-indications, warnings, etc
Contra-indications: In tuberculous and most viral lesions of the skin, particularly herpes simplex, vaccinia, varicella. The products should not be used in fungal or bacterial skin infections without suitable concomitant anti-infective therapy.

Precautions: Adrenal suppression can occur, even without occlusion.

Children: In infants, long-term, continuous topical steroid therapy should be avoided.

Pregnancy: Topical administration of corticosteroids to pregnant animals can cause abnormalities of foetal development. The relevance of this finding to humans has not been established. However, topical steroids should not be used extensively in pregnancy, i.e. in large amounts or for long periods. Topical corticosteroids should be used during pregnancy only if the potential benefit justifies the potential risk to the foetus.

Side-effects: Triamcinolone acetonide is well tolerated. Where adverse reactions occur they are usually reversible on cessation of therapy. However the following side-effects have been reported usually with prolonged usage:

Dermatologic – impaired wound healing, thinning of the skin, petechiae and ecchymoses, facial erythema and telangiectasia, increased sweating, purpura, striae, hirsutism, acneiform eruptions, lupus erythematosus-like lesions and suppressed reactions to skin tests.

These effects may be enhanced with occlusive dressings.

Signs of systemic toxicity such as oedema and electrolyte imbalance have not been observed even when high topical dosage has been used. The possibility of the systemic effects which are associated with all steroid therapy should be considered.

Overdosage: Topically applied corticosteroids can be absorbed in sufficient amounts to produce systemic effects (see Side-effects).

Pharmaceutical precautions *Storage:*
Cream: At room temperature; avoid freezing.

Ointment: At room temperature.

Adcortyl in Orabase: At room temperature.

Dilution: Cream: Cetomacrogol Cream (formula B) BPC or Aqueous Cream BP. Preservative cover may be reduced depending on diluent. Diluted creams should be stored below 25°C and should be discarded two weeks after dilution.

Ointment: White soft paraffin.

Adcortyl in Orabase: Should not be diluted. The manufacturer's advice should be sought before dilution with any other preparation.

Legal category POM.

Package quantities
Cream: Tubes of 30 g.
Ointment: Tubes of 30 g.
Adcortyl in Orabase: Tubes of 10 g.

Further information Nil.

Product licence numbers
Adcortyl Cream   0034/5000
Adcortyl Ointment   0034/5004
Adcortyl in Orabase   0034/5006

ADCORTYL* INTRA-ARTICULAR/INTRADERMAL

Presentation Sterile aqueous suspension containing triamcinolone acetonide 10 mg per ml.

Uses *Actions:* Triamcinolone acetonide is a synthetic glucocorticoid with marked anti-inflammatory and anti-allergic actions. Following local injection of Adcortyl, relief of pain and swelling and greater freedom of movement are usually obtained within a few hours; such administration avoids the more severe systemic side-effects which may accompany parenteral or oral corti-costeroid administration.

Indications: Intra-articular use: for alleviating the joint pain, swelling and stiffness associated with rheumatoid arthritis and osteoarthrosis; also for bursitis, epicondylitis, and tenosynovitis.

Intradermal use: for lichen simplex chronicus (neuro-dermatitis), granuloma annulare, lichen planus, keloids, alopecia areata and hypertrophic scars.

Dosage and administration Adcortyl injection is not for intravenous use. Strict aseptic precautions should be observed. Since the duration of effect is variable, subsequent doses should be given when symptoms recur and not at set intervals.

Adults: The dose of Adcortyl injection for intra-articular administration, and injection into tendon sheaths and bursae, is dependent on the size of the joint to be treated and on the severity of the condition. Doses of 2.5-5 mg (0.25-0.5 ml) for smaller joints and 5-15 mg (0.5-1.5 ml) for larger joints usually alleviate the symptoms. (Triamcinolone acetonide 40 mg/ml (Kenalog) is avail-able to facilitate administration of larger doses). See Precautions re Achilles tendon.

Intradermal dosage is usually 2-3 mg (0.2-0.3 ml), depending on the size of the lesion. No more than 5 mg (0.5 ml) should be injected at any one site. If several sites are injected the total dosage administered should not exceed 30 mg (3 ml). The injection may be repeated if necessary, at one or two week intervals.

Children: Adcortyl is not recommended in children under 6 years. Adcortyl intra-articular/intradermal may be used in older children in suitably adjusted dosages. Growth and development of children on prolonged corticosteroid therapy should be carefully observed.

Elderly: Treatment of elderly patients, particularly if long term, should be planned bearing in mind the more serious consequences of the common side effects of cortico-steroids in old age, especially osteoporosis, diabetes, hypertension, susceptibility to infection and thinning of the skin.

Contra-indications, warnings, etc
Contra-indications: None.

Precautions: In common with other steroids Adcortyl injection should be used with caution in patients with recent intestinal anastomoses, thrombophlebitis, psy-chotic tendencies, exanthematous disease, chronic ne-phritis, metastatic carcinoma, osteoporosis, in patients with an active peptic ulcer (or a history of peptic ulcer). Latent or healed tuberculosis; in the presence of local or systemic viral infection, systemic fungal infections or in active infections not controlled by antibiotics. In acute psychoses; in acute glomerulonephritis. Hypertension; glaucoma (or a family history of glaucoma), previous steroid myopathy or epilepsy.

Intra-articular injection should not be carried out in the presence of active infection in or near joints. The preparation should not be used to alleviate joint pain arising from infectious states such as gonococcal or tubercular arthritis.

Diabetes may be aggravated, necessitating a higher insulin dosage. Latent diabetes mellitus may be precipi-tated.

Menstrual irregularities may occur, and this possibility should be mentioned to female patients.

Patients on long-term systemic therapy with Adcortyl may require supportive corticosteroid therapy in times of stress, both during the treatment period and for a year afterwards.

During corticosteroid therapy antibody response will be reduced and therefore affect the patient's response to vaccines.

Rare instances of anaphylactoid reactions have oc-curred in patients receiving parenteral corticosteroids, especially when a patient has a history of drug allergies.

All corticosteroids increase calcium excretion.

Avoid abrupt cessation of corticosteroids.

Aspirin should be used cautiously in conjunction with corticosteroids in patients with hypoprothrombinaemia.

Corticosteroid effects may be enhanced in patients with hypothyrodism or cirrhosis.

Pregnancy: Corticosteroids are not recommended for pregnant patients, particularly in the first trimester, or for nursing mothers, except when the disease for which they are indicated warrants their use. There is inadequate evidence of safety in human pregnancy and there may be a very small risk of cleft palate and intra-uterine growth retardation in the foetus; there is evidence of harmful effects on pregnancy in animals.

Intra-articular injection: Patients should be specifically warned to avoid over-use of joints in which symptomatic benefit has been obtained. Severe joint destruction with necrosis of bone may occur if repeated intra-articular injections are given over a long period of time. Care should be taken if injections are given into tendon sheaths to avoid injection into the tendon itself.

Due to the absence of a true tendon sheath, the Achilles tendon should not be injected with depot corticosteroids.

Side-effects: Where adverse reactions occur they are usually reversible on cessation of therapy. Absorption of triamcinolone following Adcortyl injection, especially when given by the intra-articular route, is rare. However, the possibility of the systemic effects which are associ-ated with all steroid therapy should be considered. These may include:

Dyspepsia, peptic ulceration with perforation and haemorrhage, abdominal distension, oesophageal ulcer-ation, oesophageal candidiasis, acute pancreatitis.

Proximal myopathy, osteoporosis, vertebral and long bone fractures, avascular osteonecrosis, tendon rupture.

Sodium and water retention, hypertension, hypoka-laemic alkalosis.

Impaired healing, skin atrophy, bruising, striae, telan-giectasia, acne.

Suppression of the hypothalamo-pituitary adrenal axis, growth suppression in childhood and adolescence, menstrual irregularity and amenorrhoea. Cushingoid facies, hirsutism, weight gain, impaired carbohydrate tolerance with increased requirement for antidiabetic therapy, negative nitrogen balance.

Euphoria, psychological dependence, depression, in-somnia. Intracranial hypertension has been reported in children on cessation of long term steroid therapy. Aggravation of schizophrenia.

Increased intra-ocular pressure, glaucoma, papilloe-dema, cataracts, corneal or scleral thinning, exacerbation of ophthalmic viral disease.

Opportunistic infection, recurrence of dormant tuberculosis, leucocytosis, hypersensitivity, thromboembolism, increased appetite, nausea, malaise.

On withdrawal fever, myalgia, arthralgia or adrenal insufficiency may occur.

Intra-articular injection: Reactions following intra-articular administration have been rare. In a few instances transient flushing and dizziness have occurred. Pain and other local symptoms may continue for a short time before effective relief is obtained, but an increase in joint discomfort has seldom occurred. Local fat atrophy may occur if the injection is not given into the joint space, but is temporary and disappears within a few weeks to months.

Pharmaceutical precautions *Storage:* In an upright position at room temperature: avoid freezing.

Legal category POM.

Package quantities Multidose vials of 5 ml. Ampoules 5 × 1 ml.

Further information Nil.

Product licence number 0034/5002.

ADCORTYL* WITH GRANEODIN* CREAM AND OINTMENT

Presentation *Cream:* White vanishing cream.

Ointment: Smooth, soft, translucent ointment in Plastibase*.

Each gram of the cream and ointment contains:

Triamcinolone acetonide   0.1%
Neomycin (as sulphate)   0.25%
Gramicidin   0.025%

Uses *Actions:* Triamcinolone acetonide is a potent fluorinated corticosteroid with rapid anti-inflammatory, antipruritic and anti-allergic actions.

The combined action of the antibiotics neomycin and gramicidin provides comprehensive antibacterial therapy against a wide range of Gram-positive and Gram-negative bacteria, including those micro-organisms responsible for most bacterial skin infections.

Indications: For the treatment of inflammatory dermatoses, which are complicated or threatened by secondary infection such as: atopic eczema, contact eczema, follicular eczema, infantile eczema, otitis externa, anogenital pruritus (pruritus ani et vulvae), psoriasis, nummular eczema, post-traumatic infective eczema, seborrhoeic or flexural eczema, neurodermatitis.

Dosage and administration *Adults and children:* Apply to the affected areas two to four times daily.

Elderly: Natural thinning of the skin occurs in the elderly; hence corticosteroids should be used sparingly and for short periods of time.

Contra-indications, warnings, etc
Contra-indications: In tuberculous and most viral lesions of the skin, particularly herpes simplex, vaccinia, varicella. The products should not be used in fungal or bacterial skin infections without suitable concomitant anti-infective therapy.

In patients with hypersensitivity to any of the components.

Should not be applied to the external auditory canal in patients with perforated eardrums.

Precautions: Adrenal suppression can occur, even without occlusion. The use of occlusive dressings should be avoided because of the increased risk of sensitivity reactions and increased percutaneous absorption. The possibility of sensitivity to neomycin should be taken into consideration especially in the treatment of patients suffering from leg ulcers.

Children: In infants, long-term, continuous topical steroid therapy should be avoided.

Pregnancy: Topical administration of corticosteroids to pregnant animals can cause abnormalities of foetal development. The relevance of this finding to humans has not been established. However, topical steroids should not be used extensively in pregnancy, i.e. in large amounts or for long periods. Topical corticosteroids should be used during pregnancy only if the potential benefit justifies the potential risk to the foetus.

Side-effects: Triamcinolone acetonide: Is well tolerated. Where adverse reactions occur they are usually reversible on cessation of therapy. However the following side-effects have been reported, usually with prolonged usage:

Dermatologic – impaired wound healing, thinning of the skin, petechiae and ecchymoses, facial erythema and telangiectasia, increased sweating, purpura, striae, hirsutism, acneiform eruptions, lupus erythematosus-like lesions and suppressed reactions to skin tests.

These effects may be enhanced with occlusive dressings.

Signs of systemic toxicity such as oedema and electrolyte imbalance have not been observed even when high topical dosage has been used. The possibility of the systemic effects which are associated with all steroid therapy should be considered.

Neomycin: Sensitivity reactions may occur especially with prolonged use. Ototoxicity and nephrotoxicity have been reported. Large amounts of this product should be avoided in the treatment of skin infections following extensive burns, trophic ulceration and other conditions where absorption of neomycin is possible.

Gramicidin: Sensitivity has occasionally been reported.

Overdosage: Topically applied corticosteroids can be absorbed in sufficient amounts to produce systemic effects (see Side-effects).

Pharmaceutical precautions *Storage: Cream:* At room temperature; avoid freezing.

Ointment: At room temperature.

Dilution: Not recommended, as this would reduce the concentration of the antibiotics to below therapeutic levels.

Legal category POM.

Package quantities *Cream/Ointment:* 15 g tubes

Further information Nil.

Product licence numbers
Adcortyl with Graneodin Cream   0034/5015
Adcortyl with Graneodin Ointment   0034/5017

CAPOTEN* TABLETS ▼

Presentation *Capoten Tablets 12.5 mg:* Slightly mottled, white, flat-faced, bevel-edged, capsule-shaped tablets each containing captopril 12.5 mg, with a partial bisect bar on one side.

Capoten Tablets 25 mg: Slightly mottled, white, square

biconvex tablets each containing captopril 25 mg. Engraved with 'Squibb' and '452' on one side and with quadrisect bars (for identification only) on the other.

Capoten Tablets 50 mg: Slightly mottled, white, oval, biconvex tablets each containing captopril 50 mg. Engraved with 'Squibb' and '482' on one side with a bisecting bar on the other.

Uses
Actions: Captopril, 1-[(2S)-3-mercapto-2-methyl-propionyl]-L-proline, is a highly specific competitive inhibitor of angiotensin I-converting enzyme, the enzyme responsible for the conversion of angiotensin I to angiotensin II.

Until further experience has been obtained in the treatment of acute hypertensive crises, the use of Capoten should be avoided in these patients.

Indications
Hypertension: Mild to moderate hypertension as an adjunct to thiazide therapy in patients who have not responded effectively to thiazide treatment alone.

Severe hypertension where standard therapy has failed.

Congestive heart failure: Capoten is indicated for the treatment of severe, treatment-refractory congestive heart failure. The drug should be used together with diuretics and, where appropriate digitalis, but only after these agents have failed to produce a satisfactory response.

Dosage and administration
Recommended dose and dosage schedule
Hypertension: Treatment with Capoten should be at the lowest effective dose, which should be titrated according to the needs of the patient.

Mild to moderate hypertension: In mild to moderate hypertension Capoten therapy should be used as an adjunct to thiazide therapy. The starting dose is 12.5 mg twice daily. The usual maintenance dose is 25 mg twice daily which can be increased incrementally, at 2–4 week intervals, until a satisfactory response is achieved, to a maximum of 50 mg twice daily.

Severe hypertension: In severe hypertension the starting dose is 12.5 mg b.d. The dosage may be increased incrementally to a maximum of 50 mg t.i.d. Capoten should be used together with other anti-hypertensive agents but the dose of these should be individually titrated. A daily dose of 150 mg of Capoten should not normally be exceeded.

Heart failure: Capoten therapy must be started under close medical supervision. The usual dose is 25 mg three times a day. A starting dose of 6.25 mg or 12.5 mg may minimise a transient hypotensive effect. The usual maximum dose is 150 mg daily. Increases in dosage should be delayed for at least two weeks to determine if a satisfactory response has occurred.

Capoten should be used in conjunction with a diuretic and where appropriate digitalis.

Elderly: The dose should be titrated against the blood pressure response and kept as low as possible to achieve adequate control. Since elderly patients may have reduced renal function and other organ dysfunctions, it is suggested that a low dose of Capoten be used initially.

Children: Capoten is not recommended for the treatment of mild to moderate hypertension in children.

Safety and effectiveness in children have not been established. Experience in neonates and premature infants is limited.

The starting dose should be 0.3 mg per Kg bodyweight up to a maximum of 6 mg per Kg bodyweight in divided daily doses. The dose should be individualised according to the response and may be given two or three times daily.

Patients with renal impairment: Capoten is not recommended in patients with renal impairment. Where it is clinically indicated in severely hypertensive patients with impaired renal function, the dose should be kept as low as possible to maintain adequate blood pressure control. The dose can be titrated against the response but adequate time should be allowed between dosage adjustments.

In these patients a loop-diuretic rather than a thiazide should be the diuretic of choice.

Capoten is readily eliminated by haemodialysis.

Contra-indications, warnings, etc
Contra-indications: A history of previous hypersensitivity to captopril.

Pregnancy: Capoten has been shown to be lethal to rabbit and sheep foetuses. There were no foetotoxic effects to hamster or rat foetuses.

Capoten is contra-indicated in pregnancy and should not be used in women of child bearing potential unless protected by effective contraception.

Precautions: Evaluation of the hypertensive patient should include assessment of renal function prior to initiation of therapy. Patients with renal impairment should not normally be treated with Capoten.

Capoten should not be used in patients with aortic stenosis or outflow tract obstruction.

Warnings: The incidence of adverse reactions to Capoten is principally associated with renal function since the drug is excreted primarily by the kidney. The dose should not exceed that necessary for adequate control and should be reduced in patients with impaired renal function.

Haematological: Neutropenia/agranulocytosis, thrombocytopenia and anaemia have been reported in patients receiving Capoten.

In patients with normal renal function and no other complicating factors, neutropenia occurs rarely.

Capoten should not be used routinely in patients with pre-existing impaired renal function, collagen vascular disease, immunosuppressant therapy, treatment with allopurinol or procainamide, or a combination of these complicating factors, because neutropenia has been limited almost exclusively to this group. Some of these patients developed serious infections which in a few instances did not respond to intensive antibiotic therapy. If Capoten is used in such patients, it is advised that white blood cell count and differential counts should be performed prior to therapy, every 2 weeks during the first 3 months of Capoten therapy, and periodically thereafter.

During treatment, all patients should be instructed to report any sign of infection (e.g. sore throat, fever), when a differential white blood cell count should be performed. Capoten and other concomitant medication should be withdrawn if neutropenia (neutrophils less than 1000/mm^3) is detected or suspected.

In most patients neutrophil counts rapidly returned to normal upon discontinuing Capoten.

Renal: Proteinuria in patients with prior normal renal function is rare. Where PROTEINURIA has occurred it has usually been in patients with severe hypertension and evidence of prior renal disease. Nephrotic syndrome occurred in some of these patients.

In patients with evidence of prior renal disease, monthly urinary protein estimations (dip stick) are recommended for the first 9 months of therapy. If repeated determinations show increasing amounts of urinary protein a 24-hour quantitative determination should be obtained, and if this exceeds 1 g/day, the benefits and risks of continuing Capoten should be evaluated.

Although membranous glomerulopathy was found in biopsies taken from some proteinuric patients, a causal relationship to Capoten has not been established.

Some patients with renal disease, particularly those with bilateral renal artery stenosis or unilateral renal artery stenosis in a single functioning kidney, have developed increased concentrations of blood urea and serum creatinine. Capoten dosage reduction and/or discontinuation of diuretic may be required. For some of these patients it may not be possible to normalise blood pressure and maintain adequate renal perfusion.

Hypotension: With the first one or two doses some patients may experience symptomatic hypotension. In most instances, symptoms are relieved simply by the patient lying down.

In patients with severe and renin dependent hypertension (e.g. renovascular hypertension) or severe congestive heart failure, who are receiving large doses of diuretic, exaggerated hypotensive responses have occurred, usually within one hour of the initial dose of Capoten. In these patients, by discontinuing diuretic therapy or significantly reducing the diuretic dose for four to seven days prior to initiating Capoten the possibility of this occurrence is reduced. By commencing Capoten therapy with small doses (6.25 mg or 12.5 mg) the duration of any hypotensive effect is lessened. Some patients may benefit from an infusion of saline.

The occurrence of first dose hypotension does not preclude subsequent dose titration with Capoten.

Serum potassium: Since Capoten decreases aldosterone production, serum potassium is usually maintained in patients on diuretics. Potassium sparing diuretics or potassium supplements should not therefore be used routinely. In patients with marked renal impairment a significant elevation of serum potassium may occur.

Nursing mothers: Because captopril is excreted in breast milk, Capoten should not be used in nursing mothers.

Surgery/anaesthesia: In patients undergoing major surgery, or during anaesthesia with agents which produce hypotension, Capoten will block angiotensin II formation secondary to compensatory renin release. This may lead to hypotension which can be corrected by volume expansion.

Clinical chemistry: Capoten may cause a false-positive urine test for acetone.

Side-effects

Haematological: Neutropenia, anaemia and thrombocytopenia (see Warnings).

Renal: Proteinuria, elevated blood urea and creatinine, elevated serum potassium and acidosis (see Warnings).

Cardiovascular: Hypotension (see Warnings), tachycardia.

Skin: Rashes, usually pruritic, may occur. They are usually mild, transient and maculopapular, rarely urticarial. In a few cases the rash has been associated with fever and some patients have developed angio-neurotic oedema. Pruritis, flushing vesicular rash, and photosensitivity have been reported.

Gastrointestinal: Reversible and usually self-limiting taste impairment has been reported. Weight loss may be associated with the loss of taste. Stomatitis, resembling aphthous ulcers, has been reported. Elevation of liver enzymes has been noted in a few patients. Rare cases of hepatocellular injury and cholestatic jaundice have been reported. Gastric irritation and abdominal pain may occur.

Other: Paraesthesias of the hands, serum sickness, cough, bronchospasm and lymphadenopathy have been reported.

Overdosage: In the event of overdosage, blood pressure should be monitored and if hypotension develops volume expansion is the treatment of choice. Captopril is removed by dialysis.

Drug interactions

Diuretics: Diuretics potentiate the anti-hypertensive effectiveness of Capoten.

Potassium-sparing diuretics (triamterene, amiloride and spironolactone), or potassium supplements may cause significant increase in serum potassium.

Indomethacin: A reduction of anti-hypertensive effectiveness may occur. This is probably also the case with other non-steroidal anti-inflammatory drugs.

Vasodilators: Capoten has been reported to act synergistically with peripheral vasodilators such as minoxidil. Awareness of this interaction may avert an initial hypotensive response.

Clonidine: It has been suggested that the anti-hypertensive effect of Capoten can be delayed when patients treated with clonidine are changed to Capoten.

Allopurinol and procainamide: There have been reports of neutropenia and/or Stevens-Johnson syndrome in patients on Capoten plus either allopurinol or procainamide. Although a causal relationship has not been established, these combinations should only be used with caution, especially in patients with impaired renal function.

Immunosuppressants: Azathioprine and cyclophosphamide have been associated with blood dyscrasias in patients with renal failure who were also taking Capoten.

Probenecid: The renal clearance of Capoten is reduced in the presence of probenecid.

Pharmaceutical precautions Store at room temperature.

Legal category POM.

Package quantities
Tablets 12.5 mg: Bottles of 100 tablets.
Tablets 25 and 50 mg: Blister packs of 56 and 90 and bottles of 100 tablets.

Further information Nil.

Product licence numbers
12.5 mg   0034/0221
25 mg   0034/0193
50 mg   0034/0194

CORGARD* TABLETS

Presentation Pale blue, round, biconvex tablets. The 80 mg nadolol tablet is scored on one side and engraved 'Squibb' and '241' while the 40 mg nadolol tablet is unscored with 'Squibb' and '207' engraved on one side.

Uses *Actions:* Nadolol is a beta-adrenergic receptor blocking agent with a prolonged activity, permitting once-daily dosage in angina, hypertension, cardiac arrhythmias, the prophylaxis of migraine, and the relief of hyperthyroid symptoms.

Nadolol is not metabolised. It has no membrane stabilising or intrinsic sympathomimetic activity, and its only effect on the autonomic nervous system is one of beta-adrenergic blockade. Nadolol is nonselective.

Receptor blockade by nadolol results in protection from excessive inappropriate sympathetic activity. Nadolol reduces the number and severity of attacks of angina pectoris by blocking response to catecholamine stimulation and thus lowers the oxygen requirement of the heart at any given level of effort.

Nadolol reduces both supine and erect blood pressure. Like other beta-blockers nadolol exerts an antiarrhythmic action. Nadolol has been shown to reduce the rapid ventricular response which accompanies atrial fibrillation/flutter by slowing conduction through the A-V node. Beta-blockade is of particular value in arrhythmias caused by increased levels of, or sensitivity of the heart to, circulating catecholamines, e.g. arrhythmias associated with phaeochromocytoma, thyrotoxicosis, or exercise. Nadolol is effective in reducing ventricular premature beats in selected patients.

Nadolol exerts an effect in the prophylaxis of migraine by a mechanism which may involve prevention of vasoconstriction in the area served by the internal carotid artery and prevention of excessive adrenergic vasodilation in the external carotid artery.

Nadolol alleviates the symptoms of thyrotoxicosis and provides symptomatic control before and during thyroid surgery.

Beta-blocking agents have been shown in large scale studies to reduce mortality by preventing reinfarction and sudden death in patients surviving their first myocardial infarction.

Indications: Corgard is indicated in the management of:

Angina pectoris: For the long-term management of patients with angina pectoris by continuous medication.

Hypertension: For the long-term management of essential hypertension, either alone or in combination with other antihypertensive agents, especially thiazide-type diuretics.

Arrhythmias: For the treatment of cardiac tachyarrhythmias.

Migraine: For the prophylactic management of migraine headache. The efficacy of Corgard in the treatment of a migraine attack that has already started has not been established, and nadolol is not indicated for such use.

Thyrotoxicosis: For the relief of the symptoms of hyperthyroidism and the pre-operative preparation of patients for surgery. Nadolol may be used in conjunction with conventional antithyroid therapy.

Dosage and administration Dosage should be titrated gradually with at least a week between increments to assess response; individuals show considerable variation in their response to beta-adrenergic blockade.

Corgard may be given in a once daily dosage without regard to meals. The dosage interval should be increased when creatinine clearance is below 50 ml/min/1.73m².

If Corgard is to be discontinued, reduce dosage over a period of at least two weeks (see Warnings).

Angina pectoris: Initially 40 mg once daily. This may be increased at weekly intervals until an adequate response

is obtained or excessive bradycardia occurs. Most patients respond to 160 mg or less daily. The value and safety of daily doses exceeding 240 mg have not been established.

Hypertension: Initially 80 mg once daily. This may be increased by a weekly increment of 80 mg or less until an optimum response is obtained. Many patients respond to 80 mg daily and most patients respond to 240 mg or less, daily, but higher doses have been required for a few patients. In some patients it is necessary to administer a diuretic, peripheral vasodilator and/or other antihypertensive agents in conjunction with nadolol in order to achieve satisfactory response.

Treatment of hypertension associated with phaeochromocytoma may require the addition of an alpha-blocking agent.

Cardiac tachyarrhythmias: Initially 40 mg once daily. This may be increased if necessary to 160 mg once daily. If bradycardia occurs dosage should be reduced to 40 mg once daily.

Migraine: The initial dose of nadolol is 40 mg once daily. Dosage may be gradually increased in 40 mg increments until optimum migraine prophylaxis is achieved. The usual maintenance dose is 80 to 160 mg administered once daily. After 4 to 6 weeks at the maximum dose if a satisfactory response is not obtained, therapy with nadolol should be withdrawn gradually.

Thyrotoxicosis: The dosage range is 80–160 mg once daily. It has been found that most patients require a dose of 160 mg once daily. Nadolol may be used together with conventional anti-thyroid treatment. For the preparation of patients for partial thyroidectomy, nadolol should be administered in conjunction with potassium iodide for a period of 10 days prior to operation. Nadolol should be administered on the morning of operation. Post operatively nadolol dosage should be slowly reduced and then withdrawn following clinical stability.

Elderly patients: In elderly patients a low initial dose should be used so that sensitivity to side-effects may be assessed. As with all drugs, patients with impaired renal or hepatic function should be monitored.

Children: Safety and effectiveness in children have not been established.

Contra-indications, warnings, etc
Contra-indications: Like other drugs in this class, nadolol is contra-indicated in bronchial asthma or a history of asthma; sinus bradycardia and second and third degree heart block; cardiogenic shock; right ventricular failure secondary to pulmonary hypertension; congestive heart failure.

Warnings: Exacerbation of angina and myocardial infarction have occurred after abrupt discontinuation of therapy with beta-adrenergic blocking agents in patients with angina pectoris or other evidence of coronary artery insufficiency. When discontinuing long-term treatment with nadolol, the dosage should be reduced gradually over a period of at least two weeks and the patient carefully monitored.

Beta-adrenergic blockade carries the potential hazard of precipitating cardiac failure. Should this occur and it is not controlled by digitalisation, nadolol should be withdrawn, consideration being given to the foregoing warning.

Beta-blockade impairs the ability of the heart to respond to stress. It has been the usual practice to recommend withdrawal of beta-blockers several days prior to surgery.

However, this may render the patient's blood pressure unstable and difficult to control during anaesthesia and the anaesthetist may wish to advise on discontinuation of therapy. In no circumstances should beta-blockers be discontinued prior to surgery in patients with phaeo-chromocytoma or thyrotoxicosis. In the event of emergency surgery, the effects of nadolol may be reversed by isoprenaline or noradrenaline. However, such patients may be subject to protracted severe hypotension. General anaesthetics which can cause myocardial depression, such as cyclopropane, trichloroethylene, chloroform and ether, should be avoided if nadolol is continued during surgery.

Nadolol should be administered with caution to patients with chronic obstructive airways disease. Discontinue therapy if condition relapses.

Care should be exercised in the administration of nadolol to diabetic patients since early signs of acute hypoglycaemia may be masked. It may also be necessary to adjust the dosage of hypoglycaemic drugs or insulin doses.

There have been reports of skin rashes (including a psoriasiform type) and/or ocular changes (conjunctivitis and 'dry eye') associated with the use of beta-adrenergic blocking drugs. The reported incidence is small and in most cases the symptoms have cleared when the treatment was withdrawn. Discontinuance of the drug should be considered if any such reaction is not otherwise explicable. Cessation of therapy with a beta-adrenergic blocker should be gradual.

Beta-blockade may mask certain clinical signs (e.g. tachycardia) of hyperthyroidism. Patients suspected of developing thyrotoxicosis should be managed carefully to avoid abrupt withdrawal of beta-blockade which might precipitate a thyroid storm.

Precautions: Occasionally, beta-blockade with drugs such as nadolol may produce hypotension and/or marked bradycardia, resulting in vertigo, syncope or orthostatic hypotension.

Nadolol should be used with caution in patients with impaired renal or hepatic function.

Administration in renal failure: In patients with decreased renal function, dosage adjustment is necessary. The recommended dosage intervals are:

Creatinine Clearance (ml/min/1.73 m²)	Dosage Interval (Hours)
< 10	40–60
10–30	24–48
31–50	24–36
> 50	24

Use in pregnancy and nursing mothers: The safety of nadolol in pregnancy has not been established and animal studies have shown some foetotoxicity. Use of any drug in pregnancy or women of childbearing potential requires that the possible risk to the mother and/or foetus be weighed against the expected therapeutic benefit.

Nadolol is excreted in human milk; therefore nursing mothers should only receive nadolol if deemed essential.

Side-effects: Most patients tolerate nadolol well. Side-effects resemble those reported with other beta-blocking drugs and rarely require withdrawal of treatment. Those reported infrequently include gastrointestinal effects, bradycardia, fatigue, light-headedness, cold extremities, insomnia, paraesthesia, dryness of the mouth and

alopecia. Cardiac insufficiency, hypotension and AV block have occurred on rare occasions.

Overdosage or exaggerated response: Excessive brady-cardia should be treated initially with atropine. If there is no response, isoprenaline may be administered with caution.

Cardiac failure should be managed by digitalisation and diuretics. Glucagon has also been reported to be useful.

Hypotension may be managed with vasopressors such as adrenaline.

Bronchospasm may be counteracted by isoprenaline and aminophylline.

Drug interactions:

General anaesthetics: Those which cause myocardial depression such as chloroform, cyclopropane, trichloro-ethylene and ether should be avoided as the patient may be subject to protracted severe hypotension.

Myocardial depressants: Myocardial depressants such as lignocaine and procainamide may potentiate the hypotensive action of nadolol and lead to severe hypotension.

Adrenoceptor stimulants: Beta-adrenoceptor stimulants such as isoprenaline and alpha-adrenoceptor stimulants such as noradrenaline, adrenaline, will reverse the hypotensive effects and increase vasoconstrictor activity.

Catecholine depleting drugs: eg: reserpine. Excessive reduction in sympathetic drive to the heart might occur. Close observation is advised.

Antihypertensives (eg, neurone-blocking drugs, vasodilators, diuretics): Additive hypotensive effect.

Clonidine: If Corgard and clonidine are given concurrently, clonidine should not be discontinued until several days after Corgard withdrawal.

Hypoglycaemics, insulin: Possible dosage adjustment, see warnings.

Monoamine oxidase inhibitors: Administration of nadolol during and within 2 weeks of administration of adrenergic augmenting psychotropic drugs such as monoamine oxidase inhibitors, should be avoided, although the clinical significant is undetermined.

Pharmaceutical precautions Store at room temperature, protected from excessive heat and moisture in a tightly closed container.

Legal category POM.

Package quantities Calendar packs of 28.

Further information The lipid solubility of beta-blocking agents has been correlated with the extent to which these agents cross the blood-brain barrier and cause central nervous system-related side-effects. Corgard has a low lipid solubility.

Corgard has been demonstrated in both animal and clinical studies to preserve, and in some cases, increase renal blood flow upon acute and long-term administration in spite of a concurrent decrease in arterial pressure and cardiac output. Glomerular filtration rate remains unchanged, and renal vascular resistance is reduced, even in the presence of diuretic pretreatment. The exact mechanism of this effect of Corgard on the renal circulation has not been elucidated.

About 30 per cent of an oral dose of Corgard is absorbed. Peak serum concentrations usually occur in 3 to 4 hours after drug administration. The presence of food in the gastrointestinal tract does not affect the rate or extent of Corgard absorption. Approximately 30 per cent of the Corgard present in serum is reversibly bound to plasma protein. Unlike most available beta-blocking agents, Corgard is not metabolised, and is excreted unchanged principally by the kidneys. The serum half-life of therapeutic doses of Corgard is relatively long, ranging from 20 to 24 hours (permitting once daily dosage). A significant correlation between minimum steady-state serum concentrations of Corgard and total oral daily dose has been demonstrated in hypertensive patients; however, the observed dose-response range is wide and proper dosage requires individual titration.

Corgard can be efficiently removed from the general circulation by haemodialysis.

Product licence numbers
80 mg   0034/0186
40 mg   0034/0185.

CORGARETIC* TABLETS ▼

Presentation White, blue-speckled, round, biconvex tablets, in two strengths.

Corgaretic 40: nadolol 40 mg with bendrofluazide 5 mg is engraved 'Squibb' and '283' on one side with a bisect bar on the other.

Corgaretic 80: nadolol 80 mg with bendrofluazide 5 mg is engraved 'Squibb' and '284' on one side with a bisect bar on the other.

Uses *Actions:* Nadolol is a beta-adrenergic receptor blocking agent with a prolonged activity, permitting once-daily dosage.

Nadolol is not metabolised. It has no membrane stabilising or intrinsic sympathomimetic activity, and its only effect on the autonomic nervous system is one of beta-adrenergic blockade. Nadolol is nonselective.

Receptor blockade by nadolol results in protection from excessive or inappropriate sympathetic activity.

Nadolol reduces both supine and erect blood pressure.

Bendrofluazide is a thiazide diuretic which interferes with renal tubular electrolyte reabsorption, thereby increasing sodium and water excretion.

Indications: For the treatment of hypertension. The combination of a diuretic and a beta-blocker may be of particular value in patients whose blood pressure has not been adequately controlled with either component given alone.

Dosage and administration One or two tablets once daily to a maximum of 160 mg nadolol and 10 mg bendrofluazide. For doses of nadolol in excess of 160 mg, the combination product may not be appropriate because an excessive dose of the thiazide component may be administered.

The dosage should be titrated gradually with at least a week between increments to assess response; individuals show considerable variation in their response to beta-adrenergic blockade.

Corgaretic may be given in a once-daily dosage without regard to meals.

If Corgaretic is to be discontinued, reduce dosage over a period of at least two weeks (see Warnings).

Elderly patients: In elderly patients a low initial dose should be used so that sensitivity to side-effects may be assessed. As with all drugs, patients with impaired renal or hepatic function should be monitored.

Children: Safety and effectiveness in children have not been established.

Contra-indications, warnings, etc
Contra-indications: In bronchial asthma or a history of asthma; sinus bradycardia and second and third degree heart block; cardiogenic shock; right ventricular failure secondary to pulmonary hypertension; congestive heart failure, anuria, past sensitivity to thiazide diuretics or any sulphonamide-derived drugs.

Warnings: Exacerbation of angina and myocardial infarction have occurred after abrupt discontinuation of therapy with beta-adrenergic blocking agents in patients with angina pectoris or other evidence of coronary artery insufficiency. When discontinuing long-term treatment with nadolol, the dosage should be reduced gradually over a period of at least two weeks and the patient carefully monitored. If acute coronary insufficiency develops, temporarily reinstitute therapy with Corgard (nadolol) promptly.

Beta-adrenergic blockade carries the potential hazard of precipitating cardiac failure. Should this occur and it is not controlled by digitalisation, Corgaretic should be withdrawn, consideration being given to the foregoing warning.

Beta-blockade impairs the ability of the heart to respond to stress. It has been the usual practice to recommend withdrawal of beta-blockers several days prior to surgery. However, this may render the patient's blood pressure unstable and difficult to control during anaesthesia and the anaesthetist may wish to advise on discontinuation of therapy. In no circumstances should beta-blockers be discontinued prior to surgery in patients with phaeochromocytoma or thyrotoxicosis. In the event of emergency surgery, the effects of nadolol may be reversed by isoprenaline or noradrenaline. However, such patients may be subject to protracted severe hypotension. General anaesthetics which can cause myocardial depression, such as cyclopropane, trichloroethylene, chloroform and ether, should be avoided if Corgaretic is continued during surgery.

Corgaretic should be administered with caution to patients with chronic obstructive airways disease. Discontinue therapy if condition relapses.

Diabetic patients should be monitored closely as nadolol may mask the early signs of acute hypoglycaemia, and thiazide diuretics can lower insulin tolerance. Therefore, dosages of hypoglycaemic drugs or insulin doses may need adjustment.

There have been reports of skin rashes (including a psoriasiform type) and/or ocular changes (conjunctivitis and 'dry eye') associated with the use of beta-adrenergic blocking drugs. The reported incidence is small and in most cases the symptoms have cleared when the treatment was withdrawn. Discontinuance of the drug should be considered if any such reaction is not otherwise explicable. Cessation of the therapy with a beta-adrenergic blocker should be gradual.

Beta-blockade may mask certain clinical signs (e.g., tachycardia) of hyperthyroidism. Patients suspected of developing thyrotoxicosis should be managed carefully to avoid abrupt withdrawal of beta-blockade which might precipitate a thyroid storm.

Precautions: Occasionally, beta-blockade with drugs such as nadolol may produce hypotension and/or marked bradycardia, resulting in vertigo, syncope or orthostatic hypotension.

Nadolol should be used with caution in patients with impaired renal or hepatic function.

Periodic determination of serum electrolytes to detect possible imbalance, e.g. hyponatraemia, hypochloric alkalosis and hypokalaemia, should be performed at regular intervals.

Potassium depletion is a danger to digitalised patients or those with hepatic cirrhosis with ascites. In patients with renal disease, thiazides may precipitate azotaemia and cumulative effects of the drug may develop. In patients with impaired hepatic function, minor alterations of fluid and electrolyte balance may precipitate hepatic coma.

Thiazide diuretics may raise serum uric acid levels, thus exacerbating gout in susceptible patients.

Pathologic changes in the parathyroid gland with hypercalcaemia and hypophosphataemia have been observed in a few patients during prolonged thiazide therapy.

The possibility that thiazides may exacerbate or activate systemic lupus erythematosus has been reported.

Administration in renal failure: Increased blood levels of nadolol occur in the presence of renal failure. Although non-renal elimination does occur, dosage adjustments are necessary in this patient group. The total daily dose of Corgaretic should be reduced or the dose interval increased. Corgaretic, however, would not be appropriate for patients with severe renal impairment since loop diuretics (e.g. frusemide) rather than a thiazide are preferred for such patients.

Use in pregnancy and nursing mothers: The safety of nadolol in pregnancy has not been established and animal studies have shown some foetotoxicity. The use of diuretics in otherwise healthy pregnant women with or without mild oedema is contra-indicated. The hazards of using thiazides include foetal or neonatal jaundice, thrombocytopenia and possibly other adverse reactions which have occurred in the adult. Nadolol and bendrofluazide are excreted in human milk.

Corgaretic is therefore not considered suitable for pregnant patients or nursing mothers.

Side-effects: Most patients tolerate Corgaretic well.

Nadolol: Side-effects resemble those reported with other beta-blocking drugs and rarely require withdrawal of treatment. Those reported infrequently include gastrointestinal effects, bradycardia, fatigue, light-headedness, cold extremities, insomnia, paraesthesia, dryness of the mouth and alopecia. Cardiac insufficiency, hypotension and AV block have occurred on rare occasions.

Thiazides: Those reported with the use of thiazides include hypokalaemia, anorexia, gastric irritation, nausea, vomiting, cramping, diarrhoea, intrahepatic cholestatic jaundice, pancreatitis, dizziness, vertigo, headache, xanthopsia, leucopenia, agranulocytosis, thrombocytopenia, aplastic anaemia, purpura, photosensitivity, rash, urticaria, necrotising angiitis, hyperglycaemia, glycosuria, hyperuricaemia, muscle spasm, weakness and restlessness.

Overdosage or exaggerated response: Excessive bradycardia should be treated initially with atropine. If there is no response, isoprenaline may be administered with caution.

Cardiac failure should be managed by digitalisation and diuretics. Glucagon has also been reported to be useful.

Hypotension may be managed with vasopressors such as adrenaline.

Bronchospasm may be counteracted by isoprenaline and aminophylline.

Drug interactions:

General anaesthetics: Those which cause myocardial depression such as chloroform, cyclopropane, trichloroethylene and ether should be avoided as the patient may be subject to protracted severe hypotension.

Myocardial depressants: Myocardial depressants such as lignocaine and procainamide may potentiate the hypotensive action of nadolol and lead to severe hypotension.

Adrenoceptor stimulants: Beta-adrenoceptor stimulants such as isoprenaline and verapramil, or alpha-adrenoceptor stimulants such as noradrenaline, adrenaline, will reverse the hypotensive effects and increase vasoconstrictor activity. Thiazides may decrease the arterial responsiveness to noradrenaline.

Catecholine depleting drugs (eg, reserpine): Excessive reduction in sympathetic drive to the heart might occur. Close observation is advised.

Antihypertensives (eg, neurone-blocking drugs, vasodilators, diuretics): Additive hypotensive effect.

Clonidine: If Corgard and clonidine are given concurrently, clonidine should not be discontinued until several days after Corgard withdrawal.

Hypoglycaemics, insulin: Possible dosage adjustment, see warnings.

Monoamine oxidase inhibitors: Administration of nadolol during and within 2 weeks of administration of adrenergic augmenting psychotropic drugs such as monoamine oxidase inhibitors, should be avoided, although the clinical significant is undetermined.

Tubocurarine: Thiazides may increase the responsiveness to tubocurarine.

Pharmaceutical precautions Store at room temperature, protected from excessive heat and moisture in a tightly closed container.

Legal category POM.

Package quantities Calendar packs of 28.

Further information Corgaretic tablets simplify the treatment of hypertension by increasing patient acceptability and dosage flexibility. The two available strengths allow increasing the dose of the beta-blocker nadolol, without necessarily increasing the bendrofluazide dosage.

The lipid solubility of beta-blocking agents has been correlated with the extent to which these agents cross the blood-brain barrier and cause central nervous system-related side-effects. Nadolol has a low lipid solubility.

Nadolol has been demonstrated in both animal and clinical studies to preserve, and in some cases, increase renal blood flow upon acute and long-term administration in spite of a concurrent decrease in arterial pressure and cardiac output. Glomerular filtration rate remains unchanged, and renal vascular resistance is reduced, even in the presence of diuretic pretreatment.

The exact mechanism of this effect of nadolol on the renal circulation has not been elucidated. The net effect on glomerular filtration rate of the simultaneous administration of nadolol/bendrofluazide as initial therapy has not been investigated.

About 30 per cent of an oral dose of nadolol is absorbed. Peak serum concentrations usually occur in 3 to 4 hours after drug administration. The presence of food in the gastrointestinal tract does not affect the rate or extent of nadolol absorption. Approximately 30 per cent of the nadolol present in serum is reversibly bound to plasma protein. Unlike most available beta-blocking agents, nadolol is not metabolised, and is excreted unchanged. The serum half-life of therapeutic doses of nadolol is relatively long, ranging from 20 to 24 hours (permitting once daily dosage). A significant correlation between minimum steady-state serum concentrations of nadolol and total oral daily dose has been demonstrated in hypertensive patients; however, the observed dose-response range is wide and proper dosage requires individualised titration.

Bendrofluazide is almost completely absorbed from the gastro-intestinal tract. It is extensively metabolised, 30 per cent being excreted unchanged in the urine. Its plasma half-life is 3 to 4 hours, its biological half-life being much longer.

Product licence numbers
Corgaretic 40   0034/0212
Corgaretic 80   0034/0213

DOLMATIL† TABLETS ▼

Presentation Plain white round tablets with a transverse breaking line on one side and the mark D200 on the other. Each tablet contains 200 mg sulpiride.

Uses *Acute and chronic schizophrenia:* One of the characteristics of Dolmatil is its bimodal activity, as it has both antidepressant and neuroleptic properties. Schizophrenia characterised by a lack of social contact can benefit strikingly. Mood elevation is observed after a few days treatment, followed by disappearance of the florid schizophrenic symptoms. The sedation and lack of affect characteristically associated with classical neuroleptics of the phenothiazine or butyrophenone type are not features of Dolmatil therapy.

Dosage and administration *Adults:* A starting dose of 400 mg to 800 mg daily, given as one or two tablets twice daily (morning and early evening) is recommended.

Predominantly positive symptoms (formal thought disorder, hallucinations, delusions, incongruity of affect) respond to higher doses, and a starting dose of at least 400 mg twice daily is recommended, increasing if necessary up to a suggested maximum of 1200 mg twice daily. Increasing the dose beyond this level has not been shown to produce further improvement.

Predominantly negative symptoms (flattening of affect, poverty of speech, anergia, apathy), as well as depression, respond to doses below 800 mg daily; therefore, a starting dose of 400 mg twice daily is recommended. *Reducing* this dose towards 200 mg twice daily will normally *increase* the alerting affect of Dolmatil.

Patients with mixed positive and negative symptoms, with neither predominating, will normally respond to dosage of 400–600 mg twice daily.

Elderly: The same dose ranges may be required in the elderly, but should be reduced if there is evidence of renal impairment.

Children: Clinical experience in children under 14 years of age is insufficient to permit specific recommendations.

Contra-indications, warnings, etc
Contra-indications: The only absolute contra-indication is phaeochromocytoma. There are no cardiovascular contra-indications.

Warnings: Increased motor agitation has been reported at high dosage in a small number of patients: in aggressive, agitated or excited phases of the disease

process, Dolmatil may aggravate symptoms. Care should be exercised where hypomania is present.

Extrapyramidal reactions, principally akathisia have been reported in a small number of cases. If warranted, reduction in dosage or anti-parkinsonian medication may be necessary.

After over a decade of widespread use in many countries, tardive dyskinesia has occurred rarely.

Insomnia has been reported.

Many medicines, including neuroleptics, raise serum prolactin levels, which may be associated with galactorrhoea and amenorrhoea, and less frequently with gynaecomastia. In long-term animal studies with neuroleptic drugs, including sulpiride, an increased incidence of various endocrine tumours (some of which have occasionally been malignant) has been seen in some but not all strains of rats and mice studied. The significance of these findings to man is not known; there is no current evidence of an association between neuroleptic use and tumour risk in man.

Precautions: While no drug interactions are known, unnecessary polypharmacy should be avoided. Although Dolmatil only induces slight EEG modifications, caution is advised in prescribing it for patients with unstable epilepsy. Patients requiring Dolmatil who are receiving anti-convulsant therapy should continue unchanged on the latter medication. Dolmatil has no significant anticholinergic or cardiovascular activity. As with all drugs for which the kidney is the major elimination pathway, the usual precautions should be taken in cases of renal failure.

Use in pregnancy: Despite the negative results of teratogenicity studies in animals and the lack of teratogenic effects during widespread clinical use in other countries, Dolmatil should not be considered an exception to the general principle of avoiding drug treatment during pregnancy, particularly during the first 16 weeks, with potential benefits being weighed against possible hazards.

Toxicity and treatment of overdose: Dolmatil is very well tolerated and only minor side-effects occur, if at all, at the recommended doses. The range of single toxic doses is 1 to 16 g but no death has occurrred even at the 16 g dose.

The clinical manifestations of poisoning vary depending upon the size of the dose taken. After single doses of 1 to 3 g restlessness and clouding of consciousness have been reported and (rarely) extrapyramidal symptoms. Doses of 3 to 7 g may produce a degree of agitation, confusion and extrapyramidal symptoms; more than 7 g can cause, in addition, coma and low blood pressure.

The duration of intoxication is generally short, the symptoms disappearing within a few hours. Comas which have occurred after large doses have lasted up to four days.

There are no specific complications from overdose. In particular no haematological or hepatic toxicity has been reported.

Overdose may be treated with alkaline osmotic diuresis and, if necessary, anti-parkinsonian drugs. Coma needs appropriate nursing. Emetic drugs are unlikely to be effective in Dolmatil overdosage.

Pharmaceutical precautions Store at room temperature.

Legal category POM.

Package quantities Cardboard cartons containing 10 bubble blister strips, each of which contains 10 tablets.

Further information Dolmatil is a member of the group of substituted benzamides, which are structurally distinct from the phenothiazines, butyrophenones and thioxanthenes. Current evidence suggests that the actions of Dolmatil hint at an important distinction between different types of dopamine receptors or receptor mechanisms in the brain. Behaviourally and biochemically, Dolmatil shares with these classical neuroleptics a number of properties indicative of cerebral dopamine receptor antagonism. Essential and intriguing differences include lack of catalepsy at doses active in other behavioural tests, lack of effect in the dopamine sensitive adenylate cyclase systems, lack of effect upon noradrenaline or 5HT turnover, negligible anticholinesterase activity, no effect on muscarinic or GABA receptor binding, and a radical difference in the binding of tritiated sulpiride to striatal preparations in-vitro, compared with ^{3}H-spiperone or ^{3}H-haloperidol. These findings indicate a major differentiation between Dolmatil and classical neuroleptics which lack such specificity.

The plasma half-life in man is approximately 8 hours.

Product licence number 5299/0006.

† DOLMATIL-SESIF Trade Mark: Authorised User Delagrange Limited.

ECONACORT* CREAM ▼

Presentation White cream containing 1% w/w econazole nitrate and 1% w/w hydrocortisone.

Uses *Actions:* Econazole nitrate is a broad spectrum antifungal and antibiotic agent, active against dermatophytes (*Trichophyton rubrum, Trichophyton mentagrophytes, Epidermophyton floccosum* and *Malassezia furfur*); pathogenic yeasts; *Candida albicans* and other *Candida* species. It is also active against Gram-positive bacteria.

Hydrocortisone is a widely used topical anti-inflammatory agent of value in the treatment of inflammatory skin conditions including atopic and infantile eczema, contact sensitivity reactions and intertrigo.

Indications: Econacort is indicated for the topical treatment of inflammatory dermatoses where infection by susceptible organisms co-exists e.g. inflammatory fungal infections including ringworm and Candida and infected eczema where Gram-positive organisms are commonly associated with exacerbations and chronicity.

Dosage and administration
Adults and children: To be massaged gently into the affected and surrounding skin area morning and evening. The cream is particularly suitable for moist and weeping lesions.

Elderly: Natural thinning of the skin occurs in the elderly, hence corticosteroids should be used sparingly and for short periods of time.

Contra-indications, warnings, etc
Contra-indications: Hypersensitivity to either of the active ingredients.

In tuberculous and most viral lesions of the skin, particularly herpes simplex, vaccinia and varicella.

Precautions: Econacort cream should not be used in or near the eyes.

Children: As with any topical corticosteroid, care is advised with infants and children where the preparation is to be applied to extensive areas or under occlusive dressing. However, continuous prolonged treatment should not be necessary.

Pregnancy: Topical administration of corticosteroids to pregnant animals can cause foetal abnormalities. The relevance of this finding to humans has not been established. However, topical corticosteroids should not be used extensively in pregnancy, i.e. in large amounts or for long periods. Topical corticosteroids should be used during pregnancy only if the potential benefit justifies the potential risk to the foetus.

Side-effects: Econazole nitrate and hydrocortisone are well tolerated. Where adverse reactions occur they are usually reversible on cessation of therapy.

Side-effects of econazole nitrate are limited to occasional local irritation manifested by erythema, burning or stinging sensation, and pruritis, but these may be minimised by the hydrocortisone component.

The possibility of the systemic effects which are associated with all steroid therapy should be considered. These effects may be enhanced with occlusive dressings.

Overdosage: Topically applied corticosteroids can be absorbed in sufficient amounts to produce systemic effects.

Pharmaceutical precautions Store in a cool place. Dilution is not recommended, as this would reduce the concentration of the antibiotic to below therapeutic levels.

Legal category POM.

Package quantities Tubes of 30 g.

Further information Nil.

Product licence number 0034/0249.

ECOSTATIN* CREAM, LOTION, POWDER, SPRAY POWDER, AND SPRAY SOLUTION

Presentation *Cream:* White cream containing 1% w/w econazole nitrate.

Lotion: Milky white homogeneous lotion containing 1% w/w econazole nitrate.

Powder and spray powder: White powder containing 1% w/w econazole nitrate in a talc base.

Spray solution: Alcoholic solution containing 1% w/w econazole nitrate.

Uses *Actions:* Econazole nitrate is a broad spectrum antifungal agent, active against dermatophytes (*Trichophyton rubrum, Trichophyton mentagrophytes, Epidermophyton floccosum* and *Malassezia furfur*); pathogenic yeasts; *Candida albicans* and other *Candida* species. Also active against some Gram-positive bacteria, e.g. staphylococci and streptococci.

Indications All fungal skin infections due to dermatophytes (e.g. *Trichophyton* species), yeasts (e.g. *Candida* species), moulds and other fungi. These include ringworm (tinea) infections, athlete's foot, paronychia, pityriasis versicolor, erythrasma, intertrigo, fungal nappy rash, candidal vulvitis and candidal balanitis. Bacterial skin infections due to Gram-positive organisms.

Dosage and administration *Adults and Children:* *Cream:* To be massaged gently into the affected and surrounding skin area morning and evening. The cream is particularly suitable for moist or weeping lesions.

Lotion: To be applied twice daily to the affected and surrounding skin area. In the treatment of fungal infections of the nail, apply once daily with an occlusive dressing.

Powder and spray powder: To be applied to the affected area twice daily. The powder is particularly suitable for use in skin folds, e.g. inguinal and interdigital.

Spray solution: To be applied twice daily. See precautions.

Clinical improvement usually occurs promptly; however, complete disappearance of the symptoms of the disease may require prolonged treatment. Therapy should continue for several days following both clinical and mycological cure in order to prevent relapse.

Elderly: No specific dosage recommendations.

Contra-indications, warnings, etc
Contra-indications: Patients with a history of sensitivity to any of the components of the preparations.

Precautions: Ecostatin cream, lotion, powder, spray powder or spray solution should not be used in or near the eyes. Ecostatin spray solution should not be used on mucous membranes.

Pregnancy: No specific precautions apply; systemic absorption is likely to be negligible.

Side-effects: Ecostatin is well tolerated. Side-effects are limited to occasional local irritation manifested by erythema, burning or stinging sensations and pruritus.

Pharmaceutical precautions *Storage: Cream, lotion, powder:* Store at room temperature.

Spray powder, spray solution: Store in a cool place.

Legal category P.

Package quantities *Ecostatin cream:* Tubes of 30 g and 15 g.
Ecostatin lotion: 30 ml.
Ecostatin powder: 30 g.
Ecostatin spray powder: 200 g.
Ecostatin spray solution: 150 g.

Further information Nil.

Product licence numbers
Ecostatin Cream   0034/0231
Ecostatin Lotion   0034/0232
Ecostatin Powder   0034/0234
Ecostatin Spray Powder   0034/0235
Ecostatin Spray Solution 0034/0236

ECOSTATIN* PESSARIES AND TWIN PACK

Presentation *Pessaries:* White, opaque, oval pessaries each containing 150 mg econazole nitrate in an hydrogenated vegetable oil base.

Twin pack: Three Ecostatin pessaries with applicator plus 15 g Ecostatin cream (containing 1% w/w econazole nitrate).

Uses *Actions:* Econazole nitrate has a broad spectrum of antifungal activity. It is highly active against *Candida albicans* and other *Candida* species and is effective in controlling infections of the vagina and vulva caused by such organisms (thrush).

Indications: Vulvovaginal candidosis. In addition to vaginal treatment the Twin Pack contains cream for topical application to the anogenital area.

Dosage and administration *Adults: Pessaries:* One pessary to be inserted at bedtime for three consecutive nights. Administration should be continued even if menstruation occurs, and despite the disappearance of signs and symptoms of the infection.

The pessary should be inserted high into the vagina while the patient is supine.

Cream: The cream is applied twice daily, in the morning and evening, to the anogenital area.

Note: To prevent re-infection with *Candida*, the male consort should be treated concurrently with Ecostatin cream, applied twice daily to the external genital area during the treatment period.

Although a three day course of therapy usually suffices, it may be necessary to institute a second course of therapy.

Children: Vulvovaginal candidosis is not normally a problem in children, therefore there are no specific dosage recommendations.

Elderly: No specific dosage recommendations or precautions apply.

Contra-indications, warnings, etc
Contra-indications: Patients with a history of sensitivity to any of the components of the preparation.

Precautions: Avoid contact between contraceptive diaphragms and this product since the rubber may be damaged by the preparation.

Pregnancy: Ecostatin pessaries are effective in the candidal vaginitis associated with pregnancy. Safety of systemic econazole has not been established but percutaneous absorption following topical application is likely to be low. However, as with other agents, Ecostatin should not be used during the first trimester of pregnancy unless the physician deems its use essential for the welfare of the patient. In pregnancy, extra care should be taken in using an applicator to prevent the possibility of mechanical trauma.

Side-effects: Patients may rarely complain of discomfort; this is usually transitory and disappears with continued treatment. Seldom is it necessary to discontinue econazole pessary treatment.

Ecostatin cream is well tolerated. Side-effects are limited to occasional local irritation manifested by erythema, burning or stinging sensation, and pruritus.

Pharmaceutical precautions *Storage:* Store at room temperature.

Legal category Cream P.
                    Pessaries POM.

Package quantities *Pessaries:* Pack of three pessaries with applicator.
Twin pack: Three pessaries with applicator plus 15 g cream.

Further information Nil.

Product licence numbers
Ecostatin Pessaries   0034/0233
Ecostatin Cream   0034/0231

FLORINEF* TABLETS

Presentation Round, pale pink tablets, scored on one side and engraved Squibb and 429 on reverse, containing 0.1 mg fludrocortisone acetate.

Uses *Actions:* Qualitatively, the physiological action of fludrocortisone acetate is similar to hydrocortisone. In very small doses, fludrocortisone maintains life in adrenalectomised animals, enhances the deposition of liver glycogen and produces thymic involution, eosinopenia, retention of sodium and increased urinary excretion of potassium.

Indications: For partial replacement therapy for primary and secondary adrenocortical insufficiency in Addison's disease and for the treatment of salt-losing adrenogenital syndrome.

Dosage and administration
Adult dosage: A daily dosage range of 0.05–0.3 mg Florinef tablets orally. Supplementary parenteral administration of sodium-retaining hormones is not necessary. When an enhanced glucocorticoid effect is desirable, cortisone or hydrocortisone by mouth should be given concomitantly with Florinef tablets.

Children: May be used adjusted to the age and weight of the child according to the severity of the condition.

Elderly: No specific dosage recommendations or precautions.

Contra-indications, warnings, etc
Contra-indications: Because of its marked effect on sodium retention, the use of Florinef in the treatment of conditions other than those indicated, is not advised.

Since Florinef is a potent mineralocorticoid both the dosage and salt intake should be carefully monitored to avoid the development of hypertension, oedema or weight gain. Periodic checking of serum electrolyte levels is advisable during prolonged therapy; dietary salt restriction and potassium supplementation may be necessary.

Systemic corticosteroids are not indicated for patients with myasthenia gravis, diverticulitis, recent intestinal anastomoses, thrombophlebitis, psychotic tendencies, exanthematous disease, chronic nephritis, metastatic carcinoma, osteoporosis and a history of peptic ulcer.

In latent or healed tuberculosis; in the presence of local or systemic viral infection or systemic fungal infections; in acute psychoses and in patients with an active peptic ulcer; in acute glomerulonephritis and in active infections not controlled by antibiotics.

Precautions: Diabetes may be aggravated, necessitating a higher insulin dosage. Latent diabetes mellitus may be precipitated. Menstrual irregularities may occur, and this possibility should be mentioned to female patients.

Patients on long-term systemic therapy with Florinef may require supportive corticosteroid therapy in times of stress (such as trauma, surgery or severe illness), both during the treatment period and for a year afterwards.

During corticosteroid therapy antibody response will be reduced and therefore affect the patient's response to vaccines.

Rare instances of anaphylactoid reactions have occurred in patients receiving corticosteroids, especially when a patient has a history of drug allergies.

All corticosteroids increase calcium excretion.

Avoid abrupt cessation of corticosteroids.

Aspirin should be used cautiously in conjunction with corticosteroids in patients with hypoprothrombinaemia.

Corticosteroid effects may be enhanced in patients with hypothyroidism or cirrhosis.

Pregnancy: Corticosteroids are not recommended for pregnant patients, particularly in the first trimester, or for nursing mothers, except when the disease for which they are indicated warrants their use. Hypo-adrenalism may occur in the newborn of mothers receiving corticosteroid therapy.

Side-effects: Where adverse reactions occur they are usually reversible on cessation of therapy.

Patients should be watched closely for the following adverse reactions which may be associated with any corticosteroid therapy:

Fluid and electrolyte disturbances – sodium retention, fluid retention, congestive heart failure in susceptible patients, potassium loss, cardiac arrhythmias or ECG changes due to potassium deficiency, hypokalaemic alkalosis, increased calcium excretion and hypertension.

Musculoskeletal – muscle weakness, fatigue, steroid myopathy, loss of muscle mass, osteoporosis, vertebral compression fractures, delayed healing of fractures, aseptic necrosis of femoral and humeral heads, pathological fractures of long bones and spontaneous fractures.

Gastrointestinal – peptic ulcer with possible subsequent perforation and haemorrhage, pancreatitis, abdominal distension and ulcerative oesophagitis.

Dermatologic – impaired wound healing, thin fragile skin, petechiae and ecchymoses, facial erythema, increased sweating, purpura, striae, hirsutism, acneiform eruptions, lupus erythematosus-like lesions and suppressed reactions to skin tests.

Neurological – convulsions, increased intracranial pressure with papilloedema (pseudo-tumour cerebri) usually after treatment, vertigo, headache, neuritis or paraesthesias and aggravation of preexisting psychiatric conditions.

Endocrine – menstrual irregularities; development of the Cushingoid state; suppression of growth in children; secondary adrenocortical and pituitary unresponsiveness, particularly in times of stress (e.g. trauma, surgery or illness); decreased carbohydrate tolerance; manifestations of latent diabetes mellitus and increased requirements for insulin or oral hypoglycaemic agents in diabetes.

Ophthalmic – posterior subcapsular cataracts, increased intraocular pressure, glaucoma and exopthalmos.

Metabolic – hyperglycaemia, glycosuria and negative nitrogen balance due to protein catabolism.

Others – necrotising angiitis, thrombophlebitis, thromboembolism, aggravation or masking of infections, insomnia, syncopal episodes and anaphylactoid reactions, particularly where there is a history of drug allergies.

Overdosage: A single large dose should be treated with plenty of water by mouth. Careful monitoring of serum electrolytes is essential, with particular consideration being given to the need for administration of potassium chloride and restriction of dietary sodium intake.

Pharmaceutical precautions *Storage:* At room temperature.

Legal category POM.

Package quantities Bottles of 100.

Further information Nil.

Product licence numbers
Florinef Tablets 0.1 mg   0034/5027

FUNGILIN* CREAM AND OINTMENT

Presentation *Cream:* Yellow containing amphotericin 30,000 units (30 mg) per gram.

Ointment: Yellow containing amphotericin 30,000 units (30 mg) per gram in Plastibase.*

Uses *Actions:* Amphotericin is a polyene antifungal antibiotic active against a wide range of yeasts and yeast-like fungi including *Candida albicans.*

Indications: Cream and Ointment are indicated for cutaneous or mucocutaneous infections caused by susceptible fungi, particularly *C. albicans.*

Dosage and administration Should be applied two to four times daily.

Elderly: No specific dosage recommendations or precautions.

Contra-indications, warnings, etc
Contra-indications: There are no known contra-indications.

Precautions: No special precautions apply.

Pregnancy/Children: No specific precautions apply; systemic absorption is negligible.

Side-effects: There have been no substantiated reports of sensitivity associated with topical amphotericin.

Pharmaceutical precautions *Storage: Cream:* At room temperature; avoid freezing.

Ointment: At room temperature.

Dilution: Fungilin topicals should not be diluted as this may reduce therapeutic efficacy.

Legal category POM.

Package quantities Tubes of 15 g.

Further information Nil.

Product licence numbers
Fungilin Cream   0034/5032
Fungilin Ointment   0034/5035

FUNGILIN* LOZENGES, SUSPENSION AND TABLETS

Presentation *Lozenges:* Round, pale yellow, engraved 929 and Squibb, containing 10,000 units (10 mg) amphotericin.

Suspension: Orange-flavoured, viscous suspension containing 100,000 units (100 mg) amphotericin per ml.

Tablets: Yellow to tan, scored one side and engraved Squibb and 430 on reverse, containing 100,000 units (100 mg) amphotericin.

Uses *Actions:* Amphotericin is an antifungal antibiotic active against a wide range of yeasts and yeast-like fungi including *Candida albicans.* Absorption from the gastro-intestinal tract is negligible even with very large doses. Extensive clinical experience has not shown problems of toxicity or sensitisation.

Indications: Lozenges/Suspension: For the treatment of candidal lesions (thrush) of the oral and perioral areas. The suspension may be used in the treatment of denture stomatitis.

Suspension/Tablets: For the treatment of intestinal candidosis and the suppression of the intestinal reservoir of *C. albicans* which may precipitate cutaneous or vaginal candidosis.

Dosage and administration *Adult dosage: Lozenges:* Dissolve 1 slowly in the mouth four times a day.

Depending on the severity of infection, the dose may be increased to 8 lozenges daily.

To clear the condition fully may require 10-15 days' treatment.

Suspension: For denture stomatitis and oral infections caused by *C. albicans,* 1 ml should be placed in the mouth four times daily; it should be kept in contact with lesions for as long as possible.

For the treatment or suppression of intestinal candidosis, 2 ml four times daily.

Tablets: 1 or 2 tablets four times daily.

Administration of Fungilin for oral and intestinal candidosis should be continued for 48 hours after clinical cure to prevent relapse.

Infants and children: Suspension: For intestinal and oral candidosis, 1 ml should be dropped into the mouth four times daily. The suspension should be held in contact with oral lesions for as long as possible before swallowing.

For prophylaxis in the newborn, the suggested dose is 1 ml daily.

Elderly: No specific dosage recommendations or precautions.

Contra-indications, warnings, etc
Contra-indications: There are no known contra-indications to the use of these products.

Precautions: No specific precautions apply.

Pregnancy/Children: Absorption of amphotericin from the gastrointestinal tract is negligible, therefore no special precautions apply.

Side-effects: Gastro-intestinal side-effects have occasionally been reported following continuous administration of amphotericin for several months in daily doses in excess of 3 g. These have been mild in nature and have readily cleared on cessation of treatment. No systemic toxic effects or allergic reactions have been associated with its oral use.

Overdosage: Since absorption of amphotericin from the gastro-intestinal tract is negligible, overdosage causes no systemic toxicity.

Pharmaceutical precautions *Storage: Lozenges/ Tablets:* At room temperature.

Suspension: Cool place; protect from direct sunlight.

Dilution: Fungilin Suspension should not be diluted prior to use; it is formulated to coat and adhere to the oral lesions being treated.

Legal category POM.

Package quantities *Lozenges:* 20 in a tube.
Tablets: Bottles of 20.
Suspension: 12 ml bottles with graduated dropper.

Further information Nil.

Product licence numbers
Fungilin Lozenges   0034/5034
Fungilin Suspension   0034/5038
Fungilin Tablets   0034/5039

FUNGIZONE* INTRAVENOUS

Presentation Each vial contains as a yellow, fluffy powder: amphotericin 50,000 units (50 mg), sodium desoxycholate approximately 41 mg, with sodium phosphate buffer.

Uses *Actions:* Amphotericin is a polyene antifungal antibiotic active against a wide range of yeasts and yeast-like fungi including Candida albicans. Crystalline amphotericin is insoluble in water; therefore the antibiotic is solubilised by the addition of sodium desoxycholate to form a mixture which provides a colloidal dispersion for parenteral administration. Amphotericin is fungistatic rather than fungicidal in concentrations obtainable in body fluids. It probably acts by binding to sterols in the fungal cell membrane with a resultant change in membrane permeability which allows leakage of intracellular components. Mammalian cell membranes also contain sterols and it has been suggested that the damage to human and fungal cells may share common mechanisms. No strains of Candida resistant to amphotericin have been reported in clinical use, and although in vitro testing does produce a small number of resistant isolates this occurs only following repeated subcultures.

Clinical pharmacology: An initial intravenous infusion of 1 to 5 mg of amphotericin per day, gradually increased to 0.65 mg/kg daily, produces peak plasma concentrations of approximately 2 to 4 mcg/ml which can persist between doses since the plasma half-life of amphotericin is about 24 hours. (For recommended dosages, see the Dosage and Administration section.) It has been reported that amphotericin is highly bound (more than 90%) to plasma proteins and is poorly dialyzable.

Amphotericin is excreted very slowly by the kidneys with two to five per cent of a given dose being excreted in biologically active form. After treatment is discontinued the drug can be detected in the urine for at least seven weeks. The cumulative urinary output over a seven day period amounts to approximately 40 per cent of the amount of drug infused.

Details of tissue distribution and possible metabolic pathways are not known.

Indications: Fungizone Intravenous should be administered primarily to patients with progressive, potentially fatal infections. This potent drug should not be used to treat the common forms of fungal disease which show only positive skin or serological tests.

Fungizone Intravenous is specifically intended to treat cryptococcosis (torulosis); North American blastomycosis; the disseminated forms of candidosis, coccidioidomycosis and histoplasmosis; mucormycosis (phycomycosis) caused by species of the genera *Mucor, Rhizopus, Absidia, Entomophthora,* and *Basidiobolus sporotrichosis (Sporotrichum schenckii),* aspergillosis (*Aspergillus fumigatus*).

Amphotericin may be helpful in the treatment of American mucocutaneous leishmaniasis but is not the drug of choice in primary therapy.

Dosage and administration *Adults and children:* Fungizone should be administered by slow intravenous infusion over a period of six hours. Initial daily dose should be 0.25 mg/kg of body weight gradually increasing to a level of 1.0 mg/kg of body weight depending on individual response and tolerance. Within the range of 0.25-1.0 mg/kg the daily dose should be maintained at the highest level which is not accompanied by unacceptable toxicity.

In seriously ill patients the daily dose may be gradually increased up to a total of 1.5 mg/kg. Since amphotericin is excreted slowly, therapy may be given on alternate days in patients on the higher dosage schedule. Several months of therapy are usually necessary; a shorter period of therapy may produce an inadequate response and lead to relapse.

Whenever medication is interrupted for a period longer than seven days therapy should be resumed by starting with the lowest dosage level, i.e. 0.25 mg/kg of body weight, and increased gradually.

Caution: Under no circumstances should a total daily dose of 1.5 mg/kg be exceeded. The recommended concentration for intravenous infusion is 0.1 mg per ml (100 units per ml).

Elderly: No specific dosage recommendations or precautions.

Preparation of solutions: Reconstitute as follows: An initial concentrate of 5 mg amphotericin per ml is first prepared by rapidly expressing 10 ml sterile water for injection, without a bacteriostatic agent, directly into the lyophilised cake, using a sterile needle (minimum diameter: 20 gauge) and syringe. Shake the vial immediately until the colloidal solution is clear. The infusion solution, providing 0.1 mg/ml is obtained by further dilution (1:50) with 5% Dextrose Injection of pH above 4.2. The pH of each container of Dextrose Injection should be ascertained before use. Commercial Dextrose Injection usually has a pH above 4.2; however, if it is below 4.2 then 1 or 2 ml of buffer should be added to the Dextrose Injection before it is used to dilute a concentrated solution of amphotericin. The recommended buffer has the following composition:

Dibasic sodium phosphate (anhydrous)	1.59 g
Monobasic sodium phosphate (anhydrous)	0.96 g
Water for Injection BP	qs 100 ml

The buffer should be sterilised before it is added to the Dextrose Injection, either by filtration through a bacterial filter, or by autoclaving for 30 mins at 15 lb pressure (121°C).

Caution: Aseptic technique must be strictly observed in all handling, since no preservative or bacteriostatic agent is present. Do not reconstitute with saline solutions. The use of any diluent other than the ones recommended or the presence of a bacteriostatic agent in the diluent may cause precipitation of the amphotericin. Do not use the initial concentrate or the infusion solution if there is any evidence of precipitation of foreign matter.

Other preparations for injection should not be added to the infusion solution or administered via the cannula being used to administer Fungizone Intravenous.

An in-line membrane filter may be used for intravenous infusion of amphotericin; however the mean pore diameter of the filter should not be less than 1.0 micron in order to assure passage of the amphotericin dispersion.

Contra-indications, warnings, etc
Contra-indications: Those patients who are hypersensitive to amphotericin, unless, in the opinion of the physician, the condition requiring treatment is life-threatening and amenable only to such therapy.

Precautions: Prolonged therapy with amphotericin is usually necessary. Unpleasant reactions are quite common when the drug is given parenterally at therapeutic dosage levels. Some of these reactions are potentially dangerous. Hence amphotericin should be used parenterally only in hospitalised patients, or those under close clinical observation. If the BUN exceeds 6.5 mmol/l, or the serum creatinine exceeds 260 micromol/l, the drug should be discontinued or the dosage markedly reduced until renal function is improved. Weekly blood counts and serum potassium determinations are also advisable. Low serum magnesium levels have also been noted during treatment with amphotericin. Therapy should be discontinued if liver function test results (elevated bromsulphalein, alkaline phosphatase and bilirubin) are abnormal.

Corticosteroids should not be administered concomitantly unless they are necessary to control drug reactions. Other nephrotoxic antibiotics and antineoplastic agents should not be given concomitantly except with great caution.

Pregnancy: Safety for use in pregnancy has not been established; therefore it should be used during pregnancy only if the possible benefits to be derived outweigh the potential risks involved.

Side-effects: While some patients may tolerate full intravenous doses of amphotericin without difficulty, most will exhibit some intolerance, often at less than the full therapeutic dosage. They may be made less severe by giving aspirin, antihistamines or antiemetics. Administration of the drug on alternate days may decrease anorexia and phlebitis. Intravenous administration of small doses of adrenal corticosteroids just prior to or during the amphotericin infusion may decrease febrile reactions. The dosage and duration of such corticosteroid therapy should be kept to a minimum. Adding a small amount of heparin to the infusion may lessen the incidence of thrombophlebitis and coagulation problems. Extravasation may cause chemical irritation. The adverse reactions that are most commonly observed are: fever (sometimes with shaking chills), headache, anorexia, weight loss, nausea and vomiting, malaise, muscle and joint pains, dyspepsia, cramping epigastric pain, diarrhoea, local venous pain at the injection site with phlebitis and thrombophlebitis, normochromic normocytic anaemia and hypokalaemia. Abnormal renal function, including hypokalaemia, azotaemia, hyposthenuria, renal tubular acidosis or nephrocalcinosis, is also commonly observed and usually improves upon interruption of therapy; however, some permanent impairment often occurs, especially in those patients receiving large amounts (over 5 g) of amphotericin. The following adverse reactions occur less frequently or rarely: anuria (oliguria); cardiovascular toxicity including arrhythmias, ventricular fibrillation, cardiac arrest, hypotension, hypertension; coagulation defects; thrombocytopenia; leucopenia; agranulocytosis; eosinophilia; leucocytosis; melaena or haemorrhagic gastroenteritis; maculopapular rash and pruritus; hearing loss, tinnitus, transient vertigo; blurred vision, or diplopia; peripheral neuropathy, convulsions and other neurologic symptoms; anaphylactoid reactions, acute liver failure and flushing.

Pharmaceutical precautions *Storage:* Vials of powder for reconstitution should be stored in a refrigerator. The concentrate (5 mg per ml after reconstitution with 10 ml sterile Water for Injection) may be stored in the dark, at room temperature for 24 hours, or at refrigerator temperatures for one week with minimal loss of potency and clarity. Any unused material should then be discarded. Solutions prepared for intravenous infusion (0.1 mg or less amphotericin per ml) should be used promptly after preparation and should be protected from light during administration.

Legal category POM.

Package quantities Vials of 50 mg.

Further information The use of Fungizone intravenous by other routes has been documented in the published literature:

Bladder irrigation/installation (e.g. candiduria). Continuous irrigation with 50 mg Fungizone in 1 litre sterile water each day until urinary cultures are negative. Intermittent use of volumes of 100–400 ml (concentrations of 37.5–200 mcg/ml) has also been reported. The urine should be alkalinised (with potassium citrate) and antifungal ointment applied to the perineal area.

Lung inhalation (e.g. pulmonary aspergillosis). 8–40 mg amphotericin (nebulised in sterile water or 5% dextrose) has been given daily in divided doses. Concurrent eradication of oral and intestinal yeasts reservoirs is recommended.

Intrathecal (e.g. coccidioidal meningitis). Current published dosage recommendations are for maintenance 0.25–1.0 mg amphotericin 2–4 times weekly following initiation with a low dose (0.025 mg) and cautious increases. Amphotericin is irritating when injected into the CSF.

Other: Other uses of solutions prepared using Fungizone intravenous include local instillations for the treatment of fungal infections of the ear, eye, peritoneum, lung cavities and joint spaces.

Product licence number 0034/5041.

GRANEODIN* OINTMENT AND OPHTHALMIC OINTMENT

Presentation Graneodin Ointment is soft, slightly opaque, colourless, containing neomycin (as sulphate) 0.25% and gramicidin 0.025% in Plastibase*.

Graneodin Ophthalmic Ointment is sterile, pale greenish yellow, containing neomycin (as sulphate) 0.25% and gramicidin 0.025%.

Uses *Actions:* Neomycin is active against a wide range of Gram-positive and Gram-negative bacteria, including many of the organisms responsible for bacterial skin infections.

Gramicidin is active against Gram-positive bacteria and supplements the action of neomycin against the many common skin pathogens found in this group.

Indications–Topical: Superficial bacterial infections such as impetigo; impetiginised eczema; infected eczema; furuncles; sycosis barbae; folliculitis; ecthyma; chronic ulcers of the skin; scratches or abrasions; bacterial infections of the ear. (See Contra-indications.)

For prophylaxis against infections following minor surgery.

Ophthalmic: Infections of the eyelids such as hordeolum, Meibomium cysts, blepharitis. Corneal or conjunctival infections.

Dosage and administration *Adults and children– Topical:* To be applied two to four times a day. Any crusts should be removed and the ointment rubbed well in.

Ophthalmic: Half an inch of the ointment should be applied to the inside of the eyelid two to four times a day.

Elderly: No specific dosage recommendations or precautions.

Contra-indications, warnings, etc
Contra-indications: Fungal or viral infections of the skin or for the treatment of deep-seated infections. These preparations are contra-indicated in persons with known sensitivity to neomycin. Should not be applied to the external auditory canal in patients with perforated eardrums.

Precautions: The possibility of sensitivity to neomycin

should be taken into consideration especially in the treatment of patients suffering from leg ulcers. Since the use of occlusive dressings may increase the risk of sensitivity reactions such dressings should be avoided.

Pregnancy/Children: No specific precautions apply.

Side-effects: Neomycin: Sensitivity reactions may occur especially with prolonged use. Ototoxicity and nephrotoxicity have been reported. Large amounts of this product should be avoided in the treatment of skin infections following extensive burns, trophic ulceration, and other conditions where absorption of neomycin is possible.

Gramicidin: Sensitivity has occasionally been reported.

Pharmaceutical precautions *Storage:* At room temperature.

Dilution: Not recommended.

Legal category POM.

Package quantities *Ointment:* Tubes of 15 g.
Ophthalmic Ointment: Tubes of 3.6 g.

Further information Nil.

Product licence numbers
Graneodin Ointment   0034/5042
Graneodin Ophthalmic Ointment   0034/5043

HALCIDERM* TOPICAL

Presentation A white topical preparation containing halcinonide 0.1% in a water-miscible base.

Uses *Actions:* Halcinonide is a potent corticosteroid with rapid anti-inflammatory, antipruritic and anti-allergic actions.
Halciderm is suitable for both wet and dry lesions.

Indications: Halciderm is indicated in acute and chronic corticosteroid-responsive conditions which may include: psoriasis, atopic eczema, contact eczema, follicular eczema, infantile eczema, neurodermatitis, anogenital eczema (pruritus ani et vulvae), nummular eczema, seborrhoeic or flexural eczema, otitis externa.

Dosage and administration *Adults:* Halciderm should be applied to the affected area two, or occasionally three, times daily. In long-term therapy, or where lower strength preparations are required, do not dilute but use intermittently.

Children: In infants, long-term continuous topical steroid therapy should be avoided.

Elderly: Natural thinning of the skin occurs in the elderly; hence corticosteroids should be used sparingly and for short periods of time.

Contra-indications, warnings, etc
Contra-indications: Halciderm is not intended for ophthalmic use, nor should it be applied in the external auditory canal of patients with perforated eardrums.
In tuberculous and most viral lesions of the skin, particularly herpes simplex, vaccinia, varicella. The product should not be used in fungal or bacterial skin infections without suitable concomitant anti-infective therapy.

Precautions: Adrenal suppression can occur, even without occlusion.

Pregnancy: Topical administration of corticosteroids to pregnant animals can cause abnormalities of foetal development. The relevance of this finding to humans has not been established. However, topical steroids should not be used extensively in pregnancy, i.e. in large amounts or for long periods. Topical corticosteroids should be used during pregnancy only if the potential benefit justifies the potential risk to the foetus.

Side-effects: Halcinonide is well tolerated. Where adverse reactions occur they are usually reversible on cessation of therapy. However the following side-effects have been reported usually with prolonged usage:
Dermatologic – impaired wound healing, thinning of the skin, petechiae and ecchymoses, facial erythema and telangiectasia, increased sweating, purpura, striae, hirsutism, acneiform eruptions, lupus erythematosus-like lesions and suppressed reaction to skin tests. These effects may be enhanced with occlusive dressings.
Signs of systemic toxicity such as oedema and electrolyte imbalance have not been observed even when high topical dosage has been used. The possibility of the systemic effects which are associated with all steroid therapy should be considered.

Overdosage: Topically applied corticosteroids can be absorbed in sufficient amounts to produce systemic effects (see Side-effects).

Pharmaceutical precautions *Storage:* Halciderm should be stored in a cool place.

Dilution: Due to special formulation of topical Halciderm, normal dermatological diluents should not be used. For further information consult the manufacturer.

Legal category POM.

Package quantities Tubes containing 30 g.

Further information Halciderm contains halcinonide 0.1%, dissolved in the non-aqueous phase of the formulation.

Product licence number 0034/0160.

HYDREA* CAPSULES

Presentation Pink, opaque capsule body with green, opaque cap, both parts printed Squibb and 830 in black, containing hydroxyurea 500 mg.

Uses *Actions:* Hydroxyurea is an orally active antineoplastic agent. Although the mechanism of action has not yet been clearly defined, hydroxyurea appears to act by interfering with synthesis of DNA.

Indications: Active against a wide range of malignant lesions. Hydrea is particularly effective in the management of chronic myeloid leukaemia, and solid tumours particularly of the head and neck.
In the treatment of tumours of the head and neck, lung, Hodgkin's disease, astrocytoma and sarcoma, best results have been obtained with concomitant radiotherapy.

Dosage and administration Treatment regimens can be continuous or intermittent. The continuous regimen is particularly suitable for chronic myeloid leukaemia, while the intermittent regimen, with its diminished effect on the bone marrow, is more satisfactory for the management of solid tumours.
Hydrea should be started 7 days before concurrent irradiation therapy.
An adequate trial period for determining the antineoplastic effect of Hydrea is six weeks.

Continuous therapy: Hydrea 20-30 mg/kg should be given daily in single doses. Dosage should be based on the patient's actual or ideal weight, whichever is the less. Therapy should be monitored by repeat blood counts.

Intermittent therapy: Hydrea 80 mg/kg in single doses should be given every third day. Using the intermittent regimes the likelihood of WBC depression is diminished, but if low counts are produced, 1 or more doses of Hydrea should be omitted.

Children: Because of the rarity of melanoma, resistant chronic myelocytic leukaemia, carcinoma of the ovary, and carcinomas of the head and neck in children, dosage regimens have not been established.

Elderly: Elderly patients may be more sensitive to the effects of hydroxyurea, and may require a lower dosage regimen.

N.B. If the patient prefers, or is unable to swallow capsules, the contents of the capsules may be emptied into a glass of water and taken immediately.

Contra-indications, warnings, etc
Contra-indications: Marked leucopenia, thrombcytopenia, severe anaemia and previously shown hypersensitivity to Hydrea.

Precautions: The myelosuppressive activity may be potentiated by previous or concomitant radiotherapy or cytotoxic therapy.

The complete status of the blood, including bone marrow examination, if indicated, as well as kidney function and liver function should be determined prior to, and repeatedly during, treatment. The determination of haemoglobin level, total leukocyte counts, and platelet counts should be performed at least once a week throughout the course of hydroxyurea therapy.

Severe anaemia must be corrected with whole blood replacement before initiating therapy with hydroxyurea. Erythrocytic abnormalities; megaloblastic erythropoeisis, which is self-limiting, is often seen early in the course of hydroxyurea therapy. The morphologic change resembles pernicious anaemia, but is not related to Vitamin B_{12} or folic acid deficiency. Hydroxyurea may also delay plasma iron clearance and reduce the rate of iron utilisation by erythrocytes but it does not appear to alter the red blood cell survival time.

Hydroxyurea should be used with caution in patients with marked renal dysfunction.

Pregnancy: Drugs which affect DNA synthesis, such as hydroxyurea, may be potent mutagenic agents. The physician should carefully consider this possibility before administering this drug to male or female patients who may contemplate conception. Since Hydrea is a cytotoxic agent it has produced a teratogenic effect in some animal species. This product should not normally be administered to patients who are pregnant, or to mothers who are breast feeding, unless the potential benefits outweigh the possible hazards.

Side-effects: Bone-marrow suppression is the major toxic effect of Hydrea, while leucopenia, thrombocytopenia and anaemia may occur in that order. Other side-effects are generally rare, but the following have been reported; anorexia, nausea, vomiting, diarrhoea, constipation, headache, drowsiness, dizziness, stomatitis, alopecia, skin rash, melaena, abdominal pain, disorientations, pulmonary oedema, hallucinations, convulsions, potentiation of the erythema caused by irradiation, dysuria and impairment of renal tubular function

accompanied by elevation in serum uric acid, BUN, and creatinine levels. Abnormal BSP retention and fever, chills, malaise and elevation of hepatic enzymes have been reported.

Overdosage: Immediate treatment consists of gastric lavage, followed by supportive therapy for the cardio-respiratory systems if required. In the long term, careful monitoring of the haemopoietic system is essential and, if necessary, blood should be transfused.

Pharmaceutical precautions *Storage:* At room temperature. Bottles should be kept tightly closed since hydroxyurea is hygroscopic.

Legal category POM.

Package quantities Bottles of 100.

Further information Nil.

Product licence number 0034/5044.

IPRAL* TABLETS
IPRAL* PAEDIATRIC SUSPENSION

Presentation *Tablets:* Round, white tablets engraved Squibb and 513, containing 100 mg trimethoprim.

Round, white tablets engraved Squibb and 514, containing 200 mg trimethoprim.

Paediatric Suspension: White, sugar-free suspension, containing 50 mg trimethoprim per 5 ml.

Uses *Actions:* Trimethoprim is bactericidal in-vitro against most pathogenic Gram-positive and Gram-negative bacteria. Exceptions are *Nocardia* species, *Treponema pallidum, Pseudomonas aeruginosa,* anaerobic bacteria and possibly *Mycobacterium* and *Neisseria* species and *Brucella abortus.*

Indications: Urinary tract: In the treatment of acute and chronic urinary tract infections and for prophylactic treatment of patients with a tendency to recurrent urinary infections.

Respiratory tract: In the treatment of acute and chronic bronchitis, bronchopneumonia and lobar pneumonia.

Ipral is particularly useful for patients sensitive to sulphonamides.

Dosage and administration
Ipral Tablets: Adults and Children over 12 years: For acute urinary tract and respiratory tract infections, 200 mg twice daily. For long-term and prophylactic therapy of urinary tract infections, 100 mg at night.

Ipral Paediatric Suspension: Children: Acute treatment: based on a dose of approximately 8 mg/kg/day of trimethoprim:

6 to 12 years: 100 mg (10 ml suspension) twice daily
6 months to 6 years: 50 mg (5 ml suspension) twice daily
8 weeks to 6 months: 25 mg (2.5 ml suspension) twice daily

Ipral Paediatric Suspension may be diluted to half-strength with water, sorbitol or Syrup BP.

Elderly: There are no specific dosage recommendations or precautions for use in the elderly except, as with other drugs, to monitor those patients with impaired renal or hepatic function.

Contra-indications, warnings, etc
Contra-indications: Ipral should not be given to patients

with severe renal insufficiency where blood levels cannot be monitored regularly. Trimethoprim should not be given to patients with a history of sensitivity to the drug. It should not be administered to pregnant women, premature infants nor during the first two months of life. Megaloblastic anaemia.

Precautions: Care is necessary in administration to patients with impaired renal function. Regular haematological examinations should be performed during long-term therapy. Special precautions should be exercised in patients with a predisposition to folate deficiency.

Pregnancy and nursing mothers: Contra-indicated during pregnancy and in nursing mothers. Ipral is excreted in breast milk.

Side-effects: Ipral is well tolerated at therapeutic doses with few side-effects. Nausea, vomiting, gastro-intestinal upset and dermatological reactions such as pruritus and rash have been reported. Given over a prolonged period, Ipral may depress haemopoiesis due to an effect on folic acid metabolism. This effect may be reversed by calcium folinate.

Treatment of overdosage: Symptoms of overdosage include diarrhoea and vomiting. Treatment is symptomatic and gastric lavage and forced diuresis may be used. Calcium folinate may be used to counteract any effect of Ipral on bone-marrow.

Pharmaceutical precautions *Storage:* Ipral tablets and suspension should be stored in closed containers at room temperature.

Legal category POM.

Package quantities
100 mg Tablets: Packs of 100 and 500 tablets.
200 mg tablets: Packs of 100 tablets.
Suspension: Bottles of 100 ml.

Further information Absorption from the oral route is rapid, and peak plasma levels are obtained between one and four hours. Ipral is well distributed throughout the tissues and is excreted, predominantly unchanged, in the urine.

Nearly all of an oral dose of trimethoprim is excreted within 48 hours both unchanged and as metabolites.

Product licence numbers
Ipral Tablets 100 mg   0034/0190.
Ipral Tablets 200 mg   0034/0204.
Ipral Paediatric Suspension 0034/0196.

KENALOG* INTRA-ARTICULAR/INTRA-MUSCULAR

Presentation Sterile, aqueous suspension of triamcinolone acetonide 40 mg per ml.

Uses Triamcinolone acetonide is a synthetic glucocorticoid with marked anti-inflammatory and anti-allergic actions.

Intra-articular injection: Following the local injection of Kenalog, relief of pain and swelling, with greater freedom of movement, is usually obtained within a few hours.

Intramuscular injection: Provides an extended duration of therapeutic effect and fewer side-effects of the kind associated with oral corticosteroid therapy, particularly gastro-intestinal reactions such as peptic ulceration. Studies indicate that, following a single intramuscular dose of 80 mg triamcinolone acetonide, adrenal suppression occurs within 24-48 hours and then gradually returns to normal, usually in approximately three weeks. This finding correlates closely with the extended duration of therapeutic action of triamcinolone acetonide.

Indications
Intra-articular use: For alleviating the joint pain, swelling and stiffness associated with rheumatoid arthritis and osteoarthrosis with an inflammatory component; also for bursitis, epicondylitis, and tenosynovitis.

Intramuscular use: Where sustained systemic corticosteroid treatment is required: *Allergic states,* eg bronchial asthma, seasonal or perennial allergic rhinitis. In seasonal allergies, patients who do not respond to conventional therapy may achieve a remission of symptoms over the entire period with a single intramuscular injection (see Dosage); *Endocrine disorders,* eg primary or secondary adrenocortical insufficiency. *Collagen disorders,* eg during an exacerbation of maintenance therapy of selected cases of SLE or acute rheumatic carditis; *Dermatologic diseases,* eg pemphigus, severe dermatitis and Stevens Johnson Syndrome; *Rheumatic, gastrointestinal or respiratory disorders* – as an adjunctive, short-term therapy; *Haematological disorders,* eg acquired (autoimmune) haemolytic anaemia; *Neoplastic diseases,* eg palliative management of leukaemia and lymphomas; *Renal disease,* such as acute interstitial nephritis, minimal change nephrotic syndrome or lupus nephritis.

Dosage and administration
Kenalog intra-articular/intramuscular injection is not for intravenous use.

Strict aseptic precautions should be observed. Since the duration of effect is variable, subsequent doses should be given when symptoms recur and not at set intervals.

Intra-articular injection: For intra-articular administration or injection into tendon sheaths and bursae, the dose of Kenalog injection may vary from 5 mg to 10 mg (0.125-0.25 ml) for smaller joints and up to 40 mg (1 ml) for larger joints, depending on the specific disease entity being treated. Single injections into several sites for multiple joint involvement, up to a total of 80 mg, have been given without undue reactions.

It is recommended that, when injections are given into the sheaths of short tendons, Adcortyl injection (triamcinolone acetonide 10 mg/ml) should be used. (See under Precautions re Achilles tendon.)

Intramuscular injection: Adults and children over 12 years: The suggested initial dose is 40 mg (1 ml) injected deeply into the upper, outer quadrant of the gluteal muscle. Subsequent dosage depends on the patient's response and period of relief. Patients with hay fever or pollen asthma who do not respond to conventional therapy may obtain a remission of symptoms lasting throughout the pollen season after a dose of 40-100 mg given when allergic symptoms appear.

For children from 6-12 years of age: The suggested initial dose of 40 mg (1 ml) injected deeply into the gluteal muscle should be scaled according to the severity of symptoms and the age and weight of the child. Kenalog is not recommended for children under six years (see Precautions).

Elderly: Treatment of elderly patients, particularly if long term, should be planned bearing in mind the more serious consequences of the common side effects of corticosteroids in old age, especially osteoporosis, diabetes, hypertension, susceptibility to infection and thinning of the skin.

Contra-indications, warnings, etc
Contra-indications: None.

Precautions: In common with other steroids Kenalog injection should be used with caution in patients with recent intestinal anastomoses, thrombophlebitis, psychotic tendencies, exanthematous disease, chronic nephritis, metastatic carcinoma, osteoporosis, in patients with an active peptic ulcer (or a history of peptic ulcer). Latent or healed tuberculosis; in the presence of local or systemic viral infection, systemic fungal infections or in active infections not controlled by antibiotics. In acute psychoses; in acute glomerulonephritis. Hypertension; glaucoma (or a family history of glaucoma), previous steroid myopathy or epilepsy.

Intra-articular injection should not be carried out in the presence of active infection in or near joints. The preparation should not be used to alleviate joint pain arising from infectious states such as gonococcal or tubercular arthritis.

Diabetes may be aggravated, necessitating a higher insulin dosage. Latent diabetes mellitus may be precipitated.

Menstrual irregularities may occur, and this possibility should be mentioned to female patients.

Patients on long-term systemic therapy with Kenalog may require supportive corticosteroid therapy in times of stress, both during the treatment period and for a year afterwards.

During corticosteroid therapy antibody response will be reduced and therefore affect the patient's response to vaccines.

Rare instances of anaphylactoid reactions have occurred in patients receiving parenteral corticosteroids, especially when a patient has a history of drug allergies.

All corticosteroids increase calcium excretion.

Avoid abrupt cessation of corticosteroids.

Aspirin should be used cautiously in conjunction with corticosteroids in patients with hypoprothrombinaemia.

Corticosteroid effects may be enhanced in patients with hypothyroidism or cirrhosis.

Pregnancy: Corticosteroids are not recommended for pregnant patients, particularly in the first trimester, or for nursing mothers, except when the disease for which they are indicated warrants their use. There is inadequate evidence of safety in human pregnancy and there may be a very small risk of cleft palate and intra-uterine growth retardation in the foetus; there is evidence of harmful effects on pregnancy in animals.

Children: Kenalog is not recommended for children under six years. Growth and development of children on prolonged corticosteroid therapy should be carefully observed.

Intra-articular injection: Patients should be specifically warned to avoid over-use of joints in which symptomatic benefit has been obtained. Severe joint destruction with necrosis of bone may occur if repeated intra-articular injections are given over a long period of time. Care should be taken if injections are given into tendon sheaths to avoid injection into the tendon itself.

Due to the absence of a true tendon sheath, the Achilles tendon should not be injected with depot corticosteroids.

Intra-muscular injection: During prolonged therapy a liberal protein intake is essential to counteract the tendency to gradual weight loss sometimes associated with negative nitrogen balance and wasting of skeletal muscle.

N.B. To avoid the danger of subcutaneous fat atrophy, it is important to ensure that deep intramuscular injection is given into the gluteal site. The deltoid should not be used. Alternate sides should be used for subsequent injections.

Side-effects: Where adverse reactions occur they are usually reversible on cessation of therapy. Absorption of triamcinolone following injection by the intra-articular route is rare. However, the possibility of the systemic effects which are associated with all steroid therapy should be considered with both routes of administration. These may include:

Dyspepsia, peptic ulceration with perforation and haemorrhage, abdominal distension, oesophageal ulceration, oesophageal candidiasis, acute pancreatitis.

Proximal myopathy, osteoporosis, vertebral and long bone fractures, avascular osteonecrosis, tendon rupture.

Sodium and water retention, hypertension, hypokalaemic alkalosis.

Impaired healing, skin atrophy, bruising, striae, telangiectasia, acne.

Suppression of the hypothalamo-pituitary adrenal axis, growth suppression in childhood and adolescence, menstrual irregularity and amenorrhoea. Cushingoid facies, hirsutism, weight gain, impaired carbohydrate tolerance with increased requirement for antidiabetic therapy, negative nitrogen balance.

Euphoria, psychological dependence, depression, insomnia. Intracranial hypertension has been reported in children on cessation of long term steroid therapy. Aggravation of schizophrenia.

Increased intra-ocular pressure, glaucoma, papilloedema, cataracts, corneal or scleral thinning, exacerbation of ophthalmic viral disease.

Opportunistic infection, recurrence of dormant tuberculosis, leucocytosis, hypersensitivity, thromboembolism, increased appetite, nausea, malaise.

On withdrawal fever, myalgia, arthralgia or adrenal insufficiency may occur.

Intra-articular injection: Reactions following intra-articular administration have been rare. In a few instances transient flushing and dizziness have occurred. Pain and other local symptoms may continue for a short time before effective relief is obtained, but an increase in joint discomfort has seldom occurred. Local fat atrophy may occur if the injection is not given into the joint space, but is temporary and disappears within a few weeks to months.

Pharmaceutical precautions *Storage:* At room temperature; avoid freezing.

Legal category POM.

Package quantities 1 ml and 2 ml ready filled syringes (Intramuscular use only). 1 ml vials: pack of 5 (Intra-articular and Intramuscular use).

Further information Nil.

Product licence number 0034/5045.

MODECATE* INJECTION
MODECATE* CONCENTRATE INJECTION

Presentation *Modecate injection:* Straw-coloured viscous liquid containing fluphenazine decanoate 25 mg per ml in sesame oil.

Modecate Concentrate injection: Straw-coloured, viscous liquid containing fluphenazine decanoate 100 mg per ml in sesame oil. Ampoules are marked with a distinctive blue band.

Uses

Indications: For the treatment and maintenance of schizophrenic patients and those with paranoid psychoses. While Modecate injection has been shown to be effective in acute states, it is particularly useful in the maintenance treatment of chronic patients who are unreliable at taking their oral medication, and also of those who do not absorb their oral phenothiazines in adequate amounts.

Modecate Concentrate injection provides a high concentration of fluphenazine decanoate in a small volume which may be injected without discomfort to the patient and it is therefore particularly suitable for those patients who require higher doses for effective antipsychotic control.

Dosage and administration It is preferable that patients be stabilised on the injection in hospital.
Recommended dosage regimes for all indications:

1. *Modecate injection 25 mg/ml*

a) *Patients without previous exposure to a depot fluphenazine formulation:* Initially 0.5 ml (0.25 ml for patients over 60) by deep intramuscular injection into the gluteal region.

The onset of action generally appears between 24 and 72 hours after injection and the effects of the drug on psychotic symptoms become significant within 48 to 96 hours. Subsequent injections and the dosage interval are determined in accordance with the patient's response. When administered as maintenance therapy, a single injection may be effective in controlling schizophrenic symptoms up to four weeks or longer.

It is desirable to maintain as much flexibility in the dose as possible to achieve the best therapeutic response with the least side-effects; most patients are successfully maintained within the dose range 0.5 ml to 4 ml given at a dose interval of 2 to 5 weeks.

Patients previously maintained on oral fluphenazine: It is not possible to predict the equivalent dose of depot formulation in view of the wide variability of individual response.

b) *Patients previously maintained on depot fluphenazines:* Patients who have suffered a relapse following cessation of depot fluphenazine therapy may be restarted on the same dose as they were receiving formerly, although the frequency of injections may need to be increased in the early weeks of treatment until satisfactory control is obtained.

2. *Modecate Concentrate injection 100 mg/ml:* Where a smaller volume of injection is desirable, patients may be transferred directly to the equivalent dose of Modecate Concentrate on the basis that 1 ml Modecate Concentrate Injection is equivalent to 4 ml Modecate injection.

Elderly: Elderly patients may be particularly susceptible to extrapyramidal reactions. Therefore, reduced maintenance dosage may be required and a smaller initial dose (see above).

Children: Not recommended for children.

Note: The dosage should not be increased without close supervision and it should be noted that there is a variability in individual response.

The response to antipsychotic drug treatment may be delayed. If drugs are withdrawn, recurrence of symptoms may not become apparent for several weeks or months.

Contra-indications, warnings, etc

Contra-indications: Comatose states; marked cerebral atherosclerosis; phaeochromocytoma; renal failure; liver failure; severe cardiac insufficiency; and severely depressed states.

Precautions: Liver disease; cardiac arrhythmias, cardiac disease; thyrotoxicosis; severe respiratory disease; epilepsy, conditions predisposing to epilepsy (e.g. alcohol withdrawal or brain damage); Parkinson's disease; patients who have shown hypersensitivity to other phenothiazines; personal or family history of narrow angle glaucoma; in very hot weather; the elderly, particularly if frail or at risk of hypothermia; hypothyroidism; myasthenia gravis; prostatic hypertrophy.

Use in pregnancy: The safety for the use of this drug during pregnancy has not been established; therefore, the possible hazards should be weighed against the potential benefits when administering this drug to pregnant patients.

Nursing mothers: Breast feeding is not recommended during treatment with depot fluphenazines, owing to the possibility that fluphenazine is excreted in the milk of nursing mothers.

Drug interactions: The possibility should be borne in mind that phenothiazines may:
(1) Increase the central nervous system depression produced by drugs such as alcohol, hypnotics, sedatives or strong analgesics.
(2) Antagonise the action of adrenaline and other sympathomimetic agents and reverse the blood-pressure-lowering effects of adrenergic-blocking agents such as guanethidine and clonidine.
(3) Impair
    (a) the anti-Parkinsonian effect of L-Dopa
    (b) the effect of anti-convulsants
    (c) metabolism of tricyclic antidepressants
    (d) the control of diabetes
(4) Increase the effect of anticoagulants.
(5) Interact with lithium.

Anticholinergic effects may be enhanced by anti-Parkinsonian or other anticholinergic drugs.

Phenothiazines may enhance: The cardiac-depressant effects of quinidine; the absorption of corticosteroids, and digoxin, and neuromuscular blocking agents.

Side-effects: Acute dystonic reactions occur infrequently, as a rule within the first 24–48 hours, although delayed reactions may occur. In susceptible individuals they may occur after only small doses. These may include such dramatic manifestations as oculogyric crises and opisthotonos. They are rapidly relieved by intravenous administration of an anti-Parkinsonian agent such as procyclidine.

Parkinsonian-like states may occur particularly between the second and fifth days after each injection, but often decrease with subsequent injections. These reactions may be reduced by using smaller doses more frequently, or by the concomitant use of anti-Parkinsonian drugs such as benzhexol, benztropine or procyclidine. Anti-Parkinsonian drugs should not be prescribed routinely, because of the possible risks of aggravating anti-cholinergic side-effects or precipitating toxic confusional states, or of impairing therapeutic efficacy.

With careful monitoring of the dose the number of patients requiring anti-Parkinsonian drugs can be minimised

Tardive dyskinesia: As with all antipsychotic agents, tardive dyskinesia may appear in some patients on long term therapy or may occur after drug therapy has been discontinued. The risk seems to be greater in elderly patients on high dose therapy, especially females. The symptoms are persistent and in some patients appear to be irreversible.

The syndrome is characterised by rhythmical involuntary movements of the tongue, face, mouth or jaw (e.g. protrusion of tongue, puffing of cheeks, puckering of mouth, chewing movements). Sometimes these may be accompanied by involuntary movements of the extremities. There is no known effective treatment for tardive dyskinesia; anti-Parkinsonian agents usually do not alleviate the symptoms of this syndrome. It is suggested that all antipsychotic agents be discontinued if these symptoms appear. Should it be necessary to reinstitute treatment, or increase the dosage of the agent, or switch to a different antipsychotic agent, the syndrome may be masked. It has been reported that fine vermicular movements of the tongue may be an early sign of the syndrome and if the medication is stopped at that time, the syndrome may not develop.

As with other phenothiazines, drowsiness, lethargy, blurred vision, dryness of the mouth, constipation, urinary hesitancy or incontinence, mild hypotension, impairment of judgement and mental skills, and epileptiform attacks are occasionally seen.

The use of this drug may impair the mental and physical abilities required for driving a car or operating heavy machinery.

Blood dyscrasias have rarely been reported with phenothiazine derivatives. Blood counts should be performed if the patient develops signs of persistent infection. Transient leucopenia and thrombocytopenia have been reported. Antinuclear antibodies and SLE have been reported very rarely.

Jaundice has rarely been reported. Transient abnormalities of liver function tests may occur in the absence of jaundice.

A transient rise in serum cholesterol has been reported very occasionally in patients on oral fluphenazine.

Abnormal skin pigmentation and lens opacities have sometimes been seen following long-term administration of high doses of phenothiazines.

Phenothiazines are known to cause photosensitivity reactions but this has not been reported for fluphenazine. Skin rashes have occasionally been reported.

Elderly patients may be more susceptible to the sedative and hypotensive effects.

The effects of phenothiazines on the heart are dose-related. ECG changes, with prolongation of the QT interval and T-wave changes have been reported commonly in patients treated with moderate to high dosage; they are reversible on reducing the dose. In a very small number of cases, they have been reported to precede serious arrhythmias, including ventricular tachycardia and fibrillation, which have also occurred after overdosage. Sudden, unexpected and unexplained deaths have been reported in hospitalised psychotic patients receiving phenothiazines.

Phenothiazines may impair body temperature regulation. Cases of severe hypothermia or hyperpyrexia have been reported in association with moderate or high dosage of phenothiazines.

Elderly or hypothyroid patients may be particularly susceptible to hypothermia. The hazard of hyperpyrexia may be increased by especially hot or humid weather, or by drugs such as anti-Parkinsonian agents, which impair sweating.

Hormonal effects of fluphenazines include hyperprolactinaemia, which may cause galactorrhoea, gynaecomastia and oligo- or amenorrhoea. Sexual function may be impaired.

Oedema has been reported with phenothiazine medication.

Overdosage: It should be treated symptomatically and supportively. Extrapyramidal reactions will respond to oral or parenteral anti-Parkinsonian drugs such as procyclidine or benztropine. In cases of severe hypotension, all procedures for the management of circulatory shock should be instituted, e.g. vasoconstrictors and/or intravenous fluids. However, only the vasoconstrictors metaraminol or noradrenaline should be used, as adrenaline may further lower the blood pressure through interaction with the phenothiazine.

Pharmaceutical precautions *Storage:* At room temperature. Do not store in a refrigerator, since this will cause precipitation of triglycerides from the sesame oil. If precipitation does occur, warming the product to 37°C will dissolve the precipitate without harming the active ingredient. Protect from direct sunlight.

Legal category POM.

Package quantities *Modecate Injection 25 mg/ml:* Ampoules 0.5 ml, 1 ml and 2 ml; Ready-filled syringes of 1 ml, 2 ml; Multidose vials of 10 ml.
Modecate Concentrate Injection 100 mg/ml: Ampoules 0.5 ml and 1 ml.

Further information Fluphenazine decanoate is an ester of the potent neuroleptic fluphenazine, a phenothiazine derivative of the piperazine type. The ester is slowly absorbed from the intramuscular site of injection and is then hydrolysed in the plasma to the active therapeutic agent, fluphenazine.

Extrapyramidal reactions are not uncommon, but fluphenazine does not have marked sedative or hypotensive properties.

Pharmacokinetics: Plasma level profiles of fluphenazine following Modecate injection have shown half-lives of plasma clearance ranging from $2\frac{1}{2}$–16 weeks, emphasising the importance of adjusting dose and interval to the individual requirements of each patient. The slow decline of plasma levels in most patients means that a reasonably stable plasma level can usually be achieved with injections spaced at 2–4 week intervals.

Product licence numbers
Modecate Injection 25 mg/ml   0034/5046R
Modecate Concentrate Injection
100 mg/ml   0034/0189

MODITEN* ENANTHATE INJECTION

Presentation Straw-coloured viscous liquid containing fluphenazine enanthate 25 mg per ml in sesame oil.

Uses *Indications:* For the treatment and maintenance of schizophrenic patients and those with paranoid psychoses.

While Moditen Enanthate Injection has been shown to be effective in acute states, it is particularly useful in the maintenance treatment of chronic patients who are unreliable at taking their oral medication, and also in those who do not absorb their oral phenothiazines in adequate amounts.

Dosage and administration It is preferable that patients be stabilised on the injection in hospital.

Recommended dosage regimes for all indications:

(a) *Patients without previous exposure to a depot fluphenazine formulation:* Initially 0.5 ml (0.25 ml for patients over 60) by deep intramuscular injection into the gluteal region.

The onset of action generally appears between 24 and 72 hours after injection and the effects of the drug on psychotic symptoms become significant within 48 to 96 hours. Subsequent injections and the dosage interval are determined in accordance with the patient's response. When administered as maintenance therapy, a single injection may be effective in controlling schizophrenic symptoms up to three weeks or longer.

It is desirable to maintain as much flexibility in the dose as possible to achieve the best therapeutic response with the least side-effects; most patients are successfully maintained within the dose range 0.5 ml to 4.0 ml given at a dose interval of 10 days to 3 weeks.

Patients previously maintained on oral fluphenazine: It is not possible to predict the equivalent dose of depot formulation in view of the wide variability of individual response.

(b) *Patients previously maintained on depot fluphenazine:* Patients who have suffered a relapse following cessation of depot fluphenazine therapy may be restarted on the same dose as they were receiving formerly, although the frequency of injections may need to be increased in the early weeks of treatment until satisfactory control is obtained.

Elderly: Elderly patients may be particularly susceptible to extrapyramidal reactions. Therefore reduced maintenance may be required and a smaller initial dose. (See above).

Children: Not recommended for children.

Note: The dosage should not be increased without close supervision and it should be noted that there is a variability in individual response.

The response to antipsychotic drug treatment may be delayed. If drugs are withdrawn, recurrence of symptoms may not become apparent for several weeks or months.

Contra-indications, warnings, etc

Contra-indications: Comatose states; marked cerebral atherosclerosis; phaeochromocytoma; renal failure; liver failure; severe cardiac insufficiency; severely depressed states.

Precautions: Liver disease; cardiac arrhythmias, cardiac disease; thyrotoxicosis; severe respiratory disease; epilepsy, conditions predisposing to epilepsy (e.g. alcohol withdrawal or brain damage); Parkinson's disease; patients who have shown hypersensitivity to other phenothiazines; personal or family history of narrow angle glaucoma; in very hot weather; the elderly, particularly if frail or at risk of hypothermia; hypothyroidism; myasthenia gravis; prostatic hypertrophy.

Use in pregnancy: The safety for the use of this drug during pregnancy has not been established; therefore, the possible hazards should be weighed against the potential benefits when administering this drug to pregnant patients.

Nursing mothers: Breast feeding is not recommended during treatment with depot fluphenazines, owing to the possibility that fluphenazine is excreted in the milk of nursing mothers.

Drug interactions: The possibility should be borne in mind that phenothiazines may:

(1) Increase the central nervous system depression produced by drugs such as alcohol, hypnotics, sedatives or strong analgesics.

(2) Antagonise the action of adrenaline and other sympathomimetic agents and reverse the blood-pressure-lowering effects of adrenergic-blocking agents such as guanethidine and clonidine.

(3) Impair (a) the anti-Parkinsonian effect of L-Dopa; (b) the effect of anti-convulsants; (c) metabolism of tricyclic antidepressants; (d) the control of diabetes.

(4) Increase the effect of anticoagulants.

(5) Interact with lithium.

Anticholinergic effects may be enhanced by anti-Parkinsonian or other anticholinergic drugs.

Phenothiazines may enhance: The cardiac-depressant effects of quinidine; the absorption of corticosteroids, and digoxin, and neuromuscular blocking agents.

Side-effects: Acute dystonic reactions occur infrequently but nearly always within the first 24–48 hours, and may include such dramatic manifestations as oculogyric crises and opisthotonos. They are rapidly relieved by intravenous administration of an anti-Parkinsonian agent such as procyclidine.

Parkinsonian-like states may occur particularly between the second and fifth days after each injection, but often decrease with subsequent injections. These reactions may be reduced by using smaller doses more frequently, or by the concomitant use of anti-Parkinsonian drugs such as benzhexol, benztropine or procyclidine. Anti-Parkinsonian drugs should not be prescribed routinely, because of the possible risks of aggravating anti-cholinergic side-effects or precipitating toxic confusional states, or of impairing therapeutic efficacy.

With careful monitoring of the dose the number of patients requiring anti-Parkinsonian drugs can be minimised.

Tardive dyskinesia: As with all antipsychotic agents, tardive dyskinesia may appear in some patients on long term therapy or may occur after drug therapy has been discontinued. The risk seems to be greater in elderly patients on high dose therapy, especially females. The symptoms are persistent and in some patients appear to be irreversible. The syndrome is characterised by rhythmical involuntary movements of the tongue, face, mouth or jaw (e.g. protrusion of tongue, puffing of cheeks, puckering of mouth, chewing movements). Sometimes these may be accompanied by involuntary movements of the extremities. There is no known effective treatment for tardive dyskinesia; anti-Parkinsonian agents usually do not alleviate the symptoms of this syndrome. It is suggested that all antipsychotic agents be discontinued if these symptoms appear. Should it be necessary to reinstitute treatment, or increase the dosage of the agent, or switch to a different antipsychotic agent, the syndrome may be masked. It has been reported that fine vermicular movements of the tongue may be an early sign of the syndrome and if the medication is stopped at that time, the syndrome may not develop.

As with other phenothiazines, drowsiness, lethargy, blurred vision, dryness of the mouth, constipation, urinary hesitancy or incontinence, mild hypotension, impairment of judgement and mental skills, and epileptiform attacks are occasionally seen.

The use of this drug may impair the mental and physical abilities required for driving a car or operating heavy machinery.

Blood dyscrasias have rarely been reported with phenothiazine derivatives. Blood counts should be performed if the patient develops signs of persistent infection. Transient leucopenia and thrombocytopenia have been reported. Antinuclear antibodies and SLE have been reported very rarely.

Jaundice has rarely been reported. Transient abnormalities of liver function tests may occur in the absence of jaundice.

A transient rise in serum cholesterol has been reported very occasionally in patients on oral fluphenazine.

Abnormal skin pigmentation and lens opacities have sometimes been seen following long-term administration of high doses of phenothiazines.

Phenothiazines are known to cause photosensitivity reactions but this has not been reported for fluphenazine. Skin rashes have occasionally been reported.

Elderly patients may be more susceptible to the sedative and hypotensive effects.

The effects of phenothiazines on the heart are dose-related. ECG changes, with prolongation of the QT interval and T-wave changes have been reported commonly in patients treated with moderate to high dosage; they are reversible on reducing the dose. In a very small number of cases, they have been reported to precede serious arrhythmias, including ventricular tachycardia and fibrillation, which have also occurred after overdosage. Sudden, unexpected and unexplained deaths have been reported in hospitalised psychotic patients receiving phenothiazines.

Phenothiazines may impair body temperature regulation. Cases of severe hypothermia or hyperpyrexia have been reported in association with moderate or high dosage of phenothiazines.

Elderly or hypothyroid patients may be particularly susceptible to hypothermia. The hazard of hyperpyrexia may be increased by especially hot or humid weather, or by drugs such as anti-Parkinsonian agents, which impair sweating.

Hormonal effects of fluphenazines include hyperprolactinaemia, which may cause galactorrhoea, gynaecomastia and oligo- or amenorrhoea. Sexual function may be impaired.

Oedema has been reported with phenothiazine medication.

Overdosage: It should be treated symptomatically and supportively. Extrapyramidal reactions will respond to oral or parenteral anti-Parkinsonian drugs such as procyclidine or benztropine. In cases of severe hypotension, all procedures for the management of circulatory shock should be instituted, e.g. vasoconstrictors and/or intravenous fluids. However, only the vasoconstrictors metaraminol or noradrenaline should be used, as adrenaline may further lower the blood pressure through interaction with the phenothiazine.

Pharmaceutical precautions *Storage:* At room temperature. Do not store in a refrigerator, since this will cause precipitation of triglycerides from the sesame oil. If precipitation does occur, warming the product to 37°C will dissolve the precipitate without harming the active ingredient. Protect from direct sunlight.

Legal category POM.

Package quantities Ampoules of 1 ml.

Further information Fluphenazine enanthate is an ester of the potent neuroleptic fluphenazine, a phenothiazine derivative of the piperazine type. The ester is slowly absorbed from the intramuscular site of injection and is then hydrolysed in the plasma to the active therapeutic agent, fluphenazine.

Extrapyramidal reactions are not uncommon, but fluphenazine does not have marked sedative or hypotensive properties.

Product licence number 0034/5048R.

MODITEN* TABLETS

Presentation *Tablets 1.0 mg:* Round, pink, sugar-coated tablets containing 1 mg fluphenazine hydrochloride. *Tablets 2.5 mg:* Round, yellow, sugar-coated tablets containing 2.5 mg fluphenazine hydrochloride. *Tablets 5 mg:* Round, white, sugar-coated tablets containing 5 mg fluphenazine hydrochloride.

Uses *Adults:* Moditen Tablets are indicated: As an adjunct to the short-term management of anxiety, severe psychomotor agitation, excitement, violent or dangerously impulsive behaviour; in schizophrenia – treatment of symptoms and prevention of relapse; in other psychoses, especially paranoid; in mania and hypomania.

Dosage and administration
1. Adults: Anxiety and other non-psychotic behavioural disturbances: Initially 1 mg twice daily rising to 2 mg twice daily, if necessary, according to response.

Schizophrenia, mania, hypomania, and other psychoses: Initially 2.5–10 mg daily divided into 2 or 3 doses, depending on the severity and duration of symptoms, rising to 20 mg daily, as necessary. Doses exceeding 20 mg daily (10 mg in the elderly) should be used with caution.

2. Elderly: Elderly patients may be particularly susceptible to extrapyramidal reactions. Dosage at the lower end of the range is likely to be sufficient for elderly patients.

3. Children: Not recommended for children.

Note: The dosage should not be increased without close supervision and it should be noted that there is a variability in individual response.

The response to antipsychotic drug treatment may be delayed. If drugs are withdrawn, recurrence of symptoms may not become apparent for several weeks or months.

Contra-indications, warnings, etc
Contra-indications: Comatose states; marked cerebral atherosclerosis; phaeochromocytoma; renal failure; liver failure; severe cardiac insufficiency; severely depressed states.

Precautions: Liver disease; cardiac arrhythmias, cardiac disease; thyrotoxicosis; severe respiratory disease; epilepsy, conditions predisposing to epilepsy (e.g. alcohol withdrawal or brain damage); Parkinson's disease; patients who have shown hypersensitivity to other phenothiazines; personal or family history of narrow angle glaucoma; in very hot weather; the elderly, particularly if frail or at risk of hypothermia; hypothyroidism; myasthenia gravis; prostatic hypertrophy.

Use in pregnancy: The safety for the use of this drug during pregnancy has not been established; therefore, the possible hazards should be weighed against the potential benefits when administering this drug to pregnant patients.

Nursing mothers: Breast feeding is not recommended during treatment with fluphenazines, owing to the possibility that fluphenazine is excreted in the milk of nursing mothers.

Drug interactions: The possibility should be borne in mind that phenothiazines may:
(1) Increase the central nervous system depression produced by drugs such as alcohol, hypnotics, sedatives or strong analgesics.
(2) Antagonise the action of adrenaline and other sympathomimetic agents and reverse the blood-pressure-lowering effects of adrenergic-blocking agents such as guanethidine and clonidine.
(3) Impair: (a) the anti-Parkinsonian effect of L-Dopa; (b) the effect of anti-convulsants; (c) metabolism of tricyclic antidepressants; (d) the control of diabetes.
(4) Increase the effect of anticoagulants.
(5) Interact with lithium.

Tea and coffee form insoluble precipitates with fluphenazine in vitro, but there is conflicting evidence as to whether this reduces absorption in man.

Antacids may impair absorption.

Anticholinergic effects may be enhanced by anti-Parkinsonian or other anticholinergic drugs.

Phenothiazines may enhance: The cardiac-depressant effects of quinidine; the absorption of corticosteroids, digoxin and neuromuscular blocking agents.

Side-effects: Extrapyramidal reactions are common at higher doses and occasionally occur at low dosage. Acute dystonias may occur early in treatment, and oculogyric crises have been reported. Both usually respond rapidly to an i.v. or i.m. administration of an anti-Parkinsonian agent. Parkinsonian rigidity, tremor, akathisia, tend to appear less rapidly, and may be reduced by using a smaller dose or by the concomitant use of an oral anti-Parkinsonian drug such as benzhexol, benztropine or procyclidine. However, anti-Parkinsonian agents should not be prescribed routinely, because of the possible risks of aggravating anticholinergic side-effects of fluphenazine, of precipitating toxic-confusional states or of impairing its therapeutic efficacy.

Numerous surveys of schizophrenic patients receiving phenothiazine medication have reported varying prevalences of irregularly repetitive involuntary movements, which collectively have been termed 'tardive dyskinesia'. The movements most commonly involve the tongue and facial muscles, but sometimes affect the limbs and trunk. Although the only two surveys which assessed the prevalence of involuntary movements among schizophrenic patients never treated with neuroleptics found similar prevalence to that among the neuroleptic-treated patients, phenothiazines as well as other antipsychotics have been implicated in the emergence of these syndromes.

Tardive dyskinesia: As with all antipsychotic agents, tardive dyskinesia may appear in some patients on long term therapy or may occur after drug therapy has been discontinued. The risk seems to be greater in elderly patients on high dose therapy, especially females. The symptoms are persistent and in some patients appear to be irreversible. The syndrome is characterised by rhythmical involuntary movements of the tongue, face, mouth or jaw (e.g. protrusion of tongue, puffing of cheeks, puckering of mouth, chewing movements). Sometimes these may be accompanied by involuntary movements of the extremities. There is no known effective treatment for tardive dyskinesia; anti-Parkinsonian agents usually do not alleviate the symptoms of this syndrome. It is suggested that all antipsychotic agents be discontinued if these symptoms appear. Should it be necessary to reinstitute treatment, or increase the dosage of the agent, or switch to a different antispsychotic agent, the syndrome may be masked. It has been reported that fine vermicular movements of the tongue may be an early sign of the syndrome and if the medication is stopped at that time, the syndrome may not develop.

As with other phenothiazines, drowsiness, lethargy, blurred vision, dryness of the mouth, constipation, urinary hesitancy and incontinence, mild hypotension, impairment of judgement and mental skills, and epileptiform attacks are occasionally seen, but extremely rarely in doses used for non-psychotic conditions.

The use of this drug may impair the mental and physical abilities required for driving a car or operating heavy machinery.

Blood dyscrasias have rarely been reported with phenothiazine derivatives. Blood counts should be performed if the patient develops signs of persistent infection. Transient leucopenia and thrombocytopenia have been reported. Antinuclear antibodies and SLE have been reported very rarely.

Jaundice has rarely been reported. Transient abnormalities of liver function tests may occur in the absence of jaundice.

A transient rise in serum cholesterol has been reported very occasionally in patients on oral fluphenazine.

Abnormal skin pigmentation and lens opacities have sometimes been seen following long-term administration of high doses of phenothiazines.

Phenothiazines are known to cause photosensitivity reactions but this has not been reported for fluphenazine. Skin rashes have occasionally been reported.

Elderly patients may be more susceptible to the sedative and hypotensive effects.

The effects of phenothiazines on the heart are dose-related. ECG changes, with prolongation of the QT interval and T-wave changes have been reported commonly in patients treated with moderate to high dosage; they are reversible on reducing the dose. In a very small number of cases, they have been reported to precede serious arrhythmias, including ventricular tachycardia and fibrillation, which have also occurred after over-dosage. Sudden, unexpected and unexplained deaths have been reported in hospitalised psychotic patients receiving phenothiazines.

Phenothiazines may impair body temperature regulation. Cases of severe hypothermia or hyperpyrexia have been reported in association with moderate or high dosage of phenothiazines.

Elderly or hypothyroid patients may be particularly susceptible to hypothermia. The hazard of hyperpyrexia may be increased by especially hot or humid weather, or by drugs such as anti-Parkinsonian agents, which impair sweating.

Hormonal effects of fluphenazines include hyperprolactinaemia, which may cause galactorrhoea, gynaecomastia and oligo- or amenorrhoea. Sexual function may be impaired.

Oedema has been reported with phenothiazine medication.

Acute withdrawal symptoms including nausea, vomiting and insomnia, have very rarely been described after abrupt cessation of high doses of phenothiazines. Gradual withdrawal is advisable.

Overdosage: It should be treated symptomatically and supportively. Extrapyramidal reactions will respond to oral or parenteral anti-Parkinsonian drugs such as procyclidine or benztropine. In cases of severe hypotension, all procedures for the management of circulatory shock should be instituted, e.g. vasoconstrictors and/or intravenous fluids. However, only the vasoconstrictors metaraminol or noradrenaline should be used, as adrenaline may further lower the blood pressure through interaction with the phenothiazine.

Pharmaceutical precautions *Storage:* At room temperature.

Legal category POM.

Package quantities Bottles of 100.

Further information Fluphenazine hydrochloride is a salt of the potent neuroleptic fluphenazine, a phenothiazine derivative of the piperazine type. Extrapyramidal reactions, are not uncommon, but fluphenazine does not have marked sedative or hypotensive properties.

Product licence numbers
Moditen Tablets 1 mg   0034/5049R
Moditen Tablets 2.5 mg   0034/5050R
Moditen Tablets 5 mg   0034/5051R

MOTIPRESS* TABLETS
MOTIVAL* TABLETS

Presentation *Motival:* Each pink, triangular-shaped, sugar-coated tablet contains nortriptyline hydrochloride (equivalent to 10 mg nortriptyline base) and fluphenazine hydrochloride 0.5 mg.

Motipress: Each yellow, triangular-shaped, sugar-coated tablet contains nortriptyline hydrochloride (equivalent to 30 mg nortriptyline base) and fluphenazine hydrochloride 1.5 mg.

Uses *Actions:* Nortriptyline hydrochloride is a tricyclic antidepressant with more rapid activity and less sedation than the majority of the drugs of its class. It possesses some atropine-like properties. It is not a monoamine oxidase inhibitor.

Fluphenazine hydrochloride is a phenothiazine derivative of the piperazine type, its principal actions being those of tranquillization and anti-emesis.

Indications: Motival and Motipress are indicated for the treatment of patients suffering from mild to moderate mixed anxiety depressive states.

Dosage and administration *Adults:* Motival: The dose is 1 tablet three times daily.

Motipress: The dose is 1 tablet daily, preferably before retiring.

A course of treatment with either Motival or Motipress should be limited to three months. If the patient does not respond after four weeks an alternative treatment should be given.

Elderly: Elderly patients should be started on Motival one tablet twice daily. If Motival one tablet, three times

daily, is required, subsequently Motipress may be substituted.

Children: These formulations are not indicated for the treatment of children.

Contra-indications, warnings, etc
Contra-indications: Phenothiazines and tricyclic antidepressants have been shown to lower the threshold for electrically induced convulsions in animals, hence Motival and Motipress are not recommended for patients with a history of epilepsy or brain damage. It is further contra-indicated in patients with blood dyscrasias, severe cardiac insufficiency, renal or liver damage.

It is inadvisable to give monoamine oxidase inhibitors (MAOIs) with Motival or Motipress, nor should they be given within two weeks after cessation of treatment with MAOIs.

Precautions: Motival and Motipress should be given with caution to patients with glaucoma and to those who have a propensity for urinary retention. Interaction with barbiturates, alcohol and narcotic drugs may occur, so central nervous depressants should be administered with caution. Motival and Motipress may diminish the anti-hypertensive effect of adrenergic blocking agents and could potentiate the pressor response to locally injected sympathomimetic agents.

Tardive dyskinesias have been reported in association with phenothiazine therapy, usually after prolonged courses given at doses adequate to treat psychotic illness. Consequently Motival and Motipress treatment should be limited to three months (see Dosage and Administration).

The use of Motival or Motipress may impair alertness and abilities required for driving a car or operating machinery.

Motival or Motipress should be used with caution in patients with cardiac failure, especially when there is evidence of rhythm disturbance, and in patients with recent myocardial infarction.

Pregnancy: Do not use during pregnancy, especially the first and last trimesters, unless there are compelling reasons. There is no evidence as to drug safety in human pregnancy nor are the results of animal studies conclusive.

Nursing mothers: Breast feeding is not recommended in women receiving Motival and Motipress.

Side-effects: Dryness of mouth, drowsiness, faintness and constipation. Occasionally tachycardia, nasal congestion, blurred vision and excitement are seen.

Extrapyramidal reactions are unlikely to occur with this dose of fluphenazine alone, and it is probable that the anticholinergic activity of nortriptyline affords protection against such effects.

Overdosage: Overdosage should be treated symptomatically and supportively. If the patient is conscious, prompt gastric lavage, dilution of the stomach contents to delay absorption, or stimulation of vomiting should be attempted. An open airway should be maintained. Extrapyramidal symptoms are amenable to antiparkinsonian drugs. In severe hypotension, all the standard procedures for the management of circulatory shock should be instituted, e.g. vasoconstrictors and/or intravenous fluids. If vasoconstrictors are required, metaraminol, mephentermine or noradrenaline should be administered, but not adrenaline, as this will further lower the blood pressure through interaction with the phenothiazine.

Pharmaceutical precautions *Storage:* At room temperature.

Legal category POM.

Package quantities Motival: Bottles of 100 and 500 tablets.
Motipress: 28 day calendar pack. Bottles of 250 tablets.

Further information Nil.

Product licence numbers
Motival Tablets   0034/0219
Motipress Tablets   0034/0220.

MULTILIND* OINTMENT

Presentation Pale yellow ointment containing 100,000 units nystatin per gram in an emollient base (Plastibase*) thickened with 20% w/w zinc oxide.

Uses *Actions:* Nystatin is an antifungal antibiotic active against a wide range of yeasts and yeast-like fungi, including *Candida albicans.*

Indications: For the treatment of cutaneous and mucocutaneous mycoses, especially those caused by *C. albicans.* Multilind ointment is particularly indicated for the treatment of napkin rash where super-infection with *C. albicans* has occurred.

Dosage and administration *Adults and children:* To be applied liberally to the affected area two to four times daily.

Elderly: No specific dosage recommendations or precautions.

Contra-indications, warnings, etc
Contra-indications: There are no known contra-indications or special precautions for topical application of nystatin.
Side-effects: There have been no substantiated reports of sensitivity associated with the topical use of nystatin.

Pharmaceutical precautions *Storage:* At room temperature. Avoid freezing.
Dilution: Nystatin products should not be diluted as this may reduce therapeutic efficacy.

Legal category POM.

Package quantities Tubes of 50 g.

Further information Plastibase* is a specially formulated base which retains its viscosity at body temperature. This, together with the zinc oxide, makes it particularly beneficial in hot, moist areas such as the napkin area.

Product licence number 0034/0243.

MYSTECLIN* CAPSULES AND TABLETS

Presentation *Capsules:* Opaque, pink body with opaque, brown cap, both printed Squibb and 885 in white. Each capsule contains 250 mg tetracycline hydrochloride and 250,000 units nystatin.

Tablets: Orange, sugar-coated tablet containing tetracycline hydrochloride 250 mg and nystatin 250,000 units.

Uses *Actions:* Tetracycline has a broad antimicrobial activity against pathogenic organisms including many Gram-positive and Gram-negative bacteria, spirochaetes, certain rickettsiae, large viruses, *Mycoplasma*

pneumoniae and *Entamoeba histolytica.* After oral administration therapeutically effective blood and urinary levels are obtained in a short period of time. It diffuses readily into most body tissues.

Nystatin is an antifungal antibiotic active against a wide range of yeasts and yeast-like fungi, including *Candida albicans.* Following wide use over many years, no clinical isolates resistant to this compound have emerged. Repeated subculture, *in vitro,* produces a small number of resistant isolates, but with reduced growth rate and pathogenicity. The possibility of these organisms causing disease in man is remote.

Indications: For infections caused by organisms sensitive to tetracycline, particularly in patients who may be susceptible to candidal overgrowth. These may include elderly or debilitated patients, diabetics, women taking hormonal contraceptive agents, patients with malignant disease especially if receiving cytotoxic drugs and those patients receiving high doses or prolonged courses of antibiotics or corticosteroids. Representative infections due to susceptible organisms, including chronic bronchitis and other respiratory tract infections, urinary tract infections, brucellosis, acne and many mixed infections.

Dosage and administration *Adult dosage:* One Mysteclin tablet four times daily. This dose may be doubled in severe infections.

Children over 12 years: A divided daily dose equivalent to 22–44 mg tetracycline per kg should be given according to the type and severity of the infection (see 'Precautions').

Elderly: No specific dosage recommendations, but see 'Precautions' re renal and hepatic failure.

All patients: Absorption of tetracycline from the gut is diminished by milk, salts of calcium, magnesium, aluminium and iron. Lowered absorption also results from alkalis, and concomitant administration of antacids should therefore be avoided.

Mysteclin should preferably be taken one hour before, or two hours after meals.

Contra-indications, warnings, etc
Contra-indications: The tetracycline group of antibiotics is normally contra-indicated during pregnancy and childhood except in certain severe infections where tetracycline may be the drug of choice, and the risk involved is justified (see 'Precautions'). Mysteclin should not be used in patients with a history of hypersensitivity to the tetracycline group of antibiotics.

There are no known contra-indications to the use of nystatin.

Precautions: There are no special precautions for the oral use of nystatin.

If renal impairment exists, even usual oral or parenteral doses of tetracycline may lead to excessive systemic accumulation of the drug and possible liver toxicity.

During long-term therapy periodic assessment of organ system function, including renal, hepatic and haemopoeitic systems, should be made.

The effects of anticoagulants are not usually altered by concurrent treatment with tetracycline, although a few isolated cases of enhancement have been described. Therefore, occasionally, reduction in doses of concurrent anticoagulants may be required.

Pregnancy and breast feeding: Tetracycline crosses the placental barrier and, in the last half of pregnancy may cause permanent discoloration of the teeth and depression of bone growth in the foetus. Similarly, tetracycline is excreted in breast milk which may also affect the infant. Therefore tetracyclines, as a class, are contraindicated during pregnancy and breast feeding.

Infants and children: Tetracyclines may be deposited in areas of calcification in bones and teeth. The use of drugs of the tetracycline class during tooth development (last half of pregnancy, infancy and childhood to the age of twelve years) may cause permanent discoloration of the teeth (yellow-grey-brown). This reaction is more common during long-term use of the drugs but has been observed following repeated short-term courses. Enamel hypoplasia has also been reported. Tetracycline drugs, therefore, should not be used in this age group unless other drugs are not likely to be effective or are contraindicated.

Rare, reversible, increased intracranial pressure with bulging fontanelles in infants taking therapeutic doses of tetracycline has been observed.

Side-effects: Mysteclin is generally well tolerated, but a few patients may experience skin rashes or gastrointestinal side-effects such as nausea, vomiting and diarrhoea. A phototoxic reaction may be produced in some patients, although such reactions are less common with tetracycline than with other members of the group. Rise in BUN has been reported and is apparently dose-related.

No systemic effects or allergic reactions have been associated with the oral use of nystatin.

Overdosage: The most common symptoms are nausea, vomiting and diarrhoea. The possibility of liver and renal failure should be borne in mind.

Pharmaceutical precautions *Storage:* At room temperature.

Legal category POM.

Package quantities *Capsules:* Bottles of 100. *Tablets:* Bottles of 100 and 500.

Further information By the inclusion of nystatin with tetracycline, the fungal overgrowth frequently associated with broad-spectrum antibiotic therapy is avoided.

Product licence numbers
Mysteclin Capsules   0034/5054
Mysteclin Tablets   0034/5056

MYSTECLIN* SYRUP

Presentation Yellow, viscous liquid, with fruity flavour and containing per 5 ml tetracycline equivalent to tetracycline hydrochloride 125 mg and amphotericin 25 mg (25,000 units).

Uses *Actions:* Tetracycline has a broad antimicrobial activity against pathogenic organisms including many Gram-positive and Gram-negative bacteria, spirochaetes, certain rickettsiae, large viruses, *Mycoplasma pneumoniae* and *Entamoeba histolytica*. After oral administration therapeutically effective blood and urinary levels are obtained in a short period of time. It diffuses readily into most body tissues.

Amphotericin is an antifungal antibiotic active against a wide range of yeasts and yeast-like fungi, including *Candida albicans*. Following wide use over many years, no clinical isolates resistant to this compound have emerged. Repeated subculture, *in vitro*, produces a small number of resistant isolates, but with reduced growth

rate and pathogenicity. The possibility of these organisms causing disease in man is remote.

Indications: For infections caused by organisms sensitive to tetracycline, particularly in patients who may be susceptible to candidal overgrowth. These may include elderly or debilitated patients, diabetics, women taking hormonal contraceptive agents, patients with malignant disease especially if receiving cytotoxic drugs and those patients receiving high doses or prolonged courses of antibiotics or corticosteroids. Representative infections due to susceptible organisms including chronic bronchitis and other respiratory tract infections, urinary tract infections, brucellosis, acne and many mixed infections.

Dosage and administration
Adult dosage: 10 ml Mysteclin syrup four times daily. This dose may be doubled in severe infections.

Children over 12 years: A divided daily dose equivalent to 22–44 mg tetracycline per kg should be given according to the type and severity of the infection (see 'Precautions').

Elderly: No specific dosage recommendations, but see 'Precautions' re renal and hepatic failure.

All patients: Absorption of tetracycline from the gut is diminished by milk, salts of calcium, magnesium, aluminium and iron. Lowered absorption also results from alkalis, and concomitant administration of antacids should therefore be avoided.

Mysteclin Syrup should preferably be taken one hour before, or two hours after meals.

Contra-indications, warnings, etc
Contra-indications: The tetracycline group of antibiotics is normally contra-indicated during pregnancy and childhood except in certain severe infections where tetracycline may be the drug of choice and the risk involved is justified (see 'Precautions'). Mysteclin should not be used in patients with a history of hypersensitivity to the tetracycline group of antibiotics.

There are no known contra-indications to the use of amphotericin.

Precautions: There are no special precautions for the oral use of amphotericin.

If renal impairment exists, even usual oral or parenteral doses of tetracycline may lead to excessive systemic accumulation of the drug and possible liver toxicity.

During long-term therapy periodic assessment of organ system function, including renal, hepatic and haemopoeitic systems, should be made.

The effects of anticoagulants are not usually altered by concurrent treatment with tetracycline, although a few isolated cases of enhancement have been described. Therefore, occasionally, reduction in doses of concurrent anticoagulants may be required.

Pregnancy and breast feeding: Tetracycline crosses the placental barrier and, in the last half of pregnancy may cause permanent discoloration of the teeth and depression of bone growth in the foetus. Similarly, tetracycline is excreted in breast milk which may also affect the infant. Therefore tetracyclines, as a class, are contraindicated during pregnancy and breast feeding.

Infants and children: Tetracyclines may be deposited in areas of calcification in bones and teeth. The use of drugs of the tetracycline class during tooth development (last half of pregnancy, infancy and childhood to the age of twelve years) may cause permanent discoloration of the teeth (yellow-grey-brown). This reaction is more common during long-term use of the drugs but has been observed following repeated short-term courses. Enamel hypoplasia has also been reported. Tetracycline drugs, therefore, should not be used in this age group unless other drugs are not likely to be effective or are contra-indicated.

Rare, reversible, increased intracranial pressure with bulging fontanelles in infants taking therapeutic doses of tetracycline has been observed.

Side-effects: Mysteclin is generally well tolerated, but a few patients may experience skin rashes or gastro-intestinal side-effects such as nausea, vomiting and diarrhoea.

A phototoxic reaction may be produced in some patients, although such reactions are less common with tetracycline than with other members of the group. Rise in BUN has been reported and is apparently dose-related.

No systemic effects or allergic reactions have been associated with the oral use of amphotericin.

Overdosage: The most common symptoms are nausea, vomiting and diarrhoea. The possibility of liver and renal failure should be borne in mind.

Pharmaceutical precautions *Storage:* At room temperature, protected from direct sunlight. Once the bottle is opened the contents to be used within two months.

Diluent: Syrup BP. The diluted syrup to be used within two months.

Legal category POM.

Package quantities *Syrup:* Bottles of 100 ml.

Further information By the inclusion of amphotericin with tetracycline, the fungal overgrowth frequently associated with broad-spectrum antibiotic therapy is avoided.

Product licence number 0034/5055.

NOCTEC* CAPSULES

Presentation Clear, orange-red gelatin capsules, each containing 500 mg chloral hydrate in solution.

Uses *Actions:* The hypnotic, chloral hydrate, in doses of 0.5-1 g, produces sedation in approximately 15 minutes followed by sleep in about half an hour. The action of the drug is confined to the cerebral hemispheres and the drug has virtually no effect on REM sleep. It is generally believed that the central depressant effects are due to the principal pharmacologically active metabolite, trichloroethanol, which has a plasma half-life of 8–10 hours.

Blood pressure and respiration are depressed only slightly more than in normal sleep, and reflexes are not significantly depressed.

Indications: For insomnia, particularly in geriatric patients. It is a satisfactory pre-operative sedative that allays anxiety and induces sleep without depressing respiration or cough reflex. In post-operative care and control of pain, Noctec is a valuable adjunct to opiates and analgesics.

Dosage and administration *Adults and children over 12 years of age:* 500 mg to 1 g taken 15 to 30 minutes before bedtime or half-an-hour before surgery. Daily dose should not exceed 2 g. The capsules should be taken with water, to avoid gastro-intestinal upset.

Elderly: No specific dosage recommendations or precautions.

Contra-indications, warnings, etc

Contra-indications: In patients with marked hepatic or renal impairment, or in patients with severe cardiac disease. Noctec is best avoided in the presence of marked gastritis.

Precautions: Noctec should be administered with caution to patients who have previously exhibited an idiosyncrasy or hypersensitivity to chloral hydrate. As with other hypnotics, alcohol potentiates the sedative effect. Similarly there is a danger of misuse and the possibility that habituation may develop. After long term use sudden withdrawal may result in delirium.

Chloral hydrate has been reported to precipitate attacks of acute intermittent porphyria and should be used with caution in susceptible patients.

Chloral hydrate may increase the rate of metabolism of concomitantly administered coumarin or coumarin-related anticoagulants, thus reducing their effectiveness. In patients taking coumarin anticoagulants, when Noctec is withdrawn from the drug regime, or its dosage changed, careful monitoring of the prothrombin time is required.

Chloral hydrate followed by intravenous frusemide may result in sweating, hot flushes and variable blood pressure including hypertension due to a hypermetabolic state caused by displacement of thyroid hormone from its bound state.

Pregnancy and breast feeding: Chloral hydrate crosses the placental barrier. Safety has not been established; therefore, Noctec capsules should be used during pregnancy only if the possible benefits outweigh the potential risks involved. Prolonged use during pregnancy may cause withdrawal symptoms in the neonate.

Chloral hydrate is excreted in human milk; use by nursing mothers may cause sedation in the infant.

Side-effects: Few, except gastric irritation which may occur in some patients. Excitement, delirium and tolerance are rarely encountered. Allergic skin reactions, headache and ketonuria have occasionally been reported. Prolonged use of large doses could lead to habituation with resultant parenchymatous renal injury.

Overdosage: The signs and symptoms of chloral hydrate overdosage resemble those of barbiturates and especially affect the CNS and cardiovascular system. They may include: hypothermia; pin-point pupils; blood pressure falls; comatosed states or rapid and shallow breathing. Gastric irritation may result in vomiting and even gastric necrosis. If the patient survives, icterus due to hepatic damage and albuminuria from renal irritation may appear.

The toxic oral dose of chloral hydrate for adults is approximately 10 g; however death has been reported from a dose of 4 g and some patients have survived after taking as much as 30 g.

Accidental overdose should be treated with gastric lavage or inducing vomiting to empty the stomach. Supportive measures may be used. Haemodialysis is reported to be effective in promoting the clearance of trichloroethanol.

Pharmaceutical precautions *Storage:* In a cool place; avoid freezing.

Legal category POM.

Package quantities Bottles of 50 capsules.

Further information Nil.

Product licence number 0034/5057.

NYSTADERMAL* CREAM

Presentation A yellow to light buff cream containing in each gram nystatin 100,000 units and triamcinolone acetonide 0.1%.

Uses *Actions:* Triamcinolone acetonide is a potent fluorinated corticosteroid with rapid anti-inflammatory, antipruritic and anti-allergic actions. Nystatin is an antifungal antibiotic active against a wide range of yeasts and yeast-like fungi, including *Candida albicans.* The cream is formulated for use on moist weeping lesions.

Indications: Nystadermal cream is indicated for those cases of cutaneous candidosis where the addition of a corticosteroid to the antifungal antibiotic may be beneficial in controlling the commonly associated inflammation and pruritus.

Nystadermal cream will also be of benefit in those cases of eczema where *Candida* is either the precipitating cause, or present as a secondary invader.

Dosage and administration *Adults and children:* To be applied to moist weeping lesions two to four times daily.

Elderly: Natural thinning of the skin occurs in the elderly; hence corticosteroids should be used sparingly and for short periods of time.

Contra-indications, warnings, etc
Contra-indications: There are no known contra-indications or special precautions for topical application of nystatin. Corticosteroids are contra-indicated in tuberculous and most viral lesions of the skin, particularly herpes simplex, vaccinia, varicella. The products should not be used in fungal lesions not susceptible to nystatin or bacterial skin infections without suitable concomitant anti-infective therapy.

Precautions: Adrenal suppression can occur, even without occlusion.

Children: In infants, long-term continuous topical steroid therapy should be avoided.

Pregnancy: Topical administration of corticosteroids to pregnant animals can cause abnormalities of foetal development. The relevance of this finding to humans has not been established. However, topical steroids should not be used extensively in pregnancy, i.e. in large amounts or for long periods. Topical corticosteroids should be used during pregnancy only if the potential benefit justifies the potential risk to the foetus.

Side-effects: There have been no substantiated reports of sensitivity associated with topical nystatin.

Triamcinolone acetonide is well tolerated. Where adverse reactions occur they are usually reversible on cessation of therapy. However the following side-effects have been reported usually with prolonged usage:

Dermatologic – impaired wound healing, thinning of the skin, petechiae and ecchymoses, facial erythema and telangiectasia, increased sweating, purpura, striae, hirsutism, acneiform eruptions, lupus erythematosus-like lesions and suppressed reactions to skin tests.

These effects may be enhanced with occlusive dressings.

Signs of systemic toxicity such as oedema and electrolyte imbalance have not been observed even when high topical dosage has been used. The possibility of the systemic effects which are associated with all steroid therapy should be considered.

Overdosage: Topically applied corticosteroids can be absorbed in sufficient amounts to produce systemic effects (see Side-effects).

Pharmaceutical precautions *Storage:* At room temperature; avoid freezing.

Dilution: Not recommended, as this may reduce therapeutic efficacy of nystatin.

If necessary, refer to the manufacturer.

Legal category POM.

Package quantities 15 g tubes.

Further information Nil.

Product licence number
Nystadermal Cream 0034/0131

NYSTAN* CREAM, OINTMENT, GEL AND DUSTING POWDER

Presentation *Gel:* Yellow to amber, opaque, containing 100,000 units nystatin per gram.

Cream: Pale buff, containing 100,000 units per gram nystatin in a vanishing-cream base.

Ointment: Yellow to amber containing 100,000 units nystatin per gram in Plastibase*.

Dusting Powder: White to pale yellow, containing 100,000 units nystatin per gram of powder.

Uses *Actions:* Nystatin is an antifungal antibiotic active against a wide range of yeasts and yeast-like fungi, including *Candida albicans.*

Indications: For the treatment of cutaneous and mucocutaneous mycoses, particularly those caused by *C. albicans.*

Dosage and administration *Adults and children:* To be applied two to four times daily.

Elderly: No specific dosage recommendations or precautions.

Contra-indications, warnings, etc
Contra-indications: There are no known contra-indications or special precautions for topical application of nystatin.

Pregnancy/children: No specific precautions apply; systemic absorption is negligible.

Side-effects: There have been no substantiated reports of sensitivity associated with topical nystatin.

Pharmaceutical precautions *Storage:*
Gel: In a cool place; avoid freezing.

Cream: At room temperature; avoid freezing.

Ointment: At room temperature.

Dusting Powder: At room temperature, keep tightly closed.

Dilution: Nystan topicals should not be diluted as this may reduce therapeutic efficacy.

Legal category POM.

Package quantities *Cream/Ointment:* Tubes of 15 g and 30 g.
Gel: Tubes of 30 g.
Dusting Powder: Packs of 15 g.

Further information Nil.

Product licence numbers

Nystan Gel	0034/0142
Nystan Cream	0034/5058
Nystan Dusting Powder	0034/5059
Nystan Ointment	0034/0161

NYSTAN* ORAL SUSPENSION, NYSTAN* FOR SUSPENSION AND TABLETS

Presentation

Nystan Oral Suspension: Yellow, cherry-mint flavoured suspension providing 100,000 units nystatin per ml. N.B. Suspension contains sugar.

Nystan For Suspension: A powder for reconstitution to provide oral suspension containing 100,000 units nystatin per ml. N.B. Reconstituted suspension is sugar-free.

Nystan Tablets: Sugar-coated, chocolate-brown tablets containing 500,000 units nystatin.

Uses *Actions:* Nystatin is an antifungal antibiotic active against a wide range of yeasts and yeast-like fungi, including Candida albicans.

Indications: Suspension for the prevention and treatment of candidal infections of the oral cavity, oesophagus and intestinal tract. It provides effective prophylaxis against oral candidosis in those born of mothers with vaginal candidosis.

Tablets for intestinal candidosis. They may be used for the prophylaxis of candidal overgrowth during courses of broad-spectrum antibiotics.

Dosage and administration Reconstitution of Granules For Suspension: Add 22 ml water to the bottle and shake vigorously.

Adults: Suspension (Nystan Oral and Nystan For Suspensions): For the treatment of denture sores, and oral infections in adults caused by *C. albicans*, 1 ml of the suspension should be dropped into the mouth four times daily; it should be kept in contact with the affected areas as long as possible.

Tablets: For the treatment of intestinal candidosis 1 tablet four times daily, but this dose may be doubled. For prophylaxis a total daily dosage of 1 million units has been found to suppress the overgrowth of *C. albicans* in patients receiving broad-spectrum antibiotic therapy.

Older people with intestinal candidosis who are unable to swallow tablets should be given 5 ml of the suspension four times a day.

Administration should be continued for 48 hours after clinical cure to prevent relapse.

Children: Suspension: In intestinal and oral candidosis (thrush) in infants and children, 1 ml should be dropped into the mouth four times a day. The longer the suspension is kept in contact with the affected area in the mouth, before swallowing, the greater will be its effect.

For prophylaxis in the newborn the suggested dose is 1 ml once daily.

Elderly: No specific dosage recommendations or precautions.

Contra-indications, warnings, etc

Contra-indications: There are no known contra-indications to the use of nystatin.

Precautions: Nystan Oral Suspension contains sugar.

For children with disaccharide intolerance the sugar-free formulation, Nystan For Suspension, is recommended.

Pregnancy: Absorption of nystatin from the gastro-intestinal tract is negligible, therefore no special precautions apply in pregnancy.

Side-effects: Nausea, vomiting and diarrhoea have occasionally been reported with doses of nystatin exceeding 4 to 5 million units daily. No systemic effects or allergic reactions have been associated with its oral use.

Overdosage: Since the absorption of nystatin from the gastro-intestinal tract is negligible, overdosage causes no systemic toxicity.

Pharmaceutical precautions *Storage: Nystan Suspension:* At room temperature; avoid freezing. *Nystan For Suspension:* The reconstituted suspension will remain suitable for use for 7 days at room temperature or 10 days under refrigeration. Store the dry powder at room temperature. *Nystan Tablets:* At room temperature.

Dilution: Not recommended as this may reduce therapeutic efficacy.

If necessary, refer to the manufacturer.

Legal category POM.

Package quantities

Nystan Oral Suspension: Bottles of 30 ml with graduated dropper.

Nystan For Suspension: Bottles of 24 mls when reconstituted, with graduated dropper.

Nystan Tablets: Bottles of 28 and 100.

Further information Nil.

Product licence numbers

Nystan Oral Suspension	0034/0130
Nystan For Suspension	0034/5061
Nystan Tablets	0034/5063

NYSTAN* PASTILLES

Presentation Yellow-brown, aniseed flavoured soft pastille providing 100,000 units nystatin per pastille; containing sugar and cinnamon.

Uses *Actions:* Nystatin is an antifungal antibiotic active against a wide range of yeasts and yeast-like fungi, including Candida albicans.

Indications: For the treatment of oral candidosis.

Dosage and administration No food or drink should be taken for five minutes before or one hour after consumption of the pastille.

Adults and children: One pastille to be sucked slowly, four times a day for 7–14 days.

Elderly: No specific dosage recommendations or precautions.

Contra-indications, warnings, etc

Contra-indications: There are no known contra-indications to the use of nystatin.

Precautions: Pregnancy: Absorption of nystatin from the gastro-intestinal tract is negligible, therefore no special precautions apply in pregnancy.

Side-effects: Nausea, vomiting and diarrhoea have occasionally been reported with doses of nystatin exceeding 4 to 5 million units daily. No systemic effects or allergic reactions have been associated with its oral use.

Overdosage: Since the absorption of nystatin from the gastro-intestinal tract is negligible, overdosage causes no systemic toxicity.

Pharmaceutical precautions *Storage:* At room temperature.

Legal category POM.

Package quantities Packs of 28 pastilles.

Further information The pastille allows longer contact of the active ingredient nystatin with the mucous membrane than liquid formulations.

Successful treatment of oral candidosis also includes good oral hygiene. Patients with dentures are advised to remove them whilst sucking the pastilles.

Product licence number 0034/0248.

NYSTAN* PESSARIES, VAGINAL CREAM AND TRIPLE PACK

Presentation *Pessaries:* Pale yellow to tan, diamond-shaped, with Squibb logo and 457 engraved on one side, containing 100,000 units nystatin.

Vaginal Cream: Pale buff containing in each 4 g application 100,000 units nystatin.

Triple Pack: 28 Nystavescent* pessaries (containing 100,000 units nystatin in an effervescent matrix). 42 oral tablets each containing nystatin 500,000 units and 30 g Nystan Gel (containing 100,000 units nystatin per gram).

Uses *Actions:* Nystatin is an antifungal antibiotic active against a wide range of yeasts and yeast-like fungi, including *Candida albicans.*

Indications: For the treatment of candidal vaginitis. In addition to local therapy the Triple Pack contains tablets for the eradication of *Candida* from the gut and the gel for topical application in the anogenital area, thereby preventing reinfection.

Dosage and administration *Pessaries: Adults:* 1 or 2 pessaries should be inserted high into the vagina for 14 consecutive nights or longer, regardless of any intervening menstrual period.

Vaginal Cream: Adults: Insert 1 or 2 applications (of 4 g each) high into the vagina for 14 consecutive nights, or longer, regardless of any intervening menstrual period. Reinfection from the candidal content of the intestinal tract may be prevented by concomitant therapy with oral nystatin.

Nystatin Cream, Gel, Ointment or Dusting Powder should be applied to the perineal region 2–4 times daily, if necessary.

Note: To prevent reinfection with *Candida,* the male consort should be treated concurrently with Nystan Gel, applied to the external genital area 2–4 times daily during the treatment period.

Children: Vulvovaginal candidosis is rarely a problem in children. It is suggested that the vaginal cream is the most acceptable formulation for children, together with concomitant oral medication where necessary.

Elderly: No specific dosage recommendations or precautions.

Contra-indications, warnings, etc
Contra-indications: There are no known contraindications to the use of these products.

Precautions: No specific precautions apply.

Pregnancy: There is no evidence that nystatin is absorbed systemically from the vagina. However, as with all drugs, caution should be exercised in pregnancy. Care should be taken while using an applicator to prevent the possibility of mechanical trauma.

Side-effects: Nystan is well tolerated and no substantiated sensitivity reactions have been associated with its use. Some transient local discomfort may be experienced.

Overdosage of Oral Tablets: Since the absorption of nystatin from the gastro-intestinal tract is negligible, overdosage causes no systemic toxicity.

Pharmaceutical precautions *Storage: Pessaries:* At room temperature.

Triple Pack: In a cool, dry place.

Vaginal Cream: At room temperature: avoid freezing.

Dilution: Not recommended for Vaginal Cream as this may reduce therapeutic efficacy.

Legal category POM.

Package quantities *Pessaries:* Foiled, in packs of 15 and 100 with applicators.
Vaginal Cream: Tubes of 60 g with applicator.
Triple Pack: 28 Nystavescent Pessaries in foil strip with applicator. 42 Nystan Oral Tablets. 30 g Nystan Gel. Patient treatment instructions are enclosed.

Further information Nil.

Product licence numbers

Nystan Gel	0034/0142
Nystan Pessaries	0034/5062
Nystan Vaginal Cream	0034/0137
Nystan Oral Tablets	0034/5063
Nystavescent Pessaries	0034/0111

NYSTAVESCENT* PESSARIES

Presentation Pale yellow, diamond-shaped pessaries engraved with Squibb, each containing nystatin 100,000 units in an effervescent matrix.

Uses *Actions:* Nystatin is an antifungal antibiotic active against a wide range of yeasts and yeast-like fungi, including *Candida albicans.*

Indications: Local treatment of vulvovaginal candidosis.

Dosage and administration One or two pessaries should be inserted high into the vagina for 14 consecutive nights or longer regardless of any intervening menstrual period.

Re-infection from the candidal content of the intestinal tract may be prevented by the concomitant therapy with oral nystatin (Nystan*).

Similarly, Nystan Cream, Ointment or Powder should be applied to the perineal region if necessary.

Children: Vulvovaginal candidosis is rarely a problem in children. It is suggested that a vaginal cream is the most acceptable formulation for children.

Elderly: No specific dosage recommendations or precautions.

Contra-indications, warnings, etc

Contra-indications: There are no known contra-indications to the use of Nystavescent pessaries.

Side-effects: Nystavescent pessaries are well tolerated. Occasionally some transient irritation and burning have been experienced.

Precautions: Pregnancy: There is no evidence that nystatin is absorbed systemically from the vagina. However, as with all drugs, caution should be exercised in pregnancy. Care should be taken while using an applicator to prevent the possibility of mechanical trauma.

Pharmaceutical precautions *Storage:* In a cool dry place.

Legal category POM.

Package quantities 15 Pessaries in foil strip with applicator.

Further information Nil.

Product licence number 0034/0111.

OPHTHAINE* SOLUTION

Presentation Sterile, aqueous ophthalmic solution containing:

Proxymetacaine hydrochloride	0.5%
Chlorbutol	0.2%
Benzalkonium chloride	0.01%

Uses *Actions:* Proxymetacaine hydrochloride is a rapidly acting local anaesthetic. With a single drop the onset of anaesthesia occurs in an average of 13 seconds and will persist for an average of 15 minutes.

Indications: Topical anaesthesia in ophthalmic practice.

Dosage and administration *Adults and children:* Administered by topical instillation into the eye. The recommended doses are as follows:

Deep anaesthesia: Instil 1 drop every five to ten minutes for 5-7 doses.

Removal of sutures: Instil 1 or 2 drops two or three minutes before removal of stitches.

Removal of foreign bodies: Instil 1 or 2 drops prior to operating.

Tonometry: Instil 1 or 2 drops immediately before measurement.

Elderly: No specific dosage recommendations or precautions.

Contra-indications, warnings, etc

Contra-indications: Patients with known hypersensitivity to proxymetacaine or constituents.

Precautions: Ophthaine solution is not intended for long-term use.

Ophthaine Solution is not miscible with fluorescein. However, the eye can be anaesthetised with Ophthaine Solution before fluorescein is administered.

Use cautiously and sparingly in patients with known allergies, cardiac disease, or hyperthyroidism.

Regular and prolonged use of a topical ocular anaesthetic, e.g. in conjunction with contact lens insertion, may cause softening and erosion of the corneal epithelium, which could produce corneal opacification with accompanying loss of vision.

Protection of the eye from irritating chemicals, foreign bodies and rubbing during the period of anaesthesia is very important. Tonometers soaked in sterilising or detergent solutions should be thoroughly rinsed with sterile distilled water prior to use. Patients should be advised to avoid touching the eye until the anaesthesia has worn off.

Side-effects: Pupillary dilatation or cycloplegic effects have rarely been observed with Ophthaine Solution. Irritation of the conjunctiva or other toxic reactions attributable to the preparation have occurred only rarely. A severe, immediate-type apparently hyperallergic corneal reaction may rarely occur which includes acute, intense and diffuse epithelial keratitis; a grey ground-glass appearance; sloughing of large areas of necrotic epithelium; corneal filaments and sometimes, iritis with descemetitis.

Pharmaceutical precautions *Storage:* In a refrigerator. Do not freeze. Protect from light. Discard any solution which is discoloured. The product should not be used one month after first opening the container.

Legal category POM.

Package quantities Bottles of 15 ml.

Further information Nil.

Product licence number 0034/5064.

PRONESTYL* TABLETS AND SOLUTION FOR INJECTION

Presentation *Tablets:* White, engraved Squibb and 754 on one side and scored on reverse, containing 250 mg procainamide hydrochloride.

Solution for Injection: A sterile, aqueous solution containing 100 mg/ml procainamide hydrochloride.

Uses *Actions:* Procainamide depresses the excitability of cardiac muscle to electrical stimulation and slows conduction in the atrium, the bundle of His and the ventricle, thereby reversing rhythmical abnormalities. In atrial arrhythmias procainamide slows atrial rate and may re-establish normal sinus rhythm.

The action of procainamide begins almost immediately after intramuscular or intravenous administration. Following oral administration, plasma levels are comparable to those obtained parenterally and therapeutic levels are usually obtained in 30 minutes; plasma levels are maximal within an hour. Plasma levels after intramuscular injection are at their peak in 50-60 minutes.

Therapeutic plasma levels have been reported to be 3 to 10 mcg/ml, with those for a majority of patients in the range of 4 to 8 mcg/ml.

Procainamide is less readily hydrolysed than procaine and plasma levels decline slowly - about 10-20% per hour. The drug is excreted primarily in the urine, about 10% as free and conjugated p-amino-benzoic acid and about 60% in the unchanged form. The fate of the remainder is unknown.

The effects of Pronestyl are more beneficial in ventricular than in supraventricular, auricular and nodal arrhythmias.

Indications: Ventricular tachycardia, ventricular ectopic contractions, supraventricular, atrial and nodal tachycardia. Arrhythmias resulting from anaesthesia and cardiac surgery.

Dosage and administration

Adults: Oral administration of Pronestyl is preferred.

When parenteral therapy is necessary the intramuscular route of administration is the method of choice, the intravenous route being limited to emergencies and cases under direct ECG control.

Plasma concentrations correlate well with therapeutic and toxic effects; consequently plasma level assays should be carried out if facilities are available. The usual effective antiarrhythmic concentration is 4 to 8 mcg/ml. Toxic manifestations are rare in concentrations less than 12 mcg/ml.

Oral: If used in conjunction with electrical defibrillation Pronestyl 250 mg every six hours will prevent recurrence in the majority of cases.

Following intravenous therapy or for less urgent cases 250 mg by mouth every four to six hours is an alternative route to parenteral administration.

Adults – injection
Intramuscular injection: Where ECG control is not available 250 mg may be given intramuscularly supplemented by oral dosage. In less severe cases and in maintenance therapy a dose of 100–250 mg may be given by intramuscular injection every four to six hours.

Intravenous administration: Intravenous therapy for the treatment of serious arrhythmias including those following myocardial infarction should be limited to use in hospitals where monitoring facilities are available. Pronestyl Injection should be diluted prior to intravenous use to facilitate control of dosage rate.

Caution: Intravenous use of Pronestyl Injection may be accompanied by a hypotensive response, sometimes marked, if the dose is excessive or administration too rapid. Therefore, to initiate therapy, the intravenous dose should be diluted in 5% Dextrose Injection BP prior to administration to facilitate control of dosage rate; the dose should be administered at a rate no greater than 25 to 50 mg per minute by either direct intravenous administration or infusion under ECG control. Slow administration allows for some initial tissue distribution.

Direct intravenous administration: To reduce the possibility of a hypotensive response, 100 mg doses may be administered every five minutes by direct slow intravenous injection, at a rate not exceeding 50 mg in any one minute, until the arrhythmia is suppressed or the maximum dosage of 1 g has been administered. Blood pressure must be taken and the ECG read before each dose.

Some effects may be seen after the first 100 or 200 mg and it is unusual to require more than 500 to 600 mg to achieve satisfactory antiarrhythmic effects.

To maintain therapeutic levels, an infusion may then be started at a rate of 2 to 6 mg procainamide per minute (see Table) depending on the patient's body weight, circulatory conditions and renal function.

Intravenous infusion: An alternative method of achieving and then maintaining a therapeutic plasma concentration is to infuse 500 to 600 mg of procainamide at a constant rate over a period of 25 to 30 minutes and then change to another infusion for maintenance at a rate of 2 to 6 mg/min (see Table).

Note: Solutions for intravenous infusion should be prepared immediately before administration.

Intravenous therapy should be terminated as soon as the patient's basic cardiac rhythm appears to be stabilised and, if indicated, the patient should be placed on oral antiarrhythmic maintenance therapy. A period of 3 to 4 hours (one half-life) should elapse after the last intra-venous dose of procainamide before administering the first oral dose of procainamide.

Intravenous administration should be monitored by ECG. Excessive widening of the QRS complex or prolongation of the P-R interval suggests the occurrence of myocardial toxicity. Patients should be kept in a supine position and blood pressure should be measured almost continuously during administration. If the fall in blood pressure exceeds 15 mmHg, administration should be temporarily discontinued. Phenylephrine Injection BP or Noradrenaline Injection BP should be available to counteract severe hypotensive responses.

Dilutions and rates for intravenous infusions†

Approximate final concentration	Infusion bottle size (ml)	ml of Pronestyl (100 mg/ml) to be added	Infusion rate
0.2% (2 mg/ml)	500	10	1–3
	250	5	ml/min
0.4% (4 mg/ml)	500	20	0.5–1.5
	250	10	ml/min

†*Caution:* The flow rate of all intravenous infusion solutions must be closely monitored. These dilutions are calculated to deliver 2–6 mg per minute at the infusion rates listed.

Surgical use: For cardiac arrhythmias associated with anaesthesia and surgery, the suggested parenteral dose is 500 mg to 1 g, preferably given intramuscularly.

Children: Pronestyl is not recommended for use in children.

Elderly: There are no specific dosage recommendations or precautions for use in the elderly except, as with other drugs, to monitor those patients with impaired renal or hepatic function.

Contra-indications, warnings, etc
Contra-indications: Hypersensitivity to the drug is an absolute contra-indication. In this connection, cross sensitivity to procaine and related drugs must be borne in mind. Pronestyl is contra-indicated in patients with myaesthenia gravis.

Procainamide should not be administered to patients with complete atrioventricular heart block. Procainamide is also contra-indicated in cases of high degree A-V block unless an electrical pacemaker is operative.

Precautions: Hypotension may occur when Pronestyl is administered intravenously and it should not be given to conscious patients at a rate greater than 50 mg per minute up to a total of 1 g. Therefore, to initiate therapy, the intravenous dose should be diluted in 5% dextrose injection BP prior to administration to facilitate control of dosage rate. Patients should be kept in a supine position and blood pressure readings made frequently. If hypotension occurs the rate of injection should be reduced and if necessary a vasopressor agent administered cautiously. ECG tracings should be made during an injection of Pronestyl so that administration may be stopped when the arrhythmia is interrupted or if evidence of extensive depression of conduction appears.

In patients with significant impairment of renal or hepatic function, accumulation of Pronestyl may occur, leading to drug toxicity.

Use in Pregnancy: Safety has not been established: therefore, Pronestyl tablets should be used during pregnancy only if the possible benefits outweigh the potential risks involved.

Children: Pronestyl is not recommended.

Side-effects: Nausea, vomiting, diarrhoea, dizziness, headache, pruritus, chills, fever and allergic reactions are usually not sufficiently severe to discontinue treatment.

Agranulocytosis and a LE-like syndrome have been reported after prolonged courses of Pronestyl. The LE-like syndrome seldom appears in less than two months, but is very common after six months. It is virtually completely reversible and tests for antinuclear factors are usually positive before clinical signs appear. If long-term treatment is considered desirable, it is advisable to undertake serological tests at no less than monthly intervals and to continue treatment for no longer than absolutely necessary.

The patient should be instructed to report any soreness of the mouth, throat, or gums, unexplained fever or any symptoms of upper respiratory tract infection. If any of these should occur, and leucocyte counts indicate cellular depression, procainamide therapy should be discontinued, and appropriate treatment should be instituted immediately.

Hypotension may occur particularly in conscious patients (see 'Precautions').

Overdosage: Severe hypotension may be treated by placing the patient in the supine position with the feet raised. If necessary an intravenous infusion of noradrenaline 8 mcg per ml in Sodium Chloride Injection BP may be started.

Pharmaceutical precautions *Storage: Tablets/ Solution:* At room temperature.

Legal category POM.

Package quantities *Tablets:* Bottles of 100. *Solution 100 mg/ml:* 10 ml multidose vials.

Further information Nil.

Product licence numbers
Pronestyl Tablets 0034/5066
Pronestyl Solution 0034/5065

RAUTRAX* TABLETS

Presentation Red, oblong, sugar-coated tablets, containing 50 mg *Rauwolfia serpentina* whole root with hydroflumethiazide 50 mg and potassium chloride 625 mg.

Uses *Actions: Rauwolfia serpentina* is antihypertensive, tranquillising and bradycardic. The antihypertensive activity develops slowly over one to three weeks and may persist for a week after drug withdrawal. *Rauwolfia serpentina* probably produces its antihypertensive effects through depletion of the catecholamines from peripheral sites. In contrast, the sedative and tranquillising effects are thought to relate to brain 5-hydroxytryptamine depletion. It does not significantly affect normal blood pressure.

Hydroflumethiazide provides smooth reduction of elevated blood pressure.

Supplementary potassium provides protection against possible potassium depletion during long-term therapy.

Indications: Mild to moderate hypertension.

Dosage and administration
Adults: One or two tablets twice daily morning and

evening. After a period of two to three weeks a maintenance dose of one tablet daily may suffice.

Children: Not recommended.

Elderly: Dosage of Rautrax should be reduced in elderly patients.

Contra-indications, warnings, etc
Contra-indications: Severe renal failure. Patients previously demonstrating hypersensitivity to Rauwolfia. Patients with past history of depression, suicidal tendencies, peptic ulcer or ulcerative colitis. Patients receiving electroconvulsive therapy.

Precautions: Discontinue if signs of depression. Drug-induced depression may persist for several months after drug withdrawal and may be severe enough to result in suicide. Use cautiously in patients with gallstones (where biliary colic may be precipitated), renal insufficiency and in conjunction with digitalis and quinidine, as cardiac arrhythmias have occurred with Rauwolfia preparations. Care should be taken in treating patients with severely damaged kidneys and low urinary output. In patients with renal disease, thiazides may precipitate azotemia and cumulative effects of the drug may develop. In patients with impaired hepatic function, minor alterations of fluid and electrolyte balance may precipitate hepatic coma.

Periodic determination of serum electrolytes to detect possible imbalance should be performed at regular intervals.

Hypokalaemia, should it occur, can sensitise or exaggerate the response of the heart to the toxic effects of digitalis (e.g., increased ventricular irritability).

Insulin requirements in diabetic patients may be altered by thiazides and latent diabetes mellitus may emerge. Hyperuricaemia may occur or frank gout may be precipitated by thiazides in certain patients. Pathologic changes in the parathyroid gland with hypercalcaemia and hypophosphataemia have been observed in a few patients during prolonged thiazide therapy. Thiazides may decrease serum bound iodine levels without signs of thyroid disturbance.

Pre-operative withdrawal of Rauwolfia does not ensure that circulatory instability does not occur. Therefore anaesthetists should be aware of the patient's drug intake. Thiazides may increase the responsiveness to tubocurarine, and decrease arterial responsiveness to noradrenaline.

Rodent studies have shown that reserpine may cause an increased incidence of mammary fibroadenomas in female mice, malignant tumours of the seminal vesicles in male mice, and malignant adrenal medullary tumours in male rats. The breast neoplasms are thought to be related to reserpine's prolactin-elevating effect. Several other prolactin-elevating drugs have also been associated with an increased incidence of mammary neoplasia in rodents. The extent to which these findings indicate a risk to humans is uncertain. Orthostatic hypotension may occur, which may be aggravated when the drug is combined with either alcohol, barbiturates or narcotics. The antihypertensive effects of the preparation may be enhanced in the post sympathectomy patient.

Warning: Symptoms and signs which might indicate ulceration or obstruction of the small bowel in patients taking tablets or capsules containing potassium salts are indications for stopping treatment immediately. The chance of this occurring with Rautrax is slight since the formulation is not enteric-coated.

Pregnancy and breast feeding: The use of diuretics in

otherwise healthy pregnant women with or without mild oedema is contra-indicated and possibly hazardous. Therefore Rautrax is contra-indicated in pregnant women. The hazards of using thiazides include foetal or neonatal jaundice, thrombocytopenia and possibly other adverse reactions which have occurred in the adult.

Usage of Rauwolfia preparations in women of child-bearing age requires that the potential benefits of the drug be weighed against its possible hazards to the foetus. The hazards to infants born to Rauwolfia alkaloid-treated mothers include: increased respiratory secretions, nasal congestion, cyanosis and anorexia. Rauwolfia preparations cross the placental barrier and appear in cord blood and breast milk.

Side-effects: Infrequent and mild in nature, which may be controlled by modifying dosage.

Rauwolfia: Gastrointestinal: nausea, vomiting, anorexia and diarrhoea. Central nervous system: drowsiness, depression, nervousness, paradoxical anxiety, night-mares, rare Parkinsonian syndrome, deafness, glaucoma, uveitis and optic atrophy. Cardiovascular: angina-like symptoms, arrhythmias, bradycardia. Other: nasal congestion, pruritus, rash, dryness of mouth, headache, dyspnoea, purpura, impotence or decreased libido, dysuria, muscular aches, conjunctivitis, weight gain and extrapyramidal symptoms. These reactions are usually reversible.

Thiazides: Those reported with the use of thiazides include anorexia, gastric irritation, nausea, vomiting, cramping, diarrhoea, intrahepatic cholestatic jaundice, pancreatitis, dizziness, vertigo, headache, xanthopsia, leucopenia, agranulocytosis, thrombocytopenia, aplastic anaemia, purpura, photosensitivity, rash, urticaria, nec-rotising angiitis, hyperglycaemia, glycosuria, hyperuri-caemia, muscle spasm, weakness, and restlessness.

Potassium: See Warnings.

Overdosage: If conscious, emesis should be induced or the stomach emptied by aspiration or lavage. Atropine sulphate may be used to relieve parasympathomimetic side-effects. Signs of motor dysfunction may be treated with benzhexol or other anti-Parkinsonian agents. Severe hypotension may respond to placing the patient in the supine position with feet raised. Transfusions of plasma or suitable electrolyte solutions may be given slowly if necessary.

Pharmaceutical precautions *Storage:* At room tem-perature.

Legal category POM.

Package quantities Bottles of 100.

Further information Nil.

Product licence number 0034/5072.

TRI-ADCORTYL* CREAM, OINTMENT AND OTIC OINTMENT

Presentation *Cream:* Pale buff.

Ointment: Yellow to amber in Plastibase*.

Otic Ointment: Presentation for aural use in Plastibase*. This preparation is sterile.

Containing in each gram the following:

Triamcinolone acetonide	0.1%
Neomycin (as sulphate)	0.25%
Gramicidin	0.025%
Nystatin	100,000 units

Uses *Actions:* Triamcinolone acetonide is a potent fluorinated corticosteroid with rapid anti-inflammatory, antipruritic and anti-allergic actions.

The combined action of the antibiotics neomycin and gramicidin provides comprehensive antibacterial therapy against a wide range of Gram-positive and Gram-negative bacteria, including those micro-organisms responsible for most bacterial skin infections.

Nystatin is an antifungal antibiotic, active against a wide range of yeasts and yeast-like fungi, including *Candida albicans.*

Indications: The topical treatment of superficial bacterial infections, cutaneous candidosis and dermatological conditions known to respond to topical steroid therapy when threatened or complicated by bacterial or candidal superinfections. These include: atopic eczema, contact eczema, follicular eczema, infantile eczema, otitis ex-terna, anogenital pruritus (pruritus ani et vulvae), nummular eczema, post-traumatic infective eczema, seborrhoeic or flexural eczema, neurodermatitis, pso-riasis.

Dosage and administration *Adults and children:* *Cream, ointment:* Apply to the affected areas two to four times daily.

Otic Ointment: After cleaning, apply the nozzle to the aural canal and squeeze a small amount into the canal two to four times daily.

Elderly: Natural thinning of the skin occurs in the elderly; hence corticosteroids should be used sparingly and for short periods of time.

Contra-indications, warnings, etc
Contra-indications: In tuberculous and most viral lesions of the skin, particularly herpes simplex, vaccinia and varicella. Also in fungal lesions not susceptible to nystatin.

In patients with hypersensitivity to any of the com-ponents.

Should not be applied to the external auditory canal in patients with perforated eardrums.

Precautions: Adrenal suppression can occur, even with-out occlusion. The use of occlusive dressings should be avoided because of the increased risk of sensitivity reactions and increased percutaneous absorption. The possibility of sensitivity to neomycin should be taken into consideration especially in the treatment of patients suffering from leg ulcers.

Pregnancy: Topical administration of corticosteroids to pregnant animals can cause abnormalities of foetal development. The relevance of this finding to humans has not been established. However, topical steroids should not be used extensively in pregnancy, i.e. in large amounts or for long periods. Topical corticosteroids should be used during pregnancy only if the potential benefit justifies the potential risk to the foetus.

Children: In infants, long-term continuous topical steroid therapy should be avoided.

Otic ointment: Care is necessary in applying this preparation if perforation of the eardrum is suspected. Not for ophthalmic use.

Side-effects: Triamcinolone acetonide is well tolerated. Where adverse reactions occur they are usually reversible on cessation of therapy. However the following side-effects have been reported usually with prolonged usage:

Dermatologic – impaired wound healing, thinning of the skin, petechiae and ecchymoses, facial erythema and telangiectasia, increased sweating, purpura, striae, hirsutism, acneiform eruptions, lupus erythematosus-like lesions and suppressed reactions to skin tests.

These effects may be enhanced with occlusive dressings.

Signs of systemic toxicity such as oedema and electrolyte imbalance have not been observed even when high topical dosage has been used. The possibility of the systemic effects which are associated with all steroid therapy should be considered.

Neomycin: Sensitivity reactions may occur especially with prolonged use. Ototoxicity and nephrotoxicity have been reported. Large amounts of this product should be avoided in the treatment of skin infections following extensive burns, trophic ulceration and other conditions where absorption of neomycin is possible.

Gramicidin: Sensitivity has occasionally been reported.

Nystatin: There have been no substantiated reports of sensitivity associated with topical nystatin.

Overdosage: Topically applied corticosteroids can be absorbed in sufficient amounts to produce systemic effects (see Side-effects).

Pharmaceutical precautions *Storage: Cream:* At room temperature; avoid freezing.

Ointment: At room temperature.

Dilution: Not recommended, as this would reduce the concentration of the antibiotics to below therapeutic levels.

Legal category POM.

Package quantities Tubes of 15 g and 30 g.
Otic Ointment: Tubes of 10 g.

Further information Tri-Adcortyl Ointment is preservative-free, and avoids the risk of allergic reactions to preservatives.

Product licence numbers
Tri-Adcortyl Cream   0034/5093
Tri-Adcortyl Ointment   0034/5094
Tri-Adcortyl Otic Ointment   0034/5095

VELOSEF* CAPSULES
VELOSEF* SYRUP

Presentation *Capsules 250 mg:* Opaque, orange body with opaque blue cap printed Squibb and 113 in white on each half. Each capsule contains 250 mg cephradine.

Capsules 500 mg: Opaque blue printed in white with Squibb and 114 on each half. Each capsule contains 500 mg cephradine.

Syrup 125 mg: When reconstituted contains 125 mg cephradine per 5 ml.

Syrup 250 mg: When reconstituted contains 250 mg cephradine per 5 ml.

Uses *Actions:* Cephradine is a broad-spectrum, bactericidal antibiotic active against both Gram-positive and Gram-negative bacteria. It is also highly active against most strains of penicillinase-producing *Staphylococci*.

Microbiology: The following organisms have shown *in vitro* sensitivity to cephradine:

Gram-positive – *Staphylococci* (both penicillin sensitive and resistant strains), *Streptococci*, both *Streptococcus pyogenes* (beta haemolytic) and Group D *Streptococci* (enterococci) and *Streptococcus pneumoniae*.

Gram-negative – *E. coli, Klebsiella, P. mirabilis, Haemophilus influenzae, Shigella* spp., *Salmonella* spp. (including *Salmonella typhi*) and *Neisseria* spp.

Enterococci (S. faecalis) may be susceptible to the high levels of cephradine achieved in the urine.

Because cephradine is unaffected by penicillinase, many strains of *E. coli* and *Staphylococcus aureus* which produce this enzyme are susceptible to cephradine but resistant to ampicillin.

Indications: In the treatment of infections of the urinary, respiratory and gastro-intestinal tracts and of the skin and soft tissues. These include:

Upper respiratory infections – pharyngitis, sinusitis, otitis media, tonsilitis, laryngo-tracheo bronchitis.

Lower respiratory infections – acute and chronic bronchitis, lobar and bronchopneumonia.

Urinary tract infections – cystitis, urethritis, pyelonephritis.

Skin and soft tissue infections – abscess, cellulitis, furunculosis, impetigo.

Gastro-intestinal tract – bacillary dysentery, enteritis, peritonitis.

Velosef has been shown to be effective in reducing the incidence of postoperative infections in patients undergoing surgical procedures associated with a high risk of infection. It is also of value where postoperative infections would be disastrous and where patients have a reduced host resistance to bacterial infection. Protection is best ensured by achieving adequate local tissue concentrations at the time contamination is likely to occur. Thus, Velosef should be administered immediately prior to surgery and continued during the postoperative period.

Bacteriology studies to determine the causative organisms and their sensitivity to cephradine should be performed. Therapy may be instituted prior to receiving the results of the sensitivity test.

Dosage and administration Velosef may be given without regard to meals.

Adults: For urinary tract infections the usual dose is 500 mg four times daily or 1 g twice daily; severe or chronic infections may require larger doses. Prolonged intensive therapy is needed for complications such as prostatitis and epididymitis. For respiratory tract infections and skin and soft tissue infections the usual dose is 250 mg or 500 mg four times daily or 500 mg or 1 g twice daily depending on the severity and site of infections. For gastro-intestinal tract infections, 500 mg three or four times daily may be employed.

Children: The usual dose is from 25 to 50 mg/kg/day total, given in two or four equally divided doses.

For otitis media daily doses from 75 to 100 mg/kg in divided doses every 6 to 12 hours are recommended. Maximum dose 4 g per day.

Elderly: There are no specific dosage recommendations or precautions for use in the elderly except, as with other drugs, to monitor those patients with impaired renal or hepatic function.

All patients, irrespective of age and weight: Larger doses (up to 1 g four times daily) may be given for severe or chronic infections. Therapy should be continued for a minimum of 48-72 hours after the patient becomes asymptomatic or evidence of bacterial eradication has been obtained. In infections caused by haemolytic strains of streptococci, a minimum of 10 days treatment is recommended to guard against the risk of rheumatic fever or glomerulonephritis. In the treatment of chronic urinary tract infections, frequent bacteriological and clinical appraisal is necessary during therapy and may be necessary for several months afterwards. Persistent infections may require treatment for several weeks. Smaller doses than those indicated above should not be used. Doses for children should not exceed doses recommended for adults. As Velosef is available in both injectable and oral form, patients may be changed from the Velosef injectable to the Velosef oral at the same dosage level.

Renal impairment dosage: A modified dosage schedule in patients with decreased renal function is necessary. Each patient should be considered individually; the following reduced dosage schedule is recommended as a guideline, based on the creatinine clearance (ml/min/ 1.73 m²). In adults, the initial loading dose is 750 mg of Velosef and the maintenance dose is 500 mg at the time intervals listed below:

Creatinine clearance	Time interval
more than 20 ml/min	6–12 hours
15–19 ml/min	12–24 hours
10–14 ml/min	24–40 hours
5–9 ml/min	40–50 hours
less than 5 ml/min	50–70 hours

Further modification of the dosage schedule may be necessary in children.

Contra-indications, warnings, etc

Contra-indications: Patients with known hypersensitivity to the cephalosporin antibiotics.

Precautions: There is evidence of partial cross-allergenicity between the penicillins and the cephalosporins. Therefore cephradine should be used with caution in those patients with known hypersensitivity to penicillins.

After treatment with Velosef, a false positive reaction for glucose in the urine may occur with Benedict's or Fehling's solution or with reagent tablets such as Clinitest*, but not with enzyme-based tests such as Clinistix* or Diastix*.

As with all antibiotics, prolonged use may result in overgrowth of non-susceptible organisms.

Pregnancy and breast feeding: Although animal studies have not demonstrated any teratogenicity, safety in pregnancy has not been established. Cephradine is excreted in breast milk and should be used with caution in lactating mothers.

Side-effects: Limited essentially to gastro-intestinal disturbances and on occasion to hypersensitivity phenomena. The latter are more likely to occur in individuals who have previously demonstrated hypersensitivity and those with a history of allergy, asthma, hay fever or urticaria. The majority of reported side-effects have been mild. Skin reactions have occasionally been reported.

Adverse reaction reports are rare, but include glossitis, heartburn, dizziness, tightness in the chest, nausea, vomiting, diarrhoea, abdominal pain, vaginitis, candidal overgrowth. Skin and hypersensitivity reactions include urticaria, skin rashes, joint pains, oedema.

As with other cephalosporins, mild transient eosinophilia, leucopenia and neutropenia, positive direct Coombs tests and pseudomembraneous colitis have been reported.

Clinical chemistry: Isolated instances of elevated SGOT, SGPT, total bilirubin and alkaline phosphatase have been observed; in most patients, the values were only mildly elevated and tended to return to normal at the end of therapy. No consistent pattern was observed that would suggest hepatocellular damage.

Mild elevations of BUN have been reported. In most cases, however, the values tended to return to normal. In adults for whom serum creatinine determinations were performed, the rise in BUN was not accompanied by a rise in serum creatinine, which would suggest an extrarenal mechanism for the elevation of BUN.

Pharmaceutical precautions *Storage: Capsules:* In a cool place.

Powder for syrup: A cool place. After reconstitution; discard unused syrup after 14 days if stored in refrigerator, or seven days at room temperature.

Dilution: Velosef Syrup may be diluted with Syrup BP. The diluted syrup should be used within seven days.

Legal category POM.

Package quantities *Capsules:* Boxes of 20 in blisters and bottles of 100.
Syrup: Bottles of 100 ml.

Further information Cephradine has a high degree of stability to many beta-lactamases. It has a low degree of protein-binding and a large volume of distribution. Therefore, tissue levels are generally found to be high. Oral cephradine can be given twice or four times daily, and is well absorbed.

Human pharmacology: Cephradine is acid stable and is rapidly absorbed following oral administration in the fasting state. Following doses of 250 mg, 500 mg and 1000 mg average peak serum levels of approximately 9, 16.5, and 24.2 micrograms/ml, respectively, were obtained at one hour. The presence of food in the gastrointestinal tract delays the absorption but does not affect the total amount of cephradine absorbed. Measurable serum levels are present six hours after administration. Over 90% of the drug is excreted unchanged in the urine within 6 hours. Peak urine concentrations are approximately 1600 micrograms/ml following a 250 mg dose, 3200 micrograms/ml following a 500 mg dose, and 4000 micrograms/ml following a 1000 mg dose. After 48 hours' administration of 100 mg/kg/day of cephradine for the treatment of otitis media, cephradine has been measured in the middle ear exudate at an average level of 3.6 microgram/ml.

Product licence numbers
Velosef Capsules 250 mg	0034/0133
Velosef Capsules 500 mg	0034/0134
Velosef Syrup 125 mg/5 ml	0034/0135
Velosef Syrup 250 mg/5 ml	0034/0136

VELOSEF* FOR INJECTION

Presentation Velosef for Injection is a sterile powder blend of cephradine and L-arginine. After reconstitution, Velosef for Injection 500 mg and 1.0 g vials provide 500 mg and 1.0 g of cephradine activity, respectively.

Uses *Actions:* Cephradine is a broad-spectrum bactericidal antibiotic active against both Gram-positive and

Gram-negative bacteria. It is also highly active against most strains of penicillinase-producing staphylococci.

Microbiology: The following organisms have shown *in vitro* sensitivity to cephradine:

Gram-positive – *Staphylococci* (both penicillin sensitive and resistant strains), *Streptococci*, both *Streptococcus pyogenes* (beta haemolytic) and Group D *Streptococci* (enterococci) and *Streptococcus pneumoniae.*

Gram-negative – *E. coli, Klebsiella, P. mirabilis, Haemophilus influenzae, Shigella* spp., *Salmonella* spp. (including *Salmonella typhi*) and *Neisseria* spp.

Enterococci (*S. faecalis*) may be susceptible to the high levels of cephradine achieved in the urine.

Because cephradine is unaffected by penicillinase, many strains of *E. coli* and *Staphylococcus aureus* which produce this enzyme are susceptible to cephradine but resistant to ampicillin.

Indications: The treatment of infections of the urinary, respiratory and gastro-intestinal tracts and of the skin and soft tissues, bones and joints; also septicaemia and endocarditis. These include:

Upper respiratory infections – pharyngitis, sinusitis, otitis media, tonsillitis, laryngo-tracheo-bronchitis.

Lower respiratory infections – acute and chronic bronchitis, lobar and bronchopneumonia.

Urinary tract infections – cystitis, urethritis, pyelonephritis.

Skin and soft tissue infections – abscess, cellulitis, furunculosis, impetigo.

Gastro-intestinal tract – bacillary dysentery, enteritis, peritonitis.

Velosef has been shown to be effective in reducing the incidence of postoperative infections in patients undergoing surgical procedures associated with a high risk of infection. It is also of value where post-operative infection would be disastrous and where patients have a reduced host resistance to bacterial infection. Protection is best ensured by achieving adequate local tissue concentrations at the time contamination is likely to occur. Thus, Velosef should be administered immediately prior to surgery and continued during the postoperative period.

Bacteriological studies to determine the causative organisms and their sensitivity to cephradine should be performed. Therapy may be instituted prior to receiving the results of the sensitivity test.

Sterile Velosef for injection is indicated primarily for those patients unable to tolerate oral medication. It is also indicated for intravenous use either by direct injection or by intravenous infusion for the treatment of serious and life-threatening infections.

Dosage and administration Intramuscular or intravenous injection and intravenous infusion.

Adults: Treatment: The usual dose range of Velosef for injection is 2-4 g daily in four equally divided doses. This may be increased up to 8 g a day for severe infections, e.g. septicaemia and endocarditis. For the majority of infections, the usual dose is 500 mg q.i.d. in equally spaced doses; severe or chronic infections may require larger doses. Prolonged intensive therapy is needed for complications such as prostatitis and epididymitis. Patients who are severely ill and who require high serum levels of cephradine for treating their infections should be started on intravenous therapy.

Limited experience indicates that intraperitoneal administration of Velosef may be effective after surgery in cases of peritonitis where a surgical drainage system has been established.

Prophylaxis: The recommended dose for surgical prophylaxis is a single, pre-operative 1–2 g IM or IV dose. Subsequent parenteral or oral doses can be administered as appropriate.

Children: The usual dose is 50-100 mg/kg/day total given in four equally divided doses. More serious illnesses (e.g. typhoid fever) may require 200-300 mg/kg/day.

Elderly: There are no specific dosage recommendations or precautions for use in the elderly except, as with other drugs, to monitor those patients with impaired renal or hepatic function.

All patients, regardless of age and weight: Therapy should be continued for a minimum of 48-72 hours after the patient becomes asymptomatic or evidence of bacterial eradication has been obtained. In infections caused by haemolytic strains of streptococci, a minimum of 10 days of treatment is recommended to guard against the risk of rheumatic fever or glomerulonephritis. In the treatment of chronic urinary tract infections, frequent bacteriological and clinical appraisal is necessary during therapy and may be necessary for several months afterwards. Persistent infections may require treatment for several weeks. Smaller doses than those indicated above should not be used. Doses for children should not exceed doses recommended for adults. As Velosef is available in both injectable and oral form, patients may be changed from Velosef injectable to Velosef oral at the same dosage level.

Renal impairment dosage: A modified dosage schedule in patients with decreased renal function is necessary. Each patient should be considered individually; the following reduced dosage schedule is recommended as a guideline, based on the creatinine clearance (ml/min/ 1.73 m^2). In adults, the initial loading dose is 750 mg of Velosef and the maintenance dose is 500 mg at the time intervals listed below:

Creatinine clearance	Time interval
more than 20 ml/min	6–12 hours
15–19 ml/min	12–24 hours
10–14 ml/min	24–40 hours
5–9 ml/min	40–50 hours
less than 5 ml/min	50–70 hours

Further modification of the dosage schedule may be necessary in children.

Reconstitution: For intramuscular use: Aseptically add sterile water for injection or 0.9% sodium chloride injection according to the following table:

Single dose* vial size	Volume of diluent to be added
500 mg	2.0 ml
1 g	4.0 ml

* Preparation contains no bactericide and is not intended for multiple dose use.

Shake to effect solution and withdraw the entire contents. Intramuscular solutions should be used within 2 hours at room temperature; when stored in a refrigerator at 5°C, solutions retain full potency for 24 hours. Reconstituted solutions may vary in colour from light to straw yellow; however, this does not affect the potency.

For intravenous use: Velosef for injection may be administered by direct intravenous injection or by infusion. A 3 mcg/ml serum concentration can be maintained for each milligram of cephradine per kg body weight per hour of infusion.

For direct intravenous administration: Suitable intravenous injection solutions are Sterile Water for Injection, 5% Dextrose Injection or 0.9% Sodium Chloride Injection.

Aseptically add 5 ml of diluent to the 500 mg vial or 10 ml to the 1 g vial. Shake to effect solution and withdraw the entire contents. The solution may be slowly injected directly into a vein over a 3 to 5 minute period. The solution should be used within 2 hours when kept at room temperature; if stored at 5°C, solutions retain full potency for 24 hours.

For continuous or intermittent intravenous infusion: Suitable intravenous infusion solutions are Sterile Water for Injection (50 mg/ml cephradine solutions are approximately isotonic); 5% or 10% Dextrose Injection; 0.9% Sodium Chloride Injection; Sodium Lactate Injection (M/6 sodium lactate); Dextrose and Sodium Chloride Injection; Lactated Ringer's Injection; Ringer's Injection; 5% Dextrose in Lactated Ringer's Injection; 5% Dextrose in Ringer's Injection.

Aseptically add 10 ml of the diluent to the 1 g vial and shake to effect solution. Aseptically transfer the entire contents to the IV infusion diluent. Intravenous infusions prepared remain potent for 24 hours at room temperature or 1 week at 5°C at concentrations up to 10 mg/ml (1%), and for 10 hours at room temperature or 48 hours at 5°C at concentrations up to 50 mg/ml (5%). For prolonged infusion, replace 5% infusions every 10 hours and 1% infusions every 24 hours with freshly-prepared solutions.

N.B. Only cephradine solubilised with arginine may be reconstituted with solutions containing calcium salts, such as Ringer's Solutions.

For further information on compatibilities consult the manufacturer.

Protect solutions of cephradine from concentrated light or direct sunlight.

Contra-indications, warnings, etc

Contra-indications: Patients with known hypersensitivity to the cephalosporin antibiotics.

Precautions: There is evidence of partial cross-allergenicity between the penicillins and the cephalosporins. Therefore Velosef should be used with caution in those patients with known hypersensitivity to penicillins.

After treatment with Velosef a false positive reaction for glucose in the urine may occur with Benedict's solution or Fehling's solution or with reagent tablets such as Clinitest*, but not with enzyme-based tests such as Clinistix* or Diastix*.

As with all antibiotics, prolonged use may result in overgrowth of non-susceptible organisms.

Pregnancy and breast feeding: Although animal studies have not demonstrated any teratogenicity, safety in pregnancy has not been established. Cephradine is excreted in breast milk and should be used with caution in lactating mothers.

Side-effects: Limited essentially to gastro-intestinal disturbances and on occasion to hypersensitivity phenomena. The latter are more likely to occur in individual's who have previously demonstrated hypersensitivity and those with a history of allergy, asthma, hay fever or urticaria. The majority of reported side-effects have been mild. Skin reactions have occasionally been reported.

Adverse reaction reports are rare, but include glossitis, heartburn, headache, dizziness, dyspnoea, paraesthesia, nausea, vomiting, diarrhoea, abdominal pain, candidal overgrowth, vaginitis. Skin and hypersensitivity reactions include urticaria, skin rashes, joint pains, oedema.

As with other cephalosporins, mild transient eosinophilia, leucopenia and neutropenia, rarely positive direct Coombs tests and pseudomembranous colitis have been reported.

Clinical chemistry: Isolated instances of elevated SGOT, SGPT, total bilirubin and alkaline phosphatase have been observed; in most patients, the values were only mildly elevated and tended to return to normal at the end of therapy. No consistent pattern was observed that would suggest hepatocellular damage.

Mild elevations of BUN have been reported. In most cases, however, the values tended to return to normal. In adults for whom serum creatinine determinations were performed, the rise in BUN was not accompanied by a rise in serum creatinine, which would suggest an extrarenal mechanism for the elevation of BUN.

Injection: As with other parenterally administered antibiotics, transient pain may be experienced at the injection site, but is seldom the cause for discontinuing treatment. Thrombophlebitis has been reported following intravenous injection.

Since sterile abscesses have been reported following accidental subcutaneous injection, the preparation should be administered by deep intramuscular injection.

Pharmaceutical precautions *Storage (before reconstitution):* At room temperature.

Legal category POM.

Package quantities *500 mg single-dose vials:* Pack of 5.
1 g single-dose vials: Single-vial pack.

Further information Cephradine has a high degree of stability to beta-lactamases. It has a low degree of protein binding and a large volume of distribution. Therefore, tissue levels are generally found to be high.

Human pharmacology: Following intramuscular administration of a single 0.5 g dose of cephradine to normal volunteers, the average peak serum concentration was 8.41 mcg/ml with the time to peak concentration being 0.93 hours. The serum half-life averaged 1.25 hours. A single 1 g intravenous dose resulted in serum concentrations of 86 mcg/ml at 5 minutes and 12 mcg/ml at 1 hour; these concentrations declined to 1 mcg/ml at 4 hours. Continuous infusion of 500 mg per hour into a 70 kg man maintained a concentration of about 21.4 mcg/ml cephradine activity; this study showed that a serum concentration of approximately 3 mcg/ml can be obtained for each milligram of cephradine administered per kg of body weight per hour of infusion.

Cephradine is excreted unchanged in the urine. The kidneys excrete 57% to 80% of an intramuscular dose in the first six hours; this results in a high urine concentration, e.g. 880 mcg/ml of urine after a 500 mg intramuscular dose. Probenecid slows tubular secretion and almost doubles peak serum concentration.

Assays of bone obtained at surgery have shown that cephradine penetrates bone tissue.

Product licence numbers
Velosef Injection 500 mg   0034/0198
Velosef Injection 1 g   0034/0199

VERDIVITON* ELIXIR

Presentation Clear, green liquid containing in each 15 ml:

Thiamine mononitrate (vitamin B_1)	2 mg
Riboflavine (vitamin B_2)	1 mg
Pyridoxine hydrochloride (vitamin B_6)	0.5 mg
Nicotinamide	15 mg
d-Panthenol	1 mg
Cyanocobalamin (vitamin B_{12})	15 mcg
Calcium glycerophosphate	110 mg
Sodium glycerophosphate	80 mg
Potassium glycerophosphate	20 mg
Manganese glycerophosphate	10 mg
Alcohol	17% by volume

Uses *Indications:* The maintenance of adequate levels of B vitamins particularly in those conditions where such levels may be thought to be lowered.

Dosage and administration *Adults:* Three 5 ml spoonfuls three times daily.

Verdiviton should preferably be taken before meals.

Children: Not recommended.

Elderly: No specific dosage recommendations or precautions.

Contra-indications, warnings, etc
Contra-indications: Where the use of alcohol is undesirable, hepatitis and alcoholism.

Pregnancy and nursing mothers: As with other vitamin and mineral preparations no specific precautions apply, except to note alcohol content.

Pharmaceutical precautions *Storage:* Cool place, protected from light.

Legal category P.

Package quantities Bottles of 240 ml.

Further information Nil.

Product licence number 0034/5097.

*Trade Mark

Stafford-Miller Limited
Stafford-Miller House
The Common
Hatfield, Herts AL10 0NZ

ALPHOSYL*

Presentation *Lotion and Cream:* Containing refined alcoholic extract of coal tar 5%, allantoin 2%, in a greaseless vanishing-cream base.

Application PC: Refined alcoholic extract of coal tar 5%, allantoin 0.2% in a foaming shampoo base.

The lotion is a light free-flowing emulsion and the cream is smooth, homogeneous, and is light tan in colour. The application is a light green/tan soft shampoo.

Uses Dermatological stimulant for the treatment of psoriasis, psoriasis of the scalp and dandruff.

Dosage and administration *Lotion and Cream:* Apply liberally two to four times daily; massage well into the affected areas. Occlusive dressings are unnecessary.

Application PC: Wet scalp and hair, apply shampoo and vigorously massage to lather; rinse and repeat if necessary.

Contra-indications, warnings, etc For external use only. Discontinue if irritation occurs or in cases of sensitivity to coal tar.

Pharmaceutical precautions Do not refrigerate. Store at below 30°C.

Legal category P.

Package quantities *Alphosyl Lotion:* Bottles of 250 ml.
Alphosyl Cream: Tube of 75 g.
Alphosyl Application PC: Tube of 60 g.

Further information Alphosyl Lotion is the basic treatment for psoriasis of the body and scalp.

Alphosyl Cream is designed especially for lubrication in the intertriginous areas.

Alphosyl Application PC is an adjunctive therapy for patients with psoriasis of the scalp, dandruff and other scaly scalp disorders. It prevents irritation of the scalp and is used also in preparation for treatment with the Lotion.

Product licence numbers
Alphosyl Lotion   0036/5008
Alphosyl Cream   0036/5006
Alphosyl Application PC   0036/5005

ALPHOSYL* HC CREAM

Presentation A cream containing refined alcoholic extract of coal tar 5%, allantoin 2% and hydrocortisone PhEur 0.5% in a greaseless vanishing cream base. The cream is smooth, homogeneous, and is light tan in colour.

Uses Dermatological stimulant and local corticosteroid anti-inflammatory therapy for psoriasis.

Dosage and administration Apply two to four times daily, massaging well into the affected areas.

Contra-indications, warnings, etc Contra-indicated in tuberculosis or fungal lesions of the skin, herpes simplex, vaccinia or varicella, and a history of hypersensitivity to any of the ingredients.

Do not use on infected areas unless accompanied by appropriate anti-infective therapy.

Topical administration of corticosteroids to pregnant animals can cause abnormality of foetal development. The relevance of this finding to human beings has not been established. However, topical steroids should not be used extensively in pregnancy, i.e., in large amounts or for long periods.

Under occlusive dressings or in intertriginous areas, topical steroids may cause striae of the skin.

When topical steroids are used over large areas or for prolonged periods systemic side effects may possibly occur.

For external use only. Avoid contact with the eyes.

In infants, long-term continuous therapy should be avoided.

Adrenal suppression can occur even without occlusion.

Discontinue use if sensitivity occurs. Keep this and all medicines out of the reach of children.

Pharmaceutical precautions Store below 30°C. Do not refrigerate.

Legal category POM.

Package quantities Tubes of 30 g and 45 g.

Further information Alphosyl HC Cream is intended for the treatment of the acute stages of psoriasis when the basic Alphosyl action is enhanced by the addition of hydrocortisone.

Product licence number 0036/0026.

COLIFOAM*

Presentation White, odourless aerosol foam containing hydrocortisone acetate PhEur 10%. Other ingredients: propylene glycol, ethoxylated stearyl alcohol, polyoxyethylene-10-stearyl ether, cetyl alcohol, methyl and propyl hydroxybenzoate, triethanolamine and water. Inert propellants added.

Uses Anti-inflammatory corticosteroid therapy for the topical treatment of ulcerative colitis, proctosigmoiditis and granular proctitis.

Dosage and administration One applicatorful inserted into the rectum once or twice daily for two or three weeks and every second day thereafter. Shake can vigorously before use (illustrated instructions are enclosed in each pack).

Satisfactory response usually occurs within five to seven days.

Contra-indications, warnings, etc Local contra-indications to the use of intrarectal steroids include obstruction, abscess, perforation, peritonitis, fresh intestinal anastomoses and extensive fistulae.

General precautions common to all corticosteroid therapy should be observed during treatment with Colifoam. Treatment should be administered with caution in patients with severe ulcerative disease because of their predisposition to perforation of the bowel wall.

Safety during pregnancy has not been fully established.

Pharmaceutical precautions Pressurized container. Protect from sunlight and do not expose to temperatures above 50°C. Do not pierce or burn even after use.

Do not refrigerate. Shake vigorously before use. Keep out of the reach of children. For external use only.

Legal category POM.

Package quantities Aerosol canister containing 25 g (approx. 14 applications) plus a plastic applicator and illustrated leaflet.

Further information One applicatorful of Colifoam provides a dose of approximately 125 mg of hydrocortisone acetate, similar to that used in a retention enema, for the treatment of ulcerative colitis, sigmoiditis and proctitis.

Product licence number 0036/0021.

EPIFOAM*

Presentation Muco-adherent, white, odourless aerosol foam containing:

Hydrocortisone acetate PhEur   1%
Pramoxine hydrochloride USP   1%

Other ingredients: propylene glycol, ethoxylated stearyl alcohol, polyoxyethylene-10-stearyl ether, cetyl alcohol, methyl hydroxybenzoate, propyl hydroxybenzoate, triethanolamine and deionised water. Inert propellants added.

Uses For the treatment of perineal trauma including post-episiotomy pain and discomfort.

Dosage and administration A suitable quantity of foam should be dispensed onto a pad, preferably sterile, and applied to the site or affected areas 3–4 times daily.

If an absorbent pad is used, a piece of porous but non-absorbent material should be placed between the foam and the pad in order to maximise contact of the foam with the wound.

Contra-indications, warnings, etc Do not use on infected lesions unless accompanied by appropriate anti-infective agents. Should not be used extensively in pregnancy. Avoid long term therapy in infants.

Pharmaceutical precautions Pressurised container. Protect from sunlight and do not expose to temperatures above 50°C. Do not pierce or burn even after use.

Do not refrigerate. Shake vigorously before use. Use at room temperature. Keep out of the reach of children.

For external use only.

Legal category POM.

Package quantities Aerosol canister containing 12 g of foam.

Further information An illustrated instruction leaflet is enclosed with each pack.

Product licence number 0036/5002.

PHAZYME*

Presentation Pink, sugar-coated, two-phase tablet, each tablet containing:
In the outer layer,

Specially activated simethicone   20 mg

In the core, protected for release in the small intestine,

Specially activated simethicone   40 mg

Uses Deflatulent action for the relief of pain and distention due to gastro-intestinal gas.

Dosage and administration *Adults:* One or two tablets to be swallowed with meals and upon retiring or as required.

Children (6–12 years): 1 tablet as above.

Contra-indications, warnings, etc Specially activated simethicone is physiologically inert and is not absorbed and therefore has no side-effects or contra-indications.

Pharmaceutical precautions No special precautions.

Legal category P.

Package quantities Bottles of 100 tablets.

Further information Phazyme Tablets are compatible with any other therapy which may be prescribed concurrently.

Product licence number 0036/0025R.

PROCTOFOAM HC*

Presentation Muco-adherent, white, odourless aerosol foam containing:

Hydrocortisone acetate PhEur   1%
Pramoxine hydrochloride USP   1%

Other ingredients: propylene glycol, ethoxylated stearyl alcohol, polyoxyethylene-10-stearyl ether, cetyl alcohol, methyl hydroxybenzoate, propyl hydroxybenzoate, triethanolamine, deionised water, in aerosol canisters containing 24 g, with a plastic applicator. Inert propellants added.

Uses Anti-inflammatory, antipruritic, anaesthetic. For the temporary relief of inflammation, pruritus, pain and swelling associated with haemorrhoids, proctitis, cryptitis, fissures, post-operative pain and pruritus ani. For treatment of post-episiotomy pain and discomfort.

Dosage and administration One applicatorful per rectum two or three times daily and after each bowel evacuation. Perianally or for post-episiotomy use – apply as needed. Not indicated in infants and young children.

Contra-indications, warnings, etc A complete rectal examination to rule out serious pathology should be completed before instituting therapy. Do not use on infected lesions unless accompanied by appropriate anti-infective agents. Discontinue use if sensitivity develops. Steroids should not be used unnecessarily during pregnancy since safety during pregnancy has not been fully established.

Pharmaceutical precautions Pressurized container. Protect from sunlight and do not expose to temperatures above 50°C. Do not pierce or burn even after use.

Do not refrigerate. Shake vigorously before use. Use at room temperature. Keep out of reach of children

For external use only.

Legal category POM.

Package quantities Aerosol canister containing 24 g of foam (approximately 40 doses), plus a plastic applicator.

Further information One applicatorful of Proctofoam HC provides a dose of approximately 4–6 mg of both hydrocortisone acetate and pramoxine hydrochloride.

An illustrated instruction leaflet is enclosed with each pack.

Product licence number 0036/5002.

QUELLADA*

Presentation *Quellada Lotion:* Lindane BP 1% in a pleasantly perfumed lotion base, pearly white in colour.

Quellada Application PC: Lindane BP 1% in a specially formulated foaming shampoo base. Quellada Application PC is a yellow, clear liquid.

Uses Antiparasitic – ovacidal.

For the treatment of mite and lice infestations, e.g. scabies, head lice, pubic lice and body lice.

Dosage and administration *Lotion (scabies): Adults:* Apply a thin layer to the whole body surface excluding face and scalp. Leave for 24 hours, then wash thoroughly.

Babies: Do not use on babies under one month old.

Babies (1–6 months): Treat only under medical supervision. The lotion should be washed off after 8–12 hours. Repeat after 2 weeks if necessary. Precautions should be taken to prevent the baby's hands from making contact with the face during the treatment period. Swaddling in a shawl or blanket should be sufficient to do this.

Children (Over 6 months): Product may be used as per adults but parental supervision is strongly advised.

Application PC (Pediculosis): Apply a sufficient quantity of the shampoo to thoroughly wet the hair and skin of the infested and adjacent hairy areas. Work thoroughly into the hair and allow to remain in place for four minutes. Add small quantities of water until a good lather forms, and shampoo as usual. Rinse thoroughly. Towel briskly. When the hair is dry, any remaining nits or nit shells may be removed by fine tooth combing or with tweezers.

Contra-indications, warnings, etc *Lotion:* External use only. Avoid contact with eyes and other mucous membranes.

Application PC: Avoid contact with eyes. Should lather accidentally get into the eyes immediately flush with water. Do not use more than twice in any one infestation nor in any one week. Do not use on broken or infected skin.

Pharmaceutical precautions Do not refrigerate. Store at room temperature.

Legal category P.

Package quantities Both Quellada Lotion and Quellada Application PC are available in bottle of 100 ml and 500 ml.

Further information As Lindane 1% is effective against both adult and egg stages of *Sarcoptes scabiei* and *pediculus*, one application is usually sufficient to clear infestation, provided that instructions are carried out correctly. Printed instructions are issued with each pack.

Irritation and sensitivity are rare.

All insecticides penetrate human skin to some extent which, in scabies, is desirable in order to provide effective treatment. Insecticides can enter the blood stream and be distributed throughout the body prior to degradation. Organochlorine insecticides such as Lindane are highly soluble in lipids and consequently may be found in human body fat.

In the normal course of events, Lindane in body fat is rendered harmless by isolation. The rate of degradation of the insecticide continues slowly as fat cells are broken down. However, in some circumstances, the most significant of which are pregnancy and lactation, fats become mobilised with the effect that some Lindane is excreted. Small quantities of the insecticide may pass trans-placentally or be excreted in breast milk.

Use of Lindane in pregnancy and nursing mothers: In order that infants should not be unnecessarily exposed, it is now felt that some thought should be given before treatment of pregnant or nursing mothers with formulations containing Lindane. Whilst the safety of Lindane in human pregnancy and nursing mothers has not been fully established, the amount of insecticide absorbed from a single application is small and therefore likely to be of low importance.

However, where the risk of reinfection is high, further treatments with Lindane are not recommended unless other monitoring of the patient reponse is carried out.

Regular contact with Lindane: Some caution should be exercised by medical and nursing staff who carry out treatments, since they may be exposed to Lindane on a daily basis. Surgical gloves should always be worn during application.

Product licence numbers

Quellada Lotion	0036/5000
Quellada Application PC	0036/5001

TARCORTIN*

Presentation Hydrocortisone PhEur 0.5% and refined alcoholic extract of coal tar 5% in a vanishing cream base. It is a light tan, homogeneous cream.

Uses Stimulating, antipruritic. For all simple or refractory subacute and chronic skin affections, including chronic eczema, infantile eczema, localised neurodermatitis, seborrhoea, dermatitis venenata, pruritus ani and psoriasis.

Dosage and administration Apply twice daily or more frequently to the affected area by gentle massage until the cream has vanished into the skin. No dressing is needed.

Contra-indications, warnings, etc Contra-indicated in tuberculosis or fungal lesions of the skin, herpes simplex, vaccinia or varicella, and a history of hypersensitivity to any of the ingredients.

Do not use on infected areas unless accompanied by appropriate anti-infective therapy.

Topical administration of corticosteroids to pregnant animals can cause abnormality of foetal development. The relevance of this finding to human beings has not been established. However, topical steroids should not be used extensively in pregnancy, i.e., in large amounts for long periods.

Under occlusive dressings or in intertriginous areas, topical steroids may cause striae of the skin.

When topical steroids are used over large areas or for prolonged periods systemic side effects may possibly occur.

For external use only. Avoid contact with the eyes.

In infants, long-term continous therapy should be avoided. Adrenal suppression can occur even without occlusion.

Discontinue use if sensitivity occurs. Keep this and all medicines out of the reach of children.

Pharmaceutical precautions Do not refrigerate. Store at below 30°C.

Legal category POM.

Package quantities Tubes of 30 g and 45 g.

Further information Clinical studies carried out in the United States to determine the efficacy of the combination of hydrocortisone and coal tar extract in comparison with hydrocortisone alone in the topical treatment of psoriasis and atopic dermatitis, suggest that the combination of hydrocortisone and coal tar extract is superior to hydrocortisone alone in the majority of the conditions treated.

Product licence number 0036/5007.

*Trade Mark

STD Pharmaceutical Products Ltd
Fields Yard, Plough Lane
Hereford HR4 0EL

STD* INJECTION
Sodium Tetradecyl Sulphate Injection 3%

Presentation STD Injection is a sterile aqueous 3% solution of Sodium Tetradecyl Sulphate containing 2% Benzyl Alcohol and buffered to pH 7.6.

Uses The solution is designed for intravenous use and is used primarily as a sclerosant in the treatment of varicose veins of the leg by compression sclerotherapy.

The action of sodium tetradecyl sulphate in this technique is considered to be that of irritation to the intima of the vein wall, so that on compression of the vein fibrosis takes place and the vein is thus permanently occluded by a short fibrous cord therein.

Dosage and administration 0.5–1 ml at each of four sites (maximum 4 ml).

A dose of 0.5–1 ml is introduced into the superficial vein over the site of an incompetent perforating vein. It is never necessary or desirable to inject more than 1 ml at any one site and often half this volume will produce the desired effect. Three or four such injections can be given at the same visit into one limb.

The treatment of varicose veins by compression sclerotherapy is directed towards the restoration of the efficiency of the synchronised pumping systems within the leg by permanently destroying the leaking points rather than by the eradication of the superficial tortuous veins which may, in many cases, be capable of reverting to normal appearance and function after the restoration of the normal pattern of pressure within the veins of the limb.

Localisation of the perforating veins containing the injured valves is the supremely important object of diagnosis.

Treatment comprises the permanent blocking of the offending leak by producing a short fibrotic segment of vein involving the area of the junction of the perforating and superficial veins. This can be achieved by carrying out the following procedure:

1. Introducing the sclerosant into this vein after it has been emptied.
2. Maintaining the sclerosant in the empty and isolated segment for 30 seconds.
3. Applying compression immediately to the site of injection, maintaining it for a period of about six weeks, until one is quite sure that, when the patient stands erect, the internal pressure of the blood in the adjacent unobliterated vein cannot reopen the segment.
4. Application of compression is most suitably obtained by firm bandaging with a number of strong cotton crêpe bandages and by incorporating therein shaped rubber pads over the sites of injection.

An elastic stocking applied over the bandage aids compression and the retention of the bandages in position.

Contra-indications, warnings, etc The use of STD Injection of Sodium Tetradecyl Sulphate is not recommended for the treatment of varicose veins by compression sclerotherapy when any of the following factors are present:

1. *Oral contraceptives:* Until such time as the exact thromboplastic effect of the oral contraceptive tablet has been established, it is advisable not to use sclerotherapy on patients who are currently taking oral contraceptives.
2. *Inability to walk:* As the recommended treatment involves daily periods of walking by the patient it is not advisable to embark upon treatment if for any reason the patient cannot walk at least three miles each day.
3. *Obese legs:* It is recommended that patients with obese legs should not receive treatment. In many cases the obesity may be corrected by dieting, after which time treatment may be commenced.
4. *Any known allergy to sodium tetradecyl sulphate:* Treatment by injection of STD should not be continued if an allergic reaction has been experienced after a previous injection of sodium tetradecyl sulphate.

Side-effects
1. (a) Allergy and Anaphylaxis – Rarely – *see* Precautions below.
   (b) Allergy–Urticaria – *see* Precautions below.
2. Extravascular injection will give rise to pain, and may produce necrosis and ulceration (if close to surface).

Precautions
1. *Allergy and Anaphylaxis:*

(a) History of allergy should be taken from all patients prior to treatment. In particular allergic reactions to previous injections of sodium tetradecyl sulphate should be noted (see contra-indication 4, above).
(b) A higher incidence of allergic reaction is thought to result from repeated treatment involving Sodium Tetradecyl Sulphate Injection and may involve intervals of several years between courses of injection.

2. *Equipment of clinic:* The treatment of anaphylaxis may require, depending on severity of attack, some or all of the following: injection of adrenaline, injection of hydrocortisone, antihistamine injection, endotracheal tube, laryngoscope, mucus extraction pump. The treatment of varicose veins by STD injection should not be undertaken in clinics where these items are not readily available.

Pharmaceutical precautions Store in a cool place, away from direct sunlight.

Legal category POM

Package quantities STD injection.
30 ml multidose containers.
100 × 1 ml single-dose ampoules.

Further information The use of a small dose, the isolation of the injection within the vein segment and the application of immediate, adequate and lasting compression are of supreme importance in obtaining a good result.

Product licence number 0398/5000.

*Trade Mark

M. A. Steinhard Limited
32–36 Minerva Road
London NW10 7UW

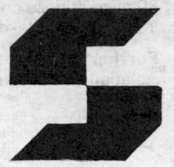

ALMAZINE* TABLETS

Presentation Almazine 1 mg tablets each contain Lorazepam 1 mg. They are presented as light green flat oval tablets, one side bearing the letters 'MAS' the other scored and bearing the letter 'L' above the score line and the figure '1' below.

Almazine 2.5 mg tablets each contain Lorazepam 2.5 mg. They are presented as pink flat oval tablets, one side bearing the letters 'MAS' and the other scored and bearing the letter 'L' above the score line and the figures '2.5' below.

Uses Almazine is used in the treatment of mild, moderate and severe anxiety and tension states, as a sedative and premedication before general surgery and operative dentistry.

Dosage and administration
Adults: Mild anxiety 1–4 mg daily in divided doses.
Moderate anxiety 4–8 mg daily in divided doses.
Severe anxiety 8–10 mg daily in divided doses.
Premedication: 2–3 mg the night before operation and 2–4 mg one to two hours before operation.
Insomnia: 1–4 mg before retiring.
Dentistry: 1–2.5 mg one to two hours before treatment.
Children: Not recommended for children.

Contra-indications, warnings, etc
1. Almazine should not be administered to patients with a previous history of sensitivity to benzodiazepines.
2. Caution should be observed should it be necessary to administer Almazine to patients with impaired renal or hepatic functions, in debilitated patients, and during pregnancy, especially during the first three months.
3. Concomitant administration with central nervous system depressants will result in an accentuated effect. Patients should be warned against driving or operating machinery until it has been established that they do not become dizzy or drowsy during treatment.
4. Careful usage does not usually develop drug dependency but after prolonged or excessive use, withdrawal of drug should be gradual.
Side-effects: Almazine is well tolerated and the occurrence of ataxia is evidence of excessive dosage. When high dosages are used, they may have a sedative effect and cause drowsiness. In such cases there is an advantage in administering the larger proportion of the daily intake at night.

Treatment of overdosage: Treatment is symptomatic, but gastric lavage may be useful if performed soon after ingestion.

Pharmaceutical precautions Protect from light, heat and moisture.

Legal category CD (Sch 4), POM.

Package quantities 1 mg and 2.5 mg tablets are supplied in Securitainers containing 50, 100, 250, 500 or 1000 tablets.

Further information Orally administered Almazine is rapidly absorbed, and steady state plasma levels are quickly reached. It is metabolised by a one-step process to the pharmacologically inactive glucuronide which is excreted in the urine.

Product licence numbers
Tablets 1 mg   0401/0050
Tablets 2.5 mg   0401/0051

ALULINE* TABLETS

Presentation Aluline 100 tablets each contain 100 mg Allopurinol BP. They are presented as biconvex white round tablets, one side bearing the name 'Steinhard' the other scored and bearing the letter 'A' above the score line and the figure '100' below.

Aluline 300 tablets each contain 300 mg Allopurinol BP. They are presented as biconvex white round tablets, one side bearing the name 'Steinhard' the other scored and bearing the letter 'A' above the score line and the figure '300' below.

Uses
1. Excess body urate including gout. Aluline reduces urate levels in the body when these are excessive.
2. Calcium renal lithiasis. Aluline is of benefit in the prophylaxis and treatment of calcium lithiasis in patients with raised serum or urinary uric acid.

Dosage and administration *Adults:* The initial dosage should be in the range 100–300 mg per day which may be taken as a single dose. Doses in excess of 300 mg should be administered in divided doses. It has rarely been found necessary to exceed 900 mg per day. The dose should be adjusted by monitoring serum uric acid and/or urinary acid levels at appropriate intervals until the desired effect is attained, which may take one to three weeks. The maintenance dose is normally 200–600 mg per day.

Children: 10–20 mg/kg bodyweight/day. Use in children is mainly indicated in malignant conditions especially leukaemia and certain enzyme disorders (e.g. Lesch-Nyhan syndrome).

Initiation of therapy: In early stages of treatment with Allopurinol, as with uricosuric agents, an acute attack of gouty arthritis may be precipitated. Therefore it is advisable to give a prophylactic dose of a suitable anti-inflammatory agent or colchicine for at least one month.

Use with uricosurics: As Allopurinol does not interfere with the action of uricosuric agents they may be given concurrently. When changing from uricosuric therapy to

Allopurinol one to three weeks overlap of treatment is recommended to ensure a continuous hypouricaemic effect.

To prevent acute uric acid nephropathy in neoplastic conditions treatment with Allopurinol should precede treatment with cytototix drugs (see also sections under Contra-indications, warnings etc.).

Dose recommendations in impaired renal function: Since Allopurinol and its metabolites are excreted via the kidney, impairment of renal function may lead to retention of the drug and its metabolites with consequent prolongation of action. Thus the amount and frequency of the dosage may require reduction as indicated by monitoring serum uric acid levels. The following schedule is provided for guidance in adults.

If creatinine clearance exceeds 20 ml/minute – give standard dose.

If creatinine clearance is between 20 and 10 ml/minute – give 100–200 mg/day.

If creatinine clearance is less than 10 ml/minute – give 100 mg/day or at longer intervals.

Dose recommendations in renal dialysis: Allopurinol and its metabolites are removed by renal dialysis. If frequent dialysis is required an alternative schedule of 300–400 mg after each dialysis, with none in the interim, should be considered.

Contra-indications, warnings, etc

Contra-indications: Known intolerance of Allopurinol. Allopurinol is contra-indicated as a treatment for the acute attack of gout. Prophylactic therapy may be started when the acute attack has completely subsided, provided anti-inflammatory agents are also taken.

Precautions: Treatment with Allopurinol should not be started during an attack of gout.

When 6-mercaptopurine or azothioprine is given concurrently with Allopurinol only one quarter of the usual dose of the cytotoxic should be given. There is no unequivocal evidence that Allopurinol potentiates the action of other cytotoxic drugs.

A reduction in dosage should be considered in the presence of renal and/or hepatic disorders.

Side- and adverse effects: Adverse reactions associated with Allopurinol are rare and mostly of a minor nature. The incidence is higher in the presence of renal and/or hepatic disorders. Treatment with Allopurinol, as with urocosuric agents, may precipitate an attack of gouty arthritis in the early stages; therefore it is advisable to give a prophylactic dose of colchicine for at least a month. When a patient on anticoagulants is given Allopurinol, the theoretical possibility of interaction should be considered. When a patient on chlorpropamide is given Allopurinol there may be a risk of prolonged hypoglycaemic activity.

Skin reactions: These are the most common reactions and may occur at any time during treatment. They may be pruritic, maculopapular, sometimes scaly or purpuric and rarely exfoliative. Allopurinol should be withdrawn immediately should such reactions occur. After recovery from mild reactions Allopurinol may, if desired, be reintroduced at a low dose (e.g. 50 mg/day) which may be gradually increased. If the rash recurs, Allopurinol should be permanently withdrawn.

Generalised hypersensitivity: Exfoliative skin reactions associated with other signs of hypersensitivity including fever, lymphadenopathy, arthralgia and eosinophilia occur rarely. If they do occur, it may be at any time during treatment. Allopurinol should then be withdrawn immediately and permanently. Corticosteroids may be beneficial in overcoming such reactions. Patients manifesting generalised hypersensitivity reactions usually have pre-existing renal and/or hepatic disorders.

Gastro-intestinal disorder: Nausea and vomiting have been reported. This reaction is not a significant problem and can be avoided by taking Allopurinol after meals.

Blood and lymphatic system: There have been occasional reports of transient reduction in the numbers of circulating formed elements of the blood, usually in association with pre-existing renal and/or hepatic disorders. The clinical significance has yet to be demonstrated.

Miscellaneous: Exacerbation of acute gouty attacks may occur in the early stages of hypouricaemic therapy (see section under dosage and administration). In those conditions where the body's miscible urate pool is greatly increased (e.g. malignant disease and its treatment: Lesch-Nyhan syndrome), the rise in xanthine concentration resulting from the action Allopurinol may lead to tissue deposition of xanthine. Fluid intake should ensure adequate urinary output. Xanthine crystals have been seen in muscle tissue of patients receiving Allopurinol, but this appears to have no clinical significance.

The following complaints have been reported occasionally, but do not appear to have a clear cause and effect relationship with Allopurinol; fever, general malaise, headache, vertigo, somnolence, taste perversion, hepatic necrosis, granulomatous hepatitis, abnormal liver function tests, hyperlipaemia, visual disorder, cataracts, macular changes, neuropathy, impotence, diabetes mellitus, furunculosis, alopecia, hypertension, haematuria, oedema.

Use in pregnancy and lactation: High dose intraperitoneal allopurinol in mice has been associated with foetal abnormalities but extensive animal studies with oral allopurinol have shown none. In human pregnancy there is no evidence that Allopurinol taken orally causes foetal abnormalities; however, as with all drugs, due caution should be exercised in the use of Allopurinol in pregnancy. No data are available on the excretion of allopurinol and its metabolites in human breast milk.

Toxicity and treatment of overdosage: No reports of overdosage or acute intoxication are available. The most likely reaction would be gastro-intestinal intolerance. Massive absorption of Allopurinol may lead to considerable inhibition of Xanthine oxidase activity which should have no untoward effect unless 6-mercaptopurine and/or azathioprine is being taken concomitantly. In this case, the risk of increased activity of these drugs must be recognised. Adequate hydration to maintain optimum diuresis facilitates excretion of alloprinol and its metabolites. Dialysis may be resorted to if considered necessary.

Pharmaceutical precautions Store in a cool dry place.

Legal category POM.

Package quantities *Aluline 100:* containers of 100. *Aluline 300:* containers of 28.

Further information Aluline presents definite advantages over uricosuric agents or simple anti-inflammatory drugs, especially in patients with gouty nephropathy, in those who form renal urate stones and those with unusually severe disease. In most patients with extensive tophaceous deposits, progressive formation of tophi has been halted and draining urate sinuses have healed.

Allopurinol and its major metabolite, oxipurinol, act by inhibiting the enzyme xanthine oxidase which catalyses the end stage of the metabolism of purines to uric acid. Allopurinol and its metabolites are excreted by the kidney but the renal handling is such that allopurinol has a plasma half-life of about one hour whereas that of oxipurinol exceeds 18 hours. Thus therapeutic effect may be achieved by once-a-day dosage.

Product licence numbers
Aluline 100   0401/0060.
Aluline 300   0401/0061.

ALUNEX* TABLETS

Presentation Alunex 4 tablets each contain 4 mg Chlorpheniramine Maleate BP. They are presented as biconvex yellow round tablets, one side bearing the name 'Steinhard' the other scored and bearing the letter 'C' above the score line and the figure '4' below.

Uses The symptomatic control of all allergic conditions which respond to antihistamines including hay fever, urticaria, vasomotor rhinitis, food allergy, drug and serum reactions, pruritus vulvae, pruritus ani, insect bites etc.

Dosage and administration *Adults:* 1 tablet three or four times daily.
Children: (6–12 years)½–1 tablet three or four times daily.

Contra-indications, warnings, etc There are no known definite contra-indications to treatment with Alunex.
Precautions: All antihistamines, given in effective dosage, may cause dizziness or drowsiness. In consequence, until the effect of the treatment is known, patients treated with Alunex should be warned not to take charge of vehicles or machinery. The sedative action of alcohol may be potentiated by antihistamines so that drowsiness can occur in patients not otherwise subject to it if alcohol is taken.
Unnecessary administration of drugs during the first trimester of pregnancy is undesirable.
Side-effects: Drowsiness and dizziness may occur.
Overdosage: The estimated lethal dose of Chlorpheniramine is 25–50 mg per kg body weight. Treatment should include gastric lavage if massive overdosage has been by the oral route. In the event of convulsions sedate with intramuscular paraldehyde. Severe respiratory depression may necessitate mechanical ventilation. Severe hypotension may require fluid replacement.

Pharmaceutical precautions Store in a cool dry place.

Legal category P.

Package quantities Containers of 50, 500 and 1000.

Further information Does not contain tartrazine.

Product licence number 0401/5042.

ALUZINE* TABLETS

Presentation Aluzine 20 tablets each containing 20 mg Frusemide BP. They are presented as flat white round tablets, one side bearing the name 'Steinhard' the other scored and bearing the letter 'F' above the score-mark and '20' below.

Aluzine 40 tablets each containing 40 mg Frusemide BP. They are presented as flat white round tablets, one side bearing the name 'Steinhard' the other scored and bearing the letter 'F' above the score-mark and '40' below.

Uses Diuretic. Oedema of cardiac, hepatic or renal origin. Pulmonary oedema. Toxaemia of pregnancy. Mild or moderate hypertension.

Dosage and administration *Adults:* The usual initial dosage is 40 mg daily, thereafter adjusted to minimum effective dose which may range from 20 mg on alternate days to 120 mg daily.
Children: From 1 to 3 mg/kg body weight.

Contra-indications, warnings, etc Frusemide is contra-indicated in the presence of electrolytic deficiency, hepatic cirrhosis or digitalis intoxication and should be used with great caution in advanced renal failure. Patients with prostatic hypertrophy or impairment of micturition have an increased risk of developing acute retention. Cephaloridine nephrotoxicity may be increased by concomitant administration of potent diuretics such as frusemide.
The dosage of concurrently administered cardiac glycosides or anti-hypertensive agents may require adjustment.
Latent diabetes may become manifest or the insulin requirements of diabetic patients may increase.
Serum acid levels tend to rise during treatment with frusemide and an acute attack of gout may occasionally be precipitated.
Other reported side-effects include nausea, gastric upset and malaise. The incidence of allergic reactions such as skin rashes is very low but when these occur treatment should be withdrawn. Bone marrow depression has been reported as a rare complication and necessitates withdrawal of treatment.
Only when it is essential should frusemide be given in the first trimester of pregnancy or to nursing mothers.
Treatment of overdosage: In cases of overdose there is a danger of dehydration and electrolyte depletion due to excessive diuresis. Treatment should therefore be aimed at fluid replacement and correction of the electrolyte imbalance.

Pharmaceutical precautions Store in a cool dry place protected from light.

Legal category POM.

Package quantities *Aluzine 20:* containers of 250. *Aluzine 40:* containers of 1000.

Further information Nil.

Product licence numbers
Aluzine 20 tablets   0401/0034
Aluzine 40 tablets   0401/0035

ALUZINE* 500 TABLETS

Presentation Aluzine 500 tablets each contain 500 mg Frusemide BP. They are presented as flat yellow round tablets, one side bearing the name 'Steinhard' the other cross-scored bearing the letter 'F' in the top quadrant and '500' in the remaining quadrants.

Uses Diuretic for the management of oliguria due to chronic or acute renal insufficiency with a GFR below 20 ml/minute.

Dosage and administration In patients with chronic renal insufficiency an initial daily dose of 250 mg ($\frac{1}{2}$ tablet) is employed. If a satisfactory diuresis is not produced then the dose may be increased in steps of 250 mg at four to six hourly intervals up to a maximum dose of 2,000 mg (4 tablets) as a single dose.

In cases of acute renal failure which have been initially controlled using Frusemide Injection oral therapy may be substituted for parenteral therapy regarding one 500 mg tablet as approximately equal to 250 mg of injection. Appropriate dosage adjustments may then be made according to the observed clinical response.

Contra-indications, warnings, etc During treatment with high-dosage forms of Frusemide fluid balance should be carefully controlled. In the case of patients with shock, steps should be taken to normalise blood pressure and circulating blood volume before commencing therapy. Regular checks of plasma electrolytes (particularly sodium, potassium, chloride and bicarbonate) should be carried out, and electrolyte replacement therapy instituted if necessary.

High dosage Frusemide is contra-indicated in renal failure as a result of poisoning by nephrotoxic or hepatoxic agents and in renal failure associated with hepatic coma. The dosage of concurrently administered cardiac glycosides or anti-hypertensive agents may require adjustment.

Cephaloridine nephrotoxicity may be increased by concomitant administration of potent diuretics such as Frusemide.

Latent diabetes may become manifest or the insulin requirements of diabetic patients may increase.

The safety of high dosage Frusemide in pregnancy has not been established and should be used with caution, weighing potential benefit to the patient against possible hazard to the foetus.

Aluzine 500 mg tablets are generally well tolerated. Side-effects of a minor nature such as nausea, malaise or gastric upset may occur but are not usually severe enough to cause withdrawal of treatment. The incidence of allergic reactions such as skin rashes is very low but when these occur treatment should be withdrawn. In common with other sulphonamide-based diuretics, hyperuricaemia may occur and, in rare cases, clinical gout can be precipitated. Bone marrow depression has been reported as a rare complication and necessitates withdrawal of treatment.

Treatment of overdosage: Correct dehydration and electrolyte depletion. Reversible deafness may occur.

Pharmaceutical precautions Store in a cool dry place protected from light.

Legal category POM.

Package quantities Containers of 100.

Further information Nil.

Product licence number 0401/0042.

FORTUNAN*

Presentation Fortunan 0.5 each contain 0.5 mg Haloperidol BP. They are presented as small white round tablets, one side bearing the name 'Steinhard' and the other the letter 'H' above the figure '0.5'.

Fortunan 1.5 each contain 1.5 mg Haloperidol BP. They are presented as small white round tablets, one side bearing the name 'Steinhard' and the other scored with the letter 'H' above the score line and the figure '1.5' below.

Fortunan 5 each contain 5 mg Haloperidol BP. They are presented as pale green round tablets, one side bearing the name 'Steinhard' and the other scored with the letter 'H' above the score line and the figure '5' below.

Fortunan 10 each contain 10 mg Haloperidol BP. They are presented as pink round tablets, one side bearing the name 'Steinhard' and the other scored with the letter 'H' above the score line and the figure '10' below.

Fortunan 20 each contain 20 mg Haloperidol BP. They are presented as white round tablets, one side bearing the name 'Steinhard' and the other scored with the letter 'H' above the score line and the figure '20' below.

Uses Fortunan is a potent neuroleptic, used for the rapid control of the symptoms of acute and chronic schizophrenia, mania and hypomania, organic psychoses, acute psychotic agitation, motor inco-ordination, behaviour disorders in children, anxiety neurosis and anxiety associated with depression.

Dosage and administration As with all neuroleptic drugs, the daily dosage of Fortunan should be titrated to the needs of the individual patient. It may be given as a single daily dose or in divided doses.

Adults: Daily dosage may range from 1 mg to as much as 200 mg, and will usually be lower for geriatric or debilitated patients. Usually, treatment may be started with 10–15 mg daily and slowly increased until control is achieved, except in anxiety states where 0.5 mg twice daily will often suffice.

Children: The usual maintenance dosage is 0.05 mg/kg body weight, but in cases of urgency treatment may be initiated at twice this level.

Contra-indications, warnings, etc Haloperidol should be used with care in patients with lesions of the basal ganglia and with patients with arteriosclerosis the possibility of occult lesions of the basal ganglia should be considered.

Haloperidol is only mildly soporific, but will potentiate the action of CNS depressants.

Should dystonic reactions or akathisia occur, they may be controlled with an anti-Parkinsonian drug.

Reports of blood dyscrasias and liver damage have been reported but are extremely rare.

Pharmaceutical precautions Store in a cool dry place.

Legal category POM.

Package quantities 0.5 mg, 1.5 mg, 5 mg and 10 mg tablets available in 50, 250 and 1,000 tablet packs. 20 mg tablets available in 50 and 250 tablet packs.

Further information Nil.

Product licence numbers

0.5 mg	0401/0021
1.5 mg	0401/0022
5 mg	0401/0023
10 mg	0401/0030
20 mg	0401/0031

METOX*

Presentation Metox tablets each contain 10 mg Metoclopramide BP. They are presented as small white round tablets, one side bearing the name 'Steinhard' the other scored and bearing the letter 'M' above the score line and the figure '10' below.

Uses To restore normal co-ordination and tone to the upper digestive tract and to relieve symptoms of gastro-duodenal dysfunction such as heartburn, nausea and vomiting in flatulent dyspepsia, gastritis and duodenitis.

As an anti-emetic for the treatment of nausea and vomiting associated with gastro-intestinal disorders, including peptic ulcers, gastritis and the results of gastrectomy, and migraine. To relieve the nausea and vomiting caused by essential drugs such as digitalis, cytotoxics and antibacterials.

Dosage and administration In normal circumstances, the total daily dose of metoclopramide should not exceed 0.5 mg/kg body weight and should be administered in divided doses. This level should not be exceeded in children and young adults.

Adults: 1 tablet (10 mg) three times daily. Young adults (15–20 years): ½–1 tablet three times daily.

Children: Metox tablets are not recommended for administration to children.

Contra-indications, warnings, etc Should not be administered concomitantly with anticholinergic drugs such as atropine, nor with phenothiazines.

The recommended dose should not be exceeded particularly in patients of low body weight and in young adults.

Although animal tests have not demonstrated any teratogenic effect, the administration of metoclopramide in pregnancy is not recommended.

Side-effects are rare with metoclopramide, but those reported include drowsiness and dystonic reactions, which are reversible and usually disappear within 24 hours of the drug being withdrawn.

Extrapyramidal reactions have been reported, including spasm of facial, extra-ocular or cervical muscles, as has generalised increase of muscle tone. Should any of these not disappear within 24 hours of the drug being withdrawn, treatment with a benzodiazepam or with an anticholinergic anti-Parkinsonian drug may be considered.

Pharmaceutical precautions Store in a cool dark place.

Legal category POM.

Package quantities Containers of 100 and 500 tablets.

Further information Nil.

Product licence number 0401/0062.

NIDAZOL*

Presentation Nidazol tablets each contain 200 mg Metronidazole BP. They are presented as round white tablets, one side bearing the name 'Steinhard' and the other scored with the letter 'M' above the score line and the figure '200' below.

Uses Nidazol is a potent antimicrobial with high activity against anaerobic bacteria and protozoa. It is indicated for the treatment of trichomonal and non-specific vaginitis, urogenital trichomoniasis in both the male and female (sexual partners should be treated concurrently), amoebiasis, giardiasis, acute dental infections (e.g. acute ulcerative gingivitis, acute pericoronitis and acute apical infections) and anaerobically infected leg ulcers and pressure sores. It's activity against colonic anaerobes makes it particularly useful in surgical and gynaecological sepsis.

Dosage and administration Nidazol tablets should be taken after meals.

In anaerobic infections: Adults and children over 10 years old: two tablets three times daily.

Children under 10 years old: 7.5 mg/kg body weight, three times daily.

In non-specific vaginitis: Adults and children over 10 years old: two tablets twice daily for 7 days or ten tablets as a single dose. No relevant dosage for younger children.

In urogenital trichomoniasis: Adults and children over 10 years old: two tablets three times a day for 7 days or four tablets each morning and six tablets each evening for 2 days or ten tablets as a single dose. Sexual partners should be treated concurrently.

Children 7–10 years old: ½ tablet three times daily for seven days.

Children 3–7 years old: ½ tablet twice daily for seven days.

Children 1–3 years old: ¼ tablet three times daily for seven days.

In amoebiasis: Adults and children over 10 years old: 10–12 tablets daily for seven days, or 4 tablets every eight hours for five days. Children 7–10 years old should be given half this adult dose, children 3–7 years old should be given one quarter the adult dose, and children 1–3 years old should be given ½–1 tablet three times daily for seven days.

In guardiasis: Adults and children over 10 years old: 10 tablets in a single daily dose for three days. Children 7–10 years old should be given half this adult dose, children 3–7 years old should be given one quarter the adult dose, and children 1–3 years old should be given 2½ tablets daily for three days.

In acute ulcerative gingivitis and dental infections: Adults and children over 10 years old: 1 tablet three times daily for three to seven days. Children 7–10 years old ½ tablet three times daily for 3 to 7 days; children 3–7 years old ½ tablet twice daily for three days.

For leg ulcers and pressure sores: Adults should be given two tablets three times daily for seven days. There is no relevant dosage for children in this indication.

Contra-indications, warnings, etc Nidazol is contra-indicated where there is a known history of allergy to metronidazole.

In those rare cases where prolonged administration of Nidazol is considered necessary, regular clinical and laboratory surveillance is recommended and clinicians are warned that there is a risk of peripheral neuropathy.

Side-effects reported include, occasionally, an unpleasant taste, nausea, leucopenia, darkening of the urine (by a metronidazole metabolite) dizziness, ataxia, and transient epileptiform seizures and peripheral neuropathy on prolonged and/or intensive dosage.

Nidazol may potentiate the action of anticoagulants. As with all medicines, metronidazole should be used during lactation or pregnancy only when considered essential, and in these circumstances short-term high-dose regimes should be avoided.

Pharmaceutical precautions Store in a cool dry place.

Legal category POM.

Package quantities In packs of 21, 250 and 1,000 tablets.

Further information Nil.

Product licence number 0401/5056.

PAXALGESIC* TABLETS

Presentation Paxalgesic tablets each contain Dextropropoxyphene Hydrochloride BP 32.5 mg and Paracetamol BP 325 mg. They are presented as biconvex white round tablets.

Uses Analgesic. For the relief of mild to moderate pain.

Dosage and administration For oral administration only to adults.

The usual dose is two tablets three or four times daily, and this should not be exceeded in normal circumstances.

In the elderly, treatment should be started with half the normal dose, particularly if renal or hepatic function is impaired.

Contra-indications, warnings, etc

Contra-indication: Hypersensitivity to dextropropoxyphene or to paracetamol.

Warnings: Dextropropoxyphene is a CNS depressant, and should be used with caution in patients taking other CNS depressant drugs; patients should be warned to avoid alcohol.

Care should be taken in prescribing dextropropoxyphene for patients with psychological or personality disorders.

Dextropropoxyphene may impair the mental and physical abilities to a varying degree depending on dosage and individual susceptability, and patients should be warned of the possible dangers in driving or operating machinery.

Overdose of paracetamol can cause hepatic necrosis.

Tolerance: Physical and psychological dependence can occur, but this is not common.

Side-effects: Side-effects such as nausea, vomiting, sedation and dizziness appear to be more common in ambulant patients, and some of these side-effects may be relieved if the patient lies down.

Other side-effects reported include constipation and abdominal pain, skin rashes, headache, weakness, euphoria and lightheadedness, dysphoria, and minor visual phenomenon.

Isolated reports suggest that dextropropoxyphene may inhibit the metabolism of some concurrently administered drugs such as anticonvulsants, anti-depressants and warfarin-like drugs.

Patients receiving these should be monitored during treatment.

Overdosage: The chronic ingestion of dextropropoxyphene in doses exceeding 720 mg (as base) per day has caused toxic psychoses and convulsions.

Symptoms of acute toxicity may be rapid in onset, with the danger of respiratory arrest. Other recognised manifestations include respiratory depression, coma, circulatory collapse, pulmonary oedema, convulsions and cardiac arrhythmias.

Deterioration may be rapid, with fatal outcome.

Treatment of overdosage: The first essential is to re-establish adequate respiratory exchange by provision of an adequate airway and controlled or assisted ventilation.

Naloxone (a narcotic antagonist) is a specific antidote to the respiratory depression produced by dextropropoxyphene. An initial intravenous dose of 0.4–2 mg should be administered with simultaneous efforts at respiratory resuscitation.

If the desired degree of improvement is not obtained, the dose should be repeated at two to three minute intervals. Subsequent doses of naloxone may be necessary for up to 24 hours due to the slow elimination of dextropropoxyphene. Naloxone may be administered by infusion. The rate of infusion should be such as to maximise the reversal of CNS depression. In addition to the use of the narcotic antagonist, the patient may require careful titration with an anticonvulsant to control seizures. Analeptics such as caffeine or amphetamine should not be used because of their tendency to precipitate convulsions.

Early assessment of the severity of paracetamol poisoning by measurement of plasma paracetamol levels is essential if treatment, which should be instituted within 10 hours of ingestion, is to be effective. Present evidence suggests that cysteamine, methionine or N-acetylcysteine given within this period are effective in greatly reducing the toxic effects of paracetamol. Oxygen, intravenous fluids, vasopressors and other supportive measures may be employed as indicated.

Gastric lavage may be helpful. Activated charcoal can absorb a significant amount of ingested dextropropoxyphene.

Pharmaceutical precautions Store in a cool dry place.

Legal category CD (Sch 5), POM.

Package quantities Cartons containing 100 tablets in blister packs (10 strips of 10 tablets).

Further information Paxalgesic tablets have the same formula as Co-proxamol tablets.

Product licence number 5783/0011.

PAXOFEN* TABLETS

Presentation Paxofen 200 each contains 200 mg Ibuprofen BP, Paxofen 400 each contains 400 mg Ibuprofen BP and Paxofen 600 each contains 600 mg Ibuprofen BP.

All are presented as pink coated, biconvex tablets.

Uses Paxofen is a non-steroid anti-inflammatory analgesic antipyretic, indicated in the treatment of pain and mild inflammation in rheumatic disease (including juvenile rheumatoid arthritis i.e. Still's disease) and other musculoskeletal disorders such as ankylosing spondylitis, osteoarthritis and other seronegative arthropathies. Paxofen is also valuable in the treatment of frozen shoulder, bursitis, tendinitis, tenosynovitis, low back pain and in other non-articular rheumatic conditions in sprains. Paxofen is useful both for the short-term treatment of mild to moderate pain (including transient musculoskeletal pain) and for the treatment of patients with chronic disease which is accompanied by pain and inflammation. Because of its ability to inhibit prostaglandin synthetase, Paxofen is particularly suitable for the relief of pain in dysmenorrhoea.

Dosage and administration

Adults: 600 mg to 1200 mg daily in divided doses; in

severe or acute conditions up to 2400 mg daily in divided doses may be used but should not be exceeded.

Children: 20 mg/kg daily, children under 30 kg never more than 500 mg in 24 hours.

Contra-indications, warnings, etc Ibuprofen should not be given to patients with active peptic ulceration or with a history of severe or active peptic ulceration, and should be prescribed with caution for patients with asthma. Great care must be exercised in prescribing for patients with a history of bronchospasm after other NSAI agents.

No teratogenic effects have been reported from animal studies, but – as with other drugs – the use of Ibuprofen during pregnancy should be avoided whenever possible.

As with other non-steroid anti-inflammatory agents, the adverse effects reported include skin rashes, gastric intolerance and bleeding, and dyspepsia; rarely, thrombocytopenia has been reported. Very rarely toxic amblyopia has been reported but recovered on withdrawal of the drug.

Overdosage: There is no specific antidote, and treatment consists of gastric lavage, attention to plasma electrolytes and symptomatic treatment.

Pharmaceutical precautions Store in a cool dry place protected from light.

Legal category POM.

Package quantities Paxofen 200 – containers of 500
Paxofen 400 – containers of 250
Paxofen 600 – containers of 100

Product licence numbers Paxofen 200   5783/001
Paxofen 400   5783/0002
Paxofen 600   5783/0003

PAXOLAX* TABLETS

Presentation Paxolax tablets each contain 5 mg bisacodyl. They are presented as yellow, sugar-enteric coated tablets.

Uses As a contact laxative for the relief of constipation and for bowel preparation before surgery, labour or radiology.

Dosage and administration
Constipation in adults and in children over 10 years old: Two tablets by mouth at night. In some rare cases, a higher dosage – up to three or four tablets at night – may be necessary.

Constipation in children under 10 years old: One tablet at night.

Pre-radiological preparation in adults and children over 10 years old: Two tablets on each of the two nights before investigation. *Children under 10 years old* should be given half this adult dose.

Warning: Because Paxolax tablets are enteric coated (so that they do not disintegrate until they reach the intestine) they should not be chewed or crushed.

Contra-indications, warnings, etc
Contra-indications: When *any* laxative is contra-indicated, e.g. suspected intestinal obstruction.

There have been no reports of teratogenic effects from bisacodyl in humans or in animal studies. However, administration of any medicines during the first trimester should be avoided unless the benefit to the mother outweighs the risk to the foetus.

Side-effects: As with all contact laxatives, griping has occasionally been reported.

Overdose: Lower abdominal colicky pain and signs of dehydration are common in overdosage with bisacodyl, particularly in the young or elderly patient. *Treatment* is by gastric lavage (where appropriate) and maintenance of adequate hydration. A watch should be kept on serum potassium. Symptomatic treatment e.g. antispasmodics may be of help.

Pharmaceutical precautions Store in a cool dry place, protected from light.

Legal category P.

Package quantities Containers of 500 and 1,000.

Further information Nil.

Product licence number 5783/0015.

*Trade Mark

Sterling Health
Sterling-Winthrop House
Onslow Street
Guildford
Surrey GU1 4YS

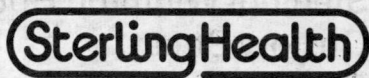

DROXALIN*

Presentation Flat, round, white, uncoated tablets with bevelled edges, 16 mm in diameter, marked 'Droxalin' on both faces, containing:

Alexitol Sodium	200 mg
Magnesium Trisilicate BP	162 mg

Uses Droxalin is an antacid. It is recommended for the relief of gastric hyperacidity, dyspepsia, and symptoms of peptic ulcer.

Dosage and administration For oral administration only.

Adults: For hyperacidity: 1 or 2 tablets as required.

Peptic ulcer: 2 or more tablets, chewed every two or four hours, or when required for relief of symptoms.

Contra-indications, warnings, etc There are no known contra-indications or adverse reactions, and no cases of overdosage have been reported.

As the ingredients of Droxalin are not significantly absorbed, systemic effects such as alkalosis due to changes in acid-base metabolism are not encountered.

The combination of aluminium and magnesium salts minimises constipating and laxative side-effects, which are rare and mild.

Pharmaceutical precautions None applicable.

Legal category GSL.

Package quantities Droxalin Tablets are available in packs of 30 and 180.

Further information The aluminium complex is rapidly activated by chewing to form a colloidal aluminium hydroxide gel, giving rapid relief of gastric hyperacidity and buffering gastric pH at an ideal non-alkaline level for long periods.

Each Droxalin tablet contains 7 to 9 mg sodium.

Product licence number 0071/5009.

*Trade Mark

Sterling Research Laboratories
Sterling-Winthrop House
Onslow Street
Guildford
Surrey GU1 4YS

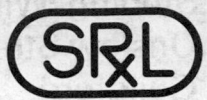

ACIDOL* PEPSIN

Presentation Near-white, bi-convex tablets, 11 mm in diameter, plain on both sides with a characteristic odour. Each tablet contains 97 mg pepsin and 388 mg betaine hydrochloride.

Uses Acidol-Pepsin Tablets provide a source of hydrochloric acid and pepsin for patients with achlorhydria.

Dosage and administration For oral administration only.

The usual adult dose is 1–3 tablets crushed and dissolved in a tumbler of water three times a day, preferably after meals.

Contra-indications, warnings, etc There are no known contra-indications or side-effects.

If Acidol-Pepsin Tablets are swallowed whole they are likely to cause irritation and symptoms of indigestion: they should therefore always be taken dissolved in water.

Because hydrochloric acid can dissolve dental enamel, the solution is best taken through a straw or a glass tube to protect the teeth.

Overdosage has not been reported. Although the ingestion of large amounts of hydrochloric acid may raise the chloride and lower the bicarbonate content of the blood it is most unlikely that metabolic acidosis would occur as a result of taking Acidol-Pepsin.

Pharmaceutical precautions Store in well-closed containers. Protect from damp.

Legal category P.

Package quantities Acidol-Pepsin is supplied in bottles of 50 tablets.

Further information In solution, betaine hydrochloride forms free hydrochloric acid. Each Acidol-Pepsin Tablet is approximately equivalent to 1 ml of Dilute Hydrochloric Acid BP.

Product licence number 0071/5017.

AT10*

Presentation A clear, deep straw-coloured, oily solution with a faint nut-like odour containing 0.25 mg/ml Dihydrotachysterol BP.

Uses AT10 is recommended for use in the acute, chronic and latent forms of hypocalcaemic tetany due to hypoparathyroidism where its action is to increase the rate of absorption and utilisation of calcium. It may also be used to treat those skin lesions such as pemphigus and impetigo herpetiformis which are associated with hypoparathyroidism.

Dosage and administration AT10 is for oral administration only.

Adults: In acute cases 3–10 ml may be given on each of the first three days of treatment, followed two to three days later by blood and urinary calcium estimations. The maintenance dose of AT10 is usually within the range of 1–7 ml each week, but the precise amount depends on the results of serum and urinary calcium determinations.

In chronic cases an initial dose of 2 ml of AT10 daily, or on alternate days, may be sufficient to maintain normocalcaemia in moderate cases. The dose of AT10 usually has to be increased during menstruation, pregnancy and periods of unusual activity.

Contra-indications, warnings, etc As with calciferol, uncontrolled, prolonged administration of AT10 can result in hypercalcaemia which may lead to nephrocalcinosis. Therefore accurate blood calcium determinations must be made at the beginning of treatment and then periodically until the required maintenance dose has been established. The serum calcium level should subsequently be kept between 2.25–2.5 mmol/litre.

If nausea and vomiting are present, serum calcium level should be checked.

The Sulkowitch test (for urinary calcium) is a convenient supplement to blood calcium determinations, but it should not be regarded as a substitute, because in hypoparathyroid patients treated with AT10 hypercalcuria can occur in the presence of hypocalcaemia.

Dihydrotachysterol is excreted in breast milk and may cause hypercalcaemia in the suckling infant.

Overdosage will result in hypercalcaemia. The symptoms (described below) usually respond to withdrawal of medication, bed rest, a liberal fluid intake, laxatives and a light diet.

Side-effects are most likely to be due to hypercalcaemia, the first signs of which are loss of appetite, listlessness and nausea. More severe manifestations include thirst, vertigo, urgency of micturition, stupor, headache, abdominal cramps and paralysis.

Pharmaceutical precautions Store in well-closed containers protected from heat and light.

Legal category P.

Package quantities AT10 is supplied in bottles containing 15 ml with a 1 ml dropper.

Further information The hypercalcaemic action of AT10 is slower in onset and more prolonged than that of parathyroid hormone, but faster in onset and less persistent in action than calciferol. In patients who have become resistant to large doses of calciferol it may be possible to control blood calcium levels with AT10.

Product licence number 0071/5020.

BENORAL*

Presentation 1. Benoral Suspension is a white suspension, 10 ml of which contains 4 g Benorylate BP.

2. Benoral Granules: sachets filled with a white, free-flowing powder which disperses readily in water. The contents of each sachet are equivalent to 2 g Benorylate BP.

3. Benoral Tablets are white, capsule-shaped tablets marked 'Benoral' on one side only, each containing 750 mg Benorylate BP.

Uses Benoral is an anti-inflammatory analgesic and antipyretic, which, after absorption, is metabolised into salicylate and paracetamol. Benoral is recommended for the treatment of rheumatoid arthritis, osteoarthritis and other painful or inflammatory musculo-skeletal conditions. It may also be used to relieve mild to moderate pain of non-rheumatic origin such as dysmenorrhoea and as an antipyretic in febrile conditions.

Dosage and administration Benoral is for oral administration only and is presented as suspension, tablet and granule dose forms.

Benoral suspension may be administered undiluted at the prescribed dose or taken in hot or cold beverages and drunk immediately.

Adults

	Suspension	Granules
Active rheumatoid arthritis	10 ml twice daily	2 sachets twice daily
Osteoarthritis Quiescent RA Soft tissue rheumatism	5 ml twice daily increasing to 10 ml depending on severity and response	1–2 sachets twice daily depending on severity and response

Tablets: Adults: Two 750 mg tablets (1.5 g benorylate) three times a day is usually adequate to relieve pain and stiffness in osteoarthritis, quiescent rheumatoid arthritis, soft tissue rheumatism and non-rheumatic pain.

Elderly: In elderly patients, especially those with impaired renal function, symptoms of salicylism may arise at dosages not normally associated with this effect. In elderly patients it is recommended that the adult dose of Benoral be reduced. For example, dose reduction of Benoral Suspension to a 5 ml (2 g benorylate) morning dose with 10 ml (4 g benorylate) at bedtime may be instituted. Further reduction to 5 ml (2 g benorylate) twice daily may be necessary in some cases.

Children: Benoral should not be given to children under the age of 3 months. Above this age the dosage requirements for children necessitate the use of a dilution of Benoral Suspension (using Syrup BP) according to the following schedule:

7–12 years: 500 mg not more than 4 times daily.
3–6 years: 500 mg not more than 3 times daily.
1–2 years: 250 mg not more than 4 times daily.
3–12 months: 25 mg/kg body weight not more than 4 times daily.

In children with Still's disease an initial dose of 200 mg/kg body weight daily has been used. Thereafter, the dose is adjusted on the basis of periodic determination

of blood salicylate and paracetamol, to maintain blood salicylate at an anti-inflammatory level (about 25 mg/100 ml).

Contra-indications, warnings, etc Benoral should not be given to patients with active peptic ulcer, or to those known to be hypersensitive to aspirin (including those with haemophilia and similar coagulation disorders).

Precautions: Patients who are taking anticoagulants should have their prothrombin time checked.

Patients taking Benoral should be advised against taking analgesics containing aspirin or paracetamol. The safety of benorylate has not been established in pregnancy, but there is clinical and epidemiological evidence that salicylate and paracetamol (which occur as metabolic products of benorylate) are safe in human pregnancy.

Overdosage: Symptoms are likely to resemble those caused by salicylate overdosage. Treatment should be based on the levels of salicylate and paracetamol found in the blood.

Side-effects: Overall tolerance is excellent. Adverse effects may include gastric intolerance (nausea, constipation or diarrhoea, indigestion or heartburn) and drowsiness and rashes have also been reported. The possibility that gastro-intestinal haemorrhage may be induced by Benoral cannot be excluded. The high salicylate levels obtained with Benoral may give rise to dizziness, tinnitus and deafness. If this happens, the dose should be reduced.

Pharmaceutical precautions No special storage requirements.

Legal category P.

Package quantities Benoral Suspension – bottles of 150 or 300 ml. Benoral Granules – cartons of 60 sachets. Benoral Tablets – bottles of 100 or 500.

Further information Benorylate is a prodrug which is metabolised to salicylate and paracetamol by esterases after absorption. Analgesic and anti-inflammatory properties are comparable to those of other antiarthritis compounds. Its antipyretic effect is similar to that of aspirin or paracetamol but more prolonged than either. Gastro-intestinal tolerance is superior to that of comparable doses of aspirin or mixtures of aspirin and paracetamol. In chemical terms, 2 g benorylate is equivalent to 1.2 g aspirin and 0.98 g paracetamol.

Carbohydrate content: Benoral Suspension contains sorbitol and each sachet of granules contains 548 mg sucrose.

Product licence numbers
Benoral Suspension 0071/5022
Benoral Granules 0071/0149
Benoral Tablets 0071/5901

BREOPRIN*

Presentation White tablets 16 mm long and 7.5 mm wide, marked ⊂⊃ on one side and scored on the other. Each tablet contains 648 mg micro-encapsulated aspirin.

Uses Breoprin Tablets may be used where aspirin is required and therefore are recommended for the relief of pain and stiffness associated with rheumatoid and osteoarthritis, rheumatism, bursitis, sprains, strains and neuralgia.

Breoprin is also recommended for the relief of symptoms of colds and influenza and in other minor painful conditions such as headache, toothache and dysmenorrhoea.

Dosage and administration *Adults:* Breoprin Tablets should be taken at approximately eight-hourly intervals, for example at 7.00 a.m., 1.00 p.m. and 9.00 p.m. Where large doses of aspirin are usually required as in acute rheumatoid conditions, each dose should consist of 2 tablets. In other cases the dose should be 1 tablet, although patients who experience pain or stiffness in the morning on rising may increase the last dose of the day to 2 tablets. No more than 6 tablets should be taken in 24 hours.

Children: Breoprin should not be given to children below the age of 14 years.

Contra-indications, warnings, etc
Contra-indications: Breoprin should not be given to patients with active peptic ulceration because aspirin may induce (occasionally major) gastro-intestinal haemorrhage. It should also be withheld from those known to be sensitive to aspirin, including those with haemophilia and similar coagulation disorders.

Precautions: There is clinical and epidemiological evidence for the safety of aspirin in human pregnancy. However, its use should be avoided at term because aspirin may prolong labour and contribute to maternal and neonatal bleeding.

Aspirin may enhance the effects of anticoagulants and inhibit the action of uricosuric agents. Because aspirin may precipitate bronchospasm, it can induce attacks of asthma in susceptible subjects.

Overdosage: Aspirin overdosage may be treated by gastric lavage with 0.5% sodium bicarbonate solution. If the condition is not serious, sodium bicarbonate and fluids by mouth will speed renal excretion of salicylate. In more serious cases, an intravenous infusion of 5% dextrose should be set up, supplemented by electrolytes and alkali as indicated by blood and urine analysis. Dialysis may be necessary. Haemorrhage may require blood transfusions. The administration of vitamin K, either orally or parenterally, will restore prothrombin time to normal.

Side-effects: The main side-effects associated with aspirin therapy are dyspepsia and other signs of gastric irritation. They are likely to occur less frequently with Breoprin than with ordinary aspirin tablets because the micro-encapsulation causes the major part of the aspirin to be released in the small intestine. If tinnitus occurs, the dose should be reduced.

Pharmaceutical precautions Protect from moisture in well-closed containers.

Legal category P.

Package quantities Bottles of 100 tablets.

Further information Nil.

Product licence number 0071/0091.

BRONCHILATOR*

Presentation Bronchilator is an aerosol inhalant in the form of an oral nebuliser, delivering 250 metered doses by finger depression of an actuator. Each metered dose contains 350 mcg isoetharine mesylate and 70 mcg Phenylephrine Hydrochloride BP.

Uses Bronchilator provides effective and relatively long-lasting relief of bronchospasm in bronchial asthma and chronic bronchitis.

Dosage and administration Bronchilator is for oral inhalation only.

Adults: The usual dose is 1 or 2 inhalations and it is not normally necessary to repeat this dose at less than half-hourly intervals. In bronchial asthma 1 or 2 inhalations more may be required, but it is important to wait one full minute after the initial 1 or 2 inhalations, to be certain that relief has not been obtained. Not more than eight treatments should be taken in 24 hours.

Children: Bronchilator should only be administered to children under the supervision of a responsible adult and strictly as recommended by the doctor.

Contra-indications, warnings, etc Bronchilator should not be given to patients taking MAO inhibitors.

As with other sympathomimetic amines, too frequent use of Bronchilator may cause tachycardia, palpitations, nausea, headache, changes in blood pressure, etc. Patients should therefore be advised not to exceed the recommended dose. Other sympathomimetic amines should be prescribed with caution in patients using Bronchilator. Dosage should be carefully adjusted in patients with hyperthyroidism, hypertension, coronary artery disease, cardiac asthma, limited cardiac reserve and in individuals sensitive to sympathomimetic amines.

Overdosage: Serious symptoms are unlikely except after massive overdosage. They may be treated in the same way as those due to adrenaline overdosage (i.e. injection of piperoxan or phentolamine). Slow intravenous procaine or procainamide should be used for fibrillation, and artificial respiration and oxygen for cyanosis and respiratory embarrassment.

Side-effects: When used as recommended, side-effects are rare. A small drop in pulse rate and blood pressure may follow inhalation of Bronchilator.

Pharmaceutical precautions Keep away from extreme heat.

Legal category POM.

Package quantities Complete nebuliser containing 12.5 ml of solution (equivalent to 250 doses).

Further information Nil.

Product licence number 0071/0196.

ERADACIN* ▼

Presentation Eradacin capsules are No. 1 opaque, red/yellow capsules filled with a white powder. Each capsule contains 150 mg acrosoxacin (rosoxacin I.N.N.)

Uses Eradacin is for the treatment of acute gonorrhoea in both male and female patients.

Dosage and administration Eradacin is for oral administration only.

Adults: Two capsules (300 mg) preferably on an empty stomach.

Children: No recommendations.

Contra-indications, warnings, etc Safe use during

human pregnancy has not yet been established and Eradacin should be used only when necessitated by the anticipated bacteriological and clinical benefits.

It should be used with caution in patients with impaired renal or hepatic function.

Eradacin may cause dizziness and drowsiness. Patients should therefore be warned not to drive or operate machinery if affected. Occasionally, headaches and gastro-intestinal upsets may occur.

Eradacin has been shown to induce lesions in weight-bearing joints of young animals receiving high, single or repeated doses. The relevance of this to man is unknown but it is recommended that frequent, repeat doses should not be given to those under 18 years of age.

Overdosage: Animal toxicity studies suggest that CNS depression is a likely symptom of overdosage. If vomiting does not occur, the drug should be removed by emesis or gastric lavage, if ingestion is recent, and symptomatic treatment applied.

Pharmaceutical precautions None.

Legal category POM.

Package quantities Eradacin is supplied in packs of 20 capsules.

Further information A single dose of 300 mg Eradacin has been shown to produce a cure rate of over 90% in cases of uncomplicated gonococcal urethritis. Treatment with Eradacin may be successful in patients infected with *N. gonorrhoeae* strains resistant to penicillin and other antibiotics.

Product licence number 0071/0168.

FORTAGESIC*

Presentation White tablets 12.7 mm diameter, marked with an ankh on one side and Fortagesic on the other. Each tablet contains Pentazocine BP 15 mg (as the hydrochloride) and Paracetamol PhEur 500 mg.

Uses Fortagesic is a compound analgesic for the relief of moderate pain associated with musculoskeletal disorders or injuries, such as bursitis, sprains, strains, fibrositis, sciatica and osteoarthritis, and for rheumatoid arthritis in patients sensitive to aspirin.

Dosage and administration Fortagesic is for oral administration only.
Adults: 2 tablets up to four times daily. *Children:* 7–12 years: 1 tablet not more frequently than every four hours. Not more than 4 doses to be taken in any 24-hour period. Not recommended for children under 7 years of age.

Contra-indications, warnings, etc There is epidemiological evidence for the safety of paracetamol in human pregnancy. No such evidence exists for pentazocine but it has been widely used for many years without apparent ill consequences. However, doses in rodents that cause maternal toxicity have produced harmful effects in the foetus.

Fortagesic should not be administered to patients with established respiratory depression, raised intracranial pressure, head injuries or pathological brain conditions where clouding of the sensorium is undesirable.

Because pentazocine is a narcotic antagonist, Fortagesic may provoke withdrawal symptoms if given to narcotic addicts and it should be given with caution to patients who have recently been treated with large doses of narcotics.

Fortagesic may produce sedation so ambulant patients should be warned not to operate machinery or drive if affected: alcohol may reinforce the sedative effect. When it is prescribed for chronic use, the physician should take precautions to avoid unnecessary increase in dose of Fortagesic by the patient. Fortagesic should be used with caution in patients who are receiving monoamine oxidase inhibitors, and in those with severe renal, hepatic or respiratory impairment.

Overdosage: In the absence of any experience of overdosage with Fortagesic it is reasonable to assume that signs and symptoms would resemble those which may occur after excessive amounts of the individual ingredients.

Means of maintaining proper oxygenation should be available and naloxone should be used to reverse any CNS depression.

Patients who have taken any overdose of paracetamol may appear well for the first three days, then succumb with liver damage. The hepatic changes produced by overdosage of paracetamol result from the accumulation of a highly active intermediate metabolite in the hepatocytes. N-acetylcysteine intravenously or 1-methionine orally protects the liver if administered within 10–12 hours of ingesting an overdose.

Side-effects: In therapeutic doses, side-effects are more likely to be due to pentazocine than to paracetamol, for adverse reactions to this latter compound are uncommon and it is without any irritant effect on the gastro-intestinal tract. The reactions to the oral administration of pentazocine which have sometimes occurred include dizziness, nausea, vomiting, headache and sedation. These effects have been self-limiting and tend to decrease after the first few doses. Less frequent reactions have included sweating, psychotomimetic effects (hallucinations, dysphoria etc) and flushing.

Dependence liability: Abrupt discontinuation of pentazocine in patients receiving large doses over a prolonged period has occasionally resulted in mild withdrawal symptoms. There have also been rare reports of a similar effect in the new-born after prolonged maternal use of pentazocine during pregnancy. This abstinence syndrome of pentazocine is not typical of opiate dependence. Symptoms include mild abdominal cramps, nausea, vomiting, nervousness or restlessness, dizziness, fever and chills, but are mild compared with opiate withdrawal symptoms. Withdrawal of pentazocine from such patients has raised few problems, only sometimes requiring treatment with tranquillisers. It should be emphasised that the majority of patients reported to have become dependent on pentazocine had previously been dependent on opiates or had misused other drugs.

Pharmaceutical precautions Nil.

Legal category CD (Sch 3), POM.

Package quantities Fortagesic is supplied in bottles of 100 and 500 tablets.

Further information Fortagesic is a logical combination of two analgesics, one (paracetamol) acting peripherally, the other (pentazocine) exerting a central action. They are presented in a ratio which has been found effective for the relief of moderate pain.

Product licence number 0071/0022.

FORTRAL*

Presentation 1. A sterile, isotonic aqueous solution for intramuscular, intravenous or subcutaneous injection containing Pentazocine BP 30 mg/ml as the lactate in 1 ml or 2 ml ampoules.

2. No. 4 hard gelatine, grey/yellow capsules marked fortral 50. Each capsule contains Pentazocine Hydrochloride BP 50 mg (equivalent to 44.3 mg base).

3. White, torpedo-shaped suppositories, average weight 1.86 g, for rectal administration. Each suppository contains Pentazocine BP 50 mg as the lactate.

4. White, bi-convex film-coated tablets, 9.5 mm diameter, marked Fortral on one face and with an ankh on the other. Each tablet contains Pentazocine Hydrochloride BP 25 mg (equivalent to 22.15 mg base).

Uses Fortral is a strong analgesic for the relief of moderate to severe pain.

Dosage and administration 1. *Fortral Ampoules: Adults:* Fortral injections may be administered subcutaneously, intramuscularly or intravenously. For severe pain, 45-60 mg. For moderate pain, 30 mg. The dose should be adjusted according to response and repeated as necessary every three to four hours.

A dose should not normally exceed 1 mg/kg body weight subcutaneously or intramuscularly or 500 mcg/kg intravenously.

Children: In the case of patients between the ages of 1 year and 12 years, the maximum single dose of parenteral Fortral should be calculated on the basis of 1 mg/kg body weight by subcutaneous or intramuscular injection or 500 mcg/kg body weight intravenously. There are no dosage recommendations for children less than one year old.

The elderly: Since impaired renal or hepatic function is often associated with ageing, elderly patients may require smaller doses of Fortral.

As with most parenteral drugs, when frequent daily injections are needed over long periods, intramuscular administration is preferable to subcutaneous. It is recommended that intramuscular sites of injection be rotated, e.g. deltoid areas, upper outer quadrants of the buttocks and mid-lateral aspects of the thighs.

2. *Fortral Capsules: Adults:* The usual recommended dosage is one to two 50 mg capsules every three to four hours after meals according to the response of the patient. Dosage is best tailored to the individual patient and to the degree of pain.

Children: For children under 12 years of age, it is recommended that other dosage forms of Fortral, tablets or injection, be used as appropriate.

3. *Fortral Suppositories: Adults:* 1 suppository at any one time. It will not normally be necessary to exceed 4 suppositories daily.

Children: Fortral Suppositories are not suitable for administration to children under 12 years of age.

4. *Fortral Tablets: Adults:* The usual starting dose is two 25 mg tablets every four hours after meals, but dosage is best tailored to the individual patient and to the degree of pain within the range of 25-100 mg every three to four hours.

Children: 6-12 years: One 25 mg tablet every three to four hours as required.

1-6 years: The recommended dosage is such that Fortral injection is considered to be a more convenient dosage form.

Contra-indications, warnings, etc There is no epidemiological evidence for the safety of pentazocine in human pregnancy but it has been widely used for many years without apparent ill consequences. However, doses in rodents that cause maternal toxicity have produced harmful effects in the foetus.

Fortral should not be administered to patients with established respiratory depression, raised intracranial pressure, head injuries or pathological brain conditions, where clouding of the sensorium is undesirable.

Because pentazocine is a narcotic antagonist, it may provoke withdrawal symptoms if given to narcotic addicts.

Fortral should be given with caution to patients with severely impaired renal or hepatic function and to those previously on large doses of narcotics. Fortral may produce sedation, so ambulant patients should be warned not to operate machinery or drive if affected; alcohol may reinforce the sedative effect.

When Fortral is prescribed for chronic use, the physician should take precautions to avoid any unnecessary increase in dose by the patient. Until further information is available Fortral, like most other strong analgesics, should be used with caution in patients who are receiving monoamine oxidase inhibitors.

If used in myocardial infarction, a small intravenous dose of pentazocine is preferable, as a larger (i.e. 60 mg) dose may cause a rise in pulmonary artery pressure.

Overdosage: Means of maintaining proper oxygenation should be available, and naloxone should be used to reverse any CNS depression.

Side-effects: No serious toxic reactions have been observed where Fortral has been given in normal therapeutic doses and side-effects are generally of a minor nature. Sedation, the most common effect, is less than that associated with morphine. Nausea, vertigo, vomiting, diaphoresis, skin flushes and visual disturbances have also been reported. Respiratory depression, though not normally of clinical significance, can occur.

The psychotomimetic effects (hallucinations, dysphoria etc.) observed with nalorphine and other narcotic antagonists occur sometimes with Fortral. Local tissue damage at injection sites has been reported, particularly after subcutaneous administration.

Dependence liability: Abrupt discontinuation of Fortral in patients receiving large parenteral doses over a prolonged period has occasionally resulted in mild withdrawal symptoms. There have also been rare reports of a similar effect in the new-born after prolonged maternal use of Fortral during pregnancy. This abstinence syndrome of Fortral is not typical of opiate dependence. Symptoms include mild abdominal cramps, nausea, vomiting, nervousness or restlessness, dizziness, fever and chills, but are mild compared with opiate withdrawal symptoms. Withdrawal of Fortral from such patients has raised few problems, only sometimes requiring treatment with tranquillisers. It should be emphasised that the majority of patients reported to have become dependent on Fortral had previously been dependent on opiates or had misused other drugs.

Pharmaceutical precautions Fortral injection appears to be compatible for up to seven days with most commonly used infusion solutions. The exceptions are those which contain sodium bicarbonate, where the high pH causes immediate precipitation of pentazocine base.

Fortral is chemically compatible with atropine sulphate, hyoscine hydrobromide and promethazine hydrochloride. Precipitation will occur if Fortral injection is mixed in the same syringe with soluble barbiturates, diazepam or with chlordiazepoxide.

Fortral Suppositories should be stored in a cool place and the ampoules should be protected from light.

Legal category CD (Sch 3), POM.

Package quantities
1. Ampoules in boxes of ten 1 ml or 2 ml.
2. Capsules in bottles of 100 or 500.
3. Suppositories in cellulose acetate strips. Boxes of 20.
4. Tablets in bottles of 100 or 500.

Further information Fortral is a strong analgesic with weak narcotic antagonist properties. In action it is comparable to morphine and other narcotics.

Product licence numbers

Fortral Ampoules	0071/5033
Fortral Capsules	0071/5034
Fortral Suppositories	0071/0064
Fortral Tablets	0071/5035

HYPAQUE* 25% AND 45% HYPAQUE* SODIUM

Presentation Hypaque is a sterile, almost colourless aqueous solution in clear glass ampoules or infusion bottles containing either 25% w/v or 45% w/v Sodium Diatrizoate BP.

Hypaque Sodium is a white, odourless powder with a saline taste consisting of Sodium Diatrizoate BP. The anhydrous material contains 59.87% of iodine.

Uses An X-ray contrast medium suitable for intravenous and retrograde urography, angiography, venography and many other specialised procedures. It may also be used orally or rectally to examine the gastro-intestinal tract.

Dosage and administration The volume and concentration of Hypaque solution used depends on the procedure being carried out. The strengths and quantities given in the table opposite are suggested.

Examination of the gastro-intestinal tract: For adults an average dose of from 100 to 150 ml of a 25–50% solution is suggested when given by mouth or tube. From 500 ml to 1,000 ml of 20–35% solution is suggested as an enema.

For infants or children the oral or tube dose may vary from 50 ml to 120 ml of a 10–25% solution, and as an enema from 100 ml to 500 ml of a 10–15% solution may be used. The following formulae may be used to make a flavoured draught from Hypaque Sodium.

	1	2	3
Hypaque Sodium	30 g*	30 g*	30 g*
Sucrose	26.41 g	—	—
Methyl p-hydroxybenzoate	0.1 g	0.08 g	0.08 g
Propyl p-hydroxybenzoate	0.01 g	—	—
Butyl p-hydroxybenzoate	0.004 g	—	—
Sodium saccharin	0.03 g	0.3 g	0.3 g
Tween 80	0.08 g	—	0.08 g
Vanillin	—	0.2 g	0.2 g
Purified water q.s. ad	75 ml	75 ml	75 ml

* Or an appropriate amount for the strength of solution required.

Contra-indications, warnings, etc Hypaque should not be used for myelography. Injection of even a small amount into the subarachnoid space may produce convulsions and result in fatality. In patients with subarachnoid haemorrhage, a rare association between contrast administration and clinical deterioration, including convulsions and death, has been reported. Therefore, administration of intravascular iodated ionic contrast media to these patients should be undertaken with caution.

It was formerly believed that the use of contrast media was contra-indicated in patients with advanced renal destruction associated with severe uraemia, and in those with severe hepatic and cardiac disorders. However, one review concludes that although there appear to be no definite contra-indications, potentially hazardous situations requiring particular care are oliguric renal failure, myeloma and combined renal and hepatic failure.

Examination	Strength (%)	Amount of medium used (ml)	
		Adults	Children
Urography:			
i.v.	45	0.5–2.0/kg	as adult
infusion	25	4 ml/kg	as adult
retrograde	25–45	5–20	as adult
Cystography	10–45	500–1500	100–300
Peripheral arteriography	45	20–40	10–20
Haemorrhoidal Portal Venography	45	30–40	15–20
Renal cyst puncture	25–45	5–60	5–20
Orbital phlebography	45	2–4	1–2
Intraosseous venography	45	20–45	—
Choledochography:			
percutaneous transhepatic	25–45	15	5
operative	25–45	5–20	5
post-op. 'T' tube	25–45	5–20	5
Hysterosalpingography	45	10	—
Arthrography	25–45	5–20	3–10
Sinography	45	20–40	—
Tube screening (gastric)	25	5–20	—
Gastro-intestinal (acute abdomen)	see above	see above	see above
Abdominal stab wounds	25	q.s.	q.s.
Dacryocystography	45	1–3	—
Vesiculography	45	1.5–2.0 to a total of 10–12 each side	—
Myography	45	3	—
Duct mammography	25	1–2	—
Discography	45	0.5 max. 2.0	—

No attempt should be made to dehydrate the uraemic patient, nor should dehydration be carried out in a patient with myeloma. Recent evidence suggests that in the latter case it is dehydration rather than the presence of myeloma protein which has been the cause of adverse effects. Prior purgation should also be avoided. X-ray examinations should be avoided during pregnancy. Because the safety of Hypaque, like some other iodine-containing contrast media, has not been established in pregnancy, examinations involving its use should be delayed until 12–16 weeks after delivery whenever possible.

Should urine be tested for albumin within four to six hours after a Hypaque injection, crystals of diatrizoic acid may separate out on acidification with mineral acid, but these crystals are easily distinguished from the amorphous albumin precipitate. Hypaque does not affect the acetic acid or heat coagulation tests.

Organic iodine contrast media are known to remain in the blood serum of patients for periods varying from two days to several years in concentrations sufficient to interfere with tests of thyroid function such as protein-bound iodine determinations. It has been reported that sodium diatrizoate remains in the serum for four days. It is therefore advisable to perform such thyroid function tests before any examination involving the use of Hypaque.

Patients with a history of allergy, especially to iodine, and those with active tuberculosis require careful consideration. Because of the possibility of inducing a temporary suppression of urine, it is wise to allow an interval of at least 24 hours before repeating excretory or retrograde pyelography in patients with unilateral reduction of normal renal function.

The precise nature of the reactions which occur with contrast media are not fully understood, although some seem to be allergic, and major reactions resemble those due to histamine release. Most minor reactions such as arm pain, giddiness, a feeling of warmth, coughing, nausea and vomiting pass off quickly. Minor allergic disturbances such as sneezing, rhinorrhoea, lacrimation and pruritus or urticarial rashes are relatively benign and respond to antihistamine treatment. Where patients complain of headache it may possibly be due to fluid deprivation.

There is no satisfactory way of pre-testing which will allow the prediction of a severe reaction, but the following precautions may help to minimise reactions, according to some workers:

1. Obtain a history of personal or familial allergies, of previous iodine studies, and of sensitivity to iodine and other drugs.
2. Make a preliminary sensitivity test by injecting intravenously a small dose (0.5–1 ml) followed by a period of observation long enough to detect delayed reactions. (Although allergic reactions generally occur quickly, on very rare occasions they may not appear for 10 or even 15 minutes.)
3. Give preliminary antihistamine medication.
4. Have drugs on hand for emergency use.

In examination of the gastro-intestinal tract, Hypaque should be used with caution in infants and debilitated elderly patients because hypovolaemia may develop due to the osmotic activity of the contrast material in the intestines.

Pharmaceutical precautions The sterile aqueous solutions are almost colourless. Hypaque is relatively thermostable and may be autoclaved if 0.0125 w/v sodium calciumeditate is added to the solution, but sterile Hypaque solutions should not be re-autoclaved because of the possibility of free amine production. Solutions should be protected from light.

Legal category Hypaque injections POM. Hypaque Sodium Powder P.

Package quantities *Hypaque 25%:* 20 ml ampoules in boxes of 5. Infusion bottles of 250 ml or 350 ml.
Hypaque 45%: 20 ml ampoules in boxes of 5 or 20.
30 ml ampoules in boxes of 20.
Hypaque Sodium: Bottles of 500 g.

Further information Nil.

Product licence numbers
Hypaque 25%   0071/5044

Hypaque 45%   0071/5045
Hypaque Sodium   0071/5048

HYPAQUE* 65% AND 85%

Presentation Sterile, almost colourless aqueous solution in clear ampoules. Hypaque 65% contains Sodium Diatrizoate BP 25.23% w/v and meglumine diatrizoate 50.46%. (The iodine content of Hypaque 65% is equivalent to that of a 65% solution of sodium diatrizoate.)

Hypaque 85% contains Sodium Diatrizoate BP 28.33% w/v and meglumine diatrizoate 56.67% w/v.

At body temperature the solutions are clear, but at lower temperatures crystals may separate out. The solid readily dissolves when heated to 40°C or 45°C and re-crystallisation does not occur for several hours.

Uses An X-ray contrast medium for angiocardiography, aortography, venography and other examinations.

Dosage and administration Hypaque is for parenteral use, oral administration for gastro-intestinal examinations and rectal administration as an enema.

The volume and concentration of Hypaque Solution used depend on the procedure being carried out.

When concentrations of Hypaque other than 85%, 65%, 45% or 25% are required, they can be obtained either by diluting a stronger medium with normal saline, or by mixing suitable amounts of two media.

The strengths and quantities given in the table on the next page are suggested.

Examination of the gastro-intestinal tract: For adults an average dose of 100–150 ml of a 25–50% solution is suggested when given by mouth or tube. From 500 ml to 1,000 ml of 20–35% solution is suggested for an enema.

For infants or children the oral or tube dose may vary from 50 ml to 120 ml of a 10–25% solution, and as an enema from 100 ml to 500 ml of a 10–15% solution may be used. The following formulae may be used to prepare a flavoured draught from Hypaque 85%:

	1	2	3
Hypaque 85%*	40 ml*	40 ml*	40 ml*
Sucrose	26.41 g	—	—
Methyl *p*-hydroxy-benzoate	0.1 g	0.08 g	0.08 g
Propyl *p*-hydroxy-benzoate	0.01 g	—	—
Butyl *p*-hydroxy-benzoate	0.004 g	—	—
Sodium saccharin	0.03 g	0.3 g	0.3 g
Tween 80	0.08 g	—	0.08 g
Vanillin	—	0.2 g	0.2 g
Purified water q.s. ad	75 ml	75 ml	75 ml

* Or an appropriate amount for the strength of solution required.

Contra-indications, warnings, etc Hypaque should not be used for myelography. Injection of even a small amount into the subarachnoid space may produce convulsions and result in fatality. In patients with subarachnoid haemorrhage, a rare association between contrast administration and clinical deterioration, including convulsions and death, has been reported. Therefore, administration of intravascular iodated ionic contrast media to these patients should be undertaken with caution.

It was formerly believed that the use of contrast media was contra-indicated in patients with advanced renal destruction associated with severe uraemia, and in severe hepatic and cardiac disorders. However, one review concludes that although there appear to be no definite contra-indications, potentially hazardous situations requiring particular care are oliguric renal failure, myeloma and combined renal and hepatic failure.

No attempt should be made to dehydrate the uraemic patient, nor should dehydration be carried out in a patient with myeloma. Recent evidence suggests that in the latter case, it is dehydration rather than the presence of myeloma protein which has been the cause of adverse effects. Prior purgation should also be avoided. X-ray examinations should be avoided during pregnancy. Because the safety of Hypaque, like some other iodine-containing contrast media, has not been established in pregnancy, examinations involving its use should be delayed until 12–16 weeks after delivery whenever possible.

Should urine be tested for albumin within four to six hours after a Hypaque injection, crystals of diatrizoic acid may separate out on acidification with mineral acid, but these crystals are easily distinguished from the amorphous albumin precipitate. Hypaque does not affect the acetic acid or heat coagulation tests.

Organic iodine contrast media are known to remain in the blood serum of patients for periods varying from two days to several years in concentrations sufficient to interfere with tests of thyroid function such as protein-bound iodine determinations. It has been reported that sodium diatrizoate remains in the serum for four days. It is therefore advisable to perform such thyroid function tests before any examination involving the use of Hypaque.

Patients with a history of allergy, especially to iodine, and those with active tuberculosis, require careful consideration. Because of the possibility of inducing a temporary suppression of urine, it is wise to allow an interval of at least 24 hours before repeating excretory or retrograde pyelography in patients with unilateral reduction of normal renal function.

Examination	Strength (%)	Amount of medium used (ml) Adults	Children
Angiocardiography	65–85	40–60	20
Abdominal aortography			
'Seldinger'	65	20	10
arch	65–85	40–60	20
translumbar	65	20	10
Selective arteriography	45–65	5–30	4–10
Portal venography:			
splenoveno-	65–85	30–40	10–15
mesenteric-	65	30–40	15–20
Peripheral venography	65	20–40	10–20
Sialography	65	1–3	1–3
Amniography	45–65	10–40	—

The precise nature of the reactions which occur with contrast media are not fully understood, although some seem to be allergic, and major reactions resemble those due to histamine release. Most minor reactions such as arm pain, giddiness, a feeling of warmth, coughing, nausea and vomiting pass off quickly. Minor allergic disturbances such as sneezing, rhinorrhoea, lacrimation and pruritus or urticarial rashes are relatively benign and respond to antihistamine treatment. Where patients complain of headache it may possibly be due to fluid deprivation.

There is no satisfactory way of pre-testing which will allow the prediction of a severe reaction, but the following precautions may help to minimise reactions, according to some workers:

1. Obtain a history of personal or familial allergies, of previous iodine studies, and of sensitivity to iodine and other drugs.

2. Make a preliminary sensitivity test by injecting intravenously a small dose (0.5–1 ml) followed by a period of observation long enough to detect delayed reactions. (Although allergic reactions generally occur quickly, on very rare occasions they may not appear for 10 or even 15 minutes.)

3. Give preliminary antihistamine medication.

4. Have drugs on hand for emergency use.

In examinations of the gastro-intestinal tract, Hypaque should be used with caution in infants and debilitated elderly patients because hypovolaemia may develop due to the osmotic activity of the contrast material in the intestines.

Pharmaceutical precautions The sterile aqueous solutions are clear and almost colourless. Hypaque is relatively stable and may be autoclaved if 0.0125% w/v sodium calciumedetate is added to the solution, but solutions should not be re-autoclaved because of the possibility of free amine production. Solutions should be protected from light.

Legal category POM.

Package quantities *Hypaque 65%:* 20 ml ampoules in boxes of 5.
Hypaque 85%: 20ml ampoules in boxes of 5.

Further information Nil.

Product licence numbers
Hypaque 65% 0071/5046
Hypaque 85% 0071/5047

INTEGRIN* CAPSULES

Presentation Integrin Capsules are No. 4 white, opaque, hard gelatine capsules marked Integrin 10 on both cap and body and filled with a fine, off-white powder. Each capsule contains 10 mg oxypertine.

Uses Integrin Capsules are recommended for the treatment of acute and chronic anxiety states and psychosomatic conditions whether or not accompanied by depressive overlay, tension, apprehension, agitation or sleep disturbance.

Dosage and administration For oral administration only.
Adults: 10 mg three or four times daily, usually after meals. In certain cases up to 60 mg daily in divided doses may be needed.

Contra-indications, warnings, etc Although tests on pregnant rabbits (Somers' test) have revealed no teratogenic effects from oxypertine the benefits of using Integrin in the first trimester of pregnancy should be weighed against the possible risks.

Because oxypertine can bring about the release of small amounts of catecholamines in experimental animals, it would be wise not to give Integrin with, or within three weeks of the use of monoamine oxidase inhibitors.

Integrin may potentiate the effect of alcohol or other tranquillisers: patients should, therefore, be warned against excessive use of alcohol and, as with all tranquillisers, patients should also be warned to observe caution in car driving and similar situations.

Overdosage: Possible effects of overdosage might include central and respiratory depression and hypotension. Gastric lavage may be indicated, otherwise treatment should be symptomatic and supportive.

Side-effects: No serious toxic reactions have been reported with Integrin treatment. Even in high doses it has been well tolerated with only minor, often transient, side-effects appearing. As would be expected from the pharmacological properties of the compound, drowsiness may occur in some patients, and a few individuals may complain of mild side-effects such as dry mouth and dizziness.

Pharmaceutical precautions Protect from moisture and heat.

Legal category POM.

Package quantities Integrin 10 mg Capsules are available in bottles of 100.

Further information Nil.

Product licence number 0071/5049.

INTEGRIN* TABLETS

Presentation Integrin 40 mg Tablets are white, slightly speckled, flat tablets with bevelled edges, 8.7 mm in diameter, marked 'int' on one side and scored on the other. Each tablet contains 40 mg oxypertine.

Uses Integrin 40 mg Tablets are recommended for the treatment of psychotics. They are particularly useful in withdrawn schizophrenics. Integrin 40 mg Tablets may also be used in acute incidents of mental disturbances such as acute agitation, behavioural disturbances, delirium, and acute and subacute psychoses, including the manic phase of manic-depressive psychoses.

Dosage and administration For oral administration only.
Adults: The usual dose is 2–3 tablets (80–120 mg) daily in divided doses. This may be varied according to the mental state and the clinical response of the patient, but the total daily dosage should not exceed 300 mg.

Contra-indications, warnings, etc Although tests on pregnant rabbits (Somers' test) have revealed no teratogenic effects from oxypertine the benefits of using Integrin in the first trimester of pregnancy should be weighed against the possible risks.

Because oxypertine can bring about the release of small amounts of catecholamines in experimental animals, it would be wise not to give Integrin with or within three weeks of the use of monoamine oxidase inhibitors. Oxypertine may potentiate the central depressant effect of alcohol and other tranquillisers.

Patients have received up to 360 mg a day and one has received a maximum of 560 mg a day without toxic effects.

Overdosage: Possible effects of overdosage might include central and respiratory depression and hypotension. Gastric lavage may be indicated, otherwise treatment should be symptomatic and supportive.

Side-effects: These are difficult to evaluate in the

psychiatric patient. Adverse reactions reported have been mostly of a minor character and include extrapyramidal effects, sedation, dizziness and vomiting. Extrapyramidal effects including restlessness may occur when high doses are used in the treatment of schizophrenia, but are rare at lower dose levels. Some observers have found that the incidence is less than with other commonly used psychotropic drugs. When these effects do occur they are readily controlled with appropriate therapy. Some patients complain of mild side-effects such as dry mouth and nasal congestion which are probably due to the autonomic effects of the drug.

There have been very few reports of hypotensive episodes such as occur with the phenothiazines. Moderately raised serum transaminase levels have been reported in some patients as well as occasional eosinophilia in high doses.

Pharmaceutical precautions Nil.

Legal category POM.

Package quantities Integrin Tablets are available in bottles of 250.

Further information Nil.

Product licence number 0071/5050.

LOBAK*

Presentation Lobak Tablets are white, flat tablets with bevelled edges, 12.7 mm in diameter marked Lobak on one side and scored on the other. Each tablet contains 450 mg Paracetamol PhEur and 100 mg chlormezanone.

Uses For the treatment of painful conditions where the combination of an analgesic and a mild tranquilliser/muscle relaxant would be of value. Such conditions include the short-term symptomatic treatment of acute musculoskeletal disorders associated with painful muscle spasm.

Dosage and administration For oral administration only.
Adults: The usual dose is 1 or 2 tablets three times daily. The dosage should be adjusted to patient's response, but should not exceed 8 tablets daily.

Elderly: Half the normal dose or less may be sufficient for a therapeutic response in the elderly.
Not recommended for children.

Contra-indications, warnings, etc There is insufficient evidence of safety of chlormezanone in human pregnancy but it has been used for many years without apparent ill consequences – animal studies have not shown ill hazard. However, do not use Lobak during pregnancy especially the first trimester, unless there are compelling reasons.

Lobak should not be given to patients with a known hypersensitivity to chlormezanone or paracetamol.

Chlormezanone at high doses may modify the patient's reactions (performance at skilled tasks, alertness, etc.) to a varying extent, depending upon individual susceptibility. Therefore patients should be advised not to drive or operate machinery during treatment, if affected. If Lobak is administered with CNS depressants, it is possible that their sedative effect may be intensified. As with other drugs acting on the central nervous system, patients should avoid alcohol while receiving Lobak since the response cannot be predicted.

Lobak should be given with caution to patients with hepatic or renal insufficiency.

Overdosage: Should be treated by gastric lavage (if the product has been recently ingested). The signs and symptoms following chlormezanone overdosage will probably resemble those seen with other central depressant drugs, for example, somnolence, prostration, muscular incoordination and memory disturbance. In severe cases hypotension, respiratory depression and loss of consciousness may occur. Symptomatic treatment is suggested for chlormezanone overdosage.

Patients who have taken an overdose of paracetamol may appear well for the first three days then succumb with liver damage. The hepatic changes produced by overdose of paracetamol result from the accumulation of a highly reactive intermediate metabolite in the hepatocytes. N-acetyl-cysteine intravenously or l-methionine orally protect the liver if administered within 10–12 hours of ingesting an overdose.

Side-effects: Drowsiness and dizziness have been the commonest side-effects, particularly at higher doses.

Other reported side-effects include nausea, lightheadedness, headache, lethargy and dryness of the mouth. Cholestatic jaundice has occurred.

Slight skin reactions of the urticaria or erythematous type can occur. Cases of fixed drug rash and various forms of exudative erythema multiforme have been reported; these are very uncommon but in certain cases can be serious.

The dependence potential of chlormezanone is not known.

Pharmaceutical precautions Nil.

Legal category POM.

Package quantities Lobak is supplied in bottles of 50 or 500.

Further information Chlormezanone acts by blocking polysynaptic reflex pathways both in the subcortical centres and in the spinal cord. It has no direct action on skeletal muscle, nor does it affect myoneural junctions or peripheral nerves. At non-toxic levels, it has no action on the autonomic nervous system, nor any direct action on smooth muscle.

Product licence number 0071/5059.

MODRENAL* ▼

Presentation Modrenal capsules are size 3, opaque, pink/black gelatin capsules, marked SRL 60, each containing 60 mg trilostane.

Uses Modrenal is for the control of the manifestations of adrenal cortical hyperfunction in such conditions as hypercortisolism and primary aldosteronism.

Dosage and administration Modrenal is for oral administration only.

Adults: One capsule (60 mg) four times a day for at least 3 days. Thereafter, the dose may be reduced or increased, according to the patient's clinical response and the results of appropriate biochemical tests. The normal dosage range is 120 mg to 480 mg per day in divided doses, but in a few patients the daily dose has been increased stepwise to 960 mg.

Children: There are no dosage recommendations for children.

Contra-indications, warnings, etc Modrenal is contra-indicated in pregnant patients. Steps should be taken to exclude pregnancy before starting treatment with Modrenal and non-hormonal contraceptive measures should be taken during the course of treatment.

As with all drugs which are metabolised by the liver and excreted by the kidney, caution should be exercised in treating patients with renal or hepatic dysfunction.

It is advisable to monitor therapeutic response by regular assay of circulating corticosteroids and blood electrolytes until the presence of an ACTH-producing tumour has been excluded. If a patient taking Modrenal develops a severe illness or needs surgery, it may be advisable to administer corticosteroids.

Information on long-term effects is not yet available.

Drug Interaction: If Modrenal is administered concurrently with thiazide or 'loop' type diuretics, its effect of inhibiting aldosterone production reduces the loss of K^+ ions in the urine usually seen with these drugs.

Overdosage: If recently ingested, the drug should be removed by emesis or gastric lavage. Subsequent treatment will depend on the effect the drug has had on blood electrolytes and circulating corticosteroids.

Side-effects: When administered as recommended above, side-effects are likely to be rare. During acute tolerance studies, side-effects were only troublesome when high *initial* doses (500–1,000 mg daily) were given; they included flushing, nausea, vomiting, diarrhoea, rhinorrhoea, and palatal oedema. All were reversible on stopping treatment.

Pharmaceutical precautions Nil.

Legal category POM.

Package quantities Modrenal capsules are supplied in bottles of 100.

Further information Modrenal selectively and reversibly reduces to normal limits both mineralo- and glucocorticoids by inhibiting an enzyme system essential for their production (3β-hydroxysteroid dehydrogenase/ $\triangle^5$-3-oxosteroid isomerase).

Product licence number 0071/0129.

MONODRAL*

Presentation Monodral Tablets are yellow, bi-convex tablets, 8 mm in diameter, marked 'W' on one side and scored on the other. Each tablet contains 5 mg penthienate methobromide.

Uses Monodral Tablets are recommended for the treatment of gastric hypermotility and hypersecretion. They may be used to relieve pain in peptic ulcer and stress dyspepsia.

Dosage and administration Monodral Tablets are for oral administration only. Dosage should be adjusted to individual needs.

Adults:

1. *Peptic ulcer:* The average dose is 1 tablet three times daily, with an additional dose at night if required. Some patients may require higher doses in the initial stages, especially when pain is severe, but a daily dose of 40 mg should be regarded as the maximum and this amount should be given for short periods only. When symptoms are controlled the dose should be reduced to the effective minimum.

2. *Stress Dyspepsia:* Small doses are often sufficient to relieve symptoms and a dosage of $\frac{1}{2}$ tablet (2.5 mg) three or four times daily is usually used.

Contra-indications, warnings, etc The safety of Monodral in pregnancy has not been established.

Monodral should not be given in the presence of glaucoma because of the possibility of a mydriatic or cycloplegic effect. Pyloric obstruction and obstruction of the neck of the urinary bladder are also contra-indications because of reduction of motility and tonus; consequently care is needed in patients with prostatic hypertrophy. Although tachycardia is rare, severe heart disease, where a possible increase in cardiac rate would be dangerous, is a further contra-indication.

Overdosage: This has not been reported with Monodral. The signs of acute toxicity would probably resemble those of atropine. Treatment should consist of gastric lavage, and physostigmine parenterally is an antidote.

Excitement may occur, but care is needed in administering sedatives because depression may occur as a late symptom of toxicity.

Side-effects: These are unusual at low doses. At higher doses, atropine-like effects such as blurring of vision, difficulty of micturition and dryness of the mouth may occur.

Pharmaceutical precautions Nil.

Legal category POM.

Package quantities Monodral is supplied in bottles of 100 tablets.

Further information Nil.

Product licence number 0071/5063.

MYTELASE*

Presentation Mytelase Tablets are white, bi-convex, film-coated tablets, 6.4 mm in diameter, marked 'MYT' and scored on one side and plain on the other side. Each tablet contains 10 mg ambenonium chloride.

Uses Mytelase Tablets are recommended for the treatment of myasthenia gravis.

Dosage and administration For oral administration only.

Adults: For the patient with moderately severe myasthenia, from 5 mg to 25 mg ($\frac{1}{2}$–2$\frac{1}{2}$ tablets) three or four times daily is recommended. Some patients require as little as 5 mg per dose: others require as much as 50 to 75 mg per dose.

It is recommended that treatment should start with a 5 mg dose, the effect of the drug in each patient being carefully observed. The dosage may be gradually increased to determine the effective and safe dose for each patient.

In addition to the individual variation in dosage requirements, the amount of cholinergic medication necessary to control symptoms may fluctuate in each patient, depending on his activity and the current status of the disease, including spontaneous remission.

A few patients may require greater doses for adequate control of the myasthenic symptoms, but increasing the dosage above 200 mg daily requires exacting supervision by a physician well aware of the signs and treatment of overdosage with cholinergic medication.

Since the warning of overdosage is minimal and the requirements of patients vary tremendously, great care and supervision are required. That a narrow margin exists between the first appearance of side-effects and serious toxic effects must be borne in mind constantly. Caution in increasing dosage is essential.

Contra-indications, warnings, etc Atropine must not be administered routinely with Mytelase. Simultaneous administration of other antimyasthenic drugs should only take place under strict medical supervision. Use with caution in patients with asthma or with mechanical intestinal or urinary obstruction.

Overstimulation with Mytelase has a clinical picture of increasing parasympathomimetic action which is more or less characteristic (when not masked by the use of atropine). The safety of Mytelase in pregnancy has not been established.

Overdosage: Signs and symptoms of overdosage, including cholinergic crises, vary considerably. They are usually manifested by increasing gastro-intestinal stimulation with epigastric distress, abdominal cramps, diarrhoea and vomiting, excessive salivation, pallor, cold sweating, urinary urgency and blurring of vision. Eventually fasciculation and paralysis of voluntary muscles including those of the tongue (thick tongue and difficulty in swallowing), shoulder, neck and arms develop. Miosis, increase in blood pressure, with or without bradycardia, and finally subjective sensations of internal trembling and often severe anxiety and panic may complete the picture. A cholinergic crisis can usually be differentiated from the weakness and paralysis of myasthenia gravis, inadequately treated with cholinergic drugs, by the fact that myasthenic weakness is not accompanied by any of the above signs and symptoms except the last two subjective ones (of anxiety and panic).

If signs of overdosage occur with Mytelase (excessive gastro-intestinal stimulation, excessive salivation, meiosis and more serious fasciculations of voluntary muscles) discontinue temporarily all cholinergic medication and administer from 0.5 to 1 mg of atropine intravenously. Give other supportive treatment as indicated (artificial respiration, tracheotomy, oxygen, etc).

Pharmaceutical precautions Nil.

Legal category POM.

Package quantities Mytelase is available in bottles of 100 tablets.

Further information Nil.

Product licence number 0071/5066.

NEGRAM*

Presentation Negram Suspension is a deep pink, viscous suspension with a raspberry odour and taste containing 300 mg Nalidixic Acid BP per 5 ml dose.

Negram Tablets are beige, bi-convex tablets, 12.7 mm in diameter, marked 'Negram' on one side and with an ankh symbol on the other. Each tablet contains 500 mg Nalidixic Acid BP.

Uses Negram is recommended for the treatment of acute or chronic infections, especially those of the urinary and gastro-intestinal tracts, caused by Gram-negative pathogens sensitive to nalidixic acid.

Dosage and administration *Adults:* For acute infections, 1 g four times daily for at least seven days, reducing to 0.5 g four times a day for chronic infections.

Children: For those over the age of three months, the maximum recommended dose is 50 mg/kg body weight per day in divided doses. When prolonged treatment is necessary it may be possible to reduce the dose to 30 mg/kg body weight without loss of therapeutic benefit.

Not recommended for babies less than three months of age.

Contra-indications, warnings, etc Although there is no evidence that nalidixic acid has any harmful effect during pregnancy, careful consideration should be given to its use during the first trimester. When treating women who are breast feeding, consideration should be given to the fact that traces of nalidixic acid are excreted in the milk.

Negram is contra-indicated for patients with a history of convulsive disorders. It should be used with caution in patients with liver disease. Patients should avoid excessive exposure to sunlight (including sunbathing).

When Negram is given to patients on anticoagulant therapy, it may be necessary to reduce the anticoagulant dosage.

Nalidixic acid has been shown to induce lesions in weight-bearing joints of young animals. The relevance of this to man is unknown. The possible risk of late degenerative joint changes in young patients receiving nalidixic acid preparations should therefore be considered. If symptoms of arthralgia occur, treatment with nalidixic acid should be stopped.

Although care should be exercised in treating patients with renal failure, the full dosage of Negram may be administered in patients with creatinine clearance of more than 20 ml/min and half the normal dosage in patients with creatinine clearance less than this. Nalidixic acid in therapeutic doses can interfere with the estimation of urinary 17-ketosteroids and may cause high results in the assay of urinary vanilmandelic acid (Pisano method).

Active proliferation of the organisms is a necessary condition for the antibacterial action of nalidixic acid: the action of Negram may therefore be inhibited by the presence of other antibacterial substances.

When testing for glycosuria in patients receiving Negram, glucose-specific methods based on glucose oxidase should be used because copper reduction methods may give false-positive results.

Overdosage: In adults, symptoms of overdosage have been noted following single doses of 20 and 25 g. These have included toxic psychosis, convulsions and metabolic acidosis.

In an emergency, it is suggested that the stomach should be emptied, and symptomatic treatment applied as necessary, a particular watch being kept for central or respiratory depression.

Side-effects: Gastro-intestinal effects, skin reactions or subjective visual disturbances may occur but are readily reversible on reduction or discontinuation of therapy. There are isolated reports of convulsive episodes usually associated with overdosage or certain predisposing factors, and of raised intracranial pressure. A few cases of sixth cranial nerve palsy have also been reported. These usually disappear rapidly with no sequelae when the drug is discontinued.

Blood dyscrasias are rare, but haemolytic anaemia (sometimes related to G-6-PD deficiency), thrombocytopenia and leucopenia have been reported.

Pharmaceutical precautions Where doses of less than 5 ml are ordered, Negram Suspension may be diluted with Syrup BP so that the standard 5 ml spoonful can be given. Such dilutions will remain stable for two to three weeks.

Legal category POM.

Package quantities *Negram Suspension:* Bottles of 150 ml or 500 ml.
Negram Tablets: Boxes of 56 tablets (7 strips of 8 tablets) and (for hospitals only) bottles of 500 tablets.

Further information Nil.

Product licence numbers
Negram Suspenion   0071/5067
Negram Tablets   0071/5068.

PLAQUENIL*

Presentation Plaquenil Tablets are orange-coloured, sugar coated tablets with no markings. Each tablet contains 200 mg Hydroxychloroquine Sulphate BP.

Uses Plaquenil Tablets are recommended for the treatment of rheumatoid arthritis, juvenile rheumatoid arthritis, discoid and systemic lupus erythematosus and light-sensitive diseases. Also recommended for the treatment and prophylaxis of malaria.

Plaquenil has been shown to have a desludging action, which may be of benefit in the prophylaxis of post-operative deep vein thrombosis.

Dosage and administration *(a) Rheumatoid arthritis, juvenile rheumatoid arthritis, discoid and systemic lupus erythematosus and light sensitive diseases.*
Adults: Initially 400 mg daily in divided doses. The dose can be reduced to 200 mg when no further improvement is evident. The maintenance dose should be increased to 400 mg daily if the response lessens.

The minimum effective dose should be employed and should not exceed 6.5 mg/kg/day (calculated from ideal body weight and not actual body weight).

Children: The minimum effective doses should be employed and should not exceed 6.5 mg/kg/day. A regimen of alternating doses may be required to provide mean daily doses other than 200 mg and 400 mg.

In rheumatoid arthritis, juvenile rheumatoid arthritis, discoid and systemic lupus erythematosus, treatment should be discontinued if there is no improvement by 6 months. In light sensitive diseases, treatment should only be given during periods of maximum exposure to light.

(b) Malaria
Adults: To treat an acute attack it is usual to give 800 mg (4 tablets) initially followed by 400 mg (2 tablets) in six to eight hours, and then 400 mg on each of two successive days. A single dose of 800 mg has been used to eradicate *Plasmodium falciparum* infection and to terminate an acute attack by *Plasmodium vivax.*

(c) Malaria prophylaxis
Adults: 6 mg/kg body weight once a week (equivalent to 400 mg weekly in most cases).

Children: 6 mg/kg body weight once a week. Plaquenil is not a convenient dosage strength for weekly administration to children of less than 30–40 kg body weight.

Prophylaxis should begin one week before arrival in a malarious area and continue for four to eight weeks after leaving the area. The dose may need to be doubled in highly malarious areas.

(d) De-sludging
Adults: 200 mg every 6–8 hours starting on the morning of the day before surgery and continuing for 14 days after.

Contra-indications, warnings, etc

Contra-indications: Plaquenil should not be used in patients with a pre-existing maculopathy or in conjunction with drugs causing adverse ocular reactions.

Precautions: All patients should have an ophthalmological examination before initiating treatment with Plaquenil. Thereafter, ophthalmological examinations should be repeated regularly, i.e. every 3–6 months. The examination should include careful ophthalmoscopy and central visual field testing with a red target. Plaquenil should be discontinued immediately in any patient who develops a pigmentary abnormality or visual field defect.

Impaired visual accommodation soon after the start of treatment has been reported and patients should be warned regarding driving or operating machinery. If the condition is not self-limiting, it will resolve on reducing the dose or stopping treatment.

A chemically-related compound, chloroquine phosphate, has been found to cause foetal cochlear damage when taken in high doses during pregnancy. Thus, use of Plaquenil in pregnancy should be avoided, except in prophylaxis of malaria when the need may outweigh the possible risks.

Plaquenil should be used with caution in patients with hepatic or renal disease, in those taking drugs known to affect those organs and in patients with severe gastrointestinal, neurological or blood disorders. Estimation of blood hydroxychloroquine levels should be undertaken in patients with severely compromised renal or hepatic function.

Although the risk of bone-marrow depression is low, periodic blood counts are advisable and Plaquenil should be discontinued if abnormalities develop.

Caution is advised if Plaquenil is to be given to a patient with a history of quinine sensitivity. Some patients with psoriasis appear to be more susceptible to skin reactions than others.

Although hydroxychloroquine has been used successfully in the treatment of porphyria cutanea tarda, exacerbation of the condition by the drug has been reported. Plaquenil should be used with caution in patients with glucose-6-phosphate dehydrogenase deficiency.

Small children are particularly sensitive to the 4-aminoquinolines; therefore, patients should be particularly warned to keep Plaquenil out of the reach of children.

Side-effects: Retinal changes can occur, but appear to be uncommon if the recommended daily dose is not exceeded. In one study, reversible retinal changes occurred in 4 of 99 patients receiving Plaquenil 400 mg a day for a median of almost 4 years. In another, no eye lesions were seen in 311 patients receiving Plaquenil up to 6.5 mg/day for at least 4 years.

Corneal opacities have occasionally been reported. They are either symptomless or may cause disturbances such as haloes, blurring of vision or photophobia. They are reversible on stopping treatment.

Skin reactions, bleaching of the hair and alopecia may also occur, but they usually clear up readily on ceasing treatment.

Other adverse effects include gastrointestinal disturbances such as nausea, diarrhoea, anorexia, abdominal cramps and, rarely, vomiting. These symptoms usually stop immediately on reducing the dose or on stopping the treatment. Less frequently, muscle weakness, vertigo, tinnitus, nerve deafness, headache, nervousness and emotional upsets have been reported. Reports of bone-marrow depression are rare. Patients should be carefully supervised in view of reports of peripheral neuropathy and toxic psychosis with other 4-aminoquinoline compounds.

Interactions: Plaquenil has been reported to increase plasma digoxin levels. Aminoglycoside antibiotics have been reported to potentiate the direct blocking action of chloroquine at the neuro-muscular junction.

Antacids given at the same time as chloroquine reduce its bioavailability. It is suggested, therefore, that Plaquenil and antacids should be given 4 hours apart.

Overdosage: Recovery under treatment has followed the ingestion of 36 Plaquenil Tablets, while an estimated dose of 54 tablets has proved rapidly fatal. Overdosage with the 4-aminoquinolines is particularly dangerous in infants, as little as 1–2 g having proved fatal.

The symptoms of overdosage may include headache, visual disturbance, cardiovascular collapse, and convulsions, followed by sudden and early respiratory and cardiac arrest. Since these effects may appear soon after taking a massive dose, treatment should be prompt and symptomatic. The stomach should be immediately evacuated, either by emesis or by gastric lavage. If convulsions are present, they should be controlled before the stomach is emptied by:

1. Parenteral diazepam if due to cerebral stimulation, or

2. The administration of oxygen, or by artificial respiration if due to anoxia, or

3. By vasopressor therapy if due to shock or hypotension.

A patient who survives the acute phase and is asymptomatic should be closely observed for at least six hours. Fluids may be forced and sufficient ammonium chloride may be administered to acidify the urine for a few days to hasten urinary excretion. Dimercaprol can be given by intramuscular injection (2.4–3 mg/kg body weight four to six times a day for three days, then every 12 hours for 10 days).

Ammonium chloride is also useful in patients who show toxic symptoms due to sensitivity to the drug.

Pharmaceutical precautions Nil.

Legal category POM.

Package quantities Plaquenil is supplied in bottles of 100 tablets.

Further information Analgesic and non-steroidal anti-inflammatory agents may be given concomitantly with Plaquenil, especially in the early stages of therapy before a response has been attained.

Product licence number 0071/5083.

SOLPADEINE*

Presentation Solpadeine Tablets are flat, white, bevelled edged tablets which effervesce vigorously when placed in water. Each tablet is 25.4 mm in diameter and contains 500 mg Paracetamol PhEur, 8 mg Codeine Phosphate PhEur and 30 mg Caffeine PhEur.

Uses Solpadeine Tablets are recommended for the relief of pain in the treatment of rheumatic pain, sciatica and lumbago as well as in sprains, headaches, sinusitis and influenza.

Dosage and administration

Adults: 2 tablets dissolved in at least half a tumblerful of water, taken three or four times a day if necessary.

Children: Children 7–12 years old may be given ½–1 tablet dissolved in water. Children should not be given doses of Solpadeine more frequently than every 4 hours and not more than 4 doses should be given in any 24-hour period.

Not suitable for children under 7 years of age.

Contra-indications, warnings, etc Apart from hypersensitivity to any of the ingredients, there are no contra-indications or precautions associated with the use of Solpadeine tablets and side-effects are unusual. Solpadeine contains 425 mg (18.5 mmol) of sodium in each tablet. This should be taken into account where the patient has been placed on a restricted sodium intake.

There is epidemiological evidence of the safety of paracetamol in human pregnancy. Codeine has been used for many years without apparent ill consequences and animal studies have not shown any hazard.

Overdosage: Nausea and vomiting are prominent symptoms of codeine toxicity and there is evidence of circulatory and respiratory depression. Suggested treatment is gastric lavage and catharsis. If CNS depression is severe, artificial respiration, oxygen and parenteral naloxone may be needed.

Patients who have taken an overdose of paracetamol may appear well for the first three days, then succumb to liver damage. The hepatic changes produced by overdosage of paracetamol result from the accumulation of a highly active intermediate metabolite in the hepatocytes. N-acetylcysteine intravenously or l-methionine orally protects the liver if administered within 10–12 hours of ingesting an overdose.

Pharmaceutical precautions Solpadeine Tablets should be protected from light and moisture.

Legal category CD (Sch 5), P.

Package quantities Solpadeine Tablets are packed in laminate strips and supplied in boxes of 12, 24 and 60 tablets.

Further information Nil.

Product licence number 0071/5091.

SOLPADEINE* FORTE

Presentation Flat, white, bevelled-edged tablets which effervesce vigorously when placed in water. Each tablet is 25.4 mm in diameter and contains Paracetamol PhEur 500 mg, Codeine Phosphate PhEur 15 mg and Caffeine PhEur 30 mg.

Uses Solpadeine Forte may be used for the treatment of moderate pain, as for example in arthritis, musculo-skeletal pain, sciatica, some post-surgical/trauma pain, dysmenorrhoea, headache (including migraine), as well as for other conditions for which an antipyretic-analgesic is often prescribed.

Dosage and administration

Adults: Two tablets dissolved in at least half a tumblerful of water up to four times a day if necessary.

Children: Not recommended.

Contra-indications, warnings, etc

Contra-indications: Hypersensitivity to paracetamol, codeine or caffeine.

Warnings: Patients should be advised not to drive or operate machinery if affected by dizziness or sedation. The effects of CNS depressants (including alcohol) may be potentiated.

Precautions: There is inadequate evidence for the safety of codeine in human pregnancy, but there is epidemiological evidence for the safety of paracetamol. Both substances have been used for many years without apparent ill consequences and animal studies have not shown any hazard.

Codeine is an opioid analgesic; tolerance and dependence can occur especially with prolonged high dosage.

Each tablet contains 425 mg (18.5 mmol) of sodium. This should be taken into account where the patient has been placed on a restricted sodium intake.

Side-effects: Adverse effects to paracetamol are rare. Codeine may cause constipation, nausea, dizziness and drowsiness, according to dosage and individual susceptibility.

Overdosage: Nausea and vomiting are prominent symptoms of codeine toxicity and there is evidence of circulatory and respiratory depression. Suggested treatment is gastric lavage and catharsis. If CNS depression is severe, artificial respiration, oxygen and parenteral naloxone may be needed.

Patients who have taken an overdose of paracetamol may appear well for the first three days, then succumb to liver damage. The hepatic changes produced by overdosage of paracetamol result from the accumulation of a highly active intermediate metabolite in the hepatocytes. N-acetylcysteine intravenously or l-methionine orally protects the liver if administered within 10–12 hours of ingesting an overdose.

Pharmaceutical precautions Protect from light and moisture.

Legal category CD (Sch 5), POM.

Package quantities Cartons of 60 in foil strips.

Further information Nil.

Product licence number 0071/0234.

STROMBA*

Presentation 1. Stromba Tablets are flat, white tablets 9.5 mm in diameter, marked Stromba on one side and scored in quarters on the other side. Each tablet contains 5 mg Stanozolol BP.

2. Stromba Injection consists of clear glass ampoules, 2 ml capacity, each containing 1 ml aqueous suspension of 50 mg Stanozolol BP.

Uses Stromba Tablets may be used for the treatment of the complications of deep vein thrombosis as in venous lipodermatosclerosis (pain, induration, pigmentation and eczema in the post-phlebitic syndrome) and for the prevention of venous thrombosis such as occurs with antithrombin III deficiency; for the control of Raynaud's phenomenon in patients with systemic sclerosis, in the vasculitis of Behçet's disease and for the control of the vascular symptoms of cutaneous vasculitis.

Stromba tablets may be used in the management of post-menopausal and senile osteoporosis and in patients suffering from weight loss and anorexia associated with chronic debilitating diseases where dietary measures alone have proved unsuccessful.

Stromba tablets may be used in the prevention of attacks of hereditary angio-oedema.

Stromba injection may be used to treat severe conditions where an anabolic effect is required to correct a negative nitrogen balance, as, for example, in major trauma, severe burns or emaciating diseases. It may also be of value in the management of anaemias (including those associated with neoplastic disease) and the management of terminal cancer patients.

Dosage and administration

Stromba Tablets

Adults: 1. Vascular complications. 10 mg daily.

2. Osteoporosis and other indications. One 5 mg tablet daily.

3. Hereditary angio-oedema. An initial dose of 2.5 to 10 mg daily may be necessary to control the occurrence of attacks. Thereafter, the dose may be reduced according to patient response. Maintenance doses as low as 2.5 mg three times a week have been achieved in selected cases.

Children: 1. Where indicated. Under 6 years – half a tablet daily. 6–10 years – half to one tablet daily. It is suggested that tablets should be administered to children in short courses of six to eight weeks. More than one course may be given with an interval of one month between courses.

2. Hereditary angio-oedema. Once control has been achieved, the lowest dose possible that maintains freedom from attacks should be used.

Stromba Injection

Adults: 50 mg (1 ml) administered by deep intramuscular injection once every two to three weeks.

Contra-indications, warnings, etc Stromba is not intended for the treatment of loss of appetite, unexplained weight loss or failure to thrive in children. Such cases should be referred to the appropriate centre for investigation.

Prolonged use in children may lead to premature closure of the epiphyses.

Because of possible virilising effects on a female foetus, Stromba should not be administered to pregnant women.

Stromba should be used with caution in the presence of impaired renal or cardiac function as it may encourage sodium and water retention that could result in cardiac failure.

Anabolic steroids increase sensitivity to warfarin type anti-coagulants; therefore, the dose of the latter should be decreased in order to maintain the prothrombin time at the desired therapeutic level.

Stromba should not be administered to patients with established liver disease. Patients with a history of jaundice should have liver function tests checked prior to commencing treatment. Stromba may raise levels of aspartate transaminase (AST) and alanine transaminase (ALT) and in some patients these may rise above laboratory normal ranges. These levels return to normal on withdrawing Stromba.

Tumours of the liver have been reported occasionally in patients subjected to prolonged treatment with androgenic anabolic steroids, especially patients with Fanconi's syndrome and aplastic anaemia. These tumours, however, are not typical of primary hepatocellular carcinoma and in some cases discontinuation of steroids has resulted in tumour regression without other therapy. The possibility that these compounds may induce or enhance the development of such hepatic tumours cannot at present be excluded and this should be considered when the use of this product is proposed for long-term treatment, particularly in young people who are not suffering from life-threatening disorders.

The use of this preparation may result in an alteration in the ratio of high and low density lipoproteins. The significance of this is not understood.

Stromba should not be used in cases of cancer of the prostate because the condition is androgen-dependent.

Stromba increases ALA synthases activity and hence porphyrin metabolism. It is therefore not recommended in patients with a history of porphyria.

Side-effects: Because of the structural relationship to the male hormones, some androgenic side-effects e.g. acne, hirsutism, amenorrhoea, are to be expected. Because the ratio of anabolic to androgenic properties is high, these effects should be minimal at the recommended dosage and those so far reported have been mild and reversible on stopping treatment. On rare occasions, usually with higher dosage, voice change has been reported; if observed, treatment should be discontinued. Other effects, such as headache, muscle cramp, dyspepsia, skin rash and occasionally hair loss, euphoria and depression have occurred. There have been occasional reports of cholestatic jaundice.

Overdosage: There are no reports of chronic or acute overdosage with Stromba. By analogy with other substances of this type, one would expect chronic overdosage to be associated with the signs and symptoms caused by excessive circulating androgens. It is unlikely that any immediate serious reactions would be seen in a single excessive dose (in animals acute toxicity cannot be measured). In such an event, however, the patient should be kept under observation and liver function monitored, in cases of delayed reactions.

Pharmaceutical precautions Each ampoule should be thoroughly shaken before use. Protect from light.

Legal category POM.

Package quantities *Stromba Tablets:* Bottles of 50 or 200 tablets and calendar packs of 56 tablets. *Stromba Injection:* Plastic boxes each containing 10 ampoules.

Further information Stromba is an anabolic agent which has been shown to enhance fibrinolysis by:

1. Increasing plasminogen activator activity.
2. Increasing free plasminogen levels.
3. Decreasing $alpha_2$ macroglobulin levels.

Important effects on the coagulation system include:

1. Decrease in fibrinogen levels.
2. Increase in antithrombin III levels.
3. Increase in protein C levels.

Product licence numbers

Stromba Tablets	0071/5092
Stromba Injection	0071/0031

TELEPAQUE*

Presentation Telepaque Tablets are off-white to buff, bi-convex tablets, 10.3 mm in diameter and plain on both sides. Each tablet contains 500 mg Iopanoic Acid BP.

Uses Telepaque Tablets are recommended for oral cholecystography and cholangiography.

Dosage and administration Telepaque Tablets are usually given 10–14 hours before cholecystography.

Adults:

1. The usual dose is 6 Telepaque Tablets swallowed whole with at least one full glass of water. Eight tablets may be given to very obese patients. For repeat examinations on the same day as the original procedure, an additional 6 tablets may be administered. However, if the repeat examination is to be performed with a double dose of Telepaque a period of five to seven days should be allowed between the two examinations. No more than 12 tablets should be taken during a 24-hour period.

2. In order to obtain better visualisation of the extra-hepatic ducts, 9–12 tablets may be given in 2 doses. Three to six tablets are given four hours after a fatty meal on the day preceding the examination, and then a full dose of 6 tablets after a fat-free meal in the evening.

Another technique is to administer a double dose (12 tablets) of Telepaque after a 12-hour fast, followed by 8 ml Camphorated Opium Tincture BP to close the sphincter of Oddi. Films may be taken 5–14 hours later, and any sphincter pain caused by the tincture may be eased with an anticholinergic. As noted above, 12 tablets is the maximum dose which should be administered in 24 hours.

3. Certain biliary calculi only become radiographically opaque after prolonged exposure to the contrast medium. Such prolonged exposure to Telepaque can be obtained by the following regimen. Patients are instructed to take two Telepaque Tablets after each of the three main meals, daily for four days. During this time the meals should be relatively fat-free. The X-ray examination is made on the morning of the fifth day, the patient fasting.

Contra-indications, warnings, etc Elective contrast radiography of the abdomen during pregnancy should be avoided.

Telepaque is contra-indicated in patients with advanced hepatorenal disease or severe impairment of renal function. It should not be given to patients with gastro-intestinal disorders which interfere with absorption and result in inadequate visualisation. Telepaque may also be contra-indicated in patients who are sensitive to iodine compounds. Caution is also necessary in patients suffering from cholangitis or marked hyperthyroidism.

In patients with severe advanced liver disease, renal function should be assessed before cholecystography, and renal output and hepatic function should be observed for a few days after the procedure. Observation of renal function after multiple doses of the contrast medium has also been recommended. Iopanoic acid has a uricosuric effect approximately equivalent to that of probenecid. Although this action cannot be definitely linked with nephrotoxicity, it has been strongly recommended that adequate hydration should be encouraged as a possible means of decreasing the risk of renal complications.

Patients with pre-existing renal disease should not receive double doses of cholecystographic media. It is possible that renal irritation in susceptible individuals could result in reflex vascular spasm with partial or complete renal shutdown. It is therefore suggested that kidney function in patients with renal disease should be assessed before administration of cholecystographic media, and for several days afterwards.

Fatal coronary occlusion in four patients with arteriosclerotic heart disease who had taken a cholecystographic agent has been reported and premedication with atropine is a reasonable prophylactic measure against vagal stimulation if cholecystography is necessary in patients with recent symptoms of coronary artery disease.

However, the connection between these fatilities and the administration of the contrast media (iopanoic acid in two cases and iodoalphionic acid in the other two) may have been wholly fortuitous. It has also been suggested that the administration of large doses of other aromatic iodine compounds like urographic and angiographic agents with or shortly following cholecystographic agents may increase the likelihood of toxic reactions.

The most frequently reported adverse reactions have been mild and transient nausea, vomiting, diarrhoea and cramps. A stinging sensation during urination occurs occasionally and has been attributed to urethal irritation. It does not indicate any renal or upper urinary tract trouble. Skin reactions such as urticaria, pruritus and flushing rarely occur.

Thrombocytopenia after two 3 g doses has been reported in a patient with a history of conjunctival haemorrhages. Acute renal failure with complete recovery has been reported in four patients, three of whom were given doses of Telepaque which were higher than those recommended.

Pharmaceutical precautions Nil.

Legal category P.

Package quantities Cartons of 36 tablets packed in aluminium foil strips of 6.

Further information Nil.

Product licence number 0071/5095.

VERIPAQUE*

Presentation Veripaque Powder is a fine, white powder containing 50 mg oxyphenisatin in 3 g.

Uses Veripaque is recommended: a) for adding to barium enemas in radiological examination of the large intestine; b) as a cleansing enema to remove colonic gas and faeces before plain abdominal radiography, intravenous pyelography, cholecystography, proctosigmoidoscopy, etc; c) for pre-operative cleansing of the large intestine.

Dosage and administration Veripaque Powder is used for the preparation of enemas for rectal administration.

Adults: Veripaque enemas should be administered slowly over a period of five to eight minutes with the fluid level 18–24 inches above the hips.

As a cleansing enema prior to diagnostic or surgical procedures, 3 g of Veripaque Powder is dissolved in 2 litres of water.

When used as an adjuvant to a barium enema, 3 g Veripaque Powder is mixed thoroughly with 2 litres of barium enema suspension.

Contra-indications, warnings, etc Care is needed in patients with an irritable colon or inflammatory diseases of the large intestine; in such cases Veripaque should be used in smaller than usual doses. As with all enemas Veripaque is not recommended in cases of appendicitis, gross bleeding from the bowel, intestinal obstruction, severe spasm or severe diarrhoea, or when there is danger of intestinal perforation. Reduced dosage is recommended for elderly or debilitated patients. Although when used in small and infrequent doses and in preparations for radiography it may well be harmless, regular, prolonged use should be discouraged because of the possibility of liver toxicity. Minor side-effects such as cramps, diarrhoea, nausea and vomiting, sweating and tachycardia may occur infrequently and can usually be obviated by decreasing the dosage. The cramps, which occur in about 8% of cases, usually produce only mild discomfort and do not interfere with completion of the procedure.

As with tannic acid, more serious side-effects such as syncope may occur occasionally; they are usually caused by administration of too large a dose.

Pharmaceutical precautions Nil.

Legal category P.

Package quantities Boxes of 6 vials each containing 3 g Veripaque Powder.

Further information Nil.

Product licence number 0071/5099.

Trade Mark

Stiefel Laboratories (UK) Limited
Holtspur Lane
Wooburn Green
High Wycombe
Buckinghamshire HP10 0AU

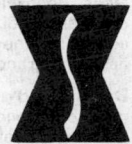

ACETOXYL* 2.5
ACETOXYL* 5

Presentation White, viscous gels containing benzoyl peroxide 2.5 and 5% w/w in an aqueous acetone base.

Uses Acetoxyl 2.5 and 5 are each indicated for use in the treatment of acne vulgaris. Benzoyl peroxide provides control of acne through its antibacterial action and also has a drying and desquamative effect.

Dosage and administration Treatment should normally commence with Acetoxyl 2.5. Apply the gel to the affected areas once daily. Washing with soap and water prior to application greatly enhances the efficacy of the preparation.

The reaction of the skin to benzoyl peroxide differs in individual patients. The higher concentration in Acetoxyl 5 may be required to ensure a satisfactory response.

Contra-indications, warnings, etc Acetoxyl should not be prescribed for patients with known hypersensitivity to benzoyl peroxide.

Avoid contact with the eyes, mouth and other mucous membranes. Care should be taken when applying the product to the neck and other sensitive areas. In normal use, a mild burning sensation will probably be felt on first application and a moderate reddening and peeling of the skin will occur within a few days. During the first weeks of treatment a sudden increase in peeling will occur in most patients, this is not harmful and will normally subside within a day or two if treatment is temporarily discontinued.

Acetoxyl may bleach dyed fabrics.

Pharmaceutical precautions Store in a cool place.

Legal category P.

Package quantities Tubes of 40 g.

Further information Nil.

Product licence numbers
Acetoxyl 2.5   0174/0041
Acetoxyl 5   0174/0039

ANTHRANOL* 0.4
ANTHRANOL* 1.0
ANTHRANOL* 2.0

Presentation Smooth soft yellow ointments containing Dithranol BP 0.4% w/w, 1.0% w/w and 2.0% w/w respectively.

Uses For the topical treatment of sub-acute and chronic psoriasis, including psoriasis of the scalp, by the *short contact therapy* method.

Dosage and administration Treatment should begin with Anthranol 0.4. Clinical response and tolerance will determine the necessity for progression to Anthranol 1.0 and subsequently Anthranol 2.0.

Apply the ointment once daily, sparingly, to the psoriatic plaques. Surrounding normal skin should be protected with white soft paraffin. Leave the ointment on for the required time then remove excess ointment with a paper tissue and wash off the remainder thoroughly.

If Anthranol has been applied to the scalp, the ointment should be removed by shampooing.

The initial daily treatment time with each strength should not exceed 10 minutes. The time may be increased gradually over a period of 7 days to a maximum of 30 minutes. The daily treatment time should not normally exceed 30 minutes.

In the event of undue irritation, stop treatment for 2 days and resume on alternate days.

Treatment should be continued at the optimum tolerated strength and leave-on time, depending on patient response.

Contra-indications, warnings, etc Anthranol ointments are contra-indicated for pustular psoriasis and are not suitable for acute psoriasis.

Anthranol ointments should not be applied to the face, the inside of the thighs, the genital region or skinfold areas. Should contact with the eyes occur, bathe immediately with water and seek medical advice.

Dithranol is a strong irritant; always wash the hands after using Anthranol ointment. The ointment will cause staining and discolouration to the skin, clothing and bathroom ware. Stains on clothing should be assumed to be permanent. Stains on bathroom ware may be removed by bleach.

Pharmaceutical precautions Store in a cool place.

Legal category POM.

Package quantity Anthranol ointments are supplied in tubes of 50 g.

Further information Anthranol 0.4 can also be used for treatment of psoriasis by the overnight method.

Product licence numbers
Anthranol 0.4 ointment   0174/0018
Anthranol 1.0 ointment   0174/0057
Anthranol 2.0 ointment   0174/0058

BENOXYL* 5
BENOXYL* 10

Presentation Benoxyl 5 is available as a white lotion or cream containing benzoyl peroxide 5% w/w.

Benoxyl 10 is a white lotion containing benzoyl peroxide 10% w/w.

Uses Benoxyl 5 and 10 are each indicated for use in the treatment of acne vulgaris. Benzoyl peroxide provides control of acne through its antibacterial action and also has a drying and desquamative effect.

Dosage and administration Treatment should normally commence with Benoxyl 5. Apply the lotion or cream to the affected areas once daily. Washing with soap and water prior to application greatly enhances the efficacy of the preparation.

The reaction of the skin to benzoyl peroxide differs in individual patients. The higher concentration in Benoxyl 10 may be required to ensure a satisfactory response.

Contra-indications, warnings, etc Benoxyl should not be prescribed for patients with a known hypersensitivity to benzoyl peroxide.

Avoid contact with the eyes, mouth and other mucous membranes. Care should be taken when applying the product to the neck and other sensitive areas. In normal use, a mild burning sensation will probably be felt on first application and a moderate reddening and peeling of the skin will occur within a few days. During the first weeks of treatment a sudden increase in peeling will occur in most patients, this is not harmful and will normally subside within a day or two if treatment is temporarily discontinued.

Benoxyl may bleach dyed fabrics.

Pharmaceutical precautions Store in a cool place.

Legal category P.

Package quantities Lotion: Bottles of 30 ml.
Cream: Tubes of 40 g.

Further information Nil.

Product licence numbers
Benoxyl 5 lotion   0174/5003
Benoxyl 5 cream   0174/5007
Benoxyl 10 lotion   0174/0034

BENOXYL* 5 WITH SULPHUR
BENOXYL* 10 WITH SULPHUR

Presentation Benoxyl 5 with Sulphur is an off-white cream containing benzoyl peroxide 5% w/w and sulphur 2% w/w.

Benoxyl 10 with Sulphur is an off white cream containing benzoyl peroxide 10% w/w and sulphur 5% w/w.

Uses Benoxyl 5 with Sulphur and Benoxyl 10 with Sulphur are each indicated in the treatment of acne vulgaris.

Benzoyl peroxide provides control of acne through its antibacterial action and also has a drying and desquamative effect.

Sulphur has antiseptic actions and enhances the keratolytic properties of benzoyl peroxide.

Dosage and administration Treatment should normally commence with Benoxyl 5 with Sulphur. Apply the cream to the affected areas once daily. Washing with soap and water prior to application greatly enhances the efficacy of the preparation.

The reaction of the skin to benzoyl peroxide and sulphur differs in individual patients. The higher concen-

trations in Benoxyl 10 with Sulphur may be required to ensure a satisfactory response.

Contra-indications, warnings, etc Benoxyl with Sulphur should not be prescribed for patients with a known hypersensitivity to benzoyl peroxide or sulphur.

Avoid contact with the eyes, mouth and other mucous membranes. Care should be taken when applying the product to the neck and other sensitive areas. In normal use, a mild burning sensation will probably be felt on first application and a moderate reddening and peeling of the skin will occur within a few days. During the first weeks of treatment a sudden increase in peeling will occur in most patients, this is not harmful and will normally subside within a day or two if treatment is temporarily discontinued.

Benoxyl with Sulphur may bleach dyed fabrics.

Pharmaceutical precautions Store in a cool place.

Legal category P.

Package quantities Tubes of 40 g.

Further information Nil.

Product licence numbers
Benoxyl 5 with Sulphur   0174/5008
Benoxyl 10 with Sulphur   0174/5009

BENOXYL* 20

Presentation Benoxyl 20 contains benzoyl peroxide 20% w/w in a stabilised lotion base.

Uses Benoxyl 20 Lotion is indicated in the management of cutaneous ulcers.

Dosage and administration Apply a protective ointment to the skin area bordering the ulcer. Cut a thick dressing such as an abdominal pad, or cotton wool between gauze layers to fit the size and shape of the ulcer exactly. Moisten the dressing with normal saline or water. Saturate the dressing with Benoxyl 20 and apply to the ulcer with sterile forceps. Apply a piece of thin plastic film over the dressing, to extend just beyond the ulcer margin.

Change the dressing every eight hours for large ulcers and every 12 hours for small ulcers. To hold the dressing in place cover it with a large pad, such as an amputation pad, and tape this firmly in place with hypoallergenic tape. For ulcers with cavities, saturate surgical ribbon gauze with Benoxyl 20 and pack into the cavities with sterile forceps, so that the Benoxyl 20 comes into contact with every area of the ulcer cavity, and then proceed as above. Renew packing at each dressing. In lesions of the legs a supporting bandage may be advantageous.

Contra-indications, warnings, etc Keep away from the mouth, eyes and other mucous membranes to avoid irritation. Avoid normal skin. Irritant dermatitis has been reported in 2.5% to 3% of cases, if undue skin irritation develops, the use of the product should be discontinued. The product may bleach dyed fabrics.

Pharmaceutical precautions Store in a cool place.

Legal category POM.

Package quantities Benoxyl 20 lotion is supplied in bottles containing 100 ml.

Further information Excess granulation growth should be treated with a dilute silver nitrate preparation to reduce it to just below epidermal level. Analgesics may be needed for the first few days of treatment.

Product licence number 0174/0036.

BRĀSIVOL*

Presentation Brāsivol is an abrasive cleansing paste in three grades, each containing graded particles of fused synthetic aluminium oxide in a non-irritant soap-detergent base.

Brāsivol No. 1 Fine is an off-white paste containing 38% aluminium oxide.

Brāsivol No. 2 Medium is a light-blue paste containing 52% aluminium oxide.

Brāsivol No. 3 Coarse is a light-green paste containing 65% aluminium oxide.

Uses Brāsivol is indicated in the treatment of acne vulgaris. Brāsivol effectively cleanses and removes debris from blocked pores and removes excess sebum from the skin, thus maintaining patency of the pore duct openings.

Dosage and administration The patient should commence treatment with Brāsivol No. 1 Fine. The abrasive cleansing paste should be applied to wetted skin and rubbed gently but firmly over the affected area with a circular motion for 15–20 seconds, then rinsed off thoroughly with water. This routine may be repeated two or three times daily, replacing ordinary soap and water.

In more severe conditions, after the use of Brāsivol No. 1 Fine for several weeks, the skin may require the slightly more abrasive action of Brāsivol No. 2 Medium and subsequently longer-term maintenance may require the use of Brāsivol No. 3 Coarse.

Contra-indications, warnings, etc Brāsivol is contra-indicated in the presence of superficial venules and telangiectasia (actinic sequelae).

Care should be taken to avoid using Brāsivol close to the eyes or mouth and male patients using an electric razor should shave before applying Brāsivol.

A degree of dryness and redness will be seen during the first few days of treatment. Over-enthusiastic use, however, can cause irritation and, if this occurs, treatment should be interrupted for a day or two and then resumed.

Pharmaceutical precautions Nil.

Legal category GSL.

Package quantities
Brāsivol No. 1 Fine. 70 g.
Brāsivol No. 2 Medium. 85 g.
Brāsivol No. 3 Coarse. 100 g.

Further information Brāsivol satisfies the patient's need to take an active part in the treatment of his condition but reduces to a minimum the desire for self-manipulation in the form of squeezing and picking of lesions.

Product licence numbers
Brāsivol No. 1 Fine   0174/5000
Brāsivol No. 2 Medium   0174/5001
Brāsivol No. 3 Coarse   0174/5002

DRICLOR*

Presentation Driclor is a clear colourless alcoholic solution containing Aluminium Chloride Hexahydrate USP 20% w/w.

Uses Driclor is indicated for the treatment of hyperhydrosis of the axillae, the hands and the feet.

Dosage and administration Apply Driclor last thing at night after drying the affected areas carefully. Wash off in the morning. Do not re-apply the product during the day.

Initially the product may be applied each night until sweating stops during the day. The frequency of application may then be reduced to twice a week. Subsequently if sweating is still absent the frequency of application may be reduced to once a week or in some cases less frequently.

Contra-indications, warnings, etc Ensure that the affected areas to be treated are perfectly dry. Do not bathe immediately before applying Driclor. Allow at least one hour following bathing.

Do not apply Driclor to broken or irritated skin. Do not shave armpits for 24 hours before or after using Driclor.

The reduction in sweating produced by Driclor may result in temporary irritation or redness. If this becomes excessive treatment should be stopped temporarily.

Keep away from the eyes.

Avoid direct contact with clothing and polished metal surfaces.

Pharmaceutical precautions Store upright in a cool place.

Replace cap tightly after use.

Inflammable – keep away from naked flame.

Legal category POM.

Package quantities 60ml in roll-on applicator plastic bottle.

Further information Driclor may cause irritation which is troublesome but not severe enough to warrant discontinuing its use. In these circumstances the irritation may be alleviated by the use of a weak corticosteroid cream.

Product licence number 0174/0044.

DUOFILM*

Presentation Duofilm is a clear mobile liquid containing:

Salicylic Acid BP   16.7% w/w
Lactic Acid BP   16.7% w/w
in Flexible Collodion BP.

Uses Duofilm is for topical application only and is indicated in the treatment of plantar and mosaic warts.

Dosage and administration The patient should be instructed as follows:

1. Soak warts in hot water for five minutes.
2. Rub surface of warts carefully with pumice stone or manicure emery board.
3. Apply Duofilm taking care to avoid normal skin.
4. Allow to dry thoroughly and cover with plaster if wart is large or on the foot.
5. Continue treatment until the wart is completely cleared and ridge lines of the skin have been restored.

Contra-indications, warnings, etc Duofilm is a product formulated for the controlled corrosion of keratin. Care must be taken to apply the product to the wart only. Avoid applying to normal skin.

Duofilm should not be used on the face or anogenital regions.

Pharmaceutical precautions Store upright in a cool place.

Replace cap tightly after use.

Highly inflammable – keep away from naked flame.

Legal category P.

Package quantities Duofilm is available in an amber screw-capped applicator bottle containing 15 ml.

Further information Nil.

Product licence number 0174/0025.

LACTICARE*

Presentation Lacticare contains lactic acid 5% w/w and sodium pyrrolidone carboxylate 2.5% w/w in an oil-in-water viscous lotion base.

Uses Lacticare is indicated for the symptomatic relief of hyperkeratotic and other chronic dry skin conditions and for dry skin conditions caused by low humidity or the use of detergents.

Dosage and administration Use as required on affected areas. Shake well before use.

Contra-indications, warnings, etc Occasionally a transient mild stinging sensation may occur. Should prolonged irritation develop when used on abraded or inflamed skin, discontinue use.

Keep away from the eyes and mucous membranes. Should contact with the eyes occur, remove with water.

Pharmaceutical precautions Nil.

Legal category P.

Package quantities Bottles containing 150 ml.

Further information Nil.

Product licence number 0174/0038.

OILATUM* CREAM

Presentation Oilatum Cream is a white, oil-in-water cream containing Arachis Oil BP, 21% w/w. Impermeability is provided by the incorporation of 1% polyvinyl pyrrolidone (PVPK 30) in the oil phase.

Mineral oil and lanolin are avoided.

Uses Oilatum Cream is indicated in cases of dry, sensitive skin, lanolin sensitivity, alkali intolerance, ichthyosis and similar conditions.

The use of Oilatum Cream in such conditions reduces moisture loss from the stratum corneum and thus restores skin flexibility.

The use of an inert plastic in the oil phase ensures a continuous residual film which tends to be more occlusive and longer-lasting than ordinary vegetable oil films.

Dosage and administration Oilatum Cream may be used as often as required. Apply to the affected area and rub in well. It is especially effective immediately after washing, when the normal acid condition of the skin may be disturbed and when the sebum content of the stratum corneum may be depleted.

Contra-indications, warnings, etc Nil.

Pharmaceutical precautions Nil.

Legal category P.

Package quantities Oilatum Cream is available in tubes containing 40 g and 80 g.

Further information The rapid symptomatic relief obtainable with Oilatum Cream is achieved by the use of an oil-in-water cream which provides a higher moisture content than is possible with water-in-oil preparations. After the evaporation and absorption of the water phase, the residual oil droplets coalesce to form an occlusive film.

Product licence number 0174/5014.

OILATUM* EMOLLIENT

Presentation Oilatum Emollient is a bath additive producing an emulsion of dispersed oil in the bath water and a homogeneous film on the surface. Active ingredients:

Acetylated wool alcohols	5.0% w/w
Liquid paraffin	63.4% w/w

Uses Oilatum Emollient is indicated in the treatment of contact dermatitis, atopic dermatitis, senile pruritus, ichthyosis and related dry skin conditions. Oilatum Emollient replaces oil and water and hydrates the keratin. Oilatum Emollient is particularly suitable for infant bathing. The preparation also overcomes the problem of cleansing the skin in conditions where the use of soaps, soap substitutes and colloid or oat-meal baths proves irritating.

Dosage and administration Oilatum Emollient should always be used with water, either added to water or applied to wet skin.

Adult bath: Add 1–3 capfuls to an 8 inch bath of water. Soak for 10–20 minutes. Pat dry.

Infant bath: Add ½–2 capfuls to a basin of water. Apply gently over entire body with a sponge. Pat dry.

Skin cleansing: Rub a small amount of oil into wet skin. Rinse and pat dry.

Where conditions permit, and particularly in cases of extensive areas of dry skin, Oilatum Emollient should be used as a bath oil, ensuring complete coverage by immersion. In addition to the therapeutic benefits, this method of use provides a means of sedating tense patients, particularly relevant in cases of acute pruritic dermatoses where relaxation of tension appears to relieve symptoms.

Contra-indications, warnings, etc The patient should be advised to use care to avoid slipping in the bath.

Pharmaceutical precautions Nil.

Legal category P.

Package quantities Oilatum Emollient is available in bottles containing 150 ml, 350 ml and 1 litre.

Further information Nil.

Product licence number 0174/5010.

PANOXYL* 5
PANOXYL* 10

Presentation White viscous gels containing benzoyl peroxide 5 and 10% w/w in an ethanolic base.

Uses PanOxyl 5 and 10 are each indicated for use in

the treatment of acne vulgaris. Benzoyl peroxide provides control of acne through its antibacterial action and also has a drying and desquamative effect, enhanced by the gel base.

Dosage and administration Treatment should normally commence with PanOxyl 5. Apply the gel to the affected areas once daily. Washing prior to application greatly enhances the efficacy of the preparation. The reaction of the skin to benzoyl peroxide differs in individual patients, and for this reason the higher percentage of benzoyl peroxide in PanOxyl 10 may be required in order to provide a satisfactory drying and desquamative action.

Contra-indications, warnings, etc PanOxyl 5 and 10 should not be prescribed for patients with a known hypersensitivity to benzoyl peroxide. Application to sensitive areas such as the neck should be made with caution; to avoid irritation there should be no contact with eyes, mouth and other mucous membranes.

In normal use, a mild burning sensation will probably be felt on first application and a moderate reddening and peeling of the skin will occur within a few days. During the first few weeks of treatment a sudden increase in peeling will occur in most patients; this is not harmful and will normally subside in a day or two if treatment is temporarily discontinued.

PanOxyl 5 and PanOxyl 10 may bleach dyed fabrics.

Pharmaceutical precautions Store in a cool place.

Legal category P.

Package quantities PanOxyl 5 and PanOxyl 10 are supplied in tubes each containing 40 g.

Further information Nil.

Product licence numbers
PanOxyl 5   0174/0019
PanOxyl 10   0174/0020

PANOXYL AQUAGEL* 2.5
PANOXYL AQUAGEL* 5
PANOXYL AQUAGEL* 10

Presentation White viscous gels containing benzoyl peroxide 2.5, 5 and 10% w/w in an aqueous, non alcoholic base.

Uses PanOxyl Aquagel 2.5, 5 and 10 are each indicated for use in the topical treatment of acne vulgaris.

Benzoyl peroxide provides control of acne through its antibacterial action and also has a drying and desquamative effect.

Dosage and administration Treatment should normally begin with PanOxyl Aquagel 2.5. Apply to the affected areas once daily. Washing prior to application enhances the efficacy of the preparation.

The reaction of the skin to benzoyl peroxide differs in individual patients. The higher concentration in PanOxyl Aquagel 5 or 10 may be required to produce a satisfactory response.

Contra-indications, warnings, etc PanOxyl Aquagel should not be prescribed for patients with a known hypersensitivity to benzoyl peroxide.

Avoid contact with the eyes, mouth and mucous membranes. Care should be taken when applying the product to the neck and other sensitive areas. In normal use, a mild burning sensation will probably be felt on first

application and a moderate reddening and peeling of the skin will occur within a few days. During the first weeks of treatment a sudden increase in peeling will occur in most patients, this is not harmful and will normally subside within a day or two if treatment is temporarily discontinued. If excessive irritation, redness or peeling occurs discontinue use.

These products may bleach dyed fabrics.

Pharmaceutical precautions Store in a cool place.

Legal category P.

Package quantities Tubes of 40 g.

Further information Nil.

Product licence numbers
PanOxyl Aquagel 2.5   0174/0049
PanOxyl Aquagel 5   0174/0050
PanOxyl Aquagel 10   0174/0051

PANOXYL* WASH

Presentation A white viscous lotion containing benzoyl peroxide 10% w/w.

Uses PanOxyl Wash is a skin cleanser for use in the topical treatment of acne vulgaris.

Benzoyl peroxide provides control of acne through its antibacterial action and also has a drying and desquamative effect.

Dosage and administration Wet the affected area with water and wash thoroughly with PanOxyl Wash. Rinse well with warm water, then rinse with cold water. Pat dry with a clean towel. Use once a day, preferably in the morning.

Contra-indications, warnings, etc PanOxyl Wash should not be prescribed for patients with a known hypersensitivity to benzoyl peroxide.

Avoid contact with the eyes, mouth and mucous membranes. Care should be taken when using the product on the neck and other sensitive areas. After a few days, the area being treated may show mild to moderate redness or peeling.

PanOxyl Wash can cause bleaching of dyed fabrics, such as towels. It is important to emphasise thorough rinsing with water after use.

Pharmaceutical precautions Store in a cool place.

Legal category P.

Package quantity 150 ml in a dispenser bottle.

Further information PanOxyl Wash can be used in conjunction with PanOxyl or PanOxyl Aquagel, or with other acne therapy.

Product licence number 0174/0048

POLYTAR* EMOLLIENT

Presentation Polytar Emollient is a concentrated tar bath additive containing a unique combination of tars. The ingredients are as follows:

Tar BP	7.5% w/w
Cade Oil BPC 1973	7.5% w/w
Coal Tar Solution USP	2.5% w/w
Arachis oil extract of crude coal tar	7.5% w/w
Liquid Paraffin	35% w/w

Uses Polytar Emollient is indicated in the treatment of psoriasis, eczema, atopic and pruritic dermatoses. The use of Polytar Emollient may be combined with ultraviolet radiation and other adjunctive therapy.

Polytar Emollient is also of value in removing loose psoriatic scales and paste following dithranol treatment.

Dosage and administration Two to four capfuls of Polytar Emollient should be added to an 8 inch bath and the patient instructed to soak for 20 minutes.

Contra-indications, warnings, etc Patients should be instructed to guard against slipping when entering or leaving the bath.

If irritation occurs and persists, discontinue use.

Pharmaceutical precautions Nil.

Legal category GSL.

Package quantities Polytar Emollient is available in bottles of 350 ml and 1 litre.

Further information Studies have confirmed that Polytar Emollient ranks highly in terms of patient acceptability.

Polytar Emollient is prescribable on FP10 for the treatment of psoriasis, eczema, atopic and pruritic dermatoses.

Product licence number 0174/5011.

POLYTAR* LIQUID

Presentation Polytar Liquid is a concentrated, antiseptic, tar-medicated scalp cleanser adjusted to pH 5.5, containing the following active ingredients:

Tar BP	0.3% w/w
Cade Oil BPC 1973	0.3% w/w
Coal Tar Solution USP	0.1% w/w
Arachis Oil extract of crude coal tar	0.3% w/w
Oleyl Alcohol	1.00% w/w

Uses Polytar Liquid is indicated in the treatment of scalp disorders such as psoriasis, dandruff, seborrhoea, eczema and pruritus. Polytar Liquid is also of value in the removal of ointments and pastes used in the treatment of psoriasis.

Dosage and administration The hair should be wetted and sufficient Polytar Liquid applied to produce an abundant lather. The scalp and adjacent areas should be vigorously massaged with the fingertips. The hair should then be thoroughly rinsed and the procedure repeated.

Polytar Liquid should be used once or twice weekly.

Contra-indications, warnings, etc Nil.

Pharmaceutical precautions Nil.

Legal category GSL.

Package quantities Polytar Liquid is available in bottles of 65 ml, 150 ml, 350 ml and 1 litre.

Further information Polytar Liquid is prescribable on FP10 for psoriasis, eczema and seborrhoea of the scalp and dandruff.

Product licence number 0174/5016.

POLYTAR PLUS*

Presentation Polytar Plus is a concentrated antiseptic, tar medicated scalp cleanser containing the following active ingredients:

Tar BP	0.3% w/w
Cade Oil BPC 1973	0.3% w/w
Coal Tar Solution USP	0.1% w/w
Arachis Oil extract of crude coal tar	0.3% w/w
Oleyl Alcohol	1.0% w/w
Hydrolysed Animal Protein	3.0% w/w

Uses Polytar Plus is indicated in the treatment of scalp disorders such as dandruff, psoriasis, seborrhoea, eczema and pruritus. Polytar Plus is also of value in the removal of ointments and pastes used in the treatment of psoriasis.

Dosage and administration The hair should be wetted and sufficient Polytar Plus applied to produce an abundant lather. The scalp and adjacent areas should be vigorously massaged with the fingertips. The hair should then be thoroughly rinsed and the procedure repeated.

Polytar Plus should be used once or twice weekly.

Contra-indications, warnings, etc Nil.

Pharmaceutical precautions Nil.

Legal category P.

Package quantities Polytar Plus is available in bottles of 150 ml and 350 ml.

Further information Polytar Plus is prescribable on FP10 for psoriasis, eczema and seborrhoea of the scalp and for dandruff.

Product licence number 0174/0037.

SPECTRABAN* 4

Presentation SpectraBAN 4 contains Padimate O 3.2% w/w in an ethanolic base. The product, which is non-greasy and invisible on the skin, is blue in colour.

Uses SpectraBAN 4 is a protective sunscreen lotion indicated in patients at risk from exposure to ultraviolet light within the UVB wavelength range (280–315 nanometres). It is this narrow waveband of ultraviolet light which is responsible for burning and tanning of the skin in man. Use of the product should allow 4 times normal exposure to sunlight before burning.

SpectraBAN 4 is indicated in sun-sensitive conditions such as polymorphic light eruptions and solar urticaria and any condition made worse by UVB light such as lupus erythematosus.

Dosage and administration Apply carefully and evenly to areas to be exposed or protected only by light clothing. Allow to dry before dressing. Allow 45 minutes before swimming or sweat producing exercise. A single application may give day long protection but the product should be re-applied during prolonged sunning or after swimming or excessive sweating.

Contra-indications, warnings, etc Sunscreen preparations occasionally produce a sensitivity reaction. Treatment should be discontinued if a skin rash or irritation develops. Do not apply to broken skin. Avoid contact with the eyes, mouth and other mucous membranes.

Pharmaceutical precautions Avoid flame.

Legal category P.

Package quantities SpectraBAN 4 is available in bottles containing 150 ml.

Further information SpectraBAN 4 is prescribable on FP 10 for patients who require protection from ultraviolet radiation in photodermatoses.

Product licence number 0174/5013.

SPECTRABAN* 15

Presentation SpectraBAN 15 contains Padimate O 3.2% w/w and Para Aminobenzoic Acid USP 5% w/w in an ethanolic base. The product, which is non-greasy and invisible on the skin, is pink in colour.

Uses SpectraBAN 15 is a protective sunscreen lotion indicated in patients at risk from exposure to ultraviolet light within the UVB wavelength range (280–315 nanometres). It is this narrow waveband of ultraviolet light which is responsible for burning and tanning of the skin in man. Use of the product should allow 15 times normal exposure to sunlight before burning.

SpectraBAN 15 is indicated in sun-sensitive conditions such as polymorphic light eruptions and solar urticaria and any condition made worse by UVB light such as lupus erythematosus.

Dosage and administration Apply carefully and evenly to areas to be exposed or protected only by light clothing. Allow to dry before dressing. Allow 45 minutes before swimming or sweat producing exercise. A single application may give day long protection but the product should be re-applied during prolonged sunning or after swimming or excessive sweating.

Contra-indications, warnings, etc Sunscreen preparations occasionally produce a sensitivity reaction. Treatment should be discontinued if a skin rash or irritation develops. Do not apply to broken skin. Avoid contact with the eyes, mouth and other mucous membranes. The product can stain clothing and other items permanently.

Pharmaceutical precautions Avoid flame.

Legal category P.

Package quantities SpectraBAN 15 is available in bottles containing 150 ml.

Further information SpectraBAN 15 is prescribable on FP 10 for patients who require protection from ultraviolet radiation in photodermatoses.

Product licence number 0174/0035.

STIEDEX* ▼

Presentation Stiedex contains 0.25% w/w desoxymethasone in an oily cream base.

Uses Stiedex contains a potent corticosteroid, desoxymethasone.

Stiedex is indicated for the treatment of severe acute inflammatory and allergic conditions and for chronic skin disorders such as psoriasis which have proved intractable to other treatment.

Stiedex is indicated for short courses of treatment only, in view of the risks of adverse steroid effects which frequently occur with the continuous administration of potent steroids.

Dosage and administration Stiedex should be applied sparingly to the affected area and rubbed gently into the skin. Initially, application should be 2–3 times daily; as the condition of the skin improves it may be possible to reduce the frequency of administration.

Contra-indications, warnings, etc
Contra-indications: Stiedex is contra-indicated for the treatment of infants or young children. Stiedex is contra-indicated in primary infective diseases of the skin, especially tuberculous conditions, fungal and viral infections. Where bacterial infection complicates an inflammatory disorder, Stiedex should be used in conjunction with antibacterial therapy.

Stiedex is not suitable for use in the treatment of inflammatory disorders of the eye.

In pregnant animals, administration of corticosteroids can cause abnormalities of foetal development. Although the relevance of this finding to human beings has not been established, Stiedex should not be used in pregnancy.

Precautions: The continuous administration of topical steroids over prolonged periods may result in adrenal suppression. The use of occlusive dressings is not recommended in view of the risks of significant steroid absorption.

The prolonged administration of potent corticosteroids may diminish skin collagen and cause subcutaneous atrophy; thinning of the epidermal layer and dilation of superficial blood vessels may occur, especially when corticosteroids are used on the face.

Warning: The product is a potent corticosteroid formulation with a greater likelihood of causing the adverse effects commonly associated with these preparations.

Pharmaceutical precautions Stiedex should be stored in a cool, dry place in containers similar to those of the manufacturer.

Legal category POM.

Package quantities Stiedex is available in tubes of 30 g.

Further information Stiedex contains no preservative. Stiedex may be diluted with Oily Cream BP.

Product licence number 0174/0052.

STIEDEX* LP ▼

Presentation Stiedex LP contains 0.05% w/w desoxymethasone in an oily cream base.

Uses Stiedex LP contains a potent corticosteroid and is indicated for the treatment of a wide range of acute inflammatory and allergic conditions, and chronic skin disorders.

Stiedex LP is specifically indicated for the treatment of eczema (including atopic, seborrhoeic and nummular eczema), intertrigo, psoriasis, pompholyx, lichen planus and discoid lupus erythematosus; acute and chronic allergic dermatoses, neurodermatitis; erythroderma, and may also be used in the non-specific treatment of sunburn, insect bites and anogenital pruritus.

Dosage and administration Stiedex LP should be applied sparingly to the affected area and rubbed gently into the skin. Initially, application should be made 2–3 times daily and the frequency of administration reduced as the conditions subsides.

Stiedex LP may be applied under an occlusive dressing. The affected area should be thoroughly cleansed prior to administration of cream and dressing to prevent infection.

Contra-indications, warnings, etc
Contra-indications: Stiedex LP is not suitable for infants and young children. Stiedex LP is contra-indicated in primary infective diseases of the skin. In particular, tuberculous, fungal and viral infections (e.g. herpes simplex and zoster, viral warts) should not be treated with topical corticosteroids. Where bacterial infection complicates an inflammatory disorder, Stiedex LP should be used in conjunction with appropriate anti-bacterial therapy, or Stiedex LPN used.

Stiedex LP is not suitable for use in the treatment of inflammatory disorders of the eye.

In pregnant animals, administration of corticosteroids can cause abnormalities of foetal development. The relevance of this finding to human beings has not been established. However, topical steroids should not be used extensively in pregnancy.

Precautions: The continuous administration of topical steroids over prolonged periods may result in adrenal suppression; in infants and children, this may cause growth retardation. The use of occlusive dressings enhances the absorption of the active substance, desoxymethasone, and in consequence systemic effects are more likely to occur. Adrenal suppression is unlikely in short courses of treatment or with doses not exceeding 10 g daily.

Prolonged administration of potent corticosteroids has been shown also to cause a reduction in skin collagen and subcutaneous atrophy, resulting in striae, thinning and dilation of superficial blood vessels. These changes are particularly liable to occur on the face.

Pharmaceutical precautions Stiedex LP should be stored in a cool, dry place, in containers similar to those of the manufacturer.

Legal category POM.

Package quantities Stiedex LP is available in tubes of 30 g.

Further information Stiedex LP contains no preservative. Stiedex LP may be diluted with Oily Cream BP.

Product licence number 0174/0053.

STIEDEX* LPN ▼

Presentation Stiedex LPN contains 0.05% w/w desoxymethasone and 0.5% w/w neomycin (as the sulphate) in an oily cream base.

Uses Stiedex LPN contains a potent corticosteroid and is indicated for the treatment of a wide range of acute inflammatory and allergic conditions, and chronic skin disorders. Neomycin sulphate is a broad spectrum antibiotic effective against the majority of bacteria commonly associated with skin infections.

Stiedex LPN is specifically indicated for the treatment of steroid-responsive dermatoses complicated by bacterial infection. Such conditions would include eczema (atopic, seborrhoeic and nummular), intertrigo, psoriasis, pompholyx, lichen planus and discoid lupus erythematosus; acute and chronic allergic dermatoses, neurodermatitis; and erythroderma, and may also be used in the non-specific treatment of insect bites, sunburn, and anogenital pruritus.

Dosage and administration Stiedex LPN should be applied sparingly to the affected area and rubbed gently into the skin. Initially, application should be made 2–3 times daily and the frequency of administration reduced as the conditions subside.

In the treatment of more resistant lesions, the effect of Stiedex LPN may be enhanced by application of occlusive dressings. The effected area should be thoroughly cleansed prior to administration of cream and dressing.

Contra-indications, warnings, etc
Contra-indications: Stiedex LPN is not suitable for infants and young children. Stiedex LPN is contra-indicated in the treatment of rosacea, acne, and perioral dermatitis, and should not be applied in the region of the external auditory meatus when the eardrum is perforated, because of the risk of ototoxicity.

Stiedex LPN is not suitable for use in the treatment of inflammatory disorders of the eye.

Stiedex LPN should not be used in the treatment of tuberculous, fungal or viral infections of the skin, in which conditions topical corticosteroids are contra-indicated.

Stiedex LPN should not be used for patients known to be allergic to neomycin.

In pregnant animals, administration of corticosteroids can cause abnormalities of foetal development. The relevance of this finding to human beings has not been established. However, topical steroids should not be used extensively in pregnancy.

Precautions: The continuous administration of topical steroids over prolonged periods may result in adrenal suppression; in infants and children, this may cause growth retardation. The use of occlusive dressings enhances the absorption of the active substance, desoxymethasone, and in consequence systemic effects are more likely to occur. Adrenal suppression is unlikely in short courses of treatment or with doses not exceeding 10 g daily.

Prolonged administration of potent corticosteroids has been shown also to cause a reduction in skin collagen and subcutaneous atrophy, resulting in striae, thinning and dilation of superficial blood vessels. These changes are particularly liable to occur on the face.

Pharmaceutical precautions Stiedex LPN should be stored in a cool, dry place, in containers similar to those of the manufacturer.

Legal category POM.

Package quantities Stiedex LPN is available in tubes of 15 g.

Further information Stiedex LPN contains no preservative.

Product licence number 0174/0054.

ZEASORB* POWDER

Presentation ZeaSORB is an off-white, highly absorbent, soft, antiseptic dusting powder containing the following:

Finely pulverised maize core	45% w/w
Chloroxylenol BPC	0.5% w/w
Aluminium dihydroxyallantoinate	0.2% w/w

Uses Intertrigo, hyperhidrosis, bromidrosis, prevention of tinea pedis and any other condition in which the absorption of fluid from the surface of the skin is desirable.

Dosage and administration The affected areas should be dried as thoroughly as possible before applying ZeaSORB Powder. The powder should be smoothed over the surface of the skin, between joints and in folds.

Contra-indications, warnings, etc Nil.

Pharmaceutical precautions Store in a cool dry place.

Legal category P.

Package quantities ZeaSORB Powder is available in sifter-top plastic containers of **30 g.**

Further information ZeaSORB Powder is non-caking and remains soft on saturation, preventing irritation.

Product licence number 0174/5015.

*Trade Mark

Stuart Pharmaceuticals Limited
50 Alderley Road
Wilmslow
Cheshire SK9 1RE

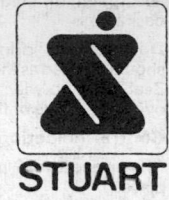

STUART

ANTASIL* LIQUID AND TABLETS

Presentation Antasil is presented as a white liquid and as white tablets, marked Stuart.

Each 5 ml of liquid contains Dried Aluminium Hydroxide Gel USP 400 mg, Magnesium Hydroxide USP 400 mg and Activated Polydimethylsiloxane 150 mg.

Each tablet contains Dried Aluminium Hydroxide Gel USP 400 mg, Magnesium Hydroxide USP 400 mg and Activated Polydimethylsiloxane 250 mg.

Uses As an antacid/deflatulent for symptomatic treatment of peptic ulcer, dyspepsia of functional or organic origin, heartburn in hiatus hernia or pregnancy, flatulence and abdominal distension, gastritis, oesophagitis and other conditions where hyperacidity or flatulence may be present.

Dosage and administration *Adults including the elderly:* Antasil liquid – 5–30 ml as required, preferably between meals and at bedtime. Antasil tablets – one or two to be sucked or chewed as required, preferably between meals and at bedtime.

Contra-indications, warnings, etc
Contra-indications: There is no known contra-indication.

Precautions: Care should be taken in patients suffering from hypophosphataemia. It is probably wise to avoid any drug, including antacids, during the first trimester of pregnancy unless there are compelling reasons for their use.

Aluminium hydroxide may form a complex with tetracyclines and reduce absorption when given concomitantly.

Although the antacids in Antasil are balanced to minimise bowel reaction, mild diarrhoea may be experienced at high doses.

Pharmaceutical precautions Store at room temperature.

Legal category P.

Package quantities Antasil liquid is supplied in bottles containing 350 ml and the tablets in cartons of 60 (6 strips of 10 tablets).

Further information The antacids in Antasil are balanced to minimise bowel reaction. Activated Polydimethylsiloxane assists in breaking down bubble-trapped gas, allowing the antacids to disperse quickly reducing hyperacidity and protecting the gastric mucosa from the inflammatory effect of high acid levels.

Product licence numbers
Tablets   0029/0118
Liquid   0029/0119

DISADINE* DP (DRY POWDER SPRAY)

Presentation Disadine DP is presented in an aerosol can which dispenses a brown powder. It is a dry powder spray containing 0.5% Povidone Iodine USP in BP propellants.

Uses Disadine DP is a wide-spectrum antiseptic for topical use. It presents all the bactericidal, fungicidal and virucidal properties of iodine with little if any risk of the skin sensitisation associated with elemental iodine. Disadine DP is indicated for topical application in the treatment and prevention of infection in wounds, including burns, varicose ulcers and bed sores.

Dosage and administration *All age groups:* The aerosol can of Disadine DP must be shaken before use. The area requiring treatment is sprayed from a distance of 6–10 inches (15–25 cm) until a light dusting of powder is deposited. When dry this forms a protective antiseptic layer over the area which has been sprayed.

Contra-indications, warnings, etc Care must be taken when Disadine DP is used on known iodine-sensitive subjects, although these do not normally react to povidone iodine.

Disadine DP must not be used on patients with non-toxic nodular colloid goitre.

In very rare cases Disadine DP may produce skin reactions with iodine-sensitive subjects. These reactions subside on cessation of treatment.

Avoid getting the powder into the eyes or nose.

Prolonged treatment with Disadine DP should be avoided in pregnant or lactating women; absorbed iodine can cross the placental barrier and is secreted into breast milk.

In cases of overdosage, treatment must be symptomatic.

Povidone iodine can be absorbed systemically during the topical treatment of burns, the degree of absorption being proportional to the depth and extent of the burn. Prolonged treatment with povidone iodine of patients with severe and extensive burns may cause metabolic acidosis, hypernatraemia, and renal impairment. In patients at risk Disadine DP should be used with caution. Excessively high serum levels may be reduced by haemodialysis. Absorption of povidine iodine may interfere with thyroid function tests by causing an increase in protein bound iodine levels.

Pharmaceutical precautions Store at room temperature. The aerosol can must be stored away from direct heat and sunlight and must not be autoclaved. The product should be used directly from the aerosol container. The container must not be punctured or destroyed by burning, even when empty.

Legal category P.

Package quantities Disadine DP is supplied in a 150 g aerosol can.

Further information Nil.

Product licence number 0029/5903.

DISPRAY* 1 QUICK PREP

Presentation Dispray 1 Quick Prep is supplied in a printed tin-plate aerosol can which dispenses a colourless liquid containing 0.5% w/v chlorhexidine gluconate (equivalent to 2.5% v/v Chlorhexidine Gluconate Solution BP) in 70% w/w total alcohols (as industrial methylated spirit) with BP propellant.

Uses Dispray 1 is a powerful disinfectant used for rapid disinfection of the skin before operations, subcutaneous or intramuscular injections or before venepuncture.

Dosage and administration *All age groups:* Dispray 1 Quick Prep is sprayed on to the surface to be disinfected from a distance of 4–8 inches (10–20 cm).

Contra-indications, warnings, etc
Contra-indications: Dispray 1 is contra-indicated for patients who have previously shown a hypersensitivity reaction to chlorhexidine. However, such reactions are extremely rare.

Precautions: For external use only. Keep out of the eyes and avoid contact with brain, meninges, or middle ear. Do not use in body cavities.

Side-effects: Irritative skin reactions can occasionally occur. Generalised allergic reactions to chlorhexidine have also been reported but are extremely rare.

Accidental ingestion: As the product is supplied in an aerosol can, it is unlikely that a significant amount will be ingested.

Pharmaceutical precautions Flammable. Store at room temperature. The aerosol can must be stored away from direct heat and sunlight and must not be autoclaved. The container must not be punctured or destroyed by burning even when empty.

The product should be used directly from its container. Hypochlorite bleaches may cause the development of brown stains in fabrics which have previously been in contact with chlorhexidine preparations. Oxidising bleaches such as sodium perborate should be used.

Legal category P.

Package quantities Dispray 1 Quick Prep is supplied as an aerosol can containing 400 ml.

Further information Nil.

Product licence number 0029/5900.

IODOSORB*

Presentation Sachets of sterile cadexomer iodine, a dry yellow-brown powder of modified starch gel microbeads containing Iodine PhEur at a concentration of 0.9% w/w for topical application.

Uses Treatment of chronic leg ulcers associated with venous disease. Treatment of decubitus ulcers. When applied to venous or decubitus ulcers, Iodosorb cleans and reduces bacterial counts at the ulcer surface, reduces pain, stimulates granulation and accelerates healing.

Dosage and administration *Adults including the elderly:* Iodosorb is applied to the wound surface to a minimum depth of 3 mm and covered with a dry, sterile non-adherent dressing. The dressing should be changed daily or when the Iodosorb has become saturated with wound exudate. Each time the dressing is changed and at the end of treatment, the remaining Iodosorb should be gently washed from the ulcer surface either with a stream of sterile water or with a wet sterile swab.

To avoid the risk of cross-contamination, it is recommended that a sachet of Iodosorb be confined to the treatment of a single patient per day.

Iodosorb is a dressing for the wound and has no influence on the underlying disturbance of circulatory function. Where considered appropriate, support bandages or stockings can be applied in conjunction with the use of Iodosorb.

Contra-indications, warnings, etc
Contra-indications: As Iodosorb contains 0.9% iodine, it should not be used in patients with known or suspected iodine sensitivity.

Warnings: Iodine is absorbed systemically especially when large ulcers are treated. The use of Iodosorb should be avoided in pregnant or lactating women; absorbed iodine can cross the placental barrier and is secreted into breast-milk.

Precautions: Systemic absorption of iodine should be taken into consideration if the thyroid function of a patient is under investigation. It has been observed occasionally that an adherent crust can form when the dressing is not changed with sufficient frequency. These crusts can be softened during dressing changes.

Side-effects: Some patients experience a transient smarting sensation during the first hour after application of Iodosorb. Mild erythema without sensitisation has also been reported.

Pharmaceutical precautions Iodosorb should be stored at room temperature protected from moisture.

Legal category POM.

Package quantities Unit dose sachet of 3 g in boxes of 7 sachets.

Further information On contact with wound exudate 1 g Iodosorb absorbs up to 6 ml of fluid removing exudate, pus and debris from the wound surface. Iodine is physically immobilised within the matrix of the dry Iodosorb and is slowly released in an active form during uptake of wound fluid. This mechanism of release provides antibacterial activity both at the wound surface and within the formed gel. The formed gel can be removed with a stream of water without damaging the fragile new epithelium beneath.

Product licence number 0029/0165.

KALTEN*

Presentation Hard gelatin capsules with opaque red caps and opaque cream bodies.

Each capsule is imprinted KALTEN and with the Stuart logo in black. Each capsule contains atenolol 50 mg, hydrochlorothiazide 25 mg and amiloride hydrochloride

BP (dihydrate) 2.85 mg (equivalent to amiloride hydrochloride 2.5 mg).

Uses Management of hypertension.

Mode of action: Kalten combines the antihypertensive effects of the cardioselective beta-adrenoceptor blocking drug atenolol (Tenormin*) and the diuretics hydrochlorothiazide and amiloride hydrochloride. The latter diuretic has potassium conserving properties.

Dosage and administration

Adults including the elderly: One capsule daily. Kalten is recommended for use in hypertensive patients where monotherapy with a beta-adrenoceptor blocker or diuretic proves inadequate. Where necessary another antihypertensive drug, such as a vasodilator, can be added. Patients can be transferred to preparations containing beta-adrenoceptor blocking drugs from other antihypertensive treatments with the exception of clonidine (see 'Warnings' below).

Kalten contains low effective doses of both a beta-adrenoceptor blocking agent and a combination of diuretics with a potassium-sparing action, and may be suited to older patients where higher doses of these drugs may be considered inappropriate.

Children: There is no paediatric experience with Kalten; therefore this is not recommended for use in children.

Contra-indications, warnings, etc

Contra-indications: Kalten should not be given to patients with second or third degree heart block, with hyperkalaemia (serum potassium over 5.5 mmol/L) or where potassium-sparing diuretics or potassium supplements are already being given. Kalten is contra-indicated in anuria, acute renal failure, severe progressive renal disease, diabetic nephropathy; patients with blood urea over 10 mmol/L or serum creatinine over 130 micro mol/L in whom serum electrolyte and blood urea levels cannot be monitored carefully and frequently.

In renal impairment, use of a potassium-conserving agent may result in rapid development of hyperkalaemia.

Kalten should not be given to those with prior sensitivity to hydrochlorothiazide or amiloride hydrochloride.

Precautions:

Cardiac: Special care should be taken with patients whose cardiac reserve is poor. Myocardial contractility must be maintained and signs of failure controlled with digitalis and diuretics.

One of the pharmacological actions of beta-adrenoceptor blocking drugs is to reduce heart rate. In the rare instance that symptoms may be attributable to the slow heart rate, the dose of the beta-adrenoceptor blocker may be reduced.

Obstructive airways disease: Kalten contains the cardioselective beta-adrenoceptor blocking drug atenolol and may therefore be used with caution in patients with chronic obstructive airways disease. However, occasionally some increase in airways resistance may occur in asthmatic patients. In contrast to that occurring with preparations containing non-selective beta-adrenoceptor blocking drugs, this bronchospasm may usually be reversed by commonly used dosage of bronchodilators such as salbutamol or isoprenaline.

Sudden withdrawal in ischaemic heart disease: Cessation of therapy with preparations containing a beta-adrenoceptor blocking drug in patients with ischaemic heart disease should be gradual.

Clonidine: Caution should be exercised when transferring patients from clonidine to beta-adrenoceptor blocking drugs. If beta-adrenoceptor blocking drugs and clonidine are given concurrently, clonidine should not be discontinued until several days after withdrawal of the beta-adrenoceptor blocking drug (also see prescribing information for clonidine).

Class I antidysrhythmic agents: Care should be taken in prescribing a beta-adrenoceptor blocking drug with Class 1 antidysrhythmic agents such as disopyramide.

Verapamil: Beta-adrenoceptor blocking drugs should be used with caution in combination with verapamil in patients with impaired ventricular function. The combination should not be given to patients with conduction abnormalities. Neither drug should be administered intravenously within 48 hours of discontinuing the other.

Lithium: Preparations containing lithium generally should not be given with diuretics because they may reduce its renal clearance.

Metabolic effects: Kalten, as with other preparations containing a potassium conserving diuretic, must be used with great caution in severely ill patients in whom metabolic or respiratory acidosis may occur (e.g. decompensated diabetes or cardiopulmonary disease). Acidosis may be associated with rapid increases in serum potassium. Kalten may be associated with minor increases in uric acid.

Measurement of potassium levels is appropriate, especially in the older patient, those receiving digitalis preparations for cardiac failure, taking abnormal (low in potassium) diet, or suffering from gastrointestinal complaints.

Diabetes: Kalten should be used with caution in diabetic patients, or those with a known pre-disposition to diabetes, particularly those with abnormal renal function. Hyperkalaemia has commonly occurred in diabetic patients on amiloride hydrochloride, especially those with chronic renal disease or pre-renal azotemia. The status of renal function should therefore be determined before Kalten is given to known or suspected diabetics. Lowering of glucose tolerance may occur and the insulin dosage of the diabetic patient may require adjustment.

Kalten should be discontinued at least 3 days before glucose tolerance testing. Kalten modifies the tachycardia of hypoglycaemia.

Hyponatraemia and hypochloraemia may occur, although the likelihood of hypochloraemic alkalosis is reduced. Any chloride deficiency may be corrected by ammonium chloride (except in hepatic disease) and largely prevented by a near normal salt intake.

Hepatic or renal impairment: Kalten should be used with caution in patients with renal or hepatic impairment and in those patients in whom fluid and electrolyte balance is critical. Hyperkalaemia or hypokalaemia may occur. Hyperkalaemia has been observed in patients receiving amiloride hydrochloride, particularly in the aged, in diabetics, and in hospital patients with hepatic cirrhosis or congestive heart failure, who had known renal impairment, were seriously ill, or were undergoing vigorous diuretic therapy. Such patients should be carefully observed for clinical, laboratory, and ECG evidence of hyperkalaemia (not always associated with an abnormal ECG). Should hyperkalaemia develop, discontinue treatment immediately, and if necessary, take active measures to reduce the serum potassium to normal.

Kalten should be used with caution in those with impaired renal function. Special care should be taken to avoid cumulative or toxic effects due to a reduced excretion of the components of Kalten. In addition, azotaemia may be precipitated or increased by hydro-chlorothiazide. If increasing azotaemia and oliguria occur, treatment should be discontinued.

In liver disease amiloride has been reported to precipitate hepatic encephalopathy, and deepening jaundice has also occurred in cirrhotic patients receiving amiloride.

Use in pregnancy and the nursing mother: As clinical experience is limited, Kalten is not recommended for use during pregnancy. Tenormin and thiazides appear in breast milk and also cross the placental barrier and appear in cord blood. In patients treated with Tenormin there were no apparent detrimental effects in the baby at birth or during breast feeding. However the use of Kalten where pregnancy is present or suspected requires that the benefits of the drug be weighed against possible hazards to the foetus. The hazards of thiazides include foetal or neonatal jaundice, thrombocytopenia, and possibly other side-effects that have occurred in the adult. If the use of the drug is deemed essential, the patient should stop nursing.

Anaesthesia: As with other preparations containing beta-adrenoceptor blocking drugs it may be decided to withdraw Kalten before surgery. In this case 48 hours should elapse between the last dose and anaesthesia. If treatment is continued, care should be taken when using anaesthetic agents such as ether, cyclopropane and trichloroethylene. Vagal dominance, if it occurs, may be corrected with atropine (1–2 mg iv).

Side-effects: With atenolol cold extremities, muscular fatigue and, in isolated cases, bradycardia may occur. Sleep disturbances of the type noted with other beta-adrenoceptor blocking drugs have rarely been reported.

There have been reports of skin rashes and/or dry eyes associated with the use of beta-adrenergic blocking drugs. The reported incidence is small and in most cases the symptoms have cleared when treatment was withdrawn. Discontinuance of the drug should be considered if any such reaction is not otherwise explicable and cessation of therapy should be gradual.

With amiloride hydrochloride and hydrochlorothiazide gastrointestinal effects including anorexia, nausea, vomiting, gastric irritation, cramps, pain, constipation and diarrhoea may occur. Dry mouth, thirst and paraesthesia, transient blurred vision, salivary gland inflammation, vertigo, fatigue, muscle cramps and orthostatic hypotension may also occur secondary to diuresis. Dizziness and headache may occur. Skin rashes with associated photosensitivity, necrotising vasculitis, acute pancreatitis and blood dyscrasias have been reported.

Treatment of overdosage/accidental and deliberate poisoning: Dehydration, electrolyte imbalance and hepatic coma are treated by the established procedures. There is no specific antidote. If ingestion is recent, emesis should be induced or gastric lavage performed. If hyperkalaemia occurs, active measures should be taken to reduce the serum potassium levels. For respiratory impairment, oxygen or artificial respiration should be administered.

Excessive bradycardia may be countered by atropine, 1–2 mg intravenously, and, if necessary this may be followed by a beta-adrenoceptor stimulant, such as isoprenaline 25 micrograms initially, or orciprenaline 0.5 mg given by slow intravenous injection. Care must be taken to ensure that the blood pressure does not fall too low if the dose of the beta-adrenoceptor agonist has to be increased.

Glucagon has also been found to be useful.

Pharmaceutical precautions Kalten capsules should be stored at room temperature, protected from light and moisture.

Legal category POM.

Package quantities Calendar packs of 28.

Further information When the combined antihypertensive effect of a beta-blocker and a potassium-conserving diuretic is required, Kalten is a simple, convenient and acceptable therapy which may be expected to improve patient compliance. The effect of Kalten following a one capsule oral dose is sustained for at least 24 hours.

Product licence number 0029/0186.

METOSYN* FAPG CREAM
METOSYN* OINTMENT

Presentation Metosyn consists of the corticosteroid fluocinonide presented as FAPG Cream and as Ointment. In Metosyn FAPG Cream, fluocinonide 0.05% w/w is dissolved completely in propylene glycol with fatty alcohols added to produce a white, homogeneous, semi-solid preparation. Metosyn Ointment contains fluocinonide 0.05% w/w completely dissolved in a petroleum base.

Uses Metosyn contains an effective topical corticosteroid, and is suitable for treating a wide variety of local inflammatory, pruritic and allergic disorders of the skin. It is indicated for topical application in the following conditions.

Eczema and dermatitis: Atopic eczema, seborrhoeic dermatitis, discoid eczema, pompholyx, contact dermatitis, neurodermatitis, intertrigo.

Non-specific ano-genital pruritus; prurigo. Psoriasis. Lichen planus. Discoid lupus erythematosus.

Metosyn FAPG Cream may be used for wet or dry lesions. Metosyn Ointment, with its emollient effects, is particularly suitable for dry scaly lesions.

Dosage and administration *All age groups:* A small quantity of Metosyn FAPG Cream or Metosyn Ointment should be applied three to four times daily to the affected area and massaged well in.

Once improvement is apparent, usage may be reduced to twice or even once daily.

It is recommended that Metosyn is used undiluted (see Pharmaceutical precautions).

Contra-indications, warnings, etc

Contra-indications: Metosyn is contra-indicated in rosacea, acne and peri-oral dermatitis, all of which can be treated with oral tetracyclines and hydrocortisone if a topical steroid is required. As with all topical steroids, Metosyn is contra-indicated in tuberculous, syphilitic, fungal and viral infections of the skin.

Precautions: Where there is bacterial infection associated with an inflammatory skin condition, Metosyn should only be administered if adequate antibacterial cover is also given. Topical administration of corticosteroids to pregnant animals has been shown to cause abnormalities of foetal development. Although the relevance of this finding to human application has not been established, when topical steroid treatment is considered necessary during pregnancy, both the amount applied and the length of treatment should be minimised. Long-term continuous topical steroid therapy should be avoided since adrenal suppression can occur, particularly when infants are being treated. Very occasionally hypersensitivity reactions may occur.

Side-effects: As with all topical steroids, striae may occur after extensive use of Metosyn. Occasionally a tingling or mild itching sensation may be noticed on application of FAPG Cream.

Overdosage: A 25 g tube of Metosyn FAPG Cream or Ointment contains 12.5 mg of fluocinonide. Toxic effects are not likely to occur following accidental oral ingestion. Similarly, the components of the vehicles, singly or collectively, have not been shown to produce toxic effects in these quantities.

Pharmaceutical precautions Metosyn should be stored in the original tube at room temperature. It is recommended that the product be used undiluted. However, if dilution of Metosyn Ointment is required, white soft paraffin should be used and special FAPG diluent should be used to dilute FAPG Cream.

Legal category POM.

Package quantities Tubes of 25 g and 100 g FAPG Cream.
Tubes of 25 g and 100 g Ointment.

Further information Metosyn FAPG Cream and Metosyn Ointment do not contain lanolin or parabens.

Product licence numbers
Metosyn FAPG Cream   0029/5071
Metosyn Ointment   0029/0133

METOSYN* SCALP LOTION

Presentation Metosyn Scalp Lotion is a clear, colourless, slightly viscous solution containing 0.05% w/v fluocinonide in a vehicle containing propylene glycol and ethanol.

Uses Steroid-responsive dermatoses of the scalp such as psoriasis, seborrhoeic dermatitis and severe dandruff.

Dosage and administration *All age groups:* A small quantity of Metosyn Scalp Lotion should be applied to the scalp morning and night until improvement is noticeable. Improvement may then be maintained with application once a day or less frequently. However, Metosyn Scalp Lotion should be prescribed for short courses of therapy and not used by patients on a continuous basis.

Contra-indications, warnings, etc
Contra-indications: Infections of the scalp. Hypersensitivity to the preparation.

Precautions: Care must be taken to keep Metosyn Scalp Lotion away from the eyes and it must not be used near a naked flame. Some patients may experience burning severe enough to warrant discontinuation of treatment.

If hypersensitivity develops treatment should be discontinued.

Long-term continuous therapy should be avoided particularly in infants and children, as adrenal suppression can occur even without occlusion.

Development of secondary infection requires withdrawal of therapy and commencement of appropriate antimicrobial therapy.

Topical administration of corticosteroids to pregnant animals has been shown to cause abnormalities of foetal development. The relevance of this finding to human application has not been established but, when topical steroid treatment is considered necessary during pregnancy, both the amount applied and the length of treatment should be minimised.

Side-effects: As with all topical steroids, treatment of large areas such as the scalp can allow sufficient absorption to give systemic steroidal effects. This is more likely with children or infants, where occlusive dressing is used or treatment is prolonged. Atrophic skin changes can take place on continued application.

A burning feeling may be noticed on application and this may, on occasion, warrant discontinuation of therapy.

Overdosage: A 30 ml bottle of Metosyn Scalp Lotion contains 15 mg of fluocinonide and 30% w/v ethanol. Toxic effects unlikely to occur following accidental oral ingestion.

Pharmaceutical precautions Metosyn Scalp Lotion should be stored in its original bottle at room temperature. The bottle should not be stored or opened near a naked flame. Use undiluted.

Legal category POM.

Package quantities Glass bottles containing 30 ml with plastic applicator.

Further information Nil.

Product licence number 0029/0163.

MONIT* TABLETS ▼

Presentation Monit tablets are white, round tablets imprinted 'Stuart 20' on one face and bisected on the reverse. Each tablet contains 20 mg isosorbide mononitrate.

Uses Prophylaxis of angina pectoris.

Mode of action: Isosorbide mononitrate is an active metabolite of isosorbide dinitrate and from an oral dose exerts qualitatively similar effects. However, unlike the dinitrate which is subject to extensive 'first pass' hepatic metabolism, it has virtually complete systemic availability from an oral dose. Isosorbide mononitrate thus achieves predictable and sustained blood levels. Onset of pharmacological effects occur within 20 minutes of an oral dose and are maintained for more than 8 hours.

Dosage and administration *Adults:* Usually one tablet twice or three times daily.

Patients already accustomed to prophylactic nitrate therapy (for example with isosorbide dinitrate) may normally be transferred directly to a therapeutic dose of Monit. For patients not receiving prophylactic nitrate therapy, it is recommended that the initial dose should be half a tablet twice daily. Maintenance dose in individual patients will be between 20 and 120 mg daily.

Elderly patients: Dosage requirements may be reduced, especially when hepatic or renal function is impaired.

The tablets should be swallowed whole with a little fluid.

Contra-indications, warnings, etc
Contra-indications: A known sensitivity to the drug or to isosorbide dinitrate.

Warnings: The following adverse effects may be seen with nitrate therapy:

1. Cutaneous vasodilation, headache, dizziness and weakness may occur. If headache is a problem, a temporary lowering of the Monit dose and the use of analgesics may be necessary. The incidence of these effects is highest at commencement of treatment and tends to decline with time.

2. Postural hypotension may occur, especially with high doses.

3. Nitrate preparations can act as physiological antagonists to noradrenaline, acetylcholine, histamine and other agents.

4. Dry rash and/or exfoliative dermatitis have been described rarely with isosorbide dinitrate and similar reactions might be expected occasionally.

Pregnancy and lactation: As with other drugs, nitrates should not be administered to pregnant women and nursing mothers unless essential.

Overdosage: Overdosage should be treated symptomatically. The main symptom is likely to be hypotension and this may be treated by elevation of the legs to promote venous return.

Pharmaceutical precautions Store at room temperature. Protect from moisture.

Legal category POM.

Package quantities Monit tablets are supplied in calendar packs of 56 tablets or bottles of 100 tablets.

Further information Isosorbide mononitrate is the British Approved Name for isosorbide-5-mononitrate.

Beta-blocking drugs have a different pharmacological action in angina and may have complementary effect co-administered with Monit.

Product licence number 0029/0174.

SORBICHEW*

Presentation Sorbichew tablets contain isosorbide dinitrate.

The chewable tablets are round, green, scored tablets embossed Stuart, each containing 5 mg isosorbide dinitrate.

Uses *Angina Pectoris:* Sorbichew tablets are to prevent or abort the acute attack.

Dosage and administration *Adults including the elderly:*

Treatment of the acute attack: Either one or two Sorbichew tablets should be chewed until dissolved completely and swallowed.

Prevention of an expected attack: Immediately prior to the stressful event either one or two Sorbichew tablets should be chewed until dissolved completely and swallowed.

Sorbichew tablets are scored for easier dose adjustment.

Contra-indications, warnings, etc
Contra-indications: A known sensitivity to the drug.

Warnings: The following adverse effects may be seen with isosorbide dinitrate.

1. Cutaneous vasodilation, headache, dizziness and weakness may occur. If headache is a problem, a temporary lowering of the dose, and the use of analgesics, may be necessary. In the majority of patients, headache diminishes or disappears after 1–3 weeks and optimum dosage may be achieved.

2. Postural hypotension.

3. The drug can act as a physiological antagonist to noradrenaline, acetylcholine, histamine and other agents.

4. Dry rash and/or exfoliative dermatitis may occasionally occur.

Pregnancy and lactation: As with other drugs, Nitrates should not be administered to pregnant women and nursing mothers unless essential.

Overdosage: Overdose should be treated symptomatically. The main symptom is likely to be hypotension and this may be treated by elevation of the legs to promote venous return.

Pharmaceutical precautions *Storage:* Although Sorbichew tablets are very stable and no special storage precautions are required, it is advised that in accordance with good pharmaceutical practice the tablets should be stored at room temperature protected from moisture.

Legal category P.

Package quantities Sorbichew: 5 mg chewable tablets are supplied in containers of 100 and 500.

Further information Unlike glyceryl trinitrate, Sorbichew tablets are very stable and therefore loss of potency when carried by the patient does not normally occur.

Sorbichew has an approximate onset of action of two minutes and duration of action up to two hours.

Product licence number
Sorbichew 5 mg   0029/0109

SORBID* S.A.

Presentation Sorbid S.A. tablets contain isosorbide dinitrate.

Sorbid S.A. tablets are yellow, round, flat, bevel-edged tablets, embossed 'Stuart' on one side and '880' on the reverse side. Each tablet contains 40 mg of isosorbide dinitrate; 10 mg for immediate release and 30 mg in a sustained action formulation.

Uses *Angina Prophylaxis:* The tablets are swallowed for protection against angina pectoris.

Dosage and administration *Adults:* 1–2 Sorbid S.A. tablets should be swallowed twice daily.

Elderly patients: Dosage requirements may be reduced, especially when hepatic or renal function is impaired.

Contra-indications, warnings, etc *Contra-indications:* A known sensitivity to the drug.

Warnings: The following adverse effects may be seen with isosorbide dinitrate.

1. Cutaneous vasodilation, headache, dizziness and weakness may occur. If headache is a problem, a temporary lowering of the Sorbid S.A. dose, and the use of analgesics, may be necessary. In the majority of patients, headache diminishes or disappears after 1–3 weeks and optimum dosage of Sorbid S.A. may be achieved.

2. Postural hypotension.

3. The drug can act as a physiological antagonist to noradrenaline, acetylcholine, histamine and other agents.

4. Dry rash and/or exfoliative dermatitis may occasionally occur.

Pregnancy and lactation: As with other drugs, Nitrates should not be administered to pregnant women and nursing mothers unless essential.

Overdosage: Overdose should be treated symptomatically. The main symptom is likely to be hypotension and this may be treated by elevation of the legs to promote venous return.

Pharmaceutical precautions *Storage:* Although Sorbid S.A. tablets are very stable and no special storage precautions are required, it is advised that in accordance with good pharmaceutical practice the tablets should be stored at room temperature protected from light and moisture.

Legal category P.

Package quantities Sorbid S.A. 40 mg tablets are supplied in containers of 60.

Further information Unlike glyceryl trinitrate. Sorbid S.A. tablets are very stable and therefore loss of potency when carried by the patient does not normally occur.

The duration of action of the Sorbid S.A. tablet is estimated to be up to 12 hours.

Product licence number
Sorbid S.A. tablets 40 mg   0029/0149

SORBITRATE*

Presentation Sorbitrate tablets contain isosorbide dinitrate. Sorbitrate tablets are available containing 10 mg and 20 mg isosorbide dinitrate. The 10 mg tablets are oval, yellow, scored tablets marked Stuart on one face and marked '780' on the reverse. The 20 mg tablets are oval, blue, scored tablets marked Stuart on one face and marked '820' on the reverse.

Uses *Angina Prophylaxis:* The tablets are taken orally for protection against angina pectoris.

Congestive Cardiac Failure: The tablets are taken as adjunctive therapy in the management of severe acute or chronic congestive cardiac failure.

Dosage and administration *Adults:*

Angina Prophylaxis: 10–40 mg, three or four times daily depending on individual requirement.

Congestive Cardiac Failure: In severe congestive cardiac failure Sorbitrate tablets may be taken in doses of 10–40 mg three or four times daily depending on patient requirements. In this situation optimal individual dose is best determined by continuous haemodynamic monitoring. The use of Sorbitrate in severe congestive cardiac failure should be considered adjunctive therapy to more conventional treatment (e.g. digitalis, diuretics, etc.).

Elderly patients: Dosage requirements may be reduced, especially when hepatic or renal function is impaired. The tablets are scored for easier dose adjustment.

Contra-indications, warnings, etc
Contra-indications: A known sensitivity to the drug.

Warnings: The following adverse effects may be seen with isosorbide dinitrate.

1. Cutaneous vasodilation, headache, dizziness and weakness may occur. If headache is a problem, a temporary lowering of the Sorbitrate dose, and the use of analgesics, may be necessary. In the majority of patients, headache diminishes or disappears after 1–3 weeks and optimum dosage of Sorbitrate may be achieved.

2. Postural hypotension.

3. The drug can act as a physiological antagonist to noradrenaline, acetylcholine, histamine and other agents.

4. Dry rash and/or exfoliative dermatitis may occasionally occur.

Pregnancy and lactation: As with other drugs, Nitrates should not be administered to pregnant women and nursing mothers unless essential.

Overdosage: Overdose should be treated symptomatically. The main symptom is likely to be hypotension and this may be treated by elevation of the patient's legs to promote venous return.

Pharmaceutical precautions *Storage:* Store at room temperature protected from moisture.

Legal category P.

Package quantities Sorbitrate tablets: 20 mg tablets are supplied in containers of 100.

10 mg tablets are supplied in containers of 100 and 500.

Further information Unlike glyceryl trinitrate, Sorbitrate tablets are very stable and therefore loss of potency when carried by the patient does not normally occur. The duration of action of the tablets is estimated to be four to six hours.

Product licence numbers
Sorbitrate Tablets 20 mg   0029/0145
Sorbitrate Tablets 10 mg   0029/0111

TENORETIC*

Presentation Tenoretic tablets are round, bi-convex, brown, film-coated tablets impressed TENORETIC on one face and with the Stuart logo on the reverse. The impressions are highlighted in white. Each tablet contains 100 mg atenolol and 25 mg chlorthalidone BP.

Uses Management of Hypertension.

Mode of action: Tenoretic combines the antihypertensive effects of the cardioselective beta-blocker atenolol (Tenormin*) and the diuretic chlorthalidone.

Dosage and administration *Adults:* One tablet daily. Most patients with hypertension will give a satisfactory response to a single tablet daily of Tenoretic. There is little or no further fall in blood pressure with increased dosage, and where necessary another antihypertensive drug, such as a vasodilator, can be added.

Elderly patients: Dosage requirements are often lower in this age group (see data sheet for Tenoret 50).

Children: There is no paediatric experience with Tenoretic, therefore this preparation is not recommended for children.

Contra-indications, warnings, etc
Contra-indications: Tenoretic should not be given to patients with second or third degree heart block.

Precautions: Cardiac: Special care should be taken with patients whose cardiac reserve is poor. Myocardial contractility must be maintained and signs of failure controlled with digitalis and diuretics.

Pulse rate: One of the pharmacological actions of beta-adrenoceptor blocking drugs is to reduce heart rate. In the rare instance when symptoms may be attributable to the slow heart rate the dose may be reduced.

Hypoglycaemia: Tenoretic modifies the tachycardia of hypoglycaemia.

Obstructive airways disease: Tenoretic contains the

cardioselective beta-adrenoceptor blocking drug atenolol and may be used with caution in patients with chronic obstructive airways disease. However, occasionally some increase in airways resistance may occur in asthmatic patients. In contrast to that occurring with non-selective beta-blockers, this bronchospasm may usually be reversed by commonly used dosage of bronchodilators such as salbutamol or isoprenaline.

Sudden withdrawal in ischaemic heart disease: In patients suffering from ischaemic heart disease, as with other beta-blocking agents, treatment should not be discontinued abruptly.

Clonidine: Caution should be exercised when transferring patients from clonidine to beta-adrenoceptor blocking drugs. If beta-adrenoceptor blocking drugs and clonidine are given concurrently, clonidine should not be discontinued until several days after withdrawal of the beta-adrenoceptor blocking drug. (See also prescribing information on clonidine.)

Class I antidysrhythmics: Care should be taken in prescribing a beta-adrenoceptor blocking drug with Class I antidysrhythmic agents such as disopyramide.

Verapamil: Beta-adrenoceptor blocking drugs should be used with caution in combination with verapamil in patients with impaired ventricular function. The combination should not be given to patients with conduction abnormalities. Neither drug should be administered intravenously within 48 hours of discontinuing the other.

Lithium: Preparations containing lithium generally should not be given with diuretics because they may reduce its renal clearance.

Metabolic effects: The metabolic effects of chlorthalidone are dose-related and, at the low dose contained in the Tenoretic tablet, are unlikely to be troublesome.

Potassium status: Tenoretic is associated with only minor changes in potassium status. Total body potassium is unaltered on chronic therapy and changes in serum potassium are minor and probably clinically unimportant. Thus, in cases of uncomplicated hypertension, concurrent potassium supplements should be unnecessary. Measurement of potassium levels is appropriate, especially in the older patient, those receiving digitalis preparations for cardiac failure, taking abnormal (low in potassium) diets, or suffering from gastro-intestinal complaints.

Serum uric acid: Tenoretic is generally associated with only a minor increase in serum uric acid. In cases of prolonged elevation the concurrent use of a uricosuric agent will reverse the hyperuricaemia.

Diabetes: Tenoretic contains chlorthalidone which may decrease glucose tolerance. During prolonged therapy regular tests for glycosuria should be carried out.

Renal impairment: In patients with severe renal impairment, a reduction in the daily dose or in frequency of administration may be necessary.

Sensitivity to chlorthalidone: Because Tenoretic contains chlorthalidone, care should be taken in patients with severe renal failure or with a history of sensitivity to chlorthalidone.

Pregnancy: Like other drugs Tenoretic should not be given during pregnancy unless its use is essential.

Anaesthesia: As with all preparations containing beta-adrenoceptor blocking drugs it may be decided to withdraw Tenoretic before surgery. In this case 48 hours should elapse between the last dose and anaesthesia. If treatment is continued care should be taken when using anaesthetic agents such as ether, cyclopropane and trichloroethylene. Vagal dominance, if it occurs, may be corrected with atropine (1–2 mg iv).

Side-effects: Tenoretic is well tolerated. Side effects associated with it are infrequent and generally mild.

Minor side effects include cold extremities, muscular fatigue and, in isolated cases, bradycardia. Sleep disturbances of the type noted with other beta-adrenoceptor blocking drugs have rarely been reported.

There have been reports of skin rashes and/or dry eyes associated with the use of beta-adrenergic blocking drugs. The reported incidence is small and in most cases the symptoms have cleared when treatment was withdrawn. Discontinuance of the drug should be considered if any such reaction is not otherwise explicable. Cessation of therapy with a beta-blocker should be gradual.

Nausea and dizziness have been reported occasionally with chlorthalidone and idiosyncratic drug reactions such as thrombocytopenia and leucopenia have occurred rarely.

Overdosage: Excessive bradycardia may be countered with atropine, 1–2 mg intravenously, followed, if necessary, by a beta-adrenoceptor stimulant, such as isoprenaline 25 micrograms initially or orciprenaline 0.5 mg, given by slow intravenous injection. Care must be taken to ensure that the blood pressure does not fall too low if the dose of beta-adrenoceptor agonist has to be increased.

Glucagon has also been reported to be useful as a cardiac stimulant in a dose of 10 mg intravenously.

Excessive diuresis should be countered by maintaining normal fluid and electrolyte balance.

Pharmaceutical precautions Tenoretic should be stored at room temperature, protected from light and moisture.

Legal category POM.

Package quantities Calendar packs of 28 tablets and blister packs of 30 tablets.

Further information When the combined antihypertensive effect of a beta-blocker and a diuretic is required, Tenoretic is a simple, convenient and acceptable therapy which may be expected to improve patient compliance. The effect of Tenoretic following a single oral dose is sustained for at least twenty-four hours.

Product licence number 0029/0139.

TENORET* 50 ▼

Presentation Tenoret 50 tablets are round, bi-convex, brown, film-coated tablets impressed TENORET 50 on one face and with the Stuart logo on the reverse. The impressions are highlighted in white. Each tablet contains 50 mg atenolol and 12.5 mg chlorthalidone BP.

Uses *Hypertension:* Particularly suited to the older patient. The combination of low effective doses of a beta-blocking drug and diuretic may be suited to older patients where full doses of both may be considered inappropriate.

Mode of action: Tenoret 50 combines the antihypertensive effects of the cardioselective beta-blocker atenolol (Tenormin) and the diuretic chlorthalidone.

Dosage and administration *Adults including the elderly:* One tablet daily. Older patients with hypertension who do not respond to low dose therapy with a single agent should have a satisfactory response to a single tablet daily of Tenoret 50. Where hypertensive control is not achieved addition of a small dose of a third agent, e.g. a vasodilator, may be appropriate.

Children: There is no paediatric experience with Tenoret 50, therefore this preparation is not recommended for children.

Contra-indications, warnings, etc

Contra-indications: Tenoret 50 should not be given to patients with second or third degree heart block.

Precautions: Cardiac: Special care should be taken with patients whose cardiac reserve is poor. Myocardial contractility must be maintained and signs of failure controlled with digitalis and diuretics.

Pulse rate: One of the pharmacological actions of beta-adrenoceptor blocking drugs is to reduce heart rate. In the rare instance when symptoms may be attributable to the slow heart rate the dose may be reduced.

Hypoglycaemia: Tenoret 50 modifies the tachycardia of hypoglycaemia.

Obstructive airways disease: Tenoret 50 contains the cardioselective beta-adrenoceptor blocking drug atenolol and may be used with caution in patients with chronic obstructive airways disease. However, occasionally some increase in airways resistance may occur in asthmatic patients. In contrast to that occurring with non-selective beta-blockers, this bronchospasm may usually be reversed by commonly used dosage of bronchodilators such as salbutamol or isoprenaline.

Sudden withdrawal in ischaemic heart disease: In patients suffering from ischaemic heart disease, as with other beta-blocking agents, treatment should not be discontinued abruptly.

Clonidine: Caution should be exercised when transferring patients from clonidine to beta-adrenoceptor blocking drugs. If beta-adrenoceptor blocking drugs and clonidine are given concurrently, clonidine should not be discontinued until several days after withdrawal of the beta-adrenoceptor blocking drug (see also prescribing information on clonidine).

Class I antidysrhythmics: Care should be taken in prescribing a beta-adrenoceptor blocking drug with Class I antidysrhythmic agents such as disopyramide.

Verapamil: Beta-adrenoceptor blocking drugs should be used with caution in combination with verapamil in patients with impaired ventricular function. The combination should not be given to patients with conduction abnormalities. Neither drug should be administered intravenously within 48 hours of discontinuing the other.

Lithium: Preparations containing lithium generally should not be given with diuretics because they may reduce its renal clearance.

Metabolic effects: The metabolic effects of chlorthalidone are dose-related and, at the low dose contained in a Tenoret 50 tablet, are most unlikely to be troublesome.

Potassium status: Experience even with a full dose of this beta-blocker and diuretic combination in Tenoretic has been associated with only minor changes in potassium status. Total body potassium is unaltered on chronic therapy, and changes in serum potassium are minor and probably clinically unimportant. Thus, in cases of uncomplicated hypertension, concurrent potassium supplements should be unnecessary. Measurement of potassium levels is appropriate, especially in the older patient, those receiving digitalis preparations for cardiac failure, taking abnormal (low in potassium) diets, or suffering from gastro-intestinal complaints.

Serum uric acid: Experience, again with Tenoretic, has generally been associated with only a minor increase in serum uric acid. In cases of prolonged elevation the concurrent use of a uricosuric agent will reverse the hyperuricaemia.

Diabetes: Tenoret 50 contains chlorthalidone which may decrease glucose tolerance. During prolonged therapy regular tests for glycosuria should be carried out.

Renal impairment: In patients with severe renal impairment a reduction in the frequency of administration may be necessary.

Sensitivity to chlorthalidone: Because Tenoret 50 contains chlorthalidone, care should be taken in patients with severe renal failure or with a history of sensitivity to chlorthalidone.

Pregnancy: Like other drugs Tenoret 50 should not be given during pregnancy unless its use is essential.

Anaesthesia: As with all preparations containing beta-adrenoceptor blocking drugs it may be decided to withdraw Tenoret 50 before surgery. In this case 48 hours should elapse between the last dose and anaesthesia. If treatment is continued care should be taken when using anaesthetic agents such as ether, cyclopropane and trichloroethylene. Vagal dominance, if it occurs, may be corrected with atropine (1–2 mg iv).

Side-effects: Tenoret 50 is well tolerated. Side effects associated with it are infrequent and generally mild.

Minor side effects include cold extremities, muscular fatigue and, in isolated cases, bradycardia. Sleep disturbances of the type noted with other beta-adrenoceptor blocking drugs have rarely been reported.

There have been reports of skin rashes and/or dry eyes associated with the use of beta-adrenergic blocking drugs. The reported incidence is small and in most cases the symptoms have cleared when treatment was withdrawn. Discontinuance of the drug should be considered if any such reaction is not otherwise explicable. Cessation of therapy with beta-adrenoceptor blocking drugs should be gradual.

Nausea and dizziness have been reported occasionally with chlorthalidone and idiosyncratic drug reactions such as thrombocytopenia and leucopenia have occurred rarely.

Overdosage: Excessive bradycardia can be countered with atropine, 1–2 mg intravenously, followed, if necessary, by a beta-adrenoceptor stimulant, such as isoprenaline 25 micrograms initially or orciprenaline 0.5 mg given by slow intravenous injection. Care must be taken to ensure that the blood pressure does not fall too low if the dose of beta-adrenoceptor agonist has to be increased.

Glucagon has also been reported to be useful as a cardiac stimulant in a dose of 10 mg intravenously.

Excessive diuresis should be countered by maintaining normal fluid and electrolyte balance.

Pharmaceutical precautions Tenoret 50 should be stored at room temperature, protected from light and moisture.

Legal category POM.

Package quantities Calendar packs of 28 tablets and blister packs of 30 tablets.

Further information When the combined antihypertensive effect of a beta-blocker and a diuretic is required, Tenoret 50 one tablet daily is a simple, convenient and acceptable therapy which may be expected to improve patient compliance.

Product licence number 0029/0156.

TENORMIN* TABLETS
TENORMIN* LS TABLETS

Presentation Tenormin tablets, containing atenolol 100 mg are round, bi-convex, orange, film-coated tablets impressed with TENORMIN on one face and the Stuart logo on the reverse. The impressions are highlighted in white.

Tenormin LS tablets, containing atenolol 50 mg are round, bi-convex, orange, film-coated tablets impressed with TENORMIN LS on one face and the Stuart logo on the reverse. The impressions are highlighted in white.

Uses
i) Management of hypertension
ii) Management of angina pectoris
iii) Management of cardiac dysrhythmias
iv) Myocardial infarction: early intervention in the acute phase.

Mode of action: Tenormin (atenolol) is a beta-adrenoceptor blocking drug which is cardioselective (i.e. acts preferentially on beta-adrenergic receptors in the heart). It is without intrinsic sympathomimetic and membrane stabilising activities. Human studies indicate that it crosses the blood brain barrier only to a negligible extent.

It is probably the action of Tenormin in reducing cardiac rate and contractility which makes it effective in eliminating or reducing the symptoms of patients with angina. As with other beta-adrenoceptor blocking drugs, its mode of action in the treatment of hypertension is unclear.

Early intervention with Tenormin in acute myocardial infarction reduces infarct size and decreases morbidity. Fewer patients with a threatened infarction progress to frank infarction; the incidence of ventricular arrhythmias is decreased and marked pain relief may result in reduced need of opiate analgesics. Early mortality may also be decreased. Tenormin is an additional treatment to standard coronary care.

Dosage and administration *Adults: Hypertension:* One tablet daily. Most patients respond to 100 mg daily given orally as a single dose. Some patients, however, will respond to 50 mg given as a single daily dose. The effect will be fully established after one to two weeks. A further reduction in blood pressure may be achieved by combining Tenormin with other antihypertensive agents. For example, co-administration of Tenormin with a diuretic, as in Tenoretic, provides a highly effective and convenient antihypertensive therapy.

Angina: Most patients with angina pectoris will respond to 100 mg given orally once daily or 50 mg given twice daily. It is unlikely that additional benefit will be gained by increasing the dose.

Dysrhythmias: A suitable initial dose of Tenormin is 2.5 mg (5 ml) injected intravenously over a 2.5 minute period (i.e. 1 mg/minute). (See also prescribing information for Tenormin Injection.) This may be repeated at 5 minute intervals until a response is observed up to a maximum dosage of 10 mg. If Tenormin is given by infusion, 0.15 mg/kg bodyweight may be administered over a 20 minute period. If required, the injection or infusion may be repeated every 12 hours. Having controlled the dysrhythmias with intravenous 'Tenormin', a suitable oral maintenance dosage is 50–100 mg daily, given as a single dose.

Myocardial infarction: For patients suitable for treatment with intravenous beta-blockade and presenting within 12 hours of the onset of chest pain. Tenormin 5 mg should be given immediately by slow intravenous injection (1 mg/minute) followed by Tenormin 50 mg orally about 15 minutes later provided no untoward effects occur from the intravenous dose. This should be followed by a further 50 mg orally 12 hours after the intravenous dose and then 12 hours later by 100 mg orally to be given once daily for up to 10 days. If bradycardia and/or hypotension requiring treatment, or any other untoward effects occur, Tenormin should be discontinued.

Elderly patients: Dosage requirements may be reduced, especially in patients with impaired renal function.

Children: There is no paediatric experience with Tenormin and for this reason it is not recommended for use in children.

Contra-indications, warnings, etc
Contra-indications: Tenormin is contra-indicated in patients with second degree or third-degree heart block.

Precautions: Special care should be taken with patients whose cardiac reserve is poor. Myocardial contractility must be maintained and signs of failure controlled with digitalis and diuretics.

One of the pharmacological actions of Tenormin is to reduce heart rate. In the rare instances when symptoms may be attributable to the slow heart rate, the dose may be reduced.

Tenormin modifies the tachycardia of hypoglycaemia.

Tenormin may be used with caution in patients with chronic obstructive airways disease. However, occasionally some increase in airways resistance may occur in asthmatic patients. In contrast to non-selective beta-blockers, this bronchospasm may usually be reversed by commonly used dosage of bronchodilators such as salbutamol or isoprenaline.

In patients suffering from ischaemic heart disease, as with other beta-blocking agents, treatment should not be discontinued abruptly.

Caution should be exercised when transferring patients from clonidine to beta-adrenoceptor blocking drugs. If beta-adrenoceptor blocking drugs and clonidine are given concurrently, clonidine should not be discontinued until several days after the withdrawal of the beta-adrenoceptor blocking drug (see also prescribing information on clonidine).

Care should be taken in prescribing a beta-adrenoceptor blocking drug with Class I antidysrhythmic agents such as disopyramide.

Beta-adrenoceptor blocking drugs should be used with caution in combination with verapamil in patients with impaired ventricular function. The combination should not be given to patients with conduction abnormalities. Neither drug should be administered intravenously within 48 hours of discontinuing the other.

Anaesthesia: As with all beta-adrenoceptor blocking drugs it may be decided to withdraw Tenormin before surgery. In this case 48 hours should be allowed to elapse between the last dose and anaesthesia. If treatment is continued care should be taken when using anaesthetic agents such as ether, cyclopropane and trichloroethylene. Vagal dominance, if it occurs, may be corrected with atropine (1–2 mg i.v.).

Renal failure: Since Tenormin is excreted via the kidneys dosage should be adjusted in cases of severe impairment of renal function. No significant accumulation of Tenormin occurs at a GFR greater than 35 ml/min/1.73 m^2 (normal range is 100–150 ml/min/1 73 m^2). For patients with a creatinine clearance of 15–35 ml/min/1.73 m^2 (equivalent to serum creatinine of 300–600 mcmol/litre) the oral dose should be 50 mg daily or 100 mg once every two days; and the intravenous dose should be 10 mg once every two days. For patients with a creatinine clearance of < 15 ml/min/1.73 m^2 (equivalent to serum creatinine of > 600 mcmol/litre) the oral dose should be 50 mg on alternate days or 100 mg once every four days; and the intravenous dose should be 10 mg once every four days.

Patients on haemodialysis should be given 50 mg orally after each dialysis; this should be done under hospital supervision as marked falls in blood pressure can occur.

Pregnancy: Tenormin has been used effectively under close supervision for the treatment of pregnancy-associated hypertension. There was no evidence of any foetal abnormalities although Tenormin was generally given after 20 weeks gestation.

Tenormin crosses the placental barrier and appears in cord blood. There is an approximate three-fold accumulation of Tenormin in the breast milk. However, there were no apparent detrimental effects in the baby at birth or during breast feeding.

The possibility of foetal injury cannot be excluded and the use of the drug in women who are, or may become pregnant or who are nursing the newborn infant, requires that anticipated benefits be weighed against possible risks.

Side-effects: In clinical studies, the side effects reported are usually attributable to its pharmacological actions and include coldness of the extremities, muscular fatigue and, in isolated cases, bradycardia. Sleep disturbances of the type noted with other beta-blockers have rarely been reported.

There have been reports of skin rashes and/or dry eyes associated with the use of beta-adrenergic blocking drugs. The reported incidence is small and in most cases the symptoms have cleared when treatment was withdrawn. Discontinuance of the drug should be considered if any such reaction is not otherwise explicable. Cessation of therapy with a beta-blocker should be gradual.

Overdosage: From first principles, excessive bradycardia may be countered by atropine, 1–2 mg intravenously, and, if necessary, this may be followed by a beta-stimulant, such as isoprenaline 25 micrograms initially, or orciprenaline 0.5 mg given by slow intravenous injection. Care must be taken to ensure that the blood pressure does not fall too low if the dose of the beta-receptor agonist has to be increased.

Glucagon has also been reported to be useful as a cardiac stimulant in a dose of 10 mg intravenously.

Pharmaceutical precautions Tenormin and Tenormin LS Tablets should be stored at room temperature, protected from light and moisture.

Legal category POM.

Package quantities Tenormin Tablets: 100 mg in Calendar packs of 28 and blister packs of 30. Tenormin LS Tablets: 50 mg in Calendar packs of 28 and blister packs of 30.

Further information Tenormin is effective for at least 24 hours after a single oral dose. The drug facilitates compliance by its acceptability to patients and simplicity of dosing. The narrow dose range and early patient response ensure that the effect of the drug in individual patients is quickly demonstrated. Tenormin is compatible with diuretics, other hypotensive agents and antianginals (but see Warnings). Since it acts preferentially on beta-receptors in the heart, Tenormin may, with care, be used successfully in the treatment of patients with respiratory disease who cannot tolerate non-selective beta-blockers.

Product licence numbers
Tenormin Tablets   0029/0122
Tenormin LS Tablets   0029/0086

TENORMIN* INJECTION ▼

Presentation Tenormin Injection containing 5 mg atenolol in 10 ml isotonic, citrate buffered aqueous solution.

Uses Management of dysrhythmias and for the early intervention treatment of acute myocardial infarction.

Tenormin (atenolol) is a beta-adrenoceptor blocking drug which is cardioselective (i.e. acts preferentially on beta-adrenergic receptors in the heart). It is without intrinsic sympathomimetic and membrane stabilising activities. Human studies indicate that it crosses the blood-brain barrier only to a negligible extent.

Early intervention with Tenormin in acute myocardial infarction reduces infarct size and decreases morbidity. Fewer patients with a threatened infarction progress to frank infarction; the incidence of ventricular arrhythmias is decreased and marked pain relief may result in reduced need for opiate analgesics. Early mortality may also be decreased. Tenormin is an additional treatment to standard coronary care.

Dosage and administration *Adults: Dysrhythmias:* A suitable initial dose of Tenormin is 2.5 mg (5 ml) injected intravenously over a 2.5 minute period (i.e. 1 mg/minute). This may be repeated at 5 minute intervals until a response is observed up to a maximum dosage of 10 mg. If Tenormin is given by infusion, 0.15 mg/kg body weight may be administered over a 20 minute period. If required, the injection or infusion may be repeated every 12 hours. Having controlled the dysrhythmias with intravenous Tenormin a suitable oral maintenance dosage is 50–100 mg daily (see prescribing information for Tenormin and Tenormin LS Tablets).

Myocardial infarction: For patients suitable for treatment with intravenous beta-blockade and presenting within 12 hours of the onset of the chest pain. Tenormin 5 mg should immediately be given by slow intravenous injection (1 mg per minute) followed by Tenormin 50 mg orally after about 15 minutes provided no untoward effects occur from the intravenous dose. This should be followed by a further 50 mg orally 12 hours after the intravenous Tenormin and then 12 hours later by 100 mg orally to be given once daily for up to 10 days. If bradycardia and/or hypotension requiring treatment or any other untoward effects occur, Tenormin should be discontinued.

Elderly patients: Dosage requirements may be reduced, especially in patients with impaired renal function.

Children: There is no paediatric experience with Tenormin and for this reason it is not recommended for children.

Contra-indications, warnings, etc

Contra-indications: Tenormin is contra-indicated in patients with second-degree or third-degree heart block.

Precautions: Special care should be taken with patients whose cardiac reserve is poor. Myocardial contractility must be maintained and signs of failure controlled with digitalis and diuretics.

One of the pharmacological actions of Tenormin is to reduce heart rate. In the rare instances when symptoms may be attributable to the slow heart rate, the dose may be reduced.

Tenormin modifies the tachycardia of hypoglycaemia.

Tenormin may be used with caution in patients with chronic obstructive airways disease. However, occasionally some increase in airways resistance may occur in asthmatic patients. In contrast to non-selective beta-blockers, this bronchospasm may usually be reversed by commonly used dosage of bronchodilators such as salbutamol or isoprenaline.

In patients suffering from ischaemic heart disease, as with other beta-blocking agents, treatment should not be discontinued abruptly.

Caution should be exercised when transferring patients from clonidine to beta-adrenoceptor blocking drugs. If beta-adrenoceptor blocking drugs and clonidine are given concurrently, clonidine should not be discontinued until several days after the withdrawal of the beta-adrenoceptor blocking drug (see also prescribing information on clonidine).

Care should be taken in prescribing a beta-adrenoceptor blocking drug with Class I antidysrhythmic agents such as disopyramide.

Beta-adrenoceptor blocking drugs should be used with caution in combination with verapamil in patients with impaired ventricular function. The combination should not be given to patients with conduction abnormalities. Neither drug should be administered intravenously within 48 hours of discontinuing the other.

Anaesthesia: As with all beta-receptor blocking drugs it may be decided to withdraw Tenormin before surgery. In this case 48 hours should be allowed to elapse between the last dose and anaesthesia. If treatment is continued care should be taken when using anaesthetic agents such as ether, cyclopropane and trichloroethylene. Vagal dominance, if it occurs, may be corrected with atropine (1–2 mg i.v.).

Renal failure: Since Tenormin is excreted via the kidneys dosage should be adjusted in cases of severe impairment of renal function. No significant accumulation of Tenormin occurs at a GFR greater than 35 ml/min/1.73 m^2 (normal range is 100–150 ml/min/1.73 m^2). For patients with a creatinine clearance of 15–35 ml/min/1.73 m^2 (equivalent to serum creatinine of 300–600 mcmol/litre) the oral dose should be 50 mg daily or 100 mg once every two days; and the intravenous dose should be 10 mg once every two days. For patients with a creatinine clearance of < 15 ml/min/1.73 m^2 (equivalent to serum creatinine of > 600 mcmol/litre) the oral dose should be 50 mg on alternate days or 100 mg once every four days; and the intravenous dose should be 10 mg once every four days.

Patients on haemodialysis should be given 50 mg orally after each dialysis; this should be done under hospital supervision as marked falls in blood pressure can occur.

Pregnancy: Tenormin has been used effectively under close supervision for the treatment of pregnancy-associated hypertension. There was no evidence of any foetal abnormalities although Tenormin was generally given after 20 weeks gestation.

Tenormin crosses the placental barrier and appears in cord blood. There is an approximate three-fold accumulation of Tenormin in the breast milk. However, there were no apparent detrimental effects in the baby at birth or during breast feeding.

The possibility of foetal injury cannot be excluded and the use of the drug in women who are, or may become pregnant or who are nursing the newborn infant, requires that anticipated benefits be weighed against possible risks.

Side-effects: In clinical studies, the side effects reported are usually attributable to its pharmacological actions and include coldness of the extremities, muscular fatigue and, in isolated cases, bradycardia. Sleep disturbances of the type noted with other beta-blockers have rarely been reported.

There have been reports of skin rashes and/or dry eyes associated with the use of beta-adrenergic blocking drugs. The reported incidence is small and in most cases the symptoms have cleared when treatment was withdrawn. Discontinuance of the drug should be considered if any such reaction is not otherwise explicable. Cessation of therapy with a beta-blocker should be gradual.

Overdosage: From first principles, excessive bradycardia may be countered by atropine, 1–2 mg intravenously, and, if necessary, this may be followed by a beta stimulant, such as isoprenaline 25 micrograms initially, or orciprenaline 0.5 mg given as a slow intravenous injection. Care must be taken to ensure that the blood pressure does not fall too low if the dose of the beta-receptor agonist has to be increased.

Glucagon has also been reported to be useful as a cardiac stimulant in a dose of 10 mg intravenously.

Pharmaceutical precautions Tenormin Injection should be stored at room temperature protected from light.

Dilutions of Tenormin Injection in Dextrose Injection BP, Sodium Chloride Injection BP, or Sodium Chloride and Dextrose Injection BP may be used.

Legal category POM.

Package quantities *Injection:* 10 ml ampoules in boxes of 10.

Further information The narrow dose range and early patient response to Tenormin ensure that the effect of the drug in individual patients is quickly demonstrated. Tenormin is fully compatible with diuretics, other hypotensive agents and antianginals (but see Warnings). Since it acts preferentially on beta-receptors in the heart, Tenormin may, with care, be used successfully in the treatment of patients with respiratory disease who cannot tolerate non selective beta blockers.

Product licence number 0029/0087.

TENORMIN* SYRUP

Presentation Tenormin Syrup is a clear, colourless, lemon and lime flavoured syrup containing 0.5% w/v atenolol (equivalent to 25 mg/5 ml).

Uses

(i) Management of hypertension.
(ii) Management of angina.
(iii) Management of cardiac dysrhythmias.
(iv) Myocardial infarction: early intervention in the acute phase.

Mode of action: Tenormin (atenolol) is a beta-adrenoceptor blocking drug which is cardioselective (i.e. acts preferentially on beta-adrenergic receptors in the heart). It is without intrinsic sympathomimetic and membrane stabilising activities. Human studies indicate that it crosses the blood brain barrier only to a negligible extent.

It is probably the action of Tenormin in reducing cardiac rate and contractility which makes it effective in eliminating or reducing the symptoms of patients with angina. As with other beta-adrenoceptor blocking drugs, its mode of action in the treatment of hypertension is unclear.

Dosage and administration

Adults: Hypertension: Two or four 5 ml spoonfuls daily i.e. 50 mg or 100 mg in patients unable to take 50 mg or 100 mg tablets.

Most patients respond to 100 mg once daily. Some patients, however, will respond to 50 mg given as a single daily dose. The effect will be fully established after one to two weeks. A further reduction in blood pressure may be achieved by combining Tenormin with other antihypertensive agents.

Angina: Most patients with angina pectoris will respond to 100 mg (four 5 ml spoonfuls) given orally once daily or 50 mg (two 5 ml spoonfuls) given twice daily. It is unlikely that additional benefit will be gained by increasing the dose.

Dysrhythmias: A suitable initial dose of Tenormin Injection is 2.5 mg (5 ml) injected intravenously over a 2.5 minute period (i.e. 1 mg/minute). (See also prescribing information for Tenormin Injection). This may be repeated at 5 minute intervals until a response is observed up to a maximum dosage of 10 mg. If Tenormin is given by infusion, 0.15 mg/kg bodyweight may be administered over a 20 minute period. If required, the injection or infusion may be repeated every 12 hours. Having controlled the dysrhythmias with intravenous Tenormin a suitable oral maintenance dosage is 50–100 mg (two to four 5 ml spoonfuls) daily given as a single dose.

Myocardial infarction: For patients suitable for treatment with intravenous beta-blockade and presenting within 12 hours of the onset of chest pain, Tenormin 5 mg should be given immediately by slow intravenous injection (1 mg/minute) followed by Tenormin 50 mg (two 5 ml spoonfuls) orally about 15 minutes later provided no untoward effects occur from the intravenous dose. This should be followed by a further 50 mg orally 12 hours after the intravenous dose and then 12 hours later by 100 mg (four 5 ml spoonfuls) orally to be given once daily for up to 10 days. If bradycardia and/or hypotension requiring treatment, or any other untoward effects occur, Tenormin should be discontinued.

Elderly patients: Dosage requirements may be reduced, especially in patients with impaired renal function.

Children: There is no paediatric experience with Tenormin and for this reason it is not recommended for use in children.

Contra-indications, warnings, etc Tenormin is contra-indicated in patients with second degree or third degree heart block.

Special care should be taken with patients whose cardiac reserve is poor. Myocardial contractility must be maintained and signs of failure controlled with digitalis and diuretics.

One of the pharmacological actions of Tenormin is to reduce heart rate. In the rare instances when symptoms may be attributable to the slow heart rate, the dose may be reduced.

Tenormin modifies the tachycardia of hypoglycaemia.

Tenormin may be used with caution in patients with chronic obstructive airways disease.

However, occasionally some increase in airways resistance may occur in asthmatic patients. In contrast to non-selective beta-blockers, this bronchospasm may usually be reversed by commonly used dosage of bronchodilators such as salbutamol or isoprenaline.

In patients suffering from ischaemic heart disease, as with other beta-blocking agents, treatment should not be discontinued abruptly.

Caution should be exercised when transferring patients from clonidine to beta-adrenoceptor blocking drugs. If beta-adrenoceptor blocking drugs and clonidine are given concurrently, clonidine should not be discontinued until several days after the withdrawal of the beta-adrenoceptor blocking drug (see also prescribing information on clonidine).

Care should be taken in prescribing a beta-adrenoceptor blocking drug with Class 1 antidysrhythmic agents such as disopyramide.

Beta-adrenoceptor blocking drugs should be used with caution in combination with verapamil in patients with impaired ventricular function. The combination should not be given to patients with conduction abnormalities. Neither drug should be administered intravenously within 48 hours of discontinuing the other.

Anaesthesia: As with all beta-adrenoceptor blocking drugs it may be decided to withdraw Tenormin before surgery. In this case 48 hours should be allowed to elapse between the last dose and anaesthesia. If treatment is continued care should be taken when using anaesthetic agents such as ether, cyclopropane and trichloroethylene. Vagal dominance, if it occurs, may be corrected with atropine (1–2 mg i.v.).

Renal failure: Since Tenormin is excreted via the kidneys dosage should be adjusted in cases of severe impairment of renal function. No significant accumulation of Tenormin occurs at a GRF greater than 35 ml/min/1.73 m^2 (normal range is 100–150 ml/min/1.73 m^2). For patients with a creatinine clearance of 15–35 ml/min/1.73 m^2 (equivalent to serum creatinine of 300–600 mcmol/litre) the dose should be 50 mg daily or 100 mg once every two days. For patients with a creatinine clearance of 15 ml/min/1.73 m^2 (equivalent to serum creatinine of >600 mcmol/litre) the dose should be 50 mg on alternate days or 100 mg once every four days.

Patients on haemodialysis should be given 50 mg after each dialysis; this should be done under hospital supervision as marked falls in blood pressure can occur.

Pregnancy: Tenormin has been used effectively under close supervision for the treatment of pregnancy-associated hypertension. There was no evidence of any foetal abnormalities although Tenormin was generally given after 20 weeks gestation.

Tenormin crosses the placental barrier and appears in cord blood. There is an approximate three-fold accumulation of Tenormin in the breast milk. However, there were no apparent detrimental effects upon the baby at birth or during breast feeding.

The possibility of foetal injury cannot be excluded and the use of the drug in women who are, or may become pregnant or who are nursing the newborn infant, requires that anticipated benefits be weighed against possible risks.

Side-effects: In clinical studies, the side effects reported are usually attributable to its pharmacological actions and include coldness of the extremities, muscular fatigue and, in isolated cases, bradycardia. Sleep disturbances of the type noted with other beta-blockers have rarely been reported.

There have been reports of skin rashes and/or dry eyes associated with the use of beta-adrenergic blocking drugs. The reported incidence is small and in most cases the symptoms have cleared when treatment was withdrawn. Discontinuance of the drug should be considered if any such reaction is not otherwise explicable. Cessation of therapy with a beta-blocker should be gradual.

Overdosage: From first principles, excessive bradycardia may be countered by atropine, 1–2 mg intravenously, and, if necessary, this may be followed by a beta-stimulant, such as isoprenaline 25 micrograms initially, or orciprenaline 0.5 mg given by slow intravenous injection. Care must be taken to ensure that the blood pressure does not fall too low if the dose of the beta-receptor agonist has to be increased.

Glucagon has also been reported to be useful as a cardiac stimulant in a dose of 10 mg intravenously.

Pharmaceutical precautions Tenormin Syrup should be stored at room temperature, protected from light.

Legal category POM.

Package quantities 300 ml bottle.

Further information Tenormin Syrup is intended for patients unable to swallow Tenormin tablets. Tenormin is effective for at least 24 hours after once daily dosing with 10 ml or 20 ml Tenormin Syrup. Tenormin Syrup facilitates compliance by its acceptability to patients and the once-daily dosing regimen. The narrow dose range and early patient response ensure that the effect of the drug in individual patients is quickly demonstrated. Tenormin is compatible with diuretics, other hypotensive agents and antianginals (but see Warnings). Since it acts preferentially on beta-receptors in the heart, Tenormin may, with care, be used successfully in the treatment of patients with respiratory disease who cannot tolerate non-selective beta-blockers.

Product licence number 0029/0195.

*Trade Mark

Syntex Pharmaceuticals Limited
St Ives Road
Maidenhead
Berkshire SL6 1RD

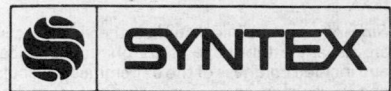

ANAPOLON* 50

Presentation Each Anapolon 50 Tablet contains oxymetholone 50 mg. The white tablets are scored and stamped with the number '50' on one side and SYNTEX on the other.

Uses Anapolon 50 is recommended for the treatment of aplastic and refractory anaemias (including acquired, idiopathic and congenital aplasias). Anapolon 50 is also recommended as adjunctive therapy in patients with malignant diseases where treatment with cytotoxic agents or radiotherapy is likely to cause bone-marrow depression.

Anapolon 50 should not replace other supportive measures such as transfusion, correction of iron, folic acid, vitamin B12 or pyridoxine deficiency, antibacterial therapy and the appropriate use of corticosteroids.

The exact mode of action of oxymetholone is as yet uncertain. It is thought, however, that oxymetholone stimulates the production of erythropoietin, which in turn acts on the primitive stem cells increasing the rate of differentiation into red cell precursors. It has also been demonstrated that oxymetholone increases the mitotic rate of the stem cells, stimulating the extension of healthy tissue into hypoplastic areas of the bone marrow. Oxymetholone has a beneficial effect on haemoglobin synthesis as shown by an increased plasma iron clearance.

Dosage and administration The recommended dosage when treating aplasias is from 2 mg to 5 mg per kg body weight daily for adults, and from 2 mg to 4 mg per kg body weight daily for children in divided doses. The selected dose will depend on the severity of the condition.

1. Initial therapy should be continued for a period of six months or until a response is seen (whichever is the shorter time). Therapy must be maintained for at least three months before a response can be expected.
2. From the time of response the same dose should be continued for a further three months.
3. At this time the dose should be halved and, if the remission is maintained, continued for three months.
4. During the next three months gradual withdrawal should be attempted.
5. Should a relapse occur at any time whilst the dose is being reduced the initial dosage regime should be re-instituted. When administering oxymetholone as an adjunctive to cytotoxic therapy and radiotherapy the recommended dosage is up to 150 mg per day.

Use in the elderly: The usual adult regimen is recommended.

Contra-indications, warnings, etc
Contra-indications: Carcinoma of the prostate or breast in male patients; pregnancy (primarily because of masculinisation of the foetus); infancy; nephrosis or the nephrotic phase of nephritis; hepatic dysfunction; hypersensitivity to oxymetholone.

Warnings and precautions: Because of serious side-effects, anabolic steroids should not be used to enhance athletic ability.

Tumours of the liver have been reported occasionally in patients subjected to prolonged treatment with androgenic-anabolic steroids. The possibility that these compounds may induce or enhance the development of hepatic tumours cannot at present be excluded and this should be considered when the use of this product is proposed, especially in young people who are not suffering from life-threatening disorders.

Hepatotoxic effects, including jaundice, are common with the prescribed dosage. Clinical jaundice may be painless, with or without pruritus. It may also be associated with acute hepatic enlargement and right-upper quadrant pain, which has been mistaken for acute (surgical) obstruction of the bile duct. Drug-induced jaundice is usually reversible when the medication is discontinued. Continued therapy has been associated with hepatic coma and death. Because of the hepato-toxicity associated with oxymetholone administration, periodic liver function tests are recommended. Disturbance of liver function tests, elevation of serum bilirubin and jaundice may occur, together with other signs of liver disturbance. Should this happen, the dosage should be halved. If liver function tests do not improve within one week then oxymetholone therapy should be withdrawn.

Caution is required in administering these agents to patients with cardiac, renal or hepatic disease. Oedema, with or without congestive heart failure, may occur occasionally. Concomitant administration with adrenal steroids or ACTH may add to the oedema. This is generally controllable with appropriate diuretic and/or digitalis therapy. Anabolic steroids should be used with caution in patients with benign prostatic hypertrophy.

When anti-coagulant therapy is used concomitantly, dosage of the anti-coagulant may have to be decreased in order to maintain the prothrombin time at the desired therapeutic level. This is because Anapolon 50, like other anabolic steroids, may enhance blood fibrinolytic activity.

Oxymetholone exhibits only slightly androgenic activity in low doses, but in the high dosage levels employed in the treatment of aplastic anaemias, it may lead to virilisation in women and pre-pubertal children.

Amenorrhoea usually occurs in the adult female, even in the presence of thrombocytopenia. Concomitant administration of large doses of progestational agents to control menorrhagia is not recommended. Hypercalcae-mia may develop both spontaneously and as a result of hormonal therapy in women with disseminated breast carcinoma. If it develops while on this agent, the drug should be stopped.

The development of iron deficiency anaemia manifested by a low serum iron and decreased percent saturation of transferrin, has been observed in some patients treated with oxymetholone. Periodic determination of the serum iron and iron binding capacity is recommended. If iron deficiency is detected, it should be appropriately treated with supplementary iron.

Leukaemia has been observed in patients with aplastic anaemia treated with oxymetholone. The role, if any, of oxymetholone is unclear since malignant transformation has been seen in blood dyscrasias and leukaemia has been reported in patients with aplastic anaemia who have not been treated with oxymetholone.

Anabolic steroids have been shown to alter glucose tolerance tests. Diabetics should be followed carefully and the insulin or oral hypoglycaemic dosage adjusted accordingly.

Serum cholesterol may increase or decrease during therapy. Therefore, caution is required in administering these agents to patients with a history of myocardial infarction or coronary artery disease. Serial determinations of serum cholesterol should be made and therapy adjusted accordingly.

Alterations in these clinical laboratory tests may occur:

(a) The metyrapone test.
(b) The fasting blood sugar and glucose tolerance test.
(c) The thyroid function tests: a decrease in the PBI, in thyroxine-binding capacity and radioactive iodine uptake and an increase in T3 uptake by the rbc's or resin may occur. Free thyroxine is normal. Altered tests usually persist for 2–3 weeks after stopping anabolic therapy.
(d) The electrolytes; retention of sodium, chlorides, water, potassium, phosphates and calcium.
(e) Increased or decreased serum cholesterol.
(f) Suppression of clotting factors II, V, VII, and X.
(g) Increased creatinine excretion lasting up to two weeks after discontinuing therapy.
(h) Decreased 17-ketosteroid excretion.

The following adverse reactions may occur:

1. Hepatotoxicity is the most serious adverse reaction associated with anabolic steroid therapy. Reversible increase in BSP retention occurs early and appears to be directly related to the dose. Increase in serum bilirubin, with or without an increase in the serum alkaline phosphatase and transaminases (SGOT and SGPT) indicate a higher degree of excretory dysfunction. Clinical jaundice, which is reversible when the drug is discontinued, may occur. The histologic picture is one of intrahepatic cholestasis with little or no cellular damage. Continued therapy may be associated with hepatic coma and death.

2. Virilisation is the most common undesirable effect associated with anabolic steroid therapy. Acne occurs frequently in all age groups.

Prepubertal male: The first signs of virilisation in the prepubertal male are phallic enlargement and an increase in frequency of erection. Hirsutism and increased skin pigmentation may also occur.

Postpubertal male: Inhibition of testicular function with oligospermia; decrease in seminal volume, alteration in libido, and impotence may occur with prolonged or intensive anabolic therapy. Gynaecomastia, and testicular atrophy may occur. Chronic priapism, hair loss, epididymitis and bladder irritability have been reported.

In females, hirsutism, hoarseness or deepening of the voice, clitoral enlargement, alteration of libido, and menstrual irregularities and male-pattern baldness may occur. The voice change and clitoral enlargement are usually irreversible even after prompt discontinuation of therapy. The use of oestrogens in combination with androgens will not prevent virilisation in females.

3. *Other adverse reactions associated with anabolic/androgenic therapy include:*
(a) Muscle cramps.
(b) Nausea.
(c) Excitation and sleeplessness.
(d) Chills.
(e) Bleeding in patients on concomitant anti-coagulant therapy.
(f) Premature closure of epiphyses in children.
(g) Vomiting.
(h) Diarrhoea.

Peliosis hepatis and hepatocellular carcinoma have been observed in patients with congenital and acquired aplastic anaemia treated with oxymetholone and other oral androgens for prolonged periods. In some cases withdrawal of the drug has been associated with regressions of the hepatic lesions.

Treatment of overdosage: There are no reports of chronic or acute overdosage with Anapolon 50. Gastric lavage may be helpful if performed soon after ingestion.

Pharmaceutical precautions Anapolon 50 should be kept under normal storage conditions.

Legal category POM.

Package quantities Anapolon 50 is available in canisters of 100 tablets.

Further information Nil.

Product licence number 0286/5009.

BREVINOR*

Presentation White, flat, circular, bevel-edged tablets inscribed B on one face. Each tablet contains norethisterone 0.5 mg and ethinyloestradiol 35 mcg.

Uses Brevinor is indicated for oral contraception, with the benefit of a low intake of oestrogen.

The mode of action of Brevinor is similar to that of other progestogen/oestrogen oral contraceptives; its activity is exerted through a combined effect on one or more of the following: hypothalamus, anterior pituitary, ovary, endometrium and cervical mucus.

Dosage and administration The dosage of Brevinor for the initial cycle of therapy is 1 tablet taken daily from the 5th to the 25th day of the menstrual cycle, counting the first day of menstrual flow as 'Day 1'. For the subsequent cycles, no tablets are taken for seven days, then a new course is started of 1 tablet daily for 21 days. This sequence of 21 days on treatment, seven days off treatment is repeated for as long as contraception is required.

When starting oral contraception with Brevinor, additional precautions must be used for the first 14 days of tablet-taking.

Tablet omissions: Tablets must be taken daily in order to maintain adequate hormone levels. If a tablet is missed, it should be taken as soon as possible, within 24 hours of the correct time even if this means that 2 tablets are taken together. If 2 tablets are missed, a tablet should be taken as soon as possible so medication is re-established. An additional method of contraception should be used for the remainder of that tablet cycle. If more than 2 tablets have been missed, oral contraceptive therapy should be discontinued immediately and a method of non-hormonal contraception should be used until menses has appeared or pregnancy has been excluded.

Changing from another oral contraceptive: Brevinor should be started seven days after completing the last course of the other product. An additional mechanical or chemical contraceptive should be used for the first 14 days of tablet-taking.

Use after childbirth, miscarriage or abortion: After childbirth, oral contraception is usually started when spontaneous menstruation has resumed. Another method of contraception should be used in the meantime, unless the first course of tablets is started within seven days of delivery. After a miscarriage or abortion, oral contraception can normally be started on the fifth day.

Contra-indications, warnings, etc

Contra-indications: As with all combined progestogen/oestrogen oral contraceptives, the following conditions should be regarded as contra-indications:

(a) Thrombophlebitis, thromboembolic disorders, cerebrovascular disorders, coronary artery disease, or a history of these conditions.
(b) Acute or severe chronic liver disease, Dubin-Johnson or Rotor syndrome, history during pregnancy of idiopathic jaundice or severe pruritus.
(c) Known or suspected breast or genital cancer.
(d) Known or suspected oestrogen-dependent neoplasia.
(e) Undiagnosed abnormal vaginal bleeding.
(f) Pregnancy.

Side-effects and precautions: As with all oral contraceptives, there may be slight nausea at first, weight gain or breast discomfort, which soon disappear.

Other side-effects known or suspected to occur with oral contraceptives include gastrointestinal symptoms, changes in libido and appetite, headache, exacerbation of existing uterine fibroid disease, depression, and changes in carbohydrate, lipid and vitamin metabolism.

Spotting or bleeding may occur during the first few cycles. Usually menstrual bleeding becomes light and occasionally there may be no bleeding during the tablet-free days.

Hypertension, which is usually reversible on discontinuing treatment, has occurred in a small percentage of women taking oral contraceptives. Oestrogen-progestogen preparations should be used with caution in patients with a history of hepatic dysfunction or hypertension.

A statistical association between the use of oral contraceptives and the occurrence of thrombosis, embolism or haemorrhage has been reported. Patients on such treatments should be kept under regular surveillance, in view of the possibility of development of such conditions as thromboembolism.

Risk of coronary artery disease in women taking oral contraceptives is increased by the presence of other predisposing factors such as cigarette smoking, hypercholesterolaemia, obesity, diabetes, history of pre-eclamptic toxaemia and increasing age. After the age of thirty-five years, the patient and physician should carefully re-assess the risk/benefit ratio of using combined oral contraceptives as opposed to alternative methods of contraception.

Benign and malignant liver tumours have been associated with oral contraceptive use. The relationship between occurrence of liver tumours and use of female sex hormones is not known at present. These tumours are very rare but they may rupture causing intra-abdominal bleeding. If the patient presents with a mass or tenderness in the right upper quadrant or an acute abdomen, the possible presence of a tumour should be considered.

The use of this product in patients suffering from epilepsy, migraine, asthma or cardiac dysfunction may result in exacerbation of these disorders, because of fluid retention. Caution should also be observed in patients who wear contact lenses.

Decreased glucose tolerance may occur in diabetic patients on this treatment, and their control must be carefully supervised.

The use of oral contraceptives has also been associated with a possible increased incidence of gallbladder disease.

An increased risk of congenital anomalies, including heart defects and limb defects, has been reported following the use of sex hormones, including oral contraceptives, in pregnancy. If the patient does not adhere to the prescribed schedule, the possibility of pregnancy should be considered at the time of the first missed period and further use of oral contraceptives should be withheld until pregnancy has been ruled out. It is recommended that for any patient who has missed two consecutive periods, pregnancy should be ruled out before continuing the contraceptive regimen. If pregnancy is confirmed the patient should be apprised of the potential risks to the foetus and the advisability of continuing the pregnancy should be discussed in the light of these risks. It is advisable to discontinue Brevinor three months before a planned pregnancy.

Gastro-intestinal upsets may interfere with the absorption of the tablets. Some drugs may modify the metabolism of Brevinor reducing its effectiveness; these include certain sedatives, antibiotics, anti-epileptic and anti-arthritic drugs. During the time such agents are used concurrently, it is advisable that mechanical contraceptives also be used.

Women taking oral contraceptives require careful observation if they have or have had any of the following conditions: breast nodules; fibrocystic disease of the breast or an abnormal mammogram; uterine fibroids; a history of severe depressive states; varicose veins; sickle-cell anaemia; diabetes; hypertension; high blood cholesterol levels; epilepsy; asthma; otosclerosis; multiple sclerosis; porphyria; tetany; disturbed liver functions; gallstones; cardiovascular disease; kidney disease; chloasma; herpes of pregnancy or any disease that is prone to worsen during pregnancy. The worsening or first appearance of any of these conditions may indicate that the oral contraceptive should be stopped. Discontinue treatment if there is a gradual or sudden, partial or complete loss of vision or any evidence of ocular changes, onset or aggravation of migraine or development of headache of a new kind which is recurrent, persistent or severe.

Brevinor should be discontinued at least six weeks before elective operations and during immobilisation.

Women with a history of oligomenorrhoea or secondary amenorrhoea or young women without regular cycles may have a tendency to remain anovulatory or to become amenorrhoeic after discontinuation of oral contraceptives. Women with these pre-existing problems should be advised of this possibility and encouraged to use other contraceptive methods.

The risk of arterial thrombosis associated with com

bined oral contraceptives increases with age, and this risk is aggravated by cigarette smoking. The use of combined oral contraceptives by women in the older age group, especially those who are cigarette smokers, should therefore be discouraged and alternative methods advised.

Use during breast-feeding: Active ingredients or their metabolites have been detected in the milk of mothers taking oral contraceptives. The effect of Brevinor on breast-fed infants has not been determined.

Treatment of overdose: Overdosage may be manifested by nausea, vomiting, breast enlargement and vaginal bleeding. There is no specific antidote and treatment should be symptomatic. Gastric lavage may be employed if the overdose is large and the patient is seen sufficiently early (within four hours).

Pharmaceutical precautions Brevinor should be stored in a cool, dry place away from direct sunlight.

Legal category POM.

Package quantities Brevinor is available in calendar packs of 3×21 tablets.

Further information Nil.

Product licence number 0286/0054.

EMKO* CONTRACEPTIVE FOAM

Presentation A pressurised metal canister which delivers into the applicator provided a foam containing nonoxynol-9 8% w/v and benzethonium chloride 0.2% w/v.

Uses Spermicidal contraceptive agent. As with other spermicidal preparations, an additional method of contraception, for example, diaphragm, cap, sheath or intrauterine device, must be used with Emko Foam.

When pregnancy is medically contra-indicated, the choice of contraceptive should be made in consultation with a doctor.

Dosage and administration The contents of the applicator to be introduced into the vagina not more than one hour before intercourse. Emko Foam must be used each time physical contact is repeated.

If a diaphragm or cap is used, Emko Foam may be used as a lubricant, spread around the rim.

Contra-indications, warnings, etc There are no known contra-indications to the use of Emko Contraceptive Foam.

On rare occasions irritation of the vagina or penis may occur; if it does, use of Emko should be discontinued and medical advice should be sought.

Douching is unnecessary; following sexual intercourse, an interval of at least six hours must elapse before douching for cleansing purposes.

Pharmaceutical precautions Store in a cool place.

Legal category GSL.

Package quantities Emko Contraceptive Foam Kit containing 40 g aerosol container and an applicator.
40 g refill aerosol pack.
90 g refill aerosol pack.

Further information In one study (1), Emko Contraceptive Foam was used by 2,932 women for 28,322 cycles; a pregnancy-rate of 3.98 pregnancies per 100 woman-years was reported. Another study (2), in 130 women who used Emko Contraceptive Foam for 2,737 women-months, showed a pregnancy-rate of 1.75 pregnancies per 100 woman-years. Both study reports emphasised the need for giving adequate, careful instructions to the patients.

References:

1. *Contraception* 1971; **3**: 37–43.
2. *Pacific Medicine and Surgery* 1965; **73**: 353–5.

Product licence number 0286/0051.

MASTERIL*

Presentation Each Masteril ampoule contains drostanolone propionate 100 mg in 1 ml of clear oily solution.

Uses Masteril is indicated for the amelioration of disseminated mammary carcinoma, used either alone or in conjunction with other medication or surgery. Masteril is thought to work by blocking the uptake of oestrogen by oestrogen-dependent carcinoma cells.

Dosage and administration *Adults (including the elderly):* The recommended dosage is 300 mg (3 ampoules) weekly given by intramuscular injection. Therapy should be continued until such time as the patient ceases to derive benefit from Masteril. 8–12 weeks of treatment should be allowed before any conclusions are drawn as to the efficacy of Masteril. If a significant progression of the disease occurs during the first 6–8 weeks of therapy another form of treatment should be considered.

Contra-indications, warnings, etc
Contra-indications: Use in pregnancy: Masteril should not be used in pregnancy, suspected pregnancy or in women who are at risk of becoming pregnant since masculinisation of the foetus could occur. Androgens are contra-indicated in carcinoma of the male breast.

Precautions: Masteril should be used with caution in the presence of any of the following: liver disease, cardiac decompensation, nephritis, nephrosis.

Side-effects: Side-effects are significantly less intense with Masteril than with comparable doses of testosterone propionate. The most likely side-effects are menstrual disorders, virilism such as deepening of the voice, acne, facial hair growth and enlargement of the clitoris. At times, marked virilism will occur after prolonged treatment. Oedema occasionally occurs. Hypercalcaemia was noted in a few cases. If it occurs the drug should be discontinued. Libido seldom seems to be affected. Local reactions at the site of injection may occur rarely.

Overdosage: Treatment should be symptomatic.

Pharmaceutical precautions Masteril should not be stored in direct sunlight.

Legal category POM.

Package quantities Masteril is available in ampoules of 1 ml (100 mg) packed in boxes of 10.

Further information Nil.

Product licence number 0286/5010.

NAPROSYN* TABLETS
NAPROSYN* 500 TABLETS
NAPROSYN* SUPPOSITORIES
NAPROSYN* SUSPENSION

Presentation Naprosyn (naproxen) is d-2(6'-methoxy-2-naphthyl) propionic acid, a non-steroidal anti-inflammatory agent, developed by Syntex Research. It is presented as:

(i) A yellow half-scored tablet containing 250 mg of naproxen, inscribed NAPROSYN on one side and SYNTEX on the other.

(ii) An oblong, scored yellow tablet containing 500 mg of naproxen, inscribed NAPROSYN 500 on one side.

(iii) Suppositories each containing 500 mg naproxen.

(iv) A flavoured yellow suspension containing 25 mg/ml naproxen.

Uses Naprosyn is indicated for the treatment of rheumatoid arthritis, osteoarthritis (degenerative arthritis), ankylosing spondylitis, juvenile rheumatoid arthritis, acute gout, and acute musculoskeletal disorders (such as sprains and strains, direct trauma, lumbosacral pain, cervical spondylitis, tenosynovitis and fibrositis).

Naprosyn has been shown to have striking anti-inflammatory analgesic and antipyretic properties when tested in classical animal test systems. It exhibits its anti-inflammatory effect even in adrenalectomised animals, indicating that its action is not mediated through the pituitary-adrenal axis. It inhibits prostaglandin synthetase, as do other non-steroidal anti-inflammatory agents. As with other agents, however, the exact mechanism of its anti-inflammatory action is not known.

Dosage and administration *Adults:* For rheumatoid arthritis, osteoarthrosis and ankylosing spondylitis, the usual dose is 500 mg to 1 g per day taken in two doses at 12-hour intervals.

Where 1 g per day is needed, the suggested regime is one Naprosyn 500 tablet twice daily.

In the following cases a loading dose of 750 mg or 1 g per day for the acute phase is recommended:

(a) In patients reporting severe night-time pain and/or morning stiffness.

(b) In patients being switched to Naprosyn from a high dose of another anti-rheumatic compound.

(c) In osteoarthrosis where pain is the predominant symptom.

For the patient who requires 750 mg per day, the size of the morning and evening doses can be adjusted on the basis of the predominant symptoms, i.e. night-time pain or morning stiffness.

Naprosyn suppositories are recommended for patients in whom rectal administration may be preferable. One suppository is to be inserted at night. If necessary another suppository or up to 500 mg oral Naprosyn therapy, can be used in the morning.

In acute gout, the recommended dosage is 750 mg at once, then 250 mg every eight hours until the attack has passed.

For the treatment of acute musculoskeletal disorders, the recommended dose is 500 mg initially followed by 250 mg at 6–8 hour intervals as needed, with a maximum daily dose after the first day of 1250 mg.

Use in the elderly: One study indicates that although total plasma concentration of naproxen is unchanged, the unbound plasma fraction of naproxen is increased in the elderly. The implication of this finding for Naprosyn

dosing is unknown, but caution is advised when high doses are required. For the effect of reduced elimination in the elderly refer to the section 'Use in patients with impaired renal function'.

Children: For the treatment of juvenile rheumatoid arthritis in children over five years of age, the usual dosage is 10 mg/kg/day taken in two doses at 12-hour intervals.

Contra-indications, warnings, etc

Contra-indications: Active peptic ulceration. Hypersensitivity to naproxen or naproxen sodium formulations. Since the potential exists for cross-sensitivity reactions, Naprosyn should not be given to patients in whom aspirin or other non-steroidal anti-inflammatory/analgesic drugs induce the syndrome of asthma, rhinitis or urticaria.

Special precautions and warnings: Episodes of gastro-intestinal bleeding have been reported in patients with Naprosyn therapy. Naprosyn should be given under close supervision to patients with a history of gastro-intestinal disease.

Bronchospasm may be precipitated in patients suffering from, or with a history of, bronchial asthma or allergic disease.

Sporadic abnormalities in laboratory tests (e.g. liver function tests) have occurred in patients on Naprosyn therapy, but no definite trend was seen in any test indicating toxicity.

Naprosyn decreases platelet aggregation and prolongs bleeding time. This effect should be kept in mind when bleeding times are determined.

Mild peripheral oedema has been observed in a few patients receiving Naprosyn. Although sodium retention has not been reported in metabolic studies, it is possible that patients with questionable or compromised cardiac function may be at a greater risk when taking Naprosyn.

Use in patients with impaired renal function: As naproxen is eliminated to a large extent (95%) by urinary excretion via glomerular filtration it should be used with great caution in patients with impaired renal function and the monitoring of serum creatinine and/or creatinine clearance is advised in these patients. Naprosyn is not recommended in patients having baseline creatinine clearance less than 20 ml/minute.

Certain patients, specifically those where renal blood flow is compromised, such as in extracellular volume depletion, cirrhosis of the liver, sodium restriction, congestive heart failure, and pre-existing renal disease, should have renal function assessed before and during Naprosyn therapy. Some elderly patients in whom impaired renal function may be expected could also fall within this category. A reduction in daily dosage should be considered to avoid the possibility of excessive accumulation of naproxen metabolites in these patients.

Use in patients with impaired liver function: Chronic alcoholic liver disease and probably also other forms of cirrhosis reduce the total plasma concentration of naproxen but the plasma concentration of unbound naproxen is increased. The implication of this finding for Naprosyn dosing is unknown, but caution is advised when high doses are required.

Interactions with other drugs: Due to the high plasma protein binding of Naprosyn, patients simultaneously receiving hydantoins, anti-coagulants or a highly protein-bound sulphonamide should be observed for signs of overdosage of these drugs. No interactions have been observed in clinical studies with Naprosyn and ant coagulants or sulphonylureas, but caution is nevertheless advised since interaction has been seen with other non-steroidal agents of this class.

The natriuretic effect of frusemide has been reported to be inhibited by some drugs of this class.

Inhibition of renal lithium clearance leading to increases in plasma lithium concentrations has also been reported.

Naprosyn and other non-steroidal anti-inflammatory drugs can reduce the anti-hypertensive effect of propranolol and other beta-blockers.

Probenecid given concurrently increases Naprosyn plasma levels and extends its plasma half-life considerably.

Caution is advised where methotrexate is administered concurrently because of possible enhancement of its toxicity, since Naprosyn, among other non-steroidal anti-inflammatory drugs, has been reported to reduce the tubular secretion of methotrexate in an animal model.

It is suggested that Naprosyn therapy be temporarily discontinued 48 hours before adrenal function tests are performed because Naprosyn may artifactually interfere with some tests for 17-ketogenic steroids. Similarly, Naprosyn may interfere with some assays of urinary 5-hydroxyindoleacetic acid.

Side-effects:

Gastro-intestinal: The more frequent reactions are nausea, vomiting, abdominal discomfort and epigastric distress. More serious reactions which may occur occasionally are gastro-intestinal bleeding and peptic ulceration (sometimes with haemorrhage and perforation).

Dermatological/hypersensitivity: Skin rashes, urticaria, angio-oedema. Anaphylactic reactions to naproxen and naproxen sodium formulations and eosinophilic pneumonitis may occur rarely.

CNS: Headache, insomnia, inability to concentrate and cognitive dysfunction have been reported.

Haematological: Thrombocytopenia, granulocytopenia, aplastic anaemia and haemolytic anaemia may occur rarely.

Other: Tinnitis, hearing impairment, vertigo, mild peripheral oedema. Jaundice, fatal hepatitis, nephropathy and ulcerative stomatitis have been reported rarely.

Naprosyn suppositories: The following minor side-effects have been reported with the use of Naprosyn Suppositories: rectal discomfort, soreness, burning and itching. Also isolated cases of rectal bleeding, tenesmus and proctitis have been reported. However, the incidence of local side-effects in clinical trials was low.

Use in pregnancy and in breast-feeding: Teratology studies in rats and rabbits, at dose levels equivalent on a human multiple basis to those which have produced foetal abnormality with certain other non-steroidal anti-inflammatory agents, e.g. aspirin, have not produced evidence of foetal damage with Naprosyn. As with other drugs of this type Naprosyn delays parturition in animals (the relevance of this finding to human patients is unknown) and also affects the human foetal cardio-vascular system (closure of the ductus arteriosus). Good medical practice indicates minimal drug usage in pregnancy, and use of this class of therapeutic agent requires cautious balancing of possible benefit against potential risk to the mother and foetus especially in the first and third trimesters.

The use of Naprosyn should be avoided in patients who are breast-feeding.

Overdosage: Significant overdosage of the drug may be characterised by drowsiness, heartburn, indigestion, nausea or vomiting. No evidence of toxicity or late sequelae have been reported 5–15 months after ingestion, for three to seven days, of doses of up to 3 g/day. One patient ingested a single dose of 25 g of naproxen and experienced mild nausea and indigestion. It is not known what dose of the drug would be life-threatening. Should a patient ingest a large amount of Naprosyn accidentally or purposefully, the stomach may be emptied and usual supportive measures employed. Animal studies indicate that the prompt administration of activated charcoal in adequate amounts would tend to reduce markedly the absorption of the drug.

Pharmaceutical precautions Protect from light.

Legal category POM.

Package quantities Naprosyn Tablets are supplied in packs of 60 and 250 tablets. Naprosyn 500 Tablets are supplied in packs of 100 tablets. Naprosyn Suppositories are supplied in packs of 10 suppositories. Naprosyn Suspension is supplied in 500 ml bottles.

Further information Nil.

Product licence numbers

Naprosyn Tablets	0286/0031
Naprosyn 500 Tablets	0286/0061
Naprosyn Suppositories	0286/0053
Naprosyn Suspension	0286/0047

NORIDAY*

Presentation Yellow, flat, circular, bevel-edged tablets inscribed NORIDAY on one side and SYNTEX on the other. Each tablet contains norethisterone 0.35 mg.

Uses Noriday is a progestogen-only oral contraceptive. It is particularly useful for women for whom oestrogens may not be appropriate. Although the mode of action of Noriday tablets has not yet been fully defined it is thought that alterations occur in the cervical mucus which inhibit the penetration of sperm, there is substantial inhibition of ovulation, and changes occur in the endometrium which inhibit implantation of the fertilised egg.

Dosage and administration The first Noriday tablet is taken on the FIRST DAY of menstrual bleeding. Thereafter, 1 tablet is taken continuously at the same time every day even during menstrual bleeding.

When starting oral contraception with Noriday, additional precautions must be used for the first 14 days of tablet-taking. Suitable methods are sheaths, caps plus spermicides, and intra-uterine devices. The rhythm, temperature and cervical-mucus methods cannot be used.

Tablet omissions: Tablets must be taken daily in order to maintain adequate hormone levels. If a tablet is missed, it should be taken as soon as possible, with the next tablet being taken at the usual time so that two tablets are taken on that date. An additional method of contraception should be used for the next 14 days. If two or more tablets are missed, Noriday should be discontinued immediately and a method of non-hormonal contraception should be used until menses has appeared or pregnancy has been excluded.

Contra-indications, warnings, etc

Contra-indications: A history during pregnancy of idiopathic jaundice or severe pruritus; Dubin-Johnson or Rotor syndrome; acute or severe chronic liver diseases; undiagnosed irregular vaginal bleeding; a history of thromboembolic disorders; pregnancy. Special caution should be observed in the presence of pre-existing breast or genital-tract cancer.

Warnings, side-effects: Hypertension, which is usually reversible on discontinuing treatment, has occurred in a small percentage of women taking oral contraceptives. Noriday should be used with caution in patients with a history of hepatic dysfunction or hypertension.

A statistical association between the use of oral contraceptives and the occurrence of thrombosis, embolism or haemorrhage has been reported. Patients on such treatments should be kept under regular surveillance, in view of the possibility of development of such conditions as thromboembolism. Risk of coronary artery disease in women taking oral contraceptives is increased by the presence of other predisposing factors such as cigarette smoking, hypercholesterolaemia, obesity, diabetes, history of pre-eclamptic toxaemia and increasing age. After the age of thirty-five years, the patient and physician should carefully re-assess the risk/benefit ratio of using oral contraceptives as opposed to alternative methods of contraception.

It is advisable to discontinue Noriday at least six weeks before elective operations and during immobilisation.

Benign and malignant liver tumours have been associated with oral contraceptive use. The relationship between occurrence of liver tumours and use of female sex hormones is not known at present. These tumours may rupture causing intra-abdominal bleeding. If the patient presents with a mass or tenderness in the right upper quadrant or an acute abdomen, the possible presence of a tumour should be considered.

An increased risk of congenital anomalies, including heart defects and limb defects, has been reported following the use of sex hormones, including oral contraceptives, in pregnancy. If the patient does not adhere to the prescribed schedule, the possibility of pregnancy should be considered at the time of the first missed period and further use of oral contraceptives should be withheld until pregnancy has been ruled out. It is recommended that for any patient who has missed two consecutive periods, pregnancy should be ruled out before continuing the contraceptive regimen. If pregnancy is confirmed the patient should be apprised of the potential risks to the foetus and the advisability of continuing the pregnancy should be discussed in the light of these risks. It is advisable to discontinue the use of oral contraceptives three months before a planned pregnancy.

Progestogen-only oral contraceptives such as Noriday may offer less protection against ectopic pregnancy than against intra-uterine pregnancy.

The incidence of side-effects in clinical trials was lower than that experienced with oestrogen-containing oral contraceptives. Side-effects which did occur included some cycle irregularity during the first few months of therapy, spotting or breakthrough bleeding, amenorrhoea, breast discomfort, gastro-intestinal symptoms, headaches, migraine, depression, fatigue, nervousness, disturbance of appetite, changes in weight and libido, rash.

Circumstances requiring additional contraceptive precautions other than the temperature, rhythm and cervical-mucus methods:

1. When changing to Noriday tablets from other hormonal contraceptives, additional contraceptive measures should be employed until 14 consecutive tablets have been taken regularly.

2. Vomiting or diarrhoea may reduce the effectiveness of the tablets by preventing them from being fully absorbed. In the case of repeated vomiting or continued diarrhoea, additional contraceptive measures should be employed for 14 days after the symptoms have subsided.

3. Interaction with other drugs. Some drugs accelerate the metabolism of oral contraceptives taken concurrently. Drugs suspected of having the capacity to reduce the efficacy of oral contraceptives include certain sedatives, antibiotics, anti-epileptic and anti-arthritic drugs.

It is therefore advisable to use non-hormonal methods of contraception during treatment with such drugs.

Menstrual pattern: A usual feature of all progestogen-only oral contraceptives is that they produce an initial irregularity of the bleeding pattern, but such irregularity tends to decrease with time. The patient should be informed before starting Noriday tablets that her menstrual pattern is likely to alter.

Irregular bleeding is, from a medical point of view, no reason for discontinuation of therapy, as long as organic causes and pregnancy can be ruled out. The patient should be instructed that if two or more consecutive periods are missed, she should consult her physician in order to rule out pregnancy.

Use after delivery or abortion: Although after delivery or abortion it is customary to start oral contraception at the end of the first biphasic menstrual cycle, Noriday tablets may be started as early as the seventh day post-partum. Additional contraceptive measures should be employed for the first 14 days of tablet-taking.

Use during breast-feeding: There is no evidence that Noriday tablets diminish the yield of breast milk. Small amounts of steroid materials appear in the milk; their effect on the breast-fed child has not been determined.

Reasons for stopping oral contraception immediately: First signs of thrombophlebitis or thromboembolism, jaundice or pregnancy.

Overdosage: Overdosage may be manifested by nausea, vomiting, breast enlargement and vaginal bleeding. There is no specific antidote and treatment should be symptomatic. Gastric lavage may be employed if the overdosage is large and the patient is seen sufficiently early (within four hours).

Pharmaceutical precautions Noriday tablets should be stored in a cool, dry place away from direct sunlight.

Legal category POM.

Package quantities Noriday tablets are available in calendar packs of 3 × 28 tablets.

Further information Nil.

Product licence number 0286/0024.

NORIMIN*

Presentation Yellow, flat, circular bevel-edged tablets inscribed SYNTEX on one face. Each tablet contains norethisterone 1.0 mg and ethinyloestradiol 35 mcg.

Uses Norimin is indicated for oral contraception, with the benefit of a low intake of oestrogen.

The mode of action of Norimin is similar to that of other progestogen/oestrogen oral contraceptives; its activity is exerted through a combined effect on one or more of the following: hypothalamus, anterior pituitary, ovary, endometrium and cervical mucus.

Dosage and administration The dosage of Norimin for the initial cycle of therapy is 1 tablet taken daily from the 5th to the 25th day of the menstrual cycle, counting the first day of menstrual flow as 'Day I'. For subsequent cycles, no tablets are taken for seven days, then a new course is started of 1 tablet daily for 21 days. This sequence of 21 days on treatment, seven days off treatment is repeated for as long as contraception is required.

When starting oral contraception with Norimin, additional precautions must be used for the first 14 days of tablet-taking.

Tablet omissions: Tablets must be taken daily in order to maintain adequate hormone levels. If a tablet is missed, it should be taken as soon as possible within 24 hours of the correct time even if this means that 2 tablets are taken together. If 2 tablets are missed, a tablet should be taken as soon as possible so medication is re-established. An additional method of contraception should be used for the remainder of that tablet cycle. If more than 2 tablets have been missed, oral contraceptive therapy should be discontinued immediately and a method of non-hormonal contraception should be used until menses has appeared or pregnancy has been excluded.

Changing from another oral contraceptive: Norimin should be started seven days after completing the last course of the other product. An additional mechanical or chemical contraceptive should be used for the first 14 days of tablet-taking.

Use after childbirth, miscarriage or abortion: After childbirth, oral contraception is usually started when spontaneous menstruation has resumed. Another method of contraception should be used in the meantime, unless the first course of tablets is started within seven days of delivery. After a miscarriage or abortion, oral contraception can normally be started on the fifth day.

Contra-indications, warnings, etc
Contra-indications: As with all combined progestogen/oestrogen oral contraceptives, the following conditions should be regarded as contra-indications:

(a) Thrombophlebitis, thromboembolic disorders, cerebrovascular disorders, coronary artery disease, or a history of these conditions.
(b) Acute or severe chronic liver disease, Dubin-Johnson or Rotor syndrome, history during pregnancy of idiopathic jaundice or severe pruritus.
(c) Known or suspected breast or genital cancer.
(d) Known or suspected oestrogen-dependent neoplasia.
(e) Undiagnosed abnormal vaginal bleeding.
(f) Pregnancy.

Side-effects and precautions: As with all oral contraceptives, there may be slight nausea at first, weight gain or breast discomfort, which soon disappear.

Other side-effects known or suspected to occur with oral contraceptives include gastro-intestinal symptoms, changes in libido and appetite, headache, exacerbation of existing uterine fibroid disease, depression, and changes in carbohydrate, lipid and vitamin metabolism.

Spotting or bleeding may occur during the first few cycles. Usually menstrual bleeding becomes light and occasionally there may be no bleeding during the tablet-free days.

Hypertension, which is usually reversible on discontinuing treatment, has occurred in a small percentage of women taking oral contraceptives. Progestogen/oestrogen preparations should be used with caution in patients with a history of hepatic dysfunction or hypertension.

A statistical association between the use of oral contraceptives and the occurrence of thrombosis, embolism or haemorrhage has been reported. Patients on such treatments should be kept under regular surveillance in view of the possibility of development of such conditions as thromboembolism.

Risk of coronary artery disease in women taking oral contraceptives is increased by the presence of other predisposing factors such as cigarette smoking, hypercholesterolaemia, obesity, diabetes, history of pre-eclamptic toxaemia and increasing age. After the age of thirty-five years, the patient and physician should carefully re-assess the risk/benefit ratio of using combined oral contraceptives as opposed to alternative methods of contraception.

Benign and malignant liver tumours have been associated with oral contraceptive use. The relationship between occurrence of liver tumours and use of female sex hormones is not known at present. These tumours are very rare but they may rupture causing intra-abdominal bleeding. If the patient presents with a mass or tenderness in the right upper quadrant or an acute abdomen, the possible presence of a tumour should be considered.

The use of this product in patients suffering from epilepsy, migraine, asthma or cardiac dysfunction may result in exacerbation of these disorders, because of fluid retention. Caution should also be observed in patients who wear contact lenses.

Decreased glucose tolerance may occur in diabetic patients on this treatment, and their control must be carefully supervised.

The use of oral contraceptives has also been associated with a possible increased incidence of gallbladder disease.

An increased risk of congenital anomalies, including heart defects and limb defects, has been reported following the use of sex hormones, including oral contraceptives, in pregnancy. If the patient does not adhere to the prescribed schedule, the possibility of pregnancy should be considered at the time of the first missed period and further use of oral contraceptives should be withheld until pregnancy has been ruled out. It is recommended that for any patient who has missed two consecutive periods, pregnancy should be ruled out before continuing the contraceptive regimen. If pregnancy is confirmed the patient should be apprised of the potential risks to the foetus and the advisability of continuing the pregnancy should be discussed in the light of these risks. It is advisable to discontinue Norimin three months before a planned pregnancy.

Gastro-intestinal upsets may interfere with the absorption of the tablets. Some drugs may modify the metabolism of Norimin reducing its effectiveness; these include certain sedatives, antibiotics, anti-epileptic and anti-arthritic drugs. During the time such agents are used concurrently, it is advisable that mechanical contraceptives also be used.

Women taking oral contraceptives require careful

observation if they have or have had any of the following conditions: breast nodules; fibrocystic disease of the breast or an abnormal mammogram; uterine fibroids; a history of severe depressive states; varicose veins; sickle-cell anaemia; diabetes; hypertension; high blood cholesterol levels, epilepsy; asthma; otosclerosis; multiple sclerosis; porphyria; tetany, disturbed liver functions; gallstones; cardiovascular disease; kidney disease; chloasma; herpes of pregnancy or any disease that is prone to worsen during pregnancy. The worsening or first appearance of any of these conditions may indicate that the oral contraceptive should be stopped. Discontinue treatment if there is a gradual or sudden, partial or complete loss of vision or any evidence of ocular changes, onset or aggravation of migraine or development of headache of a new kind which is recurrent, persistent or severe.

Norimin should be discontinued at least six weeks before elective operations and during immobilisation.

Women with a history of oligomenorrhoea or secondary amenorrhoea or young women without regular cycles may have a tendency to remain anovulatory or to become amenorrhoeic after discontinuation of oral contraceptives. Women with these pre-existing problems should be advised of this possibility and encouraged to use other contraceptive methods.

The risk of arterial thrombosis associated with combined oral contraceptives increases with age, and this risk is aggravated by cigarette smoking. The use of combined oral contraceptives by women in the older age group, especially those who are cigarette smokers, should therefore be discouraged and alternative methods advised.

Use during breast-feeding: Active ingredients or their metabolites have been detected in the milk of mothers taking oral contraceptives. The effect of Norimin on breast-fed infants has not been determined.

Treatment of overdosage: Overdosage may be manifested by nausea, vomiting, breast enlargement and vaginal bleeding. There is no specific antidote and treatment should be symptomatic. Gastric lavage may be employed if the overdose is large and the patient is seen sufficiently early (within four hours).

Pharmaceutical precautions Norimin should be stored in a cool, dry place away from direct sunlight.

Legal category POM.

Package quantities Norimin is available in calendar packs of 3 × 21 tablets.

Further information Nil.

Product licence number 0286/0059.

NORINYL*-1

Presentation White, flat, circular, bevel-edged tablets inscribed NORINYL on one side and SYNTEX on the other. Each tablet contains norethisterone 1 mg and mestranol 0.05 mg.

Uses Norinyl-1 is indicated for oral contraception and is also useful in the treatment of certain menstrual disorders, e.g. heavy, irregular or painful periods. Activity is exerted through a combined effect on one or more of the following: hypothalamus, anterior pituitary, ovary, endometrium and cervical mucus.

Dosage and administration The first tablet is taken on the *fifth* day of a menstrual period. One tablet is then taken at the same time of day, every day, until all 21 tablets are used. The next pack is started after *seven tablet-free* days: this sequence is repeated for as long as contraception is required.

When starting oral contraception with Norinyl-1, additional precautions must be used for the first 14 days of tablet-taking.

Tablet omissions: Tablets must be taken daily in order to maintain adequate hormone levels. If a tablet is missed, it should be taken as soon as possible within 24 hours of the correct time even if this means that 2 tablets are taken together. If 2 tablets are missed, a tablet should be taken as soon as possible so medication is re-established. An additional method of contraception should be used for the remainder of that tablet cycle. If more than 2 tablets have been missed, oral contraceptive therapy should be discontinued immediately and a method of non-hormonal contraception should be used until menses has appeared or pregnancy has been excluded.

Changing from another oral contraceptive: Norinyl-1 should be started seven days after completing the last course of the other product. An additional mechanical or chemical contraceptive should be used for the first 14 days of tablet-taking.

Use after childbirth, miscarriage or abortion: After childbirth, oral contraception is usually started when spontaneous menstruation has resumed. Another method of contraception should be used in the meantime, unless the first course of tablets is started within seven days of delivery. After a miscarriage or abortion, oral contraception can normally be started on the fifth day.

Contra-indications, warnings, etc
Contra-indications: As with all combined progestogen/oestrogen oral contraceptives, the following conditions should be regarded as contra-indications:

(a) Thrombophlebitis, thromboembolic disorders, cerebrovascular disorders, coronary artery disease, or a history of these conditions.
(b) Acute or severe chronic liver disease, Dubin-Johnson or Rotor syndrome, history during pregnancy of idiopathic jaundice or severe pruritus.
(c) Known or suspected breast or genital cancer.
(d) Known or suspected oestrogen-dependent neoplasia.
(e) Undiagnosed abnormal vaginal bleeding.
(f) Pregnancy.

Side-effects and precautions: As with all oral contraceptives, there may be slight nausea at first, weight gain or breast discomfort, which soon disappear.

Other side-effects known or suspected to occur with oral contraceptives include gastro-intestinal symptoms, changes in libido and appetite, headache, exacerbation of existing uterine fibroid disease, depression, and changes in carbohydrate, lipid and vitamin metabolism.

Spotting or bleeding may occur during the first few cycles. Usually menstrual bleeding becomes light and occasionally there may be no bleeding during the tablet-free days.

Hypertension, which is usually reversible on discontinuing treatment, has occurred in a small percentage of women taking oral contraceptives. Oestrogen-progestogen preparations should be used with caution in patients with a history of hepatic dysfunction or hypertension.

A statistical association between the use of oral

contraceptives and the occurrence of thrombosis, embolism or haemorrhage has been reported. Patients on such treatments should be kept under regular surveillance, in view of the possibility of development of such conditions as thromboembolism.

Risk of coronary artery disease in women taking oral contraceptives is increased by the presence of other predisposing factors such as cigarette smoking, hypercholesterolaemia, obesity, diabetes, history of preeclamptic toxaemia and increasing age. After the age of thirty-five years, the patient and physician should carefully re-assess the risk/benefit ratio of using combined oral contraceptives as opposed to alternative methods of contraception.

Benign and malignant liver tumours have been associated with oral contraceptive use. The relationship between occurrence of liver tumours and use of female sex hormones is not known at present. These tumours are very rare but they may rupture causing intra-abdominal bleeding. If the patient presents with a mass or tenderness in the right upper quadrant or an acute abdomen, the possible presence of a tumour should be considered.

The use of this product in patients suffering from epilepsy, migraine, asthma or cardiac dysfunction may result in exacerbation of these disorders, because of fluid retention. Caution should also be observed in patients who wear contact lenses.

A decreased glucose tolerance may occur in diabetic patients on this treatment, and their control must be carefully supervised.

The use of oral contraceptives has also been associated with a possible increased incidence of gallbladder disease.

An increased risk of congenital anomalies, including heart defects and limb defects, has been reported following the use of sex hormones, including oral contraceptives, in pregnancy. If the patient does not adhere to the prescribed schedule, the possibility of pregnancy should be considered at the time of the first missed period and further use of oral contraceptives should be withheld until pregnancy has been ruled out. It is recommended that for any patient who has missed two consecutive periods, pregnancy should be ruled out before continuing the contraceptive regimen. If pregnancy is confirmed the patient should be apprised of the potential risks to the foetus and the advisability of continuing the pregnancy should be discussed in the light of these risks. It is advisable to discontinue Norinyl-1 three months before a planned pregnancy.

Gastro-intestinal upsets may interfere with the absorption of the tablets. Some drugs may modify the metabolism of Norinyl-1 reducing its effectiveness; these include certain sedatives, antibiotics, anti-epileptic and anti-arthritic drugs. During the time such agents are used concurrently, it is advisable that mechanical contraceptives also be used.

Women taking oral contraceptives require careful observation if they have or have had any of the following conditions: breast nodules; fibrocystic disease of the breast or an abnormal mammogram; uterine fibroids; a history of severe depressive states; varicose veins; sickle-cell anaemia; diabetes; hypertension; high blood cholesterol levels; epilepsy; asthma; otosclerosis; multiple sclerosis; porphyria; tetany; disturbed liver functions; gallstones; cardiovascular disease; chloasma; herpes of pregnancy or any disease that is prone to worsen during pregnancy. The worsening or first appearance of any of these conditions may indicate that the oral contraceptive should be stopped. Discontinue treatment if there is a gradual or sudden, partial or complete loss of vision or any evidence of ocular changes, onset or aggravation of migraine or development of headache of a new kind which is recurrent, persistent or severe.

Norinyl-1 should be discontinued at least 6 weeks before elective operations and during immobilisation.

Women with a history of oligomenorrhoea or secondary amenorrhoea or young women without regular cycles may have a tendency to remain anovulatory or to become amenorrhoeic after discontinuation of oral contraceptives. Women with these pre-existing problems should be advised of this possibility and encouraged to use other contraceptive methods.

The risk of arterial thrombosis associated with combined oral contraceptives increases with age, and this risk is aggravated by cigarette smoking. The use of combined oral contraceptives by women in the older age group, especially those who are cigarette smokers, should therefore be discouraged and alternative methods advised.

Use during breast-feeding: Active ingredients or their metabolites have been detected in the milk of mothers taking oral contraceptives. The effect of Norinyl-1 on breast-fed infants has not been determined.

Treatment of overdose: Overdosage may be manifested by nausea, vomiting, breast enlargement and vaginal bleeding. There is no specific antidote and treatment should be symptomatic. Gastric lavage may be employed if the overdose is large and the patient is seen sufficiently early (within four hours).

Pharmaceutical precautions Norinyl-1 should be stored in a cool, dry place away from direct sunlight.

Legal category POM.

Package quantities Norinyl-1 is available in packs of 3×21 tablets.

Further information Nil.

Product licence number 0286/5000.

STAYCEPT* PESSARIES

Presentation Smooth, torpedo-shaped, solid white pessaries containing nonoxynol-9 6% w/w (equivalent to 96 mg nonoxynol-9 per pessary).

Uses Spermicidal contraceptive agent. As with other spermicidal preparations, additional methods of contraception, for example, diaphragm, cap, sheath or intra-uterine device, must be used with Staycept pessaries.

When pregnancy is medically contra-indicated, the choice of contraceptive should be made in consultation with a doctor.

Dosage and administration One to be inserted into the vagina before intercourse. When used with a diaphragm or cap, one pessary should be placed inside the diaphragm or cap before it is put into position; a second pessary is then inserted into the vagina as far as possible.

If coitus is delayed for longer than 1 hour, another pessary should be inserted. Another pessary should be used each time intercourse takes place.

Contra-indications, warnings, etc
Contra-indication: Known hypersensitivity to nonoxynol-9.

Precautions and warnings: If irritation of the vagina or penis occurs, the use of the product should be discontinued.

Pharmaceutical precautions Store in a cool place.

Legal category GSL.

Package quantities Pack of 10 pessaries.

Further information Nil.

Product licence number 0286/5012.

STAYCEPT* JELLY

Presentation A smooth, clear jelly containing octoxynol 1% w/w.

Uses Spermicidal contraceptive agent. As with other spermicidal preparations, additional methods of contraception, for example, diaphragm, cap, sheath or intrauterine device, must be used with Staycept Jelly.

When pregnancy is medically contra-indicated, the choice of contraceptive should be made in consultation with a doctor.

Dosage and administration

(a) Used with diaphragm. Two 1-inch strips of jelly to be applied to either side of diaphragm and spread in a thin layer over cap and rim.
(b) Used with intra-uterine device or sheath. Two to three inches applied into the vagina, from an applicator 10 minutes before intercourse.

If coitus is delayed for longer than 1 hour, more jelly should be used. More jelly should be used each time intercourse takes place.

Contra-indications, warnings, etc
Contra-indication: Known hypersensitivity to octoxynol.

Precautions and warnings: If irritation of the vagina or penis occurs, the use of the product should be discontinued.

Pharmaceutical precautions Store in a cool place.

Legal category GSL.

Package quantities 80 g tube.

Further information Staycept Jelly can be used as a lubricant by women who experience difficulty with intercourse because of a dry vagina.

Product licence number 0286/5011.

SYNFLEX*

Presentation Opaque, orange, film-coated oval tablet marked SYNTEX on one face, containing naproxen sodium 275 mg (equivalent to naproxen 250 mg).

Uses Synflex is an anti-inflammatory analgesic for the treatment of musculo-skeletal disorders (including sprains and strains, direct trauma and lumbo-sacral pain); post-operative pain; dysmenorrhoea

Synflex is also indicated for the relief of migraine.

Dosage and administration *Adults:* The usual dose is 550 mg initially followed by 275 mg at 6–8 hour intervals as needed. This represents a maximum daily dose of 5 tablets (1375 mg) on the first day of treatment and 4 tablets (1100 mg) thereafter.

For the relief of migraine, the recommended dose is 825 mg at the first symptom of an impending attack. 275–550 mg can be taken in addition throughout the day, if necessary, but not before half an hour after the initial dose. A total dose of 1375 mg per day should not be exceeded.

Use in the elderly: One study indicates that although total plasma concentration of naproxen is unchanged, the unbound plasma fraction of naproxen is increased in the elderly. The implication of this finding for Synflex dosing is unknown, but caution is advised when high doses are required. For the effect of reduced elimination in the elderly refer to the section 'Use in patients with impaired renal function'.

Children: As safety and efficacy studies are not yet complete, Synflex is not recommended for use in children under 16 years of age.

Contra-indications, warnings, etc
Contra-indications: Active peptic ulceration. Hypersensitivity to naproxen or naproxen sodium formulations. Since the potential exists for cross-sensitivity reactions, Synflex should not be given to patients in whom aspirin or other non-steroidal anti-inflammatory/analgesic drugs induce the syndrome of asthma, rhinitis or urticaria.

Special precautions and warnings: Episodes of gastro-intestinal bleeding have been reported in patients with Synflex therapy. Synflex should be given under close supervision to patients with a history of gastro-intestinal disease.

Bronchospasm may be precipitated in patients suffering from, or with a history of, bronchial asthma or allergic disease.

Sporadic abnormalities in laboratory tests (e.g. liver function tests) have occurred in patients on Synflex therapy, but no definite trend was seen in any test indicating toxicity.

Synflex decreases platelet aggregation and prolongs bleeding time. This effect should be kept in mind when bleeding times are determined.

Mild peripheral oedema has been observed in a few patients receiving Synflex. Although sodium retention has not been reported in metabolic studies, it is possible that patients with questionable or compromised cardiac function may be at a greater risk when taking Synflex.

Each Synflex tablet contains approximately 25 mg (about 1 m Eq) sodium. This should be considered in patients whose overall intake of sodium must be markedly restricted.

Use in patients with impaired renal function: As Synflex is eliminated to a large extent (95%) by urinary excretion via glomerular filtration it should be used with great caution in patients with impaired renal function and the monitoring of serum creatinine and/or creatinine clearance is advised in these patients. Synflex is not recommended in patients having baseline creatinine clearance less than 20 ml/minute.

Certain patients, specifically those whose renal blood flow is compromised, such as in extracellular volume depletion, cirrhosis of the liver, sodium restriction, congestive heart failure, and pre-existing renal disease, should have renal function assessed before and during Synflex therapy. Some elderly patients in whom impaired renal function may be expected could also fall within this category. A reduction in daily dosage should be considered to avoid the possibility of excessive accumulation of Synflex metabolites in these patients.

Use in patients with impaired liver function: Chronic alcoholic liver disease and probably also other forms of cirrhosis reduce the total plasma concentration of naproxen but the plasma concentration of unbound naproxen is increased. The implication of this finding for Synflex dosing is unknown, but caution is advised when high doses are required.

Interactions with other drugs: Due to the high plasma protein binding of Synflex, patients simultaneously receiving hydantoins, anti-coagulants or a highly protein-bound sulphonamide should be observed for signs of overdosage of these drugs. No interactions have been observed in clinical studies with naproxen sodium or naproxen and anti-coagulants or sulphonylureas, but caution is nevertheless advised since interaction has been seen with other non-steroidal agents of this class.

The natriuretic effect of frusemide has been reported to be inhibited by some drugs of this class.

Inhibition of renal lithium clearance leading to increases in plasma lithium concentrations has also been reported.

Synflex and other non-steroidal anti-inflammatory drugs can reduce the anti-hypertensive effect of propranolol and other beta-blockers.

Probenecid given concurrently increases Synflex plasma levels and extends its half-life considerably.

Caution is advised when methotrexate is administered concurrently because of possible enhancement of its toxicity, since Synflex, among other non-steroidal anti-inflammatory drugs, has been reported to reduce the tubular secretion of methotrexate in an animal model.

It is suggested that Synflex therapy be temporarily discontinued 48 hours before adrenal function tests are performed because Synflex may artifactually interfere with some tests for 17-ketogenic steroids. Similarly, Synflex may interfere with some assays of urinary 5-hydroxyindoleacetic acid.

Side-effects:
Gastro-intestinal: The more frequent reactions are nausea, vomiting, abdominal discomfort and epigastric distress. More serious reactions which may occur occasionally are gastro-intestinal bleeding and peptic ulceration (sometimes with haemorrhage and perforation).

Dermatological/hypersensitivity: Skin rashes, urticaria, angio-oedema. Anaphylactic reactions to naproxen and naproxen sodium formulations and eosinophilic pneumonitis may occur rarely.

CNS: Headache, insomnia, inability to concentrate and cognitive dysfunction have been reported.

Haematological: Thrombocytopenia, granulocytopenia, aplastic anaemia and haemolytic anaemia may occur rarely.

Other: Tinnitus, hearing impairment, vertigo, mild peripheral oedema. Jaundice, fatal hepatitis, nephropathy and ulcerative stomatitis have been reported rarely.

Use in pregnancy and in breast-feeding: Teratology studies in rats and rabbits, at dose levels equivalent on a human multiple basis to those which have produced foetal abnormality with certain other non-steroidal anti-inflammatory agents, e.g. aspirin, have not produced evidence of foetal damage with Synflex. As with other drugs of this type Synflex delays parturition in animals (the relevance of this finding to human patients is unknown) and also affects the human foetal cardiovascular system (closure of the ductus arteriosus). Good medical practice indicates minimal drug usage in pregnancy, and use of this class of therapeutic agent requires cautious balancing of possible benefit against potential risk to the mother and foetus especially in the first and third trimesters.

The use of Synflex should be avoided in patients who are breast-feeding.

Overdosage: Significant overdosage of the drug may be characterised by drowsiness, heartburn, indigestion, nausea or vomiting. No evidence of toxicity or late sequelae have been reported 5–15 months after ingestion, for three to seven days, of doses of up to 3 g/day. One patient ingested a single dose of 25 g of naproxen and experienced mild nausea and indigestion. It is not known what dose of the drug would be life-threatening.

Should a patient ingest a large amount of Synflex accidentally or purposefully, the stomach may be emptied and usual supportive measures employed. Animal studies indicate that the prompt administration of activated charcoal in adequate amounts would tend to reduce markedly the absorption of the drug.

Pharmaceutical precautions Synflex Tablets should be protected from light and moisture.

Legal category POM.

Package quantities Synflex Tablets are supplied in packs of 100 tablets.

Further information Nil.

Product licence number 0286/0063.

SYNPHASE*

Presentation A 21-tablet memo pack consisting of 7 white tablets containing norethisterone 0.5 mg and ethinyloestradiol 35 mcg, marked B on one side and SYNTEX on the other; then 9 yellow tablets containing norethisterone 1 mg and ethinyloestradiol 35 mcg, inscribed SYNTEX on one face; then 5 white tablets containing norethisterone 0.5 mg and ethinyloestradiol 35 mcg, marked B on one side and SYNTEX on the other.

Uses Synphase is indicated for oral contraception, with the benefit of a low intake of oestrogen.

The mode of action of Synphase is similar to that of other progestogen/oestrogen oral contraceptives; its activity is exerted through a combined effect on one or more of the following: hypothalamus, anterior pituitary, ovary, endometrium and cervical mucus.

Dosage and administration For the initial cycle of therapy one tablet is taken daily from 5th–25th day of the menstrual cycle, counting the first day of menstrual flow as 'Day 1'. No tablets are taken for 7 days, then a new course of one tablet daily for 21 days is started. Tablets must be taken in numerical order as indicated on the pack. This sequence of 21 days on treatment, 7 days off treatment is repeated for as long as contraception is required.

When starting oral contraception with Synphase, additional precautions must be used for the first 14 days of tablet-taking.

Tablet omissions: Tablets must be taken daily in order to maintain adequate hormone levels. If a tablet is missed, it should be taken as soon as possible, within 24 hours of the correct time even if this means that 2 tablets are taken together. If 2 tablets are missed, a tablet should be taken as soon as possible so medication is re-established. An additional method of contraception should be used for the remainder of that tablet cycle. If more than 2 tablets have been missed, oral contraceptive therapy should be discontinued immediately and a method of non-hormonal contraception should be used until menses has appeared or pregnancy has been excluded.

Changing from another oral contraceptive: Synphase should be started 7 days after completion of the previous course of tablets. An additional mechanical or chemical contraceptive should be used for the first 14 days of tablet-taking.

Use after childbirth, miscarriage or abortion: After childbirth, oral contraception is usually started when spontaneous menstruation has resumed. Another method of contraception should be used in the meantime, unless the first course of tablets is started within 7 days of delivery. After a miscarriage or abortion, oral contraception can normally be started as early as the fifth day.

Contra-indications, warnings, etc
Contra-indications: As with all combined progestogen/oestrogen contraceptives, the following conditions should be regarded as contra-indications:
  (i) Thrombophlebitis, thromboembolic disorders, cerebro-vascular disorders, coronary artery disease, or a history of these conditions.
  (ii) Acute or severe chronic liver disease, Dubin-Johnson or Rotor syndrome, history during pregnancy of idiopathic jaundice or severe pruritus.
  (iii) Known or suspected breast or genital cancer.
  (iv) Known or suspected oestrogen-dependent neoplasia.
  (v) Undiagnosed abnormal vaginal bleeding.
  (vi) Pregnancy.

Side-effects, precautions and warnings: As with all oral contraceptives, there may be slight nausea at first, weight gain or breast discomfort, which soon disappear.

Other side-effects known or suspected to occur with oral contraceptives include gastro-intestinal symptoms, changes in libido and appetite, headache, exacerbation of existing uterine fibroid disease, depression, and changes in carbohydrate, lipid and vitamin metabolism.

Spotting or bleeding may occur during the first few cycles. Usually menstrual bleeding becomes light and occasionally there may be no bleeding during the tablet-free days.

Hypertension, which is usually reversible on discontinuing treatment, has occurred in a small percentage of women taking oral contraceptives. Oestrogen-progestogen preparations should be used with caution in patients with a history of hepatic dysfunction or hypertension.

A statistical association between the use of oral contraceptives and the occurrence of thrombosis, embolism or haemorrhage has been reported. Patients on such treatments should be kept under regular surveillance, in view of the possibility of development of such conditions as thromboembolism.

Risk of coronary artery disease in women taking oral contraceptives is increased by the presence of other predisposing factors such as cigarette smoking, hypercholesterolaemia, obesity, diabetes, history of pre-eclamptic toxaemia and increasing age. After the age of thirty-five years, the patient and physician should carefully re-assess the risk/benefit ratio of using combined oral contraceptives as opposed to alternative methods of contraception.

Benign and malignant liver tumours have been associated with oral contraceptive use. The relationship between occurrence of liver tumours and use of female sex hormones is not known at present. These tumours are very rare but they may rupture causing intra-abdominal bleeding. If the patient presents with a mass or tenderness in the right upper quadrant or an acute abdomen, the possible presence of a tumour should be considered.

The use of this product in patients suffering from epilepsy, migraine, asthma or cardiac dysfunction may result in exacerbation of these disorders, because of fluid retention. Caution should also be observed in patients who wear contact lenses.

Decreased glucose tolerance may occur in diabetic patients on this treatment, and their control must be carefully supervised.

The use of oral contraceptives has also been associated with a possible increased incidence of gall bladder disease.

An increased risk of congenital anomalies, including heart defects and limb defects, has been reported following the use of sex hormones, including oral contraceptives, in pregnancy. If the patient does not adhere to the prescribed schedule, the possibility of pregnancy should be considered at the time of the first missed period and further use of oral contraceptives should be withheld until pregnancy has been ruled out. It is recommended that for any patient who has missed two consecutive periods, pregnancy should be ruled out before continuing the contraceptive regimen. If pregnancy is confirmed the patient should be apprised of the potential risks to the foetus and the advisability of continuing the pregnancy should be discussed in the light of these risks. It is advisable to discontinue Synphase three months before a planned pregnancy.

Gastro-intestinal upsets may interfere with the absorption of the tablets. Some drugs may modify the metabolism of Synphase reducing its effectiveness; these include certain sedatives, antibiotics, anti-epileptic and anti-arthritic drugs. During the time such agents are used concurrently, it is advisable that mechanical contraceptives also be used.

Women taking oral contraceptives require careful observation if they have or have had any of the following conditions: breast nodules; fibrocystic disease of the breast or an abnormal mammogram; uterine fibroids; a history of severe depressive states; varicose veins; sickle-cell anaemia; diabetes; hypertension; high blood cholesterol levels; epilepsy; asthma; otosclerosis; multiple sclerosis; porphyria; tetany; disturbed liver functions; gallstones; cardiovascular disease; kidney disease; chloasma; herpes of pregnancy or any disease that is prone to worsen during pregnancy. The worsening or first appearance of any of these conditions may indicate that the oral contraceptive should be stopped. Discontinue treatment if there is a gradual or sudden, partial or complete loss of vision or any evidence of ocular changes, onset or aggravation of migraine or development of headache of a new kind which is recurrent, persistent or severe.

Synphase should be discontinued at least six weeks before elective operations and during immobilisation.

Women with a history of oligomenorrhoea or secondary amenorrhoea or young women without regular cycles may have a tendency to remain anovulatory or to become amenorrhoeic after discontinuation of oral contraceptives. Women with these pre-existing problems should be advised of this possibility and encouraged to use other contraceptive methods.

The risk of arterial thrombosis associated with combined oral contraceptives increases with age, and this risk is aggravated by cigarette smoking. The use of combined oral contraceptives by women in the older age group, especially those who are cigarette smokers, should therefore be discouraged and alternative methods advised.

Use during breast feeding: Active ingredients or their metabolites have been detected in the milk of mothers taking oral contraceptives. The effect of Synphase on breast-fed infants has not been determined.

Treatment of overdosage: Overdosage may be manifested by nausea, vomiting, breast enlargement and vaginal bleeding. There is no specific antidote and treatment should be symptomatic. Gastric lavage may be employed if the overdose is large and the patient is seen sufficiently early (within four hours).

Pharmaceutical precautions Synphase should be stored in a cool dry place, away from direct sunlight.

Legal category POM.

Package quantities Synphase is available in packs of 21 tablets.

Further information Nil.

Product licence number 0286/0085.

SYNTARIS* NASAL SPRAY

Presentation A buffered, clear, colourless, slightly viscous aqueous solution in a glass bottle fitted with a metered pump device which delivers 25 mcg of flunisolide (6 α-fluoro-11 β, 16α, 17, 21-tetrahydroxypregna-1, 4-dien-3, 20-dione, 16, 17-acetonide) per actuation via a nozzle which is inserted into the nostril.

Uses Syntaris Nasal Spray is indicated for the prophylaxis and treatment of perennial and seasonal allergic rhinitis including hay fever.

Flunisolide has marked anti-inflammatory and anti-allergic activity, as shown in classical animal test systems. It is a corticosteroid which is several hundred times more potent in animal anti-inflammatory assays than the cortisol standard.

At the low doses used, clinical studies with flunisolide have shown a topical activity on the nasal mucous membrane with minimal associated systemic activity.

Dosage and administration Syntaris Nasal Spray is for administration by the intra-nasal route only.

Usual starting dose: Adults (including the elderly): 2 sprays into each nostril twice daily. If symptoms are severe, or if an exacerbation occurs, the physician may recommend 2 sprays into each nostril three times daily.
Children: For children five years of age and over, 1 spray (approximately 25 mcg) into each nostril three times daily.
Maintenance dose: After the desired clinical effect is obtained, the maintenance dose should be the smallest amount necessary to control the symptoms. Some patients may be maintained on as little as 1 spray (approximately 25 mcg) to each nostril per day.

The maximum daily dose should not exceed 6 sprays in each nostril for adults, and 3 sprays in each nostril for children five years of age and over.

Syntaris Nasal Spray is not recommended for use in children under five years of age as safety and efficacy studies are not yet completed.

The effect of Syntaris Nasal Spray, unlike that of vasoconstrictor preparations, is not immediate. Full therapeutic benefit requires regular usage. The absence of an immediate effect should be explained to the patient in order to ensure cooperation and continuation of treatment with the regular dosage schedule.

There is no evidence that exceeding the maximum recommended dosage is more effective; higher dosage should therefore be avoided.

For full information on using the device, see patient instruction insert.

Contra-indications, warnings, etc
Contra-indications:

1. Untreated fungal, bacterial or viral nasal or ocular infections.
2. Hypersensitivity to the formulation.

Warnings, precautions, side-effects: Glucocorticoids may mask some signs of infection and new infections may appear during their use.

Syntaris Nasal Spray is not recommended in the first three months of pregnancy. If used in the second or third trimester, the expected benefits should be weighed against the potential hazards to the foetus.

Since systemic activity has not been seen with therapeutic doses of Syntaris, care must be taken when transferring patients from systemic steroid therapy to Syntaris Nasal Spray if there is reason to suspect that their adrenal function is impaired.

Although adrenal suppression or atrophy of the nasal mucosa have not been observed in clinical trials, the potential for these effects should be considered with prolonged excessive usage.

Because of the inhibitory effect of corticosteroids in wound healing, in patients who have experienced recent nasal septal ulcers, recurrent epistaxis, nasal surgery or trauma, a nasal corticosteroid should be used with caution until healing has occurred.

Adverse reactions noted in clinical trials with Syntaris Nasal Spray have been consistent with what one would expect when applying topical medication to an already inflamed membrane. The most frequently observed side-effect was a mild transient nasal burning and stinging which was occasionally severe enough to warrant discontinuation of treatment. Other side-effects noted, in order of decreasing prevalence were: nasal irritation, epistaxis, runny and stuffy nose, sore throat, hoarseness and throat irritation. If severe these may require discontinuation of therapy.

Treatment of overdosage: Administration of large amounts of flunisolide over a short period may produce suppression of hypothalamic-pituitary-adrenal function. In such event, Syntaris Nasal Spray should be reduced immediately to the recommended dosage.

Pharmaceutical precautions Do not refrigerate.

Legal category POM.

Package quantities Each pack of Syntaris Nasal Spray contains one 24 ml bottle and the metered pump/nozzle device.

Further information Nil.

Product licence number 0286/0057.

SYNTEX MENOPHASE*

Presentation Syntex Menophase consists of 28 tablets in a bubble pack. This is a sequential oestrogen-progestogen product comprising six different formulations arranged so that 1 tablet is taken daily starting with 5 pink, and continuing with 8 orange, 2 yellow, 3 green, 6 blue and 4 lavender tablets.

Composition: Syntex Menophase comprises six formulations:

	(mg)	(mcg)	Tablets
1. Mestranol	0.0125	(12.5)	5 pink
2. Mestranol	0.025	(25.0)	8 orange
3. Mestranol	0.050	(50.0)	2 yellow
4. Norethisterone	1.00		
Mestranol	0.025	(25.0)	3 green
5. Norethisterone	1.50		
Mestranol	0.030	(30.0)	6 blue
6. Norethisterone	0.75		
Mestranol	0.020	(20.0)	4 lavender

Uses Syntex Menophase is designed for the treatment of hot flushes and sweats and the amelioration of symptoms associated with the climacteric. Problems which can be associated with failure of endogenous oestrogen production and which have improved in clinical studies include: hot flushes and sweats, depression, lack of concentration, emotional lability, nervousness, lethargy, insomnia, loss of libido, senile vaginitis, pruritus, dry skin, arthritis and neuralgia due to senile osteoporosis.

Dosage and administration The patient is advised to take her first tablet on a Sunday and thereafter to take one tablet at the same time each day in sequential order round the pack. She starts a new pack the day after she has taken her last lavender tablet from the previous pack.

Though menopausal symptoms are likely to improve during the first month of treatment, it will be necessary to maintain therapy for 6–12 months. If symptoms recur after discontinuation, further courses can be prescribed.

Contra-indications, warnings, etc
Contra-indications: As with other oestrogen/progestogen containing compounds, previous thromboembolism, active liver disease, pregnancy and undiagnosed irregular vaginal bleeding should be regarded as contra-indications. Caution should be observed in the presence of pre-existing breast or genital-tract cancer.

Precautions:
1. Syntex Menophase is not an oral contraceptive.
2. Syntex Menophase provides sequential graded doses of hormones; the post-menopausal patient with an intact uterus may therefore experience a small, regular monthly bleed. If forewarned of this possibility, it usually causes no distress.
3. Because Syntex Menophase has not been designed as a contraceptive agent, in the event of a tablet omission the patient should discard the tablets missed and take only that tablet appropriate to the day of the week.
4. Hypertension, which is usually reversible on discontinuing treatment, has occurred in a small percentage of women receiving oestrogen/progestogen medication. A statistical association between the use of certain oestrogen/progestogen-containing preparations and a risk of thromboembolism has been reported, although no cause and effect relationship has been proved. Foetal abnormalities have been reported to occur in the offspring of women who have taken progestogens and/or oestrogens during pregnancy. Pregnancy should be ruled out before initiating or continuing the regimen.

Side-effects: The incidence of side-effects is extremely low. Occasionally breast tenderness and nausea may occur in the first month or two, but usually improve during treatment.

Overdosage: May be manifested by: nausea, vomiting, breast enlargement and vaginal bleeding. There is no specific antidote and treatment should be symptomatic. Gastric lavage may be employed if the overdose is large and the patient is seen sufficiently early (within four hours).

Pharmaceutical precautions Syntex Menophase should be stored in a cool place.

Legal category POM.

Package quantities Push-through bubble-pack containing 28 tablets.

Further information Nil.

Product licence number 0286/0027.

TOPILAR*
TOPILAR* OINTMENT

Presentation Topilar and Topilar Ointment contain fluclorolone acetonide, which is a topical anti-inflammatory corticosteroid.

Topilar contains fluclorolone acetonide 0.025% w/w completely dissolved in the specially formulated FAPG cream base (a combination of fatty alcohols and propylene glycol). The FAPG cream base is a white, soft, non-aqueous hydrophilic, semi-solid vehicle with a slight pearly sheen.

Topilar Ointment contains fluclorolone acetonide 0.025% w/w dissolved in an emollient ointment base.

Uses Topilar and Topilar Ointment are indicated for the treatment of steroid-responsive skin conditions such as psoriasis and dermatitis (eczema), e.g. contact, atopic and seborrhoeic dermatitis.

Topilar has the advantage in that it may be used for dermatoses where, because of the character and site of the lesion and the possible use of polythene occlusion, supervening infection is a potential hazard. If *frank* infection supervenes, appropriate anti-infective therapy should be instituted.

Dosage and administration *Adults (including the elderly) and children:* A thin smear is applied to the affected areas twice daily. This regimen should be followed until the acute phase has passed. Treatment should be continued for at least one week thereafter with one application daily. The course is completed by a further short period, e.g. two weeks, during which one application is made on alternate days.

Polythene occlusion may be required for difficult cases.

Contra-indications, warnings, etc
Contra-indications: (i) Viral, tubercular and frank bacterial infections of the skin. In such cases, appropriate anti-infective therapy should be instituted according to the doctor's normal practice.
(ii) Hypersensitivity to the formulation.

Precautions and warnings: Topical administration of corticosteroids to pregnant animals can cause abnormalities of foetal development. The relevance of this finding to human beings has not been established; however, topical steroids should not be used extensively, i.e. in large amounts or for prolonged periods, in the first trimester of pregnancy.

In infants, the long-term administration of large quantities of topical steroids should be avoided as adrenal suppression may occur even without occlusion. Adrenal suppression occasionally occurs in the long-term treatment of adults, especially if occlusion is used or large areas of the body are treated, although the effect on the adrenal gland is generally transient. Similarly long-term medication with topical steroids, especially under occlusion, may result in atrophy of the skin and subcutaneous tissues. When used on the face this may occur even with short term use. As with all fluorinated topical steroids, Topilar and Topilar Ointment should be used with care in the treatment of chronic conditions.

This preparation is not for ophthalmic use.

Side-effects: The following local adverse reactions have been reported with topical corticosteroids: burning, itching, irritation, dryness, folliculitis, hypertrichosis, acneform eruptions, hypopigmentation, perioral dermatitis, allergic contact dermatitis, maceration of the skin, secondary infection, skin atrophy, striae, miliaria.

Pharmaceutical precautions Topilar and Topilar Ointment should be stored in a cool place. The propylene glycol in the FAPG base may separate at temperatures above 35°C. Topilar Ointment may be diluted in white soft paraffin when a weaker preparation is required.

Legal category POM.

Package quantities Topilar and Topilar Ointment are available in tubes of 30 g and 100 g.

Further information Nil.

Product licence numbers
Topilar 0286/0026
Topilar Ointment 0286/5002

URISPAS*

Presentation Each Urispas Tablet contains flavoxate hydrochloride 100 mg. The white, sugar-coated tablets are overprinted with the name URISPAS.

Uses Urispas is indicated for the symptomatic relief of dysuria, urgency, nocturia, vesical suprapubic pain, frequency and incontinence as may occur in cystitis, prostatitis, urethritis, urethro-cystitis and urethro-trigonitis.

In addition the preparation is indicated for the relief of vesico-urethral spasms due to catheterisation, cystoscopy or indwelling catheters, prior to cystoscopy or catheterisation and sequelae of surgical intervention of the lower urinary tract.

Urispas is an antispasmodic, selective to the urinary tract. In animal and human studies, Urispas has been shown to have a direct antispasmodic action on smooth muscle fibres. In addition, animal studies have shown Urispas to have analgesic and local anaesthetic properties.

Where evidence of urinary infection is present, appropriate anti-infective therapy should be instituted concomitantly.

Dosage and administration *Adults (including the elderly):* The recommended adult dosage is 2 tablets three times a day for as long as required.

Children: Urispas is not yet recommended for children under 12 years of age since safety and efficacy studies in this age group are not completed.

Contra-indications, warnings, etc Urispas is contra-indicated in patients who have any of the following obstructive conditions: pyloric or duodenal obstruction, obstructive intestinal lesions, or ileus, achalasia, gastro-intestinal haemorrhage and obstructive uropathies of the lower urinary tract.

Special precautions: Urispas should be used with caution in patients with suspected glaucoma.

As with all drugs, Urispas should also be used with caution in pregnant women.

Overdosage: Patients who have taken an overdosage of Urispas should have gastric lavage performed within four hours of the overdosage occurring. If overdosage is extreme, or there is delay in removing the drug from the stomach, administration of a para-sympathomimetic drug should be considered.

Side-effects: In clinical trials, comparing Urispas with other antispasmodic agents, the incidence of side-effects was low. Those adverse reactions that have been recorded include headache, nausea, fatigue, diarrhoea, blurred vision and dry mouth.

Pharmaceutical precautions No special precautions are required.

Legal category POM.

Package quantities Containers of 100.

Further information Nil.

Product licence number 0286/5005.

UTOVLAN*

Presentation Each Utovlan Tablet contains norethisterone 5 mg. The white tablets are uncoated, circular bevel-edged and with a break-line.

Uses At low dosage Utovlan is indicated for dysfunctional uterine bleeding, endometriosis, polymenorrhoea, menorrhagia, metropathia haemorrhagica, postponement of menstruation, and premenstrual syndrome. At high dosage Utovlan is recommended for disseminated carcinoma of the breast.

Dosage and administration *Low dosage*
Dysfunctional Uterine Bleeding, Polymenorrhoea, Menorrhagia, Dysmenorrhoea and Metropathia Haemorrhagica: 1 tablet three times daily for 10 days; bleeding usually stops within 48 hours. Withdrawal bleeding resembling true menstruation occurs a few days after the end of treatment. One tablet twice daily, from days 19 to 26 of the two subsequent cycles, should be given to prevent recurrence of the condition.

Endometriosis: 1 tablet three times daily for a minimum treatment period of six months. The dosage should be increased to 4 or 5 tablets a day if spotting occurs. The initial dosage should be resumed when bleeding or spotting stops.

Postponement of menstruation: 1 tablet three times daily, starting three days before the expected onset of menstruation. Menstruation usually follows within three days of finishing the treatment.

Pre-menstrual syndrome: 1 tablet daily from days 16 to 25 of the menstrual cycle.

High dosage
For disseminated breast carcinoma the starting dose is 8 tablets (40 mg) per day increasing to 12 tablets (60 mg) if no regression is noted.

Contra-indications, warnings, etc
Contra-indications: Pregnancy, disturbance of liver function, history during pregnancy of idiopathic jaundice, severe pruritus, herpes, undiagnosed irregular vaginal bleeding.

Side-effects: These rarely occur at the usual dosage levels of 15 mg per day. Mild nausea has been reported. High dosage treatment, even over long periods, is well tolerated; transitory digestive upsets and jaundice have rarely been reported.

If menstrual bleeding should fail to follow a course of Utovlan, the possibility of pregnancy must be ruled out before a further course is given.

Pharmaceutical precautions No special precautions.

Legal category POM.

Package quantities Cans of 100 and 1,000 tablets.

Further information Nil.

Product licence number 0286/5007.

Trade Mark

Tillotts Laboratories
Henlow Trading Estate
Henlow
Bedfordshire SG 16 6DS

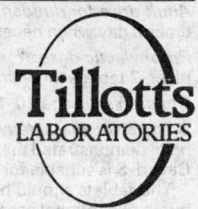

Tillotts
LABORATORIES

ASACOL* ▼
Presentation Red, oblong tablets containing 400 mg mesalazine (5-amino salicylic acid) coated with an acrylic based resin (Eudragit S) to ensure release of the active ingredient in the terminal ileum and colon.

Uses For the maintenance of remission of ulcerative colitis in patients who cannot tolerate sulphasalazine.

Dosage and administration
Adult dosage: 3 to 6 tablets daily in divided doses. There is no dose recommendation for children.

Contra-indications, warnings, etc
Contra-indications: A history of sensitivity to salicylates. Children under 2 years of age.

Precautions: Renal disorder: mesalazine is excreted rapidly by the kidney mainly as its metabolite, N-acetyl 5-amino salicylic acid. In rats, large doses of mesalazine injected intravenously produce tubular and glomerular toxicity. Although no renal toxicity has been reported in patients taking Asacol, it is not recommended in patients with renal impairment and caution should be exercised in patients with a raised blood urea or proteinuria.

Asacol should not be given with lactulose or similar preparations which lower stool pH and may prevent release of mesalazine.

Use during pregnancy: The theoretical risk of kernicterus linked to the sulphapyridine moiety of sulphasalazine is avoided with Asacol. No information is available with regard to teratogenicity, however, negligible quantities of mesalazine are transferred across the placenta and none is excreted in breast milk following sulphasalazine therapy. Use of Asacol during pregnancy should be with caution, and only if, in the opinion of the physician, the potential benefits of treatment are greater than the possible hazards.

Use in the elderly: Use in the elderly should be cautious and subject to patients having a normal renal function (see precautions).

Adverse reactions: Adverse reactions occur in a small proportion of patients who previously could not tolerate sulphasalazine. The side-effects are predominantly gastrointestinal (nausea, diarrhoea and abdominal pain) and headache. Asacol may be associated with the exacerbation of the symptoms of colitis in those patients who have previously had such problems with sulphasalazine.

Other side effects observed with sulphasalazine such as depression of bone marrow and of sperm count and function, have not been reported with Asacol.

Treatment of overdosage: Gastric lavage and intravenous transfusion of electrolytes to promote diuresis. There is no specific antidote.

Pharmaceutical precautions Store at room temperature in a dry place. Do not expose to direct sunlight.

Legal category POM.

Package quantities Cartons of 100 tablets; each carton containing 10 blister packs of 10 tablets.

Further information Mesalazine is one of the two components of sulphasalazine, the other being sulphapyridine. It is the latter which is responsible for the majority of the side effects associated with sulphasalazine therapy whilst mesalazine is known to be the active moiety in the treatment of ulcerative colitis. Asacol consists only of this active component which it releases topically in the colon.

Asacol contains 400 mg of available mesalazine. This is released in the terminal ileum and large bowel by the effect of pH. Above pH 7 the Eudragit coat disintegrates and releases the active constituent.

Asacol contains in a single tablet an equivalent quantity of mesalazine to that theoretically available from the complete azoreduction of 1 g of sulphasalazine.

Product licence number 0424/0032.

CAVED-S* TABLETS
Presentation Brown mottled tablets embossed Caved-S. Each tablet contains:

Deglycyrrhizinated liquorice	380 mg
Aluminium hydroxide gel	100 mg
Magnesium carbonate	200 mg
Sodium bicarbonate	100 mg

Uses *Action and indications:* For treatment of peptic ulcer and other allied conditions.

The main active constituent of Caved-S is deglycyrrhizinated liquorice, which has peptic ulcer healing and spasmolytic activity and is free from deoxycortone like actions (i.e. does not alter serum levels of sodium, potassium or chloride). Deglycyrrhizinated liquorice primarily enhances the defence mechanism of the mucosa by increasing the number of mucus secreting cells. The cell proliferation rate is also increased. The spasmolytic activity and the action of the added antacids, alleviates gastric distress.

The special deglycyrrhizination process of Caved-liquorice, ensures that side effects, such as oedema, hypertension and hypokalaemia, normally associated with crude liquorice or liquorice derivatives, have been eliminated.

Dosage and administration Oral administration. The tablets should be taken between meals.

Adult dose for gastric ulcer: 2 tablets three times a day.

Adult dose for duodenal ulcer: Increase to 2 tablets six times a day when necessary.

Prophylactic dose: 1 tablet three times a day for gastric ulcer, 2 tablets three times a day for duodenal ulcer.

Children's dosage 10–14 years: Half adult dose.

Dosage for the elderly: Clinical and metabolic studies have demonstrated that the recommended adult dose for Caved-S is suitable for use in elderly patients.

The tablets should be lightly chewed and swallowed but in exceptional cases of objection to taste the tablets should be broken into a few pieces and then swallowed with a drink of water. No additional antacids need be taken.

Contra-indications, warnings, etc Rare cases of mild diarrhoea can occur. No other side-effects have been reported.

Study of teratology and embryotoxicity of Caved-S in rabbits: Summary: No significant differences between treated and control groups were established in any of the parameters analysed. No skeletal or soft-tissue changes were found. The overall results of this study would indicate that the compound failed to induce teratological abnormalities in the conceptus of the animals studied. The administration of the compound (Caved-S) during days 6–18 of pregnancy did not produce signs of embryotoxicity and no teratogenic potential was demonstrated. However, Caved-S, like all drugs, should be given with caution during pregnancy.

Study of 13 weeks' subacute oral toxicity of Caved-S in dogs: Summary: The oral administration of Caved-S for 13 weeks at dose levels of 2,000, 1,000 and 500 mg/kg body weight appears to be well tolerated by beagle dogs. No significant differences were noted in parameters analysed, either during compound administration or during four-week withdrawal from the dosing schedule.

Treatment of overdosage: No cases of overdosage have been reported. If excessive amounts are taken gastric lavage and supportive symptomatic treatment are recommended.

Pharmaceutical precautions *Storage:* Protect from excessive heat and moisture.

Legal category GSL.

Package quantities Containers of 60, 240 and 600 tablets.

Further information Nil.

Product licence number 0424/5000.

CEDOCARD*-5

Presentation Round white tablets, embossed 'CC' reverse side scored, containing 5 mg isosorbide dinitrate.

Uses For the treatment and prevention of angina pectoris and for the long term management of coronary insufficiency.

Cedocard-5 is a coronary vasodilator having a marked anti-anginal effect when administered sublingually as well as orally.

The mode of action depends on the reduced work load following vasodilation and reduced venous return.

Dosage and administration *Sublingual administration:* Adult dose: For treatment of acute attack of angina pectoris – 1 tablet as required.

Oral administration: Adult dose: For prophylaxis of angina pectoris 1–2 tablets three or four times a day as required.

To prevent nocturnal attacks of angina pectoris – 1–2 tablets before retiring to sleep.

Onset of action sublingually – one to two minutes and duration of up to two hours.

Onset of action orally – 20/30 minutes and duration of four to six hours.

Dosage for the elderly: The dosage of nitrates in cardiovascular disease is usually determined by patient response and stabilisation. Clinical experience has not necessitated alternative advice for use in elderly patients. The pharmacokinetics of isosorbide dinitrate in patients with severe renal failure and liver cirrhosis are similar to those in normal subjects.

No recommended dose for children.

Contra-indications, warnings, etc Development of tolerance to this drug and cross tolerance to other nitrates and nitrites.

Adverse reaction: Cutaneous vasodilation with flushing, transient episodes of dizziness and weakness, and other signs of cerebral ischaemia, may occur with postural hypotension.

Use in pregnancy: No data have been reported which would indicate the possibility of adverse effects resulting from the use of isosorbide dinitrate in pregnancy. Safety in pregnancy, however, has not been established. Isosorbide dinitrate should only be used in pregnancy if, in the opinion of the physician, the possible benefits of treatment outweigh the possible hazards.

Treatment of overdosage: In rare cases of overdosage, gastric lavage is indicated. Passive exercise of the extremities of the recumbent patient will promote venous return.

Pharmaceutical precautions *Storage:* Protect from heat and moisture.

Legal category P.

Package quantities Containers of 60 and 180.

Further information Cedocard-5 rapidly dissolves after sublingual administration to bring quick relief from acute anginal attack.

If the tablet is swallowed a more prolonged action is achieved for prophylaxis.

Cedocard-5 is more stable than trinitrin and has a shelf life of 5 years.

Product licence number 0424/5001.

CEDOCARD-10*

Presentation Round, rose coloured tablets, scored on one side and imprinted with CC on the other side. Each tablet contains 10 mg isosorbide dinitrate.

Uses For the prophylaxis of angina pectoris.

Cedocard-10 relaxes vascular smooth muscle, dilates coronary vessels, reduces peripheral resistance and venous return, resulting in alteration of myocardial metabolism and reduction of myocardial oxygen demand.

Dosage and administration For oral administration.

Adult dose: 1–3 tablets four times daily. Onset of action 20–30 minutes and duration of four to six hours.

Dosage for the elderly: The dosage of nitrates in

cardiovascular disease is usually determined by patient response and stabilisation. Clinical experience has not necessitated alternative advice for use in elderly patients. The pharmacokinetics of isosorbide dinitrate in patients with severe renal failure and liver cirrhosis are similar to those in normal subjects.

There is no recommended dose for children.

Contra-indications, warnings, etc
Contra-indications: A history of sensitivity to the drug.

Precautions: Tolerance and cross-tolerance to other nitrates may occur.

Adverse reactions: Transient headaches, these can usually be controlled by temporary dosage reduction.

Cutaneous vasodilation with flushing, transient episodes of dizziness and weakness, and other signs of cerebral ischaemia, may occur with postural hypotension.

Use in pregnancy: No data have been reported which would indicate the possibility of adverse effects resulting from the use of isosorbide dinitrate in pregnancy. Safety in pregnancy, however, has not been established. Isosorbide dinitrate should only be used in pregnancy if, in the opinion of the physician, the possible benefits of treatment outweigh the possible hazards.

Treatment of overdosage: In rare cases of overdosage, gastric lavage is indicated. Passive exercise of the extremities of the recumbent patient will promote venous return.

Pharmaceutical precautions *Storage:* Protect from heat and moisture.

Legal category P.

Package quantity Containers of 100 and 1000 tablets.

Further information Nil.

Product licence number 0424/0015.

CEDOCARD-20*

Presentation Round, flat, bevel-edged blue tablets, scored on one side and imprinted CC on the other side, containing 20 mg isosorbide dinitrate per tablet.

Uses For the treatment of severe congestive heart failure. Cedocard-20 reduces elevated left ventricular filling pressure in patients with congestive heart failure, and lowers peripheral resistance, which leads to a reduced after load; therefore, the heart has to perform less work to overcome the peripheral resistance.

For the prophylaxis of angina pectoris.

Dosage and administration Oral administration.
Severe congestive heart failure: After determination of peripheral resistance, arterial and pulmonary pressure, and stroke volume, half a tablet of Cedocard-20 is administered. On the basis of its effect on these parameters, an effective dose of Cedocard-20 is established. This dose can vary between ½ and 2 tablets, and is then administered every 4 hours. Haemodynamic monitoring of the treatment should be carried out.

Angina prophylaxis: One half to 2 tablets three or four times daily.

Dosage for the elderly: The dosage of nitrates in cardiovascular disease is usually determined by patient response and stabilisation. Clinical experience has not necessitated alternative advice for use in elderly patients.

The pharmacokinetics of isosorbide dinitrate in patients with severe renal failure and liver cirrhosis are similar to those in normal subjects.

No recommended dose for children.

Contra-indications, warnings, etc
Contra-indications: Hypotension, cardiac shock. A known sensitivity to the drug.

Precautions: Treatment of severe congestive heart failure with Cedocard-20 should be checked haemodynamically, by measuring the intra-arterial pressure, pulmonary artery pressure, stroke volume, and peripheral resistance.

Adverse reactions: Transient headaches at the start of therapy; these can usually be controlled by temporary dosage reduction.

Use in pregnancy: No data have been reported which would indicate the possibility of adverse effects resulting from the use of isosorbide dinitrate in pregnancy. Safety in pregnancy, however, has not been established. Isosorbide dinitrate should only be used in pregnancy if, in the opinion of the physician, the possible benefits of treatment outweigh the possible hazards.

Treatment of overdosage: In rare cases of overdosage, gastric lavage is indicated. Passive exercise of the extremities of the recumbent patient will promote venous return.

Pharmaceutical precautions *Storage:* Protect from heat and moisture.

Legal category POM.

Package quantities Containers of 100 and 1000 tablets.

Further information Nil.

Product licence number 0424/0008.

CEDOCARD RETARD*-20

Presentation Round yellow sustained-release tablets, embossed CC, SR and scored on reverse side, each containing 20 mg isosorbide dinitrate.

Uses For the prophylaxis of angina pectoris.

The active principle of Cedocard Retard-20 is isosorbide dinitrate which relaxes vascular smooth muscle and produces coronary vasodilation, reduction in peripheral resistance and venous return, alteration of myocardial metabolism, and reduction of the myocardial oxygen demand.

Dosage and administration For oral administration.

Adult dose: One tablet in the morning and 1 tablet before retiring to sleep. Onset of action 20–30 minutes and the duration of action is 10–12 hours.

Dosage for the elderly: The dosage of nitrates in cardiovascular disease is usually determined by patient response and stabilisation. Clinical experience has not necessitated alternative advice for use in elderly patients. The pharmacokinetics of isosorbide dinitrate in patients with severe renal failure and liver cirrhosis are similar to those in normal subjects.

There is no recommended dose for children.

Contra-indications, warnings, etc
Contra-indication: A history of sensitivity to the drug.

Precautions: Tolerance and cross-tolerance to other nitrates may occur.

Adverse reactions: Cutaneous vasodilation with flushing, transient episodes of dizziness and weakness, and other signs of cerebral ischaemia, may occur with postural hypotension.

Use in pregnancy: No data have been reported which would indicate the possibility of adverse effects resulting from the use of isosorbide dinitrate in pregnancy. Safety in pregnancy, however, has not been established. Isosorbide dinitrate should only be used in pregnancy if, in the opinion of the physician, the possible benefits of treatment outweigh the possible hazards.

Treatment of overdosage: In rare cases of overdosage, gastric lavage is indicated. Passive exercise of the extremities of the recumbent patient will promote venous return.

Pharmaceutical precautions *Storage:* Protect from heat and moisture.

Legal category P.

Package quantities Containers of 60 and 1000 tablets.

Further information Nil.

Product licence number 0424/0007.

CEDOCARD* IV

Presentation Clear glass 10 ml ampoules, 50 ml bottles and 100 ml bottles each containing 1 mg/ml isosorbide dinitrate in colourless isotonic saline solution.

Uses For the treatment of unresponsive congestive heart failure, particularly after myocardial infarction.

Cedocard infusion reduces elevated left ventricular filling pressure in patients with congestive heart failure.

For the control of refractory angina pectoris.

Dosage and administration Administration by intravenous infusion only, or in small volumes via a syringe pump.

Adult dose: The dosage must be determined individually. Doses of 2–10 mg per hour (33–167 mcg/min) are recommended.

Dosage for the elderly: The dosage of nitrates in cardiovascular disease is usually determined by patient response and stabilisation. Clinical experience has not necessitated alternative advice for use in elderly patients. The pharmacokinetics of isosorbide dinitrate in patients with severe renal failure and liver cirrhosis are similar to those in normal subjects.

There is no recommended dose for children.

Start the infusion with 2 mg/hour and increase progressively according to the evolution of haemodynamic parameters and the clinical condition of the patient. Gradually decrease the concentration of infusion and switch to oral or sublingual isosorbide dinitrate. There should be no abrupt interruption of the infusion except for severe hypotension. Continuous haemodynamic supervision during the infusion is required.

Preparation of solution for infusion: The contents of Cedocard IV must be administered by infusion only, or in small volumes via a syringe pump.

Cedocard IV can be diluted with sodium chloride 0.9% or dextrose injection 5–30%. The diluted solution should be well mixed before administration.

Contra-indications, warnings, etc

Contra-indications: Hypotension, cardiogenic shock.

Precautions: Close supervision of the patient is necessary for safe and optimum treatment. Cedocard IV must be administered by infusion only, or in small volumes via a syringe pump.

If PVC infusion bags (e.g. Travenol Viaflex, Boots Steriflex) and administration sets are used for Cedocard infusion, 15–30% of the drug can be lost by adsorption. There is no loss of active constituent from solution in glass or polyethylene apparatus.

It is recommended that Cedocard IV is administered using a syringe pump (glass or rigid plastic) with short sections of polyethylene tubing. Alternatively, a polyethylene infusion bag (e.g. Boots Polyfusor) may be used.

Should only PVC infusion bags be available, then it is important to carry out close haemodynamic monitoring of the patient; infusion rate should be modified according to required haemodynamic response. PVC bags of 500 ml volume should be used to minimise adsorption of isosorbide dinitrate.

Adverse reactions: Headache. In the case of an excessive reduction in blood pressure, phenomena indicating a reduced blood supply to the heart may appear.

Use in pregnancy: No data have been reported which would indicate the possibility of adverse effects resulting from the use of isosorbide dinitrate in pregnancy. Safety in pregnancy, however, has not been established. Isosorbide dinitrate should only be used in pregnancy if, in the opinion of the physician, the possible benefits of treatment outweigh the possible hazards.

Treatment of overdosage: If arterial systolic blood pressure drops below 90 mm. Hg, and if heart rate increases above 10% of its initial value, the infusion should be discontinued to allow a return to pretreatment levels. Passive exercise of the extremeties of the recumbent patient will promote venous return.

Pharmaceutical precautions Protect from exposure to excessive heat. The Cedocard dilution for infusion is stable up to 24 hours.

The diluted solution should be well mixed before intravenous administration. Bottles of Cedocard IV should be used once only and discarded. (Do not multidose.)

Legal category POM.

Package quantities Packs of 10 ampoules, 5 × 50 ml bottles and 4 × 100 ml bottles.

Further information Nil.

Product licence number 0424/0012.

CHENOCEDON*

Presentation Hard gelatin capsules (size no. 1), r.p.s. lock: green cap, blue body. Each capsule contains 250 mg chenodeoxycholic acid.

Uses For the dissolution of cholesterol gallstones in a functioning gallbladder, in patients with a high surgery risk, or where surgery is contraindicated. Gallstones, which can be treated with this therapy, should be radiolucent.

Chenodeoxycholic acid, a bile acid synthesised by the liver, enhances the dissolving capacity of bile for cholesterol. Chenodeoxycholic acid also diminishes cholesterol synthesis in the liver so that the biliary concentration of cholesterol decreases. Cholesterol gallstones will dissolve when bile is no longer saturated with cholesterol.

Dosage and administration For oral administration.

Adult dose: 15 mg/kg body weight per day. Therefore, 3–5 capsules daily, depending on body weight, preferably taken during meals.

The duration of the treatment may vary from three months to two years depending on the size of the gallstones. Radiological examination should take place at six monthly intervals. When gallstones can no longer be demonstrated on two successive cholecystograms, treatment may be regarded as successful. Subsequent follow-up, however, remains necessary, as oversaturation of the bile may occur again, in which case the chenodeoxycholic acid therapy should be re-instituted.

It is recommended that treatment continues for 3–6 months after gallstone dissolution.

Dosage for the elderly: Treatment should take into consideration the stated contra-indications, precautions and warnings, with special attention to those situations prevalent in elderly patients.

There is no dose recommendation for children.

Contra-indications, warnings, etc

Contra-indications: Radio-opaque, calcified gallstones, or in patients with non-functioning gallbladders. Frequent gallstone colics with cholecystitis, cholangitis, or pancreatitis. Inflammation of the gastrointestinal tract. Chronic liver disease. Severe kidney impairment. Patients previously treated with cholestyramine. Pregnancy, or in women who may become pregnant.

Precautions: Food irritating the gallbladder should be avoided. A low calorie diet is recommended during treatment. If possible, oral contraceptives should be replaced by other methods. Liver function should be monitored during treatment.

Warnings: Chenodeoxycholic acid given in long-term studies at doses of 600 mg/kg/day to rats and 1000 mg/kg/day to mice induced malignant liver cell tumours in female rats and benign liver cell tumours in male mice and female rats. The clinical significance of these findings is not known.

Adverse reactions: Diarrhoea and transient elevation of serum transaminases have been observed particularly at the start of therapy. If diarrhoea occurs more than twice a day or serum transaminases show an increased level on more than two occasions in one month, then half the dose of chenodeoxycholic acid should be used until the side effect has disappeared. The dosage can be thereafter gradually raised to 15 mg/kg body weight. A monthly examination should be carried out during the first three months to regulate dosage, and to monitor any side effects.

Pruritus has also been reported during treatment with chenodeoxycholic acid.

Treatment of overdosage: It is unlikely that overdosage will cause serious adverse effects. Close monitoring of liver function should be carried out. If necessary, ion-exchange resins might be used to bind bile acids in the gastrointestinal tract.

Pharmaceutical precautions Store in well closed containers, in cool, dry conditions.

Legal category POM.

Package quantity 100 capsules.

Further information Nil.

Product licence number 0424/0011.

COLPERMIN*

Presentation A light blue/dark blue enteric-coated hard gelatine capsule size 1, with a green band between cap and body. Each capsule contains 0.2 ml standardised peppermint oil BP.

Uses For the treatment of symptoms of discomfort and of abdominal colic and distension experienced by patients with irritable bowel syndrome.

The enteric-coating of the capsule delays release of the peppermint oil until it reaches the distal small bowel. The oil exerts a local effect of colonic relaxation and a fall of intracolonic pressure.

Dosage and administration For oral administration.

Adult dose: One capsule three times a day, preferably before meals and taken with a small quantity of water. The capsules should *not* be taken immediately after food.

The dose may be increased to two capsules, three times a day when discomfort is more severe.

The capsules should be taken until symptoms resolve, usually within one or two weeks. At times when symptoms are more persistent, the capsules can be continued for longer periods of between 2 to 3 months.

Dosage for the elderly: The mode of action of peppermint oil is local rather than systemic. Clinical experience and known pharmacokinetics have not necessitated alternative advice for elderly patients.

There is no experience in the use of these capsules in children under the age of 15 years.

Contra-indications, warnings, etc

Precautions: The capsules should not be broken or chewed because this would release the peppermint oil prematurely, possibly causing local irritation of the mouth and oesophagus.

Patients who already suffer from heartburn, sometimes experience an exacerbation of these symptoms when taking the capsule. Treatment should be discontinued in these patients.

There are no data available to establish the safety of Colpermin in pregnancy, therefore, it should be used only if, in the opinion of the physician, the possible benefits of treatment outweigh the possible hazards.

Adverse effects: Heartburn; sensitivity reactions to menthol, which are rare, and include erythematous skin rash, headache, bradycardia, muscle tremor and ataxia.

Treatment of overdosage: If capsules have been recently ingested, the stomach should be emptied by gastric lavage. Observation should be carried out with symptomatic treatment if necessary.

Pharmaceutical precautions Store in a cool place. Avoid direct sunlight.

Legal category P.

Package quantities Containers of 100 capsules.

Further information Nil.

Product licence number 0424/0009.

MONO-CEDOCARD*-20 ▼

Presentation Round white tablets, embossed 'MONO CC', reverse side scored, containing 20 mg isosorbide 5-mononitrate.

Uses For the prophylaxis of angina pectoris.
Isosorbide mononitrate, the active constituent of Mono-Cedocard-20, is the major active metabolite of isosorbide dinitrate. It has significant vasodilator activity, the strongest effect being exerted on the venous system, and a lesser effect on the arterial circulation. As a consequence, the heart has less work to perform against diminished resistance, and therefore oxygen requirement is reduced.

Dosage and administration For oral administration.

Adult dose: One tablet two or three times a day taken after meals. The tablet should be swallowed (without chewing) with a little water. The dosage may be increased to two tablets three times a day.

Dosage for the elderly: The dosage of nitrates in cardiovascular disease is usually determined by patient response and stabilisation. Clinical experience has not necessitated alternative advice for use in elderly patients.
There is no dose recommendation for children.

Contra-indications, warnings, etc
Contra-indications: In acute myocardial infarction with low filling pressures.
In acute circulatory failure (shock, vascular collapse).
When blood pressure is very low.
During the first three months of pregnancy.

Warnings/precautions: Consumption of alcohol should be avoided during treatment, as reaction capacity may be reduced, and the vasodilator activity of isosorbide mononitrate may be enhanced.

Adverse effects: Generally, no serious adverse effects are to be expected. Headache, dizziness, fatigue, palpitations, orthostatic hypotension and flushing may occur, especially at the beginning of treatment. These reactions can usually be controlled by a temporary dosage reduction.

Treatment of overdosage: Gastric lavage; passive exercise of the extremities of the recumbent patient will promote venous return.

Pharmaceutical precautions *Storage:* Protect from heat and moisture.

Legal category POM.

Package quantities Packs of 100 tablets.

Further information The plasma half-life of isosorbide mononitrate is 4.2 hours.
After oral administration, isosorbide mononitrate is well absorbed, a haemodynamic effect being measurable within 15–20 minutes. In contrast to isosorbide dinitrate, the mononitrate is not subject to first-pass metabolism.

Product licence number 0424/0040.

MONO-CEDOCARD*-40 ▼

Presentation Round white tablets, embossed '40 MONO 40', reverse side scored, containing 40 mg isosorbide 5-mononitrate.

Uses For the prophylaxis of angina pectoris. Isosorbide mononitrate, the active constituent of Mono-Cedocard-40, is the major active metabolite of isosorbide dinitrate. It has significant vasodilator activity, the strongest effect being exerted on the venous system, and a lesser effect on the arterial circulation. As a consequence, the heart has less work to perform against diminished resistance, and therefore oxygen requirement is reduced.

Dosage and administration For oral administration.

Adult dose: One tablet twice a day taken after meals. The tablets should be swallowed (without chewing) with a little water.

Dosage for the elderly: The dosage of nitrates in cardiovascular disease is usually determined by patient response and stabilisation. Clinical experience has not necessitated alternative advice for use in elderly patients.
There is no dose recommendation for children.

Contra-indications, warnings, etc
Contra-indications: In acute myocardial infarction with low filling pressures. In acute circulatory failure (shock, vascular collapse). When blood pressure is very low. During the first three months of pregnancy.

Warnings/precautions: Consumption of alcohol should be avoided during treatment, as reaction capacity may be reduced, and the vasodilator activity of isosorbide mononitrate may be enhanced.

Adverse effects: Generally, no serious adverse effects are to be expected. Headache, dizziness, fatigue, palpitations, orthostatic hypotension and flushing may occur, especially at the beginning of treatment. These reactions can usually be controlled by a temporary dosage reduction.

Treatment of overdosage: Gastric lavage; passive exercise of the extremities of the recumbent patient will promote venous return.

Pharmaceutical precautions Storage: Protect from heat and moisture.

Legal category P.

Package quantities Packs of 60 tablets.

Further information The plasma half-life of isosorbide mononitrate is 4.2 hours.
After oral administration, isosorbide mononitrate is well absorbed, a haemodynamic effect being measurable within 15–20 minutes. In contrast to isosorbide dinitrate, the mononitrate is not subject to first-pass metabolism.

Product licence number 0424/0054.

NIFEREX*

Presentation Niferex is a non-ionic polysaccharide-iron complex.
Tablets, brown, each containing the equivalent to 50 mg elemental iron.
Elixir, brown, flavoured, containing the equivalent to 100 mg elemental iron per 5 ml teaspoonful.

Uses Haemopoietic. For the prophylaxis and treatment of uncomplicated iron-deficiency anaemia.

Dosage and administration *Prophylactic dose:*
Adults: 1 tablet or $2\frac{1}{2}$ ml elixir daily.

Therapeutic dose: Adults: 2 tablets or 5 ml elixir once or twice daily.

Children 6–12 years: 5 ml elixir daily.

Children 2–6 years: $2\frac{1}{2}$ ml elixir daily.

Infants: 1 drop elixir (paediatric) per 1 lb body weight

three times a day (one drop contains approximately 0.6 mg elemental iron).

Contra-indications, warnings, etc No specific contra-indications, but obviously Niferex should not be given to patients with known iron overload. In common with all oral iron preparations Niferex should be given with caution where there is peptic ulceration.

Use in pregnancy: As with other oral iron therapies, Niferex may be used for prophylaxis against anaemia during pregnancy.

Treatment of overdosage: Gastric lavage is recommended. Previous case reports of overdose have not resulted in serious adverse effects.

Pharmaceutical precautions Niferex Tablets should be kept in a sealed container and dispensed in moisture-proof containers. Niferex elixir can be diluted with distilled water or sorbitol to almost any concentration without stability problems, as long as the pH is maintained above 5.

Legal category P.

Package quantities *Tablets:* Plastic container of 100 tablets.
Elixir: Bottle of 240 ml.
Paediatric elixir: Dropper bottle of 30 ml.

Further information Niferex is a highly water-soluble polysaccharide-iron complex which is stable in the range pH 4.5–11.0, and disassociates only after leaving the stomach. The iron is released over a period of one hour, circumventing the nausea associated with sudden doses of free iron. In elixir form, the complex remains in solution and does not precipitate in gastric or duodenal fluid.

Product licence numbers
Tablets   5046/5000
Elixir   5046/5001

NIFEREX-150*

Presentation Size 1, hard gelatine capsule, brown opaque body and orange opaque cap, imprinted "Central" in white ink on both cap and body, containing 150 mg elemental iron (as polysaccharide-iron complex) per capsule.

Uses Haemopoietic. For the treatment of uncomplicated iron-deficiency anaemia.

Dosage and administration Oral administration.

Adults: One or two capsules daily.

Children: As directed by a physician. Niferex elixir or Niferex tablets (50 mg iron) are recommended for children.

Contra-indications, warnings, etc Niferex-150 capsules should not be given to patients with haemochromatosis and haemosiderosis, and to those with a known hypersensitivity to any of the ingredients.

Use in pregnancy: As with other oral iron preparations, Niferex-150 may be used for prophylaxis against anaemia during pregnancy.

Pharmaceutical precautions Niferex-150 capsules should be protected from heat and moisture.

Legal category P.

Package quantities Packs of 100 and 500 capsules in plastic containers.

Further information Polysaccharide-iron complex has relatively low toxicity, and few, if any, of the gastrointestinal side-effects associated with iron therapy, thus permitting full therapeutic dosage (150 to 300 mg elemental iron daily) in a single dose if desirable. There is no staining of teeth and no metallic after taste.

Product licence number 0424/0016.

ROWACHOL*

Presentation A green spherical, enteric-coated soft gelatin capsule (3 minims round). Each capsule contains the following active ingredients in Olive Oil BP:

Pinene	17 mg
Camphene	5 mg
Cineol BP	2 mg
Menthone	6 mg
Menthol BP	32 mg
Borneol	5 mg

Uses Adjunct therapy for the dispersal (by dissolution and/or expulsion) of stones in the common bile duct. To be used in combination with chenodeoxycholic acid.

It has been demonstrated that if Rowachol is combined with either low or medium dose chenodeoxycholic acid, the gallstone dissolution rate is greater than if the same dose of chenodeoxycholic acid is used alone. Combined therapy enables a reduced dose of chenodeoxycholic acid to be used and there is therefore a lower incidence of side-effects.

The treatment is particularly appropriate in the case of elderly and poor risk patients where the mortality and morbidity of surgery increases considerably, when endoscopic expertise is not available, or if endoscopic technique fails because of the presence of periampullary diverticulum, or is not technically possible because of a previous gastrectomy operation.

Rowachol increases biliary secretion, relieves spasm of the bile ducts, enhances metabolic liver function and reduces biliary stasis. By inhibiting HMGCoA reductase, endogenous cholesterol production is reduced, desaturating bile, assisting the dissolution of gallstones, and preventing the precipitation of further stones.

Dosage and administration For oral administration
Adult dose: 1–2 capsules three times daily taken before meals. A dose of one capsule three times daily is recommended at the start of treatment.
No dose recommendation for children.

Contra-indications, warnings, etc Caution should be used in patients receiving oral anticoagulants, or other agents metabolised by the liver, where the dose is critical.
Reduced cholesterol intake in the diet is advisable.
Although no teratogenic effects have been reported, Rowachol should not be given in the first trimester of pregnancy.
Conservative medical treatment for stones in the common bile duct should be initiated with the awareness that duct stones can give rise to clinical complications such as obstructive jaundice, ascending cholangitis, pancreatitis, etc. and the physician should be aware of the necessity of being promptly informed (particularly in the case of elderly patients) so that appropriate measures can be taken.

Treatment of overdosage: If capsules have been recently

ingested the stomach should be emptied by gastric lavage. Observation should be carried out with symptomatic treatment if necessary.

Pharmaceutical precautions *Storage:* Protect from heat and moisture.

Legal category POM.

Package quantities Containers of 50 and 500 capsules.

Further information Nil.

Product licence number 0007/0002.

ROWATINEX*

Presentation *Liquid:* a pale yellow liquid in a 10 ml amber, screwcap dropper bottle, containing the following active ingredients:

Pinene	31% v/v	(3.1 g)
Borneol	10% v/v	(1.0 g)
Cineole	3% v/v	(0.3 g)
Camphene	15% v/v	(1.5 g)
Fenchone	4% v/v	(0.4 g)
Anethol	4% v/v	(0.4 g)

(olive oil excipient q.s. ad 10 g)

Capsules: A yellow spherical enteric-coated soft gelatine capsule. Each capsule contains 0.1 ml of Rowatinex liquid.

Uses Urolithiasis, renal disorders and urinary tract infections. The combination of terpenes in Rowatinex promotes expulsion of calculi, and has been shown to prevent urinary stone formation. Rowatinex has a direct antispasmodic action on smooth muscle, and has also been shown to have anti-inflammatory and bactericidal properties.

Dosage and administration For oral administration.

Adult dose: Liquid: 3–5 drops 4 or 5 times daily taken thirty minutes before meals. Capsules: 1 capsule 3 or 4 times daily. No dose recommendation for children.

Contra-indications, warnings, etc
Contra-indications: None known.

Precautions: Although no teratogenic effects have been reported, Rowatinex should not be given in the first trimester of pregnancy.

Treatment of overdosage: Gastric lavage, followed by observation and symptomatic treatment if necessary.

Pharmaceutical precautions *Storage:* Protect from heat and moisture.

Legal category P.

Package quantities Liquid – 10 ml dropper bottle. Capsules – containers of 50 capsules.

Further information Nil.

Product licence numbers
Liquid   0531/6284
Capsules   0531/6283

TAMOFEN*

Presentation Round, convex, off-white tablets, scored on one side and marked T10 on the reverse. Each tablet contains 15.2 mg Tamoxifen Citrate BP equivalent to 10 mg tamoxifen.

Uses For the treatment of: (i) Breast cancer; (ii) Anovulatory infertility.

Tamoxifen is an anti-oestrogenic drug which binds to oestrogen receptors preventing the stimulating effects of oestrogen on nucleic acid synthesis. The metabolites of tamoxifen are also anti-oestrogens.

Dosage and administration For oral administration.

(1) *Breast cancer:* One tablet twice a day. This may be increased to two tablets twice a day in unresponsive cases.

(2) *Anovulatory infertility:* In women with regular menstruation but anovular cycles, treatment should start with one tablet twice a day given on the second, third, fourth and fifth days of the menstrual cycle. If treatment is unsuccessful, further courses may be given during subsequent menstrual periods, increasing the dosage to two, and then four tablets, twice daily.

In women with irregular menstruation, treatment can be initiated on any day. If there are no signs of ovulation, a subsequent course of treatment, may be started 45 days later, at the higher dosage level increased as necessary (two or four tablets twice a day). If a patient responds with menstruation then the next course of treatment is started on the second day of the cycle.

Contra-indications, warnings, etc
Contra-indications: Pregnancy.

Precautions: Tamoxifen may be given to pre-menopausal women only after thorough examination has excluded the possibility of pregnancy.

Adverse effects: Side effects are generally mild. The following effects have been reported – hot flushes, mild nausea, mild thrombocytopenia and leucopenia.

Occasionally occurring side effects are vaginal bleeding, pruritus vulvae, skin rash, fluid retention, gastrointestinal pain, pain from metastases and tumour pain.

Deep thromboses have occurred and with large doses of tamoxifen (160–200 mg per day) toxic effects on the retina have been reported. (Corneal and macular changes resulting in blurred vision have been described in a small number of cases treated continuously with these large doses for long periods).

In breast cancer patients, temporary reductions in platelet count (usually to 80,000–90,000 but sometimes lower) have been observed during treatment with tamoxifen. The platelet counts have recovered during treatment and no haemorrhagic tendency has been reported.

Hypercalcaemia has been reported in patients with bone metastases.

The adverse reactions can sometimes be controlled by a reduction of dosage.

In a proportion of pre-menopausal women treated for breast cancer, there is a suppression of menstruation; reversible cystic ovarian swelling has occasionally been observed in this group of patients receiving 40 mg of tamoxifen twice a day for short periods.

Treatment of overdosage: Overdosage causes anti-oestrogenic effects. In animals, extremely high doses (over 100 times the recommended daily dose) have caused oestrogenic effects. There is no specific antidote to overdosage, and treatment should therefore be symptomatic.

Pharmaceutical precautions *Storage:* Protect from moisture and heat (store below 25°C).

Legal category POM.

Package quantities Containers of 30 and 250 tablets.

Further information Maximum plasma levels of tamoxifen occur at 4–7 hours after administration. The elimination half-life is about 7 days. Considerable enterohepatic circulation is a probable reason for the slow elimination.

Product licence number 0424/0031.

TAMOFEN-20*

Presentation Round, convex, off-white tablets marked T20 on one side. Each tablet contains 30.4 mg Tamoxifen Citrate BP equivalent to 20 mg tamoxifen.

Uses For the treatment of: (i) Breast cancer; (ii) anovulatory infertility.

Tamoxifen is an anti-oestrogenic drug which binds to oestrogen receptors preventing the stimulating effects of oestrogen on nucleic acid synthesis. The metabolites of tamoxifen are also anti-oestrogens.

Dosage and administration For oral administration.
(1) *Breast cancer:* One tablet (20 mg) once daily. This may be increased to two tablets (40 mg) once daily in unresponsive cases.
(2) *Anovulatory infertility:* In women with regular menstruation but anovular cycles, treatment should start with one tablet (20 mg) once daily given on the second, third, fourth and fifth days of the menstrual cycle. If treatment is unsuccessful, further courses may be given during subsequent menstrual periods, increasing the dosage to two (40 mg), and then four (80 mg) tablets daily.
In women with irregular menstruation, treatment can be initiated on any day. If there are no signs of ovulation, a subsequent course of treatment, may be started 45 days later, at the higher dosage level increased as necessary (two or four tablets daily). If a patient responds with menstruation then the next course of treatment is started on the second day of the cycle.

Contra-indications, warnings, etc *Contra-indications:* Pregnancy.

Precautions: Tamoxifen may be given to pre-menopausal women only after thorough examination has excluded the possibility of pregnancy.

Adverse effects: Side-effects are generally mild. The following effects have been reported – hot flushes, mild nausea, mild thrombocytopenia and leucopenia.

Occasionally occurring side-effects are vaginal bleeding, pruritus vulvae, skin rash, fluid retention, gastrointestinal pain, pain from metastases and tumour pain.

Deep thromboses have occurred and with large doses of tamoxifen (160–200 mg per day) toxic effects on the retina have been reported. (Corneal and macular changes resulting in blurred vision have been described in a small number of cases treated continuously with these large doses for long periods).

In breast cancer patients, temporary reductions in platelet count (usually to 80,000–90,000 but sometimes lower) have been observed during treatment with tamoxifen. The platelet counts have recovered during treatment and no haemorrhagic tendency has been reported.

Hypercalcaemia has been reported in patients with bone metastases.

The adverse reactions can sometimes be controlled by a reduction of dosage.

In a proportion of pre-menopausal women treated for breast cancer, there is a suppression of menstruation; reversible cystic ovarian swelling has occasionally been observed in this group of patients receiving 40 mg of tamoxifen twice a day for short periods.

Treatment of overdosage: Overdosage causes antioestrogenic effects. In animals, extremely high doses (over 100 times the recommended daily dose) have caused oestrogenic effects. There is no specific antidote to overdosage, and treatment should therefore be symptomatic.

Pharmaceutical precautions *Storage:* protect from moisture and heat.

Legal category POM.

Package quantities Containers of 30 and 250 tablets.

Further information Maximum plasma levels of tamoxifen occur at 4–7 hours after administration. The elimination half-life is about 7 days. Considerable enterohepatic circulation is a probable reason for the slow elimination.

Product licence number 0424/0043.

TAMOFEN-40*

Presentation Round, convex, off-white tablets. Each tablet contains 60.8 mg Tamoxifen Citrate BP equivalent to 40 mg tamoxifen.

Uses For the treatment of: (1) Breast cancer; (2) anovulatory infertility.

Tamoxifen is an anti-oestrogenic drug which binds to oestrogen receptors preventing the stimulating effects of oestrogen on nucleic acid synthesis. The metabolities of tamoxifen are also anti-oestrogens.

Dosage and administration For oral administration
(1) *Breast cancer:* The daily dose is 20 to 40 mg as a single dose.
(2) *Anovulatory infertility:* In women with regular menstruation but anovular cycles, treatment should start with 20 mg once daily given on the second, third, fourth and fifth days of the menstrual cycle. If treatment is unsuccessful, further courses may be given during subsequent menstruation periods, increasing the dosage to 40 mg, and then to 80 mg daily.
In women with irregular menstruation, treatment can be initiated on any day. If there are no signs of ovulation, a subsequent course of treatment may be started 45 days later, at the higher dosage level increased as necessary (40 mg or 80 mg daily). If a patient responds with menstruation then the next course of treatment is started on the second day of the cycle.

Contra-indications, warnings, etc
Contra-indications: Pregnancy.

Precautions: Tamoxifen may be given to pre-menopausal women only after thorough examination has excluded the possibility of pregnancy.

Adverse effects: Side effects are generally mild. The following effects have been reported – hot flushes, mild nausea, mild thrombocytopenia and leucopenia.

Occasionally occurring side effects are vaginal bleeding, pruritus vulvae, skin rash, fluid retention, gastrointestinal pain, pain from metastases and tumour pain.

Deep thromboses have occurred and with large doses of tamoxifen (160–200 mg per day) toxic effects on the retina have been reported. (Corneal and macular changes resulting in blurred vision have been described in a small number of cases treated continuously with these large doses for long periods.)

In breast cancer patients, temporary reductions in platelet count (usually to 80,000–90,000 but sometimes lower) have been observed during treatment with tamoxifen. The platelet counts have recovered during treatment and no haemorrhagic tendency has been reported.

Hypercalcaemia has been reported in patients with bone metastases.

The adverse reactions can sometimes be controlled by a reduction of dosage.

In a proportion of pre-menopausal women treated for breast cancer, there is a suppression of menstruation; reversible cystic ovarian swelling has occasionally been observed in this group of patients receiving 40 mg of tamoxifen twice a day for short periods.

Treatment of overdosage: Overdosage causes anti-oestrogenic effects. In animals, extremely high doses (over 100 times the recommended daily dose) have caused oestrogenic effects. There is no specific antidote to over dosage, and treatment should therefore be symptomatic.

Pharmaceutical precautions Protect from moisture and heat. Store below 25°C.

Legal category POM.

Package quantities Containers of 30 tablets.

Further information Maximum plasma levels of tamoxifen occur at 4–7 hours after administration. The elimination half-life is about 7 days. Considerable enterohepatic circulation is a probable reason for the slow elimination.

Product licence number 0424/0055.

*Trade Mark

Typpharm Limited
14 Parkstone Road
Poole
Dorset

EFFERCITRATE* TABLETS

Presentation White, circular, flat, effervescent tablets with a slightly rough surface, weighing about 2.7 g, 19 mm in diameter and having the odour of lemon and lime.

Each tablet contains the equivalent of 1.5 g of Potassium Citrate BP and 250 mg Citric Acid BP in a pleasantly flavoured effervescent base.

Uses Effercitrate tablets provide a convenient and palatable method to administer potassium citrate to increase the alkali reserve and render the urine more alkaline when treating urinary tract infections. They may also be used to prevent crystalluria during treatment with sulphonamides. Effercitrate Tablets do not have the neutralizing effect of bicarbonate on gastric secretion and are less purgative than potassium tartrate.

Dosage and administration *Adults and children over 6 years of age:* Two tablets in a tumblerful of water up to three times daily.

Children Age 1–6 years: One tablet in a tumblerful of water up to three times daily.

Not recommended for children under 1 year.

Sufficient should be given in all cases to render and maintain the urine alkaline.

Contra-indications, warnings, etc A mild diuresis usually follows treatment with Potassium Citrate.

Each tablet contains 13.9 mmol potassium. Care should be taken to prevent hyperkalaemia particularly in patients with impaired renal function.

Side-effects: In common with other potassium salts Effercitrate may give rise to gastric irritation and the tablets must always be taken well diluted with water. Gastric effects may be minimized by giving doses with or after meals.

Overdosage: Hyperkalaemia. Below 6.5 mmol per litre poisoning is minimal, moderate up to 8 mmol per litre and severe above 8 mmol per litre. Absolute toxicity is governed by pH and sodium levels. Hyperkalaemia symptoms, may be transiently controlled with calcium gluconate, glucose or glucose and insulin, sodium bicarbonate or hypertonic sodium infusions, cationic exchange resins, or haemo and peritoneal dialysis. Patients who are digitalized may experience acute digitalis intoxication during potassium removal.

Pharmaceutical precautions Store in a cool dry place. Effercitrate tablets are hygroscopic and should be dispensed in the original containers which include a desiccant, and should be kept closed.

Legal category P.

Package quantities Tubes contain 12 tablets.

Further information Each Effercitrate tablet contains the equivalent of the Potassium Citrate and Citric acid content of 5 ml Potassium Citrate Mixture BPC 1973.

Product licence number 0051/0002.

VERACUR* GEL

Presentation Clear, water-miscible gel in a tube. Veracur Gel contains 1.5% v/v of Solution of Formaldehyde BP.

Uses Treatment of warts, particularly plantar warts (verrucae).

Dosage and administration To be applied directly on to the wart (verruca) and covered with a plaster, twice a day. Remove the outer dead layers with an emery board or pumice stone as the treatment progresses.

Contra-indications, warnings, etc If required protect surrounding skin with a thin film of Vaseline petroleum jelly before application.

For external use only.

Not to be applied to broken skin.

Pharmaceutical precautions Store in cool dry place.

Legal category GSL.

Package quantities 15 g.

Further information Nil.

Product licence number 0551/5000.

*Trade Mark

Upjohn Limited
Fleming Way
Crawley
West Sussex RH10 2NJ

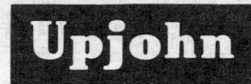

AMBAXIN*

Presentation White to off-white rod-shaped scored tablets with parallel sides and rounded ends, containing 400 mg bacampicillin hydrochloride, one side printed Upjohn, other side 130 on either side of the score.

Uses Antibacterial. Ambaxin is indicated in the treatment of infections due to susceptible strains of the following: Gram-positive organisms – Streptococci (including *S. faecalis*), pneumococci, non-penicillinase-producing staphylococci, *Clostridia* spp. and *L. monocytogenes*. Gram-negative organisms – *H. influenzae*, meningococci, *N. gonorrhoea, E. coli, P. mirabilis, Shigella* and *Salmonella*.

The indications for Ambaxin include the following: sinusitis, tonsillitis, peritonsillitis, acute and chronic bronchitis, pneumonia, skin and soft tissue infections, urinary infections, gonorrhoea, otitis media, pleurisy, acute endometritis, post-operative infections and paratyphoid fever. In vitro studies should be performed to determine causative organisms and their susceptibility to Ambaxin. Therapy may be initiated prior to obtaining results of susceptibility testing.

Penetration into the cerebrospinal fluid and brain occurs only when the meninges are inflamed.

Ampicillin, 10 mcg discs, should be used to determine the in vitro susceptibility of organisms to Ambaxin.

Ambaxin has no appreciable antibacterial activity itself but is rapidly hydrolysed to ampicillin in vivo, thus its antibacterial spectrum is the same as that of ampicillin.

Cross-resistance with cephalosporins and penicillins may occur.

Dosage and administration The usual dosage for adults is one 400 mg tablet two or three times a day. Dosage may be doubled in severe infections or where infection is caused by less sensitive pathogens. The dosage for children over 5 years is one half a 400 mg tablet (200 mg) three times daily.

The dose for uncomplicated gonorrhoea is 1600 mg plus 1 gram probenecid in a single dose.

Elderly patients: There is no information to suggest that a change in dosage is warranted in the elderly. Side effects do not appear to be more common or severe in elderly patients.

Contra-indications, warnings, etc
Contra-indications: A history of previous hypersensitivity to any of the penicillins is a contra-indication.

Warnings and precautions: The possibility of superinfection with mycotic organisms or bacterial pathogens should be kept in mind during therapy. Particular care should be taken in the treatment of atopic individuals. The risk of skin reaction is particularly high in patients with infectious mononucleosis or lymphatic leukaemia. As with other potent antibiotics, periodic assessment of

organ system function, including renal, hepatic and haemopoietic, should be made during prolonged therapy.

Safety for use in pregnancy has not been established.

Side-effects: Ambaxin is well tolerated. Since bacampicillin is hydrolysed to ampicillin in-vivo, the possibility of encountering those side-effects associated with ampicillin should be considered. Side-effects are generally mild, and of the usual penicillin type. Interruption of treatment is not usually necessary. The incidence of diarrhoea as a side-effect is lower than that seen with oral ampicillin.

Overdosage: Since Ambaxin is a penicillin, problems of overdosage are unlikely to be encountered.

Pharmaceutical precautions Store at room temperature (15–25°C).

Legal category POM.

Package quantities 100 tablets in bottles.

Further information Ambaxin is more rapidly absorbed than equimolar amounts of ampicillin, and achieves three times the serum levels of ampicillin in $\frac{1}{2}$ to 1 hour, thereby increasing its penetration into tissues and body fluids such as sinus mucosa and sputum, achieving concentrations greatly exceeding MIC's of susceptible pathogens. Ambaxin may be given without regard to time of food intake.

Product licence number 0032/0070.

ATGAM* ▼

Presentation Atgam is a transparent to slightly opalescent, colourless to light pink or brown, nearly odourless, aqueous protein solution. Atgam may develop a slight granular or flaky deposit during storage. Each 1 ml contains 50 mg equine gamma globulin.

Uses Immunosuppression. Atgam is indicated for concomitant use in immunosuppression of renal transplant patients, to delay the onset of the first rejection episode and/or, at the time of rejection, to increase the frequency of resolution of acute rejection episodes. Atgam, in addition to a regime of standard supportive care, has also induced instances of partial or complete haematological recovery and improved survival in patients with aplastic anaemia of known or suspected immunological aetiology. Anecdotal reports of benefit from concomitant immunosuppression with Atgam in non-controlled clinical studies have been published in cases of T-cell malignancies, graft-versus-host disease, or patients who have received skin, cardiac, liver or bone-marrow transplants.

Dosage and administration For intravenous use only.

The total daily dose of Atgam should be added to an inverted bottle of sterile 0.45%–0.9% saline (one mg Atgam per ml saline is optimal).

To minimise the occurrence of phlebitis and thrombosis, infusions should be given through an in-line filter (0.2–1#) into a high flow central vein although a vascular shunt or arterio-venous fistula may be used. All doses should be given under constant medical supervision. Do not infuse a dose of Atgam in less than 4 hours. Diluted solutions should be refrigerated until use and infusions should be complete within 12 hours of dilution.

Renal allograft recipients: In conjunction with azothioprine and corticosteroids it is recommended that Atgam be administered at 10 to 15 mg/kg daily for 14 days followed by alternate day therapy for a total of 21 doses in 28 days. When given to delay the onset of the first rejection episode therapy should commence within 24 hours before or after transplant.

Aplastic anaemia patients: In conjunction with standard supportive therapy, administration of Atgam at 15 to 20 mg/kg for 8 to 14 days has been beneficial. Additional alternate day therapy for another 14 days may also be given.

Contra-indications, warnings, etc

Contra-indications: Atgam should not be administered to a patient who has previously had a severe systemic reaction to it or any other equine gamma globulin preparation.

Warnings: Only physicians experienced with immunosuppressive therapy should use Atgam. Facilities equipped and staffed with adequate laboratory and supportive medical resources should be used.

Treatment with Atgam should be discontinued if anaphylaxis or severe and unremitting thrombocytopenia or leukopenia occurs. Atgam has not been evaluated in either pregnant or lactating women and experience with children is limited.

In common with products derived from, or purified with, human blood elements the possibility of transmission of some infectious diseases cannot be excluded.

Precautions: Monitor carefully for concurrent infection.

The indications for administration of Atgam must be strictly evaluated before administration, especially if the patient is atopic. Before administration, especially in patients who have previously received equine serum products, the following intracutaneous test should be carried out:

Inject 0.1 ml of a 1:1000 dilution (5 #g horse 1 gG) of Atgam in normal saline intradermally into the anterior aspect of the forearm. A contralateral saline control should also be undertaken. If a wheal or erythema greater than 10 mm develops within 1 hour infuse Atgam with caution. A systemic reaction such as generalised rash, tachycardia, dyspnoea, hypotension or anaphylaxis precludes systemic administration of Atgam. Allergic reactions can occur in patients whose skin test is negative and the patient should be observed closely for symptoms of incipient shock during infusion. Since Atgam is administered over a long period of time, the patient's serum should be regularly examined for antibodies against equine globulin.

Side-effects: The most frequently reported side effects are fever, shivering, leukopenia, thrombocytopenia, arthralgia and dermatological reactions such as rash, urticaria, pruritus. Such systemic reactions often occur 10–30 minutes after the end of infusion and are likely to be of greater severity during the first days of treatment

and if administration is too rapid. The high incidence of skin rashes and arthralgia is believed to represent serum sickness. Other reported reactions have included headache, nausea, vomiting, diarrhoea, dyspnoea, hypotension, night sweats, stomatitis, chest pain, back pain, pain at the infusion site, peripheral thrombophlebitis and clotted a–v fistula.

Reactions reported rarely have been: Dizziness, weakness or faintness, malaise, epigastric pain or hiccoughs, laryngospasm, paresthesia, lymphadenopathy, infection, herpes simplex reactivation, wound dehiscence, hyperglycemia, hypertension, edema, pulmonary edema, tachycardia, seizure, anaphylaxis, iliac vein obstruction, renal artery thrombosis and toxic epidermal necrosis.

Although anaphylaxis is rare, remedial facilities, such as adrenaline, should always be available during infusion and vaccination.

Treatment of adverse reactions

(a) Shock (anaphylaxis and allergy): Inject 1 ml (0.5 ml for children) of adrenaline 1:1,000 intramuscularly, and repeat injection of the same dose every 30 minutes until blood pressure has retured to normal. At the same time, inject 50–100 mg of prednisolone intravenously, and antihistamines intramuscularly. In cases of extremely severe collapse, 0.2–0.5 ml of adrenaline 1:10,000 can be slowly injected intravenously. Oral treatment with antihistamines should be continued for 10 days, in order to prevent the possible appearance of delayed allergic complications.

(b) Serum sickness: Antihistamines should be administered orally. Intensive pruritus can be alleviated immediately, but only temporarily, by subcutaneous injection of 1.0 ml of adrenaline 1:1,000.

Overdosage: No known antidote. Treatment should be symptomatic.

Pharmaceutical precautions Atgam should be stored in a refrigerator (2–8°C) in the manufacturer's containers. Do not freeze. Diluted solutions may be refrigerated but whether refrigerated or not must be infused within 12 hours (including time to infuse). . Dilution in dextrose infusion solutions or highly acidic infusion solutions is not recommended because of possible physical instability.

Legal category POM.

Package quantities Supplied in packs of 25 × 5 ml ampoules.

Further information The maximum tolerated dose would be expected to vary. To date the largest single daily dose administered to a patient was 7 g at a concentration of 10 mg/ml saline, with no sequelae. Repeat dosing has been used up to 50 doses in 4 months and some patients have received 28-day courses of 21 doses followed by as many as 3 more courses for acute rejection with no increase in the incidence of side-effects.

Product licence number 0032/0107.

COLESTID*

Presentation Light yellow, tasteless and odourless granules consisting of colestipol hydrochloride with 0.2% colloidal silicon dioxide.

Uses Ion-exchange resin which lowers plasma cholesterol levels through binding with bile acid in the intestinal lumen.

Colestid is indicated as adjunctive therapy to diet in the management of patients with elevated cholesterol levels. It has been shown to have no significant effect on triglyceride levels.

Although Colestid is effective in all types of hyper-cholesterolaemia, it is medically most appropriate in patients with Fredrickson's type II hyperlipoprotein-aemia.

In patients with xanthomas, the skin lesions have been reported to regress on Colestid therapy.

Dosage and administration   Colestid should be mixed with water or other fluids before ingesting.

The recommended total daily adult dosage of Colestid is 15–30 grams. This may be taken in divided doses two to four times daily.

Patients should take other drugs at least one hour before or one hour after Colestid to minimise possible interference with their absorption.

Preparation: To prepare Colestid, add the contents of a sachet to 100 ml or more of the preferred aqueous vehicle (water, orange, tomato, or other fruit juices, milk) and mix thoroughly until dispersed. Alternatively, Coles-tid may be added to soups or pulpy fruits with a high water content or to carbonated beverages.

Elderly patients: At present there are no extensive clinical studies with colestipol in patients over the age of 65. Review of available data does not suggest that the elderly are more predisposed to side effects attributable to colestipol than the general population; however, therapy should be individualized and based on each patient's clinical characteristics and tolerance to the medication.

Contra-indications, warnings, etc
Contra-indications: Colestipol is contra-indicated in individuals who have previously demonstrated hyper-sensitivity to its use.

Warnings: To avoid accidental inhalation or oesophageal distress, Colestid should not be taken in its dry form.

Safety for use in pregnant women or in children has not been established.

Precautions: In man, Colestid may interfere with the absorption of certain drugs (e.g. digitalis and its alkaloids, tetracycline hydrochloride, chlorothiazide and penicillin G). Colestid has been shown not to interfere with the absorption of clindamycin, clofibrate, aspirin, tolbuta-mide, warfarin and methyldopa. The clinical response to concomitant medication should be closely monitored and appropriate adjustments made.

Side-effects: The most common adverse reactions re-ported with Colestid have been of a functional gastro-intestinal nature. The most frequent is constipation, which is usually mild, transient and responsive to the usual adjunctive measures.

Transient and modest elevation of SGOT and of alkaline phosphatase have been observed. No medical significance is attached to these observed changes.

Overdosage: No toxic effects due to overdosage have been reported.

Pharmaceutical precautions   None.

Legal category   POM.

Package quantities   Box containing 30 × 5 gram foil sachets.

Further information   Colestid is not absorbed; its action is limited to the lumen of the gastro-intestinal tract, and it is passed in the faeces. It binds bile acids in the intestinal lumen and causes them to be excreted in the faeces together with the polymer.

When the enterohepatic circulation of bile acids is interrupted, cholesterol conversion to bile acids is enhanced and plasma cholesterol levels are thereby lowered.

Product licence number
Foil Sachet   0032/0055

CYTOSAR*

Presentation   Off-white, freeze-dried cake of 100 mg or 500 mg cytosine arabinoside (cytarabine) in a rubber-capped vial.

Uses   Cytotoxic. For induction of remission in acute myeloid leukaemia in adults and for other acute leu-kaemias of adults and children.

Dosage and administration   By intravenous infusion or injection, and subcutaneous injection. Water for Injection, 0.9% saline or 5% dextrose should be used for preparing a solution of cytarabine in the vial. When the accompanying diluent (Water for Injection containing 0.9% benzyl alcohol as preservative) is used, such solution contains 20 mg/ml (100 mg vial) or 50 mg/ml (500 mg vial) cytarabine.

The physician is reminded that in practice Cytosar has been administered in combination with a variety of other cytotoxic agents using a number of different dosage schedules, and reference to the current literature before commencing treatment is recommended.

Dosage recommendations may be converted from those in terms of bodyweight to those related to surface area by means of nomograms such as are presented in Documenta Geigy.

1.   *Remission induction: Adults:* (a) Continuous treat-ment:

(i)   Rapid injection – 2 mg/kg/day is a judicious starting dose. Administer for 10 days. Obtain daily blood counts. If no antileukaemic effect is noted and there is no apparent toxicity, increase to 4 mg/kg/day and maintain until therapeutic response or toxicity is evident. Almost all patients can be carried to toxicity with these doses.

(ii)   0.5–1.0 mg/kg/day may be given in an infusion of up to 24 hours duration. Results from one-hour infusions have been satisfactory in the majority of patients. After 10 days this initial daily dose may be increased to 2 mg/kg/day subject to toxicity. Con-tinue to toxicity or until remission occurs.

(b) Intermittent treatment:

3–5 mg/kg/day is administered intravenously on each of five consecutive days. After a two to nine-day rest period, a further course is given. Continue until response or toxicity occurs.

The first evidence of marrow improvement has been reported to occur 7–64 days (mean 28 days) after the beginning of therapy.

In general, if a patient shows neither toxicity nor remission after a fair trial, the cautious administration of higher doses is warranted. As a rule patients have been seen to tolerate higher doses when given by rapid intravenous injection as compared with slow infusion. This difference is due to the rapid metabolism of Cytosar and the consequent short duration of action of the high dose.

Children: Children appear to tolerate higher doses than adults and, where dose ranges are quoted, the children should receive tho higher dose and the adults the lower.

2. *Maintenance therapy:* Remissions which have been induced by cytarabine, or by other drugs, may be maintained by intravenous or subcutaneous injection of 1 mg/kg once or twice weekly.

Elderly patients: There is no information to suggest that a change in dosage is warranted in the elderly. Nevertheless, the elderly patient does not tolerate drug toxicity as well as the younger patient, and particular attention should thus be given to drug induced leucopenia, thrombocytopenia and anaemia with appropriate initiation of supportive therapy when indicated.

Contra-indications, warnings, etc

Contra-indications: Therapy with Cytosar should not be considered in patients with pre-existing drug-induced bone marrow suppression, unless the clinician feels that such management offers the most hopeful alternative for the patient. Cytosar should not be used in the management of non-malignant disease, except for immunosuppression.

Warning: Cytosar is a potent bone marrow suppressant. Therapy should be started cautiously in patients with pre-existing drug-induced bone marrow suppression. Patients receiving this drug must be under close medical supervision and, during induction therapy, should have leucocyte and platelet counts performed daily. Bone marrow examinations should be performed frequently after blasts have disappeared from the peripheral blood. Facilities should be available for management of complications, possibly fatal, of bone marrow suppression (infection resulting from granulocytopenia and other impaired body defences, and haemorrhage secondary to thrombocytopenia). One case of anaphylaxis that resulted in acute cardiopulmonary arrest and required resuscitation has been reported. This occurred immediately after the intravenous administration of Cytosar.

Severe and at times fatal CNS, GI and pulmonary toxicity (different from that seen with conventional therapy regimens of Cytosar) has been reported following some experimental Cytosar dose schedules. These reactions include reversible corneal toxicity; cerebral and cerebellar dysfunction, usually reversible; severe gastrointestinal ulceration, including pneumatosis cystoides intestinalis, leading to peritonitis; sepsis and liver abscess; and pulmonary oedema. Cytosar is known to be teratogenic in some animal species. The use of Cytosar in women who are, or who may become, pregnant should be undertaken only after due consideration of the potential benefits and hazards.

This product should not normally be administered to patients who are pregnant or to mothers who are breast-feeding.

Cytosar has been shown to be carcinogenic in animals. The possibility of a similar effect should be borne in mind when designing the long-term management of the patient.

Precautions: Patients receiving Cytosar (cytarabine) must be monitored closely. Frequent platelet and leucocyte counts are mandatory. Suspend or modify therapy when drug-induced marrow depression has resulted in a platelet count under 50,000 or a polymorphonuclear count under 1,000 per mm³. Counts of formed elements in the peripheral blood may continue to fall after the drug

is stopped and reach lowest values after drug-free intervals of five to seven days. If indicated, restart therapy when definite signs of marrow recovery appear (on successive bone marrow studies). Patients whose drug is withheld until 'normal' peripheral blood values are attained may escape from control.

When intravenous doses are given quickly, patients are frequently nauseated and may vomit for several hours afterwards. This problem tends to be less severe when the drug is infused.

The human liver apparently detoxifies a substantial fraction of an administered dose. Use the drug with caution and at reduced dose in patients whose liver function is poor.

Periodical checks of bone marrow, liver and kidney functions should be performed in patients receiving Cytosar.

The safety of this drug for use in infants is not established.

Like other cytotoxic drugs, Cytosar may induce hyperuricaemia secondary to rapid lysis of neoplastic cells. The clinician should monitor the patient's blood uric acid level and be prepared to use such supportive and pharmacological measures as may be necessary to control this problem.

Side-effects: Adverse reactions seen with cytarabine treatment have included those seen with cytotoxic agents having an effect on bone marrow, such as: leucopenia, thrombocytopenia, anaemia, bone marrow suppression and megaloblastosis. Other side-effects have included: nausea, vomiting, diarrhoea, oral ulceration, hepatic dysfunction. Occasional adverse experiences have been reported as follows: renal dysfunction, anorexia, sepsis, gastro-intestinal haemorrhage, irritation or sepsis at site of injection, neuritis or neurotoxicity, rash, freckling, oesophagitis, skin and mucosal bleeding, chest pain, joint pain and reduction in reticulocytes.

A Cytosar syndrome has been described. It is characterised by fever, myalgia, bone pain, occasionally chest pain, maculopapular rash, conjunctivitis and malaise. It usually occurs 6–12 hours following drug administration. Corticosteroids have been shown to be beneficial in treating or preventing this syndrome. If the symptoms of the syndrome are serious enough to warrant treatment, corticosteroids should be contemplated as well as continuation of therapy with Cytosar.

Overdosage: Cessation of therapy, followed by management of ensuing bone marrow depression including whole blood or platelet transfusion and antibiotics as required.

Pharmaceutical precautions Solutions reconstituted with Water for Injection, 0.9% saline, or 5% dextrose must be used immediately and not stored. When reconstituted with the accompanying diluent, solutions should be stored at room temperature and used within 48 hours. Discard any solution in which a slight haze develops.

Legal category POM.

Package quantities Cytosar is supplied as a single vial containing 100 mg or 500 mg cytarabine sterile powder together with an ampoule of diluent (Water for Injection with 0.9% w/v benzyl alcohol).

Cytosar is also available as 10 × 100 mg vials without diluent.

Further information Published work indicates that Cytosar is effective in the indications for which it is recommended. However, a greater treatment success has been achieved in certain studies by the combination of Cytosar with other agents. The literature should be referred to in determining whether this latter course of action should be considered.

Product licence numbers 0032/5037 (100 mg)
0032/0109 (500 mg)

DALACIN C*

Presentation Hard-filled gelatine capsules (maroon/lavender) containing 150 mg clindamycin (as clindamycin hydrochloride).

Hard-filled gelatine capsules (lavender/lavender) containing 75 mg clindamycin (as clindamycin hydrochloride).

Pink, sucrose-based granules for paediatric suspension, with pineapple flavour. Each 5 ml reconstituted suspension contains 75 mg clindamycin (as clindamycin palmitate hydrochloride).

Uses Antibacterial. Serious infections caused by susceptible Gram-positive organisms, staphylococci (both penicillinase and non-penicillinase producing), streptococci (except *Strep. faecalis),* and pneumococci. It is also indicated in serious infections caused by susceptible anaerobic pathogens.

Clindamycin does not penetrate the blood/brain barrier in therapeutically effective quantities.

Dosage and administration Oral. Absorption of Dalacin C is not appreciably modified by the presence of food.

Capsules: Adults: Moderately severe infection, 150–300 mg every six hours. Severe infection, 300–450 mg every six hours. Dalacin C Capsules should always be taken with a glass of water.

Paediatric: To each 100 ml bottle of granules add 74 ml water and shake.

Children: 3–6 mg/kg every six hours depending on the severity of the infection.

In children under one year or weighing 10 kg or less the minimum recommended dose is 2.5 ml (37.5 mg) every eight hours.

The following paediatric dose regime is recommended as a guide:

Moderately severe infection: 0–11 months: 3.5–9.0 kg: 2.5 ml every eight hours.

1–3 years: 10–15 kg: 2.5 ml every six hours.

4–7 years: 16–25 kg: 5 ml every six hours.

8–12 years: 26–38 kg: 7.5 ml every six hours.

Severe infection: 0–11 months: 3.5–9.0 kg: 2.5 ml every six hours.

1–3 years: 10–15 kg: 5 ml every six hours.

4–7 years: 16–25 kg: 7.5 ml every six hours.

8–12 years: 26–38 kg: 10 ml every six hours.

Adults: Moderately severe infection: 10 ml every six hours. *Severe infection:* 20 ml every six hours.

Note: In cases of β-haemolytic streptococcal infection, treatment with Dalacin C should continue for at least 10 days to diminish the likelihood of subsequent rheumatic fever or glomerulonephritis.

Elderly patients: The half-life, volume of distribution and clearance, and extent of absorption after administration of clindamycin hydrochloride is not altered by increased age. Analysis of data from clinical studies have not revealed any age-related increase in toxicity. Therefore, dosage requirements in elderly patients should not be influenced by age alone. See Precautions section for other factors which should be taken into consideration.

Contra-indications, warnings, etc
Contra-indications: Dalacin C is contra-indicated in patients previously found to be hypersensitive to this antibiotic. Although cross-sensitisation to lincomycin has not been demonstrated, it is recommended that Dalacin C is not used in patients who have demonstrated lincomycin sensitivity.

Warnings: Dalacin C should only be used in the treatment of serious infections. In considering the use of the product the practitioner should bear in mind the type of infection and the potential hazard of the diarrhoea which may develop since cases of colitis have been reported. The appearance of marked diarrhoea should be regarded as an indication that the product should be discontinued immediately.

Studies indicate a toxin(s) produced by *Clostridia* (especially *Clostridium difficile)* is the principal direct cause of antibiotic-associated colitis. These studies also indicate that this toxigenic *Clostridium* is usually sensitive in vitro to vancomycin. When 125 mg to 500 mg of vancomycin is administered orally four times a day, there is a rapid observed disappearance of the toxin from faecal samples and a coincident clinical recovery from the diarrhoea.

Precautions: Care should be observed in the use of Dalacin C in atopic individuals, e.g. asthma and allergy.

Clindamycin has been shown to have neuromuscular blocking properties that may enhance the action of other neuromuscular blocking agents. Therefore it should be used with caution in patients receiving such agents.

Periodic liver function tests and blood counts should be carried out during prolonged therapy. Such monitoring is also recommended in neonates and infants. Safety and appropriate dosage in infants less than one month old have not been established.

The dosage of Dalacin C may require reduction in patients with renal or hepatic impairment due to prolongation of the serum half-life of the antibiotic.

Safety for use in pregnancy has not yet been established.

Overdosage: In cases of overdosage that may have led to adverse reactions, therapy should be discontinued and the usual emergency treatment, including corticosteroids, adrenaline and antihistamines, instituted. The serum biological half-life of clindamycin is 2.4 hours. Clindamycin cannot be readily removed from the blood by dialysis or peritoneal dialysis.

Side-effects: In general Dalacin C is well tolerated. Side-effects referable to the gastro-intestinal tract include abdominal discomfort, loose stools or diarrhoea or colitis (see 'Warnings'), nausea or occasional vomiting. Hypersensitivity reactions are rare, even in patients sensitive to penicillins. A low incidence of skin rash has been observed. Dalacin C has been shown to be free from major toxicity; no direct relationship to ototoxicity, nephrotoxicity, neurotoxicity, liver disease or haematopoietic damage has been established.

Pharmaceutical precautions Dalacin C Paediatric Granules are stable at room temperature (18–25°C) for at least 24 months.

Following reconstitution the paediatric suspension is stable for up to two weeks at room temperature.

Where further dilution is required use purified water.

Legal category POM.

Package quantities 75 mg capsules in bottles of 16 and 100. 150 mg capsules in bottles of 16, 100 and 500.

Paediatric granules to make 100 ml suspension.

Further information Rapid absorption gives peak serum levels within 45 minutes and such levels exceed the in vitro minimum inhibitory concentrations for most sensitive bacteria.

Clindamycin demonstrates cross-resistance with lincomycin. When tested by in vitro methods, some staphylococcal strains originally resistant to erythromycin rapidly developed resistance to clindamycin.

Product licence numbers

Dalacin C Capsules 75 mg	0032/5006
Dalacin C Capsules 150 mg	0032/5007
Dalacin C Paediatric	0032/0023

DALACIN C* PHOSPHATE STERILE SOLUTION

Presentation Clear colourless sterile solution of clindamycin phosphate containing the equivalent of 150 mg clindamycin base per ml.

Uses Antibacterial. Dalacin C Phosphate is indicated in serious infections caused by susceptible Gram-positive organisms, staphylococci (both penicillinase and non-penicillinase-producing), streptococci (except *S. faecalis*), and pneumococci. It is also indicated in serious infections caused by susceptible anaerobic pathogens, such as, *Bacteroides* spp., *Fusobacterium* spp., *Propionibacterium, Peptostreptococcus* spp. and microaerophilic streptococci.

Clindamycin does not penetrate the blood/brain barrier in therapeutically effective quantities.

Dosage and administration Dalacin C Phosphate *must* be diluted prior to IV administration (see Package Insert) and should be infused over at least 10–60 minutes.

Adults: Parenteral (IM or IV administration).

Serious infections: 600 mg–1.2 g/day in two, three or four equal doses.

More severe infections: 1.2–2.7 g/day in two, three or four equal doses.

Single IM injections of greater than 600 mg are not recommended nor administration of more than 1.2 g in a single one-hour infusion.

For more serious infections, these doses may have to be increased. In life-threatening situations doses as high as 4.8 g daily have been given intravenously to adults.

Alternatively, the drug may be administered in the form of a single rapid infusion of the first dose followed by continuous IV infusion.

For details of dilution and infusion rates see package insert.

Children (over 1 month of age): Parenteral (IM or IV administration).

Serious infections: 15–25 mg/kg/day in three or four equal doses.

More severe infections: 25–40 mg/kg/day in three or four equal doses.

In severe infections it is recommended that children be given no less than 300 mg/day regardless of body weight.

Note: In cases of β-haemolytic streptococcal infections, treatment should continue for at least 10 days.

Elderly patients: The half-life, volume of distribution and clearance, and extent of absorption after administration of clindamycin phosphate is not altered by increased age. Analysis of data from clinical studies have not revealed any age related increase in toxicity. Therefore, dosage requirements in elderly patients should not be influenced by age alone. See Precautions section for other factors which should be taken into consideration.

Contra-indications, warnings, etc

Contra-indications: Dalacin C Phosphate is contra-indicated in patients previously found to be hypersensitive to preparations containing clindamycin. Although cross-sensitisation to lincomycin has not been demonstrated, it is recommended that Dalacin C Phosphate should not be used in patients who have demonstrated lincomycin sensitivity.

Warnings: Dalacin C Phosphate should only be used in the treatment of serious infections. In considering the use of this product the practitioner should bear in mind the type of infection and the potential hazard of the diarrhoea that may develop since cases of colitis have been reported. The appearance of marked diarrhoea should be regarded as an indication that the drug should be discontinued immediately.

Studies indicate a toxin(s) produced by *Clostridia* (especially *Clostridium difficile*) is the principal direct cause of antibiotic-associated colitis. These studies also indicate that this toxigenic *Clostridium* is usually sensitive in vitro to vancomycin. When 125 mg to 500 mg of vancomycin is administered orally four times a day, there is a rapid observed disappearance of the toxin from faecal samples and a coincident clinical recovery from the diarrhoea.

Precautions: Care should be observed in the use of Dalacin C Phosphate in atopic individuals, e.g. asthma and allergy.

Periodic liver function tests and blood counts should be carried out during prolonged therapy. Such monitoring is also recommended in neonates and infants. Safety and appropriate dosage in infants less than one month old have not been established.

The dosage of Dalacin C Phosphate may require reduction in patients with renal or hepatic impairment due to prolongation of the serum half-life of the drug.

Safety for use in pregnancy has not yet been established.

Clindamycin has been shown to have neuromuscular blocking properties that may enhance the action of other neuromuscular blocking agents. Therefore, it should be used with caution in patients receiving such agents.

Side-effects: In general Dalacin C Phosphate is well tolerated. Side-effects referable to the gastro-intestinal tract include abdominal discomfort, loose stools, diarrhoea or colitis (see Warnings), nausea or occasional vomiting. Hypersensitivity reactions are rare, even in patients sensitive to penicillins though a few cases of anaphylactoid reactions have been reported. A low incidence of skin rash has been observed.

Jaundice and abnormalities in liver function tests have been observed during clindamycin therapy. Transient neutropenia (leukopenia) and eosinophilia have been reported, and occasional reports of agranulocytosis and thrombocytopenia have been made.

Pain, induration and sterile abscess have been reported after intramuscular injection and thrombophlebitis after intravenous infusion. Reactions can be minimised or avoided by giving deep IM injections and avoiding prolonged use of indwelling intravenous catheters.

Overdosage: In cases of overdosage that may have led to adverse reactions, therapy should be discontinued and the usual emergency treatment, including corticosteroids, adrenaline and antihistamines, instituted. The serum biological half-life of clindamycin is 2.4 hours. Clindamycin cannot be readily removed from the blood by dialysis or peritoneal dialysis.

Pharmaceutical precautions In vitro compatibility studies monitored for 24 hours at room temperature using a concentration no greater than 6 mg/ml have demonstrated no inactivation or physical incompatibility with the use of Dalacin C Phosphate in IV solutions containing sodium chloride, glucose or potassium usually used clinically.

The following drugs are physically incompatible with Dalacin C Phosphate: ampicillin, diphenylhydantoin, barbiturates, aminophylline, calcium gluconate and magnesium sulphate.

Compatibility or incompatibility with other drugs besides the ones already mentioned has not been determined.

Store at room temperature. Avoid refrigeration.

Legal category POM.

Package quantities 5 × 2 ml and 5 × 4 ml ampoules.

Further information Biologically inactive clindamycin phosphate is rapidly converted to active clindamycin following injection.

Clindamycin demonstrates cross-resistance with lincomycin. When tested by in vitro methods some staphylococcal strains originally resistant to erythromycin rapidly developed resistance to clindamycin.

Product licence number 0032/0042

DEPO-MEDRONE*

Presentation White, sterile aqueous suspension for injection containing 40 mg per ml methylprednisolone acetate.

Uses Corticosteroid (glucocorticoid), Depo-Medrone is indicated in conditions requiring a glucocorticoid effect, e.g. anti-inflammatory, anti-allergic, anti-rheumatic.

Dosage and administration Depo-Medrone should not be mixed with any other suspending agent or solution. Depo-Medrone may be used by any of the following routes: intramuscular, intra-articular, periarticular, intrabursal, peribursal, intralesional, into the tendon sheath and rectal.

Intramuscular – for sustained systemic effect:

Allergic conditions (hay fever, asthma, rhinitis, drug reactions), 80–120 mg (2–3 ml).

Dermatological conditions (atopic, contact and seborrhoeic dermatitis), 40–120 mg (1–3 ml).

Collagen diseases (rheumatoid arthritis, SLE), 40–120 mg (1–3 ml) per week.

Adrenogenital syndrome, 40 mg (1 ml) every two weeks.

Note: Depo-Medrone is not intended for the prophylaxis of hay fever or other seasonal allergies and should be administered only when symptoms are present.

The frequency of intramuscular injections should be determined by the duration of clinical response.

On average the effect of a single 2 ml (80 mg) injection may be expected to last approximately two weeks.

In the case of seasonal allergic rhinitis a single injection is frequently sufficient. If necessary, however, a second injection may be given after two to three weeks.

Intra-articular: Rheumatoid arthritis, osteoarthritis. The dose of Depo-Medrone depends upon the size of the joint and the severity of the condition. Repeated injections, if needed, may be given at intervals of one to five or more weeks depending upon the degree of relief obtained from the initial injection. A suggested dosage guide is: large joint (knee, ankle, shoulder), 20–80 mg (0.5–2 ml); medium joint (elbow, wrist), 10–40 mg (0.25–1 ml); small joint (metacarpophalangeal, interphalangeal, sternoclavicular, acromioclavicular), 4–10 mg (0.1–0.25 ml).

Intrabursal: Subdeltoid bursitis, prepatellar bursitis, olecranon bursitis. For administration directly into bursae, 4–30 mg (0.1–0.75 ml). In most acute cases, repeat injections are not needed.

Intralesional: Localised neurodermatitis, hypertrophic lichen planus, nummular eczema, necrobiosis lipoidica diabeticorum, alopecia areata, discoid lupus erythematosus and insect bites. For administration directly into the lesion for local effect in dermatological conditions, 20–60 mg (0.5–1.5 ml). For large lesions, the dose may be distributed by repeated local injections of 20–40 mg (0.5–1 ml). One to four injections are usually employed. Care should be taken to avoid injection of sufficient material to cause blanching, since this may be followed by a small slough.

Periarticular: Epicondylitis. Infiltrate 4–30 mg (0.1–0.75 ml) into the affected area.

Into the tendon sheath: Tendinitis, tenosynovitis, epicondylitis. For administration directly into the tendon sheath, 4–30 mg (0.1–0.75 ml). In recurrent or chronic conditions, repeat injections may be necessary.

Rectal: Ulcerative colitis, 40–120 mg (1–3 ml). Administer in retention enemas or by continuous drip in 30–300 ml of water, three to seven times weekly for two or more weeks.

Special precautions should be observed when administering Depo-Medrone. Intramuscular injections should be made deeply into the gluteal muscles. The usual technique of aspirating prior to injection should be employed to avoid intravascular administration. Doses recommended for intramuscular injection must not be administered superficially or subcutaneously. Skin depression at the site of injection due to atrophic changes in the subcutaneous tissues has occasionally been reported following administration of corticosteroids. Intrasynovial injections should be carefully made using precise anatomical localisation. In the treatment of tendinitis care should be taken to inject Depo-Medrone into the tendon sheath rather than into the substance of the tendon.

Elderly patients: When used according to instructions, there is no information to suggest that a change in dosage is warranted in the elderly.

Contra-indications, warnings, etc

Contra-indications: The usual contra-indications to the

systemic or local use of corticosteroids should be observed. These include; latent, healed and active tuberculosis, peptic ulcer, acute psychoses, Cushing's syndrome, herpes simplex keratitis, vaccinia and varicella.

Warnings: Depo-Medrone *must not* be given by the intravenous route. Because of its inhibitory effect on fibroplasia, methylprednisolone may mask signs of infection and enhance dissemination of the infecting organism. Hence all patients receiving methylprednisolone should be watched for evidence of intercurrent infection. Should infection occur it must be brought under control by the use of appropriate antibacterial therapy, or administration of corticosteroids should be discontinued.

Injections of Depo-Medrone should be made only under aseptic conditions. At times of stress it may be necessary to increase the systemic dose when long-term therapy is involved.

Due to the absence of a true tendon sheath, the Achilles tendon should not be injected with Depo-Medrone.

Precautions: The presence of diabetes, osteoporosis, chronic psychotic reactions, predisposition to thrombophlebitis, hypertension, congestive heart failure, renal insufficiency and the presence of infection necessitate the carefully controlled use of methylprednisolone. While therapy with corticosteroids does not appear to be contra-indicated during pregnancy, caution is recommended, particularly during the first trimester. Also neonates of mothers who received such therapy during pregnancy should be observed for signs of hypoadrenalism and appropriate measures instituted if such signs exist.

Side-effects: Side-effects associated with the use of corticosteroids may be observed, including 'Cushing's syndrome, moon facies, supraclavicular pads of fat, hirsutism, striae and acne, hyperglycaemia, osteoporosis, peptic ulceration, hypertension, psychic disturbance, posterior subcapsular cataracts, suppression of growth in children, subcutaneous and cutaneous atrophy, sterile abscess, vertigo, weakness, myopathy, thrombo-embolism, pancreatitis, exophthalmos and headache.

Overdosage: No known antidote. Following overdosage the possibility of adrenal suppression should be guarded against by gradual diminution of dose levels over a period of time. In such event the patient may require to be supported during any further traumatic episode.

Pharmaceutical precautions Depo-Medrone should be protected from freezing.

Depo-Medrone should not be mixed with any other fluid.

Legal category POM.

Package quantities 1 ml, 2 ml and 5 ml rubber-capped vials packed singly and as 6-vial clinic packs, and a 2 ml pre-filled disposable syringe.

Further information Methylprednisolone, has achieved a clinically acceptable split between glucocorticoid effect and undesired mineralocorticoid effect. Methylprednisolone has five times the anti-inflammatory activity of hydrocortisone but has little tendency to cause salt and water retention. Depo-Medrone affords advantages in treatment which include high concentration in low fluid volume, greater gastric tolerance in avoidance of the GI tract and complete physician control of dosage.

Product licence numbers
2 ml syringe   0032/5015
Vials   0032/5038

DEPO-MEDRONE* WITH LIDOCAINE

Presentation White, sterile aqueous suspension for injection containing 40 mg per ml methylprednisolone acetate and 10 mg per ml lidocaine hydrochloride.

Uses Corticosteroid (glucocorticoid). Depo-Medrone with Lidocaine is indicated in conditions requiring a glucocorticoid effect: e.g. anti-inflammatory or anti-rheumatic. It is recommended for local use where the added anaesthetic effect would be considered advantageous.

Dosage and administration Depo-Medrone with Lidocaine should not be mixed with any other preparations as flocculation of the product may occur. Depo-Medrone with Lidocaine may be used by any of the following routes: intra-articular, peri-articular, intrabursal, and into the tendon sheath.

Intra-articular: Rheumatoid arthritis, osteoarthritis. The dose of Depo-Medrone with Lidocaine depends on the size of the joint and the severity of the condition. Repeated injections, if needed, may be given at intervals of one to five or more weeks depending upon the degree of relief obtained from the initial injection. A suggested dosage guide is: large joint (knee, ankle, shoulder) 0.5–2 ml (20–80 mg of steroid): medium joint (elbow, wrist) 0.25–1 ml (10–40 mg of steroid): small joint (metacarpophalangeal, interphalangeal, sternoclavicular, acromioclavicular) 0.1–0.25 ml (4–10 mg of steroid).

Peri-articular: Epicondylitis. Infiltrate 0.1–0.75 ml (4–30 mg of steroid) into the affected area.

Intrabursal: Subacromial bursitis, prepatellar bursitis, olecranon bursitis. For administration directly into bursae, 0.1–0.75 ml (4–30 mg of steroid). In most acute cases, repeat injections are not needed.

Into the tendon sheath: Tendinitis, tenosynovitis, epicondylitis. For administration directly into the tendon sheath, 0.1–0.75 ml (4–30 mg of steroid). In recurrent or chronic conditions, repeat injections may be necessary.

For infants and children, the recommended dosage should be reduced, but dosage should be governed by the severity of the condition rather than by strict adherence to the ratio indicated by age or body weight.

Special precautions should be observed when administering Depo-Medrone with Lidocaine. Intrasynovial injections should be carefully made using precise anatomical localisation. In the treatment of tendinitis, care should be taken to inject Depo-Medrone with Lidocaine into the tendon sheath rather than into the substance of the tendon.

Elderly patients: When used according to instructions, there is no information to suggest that a change in dosage is warranted in the elderly.

Contra-indications, warnings, etc
Contra-indications: Hypersensitivity to any of the components of the preparation. Depo-Medrone with Lidocaine should not be used in patients who exhibit heart block. The usual contra-indications to the systemic or local use of corticosteroids should be observed. These include; latent, healed and active tuberculosis, peptic ulcer, acute psychoses, Cushing's syndrome, herpes simplex keratitis, vaccinia and varicella.

Warnings: Depo-Medrone with Lidocaine must not be given by the intravenous or intrathecal route. Because of its inhibitory effect on fibroplasia, methylprednisolone may mask signs of infection and enhance dissemination of the infecting organism. Hence, all patients receiving methylprednisolone should be watched for evidence of intercurrent infection. Should infection occur it must be brought under control by the use of appropriate antibacterial therapy, or administration of corticosteroids should be discontinued.

Injections of Depo-Medrone with Lidocaine should only be made under strict aseptic techniques.

Due to the absence of a true tendon sheath, the Achilles tendon should not be injected with Depo-Medrone with Lidocaine.

Precautions: The presence of diabetes, osteoporosis, chronic psychotic reactions, predisposition to thrombophlebitis, hypertension, congestive heart failure, renal insufficiency and the presence of infection necessitate the carefully controlled use of methylprednisolone. While therapy with corticosteroids does not appear to be contraindicated during pregnancy, caution is recommended, particularly during the first trimester. Also neonates of mothers who received such therapy during pregnancy should be observed for signs of hypoadrenalism and appropriate measures instituted if such signs exist.

Retardation of linear growth has been noted in children receiving corticosteroids for 6 months or longer, the retardation being roughly proportional to the dose. Following cessation of therapy, the growth rate may be accelerated. For this reason the growth of children receiving prolonged steroid therapy should be observed carefully.

Side effects: Side effects associated with the use of corticosteroids may be observed, including Cushing's syndrome, moon facies, supraclavicular pads of fat, hirsutism, striae and acne, hyperglycaemia, osteoporosis, peptic ulceration, hypertension, psychic disturbance, posterior subcapsular cataracts, suppression of growth in children, subcutaneous and cutaneous atrophy, sterile abscess, vertigo, weakness, myopathy, thromboembolism, pancreatitis, exophthalmos and headache.

Overdosage: In general no positive action is required to be taken. The patient should, however, be observed closely for possible adverse reactions and appropriate steps taken.

Pharmaceutical precautions Depo-Medrone with Lidocaine should be protected from freezing. Depo-Medrone with Lidocaine should not be mixed with any other fluid.

Legal category POM.

Package quantities 2 ml rubber-capped vials and 6 × 1 ml vial clinic packs.

Further information Methylprednisolone has achieved a clinically acceptable split between glucocorticoid effect and undesired mineralocorticoid effect. Methylprednisolone has five times the anti-inflammatory activity of hydrocortisone but has little tendency to cause salt and water retention. Depo-Medrone with Lidocaine affords advantages in treatment which include high concentration in low fluid volume, greater gastric tolerance in avoidance of the GI tract and complete physician control of dosage.

Product licence number 0032/0076

DEPO-PROVERA*

Presentation White, sterile, aqueous suspension containing 50 mg/ml medroxyprogesterone acetate.

Uses Progestogen: For short-term contraception, long-term contraception and endometriosis.

a. Short-term contraception: Depo Provera may be used for short-term contraception when an oral contraceptive is contra-indicated or considered inappropriate in the following circumstances:
(i) For wives of men undergoing vasectomy, for protection until the vasectomy becomes effective.
(ii) In women who are being immunised against rubella, to prevent pregnancy during the period of activity of the virus.

b. Long-term contraception: Depo-Provera is intended for long-term use only in women in whom other contraceptives are contra-indicated or have caused unacceptable side-effects or are otherwise unsatisfactory.

It is of the greatest importance that adequate explanations of the long-term nature of the product, of its possible side-effects and of the impossibility of reversing the effects of each injection are given to potential users and that every effort is made to ensure that each patient receives such counselling as to enable her to fully understand these explanations.

Consistent with good clinical contraceptive practice a general medical as well as gynaecological examination should be undertaken before administration of Depo-Provera and at yearly intervals thereafter.

As with other long-term hormonal contraceptives, regular consideration should be given to whether the previous treatment has resulted in:
1. First time migraine or unusually severe headaches, acute visual disturbances of any kind.
2. Re-appearance of depression.
3. Pathological changes in liver function and hormone levels.

c. For the treatment of endometriosis.

Dosage and administration Doses should be given by deep intramuscular injection. It should be noted that a different dosage regime with higher overall dosage is required for endometriosis than is recommended for contraception.

Contraception: An injection of 150 mg IM should be given during the first five days of a normal menstrual cycle or before the sixth week post-partum. Further doses should be given at 3-month intervals. (N.B. For wives of men undergoing vasectomy a second injection of 150 mg IM three months after the first may be necessary in a small proportion of patients where the husband's sperm count has not fallen to zero.)

Because of the risk of heavy or prolonged bleeding in some women, the drug should be used with caution in the puerperium.

If the puerperal woman will be breast-feeding, the initial injection should be delayed until six weeks post-partum, when the infant's enzyme system is more fully developed. Further injections should be given at 3-month intervals.

Endometriosis: 50 mg IM once a week or 100 mg IM every two weeks for six months or longer.

Contra-indications, warnings, etc
Contra-indications: Depo-Provera is contra-indicated as a contraceptive at the above dosage in known or

suspected hormone-dependent malignancy of breast or genital organs, and in patients with a known sensitivity to medroxyprogesterone acetate.

Depo-Provera should not be used in pregnancy, either for diagnosis or therapy.

Warnings, precautions and side-effects: Whether administered alone or in combination with oestrogen, Depo-Provera should not be employed in patients with abnormal uterine bleeding until a definite diagnosis has been established and the possibility of genital tract malignancy eliminated.

Doctors should therefore check that patients are not pregnant before initial injection, and also if administration of any subsequent injection is overdue. Congenital anomalies, including female foetal masculinisation and clitoral hypertrophy, have been observed following larger doses of progestogens.

Medroxyprogesterone and/or its metabolites are secreted in breast milk but there is no evidence to suggest that this presents any hazard to the child.

A few cases of breast cancer have been reported in women taking Depo-Provera, but no causal relationship has been established.

Endometrial tumours have developed in monkeys given 50 × the human dose but the relevance of this to man has not been established.

A very low incidence of anaphylactoid reactions has been reported.

Patients who have a history of endogenous depression should be carefully observed and treatment discontinued if depression recurs to a significant degree.

A decrease in glucose tolerance has been observed in some patients treated with progestogens. The mechanism for this decrease is unknown. For this reason, diabetic patients should be carefully observed while receiving progestogen therapy.

Interaction with other medicinal treatment has not been reported, but the possibility should be borne in mind in patients receiving concurrent treatment with other drugs.

Patients receiving Depo-Provera may be subject to the side-effects normally associated with the use of progestogens. In addition, it is likely that some or all of the following effects may occur.

1. Delay in return to normal menstrual cycling and transient infertility lasting up to two years or longer may occur following continuous treatment with Depo-Provera.

2. Depo-Provera may be expected to cause disruption of the normal menstrual cycle. Irregular, prolonged or heavy vaginal bleeding or spotting may be experienced during the first two or three cycles of treatment. The frequency of occurrence of bleeding usually decreases with subsequent injections. After one year of treatment some women are amenorrhoeic.

3. Back pain.
4. Weight gain.
5. Fluid retention.

Overdosage: No positive action is required.

Pharmaceutical precautions Store at room temperature and protect from freezing. Do not mix with other agents.

Legal category POM.

Package quantities 1 ml, 3 ml and 5 ml vials.

Further information The contraceptive effect of 150 mg IM Depo-Provera last approximately 90 days.

Provera is a potent progestational agent with very low toxicity. Depo-Provera is ideally suited to the patient with endometriosis in whom oestrogen and androgen treatment may be considered to offer too many drawbacks on grounds of intolerance or masculinisation.

A 150 mg/ml strength of Depo-Provera is also available in a 3.3 ml vial for alternative indications.

Product licence number 0032/0056

DEPO-PROVERA* ▼

Presentation White sterile aqueous suspension. Each 1 ml contains 150 mg medroxyprogesterone acetate.

N.B. Additional strength Depo-Provera 50 mg/ml available for other indications, see Data Sheet for Depo-Provera 50 mg/ml.

Uses Progestogen. A proportion of certain classes of malignant tumours have been shown to respond to hormone administration or ablative hormonal surgery. These classes include carcinoma of endometrium, carcinoma of kidney and carcinoma of breast. Depo-Provera has been shown to be effective as adjunctive therapy in carcinoma of endometrium, carcinoma of kidney and carcinoma of breast in post-menopausal women.

Dosage and administration Doses should be given intramuscularly, deep into the gluteal muscle.

Endometrial or renal carcinoma: The normal initial dose lies in the range 400–1,000 mg per week, but doses in excess of 1,000 mg per day have been used without serious adverse effects. If improvement is noted within a few weeks or months and the disease appears stabilised, it may be possible to maintain the improvement with as little as 400 mg per month.

Breast carcinoma: The recommended schedule is 500 mg/day for 28 days. The patient should then be placed on a maintenance schedule of 500 mg twice weekly as long as the patient is responding to treatment.

Progression of disease at any time during therapy indicates treatment with Depo-Provera should be terminated, although response to hormonal therapy may not be evident until after at least 8–10 weeks of therapy.

Where large doses are being administered consideration should be given to dividing the dose between two separate sites.

Elderly patients: Depo-Provera has been extensively used in both the young (20–35) and older age groups (ages 50–75). Its use in the young has been primarily for contraception while its use in the older age group has been for the treatment of malignancies. There appears to be no evidence to suggest that the older aged patient is less well prepared to handle the drug metabolically than is the younger aged patient. Therefore the same dosage, contra-indications, and precautions would apply to either age group.

Contra-indications, warnings, etc

Contra-indications: Depo-Provera is contra-indicated in thrombophlebitis or a history of pulmonary embolism and liver dysfunction or disease and in patients with undiagnosed, irregular vaginal bleeding.

Warning: In the treatment of carcinoma of breast occasional cases of hypercalcaemia have been reported.

Any patient who develops an acute impairment of vision, proptosis, diplopia or migraine headache should be carefully evaluated ophthalmologically to exclude the presence of papilloedema or retinal vascular lesions before continuing medication.

Precautions: Animal studies show that Depo-Provera possesses adrenocorticoid activity. This has also been reported in man, therefore patients receiving large doses continuously and for long periods should be observed closely. The administration of large doses to pregnant women has resulted in the observation of some instances of female foetal masculinisation.

Because progestogens may cause some degree of fluid retention, conditions which might be influenced by this factor, such as epilepsy, migraine, asthma, cardiac or renal dysfunction, require careful observation. A very low incidence of anaphylactoid reactions has been reported. Patients who have a history of mental depression should be carefully observed and the drug discontinued if the depression recurs to a serious degree. A decrease in glucose tolerance has been observed in some patients on progestogens. The mechanism of this decrease is obscure. For this reason diabetic patients should be carefully observed while receiving progestogen therapy. Gynaecomastia, hirsutism and other evidence of virilisation may develop after prolonged courses. This form of therapy should only be administered under the direction of specialist units having facilities for appropriate surveillance of the patient.

Side-effects: Depending on the volume injected, some patients may be expected to show undesirable sequelae at the site of injection such as residual lump, change in colour of skin or sterile abscess. Other adverse reactions noted, particularly with large doses, have been:

Breast: In a few instances breast tenderness or galactorrhoea has occurred.

Psychic: An occasional patient has experienced nervousness, insomnia, somnolence, fatigue or dizziness.

Skin and mucous membranes: Sensitivity reactions ranging from pruritus, urticaria, angioneurotic oedema, to generalised rash and anaphylaxis have occasionally been reported. Acne, alopecia or hirsutism have been reported in a few cases.

Gastro-intestinal: Rarely nausea has been reported. Jaundice has been noted in a few instances.

Overdosage: No action required other than cessation of therapy.

Pharmaceutical precautions Store at room temperature and protect from freezing. Do not mix with other agents. Discard any remaining contents after use.

Legal category POM.

Package quantities 3.3 ml vial.

Further information The results of certain laboratory tests may be affected by the use of Depo-Provera; these include gonadotrophin levels, plasma progesterone levels, urinary pregnanediol levels, plasma testosterone levels (in the male), plasma oestrogen levels (in the female), plasma cortisol levels, glucose tolerance and metyrapone tests.

Product licence number 0032/0082

HALCION*

Presentation Blue flat oval tablets scored on one side and imprinted Upjohn 17 on the other side, each containing 0.25 mg triazolam.

Pale lavender flat oval tablets scored on one side and imprinted Upjohn 10 on the other, each containing 0.125 mg triazolam (for geriatric use).

Uses Halcion is an hypnotic which can be administered effectively for short-term and intermittent use in patients with recurring insomnia and poor sleeping habits. As with all hypnotics, long-term use is not recommended. Halcion may also be used in the treatment of insomnia associated with anxiety states and emotional distress.

Dosage and administration The usual dose for adults is 0.25 mg before retiring. The initial dose for geriatric patients is 0.125 mg and this may be increased to 0.25 mg if necessary.

Elderly patients: Reduced dosages are advised in the elderly, see above.

Contra-indications, warnings, etc
Contra-indications: Halcion is contra-indicated in patients with known hypersensitivity to benzodiazepines.

Warnings: As with all medicaments of this type, avoidance of alcohol in patients receiving Halcion is recommended since the individual response cannot be foreseen. Similarly, during its period of activity, Halcion may modify patients' reactions (driving, operating machinery) to a varying extent depending on dosages and individual susceptibility.

Precautions: In elderly and/or debilitated patients, it is recommended that treatment with Halcion be initiated at 0.125 mg to decrease the possibility of development of over-sedation, dizziness, or impaired co-ordination. If Halcion is to be combined with other drugs having known hypnotic properties or CNS depressant effects, consideration should be given to potential additive effects.

As with other benzodiazepines, caution should be exercised if the patient is in a depressed state or reveals evidence of a latent depression since these conditions may be intensified by hypnotic agents.

The usual precautions should be observed in patients with impaired renal or hepatic function.

Safety for use during pregnancy has not yet been established.

Use in Nursing Mothers: Human studies have not been performed; however, studies in rats have indicated that Halcion and its metabolites are secreted in milk. Therefore administration to nursing mothers is not recommended.

Safety and effectiveness in patients under the age of 18 have not been established.

Side-effects: Drowsiness, dizziness, light-headedness, confusion and impaired co-ordination have occurred. The incidence and severity of these pharmacological events are generally dose-related. Severe sedation and impaired co-ordination are indicative of drug intolerance or overdosage.

Adverse reactions: Headache has occurred in some patients. Less frequent adverse reactions which have been reported are taste alterations and depression. Adverse reactions which have been reported rarely are pruritus, skin rash, blurred vision, hiccups, palpitations, epigastric discomfort, diarrhoea, and burning eyes. As with other benzodiazepines, occasional cases of anterograde amnesia have been reported. Abnormal psychological reactions to most benzodiazepines have been reported. Rare behavioural adverse effects include paradoxical aggressive outbursts, excitement and the uncovering of depression with suicidal tendencies.

Overdosage: Manifestations of Halcion overdosage include extensions of its pharmacological activity, namely somnolence and hypnosis. As in all cases of drug overdosage, respiration, pulse, and blood pressure should be monitored and supported by general measures when necessary. Immediate gastric lavage should be performed. Intravenous fluids should be administered and an adequate airway maintained.

Experiments in animals have indicated that cardiopulmonary collapse can occur with massive intravenous doses of Halcion (over 100 mg/kg, > 20,000 times the maximum daily human dose). This could be reversed with positive mechanical respiration and the intravenous infusion of noradrenaline or metaraminol. Other animal experiments have suggested that haemodialysis and forced diuresis are probably of little value.

Pharmaceutical precautions Keep container tightly closed and protect from light.

Legal category CD (Sch 4) POM.

Package quantities Packs of 30, 250 and 1,000 tablets.

Further information Halcion has a relatively short biological half-life as do its metabolites. It does not cause enzyme induction in man. The preponderance of data from sleep laboratory studies indicates that there would be no significant tolerance development, drug accumulation or withdrawal effects after cessation of treatment.

Product licence numbers
0.25 mg Tablet   0032/0058
0.125 mg Tablet   0032/0063

KAOPECTATE*

Presentation Off-white suspension. Each 5 ml contains 1.03 g Kaolin BP in an aromatic and carminative vehicle.

Uses Antidiarrhoeal.
Diarrhoea of non-specific origin.

Dosage and administration Oral.
Adult: 10–30 ml every 4 hours.
Children:
Up to 1 year – 5 ml every 4 hours.
1–5 years – 10 ml every 4 hours.
Elderly patients: There is no information to suggest that a change in dosage is warranted in the elderly. Side-effects do not appear to be more common or severe in elderly patients.

Contra-indications, warnings, etc
Contra-indications: Intestinal obstruction.
Warnings: None.
Precautions: None.
Side-effects: None.
Overdosage: None.

Pharmaceutical precautions None.

Legal category GSL.

Package quantities Bottles of 500 ml and 180 ml.

Further information Nil.

Product licence number 0032/5040R

LINCOCIN*

Presentation Capsules (dark blue/light blue) containing 500 mg lincomycin as lincomycin hydrochloride.
Colourless sterile solution. Contains 300 mg per ml lincomycin as lincomycin hydrochloride.
Red syrup with raspberry flavour. Each 5 ml contains 250 mg lincomycin as lincomycin hydrochloride.

Uses Antibacterial.
Lincocin is indicated in serious infections caused by susceptible Gram-positive organisms, staphylococci (both penicillinase and non-penicillinase producing), streptococci (except *Strep. faecalis*) and pneumococci. It is also indicated (given parenterally) in serious infections caused by susceptible anaerobic pathogens.
Lincomycin does not penetrate the blood/brain barrier in therapeutically effective quantities.

Dosage and administration Oral. Intramuscular. Intravenous.
Oral:
Capsules: Adults: Moderately severe infections, 1 capsule three times a day. Severe infection, 1 capsule four times a day.
Syrup 250: Children 1–6 months: 1.25–2.5 ml three times a day.
6 months to 2 years: 2.5–5 ml three times a day.
3–9 years: 2.5–5 ml four times a day.
10–12 years: 5–10 ml four times a day.
For optimal absorption, it is recommended that nothing be given by mouth except water for a period of one or two hours before and after oral administration.
Intramuscular: Sterile solution. Injections should be made deeply into the gluteal muscles.
Adults: Moderately severe infection, 600 mg (2 ml) every 24 hours. Severe infection, 600 mg (2 ml) every 12 hours or more often.
Children (over 1 month): Moderately severe infection, 10 mg/kg/every 24 hours. Severe infection, 10 mg/kg/ every 12 hours or more often.
Intravenous: Sterile solution.
Adults: 600 mg (2 ml) every 8–12 hours. Administer as an infusion in 250 ml or more 5% glucose or normal saline over a period of not less than one hour.
Children (over 1 month): 10–20 mg/kg/day in 2 or 3 equal doses at 8 or 12-hourly intervals. Administer as an infusion as above.
Treatment for infections caused by β-haemolytic streptococci should be continued for at least 10 days to guard against subsequent rheumatic fever or glomerulonephritis.
Elderly patients: Specific pharmacokinetics data regarding lincomycin hydrochloride in the elderly are not available. However, there has been no indication from clinical studies or clinical use that there is any age-related increase in toxicity with regard to lincomycin. Pharmacokinetic data on the chemically-related antibiotic, clindamycin, has shown that kinetics are not altered in elderly subjects. Therefore it appears that in elderly patients dosage of lincomycin should not be influenced by age alone. See Precautions Sections for other factors which should be taken into consideration.

Contra-indications, warnings, etc
Contra-indications: Patients with a history of sensitivity to lincomycin. Although cross-sensitisation to clinda-

mycin (Dalacin C) has not been demonstrated, it is recommended that Lincocin is not used in patients who have exhibited sensitivity to clindamycin.

Warnings: Lincocin should only be used in the treatment of serious infections. In considering the use of the product the practitioner should bear in mind the type of infection and the potential hazard of the diarrhoea which may develop since cases of colitis have been reported. The appearance of marked diarrhoea should be regarded as an indication that the product should be discontinued immediately.

Studies indicate a toxin(s) produced by *Clostridia* (especially *Clostridium difficile*) is the principal direct cause of antibiotic-associated colitis. These studies also indicate that this toxigenic *Clostridium* is usually sensitive in vitro to vancomycin. When 125 mg to 500 mg of vancomycin is administered orally four times a day, there is a rapid observed disappearance of the toxin from faecal samples and a coincident clinical recovery from the diarrhoea.

Precautions: Pending further clinical experience Lincocin is not recommended in the newborn, in the prophylaxis of a recurrence of rheumatic fever, and in patients with pre-existing kidney, liver, endocrine or metabolic disease, unless special clinical circumstances so indicate. Lincomycin has been shown to have neuromuscular blocking properties that may enhance the action of other neuromuscular blocking agents. Therefore it should be used with caution in patients receiving such agents. In the case of renal impairment, a reduced dosage regime should be used. During prolonged Lincocin therapy, periodic liver function studies and blood counts should be performed. Although there is no evidence of ill effects in either the mother or foetus, Lincocin should be used with customary caution in pregnant women.

The long-term use of lincomycin may give rise to an overgrowth of non-susceptible organisms, particularly yeasts.

Side-effects: Lincocin is well tolerated. With oral administration, gastro-intestinal side-effects have been encountered, such as loose stools or diarrhoea, or colitis (see 'Warnings'), nausea, vomiting and abdominal cramps. Other minor side-effects have been observed infrequently. Leucopenia (neutropenia), agranulocytosis and hypersensitivity reactions have been reported on rare occasions.

Overdosage: In cases of overdosage that may have led to adverse reactions therapy should be discontinued and the usual emergency treatment, including corticosteroids, adrenaline and antihistamines, instituted. The serum biological half-life of lincomycin is 5.4 ± 1 hour. Lincomycin cannot be readily removed from the blood by dialysis or peritoneal dialysis.

Pharmaceutical precautions Storage temperature for capsules should not exceed 30°C. Lincocin Sterile Solution should be protected from light and freezing and stored at under 30°C.

Dilution of the Syrup 250 should be carried out using Syrup BP.

Legal category POM.

Package quantities Capsules in bottles of 12 and 100.
Syrup 250, Bottles of 100 ml.
Sterile solution 2 ml and 10×2 ml ampoules.

Further information Lincomycin exhibits cross-resistance with clindamycin. When tested by in vitro methods, some staphylococcal strains originally resistant to erythromycin rapidly developed resistance to lincomycin.

Product licence numbers
Capsules 0032/5008
Solution 0032/5009
Syrup 0032/5010

LONITEN*

Presentation Each tablet contains 2.5 mg, 5 mg, 10 mg or 25 mg minoxidil. Round, white, biconvex tablet of 25 mg with 25 imprinted on one side and scored on the other with a U above the score line and 257 below. Round white biconvex tablets of 2.5, 5, or 10 mg strength imprinted on one side and scored on the other with a U on either side of the score.

Uses Loniten is indicated for the treatment of severe hypertension.

It should not be used as the sole agent to initiate therapy. It is a peripheral vasodilator and should be given in conjunction with a diuretic, to control salt and water retention, and a beta-adrenergic blocking agent, or appropriate substitute, to control reflex tachycardia.

Dosage and administration *Adults and patients over 12 years of age:* An initial daily dose of 5 mg, which may be given as a single or divided dosage is recommended. This dose may first be increased to 10 mg daily and subsequent increases should be by increments of 10 mg in the daily dose. Dosage adjustments should be made at intervals of not less than three days, until optimum control of blood pressure is achieved. It is seldom necessary to exceed 50 mg per day although in exceptional circumstances, doses up to 100 mg per day have been used. Twice-daily dosage is satisfactory. Where diastolic pressure reduction of less than 30 mm Hg is required, once-daily dosing has been reported as effective.

Dosage requirements may be lower in dialysis patients.

Children: For patients of 12 years of age or under, the initial dose should be 0.2 mg per kilogram given as a single or divided daily dosage. Incremental increases of 0.1–0.2 mg per kilogram in the daily dose are recommended at intervals of not less than three days until optimum blood pressure control has been achieved or the maximum daily dose of 1.0 mg/kg has been reached.

Rapid reduction of blood pressure: Rapid reduction of blood pressure can be achieved using continuous blood pressure monitoring and incremental doses of 5 mg every six hours.

Concomitant antihypertensive therapy: It is recommended that, where possible, antihypertensive therapy, other than a beta-adrenergic blocking agent and a diuretic be discontinued before Loniten treatment is started. It is recognised that some antihypertensive agents should not be abruptly discontinued. These drugs should be gradually discontinued during the first week of Loniten treatment.

Loniten causes sodium retention and if used alone can result in several hundred milli-equivalents of salt being retained together with a corresponding volume of water.

Therefore, in all patients who are not on dialysis, Loniten must be given in conjunction with a diuretic in sufficient dosage to maintain salt and water balance.

Examples of the daily dosages of diuretics commonly used when starting therapy with Loniten include:

1. Hydrochlorothiazide (100 mg) – or other thiazides at equi-effective dosage.
2. Chlorthalidone (100 mg).
3. Frusemide (80 mg).

If excessive water retention results in a weight gain of more than 3 pounds when a thiazide or chlorthalidone is being used, diuretic therapy should be supplemented with spironolactone or changed to frusemide, the dose of which may be increased in accordance with the patients' requirements. Diuretic dosage in children should be proportionally less in relation to weight.

Patients will require a sympathetic nervous system suppressant to limit a Loniten-induced rise in heart rate. The preferred agent is a beta-blocker equivalent to an adult propranolol dosage of 80–160 mg/day. Higher doses may be required when pre-treated patients have an increase in heart rate exceeding 20 beats per minute or when simultaneous introduction causes an increase exceeding 10 beats per minute. When beta-blockers are contra-indicated, alternatives such as methyldopa may be used instead and should be started 24 hours prior to Loniten.

Elderly patients: At present there are no extensive clinical studies with minoxidil in patients over age 65. There is data indicating that elevated·systolic and diastolic pressures are important risk factors for cardiovascular disease in individuals over age 65. However, elderly patients may be sensitive to the blood pressure lowering effect of minoxidil and thus caution is urged in initiating therapy as orthostatic hypotension may occur. It is suggested that 2.5 mg per day be used as the initial starting dose in patients over 65 years of age.

Contra-indications, warnings, etc
Contra-indications: Loniten is contra-indicated in patients with a phaeochromocytoma.

Warnings: If used alone, Loniten can cause a significant retention of salt and water leading to positive physical signs such as oedema, and to clinical deterioration of some patients with heart failure. Diuretic treatment alone, or in combination with restricted salt intake is, therefore, necessary for all patients taking Loniten.

Patients who have had myocardial infarction should only be treated with Loniten after a stable post-infarction state has been established.

The physician should bear in mind that if not controlled by sympathetic suppressants, the rise in cardiac rate and output that follows the use of potent vasodilators may induce anginal symptoms in patients with undiagnosed coronary artery disease, or may aggravate pre-existing angina pectoris.

The effect of Loniten may be additive to concurrent antihypertensive agents. The interaction of Loniten with sympathetic-blocking agents such as guanethidine or bethanidine may produce excessive blood pressure reduction and/or orthostasis.

Precautions: The safety of Loniten in pregnancy remains to be established.

Hypertrichosis occurs in most patients treated with Loniten and all patients should be warned of this possibility before starting therapy. Spontaneous reversal to the pre-treatment state can be expected one to three months after cessation of therapy.

Soon after starting Loniten therapy approximately 60% of patients exhibit ECG alterations in the direction and magnitude of their T waves. Large changes may encroach on the ST Segment, unaccompanied by evidence of ischaemia. These asymptomatic changes usually disappear with continuing Loniten treatment. The ECG reverts to the pre-treatment state if Loniten is discontinued.

Pericardial effusion has been detected in patients treated with a Loniten-containing regime. A cause and effect relationship has not been established. Most effusions have either been present before Loniten was given, or occurred among uraemic patients. However, it is suggested that Loniten-treated patients should be periodically monitored for signs or symptoms of pericardial effusion and appropriate therapy instituted if necessary.

Salt and water retention in excess of 2 to 3 pounds may diminish the effectiveness of Loniten. Patients should therefore, be carefully instructed about compliance with diuretic therapy and a detailed record of body weight should be maintained.

Side-effects: Most patients receiving Loniten experience a diminution of pre-existing side-effects attributable to their disease or previous therapy. New events or side-effects likely to increase include peripheral oedema, associated with or independent of weight gain; increases in heart rate; hypertrichosis; and a temporary rise in creatinine and blood urea nitrogen. Gastro-intestinal intolerance, rash and breast tenderness are infrequently reported side-effects of Loniten therapy.

Overdosage: If exaggerated hypotension is encountered, it is most likely to occur in association with residual sympathetic nervous system blockade (guanethidine-like effects or alpha-adrenergic blockade). Recommended treatment is intravenous administration of normal saline. Sympathomimetic drugs, such as noradrenaline or adrenaline, should be avoided because of their excessive cardiac-stimulating action. Phenylephrine, angiotensin II and vasopressin, which reverse the effect of Loniten, should be used only if inadequate perfusion of a vital organ is evident.

Pharmaceutical precautions None.

Legal category POM.

Package quantities 2.5 mg, 5 mg, 10 mg and 25 mg Loniten tablets supplied as bottles of 100.

Further information Loniten is a potent vasodilator which probably exerts its action after binding to the smooth muscle of the blood vessel wall. At least 90% of an oral dose is rapidly absorbed and the average plasma half-life in man is 4.2 hours. The clinical duration of action is up to 72 hours. Approximately 90% of administered drug is metabolised and excreted in the urine within 24 hours. Drug-related materials can be removed by dialysis.

Product licence numbers
2.5 mg	0032/0064
5 mg	0032/0065
10 mg	0032/0066
25 mg	0032/0068

MEDRONE*

Presentation Oval double-scored white tablet 4 mg methylprednisolone: oval double-scored pink tablet 2 mg methylprednisolone; oval double-scored white tablet marked 'Upjohn 73' 16 mg methylprednisolone.

Uses Anti-inflammatory agent.

Medrone is indicated for conditions requiring glucocorticoid activity, including collagen diseases, allergic diseases, certain dermatological conditions, acute and chronic ocular inflammatory diseases, certain leukaemias and lymphatic neoplastic diseases, ulcerative colitis, nephrosis, and various metabolic diseases responsive to corticosteroid treatment

Dosage and administration Oral.

The dosage recommendations shown in the table are suggested initial daily doses and are intended as guides. The average total daily dose recommended should be given in 4 equally divided doses and given with meals and a snack at bedtime (excepting in alternate-day therapy when the minimum effective daily dose is doubled and given every other day at 8.00 a.m.)

The initial suppressive dose level is continued until a

Indications	Recommended initial daily dosage
Collagen diseases	
Rheumatoid arthritis	
Severe	12–16 mg
Moderately severe	8–12 mg
Moderate	4–8 mg
Children	4–8 mg
Systemic lupus erythematosus	20–96 mg
Acute rheumatic fever	1.1 mg per kg of body weight per day until ESR normal for one week
Allergic diseases	
Severe seasonal asthma	16–40 mg
Severe pollinosis	16–40 mg
Exfoliative dermatitis	16–40 mg
Contact dermatitis	16–40 mg
Severe intrinsic asthma	12–40 mg
Intractable allergic rhinitis	12–40 mg
Generalised atopic dermatitis	12–40 mg
Generalised infantile eczema	8–12 mg
Ocular inflammatory diseases (of the posterior segment)	
Acute	12–40 mg
Chronic	12–40 mg
Haematological disorders	
Acute granulocytic leukaemia	16–96 mg
Acute monocytic leukaemia	16–96 mg
Chronic lymphocytic leukaemia	16–96 mg
Thrombocytopenia	16–96 mg
Haemolytic anaemia	16–96 mg
	In some cases, doses of the order of 300 mg have been employed to establish control
Miscellaneous diseases	
Adrenogenital syndrome	4–12 mg
Ulcerative colitis	16–60 mg
Nephrosis	20–60 mg (for 10–14 days or until diuresis ensues)
Refractory congestive heart failure or cirrhosis of the liver with ascites	16–24 mg Medrone must be administered in conjunction with an effective diuretic

satisfactory clinical response is obtained, a period usually of three to seven days in the cases of rheumatic diseases (except for acute rheumatic carditis), allergic conditions affecting the skin or respiratory tract, and ocular inflammatory diseases. If a satisfactory response is not obtained in seven days, re-evaluation of the case to confirm the original diagnosis should be made. As soon as a satisfactory clinical response is obtained, the daily dose should be reduced gradually, either to termination of treatment in the case of acute conditions (e.g. seasonal asthma, exfoliative dermatitis, acute ocular inflammations) or to the minimal effective maintenance dose level in the case of chronic conditions (e.g. rheumatoid arthritis, systemic lupus erythematosus, bronchial asthma, atopic dermatitis). In chronic conditions, and in rheumatoid arthritis especially, it is important that the reduction in dosage from initial to maintenance dose levels be accomplished slowly. Decrements of not more than 2 mg at intervals of 7–10 days are suggested. In rheumatoid arthritis, maintenance steroid therapy should be at the lowest possible level.

In general, dosage for children should be based upon clinical response and is at the discretion of the clinician.

In alternate-day therapy, the minimum daily corticoid requirement is doubled and administered as a single dose every other day at 8.00 a.m.

Elderly patients: Elderly patients may be more prone to the problems listed in subsequent sections. In particular, calcium loss may be exaggerated.

Contra-indications, warnings, etc

Contra-indications: Medrone is contra-indicated in patients with latent, healed and active tuberculosis, Cushing's syndrome, peptic ulcer, acute psychoses, herpes simplex keratitis, vaccinia and varicella.

Warnings: Because of its inhibitory effect on fibroplasia, Medrone may mask signs of infection and enhance dissemination of the infecting organism. All patients should be watched for such intercurrent infection, which must be brought under control by use of appropriate antibacterial measures. As a general rule the administration of the corticosteroid should not be discontinued suddenly, but tailed off over a period. In certain situations involving intercurrent infection the corticosteroid dosage may require to be stepped up to counter the effects of shock.

Precautions: The presence of diabetes, osteoporosis, chronic psychotic reactions, predisposition to thrombophlebitis, hypertension, congestive heart failure and renal insufficiency necessitate the carefully controlled use of methylprednisolone. While therapy with corticosteroids during pregnancy does not appear to be contra-indicated, caution is recommended, particularly during the first trimester. Neonates of mothers who have received such therapy during pregnancy should be observed for signs of hypoadrenalism and appropriate measures instituted if such signs are present.

Medrone should be used with caution in young children as corticosteroids are known to interfere with normal growth pattern.

Side-effects: Side-effects associated with the use of corticosteroids may be observed, including Cushing's syndrome, moon facies, supraclavicular pads of fat, hirsutism, striae and acne, hyperglycaemia, osteoporosis, peptic ulceration, hypertension, psychic disturbance, posterior subcapsular cataracts, suppression of growth in children, subcutaneous and cutaneous atrophy, sterile abscess, vertigo, weakness, myopathy, thrombo-embolism, pancreatitis, exophthalmos and headache.

Overdosage: Administration of Medrone should not be discontinued abruptly but tailed off over a period of time. Appropriate action should be taken to alleviate the symptoms produced by any side-effect that may become apparent. It may be necessary to support the patient with corticosteroids during any further period of trauma occurring within two years of overdosage.

Pharmaceutical precautions No special precautions are required.

Legal category POM.

Package quantities 2 mg and 4 mg tablets in bottles of 30.
16 mg tablets in bottles of 14.

Further information Medrone has achieved a clinically acceptable split between glucocorticoid effect and undesired mineralocorticoid effect. Weight for weight, methylprednisolone has five times the anti-inflammatory activity of hydrocortisone but has little tendency to cause salt and water retention. The 16 mg tablet gives opportunity for use of alternate-day therapy in long-term use in chronic conditions.

Product licence numbers
Medrone Tablets 2 mg   0032/5017
Medrone Tablets 4 mg   0032/5018
Medrone Tablets 16 mg   0032/0024

MEDRONE* ACNE LOTION

Presentation A pale yellow emulsion containing the following active ingredients (% w/v):

Methylprednisolone acetate   0.25%
Sulphur (from colloidal sulphur)   5%
Aluminium chlorhydroxide complex   10%

Uses For topical application in the treatment of acne vulgaris, rosacea and seborrhoeic dermatitis.

Dosage and administration Apply sparingly once or twice a day. Shake well before use.

Elderly patients: This product will be seldom prescribed for the elderly. However, in elderly patients, topical corticoid side effects may be exaggerated, especially in areas where skin tends to thin, e.g., face, neck, back of hands.

Contra-indications, warnings, etc
Contra-indications: Contra-indications, warnings and precautions are those which normally apply to topical corticosteroids.

Warnings: Contact with the eyes should be avoided. Topical administration of corticosteroids to pregnant animals can cause abnormalities of foetal development. The relevance of this finding to human beings has not been established; however, topical steroids should not be used extensively in pregnancy, i.e. in large amounts or for prolonged periods.

Side-effects: Medrone Acne Lotion is designed to produce a drying effect on the skin. Should excessive drying or peeling of the skin occur, the frequency of application should be reduced. Other less frequently occurring side-effects include erythema, itching, burning, hyperpigmentation and occasional hypersensitivity or allergic reactions.

Overdosage: Unlikely to produce serious toxicity unless taken in very large amounts. Ingestion of 30 grams of aluminium chlorhydroxide complex has produced serious toxicity and an emetic should be considered, together with supportive therapy in such cases of massive ingestion.

Pharmaceutical precautions Protect from freezing. The lotion should not be diluted and should be dispensed in the original container.

Legal category POM.

Package quantities 25 ml and 75 ml polythene bottles.

Further information If infection is present the companion product Neo-Medrone Acne Lotion (which contains neomycin) is available.

Product licence number 0032/0041

MOTRIN*

Presentation Film-coated tablets containing Ibuprofen BP. 200 mg – red, debossed Upjohn and 241; 400 mg – orange tablet debossed Upjohn and 415; 600 mg – peach tablet debossed Upjohn and 742.

Uses Non-steroidal anti-inflammatory agent with analgesic and antipyretic properties. Motrin is indicated for the relief of the signs and symptoms of rheumatoid arthritis (including Still's Disease), osteoarthrosis, ankylosing spondylitis, and seronegative (non-rheumatoid) arthropathies. It may also be used in non-articular rheumatic conditions and soft tissue injuries; these include low back pain, capsulitis, bursitis, tenosynovitis, sprains and strains.

Dosage and administration
Adults: 1200–1800 mg daily in three divided doses; up to 2400 mg daily may be given in severe conditions.

Children: 20 mg/kg daily. In those children weighing less than 30 kg, the total dose in 24 hours should not exceed 500 mg.

Elderly patients: It appears that advanced age has a minimal influence on the pharmacokinetics of ibuprofen. However, the following should be considered:
Ibuprofen may increase levels of digoxin concentration presumably from reduced renal excretion of digoxin.
Ibuprofen has been reported to have an antagonistic effect on frusemide-induced diuresis in cardiac failure.
Ibuprofen has been reported to be associated with cognitive dysfunction in the elderly.
Although ibuprofen is probably one of the safer nonsteroidal anti-inflammatory drugs to use in association with anticoagulants (warfarin), it should be used with caution.

Contra-indications, warnings, etc
Contra-indications: Active peptic ulceration.

Precautions: Ibuprofen does not appear to be teratogenic in animals; however, its use in pregnancy is not recommended.

Warnings: Use with caution in patients with asthma or those who have shown hypersensitivity to other non-steroidal anti-inflammatory agents. Gastro-intestinal intolerance and bleeding have been reported. Treatment should be discontinued in patients reporting blurred or diminished vision. Thrombocytopenia has occurred infrequently.

Treatment of overdosage: Gastric lavage. No specific

antidote. It is theoretically advantageous to administer alkali and induce diuresis as the drug is acidic and excreted in the urine.

Pharmaceutical precautions Motrin tablets should be kept in a well-closed container.

Legal category POM.

Package quantities Bottles of 100 (200, 400, 600 mg), 250 (400 mg), 500 (200 mg).

Further information The absorption profile shows Motrin to be of particular value in relieving morning stiffness.

Product licence numbers
200 mg   0032/0104
400 mg   0032/0105
600 mg   0032/0106

MYCIFRADIN* SULPHATE STERILE POWDER

Presentation A white to cream, freeze-dried powder of 500 mg neomycin sulphate.

Uses Topical antibacterial.
Treatment of infections of the skin or mucous membranes caused by organisms sensitive to neomycin.

Dosage and administration The contents of the vial should be diluted before use – see section 'Preparation of Solutions', below.
Neomycin sulphate solution may be applied as wet dressings, packs or irrigations. Topical applications may be made once or twice daily.

Urological indications: For prophylaxis against infection incident to cytoscopy and retrograde pyelography, Mycifradin Sulphate has been reported to meet all the criteria for a bactericidal substance to be used for this purpose. Mycifradin Sulphate 0.1% to 1.0% solutions have been recommended for the prevention of post-catheterisation sepsis or a post-instrumental reaction. Mycifradin Sulphate 0.01% solution has been employed for irrigation in chronic bladder infections. In addition, Mycifradin Sulphate added to solution for use following several hundred transurethral resections of the prostate was reported to cause no toxic or untoward local effects.

Preparation of solutions: The addition of 5 ml of Sodium Chloride Injection to the contents of the vial of Mycifradin Sulphate Sterile Powder will produce a solution containing 100 mg per ml. The whole of this solution should be immediately diluted as required, e.g. 1:10 with saline to make up a solution containing 10 mg per ml (1%) for bladder instillation or 1:20 with saline to give a solution of 5 mg per ml (0.5%) for topical application. Any unused material should be discarded.

Elderly patients: It should be borne in mind that elderly patients may have some degree of renal impairment and thus not excrete neomycin normally. See Warnings and Precautions section for other factors which should be taken into consideration.

Contra-indications, warnings, etc
Contra-indications: Use in patients with a history of sensitivity to neomycin. Because of the dangers of ototoxicity and nephrotoxicity the product should not be used parenterally.

Warnings and precautions: Prolonged use of this product may result in overgrowth of nonsusceptible organisms – particularly monilia. Constant observation of the patient is essential. If new infections appear during therapy, appropriate measures should be taken.

When employed repeatedly on large abraded areas and/or repeatedly for irrigation of extensive wounds, significant amounts of the drug may be absorbed, with the possibility of ototoxicity and nephrotoxicity.

Not more than a total of one gram of neomycin per day should be used in solutions applied topically or for urological purposes.

Administration of solutions for urological purposes should not exceed ten consecutive days.

Neomycin should not be given concurrently or in series with other aminoglycoside antibiotics as the eighth nerve toxicity for all members of this chemical group may be additive. Potent diuretics should not be administered concurrently. Safety for use in pregnancy has not been established. Cross-resistance develops rapidly in micro-organisms with other aminoglycosides, particularly kanamycin and framycetin.

Aminoglycosides may potentiate the effects of neuro-muscular blocking agents and may cause respiratory arrest.

Side-effects: Possible ototoxicity and nephrotoxicity. See Contra-indications and Warnings above.
Hypersensitivity reactions, primarily skin rashes, have been reported.

Overdosage: If symptoms of ototoxicity or nephrotoxicity occur, discontinue treatment immediately.

Pharmaceutical precautions Store Mycifradin Sulphate Sterile Powder in a cool, dry place, protect from light. Prepared solutions should be stored in the refrigerator and used as soon as possible.

Legal category POM.

Package quantities Mycifradin Sulphate is supplied as a vial containing 500 mg neomycin sulphate (equivalent to 350 mg neomycin base) as a sterile powder.

Further information Nil.

Product licence number 0032/5011

NEO-CORTEF* EYE/EAR DROPS
NEO-CORTEF* EYE/EAR OINTMENT

Presentation White, sterile aqueous suspension containing hydrocortisone acetate 15 mg (1.5%) and neomycin sulphate 5 mg (0.5%) per ml. Yellow soft ointment containing hydrocortisone acetate 15 mg (1.5%) and neomycin sulphate 5 mg (0.5%) per gram.

Uses Inflammatory and infective ear and eye conditions susceptible to the action of the neomycin/hydrocortisone combination.
Such conditions include:
Eye: Phlyctenular keratoconjunctivitis, non-specific superficial keratitis, blepharitis, acne rosacea keratitis, allergic conjunctivitis, deep keratitis, sclerokeratitis, episcleritis, post-operative keratitis, post-operative and post-traumatic uveitis.
Ear: Otitis externa.

Dosage and administration *Drops: Eye:* 1 or 2 drops three or more times daily.
Ear: 1 or 2 drops in the external ear canal three or more times daily.
Ointment: Applications should be made one or more times daily.

Elderly patients: There is no information to suggest that a change in dosage is warranted in the elderly.

Contra-indications, warnings, etc

Contra-indications: The presence of tuberculous, fungal and acute purulent infections of the eye, viral infections of the eye such as herpes simplex, vaccinia and varicella, and in the presence of glaucoma. Hypersensitivity to any ingredient. Not to be used in the ear in patients with a perforated eardrum.

Warnings: Topical administration of corticosteroids to pregnant animals can cause abnormalities of foetal development. The relevance of this finding to human beings has not been established; however, topical steroids should not be used extensively in the first trimester of pregnancy, i.e. in large amounts or for prolonged periods.

Precautions: Corticosteroids may mask signs of infection and enhance dissemination of an infecting organism. Eye preparations containing corticosteroids can cause a serious rise in intra-ocular pressure in a small proportion of patients – usually those with a family history of glaucoma.

Side-effects: Sensitivity to neomycin has been reported in topical applications. Thinning of the cornea leading to perforation has occurred with the use of topical corticosteroids. The development of cataract has been reported to have occurred after prolonged use of topical corticosteroids in eye conditions.

Overdosage: Unlikely to produce any serious toxic effects if ingested.

Pharmaceutical precautions None.

Legal category POM.

Package quantities Neo-Cortef Eye/Ear Drops supplied as 5 ml plastic squeeze bottles with applicator tip.
Neo-Cortef Eye/Ear Ointment is supplied in tubes of 3.9 g with applicator tip.

Further information Nil.

Product licence numbers
Neo-Cortef Eye/Ear Drops   0032/5026
Neo-Cortef Eye/Ear Ointment   0032/5027

NEO-MEDRONE* ACNE LOTION

Presentation Pale yellow lotion containing suspension of methylprednisolone acetate 2.5 mg, neomycin sulphate 2.5 mg, sulphur 50 mg, alumininium chlorhydroxide complex 100 mg per ml of aqueous base.

Uses Neo-Medrone Acne Lotion is indicated for the treatment of acne vulgaris, rosacea and seborrhoeic dermatitis.

Dosage and administration Topical application to the affected area sparingly once or twice a day. Shake well before using.

Elderly patients: This product will be seldom prescribed for the elderly. However, in elderly patients, topical corticoid side effects may be exaggerated, especially in areas where skin tends to thin, e.g., face, neck, back of hands.

Contra-indications, warnings, etc

Contra-indications: Contra-indications, warnings and precautions are those which normally apply to topical corticosteroids, and the product is contra-indicated in patients with a history of sensitivity to neomycin.

Warnings: Contact with the eyes should be avoided. Topical administration of corticosteroids to pregnant animals can cause abnormalities of foetal development. The relevance of this finding to human beings has not been established; however, topical steroids should not be used extensively in pregnancy, i.e. in large amounts or for prolonged periods.

Precautions: (a) Prolonged use of antibiotic preparations may result in overgrowth of non-susceptible organisms. (b) Ototoxicity or nephrotoxicity have been reported following absorption of topically applied neomycin.

Side-effects: Neo-Medrone Acne Lotion is designed to produce a drying effect on the skin. Should excessive drying or peeling of the skin occur, the frequency of application should be reduced. Other less frequently occurring side-effects include erythema, itching, burning, hyperpigmentation and occasional hypersensitivity or allergic reactions.

Overdosage: Unlikely to produce serious toxicity unless taken in very large amounts. Ingestion of 30 grams of aluminium chlorhydroxide complex has produced serious toxicity and an emetic should be considered, together with supportive therapy in such cases of massive ingestion.

Pharmaceutical precautions Store at room temperature. Protect from freezing.

Legal category POM.

Package quantities 50 ml and 75 ml plastic squeeze bottles.

Further information Neo-Medrone Acne Lotion should be used as an adjunct to usual skin cleansing or dietary recommendations.

Product licence number 0032/5032

PROSTIN E2* STERILE SOLUTIONS

Presentation Colourless sterile solutions in ampoules containing 1 mg/ml or 10 mg/ml dinoprostone, Prostaglandin E_2, in ethanol.

Uses Oxytocic agent.
Indications for Prostin E2 are: induction of labour, foetal death in utero, therapeutic termination of pregnancy, missed abortion and hydatidiform mole.

Presentation:
1. 0.75 ml ampoule of a 1 mg/ml solution of dinoprostone in ethanol – for induction of labour and foetal death in utero (intravenous).
2. 0.5 ml ampoule of a 10 mg/ml solution of dinoprostone in ethanol – for therapeutic termination of pregnancy, missed abortion and hydatidiform mole (intravenous).
3. 0.5 ml ampoule of a 10 mg/ml solution of dinoprostone in ethanol (plus a 50 ml vial of saline diluent) – for therapeutic termination of pregnancy (extra-amniotic).

Dosage and administration Prostin E2 Sterile Solution may be administered by two routes, intravenous or extra-amniotic, depending on dose form and indication as shown above. *In each case the ampoule contents must be diluted before use and full instructions on method of dilution and dosage are given on the package insert which should be consulted prior to initiation of* *therapy.* Continuous administration of the drug for more than two days is not recommended (See Precautions). The following is a guide to dosage:

1. *Prostin E2 1 mg/ml solution (in ethanol). Intravenous for induction of labour:* Dilute with normal saline or 5% dextrose according to the package insert to produce a 1.5 mcg/ml solution. The 1.5 mcg/ml solution is infused at 0.25 mcg/minute for 30 minutes and then maintained or increased. Cases of foetal death in utero may require higher doses. An initial rate of 0.5 mcg/minute may be used with stepwise increases, at intervals of not less than one hour.

2. *Prostin E2 10 mg/ml solution (in ethanol). Intravenous for therapeutic termination of pregnancy, missed abortion and hydatidiform mole:* Dilute with normal saline or 5% dextrose according to package insert to produce a 5 mcg/ml solution. The 5 mcg/ml solution is infused at 2.5 mcg/minute for 30 minutes and then maintained or increased to 5mcg/minute. The rate should be maintained for at least four hours before increasing further.

3. *Prostin E2 10 mg/ml solution (in ethanol). Extra-amniotic for therapeutic termination of pregnancy:* Dilute with the 50 ml of diluent provided according to the package insert to produce a 100 mcg/ml solution. The 100 mcg/ml solution is instilled via a 12–14 French-gauge Foley catheter. Initial instillation is 1 ml, then, dependent on uterine response, 1 or 2 ml usually at two-hour intervals.

Contra-indications, warnings, etc

Contra-indications: There are no absolute contra-indications to the use of Prostin E2. However, its use is not recommended in the following circumstances:

1. Where the patient is sensitive to prostaglandins.

2. For patients in whom oxytocic drugs are generally contra-indicated or where prolonged contractions of the uterus are considered inappropriate, such as: cases with a history of Caesarean section or major uterine surgery; cases in which major degrees of cephalopelvic disproportion may be present; cases in which foetal malpresentation is present; cases in which there is clinical suspicion or definite evidence of pre-existing foetal distress; cases in which there is a history of difficult labour and/or traumatic delivery; grand multiparae with six or more previous term pregnancies; cases with a history of pelvic inflammatory disease.

3. In therapeutic termination of pregnancy where known pelvic infection exists, unless adequate prior treatment has been instituted.

4. The extra-amniotic route should not be employed in the presence of cervicitis or vaginal infections.

Warnings: There is some evidence in animals of a low order of teratogenicity, therefore, if abortion does not occur or is suspected to be incomplete as a result of prostaglandin therapy, the appropriate treatment for complete evacuation of the uterus should be instituted in all instances.

Since prostaglandins may potentiate the effect of oxytocin it is recommended that the use of these drugs simultaneously or in sequence be carefully monitored.

The products are available only to hospitals and clinics with specialised obstetric units and should only be used where 24-hour resident medical cover is provided.

Precautions: Caution should be exercised in the administration of Prostin E2 in patients with: (i) glaucoma or raised intra-ocular pressure; (ii) asthma or a history of asthma.

In addition, in labour induction, cephalopelvic relationships should be carefully evaluated before use of Prostin E2. During use, uterine activity, foetal status and the progression of cervical dilatation should be carefully monitored to detect possible evidence of undesired responses, e.g. hypertonus, sustained uterine contractions or foetal distress. In cases where there is a known history of hypertonic uterine contractility or tetanic uterine contractions, it is recommended that uterine activity and the state of the foetus be continuously monitored throughout labour. The possibility of uterine rupture should be borne in mind where high-tone myometrial contractions are sustained.

Animal studies lasting several weeks at high doses have shown that prostaglandins of the E and F series can induce proliferation of bone. Such effects have also been noted in newborn infants who received prostaglandin E_1 during prolonged treatment. There is no evidence that short-term administration of Prostin E2 can cause similar bone effects.

Side-effects: Clinical studies have not revealed any life-threatening adverse reactions. The incidence of side-effects is directly dose-related.

Nausea, vomiting and diarrhoea have been reported as commonly encountered at dose levels required to induce therapeutic termination of pregnancy by the intravenous route; however, these side-effects are markedly less frequent with doses used by either the extra-amniotic route for therapeutic termination of pregnancy, or intravenously for induction of labour. Transient vasovagal symptoms, including flushing, shivering, headache and dizziness, have been recorded. On intravenous use of Prostin E2 local tissue irritation and erythema have occurred.

No evidence of thrombophlebitis has been recorded and local tissue erythema at the infusion site has disappeared within two to five hours after infusion. A temporary pyrexia and elevated WBC are not unusual, but both have reverted after termination of infusion. In extra-amniotic therapy the possibility of local infection must be considered and appropriate therapy initiated if necessary.

Overdosage: Treatment of overdosage must be, at this time, symptomatic, as clinical studies with prostaglandin antagonists have not progressed to the point where recommendations may be made. However, the following guidelines are recommended.

If evidence of excessive uterine activity or side-effects appear, the rate of infusion should be decreased or discontinued.

In cases of massive overdosage resulting in extreme uterine hypertonus appropriate obstetric procedures are indicated.

Pharmaceutical precautions Prostin E2 Sterile Solutions (in ethanol) must be refrigerated at 4°C. They should be diluted before use only with the diluents stated. Diluted solutions should be used within 24 hours (48 hours for extra-amniotic).

Legal category POM.

Package quantities
1. Pack containing 1 × 0.75 ml ampoule of Prostin E2 Sterile Solution 1 mg/ml (IV induction).
2. Pack containing 1 × 0.5 ml ampoule of Prostin E2 Sterile Solution 10 mg/ml (IV termination).

3. Pack containing 1 × 0.5 ml ampoule of Prostin E2 Sterile Solution 10 mg/ml plus 50 ml diluent (EA termination).

Further information Oral Prostin E2 Tablets and Prostin E2 Vaginal Tablets are also available for the induction of labour.

Product licence numbers

0.75 ml ampoule (1 mg/ml i.v.)	0032/0020
0.5 ml ampoule (10 mg/ml i.v.)	0032/0021
0.5 ml ampoule (10 mg/ml e.a.)	0032/0026

PROSTIN E2* TABLETS

Presentation Prostin E2 tablets are presented as white, roughly rectangular tablets embossed on one side to resemble the letter 'U' and on the other side '76'. Each tablet contains 0.5 mg dinoprostone.

Uses Oxytocic agent. Prostin E2 tablets are indicated for the induction of labour when there are no foetal or maternal contra-indications.

Dosage and administration The dosage of Prostin E2 must be adapted to the patient's response and should always be maintained at the lowest level which will produce satisfactory uterine response. All doses should be taken with a small glass of water.

An initial dose of 0.5 mg (1 tablet) should be given. Thereafter, doses should be given hourly. The usual dose will be 0.5 mg (1 tablet), but if uterine activity is inadequate, 1 mg (2 tablets) may be given hourly until such time as adequate uterine activity is established. Thereafter it may be possible to reduce the dosage to 0.5 mg (1 tablet) hourly. It is recommended that a total single dose of 1.5 mg (3 tablets) not be exceeded.

Continuous administration of the drug for more than two days is not recommended. (See Precautions.)

Contra-indications, warnings, etc
Contra-indications: There are no absolute contra-indications to the use of Prostin E2. However, its use is not recommended in the following circumstances:

1. Where the patient is sensitive to prostaglandins.
2. For patients in whom oxytocic drugs are generally contra-indicated or where prolonged contractions of the uterus are considered inappropriate, such as:

Cases with a history of Caesarean section or major uterine surgery;
Cases in which major degrees of cephalopelvic disproportion may be present;
Cases in which there is clinical suspicion or definite evidence of pre-existing foetal distress;
Cases in which there is a history of difficult labour and/or traumatic delivery;
Grand multiparae with six or more previous term pregnancies.
3. Cases with a history of pelvic inflammatory disease.

Warnings: Since it has been found that prostaglandins may potentiate the effect of oxytocin, it is recommended that these drugs should not be used together, and, if used in sequence, that the patient's uterine activity should be carefully monitored.

The product is available only to hospitals, and clinics with specialised obstetric units and should only be used where 24-hour resident medical cover is provided.

Precautions: Caution should be exercised in the administration of Prostin E2 tablets for the induction of labour

in patients with: (i) glaucoma or raised intra-ocular pressure; (ii) asthma or a history of asthma. In addition, in labour induction, cephalopelvic relationships should be carefully evaluated before use of Prostin E2. During use, uterine activity, foetal status, and the progression of cervical dilatation should be carefully monitored to detect possible evidence of undesired responses, e.g. hypertonus, sustained uterine contractions, or foetal distress. In cases where there is a known history of hypertonic uterine contractility or tetanic uterine contractions, it is recommended that uterine activity and the state of the foetus should be continuously monitored throughout labour. The possibility of uterine rupture should be borne in mind where high-tone myometrial contractions are sustained.

Animal studies lasting several weeks at high doses have shown that prostaglandins of the E and F series can induce proliferation of bone. Such effects have also been noted in newborn infants who received prostaglandin E_1 during prolonged treatment. There is no evidence that short-term administration of Prostin E2 can cause similar bone effects.

Side-effects: Clinical studies have not revealed any life-threatening adverse reactions. The incidence of side-effects is directly dose-related. Nausea, vomiting and diarrhoea have been noted following oral administration of Prostin E2, but have seldom been severe enough to necessitate discontinuation of medication.

Overdosage: Uterine hypertonus or unduly severe uterine contractions have rarely been encountered, but might be anticipated to result from overdosage. In the rare instance where temporary discontinuation of therapy is not effective in reversing foetal distress or uterine hypertonus then prompt delivery is indicated. Treatment of overdosage must be, at this time, symptomatic, since clinical studies with prostaglandin antagonists have not progressed to the point where recommendations may be made. It is currently believed that vomiting produced by overdosage may act as a self-limiting factor in protecting the patient.

Pharmaceutical precautions Prostin E2 tablets have a shelf-life of two years when stored at 4°C. Store in a refrigerator. The tablets should be used within three months of opening the bottle.

Legal category POM.

Package quantities Prostin E2 tablets are packed in bottles of 10.

Further information Unlike other oxytocics, Prostin E2 exhibits the capacity of the prostaglandins to influence uterine activity at any stage of gestation. Other Prostin E2 dose forms are available for a number of indications, including induction of labour.

Product licence number 0032/0040

PROSTIN E2* VAGINAL GEL

Presentation Translucent thixotropic gel containing 1 or 2 mg dinoprostone per 3 g (2.5 ml).

Uses Oxytocic. Prostin E2 Vaginal Gel is indicated for the induction of labour, especially in patients with favourable induction features, when there are no foetal or maternal contra-indications.

Dosage and administration One milligram to be administered vaginally. If labour is not established a second dose of one or two milligrams may be administered after 6 hours as follows:

One milligram should be used where uterine activity is insufficient for satisfactory progress of labour.

Two milligrams may be used where response to the initial dose has been minimal.

Maximum dose 3 mg (see 'Precautions').

The gel should be inserted high into the posterior fornix avoiding administration into the cervical canal. The patient should be instructed to remain supine for at least 30 minutes.

Contra-indications, warnings, etc

Contra-indications: There are no absolute contra-indications to the use of Prostin E2. However, its use is not recommended in the following circumstances:

1. For patients in whom oxytocic drugs are generally contra-indicated or where prolonged contractions of the uterus are considered inappropriate such as:

Cases with a history of Caesarean section or major uterine surgery;

Cases in which major degrees of cephalopelvic disproportion may be present;

Cases in which there is clinical suspicion or definite evidence of pre-existing foetal distress;

Cases in which there is a history of difficult labour and/or traumatic delivery;

Grand multiparae with six or more previous term pregnancies.

2. Patients with ruptured membranes.

3. Patients with a known sensitivity to prostaglandins.

Warnings: Since it has been found that prostaglandins may potentiate the effect of oxytocin, it is recommended that, if these drugs are used together or in sequence, the patient's uterine activity should be carefully monitored. The product is available only to hospitals and clinics with specialised obstetric units.

Precautions: Prostin E2 Vaginal Gel and Prostin E2 Vaginal Tablets are not bioequivalent.

Caution should be exercised in the administration of Prostin E2 Vaginal Gel for the induction of labour in patients with:

(i) glaucoma or raised intra-ocular pressure;

(ii) asthma or history of asthma.

In addition, in labour induction, cephalopelvic relationships should be carefully evaluated before use of Prostin E2. During use, uterine activity, foetal status and the progression of cervical dilatation should be carefully monitored to detect possible evidence of undesired responses, e.g. hypertonus, sustained uterine contractions, or foetal distress. In cases where there is a known history of hypertonic uterine contractility or tetanic uterine contractions, it is recommended that uterine activity and the state of the foetus should be continuously monitored throughout labour. The possibility of uterine rupture should be borne in mind where high-tone myometrial contractions are sustained. Animal studies lasting several weeks at high doses have shown that prostaglandins of the E and F series can induce proliferation of bone. Such effects have also been noted in newborn infants who have received prostaglandin E1 during prolonged treatment. There is no evidence that short-term administration of Prostin E2 Vaginal Gel can cause similar bone effects.

Side-effects: Very occasional gastrointestinal disturbance. Uterine hypertonus or unduly severe uterine contractions have rarely been encountered.

Overdosage: Treatment of overdosage must be, at this time, symptomatic since clinical studies with prostaglandin antagonists have not progressed to the point where recommendations may be made.

Pharmaceutical precautions Store in a refrigerator at 2–8°C. The contents of one syringe to be used for one patient. Discard after use.

Legal category POM.

Package quantities Prostin E2 Vaginal Gel is available in single packs of 1 mg or 2 mg.

Further information Unlike other oxytocics, Prostin E2 exhibits the capacity of the prostaglandins to influence uterine activity at any stage of gestation. Other Prostin E2 dosage forms are available for induction of labour (oral, vaginal and i.v. routes), foetal death in utero (i.v. route), therapeutic termination of pregnancy (i.v. and extra-amniotic routes), missed abortion and hydatidiform mole (i.v. route).

Product licence numbers
1 g   0032/0123
2 g   0032/0124

PROSTIN E2* VAGINAL TABLETS

Presentation Prostin E2 Vaginal Tablets are presented as white biconvex oblong tablets with radiused corners debossed with 'UPJOHN' and '715' on one side. Each tablet contains 3 mg dinoprostone.

Uses Oxytocic. Prostin E2 Vaginal Tablets are indicated for the induction of labour, especially in patients with favourable induction features, when there are no foetal or maternal contra-indications.

Dosage and administration One tablet (3 mg) to be inserted high into the posterior fornix. A second tablet may be inserted after six to eight hours if labour is not established. Maximum dose 6 mg.

Contra-indications, warnings, etc

Contra-indications: There are no absolute contra-indications to the use of Prostin E2. However, its use is not recommended in the following circumstances:

1. For patients in whom oxytocic drugs are generally contra-indicated or where prolonged contractions of the uterus are considered inappropriate such as:

Cases with a history of Caesarian section or major uterine surgery;

Cases in which major degrees of cephalopelvic disproportion may be present;

Cases in which there is clinical suspicion or definite evidence of pre-existing foetal distress;

Cases in which there is a history of difficult labour and/or traumatic delivery;

Grand multiparae with six or more previous term pregnancies.

2. Patients with ruptured membranes.

3. Patients with known hypersensitivity to prostaglandin.

Warning: Since it has been found that prostaglandins may potentiate the effect of oxytocin, it is recommended that, if these drugs are used together or in sequence, the patient's uterine activity should be carefully monitored.

The product is available only to hospitals and clinics with specialised obstetric units.

Precautions: Caution should be exercised in the administration of Prostin E2 Vaginal Tablets for the induction of labour in patients with:

    (i) glaucoma or raised intra-ocular pressure;
    (ii) asthma or a history of asthma.

In addition, in labour induction, cephalopelvic relationships should be carefully evaluated before use of Prostin E2. During use, uterine activity, foetal status, and the progression of cervical dilatation should be carefully monitored to detect possible evidence of undesired responses, e.g. hypertonus, sustained uterine contractions, or foetal distress. In cases where there is a known history of hypertonic uterine contractility or tetanic uterine contractions, it is recommended that uterine activity and the state of the foetus should be continuously monitored throughout labour. The possibility of uterine rupture should be borne in mind where high-tone myometrial contractions are sustained. Animal studies lasting several weeks at high doses have shown that prostaglandins of the E and F series can induce proliferation of bone. Such effects have also been noted in newborn infants who have received prostaglandin E_1 during prolonged treatment. There is no evidence that short-term administration of Prostin E2 Vaginal Tablets can cause similar bone effects.

Side Effects: Very occasional nausea and vomiting. Uterine hypertonus or unduly severe uterine contractions have rarely been encountered.

Overdosage: Treatment of overdosage must be, at this time, symptomatic, since clinical studies with prostaglandin antagonists have not progressed to the point where recommendations may be made.

Pharmaceutical precautions Prostin E2 Vaginal Tablets have a shelf-life of 24 months when stored in a refrigerator at 4°C. The tablets should be used within 1 month of opening the bottle.

Legal category POM.

Package quantities Prostin E2 Vaginal Tablets are packed in bottles of 4.

Further information Tablet disintegration and release of prostaglandin is moisture dependent. In a small proportion of women tablet remains may be seen in the vagina a few hours after insertion and may contain some prostaglandin. However this is rarely of clinical significance.

Unlike other oxytocics, Prostin E2 exhibits the capacity of the prostaglandins to influence uterine activity at any stage of gestation.

Other Prostin E2 dose forms are available for a number of indications, including induction of labour.

Product licence number 0032/0074

PROSTIN F2 alpha*
STERILE SOLUTIONS

Presentation Colourless, sterile aqueous solution containing 5 mg per ml dinoprost (Prostaglandin F_2 alpha). Dinoprost is presented as the tromethamine (THAM) salt.

1. Prostin F2 alpha Sterile Solution 5 mg/ml, 1.5 ml ampoule (intravenous).
2. Prostin F2 alpha Sterile Solution 5 mg/ml, 4 ml and 8 ml ampoules (intra-amniotic).
3. Prostin F2 alpha Sterile Solution 5 mg/ml, 5 ml ampoule (intravenous).

Uses Oxytocic agent. Prostin F2 alpha is indicated for induction of labour, foetal death in utero, therapeutic termination of pregnancy, missed abortion and hydatidiform mole.

Dosage and administration Prostin F2 alpha may be administered by the intravenous and intra-amniotic routes as follows:

1. Intravenous: for induction of labour and foetal death in utero.
2. Intra-amniotic: for therapeutic termination of pregnancy during the second trimester.
3. Intravenous: for therapeutic termination of pregnancy, missed abortion and hydatidiform mole.

For each route of administration except the intra-amniotic route, the ampoule contents must be diluted before use and full instructions on method of dilution and dosage are given on the package insert which should be consulted prior to initiation of therapy. The dose of Prostin F2 alpha used normally depends not only upon the indication but also on patient response. Increase in dosage above that recommended is possible but may produce excessive uterine activity and be governed by the unacceptable appearance of dose-related side-effects, such as nausea and vomiting. Continuous administration of the drug for more than two days is not recommended. (See Precautions.)

The following is a guide to dosage:

1. *Prostin F2 alpha 5 mg/ml (1.5 ml ampoule) intravenous for induction of labour and foetal death in utero:* 15 mcg/ml solution is infused at 2.5 mcg/minute for at least 30 minutes and then maintained or increased. Cases of foetal death in utero may require higher doses than those given above. An initial rate of 5 mcg/minute may be used with step-wise increases, at intervals of not less than one hour.

2. *Prostin F2 alpha 5 mg/ml (4 and 8 ml ampoules) intra-amniotic for therapeutic termination of pregnancy:* 8 ml of undiluted solution (40 mg initial dose) should be withdrawn from the ampoule(s) and should be injected slowly into the amniotic sac.

3. *Prostin F2 alpha 5 mg/ml (5 ml ampoule) intravenous for therapeutic termination of pregnancy, missed abortion and hydatidiform mole:* 50 mcg/ml solution is infused at 25 mcg/minute for at least 30 minutes and then maintained or increased to 50 mcg/minute. This rate should be maintained for at least four hours before increasing further.

Contra-indications, warnings, etc
Contra-indications: There are no absolute contra-indications to the use of Prostin F2 alpha. However, its use is not recommended in the following circumstances:

1. Where the patient is sensitive to prostaglandins.
2. For patients in whom oxytocic drugs are generally contra-indicated or where prolonged contractions of the uterus are considered inappropriate, such as: cases with a history of Caesarean section or major uterine surgery; cases in which major degrees of cephalopelvic disproportion may be present; cases in which foetal malpresentation is present; cases in which there is clinical suspicion or definite evidence of pre-existing foetal distress; cases in which there is a history of difficult labour and/or traumatic delivery; grand multiparae with six or more previous term pregnancies; cases with a history of pelvic inflammatory disease.
3. In therapeutic termination of pregnancy where

known pelvic infection exists, unless adequate prior treatment has been instituted.

4. The intra-amniotic route should not be employed in patients with a history of Caesarean section or prior major uterine surgery.

Warnings: There has been some evidence in animals of a low order of teratogenic activity, therefore, if abortion does not occur or is suspected to be incomplete as a result of prostaglandin therapy, the appropriate treatment for complete evacuation of the pregnant uterus should be instituted in all instances. Since it has been found that prostaglandins may potentiate the effect of oxytocin, it is recommended that these drugs should not be used together, and if used in sequence, that the patient's uterine activity should be carefully monitored.

The products are available only to hospitals and clinics with specialised obstetric units and should only be used where 24-hour resident medical cover is provided.

Precautions: Caution should be exercised in the administration of Prostin F2 alpha for induction of labour or therapeutic termination of pregnancy in patients with: (i) glaucoma or raised intra-ocular pressure; (ii) asthma or history of asthma. In addition, in labour induction, cephalopelvic relationships should be carefully evaluated before use of Prostin F2 alpha. During infusion, uterine activity, foetal status and the progression of cervical dilatation should be carefully monitored to detect possible evidence of undesired response, e.g. hypertonus, sustained uterine contractions or foetal distress. In cases where there is a known history of hypertonic uterine contractility or tetanic uterine contractions, it is recommended that uterine activity and the state of the foetus be continuously monitored throughout labour. The possibility of uterine rupture should be borne in mind where high-tone myometrial contractions are sustained.

Very rare cases of sudden and sometimes fatal collapse, of unknown aetiology, have been reported with intra-amniotic administration of Prostin F2 alpha. Animal studies lasting several weeks at high doses have shown that prostaglandins of the E and F series can induce proliferation of bone. Such effects have also been noted in newborn infants who received prostaglandin E_1 during prolonged treatment. There is no evidence that short-term administration of Prostin F2 alpha can cause similar bone effects.

Side-effects: Clinical studies have not revealed any life threatening adverse reactions. The incidence of side-effects is directly dose-related. Nausea, vomiting and diarrhoea have been reported as commonly encountered at dose levels required to induce therapeutic termination of pregnancy by the intravenous route; however, these side-effects are markedly less frequent with doses used by either the intra-uterine route for termination of pregnancy or intravenously for the induction of labour. Transient vasovagal symptoms including flushing, shivering, headache and dizziness have been recorded. On intravenous use of Prostin F2 alpha local tissue irritation and erythema have occurred. No evidence of thrombophlebitis has been recorded and erythema has disappeared within two to five hours after infusion. A temporary pyrexia and elevated WBC are not unusual, but both generally revert to normal shortly after termination of infusion. In intra-amniotic therapy the possibility of local infection must be considered and appropriate therapy initiated if necessary.

Overdosage: Treatment of overdosage must be, at this time, symptomatic, as clinical studies with prostaglandin antagonists have not progressed to the point where recommendations may be made. If evidence of excessive uterine activity or side-effects appears, the rate of infusion should be decreased or discontinued. In cases of massive overdosage resulting in extreme uterine hypertonus, appropriate obstetric procedures are indicated.

Pharmaceutical precautions Prostin F2 alpha has a shelf-life of 36 months at room temperature. Prostin F2 alpha should be mixed only with diluents as stated. Diluted solutions should be used within 24 hours.

Legal category POM.

Package quantities Prostin F2 alpha is supplied as an aqueous solution of 5 mg/ml of dinoprost presented as the THAM salt:

1. Pack containing a 1.5 ml ampoule (intravenous induction of labour and foetal death in utero).
2. Pack containing a 4 ml or 8 ml ampoule (intra-amniotic termination of pregnancy).
3. Pack containing a 5 ml ampoule (intravenous termination of pregnancy, missed abortion and hydatidiform mole).

Further information The exact mode of action of the prostaglandins is not completely understood. Prostin F2 alpha has been shown to have a local action on isolated uterine musculature and clinically its main action is oxytocic. Unlike other oxytocics, prostaglandins do not cause water retention. Prostin F2 alpha exhibits the capacity of the prostaglandins to influence uterine activity at any stage of gestation.

Product licence numbers

1.5 ml ampoule	0032/0037
4 and 8 ml ampoules	0032/0051 (intra-amniotic)
5 ml ampoule	0032/0038

PROSTIN VR* STERILE SOLUTION ▼

Presentation Ampoule containing 0.5 mg alprostadil in 1 ml dehydrated ethanol.

Uses Prostin VR is indicated to temporarily maintain the patency of the ductus arteriosus until corrective or palliative surgery can be performed in infants who have congenital defects and who depend upon the patent ductus for survival. Such congenital heart defects include pulmonary atresia, pulmonary stenosis, tricuspid atresia, tetralogy of Fallot, interruption of the aortic arch, coarctation of the aorta, aortic stenosis, aortic atresia, mitral atresia, or transposition of the great vessels with or without other defects.

Dosage and administration For administration by intravenous drip or constant-rate infusion pump.

In infants with lesions restricting pulmonary blood flow (blood is flowing through the ductus arteriosus from the aorta to the pulmonary artery), Prostin VR may be administered by continuous infusion through an umbilical artery catheter placed at or just above the junction of the descending aorta and the ductus arteriosus, or intravenously. Adverse effects have occurred with both routes of administration, but the types of reactions are different. A higher incidence of flushing has been associated with intra-arterial than with intravenous administration.

Infusion should begin with 0.1 micrograms alprostadil per kilogram of body weight per minute. If the aorta can not be catheterised via the umbilical artery, the infusion may be given through a catheter advanced from the periphery into a larger vein.

In infants with lesions restricting systemic blood flow (blood is flowing through the ductus arteriosus from the pulmonary artery to the aorta), Prostin VR may be administered by continuous infusion through an umbilical artery catheter passed across the ductus arteriosus and into the pulmonary artery proximal to the ductus arteriosus, or intravenously. Infusion should begin with 0.1 micrograms alprostadil per kilogram of body weight per minute. If the pulmonary artery cannot be catheterised via the umbilical artery, the infusion may be given through a catheter advanced from the periphery into a large vein.

When an effect is achieved, decrease the infusion to the lowest possible dose while maintaining the desired effects.

Dilution Instructions. To prepare infusion solutions, dilute 1 ml of Prostin VR Sterile Solution with sterile 0.9% Sodium Chloride Intravenous Infusion or sterile 5% Dextrose Intravenous Infusion. Dilute to volumes appropriate for the delivery system available. Prepare fresh infusion solutions every 24 hours. Discard any solution more than 24 hours old.

Examples: Dissolve 1 ml Prostin VR Sterile Solution (500 micrograms alprostadil) in 25 to 100 ml sterile 0.9% Sodium Chloride Intravenous Infusion or sterile 5% Dextrose Intravenous Infusion to provide a solution containing 500 micrograms alprostadil. The infusion rate can be calculated as follows:

Infusion rate (ml/hr) =

$$\frac{\text{Vol. containing 500 mcg alprostadil} \times \text{body weight (kg)}}{83.3}$$

With an infusion pump limited to discrete infusion rates, infuse 2 or 4 ml per hour. Calculate the volume of 0.9% saline or 5% dextrose to add to 1 ml Prostin VR Sterile Solution to deliver 0.1 micrograms alprostadil per kilogram of body weight per minute at the chosen pump rate as follows:

Volume of saline or dextrose needed (ml) =

$$\frac{\text{Pump rate (ml/hour)} \times 83.3}{\text{body weight (kg)}} - 1$$

The infusion solution may be mixed conveniently in a graduated mixing chamber inserted between the IV bottle and the pump.

Change the dosage from 0.1 micrograms per kilogram of body weight per minute to 0.05 micrograms per kilogram of body weight per minute by reducing the pump rate to one-half the original rate.

PARTICULAR CARE SHOULD BE TAKEN IN CALCULATING AND PREPARING DILUTIONS OF PROSTIN VR

Contra-indications, warnings, etc
Contra-indications: None.

Warnings: Only the recommended Prostin VR dosages should be administered and only by medically trained personnel in hospitals or other facilities with immediately available intensive care.

Approximately 10–12% of neonates with congenital heart defects treated with Prostin VR Sterile Solution (alprostadil) experienced apnoea. Apnoea is most often seen in neonates weighing less than 2 kg at birth and usually appears during the first hour of drug infusion.

Therefore, Prostin VR Sterile Solution should be used where ventilatory assistance is immediately available.

Precautions: Prostin VR Sterile Solution (alprostadil) should be infused for the shortest time and at the lowest dose which will produce the desired effects. The risk of long-term infusion of Prostin VR should be weighed against the possible benefits that critically ill infants may derive from its administration.

Cortical proliferation of the long bones has followed long-term infusions of alprostadil in infants and dogs. The proliferation in infants regressed after withdrawal of the drug.

Use Prostin VR Sterile Solution (alprostadil) cautiously in neonates with histories of bleeding tendencies.

Care should be taken to avoid the use of Prostin VR Sterile Solution in neonates with respiratory distress syndrome (hyaline membrane disease), which sometimes can be confused with cyanotic heart disease. If full diagnostic facilities are not immediately available, cyanosis (pO_2 less than 40 mmHg) and restricted pulmonary blood flow apparent on an X-ray are good indicators of congenital heart defects.

In all infants, commencing when infusion starts, intermittently monitor arterial pressure by umbilical artery catheter, auscultation, or with a Doppler transducer. Should arterial pressure fall significantly, decrease the rate of infusion immediately.

A weakening of the wall of the ductus arteriosus and pulmonary artery has been reported, particularly during prolonged administration.

Side-effects and Adverse reactions: The most frequent adverse reactions observed with Prostin VR are related to its known pharmacological effects. These include flushing, bradycardia, hypotension, tachycardia, cardiac arrest, oedema, apnoea, diarrhoea, fever, convulsions, disseminated intravascular coagulation, and hypokalaemia.

Overdosage: The effects of Prostin VR abate quickly when infusion is stopped.

Pharmaceutical precautions Prostin VR must be stored in a refrigerator. See dilution instructions for shelf-life of diluted solutions.

Diluted solutions of Prostin VR should be infused from glass or hard plastic containers; use with soft plastic such as PVC has not been established.

Legal category POM.

Package quantities Pack containing 5 × 1 ml ampoules Prostin VR Sterile Solution.

Further information Alprostadil (formerly known as prostaglandin E1) dilates the ductus arteriosus in neonates, probably by relaxing smooth muscle, thereby helping to maintain patency. It also relaxes smooth muscle in other parts of the vascular system, and can thus lower blood pressure.

Product licence number 0032/0083

PROVERA*

Presentation White compressed tablets scored on one face, embossed 286 on either side of score, and marked U on other face, containing 5 mg medroxyprogesterone acetate.

Uses Progestogen.

Indicated for secondary amenorrhoea and for functional uterine bleeding.

Dosage and administration Oral.

Secondary Amenorrhoea: 2.5–10 mg daily for 5–10 days beginning on the assumed or calculated sixteenth to twenty-first day of the cycle. Repeat treatment for three consecutive cycles. In amenorrhoea associated with a poorly developed proliferative endometrium, conventional oestrogen therapy may be employed in conjunction with medroxyprogesterone acetate in doses of 5–10 mg for 10 days.

Functional uterine bleeding: 2.5–10 mg daily for 5–10 days commencing on the assumed or calculated sixteenth to twenty-first day of the cycle. Treatment should be given for two consecutive cycles. When bleeding occurs from a poorly developed proliferative endometrium, conventional oestrogen therapy may be employed in conjunction with medroxyprogesterone acetate, in doses of 5–10 mg for 10 days.

Contra-indications, warnings, etc

Contra-indications: Use in patients with a known sensitivity to medroxyprogesterone acetate. Use in patients with a history of, or existing thromboembolic disorders, or, at the above dosage, with breast or genital cancer (known or suspected to be oestrogen-dependent). Use in patients with impaired liver function, or with active liver disease; in patients with undiagnosed, irregular vaginal bleeding, or with undiagnosed breast pathology. Use during pregnancy.

Precautions: A negative pregnancy test should be demonstrated before starting therapy for secondary amenorrhoea. Whether administered alone or in conjunction with oestrogens, Provera should not be employed in patients with abnormal uterine bleeding until a definite diagnosis has been established and the possibility of genital malignancy eliminated.

Side-effects: No significant untoward effects or intolerance have been reported.

Overdosage: In animals Provera has been shown to be capable of exerting an adreno-corticoid effect but this has not been reported in the human, following usual dosages. The oral administration of Provera at a rate of 100 mg per day has been shown to have no effect on adrenal function.

Pharmaceutical precautions None.

Legal category POM.

Package quantities Bottles of 100.

Further information Provera is a highly active progestational agent. During its years of clinical use no significant toxicity has been recorded and it appears to be free of androgenic and oestrogenic effects.

Product licence number 0032/5035

PROVERA* TABLETS 100 mg and 200 mg

Presentation *100 mg:* White, circular, flat bevelled tablets marked 'U 467' on one side and scored on the reverse, containing 100 mg medroxyprogesterone acetate.

200 mg: White, circular, biconvex tablets marked 'U 320' on one side and scored on the reverse, containing 200 mg medroxyprogesterone acetate.

Uses Progestogen.

Indicated for the treatment of certain hormone dependent neoplasms, such as endometrial carcinoma, renal cell carcinoma and carcinoma of breast in postmenopausal women.

Dosage and administration Oral.

For endometrial and renal cell carcinoma: 200–400 mg daily.

For breast carcinoma: 400–800 mg per day. Doses of 1000 mg daily have been given although the incidence of minor side effects, such as indigestion and weight gain, increase with the increase in dose.

Response to hormonal therapy may not be evident until after at least 8–10 weeks of therapy.

Elderly patients: This product has been used primarily in the older age group for the treatment of malignancies. We have no evidence to suggest that the older group is any less prepared to handle the drug metabolically than is the younger aged patient. Therefore, the same dosage, contra-indications and precautions would apply to either age group.

Contra-indications, warnings, etc

Contra-indications: Provera is contraindicated in thrombophlebitis or a history of pulmonary embolism and liver dysfunction or disease.

Warnings: In the treatment of carcinoma of the breast, occasional cases of hypercalcaemia have been reported. Any patient who develops an acute impairment of vision, proptosis, diplopia or migraine headache should be carefully evaluated ophthalmologically to exclude the presence of papilloedema or retinal vascular lesions before continuing medication.

Precautions: Animal studies show that Provera possesses adrenocorticoid activity. This has also been reported in man, therefore, patients receiving large doses continuously and for long periods should be observed closely. The administration of large doses to pregnant women has resulted in the observation of some instances of female foetal masculinisation. Because progestogens may cause some degree of fluid retention, conditions which might be influenced by this factor, such as epilepsy, migraine, asthma, cardiac or renal dysfunction, require careful observation.

Patients who have a history of mental depression should be carefully observed and the drug discontinued if the depression recurs to a serious degree. A decrease in glucose tolerance has been observed in some patients on progestogens. The mechanism of this decrease is obscure. For this reason, diabetic patients should be carefully observed while receiving progestogen therapy.

This product should be used under the supervision of a specialist and the patients kept under regular surveillance.

Side-effects: Reactions occasionally noted with large doses are:

Breast: tenderness or galactorrhoea.

Psychic: nervousness, insomnia, somnolence, fatigue, dizziness.

Skin and Mucous Membranes: sensitivity reactions ranging from pruritus, urticaria, angioneurotic oedema, to generalised rash and anaphylaxis have occasionally been reported. Acne, alopecia or hirsutism have been reported in a few cases.

Gastro-intestinal: nausea and indigestion have been noted particularly with the higher doses.

Miscellaneous: hyperpyrexia, weight gain and moon facies.

Overdosage: No action required other than cessation of therapy.

Pharmaceutical precautions Keep container tightly closed. Store at controlled room temperature 15–30°C.

Legal category POM.

Package quantities Bottles of 100 × 100 mg and 60 × 200 mg.

Further information The results of certain laboratory tests may be affected by the use of Provera; these include gonadotrophin levels, plasma progesterone levels, urinary pregnanediol levels, plasma testosterone levels (in the male), plasma oestrogen levels (in the female), plasma cortisol levels, glucose tolerance and metyrapone tests.

Product licence numbers
100 mg tablet   0032/0111
200 mg tablet   0032/0112

SOLU-CORTEF*

Presentation White, freeze-dried powder of hydrocortisone sodium succinate, equivalent to 100 mg hydrocortisone, in rubber-capped vials.

Uses Anti-inflammatory agent.

Indicated for acute adrenocortical insufficiency, bilateral adrenalectomy, severe shock, acute hypersensitivity reactions, overwhelming infections with severe toxicity, systemic lupus erythematosus in relapse, aspiration pneumonitis and other conditions requiring the metabolic and anti-inflammatory actions of hydrocortisone.

Dosage and administration Intravenous injection, intravenous infusion or intramuscular injection.

Preparation of solutions for intravenous or intramuscular use:

For intravenous and intramuscular injection add 2 ml sterile water for injection from accompanying ampoule to the vial, shake and withdraw for use.

For intravenous infusion, prepare a primary solution as above and then add to 100–1,000 ml (not less than 100 ml) of 5% dextrose in water, or isotonic saline or 5% dextrose in isotonic saline solution, if patient is not on sodium restriction.

When reconstituted as directed, the pH of solution will range from 7.0 to 8.0.

Dosage usually ranges from 100 mg to 500 mg, depending on the severity of the condition, and should be administered by intravenous injection over a period of one to several minutes.

In infants and children dose may be reduced but should not be less than 25 mg daily.

In critically ill patients, particularly in shock, it has been recommended that a dose of 1 g administered intravenously over several minutes be given, followed by 500 mg every four to eight hours for three to five days if necessary.

Elderly patients: Solu-Cortef is primarily used in acute short-term conditions. There is no information to suggest that a change in dosage is warranted in the elderly. See Contra-indications, Warnings and Precautions sections for other factors which should be taken into account.

Contra-indications, warnings, etc

Contra-indications: The usual contra-indications to the use of systemic corticosteroids apply (excepting in the case of treatment of bilateral adrenalectomy) and include latent, healed and active tuberculosis, herpes simplex, chronic nephritis, acute psychosis, Cushing's syndrome, peptic ulcer and predisposition to thrombophlebitis.

Warnings: Due to its inhibitory effect on fibroplasia hydrocortisone may mask signs of infection and enhance dissemination of the infecting organism.

Precautions: The existence of congestive heart failure, hypertension, diabetes, osteoporosis, or chronic psychotic reactions necessitate caution in the administration of Solu-Cortef.

Injection into the deltoid muscle should be avoided because of a high incidence of subcutaneous atrophy.

Side-effects: Since Solu-Cortef is normally employed on a short-term basis it is unlikely that side-effects will occur; however, the possibility of side-effects attributable to corticosteroid therapy should be recognised.

Overdosage: No known antidote. Following overdosage the possibility of adrenal suppression should be guarded against by gradual diminution of dose levels over a period of time. In such event the patient may require to be supported during any further traumatic episode.

Pharmaceutical precautions Store at room temperature. No diluents, other than referred to, are recommended.

Legal category POM.

Package quantities Solu-Cortef is supplied as: 100 mg vial with an ampoule containing 2 ml of water for injection with 0.9% w/v benzyl alcohol.

Further information In the treatment of shock, massive, pharmacological, doses of corticosteroid of the order of equivalents of 1 g hydrocortisone are accepted therapy. It is considered that the corticosteroid assists in resensitising the capillary bed, thus helping to prevent blood stagnation and the onset of irreversible shock.

Product licence number
100 mg vial   0032/5019

SOLU-MEDRONE*

Presentation Mix-O-Vials* of 40 mg and 125 mg methylprednisolone (as the sodium succinate). Each Mix-O-Vial consists of adjoining compartments of lyophilised powder and solvent. Also 500 mg, 1 g and 2 g vials of methylprednisolone (as the sodium succinate).

Uses Medrone is a potent corticosteroid with an anti-inflammatory activity at least five times that of hydrocortisone. An enhanced separation of glucocorticoid and mineralocorticoid effect results in a reduced incidence of sodium and water retention.

Solu-Medrone is indicated for any condition in which rapid and intense corticosteroid effect is required such as:

1. Hypersensitivity reactions.
2. Severe shock, i.e. haemorrhagic, septic, surgical, traumatic, or cardiogenic.
3. Overwhelming infection with severe toxaemia.
4. Acute adrenal insufficiency.
5. Suppression of graft rejection reactions following transplantation.
6. Cerebral oedema.

7. The treatment of certain emergency situations in advanced cancer patients such as acute dyspnoea due to pulmonary or mediastinal metastases or the obstruction of other hollow viscera.

Dosage and administration Solu-Medrone may be administered intravenously or intramuscularly, the preferred method for emergency use being intravenous injection given over a suitable time interval (see 'Precautions'). For intravenous infusion the initially prepared solution may be diluted with 5% dextrose, isotonic saline or dextrose saline. Dosage should be varied according to the severity of the condition. In general not less than 0.5 mg/kg/day. In the treatment of shock and graft rejection reactions a dose of up to 30 mg/kg may be required for limited periods. For detailed recommendations on dosage see Package Insert.

Elderly patients: Solu-Medrone is primarily used in acute short-term conditions. There is no information to suggest that a change in dosage is warranted in the elderly. See Contra-indications, Warnings and Precautions section for other factors which should be taken into account.

Contra-indications, warnings, etc
Contra-indications: Like all corticosteroids Solu-Medrone is contra-indicated in herpes simplex keratitis, acute psychoses, and latent, healed or active tuberculosis. Relative contra-indications include active or latent peptic ulcer, Cushing's syndrome, diverticulitis, osteoporosis, renal insufficiency, thromboembolic tendencies, diabetes mellitus, hypertension, local or systemic infection including viral, fungal and other exanthematous diseases. Pregnancy is included as a relative contra-indication.

Warnings and precautions: There have been a few reports of cardiovascular collapse associated with the rapid intravenous administration of large doses of Solu-Medrone (greater than 500 mg) in organ transplant recipients. The cause and relation to other medications (e.g. diuretics) are not known at this time, but physicians and surgeons should be alert to this possibility. When administering Solu-Medrone in high doses intravenously, it should be given over a period of 10–20 minutes. It should be remembered that prolonged high-dose corticosteroid therapy can cause serious corticosteroid-induced side-effects, and high dose therapy should, in general, be continued only until the patient's condition has stabilised: usually not beyond 48–72 hours.

Solu-Medrone should not be used for the treatment of cardiogenic shock if the central venous pressure is under 10 cm water.

In the treatment of acute adrenal insufficiency a sodium-retaining corticosteroid, in addition to Solu-Medrone, will be needed.

When used to treat cerebral oedema due to brain trauma, gastro-intestinal bleeding may occur and daily stool guaiac tests may be diagnostically helpful. Prophylactic peptic ulcer therapy (i.e. antacids, etc) should be considered.

Injection into the deltoid muscle should be avoided because of a high incidence of subcutaneous atrophy.

The normal precautions to the use of systemic corticosteroids should be observed.

Reproduction studies in rats and mice at several times the human dose have revealed no evidence of impaired fertility or harm to the foetus. There are, however, no well controlled studies in pregnant women, so Solu-Medrone should only be used in pregnancy if clearly needed.

Because prednisolone is excreted in breast milk, it is reasonable to assume that all corticosteroids are. No specific data are known for methylprednisolone sodium succinate.

Monitoring and resuscitation facilities should be available, particularly when high doses of methylprednisolone sodium succinate are used intravenously.

Convulsions have been reported in patients receiving high dose methylprednisolone sodium succinate and cyclosporin.

The solvent for Solu-Medrone contains benzyl alcohol.

Adverse reactions and side-effects: Under normal circumstances Solu-Medrone therapy would be considered as short-term. However, the possibility of side-effects and adverse reactions common to corticosteroids must be considered, particularly when high-dose therapy is being used.

Overdosage: No known antidote. Following overdosage the possibility of adrenal suppression should be guarded against by gradual diminution of dose levels over a period of time. In such event the patient may require to be supported during any further traumatic episode.

Pharmaceutical precautions The Mix-O-Vial should be protected from freezing. No special requirement for syringes or infusion solution containers. Solutions prepared using sterile water for injection should be used immediately. Those solutions that also incorporate a suitable preservative concentration (e.g., benzyl alcohol 9 mg/ml) should be used within 48 hours.

Legal category POM.

Package quantities In a 40 mg/1 ml, and 125 mg/2 ml Mix-O-Vial.
Vials of 500 mg, 1 g and 2 g.

Further information The following instructions for the use of the Mix-O-Vials should be observed. Remove the protective cap from the Mix-O-Vial. Give a half-turn to the piston and press it down as far as possible to allow the diluent to pass into the lower powder chamber. Shake well until solution is complete. Sterilise the surface of the rubber piston. Hold the vial up at 45° and insert the syringe needle through the centre of the piston to withdraw the required quantity of solution.

Product licence numbers

40 mg/1 ml	0032/0033
125 mg/2 ml	0032/0034
500 mg/8 ml	0032/0035
1 g/16 ml	0032/0039
2 g/32 ml	0032/0073

TOLANASE*

Presentation White, scored, convex tablets marked 'UPJOHN 70' on the opposite side, containing 100 mg tolazamide.
White, scored, convex tablet marked 'UPJOHN 114' on other side, containing 250 mg tolazamide.

Uses Sulphonylurea.
Indicated in maturity-onset diabetes of mild to moderate severity.

Dosage and administration Oral.
100–250 mg daily, or up to 1 g daily in divided doses if necessary. It is doubtful whether doses greater than 1 g daily will result in improved control. (For dose

conversion from other oral hypoglycaemic agents see literature.)

Depending on the results of urinary glucose tests and blood sugar determinations the daily dose should be either raised or lowered by amounts of one tablet (100 mg or 250 mg) at weekly intervals.

Elderly patients: These agents have had their primary use in the older aged group. The contra-indications and precautions that appear in the data sheet should be carefully observed for all aged patients and any patient with significantly compromised liver or renal function should be very carefully followed if it is the election of the physician to use oral agents.

Contra-indications, warnings, etc

Contra-indications: Tolanase is not indicated in juvenile or labile (brittle) diabetes, or in patients with infections or those undergoing surgery or trauma. It is contra-indicated in patients with ketosis, acidosis or in coma, and who have a history of such.

Since Tolanase has not been studied extensively in diabetes complicated by pregnancy or in diabetics with liver, kidney or endocrine disease, it is not recommended in these instances.

Warnings: The appearance of significant acetonuria in a patient transferred from insulin to tolazamide makes return to insulin therapy mandatory.

Interactions: The hypoglycaemic action of sulphonylureas may be potentiated by certain drugs including phenylbutazone, oxyphenbutazone, salicylates, sulphonamides, chloramphenicol, probenecid, coumarins, monoamine oxidase inhibitors, and beta adrenergic blocking agents. When such drugs are administered to a patient receiving Tolanase, the patient should be closely observed for hypoglycaemia. When such drugs are withdrawn from a patient receiving Tolanase, the patient should be observed closely for loss of control.

Certain drugs tend to produce hyperglycaemia and may lead to loss of control. These drugs include the thiazides and other diuretics, corticosteroids, phenothiazines, thyroid products, oestrogens, oral contraceptives, phenytoin, nicotinic acid, sympathomimetics and isoniazid. When such drugs are administered to a patient receiving Tolanase, the patient should be observed for loss of control. When such drugs are withdrawn from a patient receiving Tolanase, the patients should be observed closely for hypoglycaemia.

Side-effects: The most commonly encountered symptoms are gastro-intestinal (1.8%), including nausea, anorexia, diarrhoea. Other minor occurrences, such as dizziness, weakness, insomnia, lethargy, have been reported. A disulfiram-like action after taking alcohol has not been reported.

Overdosage: Action should be taken to counteract the ensuing hypoglycaemic period. No known antidote.

Pharmaceutical precautions Store at room temperature.

Legal category POM.

Package quantities Tolanase is supplied as tablets containing 100 mg or 250 mg tolazamide in bottles of 100.

Further information The half-life of seven hours makes Tolanase an ideal agent for a single or twice-daily dose regime.

Product licence numbers
Tablets 100 mg   0032/5043
Tablets 250 mg   0032/5044

TROBICIN*

Presentation Vial containing spectinomycin dihydrochloride pentahydrate equivalent to spectinomycin 2 g. Also ampoule of diluent containing benzyl alcohol 0.9%. When reconstituted with diluent each vial yields 5 ml containing the equivalent of 400 mg spectinomycin per millilitre.

Uses Antibiotic for intramuscular injection in the treatment of gonorrhoea.

Dosage and administration For adults a single dose of 2 grams by deep intramuscular injection. Up to 4 grams have been administered in difficult-to-treat cases and in areas where antibiotic resistance is known to occur. Intramuscular injection should be made deep into the upper outer quadrant of the gluteal muscle. The dose may be divided between two injection sites.

Contra-indications, warnings, etc

Contra-indications: As with all drugs, the use of Trobicin is contra-indicated in patients previously found hypersensitive to it. Trobicin is not indicated for the treatment of syphilis.

Warnings: Antibiotics used in high doses for short periods of time to treat gonorrhoea may mask or delay the symptoms of incubating syphilis. Since the treatment of acute syphilis demands prolonged therapy with any effective antibiotic, patients being treated for gonorrhoea should be closely observed clinically for a period of four to six weeks. Appropriate serological follow-up for at least four months should be instituted if a diagnosis of syphilis is suspected.

Safety for use in pregnancy has not been established.

Precautions: Development of resistance to antibiotics has been observed with Neisseria gonorrhoea. This appears so far to occur only rarely with Trobicin, however, the clinical effectiveness of Trobicin should be monitored to detect evidence of resistance development.

Side-effects: During clinical trials no anaphylactic reactions or other serious side-effects were encountered. However, the usual precautions should be observed with atopic individuals. The following minor side-effects have been observed: dizziness, nausea, chills-fever, urticaria and (rarely) mild to moderate discomfort at the injection site.

Overdosage: Overdosage is unlikely to be a problem in practice.

Pharmaceutical precautions Shake vial vigorously immediately after adding diluent and before withdrawing dose. Dilution of the reconstituted suspension should not be necessary. Prepared suspension should be stored at room temperature and used within 24 hours. Otherwise no special storage precautions.

Legal category POM.

Package quantities 1 × 2 g vial plus diluent.

Further information Trobicin bears no structural or antigenic relationship to the penicillins. It is an inhibitor of protein synthesis in the bacterial cell, the site of action being the 30 S ribosomal subunit. Trobicin is rapidly absorbed after intramuscular injection, a single 2 g dose producing peak serum concentrations averaging 103 mcg/ml at one hour. Serum concentrations inhibitory to most gonococcal strains persist for up to eight hours. Up to 100% of the administered dose is excreted in the urine within 48 hours in a biologically active form.

Product licence number 0032/0032

XANAX* ▼

Presentation White ovoid-shaped tablets containing 0.25 mg alprazolam, scored on one side and marked 'Upjohn 29' on the other. Pink, ovoid-shaped tablets containing 0.5 mg alprazolam, scored on one side and marked 'Upjohn 55' on the other.

Uses Xanax is indicated for the short-term treatment of symptoms of anxiety and anxiety associated with depression. As the efficacy of Xanax in depression has yet to be established, specific treatment may have to be considered.

Dosage and administration The optimum dosage of Xanax should be based upon the severity of the symptoms and individual patient response. The usual dosage is stated below; in the few patients who require higher doses, the dosage should be increased cautiously to avoid adverse effects. When higher dosage is required, the evening dose should be increased before the daytime doses. In general, patients who have not previously received psychotropic medications will require lower doses than those so treated, or those with a history of chronic alcoholism. There is a reduced clearance of the drug and, as with other benzodiazepines, an increased sensitivity to the drug in elderly patients.

Anxiety: 0.25 mg to 0.5 mg three times daily increasing if required to a total of 3 mg daily.

Geriatric patients or in the presence of debilitating disease: 0.25 mg two to three times daily to be gradually increased if needed and tolerated.

If side-effects occur, the dose should be lowered. It is advisable to review treatment regularly and to discontinue use as soon as possible.

Contra-indications, warnings, etc

Contra-indications: Known sensitivity to benzodiazepines. Acute pulmonary insufficiency.

Precautions: 1. Xanax is not recommended as the primary treatment for psychotic patients and should not be used in lieu of appropriate treatment for psychosis.

2. There is no evidence as to drug safety in human pregnancy nor is there evidence from animal work that it is free from hazard. Do not use during pregnancy, especially during the first and last trimesters, unless there are compelling reasons.

3. Chronic pulmonary insufficiency.

4. In chronic renal or hepatic disease.

5. In labour. High single doses or repeated low doses have been reported to produce hypotonia, poor sucking and hypothermia in the neonate and irregularities in the foetal heart.

6. Avoid if possible in lactation.

7. The concurrent use of other CNS depressant drugs should be avoided.

Warnings and adverse effects: Common adverse effects include drowsiness, sedation, blurring of vision, unsteadiness and ataxia. These effects occur following single as well as repeated dosage and may persist well into the following day. Performance at skilled tasks and alertness

may be impaired. Patients should be warned of this hazard and advised not to drive or operate machinery during treatment. These effects are potentiated by alcohol. The elderly are particularly liable to experience these symptoms together with confusion especially if organic brain symptoms are present. See also Dependence potential and withdrawal symptoms below.

Abnormal psychological reactions to benzodiazepines have been reported. Rare behavioural adverse effects include paradoxical aggressive outbursts, excitement, and confusion.

Other rare adverse effects including hypotension, gastrointestinal and visual disturbances, skin rashes, urinary retention, headache, vertigo, changes in libido, blood dyscrasias and jaundice have also been reported.

The safety and efficacy of Xanax in patients less than 18 years old has not been established.

Dependence potential and withdrawal symptoms: In general the dependence potential of benzodiazepines is low but this increases when high dosage is attained, especially when given over long periods. This is particularly so in patients with a history of alcoholism, drug abuse or in patients with marked personality disorders. Regular monitoring of treatment in such patients is essential and routine repeat prescriptions should be avoided.

Treatment in all patients should be withdrawn gradually as symptoms such as depression, nervousness, rebound insomnia, irritability, sweating and diarrhoea have been reported following abrupt cessation of treatment in patients receiving even normal therapeutic doses for short periods of time.

Abrupt withdrawal following excessive dosage may produce confusion, toxic psychosis, convulsions or a condition resembling delirium tremens.

Overdosage: Manifestations of Xanax overdosage include extensions of its pharmacological activity, namely ataxia and somnolence. Induced vomiting and/or gastric lavage are indicated. As in all cases of drug overdosage, respiration, pulse, and blood pressure should be monitored and supported by general measures when necessary. Intravenous fluids may be administered and an adequate airway maintained.

Animal experiments have suggested that forced diuresis or haemodialysis are probably of little value in treating overdosage.

As with the management of any overdosage, the physician should bear in mind that multiple agents may have been ingested.

Pharmaceutical precautions Protect from light.

Legal category CD (Sch 4) POM.

Package quantities Packs of 60.

Further information Alprazolam is readily absorbed. Following oral administration, peak concentrations in the plasma occur after 1–2 hours. The mean half-life is 12–15 hours. Repeated dosage may lead to accumulation and this should be borne in mind in elderly patients and those with impaired renal or hepatic function. Alprazolam and its metabolites are excreted primarily in the urine. Xanax did not affect the prothrombin times or plasma warfarin levels in male volunteers administered sodium warfarin orally.

Product licence numbers
Tablets 0.25 mg   0032/0092
Tablets 0.5 mg   0032/0093

*Trade Mark

Wellcome Medical Division
The Wellcome Foundation Limited
Crewe Hall
Crewe, Cheshire CW1 1UB

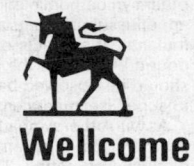

Wellcome

ACTIDIL* TABLETS AND ELIXIR

Presentation Each tablet contains 2.5 mg Triprolidine Hydrochloride BP. Scored and coded Wellcome L2A. White in colour.

Each 5 ml of orange-coloured elixir contains 2 mg Triprolidine Hydrochloride BP and has a flavour of mandarin orange.

Uses Antihistamine.
Symptomatic relief of allergic conditions.
Actidil elixir is particularly suitable for use in children.

Dosage and administration *Adults:* 1–2 tablets or 5–10 ml elixir three times a day.

Children: Over 12 years: As for adults.

6–12 years: 7.5 ml three times a day.

1–6 years: 5 ml three times a day.

Under 1 year: 2.5 ml three times a day.
Actidil Elixir may be diluted with Syrup BP.

Use in the elderly: No specific studies have been carried out in the elderly, although Actidil has been widely used in older people. However, it may be advisable to monitor renal or hepatic function and if there is serious impairment then caution should be exercised.

Contra-indications, warnings, etc

Contra-indications: Contra-indicated in patients with known hypersensitivity to triprolidine.

Precautions: May cause drowsiness. Patients should not drive a vehicle or operate machinery until they have determined their own response. In some patients the drowsiness induced by antihistamines may be potentiated by alcohol or other central sedatives.

In severe hepatic or renal dysfunction a single dose of Actidil should be given initially and the response to it used as a guide to the patient's requirement for further administration of the product.

Side- and adverse effects: Triprolidine may cause drowsiness. Lichenoid skin eruptions due to triprolidine have rarely been reported

Use in pregnancy and lactation: No data are available on the use of Actidil in human pregnancy. Triprolidine is excreted in human milk.

Toxicity and treatment of overdosage: Drowsiness, dizziness, inco-ordination, weakness, convulsions and respiratory depression may occur.

Necessary measures should be taken to maintain and support respiration. Gastric lavage should be performed if indicated and convulsions controlled with diazepam. There are theoretical grounds for believing that the elimination of triprolidine and its metabolites could be accelerated by dialysis.

Pharmaceutical precautions *Tablets and elixir:* Store below 25°C. Protect from light.

Legal category P.

Package quantities Bottle of 100 tablets. Bottle of 500 ml elixir.

Further information Nil.

Product licence numbers
Tablets   0003/5001
Elixir   0003/5002

ACTIFED* COMPOUND LINCTUS

Presentation Each 5 ml of bright-red-coloured linctus contains 10 mg Dextromethorphan Hydrobromide BP, 30 mg Pseudoephedrine Hydrochloride BP, and 1.25 mg Triprolidine Hydrochloride BP and has a fruity flavour.

Uses Relief of unproductive cough accompanied by congestion of the upper respiratory tract, including congestion with an allergic component.

Dosage and administration

Adults and children over 12 years: 10 ml three times a day.

Children 6–12 years: 5 ml three times a day.

2–5 years: 2.5 ml three times a day.
May be diluted with Syrup BP.

Use in the elderly: No specific studies have been carried out in the elderly, however, it may be advisable to monitor renal or hepatic function and if there is serious impairment then caution should be exercised.

Pharmacology: Pseudoephedrine has direct and indirect sympathomimetic activity and is an orally effective upper respiratory tract decongestant. Pseudoephedrine is substantially less potent than ephedrine in producing both tachycardia and elevation in systolic blood pressure, and is considerably less potent in causing stimulation of the central nervous system. Triprolidine provides antihistamine activity by antagonising H_1 receptors. Dextromethorphan provides antitussive activity by acting on the medullary cough centre.

Contra-indications, warnings, etc

Contra-indications: Contra-indicated in patients with a known hypersensitivity to pseudoephedrine, triprolidine, or dextromethorphan. Contra-indicated in persons under treatment with monoamine oxidase inhibitors or within 2 weeks of stopping such treatment.

Precautions: Actifed Compound Linctus should be used with caution in patients with cardiovascular disorders, including hypertension. The effect of anti-hypertensive agents that modify sympathetic activity may be partially reversed by Actifed Compound Linctus.

Also, caution should be exercised in patients taking other sympathomimetic agents, such as decongestants, appetite suppressants and amphetamine-like psychostimulants. The effects of a single dose of Actifed Compound Linctus on the blood pressure of these patients should be observed before recommending repeated or unsupervised treatment.

As with other sympathomimetic agents, caution should be exercised in patients with prostatic enlargement or bladder dysfunction.

In severe hepatic or renal dysfunction, a single dose of Actifed Compound Linctus should be given, and the patient's response used as a guide to the dosage requirement for further administration.

The antibacterial agent furazolidone is known to cause a progressive inhibition of monoamine oxidase and although there are no reports of a hypertensive crisis having occurred, it should not be administered concurrently with Actifed Compound Linctus.

Side- and adverse effects: In some patients, pseudoephedrine may occasionally cause insomnia. Rarely, sleep disturbance and hallucinations have been reported. Triprolidine may cause drowsiness and patients should not drive a vehicle or operate machinery until they have determined their own response. In some patients, the drowsiness induced by antihistamines may be potentiated by alcohol or other central sedatives. Fixed drug eruption due to pseudoephedrine, taking the form of erythematous nummular patches, and lichenoid skin eruption due to triprolidine, have been reported but both these reactions should be regarded as rare events.

Use in pregnancy and lactation: No data are available on the use of Actifed Compound Linctus in human pregnancy. Pseudoephedrine and triprolidine are excreted in breast milk.

Toxicity and treatment of overdosage: As with other sympathomimetic agents, symptoms of overdosage include irritability, convulsions, palpitations, hypertension and difficulty in micturition. In severe cases, respiratory depression may occur from the dextromethorphan. Catheterisation of the bladder may be necessary. Alpha-adrenergic blockade may be required to treat hypertensive crises, and beta-adrenergic blockade for the control of supraventricular dysrhythmias.

If desired, the elimination of pseudoephedrine can be accelerated by acid diuresis or by dialysis.

Pharmaceutical precautions   Store below 25°C. Protect from light.

Legal category   P.

Package quantities   Bottles of 100 ml and 2 litres.

Further information   Nil.

Product licence number   0003/0160.

ACTIFED* EXPECTORANT

Presentation   Each 5 ml of clear orange syrup contains 1.25 mg Triprolidine Hydrochloride BP, 30 mg Pseudoephedrine Hydrochloride BP and 100 mg Guaiphenesin BP.

Uses   Conditions where an expectorant and upper respiratory tract decongestant are required.

Dosage and administration
Adults and children over 12 years: 10 ml three times a day

Children 6–12 years: 5 ml three times a day
Children 2–5 years: 2.5 ml three times a day
Actifed Expectorant may be diluted with Syrup BP.

Use in the elderly: No specific studies have been carried out in the elderly, although Actifed Expectorant has been widely used in older people. However, it may be advisable to monitor renal or hepatic function and if there is serious impairment then caution should be exercised.

Pharmacology: Pseudoephedrine has direct and indirect sympathomimetic activity and is an orally effective upper respiratory tract decongestant. Pseudoephedrine is substantially less potent than ephedrine in producing both tachycardia and elevation in systolic blood pressure and considerably less potent in causing stimulation of the central nervous system. On the basis of widespread and long established clinical use, guaiphenesin is recognised as an expectorant in bronchitis. Triprolidine provides antihistamine activity by antagonising H_1 receptors.

Contra-indications, warnings, etc
Contra-indications: Contra-indicated in patients with a known hypersensitivity to pseudoephedrine, triprolidine or guaiphenesin. Contra-indicated in persons under treatment with monoamine oxidase inhibitors and within 2 weeks of stopping such treatment.

Precautions: Although pseudoephedrine causes virtually no pressor effect in patients with normal blood pressure, Actifed Expectorant should be used with caution in patients with cardiovascular disorders, including hypertension. The effect of anti-hypertensive agents that modify sympathetic activity may be partially reversed by Actifed Expectorant.

Also caution should be exercised in patients taking other sympathomimetic agents, such as decongestants, appetite suppressants and amphetamine-like psychostimulants. The effects of a single dose on the blood pressure of these patients should be observed before recommending repeated or unsupervised treatment.

As with other sympathomimetic agents caution should be exercised in patients with prostatic enlargement or bladder dysfunction.

In severe hepatic or renal dysfunction a single dose of Actifed Expectorant should be given and the patient's response used as a guide to the dosage requirement for further administration.

The antibacterial agent furazolidone is known to cause a progressive inhibition of monoamine oxidase and although there are no reports of a hypertensive crisis having occurred, it should not be administered concurrently with Actifed Expectorant.

Side- and adverse effects: In some patients, pseudoephedrine may occasionally cause insomnia. Rarely, sleep disturbance and hallucinations have been reported. Triprolidine may cause drowsiness. Patients should not drive a vehicle or operate machinery until they have determined their own response. In some patients the drowsiness induced by antihistamines may be potentiated by alcohol or other central sedatives. Fixed drug eruption due to pseudoephedrine taking the form of nummular patches and lichenoid skin eruption due to triprolidine have been reported but these are rare events.

Use in pregnancy and lactation: No data are available on the use of Actifed Expectorant in human pregnancy. Pseudoephedrine and triprolidine are excreted in breast milk.

Toxicity and treatment of overdosage: Probable symptoms may comprise drowsiness, inco-ordination, weakness, palpitations, irritability, hypertension, convulsions and difficulty in micturition. Gastric lavage and supportive measures for respiration and circulation should be performed if indicated. Convulsions should be controlled with an anticonvulsant. Catheterisation of the bladder may be necessary. Alpha-adrenergic blockade may be required to treat hypertensive crisis and beta-adrenergic blockade for the control of supraventricular dysrhythmias.

If desired, the elimination of pseudoephedrine can be accelerated by acid diuresis or by dialysis.

Pharmaceutical precautions Store below 25°C. Do not refrigerate. Protect from light.

Legal category P.

Package quantities Bottles of 100 ml and 1 litre.

Further information Nil.

Product licence number 0003/0152.

ACTIFED* TABLETS AND SYRUP

Presentation Each tablet contains 2.5 mg Triprolidine Hydrochloride BP and 60 mg Pseudoephedrine Hydrochloride BP. Scored and coded Wellcome M2A. White in colour.

Each 5 ml of clear, golden-yellow syrup contains 1.25 mg Triprolidine Hydrochloride BP and 30 mg Pseudoephedrine Hydrochloride BP, and has a pleasant flavour.

Uses Decongestant and antihistamine.

For decongestion of the upper respiratory tract including the sinuses, antra and Eustachian tubes in the common cold, hay fever, allergic and vasomotor rhinitis and aerotitis (otitis barotrauma).

Dosage and administration *Adults, and children over 12 years:* 1 tablet or 10 ml three times a day.

6–12 years: 5 ml three times a day.

2–5 years: 2.5 ml three times a day.

Actifed Syrup may be diluted with Syrup BP.

Use in the elderly: No specific studies have been carried out in the elderly, although Actifed has been widely used in older people. However, it may be advisable to monitor renal or hepatic function and if there is serious impairment then caution should be exercised.

Pharmacology: Pseudoephedrine has direct and indirect sympathomimetic activity and is an orally effective upper respiratory tract decongestant. Pseudoephedrine is substantially less potent than ephedrine in producing both tachycardia and elevation in systolic blood pressure and considerably less potent in causing stimulation of the central nervous system. Triprolidine provides antihistamine activity by antagonising H_1 receptors.

Contra-indications, warnings, etc
Contra-indications: Contra-indicated in patients with known hypersensitivity to pseudoephedrine or triprolidine.

Contra-indicated in persons under treatment with monoamine oxidase inhibitors, and within two weeks of stopping such treatment.

Precautions: Although pseudoephedrine causes virtually no pressor effect in patients with normal blood pressure, Actifed should be used with caution in patients with cardiovascular disorders, including hypertension. The effect of antihypertensive agents which modify sympathetic activity may be partially reversed by Actifed.

Caution should also be exercised in patients taking other sympathomimetic agents, such as decongestants, appetite suppressants and amphetamine-like psychostimulants. The effects of a single dose on the blood pressure of these patients should be observed before recommending repeated or unsupervised treatment.

As with other sympathomimetic agents, caution should be exercised in patients with prostatic enlargement or bladder dysfunction.

In severe hepatic or renal dysfunction a single dose of Actifed should be given initially and the response to it used as a guide to the patient's requirement for further administration of the product.

The antibacterial agent furazolidone is known to cause a progressive inhibition of monoamine oxidase and although there are no reports of hypertensive crises having occurred, it should not be administered concurrently with Actifed.

Side- and adverse effects: In some patients, pseudoephedrine may occasionally cause insomnia. Rarely, sleep disturbance and hallucinations have been reported. Triprolidine may cause drowsiness. Patients should not drive a vehicle or operate machinery until they have determined their own response. In some patients the drowsiness induced by antihistamines may be potentiated by alcohol or other central sedatives. Fixed drug eruption due to pseudoephedrine taking the form of nummular patches and lichenoid skin eruption due to triprolidine have been reported but these are rare events.

Use in pregnancy and lactation: No data are available on the use of Actifed in human pregnancy. Pseudoephedrine and triprolidine are excreted in breast milk.

Toxicity and treatment of overdosage: Probable symptoms include drowsiness, inco-ordination, weakness, palpitation, irritability, hypertension, convulsions and difficulty in micturition. Gastric lavage and supportive measures for respiration and circulation should be performed if indicated. Convulsions should be controlled with an anticonvulsant. Catheterisation of the bladder may be necessary. Alpha-adrenergic blockade may be required to treat hypertensive crises and beta-adrenergic blockade for the control of supra-ventricular dysrhythmias.

If desired, the elimination of pseudoephedrine can be accelerated by acid diuresis or by dialysis.

Pharmaceutical precautions *Tablets and syrup:* Store below 25°C in a dry place. Protect from light.

Legal category P.

Package quantities Bottles of 100 and 500 tablets. Pack of 12 tablets. Bottles of 100 ml, 500 ml and 2 litres syrup.

Further information Nil.

Product licence numbers
Tablets   0003/5003
Syrup   0003/5004

ALCOPAR* DISPERSIBLE GRANULES

Presentation 5 g of the dispersible yellow-green granules contain the equivalent of 2.5 g bephenium (base) as Bephenium Hydroxynaphthoate BP.

Uses For the treatment of hookworm infestation by

Ancylostoma duodenale (but not Necator americanus). Also concurrent ascariasis (roundworm infection), trichostrongyliasis, and heterophyidiasis.

Dosage and administration The required dose of Alcopar should be mixed in water or in a flavoured drink and swallowed immediately.

Adults: The contents of 1 sachet.

Children: Over 2 years: The contents of 1 sachet.

Under 2 years or under 10 kg body weight: Half the contents of 1 sachet.

In the presence of heavy infestations it is recommended that treatment be repeated after three days.

No purgation or dietary restriction is necessary.

Oral iron may be given concurrently with Alcopar to patients with iron deficiency anaemia.

Use in the elderly: No special comment. Alcopar is poorly absorbed from the intestinal tract, it is, therefore, unlikely to affect elderly patients in apparently good health.

Contra-indications, warnings, etc
Contra-indications: Alcopar should not be given to patients with persistent vomiting.

Side- and adverse effects: No serious side-effects have been reported. Nausea, vomiting, abdominal discomfort and diarrhoea have occasionally been observed.

Use in pregnancy and lactation: Alcopar can be administered during pregnancy, and to the lactating mother.

Toxicity and treatment of overdosage: No data available. When administered orally, only a small fraction is absorbed from the gastro-intestinal tract. Thus symptoms are likely to be similar to those listed under side- and adverse effects. Gastric lavage followed by symptomatic and general supportive therapy is recommended.

Pharmaceutical precautions Nil.

Legal category P.

Package quantities Box of 25 × 5 g sachets.

Further information Nil.

Product licence number 0003/5007.

ALMEVAX* RUBELLA VACCINE, LIVE BP

Presentation A live attenuated Wistar RA 27/3 rubella virus strain, propagated in human diploid cells, and freeze-dried. The vaccine is manufactured and tested in accordance with the requirements of the United Kingdom control authorities and the World Health Organization. It also complies with the European Pharmacopoeia (1982).

0.5 ml of the reconstituted vaccine contains not less than 1,000 TCID$_{50}$ (tissue culture infective dose, 50).

This vaccine contains not more than 2 i.u. neomycin sulphate and 5 i.u. polymyxin B sulphate per 0.5 ml reconstituted vaccine.

Uses For active immunisation against rubella. Vaccination may be carried out at any age; preferably, however, it should be postponed beyond the first year of life since, below one year, the presence of maternal antibodies may impair the immune response. It should be noted that a past history of clinical rubella is an unreliable guide to immune status.

As with any other live attenuated virus vaccine, vaccination does not always result in seroconversion of 100% of susceptible subjects.

Dosage and administration *Adults:* 0.5 ml of the reconstituted vaccine.

Children: As for adults.

A single dose constitutes a full immunising course.

0.5 ml of the reconstituted vaccine is injected subcutaneously. If the injection site is swabbed, only acetone, ether or isopropyl alcohol should be used and allowed to dry before the injection is made.

Use in the elderly: No special comment.

Method of use: For reconstitution, use only the special sterile diluent. Almevax diluent has been tested to ensure that it does not inhibit the live attenuated virus.

Use only sterile disposable syringes and needles which are free from traces of disinfectants or spirits. Use a fresh syringe and needle for each injection.

To ensure satisfactory reconstitution add the diluent slowly. The reconstituted vaccine should be colourless to light pink. See *Pharmaceutical Precautions* for handling of reconstituted vaccine.

Do not attempt to obtain more than the stated number of doses from the vial. It is good practice to record the title, dose and lot numbers of all vaccines and dates of administration. Any untoward reactions should be reported to the regulatory authorities and to the manufacturer.

Reconstitution: Pack size – volume of special sterile diluent required for reconstitution of vaccine.
One-dose: The contents of the diluent container.
Ten-dose: The contents of the diluent container.

Contra-indications, warnings, etc
Contra-indications: Pregnant women must not be vaccinated. Vaccination should not be carried out within three weeks of other live vaccines or within 3 months following administration of human immune serum globulin, whole blood or plasma.

In the rare cases where anti-D immunoglobulin and rubella vaccine are required in the immediate postpartum period, it is advisable to test for rubella antibodies at 6–8 weeks after vaccination to ensure that the anti-D immunoglobulin has not interfered with the response to the vaccine. Data on the persistence of antibody following concurrent administration of rubella vaccine and anti-D immunoglobulin are not available.

The vaccine should not be given to persons suffering from febrile conditions, any active or suspected infection, malignant disease, severe chronic disease, gammaglobulin deficiency or to those with impaired immune responsiveness, whether idiopathic or as a result of treatment with steroids, radiotherapy, cytotoxic drugs or other agents. Vaccination of subjects with thrombocytopenia should be avoided. The vaccine should not be administered to a subject who has experienced a serious reaction (e.g. anaphylaxis) to a previous dose of this vaccine or who is known to be hypersensitive to any component thereof. The vaccine contains a small amount of neomycin and polymyxin and should not be given to individuals known to be sensitive to either of them.

Precautions: Attenuated rubella virus vaccine may temporarily depress tests for cell-mediated immunity.

Caution should be exercised should it become necessary to administer a second dose of rubella vaccine, if there has been a severe local or general reaction to a previous injection of the vaccine.

Rubella virus has been implicated as a possible aetiological factor in juvenile rheumatoid arthritis. The rubella immune status of any child with a history of juvenile arthritis should be determined by serological testing before vaccination. Vaccine should be withheld from seropositive children. Vaccination of seronegative children should be deferred until the disease is in remission since, as with other chronic illness, juvenile rheumatoid arthritis may be exacerbated by intercurrent infection.

Although anaphylaxis is rare, facilities for its management should always be available during vaccination.

Side- and adverse effects: Side-effects are uncommon, but mild symptoms may occur about the ninth day after vaccination. Symptoms relate to those seen following natural infection, but in the majority of cases are slight and transient. They include lymphadenopathy, rash, malaise, sore throat, mild fever, headache and occasionally temporary arthràlgia, infrequently associated with signs of inflammation. Marked joint symptoms are more often seen in adult females than in children or adolescents. Nevertheless, even in adults, joint symptoms do not usually interfere with normal activities. Local pain and, rarely, erythema at the site of injection may occur.

Falls in platelet counts, unassociated with symptoms, have been described after vaccination. Serious neurological symptoms have been reported rarely following vaccination. However, a cause and effect relationship has not been established.

Use in pregnancy and lactation: There is a possibility that live attenuated virus administered during pregnancy could infect and damage the foetus, producing congenital abnormalities. Therefore, *pregnant women must not be vaccinated* and pregnancy should be excluded before vaccination is undertaken. This danger to the developing foetus equally applies in the case of a pregnancy conceived within three months following vaccination. Women of childbearing age must be warned that, for at least three months after vaccination, they must take strict contraceptive precautions. If there is any possibility that they may become pregnant within this period, they should not be vaccinated.

Toxicity and treatment of overdosage: Not applicable.

Pharmaceutical precautions Store at 2–8°C. Use special Almevax diluent for reconstitution. After reconstitution the vaccine should be kept cool (2–20°C), protected from light, and used within one hour.

Legal category POM.

Package quantities Ampoule of 1 dose, with container of special diluent.

Rubber-capped vial of 10 doses, with container of special diluent.

Further information Rubella vaccination policy differs from country to country. In the UK the vaccine is offered routinely to all girls between their 11th and 14th birthdays and to susceptible adult females of childbearing age, including post-partum women.

Product licence number 0003/5123.

ANTEPAR* TABLETS AND ELIXIR

Presentation Each tablet contains Piperazine Phosphate BP equivalent to 500 mg Piperazine Hydrate BP, coloured yellow and scored, with the word Antepar embossed on the reverse side.

The elixir is a pineapple-flavoured, clear, orange-coloured syrup containing a stable combination of Piperazine Hydrate BP and Piperazine Citrate BP equivalent to 750 mg Piperazine Hydrate BP in each 5 ml.

Uses For the treatment of enterobiasis (pinworm, threadworm infection) and ascariasis (roundworm infection).

Antepar Elixir is especially suitable for administration to infants and children.

Dosage and administration The tablets should be chewed.

Antepar Elixir may be diluted with Syrup BP.

Enterobiasis: The dose should be calculated according to age or weight and given once daily for seven days.

Age (years)	Approx. weight	Elixir	Tablets
Adults	Over 55 kg	15 ml	4
Children:			
Over 12	Over 40 kg	15 ml	4
5–12	17–40 kg	10 ml	3
2–4	13–16 kg	5 ml	1½
Under 2	Under 13 kg	50–75 mg piperazine hydrate/kg bodyweight	

It may be necessary to repeat the course after a week's interval.

No special dietary regimen is needed.

Attention to general cleanliness is essential in order to prevent reinfection.

Owing to the facility with which pinworm infection is transmitted, it is advisable to examine all other members of a household since one is known to be infected. Treatment of all positive cases should be carried out simultaneously.

Ascariasis: A single dose taken preferably in the morning will usually produce complete clearance of worms from the gut.

Age (years)	Approx. weight	Elixir	Tablets
Adults	Over 55 kg	30 ml	8
Children:			
Over 10	Over 34 kg	30 ml	8
6–10	21–33 kg	20 ml	6
5–6	17–20 kg	15 ml	4½
2–4	13–16 kg	10 ml	3
Under 2	Under 13 kg	120 mg piperazine hydrate/kg bodyweight	

Use in the elderly: No specific studies have been carried out in the elderly, although Antepar has been widely used in older people. However, it may be advisable to monitor renal or hepatic function and if there is serious impairment then caution should be exercised. Antepar should not be given to elderly patients with symptomatic abnormalities of the kidney or CNS.

Contra-indications, warnings, etc

Contra-indications: Patients with a history of piperazine hypersensitivity or patients with renal failure.

Precautions: Caution should be exercised in treating patients with renal or significant hepatic impairment, or chronic disorders of the central nervous system.

Precipitation of grand mal attacks in patients with a known history of epilepsy has been reported.

Care should be taken in administration of piperazine to patients receiving phenothiazines as it has been suggested that piperazine potentiates the extrapyramidal effects of chlorpromazine in man and animals.

Side- and adverse effects: These are uncommon when Antepar is given at the recommended dosage but the following reactions have been reported:

Gastro-intestinal: nausea, vomiting, colic and diarrhoea.

Central nervous system: transient headache and dizziness. More severe reactions, including ataxia, muscle hypotonia, clonic contractions, drowsiness and impaired consciousness, seldom occur at the recommended dosage in individuals without a previous history of neurological abnormalities or renal disease.

Hypersensitivity reactions: urticaria, bullous eruptions, oedema, arthralgia, fever and tachycardia.

Case reports of purpura, a viral hepatitis-like disorder and acute haemolysis in a glucose-6-phosphate dehydrogenase deficient individual after piperazine administration, appear in the medical literature.

Use in pregnancy and lactation: The safety of Antepar for use during pregnancy has not been established but foetal toxicity studies in animals and extensive clinical experience have not revealed evidence that its use is associated with a risk to the foetus. Unless symptoms warrant immediate treatment it is advisable to postpone administration of Antepar until after parturition. No information is available on the excretion of piperazine or its metabolites in breast milk.

Toxicity and treatment of overdosage: Symptoms of overdosage are likely to be similar in character to the side-effects listed above. These may be expected to resolve spontaneously. Gastric lavage should be carried out only if Antepar has been recently ingested. Adequate fluids and routine supportive measures should be given, including the administration of anti-convulsants when necessary.

Pharmaceutical precautions *Tablets:* Store below 25°C. Keep dry. Protect from light.

Elixir: Store below 25°C. Protect from light.

Legal category P.

Package quantities Strip pack of 28 tablets. Bottles of 100 ml and 500 ml elixir.

Further information Nil.

Product licence numbers
Tablets 0003/5016
Elixir 0003/5015

ARILVAX* YELLOW FEVER VACCINE, LIVE BP
(17D strain live freeze-dried)
(Yel/Vac)

Presentation A specially stabilised freeze-dried preparation of the living attenuated 17D strain of yellow fever virus. The strain of virus used in this preparation is free of avian leucosis viruses and is propagated in leucosis-free chick embryos. The vaccine fulfils the requirements of the World Health Organisation.

Each 0.5 ml dose of reconstituted vaccine contains the equivalent of not less than 1,000 mouse LD_{50} units as defined by the World Health Organisation requirements, and not more than 2 i.u. of neomycin sulphate and 5 i.u. of polymyxin B sulphate.

The diluent consists of sterile water which has been specially tested to ensure that it does not inhibit the vaccine virus.

Uses For active immunisation of residents in yellow fever endemic areas and travellers to and from such areas, for the issue of an International Certificate of Vaccination, as required by the national health authorities of certain countries which consider these zones as infected areas (although the 'yellow-fever endemic zones' are in fact no longer included in the International Health Regulations). Yellow fever endemic areas are limited to the African and South American continents and Central America. The International Health Regulations define the form of certificate of vaccination to be used which, in the case of primary vaccination, is valid for a period of 10 years from the 10th day after vaccination. In the case of revaccination within 10 years, the certificate is valid at once.

Dosage and administration *Adults and children over age of 9 months:* The dose shall be the same for persons of all ages, 0.5 ml of reconstituted vaccine, given subcutaneously.

Use in the elderly: No special comment.

For reconstitution use only the special sterile diluent supplied.

Arilvax diluent has been tested to ensure that it does not inhibit the vaccine virus. Using a sterile syringe and needle inject the contents of the appropriate Arilvax diluent container into the vaccine vial and gently agitate to ensure reconstitution. The vaccine vial is sealed under vacuum to enhance stability and some users may prefer to break this vacuum to facilitate withdrawal of the vaccine solution. Any frothing will then subside.

See *Pharmaceutical precautions* for handling of reconstituted vaccine.

Use a fresh sterile disposable syringe and needle free from traces of spirit and disinfectants for each injection.

Do not attempt to obtain more than the stated number of doses from the vial. It is good practice to record the title, dose and lot numbers of all vaccines and dates of administration. Any untoward reactions should be reported to the regulatory authorities and to the manufacturer.

Contra-indications, warnings, etc
Contra-indications: The vaccine should not be administered to a subject who has experienced a serious reaction (e.g. anaphylaxis) to a previous dose of this vaccine or who is known to be hypersensitive to any component thereof. It is advisable to avoid vaccination during an acute infection. Since the vaccine is prepared in chick embryos and contains small quantities of neomycin and polymyxin, it should not be administered to individuals who are hypersensitive to egg or chick protein or to these antibiotics.

The vaccine should not be given to those with impaired immune responsiveness, whether idiopathic or as a result of treatment with steroids, radiotherapy, cytotoxic drugs or other agents.

Precautions: The vaccine is not recommended for use in children under the age of 9 months. The decision to vaccinate infants under this age must depend on the anticipated risk of exposure to the disease, since the small number of cases of encephalitis that have been reported have nearly all occurred in infants under this age.

It is advisable to avoid administration of the vaccine within 6 weeks following the administration of immune globulin on general principles. Similarly, on theoretical grounds it is advisable to avoid the administration of immune globulin within 2 weeks following vaccination.

Although anaphylaxis is rare, facilities for its management should always be available during vaccination.

An interval of not less than 3 weeks should normally be allowed to lapse between the administration of any two live vaccines. If time does not permit then they might be given simultaneously at separate sites.

Side- and adverse effects: Reactions to the vaccine are extremely rare. Occasionally some redness and swelling may occur at the site of injection, and headache has been reported.

One or two cases of urticaria, bursitis, jaundice and neuritis have been reported in a temporal relationship to vaccination.

Use in pregnancy and lactation: On theoretical grounds the vaccine should not be administered during pregnancy.

Toxicity and treatment of overdosage: Not applicable.

Pharmaceutical precautions The freeze-dried vaccine should be stored at temperatures below 8°C and protected from light. Diluent should not be frozen but should be stored upright in a cool place (below 15°C).

After reconstitution the vaccine should be kept cool, protected from light and used within one hour.

Any remaining vaccine should be disposed of by incineration or by treatment with disinfectant such as strong hypochlorite solution.

Legal category POM.

Package quantities Freeze-dried vaccine in packs of 10 × 1-dose vials with separate diluent; 10 × 5-dose vials with separate diluent; 10 × 10-dose vials with separate diluent.

Further information Nil.

Product licence number 0003/0100.

BANOCIDE* TABLETS

Presentation Each tablet contains 50 mg Diethylcarbamazine Citrate BP. Each tablet is scored, coded 'Wellcome S2A' and is white in colour.

Uses For the treatment of filarial infections due to: *Wuchereria bancrofti, Brugia malayi, Onchocerca volvulus, Loa loa.*

For the prophylaxis of bancroftian and malayan filariasis and loiasis.

Dosage and administration *Adults: Treatment:* 6 mg/kg body weight daily in 3 divided doses for three weeks. In order to reduce the incidence and severity of allergic manifestations (see below), an initial dose of 1 mg/kg body weight, gradually increased over three days, is recommended.

Prophylaxis: Bancroftian and malayan filariasis – 50 mg monthly.

Loiasis – 4 mg/kg for three successive days each month.

Children: As for adults.

Use in the elderly: There is no information on the effect of Banocide on elderly individuals. Older patients suffering from loiasis or lymphatic filariasis should be treated with careful attention to the normal precautions. In view of the severe side-effects associated with onchocerciasis and the limited benefit associated with treatment of this disease in the elderly, each individual should be assessed carefully before treatment is given.

In particular the benefit of treatment to elderly patients likely to return to a hyperendemic area is likely to be outweighed by the risk.

Contra-indications, warnings, etc
Contra-indications: None.

Precautions: Onchocerciasis patients receiving diethylcarbamazine should be carefully monitored for eye changes.

Side- and adverse effects: Allergic reactions, arising from the destruction of microfilariae, are common and may be severe – particularly during treatment of onchocerciasis and malayan filariasis. They take the form of generalised pruritus and conjunctival congestion and may be modified by the concurrent administration of antihistamines or corticosteroids.

Eye changes, including reduction in visual field and acuity, optic atrophy and optic disc leakage have been observed during administration of diethylcarbamazine for the treatment of onchocerciasis. The frequency and duration of the changes and the roles of the parasite and drug in their aetiology are, at present, unknown. Investigations have not shown eye changes during treatment of other filarial infections.

Use in pregnancy and lactation: In view of the severe reactions that may follow diethylcarbamazine administration, it is advisable to postpone treatment of pregnant women until after parturition. No information is available on the excretion of diethylcarbamazine in breast milk.

Toxicity and treatment of overdosage: Symptoms are likely to be those of nausea, vomiting, headache, dizziness and drowsiness. In severe cases convulsions and coma may occur. In view of the rapid absorption of diethylcarbamazine, gastric lavage should be considered only if the patient is seen within 2 hours of excessive ingestion of Banocide. Adequate fluids should be given to ensure optimal diuresis. Acidification of urine should enhance the excretion of diethylcarbamazine. Anticonvulsants may be required in cases of convulsions and coma. Routine supportive measures should be given when necessary.

Pharmaceutical precautions Store below 25°C. Keep dry.

Legal category P.

Package quantities Bottle of 100 tablets.

Further information Nil.

Product licence number 0003/5018.

BRETYLATE* INJECTION

Presentation Each 2 ml ampoule contains 100 mg bretylium tosylate.

Uses Bretylate Injection is indicated for the treatment of severe or life-threatening ventricular arrhythmias, principally ventricular fibrillation and ventricular tachycardia, which are refractory to conventional antiarrhythmic agents such as lignocaine.

In patients with ventricular fibrillation, bretylium may produce pharmacological defibrillation but more usually facilitates electrical cardioversion to sinus rhythm. Bretylium is effective in the treatment of dysrhythmias associated with acute myocardial infarction and may also be useful in the treatment of post-operative arrhythmias.

Dosage and administration The use of Bretylate Injection should be limited to coronary or intensive-care units where there are facilities for monitoring cardiac rhythm and blood pressure. Patients should be supine or closely monitored for orthostatic hypotension.

Bretylium may be administered either intramuscularly or intravenously but a more rapid antifibrillatory action may be achieved by intravenous injection. An initial dose of 5–10 mg/kg may be repeated after 1–2 hours if the arrhythmia persists. Further doses of 5–10 mg/kg may be given at 6–8 hourly intervals for up to 5 days. The anti-arrhythmic effects of a single dose of bretylium last for 6–12 hours. The anti-arrhythmic action against some ventricular arrhythmias appears 20–40 minutes after intramuscular or intravenous administration and in some patients may require several hours to develop. The site of intramuscular injection should be varied and not more than 5 ml should be given into any one site.

Bretylium has been administered by slow IV infusion (10 mg/kg/24 hours) but the clinical efficacy of this mode of administration has not been established. Rapid IV injection of bretylium (10–30 mg/kg and repeated after 20 minutes) has been shown to reverse ventricular fibrillation but in these cases it was used as a first line anti-arrhythmic agent and the efficacy in such practice is not extensively documented.

Bretylium Injection may be diluted down to 10 mg/ml with Glucose Intravenous Infusion BP (5% w/v) or Sodium Chloride Intravenous Infusion BP (0.9% w/v).

Use in children: No data available.

Use in the elderly: The use of Bretylate Injection in the elderly depends on the degree of reduction in cardiac and renal function. The decision to treat rests on the balance between the expected anti-arrhythmic effect and the disadvantages of inappropriate dosing.

Contra-indications, warnings, etc
Contra-indications: There is no evidence that prophylactic administration of Bretylate Injection confers clinical benefit in patients with recent but uncomplicated myocardial infarction. Not to be used in the primary treatment of cardiac dysrhythmias, nor in digitalis induced arrhythmias.

Precautions: The use of bretylium is safer in intensive-care units where facilities for monitoring cardiac rhythm and blood pressure are available. Hypotension is a common troublesome adverse effect but not if the patients remain supine. However, hypotension can occur in the supine position in patients with severely compromised cardiac function. If vital organs become under-perfused, blood volume should be re-expanded by suitable intravenous infusions.

An initial transient increase in blood pressure and heart rate with worsening of arrhythmias may follow the first administration of bretylium, probably because of neuronal noradrenaline release. Until sympathetic blockade supervenes, patients should be observed closely for possible deterioration of the arrhythmia.

Bretylium for patients with severe renal damage should be carefully considered because its elimination is substantially by this route. Dosing of patients with renal impairment should be submaximal and related to endogenous creatinine clearance. Bretylium accumulates with inadequate renal function but can be eliminated by haemodialysis.

Drug interactions: Patients generally receive bretylium after many other anti-arrhythmic agents have failed. Nevertheless, clinical observations suggest that bretyl-ium is a more effective anti-arrhythmic and anti-fibrillatory agent when given alone rather than in combination with other anti-arrhythmics.

Parenteral administration of bretylium may exacerbate ventricular tachyarrhythmias caused by digitalis toxicity. Bretylium is therefore not indicated in such disturbances of rhythm (see also *Contra-indications*).

Hypersensitivity to infused catecholamines would be expected after bretylium administration because of their uptake and subsequent degradation by monoamine oxidase. For this reason, when it is necessary to increase perfusion pressure to vital organs after bretylium induced hypotension, noradrenaline or other sympathomimetics should only be given under expert supervision.

Side- and adverse effects: Administration of bretylium may have to be discontinued because of possible adverse effects in approximately 7% of patients. Moderate increases in blood pressure, heart rate and a positive inotropic effect may occur on commencement of therapy.

The most common side-effect following bretylium administration is hypotension, especially in patients whose initial haemodynamic state and cardiac function is poor. Hypotension with increased pulmonary vascular resistance has also been reported.

Immediately after commencement of bretylium administration, more ectopic beats may arise, but such effects do not usually lead to serious problems. Nausea and vomiting may occur occasionally when bretylium is administered rapidly by the intravenous route, but this effect may be overcome by administering the drug over periods of 8–15 minutes or by using the intramuscular route.

Intramuscular administration of bretylium may cause tissue necrosis at the site of injection. This is rare if the site of injection is varied and the injection volume limited to 5 ml.

Use in pregnancy and lactation: No data are available on the use of bretylium in pregnancy nor on its excretion into breast milk.

Toxicity and treatment of overdosage: The symptoms of acute overdosage are likely to be marked hypotension with syncope.

Treatment is by means of general supportive measures with intravenous infusion of plasma. *Slow* intravenous injection of noradrenaline or phenylephrine may be given under expert supervision.

Pharmaceutical precautions Store below 25°C. Do not freeze. Protect from light.

Legal category POM.

Package quantities Box of 5 ampoules.

Further information Nil.

Product licence number 0003/0038.

CEFIZOX* INJECTION ▼

Presentation Vials containing 500 mg, 1 g and 2 g of ceftizoxime as its sterile sodium salt. Ceftizoxime sodium is a white to pale yellow crystalline powder. For each gram of ceftizoxime there is approximately 60 mg (2.6 mmol) of sodium.

Uses Broad-spectrum, bactericidal, cephalosporin antibiotic indicated for the treatment of infections either before the infecting organism has been identified, or when caused by bacteria of known sensitivity. Indications include lower respiratory tract infections, genitourinary tract infections including gonorrhoea, intraabdominal infections, septicaemia, skin and soft tissue infections.

Many infections caused by aerobic and anaerobic, Gram-negative and Gram-positive organisms resistant to other cephalosporins, aminoglycosides, or penicillins, have responded to treatment with Cefizox. Cefizox has been effective in the treatment of seriously ill, immunocompromised patients e.g. those with neutropenia and granulocytopenia.

Bacteriology: Cefizox is active *in vitro* against a wide range of Gram-positive and Gram-negative organisms. These include the following:

Gram-positive aerobes – staphylococci including *Staph. pyogenes* and *Staph. epidermidis,* streptococci including *Strep. pneumoniae* and *Strep. pyogenes, Corynebacterium diphtheriae.* Most strains of enterococci are resistant.

Gram-negative aerobes – *Esch. coli,* Klebsiella spp., Proteus spp. both indole positive and negative, Serratia spp., Enterobacter spp., Providencia spp., many strains of Pseudomonas spp., Citrobacter spp., *Haemophilus influenzae* including ampicillin-resistant strains, Neisseria spp. including β-lactamase-producing strains, Salmonella spp., Shigella spp., *Aeromonas hydrophila, Yersinia enterocolitica.*

Anaerobes – Bacteroides spp. including many, but not all strains of *B.fragilis.,* Peptococcus spp., Eubacterium spp., Clostridium spp.

Cefizox is stable to a broad spectrum of beta-lactamases produced by both aerobic and anaerobic organisms.

Dosage and administration Cefizox may be given by slow intravenous injection, by continuous or intermittent intravenous infusion or by deep intramuscular injection. Dosage and route of administration should be determined by the condition of the patient, severity of the infection and susceptibility of the causative organisms.

General guidelines: Adults:

Type of infection	Dosage	Route
Urinary tract	0.5–1 g 12-hourly	IM or IV
Gonorrhoea	1 g single dose	IM
Other infections	1–2 g 8–12 hourly	IM* or IV
Severe or life-threatening infections	2–3 g 8-hourly	IM* or IV

* When administering 2 g intramuscularly, the dose should be divided and given in different large muscle masses.

Dosages in excess of 4 g daily are rarely necessary but, exceptionally, dosages up to 8 g per day have been given and were well tolerated.

Children over the age of 3 months: 30–60 mg/kg bodyweight/day in 2–4 divided doses, increased in severe or life-threatening infections to 100–150 mg/kg bodyweight/day. The total dose should not exceed the adult dose.

Children under the age of 3 months: There are insufficient data to recommend the use of Cefizox.

Dosage in renal impairment: Modification of dosage is necessary in patients with impaired renal function. For an adult, following an initial loading dose of 500 mg–1.0 g, IM or IV, the maintenance dosing schedule shown below should be followed (no data are available for children):

Creatinine clearance ml/min.	Less severe infections	Severe or life-threatening infections
50–79	500 mg 8-hourly	0.75–1.5 g 8-hourly
5–49	250–500 mg 12-hourly	0.5–1.0 g 12-hourly
0–4 (dialysis patients)	500 mg 48-hourly or 250 mg 24-hourly	0.5–1.0 g 48-hourly or 0.5 g 24 hourly

In patients undergoing haemodialysis, no additional supplemental dosing is required following haemodialysis; however, dosing should be timed so that the patient receives the dose (according to the table above), at the end of the dialysis.

Preparation of parenteral solutions: Reconstitute with Water for Injections BP in the minimum volumes shown below. Shake well. Further dilutions may be used. See 'Administration'.

Vial size	Vol. diluent
500 mg	2.0 ml
1 g	3.0 ml
2 g	6.0 ml

These solutions are stable for 8 hours at room temperature. When freshly reconstituted, Cefizox is a colourless to pale yellow solution with a pH of 6.0 to 8.0. Reconstituted solutions may discolour. Yellow discolouration will not alter potency or therapeutic efficacy. Discard solution if markedly discoloured.

Administration: IM injection: Inject deep within the body of a relatively large muscle. When administering 2 g, the dose should be divided and given in different large muscle masses. For intramuscular injection, Cefizox may be diluted with 0.5% lignocaine.

IV injection: Inject slowly over 3 to 5 mins. either directly or via the tubing of an established intravenous infusion (see list below).

IV infusion: For intermittent or continuous infusion, dilute Cefizox reconstituted with Water for Injections BP, or Sodium Chloride Injection BP in 50 to 100 ml of one of the following solutions:

Glucose Intravenous Infusion BP (5% and 10% w/v)
Sodium Chloride Intravenous Infusion BP
Sodium Chloride and Glucose Intravenous Infusion BP (0.18% and 4% w/v, 0.45% or 0.9% and 5% w/v)
Compound Sodium Chloride Injection BPC 1959 (Ringer's Solution for Injection)
Compound Sodium Lactate Intravenous Infusion BP

Cefizox in these fluids is stable for 8 hours at 25°C and for 24 hours at 5°C.

Use in the elderly: It is recommended that the dose is reduced even though the serum creatinine level shows a normal value. In the presence of renal impairment doses should be reduced according to the table above, on the basis of creatinine clearance values.

Contra-indications, warnings, etc
Contra-indications: Hypersensitivity to cephalosporin antibiotics.

Precautions: Cefizox should be given cautiously to penicillin-sensitive patients. Although cephalosporin antibiotics may usually be given safely to such patients, cross reactions have been reported. Special care is required in patients who have had an anaphylactic reaction to penicillin.

Patients with impaired renal function – see 'Dosage and Administration'.

Cefizox has not been shown to alter renal function, but renal status should be monitored, especially in seriously ill patients receiving maximum dose therapy and co-administration of aminoglycoside antibiotics. Although the occurrence has not been reported with Cefizox, nephrotoxicity has been reported following concomitant administration of other cephalosporins and aminoglycosides.

As with any antibiotic, prolonged use may result in overgrowth of non-susceptible organisms.

Side- and adverse effects: Cefizox is generally well tolerated. The most common adverse reactions have been local following IM or IV injection. These include burning, cellulitis, pain, induration, tenderness, paraesthesia and phlebitis. Other adverse reactions include hypersensitivity reactions (rash, pruritus, fever), gastrointestinal disturbance (diarrhoea, nausea and vomiting), vaginitis, transient eosinophilia, and thrombocytosis. Neutropenia, leucopenia and thrombocytopenia have been reported rarely. Some individuals have developed a positive Coombs' test. Transient elevation in SGOT, SGPT, alkaline phosphatase, BUN and serum creatinine have occasionally been observed.

Use in pregnancy and lactation: Animal studies have not revealed evidence of an adverse effect on the developing foetus but there are no data in pregnant women. Thus the benefit of using Cefizox in pregnancy should be weighed against the possible hazard. Ceftizoxime is excreted in human milk in low concentrations. Caution should therefore be exercised if Cefizox is administered to a nursing mother.

Toxicity: None has been reported.

Treatment of overdosage: Not applicable.

Pharmaceutical precautions Store below 25°C. Protect from light.

Legal category POM.

Package quantities Individual vials containing 500 mg, 1 gram and 2 gram packed singly.

Further information Ceftizoxime is not metabolised and is excreted virtually unchanged by the kidneys within 24 hours, thus providing high urinary concentrations. It passes readily into various body fluids and tissues including those of the full-term foetus.

Interference with laboratory tests: a false-positive reaction to glucose may occur with reducing substances but not with the use of specific glucose oxidase methods.

Product licence numbers
500 mg   0003/0174
1 g, 2 g   0003/0175

CHOLERA VACCINE BP WELLCOME* (Cho/Vac)

Presentation Cholera vaccine contains heat-killed phenol-preserved *Vibrio cholerae,* serotypes Inaba and Ogawa, at a concentration of not less than 8,000 million per ml. The phenol concentration is 0.5% w/v.

Uses Immunisation against cholera including cholera El Tor. Although this vaccine does not contain the El Tor biotypes of the classical Inaba and Ogawa serotypes, carefully controlled field studies have shown that the classical biotype equally protects against both classical and El Tor.

Dosage and administration Primary vaccination consists of two doses of vaccine given subcutaneously or intramuscularly, preferably separated by a period of over a month. This interval may be reduced even to seven days, though the response may be poorer, when rapid immunisation is necessary.

Age	First dose	All subsequent doses
1–5 years	0.1 ml	0.3 ml
5–10 years	0.3 ml	0.5 ml
Over 10 years	0.5 ml	1.0 ml

The container should on all occasions be well shaken before withdrawing material for injection.

Immunity is short-lived so that booster doses are required every six months under conditions of continued exposure. A single booster dose will suffice even if considerably longer than six months has elapsed since the last dose was administered.

For second and subsequent doses, particularly if there has been some reaction to a previous dose, it may be preferable to give the vaccine intradermally, in a volume of 0.1 ml where the subcutaneous dose is 0.5 ml or less, and 0.2 ml in other cases. However, it is possible that some countries may be unwilling to accept travellers who have not received the larger subcutaneous doses.

Travellers to or from certain countries which have reported cholera infection may be required to produce written evidence of cholera vaccination during the previous six months. A single dose normally meets these requirements and the International Certificate becomes valid six days after the first dose of vaccine was administered, but some countries may demand two doses. The certificate becomes valid immediately after a booster dose within six months of primary immunisation.

It is good practice to record the title, dose and lot numbers of all vaccines and dates of administration. Any untoward reactions should be reported to the regulatory authorities and to the manfacturer.

Use in the elderly: No special comment.

Contra-indications, warnings, etc

Contra-indications: The vaccine should not be administered to a subject who has experienced a serious reaction (e.g. anaphylaxis) to a previous dose of this vaccine or who is known to be hypersensitive to any component thereof. It is advisable to avoid vaccination during acute infection or chronic illness.

Precautions: Repeated vaccination may result in the development of hypersensitivity to protein constituents of the vaccine. Although anaphylaxis is rare, facilities for its management should always be available during vaccination.

Cholera vaccine is not recommended for administration to infants under the age of one year as reactions are more frequent in this age group.

Intradermal administration of the first dose of a primary course is not recommended.

Side- and adverse effects: Local reactions consisting of pain, redness and swelling may develop within hours of vaccination resulting in discomfort at the site of injection for one or two days. They may be accompanied by fever, malaise and headache. Persons who have received numerous doses of cholera vaccine are particularly susceptible to such reactions even if many years have elapsed since the last vaccination was carried out. Occasionally delayed reactions occur. Serious reactions are uncommon but may include collapse, and rarely neurological symptoms such as neuritis, polyneuritis and various other manifestations of cerebral and meningeal involvement.

Use in pregnancy and lactation: This vaccine has been in wide use for many years without apparent ill consequence. However, as with any agent which may produce a systemic reaction, such as pyrexia, vaccination is, if possible, to be avoided in pregnancy.

Toxicity and treatment of overdosage: Not applicable.

Pharmaceutical precautions Store at 2–8°C. Protect from light. *Do not freeze.* When multidose containers are employed it is good practice to discard any partly used vaccine vials at the end of the vaccinating session.

This preparation on standing has a tendency to settle out in a gelatinous form. This is the nature of the organism in the vaccine and vigorous shaking as a rule will yield a homogenous suspension for injection. The container should on all occasions be well shaken before withdrawing material for injection.

Legal category POM.

Package quantities Vials of 1.5 ml and 10 ml.

Further information Nil.

Product licence number 0003/5126.

DARAPRIM* TABLETS

Presentation Each tablet contains 25 mg of Pyrimethamine BP, Scored and coded A3A and white in colour.

Uses Daraprim acts as a causal prophylactic and suppressive agent against malaria caused by Plasmodium falciparum. It also acts as a suppressant against Plasmodium vivax infections. In areas of known or suspected resistance to pyrimethamine or related compounds, another prophylactic should be used.

Dosage and administration *Adults:* 1 tablet regularly each week.

Children: Over 10 years: 1 tablet regularly each week.

5–10 years: ½ tablet regularly each week.

Under 5 years: Formulation not applicable.

Daraprim is rapidly absorbed and therefore prophylactic cover can be expected shortly after the first dose. Prophylaxis should commence before arrival in an endemic area and be continued once weekly. On returning to a non-malarious area dosage should be maintained for a further four weeks.

Use in the elderly: No specific studies have been carried out in the elderly, however, it may be advisable to monitor renal or hepatic function and if there is serious impairment then caution should be exercised.

Daraprim, at the doses recommended for the prevention of Malaria is unlikely to have any adverse effect on older people normally of good health.

Contra-indications, warnings, etc
Contra-indications: Daraprim should not be given to patients with a history of pyrimethamine sensitivity.

Precautions: The recommended dosage should not be exceeded.

Daraprim should be used with caution in patients with hepatic or renal disorders.

During pregnancy and in other conditions predisposing to folate deficiency, a folate supplement should be given.

Daraprim, by its mode of action, may further depress folate metabolism in patients receiving treatment with other folate inhibitors. Occasional reports suggest that individuals taking pyrimethamine as malarial prophylaxis at doses in excess of 25 mg weekly may develop megaloblastic anaemia if co-trimoxazole is prescribed concurrently.

The concurrent administration of lorazepam and Daraprim may induce hepatotoxicity.

Daraprim may exacerbate folate deficiency due to innate disease or malnutrition.

Side- and adverse effects: At the recommended dose, side-effects are rare. Occasionally, rashes have been observed which disappeared when the administration of Daraprim was stopped. Excessive doses may produce a macrocytic anaemia resembling that of folic acid deficiency. Insomnia has been reported when pyrimethamine has been given at weekly doses above those recommended.

Use in pregnancy and lactation: While there is a theoretical risk of foetal abnormality with all folate inhibitors given during pregnancy, no such adverse effects have been reported with Daraprim in humans. A folate supplement should be given to pregnant women receiving Daraprim. The amount of pyrimethamine excreted in breast milk is insufficient to contra-indicate its use in lactating mothers, but breast-fed infants should not receive other anti-folate agents.

Toxicity and treatment of overdosage: Symptoms reported have included vomiting, cyanosis, respiratory distress, convulsions and tachycardia. Routine supportive treatment , including maintenance of a clear airway and control of convulsions, should be given. Adequate fluids should be given to ensure optimal diuresis. Gastric lavage may be of value only if instituted within two hours of ingestion, in view of the rapid absorption of Daraprim. Fresh blood transfusions to counteract blood dyscrasias should be available.

To counteract possible folate deficiency, calcium folinate 9 to 15 mg daily should be given until the signs of toxicity have subsided. There may be a delay of 7 to 10 days before the full leucopenic side-effects become evident, therefore calcium folinate therapy should be continued for the period at risk.

Pharmaceutical precautions Store below 35°C. Protect from light.

Legal category P.

Package quantities Strip pack of 30 tablets.

Further information When taken as directed Daraprim is an effective antimalarial, but it may be rendered ineffective by the development of drug resistance from time to time in certain regions. Local medical advice about the suitability of the product should, therefore, be obtained immediately on arrival in a malarious region.

Product licence number 0003/5026.

DIGIBIND* ▼
Digoxin-specific antibody fragments (F(ab))

Presentation Each vial of Digibind contains a sterile, lyophilised, crystalline, off-white powder, comprising 40 mg of antigen-binding fragments (F(ab)) derived from specific antidigoxin antibodies raised from sheep, approximately 75 mg Sorbitol BP and approximately 28 mg Sodium Chloride BP.

Uses Digoxin-specific antibody fragments are at present indicated for the reversal of life-threatening manifestations of intoxication by digoxin or by digitoxin. Although designed specifically to treat digoxin overdose, the product has successfully reversed digitoxin overdose.

Dosage and administration F(ab) dosage is governed by the body load of digoxin (or digitoxin) to be counteracted. The load can be estimated in two ways:

either (i) from information on the acutely ingested dose, the amount of which, in mg, should be multiplied by 0.80 to take account of incomplete absorption;

or (ii) from the plasma or serum concentration in the quasi-steady state, which can be assumed for any interval longer than 6 hours after ingesting a dose.

Using the latter method, the following formulae are employed:

digoxin
plasma (serum) concentration (ng/ml)
$\times\ 0.0056 \times$ bodyweight (kg)
= estimated total body load (mg)

Thus, for a plasma (serum) concentration of 20 ng/ml in a patient weighing 70 kg: body load $= 20 \times (0.0056 \times 70) = 7.84$ mg

digitoxin
plasma (serum) concentration (ng/ml)
$\times\ 0.00056 \times$ bodyweight (kg)
= estimated total body load (mg)

Thus, for a plasma (serum) concentration of 250 ng/ml in a patient weighing 65 kg: body load $= 250 \times (0.00056 \times 65) = 9.1$ mg
The plasma concentration factor is derived from the volume of distribution (L/kg body weight) divided by 1000 to reduce the body load estimate to mg.

The approximate molecular weight ratio of F(ab) and digoxin (or digitoxin) is 60. Hence the approximate dose of F(ab) required is 60 times the load, rounded up to the nearest 40 mg, since this is the amount of F(ab) contained in a single vial. Hence, in the examples above, 480 mg (12 vials) and 560 mg (14 vials) would be required respectively.

The content of each vial to be used should be dissolved in 4 ml of Water for Injections BP, thus producing an approximately isosmotic solution with a protein concentration of between 9 and 11 mg/ml. This may then be diluted further to any convenient volume with Sodium Chloride Intravenous Infusion BP. The final solution of F(ab) should be administered intravenously over a 20-minute period through a 0.22 micron Millipore filter, which is recommended to remove any incompletely dissolved aggregates.

If there is incomplete reversion, or a recurrence of toxicity, further F(ab) can be given after a few hours at a dose suggested from the earlier clinical experience.

Use in children and the elderly: There is no information to suggest that the treatment of children or the elderly presents any special risk in an already grave situation – thus they should be dosed in the same way.

Pharmacology: The affinity constant (K_D) of F(ab) for digoxin is high (10^{-10}M) and greater than that of digoxin for its receptor (Na-K ATPase), which is implicated in the digoxin toxic effects. The affinity constant of F(ab) for digitoxin is also high (10^{-9}M). Digoxin (and digitoxin) are therefore attracted away from the receptor on heart tissue (and presumably other tissues as well, though this has not been studied) and their rate of elimination is changed from that governed by the kinetics of receptor binding to that governed by the kinetics of access and elimination of F(ab).

In animals F(ab) reverses digoxin effects much more quickly than does IgG. There is a suggestion that reversal of inotropy with F(ab) lags behind reversal of electrical dysrhythmic effects. This could possibly be due to cellular differences between contractile and conducting tissue, or to differences in accessibility.

The plasma disappearance half-life of F(ab) in the baboon is 9–13 h and that of the parent IgG antibody is 61 h. The total volume of distribution of F(ab) in the baboon is 8.7 times greater than that of IgG and the readier diffusion of the smaller moiety sufficiently accounts for this.

About 93% of radioactively labelled F(ab), injected into baboons, appeared in the urine within 24 h and the corresponding amount of digoxin-specific IgG was less than 1%. However, much of the urinary F(ab) was not intact. Small molecular weight proteins are catabolised by the kidney, as after filtration they are taken up into proximal tubular cells. F(ab) elimination is greatly prolonged in nephrectomised rats, but is actually enhanced in rats whose renal tubules have been damaged by the specific toxin maleate.

Corresponding information on human patients is sparse, but the close relationship of the therapeutic performance to predictions suggests that the animal data will be helpful. The human plasma disappearance half-life after intravenous administration of F(ab) is about 16 h with good renal function.

Several patients with renal dysfunction have received digoxin-specific F(ab). The time course of therapeutic effect was not distinguishable from that in patients with good function. In the patient with virtually no renal excretory function, the reticuloendothelial system might be expected to eliminate the complex. Whether elimination would be accomplished with the digoxin still bound, rendered inactive, is not known.

Ordinarily, following administration of F(ab), improvements in signs and symptoms begin within 30 minutes. At the same time, the plasma digoxin concentration rises sharply. The digoxin is protein-bound and pharmacologically inactive. The free digoxin remains less than 0.2 ng/ml in intoxicated dogs treated with IgG.

Contra-indications, warnings, etc
Contra-indications: None known.

Precautions: Digibind has been used in only a small number of humans. Therefore it should be used with care and only when other modes of therapy have proved inadequate or are anticipated to be inadequate.

Although no allergic responses have yet occurred in man, the possibility of anaphylactic, hypersensitivity or febrile reactions should be borne in mind. Patients known to be allergic to ovine proteins would be particularly at risk, as would individuals who have previously received digoxin-specific antibody fragments raised from sheep.

Since the F(ab) fragment of the antibody lacks the antigenic determinants of the F(c) fragment, it should pose less of an immunogenic threat to patients than does an intact immunoglobulin molecule.

Several patients with mild to moderate renal dysfunction have been successfully treated with digoxin-specific antibody fragments. The elimination half-life in the presence of renal failure has not been clearly defined but is expected to be substantially prolonged. The time course of therapeutic effect has not been different in these patients, but excretion of the antibody fragment-digoxin complex from the body should be delayed.

Patients previously dependent on the inotropism of digoxin could develop signs of heart failure when treated with Digibind. After successful management of poisoning, digoxin has had to be reinstituted in some cases. During management, additional inotropic support can be obtained from intravenous dopamine or dobutamine, but caution is required as catecholamines can aggravate dysrhythmias caused by cardiac glycosides.

Laboratory tests: Patients should be closely monitored, including blood pressure and electrocardiogram, at all times during and after administration of Digibind. Presence of the exogenous antibody fragments will interfere with radioimmunoassay measurements of digoxin.

Potassium concentrations should be followed carefully, since severe digitalis intoxication can cause life-threatening elevation in serum potassium concentration by shifting it from within the cells. Such patients often have a total body deficit of potassium, and when the effect of digitalis is reversed by Digibind, potassium returns to the cell causing hypokalaemia.

Side- and adverse effects: None so far observed.

Use in pregnancy and lactation: Animal reproduction studies have not been conducted with Digibind. Whether Digibind can cause foetal damage when administered to a pregnant woman or can affect reproductive capacity is not known. Hence digoxin-specific antibody fragments should be given to a pregnant woman only if clearly needed.

Carcinogenesis, multagenesis, impairment of fertility: There have been no long-term studies performed in animals to evaluate carcinogenic or mutagenic potential or effects on fertility.

Toxicity and treatment of overdosage: Not relevant.

Pharmaceutical precautions Store at 2–8°C. Protect from light.

Legal category POM.

Package quantities Single vial of lyophilised powder containing 40 mg of antigen-binding fragments (F(ab)).

Further information Digoxin-specific antibody fragments (F(ab)) have been used successfully to treat a case of lanatoside C intoxication.

The scale of usage in man has been small and the safety of Digibind is not well established, hence Digibind should only be considered when the response to conventional measures is inadequate or when the response to such measures would be expected to be inadequate. Ordinarily, these measures will have included withdrawal of the glycoside, attempts to control cardiac dysrhythmias by potassium supplements, beta-blockade, class 1 antidysrhythmics or possibly direct current electro-shock, attempts to control sinus bradycardia or atrioventricular block by atropine or pacemaker and attempts to mitigate aggravating factors such as electro-lyte disturbances, hypoxia, acid-base imbalance or catecholamine excess.

Product licence number 0003/0207.

ADSORBED DIPHTHERIA VACCINE BP, WELLCOME* (Dip/Vac/Ads)

Presentation Adsorbed Diphtheria Vaccine is a suspension of highly purified toxoid prepared from the exotoxin of *Corynebacterium diphtheriae* adsorbed onto hydrated aluminium phosphate. The aluminium content does not exceed 1.25 mg/dose. Thiomersal BP is added as a preservative to a concentration of 0.01%

Each 0.5 ml dose has an immunising potency of not less than 30 International Units (IU).

The immunising potency of this vaccine is now expressed in International Units in accordance with the requirements of the European and British Pharmacopoeias. These units measure the immunising activity of the vaccine whereas the previously used Lf units expressed the quantity of toxoid present. There is no simple numerical relationship between IU and Lf. No change has been made to the potency although it is now expressed in IU.

Uses For active immunisation against diphtheria.

Primary immunisation against diphtheria in infancy is usually carried out by the administration of combined adsorbed diphtheria and tetanus (DT/Vac/Ads) or Trivax* (DTPer/Vac) or Trivax-Ad* (DTPer/Vac/Ads). Primary immunisation against diphtheria alone for children under the age of 10 years may be carried out with adsorbed diphtheria vaccine. It may also be used in Schick-positive adults and children over the age of 10 years who are at particular risk.

Dosage and administration The primary course of immunisation is two doses given by intramuscular or deep subcutaneous injection separated by an interval of at least four weeks.

In the UK and many other countries a third dose is advised in order to ensure long-lasting immunity.

Adults and children over 10 years of age: Two doses of 0.2 ml.

Children under 10 years of age: Two doses of 0.5 ml.

A reinforcing dose of 0.5 ml should be administered at about five years of age to children immunised in infancy.

Oral Poliomyelitis Vaccine BP may be given at the same time as Diphtheria Vaccine.

Shake well before each dose is withdrawn. It is good practice to record the title, dose and lot numbers of all vaccines and the dates of administration. Any untoward reactions should be reported to the regulatory authorities and to the manufacturer.

Use in the elderly: No special comment.

Contra-indications, warnings, etc

Contra-indications: Adsorbed diphtheria vaccine should not be administered intradermally. The vaccine should not be administered to a subject who has experienced a serious reaction (e.g. anaphylaxis) to a previous dose of this vaccine or who is known to be hypersensitive to any component thereof. It is advisable to avoid vaccination during an acute infection.

Precautions: Adsorbed Diphtheria Vaccine should not be administered to children over the age of 10 years or to adults without a preliminary Schick test, to avoid giving vaccine to persons who are already immune or to those who are hypersensitive, i.e. those who show a negative-or-pseudo-Schick reaction.

Although anaphylaxis is rare, facilities for its management should always be available during vaccination.

Side- and adverse effects: Local reactions consisting of swelling, redness and tenderness at the injection site may occur and occasionally may be severe. They may be more frequent and severe after the second than the first injection. Local reactions are uncommon in children under two years of age.

General reactions consisting of transient fever, malaise and headache may occur.

Allergic reactions, urticaria, pallor and dyspnoea have been reported following injection of adsorbed diphtheria vaccine.

A small painless nodule may form at the injection site but usually disappears without sequelae. However, persistent nodules at the injection site may occasionally follow the administration of this vaccine especially if the inoculation is introduced into the superficial layers of subcutaneous tissue.

Use in pregnancy and lactation: Accurate information is not available on the safety of the vaccine in pregnancy.

Toxicity and treatment of overdosage: Not applicable.

Pharmaceutical precautions Store at 2–8°C. Protect from light.
   Do not freeze.

Legal category POM.

Package quantities Box of 5 × 0.5 ml ampoules.

Further information Nil.

Product licence number 0003/5128.

DIPHTHERIA AND TETANUS VACCINE BP, WELLCOME* (DT/Vac/FT)

Presentation Diphtheria and tetanus vaccine is a mixture of purified diphtheria and tetanus toxoids which are prepared by formalin detoxification of *Corynebacterium diphtheriae* and *Clostridium tetani* exotoxins. Thiomersal BP is added as a preservative to a concentration of 0.01%. Each 0.5 ml dose contains 25 Lf diphtheria toxoid and 3.5 Lf tetanus toxoid.

The antigenic content and formulation of this vaccine has not been changed, although the labelled content of the tetanus component has been altered to conform with the flocculation equivalence of the new British reference antitoxin preparation.

Uses For reinforcement of immunity at five years or over in children who were immunised in infancy with either adsorbed diphtheria-tetanus vaccine (DT/Vac/Ads) or with Trivax* (DTPer/Vac) or Trivax-Ad* (DTPer/Vac/Ads) and who do not require continued immunisation against whooping cough.

The more potent antigen, Adsorbed Diphtheria and Tetanus Vaccine is preferred for primary immunisation against diphtheria and tetanus, but either preparation of combined diphtheria-tetanus vaccine may be used for reinforcement of immunity.

Simultaneous reinforcement of immunity to diphtheria and tetanus in adults and children over 10 years of age is rarely needed. Diphtheria-containing vaccines should not be given unless a Schick test has been carried out to avoid giving the vaccine to persons who are already immune or to those who are hypersensitive, i.e. those who show a negative-or-pseudo-Schick reaction.

Dosage and administration The vaccine is given by intramuscular or deep subcutaneous injection.

Children under 10 years: 0.5 ml.

Adults and children over 10 years: 0.2 ml.

Use in the elderly: No special comment.

In subjects who suffered a reaction to a previous dose of adsorbed vaccine it may be preferable to administer 0.1 ml of Diphtheria and Tetanus vaccine in Simple Solution intradermally. Oral Poliomyelitis Vaccine BP may be given at the same time as Diphtheria Tetanus Vaccine.

Shake well before withdrawing a dose. It is good practice to record the title, dose and lot numbers of all vaccines and the dates of administration. Any untoward reactions should be reported to the regulatory authorities and to the manufacturer.

Contra-indications, warnings, etc

Contra-indications: The vaccine should not be administered to a subject who has experienced a serious reaction (e.g. anaphylaxis) to a previous dose of this vaccine or who is known to be hypersensitive to any component thereof. It is advisable to avoid vaccination during an acute infection.

Precautions: Although anaphylaxis is rare, facilities for its management should always be available during vaccination.

Side- and adverse effects: Local reactions, swelling, redness and tenderness at the injection site, and general reactions, transient fever, malaise and headache may be caused by either or both component toxoids. Acute allergic reactions – anaphylaxis, urticaria, angioneurotic oedema, pallor and dyspnoea, serum sickness and peripheral neuropathy have been reported following administration of diphtheria or tetanus vaccines.

Transverse myelitis has been reported after simultaneous administration of diphtheria and tetanus vaccine and oral polio vaccine, but a cause and effect relationship has not been established.

Use in pregnancy and lactation: Since simultaneous vaccination against diphtheria and tetanus in adults is uncommon, there is no accurate information on the safety of this vaccine in pregnancy.

Toxicity and treatment of overdosage: Not applicable.

Pharmaceutical precautions Store at 2–8°C. Protect from light.
   Do not freeze.
   When multi-dose containers are employed it is good practice to discard any partly used vaccine vials at the end of the vaccinating session.

Legal category POM.

Package quantities Vial of 5 ml.

Further information Nil.

Product licence number 0003/5130.

ADSORBED DIPHTHERIA AND TETANUS VACCINE BP, WELLCOME* (DT/Vac/Ads)

Presentation Adsorbed diphtheria and tetanus vaccine is a mixture of highly purified diphtheria and tetanus toxoids which are prepared by formalin detoxification of

Corynebacterium diphtheriae and *Clostridium tetani* exotoxins. The toxoids are adsorbed onto aluminium hydroxide. The aluminium content does not exceed 1.25 mg/dose. Thiomersal BP is added as a preservative to a concentration of 0.01%. Each 0.5 ml dose contains not less than 30 i.u. diphtheria toxoid and 40 i.u. tetanus toxoid.

The immunising potency of this vaccine is now expressed in International Units in accordance with the requirements of the European and British Pharmacopoeias. These units measure the immunising activity of the vaccine whereas the previously used Lf units expressed the quantity of toxoid present. There is no simple numerical relationship between IU and Lf. No change has been made to the potency although it is now expressed in IU.

Uses For active immunisation against diphtheria and tetanus.

Adsorbed diphtheria and tetanus vaccine is used principally for the primary immunisation of infants and children under ten years of age against tetanus and diphtheria where the use of pertussis-containing vaccines (DTPer/Vac, DTPer/Vac/Ads) is contra-indicated or not required. It is also given to reinforce immunity in children under 10 years of age immunised in infancy with diphtheria and tetanus vaccine. Trivax* or Trivax-Ad* (DT/Vac/Ads, DTPer/Vac, DTPer/Vac/Ads).

Simultaneous primary immunisation or reinforcement of immunity to diphtheria and tetanus in adults and children over 10 years of age is rarely needed. Diphtheria-containing vaccines should not be given to these subjects unless a Schick test has been carried out to avoid immunising persons who are already immune and/or hypersensitive, i.e., those who show a negative-and/or-pseudo-Schick reaction.

Dosage and administration For primary immunisation two intramuscular or deep subcutaneous injections separated by an interval of at least four weeks are recommended.

In the UK and many other countries a third dose is advised in order to ensure long-lasting immunity.

Children under 10 years: Two doses of 0.5 ml.

Adults and children over 10 years: Two doses of 0.2 ml.

A single dose of adsorbed tetanus vaccine should be administered 6 to 12 months after the second dose of the combined diphtheria and tetanus vaccine to complete the primary course of immunisation against tetanus.

A reinforcing dose of 0.5 ml of adsorbed or simple diphtheria and tetanus vaccines should be administered at about five years of age to children immunised in infancy with diphtheria and tetanus vaccine or combined diphtheria, tetanus and pertussis vaccine.

It may be preferable to administer 0.1 ml of Diphtheria and Tetanus vaccine in simple solution intradermally to adults and children who have suffered a reaction to a previous dose of adsorbed vaccine.

Poliomyelitis vaccine (oral) may be given at the same time as diphtheria and tetanus vaccine.

Shake thoroughly before withdrawing each dose. It is good practice to record the title, dose and lot numbers of all vaccines and the dates of administration. Any untoward reactions should be reported to the regulatory authorities and to the manufacturer.

Use in the elderly: No special comment.

Contra-indications, warnings, etc

Contra-indications: Adsorbed Diphtheria and Tetanus vaccine should not be administered intradermally.

The vaccine should not be administered to a subject who has experienced a serious reaction (e.g. anaphylaxis) to a previous dose of this vaccine or who is known to be hypersensitive to any component thereof. It is advisable to avoid vaccination during an acute infection.

Precautions: Although anaphylaxis is rare, facilities for its management should always be available during vaccination.

Side- and adverse effects: Local reactions, swelling, redness and tenderness at the injection site, and general reactions, transient fever, malaise and headache may be caused by either or both component toxoids. Acute allergic reactions – anaphylaxis, urticaria, angioneurotic oedema, pallor and dyspnoea, serum sickness and peripheral neuropathy have been reported following administration of diphtheria or tetanus vaccines.

Persistent nodules at the injection site may occasionally follow administration of adsorbed vaccine, especially if the inoculation is into the superficial layers of subcutaneous tissue.

Transverse myelitis has been reported after simultaneous administration of diphtheria and tetanus vaccine and oral polio vaccine, but a cause and effect relationship has not been established.

Use in pregnancy and lactation: Since simultaneous vaccination against diphtheria and tetanus in adults is uncommon there is no accurate information on the safety of this vaccine in pregnancy.

Toxicity and treatment of overdosage: Not applicable.

Pharmaceutical precautions Store at 2–8°C. Protect from light.

Do not freeze.

It is good practice to discard any partly used vaccine vials at the end of the vaccinating session.

Legal category POM.

Package quantities Box of 5 × 0.5 ml ampoules. Vial of 5 ml.

Further information Nil.

Product licence number 0003/5131.

FLOLAN* ▼

Presentation Each vial contains 500 mcg (500,000 nanograms (ng)) freeze-dried epoprostenol (formerly known as prostacyclin) as the sodium salt. The contents of the vial will have the appearance of a white, or off-white fluffy solid.

Each 50 ml vial of sterile diluent for Flolan contains Sodium Chloride BP 0.147% w/v and Glycine BP 0.188% w/v in clear solution. The alkalinity of the diluent has been adjusted to pH 10.5 ± 0.3 by the addition of sodium hydroxide.

A filter unit is provided for use during reconstitution.

Uses *Cardiopulmonary bypass:* Flolan is indicated for the preservation of platelet numbers and function during cardiopulmonary bypass. It may therefore improve post-operative haemostasis.

Charcoal haemoperfusion: Flolan is indicated for the prevention of platelet activation during charcoal haemoperfusion of patients in fulminant hepatic failure.

Renal dialysis: Flolan is indicated as an alternative to

heparin during renal dialysis, especially when a high risk of bleeding problems due to heparin exists.

Pharmacology:
Epoprostenol is a naturally occurring prostaglandin produced by the intima of blood vessels and is the most potent inhibitor of platelet aggregation known. The inhibition is dose-related. Unlike many other prostaglandins, it is not metabolised during passage through the pulmonary circulation.

Epoprostenol sodium is a potent vasodilator. The cardiovascular effects disappear within 30 minutes of the end of infusion.

It inhibits platelet aggregation by elevating platelet cyclic adenosine monophosphate. The action is dose-related above 2 nanograms/kg/min, following intravenous administration. Significant inhibition of aggregation induced by adenosine diphosphate is observed after intravenous administration of 4 or more nanograms/kg/min. Effects on platelets usually disappear within 30 minutes of discontinuing infusion of epoprostenol sodium.

Higher doses of epoprostenol sodium (20 nanograms/kg/min) disperse circulating platelet aggregates and increase by up to twofold the cutaneous bleeding time.

Epoprostenol sodium reduces platelet procoagulant activity and the release of heparin neutralising factor.

The fate of epoprostenol sodium in man is not fully established. At normal physiological pH and temperature, epoprostenol sodium is hydrolysed with a half-life of 2–3 minutes to 6-keto prostaglandin $F_{1\alpha}$.

Dosage and administration Flolan is suitable for continuous infusion only, either intravascularly or into the blood supplying the extracorporeal circulation.

The following schedules of infusion have been found effective in adults:

Cardiopulmonary bypass: After induction of anaesthesia, until the start of bypass: 10 nanograms/kg/min intravenously by central venous catheter. During bypass: 20 nanograms/kg/min intravenously by central venous catheter.

The infusion should be stopped at the end of bypass.

Charcoal haemoperfusion: Prior to the start of charcoal haemoperfusion: 2–16 nanograms/kg/min intravenously. During charcoal haemoperfusion: 16 nanograms/kg/min into the proximal line of the charcoal column.

The infusion should be stopped at the end of haemoperfusion.

Renal dialysis: Prior to dialysis: 5 nanograms/kg/min intravenously. During dialysis: 5 nanograms/kg/min into the arterial inlet of the dialyser.

The recommended doses should be exceeded only with appropriate patient monitoring.

Use in children:
There is no information on the use of Flolan in children for cardiopulmonary bypass, charcoal haemoperfusion or renal dialysis.

Use in the elderly: There is no evidence to indicate whether modification of dosage in the elderly is required.

Reconstitution:
Only the diluent provided for the purpose should be used. The enclosed filter unit must be used once only and then discarded after use.

To reconstitute Flolan, a strict aseptic technique must be used. *Particular care should be taken in calculating dilutions,* and in diluting Flolan the following procedure is recommended:

1. Withdraw approximately 10 ml of the sterile diluent into a sterile syringe.
2. Inject the contents of the syringe into the vial containing Flolan and dissolve the contents completely.
3. Draw up all the Flolan solution into the syringe.
4. Re-inject the entire contents into the residue of the original 50 ml of sterile diluent.
5. Mix well. This solution is now referred to as the *concentrated solution* and contains Flolan 10,000 nanograms per millilitre. The *concentrated solution* is normally further diluted before use. It may be diluted with physiological saline (0.9%), provided a ratio of 6 volumes of saline to 1 volume of *concentrated solution* is not exceeded; e.g. 50 ml of *concentrated solution* further diluted with a maximum of 300 ml saline.
6. Before further dilution, draw up the *concentrated solution* into a larger syringe.
7. The filter provided should then be attached to the syringe and the *concentrated solution* is dispensed by filtration using firm but not excessive pressure. The typical time taken for filtration of 50 ml of solution is 70 seconds.

In general, the infusion rate may be calculated by the following formula:

Infusion rate (ml/min)

$$= \frac{\text{Dosage (ng/kg/min)} \times \text{body weight (kg)}}{\text{Concentration of infusion (ng/ml)}}$$

For administration using a pump capable of delivering small volume constant infusions, suitable aliquots of concentrated solution may be diluted with sterile physiological saline. For example, 35 ml of *concentrated solution* made up to 50 ml with sterile saline to give a solution containing epoprostenol 7,000 nanograms/ml will, when infused at 0.1 ml/min, deliver a dose of 10 nanograms/kg/min to a 70 kg patient.

Other common intravenous fluids are unsatisfactory for the dilution of the *concentrated solution* as the required pH is not attained. Flolan solutions are less stable at low pH.

Contra-indications, warnings, etc
Contra-indications:
There are no recognised contra-indications to the administration of Flolan in cardiopulmonary bypass, charcoal haemoperfusion or renal dialysis.

Precautions:
Epoprostenol sodium is a potent vasodilator. The cardiovascular effects disappear within 30 minutes of the end of the infusion.

Epoprostenol sodium is not a conventional anticoagulant and should not be used to replace heparin in cardiopulmonary bypass or charcoal haemoperfusion. Flolan has been successfully used instead of heparin in renal dialyses, but in a small proportion of dialyses clotting has developed in the dialysis circuit, requiring termination of dialysis.

Haemorrhagic complications have not been encountered when Flolan has been administered during surgery but the possibility should be considered when the drug is administered to patients with spontaneous or drug-induced haemorrhagic diatheses.

The vasodilator effect of Flolan may augment or be augmented by concomitant use of other vasodilators.

The effects of epoprostenol sodium on heart-rate may

be masked by concomitant use of drugs which affect cardiovascular reflexes.

If excessive hypotension occurs during administration of epoprostenol sodium, the dose should be reduced or the infusion discontinued. The hypotensive effect of epoprostenol may be enhanced by the use of acetate buffer in the dialysis bath during renal dialysis.

Elevated serum glucose levels have been reported during infusion of epoprostenol sodium in man.

Use in pregnancy and lactation:
In the absence of adequate experience of administration of Flolan to pregnant or lactating women, the potential benefit to the mother must be weighed against the unknown risks to the foetus and infant.

Side- and adverse effects:
Facial flushing is commonly seen, even in the anaesthetised patient.

Headache and gastro-intestinal symptoms including nausea, vomiting and abdominal colic have occurred in some conscious individuals.

Jaw pain, dry mouth, lassitude, reddening over the infusion site, chest pain and tightness have been reported with varying frequency.

Bradycardia associated with a considerable fall in systolic and diastolic blood pressure has followed intravenous administration of a dose of epoprostenol sodium equivalent to 30 nanograms/kg/min in healthy conscious volunteers. Bradycardia, accompanied by pallor, nausea, sweating and sometimes abdominal discomfort and orthostatic hypotension, has occurred in healthy volunteers at doses of epoprostenol greater than 5 nanograms/kg/min.

Toxicity and treatment of overdosage:
The main feature of overdosage is likely to be hypotension.

Reduce the dose or discontinue the infusion and initiate appropriate supportive measures as necessary; for example, plasma volume expansion and/or adjustment to bypass pump flow.

Pharmaceutical precautions Concentrated solutions of Flolan (10,000 nanograms per millilitre) in glycine buffer, when diluted to a maximum of 1:6 with Sodium Chloride Intravenous Infusion BP 0.9% w/v, will retain 90% of initial potency for at least 12 hours at room temperature. No other concentration of reconstituted Flolan should be diluted and no other intravenous fluid should be used for dilution of the concentrated solution.

Flolan should be reconstituted only with the glycine buffer supplied.

Flolan should not be used if more than 12 hours have elapsed since reconstitution. Glycine buffer vials contain no preservative, consequently they should be used once and then discarded. Vials of Flolan should be stored between 2–8°C and protected from light. Vials of sterile diluent should be stored between 2–8°C and should not be frozen.

Legal category POM.

Package quantities 1 vial of 500 mcg epoprostenol with 1 vial of diluent.

Further information Flolan may potentiate the action of heparin, and standard anticoagulant monitoring is advisable when Flolan is administered to patients receiving concomitant anticoagulants.

Product licence number 0003/0151.

HUMOTET* ANTITETANUS IMMUNOGLOBULIN INJECTION BP

Presentation Purified immunoglobulin obtained from the sera of healthy human donors known to have high levels of tetanus antitoxin following active immunisation with tetanus vaccine.

Humotet is a clear, colourless, semi-viscous liquid containing thiomersal 0.01% as a preservative, and glycine 2.25%. Each vial contains 250 i.u. of tetanus antitoxin in 1.0 ml solution.

Uses For passive immunisation against tetanus, in conjunction with adsorbed tetanus vaccine as soon as practicable after a tetanus-susceptible person has sustained a wound. Also for the treatment of tetanus.

Dosage and administration *Prevention of tetanus following injury: Adults and children:* Humotet should be administered by intramuscular injection usually in a dose of 250 i.u. – see table below.

Persons not immunised, or inadequately immunised, with tetanus vaccine are susceptible to tetanus and all wounds are prone to tetanus infection. In cases of doubt a person should be regarded as inadequately immunised.

Administration of immunoglobulin does not obviate the need for debridement and wound cleansing, nor does it contra-indicate the use of antibiotics.

The prophylactic immunisation schedule against tetanus (see table) should be carried out as soon as possible after a person has sustained a wound. Passive immunisation with immunoglobulin should be accompanied by simultaneous active immunisation with adsorbed tetanus vaccine.

If more than 24 hours have elapsed since the wound was sustained or if there is a risk of heavy contamination with *Clostridium tetani* 2 ml (500 i.u.). Humotet should be given, irrespective of immunisation history.

Humotet and adsorbed tetanus vaccine should be administered with separate syringes and into separate sites. Tetanus vaccine in simple solution is unsuitable for administration concurrently with Humotet.

A single dose of Humotet usually provides a protective level of tetanus antitoxin, over 0.01 i.u. per ml serum, for a period of four weeks. Long-term immunity against tetanus is conferred by giving further doses of vaccine; see table above.

Treatment of tetanus: Adults and children: 30–300 i.u. per kilogram body weight given intramuscularly.

Use in the elderly: No special comment.

Contra-indications, warnings, etc
Contra-indications: Humotet should not be given intravenously. The administration of immunoglobulin may be contra-indicated by a history of anaphylaxis resulting from administration of a previous dose of human gamma-globulin.

Precautions: Humotet should not be given concurrently with tetanus in simple solution.

Although anaphylaxis is rare, facilities for its management should always be available during vaccination.

Side- and adverse effects: A local reaction, consisting of a small area of inflammation and tenderness, may occur after administration of the immunoglobulin, but this rarely constitutes more than a temporary inconvenience. Constitutional upsets, and particularly anaphylactic reactions, are uncommon. Patients with antibody deficiency syndromes may be liable to have local reactions after administration of the immunoglobulin.

Patient's history	Immediate action		Follow-up action
Previous record of receiving tetanus vaccine	Administer Humotet	Administer adsorbed tetanus vaccine	Administer tetanus vaccine (adsorbed or in simple solution)
None or Not known	1.0 ml (250 i.u.)	0.5 ml	0.5 ml after 6–12 weeks and 6–12 months
One dose (during last 6 weeks)	1.0 ml (250 i.u.)	0.5 ml to be given 4–6 weeks after first dose of vaccine	0.5 ml 6–12 months after second dose
One dose (more than 6 weeks ago)	1.0 ml (250 i.u.)	0.5 ml	0.5 ml 6–12 months after second dose
Two doses	Nil	0.5 ml to be given if more than 6 weeks after second dose of vaccine	Nil
Three doses	Nil	0.5 ml if more than 1 year since third dose of vaccine	Nil

Use in pregnancy and lactation: Accurate information is not available on the safety of Humotet in pregnancy.

Toxicity and treatment of overdosage: Not applicable.

Pharmaceutical precautions Store at 2–8°C.
Do not freeze. Protect from light.

Legal category POM.

Package quantities Vial containing 250 i.u. in 1.0 ml.

Further information Nil.

Product licence number 0003/0087.

INSULINS – NORDISK WELLCOME

HUMAN VELOSULIN* ▼
HUMAN INSULATARD* ▼
HUMAN MIXTARD* 30/70 ▼
HUMAN INITARD* 50/50. ▼

Presentation Human Velosulin (Neutral Insulin Injection) is a neutral solution of highly purified human insulin (emp).

Human Insulatard (Isophane Insulin Injection [NPH]) is a neutral suspension of highly purified microcrystalline human insulin (emp).

Human Mixtard 30/70 is a neutral suspension of highly purified human insulin (emp) comprising 30% Neutral Insulin in solution and 70% Isophane Insulin in microcrystalline form.

Human Initard 50/50 is a neutral suspension of highly purified human insulin (emp) comprising 50% Neutral Insulin in solution and 50% Isophane Insulin in microcrystalline form.

All the above insulins are available in 100 iu/ml strength. The vials are fitted with orange-coloured disposable plastic caps as a security safeguard. No attempt should be made to refit the caps after removal. Additionally, to aid identification, Human Velosulin has one, Human Insulatard two, Human Mixtard 30/70 three and Human Initard 50/50 four raised tactile marks on the aluminium closure ring.

Uses The treatment of insulin-requiring diabetic patients. Human Velosulin has a rapid onset and a short duration of action making it particularly suitable for the treatment of diabetic coma and pre-coma.

Dosage and administration The dosage of insulin is determined by the physician according to the needs of the patient. Human Velosulin, Human Insulatard, Human Mixtard 30/70 and Human Initard 50/50 may be mixed in all proportions without changing the characteristic effect of any of the types of insulin.

Human Velosulin may be given by subcutaneous, intramuscular or intravenous injection or infusion. It has an onset of action of approximately 30 minutes after subcutaneous injection with duration of about 8 hours, the maximum effect being 1 to 3 hours after injection.

Human Insulatard, Human Mixtard 30/70 and Human Initard 50/50 should be well mixed by gently inverting the vial several times before being given either once or twice daily by subcutaneous or intramuscular injection. Human Insulatard, Human Mixtard 30/70 and Human Initard 50/50 should not be given intravenously.

Human Insulatard has an onset of action of approximately $1\frac{1}{2}$ hours after subcutaneous injection with an overall duration of action which may extend to 24 hours, the maximum effect occurring 4 to 12 hours after injection.

Human Mixtard 30/70 and Human Initard 50/50 each have a duration of action of some $\frac{1}{2}$ to 24 hours after subcutaneous injection, the maximum effect occurring 4 to 8 hours after injection. Human Initard 50/50 has a stronger initial effect than Human Mixtard 30/70.

Onset of action is more rapid and overall duration of action shorter following intramuscular injection than with the subcutaneous route assuming adequate vascular perfusion.

Use in pregancy and lactation: It is essential to maintain continuous good control of the insulin-requiring diabetic patient throughout pregnancy. In the insulin-treated (gestational or insulin-dependent) pregnant diabetic patient, the insulin requirements fall during the first trimester and increase during the second and third trimesters.

Use in the elderly: Clearance rates may be reduced in the elderly due to falling renal function. Insulin may therefore have a more prolonged action. Dose requirements should be regularly reviewed.

Contra-indications, warnings, etc
Contra-indications: Insulin is contra-indicated in hypoglycaemia.

Precautions: Variations in lifestyle and other factors, eg, infection and pregnancy, can affect insulin requirements.

Patients previously treated with insulin of beef or mixed beef/pork origin may require a dosage adjustment on transfer to highly purified human insulin (emp).

Hypoglycaemia can be enhanced by drugs including the following: aspirin; sulphonylureas and agents affecting them; certain steroids.

Hyperglycaemia can be enhanced by drugs including the following: triiodothyronine; thyroxine; various natural and synthetic steroids, including some oral contraceptives; diuretics, including thiazides; cyclophosphamide.

Certain β-blockers, especially propranolol, may affect insulin requirements and mask the signs of hypoglycaemia mediated by the sympathetic nervous system.

Monoamine oxidase inhibitors (MAOI) may potentiate the action of insulin.

Side-and adverse effects: The most important side-effect is hypoglycaemia. Reduction of hyperglycaemia in newly diagnosed diabetics may alter visual refraction.

Insulin, and protamine, like any other injected proteins, are potentially immunogenic. This may or may not have clinical implications. Local reactions at the injection site may include transient erythema, induration, urticaria and oedema. The incidence is minimal with highly purified human insulin (emp). These usually resolve with continuing usage of insulin. True generalised hypersensitivity reactions approaching anaphylaxis are very rare.

Clinical evidence suggests that highly purified human insulins (emp) are unlikely to cause localised lipodystrophies, However, at present, this possibility cannot be totally excluded.

Toxicity and treatment of overdosage: The symptoms and signs of hypoglycaemia depend on the patient's clinical state and on the rate and extent of the fall in blood glucose levels.

If possible, glucose, sucrose, or rapidly absorbable carbohydrate should be taken by mouth. Failing this, hypoglycaemia should be reversed as rapidly as possible by intravenous injection of glucose 50% solution. Alternative emergency treatments include the subcutaneous injection of up to 1 ml of adrenaline solution 1:1000 or the subcutaneous, intramuscular or intravenous injection of lyophilised glucagon 0.5–1.0 mg (1 unit= 1.0 mg). Both adrenaline and glucagon injections mobilise hepatic glycogen, but the effect is short lived and must be supplemented by freely available carbohydrate as soon as possible.

Pharmaceutical precautions Nordisk Wellcome highly purified human insulins (emp) should be stored between 2 and 8°C, protected from sunlight. Insulin which has been frozen should not be used.

Legal category P.

Package quantities 10 ml glass vials.

Further information Mixing of these highly purified human insulins (emp) with preparations of other species is not recommended.

Product licence numbers

Nordisk-UK Ltd		The Wellcome Foundation Ltd
Human Velosulin	3132/0031	0003/0211
Human Insulatard	3132/0034	0003/0212
Human Mixtard 30/70	3132/0037	0003/0213
Human Initard 50/50	3132/0040	0003/0214

VELOSULIN*
INSULATARD*
MIXTARD* 30/70
INITARD* 50/50

Presentation Velosulin (Neutral Insulin Injection BP) is a neutral solution of highly purified pork insulin.

Insulatard (Isophane Insulin Injection BP [NPH]) is a neutral suspension of highly purified microcrystalline pork insulin.

Mixtard 30/70 is a neutral suspension of highly purified pork insulin comprising 30% Neutral Insulin in solution and 70% Isophane Insulin in microcrystalline form.

Initard 50/50 is a neutral suspension of highly purified pork insulin comprising 50% Neutral Insulin in solution and 50% Isophane Insulin in microcrystalline form.

All the above insulins are available in 100 iu/ml strength. The vials are fitted with orange coloured disposable plastic caps as a security safeguard. No attempt should be made to refit the caps after removal. Additionally, to aid identification, Velosulin has one, Insulatard two, Mixtard 30/70 three and Initard 50/50 four raised tactile marks on the aluminium closure ring.

Uses The treatment of insulin-requiring diabetic patients. Velosulin has a rapid onset and a short duration of action making it particularly suitable for the treatment of diabetic coma and pre-coma.

Dosage and administration The dosage of insulin is determined by the physician according to the needs of the patient. Velosulin, Insulatard, Mixtard 30/70 and Initard 50/50 may be mixed in all proportions without changing the characteristic effect of any of the types of insulin.

Velosulin may be given by subcutaneous, intramuscular or intravenous injection or infusion. It has an onset of action of approximately 30 minutes after subcutaneous injection with duration of about 8 hours, the maximum effect being 1 to 3 hours after injection.

Insulatard, Mixtard 30/70 and Initard 50/50 should be well mixed by gently inverting the vial several times before being given either once or twice daily by subcutaneous or intramuscular injection. Insulatard, Mixtard 30/70 and Initard 50/50 should not be given intravenously.

Insulatard has an onset of action of approximately 1½ hours after subcutaneous injection with an overall duration of action which may extend to 24 hours, the maximum effect occurring 4 to 12 hours after injection.

Mixtard 30/70 and Initard 50/50 each have a duration of action of some ½ to 24 hours after subcutaneous injection, the maximum effect occurring 4 to 8 hours after injection. Initard 50/50 has a stronger initial effect than Mixtard 30/70.

Onset of action is more rapid and overall duration of action shorter following intramuscular injection than with the subcutaneous route assuming adequate vascular perfusion.

Use in pregnancy and lactation: It is essential to maintain continuous good control of the insulin-requiring diabetic patient throughout pregnancy. In the insulin-treated (gestational or insulin-dependent) pregnant diabetic patient, the insulin requirements fall during the first trimester and increase during the second and third trimesters.

Use in the elderly: Clearance rates may be reduced in the elderly due to falling renal function. Insulin may therefore have a more prolonged action. Dose requirements should be regularly reviewed

Contra-indications, warnings, etc
Contra-indications: Insulin is contra-indicated in hypoglycaemia.

Precautions: Variations in lifestyle and other factors, eg. infection and pregnancy, can affect insulin requirements.

Patients previously treated with insulin of beef or mixed beef/pork origin may require a dosage adjustment on transfer to highly purified pork insulin.

Hypoglycaemia can be enhanced by drugs including the following: aspirin; sulphonylureas and agents affecting them; certain steroids.

Hyperglycaemia can be enhanced by drugs including the following: triiodothyronine; thyroxine; various natural and synthetic steroids, including some oral contraceptives; diuretics, including thiazides; cyclophosphamide.

Certain β-blockers, especially propranolol, may affect insulin requirements and mask the signs of hypoglycaemia mediated by the sympathetic nervous system.

Monoamine oxidase inhibitors (MAOI) may potentiate the action of insulin.

Side-and adverse effects: The most important side-effect is hypoglycaemia. Reduction of hyperglycaemia in newly diagnosed diabetics may alter visual refraction.

Insulin, and protamine, like any other injected proteins, are potentially immunogenic. This may or may not have clinical implications. Local reactions at the injection site may include transient erythema, induration, urticaria and oedema. The incidence is minimal with highly purified pork insulin. These usually resolve with continuing usage of insulin. True generalised hypersensitivity reactions approaching anaphylaxis are very rare.

Clinical evidence suggests that highly purified pork insulins are unlikely to cause localised lipodystrophies. However, at present, this possibility cannot be totally excluded.

Toxicity and treatment of overdosage: The symptoms and signs of hypoglycaemia depend on the patient's clinical state and on the rate and extent of the fall in blood glucose levels.

If possible, glucose, sucrose, or rapidly absorbable carbohydrate should be taken by mouth. Failing this, hypoglycaemia should be reversed as rapidly as possible by intravenous injection of glucose 50% solution. Alternative emergency treatments include the subcutaneous injection of up to 1 ml of adrenaline solution 1:1000 or the subcutaneous, intramuscular or intravenous injection of lyophilised glucagon 0.5–1.0 mg (1 unit = 1.0 mg). Both adrenaline and glucagon injections mobilise hepatic glycogen, but the effect is short lived and must be supplemented by freely available carbohydrate as soon as possible.

Pharmaceutical precautions
Nordisk Wellcome highly purified pork insulins should be stored between 2 and 8°C, protected from sunlight. Insulin which has been frozen should not be used.

Legal category
P.

Package quantities
10 ml glass vials.

Further information
Mixing of these highly purified pork insulins with preparations of other species is not recommended.

Product licence numbers

Nordisk-UK Ltd		The Wellcome Foundation Ltd
Velosulin	3132/0019	0003/0188
Insulatard	3132/0018	0003/0191
Mixtard 30/70	3132/0021	0003/0194
Initard 50/50	3132/0020	0003/0197

VELOSULIN* CARTRIDGE ▼
Neutral Insulin Injection BP, highly purified pork

Presentation Velosulin Cartridge is a neutral solution of highly purified pork insulin available in 5.7 ml glass cartridge vials containing 100 iu/ml for use only in the Nordisk Infuser.

Uses The treatment of insulin-requiring diabetic patients. To be used only with the Nordisk Infuser.

Dosage and administration Velosulin Cartridge is intended to be administered as subcutaneous infusion using the Nordisk Infuser System.

Basal rate and prandial doses are to be determined by the physician.

Velosulin Cartridge should only be used with the infusion set supplied with the Nordisk Infuser. No attempt should be made to refill the cartridges. When empty, they should be discarded and a fresh cartridge inserted. In order to minimise the risk of infusion site irritation or infection, it is recommended that the infusion set is changed every 2–3 days. The infusion site should be cleansed thoroughly and the needle taped securely in place. The infusion site should be changed according to a suitable routine and should be cleansed regularly. The procedure (given in the User's Manual) should be followed when the cartridge or infusion set is changed. The maximum in-use life of Velosulin Cartridge used in the Nordisk Infuser is 14 days.

Velosulin Cartridge is stable at normal Infuser operating temperatures (30–37°C if worn under outdoor clothing), although care must be taken to avoid extremes of temperature, eg. when sunbathing, winter sports, etc.

Use in pregnancy and lactation: It is essential to maintain continuous good control of the insulin-requiring diabetic patient throughout pregnancy. In the insulin-treated (gestational or insulin-dependent) pregnant diabetic patient, the insulin requirements fall in the first trimester and increase during the second and third trimesters.

Use in the elderly: No specific studies regarding continuous subcutaneous insulin infusion (CSII) in the elderly have yet been conducted. Clearance rates may be reduced in the elderly due to falling renal function. Insulin may therefore have a more prolonged action. Dose requirements should be regularly reviewed.

Contra-indications, warnings, etc
Contra-indications: Insulin is contra-indicated in hypoglycaemia.

Precautions: Variations in lifestyle and other factors, eg. infection and pregnancy, can affect insulin requirements.

Patients previously treated by subcutaneous insulin injection may require a dosage adjustment when transferred to subcutaneous infusion.

Hypoglycaemia can be enhanced by drugs including the following: aspirin; sulphonylureas, and agents affecting them; certain steroids.

Hyperglycaemia can be enhanced by drugs including the following: triiodothyronine; thyroxine; various natural and synthetic steroids, including some oral contraceptives; diuretics, including thiazides; cyclophosphamide.

Certain β-blockers, especially propranolol, may affect insulin requirements and mask the signs of hypoglycaemia mediated by the sympathetic nervous system.

Monoamine oxidase inhibitors (MAOI) may potentiate the action of insulin.

Side-and adverse effects: The most important side-effect is hypoglycaemia. Reduction of hyperglycaemia in newly diagnosed diabetics may alter visual refraction.

Insulin, like many other injected substances, is potentially immunogenic. This may or may not have clinical implications. Local reactions at the infusion site may include transient erythema, induration, urticaria and oedema. The incidence is minimal with highly purified pork insulin. These usually resolve with continuing usage of insulin. True generalised hypersensitivity reactions approaching anaphylaxis are very rare.

Clinical evidence suggests that highly purified pork insulins are unlikely to cause localised lipodystrophies. However, at present, this possibility cannot be totally excluded.

Toxicity and treatment of overdosage: The symptoms and signs of hypoglycaemia depend on the patient's clinical state and on the rate and extent of the fall in blood glucose levels.

Infusion with Velosulin Cartridge should be reduced or suspended until normal blood glucose levels are restored.

If possible, glucose, sucrose, or rapidly absorbable carbohydrate should be taken by mouth. Failing this, hypoglycaemia should be reversed as rapidly as possible by intravenous injection of glucose 50% solution. Alternative emergency treatments include the subcutaneous injection of up to 1 ml of adrenaline solution 1:1000 or the subcutaneous, intramuscular or intravenous injection of lyophilised glucagon 0.5–1.0 mg (1 unit = 1.0 mg). Both adrenaline and glucagon injections mobilise hepatic glycogen, but the effect is short lived and must be supplemented by freely available carbohydrate as soon as possible.

Pharmaceutical precautions Velosulin Cartridge should be stored between 2 and 8°C, protected from sunlight. Insulin which has been frozen should not be used. Velosulin Cartridge insulin which appears turbid (cloudy) should not be used.

Legal category P.

Package quantities 1 × 5.7 ml glass cartridge vials.

Further information Nil.

Product licence numbers
Nordisk-UK Ltd   The Wellcome Foundation Ltd
3132/0043   0003/0208

INSULINS – WELLCOME

NEUSULIN*
Neutral Insulin Injection BP WELLCOME*

Presentation Neusulin insulin is a clear neutral solution of purified crystalline insulin.
pH 7.3 ± 0.7.
It is available in a strength of 100 units per ml.
This insulin is prepared from ox pancreas.

Uses For the management of diabetes mellitus. Wellcome purified insulin may be helpful in obviating or resolving problems sometimes encountered with standard insulin therapy; local skin reactions, lipoatrophy, generalised insulin allergy, and insulin resistance/high daily dose requirement.

Dosage and administration *Adults and children:* The daily unit dosage of insulin is determined by the physician in accordance with the patient's requirements.

Neusulin is administered by subcutaneous, intramuscular or intravenous injection. The site of each injection should be changed according to a suitable routine.

Accidental intravascular injection should be avoided.

Use in the elderly: Insulin clearance rates may be reduced in the elderly due to a falling renal function. Insulin may therefore have a more prolonged action. Dose requirements should be regularly reviewed.

Subcutaneous: Onset of action occurs within 30–60 minutes, with an overall duration of action of approximately 6–8 hours. Consequently, 2 or 3 injections daily before meals may be appropriate if not used in combination with other insulins.

Intramuscular: Onset of action is more rapid and overall duration of action shorter than with the subcutaneous route, assuming adequate vascular perfusion.

Intravenous: Onset of action is most rapid and duration of action shortest with this route. It is usually reserved either for investigational purposes, or for the management of diabetic ketoacidosis. See literature for details of continuous low-dose insulin infusion.

Note: Insulin may adsorb to surfaces of the infusion apparatus and other infusion constituents.

Transfer from standard insulin: When patients treated with standard bovine insulin are transferred to Wellcome purified bovine insulin, there is no general decrease in dose requirement in the short term. Neusulin may therefore be conveniently given in similar unit dosage to the corresponding standard insulins, without risk of provoking sudden hypoglycaemia.

Contra-indications, warnings, etc
Contra-indications: Hypoglycaemia is an absolute contra-indication.

Precautions: Variation in lifestyle and other factors, e.g. infection and pregnancy, can affect insulin requirements.

Insulin dosage requirement may change if the species of origin, type, or purity of insulin is changed.

Hypoglycaemia can be enhanced by drugs including the following: aspirin, sulphonylureas and agents affecting them; certain steroids.

Hyperglycaemia can be enhanced by drugs including the following: triiodothyronine; thyroxine; various natural and synthetic steroids, including some oral contraceptives; diuretics, including thiazides; certain psychotherapeutic agents, including benzodiazepines; cyclophosphamide.

Certain β-blockers, especially propranolol, may affect insulin requirements and mask the signs of hypoglycaemia mediated by the sympathetic nervous system.

Monoamine oxidase (M.A.O.) inhibitors may potentiate the action of insulin.

Side- and adverse effects: The most important side-effect is hypoglycaemia.

Reduction of hyperglycaemia in newly diagnosed diabetics may alter visual refraction.

Local reactions at the injection site may include,

among others, transient erythema, induration, urticaria and oedema. These usually resolve with continuing usage of insulin.

True generalised hypersensitivity reactions approaching anaphylaxis are very rare.

Clinical evidence suggests that purified insulins are unlikely to cause localised lipodystrophies. However, at present this possibility cannot be totally excluded.

Use in pregnancy and lactation: It is essential to maintain continuous good control of the insulin-requiring diabetic patient throughout pregnancy. In the insulin-treated (gestational or insulin-dependent) pregnant diabetic patient, the insulin requirements fall in the first trimester and increase during the second and third trimester.

Breast-feeding is probably best avoided in insulin-dependent diabetic mothers because of their metabolic instability.

Toxicity and treatment of overdosage: The symptoms and signs of hypoglycaemia depend on the patient's clinical state and on the rate and extent of the fall in blood glucose.

If possible, glucose, sucrose or rapidly available carbohydrate should be taken by mouth. Failing this, hypoglycaemia should be reversed as rapidly as possible by intravenous injection of glucose 50% solution. Alternative emergency treatments include the subcutaneous injection of up to 1 ml of adrenaline solution 1:1000, or the subcutaneous, intramuscular or intravenous injection of lyophilised glucagon 0.5–1.0 mg (1 unit = 1.0 mg). Both adrenaline and glucagon injections mobilise hepatic glycogen, but the effect is short-lived, and must be supplemented by freely available carbohydrate as soon as possible.

Pharmaceutical precautions Store at 2–8°C.
Do not freeze.
Avoid direct sunlight.

Legal category P.

Package quantities 100 units/ml vial of 10 ml

Further information *Mixing in the syringe:* Neusulin insulin can be mixed with Neuphane or Neulente insulin. If, *on medical advice,* Neusulin insulin is to be mixed in the syringe with one of these long-acting purified insulins, the following procedure should be adopted:
1. Inject a volume of air equivalent to the dose into the bottle of long-acting insulin, without inverting the bottle or withdrawing the dose.
2. Inject the appropriate volume of air into the bottle of Neusulin insulin and withdraw the dose in the usual way.
3. Re-insert the needle into the long-acting insulin and withdraw the appropriate dose.
4. Inject the mixture immediately.

Mixing of purified with standard preparations is not recommended, since this would result in the loss of their special advantages.

Further information is available on request.

Product licence number
Neusulin 100 units/ml 0003/0161

NEUPHANE*
Isophane Insulin Injection BP WELLCOME*

Presentation Neuphane insulin is a cloudy neutral suspension of an insulin (purified)/protamine complex.

pH 7.2 ± 0.3
It is available in a strength of 100 units per ml.
This insulin is prepared from ox pancreas.

Uses For the management of diabetes mellitus. Wellcome purified insulins may be helpful in obviating or resolving problems sometimes encountered with standard insulin therapy; local skin reactions, lipoatrophy, generalised insulin allergy and insulin resistance/high daily dose requirement.

Dosage and administration *Adults and children:* The daily unit dosage of insulin is determined by the physician in accordance with the patient's requirements.

Neuphane insulin should be well mixed by inverting the vial several times before use. It is administered by subcutaneous or intramuscular injection.

The site of each injection should be changed according to a suitable routine.

Accidental intravascular injection should be avoided.

Use in the elderly: Insulin clearance rates may be reduced in the elderly due to a falling renal function. Insulin may therefore have a more prolonged action. Dose requirements should be regularly reviewed.

Subcutaneous: Onset of action occurs within 2 hours, with an overall duration of action which may extend to 20–24 hours.

Intramuscular: Onset of action is more rapid and overall duration of action shorter than with the subcutaneous route, assuming adequate vascular perfusion.

Neuphane insulin should not be given intravenously.

Transfer from standard insulin: When patients treated with standard bovine insulin are transferred to Wellcome purified bovine insulin, there is no general decrease in dose requirement in the short term. Neuphane may therefore be conveniently given in similar unit dosage to the corresponding standard insulin, without risk of provoking sudden hypoglycaemia.

Contra-indications, warnings, etc
Contra-indications: Hypoglycaemia is an absolute contra-indication.

Precautions: Variation in lifestyle and other factors, e.g. infection and pregnancy, can affect insulin requirements.

Insulin dosage requirement may change if the species of origin, type, or purity of insulin is changed.

Hypoglycaemia can be enhanced by drugs including the following: aspirin, sulphonylureas and agents affecting them; certain steroids.

Hyperglycaemia can be enhanced by drugs including the following: triiodothyronine; thyroxine; various natural and synthetic steroids, including some oral contraceptives; diuretics, including thiazides; certain psychotherapeutic agents, including benzodiazepines; cyclophosphamide.

Certain β-blockers, especially propranolol, may affect insulin requirements and mask the signs of hypoglycaemia mediated by the sympathetic nervous system.

Monoamine oxidase (M.A.O.) inhibitors may potentiate the action of insulin.

Side- and adverse effects: The most important side-effect is hypoglycaemia.

Reduction of hyperglycaemia in newly diagnosed diabetics may alter visual refraction.

Local reactions at the injection site may include, among others, transient erythema, induration, urticaria and oedema. These usually resolve with continuing usage of insulin.

True generalised hypersensitivity reactions approaching anaphylaxis are very rare.

Clinical evidence suggests that purified insulins are unlikely to cause localised lipodystrophies. However, at present this possibility cannot be totally excluded.

Use in pregnancy and lactation: it is essential to maintain continuous good control of the insulin-requiring diabetic patient throughout pregnancy. In the insulin-treated (gestational or insulin-dependent) pregnant diabetic patient, the insulin requirements fall in the first trimester and increase during the second and third trimester.

Breast-feeding is probably best avoided in insulin-dependent diabetic mothers because of their metabolic instability.

Toxicity and treatment of overdosage: The symptoms and signs of hypoglycaemia depend on the patient's clinical state and on the rate and extent of the fall in blood glucose.

If possible, glucose, sucrose or rapidly available carbohydrate should be taken by mouth. Failing this, hypoglycaemia should be reversed as rapidly as possible by intravenous injection of glucose 50% solution. Alternative emergency treatments include the subcutaneous injection of up to 1 ml of adrenaline solution 1:1000, or the subcutaneous, intramuscular or intravenous injection of lyophilised glucagon 0.5–1.0 mg (1 unit = 1.0 mg). Both adrenaline and glucagon injections mobilise hepatic glycogen, but the effect is short-lived and must be supplemented by freely available carbohydrate as soon as possible.

Pharmaceutical precautions Store at 2–8°C.
Do not freeze.
Avoid direct sunlight.

Legal category P.

Package quantities 100 units/ml vial of 10 ml

Further information *Mixing in the syringe:* Neuphane insulin can be mixed with Neusulin insulin.

If, *on medical advice*, Neuphane insulin is to be mixed in the syringe with Neusulin insulin, the following procedure should be adopted:

1. Inject a volume of air equivalent to the dose into the bottle of Neuphane insulin without inverting the bottle or withdrawing the dose.
2. Inject the appropriate volume of air into the bottle of Neusulin insulin and withdraw the dose in the usual way.
3. Re-insert the needle into the Neuphane insulin and withdraw the appropriate dose.
4. Inject the mixture immediately.

Mixing of purified with standard preparations is not recommended, since this would result in the loss of their special advantages.

Further information is available on request.

Product licence number
Neuphane 100 units/ml 0003/0162

NEULENTE*
Insulin Zinc Suspension BP WELLCOME*

Presentation Neulente insulin is a neutral suspension of purified insulin consisting of 3 parts Semilente and 7 parts Ultralente insulin.
Appearance is cloudy after shaking.
pH 7.2 ± 0.3

It is available in a strength of 100 units per ml.
This insulin is prepared from ox pancreas.

Uses For the management of diabetes mellitus. Wellcome purified insulins may be helpful in obviating or resolving problems sometimes encountered with standard insulin therapy; local skin reactions, lipoatrophy, generalised insulin allergy and insulin resistance/high daily dose requirement.

Dosage and administration *Adults and children:* The daily unit dosage of insulin is determined by the physician in accordance with the patient's requirements.

Neulente insulin should be well mixed by gently inverting the vial several times before use. It should be administered by subcutaneous or intramuscular injection.

The site of each injection should be changed according to a suitable routine.

Accidental intravascular injection should be avoided.

Use in the elderly: Insulin clearance rates may be reduced in the elderly due to a falling renal function. Insulin may therefore have a more prolonged action. Dose requirements should be regularly reviewed.

Subcutaneous: Onset of action occurs within 2 hours, with an overall duration of action which may extend to 24–28 hours.

Intramuscular: Onset of action is more rapid and overall duration of action shorter than with the subcutaneous route, assuming adequate vascular perfusion.

Neulente insulin should not be given intravenously.

Transfer from standard insulin: When patients treated with standard bovine insulin are transferred to Wellcome purified bovine insulin, there is no general decrease in dose requirement in the short term, Neulente may therefore be conveniently given in similar unit dosage to the corresponding standard insulin, without risk of provoking sudden hypoglycaemia.

Contra-indications, warnings, etc
Contra-indications: Hypoglycaemia is an absolute contra-indication.

Precautions: Variation in lifestyle and other factors, e.g. infection and pregnancy, can affect insulin requirements.

Insulin dosage requirement may change if the species of origin, type, or purity of insulin is changed.

Hypoglycaemia can be enhanced by drugs including the following: aspirin, sulphonylureas and agents affecting them; certain steroids.

Hyperglycaemia can be enhanced by drugs including the following: triiodothyronine; thyroxine; various natural and synthetic steroids including some oral contraceptives; diuretics, including thiazides; certain psychotherapeutic agents, including benzodiazepines; cyclophosphamide.

Certain β-blockers, especially propranolol, may affect insulin requirements and mask the signs of hypoglycaemia mediated by the sympathetic nervous system.

Monoamine oxidase (M.A.O.) inhibitors may potentiate the action of insulin.

Side- and adverse effects: The most important side-effect is hypoglycaemia.

Reduction of hyperglycaemia in newly diagnosed diabetics may alter visual refraction.

Local reactions at the injection site may include, among others, transient erythema, induration, urticaria and oedema. These usually resolve with continuing usage of insulin.

True generalised hypersensitivity reactions approaching anaphylaxis are very rare.

Clinical evidence suggests that purified insulins are unlikely to cause localised lipodystrophies. However, at present this possibility cannot be totally excluded.

Use in pregnancy and lactation: It is essential to maintain continuous good control of the insulin-requiring diabetic patient throughout pregnancy. In the insulin-treated (gestational or insulin-dependent) pregnant diabetic patient, the insulin requirements fall in the first trimester and increase during the second and third trimester.

Breast-feeding is probably best avoided in insulin-dependent diabetic mothers because of their metabolic instability.

Toxicity and treatment of overdosage: The symptoms and signs of hypoglycaemia depend on the patient's clinical state and on the rate and extent of the fall in blood glucose.

If possible, glucose, sucrose or rapidly available carbohydrate should be taken by mouth. Failing this, hypoglycaemia should be reversed as rapidly as possible by intravenous injection of glucose 50% solution. Alternative emergency treatments include the subcutaneous injection of up to 1 ml of adrenaline solution 1:1000, or the subcutaneous, intramuscular or intravenous injection of lyophilised glucagon 0.5–1.0 mg (1 unit = 1.0 mg). Both adrenaline and glucagon injections mobilise hepatic glycogen, but the effect is short-lived and must be supplemented by freely available carbohydrate as soon as possible.

Pharmaceutical precautions Store at 2–8°C.
Do not freeze.
Avoid direct sunlight.

Legal category P.

Package quantities 100 units/ml vial of 10 ml

Further information *Mixing in the syringe:* Neulente insulin can be mixed with Neusulin insulin. If, *on medical advice,* Neulente insulin is to be mixed in the syringe with Neusulin insulin, the following procedure should be adopted:

1. Inject a volume of air equivalent to the dose into the bottle of Neulente insulin, without inverting the bottle or withdrawing the dose.
2. Inject the appropriate volume of air into the bottle of Neusulin insulin and withdraw the dose in the usual way.
3. Re-insert the needle into the Neulente insulin and withdraw the appropriate dose.
4. Inject the mixture immediately.

Mixing of purified with standard preparations is not recommended, since this would result in the loss of their special advantages.

Further information is available on request.

Product licence number
Neulente 100 units/ml 0003/0171

INSULIN INJECTION BP (PURIFIED) WELLCOME*

Presentation Insulin Injection is a clear acidic solution of purified crystalline insulin. pH 3.25 ± 0.25.

It is available in a strength of 100 units per ml. This insulin is prepared from ox pancreas.

Uses For the management of diabetes mellitus. Well-come purified insulins may be helpful in obviating or resolving problems sometimes encountered with standard insulin therapy: local skin reactions, lipoatrophy, generalised insulin allergy and insulin resistance/high daily dose requirement.

Dosage and administration
Adults and children: The daily unit dosage of insulin is determined by the physician in accordance with the patient's requirements.

Insulin Injection is administered by subcutaneous, intramuscular or intravenous injection.

The site of each injection should be changed according to a suitable routine.

Accidental intravascular injection should be avoided.

Use in the elderly: Insulin clearance rates may be reduced in the elderly due to a falling renal function. Insulin may therefore have a more prolonged action. Dose requirements should be regularly reviewed.

Subcutaneous: Onset of action occurs within 30–60 minutes, with an overall duration of action of approximately 6–8 hours. Consequently, 2 or 3 injections daily before meals may be appropriate if not used in combination with other insulins.

Intramuscular: Onset of action is more rapid and overall duration of action shorter than the subcutaneous route, assuming adequate vascular perfusion.

Intravenous: Onset of action is most rapid and duration of action shortest with this route. It is usually reserved either for investigational purposes, or for the management of diabetic ketoacidosis. See literature for details of continuous low-dose insulin infusion.

Note: Insulin may adsorb to surfaces of infusion apparatus and other infusion constituents.

Transfer from standard insulin: When patients treated with standard bovine insulin are transferred to Wellcome purified bovine insulin, there is no general decrease in dose requirement in the short term. Insulin Injection may therefore be conveniently given in similar unit dosage to the corresponding standard insulins (soluble or neutral soluble insulin), without risk of provoking sudden hypoglycaemia.

Contra-indications, warnings, etc
Contra-indications: Hypoglycaemia is an absolute contra-indication.

Precautions: Variation in lifestyle and other factors, e.g. infection and pregnancy, can affect insulin requirements.

Insulin dosage requirements may change if the species of origin, type, or purity of insulin is changed.

Hypoglycaemia can be enhanced by drugs including the following: aspirin; sulphonylureas and agents affecting them; certain steroids.

Hyperglycaemia can be enhanced by drugs including the following: triiodothyronine; thyroxine; various natural and synthetic steroids, including some oral contraceptives; diuretics, including thiazides; certain psychotherapeutic agents, including benzodiazepines; cyclophosphamide.

Certain β-blockers, especially propranolol, may affect insulin requirements and mask the signs of hypoglycaemia mediated by the sympathetic nervous system.

Monoamine oxidase (M.A.O) inhibitors may potentiate the action of insulin.

Side- and adverse effects: The most important side-effect is hypoglycaemia.

Reduction of hyperglycaemia in newly diagnosed diabetics may alter visual refraction.

Bovine insulin, like any other foreign protein, is potentially immunogenic. This may, or may not, have clinical implications.

Local reactions at the injection site may include, among others, transient erythema, induration, urticaria and oedema. These usually resolve with continuing usage of insulin.

True generalised hypersensitivity reactions approaching anaphylaxis are very rare.

Use in pregnancy and lactation: It is essential to maintain continuous good control of the insulin-requiring diabetic patient throughout pregnancy. In the insulin-treated (gestational or insulin-dependent) pregnant diabetic patient, the insulin requirements fall in the first trimester and increase during the second and third trimesters.

Breast-feeding is probably best avoided in insulin-dependent diabetic mothers because of their metabolic instability.

Toxicity and treatment of overdosage: The symptoms and signs of hypoglycaemia depend on the patient's clinical state and on the rate and extent of the fall in blood glucose.

If possible, glucose, sucrose or rapidly available carbohydrate should be taken by mouth. Failing this, hypoglycaemia should be reversed as rapidly as possible by intravenous injection of glucose 50% solution. Alternative emergency treatments include the subcutaneous injection of up to 1 ml of adrenaline solution 1:1000, or the subcutaneous, intramuscular or intravenous injection of lyophilised glucagon 0.5–1.0 mg (1 unit = 1.0 mg). Both adrenaline and glucagon injections mobilise hepatic glycogen, but the effect is short-lived and must be supplemented by freely available carbohydrate as soon as possible.

Pharmaceutical precautions Store at 2–8°C.
Do not freeze.
Avoid direct sunlight.

Legal category P.

Package quantities 100 units/ml. Vial of 10 ml.

Further information *Mixing in the syringe:* Although Insulin Injection can be mixed with Neuphane or Neulente insulin, it is preferable to avoid mixing insulins of different pH. If, *on medical advice*, Insulin Injection is to be mixed in the syringe with one of these long-acting purified insulins, the following procedure should be adopted:

1. Inject a volume of air equivalent to the dose into the bottle of long-acting insulin, without inverting the bottle or withdrawing the dose.
2. Inject the appropriate volume of air into the bottle of Insulin Injection and withdraw the dose in the usual way.
3. Re-insert the needle into the long-acting insulin and withdraw the appropriate dose.
4. Inject the mixture immediately.

Mixing of purified with standard preparations is not recommended, since this would result in the loss of their special advantages.

Additional information is available on request.

Product licence number 100 units/ml. 0003/0165.

KEMADRIN* TABLETS AND INJECTION

Presentation *Tablets:* Each white tablet containing 5 mg Procyclidine Hydrochloride BP is scored and coded Wellcome S3A.

Injection: Each 2 ml ampoule contains 10 mg Procyclidine Hydrochloride BP.

Uses Kemadrin is indicated in all forms of Parkinson's disease: idiopathic (paralysis agitans), postencephalitic and arteriosclerotic.

Symptoms often responding well to Kemadrin include: rigidity, akinesia, tremor, speech and writing difficulties, gait, sialorrhoea and drooling, sweating, oculogyric crises and depressed mood.

Kemadrin is also used to control troublesome extrapyramidal symptoms induced by neuroleptic drugs including pseudo-parkinsonism, acute dystonic reactions and akathisia.

Dosage and administration The variation in optimum dosage from one patient to another should be taken into consideration by the physician. Treatment is usually started at 2.5 mg three times a day, increasing by 2.5–5 mg daily at intervals of two or three days until the optimum clinical response is achieved. The usual maximum total daily dose is 30 mg. However, at the discretion of the attending physician where appropriate this total may be as high as 60 mg.

The daily dosage used in the control of neuroleptic-induced extrapyramidal symptoms is usually not more than 20 mg daily. After a period of 3–4 months, Kemadrin should be stopped and the patient observed to see if the neuroleptic-induced extrapyramidal symptoms recur. Cessation of treatment periodically is to be recommended even in patients who appear to require the drug for longer periods.

Avoid abrupt discontinuation of treatment.

Kemadrin may be combined with levodopa or amantadine in patients who are inadequately controlled on a single agent.

In acute dystonia 5 mg Kemadrin intravenously is frequently effective within 5 minutes. An occasional patient may need 10 mg or more and may require up to half an hour to obtain relief.

Children: Not applicable.

Use in the elderly: Elderly patients are more sensitive to anticholinergics, and a reduced dose may be required.

Pharmacology: Procyclidine is a synthetic anticholinergic agent which blocks the excitatory effects of acetylcholine at the muscarinic receptor.

Idiopathic Parkinson's disease is now thought to result from degeneration of neurones in the substantia nigra whose axons project and inhibit cells in the corpus striatum. Blockade by neuroleptic drugs of the dopamine released by these terminals produces a similar clinical picture. The cell bodies in the corpus striatum also receive cholinergic innervation which is excitatory. Relief of the parkinsonian syndrome can be achieved either by potentiation of the dopaminergic system or blockade of the cholinergic input by anticholinergics. It is by a central action of this latter type that procyclidine exerts its effect.

Procyclidine is adequately absorbed from the gastro-intestinal tract and disappears rapidly from the tissues. After intravenous administration it acts within 5 to 20 minutes with a duration of up to 4 hours. After both oral and IV dosing the mean values for volume of distribution, total body clearance and plasma elimination half-life of procyclidine were of the order of 1 litre/kg, 68 ml/min and 12 hours respectively.

Contra-indications, warnings, etc
Contra-indications: Tardive dyskinesias.

Precautions: As with all anticholinergics such as Kemadrin, cautious prescribing is indicated in patients predisposed to glaucoma, obstructive disease of the gastro-intestinal tract, those with urinary symptoms associated with prostatic hypertrophy and in hepatic and renal impairment.

In a proportion of patients undergoing neuroleptic treatment, tardive dyskinesias will occur. While anticholinergic agents do not cause this syndrome, when given in combination with neuroleptics they may reduce the threshold at which dyskinesias appear in patients predisposed to this abnormality. In such individuals subsequent adjustment of neuroleptic therapy is indicated.

Drug interactions: The anticholinergic activity of Kemadrin may be increased by agents having anticholinergic activity, e.g. antidepressants (e.g. amitriptyline), phenothiazines, (e.g. thioridazine), amantadine and disopyramide. The absorption of ketoconazole may be reduced by concomitant administration of Kemadrin.

Use in pregnancy and lactation: The safety of using Kemadrin during pregnancy has not been established. However, extensive clinical use has not given any evidence that it in any way compromises the normal course of pregnancy. No data are available on the excretion of this drug in breast milk.

Side- and adverse effects: The main side-effects are those to be expected from any anticholinergic agent. Dry mouth, blurring of vision and constipation are most commonly recorded. At higher doses dizziness, mental confusion and hallucinations may occur. The unwanted anticholinergic effects are easily reversed by reducing the dosage.

In rare instances, Kemadrin administered for the treatment of neuroleptic-induced symptoms was associated with an apparent worsening of the patient's state.

Toxicity and treatment of overdosage: Reports of overdosage are relatively rare. Symptoms of overdosage are agitation, restlessness and confusion with severe sleeplessness lasting up to 24 hours or more. Visual and occasionally auditory hallucinations are likely. Most subjects are euphoric but the occasional patient may be anxious and aggressive. The pupils are widely dilated and unreactive to light. In recorded cases, the disorientation has lasted 1 to 4 days and ended in recuperative sleep.

If procyclidine has been ingested within the previous hour or two (or possibly longer in view of its likely effects on gastric motility) then gastric lavage is probably indicated. Other active measures such as the use of cholinergic agents or haemodialysis are extremely unlikely to be of clinical value, although if convulsions occur they should be controlled by injections of diazepam.

Pharmaceutical precautions *Tablets and injection:* Store below 25°C.

Legal category POM.

Package quantities Bottles of 100 and 500 tablets. Ampoule of 10 mg in 2 ml. Box of 5 ampoules.

Further information Nil.

Product licence numbers
Tablets   0003/5255
Injection 0003/5256

LANOXIN* TABLETS
LANOXIN-125* TABLETS
LANOXIN-PG* TABLETS
LANOXIN* INJECTION
LANOXIN-PG* ELIXIR

Presentation Lanoxin tablets each contain 250 mcg (0.25 mg) of Digoxin BP, scored and coded Wellcome X3A, white in colour.

Lanoxin-125 Tablets each contain 125 mcg (0.125 mg) of Digoxin BP coded Wellcome Y3B, white in colour.

Lanoxin-PG (Paediatric/Geriatric) Tablets each contain 62.5 mcg (0.0625 mg) of Digoxin BP, coloured blue and coded Wellcome U3A.

Lanoxin Injection contains 250 mcg (0.25 mg) of Digoxin BP per ml in each 2 ml ampoule.

Lanoxin-PG (Paediatric/Geriatric) Elixir contains 50 mcg (0.050 mg) of Digoxin BP in each ml. Clear bright yellow in colour and lime flavoured.

Uses Lanoxin is indicated for the management of certain supraventricular dysrhythmias, and is particularly valuable when they are accompanied by the manifestations of heart failure.

Dosage and administration The dose of Lanoxin has to be adjusted for each patient and the suggested doses are only intended as an initial guide. Factors which may be considered include the patient's age, lean body mass, renal and thyroid status, electrolyte balance, degree of tissue oxygenation and the nature of the underlying cardiac or pulmonary disease.

Parenteral Lanoxin
Intravenous Lanoxin is indicated when emergency parenteral digitalisation is necessary. Patients should not have been taking cardiac glycosides within the previous two weeks. An appreciable electro-physiological effect is detectable within 10 minutes of administration, with maximum effect at 2 hours. After loading with parenteral Lanoxin, maintenance is continued with oral therapy.

Lanoxin Injection can be administered undiluted by *slow* intravenous injection or diluted, by intravenous infusion. When given intravenously it may be diluted with:
Sodium Chloride Intravenous Infusion B.P. (0.9% w/v)
Glucose Intravenous Infusion BP (5% w/v) or
Sodium Chloride (0.18% w/v) and Glucose (4% w/v) Intravenous Infusion BP.

The infusion period should be at least 10 minutes. Dilutions down to 0.5 mg/500 ml may be made in the above infusion fluids but any unused solution should be discarded after 24 hours.

Rapid intravenous injection can cause vasoconstriction, producing hypertension and/or reduced coronary flow. The slow injection rate is particularly important in hypertensive heart failure and acute myocardial infarction.

In cases where cardiac glycosides have been taken in the preceding 2 weeks the recommendations for initial dosing of a patient should be reconsidered and a reduced dose advised. *In such cases if the intravenous dose is chosen, doses should be approximately 30% lower than the previous oral digoxin dose.*

Intramuscular Lanoxin offers no advantage over oral

Lanoxin in terms of speed of onset of action or effectiveness. The injection may be given undiluted. It may cause local pain, and cannot be recommended if another route is available.

Subcutaneous injection is not recommended as it causes intense local irritation.

Infants and children up to 10 years (Parenteral routes).

Digitalisation: 10–20 mcg/kg boy weight repeated 6 hourly until therapeutic result is obtained, usually 2–4 doses being sufficient.

Maintenance: 10–20 mcg/kg bodyweight daily in divided doses. The lower dosage applies to premature neonates and infants who may be more sensitive to the effects of Lanoxin.

Adults and children over 10 years: The total digitalising dose with parenteral Lanoxin is 0.5–1.0 mg, depending upon body size and other sensitising factors, such as age. This may be given slowly by the intravenous route either as a single dose or in divided doses of 0.25–0.5 mg at intervals of 4–6 hours.

Oral Lanoxin

Lanoxin-PG Elixir is indicated in circumstances where a smaller dose of Lanoxin than usual is needed, especially in children and the elderly.

Lanoxin tablets: Infants and children up to 10 years: Digitalisation: 10–20 mcg/kg body weight repeated 6-hourly until therapeutic effect is obtained, 2–4 doses usually being sufficient.

Maintenance: 10–20 mcg/kg body weight daily. The lower dosage applies to premature infants and neonates who may be more sensative to the effects of Lanoxin.

Children over 10 years and adults: Rapid oral digitalisation: 0.75–1.5 mg as a single dose, followed by 0.25 mg every 6 hours until the desired effects are obtained.

In elderly patients and where there is less urgency or more risk of toxicity a small initial dose of 0.5–0.75 mg may be given.

Slow oral digitalisation: 0.125–0.75 mg daily for one week, followed by the appropriate maintenance dose.

Maintenance: 0.25–0.5 mg daily is the range for patients with relatively normal renal function. A maintenance dose of 0.125–0.25 mg per day is usually sufficient in the elderly.

Use in the elderly: The dosage of Lanoxin should be reduced if the patients are elderly or have other reasons for reduced renal clearance of Lanoxin such a renal disease or renal impairment secondary to cardiovascular disease. The prolongation of excretion in these cases enjoins a reduction in both initial and maintenance doses and also a greater awareness of the possibility of intoxication.

Contra-indications, warnings, etc The only absolute contra-indication to Lanoxin is toxicity due to cardiac glycosides. Lanoxin is contra-indicated in supraventricular dysrhythmias caused by Wolff-Parkinson-White syndrome.

Precautions: Lanoxin intoxication produces a variety of cardiac dysrhythmias, some of which can resemble those for which the product was intended. Atrial tachycardia with intermittent AV block although not the commonest dysrhythmia resulting from Lanoxin overdosage requires particular care as the irregular rhythm clinically resembles atrial fibrillation.

In acute myocarditis with failure, the heart is especially sensitive to digoxin-induced arrhythmias. Renal failure

calls for decreased dosage and close monitoring of effects. Caution should be taken when given concurrently with drugs which depress the AV node.

Hypokalaemia sensitises the myocardium to the cardiac glycosides. Care should be taken with patients who may be hypokalaemic, including those treated with diuretics, corticosteroids, peritoneal or haemodialysis, suction of gastroenteric secretion, ion exchange resins and carbenoxolone treatments. Hypokalaemia may accompany malnutrition, diarrhoea, vomiting and long standing wasting diseases. In these cases the dose may need to be reduced.

Hypercalcaemia and hypomagnnesaemia may also increase myocardial sensitivity.

Hypothyroidism renders a patient more sensitive to Lanoxin and the dose should be reduced. In hyperthyroidism there is relative Lanoxin resistance and the dose may have to be reduced when thyroid activity is brought under control.

D.C. shock for cardioversion appears to enhance cardiac excitability possibly by inducing an abrupt reduction in intracellular potassium concentration of the myocardium. Thus cardioversion may induce signs of toxicity if digoxin is already present. Lanoxin should be witheld for 24–28 hours before electro-conversion is performed depending on the likely excretion of the drug. In emergencies such as cardiac arrest, the smallest possible shock should be given.

Electro-conversion is inappropriate treatment of arrythmia thought to be caused by cardiac glycosides.

Immediately after an infarct the myocardium is electrically unstable and may develop dysrhythmias of shorter or longer duration. Whilst prospective studies do not support the impression that infarction sensitises the myocardium to digoxin's toxic actions, and that normal doses may be administered if the drug is thought indicated, it must be remembered that the action of Lanoxin will persist for a large part of the electrically vulnerable period. The resultant limitations of possible electric cardioversion should be considered.

Lanoxin is not recommended in supraventricular dysrhythmias caused by the Wolff-Parkinson-White syndrome.

Premature infants and neonates are particularly sensitive to digoxin, whereas children between one month and two years may require relatively larger doses than older children.

Use in pregnancy and lactation: Digoxin has been available since 1929 and there have been no reports to date of any teratogenic effects. Although digoxin is excreted in breast milk, the quantities are minute and breast feeding is not contra-indicated.

Drug interactions: Oral Lanoxin: Antacids may reduce absorption of digoxin. Neomycin may decrease digoxin absorption. Metoclopramide is without effect. The use of bran may reduce the absorption of digoxin as may kaolin-pectin mixtures. The concurrent administration of erythromycin or tetracyline can increase the bioavailability of digoxin from tablets in certain subjects who harbour enteric organisms capable of inactivating a proportion of ingested digoxin.

All forms of Lanoxin: Anti-arrhythmic agents: Concurrent administration of quinidine increases the serum digoxin concentration. The steady state serum digoxin concentration starts to rise on the first day of quinidine treatment and resettles at about day 5. The level will remain elevated for as long as quinidine is given. The magnitude of the increase is variable, but on average a two-fold increase can be expected.

Verapamil, nifedipine and amiodarone also increase serum digoxin levels by approximately 75, 45 and 70% respectively. The clinical significance is uncertain. Diazepam may also increase the plasma level of digoxin.

Drugs which cause hypokalaemia, especially thiazide and loop diuretics may sensitise the myocardium to toxic effects of digoxin. Amphotericin and corticosteroids may have a similar effect. Beta-adrenergic agonists or suxamethonium may increase the likelihood of arrhythmia in digitalised patients.

Beta-blockers and other drugs which suppress AV conduction may be hazardous with digoxin especially if given intravenously.

Lithium may sensitise the myocardium to the effects of Lanoxin.

Side- and adverse effects: The margin between digoxin's therapeutic and toxic dose is small; side-effects are common and fatalities have occurred. Nausea, vomiting and anorexia may be among the earlier symptoms of digoxin overdosage.

Diarrhoea, abdominal pains, salivation and sweating may also occur.

Certain cerebral effects are also early symptoms with digoxin overdosage and include headache, facial pain, malaise, fatigue, drowsiness, depression, disorientation, mental confusion, asphasia, delirium and hallucinations. Visual disturbances including blurred vision may occur. Colour vision may be affected with objects appearing yellow or green or less frequently red, brown, blue or white. Allergic skin reactions are rare. Thrombocytopenia has been reported. Gynaecomastia may occasionally occur.

The most serious adverse effects are those on the heart. Frequent ectopic beats may indicate poisoning of the myocardium. Atrial or ventricular arrhythmias and conduction defects are common and may indicate overdosage. In general, the incidence and severity of arrhythmias is related to the severity of the underlying heart disease. Almost any arrhythmia may ensue, but particular note should be made of multi-focal ventricular ectopic beats, bigemini, ventricular tachycardia, conduction defects, bradycardia and paroxysmal atrial tachycardia with heart block.

Hypokalaemia is associated with chronic digoxin toxicity and adverse reactions to digoxin may be precipitated if there is potassium depletion such as may be caused by prolonged administration of diuretics. Hyperkalaemia occurs in acute overdosage.

The adverse effects of digoxin are similar to the symptoms of cardiac disease and measurement of plasma concentration is of value in diagnosing overdosage. In general, toxicity is likely with plasma concentrations of digoxin above 2 ng/ml, but while mean plasma digoxin concentrations appear to distinguish between patients who are and are not suffering from digoxin toxicity, marked individual variations exist. Also, a value below 2 ng/ml may still be accompanied by signs of toxicity if the patient is for example, hypokalaemic. If overdosage is suspected, digoxin should be withdrawn.

Toxicity and treatment of overdosage: Common symptoms include nausea and vomiting, whilst the commonest cardiac features of toxicity are ventricular bigemini and trigemini. Other ectopic arrhythmias are ventricular tachycardia, multiform ventricular ectopics, paroxysmal atrial tachycardia, particularly with block. Ventricular tachycardia is usually fatal. There may be atrial ventricular

conduction disturbance such as Wenckebach phenomenon, complete heart block and junctional escape rhythms. Sinus arrest is uncommon and in children arrhythmias tend to be atrial rather than ventricular.

Gastric lavage and ECG monitoring are appropriate for recent ingestion of Lanoxin as in situations of accidental or deliberate self-poisoning.

For insidious toxicity, when merely discontinuing Lanoxin is considered insufficient, the next most useful step is to correct hypokalaemia. A slow intravenous infusion of 20–80 mEq as potassium chloride solution (60 mEq/l) in about 3 hours is recommended if such haste is required. Otherwise oral supplements of potassium chloride can be given.

In severe poisoning fatal hyperkalaemia can occur from skeletal muscle release. A plasma measurement should be made before prescribing potassium. Atropine may be given for bradycardia. Atrial tachyarrhythmias are often associated with AV block and may not require active treatment if the ventricular rate is not too fast. They may respond to phenytoin, although they do not often respond to lignocaine which is more useful in ventricular tachyarrhythmias.

Pharmaceutical precautions *Tablets:* Store below 25°C.

Elixir: Store below 25°C. Protect from light.

Injection: Store below 25°C. Protect from light.

Legal category POM.

Package quantities *Lanoxin tablets:* Bottles of 500 and 1,000; container of 5,000.
Lanoxin-125 Tablets: Bottle of 500.
Lanoxin Injection: Ampoule of 2 ml; box of 5 ampoules.
Lanoxin-PG Elixir: Bottle of 60 ml.
Lanoxin-PG Tablets: Bottles of 100 and 500.

Further information Absorption of Lanoxin digoxin is uniform and almost complete. Duration of action is short. These characteristics improve control during digitalisation and offer an increased measure of safety.

Product licence numbers

Tablets	0003/0090
125 Tablets	0003/0102
PG Tablets	0003/0091
PG Elixir	0003/5260
Injection	0003/5259

LINCTIFED* EXPECTORANT
LINCTIFED* EXPECTORANT PAEDIATRIC

Presentation Linctifed Expectorant contains:

Triprolidine Hydrochloride BP	1.25 mg
Pseudoephedrine Hydrochloride BP	20 mg
Codeine Phosphate BP	7.5 mg
Guaiphenesin BP	100 mg

in each 5 ml of orange-coloured syrup. It has an aromatic flavour.

Linctifed Expectorant Paediatric contains:

Triprolidine Hydrochloride BP	0.6 mg
Pseudoephedrine Hydrochloride BP	12 mg
Codeine Phosphate BP	3 mg
Guaiphenesin BP	50 mg

in each 5 ml of red-coloured syrup. It has a sweet, fruity flavour.

Uses Expectorant.

To aid expectoration in bronchitis and other conditions where tenacious mucoid secretions are a problem.

Dosage and administration *Linctifed Expectorant: Adults:* 10 ml three times a day.

Children: Over 12 years: 10 ml three times a day.

Under 12 years: Linctifed Expectorant Paediatric is recommended.

Linctifed Expectorant Paediatric: Children: 6–12 years: 10 ml three times a day.

1–6 years: 5 ml three times a day.

May be diluted with Syrup BP.

Use in the elderly: No specific studies have been carried out in the elderly, however, it may be advisable to monitor renal or hepatic function and if there is serious impairment then caution should be exercised. Caution is also necessary in patients with prostatic enlargment.

Pharmacology: Pseudoephedrine has direct and indirect sympathomimetic activity and is an orally effective upper respiratory tract decongestant. Pseudoephedrine is substantially less potent than ephedrine in producing both tachycardia and elevation in systolic blood pressure and considerably less potent in causing stimulation of the central nervous system. On the basis of widespread and long established clinical use, guaiphenesin is recognised as an expectorant in bronchitis. Triprolidine provides antihistamine activity by antagonising H_1 receptors whilst codeine provides analgesic and antitussive actions, decreasing cough frequency but not totally suppressing it.

Contra-indications, warnings, etc
Contra-indications: Contra-indicated in patients with known hypersensitivity to any of the constituents.

Contra-indicated in persons under treatment with monoamine oxidase inhibitors and within two weeks of stopping such treatment.

Precautions: Although pseudoephedrine causes virtually no pressor effect in patients with normal blood pressure, Linctifed should be used with caution in patients with cardiovascular disorders, including hypertension. The effect of antihypertensive agents which modify sympathetic activity may be partially reversed by Linctifed.

Caution should also be exercised in patients taking other sympathomimetic agents, such as decongestants, appetite suppressants and amphetamine-like psychostimulants. The effects of a single dose on the blood pressure of these patients should be observed before recommending repeated or unsupervised treatment.

As with other sympathomimetic agents, caution should be exercised in patients with prostatic enlargement or bladder dysfunction.

In severe hepatic or renal dysfunction a single dose of Linctifed Expectorant or Linctifed Expectorant Paediatric should be given initially and the response to it used as a guide to the patient's requirement for further administration of the product.

The antibacterial agent furazolidone is known to cause a progressive inhibition of monoamine oxidase and although there are no reports of hypertensive crises having occurred, it should not be administered concurrently with Linctifed Expectorant or Linctifed Expectorant Paediatric.

Side- and adverse effects: In some patients pseudoephedrine may occasionally cause insomnia. Triprolidine may cause drowsiness. Patients should not drive a vehicle or operate machinery until they have determined their own response. In some patients the drowsiness induced by antihistamines may be potentiated by alcohol or other central sedatives. Codeine may cause constipation. Fixed drug eruption due to pseudoephedrine taking the form of nummular patches and lichenoid skin eruption due to triprolidine have been reported but these are rare events.

Use in pregnancy and lactation: No data are available on the use of Linctifed Expectorant during pregnancy nor on the excretion of it or its metabolites in human milk.

Toxicity and treatment of overdosage: Probable symptoms include drowsiness, inco-ordination, weakness, palpitation, irritability, hypertension, convulsions and difficulty in micturition. In severe cases there may be respiratory depression due to the codeine component. Gastric lavage and supportive measures for respiration and circulation should be performed if indicated. Convulsions should be controlled with an anticonvulsant. Catheterisation of the bladder may be necessary. Alpha-adrenergic blockade may be required to treat hypertensive crises and beta-adrenergic blockade for the control of supra-ventricular dysrhythmias. Pseudoephedrine has a renal excretion half-life of approximately seven hours and if desired the elimination can be accelerated by acid diuresis or by dialysis.

Pharmaceutical precautions Store below 25°C. Protect from light. Do not refrigerate.

Legal category CD (Sch 5), P.

Package quantities *Linctifed Expectorant:* Bottles of 500 ml and 2 litres.
Linctifed Expectorant Paediatric: Bottles of 500 ml and 2 litres.

Further information Nil.

Product licence numbers
Expectorant 0003/5266
Expectorant Paediatric 0003/5267

MALOPRIM* TABLETS

Presentation *Tablets:* Each white tablet is scored and contains 12.5 mg Pyrimethamine BP and 100 mg Dapsone BP, coded Wellcome H9A.

Uses Maloprim is effective as a causal prophylactic and suppressive agent against malaria caused by *Plasmodium falciparum* and probably other malaria parasites, notably *P. vivax*. Since potentiation takes place between its two active constituents Maloprim is recommended particularly when resistance to pyrimethamine or other anti-folate preparations is known or suspected. It is also effective in chloroquine-resistant areas.

Note: Maloprim should not be used for treatment of the acute attack.

Dosage and administration *Adults:* 1 tablet each week.

Children: Over 10 years: 1 tablet each week.

5–10 years: ½ tablet each week.

Under 5 years: Formulation not applicable.
THE RECOMMENDED DOSE MUST NOT BE EXCEEDED.

The constituents are rapidly absorbed and prophylactic cover can be expected shortly after taking the first dose. Prophylaxis should commence before arrival in an endemic area and be continued once weekly. On returning to a non-malarious area dosage should be maintained for a further four weeks.

Use in the elderly: No specific studies have been carried out in the elderly, however, it may be advisable to monitor renal or hepatic function and if there is serious impairment then caution should be exercised.

Maloprim, at the doses recommended for the prevention of Malaria is unlikely to have any adverse effect on older people normally of good health.

Contra-indications, warnings, etc

Contra-indications: Maloprim should not be given to individuals with a known history of sensitivity to sulphonamides or sulphones or pyrimethamine.

Precautions: Maloprim should be used with caution in patients with hepatic or renal disorders.

During pregnancy and in the presence of other conditions predisposing to folate deficiency a folic acid supplement should be given.

Maloprim, through its mode of action, may further depress folate metabolism in patients already receiving treatment with other folate inhibitors, including combinations of trimethoprim and sulphonamides.

Maloprim may exacerbate folate deficiency due to innate disease or malnutrition.

Side- and adverse effects: Side-effects caused by Maloprim at the recommended doses are rare. Agranulocytosis has been reported, particularly in association with doses of one tablet twice weekly.

Cyanosis, attributable to methaemoglobinaemia, has occurred.

Excessive doses over a prolonged period may produce megaloblastic or haemolytic anaemia.

Acute haemolysis may also occur in individuals with glucose-6-phosphate dehydrogenase deficiency.

Skin sensitivity reactions have occurred.

Insomnia has been reported when pyrimethamine has been given at weekly doses above those recommended.

Use in pregnancy and lactation: While there is a theoretical risk of foetal malformation with all folate inhibitors given during pregnancy, no such adverse effects have been reported with Maloprim in humans. A folate supplement should be given to pregnant women receiving Maloprim. The amount of the components of Maloprim excreted in breast milk is insufficient to contra-indicate its use in lactating mothers, but breast-fed infants should not receive other anti-folate agents.

Toxicity and treatment of overdosage: Symptoms are likely to be nausea, vomiting, hyperexcitability, methaemoglobinaemia and haemolytic anaemia. Convulsions may be apparent and megaloblastic anaemia may ensue. Routine supportive treatment, including maintenance of a clear airway and control of convulsions should be given. Adequate fluids should be given to enhance optimal diuresis. Gastric lavage may be of value only if instituted within two hours in view of the rapid absorption of Maloprim. Provision should be made for fresh blood transfusions. To counteract possible folate deficiency calcium folinate 9–15 mg daily should be administered. There may be a delay of 7 to 10 days before the full leucopenic side effects become evident, therefore calcium folinate should be continued for the period at risk. Methaemoglobinaemia should be treated with ascorbic acid, 200 mg three times daily, or, except in patients with G-6-PD deficiency, by intravenous administration of methylene blue, 2 mg/kg body weight.

Pharmaceutical precautions Store below 25°C. Protect from light.

Legal category POM.

Package quantities Strip pack of 30 tablets.

Further information Nil.

Product licence number 0003/5117.

MIGRIL* TABLETS

Presentation White, round, biconvex compression-coated tablets with a pink core, scored and impressed WELLCOME A4A, with each tablet containing 2 mg Ergotamine Tartrate BP, 50 mg Cyclizine Hydrochloride BP and Caffeine BP equivalent to 100 mg Caffeine Hydrate BP.

Uses MIGRIL is indicated for the relief of the acute migraine attack.

Dosage and administration

Adults: Migril should be taken as soon as possible after the first warning of an attack of migraine and repeated if necessary at the prescribed intervals.

The usual initial dose is one tablet.

Additional doses of a half to one tablet may then be required at half-hourly intervals.

No more than 4 tablets (8 mg ergotamine) should be taken in any one attack.

No more than 6 tablets (12 mg ergotamine) should be given in any one week.

Children: There is no absolute contra-indication to the use of Migril in children but its use is not recommended.

Use in the elderly: There is no absolute contra-indications to the use of Migril in the elderly but see 'Contra-indications' and 'Precautions'.

Contra-indications, warnings, etc

Contra-indications: Migril is contra-indicated during pregnancy because of a direct effect of ergotamine on the uterus. In animals ergotamine has been reported to inhibit implantation, cause peri-natal mortality and foetal retardation.

Migril is contra-indicated during lactation and breast-feeding; it may suppress milk production and may also be excreted in milk at levels high enough to cause pharmacological effects in breast-fed infants.

Migril is contra-indicated in pre-existing vascular disease including angina, claudication, peripheral ischaemia, Raynaud's syndrome and hypertension.

Migril should not be taken if there is a hypersensitivity to any of its constituents.

Precautions: Migril should not be used for migraine prophylaxis because of the risk of inducing ergotism.

The use of ergotamine-containing compounds carries the risk of precipitating arterial constriction and other manifestations of ergotism.

Use the *minimum* effective dosage of Migril necessary since individual sensitivity to the arterial effects of ergotamine varies considerably.

Discontinue the use of Migril if symptoms of arterial insufficiency develop.

Doses of ergotamine as small as 2 mg have caused signs of arterial insufficiency but this is a very rare occurrence.

Migril should be used with caution in patients with infective hepatitis because of an increased risk of precipitating peripheral ischaemia.

Repeated doses of egotamine have occasionally been associated with renal artery spasm and loss of renal function.

Alcohol and Migril should not be taken concurrently.

Ergotamine should be used with care when hyperthyroidism, sepsis and anaemia are present.

Cyclizine, in common with other antihistamines, may cause sedation; patients should be cautioned about driving or operating machinery.

Drug interactions: The concomitant use of ergot alkaloids and beta-blocking agents increases the risks of peripheral vasoconstriction.

Vomiting and peripheral ischaemia have been reported after concomitant use of ergot alkaloids and the antibiotics erythromycin and oleandomycin.

Side- and adverse effects: Habitual use of ergotamine-containing preparations can produce a syndrome of non-migrainous rebound headaches in which case Migril should be discontinued.

Side-effects seen with Migril are usually due to the ergotamine components of the preparation and are more common if the dosage recommendations are exceeded. They include intermittent claudication, coldness and whiteness of the extremities, dysaesthesia, paraesthesia, formication and precordial pain.

Other side-effects seen with ergotamine include muscle cramps, joint pains, raised blood pressure, pulselessness, cyanosis, thrombophlebitis, peripheral arterial thrombosis, gangrene, abdominal pain, coronary infarction, cerebral thrombosis, nausea, dyspnoea, decreased visual acuity, vertigo and diarrhoea. These effects have mostly occurred following habitual chronic use exceeding the recommended dose; they may occasionally occur however at the therapeutic dose.

Arterial vasospasm severe enough to threaten the viability of the limbs has been reported after routine therapy but it is more normally to be expected after prolonged overdosage.

Use in pregnancy and lactation: See 'Contra-indications'.

Toxicity and treatment of overdosage
Acute overdosage:
Symptoms; Acute overdosage with an ergotamine-containing preparation is characterised by nausea, vomiting, tachycardia, hypotonia and peripheral ischaemia. Blood pressure may be difficult to measure.

Treatment: If vomiting has not occurred, efforts should be made to clear the stomach contents. General supportive measures should be applied and intravenous vasodilators may be necessary to relieve vasospasm.

Peritoneal dialysis and forced diuresis may help to eliminate ergotamine from the body.

Chronic overdosage:
Symptoms:
Chronic overdosage with ergotamine-containing preparations usually presents as peripheral ischaemia threatening the viability of the affected limb.

Treatment: Withdraw Migril immediately.

Intravenous vasodilators such as nitroprusside and nitroglycerin may be used to re-establish normal blood flow. Captopril has also been used to reverse the effects of chronic overdosage with ergotamine.

Re-establishment of blood flow may be associated with intense burning sensations in the affected areas but these usually resolve after several weeks.

Pharmaceutical precautions Store below 25°C. Keep dry. Protect from light.

Legal category POM.

Package quantities Bottle of 100 tablets.

Further information Nil.

Product licence number 0003/5114

PENTOSTAM* INJECTION

Presentation Pentostam is a sterile faintly straw-coloured solution of Sodium Stibogluconate BP containing the equivalent of 100 mg pentavalent antimony per ml.

Uses Pentostam is indicated in the following infections caused by Leishmania organisms:

Visceral leishmaniasis (kala-azar)
Cutaneous leishmaniasis (oriental sore) – both dry and moist forms, but excluding diffuse leishmaniasis.
American muco-cutaneous leishmaniasis (espundia).

Dosage and administration *Visceral leishmaniasis (kala-azar): Adults:* 6 ml daily for 7–10 days by intramuscular or intravenous injection. Two or three further courses, separated by an interval of 10 days, may be necessary.
Children: 0.1 ml/kg body weight for 21 days or 0.25 ml/kg body weight for 12–14 days by intravenous or intramuscular injection up to a maximum of 6 ml in a day.

Use in the elderly: No specific studies have been carried out in the elderly, however, it may be advisable to monitor ECG and if there is abnormal ECG extreme caution should be exercised.

If treatment of cutaneous lesions is necessary, local infiltration should be used. The normal precautions should be strictly adhered to when treating older patients for visceral leishmaniasis.

Inadequate treatment may lead to relapse. Therefore a full course of treatment should be given where possible.

All patients should be re-examined regularly for two years after treatment.

Cutaneous leishmaniasis (oriental sore): The dosage regime outlined for visceral leishmaniasis is recommended. Alternatively Pentostam can be infiltrated around the edge of the lesions.

Muco-cutaneous leishmaniasis (espundia): Improvement or complete resolution may occur after a course of 6 ml Pentostam daily for 10 days given intravenously or intramuscularly. A similar course can be repeated, if necessary, on two occasions at monthly intervals.

Intravenous injections should be administered very slowly and discontinued immediately if coughing, vomiting or substernal pain occurs. In such cases extreme care should be taken if Pentostam is readministered by this route.

Contra-indications, warnings, etc
Contra-indications: Pentostam is contra-indicated in myocarditis, hepatitis, pneumonia and nephritis.

Precautions: Very rarely anaphylactic shock may develop during treatment, for which Adrenaline Injection BP and appropriate supportive measures should be given immediately.

Antimonial compounds should be used with extreme caution in patients with an abnormal ECG. Accumulation of antimony in the cardiac conducting tissue may give rise to disturbances in cardiac rhythm. In such circumstances further treatment with Pentostam may be contra-indicated.

Care should be taken in the administration of Pentostam to patients who have recently received other antimonial drugs.

Side- and adverse effects: Documented side-effects include anorexia, substernal or abdominal pain, coughing, nausea, vomiting, weakness, diarrhoea, rash, bleeding from nose or gum and weakness.

Other reported reactions include rigor, fever, vertigo, facial flushing, myalgia and jaundice.

Use in pregnancy and lactation: Although no effects on the foetus have been reported, Pentostam should be withheld during pregnancy unless the potential benefits to the patient outweigh the possible risk to the foetus.

Children should not be breast-fed by mothers receiving antimony.

Toxicity and treatment of overdosage: Main symptoms of antimony poisoning are gastro-intestinal disturbances (nausea, vomiting and severe diarrhoea). Haemorrhagic nephritis and hepatitis may also occur. After oral ingestion gastric lavage should be carried out.

There is only limited information on the use of chelating agents in the treatment of intoxication with antimony compounds. Dimercaprol has been reported to be effective. A dose of 200 mg by intramuscular injection, every six hours until recovery is complete, is suggested.

Pharmaceutical precautions Store below 25°C and protect from light.

Legal category POM.

Package quantities Rubber-capped bottle of 100 ml.

Further information Nil.

Product licence number 0003/5105.

POLIOMYELITIS VACCINE, LIVE (ORAL) BP
WELLCOME* 10 DOSE OPV
TRIVALENT SABIN TYPE (Pol/Vac (Oral))

Presentation This vaccine is a stabilised sterile aqueous suspension of suitable live attenuated strains of poliomyelitis virus, types 1, 2 and 3, grown in cultures of human diploid cells.

The attenuated vaccine strain of each type of poliovirus has antibody-inducing characteristics similar to its virulent counterpart. Extensive studies have shown that there is little risk of Sabin attenuated virus reverting to a virulent condition.

The vaccine may vary in colour from clear to light pink.

Each dose of Poliomyelitis Vaccine, Live (Oral) contains up to 6 i.u. polymyxin and up to 3 i.u. neomycin. In common with all vaccine derived from Sabin seed, it may also contain traces of penicillin and streptomycin.

Use For active immunisation against poliomyelitis.

Dosage and administration *Dosage: Adults and children:* Three drops constitute one dose. The primary course consists of three doses of poliomyelitis vaccine at intervals of not less than four weeks.

Use in the elderly: No special comment.

Administration: For oral use only. The container should be shaken. To ensure the correct drop size is obtained, the container should be held vertically with the nozzle pointing downwards. Although between batches of containers the drop size, and hence the fill volume, may vary, the virus dose provided remains constant.

In the United Kingdom, oral polio vaccine is usually given in infancy at the same time as routine immunisation against diphtheria, tetanus and pertussis. Thereafter it is recommended that all immunised children be given a single reinforcing dose of oral poliomyelitis vaccine at school entry at the time they receive their reinforcing dose of diphtheria/tetanus vaccine, and again at 15 to 19 years of age or on leaving school. Further reinforcing doses are given to adults if they are likely to be exposed to special risk of contracting the disease.

Administration of oral poliomyelitis vaccine induces circulating antibodies and local antibody responses in the intestine. However, one type of poliovirus in the vaccine may inhibit another from establishing immunity. Thus, when only a single dose of trivalent oral polio vaccine is given successful immunisation against all three types of poliovirus may not occur. Therefore in the primary course the vaccine is administered on at least three occasions to ensure that each type of vaccine poliovirus is given an opportunity of establishing immunity.

If parents or siblings of an infant due for immunisation have never been immunised then, provided there is no contra-indication, it is preferable to vaccinate them with Poliomyelitis Vaccine, Live (Oral) at the same time in order to reduce the remote risk of contact paralysis.

Alternatively, two doses of inactivated poliomyelitis vaccine, one month apart, may be given to the adults *before* administration of Poliomyelitis Vaccine, Live (Oral) to the infant.

It is good practice to record the title, dose and lot numbers of all vaccines and dates of administration. Any untoward reactions should be reported to the regulatory authorities and to the manufacturer.

Contra-indications, warnings, etc

Contra-indications: The antibiotic content of the vaccine does not normally contra-indicate use except in cases of extreme hypersensitivity, e.g. anaphylaxis following its administration.

The efficacy of the vaccine may be impaired if given while the subject has diarrhoea or vomiting. In common with other live vaccines, it should not be administered to subjects with an acute febrile illness or impaired immune responsiveness whether idiopathic, or as a result of treatment with steroids, radiotherapy, cytotoxic drugs or other agents.

Vaccinees, parents and other household contacts should be made aware of the possible risk of recipient and contact paralysis prior to vaccination.

Any patient who has previously experienced a serious reaction to the vaccine or any component thereof should not be re-vaccinated.

Precautions: Although anaphylaxis is rare, facilities for its management should always be available during vaccination.

Side- and adverse effects: Vaccine-related paralysis in recipients or contacts may occur on very rare occasions.

Use in pregnancy and lactation: Routine oral poliomyelitis vaccination in pregnancy should be avoided, particularly in the first 4 months. If rapid protection must be achieved during pregnancy because of exposure to poliomyelitis, then oral poliomyelitis vaccine may be given. There is some evidence that polio virus is not teratogenic and does not cross the placental barrier.

Poliomyelitis Vaccine Live (Oral) may be administered

as early as six weeks of age and the response has been shown to be unaffected by breast feeding from this age onwards.

Toxicity and treatment of overdosage: Not applicable.

Pharmaceutical precautions If stored between 0° and 4°C oral poliomyelitis vaccine can be expected to retain its potency for six months. If stored at or just below 25°C, oral poliomyelitis vaccine can be expected to retain its potency for one week. When tubes of vaccine have been opened there is a risk of contamination with bacteria and moulds which may result in a reduction of vaccine potency. It is good practice, therefore, to discard vaccine remaining in opened tubes at the end of the vaccinating session.

Legal category POM.

Package quantities Polythene dropper tubes of 10 doses.

Product licence number 0003/0116

POLIOMYELITIS VACCINE, LIVE (ORAL) BP, WELLCOME* SINGLE DOSE OPV TRIVALENT SABIN TYPE (Pol/Vac (Oral))

Presentation This vaccine is a stabilised sterile aqueous suspension of suitable live attenuated strains of poliomyelitis virus, types 1, 2 and 3, grown in cultures of human diploid cells.

The attenuated vaccine strain of each type of poliovirus has antibody-inducing characteristics similar to its virulent counterpart. Extensive studies have shown that there is little risk of Sabin attenuated virus reverting to a virulent condition.

The vaccine may vary in colour from clear to light pink.

Each dose of Poliomyelitis Vaccine, Live (Oral) contains up to 6 i.u. polymyxin and up to 3 i.u. neomycin. In common with all vaccine derived from Sabin seed, it also may contain traces of penicillin and streptomycin.

Uses For active immunization against poliomyelitis.

Dosage and administration

Dosage: Adults and children: The contents of one single dose polythene tube constitute one dose. The primary course consists of three doses of poliomyelitis vaccine at intervals of not less than four weeks.

Use in the elderly: No special comment.

Administration: For oral use only. Separate a single-dose tube from the strip. The tube should be held by the tapered end and shaken down, as with a thermometer, to propel the entire contents to the corrugated end. The tube should be held upright without applying pressure to the tube and cut across the tapered end at the narrowest point. Incline tube gently to move the vaccine to the cut end. It may be necessary to shake the tube gently. The contents are then expelled by exerting gentle pressure to the tube just above the surface of the liquid. Since the vaccine contains live attenuated poliomyelitis virus, care should be taken to avoid transfer of virus to immunodeficient subjects. Both parts of the container should be subject to disposal, e.g. by incineration, while the spoon may be either incinerated or sterilised in Milton. Scissors may be decontaminated at the end of a vaccinating session by boiling in water or by soaking them for 5 minutes in 1:10 Milton 1% and then rinsing in water.

In the United Kingdom, oral polio vaccine is usually given in infancy at the same time as routine immunization against diphtheria, tetanus and pertussis. Thereafter it is recommended that all immunized children be given a single reinforcing dose of oral poliomyelitis vaccine at school entry at the time they receive their reinforcing dose of diphtheria/tetanus vaccine, and again at 15 to 19 years of age or on leaving school. Further reinforcing doses are given to adults if they are likely to be exposed to special risk of contracting the disease.

Administration of oral poliomyelitis vaccine induces circulating antibodies and local antibody responses in the intestine. However, one type of poliovirus in the vaccine may inhibit another from establishing immunity. Thus, when only a single dose of trivalent oral polio vaccine is given, successful immunization against all three types of poliovirus may not occur. Therefore in the primary course the vaccine is administered on at least three occasions to ensure that each type of vaccine poliovirus is given an opportunity of establishing immunity.

If parents or siblings of an infant due for immunization have never been immunized then, provided there is no contra-indication, it is preferable to vaccinate them with Poliomyelitis Vaccine, Live (Oral) BP at the same time in order to reduce the remote risk of contact paralysis.

Alternatively, two doses of inactivated poliomyelitis vaccine, one month apart, may be given to the adults *before* administration of Poliomyelitis Vaccine, Live (Oral) BP to the infant.

It is good practice to record the title, dose and lot numbers of all vaccines and dates of administration. Any untoward reactions should be reported to the regulatory authorities and to the manufacturer.

Contra-indications, warnings, etc

Contra-indications: The antibiotic content of the vaccine does not normally contra-indicate use except in cases of extreme hypersensitivity, e.g. anaphylaxis following its administration.

The efficacy of the vaccine may be impaired if given while the subject has diarrhoea or vomiting. In common with other live vaccines, it should not be administered to subjects with an acute febrile illness or impaired immune responsiveness whether idiopathic, or as a result of treatment with steroids, radiotherapy, cytoxic drugs or other agents.

Vaccines, parents and other household contacts should be made aware of the possible risk of recipient and contact paralysis prior to vaccination.

Any patient who has previously experienced a serious reaction to the vaccine or any component thereof should not be re-vaccinated.

Precautions: Although anaphylaxis is rare, facilities for its management should always be available during vaccination.

Side- and adverse effects: Vaccine-related paralysis in recipients or contracts may occur on very rare occasions.

Use in pregnancy and lactation: Routine oral poliomyelitis vaccination in pregnancy should be avoided particularly in the first 4 months, but it may be given if rapid protection during pregnancy is indicated because of exposure to poliomyelitis. There is some evidence that polio virus is not teratogenic and does not cross the placental barrier.

Poliomyelitis Vaccine Live (Oral) BP may be administered as early as six weeks of age and the response has been shown to be unaffected by breast feeding from this age onwards.

Toxicity and treatment of overdosage: Not applicable.

Pharmaceutical precautions If stored between 0° and 4°C, oral poliomyelitis vaccine can be expected to retain its potency for six months. If stored at or just below 25°C, oral poliomyelitis vaccine can be expected to retain its potency for one week.

Legal category POM.

Package quantities 10 polythene dropper tubes each containing one dose.

Product licence number 0003/0116.

POLYTRIM* EYE DROPS

Presentation A clear, colourless, sterile, aqueous solution containing in each ml: Trimethoprim BP 1 mg; Polymyxin B Sulphate BP 10,000 units. Thiomersal BP (0.05 mg per ml) is included as a preservative.

Uses Antibacterial agent. For the treatment and prophylaxis of external bacterial infections of the eye including conjunctivitis, keratitis, corneal ulceration, ulcerative blepharitis with associated conjunctivitis, and chronic dacryocystitis. Prophylactically, it is useful following removal of foreign bodies, and before and after ophthalmic surgery to help provide and maintain a sterile field. Use of Polytrim does not exclude concomitant systemic therapy or other forms of local therapy, where appropriate.

Dosage and administration *Adults:* 1 drop in the affected eye four times daily. *Children:* As for adults.

More frequent administration may be required, depending on the severity of the condition. Treatment should normally be continued for at least forty-eight hours after the eye has apparently returned to normal.

Use in the elderly: No special precautions.

Contra-indications, warnings, etc
Contra-indications: Contra-indicated in individuals who have a history of hypersensitivity to trimethoprim, polymyxins, or cross-sensitising substances.

Precautions: As with all antibacterial preparations, prolonged use may result in the overgrowth of non-susceptible organisms including fungi.

Side- and adverse effects: Polytrim is isotonic with tear fluid and is well tolerated in the eye. No local adverse effects are to be expected, except rarely, a hypersensitivity reaction. If one is suspected during treatment, administration should be discontinued.

Toxicity and treatment of overdosage: Not applicable.

Pharmaceutical precautions Do not use if the container seal has been broken. Use within one month of opening container: Store in a dry place, below 25°C, and protect from light. Not suitable for injection.

Legal category POM.

Package quantities Screw-capped plastic dropper bottle containing 5 ml.

Further information There is *in vitro* evidence of synergy between trimethoprim and polymyxin. The combination is effective against a wide variety of Gram-positive and Gram-negative bacterial ocular pathogens, including *Pseudomonas aeruginosa*.

Product licence number 0003/0153.

PRO-ACTIDIL* TABLETS

Presentation Each tablet contains 10 mg of Triprolidine Hydrochloride BP divided between three layers to give a rapid onset of action, followed by a sustained release of the drug to give a therapeutic effect lasting up to 24 hours in most patients. Each tablet is coded Wellcome M4A and is white with blue core and pink middle layer.

Uses Prolonged action antihistamine.

In allergic dermatoses, urticaria, seborrhoeic eczema, angioneurotic oedema, pruritus, vasomotor rhinitis, hay fever.

Dosage and administration *Adults:* 1 tablet swallowed whole with a little water in the early evening, or five to six hours before retiring. A few patients with very severe symptoms may need two tablets during 24 hours.

Children: Over 10 years: 1 tablet a day.

Under 10 years: It is recommended that Actidil Elixir is used.

Use in the elderly: No specific studies have been carried out in the elderly, however, it may be advisable to monitor renal or hepatic function and if there is serious impairment then caution should be exercised.

Contra-indications, warnings, etc
Contra-indications: Contra-indicated in patients with known hypersensitivity to triprolidine.

Precautions: Caution in severe hepatic or renal dysfunction.

May cause drowsiness. Patients should not drive a vehicle or operate machinery until they have determined their own response. In some patients the drowsiness induced by antihistamines may be potentiated by alcohol or other central sedatives.

Side- and adverse effects: Triprolidine may cause drowsiness. Lichenoid skin eruptions due to triprolidine have rarely been reported.

Use in pregnancy and lactation: No data are available on the use of Pro-Actidil in human pregnancy. Triprolidine is excreted in human milk.

Toxicity and treatment of overdosage: Drowsiness, dizziness, inco-ordination, weakness, convulsions and respiratory depression may occur.

Necessary measures should be taken to maintain and support respiration. Gastric lavage should be performed if indicated and convulsions controlled with diazepam. There are theoretical grounds for believing that the elimination of triprolidine and its metabolites could be accelerated by dialysis.

Pharmaceutical precautions Store below 15°C. Protect from light.

Legal category P.

Package quantities Bottle of 100 tablets.

Further information Nil.

Product licence number 0003/5228.

SCHICK TEST TOXIN BP AND
SCHICK CONTROL BP WELLCOME*

Presentation Schick Test Toxin is the sterile diluted filtrate from a culture of *Corynebacterium diphtheriae*. The Control Fluid is the same material heated sufficiently to inactivate the toxin but not sufficiently to destroy the more heat-stable bacterial proteins and broth constituents.

Schick Test Toxin contains thiomersal 0.004% as preservative.

Uses The Schick test is used to demonstrate whether or not a certain degree of immunity to diphtheria is present, either initially or after immunisation. The toxin produces a local skin reaction in those who are susceptible to the disease, while in those who are satisfactorily immune it is neutralised by the subject's antitoxin and no reaction results. The concurrent injection of Control Fluid at another, comparable site provides a means of distinguishing between true, positive reactions due to toxin and other reactions of an allergic nature due to non-specific constituents. During the first few months of life babies usually have maternally derived immunity. Those between 6 months and 8 years old rarely suffer from untoward reactions after primary immunisation. Therefore, the Schick test is not usually given to infants or children up to 8 or even 10 years of age. In children over 10 years and adults, the state of immunity varies, so a preliminary Schick test should always be performed before injection of a vaccine, the main purpose being to detect those giving a negative-and-pseudo reaction, for they may experience a reaction after a dose of vaccine.

Dosage and administration *Technique:* A dose of 0.2 ml of the Toxin is injected *intradermally* into the anterior surface of the left forearm, and 0.2 ml of the Control Fluid into the corresponding position on the right forearm.

Separate syringes and needles should be used for the Toxin and Control Fluid. It is a practical advantage, when dealing with groups of subjects, to identify each syringe; a rubber band around the barrels of, say, those for the Control Fluid is suggested. Any unused portion of a container should be discarded.

Readings: Results may be read at 24–48 (possibly up to 72) hours, and again at five to seven days to detect late reactors and to reconsider earlier, doubtful readings. By comparing the appearance of the two arms it is possible to judge how far any reaction is due to the toxin and how far to the other constituents. Four types of result may be seen:

Negative (= immune). No reaction visible on either arm.

Negative-and-pseudo (= immune). Both arms show somewhat similar flushes which usually fade more rapidly than that of a true positive reaction. They are due to non-specific constituents and not to toxin.

Positive (= susceptible). The left arm shows a flush from 10–50 mm in diameter; this fades and becomes brown and fine desquamation may occur. The staining may persist for several weeks.

Positive-and-pseudo (= susceptible) (also called 'combined'). Both arms show a flush but the left is larger, deeper and more persistent than the right. The pseudo effect develops more rapidly than any positive response and may be at its maximum at 24–72 hours. By the fifth to sixth day, the pseudo effect has faded considerably or disappeared, whereas the positive reaction has increased in size and intensity.

Distinction must be made between those with a well-marked pseudo reaction, which may be slightly greater on the left arm, and those with a positive-and-pseudo result, which will be markedly greater on the left arm. The true positive-and-pseudo reaction is extremely rare

and most subjects showing a large flush on both arms are immune, even if there is some difference between the two arms. Persons showing a well-marked pseudo reaction are almost invariably immune to diphtheria and should not be immunised further because they may react severely to the vaccine.

The Schick test may be vitiated by the following: the reading of Schick tests performed from 12 hours before to four weeks after the administration of diphtheria, tetanus or of any other equine antitoxin or of convalescent human serum or gammaglobulin may be erroneous and should, if negative, be disregarded.

Use in the elderly: No special comment.

Contra-indications, warnings, etc
Contra-indications: Subjects with a history of hypersensitivity to previous doses of Schick Test materials or with a known hypersensitivity to diphtheria vaccine should not be tested.

Precautions: Although anaphylaxis associated with the Schick Test is extremely rare, facilities for the management of anaphylaxis should be available during its administration.

The validity of the Schick Test may be impaired if the test is performed within 12 hours to 4 weeks following the administration of any equine antitoxin or of human sera or gamma globulin. Negative results obtained during this period are not indicative of immunity to diphtheria and should be disregarded.

Use in pregnancy and lactation: The Schick Test has been in wide use for many years without apparent ill consequence.

Toxicity and treatment of overdosage: Not applicable.

Pharmaceutical precautions Store at 2–8°C. *Do not freeze.*

Legal category POM.

Package quantities Set of 2 ml.

Further information Nil.

Product licence number 0003/5139.

SEPTRIN* TABLETS
SEPTRIN* DISPERSIBLE TABLETS
SEPTRIN* FORTE TABLETS
SEPTRIN* ADULT SUSPENSION
SEPTRIN* PAEDIATRIC SUSPENSION
SEPTRIN* PAEDIATRIC TABLETS

Presentation Septrin Tablets (Co-trimoxazole Tablets BP) each contain 80 mg Trimethoprim BP and 400 mg Sulphamethoxazole BP. Coded Septrin Y2B Wellcome. White in colour.

Septrin Dispersible Tablets (Dispersible Co-trimoxazole Tablets BP) each contain 80 mg Trimethoprim BP and 400 mg Sulphamethoxazole BP. Coded Septrin Y2B Wellcome. Orange in colour.

Septrin Forte Tablets (Co-trimoxazole Tablets BP) each contain 160 mg Trimethoprim BP and 800 mg Sulphamethoxazole BP. Scored and coded Septrin Forte O2C. White in colour.

Septrin Adult Suspension (Co-trimoxazole Mixture BP) contains 80 mg Trimethoprim BP and 400 mg Sulphamethoxazole BP in each 5 ml. Off-white in colour.

Septrin Paediatric Suspension (Paediatric Co-trimoxazole Mixture BP) contains 40 mg Trimethoprim BP and

200 mg Sulphamethoxazole BP in each 5 ml. Pale pink in colour.

Septrin Paediatric Tablets (Paediatric Co-trimoxazole Tablets BP) each contain 20 mg Trimethoprim BP and 100 mg Sulphamethoxazole BP. Scored and coded Wellcome H4R. White in colour.

Uses Septrin is an antibacterial agent. Septrin is effective *in vitro* against a wide range of Gram-positive and Gram-negative organisms. It is not active against *Mycobacterium tuberculosis, Mycoplasma* or *Treponema pallidum, Pseudomonas aeruginosa* is usually insensitive.

Septrin is of value in the treatment of the following:

Respiratory tract: Acute and chronic bronchitis, bronchiectasis, lobar and broncho-pneumonia, *Pneumocystis carinii* pneumonitis, otitis media and sinusitis.

Genito-urinary tract: Urethritis, cystitis, pyelitis, pyelonephritis, and prostatitis. Male and female gonorrhoea.

Gastro-intestinal tract: Typhoid and paratyphoid fevers, chronic carriage of *Salmonella typhi* and *paratyphi,* cholera and shigellosis.

Skin infections: Pyoderma, abscesses and wound infections.

Other bacterial infections: Acute and chronic osteomyelitis, acute brucellosis, septicaemias and other infections caused by sensitive organisms.

Dosage and administration *Septrin Tablets* and *Septrin Dispersible Tablets – Adults:* Standard dosage: 2 twice daily.

For severe infections: 3 twice daily.
Children over 12 years: As for adults.
6–12 years: 1 twice daily.

Septrin Dispersible Tablets should be taken in a little water or swallowed whole.

Septrin Forte Tablets – Adults: Standard dosage: 1 twice daily.

For severe infections: 1½ twice daily.
Children over 12 years: As for adults.
Children under 12 years: Not applicable.

Septrin Adult Suspension – Adults: Standard dosage: 10 ml twice daily.

For severe infections: 15 ml twice daily. For long-term treatment (more than 14 days): 5 ml twice daily.
Children over 12 years: As for adults.

Septrin Paediatric Suspension
Children 6–12 years: 10 ml twice daily.
6 months to 6 years: 5 ml twice daily.
6 weeks to 6 months: 2.5 ml twice daily.

Septrin Adult and Paediatric Suspensions may be diluted with Syrup BP but should be used within 14 days as maintenance of stability cannot be guaranteed.

Septrin Paediatric Tablets
Children 6–12 years: 4 twice daily.
2–6 years: 2 twice daily.

Paediatric dosage may be increased by 50% for severe infections.

Septrin may be taken with some food to minimise the possibility of GI disturbances.

Special Dosage Recommendations: Unless stated, standard dosage applies.

In acute infections, Septrin should be given for at least five days or until the patient has been symptom-free for two days.

Impaired renal function: If Septrin is given to patients with renal impairment then the following dosage scheme is suggested (no information is available for children with renal failure).

Creatinine clearance (ml/min)	Serum creatinine (μmol/l)		Dosage
Above 25	men women	<265 <175	Standard dosage.
15–25	men women	265–620 175–400	Standard dosage for a maximum of three days followed by half the standard dosage.
Below 15	men women	>620 >400	Not to be administered unless haemodialysis facilities are available. Under this condition half the standard dosage may be given.

Measurements of plasma concentrations of sulphamethoxazole at intervals of two to three days are recommended in samples obtained 12 hours after administration of Septrin. If the concentration of total sulphamethoxazole exceeds 150 mcg/ml, then treatment should be interrupted until the value falls below 120 mcg/ml.

Long-term prophylaxis of recurrent or suppression of chronic infection following sterilisation of the urine:

Adults and children over 12 years: 1 tablet nightly.

Children under 12 years: A single nightly dose of 2 mg trimethoprim and 10 mg sulphamethoxazole per kg body weight.

Treatment may be continued for 3 to 12 months or more as appropriate.

Chronic prostatitis: It may be advisable to use a *higher* than standard dose initially. The course of treatment should last for three months to reduce the risk of relapse.

Pneumocystis carinii *pneumonitis:*

Treatment: 20 mg trimethoprim and 100 mg sulphamethoxazole per kg body weight per day in two or more divided doses for two weeks. The steady state or serum level of trimethoprim should be maintained at 5 mcg/ml or higher for maximum efficacy.

Prevention: Standard dosage for the duration of the period at risk.

Gonorrhoea: In uncomplicated cases 4 tablets every 12 hours for two days *or* 5 tablets followed by a further dose of 5 tablets eight hours later.

Acute brucellosis: It may be advisable to use a *higher* than standard dose initially. Treatment should continue for a period of at least four weeks and repeated courses may be beneficial.

Typhoid and paratyphoid carriage: Treatment should be continued for at least 1–3 months.

Use in the elderly: No specific studies have been carried out in the elderly, although Septrin has been widely used in older people. However, care is advised when treating the elderly because, as a group, they are more susceptible to adverse reactions.

Contra-indications, warnings, etc

Contra-indications: Septrin should not be given to

patients with a history of sulphonamide, trimethoprim or co-trimoxazole hypersensitivity.

Contra-indicated in patients showing marked liver parenchymal damage.

Except in certain circumstances it should not be given to patients with serious haematological disorders. The combination has been administered to patients receiving cytotoxic agents without evidence of an adverse effect on the bone marrow or peripheral blood.

Contra-indicated in severe renal insufficiency where repeated measurements of the plasma concentration cannot be performed.

Septrin should be taken to premature babies nor to full-term infants during the first six weeks of life. The drug should not be given during pregnancy. (See below.)

Precautions: Septrin should be discontinued if a skin rash appears.

In cases with renal impairment a modified dosage schedule as described above is indicated. In such patients, measurements of the plasma concentration of the drug is advisable.

An adequate urinary output should be maintained.

A folate supplement should be considered when treating potentially folate deficient patients or with prolonged high dosage of Septrin.

If Septrin treatment is prolonged, especially in patients with suspected impairment of folate metabolism, it is suggested that complete blood counts including thrombocytes be performed at monthly intervals.

The usual caution in prescribing any drug for women of child-bearing age should be exercised with Septrin.

Care should be taken when giving Septrin to patients receiving sulphonylurea hypoglycaemics, warfarin, or phenytoin as the action of these agents may be increased.

Patients receiving pyrimethamine in doses in excess of 25 mg weekly who are also receiving Septrin should have their blood pictures monitored because of the occasional report of megaloblastic anaemia apparently occurring in these circumstances.

In elderly patients concurrently receiving diuretics, mainly thiazides, there appears to be an increased risk of thrombocytopenia with or without purpura.

Side- and adverse effects: As Septrin contains trimethoprim and a sulphonamide, the type and frequency of adverse effects associated with such compounds may be expected.

Nausea, vomiting, diarrhoea, glossitis and skin rashes can occur. Pseudomembranous colitis has been reported rarely. Severe skin sensitivity reactions such as erythema multiforme bullosa (Stevens-Johnson syndrome) and toxic epidermal necrolysis (Lyell syndrome) have occurred infrequently and, rarely, have been associated with a fatality.

As Septrin contains a sulphonamide, the possibility of blood dyscrasias like those associated with sulphonamides should be borne in mind. The changes reported with Septrin mainly consist of thrombocytopenia, purpura, leucopenia, neutropenia and very rarely agranulocytosis. They have usually proved to be reversible on withdrawal of the drug. Elderly patients are more susceptible to these blood changes. Septrin may induce haemolysis in certain susceptible glucose-6-phosphate dehydrogenase deficient patients. Jaundice and, very rarely, hepatic necrosis have been reported.

There have been a few reports of subjective experiences such as headache, depression, dizziness and hallucinations but their relationship to therapy remains unproven.

During long-term therapy, isolated cases of megaloblastic changes in the bone marrow have been reported; these are reversible by folinic acid therapy.

Use in pregnancy and lactation: The safety of Septrin in human pregnancy has not been established. Animal studies have shown teratogenic effects typical of a folate antagonist in rats but not rabbits at high doses; these were prevented by administration of dietary folates. Sulphonamide-containing products should not be administered in late pregnancy because of the risk of kernicterus.

Both sulphamethoxazole and trimethoprim may be found in breast milk but the administration of Septrin represents a negligible risk to the suckling infant.

Toxicity and treatment of overdosage: Symptoms of acute overdosage are likely to be nausea, vomiting, abdominal pain, dizziness and confusion. Treatment should consist of gastric lavage if within an hour of ingestion. Absorption of trimethoprim from the gastrointestinal tract is normally complete in approximately 2 hours, but this may not be the case in gross overdosage. Increased fluid intake will increase the elimination of sulphamethoxazole. Alkalinisation of the urine will also increase the elimination of sulphamethoxazole but decrease that of the trimethoprim. Calcium folinate (3–6 mg/day) should reverse any folate deficiency effect of trimethoprim. General supportive measures are recommended.

Both trimethoprim and sulphamethoxazole are dialysable by renal dialysis.

Pharmaceutical precautions *Tablets:* Store below 25°C. Protect from light.

Dispersible Tablets: Store below 25°C. Keep dry, protect from light.

Adult and Paediatric Suspension: Store below 25°C. Protect from light.

Legal category POM.

Package quantities *Septrin Tablets:* packs of 100 and 500 tablets.

Septrin Dispersible Tablets: packs of 100 and 500 tablets.

Septrin Forte Tablets: pack of 100 tablets.

Septrin Adult Suspension: bottle of 100 ml.

Septrin Paediatric Suspension: bottle of 100 ml.

Septrin Paediatric Tablets: pack of 100 tablets.

Further information Absorption by the oral route is rapid: significant plasma levels are obtained within an hour. Peak levels are reached between two and four hours and are maintained over a period of 12 hours.

In the treatment of tonsillo-pharyngitis due to Group A beta-haemolytic streptococci, eradication of these organisms from the oro-pharynx is less rapid than with some other antibiotics.

Trimethoprim may cause an apparent rise in serum creatinine levels due to (a) competition for the tubular secretory mechanisms; (b) chemical interference with the visual auto-analyser method of estimating creatinine.

Co-trimoxazole may cause a fall in circulating thyroid hormone levels but the clinical significance requires confirmation.

Trimethoprim has been noted to impair phenylalanine metabolism but this is of no significance in phenylketonuric patients on appropriate dietary restriction.

Plasma or serum levels of sulphamethoxazole and

trimethoprim may be determined by high performance liquid chromatography.

Septrin for Infusion and Septrin Intra-muscular Injection are also available.

Product licence numbers

Tablets	0003/0109
Dispersible Tablets	0003/0099
Forte Tablets	0003/0121
Adult Suspension	0003/5223
Paediatric Suspension	0003/5222
Paediatric Tablets	0003/0108

SEPTRIN* FOR INFUSION

Strong Sterile Co-trimoxazole Solution
To make Co-trimoxazole Intravenous Infusion BP.

Presentation Septrin for Infusion contains 80 mg Trimethoprim BP and 400 mg Sulphamethoxazole BP in each 5 ml ampoule. The infusion is faintly yellow and contains 40 per cent w/v propylene glycol together with ethyl alcohol and a small amount of benzyl alcohol. It has a pH of approximately 10.

Uses Septrin is an antibacterial agent. Septrin is effective *in vitro* against a wide range of Gram-positive and Gram-negative organisms. It is not active against *Mycobacterium tuberculosis, Mycoplasmata* or *Treponema pallidum. Pseudomonas aeruginosa* is usually insensitive.

In general, the indications for the use of Septrin for Infusion are the same as those for oral presentations. Septrin for Infusion is for use when oral dosage is not possible.

Clinical experience with oral Septrin indicates its value in the following:

Respiratory tract: Acute and chronic bronchitis, bronchiectasis, lobar and broncho-pneumonia, *Pneumocystis carinii* pneumonitis, otitis media and sinusitis.

Genito-urinary tract: Urethritis, cystitis, pyelitis, pyelonephritis and prostatitis. Male and female gonorrhoea.

Gastro-intestinal tract: Typhoid and paratyphoid fevers, chronic carriage of *Salmonella typhi* and *paratyphi*, cholera, and shigellosis.

Skin infections: Pyoderma, abscesses and wound infections.

Other bacterial infections: Acute and chronic osteomyelitis, acute brucellosis, septicaemias and other infections caused by sensitive organisms.

Dosage and administration
Adults and children over 12 years: Standard dosage: 10 ml twice daily, morning and evening.

For severe infections: 15 ml twice daily, morning and evening.

Children up to 12 years: The recommended dosage is approximately 6 mg trimethoprim and 30 mg sulphamethoxazole per kg body weight per 24 hours, divided into two equal doses. As a guide the following doses of Septrin for Infusion may be used:

6 weeks to 6 months: 1.25 ml twice daily.
6 months to 6 years: 2.5 ml twice daily.
6–12 years: 5.0 ml twice daily.

Paediatric dosage may be increased by 50% for severe infections.

It is intended that Septrin for Infusion should be used only during such a period as the patient is unable to accept oral therapy.

Dosage in Pneumocystis carinii *pneumonitis:* The dosage is 20 mg trimethoprim, 100 mg sulphamethoxazole/kg/day in two or more divided doses. The course is two weeks, but oral therapy should be substituted as soon as it is appropriate. The steady state or serum level of trimethoprim should be maintained at 5 mcg/ml or higher for maximum efficacy.

Dosage recommendations in renal impairment: If Septrin is given to patients with renal impairment then the following dosage scheme is suggested (no information is available for children with renal failure); see table below.

Creatinine clearance (ml/min)	Serum creatinine (μmol/l)		Dosage
Above 25	men women	< 265 < 175	Standard dosage.
15–25	men women	265–620 175–400	Standard dosage for a maximum of three days followed by half the standard dosage.
Below 15	men women	> 620 > 400	Not to be administered unless haemodialysis facilities are available. Under this condition half the standard dosage may be given.

Measurements of plasma concentrations of sulphamethoxazole at intervals of two to three days are recommended in samples obtained 12 hours after administration of Septrin. If the concentration of total sulphamethoxazole exceeds 150 mcg/ml then treatment should be interrupted until the value falls below 120 mcg/ml.

Use in the elderly: No specific studies have been carried out in the elderly, although Septrin has been widely used in older people. However, care is advised when treating the elderly because, as a group, they are more susceptible to adverse reactions.

Administration: Septrin for Infusion must be given by the intravenous route ONLY and MUST BE DILUTED before administration, according to the following schedules:

One ampoule Septrin for Infusion (5 ml) to 125 ml infusion solution.

Two ampoules Septrin for Infusion (10 ml) to 250 ml infusion solution.

Three ampoules Septrin for Infusion (15 ml) to 500 ml infusion solution.

DILUTION SHOULD BE CARRIED OUT DIRECTLY BEFORE USE. After the addition of Septrin for Infusion to the infusion solution the mixture should be shaken to ensure thorough mixing. Should visible turbidity or crystallisation appear in the solution at any time before or during an infusion the mixture should be discarded.

Septrin for Infusion is known to be compatible, when diluted in accordance with the schedules above, with the following fluids:

Glucose Intravenous Infusion BP 5% and 10%.
Fructose Intravenous Infusion BP 5%.
Sodium Chloride Intravenous Infusion BP (0.9%).

Sodium Chloride (0.18%) and Glucose (4%) Intravenous Infusion BP.

Dextran 70 Injection BP 6% in glucose 5% or normal saline.

Dextran 40 Injection BP 10% in glucose 5% or normal saline.

Ringer' Solution for Injection BPC 1959.

No other substance should be mixed with the infusion.

It is suggested that the duration of the infusion should be approximately one and a half hours, but this should be balanced against the fluid requirements of the patient.

When fluid restriction is necessary, Septrin for Infusion may be given in a higher concentration such as one 5 ml ampoule in 50 ml or 75 ml of 5% w/v glucose in water.

Contra-indications, warnings, etc

Contra-indications: Septrin should not be given to patients with a history of sulphonamide, trimethoprim or co-trimoxazole hypersensitivity.

Contra-indicated in patients showing marked liver parenchymal damage.

Except in certain circumstances it should not be given to patients with serious haematological disorders. The combination has been administered to patients receiving cytotoxic agents without evidence of an adverse effect on the bone marrow or peripheral blood.

Contra-indicated in severe renal insufficiency where repeated measurements of the plasma concentration cannot be performed.

Septrin should not be given to premature babies nor to full-term infants during the first six weeks of life. The drug should not be given during pregnancy. (See below.)

Precautions: Septrin for Infusion should be discontinued if a skin rash appears.

Fluid overload is possible, especially when very high doses are being administered to patients with underlying cardiopulmonary disease. In cases with renal impairment a modified dosage schedule as described above is indicated. In such patients, measurement of the plasma concentration of the drug is advisable. An adequate urinary output should be maintained.

A folate supplement should be considered when treating potentially folate deficient patients or with prolonged high dosage of Septrin.

If Septrin treatment is prolonged, especially in patients with suspected impairment of folate metabolism, it is suggested that complete blood counts including thrombocytes be performed at monthly intervals.

The usual caution in prescribing any drug for women of child-bearing age should be exercised with Septrin.

Care should be taken when giving Septrin to patients receiving sulphonylurea hypoglycaemics, warfarin, or phenytoin as the action of these agents may be increased.

Patients receiving pyrimethamine in doses in excess of 25 mg weekly who are also receiving Septrin should have their blood pictures monitored because of the occasional report of megaloblastic anaemia apparently occurring in these circumstances.

In elderly patients concurrently receiving diuretics, mainly thiazides, there appears to be an increased risk of thrombocytopenia with or without purpura.

Side- and adverse effects: As Septrin contains trimethoprim and a sulphonamide, the type and frequency of adverse effects associated with such compounds may be expected.

Nausea, vomiting, diarrhoea, glossitis and skin rashes can occur. Pseudomembranous colitis has been reported rarely. Severe skin sensitivity reactions such as erythema

multiforme bullous (Stevens-Johnson syndrome) and toxic epidermal necrolysis (Lyell syndrome) have occurred infrequently and, rarely, have been associated with a fatality.

As Septrin contains a sulphonamide, the possibility of blood dyscrasias like those associated with sulphonamides should be borne in mind. The changes reported with Septrin mainly consist of thrombocytopenia, purpura, leucopenia, neutropenia and very rarely agranulocytosis. They have usually proved to be reversible on withdrawal of the drug. Elderly patients are more susceptible to these blood changes. Septrin may induce haemolysis in certain susceptible glucose-6-phosphate dehydrogenase deficient patients.

Jaundice and, very rarely hepatic necrosis have been reported.

There have been a few reports of subjective experiences such as headache, depression, dizziness and hallucinations but their relationship to therapy remains unproven.

During long-term therapy, isolated cases of megaloblastic changes in the bone marrow have been reported; these are reversible by folinic acid therapy.

Use in pregnancy and lactation: The safety of Septrin in human pregnancy has not been established. Animal studies have shown teratogenic effects typical of a folate antagonist in rats but not rabbits at high doses; these were prevented by administration of dietary folates. Sulphonamide-containing products should not be administered in late pregnancy because of the risk of kernicterus.

Both sulphamethoxazole and trimethoprim may be found in breast milk, but the administration of Septrin represents a negligible risk to the suckling infant.

Toxicity and treatment of overdosage: The maximum tolerated dose in humans is unknown.

Nausea, vomiting, dizziness and confusion are likely symptoms of overdosage.

In cases of known, suspected, or accidental overdosage stop therapy.

Acidification of the urine will increase the elimination of trimethoprim. Inducing diuresis plus alkalinisation of urine will enhance the elimination of sulphamethoxazole. Alkalinisation will reduce the rate of elimination of trimethoprim. Calcium folinate (3–6 mg/day) should reverse any folate deficiency effect of trimethoprim. General supportive measures are recommended.

Both trimethoprim and sulphamethoxazole are dialysable by renal dialysis.

Pharmaceutical precautions Store below 25°C. Protect from light.

Legal category POM.

Package quantities Box of 10 ampoules.

Further information In the treatment of tonsillopharyngitis due to Group A beta-haemolytic streptococci, eradication of these organisms from the oropharynx is less rapid than with some other antibiotics.

Trimethoprim may cause an apparent rise in serum creatinine levels due to (a) competition for the tubular secretory mechanisms; (b) chemical interference with the visual auto-analyser method of estimating creatinine.

Co-trimoxazole may cause a fall in circulating thyroid hormone levels but the clinical significance requires confirmation.

Trimethoprim has been noted to impair phenylalanine

metabolism but this is of no significance in phenylketon-uric patients on appropriate dietary restriction.

Plasma or serum levels of sulphamethoxazole and trimethoprim may be determined by high performance liquid chromatography.

Septrin is available also as: Tablets, Dispersible Tablets, Forte Tablets, Adult Suspension, Paediatric Suspension, Paediatric Tablets, and Intramuscular Injection.

Product licence number 0003/0095.

SEPTRIN* INTRAMUSCULAR INJECTION

Presentation Septrin IM Injection contains 160 mg Trimethoprim BP and 800 mg Sulphamethoxazole BP in each 3 ml ampoule.

The sterile solution is faintly yellow and contains the active substances in a 52 per cent v/v solution of glycofurol.

The pH of the solution is approximately 9.0–10.5.

Uses Septrin is an antibacterial agent. Septrin is effective *in vitro* against a wide range of Gram-positive and Gram-negative organisms. It is not active against *Mycobacterium tuberculosis, Mycoplasmata* or *Treponema pallidum. Pseudomonas aeruginosa* is usually insensitive.

In general, the indications for the use of Septrin Intramuscular are the same as for oral presentations. Septrin Intramuscular should be used when the intramuscular route is considered preferable.

Clinical experience with oral Septrin indicates its value in the following:

Respiratory tract: Acute and chronic bronchitis, bronchiectasis, lobar and broncho-pneumonia, *Pneumocystis carinii* pneumonitis, otitis media and sinusitis.

Genito-urinary tract: Urethritis, cystitis, pyelitis, pyelonephritis and prostatitis. Male and female gonorrhoea.

Gastro-intestinal tract: Typhoid and paratyphoid fevers, chronic carriage of *Salmonella typhi* and *paratyphi*, cholera and shigellosis.

Skin infections: Pyoderma, abscesses and wound infections.

Other bacterial infections: Acute and chronic osteomyelitis, acute brucellosis, septicaemias and other infections caused by sensitive organisms.

Dosage and administration *Adults and children over 12 years:* Standard dosage: One 3 ml ampoule 12-hourly, morning and evening.

Maximum dosage (for severe infections): One and a half ampoules (4.5 ml) 12-hourly, morning and evening, or one 3 ml ampoule three times daily.

Children aged 6–12 years: The usual recommended dose is half an ampoule (1.5 ml) 12-hourly, morning and evening (this dose is based on an average of 6 mg trimethoprim plus 30 mg sulphamethoxazole per kg body weight daily). Paediatric dosage may be increased by 50% for severe infections.

Slight adjustment of this dose may be necessary for children whose body weights approach the extremes of the range for their height and age.

It is NOT recommended that Septrin Intramuscular Injection be given to children under the age of six years because of their small muscle mass.

It is intended that Septrin IM Injection should be used only during such a period as the patient is unable to accept oral therapy. It is recommended that the standard dosage (above) should not normally be administered for more than five successive days nor the maximum dosage (above) for more than three successive days.

Dosage in *Pneumocystis carinii* pneumonitis: Since the volume containing the suggested dose exceeds the maximum recommended, the use of Septrin Intramuscular is inappropriate. Septrin for Infusion should be administered if parenteral therapy is required.

Dosage recommendations in renal impairment: If Septrin is given to patients with renal impairment then the dosage scheme below is suggested (no information is available for children with renal failure).

Creatinine clearance (ml/min)	Serum creatinine (µmol/l)		Dosage
Above 25	men women	< 265 < 175	Standard dosage.
15–25	men women	265–620 175–400	Standard dosage for a maximum of three days followed by half the standard dosage.
Below 15	men women	> 620 > 400	Not to be administered unless haemodialysis facilities are available. Under this condition half the standard dosage may be given.

Measurements of plasma concentration of sulphamethoxazole at intervals of two to three days are recommended in samples obtained 12 hours after administration of Septrin. If the concentration of total sulphamethoxazole exceeds 150 mcg/ml, then treatment should be interrupted until the value falls below 120 mcg/ml.

Use in the elderly: No specific studies have been carried out in the elderly, although Septrin has been widely used in older people. However, care is advised when treating the elderly because, as a group, they are more susceptible to adverse reactions.

Administration: Septrin IM Injection must be given by this route ONLY and ONLY when an intramuscular formulation is indicated by the clinical condition.

The injection should be made deep into the upper and outer quadrant of the buttock, and injections should be given into each buttock alternately.

If the total contents of an ampoule are not used after opening then the remainder should be destroyed.

Contra-indications, warnings, etc

Contra-indications: Septrin should not be given to patients with a history of sulphonamide, trimethoprim or co-trimoxazole hypersensitivity.

Contra-indicated in patients showing marked liver parenchymal damage.

Except in certain circumstances it should not be given to patients with serious haematological disorders. The combination has been administered to patients receiving cytotoxic agents without evidence of an adverse effect on the bone marrow or peripheral blood.

Contra-indicated in severe renal insufficiency where repeated measurements of the plasma concentration cannot be performed.

Septrin should not be given to premature babies nor

to full-term infants during the first six weeks of life. The drug should not be given during pregnancy. (See below.)

Precautions: Septrin Intramuscular Injection should be discontinued if a skin rash appears.

In cases with renal impairment a modified dosage schedule as described above is indicated. In such patients, measurements of the plasma concentration of the drug is advisable. An adequate urinary output should be maintained.

A folate supplement should be considered when treating potentially folate deficient patients or with prolonged high dosage of Septrin.

The usual caution in prescribing any drug for women of child-bearing age should be exercised with Septrin.

If Septrin treatment is prolonged, especially in patients with suspected impairment of folate metabolism, it is suggested that complete blood counts including thrombocytes be performed at monthly intervals.

Care should be taken when giving Septrin to patients receiving sulphonylurea hypoglycaemics, warfarin, or phenytoin as the action of these agents may be increased.

Patients receiving pyrimethamine in doses in excess of 25 mg weekly who are also receiving Septrin should have their blood pictures monitored because of the occasional report of megaloblastic anaemia apparently occurring in these circumstances.

In elderly patients concurrently receiving diuretics, mainly thiazides, there appears to be an increased risk of thrombocytopenia with or without purpura.

Side- and adverse effects: Local reactions mainly vary from mild to moderate pain at the injection site; induration is uncommon. As Septrin contains trimethoprim and a sulphonamide, the type and frequency of adverse effects associated with such compounds may be expected.

Nausea, vomiting, diarrhoea, glossitis and skin rashes can occur. Pseudomembranous colitis has been reported rarely. Severe skin sensitivity reactions such as erythema multiforme bullosa (Stevens-Johnson syndrome) and toxic epidermal necrolysis (Lyell syndrome) have occurred infrequently and, rarely, have been associated with a fatality.

As Septrin contains a sulphonamide, the possibility of blood dyscrasias like those associated with sulphonamides should be borne in mind. The changes reported with Septrin mainly consist of thrombocytopenia, purpura, leucopenia, neutropenia and very rarely agranulocytosis. They have usually proved to be reversible on withdrawal of the drug. Elderly patients are more susceptible to these blood changes. Septrin may induce haemolysis in certain susceptible glucose-6-phosphate dehydrogenase deficient patients.

Jaundice and, very rarely, hepatic necrosis have been reported.

There have been a few reports of subjective experiences such as headache, depression, dizziness and hallucinations but their relationship to therapy remains unproven.

During long-term therapy, isolated cases of megaloblastic changes in the bone marrow have been reported: those are reversible by folinic acid therapy.

Use in pregnancy and lactation: The safety of Septrin in human pregnancy has not been established. Animal studies have shown teratogenic effects typical of a folate antagonist in rats but not rabbits at high doses; these were prevented by administration of dietary folates. Sulphonamide-containing products should not be administered in late pregnancy because of the risk of kernicterus.

Both sulphamethoxazole and trimethoprim may be found in breast milk, but the administration of Septrin represents a negligible risk to the suckling infant.

Toxicity and treatment of overdosage: Nausea, vomiting, dizziness and confusion are likely symptoms of overdosage.

In cases of known, suspected or accidental overdosage, stop therapy.

Acidification of the urine will increase the elimination of trimethoprim. Inducing diuresis plus alkalinisation of urine will enhance the elimination of sulphamethoxazole. Alkalinisation will reduce the rate of elimination of trimethoprim. Calcium folinate (3–6 mg/day) should reverse any folate deficiency effect of trimethoprim. General supportive measures are recommended.

Both trimethoprim and sulphamethoxazole are dialysable by renal dialysis.

Pharmaceutical precautions Do not use if the injection solution is cloudy or if precipitation has occurred. Store below 25°C. Do not freeze. Protect from light.

Legal category POM.

Package quantities Box of 10 ampoules.

Further information In the treatment of tonsillopharyngitis to Group A beta-haemolytic streptococci, eradication of these organisms from the oropharynx is less rapid than with some other antibiotics.

Trimethoprim may cause an apparent rise in serum creatinine levels due to (a) competition for the tubular secretory mechanisms; (b) chemical interference with the visual auto-analyser method of estimating creatinine.

Co-trimoxazole may cause a fall in circulating thyroid hormone levels but the clinical significance requires confirmation.

Trimethoprim has been noted to impair phenylalanine metabolism but this is of no significance in phenylketonuric patients on appropriate dietary restriction.

Plasma or serun levels of sulphamethoxazole and trimethoprim may be determined by high performance liquid chromatography.

Septrin is available also as: Tablets, Dispersible Tablets, Forte Tablets, Adult Suspension, Paediatric Suspension, Paediatric Tablets and Septrin for Infusion.

Product licence number 0003/0124.

SYRAPRIM* TABLETS

Presentation White scored tablets coded 'Y3C' containing 300 mg Trimethoprim BP. White scored tablets coded '09A' containing 100 mg Trimethoprim BP.

Uses Syraprim is an antibacterial agent indicated for the treatment of infections due to trimethoprim-sensitive organisms, particularly those affecting the urinary and respiratory tracts. Also for the long-term prophylaxis of recurrent, or suppression of chronic, urinary tract infections caused by sensitive organisms.

Syraprim is active *in vitro* against a wide range of Gram-negative and Gram-positive organisms. It is not active against *Pseudomonas* spp., *Mycobacterium tuberculosis, Mycoplasmata, Clostridia, Treponema pallidum* and anaerobes. It is relatively inactive against *Brucella* and *Neisseria.*

Dosage and administration *Urinary Tract Infections: Treatment:*

Adults: 300 mg once daily.
Children over 12 years: as for adults.
6–12 years: 150 mg once daily.
Under 6 years: formulation inapplicable.

Prophylaxis:

Adults: 100 mg once daily.
Children over 12 years: as for adults.
6–12 years: 50 mg once daily.
Under 6 years: formulation inapplicable.

To ensure maximal urinary concentrations it may be advantageous to take the dose at bedtime.

Respiratory Infections:

Adults: 200 mg twice daily.
Children over 12 years: as for adults.
6–12 years: 100 mg twice daily.
6 months–6 years: 50 mg twice daily.

In acute infections, Syraprim should be given for at least five days or until the patient has been symptom-free for two days. Long-term administration may be continued for 3 to 12 months or more as appropriate.

Dosage recommendations in renal impairment: When creatinine clearance is below 15–20 ml/minute, trimethoprim levels should be monitored after approximately 3 days' treatment to provide guidance on the appropriate dosage reduction. When the clearance is below 10 ml/minute Syraprim should not be administered unless plasma concentrations can be estimated regularly and haemodialysis facilities are available.

Use in the elderly: No specific studies have been carried out in the elderly, although Septrin has been widely used in older people. However, care is advised when treating the elderly because, as a group, they are more susceptible to adverse reactions.

Contra-indications, warnings, etc
Contra-indications: Syraprim should not be given to patients with a history of hypersensitivity to trimethoprim.

Contra-indicated in patients with severe impairment of renal function where repeated estimations of the plasma concentration, or haemodialysis, cannot be carried out.

Precautions: Care should be taken when giving the drug to patients with blood dyscrasias.

Caution should be exercised in the administration of Syraprim to patients with actual or potential folate deficiency and administration of a folate supplement should be considered.

Care should be taken if Syraprim and warfarin or phenytoin are co-administered as occasional potentiation of the effects of these agents may occur.

Patients receiving pyrimethamine in doses in excess of 25 mg weekly for malarial prophylaxis and who are given Syraprim should have their blood pictures monitored because of the possibility of megaloblastic anaemia developing.

During prolonged administration regular blood counts are advised. It is suggested that blood counts be performed at approximately monthly intervals.

Trimethoprim has been noted to impair phenylalanine metabolism but this is of no significance in phenylketon-uric patients on appropriate dietary restriction.

Side- and adverse effects: Minor gastro-intestinal disturbances including nausea and vomiting, sore mouth/tongue, pruritus and skin rashes may occasionally occur. Although an effect on folate metabolism is possible, interference with haematopoiesis rarely occurs at the recommended dose. If any such change is seen, folinic acid should reverse the effect. Elderly patients may be more susceptible and a lower dosage may be advisable.

Use in pregnancy and lactation: The safety of trimethoprim in human pregnancy has not been established. Animal studies have shown, at high doses, teratogenic effects typical of a folate antagonist in rats but not rabbits; these were prevented by administration of dietary folates. The benefit of using Syraprim in pregnancy should be weighed against the possible hazard.

Despite its excretion in breast milk the administration of Syraprim to a lactating woman represents a negligible risk to the suckling infant.

Toxicity and treatment of overdosage: Nausea, vomiting, abdominal pain, dizziness and confusion are likely symptoms of overdosage. Gastric lavage may be useful although absorption of trimethoprim from the gastro-intestinal tract is normally complete in approximately 2 hours. This may not be the case in gross overdosage. Calcium folinate 3–6 mg given for five to seven days should counteract any effect on the bone marrow. Acidification of the urine will increase the elimination of trimethoprim. General supportive measures are recommended.

Pharmaceutical precautions Store below 25°C and protect from light.

Legal category POM.

Package quantities
Bottle of 100 × 300 mg tablets.
Bottle of 100 × 100 mg tablets.

Further information Absorption by the oral route is rapid; significant plasma levels are obtained within half an hour; peak levels may be reached as early as one hour.

Excretion is predominantly in the urine in the form of unchanged drug. Urinary concentrations are generally well above the MIC of common pathogens for more than 24 hours after the last dose.

Trimethoprim may cause an apparent rise in serum creatinine levels due to (a) competition for the tubular secretory mechanisms; (b) chemical interference with the visual auto-analyser method of estimating creatinine.

Product licence numbers
300 mg tablets 0003/0148
100 mg tablets 0003/0147

SYRAPRIM* INJECTION

Presentation Syraprim Injection is a sterile aqueous solution of trimethoprim lactate equivalent to 20 mg trimethoprim base in 1 ml of water. Each ampoule contains 5 ml. The pH is 4.0.

Uses Syraprim is an antibacterial agent indicated for the treatment of infections due to sensitive organisms, in particular for Gram-negative infections. Trimethoprim is effective *in vitro* against a wide range of Gram-negative and Gram-positive organisms. It is not active against *Pseudomonas* spp., *Mycobacterium tuberculosis, Mycoplasmata, Clostridia, Treponema pallidum,* and anaerobes. It is relatively inactive against *Brucella* and *Neisseria.*

Dosage and administration *Dosage: Adults and children over 12 years:* 150–250 mg every 12 hours. *Children under 12 years:* The total daily dose should approximate to 6–9 mg/kg of body weight divided into two or three equal doses and administered either 12-hourly or 8-hourly.

The severely ill patient may require initially higher, or more frequent, doses as may a person considerably in excess of the average weight for his/her height. Total daily doses up to 20 mg/kg of body weight in divided doses have been well tolerated.

Dosage recommendations in renal impairment: When creatinine clearance is below 15–20 ml/minute, trimethoprim levels should be monitored after approximately 3 days' treatment to provide guidance on the appropriate dosage reduction. When the clearance is below 10 ml/minute Syraprim should not be administered unless plasma concentrations can be estimated regularly and haemodialysis facilities are available.

Use in the elderly: No specific studies have been carried out in the elderly, although Syraprim has been widely used in older people. However, care is advised when treating the elderly because, as a group, they are more susceptible to adverse reactions.

Administration: Syraprim Injection should be administered slowly.

1. By direct intravenous injection, or
2. via the tubing (close to the vein) of an established intravenous infusion.

If it is necessary to add Syraprim Injection to the infusion fluid it is compatible with the following:

Glucose Intravenous Infusion BP 5% w/v.

Fructose Intravenous Infusion BP 5% w/v.

Sodium Lactate Intravenous Infusion BP.

Any chloride-containing solution is likely to cause precipitation of trimethoprim hydrochloride when used with Syraprim injection.

Contra-indications, warnings, etc

Contra-indications: Syraprim should not be given to patients with a history of hypersensitivity to trimethoprim.

Contra-indicated in patients with severe impairment of renal function where repeated estimations of the plasma concentration, or haemodialysis cannot be carried out.

Precautions: Care should be taken when giving the drug to patients with blood dyscrasias.

A folate supplement should be given when high doses of Syraprim are administered intravenously.

Caution should be exercised in the administration of Syraprim to patients with actual or potential folate deficiency, and administration of a folate supplement should be considered.

Care should be taken if Syraprim and warfarin or phenytoin are co-administered as occasional potentiation of the effects of these agents may occur.

Patients receiving pyrimethamine in doses in excess of 25 mg weekly for malarial prophylaxis and who are given Syraprim should have their blood pictures monitored because of the possibility of megaloblastic anaemia developing.

Side- and adverse effects: Minor gastro-intestinal disturbances including nausea and vomiting, sore mouth/tongue, pruritus and skin rashes may occasionally occur. An effect on folate metabolism is possible but rarely occurs. Interference with haematopoiesis may occur particularly if the daily dose exceeds 500 mg in adults. Folinic acid should reverse any such effect. Elderly patients may be more susceptible and a lower dosage may be advisable.

Nausea due to too rapid injection may occur and if so the time over which the injection is given should be prolonged.

Use in pregnancy and lactation: The safety of trimethoprim in human pregnancy has not been established. Animal studies have shown, at high doses, teratogenic effects typical of a folate antagonist in rats but not rabbits; these were prevented by administration of dietary folates. The benefit of using Syraprim in pregnancy should be weighed against its possible hazard.

Despite its excretion in breast milk the administration of Syraprim to a lactating woman represents a negligible risk to the suckling infant.

Toxicity and treatment of overdosage. Nausea, vomiting, abdominal pain, dizziness and confusion are likely symptoms of overdosage. Stop therapy. Calcium folinate 3–6 mg given for five to seven days should counteract any effect on the bone marrow. Acidification of the urine will increase the elimination of trimethoprim. General supportive measures are recommended.

Pharmaceutical precautions Store below 25°C and protect from light.

Syraprim Injection should not be added to any chloride-containing infusion fluid.

Syraprim Injection is incompatible with solutions of sulphonamides and the two should not be mixed.

Legal category POM.

Package quantities Box of 10 ampoules.

Further information Excretion is predominantly in the urine in the form of unchanged drug.

Trimethoprim may cause an apparent rise in serum creatinine levels due to (a) competition for the renal tubular secretory mechanism, (b) chemical interference with the usual auto-analyser method of estimating creatinine.

Syraprim Injection may be given in conjunction with, but separately from, parenteral aminoglycosides, metronidazole, or sulphonamides depending on the organism responsible for the infection.

Product licence number 0003/0149.

TETANUS VACCINE BP (IN SIMPLE SOLUTION) WELLCOME* (Tet/Vac/FT)

Presentation Tetanus vaccine is prepared by formalin detoxification of *Clostridium tetani* exotoxin. Thiomersal BP is added as a preservative to a concentration of 0.01%. Each 0.5 ml dose contains 14Lf toxoid.

The antigenic content and formulation of this vaccine has not been changed, although the labelled content has been altered to conform with the flocculation equivalence of the new British reference antitoxin preparation.

Uses For active immunisation against tetanus.

Administration of the antigenically more potent adsorbed vaccine is usually preferred for all injections. Tetanus vaccine in simple solution is insufficiently antigenic to be used as the first immunising dose but may be used instead of adsorbed tetanus vaccine if necessary for the second, third or later reinforcing injections. Tetanus vaccine in simple solution is now often reserved for administration to patients who have had some reaction to a previous dose of adsorbed vaccine and who are not thought to be adequately protected against infection.

Dosage and administration The dose of tetanus

vaccine in simple solution is 0.5 ml given by deep subcutaneous or intramuscular injection. When Tetanus vaccine in simple solution is used for second or third doses in an immunising course, intervals of 6 to 12 weeks and 6 to 12 months respectively are recommended between the first and second and the second and third doses.

The United Kingdom Department of Health and Social Security recommend the administration of reinforcing doses after five years and after a further 5 to 15 years with the administration of additional doses in the event of injuries which may give rise to tetanus. Tetanus vaccine should not be given to any patient who has received a booster dose in the preceding year.

A single dose of vaccine given several years after the completion of a primary course will rapidly stimulate the production of tetanus antitoxin in the circulation.

In subjects who have suffered a reaction to a previous dose of adsorbed vaccine it may be preferred to administer 0.1 ml of tetanus vaccine in simple solution intradermally.

Oral Poliomyelitis Vaccine BP may be given at the same time as tetanus vaccine.

Shake well before each dose is withdrawn. It is good practice to record the title, dose and lot numbers of all vaccines and dates of administration. Any untoward reactions should be reported to the regulatory authorities and to the manufacturer.

Use in the elderly: No special comment.

Contra-indications, warnings, etc
Contra-indications: The vaccine should not be administered to a subject who has experienced a serious reaction (e.g. anaphylaxis) to a previous dose of this vaccine or who is known to be hypersensitive to any component thereof. It is advisable to avoid vaccination during an acute infection. Tetanus vaccine in simple solution should not be given simultaneously with human tetanus immunoglobulin or tetanus antitoxin which may markedly depress its antigenicity.

Precautions: Although anaphylaxis is rare, facilities for its management should always be available during vaccination.

Side- and adverse effects: Local reactions consisting of swelling, redness and pain may develop at the injection site and persist for several days. Delays of up to 10 days before symptoms develop are reported. Occasionally these local reactions may be quite marked, with tenderness and swelling of a large area. Local reactions are rare in children and the incidence increases with age and according to the number of previously administered doses, but reactions may occur after the first dose. Subjects who develop reactions frequently have high titres of circulating antitoxin. Women develop reactions more frequently than men. General reactions are uncommon but may include headache, lethargy, malaise, myalgia and pyrexia. Acute anaphylactic reactions, urticaria, angioneurotic oedema, serum sickness and peripheral neuropathy occasionally occur.

Use in pregnancy and lactation: In developing countries tetanus vaccines are widely administered during pregnancy to prevent neonatal tetanus without significant apparent adverse effects on pregnancy or foetal development.

Toxicity and treatment of overdosage: Not applicable.

Pharmaceutical precautions Store at 2–8°C. Protect from light. *Do not freeze.* When multidose containers are

employed it is good practice to discard any partly used vaccine vials at the end of the vaccinating session.

Legal category POM.

Package quantities Pack of 5 × 0.5 ml ampoules. Vial of 5 ml.

Further information Persons of all ages are susceptible to tetanus unless they have been immunised with tetanus vaccine. Rarely, if ever, does natural immunity develop even in persons who have recovered from severe tetanus. Since most tetanus cases follow trivial wounds all persons should be actively immunised against the disease.

Product licence number 0003/5190.

ADSORBED TETANUS VACCINE BP WELLCOME* (Tet/Vac/Ads)

Presentation Adsorbed tetanus vaccine is a suspension of highly purified toxoid prepared by formalin detoxification of *Clostridium tetani* exotoxin. The toxoid is adsorbed onto aluminium hydroxide. Thiomersal BP is added as a preservative to a concentration of 0.01%. Each 0.5 ml dose has an immunising potency of not less than 40 International Units (IU).

The immunising potency of this vaccine is now expressed in International Units in accordance with the requirements of the European and British Pharmacopoeias. These units measure the immunising activity of the vaccine whereas the previously used Lf units expressed the quantity of toxoid present. There is no simple numerical relationship between IU and Lf. No change has been made to the potency although it is now expressed in IU.

Uses For active immunisation against tetanus.

Dosage and administration Primary immunisation consists of three deep subcutaneous or intramuscular doses of adsorbed vaccine each of 0.5 ml administered at intervals of 6 to 12 weeks and 6 to 12 months respectively. Adsorbed tetanus vaccine may be used for the routine anti-tetanus immunisation of persons of all ages although it is usual to employ plain or adsorbed combined diphtheria/tetanus/pertussis vaccine (DTPer/Vac or DTPer/Vac/Ads) or adsorbed diphtheria and tetanus vaccine (DT/Vac/Ads) for immunisation of infants.

The United Kingdom Department of Health and Social Security recommend the administration of reinforcing doses after five years and after a further 5 to 15 years with the administration of additional doses in the event of injuries which may give rise to tetanus. Tetanus vaccine should not be given to any patient who has received a booster dose in the preceding year.

A single dose of vaccine given several years after the completion of a primary course will rapidly stimulate the production of tetanus antitoxin in the circulation.

Adsorbed tetanus vaccine may be administered simultaneously with human tetanus immunoglobulin or tetanus antitoxin but must be given at separate sites. The antibody response of subjects to subsequent doses of vaccine is not significantly impaired by this procedure.

Oral Poliomyelitis Vaccine BP may be given at the same time as Tetanus Vaccine.

Shake well before each dose is withdrawn. It is good practice to record the title, dose and lot numbers of all vaccines and dates of administration. Any untoward reactions should be reported to the regulatory authorities and to the manufacturer.

Use in the elderly: No special comment.

Contra-indications, warnings, etc
Contra-indications: Adsorbed tetanus vaccine should not be administered intradermally.

The vaccine should not be administered to a subject who has experienced a serious reaction (e.g. anaphylaxis) to a previous dose of this vaccine or who is known to be hypersensitive to any component thereof. It is advisable to avoid vaccination during an acute infection.

Precautions: Although anaphylaxis is rare, facilities for its management should always be available during vaccination.

Side- and adverse effects: Local reactions consisting of swelling, redness and pain may develop at the injection site and persist for several days. Delays of up to 10 days before symptoms develop are reported. Occasionally these local reactions may be quite marked, with tenderness and swelling of a large area. Local reactions are rare in children and the incidence increases with age and according to the number of previously administered doses, but reactions may occur after the first dose. Subjects who develop reactions frequently have high titres of circulating antitoxin. Women develop reactions more frequently than men. General reactions are uncommon but may include headache, lethargy, malaise, myalgia and pyrexia. Acute anaphylactic reactions, urticaria, angioneurotic oedema, serum sickness and peripheral neuropathy occasionally occur.

Persistent nodules at the site of injection may occasionally follow administration of adsorbed vaccines especially if the inoculation is into the superficial layers of subcutaneous tissue.

Use in pregnancy and lactation: In developing countries tetanus vaccines are widely administered during pregnancy to prevent neonatal tetanus without significant apparent adverse effects on pregnancy or foetal development.

Toxicity and treatment of overdosage: Not applicable.

Pharmaceutical precautions Store at 2–8°C. Protect from light. *Do not freeze.* When multidose containers are employed it is good practice to discard any partly used vaccine vials at the end of the vaccinating session.

Legal category POM.

Package quantities Pack of 5 × 0.5 ml ampoules. Vial of 5 ml.

Further information Persons of all ages are susceptible to tetanus unless they have been immunised with tetanus vaccine. Rarely, if ever, is natural immunity developed even in persons who have recovered from severe tetanus. Since most tetanus cases follow trivial wounds all persons should be actively immunised against the disease.

Product licence number 0003/5191.

TINEAFAX* OINTMENT

Presentation Zinc Undecenoate BP 80 mg and zinc naphthenate solution 80 mg (10% zinc) in a non-greasy base. Cream in colour.

Uses To eradicate 'athlete's foot' and other ringworm infections of the skin.

Dosage and administration *Adults:* The affected parts must first be washed with soap and water and thoroughly dried. Dead or loose skin should be removed. The ointment is then rubbed into and around the lesions. This treatment is, at first, repeated night and morning then, as healing progresses, one treatment daily is sufficient. It is important to keep the feet free from moisture; a daily change of stockings is advisable.

Children: As for adults.

Use in the elderly: No special comment.

Contra-indications, warnings, etc
Contra-indications: No special comment.

Treatment of overdosage: Not applicable.

Pharmaceutical precautions Store below 25°C.

Legal category P.

Package quantities Tube of 25 g.

Further information Nil.

Product licence number 0003/5216.

TINEAFAX* POWDER

Presentation Zinc Undecenoate BP 100 mg per gram of white powder.

Uses Prophylactic against 'athlete's foot'.

Dosage and administration *Adults:* To avoid either initial infection or reinfection with the fungi responsible for 'athlete's foot', hosiery and shoes should be dusted inside with Tineafax Powder. The feet should be kept dry, and walking barefooted in public dressing rooms should be avoided.

Children: As for adults.

Use in the elderly: No special comment.

Contra-indications, warnings, etc
Contra-indications: No special comment.

Pharmaceutical precautions Store below 25°C.

Legal category GSL.

Package quantities Puffer pack of 50 g.

Further information Nil.

Product licence number 0003/5215.

TRIVAX* DIPHTHERIA, TETANUS AND PERTUSSIS VACCINE BP (DTPer/Vac)

Presentation Trivax is a sterile preparation consisting of a mixture of diphtheria and tetanus toxoids and killed whole *Bordetella pertussis.*

Each 0.5 ml of vaccine contains 25 Lf of purified diphtheria toxoid, 3.5 Lf of purified tetanus toxoid and not more than 20,000 million chemically killed Bordetella pertussis organisms with a potency of not less than 4 i.u., in an isotonic buffer solution. Organisms bearing all three pertussis agglutinogens are included. Vaccine of this composition has been shown to provide adequate immunising potency against each of the three diseases. Thiomersal is added as a preservative to a final concentration of 0.01%.

The antigenic content and formulation of this vaccine has not been changed, although the labelled content of the tetanus component has been altered to conform with the flocculation equivalence of the new British reference antitoxin preparation.

Uses For active immunisation against diphtheria, tetanus and whooping cough in infants and pre-school children. It is not recommended that pertussis-containing vaccines be used in older children except in areas where whooping cough is a serious problem.

Dosage and administration *Dosage: Adults:* Not recommended.

Children up to 5 years: Each dose is 0.5 ml, given by deep subcutaneous or intramuscular injection. The primary course consists of 3 doses of vaccine at intervals of not less than four weeks.

Use in the elderly: No special comment.

Administration: Since whooping cough can often be a serious disease in the early months of life the primary course should preferably be started between the third and sixth month of life. It is believed that immune responses are better if the interval between the first and second dose is extended to six to eight weeks and the interval between the second and third dose is four to six months. It is not considered necessary to repeat the full course of immunisation if these intervals are exceeded.

Reinforcing doses: Where primary immunisation was completed during the first six to eight months of life one reinforcing dose of 0.5 ml Diphtheria and Tetanus Vaccine (DT/Vac/FT or DT/Vac/Ads) should be given about 12 months later in order to boost immunity. Children over the age of five years do not normally require further immunisation with pertussis vaccine since whooping cough is rarely a problem in older children. However, reinforcement of immunity against diphtheria and tetanus is necessary. This can be achieved by giving 1 dose (0.5 ml) of Diphtheria and Tetanus Vaccine (DT/Vac/FT or DT/Vac/Ads) to five-year-old children and 1 dose (0.5 ml) of Tetanus Vaccine (Tet/Vac/Ads) at 15/19 years of age or on leaving school.

Shake well before withdrawing a dose. It is good practice to record the title, dose and lot numbers of all vaccines and dates of administration. Any untoward reactions should be reported to the regulatory authorities and to the manufacturer.

Contra-indications, warnings, etc

Contra-indications: Not for intradermal use. The administration of pertussis-containing vaccine is contra-indicated in children with a personal or family history of epilepsy or other familial or hereditary diseases of the central nervous system. Administration of pertussis vaccine is also contra-indicated in children with a history of seizures, convulsions, cerebral irritation in the neonatal period, developmental neurological defect or other disorder of the central nervous system. Children with acute infection or illness, particularly those with respiratory symptoms should not be immunised until they are fully recovered. Any child exhibiting a severe local or significant general reaction to a previous dose of a pertussis-containing vaccine should not be given a further dose. However, protection against diphtheria and tetanus is advisable and can be accomplished by giving Adsorbed Diphtheria and Tetanus Vaccine.

Precautions: Since combined diphtheria, tetanus and pertussis vaccines are widely used in a population in which sudden illnesses of undefined origin are not uncommon, intercurrent illness bearing a temporal but not a causal relationship to vaccination may be expected.

Although anaphylaxis is rare, facilities for its management should always be available during vaccination.

Side- and adverse effects: Local reactions, particularly erythema at the site of injection, are commonly seen during the 24 hours following vaccination. They normally subside without treatment. A nodule may be found at the site of injection; this occurs less frequently and is less persistent following the administration of plain vaccine.

A transient rise in temperature, restlessness, irritability, crying or loss of appetite may sometimes occur a few hours after vaccination, but does not generally call for treatment. The incidence of these systemic reactions is lower following the administration of adsorbed vaccine. Allergic manifestations including pallor, dyspnoea and collapse have been observed rarely. Convulsions, infantile spasms and encephalopathy have been reported as rare complications after pertussis vaccination.

Convulsions may be precipitated by a febrile response to the pertussis component. In an individual case it may be difficult to distinguish between spontaneously occurring convulsions and those associated with vaccination.

Abnormal crying and persistent screaming have also been described as reactions which may be encountered after vaccination.

An increased incidence of reactions may occur due to failure to shake the container and re-suspend the vaccine before withdrawing a dose, to inadvertent intravenous administration or to an over-rapid injection.

Since combined diphtheria, tetanus and pertussis vaccines are widely used in a population in which sudden illnesses of undefined origin are not uncommon, intercurrent illness bearing a temporal but not a causal relationship to vaccination may be expected.

Use in pregnancy and lactation: Since simultaneous vaccination against diphtheria, tetanus and pertussis in adults is uncommon there is no accurate information on the safety of this vaccine in pregnancy.

Toxicity and treatment of overdosage: Not applicable.

Pharmaceutical precautions Store between 2°C and 8°C, protected from light. *Do not freeze.*

When multi-dose containers are employed, it is good practice to discard any partly used vaccine vials at the end of the vaccinating session.

Legal category POM.

Package quantities Pack of 5 × 0.5 ml ampoules. Vial of 5 ml.

Further information Oral Poliomyelitis Vaccine BP may be given at the same time as Trivax.

Product licence number 0003/5192.

TRIVAX-AD* ADSORBED DIPHTHERIA, TETANUS AND PERTUSSIS VACCINE BP (DTPer/Vac/Ads)

Presentation Trivax-AD is a sterile preparation consisting of a mixture of diphtheria and tetanus toxoids and killed whole *Bordetella pertussis*.

Each 0.5 ml of vaccine has an immunizing potency of not less than 30 International units (IU) purified diphtheria toxoid and not less than 60 IU (mouse assay) purified tetanus toxoid, with not more than 20,000 million chemically killed *Bordetella pertussis* organisms with a potency of not less than 4 IU adsorbed onto aluminium hydroxide in an isotonic buffer solution. The aluminium content does not exceed 1.25 mg per dose. Organisms bearing all three pertussis agglutinogens are included. Vaccine of this composition has been shown to provide adequate immunizing potency against each of the three diseases. Thiomersal is added as a preservative to a final concentration of 0.01%

The potency of this vaccine is now expressed in International Units in accordance with the requirements of the European and British Pharmacopoeias. These units measure the immunizing activity of the vaccine, whereas the previously used Lf units expressed the quantity of toxoid present. There is no simple numerical relationship between IU and Lf. No change has been made to the potency although it is now expressed in IU.

Uses For active immunisation against diphtheria, tetanus and whooping cough in infants and pre-school children. It is not recommended that pertussis-containing vaccines be used in older children except in areas where whooping cough is a serious problem.

Dosage and administration *Dosage: Adults:* Not recommended.

Children up to 5 years: Each dose is 0.5 ml, given by deep subcutaneous or intramuscular injection. The primary course consists of 3 doses of vaccine at intervals of not less than four weeks.

Use in the elderly: No special comment.

Administration: Since whooping cough can often be a serious disease in the early months of life the primary course should preferably be started between the third and sixth month of life. It is believed that immune responses are better if the interval between the first and second dose is extended to six to eight weeks and the interval between the second and third dose is four to six months. It is not considered necessary to repeat the full course of immunisation if these intervals are exceeded.

Reinforcing doses: Where primary immunisation was completed during the first six to eight months of life one reinforcing dose of 0.5 ml Diphtheria and Tetanus Vaccine (DT/Vac/FT or DT/Vac/Ads) should be given about 12 months later in order to boost immunity. Children over the age of five years do not normally require further immunisation with pertussis vaccine since whooping cough is rarely a problem in older children. However, reinforcement of immunity against diphtheria and tetanus is necessary. This can be achieved by giving 1 dose (0.5 ml) of Diphtheria and Tetanus Vaccine (DT/Vac/FT or DT/Vac/Ads) to five-year-old children and 1 dose (0.5 ml) of Tetanus Vaccine (Tet/Vac/Ads) at 15–19 years of age or on leaving school.

Shake well before withdrawing a dose. It is good practice to record the title, dose and lot numbers of all vaccines and dates of administration. Any untoward reactions should be reported to the regulatory authorities and to the manufacturer.

Contra-indications, warnings, etc
Contra-indications: Not for intradermal use. The administration of pertussis-containing vaccine is contra-indicated in children with a personal or family history of epilepsy or other familial or hereditary diseases of the central nervous system. Administration of pertussis vaccine is also contra-indicated in children with a history of seizures, convulsions, cerebral irritation in the neonatal period, developmental neurological defect or other disorder of the central nervous system. Children with acute infection or illness, particularly those with respiratory symptoms should not be immunised until they are fully recovered. Any child exhibiting a severe local or significant general reaction to a previous dose of a pertussis-containing vaccine should not be given a further dose. However, protection against diphtheria and tetanus is advisable and can be accomplished by giving Adsorbed Diphtheria and Tetanus Vaccine.

Precautions: Since combined diphtheria, tetanus and pertussis vaccines are widely used in a population in which sudden illnesses of undefined origin are not uncommon, intercurrent illness bearing a temporal but not a causal relationship to vaccination may be expected.

Although anaphylaxis is rare, facilities for its management should always be available during vaccination.

Side and adverse effects: Local reactions, particularly erythema at the site of injection, are commonly seen during the 24 hours following vaccination. They normally subside without treatment. A nodule may be found at the site of injection; this occurs less frequently and is less persistent following the administration of plain vaccine.

A transient rise in temperature, restlessness, irritability, crying or loss of appetite may sometimes occur a few hours after vaccination, but does not generally call for treatment. The incidence of these systemic reactions is lower following the administration of adsorbed vaccine. Allergic manifestations including pallor, dyspnoea and collapse have been observed rarely. Convulsions, infantile spasms and encephalopathy have been reported as rare complications after pertussis vaccination.

Convulsions may be precipitated by a febrile response to the pertussis component. In an individual case it may be difficult to distinguish between spontaneously occurring convulsions and those associated with vaccination.

Abnormal crying and persistent screaming have also been described as reactions which may be encountered after vaccination.

An increased incidence of reactions may occur due to failure to shake the container and re-suspend the vaccine before withdrawing a dose, to inadvertent intravenous administration, or to an over-rapid injection.

Since combined diphtheria, tetanus and pertussis vaccines are widely used in a population in which sudden illnesses of undefined origin are not uncommon, intercurrent illness bearing a temporal but not a causal relationship to vaccination may be expected.

Use in pregnancy and lactation: Since simultaneous vaccination against diphtheria, tetanus and pertussis in adults is uncommon there is no accurate information on the safety of this vaccine in pregnancy.

Toxicity and treatment of overdosage: Not applicable.

Pharmaceutical precautions Store between 2°C and 8°C, protected from light. *Do not freeze.*

When multi-dose containers are employed, it is good practice to discard any partly used vaccine vials at the end of the vaccinating session.

Legal category POM.

Package quantities Pack of 5 × 0.5 ml ampoules. Vial of 5 ml.

Further information Oral Poliomyelitis Vaccine BP may be given at the same time as Trivax-AD.

Product licence number 0003/5193.

TYPHOID VACCINE BP (MONOVALENT) WELLCOME* (Typhoid/Vac)

Presentation Typhoid (Monovalent) Vaccine contains heat-killed, phenol-preserved, *Salmonella typhi* organisms at a concentration of not less than 1,000 million organisms per ml.

Uses For active immunisation against typhoid fever.

Typhoid vaccine protects 70–90% of recipients against typhoid.

Dosage and administration

Wellcome Typhoid Vaccine (Monovalent) may be administered subcutaneously, intramuscularly or intradermally. Subcutaneous or intramuscular injection should be used for the first dose but intradermal injection reduces systemic reactions and may therefore be preferred for the second dose, particularly for persons who have experienced reactions in the past.

Shake well before withdrawing dose.

The interval between the first and second doses should be four to six weeks.

Initial dose to be administered by deep subcutaneous or intramuscular injection	Time interval between administration of initial dose and second dose	Second dose
Children 1–10 years 0.25 ml	4–6 weeks	0.25 ml by i.m. or s.c. injection or 0.1 ml by intradermal injection
Children over 10 years and adults 0.5 ml	4–6 weeks	0.5 ml by i.m. or s.c. injection or 0.1 ml by intradermal injection

Although two doses of vaccine are recommended for primary immunisation, the results of field trials indicate that one dose of typhoid vaccine is almost as effective, for a short period, as two doses.

Use in the elderly: No special comment.

Reinforcing doses: Under conditions of continued or repeated exposure to infection a reinforcing dose of vaccine should be given at least every three years. When more than three years have elapsed since the last dose, a single dose is sufficient to boost immunity.

It is good practice to record the title, dose and lot numbers of all vaccines and dates of administration. Any untoward reactions should be reported to the regulatory authorities and to the manufacturer.

Contra-indications, warnings, etc

Contra-indications: The vaccine should not be administered to a subject who has experienced a serious reaction (e.g. anaphylaxis) to a previous dose of this vaccine or who is known to be hypersensitive to any component thereof. It is advisable to avoid vaccination during an acute infection.

Precautions: Typhoid vaccine produces in some people constitutional or local reactions. These are often more marked in adults over the age of 35 years, especially where there is a history of previous vaccination against typhoid.

It is prudent to avoid administering vaccine to subjects with acute infections or chronic illness.

Vaccination of children under 12 months of age is not advised because of the risk of adverse reactions, the relatively low incidence of typhoid in this age group and the relatively mild course of the disease in infants.

Although anaphylaxis is rare, facilities for its management should always be available during vaccination.

Side- and adverse effects: Local redness, swelling, pain and tenderness may appear in two or three hours.

Systemic reactions, such as malaise, nausea, headache, or pyrexia may occur, but usually disappear in 36 hours, when they are severe the patient is best kept in bed. The incidence of systemic reactions is considerably reduced by giving the vaccine intradermally, but local reactions may still occur.

Neurological complications including polyneuritis, neuritis, myelitis or various manifestations of cerebral and meningeal disease have been described following the administration of typhoid-containing vaccines.

Use in pregnancy and lactation: While no specific effects on the foetus have followed the administration of Typhoid Vaccine, it is not considered advisable to administer vaccines which may cause pyrexia during pregnancy.

Toxicity and treatment of overdosage: Not applicable.

Pharmaceutical precautions Store at 2–8°C. Protect from light. *Do not freeze.* When multi-dose containers are employed it is good practice to discard any partly used vaccine vials at the end of the vaccinating session.

Legal category POM.

Package quantities Vial of 1.5 ml.

Further information Nil.

Product licence number 0003/5195.

ZOVIRAX* CREAM ▼

Presentation Zovirax cream is white and contains 5% w/w acyclovir in an aqueous cream base. It is supplied in tubes containing 2 g or 10 g.

Uses Zovirax cream is indicated for the treatment of herpes simplex virus infections of the skin including initial and recurrent genital herpes and herpes labialis.

Do not use in eyes.

Dosage and administration Zovirax cream should be applied five times daily at approximately four hourly intervals. Treatment should be continued for 5 days. If, after 5 days, healing is not complete then treatment may be continued for a further 5 days. Therapy should begin as early as possible after the start of an infection, and for recurrent episodes this should preferably be during the prodromal period or when the lesions first appear.

Use in the elderly: No special comment.

Pharmacology: Acyclovir is an antiviral agent which is highly active *in vitro* against herpes simplex virus (HSV) types I and II and varicella zoster virus. Toxicity to mammalian host cells is low.

Acyclovir is phosphorylated after entry into herpes infected cells to the active compound acyclovir triphosphate. The first step in this process is dependent on the presence of the HSV-coded thymidine kinase. Acyclovir triphosphate acts as an inhibitor of, and substrate for, the herpes-specified DNA polymerase, preventing further viral DNA synthesis without affecting normal cellular processes.

Contra-indications, warnings, etc

Contra-indications: Hypersensitivity to propylene glycol.

Zovirax cream is contra-indicated in patients known to be hypersensitive to acyclovir.

Precautions: Zovirax cream is not recommended for application to buccal or vaginal mucous membranes.

Particular care should be taken to avoid accidental introduction into the eye.

Animal studies indicate that reversible irritation may result from introduction of Zovirax cream into the vagina.

Side- and adverse effects: Transient burning or stinging following application of Zovirax cream may occur. Erythema or mild drying and flaking of the skin have been reported in a small proportion of patients.

The results of a wide range of mutagenicity tests *in vitro* and *in vivo* indicate that acyclovir does not pose a genetic risk to man.

Acyclovir was not found to be carcinogenic in long-term studies in the rat and the mouse.

Use in pregnancy and lactation: No information is available on the effects of administration of Zovirax cream during human pregnancy. Systemic administration of acyclovir to rats and rabbits did not produce embryotoxic or teratogenic effects. No information is available on levels of acyclovir which may appear in breast milk after administration of Zovirax cream.

There has been no experience of the effect of Zovirax cream on human fertility. However, in two-generation mouse studies no effects of systemic acyclovir on fertility have been demonstrated.

Drug interactions: Probenecid increases the mean half-life and area under the plasma concentration curve of systemically administered acycloir. Clinical experience has not identified other drug interactions with acyclovir.

Toxicity and treatment of overdosage: No untoward effects would be expected if the entire contents of a Zovirax cream 10 g tube containing 500 mg of acyclovir were ingested orally. Doses of 800 mg five times daily (4 g per day), have been administered for five days without adverse effects. Single intravenous doses of up to 80 mg/kg have been inadvertently administered without adverse effects. Acyclovir is dialysable.

Pharmaceutical precautions Store below 25°C.

Legal category POM.

Package quantities Tubes of 2 g and 10 g.

Further information Nil.

Product licence number 0003/0180.

ZOVIRAX* I.V. for intravenous infusion ▼

Presentation Each vial contains the equivalent of 250 mg sterile acyclovir as the freeze-dried sodium salt. It is a white to off-white powder. When reconstituted as directed, Zovirax I.V. has a pH of about 11.

Uses

Non Immuno-compromised Patients	Immuno-compromised Patients	Severely Immuno-compromised Patients
Severe initial genital herpes	Herpes simplex infection	Prophylaxis of herpes simplex infection
Recurrent VZV infection	Primary and recurrent VZV infection	

Dosage and administration *Dosage:* In patients with herpes simplex infections (with normal or impaired immune responses) and in patients with recurrent shingles (with normal immune responses) Zovirax I.V. should be given in doses of 5 mg/kg every 8 hours in patients with normal renal function. Each dose should be administered by slow intravenous infusion *over a one-hour period.*

In patients with varicella zoster infections (with impaired immune responses) Zovirax I.V. should be given in doses of 10 mg/kg every 8 hours in patients with normal renal function. Each dose should be administered by slow intravenous infusion *over a one-hour period.*

In patients with renal impairment, Zovirax I.V. should be administered with caution because the drug is excreted by the kidneys.

As transient rises in serum creatinine or urea have been reported during use of Zovirax, monitoring of renal function is recommended, particularly in patients with renal transplants where, should this occur, it could be confused with graft rejection.

The following modifications in dosage are recommended:

Creatinine clearance	Dosage
25–50 ml/min	5 mg/kg every 12 hours
10–25 ml/min	5 mg/kg every 24 hours
0 (Anuric) – 10 ml/min	2.5 mg/kg every 24 hours and after dialysis

Dosage in children: The dosage of Zovirax I.V. can be calculated on the basis of the body surface area. In children between 3 months and 12 years this provides a more accurate method of calculating the dosage. 5 mg/kg is approximately equal to 250 mg per square metre body surface area. 10 mg/kg is approximately equal to 500 mg per square metre body surface area. The dose in children should therefore be based on the equivalent dose in adults calculated according to the child's body surface area.

Dosage in the elderly: In the elderly, total acyclovir body clearance declines along with creatinine clearance. Special attention should be given to dosage reduction in elderly patients with impaired creatinine clearance.

The duration of prophylactic administration of Zovirax I.V. is determined by the duration of the period at risk.

For acute infections with herpes simplex virus, 5 days' treatment should be adequate. However, this should be judged in the light of the patient's illness, and the response to treatment.

Method of administration: In all cases the total dose should be administered slowly over a period of one hour. Zovirax I.V. must be given by the intravenous route only and must be reconstituted and used as directed.

Each vial (containing the equivalent of 250 mg acyclovir) should be reconstituted by the addition of 10 ml of either Water for Injections BP or Sodium Chloride Intravenous Infusion BP (0.9% w/v). The required dose/volume should be calculated on the basis of 25 mg per ml of reconstituted solution.

Zovirax I.V., after reconstitution, may be injected directly into a vein over 1 hour by a controlled rate infusion pump, or be further diluted for administration by infusion. For intravenous injection by controlled rate infusion pump, a solution containing 25 mg acyclovir/ml is used.

For intravenous infusion, each vial of Zovirax I.V. should be reconstituted and then, wholly or in part (according to dosage required), added to and mixed with at least 50 ml of infusion solution. The contents of two vials (500 mg of acyclovir) may therefore be added to 100 ml of infusion solution. Where the dose required for infusion is greater than 500 mg, a second volume of infusion solution must be used.

Zovirax I.V., when diluted in accordance with the above schedules to give a concentration not greater than 0.5% w/v of acyclovir, is known to be compatible with the following infusion fluids and stable for up to 12 hours at room temperature (15–25°C).

Sodium Chloride Intravenous Infusion BP (0.45% and 0.9% w/v).

Sodium Chloride (0.18% w/v) and Glucose (4% w/v) Intravenous Infusion BP.

Sodium Chloride (0.45% w/v) and Glucose (2.5% w/v) Intravenous Infusion BP.

Compound Sodium Lactate Intravenous Infusion BP (Hartmann's solution).

After addition of Zovirax I.V. to an infusion solution, the mixture should be shaken to ensure thorough mixing.

Reconstitution or dilution should be carried out immediately before use and, as no preservative is included, any unused solution should be discarded. Should visible turbidity or crystallisation appear in the solution, before or during the infusion, the mixture should be discarded. The solution should not be refrigerated.

Pharmacology: Zovirax is an antiviral agent which is highly active *in vitro* against herpes simplex types I and II, and varicella zoster viruses. Toxicity to mammalian host cells is low.

Zovirax is phosphorylated to the active triphosphate after entry into a herpes-infected cell. The first step in this process requires the presence of the HSV-coded thymidine kinase. Acyclovir triphosphate acts as an inhibitor of, and substrate for, the herpes-specified DNA polymerase, preventing further viral DNA synthesis without affecting normal cellular processes.

In adults, the terminal plasma half-life of acyclovir after administration of Zovirax I.V. is about 2.9 hours. Most of the drug is excreted unchanged by the kidney. Renal clearance of acyclovir is substantially greater than creatinine clearance, indicating that tubular secretion, in addition to glomerular filtration, contributes to the renal elimination of the drug. 9-carboxymethoxymethylguanine is the only significant metabolite of acyclovir and accounts for 10–15% of the dose excreted in the urine. When acyclovir is given one hour after 1 gram of probenecid the terminal half-life, and the area under the plasma concentration time curve, is extended by 18% and 40% respectively.

Mean steady peak plasma concentrations ($C^{ss}max$) following a one-hour infusion of 5 mg/kg or 10 mg/kg were 9.8 and 20.7 micrograms/ml respectively. The equivalent trough levels 7 hours later were 0.7 and 2.3 micrograms/ml respectively. In children over 1 year of age similar mean peak ($C^{ss}max$) and trough ($C^{ss}min$) levels were observed when a dose of 250 mg/m^2 was substituted for 5 mg/kg, and a dose of 500 mg/m^2 was substituted for 10 mg/kg. In neonates (0–3 months of age) treated with doses of 10 mg/kg administered over a one-hour infusion every 8 hours, the $C^{ss}max$ was found to be 13.8 micrograms/ml and the $C^{ss}min$ to be 2.3 micrograms/ml. The terminal plasma half-life in these

patients was 3.8 hours. In the elderly, total body clearance falls with increasing age and is associated with decreases in creatinine clearance although there is little change in the terminal plasma half-life.

In patients with chronic renal failure the mean terminal half-life was found to be 19.5 hours. The mean acyclovir half-life during haemodialysis was 5.7 hours. Plasma acyclovir levels dropped approximately 60% during dialysis.

Cerebrospinal fluid levels are approximately 50 per cent of corresponding plasma levels. Plasma protein binding is relatively low (9 to 33%) and drug interactions involving binding site displacement are not anticipated.

Contra-indications, warnings, etc

Contra-indications: Zovirax I.V. is contra-indicated in patients known to be previously hypersensitive to acyclovir.

Precautions: Care should be observed when administering Zovirax to patients with abnormal renal function (see above), in order to avoid accumulation. The drug should not be given as a bolus intravenous injection, but by slow infusion over one hour.

Reconstituted Zovirax I.V. has a pH of approximately 11 and should not be administered by mouth.

Side- and adverse effects: Rapid increases in blood urea and creatinine levels may occasionally occur in patients given Zovirax I.V.

Renal impairment developing during treatment with Zovirax I.V. usually responds rapidly to hydration of the patient and/or dosage reduction or withdrawal of the drug. Progression to acute renal failure, however, can occur in exceptional cases.

Severe inflammation sometimes leading to ulceration has occurred when Zovirax I.V. has been accidentally infused into extravascular tissues. Mechanical infusion pumps pose a greater risk than infusion by gravity feed.

The following events have been reported whilst patients have been receiving Zovirax I.V.: increased liver related enzymes, decreases in haematological indices, neurological reactions, and rashes. There is no evidence to suggest that these events are directly related to Zovirax therapy.

Use in pregnancy and lactation: Studies in animals with systemically administered Zovirax have not demonstrated an effect on the foetus. However, as there has been no clinical experience of the effects of Zovirax intravenous infusion on human pregnancy, or the foetus, caution should be exercised in prescribing Zovirax to pregnant women. No information is available on levels of Zovirax which may appear in breast milk after administration of Zovirax I.V.

There is no experience of the effect of Zovirax I.V. on human fertility. Two-generation studies in mice did not reveal any effect on fertility.

Drug interactions: Probenecid increases the acyclovir mean half-life and area under the plasma concentration curve. Clinical experience has not identified other drug interactions with acyclovir.

Toxicity and treatment of overdosage: Single doses of up to 80 mg/kg have been accidentally administered with no adverse consequences. Zovirax I.V. is dialysable.

Pharmaceutical precautions Store below 25°C. The injection contains no preservative. Reconstitution and dilution should therefore be carried out immediately before use and any unused solution should be discarded.

The reconstituted or diluted solution should not be refrigerated.

Legal category POM.

Package quantities Pack of 5 vials.

Further information Nil.

Product licence number 0003/0159.

ZOVIRAX* OPHTHALMIC OINTMENT ▼

Presentation White to pale yellow sterile ointment containing 3 per cent w/w acyclovir in a white soft paraffin base.

Uses Treatment of herpes simplex keratitis. Acyclovir is an antiviral agent which is highly active *in vitro* against herpes simplex (HSV) types I and II.

Dosage and administration *Adults:* 1 cm ribbon of ointment should be placed inside the lower conjunctival sac five times a day at approximately four hourly intervals. Treatment should continue for at least 3 days after healing is complete.

Children: As for adults.

Use in the elderly: No special comment.

Pharmacology: Acyclovir is phosphorylated to the active compound acyclovir triphosphate after entry into a herpes infected cell. The first step in this process requires the presence of the HSV coded thymidine kinase. Acyclovir triphosphate acts as an inhibitor of, and substrate for, the herpes specified DNA polymerase, preventing further viral DNA synthesis without affecting normal cellular processes. Acyclovir is rapidly absorbed through the corneal epithelium and superficial ocular tissues. In animals, it achieves antiviral concentrations in aqueous humor. It has not been possible by existing methods to detect acyclovir in the blood after topical application to the eye. However, trace quantities may be measured in the urine. These levels are not clinically significant.

Contra-indications, warnings, etc *Contra-indications:* Patients with a known hypersensitivity to acyclovir.

Side- and adverse effects: For ophthalmic use only. Transient mild stinging immediately following administration occurs in a small proportion of patients. Superficial punctate keratopathy has been reported but has not resulted in patients being withdrawn from therapy, and healing has occurred without apparent sequelae. Blepharitis has also been reported.

The results of a wide range of mutagenicity tests *in vitro* and *in vivo* indicate that acyclovir does not pose a genetic risk to man. Acyclovir was not found to be carcinogenic in long-term studies in the rat and the mouse.

Drug interactions: Probenecid increases the mean half-life and area under the plasma concentration curve of systemically administered acyclovir. Clinical experience has not identified other drug interactions with acyclovir.

Use in pregnancy and lactation: No teratogenicity, embryo-toxicity or effects on fertility have been demonstrated following systemic administration of acyclovir in animal studies.

The results of tests in animals indicate that Zovirax ophthalmic ointment does not affect human fertility. In two-generation mouse studies no effects on fertility have been demonstrated.

No information is available on levels of acyclovir which may appear in breast milk after administration of Zovirax ophthalmic ointment.

Toxicity and treatment of overdosage: No untoward effects would be expected if the entire contents of the tube containing 135 mg of acyclovir were ingested orally. Doses of 800 mg five times daily (4 g per day), have been administered for five days without adverse effects. Single intravenous doses of up to 80 mg/kg have been inadvertently administered without adverse effects. Acyclovir is dialysable.

Pharmaceutical precautions When stored below 25°C Zovirax ophthalmic ointment can be expected to have a shelf life of 3 years. Discard one month after opening.

Legal category POM.

Package quantities 4.5 g tube.

Further information Nil.

Product licence number 0003/0150.

ZOVIRAX* TABLETS ▼
ZOVIRAX SUSPENSION ▼

Presentation Each pale-blue, shield-shaped tablet is impressed with the word 'Zovirax' and contains 200 mg acyclovir.

Zovirax Suspension is an off-white, viscous suspension with a banana odour and taste, and contains 200 mg acyclovir per 5 ml.

Uses Zovirax Tablets and Suspension are indicated for the treatment of herpes simplex virus (HSV) infections of the skin and mucous membranes, including initial and recurrent genital herpes.

Zovirax Tablets and Suspension are also indicated for the prophylaxis of herpes simplex infections in immunocompromised patients.

Pharmacokinetics: Acyclovir is only partially absorbed from the gut. Mean steady state peak plasma concentrations ($C^{ss}max$) following doses of 200 mg administered four hourly were 0.68 micrograms/ml and the equivalent trough plasma levels ($C^{ss}min$) were 0.36 micrograms/ml.

From studies with intravenous acyclovir, the terminal plasma half-life has been determined as about 2.9 hours. Most of the drug is excreted unchanged by the kidney. Renal clearance of acyclovir is substantially greater than creatinine clearance, indicating that tubular secretion, in addition to glomerular filtration, contributes to the renal elimination of the drug. 9-carboxymethoxymethylguanine is the only significant metabolite of acyclovir, and accounts for 10–15% of the dose excreted in the urine. In patients with chronic renal failure, the mean terminal half-life was found to be 19.5 hours. The mean acyclovir half-life during haemodialysis was 5.7 hours. Plasma acyclovir levels dropped approximately 60% during dialysis. In the elderly, total body clearance falls with increasing age and is associated with decreases in creatinine clearance, although there is little change in the terminal plasma half-life.

Pharmacology: Acyclovir is an antiviral agent that is highly active *in vitro* against herpes simplex virus (HSV) types I and II and varicella zoster virus. Toxicity to mammalian host cells is low.

After entry into herpes-infected cells, acyclovir is

phosphorylated to the active compound acyclovir triphosphate. The first step in this process is dependent on the presence of the viral-coded thymidine kinase. Acyclovir triphosphate acts as an inhibitor of, and substrate for, the herpes-specified DNA polymerase, preventing further viral DNA synthesis without affecting normal cellular processes.

Dosage and administration

Dosage in adults: For *treatment* of herpes simplex infections, one 200 mg Zovirax Tablet or 5 ml Zovirax Suspension should be taken five times daily at approximately four-hourly intervals, omitting the night-time dose. Treatment should continue for 5 days, but in severe initial infections may have to be extended.

Dosing should begin as early as possible after the start of an infection; for recurrent episodes this should preferably be during the prodromal period or when lesions first appear.

For *prophylaxis* of herpes simplex infections in the immunocompromised, one 200 mg Zovirax Tablet or 5 ml Zovirax Suspension should be taken FOUR times daily at approximately six-hourly intervals. In severely immunocompromised patients (e.g. after marrow transplant) or in patients with impaired absorption from the gut, the dose can be doubled to 400 mg or alternatively intravenous dosing could be considered. The duration of prophylactic administration is determined by the duration of the period at risk.

Dosage in children: For treatment of herpes simplex infections and for prophylaxis in the immunocompromised, children over the age of 2 years should be given adult dosages, and children below the age of 2 years should be given *half* the adult dose.

Zovirax Suspension may be diluted 50:50 with either Syrup BP or Sorbitol Solution 70% BPC. The freshly prepared dilution is stable for up to 4 weeks at 25°C.

In patients with impaired renal function, the recommended oral dose will not lead to accumulation of acyclovir above levels that have been established safe by intravenous infusion. However, for patients with severe renal impairment (creatinine clearance less than 10 ml/minute) a dosage adjustment to 200 mg every 12 hours is recommended.

Dosage in the elderly: In the elderly, total acyclovir body clearance declines along with creatinine clearance. Special attention should be given to dosage reduction in elderly patients with impaired creatinine clearance.

Contra-indications, warnings, etc

Contra-indications: Zovirax Tablets and Zovirax Suspension are contra-indicated in patients known to be hypersensitive to acyclovir.

Side- and adverse effects: Events occurring during oral acyclovir treatment or prophylaxis were no different in nature, incidence or severity from events occurring in patients receiving placebo.

The results of a wide range of mutagenicity tests *in vitro* and *in vivo* indicate that acyclovir does not pose a genetic risk to man.

Acyclovir was not found to be carcinogenic in long-term studies in the rat and the mouse.

Use in pregnancy and lactation: Studies with systemically administered Zovirax in animals have not demonstrated any embryotoxic or teratogenic effects. No information is available on the effects of administration of Zovirax Tablets or Suspension during human pregnancy, and therefore caution should be exercised in prescribing Zovirax Tablets or Suspension in pregnancy. No information is available on levels of acyclovir which may appear in human breast milk after administration of Zovirax Tablets or Suspension.

Fertility: There is no experience of the effect of Zovirax Tablets or Zovirax Suspension on human fertility. Two-generation studies in mice did not reveal any effect of acyclovir on fertility.

Drug interactions: Probenecid increases the acyclovir mean half-life and area under the plasma concentration curve. Clinical experience has not identified other drug interactions with acyclovir.

Toxicity and treatment of overdosage: Acyclovir is only partially absorbed in the gastrointestinal tract (approximately 20% at the recommended dosage). It is unlikely that serious toxic effects would occur if an entire treatment course of 25 Zovirax Tablets or 125 ml Zovirax Suspension were taken on a single occasion. Doses of 800 mg five times a day (4 grams per day) have been administered for 5 days without adverse effects.

Single intravenous doses of up to 80 mg/kg have been inadvertently administered without adverse effects. Acyclovir is dialysable.

Pharmaceutical precautions *Tablets and Suspension:* Store at a temperature not exceeding 25°C, in a dry place.

Legal category POM.

Package quantities
Zovirax Tablets: Pack of 25 tablets.
Zovirax Suspension: Bottle of 125 ml.

Further information Nil.

Product licence numbers
Zovirax Tablets   0003/0173
Zovirax Suspension   0003/0202

*Trade Mark

Winthrop Laboratories
Sterling-Winthrop House
Onslow Street
Guildford
Surrey GU1 4YS

WIN♀HROP

ACTAL*

Presentation 1. Flat, white tablets with bevelled edges. 12.7 mm in diameter, marked Actal on both faces, containing 360 mg alexitol sodium.
2. A white suspension with a slight odour and a sweet taste. Each 5 ml contains 360 mg alexitol sodium.

Uses Actal is an antacid. It is recommended for the relief of hyperacidity, dyspepsia and pain due to peptic ulcer.

Dosage and administration For oral administration only.

Adults: Tablets – 1 or 2 to be sucked. Suspension – one or two 5 ml spoonfuls. The dose may be repeated as required.

Contra-indications, warnings, etc There are no known contra-indications or adverse reactions and no cases of overdosage have been reported. If a large amount is taken it should be sufficient to empty the stomach by emesis.

Pharmaceutical precautions Store the tablets in a dry place.

Legal category Actal Tablets GSL
Actal Suspension P.

Package quantities Actal tablets are available in packs of 12, 24, 48 and 96.
Actal Suspension is supplied in white polyethylene bottles containing 300 ml.

Further information Each Actal tablet (or 5 ml of Suspension) contains 14 mg sodium.

Product licence numbers
Actal Tablets   0071/5018
Actal Suspension   0071/0089

ALEVAIRE*

Presentation A clear, colourless solution which foams on shaking, containing tyloxapol 0.125% w/v. Alevaire has a slight characteristic odour.

Uses Alevaire is recommended for use as a mucolytic agent in the treatment of lung conditions accompanied or complicated by excessive or thickened bronchopulmonary secretions. It may also be used as a vehicle for aerosol medication. Alevaire containing one or more antibiotics may be used in a closed irrigation system for the treatment of pyogenic bone or joint infections.

Dosage and administration
1. *As a mucolytic agent:* In continuous therapy the dose

of Alevaire delivered will depend on the nebuliser used and the oxygen/air flow rate, but daily dosages ranging from 144 to 360 ml with gas flows of 4–8 litres per minute have been employed. In intermittent therapy, Alevaire is inhaled three or four times a day for periods of 20 minutes, resulting in the administration of from 6 ml to 20 ml of Alevaire in a 24-hour period. Infants and small children are best treated in an oxygen tent or incubator, the mist being led into the tent through one of the nursing apertures. Treatment should be maintained for one or two days or until improvement is apparent.
2. *As a vehicle for aerosol medication:* Because of its stability and carrying properties, Alevaire mist can be used to deliver certain medicaments to the lungs. The use of Alevaire enables the drugs to reach the fine subdivisions of the bronchioles and facilitates their distribution over a wide area.
3. *In pyogenic bone or joint infections:* A suitable irrigation solution may be prepared by mixing 200 ml Alevaire with 800 ml physiological saline in which one or more appropriate antibacterial agents are dissolved. This solution is run into the wound at the rate of 80 ml per hour (about 2 litres in 24 hours).

Contra-indications, warnings, etc There are no known contra-indications.
After prolonged therapy, slight inflammation of the eyelids may develop, but this clears rapidly when treatment is discontinued.

Pharmaceutical precautions Containers of Alevaire which have been opened are easily contaminated by mould or bacteria which grow readily in the solution. If only small amounts of Alevaire are required they should be removed from the original containers with aseptic precautions. Alternatively, any unused solution in containers should be discarded after 24 hours. Alevaire should not be used if it becomes cloudy or develops a sediment.
Any Alevaire Solution remaining in a nebuliser after use should be discarded and the nebuliser rinsed and cleaned. If nebulisers are left uncleaned the Alevaire evaporates leaving a gummy residue. Alevaire should not be allowed to come into contact with brass or copper because of possible damage to the metal surface.
As a general rule, the addition of supplementary drugs to bulk containers of Alevaire is not recommended, as it may prove wasteful and difficult to determine the amount of nebulised drug received by the patient. It is preferable to dissolve the medication in a small quantity of Alevaire for administration over a short period.

Legal category P.

Package quantities Alevaire is supplied in non-reclosable amber glass bottles containing 60 or 200 ml.

Further information Alevaire is best administered as a fine mist produced by a nebuliser activated by oxygen or a motor-driven air compressor capable of reducing particle size to 0.5–5 μm.

Product licence number 0071/5019.

BIOGASTRONE*

Presentation White, flat, round, bevelled-edged tablets 9.6 mm in diameter, marked BG and scored on one side and unmarked on the other. Each tablet contains Carbenoxolone Sodium BP 50 mg.

Uses For the treatment of gastric ulcers.

Dosage and administration For oral administration only. Adults should take 2 tablets three times daily after meals for the first week. Thereafter, 1 tablet should be taken three times a day until the ulcer has healed. Four to six weeks' treatment is usually needed but up to 12 weeks may be required in resistant cases; Lower doses may be needed in the elderly (see under Precautions).

Contra-indications, warnings, etc
Contra-indications: Biogastrone should not be prescribed for patients suffering from severe cardiac, renal and hepatic failure, Nor should it be prescribed for patients on digitalis glycosides unless serum electrolyte levels are monitored at weekly intervals and measures taken to avoid the development of hypokalaemia.

Precautions: Special care should be exercised with patients predisposed to sodium and water retention, potassium loss and hypertension (e.g. the elderly and those with cardiac, renal and hepatic disease) since carbenoxolone can induce similar changes.

Potassium supplements should be considered for those at risk from developing hypokalaemia.

A slower clearance rate and decreased protein binding of carbenoxolone may explain the higher incidence of side effects in the elderly and justify a reduction in dosage.

Regular monitoring of weight and blood pressure is advisable for all patients. A thiazide diuretic should be administered if oedema or hypertension occurs (spironolactone or amiloride should not be used because they hinder the therapeutic action of carbenoxolone). Potassium loss should be corrected by the administration of oral supplements.

No teratogenic effects have been reported with carbenoxolone sodium but careful consideration should be given before prescribing Biogastrone for women who may become pregnant.

Overdosage: If the tablets have been recently ingested, the stomach should be emptied by gastric lavage. Serum electrolytes should be monitored and any deficiency in potassium should be corrected, using the intravenous route if necessary, or slow-release or effervescent potassium chloride tablets. Water retention and sodium balance should be corrected by means of a diuretic (spironolactone or amiloride would appear to be a logical choice).

Pharmaceutical precautions Nil.

Legal category POM.

Package quantities Bottles of 100 tablets.

Further information Carbenoxolone has been shown to exert a healing effect on gastric ulcers, possibly by improving mucus synthesis and by prolonging the lifespan of gastric epithelium.

Made under licence from Biorex Laboratories Ltd, England.

Product licence number 0071/5902.

BIORAL GEL*

Presentation A buff-coloured gel containing 2% Carbenoxolone Sodium BP.

Uses For the treatment of mouth ulcers

Dosage and administration Adults and children. Apply thickly to the lesion after meals and at bedtime. The gel should be allowed to remain on the ulcer as long as possible.

Contra-indications, warnings, etc There are no known contra-indications and no side-effects have been reported.

If the lesion is infected, additional appropriate therapy should be used. If the ulcer fails to heal within three weeks, treatment and diagnosis should be reviewed.

Pharmaceutical precautions Tubes should be kept well closed to avoid deterioration.

Legal category P.

Package quantities Tubes containing 5 g.

Further information Bioral Gel contains carbenoxolone sodium in a specially formulated base which adheres to the moist oral mucosa and ensures prolonged contact with the ulcer.

Made under licence from Biorex Laboratories Ltd, England.

Product licence number 0071/5904.

CALCIUM RESONIUM*

Presentation Calcium Resonium is ground and flavoured calcium polystyrene sulphonate and is a yellow to golden brown fine powder with a pleasant vanilla odour and sweet taste. It contains about 8% w/w of calcium.

Uses Calcium Resonium is an ion-exchange resin. It is recommended for the treatment of hyperkalaemia associated with anuria or severe oliguria. It is also used to treat hyperkalaemia in patients requiring dialysis and in patients on regular haemodialysis or on prolonged peritoneal dialysis.

Dosage and administration Calcium Resonium is for oral or rectal administration only. The dosage recommendations detailed below are a guide only; the precise requirements should be decided on the basis of regular serum electrolyte determinations.

Adults:
1. *Oral:* Usual dose 15 g three or four times a day. The resin is given by mouth in a little water, or it may be made into a paste with some sweetened vehicle.

2. *Rectal:* In cases where vomiting may make oral administration difficult the resin may be given rectally as a suspension of 30 g resin in 100 ml 2% Methylcellulose 450 BP (medium viscosity) and 100 ml water, as a daily retention enema. In the initial stages administration by

this route as well as orally may help to achieve a more rapid lowering of the serum potassium level.

The enema should if possible be retained for at least nine hours. If both routes are used initially it is probably unnecessary to continue rectal administration once the oral resin has reached the rectum.

Elderly: No specific dosage recommendations.

Children: 1 g/kg body weight daily in divided doses in acute hyperkalaemia. Dosage may be reduced to 0.5 g/kg body weight daily in divided doses for maintenance therapy.

The resin is given orally, preferably with a drink (not a fruit squash) or a little jam or honey. When refused by mouth it should be given rectally using a dose at least as great as that which would have been given orally, diluted in the same ratio as described for adults.

Contra-indications, warnings, etc

Contra-indications: Calcium Resonium should not be used to treat patients with hyperparathyroidism, multiple myeloma, sarcoidosis or metastatic carcinoma who may present with renal failure and hypercalcaemia.

Precautions: The possibility of severe potassium depletion should be considered, and adequate biochemical control is essential during treatment.

Administration of the resin should be stopped when the serum potassium falls to 5 mmol/litre. Serum calcium levels should be estimated at weekly intervals to detect the early development of hypercalcaemia, and the dose of resin adjusted to levels at which hypercalcaemia and hypokalaemia are prevented.

In children, particular care is needed with rectal administration as excessive dosage or inadequate dilution could result in impaction of the resin.

Overdosage: In the event of overdosage the resin should be removed from the alimentary tract by the use of laxatives or enemas, and appropriate measures should be taken to restore serum potassium levels to normal, and to reduce blood calcium levels if these are raised.

Side-effects: Hypercalcaemia has been reported in well-dialysed patients receiving calcium resin, and in the occasional patient with chronic renal failure. Many patients in chronic renal failure have low serum calcium and high serum phosphate, but some, who cannot be screened out beforehand, show a sudden rise in serum calcium to high levels after therapy. The risk emphasises the need for adequate biochemical control.

Pharmaceutical precautions It is suggested that Calcium Resonium should not be administered in fruit squashes since these have a high potassium content.

Legal category P.

Package quantities Polystyrene containers of 300 g each containing a plastic scoop which, when filled level, contains 15 g.

Further information Nil.

Product licence number 0071/5025.

DANOL*

Presentation

1. *Danol:* pink/white No. 1 hard gelatin capsules printed in black ink with Danol 200 and filled with a white or almost white powder containing 200 mg danazol.
2. *Danol-½ (Half Strength):* grey/white No. 3 hard gelatin capsules printed in black ink with Danol 100 and filled with a white or almost white powder containing 100 mg danazol.

Uses Danol is recommended for the treatment of endometriosis and associated infertility, benign breast disease (e.g. fibrocystic mastitis), primary menorrhagia and the premenstrual syndrome. Danol has also been used to treat virginal breast hypertrophy, primary constitutional precocious puberty, gynaecomastia and other similar endocrine disorders where regulation of the release of pituitary gonadotrophins LH and FSH would be of therapeutic value.

Dosage and administration Danol is for oral administration only. To guard against administration to pregnant patients it is recommended that Danol therapy in adult females should start during menstruation, preferably on the first day. Thereafter, Danol should be given continuously. Dosage depends on the condition being treated and the patients' response. In some patients, once a satisfactory response has been obtained it may be possible to maintain improvement with a reduced dose. The need for treatment should be reviewed at regular intervals.

1. *Adults:* The usual range of dosage is 200 mg to 800 mg daily in two to four divided doses.

In endometriosis it is recommended that a starting dose of 400 mg daily be used reducing or increasing as necessary.

Treatment should normally be continued for six months or until the condition resolves, whichever is the shorter period of time.

In benign breast disorders a starting dose of 300 mg daily is recommended and treatment is normally continued for three to six months.

In primary menorrhagia daily doses of 100–400 mg have been found effective but 200 mg daily is usually sufficient to reduce menstrual blood loss to acceptable levels. In the premenstrual syndrome 200 mg/day is recommended. The need to continue treatment should be reviewed after three months in these conditions.

2. *Children:* The recommended dose in precocious puberty is 100–400 mg daily, depending on the patient's age, weight and clinical response.

Contra-indications, warnings, etc

Contra-indications: Although no teratogenic effects have been observed in animal studies, it is recommended that Danol should not be given to patients who are pregnant. In patients with amenorrhoea before treatment, tests should be considered to establish that they are not pregnant. Administration should be stopped if a patient is found to be pregnant after starting a course of treatment. Continuing treatment may result in an androgenic effect on the foetus. Danol should not be given to mothers who are breast-feeding.

Since Danol may increase ALA synthetase activity and hence porphyrin metabolism, it should not be given to patients with porphyria.

Precautions: Contraception: Although Danol can inhibit ovulation, it must not be relied upon for contraception and non-hormonal methods should be advised during the course of treatment. This is because the concurrent administration of oestrogens and/or progestogens, including oral contraceptives may modify the action of Danol.

Because Danol may cause some degree of fluid retention, patients with conditions which may be influenced by this factor, such as cardiac or renal dysfunction or migraine, require careful observation.

Anticonvulsant therapy in epileptic patients should be carefully monitored when introducing or discontinuing Danol. Danol should be administered with caution in patients with hepatic dysfunction. Occasionally, increases in liver transaminases may occur. Very rarely hepatocellular jaundice in association with Danol has been reported.

Care is needed in patients with diabetes mellitus because Danol may increase insulin resistance and thus aggravate the condition.

Danol may potentiate the action of anticoagulants.

There is some evidence that danazol has fibrinolytic properties, therefore the thrombo-embolic complications sometimes seen in patients taking oestrogen/progestogen combinations are not to be expected. However, until more information is available it would be wise to avoid high doses of Danol and prolonged treatment in patients with a history of thrombosis.

Overdosage: In animal tests, doses of 16,000 mg/kg body weight produced no fatalities, and it is unlikely that any immediate serious reactions would be seen from a single excessive dose in man.

In the case of acute overdosage, the drug should be removed by emesis or stomach pump (if ingestion is recent) and the patient should be kept under observation in case of any delayed reactions.

Side-effects: Acne, oily-skin, fluid retention, mild hirsutism and, rarely, clitoral hypertrophy, all of which can be attributed to the mild androgenic activity of Danol, have been reported on occasions, particularly in patients where such tendencies were already present. Flushing and reduction in breast size have also been noted. If signs of virilisation (e.g. voice changes) develop, Danol should be discontinued.

Other adverse reactions which have been reported include rashes, nervousness and nausea, headache, dizziness, vertigo, emotional lability, backache, skeletal muscle spasm and hair loss.

A small increase in weight is not uncommon and reflects mild anabolic activity. Increases greater than 4 or 5 kg (10 lbs) however are not common and tend to be associated with higher doses and longer periods of treatment. Control of diet may be beneficial in some susceptible patients.

HDL cholesterol is likely to fall during Danol and return to pretreatment levels after discontinuing therapy. The biological significance of this is not established.

In long-term high-dosage toxicity studies in the rhesus monkey, although no change was seen in the activity of the drug-metabolising enzymes, azoreductase and p-nitroanisole O-demethylase, a decrease was observed in aminopyrine N-demethylase and aniline hydroxylase.

Pharmaceutical precautions Nil.

Legal category POM.

Package quantities Danol capsules are supplied in cartons of 50 and 100 in blisters and as Danol 200 C-Pak in calendar packs of 56.
Danol -½ (Half Strength) capsules are supplied in cartons of 50 and 100 in blisters.

Further information The effect of Danol on the hypothalamic-pituitary-gonadal axis is reversible when treatment is stopped. In those patients who have conceived after treatment, there is no evidence to suggest that the compound has any effect on the course or outcome of pregnancy. There is no clinical or laboratory evidence that Danol affects other pituitary-endocrine axes. It should be noted, however, that while T.S.H. levels are unaffected by Danol, some patients who are clinically euthyroid may show increased T_3 uptake, decreased T_4 levels, and a decrease in thyroxine binding globulin.

Product licence numbers
Danol 200 mg   0071/0095
Danol-½ (Half Strength) 100 mg   0071/0094

DUOGASTRONE*

Presentation Colourless, transparent, unmarked position-release capsules filled with a white powder. Each contains 50 mg Carbenoxolone Sodium BP.

Uses For the treatment of duodenal ulcers.

Dosage and administration *Adults:* One capsule to be swallowed *whole and unbroken* with liquid, four times daily, *15–30 minutes before meals*. Patients taking antacids should continue to do so until symptoms disappear but anticholinergic drugs should be discontinued. Despite early relief of symptoms, treatment should continue for at least six weeks and should usually be extended to 12 weeks to ensure maximum healing effect.

The elderly may need less frequent dosage (see under Precautions).

Contra-indications, warnings, etc
Contra-indications: Duogastrone should not be prescribed for patients suffering from severe cardiac, renal or hepatic failure. Nor should it be given to patients on digitalis glycosides unless serum electrolyte levels are monitored at weekly intervals, and measures taken to avoid the development of hypokalaemia.

Precautions: Special care should be exercised with patients predisposed to sodium and water retention, potassium loss and hypertension (e.g. the elderly and those with cardiac, renal or hepatic disease) since carbenoxolone can induce similar changes. Potassium supplements should be considered for those at risk from developing hypokalaemia.

A slower clearance rate and decreased protein binding of carbenoxolone may explain the higher incidence of side effects in the elderly and justify a reduction in dosage.

Regular monitoring of weight and blood pressure is advisable for all patients. A thiazide diuretic should be administered if oedema or hypertension occurs (spironolactone or amiloride should not be used because they hinder the therapeutic action of carbenoxolone). Potassium loss should be corrected by the administration of oral supplements.

No teratogenic effects have been reported with carbenoxolone sodium but careful consideration should be given before prescribing Duogastrone for women who may become pregnant.

Overdosage: If the capsules have been recently ingested, the stomach should be emptied by gastric lavage. Serum electrolytes should be monitored and any deficiency in potassium should be corrected, using the intravenous route if necessary, or slow-release or effervescent tablets of potassium chloride. Water retention and sodium balance should be corrected by means of a diuretic. (Spironolactone or amiloride would appear to be a logical choice).

Pharmaceutical precautions Care should be taken not to damage the capsules. Store in a cool, dry place.

Legal category POM.

Package quantities Bottles of 28 capsules.

Further information Duogastrone is a unique 'position-release' capsule designed to deliver carbenoxolone sodium into the duodenum. The capsule contents are released only when it is ruptured by the pressure of the antral or pyloric contractions. Carbenoxolone sodium exerts a local healing effect on the ulcer possibly by improving mucus synthesis and by prolonging the life span of epithelium cells of the duodenum.

Made under licence from Biorex Laboratories Ltd, England. Brit Pat. No. 1093286.

Product licence number 0071/5903.

FERGON*

Presentation Fergon Tablets are smoothly polished, red, sugar-coated tablets with no markings, each containing 300 mg Ferrous Gluconate PhEur.

Uses Fergon Tablets are recommended for the treatment of hypochromic anaemia caused by deficient iron intake, excessive iron loss as in menorrhagia, or chronic bleeding from the gastro-intestinal tract. They are also used as a supplement during pregnancy, in idiopathic hypochromic anaemia and in the treatment of iron deficiency in childhood.

Dosage and administration Fergon is for oral administration. It is best administered about one hour before meals.

Adults and the Elderly Prophylactic: 2 tablets (600 mg) daily.

Therapeutic: 4–6 tablets (1.2–1.8 g) daily in divided doses.

Children: Children aged 6–12 years may be given 1–3 tablets daily for therapeutic or prophylactic purposes.

Contra-indications, warnings, etc There are no recorded contra-indications to Fergon but it should be used with caution in patients with haemochromatosis or haemolytic anaemia.

Patients should be warned to keep Fergon Tablets out of the reach of young children. The absorption of iron salts is decreased in the presence of antacids. Fergon will also diminish the absorption of concurrently administered tetracyclines.

Overdosage: It is well known that overdosage of ferrous salts is particularly dangerous to small children.

The following treatment is suggested. Gastric lavage with 5% sodium bicarbonate and saline cathartics (e.g. sodium sulphate 30 g for adults). Milk and eggs with 5 g bismuth carbonate every hour as demulcents. Blood or plasma transfusion for shock, oxygen for respiratory embarrassment. Chelating agents such as disodium calcium edetate may be tried (500 mg in 500 ml by continuous i.v. infusion). Dimercaprol should not be used since it forms a toxic complex with iron. Desferrioxamine is a specific iron chelating agent.

Side-effects: are mainly gastro-intestinal. They appear to occur less frequently than with ferrous sulphate, and patients are therefore less likely to default during treatment.

Pharmaceutical precautions Store in well-closed containers. Protect from light.

Legal category P.

Package quantities Fergon is supplied in bottles of 50 or 100 tablets.

Further information Nil.

Product licence number 0071/5032.

FRANOL*

Presentation Franol Tablets are flat, white tablets with bevelled edges, 8.7 mm in diameter, marked F on one side and plain on the other side. Each tablet contains 120 mg Theophylline PhEur, 8 mg Phenobarbitone PhEur and 11 mg Ephedrine Hydrochloride PhEur.

Uses Franol Tablets are recommended for the treatment of bronchial asthma and bronchitis.

Dosage and administration Franol Tablets are for oral administration only.

Adults:
1. *Bronchial asthma:* Dosage varies with individual requirements and should be adjusted accordingly. The usual dosage is 3 tablets a day (morning, midday and evening). For the patient who suffers nocturnal attacks, an extra tablet taken at bedtime is recommended.

In order to avoid recurrences, it is important that treatment should be continued for a considerable time after attacks have stopped.
2. *Bronchitis:* Usual dosage 3 tablets a day. This may be increased if necessary.

Elderly: No specific dosage recommendation.

Children: The usual dose is one-third to one-half the adult dose, though full doses may be used should these be needed. The dose will depend on the severity of the condition, on individual tolerance and on the response obtained.

Contra-indications, warnings, etc Franol should not be used during pregnancy or lactation. It should not be given to patients with acute intermittent porphyria or to those who are hypersensitive or exhibit idiosyncrasy to barbiturates or sympathomimetic amines.

It should not be given to those who are taking MAO inhibitors or have received them during the previous 14 days. Franol should be used with caution in patients with cardiovascular disease, hypertension, hyperthyroidism, prostatic hypertrophy or glaucoma.

Overdosage: The symptoms of overdosage are likely to be those attributable to ephedrine and include excessive irritability, fever, nausea and vomiting, cyanosis, tachycardia, dilated pupils, opisthotonus, spasm, convulsion and respiratory embarrassment. If recently ingested and vomiting (due to the theophylline) has not occurred, the stomach should be emptied. Subsequent treatment should be symptomatic.

Side-effects: The phenobarbitone in the formula will usually overcome any stimulation due to the ephedrine. Any minor gastric disturbances can be avoided by taking the tablets with meals.

Pharmaceutical precautions Nil.

Legal category CD (Sch 3) POM.

Package quantities Franol Tablets are supplied in bottles of 100, 500 and 1,000.

Further information Nil.

Product licence number 0071/5036.

FRANOL* EXPECT.

Presentation Franol Expect. is a clear, deep red, viscous solution with an odour of aniseed. Each 10 ml dose contains 120 mg Theophylline PhEur (equivalent to 130 mg Theophylline Hydrate PhEur), 8 mg Phenobarbitone, PhEur, 9.5 mg Ephedrine PhEur and 50 mg Guaiphenesin PhEur.

Uses Franol Expect. is recommended for the treatment of chronic bronchitis, bronchial asthma associated with productive bronchitis, and coughs associated with tracheobronchitis and influenza.

Dosage and administration Franol Expect. is for oral administration only. Dosage depends on individual needs and tolerance.

Adults: 10 ml (2 × 5 ml spoonfuls) three times a day, with an additional dose before retiring, if required.

Elderly: No specific dosage recommendation.

Children: The usual dose is one-third to one-half the adult dose, though older children will tolerate full doses, should these be needed.

Contra-indications, warnings, etc Franol Expect should not be used during pregnancy or lactation. It should not be given to patients with acute intermittent porphyria or to those who are hypersensitive or exhibit idiosyncrasy to barbiturates or sympathomimetic amines.

It should not be given to those who are taking MAO inhibitors or have received them during the previous 14 days. Franol Expect should be used with caution in patients with cardiovascular disease, hypertension, hyperthyroidism, prostatic hypertrophy or glaucoma.

Overdosage: The symptoms of overdosage are likely to be those attributable to ephedrine and include excessive irritability, fever, nausea and vomiting, cyanosis, tachycardia, dilated pupils, opisthotonus, spasm, convulsions and respiratory embarrassment. If recently ingested and vomiting (due to the theophylline) has not occurred, the stomach should be emptied. Subsequent treatment should be symptomatic.

Side-effects: The phenobarbitone in the formula will usually overcome any stimulation due to the ephedrine. Minor gastric disturbances can be overcome by taking the dose with meals.

Pharmaceutical precautions When doses of less than 5 ml are ordered Franol Expect. may be diluted with Syrup BP. A 50:50 dilution is stable for at least two to three weeks.

Legal category CD (Sch 3) POM.

Package quantities Franol Expect. is supplied in bottles containing 150 ml or 1 litre.

Further information Nil.

Product licence number 0071/5038.

FRANOL* PLUS

Presentation Franol Plus Tablets are flat, white tablets with bevelled edges, 8.7 mm in diameter, marked F + on one side and W on the other. Each tablet contains 120 mg Theophylline PhEur, 8 mg Phenobarbitone PhEur, 15 mg ephedrine sulphate and 10 mg thenyldiamine hydrochloride.

Uses Franol Plus Tablets are recommended for the treatment of asthma and bronchitis, especially where exacerbated by allergy and hay fever.

Dosage and administration *Adults:*
1. *Bronchial asthma:* Dosage varies with individual requirements and should be adjusted accordingly. The usual dosage is 3 tablets a day (morning, midday and evening). For the patient who suffers from nocturnal attacks, an extra tablet taken at bedtime is recommended.

In order to avoid recurrences, it is important that treatment should be continued for a considerable time after attacks have stopped.
2. *Bronchitis:* Usual dosage 3 tablets a day. This may be increased if necessary.
3. *Hay fever:* 1 tablet three times a day.

Elderly: No specific dosage recommendations.

Children: The usual dose is one-third to one-half the adult dose, though full doses may be used should these be needed. The dose will depend on the severity of the condition, on individual tolerance and on the response obtained.

Contra-indications, warnings, etc Franol Plus should not be used during pregnancy or lactation. It should not be given to patients with acute intermittent porphyria or to those who are hypersensitive or exhibit idiosyncracy to barbiturates or sympathomimetic amines.

It should not be given to those who are taking MAO inhibitors or have received them during the previous 14 days. Franol Plus should be used with caution in patients with cardiovascular disease, hypertension, hyperthyroidism, prostatic hypertrophy or glaucoma.

Overdosage: The symptoms of overdosage are likely to be those attributable to ephedrine and include excessive irritability, fever, nausea and vomiting, cyanosis, tachycardia, dilated pupils, opisthotonus, spasm, convulsions and respiratory embarrassment. If recently ingested and vomiting (due to the theophylline) has not occurred, the stomach should be emptied. Subsequent treatment should be symptomatic.

Side-effects: Any minor gastric disturbances can be avoided by taking the tablets with meals. The principal side-effects of thenyldiamine when used alone is sedation, but in Franol Plus, this effect is counteracted by the increased dose of ephedrine.

Pharmaceutical precautions Nil.

Legal category CD (Sch 3) POM.

Package quantities Franol Plus is supplied in bottles of 50 and 250 tablets.

Further information Franol Plus consists of the Franol formulation with the addition of the antihistamine thenyldiamine hydrochloride and an increased dose of ephedrine.

Product licence number 0071/5037.

GLURENORM*

Presentation Flat, white, bevelled-edged tablets, 9 mm in diameter, scored on one side and with G on the other, each containing 30 mg gliquidone.

Uses For the treatment of non-insulin dependent diabetics, including those with impaired renal function, who do not respond adequately to dietary control.

Dosage and administration Glurenorm should be

taken up to half an hour before a meal. The daily dose should be adjusted according to the patient's metabolic state, and the frequency of administration may be varied to obtain the best possible control of the diabetes throughout the day.

Adults: Most patients respond to a total daily dose of 45–60 mg given in two or three divided doses, of which the largest dose is usually taken in the morning with breakfast. The recommended maximum single dose is 60 mg (2 tablets) and the maximum daily dose 180 mg (6 tablets).

During stabilisation, dosage adjustment should be based on frequent blood (random and postprandial) and urinary sugar determinations.

Elderly: No specific dosage recommendation.

Stabilisation of previously untreated cases: Normally, treatment should begin with 15 mg (half a tablet) before breakfast and this should be gradually increased by 15 mg increments prior to mealtimes.

Change-over in patients previously treated with other oral anti-diabetic agents: Patients can be changed over from other sulphonylureas to Glurenorm without interruption. It is usual to start with 30 mg Glurenorm before breakfast, increasing as necessary by increments of 15 mg at mealtimes. In terms of comparative potency of single doses, 30 mg Glurenorm corresponds approximately to 1,000 mg tolbutamide, 5 mg glibenclamide, 250 mg chlorpropamide or 500 mg acetohexamide. However, in estimating equivalent total daily doses, the half-lives and duration of action of the respective sulphonylureas must be taken into consideration. Thus it is usually necessary to administer Glurenorm more frequently than a long-acting sulphonylurea.

Change-over in non-insulin dependent diabetics previously treated with insulin: In patients treated with up to 30 i.u. of insulin daily, change-over to Glurenorm may be attempted with an initial dose of 30 mg accompanied by a simultaneous gradual reduction of the amount of insulin, provided the pancreas still contains some functioning β cells. Patients who change from insulin to Glurenorm should be strictly supervised and response assessed by frequent and regular blood-sugar determinations.

It may be possible to reduce the insulin requirements of patients who require more than 30 i.u. daily by the concurrent administration of Glurenorm. Blood-sugar should be monitored frequently during the change-over period.

Combined treatment: The administration of a biguanide with Glurenorm to patients who cannot be adequately controlled by Glurenorm alone will often achieve satisfactory stabilisation of blood-sugar levels.

Contra-indications, warnings, etc

Contra-indications: Do not use for diabetes complicated by acidosis or ketosis nor in patients subject to the stress of surgery or acute infections. Glurenorm should not be used in pregnancy or in patients with severe hepatic or renal failure.

Precautions: Patients who miss a meal (particularly the elderly or debilitated) should be warned not to take their dose of Glurenorm, in order to reduce the risk of a hypoglycaemic reaction.

The effect of Glurenorm may be increased by physical exertion, alcohol, salicylates, sulphonamides, phenylbutazone, ethionamide, coumarin anticoagulants, chloramphenicol, tetracyclines, cyclophosphamide, MAO inhibitors, tuberculostatics and β-adrenergic blocking agents.

It may be necessary to increase the dose of Glurenorm when any of the following are administered concurrently: oral contraceptives, chlorpromazine, sympathomimetic agents, corticosteroids, thyroid hormones and nicotinic acid preparations.

The effect of barbiturates, vasopressin and oral anticoagulants are potentiated by the administration of Glurenorm.

Side-effects: Glurenorm is well tolerated. There have been some reports of minor skin allergies, gastric upsets and other non-specific side-effects. Reversible leucopenia has been reported on one occasion and reversible thrombocytopenia twice, but a causal connection with Glurenorm was not established.

Hypoglycaemic reactions should be infrequent, but may be accompanied by malaise, impaired concentration and altered consciousness. They may be treated with oral carbohydrate or with intravenous dextrose if the oral route is impractical. Glucagon (1 mg subcutaneously) could also be given.

Overdosage: In the conscious patient, hypoglycaemia may be managed by the oral administration of glucose. In the comatose patient, parenteral administration of glucose by intravenous infusion should be instituted. The patient should be kept under observation for further signs of hypoglycaemia. Consideration may be given to the recovery of ingested tablets by gastric lavage.

Pharmaceutical precautions Nil.

Legal category POM.

Package quantities Bottles of 100 tablets.

Further information Glurenorm is a sulphonylurea hypoglycaemic agent which is rapidly absorbed, its action starts within one hour and its optimum effect lasts two to three hours (plasma half-life 1.4 hours). It is almost completely metabolised in the liver by hydroxylation and demethylation. Only 5% of the pharmacologically inactive metabolites is excreted by the kidneys, the remainder is eliminated in the faeces via the bile. There is thus little risk of hypoglycaemia due to drug accumulation in patients with impaired renal function.

Sold under licence from Boehringer Ingelheim International GmbH.

Product licence number 0071/0155.

HAYPHRYN* NASAL SPRAY

Presentation Hayphryn Nasal Spray is a clear, colourless solution containing 0.5% w/v Phenylephrine Hydrochloride BP and 0.1% w/v thenyldiamine hydrochloride in a plastic spray bottle presentation. The solution has a faint odour and foams when shaken.

Uses Hayphryn Nasal Spray is recommended for the relief of nasal congestion in such conditions as the common cold, sinusitis and vasomotor rhinitis, particularly when an allergic factor is present as, for example, in hay fever and allergic rhinitis.

Dosage and administration For nasal administration only.

Adults: The tip of the atomiser should be inserted into each nostril in turn and the container squeezed twice, sharply, as the patient breathes in. The application may be repeated in three to four hours if necessary.

Children: For children the product may be administered as for adults, except that the container is squeezed once only into each nostril.

Contra-indications, warnings, etc Because it contains a sympathomimetic amine, Hayphryn Nasal Spray should not be used by patients taking monoamine oxidase inhibitors and it should be used with caution in patients taking β-adrenergic blocking agents. Hayphryn Nasal Spray should not be used for longer than three weeks, and should not be used for chronic nasal congestion.

Excessive or too prolonged use of Hayphryn Nasal Spray may lead to secondary congestion. Oral overdosage is unlikely to be a problem since the quantities of active ingredients in each spray are insufficient to cause any serious reaction.

Adverse effects are uncommon when the spray is used as recommended.

Pharmaceutical precautions Nil.

Legal category P.

Package quantities Plastic spray bottles containing 15 ml.

Further information Nil.

Product licence number 0071/5041.

HEXOPAL* TABLETS AND SUSPENSION HEXOPAL FORTE

Presentation 1. Hexopal Suspension is a smooth white fluid with a sweet odour and taste which contains 1000 mg Inositol Nicotinate BP in each 5 ml.

2. Hexopal Forte. White or almost white, oval, biconvex tablets marked HEX750 on one side and scored on the other. Each tablet contains 750 mg Inositol Nicotinate BP.

3. Hexopal Tablets are white or almost white, flat tablets with bevelled edges, 12.7 mm in diameter and marked with a symbol on one side and scored on the other. Each tablet contains 500 mg Inositol Nicotinate BP.

Uses Hexopal is recommended for the symptomatic treatment of conditions arising from arterial insufficiency, such as intermittent claudication, and in peripheral arteriosclerosis.

It is also recommended for the treatment of vasospastic conditions including chilblains, primary and secondary Raynaud's phenomenon, night cramps, 'restless legs', acrocyanosis and erythrocyanosis, and other conditions where a peripheral vasodilator is required.

Dosage and administration Hexopal is for oral administration only.

Adults: For the symptomatic treatment of conditions arising from arterial insufficiency, such as intermittent claudication or peripheral arteriosclerosis, the usual starting dose is 3 g daily (5 ml Hexopal Suspension or two Hexopal tablets three times a day or two Hexopal Forte tablets twice daily). The dose may be increased to 4 g daily if necessary. For patients with vasospastic conditions an initial dose of 1.5 g daily is recommended, but dosage depends on response to treatment and may be increased to 3 or 4 g daily in divided doses if necessary.

Contra-indications, warnings, etc There are no known contra-indications or precautions associated with the use of Hexopal, and side-effects are uncommon.

Hexopal appears to be virtually non-toxic to animals even in doses up to 100 times the normal therapeutic level. Despite extensive clinical experience in Britain since 1959, no case of poisoning or overdosage with Hexopal has been reported. In an emergency, it is suggested that the stomach should be emptied by gastric lavage and symptomatic treatment given.

Pharmaceutical precautions When doses of less than 5 ml are ordered, Hexopal Suspension may be diluted with Syrup BP so that the standard 5 ml spoonful may be given.

Legal category Hexopal Tablets GSL; Hexopal Suspension and Hexopal Forte P.

Package quantities Hexopal Tablets: Bottles of 100 or 500. Hexopal Suspension: Bottles of 300 ml. Hexopal Forte: Bottles of 100 and as Hexopal Forte C-Pak in calendar packs of 112.

Further information Hexopal appears to protect against vasospasm and has been reported to reduce fibrinogen and blood viscosity and to have a beneficial effect on the fibrinolytic systems and on raised blood lipids.

Product licence numbers
Hexopal Tablets   0071/5043
Hexopal Suspension   0071/0090
Hexopal Forte   0071/0164

KANNASYN*

Presentation Kannasyn Powder is a white, or almost white, crystalline powder. The powder is filled into vials containing Kanamycin Acid Sulphate PhEur equivalent to 1 g kanamycin base.

Kannasyn Solution is a sterile aqueous solution containing Kanamycin Sulphate equivalent to 250 mg/ml kanamycin base in clear glass vials. The vials are of 4 ml nominal fill to provide doses of 1.0 g kanamycin base as the sulphate.

Uses Kannasyn is recommended for the treatment of infections due to Gram-negative organisms resistant to other antibotics. It may also be used in the treatment of certain staphylococcal infections due to multiple-resistant strains, and in gonorrhoea.

Dosage and administration
1. *Intramuscular injection: Adults:* In acute infections: 1 g daily in two to four equally divided doses. Therapy should be limited to either a total dosage of 10 g or six days' treatment, whichever represents the greater quantity of antibiotic.

In chronic infections: 3 g weekly (1 g on alternate days) or 1 g twice a day, twice weekly (4 g weekly). The total amount administered should not exceed 50 g.

Elderly: A reduced dosage may be required. See under warnings.

Children: In acute infections: 15 mg/kg body weight daily in 2–4 equally divided doses.

In chronic infections: there are no specific dosage recommendations.

2. *Intravenous use:* This route is recommended only for gravely ill patients with overwhelming infections or with impending vascular collapse. Kannasyn may be given as a solution containing 2.5 mg/ml by slow intravenous

infusion at the rate of 3–4 ml per minute. The dosage for both adults and children is 15–30 mg/kg body weight daily in 2 or 3 divided doses.

3. *Intrathecal administration: Adults:* 100 mg in 10 ml saline once per day.

Children: Under 1 year: 25 mg in 10 ml saline once per day.

Over 1 year: 50 mg in 10 ml saline once per day.

It should be noted, however, that 7.5 mg/kg *intramuscularly* has produced CSF concentrations of 9 mcg/ml in infants with bacterial meningitis. This is about double the CSF concentration produced in normal infants and exceeds the MIC of many pathogens.

Contra-indications, warnings, etc Kanamycin should not be used during pregnancy. Local intolerance to intramuscular injection has sometimes been reported, but it is transient and does not require interruption of therapy. Ecchymoses have also been observed at the site of injection in a few patients. It has been suggested that high concentrations of kanamycin have anticoagulant properties, and this may explain these local haematomas at the injection site. It should, however, be noted that anticoagulant levels of kanamycin are not obtained in the blood with therapeutic doses. Sensitivity rashes appear to be uncommon. Intravenous injections are well tolerated and pain is not a problem. Thrombophlebitis has only been reported once in a patient who was receiving 50 million units of penicillin with the kanamycin.

As with other aminoglycoside antibiotics, apnoea and respiratory depression has been reported following the intraperitoneal use of kanamycin because of a curarelike effect. In addition, motor and sensory neuropathy has occurred following local application of kanamycin during spinal surgery, it has also produced slight weakening in muscle strength in a patient with myasthenia gravis. Because of these effects, it has been suggested that kanamycin should not be given intraperitoneally during surgery to patients who have received neuromuscular blocking agents.

Calcium gluconate has been suggested to counteract this curare-like action of kanamycin, but neostigmine appears to be more effective.

It has been shown that calcium can inhibit the antibacterial activity of kanamycin against certain organisms and for this reason the routine prophylactic use of calcium solutions with intraperitoneal kanamycin should be discouraged. In common with certain other antibiotics, kanamycin can affect the hearing when used in large doses or for long periods. This auditory damage, which may be permanent, is usually but not always preceded by tinnitus. Should this appear, the dose of kanamycin should be reduced or it should be discontinued. This antibiotic should always be administered with caution and preferably only in severe or resistent infections caused by organisms known to be sensitive to the compound, and blood levels should not be allowed to rise above 30 mcg/ml.

Hyaline and granular casts are sometimes observed in urine samples collected in the first 16 hours after administration in patients who have been given high doses of kanamycin. In these cases no permanent impairment of renal function occurs and the casts disappear within a few days of stopping treatment. Although nephrotoxic effects have been reported in some studies serious renal toxicity is not a frequent problem with the doses now used. It should be noted that prior treatment with streptomycin or viomycin may increase the likelihood of a nephrotoxic reaction with kanamycin.

In cases of impaired renal function, the kidney may be unable to eliminate kanamycin effectively and as a result the serum level will rise quickly. In these conditions reduced doses are necessary to avoid toxic effects. It has been reported that kanamycin is retained in the serum of patients with renal disease for a considerable time. If it is necessary to give the antibiotic to anuric patients, they should not receive increments more frequently than every three to four days and these increments should be one-half the loading dose used. The safest procedure, however, is to control the dosage by blood-level studies to prevent a rise above 30 mcg per ml.

The use of potent diuretics such as ethacrynic acid or frusemide with kanamycin should be avoided because they are known to potentiate the toxic action of aminoglycoside antibiotics.

Kanamycin is poorly absorbed from the gastrointestinal tract and oral administration does not normally give rise to systemic side-effects.

Pharmaceutical precautions Kannasyn should be protected from light. The powder may be stored at room temperature but should be used within three years of assay. When dissolved in water, the solution will keep for two to three weeks at room temperature and for three weeks to one month if refrigerated. Solutions left at room temperature may discolour slightly, but there is no loss of activity for 24 days. This colour change may be prevented or retarded by adjusting the pH to 5.5. A bacteriostat such as a 0.5% phenol or 0.1% chlorocresol may be added.

Kannasyn Solution (4 ml vials) may also be stored at room temperature but should be used within two years of assay. There is no loss of potency when it is subjected to a temperature of 100°C for one hour. Dilutions of Kannasyn Solution may be made with normal saline or 5% dextrose and these remain stable for two to three months at room temperature. It should be noted, however, that such dilution may reduce the amount of bacteriostats to ineffective levels, and the reduction in concentration of sodium metabisulphite could lead to the solution developing a yellowish tint.

Infusion solutions containing kanamycin have been reported to be incompatible with the following substances: amphotericin, barbiturates, cephalothin sodium, chlorpromazine, electrolytes (Ca^{++} Mg^{++}, citrate or phosphate ions), heparin, hydrocortisone, methicillin sodium, methohexitone, nitrofurantoin, phenytoin, prochlorperazine, sulphafurazole.

Legal category POM.

Package quantities *Kannasyn Powder:* Boxes of 5 vials.
Kannasyn Solution: Boxes of 5 vials each containing 4 ml.

Further information Nil.

Product licence numbers
Kannasyn Powder   0071/5052
Kannasyn Solution   0071/5053

LENIUM*

Presentation Lenium is an orange-yellow cream which, on mixing with water, gives a copious soft foam and leaves a fine red to orange coloured precipitate. It has a characteristic lavender odour, and contains 2.5% w/w Selenium Sulphide BP.

Uses Lenium is recommended for the control of pityriasis capitis and seborrhoeic dermatitis of the scalp and dandruff.

Dosage and administration Lenium is for topical use only for adults or children. The amount of Lenium required varies from person to person; sufficient should be used to allow the lather to penetrate to the scalp.

Lenium should be applied twice a week for two weeks, once a week for a further two weeks, then as required to maintain control of dandruff (every three to to six weeks). After initial treatment it is neither necessary nor desirable to use Lenium weekly to maintain control.

Selenium sulphide has a low index of sensitivity and a low toxicity when applied to the intact skin. When used in accordance with the instructions it should not discolour grey or light hair and it can be used on hair which has been waved or tinted.

Contra-indications, warnings, etc Lenium may cause an increase in the secretion of the natural oil of the scalp. If this becomes excessive an ordinary shampoo should be used between Lenium treatments.

Precautions: Wash the hands thoroughly after use. Keep out of reach of children. Do not apply to broken or denuded skin. Selenium sulphide may discolour some metals. Do not apply at the time hot or cold permanent waves are being given. Do not allow to enter the eyes. More than 48 hours should elapse between the use of Lenium and the application of hair-tinting agents.

Accidental ingestion: Although insoluble selenium sulphide is less toxic than soluble selenium compounds it may produce signs of acute toxicity if swallowed. Apart from symptomatic measures treatment consists of gastric lavage and saline cathartics. Ascorbic acid orally may increase the rate of excretion in the urine. BAL should not be used as an antidote since it may aggravate symptoms.

Pharmaceutical precautions Nil.

Legal category P.

Package quantities Lenium is available in 9 g sachets and flexible plastic tubes containing 42 g or 100 g.

Further information Nil.

Product licence number 0071/5055.

LEVOPHED*
LEVOPHED* SPECIAL

Presentation Levophed is a clear, colourless or almost-colourless solution containing 2 mg/ml Noradrenaline Acid Tartrate PhEur (equivalent to 1 mg/ml noradrenaline base).

Levophed Special is a clear, colourless or almost colourless, sterile solution containing 200 mcg/ml Noradrenaline Acid Tartrate PhEur (equivalent to 100 mcg/ml of noradrenaline base).

Uses Levophed is recommended for use as an emergency measure to restore the blood pressure to normal in cases of acute hypotension.

Dosage and administration Levophed Solution should be diluted and administered as an intravenous infusion, preferably through a fine polythene catheter inserted into an arm or leg vein where blood flow is rapid. It is recommended that Levophed be administered in 5% dextrose or dextrose-saline solution.

Adults: A suitable initial concentration is obtained by adding 4 ml Levophed to a litre of infusion fluid to give a drug concentration of 4 mcg per ml. There is a direct relationship between the drip rate and the blood pressure. After observing the response to an initial dose of 2 ml or 3 ml per minute, the rate of flow should be adjusted to establish and maintain a low normal blood pressure (100–120 mm Hg systolic), or somewhat higher in previously hypertensive patients. In patients with severe haemorrhagic or hypovolaemic shock, when blood or fluid replacement has not been completed, it is preferable to maintain the pressure at a lower level sufficient to maintain the circulation to vital organs. The average maintenance dose ranges from 0.5 ml to 1 ml per minute, but there is great individual variation in the dose required to attain and maintain normotension. Infusion should be continued until adequate blood pressure is maintained without the help of Levophed. The concentration of the solution employed depends on the clincal needs. If larger volumes of fluid are required at a flow rate which would involve an excessive dose of pressor agent, the solution may be used more diluted than the 4 mcg/ml suggested. Conversely, where fluid volume should be restricted as in congestive heart failure, higher concentrations may be used.

Levophed Special: In cases of cardiac standstill the rapid intravenous or intracardiac injection of 0.50–0.75 ml of undiluted Levophed Special may restore a recordable blood pressure for one to four minutes. After intravenous injection the solution should be massaged towards the heart.

A similar dose may be repeated when the blood pressure starts to fall again or blood pressure can be maintained with a normal Levophed drip. If there is no response to Levophed Special Solution administration intravenously, cardiac massage should be started with the injection of 0.50–0.75 ml Levophed Special into the ascending aorta or into the left auricle. Injection into the ventricle should be avoided because of the possible risk of inducing fibrillation. If the myocardium is fibrillating, a dose of Levophed Special may be injected after normal rhythm has been restored by massage or by electrical defibrillation.

Contra-indications, warnings, etc Check blood pressure frequently during administration to avoid hypertension. Extravasation of the solution may cause local tissue necrosis. It has been suggested that phentolamine may be added directly to the infusion flask to act as an antidote against sloughing without affecting the vasopressor activity of the Levophed.

The use of pressor amines during halothane anaesthesia may cause serious cardiac arrhythmias. Because of the possibility of increasing the risk of ventricular fibrillation, Levophed should be used with caution in patients receiving cyclopropane or any other cardiac sensitising agent.

Pharmaceutical precautions Protect from light. Store below 25°C. The solution should not be used if it is brown in colour. Levophed is best administered in 5% dextrose or dextrose saline solution because the dextrose protects against significant loss of potency due to oxidation. Deterioration occurs more rapidly in normal saline, but plasma, blood and blood substitutes can be used as diluents, though Levophed is less stable in these than in dextrose solution. If Levophed is administered in blood, ascorbic acid (10^{-6}) should be added to reduce the rate of oxidation.

Infusion solutions containing noradrenaline acid tartrate have been reported to be incompatible with the following substances: alkalis and oxidising agents, barbiturates, chlorpheniramine, chlorothiazide, nitrofurantoin, novobiocin, phenytoin, sodium bicarbonate, sodium iodide, streptomycin.

Legal category POM.

Package quantities *Levophed:* Boxes of six 2 ml or 4 ml ampoules.
Levophed Special: Boxes of five 2 ml ampoules.

Further information Nil.

Product licence numbers
Levophed   0071/5056
Levophed Special   0071/5057

LINGRAINE*

Presentation Lingraine Tablets are bright green, bi-convex tablets, 6.4 mm in diameter, with no markings. Each tablet contains 2.0 mg Ergotamine Tartrate PhEur.

Uses Lingraine Tablets are recommended for the relief of migraine and other vascular headaches.

Dosage and administration Lingraine Tablets are for sublingual administration only.

Adults: 1 tablet to be taken at the first sign of an attack of migraine. If necessary another tablet may be taken half an hour to an hour later. No more than 3 tablets should be taken in 24 hours and not more than 6 tablets in any one week.

Elderly: No specific dosage recommendations.

Children: Not recommended.

Contra-indications, warnings, etc Because ergotamine brings about constriction of peripheral blood vessels it should not be used in the presence of severe arteriosclerosis, coronary artery disease thrombophlebitis, Raynaud's syndrome or Buerger's disease. The concomitant administration of erythromycin may increase the risk of peripheral ischaemia. Lingraine should not be used where there is liver or kidney dysfunction, and since (like other ergot alkaloids) it causes contraction of uterine muscle it should not be used during pregnancy. Avoid where possible during breast feeding.

Overdosage: Like all the natural amino-acid alkaloids of ergot, ergotamine is a highly toxic substance which may cause chronic or acute poisoning, although the latter is less frequent. The oral administration of 26 mg over several days has proved fatal, and there have also been deaths from as little as 0.5 mg to 1.5 mg in a single injection.

The principal signs of overdosage are convulsions and severe peripheral vasoconstriction, leading to gangrene of the extremities.

The main symptoms consist of vomiting, diarrhoea, unquenchable thirst, tingling, itching and coldness of the skin, a rapid and weak pulse, confusion and unconsciousness. Amyl nitrate inhalations (0.2–0.3 ml) are suggested to counteract arterial spasm.

Side-effects: These are a relatively minor problem if the dose is carefully regulated. Nausea and vomiting are most frequently reported; other side-effects encountered include abdominal pain, leg cramps, vertigo, diarrhoea and, occasionally, increased headache.

Pharmaceutical precautions Nil.

Legal category POM.

Package quantities Lingraine Tablets are available in P.F.P. laminate strips in boxes of 12 tablets.

Further information Nil.

Product licence number 0071/5058.

LUMINAL*

Presentation Luminal Tablets are white, bi-convex tablets, 6.0 mm in diameter, marked III on one side and either LUM 15, LUM 30 or LUM 60 on the other. Each tablet contains 15 mg, 30 mg or 60 mg Phenobarbitone Ph Eur respectively.

Uses Luminal Tablets are for use in the treatment of grand mal and focal epilepsies.

Dosage and administration For oral administration only.

Adults: Dosage will depend upon the need of the individual patient. Maintenance doses in the range 60 to 200 mg/day (average 90 mg/day) in divided doses have proven adequate. The dose should not exceed 600 mg in 24 hours, and the effect of such large doses should be carefully monitored.

Elderly: No special doseage recommendations (but see 'Precautions').

Children: Dosage will be in the range 2 to 10 mg/kg/day in divided doses depending upon the age and condition of the patient.

Dosage should be adjusted carefully and with gradual increment until fits are controlled or there are overdose effects. Frequency of administration may be twice daily or often once daily at bedtime. Once a regimen is established it should be maintained until there is freedom from fits for at least two years. Treatment should not be withdrawn abruptly.

Contra-indications, warnings, etc

Contra-indications: Acute intermittent porphyria and patients who are hypersensitive or who exhibit idiosyncrasy to barbiturates.

Avoid during pregnancy and lactation, in debilitated or senile patients and in those with a history of alcohol or drug abuse.

Precautions: Barbiturates should be avoided or used only with particular caution and appropriate supervision in children and the elderly.

Phenobarbitone in daily doses is cumulative and its effects will eventually extend into the day if used on many successive nights. Continuous use of excessive amounts may result in ataxia, stupor and delirium, and the possibility of tolerance and drug dependence of the barbiturate-alcohol type should always be borne in mind.

Some patients exhibit idiosyncrasy to barbiturates, and such individuals' response to these compounds is likely to be restlessness and excitement even in the absence of pain.

Large doses should not be given to patients with renal impairment or with diseases of the liver. A reduced dose will be necessary in patients with renal or hepatic failure. In severe pulmonary insufficiency even hypnotic doses of barbiturates will depress the respiration. Barbiturates may potentiate the central depressant effect of alcohol and other sedatives and affect the action of a number of other drugs, by hepatic enzyme induction, including coumarin type anticoagulants, systemic steroids (including oral contraceptives), phenytoin, griseofulvin, rifampicin, phenothiazines and tricyclic antidepressants. Prolonged treatment may produce dependence; abrupt withdrawal may provoke convulsions.

Adverse effects: Common adverse effects include drowsiness, sedation, unsteadiness, vertigo and inco-ordination. Performance and alertness may be impaired during the first week of administration. Patients should be warned of the possible hazard when driving or operating machinery.

Other adverse reactions may include a 'hangover' effect, paradoxical excitement, restlessness, confusion, particularly in the elderly and in children, skin rashes in patients who may be sensitive to this type of drug, and megaloblastic anaemia.

Overdosage: Where patients are seen within four hours of taking an overdose, gastric aspiration or lavage may be beneficial in adults, while children who are conscious may be given an emetic (e.g. Ipecacuanha Emetic Mixture Paediatric BP).

The prime objective in treating phenobarbitone overdosage is to maintain vital functions (respiration, cardiovascular and renal function, and electrolyte balance) while the majority of the drug is metabolised by hepatic enzymes. At the same time some of the drug is excreted unchanged by the kidneys. Given normal renal function, this latter process may be enhanced by alkaline diuresis, maintaining the urinary pH at about 8 by appropriate intravenous infusion. In severe cases, haemodialysis may help but extracorporeal haemoperfusion is probably more effective.

Pharmaceutical precautions Nil.

Legal category CD (Sch 3) POM.

Package quantities Luminal Tablets 15 mg: Bottles of 100.
Luminal Tablets 30 mg: Bottles of 100 or 500.
Luminal Tablets 60 mg: Bottles of 250.

Further information Barbiturates have a high addiction potential. Long term use or use of high dosage for short periods may lead to tolerance and subsequently to physical and psychological dependence. Symptoms of dependence include confusion, defective judgement and loss of emotional control. Withdrawal symptoms occur after long-term use (and particularly after abuse) on rapid cessation of barbiturate treatment. Symptoms include nightmares, irritability and insomnia and in severe cases, tremors, delirium, convulsions and death. Withdrawal symptoms have been reported in neonates after barbiturate treatment during pregnancy and labour.

Product licence numbers
Luminal 15 mg   0071/5060
Luminal 30 mg   0071/5061
Luminal 60 mg   0071/5062

MICTRAL*

Presentation A mixture of granules containing particles varying in colour from white to yellow. When added to water, they disperse with slight effervescence, yielding a citrus-flavour suspension. Each 7 g of granules contains Nalidixic Acid BP 660 mg, Sodium Citrate PhEur 3.75 g, Citric Acid PhEur 250 mg and Sodium Bicarbonate PhEur 250 mg.

Uses For the treatment of cystitis and lower urinary tract infections caused by pathogens sensitive to nalidixic acid.

Dosage and administration For oral administration only.

Adults: The contents of one sachet should be dissolved in a tumblerful of water and taken three times a day. A 3-day course is normally sufficient.

Elderly: No specific dosage recommendations.

Children: Not recommended.

Contra-indications, warnings, etc Nalidixic acid should not be given to patients with a history of convulsive disorders. It should be used with caution in patients with liver disease. Patients should avoid excessive exposure to sunlight. Although there is no evidence that nalidixic acid has any harmful effect during pregnancy, careful consideration should, as with all drugs, be given to the use of Mictral granules during the first trimester. Small amounts of nalidixic acid may be excreted in human milk. When nalidixic acid is given to patients on anticoagulant therapy, it may be necessary to reduce the anticoagulant dosage. Each sachet contains the equivalent of 950 mg (41.3 mmol) of sodium. This should be taken into account when prescribing for patients for whom sodium restriction is indicated.

Active proliferation of the organisms is a necessary condition for the antibacterial action of nalidixic acid; the action of Mictral may therefore be inhibited by the presence of other antibacterial substances.

When testing for glycosuria in patients receiving Mictral, 'Clinistix' or 'Tes-Tape' should be used since other reagents may give a false-positive result.

Nalidixic acid, in therapeutic doses, can interfere with the estimation of urinary 17-ketosteroids and may cause high results in the assay of urinary vanilmandelic acid (Pisano method).

Overdosage: Because of the nature of the product, serious overdosage is unlikely. An excessive amount of granules is likely to cause vomiting.

Side Effects: Gastro-intestinal effects (constipation or diarrhoea, anorexia, nausea or vomiting) and subjective visual disturbances have been reported with nalidixic acid. They have resolved on reducing the dose or discontinuing treatment. If skin rashes occur, administration of Mictral should be stopped.

Blood dyscrasias are rare, but haemolytic anaemia (sometimes related to G-6-PD deficiency), thrombocytopenia and leucopenia have been reported.

Pharmaceutical precautions Nil.

Legal category POM.

Package quantities Cartons containing nine 7 g sachets.

Further information Sodium citrate raises the urinary pH. In these conditions, it has been shown that the amount of free nalidixic acid and of its active metabolite which appears in the urine is more than doubled as a result of a corresponding reduction in inactive glucuronides.

Product licence number 0071/0126.

MYCARDOL*

Presentation Mycardol Tablets are white, flat tablets with bevelled edges, 7.9 mm in diameter, marked M on one side and scored on the other. Each tablet contains 30 mg pentaerythritol tetranitrate.

Uses Mycardol Tablets are recommended for the symptomatic treatment of angina pectoris. They are not recommended as a single measure for the treatment of anginal attacks, but rather as an adjunct to glyceryl trinitrate.

Dosage and administration For oral administration only.

Adults: The usual dosage is 2 tablets three times a day, though some may need 2 tablets four times daily. If there is nocturnal pain, the last dose should be taken before retiring. The tablets should be taken before meals.

Elderly: No specific dosage recommendations.

Contra-indications, warnings, etc Mycardol should not be used immediately following a coronary thrombosis or in patients with marked anaemia or cerebral haemorrhage. It should be used with caution in cases of glaucoma.

Overdosage: There have been no reports of Mycardol overdosage.

The possible effects of pentaerythritol tetranitrate toxicity are reported as being; cyanosis, methaemoglobinaemia, severe headache, fall in blood pressure, muscular weakness, dizziness, palpitation, vomiting and diarrhoea. Chronic overdosage may result in confusion and collapse, particularly in sensitive patients.

Methylene blue is usually recommended for the correction of methaemoglobinaemia: it is also indicated in the event of cyanosis (up to 50 ml of 1% solution i.v.).

Treatment of other serious toxic effects will consist of gastric lavage and saline cathartics (e.g. sodium sulphate, 30 g in 250 ml). Blood pressure should be restored by postural means (prone position with feet raised) or by an appropriate pressor agent.

Side-effects: No serious side-effects have been encountered following normal dosage, even over long periods. Headache, lethargy and nausea can occur during the first few days of treatment. If palpitations or vomiting occur, treatment should be stopped.

Methaemoglobinaemia is rarely seen with therapeutic dosage. Tolerance to Mycardol does not appear to develop.

Pharmaceutical precautions Store in a cool place and protect from light.

Legal category P.

Package quantities Mycardol Tablets are supplied in bottles of 100.

Further information Nil.

Product licence number 0071/5065.

NEOPHRYN*

Presentation Neophryn Nasal Drops consist of a clear, colourless solution containing 0.25% w/v Phenylephrine Hydrochloride BP.

Neophryn Nasal Spray is a clear, colourless solution containing 0.5% w/v Phenylephrine Hydrochloride BP in a plastic spray bottle presentation. The solution has a faint aromatic odour and foams when shaken.

Uses Neophryn Nasal Drops and Neophryn Nasal Spray are recommended for the relief of nasal congestion in such conditions as the common cold, sinusitis and vasomotor rhinitis.

Dosage and administration
1. *Neophryn Nasal Drops: Adults:* 2–3 drops in each nostril. In sinusitis, Neophryn Drops are well adapted to the Proetz displacement technique, but the alternative lateral head low method may equally well be used.

Children: 1–2 drops in each nostril.

2. *Neophryn Nasal Spray: Adults:* The tip of the atomiser should be inserted into each nostril in turn and the container squeezed twice, sharply, as the patient breathes in. The application may be repeated in three to four hours if necessary.

Contra-indications, warnings, etc Because Neophryn contains a sympathomimetic amine it should not be used by patients taking monoamine oxidase inhibitors and it should be used with caution by patients taking β-adrenergic blocking agents. Neophryn appears to be remarkably free from side-effects, but like all solutions for nasal application, it should be used for short periods only, because prolonged use may permanently damage the respiratory mucosa, and may even induce hypersensitivity. It is therefore suggested that Neophryn should not be used for longer than three weeks and that it should not be used for chronic nasal obstruction. As with all drugs, Neophryn should not be used in pregnancy unless strictly necessary.

Toxicity resulting from local use is practically unknown because the local vasoconstrictor action of phenylephrine retards its absorption. In the alimentary tract, phenylephrine is hydrolysed and absorption is unpredictable. This, combined with the small amount in each pack, makes acute overdosage highly unlikely.

Pharmaceutical precautions Nil.

Legal category P.

Package quantities *Neophryn Nasal Drops:* Bottles of 15 ml complete with dropper.
Neophryn Nasal Spray: Plastic spray bottles each containing 15 ml.

Further information Nil.

Product licence numbers
Neophryn Nasal Drops 0071/5069
Neophryn Nasal Spray 0071/5070

PAMETON*

Presentation White, unmarked, capsule-shaped tablets 19.05 mm long and 8 mm wide, with a characteristic odour of methionine. Each tablet contains Paracetamol PhEur 500 mg and D.L-methionine 250 mg.

Uses A mild analgesic and antipyretic suitable for use in most painful and febrile conditions: for example headache, toothache, colds, influenza, rheumatic pain and dysmenorrhoea. This formulation should prove particularly useful where the possibility of misuse or overdosage exists.

Dosage and administration
Adults: Two tablets up to four times a day as required.

Elderly: No specific dosage recommendations.

Children: 6–12 years: Half to one tablet. Children should not be given doses more frequently than every 4 hours and not more than four doses should be given in any 24-hour period. Not suitable for children under 6 years of age.

Contra-indications, warnings, etc Concurrent administration of methionine and levodopa may inhibit the effect of the latter drug.

Because of their methionine content, these tablets should be used with care in patients with severe liver damage.

There is epidemiological evidence of the safety of paracetamol in human pregnancy and methionine is an essential amino acid.

Overdosage: Death from paracetamol overdosage invariably results from hepatic necrosis caused by a reactive metabolite of paracetamol which only becomes toxic when liver glutathione stores are exhausted. Concurrent ingestion of methionine (a precursor of glutathione) in these tablets is designed to help protect the liver against the hepatotoxic effect of excessive amounts of paracetamol. If a patient is seen within 4 hours of ingestion of an overdose of Pameton, the stomach should be emptied by gastric lavage or emesis and, if indicated by blood levels of paracetamol, treatment should be continued with either oral methionine or N-acetyl-cysteine intravenously taking into account the amount of methionine already ingested by the patient.

Pharmaceutical precautions Protect from light.

Legal category P.

Package quantities Cartons of 60 tablets in blisters.

Further information Nil.

Product licence number 0071/0216.

PANADEINE*

Presentation Panadeine Tablets are flat, white tablets with bevelled edges, 12.7 mm in diameter, marked with the product name on one side and scored on the other. Each tablet contains 500 mg Paracetamol PhEur and 8 mg Codeine Phosphate PhEur.

Uses Panadeine Tablets are recommended for the treatment of most painful and febrile conditions such as headache, toothache, colds, influenza, dysmenorrhoea, arthritic and rheumatic pain.

Dosage and administration For oral administration only.

Adults: 2 tablets taken with a draught of water up to four times daily as required.

Elderly: No specific dosage recommendations.

Children: 7–12 years: ½–1 tablet. This dose should not be repeated more frequently than every 4 hours and not more than 4 doses should be given in any 24-hour period.

Under 7 years: Panadeine is not recommended.

Contra-indications, warnings, etc Apart from hypersensitivity to paracetamol or codeine which is rare, there are no contra-indications or special precautions associated with the use of Panadeine. There is epidemiological evidence of the safety of paracetamol in human pregnancy. Codeine has been used for many

years without apparent ill consequences and animal studies have not shown any hazard.

Overdosage: Nausea and vomiting are prominent symptoms of codeine toxicity and there is evidence of circulatory and respiratory depression. Suggested treatment is gastric lavage and catharsis, e.g. sodium sulphate 30 g. If CNS depression is severe, artificial respiration and oxygen may be necessary. Naloxone can be used to combat the depression.

Patients who have taken an overdose of paracetamol may appear well for the first three days, then succumb to liver damage. The hepatic changes produced by overdosage of paracetamol result from the accumulation of a highly active intermediate metabolite in the hepatocytes. N-acetyl-cysteine intravenously, or l-methionine orally protects the liver if administered within 10–12 hours of ingesting an overdose.

Pharmaceutical precautions Panadeine should be stored in well-closed containers protected from light and moisture.

Legal category CD (Sch 5), P.

Package quantities Blister packs of 12, 24 and 48 tablets and bottles containing 100 or 1,000 tablets.

Further information Nil.

Product licence number 0071/5073.

PANADEINE* FORTE

Presentation Red, film-coated, capsule-shaped tablets 17.7 mm long and 7.3 mm wide which contain Paracetamol PhEur 500 mg and Codeine Phosphate PhEur 15 mg.

Uses Panadeine Forte may be used for the relief of moderate pain, such as sciatica, arthritic and rheumatic pain, and headache (including migraine) as well as other conditions for which an antipyretic analgesic is required, including the pains and febrile symptoms of influenza.

Dosage and administration

Adults: Two tablets up to four times a day.

Elderly: No specific dosage recommendations.

Children: Not recommended.

Contra-indications, warnings, etc Apart from hypersensitivity to paracetamol or codeine, which is rare, there are no contra-indications or special precautions associated with the use of Panadeine Forte.

Warnings: Patients should be advised not to drive or operate machinery if affected by dizziness or sedation. The effects of CNS depressants (including alcohol) may be potentiated.

There is inadequate evidence for the safety of codeine in human pregnancy, but there is epidemiological evidence for the safety of paracetamol. Both substances have been used for many years without apparent ill consequences and animal studies have not shown any hazard.

Codeine is an opioid analgesic; tolerance and dependence can occur especially with prolonged high dosage.

Side-effects: Adverse effects to paracetamol are rare. Codeine may cause constipation, nausea, dizziness and drowsiness, according to dosage and individual susceptibility.

Overdosage: Nausea and vomiting are prominent symptoms of codeine toxicity and there is evidence of circulatory and respiratory depression. Suggested treatment is gastric lavage and catharsis. If CNS depression is severe, artificial respiration, oxygen and parenteral naloxone may be needed.

Patients who have taken an overdose of paracetamol may appear well for the first three days, then succumb to liver damage. The hepatic changes produced by overdosage of paracetamol result from the accumulation of a highly reactive intermediate metabolite in the hepatocytes.

N-acetylcysteine intravenously or l-methionine orally protects the liver if administered within 10–12 hours of ingesting an overdose.

Pharmaceutical precautions Nil.

Legal category CD (Sch 5), POM.

Package quantities Cartons of 100 (10 blister packs of ten tablets).

Further information Nil.

Product licence number 0071/0233.

PANADEINE* SOLUBLE

Presentation Flat, white, scored, bevelled-edge tablets which effervesce vigorously when placed in water. Each tablet is 25.4 mm in diameter and contains 500 mg Paracetamol PhEur and 8 mg Codeine Phosphate PhEur.

Uses For quick relief of headache, including migraine, toothache, period pains, sore throat, rheumatic pains and symptoms of cold and influenza.

Dosage and administration
Adults: Two tablets dissolved in a tumblerful of water to be taken up to 4 times a day if required.

Elderly: No specific dosage recommendations, but see 'Warnings'.

Children: 7–12 years: Half to one tablet dissolved in water not more frequently than every 4 hours. No more than 4 doses should be given in any 24-hour period.

Not recommended for children under 7 years of age.

Contra-indications, warnings, etc Apart from hypersensitivity to paracetamol or codeine, which is rare, there are no contra-indications or special precautions associated with the use of Panadeine Soluble.

Warnings: Each tablet contains 425 mg sodium (18.5 m mol). This sodium content should be taken into account when prescribing for patients for whom sodium restriction is indicated.

There is epidemiological evidence of the safety of paracetamol in human pregnancy. Codeine has been used for many years without apparent ill consequences and animal studies have not shown hazard.

Overdosage: Naloxone can be used to counteract central depression due to codeine overdosage. An overdose of paracetamol can cause hepatic necrosis. Patients appear well for the first three days, then succumb to liver damage. The hepatic changes produced by an overdose of paracetamol result from the accumulation of a highly reactive metabolite in the hepatocytes. N-acetylcysteine intravenously or l-methionine orally protects the liver if administered within 10–12 hours of ingesting an overdose.

Pharmaceutical precautions Protect from light and moisture.

Legal category CD (Sch 5), P.

Package quantities Cartons of 12, 24 and 60 tablets in foil strips.

Further information Nil.

Product licence number 0071/0235.

PANADOL*

Presentation Panadol Tablets are flat, white tablets with bevelled edges, 12.7 mm in diameter, marked Panadol on both sides. Each tablet contains 500 mg Paracetamol PhEur.

Panadol Caplets*. Capsule-shaped tablets, 17 mm long and 8 mm wide, marked Panadol on one face, each containing 500 mg Paracetamol PhEur.

Panadol Soluble consists of white, bevelled-edged, unmarked, scored tablets which effervesce vigorously when placed in water. Each is 25.4 mm in diameter and contains 500 mg Paracetamol PhEur.

Panadol Elixir is a clear, yellow, viscous solution with a characteristic odour of passion fruit and containing 120 mg Paracetamol PhEur per 5 ml dose.

Uses Panadol is a mild analgesic and antipyretic. The tablets are recommended for the treatment of most painful and febrile conditions, for example, headache, toothache, colds, influenza, rheumatic pain and dysmenorrhoea.

Panadol Elixir is recommended for the treatment of painful and febrile conditions of childhood such as teething, headache, toothache, earache, general aches and pains. colds, influenza and reactions after immunisation and vaccination.

Dosage and administration For oral administration only. Panadol Soluble should be dissolved in a tumbler of water before taking. Panadol tablets, caplets and Panadol Soluble:

Adults: Two tablets up to 4 times a day, as required.

Elderly: No specific dosage recommendations but see warnings.

Children: 6–12 years: Half to one tablet. For younger children, use Panadol Elixir as follows:

3 months–1 year: Half to one 5 ml spoonful (preferably in milk).

1 year–6 years: One or two 5 ml spoonfuls.

6 years–12 years: Two to four 5 ml spoonfuls. Children should not be given doses of Panadol more frequently than every 4 hours and not more than 4 doses should be given in any 24-hour period.

Contra-indications, warnings, etc Apart from hypersensitivity to paracetamol, which is rare, there are no known contra-indications or precautions associated with the use of Panadol and side-effects are unusual. There is epidemiological evidence of the safety of paracetamol in human pregnancy. Each Panadol Soluble tablet contains 421 mg (18.3 mmol) of sodium. This sodium content should be taken into account when prescribing for patients for whom sodium restriction is indicated.

Overdosage: It should be noted that patients who have taken an overdose of paracetamol may appear well for the first three days then succumb with liver damage. The hepatic changes produced by overdosage of paracetamol result from the accumulation of a highly reactive intermediate metabolite in the hepatocytes. N-acetyl-cysteine intravenously, or l-methionine orally protects the liver if administered within 10–12 hours of ingesting the overdose.

Pharmaceutical precautions Where doses of less than 5 ml are ordered Panadol Elixir may be diluted with Syrup BP so that the standard 5 ml spoonful can be given. Such dilutions will remain stable for two to three weeks. Protect tablets from light and moisture.

Legal category 12, 24 GSL. Other packs P. Panadol Elixir P.

Package quantities *Panadol Tablets:* Blister packs of 12, 24, 48 and 96 tablets and dispensing packs of 500 and 2,500. Special hospital packs of 100.
    Panadol Caplets are supplied in opaque blisters in cartons of 16 and 48.
    Panadol Soluble tablets are packed in PFP laminate strips in cartons of 12, 24 and 60 tablets.
    Panadol Elixir: Bottles containing 60 ml, 100 ml or 1 litre.

Further information Nil.

Product licence numbers
Panadol Tablets and Caplets   0071/5074
Panadol Elixir   0071/5075
Panadol Soluble Tablets   0071/0072

PANASORB*

Presentation Panasorb Tablets are flat, white tablets with bevelled edges, 12.7 mm in diameter, marked Panasorb on both faces. Each tablet contains 500 mg Paracetamol PhEur.

Uses Panasorb Tablets are recommended for the treatment of most painful and febrile conditions, for example, headache (including migraine), toothache, neuralgia, colds, influenza, sore throat, rheumatic pain and dysmenorrhoea.

Dosage and administration For oral administration only.
Adults: 2 tablets up to four times daily.
Elderly: No specific dosage recommendations.
Children: Not suitable for children under 6 years old.
6–12 years: Half to one tablet.
    These doses should not be repeated more frequently than every 4 hours, nor should more than 4 doses be given in any 24-hour period.
    For younger children, it is recommended that Panadol Elixir be used.

Contra-indications, warnings, etc Apart from hypersensitivity to paracetamol, which is rare, there are no known contra-indications or precautions associated with the use of Panasorb and side effects are unusual. There is epidemiological evidence of the safety of paracetamol in pregnancy.
Overdosage: It should be noted that patients who have taken an overdose of paracetamol may appear well for the first three days, then succumb with liver damage. The hepatic changes produced by overdosage of paracetamol result from the accumulation of a highly reactive intermediate metabolite in the hepatocytes. N-acetyl-cysteine intravenously, or l-methionine orally protects

the liver if administered within 10–12 hours of ingesting an overdose.

Pharmaceutical precautions Panasorb should be stored in well-closed containers protected from light and moisture.

Legal category 12s and 24s GSL, 250s and 1,000s P.

Package quantities Panasorb is available in blister packs of 12 or 24 tablets and in bottles of 250 and tins of 1,000 tablets.

Further information Panasorb Tablets are formulated with a special sorbitol-containing base. Average blood levels of paracetamol with Panasorb are higher than those with crushed paracetamol tablets. Because of better absorption in poor paracetamol absorbers relief of symptoms may be more effective.

Product licence number 0071/5076.

PHANODORM*

Presentation Phanodorm Tablets are white, bi-convex tablets, 10.3 mm in diameter, marked with a triangle on one side and plain on the other side. Each tablet contains 200 mg Cyclobarbitone Calcium PhEur.

Uses Phanodorm Tablets are recommended for the treatment of severe, intractable insomnia.

Dosage and administration For oral administration only.
Adults: $\frac{1}{2}$–2 tablets before retiring.
Elderly: Not recommended.
Children: Not recommended.

Contra-indications, warnings, etc
Contra-indications: Barbiturate hypnotics should not be used in children, young adults, the elderly or in patients who are debilitated, or in those who have a history of alcohol or drug abuse. They are also contra-indicated in the presence of uncontrolled pain, pregnancy or breast feeding and porphyria.
Precautions: In patients with renal or hepatic failure, the dose should be reduced. Because barbiturates can increase the activity of hepatic enzymes involved in drug metabolism, the availability and blood concentration of concurrently administered drugs may be altered. Among the compounds known to be affected are coumarin-type anticoagulants, systemic steroids (including oral contraceptives), phenytoin, griseofulvin, rifampicin, phenothiazines and tricyclic antidepressants.
Overdosage: Where patients are seen within four hours of taking an overdose, gastric aspiration or lavage may be beneficial in adults, while children who are conscious may be given an emetic (e.g., Ipecacuanha Emetic Mixture Paediatric BP).
    The prime objective in treating barbiturate overdosage is to maintain vital functions (respiration, cardiovascular and renal function and electrolyte balance) while the majority of the drug is metabolised by hepatic enzymes. At the same time some of the drug is excreted unchanged by the kidneys. Given normal renal function, this latter process may be enhanced by alkaline diuresis, maintaining the urinary pH at about 8 by appropriate intravenous infusion. In severe cases, haemodialysis may help, but extracorporeal haemoperfusion is probably more effective.

Side Effects: Drowsiness, sedation, unsteadiness, vertigo and inco-ordination may occur. During the first week of administration, performance and alertness may be impaired; patients should be warned not to drive or operate machinery if affected. These effects may be potentiated by alcohol. Other adverse reactions may include a 'hangover' effect, paradoxical excitement, confusion, memory defects and skin rashes in patients who may be sensitive to this type of drug.

Pharmaceutical precautions Nil.

Legal category CD (Sch 3) POM.

Package quantities Phanodorm is available in bottles of 50 tablets.

Further information Barbiturates have a high addiction potential. Long-term use or use of high doses for short periods may lead to tolerance and subsequently to physical and psychological dependence. Symptoms of dependence include confusion, defective judgement and loss of emotional control. Withdrawal symptoms occur after long-term normal use (and particularly after abuse) if barbiturate treatment is stopped abruptly. These include nightmares, irritability and insomnia and, in severe cases, tremors, delirium, convulsions and death. Withdrawal symptoms have been reported in neonates after barbiturate treatment during pregnancy and labour.

Product licence number 0071/5077.

pHiso-MED*

Presentation A white solution which forms suds when added to water. It contains 21.1% w/w Chlorhexidine Gluconate Solution BP (equivalent to 4% w/w chlorhexidine gluconate) and 2% Benzyl Alcohol BP as preservative.

Uses 1. Pre-operative preparation of surgeons' and nurses' hands and the skin of patients.
2. As an antiseptic skin cleanser for routine hand washing and for spots and acne on the face, shoulders and chest.
3. For use in maternity units by nurses and mothers, and for bathing babies, as a measure to prevent cross-infection.

Dosage and administration 1. *Pre-operative hand preparation:* Wet the hands and forearms, apply about 5 ml of solution and wash for one minute. Thoroughly clean finger-nails with a brush or scraper. Rinse, and repeat the wash for two minutes. Rinse thoroughly and dry. 2. *Preparation of patients for elective surgery:* Using a sterile swab, the solution is rubbed over the site and surrounding skin for two minutes, adding a little sterile water to work up a lather. Wipe off and dry thoroughly with fresh sterile swabs. Subsequently, at the time of operation, a 0.5% solution of chlorhexidine in alcohol should be applied to the site with sterile gauze swabs. The site and the surrounding skin should be rubbed vigorously for two minutes and until dry. 3. *As an antiseptic skin cleanser:* Wet the area to be cleaned, apply 5 ml of solution and wash for one minute. Rinse thoroughly and dry. 4. *For bathing infants in maternity unit:* A 1 in 10 dilution of the solution is applied over the baby's body with a swab or with the palm of the hand. Rinse thoroughly with warm water and dry in the usual way.

Contra-indications, warnings, etc Chlorhexidine should not be allowed to come into contact with the brain, meninges or middle ear. During use, ensure that the solution is kept away from the eyes and ears. Material which has been in contact with the solution may be stained brown by hypochlorite bleaches.

Overdosage: If the solution is swallowed, it should be removed from the stomach by gastric lavage and symptomatic treatment applied as necessary.

Pharmaceutical precautions Protect from heat and light.

Legal category GSL.

Package quantities Containers of 150 ml.

Further information Nil.

Product licence number 0071/0178.

PROMINAL*

Presentation Prominal Tablets 30 mg are white, bi-convex tablets, 6.4 mm in diameter, marked P30 on one side and plain on the other. Each tablet contains 30 mg Methylphenobarbitone PhEur.

Prominal Tablets 60 mg are white, biconvex tablets, 8 mm in diameter, marked P60 on one side and plain on the other. Each tablet contains 60 mg Methylphenobarbitone PhEur.

Prominal Tablets 200 mg are white, bi-convex tablets, 10.3 mm diameter, marked P200 on one side and plain on the other. Each tablet contains 200 mg Methylphenobarbitone PhEur.

Uses Prominal Tablets are recommended for the treatment of epilepsy.

Dosage and administration *Adults:* The daily dosages, which must be fixed individually, range from 100 to 600 mg, the average being 200–400 mg.

Elderly: No specific dosage recommendations but see Precautions.

Children: 5–15 mg/kg/day.

Contra-indications, warnings, etc
Contra-indications: Acute intermittent porphyria and patients who are hypersensitive or who exhibit idiosyncrasy to barbiturates.

Precautions: The possibility of tolerance or dependence developing should be considered. Abrupt cessation of treatment may give rise to withdrawal symptoms. Use with caution in senile or debilitated patients. Large doses should not be given to those with renal or liver damage. In severe pulmonary insufficiency, even normal therapeutic doses may depress respiration. Barbiturates may potentiate the central depressant effect of alcohol and affect the action of a number of other drugs.

Anticonvulsant drugs are as useful to an epileptic during pregnancy as they are at other times and for the individual epileptic mother the chance of an abnormal baby due to drug treatment is small. However, a number of reports have appeared in the literature suggesting possible implication of the epileptic state, anticonvulsants and folic acid deficiency as causative agents in certain congenital abnormalities. Scientific knowledge does not yet permit an adequate definition to be made of the respective roles of these three factors. It is recommended, therefore, that if anticonvulsants are judged necessary during pregnancy, adequate folic acid supplements should be given and the epilepsy controlled as completely as possible.

Overdosage: Where patients are seen within four hours of taking an overdose, gastric aspiration or lavage may be beneficial in adults, while children who are conscious may be given an emetic (e.g., Ipecacuanha Emetic Mixture Paediatric BP).

The prime objective in treating methylbarbitone overdosage is to maintain vital function (respiration, cardiovascular and renal function, and electrolyte balance) while the majority of the drug is metabolised by hepatic enzymes. At the same time some of the drug is excreted unchanged by the kidneys. Given normal renal function, this latter process may be enhanced by alkaline diuresis, maintaining the urinary pH at about 8 by appropriate intravenous infusion. In severe cases, haemodialysis may help, but extracorporeal haemoperfusion is probably more effective.

Side Effects: Drowsiness, sedation unsteadiness, vertigo and inco-ordination may occur. During the first week of administration, performance and alertness may be impaired; patients should be warned not to drive or operate machinery if affected. These effects may be potentiated by alcohol. Other adverse reactions may include a 'hangover' effect, paradoxical excitement, confusion, memory defects and skin rashes in patients who may be sensitive to this type of drug.

Pharmaceutical precautions Nil.

Legal category CD (Sch 3) POM.

Package quantities Prominal Tablets (30 mg, 60 mg and 200 mg) are supplied in bottles of 100.

Further information Nil.

Product licence numbers
Prominal Tablets 30 mg	0071/5084
Prominal Tablets 60 mg	0071/5085
Prominal Tablets 200 mg	0071/5086

PYROGASTRONE*

Presentation White, round, strawberry-flavoured chewable tablets. 22.2 mm in diameter, marked with a symbol on one side and PG on the other. Each tablet contains:

Dried Aluminium Hydroxide PhEur	240 mg
Magnesium Trisilicate PhEur	60 mg
Carbenoxolone Sodium PhEur	20 mg

in a base containing 210 mg Sodium Bicarbonate BP and 600 mg Alginic Acid BPC.

Uses For the treatment of oesophageal inflammation, erosions and ulcers due to hiatus hernia or other conditions causing gastric reflux and for the relief of heartburn, flatulence and other symptoms associated with reflux oesophagitis.

Dosage and administration For oral administration only.
Adults: 1 tablet to be chewed three times daily immediately after meals and 2 tablets to be chewed at bedtime.

Treatment should be continued for at least six weeks, but up to 12 weeks treatment may be necessary to ensure maximum healing effect.

Elderly: No specific dosage recommendations but see warnings.

Children: Not recommended.

Contra-indications, warnings, etc Pyrogastrone should not be prescribed for patients suffering from severe cardiac, renal or hepatic failure. Nor should it be prescribed for patients on digitalis glycosides unless serum electolyte levels are monitored at weekly intervals to detect promptly the development of hypokalaemia. Each tablet contains 59.2 mg (2.6 mmol) Sodium.

Special care should be exercised with patients predisposed to sodium and water retention, potassium loss and hypertension (e.g. the elderly and those with cardiac, renal and hepatic disease) since the carbenoxolone content of Pyrogastrone can induce similar changes. Potassium supplements should be considered for those at risk from developing hypokalaemia.

Regular monitoring of weight and blood pressure which should indicate the development of such effects is advisable for all patients. A thiazide diuretic should be administered if oedema or hypertension occurs (spironolactone or amiloride should not be used because they hinder the therapeutic action of carbenoxolone). Potassium loss should be corrected by the administration of oral supplements.

No teratogenic effects have been reported with carbenoxolone sodium, but careful consideration should be given before prescribing Pyrogastrone for women who may become pregnant.

Overdosage: If the tablets have been recently ingested, the stomach should be emptied by gastric lavage. Serum electolytes should be monitored and any deficiency in potassium should be corrected, using the intravenous route if necessary or slow-release or effervescent tablets of potassium chloride. Water retention and sodium balance should be corrected by means of a diuretic. (Spironolactone or amiloride would appear to be a logical choice).

Pharmaceutical precautions Store in a dry place.

Legal category POM.

Package quantities Boxes containing 25 foil strips of 4 tablets.

Further information The alginate antacid base of Pyrogastrone tablets forms a clinging viscous foam which has buffering capacity. This relieves symptoms, either by coating the oesophageal wall, by impeding oesophageal reflux, or the foam may reflux instead of the acid gastric contents. The incorporation of carbenoxolone into the formulation has been shown to exert an additional healing effect on oesophageal ulcers possibly by improving mucus synthesis and/or by increasing the life-span of oesophageal epithelium.

Although Pyrogastrone quickly relieves symptoms, treatment should be continued for at least six weeks, but up to 12 weeks' treatment may be necessary to ensure a maximum healing effect.

Made under licence from Biorex Laboratories, England. Brit. Pat. No. 1390683.

Product licence number 0071/0138.

PYROGASTRONE* LIQUID

Presentation Bottles containing a white powder for the preparation of 500 ml of suspension. When prepared as instructed, each 10 ml contains Carbenoxolone Sodium PhEur 20 mg and Dried Aluminium Hydroxide PhEur 300 mg in a vehicle with sodium alginate and potassium bicarbonate.

Uses For the treatment of oesophageal inflammatory erosions and ulcers due to hiatus hernia or other conditions causing gastric reflux and for the relief of heartburn, flatulence and other symptoms associated with reflux oesophagitis.

Dosage and administration
Adults: 10 ml to be taken three times daily immediately after meals and 20 ml at bedtime.

Treatment should be continued for at least six weeks, but up to 12 week's treatment may be necessary to ensure maximum healing effect.

Elderly: No specific dosage recommendations but see warnings.

Children: Not recommended.

Contra-indications, warnings, etc Pyrogastrone Liquid should not be prescribed for patients suffering from severe cardiac, renal or hepatic failure. Nor should it be prescribed for patients on digitalis glycosides unless serum electrolyte levels are monitored at weekly intervals to detect promptly the development of hypokalaemia. It should be noted however that, unlike Pyrogastrone tablets, each 10 ml of Pyrogastrone liquid provides 117 mg (3.0 mmol) potassium. Sodium content is 38.8 (1.7 mmol) per 10 ml dose.

Special care should be exercised with patients predisposed to sodium and water retention, potassium loss and hypertension (e.g. the elderly and those with cardiac, renal or hepatic disease) since carbenoxolone can induce similar changes.

Regular monitoring of weight and blood pressure which should indicate the development of such effects is advisable in all patients. A thiazide diuretic should be administered if oedema or hypertension occurs (spironolactone or amiloride should not be used because they hinder the therapeutic action of carbenoxolone.) If potassium loss occurs it may be corrected by the administration of oral supplements.

No teratogenic effects have been reported with carbenoxolone sodium, but careful consideration should be given before prescribing Pyrogastrone Liquid for women who may become pregnant.

Overdosage: If recently ingested the stomach should be emptied by gastric lavage. Serum electrolytes should be monitored and any deficiency in potassium should be corrected using the intravenous route if necessary or slow-release or effervescent tablets of potassium chloride. Water retention and sodium balance should be corrected by means of a diuretic. (Spironolactone or amiloride would appear to be a logical choice.)

Pharmaceutical precautions Nil.

Legal category POM.

Package quantities Bottles containing sufficient powder to prepare 500 ml Pyrogastrone Liquid.

Further information In contact with the acid stomach contents, the alginate antacid base of Pyrogastrone Liquid forms a clinging viscous foam with buffering capacity. This relieves symptoms, either by coating the oesophageal wall, by impeding oesophageal reflux, or the foam may reflux instead of the acid gastric contents. The incorporation of carbenoxolone into the formulation has been shown to exert an additional healing effect on oesophageal ulcers possibly by improving mucus synthesis and/or by increasing the life-span of oesophageal epithelium.

Although Pyrogastrone quickly relieves symptoms, treatment should be continued for at least six weeks, but up to 12 weeks' treatment may be necessary to ensure a maximum healing effect.

Carbohydrate content: Pyrogastrone Liquid contains 10% sucrose.

Made under licence from Biorex Laboratories, England.

Product licence number 0071/0236.

RESONIUM* A

Presentation Resonium A is ground and flavoured sodium polystyrene sulphonate. It is a buff-coloured powder with a pleasant vanilla odour and sweet taste.

Uses Resonium A is an ion-exchange resin which is recommended for the treatment of hyperkalaemia associated with anuria or severe oliguria. It is also used to treat hyperkalaemia in patients requiring dialysis and in patients on regular haemodialysis or on prolonged peritoneal dialysis.

Dosage and administration Resonium A is for oral or rectal administration only. The dosage recommendations detailed in this section are a guide only, the precise requirements should be decided on the basis of regular serum electrolyte determinations.

Adults:
1. *Oral:* Usual dose 15 g three or four times a day. The resin is given by mouth in a little water, or it may be made into a paste with some sweetened vehicle.
2. *Rectal:* In cases where vomiting may make oral administration difficult, the resin may be given rectally as a suspension of 30 g resin in 100 ml 2% Methylcellulose 450 BP (medium viscosity) and 100 ml water, as a daily retention enema. In the initial stages administration by this route as well as orally may help to achieve a more rapid lowering of the serum potassium level.

The enema should if possible be retained for at least nine hours. If both routes are used initially it is probably unnecessary to continue rectal administration once the oral resin has reached the rectum.

Elderly: No specific dosage recommendations.

Children: 1 g/kg body weight daily in divided doses in acute hyperkalaemia. Dosage may be reduced to 0.5 g/kg body weight in divided doses for maintenance therapy.

The resin is given orally, preferably with a drink or a little jam or honey. When refused by mouth it should be given rectally using a dose at least as great as that which would have been given orally, diluted in the same ratio as described for adults.

Contra-indications, warnings, etc The possibility of potassium depletion should be considered and adequate biochemical control is essential during treatment. Administration of the resin should be stopped when the serum potassium level falls to 5 mmol/litre. In children particular care is needed with rectal administration as excessive dosage or inadequate dilution could result in impaction of the resin.

Overdosage: In the event of overdosage the resin should be removed from the alimentary tract by the use of laxatives or enemas and appropriate measures taken to restore serum potassium levels to normal.

In patients with severe renal damage the sodium ions liberated by Resonium A may lead to sodium overloading and congestive heart failure. In such cases Calcium

Resonium (calcium polystyrene sulphonate) may be used in place of Resonium A.

Pharmaceutical precautions It is suggested that Resonium A should not be administered in fruit squashes since these have a high potassium content.

Legal category P.

Package quantities Lever-lid tins containing 454 g Resonium A together with a plastic scoop which, when filled level, contains 15 g.

Further information Nil.

Product licence number 0071/5087.

ROCCAL* ANTISEPTIC
ROCCAL* CONCENTRATE 10X

Presentation Roccal Antiseptic and Roccal Concentrate 10X are clear blue solutions containing 1% or 10% benzalkonium chloride respectively. The solutions foam when shaken, have a characteristic antiseptic odour and are miscible with water in all proportions.

Uses Roccal is recommended for use as an antiseptic in wound cleansing (including cuts, bites and abrasions), for sterilisation of dressings, breast and nipple shield hygiene, vaginal douching and as a bladder washout. It may also be used as a skin antiseptic and as a general disinfectant.

Dosage and administration Roccal is for topical use only. Appropriate dilutions for the recommended uses are shown in the table on the next page.

Roccal Concentrate 10% is intended for the preparation of Roccal Antiseptic only, by diluting 1 in 10 with water.

Contra-indications, warnings, etc Roccal should not be mixed with strong soap solution or with antiseptics containing soap such as solutions of chloroxylenol, lysol, the black and white fluids or with products containing anionic detergents such as pHiso-MED.

Roccal appears to be relatively non-irritant to skin and mucous membranes. Although benzalkonium chloride may be used as a preservative for eye drops Roccal is not recommended for use in the eyes because of the additives it contains. The presence of benzalkonium chloride in a urine sample may give rise to a false-positive result in tests for protein.

Accidental ingestion: The oral toxic dose of benzalkonium chloride is estimated to be between 1 and 3 g. The main signs of poisoning are vomiting, collapse and coma. Roccal acts primarily as a local irritant on the throat, oesophagus and gastro-intestinal tract. Toxic doses lead to restlessness, apprehension, dyspnoea, cyanosis, convulsions, muscle weakness and death due to paralysis of respiratory muscles.

Treatment consists of giving milk, egg whites or even a mild soap solution by mouth, followed by emesis or gastric lavage with a weak soap solution. Respiration should be supported by oxygen or artificial respiration if necessary.

Convulsions should be treated by short-acting barbiturates or intravenous diazepam.

Pharmaceutical precautions The potency of a 10% solution of benzalkonium chloride is unchanged even after 10 years of storage. Roccal may be boiled or autoclaved without loss of bactericidal activity as shown

Use	Concentration of benzalkonium chloride	Dilution of Roccal
Bladder washout	1:5,000 to 1:20,000	1:50 to 1:200
Breast and nipple shield hygiene etc.	1:1,000 to 1:2,000	1:10 to 1:20
Dressings	1:4,000	1:40
General disinfectant	1:1,000 to 1:8,000	1:10 to 1:80
Skin disinfectant	1:1,000 to 1:2,000	1:10 to 1:20
Vaginal douching	1:2,000 to 1:5,000	1:20 to 1:50
Wound cleansing including cuts, bites and abrasions	1:1,000 to 1:5,000	1:10 to 1:50

by phenol coefficient determinations. The efficacy of solutions of Roccal is not affected by freezing and subsequent thawing.

Dilutions of Roccal should not be prepared with tap water due to possible interference by certain cations such as calcium, magnesium, iron and aluminium.

Roccal 1:10 (benzalkonium chloride 1:1,000) is compatible with the following substances:

Acriflavine	Oil of sassafras 1.5–2.5%
Adrenaline	Oxytetracycline
Alcohol	Penicillin
Amethocaine HCl	Phenol
Benzocaine	Phenylephrine HCl
Boroglycerin	Pilocarpine (2% solution
Camphor	or less)
Carbachol	Polyethylene glycol
Chlorbutol 1:5,000	Procaine HCl
Cocaine	Resorcin (cloudy when
Cresol	mixed)
Eosin	Rose water
Ephedrine HCl	Scopolamine
Eserine sulphate (not	Sodium bicarb. and
salicylate salt)	phosphate
Formaldehyde 1%	Sodium carbonate and
Fuchsin	sodium nitrate
Glycerin 5–15%	Sulphadiazine sodium
Homatropine 5%	Sulphanilamide
Hydrazine hydrate 0.1–	Trisodium phosphate
0.5%	Urea
Lime water	Urethane
Mercurial salts 1%	Zinc chloride (up to and
Methylene blue	including 1%)
Methylparaben	
Natural rubber	

But incompatible with these substances:

Aluminium	Pilocarpine nitrate (3% or
Benzylephedrine	more)
Boric acid 5%	Pine oil
Caramel	Potassium iodine
Citric acid	Potassium permanganate
Ethylparaben	Saponin 0.1–0.5%
Fluorescein sodium	Silicates
Hydrogen peroxide	Silver salts
Iodine	Sodium citrate and tartrate
Kaolin	Sodium lauryl sulphate
Lanolin	Sulphapyridine
Mild silver proteinate	Sulphathiazole
Physostigmine	Sulphathiazole sodium

Synthetic rubber (some)	Zinc oxide
Tartaric acid	Zinc peroxide
Yellow oxide of mercury	Zinc sulphate

Legal category GSL.

Package quantities Roccal Antiseptic is supplied in clear plastic bottles containing 250 ml or 500 ml, or in translucent plastic bottles containing 2.25 litres.

Roccal Concentrate 10X is supplied in translucent plastic bottles containing 2.25 litres.

Further information Nil.

Product licence numbers
Roccal Antiseptic   0071/5088
Roccal Concentrate   0071/5089

SEOMINAL*

Presentation Seominal Tablets are pale yellow. biconvex tablets, 10.3 mm in diameter, marked III on one side and scored on the other. Each tablet contains 10 mg Phenobarbitone PhEur, 325 mg Theobromine PhEur and 200 mg Reserpine PhEur.

Uses Seominal Tablets are recommended for the treatment of mild to moderate essential hypertension.

Dosage and administration *Adults:* The average initial dosage of Seominal is 1 tablet twice daily, or for the more severe cases, three times daily, but the possibility of excessive sedation must be borne in mind. This dosage is continued until improvement has been maintained for some time.

Thereafter the daily dosage may be reduced to 1 tablet. Some patients may even dispense with the drug for a time.

It must be emphasised that, because of the slow onset of hypotensive action, no improvement in blood pressure readings may be observed for a month or so, although a tranquillising effect may be apparent within a few days. Thereafter Seominal should be continued for some weeks in full dosages.

Children: Not recommended.

Contra-indications, warnings, etc

Contra-indications: Seominal should not be used for patients with anxiety, depression or confusional states or in those with peptic ulceration, ulcerative colitis, Parkinson's disease, phaeochromocytoma, cardiac arrhythmia, myocardial infarction or renal failure. It should not be given with MAO inhibitors. It may cause severe hypotension in patients who have recently suffered strokes. It is also contra-indicated in acute intermittent porphyria, in those who are hypersensitive or exhibit an idiosyncrasy to barbiturates and during pregnancy and lactation.

Precautions: Some patients exhibit idiosyncrasy to barbiturates, and such individuals' response to these compounds is likely to be restlessness and excitement even in the absence of pain. Skin reactions are the most common type of allergic manifestation. Barbiturates should be used with caution in debilitated or senile patients. Large doses should not be given to patients with renal impairment or with diseases of the liver. In severe pulmonary insufficiency, even normal doses of barbiturates may depress respiration.

The possibility of tolerance or dependence developing should be considered. Abrupt cessation of treatment in these circumstances may give rise to withdrawal symptoms. Barbiturates may potentiate the central depressant effect of alcohol and affect the action of a number of other drugs, by hepatic enzyme induction including coumarin type anticoagulants, systemic steroids (including oral contraceptives), phenytoin, griseofulvin, rifampicin, phenothiazines and tricylic antidepressants.

Caution is advised in patients with a history of depression and in those taking digitalis or quinidine.

Overdosage: There have been no reports of overdosage with Seominal. Symptoms of acute toxicity would probably be those caused by the individual ingredients. Theobromine could cause gastro-intestinal disturbances, haemorrhage, insomnia, tremor and convulsions. An overdosage of reserpine may produce diarrhoea, dizziness, fatigue, headache, nasal stuffiness, flushing, hypotension and bradycardia or tachycardia, Parkinsonism, convulsions, etc. Diphenhydramine may be used for the Parkinsonism and noradrenaline or dopamine for the hypotension.

Where patients are seen within four hours of taking an overdose, gastric aspiration or lavage may be beneficial in adults, while children who are conscious may be given an emetic (e.g., Ipecacuanha Emetic Mixture Paediatric BP).

The prime objective in treating phenobarbitone overdosage is to maintain vital functions (respiration, cardiovascular and renal function, and electrolyte balance) while the majority of the drug is metabolised by hepatic enzymes. At the same time some of the drug is excreted unchanged by the kidneys. Given normal renal function, this latter process may be enhanced by alkaline diuresis, maintaining the urinary pH at about 8 by appropriate intravenous infusion. In severe cases, haemodialysis may help, but extracorporeal haemoperfusion is probably more effective.

Diuresis will not hasten the excretion of theobromine or reserpine. Measures may be required to correct the hypotensive effect of reserpine. Supportive measures, including the head-down position, the intravenous infusion of plasma expanders and the administration of a vasopressor agent such as noradrenaline or dopamine may be indicated.

Side-effects: Minor reactions include excessive sedation, headache, dizziness, nasal stuffiness, dry mouth, nausea, diarrhoea or cutaneous eruptions. Lowering the dose or halting medication for a short time generally results in their disappearance. Mental depression is the most serious side-effect associated with reserpine. If depressive symptoms develop during treatment with Seominal the drug must be stopped, and if the depression does not resolve within a few days psychiatric advice should be sought.

Pharmaceutical precautions Nil.

Legal category CD (Sch 3) POM.

Package quantities Seominal is available in bottles of 100 or 500 tablets.

Further information Nil.

Product licence number 0071/5090

SULFAMYLON* CREAM

Presentation Sulfamylon Cream is a smooth, white to pale yellow, water-miscible cream with a slight acetous odour and containing 8.5% w/w mafenide as the acetate, with methyl and propyl hydroxybenzoates, sodium metabisulphite and disodium edetate as preservatives.

Uses Sulfamylon Cream is recommended for the prophylaxis and treatment of infection, particularly that due to Pseudomonas species in second and third degree burns.

Dosage and administration Sulfamylon Cream is for topical use only.

Adults: Sulfamylon Cream should be applied to a thickness of 1–2 mm (a layer sufficient to prevent seeing the burn surface), once or twice daily with a sterile gloved hand. Any covering lost owing to a change of body linen or a shift of position should be replaced by further applications. In the first 24 hours of the post-burn period the wound is moist and exudative and may require more frequent applications. Dressings are not usually required, but if necessary a thin layer of gauze may be used.

The length of treatment will depend on the rate of separation of the eschar and the appearance of the granulating surface necessary for skin grafting. Duration of treatment may vary from five days to three to four weeks.

Elderly: No specific dosage recommendations.

Children: The product should be applied according to the recommendations for adults.

Contra-indications, warnings, etc
Contra-indications: Sulfamylon Cream should not be used if the patient has a known sensitivity to mafenide or any other sulphonamide. It is not known if there is cross-sensitivity to other sulphonamides.

Precautions: Sulfamylon and its ρ-carboxybenzene-sulphonamide metabolite are absorbed systemically. In the presence of impaired renal function, high blood levels may result which may exaggerate carbonic anhydrase inhibition. Close monitoring of the acid-base balance is therefore necessary, particularly in patients with extensive burns. If persistent acidosis occurs, treatment should be suspended for 24–48 hours, when continuous fluid therapy will usually restore acid-base balance.

Fungal colonisation in and below the eschar may occur concomitantly with reduction of bacterial growth in the burn wound. However, fungal dissemination through the infected burn wound is rare.

Sulfamylon should be avoided in pregnancy unless its use is judged to be strictly necessary. Occasionally application of the cream may be accompanied by pain or a burning sensation severe enough to require an analgesic or sedation. Allergic manifestations, such as maculopapular rash, oedema, erythema and eosinophila, also occur in a small portion of patients.

Warnings: An unexplained syndrome of marked hyperventilation with resulting respiratory alkalosis has occasionally been reported.

Pharmaceutical precautions Store in cool, not refrigerated conditions, and protect from light. The cream has an estimated shelf-life of 12 months. The normal precautions involved in aseptic dressing should be observed to prevent contamination. It is recommended that each patient should have an individual jar of cream and any cream remaining after 24 hours should be discarded.

Legal category POM.

Package quantities Black plastic jars each containing 500 g.

Further information Nil.

Product licence number 0071/5093.

SULFOMYL*

Presentation Sulfomyl is a clear, colourless solution in a dropper-bottle presentation. The solution contains 5% w/v mafenide propionate with phenylmercuric acetate 0.002% and not more than 0.4% chlorbutol as preservatives.

Uses Sulfomyl is recommended for the treatment of superficial eye infections.

Dosage and administration *Adults: First-aid for minor eye injuries:* 3 or 4 drops are instilled into the injured eye.

Established infection: 3 or 4 drops are instilled into the eye three or four times a day.

Children: The adult dosage recommendations may be followed for children.

Contra-indications, warnings, etc Although no instances of allergy or irritation have been reported with Sulfomyl Eye Drops, they should not be used in patients known to be sensitive to other sulphonamides.

Pharmaceutical precautions Nil.

Legal category P.

Package quantities Polythene drop bottles each containing 10 ml.

Further information Nil.

Product licence number 0071/5094.

TRANCOPAL

Presentation Trancopal tablets are flat, yellow tablets with bevelled edges 9.5 mm in diameter, marked with a symbol on one side and plain on the reverse. Each tablet contains 200 mg chlormezanone.

Uses Trancopal tablets are recommended for the short-term treatment of insomnia. They are also recommended for the symptomatic treatment of anxiety states where muscle tension is prominent and as an adjunct to the treatment of acute musculo-skeletal disorders associated with painful muscle spasm.

Dosage and administration For oral administration only.

Adults: Sleep disturbances: usually 400 mg at night.

States of anxiety and skeletal muscle tension: usually 200 mg repeated up to 3 or 4 times daily or a single dose of 400 mg at night.

Elderly: Half the normal adult dose or less may be sufficient for a therapeutic response in the elderly.

Children: Not recommended.

Contra-indications, warnings, etc Trancopal tablets are contra-indicated in patients sensitive to chlormezanone. There is insufficient evidence of safety of chlormezanone in human pregnancy but it has been in use for many years without apparent ill consequences; animal studies have not shown hazard. However, do not use during pregnancy, especially the first trimester, unless there are compelling reasons.

Trancopal at high doses may modify the patient's reactions (performance at skilled tasks, alertness, etc.) to a varying extent, depending on individual susceptibility. Therefore, patients should be advised not to drive or operate machinery during treatment, if affected. If Trancopal is administered with CNS depressants, it is possible that their sedative effect may be intensified. As with other drugs acting on the central nervous system, patients should avoid alcohol while receiving Trancopal since the response cannot be predicted.

Trancopal should be given with caution to patients with hepatic or renal insufficiency.

Overdosage: The signs and symptoms of overdosage with chlormezanone resemble those seen with other central depressant drugs, for example, somnolence, prostration, muscular incoordination and memory disturbances. In severe cases, there may be hypotension, respiratory depression and loss of consciousness.

Symptomatic treatment should follow gastric lavage.

Side effects: Drowsiness and dizziness have been the commonest side effects, particularly at higher doses. Other reported side effects include nausea, lightheadedness, headache, lethargy and dryness of the mouth. Very rarely, cholestatic jaundice has been reported in patients who have taken chlormezanone. Slight skin reactions of the urticaria or erythematous type can occur. Cases of fixed drug rash and various forms of exudative erythema multiforme have been reported; these are very uncommon but in certain cases can be serious.

The dependence potential of chlormezanone is not known.

Pharmaceutical precautions Nil.

Legal category POM.

Package quantities Trancopal tablets are available in bottles of 60.

Further information Nil.

Product licence number 0071/5098.

TRANCOPRIN*

Presentation White, flat, bevelled-edge tablets 11 mm in diameter, marked with a 'T' on one face and scored on the other. Each tablet contains Aspirin BP 300 mg and chlormezanone 100 mg.

Uses For the treatment of painful conditions where the combination of an analgesic and a mild tranquilliser/muscle relaxant would be of value. Such conditions include musculoskeletal disorders associated with muscle spasm, headache and painful menstrual disorders.

Dosage and administration Trancoprin tablets are for oral administration only. The usual adult dose is 1 or 2 tablets three times a day. Not more than 8 tablets should be taken daily. There are no specific recommendations for children. Half the adult dose or less may be sufficient for a therapeutic response in the elderly.

Contra-indications, warnings, etc Trancoprin tablets should not be given to patients with a known hypersensitivity to chlormezanone or aspirin (including those with haemophilia and similar coagulation disor-

ders). They should not be taken by patients with a history of peptic ulcer because aspirin may induce (occasionally major) intestinal haemorrhage and it should be given with caution to patients with hepatic or renal insufficiency. Chlormezanone in high doses may modify the patient's reactions (performance of skilled tasks, alertness, etc.) to a varying extent, depending upon individual susceptibility. Therefore, patients should be advised not to drive or operate machinery during treatment if affected. If Trancoprin is administered with CNS depressants, it is possible that their sedative effect may be intensified. As with other drugs acting on the central nervous system, patients should avoid alcohol while receiving Trancoprin since the response cannot be predicted.

There is clinical and epidemiological evidence of the safety of aspirin in human pregnancy. There is insufficient evidence of safety of chlormezanone in pregnancy but it has been used for many years without apparent ill consequences. Animal studies have not shown hazard. However, do not use during pregnancy, especially the first trimester unless there are compelling reasons. Because aspirin may prolong labour and contribute to maternal and neonatal bleeding, the use of Trancoprin is best avoided at term. Aspirin may enhance the effect of anticoagulants and inhibit the action of uricosuric agents. Because it may precipitate bronchospasm, it may induce attacks of asthma in susceptible subjects.

Overdosage: Should be treated by gastric lavage (if the product has been recently ingested) together with the usual measures taken for salicylate toxicity. There are likely to be additional symptoms due to the excessive amount of chlormezanone absorbed, such as somnolence, depression and prostration. There may also be muscular incoordination, blurred vision, weakness and memory disturbances. In severe cases, hypotension, respiratory depression and loss of consciousness may occur. Symptomatic treatment is suggested for chlormezanone overdosage.

Side-effects: Adverse effects have been infrequent with Trancoprin. As would be expected with chlormezanone, a compound having mild tranquillising properties, drowsiness and dizziness have been the commonest.

There have also been occasional reports of constipation, flushing, dry mouth, nausea and weakness. Very rarely reversible cholestatic jaundice has been reported in patients who have taken chlormezanone. Slight skin reactions of the urticaria or erythematous type can occur. Cases of fixed drug rash and various forms of exudative erythema multiforme have been reported; these are very uncommon but in certain cases can be serious.

The dependence potential of chlormezanone is not known.

Pharmaceutical precautions Trancoprin tablets should be kept in well-closed containers protected from moisture.

Legal category POM.

Package quantities Amber glass bottles, each containing 100 tablets.

Further information Nil.

Product licence number 0071/0093.

Trade Mark

Wyeth Laboratories
Huntercombe Lane South
Taplow
Maidenhead, Berks

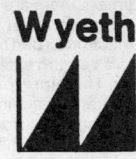

ALUDROX*

Presentation Aludrox consists of Aluminium Hydroxide Mixture BP containing the equivalent of 3.5–4.4% w/w Al_2O_3 presented as a white gel with the odour and flavour of peppermint.

Uses Aludrox is an antacid preparation indicated for the relief of hyperacidity, particularly that associated with peptic ulceration and dyspepsia. It may also be prescribed in the treatment of hyperphosphataemia.

Dosage and administration *Route of administration:* Oral.

Dosage – Adults: For antacid use:

One to two 5 ml doses either four times daily between meals and on retiring or as required.

In hyperphosphataemia: Larger doses may be given according to the requirements of the patient.

Elderly: The adult dosage schedule can be used in the elderly.

Children: Not recommended in infancy. Otherwise in childhood, proportional to adult dosage for 70 kg adult.

Contra-indications, warnings, etc
Contra-indications: The aluminium ion combines with phosphate to form an insoluble complex which is not absorbed, and when high doses are given together with a low phosphorus diet phosphate depletion occurs. This regime is used in the treatment of phosphate calculi and hyperphosphataemia associated with chronic renal failure. Phosphate depletion does not occur in patients on a normal diet. Aludrox is contra-indicated in patients with hypophosphataemia.

Precautions:
1. Aluminium hydroxide may form a complex with tetracyclines and reduce their absorption when given concomitantly.
2. Aluminium hydroxide may reduce absorption of digoxin.

Side-effects: Few side effects are to be expected. In some patients constipation may develop, but this is easily overcome by the administration of a suitable laxative preparation or by the joint administration of magnesium hydroxide.

Pharmaceutical precautions Store in a cool place. Where necessary dispense Aludrox into suitable well-closed glass or polythene bottles.

Legal category GSL.

Package quantities *Polythene bottles of 200 ml, 500 ml and 2 litres.*

Further information There is no evidence to suggest that Aludrox should not be given to breast-feeding mothers.

Product licence number 0011/5000

ALUDROX* TABLETS

Presentation Aludrox tablets are round, white, flat, bevelled edge tablets, 12.6 mm in diameter, one face marked WYETH and the other face plain. Each tablet contains:

Aluminium hydroxide, magnesium carbonate Co-dried gel 282 mg
Magnesium hydroxide BP 85 mg

Uses Aludrox tablets are an antacid preparation indicated for the relief of hyperacidity, particularly that associated with peptic ulceration and dyspepsia. Magnesium hydroxide is included to avoid development of constipation.

Dosage and administration *Route of administration:* Oral.

Dosage: Adults: One to two tablets either four times daily between meals and on retiring or as required. The tablets should be chewed before swallowing.

Elderly: The adult dosage schedule can be used in the elderly.

Children: Not recommended in infancy. Otherwise in childhood, proportional to adult dosage for 70 kg adult.

Contra-indications, warnings, etc
Contra-indications: The aluminium ion combines with phosphate to form an insoluble complex which is not absorbed, and when high doses are given together with a low phosphorus diet phosphate depletion occurs. Phosphate depletion does not occur in patients on a normal diet. Aludrox tablets are contra-indicated in patients with hypophosphataemia and patients on dialysis or with renal failure.

Precautions: 1. Aluminium hydroxide may form a complex with tetracyclines and reduce their absorption when given concomitantly.
2. Aluminium hydroxide may reduce absorption of digoxin.

Side-effects: Few side-effects are to be expected at the recommended dosage.

Pharmaceutical precautions Nil.

Legal category GSL.

Package quantities Blister packs of 60.

Further information There is no evidence to suggest

that Aludrox tablets should not be given to breast-feeding mothers.

Product licence number 0011/0090.

APISATE*

Presentation Apisate tablets are two-layer tablets of 11.0 mm diameter. Both layers are yellow, the lighter coloured face is marked WYETH, the other face is plain. Each tablet contains:

Diethylpropion hydrochloride (in a sustained action formulation)	75 mg
Thiamine Hydrochloride BP	5 mg
Riboflavine BP	4 mg
Pyridoxine Hydrochloride BP	2 mg
Nicotinamide BP	30 mg

Uses Apisate, containing diethylpropion hydrochloride, in a sustained action formulation, with a supplement of B-complex vitamins, is designed to give anorectic activity throughout the waking hours.

Apisate is suitable for short term use as an adjunct to the treatment of patients with moderate to severe obesity for whom close support and dietary supervision are also provided.

Dosage and administration *Route of administration:* Oral.

Dosage – Adults: Dosage depends on eating habits. Most patients require only one tablet a day, taken early morning or mid-afternoon. Some patients however, may require 2 tablets; one at each of these two times.

Elderly: Not recommended for the elderly.

Children: Not recommended for children.

Current medical opinion supports intermittent use of appetite suppressants. Apisate may be given for 4–8 weeks followed by a similar period without medication. This may reduce the risk of dependence. The stated dose should not be exceeded. Efficacy if used for more than 3–6 months, and safety in long-term use have not been established. Apisate should be discontinued if weight loss does not occur, or when patients stop losing weight.

Contra-indications, warnings, etc
Contra-indications:

1. Use in emotionally unstable individuals, including psychotics, who are known to be susceptible to alcohol or drug abuse.

2. Use in patients concomitantly treated with MAOIs or within two weeks of such treatment.

3. Use of diethylpropion is also contra-indicated in patients with advanced arteriosclerosis, hyperthyroidism, severe hypertension, glaucoma or idiosyncrasy to sympathomimetic amines.

4. Concurrent use with other appetite suppressant drugs.

Precautions: 1. Prolonged use of diethylpropion may induce dependence with a withdrawal syndrome on cessation of therapy. Several cases of toxic psychoses have been reported after excessive use of diethylpropion and a very small number have been reported in which the recommended dosage appears not to have been exceeded. The psychosis was temporary and cleared up when the drug was discontinued.

Since its introduction in 1958, diethylpropion has been used by at least 33,000,000 patients. Against this background of extensive clinical use, reports of abuse have been very rare. Most of the subjects who abused diethylpropion had previously misused other drugs, e.g. amphetamine or phenmetrazine, and many were described as having unstable personalities.

2. Diethylpropion should be used with caution in patients with hypertension, angina pectoris, cardiac arrhythmias and peptic ulceration. Caution should also be observed in patients with epilepsy, anxiety or tension states or severe depression.

3. Diethylpropion may interact with sympathomimetic agents. Care should be taken when treating hypertensive patients receiving anti-hypertensive drugs. Animal experiments suggest that anti-obesity agents can block or reverse the actions of such agents when taken together. Diethylpropion should not be given concurrently with psychotropic drugs, including sedatives.

4. Apisate should not be administered during pregnancy or lactation unless in the judgement of the physician such administration is clinically justifiable. Special care should be taken in the first three months of pregnancy.

5. Patients should be warned against driving or operating machinery until it is established that they are not over-stimulated while taking Apisate.

Side-effects: Diethylpropion has negligible effect on blood pressure, pulse rate or cardiac activity. Side-effects are infrequent and rarely severe enough to require discontinuation of treatment. They include sleeplessness, restlessness, increased nervousness, euphoria, agitation, palpitations, depression, psychosis, hallucinations, dependence, nausea, vomiting, dry mouth, headache, tachycardia, constipation and allergic rashes. Gynaecomastia has been reported rarely.

Overdosage: A few unsuccessful suicide attempts by deliberate overdosage of diethylpropion hydrochloride have been reported in adults. Dosage ranged from 450 to 2,250 mg. Transient sequelae included semi-coma or coma, lethargy, increased irritability and nausea.

A number of cases of accidental overdosage have been reported in children aged 6 months to $3\frac{1}{2}$ years. Known doses taken were from 50 to 1,100 mg. The most frequent effects were motor hyperactivity, excitability, tachycardia, rapid respiration, pupillary dilatation, and flushing.

Treatment of overdosage is initially by gastric lavage and close observation. The foregoing reports show that individual reactions may differ and further treatment will be symptomatic.

Recovery occurred in all patients with overdosage except one, in whom treatment with a large intravenous dose of sodium amobarbital was implicated.

Pharmaceutical precautions Store in a cool dry place, keep tightly closed. Where necessary dispense into suitable, well-closed glass bottles.

Legal category CD (Sch 3), POM.

Package quantities Bottles of 100.

Further information Diethylpropion, including illegally manufactured tablets have been the subject of social abuse for euphoriant effect.

Product licence number 0011/5004.

ATIVAN* TABLETS

Presentation Ativan tablets are capsule shaped containing 1 mg or 2.5 mg lorazepam BP, and are approximately 4 × 8 mm. The 1 mg tablets are blue with A1 on one side and a breakbar on the other. The 2.5 mg tablets are yellow with A2.5 on one side and a breakbar on the other.

Uses Ativan is indicated for the following: mild, moderate and severe anxiety states, phobic or obsessional states, moderate to severe tension states, anxiety in psychosomatic, organic or psychotic illness, short term treatment of insomnia associated with anxiety, premedication before operative dentistry and as a sedative for the anxious dental patient, premedication before general surgery.

Dosage and administration Route of administration: Oral.

Dosage: Adults: Mild anxiety – 1–4 mg daily in divided doses.

Moderate/severe anxiety – up to 8 mg daily in divided doses.

Severe anxiety, phobic or obsessional/compulsive state – up to 10 mg daily.

Insomnia – 1–4 mg before retiring.

Premedication – 2–3 mg the night before operation, 2–4 mg one to two hours before operation.

Elderly: The elderly may respond to lower doses and half the normal adult dose or less may be sufficient.

Children: Premedication – aged 5–13 years, 0.5–2.5 mg at 0.05 mg/kg to the nearest 0.5 mg according to weight, not less than one hour before operation.

Dentistry: 1–2.5 mg, 1½–2 hours before dental treatment. For operative dentistry dosage as for premedication.

Contra-indications, warnings, etc
Contra-indication: Ativan should not be given to patients with a previous history of sensitivity to benzodiazepines or patients with acute pulmonary insufficiency.

Use in pregnancy: Ativan tablets should not be administered during pregnancy or lactation unless in the judgement of the physician such administration is clinically justifiable. Special care should be taken in the first three months of pregnancy.

Precautions and warnings: 1. Concomitant administration with central nervous system depressants, including alcohol, general anaesthetics, narcotic analgesics, monoamine oxidase inhibitors and antidepressants will result in an accentuation of their effects.

2. Prolonged or excessive use of benzodiazepines may occasionally result in the development of some psychological dependence with withdrawal symptoms on sudden discontinuation. This is more likely in patients with a history of alcoholism, drug abuse or in patients with marked personality disorders.

Treatment in all patients should be withdrawn gradually. Careful monitoring of all patients is essential.

3. As with other drugs acting on the central nervous system, patients should be cautioned against driving or operating machinery until it is established that they do not become dizzy or drowsy while taking lorazepam.

4. This product should be used with caution in patients with impairment of renal or hepatic function.

5. Elderly patients or those suffering from cerebral vascular changes such as arteriosclerosis are likely to respond to smaller doses.

6. Ativan should be used with caution during labour. Respiratory depression, poor sucking and hypothermia in the neonate have occasionally been reported especially in patients who are at high risk.

7. Ativan does not depress respiration in most patients but the drug should be used with caution in patients with chronic pulmonary insufficiency.

8. The use of benzodiazepines may release suicidal tendencies in depressed patients. Other rarely reported behavioural effects of the benzodiazepines include paradoxical aggressive outbursts, excitement and confusion.

Overdosage: As with other benzodiazepines, overdosage should not present a threat to life. General supportive measures should be used. Treatment is symptomatic and gastric lavage may be of use if performed shortly after ingestion. If the patient is conscious, an emetic such as ipecacuanha may be given. The patient is likely to sleep and a clear airway should be maintained.

Side-effects: Ativan is well tolerated and imbalance or ataxia is an indication of excessive dosage. Daytime drowsiness may be seen initially and is to be anticipated in the effective treatment of anxiety. It will normally diminish rapidly and may be minimised in the early days of treatment by giving the larger proportion of the day's dose before retiring.

Occasional confusion, hangover, headache on waking, dizziness, blurred vision and nausea have been reported.

On rare occasions visual disturbances, hypotension, gastrointestinal disturbances and mild, transient skin rashes have also been reported.

Pharmaceutical precautions Store in a cool dry place.

Legal category CD (Sch 4), POM.

Package quantities 1 mg and 2.5 mg tablets: boxes of 100 (5 × 20 blister strips) and containers of 1000.

Further information Ativan is a short acting benzodiazepine. It is rapidly absorbed from the gastro-intestinal tract and is metabolised by a simple one-step process to a pharmacologically inactive glucuronide. The elimination half-life of Ativan is about 12 hours so that steady state plasma levels are quickly reached and there is minimal risk of excessive accumulation, giving a wide margin of safety.

Product licence numbers
Tablets 1 mg   0011/0034R
Tablets 2.5 mg   0011/0036R

ATIVAN* INJECTION ▼

Presentation Ativan injection is a clear, colourless solution containing Lorazepam BP at a concentration of 4 mg/ml supplied in 1 ml quantities in clear glass ampoules.

Uses Ativan injection is indicated for:

Pre-operative medication or premedication for uncomfortable or prolonged investigations, e.g. bronchoscopy, arteriography, endoscopy.

The treatment of acute anxiety states, acute excitement or acute mania. The control of status epilepticus.

Dosage and administration *Route of administration:* Ativan injection can be given intravenously or intramuscularly. However, the intravenous route is to be preferred. Care should be taken to avoid injection into small veins and intra-arterial injection.

Absorption from the injection site is considerably slower if the intramuscular route is used and as rapid an effect may be obtained by oral administration of Ativan tablets.

Preparation of the injection: Ativan injection is slightly viscid when cool. To facilitate injection it may be diluted 1:1 with normal Saline or Water for Injections BP immediately before administration. If given intramuscularly it should always be diluted.

Ativan injection is presented as a 1 ml solution in a 2 ml ampoule to facilitate dilution.

Ativan injection should not be mixed with other drugs in the same syringe.

Dosage:
1. *Premedication: Adults:* 0.05 mg/kg (3.5 mg for an average 70 kg man). By the intravenous route the injection should be given 30–45 minutes before surgery when sedation will be evident after 5–10 minutes and maximal loss of recall will occur after 30–45 minutes. By the intramuscular route the injection should be given 1– $1\frac{1}{2}$ hours before surgery when sedation will be evident after 30–45 minutes and maximal loss of recall will occur after 60–90 minutes.
Children: Ativan injection is not recommended in children under 12.
2. *Anxiety: Adults:* 0.025–0.03 mg/kg (1.75–2.1 mg for an average 70 kg man). Repeat 6 hourly.
Children: Ativan injection is not recommended in children under 12.
3. *Status epilepticus: Adults:* 4 mg intravenously. *Children:* 2 mg intravenously.
Elderly: The elderly may respond to lower doses and half the normal adult dose may be sufficient.

Contra-indications, warnings, etc
Contra-indications:
1. Ativan injection should not be given to patients with a previous history of sensitivity to the benzodiazepines.
2. Ativan injection is not recommended for outpatient use unless the patient is accompanied.

Precautions and warnings:
1. Patients should remain under observation for at least eight hours and preferably overnight.
2. Patients should not drive or operate machinery within 24 hours of administration of Ativan injection and should be advised not to take alcohol.
3. The effects of centrally acting cerebral depressant drugs may be potentiated.
4. This product should be used with caution in patients with impairment of renal or hepatic function.
5. The injection should be given slowly except in the control of status epilepticus where rapid injection is required.
6. Elderly patients may require a lower dosage.
7. Ativan injection should not be administered during pregnancy or lactation unless in the judgement of the physician such administration is clinically justifiable. Special care should be taken in the first three months of pregnancy.
Overdosage: As with other benzodiazepines, overdosage should not present a threat to life. General supportive measures should be used and the treatment of overdosage is symptomatic. The patient is likely to sleep and a clear airway should be maintained.

Side-effects: Ativan injection is well tolerated and imbalance or ataxia are signs of excessive dosage. Drowsiness may be an initial effect and is to be anticipated in the effective treatment of anxiety. It will normally diminish as treatment continues. Occasional confusion, hangover, headache on waking, drowsiness or dizziness, blurred vision and nausea have also been reported.

Pharmaceutical precautions Store in a refrigerator between 0°C and 4°C. Protect from light.

Legal category CD (Sch 4), POM.

Package quantities 10 × 1 ml solution (in 2 ml ampoules) per pack.

Further information As with other benzodiazepines, Ativan crosses the placental barrier and foetal concentration will be the same as that in the mother. Ativan will be present in the milk of nursing mothers, but as with other benzodiazepines this is not significant if the mother is receiving Ativan injection within the recommended doses.

Ativan is metabolised by a simple one-step process to a pharmacologically inactive glucuronide. There is minimal risk of accumulation after repeated doses, giving a wide margin of safety. Ativan injection can be administered concurrently with a wide range of other drugs and has minimal effect on blood pressure and respiration. Tolerance at the injection site is good.

Product licence number 0011/0051.

BARATOL* ▼

Presentation Baratol tablets are round, convex, film coated tablets containing indoramin hydrochloride equivalent to 25 or 50 mg indoramin base. The 25 mg tablets are blue, 8.00 mm in diameter and marked WYETH on one face and '25' on the other. The 50 mg tablets are green, 9.5 mm in diameter, marked WYETH on one face and '50' on the other face which is also scored.

Uses *Actions:* Baratol is an alpha adrenoceptor blocking agent which acts selectively and competitively on post-synaptic alpha-1 receptors, causing a decrease in peripheral resistance.

Indications: Baratol tablets are indicated for the treatment of all grades of essential hypertension.

Dosage and administration
Adults: Initial dose: 25 mg twice daily for all patients.

Dose titration: The dosage of Baratol should be titrated as necessary to control blood pressure to a maximum of 200 mg daily in two or three divided doses. The daily dosage may be increased by the progressive addition of 25 mg or 50 mg, made at intervals of two weeks. When unequal doses are used, the largest dose should be given at night in order to avoid daytime sedation.

Elderly: Clearance of indoramin may be affected in the elderly. A reduced dose and/or reduced frequency of dosing may be sufficient for effective control of blood pressure in some elderly patients.

Combination with other anti-hypertensive agents: Baratol is effective in lowering blood pressure in all grades of hypertension, either used alone or when combined with other anti-hypertensive agents. The anti-hypertensive effect of Baratol is enhanced by concomitant administration of a thiazide diuretic or a beta-adrenoceptor blocking drug. Control of most cases of mild and moderate hypertension should be achieved by using Baratol alone or by adding Baratol to the regimen of a patient already under treatment with a thiazide diuretic. In severe hypertension, a combination of Baratol, a thiazide diuretic and a beta-adrenoceptor blocking drug is effective in many such patients.

When Baratol is used in combination with other antihypertensive agents, the dose of Baratol should be titrated in the same way as when it is used alone.

Contra-indications, warnings, etc

Contra-indications: Baratol tablets should not be prescribed for:

1. Patients with established heart failure.
2. Patients already under treatment with MAOIs.

Precautions and warnings:

1. Drowsiness is sometimes seen in the initial stages of treatment with Baratol or when dosage is increased too rapidly. Patients should be warned not to drive or operate machinery until it is established that they do not become drowsy while taking Baratol.
2. Incipient cardiac failure should be controlled with diuretics and digitalis before treatment with Baratol.
3. Caution should be observed in prescribing Baratol for patients with hepatic or renal insufficiency.
4. A few cases of extrapyramidal disorders have been reported in patients treated with Baratol. Caution should be observed in prescribing Baratol in patients with Parkinson's disease.
5. In animals and in the one reported case of overdose in humans, convulsions have occurred. Due consideration should be given and great caution exercised in the use of Baratol in patients with epilepsy.
6. Caution should be observed in prescribing Baratol for patients with a history of depression.
7. Animal experiments indicate no teratogenic effects but Baratol tablets should not be prescribed for pregnant women unless considered essential by the physician.
8. There is no data available on the excretion of Baratol in human milk but the drug should not be administered during lactation unless in the judgement of the physician such administration is clinically justifiable.
9. Clearance of indoramin may be affected in the elderly. A reduced dose, and/or reduced frequency of dosing may be sufficient for effective control of blood pressure in some elderly patients.

Side-effects: Sedation occurs in some patients but is rarely intolerable and is usually overcome by a modest reduction in dosage. Less commonly, dry mouth, nasal congestion, weight gain, dizziness, failure of ejaculation and depression have also been noted.

Treatment of overdosage: The information available at present of the effects of acute overdosage in humans with Baratol is limited to one case. Effects seen in this case included deep sedation leading to coma, hypotension and fits. Results of animal work suggest that hypothermia may also occur.

Suggested therapy is along the following lines:

1. Recent ingestion of large numbers of tablets would require gastric lavage or a dose of ipecacuanha to remove any of the product still in the stomach of the conscious patient.
2. Ventilation should be monitored and assisted if necessary.
3. Circulatory support and control of hypotension should be maintained.
4. If convulsions occur diazepam may be tried.
5. Temperature should be closely monitored. If hypothermia occurs, rewarming should be carried out very slowly to avoid possible convulsions.

Legal category POM.

Pharmaceutical precautions Store below 25°C and protect from light.

Package quantities Bottles of 100.

Further information Baratol may be especially suitable for patients for whom beta-adrenoceptor blockade is contra-indicated, for example, in patients with a history of obstructive airways disease.

Reflex tachycardia is not associated with treatment with Baratol.

Postural hypotension is not a problem.

In one study, patients on Baratol who were treated with a tricyclic antidepressant showed no adverse effect on their blood pressure control.

Baratol has been used concomitantly with cardiac glycosides and other anti-hypertensive drugs with no interaction.

Rebound hypertension has not been observed after withdrawal of Baratol.

Selective alpha-1-blockade has been shown to be useful in the treatment of congestive heart failure. As yet, there is insufficient data to determine whether Baratol can also be indicated in this disorder.

Product licence numbers
25 mg tablets   0011/0071
50 mg tablets   0011/0058

EQUAGESIC*

Presentation Equagesic Tablets are three layer, flat bevel-edged tablets, 12.0 mm in diameter. A white layer is sandwiched between a yellow layer and a pink layer. The yellow face is marked WYETH and the pink face is plain. Each tablet contains:

Ethoheptazine citrate	75 mg
Meprobamate BP	150 mg
Aspirin BP	250 mg

Uses Equagesic is an analgesic with muscle-relaxant properties indicated for short-term symptomatic treatment of pain occurring in musculo-skeletal disorders.

Dosage and administration Route of administration: Oral.

Dosage – Adults: 2 tablets three or four times daily as needed for the relief of pain.

Elderly: The elderly may respond to lower doses and half the normal adult dose or less may be sufficient.

Children: Not recommended for children.

Contra-indications, warnings, etc

Contra-indications:

1. Equagesic should not be used in patients known to be hypersensitive to the active ingredients or to compounds related to meprobamate such as carisoprodol or carbromal.
2. Meprobamate should not be used in patients with a known propensity for dependence on drugs including alcohol and in patients susceptible to attacks of acute intermittent porphyria.
3. Aspirin should not be used in patients with active peptic ulceration, haemophilia or in renal disease.
4. Equagesic should not be used during lactation.
5. Equagesic should not be used concurrently with coumarin-type anticoagulants.
6. *Pregnancy:* There is no evidence as to drug safety in human pregnancy nor is there evidence that it is free from hazard. Do not use during pregnancy, especially

during the first three months, unless there are compelling reasons.

Precautions and warnings:

1. This product may cause drowsiness. Patients receiving this medication should not drive or operate machinery unless the drug has been shown not to interfere with physical or mental ability.

2. Meprobamate may increase the effects of concurrently administered central nervous system depressants including alcohol.

3. The concurrent use of CNS depressant drugs should be avoided in hepatic or renal insufficiency.

4. Meprobamate may induce seizures in epileptic patients and meprobamate withdrawal may precipitate convulsions.

5. Like barbiturates, meprobamate causes induction of liver enzymes, so that the availability and blood levels of drugs given concurrently that are metabolised in the liver may be affected. These include the following: systemic steroids (including oral contraceptives), phenytoin, griseofulvin, rifampicin, phenothiazines (such as chlorpromazine) and tricyclic antidepressants. The clinical importance of the effect of enzyme induction by meprobamate on concurrently administered agents has not been established.

6. Individual response in overdosage with meprobamate is variable but in some cases the symptoms may be severe. It is therefore advisable that caution should be observed in prescribing drugs which contain meprobamate to patients with depression or to others who may be liable to suicidal ideation or intent.

7. Some degree of dependence may occasionally occur with meprobamate in certain cases if dosage recommendations are exceeded with withdrawal symptoms on sudden discontinuation. This is more likely in individuals with emotionally unstable personalities if the drug is taken over long periods, or in others liable to alcohol or other drug dependence. Treatment in these cases should be withdrawn gradually.

Equagesic is recommended for use for short periods only and therefore the risk of dependence occurring with this product is very small.

Aspirin: 8. (a) Aspirin may prolong labour and contribute to maternal and neonatal bleeding and is best avoided at term. It may precipitate bronchospasm and may induce attacks of asthma in susceptible subjects. Aspirin should only be used with great caution in patients with a history of peptic ulceration.

(b) Concomitant administration with certain other medications such as corticosteroids or oral hypoglycaemics may require adjustment of dosage of the various drugs. The action of uricosuric agents may be inhibited.

Overdosage: Meprobamate: Acute poisoning with meprobamate produces coma, shock, vasomotor and respiratory collapse. Very few suicide attempts have proved successful and documented fatal doses have ranged from 12 gm to 47.6 gm. Recovery has occurred after ingestion of similar large amounts (20–40 gm). Gastric lavage is only effective within a short period of drug ingestion as meprobamate is rapidly absorbed from the gastrointestinal tract. Blood concentrations may be reduced by a regime of forced alkaline diuresis or haemodialysis. Respiration may require assistance.

Aspirin: Overdosage with aspirin will result in the appearance of the signs and symptoms of salicylism. Treatment of aspirin poisoning is largely symptomatic and directed towards correction of the acid-base balance and electrolyte balance of the plasma.

Side-effects: Drowsiness, dizziness and nausea may be experienced with Equagesic but these symptoms usually disappear as treatment continues. Ataxia, vomiting, hypotension, paraesthesia and paradoxical excitement may also occur.

Hypersensitivity reactions have been reported in about 2% of patients being treated with meprobamate. These reactions include skin rashes, and may arise after one to four doses of the drug. They may be generalised or local, and include urticaria, itchy maculopapular rashes or erythema. Severe systemic reactions with shaking, chills and fever, nausea and vomiting, hypotension and collapse have occasionally occurred.

Blood disorders, including non-thrombocytopenic purpura, and rarely, thrombocytopenia, agranulocytosis, aplastic anaemia and pancytopenia have occurred. Rarely reported reactions, usually occurring as part of a generalised hypersensitivity reaction, include hyperpyrexia, angioneurotic oedema, bronchospasm, oliguria and anuria. Anaphylaxis, erythema multiforme, exfoliative dermatitis, stomatitis, proctitis, Stevens Johnson syndrome and bullous dermatitis have also been reported.

Hypersensitivity reactions to aspirin may manifest themselves as asthma, skin reactions and shock. Aspirin may induce gastro-intestinal haemorrhage, which is occasionally severe but in most cases blood loss is not significant.

Pharmaceutical precautions Store in a cool dry place. Keep tightly closed. Where necessary dispense Equagesic Tablets into suitable well-closed glass bottles.

Legal category CD (Sch 3), POM.

Package quantities Bottles of 100.

Further information Safety and efficacy have not been established beyond short-term use.

Product licence number 0011/5009R.

LORAMET* ▼

Presentation Loramet capsules are orange No. 4 liquid filled soft gelatin capsules containing 1 mg lormetazepam printed with WYETH on one side and 1 on the reverse side in black lettering.

Uses Loramet is indicated for the short term treatment of insomnia, including difficulty in falling asleep and/or frequent nocturnal awakenings.

Dosage and administration

Route of administration: oral.

Dosage: Adults: 1–2 mg before retiring.

Elderly: Usually 0.5 mg but if 1 mg is required this formulation may be used.

Children: Loramet has not been evaluated for the treatment of children.

Contra-indications, warnings, etc

Contra-indications: 1. Sensitivity to benzodiazepines.
2. Myasthenia gravis.

Precautions and warnings: 1. Concomitant administration with central nervous system depressants, including alcohol, general anaesthetics, narcotic analgesics, monoamine oxidase inhibitors and antidepressants may result in an accentuation of their effects.

2. Prolonged or excessive use of benzodiazepines may occasionally result in the development of some psychological dependence with withdrawal symptoms

on sudden discontinuation. This is more likely in patients with a history of alcoholism, drug abuse or in patients with marked personality disorders. Treatment in these cases should be withdrawn gradually. Careful usage seldom results in the development of dependence.

3. As with other drugs acting on the central nervous system, patients should be cautioned against driving or operating machinery until it is established that they do not become dizzy or drowsy while taking lormetazepam.

4. Loramet capsules should not be administered during pregnancy unless in the judgement of the physician such administration is clinically justifiable. Special care should be taken in the first three months of pregnancy.

5. Patients suffering from cerebral vascular changes such as arteriosclerosis are likely to respond to smaller doses.

Side-effects: Loramet is generally well tolerated. However, in occasional sensitive patients, or because of overdosage, headaches, drowsiness, dizziness and nausea may occur on the following morning.

Rare behavioural adverse effects of benzodiazepines include paradoxical aggressive outbursts, excitement, confusion, and the uncovering of depression with suicidal tendencies. Even more rarely hypotension, gastrointestinal and visual disturbances, skin rashes, urinary retention, changes in libido, blood dyscrasias, and jaundice have been reported with some benzodiazepines. They have not been reported with Loramet.

Overdosage: As with other benzodiazepines, overdosage should not present a threat to life. General supportive measures should be used. Treatment is symptomatic and gastric lavage may be of use if performed shortly after ingestion. If the patient is conscious, an emetic such as ipecacuanha may be given. The patient is likely to sleep and a clear airway should be maintained.

Pharmaceutical precautions Store in a cool dry place.

Legal category CD (Sch 4), POM.

Package quantities 1 mg capsules are supplied in glass bottles of 100.

Further information Loramet is rapidly absorbed from the liquid-filled soft gelatin capsules and peak plasma levels are usually reached in about 60 minutes. Loramet has a terminal phase half life of about 11 hours. Loramet is principally metabolised by a simple one-step process to a pharmacologically inert glucuronide. There are no major active metabolites and little risk of accumulation. Clinical studies have shown minimal effects on REM sleep and on psychomotor performance on the day after treatment with Loramet.

Product licence number 1 mg capsules 0011/0088.

LORAZEPAM TABLETS

Presentation Lorazepam tablets are capsule shaped containing 1 mg or 2.5 mg Lorazepam BP, and are approximately 4 × 8 mm. The 1 mg tablets are blue with WYETH on one side and WY breakbar 19 on the other. The 2.5 mg tablets are yellow with WYETH on one side and WY breakbar 20 on the other.

Uses Lorazepam is indicated for the following: Mild, moderate and severe anxiety states, phobic or obses-

sional states, moderate to severe tension states, anxiety in psychosomatic, organic or psychotic illness, short term treatment of insomnia associated with anxiety, premedication before operative dentistry and as a sedative for the anxious dental patient, premedication before general surgery.

Dosage and administration
Route of administration: Oral.

Dosage: Adults: Mild anxiety – 1–4 mg daily in divided doses.

Moderate/severe anxiety – up to 8 mg daily in divided doses.

Severe anxiety, phobic or obsessional/compulsive state – up to 10 mg daily.

Insomnia – 1–4 mg before retiring.

Premedication – 2–3 mg the night before operation; 2–4 mg one to two hours before operation.

Elderly: The elderly may respond to lower doses and half the normal adult dose or less may be sufficient.

Children: Premedication – aged 5–13 years, 0.5–2.5 mg at 0.05 mg/kg to the nearest 0.5 mg according to weight, not less than one hour before operation.

Dentistry: 1–2.5 mg, 1½–2 hours before dental treatment. For operative dentistry dosage as for premedication.

Contra-indications, warnings, etc
Contra-indications: Lorazepam should not be given to patients with a previous history of sensitivity to benzodiazepines or patients with acute pulmonary insufficiency.

Use in pregnancy: Lorazepam tablets should not be administered during pregnancy or lactation unless in the judgment of the physician such administration is clinically justifiable. Special care should be taken in the first three months of pregnancy.

Precautions and warnings:

1. Concomitant administration with central nervous system depressants, including alcohol, general anaesthetics, narcotic analgesics, monoamine oxidase inhibitors and antidepressants will result in an accentuation of their effects.

2. Prolonged or excessive use of benzodiazepines may occasionally result in the development of some psychological dependence with withdrawal symptoms on sudden discontinuation. This is more likely in patients with a history of alcoholism, drug abuse or in patients with marked personality disorders.

Treatment in all patients should be withdrawn gradually. Careful monitoring of all patients is essential.

3. As with other drugs acting on the central nervous system, patients should be cautioned against driving or operating machinery until it is established that they do not become dizzy or drowsy while taking Lorazepam tablets.

4. This product should be used with caution in patients with impairment of renal or hepatic function.

5. Elderly patients or those suffering from cerebral vascular changes such as arteriosclerosis are likely to respond to smaller doses.

6. Lorazepam tablets should be used with caution during labour. Respiratory depression, poor sucking and hypothermia in the neonate have occasionally been reported especially in patients who are at high risk.

7. Lorazepam does not depress respiration in most patients but the drug should be used with caution in patients with chronic pulmonary insufficiency.

8. The use of benzodiazepines may release suicidal

tendencies in depressed patients. Other rarely reported behavioural effects of the benzodiazepines include paradoxical aggressive outbursts, excitement and confusion.

Overdosage: As with other benzodiazepines, overdosage should not present a threat to life. General supportive measures should be used. Treatment is symptomatic and gastric lavage may be of use if performed shortly after ingestion. If the patient is conscious, an emetic such as ipecacuanha may be given. The patient is likely to sleep and a clear airway should be maintained.

Side-effects: Lorazepam is well tolerated and imbalance or ataxia is an indication of excessive dosage. Daytime drowsiness may be seen initially and is to be anticipated in the effective treatment of anxiety. It will normally diminish rapidly and may be minimised in the early days of treatment by giving the larger proportion of the day's dose before retiring.

Occasional confusion, hangover, headache on waking, dizziness, blurred vision and nausea have been reported. On rare occasions visual disturbances, hypotension, gastro-intestinal disturbances and mild, transient skin rashes have also been reported.

Pharmaceutical precautions Store in a cool dry place.

Legal category CD (Sch 4), POM.

Package quantities 1 mg and 2.5 mg tablets: boxes of 100 (5 × 20 blister strips) and containers of 1000.

Further information Lorazepam is a short-acting benzodiazepine. It is rapidly absorbed from the gastrointestinal tract and is metabolised by a simple one-step process to a pharmacologically inactive glucuronide. The elimination half-life of Lorazepam is about 12 hours so that steady state plasma levels are quickly reached and there is minimal risk of excessive accumulation, giving a wide margin of safety.

Product licence numbers
Tablets 1 mg   0011/0108
Tablets 2.5 mg   0011/0109

MEPTID* INJECTION ▼

Presentation Meptid injection is a clear solution, containing meptazinol hydrochloride at a concentration equivalent to 100 mg meptazinol base per ml, supplied in 1 ml quantities in clear glass ampoules.

Uses Meptid injection is indicated for the treatment of moderate to severe pain, including post-operative pain, obstetric pain and the pain of renal colic.

Dosage and administration *Adults: Intramuscular dosage:* 75–100 mg Meptid. The injection may be repeated 2–4 hourly as required. For obstetric pain a dose of 100–150 mg should be used according to weight. This dose should approximate 2 mg/kg.

Intravenous dosage: 50–100 mg Meptid by slow intravenous injection. The injection may be repeated 2–4 hourly as required. If vomiting occurs, a suitable antiemetic should be given.

Epidural/Intrathecal use: This formulation is *not* suitable for these routes.

Elderly: The adult dosage schedule can be used in the elderly.

Children: Meptid Injection has not been evaluated for use in children.

Contra-indications, warnings, etc
Contra-indications: None known.

Precautions:
1. Caution should be observed in treating patients with hepatic or renal insufficiency.
2. Clinical studies have indicated absence of clinically significant respiratory depression but caution should be exercised in patients already severely compromised.
3. Safety for use in myocardial infarction has not been established.
4. Meptid injection is a useful analgesic in labour but in accordance with general medical principles it should not be given in other stages of pregnancy unless considered essential by the physician. There is no evidence from animal reproductive studies to anticipate a teratogenic risk.

Treatment of overdosage: Overdosage with Meptid injection has not been reported. Large doses, including seven times the recommended therapeutic dose, have been given in balanced and total intravenous anaesthesia, without significant respiratory depressant effects.

In the event of cardiovascular and respiratory collapse, normal resuscitative procedures should be employed. Respiratory depression caused by overdosage with meptazinol may be reversed in part with therapeutic doses of Naloxone.

Side-effects: No serious adverse reactions have been reported after treatment with Meptid injection. Dizziness, nausea and vomiting have been noted in some cases.

Pharmaceutical precautions Store below 25°C.

Meptid injection should *not* be mixed with other drugs in the same infusion solution or in the same syringe. Meptid injection is an acidic solution of the hydrochloride salt of meptazinol and is therefore pharmaceutically incompatible with injection solutions known to be strongly basic (for example thiopentone) as precipitation of the meptazinol base may occur.

Meptid at concentrations of 200 mg in 500 ml and 500 mg in 500 ml has been shown to be compatible with the following intravenous infusion fluids when added immediately prior to use:

Dextrose 5% w/v
Dextrose 10% w/v
Sodium chloride 0.9% w/v
Ringers solution
Hartmanns solution
Sodium chloride 0.9% w/v and dextrose 5% w/v

If Meptid is administered through an intravenous cannula, it is essential to flush the system with saline before and after administration.

Legal category POM.

Package quantities Cartons of 10 ampoules.

Further information Meptid injection at a dose of 100 mg has equivalent analgesic potency to 15 mg morphine or 100 mg pethidine. Meptid has little sedative effect. Because treatment with Meptid is not associated with clinically significant respiratory depression, it is particularly useful for post-operative pain reducing the risk of chest complications.

Product licence number 0011/0046.

MEPTID* TABLETS ▼

Presentation Meptid tablets are oval orange film coated tablets marked WYETH on one side, 14.5 mm in length and containing 200 mg meptazinol.

Uses Meptid tablets are indicated for the short term treatment of moderate pain, including the pain associated with rheumatoid and osteo-arthritis, post-traumatic pain, dysmenorrhoea, post-operative pain and musculoskeletal pain.

Dosage and administration *Route of administration:* oral.

Dosage – Adults: 200 mg 3–6 hourly as required. Usually one tablet four hourly.

Elderly: The adult dosage schedule should be used in the elderly.

Children: Meptid tablets have not been evaluated for use in children.

Contra-indications, warnings, etc

Contra-indications: None known.

Precautions:

1. Caution should be observed in treating patients with hepatic or renal insufficiency.

2. Clinical studies have indicated absence of clinically significant respiratory depression but caution should be exercised in patients already severely compromised.

3. In accordance with general medical principles Meptid tablets should not be given to pregnant or lactating women unless considered essential by the physician. There is no evidence from animal reproductive studies to anticipate a teratogenic risk.

Treatment of overdosage: Meptid tablets are subject to a hepatic first pass metabolism which prevents systemic concentrations of the drug reaching levels achieved by parenteral administration. In the unlikely event of overdose producing respiratory depression naloxone is the treatment of choice.

Recommended treatment includes gastric lavage, supportive therapy and naloxone if required.

Side-effects: No serious adverse reactions have been reported after treatment with Meptid tablets. Dizziness, nausea and vomiting have been reported.

Pharmaceutical precautions None.

Legal category POM.

Package quantities Cartons of 100 tablets (5 blister packs of 20 tablets).

Further information Meptazinol is an analgesic compound with no anti-inflammatory effects. It has little sedative effect, few CNS effects in general and a volunteer study indicates no interaction with alcohol. Constipation is rare. Available evidence indicates no significant addiction potential and no euphoric effects. Meptazinol is eliminated rapidly via the kidney. The main metabolite is a glucuronide conjugate and there is no accumulation of the drug or of active metabolites.

Mode of action: Meptazinol is a centrally-acting analgesic which acts as a mixed agonist-antagonist at opioid receptors. It is selective for one of several opioid binding sites (μ_1) and this may be responsible for the unusually low incidence of some common side effects (for example respiratory depression) of conventional centrally acting analgesics.

Product licence number 0011/0079.

MICROVAL*

Presentation Microval tablets are round white lustrous coated, convex tablets 5.0 mm in diameter. Each tablet contains 30 mcg levonorgestrel.

Uses Oral contraception. Microval is particularly indicated for the older woman changing from combined oral contraceptives and for women for whom oestrogen treatment is considered unsuitable.

Dosage and administration The tablets are started on the first day of menstruation and taken daily without interruption for as long as contraception is desired. They should be taken at the same time each day, preferably after the evening meal or at bedtime so that the interval between tablets is always about 24 hours. Protection may be reduced when the interval increases beyond 27 hours.

During the first cycle additional contraceptive precautions should be taken for the first 14 days.

If a tablet is not taken at the usual time it should be taken as soon as possible and the next tablet taken at the usual time. If the interval between tablets is more than 27 hours protection may be impaired. The patient should take one tablet as soon as she remembers and thereafter one tablet daily as before but should use additional contraceptive measures until the tablets have been taken regularly for 14 days. If a tablet is missed, the patient should take 1 tablet daily as before but should use additional contraceptive measures until the tablets have been taken regularly for 14 days.

If vomiting occurs shortly after a tablet has been taken contraceptive protection can be maintained by taking another tablet, provided that it is taken within three hours of the normal time. The last tablet in the pack may be used for this purpose. If repeated vomiting or diarrhoea endanger absorption additional contraceptive precautions should be used for 14 days after the symptoms have disappeared.

Irregular spotting or bleeding may occur with a proportion of women initially but menstrual regularity is usually re-established after the first few cycles. Those patients whose menstrual patterns do not become reasonably regular after three to four cycles or who have prolonged bleeding or amenorrhoea lasting for two months should be instructed to return for advice.

Women who change from a combined oral contraceptive to Microval should stop taking the previous product, leave seven clear days and take the first Microval tablet on the eighth day, then continue to take 1 tablet daily. Additional contraceptive precautions should be taken until the fourteenth tablet has been taken.

Microval does not diminish the yield of breast milk and can be used from the seventh post-partum day.

Contra-indications, warnings, etc

Contra-indications: Microval should not be given –

1. To patients with established hepatic disease or to those in whom there is evidence of persistently abnormal liver function such as the Dubin–Johnson and Rotor syndromes, or to those who have idiopathic recurrent jaundice of pregnancy.

2. To patients with a history of infectious hepatitis until the liver function tests have returned to normal values.

3. To patients with abnormal vaginal bleeding of unknown aetiology.

4. To patients with suspected pregnancy.

5. Although the risk of thromboembolism has not been associated with progestogen-only contraceptives,

it is at present required that a history of thromboembolic disorders should be regarded as a contra-indication.

Precautions:

1. Oral contraceptive medication should be discontinued if there is a gradual or sudden, partial or complete loss of vision, proptosis or diplopia, papilloedema or any evidence of retinal or vascular lesions.

2. Caution should be observed in prescribing oral contraceptives for any patients with a history of migraine, or if migraine is being treated with vasoconstrictor drugs. If migraine worsens or migraine or severe headache develops for the first time during treatment, medication should be discontinued immediately.

3. A small fraction of the progestogen has been identified in the milk of mothers receiving the drug. The long-range effects to the nursing infant is currently unknown.

4. Examination of the pelvic organs, breasts and blood pressure should precede prescription of Microval and should be repeated regularly.

5. Ectopic pregnancies appear to occur more frequently on progestogen-only oral contraceptives.

Side-effects: Microval is well tolerated but certain endocrine effects which are also characteristic of ovulatory cycles may occur. Those noted are headache, slight weight gain, nausea, breast tenderness and spotting between periods. The incidence of such effects with Microval is low and tends to decrease as treatment continues.

Drug interactions: Caution should be observed in prescribing oral contraceptives for patients taking other drugs since various interactions have been reported. Pregnancies have been reported in women taking oral contraceptives concurrently with rifampicin and other antibiotics, anti-epileptic drugs, barbiturates and other sedative drugs.

Steroids affect drug metabolism and the therapeutic or toxic effects of other drugs may be modified. Interactions have been reported between oral contraceptives and tricyclic antidepressants, anticoagulants and corticosteroids.

Overdosage: No reports of serious ill-effects from overdosage with oral contraceptives have been reported. In general, therefore, treatment of overdosage is not necessary. If overdosage is, however, discovered within one hour and is so large that treatment seems desirable, gastric lavage or a suitable dose of ipecacuanha can be used. There are no specific antidotes and further treatment should be symptomatic.

Pharmaceutical precautions Store at or below room temperature.

Legal category POM.

Package quantities Microval tablets are supplied in memo packs of 35 tablets.

Further information Estimates from clinical trials show that, if the tablets are taken correctly, out of 100 women taking them for one year, on average one woman may become pregnant during that year. Microval although not quite as effective as combined oral contraceptives, provides an extremely high degree of protection and is very much more effective than withdrawal, condom, rhythm method or chemicals and comparable to the I.U.C.D. and diaphragm.

Levonorgestrel is a totally synthetic progestogen which possesses no inherent oestrogenicity. It has anti-oestrogenic properties and has minimal effects on metabolic functions.

Product licence number 0011/0040.

MUCAINE*

Presentation Mucaine Suspension is a white suspension with the odour and flavour of peppermint. Each 5 ml contains:

Oxethazaine	10 mg
Magnesium Hydroxide BP	100 mg
Aluminium Hydroxide Mixture BP	4.75 ml

Uses Mucaine is an antacid mixture containing a topical anaesthetic and is indicated for oesophagitis whatever its cause, including peptic oesophagitis with or without hiatus hernia, radiation oesophagitis and the heartburn of late pregnancy.

The relief obtained in the symptomatic treatment of oesophagitis is due to the surface anaesthetic, oxethazaine, aided by the physical and antacid properties of the vehicle. Oxethazaine is stable at the levels of acidity or alkalinity found in the upper gastrointestinal tract and has relatively prolonged action.

Dosage and administration *Route of administration:* Oral.

Dosage – Adults: One to two 5 ml doses should be taken three or four times daily, 15 minutes before meals, and at bedtime, or as required. The dose should not be washed down with a drink.

Elderly: The adult dosage schedule can be used in the elderly.

Children: Not recommended for children.

Contra-indications, warnings, etc

Contra-indications: The aluminium ion combines with phosphate to form an insoluble complex which is not absorbed. When high doses are given together with a low phosphorus diet, phosphate depletion occurs. Phosphate depletion does not occur in patients on a normal diet. Mucaine is contra-indicated in patients with hypophosphataemia.

Side-effects: Mucaine is well tolerated and the side-effects which have been reported are almost invariably mild and transient in nature, consisting principally of constipation, dryness of the mouth and nausea.

Precautions:

1. Magnesium and aluminium hydroxides may form complexes with tetracyclines and reduce their absorption when given concomitantly.

2. Aluminium hydroxide may reduce absorption of digoxin.

3. Mucaine suspension should not be given during the first three months of pregnancy unless in the judgement of the physician such administration is clinically justifiable.

Action in case of overdosage: Not reported. Treatment should be symptomatic.

Pharmaceutical precautions Store in a cool place. Where necessary dispense Mucaine Suspension into suitable well-closed glass or polythene bottles.

Legal category POM.

Package quantities Polythene bottles of 500 ml.

Further information It is important to stress that

Mucaine should not be washed down with a drink because maximal relief depends on good contact between the affected mucosal surface and the suspension as it passes down the oesophagus.

Product licence number 0011/5014.

NORMISON*

Presentation Normison capsules are yellow, opaque soft gelatin capsules containing 10 mg or 20 mg temazepam. The 10 mg capsules are No. 4 capsules printed with N10 in black lettering. The 20 mg capsules are No. 10 capsules printed N20 in red lettering.

Uses Normison is indicated for the short term treatment of insomnia, and for premedication before minor surgery or other procedures especially when hospital admission is not essential.

Dosage and administration *Route of administration:* Oral.

Insomnia: Adults: 10–30 mg half an hour before retiring. The dose may be increased to 40 or 60 mg in patients who do not respond to the lower dose because of severe or persistent insomnia.

Elderly: Elderly patients or those suffering from cerebral vascular changes such as arteriosclerosis are likely to respond to smaller doses, possibly half the normal adult dose.

Children: Not recommended.

Premedication:
Adults: 20–40 mg, 30–60 minutes before surgical or other procedures.

Elderly: Elderly patients are likely to respond to smaller doses, possibly half the normal adult dose.

Children: Not evaluated.

Contra-indications, warnings, etc
Contra-indications: Normison should not be given to patients with a previous history of sensitivity to benzodiazepines.

Use in pregnancy: Animal experiments show no teratogenic effects, but the safety for use in pregnancy has not been established. Normison should not be administered during pregnancy or lactation unless in the judgement of the physician such administration is clinically justifiable. Normison is not recommended for use in the first three months of pregnancy.

Precautions:
1. Concomitant administration with central nervous system depressants, including alcohol, general anaesthetics, narcotic analgesics, monoamine oxidase inhibitors and antidepressants will result in an accentuation of their effects.
2. Prolonged or excessive use of benzodiazepines may occasionally result in the development of some psychological dependence with withdrawal symptoms on sudden discontinuation. Treatment in these cases should be withdrawn gradually. Careful usage seldom results in the development of dependence.
3. When used as a hypnotic, daytime drowsiness is unlikely to be a problem with Normison since the short half-life usually ensures that the effects disappear by the morning. As with other drugs acting on the central nervous system, however, patients should be cautioned against driving or operating machinery until it is estab-

lished that they do not become dizzy or drowsy while taking Normison.
4. Elderly patients or those suffering from cerebral vascular changes such as arteriosclerosis are likely to respond to smaller doses.
5. After medication with Normison before surgical or other procedures, patients should be accompanied home.

Side-effects: Because of its short half-life, the effects of temazepam are usually restricted to the night of ingestion. Drowsiness or dizziness on waking is rare. Morning headaches, transient rashes and mild gastro-intestinal disturbances have occasionally been reported.

Overdosage: As with other benzodiazepines, overdosage should not present a threat to life. General supportive measures should be used. Treatment is symptomatic and gastric lavage may be of use if performed shortly after ingestion. If the patient is conscious, an emetic such as ipecacuanha may be given. The patient is likely to sleep and a clear airway should be maintained.

Pharmaceutical precautions Store in a cool, dry place. Dispense Normison capsules into well-closed amber glass or amber/opaque plastic containers.

Legal category CD (Sch 4), POM.

Package quantities 10 mg: bottles of 50 and 100, securitainers of 500 and 1000. 20 mg: bottles of 100, securitainers of 500.

Further information Normison is a short acting benzodiazepine. It is rapidly absorbed from the liquid-filled soft gelatin capsules and peak plasma levels are usually reached in 20 to 40 minutes. Normison has a plasma half life of about eight hours. Normison is metabolised by a simple one-step process to a pharmacologically inert glucuronide. There are no major active metabolites and virtually no risk of accumulation. Clinical studies have shown minimal effects on REM sleep patterns and on psychomotor performance on the day after treatment with Normison.

Product licence numbers
10 mg capsules   0011/0060
20 mg capsules   0011/0063

OVRAN*
OVRAN 30*
OVRANETTE*

Presentation Ovran tablets are round, white, convex tablets, 6.5 mm in diameter, both faces marked WYETH. Each tablet contains 250 mcg levonorgestrel (d-norgestrel) and 50 mcg Ethinyloestradiol BP.

Ovran 30 tablets are round, white, convex tablets, 6.5 mm in diameter, one face marked WYETH and the other plain. Each tablet contains 250 mcg levonorgestrel (d-norgestrel) and 30 mcg Ethinyloestradiol BP.

Ovranette tablets are round, white, convex tablets, 6.5 mm in diameter, one face marked WYETH and the other face marked '30'. Each tablet contains 150 mcg levonorgestrel (d-norgestrel) and 30 mcg Ethinyloestradiol BP.

Uses Oral contraception. Treatment of endometriosis, spasmodic dysmenorrhoea, pre-menstrual tension, oligomenorrhoea. Treatment of abnormal uterine bleeding such as menorrhagia, metropathia haemorrhagica. Emergency treatment of acute uterine bleeding.

Dosage and administration *Contraception:* For the

first course of medication the tablets are started on the fifth day of the cycle, counting the first day of menstruation as day one. One tablet is taken at the same time each day for 21 days followed by seven days without medication. On the eighth day the tablets are started again. Additional contraceptive precautions should be taken until the fourteenth tablet of the first cycle has been taken. In subsequent cycles the protection covers every day of the cycle, provided that the tablets are taken correctly. During the seven clear days, withdrawal bleeding should occur. If a cycle with amenorrhoea occurs the patient should seek medical advice.

Women who change from another oral contraceptive to Ovran, Ovran 30 or Ovranette should stop taking the previous product, at the end of the pack leave seven clear days and take the first Ovran, Ovran 30 or Ovranette tablet on the eighth day, then continue to take 1 tablet daily for 21 days. Additional contraceptive precautions should be taken until the fourteenth tablet of the first cycle has been taken.

Occasionally spotting or bleeding may occur in some women initially, but menstrual regularity is usually re-established after the first few cycles. If medication is discontinued because of severe breakthrough bleeding a new course should be started on the fifth day from the start of bleeding. Additional contraceptive precautions should be taken until the fourteenth tablet of the new course has been taken.

If a tablet is forgotten the woman should take two on the following day at the usual time. If more than one tablet is missed, tablet taking should be resumed when remembered with the tablet appropriate for that day and additional precautions should be taken until the next withdrawal bleed. Withdrawal bleeding may occur as a result of missed tablets, but the patient should continue to take the tablets as directed.

Treatment with Ovran, Ovran 30 or Ovranette should be withdrawn six weeks before elective surgery or treatment of varicose veins by injection of sclerosant.

After childbirth oral contraception is usually started as soon as spontaneous menstruation has been resumed. Another method of contraception should be used in the interval between delivery and the first course, unless it is started within seven days of delivery.

Oral contraception may be started on the fifth day after an abortion or miscarriage.

If vomiting or diarrhoea impair absorption additional contraceptive precautions should be taken until the next withdrawal bleed.

Other indications: Ovran and Ovranette can be used for the indications listed below, but Ovran usually provides the more convenient dosage unit.

Endometriosis: Treatment should be continuous with 1 Ovran tablet daily. If spotting or breakthrough bleeding occurs it may be necessary to give 2 tablets daily or rarely 3 tablets daily in divided doses.

Spasmodic dysmenorrhoea, premenstrual tension, oligomenorrhoea: Dosage as for oral contraception.

Postponement of menstruation: If postponement of a withdrawal bleed is considered desirable, the woman should continue taking the tablets for the period during which delay is required. A seven-day gap should then be left before starting a new pack. If spotting or break-through bleeding occurs dosage should be increased to 2 tablets daily.

Functional uterine bleeding: When the diagnosis has been established dosage is similar to the dosage for oral contraception, but in the first one or two cycles it may be necessary to give 2 Ovran tablets (or in exceptional cases), 3 tablets daily in order to control the regularity of the cycle.

Emergency treatment of the acute uterine bleeding: 2 Ovran tablets are given immediately. If bleeding continues medication is continued at a dose of 4 tablets daily in divided doses. This can usually be reduced to 2 tablets within two to four days. Treatment should continue for 10 days and after this time it can either be discontinued to be followed after seven days by a complete course of 1 tablet daily for 21 days (see 'Functional uterine bleeding') or it can be continued for one to three months to inhibit the menses (see 'Postponement of menstruation'). In the latter case it should be possible to reduce the dosage to 1 tablet daily.

Contra-indications, warnings, etc

Contra-indications: Ovran, Ovran 30 and Ovranette, like other progestogen-oestrogen combinations, should not be given:

1. To patients with established hepatic disease or to those in whom there is evidence of persistently abnormal liver function such as the Dubin–Johnson and Rotor syndromes, or to those who have idiopathic recurrent jaundice of pregnancy.

2. To patients with a history or suspicion of carcinoma of the reproductive organs or breasts.

3. To patients with a history or evidence suggestive of thromboembolic or cerebrovascular disease or phlebitis.

4. To patients with cardiovascular disease.

5. To patients with a history of infectious hepatitis until the liver function tests have returned to normal values.

6. To patients with abnormal, vaginal bleeding of unknown aetiology.

7. To patients with known or suspected oestrogen-dependent neoplasia.

8. To patients with suspected pregnancy.

9. To patients with sickle cell anaemia.

10. To patients with deterioration of otosclerosis during pregnancy.

11. To patients with a history of herpes gestationis.

Precautions:

1. Under the influence of oestrogen-progestogen preparations, pre-existing uterine fibromyomata may increase in size.

2. Oestrogen-progestogen preparations may cause some degree of fluid retention. Conditions which might be influenced by this factor, such as epilepsy, migraine, asthma, cardiac or renal dysfunction, require careful observation.

3. Patients with a history of psychic depression should be carefully observed and the drug discontinued if the depression recurs to a serious degree.

4. A decrease in glucose tolerance has been observed in a significant percentage of patients on oral contraceptives. Diabetic patients should be carefully observed while receiving therapy.

5. Susceptible women may experience an increase in blood pressure following administration of contraceptive steroids. Caution should therefore be exercised in prescribing oral contraceptives for women with a history of hypertension.

6. Oral contraceptive medication should be discontinued if there is a gradual or sudden, partial or complete

loss of vision, proptosis or diplopia, papilloedema or any evidence of retinal or vascular lesions.

7. Caution should be observed in prescribing oral contraceptives for any patient with a history of migraine, or if migraine is being treated with vasoconstrictor drugs. If migraine worsens or migraine or severe headache develops for the first time during treatment, medication should be discontinued immediately.

8. A small fraction of the hormonal agents in oral contraceptives has been identified in the milk of mothers receiving these drugs. The long-range effect to the nursing infant is currently unknown.

9. Hepatic lesions (adenomas, hepatomas, hamartomas, regenerating nodules, etc.), occasionally fatal, have been reported in women taking oral contraceptives. Such lesions may present as an abdominal mass or with the signs and symptoms of an acute abdomen. These lesions should be considered if the patient has abdominal pain or evidence of intra-abdominal bleeding. Such lesions have been reported in short-term as well as long-term users of oral contraceptives.

10. In breakthrough bleeding or irregular vaginal bleeding, non-functional causes should be borne in mind.

11. The risk of arterial thrombosis associated with combined oral contraceptives increases with age, and this risk is aggravated by cigarette smoking. The use of combined oral contraceptives by women in the older age group, especially those who are cigarette smokers, should therefore be discouraged and alternative methods advised.

12. Examination of the pelvic organs, breasts and blood pressure should precede prescription of an oral contraceptive and should be repeated regularly.

13. Certain conditions require careful observation during treatment with oral contraceptives. These are: a history of depression, varicose veins, diabetes, hypertension, epilepsy, otosclerosis, multiple sclerosis, porphyria, tetany, disturbed liver function, gall-stones, renal diseases, chloasma, uterine fibroids, asthma, the wearing of contact lenses or any condition prone to worsen during pregnancy.

Side-effects: Oral contraceptives produce certain endocrine effects characteristic of ovarian oestrogens and progesterone. The hormones secreted during an ovulatory cycle may produce similar effects including headache, slight weight gain, nausea, breast tenderness, changed libido, depressive moods, and spotting between periods. The overall incidence of such effects with Ovran, Ovran 30 and Ovranette is low and tends to decrease as treatment cycles continue. Cycle control is good and spotting and breakthrough bleeding occur only rarely. Extensive studies on considerable numbers of women taking oral contraceptives indicate some increased risks over non-pregnant women who are not taking oral contraceptives. These include thromboembolism, impaired glucose tolerance and even more rarely, liver dysfunction, hypertension and raised serum lipids.

Drug interactions: Caution should be observed in prescribing oral contraceptives for patients taking other drugs since various interactions have been reported. Pregnancies have been reported in women taking oral contraceptives concurrently with rifampicin and other antibiotics, anti-epileptic drugs, barbiturates and other sedative drugs.

Steroids affect drug metabolism and the therapeutic or toxic effects of other drugs may be modified.

Interactions have been reported between oral contraceptives and tricyclic anti-depressants, anticoagulants and corticosteroids.

Overdosage: No reports of serious ill-effects from overdosage with combined oral contraceptives have been reported. In general, therefore, treatment of overdosage is not necessary. If overdosage is, however, discovered within one hour and is so large that treatment seems desirable, gastric lavage or a suitable dose of ipecacuanha can be used. There are no specific antidotes and further treatment should be symptomatic.

Pharmaceutical precautions Store at, or below, room temperature.

Legal category POM.

Package quantities Ovran, Ovran 30, and Ovranette are supplied in memo packs of 21 tablets.

Further information Levonorgestrel is a totally synthetic progestogen which possesses no inherent oestrogenicity. It has anti-oestrogenic properties and has minimal effects on metabolic functions.

Pearl Index: Ovran, 0.19. Ovran 30, 0.13. Ovranette, 0.35.

Product licence numbers
Ovran   0011/0015
Ovran 30   0011/0050
Ovranette   0011/0041

OXAZEPAM TABLETS 10 and 15 mg

Presentation Oxazepam Tablets BP containing 10 or 15 mg oxazepam.

Oxazepam 10 mg tablets are white flat bevel edged tablets 6.5 mm in diameter, marked WYETH on one face and '10' on the other.

Oxazepam 15 mg tablets are white, flat, bevel edged tablets, 8.0 mm in diameter, marked '15' on one face and WYETH on the other.

Uses Treatment of the symptoms of anxiety.

Dosage and administration Route of administration: Oral.

Dosage: Adults: Mild to moderate anxiety – one to two 15 mg tablets three (or four) times daily.

Elderly patients or those who are particularly sensitive to the effects of benzodiazepines – 10–20 mg three or four times daily.

Children: Oxazepam is not recommended for the treatment of children.

Contra-indications, warnings, etc
1. Oxazepam should not be given to patients with a previous history of sensitivity to benzodiazepines.
2. Acute pulmonary insufficiency.

Use in pregnancy: There are no human or animal studies which establish safety in pregnancy. Oxazepam should not be administered during pregnancy or lactation unless in the judgment of the physician such administration is clinically justifiable. Special care should be taken in the first and last trimesters.

Precautions and warnings:
1. Concomitant administration with central nervous system depressants, including alcohol, general anaesthetics, narcotic analgesics, monoamine oxidase inhibitors

and antidepressants will result in an accentuation of their effects.

2. In general, the dependence potential of benzodiazepines is low, but this increases when high dosages are attained, especially when given over long periods. This is particularly so in patients with a history of alcoholism, drug abuse or in patients with marked personality disorders. Regular monitoring of treatment in such patients is essential and routine repeat prescriptions should be avoided.

3. As with other drugs acting on the central nervous system, patients should be cautioned against driving or operating machinery until it is established that they do not become dizzy or drowsy while taking oxazepam.

4. The use of anxiolytic drugs may uncover covert suicidal tendencies in patients with a psychological depressive component of the illness.

5. Oxazepam should not be used in labour unless considered essential. High single doses or repeated low doses of other benzodiazepines have been reported to produce hypotonia, poor sucking and hypotension in the neonate and irregularities in the foetal heart.

6. Caution should be observed in using oxazepam in chronic pulmonary insufficiency.

7. The pharmacokinetics of oxazepam in patients with liver disease differs little from that in normal subjects but caution should be observed in patients with liver damage. Oxazepam is conjugated in the liver.

Side-effects: Transient mild drowsiness is commonly seen in the first few days of therapy. If it becomes troublesome dosage should be reduced. In a few cases dizziness, ataxia, vertigo and headache have occurred either alone or with drowsiness. Mild excitatory effects with stimulation of affect have sometimes been reported in psychiatric patients; these reactions usually appear in the first two weeks of therapy.

Other side effects include rare cases of minor diffuse skin rashes (morbilliform, urticarial and maculopapular), altered libido and nausea. Blood dyscrasias and jaundice have been rarely reported.

Overdosage: A few cases of attempted suicide with oxazepam have been reported, but none has been successful with oxazepam alone. Records show that up to 540 mg have been taken without long-term ill-effects. As with other benzodiazepines, overdosages should not present a threat to life. General supportive measures should be used.

Treatment is symptomatic and gastric lavage may be of use if performed shortly after ingestion. If the patient is conscious, an emetic such as ipecacuanha may be given. The patient is likely to sleep and a clear airway should be maintained.

Pharmaceutical precautions Store in a cool, dry place.

Legal category CD (Sch 4), POM.

Package quantities Oxazepam Tablets 10 mg and 15 mg – Packs of 100.

Further information Oxazepam may offer advantages in the treatment of the elderly because of its short half-life and lack of accumulation.

Oxazepam is a short-acting benzodiazepine. It is metabolised by a simple one-step process to a pharmacologically inert glucuronide. There are no major active metabolites. The elimination half-life is 6–8 hours and there is minimal risk of excessive accumulation. Little is known regarding efficacy and safety of benzodiazepines in long term use. It is advisable to review treatment regularly and to discontinue use as soon as possible.

Product licence numbers
Oxazepam Tablets 10 mg   0011/0110
Oxazepam Tablets 15 mg   0011/0111

PENIDURAL* (ORAL)

Presentation Penidural Oral Suspension is a smooth, pink suspension with a sweet cherry flavour. Each 5 ml dose contains: 229 mg Benzathine Penicillin BP (equivalent to 300,000 units Penicillin G).

Penidural Oral Drops is a smooth pink suspension with a sweet cherry flavour. Each 1 ml contains 115 mg Benzathine Penicillin BP (equivalent to 150,000 units Penicillin G).

Uses Penidural Oral presentations are indicated for the treatment of mild to moderately severe penicillin-sensitive infections and prophylaxis of penicillin-sensitive secondary infections especially in children.

Dosage and administration *Route of administration:* Oral.

Dosage: Benzathine penicillin is a repository penicillin which gives effective blood levels for a long period, six- to eight-hourly dosage being adequate in most patients.

Penidural oral suspension: Adults: Two 5 ml doses three to four times daily.

Elderly: The adult dosage schedule should be used in the elderly.

Children: One 5 ml dose three to four times daily.

Penidural oral drops: Adults: Not recommended.

Children: up to 5 years of age: 1 or 2 dropperfuls three or four times daily. Each dropperful contains the equivalent of 100,000 units of Penicillin G.

Contra-indications, warnings, etc
Contra-indications: Benzathine penicillin is contra-indicated in patients with a previous history of penicillin hypersensitivity and in small babies whose mothers have such a history.

Precautions and warnings: 1. Prolonged use of an antibiotic may result in the development of super infection due to organisms resistant to that anti-biotic.

2. Penidural oral suspension should not be administered during pregnancy or lactation unless in the judgement of the physician such administration is clinically justifiable. Special care should be taken in the first three months of pregnancy.

3. High doses of Penidural should be used with caution in patients with renal failure.

Side-effects: Pencillin may cause an acute anaphylactic reaction which can be fatal. This reaction appears to occur more frequently in patients with bronchial asthma or other allergic disorders. Reactions have been reported after the use of all forms of penicillin by all routes of administration but are less likely after oral penicillin because of slower absorption.

Penidural is otherwise virtually free from side-effects apart from occasional loose stools or borborygmi.

Pharmaceutical precautions *Penidural Oral Suspension:* Store in a cool place. Where necessary dispense Penidural Oral Suspension into suitable well-closed glass bottles. When required Penidural Oral Suspension may be diluted with Syrup BP (unpreserved or preserved with parahydroxybenzoates).

Penidural Oral Drops: Store in a cool place.

Legal category POM.

Package quantities Penidural Oral Suspension. Bottles of 100 ml.
Penidural Oral Drops: Bottles of 10 ml.

Further information Nil.

Product licence numbers
Suspension 0011/5019R
Drops 0011/5018R

SPARINE* (ORAL)

Presentation Sparine is presented as tablets containing 25 mg, 50 mg or 100 mg Promazine Hydrochloride BP per tablet and as an oral suspension. Each 5 ml suspension contains promazine embonate equivalent to 50 mg Promazine Hydrochloride BP.

Sparine Tablets 25 mg: Yellow, sugar-coated tablets, 7.5 mm in diameter.

Sparine Tablets 50 mg: Orange, sugar-coated tablets, 10 mm in diameter.

Sparine Tablets 100 mg: Red, sugar-coated tablets, 11 mm in diameter.

Sparine Suspension: Yellow suspension with an odour of pineapple.

Uses 1. As an adjunct to the short term management of moderate to severe psychomotor agitation.
2. Agitation and restlessness in the elderly.

Dosage and administration *Route of administration:* Oral.

Dosage: Psychomotor agitation: Adults: 100–200 mg four times daily.

Elderly: Half the normal dose may be sufficient for a therapeutic response in elderly patients.

Agitation and restlessness: Elderly: 25 mg initially. Increase if necessary up to 50 mg four times daily.

Children: Oral Sparine is not recommended for children.

Contra-indications, warnings, etc
Contra-indications: 1. Use in patients hypersensitive to the active ingredient or other phenothiazines.
2. Sparine should not be used during lactation.
3. *Use in pregnancy:* Do not use during pregnancy, especially during the first three months, unless there are compelling reasons. There is insufficient evidence of the safety of promazine in human pregnancy nor is there evidence from animal studies that it is free from hazard.

Precautions and warnings:
1. Phenothiazines should only be used with great caution in patients with a history of jaundice or with existent liver dysfunction, or blood dyscrasias, coronary insufficiency or cardiac disease.
2. Respiratory depression may occur in patients with severe respiratory disease.
3. Promazine should be used with caution in patients with renal failure.
4. Patients receiving phenothiazines over a prolonged period require regular and careful surveillance with particular attention to potential for inducing eye changes, effects on haemopoiesis, liver dysfunction, myocardial conduction effects, particularly if other concurrently administered drugs also have potential effects on these systems.
5. Phenothiazines may impair alertness and induce drowsiness especially at the start of treatment. Persons taking these drugs should not drive or operate machinery unless the drug has been shown not to interfere with physical or mental ability.
6. Use of phenothiazines at high (relative or absolute) doses may induce extrapyramidal side-effects, dyskinesia, akathisia, dystonia. These are likely to be particularly severe in children. Caution should be exercised in patients with Parkinson's disease. Anti-Parkinson agents should not be prescribed routinely because of the risk of aggravating anticholinergic side-effects of promazine, of precipitating toxic-confusional states or of impairing its therapeutic efficacy. They should be given only as required.
7. Prolonged administration of phenothiazines may result in persistent or tardive dyskinesias particularly in the elderly.
8. Care should be exercised if Sparine is used for the treatment of patients with cerebral arteriosclerosis, coronary heart disease or other conditions in which a fall in blood pressure might be undesirable.
9. Caution should be observed with patients suffering from epilepsy or conditions predisposing to epilepsy.
10. Personal or family history of narrow angle glaucoma.
11. Phenothiazines may impair body temperature regulation. Caution should be observed in very hot weather.
12. Hypothyroidism.
13. Myasthenia gravis.
14. Phaeochromocytoma.
15. Prostatic hypertrophy.
16. Antipsychotic drugs may increase prolactin secretion.
17. Sparine suspension is formulated with aluminium hydroxide which may complex tetracyclines if given concomitantly.
18. *Drug interactions:* The concomitant administration of this product with other medication such as central nervous system depressants (including alcohol and anaesthetics) or antihypertensives, anticholinergic or dopaminergic drugs will result in accentuation of their effects, while potentiation of action will also occur with monoamine oxidase inhibitors, antidepressants and analgesics. Promazine may impair the effects of anticonvulsants.

Promazine may affect the control of diabetes. Undesirable anti-cholinergic effects can be enhanced by anti-Parkinson or other anticholinergic drugs.

Side-effects: Sparine is a member of the phenothiazine group of drugs and the side-effects associated with that group have been noted. These include drowsiness, sedation, dry mouth, nasal stuffiness. Other possible anticholinergic side-effects are blurred vision, tachycardia, constipation and urinary hesitancy or retention when due to enlarged prostate.

Confusional states, or epileptic fits can occur. Sexual function may be impaired. Agranulocytosis and transient leucopenia have rarely been reported. Allergic skin reactions have also been reported.

Promazine rarely causes obstructive jaundice associated with stasis in biliary canaliculi. Promazine treatment should be withdrawn and not given again. Transient abnormalities of liver function tests may occur without jaundice.

Some individuals may be susceptible to the drug in low dosage and show paradoxical effects of excitement, agitation, or insomnia and other minor side effects.

The elderly are particularly susceptible to side-effects of promazine, especially to the sedative, hypotensive and temperature regulation effects. These effects may be dose related.

Treatment of overdosages: Ingestion of large amounts of promazine is followed by deep sleep, with or without a pronounced fall in blood pressure and without particular change in respiration rate, other than the slowing attendant upon sedation. Occasionally an initial period of excitement may precede coma, followed by grand mal seizures.

In the absence of any specific antidote, treatment should be based on ordinary therapeutic principles with special emphasis on the following measures: (1) gastric lavage; (2) treat convulsions if present; (3) correction of acute hypotension if necessary; (4) counteraction of the effects of an excess of promazine hydrochloride on the central nervous system; (5) control and natural recovery of hypothermia.

Pharmaceutical precautions Store Sparine Suspension in a cool place and protect from light. When required Sparine Suspension may be diluted with Syrup BP (unpreserved or preserved with p-hydroxybenzoates).

Legal category POM.

Package quantities
Sparine Tablets 25 mg,
  50 mg and 100 mg   Bottles of 250.
Sparine Suspension   Bottles of 150 ml and 1
                       litre

Further information Nil.

Product licence numbers
Sparine Tablets   25 mg   0011/5050
Sparine Tablets   50 mg   0011/5056
Sparine Tablets 100 mg   0011/5057
Sparine Suspension   0011/5045

SPARINE* (PARENTERAL)

Presentation Sparine injection is a clear, colourless aqueous solution containing 50 mg Promazine Hydrochloride BP per millilitre.

Uses 1. As an adjunct to the short term management of moderate to severe psychomotor agitation.
  2. Agitation and restlessness in the elderly.
  3. Intractable hiccup.
  4. Alleviation of nausea and vomiting, including that in labour.
  5. Investigations in children, including cardiac and EEG examinations.

Dosage and administration *Route of administration:* Parenteral.

Dosage: Adults: Psychomotor agitation, 50 mg Sparine intramuscularly. Repeat if necessary after six to eight hours.

Intractable hiccup, 50 mg intramuscularly. Repeat if necessary with doses up to 100 mg 4 hourly. The daily dose should not exceed 1 g.

Labour, 50 mg Sparine intramuscularly. For convenience 50 mg Sparine may be mixed with 50 mg pethidine in the same syringe.

Elderly: Half the normal dose may be sufficient for a therapeutic response in elderly subjects.

Children: 0.7 mg/kg intramuscularly.

If Sparine is injected intravenously it should be diluted with an equal volume of saline.

Contra-indications, warnings, etc
Contra-indications: 1. Use in patients in coma.
  2. Use in patients hypersensitive to the active ingredient or other phenothiazines.
  3. Sparine should not be used during lactation.
  4. *Use in pregnancy.* Do not use during pregnancy, especially during the first three months, unless there are compelling reasons. There is insufficient evidence of the safety of promazine in human pregnancy nor is there evidence from animal studies that it is free from hazard.

Precautions and warnings:
  1. Phenothiazines should only be used with great caution in patients with a history of jaundice or with existent liver dysfunction, or blood dyscrasias, coronary insufficiency or cardiac disease.
  2. Respiratory depression may occur in patients with severe respiratory disease.
  3. Promazine should be used with caution in patients with renal failure.
  4. Patients receiving phenothiazines over a prolonged period require regular and careful surveillance with particular attention to potential for inducing eye changes, effects on haemopoiesis, liver dysfunction, myocardial conduction effects, particularly if other concurrently administered drugs also have potential effects on these systems.
  5. Phenothiazines may impair alertness and induce drowsiness, especially at the start of treatment. Persons taking these drugs should not drive or operate machinery unless the drug has been shown not to interfere with physical or mental ability.
  6. Use of phenothiazines at high (relative or absolute) doses may induce extrapyramidal side-effects, dyskinesia, akathisia, dystonia. These are likely to be particularly severe in children. Caution should be exercised in patients with Parkinson's disease. Anti-Parkinson agents should not be prescribed routinely because of the risk of aggravating anticholinergic side-effects of promazine, of precipitating toxic-confusional states or of impairing its therapeutic efficacy. They should be given only as required.
  7. Prolonged administration of phenothiazines may result in persistent or tardive dyskinesias particularly in the elderly.
  8. Administration by the intravenous route may induce local vascular spasm or thrombophlebitis. The preparation must be diluted before use. Arteriolar spasm and gangrene have been reported following accidental intra-arterial injection of high concentrations.
  9. Care should be exercised if Sparine is used for the treatment of patients with cerebral arteriosclerosis, coronary heart disease or other conditions in which a fall in blood pressure might be undesirable.
  10. Caution should be observed with patients suffering from epilepsy or conditions predisposing to epilepsy.
  11. Personal or family history of narrow angle glaucoma.
  12. Phenothiazines may impair body temperature regulation. Caution should be observed in very hot weather.
  13. Hypothyroidism.

14. Myasthenia gravis.

15. Phaeochromocytoma.

16. Prostatic hypertrophy.

17. Antipsychotic drugs may increase prolactin secretion.

18. *Drug interactions:* The concomitant administration of this product with other medication such as central nervous system depressants (including alcohol and anaesthetics) or antihypertensives, anticholinergic or dopaminergic drugs will result in accentuation of their effects, while potentiation of action will also occur with monoamine oxidase inhibitors, antidepressants and analgesics. Promazine may impair the effects of anticonvulsants.

Promazine may affect the control of diabetes. Undesirable anti-cholinergic effects can be enhanced by anti-Parkinson or other anticholinergic drugs.

Side-effects: Sparine is a member of the phenothiazine group of drugs and the side effects associated with that group have been noted. These include drowsiness, sedation, dry mouth, nasal stuffiness. Other possible anticholinergic side-effects are blurred vision, tachycardia, constipation and urinary hesitancy or retention when due to enlarged prostate.

Confusional states, or epileptic fits can occur. Sexual function may be impaired. Agranulocytosis and transient leucopenia have rarely been reported. Allergic skin reactions have also been reported.

Promazine rarely causes obstructive jaundice associated with stasis in biliary canaliculi. Promazine treatment should be withdrawn and not given again. Transient abnormalities of liver function tests may occur without jaundice.

Some individuals may be susceptible to the drug in low dosage and show paradoxical effects of excitement, agitation or insomnia and other minor side effects.

The elderly are particularly susceptible to side-effects of promazine, especially to the sedative, hypotensive and temperature regulation effects. These effects may be dose related.

Treatment of overdosages: Injection of large amounts of promazine is followed by deep sleep, with or without a pronounced fall in blood pressure and without particular change in respiration rate, other than the slowing attendant upon sedation. Occasionally an initial period of excitement may precede coma, followed by grand mal seizures.

In the absence of any specific antidote, treatment should be based on ordinary therapeutic principles with special emphasis on the following measures: (1) treat convulsions if present; (2) correction of acute hypotension if necessary; (3) counteraction of the effects of an excess of promazine hydrochloride on the central nervous system; (4) control and natural recovery of hypothermia.

Pharmaceutical precautions Sparine Injection should not be mixed with other injections with the exception of Pethidine Injection BP.

Legal category POM.

Package quantities Boxes of 10 by 1 ml or 2 ml ampoules.

Further information Nil.

Product licence number 0011/5043R.

TEMAZEPAM CAPSULES

Presentation Temazepam capsules are opaque yellow, oval, soft gelatin capsules containing 10 mg or 20 mg temazepam. The 10 mg capsules are No. 4 capsules imprinted WYETH on one side in black lettering. The 20 mg capsules are No. 10 oval capsules imprinted WYETH on one side and 20 on the reverse side in red lettering.

Uses Temazepam is indicated for the short term treatment of insomnia, and for premedication before minor surgery or other procedures especially when hospital admission is not essential.

Dosage and administration Route of administration: Oral.

Insomnia
Adults: 10–30 mg half an hour before retiring. The dose may be increased to 40 or 60 mg in patients who do not respond to the lower dose because of severe or persistent insomnia.

Elderly: Elderly patients or those suffering from cerebral vascular changes such as arteriosclerosis are likely to respond to smaller doses, possibly half the normal adult dose.

Children: Not recommended.

Premedication
Adults: 20–40 mg, 30–60 minutes before surgical or other procedures.

Elderly: Elderly patients are likely to respond to smaller doses, possibly half the normal adult dose.

Children: Not evaluated.

Contra-indications, warnings, etc
Contra-indications: Temazepam should not be given to patients with a previous history of sensitivity to benzodiazepines.

Use in pregnancy: Animal experiments show no teratogenic effects, but the safety for use in pregnancy has not been established. Temazepam should not be administered during pregnancy or lactation unless in the judgment of the physician such administration is clinically justifiable. Temazepam is not recommended for use in the first three months of pregnancy.

Precautions:
1. Concomitant administration with central nervous system depressants, including alcohol, general anaesthetics, narcotic analgesics, monoamine oxidase inhibitors and antidepressants will result in an accentuation of their effects.

2. Prolonged or excessive use of benzodiazepines may occasionally result in the development of some psychological dependence with withdrawal symptoms on sudden discontinuation. Treatment in these cases should be withdrawn gradually. Careful usage seldom results in the development of dependence.

3. When used as a hypnotic, daytime drowsiness is unlikely to be a problem with temazepam since the short half-life usually ensures that the effects disappear by the morning. As with other drugs acting on the central nervous system, however, patients should be cautioned against driving or operating machinery until it is established that they do not become dizzy or drowsy while taking temazepam.

4. Elderly patients or those suffering from cerebral vascular changes such as arteriosclerosis are likely to respond to smaller doses.

5. After medication with temazepam before surgical or other procedures, patients should be accompanied home.

Side-effects: Because of its short half-life, the effects of temazepam are usually restricted to the night of ingestion. Drowsiness or dizziness on waking is rare. Morning headaches, transient rashes and mild gastro-intestinal disturbances have occasionally been reported.

Overdosage: As with other benzodiazepines, overdosages should not present a threat to life. General supportive measures should be used. Treatment is symptomatic and gastric lavage may be of use if performed shortly after ingestion. If the patient is conscious, an emetic such as ipecacuanha may be given. The patient is likely to sleep and a clear airway should be maintained.

Pharmaceutical precautions Store in a cool, dry place. Dispense Temazepam capsules into well closed amber glass or amber/opaque plastic containers.

Legal category CD (Sch 4), POM.

Package quantities 10 mg: securitainers of 250, 500 and 1000, bottles of 50.
20 mg: securitainers of 250 and 500.

Further information Temazepam is a short acting benzodiazepine. It is rapidly absorbed from the liquid-filled soft gelatin capsules and peak plasma levels are usually reached in 20 to 40 minutes. Temazepam has a plasma half life of about eight hours. Temazepam is metabolised by a simple one-step process to a pharmacologically inert glucuronide. There are no major active metabolites and virtually no risk of accumulation. Clinical studies have shown minimal effects on REM sleep patterns and on psychomotor performance on the day after treatment with temazepam.

Product licence numbers
10 mg capsules   0011/0106
20 mg capsules   0011/0107

TRINORDIOL* ▼

Presentation The memo pack holds six light brown tablets, containing 50mcg levonorgestrel and 30 mcg Ethinyloestradiol BP, five white tablets containing 75 mcg levonorgestrel and 40 mcg Ethinyloestradiol BP and ten ochre tablets containing 125 mcg levonorgestrel and 30 mcg Ethinyloestradiol BP.
All tablets are round 5.6 mm in diameter with a lustrous sugar coating.

Uses Oral contraception.

Dosage and administration *Contraception:* For the first course of medication the tablets are started on the first day of the cycle, counting the first day of menstruation as day one. One tablet is taken at the same time each day for 21 days followed by seven days without medication. On the eighth day the tablets are started again. The protection covers every day of the cycle, provided that the tablets are taken correctly. During the seven clear days withdrawal bleeding should occur. If a cycle with amenorrhoea occurs the patient should seek medical advice.

Women who change from another oral contraceptive to Trinordiol should stop taking the previous product at the end of the pack and take the first tablet of Trinordiol on the day after taking the last tablet of their old pack, then continue to take 1 tablet daily for 21 days. If it is preferred to leave a seven-day gap before starting Trinordiol, then additional contraceptive precautions should be taken for the first 14 days of the first cycle.

Occasionally spotting or bleeding may occur in some women initially, but menstrual regularity is usually re-established after the first few cycles. If medication is discontinued because of severe breakthrough bleeding a new course should be started on the fifth day from the start of bleeding. Additional contraceptive precautions should be taken until the fourteenth tablet of the new course has been taken.

If a tablet is forgotten the woman should take it as soon as possible. If the delay is more than 12 hours additional precautions should be taken until the next withdrawal bleed. If more than one tablet is missed, tablet taking should be resumed when remembered with the tablet appropriate for that day and additional precautions should be taken until the next withdrawal bleed. Withdrawal bleeding may occur as a result of missed tablets, but the patient should continue to take the tablets as directed.

Treatment with Trinordiol should be withdrawn six weeks before elective surgery or treatment of varicose veins by injection of sclerosant.

After childbirth oral contraception is usually started as soon as spontaneous menstruation has been resumed. Another method of contraception should be used in the interval between delivery and the first course, unless it is started within seven days of delivery.

Oral contraception may be started on the fifth day after an abortion or miscarriage.

If vomiting or diarrhoea impair absorption, additional contraceptive precautions should be taken until the next withdrawal bleed.

Contra-indications, warnings, etc
Contra-indications: Trinordiol like other progestogen-oestrogen combinations, should not be given:

1. To patients with established hepatic disease or to those in whom there is evidence of persistently abnormal liver functions such as Dubin–Johnson and Rotor syndromes, or to those who have idiopathic recurrent jaundice of pregnancy.

2. To patients with a history or suspicion of carcinoma of the reproductive organs or breasts.

3. To patients with a history or evidence suggestive of thromboembolic or cerebrovascular disease or phlebitis.

4. To patients with cardiovascular disease.

5. To patients with a history of infectious hepatitis until the liver function tests have returned to normal values.

6. To patients with abnormal vaginal bleeding of unknown aetiology.

7. To patients with known or suspected oestrogen-dependent neoplasia.

8. To patients with suspected pregnancy.

9. To patients with sickle cell anaemia.

10. To patients with deterioration of otosclerosis during pregnancy.

11. To patients with a history of herpes gestationis.

Precautions:
1. Under the influence of oestrogen-progestogen preparations, pre-existing uterine fibromyomata may increase in size.

2. Oestrogen-progestogen preparations may cause some degree of fluid retention. Conditions which might

be influenced by this factor, such as epilepsy, migraine, asthma, cardiac or renal dysfunction, require careful observation.

3. Patients with a history of psychic depression should be carefully observed and the drug discontinued if the depression recurs to a serious degree.

4. A decrease in glucose tolerance has been observed in a significant percentage of patients on oral contraceptives. Diabetic patients should be carefully observed while receiving therapy.

5. Susceptible women may experience an increase in blood pressure following administration of contraceptive steroids. Caution should therefore be exercised in prescribing oral contraceptives for women with a history of hypertension.

6. Oral contraceptive medication should be discontinued if there is a gradual or sudden, partial or complete loss of vision, proptosis or diplopia, papilloedema or any evidence of retinal or vascular lesions.

7. Caution should be observed in prescribing oral contraceptives for any patient with a history of migraine, or if migraine is being treated with vasoconstrictor drugs. If migraine worsens or migraine or severe headache develops for the first time during treatment, medication should be discontinued immediately.

8. A small fraction of the hormonal agents in oral contraceptives has been identified in the milk of mothers receiving these drugs. The long-range effect to the nursing infant is currently unknown.

9. Hepatic lesions (adenomas, hepatomas, hamartomas, regenerating nodules, etc) occasionally fatal, have been reported in women taking oral contraceptives. Such lesions may present as an abdominal mass or with the signs and symptoms of an acute abdomen. These lesions should be considered if the patient has abdominal pain or evidence of intra-abdominal bleeding. Such lesions have been reported in short-term as well as long-term users of oral contraceptives.

10. In breakthrough bleeding or irregular vaginal bleeding, non-functional causes should be borne in mind.

11. The risk of arterial thrombosis associated with combined oral contraceptives increases with age, and this risk is aggravated by cigarette smoking. The use of combined oral contraceptives by women in the older age group, especially those who are cigarette smokers, should therefore be discouraged and alternative methods advised.

12. Examination of the pelvic organs, breasts and blood pressure should precede prescription of an oral contraceptive and should be repeated regularly.

13. Certain conditions require careful observation during treatment with oral contraceptives. These are: history of depression, varicose veins, diabetes, hypertension, epilepsy, otosclerosis, multiple sclerosis, porphyria, tetany, disturbed liver function, gall-stones, renal disease, chloasma, uterine fibroids, asthma, the wearing of contact lenses or any condition prone to worsen during pregnancy.

Side-effects: Oral contraceptives produce certain endocrine effects characteristic of ovarian oestrogens and progesterone. The hormones secreted during an ovulatory cycle may produce similar effects including headache, slight weight gain, nausea, breast tenderness, changed libido, depressive moods and spotting between periods. The overall incidence of such effects with Trinordiol is low and tends to decrease as treatment cycles continue. Cycle control is good and spotting and breakthrough bleeding occur only rarely. Extensive studies on considerable numbers of women taking oral contraceptives indicate some increased risks over non-pregnant women who are not taking oral contraceptives. These include thromboembolism, impaired glucose tolerance and even more rarely, liver dysfunction, hypertension and raised serum lipids.

Drug interactions: Caution should be observed in prescribing oral contraceptives for patients taking other drugs since various interactions have been reported. Pregnancies have been reported in women taking oral contraceptives concurrently with rifampicin and other antibiotics, anti-epileptic drugs, barbiturates and other sedative drugs.

Steroids affect drug metabolism and the therapeutic or toxic effects of other drugs may be modified. Interactions have been reported between oral contraceptives and tricyclic antidepressants, anticoagulants and corticosteroids.

Overdosage: No reports of serious ill-effects from overdosage with combined oral contraceptives have been reported. In general, therefore, treatment of overdosage is not necessary. If overdosage is, however, discovered within one hour and is so large that treatment seems desirable, gastric lavage or a suitable dose of ipecacuanha can be used. There are no specific antidotes and further treatment should be symptomatic.

Pharmaceutical precautions Store at, or below, room temperature.

Legal category POM.

Package quantities Trinordiol is supplied in packs of 3 blisters of 21 tablets.

Further information Levonorgestrel is a totally synthetic progestogen which possesses no inherent oestrogenicity. It has anti-oestrogenic properties and has minimal effects on metabolic functions.

Research has shown that it is unnecessary to give the same doses of hormones throughout the cycle. The three-phase dosage mimics the secretion of hormones in a natural cycle and allows the total intake of steroids to be reduced while maintaining contraceptive efficacy and good cycle control.

Product licence number 0011/0066.

*Trade Mark

Zyma (United Kingdom) Limited
Westhead
10 West Street
Alderley Edge
Cheshire SK9 7XP

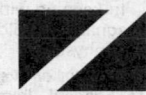

FABROL* ▼

Presentation Pale yellow, orange-flavoured granules in sachets containing 200 mg acetylcysteine.

Uses
Mode of action: Fabrol has an intense mucolytic action on mucoid and mucopurulent secretions due to its ability to split disulphide bonds in mucus glycoprotein. This property allows it to be used as adjuvant therapy in many clinical conditions characterised by the presence of viscous mucoid or mucopurulent secretions, particularly in the respiratory tract.

Indications: Fabrol is indicated in acute and chronic bronchitis and other respiratory conditions associated with the production of viscous mucus. Given on a long term basis in chronic bronchitis, it progressively improves symptoms due to mucus hypersecretion and substantially reduces the rate of infectious exacerbations.

Fabrol is also indicated for use in patients with abdominal complications associated with cystic fibrosis.

Dosage and administration The following dosage is recommended for the treatment of respiratory conditions:

Children up to 2 years: 1 sachet (200 mg) daily.

Children aged 2–6 years: 1 sachet (200 mg) twice daily.

Adults: 1 sachet (200 mg) three times daily.

Use in the elderly: There is no evidence to suggest that the dosage should be different in elderly patients.

In acute cases, a treatment period of 5–10 days is usually adequate but may be extended if necessary.

In chronic bronchitis, relief of symptoms may be noticeable after treatment for 1–2 months but treatment may be continued for up to six months, e.g. during the winter season.

For maintenance therapy in cystic fibrosis, the following dosage ranges are recommended:

Children up to 2 years: ½ to 1 sachet (100 to 200 mg) three times daily.

Children aged 2–6 years: 1 sachet (200 mg) three times daily.

Adults: 1 or 2 sachets (200 or 400 mg) three times daily. In adults, a higher starting dose of 4 sachets (800 mg) three times daily is recommended for the acute treatment of abdominal complications associated with cystic fibrosis and, in severe cases, doses of up to 18 g acetylcysteine daily have been used and were well tolerated.

The granules should be dissolved before administration in a glass of water.

Fabrol can be administered concurrently with amoxycillin, doxycillin and erythromycin. When other oral antibiotics or drugs are required, they should be administered 1–2 hours apart from Fabrol.

Contra-indications, warnings, etc
Contra-indications: Hypersensitivity to acetylcysteine.

Precautions: Each Fabrol sachet contains the equivalent of 2.70 g sucrose. This should be taken into account when treating diabetic patients.

Side-effects: Nausea, heart-burn, vomiting, urticaria, headache and tinnitus have infrequently been reported but these rarely necessitate withdrawal of treatment.

Allergic skin reactions and bronchospasm, especially in asthmatic patients, have been reported rarely in patients taking oral acetylcysteine. High doses of acetylcysteine given intravenously have caused anaphylactoid reactions.

Pregnancy: The administration of acetylcysteine during pregnancy is advised only if there are compelling reasons.

Accidental overdosage: There is no specific antidote for acetylcysteine and treatment is symptomatic. It consists of postural drainage, bronchial suction and supportive therapy as indicated.

Pharmaceutical precautions The addition of other drugs to the Fabrol solution should be avoided.

Legal category POM.

Package quantities Pack of 30 sachets.

Further information Nil.

Product licence number 0030/0038.

FENOSTIL*

Presentation *Fenostil-Retard Tablets:* Round, biconvex, greyish-white in colour, stamped on one face with the Zyma logo and on the reverse with the initials KA; diameter 9 mm, thickness 4.4 mm. Each tablet contains 2.5 mg dimethindene maleate in an inert slow release matrix.

Uses Antihistamine.

Indicated for allergic conditions including hay fever, allergic rhinitis, urticaria, allergic dermatoses and pruritus.

Dosage and administration For oral administration.

Adults: 1 tablet, swallowed whole, morning and evening.

Children: No formulation of a dose suitable for children is available.

Use in the elderly: Since dimethindene maleate has a wide therapeutic index there are no specific precautions required when Fenostil Retard tablets are administered to elderly patients. The usual recommended adult dose is therefore considered suitable.

Contra-indications, warnings, etc There are no known contra-indications.

Warnings: May cause drowsiness: if affected do not drive or operate machinery. Avoid alcoholic drink.

In keeping with current medical practice, use during pregnancy should be avoided unless considered essential by a physician.

Treatment of overdosage: There is no specific antidote to Fenostil. Immediate treatment consists of forced emesis followed by gastric lavage with luke-warm water and instillation of approximately 10 g activated charcoal and 20–30 g sodium sulphate dissolved in water. Should convulsions or hypertonicity occur these may be treated with diazepam or phenobarbitone injection. Severe respiratory depression may necessitate mechanical respiration.

Pharmaceutical precautions Store in a cool, dry place protected from light.

Legal category P.

Package quantities Containers of 100.

Further information Pharmacological studies show Fenostil to have a specific, potent, antihistaminic activity with low toxicity, long duration of action and one of the highest reported therapeutic ratios for an antihistaminic substance.

Product licence number 0030/5000.

ISMELIN* EYE DROPS

Presentation A clear colourless odourless solution containing guanethidine sulphate 5% w/v, with Benzalkonium Chloride BP as a preservative.

Uses *Mode of Action:* The precise mechanism of action of Ismelin in reducing intra-ocular tension has not yet been fully determined but a working hypothesis could be envisaged in which the therapeutic benefits are mediated by a local effect on the release of catecholamines, particularly those involved in the transmission of sympathetic impulses from terminal nerve fibres to target organs. This would be in line with the generally accepted concept of Ismelin activity in anti-hypertensive therapy. In relation to the eye one would have to postulate that to a greater or lesser extent the following ocular conditions are related to sympathetic overactivity: exophthalmos, lid retraction and lid lag in thyrotoxicosis and secretion of aqueous humor in glaucoma.

Indications: The reduction of intra-ocular pressure in glaucoma of the open angle type.

The treatment of lid retraction following exophthalmos and endocrine imbalance.

Dosage and administration Ismelin Eye Drops are intended for local administration to the eye.

The recommended adult dosages are as follows:

Open angle glaucoma: Initially one drop twice daily for at least a week. Dosage should then be adjusted according to the patient's needs, which may be one drop once or twice daily, or if necessary two drops once or twice daily, but rarely in excess of this.

Lid retraction: Initially one drop twice daily for at least one week, reducing thereafter to one drop daily. The dosage should be reduced as soon as possible to the minimum required to maintain the initial response – one drop on alternate days may be adequate.

Use in children: Ismelin Eye Drops are not recommended for use in children.

Use in the elderly: No specific studies have been performed in the elderly. Dosage in these patients is therefore at the discretion of the physician.

Contra-indications, warnings, etc *Contra-indications:* Use in narrow angle glaucoma or in patients with a shallow anterior chamber. Hypersensitivity to any of the components of the formulation. Ismelin Eye Drops should not be used during or within 14 days of treatment with a monoamine oxidase inhibitor.

Precautions: Soft contact lenses (hydrophilic lenses) should not be worn during treatment with Ismelin Eye Drops.

Side-effects: Conjunctival vasodilation is regarded as a pharmacological side effect of Ismelin, but does not generally prove troublesome at the recommended dosage. Hyperaemia with discomfort is usually a sign of overdosage. Some degree of ptosis, valuable in the management of exophthalmos, may represent an adverse effect in glaucoma but will usually respond to a reduction in dosage or frequency of administration. The slight miosis which occurs in most cases during Ismelin treatment causes little or no inconvenience and accommodation is not usually affected. At prolonged high dosage a tendency to superficial punctate keratitis has been reported, responding either to a reduction in dosage or interruption of treatment.

No systemic effects have been reported with Ismelin eye drops, even at maximum dosage.

Pharmaceutical precautions Protect from heat.

Do not exceed the stated dose.

The drops should not be used later than one month after first breaking the seal.

Legal category POM.

Package quantities Ismelin eye drops 5 ml.

Further information The results of therapy with Ismelin eye drops have been in many cases dramatic, particularly in terms of cosmetic improvement of the unsightly eye manifestations such as lid retraction which occur in a high proportion of patients with exophthalmos and thyrotoxicosis.

There is minimal local irritation when the eye drops are used carefully according to the recommended dosage. Also considerable subjective relief of symptoms has been afforded even when the reduction in physical signs has been minimal.

Product licence number 0030/5901.

OTRIVINE-ANTISTIN* STERILE EYE DROPS

Presentation A clear colourless odourless solution containing xylometazoline hydrochloride 0.05% w/v and antazoline sulphate 0·5% w/v, with Benzalkonium Chloride BP as a preservative.

Uses Otrivine-Antistin is a combination of a long acting vasoconstrictor and an antihistamine. The eye drops are suitable for use in the relief of conjunctivitis associated with seasonal and perennial allergies, such as hay fever, and in all non-infective conditions of the conjunctiva, such as irritation caused by smoke or dust or following the removal of foreign bodies.

Dosage and administration Otrivine-Antistin Eye Drops are intended for local administration to the eye.

Adults: 1 or 2 drops instilled 2-4 times per day into the conjunctival sac will be found to be effective. Mydriatics and miotics may be administered simultaneously with Otrivine-Antistin Eye Drops when necessary.

Use in children and in the elderly: No specific studies have been performed in these patients. Due to possible systemic adverse effects on the central nervous system, caution must be exercised and the dosage (i.e. number of drops per day) should be reduced.

Contra-indications, warnings, etc *Contra-indications:* Hypersensitivity to any of the components of the formulation. Presence of narrow angle glaucoma. Otrivine-Antistin Eye Drops should not be used during or within 14 days of treatment with a monoamine oxidase inhibitor.

Precautions: Use with caution in the presence of hypertension, cardiac irregularities, hyperthyroidism or hyperglycaemia (diabetes). Rebound congestion may follow prolonged frequent use. Soft contact lenses (hydrophilic lenses) should not be worn during treatment with Otrivine-Antistin Eye Drops. Inflammation arising from infection should receive appropriate antibacterial therapy.

Side effects: Both Otrivine and Antistin are well tolerated in the eye and for the majority of patients will be non-irritant, but in a few cases, slight transient local stinging may occur. Other side effects which may occur include headache, insomnia, drowsiness and in sensitive patients, tachycardia.

Pharmaceutical precautions Protect from heat.

The drops should not be used later than one month after first breaking the seal.

Legal category P.

Package quantities Otrivine-Antistin Sterile Eye Drops 10 ml.

Further information Nil.

Product licence number 0030/5900.

PAROVEN*

Presentation Greyish-yellow, opaque, hard gelatin capsule (size No. 2) printed 'Paroven Zyma'. Each capsule contains 250 mg oxerutins.

Uses Paroven improves capillary function by reducing abnormal leakage, probably by maintaining the integrity of endothelial cell junctions. Improved tissue perfusion increases the O_2 content of venous blood.

For long-term relief of the symptoms of capillary impairment (fragility and permeability) associated with venous insufficiency, especially of the lower limb, for example painful heavy tired legs, night cramps, paraesthesia, restless legs, ankle oedema, varicose states with or without ulceration, post-phlebitic syndrome. Haemorrhoids.

Dosage and administration For oral administration.

Adults: Initially 3-4 capsules per day. This dosage may be reduced as improvement occurs. The capsules are best taken at mealtimes.

Children: No known indication, therefore not recommended for children.

Use in the elderly: No specific studies have been performed in these patients. However, as venous insufficiency is a disease of ageing, many elderly patients have been successfully treated with Paroven at the recommended adult dose.

Contra-indications, warnings, etc There are no known contra-indications.

Side-effects: Minor complaints such as slight gastro-intestinal upsets, flushes and headaches have been reported, although in most trials authors remarked on freedom from side-effects.

Precautions: Teratogenic studies in animals have revealed no adverse effects. However, in keeping with current medical practice, the use of Paroven during the first trimester of pregnancy should be avoided.

Pharmaceutical precautions Protect from moisture.

Legal category P.

Package quantities Packs of 120 capsules.

Further information Nil.

Product licence number 0030/5002.

SABIDAL* SR

Presentation *Sabidal SR 270 tablets:* Round, convex, light yellow tablets, diameter 12 mm, thickness 6 mm. Each tablet contains 424 mg Choline Theophyllinate BP, equivalent to 270 mg anhydrous theophylline, in a sustained release formulation.

Uses For the relief and prevention of bronchospasm in asthma, chronic bronchitis and emphysema.

Dosage and administration For oral administration. The tablets should be swallowed whole and not chewed. The dosage should be adjusted to suit the individual patient, preferably on the basis of plasma theophylline levels (plasma concentrations of 10–20 mg/l are required for maximum therapeutic effect). The following initial dosage scheme is recommended:

The recommended adult dose is one tablet in the morning and two tablets at night. As with all theophylline preparations, it may be advisable in certain patients to commence treatment with one tablet twice daily for three days and then add the additional tablet at night. Sabidal SR 270 tablets are not recommended for children.

Initially, treatment should be started at the above dose, which may be increased gradually if optimal bronchodilator effects are not achieved. If a higher dose is required, it is recommended that plasma theophylline levels should be monitored, since there is considerable individual variation in the rate of drug elimination. A plasma concentration of 20 mg/l should not be exceeded.

Use in the elderly: As with all theophylline-containing products, elimination of theophylline may be slightly retarded in elderly patients. However, the observed inter-individual variations at any age are far more important and, as with all patients, the dosage should be individually adjusted.

Contra-indications, warnings, etc There are no known contra-indications.

Precautions: Caution should be exercised during use in patients with cardiac disease. The actions of theophylline and beta-2-adrenergic agents are additive and the dosage should, therefore, be individually adjusted when these agents are co-administered. As with all methylxanthine preparations, some patients may experience gastro-intestinal side-effects.

Great caution must be exercised if intravenous aminophylline is administered and plasma theophylline concentrations should be monitored.

As with all sustained release methylxanthine preparations, tablets in the intestine will continue to release the drug over a period of hours.

Overdosage: This is characterised by nausea, vomiting, gastro-intestinal irritation, unusual thirst, tachycardia, fall in blood pressure and collapse. Treatment should be by gastric lavage or in severe cases (usually, serum theophylline concentrations of 40 mg/l or more) by charcoal haemoperfusion. For fall in blood pressure, nurse in head-down position and give pressor drugs intravenously with general supportive measures. The physician should be aware that tablets in the intestine will continue to release the drug over a period of hours.

Pharmaceutical precautions Protect from moisture.

Legal category P.

Package quantities Containers of 100 tablets.

Further information The sustained release properties of Sabidal SR tablets are due to pores in the membrane surrounding the tablet. Choline theophyllinate is released through these pores at a controlled rate as the tablet passes through the alimentary canal, where the active substance is completely absorbed. As a result of these features, effective plasma theophylline concentrations are obtained throughout the 12 hour dosage interval whilst the risk of side-effects associated with high-peaking formulations is reduced to a minimum.

Product licence number 0030/0023.

TANDERIL* EYE OINTMENT

Presentation A white to yellowish-white soft ointment, containing 10% Oxyphenbutazone BP as active ingredient and phenyl ethyl alcohol 0.5% as a preservative in a special paraffin base.

Uses Anti-inflammatory.

Disease of the anterior segment of the eye and conjunctival sac: blepharitis, conjunctivitis, kerato-conjunctivitis, episcleritis, keratitis and disease of the anterior uveal tract.

Inflammation following trauma: Traumatic injury, penetrating and non-penetrating.

Post Operative: Following cataract, squint or other surgical procedures.

Note: Herpes Simplex:

While Tanderil eye ointment is not recommended for the treatment of a simple dendritic ulcer it may prove particularly valuable in treating other stages of the disease which may develop, e.g. metaherpetic ulcer, disciform keratitis or anterior uveitis. In view of the serious nature of this disease, it is recommended that these patients be under close medical supervision and if necessary additional therapy be instituted.

Dosage and administration Apply to the inner surface of the lower lid of the affected eye two to five times a day.

Use in the elderly: No specific studies have been performed in the elderly. Dosage in these patients is therefore at the discretion of the physician.

Contra-indications, warnings, etc *Contra-indications:* Previous local or systemic sensitivity to pyrazole compounds such as phenylbutazone and oxyphenbutazone.

Side-effects: Intolerance to the eye ointment may develop after continued use, the signs being: oedema of the eyelid, epiphora (minimal), redness of the conjunctiva.

Precautions: In the treatment of purulent inflammatory eye conditions, appropriate anti-infective therapy should be given concurrently with Tanderil eye ointment.

Although there is no evidence that Tanderil eye ointment increases intra-ocular pressure, it should be used with caution in cases of glaucoma secondary to injury or infection.

To ensure maximum therapeutic benefit in the treatment of conditions involving the posterior uveal tract, retina or choroid, Tanderil Eye Ointment may be used in conjunction with a suitable systemic non-steroidal anti-inflammatory agent.

Pharmaceutical precautions Store in a cool place. Use within one month of opening the tube. Dilution of this formulation is not recommended.

Legal category POM.

Package quantities Ophthalmic tubes of 5 g.

Further information Experimental studies confirm that following local application of the ointment to the eye, Tanderil penetrates the corneoscleral barrier and is present in therapeutic concentrations in the aqueous humor, iris and ciliary body.

In therapeutic concentrations Tanderil does not affect lens metabolism, intra-ocular pressure in the normal eye or in latent glaucoma, nor does it impede tissue healing or promote cataract formation.

Furthermore, in contrast to the anti-inflammatory corticosteroids, Tanderil does not enhance viral replication or the invasiveness of bacterial pathogens.

Product licence number 0030/0017.

TANDERIL* CHLORAMPHENICOL EYE OINTMENT

Presentation A white to yellowish white soft ointment containing 10% Oxyphenbutazone BP and 1% Chloramphenicol BP as active ingredients and phenyl ethyl alcohol 0.5% as a preservative.

Uses Anti-inflammatory and antibacterial.

Disease of the anterior segment of the eye and conjunctival sac: blepharitis, conjunctivitis, episcleritis, keratitis and disease of the anterior uveal tract.

Inflammation of the eye following trauma and prophylaxis of secondary bacterial infection.

Post Operative: Following squint, cataract or other surgical procedures.

Note: Herpes Simplex:

The ointment is not contraindicated in the treatment of simple dendritic ulcer, but in view of the serious nature of this disease it is recommended that these patients be under close medical supervision and the necessary additional therapy be instituted.

Dosage and administration Apply to the inner surface of the lower lid of the affected eye two to five times daily.

Use in the elderly: No specific studies have been performed in the elderly. Dosage in these patients is therefore at the discretion of the physician.

Contra-indications, warnings, etc *Contra-indications:* Previous local or systemic sensitivity to pyrazole compounds such as phenylbutazone and oxyphenbutazone. Sensitivity to chloramphenicol.

Side-effects: Intolerance to the eye ointment may develop after continued use, the signs being: oedema of the eyelid, epiphora (minimal), redness of the conjunctiva.

Pharmaceutical precautions Store in a cool place.
Use within one month of opening the tube.
Dilution of this formulation is not recommended.

Legal category POM.

Package quantities Ophthalmic tubes of 5 g.

Further information Nil.

Product licence number 0030/0018.

VIBROCIL*

Presentation *Nasal Spray and Nasal Drops:* A clear colourless solution with slight odour of lavender. Each 100 ml of solution contains:

Dimethindene maleate	0.025 g
Phenylephrine base	0.250 g
Neomycin sulphate	0.350 g

with Benzalkonium Chloride BP as a preservative.

Nasal Gel: A colourless gel with slight odour of lavender. Each 100 g of Nasal Gel contains:

Dimethindene maleate	0.025 g
Phenylephrine base	0.250 g
Neomycin sulphate	0.350 g

with Benzalkonium Chloride BP as a preservative.

Uses Vibrocil has decongestant, antihistaminic and antibiotic properties. It is indicated for use in common colds, acute and chronic rhinitis, allergic and vasomotor rhinitis, pollenosis (hay fever), acute and chronic sinusitis in children and adults.

Vibrocil does not interfere with the activity of the cilia.

Dosage and administration For topical application to the nasal mucosa.

Spray: Adults: 3 sprays in each nostril three to four times a day. For children the use of Drops or Gel is recommended.

Drops: Infants and children under six years: 1–2 drops in each nostril three to four times a day.

Children over six and adults: 3–4 drops in each nostril three to four times a day.

Gel: Apply a small quantity as high up the nostril as possible.

Adults: Three to four times a day.

Children: Two to three times a day.

Contra-indications, warnings, etc

Contra-indications: Hypersensitivity to any of the components. Concurrent use in patients who are receiving monoamine oxidase inhibitors or have received them in the previous 14 days.

Precautions: The following precautions concerning the constituents should be noted:

Prolonged use of neomycin may result in the development of super-infection due to organisms, including fungi, resistant to neomycin. Neomycin may be toxic if absorbed from extensive open surfaces when symptoms of nephrotoxicity and ototoxicity could occur, particularly in patients with impaired renal function. Phenylephrine should be used with caution in patients with hypertension, cardiovascular disease or thyrotoxicosis. Prolonged or excessive use may induce tachyphylaxis and rebound congestion.

Dimethindene maleate has potent antihistamine activity with low toxicity and a high therapeutic ratio but the possibility of drowsiness, as with other antihistamines in hypersensitive patients, should be observed. If affected, the patient should not drive or operate machinery. Avoid alcoholic drink.

Side-effects: Vibrocil is very well tolerated and does not interfere with the activity of the nasal cilia.

Pharmaceutical precautions Protect from heat and light.

Legal category POM.

Package quantities *Spray:* 10 ml nebulisers – plastic. *Drops:* 15 ml amber glass dropper bottles with plastic screw cap.
Gel: 12 g in aluminium tubes with lacquered interior.

Further information Nil.

Product licence numbers

Gel	0030/5008
Spray	0030/5009
Drops	0030/5010

ZYMAFLUOR*

Presentation *Zymafluor 1.00 mg:* Round, bi-convex tablets with bevelled edge, greyish-yellow in colour, diameter 5.0 mm, thickness 2.1 mm. Each tablet contains 2.21 mg sodium fluoride equivalent to 1.00 mg available fluoride.

Zymafluor 0.25 mg: Round, bi-convex, white tablets, slightly sweet to the taste with odour of peppermint, diameter 4.0 mm, thickness 2.6 mm. Each tablet contains 0.55 mg sodium fluoride equivalent to 0.25 mg available fluoride.

Uses Prophylaxis of dental caries. Fluoride enhances the resistance of teeth to caries. The protective action of fluoride is due especially to its accumulation in the outer layers of the dental enamel. This process should begin before eruption of the teeth and continue for a long time afterwards.

Before eruption, Zymafluor when swallowed is carried to the developing teeth by the blood stream and thus permits effective pre-eruptive fluoridation. After their eruption the teeth take up fluoride both by internal channels and especially by way of direct contact with the fluoride contained in the saliva. Zymafluor Tablets should thus not be swallowed whole: it is extremely important that they are allowed to dissolve slowly in the mouth.

Dosage and administration For oral administration. Not to be taken except on the advice of a dentist, doctor or pharmacist. Zymafluor should be given regularly, without interruption, from birth until about 16 years.

Intake of Zymafluor during pregnancy and feeding will protect the mother's teeth and lay down optimum conditions for a resistant set of milk teeth in her infant.

As soon as the age of the child permits, Zymafluor Tablets should no longer be swallowed, but sucked slowly in the mouth, between the cheek and gum, sometimes on the left and sometimes on the right side. They are best taken in the evening before bedtime. For smaller infants 1 tablet should be crushed and dissolved in a little boiled and cooled water and added to one bottle or solid meal a day, or administered alone.

Zymafluor 0.25 mg: If not otherwise prescribed by the doctor or dentist.

From birth to two years of age: 1 tablet daily.

From two to four years: 2 tablets daily.

After the age of 4 years Zymafluor is best administered in the form of 1.00 mg tablets.

Zymafluor 1.00 mg: From the age of 4 years, adults and pregnant women: 1 tablet daily or as prescribed by the doctor or dentist.

In areas where there is fluoridation of the drinking water, the following doses are recommended:

Recommended Dose (mg of fluoride/day)

Concentration of fluoride in drinking water (ppm)	<0.3	0.3 0.7	>0.7
Age			
2 weeks to 2 years	0.25	0	0
2 to 4 years	0.50	0.25	0
4 to 16 years	1.00	0.50	0

Use in the elderly: The indication for Zymafluor is not applicable to elderly patients.

Contra-indications, warnings, etc There are no known contra-indications.

Precautions: The reduced doses recommended above should be given in areas where there is fluoridation of the drinking water.

Pharmaceutical precautions Store in a cool dry place.

Legal category P.

Package quantities *0.25 mg strength:* Packs of 400. *1.00 mg strength:* Packs of 100.

Further information Nil.

Product licence numbers
0.25 mg strength   0030/5011
1.00 mg strength   0030/5012

*Trade Mark

Physiological Values for some Body Fluids

This information concerning physiological values for certain body fluids is reproduced, by permission, from the Pharmaceutical Handbook, Nineteenth Edition, The Pharmaceutical Press, London, 1980.

The values given in the following pages have been taken from many sources and represent approximate normal ranges or typical normal values. In practice 'normal' values can vary considerably from laboratory to laboratory depending on the reagents and analytical methods used. Therefore when evaluating the results of laboratory tests the normal values from the laboratory which performed the test should be consulted.

Many factors affect the reliability of laboratory tests. The specimen must be withdrawn and stored in the correct manner, an appropriate preservative being used if necessary. Certain values fluctuate in every person according to diurnal, nocturnal, or seasonal influences. Other factors, such as exercise, posture, stress, or emotional disturbances, and the age and sex of the patient may also influence the results of laboratory tests.

Many drugs and foods can interfere with laboratory tests. This interference may be physical, chemical, or pharmacological. Dyes may interfere with colorimetric or spectrometric determinations. For example, ingestion of carrots, riboflavine, or foods containing yellow pigment prior to withdrawal of a sample will elevate estimates of total bilirubin in plasma. Many chemicals can cause test results to appear abnormally high or low. High values for catecholamines in urine may be obtained if the patient is taking drugs such as methyldopa. The pharmacological effects of drugs may interfere with laboratory test results. Antihistamines interfere with tests for allergies and mask hypersensitivities.

In the following tables these abbreviations are used: B = Blood; P = Plasma; S = Serum.

BLOOD

Physical Values

Circulation time	3 to 8 seconds (arm to lung)
Freezing-point	$-0.52°$
Osmolality, plasma	280 to 295 mmol per kg
pH, arterial	7.35 to 7.45
Pressure, arterial	
Systolic	<140 mmHg
Diastolic	<90 mm Hg
Specific gravity	1.05 to 1.06
Volume, blood	50 to 80 ml per kg body-weight
Volume, plasma	31 to 55 ml per kg body-weight

Haematological Values

Blood count, complete	
Haematocrit (Packed cell volume)	Male: 40 to 54%
	Female: 35 to 47%
Haemoglobin	Male: 13 to 18 g per 100 ml
	Female: 12 to 16 g per 100 ml
Red cell count	Male: 4.5 to 6.5 million per mm^3
	or 4.5 to 6.5×10^{12} per litre
	Female: 3.9 to 5.6 million per mm^3
	or 3.9 to 5.6×10^{12} per litre
White cell count	4000 to 11 000 per mm^3
Coagulation tests	
Bleeding time	
Duke's method	<7 minutes
Ivy method	<7 minutes
Clotting time, Lee White method	5 to 11 minutes
Partial thromboplastin time, activated	35 to 60 seconds
Prothrombin time, Quick one stage	12 to 20 seconds
Erythrocyte sedimentation rate (ESR),	Male: 3 to 5 mm in 1 hour
Westergren method	Female: 4 to 7 mm in 1 hour
Haemoglobin A_2	1.5 to 3.5%
Haemoglobin F	$<2\%$
Haptoglobin	0.3 to 2.0 g per litre
Platelet count	150 000 to 400 000 per mm^3 or per µl
Red cell diameter	6.7 to 7.7 µm
	average 7.2 µm
Red cell thickness	1.7 to 2.5 µm
Red cell volume	23 to 35 ml per kg body-weight
Reticulocyte count	0.5 to 2.0% of red cells
White cell count, differential	
Neutrophils, segmented	2500 to 7500 per mm^3 or per µl
Lymphocytes	1500 to 3500 per mm^3 or per µl
Monocytes	200 to 800 per mm^3 or per µl
Eosinophils	40 to 440 per mm^3 or per µl
Basophils	15 to 100 per mm^3 or per µl

BLOOD—*continued*

Blood Gases and Acid–Base Values

Base excess	±2.3 mmol per litre
Bicarbonate	
Plasma	21 to 30 mmol per litre
Standard	22 to 28 mmol per litre
Buffer base	45 to 50 mmol per litre
Carbon dioxide	
Arterial pCO_2	36 to 44 mmHg
Total CO_2	23 to 33 mmol per litre
Oxygen	
Arterial pO_2	90 to 110 mmHg

Chemical Values

		Metric	SI
Alpha-amino acid nitrogen	P	30 to 55 mg per litre	2.1 to 4 mmol per litre
Ammonium nitrogen (enzymatic method)	B	400 to 800 µg per litre	29 to 57 µmol per litre
Amylase	S	0.8 to 1.8 Somogyi units per ml	—
		3 to 10 Wohlgemuth units per ml	—
		86 to 268 iu per litre	—
Angiotensin II	B	12 to 36 ng per litre	11.6 to 34.9 pmol per litre
Ascorbic acid	B	5 to 20 mg per litre	28 to 114 µmol per litre
Bicarbonate	P	—	21 to 28 mmol per litre
Bilirubin,			
total	S	1 to 15 mg per litre	1.7 to 25 µmol per litre
total newborn	S	10 to 120 mg per litre	17 to 205 µmol per litre
Caeruloplasmin,			
adult	S	300 to 600 mg per litre	—
child	S	130 to 300 mg per litre	—
Calcium,			
total	S	85 to 105 mg per litre	2.1 to 2.6 mmol per litre
ionised	S	40 to 50 mg per litre	1 to 1.25 mmol per litre
Catecholamines, at rest			
Adrenaline	P	55 ng per litre	0.3 nmol per litre
Nor-adrenaline	P	254 ng per litre	1.5 nmol per litre
Chloride	S or P	3.368 to 3.723 g per litre (as chloride)	95 to 105 mmol per litre
Copper	S or P	0.7 to 1.5 mg per litre	11 to 24 µmol per litre
Cortisol 9 am	P	50 to 260 µg per litre	138 to 717 nmol per litre
5 pm	P	20 to 180 µg per litre	55 to 497 nmol per litre
Creatinine	S or P	6 to 15 mg per litre	53 to 133 µmol per litre
Cyanocobalamin	S	100 to 800 ng per litre	74 to 590 pmol per litre
Fibrinogen	P	2 to 4 g per litre	—
Folate	S	3 to 25 µg per litre	—
Gastrin	S, or P	5 to 290 ng per litre	—
Glucagon	P	0.4 to 1.4 µg per litre	115 to 402 pmol per litre
Glucose, fasting	S or P	0.7 to 1.1 g per litre	3.9 to 6.1 mmol per litre
Growth hormone	S	<10 µg per litre	—
Immunoglobulins	S		
IgA		0.5 to 4 g per litre	—
IgD		5 to 50 mg per litre	—
IgE		0.1 to 1.3 mg per litre	—
IgG		8 to 16 g per litre	—
IgM		0.4 to 2.9 g per litre	—
Insulin	S	4 to 30 milliunits per litre	—
Iodine, protein-bound (PBI)	S	35 to 80 µg per litre	276 to 630 nmol per litre
Iron, total	S	0.5 to 1.8 mg per litre	9 to 32 µmol per litre
Iron-binding capacity	S	2.5 to 4.5 mg per litre	45 to 81 µmol per litre

BLOOD—*continued*

		Metric	SI
Ketones (acetoacetate and acetone)	B	<30 mg per litre	—
Lactic acid,			
arterial	B	30 to 70 mg per litre	0.3 to 0.8 mmol per litre
venous	B	50 to 200 mg per litre	0.56 to 2.2 mmol per litre
Lead	B	<800 µg per litre	<3.9 µmol per litre
Lipids,			
total	S	4 to 10 g per litre	
cholesterol	S	1.1 to 3.0 g per litre	2.8 to 7.8 mmol per litre
triglycerides	S	0.4 to 1.5 g per litre	
Magnesium	S	18 to 30 mg per litre	0.7 to 1.2 mmol per litre
Phenylalanine	S	<40 mg per litre	<242 µmol per litre
Phosphatase,			
acid, total	S	0.5 to 4 King-Armstrong units per 100 ml	—
alkaline, total	S	4 to 13 King-Armstrong units per 100 ml	—
Phosphorus, inorganic adults	S or P	25 to 45 mg per litre	0.8 to 1.5 mmol per litre
Potassium	P	137 to 196 mg per litre	3.5 to 5 mmol per litre
Prolactin	S	2 to 15 µg per litre	—
Proteins,			
total serum	S	60 to 84 g per litre	—
albumin	S	30 to 52 g per litre	—
globulin	S	23 to 37 g per litre	—
Pyruvic acid	B	3 to 10 mg per litre	34 to 114 µmol per litre
Sodium	P	3.1 to 3.4 g per litre	135 to 148 mmol per litre
Sulphate, inorganic	S	9 to 60 mg per litre	94 to 625 µmol per litre
Transaminases			
SGOT	S	0 to 30 iu per litre	—
SGPT	S	0 to 24 iu per litre	—
Thyroid hormone tests			
Thyroid stimulating hormones (TSH)	S	0.5 to 3.5 milliunits per litre	—
T_3 (Radio-immuno-assay)	S	0.7 to 1.9 µg per litre	—
T_4 (radio-immuno-assay)	S	40 to 120 µg per litre	—
T_4 Free	S	10 to 40 ng per litre	—
Urea nitrogen (BUN)	B or S	80 to 250 mg per litre	5.7 to 17.9 mmol per litre
Urea	B	171 to 535 mg per litre	2.9 to 8.9 mmol per litre
Uric acid	S	15 to 70 mg per litre	89 to 417 µmol per litre
Vitamin A	S	150 to 900 µg per litre	0.5 to 3.1 µmol per litre
Zinc	S	0.5 to 1.5 mg per litre	8 to 23 µmol per litre

CEREBROSPINAL FLUID

Physical Values

Freezing-point	−0.540° to −0.603°
Osmolality	306 mmol per kg
pH	7.33 to 7.37
Pressure	60 to 180 mm of water
Specific gravity	1.0062 to 1.0082
Volume, adults	100 to 160 ml

Chemical Values

Calcium	1 to 1.5 mmol per litre
Chloride	120 to 130 mmol per litre
Glucose	2.5 to 4.5 mmol per litre
Lactate dehydrogenase	0.2 to 4 iu per ml
Protein	
Lumbar	150 to 500 mg per litre
Cisternal	100 to 300 mg per litre
Ventricular	0 to 150 mg per litre
Albumin/Globulin ratio	2:1
Infants <1 year	1:1
Albumin	100 to 300 mg per litre
Globulin	60 to 160 mg per litre
Urea	2 to 7 mmol per litre

URINE

Physical Values

Glomerular filtration rate	100 to 150 ml per minute
Osmolality	100 to 1000 mmol per kg
pH	4.5 to 8.0
Specific gravity	1.010 to 1.025
Volume, normal adult	800 to 2000 ml per 24 hours

Chemical Values

	Metric	SI
α Amino acid nitrogen	50 to 300 mg per 24 h	3.6 to 21.4 mmol per 24 h
δ Aminolaevulinic acid	0.1 to 7.5 mg per 24 h	0.8 to 57 µmol per 24 h
Calcium	100 to 300 mg per 24 h	2.5 to 7.5 mmol per 24 h
Catecholamines		
Adrenaline	<20 µg per 24 h	<109 nmol per 24 h
Nor-adrenaline	<100 µg per 24 h	<591 nmol per 24 h
Chloride	3.545 to 8.863 g per 24 h	100 to 250 mmol per 24 h
Creatine, adults	0 to 100 mg per 24 h	0 to 763 µmol per 24 h
Creatinine	1 to 2 g per 24 h	8 to 18 mmol per 24 h
Formiminoglutamic		
acid (FIGLU)	0 to 3 mg per 24 h	0 to 17 µmol per 24 h
After 15 g of L-Histidine	4 mg per 8 h	23 µmol per 8 h
Homovanillic acid (HVA)	0 to 15 mg per 24 h	0 to 82 µmol per 24 h
Hydroxyindole acetic acid (HIAA)	3 to 14 mg per 24 h	16 to 73 µmol per 24 h
Lead	<100 µg per 24 h	<483 nmol per 24 h
Magnesium	49 to 243 mg per 24 h	2 to 10 mmol per 24 h
Oxalate	15 to 40 mg per 24 h	167 to 444 µmol per 24 h
Phosphate, inorganic	0.5 to 1.5 g per 24 h	16 to 48 µmol per 24 h
Potassium	1.4 to 3.5 g per 24 h	35 to 90 mmol per 24 h
Protein	<100 mg per 24 h	—
Urea	10 to 30 g per 24 h	167 to 500 mmol per 24 h
Uric acid,		
normal diet	0.2 to 0.5 g per 24 h	1.2 to 3 mmol per 24 h
high purine diet	up to 2 g per 24 h	up to 12 mmol per 24 h
Vanillylmandelic acid (VMA)	up to 9 mg per 24 h	up to 45 µmol per 24 h

Clearance Values

Serum and Urine

Aminohippuric acid (PAH) clearance	600 to 750 ml per min
Creatinine clearance (endogenous)	95 to 135 ml per min
Inulin clearance	100 to 150 ml per min
Urea clearance	
average standard	41 to 65 ml per min
average maximum	64 to 99 ml per min

Physiological Values During Pregnancy

The following table giving physiological values during pregnancy has been provided by Professor Geoffrey Chamberlain of the Department of Obstetrics and Gynaecology, St George's Hospital Medical School, London.

Haematological Functions	Prepregnancy	Weeks of pregnancy		
		20	30	40
Total Blood Volume (ml)	4000	4600	5500	5700
Erythrocyte Volume (ml)	1400	1500	1650	1800
Red Blood Cells (million/ml)	4.5	4.0	3.7	4.0
White Blood Cells (per ml)	7200	9400	10700	10400
Haemoglobin (g/dl)	13.5	12.0	11.5	12.0
Serum Iron (mg/l)	1.2	1.0	0.9	0.9
Serum Folate (μg/l)	10	7	6	6
Total Iron Binding capacity (μmol/l)	50	40	60	70

Biochemical Functions	Prepregnancy	Weeks of pregnancy		
		20	30	40
Sodium (m Eq/l)	138	136	137	136
Potassium (m Eq/l)	4.26	4.00	4.10	4.21
Calcium (m Eq/l)	5.00	4.90	4.55	4.60
Colloid osmotic plasma (cm H_2O)	37	32	31	31
Albumen (g/l)	35	28	26	25
Total protein (g/l)	70	60	61	62
Plasma Osmolality (mπ/Kg)	281	283	280	280

Liver Function Tests	Prepregnancy	Weeks of pregnancy		
		20	30	40
Total Bilirubin (μmol/l)	4–16	0.5–16	0.5–16	0.5–16
Cholesterol (μmol/l)	4–8	6–8	7–9	8–10
Alkaline phosphatase (I.U./l)	16–24	16–44	16–60	20–100

Note: Pregnancy is a great physiological change and many normal ranges of laboratory tests are changed, some greatly. In these simplified charts, means are used from large series of normal pregnant women. This shows the trend of changes in later pregnancy; to include all ranges would have clouded the tables. For fuller and further details, the reader is referred to:

Hytten, F. & Lind, T. (1973) Diagnostic Indices in Pregnancy, Documenta Geigy, Basle.
Hytten, F. & Chamberlain, G. (1984) Clinical Physiology in Pregnancy, Blackwells, Medical Publishers, Oxford.

1983 Metropolitan Height and Weight Tables for Men and Women

Weights at ages 25–59 based on lowest mortality. Weight in pounds according to frame (in indoor clothing weighing 5 lbs for men and 3 lbs for women; shoes with 1" heels). Source of basic data: 1979 Build Study, Society of Actuaries and Association of Life Insurance Medical Directors of America, 1980.

MEN. Weight in pounds (in indoor clothing).

Height (in shoes)	Small frame	Medium frame	Large frame
5 ft. 2 in.	128 – 134	131 – 141	138 – 150
5 ft. 3 in.	130 – 136	133 – 143	140 – 153
5 ft. 4 in.	132 – 138	135 – 145	142 – 156
5 ft. 5 in.	134 – 140	137 – 148	144 – 160
5 ft. 6 in.	136 – 142	139 – 151	146 – 164
5 ft. 7 in.	138 – 145	142 – 154	149 – 168
5 ft. 8 in.	140 – 148	145 – 157	152 – 172
5 ft. 9 in.	142 – 151	148 – 160	155 – 176
5 ft. 10 in.	144 – 154	151 – 163	158 – 180
5 ft. 11 in.	146 – 157	154 – 166	161 – 184
6 ft. 0 in.	149 – 160	157 – 170	164 – 188
6 ft. 1 in.	152 – 164	160 – 174	168 – 192
6 ft. 2 in.	155 – 168	164 – 178	172 – 197
6 ft. 3 in.	158 – 172	167 – 182	176 – 202
6 ft. 4 in.	162 – 176	171 – 187	181 – 207

WOMEN. Weight in pounds (in indoor clothing).

Height (in shoes)	Small frame	Medium frame	Large frame
4 ft. 10 in.	102 – 111	109 – 121	118 – 131
4 ft. 11 in.	103 – 113	111 – 123	120 – 134
5 ft. 0 in.	104 – 115	113 – 126	122 – 137
5 ft. 1 in.	106 – 118	115 – 129	125 – 140
5 ft. 2 in.	108 – 121	118 – 132	128 – 143
5 ft. 3 in.	111 – 124	121 – 135	131 – 147
5 ft. 4 in.	114 – 127	124 – 138	134 – 151
5 ft. 5 in.	117 – 130	127 – 141	137 – 155
5 ft. 6 in.	120 – 133	130 – 144	140 – 159
5 ft. 7 in.	123 – 136	133 – 147	143 – 163
5 ft. 8 in.	126 – 139	136 – 150	146 – 167
5 ft. 9 in.	129 – 142	139 – 153	149 – 170
5 ft. 10 in.	132 – 145	142 – 156	152 – 173
5 ft. 11 in.	135 – 148	145 – 159	155 – 176
6 ft. 0 in.	138 – 151	148 – 162	158 – 179

Obstetric Table

Calculated from the first day of the last menstrual period.

LMP month	1	2	3	4	5	6	7	8	9	10	11	12	13	14	15	16	17	18	19	20	21	22	23	24	25	26	27	28	29	30	31	Due month
January / *October*	8	9	10	11	12	13	14	15	16	17	18	19	20	21	22	23	24	25	26	27	28	29	30	31	1	2	3	4	5	6	7	**January** / *November*
February / *November*	8	9	10	11	12	13	14	15	16	17	18	19	20	21	22	23	24	25	26	27	28	29	30	1	2	3	4	5				**February** / *December*
March / *December*	6	7	8	9	10	11	12	13	14	15	16	17	18	19	20	21	22	23	24	25	26	27	28	29	30	31	1	2	3	4	5	**March** / *January*
April / *January*	6	7	8	9	10	11	12	13	14	15	16	17	18	19	20	21	22	23	24	25	26	27	28	29	30	31	1	2	3	4		**April** / *February*
May / *February*	5	6	7	8	9	10	11	12	13	14	15	16	17	18	19	20	21	22	23	24	25	26	27	28	1	2	3	4	5	6	7	**May** / *March*
June / *March*	8	9	10	11	12	13	14	15	16	17	18	19	20	21	22	23	24	25	26	27	28	29	30	31	1	2	3	4	5	6		**June** / *April*
July / *April*	7	8	9	10	11	12	13	14	15	16	17	18	19	20	21	22	23	24	25	26	27	28	29	30	1	2	3	4	5	6	7	**July** / *May*
August / *May*	8	9	10	11	12	13	14	15	16	17	18	19	20	21	22	23	24	25	26	27	28	29	30	31	1	2	3	4	5	6	7	**August** / *June*
September / *June*	8	9	10	11	12	13	14	15	16	17	18	19	20	21	22	23	24	25	26	27	28	29	30	1	2	3	4	5	6	7		**September** / *July*
October / *July*	8	9	10	11	12	13	14	15	16	17	18	19	20	21	22	23	24	25	26	27	28	29	30	31	1	2	3	4	5	6	7	**October** / *August*
November / *August*	8	9	10	11	12	13	14	15	16	17	18	19	20	21	22	23	24	25	26	27	28	29	30	31	1	2	3	4	5	6		**November** / *September*
December / *September*	7	8	9	10	11	12	13	14	15	16	17	18	19	20	21	22	23	24	25	26	27	28	29	30	1	2	3	4	5	6	7	**December** / *October*

Data sheets new to this edition

The following list comprises products which are the subject of data sheets in this edition of the Compendium but which were not included in the 1985–86 edition. It does not necessarily follow that they are recently introduced products.

Anthranol Ointment 1539
Asacol 1579
Aspav 376
Atgam 1590
Atrovent Forte 217
Azathioprine Tablets BP 188

Bactroban Ointment 147
Benzagel 214
Bezalip-Mono 889

Calmurid Solution 1201
Carbo Cort Cream 722
Carbo Dome Cream 723
Cervagem 853
Clinitar Gel 1432
Creon 447

Debrisan Absorbent Pad 1202
Deponit 5 1410
Dermalex 714
Didronel 1056
Digibind 1630
Dimotane with Codeine 1259
Dimotane with Codeine
  Paediatric 1259
Dioralyte Pineapple 88
Diprivan 617
Disprol Paediatric 1228
Dome Acne Cream 723
Dome Acne Medicated
  Cleanser 723
Dome Cort Cream 724
Dopamine Hydrochloride in 5%
  Dextrose Injection 2

Erymax 1147
Erythroped Sugar-free 8

Fabrol 1713
Factorate Heat Treated 88
Factorate Heat Treated, High
  Potency 90

Glibenclamide Tablets BP 200
Guarina 1047
Gx Allopurinol Tablets 578
Gx Amitriptyline Tablets 579
Gx Ampicillin Capsules 580
Gx Ampicillin Syrup 580
Gx Chlorpropamide Tablets 581

Gx Co-trimoxazole Tablets 582
Gx Frusemide Tablets 582
Gx Glibenclamide Tablets 583
Gx Ibuprofen Tablets 584
Gx Indomethacin Capsules 584
Gx Indomethacin
  Suppositories 585
Gx Methyldopa Tablets 585
Gx Oxprenolol Tablets 586
Gx Propranolol Tablets 587
Gx Salbutamol Inhaler 588
Gx Salbutamol Tablets 589
Gx Spironolactone Tablets 589
Gx Tamoxifen Tablets 590
Gynatren 307
Gynol II 1104
Gyno-Pevaryl 1 Vaginal
  Pessary 1378

Hamarin 100 Tablets 1031
Hamarin 300 Tablets 1031
Heparinised Saline 1127
Heplok 778
Hespan 61
Hibitane Tincture 625
Human Actraphane 1067
Human Actrapid Penfill 1066
Human Initard 1041, 1636
Human Mixtard 1041, 1636
Human Velosulin 1041, 1636

Ibuprofen Tablets BP 201
Intal 5 Inhaler 494

Kalten 1549
Kerecid 58

Lactulose Solution BP 1358
Lipobase 294
Lodine 122
Lorazepam Tablets BP
  (Berk) 203

Maxtrex 476
Metramid 1033
Metrodin 1421
Micro K 908
Minilok 301
Modrasone 701
Moduret 25 1003
Mucogel Suspension 1218
Myotonine 565

Nericur Gel 1395
Nitronal 826
Nizoral Tablets and
  Suspension 672
Noltam 757
Normacol 1048
Normetic 15

Octovit 1455
Oxprenolol Tablets BP
  (Berk) 205

Pancrease Capsules 1117
PanOxyl Wash 1543
Paraplatin 276
Paxalgesic 1519
Paxofen 1519
Paxolax 1520
Plegisol 17
Poliomyelitis Vaccine, Single
  Dose 1651
Potaba 565
Prempak 127
Primalan 877
Prostin E2 Vaginal Gel 1609

Quinocort 1223

Refolinon 481

Sential 1208
Softgut 397
Solco Hida Kit 307
Somatonorm 690
Suprefact Injection 609
Suprefact Nasal Spray 609

Tamofen-40 1587
Temazepam (Berk) 210
Temazepam (Farmitalia) 483
Tenormin Syrup 1559
Tetralysal 300 484
Topal 646
Topicycline 1061
Tridesilon 730
Tutoplast Dura 919

Vancocin Matrigel Capsules 818
Velosulin Cartridge 1043
Videne Powder 1256
Videne Solution 1256
Videne Surgical Scrub 1257
Videne Tincture 1257

Index of Products

Non-proprietary/Proprietary Names Index

This index of non-proprietary names is provided to enable users of the Compendium to identify the brand names of relevant products when only non-proprietary names are known.

It should be noted that although different products may contain the same active ingredient this does not imply that they are equivalent in regard to bio-availability or therapeutic activity.

Some products contain a number of ingredients and it has not been possible in every instance to identify such products by a reference in this index to each ingredient.

* Products with an asterisk contain a number of active ingredients and may be available in more than one formulation.

Products without an asterisk contain a single active ingredient; in certain instances such products may also be available with added constituents and these formulations are often designated by the principal brand name with the addition of a suffix or other mark of distinction.

Where a number of presentations of a product bear the same proprietary name, the page number given below is that of the first of the respective entries.

Non-proprietary name in bold type   Proprietary name in ordinary type

Acebutolol
Sectral 879
Secadrex* 878
Acetazolamide
Diamox 743
Acetic Acid
Aci-Jel 1101
Acetohexamide
Dimelor 792
Acetomenaphthone
Pernivit* 440
Ketovite Tablets* 1128
Acetylcysteine
Fabrol 1713
Parvolex 439
Airbron 428
Ilube* 434
Acrosoxacin
Eradacin 1524
Actinomycin
Cosmegen Lyovac 938
Acyclovir
Zovirax 1667
Adrenaline
Eppy 1433
Isopto Epinal 23
Medihaler-Epi 1244
Epifrin 57
Simplene 1440
Marcain with Adrenaline* 105
Ganda* 1434
Brovon* 1014, 1021
Rybarvin* 1353
Lignostab A* 249
Xylocaine with Adrenaline* 110
Xylotox* 1200
Adrenocortical Extract
Movelat* 835
Aesculin
Proctosedyl* 1347
Agar
Agarol* 1132
Albumin Fraction Saline, Human
(Immuno) 655
Albumin, Human
(Merieux) 1428
Albuminar 78

(Immuno) 652
Alclometasone
Modrasone 701
Alcuronium Chloride
Alloferin 1268
Alexitol Sodium
Actal 1671
Droxalin* 1521
Alfacalcidol
One-Alpha 780
Alfentanil
Rapifen 675
Alginic Acid
Gaviscon* 1228
Gastrocote* 891
Topal* 646
Allantoin
Alphosyl* 1508
Actinac* 1338
Dermalex* 714
Allergens
Conjuvac 424
Merck Skin Testing Solutions 907
Allpyral 422
Bencard Skin Testing Solutions 168
Migen 172
Pharmalgen 1210
SDV 180
Norisen 911
Pollinex 178
Alavac 160
Spectralgens 1211
Allopurinol
Zyloric 337
Caplenal 192
Aluline 1514
GX Allopurinol 578
Hamarin 1031
Allylestranol
Gestanin 1075
Almasilate
Malinal 1261
Aloes
Opobyl* 186
Aloin
Alophen* 1133
Aloxiprin
Palaprin Forte 1037

Alprazolam
Xanax 1618
Alprostadil
Prostin VR 1612
Aluminium Acetate
Xyloproct* 113
Aluminium Chlorhydroxide Complex
Neo-Medrone Acne Lotion* 1607
Medrone Acne Lotion* 1605
Aluminium Chloride Hexahydrate
Anhydrol Forte 404
Driclor 1541
Aluminium Dihydroxyallantoinate
Rikospray Silicone* 1251
Zeasorb* 1546
Aluminium Glycinate
Prodexin* 180
Aluminium Hydroxide
Aludrox 1694
Alu-Cap 1235
Asilone* 187
Gelusil* 1148
Polycrol* 1038
Andursil* 501
Topal* 646
Mucogel* 1218
Antasil* 1548
Kolanticon* 979
APP* 371
Pyrogastrone* 1688
Gastrocote* 891
Caved-S* 1579
Gaviscon* 1229
Theodrox* 1254
LoAsid* 323
Maalox* 1335
Mucaine* 1703
Kolantyl* 980
Aluminium Hydroxide/ Magnesium Carbonate Co-Dried Gel
Andursil* 501
Polycrol Tablets* 1038
Aluminium Oxide
Brasivol 1541

Directory of participants

This directory is included in the Compendium so that doctors and other professional people may obtain additional information about products from participating companies.

page

The Medical Information Executive
Duphar Laboratories Ltd
Gaters Hill
West End
Southampton SO3 3JD

Southampton (0703) 472281
447

Medical Information Department
Du Pont (U.K.) Ltd
Pharmaceuticals
Wedgwood Way
Stevenage
Hertfordshire SG1 4QN

Stevenage (0438) 734549   **455**

Ethicon Ltd
PO Box 408
Bankhead Avenue
Edinburgh EH11 4HE

031-453 5555   **458**

Evans Medical Ltd
318 High Street North
Dunstable
Bedfordshire LU6 1BE

Dunstable (0582) 608308   **463**

Medical Information
Farmitalia Carlo Erba Ltd
Italia House
23 Grosvenor Road
St Albans
Hertfordshire AL1 3AW

St Albans (0727) 40041   **470**

Medical Department
Fisons plc
Pharmaceutical Division
12 Derby Road
Loughborough
Leicestershire LE11 0BB

Loughborough (0509)
263113   **486**

Information Services
Geigy Pharmaceuticals
Wimblehurst Road
Horsham
West Sussex RH12 4AB

Horsham (0403) 50101   **500**

page

Geistlich Sons Ltd
Newton Bank
Long Lane
Chester CH2 3QZ

Chester (0244) 47534   **522**

Medical Information
Glaxo Laboratories Ltd
Greenford Road
Greenford
Middlesex UB6 0HE

01-422 3434   **531**

Glenwood Laboratories Ltd
19 Wincheap
Canterbury
Kent CT1 3TB

Canterbury (0227) 60139   **565**

Medical Information Department
Gold Cross Pharmaceuticals
Division of G. D. Searle & Co Ltd
PO Box 53
Lane End Road
High Wycombe
Buckinghamshire HP12 4HL

High Wycombe (0494) 21124
567

GX Ltd
The Old Post House
London End
Beaconsfield
Buckinghamshire HP9 2JH

Beaconsfield (04946) 78501
578

Medical Information Department
Hoechst UK Ltd
Pharmaceutical Division
Hoechst House
Salisbury Road
Hounslow
Middlesex TW4 6JH

01-570 7712   **591**

Medical Information Department
Hough, Hoseason & Co Ltd
20–22 Chapel Street
Levenshulme
Manchester M19 3PT

061- 224 3271   **612**

page

Medical Information
ICI Pharmaceuticals (UK)
Alderley House
Alderley Park
Macclesfield
Cheshire SK10 4TF

Alderley Edge (0625)
582828   **614**

The Marketing Department
Immuno Ltd
Arctic House
Rye Lane
Dunton Green
Nr. Sevenoaks
Kent TN14 5HB

Sevenoaks (0732) 458101   **649**

Medical Information Department
International Laboratories Ltd
Charwell House
Wilsom Road
Alton
Hampshire GU34 2TJ

Alton (0420) 88174   **658**

The Medical Information
Department
Janssen Pharmaceutical Ltd
Grove
Wantage
Oxon OX12 0DQ

Wantage (02357) 2966   **660**

Technical and Medical Services
Department
KabiVitrum Ltd
KabiVitrum House
Riverside Way
Uxbridge
Middlesex UB8 2YF

Uxbridge (0895) 51144   **681**

The Medical Information Officer
Kirby-Warrick
Pharmaceuticals Ltd
Mildenhall
Bury St Edmunds
Suffolk IP28 7AX

Mildenhall (0638) 716321   **697**

page

A. H. Robins Company Ltd
Langhurst
Horsham
West Sussex RH13 5QP

Horsham (0403) 60361/4 **1258**

Medical Information Department
Roche Products Ltd
PO Box 8
Welwyn Garden City
Hertfordshire AL7 3AY

Welwyn Garden (0707)
328128 **1267**

Product Information Department
Rorer Pharmaceuticals
Stepfield
Witham
Essex CM8 3AG

Witham (0376) 512538 **1333**

Medical Information Department
Roussel Laboratories Ltd
Broadwater Park
North Orbital Road
Uxbridge
Middlesex UB9 5HP

Uxbridge (0895) 834343 **1338**

Rybar Laboratories Ltd
Amersham
Buckinghamshire HP6 5BX

Amersham (02403) 22741 **1352**

Medical Information Services
Department
Sandoz Products Ltd
Sandoz House
98 The Centre
Feltham
Middlesex TW13 4EP

01-890 1366 **1354**

Medical Information Department
Schering Pharmaceuticals
(Division of Schering Chemicals
Ltd)
The Brow
Burgess Hill
West Sussex RH15 9NE

Burgess Hill (04446) 6011 **1377**

page

Technical Services Manager
Schwarz Pharmaceuticals Ltd
Schwarz House
East Street
Chesham
Buckinghamshire HP5 1DG

Chesham (0494) 772071 **1410**

Medical Information Department
Searle Pharmaceuticals
Division of G. D. Searle & Co Ltd
PO Box 53
Lane End Road
High Wycombe
Buckinghamshire HP12 4HL

High Wycombe (0494) 21124
1414

Serono Laboratories (U.K.) Ltd
2 Tewin Court
Welwyn Garden City
Hertfordshire AL7 1AU

Welwyn Garden (0707) 331972
1421

Medical Department
Servier Laboratories Ltd
Fulmer Hall
Windmill Road
Fulmer
Slough
Buckinghamshire SL3 6HH

Fulmer (02816) 2744 **1426**

Technical Services Department
**Smith & Nephew
Pharmaceuticals Ltd**
Bampton Road
Harold Hill
Romford
Essex RM3 8SL

Ingrebourne (04023)
49333 **1432**

Medical Information Department
**Smith Kline & French
Laboratories Ltd**
Welwyn Garden City
Hertfordshire AL7 1EY

Welwyn Garden (0707)
325111 **1443**

page

Medical Information
E. R. Squibb & Sons Ltd
Squibb House
141/149 Staines Road
Hounslow
Middlesex TW3 3JA

01-572 7422 **1467**

Medical Products Manager
Stafford-Miller Ltd
Stafford-Miller House
The Common
Hatfield
Hertfordshire AL10 0NZ

Hatfield (07072) 61151 **1508**

**STD Pharmaceutical Products
Ltd**
Fields Yard
Plough Lane
Hereford HR4 0EL

Hereford (0432) 53684 and
272152 **1512**

Medical Information Department
M. A. Steinhard Ltd
32–36 Minerva Road
London NW10 6HJ

01-965 0194 **1514**

Medical Information Department
Sterling Health
Sterling Winthrop House
Onslow Street
Guildford
Surrey GU1 4YS

Guildford (0483) 505515 **1521**

Medical Information Department
Sterling Research Laboratories
Sterling Winthrop House
Onslow Street
Guildford
Surrey GU1 4YS

Guildford (0483) 505515 (including 24-hour emergency service)
1522

Stiefel Laboratories (UK) Ltd
Holtspur Lane
Wooburn Green
High Wycombe
Buckinghamshire HP10 0AU

Bourne End (06285) 24966 **1539**

page

Medical Information
Stuart Pharmaceuticals Ltd
50 Alderley Road
Wilmslow
Cheshire SK9 1RE

Wilmslow (0625) 535999 **1548**

Information Services Department
Syntex Pharmaceuticals Ltd
Syntex House
St Ives Road
Maidenhead
Berkshire SL6 1RD

Maidenhead (0628) 33191
1562

Medical Information
Tillotts Laboratories
Unit 24
Henlow Trading Estate
Henlow
Bedfordshire SG16 6DS

Hitchin (0462) 813933 **1579**

page

Typharm Ltd
14 Parkstone Road
Poole
Dorset BH15 2PG

Ringwood (04254) 79711 **1589**

Medical Information
Upjohn Ltd
Fleming Way
Crawley
West Sussex RH10 2NJ

Crawley (0293) 31133 **1590**

Scientific Services Division
Wellcome Medical Division
The Wellcome Foundation Ltd
Crewe Hall
Crewe
Cheshire CW1 1UB

Crewe (0270) 583151 **1619**

page

Medical Information Department
Winthrop Laboratories
Sterling Winthrop House
Onslow Street
Guildford
Surrey GU1 4YS

Guildford (0483) 505515 (including 24-hour emergency service)
1671

Medical Information Department
Wyeth Laboratories
Huntercombe Lane South
Taplow
Maidenhead
Berkshire SL6 0PH

Burnham (Bucks) (06286)
4377 **1694**

Zyma (UK) Ltd
Westhead
10 West Street
Alderley Edge
Cheshire SK9 7XP

Alderley Edge (0625)
584788 **1713**